Stocker & Dehner's

Pediatric Pathology

THIRD EDITION

EDITORS

J. Thomas Stocker, MD
Professor of Pathology, Pediatrics and Emerging Infectious Disease
Department of Pathology
Uniformed Services University of the Health Sciences
Bethesda, Maryland

Louis P. Dehner, MD
Professor
Division of Anatomy and Molecular Pathology
Department of Pathology and Immunology
Washington University in St. Louis
Attending Surgical Pathologist
Lauren V. Ackerman Laboratory of Surgical Pathology
Barnes-Jewish and St. Louis Children's Hospitals at the Washington University Medical Center
St. Louis, Missouri

Aliya N. Husain, MD
Professor
Department of Pathology
University of Chicago
Chicago, Illinois

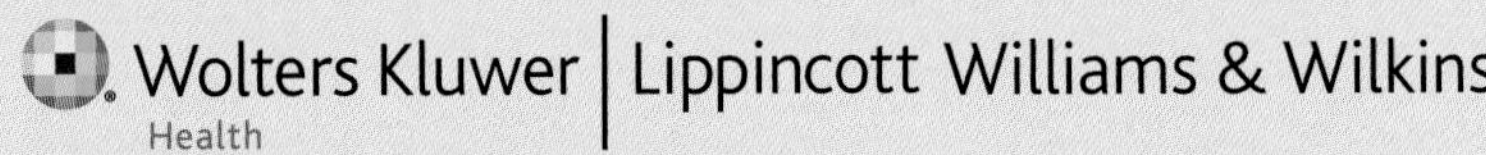
Wolters Kluwer | Lippincott Williams & Wilkins
Health

Philadelphia • Baltimore • New York • London
Buenos Aires • Hong Kong • Sydney • Tokyo

Senior Executive Editor: Jonathan W. Pine, JR.
Product Manager: Marian Bellus
Production Manager: Alicia Jackson
Senior Manufacturing Manager: Benjamin Rivera
Senior Marketing Manager: Angela Panetta
Creative Director: Doug Smock
Production Service: SPi Technologies

Two Commerce Square
2001 Market Street
Philadelphia, PA 19103 USA
LWW.com

Printed in the People's Republic of China

Library of Congress Cataloging-in-Publication Data
Stocker & Dehner's pediatric pathology / [edited by] J. Thomas Stocker, Louis P. Dehner, Aliya N. Husain. — 3rd ed.
p. ; cm.
Other title: Pediatric pathology
Rev. ed. of: Pediatric pathology / editors, J. Thomas Stocker, Louis P. Dehner. 2nd ed. c2001.
Includes bibliographical references and index.
Summary: "Revised and updated for its Third Edition, Stocker & Dehner's Pediatric Pathology provides encyclopedic coverage of the diagnosis of pediatric disorders from the neonatal period through adolescence. It covers all major aspects of the pathologic anatomy of childhood disorders ranging from chromosomal syndromes and neoplasms to forensic pathology. Sections are organized by disease classification and by organ system. The book contains more than 1,300 gross and microscopic images, including 1,200 in full color. This edition includes a new chapter on transplantation pathology. Other highlights include significant updates in the areas of pediatric autopsy, imaging techniques, molecular techniques, embryonic and fetal wastage, congenital abnormalities, metabolic disorders, SIDS and forensic pathology, the placenta, and the nervous system"—Provided by publisher.
ISBN 978-0-7817-6669-2
1. Pediatric pathology. I. Stocker, J. Thomas. II. Dehner, Louis P., 1940- III. Husain, Aliya N. IV. Pediatric pathology.
V. Title: Pediatric pathology.
[DNLM: 1. Pathologic Processes. 2. Pediatrics. WS 200]
RJ49.P413 2011
618.92'007—dc22

2010029168

To purchase additional copies of this book, call our customer service department at (800) 638-3030 or fax orders to (301) 223-2320. International customers should call (301) 223-2300.

Visit Lippincott Williams & Wilkins on the Internet: at LWW.com. Lippincott Williams & Wilkins customer service representatives are available from 8:30 am to 6 pm, EST.

10 9 8 7 6 5 4 3 2 1

CCS1110

To my children and grandchildren—Louis, Jr., Carl, Christopher, Elizabeth, Rebecca, Rachael, Jennifer, and Charlie.

Louis P. Dehner

To my mother, Khadija Omar, who has inspired me throughout my life and in memory of my father, Zahid Omar, who saw only the beginnings of his children's lives.

Aliya N. Husain

To my wife, Pat, the Center of my life, at 44 years together and counting: to our children; Rick, his wife Cathy and sons Jack and Joseph; David, his wife Carol and daughter Sydney; and Meg. How full they make our lives!

J. Thomas Stocker

Contents

Dedication v
Contributors viii
Preface xi
Preface to the First Edition xii
Acknowledgements xiii

SECTION I

General Pathology Techniques in Pediatric Pathology........ 1

CHAPTER 1A
The Pediatric Autopsy 1
J. Thomas Stocker

CHAPTER 1B
Fine-Needle Aspiration 18
John J. Buchino and Robert F. Debski

CHAPTER 1C
Molecular Techniques in Pediatric Pathology 21
Jason A. Jarzembowski and D. Ashley Hill

CHAPTER 1D
Electron Microscopy 47
Gary W. Mierau

CHAPTER 2
First and Second Trimester Pregnancy Loss 56
Deborah E. McFadden

CHAPTER 3
Chromosomal Abnormalities 72
Raj P. Kapur and Joseph R. Siebert

CHAPTER 4
Congenital Anomalies and Malformation Syndromes 94
Joseph R. Siebert

CHAPTER 5
Inborn Errors of Metabolism 126
Carole A. Vogler, David S. Brink and Dorothy K. Grange

CHAPTER 6
Congenital and Acquired Systemic Infectious Diseases 186
Haresh Mani and J. Thomas Stocker

CHAPTER 7
Pediatric Forensic Pathology 252
Tracey S. Corey and Kim A. Collins

CHAPTER 8
Transplant Pathology 291
Rish Pai, Theodore J. Pysher and Aliya N. Husain

SECTION II

Organ System Pathology................................. 323

CHAPTER 9
The Placenta 323
Raymond W. Redline

CHAPTER 10
The Nervous System 352
Christopher Dunham and Arie Perry

CHAPTER 11
Pediatric Ophthalmic Pathology 406
J. Douglas Cameron

CHAPTER 12
The Respiratory Tract 441
J. Thomas Stocker, Haresh Mani and Aliya N. Husain

CHAPTER 13
The Cardiovascular System 516
Kathleen Patterson

CHAPTER 14
The Gastrointestinal Tract 574
John Hart, Rebecca Wilcox and Christopher R. Weber

CHAPTER 15
The Liver, Gallbladder, and Biliary Tract 640
John Hicks, Haresh Mani and J. Thomas Stocker

CHAPTER 16
The Pancreas 743
Mariko Suchi

CHAPTER 17
The Kidney and Lower Urinary Tract 779
Aliya N. Husain and Theodore J. Pysher

CHAPTER 18
The Female Reproductive System 837
Elizabeth J. Perlman and Michael K. Fritsch

CHAPTER 19
The Male Reproductive System, Including Intersex Disorders 865
Hikmat A. Al-Ahmadie

CHAPTER 20
The Breast 897
Jeffrey Mueller, Rebecca Wilcox and Jerome B. Taxy

CHAPTER 21
The Pineal, Pituitary, Parathyroid, Thyroid, and Adrenal Glands 911
Richard M. Conran, Ellen Chung, Louis P. Dehner and Hiroyuki Shimada

CHAPTER 22
The Lymph Nodes, Spleen, and Thymus 975
Thomas L. McCurley, Mary M. Zutter, and Andrea M. Sheehan

CHAPTER 23
The Bone Marrow 1010
Jochen K.M. Lennerz and Anjum Hassan

CHAPTER 24
Soft Tissue 1040
Louis P. Dehner

CHAPTER 25
The Skin 1105
Vijaya B. Reddy and Aliya N. Husain

CHAPTER 26
Neuromuscular Diseases 1147
Kevin E. Bove and Lili Miles

CHAPTER 27
Skeletal System 1190
Louis P. Dehner

Index 1271

Contributors

Hikmat A. Al-Ahmadie, MD Assistant Attending, Department of Pathology, Memorial Sloan-Kettering Cancer Center, New York, New York

Kevin E. Bove, MD Professor, Department of Pathology and Laboratory Medicine, University of Cincinnati, College of Medicine
Staff Pathologist, Division of Pathology and Laboratory Medicine, Cincinnati Children's Hospital Medical Center, Cincinnati, Ohio

David S. Brink, MD Associate Professor, Departments of Pathology and Pediatrics, St. Louis University School of Medicine
Associate Pathologist, Department of Pathology, SSM Cardinal Glennon Children's Medical Center, St. Louis, Missouri

John J. Buchino, MD Emeritus Professor, Department of Pathology, Department of Pediatrics, University of Louisville
Emeritus Chief, Department of Pathology, Kosair Children's Hospital, Louisville, Kentucky

J. Douglas Cameron, MD Professor of Ophthalmology, Departments of Ophthalmology and Pathology, Mayo Clinic, Rochester, Minnesota

Ellen Chung Assistant Professor, Department of Radiology and Radiological Sciences and Department of Pediatrics, Uniformed Services University of the Heath Sciences
Integrated Chief, Diagnostic Radiology Service, Department of Radiology, Walter Reed National Military Medical Center, Bethesda, Maryland

Kim A. Collins, MD Professor, Department of Pathology and Laboratory Medicine, Medical University of South Carolina, Charleston, South Carolina

Richard M. Conran, MD, PhD, JD Professor of Pathology and Emerging Infectious Diseases, Department of Pathology, Uniformed Services University of the Health Sciences, Bethesda, Maryland

Tracey S. Corey Clinical Professor, Division of Forensic Pathology, University of Louisville School of Medicine
Chief Medical Examiner, Kentucky Medical Examiner Program, Commonwealth of Kentucky, Louisville, Kentucky

Robert F. Debski, MD Assistant Professor, Department of Pathology, Department of Pediatrics, University of Louisville
Chief, Department of Pathology, Kosair Children's Hospital, Louisville, Kentucky

Louis P. Dehner, MD Professor, Division of Anatomic and Molecular Pathology, Department of Pathology and Immunology, Washington University in St. Louis
Attending Surgical Pathologist, Lauren V Ackerman Laboratory of Surgical Pathology, Barnes-Jewish and St. Louis Children's Hospitals at the Washington University Medical Center, St. Louis, Missouri

Christopher Dunham, MD Clinical Fellow, Department of Pathology and Immunology, Washington University
Clinical Fellow, Department of Pathology and Immunology, Barnes-Jewish Hospital, St. Louis, Missouri

Michael K. Fritsch, MD, PhD Associate Professor, Department of Pathology and Laboratory Medicine, University of Wisconsin, Madison, Wisconsin

Dorothy K. Grange, MD Professor of Pediatrics, Department of Pediatrics, Division of Genetics and Genomic Medicine, Washington University School of Medicine
Professor of Pediatrics, Department of Pediatrics, St. Louis Children's Hospital, St. Louis, Missouri

John Hart, MD Professor, Department of Pathology, University of Chicago, Chicago, Illinois

Anjum Hassan, MD Assistant Professor, Division of Anatomic and Molecular Pathology, Washington University School of Medicine
Assistant Director FISH Laboratory, Department of Pathology, Washington University Medical Center, Barnes Jewish Hospital, St. Louis, Missouri

M. John Hicks MD, DDS, MS, PhD Professor of Pathology, Department of Pathology and Immunology, Baylor College of Medicine
Attending Pathologist, Department of Pathology, Texas Children's Hospital, Houston, Texas

D. Ashley Hill, MD Associate Professor, Department of Pathology and Pediatrics, The George Washington University
Chief, Department of Pathology, Children's National Medical Center, Washington, DC

Aliya N. Husain, MD Professor, Department of Pathology, University of Chicago, Chicago, Illinois

Jason A. Jarzembowski, MD, PhD Assistant Professor, Department of Pathology, Medical College of Wisconsin
Program Director, Perinatal Pathology, Department of Pathology, Children's Hospital of Wisconsin, Milwaukee, Wisconsin

Raj P. Kapur, MD, PhD Professor, Department of Pathology, University of Washington
Staff Pathologist, Department of Laboratories, Seattle Children's Hospital, Seattle, Washington DC

Jochen K. M. Lennerz, MD, PhD Division of Anatomic and Molecular Pathology, Department of Pathology and Immunology, Washington University School of Medicine, St. Louis, Missouri

Haresh Mani, MD Assistant Professor, Department of Pathology, Northwestern University's Feinberg School of Medicine
Pathologist-in-Chief, Children's Memorial Hospital, Chicago, Illinois

Thomas L. McCurley, MD Associate Professor, Department of Pathology, Vanderbilt University
Director, Department of Immunopathology Laboratory, Nashville, Tennessee

Deborah E. McFadden, MD Clinical Professor, Department of Pathology and Laboratory Medicine, University of British Columbia
Head and Medical Director, Department of Pathology and Laboratory Medicine, BC Children's Hospital and BC Women's Hospital and Health Centre, Vancouver, British Columbia

Gary W. Mierau, PhD Electron Microscopist, Department of Pathology and Laboratory Medicine, The Children's Hospital, Aurora, Colorado

Lili Miles, MD Associate Professor, Department of Pathology and Laboratory Medicine, University of Cincinnati, College of Medicine
Staff Pathologist, Division of Pathology and Laboratory Medicine, Cincinnati Children's Hospital Medical Center, Cincinnati, Ohio

Jeffrey Mueller, MD Assistant Professor, Department of Pathology, University of Chicago, Chicago, Illinois

Rish K. Pai, MD, PhD Associate Staff, Department of Anatomic Pathology, Cleveland Clinic Foundation, Cleveland, Ohio

Kathleen Patterson, MD Associate Professor, Department of Pathology, University of Washington
Associate Pathologist, Department of Pathology, Seattle Children's Hospital, Seattle, Washington DC

Elizabeth J. Perlman, MD Pathologist-in-chief, Children's Memorial Hospital
Professor of Pathology, Northewestern University's Feinberg School of Medicine, Chicago, Illinois

Arie Perry, MD Professor of Pathology and Neurological Surgery, Director of Neuropathology and Vice Chair of Pathology, Department of Pathology, Division of Neuropathology, University of California, San Francisco (UCSF), San Francisco, California

Theodore J. Pysher, MD Professor of Pathology, Department of Pathology, University of Utah School of Medicine
Division Chief of Pediatric Pathology and Director of Laboratories, Primary Children's Medical Center, Salt Lake City, Utah

Vijaya B. Reddy, MD Professor, Department of Pathology, Rush Medical College
Senior Attending, Department of Pathology, Rush University Medical Center, Chicago, Illinois

Raymond W. Redline, MD Professor, Pathology and Reproductive Biology, Case Western Reserve University School of Medicine, Cleveland, OH
Co-director, Pediatric Pathology, Pathology, University Hospitals Case Medical Center, Cleveland, OH

Andrea M. Sheehan, MD Assistant Professor, Department of Pathology and Immunology, Department of Pediatrics, Section of Hematology and Oncology, Baylor College of Medicine
Director of Hematology and Flow Cytometry, Department of Hematopathology, Department of Pathology, Texas Children's Hospital, Houston, Texas

Hiroyuki Shimada, MD, PhD Professor, Department of Pathology, University of Southern California Keck School of Medicine
Pathologist, Department of Pathology and Laboratory Medicine, Children's Hospital Los Angeles, Los Angeles, California

Joseph R. Siebert, PhD Professor of Pathology, Adjunct Professor of Pediatrics, Departments of Pathology, Pediatrics, University of Washington
Director of Autopsy Services, Department of Laboratories, Seattle Children's Hospital, Seattle, Washington

J. Thomas Stocker, MD Professor of Pathology, Pediatrics and Emerging Infectious Disease, Department of Pathology, Uniformed Services University of the Health Sciences, Bethesda, Maryland

Mariko Suchi, MD, PhD Assistant Professor, Department of Pathology, Medical College of Wisconsin
Department of Pathology and Laboratory Medicine, Children's Hospital of Wisconsin, Milwaukee, Wisconsin

Jerome B. Taxy, MD Professor, Department of Pathology, University of Chicago, Chicago, Illinois

Carole A. Vogler, MD Professor and Chair, Department of Pathology, Saint Louis University School of Medicine
Pathologist, Department of Pediatric Pathology, SSM Cardinal Glennon Children's Medical Center, St. Louis, Missouri

Christopher R. Weber, MD, PhD Instructor, Department of Pathology, The University of Chicago, Chicago, Illinois

Rebecca Wilcox, MD Assistant Professor, School of Medicine, The University of Vermont
Assistant Professor, Department of Pathology, Fletcher Allen Hospital, Burlington, Vermont

Mary M. Zutter, MD Professor of Pathology and Cancer Biology, Department of Pathology, Vanderbilt University
Director of Hematopathology, Scientific Director, HTAP Shared Resource, Department of Pathology, Vanderbilt University Medical Center, Nashville, Tennessee

Preface

There is no other way to put it, a book, especially one that is now in its third edition, has long since become an enduring burden. Almost 10 years have elapsed since the last edition and no decade passes without advances being made and old "truths" being dismissed as folly. We have attempted to capture within the front and back covers of this book a reasonable approximation of the latest truths as they relate to our understanding of those unique disorders of maldevelopmental, infectious, and neoplastic nature that are found predominantly in children and in the period of 9 months preceding childhood.

The codex of pediatric pathology is still largely based upon morphologic features that are apparent in their gross manifestations as in the case of congenital heart disease and skeletal dysplasias or on visualizing microscopic features. Immunohistochemistry has become as routine today as the trichrome and Gomori methenamine-silver stains. However, we have now moved into the era of application of molecular diagnostic methodologies that have admitted us into an unseen world in a sense. The pace of discoveries has created a world where yesterday becomes a part of the deep past as we catapult through today. In the microcosm of pediatric pathology, the current endeavor is our attempt to capture what is reasonably stable as the foundation of morphologic pediatric pathology. In the yesterdays, we may have speculated about the pathogenesis or puzzled over the morphologic findings, but today, we have the ability to test those speculations and begin the process of diagnostic discovery and investigation. As we have all experienced, this process is oftentimes one door leading to another. An attempt has been made in this edition to not only lay out the foundation of pediatric pathology but also convey the idea that another door awaits to be opened. It is to our younger colleagues in pediatric pathology that we address this latter challenge.

For the majority of the chapters, about 200 of the most important references are in the printed book; the rest are available as eReferences as indicated in the text. Similarly, some additional photomicrographs are available as eFigures.

We have gathered a distinguished group of contributors to this tome whose collective efforts are every bit as worthy as the three names that appear on the front cover. It is very difficult to find individuals as knowledgeable as they are who choose to devote their precious time to the arduous task of writing a chapter that conforms to the goals of this volume as discussed in the preceding paragraph. These authors met and exceeded those aspirations. Some authors questioned whether the third edition would ever become a reality with legitimate cause since we all recognize the prolonged gestation of this enterprise. One of us (LPD) had to be coaxed and even harangued into the yoke but here we are through the monumental efforts of another one of us (ANH). We are grateful to our authors who are also our colleagues, both past and present. Your patience and perseverance are appreciated well beyond this acknowledgment.

J. Thomas Stocker, MD
Louis P. Dehner, MD
Aliya N. Husain, MD

Preface to the First Edition

Several years ago, the editors of this volume were lamenting the fact that a third edition of Kissane's *Pathology of Infancy and Childhood* was unlikely because John Kissane had committed himself to another formidable publishing enterprise. Our British colleagues in pediatric pathology have authored two fine references (Keeling's *Fetal and Neonatal Pathology* and Berry's *Paediatric Pathology*), but it was our opinion that a comprehensive volume on all major aspects of the pathologic anatomy of chlldhood disorders ranging from chromosomal syndromes and neoplasms to forensic pathology was needed. At this juncture in our deliberations, we were confronted with the daunting nature of the potential task at hand given the required range of expertise necessary to cover all of these areas. Our attention turned to the reservoir of such abilities that exists in an organization of which we are privileged to be members, the Society for Pediatric Pathology, formerly known as the Pediatric Pathology Club. Many of the contributors to this volume are friends and colleagues whom we met through the Society for Pediatric Pathology.

It was Albert Einstein who acknowledged the fact that we all stand on the shoulders of giants, and certainly pediatric pathology has evolved to its present state through the seminal contributions of the "first" generation of North American pediatric pathologists. Some of these include Maude Abbott, Dorothy Andersen, James B. Arey, J. Bruce Beckwith, Jay Bernstein, William A. Blanc, Robert P. Bolande, John Craig, John R. Esterly, Sidney Farber, George Fetterman, Enid Gilbert-Barness, M. Daria Haust, John M. Kissane, Benjamin H. Landing, A. James McAdams, Harry B. Neustein, William A. Newton, Ella Oppenheimer, Eugene V. Perrin, Edith Potter, Harvey S. Rosenberg, Marie Valdes-Dapena, Gordon Vawter, and F.W. Wigglesworth, to mention only a few. Virtually all of us in the second and now third generation of pediatric pathologists can call one of these extraordinary individuals our mentor.

Because we the editors are also the co-authors of several chapters in this textbook, we appreciate firsthand the many hours that our contributors have invested in the completion of their manuscripts. The time, experience, and patience necessary to compile information into the concise prose required by a textbook of this type are greatly appreciated. This textbook belongs to all of these authors collectively, despite the connotations of the cover and title page.

We also thank our colleagues and friends at our respective institutions for their understanding and support during the prolonged gestation and difficult delivery of this textbook. At the Armed Forces Institute of Pathology, these include Robert McMeekin, MD, Robert F. Karnei, MD, Vernon Armbrustmacher, MD, Nancy Roberts, Luther Duckett, Lisa Penalver, and Venetia Valiga. At the University of Minnesota, Ellis S. Benson, MD, Dale Snover, MD, and Diane Perez, and at the Washington University Medical Center, Emil Unanue, MD, Mark R. Wick, MD; Eleanor Grob, and Patricia Dixon are recognized for their special support.

J. Thomas Stocker, MD
Louis P. Dehner, MD

Acknowledgments

Dr. Stocker would like to acknowledge the authors of prior editions who are no longer with us: Drs. Laurence E. Becker and Patricia A. O'Shea.

Dr. Dehner would like to acknowledge Jeannie Doerr, Margaret Chesney, and Walter Clermont whose tireless efforts and encouragement brought him back from the lip of the abyss.

Dr. Husain would like to acknowledge the strong support and advice given by Drs. Thomas Krausz and Vinay Kumar and the excellent secretarial service provided by Dorothy Peoples and Margaret Rietman.

SECTION I
General Pathology Techniques in Pediatric Pathology

CHAPTER 1A

The Pediatric Autopsy

J. THOMAS STOCKER

As described by the Autopsy Committee of the College of American Pathologists, the autopsy is "a medical-surgical procedure by a physician for the welfare of the living through the study of those patients for whom all our current knowledge and technology were inadequate"(1). The use of the autopsy in medicine as a tool of discovery and education has declined frighteningly in the past 25 years, with some newer hospitals not even including an autopsy suite in their design. In many hospitals, including university hospitals, the autopsy incidence (autopsies compared to number of deaths) has dropped well below 20%, often reaching as low as 2% to 5%. Pediatric hospitals have historically had a higher incidence, often as high as 75% or more, but in recent years this incidence has declined as well. In a survey in 2005 (by the author) of 15 children's hospitals, the autopsy rate for in-hospital deaths varied from 15% to 48% with an average of 32%, and that figure represented a 5% to 10% drop from the rate in 2000 at these same children's hospitals.

Many excellent textbooks and protocols have been written describing methods for performing an autopsy. The following is a technique the author has developed over the past 40 years, often incorporating many techniques from these textbooks and colleagues' experience. This type of autopsy has proven useful to the author, but is by no means the only procedure that might be used.

THE STANDARD PEDIATRIC AUTOPSY

Autopsy Permit

The first step with any autopsy is examination of the autopsy permit for its completeness. This includes a determination of the nature of the death of the patient and whether it may be under medical examiner jurisdiction (i.e., a coroner's case). It is imperative that the pathologist performing the autopsy be intimately familiar with the criteria for medical examiner jurisdiction in the community in which the patient died. The College of American Pathology maintains a state-by-state file of these criteria (www.CAP.org).

Following examination of the autopsy permit, the clinical chart of the patient should be reviewed and a call placed (if possible) to the attending physician or other members of the medical team responsible for the patient. In addition to a review of the clinical or hospital course of the patient, the medical team should be asked what questions they might have that the autopsy should address.

A variety of forms and protocols are available for the pediatric autopsy and one of these might be used (see Appendix) or one designed specifically to address the types of patients in a particular hospital.

Instrumentation

The instruments used in performing the pediatric autopsy are often quite different than those used in adult autopsies, both in type and the size (Figure 1A-1). Pediatric autopsies, particularly those done on fetuses and neonates, require smaller and more delicate instruments than the "full-sized" instruments used on larger children or adults (Table 1A-1). In morgues where adult autopsies are also done, it is often wise to keep the instruments used for the pediatric autopsy in a separate area, even under lock and key, if necessary, to assure they are not used (and abused) doing autopsies on adults.

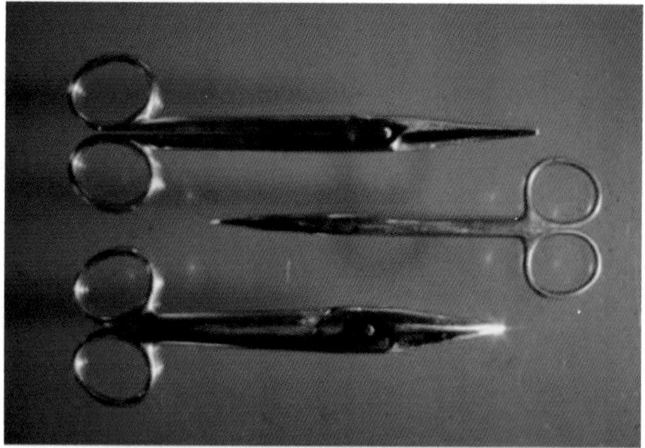

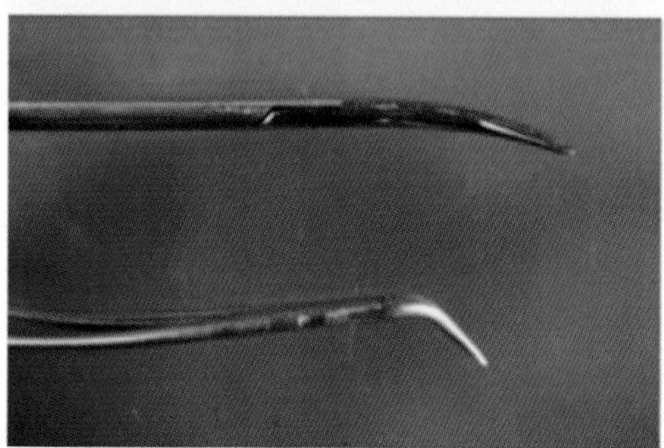

FIGURE 1A-1 ■ **Top**: Small instruments such as these scissors, that are proportional to the size of the infant are vital to the performance of the autopsy. **Bottom**: Curved and tapered ends are helpful in dissecting and holding tissues.

External Examination

The external examination of the body is one of the most important aspects of the pediatric autopsy for it offers information about the general health of the infant/child, evidence of therapy, and portends what might be expected when the body is opened. And since, with the exception of skin sections taken for microscopic examination, the "shell" of the patient will be documented and recorded only as measurements, photographs and descriptive phrases, accuracy and completeness of the examination are all the more important.

General measurements include body weight, body length (crown-heel and crown-rump [in neonates]) (Figure 1A-2), arm span from the tip of the fingers of one hand to the tip of the fingers on the other hand (which in most cases approximates the crown-heel length) (eFigure 1A-1), and head (occiput to frontal) (Figure 1A-3), chest (at level of nipples) (eFigure 1A-2), and abdominal (at level of umbilicus) circumference (eFigure 1A-3). This information can be recorded in the autopsy description or on drawings included in the final autopsy report. External markings such as needle marks, IV tubes, chest tubes, incisions, abrasions, etc. also need to be recorded and can be illustrated on standard drawings (Figure 1A-4).

FACE, EYES, EARS, MOUTH (EXTERNAL AND INTERNAL)

Examination of the *face* begins with an overall view to determine symmetry and gross abnormalities. As facial abnormalities often predict brain abnormalities, special attention should be paid to midfacial development (hypertelorism/hypotelorism, nasal bridge deformities) and hair patterns. The hair growth pattern usually consists of one or two whorls in the upper occipital/parietal area. More than two whorls or actual defects in the scalp (eFigure 1A-4) are associated with underlying CNS abnormalities. The anterior and posterior fontanelles should be examined for their size (maximum length and width), shape, and "fullness" (i.e., bulging, depressed) (Figure 1A-5). The *neck* should be

Table 1A-1 ■ INSTRUMENTS USED IN PERFORMING THE PEDIATRIC AUTOPSY

Scissors
- a. Thin, small, with tapered points and curved tip, used more for dissection than cutting. Limit their use to soft tissues, and organs, not for bone, cartilage, or dense tissues.
- b. Medium sized, straight or curved for opening bowel.
- c. Large or heavier ones for opening calvarium and vertebral column.

Forceps
- a. Small and medium sized, but WITHOUT teeth (which only tears tissue)

Hemostats
- a. Small and medium sized
- b. Straight and curved

Scalpels
- a. No. 10 size curved for most routine work
- b. No. 1 size with pointed tip for delicate cutting
- c. Double edged, rectangular for sectioning organs such as spleen, lung, liver, kidneys

Knives
- a. Straight, of various sizes for sectioning larger organs such as liver, brain, or organs of larger children

Balances for weighing
- a. Standard hanging balance for weighing neonates or small children
- b. Electronic balance (accurate to 0.1 g) for weighing organs

Probes of various diameters to establish patency of various openings including nares, ears, ureters, urethra, biliary tract, heart valves, patency of foramen ovale, and ductus arteriousus.

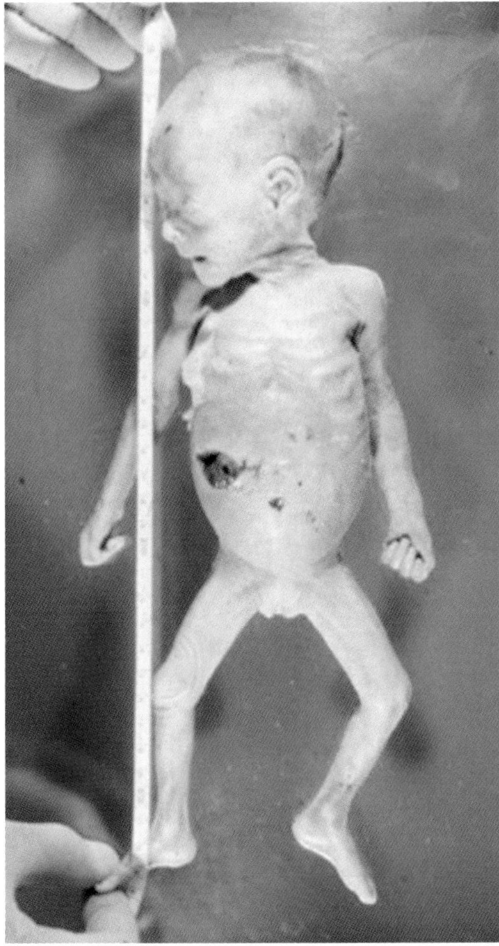

FIGURE 1A-2■ Fullbody view showing crown-hell measurement.

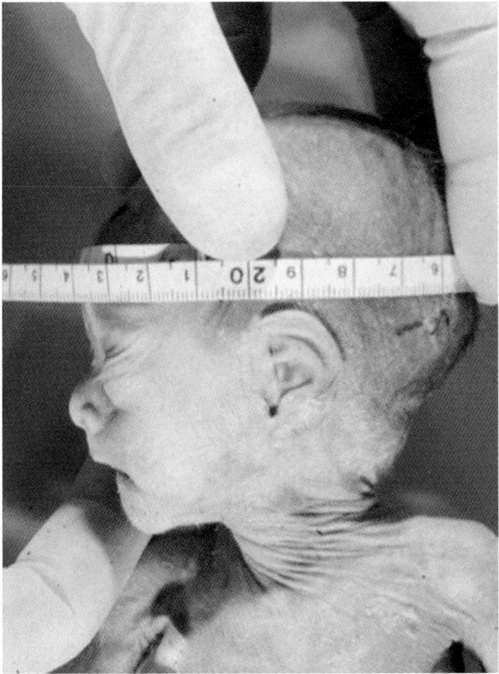

FIGURE 1A-3■ Head circumference is measured in the frontal-occipital plane.

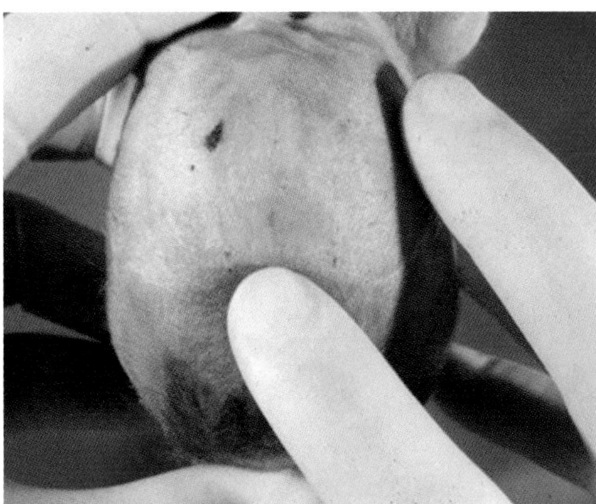

FIGURE 1A-4■ Head examination includes palpation and measurement of the anterior fontanel.

flexed and extended as far as possible to determine its range of motion (eFigure 1A-5A,B).

The *eyes* are examined for both size and location. The measurement of each palpebral fissure should, in a normal infant, equal the intercanthal distance (eFigure 1A-6, Figure 1A-6) effectively dividing the face at the level of the eyes into three equal expanses. If the fissure length exceeds the intercanthal distance, the eyes are closer together than normal (hypotelorism), and conversely, if the intercanthal distance exceeds the palpebral fissure length, the eyes are too far apart (hypertelorism).

Examination of the eye itself includes the diameter of each pupil and comparison with each other to determine if the eyes are of equal size (eFigure 1A-7). If one is smaller than the other, microphthalmia may be present. If there is a question, the eyeballs may be removed from within the cranium after the brain is removed (see CNS examination). The pupils are also examined for their symmetry and completeness (vs. aniridia) and their color (which may be difficult to determine in a premature infant).

The *nose* examination includes its position and shape (e.g., upturned, flat) with evaluation of cartilage development. A curved probe can be used to determine the patency of the choanae (posterior nasal apertures) (Figure 1A-7). The lip beneath the nose (the prolabium) should be observed and determined if longer that usual (associated with the fetal alcohol syndrome).

Examination of the *ears* begins with determining their position on the side of the head relative to the level of the palpebral fissures. In near-term and term infants, the tip of the ears should be above the level of the palpebral fissures (Figure1A-8) or they are considered to be "lowset." As the ears develop in utero, they "move" upward as the lower face and jaw develop and expand, reaching and then rising above the palpebral fissure level in late third trimester.

The ears are also examined for patency of the external auditory canal (via small caliber probe) by pulling down on the earlobe as the probe is inserted (eFigure 1A-8). The external ear should be evaluated for its shape and completeness and for the presence of cartilage.

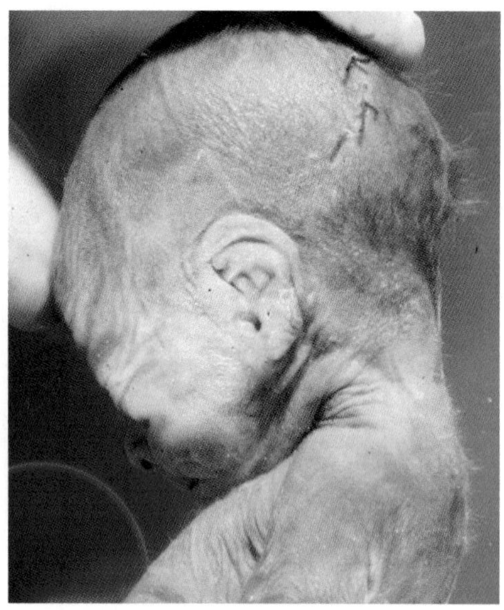

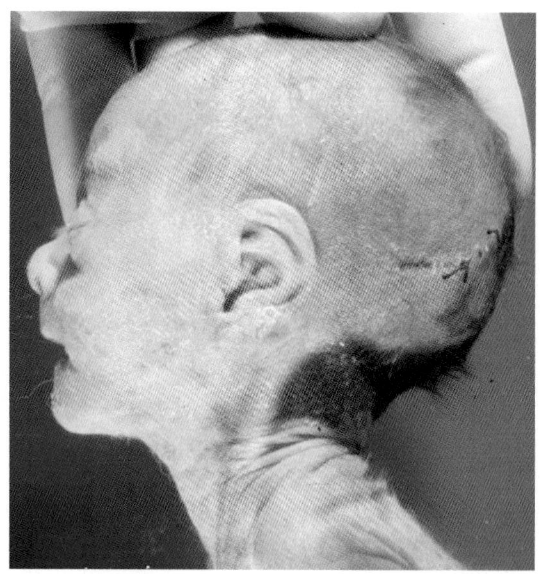

A B

FIGURE 1A-5 ■ Check the mobility of the neck by flexing (**A**) and extending (**B**) it.

The *mouth* should be inspected both externally and internally. A finger can be inserted into the mouth to examine the alveolar ridges of the jaw for the presence (or absence) of teeth and for determination of the shape and completeness of the palate (eFigure 1A-9). The tongue can be palpated as well, but may also be removed intact after the thoracic organs have been removed (see below).

ARMS, HANDS, FINGERS

The *upper extremities* are examined for symmetry, mobility, and the presence of skin lesions. The *axilla* should be palpated for the presence of lymph nodes or other masses. The positioning and mobility of the fingers should be noted along with their length. Some chromosomal anomalies (e.g., trisomies 13 and 18) may produce an overlapping of the little finger over the fourth finger and the index finger over the third finger (eFigure 1A-10). Children with Down syndrome (trisomy 21) often display short metacarpals and phalanges, and hypoplasia of the midphalanx of the fifth finger (eFigure 1A-11). Nails should be examined for the presence of hypoplasia or dysplasia. Radiographs of the extremities may be helpful in identifying skeletal abnormalities (e.g., radial hypoplasia of the VATER association) or recent or old fractures. In fact, in cases of suspected nonaccidental trauma (NAT), a full skeletal survey would be important.

The *palms of the hands* should be examined for aberrant patterning, most notably for the presence of a Simian crease or a malpositioned axial triradius, common findings in Down syndrome but also seen in a wide variety of other syndromes.

FIGURE 1A-6 ■ Measuring the intercanthal distance.

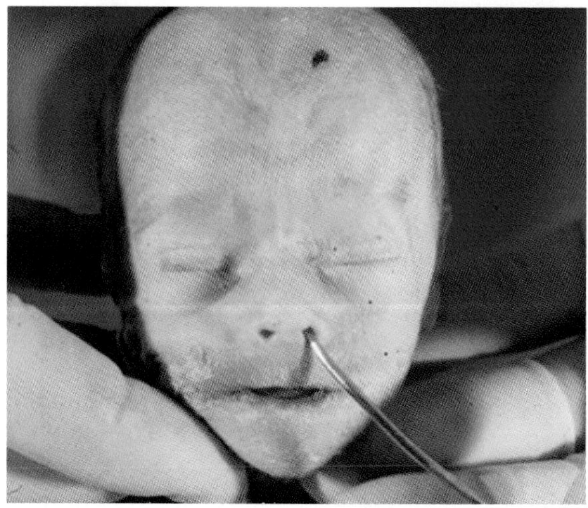

FIGURE 1A-7 ■ Examination of the nose includes checking for the patency of each nares into the upper pharynx with a probe or curved suturing needle.

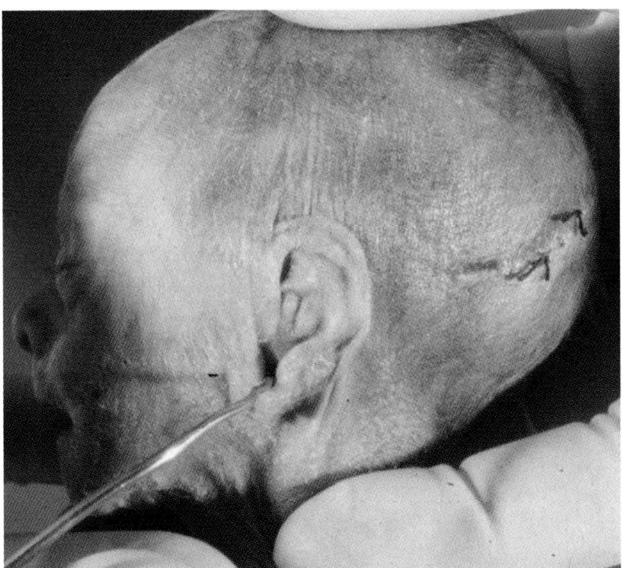

FIGURE 1A-8 Probing the external auditory canal.

CHEST: FRONT AND BACK

Examination of the chest begins with the determination of its symmetry, position of the nipples, and length and positioning of the sternum (e.g., pectus excavatum or carinatum). The junction of the neck with the chest should be examined to note the shape and the length of the neck (short neck or webbed skin). The clavicles should be palpated for degree of development (e.g., hypoplasia) and the presence of fractures. Breast development should be determined using a system such as the Tanner stage I to V system (2).

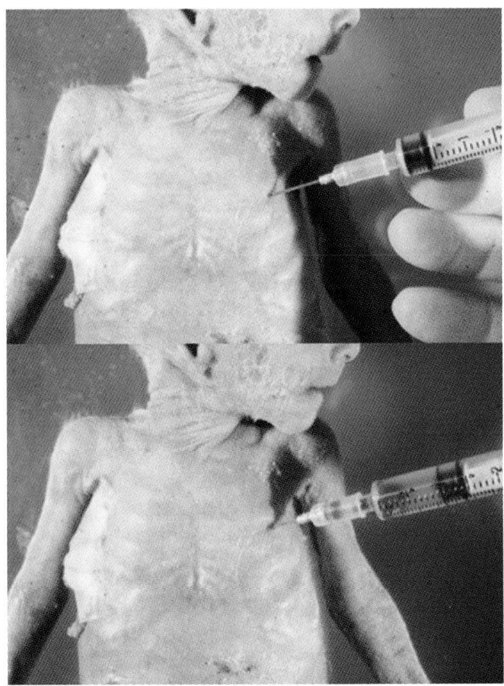

FIGURE 1A-9 **Top**: A needle is inserted between the upper ribs at an angle parallel to the sternum. **Bottom**: If air or fluid is present in the thorax it can be withdrawn and measured (or cultured, if appropriate cleansing is performed).

Turning the body over or rolling it on its side allows examination of the back for symmetry (e.g., scoliosis, lordosis) and the presence of lesions. Particularly important in infants is the presence of spinal and vertebral column defects indicative of meningomyelocele and spina bifida, remembering that one form, spinal bifida occulta, may not be visible as a skin defect.

At this point, prior to the opening of the chest and abdomen, aspiration of the thorax for air, blood and/or fluid can be performed. In young children, in particular, the presence of air or fluid in each hemithorax can be determined as well as its amount. With the body in the supine position, a 12- to 14-gauge needle on a 5- to 25-mL syringe (depending on the size of the child), can be inserted parallel to the autopsy table at the rib-sternal junction between the 4th and 5th or 5th and 6th ribs, being careful to avoid the heart (Figure 1A-9). When inserted through the parietal pleura, aspiration of air or fluid within the free space of the hemithorax can be attempted. If nothing is present as the syringe plunger is pulled back, the plunger when released will move back toward the needle. If air or fluid is present, it will be withdrawn as the plunger is pulled back until it can no longer be done. At this point, the amount of fluid/air in the syringe can be measured and, if a sterile draw has been done, the fluid may be sent for culture. If the plunger is pulled back to its maximum length, the needle and/or syringe can be removed, the amount of air/fluid measured and expelled from the syringe, and then reinserted into the same needle hole for aspiration of as much air/fluid as is left (repeating as many times as needed). The same procedure can then be performed on the other hemithorax. This allows for an accurate measurement of the amount of pneumothorax, hemithorax, or transudate/exudate present on each side.

ABDOMEN: FRONT AND BACK INCLUDING ANUS/VAGINA, URETHRA

The shape of the abdomen should be evaluated looking for distension (e.g., ascites or abdominal air), depression (e.g., secondary to dehydration), and wall thickness (edema, muscular atrophy, etc.). Sterile aspiration of abdominal fluid may be performed for culture prior to incising the abdominal wall. Signs of premortem medical intervention such as needle marks or incisions should be recorded. In newborn infants, the umbilicus should be examined for evidence of inflammation or necrosis and, if present, the stump of the umbilical cord may be examined for the presence of two umbilical arteries and one umbilical vein. Discoloration of the abdominal wall may indicate underlying hemorrhage, infection, or gastrointestinal necrosis as in neonatal necrotizing enterocolitis (eFigure 1A-12).

The external genitalia can be examined for anatomic development and, in infant boys, the presence or absence of testes in the scrotum should be noted along with the size and development of the penis. A staging system can be used to describe pubic hair growth in male and females. In females,

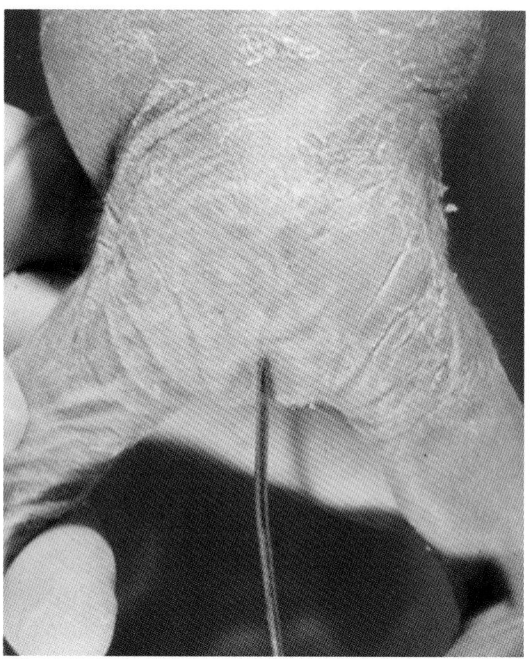

FIGURE 1A-10 ■ The anus (and penis of vagina) should be probed for patency.

the patency of the vaginal opening may be determined with a probe (eFigure 1A-13). Similarly, the anus should be probed for patency in neonates, recognizing that anal atresia may be higher that the anal opening (Figure 1A-10). The presence of meconium is a clear sign of anal patency.

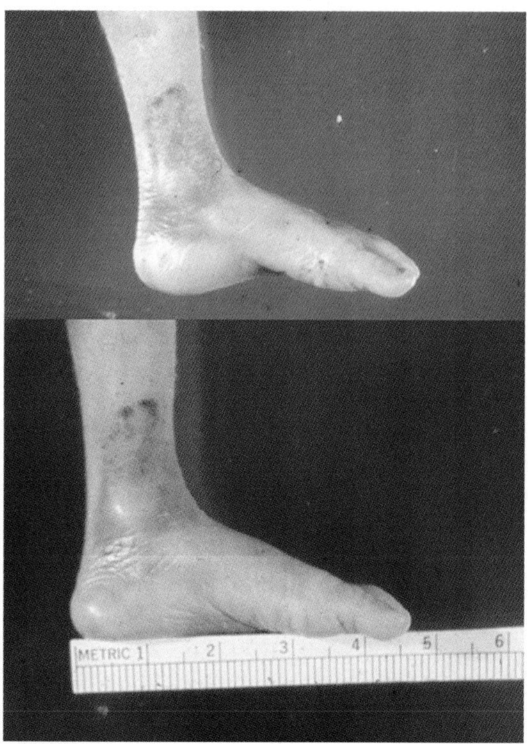

FIGURE 1A-11 ■ Examination of the foot includes its overall development and configuration (arched versus "rocker-bottom") (**top**) as well as it length (**bottom**) which correlates with gestational age.

LEGS, FEET, TOES

The lower extremities should be examined for symmetry and length (i.e., in proportion to trunk and arm length). In infants, the hips can be rotated to determine laxity. Feet should be examined for the presence of an arch to the sole (Figure 1A-11), versus a "rocker-bottom" configuration as may be seen with certain trisomies (eFigure 1A-14). Five toes should be present on each foot and the spaces between toes should be of equal depth.

Special Techniques and Studies

Photography. Photography is an integral and highly important part of any autopsy, particularly images of abnormalities or gross pathology for which microscopic sections may be inadequate documentation. And with the availability of digital technology, many photographs can be taken with the "excess or unnecessary" images easily removed at no cost. While fixed photography equipment is useful, a handheld camera is more easily utilized and encourages the taking of images throughout the performance of the autopsy.

Basic images should include the external surface of the body (front and back) and anterior and lateral views of the face. Incisions and other surface marks on the face trunk and extremities may be photographed and documented particularly in cases of suspected NAT. A ruler placed at the edge of the picture helps define the dimensions of a lesion. Images of internal organs are taken as needed to document anatomic abnormalities or specific pathologic changes (e.g., necrosis, hemorrhage).

Radiography. Imaging via x-rays, MRI, or CT can be important in diagnosing and documenting skeletal abnormalities from chondrodyplasias to fractures. They may also be helpful in recording the presence of such things as pneumothorax, pneumopericardium, and pneumoperitonium, along with documenting the extent of tumor involvement in metastatic diseases.

LABORATORY TECHNIQUES

Cultures. "Standard" cultures (aerobic and anaerobic bacterial) of blood, lung, and CSF may be taken, or appropriate cultures (fungal and/or viral) might be determined as the clinical history suggests or as the autopsy progresses and signs of infection are noted (e.g., cloudy abdominal fluid in peritonitis or aspirated fluid from an unsuspected cyst or abscess).

Unusual studies are those that extend beyond the limits of the standard autopsy as described in the autopsy permit, for example, examination of the organs of the chest and abdomen, and the brain. Removal of the eyes or long bones of the arms and legs might be needed to diagnose diseases of the eyes or to define a particular type of musculoskeletal dysplasia. (Special permission for these procedures may be needed.)

Cytogenetics. Tissue for cell culture should be taken as soon as possible after death (and having the autopsy permit signed and witnessed). Chromosome studies should be considered in embryos and fetuses when the maternal history or the appearance of the embryo/fetus suggests the presence of chromosomal abnormalities. "Large" chromosomal abnormalities such as trisomies or deletion of a major portion of a long or a short arm are often associated with significant external abnormalities such as midline defects (facial dysmorphia), hand or feet changes (syndactyly, "rocker-bottom" feet), and scalp defects (see Chapters 3 and 4).

The source of the tissue is dependent on the time after death in which the sample is obtained (see below).

Internal Examination

Chest and Abdomen

Unless the clinical history or appearance of the body suggests otherwise (e.g., a large gastroschisis or previous thoracic or abdominal surgery with sutured incisions still present), the opening of the body is most commonly done via a "Y"-shaped incision (Figure 1A-12) or some variation (e.g., "U"-shaped over chest with extension to the symphysis pubis). In either case, the incision begins in the anterior axillary line at the level of the clavicle and extends to the xyphoid just below the sternum then up to the opposite anterior axillary line. In a neonate or infant, the chest incision can be positioned through or adjacent to the nipples to allow sampling of breast tissue while obtaining a section of skin. Subcutaneous tissue may also be measured (thickness) (eFigure 1A-15) and observed to determine the state of nutrition of the infant or the state of hydration. Edema can often be noted in the subcutaneous tissue of the chest. From the point below the xyphoid, the incision is extended toward the symphysis pubis on either side of the umbilicus.

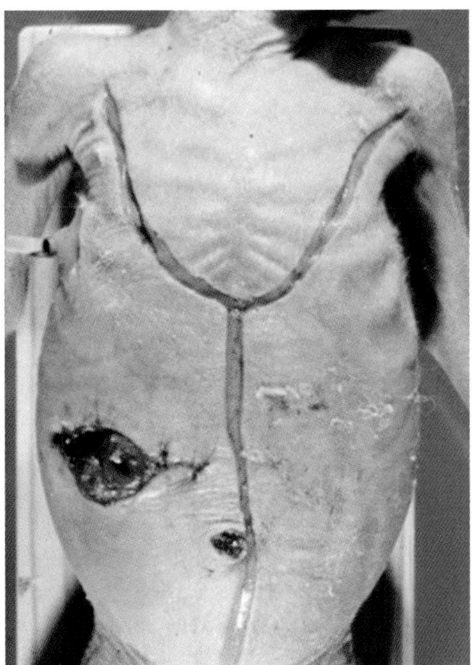

FIGURE 1A-12 ■ A "standard" Y-shaped incision is used to gain access to the thorax and abdomen. Note the gastronomy site in the right upper quadrant.

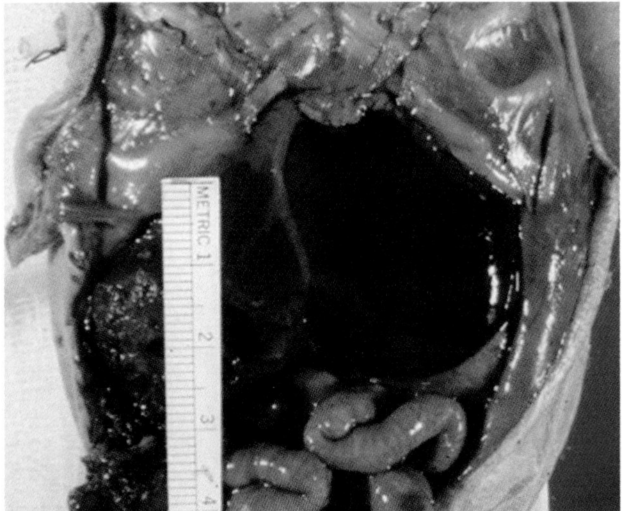

FIGURE 1A-13 ■ With the abdomen open, but before removal of the chest plate, the abdominal organs can be examined. Here the size of the liver is determined by measuring its extension below the lower sternal border, in this measurment in the right midclavicular line.

The skin of the chest and abdomen is reflected to either side after dissecting it free from the sternum and thoracic cage (eFigure 1A-16). The abdominal skin is freed along the lower rib margin.

The following measurements may be made prior to removing the chest plate (Figure 1A-13). The size of the liver is judged by measuring the distance that it extends below the rib margin (assuming no diaphragmatic hernia is present). Measurements are made in the anterior axillary lines, the midclavicular line, and the midline (eFigures 1A-17 and 1A-18). If the liver does not extend to the left anterior axillary line, the distance it does extend to the left can be recorded by measuring the distance from the midline to where it disappears beneath the rib margin (eFigure 1A-19). Other measurements include

1. The distance the spleen tip extends below (or above) the rib margin.
2. The distance the gallbladder extends above or below the margin of the liver—done primarily to see that a gallbladder is present.
3. The distance the urinary bladder extends above the symphysis pubis.
4. The root and the radius of the mesentery. The root is determined by moving the bowel toward the upper right quadrant and measuring the length of its attachment to the vertebral column (eFigure 1A-20). The radius is determined by placing one end of a ruler on the vertebral column where the mesentery attaches and pulling up a segment of small bowel and measuring the distance from the vertebral column to where it attaches at the mesenteric border of the bowel (eFigure 1A-21).
5. The amount the diaphragm leaflets are pushed up into the thorax by the abdominal organs. This is done by placing a finger beneath the rib margin in the right and left

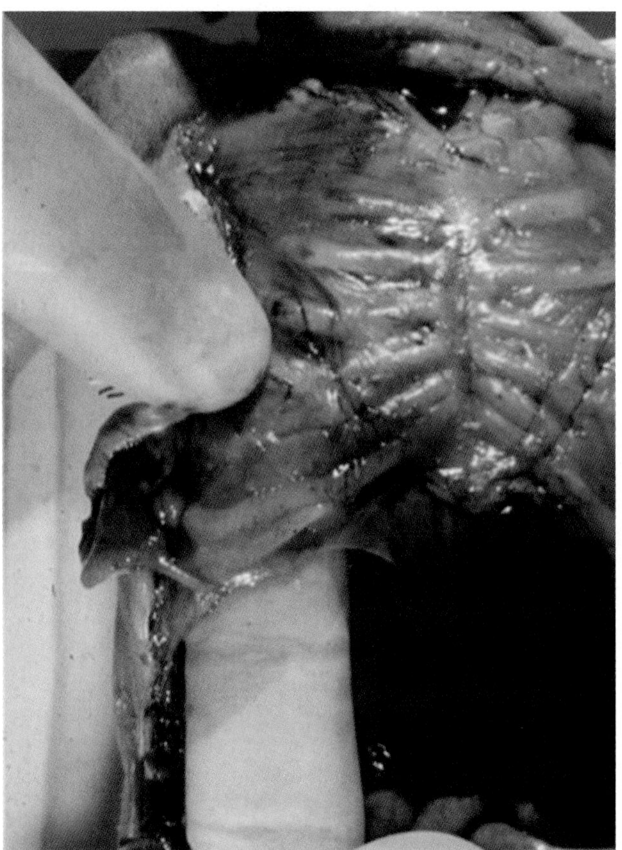

FIGURE 1A-14 ■ The height of the diaphragm is measured by inserting a finger up under the lower sternal border and palpating its upward extension to the highest rib or intercostal space.

midclavicular line and feeling how high the leaflets extend (Figure 1A-14). This is determined by noting where one can feel one's finger in relationship to a rib or intercostal space (e.g., 5th intercostal space or 6th rib) (eFigure 1A-22). This measurement is significant for determining whether the diaphragm leaflets are intact, and whether air or fluid (e.g., blood, pus) in the thorax have forced the leaflets down.

THYMUS

The thymus in infants is often quite large and may obstruct the view of the pericardium and great vessels of the heart. It is usually helpful to dissect the thymus free from the other chest organs and weigh it before proceeding to the examination of the heart and lungs. Care must be taken to include the portion of the thymus that extends "outside" the chest into the cervical tissues of the neck.

BLOOD CULTURE

When a blood-borne infection is suspected, a blood culture may be obtained prior to dissecting the cardiovascular system. An easy approach is to open the pericardial sac and, after measuring any fluid that may be present, use a needle and syringe (after searing the surface of the right atrium with a heated spatula) (eFigure 1A-23A,B) to withdraw blood for culture (Figure 1A-15). *Caution*: if a cardiac anomaly is suspected, one may choose to sterilize and withdraw blood from the inferior vena cava just prior to its entering the heart, thus avoiding damage to the atrium by the heated spatula.

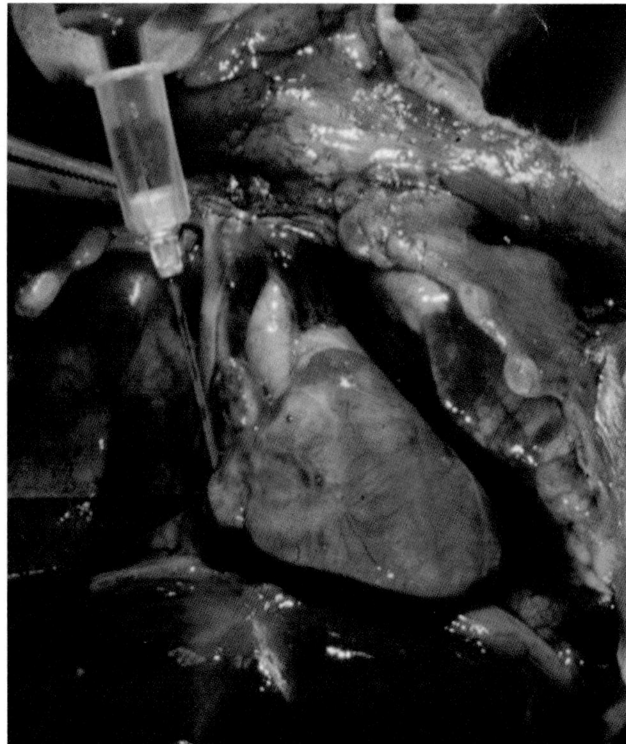

FIGURE 1A-15 ■ A blood culture can be taken from the inferior vena cava or the right atrium after searing the appropriate area with a heated spatula.

LUNG CULTURE

Lung tissue for culture may easily be obtained from the right or left lower lobe by immobilizing it with a forceps or hemostat, searing the surface with a heated spatula, and, using a sterile scalpel, excising a piece of lung tissue (eFigure 1A-24A to C).

TISSUE FOR CYTOGENETICS

Before taking tissue for examination and culture, contact the laboratory performing the analysis and obtain appropriate media (such as RPMI) for transportation. Tissues that may be used for cell culture include the amniotic membranes of the placenta, spleen, and blood for lymphocytes and skin, fascia, pericardium, pleura, and retroperitoneal tissue for fibroblasts. The sooner this tissue can be placed in the appropriate media, the better chance for successful growth, but fibroblasts from fascia and skin may often still be successfully harvested 24 to 48 hours after death.

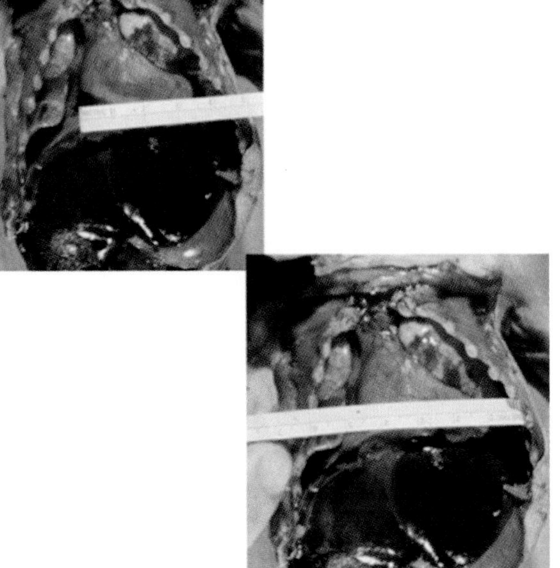

FIGURE 1A-16 ■ The cardiac-thoracic ratio is determined by measuring the width of the heart (**top**) at its widest point and the width of the thoracic cavity (**bottom**) at its widest internal point.

CARDIAC/THORACIC RATIO

Prior to removal of the organs of the chest, the width of the heart at its widest point should be measured and compared to the width of the thorax at the same point (Figure 1A-16). The ratio is helpful in detecting cardiac anomalies since a ratio of greater than 0.5 is often associated with many of these anomalies. With this initial suspicion, a "nonstandard" approach to the heart's dissection may be employed (see later).

REMOVING THE ORGANS

Organ-by-organ versus Rokitansky. Removal and examination of the chest and abdominal organs can be done one organ at a time or by removing the neck, chest, and abdominal organs as one unit (Rokitansky technique). The latter technique is best performed by beginning in the area of the neck and working caudally. The neck organs are dissected by working around the larynx, esophagus, and descending aorta, freeing them with blunt dissection from the soft tissues laterally and behind. Anteriorly, the left brachial artery, the left carotid artery, and the right brachiocephalic artery may be tied off and transected to allow access to them by the mortician (eFigure 1A-25). When dissection has extended behind and laterally above the larynx, the region above the epiglottis can be transected allowing the complete larynx with attached esophagus to be pulled inferiorly (eFigure 1A-26A,B). Following this, the left lung can be pulled aside to allow an incision to be made along the spinal column just behind the esophagus and aorta. When this procedure is repeated on the right side, the neck organs along with the heart/lung/esophagus can be pulled forward (eFigure 1A-27). The abdominal organs are mobilized by cutting the diaphragm (a good time to take a section for microscopic examination) along the contour of the body wall and dissecting inferiorly along the spinal canal, freeing up the spleen and kidney on the left and the liver and kidney on the right. Care must be taken to avoid cutting across the ureters as they pass along the sides of the spinal column before entering the bladder. At this point, the urethra and rectum (and vagina in a female) must be transected (eFigure 1A-28A,B) and freed from the soft tissue of the pelvis allowing the entire neck, chest, and abdominal block to be removed intact.

Note: In a premature infant, it is often prudent to remove the ovaries or testes (if undescended) prior to performing the Rokitansky technique in order to not "lose" them during the dissection (eFigure 1A-29).

It may also be helpful in some cases to perform a *"modified" Rokitansky technique* and remove one or more of the organs before removing the entire block (e.g., remove the spleens in cases of polysplenia, or the bowel in cases of intestinal atresia or duplication).

TESTES/OVARIES

As noted above, it is often easier to remove the ovaries (and testes if undescended) shortly after opening the abdomen. The small size of an infant's ovaries may make locating them difficult. By finding the uterus and fallopian tubes behind the urinary bladder, one can locate the ovaries adjacent to the tubes. They can then be removed, weighed, and often submitted in toto for microscopic examination. Larger ovaries from older infants and young girls may be hemisected. These often contain small fluid-filled cysts.

Testes that are present in the scrotum may be removed by pressure on the scrotum in the direction of the inguinal canal, then inserting a forceps into the canal from the open abdomen, pulling on the vas deferens, and extracting both the vas deferens and testis. This can then be examined for the presence of a vascular malformation or a hydrocele before dissecting the testis free from the vas deferens and attached soft tissue, weighing it and submitting a section for microscopic examination.

EXAMINATION OF THE BODY CAVITY

Following removal of the chest and abdominal organs, the body cavity can be examined for abnormalities of the *ribs* and spinal cord (Figure 1A-17). *Vertebral bodies* may be noted to be irregular, for example, butterfly vertebrae in the VATER association (Vertebral or Vascular anomaly, Anal atresia, TracheoEsophageal fistula, Renal or Radial abnormality), or out of alignment, for example, scoliosis or lordosis (eFigure 1A-30). Special attention should be given to the area in which the ribs abut the spinal column as this is a region in which rib

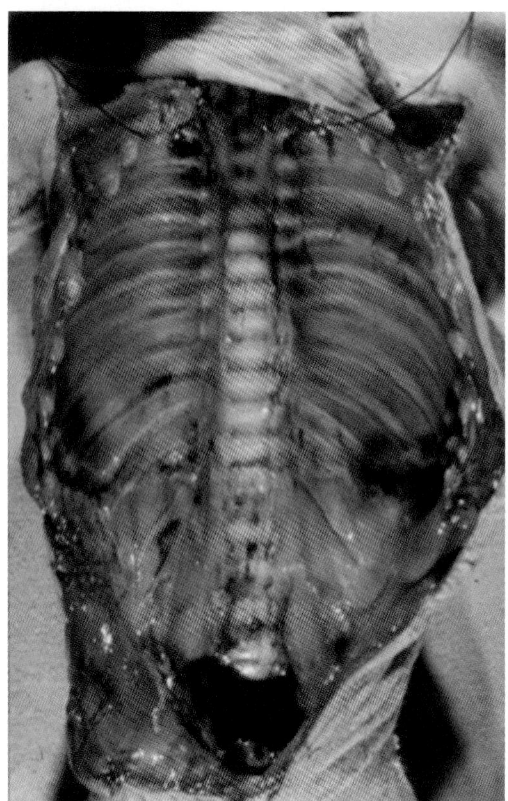

FIGURE 1A-17 ■ With all organs removed the ribs and vertebral column can be examined for developmental abnormalities and the psoas muscle can be sampled for histological sections.

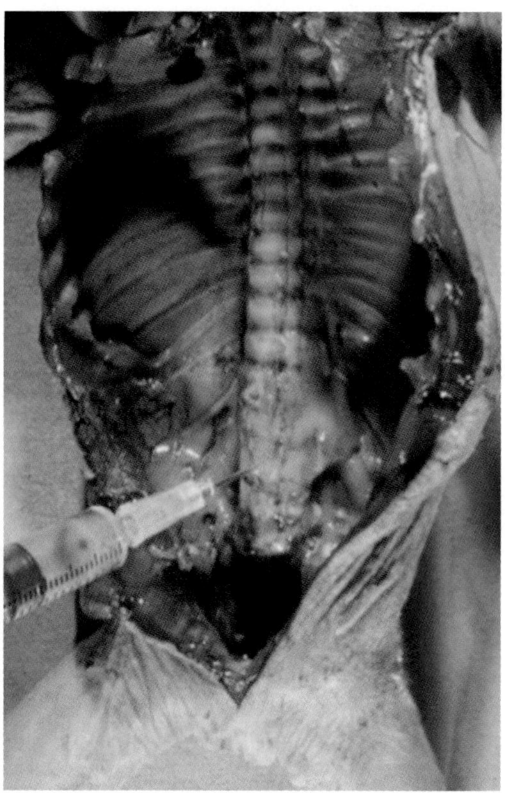

FIGURE 1A-18 ■ CSF can be obtained for culture and other purposes by inserting a long needle through the intervertebral disc of a lumbar vertebra after sterilizing the area.

fractures, both old and recent, may be observed. A section of rib including the costo-chondral junction may be taken for microscopic examination of bone and bone marrow.

VERTEBRAL COLUMN/SPINAL CORD

CSF culture. A culture of the cerebral spinal fluid is relatively easy in an infant and a young child. Once all the abdominal organs have been removed, the intervertebral disc region of one of the lumbar discs can be seared with a hot spatula (eFigure 1A-31), and a long needle (in an infant) or a spinal tap needle may be inserted through the disc into the spinal canal (Figure 1A-18). Aspiration not only supplies fluid for culture but can also be used for documenting hemorrhage (eFigure 1A-32). In a small infant, the head may need to be elevated to provide enough fluid in the spinal canal for aspiration.

Section of psoas muscle. The psoas muscles provide an easily accessible source of skeletal muscle and often include ganglion cells from the paraspinal ganglia (eFigure 1A-33).

Removing the vertebral column. While older children may require spinal cord removal similar to that of an adult, infants, particularly neonates, have vertebral columns easily removed from an abdominal approach to provide ready access to the spinal cord. This is accomplished by *making* an incision through two of the lowest intervertebral discs and then bending the pelvis backward to allow a pair of round-ended scissors into the vertebral canal to transect the pedicles on both sides of the vertebral columns (eFigure. 1A-34A to D). As one moves caudally, the vertebral column can be lifted to allow the thoracic and cervical vertebral to be freed up by cutting their pedicles. To remove the vertebral column completely, the highest cervical intervertebral disc accessible can be transected. Upon removal of the vertebral column, vertebral body anomalies may again be noted and a vertebral body may be taken for microscopic examination following fixation and decalcification.

Removing the spinal cord. With the vertebral column removed, the spinal cord in its dura can be dissected free by cutting across the spinal nerves exiting through the dura (Figure 1A-19). The spinal cord may be dissected at this time with cross sections taken from the upper, mid, and lower levels or may be placed in fixative with the brain for dissection after fixation (eFigure 1A-35A,B).

SEPARATION AND EXAMINATION OF HEART/LUNG

Prior to separating the heart lung block from the abdominal organs, assuming the Rokitansky technique was used to remove the organs, an examination of the *esophagus* should be performed. This is done by placing the block, so its posterior surface is exposed. The entrance to the esophagus

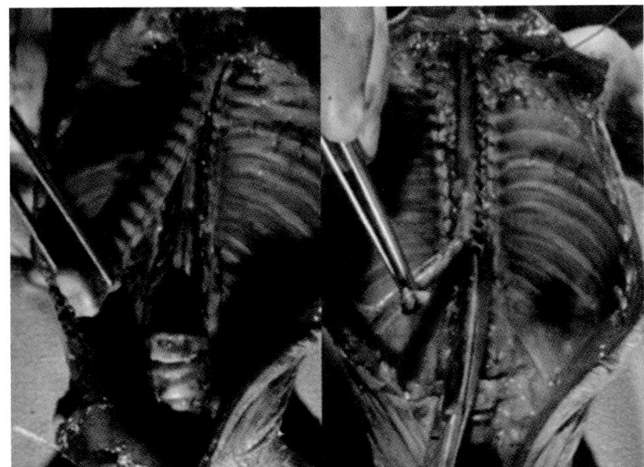

FIGURE 1A-19 ■ Following removal of the vertebral column (**left**) the spinal cord along with it dura can be removed from the spinal canal (**right**).

behind the larynx can then be entered with a pair of scissors and an incision made from the opening to the point the esophagus passed through the diaphragm. This posterior exposure allows examination of the internal surface of the esophagus with particular attention paid to the portion of the anterior wall of the esophagus lying adjacent to the trachea. Esophageal atresia will be easily discovered if present, and the presence of tracheoesophageal fistula, particularly of the "H" type (see Chapter 12), can be established prior to the esophagus being separated from the trachea. Following this examination, the upper portion of the esophagus is separated from the larynx and the mediastinal tissue and left intact for examination with the remainder of the gastrointestinal tract.

Section thoracic/abdominal aorta and inferior vena cava. With the esophagus separated from the thoracic organs, the descending aorta can be examined for abnormalities (Figure 1A-20) and, if none are present, transected beyond the arch and freed from the mediastinal tissues to be left with the abdominal organs. This leaves the chest and abdominal organs attached by only the inferior vena cava, which, when transected as near to the diaphragm/liver as possible, separates the two blocks.

Examination of the chest block. If the clinical history suggests a cardiac malformation, if the cardiac/thoracic ratio is greater than 0.5, or if external examination of the heart is noticeably abnormal, consideration should be given to a "fixed inflation" of the heart (see below) prior to opening the atria and ventricles. If no abnormality is suspected, the heart may be opened in a standard fashion.

Standard examination of the heart. The heart should be separated from the lungs following identification and transection of the pulmonary arteries and veins, noting their anatomic relationships (i.e., origin and position). The heart may then be weighed and examined by opening the chambers along the line of blood flow. This is most easily accomplished by opening the right atrium between the inferior vena cava and the atrial appendage. This incision leaves intact the sinoatrial node that is located in the anterior wall of the right atrium just below the entrance of the superior vena cava.

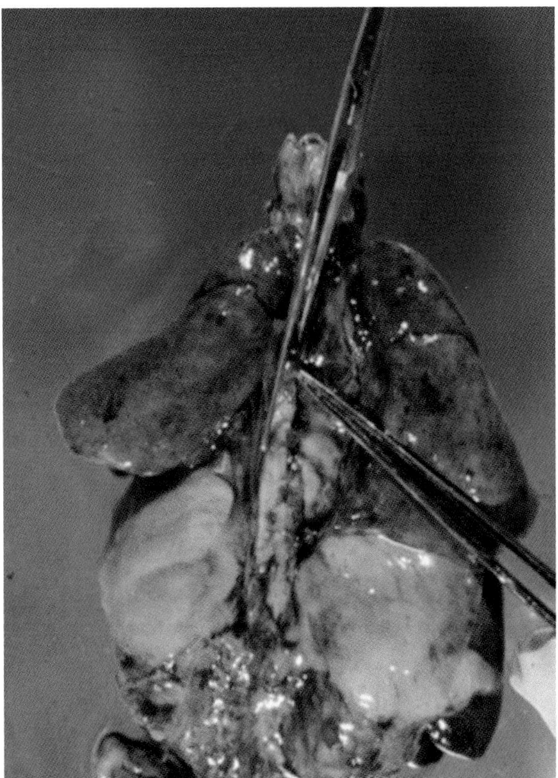

FIGURE 1A-20 ■ The thoracic aorta and the esophagus can be opened while the abdominal and thoracic organ block is still intact. Here the aorta is opened along the posterior aspect of the organ block.

A pair of scissors can be used to cut through the lateral wall of the right atrium, through the tricuspid valve and along the lateral portion of the right ventricular wall. With the right side of the heart thus opened, the atrium can be examined for completeness of the foramen ovale and the entrance of the coronary sinus. The tricuspid can be measured (circumference) and the leaflets inspected, and the right ventricle can be measured for the thickness of the free wall.

The next incision, most easily accomplished with a pair of blunt-nosed scissors, extends up the anterior wall of the right ventricle adjacent to the septum and along the outflow tract into and then through the pulmonary valve. This allows examination of the septum for ventricular septal defects and for measurement of the pulmonary valve circumference and presence of three cusps. With the pulmonary valve opened, the right and left pulmonary artery branches can be identified as can the ductus arteriosus (for patency, circumference, and length).

The left side of the heart is examined by cutting between the openings of the pulmonary veins and then down the lateral wall of the left atrium, through the mitral valve and along the wall of the left ventricle. The mitral valve circumference can be measured and the leaflets observed for orientation and completeness. The left ventricular wall thickness is determined and the septum is examined for defects. The systemic outflow tract is then opened with an incision through the anterior wall of the left ventricle adjacent to the septum and behind the mitral leaflet into the aorta. When opening the aorta, care must be taken to move the opened pulmonary trunk aside and make an incision through the aortic valve. The opened valve circumference may be measured and the three cusps observed, noting the position of the origin of the coronary arteries above and behind two of the cusps (the right and left coronary sinuses). Finally, the arch of the aorta is examined for anomalies (e.g., coarctation, patent ductus, etc.). If myocardial infarction is suspected, the right and left ventricles may be "bread-loafed" remembering that the papillary muscles are often affected first in infants with myocardial damage.

Fixed inflation and dissection of the heart—Figures EP1–48 The study of an organ by removing, inflating, and fixing prior to its dissection is useful primarily for examining (and retaining for teaching) the heart but could also be used for other "hollow" organs such as the small or large bowel and the urinary or gallbladder.

The technique for the heart involves separating the heart from the lungs by tying off (as far from the heart as possible) all the vessels including the pulmonary arteries, pulmonary veins, superior and inferior vena cavas, and arteries of the aortic arch, then attaching the heart via canullas to the superior vena cava and a pulmonary vein, and inflating it under mild pressure (e.g., 20-cm water) with a mixture in four parts to one of 100% alcohol and 37% formalin. Following approximately 24 hours in this fixative, the heart is "opened" by transecting each of the vessels that have been tied off and opening a series of "windows" in the atria, ventricles, and pulmonary trunk and aorta above the valves.

The windows begin with a square or rectangular opening in the right atrium, and after examination of the interior of the atrium and the tricuspid valve, continue with a triangular opening in the right ventricle dictated by any anomalies that may be observed, for example, an incomplete tricuspid valve or a high ventricular septal defect. After observing the anatomy of the right ventricle, its outflow tract can be examined from the window into the right ventricle as well as from a rectangular window opening in the pulmonary trunk just above the pulmonary valve.

The left side of the heart is approached with a window in the left atrium made from incisions connecting the openings for the pulmonary veins, or, to spare the veins, a window just "inside" the locations of the pulmonary veins. With the atrium open, the upper aspect of the mitral valve can be observed and, if normal, the left ventricle can be opened with an incision from the apex of the ventricle, parallel to the ventricular septum, and upward through the anterior and posterior wall, creating a hinge-like opening through which the interior of the ventricle and the lower portion of the mitral valve can be examined. The outflow tract through the aorta can also be observed from the ventricular side and, with a rectangular window cut into the aorta above the aortic valve, from the aortic side.

The incisions involved in creating the windows also allow access to atrial and ventricular myocardial tissue, as well as aortic and pulmonary artery wall for microscopic sections.

Following dissection, the heart can be processed through various concentrations of alcohol and then xylene as is performed with other tissues submitted for processing for microscopic sections. The processing may take a day or more in each solution, and then when the xylene has cleared the heart, it is placed in a paraffin bath under a slight vacuum, which will help speed the impregnation of the tissue. When removing the heart from the heated paraffin, it should be rotated in all planes to clear the paraffin from the heart chambers and vessel openings. Doing this over Bunsen burner with a low flame allows the excess paraffin to exit more rapidly. The heart can then be cooled slowly and retained for future study or teaching purposes.

Examination of the thymus. This includes weighing and describing it and submitting a representative section for microscopic examination.

Examination/removal of thyroid and parathyroids. The thyroid is usually readily visible adjacent to the lower larynx and can be dissected free intact. The weight should be taken and a representative section submitted for microscopic examination. The parathyroid glands may only rarely be visible in an infant, and to ensure that they are available for microscopic examination (if clinical history warrants), the entire thyroid gland and adjacent soft tissue may need to be submitted.

Removal/examination of the tongue. While not necessary or feasible in most cases, removal of the tongue not only allows more extensive examination of the mouth and nasopharynx but also provides another specimen of skeletal muscle for microscopic examination. Once the larynx has been removed (or in continuity with the removal of the chest organs), the tongue may be freed from the mandible by cutting with a scalpel (or preferably a pair of scissors) along the inner edge of the mandible. Care must be taken to not cut the lips or outside of the mouth (Figure 1A-21). A safe way to

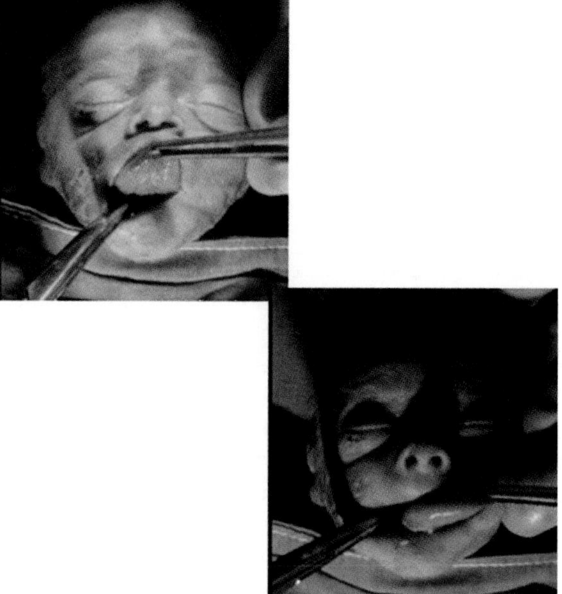

FIGURE 1A-21 ■ The tongue is removed by lifting it with a forceps toward the top of the mouth (**top**) and then incision and separating the base and lateral surfaces of the tongue from the floor of the mouth (**bottom**).

avoid this possibility is to use a pair of scissors (rather than a scalpel) and only opening the blades after inserting the pair of scissors inside the mouth.

EXAMINATION OF THE RESPIRATORY SYSTEM

Following removal of the heart from the heart/lung block as described above, the respiratory system can be examined. The pulmonary arteries and veins should be identified and examined for the presence of clots (emboli). If present, the arteries or veins should be opened along their length into the lung to determine the extent of the vascular obstruction.

The *larynx* (with thyroid and parathyroids removed) should be separated from the trachea and then examined for patency from above and below. It may then be hemisected from anterior to posterior, allowing a view of the vocal cords and laryngeal mucosa.

The *trachea* should also be probed for patency and for the size of the lumen throughout. Externally, the cartilage plates along its circumference should be examined for the presence of complete rings. The trachea may then be resected at the carina leaving as much as possible of the right and left main stem bronchi.

Lung examination begins by weighing the right and the left lungs separately and noting the lobation of the lobes (two on the left and three on the right) and their color and consistency (eFigure 1A-36). At this point, it is often helpful to inflate one of the lungs with formalin by inserting a syringe in the mainstem bronchus and slowly injecting 10 to 50 mL of formalin depending on the size of the lungs. A hemostat may then be used to close off the bronchus and the lung placed in formalin for an hour or two (or overnight if possible) before dissecting. The other lung is examined by gently probing the bronchi and vessels and then sectioning the lung perpendicular to the hilum. This allows examination of the parenchyma for lesions (cysts, abscesses, areas of consolidation and hemorrhage). Sections should be taken from obvious areas of pathology as well as from pleural and hilar regions. While a section may be taken from each of the five lobes, in small lungs a slice of the entire lung may fit into one cassette.

EXAMINATION OF THE ABDOMINAL ORGANS

In females, separate the *uterus and fallopian tubes* from the abdominal block (ovaries already removed and weighed).

Spleen. The spleen may have been removed earlier (see above), but if not, should now be dissected from the abdominal block with special attention paid to the areas adjacent to the spleen and liver for smaller "accessory" spleens. If none are present, the spleen can be weighed, sectioned and a sample taken for microscopic examination (eFigure 1A-37).

Liver. From the anterior portion of the abdominal block, the diaphragm can be removed and the liver examined. The biliary tract is difficult to dissect in a small infant, but its patency can be demonstrated by making an incision in the duodenum in the region of the ampulla of Vater. The gallbladder can then be compressed against the liver, and if the biliary tree is patent, bile can be expressed through the ampulla (Figure 1A-22). Following this, the liver can be removed from the block, weighed, and sectioned at 1.0-cm intervals with representative tissue taken for microscopic examination.

Adrenals and kidneys. From the rear of the abdominal block, the aorta can be opened to observe the origin and patency of the celiac axis, mesenteric arteries, and renal/adrenal arteries as wall as the iliac arteries. The renal veins can also be observed entering the inferior vena cava and their patency observed. The adrenals can be dissected from the kidneys, weighed, and sectioned with a cross section taken from each adrenal for microscopic examination.

The kidneys, ureters, and bladder can be dissected en bloc either with or without the renal arteries and section of the aorta (eFigure 1A-38). After identifying the origin, course, and entrance into the bladder of each ureter, each kidney can be removed, weighed, and examined by clearing off the soft tissue from the capsule (without stripping the capsule) and bisecting the kidney. The cortex and medullary thicknesses are measured and examined for lesions before sections are taken for microscopic examination. The renal pelvis should be opened and the entrance to the ureters examined, followed by opening the entire length of the ureters into the bladder. The bladder itself should be opened and the mucosa examined before a section is taken for microscopic examination. The urethra can be probed for patency and when opened in a male the prostate can be examined and a section submitted for microscopic examination.

Note: In cases of suspected *urethral stricture or atresia*, it may be helpful to remove the urethra along with the external genitalia, most noticeably the penis in male infants.

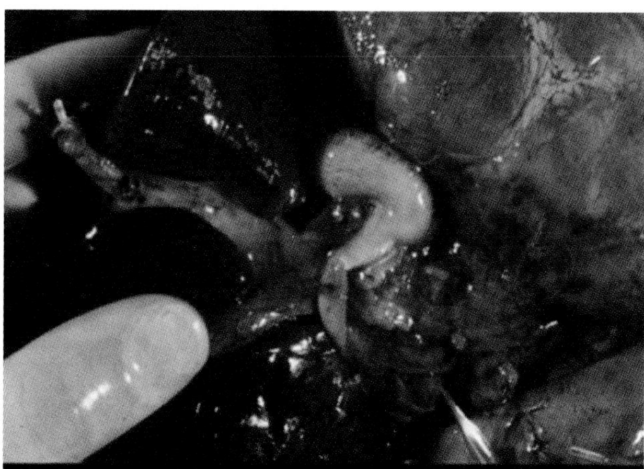

FIGURE 1A-22 ▪ The biliary tree can be examined for patency by first opening the duodenum in the region of the ampulla of Vater then compressing the gallbladder (note thumb over gallbladder) and observing the flow of bile from the ampulla (at tip of scissors).

This is accomplished by separating the symphysis pubis and dissecting the penis in continuity with the bladder. It may also be helpful to fix the penis and distal portion of the bladder and then cross section the specimen and submit it in its entirety.

Removing, measuring, and sectioning the bowel. The bowel may be removed prior to removing the chest/abdomen block or when dissecting the abdominal organs. In either event, the bowel is best separated from the other organs by beginning in the area of the sigmoid/rectum and working toward the stomach, using a pair of curved scissors to cut along the mesenteric attachment as close to the bowel wall as possible, being careful to identify (and not cut across) the appendix when working near the cecum. In a small infant, the bowel may be wrapped around one's fingers as one progresses from the sigmoid to the duodenum. The bowel may be transected at the duodenum at the point it passes beneath the inferior duodenal fold. The entire bowel can then be laid out on a cutting board for measuring the length and width of the small intestine, colon, and appendix. If lesions are identified along the length of the bowel, they may be cross-sectioned and examined, or the entire length of the bowel may be opened for inspection before sectioning (eFigure 1A-39).

The most proximal part of the gastrointestinal tract (esophagus, stomach, and upper duodenum) along with the pancreas is then (if not previously done) separated from the diaphragm and liver. The incision in the previously opened esophagus (see under "Separation and Examination of Heart/Lung") can be extended through the gastroesophageal junction, along the edge of the stomach and through the pylorus into the duodenum. Gastric contents can be observed and a portion saved for further analysis if appropriate. Beyond the pylorus, the ampulla of Vater is again identified (see liver above) and its relationship to the pancreas observed. The pancreas can then be dissected from its attachment to the duodenum, weighed, and sections taken from the head and tail for microscopic examination. With the entire gastrointestinal tract now opened, portions along its length (2 × 1 cm) may be taken (esophagus ×1, esophageal-gastric junction ×1, stomach ×2, small bowel ×3, appendix ×1 and colon ×2) and placed on paper (Figure 1A-23) for fixation and sectioning at a later time (overnight is best, but only 1 to 3 hours in 37% formalin is usually sufficient).

Note: In situations in which the bowel is extremely fragile, particularly in cases of necrotizing enterocolitis, it may be best to leave the small bowel and colon intact with the mesentery, and fix the entire specimen in formalin prior to dissection.

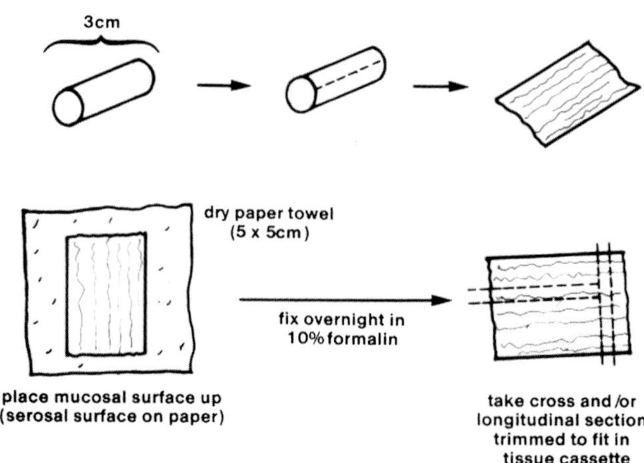

FIGURE 1A-23■ Technique for fixing thin-walled tissue on paper towels before sectioning.

Central Nervous System

Examination of the scalp. The scalp should be examined for abnormalities in the pattern of the growth of the hair, looking for two or more swirls of growth; the more swirls or defects in hair growth, the more likely there will be abnormalities in the structure of the brain. The anterior and the posterior fontanels should be palpated in infants to check for fullness or depression.

Opening the scalp. An intermastoid, suboccipital incision (Figure 1A-24) allows reflection of the scalp anteriorly to the level of the eyebrows and posteriorly to below the posterior fontanel (eFigure 1A-40A,B). In young infants, pushing a finger between the scalp and the calvarium and rolling the skin forward may accomplish this. In older children, dissection of the tissue between the scalp and calvarium may require a pair of scissors or a scalpel.

Measuring the calvarium. With the fontanels exposed, they may again be palpated and measured (length and width) (eFigure 1A-41). The calvarium can also be examined for developmental defects, fractures, or hemorrhage.

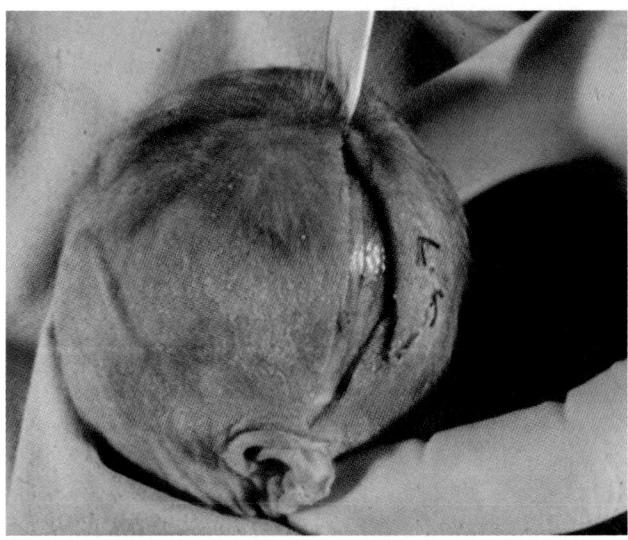

FIGURE 1A-24■The scalp is opened with an incision between the ears at the level below (posterior to) the crown of the head, that is, an intermastoid suboccipital incision.

Opening the calvarium. In infants whose calvarium has not completely ossified, the calvarium may be opened with a scalpel and a pair of scissors along the unfused sutures. Examination of the saggital sinus may be done by cutting with a pair of scissors through the parietal bone from the anterior fontanel to the posterior fontanel about one centimeter to each side of the saggital suture. Lifting the edge of the strip left in the middle allows a view of the intact sinus (eFigure 1A-42A to C).

Extending the incisions parallel to the saggital suture to the anterior and the posterior portions of the calvarium and then laterally from both ends of the incision into the parietal bone (on both the right and the left sides) until they are 1 to 4 cm apart (depending on the size of the head), allow both parietal/frontal bones to be reflected laterally (Figure 1A-25, eFigure 1A-43). By cutting across the anterior extension of the saggital suture and reflecting it posteriorly, the brain is exposed. The calvarium of older infants and children is removed as one would for an adult.

Removing the brain. The brain of a small infant is removed from anterior to posterior by placing one's hand behind the head (with the reflected saggital suture between the middle and the ring fingers and tilting the head backward (Figure 1A-26)). As the brain falls away from the base of the skull, the cranial nerves, pituitary stalk, and tentorium can be cut across as they come into view. Eventually, one can see into the spinal canal and insert a pair of scissors to cut across the spinal cord well below the brainstem. At this point, the brain should easily be "delivered" into the hand held beneath the head.

Examination of the external brain. Following removal, the brain should be weighed and the external features examined including the basic development of the cerebral cortex related to the infant's gestation age (see Addendum), The vessels at the base of the brain may also be examined, but further

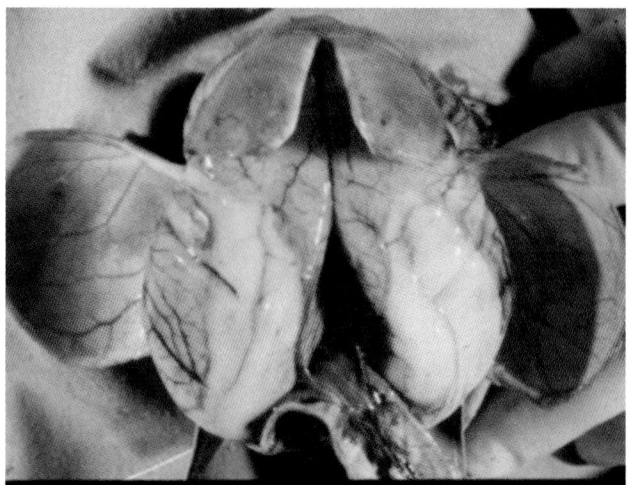

FIGURE 1A-25■The calvarium can be opened by cutting lateral to each side of the saggital suture and then along the sutures between the frontal-parietal and parietal-occipital bones. After examining the saggital vein the suture line is reflected posteriorly (bottom) and the parietal bones are reflected laterally to expose the brain.

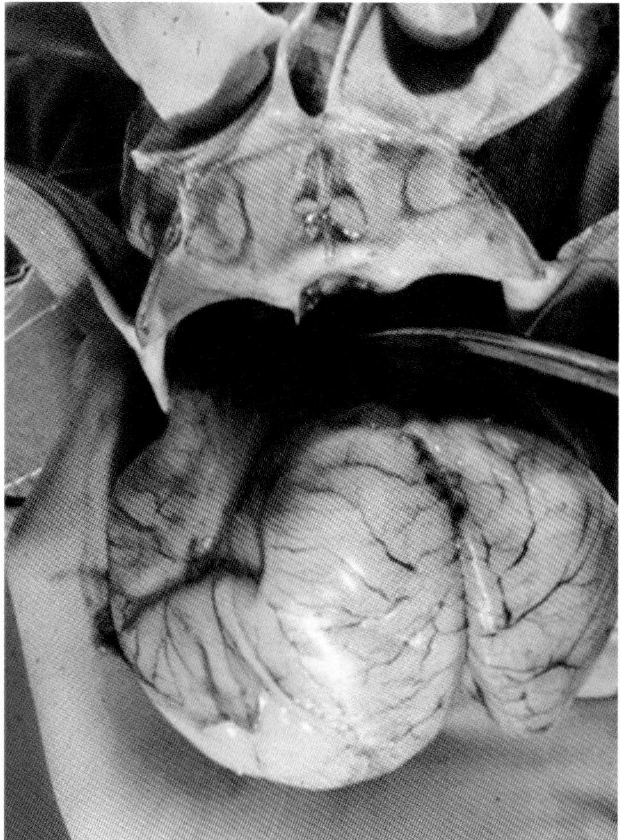

FIGURE 1A-26■Remove the brain by tipping the head posteriorly and transecting the cranial nerves, tentorium, and spinal cord.

manipulation of the brain should be put off until it can be made more firm by fixing in formalin (10% to 37%) for 1 to 2 weeks. Placing the container with the brain near a source of low heat (e.g., a radiator or a heat vent) may hasten the fixation.

Sectioning the brain and spinal cord. The spinal cord, if removed via the abdominal approach, can be fixed along with the brain. Examination consists of opening the dura along its length and then sectioning the cord at 0.5- to 1.0-cm intervals saving two or more sections for microscopic examination.

The *brain after fixation* should be examined for gross abnormalities (e.g., area of hemorrhage or necrosis, developmental anomalies such as holoprosencephaly) and a unique approach to dissection determined by the abnormalities. In most instances, however, major anomalies are not seen and a more "standard" approach may be taken. This consists first of examining the vessels at the base of the brain after gently removing the meninges. The circle of Willis should be identified and any variations recorded. The cerebellum and brainstem can be removed from the rest of the brain by making a transverse section in the region of the cerebral peduncles (eFigure 1A-44A,B). In a small infant's brain, this cerebellar/brainstem block may be cut transversely at 0.5- to 1.0-cm intervals to view the cerebellar folia and dentate nucleus along with the lower brainstem (eFigure 1A-45A to C). In larger brains, the brainstem might be separated from the cerebellum prior to sectioning.

If significant hemorrhage is present in the cerebral hemispheres, the meningeal arteries may be followed into the cerebrum to search for a site of an aneurysm or rupture. After the exterior of the cerebral hemispheres has been examined, the brain is placed "base up" and transverse (coronal) sections made at 1.0- to 1.5-cm intervals (depending on the size of the brain) from the anterior lobe through the occipital lobe (eFigure 1A-46). If possible, these sections (often only five or six in infants but as many as 12 to 15 in older children) should include ones through the stalk of the pituitary, the mammillary bodies, the apex of the interpeduncular fossa, and the top of the cerebral peduncles. This allows close examination of the numerous nuclei of the deep gray matter.

CNS Microscopic sections. Routine sections of the central nervous system include, but are not limited to, the following (Figure 1A-27):

1. Brainstem—pons
2. Cerebellum including dentate nucleus
3. Frontal (or occipital) cortex and white matter
4. Hippocampus
5. Internal capsule/posterior limb/thalamus
6. Cervical, thoracic, and lumbar spinal cord
7. Additional sections of specific lesions—for example, tumor, necrosis, hemorrhage

Examination of the inside of the cranium

Removal of the pituitary. The pituitary can easily be removed from the hypophyseal fossa of the sella turcica after the brain has been removed. The gland is usually quite soft and delicate, and the best approach is made by using a pair of small curved scissors to dissect around and beneath the gland.

Opening of middle ear. The middle ear can be visualized by removing the petrous portion of the temporal bone with a pair of heavy (bone) scissors or with saw cuts on either side of the petrous protrusion (Figure 1A-28). With removal of the bone, the middle ear can be examined for infection (pus or cloudy fluid) and a culture performed if indicated. The bones of the middle ear (maleus, incus, and stapes) can also be seen.

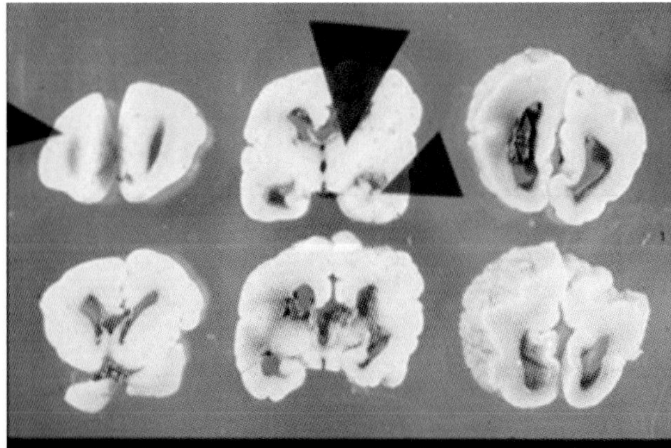

FIGURE 1A-27 ■ Standard histological sections from the brain include portions of the cerebrum, hippocampus, and basal nuclei (*arrows*) along with sections of cerebellum and brain stem.

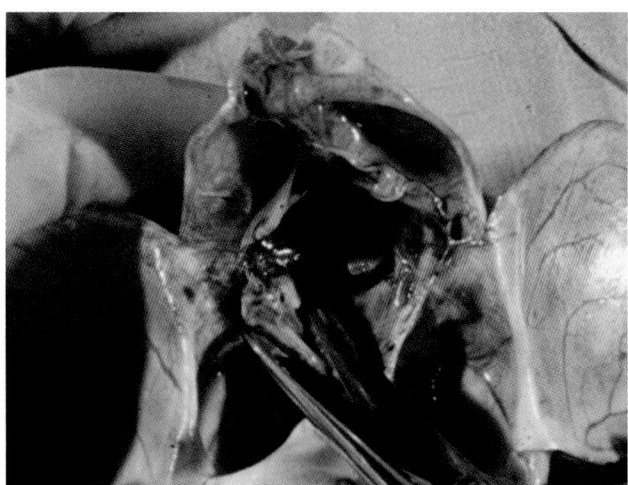

FIGURE 1A-28 ■ The middle ear is exposed by removing the petrous portion of the temporal bone.

Removal of eye/s can be performed from beneath the eyelids by cutting around the orbital septum and palpebral ligaments holding the eyeball to the bones of the orbit, then dissecting posteriorly to separate the ocular muscles and transect the optic nerve. Care must be taken to avoid damage to the eyelid and skin of the face.

A less potentially damaging approach is through the opened skull following removal of the brain. Access to the eye is made by cutting an opening in the superior surface of the orbital plate of the frontal bone (Figure 1A-29). In a newborn, this can often be done with a scalpel and a pair of scissors but may require a saw in older patients. When the opening is large enough to accommodate the size of the eyeball, the optic nerve and orbital muscles can be dissected and visualized, then transected. As the eye is moved posteriorly, the ligaments holding the eye to the orbit can be cut across

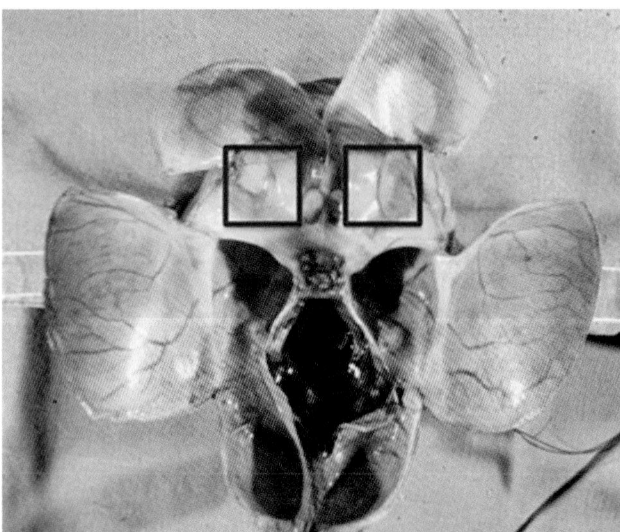

FIGURE 1A-29 ■ The opened calvarium provides access to the eyes through the roof of the orbits (*indicated with squares*).

(with special care taken to avoid cutting the eyelid) and the eye pulled through the opening in the orbital plate.

Preparing the Remains for Disposition

Following the completion of the gross autopsy examination, all tissues NOT taken for microscopic examination, long-term storage, or teaching purposes (in accordance with the autopsy permit) should be returned to the body in a plastic bag of appropriate size. This includes the chest plate and vertebral column. The body and scalp over the calvarium can be sewn closed, as might be the custom in your area. Consulting with morticians as to their preference is often helpful. The outside of the body should be appropriately tagged for identification, washed, dried, and wrapped in appropriate material for transfer to the funeral home.

REFERENCES

1. College of American Pathologists Pamphlet. *Autopsy: aiding the living by understanding death*. Northfield, IL.
2. Marshall WA, Tanner JM. Variations in pattern of pubertal changes in girls. *Arch Dis Child* 1969;44:291–303.

CHAPTER 1B

Fine-Needle Aspiration

JOHN J. BUCHINO
ROBERT F. DEBSKI

Fine-needle aspiration (FNA) was first reported in the early 1930s by Martin and Ellis (10) and Stewart (12), but the procedure did not gain widespread acceptance until after Zajicek published his monograph in 1974 (15). Although several studies and monographs have established the usefulness of FNA in pediatrics, many pediatric centers have been slow to adopt this technique. However, those that have adopted this technique have found it to be a relatively easy, low-cost diagnostic procedure that can provide a great deal of information (9). Several important advantages of FNA are listed in Table 1B-1. It is important that clinicians recognize that FNA is most applicable in mass lesions, generally not in diffuse processes such as a pulmonary infiltrate. However, Their et al. have advocated the use of FNA for the evaluation of rejection in children after liver transplantation (13). Indications for the use of FNA in children are summarized in Table 1B-2. For several reasons, we strongly believe that a pathologist should perform FNA of all palpable lesions, and that a pathologist should be present when a radiologist performs image-guided FNA of deep-seated lesions. The pathologist is able to obtain an accurate history and observe the exact size and location of the lesion. The person performing the aspiration is best able to evaluate whether the lesion has been penetrated. As one gains experience, the texture of the lesion and consistency of the aspirated material help in the formulation of a differential diagnosis. The pathologist is also best able to prepare the smears and triage the aspirated material for other studies.

The equipment required for FNA is listed in Table 1B-3. If need be, it can easily be carried in a phlebotomy tray to the patient's bedside or, preferably, to a treatment room. For outpatient FNA, we recommend a setting with adequate room for the patient, parents, and assistants as well as the pathologist. An adjacent area in which rapid staining and microscopic evaluation can be performed is highly desirable. Although untoward complications are extremely rare when a superficial lesion is aspirated, the area in which the procedure is performed should be equipped to handle emergencies, just like any other area in which clinical procedures are carried out.

Relatively few complications are associated with FNA. The most common is bruising or swelling at the site. Inadvertent puncture of a vessel may result in a small hematoma. However, a history of a possible bleeding diathesis should always be obtained. A vasovagal response or a light-headedness may occur in a small percentage of patients. (We have also experienced parents feeling faint when observing the procedure.) A pneumothorax is possible when a chest wall lesion or a lesion in the supraclavicular space is aspirated. Seeding of tumor in the needle tract is a markedly rare occurrence (11).

The technique of FNA is outlined in Figure 1B-1. This is essentially the same as the technique used for adults. It should be noted that use of an aspiration gun and the specific type of gun are optional. In children, the standard size of the needle for superficial FNA is 1 inch, 23 gauge. A 23-gauge needle recovers adequate material for diagnosis in more than 90% of cases and is unlikely to cause any significant organ or vessel trauma. A 22-gauge needle may facilitate the drainage of purulent material but should not be used in regions where a major vessel in an infant might be sheared (e.g., near the carotid artery). One must also be mindful of spatial differences, such as decreased chest wall thickness in infants and small children.

Table 1B-1 ■ ADVANTAGES OF FNA
Can be performed on outpatient basis
Low cost
Rapid diagnosis
No general anesthesia necessary
Minimal trauma with little morbidity
Can be used in conjunction with other diagnostic modalities (e.g., immunocytochemistry, electron microscopy, microbiologic culture, flow cytometry)
Allows pathologist to have direct patient interaction

Table 1B-2 ■ INDICATIONS FOR FNA

Indication	Example
Mass lesion of unknown cause	Any tumor >0.5 cm
Alternative to surgery	High-risk surgical candidate Child in respiratory distress secondary to an anterior mediastinal mass
Documentation of a nonresectable tumor	Large neuroblastoma-tissue diagnosis necessary before chemotherapy
Confirmation of a metastasis	Pulmonary lesion in a child with previous Wilms tumor
Support of a clinical diagnosis	Persistent lymphadenopathy
Preoperative planning	Salivary gland lesion

Table 1B-3 ■ EQUIPMENT NEEDED FOR FNA

Needles (22- to 25-gauge)
Local anesthetic
Syringe
Betadine, alcohol
Aspiration gun (optional)
Gauze
Glass slides
Paper clips
Fixatives
Adhesive bandage
Gloves
Nonbacteriostatic normal saline solution
Flow cytometry medium with heparin

When FNA is performed in children, adequate control of the patient must be maintained so that the need to attempt to aspirate a moving target does not arise. A skilled assistant is invaluable in this situation. The assistant is usually able to hold infants less than 1 year of age in the desired position. Children older than 6 years can generally cooperate well when talked through the procedure. However, children between 12 months and 6 years can be difficult because of their lack of comprehension of what is happening and their strength. We advocate the use of sedation whenever possible. Most tertiary-care pediatric services now have sedation teams that are adept at sedating children for procedures. The choice of sedatives may vary and is somewhat dependent on the personal preference of the anesthesiologist and/or the pathologist. When sedation is used, the child must be monitored in the appropriate fashion. If sedation is not available, a papoose wrap may be employed to immobilize the child. We also use a local anesthetic whenever possible. The only exceptions to the use of a local anesthetic are a known allergy or a lesion so small that the injected anesthetic will make it difficult to palpate the lesion.

Prior to actually performing the aspiration, we recommend a "time out." During this time out, the pathologist and assistant should verify patient identification, the site to be

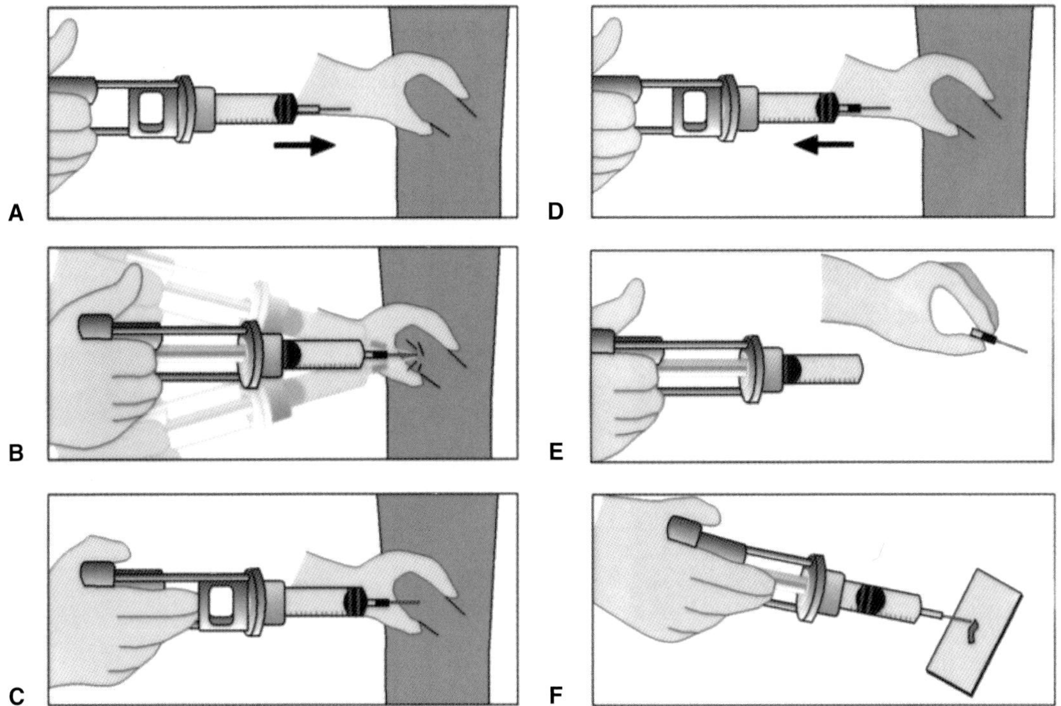

FIGURE 1B-1 ■ Aspiration technique. **A**: Insert needle attached to syringe/gun into mass while stabilizing mass with the other hand. **B**: Create negative pressure while moving needle back and forth until aspirate is present on the needle hub. **C**: Release negative pressure. **D**: Remove needle from mass. **E**: Detach needle from syringe and fill syringe with air. **F**: Attach needle to syringe and express aspirate onto slide or into medium.

aspirated, and that a consent form for the procedure has been signed. The site to be aspirated should have been marked in the presence of the patient's parents/guardians.

Typically, we perform three separate aspirations to obtain adequate material for cytologic evaluation. The number of aspirates may vary somewhat depending on the amount and type of material obtained. One of the significant advantages of FNA is that it can be used to obtain material for studies in addition to cytomorphology. However, each ancillary study usually requires an additional aspiration, which may be difficult in a child.

The most common condition for which children are referred for FNA is persistent lymphadenopathy. In contrast to the adult population, malignancy is present in only a very small percentage of children with enlarged lymph nodes (7). Because infections are the most common cause of enlarged lymph nodes in children, microbiologic culture, including culture for acid-fast bacilli, of the aspirate can have a significant positive yield (3). Other studies, such as flow cytometry for the immunophenotyping of lymphoid populations or the determination of the ploidy of tumors, immunocytochemistry, cytogenetics, electron microscopy, and polymerase chain reaction, may be performed if warranted by the clinical situation (1,4).

Several articles and monographs have described various lesions encountered in the pediatric population and diagnosed by FNA (2,6,14). Although it is helpful to be familiar with these, the algorithmic approach offered by Howell et al. (8) serves as an excellent starting point in the evaluation of FNA smears. For those pathologists considering initiating an FNA service, practicing on fresh surgical specimens can be helpful to gain experience with little risk.

One should be mindful of common pitfalls in the diagnosis of lesions by FNA in children. These include (a) obtaining inadequate material because of inadequate patient control; (b) attempting to aspirate an ill-defined swelling rather than a discrete, palpable mass; and (c) lacking familiarity with the differential diagnosis of lesions in children.

The accuracy of an FNA diagnosis in pediatrics varies depending on the type of lesion aspirated and the experience of the pathologist obtaining and interpreting the specimen. In several published series of pediatric FNA, the sensitivity has been greater than 90% and the specificity greater than 95% in distinguishing benign from malignant lesions (5). The percentage of samples inadequate for diagnosis typically ranges from 5% to 10%.

Finally, essential to achieving a sound diagnosis by FNA is clear communication between the clinician and the pathologist, both before and after the procedure. This was best stated by Dr. Fred Stewart in 1933: "Diagnosis by aspiration is as reliable as the combined intelligence of the clinician and the pathologist make it" (12).

REFERENCES

1. Barroca H, Carvalho J, Gil da Costa M, et al. Detection of N-myc amplification in neuroblastomas using Southern blotting on fine needle aspirates. *Acta Cytol* 2001;45:169–172.
2. Buchino JJ. Cytopathology in pediatrics. In: Wied GL, ed. *Monographs in clinical cytology*, Vol. 13. Basel, Switzerland: Karger, 1991:1–7.
3. Buchino JJ, Jones VF. Fine-needle aspiration in the evaluation of children with lymphadenopathy. *Arch Pediatr Adolesc Med* 1994;48:1327–1330.
4. Buchino JJ, Lee HK. Specimen collection and preparation in fine-needle aspirations in children. *Am J Clin Pathol* 1998;109:54–58.
5. Drut R, Drut R, Pollono D, et al. Fine-needle aspiration biopsy in pediatric oncology patients. *J Pediatr Hematol Oncol* 2005;27:370–376.
6. Geisinger KR, Silverman JF, Wakely PE. *Pediatric cytopathology*. Chicago, IL: ASCP Press, 1994:4–5.
7. Handa U, Mohan H, Bal A. Role of fine needle aspiration cytology in evaluation of paediatric lymphadenopathy. *Cytopathology* 2003;14:66–69.
8. Howell L, Russell LA, Howard PH, et al. The cytology of pediatric masses: a differential diagnostic approach. *Diagn Cytopathol* 1992;8:107–115.
9. Howell L. Changing role of fine-needle aspiration in the evaluation of pediatric masses. *Diagn Cytopathol* 2001;24(1):65–70.
10. Martin HE, Ellis EB. Biopsy by needle puncture and aspiration. *Am Surg* 1930;92:169–181.
11. Postovsky S, Elhasid R, Weyl Ben Arush M, et al. Local dissemination of hepatocellular carcinoma in a child after fine-needle aspiration (Letter to the Editor). *Med Pediatr Oncol* 2001;36:667–668.
12. Stewart FW. The diagnosis of tumors by aspiration biopsy. *Am J Pathol* 1933;9:801–812.
13. Their M, Lautenschlager I, Willenbrand E, et al. The use of fine-needle aspiration biopsy in detection of acute rejection in children in after liver transplantation. *Transpl Int* 2002;15:240–247.
14. Vielh P, Howell LP. Techniques. In: Kline TS, ed. *Guides to clinical aspiration biopsy*. Pediatrics. New York, NY: Igaku-Shoin; 1994:5–8.
15. Zajicek J. *Aspiration biopsy cytology. Part I: cytology of supradiaphragmatic organs*. New York, NY: Karger, 1974.

CHAPTER 1C

Molecular Techniques in Pediatric Pathology

JASON A. JARZEMBOWSKI
D. ASHLEY HILL

INTRODUCTION

Rapid advances in the understanding of the molecular and genetic basis of disease have led to an increasingly information-rich and complex working environment for the pediatric pathologist. In addition to providing insight into the pathology and biology of disease, these advances have led to improvements and refinements in diagnosis, risk stratification, prediction of outcome, determination of eligibility for new targeted therapies, and gene-based screening for disease risk. Molecular techniques have become the standard of care in the pathologic evaluation of hematopoietic diseases, pediatric tumors, infectious diseases, immunodeficiencies, metabolic diseases, and chromosomal/genetic disorders. Pediatricians and surgeons, armed with the latest literature on the gene expression profile of a given set of tumors or a newly described mutation associated with a congenital defect, are anxious to apply these new discoveries to their patients' specimens. With a solid understanding of disease morphology and pathogenesis coupled with access to advanced technology and tissue resources, pediatric pathologists are in an advantageous position to utilize this wealth of information in a manner that is clinically important to today's patients. Here, we discuss several molecular techniques focusing on relevance to the standard practice of a pediatric pathologist. We include a broad overview of the technical aspects of each methodology with the utility of each method illustrated by applications to specific pediatric diseases. Because detailed descriptions of all techniques and all relevant diseases are beyond the scope of this chapter, we refer the reader to key references and helpful websites for a more in-depth discussion.

Tissue Handling

The appropriate management of complicated pediatric specimens submitted to the pathology laboratory begins well before the slides cross the microscope stage. Even before the child is in the operative suite, it is fundamental that pathologists participate in the preoperative treatment planning. Establishing an open line of communication with the referring physicians and surgeons will ensure that the pathology team is well prepared for special handling requirements. This is a good opportunity to consider the differential diagnosis and plan ahead for appropriate specimen transport; intraoperative assessment of tissue adequacy, preliminary diagnosis, and margin evaluations when necessary; and tissue requirements for potential ancillary testing and clinical trial enrollment (Table 1C-1). Debski and colleagues have written an excellent review on the approach to handling pediatric tumors that applies to other specimen types as well (Figure 1C-1) (9).

Specific Molecular Techniques

Most pathology laboratories today have a sizeable arsenal of molecular tools that can be deployed to assist in diagnosis, predict treatment efficacy, or provide other pertinent clinicopathologic information. The first group of assays described—flow cytometry, immunohistochemistry (IHC), and immunofluorescence—are all protein based and predicated on the specific recognition of antigen by antibody. Those in the second group are all nucleic acid dependent and include traditional cytogenetics, *in situ* hybridization, polymerase chain reaction (PCR), and the recently developed and continually evolving worlds of microarray technology and next-generation sequencing (NGS).

FLOW CYTOMETRY

Background

Since its inception in the 1970s, flow cytometry has gained widespread acceptance and is today considered an essential component of the diagnostic workup of hematopoietic neoplasms and immunodeficiency disorders. This methodology allows for rapid identification of cell surface molecules and

Table 1C-1 ■ TYPICAL TISSUE REQUIREMENTS FOR COMMONLY USED MOLECULAR DIAGNOSTIC TECHNIQUES

Methodology	Tissue Amount	Tissue Format		
		Fresh	Frozen	FFPE
Flow cytometry	<1 cm^3	✓		
FISH/ISH	4–10-μm sections			✓
Immunofluorescence	4–10-μm sections		✓	
Immunohistochemistry	4–10-μm sections		Some	✓
Cytogenetics	<1 cm^3	✓		
PCR	Varies	✓	✓	✓
Microarray	<1 cm^3	✓	✓	

FFPE, formalin-fixed paraffin-embedded; PCR, polymerase chain reaction

their coexpression patterns, thus separating subpopulations of cells such as monocytes from lymphocytes, B- from T-lymphocytes, or CD4$^+$ from CD8$^+$ T-lymphocytes. Aberrant marker profiles or absolute cell counts can also be easily determined. The diagnosis and classification of leukemias and lymphomas are thoroughly discussed elsewhere in this book. Herein we describe the general theory and method with special attention to specimen processing and practical applications.

Method

The most common specimens submitted for flow cytometry are peripheral blood, bone marrow aspirates, cerebrospinal fluid, and lymph nodes. For peripheral blood (except for paroxysmal nocturnal hematuria [PNH] studies) and bone marrow specimens, erythrocytes are removed by lysis or differential centrifugation. A portion of the sample is spun onto a slide for assessment of cell viability and possible contaminating debris. From this, total cell counts can be estimated, which determines how many analysis tubes can be run; approximately 10^6 cells are needed for optimal results from a typical reaction tube. When testing will be applied to solid samples, the tissue should be immediately transported on saline-moistened gauze or in fresh RPMI medium to the laboratory. Touch preparations for cytological evaluation are useful in guiding the triage of the sample for light microscopy, flow cytometry, cytogenetics, and storage in a −80°C freezer for subsequent studies. Flow cytometry requires a small (3 to 5 mm^3) piece of viable tissue placed in fresh RPMI or similar medium. If subsequent processing will be delayed for more than an hour or so, the tissue should be finely diced to maximize exposure to the nutritive medium and prolong viability (10). Once at the flow cytometry laboratory, the tissue is carefully teased apart and separated into a single-cell suspension (23,24,57).

For the next step, cell aliquots are mixed with surface antigen-specific antibodies that have been conjugated to fluorescent dyes, such as phycoerythrin (PE), fluorescein isothiocyanate (FITC), and phthalocyanines (PC5, PC7). After a short incubation to allow the conjugated antibodies to bind their target surface antigens on the cells in the aliquot, the sample is loaded into the flow cytometer (Figure 1C-2). The cell suspension flows through capillary tubing, eventually streaming single file through the detection chamber. Here,

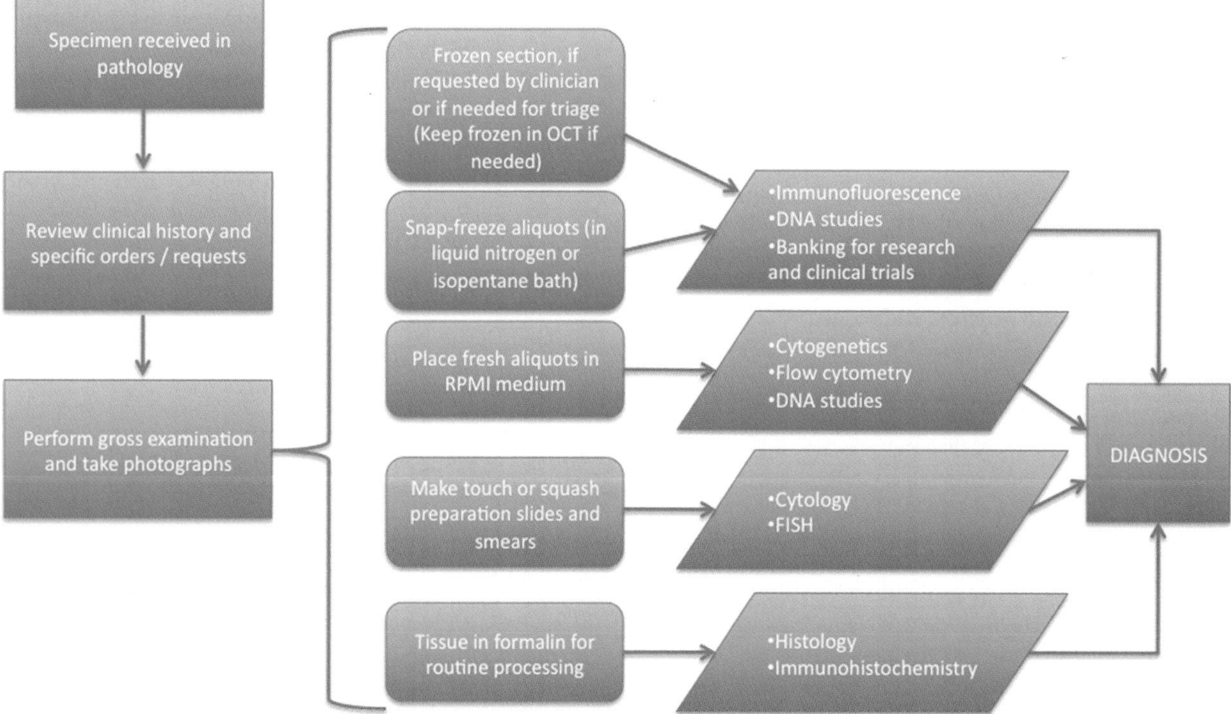

FIGURE 1C-1 ■ Recommended triage and sampling protocol for pediatric specimens.

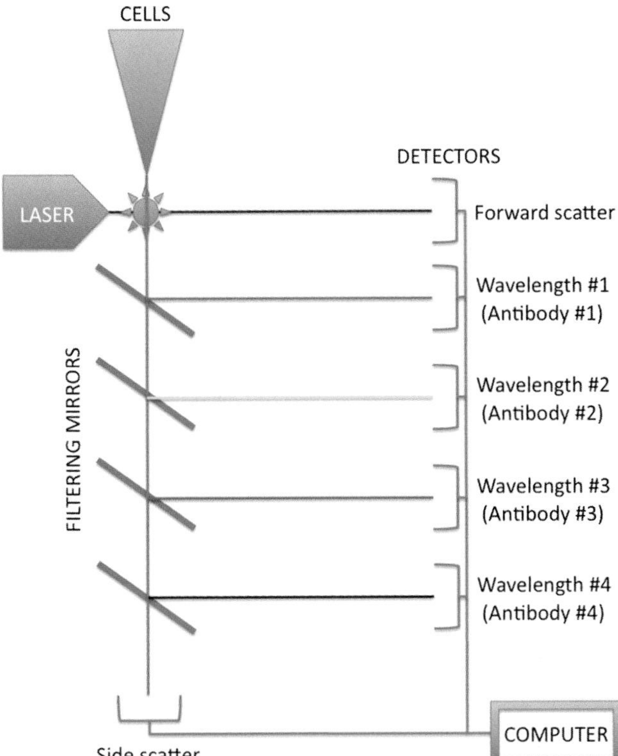

FIGURE 1C-2 ■ Overview of a typical four-channel flow cytometry setup. The antibody-bound cell suspension flows through the cytometer with cells passing singly through the laser beam(s). Forward scatter (**to the right**) is determined by the intensity of the light passing directly through the cell, whereas side scatter (**to the bottom**) depends on the intensity of reflected light. A series of filtering mirrors (**left**) selectively reroute light of the desired wavelength toward the detectors and allow the remainder of the beam to pass. Each antibody under investigation is conjugated to a tag that fluoresces at a different wavelength. Thus, each detector effectively measures a specific antibody and, together, four antibodies, forward scatter, and side scatter are measured simultaneously for each cell. Data are compiled by a computer processor and presented as interactive scattergrams.

one or more lasers "interrogate" each cell, determining the forward scatter (roughly correlating with size), the side scatter (roughly correlating with cytoplasmic complexity or granularity), and a measurement of fluorescent dyes reflecting expression of a particular protein by the cell. Multiple antibodies can be combined in each tube to the extent that they each have a distinct fluorescent tag. For example, a single tube for profiling lymphocytes might contain CD3-PE, CD19-PC5, and kappa-FITC; the expression profile of these four surface markers can be quantitated separately because each has a different associated dye. Detection of each fluorescent signal requires a separate channel on the device, so that a four-channel flow cytometer can analyze four markers per tube, and a five-channel machine can observe five molecules in concert. In addition to demonstrating the coexpression patterns of these markers on distinct cellular populations, multichannel technology also minimizes the necessary sample size and shortens analysis time by reducing the number of tubes needing to be run. Nonetheless, modern cytometers can analyze cells at flow rates exceeding 1,000 cells/second.

The data obtained from each cell are recorded as an event, theoretically allowing the user to look at the individual profile of each cell in the specimen. By selecting populations of cells with a certain range of expression for a particular marker ("gating"), the relative frequency and coexpressed markers can be visualized (see Figure 1C-3, panel D). For example, one might initially gate on $CD45^+$ cells (leukocytes only), and then observe the $CD3^+$ and $CD20^+$ cell populations to assess the relative B- and T-cell numbers. T-cells might be gated into $CD4^+$ and $CD8^+$ groups. If the T-cells coexpressed both markers, one might suspect an immature T-cell neoplasm such as pre-T-ALL, and would then investigate other markers such as CD5, CD10, and TdT. In such a stepwise fashion, each cell subpopulation can be examined for abnormalities.

The interpretation of flow cytometric data is a dynamic process (19). Tabular reports that list the markers analyzed and the percentage of cells positive are unable to capture the complexity of such data. It is good clinical practice to review the expression patterns of the cells of interest, seeing where they lie on each plot and correlating the flow cytometric patterns with the microscopic appearance and results of other ancillary studies.

Applications

Flow cytometric analysis is invaluable, not only in the diagnostic workup of leukemias and lymphomas, but in a myriad of other applications, as well. For example, in lieu of the traditional Kleihauer-Betke test, the degree of fetomaternal hemorrhage can be accurately determined using flow cytometry with antibodies directed against fetal hemoglobin (7,12). The diagnosis of PNH can be made by demonstrating an absence of GPI-linked proteins such as CD55 and CD59 (25,39). For some diseases, it is important to enumerate classes of lymphocytes such as monitoring $CD4^+$ cell counts in HIV-infected patients, or other specific subtypes that may be lacking (such as in various immunodeficiencies) or present in excessive numbers (such as $CD3^+$, $CD4^-$, $CD8^-$, "double negative" T-cells in autoimmune lymphoproliferative disorder) (47,51).

IMMUNOHISTOCHEMISTRY

Background

Over the course of a single decade, IHC has rapidly gained acceptance and became standard of care in most anatomic pathology laboratories. IHC boasts high sensitivity, specificity, and resiliency. Unlike immunofluorescence or many molecular techniques, IHC can be performed on formalin-fixed, paraffin-embedded tissue (FFPE). This greatly enhances its utility, especially on cases with limited material and in retrospective studies. Finally, automated stainers can easily perform IHC with minimal human hands-on time. Such machines have reduced the relative cost of IHC in many laboratories.

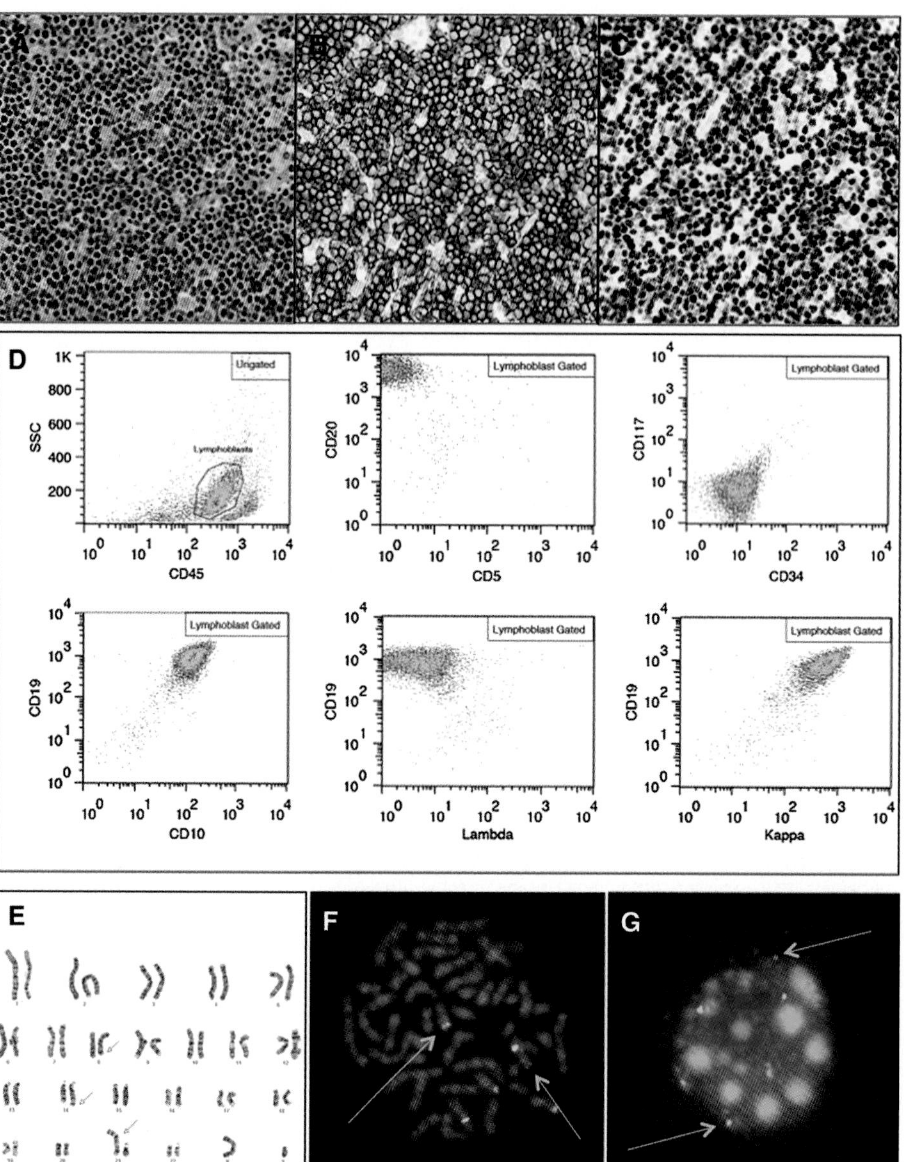

FIGURE 1C-3 ■ **Burkitt lymphoma.** Although just a small round blue cell tumor at first glance, the H&E-stained section (**A**) shows uniform cells with scant cytoplasm and a high mitotic rate along with interspersed tingible body macrophages. The lesional cells are positive for CD19 (**B**), identifying them as B-lymphocytes with a near-100% proliferation rate (**C**, MIB-1 IHC). Flow cytometry (**D**) shows lymphoblasts that are negative for CD34 and CD117 (blastic and myeloblastic markers, respectively), but positive for the B-cell markers CD10 (moderate), CD19, and CD20 (bright) and kappa-restricted (suggesting monoclonality). Conventional cytogenetic analysis (**E**) revealed an abnormal karyotype with a t(8;14) characteristic of Burkitt lymphoma, as well as an extra copy of 1q attached to the short arm of 21. FISH was performed on both metaphase (**F**) and interphase nuclei (**G**) using *MYCC* (chr 8, *red*) and *IGH* probes (chr 14, *green*) and demonstrates several fusion genes (*in yellow*). Extra green signals indicate occasional gain of chromosome 14. (Flow cytometry plots kindly provided by Dennis W. Schauer, Clinical Immunodiagnostic and Research Laboratory, Department of Pediatrics, Medical College of Wisconsin. Karyotype and FISH analysis courtesy of Dr. Peter vanTuinen, Dynacare Clinical Cytogenetics Laboratory, Medical College of Wisconsin.)

Method

The principle of IHC is simple enough and involves a primary antibody specific for the antigen of interest, a secondary antibody that not only binds the first antibody but is also conjugated to an enzyme, and a colorimetric indicator such as a dye that is formed or changes color via the action of the aforementioned enzyme. Thus, a molecular linkage is formed that localizes a readily discernible color (typically, brown or red) to the vicinity of the antigen of interest (Figure 1C-4) (31).

For most diagnostic and research applications of IHC, FFPE tissue is used (3,14). The application of microwave or steam heat to the tissue prior to the staining process ("antigen retrieval" or "unmasking") can improve sensitivity of the technique by reducing or reversing formalin-induced crosslinking of proteins (which modifies or blocks some epitopes required for antibody recognition). A few special antibodies have been optimized for use with frozen tissue sections, and these require the forethought to reserve a piece of the specimen for this purpose.

The primary antibody is the primary determinant of IHC reactivity. The choice of antibody is guided not only by the target antigen, but also by the desired sensitivity/specificity, the reaction conditions, and the cost and reliability of product from a given manufacturer. Different antibody clones react with different portions of proteins and may yield strikingly different IHC results. Monoclonal antibodies (where all antibody molecules recognize a single epitope) are usually more specific than polyclonal sera (where the antibody molecules recognize a variety of antigenic epitopes on a single protein); however, the former are therefore more vulnerable

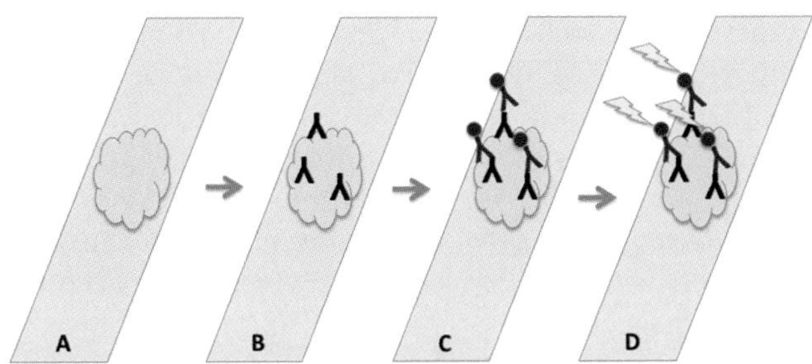

FIGURE 1C-4▪Overview of immunohistochemical staining. Tissue slides (**A**) are incubated with a primary antibody specific for the antigen of interest (**B**), to which a secondary antibody conjugated to a marker is then bound (**C**). Detection is then achieved by a colorimetric or light-producing assay (**D**).

to false-negative results when the epitope is obscured (by protein interactions or misfolding) or absent (via mutations). Perhaps the most pronounced difference between monoclonal and polyclonal antibodies is seen with carcinoembryonic antigen (CEA); fewer than 5% of all hepatocellular carcinomas stain with monoclonal CEA antibodies, whereas roughly 70% stain with polyclonal CEA antibodies in a cytoplasmic or canalicular pattern (34).

The optimal reaction conditions, such as antibody concentration and incubation time, must be determined for each new antibody and existing protocols should be tested with each new lot of an established antibody. Excessive concentrations of antibody or prolonged incubation times may allow nonspecific binding, whereas insufficient antibody or time can yield false-negative results (21).

The choice of secondary antibody is in large part dictated by the primary antibody; the two must originate from different species so that the secondary antibody recognizes the constant portions of the primary antibody. Some manufacturers offer a secondary antibody that reacts against primary antibodies from multiple species. The variety of signaling methods and permutations thereof is too numerous to describe here. Suffice it to say, the secondary antibody is conjugated to a signal molecule—a dye, an enzyme, or a fluorescent marker—such that the location of the antibody "sandwich" can in some way be visualized.

One of the most common detection reactions involves horseradish peroxidase (HRP), which can convert a chromogen (such as TMB or DAB) into a brown-colored product. This method is susceptible to high background signal created by endogenous peroxidases found especially in erythrocytes and granulocytes; these cytoplasmic enzymes can react with the dye precursors to produce a signal indistinguishable from the intended one, except for its localization. In order to quench these enzymes and lower the background noise, pretreatment with methanol and dilute hydrogen peroxide (or other related methods) is used to denature these culprits without significantly inhibiting the subsequently used HRP. However, endogenous peroxidase activity may still hinder interpretation in enzyme-rich tissues such as spleen and bone marrow. Regardless of the specific methods employed, the end result is a color change localized to the antigenic sites of interest. A light counterstain, such as hematoxylin alone, hematoxylin and eosin, methyl green, or periodic acid Schiff, is often employed to allow background architecture and unstained cells to be discerned.

The final step is careful interpretation. The positive control should show strong, specific staining on a section of tissue known to contain the antigen of interest. Ideally, this positive control tissue should be present on the same slide as the case tissue section. Likewise, the negative control, usually performed on an additional slide of the actual case material, omits the primary antibody and should demonstrate the lack of nonspecific binding of secondary antibody. Each case tissue section has internal controls built in, as well, in the form of adjacent normal constituents—blood vessels, connective tissue, or epithelium. The staining patterns of these should be confirmed before interpreting the staining of the areas of interest. Interpretation should include consideration of the quality, quantity, and patterns of staining. Proteins can be nuclear, cytoplasmic, and/or cytoplasmic membranous. Knowledge of the expected pattern of antibody staining in particular tissues is important for quality control.

As an ancillary diagnostic method, IHC results are usually reported as part of a more comprehensive report. Within the "Microscopic Description" or "Comment" section, the performed IHC stains should be described (in tabular or textual format) including the name of the stain, the results with lesional cells, and verification of controls. For example, "Properly controlled immunohistochemical stains demonstrate that the lesional cells are positive for a, b, and c, but negative for x, y, and z." Depending on personal and institutional preference, an explanation of these results and how they support the diagnosis may then be appended. Most laboratories automatically add a note detailing whether these stains are FDA approved for clinical use or are investigational only, which may affect the interpretation of, or payment for, these services.

Applications

The most common use for IHC is as an ancillary method in the diagnosis and detection of tumors and identification of tissue. Sometimes, its purpose is to detect or highlight a single population of cells—for example, ganglion cells (for the ret protein, in biopsies of suspected Hirschsprung disease) or endodermal sinus tumor components (by α-fetoprotein staining) of mixed germ cell tumors or teratomas (44,48,50). Some IHC stains lend insight into the origin and portend outcome of tumors, such as EGFR and p53 expression patterns, which distinguish *de novo* pediatric and adult glioblastomas, and differ between *de novo* and progressive glioblastoma in adults (35,56). The results of other IHC tests can direct and optimize treatment by confirming the presence of target molecules, for example, estrogen and progesterone receptor status for antihormonal therapy in adult breast carcinoma, and CD20 surface expression for rituximab in leukemia/lymphoma and autoimmune disease

(52,58). As with any ancillary technique, the results of IHC alone should not determine the diagnosis or treatment but, rather, should be interpreted in the context of the morphologic appearance and clinical history.

ANTIGENS

Cytoskeleton

Three main groups constitute the cytoskeleton of human cells: thin, intermediate, and thick filaments. *Thin filaments* (5 to 6 nm) are composed of α-, β-, and γ-actins; the former are exclusively found in muscle cells and can be distinguished by antibodies such as muscle-specific actin (MSA; HHF35), smooth muscle actin (SMA), and smooth muscle myosin heavy chain (SMMS-1). For example, the IHC staining pattern differentiates between nonmuscle cells and tumors (MSA- SMA− SMMS-1−), skeletal muscle myocytes and rhabdomyosarcomas (MSA+ SMA− SMMS-1−), and smooth muscle myocytes and leiomyosarcomas (MSA+ SMA+ SMMS-1+). Myoepithelial cells and myofibroblasts also stain positively for all three markers, although to varying degrees.

Diagnostically speaking, the most useful cytoskeletal proteins are the *intermediate filaments* (10 nm). The relative composition of intermediate filaments varies by cell type and allows distinction by IHC. The major intermediate filaments include vimentin, desmin, glial fibrillary acidic protein (GFAP), and cytokeratins.

Vimentin can be found in all mesenchyme-derived cells—fibroblasts, myocytes, osteocytes, chondrocytes, Schwann cells, endothelial cells, and hematopoietic elements—often leading to its dismissal as "nonspecific." Nonetheless, a vimentin stain serves well to distinguish sarcomas and lymphomas from carcinomas. Even with the most poorly differentiated neoplasms, this distinction can usually be made. Vimentin IHC is also of great utility in confirming that tissue antigenicity has been preserved; most sections have at least focal areas of vimentin-positive cells. Necrotic tissue can be surprisingly informative, as it often maintains some degree of reactivity, often in the original pattern of distribution. In these cases, careful comparison with control tissue and nontumoral tissue in the section is necessary to ensure accurate interpretation.

Desmin shares sequence homology with vimentin and is likewise restricted to mesenchymal cells. However, unlike vimentin, desmin is only expressed at significant levels in smooth, skeletal, and cardiac myocytes. Thus, in a sense, desmin is a marker of myogenic differentiation; although the aforementioned cells contain desmin, primitive mesenchymal cells and neoplasms do not. Desmin-positive tumors include leiomyomas, leiomyosarcomas, and rhabdomyosarcomas. Of special note, desmin expression in most cardiac myocytes is limited to the intercalated discs, whereas the Purkinje fibers show diffuse cytoplasmic staining.

Glial fibrillary acidic protein (GFAP) is relatively specific for astrocytes and their corresponding neoplasms—astrocytomas, glioblastomas, and other gliomas (5). Reactive astrocytes are markedly positive and care must be taken to ensure that such a population of cells is not mistaken for the actual neoplasm (5,11,60). Ependymal cells and their derivative neoplasms show variable reactivity for GFAP. *Neurofilament* is actually a set of three related proteins that form fibers within the cell bodies and processes of neurons; the main diagnostic utility of a neurofilament IHC stain is to highlight neurons within tissue or tumor.

Epithelial cells are easily distinguishable by the presence of distinct *cytokeratin* profiles. Carcinomas are positive when using broad-spectrum cytokeratin antibody "cocktails" such as *AE1/AE3* or *CK7/CK20*, which can rule out most lymphomas and sarcomas. Important exceptions include the glandular component of biphasic synovial sarcoma (Figure 1C-5, panel C) and the characteristic cytoplasmic inclusions of malignant rhabdoid tumors; the latter stain for cytokeratin, not muscle markers, belying their epithelial origin. More specific antibodies can help highlight organ-specific epithelium, for example, *CK19* in breast or biliary tract.

Thick filaments (20 to 25 nm) are composed of β-tubulin and are ubiquitous to all cell types. Thus, their diagnostic utility is limited.

Cell Surface Markers

Cell surface antigens have proven utility not only in IHC, but also in flow cytometry and cell sorting. However, while flow cytometry requires fresh tissue or cell-rich fluid, the same markers can be evaluated on FFPE tissue by IHC. These antigens are indispensable in the diagnosis of hematopoietic neoplasms, and such use is detailed elsewhere in this book (see Chapter 22).

Many of these cell surface molecules are numerically designated as a "cluster of differentiation," or "CD." For example, the normal constituent cells of the immune system can be roughly grouped by their expression of these proteins: B-lymphocytes (positive for CD19, CD20 [L26], CD79a; Figure 1C-3), T-lymphocytes (positive for CD3, CD4, CD8), and natural killer cells (positive for CD56). Myeloblasts stain for CD34 and CD117 (c-kit), two markers also associated with other neoplasms; a CD34 stain is positive in synovial sarcoma and some vascular tumors, and CD117 positivity is an important finding in gastrointestinal stromal tumors (26).

Macrophages and histiocytes exhibit granular staining in their cytoplasm for CD68, a component of lysosomal membranes (more accurately, a *lysosomal* surface marker); CD1a is specific for Langerhans cells and T-lymphoblasts (6,22,29,46). Mast cells have membrane positivity for CD138, as well as cytoplasmic positivity for a characteristic enzyme, tryptase (30). This enzyme can also be detected by histochemical methods that require frozen tissue.

Endothelial cells, both nascent and tumoral, can be marked with CD31 and CD34, although these antibodies mark some other cells, as well. GLUT-1 is a relatively specific marker for the endothelial cells of infantile hemangiomas (45).

Pathogens

A wide variety of viruses can be detected by antibodies specific for well-conserved antigens, including adenovirus, cytomegalovirus (CMV), herpes simplex virus (HSV) types I and II, parvovirus B19, human herpesvirus 8 (HHV8), human papilloma virus, BK virus (via large T antigen), hepatitis B (via surface antigen), and Epstein-Barr virus (EBV, via the latent membrane protein [LMP]). Typically, clinical suspicion, positive serologic testing, or viral cytopathic change seen on routine H&E-stained slides serves as a trigger for further workup by IHC. Companion *in situ* hybridization tests are available for both HPV and EBV (Figure 1C-6, panel D); these tests can identify the former as high- or low-risk subtypes. Whenever possible, viral IHC should be performed in tandem with culture and serologic testing (64).

IHC is less commonly used to identify bacteria, both because of these organisms' patchy and often sparse distribution in tissue and the greater detection sensitivity of microbiologic culture methods (2,64). However, antibodies against *Helicobacter pylori* have supplanted more traditional Steiner, Giemsa, or Alcian Yellow stains at some institutions (16,33). Also, *Pneumocystis jiroveci*, once thought to be protozoal but now formally classified as a fungus, can be easily highlighted by appropriate antibodies in IHC (38,62).

Hormones

IHC can assist in confirming the diagnosis and hormone secretion profile of many endocrine tumors. For example, pancreatic endocrine neoplasms (islet cell tumors) can be categorized as derived from alpha, beta, delta, or G cells based on immunohistochemically verifiable expression of glucagon, insulin, somatostatin, or gastrin, respectively. Likewise, VIP-producing tumors and serotonin-secreting carcinoids can be demonstrated by IHC.

In conjunction with clinical presentation, pituitary adenomas can be easily classified by IHC profiling for prolactin, adrenocorticotrophin hormone (ACTH), thyroid-stimulating hormone, growth hormone, follicle-stimulating hormone, and luteinizing hormone (1,32). This approach is especially useful with silent adenomas, which have

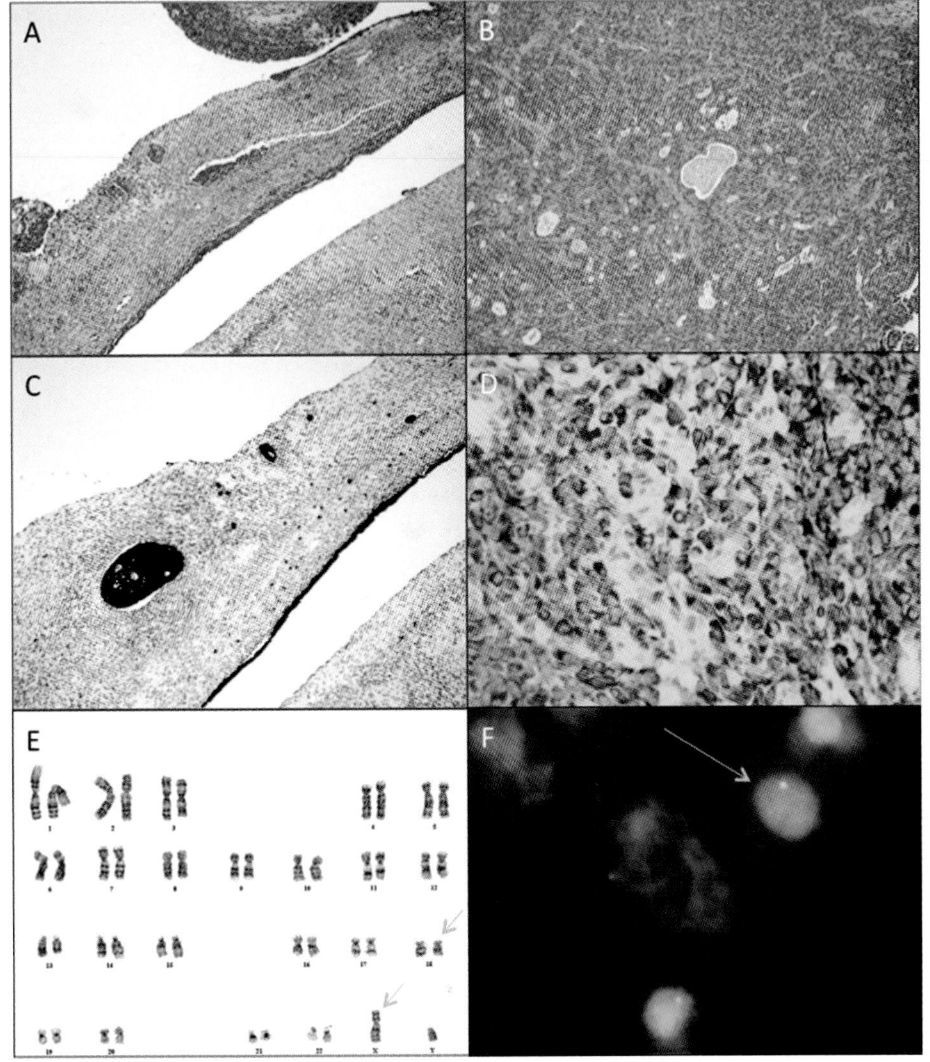

FIGURE 1C-5 ■ **Biphasic synovial sarcoma.** The H&E-stained sections (**A,B**) demonstrate a spindle cell sarcoma with areas of glandular differentiation; the latter are immunohistochemically positive for mixed cytokeratins (**C**) and the majority of the tumor cells are positive for bcl-2 (**D**). Conventional cytogenetic analysis (**E**) demonstrated t(X;18) pathognomonic for the *SYT-SSX* fusion gene of synovial sarcoma. Breakapart FISH probes (*one red, one green* from opposite ends [5′ and 3′, respectively] of the *SYT* gene) are seen separately instead of together as a single intact yellow signal (as seen in the surrounding normal cells) (**F**). (Karyotype and FISH analysis courtesy of Dr. Peter vanTuinen, Dynacare Clinical Cytogenetics Laboratory, Medical College of Wisconsin.)

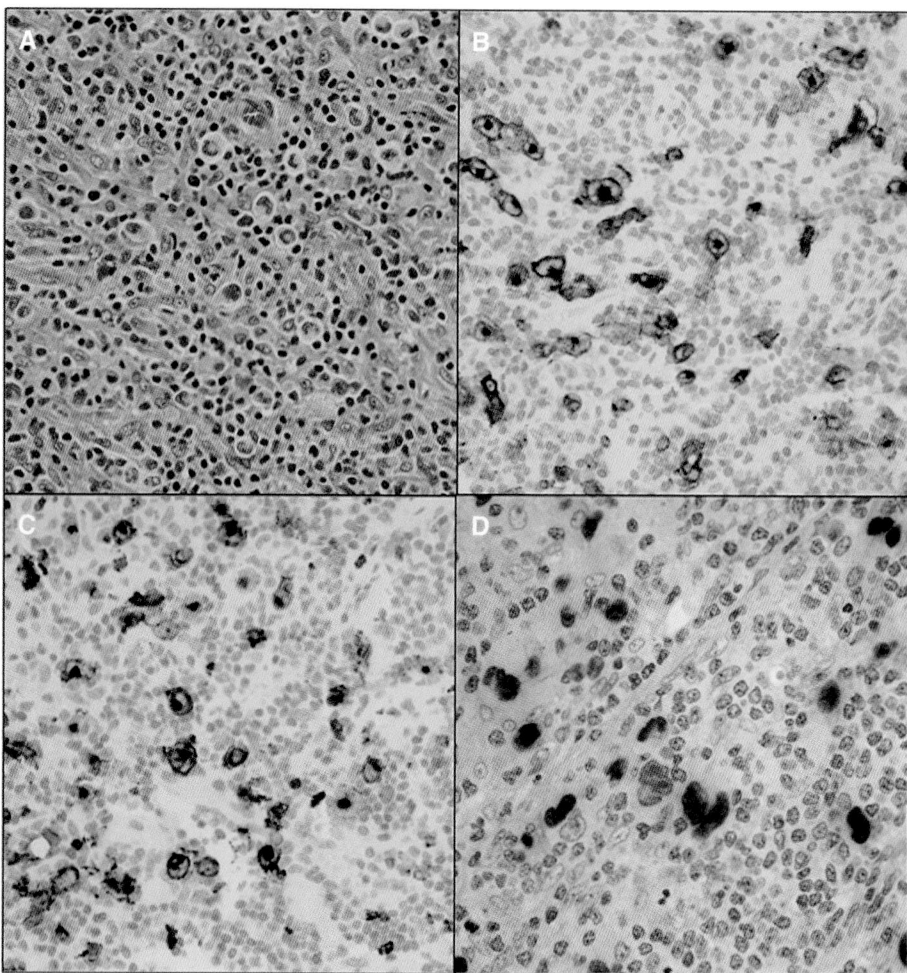

FIGURE 1C-6 ■ **Classic Hodgkin lymphoma.** The H&E-stained section (**A**) reveals scattered large cells with atypical, convoluted nuclei in a mixed inflammatory background. At lower power, fibrous bands were seen entrapping nodules of tumor. By IHC, the Hodgkin cells are positive for CD15 (**B**) and CD30 (**C**). *In situ* hybridization for EBV encoded RNA (EBER) is positive in many of these cells (**D**, *red staining*).

detectable hormone(s) in the tumor cells' cytoplasm, but not in the patient's serum.

Medullary thyroid carcinoma stains positively for calcitonin, as do normal C-cells and the hyperplastic foci of multiple endocrine neoplasia syndrome. More generally, thyroid epithelial cells can be highlighted by antibodies to thyroglobulin or thyroid transcription factor-1 (TTF-1). Parathyroid hormone stains are useful in identifying parathyroid tissue, although normal, hyperplastic, and neoplastic tissues react identically.

Although less often useful in the pediatric realm, IHC for estrogen and progesterone receptors has become standard of care in the evaluation of breast cancer, serving to guide the choice of chemotherapy. Germ cell and sex cord tumors can express α-inhibin and β-human chorionic gonadotrophin (β-hCG), and the serum levels of these markers are sometimes used to monitor patients for recurrence.

Embryonal and Cancer Markers

Fetal tissues and neoplasms share expression of primitive traits, including a subset of proteins normally restricted to developmental periods. For example, α-fetoprotein can be found in fetal liver as well as hepatoblastomas, hepatomas, and endodermal sinus tumors. Placental alkaline phosphatase (PLAP) stains germ cell tumors and some carcinomas. The stem cell marker OCT4 is now replacing PLAP as a more sensitive and specific marker of germ cell neoplasms, specifically seminoma/germinoma, embryonal carcinoma, and intratubular germ cell neoplasia. Among the so called cancer markers, CA-125 is more specific for genitourinary neoplasms, whereas CA19-9 is preferentially expressed in gastrointestinal cancers. Both these markers are also detectable in patient serum.

Protooncogenes

Anaplastic lymphoma kinase-1 (ALK-1) is the fusion product of a characteristic t(2;5) translocation found in most anaplastic large cell lymphomas and inflammatory myofibroblastic tumors; its expression in the former is thought to portend favorable prognosis. Tyrosine kinases, such as *c-kit* (CD117), can help diagnose tumors such as gastrointestinal stromal tumors, as well as predict which lesions might respond to monoclonal antibody therapy (in this case, imatinib).

Cell Cycle and Apoptotic Markers

The most commonly used antibody in this category is MIB-1 (Ki67), a proliferation marker frequently used to assess the proliferative activity of lesions. Although a high MIB-1 index does not define something as neoplastic, it can be used as a corroborating piece of evidence in making such a decision, or in determining the histologic grade of a tumor (Figure 1C-3, panel C). Some apoptotic markers, such as Bcl-2 and Bcl-6, have utility in identifying the lineage of hematopoietic neoplasms and other tumors (Figure 1C-5, panel D). β-Catenin, a molecule involved in the Wnt signaling pathway, is highly expressed in desmoid tumors, as well as colorectal lesions with aberrations of the APC pathway.

Other

Alpha-1-antitrypsin (A1AT) is expressed in normal and neoplastic liver tissue, as well as in yolk sac tumors. Its primary diagnostic utility, however, is in identifying A1AT deficiency manifest as strong cytoplasmic positivity in the setting of hepatic or pulmonary disease; recall that the disorder affects A1AT export, not production, so the mutated protein accumulates intracellularly. Alpha-1-antichymotrypsin is also a serine protease inhibitor (serpin), and is found in histiocytes and pancreatic and salivary duct epithelium.

Limitations

As mentioned previously, immunohistochemical stains are only useful when done properly and in a well-controlled fashion. Evaluation of appropriate positive and negative controls, as well as internal controls, is required every time a stain is run in order to ensure validity. Minor changes in reaction conditions or the antibody supplier can lead to major changes in results.

IHC staining patterns can only be interpreted in the context of the H&E morphology, the clinical scenario, and the results of other ancillary tests. Basing a diagnosis on a single immunostain can be risky. Performing a panel of five stains that are 80% specific is bound to result in at least one stain with spurious results.

IMMUNOFLUORESCENCE

Background

Direct immunofluorescence (DIF) is a molecular technique that provides ancillary information in the diagnosis of dermatologic, renal, and transplant organ disease. DIF relies on the same antibody-antigen recognition as flow cytometry and IHC. The most common uses in pathology include detection of immunoglobulins, complement proteins, and fibrinogen in patient tissue sections or infectious organisms in other samples (*Pneumocystis* spp.) (40).

Method

DIF requires fresh or snap frozen tissue as formalin and other aldehyde-derived fixatives alter the antigenicity of immunoglobulins, complement proteins, and other molecules of interest (27). Ammonium sulfate–based buffers that inhibit

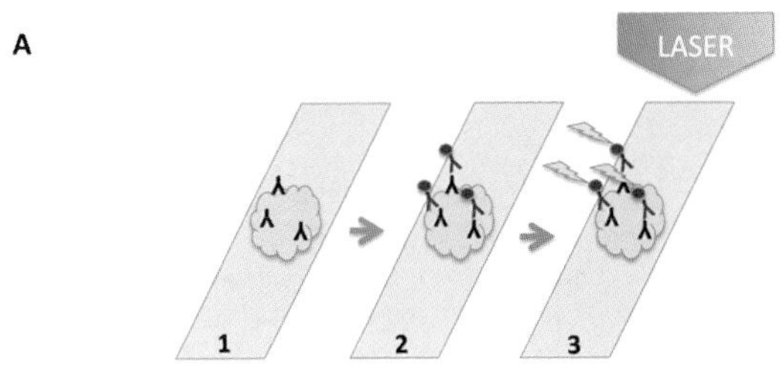

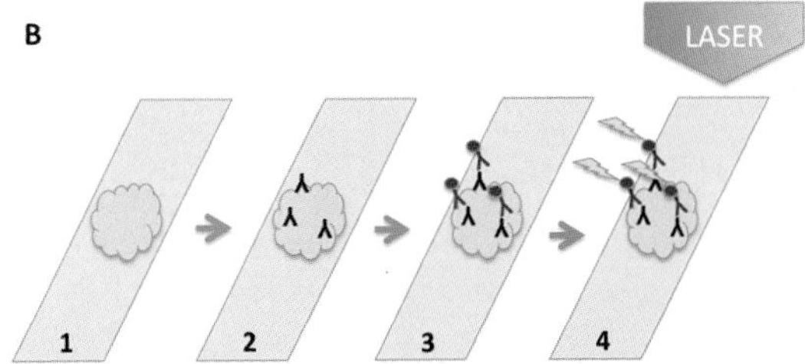

FIGURE 1C-7 ■ Overview of immunofluorescent staining. For DIF (**A**), slides bear tissue with native antibody of interest already bound (*1*). A secondary antibody conjugated to a fluorescent tag is then bound to the original antibodies (*2*), and then detected by laser-induced fluorescence (*3*). DIF (**B**) is nearly identical to IHC (see Figure 1C-4), except detection requires laser excitation.

tissue proteases can be used to transport specimens from the procedure areas to the testing laboratory (13,20,41,43,54,59). Tissue is then snap frozen in OCT, sectioned in a cryostat, air dried, rehydrated, and incubated with the appropriate antibody solution. If DIF is not needed immediately, it is helpful to know that tissue antigens are stable in OCT for up to 4 months at either −20°C or −70°C (40).

For most renal and skin biopsies, a typical immunofluorescence panel will include antibodies directed against IgG, IgA, IgM, C1, C3, fibrinogen, C4d (in renal transplant), properdin, and albumin—the latter as a positive control. Antibody binding and staining is similar to that for IHC but uses a fluorochrome rather than a dye for detection (Figure 1C-7). Stained slides are stored in a dark refrigerator until reading, which should occur as promptly as possible (within 24 hours) as fluorescence intensity diminishes with time.

Applications

The most common specimens that routinely involve immunofluorescence staining are for medical kidney disease and autoimmune skin disorders (Figure 1C-8). In addition to the particular stains that are positive (e.g., IgG versus IgM), the pattern (linear versus granular) and the location (basement membrane versus dermal-epidermal junction) of staining are also important in distinguishing between specific entities. (*See Chapters 17 and 25 for detailed information about DIF in kidney and skin lesions.*) Ultimately, the simultaneous consideration of all available information—clinical presentation, laboratory studies, H&E-stained sections, and DIF—is required to maximize diagnostic sensitivity and accuracy.

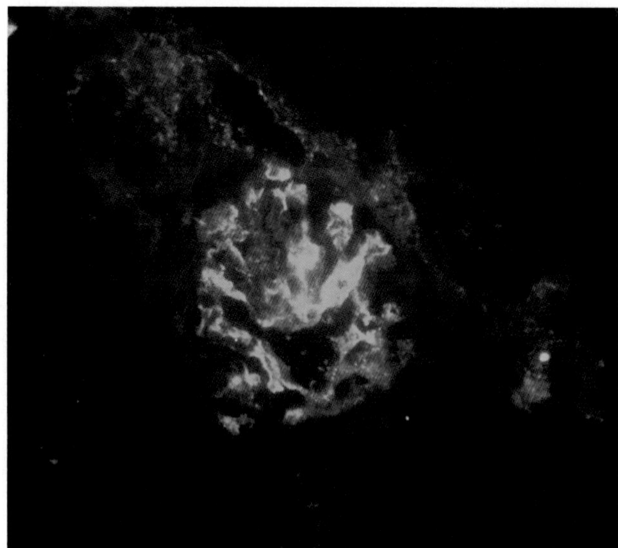

FIGURE 1C-8 ■ DIF for IgA in a renal core biopsy from an 11-year-old girl with gross hematuria and nephrotic-range proteinuria. Glomeruli showed diffuse IgA deposits in the mesangium and granular deposition in the capillary loops which, in conjunction with the light and electron microscopic findings, was consistent with IgA nephropathy.

FLUORESCENCE *IN SITU* HYBRIDIZATION (FISH/ISH)

Background

Increasing numbers of tumors and congenital disorders are being identified as monogenic in nature, and their underlying genetic alterations are being discovered. In turn, this has yielded a large number of genetic targets that can be used in the diagnosis, prognosis, and therapeutic selection of these diseases. As such, a variety of molecularly based genetic assays have been developed to investigate and analyze these targets. Instead of relying on the specificity of an antibody-antigen reaction, as in IHC and IF, FISH and ISH instead utilize the base complementarity between a labeled oligonucleotide probe and a DNA or RNA sequence of interest.

One of the main advantages of FISH/ISH is its *in situ* nature—target sequences of interest are precisely localized within specific cells, the nuclear/cytoplasmic distribution can be compared, and the relative chromosomal location of two genes can be identified. This is in contrast to techniques such as PCR, microarrays, or cytogenetics, which by necessity destroy the architecture to get at the DNA, RNA, or chromosomes, respectively. Another benefit of FISH/ISH is the high specificity of nucleic acid strand interactions, which can easily distinguish between closely related gene products. Alternatively, probes can be designed against conserved sequences to detect multiple isoforms or products, for example, multiple strains of a single virus or common population variants of a polymorphous locus. Linking the probes to a fluorescent tag (in FISH) amplifies the signal and increases the sensitivity of the assay without affecting the specificity. Finally, these methods are usually suitable for use with formalin-fixed, paraffin-embedded tissue, allowing their application in cases with limited material as well as in retrospective research studies.

Methods

The optimal tissue source for FISH/ISH assays depends on the target molecule; frozen tissue is preferable for RNA studies, whereas formalin-fixed, paraffin-embedded tissue is suitable for DNA work as well as for some small, stable RNAs. Standard 4- to 10-μm sections are cut on a cryostat or microtome and, for FFPE, deparaffinized and rehydrated. Other potential specimen sources include touch preparations and nuclear spreads from conventional cytogenetics (Figures 1C-3, 1C-5, and 1C-9); in both instances nuclei are fixed by alcohol- or aldehyde-based methods.

Slides are overlaid with a small amount of buffer containing the desired probe, and incubated from several hours to overnight. Probes can be RNA or DNA, and can be synthesized in-house from templates or purchased from a variety of commercial vendors; some of the latter sell kits with multiple probes and controls appropriately packaged together for a particular disease entity or differential diagnostic workup.

Sections are then washed to remove unbound and nonspecifically bound probe. Then, for ISH, the detection reaction is run to create a color change at the site of binding, akin to that described for IHC (Figure 1C-6, panel D). For FISH, sections are examined under a fluorescent microscope to detect the labeled probe (Figure 1C-3, panels F and G; Figure 1C-5, panel F; Figure 1C-9, panel F; and Figure 1C-10, panels B and C). Appropriate controls include probes against "housekeeping" genes, or the centromeres of uninvolved chromosomes, as well as evaluation of the analytic probes in "normal" or uninvolved cells.

Applications

FISH and ISH have wide utility in a broad range of applications. The most common may be in the detection of chromosomal translocations in solid and hematopoietic neoplasms. This analysis can be approached in two ways: looking for the fusion product, or looking for the destruction of the original gene ("breakapart"). For example, in some cases of Burkitt lymphoma (Figure 1C-3, panels F and G), the *MYCC* and *IGH* genes are involved in a t(8;14) translocation. In the assay pictured, the *MYCC* probe is conjugated to a red tag and the *IGH* probe to a green tag. In normal cells, two separate red signals and two separate green signals should be present. However, in Burkitt cells harboring the translocation, one set of red and green signals overlaps producing a yellow fusion signal. For the breakapart strategy, the principle is reversed: normal cells should have two intact signals, but translocation will destroy one of those signals and create two new signals. For example, in synovial sarcoma (Figure 1C-5, panel F), the central tumor cell has two separate *SYT* signals (one red and one green, from opposite

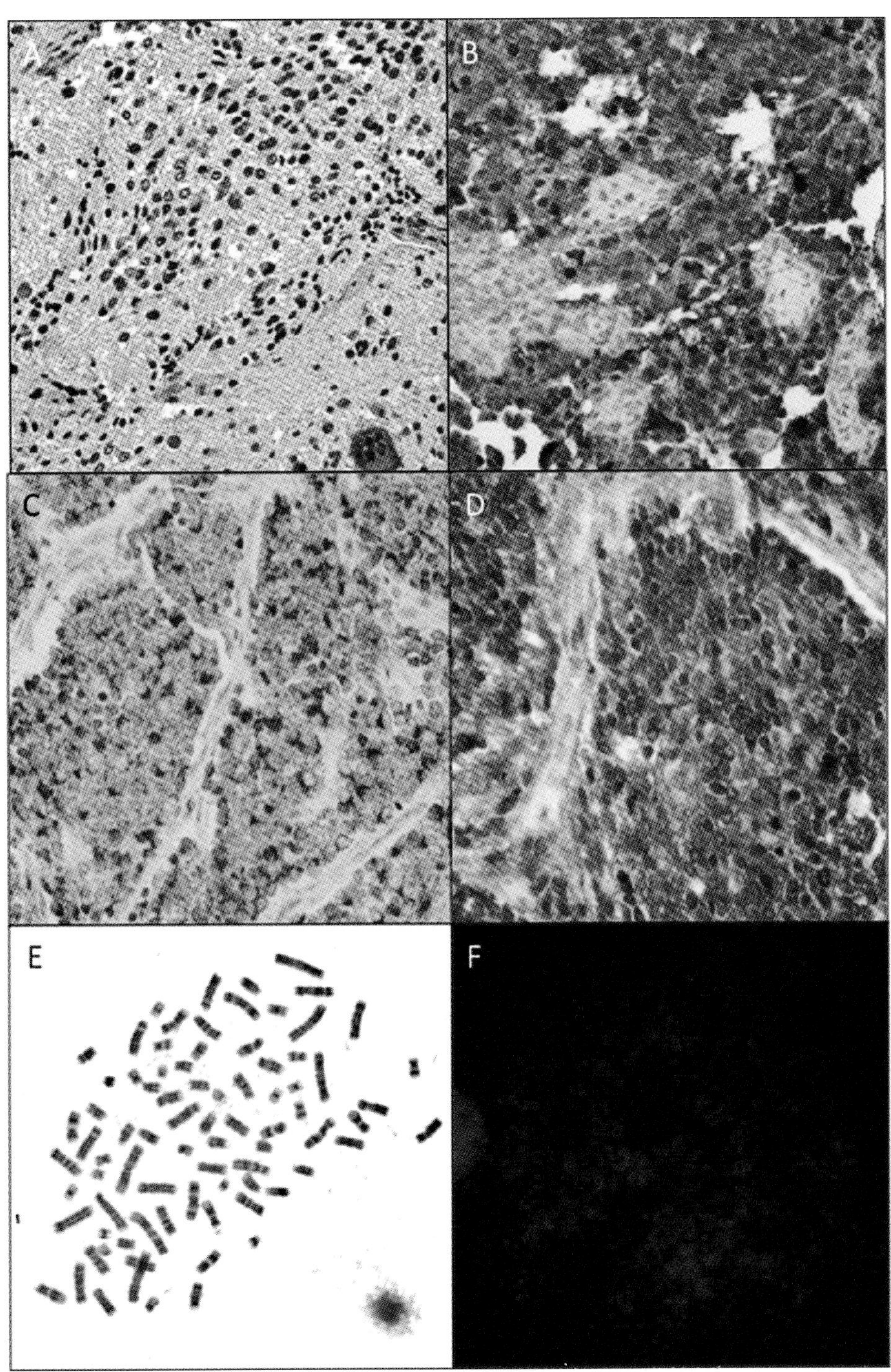

FIGURE 1C-9 ■ **Neuroblastoma.** On an H&E-stained section (**A**), small round blue cells with occasional early gangliocytoid differentiation, copious neuropil, and a low mitotic-karyorrhectic index are seen. The tumor cells are immunohistochemically positive for PGP9.5 (**B**), NB84 (**C**), and synaptophysin (**D**), confirming the diagnosis of neuroblastoma. A metaphase chromosomal spread (**E**) shows numerous double minutes in the background, which are FISH-positive for *MYCN* (**F**), indicating amplification. (Chromosomal and FISH analyses courtesy of Dr. Peter vanTuinen, Dynacare Clinical Cytogenetics Laboratory, Medical College of Wisconsin.)

ends of the gene) instead of a single intact yellow signal as seen in the surrounding normal cells.

FISH can also be used to detect copy number changes of a gene or locus, such as *MYCN* amplification in neuroblastoma (Figure 1C-9, panel F) or loss of one copy of the *hSNF5/INI1* locus in malignant rhabdoid tumor (4). In the case of *MYCN* amplification, this method is able to detect amplification whether via intrachromosomal sequence duplication or extrachromosomal double minutes (as shown).

FISH is invaluable in the examination of stillbirth and intrauterine death, especially in cases of delayed delivery where tissue quality is compromised. In the example case of a fetal demise with dysmorphic features (Figure 1C-10), the bottom two panels (B and C) show a standard FISH workup for common cytogenetic abnormalities in this setting—analysis of chromosomes 13, 18, 21 (most commonly implicated in stillborn trisomies), and X and Y. As shown, the fetus is triploid with three clear signals for chromosomes 13,

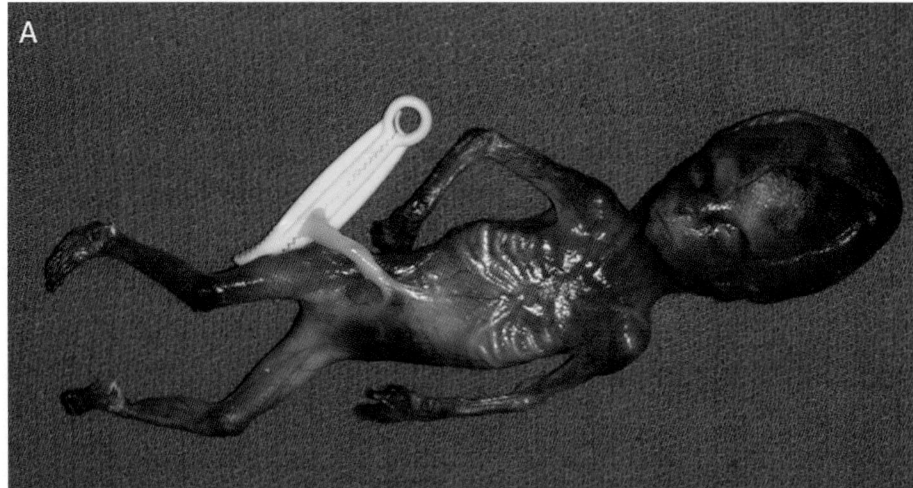

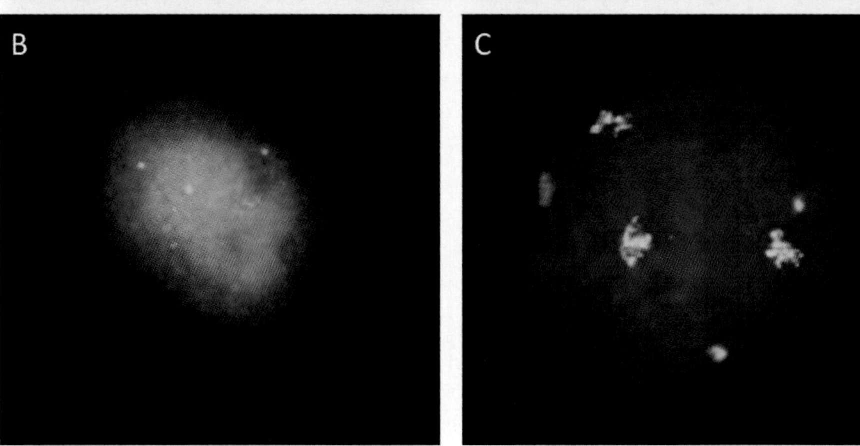

FIGURE 1C-10 ■ **Fetal triploidy.** A 29-year-old G1P0 female underwent medical pregnancy termination at 20 weeks' gestation following ultrasound diagnosis of intrauterine growth retardation, Dandy-Walker malformation, and ventricular septal heart defect (**A**) (Courtesy of Pat Rogers, Children's Hospital of Wisconsin, Audio Visual Services). Amniocentesis and FISH analysis had been performed, demonstrating triploidy (69,XXX). FISH probes in (**B**) include chromosomes 13 (*red*) and 21 (*green*) and, in (**C**), chromosomes 18 (*aqua*) and X (*green*); three copies of each chromosome are present, and no copies of the Y chromosome [*red probe* in (**C**)] are identified. (FISH analysis courtesy of Dr. Peter vanTuinen, Dynacare Clinical Cytogenetics Laboratory, Medical College of Wisconsin.)

18, 21, and X. Not only is this study diagnostic, but essential because cells did not grow for conventional cytogenetics and karyotyping (see Chapter 3).

Nonfluorescent (colorimetric) ISH is often used as a nucleic acid version of IHC with otherwise similar techniques and applications. Most commonly, ISH is used for detecting nucleic acids of infectious agents, such as HPV, HSV, and EBV (Figure 1C-6, panel D). ISH tends to have higher sensitivity and specificity than IHC for the companion viral proteins (18).

CYTOGENETICS

Background

Conventional cytogenetic analysis, or karyotyping, is a well-established technique that gives a broad genetic overview at a chromosomal level. It can identify constitutional disorders and demonstrate abnormalities that aid in diagnosis with or without providing insight into prognosis and therapeutic effectiveness. Despite the development of increasingly sophisticated and sensitive molecular assays, cytogenetics maintains a crucial diagnostic role because of its capability to detect a wide range of abnormalities at once using a simple and cost-effective procedure.

Method

Typical specimens submitted for cytogenetic analysis include tumor or lymph node tissue, skin biopsy as a source of fibroblasts, whole blood or peripheral blood mononuclear cells, and prenatal samples from chorionic villus sampling or amniocentesis. For conventional cell culture and karyotyping, fresh viable tissue is required. For tumors and lymph nodes, a small (1 cm^3) piece of grossly viable lesional tissue usually suffices. For fetuses or neonates, a placental biopsy, taken superficially from the cleansed fetal surface, is usually an acceptable surrogate; however, care must be taken to prevent contamination of the sample with maternal cells (decidua or blood).

Samples should be immediately placed in standard tissue culture medium (such as RPMI) and kept at room temperature until transport to the cytogenetics laboratory. Often, testing can be delayed until initial workup of the case is completed—for example, with most tumors we routinely save a tissue sample in medium until the H&E-stained slides can be reviewed, and the necessity of cytogenetic testing can be evaluated. Most tissue is stable and viable for several days in culture medium at 4°C, although the risk of bacterial or fungal contamination increases over time unless antibiotics are included in the formulation of the medium. Another alternative is to submit the tissue to the cytogenetics lab for tissue culture and to make the decision about proceeding with karyotyping at a later date.

Upon receipt in the laboratory, specimens are disaggregated and the cells are allowed to grow in culture for several days until they reach a sufficient number of actively dividing cells. At this point, a mitotic inhibitor is added that arrests the cells in metaphase with chromosomes neatly condensed and separated. Cells are cultured long enough for as many cells as possible to reach the stage of mitotic arrest, without reducing viability. The cells are then chemically treated to preserve the chromosomal integrity, fix the nuclei, and remove the cell membrane and cytoplasm. The nuclear preparation is then placed onto slides for staining and analysis.

Several different stains and procedures can be employed, but the most commonly used method is Giemsa staining (G-banding; see Figure 1C-3, panel E, and Figure 1C-5, panel E), which utilizes a limited trypsin digestion before staining with the same DNA-binding dye used elsewhere in histology, thereby producing light-and-dark bands across each chromosome. Other protocols utilize other chemical treatments and other dyes to specifically stain telomeres (T-banding), heterochromatin (C-banding), or AT-rich sequences (Q-banding). Each method produces a characteristic banding pattern that can be compared to known reference standards. G-banding typically yields roughly 400 bands across the genome for analysis, but higher resolution banding can discriminate smaller regions but requires preparation of less condensed chromosomes, such as those in prometaphase instead of metaphase, and involves a more lengthy analysis. Standard G-banding has a detection limit of about four megabases; deletions or additions of smaller amounts of DNA may not be identified by this method.

Regarding terminology, the pattern produced by a particular method is compared to a standard reference (the Paris nomenclature) where bands are numbered according to their location on the chromosome – arm, region, band, sub-band, sub-sub-band, etc. The short arm is dubbed p (petit) and the long arm is q (queue). Bands (p11, p12, p13,...), sub-bands (p12 divided into p12.1, p12.2, p12.3,...), and sub-sub-bands (p12.2 divided into p12.21, p12.22, p12.23,...) are numbered from the centromere outward (the centromere can be considered to be both p10 and q10); p21.23 would be more telomeric than p21.22. Note that this terminology places band p3.25 between p3.1 and p3.3, as a sub-sub-band belonging to sub-band p3. A band's location is preceded by its host chromosome, such as 5q23.1, which is an area located roughly halfway out on the long arm of chromosome 5, and is properly described as "five q two three point one." Karyotypes are denoted in writing as the total diploid number of chromosomes, followed by the identities of the sex chromosomes, and then details regarding abnormalities. For example, boys and girls would usually have constitutional karyotypes of 46,XY, and 46,XX, respectively, while a female patient with Cri du chat syndrome might instead have a 46,XX,del(5p) karyotype.

Chromosomes are examined under a microscope and their banding patterns are compared within each chromosomal pair (22 autosomal pairs and 2 sex chromosomes in each examined mitotic spread) and to the reference standards looking for aberrations in number, size, and/or composition. Standard karyotyping can detect numerical changes in chromosomes (e.g., monosomy or trisomy), duplication or loss of chromosomal material, translocations, and other disorders. Typically, the chromosomes from 20 different nuclei are examined, assuring a representative sampling in order to exclude mosaicism or a small percentage of abnormal cells, such as occasional tumor cells within a preponderance of normal cells.

Chromosomal abnormalities detectable by conventional cytogenetics are numerical or structural in nature. The former includes common constitutional disorders such as Down syndrome (trisomy 21), Edwards syndrome (trisomy 18), and Patau syndrome (trisomy 13), in all of which patients have a third, additional copy of an autosome (e.g., a girl with Down syndrome would have a 47,XX,+21 karyotype). Constitutional triploidy, three copies of all chromosomes (e.g., 69,XXX) is much less common than isolated trisomies, and is almost always embryonic lethal (Figure 1C-10). Monosomies, such as Turner syndrome (45,XO), are readily detected. Again, standard analysis includes 20 cells because sporadic loss of a chromosome (or other aberration) can occur during sample preparation; an abnormality should be consistently seen in multiple cells before it is considered real. Tumors often show aneuploidy with varying numbers of each chromosome, in addition to structural aberrations.

Structural chromosomal problems occur in many different forms and appear to be the result of DNA damage and/or faulty repair. Some are balanced, in which no net material is lost, but sequences are simply rearranged; this includes translocations and inversions. Others are unbalanced, with net loss (deletions) or gain (duplications) of genetic material. These include inversions, deletions, additions, ring chromosomes, translocations with loss of one derivative chromosome and combinations thereof.

Translocations involve swapping of material between two or more chromosomes, usually without net loss (reciprocal and balanced). However, the rearranged genes can be separated from their regulatory sequences and be aberrantly expressed, or can instead be combined to produce a novel fusion protein. The former is exemplified by common translocations involving the *MYC* proto-oncogene in Burkitt lymphoma, such as t(8;14)(q24;q32), which places *MYC* under constitutive expression of the immunoglobulin heavy chain promoter, instead of its usual tightly controlled regulation (Figure 1C-3). A classic example of the latter mechanism is the Philadelphia chromosome, t(9;22)(q34;q11), seen in a subset of adult and pediatric leukemias, which juxtaposes the *BCR* and *ABL* genes to create a novel BCR-ABL fusion protein with dysregulated tyrosine kinase activity that drives oncogenesis. Note the terminology used for such events: "t" for translocation, followed by the involved chromosomes (9 and 22), and the regions or bands involved (q34 from chromosome 9 and q11 from chromosome 11); thus, the karyotype of a Philadelphia chromosome-positive pediatric ALL might be 46,XY,t(9;22)(q34;q11). Some balanced translocations are constitutional, but because the overall genetic content of the cells is unchanged, there is no problem detected in the carrier of a particular translocation. The problem occurs when offspring inherit only one of the abnormal parental chromosomes incurring an unbalanced genotype and, therefore, disease. A good example of this is a subset of Robertsonian translocations implicated in some cases of Down syndrome.

Applications

Probably the most common application of conventional cytogenetics is analyzing constitutional karyotype. This usually occurs prenatally, using fetal cells obtained by chorionic villus sampling or amniocentesis, or in the neonatal period using a blood sample. Such information may guide prenatal care, anticipate difficulties in the neonatal period, portend outcomes, or guide future family planning. In instances of fetal loss or stillbirth, samples of skin or placenta should be sent for cytogenetics as part of the standard workup, especially if dysmorphic features are noted. In all cases with abnormal genetic results, and in many cases with normal karyotypes, parental referral to a genetic counselor is helpful.

Cytogenetic analysis can also provide important information in the evaluation of many neoplasms. A particular translocation may be identified that is pathognomonic for a given tumor (Figures 1C-3 and 1C-5), while other genetic aberrations may provide information on prognosis or therapeutic efficacy. For example, 95% of cases of acute promyelocytic leukemia bear a t(15;17)(q22;q12) abnormality that, besides being a diagnostic finding, can be used in molecular tests to monitor recurrence and also offers a therapeutic target—the fusion protein that results from this translocation, PML-RARα, appears to convey sensitivity to all-trans retinoic acid. (37) Other prognostic genetic markers include 1p/19q loss in oligodendrogliomas, 1p/16q loss in Wilms' tumor, 6q/17q loss in medulloblastoma, and 1p loss and the previously mentioned *MYCN* amplification in neuroblastoma.

Limitations

The major limitations of conventional cytogenetic analysis are threefold: the requirement for fresh, viable tissue with cells that can grow in a culture environment, the variable length of time for cells to grow and be analyzed, and the relatively low resolution of detection (four megabases). Assays such as FISH and PCR can circumvent the need for growing cells, can be done in 1 day, and provide higher resolution than cytogenetics. On the other hand, they are considerably more expensive and are designed for targeting precise molecular abnormalities. In many cases, the methods may be more complementary than competing. Despite continued methodological advances in molecular pathology (see below), karyotyping still has a major role as a simple, cost-effective method of examining the entire genome at low-resolution for numerical or structural abnormalities.

POLYMERASE CHAIN REACTION

Background

The purpose of PCR is to create millions of copies of a specific segment of DNA so that it can be analyzed by its sequence, size, and complementarity to other sequences. It is used regularly in molecular diagnostics, forensic science, and research laboratories. Variations of the basic principles of PCR have led to numerous advancements in our ability to quickly and cost-effectively detect DNA sequence variants associated with specific diseases.

Methods

PCR sensitivity is best on fresh, snap frozen samples but the technique can also be applied to formalin-fixed paraffin embedded tissue. First, DNA is extracted from the sample of interest. If starting with RNA, total RNA is extracted and then converted into cDNA (complementary DNA) by an enzyme called *reverse transcriptase* (RT), the so-called RT-PCR. This DNA or cDNA is then mixed with free nucleotides (dNTPs), buffer, thermostable DNA polymerase, and two short, sequence-specific oligonucleotides called *primers* (Figure 1C-11). Primers are approximately 20 base pairs long and are designed so that one primer is complementary to the top strand of DNA at one end of the target segment and a second primer is complementary to the bottom strand of DNA at the other end of the target segment. Within this mixture, the target DNA or cDNA is then amplified through cycles of denaturation (at high temperatures such as 95°C), annealing (at lower temperatures defined by primer-template nucleotide sequence, 55°C to 65°C), and elongation (70°C). The denaturation stage separates the DNA into single strands, to which the primers can then bind during the annealing phase. During elongation, the polymerase uses the target DNA strand as a template to lengthen the primers, creating complementary double-stranded molecules; these products then serve as additional targets in the next round, allowing exponential amplification.

The amplified product is then subjected to gel electrophoresis and staining (with ethidium bromide or fluorescent analogues) where the relative size of the DNA can be determined by comparison to known standards. Confirmation that this product is the sequence of interest can be done by transferring the DNA from the gel to a nylon or nitrocellulose membrane, applying a radioactively or fluorescently labeled probe

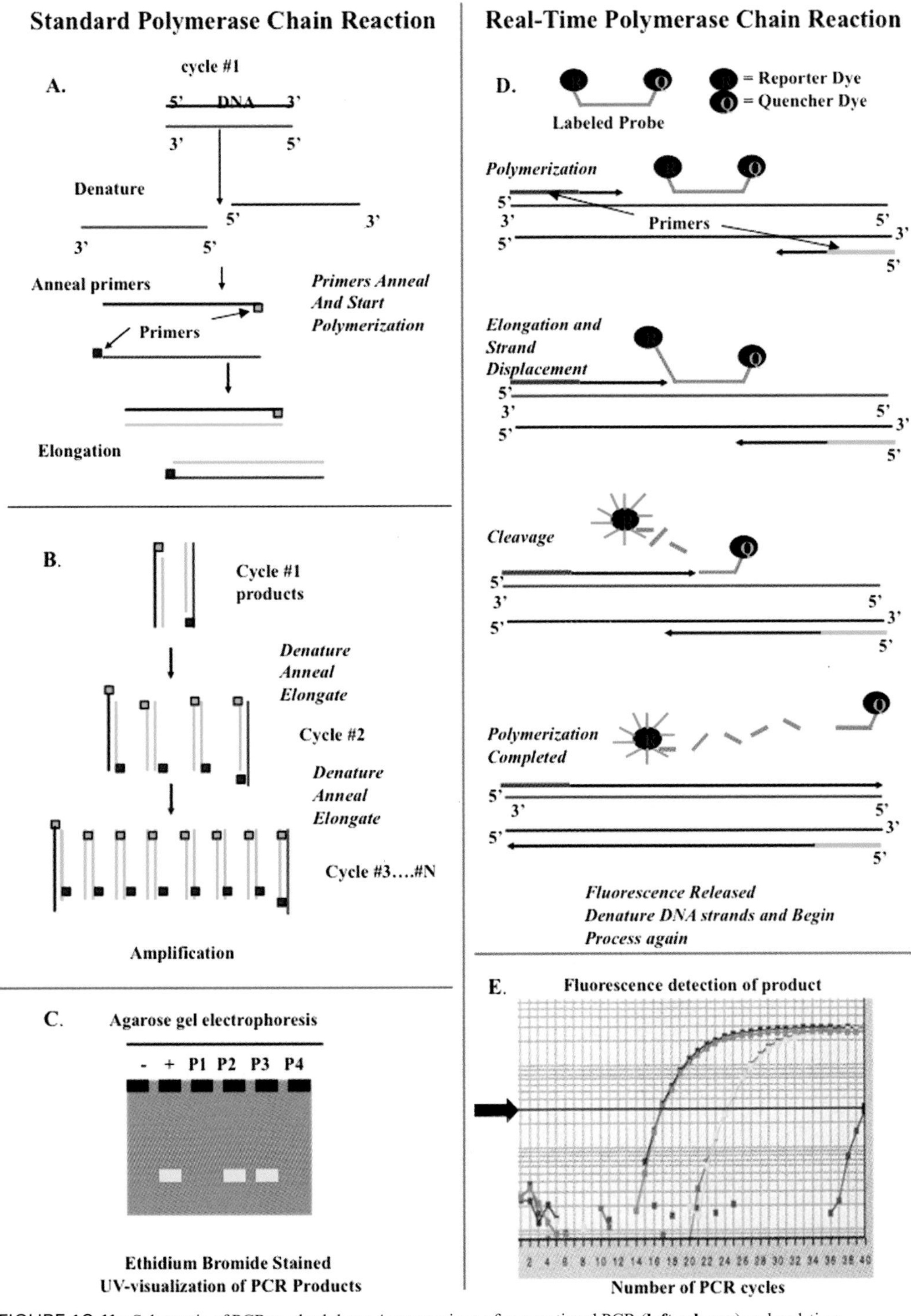

FIGURE 1C-11 ■ Schematic of PCR methodology. A comparison of conventional PCR (**left column**) and real-time PCR (**right column**). Conventional PCR involves denaturing of double-stranded DNA (or cDNA), annealing of primers, and elongation steps (**A,B**). The detection of amplified product typically involves agarose gel electrophoresis (**C**). **D, E:** Real-time PCR uses the same features of denaturation, annealing of primers, and elongation but adds a probe complementary to sequence in between the two end primers. This probe is labeled with both fluorescent reporter and quencher dyes that when in close proximity do not emit a signal. As the strand elongates from the 5′ primer, the probe is disrupted and cleaved, releasing the reporter dye into the solution. Once the reporter is no longer in proximity to the quencher dye, its fluorescent signal is detectable. Additional reporter dye will be released with each cycle and is proportional to the accumulated amount of amplified product. A detector measures fluorescence in real time and the results are viewed in graphical form with quantity of signal on the y-axis and number of PCR cycles on the x-axis. The horizontal line indicates a threshold level beyond which there is exponential accumulation of signal, confirming that the specific DNA product is obtained. (**D** and **E** adapted from Applied Biosystems' TaqMan literature.)

(similar to a primer, a probe is a short sequence of DNA designed to match a sequence internal to that of the primer pairs), and then placing the membrane on x-ray film. If the probe matches the sequence on the membrane, the label will expose the x-ray film at the location of the band. This process is known as *Southern blotting*. Some laboratories choose to clone and sequence PCR products for confirmation rather than blotting. Other laboratories do not perform either of these confirmatory steps; these laboratories may be at risk for reporting false positives.

Real-Time Polymerase Chain Reaction

Real-time or quantitative PCR is a variation on standard PCR that was first described by Holland et al. (28,55). It follows the same basic principles of standard RT-PCR, but utilizes the 5′ exonuclease activity of the *Thermus aquaticus* (Taq) DNA polymerase coupled with fluorescence energy transfer (Figure 1C-6). First DNA is extracted from the sample of interest. If starting with RNA, the RNA is extracted and reverse transcribed into cDNA. The target cDNA or DNA is amplified in a mix containing not only a set of forward and reverse oligonucleotide primers designed to amplify sequences specific to the gene of interest but also a probe designed to match a sequence internal to that of the primer pairs. The probe is labeled with a reporter fluorescent dye at the 5′ end and a quencher fluorescent dye at the 3′ end. The quencher dye acts to decrease emission of the reporter dye as long as they are in close proximity to each other (on the ends of the same molecule). During the elongation phase of PCR, both primers and probe anneal to the target sequence if present. As the 5′ primer is extended, the 5′ exonuclease activity of the *Taq* DNA polymerase releases the fluorescent reporter dye once it reaches the 5′ end of the annealed probe; now separated from the 3′ quencher, fluorescence from the 5′ dye increases. As the specific product accumulates, additional probes anneal and then release more fluorescent signal with each PCR cycle. Rather than visualizing the PCR product after agarose gel electrophoresis and staining, the product is visualized in real time on a computer that plots the intensity of the reporter's fluorescent signal. Signal intensity is directly proportional to the amount of specific amplicon produced with each cycle of amplification. This method is capable of providing highly sensitive detection of target DNA and rapid results. Because of the elimination of postprocessing steps such as nested PCR or Southern blot confirmation, the risk of cross contamination in association with carryover PCR product is reduced and there is no need for radioactive materials.

Applications

PCR has numerous applications for pediatric pathologists primarily in tumor pathology, microbiologic speciation of organisms, genetic testing for mutations and forensic identification.

Detection of Fusion Gene Transcripts

One of the first applications developed for pathology was detection of fusion gene transcripts resulting from translocations in hematopoietic and solid tumors (Table 1C-2). Although many of these translocations are also detectable by cytogenetics, the latter technique requires fresh tissue and growing cells. FISH is another method for detecting gene fusions/translocations and may perform superiorly to RT-PCR when only FFPE is available. The benefit of RT-PCR over both those techniques is that it preserves the ability to obtain sequence information from the fusion gene product. A few studies have suggested that in some tumors, the fusion type may have prognostic importance, thus designing the test to distinguish between variants may have some additional clinical utility (36,55). Also, RT-PCR can detect fusion genes in the setting of complex translocations involving small amounts of DNA (<400 kb) below the resolution of conventional chromosomal banding and karyotyping.

Molecular Microbiology

The use of PCR technology has transformed the clinical microbiology laboratory. For many microbial infections, PCR techniques have replaced standard culture or immunoassay identification (17). Real-time PCR is particularly appealing for use in microbiology for its speed over current methods (results in hours rather than days), efficacy (the ability of an organism to grow in culture is not an issue with PCR), and accuracy for speciation. Further, because real-time PCR is performed in a closed system, meaning that there is no open handling of amplified DNA products, there is a greatly decreased risk of crosscontamination. PCR-based sequencing can add additional utility to the microbiology laboratory. The sequence of 16S ribosomal RNA appears to be unique among microbial species and can be used to accurately identify organisms such as mycobacteria as well as to identify new pathogens (53). Further, PCR-based assessment of antimicrobial resistance genes may become more commonplace as information from microbial research laboratories makes its way to clinical application (63).

Genetic Testing for Mutations

In the last decade, hundreds of diseases have been attributed to abnormalities in the DNA sequence code. Base substitutions and insertions and deletions of coding sequences alter the production of or change the nature of proteins in a manner that is associated with particular diseases. Duchenne muscular dystrophy, cystic fibrosis, and neurofibromatosis type 1 are common examples of monogenic diseases that are amenable to PCR-based genetic testing, but there are many more in the categories of metabolic diseases, neurologic and muscular diseases, and cancer predisposition syndromes. Sequencing for commonly mutated exons (so-called mutational hot spots) in affected children or offspring of affected or carrier parents provides important information

Table 1C-2 ■ MOLECULAR TESTING IN PEDIATRIC DISEASES

System	Tumor	Genetic Aberration	Immunohistochemistry		Notes
			Pertinent Positives	Pertinent Negatives	
Head and Neck	Congenital epulis	—	—	S100	S100(−) unlike other granular cell tumors
	Sinonasal papillomas	—	HPV, in a subset	—	—
	Nasopharyngeal angiofibroma	Some associated with *APC* mutations and/or FAP	β-catenin	—	—
	Osteomas	May be associated with Gardner syndrome	—	—	—
	Teratoma	—	Varies by component	AFP to rule out yolk sac tumor component	—
	Nasopharyngeal carcinoma	HLA associations	EBV/EBER; mixed cytokeratins	Cytokeratins 7 and 20	—
	Adenoid cystic carcinoma	Some have t(6;9) (q21-24;p13-23), others have LOH at 6q.	Ductal cells: cytokeratin, EMA, and CEA. Myoepithelial cells: cytokeratin, p63, S100.	—	IHC helps identify different components.
	Pleomorphic adenoma	FLAG 1 t(3:8) (p21;q21)	Ductal cells: cytokeratin, EMA, and CEA. Myoepithelial cells: cytokeratin, p63, S100.	—	IHC helps identify different components.
	Salivary gland anlage tumor	—	Epithelial cells: cytokeratin; stromal cells: vimentin, actin, and cytokeratin	—	—
	Mucoepidermoid carcinoma	***MECT1/MAML2*** translocations	Cytokeratin, including CK7	—	—
	Sialoblastoma	—	Ductal cells: cytokeratin; basaloid cells: S100 and actin	—	—
Cardiovascular	Fibroma	May be associated with Gorlin syndrome	—	—	—
	Rhabdomyoma	May be associated with tuberous sclerosis	Myoglobin, actin, desmin	S100	—
	Myxoma	May be associated with Carney syndrome	Vimentin	—	—
	Teratoma	—	Varies by component	AFP to rule out yolk sac tumor component	—
	Juvenile hemangioma	—	GLUT1, LeY	—	—
	Kaposiform hemangioendothelioma	—	CD31, CD34	GLUT1, LeY	—
	Epithelioid hemangioendothelioma	—	CD31, vWF; substantial fraction show cytokeratin staining	EMA	—
	Lymphangioma	—	D240	—	—

(Continued)

Table 1C-2 ■ MOLECULAR TESTING IN PEDIATRIC DISEASES *(Continued)*

System	Tumor	Genetic Aberration	Immunohistochemistry: Pertinent Positives	Immunohistochemistry: Pertinent Negatives	Notes
Respiratory	Juvenile papillomatosis	—	HPV 6 and 11, cytokeratins	—	—
	Pleuropulmonary blastoma	Germline loss-of-function *DICER1* mutations in familial cases	Primitive stromal component similar to embryonal RMS: desmin, myogenin, MyoD1, myoglobin	Loss of Dicer1 staining in epithelium	—
	Pulmonary blastoma	—	Cytokeratin, EMA; morule positive for CGA	—	—
	Midline poorly differentiated carcinoma	NUT translocation t(15;19) (q14;p13.1)	—	—	—
	Embryonal rhabdomyosarcoma	LOH at 11p15	Muscle markers: desmin, myogenin, MyoD1, myoglobin	Rule out other SRBCTs: PGP9.5, WT1, CD99, CD45	Myogenin usually <50% (as opposed to alveolar RMS)
	Inflammatory myofibroblastic tumor	*ALK* rearrangements in some	ALK; myofibroblastic markers	—	—
Gastrointestinal	Granular cell tumor	—	S100	—	—
	Gastrointestinal stromal tumor	Mutations in *KIT* or *PDGFRA*	c-kit (CD117), vimentin, bcl-2, CD34	—	KIT staining may identify tumors suitable for monoclonal antibody therapy
	Adenocarcinoma	—	Cytokeratins, CEA, CA19.9	—	—
	Inflammatory myofibroblastic tumor	*ALK* rearrangements in some	ALK; myofibroblastic markers	—	—
	Schwannoma	—	S100, GFAP	KIT, desmin, smooth muscle actin	—
	Leiomyoma	—	Desmin, smooth muscle actin	S100, KIT	—
	Fundic gland gastric polyps	Some associated with FAP (*APC* mutations)	—	—	—
	Juvenile polyps	Cronkhite-Canada syndrome; some with *SMAD4/DPC4* mutations	—	—	—
	Peutz-Jeghers polyps	Mutations in *LKB1* gene	—	—	—
	Carcinoid tumors	—	Chromogranin, NSE, PGP 9.5, specific polypeptide hormones	—	—
Hepatobiliary	Adenoma	None known	Hep Par 1, CAM5.2, polyclonal CEA; CD34 in endothelial lining	AFP	IHC does not help distinguish adenoma from carcinoma
	Focal nodular hyperplasia	None known	Hep Par 1, CAM5.2, polyclonal CEA; CD34 in endothelial lining	—	—
	Hepatocellular carcinoma	Gains of 1q, 7q, 8q; losses of 16q	Hep Par 1, CAM5.2, polyclonal CEA; CD34 in endothelial lining	—	—

	Hepatoblastoma	Variable; some associated with BWS	AFP, hCG, Hep Par 1, polyclonal CEA	—	—
	Infantile hemangioendothelioma	—	CD31, CD34, factor VIII	—	—
	Mesenchymal hamartoma	Translocations involving 11, 17, and 19 t(11;19) (q11;q13.4)	Cytokeratins in ductal component; smooth muscle actin in stromal cells	—	—
	Desmoplastic small round cell tumor	t(11;22)(p13;q12) creating ***EWS-WT1*** fusion gene	Cytokeratin, EMA, WT1, CD99, NSE, PLAP	—	—
	Undifferentiated embryonal sarcoma	May have same translocation as mesenchymal hamartoma	Not much: sometimes vimentin and bcl-2	—	—
Pancreatic	Acinar cell carcinoma	—	Enzymes: lipase, trypsin, chymotrypsin	Chromogranin, synaptophysin	—
	Solid pseudopapillary tumor	Mutations in β-catenin	Vimentin, NSE, CD10, CD56, α_1-antitrypsin; nuclear β-catenin expression	Cytokeratins usually negative	—
	Pancreatoblastoma	Mutations in β-catenin/APC pathways	Enzymes: lipase, trypsin, chymotrypsin; also CEA and CA19.9	—	—
Genitourinary	Nephroblastoma (Wilms tumor)	Deletions or mutations in WT1, WT2, WT3, or WTX	WT1	—	—
	Cellular mesoblastic nephroma	t(12;15)(p13;q25) creating ***ETV6-NTRK3*** fusion	—	—	Same genetic aberration as congenital infantile fibrosarcoma
	Ewing sarcoma/PNET	Translocations of ***EWS*** on 22q11; partners vary	CD99	—	—
	Clear cell sarcoma	t(10;17) and del 14q have been described	—	—	—
	Malignant rhabdoid tumor	***hSNF5*** mutations/deletions (22q11)	Cytokeratin	Loss of nuclear INI1 staining, BAF47	—
	"Translocation" carcinomas	t(X;1)(p11.2;q25) and ***APSL-TFE*** fusion or t(6;11)(p21;q12) involving ***TFEB***	Cytokeratins; overexpression of TFE	—	—
	Renal medullary carcinoma	Sickle cell carriers (11p15.5 mutation = HbS); possible 22q11 involvement	Cytokeratin	Loss of nuclear INI staining	—
	Angiomyolipoma	***TSC1*** and ***TSC2*** genes—9q34 or 16p13.3 mutations	HMB45, smooth muscle actin, Melan-A	—	—
	Inflammatory myofibroblastic tumor	***ALK*** rearrangements such as t(2;5)	ALK, vimentin,smooth muscle actin, desmin; variably for cytokeratin	—	—

(Continued)

TABLE 1C-2 ■ MOLECULAR TESTING IN PEDIATRIC DISEASES *(Continued)*

System	Tumor	Genetic Aberration	Immunohistochemistry: Pertinent Positives	Immunohistochemistry: Pertinent Negatives	Notes
	Embryonal rhabdomyosarcoma	LOH at 11p15	Muscle markers: desmin, myogenin, MyoD1, myoglobin	Rule out other SRBCTs: PGP9.5, WT1, CD99, CD45	Myogenin usually <50% (as opposed to alveolar RMS)
Female Reproductive System	Condyloma accuminata	—	HPV 6,11	—	—
	Clear cell adenocarcinoma	—	Cytokeratin	—	—
	Embryonal rhabdomyosarcoma	LOH at 11p15	Muscle markers: desmin, myogenin, MyoD1, myoglobin	Rule out other SRBCTs: PGP9.5, WT1, CD99, CD45	Myogenin usually <50% (as opposed to alveolar RMS)
	Dysgerminoma	I(12p)	PLAP, hCG	—	—
	Embryonal carcinoma	—	CD30, cytokeratin; less often PLAP and AFP	—	—
	Endodermal sinus tumor (yolk sac tumor)	I(12p)±	AFP	—	—
	Mature teratoma	>95% karyotypically normal	Component-specific	Rule out yolk sac tumor component: AFP	—
	Immature teratoma	60% with nonrecurrent cytogenic abnormalities	Component-specific	Rule out yolk sac tumor component: AFP	—
	Struma ovarii	—	Thyroglobulin, TTF-1	—	—
	Granulosa cell tumor	—	Inhibin, vimentin, CD99, cytokeratin	—	—
	Sertoli-Leydig cell tumor	—	CD99, WT1, inhibin, calretinin, cytokeratin	—	—
	Gonadoblastoma	Phenotypic females with 46,XY karyotype	—	—	—
	Small cell carcinoma	—	Cytokeratin, NSE, chromogranin	—	—
	Complete hydatidiform mole	46,XX or 46,XY by dispermy	—	Negative for p57/KIP2 in the cytotrophoblast	Cytogenetics and p57 staining are far superior to histology for distinguishing partial versus complete moles
	Partial hydatidiform mole	Triploid: usually 69,XXY, but also 69,XXX and 69,XYY	—	Positive for p57/KIP2 in the cytotrophoblast	—
	Choriocarcinoma	—	hCG	Only weak hPL staining	—

Male Reproductive System	Condyloma accuminata	—	HPV 6,11	—	—
	Intratubular germ cell neoplasia	I(12p)	PLAP, OCT4, NSE, p53, ferritin, CD117, D2-40	—	—
	Embryonal rhabdomyosarcoma	LOH at 11p15	Muscle markers: desmin, myogenin, MyoD1, myoglobin	Rule out other SRBCTs: PGP9.5, WT1, CD99, CD45	Myogenin usually <50% (as opposed to alveolar RMS)
	Seminoma	I(12p)	PLAP, focal cytokeratin, vimentin, CD30, CD44	—	—
	Embryonal carcinoma	—	CD30, cytokeratin, OCT4, less often PLAP and AFP	—	—
	Endodermal sinus tumor (yolk sac tumor)	—	AFP, SALL4	PLAP±	—
	Mature teratoma	>95% karyotypically normal	Component-specific	Rule out yolk sac tumor component: AFP	—
	Immature teratoma	60% with nonrecurrent cytogenic abnormalities	Component-specific	Rule out yolk sac tumor component: AFP	—
	Granulosa cell tumor	—	Inhibin, vimentin, CD99, cytokeratin	—	—
	Sertoli cell tumor	—	Inhibin, vimentin, cytokeratin, variably for S100	PLAP, CEA	—
	Leydig cell tumor	—	Inhibin, melan A, vimentin, S100, chromogranin, synaptophysin; variably for cytokeratin, EMA, desmin	PLAP, CEA	—
Endocrine	Pituitary adenomas	—	Mono/oligoclonal hormone production	Decreased type IV collagen matrix	—
	Papillary thyroid carcinoma	*RET* gene mutations; also *BRAF*, *APC*, *RAS*, *TRK*	Cytokeratin, TTF-1, thyroglobulin	—	—
	Medullary thyroid carcinoma	*RET* mutations	Calcitonin, cytokeratin, chromogranin, TTF-1, synaptophysin, CEA	—	—
	Spindle epithelial tumor with thymus-like differentiation (SETTLE)	—	Cytokeratin	—	—
	Parathyroid adenomas/ hyperplasia	*MEN1* (11q13), *RET* (10q11), or *HRPT2* (1q25)	Cytokeratin, PTH	—	—
	Pheochromoytoma	*RET* in MEN2-related cases; 1p losses	NSE, chromogranin, synpatophysin; S100 in su stentacular cells	Cytokeratin, EMA	—

(Continued)

Table 1C-2 ■ MOLECULAR TESTING IN PEDIATRIC DISEASES *(Continued)*

System	Tumor	Genetic Aberration	Immunohistochemistry		Notes
			Pertinent Positives	**Pertinent Negatives**	
	Neuroblastoma	*MYCN* amplification, *ALK* amplification or mutation	PGP9.5, NSE, synpatophysin, NB84	CD99, CD45	—
	Pancreatic endocrine tumors	Variable	Chromogranin, synaptophysin, NSE, specific hormones	—	—
Skin	Verruca vulgaris	—	HPV	—	—
	Tricholemmoma	Multiple in Cowden syndrome	CD34 in lesional cells	—	—
	Epidermoid cyst	Multiple in Gardner syndrome	—	—	—
	Sebaceous adenoma	Muir-Torre syndrome	—	—	—
	Melanocytic nevi	—	S100, Melan A, HMB4	—	—
	Cellular blue nevus	Carney complex	HMB45	S100	—
	Dermatofibroma	—	Factor XIIIa	CD34	—
	Dermatofibrosarcoma protuberans	Translocation COLIA1 – PDFGB t(17;22) (q22;q13)	CD34, p53	Factor XIIIa	Same translocation as giant cell fibroblastoma
	Juvenile xanthogranuloma	—	CD68, vimentin, S100 (variable)	CD1a	—
	Langerhans cell histiocytosis	—	S100, CD1a	—	—
	Neurothekeoma	—	S100, vimentin; cellular variant positive for NKI/C3 and negative for S100	CD68	—
Soft tissue	Lipoblastoma	*PLAG1* rearrangements	—	—	—
	Liposarcoma	*FUS-CHOP* fusion gene from t(12;16) or variant translocation	—	—	—
	Gardner fibroma	*APC* mutations	β-catenin	—	—
	Desmoid fibromatosis	*APC* mutations	β-catenin	—	—
	Inflammatory myofibroblastic tumor	*ALK* rearrangements in some	ALK; myofibroblastic markers	—	—
	Infantile fibrosarcoma	t(12;15)(p13;q25) creating *ETV6-NTRK3* fusion	—	—	Same translocation as cellular mesoblastic nephroma
	Low-grade fibromyxoid sarcoma	Some with t(7;16) (q34;p11) translocation and *FUS-CREB3L2* fusion	—	—	—
	Embryonal rhabdomyosarcoma	LOH at 11p15	Muscle markers: desmin, myogenin, MyoD1, myoglobin	Rule out other SRBCTs: PGP9.5, WT1, CD99, CD45	Myogenin usually <50% (as opposed to alveolar RMS)
	Alveolar rhabdomyosarcoma	t(2;13) or t(1;13) translocations fusing *PAX3* or *PAX7*, respectively, with *FOXO1*	Muscle markers: desmin, myogenin, MyoD1, myoglobin	Rule out other SRBCTs: PGP9.5, WT1, CD99, CD45	Myogenin usually >50% (as opposed to embryonal RMS)

	Ossifying fibromyxoid tumor	—	S100; rarely, desmin, GFAP, and cytokeratins	—	—
	Soft tissue myoepithelioma	—	Cytokeratin, S100, calponin	—	—
	Synovial sarcoma	t(X;18)(p11.2;q11.2) fusing ***SYT*** and ***SSX1*** or ***SSX2***	Cytokeratin and EMA in the epithelial phase	—	—
	Epithelioid sarcoma	—	Vimentin, keratin, and EMA	Loss of nuclear INI expression	—
	Alveolar soft part sarcoma	***TFE3-ASPL*** fusion gene	—	—	—
	Clear cell sarcoma (melanoma of soft parts)	t(12;22)(q13;q13) with ***EWS-ATF1*** fusion	S100, HMB45	—	—
	Ewing sarcoma/PNET	Translocations of ***EWS*** on 22q11; partners vary	CD99	—	—
Bone	Osteochondroma	***EXT1*** and ***EXT2*** gene mutations in multiple hereditary exostoses	—	—	—
	Chondromyxoid fibroma	6q13 rearrangements	—	—	—
	Osteomas	May be associated with Gardner syndrome	—	—	—
	Chordoma	—	S100 and epithelial markers	—	—
	Fibrous dysplasia	Seen in McCune-Albright syndrome and with ***GNAS*** mutations	—	—	—
Central Nervous System	Medulloblastoma	i(17q) most common, other various ones. Some cases associated with Gorlin syndrome and ***PTCH*** gene.	—	—	—
	Retinoblastoma	Rb loss-of-function	—	—	—
	Atypical teratoid/rhabdoid tumors	***hSNF5*** gene—22q11 mutations/deletions	—	Loss of nuclear INI1 expression, BAF47	—
	Hemangioblastoma	von Hippel-Lindau syndrome	Vimentin, NSE, GFAP, inhibin A	Epithelial markers	—
	Dysplastic gangliocytomas	Cowden syndrome	—	—	—
Peripheral Nervous System	Schwannoma	Monosomy 22 or 22q loss (NF2 gene)	S100	—	—
	Neurofibroma	NF1	S100	—	—
	MPNST	Associated with NF1	Only a minority are S100-positive	—	—
Lymph nodes	Hodgkin lymphoma	—	CD15, CD30, EBER ISH	ALK	—
	Anaplastic large cell lymphoma	—	ALK, CD30	—	—
	Burkitt lymphoma	***MYC*** translocations	CD10, CD19, near-100% MIB-1 positivity	—	—
	Precursor B- or T-cell lymphoblastic lymphoma/leukemia	—	TdT, lineage specific markers (may be mixed)	—	—

to the treating physician and parents, but full sequencing of large genes can be complex and arduous with routine PCR technology.

Forensic Identification

PCR is commonly used to amplify specific segments of DNA for forensic analysis such as for identification of victims of natural disasters, victims of crimes, and also identification of perpetrators leaving DNA evidence at a crime scene. PCR-based identification methods include analysis of sequence and length polymorphisms and mitochondrial DNA sequences. The most common method used to identify individuals is examination of 13 different loci that show variability among humans to create a "DNA fingerprint." (49).

Limitations

While PCR has become one of the most commonly used tools in molecular medicine, it is important to note its limitations. The assay is extremely sensitive and care must be taken to avoid contamination from nucleic acids in the environment, particularly in the microbiology laboratory. Laboratory technicians performing PCR testing should have adequate training and experience and understand the importance of good technique. PCR detection of sequence variants in mutation analysis is limited to base substitutions and small insertion/deletions. Detection of larger intragenic deletions currently requires other supporting methodology (8,15). PCR applications in detecting and identifying new organisms can lead to dilemmas about whether or not a newly sequenced isolate is clinically relevant. Finally, PCR testing is not "agnostic." It is not a screening test for unknown abnormalities; rather, it is applied in a target-specific manner.

ARRAY TECHNOLOGY

DNA microarrays are used as a tool to evaluate and quantify sequence information for tens of thousands to a million sequences in a single experiment. The development of microarrays required the advances of miniaturization and computer technology coupled with the knowledge of DNA sequence among multiple species. The basic methodology involves thousands/millions of small chemically generated oligonucleotide sequences representing portions of the genomic DNA sequence that are fixed to a platform such as a glass slide or silicon wafer. These sequences are "arrayed" in a manner such that the location and sequence of each probe is known and millions of probes can fit in a small area. The patient DNA (or cDNA reverse transcribed from RNA) is then labeled with a fluorescent dye and hybridized to the array. Patient DNA that has sequence identity to a probe on the array binds there and can be detected by a fluorescence detector.

There are currently three main applications of microarray technology: (a) comparative genomic hybridization (CGH), which compares the amount of patient DNA at a given locus to a reference standard, (b) Single nucleotide polymorphism (SNP) detection, which assays the genotype of an individual at hundreds of thousands of sites known to be polymorphic among individuals, and (c) gene expression, which is a reflection of which genes are actively transcribed in a given sample in a relatively quantifiable manner. CGH arrays can provide information on genomic gains and losses just as in standard karyotyping albeit at a much higher resolution and without the requirement for growing cells. Karyotyping has one big advantage over CGH in that karyotyping can detect balanced translocations whereas CGH cannot. SNP arrays can detect SNPs or mutations that can link someone to a specific disease state, determine suitability to targeted therapy, or determine individual variations in drug metabolism. SNP arrays can also measure copy number changes including uniparental disomy. It is clear that microarray technology has transformed molecular biology and genetic research and for the same reasons it is valuable in research, there is no shortage of potential applications in clinical molecular diagnostics.

NEXT-GENERATION SEQUENCING

For the last three decades, the Sanger method of sequencing has been the favored method of reading the base code sequence of DNA. This method using capillary sequencer machines has high fidelity and is still considered the gold standard. It was used to sequence the first human genome in a 13-year effort ending in 2003. Since the completion of that first human genome sequence, new powerful technology has emerged. These so-called *next-generation* sequencers can perform massively parallel DNA sequencing of clonally amplified or single DNA molecules. This technology has made sequencing entire genomes possible in a matter of days to weeks rather than years and has also substantially brought down the price of sequencing large areas of DNA.

NGS may soon replace standard PCR-based methods for mutation detection and screening. Advances in the preparation and enrichment of specific regions of DNA for subsequent sequencing will facilitate the use of this technology in disease-specific manner both for diagnosis and management. Sequencing large numbers of genes for clinical conditions such as hypertrophic cardiomyopathy (42), and neuromuscular diseases becomes possible with this new technology. Testing genomes of viral populations in sera for therapeutic sensitivity or resistance can guide choice of antiretrovirals in HIV infection (61). One can envision routine testing of tumor cells for genes predicting responses or lack thereof to common chemotherapeutic agents as well as targeted therapies.

More advances are needed in streamlining and automating the technical procedures and data analysis steps before a complete transition of NGS from research to clinical laboratories is possible. In addition, at the present in 2010, its cost remains prohibitive for routine clinical use. But, considering how powerful this technology is and how rapidly it has evolved, it is likely only a matter of time before these technical issues are addressed and these platforms become more affordable and ready for use in molecular diagnostics.

FUTURE DIRECTIONS FOR MOLECULAR METHODS IN PEDIATRIC PATHOLOGY

Technology and its applications to medical sciences will inevitably continue to advance at an extremely rapid pace. The era of personalized medicine is coming, but that does not mean that the hematoxylin and eosin stain is no longer sufficient and cost effective for diagnosing the vast majority of diseases. Pathologists have an important role ensuring that new methodologies are subjected to validation, quality control, and quality assurance measures just as one would naturally expect from any clinical chemistry test or immunohistochemical stain. And, pathologists and laboratory managers are especially qualified to determine the cost-benefit ratio of introducing new tests. These are very important responsibilities. Far from being at risk of replacement by technological machinery, as pathologists we are uniquely positioned to determine which new technologies will be beneficial to the patient in terms of improving accuracy or timeliness of diagnosis, reducing costs, improving quality, or providing added benefit over currently used diagnostic methods.

REFERENCES

1. Asa SL. *Tumors of the pituitary gland. Atlas of Tumor Pathology*, Third Series, Vol. 22. Washington, DC: Armed Forces Institute of Pathology, 1998.
2. Bacchi CE, Gown AM, Bacchi MM. Detection of infectious disease agents in tissue by immunocytochemistry. *Braz J Med Biol Res* 1994;27(12):2803–2820.
3. Bhan AK. Immunoperoxidase. In: Colvin RB, Bhan AK, McCluskey RT, eds. *Diagnostic immunopathology*. New York, NY: Raven Press, 1994.
4. Biegel JA, Rorke LB, Emanuel BS. Monosomy 22 in rhabdoid or atypical teratoid tumors of the brain. *N Engl J Med* 1989;321(13):906.
5. Bignami A, Schoene W. Glial fibrillary acidic protein in human brain tumors. In: DeLellis R, ed. *Diagnostic immunohistochemistry*. New York, NY: Masson Publishing, 1981.
6. Chu T, Jaffe R. The normal Langerhans cell and the LCH cell. *Br J Cancer Suppl* 1994;23:S4–S10.
7. Davis BH, Olsen S, Bigelow NC, et al. Detection of fetal red cells in fetomaternal hemorrhage using a fetal hemoglobin monoclonal antibody by flow cytometry. *Transfusion* 1998;38(8):749–756.
8. De Lellis L, Curia MC, Catalano T, et al. Combined use of MLPA and nonfluorescent multiplex PCR analysis by high performance liquid chromatography for the detection of genomic rearrangements. *Hum Mutat* 2006;27(10):1047–1056.
9. Debski R, Rutledge J, Kapur R. A plea for the masses: a gross room approach to pediatric tumors. *J Histotechnol* 2004;27:221–228.
10. Dressler LG, Visscher D. Handling, storage, and preparation of human tissues. *Curr Protoc Cytom* 2001;Chapter 5:Unit 5 2.
11. Duffy PE, Huang YY, Rapport MM, et al. Glial fibrillary acidic protein in giant cell tumors of brain and other gliomas. A possible relationship to malignancy, differentiation, and pleomorphism of glia. *Acta Neuropathol* 1980;52(1):51–57.
12. Dziegiel MH, Nielsen LK, Berkowicz A. Detecting fetomaternal hemorrhage by flow cytometry. *Curr Opin Hematol* 2006;13(6):490–495.
13. Elias J, Boss E, Kaplan AP. Studies of the cellular infiltrate of chronic idiopathic urticaria: prominence of T-lymphocytes, monocytes, and mast cells. *J Allergy Clin Immunol* 1986;78(5 Pt 1):914–918.
14. Elias JM. *Immunohistopathology: a practical approach to diagnosis*. Chicago, IL: American Society of Clinical Pathologists, 1990.
15. Engert S, Wappenschmidt B, Betz B, et al. MLPA screening in the BRCA1 gene from 1,506 German hereditary breast cancer cases: novel deletions, frequent involvement of exon 17, and occurrence in single early-onset cases. *Hum Mutat* 2008;29(7):948–958.
16. Eshun JK, Black DD, Casteel HB, et al. Comparison of immunohistochemistry and silver stain for the diagnosis of pediatric Helicobacter pylori infection in urease-negative gastric biopsies. *Pediatr Dev Pathol* 2001;4(1):82–88.
17. Espy MJ, Uhl JR, Sloan LM, et al. Real-time PCR in clinical microbiology: applications for routine laboratory testing. *Clin Microbiol Rev* 2006;19(1):165–256.
18. Fanaian NK, Cohen C, Waldrop S, et al. Epstein-Barr virus (EBV)-encoded RNA: automated in-situ hybridization (ISH) compared with manual ISH and immunohistochemistry for detection of EBV in pediatric lymphoproliferative disorders. *Pediatr Dev Pathol* 2009;12(3):195–199.
19. Finn WG. Beyond gating: capturing the power of flow cytometry. *Am J Clin Pathol* 2009;131(3):313–314.
20. Fischer EG. To fix or not to fix: Michel's is the solution. *Int J Surg Pathol* 2006;14(1):108.
21. Fritschy JM. Is my antibody-staining specific? How to deal with pitfalls of immunohistochemistry. *Eur J Neurosci* 2008;28(12):2365–2370.
22. Gloghini A, Rizzo A, Zanette I, et al. KP1/CD68 expression in malignant neoplasms including lymphomas, sarcomas, and carcinomas. *Am J Clin Pathol* 1995;103(4):425–431.
23. Gudgin EJ, Erber WN. Immunophenotyping of lymphoproliferative disorders: state of the art. *Pathology* 2005;37(6):457–478.
24. Haferlach T, Kern W, Schnittger S, et al. Modern diagnostics in acute leukemias. *Crit Rev Oncol Hematol* 2005;56(2):223–234.
25. Hall SE, Rosse WF. The use of monoclonal antibodies and flow cytometry in the diagnosis of paroxysmal nocturnal hemoglobinuria. *Blood* 1996;87(12):5332–5340.
26. Hasegawa T, Matsuno Y, Shimoda T, et al. Gastrointestinal stromal tumor: consistent CD117 immunostaining for diagnosis, and prognostic classification based on tumor size and MIB-1 grade. *Hum Pathol* 2002;33(6):669–676.
27. Holden CA, MacDonald DM. Immunoperoxidase techniques in dermatopathology. *Clin Exp Dermatol* 1983;8(5):443–457.
28. Holland PM, Abramson RD, Watson R, et al. Detection of specific polymerase chain reaction product by utilizing the 5′—3′ exonuclease activity of Thermus aquaticus DNA polymerase. *Proc Natl Acad Sci U S A* 1991;88(16):7276–7280.
29. Holness CL, Simmons DL. Molecular cloning of CD68, a human macrophage marker related to lysosomal glycoproteins. *Blood* 1993;81(6):1607–1613.
30. Horny HP, Valent P. Diagnosis of mastocytosis: general histopathological aspects, morphological criteria, and immunohistochemical findings. *Leuk Res* 2001;25(7):543–551.
31. Hsu SM, Raine L, Fanger H. Use of avidin-biotin-peroxidase complex (ABC) in immunoperoxidase techniques: a comparison between ABC and unlabeled antibody (PAP) procedures. *J Histochem Cytochem* 1981;29(4):577–580.
32. Jarzembowski J, McKeever P. The pathologic perspective on the pituitary. *Rev Endocrinol* 2008;30–35.
33. Jonkers D, Stobberingh E, de Bruine A, et al. Evaluation of immunohistochemistry for the detection of Helicobacter pylori in gastric mucosal biopsies. *J Infect* 1997;35(2):149–154.
34. Kakar S, Gown AM, Goodman ZD, et al. Best practices in diagnostic immunohistochemistry: hepatocellular carcinoma versus metastatic neoplasms. *Arch Pathol Lab Med* 2007;131(11):1648–1654.

35. Kleihues P, Ohgaki H. Primary and secondary glioblastomas: from concept to clinical diagnosis. *Neuro Oncol* 1999;1(1):44–51.
36. Ladanyi M, Antonescu CR, Leung DH, et al. Impact of SYT-SSX fusion type on the clinical behavior of synovial sarcoma: a multi-institutional retrospective study of 243 patients. *Cancer Res* 2002;62(1):135–140.
37. Licht JD. Acute promyelocytic leukemia–weapons of mass differentiation. *N Engl J Med* 2009;360(9):928–930.
38. Linder J, Radio SJ. Immunohistochemistry of Pneumocystis carinii. *Semin Diagn Pathol* 1989;6(3):238–244.
39. Luzzatto L, Gianfaldoni G. Recent advances in biological and clinical aspects of paroxysmal nocturnal hemoglobinuria. *Int J Hematol* 2006;84(2):104–112.
40. Mackie RM, Young H, Campbell IA. Studies in cutaneous immunofluorescence. I. The effect of storage time on direct immunofluorescence of skin biopsies from bullous disease and lupus erythematosus. *J Cutan Pathol* 1980;7(4):236–243.
41. Michel B, Milner Y, David K. Preservation of tissue-fixed immunoglobulins in skin biopsies of patients with lupus erythematosus and bullous diseases–preliminary report. *J Invest Dermatol* 1972;59(6):449–452.
42. Morita H, Rehm HL, Menesses A, et al. Shared genetic causes of cardiac hypertrophy in children and adults. *N Engl J Med* 2008;358(18):1899–1908.
43. Mutasim DF, Pelc NJ, Supapannachart N. Established methods in the investigation of bullous diseases. *Dermatol Clin* 1993;11(3): 399–418.
44. Nogueira AM, Barbosa AJ, Carvalho AA, et al. Usefulness of immunocytochemical demonstration of neuron-specific enolase in the diagnosis of Hirschsprung's disease. *J Pediatr Gastroenterol Nutr* 1990;11(4):496–502.
45. North PE, Waner M, Mizeracki A, et al. GLUT1: a newly discovered immunohistochemical marker for juvenile hemangiomas. *Hum Pathol* 2000;31(1):11–22.
46. Ornvold K, Ralfkiaer E, Carstensen H. Immunohistochemical study of the abnormal cells in Langerhans cell histiocytosis (histiocytosis x). *Virchows Arch A Pathol Anat Histopathol* 1990;416(5):403–410.
47. Pattanapanyasat K, Thakar MR. CD4+ T cell count as a tool to monitor HIV progression & anti-retroviral therapy. *Indian J Med Res* 2005;121(4):539–549.
48. Perrone T, Steeper TA, Dehner LP. Alpha-fetoprotein localization in pure ovarian teratoma. An immunohistochemical study of 12 cases. *Am J Clin Pathol* 1987;88(6):713–717.
49. Project, USDHG. *DNA Forensics*. 2009 6/16/2009 [cited 2009 11/1/2009]; Available from: http://www.ornl.gov/sci/techresources/Human_Genome/elsi/forensics.shtml
50. Robey SS, Kuhajda FP, Yardley JH. Immunoperoxidase stains of ganglion cells and abnormal mucosal nerve proliferations in Hirschsprung's disease. *Hum Pathol* 1988;19(4):432–437.
51. Sherman GG, Galpin JS, Patel JM, et al. CD4+ T cell enumeration in HIV infection with limited resources. *J Immunol Methods* 1999;222(1–2):209–217.
52. Smith MR. Rituximab (monoclonal anti-CD20 antibody): mechanisms of action and resistance. *Oncogene* 2003;22(47):7359–7368.
53. Sontakke S, Cadenas MB, Maggi RG, et al. Use of broad range16S rDNA PCR in clinical microbiology. *J Microbiol Methods* 2009;76(3): 217–225.
54. Sorelli P, Gratian MJ, Bhogal BS, et al. Immunogold electron microscopy using skin in Michel's medium intended for immunofluorescence analysis. *Clin Dermatol* 2001;19(5):638–641.
55. Sorensen PH, Lynch JC, Qualman SJ, et al. PAX3-FKHR and PAX7-FKHR gene fusions are prognostic indicators in alveolar rhabdomyosarcoma: a report from the children's oncology group. *J Clin Oncol* 2002;20(11):2672–2679.
56. Sung T, Miller DC, Hayes RL, et al. Preferential inactivation of the p53 tumor suppressor pathway and lack of EGFR amplification distinguish de novo high grade pediatric astrocytomas from de novo adult astrocytomas. *Brain Pathol* 2000;10(2):249–259.
57. Szczepanski T, van der Velden VH, van Dongen JJ. Flow-cytometric immunophenotyping of normal and malignant lymphocytes. *Clin Chem Lab Med* 2006;44(7):775–796.
58. Teng YK, Levarht EW, Hashemi M, et al. Immunohistochemical analysis as a means to predict responsiveness to rituximab treatment. *Arthritis Rheum* 2007;56(12):3909–3918.
59. Vaughn Jones SA, Palmer I, Bhogal BS, et al. The use of Michel's transport medium for immunofluorescence and immunoelectron microscopy in autoimmune bullous diseases. *J Cutan Pathol* 1995;22(4): 365–370.
60. Velasco ME, Dahl D, Roessmann U, et al. Immunohistochemical localization of glial fibrillary acidic protein in human glial neoplasms. *Cancer* 1980;45(3):484–494.
61. Wang C, Mitsuya Y, Gharizadeh B, et al. Characterization of mutation spectra with ultra-deep pyrosequencing: application to HIV-1 drug resistance. *Genome Res* 2007;17(8):1195–1201.
62. Wazir JF, Macrorie SG, Coleman DV. Evaluation of the sensitivity, specificity, and predictive value of monoclonal antibody 3F6 for the detection of Pneumocystis carinii pneumonia in bronchoalveolar lavage specimens and induced sputum. *Cytopathology* 1994;5(2):82–89.
63. Weile J, Knabbe C. Current applications and future trends of molecular diagnostics in clinical bacteriology. *Anal Bioanal Chem* 2009;394(3):731–742.
64. Woods GL, Walker DH. Detection of infection or infectious agents by use of cytologic and histologic stains. *Clin Microbiol Rev* 1996;9(3):382–404.

FURTHER READING

Arch Pathol Lab Med 2008;132(3). A special issue devoted to immunohistochemistry, with individual articles devoted to various organ systems.

Dabbs DJ. *Diagnostic immunohistochemistry: theranostic and genomic applications*, 3rd ed. Philadelphia, PA: Saunders, 2010.

Li MM, Andersson HC. Clinical application of microarray-based molecular cytogenetics: an emerging new era of genomic medicine. *J Pediatr* 2009;155(3):311–317.

Miller MB, Tang YW. Basic concepts of microarrays and potential applications in clinical microbiology. *Clin Microbiol Rev* 2009;22(4): 611–633.

Roulston D, Le Beau MM. Cytogenetic analysis of hematologic malignant disease. In: Barch MJ, Knutsen T, Spurbeck J, ed. *The AGT cytogenetics laboratory manual*, 3rd ed. Philadelphia, PA: Lippincott-Raven, 1997.

Speicher M, Antonara SE, Motulsky AG (eds). *Vogel and Motulsky's human genetics: problems and approaches*, 4th ed. New York, NY: Springer, 2010.

Strachan T, Read AP. *Human molecular genetics*, 2nd ed. New York, NY: Wiley-Liss, 1999.

Voelkerding KV, Dames SA, Durtschi JD. Next generation sequencing: from basic research to diagnostics. *Clin Chem* 2009;55;4:1–18.

CHAPTER 1D

Electron Microscopy

GARY W. MIERAU

Electron microscopy remains an essential tool for today's pediatric pathologist. The technique continues to provide for a significant number of childhood diseases the best, and sometimes the only, means of establishing a definitive diagnosis. Offering a direct morphologic approach, it is arguably the most powerful and least treacherous of the many ancillary diagnostic techniques currently available. This having been said, it must also be stressed that each special technique has its relative strengths and weaknesses in particular situations. These should not be regarded as competitive techniques but rather as complementary tools, which are best employed using a highly selective but fully integrated approach.

We have found ancillary electron microscopic studies to be warranted in approximately 5% of the surgical specimens submitted for histologic examination. In contrast to our experience with the adult population, where renal specimens predominate, a very broad mix of specimens is received from pediatric patients. Presented in Figure 1D-1 are workload distribution statistics derived from an analysis of 1,000 consecutive diagnostic studies performed on patients from our institution. Tumors comprise the largest proportion of cases, followed closely by muscle and cilia, not too distantly by liver and skin, and then in gradually diminishing numbers by a wide variety of other tissue types.

Increasing recognition of the fact that immunohistochemical studies, even when properly performed and interpreted, will sometimes produce misleading information (5,9,12–15, 18,21,24,31) has led to a resurgence in the popularity of electron microscopy for tumor diagnosis. Ultrastructural studies of muscle biopsy specimens are of particular utility in diagnosing mitochondriopathies, storage diseases, and causes of infantile hypotonia. With respiratory tract specimens, electron microscopy offers the only readily available means of demonstrating defects in ciliary structure, and is also useful in the diagnosis of surfactant deficiency states, pulmonary interstitial glycogenosis, and some infectious diseases. Liver specimens are examined, among other things, to look for early evidence of metabolic disease. Electron microscopy often offers the fastest, cheapest, easiest, and sometimes the only means of screening for metabolic storage diseases. Skin biopsies are utilized for diagnosis of the inherited epidermolyses. Bowel biopsies are examined to diagnose microvillous inclusion disease and to detect furtive organisms such as microsporidia. A substantial number of renal diseases (e.g., minimal change lesion, thin basement membrane nephropathies, dense deposit disease) can only be diagnosed with confidence using this technology. Making up the remainder of the workload is a smattering of almost every type of specimen imaginable. Specific examples demonstrating some of the many applications of electron microscopy will be found in the chapters that follow.

It is not just in surgical pathology, however, that electron microscopy has a role to play. Collaborative endeavors involving the clinical pathology services account for a substantial portion of our total workload. During that same period when the previously alluded to 1,000 surgical pathology specimens were examined, 3,206 stool specimens were received for viral diagnosis. As a component of our departmental quality assurance program, we also at that time performed 266 ultrastructural studies on a random selection of the tumor specimens for which special studies had not been considered necessary for diagnosis, with the resulting information being used to help establish appropriate levels of test utilization and to stimulate a review of the diagnosis in cases with discordant findings. An additional 37 cases were studied to support the autopsy service, where the technique can be useful with questions arising after the option to perform alternative procedures (e.g., virus culture) has already been lost. Research activity was at an ebb during this interval, with only 21 such specimens being examined, but it is worth emphasizing that opportunities do abound for the use of electron microscopy in this setting.

THE ELECTRON MICROSCOPY LABORATORY

The central element in any electron microscopy laboratory is, of course, the electron microscope itself. A basic transmission electron microscope is all that is needed for diagnostic applications. Ease of operation, reliability, and

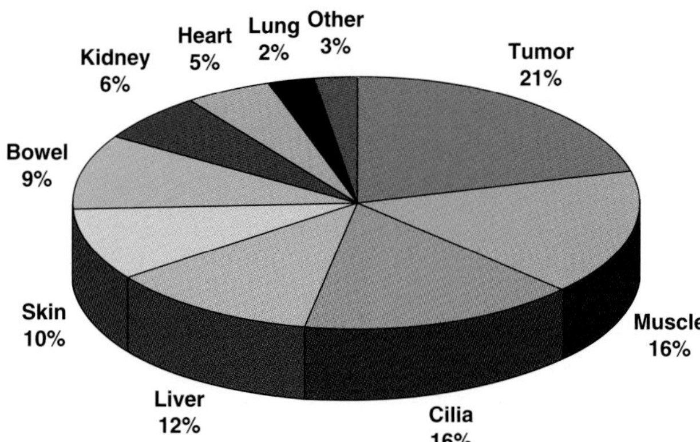

FIGURE 1D-1 ■ Distribution of pediatric surgical pathology workload by specimen type.

optimal performance at low magnifications are of far greater importance in this setting than are the advanced features offered by the more expensive and more demanding "analytical" microscopes. Electron microscopes have achieved a relatively mature state of technological development, and several manufacturers produce excellent (100 to 120 kV) instruments suitable for this application. In contrast to the situation with respect to electron microscopes, the technology associated with integrated digital imaging systems presently remains in a state of rapid evolution. Digital cameras offer many advantages over film cameras. They are, however, comparatively expensive and tend to perform least well at the lower magnifications generally employed for diagnostic studies. Alternatively, most of the benefits afforded by this new technology can also be attained by the means of scanning negatives produced by a film camera. Other than the electron microscope, the only specialized equipment needed is an ultramicrotome. Because ultimate success with this technique depends so heavily upon the capacity to obtain quality ultrathin sections in a reliable and rapid manner, it is more important to possess a modern ultramicrotome than a modern electron microscope.

The space requirements for an electron microscopy facility are quite modest. Following the changeover from photographic to electronic image processing, which eliminated the need for a darkroom, just 185 square feet of floor space in our current facility remained dedicated to this enterprise. Some activities, such as specimen processing, can be integrated into the workflow of the routine histology laboratory. This sharing of equipment, space, and personnel serves not only to reduce costs but also to enhance overall productivity. If occasional assistance can be provided by other team members, one dedicated technologist for every 250 specimens examined annually would seem a reasonable guide for staffing the EM laboratory. Generating results within a clinically relevant time frame is crucial to a successful operation. It is a reasonable expectation to have an interpretive report, complete with illustrations, available within two working days of specimen receipt.

In providing the interpretive component of the ultrastructural studies, a number of organizational models have been shown effective. Which is best in a given situation will depend upon the particular circumstances and personnel available. In some institutions, each pathologist while on service assumes full responsibility for the submission, examination, and interpretation of their cases. In others, a designated pathologist carries the responsibility for the examination and interpretation of all cases. In the majority of laboratories, however, technical personnel (with appropriate training and guidance) do much of the examination and may even assist with the interpretation of results.

It is often assumed that the electron microscopy laboratory will be a financial liability for its parent institution. This need not be true. With some attentiveness to basic business practices, an electron microscopy laboratory can be a profitable enterprise. Electron microscopy is sometimes still thought of as being a very expensive and extremely slow technique, but its modern-day cost and speed is actually quite comparable to that of most other ancillary diagnostic techniques. The cost savings to be derived from using the most powerful techniques available to obtain a fast and accurate diagnosis, necessary for minimizing the length of a hospital stay, should be obvious. Certainly for health care facilities already maintaining an electron microscopy laboratory, there is no economic reason not to use the technique to its fullest advantage. The major expenses associated with this endeavor are fixed rather than incremental, so its actual cost to the institution will remain virtually the same whether it is used a little or used a lot.

THE ELECTRON MICROSCOPY TECHNIQUE

While most other ancillary techniques (e.g., IHC, FISH, PCR) are restricted in application to hypothesis testing, electron microscopy can provide the right answer even when the wrong question, or no specific question, is being asked. Preserving the option to perform electron microscopy is therefore an important habit to develop. Placing a bit of tissue into an appropriate fixative as a matter of routine takes little extra time and costs next to nothing—but provides excellent insurance should a diagnostic issue arise later.

Electron microscopy is not so much a different technology as a modification, and extension, of a most familiar one. Specimens for electron microscopy are handled in almost the same way as for light microscopy. Here the standard fixative, instead of formaldehyde, is glutaraldehyde (to better preserve proteins) followed by osmium tetroxide (to better preserve lipids). Ordinary formalin preparations, if they are properly buffered (pH 7.2 to 7.4 range) and adjusted to moderate hypertonicity (400 to 500 milliosmols), actually serve quite well as a primary fixative for electron microscopy and can be substituted when necessary. The tissues are dehydrated in a similar fashion but then are embedded in an epoxy resin to enable the cutting of thinner sections than would be possible with the softer paraffin wax used for routine histology. To cut the necessary (~80-nm thick) ultrathin sections requires a similar but more refined "ultra" microtome and the use of a diamond blade. An electron beam cannot penetrate glass, so the sections are mounted on a fine-meshed screen (referred to as a grid) rather than on a glass slide. The sections are not stained in the true sense of the word (as color reactions cannot be detected with an electron microscope) but are incubated in similar fashion in heavy metal solutions (usually of uranium and lead) to selectively add contrast to various substructural components. Methodological details for all these procedures can be found in many standard texts (3,17). Except in its use of a beam of electrons, rather than a beam of light, the electron microscope is not very different in design or operation from that of an ordinary light microscope. It is the shorter wavelength of electrons that enables the superior point-to-point resolution and, thus, higher working magnifications offered by this instrumentation. The two techniques form a strong partnership, with the light microscope being best suited for the study of collections of cells and the electron microscope being best suited for the study of individual cells.

Under ideal conditions, specimens submitted for electron microscopy will consist of a representative sampling of appropriately sized (~1 mm^3) tissue cubes placed, upon removal from the patient, into the most suitable fixative immediately. Real-life conditions will not always be ideal but all is not necessarily lost if they are not. Just as an experienced automobile mechanic can still usually identify the make and model of a car after it has been involved in an accident, so can an experienced electron microscopist still usually identify the cell type and disease process involved in a partially wrecked tissue specimen. One has to be more cautious when dealing with suboptimal specimens, however, as there is a strong inverse relationship between the quality of specimen preservation and the probability of making a significant interpretive error. The safest strategy when dealing with suboptimally preserved specimens is to restrict electron microscopy to the search for some particular feature(s) predetermined to be of diagnostic relevance.

A demonstration of the deleterious effects associated with suboptimal specimen processing is presented in Figure 1D-2, which shows subsamples from the same case of Langerhans cell histiocytosis after being subjected to progressively harsher treatments. Here it can be seen that, though the diagnosis can still be made, the degree of difficulty increases (and the degree of confidence decreases) as the quality of cellular preservation is diminished. With optimal processing (Figure 1D-2A), the richness of cytoplasmic detail almost obscures the diagnostic Birbeck granules. Substitution of formaldehyde for glutaraldehyde as the primary fixative (Figure 1D-2B) results in a significant loss of cytoplasmic detail but, at least in this instance, this does not interfere with identification of the critical feature. Often, it is the case that in order to perform additional specialized procedures, such as the immunohistochemical reaction for S100 protein shown here, it becomes necessary to trade-off some degree of cellular preservation to maintain an adequate degree of tissue reactivity. Such applications, however, will fall mainly within the domain of research. For general purposes, when using formalin fixed tissues for electron microscopy, it is best to refix the specimen in glutaraldehyde before proceeding with the tissue processing. As a last resort, one can retrieve and reprocess for electron microscopy tissue that has already been embedded in paraffin. The technique is simple (20). Following removal of a carefully selected appropriately sized tissue sample from the paraffin block using a sharply pointed scalpel blade, the specimen is dewaxed overnight in xylene. Best results are obtained if, following rehydration in graded alcohols, the tissue is refixed both with glutaraldehyde and with osmium tetroxide prior to further processing. Because much of the lipid will have been extracted during the earlier processing events, one can expect poor preservation of membranes and other structures of high lipid content. Nevertheless, as shown in Figure 1D-2C, the features of key interest may still remain clearly identifiable. Structures composed largely of proteins (e.g., filaments, granules, intercellular junctions, immune deposits) are most likely to remain identifiable but sometimes membranous structures also are preserved. We were, for example, in a correlative study able to demonstrate Birbeck granules in deparaffinized material from 11 of 14 cases in which they were known to exist (25). In some situations, for example in attempting to identify a focally distributed virus, this approach may actually prove more efficacious than would an unfocused search through optimally preserved tissue. Utilization of deparaffinized tissue preserved with a nonaldehyde type fixative (e.g., alcohol, B5, Bouin's) will generally be unrewarding for, without crosslinking of proteins, nearly all substructural features are lost during processing (Figure 1D-2D).

It is often assumed that autopsy specimens will not be suitable for electron microscopic study. This is not always the case. While some autolytic degradation is inevitable, its severity and speed of occurrence is not entirely predictable. Sometimes, as illustrated in Figure 1D-3, cellular preservation remains surprisingly good even after an extended postmortem interval. The appearance of certain organelles, such as mitochondria, is very quickly altered by anoxic conditions. One would not, therefore, want to attempt assessment of a mitochondrial disorder using autopsy material. On the other hand, many structures are quite durable and can be confidently identified even in a specimen that is very degenerate. Here again, the denser the structure, and the greater its protein content, the more likely it is to remain recognizable.

Frozen tissue as well can be used for electron microscopy. Best results are obtained when the frozen tissue is placed directly into cold glutaraldehyde and allowed to fix as it thaws. The quality of cellular preservation, particularly with respect to ice crystal damage, varies regionally within a specimen. Examination of multiple sites may therefore prove beneficial. This recovery technique is especially useful in renal pathology, in circumstances where the initial specimen

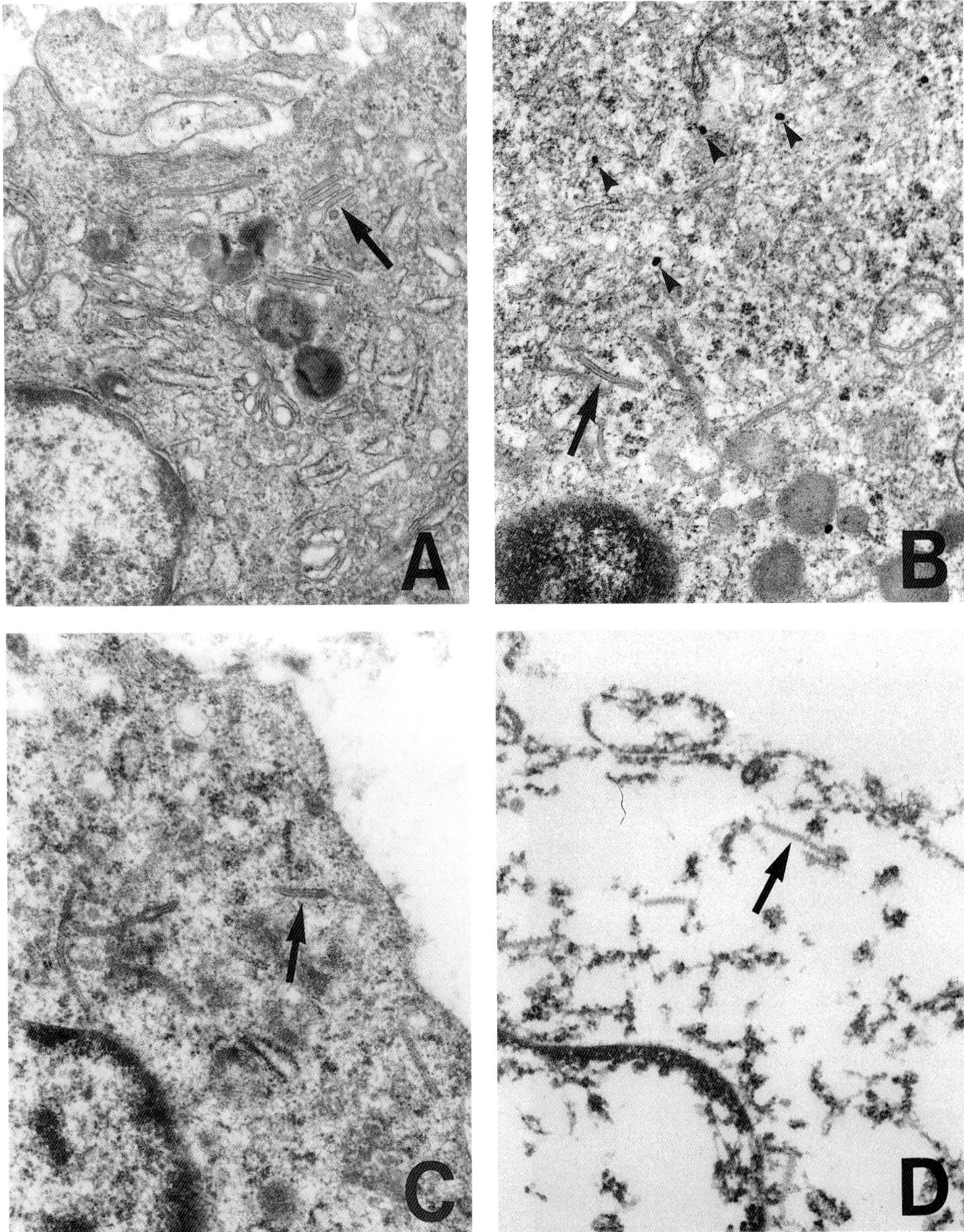

FIGURE 1D-2 ■ Subsamples from the same case of Langerhans cell histiocytosis subjected to variations in processing technique. **A**: Routine processing, utilizing glutaraldehyde fixation, results in optimal preservation of Birbeck granules (*arrow*) and other subcellular components. **B**: Substitution of formaldehyde for glutaraldehyde results in swelling of the mitochondria and some loss of cytoplasmic detail but has little effect on the Birbeck granules (*arrow*). The less intense fixation enables immunogold labeling of S100 protein (*arrowheads*). **C**: Birbeck granules (*arrow*) display an altered appearance but remain clearly identifiable in formalin-fixed tissue retrieved from a paraffin block. The mitochondria are reduced to smudges and most other cytoplasmic detail is lost. **D**: In B5-fixed tissue retrieved from paraffin, the Birbeck granules (*arrow*) are hardly recognizable and nearly all other components have been lost.

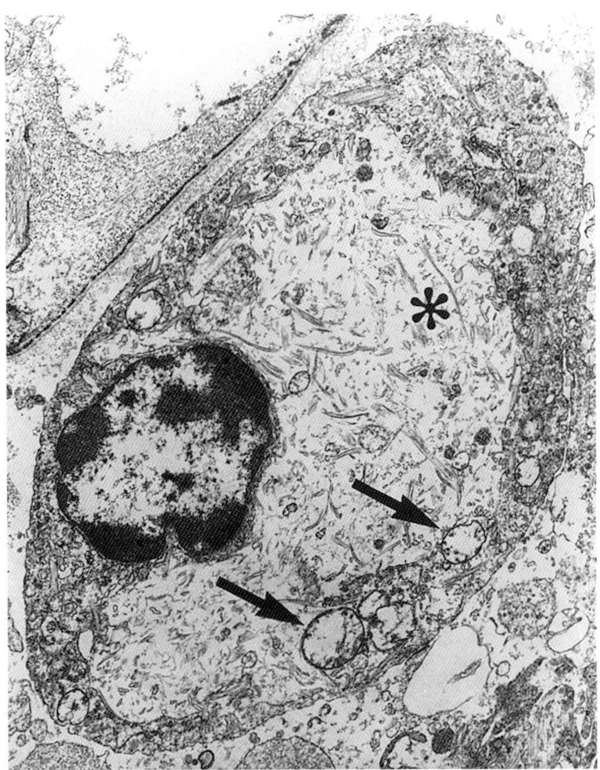

FIGURE 1D-3 ■ Autopsy specimen of brain showing perivascular cell with large cytoplasmic inclusion (*asterisk*). The mitochondria (*arrows*) exhibit degenerative changes but the material within the inclusions remains well enough preserved to enable a confident diagnosis of Krabbe disease.

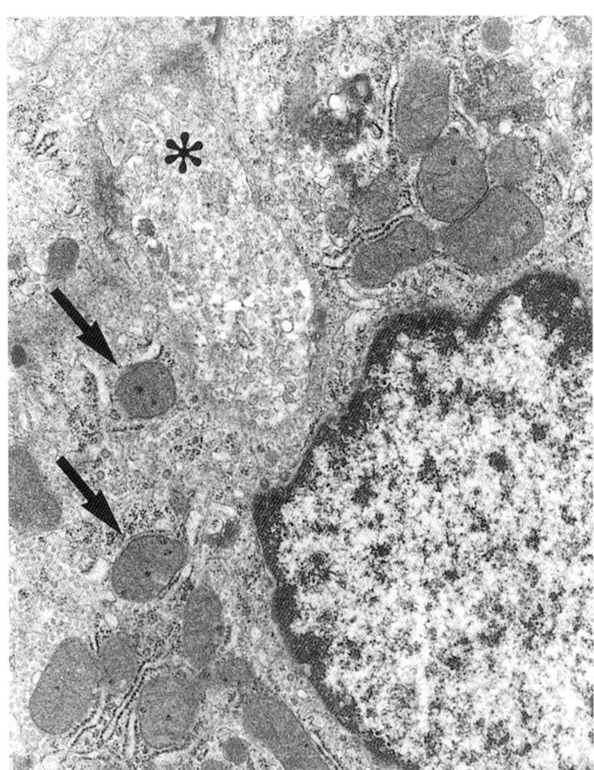

FIGURE 1D-4 ■ Snap frozen specimen of liver thawed in chilled glutaraldehyde shows excellent preservation of mitochondria (*arrows*) and other cellular structures, and allows demonstration of the "granular" bile (*asterisk*) characteristic of Byler disease.

submitted for electron microscopy happens not to contain any glomeruli. The technique may serve other purposes as well, as demonstrated in Figure 1D-4.

Electron microscopy is very well suited for the examination of fine-needle aspirate specimens (30,35). The aspiration biopsy technique is not as frequently employed in pediatric medicine but has been shown useful in this setting as well (4,32–34). We, along with others (1), have found an electron microscopic approach to the examination of fine-needle aspirates to be especially useful in the diagnosis of childhood round-cell tumors. Since with electron microscopy it is normally the situation that relatively small numbers of cells are examined individually for identifying characteristics, the technique is not much compromised by the small disrupted samples produced by the aspiration procedure. Figure 1D-5A shows how a confident diagnosis can be established even with just a few neoplastic cells being present. Demonstrated in Figure 1D-5B is an ultrastructural "special stain" for glycogen that can be of particular usefulness in circumstances like these (7), as it can be applied directly to an existing ultrathin section and does not require the processing of any additional material.

With lower risk of loss during the embedding process, and within approximately the same time frame, tiny specimens of other sorts (for instance, from an endomyocardial biopsy procedure) can be embedded in epoxy resin instead of paraffin wax. More specimen detail than usual will be observed by light microscopy because of the enhanced resolution offered by the 1-μm-thick resin-embedded sections. The array of special stains utilizable with these sections is somewhat limited, but this strategy does preserve the option to use electron microscopy, which might be considered the most powerful "special stain" of all.

The introduction of flow cytometric, immunocytochemical, and molecular diagnostic techniques has greatly diminished the role for electron microscopy in the diagnosis of hematological disorders. Nevertheless, it remains for the diagnosis of certain conditions (e.g., platelet storage pool disorders) an indispensable tool. Ultrastructural studies continue furthermore to be helpful in the diagnosis of leukemias, especially when routine cytochemical and/or flow cytometric studies produce conflicting, confusing, or equivocal results; insufficient or aberrant leukemic cell differentiation causes diagnostic uncertainty; or where an unusual or uncommon diagnosis is under consideration (11,29). To meet the challenges presented by the minuscule specimens obtainable from pediatric patients, we have developed the following procedure (22). Specimens for electron microscopy are procured in two or three heparinized glass microhematocrit tubes. Immediately upon transport to the laboratory (or the next morning, in

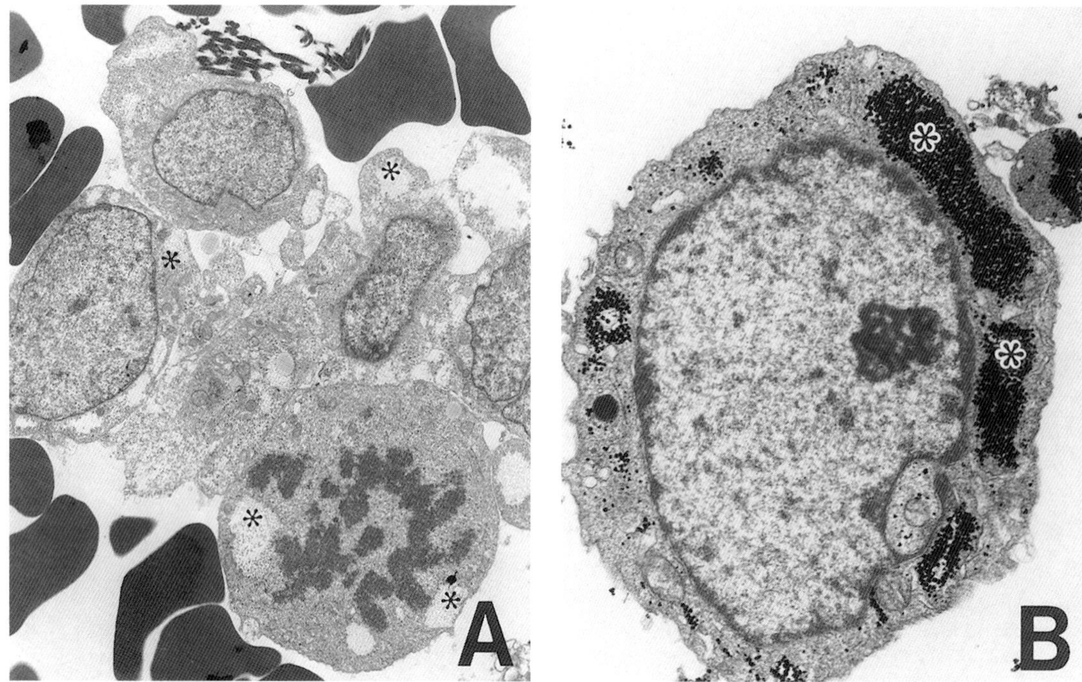

FIGURE 1D-5 ■ Fine-needle aspirate specimen displaying focal deposits of cytoplasmic glycogen (*asterisk*) characteristic of Ewing sarcoma. That the "moth-eaten" areas represent glycogen deposits (**A**) is easily confirmed by incubating the sections in a weak tannic acid solution prior to staining with uranyl acetate and lead citrate (**B**).

the case of late arriving specimens), the hematocrit tubes are centrifuged and then scored and broken just below the buffy coat layer (Figure 1D-6A). The buffy coat samples are then gently expelled into a vial of glutaraldehyde. As the droplet settles through the fixative, it consolidates into a single small firm pellet, which can subsequently then be processed with the ease of a solid tissue specimen. After about an hour, the fixative is replaced with a buffer "holding" solution and, at this point, further processing can be suspended. We normally proceed next to performing the Graham/Karnovsky reaction (16) for myeloperoxidase (MPO) and then embedding the specimen, holding in reserve whenever possible a bit of the fixed tissue for additional or repeat studies. The technical performance of the MPO reaction can be satisfactorily evaluated simply by examining the accompanying granulocytes that will almost invariably be present within the specimen. For our basic morphologic studies, we simply perform the customary uranyl acetate/lead citrate stain over the peroxidase stain. This produces no interpretive difficulty (Figure 1D-6B). Neither does subjecting the tissue to the peroxidase reaction interfere with a subsequent tannic acid stain that might be employed for the demonstration of glycogen. Performing the MPO reaction (Figure 1D-6C) enables us at least to determine whether it is a case of lymphogenous or nonlymphogenous leukemia that we are dealing with. The majority of cases can be confidently identified at this point but, occasionally, we do find it necessary to proceed with some additional techniques (11). The tannic acid procedure for demonstration of glycogen mentioned previously (Figure 1D-5B), which is more sensitive than the light microscopic PAS stain, can be useful in a number of situations and is of particular value in establishing a diagnosis of erythroleukemia. The acid phosphatase stain, which can be performed on the remaining unprocessed fixed tissue, is sometimes helpful in identifying immature or aberrant granules (2). The fixed tissue being held in reserve can also be used for the NTA (nonspecific esterase) reaction, which is a bit capricious but sometimes useful in the identification of monocytic precursors (Figure 1D-6D) (26). The routine MPO technique will sometimes enable the identification of platelet peroxidases (PPO) but, generally, when a diagnosis of megakaryoblastic leukemia is being considered another specimen must be procured to perform the more sensitive PPO procedure (Figure 1D-6E) (19). Cryopreserved cells can be used for this or any other purpose requiring special fixation or handling, such as the immunogold/MPO procedures that are helpful in dealing with "mixed" or "hybrid" cell leukemias (Figure 1D-6F) (17).

In the diagnosis of peroxisomal disorders, ultrastructural studies are often needed to determine whether these organelles are normal, abnormal, reduced in number, or absent (6). Usually, this can be accomplished without the application of any special techniques. Occasionally, however, we have found it necessary to employ the alkaline-diaminobenzidine reaction for catalase activity (10) to verify the identity of morphologically abnormal peroxisomes.

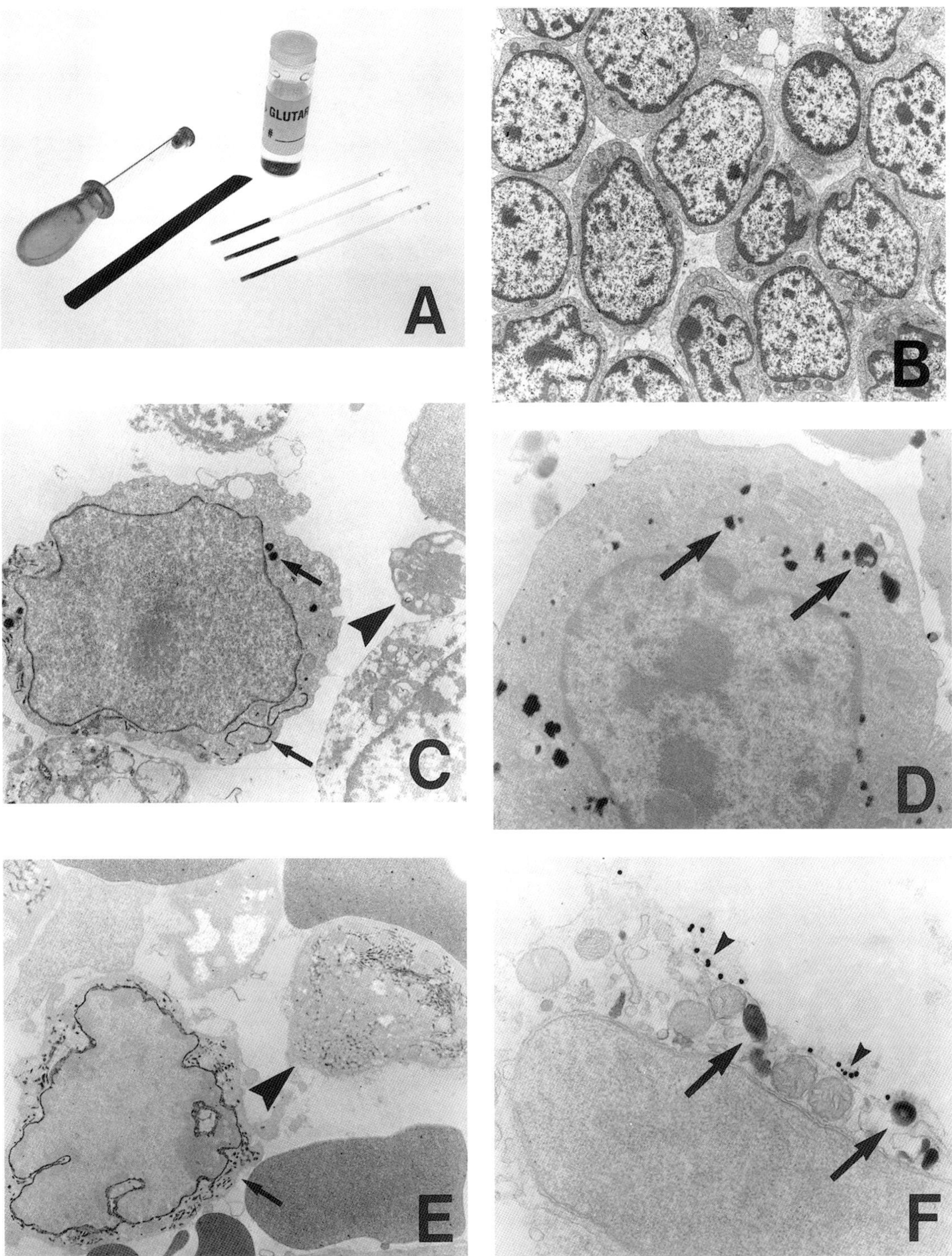

FIGURE 1D-6 ■ Special procedures for the diagnosis of acute leukemias. **A**: The capillary tube technique (described in text) provides an easy and utilitarian means of specimen collection that yields consistent high-quality results. **B**: Performing the MPO reaction prior to routine staining with uranyl acetate and lead citrate, as illustrated with this case of acute myeloid leukemia, does not affect the morphology. This example demonstrates also that, provided the capillary tubes are not first subjected to centrifugation, these specimens suffer little from an overnight delay in fixation. **C**: Detection of MPO (*arrows*), as shown in this case of acute "undifferentiated" leukemia, can be achieved by electron microscopy when not possible by light microscopy. Note that accompanying normal platelet (*arrowhead*) is not stained. **D**: Ultrastructural demonstration of nonspecific esterase activity (*arrows*) can be useful in the identification of early monocytic precursors. **E**: Identification of megakaryoblasts is enabled by the demonstration of PPO (*arrow*) within the endoplasmic reticulum. Note that the accompanying abnormal platelet (*arrowhead*) shows similar staining. **F**: Cryopreserved cells offer a convenient source of material for procedures with special processing requirements. Shown is a leukemic cell that, after retrieval, was subjected both to immunogold labeling with MY7 cell surface marker (*arrowheads*) and the MPO reaction (*arrows*).

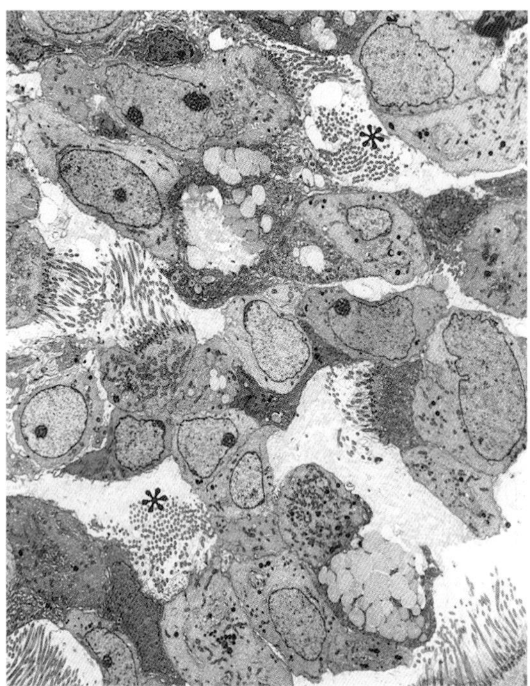

FIGURE 1D-7 ■ Brush biopsy specimen of nasal respiratory epithelium showing numerous favorably oriented cilia (*asterisks*).

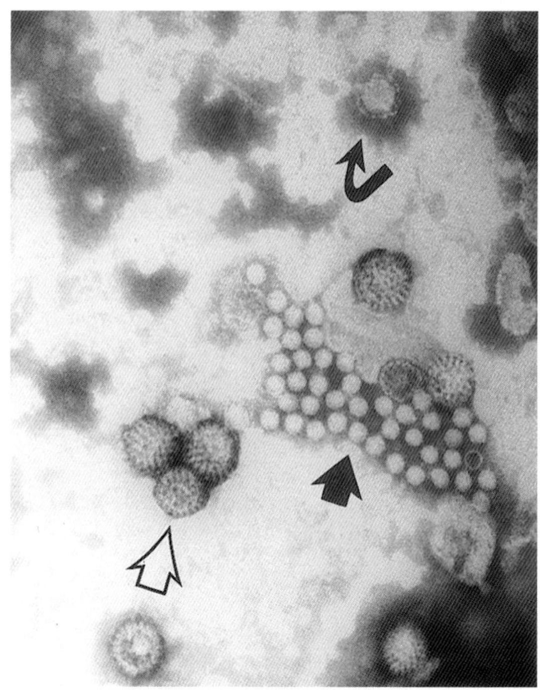

FIGURE 1D-8 ■ Negative stained stool specimen from a patient infected simultaneously with rotavirus (*open arrow*), coronavirus (*curved arrow*), and a small round virus (*solid arrow*).

Another easily performed ultrastructural special stain that has upon occasion proved very helpful is the uranaffin reaction. It can be used, among other things, to establish the identity of neuroendocrine granules in tumors (28) and serotonin granules in platelets (27).

Evaluation of cilia morphology requires electron microscopy. Nasal brush or curette specimens are recommended for this purpose because they generally produce a better yield of favorably oriented cilia than do traditional biopsy methods (Figure 1D-7). These techniques also offer the advantages of being less expensive to perform and easier for the patient to endure. We have found little need here for the use of any special fixatives or techniques (23).

Electron microscopy, while losing popularity as a means for detecting viruses in solid tissue specimens, has been gaining in utilization for detection of viruses in body fluids and fecal specimens. The techniques used for this purpose are fast and easy to perform, and need not be very elaborate. We routinely use a Beckman Airfuge ultracentrifuge to help concentrate the virus onto the grid surface but have found the agar diffusion method, which requires no special equipment, to work almost as well (8). The more cumbersome immunological techniques have not performed as well for us in this regard but have occasionally proved useful in confirming the identity of a detected virus. The negative staining technique can be used with a variety of specimens (e.g., urine, blood, vesicle fluid, cerebrospinal fluid, amniotic fluid, respiratory tract secretions), but its major application in pediatrics lies in the diagnosis of acute viral gastroenteritis. This very practical and cost-effective approach is being employed as the primary method for detection of stool viruses in a growing number of institutions. Not only does it provide the most reliable means for detecting rotavirus but concurrently enables detection of all the other viral pathogens, which together account for nearly as many cases of pediatric gastroenteritis as does rotavirus. Multiple agent infections are readily detected using this methodology (Figure 1D-8), which can be important when isolation procedures to stem a nosocomial outbreak are being implemented. The technique can be performed in just a matter of minutes, which may be of importance when initiation of therapy awaits establishment of a firm diagnosis or, in the event of a bioterrorism attack, an infectious organism requires quick identification.

It is emphasized in concluding that electron microscopy remains today an extremely powerful, highly versatile, absolutely indispensable diagnostic technique for the practice of pediatric pathology. Ideally, every pathologist would have an electron microscope located just down the hall. Fortunately, when such is not the case, modern-day transportation and communication systems allow consultative arrangements to be developed, almost anywhere in the world, that are virtually as fast, convenient, and effectual. Barriers to its utilization do not exist.

REFERENCES

1. Akhtar M, Ali MA, Sabbah R, et al. Fine-needle aspiration biopsy diagnosis of round cell malignant tumors of childhood. A combined light and electron microscopic approach. *Cancer* 1985;55:1805–1817.
2. Bainton DF, Farquhar MG. Differences in enzyme content of azurophil and specific granules of polymorphonuclear leukocytes. II. Cytochemistry and electron microscopy of bone marrow cells. *J Cell Biol* 1968;39:299–317.

3. Bozzola JJ, Russell LD. *Electron microscopy. Principles and techniques for biologists*, 2nd ed. Sudbury, MA: Jones and Bartlett Publishers, 1998.
4. Buchino JJ. Cytopathology in pediatrics. In: Wied GL, ed. *Monographs in clinical cytology*, Vol. 13. Basel, Switzerland: Karger, 1991:1–7.
5. Dehner LP. On trial: a malignant small cell tumor in a child. Four wrongs do not make a right. *Am J Clin Pathol* 1998;109:662–668.
6. Dimmick JE, Applegarth DA. Pathology of peroxisomal disorders. In: Landing BH, Haust MD, Bernstein J, et al., eds. *Genetic metabolic diseases*, Vol. 17 Basel, Switzerland: Karger, 1993:45–98. (Rosenberg HS, Bernstein J, eds. *Perspectives in Pediatric Pathology Series*.)
7. Dingemans KP, van den Bergh Weerman MA. Rapid contrasting of extracellular elements in thin sections. *Ultrastruct Pathol* 1990;14:519–527.
8. Doane FW, Anderson N. *Electron microscopy in diagnostic virology. A practical guide and atlas*. Cambridge, UK: Cambridge University Press, 1987.
9. Erlandson RA. *Diagnostic transmission electron microscopy of tumors: with clinicopathological, immunohistochemical, and cytogenetic correlations*. New York, NY: Raven Press, 1994.
10. Fahimi HD. Cytochemical localization of peroxidatic activity of catalase in rat hepatic microbodies (peroxisomes). *J Cell Biol* 1969;43:275–288.
11. Favara BE, Mierau GW, McCarthy RC, et al. The leukemias of childhood. In: Rosenberg HS, Berstein J, Newton WA Jr, eds. *Neoplasia in infancy and childhood*, Vol. 9. Basel, Switzerland: Karger, 1987:75–132. (Rosenberg HS, Bernstein J, eds. *Perspectives in Pediatric Pathology Series*.)
12. Franke FE, Schechenmayr W, Osborn M, et al. Unexpected immunoreactivities of intermediate filament antibodies in human brain and brain tumors. *Am J Pathol* 1991;139:67–79.
13. Friedman HD, Tatum AH. HMB-45-positive malignant lymphoma. A case report with literature review of aberrant HMB-45 reactivity. *Arch Pathol Lab Med* 1991;115:826–830.
14. Frierson HF Jr, Bellafiore FJ, Gaffey MJ, et al. Cytokeratin in anaplastic large cell lymphoma. *Mod Pathol* 1994;7:317–321.
15. Gown AM, Boyd HC, Chang Y, et al. Smooth muscle cells can express cytokeratins of "simple" epithelium. Immunocytochemical and biochemical studies in vitro and in vivo. *Am J Pathol* 1988;132:222–232.
16. Graham RC, Karnovsky MJ. The early stages of absorption of injected horseradish peroxidase in the proximal tubules of mouse kidney. Ultrastructural cytochemistry by a new technique. *J Histochem Cytochem* 1966;14:291–302.
17. Hayat MA. *Principles and techniques of electron microscopy. Biological applications*, 3rd ed. Boca Raton, FL: CRC Press, 1989.
18. Heyderman E, Warren PJ, Haines AMR. Immunohistochemistry today—problems and practice [Commentary]. *Histopathology* 1989;15:653–658.
19. Heynen MJ, Tricot G, Verwilghen RL. A reliable method with good cell preservation for the demonstration of peroxidase activity in human platelets and megakaryocytes. *Histochemistry* 1984;80:79–84.
20. Johannessen JV. Use of paraffin material for electron microscopy. *Pathol Annu* 1977;12:189–224.
21. Mechtersheimer G, Moller P. Expression of Ki-1 antigen (CD30) in mesenchymal tumors. *Cancer* 1990;66:1732–1737.
22. Mierau GW. New approaches to the diagnosis of childhood leukemias. Proceedings of the 47th annual meeting of the Electron Microscopy Society of America. San Antonio, TX: San Francisco Press, 1989: 870–871.
23. Mierau GW, Agostini R, Beals TF, et al. The role of electron microscopy in evaluating ciliary dysfunction: Report of a workshop. *Ultrastruct Pathol* 1992;16:245–254.
24. Mierau GW, Berry PJ, Malott RL, et al. Appraisal of the comparative utility of immunohistochemistry and electron microscopy in the diagnosis of childhood round cell tumors. *Ultrastruct Pathol* 1996;20: 507–517.
25. Mierau GW, Favara BE, Brenman JM. Electron microscopy in histiocytosis X. *Ultrastruct Pathol* 1982;3:137–142.
26. Payne BC, Kim H, Pangalis GA, et al. A method for the ultrastructural demonstration of non-specific esterase in human blood and lymphoid tissue. *Histochem J* 1980;12:71–86.
27. Payne CM. A quantitative ultrastructural evaluation of the cell organelle specificity of the uranaffin reaction in normal human platelets. *Am J Clin Pathol* 1984;81:62–70.
28. Payne CM, Nagle RB, Borduin VF, et al. An ultrastructural evaluation of the cell organelle specificity of the uranaffin reaction in two human endocrine neoplasms. *J Submicrosc Cytol* 1983;15:833–841.
29. Stork L, Wilson H, Mierau GW, et al. Heterogeneity of acute "undifferentiated" leukemia of childhood: Ultrastructural, immunophenotypic, and karyotypic analyses. *Am J Ped Hematol Oncol* 1990;12:34–44.
30. Strausbauch P, Neill J, Dabbs DJ, et al. The impact of fine needle aspiration biopsy on a diagnostic electron microscopy laboratory. *Arch Pathol Lab Med* 1989;113:1354–1356.
31. Swanson PE, Dehner LP, Sirgi KE, et al. Cytokeratin immunoreactivity in malignant tumors of bone and soft tissue. A reappraisal of cytokeratin as a reliable marker in diagnostic immunohistochemistry. *Appl Immunohistochem* 1994;2:103–112.
32. Taylor SR, Nunez C. Fine-needle aspiration biopsy in a pediatric population. *Cancer* 1984;54:1449–1453.
33. Vielh P, Howell LP. Techniques. In: Kline TS, ed. *Guides to clinical aspiration biopsy. Pediatrics*. New York, NY: Igaku-Shoin, 1994:5–8.
34. Wakely PE Jr, Kardos TF, Frable WJ. Application of fine needle aspiration biopsy to pediatrics. *Hum Pathol* 1988;19:1383–1386.
35. Yazdi HM, Dardick I. Diagnostic immunocytochemistry and electron microscopy. In: Kline TS, ed. *Guides to clinical aspiration biopsy*. New York, NY: Igaku-Shoin, 1992:1.

CHAPTER 2

First and Second Trimester Pregnancy Loss

DEBORAH E. MCFADDEN

Pathologic examination of the products of embryos and fetuses, both from spontaneous abortions (SAs) and terminations of pregnancy, has become increasingly important over the past few decades. While such examination was once performed primarily for the purpose of furthering scientific understanding of prenatal human development, the practical medical applications of this knowledge have become clear and now form an integral part of the medical assessment and management of fertility issues (30,52,65,68). As an understanding of the factors involved in successful pregnancies has developed and as patient demand for information has increased, the role of pathologic examination has grown. Increased use of assisted fertilization techniques has heightened the interest of physicians and patients alike in understanding why pregnancies fail. This chapter will address the examination of disorders encountered in those pregnancies that end spontaneously in the first and second trimesters of gestation; the pathology of fetuses delivered after pregnancy termination after prenatal ultrasound diagnosis is beyond the scope of this chapter.

It is recognized that many conceptions do not end in livebirths but, rather, that there is a high rate of loss, especially early in gestation. It is estimated that 10% to 20% of recognized pregnancies end as SAs, with most losses occurring in the first trimester or first 12 to 14 weeks of gestation. With the demonstration of fetal cardiac activity, the miscarriage rate drops somewhat to approximately 3% to 12% (38). In a study of women who had had a normal prenatal visit at 6 to 11 weeks of gestational age (GA), the risk of subsequent SA was 1.6% or less, considerably lower than for pregnancies overall (69). After the first trimester, approximately 1% to 2% of pregnancies are spontaneously aborted (56). The incidence of stillbirth at term gestation is in the order of 0.1% to 0.5%. This high loss rate, together with changing or changed societal approaches and expectations of pregnancy such as delaying childbearing until later in a woman's reproductive life and increased access to assisted reproduction methods, has led to an intense interest in understanding the cause of pregnancy loss and the implications for future reproductive success.

GA refers to the number of weeks since the last menstrual period (equivalent to menstrual dates), while developmental age (DA) refers to the age as determined from the time of fertilization, generally considered to be approximately 2 weeks after the last menstrual period. Embryos are assessed by developmental features that correlate with age, usually given as DA. Thus, in a normal gestation, GA is DA plus 2 weeks.

The first trimester of pregnancy is the period of implantation and embryogenesis, with the completion of embryogenesis by 8 weeks of DA (10 weeks of gestational age). Upon completion of embryogenesis with development of all organ systems, the conceptus is referred to as a fetus. Definitions of fetus and infant vary with locale; in Canada, a fetus is considered an infant once it has reached the GA of 20 weeks or is liveborn at any GA. Stillbirth is defined as delivery of a deceased infant at or after 20 weeks of GA.

CAUSES OF EARLY SPONTANEOUS ABORTION

It is well recognized that the major cause of early SA is chromosome abnormality, usually aneuploidy. The use of techniques such as comparative genomic hybridization (CGH) and quantitative fluorescence-polymerase chain reaction (QF-PCR) to supplement conventional cytogenetic analysis has increased the detection of chromosome abnormalities because these techniques do not require cell culture and can address the issue of maternal cell contamination.

Numerous studies have shown that at least half of early SAs are chromosomally abnormal; in our laboratory, 70% of cases are chromosomally abnormal, somewhat higher than reported rates. Some of this may be attributable to our routine use of cytogenetic analysis supplemented by CGH with flow cytometry in cases in which tissue culture for cytogenetic analysis has failed or in which maternal cell contamination is suspected (36) and some is attributable to the fact that the average maternal age in our population is higher than in other published reports.

The distribution of chromosome abnormalities is consistent between various studies, with trisomy accounting for nearly half of all chromosomally abnormal SAs, triploidy accounting for 6% to 8%, and monosomy X accounting for another 8% to 10%. Autosomal monosomy (primarily monosomy 21) and structural rearrangements account for an additional 5% of abnormal cases. The structural abnormalities are an important subgroup because of the possibility that they have arisen from a parent who carries a rearrangement predisposing to an unbalanced karyotype in offspring. Studies of couples who have had recurrent miscarriages show that 5% have balanced rearrangements such as reciprocal translocations (67). These individuals have an increased risk of having chromosomally abnormal pregnancies, with the actual risk depending on the type of rearrangement and the chromosomes involved (66).

Thus, the vast majority of early pregnancy loss is due to trisomy. Studies of parental origin of trisomies have demonstrated that the largest proportion of trisomy is maternal in origin. There is a strong association with maternal age, with the births of trisomic infants rising with increasing maternal age. Trisomy affects 3% of pregnancies in 25-year-old women but affects 35% of pregnancies in women aged 42 years (58). Most trisomies are the result of errors in meiosis I (26), although this varies for individual chromosomes. For example, trisomy 18 is more typically the result of errors in the second meiotic division, while trisomy 21 is predominantly the result of errors in the first meiotic division.

With the predominance of chromosome abnormality in SA, it is clear that in order to ensure clinical relevance of examination of SAs, the examination must include determination of the karyotype. In the event that the examination proves normal, with normal karyotype and normal villus histology, management of persons having SAs, especially recurrent SAs, shifts and other etiologies for pregnancy loss must be considered.

The investigation of those who have had chromosomally normal miscarriages with no other pathology is dependent upon the proposed nonchromosome mechanisms for fetal loss. These proposed associations include exogenous environmental exposures (77), skewed X-inactivation (5,28), disorders of endocrine function, immune disorders including conditions with autoantibodies, and thrombophilic conditions (56). The roles of these factors in miscarriage remain under investigation, and the significance of each has not been established with certainty. Antiphospholipid antibodies are found more in women who have recurrent miscarriages (RSA) than in other women. The mechanism by which an antiphospholipid antibody causes pregnancy loss is not known. There are no specific pathologic features identified in the first trimester SA from women who are positive for this antibody (61,63,73). There is some evidence to suggest that those with recurrent miscarriages are more likely to have thrombophilia mutations such as antiphospholipid antibody, factor V Leiden deficiency, prothrombin gene mutations, or methylene tetrahydrofolate reductase (MTHFR) gene, although the studies of small series of affected individuals have shown conflicting results (15,21,33,56,59). Some studies have demonstrated that the incidence of factor V Leiden, MTHFR, and prothrombin gene mutations is no different in a population with recurrent miscarriages than in parous controls (15,31), and one review points out that while there is an association between thrombophilia and pregnancy loss, a causal relationship has not been established (59). Others suggest that there are insufficient data to recommend that all women who have recurrent pregnancy loss should be screened for a broad range of inherited thrombophilias in the absence of other clinical features (1). There is possibly less controversy about the role of antiphospholipid antibody in recurrent pregnancy loss, and some advocate screening for this antibody (only) in those with recurrent miscarriages (9). The management of those diagnosed with one of the thrombophilic disorders remains controversial. This area of investigation in recurrent pregnancy loss is confounded by the fact that many reported series and treatment trials are compromised by methodological problems (13).

With changing reproductive patterns such as women starting their families later in life and having fewer children, there is a desire to diagnose and manage causes of miscarriage. Given that cytogenetic abnormalities account for the majority of first trimester abortions, it has been suggested that the evaluation of first trimester SA with cytogenetic analysis may prove more cost effective than a standard battery of tests such as thyroid function tests, endometrial biopsy, or thrombophilia testing (35). Such examination also serves to identify those conditions not associated with abnormal karyotype that may require additional investigation or treatment to increase the chance of successful pregnancy and to diagnose conditions in which there is a risk of neoplasia, as with complete hydatidiform mole (CHM) and its attendant risk of gestational trophoblastic neoplasia (GTN) (30).

Examination of fetal losses in the second trimester is similar to the investigation of intrauterine death in later gestation and requires a complete autopsy examination. This examination is performed in the same way as autopsies in older fetuses and infants, with the intent of identifying a cause of intrauterine death, making a diagnosis, and assessing risks of recurrence. The rate of chromosome abnormality in the second trimester is approximately 5% to 10%, less than observed in first trimester SAs, and an indication that other processes play a more significant role in the second trimester intrauterine death or SA. The identification of these other causes of pregnancy loss can not only provide some understanding and comfort to the affected individual but also be important in assessing risks of adverse outcomes in future pregnancies and in determining management options.

FIRST TRIMESTER SPONTANEOUS ABORTION

Indication for Cytogenetic Analysis

Given that chromosome abnormality accounts for the majority of first trimester SAs, an argument can be made for performing cytogenetic analysis in all cases. The proportion of cases in which morphological abnormalities that account for the SA are identified is small. To assist in the reproductive counseling regarding cause of the SA and risks for recurrence, karyotype is a vital piece of information. Where embryopathology examination was once performed only in cases of recurrent SAs, changes in reproductive patterns and practices have altered, resulting in a broader range of cases referred for embryopathologic examination. Those who treat women who have had difficulty conceiving or who have had previous miscarriage(s) are anxious to know whether the pregnancy failure was the result of chromosome abnormality or if there is perhaps another etiology necessitating further investigation. Increasingly, assisted reproductive technologies (ARTs) such as *in vitro* fertilization (IVF) or intracytoplasmic sperm injection (ICSI) are utilized. There are concerns that ARTs are associated with increased incidence of chromosome abnormalities at prenatal diagnosis and at birth, specifically for sex chromosome abnormalities in pregnancies that are the result of ICSI (3,22). In a comparison of 133 cases of SAs occurring after ARTs with 144 cases of SAs in naturally conceived pregnancies, there was no significant difference in the rate of chromosome abnormality between the two groups, with 63.2% of the ART group abnormal as compared to 71.5% of the naturally conceived group (8). This suggests that the increased rate of chromosome abnormality in the ICSI population does not translate to an increased rate of miscarriage of chromosomally abnormal pregnancies.

Until the natural history of ART pregnancies is delineated, the use of these technologies should be considered as an indication for cytogenetic analysis in cases of SA. In some laboratories, the fact that the majority of first trimester SAs are the result of chromosome abnormality is sufficient indication to perform cytogenetic analysis of *all* cases examined morphologically. In other laboratories, constraints imposed by funding structures may impose the necessity of specific clinical indication before cytogenetic studies will be funded. These other indications include a history of recurrent miscarriages (variably defined as two or more losses or three or more losses), abnormal villus morphology, abnormal or normal embryo, parental chromosome rearrangement, and maternal age 35 years or greater.

Examination

Examination of the early pregnancy loss or embryo specimen is quite different from that of a fetal specimen as the latter represents an autopsy examination of a fetus and its placenta. Examination of the products of an early pregnancy loss (spontaneous or missed abortion) is performed to identify pregnancy-related tissues (embryo and/or placental tissue) to confirm intrauterine pregnancy and to assess their morphology. This examination includes sampling of tissues for additional studies, including for cytogenetic analysis or other means of determining the chromosome complement of the conceptus. Thus, it is imperative that all specimens for embryopathology examination are submitted in the fresh state, not in fixative.

An assessment of the products of conception is best accomplished by examining the specimen under a dissecting microscope equipped with a camera. The presence of any placental or embryonic tissue allows confirmation of intrauterine pregnancy. In the absence of pregnancy-related tissues, intrauterine pregnancy cannot be confirmed, and the report must reflect that. Decidualized endometrium may be seen in estrogen effect, including with ectopic pregnancy, and is therefore insufficient for confirmation of intrauterine pregnancy.

The morphology of the chorionic villi is characterized—their individual morphology and their distribution over the chorionic sac. Attention to whether the villi appear overly abundant and/or cystic is important because of concerns for CHM or partial hydatidiform mole (PHM). Other features of embryonic development, such as presence of amnion, yolk sac, and umbilical cord, are assessed.

Tissues are sampled for cytogenetic analysis and to be retained frozen for additional studies as required. Our practice is to submit amnion and chorion for cytogenetic analysis as the amnion is thought to be most reflective of the embryo itself. Cytogenetic cultures from chorion are more likely to be complicated by maternal cell contamination, necessitating further examination by other means, such as CGH, to confirm the karyotype of the conceptus, but amnion is not present in all cases and chorion must be sampled. Chorion and amnion seem to grow in culture more readily than do chorionic villi and are preferred. In all cases, chorionic villi are frozen and are available in the event that the tissue submitted for cytogenetic analysis fails to grow in culture and additional testing such as CGH is required, for assessment in cases where maternal cell contamination is of concern, or for additional genetic studies as indicated. In the case of pronounced maceration, the decision is made to proceed directly to CGH, rather than attempting tissue culture for cytogenetic analysis. With the introduction of array CGH techniques, subtle abnormalities that cannot be detected by cytogenetic analysis will be diagnosed; an argument can be made to utilize array CGH in all cases of SAs to eliminate the labor and risk of culture failure associated with conventional cytogenetic analysis (7,36,62).

The presence of embryonic tissue confirms intrauterine pregnancy and is a feature in favor of a diagnosis other than CHM, a frequent concern as edematous villi are often identified on ultrasound or at gross examination. In determining the developmental stage and thus age of the embryo, standard developmental criteria are used (24,48). Embryos may be normally developed (Figure 2-1) according to established criteria, but this does not exclude chromosome abnormality. Most developmental tables were established without karyotype determination. Some cases do not show regularly

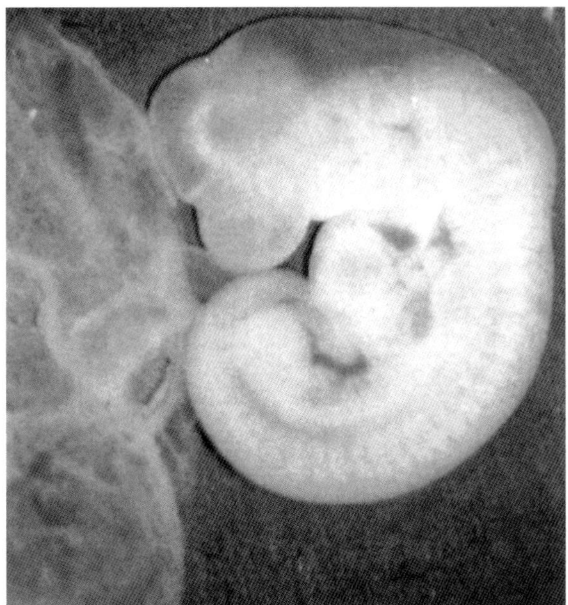

FIGURE 2-1 ■ Normally developed human embryo, stage 14 of development.

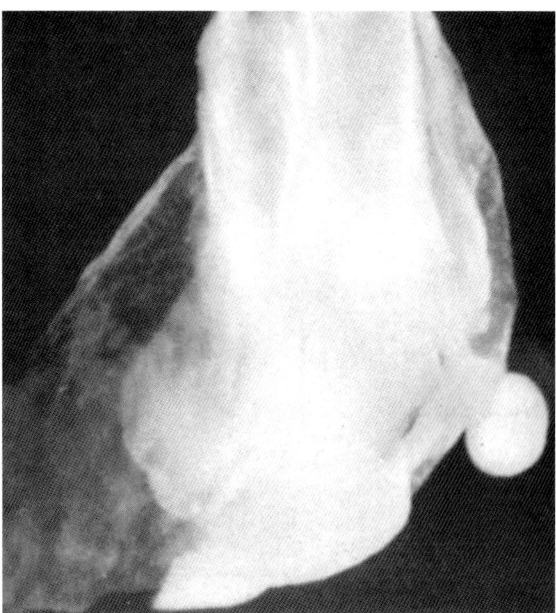

FIGURE 2-3 ■ Growth-disorganized embryo, GD2—1 mm nodular embryo in opened amniotic and chorionic sac.

developed embryos but rather embryos or embryonic tissues in which normal developmental features are not present, a state referred to as growth disorganization. In our experience, when embryos are identified, slightly less than half of them show features of growth disorganization. Growth disorganization has been divided into four categories: a type I growth-disorganized embryo (GD1) refers to an intact empty sac (Figure 2-2), type II refers to a nodular embryo in which cranial and caudal ends cannot be distinguished (Figure 2-3), type III refers to a cylindrical embryo in which there is some cranial-caudal differentiation with retinal pigment (Figure 2-4), and type IV refers to an embryo in which there is more recognizable embryonic development but delayed growth of limbs and other developmental features (Figure 2-5). While growth disorganization is readily identified and classified, the findings are nonspecific—in all types of growth-disorganized embryos, the incidence of chromosome abnormality is similar to that encountered in SAs in general, with the same types of chromosome abnormalities identified. Ultrasound detection of an embryo does not strictly correlate with the morphological detection of embryonic tissue, but it has been demonstrated that the rates of abnormal karyotypes are not

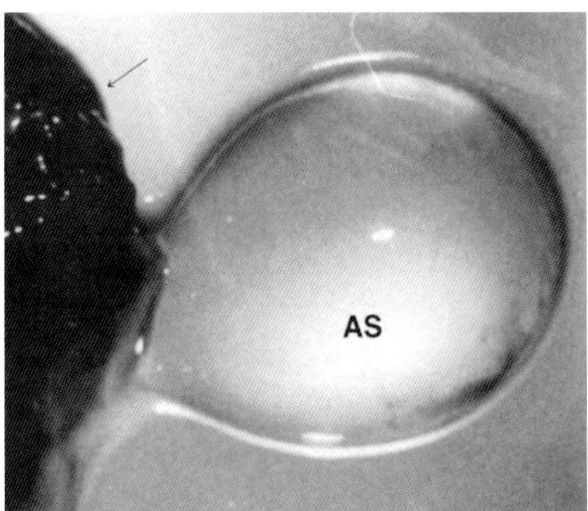

FIGURE 2-2 ■ Growth-disorganized embryo, GD1—intact empty amniotic sac (AS). Opened chorionic sac (*arrow*).

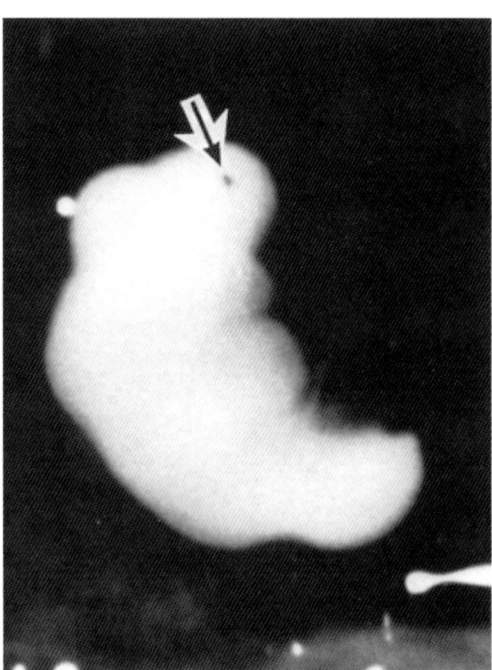

FIGURE 2-4 ■ Growth-disorganized embryo, GD3—cylindrical embryo with retinal pigment (*arrow*).

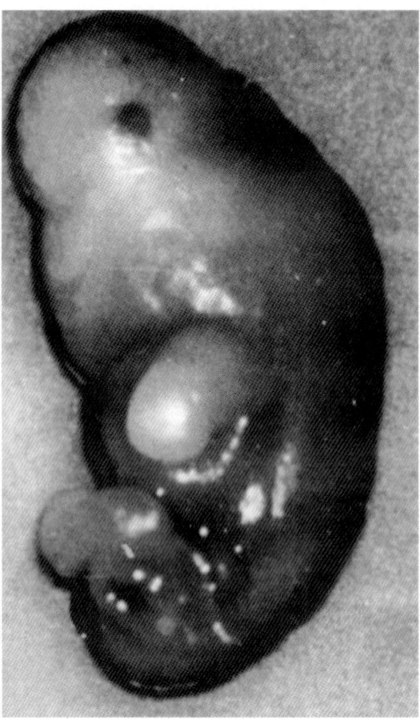

FIGURE 2-5 ■ Growth-disorganized embryo, GD4—delayed development of head, trunk, and limbs relative to crown-rump length.

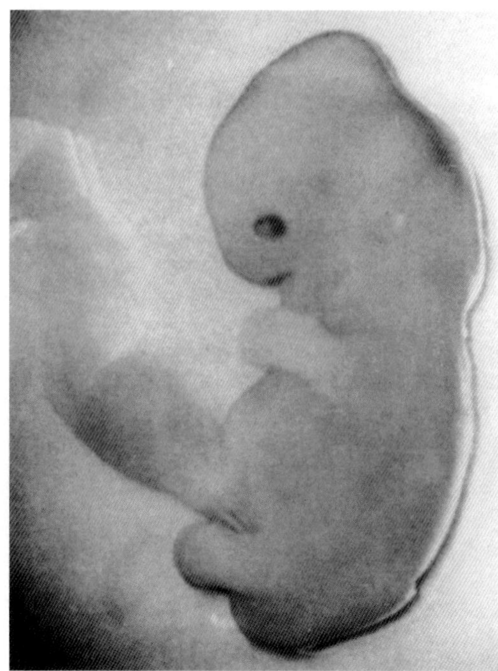

FIGURE 2-7 ■ Monosomy X embryo with parietal encephalocele.

significantly different between SAs in which an embryonic pole is identified on ultrasound examination and those that appear anembryonic (35). This corresponds to our experience: 63% of anembryonic specimens are chromosomally abnormal and 71% of embryonic specimens are chromosomally abnormal. Of embryonic specimens, 58% of growth-disorganized embryos are abnormal and 79% of regularly developed embryos are abnormal.

Embryos may show isolated or focal abnormalities such as neural tube defects, facial clefts, or limb anomalies (Figures 2-6 to 2-8). Many of these abnormalities, such as neural tube defects, occur in the setting of chromosome

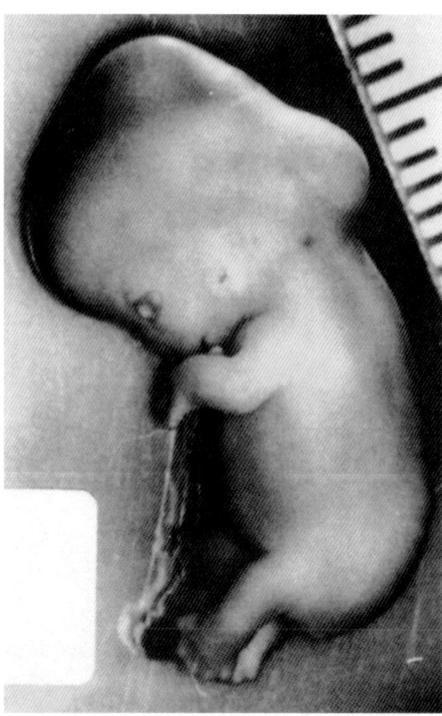

FIGURE 2-6 ■ Stage 20 embryo with parietal and occipital encephaloceles.

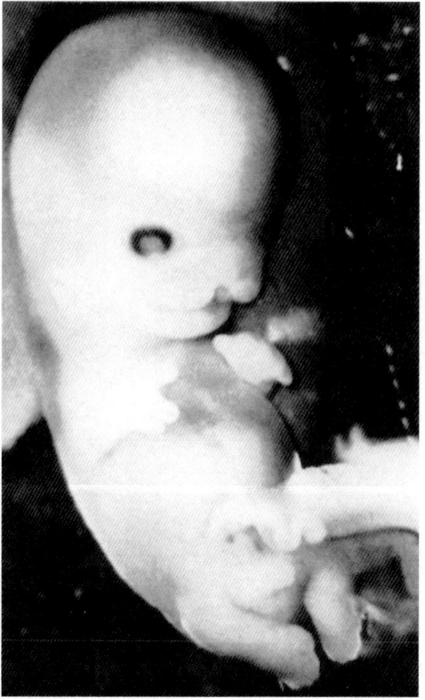

FIGURE 2-8 ■ Stage 18 embryo with cleft lip, absent digit in the right hand, and coloboma.

abnormality (41). In the setting of a normal karyotype, the focal defects likely have the same significance as in later gestation, and genetic counseling to discuss the findings and possible recurrence risks is indicated. Chromosomally abnormal embryos may show a number of nonspecific abnormalities, such as delay of normal limb development, abnormal tan deposits, and various types of growth disorganizations. Embryos with the trisomies more commonly encountered in later gestation and livebirths, such as trisomy 13, 18, and 21, may show some features in common with the phenotypes observed in the fetal period. Most often, however, embryonic phenotypic manifestations of these trisomies are nonspecific (Figure 2-9).

Triploidy is encountered in approximately 6% of early SAs, and embryos are often identified. A phenotype thought to be characteristic of triploidy has been described by Harris et al. (25) (Figure 2-10). With the identification of imprinting effect in fetal triploid phenotypes, the possibility of imprinting effect in the triploid embryo population has been assessed and there has been no correlation with embryo phenotype and parental origin of the triploidy. In triploid embryos, a variety of appearances are encountered, ranging from growth-disorganized to apparently normal embryos. These apparently normal embryos are most often at approximately stage 16 of development (37 to 42 days), equivalent to approximately 7 to 8 weeks of GA (Figure 2-11). The normal phenotype and the growth-disorganized phenotypes were seen in triploids of both maternal origin and paternal origin. In this series of triploids with embryonic tissue present, digynic triploidy accounted for 67% of cases. Of the nine cases of diandric origin, eight showed features of PHM (43).

Histological examination of placental tissues and decidua is routinely performed in all cases. Microscopic examination of the chorionic villi allows detection of infection, including viral infections such as cytomegalovirus (CMV) and bacterial infections such as listeriosis. In addition, disorders of uncertain etiology such as intervillositis or conditions with increased intervillus fibrin are occasionally detected. Villus infarction is distinctly unusual and should raise concerns of maternal vascular/thrombophilic disease. Routine histological examination of decidua allows for assessment of decidual (maternal) vasculature. In a review of the histopathology of SAs with known karyotype, 19% of SAs with a normal karyotype showed evidence of chronic inflammation or perivillus fibrin deposition in contrast to 8% of those with an abnormal

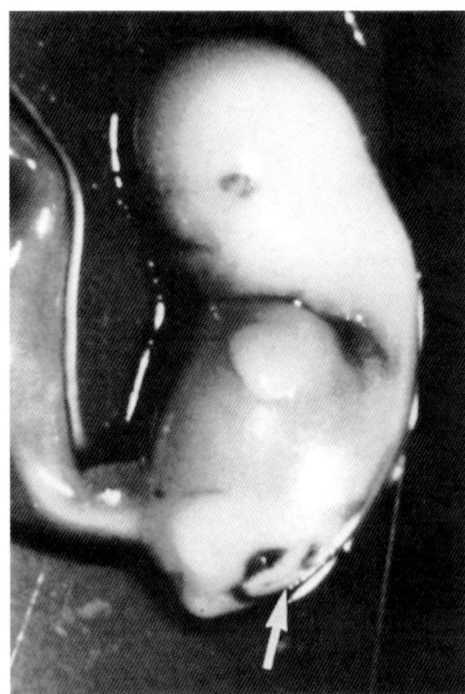

FIGURE 2-10 ■ Triploid embryo showing dysplastic face, delayed limb development, and defect in lumbosacral region (*arrow*).

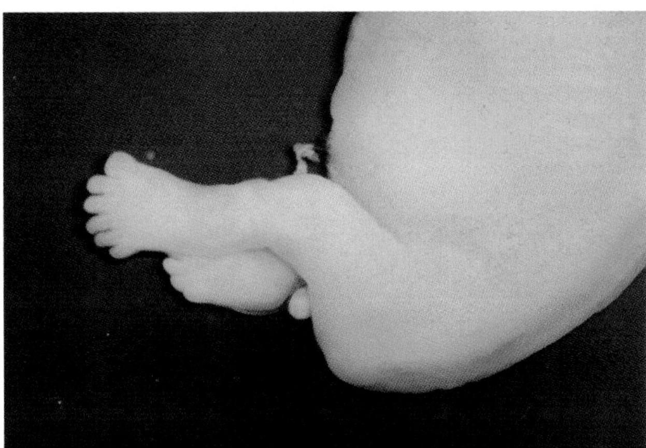

FIGURE 2-9 ■ Embryo with trisomy 13—postaxial polydactyly of feet.

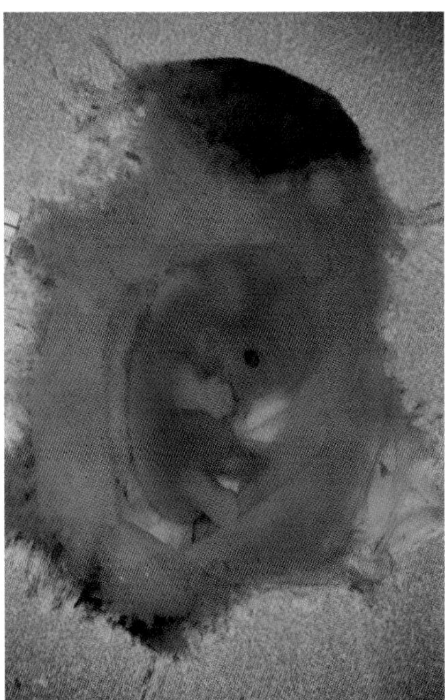

FIGURE 2-11 ■ Triploid embryo showing normal stage 18 phenotype, approximately 41 days DA.

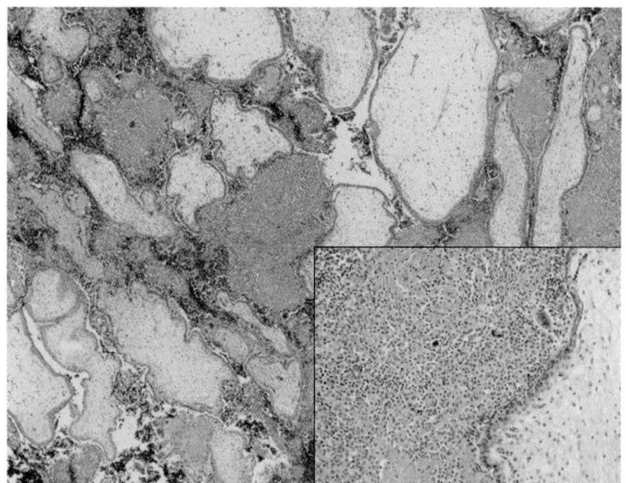

FIGURE 2-12 ■ Chronic (mononuclear) intervillositis in SA at 10 weeks' GA.

karyotype. The findings were even more frequent (31%) in the subset of SAs that were chromosomally normal and occurred in a population with recurrent SAs (55).

Intervillositis is a disorder of unknown etiology in which there is either focal or diffuse increase in mononuclear cells within the intervillus (maternal) space (Figure 2-12). The lesion is thought to be possibly an immune disorder and may recur in subsequent pregnancies (11,16). With focal intervillositis, it may be difficult to distinguish between focal intervillositis and an infectious process characterized by intervillus inflammation and villus abscess; special stains for organisms should be performed to exclude Listeria and syphilis.

Increased perivillus fibrin is another disorder of unknown etiology in which it has been suggested that immune disorder may play a role. Perivillus fibrin may be increased as a degenerative change in response to intrauterine death of the embryo; distinguishing between degenerative changes and subtle increases in perivillus fibrin is difficult. When there is obvious increase in perivillus fibrin, the lesion may be considered to account for the loss; some suggest that an arbitrary threshold of 50% villus involvement be used to make this diagnosis (75). Although probably etiologically heterogeneous, this entity may also recur and has been associated with recurrent SAs.

Infection is a clear cause of pregnancy loss, with viruses, spirochetes, and bacteria all playing significant roles. Syphilis has increased in frequency over the past few years, and it has been encountered with increasing frequency in pediatric pathology, including in the pregnancy loss specimens. Although first trimester loss may occur with syphilis, it is seen more often in losses occurring in later gestation.

Listeriosis, by contrast, causes pregnancy loss throughout gestation. Listeriosis may occur as outbreaks in a community related to improper food handling or may occur as sporadic events related to ingestion of foods known to be at higher risk of containing Listeria, such as soft or unpasteurized cheeses (10). Listeriosis in the first trimester SA is characterized, histologically, by acute villus abscesses, with abundant neutrophils in the intervillus spaces (Figure 2-13). There is usually

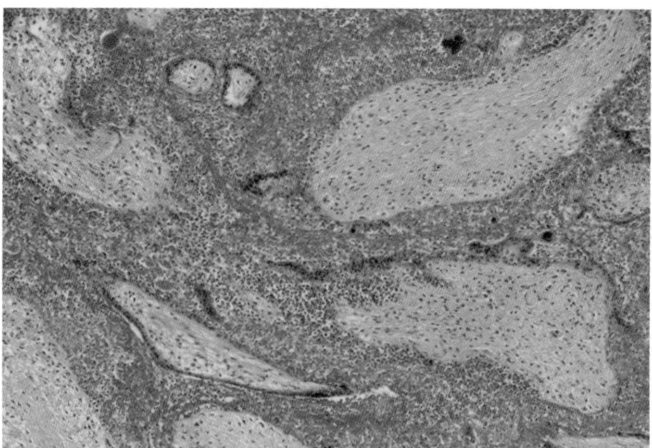

FIGURE 2-13 ■ Villus abscesses of listeriosis. SA at 14 weeks' GA.

also an acute chorioamnionitis. Gram-positive bacilli may be demonstrated on Gram stain; the histology is usually sufficiently characteristic to allow diagnosis.

Excluding the small number of cases in which infectious, immune, or vascular causes of first trimester SA are identified, the majority of SAs are shown to be chromosomally abnormal. Although there are histological features that have been suggested as being more commonly observed in aneuploid pregnancies, such as irregular villus outlines, trophoblast inclusions, or invaginations, in general, the predictive value of these findings is low (20,47,57,74). Our experience, similar to that of others (54), is that some trisomies, such as trisomy 22, are more likely to show these features (Figure 2-14).

The most commonly encountered chromosome abnormalities are trisomy, and there are reports for trisomies of all chromosomes encountered in SAs. Trisomy 16 is the single most commonly encountered trisomy. Trisomy for two chromosomes (double trisomy) is seen in 3% of the chromosomally abnormal SAs.

Concern for GTN is heightened in the SA population as CHM may present as spontaneous or missed abortion. It has been shown that fewer than 44% of CHMs or PHMs are detected at routine first trimester ultrasound (18), providing

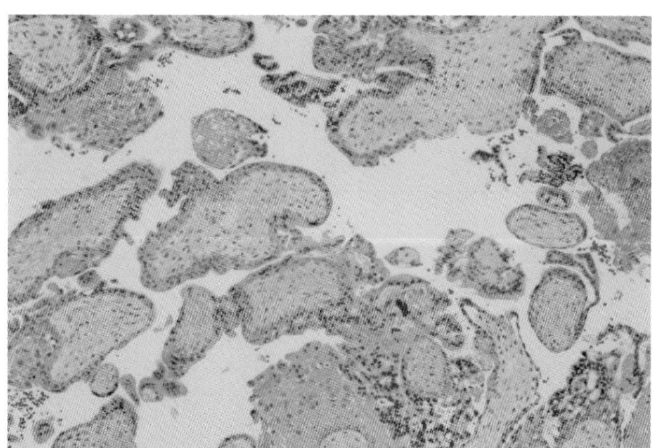

FIGURE 2-14 ■ Irregular ("busy") appearing trophoblastic epithelium in trisomy 22.

an indication for the necessity of histological examination of SAs, even when a gestation is apparently normal at ultrasound or at the time of evacuation. The risk of GTN requiring chemotherapy is 15% to 28% after diagnosis of CHM (78), making the diagnosis imperative. The risk of GTN after triploid PHM is less well-defined; there are case reports of choriocarcinoma occurring after triploid PHM (12,39,45,64), but others have shown that the risk of persistent GTN is rare, occurring in fewer than 5% of cases (22). Given the risks, some recommend that these cases be managed as would women who have had a CHM (76).

The diagnosis of early CHM and PHM can be difficult in specimens from early SAs, perhaps more so than in the past when these pregnancies presented later in gestation. Gross examination of early hydatidiform moles may show cystic change of chorionic villi—grossly this may be impossible to differentiate from the cystic change in partial moles and the hydropic degeneration occurring in nonmolar SAs. Histological diagnosis is readily achieved by pathologists experienced with this type of pathology, but there have been studies that demonstrate considerable interobserver and intraobserver variability in the diagnosis of both CHM and PHM (19), and concerns about the ability to consistently diagnose these entities have been raised by those practicing in a less specialized environment (53). With recognition that the features in early CHM may be subtle and with the availability of karyotype determination, ploidy determination, and immunohistochemical staining for p57kip2, diagnostic accuracy is increased (20). A major problem that occurs in routine practice is to distinguish between hydropic abortion (degenerative change) and molar gestation.

CHMs are diploid, with both haploid complements being paternal in origin. Thus, CHMs are androgenetic, with no maternal contribution present. The abnormal development in this situation is considered to be a reflection of abnormal imprinting (see Chapter 3), since both maternal and paternal genetic contributions are required for normal embryo and placenta development.

The histopathological features of CHM are diffuse villus edema (hydropic change), cistern formation, and circumferential trophoblastic hyperplasia. Rudimentary fetal vessels may be identified, but ordinarily fetal blood cells are not seen within such vessels. Stromal karyorrhexis is a feature of early CHM, thought to be related to increased stromal proliferation and apoptosis (Figure 2-15) (76). Immunohistochemical staining for p57kip2 is useful in the assessment of possible molar gestations because of its expression from the maternal allele only. Thus, in a CHM by definition androgenetic, the normal p57kip2 staining of cytotrophoblast and villus stroma is absent (46). p57kip2 staining of triploid PHM is normal because of the maternal haploid contribution.

Triploidy may be either paternal (diandric) or maternal (digynic) in origin. Older studies demonstrated that diandry was the predominant origin of triploidy, while more recent studies have shown that the distribution of diandric triploidy and digynic triploidy is somewhat more complex than that. In very early gestation, digyny is at least as common as diandry, while in cases presenting as later missed abortion with grossly cystic villi, diandry is more common; in the fetal and

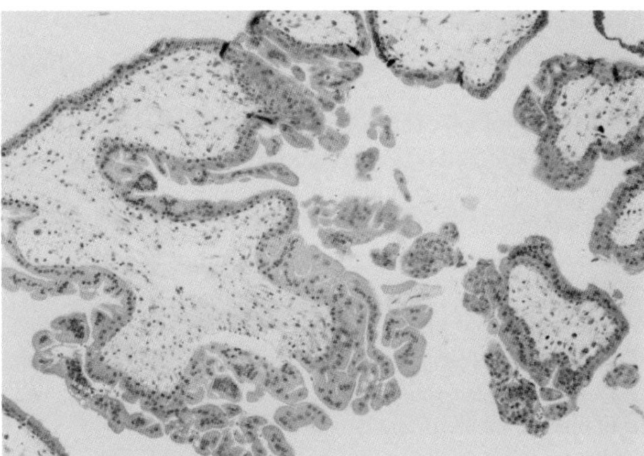

FIGURE 2-15 ■ Early CHM with stromal karyorrhexis.

infant population, digyny is clearly predominant. In early pregnancy, the incidence of diandric triploidy is in the range of 50% to 65% (40,42,79). Of the two origins, it is diandric triploidy that presents as PHM.

PHM is characterized, classically, by two populations of villi, some with hydropic change and cistern formation and others that are small and not hydropic. The trophoblastic profile is irregular and has been described as fjord-like. Invaginations or inclusions of trophoblast are common. There may be a lacey appearance to the syncytiotrophoblast and the trophoblast hyperplasia is focal. Unlike CHM, there may be extensive fetal vasculature with fetal blood cells present.

In our practice, any case in which cystic villi are identified grossly is submitted for histological examination, flow cytometry, and cytogenetic analysis. Tissue is retained frozen at −70°C in the event that additional studies are required. The slides are examined, and if a diagnosis of CHM is made on morphological grounds, a p57 stain is ordered to support that diagnosis. The case is reported on histopathological grounds, and the results of additional studies are reported as they become available. Similarly, if the histological diagnosis is of PHM, the diagnosis is issued and flow cytometry and/or cytogenetic results are added later. If the case appears to be a hydropic abortus, with no evidence of trophoblastic hyperplasia, p57 is ordered and the results of flow cytometry and cytogenetic analysis are awaited.

Second Trimester Pregnancy Loss

With completion of the embryonic phase of life, all organ systems are developed. The forces that lead to loss of pregnancy during fetal life are somewhat different than during embryonic life—while chromosome abnormality remains a significant factor, it is considerably less so than in first trimester losses, and the types of chromosome abnormalities more closely resemble those seen in third trimester losses and neonates. Nonchromosomal factors such as twinning and placental pathology assume a larger role, and thus the causes of second trimester loss are more heterogeneous with a broader range of implications for counseling and management of future pregnancy.

As many of the cases examined in the fetal pathology service come after diagnosis of intrauterine fetal death, maceration of tissues is a problem that must be addressed. The characteristic features of various disorders are present but may be altered or obscured by the effects of maceration. Maceration is not a diagnosis and should not be considered a limitation to the examination of affected fetuses. The extent of examination varies between institutions, with external examination of a formalin-fixed fetus sufficing in some laboratories, while others provide complete autopsy examination. The latter is the only way of adequately assessing such specimens, and examination other than complete autopsy with examination of the placenta should be considered incomplete.

The autopsy of fetal specimens is conducted exactly as in all other perinatal cases: a complete external examination is performed, skeletal survey is done as indicated, and internal examination with dissection of all organ systems, including central nervous system (CNS), is performed. The external examination includes an assessment of all growth parameters and comparison to established normal values for the determination of DA and detection of intrauterine growth restriction (IUGR). Sections from all organ systems are submitted for histological examination. Cytogenetic studies are initiated in all cases of intrauterine death, abnormal maternal serum screening, hydrops fetalis, fetal anomaly, cystic placental abnormality, and maternal age 35 years or more. Fetal and placental tissues are frozen in all cases in the event that the tissue is required for CGH or other genetic studies. When indicated, tissues are submitted for molecular genetic analysis for disorders such as hemoglobinopathies and for viral cultures. In cases of suspected skeletal dysplasia, skeletal survey is performed, fibroblast cultures are initiated, and the resultant cell line is frozen and retained.

It is not possible to outline all of the disorders encountered in the pathology of second trimester losses. Suffice it to say that with the possible exception of a greater proportion of cases showing chromosome abnormality in the second trimester, one has to be prepared to see all of the pathology encountered in later gestation intrauterine deaths and pregnancy losses (see Chapter 4).

In general, the losses occurring in the second trimester can be considered as fetal deaths (missed abortions) or SAs. In the latter setting, the fetuses are well preserved and the findings raise concerns for uterine anomalies, cervical incompetence, and/or ascending infection.

Uterine anomalies are present in approximately 15% of women who have recurrent miscarriages (14). Pathologic examination of the aborted fetus and placenta cannot make this diagnosis, but the finding of a nonmacerated, anatomically and chromosomally normal fetus with no evidence of ascending infection may lead to clinical consideration of anatomic or mechanical uterine factors.

Ascending infection is a common cause of second trimester pregnancy loss (27,65). There may be no antecedent history. Examination of the fetus shows a well-preserved, anatomically normal fetus. Histological examination of fetal organs may show neutrophils within the gastrointestinal tract and lungs, with pulmonary neutrophils seen more often in later gestation. Gross examination of the placenta may show opaqueness of the fetal membranes, and histological examination shows neutrophils in the chorion and amnion. Fetal response may be present in the form of neutrophils in the fetal surface vessels and in the vessels of the umbilical cord.

Ascending infection has been associated with intrauterine death though this presentation is less common before 20 weeks of GA. It is not clear what the mechanism of intrauterine death is in these cases; death has been reported to be more likely when there is fetal response to intrauterine infection (34,60).

Although a broad range of organisms is responsible for chorioamnionitis, routine culturing of the products of SA is not performed. When there is clinical concern for specific notifiable diseases, such as listeriosis or syphilis, confirmatory cultures are indicated. Listeriosis may occur as outbreaks, and thus knowledge of its role in infection of pregnancy is important from an epidemiological perspective as well as from a clinical one.

Listeriosis is caused by *Listeria monocytogenes*. Infection may be caused by exposure to foods such as unpasteurized or soft cheeses as well as processed meats. Outbreaks may occur and have been related to contaminated processes such as cheese making or machines used in processing meats. Listeriosis may be subclinical or may be associated with gastrointestinal diseases such as vomiting and diarrhea or generalized malaise that includes fever and myalgias. Infection in pregnant women is associated with an increased risk of intrauterine death and SA, including both first and second trimester SAs.

Pathologically, listeriosis may be suspected when external examination of a fetus shows small white lesions on the skin, which are confirmed to be small abscesses in which organisms abound. Similar abscesses may be identified in fetal organs. Gross examination of the placenta may be normal or show characteristic gross features of ascending infection. Histological examination usually shows chorioamnionitis that may be severe. The characteristic lesion of listeriosis is acute villus abscess. Gram-positive bacilli are abundant on tissue Gram stain (Figures 2-16 [skin] and 2-17 [villus abscess]).

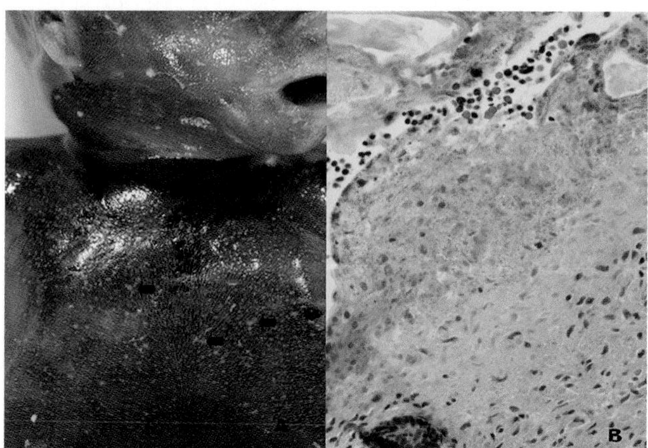

FIGURE 2-16 ■ Listeriosis. **A:** Gross examination shows small white nodules/plaques on the skin of second trimester fetus (*arrows*). **B:** Histological examination shows necrosis with abundant bacteria, shown to be Gram-positive bacilli, culture positive for *Listeria monocytogenes*.

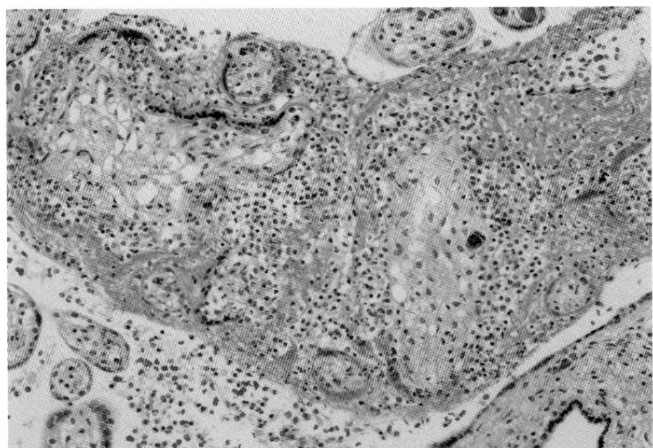

FIGURE 2-17 ■ Villus abscesses of listeriosis associated with severe, acute chorioamnionitis.

Other infections, including viral infections, can account for intrauterine death in the second trimester, with CMV being the viral infection most commonly encountered in fetal death (2). Fetuses affected by CMV may be grossly morphologically normal aside from the effects of retention after fetal death but may also show hepatic calcification and CNS abnormalities. Histological examination of fetal organs may show mononuclear inflammatory infiltrates, ranging in severity, and CMV inclusions may be identified. Destructive lesions may be seen in affected organs. The placenta will show lymphoplasmacytic villitis, and CMV inclusions are often readily identifiable on routine H&E stains (Figure 2-18). *In situ* hybridization with appropriate probes can be used for confirmation, as necessary. There may be a discrepancy between the severity of placental manifestations and those of the fetal organs—it often appears that the fetal organs are more likely to show inclusions and inflammation when the placental inflammation is milder.

Syphilis is encountered with increasing frequency in the obstetric population, including in fetal deaths. Spirochetes may be readily identified in fetal organs, and the placenta shows the features described elsewhere (see Chapter 9), including villitis, villus edema, and vascular changes.

Chromosome abnormality is encountered less often in second trimester losses than in those occurring in the first trimester, and the type of aneuploidy encountered is less varied, bearing a closer resemblance to the range observed nearer term (see Chapter 3). The trisomies encountered during life, trisomy 21, 13, and 18, as well as monosomy X and triploidy are the most commonly identified abnormalities. These abnormalities are expected to be encountered in second trimester miscarriages because intrauterine survival is profoundly affected, with only a minority of chromosomally abnormal cases surviving to term; it is estimated that only 20% of trisomy 21 conceptions, 5% of trisomy 18 conceptions, and 1% of monosomy X conceptions survive to be liveborn. The mechanism allowing some of the chromosome abnormalities, such as trisomy 13 and 18, to survive into later gestation has been suggested to be the presence of a normal cell line in trophoblast. Placental mosaicism has not been shown to account for the survival of trisomy 21 concepti.

Trisomy 21

Trisomy 21 syndrome in the fetus shows the same range of developmental anomalies observed in liveborns and may be associated with abnormalities of maternal serum markers (Table 3-5). In addition, it is common for trisomy 21 (+21) to present as hydrops fetalis, with generalized subcutaneous edema and nuchal hygroma (Figure 2-19). The only feature observed more commonly in those +21 cases presenting as intrauterine death as opposed to those terminated after prenatal cytogenetic diagnosis is hydrops fetalis; the other anomalies do not appear to be different between the two

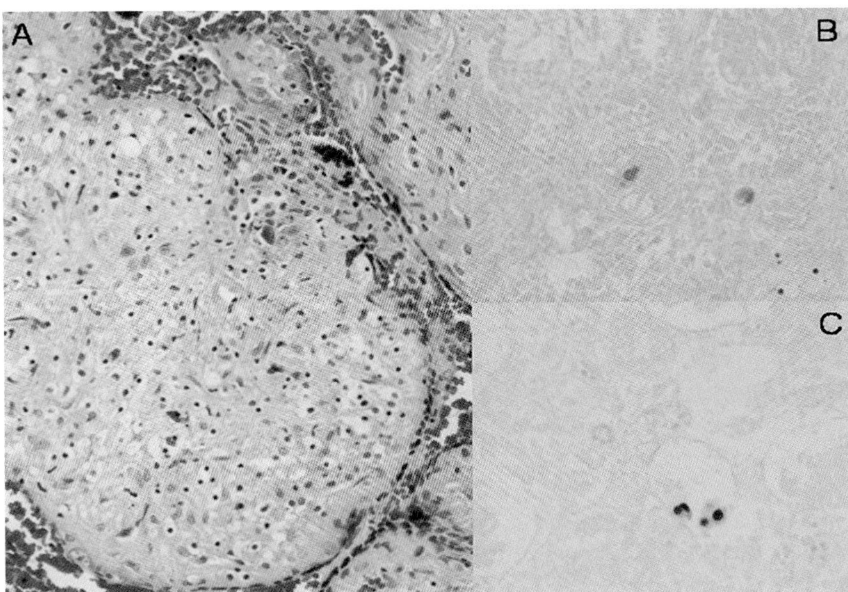

FIGURE 2-18 ■ CMV in macerated second trimester fetus. **A:** Villitis with viral inclusions. **B:** Viral inclusions in kidney. **C:** *In situ* hybridization for CMV highlights inclusions.

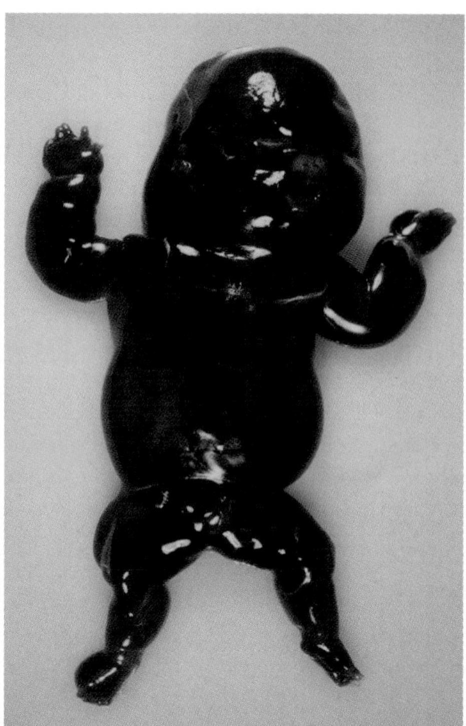

FIGURE 2-19■Trisomy 21 syndrome. Hydropic fetus confirmed by cytogenetic analysis to have trisomy 21. No other internal anomalies.

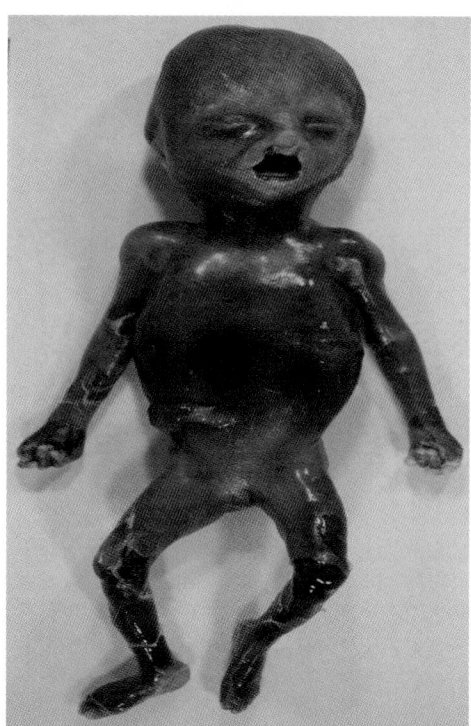

FIGURE 2-20■Trisomy 18 syndrome. Fetus showing rounded head and rather small face with bilateral cleft lip and palate. Hands show characteristic clenched appearance. Internal examination showed horseshoe kidney, single umbilical artery, ventricular septal defect (VSD), and dysplasia of the cardiac valves.

groups and thus do not provide an explanation to account for the survival of only some +21 conceptions until later gestation. The presence of features such as atrioventricular cardiac defect suggests trisomy 21 syndrome, but cytogenetic analysis is required for confirmation. Occasionally, myeloproliferative syndrome with hepatic fibrosis is identified in a hydropic +21 fetus, but this does not account for all hydrops fetalis observed in trisomy 21. Identification of the specific chromosome abnormality is necessary as diagnosis will affect management of subsequent pregnancies. There is an empiric risk of recurrence of trisomy on the order of 1% after a pregnancy (second trimester or later) is affected by trisomy, whereas other chromosome abnormalities, such as monosomy X, are not associated with the increased risk of recurrence. In addition, if the trisomy 21 is the result of a robertsonian translocation carried in balanced form by one parent, the risk for recurrent trisomy 21 is even higher.

Trisomy 18

Fetuses with trisomy 18 syndrome may present as intrauterine death with no external anomalies and may have been associated with abnormal maternal serum screening, including very low estriol levels. The assessment of IUGR can be difficult in a case where there is maceration, as retention after fetal death may account for some of the discrepancy in fetal growth parameters. Trisomy 18 syndrome fetuses often show a somewhat rounded appearance to the head with a small face (Figure 2-20). The hands show flexion of the fingers, with the second and fifth fingers clasped over the third and fourth, respectively. Feet may show prominent heels and rocker bottom feet, though these features are subjective and often overstated. Internal examination may be normal or may show the internal abnormalities described in liveborns, with renal anomalies such as horseshoe kidney being one of the most commonly observed (See Chapter 3, Table 3-6). Dysplasia of cardiac valves is encountered in most cases and has been referred to as "diaphanous dysplasia." Although it has been suggested that there are more female than male fetuses with trisomy 18, a review of our data of trisomy 18 fetuses, either spontaneously or therapeutically aborted, showed no variation from the expected sex chromosome ratio and no difference between those miscarried and those therapeutically aborted.

Trisomy 13

Trisomy 13 may also present as otherwise unanticipated fetal death, with only 5% of all trisomy 13 conceptions surviving to be liveborn. There is often cleft lip and palate, and the facial abnormalities may include those reflective of the characteristic brain anomaly, holoprosencephaly, and include proboscis and synophthalmia (Figure 2-21). There is often postaxial polydactyly. There may be an omphalocele and internal anomalies affecting a variety of systems including the kidneys, which may be enlarged and show cystic change, and the heart, which characteristically shows a tetralogy of Fallot or truncus arteriosus (See Chapter 3, Table 3-7). At gross examination, the differential diagnosis includes Meckel-Gruber and pseudo–trisomy 13 syndromes.

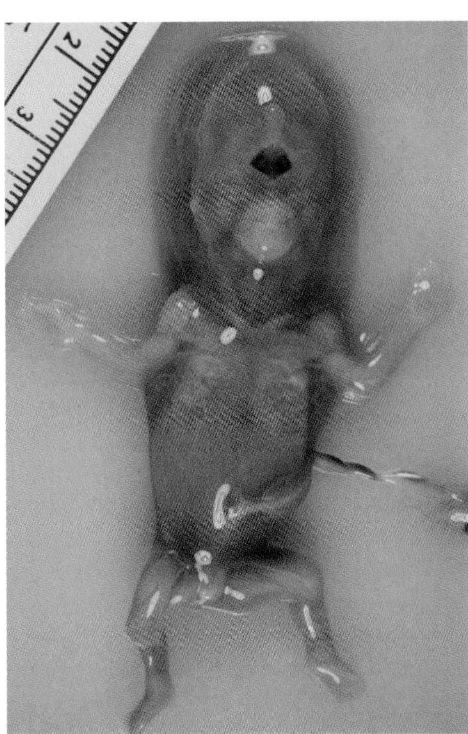

FIGURE 2-21 ■ Trisomy 13 syndrome. Macerated fetus showing synophthalmia with proboscis. Bilateral postaxial polydactyly of feet. Internal examination showed VSD.

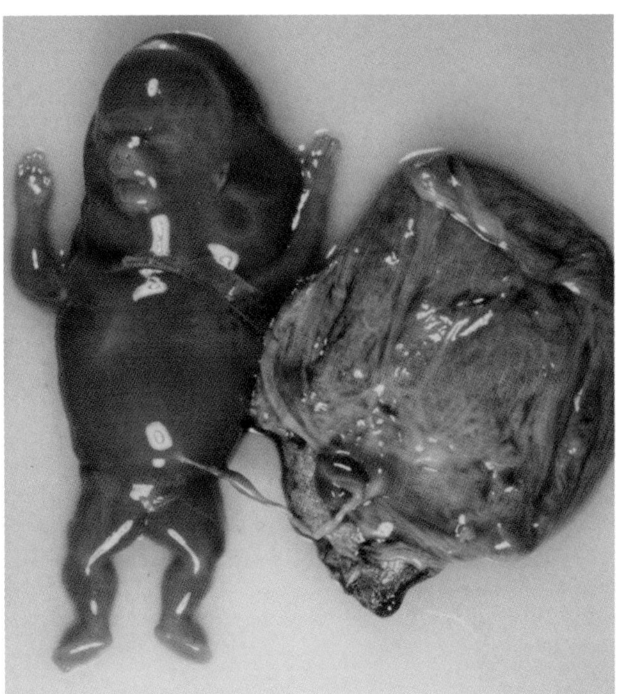

FIGURE 2-22 ■ Monosomy X syndrome. Macerated female fetus showing hydrops fetalis with large cystic nuchal hygroma. Internal examination showed hypoplasia of the aorta.

Monosomy X

Monosomy X is also known as Turner syndrome. In the fetal period, this most commonly presents as hydrops fetalis, often with a very large cystic hygroma. Accentuation of the subcutaneous edema on the dorsal aspects of the hands and feet is characteristic but nonspecific. These fetuses are female and show normal female genitalia, internally and externally. Characteristic anomalies include left-sided cardiac anomalies such as hypoplasia of the aortic arch and/or left ventricle. Renal anomalies include horseshoe kidney (Figure 2-22).

Triploidy

Triploidy is the presence of an entire extra haploid set of chromosomes, which may be of maternal (digynic) or paternal (diandric) origin. In the fetal period, digynic triploidy predominates, accounting for the majority of cases (42). Although the chromosome abnormality is numerically the same, an epigenetic phenomenon known as imprinting causes the fetal and placental phenotypes to vary quite significantly from each other.

In general, triploidy is characterized by anomalies that affect almost every organ system and can be present in both digynic triploidy and diandric triploidy. Complete syndactyly of the third and fourth fingers is a characteristic feature of triploidy, independent of parental origin. Thus far, only adrenal hypoplasia has been shown to be dependent on parental origin, being found in digynic triploids. The parental origin effects appear to be limited to growth patterns in both the fetus and the placenta. Digynic triploidy is characterized by marked asymmetric IUGR, with the head size being relatively well preserved compared to the trunk and extremities, which are very thin (Figure 2-23). There is marked adrenal hypoplasia as observed in other cases of

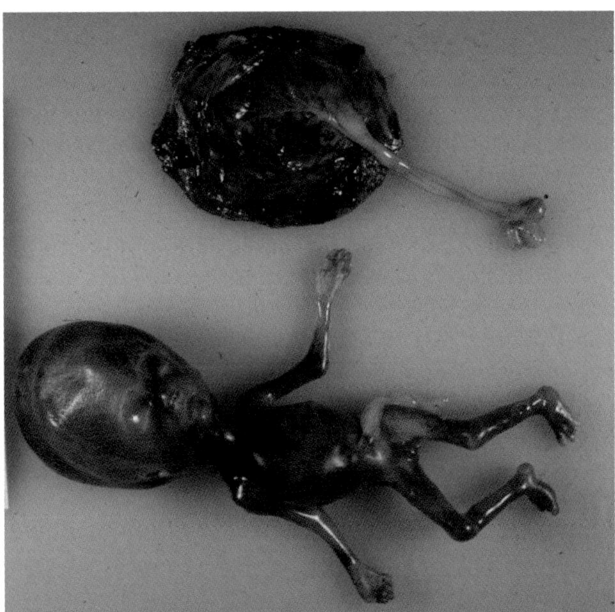

FIGURE 2-23 ■ Digynic triploid phenotype—the phenotype most often encountered in triploid fetuses. Asymmetric IUGR, with relative sparing of the head and thin extremities. No molar change is seen in the placenta.

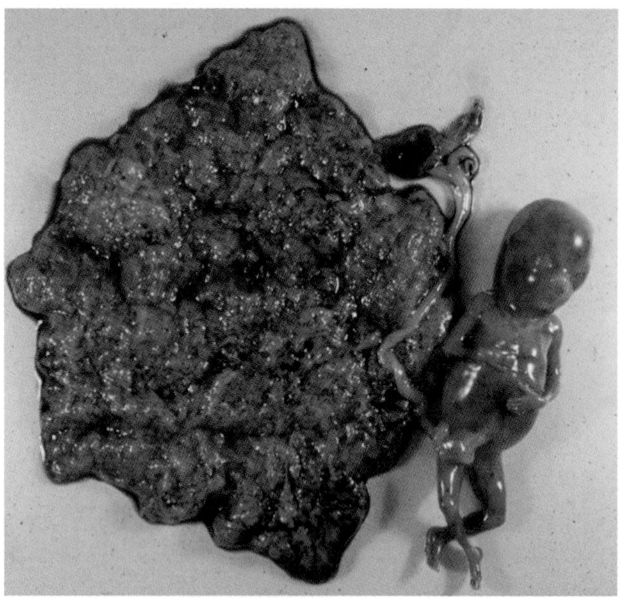

FIGURE 2-24 ■ Diandric triploid phenotype—the phenotype seen only rarely in triploid fetuses. Growth parameters better preserved. Large placenta shows changes of PHM.

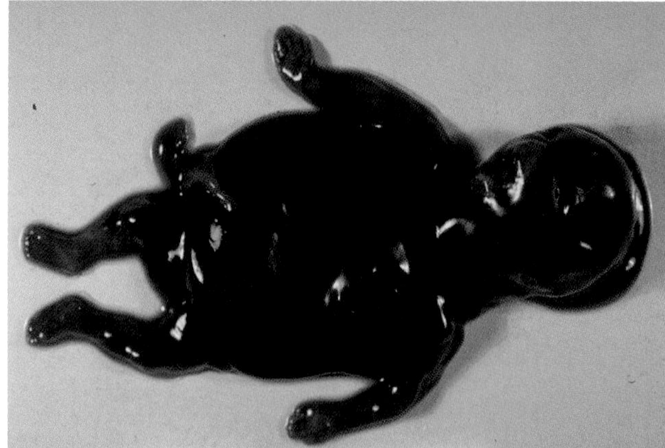

FIGURE 2-25 ■ Hydrops fetalis, cause not determined, after extensive investigation. Genetic counseling should include possibility of undiagnosed genetic conditions, with recurrence risks as high as 25%.

severe IUGR, consistent with the role of placental function in intrauterine adrenal growth and development. Other anomalies are varied and affect all organ systems. The placenta is abnormally small and shows no villus edema or trophoblastic hyperplasia. In diandric triploidy, growth is better preserved, but there may be symmetric IUGR (Figure 2-24). The placenta shows changes of PHM with villus edema and cistern formation, with focal trophoblastic hyperplasia involving the syncytiotrophoblast, which can have a lacey appearance with invaginations into the villus stromal core. The growth and placental differences are reflected in the abnormalities observed in maternal serum screening with digynic triploids showing markedly decreased estriol and human chorionic gonadotropin (hCG), while the diandric triploids can show markedly increased levels of alpha-fetoprotein (AFP) and hCG.

Hydrops Fetalis

Hydrops fetalis is a common presentation in second trimester fetal deaths and warrants complete evaluation for diagnosis, as in those cases diagnosed as stillbirths (Figure 2-25). The differential diagnosis is extensive and includes chromosome abnormality, infection such as CMV and parvovirus B19, hemoglobinopathies such as thalassemia, antibodies such as Rh isoimmunization, fetal arrhythmias, congenital pulmonary airway malformations of the lung, tumors, and metabolic disorders (see Chapter 4) (37,44). Accordingly, the approach to hydrops fetalis includes complete autopsy examination with cytogenetic analysis, viral cultures, PCR for parvovirus, initiation of fibroblast cultures, and retention of a variety of tissues for freezing at −70°C in the event that additional studies such as alpha-thalassemia gene studies are required. With the exclusion of these entities, one is left with a diagnosis of hydrops fetalis, etiology undetected. Because of the possibility of an undetected metabolic condition leading to the hydrops, genetic counseling considers the risk of an undiagnosed autosomal recessive condition; thus, the risk of recurrence may be as high as 25% for each subsequent pregnancy.

Twinning

Monozygous twinning is associated with an increased risk of intrauterine fetal death and may occur on the basis of vascular anastomoses, leading to twin-twin transfusion syndrome (Figure 2-26) or twin reversed arterial perfusion (TRAP)

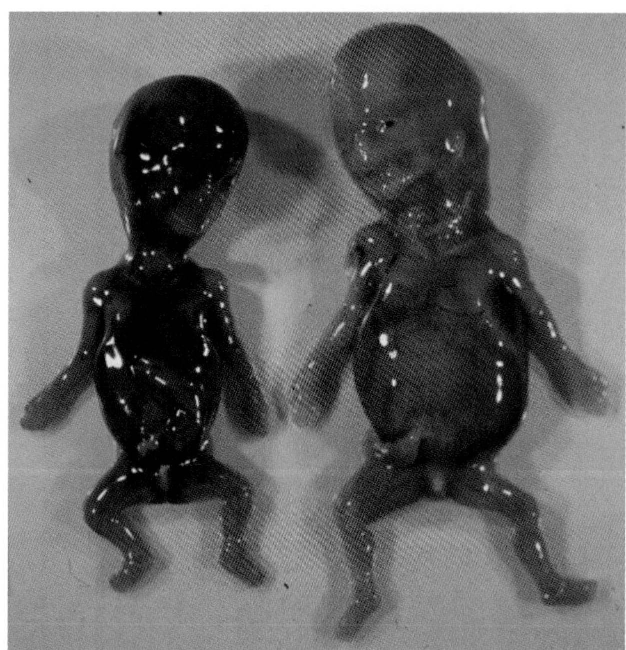

FIGURE 2-26 ■ Twin-twin transfusion syndrome in intrauterine death. Monochorionic twin fetuses show size difference as well as differences in the degree of congestion, consistent with circulatory imbalance.

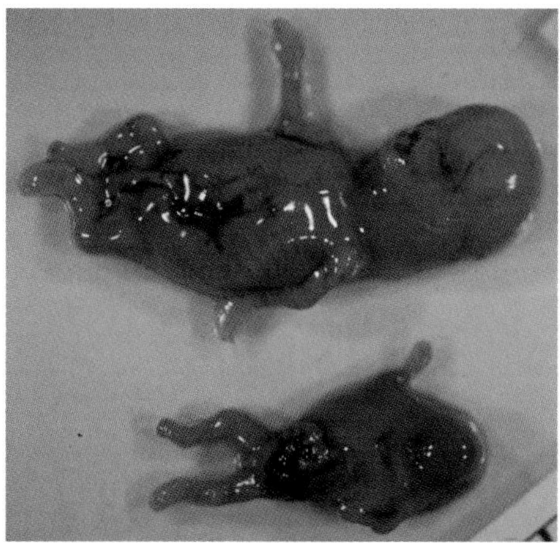

FIGURE 2-27 ■ TRAP sequence, with normal pump twin and acardiac recipient twin.

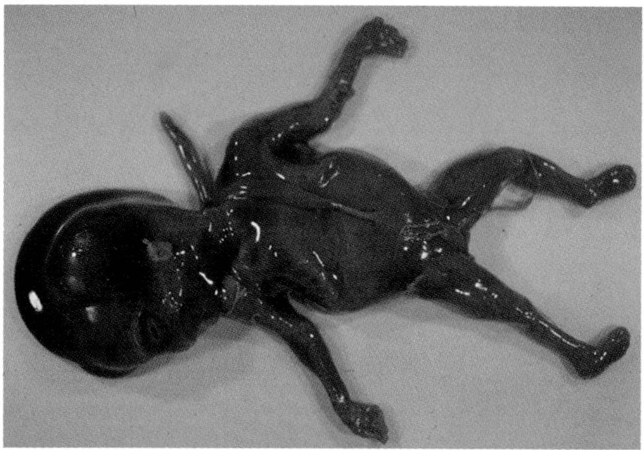

FIGURE 2-28 ■ Probable cord entanglement in intrauterine fetal death.

sequence (23,70–72). The former cannot be diagnosed conclusively but can be suggested if there are growth and/or perfusion discrepancies between the two fetuses. TRAP is a condition in which the umbilical cords of monochorionic monoamniotic twins are implanted very close to one another, establishing large vascular anastomoses. It is hypothesized that some event leads to an imbalance in the shunting of blood, resulting in reversed perfusion such that one twin receives deoxygenated blood from the other via retrograde flow through its umbilical artery. This results in hypoxia in the recipient twin with resultant tissue necrosis, most severe in the cranial aspect. Thus, the tissues of the perfused twin regress, leading to an acardiac, acephalic twin (Figure 2-27). This perfusion abnormality may result in the death of both twins, or the acardiac twin may be delivered at term with the coexisting twin. Monoamniotic twins are also more likely to have cord entanglement that can lead to compromise of umbilical cord blood flow, resulting in the death of both twins.

Umbilical Cord Compromise

Umbilical cord compromise can occur in a variety of settings and results in the death of the fetus (4,6,29,32,51). In some cases, there may be no gross features to suggest the cause of death, whereas other cases show features, such as entanglement that could not have occurred postmortem, that suggest the diagnosis (Figure 2-28). Some have identified histological features that support a diagnosis of cord blood flow restriction (50); some of the features are difficult to assess in the very macerated fetus. There has been considerable controversy as to whether the twist at the junction of the umbilical cord with the abdominal wall often observed in macerated fetuses is a cause of cord compromise or a postmortem artifact; we have observed this finding in cases of pregnancy termination in which death has been caused by potassium chloride injection prior to delivery, and thus we consider it usually to be a postmortem artifact.

Limb–Body Wall Complex

Limb–body wall complex (LBWC) is a disorder within the spectrum of short cord or placental adhesion sequence, is characterized usually by limb anomalies, often absence of an entire limb, associated with a large body wall defect and an abnormally short umbilical cord, and is usually chromosomally normal (Figure 2-29) (70,71). With the routine use of detailed ultrasound examination in pregnancy, these cases are now more often encountered as products of pregnancy termination but may present as early intrauterine death, presumably on the basis of compromise of umbilical cord blood flow.

Postprocedure Pregnancy Loss

Loss of pregnancy can occur after invasive prenatal procedures such as chorionic villus sampling and amniocentesis. The rate varies with institution, usually being on the order of 0.5%, although some studies show no significant increase in fetal loss in those who had amniocentesis than in those who did not (17,49). The loss can take the form of SA or fetal death. Ascending infection is one cause of SA, while placental circulatory abnormalities have been hypothesized to account for fetal death. For quality assurance purposes, losses occurring within a month of an invasive procedure are considered postprocedure losses.

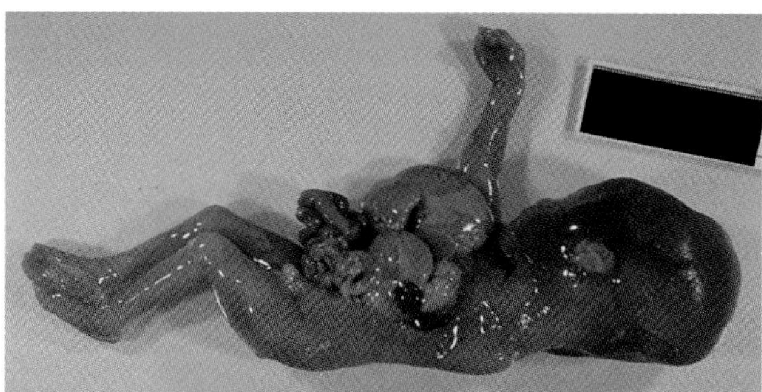

FIGURE 2-29 ■ LBWC in intrauterine death. Large body wall defect, absence of limb, and abnormally short umbilical cord.

REFERENCES

1. Adelberg AM, Kuller JA. Thrombophilias and recurrent miscarriage. *Obstet Gynecol Surv* 2002;57(10):703–709.
2. Al-Adnani M, Sebire NJ. The role of perinatal pathological examination in subclinical infection in obstetrics. *Best Pract Res Clin Obstet Gynaecol* 2007;21(3):505–521.
3. Allen VM, Wilson RD, Cheung A. Pregnancy outcomes after assisted reproductive technology. *J Obstet Gynaecol Can* 2006;28(3): 220–250.
4. Baergen RN. Cord abnormalities, structural lesions, and cord "accidents." *Semin Diagn Pathol* 2007;24(1):23–32.
5. Beever CL, Stephenson MD, Penaherrera MS, et al. Skewed X-chromosome inactivation is associated with trisomy in women ascertained on the basis of recurrent spontaneous abortion or chromosomally abnormal pregnancies. *Am J Hum Genet* 2003;72(2):399–407.
6. Bendon RW. Articles on umbilical cord torsion and fetal death. *Pediatr Dev Pathol* 2007;10(2):165–166.
7. Benkhalifa M, Kasakyan S, Clement P, et al. Array comparative genomic hybridization profiling of first-trimester spontaneous abortions that fail to grow in vitro. *Prenat Diagn* 2005;25(10):894–900.
8. Bettio D, Venci A, Levi Setti PE. Chromosomal abnormalities in miscarriages after different assisted reproduction procedures. *Placenta* 2008;29(Suppl B):126–128.
9. Bick RL. Antiphospholipid syndrome in pregnancy. *Hematol Oncol Clin North Am* 2008;22(1):107–120, vii.
10. Bortolussi R. Listeriosis: a primer. *CMAJ* 2008;179(8):795–797.
11. Boyd TK, Redline RW. Chronic histiocytic intervillositis: a placental lesion associated with recurrent reproductive loss. *Hum Pathol* 2000;31(11):1389–1396.
12. Cheung AN, Khoo US, Lai CY, et al. Metastatic trophoblastic disease after an initial diagnosis of partial hydatidiform mole: genotyping and chromosome in situ hybridization analysis. *Cancer* 2004;100(7): 1411–1417.
13. Christiansen OB, Nielsen HS, Kolte A, et al. Research methodology and epidemiology of relevance in recurrent pregnancy loss. *Semin Reprod Med* 2006;24(1):5–16.
14. Devi Wold AS, Pham N, Arici A. Anatomic factors in recurrent pregnancy loss. *Semin Reprod Med* 2006;24(1):25–32.
15. Dilley A, Benito C, Hooper WC, et al. Mutations in the factor V, prothrombin and MTHFR genes are not risk factors for recurrent fetal loss. *J Matern Fetal Neonatal Med* 2002;11(3):176–182.
16. Doss BJ, Greene MF, Hill J, et al. Massive chronic intervillositis associated with recurrent abortions. *Hum Pathol* 1995;26(11): 1245–1251.
17. Eddleman KA, Malone FD, Sullivan L, et al. Pregnancy loss rates after midtrimester amniocentesis. *Obstet Gynecol* 2006;108(5): 1067–1072.
18. Fowler DJ, Lindsay I, Seckl MJ, et al. Routine pre-evacuation ultrasound diagnosis of hydatidiform mole: experience of more than 1000 cases from a regional referral center. *Ultrasound Obstet Gynecol* 2006;27(1):56–60.
19. Fukunaga M, Katabuchi H, Nagasaka T, et al. Interobserver and intraobserver variability in the diagnosis of hydatidiform mole. *Am J Surg Pathol* 2005;29(7):942–947.
20. Genest DR. Partial hydatidiform mole: clinicopathological features, differential diagnosis, ploidy and molecular studies, and gold standards for diagnosis. *Int J Gynecol Pathol* 2001;20(4):315–322.
21. ESHRE Capri Workshop Group. Genetic aspects of female reproduction. *Hum Reprod Update* 2008;14(4):293–307.
22. Gjerris AC, Loft A, Pinborg A, et al. Prenatal testing among women pregnant after assisted reproductive techniques in Denmark 1995–2000: a national cohort study. *Hum Reprod* 2008;23(7):1545–1552.
23. Hanafy A, Peterson CM. Twin-reversed arterial perfusion (TRAP) sequence: case reports and review of literature. *Aust N Z J Obstet Gynaecol* 1997;37(2):187–191.
24. Harkness LM, Baird DT. Morphological and molecular characteristics of living human fetuses between Carnegie stages 7 and 23: developmental stages in the post-implantation embryo. *Hum Reprod Update* 1997;3(1):3–23.
25. Harris MJ, Poland BJ, Dill FJ. Triploidy in 40 human spontaneous abortuses: assessment of phenotype in embryos. *Obstet Gynecol* 1981;57(5):600–606.
26. Hassold T, Hall H, Hunt P. The origin of human aneuploidy: where we have been, where we are going. *Hum Mol Genet* 2007;16(2): R203–R208.
27. Heller DS, Moorehouse-Moore C, Skurnick J, et al. Second-trimester pregnancy loss at an urban hospital. *Infect Dis Obstet Gynecol* 2003;11(2):117–122.
28. Hogge WA, Prosen TL, Lanasa MC, et al. Recurrent spontaneous abortion and skewed X-inactivation: is there an association? *Am J Obstet Gynecol* 2007;196(4):384, e381–386; discussion 384, e386–388.
29. Horn LC, Faber R, Stepan H, et al. Umbilical cord hypercoiling and thinning: a rare cause of intrauterine death in the second trimester of pregnancy. *Pediatr Dev Pathol* 2006;9(1):20–24.
30. Jindal P, Regan L, Fourkala EO, et al. Placental pathology of recurrent spontaneous abortion: the role of histopathological examination of products of conception in routine clinical practice: a mini review. *Hum Reprod* 2007;22(2):313–316.
31. Jivraj S, Rai R, Underwood J, et al. Genetic thrombophilic mutations among couples with recurrent miscarriage. *Hum Reprod* 2006;21(5):1161–1165.
32. Kaplan C. Twist and shout: the excitement over coils in the umbilical cord. *Pediatr Dev Pathol* 2006;9(1):1–2.
33. Kutteh WH, Triplett DA. Thrombophilias and recurrent pregnancy loss. *Semin Reprod Med* 2006;24(1):54–66.
34. Lahra MM, Gordon A, Jeffery HE. Chorioamnionitis and fetal response in stillbirth. *Am J Obstet Gynecol* 2007;196(3):229, e221–224.
35. Lathi RB, Mark SD, Westphal LM, et al. Cytogenetic testing of anembryonic pregnancies compared to embryonic missed abortions. *J Assist Reprod Genet* 2007;24(11):521–524.
36. Lomax B, Tang S, Separovic E, et al. Comparative genomic hybridization in combination with flow cytometry improves results of cytogenetic analysis of spontaneous abortions. *Am J Hum Genet* 2000;66(5):1516–1521.
37. Machin GA. Hydrops revisited: literature review of 1,414 cases published in the 1980s. *Am J Med Genet* 1989;34(3):366–390.
38. Makrydimas G, Sebire NJ, Lolis D, et al. Fetal loss following ultrasound diagnosis of a live fetus at 6–10 weeks of gestation. *Ultrasound Obstet Gynecol* 2003;22(4):368–372.
39. Matsui H, Iizuka Y and Sekiya S. Incidence of invasive mole and choriocarcinoma following partial hydatidiform mole. *Int J Gynaecol Obstet* 1996;53(1):63–64.
40. McFadden DE, Jiang R, Langlois S, et al. Dispermy—origin of diandric triploidy: brief communication. *Hum Reprod* 2002;17(12): 3037–3038.
41. McFadden DE, Kalousek DK. Survey of neural tube defects in spontaneously aborted embryos. *Am J Med Genet* 1989;32(3): 356–358.
42. McFadden DE, Langlois S. Parental and meiotic origin of triploidy in the embryonic and fetal periods. *Clin Genet* 2000;58(3):192–200.
43. McFadden DE, Robinson WP. Phenotype of triploid embryos. *J Med Genet* 2006;43(7):609–612.
44. McGillivray BC, Hall JG. Nonimmune hydrops fetalis. *Pediatr Rev* 1987;9(6):197–202.
45. Medeiros F, Callahan MJ, Elvin JA, et al. Intraplacental choriocarcinoma arising in a second trimester placenta with partial hydatidiform mole. *Int J Gynecol Pathol* 2008;27(2):247–251.
46. Merchant SH, Amin MB, Viswanatha DS, et al. p57KIP2 immunohistochemistry in early molar pregnancies: emphasis on its complementary role in the differential diagnosis of hydropic abortuses. *Hum Pathol* 2005;36(2):180–186.

47. Minguillon C, Eiben B, Bahr-Porsch S, et al. The predictive value of chorionic villus histology for identifying chromosomally normal and abnormal spontaneous abortions. *Hum Genet* 1989;82(4):373–376.
48. O'Rahilly R, Muller F. *Developmental Stages in Human Embryos, Publication 637*. Washintgon, DC: Carnegie Institute of Washington; 1987.
49. Odibo AO, Gray DL, Dicke JM, et al. Revisiting the fetal loss rate after second-trimester genetic amniocentesis: a single center's 16-year experience. *Obstet Gynecol* 2008;111(3):589–595.
50. Parast MM, Crum CP, Boyd TK. Placental histologic criteria for umbilical blood flow restriction in unexplained stillbirth. *Hum Pathol* 2008;39(6):948–953.
51. Peng HQ, Levitin-Smith M, Rochelson B, et al. Umbilical cord stricture and overcoiling are common causes of fetal demise. *Pediatr Dev Pathol* 2006;9(1):14–19.
52. Poland BJ, Lowry RB. The use of spontaneous abortuses and stillbirths in genetic counseling. *Am J Obstet Gynecol* 1974;118(3):322–326.
53. Poller DN. When trophoblastic disease is suspected. *Lancet* 2000;356(9239):1443–1444.
54. Redline RW, Hassold T, Zaragoza M. Determinants of villous trophoblastic hyperplasia in spontaneous abortions. *Mod Pathol* 1998;11(8):762–768.
55. Redline RW, Zaragoza M, Hassold T. Prevalence of developmental and inflammatory lesions in nonmolar first-trimester spontaneous abortions. *Hum Pathol* 1999;30(1):93–100.
56. Regan L, Rai R. Epidemiology and the medical causes of miscarriage. *Baillieres Best Pract Res Clin Obstet Gynaecol* 2000;14(5):839–854.
57. Rehder H, Coerdt W, Eggers R, et al. Is there a correlation between morphological and cytogenetic findings in placental tissue from early missed abortions? *Hum Genet* 1989;82(4):377–385.
58. Robinson WP, McFadden DE. Chromosomal genetic disease: numerical aberrations. In: *Encyclopedia of Life Sciences*. 2000, Macmillan Reference Ltd, United Kingdom.
59. Rodger MA, Paidas M, McLintock C, et al. Inherited thrombophilia and pregnancy complications revisited. *Obstet Gynecol* 2008;112 (2 Pt 1):320–324.
60. Romero R, Espinoza J, Goncalves LF, et al. The role of inflammation and infection in preterm birth. *Semin Reprod Med* 2007;25(1):21–39.
61. Salafia CM, Cowchock FS. Placental pathology and antiphospholipid antibodies: a descriptive study. *Am J Perinatol* 1997;14(8):435–441.
62. Schaeffer AJ, Chung J, Heretis K, et al. Comparative genomic hybridization-array analysis enhances the detection of aneuploidies and submicroscopic imbalances in spontaneous miscarriages. *Am J Hum Genet* 2004;74(6):1168–1174.
63. Sebire NJ, Backos M, El Gaddal S, et al. Placental pathology, antiphospholipid antibodies, and pregnancy outcome in recurrent miscarriage patients. *Obstet Gynecol* 2003;101(2):258–263.
64. Seckl MJ, Fisher RA, Salerno G, et al. Choriocarcinoma and partial hydatidiform moles. *Lancet* 2000;356(9223):36–39.
65. Srinivas SK, Ma Y, Sammel MD, et al. Placental inflammation and viral infection are implicated in second trimester pregnancy loss. *Am J Obstet Gynecol* 2006;195(3):797–802.
66. Stephenson MD, Sierra S. Reproductive outcomes in recurrent pregnancy loss associated with a parental carrier of a structural chromosome rearrangement. *Hum Reprod* 2006;21(4):1076–1082.
67. Sugiura-Ogasawara M, Aoki K, Fujii T, et al. Subsequent pregnancy outcomes in recurrent miscarriage patients with a paternal or maternal carrier of a structural chromosome rearrangement. *J Hum Genet* 2008;53(7):622–628.
68. Szulman AE. Examination of the early conceptus. *Arch Pathol Lab Med* 1991;115(7):696–700.
69. Tong S, Kaur A, Walker SP, et al. Miscarriage risk for asymptomatic women after a normal first-trimester prenatal visit. *Obstet Gynecol* 2008;111(3):710–714.
70. Van Allen MI, Curry C, Gallagher L. Limb body wall complex: I. Pathogenesis. *Am J Med Genet* 1987;28(3):529–548.
71. Van Allen MI, Curry C, Walden CE, et al. Limb-body wall complex: II. Limb and spine defects. *Am J Med Genet* 1987;28(3):549–565.
72. Van Allen MI, Smith DW, Shepard TH. Twin reversed arterial perfusion (TRAP) sequence: a study of 14 twin pregnancies with acardius. *Semin Perinatol* 1983;7(4):285–293.
73. Van Horn JT, Craven C, Ward K, et al. Histologic features of placentas and abortion specimens from women with antiphospholipid and antiphospholipid-like syndromes. *Placenta* 2004;25(7):642–648.
74. van Lijnschoten G, Arends JW, De La Fuente AA, et al. Intra- and inter-observer variation in the interpretation of histological features suggesting chromosomal abnormality in early abortion specimens. *Histopathology* 1993;22(1):25–29.
75. Waters BL, Ashikaga T. Significance of perivillous fibrin/oid deposition in uterine evacuation specimens. *Am J Surg Pathol* 2006;30(6): 760–765.
76. Wells M. The pathology of gestational trophoblastic disease: recent advances. *Pathology* 2007;39(1):88–96.
77. Weselak M, Arbuckle TE, Walker MC, et al. The influence of the environment and other exogenous agents on spontaneous abortion risk. *J Toxicol Environ Health B Crit Rev* 2008;11(3–4):221–241.
78. Wolfberg AJ, Berkowitz RS, Goldstein DP, et al. Postevacuation hCG levels and risk of gestational trophoblastic neoplasia in women with complete molar pregnancy. *Obstet Gynecol* 2005;106(3):548–552.
79. Zaragoza MV, Surti U, Redline RW, et al. Parental origin and phenotype of triploidy in spontaneous abortions: predominance of diandry and association with the partial hydatidiform mole. *Am J Hum Genet* 2000;66(6):1807–1820.

CHAPTER 3

Chromosomal Abnormalities

RAJ P. KAPUR
JOSEPH R. SIEBERT

Chromosomal abnormalities are defined as alterations that can be resolved by microscopic examination of banded chromosome preparations. The primary means to recognize chromosomal disorders is a karyotype—organization of all the individual chromosomes from largest to smallest with the shorter chromosomal arms oriented upward. Karyotype analysis has led to the recognition of a wide range of chromosomal abnormalities and corresponding clinical-pathological features. The growth of this discipline is apparent from the rich lexicon that is used to characterize specific types of chromosomal disorders and their consequences. Some of the terms commonly encountered in the practice of pediatric pathology are defined in Table 3-1.

A traditional definition distinguishes chromosomal abnormalities from more subtle genetic alterations (e.g., single base pair changes, microdeletions, epigenetic modifications), despite the fact that chromosomes are the common substrate for all these events. The use of fluorescent molecular probes to interrogate specific genetic sequences blurs this distinction because methods such as fluorescence in situ hybridization (FISH), comparative genomic hybridization (CGH), and spectral karyotyping (SKY) are being used to identify and/or clarify chromosomal rearrangements that frequently encompass more than an individual gene but cannot be resolved in a routine karyotype. At present, it seems reasonable to subclassify genetic defects into microscopically visible chromosomal abnormalities and "submicroscopic" alterations. In addition to changes that affect the nucleotide sequence, submicroscopic alterations also include epigenetic DNA modifications (e.g., methylation, histone acetylation), which influence gene expression without changing the primary sequence. These covalent modifications are involved intimately in parental imprinting, X-chromosome inactivation, and the physiological silencing/activation of genes. Defects in epigenetic regulation are associated with developmental disorders, neoplastic transformation, and other disease states.

The focus of this chapter is traditional karyotypic and selected submicroscopic disorders, which are particularly relevant to the practice of pediatric and surgical pathology. Emphasis is placed on conditions that arise during gametogenesis or prenatally, most of which have developmental consequences. Related topics that are not covered in this chapter include chromosomal rearrangements associated with pediatric neoplasms and mutations that affect mitochondrial DNA. Cytogenetic changes characteristic of childhood tumors are introduced as part of the discussion of specific neoplasms in other chapters and have been the subject of several excellent reviews (42,67,100,105). For information about the mitochondrial genome and related diseases, the reader is referred to the review by Schapira (108).

TRADITIONAL CYTOGENETIC ANALYSIS (THE KARYOTYPE)

Routine cytogenetic studies require mitotically active cells. The goal is to visualize chromosomes in their most elongate forms (prophase or early metaphase), identify each one, and assess its integrity. Distinctive features for each chromosome include size, centromere position, and banding pattern, which refers to characteristic zones of GC- or AT-rich sequences that are resolved by specific stains (Table 3-2) (89). Giemsa (G)-banding is the routine procedure employed by most laboratories. Recognition of subtle structural defects is limited ultimately by the number of chromosomal bands that can be unambiguously identified, which varies with cell type, staining procedures, culture conditions, and laboratory technique (Table 3-3) (64). The conventional range of reportable karyotypes extends from 300–450 (low resolution) to 650–850 (high resolution) bands. Explicit statement of the band resolution is an integral part of a cytogenetics report.

An international standardized nomenclature exists for cytogenetic results (111). The format and abbreviations are designed to encompass the broad range of observable chromosomal aberrations and the methods by which they are resolved. Some of the more frequently used abbreviations are summarized in Table 3-4 with some examples of their use.

Table 3-1 ■ GLOSSARY OF TERMS USED FREQUENTLY IN CYTOGENETICS

Aneuploidy—numerical deviations of just one or a few chromosomes. Usually includes trisomies and monosomies, but not polyploidy. Does not encompass other types of genetic imbalance (e.g., partial deletions or duplications of a specific chromosome).
Chimerism—coexistence, within one conceptus, of more than one cell lineage due to the union of two originally separate embryos.
Chromosomal mosaicism—coexistence, within one conceptus, of two or more chromosomally distinct cell lines that derived from a single zygote.
Deletion—loss of a portion of a chromosome.
Duplication—gain of a portion of a chromosome.
Insertion—intercalation of a portion of one chromosome into a second chromosome (interchromosomal) or into a new location on the original chromosome (intrachromosomal).
Inversion—180-degree rotation of an intrachromosomal segment.
Pericentric—the inverted segment encompasses the centromere.
Paracentric—the centromere is excluded from the inverted segment.
Nondisjunction—failure of homologous chromosomes or sister chromatids to segregate properly during cell division.
Parental imprinting—differential expression of alleles acquired from each parent.
Polyploidy—one or more complete extra set of chromosomes (triploidy, tetraploidy, etc.).
Ring chromosome—circular chromosome, which is formed from a chromosome by end-to-end fusion of either the telomeres or subtelomeric sites which are exposed by chromosomal breaks in the long and short arms.
Translocation—recombination of nonhomologous parts of two chromosomes.
Balanced—reciprocal translocation with no net gain or loss of the diploid chromosomal content.
Unbalanced—net gain and loss of translocated portions of specific chromosomes due to segregation of a balanced translocation during meiosis.
Robertsonian—centric or pericentric translocation of acrocentric chromosomes (e.g., t[13q14q]).
Uniparental disomy—both chromosomes of a homologous pair are derived from the same parent.
Heteroisodisomy—UPD in which the two homologues differ.
Isodisomy—UPD in which the homologues are identical.

Common tissue sources for routine cytogenetic study include blood (phytohemagglutinin-stimulated T lymphocytes), amniotic fluid (amniotic epithelial cells), chorionic villous biopsy (trophoblast and/or fibroblasts), and skin (fibroblasts). For most samples, days to weeks of tissue culture is required to produce a cohort of cells that can be pharmacologically arrested in metaphase, harvested, stained, and analyzed. These cell culture preparations differ from *direct preps*, which can be obtained within 48 hours from tissue samples with high basal rates of proliferation (e.g., leukemic blasts, chorionic trophoblast). It is important to realize that tissue culture may select for subsets of mitotically active cells in the original sample and/or cytogenetic changes that arise *in vitro*. Biased selection in cell culture may yield a karyotype that does not represent particular cells of interest. In this respect, direct preps are more reliable.

Sampling also affects interpretation of cytogenetic results. Some tissue sources contain a mixture of cell types with different chromosomal compositions. Depending on the clinical situation, it may be critical to obtain karyotypic information from one or more of the sampled populations. For example, some individuals are mosaics, whose tissues contain chromosomally different lineages. In the case of a diploid:aneuploid mosaicism, sampling and successful culture of both cell populations are essential to establish the diagnosis cytogenetically. Placental samples can be particularly confusing in this regard. The placenta contains a mixture of cell types that are closely (chorionic stroma, amniocytes), remotely (trophoblast), or not (decidualized endometrium) related to cell lineages of the fetus. Decidualized endometrium is most concentrated at the maternal surface of the placenta. Stromal cells, not trophoblast, are propagated selectively in cultures of chorionic villus samples. Appropriate tissue sampling (fetal versus maternal surface) and culture methods (direct versus prolonged growth *in vitro*) can bias cytogenetic studies toward desired cell types.

Because routine cytogenetic analysis requires successful cell culture, autolysis or contamination by microorganisms may also compromise results. Rapid handling and sterile technique minimize these risks, but for postmortem specimens, particularly stillborn fetuses, significant autolysis may be unavoidable. Several studies have shown that the likelihood of successful culture is inversely related to postmortem interval, particularly the period of time a dead fetus is retained in the uterus (65,74). It is unlikely that a karyotype can be obtained from fetal samples acquired more than 3 days after intrauterine demise (116). Refrigeration slows autolysis considerably, and Macpherson et al. reported

Table 3-2 ■ CYTOGENETIC BANDING TECHNIQUES

Technique	Reagent	Principle Target	Properties
Q (Quinacrine)-banding	Quinacrine fluorophore	AT-rich areas	Fades with time
C (Constitutive heterochromatin)-banding	Acid/alkali-pretreatment prior to Giemsa stain	Stains heterochromatin	Permanent
G (Giemsa)-banding	Proteolytic pretreatment prior to Giemsa stain	AT-rich areas	Permanent
R (Reverse)-banding	Hot alkali prior to Giemsa	GC-rich areas	Permanent (inverse of Q- or G-banding)

Table 3-3 ■ TISSUE SOURCES, CELL TYPES, APPROXIMATE INCUBATION TIMES, AND BAND RESOLUTION FOR TRADITIONAL CYTOGENETIC ANALYSES

Tissue Source	Cell Type	Approximate Incubation Time (64)	Typical Band Resolution
Amniotic fluid	Amniocytes	5–21 days	450–500
Chorionic villi			
Direct preparation	Trophoblast	0–2 days	400–450
Culture		5–21 days	
Peripheral blood	Lymphoblasts	2–4 days	500–650[a]
Skin or soft tissue	Fibroblasts	1–6 weeks	450–500

[a]Higher resolution (>650 bands) is possible with prometaphase preparations.

successful cultures from the tissues of a refrigerated neonate 144 hours after demise (74). In general, fibroblasts seem to be the heartiest cells in most organs. Therefore, fibroblast-rich tissues (e.g., dermis, fascia) are favored sites. Chondrocytes also are reported to fare well despite generalized fetal autolysis (34). Organs such as lung and gastrointestinal tract are less reliable since they may be colonized by microorganisms. If subcutaneous tissue is sampled, it is generally best to procure a sample immediately after the skin has been incised to avoid contamination during subsequent dissection. The skin does not need to be sterilized, but the sample should be taken with a sterile blade, deep to the epidermis and away from the initial incision to exclude surface microbes. If chemicals are used to sterilize the skin, care should be taken not to contaminate the transport medium with toxic agents that may prevent cell culture. For very autolyzed stillborn fetuses, placenta may be the tissue of choice, because it is kept viable by the maternal circulation after the fetus dies (3,27).

Table 3-4 ■ CYTOGENETIC NOMENCLATURE

Common abbreviations:
del, deletion; inv, inversion; dup, duplication; mar, marker chromosome; t, translocation; rob, Robertsonian translocation; pter, terminus of short arm; qter, terminus of long arm; der, derivative (of abnormal recombination)

Normal karyotype

46,XX [20]
- 46: total number of chromosomes
- XX: sex chromosome constitution
- [20]: No. of cells evaluated (often omitted for single cell lines)

Autosomes are specified only when an abnormality is present:

47,XX,+21	**45,XY,-5**	**45,X**
An extra (+) chromosome 21 (*Trisomy 21*)	Missing (-) one copy of chromosome 5 (*Monosomy 5*)	Missing one sex chromosome (*Monosomy X*)

Symbols and band numbers are used to denote complex rearrangements between chromosomes:

46,XX,t(9;22)(q34;q11.2)
- t: Balanced translocation between chromosomes 9 and 22
- ;: Breakpoint in first and second chromosomes are separated by a semicolon

46,XX,der(9)t(9;22)(q34;q11.2)
- der(9): Derivative formed by translocation between chromosomes 9 and 22

KARYOTYPIC DISORDERS

Constitutive karyotypic disorders are extremely common during all stages of development. The results of several studies suggest that 5% to 25% of conceptions are aneuploid, of which 99% are spontaneously aborted (46). Rates and types of chromosomal abnormalities detected in spontaneous abortions differ through gestation: 78% at 2 weeks post conception, 35% to 62% between the first missed menses and 20 weeks, and 4% to 6% for stillborn infants (Table 3-5). The pathology of early embryonic loss and its poor correlation with cytogenetic findings are discussed in Chapter 2. The rate of aneuploidy among all liveborn infants is approximately 0.5%, although the rate in malformed infants is significantly higher (4,73).

The most common karyotypic anomalies are forms of chromosomal aneuploidy (Table 3-6) in which one or a few complete chromosomes are lost or gained during cell division. The underlying basis for aneuploidy is nondisjunction, failure of paired chromatids or homologous chromosomes to segregate appropriately during mitosis or meiosis (17). Premature separation of a chromatid pair during the first meiotic division is another theoretical mechanism to produce an aneuploid gamete, but nondisjunction has received more experimental support (83). Meiotic nondisjunction produces an aneuploid gamete and zygote, which is the basis for most nonmosaic aneuploid conceptuses (33). Autosomal nondisjunction is far more common during oogenesis than spermatogenesis and typically occurs during the first meiotic division (when bivalent chromosomes segregate). By contrast, sex chromosome nondisjunction occurs more commonly during male gametogenesis in the second meiotic division (separation of chromatids). Postzygotic chromosomal nondisjunction during mitosis is the basis for diploid:aneuploid mosaicism, either because an aneuploid clone arises from a diploid zygote or vice versa. Examination of human embryos conceived by *in vitro* fertilization suggests that rates of spontaneous postzygotic nondisjunction are very high (20% to 50% of preimplantation embryos) (8,46).

Chromosomal segregation and cytokinesis are synchronized by meiotic and mitotic checkpoints. The molecules that influence these cellular events have been partially characterized (17). Not surprisingly, genetic or pharmacologic alterations

Table 3-5 ■ INCIDENCE OF ANEUPLOIDY DURING DEVELOPMENT

Gestation (weeks):			0		6–8	20	40
	Sperm	Oocytes	Preimplantation Embryos	Preclinical Abortions	Spontaneous Abortions	Stillbirths	Livebirths
Incidence of aneuploidy	1%–2%	~20%	~20%	?	35%–54%	4%–6%	0.3%–0.6%
Most common aneuploidies	Various	Various	Various	?	45,X; +16, +21, +22, polyploidy	45,X, +13, +18, +21, polyploidy	45X, +13, +18, +21 XXX, XXY, XYY

From reference (49), modified to include data from references (12,62,92).

that disrupt these proteins predispose to nondisjunction and aneuploidy (33). However, most instances of human meiotic nondisjunction are sporadic; in one population-based study, aneuploid spontaneous abortion was not associated with an increased risk of aneuploidy in a subsequent spontaneous abortion (102).

Karyotypic disorders other than aneuploidy involve structural rearrangements (deletions, duplications, and translocations) that alter the normal banding pattern, but not necessarily the total number, of chromosomes. Most of these structural changes arise from recombination between or within individual chromosomes, as discussed later in this chapter (33).

Mosaicism

In the context of human chromosomal disorders, mosaicism refers to the presence of more than one karyotypically distinct cell lineage, derived from a single zygote. Usually, two cell populations are present, one with a normal, diploid chromosome content and another aneuploid cohort. In cytogenetic reports, mosaicism is denoted by a slash that separates the karyotype of each cell population and brackets that indicate the number of cells observed with each karyotype (e.g., 45,X[15]/46XY[5]). Occasionally, both populations are aneuploid. The relative abundance of the two cell populations is highly variable, between individuals and between organs. Interorgan differences may reflect origin of a cytogenetic abnormality in a cell lineage with restricted embryological fates and/or selective pressures that favor a cytogenetically distinct cell population. Because of interorgan differences and the possibility that cytogenetically distinct cell populations may have very different growth properties *in vitro*, routine cytogenetic studies cannot completely exclude low level mosaicism. Evaluation of multiple tissues (skin, blood, and amniocytes) or application of sensitive techniques (e.g., FISH) increases the likelihood of detecting mosaicism. Because aneuploid populations can arise during tissue culture, accepted standards for the diagnosis of mosaicism require 3/100 monosomic cells and 2/100 trisomic cells (118).

Chromosomal mosaicism is a consequence of postzygotic mitotic errors, which can occur at any stage of prenatal development. Empirical data suggest that such errors occur frequently in mitotically active cell populations (e.g., hematopoietic precursors), but the majority of aneuploid cells are eliminated by unknown mechanisms (17). Many neoplasms are complex mosaics, often comprised of several cytogenetically distinct cell populations.

Conceptuses with aneuploid:diploid mosaicism can arise from either a diploid or aneuploid zygote. In a diploid embryo, nondisjunction of a single chromatid pair during mitosis will give rise to daughter cells that are trisomic and monosomic. Aneuploid:diploid mosaicism results from survival and clonal expansion of either the trisomic or monosomic lineages. Excluding monosomy X, trisomy:diploid mosaicism is far more common than monosomy:diploid mosaicism, probably because autosomal monosomies are not compatible with cell lineage survival. The other origin for aneuploid:diploid mosaics is a nondisjunction event during cell division in an aneuploid embryo. In the case of a trisomic or monosomic embryo, nondisjunction may restore a diploid chromosome content (trisomic rescue) to one of the daughter cells and its descendants. The most frequent mosaics are trisomy:diploid and 45X:diploid combinations. However, monosomy:diploid, polyploid (one or more complete extra set of chromosomes):diploid mosaics and mosaicism involving structurally abnormal chromosomes also occur.

The phenotype of mosaic individuals is largely influenced by the relative number of aneuploid and diploid cells in each tissue lineage. Large numbers of aneuploid cells are more likely to alter development. For monosomy X or trisomies associated with syndromes, longer survival or mild clinical features are often an indication of underlying mosaicism. If

Table 3-6 ■ CHROMOSOMAL ANOMALIES IN SPONTANEOUS ABORTIONS

Abnormality	Reported Rate of Occurrence (%)[a]
Autosomal trisomy	50–60
Polyploidy	20–25
Monosomy X	10–20
Translocations	2–5

[a]Pooled results from references (7, 12, 57, 62, 73).

mosaicism arises in the cleavage-stage embryo, both aneuploid and diploid cell populations are likely to contribute to the embryonic (embryo, amnion) and extraembryonic lineages. Mitotic errors occurring later in development produce more restricted mosaicism that may be confined to either the fetus or placenta.

Confined Placental Mosaicism

Confined placental mosaicism (CPM) appears to be a relatively common phenomenon. Discrepant fetal and placental karyotypes have been observed in 0.5% to 2% of chorionic villus samples, with a placental aneuploid population in 80% to 90% (118). CPM can be subclassified into three types depending on whether the aneuploid population is confined to the trophoblast (type I), chorionic stroma (type II), or both cell lineages (type III) (59). Specific trisomies are more commonly associated with particular types of CPM (70). It is important to understand that chorionic stromal cells, but not trophoblast, replicate efficiently in cell culture. Therefore, type I CPM will not be detected by routine karyotype of indirect preparations. Type I CPM can be ascertained by direct analysis of cytotrophoblast cells or by *in situ* methods like FISH that target specific chromosomes.

Prospective studies indicate that the vast majority of placentas with confined aneuploid mosaicism detected by chorionic villus sampling early in gestation have no clinical significance (118). However, the remaining cases represent important causes of miscarriage, intrauterine growth restriction (IUGR), intrauterine demise, and postnatal morbidity. Risks for each of these outcomes differ depending on the type of CPM (Figure 3-1) (70).

Lestou and Kalousek recommend testing the placenta for CPM in cases of idiopathic IUGR (birth weight < 5th percentile) without obvious maternal, fetal, or placental causes (70). The contemporary approach of most perinatal services is to perform traditional indirect cytogenetic analysis of one or more biopsies of the placenta, an approach that will only detect CPM types II or III. CGH or array-based CGH is less expensive and can detect all three forms of CPM, but is not widely available. Although CGH will not detect low-level mosaicism, only high levels of mosaicism (CGH-detectable) are thought to be clinically significant. For this reason, a single placental biopsy may be adequate to exclude "clinically relevant" mosaicism by traditional cytogenetics or CGH. The practice of screening all placentas from newborns with idiopathic growth restriction has yet to be adopted as the standard of care in the United States or many other countries.

A strong reason to test for CPM in the placentas of liveborn growth-restricted infants is to identify uniparental disomy (UPD) (128). Some infants with constitutive UPD appear to arise from a trisomic zygote when an early progenitor of the embryonic lineage undergoes a nondisjunction event that restores a diploid chromosome content. Descendants of the diploid lineage populate the entire embryo, but the placenta

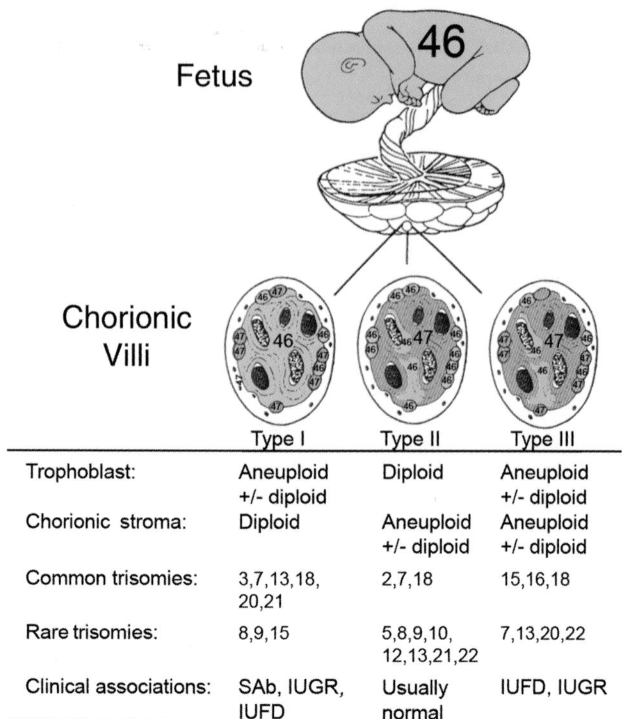

	Type I	Type II	Type III
Trophoblast:	Aneuploid +/- diploid	Diploid	Aneuploid +/- diploid
Chorionic stroma:	Diploid	Aneuploid +/- diploid	Aneuploid +/- diploid
Common trisomies:	3,7,13,18, 20,21	2,7,18	15,16,18
Rare trisomies:	8,9,15	5,8,9,10, 12,13,21,22	7,13,20,22
Clinical associations:	SAb, IUGR, IUFD	Usually normal	IUFD, IUGR

FIGURE 3-1 ■ Three types of CPM in which the fetus is diploid are distinguished based on whether aneuploid cells are either restricted to the trophoblast (type I), chorionic stroma (type II), or both trophoblast and chorionic stroma (type III). Trisomies commonly or rarely associated with each type and their clinical correlates are indicated in the table. (Modified from Tyson RW, Kalousek DK. Chromosomal abnormalities in stillbirth and neonatal death. In: Dimmick JE, Kalousek DK, eds. *Pathology of the embryo and fetus*, JB Lippincott, Philadelphia, PA, 1992, with permission.)

retains some of the original aneuploid cell lineage. In this scenario, the aneuploid zygote contains two chromosomal homologues that were derived from one parent and a third homologue derived from the other parent. In theory, a one-in-three chance exists that postzygotic nondisjunction will eliminate the latter chromosome, creating a diploid daughter cell with a chromosome pair from a single parent—UPD. If embryonic tissues descend from the diploid cell lineage, the fetus/infant is at risk for syndromes or other complications of UPD for the chromosome in question (70). In some instances, the clinical features may be nonspecific and/or not apparent until childhood, at which point screening for UPD is impractical using contemporary methods. Therefore, testing for placental CPM in infants at risk (growth restricted) may be worthwhile, even though the majority of studies will exclude CPM and only a small fraction of those with CPM will have UPD (128).

Trisomy 16 may be the most common and best studied aneuploidy associated with CPM, long-term fetal survival, and UPD. Langlois and colleagues provided follow-up data for 36 cases of trisomy 16 mosaicism, 19 diagnosed by chorionic villus sampling, and 17 by amniocentesis (66). UPD was only observed in a subset (10/18 tested) of cases diagnosed by chorionic villus sampling, six of which had major anomalies. None of the ten chromosome 16 UPD patients in this series exhibited developmental delay.

No specific gross or microscopic placental findings exist for CPM, although very few case series include these data. Although Lestou and Kalousek do not recommend testing for CPM if maternal or placental disorder can explain fetal growth restriction, maternal hypertension sometimes complicates CPM pregnancies and corresponding placental pathology can be present (57,70,128,139).

Mosaic Variegated Aneuploidy

As described previously, mitotic nondisjunction can lead to somatic aneuploidy. Premature chromatid separation with mosaic variegated aneuploidy (PCS-MVA) is a fascinating rare disorder that highlights this mechanism (15). Individuals with PCS-MVA have several different aneuploid cell populations in their tissues. Their clinical findings include IUGR, neurological deficits, ocular malformations, and high rates of neoplasia. Cytogenetic studies demonstrate premature separation of chromatids in ≥50% of stimulated lymphocytes from these patients due to mutations in the *BUB1B* gene, which encodes a mitotic checkpoint protein (45,79).

Autosomal Trisomies

Most nonmosaic autosomal trisomies lead to early embryonic demise. Only trisomies 21, 13, and 18 appear to be compatible with survival to term, though each has a high rate of embryo and fetal wastage (Table 3-5). Although trisomies for each of the nonsex chromosomes have been identified in spontaneous abortuses, the pattern is not random. Trisomies 16, 21, and 22 are particularly common. Most trisomic abortuses manifest as highly disorganized embryos. The reader should consult Chapter 2 for a discussion of the anatomic pathology of early abortuses.

The vast majority of nonmosaic autosomal trisomies arise from errors during the first meiotic division in the maternal germline (83). In human female fetuses, oogenesis arrests in late prophase of the first meiotic division and oocytes remain in a "dormant" state from the second trimester until one to five decades after birth. During this period of meiotic arrest, recombination between homologous chromosomes occurs (46). The physical sites of recombination, termed chiasmata, stabilize the chromosomal pairs through metaphase (103). It is believed that the prolonged first meiotic division increases the risk of nondisjunction, possibly due to age-related loss of chiasmata.

The three autosomal trisomies compatible with postnatal survival (trisomies 21, 18, and 13) are associated with clinically defined syndromes that include malformations of multiple organ systems. Tables 3-7, 3-8, and 3-9 list many of the phenotypic features of these "surviving" trisomies, some of which are illustrated in Figures 3-2 to 3-4. Some of the findings (e.g., appendiceal diverticula in trisomy 13) are fairly specific, though relatively insensitive markers of a particular trisomy (31). Mental retardation is common to all three.

Two theories have been developed to explain the syndromes associated with specific trisomies (98). The "critical region" hypothesis asserts that a subset of syndromic anomalies are due to a 1.5-fold increase in the dose of a small set of genes on the trisomic chromosome. The resemblance of individuals with partial trisomies (due to duplication or translocation of portions of a chromosome) as well as transgenic mouse models, support this model. Based on such data, a 1.6 to 2.5 megabase critical region in chromosome 21 has been postulated to contain all of the genes necessary to produce the Down syndrome (122). Critical regions have been proposed for trisomies 18 and 13 as well (10,49,130). However, the critical region theory for Down syndrome remains controversial and is not consistent with data from other sources (94). An alternative hypothesis, termed "amplified developmental instability," contends that developmental defects are the effect of triplicated genes in general, related more to the number of triplicated genes than their specific functions (98).

A significant fraction of nonmosaic trisomy 21 and possibly all nonmosaic trisomy 13 or 18 conceptions die spontaneously *in utero* (Table 3-10). A retrospective examination of fetuses with trisomy 21 or trisomy 18 established a relatively constant rate of spontaneous demise in each group after diagnostic amniocentesis (134). In total, 10% of trisomy 21 and 32% of trisomy 18 died *in utero*, although higher rates of demise were observed in a different series of fetuses with trisomy 21 (50). In an independent study, analysis of placentas from fetuses and infants with apparent nonmosaic trisomy 13 or 18 suggests that those surviving to term are placental mosaics (56). It is possible that fetal demise is a consequence of placental trisomy 13 or 18 and that formation of diploid placental cells, presumably by postzygotic rescue in the cytotrophoblast lineage, permits survival.

Prenatal diagnosis and elective termination of pregnancy also impact the rate of liveborn trisomies. Definitive prenatal diagnosis requires amniocentesis, chorionic villus sampling, or another invasive procedure to obtain tissue for cytogenetic studies (karyotype, FISH, or another approach). To reduce unnecessary risks and cost associated with prenatal diagnosis, screening methods have been developed, which identify pregnancies at greatest risk (Table 3-10). Contemporary studies suggest that an "integrated test" affords an 80% to 85% detection rate of trisomy 21, with a false positive rate of less than 1% to 5% (13,129). The integrated test includes quantitative measurement of pregnancy-associated plasma protein A, alpha-fetoprotein, unconjugated estriol, free β–human chorionic gonadotropin, and/or inhibin A in maternal serum, early second trimester ultrasound evaluation of nuchal translucency, and maternal age. Similar sensitivity and specificity have been reported for trisomy 18 based on a two-stage screening approach using maternal serum markers.

Table 3-7 ■ MALFORMATIONS AND POSTNATAL DISORDERS ASSOCIATED WITH TRISOMY 21/DOWN SYNDROME (DS)

Malformation	% of DS[a]	Postnatal Disorder	% of DS[a]
Craniofacial[b]		**Central nervous system**	
Upslanted palpebral fissures	>50	Mental retardation	100
Ear anomalies	>50	Early-onset Alzheimer dementia	>50[c]
Epicanthal folds	>50	Seizures	
Flat midface	>50	**Cancer (relative risk)**	
Hypertelorism	25–50	Acute lymphoblastic leukemia (22)	
Other: brachycephaly, midline parietal hair whorl, mild		Acute myeloid leukemia (17)	
microcephaly, choanal stenosis, cleft palate without cleft lip		Lymphoma (3)	
Cardiovascular	>50	Colon (3)	
Atrioventricular canal	10–25	Testicular (12)	
Patent ductus arteriosus	10–25	**Transient myeloproliferative**	
Tricuspid valve defects	10–25	**disease**	5–10
Ventricular septal defect	5–10	**Autoimmune (relative risk):**	
Atrial septal defect	5–10	Crohn disease (3)	1–5
Tetralogy of Fallot	1–5	Ulcerative colitis (3)	
Other: coronary valve defects, hypoplastic right heart, hypoplastic		Celiac disease (5)	
left heart, anomalies of coronary circulation, coarctation of		Early-onset diabetes mellitus (3)	
the aorta, other aortic anomalies, pulmonary artery stenosis,		Thyroiditis (44)	
anomalies of great veins, single umbilical artery		Autoimmune hepatitis (47)	
Digestive tract	10–25	Psoriasis (4)	
Duodenal stenosis	5–10	**Musculoskeletal**	
Hirschsprung disease	1–5	Hypotonia	>50
Anal atresia/stenosis	1–5	Joint hyperextensibility	>50
Other: tracheoesophageal fistula, esophageal atresia/stenosis,		**Other**	
nonduodenal intestinal atresia/stenosis, intestinal malrotation,		Testicular microlithiasis	25–50
ectopic anus, annular pancreas		Enlarged thymic Hassall corpuscles	10–25
Respiratory		Abnormal lymphocyte subsets	10–25
Anomalies of larynx, trachea, or bronchi		Ocular:	10–25
Pulmonary anomalies		Glaucoma	5–10
Genitourinary		Strabismus	25–50
Obstructive defects of renal pelvis, ureter, bladder neck, or urethra	1–5	Nystagmus	
Cryptorchidism	5–10	Scoliosis	
Hypospadias/epispadias	1–5	Hearing loss[d]	
Central nervous system			
Hypoplastic superior temporal gyrus			
Flat frontal poles, retarded myelination			
Hydrocephalus			
Limb			
Clinodactyly (fifth finger)	25–50		
Single transverse palmar crease	25–50		
Syndactyly	1–5		
Other: clubfoot, polydactyly, limb reduction defects,			
rhizomelic shortening			
Ocular			
Brushfield spots	1–5		
Cataract	1–5		
Keratoconus	5–10		

[a]Data pooled from multiple references (1,26,36,38,44,47,55,60,76,77,88,96,109,114,121,125,126,138,140).
[b]Many of the craniofacial features are less distinct in fetuses than in infants or children.
[c]Onset of Alzheimer dementia is age dependent. Hundred percent have pathological changes by age 40 years and >50% have clinical findings by age 50 years.
[d]The incidence of hearing loss varies with age and aggressive treatment of middle ear infections.

Approximately 50% of infants born with either trisomy 13 or trisomy 18 die within the 1st year and less than 5% survive to 10 years (6). Most deaths are secondary to cardiac malformations, and these infants have significant neurocognitive deficits and multiple other medical complications. By contrast, the life expectancy of infants with trisomy 21 is much better. In developed countries, more than 90% of Down syndrome children born after 1990 live beyond 10 years and the average lifespan for present-day populations of Down patients is approximately 60 years (9). In addition

Table 3-8 ■ MALFORMATIONS ASSOCIATED WITH TRISOMY 18/EDWARDS SYNDROME (ES)

Malformation	% of ES[a]
General	
Intrauterine growth restriction	25–50[b]
Fetal hydrops	5–10
Craniofacial[b]	
Microcephaly	25–50[b]
Choroid plexus cyst	
Other: triangular facies, abnormal calvarial shape ("strawberry" skull), hydrocephalus, micrognathia, hypotelorism, cleft lip/palate, small ears, wide fontanels, narrow nasal bridge, microstomia, short sternum	
Cardiovascular	>50
Ventricular septal defect	25–50
Atrioventricular communis	
Other: ectopia cordis (pentalogy of Cantrell), hypoplastic left or right heart, overriding aorta, single umbilical artery, patent ductus arteriosus, tetralogy of Fallot, double-outlet right ventricle, transposition of the great arteries, mitral valvular disease	
Digestive tract	
Omphalocele	10–25
Meckel diverticulum	>50
Other: anorectal atresia, esophageal atresia, pyloric stenosis, ectopic pancreas, abnormal liver lobation	
Respiratory	
Abnormal lung lobation, tracheal stenosis, tracheoesophageal fistula	
Genitourinary	
Abnormal genitalia, cloacal exstrophy, obstructive uropathy, horseshoe kidney, renal a/hypoplasia, renal/ureteral duplication, cryptorchidism, bifid uterus	
Central nervous system	
Cerebellar and pontine hypoplasia	>50
Meningomyelocele ± Chiari malformation	10–25
Other: anencephaly, craniorrhachischisis, hippocampal dysplasia, agenesis of the corpus callosum, neural migration defects	
Limb	
Clenched hand with overlapping digits	>50
Radial ray defects	5–10
Rocker-bottom feet	25–50
Other: arthrogryposes, polydactyly, phocomelia, syndactyly, hypoplastic nails, ectrodactyly	
Ocular	
Coloboma, cataract, cloudy cornea, retinal hypopigmentation, microphthalmia, iridial hypoplasia	
Musculoskeletal	
Other: diaphragmatic defect, absent 12th ribs, malformed occipital bones	
Other viscera	
Hypoplasia of adrenals, thymus, thyroid, and/or gallbladder, accessory spleen	
Placenta/Cord	
Umbilical cord cysts	
Small placenta	

[a]Data pooled from multiple references (12,14,24,37,61,75,92,93,113,115,131,137).
[b]Frequency as a second trimester ultrasound finding.

to mental retardation and malformations, postnatal health issues often associated with trisomy 21 include acute leukemia, early-onset Alzheimer disease, hearing loss, and other conditions (Table 3-7).

Autosomal Monosomies

In theory, meiotic nondisjunction events that lead to trisomic embryos should produce an equal number of monosomic embryos. This is not the case because monosomic embryos, with the exception of monosomy 21 (1/1,000 karyotyped abortions) or monosomy X, die prior to implantation (91). Empiric data to support this concept come from studies of embryos conceived *in vitro* (91,106). Mosaic autosomal monosomy:diploidy is compatible with long-term survival, and phenotype/genotype correlations have been established for some autosomes (81,97).

Sex Chromosome Aneuploidies

At least one X chromosome is required for survival of the preimplantation embryo. Therefore, monosomy Y conceptuses are not observed. However, other forms of sex chromosome aneuploidy, including monosomy X or extra copies of either the X or Y chromosomes, are compatible with long-term

Table 3-9 ■ MALFORMATIONS ASSOCIATED WITH TRISOMY 13/PATAU SYNDROME (PS)

Malformation	% of PS[a]
General	
Intrauterine growth restriction	10–50[b]
Fetal hydrops	5–10
Craniofacial	
Microcephaly	10–50
Holoprosencephalic facies (cyclopia, ethmocephaly, cebocephaly, premaxillary agenesis/dysgenesis)	>50
Cleft lip/palate (midline/bilateral > unilateral)	
Ocular hypotelorism	
Other: malformed ears, absent ear canal, aplasia cutis of scalp, choanal stenosis or atresia; hemangiomas, receding forehead, sparse curled eyelashes, natal teeth, micrognathia	
Cardiovascular	>50
Ventricular septal defect	25–50
Patent ductus arteriosus	25–50
Echogenic intracardiac foci (myocardial calcifications)	10–25
Other: dextrocardia, tetralogy of Fallot, atrial septal defect, truncus arteriosus, aortic coarctation, pulmonary atresia/stenosis, bicuspid aortic valve, single umbilical artery	
Digestive tract	
Pancreatic-splenic fusion	
Appendiceal diverticulum	
Other: omphalocele, abnormal liver lobation, intestinal atresia, Meckel diverticulum	
Respiratory	
Abnormal lung lobation	
Genitourinary	
Obstructive dysplasia	25–50
Renal/ureteral duplications	25–50
Other: cryptorchidism, double vagina, bicornuate uterus, abnormal Fallopian tubes, small penis, abnormal scrotum	
Central nervous system	
Holoprosencephaly	25–50
Arrhinencephaly	>50
Cerebellar malformations	25–50
Other: anencephaly, meningomyelocele, agenesis of the corpus callosum, hydrocephaly, hippocampal dysplasia, neural migratory defects, choroid plexus cyst	
Limb	
Postaxial polydactyly	~50
Other: syndactyly, rocker-bottom feet, hypoplastic nails, clubbed feet, hypoplastic nails, single transverse palmar crease, radial aplasia	
Ocular	
Microphthalmia	25–50
Coloboma of iris or retina	25–50
Other: retinal dysplasia, aniridia, anophthalmia, cataract, premature vitreous body, hypoplasia of optic nerve	
Musculoskeletal	
Dysplastic/fused lumbosacral ± thoracic vertebra, absent 12th ribs, hypoplastic sphenoid bone, diaphragmatic defect	>50
Hematologic	
Irregular neutrophil nuclei	
Increased fetal and Gower-2 hemoglobin	

[a]Data pooled from multiple references (32,37,62,69,115,131).
[b]Reported rates of IUGR appear to be higher in populations that were studied later in gestation.

survival and account for the majority of liveborn aneuploid infants.

Monosomy X (Turner Syndrome)

A 45,X karyotype is one of the most frequently encountered forms of aneuploidy in spontaneously aborted embryos. In contrast with autosomies, for which maternal meiotic nondisjunction events predominate, loss of either the maternal or paternal sex chromosome appears to occur more often during postzygotic mitosis. Hence, mosaic monosomy X is very frequent, and occult mosaicism has been speculated to exist in all "pure" 45,X patients (124). Pure 45,X or high 45,X mosaicism produces a fairly distinct syndrome characterized by female genitalia, short stature, and a high prevalence of specific anomalies (Table 3-11). Intelligence is usually in the normal range.

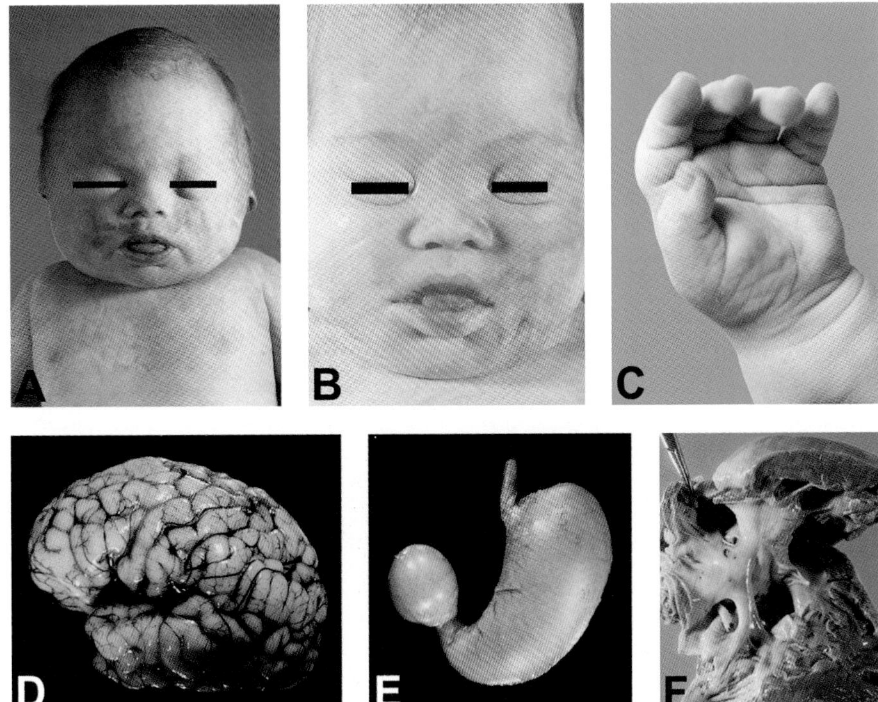

FIGURE 3-2 ■ Trisomy 21: **A:** 35-week fetus with typical late gestation facies (epicanthal folds, broad nose, bulging tongue). **B:** Similar facial changes are apparent in 2-month-old infant (note increased 'Mongoloid' slant of palpebral fissures). **C:** Single palmar crease. **D:** Lateral view of brain showing small superior temporal gyrus and enlarged middle temporal gyrus. **E:** Duodenal atresia. **F:** Atrioventricular canal, with large primum atrial septal defect, large ventricular septal defect in position of AV canal, and cleft septal leaflet of the tricuspid valve.

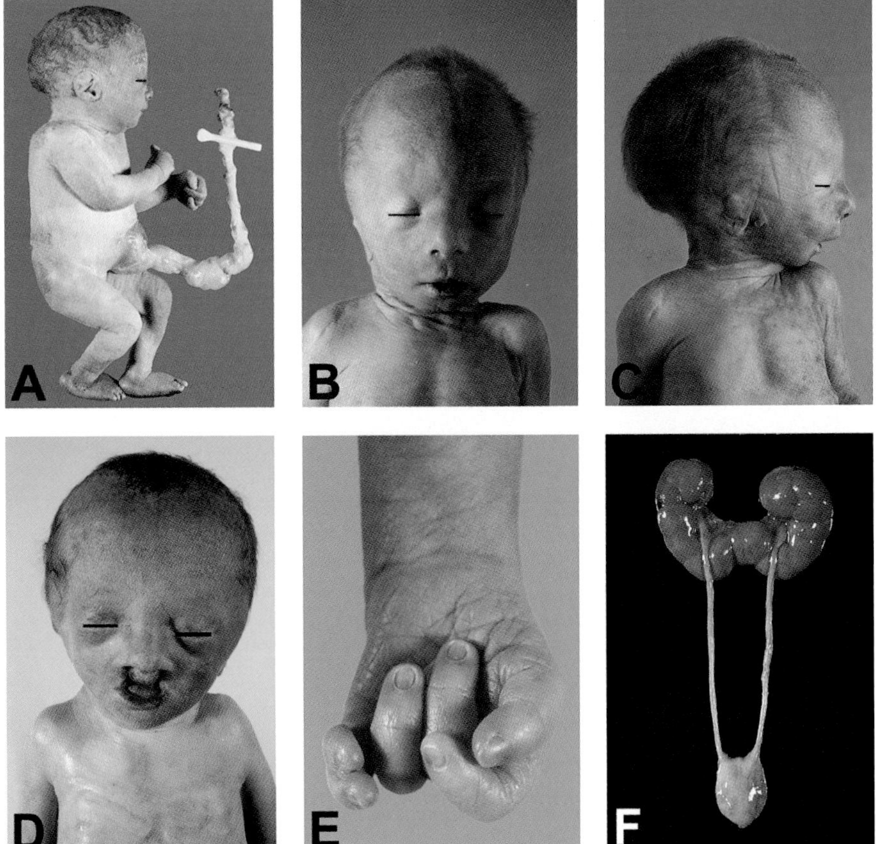

FIGURE 3-3 ■ Trisomy 18. **A:** Late gestational fetus with omphalocele and rocker bottom feet. **B:** Young infant with widely separated eyes and mild trigonocephaly. **C:** Infant shown in (**B**), with dysplastic ear and micrognathia. **D:** Infant with triangular facies, ocular hypertelorism, and bilateral cleft lip. **E:** Overlapping digits in pattern common to trisomy 18. **F:** Horseshoe kidney (with ureters and urinary bladder).

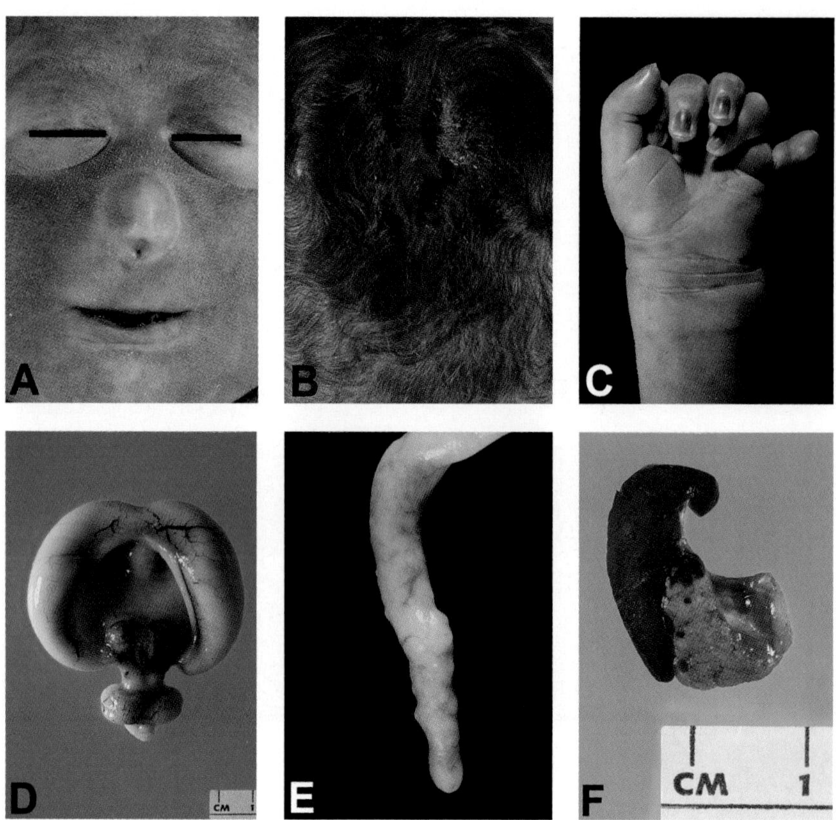

FIGURE 3-4 ■ Trisomy 13. **A:** Infant with cebocephaly (ocular hypotelorism and single nostril nose), one of the facial changes associated with holoprosencephaly. **B:** Aplasia cutis of the scalp. **C:** Postaxial polydactyly. **D:** Alobar holoprosencephaly. **E:** Appendiceal diverticula ("dinosaur tail") are pathognomonic for trisomy 13, although not present in every case. **F:** Fusion of spleen (**left**) and tail of pancreas (note tiny splenic islands within the pancreas).

Only 1% of 45,X embryos survive to term. Many are lost in the first trimester, but late fetal loss is also common. Severe hydrops with massive nuchal edema is common *in utero* (Figure 3-5) and usually portends a poor outcome. Extravascular fluid in the neck collects as a multiloculated cystic hygroma, a lymphatic malformation characterized by thin membranous septa and inconspicuous endothelial linings (16). Gross and microscopic studies of cystic hygroma in Turner syndrome suggest hypoplasia/agenesis of lymphatic vessels and failure of the lymphatics to connect to the venous system (127). Resolution of transient nuchal edema is proposed as the basis for the webbed neck commonly observed in Turner syndrome. Other common malformations (Table 3-11) include aortic coarctation, hypoplastic left heart, "horseshoe" kidney, and streak ovaries (Figure 3-5).

Table 3-10 ■ PRENATAL SCREENING MARKERS FOR COMMON TRISOMIES

	Prenatal Screening Markers[a]		**Rate of IUFD or Stillbirth**[b,c]	**Percentage of Liveborns Surviving to**[b]		
Trisomy	Maternal serum analytes[a]	Ultrasound[d]		1 month	1 year	10 year
21	↓ AFP ↓ PAPP-A, ↑ fβ-HCG ↑ inhibin	1st trimester: nuchal translucency, nasal bone hypoplasia 2nd trimester: echogenic intracardiac foci, echogenic bowel, rhizomelic limb shortening; mild pyelectasis	10%–30%	>95	95	>90
18	↓ AFP ↓ ↓ PAPP-A ↓ ↓ fβ-HCG ↓ uE3	1st trimester: nuchal translucency 2nd trimester: choroid plexus cyst, clenched hands, echogenic bowel, IUGR, mild pyelectasis, mild ventriculomegaly	45%–70%	50%	5%–30%	1%
13	↓ AFP ↓ ↓ PAPP-A ↓ ↓ fβ-HCG	2nd trimester: mild pyelectasis, echogenic intracardiac foci, IUGR, mild ventriculomegaly	20%–40%	50%	15%–30%	1%

[a]References (100,109,123).
[b]References (6,9,29,51,58,73,90,95,104,117,134–136).
[c]After diagnosis by amniocentesis or ultrasound; does not include first trimester losses or elective terminations of pregnancy.
[d]Nonspecific findings that significantly increase the risk for trisomy.
AFP, α-fetoprotein; PAPP-A, pregnancy-associated plasma protein A, increased inhibin A; fβ-HCG, free β-human chorionic gonadotropin; uE3, unconjugated estriol; IUGR, intrauterine growth restriction; VSD, ventricular septal defect; IUFD, intrauterine fetal demise.

Table 3-11 ■ MALFORMATIONS AND POSTNATAL ABNORMALITIES ASSOCIATED WITH MONOSOMY X/TURNER SYNDROME (TS)

Malformation	% of TS[a]	Postnatal Abnormality	% of TS
General		**External**	
Intrauterine growth restriction	>80	Short stature	>90
Fetal hydrops (may be transient)	>80	Webbed neck	>80
Broad chest		Short neck/low hairline	>70
Widely spaced nipples		Cubitus valgus	
Inverted and/or hypoplastic nipples		Infantile external genitalia	
		Scant pubic/axillary hair	
		Failure to develop secondary sex characteristics	
Craniofacial		**Endocrine**	
Nuchal cystic hygroma		Low estrogen and progesterone	15–30
Triangular face			
Down-slanted palpebrae		Elevated follicle stimulating hormone (FSH)	
Other: epicanthus, ptosis, high-arched narrow palate, micrognathia, hypertelorism, low-set ears, dysmorphic ears		Autoimmune thyroiditis Diabetes mellitus	
Cardiovascular	17–45	**Other**	
Coarctation of the aorta Hypoplastic left heart Bicuspid aortic valve Cystic medial necrosis of aorta Other: mitral valvular dysplasia, ventricular septal defect, anomalous pulmonary venous return		Aortic dissection, myopia. deafness, hypertension, Crohn disease, cardiac conduction defects, chondrodysplasia of the distal radius (Madelung deformity)	
Genitourinary		**Increased risk for neoplasia[b]**	>50
Gonadal dysgenesis (streak gonads)	>90	Melanocytic nevi	
Horseshoe kidney or other renal malformations	40	Gonadoblastoma (if portion of Y chromosome is present)	
Hypoplastic uterus			
Clitoral hypertrophy			
Central nervous system			
Mild cortical dysplasia			
Neuroglial heterotopia			
Hydrocephalus			
Limb			
Short 4th and 5th metacarpals	>50		
Other: narrow hyperconvex nails			
Ocular			
Cataracts			
Musculoskeletal			
Raised semilunar carpal bones	>60		
Inferior displacement of inner tibial growth			
Other: bone dysplasia with coarse trabeculae, scoliosis, spina bifida, vertebral fusion, cervical rib, abnormal sella turcica, dislocated hip			

[a]Data pooled from multiple references (37,54,80,119,120,133).
[b]Although a study suggested that Turner syndrome patients may be at risk for a wide variety of nongonadal neoplasms (143), this has not been supported by recent large reviews (126).

One half of all individuals with Turner syndrome have a 45,X karyotype; various forms of 45,X mosaicism account for most of the rest (120). Those with 45,X/46,XY mosaicism or retained portions of a Y chromosome exhibit a range of phenotypic features from normal male to Turner syndrome. Within this continuum, genitalia and gonads may show ambiguous differentiation. Ovotestes or other forms of gonadal dysgenesis are common and 7% to 30% of patients develop gonadoblastoma (43).

Sex Chromosome Polysomy

In general, all the genes of only one X chromosome remain active beyond the blastocyst stage (48). After this stage, most genes of all but one X chromosome in each cell are inactivated (silenced) by epigenetic modifications. The process of X-inactivation appears random in each cell of the inner cell mass. Therefore, each cell in a 46,XX embryo has an equal chance of inactivating the paternal or maternal X chromosome.

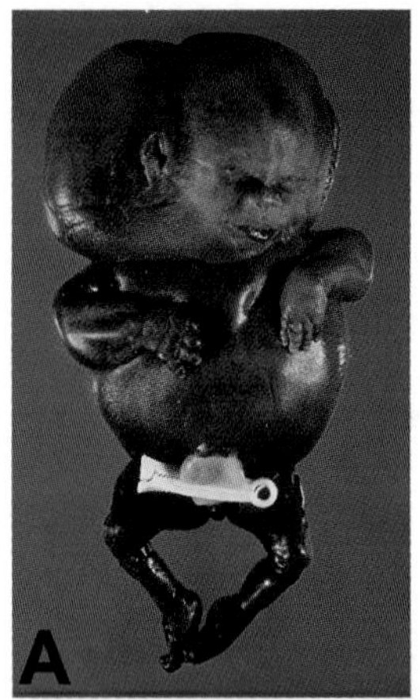
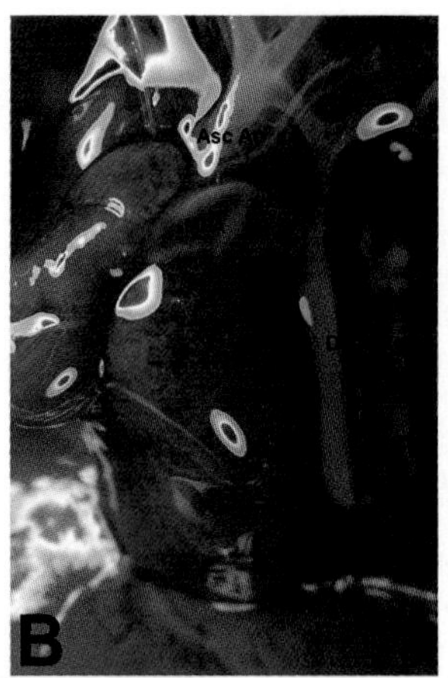
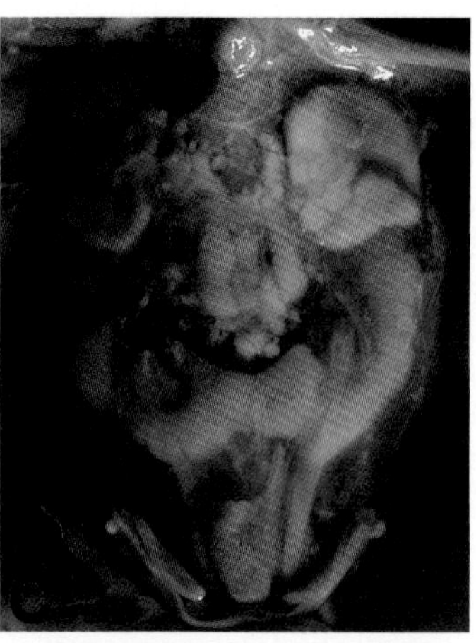
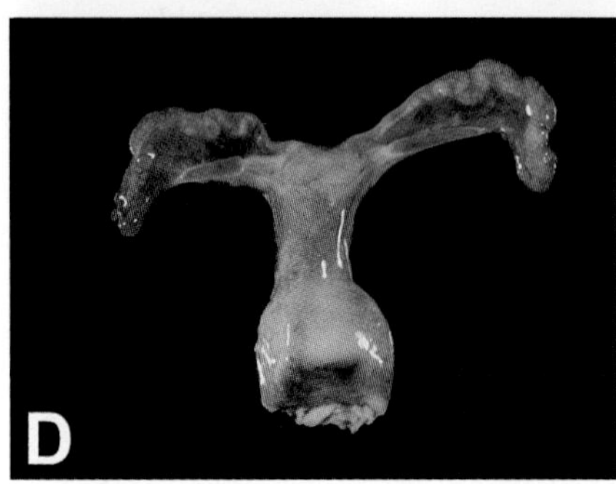
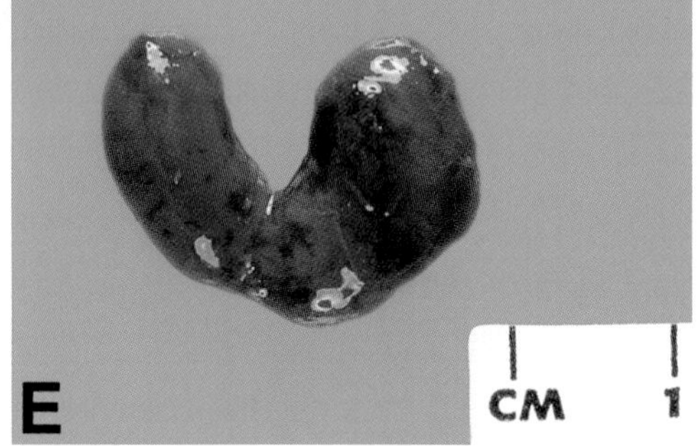

FIGURE 3-5 ■ 45X. **A:** Fetus with massive cystic hygroma and hydrops. **B:** Left anterior oblique view of heart *in situ*; arrow indicates region of narrowing (coarctation) of the preductal aorta (Asc Ao, ascending aorta; MPA, main pulmonary artery; Desc Ao, descending aorta)—17 weeks. **C:** *In situ* view of low-set horseshoe kidneys and small but histologically normal ovaries—18 weeks. **D:** Streak ovaries in specimen from newborn; prominent cervix is normal for age. **E:** Small horseshoe kidney—17 weeks.

In embryos that carry three or more X chromosomes, genes on all but one are silenced, except for the subset of X-linked genes that normally escape X inactivation. The latter seem to have little impact on the development of females with a 47,XXX karyotype. However, dose-related effects are observed in males and females with tetrasomy or pentasomy X, who exhibit mental deficiency and mild dysmorphic features (Table 3-12). A 47,XXY karyotype causes Klinefelter syndrome (mild neurocognitive deficits, behavioral problems, hypogonadism, and hypogenitalism) (132).

One of every thousand liveborn males has an extra Y chromosome (47,XYY). Associated features are highly variable, but aggressive behavior, mild cognitive defects, and minor dysmorphic features have been reported (54).

Polyploidy

Polyploidy refers to complete extra haploid sets of chromosomes, as with triploidy (69 chromosomes) or tetraploidy (96 chromosomes). Triploidy is common (1% of human embryos), and usually leads to spontaneous abortion between 7 and 17 weeks (23). The extra chromosomal set is more often of maternal (digyny) than paternal (diandry) origin (6). However, diandry predominates in triploid early spontaneous abortions. Most, if not all, diandric triploid conceptions result from dispermic fertilization of a single oocyte (84,123). Maternal origin of the extra chromosomes in triploid conceptuses (digyny) is caused by errors in the first, or less often the second, meiotic division.

Most triploid embryos are miscarried (141). Liveborn triploid infants are rare and generally die within a few hours (25). Diandric and digynic triploid conceptuses exhibit distinct phenotypes, which are referred to as type I and type II

Table 3-12 ■ SEX CHROMOSOME POLYSOMIES

Polysomy	Clinical/Pathological Features[a]
47,XXX	Normal
47,XYY	Accelerated growth, prominent glabella, "dull" mentality, behavioral problems, severe acne
47,XXY	*Klinefelter syndrome*: hypogonadism, hypogenitalism, infertility (testicular fibrosis), long limbs, gynecomastia, mental retardation (15%–20%), neoplasia (1%–2%) including breast cancer, leukemia/lymphoma, testicular tumors, and extragonadal germ cell tumors
48,XXXX	Mental retardation, mild facial anomalies, 5th finger clinodactyly
49,XXXXX	*Penta X syndrome*: microcephaly, mental retardation, small hands with 5th finger clinodactyly, abnormal facies, growth deficiency, patent ductus arteriosus
48,XXXY	Klinefelter syndrome with mental retardation, growth deficiency, radioulnar synostosis
48,XXYY	Klinefelter-like syndrome with higher incidence of mental retardation and behavioral abnormalities

[a]References (2,37,54).

triploidy, respectively (85). Diandric fetuses that survive into the second trimester typically show normal fetal growth to moderate symmetrical growth restriction and partial molar transformation of their placentas, with large cystic villi and trophoblast hyperplasia (18). Survival of digynic embryos into the second and third trimesters is associated with severe asymmetrical growth restriction and small placentas that do not exhibit molar change. These phenotypic differences have been attributed to parental imprinting of genes that influence placental and fetal growth (21).

Common malformations observed in triploid fetuses include adrenal hypoplasia, syndactyly (particularly digits 3 and 4), hydrocephalus, and other defects (Table 3-13). Apart from partial mole formation, no specific malformations have been found to distinguish diandric versus digynic triploidy (18,86). If triploidy is suspected, the diagnosis can be confirmed less expensively and faster by flow cytometry than traditional cytogenetics.

Partial Chromosomal Aneuploidies

A variety of structural chromosomal anomalies result in partial duplication (trisomy) or deletion (monosomy) of portions of chromosomes (Figure 3-6). The initiating event for most of these aberrations is abnormal recombination between homologous and heterologous chromosomes during gametogenesis. As a consequence, portions of chromosomes may be translocated, duplicated, or lost. Reciprocal translocations between heterologous chromosomes are often "balanced," with two abnormal chromosomes but no net gain or loss of genetic material. Individuals who constitutively harbor balanced translocations are likely to be normal, unless a translocation breakpoint results in a microdeletion/duplication or disrupts coding or regulatory elements of a particular gene. However, carriers of balanced translocations are at risk for transmitting an unbalanced translocation (one of their abnormal derivative chromosomes) to their offspring, who will be partially monosomic and partially trisomic for portions of the two chromosomes involved in the translocation.

Schinzel has cataloged numerous translocations, duplications, and deletions in an effort to identify phenotypes associated with the gain or loss of specific chromosomal segments (110). As expected, a myriad of unbalanced chromosomal rearrangements have been reported, many of which are unique with regard to the specific DNA sequences that are lost or gained. However, partial chromosomal aneuploidies that involve overlapping portions of the genome have been correlated with recognizable syndromes, including those listed in Table 3-14.

Robertsonian translocations are those that involve the diminutive short (p) arms of acrocentric chromosomes (33). The acrocentric chromosomes in humans are numbers 13, 14, 15, 21, and 22. The product of a Robertsonian translocation is a composite chromosome containing two closely spaced centromeres and q arms of both "donor" chromosomes, but lacking portions of the donor p arms. Robertsonian translocations can be homologous (e.g., 13q13q) or heterologous (e.g., 13q14q). Loss of DNA from the miniscule short arms of these chromosomes is not clinically significant, so carriers of "balanced" Robertsonian translocations are generally normal. Diploid cells of heterologous Robertsonian translocation carriers also contain one normal copy of each chromosome involved in the translocation. If one of these normal chromosomes segregates with the Robertsonian translocation product during meiosis, the resulting zygote will be trisomic. Therefore, carriers of Robertsonian translocations are at significant risk for producing a conceptus with trisomy of either chromosome involved in the translocation, as well as recurrent trisomy.

Sites of the interchromosomal and intrachromosomal recombination events that occur during gametogenesis and

Table 3-13 ■ DIGYNIC VERSUS DIANDRIC TRIPLOIDY[a]

	Digynic	Diandric
Fetus		
Growth	Asymmetric IUGR	Usually normal or symmetric IUGR
Craniofacial	Macrocephaly, hypertelorism, ventriculomegaly, low-set ears, microphthalmia, coloboma	Usually normal or microcephaly, ventriculomegaly
Cardiac	Normal, ventricular septal defect	Normal, ventricular septal defect
Extremities	Syndactyly between 3rd and 4th digits	Syndactyly between 3rd and 4th digits
Other	Adrenal hypoplasia, micropenis, renal malformations, pulmonary hypoplasia, Leydig cell hyperplasia	Adrenal hypoplasia, ambiguous genitalia
Placenta	Hypoplastic with no features of partial mole	Partial mole edematous with cisternae in terminal villi trophoblast hyperplasia scalloped villus contours
Common mechanism	Error in meiosis II	Fertilization of normal oocyte by two spermatozoa
Usual outcome	Spontaneous abortion or stillbirth	Spontaneous abortion or stillbirth

[a]References (18,21,25,46,53,123,141).

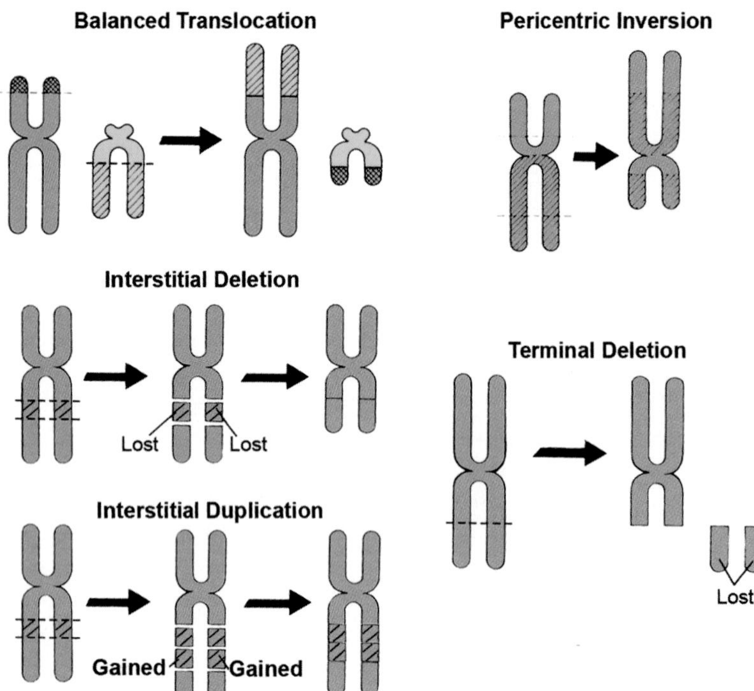

FIGURE 3-6 ■ Examples of chromosomal rearrangements.

underlie many constitutional translocations are not randomly distributed (28). Instead, "hot spots" appear to exist that are prone to recombination. In some instances, these produce submicroscopic duplications or deletions that are below the resolution of standard cytogenetic analysis. Application of array-based CGH and other methods to screen for these rearrangements is likely to uncover hitherto unrecognized disorders that have their basis in structural chromosomal anomalies (112).

Chromosomal Instability Disorders

Several human syndromes and diseases are due in part to chromosomal instability that can be resolved by karyotype analysis using normal or specialized culture and/or staining techniques (Table 3-15). Most chromosomal instability disorders are genetic conditions that predispose to congenital malformations and/or cancer because of an underlying

Table 3-14 ■ SELECTED SYNDROMES ASSOCIATED WITH PARTIAL ANEUPLOIDY

Partial Aneuploidy	Clinical and Pathological Features[a,b]
del 4p16-ter	*Wolf-Hirschhorn syndrome*: IUGR, microcephaly, hypotonia, seizures, "Greek warrior helmet" facies (prominent glabella, ocular hypertelorism, high-arched eyebrows, broad nasal bridge), cleft lip ± palate (47%), strabismus, epicanthal folds, micrognathia, "fish" mouth, short upper lip and philtrum, preauricular skin tag or pit, talipes equinovarus, single transverse palmar crease, hypospadias (50% of males), renal hypoplasia, malformed toes, cryptorchidism, cardiac malformation (33%), mental retardation
del 5p15.2-ter	*Cri du chat syndrome*: IUGR (72%), catlike cry (100%), mental retardation (100%), hypotonia (78%), microcephaly (100%), abnormal facies, cardiac malformation (30%), single transverse palmar crease, CNS malformations (arachnoid cyst, hydrocephalus, cerebellar hypoplasia), renal malformations
del 9p21-ter	Mental retardation, trigonocephaly, abnormal facies (upslanting palpebrae, midfacial hypoplasia, anteverted nares, depressed nasal bridge, long philtrum), hypoplastic ear lobes, long middle and short distal phalanges, cardiac defects (33%–50%), scoliosis, abnormal external genitalia
dup 10q24-ter	Mental retardation, IUGR, microcephaly, abnormal facies (flat with high forehead, high-arched eyebrows, ptosis, microphthalmia, broad nasal bridge, bow-shaped mouth, cleft palate, posteriorly rotated ears), camptodactyly, proximally placed thumbs, two to three pedal syndactyly, cardiac (50%) and renal (50%) malformations, absent 12th ribs, kyphoscoliosis
tetrasomy 22q11-pter	*Cat eye syndrome*: iris coloboma, mild mental retardation, ocular hypertelorism, preauricular skin tags or pits, micrognathia, downslanting palpebral fissures, cardiac malformations (>33%), anal atresia, renal agenesis

[a]Numbers in parentheses are frequencies of selected findings.
[b]References (15,22,54,82).
IUGR, intrauterine growth restriction; CNS, central nervous system.

Table 3-15 ■ CYTOGENETICS AND MOLECULAR GENETICS OF SELECTED CHROMOSOMAL INSTABILITY SYNDROMES

Syndrome	Clinical Features	Cytogenetic Finding	Genetic Defect(s)	Comment
Fanconi (FA)	Pancytopenia, IUGR, abnormal skin pigmentation, radial ray defects, VACTERL- like malformations, increased cancer risk (AR)	Increased chromosomal breakage after exposure to a clastogenic agent	*FANCA, FANCB, FANCC, FANCD1/BRCA2, FANCD2, FANCE, FANCF, FANCG, FANCJ/BRIP1, FANCL, FANCM/Hef*	Mutations in at least 12 different genes (complementation groups) can cause Fanconi anemia. Molecular genetic testing for every complementation group is not available. Diagnosis and determination of complementation group by cytogenetic analysis of somatic cell hybrids facilitate targeted DNA testing.
Robert-SC (R-SC)	Symmetric limb reduction defects, IUGR, cleft lip/palate, other craniofacial malformations, mental retardation (AR)	Repulsion of heterochromatic regions near centromeres ("puffing") and delayed progression through metaphase ("anaphase lag")	*ESCO2*	
Nijmegen breakage (NB)	Characteristic facies, microcephaly, immunodeficiency, growth retardation, radiosensitivity, increased cancer risk (AR)	Increased chromosomal breakage with normal culture or after exposure to a clastogenic agent	*NBS1*	Nijmegen breakage syndrome is observed primarily in patients of Slavic descent due to the founder effect of a single mutation. *NBS1, FANCD2,* and *ATM* may interact with one another.
Fragile X (FRAX)	Macrocephaly, large testes, mental retardation (X-linked)	"Fractured" appearance of the X chromosome induced by one of several culture methods	*FRM1*	Clinical disease is associated with expansion of a trinucleotide repeat (>200 repeats) in the 5′-untranslated region of exon 1. Molecular genetic testing has replaced cytogenetic testing.
Ataxia-Telangiectasia (AT)	Ataxia, telangiectasia, dysarthria, abnormal ocular movements, recurrent infections, increased cancer risk (AR)	Radiation-induced nonrandom rearrangements of chromosomes 7, 14, and X ± nonspecific chromosome breakage in fibroblasts	*ATM*	AT-like disorders have been described due to mutations in other genes (e.g., *MRE11*).

AR, autosomal recessive; IUGR, intrauterine growth restriction; VACTERL, *v*ertebral-*a*norectal-*c*ardiac-*t*racheo-*e*sophageal-*r*enal-*l*imb malformation association.
References: FA (83), R-SC (116,135), NB (138), FRAX (26,128), AT (36,127).

defect in molecular systems that mediate DNA replication or repair. Medical professionals who deal with these conditions need to be aware that cytogenetic evaluation of specimens for chromosomal instability is somewhat specialized and not available in every laboratory. Many of the assays require quantitative measurements with appropriate controls. For many of the conditions listed in Table 3-15, mutational analysis of specific genes has replaced cytogenetic studies.

For Fanconi anemia, however, chromosomal breakage studies remain diagnostically useful. Fanconi anemia, a multigene disorder, is manifest by pancytopenia, IUGR, and high incidence of congenital malformations (Figure 3-7) that overlap with the anomalies of the VACTERL (*v*ertebral-*a*norectal-*c*ardiac-*t*racheo-*e*sophageal-*r*enal-*l*imb) association (35). Because of this phenotypic overlap, some authors have recommended testing for Fanconi anemia of any individual with VACTERL association including a radial ray defect (30). At least 12 different "complementation groups" for Fanconi anemia are recognized and the specific genes responsible for many of these groups have been identified (Table 3-15) (78). To determine a

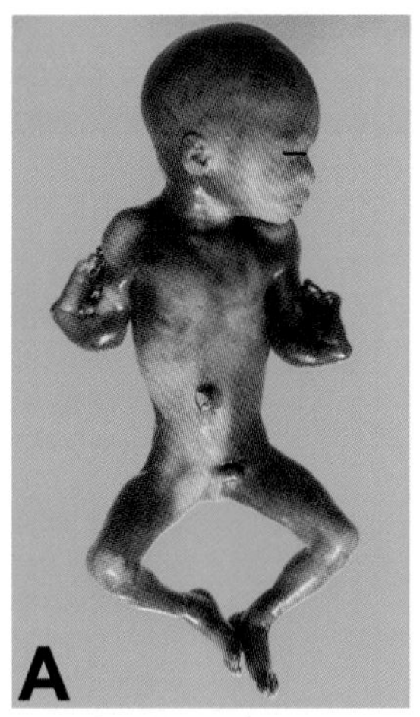

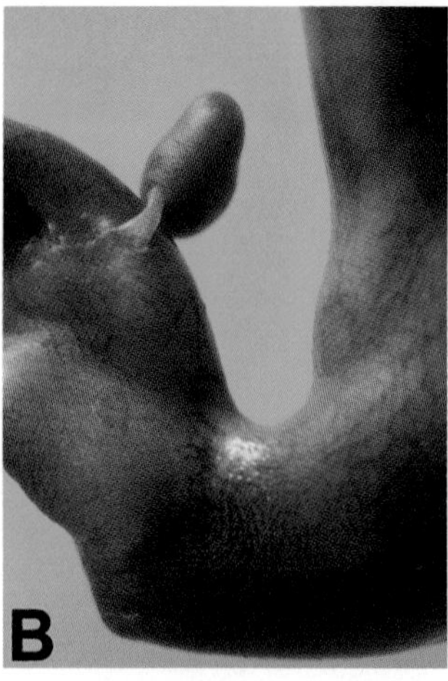

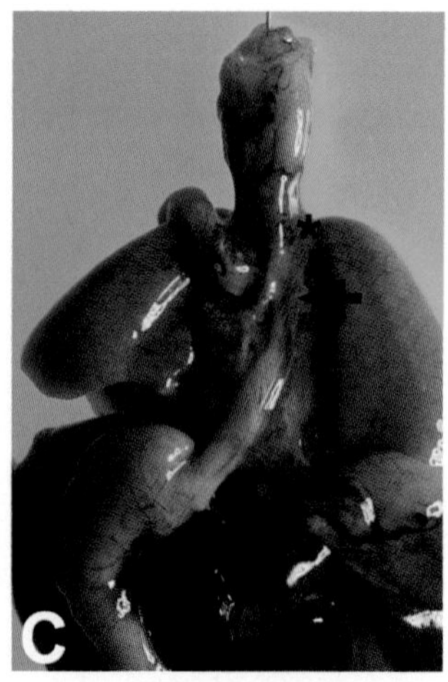

FIGURE 3-7 ■ Fanconi syndrome. **A:** Fetus with bilateral radial aplasia. **B:** Close view of right arm and hand, showing marked deviation of wrist, secondary to radial aplasia, and tiny remnant of thumb. **C:** Posterior view of viscera, showing proximal atresia of esophagus (*) with distal tracheoesophageal fistula (*arrow*). Thoracic aorta is reflected to left.

patient's complementation group, his/her cells are fused with cells of established complementation groups and then chromosomal breakage rates are examined in the somatic cell hybrids (Figure 3-8). The patient is assigned to the complementation group that fails to rescue the breakage phenotype in these somatic cell hybrid assays. Approximately 66% of cases fall into complementation group A (FANCA) (78).

Most of the genes that are disrupted in patients with Fanconi syndrome encode proteins that mediate DNA repair. Mutational analysis of one or more of these genes is a potential alternative to complementation studies, but is less efficient and will miss cases of Fanconi anemia due to complementation groups for which mutational analysis is not yet possible. Novel techniques have been introduced to replace somatic cell hybridization for complementation group determination, but at present these are only available for select complementation groups.

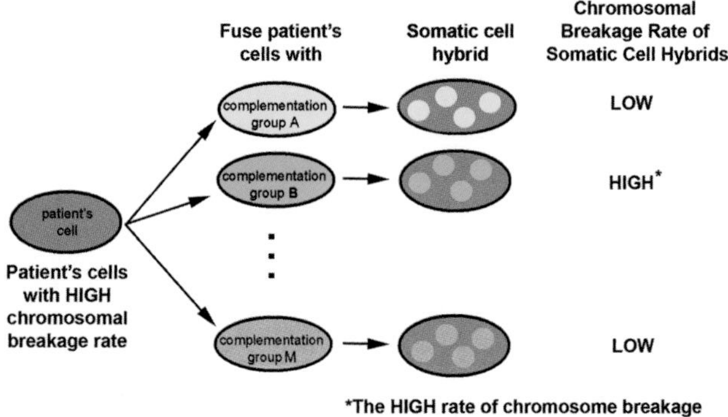

FIGURE 3-8 ■ Identification of Fanconi complementation group by somatic cell hybridization. Cells from the patient with Fanconi anemia are fused with cells from established complementation groups to create somatic cell hybrids. The hybrids are exposed to clastogenic agents *in vitro* and chromosomal breakage rates are observed. Only hybrids of the same complementation group retain the high rate of chromosome breakage that characterizes Fanconi anemia.

SUBMICROSCOPIC DISORDERS

Development of sensitive methods to resolve small chromosomal aberrations has expanded the scope of cytogenetic disorders to include microdeletions, microduplications, and other structural changes that cannot be elucidated by traditional karyotype analysis. This is a rapidly evolving field in which targeted FISH probes and targeted or global array-based CGH are important techniques. Some of the more common applications in fetal and pediatric medicine are listed in Table 3-16. As examples of this class of disorders, the 22q11 microdeletions associated with velocardiofacial (VCF)/DiGeorge syndrome and subtelomeric deletions are discussed in more detail.

Velocardiofacial/DiGeorge Syndrome

VCF/DiGeorge syndrome (also referred to as the 22q11 deletion syndrome) is a convenient designation for two clinical entities that share pathogenic and phenotypic features including craniofacial and cardiovascular anomalies (39,63). In addition to these common elements, DiGeorge patients classically exhibit agenesis or hypoplasia of the thymus and parathyroid glands. VCF/DiGeorge syndrome is an autosomal dominant disorder with variable penetrance and expressivity. Palatal insufficiency or clefts are common. Cardiac malformations usually involve the conotruncal region (truncus arteriosus, tetralogy of Fallot, interrupted aortic arch, ventricular septal defect, or others). In addition, the 22q11 deletion is frequently detected in patients with the same spectrum of isolated heart anomalies (40).

The VCF/DiGeorge syndrome critical region (DGCR), a 3-MB segment on chromosome 22q11, is deleted in 90% of patients with DiGeorge syndrome. The overwhelming majority of these deletions are not detected by routine karyotype, but are readily identified by FISH. The DGCR contains more than 20 genes. Of these, *TBX1* is afforded considerable

Table 3-16 ■ SELECTED SUBMICROSCOPIC CHROMOSOMAL ANOMALIES

Syndrome or Disorder	Genetic Locus [affected gene(s)]	Alteration
Velocardiofacial syndrome (VCFS)/DiGeorge	22q11.2 (*TBX1* and contiguous genes)	Microdeletion
X-linked congenital adrenal hypoplasia/ Glycerol kinase deficiency/Duchenne myopathy	Xp21 (*DAX1, GK, DMD*)	Microdeletion
Tuberous sclerosis/Autosomal dominant polycystic kidney disease	16p13 (*TSC2, PKD1*)	Microdeletion
Maturity-onset diabetes of the young type 5	17q12 (*TCF2*)	Microdeletion
WAGR	11p13.3 (*PAX6, D11S2163, PER, WT-1*)	Microdeletion
Smith-Magenis	17p11.2 (*RAI1*)	Microdeletion[a]
Rubinstein-Taybi	16p13.3 (*CBP*)	Microdeletion[a]
Alagille	20p12 (*JAG1*)	Microdeletion[a]
Williams	7q11.23 (*ELN* + >20 contiguous genes)	Microdeletion
Prader-Willi/Angelman	15q11-13 (*SNURF-SNRPN* and contiguous genes)	Microdeletion (70% of cases)
Miller-Dieker	17p13.3 (*LIS1* and contiguous genes)	Microdeletion
Monosomy 1p36	1p36 (*KIAA1273* and contiguous genes)	Microdeletion
Microduplication 22q11.2	22q11.2 (same as VCFS/DiGeorge)	Microduplication
Hereditary neuropathy with liability to pressure palsies (HNPP)	17p11.2 (*PMP22*; same as CMT1A)	Microdeletion
Charcot-Marie-Tooth 1A (CMT1A)	17p11.2 (*PMP22*; same as HNPP)	Microduplication

[a]Point mutations have also been observed in a small subset of patients, but FISH is often used as an initial diagnostic test.

attention because disruption of the murine homologue is associated with conotruncal defects, and some humans with VCF/DiGeorge syndrome and no 22q11 deletion have point mutations in *TBX1* (41). *TBX1* encodes a transcription factor that is expressed in embryonic pharyngeal arch mesoderm and the cardiac outflow tracts. The current standard of care is to perform FISH testing for the DGCR in any patient with VCF/DiGeorge syndrome or an isolated conotruncal cardiac malformation (63).

Subtelomeric Deletions

Telomeres are short repetitive sequences found at the very ends of chromosomes. The adjacent subtelomeric regions are gene-rich areas that are difficult to evaluate by traditional cytogenetic methods because subtelomeres contain indistinct G-bands that look similar from one chromosome to the next. Therefore, small subtelomeric deletions or terminal translocations are often undetectable in routine or high-resolution karyotypes. In many instances, subtelomeric rearrangements are heritable and a subset appears as benign variants (99). Therefore, the genetic implications are quite variable.

FISH with subtelomere-specific probes and array-based CGH permit screening for deletions or translocations involving subtelomeres (52). These methods have shown that deletions are relatively common, particularly among individuals with unexplained mental retardation and/or malformations. For some chromosomal arms, subtelomeric deletions result in well-known syndromes that are associated with larger deletions (e.g., Wolf-Hirschhorn (4p-) syndrome; Table 3-14); thereby narrowing the critical regions responsible for these phenotypes. In other instances, new syndromes are being defined based on large series of patients with the same subtelomeric deletions and similar phenotypic features. An outstanding review of specific subtelomeric deletions and their associated findings was written by de Vries et al. (19).

The "del 1p36 syndrome" is a prime example of how FISH-based diagnosis of subtelomeric deletions has helped define a clinical-pathological syndrome and shown it to be more common than believed (5). The current literature suggests that 1p36.3 deletions account for up to 0.5% to 0.7% of idiopathic mental retardation. The syndrome also includes high rates of structural heart defects (>50%), dysmorphic facies, hypothyroidism (15% to 20%), deafness, and other neurological anomalies. Brains of these patients show a variety of nonspecific findings including cortical dysplasia, hydrocephalus, and leukodystrophy. This syndrome poses a difficult and more frequently encountered problem for perinatal pathologists because only nonspecific findings (e.g., isolated heart defect) may be evident in a fetus. The yield for 1p36 deletion studies is likely to be very low in this scenario, and FISH analysis is not the standard of care at present. However, the situation is likely to change as array-based CGH or other techniques for targeted or global microdeletion analysis become less expensive and more readily available.

EPIGENETIC CHROMOSOMAL MODIFICATIONS AND ASSOCIATED DISORDERS

Each human chromosome is a linear sequence of nucleotides surrounded by proteins and RNA. Nucleotide sequence is crucial to genetic integrity, and gain, loss, and alteration of nucleotides are the primary bases for many pediatric disorders. However, a large and growing number of disease states result from epigenetic chromosomal modifications that influence gene expression without mutations of genes themselves (101). Pediatric disorders associated with abnormal parental imprinting are listed in Table 3-17. Recent case reports

TABLE 3-17 ■ PEDIATRIC IMPRINTING DISORDERS

Disorder or Syndrome	Chromosomal Locus [*Affected Gene(s)*]	Phenotypic Features
Beckwith-Wiedemann	11.15.5 (*IGF2, H19, KCNQ1,* and others)	Macrosomia, large tongue, hemihypertrophy, omphalocele, ear pits, adrenocytomegaly, placental mesenchymal dysplasia, neoplasia (Wilms tumor, hepatoblastoma)
Pseudohypoparathyroidism/Albright hereditary osteodystrophy	20q13 (*GNAS*)	Developmental delay, mental retardation, obesity, short stature, ± hypocalcemia
Prader-Willi	15q11.2 (*MKRN3, MAGEL2, NDN, and others*)	Mental retardation, obesity, short stature, behavioral problems
Angelman	15q12 (*UBE3A, ATPC10C*)	Mental retardation, dysmorphic facies, behavioral and speech problems
Transient neonatal diabetes mellitus	6q24 (*PLAG1*)	Growth retardation, low fetal/infantile insulin levels
Russell-Silver syndrome	7p11.2	Short stature, asymmetric skull, triangular facies, incurved 5th fingers

suggest that disorders of imprinting may be more common among individuals conceived *in vitro* by assisted reproductive technologies (72). However, more data is needed to substantiate this hypothesis.

Epigenetic chromosomal modifications affect the secondary and/or tertiary structure of chromosomes, but do not alter the chromosomal bands that are visualized by traditional cytogenetic methods. For example, chromosomal DNA is intimately wound around histone proteins, which are particularly dense in transcriptionally silent portions of the genome. Histones are subject to phosphorylation, methylation, and acetylation, which modify their interaction with the DNA and other proteins to facilitate or reduce transcriptional activity (87). The nucleotides of chromosomes are also subject to covalent modifications that correlate with local gene activity, including methylation of cytosine bases. Epigenetic modifications differ between individuals, cell types, and maternally versus paternally derived chromosomes (11). Gene silencing, such as X-chromosome inactivation, is often correlated with high levels of cytosine methylation. The molecular bases for X-chromosome inactivation are partially worked out, but the mechanisms that regulate epigenetic modification of many autosomal genes remain poorly understood (71).

Parental imprinting, a type of epigenetic regulation already referred to in this chapter, refers to differential "marking" of genes in the maternal and paternal germlines, which influences gene expression in tissues of resulting offspring. Imprinting generally involves clusters of closely spaced genes, which are regulated coordinately by discrete DNA elements termed imprinting centers (71). The *IGF2/H19* imprinting cluster, one of the best studied, is located on chromosome 11p15, where improper imprinting has been associated with Beckwith-Wiedemann syndrome (20). Paternal imprinting is associated with methylation of the *IGF2/H19* imprinting center, expression of *IGF2*, and silencing of *H19*, whereas the reverse methylation and expression patterns occur for the maternal allele. In a subset of patients with Beckwith-Wiedemann syndrome, *IGF2* is overexpressed due to either paternal uniparental isodisomy of 11p15 (replacement of the maternal locus by a paternal locus) or loss of imprinting (activation of the normally silent maternal locus).

Unfortunately, neither UPD nor other alterations of imprinting are detected by traditional cytogenetic methods. Instead, sophisticated molecular genetic studies are required.

Future Directions

For several decades, karyotype analysis has been the basis for defining chromosomal disorders. However, the advent of molecular diagnostic approaches is revolutionizing this field to encompass smaller and more subtle chromosomal alterations, a small subset of which are discussed above. In the future, approaches such as array-based CGH are likely to replace the karyotype as a screen for cytogenetic defects (7). Pilot studies suggest that CGH is faster, as sensitive to most and more sensitive to some unbalanced chromosomal alterations, and may be more economical than traditional cytogenetic methods (68,107). As these approaches are applied, recognition of submicroscopic abnormalities will expand the range of chromosomal disorders and probably define genotype-phenotype correlations. As in the past, accurate and comprehensive anatomic pathology, including pathology of the embryo and fetus, will be vital to the evolution of this field.

ACKNOWLEDGMENTS

The authors thank Dr. Kent Opheim for his thoughtful comments.

REFERENCES

1. Abbag FI. Congenital heart diseases and other major anomalies in patients with Down syndrome. *Saudi Med J* 2006;27(2):219–222.
2. Aguirre D, Nieto K, Lazos M, et al. Extragonadal germ cell tumors are often associated with Klinefelter syndrome. *Hum Pathol* 2006;37(4):477–480.
3. Baena N, Guitart M, Ferreres JC, et al. Fetal and placenta chromosome constitution in 237 pregnancy losses. *Ann Genet* 2001;44(2):83–88.

4. Baldwin VJ, Kalousek DK, Dimmick JE, et al. Diagnostic pathologic investigation of the malformed conceptus. *Perspect Pediatr Pathol* 1982;7:65–108.
5. Battaglia A. Del 1p36 syndrome: a newly emerging clinical entity. *Brain Dev* 2005;27(5):358–361.
6. Baty BJ, Blackburn BL, Carey JC. Natural history of trisomy 18 and trisomy 13: I. Growth, physical assessment, medical histories, survival, and recurrence risk. *Am J Med Genet* 1994;49(2):175–188.
7. Bejjani BA, Shaffer LG. Application of array-based comparative genomic hybridization to clinical diagnostics. *J Mol Diagn* 2006;8(5):528–533.
8. Bielanska M, Tan SL, Ao A. Chromosomal mosaicism throughout human preimplantation development in vitro: incidence, type, and relevance to embryo outcome. *Hum Reprod* 2002;17(2):413–419.
9. Bittles AH, Bower C, Hussain R, et al. The four ages of Down syndrome. *Eur J Public Health,* 2007;17(2):221–225.
10. Boghosian-Sell L, Mewar R, Harrison W, et al. Molecular mapping of the Edwards syndrome phenotype to two noncontiguous regions on chromosome 18. *Am J Hum Genet* 1994;55(3):476–483.
11. Brena RM, Huang TH, Plass C. Toward a human epigenome. *Nat Genet* 2006;38(12):1359–1360.
12. Bronsteen R, Lee W, Vettraino IM, et al. Second-trimester sonography and trisomy 18. *J Ultrasound Med* 2004;23(2):233–240.
13. Canick JA, MacRae AR. Second trimester serum markers. *Semin Perinatol* 2005;29:203–208.
14. Chen CP. Congenital heart defects associated with fetal trisomy 18. *Prenat Diagn* 2006;26(5):483–485.
15. Chen CP, Lee CC, Chen WL, et al. Prenatal diagnosis of premature centromere division-related mosaic variegated aneuploidy. *Prenat Diagn* 2004;24(1):19–25.
16. Chervenak FA, Isaacson G, Blakemore KJ, et al. Fetal cystic hygroma. Cause and natural history. *N Engl J Med* 1983;309(14):822–825.
17. Cimini D, Degrassi F. Aneuploidy: a matter of bad connections. *Trends Cell Biol* 2005;15(8):442–451.
18. Daniel A, Wu Z, Bennetts B, et al. Karyotype, phenotype and parental origin in 19 cases of triploidy. *Prenat Diagn* 2001;21(12):1034–1048.
19. De Vries BB, Winter R, Schinzel A, et al. Telomeres: a diagnosis at the end of the chromosomes. *J Med Genet* 2003;40(6):385–398.
20. DeBaun MR, Feinberg AP. *IGF2, H19, p57*^{KIP2}, and *LIT1* and the Beckwith-Wiedemann syndrome. In: Epstein CJ, Erickson RP, Wynshaw-Boris A, eds. *Inborn Errors of Development*. Oxford, UK: Oxford University Press, 2004:758–765.
21. Devriendt K. Hydatidiform mole and triploidy: the role of genomic imprinting in placental development. *Hum Reprod Upd* 2005;11:137–142.
22. Dietze I, Fritz B, Huhle D, et al. Clinical, cytogenetic and molecular investigation in a fetus with Wolf-Hirschhorn syndrome with paternally derived 4p deletion. Case report and review of the literature. *Fetal Diagn Ther* 2004;19(3):251–260.
23. Dietzsch E, Ramsay M, Christianson AL, et al. Maternal origin of extra haploid set of chromosomes in third trimester triploid fetuses. *Am J Med Genet* 1995;58(4):360–364.
24. Donaldson SJ, Wright CA, de Ravel TJ. Trisomy 18 with total cranio-rachischisis and thoraco-abdominoschisis. *Prenat Diagn* 1999;19(6):580–582.
25. Doshi N, Surti U, Szulman AE. Morphologic anomalies in triploid liveborn fetuses. *Hum Pathol* 1983;14(8):716–723.
26. Douglas SD. Down syndrome: immunologic and epidemiologic associations-enigmas remain. *J Pediatr* 2005;147(6):723–725.
27. Doyle EM, McParland P, Carroll S, et al. The role of placental cytogenetic cultures in intrauterine and neonatal deaths. *J Obstet Gynaecol* 2004;24(8):878–880.
28. Emanuel BS, Shaikh TH. Segmental duplications: an 'expanding' role in genomic instability and disease. *Nat Rev Genet* 2001;2(10): 791–800.
29. Embleton ND, Wyllie JP, Wright MJ, et al. Natural history of trisomy 18. *Arch Dis Child Fetal Neonatal Ed* 1996;75(1):F38–F41.
30. Faivre L, Portnoi MF, Pals G, et al. Should chromosome breakage studies be performed in patients with VACTERL association? *Am J Med Genet A* 2005;137(1):55–58.
31. Favara BE. Multiple congenital diverticula of the vermiform appendix. *Am J Clin Pathol* 1968;49(1):60–64.
32. Fujinaga M, Shepard TH, Fitzsimmons J. Trisomy 13 in the fetus. *Teratology* 1990;41(2):233–238.
33. Gardner RJM, Sutherland GR. *Chromosome Abnormalities and Genetic Counseling*, 3rd ed. Oxford, UK: Oxford University Press, 2004:577.
34. Gelman-Kohan Z, Rosensaft J, Ben-Hur H, et al. Cytogenetic analysis of fetal chondrocytes: a comparative study. *Prenat Diagn* 1996;16(2):165–168.
35. Giampietro PF, Adler-Brecher B, Verlander PC, et al. The need for more accurate and timely diagnosis in Fanconi anemia: a report from the International Fanconi Anemia Registry. *Pediatrics* 1993;91(6):1116–1120.
36. Gilbert-Barness E, Opitz JM. Chromosome abnormalities. In: Stocker JT, Dehner LP, eds. *Pediatric Pathology*. Philadelphia, PA: J. B. Lippincott, 1992:41–71.
37. Gilbert EF, Opitz JM. Developmental and other pathologic changes in syndromes caused by chromosome abnormalities. *Persp Pediatr Pathol* 1973;7:1–63.
38. Goldacre MJ, Wotton CJ, Seagroatt V, et al. Cancers and immune related diseases associated with Down's syndrome: a record linkage study. *Arch Dis Child* 2004;89(11):1014–1017.
39. Goldmuntz E. DiGeorge syndrome: new insights. *Clin Perinatol* 2005;32(4):963–978, ix-x.
40. Goldmuntz E, Clark BJ, Mitchell LE, et al. Frequency of 22q11 deletions in patients with conotruncal defects. *J Am Coll Cardiol* 1998;32(2):492–498.
41. Gong W, Gottlieb S, Collins J, et al. Mutation analysis of TBX1 in non-deleted patients with features of DGS/VCFS or isolated cardiovascular defects. *J Med Genet* 2001;38(12):E45.
42. Graux C, Cools J, Michaux L, et al. Cytogenetics and molecular genetics of T-cell acute lymphoblastic leukemia: from thymocyte to lymphoblast. *Leukemia* 2006;20(9):1496–1510.
43. Gravholt CH, Fedder J, Naeraa RW, et al. Occurrence of gonadoblastoma in females with Turner syndrome and Y chromosome material: a population study. *J Clin Endocrinol Metab* 2000;85(9):3199–3202.
44. Haargaard B, Fledelius HC. Down's syndrome and early cataract. *Br J Ophthalmol* 2006;90(8):1024–1027.
45. Hanks S, Coleman K, Reid S, et al. Constitutional aneuploidy and cancer predisposition caused by biallelic mutations in BUB1B. *Nat Genet* 2004;36(11):1159–1161.
46. Hassold T, Hunt P. To err (meiotically) is human: the genesis of human aneuploidy. *Nat Rev Genet* 2001;2(4):280–291.
47. Head E, Lott IT. Down syndrome and beta-amyloid deposition. *Curr Opin Neurol* 2004;17(2):95–100.
48. Heard E, Disteche CM. Dosage compensation in mammals: fine-tuning the expression of the X chromosome. *Genes Dev* 2006;20(14):1848–1867.
49. Helali N, Iafolla AK, Kahler SG, et al. A case of duplication of 13q32→qter and deletion of 18p11.32→pter with mild phenotype: Patau syndrome and duplications of 13q revisited. *J Med Genet* 1996;33(7):600–602.
50. Hook EB, Mutton DE, Ide R, et al. The natural history of Down syndrome conceptuses diagnosed prenatally that are not electively terminated. *Am J Hum Genet* 1995;57(4):875–881.
51. Hook EB, Topol BB, Cross PK. The natural history of cytogenetically abnormal fetuses detected at midtrimester amniocentesis which are not terminated electively: new data and estimates of the excess and relative risk of late fetal death associated with 47,+21 and some other abnormal karyotypes. *Am J Hum Genet* 1989;45(6):855–861.
52. Irons M. Use of subtelomeric fluorescence in situ hybridization in cytogenetic diagnosis. *Curr Opin Pediatr* 2003;15(6):594–597.

53. Jacobs PA, Szulman AE, Funkhouser J, et al. Human triploidy: relationship between parental origin of the additional haploid complement and development of partial hydatidiform mole. *Ann Hum Genet* 1982;46(Pt 3):223–231.
54. Jones KL. *Smith's Recognizable Patterns of Human Malformation*. Philadelphia, PA: W.B. Saunders Co.; 2006:778.
55. Kallen B, Mastroiacovo P, Robert E. Major congenital malformations in Down syndrome. *Am J Med Genet* 1996;65(2):160–166.
56. Kalousek DK, Barrett IJ, McGillivray BC. Placental mosaicism and intrauterine survival of trisomies 13 and 18. *Am J Hum Genet* 1989;44(3):338–343.
57. Kalousek DK, Langlois S, Barrett I, et al. Uniparental disomy for chromosome 16 in humans. *Am J Hum Genet* 1993;52(1):8–16.
58. Kalousek DK, Lau AE. Pathology of spontaneous abortion. In: Dimmick JE, Kalousek DK, eds. *Developmental Pathology of the Embryo and Fetus*. J. B. Lippincott, Philadelphia, PA: 1992:55–82.
59. Kalousek DK, Vekemans M. Confined placental mosaicism and genomic imprinting. *Baillieres Best Pract Res Clin Obstet Gynaecol* 2000;14(4):723–730.
60. Kava MP, Tullu MS, Muranjan MN, et al. Down syndrome: clinical profile from India. *Arch Med Res* 2004;35(1):31–35.
61. Kinoshita M, Nakamura Y, Nakano R, et al. Thirty-one autopsy cases of trisomy 18: clinical features and pathological findings. *Pediatr Pathol* 1989;9(4):445–457.
62. Kjaer I, Keeling JW, Fischer Hansen B. Pattern of malformations in the axial skeleton in human trisomy 13 fetuses. *Am J Med Genet* 1997;70(4):421–426.
63. Klewer SE, Runyan RB, Erickson RP. *TBX1* and the DiGeorge syndrome critical region. In: Epstein CJ, Erickson RP, Wynshaw-Boris A, eds. *Inborn Errors of Development*. Oxford, UK: Oxford University Press, 2004:699–704.
64. Knutsen T. Laboratory safety, quality control, and regulations. In: Barch MJ, Knutsen T, Spurbeck J, eds. *The AGT Cytogenetics Laboratory Manual*, 3rd ed. Philadelphia, PA: Lippincott-Raven, 1997:597–646.
65. Kyle PM, Sepulveda W, Blunt S, et al. High failure rate of post-mortem karyotyping after termination for fetal abnormality. *Obstet Gynecol* 1996;88(5):859–862.
66. Langlois S, Yong PJ, Yong SL, et al. Postnatal follow-up of prenatally diagnosed trisomy 16 mosaicism. *Prenat Diagn* 2006;26(6): 548–558.
67. Lazar A, Abruzzo LV, Pollock RE, et al. Molecular diagnosis of sarcomas: chromosomal translocations in sarcomas. *Arch Pathol Lab Med* 2006;130(8):1199–1207.
68. Le Caignec C, Boceno M, Saugier-Veber P, et al. Detection of genomic imbalances by array based comparative genomic hybridisation in fetuses with multiple malformations. *J Med Genet* 2005;42(2):121–128.
69. Lehman CD, Nyberg DA, Winter TC III, et al. Trisomy 13 syndrome: prenatal US findings in a review of 33 cases. *Radiology* 1995;194(1):217–222.
70. Lestou VS, Kalousek DK. Confined placental mosaicism and intrauterine fetal growth. *Arch Dis Child Fetal Neonatal Ed* 1998;79(3):F223–F226.
71. Lewis A, Reik W. How imprinting centres work. *Cytogenet Genome Res* 2006;113(1–4):81–89.
72. Lidegaard O, Pinborg A, Andersen AN. Imprinting disorders after assisted reproductive technologies. *Curr Opin Obstet Gynecol* 2006;18(3):293–296.
73. Machin GA, Crolla JA. Chromosome constitution of 500 infants dying during the perinatal period. With an appendix concerning other genetic disorders among these infants. *Humangenetik* 1974;23(3):183–198.
74. Macpherson TA, Garver KL, Turner JH, et al. Predicting in vitro tissue culture growth for cytogenetic evaluation of stillborn fetuses. *Eur J Obstet Gynecol Reprod Biol* 1985;19(3):167–174.
75. Makrydimas G, Papanikolaou E, Paraskevaidis E, et al. Upper limb abnormalities as an isolated ultrasonographic finding in early detection of trisomy 18. A case report. *Fetal Diagn Ther* 2003;18(6):401–403.
76. Malaga S, Pardo R, Malaga I, et al. Renal involvement in Down syndrome. *Pediatr Nephrol* 2005;20(5):614–617.
77. Massey GV, Zipursky A, Chang MN, et al. A prospective study of the natural history of transient leukemia (TL) in neonates with Down syndrome (DS): Children's Oncology Group (COG) study POG-9481. *Blood* 2006;107(12):4606–4613.
78. Mathew CG. Fanconi anaemia genes and susceptibility to cancer. *Oncogene* 2006;25(43):5875–5884.
79. Matsuura S, Matsumoto Y, Morishima K, et al. Monoallelic BUB1B mutations and defective mitotic-spindle checkpoint in seven families with premature chromatid separation (PCS) syndrome. *Am J Med Genet A* 2006;140(4):358–367.
80. Mazzanti L, Cacciari E. Congenital heart disease in patients with Turner's syndrome. Italian Study Group for Turner Syndrome (ISGTS). *J Pediatr* 1998;133(5):688–692.
81. McConnell V, Derham R, McManus D, et al. Mosaic monosomy 14: clinical features and recognizable facies. *Clin Dysmorphol* 2004;13(3):155–160.
82. McDermid HE, Morrow BE. Genomic disorders on 22q11. *Am J Hum Genet* 2002;70(5):1077–1088.
83. McFadden DE, Friedman JM. Chromosome abnormalities in human beings. *Mutat Res* 1997;396(1–2):129–140.
84. McFadden DE, Jiang R, Langlois S, et al. Dispermy—origin of diandric triploidy: brief communication. *Hum Reprod* 2002; 17(12):3037–3038.
85. McFadden DE, Kalousek DK. Two different phenotypes of fetuses with chromosomal triploidy: correlation with parental origin of the extra haploid set. *Am J Med Genet* 1991;38(4):535–538.
86. McFadden DE, Robinson WP. Phenotype of triploid embryos. *J Med Genet* 2006;43(7):609–612.
87. Mellor J. Dynamic nucleosomes and gene transcription. *Trends Genet* 2006;22(6):320–329.
88. Milbrandt TA, Johnston CE II. Down syndrome and scoliosis: a review of a 50-year experience at one institution. *Spine* 2005;30(18):2051–2055.
89. Miller OJ, Therman E. *Human Chromosomes*, 4th ed. New York, NY: Springer-Verlag, 2001:501.
90. Morris JK, Wald NJ, Watt HC. Fetal loss in Down syndrome pregnancies. *Prenat Diagn* 1999;19(2):142–145.
91. Munne S, Cohen J. Chromosome abnormalities in human embryos. *Hum Reprod Upd* 1998;4:842–855.
92. Nakamura Y, Hashimoto T, Sasaguri Y, et al. Brain anomalies found in 18 trisomy: CT scanning, morphologic and morphometric study. *Clin Neuropathol* 1986;5(2):47–52.
93. Nyberg DA, Kramer D, Resta RG, et al. Prenatal sonographic findings of trisomy 18: review of 47 cases. *J Ultrasound Med* 1993;12(2):103–113.
94. Olson LE, Richtsmeier JT, Leszl J, et al. A chromosome 21 critical region does not cause specific Down syndrome phenotypes. *Science* 2004;306(5696):687–690.
95. Oyelese Y, Vintzileos AM. Is second trimester genetic amniocentesis for trisomy 18 ever indicated in the presence of a normal genetic sonogram? *Ultrasound Obstet Gynecol* 2005;26:691–694.
96. Papp C, Ban Z, Szigeti Z, et al. Prenatal sonographic findings in 207 fetuses with trisomy 21. *Eur J Obstet Gynecol Reprod Biol* 2007;133(2):186–190.
97. Pinto-Escalante D, Ceballos-Quintal JM, Castillo-Zapata I, et al. Full mosaic monosomy 22 in a child with DiGeorge syndrome facial appearance. *Am J Med Genet* 1998;76(2):150–153.
98. Pritchard MA, Kola I. The "gene dosage effect" hypothesis versus the "amplified developmental instability" hypothesis in Down syndrome. *J Neural Transm Suppl* 1999;57:293–303.
99. Ravnan JB, Tepperberg JH, Papenhausen P, et al. Subtelomere FISH analysis of 11 688 cases: an evaluation of the frequency and pattern of subtelomere rearrangements in individuals with developmental disabilities. *J Med Genet* 2006;43(6):478–489.

100. Roberts P, Chumas PD, Picton S, et al. A review of the cytogenetics of 58 pediatric brain tumors. *Cancer Genet Cytogenet* 2001;131(1):1–12.
101. Robertson KD. DNA methylation and human disease. *Nat Rev Genet* 2005;6(8):597–610.
102. Robinson WP, McFadden DE, Stephenson MD. The origin of abnormalities in recurrent aneuploidy/polyploidy. *Am J Hum Genet* 2001;69(6):1245–1254.
103. Roeder GS. Meiotic chromosomes: it takes two to tango. *Genes Dev* 1997;11(20):2600–2621.
104. Rosen T, D'Alton ME. Down syndrome screening in the first and second trimesters: what do the data show? *Semin Perinatol* 2005;29:367–375.
105. Rowland JM. Molecular genetic diagnosis of pediatric cancer: current and emerging methods. *Pediatr Clin North Am* 2002;49(6):1415–1435.
106. Rubio C, Simon C, Vidal F, et al. Chromosomal abnormalities and embryo development in recurrent miscarriage couples. *Hum Reprod* 2003;18(1):182–188.
107. Sahoo T, Cheung SW, Ward P, et al. Prenatal diagnosis of chromosomal abnormalities using array-based comparative genomic hybridization. *Genet Med* 2006;8(11):719–727.
108. Schapira AH. Mitochondrial disease. *Lancet* 2006;368(9529): 70–82.
109. Schepis C, Barone C, Siragusa M, et al. An updated survey on skin conditions in Down syndrome. *Dermatology* 2002;205(3): 234–238.
110. Schinzel A. *Catalogue of Unbalanced Chromosomal Aberrations in Man*, 2nd ed. Berlin, Germany: Walter de Gruyer GmbH & Co.; 2001:966.
111. Shaffer LG, Tommerup N. *ISCN (2005): An International System for Human Cytogenetic Nomenclature*. Basel, Switzerland: S. Karger; 2005:130.
112. Sharp AJ, Hansen S, Selzer RR, et al. Discovery of previously unidentified genomic disorders from the duplication architecture of the human genome. *Nat Genet* 2006;38(9):1038–1042.
113. Shaw SW, Cheng PJ, Chueh HY, et al. Ectopia cordis in a fetus with trisomy 18. *J Clin Ultrasound* 2006;34(2):95–98.
114. Shott SR. Down syndrome: common otolaryngologic manifestations. *Am J Med Genet C Semin Med Genet* 2006;142(3): 131–140.
115. Siebert JR. CNS manifestations of chromosomal change. In: Golden JA, Harding BN, eds. *Developmental Neuropathology*. Basel, Switzerland: International Society of Neuropathology, 2004:132–141.
116. Smith A, Bannatyne P, Russell P, et al. Cytogenetic studies in perinatal death. *Aust N Z J Obstet Gynaecol* 1990;30(3):206–210.
117. Spencer K, Heath V, Flack N, et al. First trimester maternal serum AFP and total hCG in aneuploidies other than trisomy 21. *Prenat Diagn* 2000;20(8):635–639.
118. Stetten G, Escallon CS, South ST, et al. Reevaluating confined placental mosaicism. *Am J Med Genet A* 2004;131(3):232–239.
119. Sybert VP. Cardiovascular malformations and complications in Turner syndrome. *Pediatrics* 1998;101(1):E11.
120. Sybert VP, McCauley E. Turner's syndrome. *N Engl J Med* 2004;351(12):1227–1238.
121. Torfs CP, Christianson RE. Anomalies in Down syndrome individuals in a large population-based registry. *Am J Med Genet* 1998;77(5):431–438.
122. Toyoda A, Noguchi H, Taylor TD, et al. Comparative genomic sequence analysis of the human chromosome 21 Down syndrome critical region. *Genome Res* 2002;12(9):1323–1332.
123. Uchida IA, Freeman VC. Triploidy and chromosomes. *Am J Obstet Gynecol* 1985;151(1):65–69.
124. Uematsu A, Yorifuji T, Muroi J, et al. Parental origin of normal X chromosomes in Turner syndrome patients with various karyotypes: implications for the mechanism leading to generation of a 45,X karyotype. *Am J Med Genet* 2002;111(2):134–139.
125. Uibo O, Teesalu K, Metskula K, et al. Screening for celiac disease in Down's syndrome patients revealed cases of subtotal villous atrophy without typical for celiac disease HLA-DQ and tissue transglutaminase antibodies. *World J Gastroenterol* 2006;12(9): 1430–1434.
126. Vachon L, Fareau GE, Wilson MG, et al. Testicular microlithiasis in patients with Down syndrome. *J Pediatr* 2006;149(2):233–236.
127. van der Putte SC. Lymphatic malformation in human fetuses. A study of fetuses with Turner's syndrome or status Bonnevie-Ullrich. *Virchows Arch A Pathol Anat Histol* 1977;376(3):233–246.
128. Van Opstal D, Van den Berg C, Deelen WH, et al. Prospective prenatal investigations on potential uniparental disomy in cases of confined placental trisomy. *Prenat Diagn* 1998;18(1):35–44.
129. Wald NJ, Rodeck C, Hackshaw AK, et al. SURUSS in perspective. *Semin Perinatol* 2005;29(4):225–235.
130. Warburton PE, Dolled M, Mahmood R, et al. Molecular cytogenetic analysis of eight inversion duplications of human chromosome 13q that each contain a neocentromere. *Am J Hum Genet* 2000;66(6):1794–1806.
131. Warkany J. *Congenital Malformations*. Chicago, IL: Year Book Medical Publishers, 1971:1309.
132. Wattendorf DJ, Muenke M. Klinefelter syndrome. *Am Fam Physician* 2005;72(11):2259–2262.
133. Wertelecki W, Fraumeni JF Jr, Mulvihill JJ. Nongonadal neoplasia in Turner's syndrome. *Cancer* 1970;26(2):485–488.
134. Won RH, Currier RJ, Lorey F, et al. The timing of demise in fetuses with trisomy 21 and trisomy 18. *Prenat Diagn* 2005;25(7): 608–611.
135. Wyllie JP, Wright MJ, Burn J, et al. Natural history of trisomy 13. *Arch Dis Child* 1994;71(4):343–345.
136. Yamanaka M, Setoyama T, Igarashi Y, et al. Pregnancy outcome of fetuses with trisomy 18 identified by prenatal sonography and chromosomal analysis in a perinatal center. *Am J Med Genet A* 2006;140(11):1177–1182.
137. Yeo L, Guzman ER, Day-Salvatore D, et al. Prenatal detection of fetal trisomy 18 through abnormal sonographic features. *J Ultrasound Med* 2003;22(6):581–590; quiz 591–582.
138. Yokoyama T, Tamura H, Tsukamoto H, et al. Prevalence of glaucoma in adults with Down's syndrome. *Jpn J Ophthalmol* 2006;50(3):274–276.
139. Yong PJ, Langlois S, von Dadelszen P, et al. The association between preeclampsia and placental trisomy 16 mosaicism. *Prenat Diagn* 2006;26:956–961.
140. Yurdakul NS, Ugurlu S, Maden A. Strabismus in Down syndrome. *J Pediatr Ophthalmol Strabismus* 2006;43(1):27–30.
141. Zaragoza MV, Surti U, Redline RW, et al. Parental origin and phenotype of triploidy in spontaneous abortions: predominance of diandry and association with the partial hydatidiform mole. *Am J Hum Genet* 2000;66(6):1807–1820.

CHAPTER 4

Congenital Anomalies and Malformation Syndromes

JOSEPH R. SIEBERT

The study of congenital anomalies continues to be hampered by misunderstandings at a number of levels. In many circles, for example, the statement that "the baby was born with a genetic deformity" is often heard. In fact, this is often not the case, for many congenital anomalies are not genetic in origin nor do they constitute a physical deformation per se. Another common, but erroneous, opinion is that hundreds or even thousands of substances in the environment cause birth defects. In fact, only 30 to 40 exogenous substances (i.e., teratogens) have been proven to have this potential. But if these issues continue to hamper our dealings professionally, they also tug at the souls of grieving parents who ask "What caused my baby's problem?" "How did this happen?" or "Will it happen again?" These questions take on added complexity when multiple anomalies are encountered in a single patient. It can fall to the pathologist, as well as clinical specialists, to help explain these findings. The purpose of this chapter, then, is to provide a broad context for understanding the basic *patterns* of anomalies. As such, descriptions will emphasize gross features over microscopic appearances or discussions of intricate pathologic processes. For help with these latter matters, the reader is referred to chapters that cover specific organ systems.

ETIOLOGY AND PATHOGENESIS

The question of causation—etiology—is not at all simple, for etiology may be heterogeneous, that is, multiple factors may bring about a given defect. Holoprosencephaly is a powerful example, for it arises sporadically or is associated with several gene mutations, aneuploidies (i.e., trisomy 13), and teratogens (e.g., ethyl alcohol). Robin sequence (micrognathia, cleft palate, glossoptosis) is another example, in which causes may be chromosomal, teratogenic, monogenic, disruptive (i.e., amniotic bands), or unknown (45).

The mechanism—or pathogenesis—responsible for a defect may be varied as well. In Robin sequence, for example, deformations may occur secondary to intrauterine constraint produced by oligohydramnios. However, reduced amniotic fluid volume may occur from premature rupture of membranes (particularly chronic leakage), renal anomalies, placental, or maternal factors.

CONCEPTS AND TERMS OF MORPHOGENESIS

In 1982, a set of standardized terms for describing human developmental abnormalities was established (235). The definitions are essential for pediatric pathologists, pediatricians, medical geneticists, and others dealing with congenital anomalies. Several discussions of the terminologic, historic, diagnostic, nosologic, and morphologic aspects of congenital anomalies in humans are available (45,180).

Hypoplasia refers to underdevelopment and *hyperplasia* to overdevelopment of an organism, organ, or tissue and result from a change in cell number. *Hypotrophy* and *hypertrophy* refer to a decrease and increase, respectively, in the size of an organ, tissue, or cells. *Agenesis* is the absence of a part of the body caused by a presumed absence of the anlage, or primordium. *Aplasia* refers to absence of a rudimentary structure caused by failure of the anlage to develop completely. Aplasia can be regarded as an extreme degree of hypoplasia. *Atrophy* describes the shrinkage of a previously normally developed tissue mass or organ because of a decrease in cell size or cell number.

A *developmental field* is the portion of the embryo that reacts as a coordinated unit to inductive effects with differentiation and growth (178). Developmental fields represent, then, the major branches on the morphogenetic tree. It has been suggested that the embryo itself constitutes the *primary developmental field* (177) and that other more constricted ones are operational at later stages of development. A *monotopic field defect* represents a defect in organogenesis and includes contiguous anomalies (e.g., cyclopia and holoprosencephaly; cleft lip and cleft palate). Such alterations are more likely to arise late in gestation and produce more confined defects (151). By contrast, a *polytopic field defect* is thought to result from an earlier defect during blastogenesis—the first 4 weeks of development—and occurs if abnormal inductive processes produce more distantly located and diverse defects (151,152).

The midline also acts as a developmental field (179). It represents the normal plane of cleavage in monozygotic twinning and the plane around which symmetry of visceral position is determined. It is an especially vulnerable site in terms of developmental anomalies. Morphogenetic events involving the midline include fusions, segmentation, programmed cell death with morphogenetic "necroses" or resorptions, rotations, and other developmental movements. In some anomalies involving the midline, the incidence of monozygotic twinning may be increased (e.g., sirenomelia, cloacal anomalies). Other examples of midline anomalies include the holoprosencephaly complex, agenesis of the corpus callosum, cleft lip, cleft palate, midface cleft complex, spina bifida, omphalocele, congenital heart defects, hypospadias, and imperforate anus.

A *malformation* is "a morphologic defect of an organ, part of an organ, or larger region of the body resulting from an intrinsically abnormal developmental process" (235).

A *disruption*, or secondary malformation, is "a morphologic defect of an organ, part of an organ, or a larger region of the body, resulting from the extrinsic breakdown of, or interference with, an originally normal developmental process" (235). Disruptions are causally heterogeneous and may bear close resemblance to malformations anatomically. In a given case, the distinction between a disruption and a malformation may be made on the basis of the associated malformations or the history of gestational exposure to a teratogenic agent or event. The general prevalence of birth defects is given as 3% to 5%.

A *deformation* is "an abnormal form, shape, or position of a part of the body caused by mechanical forces." It may be extrinsic, due to intrauterine constraint (e.g., lack of amniotic fluid), or intrinsic, due to a defect of the nervous system that causes hypomobility (235). Examples of deformities are talipes equinovarus and arthrogryposis. About 1% to 2% of newborn infants have deformations of some sort.

Dysplasia represents "an abnormal organization of cells into tissue(s) and its morphologic result(s)" (235). Dysplasia is therefore a process and the consequence of *dyshistogenesis*, an abnormal differentiation of tissue structure. This is in contrast to a malformation, which is a defect in morphogenesis of the organ structure. Dysplasias may or may not be metabolically induced, may involve one or several germ layers, and may be generalized or localized; they often demonstrate a sporadic pattern of occurrence (235).

Mild dysplasias, common in the normal population, include freckling, capillary hemangioma over the glabella and metopic suture area of the forehead, café au lait spots, moles, and nevi. If they are Mendelian traits, they usually represent autosomal dominant mutations. Dysplasias are components of every aneuploidy syndrome and probably are one reason for the increased incidence of associated cancers. Dysplasias can be induced environmentally by radiation, viruses, and carcinogens.

Anomalies sometimes occur as groups of defects, which require additional classification. The terms described below help in categorizing anomalies, but are only aids. Placing a name on a cluster of anomalies helps in organizing thoughts about a given condition, but does not identify cause or mechanism or suggest recurrence risk. In general, "the classification and terminology of infants with birth defects remain confusing. Terms such as syndromes, associations, phenotypes, patterns, fields, and spectra often appear to be used as convenient labels and do not help clarify the underlying cause or pathogenesis" (125).

That being said, a *syndrome* is "a pattern of multiple anomalies thought to be pathogenetically related and not known to represent a single sequence or a polytopic field defect" (235). No structural component anomaly of any malformation syndrome is obligatory, and no one component is pathognomonic of any syndrome.

A *sequence* is a "pattern of multiple anomalies derived from a single known or presumed prior anomaly or mechanical factor" (235). In the Potter sequence, the pathogenetic event is oligohydramnios arising from a genetic or nongenetic cause; the causal event represents a malformation (e.g., renal agenesis or dysplasia, as in polycystic kidney) or a mechanical factor (e.g., amniotic fluid leakage). Lack of amniotic fluid restricts fetal movement and causes fetal compression, producing the typical changes of Potter sequence (Figure 4-1).

A *malformation complex* consists of "those groups of heterogeneous disorders with overlapping characteristics that are difficult to separate into specific conditions," for example, facio-auriculo-vertebral spectrum and hypoglossia-hypodactylia.

An *association* consists of "a nonrandom occurrence in two or more individuals of multiple anomalies not known to be a polytopic field defect, sequence, or syndrome" (235). Associations have also been defined as the results of "disruptive events acting on developmental fields" (144). However, the diversity of findings in such associations as CHARGE highlight how much remains unknown about possible developmental fields. In a sense, the term "association" is a temporary category that should change as conditions become better understood.

Jones has offered a valuable policy for naming patterns of malformations (118):

1. When the etiology is known and easily remembered, the appropriate term should be used to designate the disorder.
2. Time-honored designations should be continued unless there is good reason to change.
3. In the absence of a reasonably descriptive designation, eponyms, some of them multiple, may be used until the basic defect for the disorder is recognized. However, use of an eponym should thereafter be limited to one proper name.

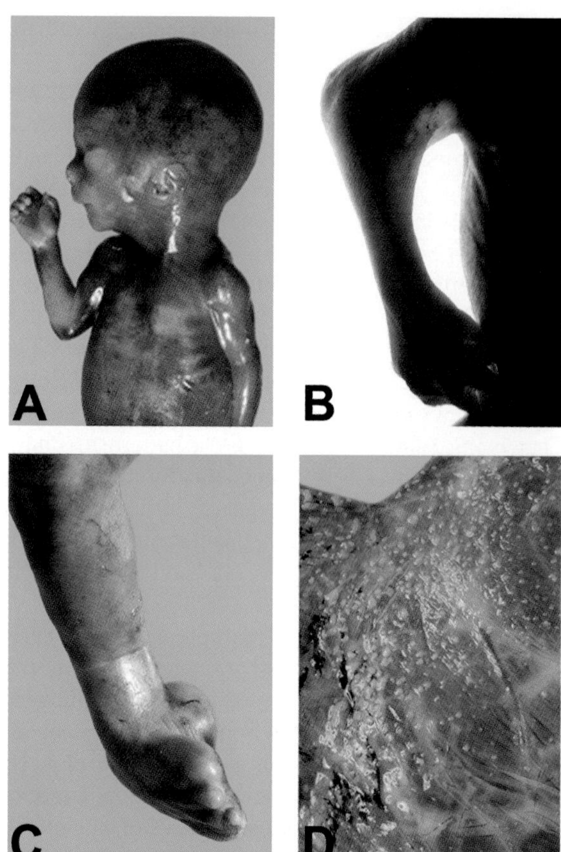

FIGURE 4-1 ■ Potter sequence. **A:** 22-week fetus with history of severe oligohydramnios (renal system normal; no history of premature rupture of membranes). Note the blunt nose, small mandible, and flattened ear. **B:** Marked skin webbing (pterygium) of right elbow developed secondary to prolonged immobilization of joint. **C:** Medial rotation of foot at ankle joint (talipes equinovarus) resulted from intrauterine constraint. **D:** Fetal surface of placenta shows amnion nodosum, a finding common in cases of oligohydramnios.

4. The use of the possessive form of an eponym should be discontinued, because the author neither had nor owned the disorder.
5. Designation of a disorder by one or more of its manifestations does not necessarily imply that they are either specific or consistent components of that disorder.
6. Names that may have an unpleasant connotation for the family or affected individual should be avoided.
7. The syndrome should not be designated by the initials of the originally described patients.
8. Names that are too general for a specific syndrome should be avoided.
9. Unless acronyms are extremely pertinent or appropriate, they should be avoided.

DEFORMATIONS

Amniotic Fluid Volume

Oligohydramnios, or anhydramnios, effectively reduces the space available to the fetus and is associated with a wide variety of fetal deformations involving the limbs and the craniofacial complex. With reduced inhalation of fluid comes pulmonary hypoplasia, which is lethal when severe. Reduced fluid volume comes about primarily from leakage (i.e., premature rupture of membranes) or renal anomalies with reduced production of fetal urine.

Uterine and Placental Implantation Abnormalities

A bicornate uterus may cause fetal compression and constraint, resulting in a deformed fetus. Uterine malformations may also predispose the fetus to malformations arising from abnormalities in implantation, placentation, body stalk formation, and late fetal cord compression or torsion. With these occurrences comes an increased risk of stillbirth (see Chapter 18).

Neurogenic, Skeletal, and Other Causes of Deformations

Central nervous system (CNS) and skeletal muscle defects (e.g., amyoplasia) may result in deformations. The most common congenital limb deformities are tibial bowing, mild metatarsus varus, talipes equinovalgus and varus, and the flexural contractures of arthrogryposis (Figure 4-2). Skeletal dysplasias may be associated with deformities of prenatal or postnatal onset. Twins and multiple fetuses may effectively interfere with each other's physical development and manifest deformities.

DISRUPTIONS

Ionizing Radiation

Studies of radiation exposure to pregnant women during medical treatments or warfare have provided valuable information regarding radiation-induced fetal anomalies.

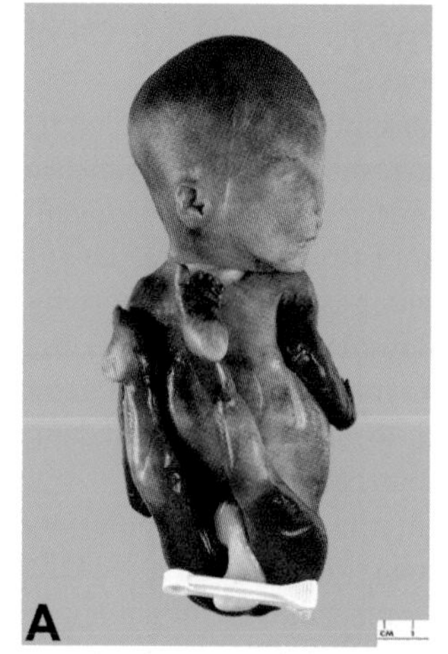

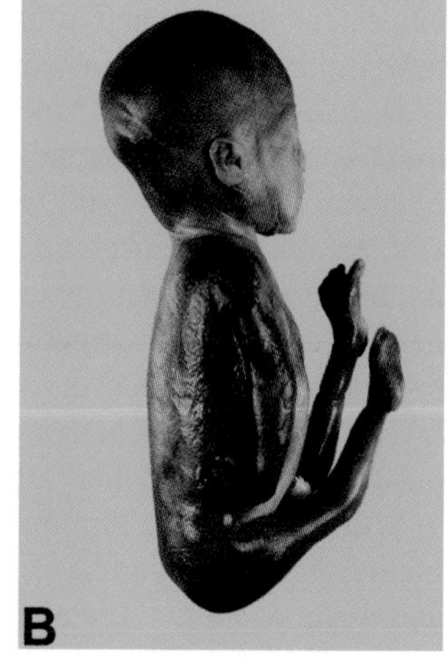

FIGURE 4-2 ■ Severe arthrogryposis in 23-week fetus. Extraordinary flexion and contracture deformities and marked flattening of the face are apparent. Autopsy revealed no other fetal anomalies (karyotype 46,XX). Etiology is heterogeneous in this condition.

It is commonly held that pregnant women should avoid all unnecessary radiation exposure. However, data regarding exact doses of radiation are often unavailable, and so fears and actions based upon those fears (i.e., elective abortion after an exposure or suspected exposure) are often unwarranted. Counselors must use extreme caution when dealing with questions regarding radiation exposure.

Guidelines are widely available for this purpose (9,13,32,255). During pregnancy, the acceptable cumulative dose of ionizing radiation during pregnancy is 5 rads. With few exceptions, diagnostic studies produce dosages less than this level. A two-view radiograph of mother's chest, for example, exposes the fetus to just 0.00007 rads. Therefore, a mother would need the equivalent of 500 chest examinations before the fetus would be exposed to a harmful level of radiation. Because 8 to 25 weeks, and especially 10 to 17 weeks, of gestation is a highly sensitive period for CNS teratogenesis, unnecessary exposures directly to the fetus should be avoided during this time. Prenatal radiation exposure may produce a slight increase in the risk of childhood leukemia or small change in the frequency of gene mutations, but these are quite rare and not an indication for pregnancy termination.

Fetal irradiation is associated with generalized growth retardation, microcephaly, skull defects, spina bifida, microphthalmia, cleft palate, micromelia, clubfoot, and other anomalies following maternal exposure to high-dose radiation (83). Altered mental status, ranging from reduced intelligence quotient (IQ) to frank mental retardation and seizures, are recognized; MRI examinations are suggestive of neuronal migration defects (184,185, 198).

Teratogenic Disruptions

A list of teratogenic agents in humans is shown in Table 4-1 and the specific time of action in embryonic development is shown in Table 4-2. Excellent resources on this topic are available (73,225).

Thalidomide Embryopathy

Thalidomide was first recognized as a teratogen by Lenz and McBride in separate reports in 1961. Maternal administration of thalidomide during the critical period (day 23 to 28 of gestation) results in a number of defects, the most notable of which are limb defects ranging from triphalangeal thumb to tetra-amelia or phocomelia of the upper and lower limbs, at times with preaxial polydactyly of six or seven toes per foot. Congenital heart defects, urinary tract anomalies, genital defects, gastrointestinal anomalies, eye defects, ear malformations, and dental anomalies have been observed. The mechanism of action continues to be studied. Some have suggested that defective angiogenesis in developing limb buds may be operational (238). This hypothesis may also have application to the sensitivity of certain neoplasias to thalidomide.

Table 4-1 ■ TERATOGENIC AGENTS IN HUMANS

Radiation
- Atomic weapons
- Radioiodine
- Therapeutic

Infections
- Cytomegalovirus
- Herpes simplex virus 1 and 2
- Lymphocytic choriomeningitis virus (LCMV)
- Parvovirus B-19 (erythema infectiosum)
- Rubella virus
- Syphilis
- Toxoplasmosis
- Varicella virus
- Venezuelan equine encephalitis virus

Maternal and Metabolic Imbalance
- Alcoholism
- Amniocentesis, early
- Chorionic villus sampling (before day 60)[a]
- Cretinism, endemic
- Diabetes mellitus
- Folic acid deficiency
- Hyperthermia
- Myasthenia gravis
- Phenylketonuria
- Rheumatic disease and congenital heart block
- Sjogren syndrome
- Virilizing tumors

Drugs and Environmental Chemicals
- Aminopterin and methylaminopterin
- Androgenic hormones
- Captopril (renal failure)
- Carbamazepine[a]
- Chlorobiphenyls
- Cigarette smoke (nicotine)
- Cocaine
- Corticosteroids[a]
- Coumarin anticoagulants
- Cyclophosphamide
- Diethylstilbestrol
- Diphenylhydantoin
- Enalapril (renal failure)
- Etretinate
- Fluconazole, high dose
- Iodides and goiter
- Lithium[a]
- Mercury, organic
- Methimazole (scalp defects and choanal atresia)[a]
- Methylene blue via intra-amniotic injection
- Misoprostol[a]
- Penicillamine
- Phenobarbitol[a]
- 1,3-*cis*-Retinoic acid (Isotretinoin and Accutane)
- Sartans
- Tetracyclines
- Thalidomide
- Toluene abuse
- Trimethadione
- Valproic acid

[a]Agents produce less than 10 defects per 1,000 exposures.
From Shepard and Lemire (225), with permission.

Table 4-2 ■ TIME OF ACTION OF HUMAN TERATOGENS

Teratogen	Gestational Age (Days)	Malformation
Rubella virus	0–60	Cataract or heart defect more likely
	0–129+	Deafness
Thalidomide	21–40	Reduction defects of extremities
Hyperthermia	18–30	Anencephaly
Male hormones (androgens, tumors)	Before 90	Clitoral hypertrophy and labial fusion only
	After 90	Clitoral hypertrophy
Coumadin anticoagulants	Before 100	Hypoplasia of nose and stippling of epiphyses
	After 100	Possible mental retardation
Diethylstilbestrol	After 14	Vaginal adenosis (50%)
	After 98	Vaginal adenosis (30%)
	After 126	Vaginal adenosis (10%)
Radioiodine therapy	After 65–70	Fetal "thyroidectomy"
Goitrogens, iodides	After 180	Fetal goiter
Tetracycline	After 120	Dental enamel staining of primary teeth
	After 250	Staining of crowns of permanent teeth

From Shepard (224), with permission.

Folic Acid Deficiency

Deficiency of folic acid results in up to 70% of neural tube deficits (NTDs), particularly anencephaly. Preconceptional intake of 0.4-mg folic acid daily reduces the incidence of NTDs by approximately 60% (140,271). The fortification of wheat flour with folic acid in the United States has resulted in a decrease in the incidence of NTDs; a similar success might also be expected with similar fortification and surveillance worldwide (14,25). In addition to aiding in the prevention of NTDs, prenatal supplementation with folic acid prevents pregnancy-induced megaloblastic anemia (245).

Folic Acid Antagonists and Derivatives

Aminopterin and methotrexate, its methyl derivative, are folic acid antagonists that may cause a variety of anomalies. Because of the use of methotrexate to end an unwanted or ectopic pregnancy, exposure during early pregnancy is possible (3). Craniofacial anomalies include severe hypoplasia of frontal, parietal, temporal, or occipital bones; wide fontanelles; upsweep of frontal scalp hair; broad nasal bridge; shallow supraorbital ridges; prominent eyes; cleft palate; apparently low-set ears; micrognathia; maxillary hypoplasia; and epicanthal folds. The limbs are relatively short, and dislocation of hips, short thumbs, partial syndactyly of third and fourth fingers, dextroposition of the heart, and hypotonia may occur (163,223,252).

Fetal Iodine Deficiency

The pregnant woman and her developing fetus both have an increased need for iodine. The woman deficient in dietary intake of iodine therefore puts both herself and her fetus at risk (81). The use of iodized salt has done much to reduce the risk of associated mental retardation worldwide but is of little help to women who do not have access to this food or those who must reduce their salt intake during pregnancy.

Fetal iodine deficiency results in mental retardation, spastic diplegia, deafness, and strabismus (48,106). It develops from severe maternal iodine deficiency (<20 μg/day) during the first half of gestation, which occurs primarily in a number of European countries and in some mountainous areas, such as New Guinea, the Himalayas, and the Andes (169). The World Health Organization recommends a daily iodine intake of between 150 and 300 μg (12).

Trimethadione Syndrome

In one report of 53 cases, 87% were associated with pregnancy loss or abnormalities in offspring, most commonly delayed growth and mental development, skeletal, cardiac, or urogenital anomalies, malformed ears, and cleft palate (71). Infants with the trimethadione or paramethadione syndrome may also have changes that include unusual eyebrows, high-arched palate, and irregular teeth (76,124,279).

Valproic Acid Embryopathy

The teratogenicity of valproic acid has been well documented (43,51,172,206). Although valuable as an antiepileptic drug, valproic acid administration during pregnancy is associated with a host of anomalies, including microcephaly, porencephaly, spina bifida, and other CNS defects, facial anomalies, cardiac defects, limb reduction anomalies, and hypospadias (17). Dosages associated with malformations have generally been 750 to 1,000 mg per day and exposures verified during the first trimester.

Warfarin Embryopathy

Although the contraindications of Warfarin during pregnancy are well recognized, women may take the drug during the first trimester, before pregnancy is recognized. Such exposure produces an embryopathy characterized by reduced growth, hypoplastic nose, limb defects (shortening, brachydactyly, nail hypoplasia), gastroschisis, cardiac defects, and stippled epiphyses or chondrodysplasia punctata (21,36,190,218,222). If the drug is administered late in pregnancy, brain damage with mental retardation may be caused by CNS bleeding in the fetus (268). Death may occur from respiratory failure.

Synthetic Progestin Embryopathy

Exposure to synthetic progestins (e.g., 17-α-ethinyl-19-nortestosterone) early in gestation can induce enlargement of the clitoris or labioscrotal fusion in female fetuses and hypospadias in boys (2,273). The incidence of ectopic pregnancy is increased in women who experience contraception failure from either oral progestins or implants (74). Diethylstilbestrol may cause vaginal adenosis in prenatally exposed girls and reproductive anomalies in similarly exposed boys (98,272). The use of a variety of exogenous sex hormones is not associated with increased risk of major malformations, with the exception of esophageal atresia, which carries a risk ratio of 2.87, which translates to approximately 6 per 10,000 live births (134).

Mercury Embryopathy

Exposure of the developing human to mercury compounds has serious effects, most notably an increased incidence of growth retardation, microcephaly, and CNS damage, with consequent deficits that include blindness, hypotonia or spasticity, deafness, dysarthria, chorea, athetosis, and strabismus. Both maternal ingestion and occupational exposure are recognized routes of exposure. The classic condition is Minamata disease, an epidemic that affected women living on the island of Minamata, Japan, who ingested shellfish contaminated with methyl mercury (153,225). Women continue to be exposed by this route, especially those living in areas of heavy industrial pollution, where contamination of soil and water occurs (154), or those ingesting contaminated marine food in the Arctic (92). In one study of maternal exposure to inorganic mercury, significant increases were noted in structural anomalies of the CNS, but not miscarriage or stillbirth (68).

Isotretinoin Embryopathy

Isotretinoin (of which the drug Accutane is a prime example) is a synthetic vitamin A analog, 13-*cis*-retinoic acid; because it inhibits sebaceous gland function, the drug is valuable in the treatment of cystic acne (133,192). Administration to pregnant women is associated with a variety of serious anomalies. Miscarriage, perinatal mortality, and premature birth are reported, and survivors may have a variety of malformations or decreased mental status. Ear anomalies are common, including dysplastic, hypoplastic, or absent ears; agenesis of the external ear canal is variable. CNS abnormalities (microcephaly, hydrocephalus, porencephaly, Dandy-Walker malformation, neuronal migration defects) and conotruncal congenital heart defects have been reported (211). The association of isotretinoin administration with adverse psychiatric effects has been described, but remains controversial (240).

Alcohol Embryopathy

Alcohol is a common and important teratogen in humans, but its influence was not fully appreciated until 1968 (138). In 1973, Jones and Smith named the condition "fetal alcohol syndrome" (FAS) (120). Effects are broad, including structural, behavioral, and neurocognitive deficits, and so a number of other designations have been used, including the earlier "fetal alcohol effect" and current "fetal alcohol spectrum disorders" (34,111). In a sense, the term "fetal alcohol syndrome" is unfortunate, for, although popular, it implies that alcohol exerts its primary influence on the fetus; in fact, teratogenic damage to the embryo is far more significant, hence the term "alcohol embryopathy."

A maternal history of alcohol consumption is often difficult to ascertain, but nevertheless, clinical criteria for making the diagnosis are available (111). Major characteristics of affected infants and children include distinctive facies (epicanthal folds, short palpebral fissures, midface hypoplasia, thin vermilion border of the upper lip, absent to indistinct philtrum, and short, upturned nose), growth retardation, malformations, and psychomotor abnormalities (42,120). Patients generally present with prenatal and postnatal growth retardation and CNS dysfunction, including mental retardation, hyperactivity, sleep disorders, spastic tetraplegia, seizures, and behavioral difficulties (Table 4-3). Joint, limb, and conotruncal cardiac anomalies are often present; limb defects include shortness of the metatarsals and metacarpals or severe ectrodactyly (101). The unusual hirsutism that is present at birth may disappear with age. Structural brain malformations, chiefly hypoplasia or agenesis of the corpus callosum, lissencephaly, and holoprosencephaly, as well as ocular abnormalities, have been described (41). Cystic hygromas are found in patients with FAS, but also with a number of other conditions (Table 4-4). FAS has been reported in both monozygotic and dizygotic twins; the higher incidence in the former has suggested a genetic influence (40,242). Despite small head circumference and initially slow psychomotor maturation, some infants with FAS may progress and develop intelligence within the normal range. Endocrine investigations usually show normal or near-normal levels of growth hormone, cortisol, and gonadotropins (see Chapter 21) (99,258). FAS is also a carcinogenic syndrome and is associated with tumors virtually identical to those seen in the fetal diphenyl-hydantoin (Dilantin) syndrome.

Diphenylhydantoin Embryopathy

Diphenylhydantoin (Dilantin) is associated with a syndrome of microcephaly and mental retardation, cleft palate, congenital heart defect, and a characteristic facial appearance (93). Human exposure during the 5th to 6th week results in cleft lip and maxillary hypoplasia (270). Changes produced experimentally are due to embryonic bradycardia or other arrhythmia and resulting hypoxia, stemming from phenytoin-induced blockage of potassium ion channels and delayed cardiac repolarization (19,52).

Table 4-3 ■ CHARACTERISTICS OF FAS

Somatic and Cutaneous Findings
- Prenatal and postnatal growth retardation, with diminished adipose
- Hirsutism
- Cutaneous hemangiomas

Central Nervous System
- Micrencephaly
- Neuronal migration defects (heterotopia)
- Absent or hypoplastic corpus callosum
- Ventriculmegaly
- Holoprosencephaly
- Hypoplastic cerebellum
- Dysplastic brainstem
- Lissencephaly

Craniofacial
- Microcephaly
- Ocular hypertelorism
- Short palpebral fissures, sometimes downslanting or with epicanthal folds
- Microphthalmia, other eye anomalies
- Posteriorly rotated ears, with hypoplastic concha
- Low nasal bridge
- Hypoplastic midface, with hypoplastic maxillae
- Retro- or micrognathia
- Cleft lip and/or palate
- Smooth vermillion border
- Long, indistinct philtrum
- Small teeth

Cardiovascular
- Congenital heart disease, often conotruncal (e.g., tetralogy of Fallot)
- Atrial and/or ventricular septal defects

Gastrointestinal tract
- Esophageal, duodenal, or anal atresia
- Tracheoesophageal fistula
- Pyloric stenosis

Urogenital System
- Hypospadias
- Hypoplastic labia
- Small rotated kidneys
- Hydronephrosis

Musculoskeletal Systems
- Abnormal palmar creases
- Hypoplastic nails
- Reduction defects of limbs and digits
- Pectus excavatum or carinatum
- Scoliosis
- Klippel-Feil anomaly
- Diaphragmatic hernia
- Umbilical hernia

Behavioral
- Developmental delay, mental retardation
- Irritability (in infancy)
- Hyperactivity (in childhood)
- Hypotonia, reduced coordination

From Clarren et al. (41,42); Potter and Hetzel (198).

Fetal exposure to diphenylhydantoin is also known to be carcinogenic. Neuroblastoma, ganglioneuroblastoma, and malignant mesenchymoma have been observed in individuals exposed to diphenylhydantoin *in utero* (77). A newborn infant has been described with fetal hydantoin syndrome and extrarenal Wilms tumor (248).

Table 4-4 ■ CONDITIONS ASSOCIATED WITH CYSTIC NUCHAL HYGROMA

Single Gene Disorders
- Familial neck webbing (autosomal dominant)
- Lymphedema distichiasis syndrome (autosomal dominant)
- Roberts syndrome (autosomal recessive)
- Bieber syndrome (autosomal recessive?)

Chromosome Disorders
- 45X (Ullrich-Turner syndrome or monosomy X)
- X-chromosome polysomy
- 13q–
- 18p–
- Trisomy 18
- Trisomy 21
- Trisomy 22 mosaicism

Teratogenic Disorders
- Alcohol embryopathy
- Fetal amethopterin syndrome
- Fetal trimethadione syndrome

Disorders of Unknown Cause
- Noonan syndrome (autosomal dominant?)

Adapted from Gilbert-Barness and Opitz (78).

Metabolic Disruptions

Phenylketonuria

Maternal phenylketonuria (PKU) leads to intrauterine and postnatal growth retardation, microcephaly and mental retardation, cardiovascular defects, dislocated hips, and other anomalies. The incidence of fetal defects is greatly decreased in mothers whose PKU is well controlled during pregnancy. It has been suggested that impaired accretion of two fatty acids, arachidonic and docosahexaenoic acids (structural components of the CNS), contributes to the small head, reduced vision, and mental retardation (114,115). Infants of phenylketonuric mothers are heterozygous, and because phenylketonuric heterozygotes are generally normal, the defect in the fetus must be attributed to the maternal metabolic disturbance.

Diabetes Mellitus

A large number of complications are recognized in pregnant women suffering from diabetes mellitus. Stillbirth and perinatal mortality in insulin-dependent women occur at five times the background rate; neonatal mortality is increased 15 times and infant mortality three times over the general population (230). Macrosomia complicates vaginal delivery. Type I maternal diabetes is also associated with an increased incidence of preeclampsia and pregnancy-induced hypertension (135). The effects of gestational diabetes remain under scrutiny.

Maternal diabetes mellitus is associated with a number of fetal anomalies, with an incidence variably estimated at two to eleven times that of the normal population (64,84,276).

In diabetic embryopathy, defects include those of the CNS (anencephaly, holoprosencephaly, arhinencephaly, and myelomeningocele), congenital heart defect, caudal regression anomaly, sirenomelia, imperforate anus, radial aplasia, and renal abnormalities, including renal agenesis and dysplasia (Figure 4-3). Malformations (Table 4-5) are the most important cause of mortality in infants of diabetic mothers (127).

The exact role of glucose metabolism in diabetic embryopathy is unclear, and workers continue to discuss the possible effects—and interrelationships—of both hyperglycemia and hypoglycemia (251). Hyperglycemia is associated with a number of metabolic derangements, including myo-inositol and arachidonic acid deficiency and altered prostaglandin metabolism, which in turn influences the formation and function of cell membranes (276). The dramatic influx of glucose through faulty membranes induces the generation of free oxygen radicals, altered mitochondrial function, and increased peroxidation of lipids, all of which can cause malformations in the developing embryo.

The correlation between hemoglobin A1C (HbA1C), maternal microvascular disease, and the incidence of major congenital anomalies in infants of diabetic mothers is high (147). HbA1C is a normal, minor hemoglobin, whose glycosylation depends upon glucose concentration. Measurement of HbA1C thus provides an index of glucose, and therefore, of diabetes control; a higher incidence of major anomalies has been observed in the offspring of women with elevated HbA1C (see also Chapter 27).

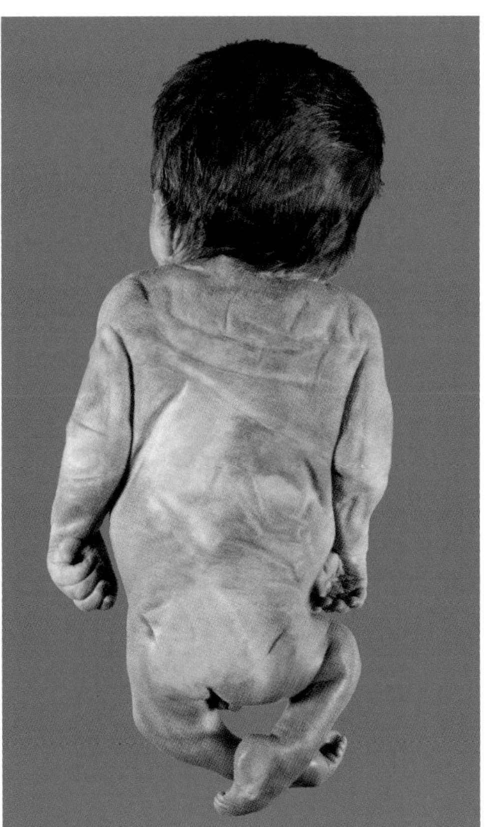

FIGURE 4-3 ■ Infant of diabetic mother. Pelvic girdle is reduced noticeably in this 31-week-old male with absent lumbosacral spine and malformed pelvis (caudal regression syndrome).

Table 4-5 ■ FETAL ANOMALIES ASSOCIATED WITH MATERNAL DIABETES

Central Nervous System
Anencephaly
Holoprosencephaly
Arhinencephaly
Occipital encephalocele
Cardiovascular System
Atrial, ventricular septal defect
Transposition of the great vessels
Tetralogy of Fallot
Single ventricle, hypoplastic left heart
Ebstein anomaly of tricuspid valve
Pulmonic stenosis, mitral atresia
Other Abnormalities
Bilateral auricular atresia
Cleft lip
Omphalocele
Unilateral renal agenesis
Hypoplastic lungs
Caudal regression
Amelia of upper limbs

Adapted from Gilbert-Barness and Opitz (78).

Infectious Disruptions

Infections, particularly toxoplasmosis, rubella, cytomegalovirus (CMV), herpes simplex, varicella, syphilis, and others (TORCHS) may cause fetal disruptions (see Chapter 6). The earlier in pregnancy the infection occurs, the greater is the likelihood of embryonic death or fetal anomalies. The most frequent fetal abnormalities are intrauterine growth retardation, microcephaly and mental retardation, deafness, cataracts, retinopathy, microphthalmia, glaucoma, myopia, and congenital heart defects.

Periventricular calcifications and chorioretinitis are frequent in toxoplasmosis. Other organisms that may be implicated in human congenital anomalies are herpes hominis type 2, which is associated with a severe congenital brain defect, varicella (119), Venezuelan equine encephalitis, coxsackie virus, and syphilis. Acquired immune deficiency syndrome (AIDS) is transmitted transplacentally or during labor, delivery, or breast feeding and constitutes an enormous problem worldwide (160). In 2005 in the United States, 92% of cases of children with AIDS were attributed to maternal transmission of the human immunodeficiency virus (HIV) (1). The incidence of neonatal HIV infection has fallen substantially in the United States with the implementation of prenatal testing, antiretroviral therapy, C-section, and avoidance of breast feeding (1).

Amnion Rupture Disruption Sequence

Early amnion rupture (or ADAM complex) may result in severe defects of the fetus, including asymmetric clefts, body wall defects, with extrusion of viscera, and highly variable amputations (Figure 4-4). When amnion adheres to the head, marked distortions of craniofacial structures are found, with widely separated eyes, displacement of the nose onto the forehead, and exencephaloceles; swallowing of amniotic bands may produce bizarre orofacial clefts. Marked deformations, growth deficiency, and a short umbilical cord are also observed in this condition (161). The fetus may also be adherent to the placenta, making diagnosis straightforward. However, when strands of amnion are not identified, diagnosis is hampered, although the pattern of defects may still imply this mode of pathogenesis. In the macerated fetus, strands of tissue resembling sloughed epidermis may be identified as amnion by microscopy. Amnion may also be absent from the fetal surface of the placenta, or free membranes. The least severe form of amniotic band disruption is a constriction groove (Streeter band) on a limb. The temporal relationship of abnormalities in early amnion rupture sequence is shown in Table 4-6.

The phenomenon of amnion rupture is thought to be rather common, affecting perhaps 1 of every 1,200 liveborn and stillborn fetuses. If this is the case, many cases apparently have few or no sequelae. Rare families with amniotic bands in relatives have been reported, but the recurrence risk appears to be negligible (145). Causes for premature rupture are not understood. The forces of uterine contraction have been implicated, but recent studies have suggested that a process of programmed weakening of membranes may operate prior to delivery (165). This observation could help explain familial recurrences (see Chapter 27 for additional details).

Chorion and Yolk Sac Rupture Sequence

While rupture of the amnion is well recognized, others have hypothesized that similar defects might arise from rupture of the chorion or yolk sac. Rupture during the 3rd week of gestation and the subsequent mechanical compression of the fetus could interfere with normal cardiac descent, resulting in cleft sternum, ectopia cordis, and thoracic and pulmonary hypoplasia (122). Such cases reflect the complex nature of embryogenesis in the region. Another published example involved an infant with rudimentary occipital meningocele and transverse defects of the hands, who, by microscopy, had intestinal mucosa adherent to the scalp (250). Possible explanations included a genetic defect similar to disorganization in the rodent; homeotic transformation; abnormal juxtaposition of epidermis and yolk sac remnant (or omphaloenteric duct); or adhesion of endoderm and ectoderm to the embryo.

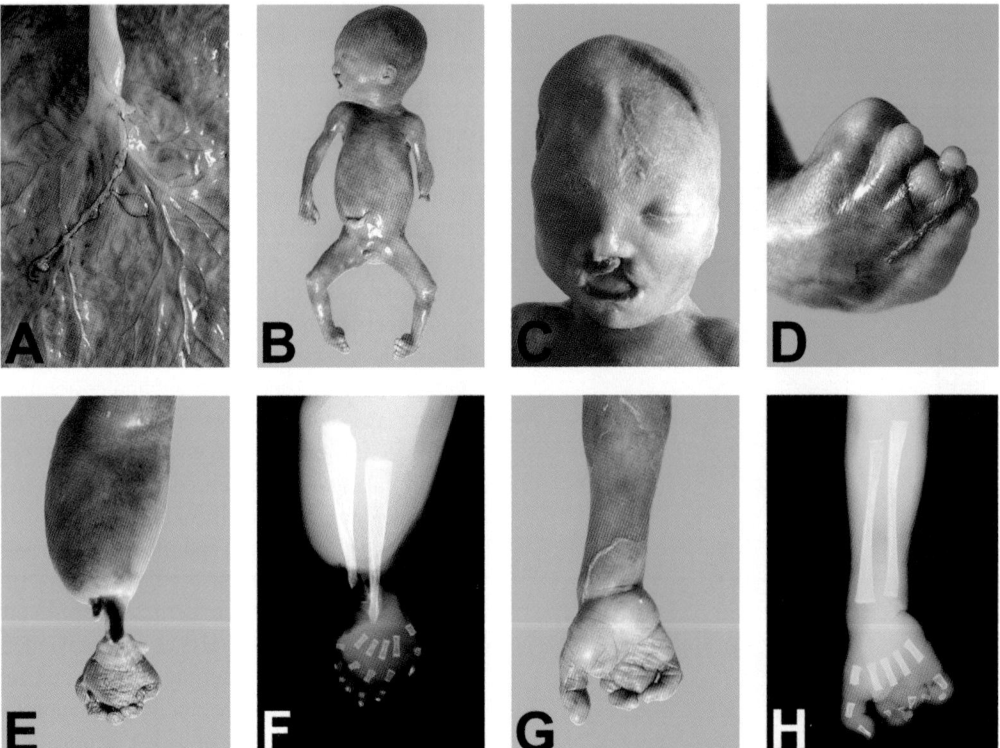

FIGURE 4-4■Amnion rupture sequence. **A:** Close-up view of fetal surface of placenta shows tiny remnant of amnion. **B:** 22-week male fetus with multiple amputation defects. **C:** Face with unilateral cleft lip. **D:** Right foot with syndactyly and multiple amputations of the digits. **E:** Exposed radius and ulna and necrosis of hand reflect the evolution of a band-induced amputation. **F:** Radiograph corresponding to **E**. **G:** Right hand with multiple amputation defects. **H:** Radiograph corresponding to **G**.

Table 4-6 ▪ TEMPORAL RELATIONSHIP OF ABNORMALITIES IN EARLY AMNION RUPTURE

Fetal Age at Occurrence	Craniofacial Defects	Limb Defects	Other Abnormalities
3 weeks	Anencephaly Encephalocele Meningocele Facial distortion Clefting Proboscis Eye defects		Placenta adherent to head or abdomen Short umbilical cord
5 weeks	Cleft lip Choanal atresia	Limb deficiency	Abdominal wall defect
7 or more weeks	Cleft palate Micrognathia Ear deformities Craniostenosis	Polydactyly Syndactyly Amniotic bands Amputation Hypoplasia Pseudosyndactyly Distal lymphedema Foot deformities Dislocation of hip	Thoracic wall defect Scoliosis Short umbilical cord Omphalocele
Third trimester	Oligohydramnios, with associated deformations		

Adapted from Gilbert-Barness and Opitz (78).

Ischemic and Vascular Disruptions

Interference with blood supply may result in ischemic disruptions. Cutis marmorata telangiectatica congenita is a vascular disruption characterized by atypical capillaries, venules, and veins in different cutaneous layers. Clinically, the lesions manifest as telangiectasia, capillary hemangiomata, cutis marmorata, venous hemangiomata, and varicose veins, depending on the type of vessels involved and the layer of skin affected. Secondary thrombosis with subsequent localized atrophy and ulceration may occur. Cutis marmorata telangiectatica congenita occurs sporadically, with female preponderance and occasional minor manifestations in close relatives.

In the Klippel-Trenaunay-Weber syndrome (see below), which usually occurs sporadically, dysplasia and capillary or cavernous hemangiomatosis and phlebectasia and varicosities with oligodactyly, syndactyly, and gigantism of digits have been observed. Congenital or postnatal hypertrophy of one or more limbs is frequent. Visceral hemangiomata may occur.

In addition to the well-recognized difficulties that arise in singletons, twins or other multiple gestations are especially at risk. Cord entanglement occurs in twins and may disrupt blood flow. Because of the variability in distance between cord insertion sites, more complications are observed in monochorionic monoamniotic than in monochorionic diamniotic placentas (20). Two additional examples of vascular disruption involve monochorionic twinning, namely twin-twin transfusion syndrome and twin reversed arterial perfusion (TRAP).

Twin-Twin Transfusion Syndrome

Twinning within the context of a shared placental disc is complicated by the presence of intraplacental vascular anastomoses. These may be small and mild or quite large, allowing significant sharing of blood between fetuses. Problems arise when blood flow is unbalanced and unidirectional, creating "pump" and "recipient" twins (Figure 4-5A). In such circumstances, the pump twin is pale and anemic, while the recipient or perfused twin is congested, possibly hydropic, and polycythemic. Differences in amniotic fluid volume can create the "stuck twin" phenomenon, with oligohydramnios in one amniotic sac (with consequent fetal deformation) and polyhydramnios in the other. The death of one twin quickly affects the well-being of the other, resulting in death or embolization of decay products, resulting in disseminated intravascular coagulation or visceral infarcts (155).

Twin Reversed Arterial Perfusion

Artery-to-artery anastomoses have a particularly striking effect when flow in one umbilical artery and aorta is reversed, a phenomenon that can be diagnosed *in utero* by Doppler flow studies. In such a circumstance, the lower body is perfused, but upper regions are not (Figure 4-5B). The heart may fail to develop (acardia); absence of the head (acardia-acephalus), upper limbs, or other viscera lungs often occur.

Dysplastic Disruptions

Dysplastic disruptions include the presacral teratoma that may be associated with anencephaly, spina bifida, meningocele, or imperforate anus; duplication of the lower intestinal tract, uterus, vagina, and ureter/renal pelvis; patent urachus; cleft palate; and esophageal and duodenal atresia. Imperforate anus and sacral defects may be inherited on an autosomal dominant basis.

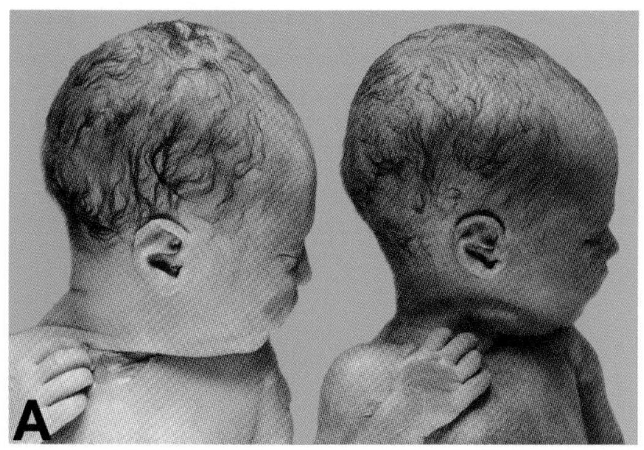

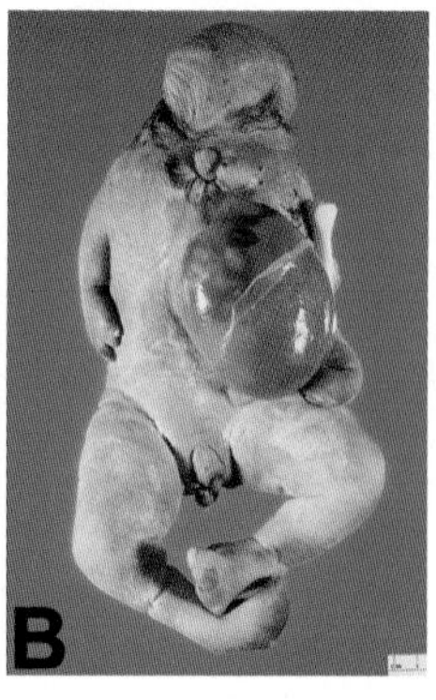

FIGURE 4-5 ■ Complications of monochorionic twinning. **A:** Pale, donor twin (**left**) and congested, recipient co-twin (**right**) in twin-twin transfusion syndrome. **B:** Acardiac co-twin in TRAP. Note the absence or malformation of structures of the upper body, omphalocele, and more normal lower extremities (but with anomalies of numerous digits).

Hyperthermia as a Disruption

Smith and colleagues were the first to make a systematic study of the effects of hyperthermia caused by infections or sauna bathing during pregnancy (232). Hyperthermia is an antimitotic teratogen that interferes mostly with CNS development, producing neural tube defects (NTDs), microcephaly, micrencephaly, microphthalmia, and neurogenic contractures (66). Other anomalies associated with hyperthermia include neuronal heterotopia, polymicrogyria, small midface, micrognathia, cleft lip and palate, ear defects, and limb defects (e.g., arthrogryposis and syndactyly). Severe mental deficiency and seizures in infancy have also been described (232).

The presence and severity of anomalies depend upon the duration of hyperthermic episode, maximum temperature reached, and stage of development (66). Both mild temperature elevation during the preimplantation period and more significant elevations during embryonic and fetal development may manifest as anomalies (67). At weeks 7 to 16 of gestation, hyperthermia may be associated with hypotonia, neurogenic arthrogryposis, or CNS dysgenesis. In one study, some 18% of women who delivered anencephalic embryos had experienced hyperthermia at a critical embryonic stage (226). Most mothers experienced febrile illnesses with temperatures of 38.9°C or higher, commonly 40°C or above. Embryonic studies in a number of animal species have highlighted the sensitivity of brain development to elevated temperatures and identified NTDs, microphthalmia, cataract, craniofacial clefts, and defects of the body wall, skeleton, heart, and teeth (67).

NONMETABOLIC DYSPLASIA SYNDROMES

The most common dysplasia syndromes are the autosomal dominant conditions: neurofibromatosis 1, von Hippel–Lindau disease, Marfan syndrome, and the osteochondrodysplasias, most of the lethal forms of which are autosomal recessive traits. These conditions are discussed in various chapters including Chapters 12, 24 and 27.

Beckwith-Wiedemann Syndrome

In the early 1960s, Beckwith and Wiedemann reported a syndrome of exomphalos (i.e., omphalocele), macroglossia, and gigantism. In one review, Beckwith-Wiedemann syndrome (BWS) accounted for nearly 12% of all cases of omphalocele. Craniofacial abnormalities (Figure 4-6) include microcephaly, macroglossia (which may interfere with respiration or swallowing), prominent eyes with relative infraorbital hypoplasia, capillary nevus flammeus of the central forehead and eyelids, metopic ridge in the central forehead, large fontanelles, prominent occiput, and malocclusion, with a tendency toward mandibular prognathism. A marker for the

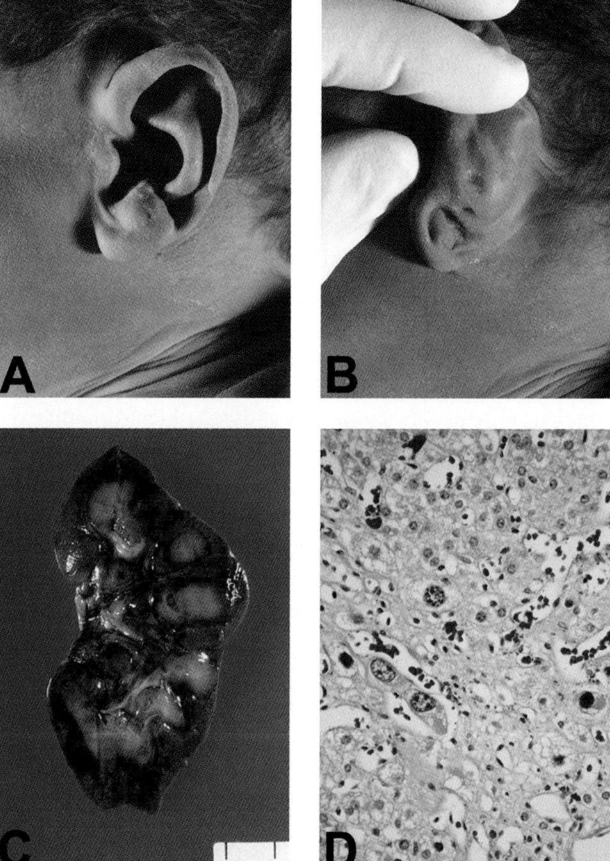

FIGURE 4-6 ■ Beckwith-Wiedemann syndrome. **A,B:** Ear pits were identified in this 9-month-old infant, who had a large omphalocele excised shortly after birth (46,XY, no deletion recognized). **C:** Note the distorted architecture in this dysplastic kidney. **D:** Microscopic view of adrenal gland, showing marked cytomegaly.

syndrome is the unusual linear fissures or pits in the lobule of the external ear and semilunar indentations of the posterior rim of the helix. Hemihypertrophy, clitoromegaly, large ovaries, hyperplastic uterus and bladder, bicornuate uterus, hypospadias, and immunodeficiency are recognized. Interstitial cell hyperplasia of the testis, pituitary hyperplasia, neonatal polycythemia, diastasis recti, posterior diaphragmatic eventration, and cryptorchidism may also occur. BWS also includes neonatal hypoglycemia, organomegaly, and cytomegaly of the adrenal cortex and islet cells of the pancreas. The placenta in BWS may exhibit mesenchymal dysplasia, a rare change that may be mistaken for partial hydatidiform mole. In one study, over 20% of placentas with this change were from patients with BWS (195).

The predisposition to the development of malignant tumors such as Wilms tumor, adrenocortical carcinoma, hepatoblastoma, gonadoblastoma, and brain stem glioma is widely recognized. Wilms tumor may be bilateral when it is associated with this syndrome (see Chapter 17). Even when free of tumor, the kidneys may be strikingly enlarged, and their surfaces traversed by numerous, irregularly disposed, shallow fissures that markedly increase the number of lobulations. The parenchyma is disorganized; minute lobulations crowd one another, each with a distinctly demarcated cortex and medulla. Other renal changes include persistent glomerulogenesis, medullary dysplasia, diffuse bilateral nephroblastomatosis, metanephric hamartomas, hydronephrosis and hydroureters, and duplications.

The incidence of polyhydramnios and prematurity is relatively high in BWS. Most cases are sporadic, but familial and dominantly inherited cases have been reported. BWS is caused by disruption of the cycle of genomic imprinting (i.e., germline erasure and establishment, somatic maintenance) within the 11p15 region (16). This mechanism has been exhibited in dramatic fashion by the increased incidence of BWS in families utilizing assisted reproductive technologies, namely *in vitro* fertilization and intracytoplasmic sperm injection (8).

Perlman Syndrome

Perlman syndrome is an autosomal recessive disorder comprising macrosomia, nephromegaly with renal dysplasia (persistent fetal lobation, nephrogenic rests, immature glomeruli, sclerotic glomeruli, primitive tubular structures, and medullary hamartomatous dysplasia), Wilms tumor, hyperplasia of the endocrine pancreas with resultant hypoglycemia, cryptorchidism, multiple congenital anomalies (mostly infrequent and nonspecific ones, such as facial dysmorphia, cleft lip, and cardiac anomalies), and mental retardation. The frequent occurrence of Wilms tumor has led to the speculation that persistent foci of renal dysplasia, blastema, or nephroblastomatosis constitute predisposing lesions (100). The condition resembles BWS, but is distinguished on the basis of inheritance (e.g., BWS is autosomal dominant), differences in specific anomalies or appearance, and different natural histories and associated malformations. Death by 1 year of age is common.

METABOLIC DYSPLASIA SYNDROMES

Williams Syndrome

Williams syndrome is an autosomal dominant disorder manifest by characteristic facial features, supravalvular and aortic stenosis, infantile hypercalcemia, and behavioral and neurological abnormalities. Specific characteristics include growth and mental retardation, microcephaly, congenital hypotonia, and elfin face with short palpebral fissures, depressed nasal bridge, epicanthal folds, and anteverted nares. Many neonates have a symptom complex of irritable failure to thrive with spitting up; in more severely affected infants, manifestations of hypercalcemia may be life threatening or lethal. Cardiovascular defects include supravalvular aortic stenosis, peripheral pulmonary artery stenosis, pulmonary valvular stenosis, and ventricular and atrial septal defect. Renal artery stenosis with hypertension, hypoplasia of the aorta, and other arterial anomalies have been reported.

Culler and colleagues studied the hormonal control of calcium metabolism in patients with Williams syndrome, noting delayed calcium clearance following intravenous loading. No abnormalities of vitamin D metabolism were found either before or after parathyroid hormone stimulation. Immunoradioactive studies suggested that patients with Williams syndrome may have a defect in the synthesis or release of calcitonin. A heterozygous deletion of a region on chromosome 7q11.23, the Williams syndrome critical region, encompasses genes which encode for proteins that regulate the cellular cytoskeleton; defects in the cytoskeleton are thought to relate to the neurological symptoms of the syndrome (110).

Zellweger Syndrome

Zellweger syndrome (cerebrohepatorenal syndrome) belongs to a group of some 17 inherited peroxisomal disorders (266). Genetic diseases involving peroxisomes (single-membrane–bound organelles involved in multiple metabolic processes) include those in which only a single peroxisomal function is impaired—acatalasemia, X-linked adrenoleukodystrophy, and the adult form of Refsum disease—and those with impaired peroxisome biogenesis—the so-called Zellweger spectrum (consisting of Zellweger syndrome, infantile Refsum disease, and neonatal adrenoleukodystrophy) and rhizomelic chondrodysplasia punctata (267).

An autosomal recessive trait, Zellweger syndrome results from mutations in at least 12 PEX genes encoding for peroxins (33). The syndrome is lethal in infancy and dominated clinically by severe CNS dysfunction (234). Affected infants are usually born at term and do not manifest intrauterine growth retardation. The clinical manifestations are listed in Table 4-7 and include a pear-shaped or light bulb–shaped head, large fontanelles, flat occiput, high forehead with shallow supraorbital ridges, a flat face, minor ear anomalies, inner epicanthal folds, Brushfield spots, mild micrognathia, and redundant neck skin.

Table 4-7 ■ CLINICAL FINDINGS IN ZELLWEGER SYNDROME

Craniofacial Anomalies
Macrocephaly; high forehead; dolichocephaly
Large anterior fontanel; open metopic suture
Mongoloid slant of palpebral fissures; hypertelorism; shallow supraorbital ridges; epicanthal folds
High-arched palate; posterior cleft of palate
Minor anomalies of ears
Limbs
Talipes equinovarus
Camptodactyly
Contractures
Central Nervous System
Hypotonia, rarely hypertonia
Severe mental retardation
Seizures
Nystagmus; oculogyric fits
Absent neonatal reflexes
Eyes
Cataract
Glaucoma
Corneal clouding
Brushfield spots
Pigmentary retinopathy
Optic nerve "dysplasia" or hypoplasia
Skeletal Anomalies
Chondrodysplasia calcificans (especially of the patellae)
Delayed skeletal maturation
Bell-shaped thorax
Large fontanels
Other Abnormalities
Cardiac defect
Jaundice with hepatomegaly
Cryptorchidism; clitoromegaly
Single palmar crease
DiGeorge anomaly

Adapted from Gilbert-Barness and Opitz (78).

Table 4-8 ■ PATHOLOGIC FINDINGS IN ZELLWEGER SYNDROME

Brain
Cerebellar, olivary hypoplasia
Abnormal cerebral convolutions (microgyria, pachygyria)
Partial lissencephaly
Agenesis or hypoplasia of the corpus callosum
Cerebral or cerebellar heterotopias
Enlarged lateral ventricles
Sudanophilic leukoencephalomyelopathy
Gliosis
Heart
Ventricular septal defect
Patent ductus arteriosus
Patent foramen ovale
Liver
Biliary dysgenesis
Cirrhosis
Siderosis
Absent peroxisomes
Abnormal mitochondria
Diminished smooth endoplasmic reticulum
Kidney
Multiple cortical microcysts; glomerular and tubular cystic dysplasia
Hydronephrosis
Horseshoe kidney
Pancreas
Islet cell hyperplasia
Thymus
Thymic hypoplasia

Adapted from Gilbert-Barness and Opitz (78).

The infant with Zellweger syndrome is severely hypotonic, with an inability to suck, reduced deep tendon reflexes, and total lack of psychomotor development (31,247). Because of the hypotonia and physical appearance, infants are sometimes thought to have Down syndrome. Other manifestations include congenital heart defects (e.g., anomalies of aortic arch, patent ductus arteriosus, ventricular septal defect), stippled calcification of the epiphyses, and hepatomegaly with signs of hepatic dysfunction and occasional jaundice. Increased serum iron and tissue siderosis aid diagnosis, but do not appear to be related to disease progression (264). Death before 1 year of age usually occurs from respiratory complications.

Autopsy findings of patients with Zellweger syndrome are listed in Table 4-8. Brain abnormalities include focal lissencephaly and other cerebral gyral abnormalities, heterotopic cerebral cortex, olivary nuclear dysplasia, defects of the corpus callosum, numerous lipid-laden macrophages and histiocytes in cortical and periventricular areas, and dysmyelination (265). The liver is characterized by hepatic lobular disarray, or micronodular cirrhosis, biliary dysgenesis, and siderosis. The kidneys show persistent fetal lobulations with cortical cysts. Albuminuria and aminoaciduria may be observed. Other abnormalities include hypoglycemia, elevated serum iron, siderosis, hyperpipecolic acidemia, hepatic and cerebral glycogen storage, elevated very long chain fatty acids, abnormal bile acids, dicarboxylic aciduria, and hypocarnitinemia. Renal cysts have been a consistent finding and may be a pathologic marker for this condition. They are often macroscopic and both glomerular and tubular by microscopy. Occasionally, cysts appear to connect directly to terminal ends of collecting tubules without an intervening tubular segment, suggesting focally deficient metanephric differentiation. More classic cystic dysplastic changes may also be observed (26), and horseshoe kidneys and ureteral duplication have been noted (79). Immunodeficiency may develop, and some patients have been diagnosed mistakenly with DiGeorge syndrome (109). Atypical cases of Zellweger syndrome (Versmold variant) have hypertonia and may live longer (262). (See Chapter 5.)

SEQUENCES

Robin Sequence

The defects in Robin sequence include micrognathia, glossoptosis, and cleft soft palate. Hypoplasia of the mandibular area before week 9 of gestation causes the tongue to be posteriorly located, presumably preventing closure of the posterior palatal shelves. It may also be a result of early mechanical constraint *in utero*, limiting growth before palatine closure. The Robin sequence should alert the clinician to the possible presence of the Stickler syndrome (see below) and the possibility of blindness due to high myopia.

Prune Belly Sequence

Prune belly sequence occurs as a triad of absent or hypoplastic abdominal muscles, urinary tract defects, and cryptorchidism (65). The umbilicus may be displaced cephalad, with flaring of rib margins, Harrison groove, and pectus deformities, all apparently secondary to the muscle defect. Nearly three quarters of patients have additional defects of the cardiac, pulmonary, gastrointestinal, or musculoskeletal systems. Most cases are sporadic, but some familial cases have been autosomal recessive.

Renal anomalies are a critical part of the spectrum. With urethral or bladder neck obstruction, more proximal segments of the urinary tract become dilated, resulting in megalourethra, megacystis, hydroureter, and hydronephrosis, the latter with consequent renal hypoplasia. Urinary ascites may occur from overdistention and prenatal rupture of the bladder. Thus, the abdomen tends to be tense and glassy in the fetus, and, after collapse of the bladder and/or absorption of intraabdominal fluid, lax and wrinkled in the newborn (Figure 4-7). Neonatal death occurs in 20% of infants, usually from pulmonary hypoplasia, a sequel of oligohydramnios or abdominal pressure on the diaphragm. However, long-term survival is possible, especially in patients with mild or no changes of the abdominal musculature or urinary tract. Complications in survivors include decreased spermatogenesis/absence of spermatogonia and salt-wasting nephritis (49).

Pathogenesis continues to receive attention. One hypothesis is that an early insult to developing mesenchyme is responsible for the condition (94). A different view is that massive distention of the urinary bladder causes stretching and thinning of abdominal skeletal muscles (186). Some have attributed a major role to hypoplasia of the prostate gland (107).

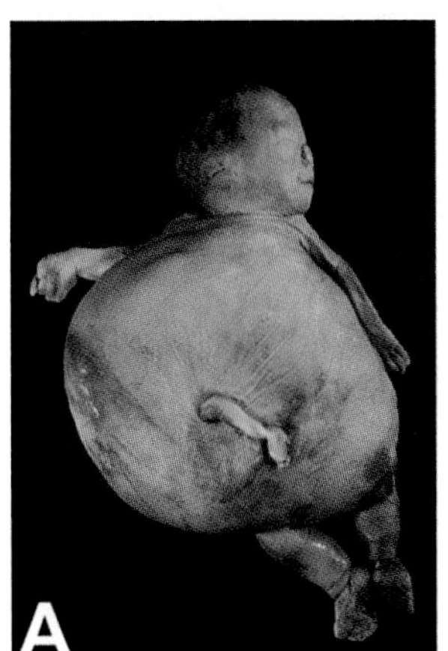

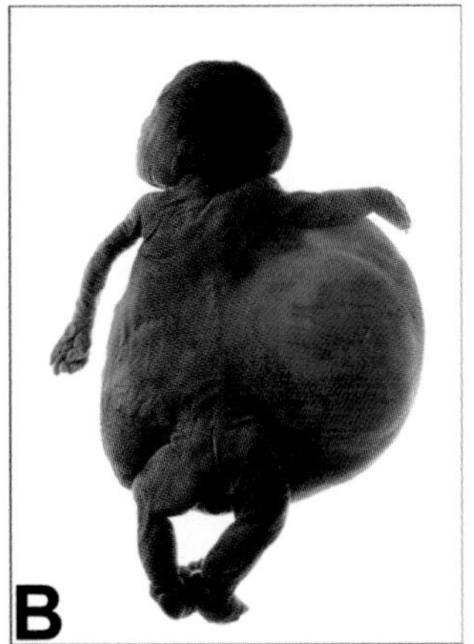

FIGURE 4-7 ■ Prune belly sequence. **A:** Anterior view of 32-week male fetus with marked distention of the abdomen secondary to megacystis and bladder outlet obstruction from posterior urethral valves. Used with permission (231). Note flattened face, a result of intrauterine constraint. **B:** Posterior view of fetus, transilluminated to demonstrate fluid-filled abdomen. Abdominal skin takes on a very wrinkled appearance when/if fluid is resorbed.

ASSOCIATIONS

Because of shared molecular determinants, spatial contiguity, and close timing of morphogenetic events during blastogenesis, it is thought that most malformations arising during this period are polytopic, that is, involving two or more developmental fields. Some have suggested, therefore, that associations (e.g., VATER, schisis association) be designated polytopic field defects (152). Regardless of nomenclature, it is evident that certain malformation complexes, of which VATER and schisis feature prominently, develop from a widespread insult or insults during early development.

VATER Association

In 1973, Quan and Smith coined the acronym VATER to represent the association of vertebral defects, anal atresia, tracheoesophageal fistula, esophageal atresia, and radial and renal abnormalities (Figure 4-8). Genitourinary defects

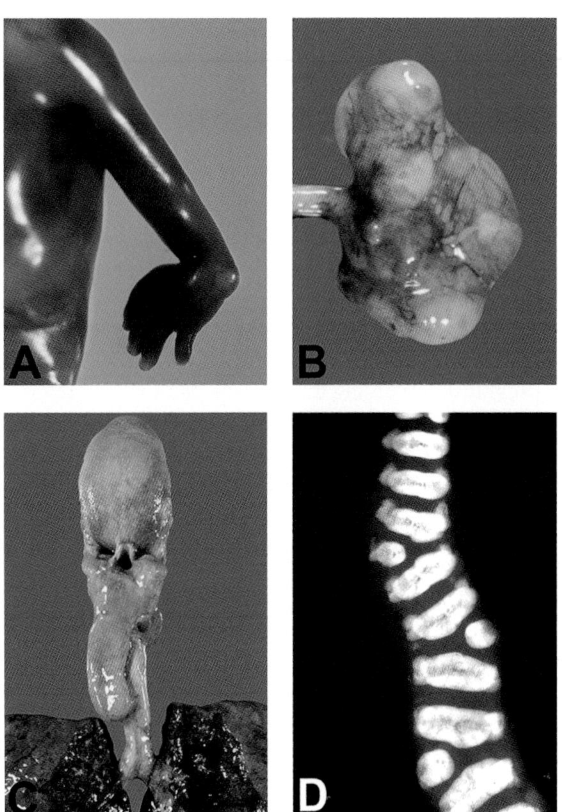

FIGURE 4-8 ■ VATER/VACTERL association. **A:** Marked deviation of wrist and hand; thumb and radius are absent. **B:** Cystic renal dysplasia. **C:** Esophageal atresia (without tracheoesophageal fistula) from infant with VACTERL association. **D:** Radiograph of excised vertebral column with hemivertebrae. Latter image used with permission (231).

include renal dysplasia or agenesis, renal ectopia, persistent urachus, hypospadias, and caudally displaced, hypoplastic penis. Prenatal growth deficiency, ear anomalies, large fontanels, cleft palate, cloacal exstrophy, and rib anomalies are also recognized. This pattern of malformations occurs sporadically.

The phenotypic variability of VATER association complicates both diagnosis and classification. VACTERL is an expansion of VATER that includes cardiac and limb defects. The overlap with Müllerian duct, renal, and cervicothoracic somite malformations (MURCS) with tracheal agenesis, hemifacial microsomia, and other facial asymmetry syndromes has been recognized (63). The VATER phenotype also overlaps with Fanconi syndrome and to a lesser degree with sirenomelia. Some have recommended performing chromosomal breakage studies on patients with features of both VATER association and Fanconi syndrome (70).

The etiology and pathogenesis of VATER association remain unknown. It has been hypothesized that anomalies derive from a common pathogenetic mechanism, namely a defect of blastogenesis prior to day 35 of gestation. Evidence comes from the fact that several critical tissues develop before 35 days, including the septa that divide rectum/anus and trachea/esophagus, radial limb bud, and mesoderm that form the vertebral bodies (77). The adriamycin animal model may contribute to future understanding of these issues (167) (see Chapters 12, 17 and 27 for additional details).

MURCS Association

MURCS is an acronym for Müllerian duct aplasia, renal aplasia, and cervicothoracic somite malformations, which cause cervicothoracic vertebral defects, especially from C5 to T1 (63). This condition is sporadic and not associated with abnormal karyotype. Absence of the vagina, absence or hypoplasia of the uterus, and renal abnormalities (in up to 40% of patients), also occur (23). A variety of additional anomalies, including those involving the skeletal, cardiac, and renal systems, complicate diagnosis (196). A male form of MURCS has been postulated; findings are azoospermia, renal anomalies, and cervicothoracic spinal abnormalities (156).

Schisis Association and Variants

Midline defects such as NTDs (i.e., anencephaly, encephalocele, meningomyelocele), oral clefts, omphalocele, and diaphragmatic hernia occur more frequently than expected (50). This so-called schisis association is frequently a lethal abnormality. It occurs more often in girls, in twins (4.6%), and in breech presentations (13.7%), and it is associated with lower mean birth weight and a shorter gestational period. Congenital cardiac defects, limb deficiencies, and defects of the urinary tract, mainly renal agenesis, are defects that have a high association (50). Schisis-type abnormalities appear to occur in a nonrandom fashion and have been postulated to arise during blastogenesis (105).

AUTOSOMAL DOMINANT CONDITIONS

Nail-Patella Syndrome

In nail-patella syndrome, or hereditary onycho-osteodysplasia, fingers and toes, especially thumbs and great toes, show onychodysplasia, hypoplasia, longitudinal ridging, and hemiatrophy. The patellae are small or absent and the elbows are dysplastic; small osseous spurs or horns on the iliac bones are pathognomonic for the condition. Glaucoma may develop or progress after birth, and a peculiar heterochromia may be seen in the iris. Subtle impairment of hearing and peripheral neurological symptoms such as sensory dysfunction are also recognized. A nephropathy is more frequent in females and varies from proteinuria, which may be transient and asymptomatic, to renal failure (29). Thickening of the glomerular basement membrane that contains focal collections of collagen fibers and mesangial thickening is present. Immunofluorescence shows a nonspecific focal distribution of IgM or complement (additional details are found in Chapters 17 and 27).

One gene identified to date, *LMX1B*, on chromosome 9q34.1, is a transcription factor important to limb patterning and morphogenesis of the glomerular basement membrane (28). However, the interfamilial and intrafamilial variability in phenotypes is highly suggestive of additional genetic involvement (29,30,149).

Orofaciodigital Syndrome Type I (OFD1)

Orofaciodigital syndrome is an extremely variable constellation of congenital disorders, and as such has engendered both attention and debate. Major changes in the group of conditions include hypertrophic frenula, lingual hamartomas, cleft lip or palate, ocular hypertelorism, brachydactyly, polydactyly, and syndactyly. Recent investigations have emphasized the OFD1 protein, a core component of the centrosome and thus influential to development in numerous ways. OFD1 is an X-linked dominant trait, lethal in hemizygous males prenatally and characterized by webbing between the buccal mucous membrane and alveolar ridge, partial clefts in the mid-upper lip, hypoplasia of nasal cartilages, absent lateral incisors, asymmetric shortening of the digits with clinodactyly, bifid hallux with or without syndactyly, and variable mental deficiency (175).

Branchiootorenal Syndrome

The branchiootorenal syndrome is an autosomal dominant disorder characterized by branchial arch anomalies (i.e., preauricular pits, branchial fistulas, anomalies of the external ear), hearing loss, and renal hypoplasia and dysplasia. A preauricular pit at birth is a marker for this syndrome and suggests 1 chance in 200 of severe hearing loss. The renal anomalies range from minor defects to marked hypoplasia with renal failure. Mutations in the *EYA1* gene have been identified in families with the complete syndrome, but not those lacking branchial fistulae, suggesting genetic heterogeneity (208,209).

Townes-Brocks Syndrome

Townes-Brocks syndrome is an autosomal dominant disorder with variable expressivity (199). Major changes include thumb anomalies (i.e., triphalangeal thumb), preaxial polydactyly, auricular anomalies, imperforate anus, cardiac defects, and anomalies of other internal organs, including renal hypoplasia and cysts. Mental retardation has been reported in a minority of patients (199). Anomalies overlap with the VATER association and hemifacial microsomia. It may be particularly difficult, but also important, to distinguish Townes-Brocks syndrome from the latter condition, which occurs sporadically from mutations in *SALL1* (123).

Holt-Oram Syndrome

This syndrome is characterized by certain skeletal and cardiovascular abnormalities (108) and appears as an autosomal dominant trait with variable expressivity. Skeletal abnormalities in the upper limbs range from thumb hypoplasia to phocomelia and have a preponderance of left-sided involvement. Hypoplasia or absence of the first metacarpal and radius, and defects of the ulna, humerus, clavicle, scapula, and sternum may be present. The most frequently described cardiac anomaly is a secundum-type atrial septal defect. However, a variety of other cardiac defects and anomalies of the coronary arteries have been recognized. To date, some 37 mutations of the gene responsible for Holt-Oram syndrome, *TBX5*, have been identified (112); missense mutations are associated with distinct phenotypes. Variability within affected families suggests that the genetic background, environmental or stochastic modifiers, or modifier genes may be important (112).

Mandibulofacial Dysostosis

Mandibulofacial dysostosis, also known as Treacher Collins or Franceschetti-Klein-Zwahlen syndrome, is also viewed as a nonspecific developmental field defect that is inherited as an autosomal dominant condition. The main characteristics of this disorder are malar hypoplasia with downslanting palpebral fissures, defects of the lower lid, mandibular hypoplasia, and malformations of the external ear (228). Other abnormalities include partial to total absence of the lower eyelashes, external ear canal defects, conductive deafness, cleft palate, incompetent soft palate, and a projection of scalp hair onto the lateral cheek. Pharyngeal hypoplasia, microphthalmia, macrostomia or microstomia, choanal atresia, blind fistulas and skin tags between the auricle and the angle of the mouth, absence of the parotid gland, congenital heart defects, and cryptorchidism are occasionally reported. Because the majority (over 60%) of cases arise *de novo* and expression is highly variable, diagnosis and counseling can be challenging (60). Some 51 mutations in the *TCOF1* gene, which encodes the protein "treacle," have been identified, and the Treacher Collins locus mapped to chromosome 5q31.3-32 (150).

Opitz-Frias Syndrome

A heterogenous condition, Opitz-Frias syndrome, also known as hypertelorism-hypospadias or GBBB syndrome, was described and named using the initials of the surnames of the three families (183). Affected males usually have ocular hypertelorism and hypospadias, but affected females have only hypertelorism. Cardiac anomalies, cleft lip or palate, cranial asymmetry, strabismus, and downslanting palpebral fissures may be present. Because of the overlap between G and BBB syndrome manifestations, some investigators have suggested that they are the same entity and should be called Opitz or Opitz-Frias syndrome. Neonatally, infants can be recognized by their hypertelorism, hypospadias, and other anomalies, such as cleft lip or palate and congenital heart defects. The syndrome is genetically heterogeneous, with both X-linked and autosomal dominant forms recognized. The former maps to Xp22 and is designated type I; the latter maps to 22q11 and is designated type II. Mutations in the *MID1* gene have been demonstrated in X-linked cases. Patients with the two forms are not easily differentiated by phenotypic means.

ACROCEPHALOSYNDACTYLY SYNDROMES

Acrocephalosyndactyly syndromes are caused by autosomal dominant mutations. The numeric designations of these entities derive from earlier classifications and are more commonly known by their proper names. The abnormalities that occur in these syndromes are listed in Table 4-9.

Apert Syndrome

Apert syndrome, or acrocephalosyndactyly type I (27), was formerly called acrocephalosyndactyly type II, Vogt cephalodactyly, or Apert-Crouzon disease. The disorder is characterized by irregular craniosynostosis (especially of coronal sutures), midface hypoplasia, syndactyly, and a broad distal phalanx of the thumb and hallux. Patients may have mental retardation. Craniofacial anomalies include short anteroposterior skull diameter with a high, full forehead and flat occiput, flat face, supraorbital horizontal groove, shallow orbits, ocular hypertelorism, downslanting palpebral fissures, small nose, and maxillary hypoplasia. Cutaneous syndactyly of all toes occurs with or without osseous syndactyly. Synostosis of the radius and humerus, pyloric stenosis, ectopic anus, pulmonary aplasia, anomalous tracheal cartilages, pulmonary stenosis, cardiac malformations, cystic kidneys, hydronephrosis, and bicornuate uterus may occur.

The condition is easily diagnosed at birth, although the possibility has been raised that infants with Apert syndrome with polydactyly, especially of the toes, represent a nosologically different entity. Two point mutations in the fibroblast growth factor receptor 2 gene (*FGFR2*) are the cause of most cases, even though they differ phenotypically (113). It has been suggested that changes in the composition of extracellular matrix could be responsible for such variability (35). (See Chapter 27 for additional details.)

Table 4-9 ■ MAJOR FEATURES OF THE ACROCEPHALOSYNDACTYLY SYNDROMES

Apert Syndrome (Type I)	Saethre-Chotzen (Type III)	Pfeiffer Syndrome (Type V)
Irregular thumb and toe	Brachycephaly, high forehead	Craniosynostosis of coronal and sagittal sutures
Mental retardation or normal intelligence	Synostosis of coronal sutures	Cloverleaf skull[a]
Short anteroposterior skull diameter, with high forehead and flat occiput	Maxillary hypoplasia	Ocular hypertelorism
Supraorbital horizontal groove	Facial asymmetry	Antimongoloid palpebral fissures
Flat face	Shallow orbits	Small nose
Shallow orbits	Ocular hypertelorism	Radiohumeral synostosis[a]
Ocular hypertelorism	Small ears	Broad distal phalanges of thumb and great toe
Downslanted palpebral fissures	Large fontanels	Partial syndactyly of fingers and toes
Small nose	Ptosis of eyelids	
Maxillary hypoplasia	Cutaneous syndactyly	
Cutaneous syndactyly of all toes, with or without syndactyly	Single upper palmar crease	
Synostosis of the radius and humerus	Broad thumbs, great toes	
Pyloric stenosis	Mental deficiency[a]	
Ectopic anus	Small stature[a]	
Pulmonary aplasia	Deafness[a]	
Anomalous tracheal cartilages	Vertebral anomaly[a]	
Pulmonic stenosis, other cardiac malformations	Cryptorchidism[a]	
Cystic kidneys	Renal anomalies[a]	
Hydronephrosis		
Bicornuate uterus		

[a]Occasional abnormality.
Table adapted from Reference (77).

Pfeiffer Syndrome

Pfeiffer syndrome, also known as acrocephalosyndactyly type V, arises on an autosomal dominant basis, with most cases representing new mutations. Mutations in *FGFR1* have been identified (168), as well as *FGFR2* (213). Craniosynostosis of coronal or sagittal sutures, ocular hypertelorism, downward slant of palpebral fissures, small nose, broad distal phalanges of thumbs and big toes, partial syndactyly of fingers and toes, and sometimes radiohumeral synostosis and cloverleaf skull (Kleeblattschädel) characterize this syndrome. Craniofacial abnormalities tend to improve with age. Intelligence is usually normal, although severe secondary brain defects occur with the Kleeblattschädel anomaly (see Chapter 27 for additional details).

Other Related Conditions

Crouzon Craniofacial Dysostosis

Inherited as an autosomal dominant trait, Crouzon craniofacial dysostosis occurs from a *FGFR2* mutation (204). It is a relatively common disorder that includes craniofacial anomalies with shallow orbits and ocular proptosis, hypertelorism, frontal bossing, and maxillary hypoplasia with a curved parrotlike nose (61). Craniosynostosis may involve coronal, lambdoid, and sagittal sutures. The teeth are peg-shaped and widely spaced, and associated with a large tongue, deviated nasal septum, atretic auditory meatus, and deafness. Facial operations may be required to correct extreme midface hypoplasia and proptosis.

Robinow Syndrome

Robinow syndrome, or "fetal face" syndrome, is heterogeneous, with both autosomal dominant and autosomal recessive forms recognized. The gene for the recessive form is *ROR2* and located on chromosome 9q22; the relationship of this gene to the dominant form is unclear (189). Abnormalities include macrocephaly, large anterior fontanelle, frontal bossing, hypertelorism, small upturned nose, small mouth, and micrognathia. The latter findings resemble a fetal face (207). The forearms are short with brachydactyly; pectus excavatum, rib anomalies, hemivertebrae, inguinal hernia, and cardiac anomalies may occur, along with a small penis and cryptorchidism in boys and small clitoris and labia majora in girls.

Stickler Syndrome

Stickler syndrome, or hereditary arthroophthalmopathy, is characterized by depressed nasal bridge, epicanthal folds, midface hypoplasia, cleft of hard palate, micrognathia, deafness, and myopia complicated by frequent retinal detachment or cataracts (239). Hypotonia, marfanoid habitus, prominence of large joints, and spondyloepiphyseal dysplasia are also present in Stickler syndrome. Fifty percent of girls and 40% of boys have mitral valve prolapse. The syndrome should be considered in every newborn infant with the Pierre Robin sequence—in one study, one-third of patients with Robin sequence were diagnosed subsequently with Sticker syndrome (261). Stickler syndrome is heterogenous and autosomal dominant with highly variable expression (139).

Two genes have been mapped, and two *COL2A1* mutations identified. Only mutations in the *COL2A1* lead to the full syndrome with recognizable features.

Noonan Syndrome

Edema of the dorsum of the hands and feet in the newborn may simulate that seen in the infant with Ullrich-Turner (45X) syndrome. Webbing of the neck, pectus excavatum, cryptorchidism, and pulmonic stenosis characterize this syndrome (173). Short stature, epicanthal folds, ptosis of eyelids, ocular hypertelorism, myopia, low-set or abnormal ears, anomalous vertebrae, and mental retardation are common. The condition is genetically heterogeneous, with mutations in the gene *PTPN11* identified in approximately 40% of patients (176). Somatic *PTPN11* mutations are also found in several childhood malignancies, including juvenile myelomonocytic, acute myeloid, and acute lymphoblastic leukemias (246).

Brachmann–de Lange Syndrome

Cornelia de Lange, or Brachmann–de Lange syndrome (BDLS), has as major manifestations growth deficiency, profound mental retardation, synophrys, hirsutism, and thin, downturned vermilion borders (Figure 4-9). Other common anomalies are microcephaly, micrognathia, limb anomalies, dental abnormalities, such as late eruption of widely spaced teeth, and male genital abnormalities, such as cryptorchidism and hypospadias (97). Less common anomalies involve the eye (myopia, microcornea, astigmatism, optic atrophy, coloboma of the optic nerve, strabismus, and proptosis), choanal atresia, low-set ears, cleft palate, congenital heart defects (most commonly a ventricular septal defect), hiatus hernia, gastrointestinal anomalies (e.g., duplication of the gut, malrotation of the colon, short esophagus, and pyloric stenosis), inguinal hernia, small labia majora, and absent second to third interdigital triradius. BDLS, dup(3q), and FASs show some phenotypic overlap, but are distinguishable (24,275).

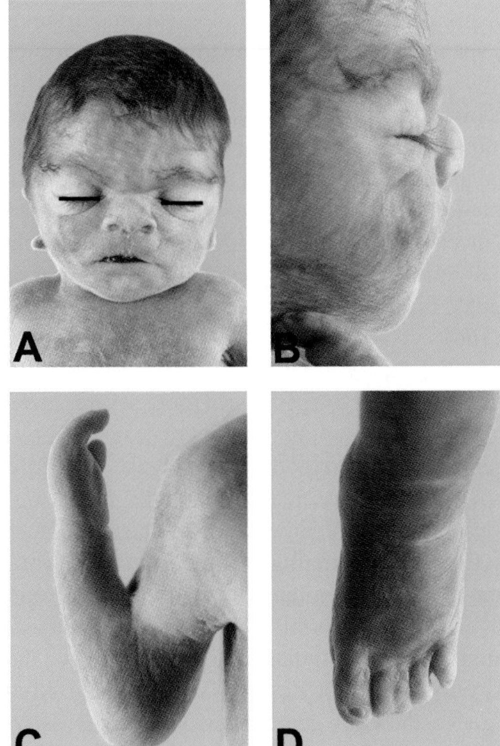

FIGURE 4-9 ▪ Brachmann–de Lange syndrome. This 30-week fetus was born spontaneously and lived several hours, dying of respiratory failure secondary to congenital diaphragmatic hernia. **A:** Characteristic facies, with hirsutism, synophrys, ocular hypertelorism, and elongated philtrum. **B:** Lateral view showing elongated eyelashes, blunt nose, and small mandible. **C:** Severe reduction anomaly of right arm (absent ulna, third, fourth, and fifth fingers), with pterygium at elbow. **D:** Syndactyly of second and third toes.

Both dominant and X-linked forms are recognized. Dominant cases are associated with *NIPBL* (130). To date, about 50% of patients with BDLS or BDLS-like phenotypes have had heterozygous mutations in the *NIPBL* gene (219); about one-half of cases of X-linked BDLS are estimated to occur from *SMC1L1* mutations (170).

AUTOSOMAL RECESSIVE CONDITIONS

Meckel Syndrome

Meckel first described this syndrome in 1822, and in 1934, Gruber coined the term *dysencephalia splanchnocystica* (181). Meckel, or Meckel-Gruber, syndrome is recessively inherited and generally leads to death in the perinatal period or early infancy from respiratory or renal failure; prolonged survival to 28 months has been reported (143). The sex ratio is equal, and incidence estimated at 1 in 13,250 to 1 in 140,000 live births worldwide; regional incidences can be considerably higher, for example, 1 in 3,000 in Belgium and 1 in 9,000 in Finland (216).

The classic diagnostic triad is occipital encephalocele, cystic kidneys, and polydactyly (Figure 4-10). Cranial rachischisis, Chiari malformation, hydrocephalus, polymicrogyria, ocular anomalies, cleft palate, congenital heart defects, hypoplasia of the adrenal glands, pseudohermaphroditism in males, and other malformations may be present. Excessively large, cystic, dysplastic kidneys cause marked abdominal distension. The cysts are spherical, glomeruli are absent, and interstitial fibrosis is prominent. The cysts display an orderly, progressive increment in size from capsule to calyx (10). Other genitourinary anomalies include agenesis, atresia, hypoplasia, and duplication of ureters and absence or hypoplasia of the urinary bladder (see Chapter 17). Cysts of the liver and pancreas are encountered; hepatic fibrosis and proliferation of bile ducts (i.e., ductal plate malformation) are seen in portal tracts and the pancreas may exhibit fibrosis as well. Severe hypoplasia of male genitalia with cryptorchidism, epididymal cysts, and ductal dilatation are common (202). Bilateral multicystic kidneys, fibrotic changes in the liver, and occipital encephalocele or other CNS malformation have been offered as minimum diagnostic criteria (7,214).

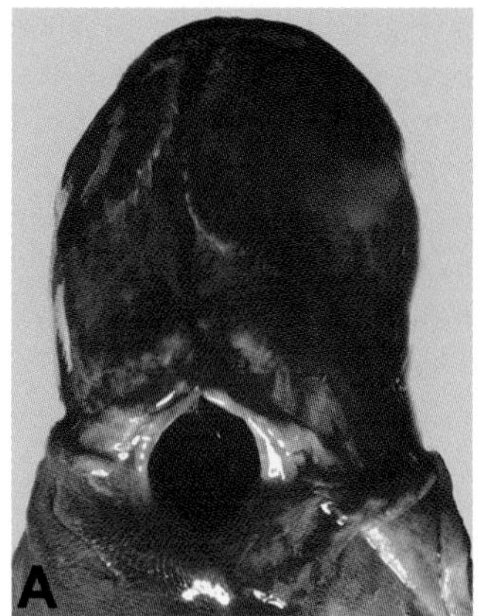

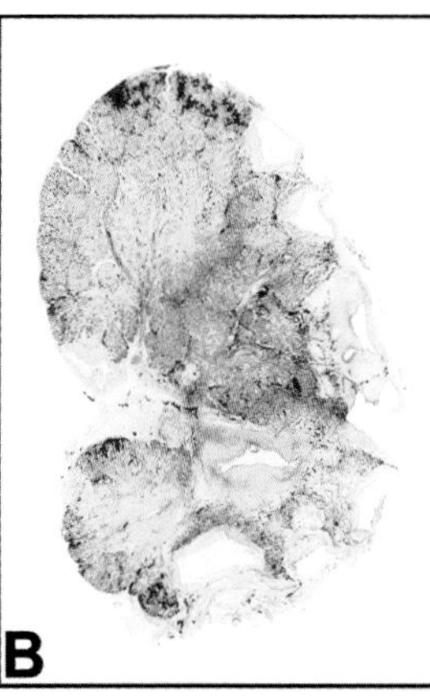

FIGURE 4-10 ■ Meckel-Gruber syndrome. **A:** Occipital defect marks location of encephalocele, absent at autopsy (secondary to autolysis) but identified by prenatal ultrasound. **B:** Microscopic view of cystic renal dysplasia, associated with atretic ureter; large cysts are mostly collecting tubules; other changes include tubular loss and peritubular and medullary fibrosis.

Maternal serum alpha-fetoprotein levels may be elevated due to the encephalocele. Prenatal diagnosis may also be made by ultrasonography, often before the 11th to 12th week (7,217). Clinical and genetic heterogeneity are recognized, and three loci, MKS (or MKS1), MKS2, and MKS3, have been localized to 17q, 11q, and 8q respectively. Mutations in a gene designated *MKS1* have been identified at 17q (132) (see Chapter 10 for details).

Smith-Lemli-Opitz Syndrome

This autosomal recessive disorder was the first true malformation complex to be associated with a metabolic derangement and the first associated with abnormal synthesis of cholesterol. Deficient cholesterol levels result from reduced activity of the final enzyme in the synthetic pathway, 7-dehydrocholesterol reductase (DHCR7). As a result, plasma concentrations of intermediate products are elevated (e.g., 7-dehydrocholesterol).

A distinctive craniofacial appearance with microcephaly, anteverted nostrils, ptosis of eyelids, inner epicanthal folds, strabismus, micrognathia, syndactyly of second and third toes, hypospadias, cryptorchidism, growth retardation, and mental deficiency are the main characteristics of Smith-Lemli-Opitz syndrome (75,233). Defects in brain morphogenesis include micrencephaly, holoprosencephaly, hypoplasia of the frontal lobes, hypoplasia of cerebellum and brain stem, dilated ventricles, and irregular gyral patterns and neuronal organization.

Less frequent anomalies are rudimentary postaxial hexadactyly, congenital heart defect, and defects of renal and spinal cord development. Cystic renal disease, hypoplasia, hydronephrosis, and abnormalities of the ureters are frequent. Rarely, severe perineoscrotal hypospadias may be seen. The reported higher frequency of boys affected than girls may be related to a bias in ascertaining the genital anomaly. A number of mutations have been identified in the delta-7-dehydrocholesterol reductase gene (*DHCR7*), which is localized to 11q12-q13 (117,278).

Leprechaunism

Individuals with leprechaunism, also known as Donohue or Donohue-Uchida syndrome, have a strikingly characteristic ("elflike") facial appearance with prominent ears, hirsutism, excessive skin folding with decreased subcutaneous adipose, acanthosis nigricans, skeletal involvement (large hands and feet), enlarged genitalia, and hyperinsulinemia (69). Intrauterine growth restriction, failure to thrive, and postnatal mental retardation are recognized, and marked hyperplasia of pancreatic islet cells is apparent by microscopy. Leprechaunism is an autosomal recessive congenital disorder of extreme insulin resistance. Some patients have had a limited response to growth hormone administration, suggesting that other defects account for growth failure. Mutations in the insulin receptor gene (*INSR*), located at 19p, are the cause of this condition. Prenatal diagnosis is thus possible. Another condition with phenotypic similarity, termed leprechaunoid syndrome or pseudoleprochaunism, is poorly understood (56).

Cockayne and Related Syndromes

Cockayne syndrome (CS) is an autosomal recessive disorder characterized by retarded growth and development, short stature, premature aging, neurological impairment (e.g., ataxia, spasticity, dementia), hearing loss, chorioretinitis, dental abnormalities, and photosensitivity (15,44). It generally becomes manifest in early infancy and leads to death from intercurrent infections or development of hypertension and atherosclerosis before adulthood. CNS abnormalities include microcephaly, hydrocephalus, patchy irregular loss of myelin, axons in a tigroid pattern, focal calcification (especially in basal ganglia), cerebellar atrophy, peripheral neuropathy, bizarre astrocytosis, and oligodendroglial dysplasia (166).

Two forms of the disorder are recognized. CSA is the classic form described above; CSB is a more severe, early-onset form that progresses rapidly, leading to death at 6 or 7 years. Pathogenesis is understood incompletely. The growth of patient fibroblasts is decreased markedly following ultraviolet (UV) irradiation. However, subsequent DNA synthesis is normal, demonstrating that the defects are not due to abnormal DNA excision repair (as is the case in xeroderma pigmentosum). Cells do fail to recover RNA synthesis post irradiation (11). Prenatal diagnosis can be made on the basis of sensitivity of amniocytes to UV light (136). Mutations in two genes, the CSA gene (excision-repair cross-complementing gene, *ERCC8*, type A or I, located on 5q) and the CSB gene (*ERCC6*, type B or II, on 10q) are most common, but others in the xeroderma pigmentosum genes *XPB*, *XPD*, and *XPG* are recognized (15,137).

Other conditions bear some resemblance to CS and may in fact constitute a Cockayne spectrum. CAMFAK syndrome (congenital cataracts, microcephaly, failure to thrive, kyphoscoliosis) is an autosomal recessive disease with central and peripheral demyelination that is similar to that seen in CS (244). A less severe variety, without failure to thrive, is termed CAMAK (57). MICRO syndrome, also autosomal recessive, is characterized by microcephaly, cataracts, and microcornea, should be distinguished from Cockayne and CAMFAK syndromes, but also cerebro-oculo-facial-skeletal (COFS) syndrome (87). Cultured cells from patients with COFS and Cockayne syndromes manifest hypersensitivity to UV light (in contrast to those with CAMFAK, CAMAK, or MICRO syndromes), and mutations in *CSB* and *XPD* have been reported in patients diagnosed with COFS (86).

Seckel Syndrome

Seckel syndrome, or "bird-headed" dwarfism, is inherited as an autosomal recessive trait. It is associated with severe prenatal growth and mental deficiency with microcephaly and premature synostosis, hypoplasia of maxilla with prominent nose, malformed ears, sparse hair, clinodactyly of fifth finger, hypoplasia of proximal radius, dislocation of hip and hypoplasia of proximal fibula, 11 pairs of ribs, and cryptorchidism in boys (95,221). Malignant hypertension has been reported to cause rupture of a cerebral aneurysm in one patient (59). Loci for three forms of the syndrome are recognized: SCKL1 (caused by mutations in the gene *ATR*, which maps to 3q22-24), SCKL2 at18p11-q11, and SCKL3 at 14q (126).

Dubowitz Syndrome

Dubowitz syndrome is an autosomal recessive, but possibly heterogeneous, disorder characterized by an unusual facial appearance, infantile eczema, small stature, and mild microcephaly (62). Infants with this syndrome are usually small for their gestational age and demonstrate retarded osseous maturation. The clinical manifestations include mild mental deficiency, mild microcephaly, small face, shallow supraorbital ridges, ocular hypertelorism, and micrognathia. In this regard, facial characteristics may resemble those of FAS. Other abnormalities include submucous cleft palate, pes planus, metatarsus adductus, hypospadias, cryptorchidism, clinodactyly of the fifth finger, and pilonidal dimple (274). Multiple chromosome breakage and malignancy are complications (5). A number of behavioral changes have been described, including hyperactivity and shyness; some patients like music, rhythm, and the vibrations produced by music; others dislike crowds (257). No gene has been identified.

Orofaciodigital syndrome Type II (Mohr Syndrome)

The orofaciodigital syndrome type II is characterized by shortness of stature, conductive deafness, midline partial cleft lip, midline cleft of the tongue, hypoplasia of the maxilla and mandible, relatively short hands, partial duplication of the hallux and first metatarsal, cuneiform and cuboid bones, and normal intelligence (256). The condition is autosomal recessive.

Pena-Shokeir Phenotype

Pena-Shokeir Type I Sequence (Fetal Akinesia Deformation Sequence)

In 1974, Pena and Shokeir first described early lethal neurogenic arthrogryposis and pulmonary hypoplasia (Pena-Shokeir I syndrome or fetal akinesia deformation). Facial abnormalities include prominent eyes, hypertelorism, telecanthus, epicanthal folds, malformed ears, depressed tip of the nose, small mouth, high arched palate, and micrognathia (194). Polyhydramnios, small placenta, and relatively short umbilical cord are frequent findings. Infants are small for their gestational age; approximately 30% are stillborn. Most die from the complications of pulmonary hypoplasia within the first few weeks.

The sequence has an estimated frequency of 1 in 12,000 births, with a heterozygote frequency of 1 in 55. The phenotypic malformations appear to be nonspecific and caused by decreased or absent *in utero* movements, resulting in the fetal akinesia deformation sequence. Genetic heterogeneity is recognized. One-half of the cases are sporadic, and one-half are familial and autosomal recessive or X-linked (193). Hall proposed the term Pena-Shokeir "phenotype," because the condition is not a specific syndrome but rather a physical change produced by lack of movement *in utero* (89).

Polyhydramnios occurs due to failure of normal deglutition. Neuromuscular deficiency in the function of the diaphragm and intercostal muscles causes pulmonary hypoplasia. Multiple ankyloses at elbows, knees, hips, and ankles, rocker-bottom feet, talipes equinovarus, and camptodactyly are present. Absence of the flexion creases on the fingers and palms, and sparse dermatoglyphic ridges are frequent. The phenotype may resemble that of trisomy 18, from which it should be distinguished.

Neuropathologic findings include thin cerebral and cerebellar cortices, polymicrogyria, and multiple foci of encephalomalacia, with loss of neurons and gliosis. The spinal cord is usually involved, with reduction in anterior motor horn cells. Skeletal muscles show diffuse and group atrophy consistent with neurogenic atrophy.

Prenatal diagnosis may be possible with prior occurrence and a high index of suspicion. Pterygium formation is one of the manifestations of the Pena-Shokeir phenotype. The lethal form of recessive multiple pterygium syndrome may represent a severe form of the Pena-Shokeir phenotype (38). (see chapter 27 for additional discussion).

Pena-Shokeir Type II Sequence (Cerebro-Oculo-Facio-Skeletal Syndrome)

COFS syndrome is recognized as an autosomal recessive disorder with degenerative brain and spinal cord defects that are usually manifest at birth. Reduced white matter of the brain with mottling of the gray matter associated with generalized hypotonia and hyporeflexia or areflexia are characteristic. The usual postnatal course is characterized by progressive psychomotor deterioration and death before 5 years of age (200).

Robert Syndrome

Robert syndrome has been described under the names pseudothalidomide or SC syndrome, SC-phocomelia syndrome, total phocomelia, hypomelia-hypotrichosis-facial hemangioma syndrome, and others (104). This malformation syndrome includes as the most prominent characteristics nearly symmetric phocomelia-like limb deficiency, often with radial defects, prenatal and postnatal growth retardation, microbrachycephaly, eye abnormalities (i.e., shallow orbits, prominent globes, cloudy cornea), cleft lip with or without cleft palate, and prominent premaxilla (Figure 4-11). The upper limbs may be affected more severely than the lower ones, the latter sometimes being altered by absent or hypoplastic fibulae (249). Minor craniofacial abnormalities include sparse, silver-blond hair, extensive hemangiomas, micrognathia, hypoplastic nasal cartilages, and malformed ears with hypoplastic lobules (102). Nuchal cystic hygromas have been described (85). Autopsy studies have shown cystic dysplastic kidneys, horseshoe kidney, and ureterostenosis with hydronephrosis. The condition is inherited as an autosomal recessive trait. Infants are stillborn or die in early infancy. Premature centromere separation with puffing and splitting and heterochromatin repulsion are diagnostic markers for this syndrome (249).

Familial Agnathia: Holoprosencephaly

Agnathia may occur alone or in association with other anomalies. The association with holoprosencephaly has been described in siblings, suggesting autosomal recessive inheritance; other cases are due to unbalanced translocations (131,197) or appear to occur sporadically (191,197). Associations of agnathia with situs inversus, renal agenesis, ectopia cordis, rib, and vertebral anomalies have been reported (191), as have occurrences with tetramelia (4) and anal atresia/situs inversus (158). Some of these associations raise fundamental questions regarding embryogenetic control of the midline (18).

Thrombocytopenia and Absent Radius Syndrome

The thrombocytopenia absent radius (TAR) syndrome is inherited as an autosomal recessive trait; almost half of patients die during early infancy. Limb defects include absence or hypoplasia of the radius, despite the presence of thumbs. These defects are usually bilateral and occur with associated ulnar hypoplasia and defects of the hands, legs, and feet. Other abnormalities include congenital heart

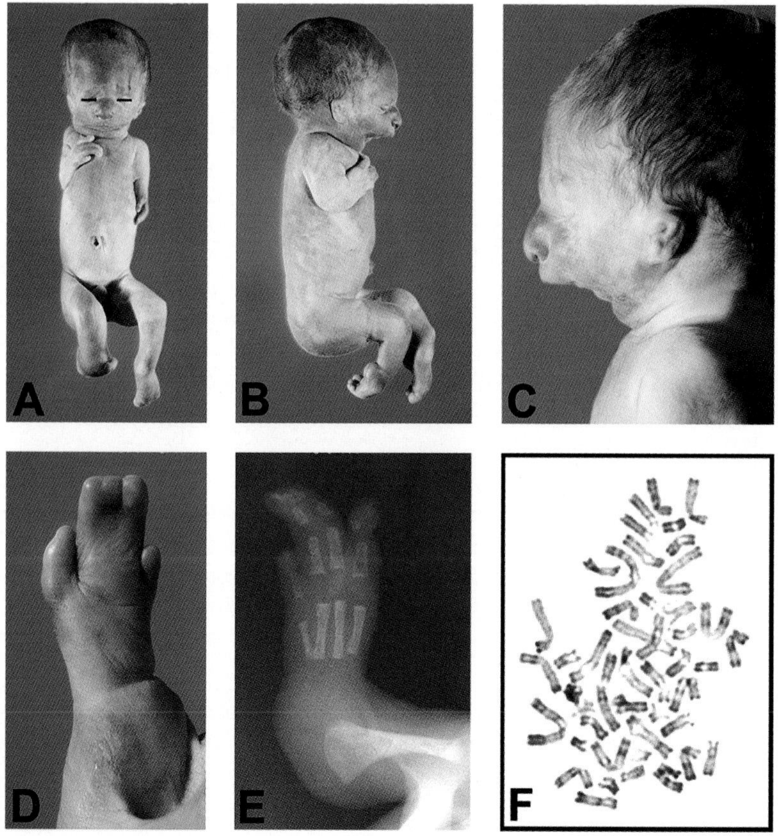

FIGURE 4-11 ■ Robert (pseudothalidomide) syndrome. **A:** Fetus with multiple limb malformations. **B:** Lateral view. **C:** Agnathia and severely hypoplastic ear. **D:** Phocomelia and syndactyly of upper limb. **E:** Radiograph of foot. **F:** Metaphase spread, showing prominent centromeres.

defect, spina bifida, brachycephaly, strabismus, micrognathia, syndactyly, short humerus, and dislocation of the hips. In one review of 34 patients, a host of additional anomalies were recognized: lower limb, renal, and cardiac anomalies, capillary hemangiomas of the face, intracranial vascular malformations, sensorineural hearing loss, and scoliosis (88). Mental retardation occurs in a small percentage (i.e., 7%) of patients. Prenatal diagnosis can be suggested by ultrasonography when defects of the upper limbs are recognized. Thrombocytopenia with absence or hypoplasia of megakaryocytes, leukemoid granulocytosis, eosinophilia, and anemia comprise the major hematologic abnormalities. A pronounced intolerance to cow's milk is probably related to disturbances in eosinophils. Leukemoid granulocytosis is present in over half of the patients, particularly during bleeding episodes. The development of acute myeloid leukemia has been described in an adult patient (82). (see Chapter 27 for details).

Hydrolethalus Syndrome

Hydrolethalus syndrome is characterized by hydrocephalus, midline defects of the brain (e.g., absent or hypoplastic corpus callosum, absent pituitary gland), micrognathia, limb anomalies including polydactyly, abnormal lobation of the lungs, microphthalmia, cleft lip or palate, small or absent tongue, wide or bifid nose, and low-set, malformed ears. The occipital bone may be altered by a keyhole-shaped defect at the posterior margin of the foramen magnum. Bilateral pulmonary agenesis and renal anomalies including unilateral agenesis and hypoplasia or tubular cysts are associated manifestations (215). The syndrome is autosomal recessive and tends to be lethal in the fetal or newborn period (227). It occurs with increased frequency in Finland, where the gene has been mapped to 11q23.25 in a number of affected families (263).

HETEROGENOUS AUTOSOMAL DOMINANT AND RECESSIVE DYSPLASIAS

Osteochondrodysplasias and Other Skeletal Dysplasias

Spranger et al. (237) have identified three basic constitutional errors of bone development: dysostoses ("malformations of single bones, alone or in combination"), disruptions ("secondary malformations of bones"), and skeletal dysplasias ("developmental disorders of chondro-osseous tissue"). Pathologic diagnosis of these conditions requires both radiographic and histologic techniques (277). The latter should involve samples of affected bone and cartilage, and generally includes rib (to include costochondral junction), vertebral body, and proximal and distal ends of major long bones (again to include osteochondral junctions).

Dysostoses may arise from defects in signaling factors, expressed only temporarily during development. Examples include those described elsewhere in this chapter, that is, Holt-Oram and Smith-Lemli-Opitz syndromes, as well as the brachydactylies, Greig polysyndactyly, and Pallister-Hall syndrome. Lesions may be asymmetric, and in general do not lead to dwarfism unless the axial bones are involved.

Disruptions may arise from the action of teratogens or infectious agents. Thalidomide and warfarin embryopathies are examples presented in this chapter.

Dysplasias comprise a larger group of disorders, and may be subcategorized as "primary dysplasias," which result from mutated genes that are expressed in cartilage or bone, or "secondary dysplasias," abnormalities arising from hormonal disease (e.g., hypothyroidism) or metabolic errors (e.g., hypophosphatasia). In these conditions, effects are widespread and sufficiently severe to cause dwarfism.

The osteochondrodysplasias, in order of increasing lethality, include osteogenesis imperfecta, thanatophoric dysplasia, achondrogenesis, and the short rib polydactyly syndromes (Figure 4-12). Even combined, these disorders are encountered infrequently, on the order of 16 per 100,000 births (237). However, because of the often striking changes in bones, the conditions are rather easily recognized by prenatal ultrasound, undergo therapeutic termination of pregnancy, and are seen with some frequency by fetal pathologists.

Chondrodysplasias

These are defects of collagen synthesis, principally type 2 collagen. The classification of chondrodysplasias has been approached in somewhat different manners by various authors: early clinical manifestations (lethal versus nonlethal), gross phenotype (short trunk versus normally proportioned trunk with platyspondyly versus short rib polydactyly), and predominant site of bone involvement (epiphysis, metaphysis, or spine) (237,269). The chondrodysplasias are associated with short stature; the major cause of death among lethal forms is pulmonary hypoplasia, resulting from rib anomalies and reduced intrathoracic volume.

Those chondrodysplasias with predominant metaphyseal involvement of tubular bones and, in some cases, the spine, also include many of the same disorders that cause death *in utero* or shortly after birth (236). The physis, which is composed of resting and proliferating cartilage, enlarged chondrocytes, and calcified regions within the zone of enchondral ossification, is the site of the major histologic abnormalities. Deficiency of chondroid matrix, disorganization of chondrocytes, deviations in individual chondrocytic cytology, absence of proliferating chondrocytes, degeneration of matrix, and absence or alteration of chondrocytic columnation are some of the specific microscopic features that, in different combinations, represent the principal histopathologic findings among the various types of short trunk and non–short trunk chondrodysplasias. Nodules of immature mesenchymal tissue are interposed at the disorganized and attenuated physeal growth zone in thanatophoric dysplasia. (see Chapters 12 and 27 for additional discussion).

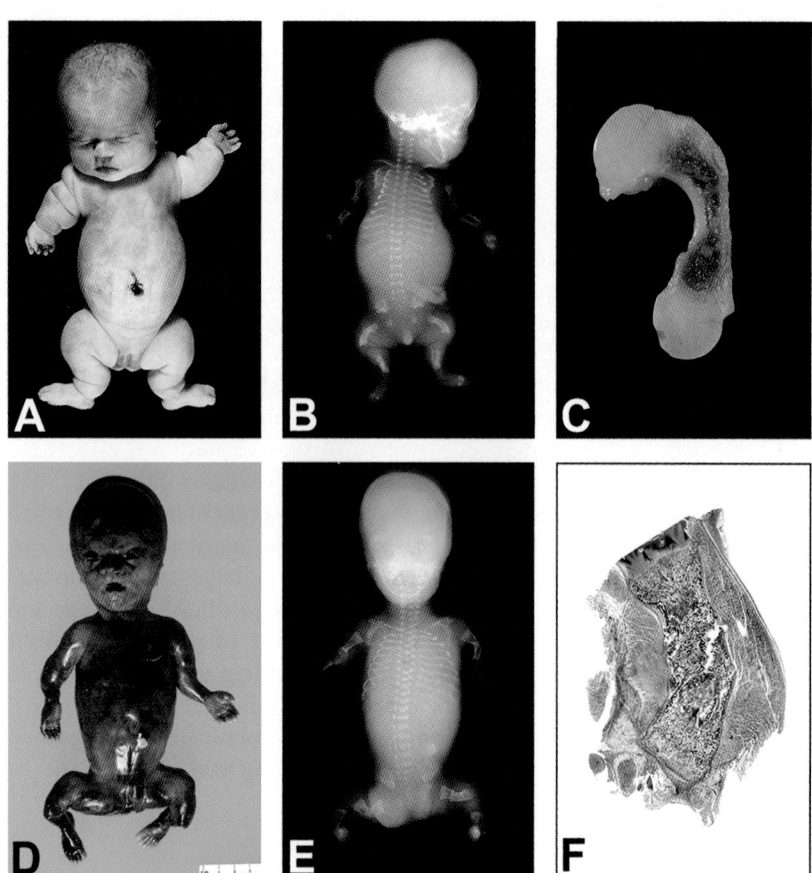

FIGURE 4-12 ■ Skeletal dysplasia. **A:** Full-term infant with thanatophoric dwarfism type I. **B:** Radiograph of 24-week male fetus with the same condition. Note short limbs, flat vertebral bodies, short ribs, and curved long bones, especially humeri and femora. **C:** Excised "telephone-receiver" femur is characteristic of thanatophoric dwarfism type I. **D:** 22-week male fetus with osteogenesis imperfecta, type 2. **E:** Radiograph of same fetus. Note multiple telescoping fractures of long bones, multiple rib fractures, and poorly mineralized calvaria. **F:** Microscopic section of femur, showing multiple compression fractures.

Other Osteochondrodysplasias

Except for some very general phenotypic similarities, the nonchondrodysplasias constitute a heterogeneous group of conditions due to defects in collagen. Osteogenesis imperfecta represents a group of inherited connective tissue disorders associated with fragile bones and a number of other nonosseous abnormalities of connective tissues (148). Its prevalence is approximately 1 case per 100,000 births. The most severe form of osteogenesis imperfecta is type II, which is typically lethal in the perinatal period.

Osteopetrosis is heterogenous and either an autosomal recessive or dominant condition that is characterized by a generalized increase in bone density, especially affecting the pelvis and skull. A defect in osteoclast function has been demonstrated, particularly in the "malignant" or autosomal recessive form, with death occurring in the first decade of life. The histologic findings are diagnostic in most cases.

X-LINKED MUTATIONS

Lowe Syndrome

Hypotonia, congenital cataract, renal tubular dysfunction, and mental retardation manifest as Lowe syndrome or oculocerebrorenal syndrome of Lowe (141). The disorder may represent an inborn error of inositol phosphate metabolism, for such metabolism is abnormal in cultured cells (142). The renal tubular defect causes limited ammonium production, hyperchloremic acidosis, phosphaturia, hypophosphatemia, generalized aminoaciduria, albuminuria, osteoporosis, sometimes rickets, and organic aciduria (205). Protein trafficking between endosomes and the trans-Golgi network is disrupted and may be responsible for some of the phenotypic changes (39). Death is usually due to renal failure. Mutations in the Lowe syndrome gene *OCRL1* (mapped to Xq24-26) are recognized (142).

Menkes Syndrome

Menkes, or Menkes kinky hair, syndrome is distinguished by progressive cerebral deterioration with seizures, twisted and fractured hair (pili torti), and systemic copper deficiency (53,159). Affected infants have pudgy cheeks and sparse, coarse, and lightly pigmented hair that, when magnified, shows pronounced twisting and breakage. Hair changes are thought to be due to defective disulfide bonds in keratin (which are copper dependent). Nervous system findings include reduced numbers of noradrenergic fibers in the forebrain and peculiar torpedo-like swellings of catecholamine-containing axons in peripheral nerve tracts, which may relate to vascular disturbances, deterioration of the viscera, and eventual death (260). Skeletal changes in Menkes syndrome include wormian bones, metaphyseal widening, particularly of ribs and femora, and lateral spurs. Arteriograms show widespread arterial elongation and tortuosity due to reduced copper-dependent cross-linking in the internal elastic membrane of vessel walls. The condition is X-linked recessive. The gene for Menkes disease (*MNK*) codes for a copper-transporting ATPase that controls copper homeostasis in virtually every tissue except the liver (96). Copper transporters are impaired, limiting copper uptake, primarily in the small intestine. First-trimester prenatal diagnosis is possible with a DNA probe.

Lesch-Nyhan Syndrome

Lesch-Nyhan syndrome is caused by an X-linked recessive trait that produces a deficiency of the enzyme involved in purine synthesis—hypoxanthine guanine phosphoribosyl transferase. Patients produce excessive amounts of uric acid and suffer from profound mental retardation, characteristic self-mutilation, and motor disability, the latter primarily a severe action dystonia overlying a baseline hypotonia (116). The gene has been cloned and mapped to the long arm of the X chromosome at Xq26; a large number of mutations are recognized (174).

Opitz-Kaveggia (FG) Syndrome

This syndrome is X-linked and associated with mental retardation, hypotonia, and anal malformation, sometimes with constipation (58,182). Other prominent findings are megalencephaly, midline fusion of the mammillary bodies, heterotopia of cranial nerve nuclei, and pachygyria or other dysgenesis of the cerebral cortex (182). Affected patients have lived up to 18 years of age (182). Five loci (FGS1-5) have been mapped to the X chromosome. X inactivation has been reported but not correlated with specific loci (203).

Pallister (W) Syndrome

Pallister and colleagues described two brothers with mental retardation and unusual appearances including frontal prominence, anterior cowlick, hypertelorism, antimongoloid orbital slant, broad, flat nasal bridge, midline notch of the upper lip, submucosal cleft of the hard palate, absent upper central incisors, elbow subluxation, camptodactyly, and pes cavus (187). These children had grand mal seizures. The mother and a sister were mildly afflicted, consistent with heterozygous manifestations of an X-linked trait. The sister is known to have had an affected boy.

SPORADIC ABNORMALITIES

Klippel-Trenaunay-Weber Vascular Malformation

Features of this malformation complex include limb hypertrophy; hemangiomata that may be capillary; cavernous phlebectasias; and varicosities (128,188). The legs, buttocks, abdomen, and lower trunk are the usual sites of vascular lesions. Less common abnormalities include arteriovenous fistulas, lymphangiomas, macrodactyly, syndactyly, polydactyly, hyperpigmented nevi, and telangiectasia. Craniofacial abnormalities include asymmetric facial hypertrophy, hemangiomata, intracranial calcifications, and eye abnormalities. Visceromegaly and hemangiomata of the intestinal tract, urinary system, and mesentery may be present. Mental deficiency and seizures may occur with facial hemangiomatosis. A susceptibility gene, *VG5Q* (formerly *AGGF1*), encodes for an angiogenic factor, that, when mutated, enhances angiogenic activity (253,254).

Sturge-Weber Dysplasia

The association of hemangiomata in the facial skin, eyes, and meninges in this condition may be related to an early defect in vascular morphogenesis. Aberrant vascular innervation and expression of vasoactive and extracellular matrix molecules may play important roles in pathogenesis (46). Cutaneous hemangiomata may occur in the trigeminal distribution, but this is not obligatory; meningeal hemangiomata may present in occipital and temporal areas (6,37). Progressive neurological deficits are complicated by seizures and may develop from impaired cerebral perfusion (47). Pathologic findings include cerebral cortical atrophy, sclerosis, and calcification.

Hallermann-Streiff Syndrome

Oculomandibulodyscephaly with hypotrichosis was first reported by Audry in 1893; Hallermann and Streiff independently described three cases later (91,241). The syndrome is rare, with only 150 cases reported, and characterized by microphthalmia, a small, pinched, birdlike nose, and hypotrichosis (55,72,121,164). Infants with this syndrome have proportionately small stature, brachycephaly with frontal and parietal bossing, thin calvaria, malar hypoplasia, micrognathia, and anterior displacement of the temporomandibular joint. Other facial anomalies are microstomia and high, narrow, arched palate. Hair is sparse, and skin is thin and atrophic, most prominently over the nose and suture areas of the scalp. Additional ocular manifestations include spherophakia, blue sclerae, nystagmus, strabismus, colobomata, glaucoma, and various chorioretinal pigment alterations; cataracts may resorb spontaneously. Nasal and mandibular anomalies may compromise respiration and feeding, requiring rhinoplasty, facial augmentation, or mandibular surgery (55). Reported karyotypes have been normal, and possible inheritance patterns remain unknown.

Hypomelanosis of Ito

Hypomelanosis of Ito (systematized achromic nevus or incontinentia pigmenti achromians) appears to be a manifestation of mosaicism rather than a distinct entity, most likely involving a number of chromosomes, that disrupts pigmentary genes (243). Thus, the condition has been termed "pigmentary mosaicism" and consists of a triad of scattered, streaked, whorled, or mottled areas of cutaneous hypopigmentation that fluoresce, mental deficiency, and severe intractable seizures present from birth (201,220). Skin manifestations bear a resemblance to those of incontinentia pigmenti and the ash leaf macule of tuberous sclerosis. Pathologic changes in the brain are variable and include cortical dysplasias, heterotopias, and hamartomas (201,220). Recognition of the cutaneous changes may alert clinicians to defects in other organ systems (220).

Rubinstein-Taybi Syndrome

The Rubinstein-Taybi mental retardation syndrome (RTS) is a rare condition characterized by mental retardation and a number of physical anomalies. RTS is characterized by broad thumbs and toes, bulbous fingers, slanted palpebral fissures, and hypoplastic maxilla (212). Other abnormalities include short stature and small cranium, mental retardation, beaked nose with nasal septum extending below nasal alae, epicanthal folds, strabismus, low-set or malformed auricles, excess dermal ridge patterning in the thenar and first interdigital areas of the palm, cryptorchidism, and cardiac defects (particularly ventricular septal defect and patent ductus arteriosus). Cataract, colobomata, ptosis of eyelids, long eyelashes and hypertrichosis, polydactyly, simian crease, and renal anomalies have been described (103). A large number of mutations in *CBP*, the gene encoding the cyclic AMP response element binding protein (CREB), a coactivator important to gene transcription and cognitive functioning (90). A second gene, *EP300*, has also been identified in patients (210).

ABNORMALITIES OF UNKNOWN ORIGIN

Short-Cord Syndrome

The length of the normal umbilical cord varies, but averages about 60 cm (±13 cm) at term (171). Cord length is static during the third trimester, presumably because the fetus is constrained during this period. This observation supports the notion that cord length is determined in large part by fetal activity and the tension placed on the cord during growth (162). Both short and long cords are associated with an increased risk of complications during labor and delivery. The former may complicate delivery (129,229), while the latter is more easily obstructed. Short umbilical cords are associated with a variety of severe fetal anomalies. Factors that retard fetal movement (e.g., intrauterine compression, uterine anomaly, amniotic bands, CNS or musculoskeletal anomaly, other fetal malformation) are associated with a short umbilical cord. While some cases appear to be due to reduced fetal motion, others are thought to develop as part of an early defect involving the body stalk or the cord itself (22,54,259).

Nonimmune Hydrops Fetalis

Fetal hydrops is a generalized increase in fluid accumulation in serous cavities, causing edema of the soft tissues in a fetus (Figure 4-13). At birth, the affected infant shows gross edema and may be difficult to resuscitate because of pleural effusions, ascites, and associated lung hypoplasia. Fetal hydrops is divided into immune and nonimmune types. The most common cause of immune hydrops was once Rh isoimmunization. Since the advent of anti-D globulin (i.e., RhoGAM), most cases of fetal hydrops are nonimmune in nature (Table 4-10). The incidence of nonimmune hydrops is thought to be between 1 in 2,500 and 1 in 3,500 newborns. The pathogenetic mechanisms leading to fetal hydrops are increased intracapillary hydrostatic pressure, decreased intracapillary osmotic pressure, and damage to the peripheral capillary or vascular integrity. Machin has extensively reviewed the differential diagnosis and pathogenesis of hydrops fetalis (146).

Chronic and severe anemia leading to hydrops may be caused by a variety of conditions, most commonly homozygous alpha-thalassemia, twin-to-twin transfusion, chronic fetomaternal transfusion, or infection by parvovirus B19. Severe, progressive anemia leads to congestive heart failure. Fetomaternal transfusion is thought to occur in at least half of all pregnancies, but the quantity of transfused blood is usually small. A Kleihauer-Betke acid elution test of the mother's blood is used to demonstrate the presence of fetal erythrocytes. The presence of fetal cells indicates bleeding from the fetal circulation into maternal circulation; by knowing the percentage of fetal cells in the maternal circulation, one can estimate the amount of blood lost by the fetus. If this quantity reaches significant proportions, it can be a cause of

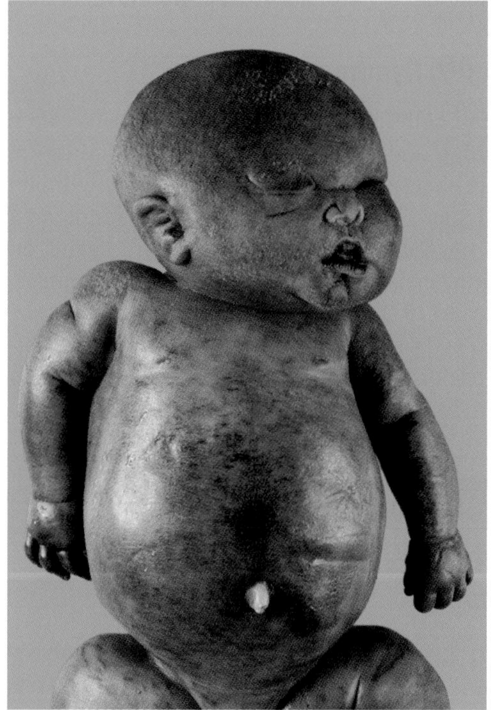

FIGURE 4-13 ■ Nonimmune hydrops fetalis. This 25-week female fetus suffered intrauterine fetal demise. The heart was enlarged and showed biventricular endocardial fibroelastosis. The cause of fetal hydrops was not ascertained but may have been related to maternal antiphospholipid antibody syndrome.

Table 4-10 ■ CONDITIONS ASSOCIATED WITH NONIMMUNE HYDROPS FETALIS

CAUSAL CONDITIONS
Fetal conditions
Severe chronic anemia *in utero*
Fetomaternal transfusion
Twin-to-twin transfusion
Homozygous thalassemia
Acardius
Atrioventricular shunts
Hemorrhage or thrombosis
Maternal drugs (e.g., chloramphenicol)
Placental conditions
Chorionic vein thrombosis
Umbilical vein thrombosis
Angiomyxoma of umbilical cord
Aneurysm of umbilical cord
Chorioangioma of placenta
Maternal conditions
Maternal diabetes mellitus
Maternal nephritis
EFFECTS ON BODY SYSTEMS
Cardiovascular system
Severe congenital heart disease
Large arteriovenous malformation
Premature closure of foramen ovale
Hypoplastic left heart
Hypoplastic right heart
Cardiopulmonary hypoplasia with bilateral hydrothorax
Premature closure of ductus arteriosus, with pulmonary hypoplasia
Fetal arrhythmias
Myocarditis
Cardiac tumors (rhabdomyomas)
Pulmonary system
Congenital cystic adenomatoid malformation of the lung
Pulmonary hypoplasia
Pulmonary lymphangiectasia
Intrathoracic mass
Diaphragmatic hernia
Gastrointestinal system
Bowel atresia
Duplications of the gut
Peritonitis
Liver
Congenital hepatitis
Kidney
Congenital nephrosis
Renal vein thrombosis
ASSOCIATED CONDITIONS
Developmental or genetic disorders
Ullrich-Turner syndrome
Trisomy 18
Meckel syndrome
Pena-Shokeir syndrome
Noonan syndrome
Neu-Laxova syndrome
Multiple pterygium syndrome
Skeletal dysplasias (lethal congenital short limb dysplasias)
Multiple congenital abnormalities
Intrauterine infections
Syphilis
Toxoplasmosis
Cytomegalovirus
Coxsackie B virus pancarditis
Chagas disease
Leptospirosis
Lysosomal storage diseases
Mucopolysaccharidosis
Gaucher disease
Gangliosidosis
Sialidosis
Other conditions
Fetal neuroblastoma
Hemangioendothelioma
Tuberous sclerosis
Dysmaturity
Amniotic band syndrome
Fetal tumors (teratoma, neuroblastoma, angiomas)

From McGillivray and Hall (157), with permission.

fetal death. In twin-to-twin transfusion, nonimmune hydrops may be seen in the donor twin secondary to anemia (where it causes congestive heart failure), but more often the condition occurs in the recipient twin, secondary to volume overload.

Cardiovascular causes of fetal hydrops include transient arrhythmias during pregnancy. When arrhythmias persist, they lead to fluid accumulation and congestive failure in the fetus. Congenital heart block with bradycardia should suggest a possible diagnosis of autoimmune disease in the mother (especially systemic lupus erythematosus). A number of cardiovascular abnormalities can lead to intrauterine congestive heart failure, including septal defects, premature closure of the foramen ovale, premature closure of the ductus arteriosus, agenesis of the ductus venosus, and hypoplastic left ventricle.

Respiratory causes of fetal hydrops include diaphragmatic hernia, pulmonary lymphangiectasis, and congenital pulmonary airway malformation of the fetal lung. Within the context of mediastinal shift, obstruction of the lymphatic duct and major blood vessels occurs, producing excess accumulation of fluid. Gastrointestinal atresia, midgut volvulus, and duplication are thought to cause hydrops because of decreased intravascular colloid osmotic pressure. Obstruction of the fetal urinary tract at the ureteropelvic junction or by posterior urethral valves or renal abnormalities causing nephrosis may also be associated with fetal hydrops. In this latter case, hypoalbuminemia develops, with subsequent cardiac failure and fluid accumulation.

Chromosomal defects may be associated with cystic hygroma and often with generalized hydrops fetalis. This is commonly seen with Ullrich-Turner syndrome. Bieber syndrome manifests as a familial cystic hygroma simulating an encephalocele. Incomplete formation of the lymphatic system delays drainage into the thoracic duct. The cause of nuchal cysts and hydrops is not clear, but the condition is relatively common and its associated conditions have been reported.

Placental abnormalities, including chorioangioma, torsion of the cord, or umbilical vein thrombosis, may also be the primary cause of fetal hydrops. Intrauterine infection, particularly the toxoplasmosis, rubella, CMV, and herpes simplex (TORCH) syndrome, may also have associated hydrops. The likely mechanism for ascites and more extreme fluid collections is usually the severe hepatic injury caused by the infection and consequent hypoalbuminemia and portal hypertension.

The lethal chondrodysplasias may be associated with hydrops. Syndromes involving absent or abnormal fetal movement, including syndromes exhibiting the Pena-Shokeir phenotype, may exhibit fetal hydrops. The mechanism leading to fluid collection is unknown. Transient *in utero* hydrops early in the second trimester is characteristic of the Noonan syndrome. Lysosomal storage diseases, including Gaucher disease, GM1 gangliosidosis, mucopolysaccharidoses, disorders of sialic acid, and others, have been described with fetal hydrops (80). Hypoproteinemia and sinusoidal obstruction of the liver by Kupffer cells swollen with storage material have been suggested as causes for the fluid accumulation.

ACKNOWLEDGMENT

The contributions of Drs. Enid Gilbert-Barness and John Opitz to the previous edition are gratefully acknowledged.

REFERENCES

1. (CDC). CfDCaP. Achievements in public health. Reduction in perinatal transmission of HIV infection—United States, 1985–2005. *MMWR* 2006;55:592–597.
2. Aarskog D. Maternal progestins as a possible cause of hypospadias. *N Engl J Med* 1979;300:75–78.
3. Adam MP, Manning MA, Beck AE, et al. Methotrexate/misoprostol embryopathy: report of four cases resulting from failed medical abortion. *Am J Med Genet A* 2003;123:72–78.
4. Ades LC, Sillence DO. Agnathia-holoprosencephaly with tetramelia. *Clin Dysmorphol* 1992;1:182–184.
5. Al-Nemri AR, Kilani RA, Salih MA, et al. Embryonal rhabdomyosarcoma and chromosomal breakage in a newborn infant with possible Dubowitz syndrome. *Am J Med Genet* 2000;92:107–110.
6. Alexander GL, Norman RM. *The Sturge-Weber Syndrome*. Bristol, UK: John Wright and Sons, 1960.
7. Alexiev BA, Lin, X, Sun CC, et al. Meckel-Gruber syndrome: pathologic manifestations, minimal diagnostic criteria, and differential diagnosis. *Arch Pathol Lab Med* 2006;130:1236–1238.
8. Allen C, Reardon W. Assisted reproduction technology and defects of genomic imprinting. *BJOG* 2005;112:1589–1594.
9. American College of Obstetricians and Gynecologists CoOP. Guidelines for diagnostic imaging during pregnancy. 1995; Washington, D.C.: ACOG, 1995.
10. Anderson VM. Meckel syndrome: morphologic considerations. *Birth Defects Orig Artic Series* 1982;18:145–160.
11. Andrews AD, Barrett SF, Yoder FW, et al. Cockayne's syndrome fibroblasts have increased sensitivity to ultraviolet light but normal rates of unscheduled DNA synthesis. *J Invest Dermatol* 1978;70: 237–239.
12. Anonymous. Goitre and iodine deficiency in Europe. Report of the Subcommittee for the Study of Endemic Goitre and Iodine Deficiency of the European Thyroid Association. *Lancet* 1985;1: 1289–1293.
13. Anonymous. Possible health effects of radiation exposure on unborn babies (CDC). In: Services. DoHaH, ed., 2005.
14. Anonymous. Spina bifida and anencephaly before and after folic acid mandate—United States, 1995–1996 and 1999–2000. *MMWR* 2004;53:362–365.
15. Arenas-Sordo Mde L, Hernandez-Zamora E, Montoya-Perez LA, et al. Cockayne's syndrome: a case report. Literature review. *Med Oral Patol Oral Cir Bucal* 2006;11:E236–E238.
16. Arnaud P, Feil R. Epigenetic deregulation of genomic imprinting in human disorders and following assisted reproduction. *Birth Defects Res C Embryo Today* 2005;75:81–97.
17. Arpino C, Brescianini S, Robert E, et al. Teratogenic effects of antiepileptic drugs: use of an International Database on Malformations and Drug Exposure (MADRE). *Epilepsia* 2000;41:1436–1443.
18. Aylsworth AS. Clinical aspects of defects in the determination of laterality. *Am J Med Genet* 2001;101:345–355.
19. Azarbayjani F, Danielsson BR. Phenytoin-induced cleft palate: evidence for embryonic cardiac bradyarrhythmia due to inhibition of delayed rectifier K+ channels resulting in hypoxia-reoxygenation damage. *Teratology* 2001;63:152–160.
20. Bajoria R. Abundant vascular anastomoses in monoamniotic versus diamniotic monochorionic placentas. *Am J Obstet Gynecol* 1998;179:788–793.
21. Barr M, Burdi AR. Warfarin-associated embryopathy in a 17-week abortus. *Teratology* 1976;14:129–134.
22. Barr M, Heidelberger KP. Short umbilical cord: cause or effect of fetal anomalies. *Proc Greenwood Genetics Center* 1983;2:100–101.
23. Basile C, De Michele V. Renal abnormalities in Mayer-Rokitanski-Kuster-Hauser syndrome. *J Nephrol* 2001;14:316–318.
24. Beck B, Mikkelson M. Chromosomes in the Cornelia de Lange syndrome. *Hum Genet* 1981;59:271–276.
25. Bell KN, Oakley GP Jr. Tracking the prevention of floic acid-preventable spina bifida and anencephaly. *Birth Defects Res A Clin Mol Teratol* 2006;76:654–657.
26. Bernstein J, Brough, AJ, McAdams AJ. The renal lesion in syndromes of multiple congenital malformations. Cerebrohepatorenal syndrome; Jeune asphyxiating thoracic dystrophy; tuberous sclerosis; Meckel syndrome. *Birth Defects Orig Art Ser* 1974;10:35–43.
27. Blank CE. Apert syndrome (a type of acrocephalosyndactyly): observations on a British series of thirty-nine cases. *Ann Hum Genet* 1960;24:151–164.
28. Bongers EM, Gubler MC, Knoers NV. Nail-patella syndrome. Overview on clinical and molecular findings. *Pediatr Nephrol* 2002;17:703–712.
29. Bongers EM, Huysmans FT, Levtchenko E, et al. Genotype-phenotype studies in nail-patella syndrome show that LMX1B mutation location is involved in the risk of developing nephropathy. *Eur J Hum Genet* 2005;13:935–946.
30. Bongers EM, van Kampen A, van Bokhoven H, et al. Human syndromes with congenital patellar anomalies and the underlying gene defects. *Clin Genet* 2005;68:302–319.
31. Bowen P, Lee CSN, Zellweger H, et al. A familial syndrome of multiple congenital defects. *Bull Johns Hopkins Hosp* 1964;114:402–414.
32. Brent RL. The effect of embryonic and fetal exposure to x-ray, microwaves, and ultrasound: counseling the pregnant and nonpregnant patient about these risks. *Semin Oncol* 1989;16:347–368.
33. Brosius U, Gartner J. Cellular and molecular aspects of Zellweger syndrome and other peroxisome biogenesis disorders. *Cell Mol Life Sci* 2002;59:1058–1069.
34. Calhoun F, Attilia ML, Spagnolo PA, et al. National Institute on Alcohol Abuse and Alcoholism and the study of fetal alcohol spectrum disorders. The International Consortium. *Ann Ist Super Sanita* 2006;42:4–7.
35. Carinci F, Pezzetti F, Locci P, et al. Apert and Crouzon syndromes: clinical findings, genes and extracellular matrix. *J Craniofac Surg* 2005;16:361–368.

36. Chan KY, Gilbert-Barness E, Tiller G. Warfarin embryopathy. *Pediatr Pathol Mol Med* 2003;22:277–283.
37. Chao DH-C. Congenital neurocutaneous syndromes of childhood. III. Sturge-Weber disease. *J Pediatr* 1959;55:635–649.
38. Chen H, Chang CH, Misra RP, et al. Multiple pterygium syndrome. *Am J Med Genet* 1980;7:91–102.
39. Choudhury R, Diao A, Zhang F, et al. Lowe syndrome protein OCRL1 interacts with clathrin and regulates protein trafficking between endosomes and the trans-Golgi network. *Mol Biol Cell* 2005;16:3467–3479.
40. Christoffel KK, Salafsky I. Fetal alcohol syndrome in dizygotic twins. *J Pediatr* 1975;87:963–967.
41. Clarren SK, Alvord EC, Sumi SM, et al. Brain malformations related to prenatal exposure to ethanol. *J Pediatr* 1978;92:64–67.
42. Clarren SK, Smith DW. The fetal alcohol syndrome. *N Engl J Med* 1978;298:1063–1067.
43. Clay SA, McVie R, Chen H. Possible teratogenic effect of valproic acid. *J Pediatr* 1981;99:828.
44. Cockayne EA. Dwarfism with retinal atrophy and deafness. *Arch Dis Child* 1936;11:1–8.
45. Cohen MM Jr. *The child with multiple birth defects*, 2nd ed. Oxford, UK: Oxford University Press, 1997.
46. Comi AM. Advances in Sturge-Weber syndrome. *Curr Opin Neurol* 2006;19:124–128.
47. Comi AM. Pathophysiology of Sturge-Weber syndrome. *J Child Neurol* 2003;18:509–516.
48. Connolly KJ, Pharoah POD, Hetzel BS. Fetal iodine deficiency and motor performance during childhood. *Lancet* 1979;2:1149–1151.
49. Cremin BJ. The urinary tract anomalies associated with agenesis of the abdominal wall. *Br J Radiol* 1971;44:767–772.
50. Czeizel A. Schisis-association. *Am J Med Genet* 1981;10:25–35.
51. Dalens B, Raynaud EJ, Gaulme J. Teratogenicity of valproic acid. *J Pediatr* 1980;97:332–333.
52. Danielsson BR, Skold AC, Johansson A, et al. Teratogenicity by the hERG potassium channel blocking drug almokalant: use of hypoxia marker gives evidence for a hypoxia-related mechanism mediated via embryonic arrhythmia. *Toxicol Appl Pharmacol* 2003;193:168–176.
53. Danks DM, Campbell PE, Stevens BJ, et al. Menkes kinky hair syndrome. An inherited defect in copper absorption with widespread effects. *Pediatrics* 1972;50:188–201.
54. Daskalakis G, Pilalis A, Papadopoulos D, et al. Body stalk anomaly diagnosed in the 2nd trimester. *Fetal Diagn Ther* 2003;18:342–344.
55. David LR, Finlon M, Genecov D, et al. Hallermann-Streiff syndrome: experience with 15 patients and review of the literature. *J Craniofac Surg* 1999;10:160–168.
56. David TJ, Webb BW, Gordon IRS. The Patterson syndrome, leprechaunism, and pseudoleprechaunism. *J Med Genet* 1981;18:294–298.
57. Derbent M, Agras PI, Gedik S, et al. Congenital cataract, microphthalmia, hypoplasia of corpus callosum and hypogenitalism: report and review of Micro syndrome. *Am J Med Genet A* 2004;128:232–234.
58. Dessay S, Moizard MP, Gilardi JL, et al. FG syndrome: linkage analysis in two families supporting a new gene localization at Xp22.3. *Am J Med Genet* 2002;112:6–11.
59. Di Bartolomeo R, Polidori G, Piastra M, et al. Malignant hypertension and cerebral haemorrhage in Seckel syndrome. *Eur J Pediatr* 2003;162:860–862.
60. Dixon J, Ellis I, Bottani A, et al. Identification of mutations in TCOF1: use of molecular analysis in the pre- and postnatal diagnosis of Treacher Collins syndrome. *Am J Med Genet A* 2004;127:244–248.
61. Dodge HW, Wood MW, Kennedy RL. Craniofacial dysostosis: Crouzon disease. *Pediatrics* 1959;23:98–106.
62. Dubowitz V. Familial low birth weight dwarfism with an unusual facies and a skin eruption. *J Med Genet* 1965;2:12–17.
63. Duncan PA, Shapiro LR, Stangel JJ, et al. The MURCS association: mullerian duct aplasia, renal aplasia, and cervicothoracic somite dysplasia. *J Pediatr* 1979;95:399–402.
64. Dunne F, Brydon P, Smith K, et al. Pregnancy in women with type 2 diabetes: 12 years outcome data 1990–2002. *Diabet Med* 2003;20:734–738.
65. Eagle JF, Barrett GS. Congenital deficiency of abdominal musculature with associated genitourinary abnormalities: a syndrome; report of nine cases. *Pediatrics* 1950;6:721–736.
66. Edwards MJ. Apoptosis, the heat shock response, hyperthermia, birth defects, disease and cancer. Where are the common links? *Cell Stress Chaperones* 1998;3:213–220.
67. Edwards MJ. Review: hyperthermia and fever during pregnancy. *Birth Defects Res A Clin Mol Teratol* 2006;76:507–516.
68. Elghany NA, Stopford W, Bunn WB, et al. Occupational exposure to inorganic mercury vapour and reproductive outcomes. *Occup Med* 1997;47:333–336.
69. Elsas LJ, Endo F, Strumlauf E, et al. Leprechaunism: an inherited defect in a high-affinity insulin receptor. *Am J Hum Genet* 1985;37:73–88.
70. Faivre L, Portnoi MF, Pals G, et al. Should chromosome breakage studies be performed in patients with VACTERL association? *Am J Med Genet A* 2005;137:55–58.
71. Feldman GL, Weaver DD, Lovrien EW. The fetal trimethadione syndrome: report of an additional family and further delineation of this syndrome. *Am J Dis Child* 1977;131:1389–1392.
72. Francois J. A new syndrome: dyscephalia with bird face and dental anomalies, nanism, hypotrichosis, cutaneous atrophy, microphthalmia and congenital cataract. *Arch Ophthalmol* 1958;60:842–862.
73. Friedman JM, Polifka JE. *Teratogenic effects of drugs*, 2nd ed. Baltimore, MD: The Johns Hopkins University Press, 2000.
74. Furlong LA. Ectopic pregnancy risk when contraception fails. A review. *J Reprod Med* 2002;47:881–885.
75. Garcia CA, McGarry PA, Voirol M, et al. Neurological involvement in the Smith-Lemli-Opitz syndrome. *Dev Med Child Neurol* 1973;15:48–55.
76. German J, Kowal A, Ehlers KHY. Trimethadione and human teratogenesis. *Teratology* 1970;3:349–362.
77. Gilbert-Barness EF, Opitz JM. Congenital anomalies and malformation syndromes. In: Stocker JT, Dehner LP, eds. *Pediatric pathology*. Philadelphia, PA: Lippincott Williams & Wilkins, 2001.
78. Gilbert–Barness EF, Opitz JM. Congenital anomalies and malformation syndromes. In: Wigglesworth JS, Singer DB, eds. *Textbook of fetal and perinatal pathology*. Oxford, UK: Blackwell Scientific Publications, 1991.
79. Gilchrist KW, Gilbert EF, Goldfarb S, et al. Studies of malformation syndromes of man XIB: The cerebro-hepato-renal syndrome of Zellweger: comparative pathology. *Eur J Pediatr* 1976;121:99–118.
80. Gillan JE, Lowden JA, Gaskin K, et al. Congenital ascites as a presenting sign of lysosomal storage disease. *J Pediatr* 1984;104:225–231.
81. Glinoer D. Feto-maternal repercussions of iodine deficiency during pregnancy. An update. *Ann Endocrinol (Paris)* 2003;64:37–44.
82. Go RS, Johnston KL. Acute myelogenous leukemia in an adult with thrombocytopenia with absent radii syndrome. *Eur J Haematol* 2003;70:246–248.
83. Goldstein L, Murphy DP. Microcephalic idiocy following radium therapy for uterine cancer during pregnancy. *Am J Obstet Gynecol* 1929;18:189.
84. Goto MP, Goldman AS. Diabetic embryopathy. *Curr Opin Pediatr* 1994;6:486–491.
85. Graham JM, Stephens TD, Shepard TH. Nuchal cystic hygroma in a fetus with presumed Roberts syndrome. *Am J Med Genet* 1983;15:163–167.
86. Graham JMJ, Anyane-Yeboa K, Raams A, et al. Cerebro-oculo-facio-skeletal syndrome with a nucleotide excision-repair defect and a mutated XPD gene, with prenatal diagnosis in a triplet pregnancy. *Am J Hum Genet* 2001;69:291–300.
87. Graham JMJ, Hennekam R, Dobyns WB, et al. MICRO syndrome: an entity distinct from COFS syndrome. *Am J Med Genet A* 2004;128:235–245.
88. Greenhalgh KL, Howell RT, Bottani A, et al. Thrombocytopenia-absent radius syndrome: a clinical genetic study. *J Med Genet* 2002;39:876–881.

89. Hall JG. Analysis of Pena Shokeir phenotype (Invited editorial comment). *Am J Med Genet* 1986;25:99–117.
90. Hallam TM, Bourtchouladze R. Rubinstein-Taybi syndrome: molecular findings and therapeutic approaches to improve cognitive dysfunction. *Cell Mol Life Sci* 2006;63:1725–1735.
91. Hallermann W. Vogelgesicht und cataracta congenita. *Klin Monatsbl Augenheilkd* 1948;113:315–318.
92. Hansen JC, Gilman AP. Exposure of Arctic populations to methylmercury from consumption of marine food: an updated risk-benefit assessment. *Int J Circumpolar Health* 2005;64:121–136.
93. Hanson JW, Myrianthopoulos NC, Harvey MA, et al. Risks to the offspring of women treated wtih hydantoin anticonvulsants, with emphasis on the fetal hydantoin syndrome. *J Pediatr* 1976;89: 662–668.
94. Harley LM, Chen Y, Rattner WH. Prune belly syndrome. *J Urol* 1972;108:174–176.
95. Harper RG, Orti E, Baker RK. A familial pattern of developmental, dental, skeletal, genital, and central nervous system anomalies. *J Pediatr* 1967;70:799–804.
96. Harris ED, Reddy MC, Majumdar S, et al. Pretranslational control of Menkes disease gene expression. *Biometals* 2003;16:55–61.
97. Hawley PP, Jackson LG, Kurnit DM. Sixty-four patients with Brachmann-de Lange syndrome: a survey. *Am J Med Genet* 1985;20:453–459.
98. Heinonen OP. Diethylstilbestrol in pregnancy. Frequency of exposure and usage patterns. *Cancer* 1973;31:573–577.
99. Hellstrom A, Jansson C, Boguszewski M, et al. Growth hormone status in six children with fetal alcohol syndrome. *Acta Paediatr* 1996;85:1456–1462.
100. Henneveld HT, van Lingen RA, Hamel BC, et al. Perlman syndrome: four additional cases and review. *Am J Med Genet* 1999;86:439–446.
101. Hermann J, Pallister PD, Opitz JM. Tetraectrodactyly and other skeletal manifestations in the fetal alcohol syndrome. *Eur J Pediatr* 1980;133:221–226.
102. Herrmann J, Feingold M, Tuffli GA, et al. A familial dysmorphogenetic syndrome of limb deformities, characteristic facial appearance and associated anomalies: the 'pseudothalidomide' or SC-syndrome. *Birth Defects Orig Art Ser* 1969;5:81–89.
103. Herrmann J, Opitz JM. Dermatoglyphic studies in a Rubinstein-Taybi patient, her unaffected dizygous twin sister and other relatives. *Birth Defects Orig Art Ser* 1969;5:22–24.
104. Herrmann J, Opitz JM. The SC phocomelia and the Roberts syndrome: nosologic aspects. *Eur J Pediatr* 1977;125:117–134.
105. Hersh JH, Angle B, Fox TL, et al. Developmental field defects: coming together of associations and sequences during blastogenesis. *Am J Med Genet* 2002;110:320–323.
106. Hetzel BS, Hay ID. Thyroid function, iodine nutrition, and fetal brain development. *Clin Endocrinol* 1979;11:445–460.
107. Hoagland MH, Hutchins GM. Obstructive lesions of the lower urinary tract in the prune belly syndrome. *Arch Pathol Lab Med* 1987;111:154–156.
108. Holt M, Oram S. Familial heart disease with skeletal malformations. *Br Heart J* 1960;22:236–242.
109. Hong R, Horowitz SD, Borzy MF, et al. The cerebro-hepato-renal syndrome of Zellweger: similarity to and differentiation from the DiGeorge syndrome. *Thymus* 1981;3:97–104.
110. Hoogenraad CC, Akhmanova A, Galjart N, et al. LIMK1 and CLIP-115: linking cytoskeletal defects to Williams syndrome. *Bioessays* 2004;26:141–150.
111. Hoyme HE, May PA, Kalberg WO, et al. A practical clinical approach to diagnosis of fetal alcohol spectrum disorders: clarification of the 1996 Institute of Medicine criteria. *Pediatrics* 2005;115:39–47.
112. Huang T. Current advances in Holt-Oram syndrome. *Curr Opin Pediatr* 2002;14:691–695.
113. Ibrahimi OA, Chiu ES, McCarthy JG, et al. Understanding the molecular basis of Apert syndrome. *Plast Reconstr Surg* 2005;115: 264–270.
114. Infante JP, Huszagh VA. Impaired arachidonic (20:4n-6) and docosahexaenoic (22:6n-3) acid synthesis by phenylalanine metabolites as etiological factors in the neuropathology of phenylketonuria. *Mol Gen Metab* 2001;72:185–198.
115. Innis SM. Essential fatty acid transfer and fetal development. *Placenta* 2005;26(suppl A):S70–S75.
116. Jinnah HA, Visser JE, Harris JC, et al. Delineation of the motor disorder of Lesch-Nyhan disease. *Brain* 2006;129:1201–1217.
117. Jira PE, Waterham HR, Wanders RJ, et al. Smith-Lemli-Opitz syndrome and the DHCR7 gene. *Ann Hum Genet* 2003;67:269–280.
118. Jones KL. *Smith's recognizable patterns of human malformation*, 6th ed. Philadelphia, PA: Elsevier Saunders, 2006.
119. Jones KL, Johnson KA, Chambers CD. Offspring of women infected with varicella during pregnancy: a prospective study. *Teratology* 1994;49:29–32.
120. Jones KL, Smith DW. Recognition of the fetal alcohol syndrome in early infancy. *Lancet* 1973;2:999–1001.
121. Judge C, Chakanovskis JE. The Hallermann-Streiff syndrome. *J Ment Defic Res* 1971;15:115–120.
122. Kaplan LC, Matsuoka R, Gilbert EF, et al. Ectopia cordis and cleft sternum: evidence for mechanical teratogenesis following rupture of the chorion or yolk sac. *Am J Med Genet* 1985;21:187–202.
123. Keegan CE, Mulliken JB, Wu BL, et al. Townes-Brocks syndrome versus expanded spectrum hemifacial microsomia: review of eight patients and further evidence of a "hot spot" for mutation in the SALL1 gene. *Genet Med* 2001;3:310–313.
124. Kelly TE. Teratogenicity of anticonvulsant drugs. I: A review of the literature. *Am J Med Genet* 1984;19:413–434.
125. Khoury MJ, Moore CA, Evans JA. On the use of the term "syndrome" in clinical genetics and birth defects epidemiology. *Am J Med Genet* 1994;49:26–28.
126. Kilinc MO, Ninis VN, Ugur SA, et al. Is the novel SCKL3 at 14q23 the predominant Seckel locus? *Eur J Hum Genet* 2003;11:851–857.
127. Kitzmiller JL, Cloherty JP, Younger MD, et al. Diabetic pregnancy and perinatal morbidity. *Am J Obstet Gynecol* 1978;131:560–580.
128. Klippel M, Trenaunay P. Du naevus variqueux osteo-hypertrophique. *Arch Gen Med* 1900;185:641–672.
129. Krakowiak P, Smith EN, de Bruyn G, et al. Risk factors and outcomes associated with a short umbilical cord. *Obstet Gynecol* 2004;103:119–127.
130. Krantz ID, McCallum J, DeScipio C, et al. Cornelia de Lange syndrome is caused by mutations in NIPBL, the human homolog of Drosophila melanogaster Nipped-B. *Nat Genet* 2004;36:631–635.
131. Krassikoff N, Sekhon GS. Familial agnathia-holoprosencephaly caused by an inherited unbalanced translocation and not autosomal recessive inheritance. *Am J Med Genet* 1989;34:255–257.
132. Kyttala M, Tallila J, Salonen R, et al. MKS1, encoding a component of the flagellar apparatus basal body proteome, is mutated in Meckel syndrome. *Nat Genet* 2006;38:155–157.
133. Lammer EJ, Chen DT, Hoar RM, et al. Retinoic acid embryopathy. *N Engl J Med* 1985;313:837–841.
134. Lammer EJ, Cordero JF. Exogenous sex hormone exposure and the risk for major malformations. *JAMA* 1986;255:3128–3132.
135. Leguizamon GF, Zeff NP, Fernandez A. Hypertension and the pregnancy complicated by diabetes. *Curr Diab Rep* 2006;6:297–304.
136. Lehmann AH, Francis AJ, Giannelli F. Prenatal diagnosis of Cockayne syndrome. *Lancet* 1985;1:486–488.
137. Lehmann AR. DNA repair-deficient diseases, xeroderma pigmentosum, Cockayne syndrome and trichothiodystrophy. *Biochimie* 2003;85:1101–1111.
138. Lemoine P, Harousseau H, Borteyru JP, et al. Les enfants de parents alcoholiques: anomalies observees. *Quest Med* 1968;25:476–482.
139. Liberfarb RM, Levy HP, Rose PS, et al. The Stickler syndrome: genotype/phenotype correlation in 10 families with Stickler syndrome resulting from seven mutations in the type II collagen gene locus COL2A1. *Genet Med* 2003;5:21–27.

140. Lin-Fu JS, Anthony M. Folic acid and neural tube defects: a fact sheet for health care providers. In: Maternal and Child Health Bureau HRaSA, Washington, DC: Public Health Service, 1993.
141. Lowe CU, Terrey M, MacLachland EA. Organic-aciduria, decreased renal ammonia production, hydrophthalmos, and mental retardation. *Am J Dis Child* 1952;83:164–184.
142. Lowe M. Structure and function of the Lowe syndrome protein OCRL1. *Traffic* 2005;6:711–719.
143. Lowry RB, Hill RH, Tischler B. Survival and spectrum of anomalies in the Meckel syndrome. *Am J Med Genet* 1983;14:417–421.
144. Lubinsky M. VATER and other associations: historical perspectives and modern interpretations. *Am J Med Genet* 1986;2:9–16.
145. Lubinsky M, Sujansky E, Sanger W, et al. Familial amniotic bands. *Am J Med Genet* 1983;14:81–87.
146. Machin GA. Hydrops revisited: literature review of 11,414 cases published in the 1980s. *Am J Med Genet* 1989;34:366–390.
147. Manley S. Haemoglobin A1c—a marker for complications of type 2 diabetes: the experience from the UK Prospective Diabetes Study (UKPDS). *Clin Chem Lab Med* 2003;41:1182–1190.
148. Marini JC. Osteogenesis imperfecta: comprehensive management. *Adv Pediatr* 1988;35:391–426.
149. Marini M, Giacopelli F, Seri M, et al. Interaction of the LMX1B and PAX2 gene products suggests possible molecular basis of differential phenotypes in nail-patella syndrome. *Eur J Hum Genet* 2005;13:789–792.
150. Marszalek B, Wojcicki P, Kobus K, et al. Clinical features, treatment and genetic background of Treacher Collins syndrome. *J Appl Genet* 2002;43:223–233.
151. Martinez-Frias ML, Frias JL. Primary developmental field III: clinical and epidemiological study of blastogenetic anomalies and their relationship to different MCA patterns. *Am J Med Genet* 1997;70:11–15.
152. Martinez-Frias ML, Frias JL, Opitz JM. Errors of morphogenesis and developmental field theory. *Am J Med Genet* 1998;76:291–296.
153. Matsumoto H, Koya G, Takeuchi T. Fetal Minamata disease: a neuropathological study of two cases of intrauterine intoxication by a methyl mercury compound. *J Neuropathol Exp Neurol* 1965;24:563–574.
154. Matsuyama A, Yasuda Y, Yasutake A, et al. Detailed pollution map of an area highly contaminated by mercury containing wastewater from an organic chemical factory in People's Republic of China. *Bull Environ Contam Toxicol* 2006;77:82–87.
155. McCulloch K. Neonatal problems in twins. *Clin Perinatol* 1988;15:141–158.
156. McGaughran J. MURCS in a male: a further case. *Clin Dysmorphol* 1999;8:77.
157. McGillivray BC, Hall JG. Nonimmune hydrops fetalis. *Pediatr Rev* 1987;9:197–202.
158. Meinecke P, Padberg B, Laas R. Agnathia, holoprosencephaly, and situs inversus: a third report. *Am J Med Genet* 1990;37:286–287.
159. Menkes JH, Alter M, Steigleder GK, et al. A sex-linked recessive disorder with retardation of growth, peculiar hair, and focal cerebral and cerebellar degeneration. *Pediatrics* 1962;29:764–779.
160. Merchant RH, Lala MM. Prevention of mother-to-child transmission of HIV—an overview. *Indian J Med Res* 2005;121:489–501.
161. Miller ME, Graham JM, Higginbottom MC, et al. Compression-related defects from early amnion rupture: evidence for mechanical teratogenesis. *J Pediatr* 1981;98:292–297.
162. Miller ME, Higginbottom M, Smith DW. Short umbilical cord: its origin and relevance. *Pediatrics* 1981;67:618–621.
163. Milunsky A, Graef JW, Gaynor MF. Methotrexate-induced congenital malformations, with a review of the literature. *J Pediatr* 1968;72:790–795.
164. Mirshekari A, Safar F. Hallermann-Streiff syndrome: a case review. *Clin Exp Dermatol* 2004;29:477–479.
165. Moore RM, Mansour JM, Redline RW, et al. The physiology of fetal membrane rupture: insight gained from the determination of physical properties. *Placenta* 2006;27:1037–1051.
166. Moossy J. The neuropathology of Cockayne syndrome. *J Neuropathol Exp Neurol* 1967;26:654–660.
167. Mortell A, O'Donnell AM, Giles S, et al. Adriamycin induces notochord hypertrophy with conservation of sonic hedgehog expression in abnormal ectopic notochord in the adriamycin rat model. *J Pediatr Surg* 2004;39:859–863.
168. Muenke M, Schell U, Hehr A, et al. A common mutation in the fibroblast growth factor receptor 1 gene in Pfeiffer syndrome. *Nature Genet* 1994;8:269–274.
169. Murdoch DR, Harding EG, Dunn JT. Persistence of iodine deficiency 25 years after initial correction efforts in the Khumbu region of Nepal. *NZ Med J* 1999;112:266–268.
170. Musio A, Selicorni A, Focarelli ML, et al. X-linked Cornelia de Lange syndrome owing to SMC1L1 mutations. *Nature Genet* 2006;38:528–530.
171. Naeye RL. Umbilical cord length: clinical significance. *J Pediatr* 1985;107:278–281.
172. Nau H, Rating D, Koch S, et al. Valproic acid and its metabolites: placental transfer, neonatal pharmacokinetics, transfer via mother's milk, and clinical status in neonates of epileptic mothers. *Pharmacol Exp Ther* 1981;219:768–777.
173. Noonan J, Ehmke DA. Associated noncardiac malformations in children with congenital heart disease. *J Pediatr* 1963;63:468–470.
174. Nyhan WL. Lesch-Nyhan disease. In: *Atlas of metabolic diseases*. London, UK: Chapman and Hall, 1998:376.
175. Odent S, LeMarec B, Toutain A, et al. Central nervous system malformations and early end-stage renal disease in oro-facio-digital syndrome type I: a review. *Am J Med Genet* 1998;75:389–394.
176. Ogata T, Yoshida R. PTPN11 mutations and genotype-phenotype correlations in Noonan and LEOPARD syndromes. *Pediatr Endocrinol Rev* 2005;2:669–674.
177. Opitz JM. Blastogenesis and the "primary field" in human development. *Birth Defects Orig Artic Series* 1993;29:3–37.
178. Opitz JM. The developmental field concept in pediatrics. *J Pediatr* 1982;101:805–809.
179. Opitz JM, Gilbert EF. CNS anomalies and the midline as a "developmental field." *Am J Med Genet* 1982;12:443–455.
180. Opitz JM, Herrmann J, Pettersen JC, et al. Terminological, diagnostic, nosological, and anatomical-developmental aspects of developmental defects in man. *Adv Hum Genet* 1979;9:71–164.
181. Opitz JM, Howe JJ. The Meckel syndrome (dysencephalia splanchnocystica, the Gruber syndrome). *Birth Defects Orig Artic Series* 1969;5:167.
182. Opitz JM, Kaveggia EG, Adkins WN Jr, et al. Studies on malformation syndromes of humans. XXXIIC: the FG syndrome—further studies on three affected individuals from the FG family. *Am J Med Genet* 1982;12:147–154.
183. Opitz JM, Smith DW, Summitt RL. Hypertelorism and hypospadias. *J Pediatr* 1965;67(969 [abstract]).
184. Otake M, Schull WJ. Radiation-related brain damage and growth retardation among the prenatally exposed atomic bomb survivors. *Int J Radiat Biol* 1998;74:159–171.
185. Otake M, Schull WJ, Yoshimaru H. A review of forty-five years study of Hiroshima and Nagasaki atomic bomb survivors. Brain damage among the prenatally exposed. *J Radiat Res* 1991;32(suppl.):249–264.
186. Pagon RA, Smith DW, Shepard TH. Urethral obstruction malformation complex: a cause of abdominal muscle deficiency and the "prune belly." *J Pediatr* 1979;94:900–906.
187. Pallister PD, Herrmann J, Spranger JW, et al. The W syndrome. *Birth Defects Orig Art Ser* 1974;10:51–60.
188. Parkes-Weber F. Angioma formation in connection with hypertrophy of limbs and hemi-hypertrophy. *Br J Dermatol* 1907;19:231.
189. Patton MA, Afzal AR. Robinow syndrome. *J Med Genet* 2002; 39:305–310.
190. Pauli RM, Lian JB, Mosher DF, et al. Association of congenital deficiency of multiple vitamin K-dependent coagulation factors and the

phenotype of the warfarin embryopathy: clues of the mechanism of teratogenicity of coumarin derivatives. *Am J Hum Genet* 1987;41:566–583.

191. Pauli RM, Pettersen JC, Arya S, et al. Familial agnathia-holoprosencephaly. *Am J Med* 1983;14:677–698.
192. Peck GL, Olson TG, Yoder FW, et al. Prolonged remission of cystic and conglobate acne with 13-cis-retinoic acid. *N Engl J Med* 1979;300:329–333.
193. Pena SDJ, Shokeir MHK. Syndrome of camptodactyly, multiple ankyloses, facial anomalies and pulmonary hypoplasia—further delineation and evidence for autosomal recessive inheritance. *Birth Defects Orig Art Ser* 1976;12:201–208.
194. Pena SDJ, Shokeir MHK. Syndrome of camptodactyly, multiple ankyloses, facial anomalies and pulmonary hypoplasia: a lethal condition. *J Pediatr* 1974;85:373–375.
195. Pham T, Steele J, Stayboldt C, et al. Placental mesenchymal dysplasia is associated with high rates of intrauterine growth restriction and fetal demise: a report of 11 new cases and a review of the literature. *Am J Clin Pathol* 2006;126:67–78.
196. Pittock ST, Babovic-Vuksanovic D, Lteif A. Mayer-Rokitansky-Kuster-Hauser anomaly and its associated malformations. *Am J Med Genet A* 2005;135:314–316.
197. Porteous ME, Wright C, Smith D, et al. Agnathia-holoprosencephaly: a new recessive syndrome? *Clin Dysmorphol* 1993;2:161–164.
198. Potter BJ, Hetzel BS. Fetal alcohol syndrome. In: Hetzel BS, Smith RM, eds. *Fetal brain disorders: recent approaches to the problem of mental deficiency*. New York, NY: Elsevier North Holland, 1981.
199. Powell CM, Michaelis RC. Townes-Brocks syndrome. *J Med Genet* 1999;36:89–93.
200. Preus M, Fraser FC. The cerebro-oculo-facio-skeletal syndrome. *Clin Genet* 1974;5:294–297.
201. Quigg M, Rust RS, Miller JQ. Clinical findings of the phakomatoses: hypomelanosis of Ito. *Neurology* 2006;66:E45.
202. Rapola J, Salonen R. Visceral anomalies in the Meckel syndrome. *Teratology* 1985;31:193–201.
203. Raynaud M, Dessay S, Ronce N, et al. Skewed X chromosome inactivation in carriers is not a constant finding in FG syndrome. *Eur J Hum Genet* 2003;11:352–356.
204. Reardon W, Winter RM, Rutland P, et al. Mutations in the fibroblast growth factor receptor 2 gene cause Crouzon syndrome. *Nature Genet* 1994;8:98–103.
205. Richards W, Donnell GN, Wilson WA, et al. The oculo-cerebro-renal syndrome of Lowe. *Am J Dis Child* 1965;109:185–203.
206. Robert E, Guiband P. Maternal valproic acid and congenital neural tube defects. *Lancet* 1982;2:937.
207. Robinow M, Silverman FN, Smith HD. A newly recognized dwarfing syndrome. *Am J Dis Child* 1969;117:645–651.
208. Rodriguez-Soriano J. Branchio-oto-renal syndrome. *J Nephrol* 2003;16:603–605.
209. Rodriguez-Soriano J, Vallo A, Bilbao JR, et al. Branchio-oto-renal syndrome: identification of a novel mutation in the EYA1 gene. *Pediatr Nephrol* 2001;16:550–553.
210. Roelfsema JH, White SJ, Ariyurek Y, et al. Genetic heterogeneity in Rubinstein-Taybi syndrome: mutations in both the CBP and EP300 genes cause disease. *Am J Hum Genet* 2005;76:572–580.
211. Rosa FW. Isotretinoin: a newly recognized human teratogen. *MMWR* 1984;33:71.
212. Rubenstein JH. T, H. Broad thumbs and toes and facial abnormalities. A possible mental retardation syndrome. *Am J Dis Child* 1963;105:588–603.
213. Rutland P, Pulleyn LJ, Reardon W, et al. Identical mutations in the FGFR2 gene cause both Pfeiffer and Crouzon syndrome phenotypes. *Nature Genet* 1995;9:173–176.
214. Salonen R. The Meckel syndrome: clinicopathological findings in 67 patients. *Am J Med Genet* 1984;18:671–689.
215. Salonen R, Herva R, Norio R. The hydrolethalus syndrome: delineation of a "new" lethal malformation syndrome based on 28 patients. *Clin Genet* 1981;19:321–330.
216. Salonen R, Norio R. The Meckel syndrome in Finland: epidemiologic and genetic aspects. *Am J Med Genet* 1984;18:691–698.
217. Salonen R, Paavola P. Meckel syndrome. *J Med Genet* 1998;35:497–501.
218. Sathienkijkanchai A, Wasant P. Fetal warfarin syndrome. *J Med Assoc Thai* 2005;88(suppl. 8):S246–S250.
219. Schoumans J, Wincent J, Barbaro M, et al. Comprehensive mutational analysis of a cohort of Swedish Cornelia de Lange syndrome patients. *Eur J Hum Genet* 2007;15(2):143–149.
220. Schwartz MFJ, Esterly NB, Fretzin DF, et al. Hypomelanosis of Ito (incontinentia pigmenti achromians): a neurocutaneous syndrome. *J Pediatr* 1977;90:236–240.
221. Seckel HPG. *Bird-headed dwarfs*. Springfield, IL: Charles C. Thomas, 1960.
222. Shaul WL, Emery H, Hall JG. Chondrodysplasia punctata and maternal warfarin use during pregnancy. *Am J Dis Child* 1975;129:360–362.
223. Shaw EB, Steinback HL. Aminopterin-induced fetal malformation. Survival of infant after attempted abortion. *Am J Dis Child* 1968;115:477–482.
224. Shepard TH. Human teratogenicity. *Adv Pediatr* 1986;33:225–268.
225. Shepard TH, Lemire RJ. *Catalog of teratogenic agents*, 11th ed. Baltimore, MD: The Johns Hopkins University Press, 2004.
226. Shiota K. Neural tube defects and maternal hyperthermia in early pregnancy: epidemiology in a human embryonic population. *Am J Med Genet* 1982;12:281–288.
227. Shotelersuk V, Punyavoravud V, Phudhichareonrat S, et al. An Asian girl with a 'milder' form of the hydrolethalus syndrome. *Clin Dysmorphol* 2001;10:51–55.
228. Shprintzen RJ, Croft C, Berkman MD, et al. Pharyngeal hypoplasia in Treacher Collins syndrome. *Arch Otolaryngol* 1979;105:127–131.
229. Shukunami K, Hirabuki S, Kaneshima M, et al. Face presentation caused by a short umbilical cord round the fetal neck. *J Obstet Gynaecol* 1999;19:668.
230. Siddiqui F, James D. Fetal monitoring in type 1 diabetic pregnancies. *Early Hum Dev* 2003;72:1–13.
231. Siebert JR, Kapur RP. Back and perineum. In: Gilbert-Barness EF, Oligny L, Kapur RP, et al., eds. *Potter's pathology of the fetus, infant, and child*. Edinburgh, UK: Elsevier, 2007.
232. Smith DW, Clarren SK, Harvey MA. Hyperthermia as a possible teratogenic agent. *J Pediatr* 1978;92:878–883.
233. Smith DW, Lemli L, Opitz JM. A newly recognized syndrome of multiple congenital anomalies. *J Pediatr* 1964;64:210–217.
234. Smith DW, Opitz JM, Inhorn SL. A syndrome of multiple developmental defects including polycystic kidneys and intrahepatic biliary dysgenesis in two siblings. *J Pediatr* 1965;67:617–624.
235. Spranger J, Benirschke K, Hall JG, et al. Errors of morphogenesis: concepts and terms. Recommendations of an International Working Group. *J Pediatr* 1982;100:160–165.
236. Spranger JM, P. The lethal osteochondrodysplasias. *Adv Hum Genet* 1991;19:1–103.
237. Spranger JW, Brill PW, Poznanski AK. *Bone dysplasias: an atlas of genetic disorders of skeletal development*. Oxford, UK: Oxford University Press, 2002.
238. Stephens TD, Bunde CJ, Fillmore BJ. Mechanism of action in thalidomide teratogenesis. *Biochem Pharmacol* 2000;59:1489–1499.
239. Stickler GB, Belau PG, Farrel FJ, et al. Hereditary progressive arthro-ophthalmopathy. *Mayo Clin Proc* 1965;40:433–455.
240. Strahan JE, Raimer S. Isotretinoin and the controversy of psychiatric adverse effects. *Int J Dermatol* 2006;45:789–799.
241. Streiff EB. Dysmorphie mandibulo-faciale (tete d'oiseau) et alteration oculaires. *Ophthalmologica* 1950;120:79–83.
242. Streissguth AP, Dehaene P. Fetal alcohol syndrome in twins of alcoholic mothers: concordance of diagnosis and IQ. *Am J Med Genet* 1993;47:857–861.
243. Taibjee SM, Bennett DC, Moss C. Abnormal pigmentation in hypomelanosis of Ito and pigmentary mosaicism: the role of pigmentary genes. *Br J Dermatol* 2004;151:269–282.

244. Talwar D, Smith SA. CAMFAK syndrome: a demyelinating inherited disease similar to Cockayne syndrome. *Am J Med Genet* 1989;34:194–198.
245. Tamura T, Picciano MF. Folate and human reproduction. *Am J Clin Nutr* 2006;83:993–1016.
246. Tartaglia M, Gelb BD. Noonan syndrome and related disorders: genetics and pathogenesis. *Annu Rev Genomics Hum Genet* 2005;6:45–68.
247. Taylor JC, Zellweger H, Hanson JW. A new case of the Zellweger syndrome. *Birth Defects Orig Art Ser* 1969;5:159–160.
248. Taylor WF, Myers M, Taylor WR. Extrarenal Wilms tumour in an infant exposed to intrauterine phenytoin. *Lancet* 1980;2:481–482.
249. Temtamy SA, Ismail S, Helmy NA. Roberts syndrome: study of 4 new Egyptian cases with comparison of clinical and cytogenetic findings. *Genet Couns* 2006;17:1–13.
250. ten Donkelaar HJ, Hamel BC, Hartman E, et al. Intestinal mucosa on top of a rudimentary occipital meningocele in amniotic rupture sequence: disorganization-like syndrome, homeotic transformation, abnormal surface encounter or endoectodermal adhesion? *Clin Dysmorphol* 2002;11:9–13.
251. ter Braak EW, Evers IM, Willem Erkelens D, et al. Maternal hypoglycemia during pregnancy in type 1 diabetes: maternal and fetal consequences. *Diabetes Metab Res Rev* 2002;18:96–105.
252. Thiersch JB. Therapeutic abortions with a folic acid antagonist, 4-aminopteroylglutamic acid (4-amino PGA) administered by the oral route. *Am J Obstet Gynecol* 1952;63:1298–1304.
253. Tian XL, Kadaba R, You SA, et al. Identification of an angiogenic factor that when mutated causes susceptibility to Klippel-Trenaunay syndrome. *Nature* 2004;427:640–645.
254. Timur AA, Driscoll DJ, Wang Q. Biomedicine and diseases: the Klippel-Trenaunay syndrome, vascular anomalies and vascular morphogenesis. *Cell Mol Life Sci* 2005;62:1434–1447.
255. Toppenberg KS, Hill DA, Miller DP. Safety of radiographic imaging during pregnancy. *Am Fam Physician* 1999;59:1813–1818.
256. Toriello HV. Review. Oral-facial-digital syndromes. *Clin Dysmorphol* 1992;2:95–105.
257. Tsukahara M, Opitz JM. Dubowitz syndrome: review of 141 cases including 36 previously unreported patients. *Am J Med Genet* 1996;63:277–289.
258. Tze WJ, Friesen HG, MacLeod PM. Growth hormone response in fetal alcohol syndrome. *Arch Dis Child* 1976;51:703–706.
259. Ullrich K, Bohm N. Early embryonal maldevelopment of the umbilical cord with defect of the abdominal wall and severe body malformations (dysplasia umbilico-fetalis). *Beitr Pathol* 1977;160:286–297.
260. Uno H, Arya S, Laxova R, et al. Menkes syndrome with vascular and adrenergic nerve abnormalities. *Arch Pathol Lab Med* 1983;107:286–289.
261. van den Elzen AP, Semmekrot BA, Bongers EM, et al. Diagnosis and treatment of the Pierre Robin sequence: results of a retrospective clinical study and review of the literature. *Eur J Pediatr* 2001;160:47–53.
262. Versmold HT, Bremer HJ, Herzog V, et al. A metabolic disorder similar to Zellweger syndrome with hepatic acatalasia and absence of peroxisomes, altered content and redox state of cytochromes, and infantile cirrhosis with hemosiderosis. *Eur J Pediatr* 1977;124:261–275.
263. Visapaa I, Salonen R, Varilo T, et al. Assignment of the locus for hydrolethalus syndrome to a highly restricted region on 11q23–25. *Am J Hum Genet* 1999;65:1086–1095.
264. Vitale L, Opitz JM, Shahidi NT. Congenital and familial iron overload. *N Engl J Med* 1969;280:642–645.
265. Volpe JJ, Adams RD. Cerebro-hepato-renal syndrome of Zellweger: an inherited disorder of neuronal migration. *Acta Neuropathol* 1972;20:175–198.
266. Wanders RJ. Metabolic and molecular basis of peroxisomal disorders: a review. *Am J Med Genet A* 2004;126:355–375.
267. Wanders RJ, Waterham HR. Peroxisomal disorders I: biochemistry and genetics of peroxisome biogenesis disorders. *Clin Genet* 2005;67:107–133.
268. Warkany J. Warfarin embryopathy. *Teratology* 1976;14:205–209.
269. Weaver DD. Skeletal dysplasias. In: Oski FA, DeAngelis CD, Feigin RD, et al., eds. *Principles and practice of pediatrics*. Philadelphia, PA: J.B. Lippincott, 1990.
270. Webster WS, Howe AM, Abela D, et al. The relationship between cleft lip, maxillary hypoplasia, hypoxia and phenytoin. *Curr Pharm Des* 2006;12:1431–1448.
271. Werler MM, Shapiro S, Mitchell AA. Periconceptional folic acid exposure and risk of occurrent neural tube defects. *JAMA* 1993;269:1257–1261.
272. Whitehead ED, Leiter E. Genital abnormalities and abnormal semen analysis in male patients exposed to diethylstilbestrol in utero. *J Urol* 1981;125:47–50.
273. Wilkins L, Jones HW, Holman GH, et al. Masculinization of the female fetus associated wtih administration of oral and intramuscular progestins during gestation: non-adrenal female pseudohermaphrodism. *J Clin Endocrinol Metabol* 1958;18:559.
274. Wilroy RS, Tipton RE, Summitt RL. The Dubowitz syndrome. *Am J Med Genet* 1978;2:275–284.
275. Wilson G, Hicher VC, Schmickel RD. The association of chromosome 3 duplications and the Cornelia de Lange syndrome. *J Pediatr* 1978;93:783–788.
276. Wiznitzer A, Furman B, Mazor M, et al. The role of prostanoids in the development of diabetic embryopathy. *Semin Reprod Endocrinol* 1999;17:175–181.
277. Yang SS. The skeletal system. In: Wigglesworth JS, Singer DB, eds. *Textbook of fetal and perinatal pathology*. Boston, MA: Blackwell Scientific, 1991.
278. Yu H, Patel SB. Recent insights into the Smith-Lemli-Opitz syndrome. *Clin Genet* 2005;68:383–391.
279. Zackai EH, Mellman WJ, Neiderer B, et al. The fetal trimethadione syndrome. *J Pediatr* 1975;87:280–284.

CHAPTER 5

Inborn Errors of Metabolism

CAROLE A. VOGLER
DAVID S. BRINK
DOROTHY K. GRANGE

In the early 1900s, Garrod defined a group of four inherited disorders, each characterized by blocked metabolic pathways, as *inborn errors of metabolism* (IEM) (98). Since that time, knowledge of the human genome and understanding of IEM have increased dramatically. This, along with improved technology, has resulted in refinement in diagnosis and classification of IEM (285,302). Early diagnosis is increasingly important as treatments, such as dietary management and enzyme replacement, become a reality for these disorders (303). Although individually rare, the collective incidence of IEM is approximately 1/1,500 persons (304).

Online genetic/metabolic disease databases such as OMIM (Online Mendelian Inheritance in Man http://www.ncbi.nlm.nih.gov/entrez/query.fcgi?db=OMIM), MetaGene (http://www.metagene.de/index.html), Human Genetic Disease Data base (http://life2.tau.ac.il/GeneDis/), Japan Metabolic Disease Database (http://www.jmdbase.jp/JmdBaseExt/Top.aspx), Genetests (http://www.genetests.org/), Gene Reviews (www.genere-views.org) and NORD (http://www.rare-diseases.org/) are ideal sources for current information on IEM.

CLINICAL PRESENTATION OF INBORN ERRORS OF METABOLISM

Most metabolic diseases are autosomal recessive disorders, some are X-linked, and a few are inherited as dominant traits (102). Heterozygotes are usually asymptomatic, while homozygous (autosomal) or hemizygous (X-linked) patients are symptomatic. IEM may present at any age and in a variety of ways (Table 5-1). Symptoms may begin before birth (for example with hydrops fetalis or fetal ascites), at birth, with sudden death in infancy, or with deterioration after a symptom-free interval (80,255). Symptoms may suggest sepsis and infection can lead to decompensation in IEM (80).

IEM can cause dysmorphism. Peroxisomal biogenesis disorders such as Zellweger syndrome, disorders of lipid metabolism such as Smith-Lemli-Opitz and Conradi-Hunermann syndromes, desmosterolosis, mevalonic aciduria, and glutaric acidemia type II are examples of metabolic dysplasias. Lysosomal storage diseases (LSD) can cause abnormal facies and skeletal abnormalities that are present at birth (80,259).

DIAGNOSIS OF INBORN ERRORS OF METABOLISM

Biochemical studies may allow definitive diagnosis: Evaluations of blood glucose, lactate, ammonia, and ketones

Table 5-1 ■ CLINICAL SYMPTOMS IN PATIENTS WITH INBORN ERRORS OF METABOLISM

Nonimmune hydrops fetalis, fetal ascites
Sudden unexpected death in infancy
Episodic illness
Failure to thrive
Loss of cognitive milestones or motor skills
Lethargy
Vomiting
Respiratory distress and tachypnea
Shock
Coma
Seizures
Macrocephaly or microcephaly
Hepatomegaly
Splenomegaly
Cardiomyopathy and arrhythmias
Acute parenchymal liver disease
Chronic liver disease/cirrhosis
Hypotonia or hypertonia
Exercise intolerance, cramps, fatigue, and rhabdomyolysis
Corneal clouding
Macular and retinal changes
Deafness
Skeletal abnormalities
Dysostosis multiplex
Coarse facial features
Macroglossia
Unusual odor
Burnt sugar—maple syrup urine disease
Mousy—phenylketonuria
Cabbage, fishy—tyrosinemia type 1
Sweaty feet—isovaleric acidemia and glutaric acidemia type II
Cat urine—multiple carboxylase deficiency

may provide important information (80). Enzymes and metabolites including organic, fatty, and amino acids can be evaluated. Molecular analysis is important for disorders in which a specific mutation is common or has been identified in a family.

Morphology of tissues, including liver, muscle, skin, conjunctiva, or placenta, may show characteristic findings by light microscopy (LM). Brain, lymph nodes, spleen, kidney, and heart may also show findings in IEM, but biopsies of these sites are not evaluated as commonly. Transmission electron microscopy (EM) of skin, conjunctiva, rectal mucosa, liver, peripheral nerve, muscle, bone marrow, or peripheral blood leukocytes is important in evaluation of some IEM. Particularly for LSD, ultrastructural study of these sites is a sensitive screen that can provide valuable information about stored material (see LSD below) (10,44,83,144,248,272,301,340).

Many IEM affect the liver; in some cases (cystinosis, metachromatic leukodystrophy, Fabry disease), morphologic alterations have no apparent clinical consequence. In other disorders—such as tyrosinemia, Wilson disease, and GSD IV—progressive liver disease is common (70,94). A variety of histologic alterations—including hepatitis, steatosis, cirrhosis, cholestasis, ductopenia, ductular proliferation, neoplasia, and storage—can be seen in IEM, and many IEM cause similar morphological alterations (169,300).

We receive liver biopsies at the bedside on a Telfa-coated pad, and divide and fix the tissue for LM and EM. Placing the liver biopsy on gauze or handling it with forceps with teeth causes artifacts. For LM, at least a 1-cm core of liver is fixed in 10% buffered formalin (170,300). There are many special stains useful for evaluating liver biopsies (254) (Table 5-2). Fixation in 95% alcohol allows preservation of cystine crystals and glycogen. If indicated, tissue for biochemical or molecular analysis should be snap frozen in liquid nitrogen and stored at −70°C in a metal-free container. With a 16-gauge needle, a 2-cm core yields approximately 45 mg of tissue, and in general, 20 mg of tissue is adequate for biochemical diagnosis of most IEM (171). Exceptions include investigation of GSDs of unknown type or nonketotic hyperglycinemia, either of which may require 100 mg of tissue and an open biopsy for diagnosis (172). For EM, several 1-mm^3 samples of tissue are fixed at the bedside in 2.5% glutaraldehyde. Transmission EM of liver and other tissues, such as skin or conjunctiva, may be useful in the evaluation of patients with a variety of disorders, particularly the LSD (Tables 5-3 and 5-4) (300). Placenta alterations may suggest an LSD (Table 5-5) (37,46,107,250,253,306,327,337).

Muscle biopsy is useful for evaluation of mitochondrial myopathies and LSD. Increased mitochondria, with "ragged-red fibers," subsarcolemmal mitochondria collections, and structurally abnormal mitochondria, occur in mitochondrial myopathies. Increased muscle fiber glycogen, sometimes in vacuoles, may be present in the glycogen storage diseases. Increased lipid occurs with abnormal fatty acid metabolism and with mitochondrial dysfunction (85).

Newborn screening began in the 1960s with testing for phenylketonuria, and additional tests have been added since then. Disorders evaluated in newborn screening have generally been those that have a treatment available and for which early detection and therapy can prevent morbidity and mortality (Table 5-6). Congenital hypothyroidism, galactosemia, phenylketonuria, and hemoglobinopathies are now screened for in all states in the United States, and congenital adrenal hyperplasia (21-hydroxylase deficiency form) has been added in 46 states thus far. With the development of tandem mass spectrometry (MS/MS) for newborn screening, it has become possible to detect many more metabolic disorders via a rapid-throughput methodology. As of April, 2007, 47 states in the United States have added expanded newborn screening using MS/MS. Information on each state's IEM screening program is available through Genes-R-Us, http://genes-r-us.uthscsa.edu. The March of Dimes and the American College of Medical Genetics have recommended that all newborns should be screened for 29 core conditions, with detection of an additional 22 secondary target conditions.

Table 5-2 ■ LIVER BIOPSY SPECIAL STAINS

Stain	Material Highlighted
Periodic acid-Schiff (PAS)	Glycoproteins, glycolipids, amylopectin, glycogen
PAS after diastase digestion	Glycoproteins, glycolipids, amylopectin
Prussian blue (Perls')	Hemosiderin
Fontana	Lipomelanin, lipofuscin
Acid fast	Lipofuscin
Colloidal iron	Glycosaminoglycans
Reticulin	Reticulin fibers
Masson trichrome	Collagen and bile ducts
Hall	Bilirubin
Oil Red O and Sudan black	Neutral lipids, triglyceride, cholesterol phospholipid (frozen tissue)
Schultz modification	Cholesterol of Lieberman-Burchard stain
Orcein	Copper-associated protein
Victoria blue	Copper-associated protein
Aldehyde fuchsin	Copper-associated protein
Rubeanic acid	Copper
Rhodanine	Copper

Table 5-3 ■ TRANSMISSION EM IN DIAGNOSIS OF INBORN ERRORS OF METABOLISM

Lysosomal storage diseases (LSD)
Glycogen storage diseases (GSD)
Hereditary fructose intolerance
Peroxisomal disorders
Hyperammonemia/Urea cycle disorders
Mitochondriopathies
Wilson disease
Alpha-1-antitrypsin deficiency

Table 5-4 ■ ULTRASTRUCTURAL APPEARANCE OF LYSOSOMAL STORAGE IN SKIN AND CONJUNCTIVAL BIOPSIES

Disorder	Ultrastructural Appearance of Predominant Storage	Stored Material	Cells Affected
Disorders with ultrastructurally characteristic storage			
Pompe disease	Electron-dense glycogen granules	Glycogen	Lymphocytes, endothelium, fibroblasts, epithelium, nerves
Cholesterol ester storage disease, Wolman disease	Cholesterol, lipids	Cholesterol ester	Fibroblasts
Infantile ceroid lipofuscinosis	Granular osmiophilic	Saposin A, D	Perithelial and endothelial cells, smooth muscle, sweat gland epithelial cells, lymphocytes
Late infantile ceroid lipofuscinosis	Curvilinear	Mitochondrial subunit c of ATPase synthase	Perithelial and endothelial cells, smooth muscle, sweat gland epithelial cells, lymphocytes
Juvenile ceroid lipofuscinosis	Curvilinear and fingerprint profiles	Mitochondrial subunit c of ATPase synthase	Perithelial and endothelial cells, smooth muscle, sweat gland epithelial cells, lymphocytes
Cystinosis	Rectangular, rhomboid, polymorphic crystals	Cystine	Fibroblasts
Metachromatic leukodystrophy	Tuffstone or herringbone	Sulfatide, cholesterol, phosphatides	Peripheral nerve Schwann cells, histiocytes
Krabbe disease (globoid leukodystrophy)	Crystals with sharp corners	Galactosylceramide	Peripheral nerve Schwann cells
Fabry disease	Pleomorphic leaflets, lamellae, tubular structures	Globotriaosylceramide-containing substrates	Epithelium, fibroblasts, endothelium, lymphocytes
Disorders with ultrastructurally nonspecific storage			
Mucopolysaccharidoses (MPS), Mucolipidoses, Aspartylglycosaminuria, Alpha-mannosidosis, Beta-mannosidosis, G_{M1} Gangliosidosis, I-cell disease	Lucent or fine fibrillogranular	Oligosaccharides, glycosaminoglycans	Eccrine gland epithelium, endothelial cells (may be spared in MPS), fibroblasts, lymphocytes, macrophages, pericytes, Schwann cells, smooth muscle cells. Mucolipidosis III affects primarily fibroblasts with normal lymphocytes.
Fucosidosis, G_{M1} and G_{M2} gangliosidosis, galactosialidosis, MPS, Mucolipidosis IV and sialidosis	Fine lamellated membranous cytoplasmic bodies, zebra bodies	Gangliosides and glycolipids	Peripheral nerve Schwann cells, endothelial cells, pericytes, smooth muscle cells in Fabry disease. In Niemann Pick and ML IV lymphocytes have storage

Table 5-5 ■ PLACENTAL LYSOSOMAL STORAGE

Lysosomal Storage Disease	Affected Cells	Hydrops Fetalis
Sialidosis (Mucolipidosis type I)	Syncytiotrophoblasts, Hofbauer and stromal cells	yes
Mucolipidosis II (I-Cell Disease)	Syncytiotrophoblasts, Hofbauer and stromal, X-cells	yes
Mucolipidosis IV	Hofbauer and stromal cells	yes
Sialic acid storage disease	Syncytiotrophoblasts, Hofbauer cells, endothelium, amniocytes	yes
Galactosialidosis	Syncytiotrophoblasts	yes
MPS I (Hurler)	Villous stromal cells	yes
MPS III (Sanfilippo)	Syncytiotrophoblasts, Hofbauer and stromal cells	
MPS IVA (Morquio A)	Villous stromal cells	yes
MPS VII (Sly)	Villous stromal cells	yes
G_{M1} gangliosidosis	Syncytiotrophoblasts, Hofbauer cells,	yes
G_{M2} gangliosidosis (Tay Sachs)	Syncytiotrophoblasts	
Cholesterol ester storage disease	Syncytiotrophoblasts	
Wolman disease	Syncytiotrophoblasts	yes
GSD II	Amniocytes, endothelial cells, stromal cells	
GSD IV	Amniocytes	
Niemann-Pick A	Syncytiotrophoblasts, Hofbauer cells, fibrocytes in cord	yes
Gaucher disease type 2	Vessels	yes
Fabry disease	Endothelial cells, perithelial cells, vascular smooth muscle cells	yes

Table 5-6 ■ DISORDERS COMMONLY SCREENED FOR IN NEWBORNS

- Cystic fibrosis (immunoreactive trypsinogen (IRT), CFTR DNA analysis)
- Hemoglobinopathies, including sickle cell disease, sickle/beta-thalassemia disease and sickle-C disease (hemoglobin electrophoresis)
- Congenital adrenal hyperplasia (17-OH-progesterone for 21-hydroxylase deficiency)
- Congenital hypothyroidism (T4, TSH)
- Galactosemia (total galactose level and/or galactose-1-phosphate, galactose-1-phosphate uridyl transferase activity)
- Biotinase deficiency (biotinidase activity)
- Amino acid disorders (MS/MS technology used)
  - Phenylketonuria
  - Maple syrup urine disease
  - Tyrosinemia I and II
  - Homocystinuria
- Urea cycle defects (MS/MS technology used)
  - Citrullinemia (argininosuccinate synthase deficiency)
  - Argininosuccinic aciduria (argininosuccinate lyase deficiency)
  - Argininemia (arginase deficiency)
- Organic acid disorders (MS/MS technology used)
  - Methylmalonic acidemia (mutase deficiency)
  - Methylmalonic acidemia due to cobalamin A or cobalamin B defect
  - Propionic acidemia
  - Isovaleric acidemia
  - Glutaric acidemia type I
  - 3-Methylcrotonyl CoA carboxylase deficiency (3-MCC)
  - HMG CoA lyase deficiency
  - Beta-ketothiolase deficiency
  - Multiple carboxylase deficiency
- FAO defects (MS/MS technology used)
  - MCAD
  - SCAD
  - LCHAD/trifunctional protein deficiency
  - VLCAD
  - Glutaric acidemia type II (MADD)
  - CPT I deficiency
  - CPT II deficiency
  - Carnitine transporter deficiency
  - Carnitine acylcarnitine translocase deficiency

HMG = hydroxy-methyl-glutaryl; MCAD = medium chain acyl-coenzyme deficiency; SCAD = short chain acyl-CoA dehydrogenase deficiency; LCHAD = long chain 3-hydroxyacyl-CoA dehydrogenase deficiency; VLCAD = very long chain acyl-CoA dehydrogenase deficiency; MADD = multiple acyl-CoA dehydrogenase deficiency; CPT = carnitine palmitoyltransferase.

LYSOSOMAL STORAGE DISEASES

The LSD are a group of some 50 genetic disorders with a combined incidence of approximately 1/5,000 to 8,000 live births (375). In the United States, 500 to 800 patients with LSD are born each year (354). As a group, LSD are among the most commonly diagnosed metabolic disorders. Most LSD result from a mutation in a gene that encodes a single hydrolyzing lysosomal enzyme (Table 5-7). A few are caused by mutations in genes coding for an activator or transport protein or for an enzyme required for posttranslational processing of lysosomal enzymes (11,357).

In LSD, the enzyme's substrates progressively accumulate in lysosomes in many tissues, resulting in progressive cellular and organ dysfunction by virtue of disruption of cytoplasm, metabolic imbalance, or metabolite toxicity. Perturbation in complex cell signaling mechanisms with secondary structural and biochemical changes may be central to the pathogenesis of LSD (339). Phenotypic variability is common in LSD, and clinical features depend on what cell or organ is dependent on the deficient enzyme for normal function. For most LSD patients, symptoms begin in the first months of life and are progressive. Symptoms can include nonimmune hydrops fetalis, dysmorphic facies, dysostosis multiplex, organomegaly, psychomotor delay, and progressive loss of developmental milestones (16,41,46,252,374).

Six to fifteen percent of cases of nonimmune hydrops fetalis are due to LSD (37,227,250,253). The pathogenesis of hydrops fetalis in LSD is debated. Storage in liver, spleen, and marrow may cause decreased hematopoiesis and/or hypoproteinemia. Visceromegaly and myocardial damage by storage may cause decreased venous drainage and ascites. In hydrops due to LSD, the placenta may be pale and bulky (327).

Classification of LSD is based on the character of the stored material. Individual disorders are defined by the deficient enzyme. Most LSD are autosomal recessive traits. The exceptions—Hunter (MPS II), Fabry, and Danon diseases—are inherited as X-linked traits.

Diagnosis of Lysosomal Storage Diseases

Diagnosis is established by a biochemical assay for the deficient enzyme. Leukocytes, fibroblasts, or amniocytes can be assessed for enzyme levels, and the degree of enzyme deficiency impacts prognosis. These assays are generally based on catabolism of simple water soluble substrates that incorporate colored or fluorescent groups (373).

Ultrastructural evaluation of tissue for morphological evidence of stored material may be used as a screening tool or if an unusual or as yet unrecognized enzyme deficiency is suspected. Skin, conjunctiva, peripheral blood lymphocytes, liver, marrow, muscle, rectal biopsy (including neurons), or placenta can provide confirmation of LSD. The morphological character of the stored material and its distribution may suggest a specific diagnosis or a group of LSD. Ultrastructurally characteristic storage occurs in some of the LSD, while others show less specific storage, with diagnosis resting on biochemical analysis (100) (Table 5-4). The presence of storage may allow for rapid identification of LSD and may help to direct the diagnostic evaluation.

Methods for newborn screening for LSD are being developed. As therapeutic options for these disorders become a reality, early diagnosis becomes more critical to ensure that treatment is instituted as soon as possible after birth. Enzyme replacement is an established therapy for Type I Gaucher

Table 5-7 ■ LYSOSOMAL STORAGE DISEASES

Disease	Deficient Protein
Gaucher disease	Beta-glucocerebrosidase
Fabry disease (angiokeratoma corporis diffusum universale)	Alpha-galactosidase A (ceramide trihexosidase)
Mucopolysaccharidosis	
MPS I Hurler	Alpha-L-iduronidase
MPS II Hunter	Iduronate sulfatase
MPS III Sanfilippo A	Heparan *N*-sulfatase (Sulfamidase)
MPS III Sanfilippo B	*N*-acetyl-alpha-D-glucosaminidase
MPS III Sanfilippo C	Acetyl-CoA: alpha-glucosaminidase *N*-acetyl transferase
MPS III Sanfilippo D	*N*-acetylglucosamine-6-sulfatase
MPS IV Morquio A	Galactosamine-6-sulfatase
MPS IV Morquio B	Beta-galactosidase
MPS VI Morateau Lamy	*N*-acetylgalactosamine 4-sulfatase (arylsulfatase B)
MPS VII Sly	Beta-glucuronidase
MPS IX	Hyaluronidase
Neuronal Ceroid Lipofuscinoses (NCL)	
Infantile (INCL, CLN1)	Palmitoyl-protein thioesterase 1 (PPT 1), Cathepsin D
Late infantile (LICL, LINCL, CLN2)	Tripeptidyl peptidase 1 (TPP1)
Juvenile (JNCL, CLN3)	Battenin (a lysosomal transmembrane protein)
Adult (ANCL, CLN4)	Unknown
Pompe disease (glycogen storage disease type II, GSD-II)	Alpha-glucosidase (acid maltase)
Danon disease, X-linked vacuolar myopathy	Lysosome-associated membrane protein-2 (LAMP-2)
Disorders of lysosomal enzyme phosphorylation and localization	
Mucolipidoses II (ML II, I-cell disease)	*N*-acetylglucosamine 1-phosphotransferase (phosphotransferase)
Mucolipidoses III (ML III, pseudo-Hurler polydystrophy)	*N*-acetylglucosamine 1-phosphotransferase (phosphotransferase)
Mucolipidosis type IV	Mucolipidin 1
Disorders of Glycoprotein Degradation (Oligosaccharidoses/ Glycoproteinoses)	
Alpha-Mannosidosis	Alpha-mannosidase
Beta-Mannosidosis	Beta-mannosidase
Fucosidosis	Alpha-L-fucosidase
Sialidosis (formally ML I)	Neuraminidase
Aspartylglycosaminuria	Aspartylglucosaminidase
Gangliosidoses	
G_{M1} gangliosidosis	Beta galactosidase
G_{M2} gangliosidosis	
G_{M2} Type 1, Tay-Sachs disease, B variant	Hexosaminidase A
G_{M2} Type II, Sandhoff disease, O variant	Hexosaminidase A and B
G_{M2} activator deficiency, AB variant	G_{M2} activator protein
Niemann-Pick disease (Sphingolipidoses, sphingomyelin lipidosis, sphingomyelin-cholesterol lipidosis, NPD) type A, B	Sphingomyelinase
Niemann-Pick disease type C, D	*NPC-1* or *NPC-2* mutation, protein not identified
Metachromatic leukodystrophy (Sulfatide Lipidosis, MLD)	Arylsulfatase A or Saposin
Wolman disease and cholesterol ester storage disease (CESD)	Acid lipase
Farber disease (disseminated lipogranulomatosis)	Acid ceramidase
Krabbe disease (galactosylceramide lipidosis, globoid cell leukodystrophy)	Galactocerebroside beta-galactosidase
Cystsinosis	Cystinosin

disease, Fabry disease, MPS I, II, VI, and Pompe disease. Stem cell transplantation and substrate inhibition have utility in some clinical settings.

Gaucher Disease

Gaucher disease is the most common LSD and is classified as a sphingolipidosis. The three clinical types (Table 5-8) are allelic disorders due to autosomal recessive mutations in the beta-glucocerebrosidase gene, leading to failure of cleavage of glucose from ceramide. Glucocerebroside derived from glycolipids in white and red cell membranes accumulates in lysosomes mainly in reticuloendothelial tissues. There are more than 150 allelic mutations that cause Gaucher disease.

Type 1 Gaucher disease is the most common LSD with an incidence of 1/855 among Ashkenazi Jewish individuals (228,327). Patients typically present with painless splenomegaly and pancytopenia (100). Type 2, the infantile, acute neuronopathic type (the most severe form (228), is panethnic, and patients have virtually no detectable enzyme activity.

Table 5-8 ■ CLINICAL FORMS OF GAUCHER DISEASE

Type	Onset/Survival	Hepatosplenomegaly	CNS Disease	Storage/Pathology
1. Chronic nonneuronopathic	Childhood to adulthood	+ to +++	None	Limited to phagocytes, hepatosplenomegaly, pancytopenia (due to marrow storage, hypersplenism), destructive osteoporotic bone disease
2. Infantile, acute neuronopathic	Infancy to <2 years	+	+++	Neuronal loss, gliosis, perivascular cell storage, hydrops fetalis rarely
3. Juvenile, chronic neuronopathic (Norrbottnian)	Childhood to second to fourth decade	+ to +++	+ to ++	3a: primarily neurologic disease 3b: marked visceral disease

Type 3, the juvenile (Norrbottnian) form, is clinically intermediate between types 1 and 2 (80,311,324,327).

Glucocerebrosides accumulate in phagocytic cells in the three types. Characteristic Gaucher cells are large, 20- to 100-µm eosinophilic phagocytes with wrinkled or striated cytoplasm (Figure 5-1A to C) and are present in liver, marrow, spleen, nodes, tonsils, thymus, Peyer patches, alveolar septa and airspaces, and Virchow-Robin space. Gaucher cells are capable of erythrophagocytosis, are acid phosphatase positive, and label with antibody to CD68. The striations can be highlighted with Masson trichrome, aldehyde fuscin, and PAS after diastase (228). By EM, lysosomal rod-shaped or tubular lipid bilayer stacks with a diameter of up to 4 µm distend cytoplasm (Figure 5-1D,E).

The liver is enlarged in all three types, and storage accumulates in Kupffer cells, most prominent in zone 3, but hepatocytes are not affected (69,220). Fibrosis may progress to cirrhosis. The spleen is enlarged, weighing as much as 10 kg, and may be uniformly pale or mottled due to storage accumulation. In marrow, infiltrating Gaucher cells lead to osteopenia, sclerosis, necrosis, and pathologic fractures (80). Erlenmeyer flask deformity of the distal femur is considered diagnostic of Gaucher disease (100). The brain has storage in cells in Virchow-Robin space but no neuronal storage, although neurons are progressively lost. It is suspected that lipids that accumulate in brain phagocytes are toxic to neurons in patients with type 2 and 3 Gaucher disease. The placenta may be involved with Gaucher cells in villous vessels (80).

Diagnosis is based on quantitating beta-glucocerebrosidase activity in leukocytes or fibroblasts or by DNA analysis. Enzyme replacement therapy effectively treats the pancytopenia and hepatosplenomegaly in Type 1 patients, but the bone disease responds slowly, if at all (39).

Fabry Disease (Angiokeratoma Corporis Diffusum Universale)

Fabry disease is due to alpha-galactosidase A (ceramide trihexosidase) deficiency leading to disordered glycosphingolipid metabolism with accumulation of globotriaosylceramide (ceramide trihexoside, ceramide digalactoside, blood group B glycolipid) containing substrates (56,91). Fabry disease is X-linked, and 1:40,000 to 1:60,000 males are affected. Over 150 mutations have been identified (56,92). Clinical manifestations include extremity pain and paresthesias, skin and mucous membrane angiokeratomas, and corneal opacities; renal impairment leads to end-stage renal disease by 20 to 40 years of age. Death is due to renal failure, cardiac disease, or cerebrovascular disease. Female heterozygotes have an intermediate level of alpha-galactosidase A; they may be asymptomatic or have corneal opacity, though rarely they are as severely affected as hemizygous males (56,80). Hemizygotes and heterozygotes with B or AB blood type are more severely affected due to the additional accumulation of B-specific glycolipid (100).

Renal, cardiac, and cerebral dysfunction relates to endothelial storage. PAS-positive glycolipid and cholesterol accumulate in lysosomes in endothelial cells, reticuloendothelial cells, and macrophages, and, by EM, osmiophilic lamellated leaflets and tubules are seen in endothelial, perithelial, and smooth muscle cells (7,56,87,263). Glomerular podocytes, endothelial, mesangial, interstitial, and tubular epithelial cells all can contain storage. Podocyte storage causes cellular injury, followed by glomerular capillary wall thickening, progressive mesangial matrix expansion, glomerulosclerosis, and, eventually, end-stage renal disease (Figure 5-2A to C) (93). Some patients with Fabry disease develop hypertrophic obstructive cardiomyopathy. Liver lysosomal storage is of little clinical significance. Kupffer cells have a tan appearance in H & E sections, and storage is birefringent and crystalline in frozen sections stained with the Schultz method (219).

Diagnosis is based on identifying decreased alpha-galactosidase A in leukocytes or fibroblasts or by DNA analysis for the mutation. Enzyme replacement therapy may have benefit in Fabry patients.

Neuronal Ceroid Lipofuscinoses (NCL, Batten Disease)

These progressive encephalopathies affect patients at any age causing seizures, blindness, psychomotor deterioration,

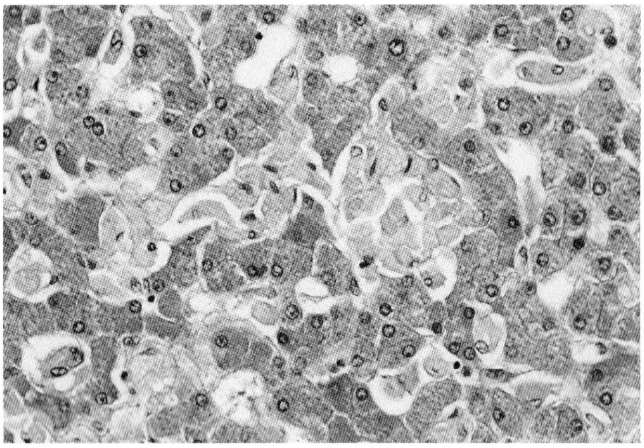

A

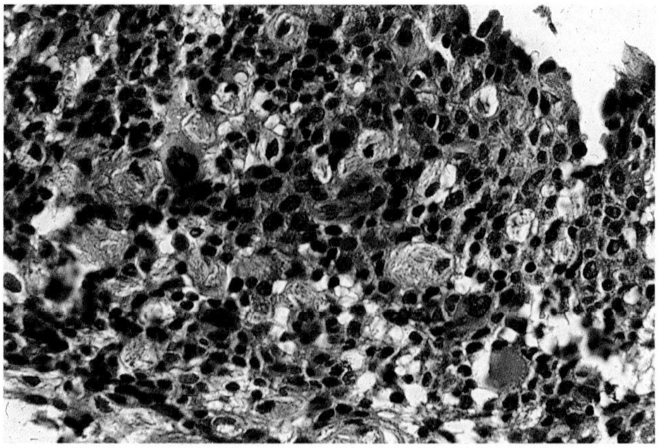

B

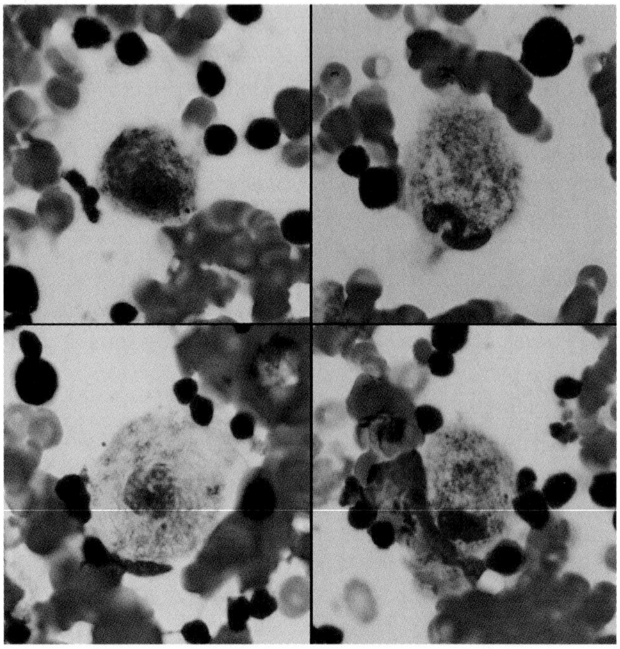

C

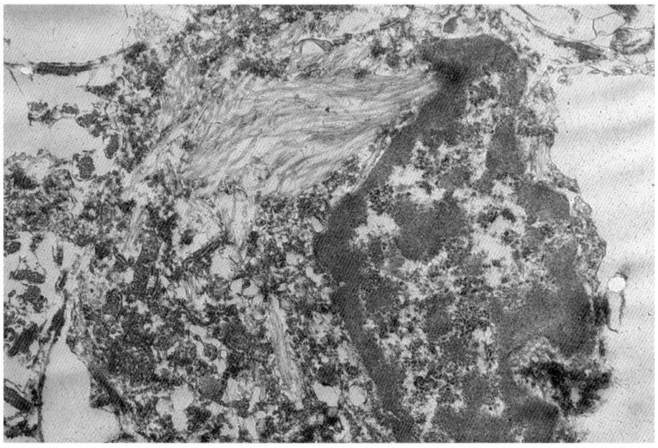

D

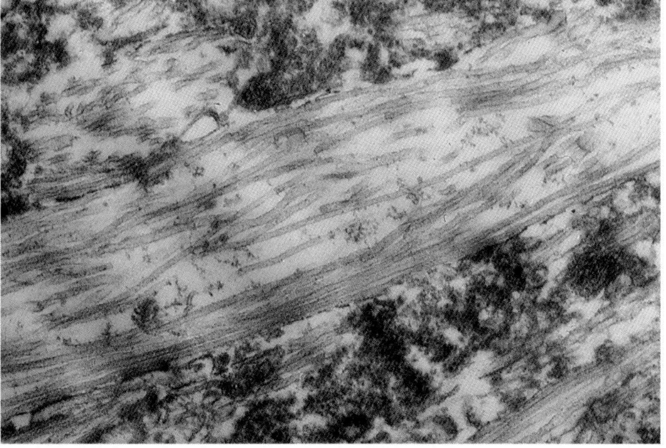

E

FIGURE 5-1 ■ **Gaucher disease. A:** The liver of a patient with Gaucher disease has prominent Kupffer cells due to pale eosinophilic expansion of the cytoplasm by lysosomal glucocerebroside storage material (H&E). **B:** Enlarged phagocytes in the spleen have a "wrinkled tissue paper" appearance of their cytoplasm because of the glucocerebroside storage (H&E). **C:** Wright stained bone marrow aspirate from a patient with Gaucher disease showing "Gaucher cells" with a "wrinkled tissue paper" appearance of cytoplasm due to glucocerebroside storage (Wright). **D:** Ultrastructural appearance of Gaucher cell from the spleen, obtained at autopsy, showing cytoplasmic storage in upper middle and lower middle of the image, to the left of the nucleus (Uranyl acetate, lead citrate). **E:** Ultrastructurally, glucocerebroside storage material in Gaucher disease comprises rod-shaped or tubular lipid bilayer stacks with diameter of up to 4 μm (Uranyl acetate, lead citrate).

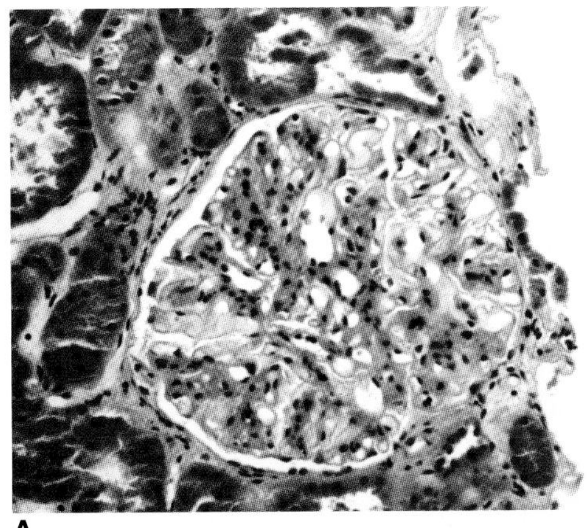

A

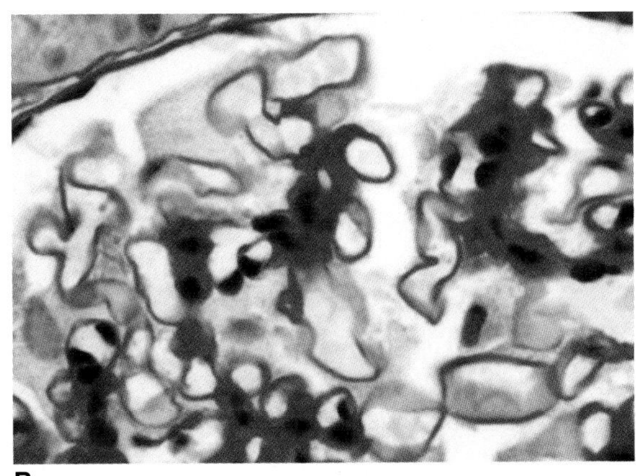

B

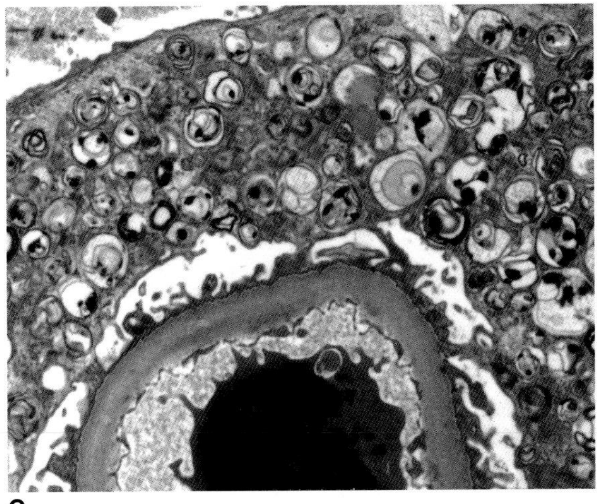

C

FIGURE 5-2 ▪ **Fabry disease. A:** By LM, glomeruli in Fabry disease show mesangial expansion with prominence of pale-staining visceral epithelial cells (podocytes) (H&E). **B:** At higher magnification, podocyte cytoplasm is markedly expanded by PAS-positive storage material (PAS). **C:** Ultrastructurally, visceral epithelial cell cytoplasm is expanded by osmiophilic, lamellated leaflets and tubules, representing glycolipid and cholesterol storage (Uranyl acetate, lead citrate). (Images' courtesy of Helen Liapis, M.D., Washington University Department of Pathology & Immunology, St. Louis, Missouri.)

and premature death. The incidence is 1/10,000, and carrier frequency is approximately 1%. Collectively, the NCL are the most common inherited progressive encephalopathies of childhood. The NCL have been divided into nine forms based on age of onset, character of storage, and deficient enzyme. The most common and best characterized are infantile, late infantile, juvenile, and adult NCL (Table 5-9). The infantile and the late infantile forms have deficient lysosomal enzyme activity; other types have abnormal lysosomal membrane proteins (6,108,116,322).

Table 5-9 ▪ THE MORE COMMON NEURONAL CEROID LIPOFUSCINOSES

Type	Eponym	Age at Presentation	Predominant Storage[a]	Protein Defect
Infantile (INCL, CLN1)	Santavuori-Haltia	6–12 months	Granular osmiophilic (GROD), saposin A, D	Palmitoyl-protein thioesterase 1 (PPT 1), Cathepsin D
Late infantile (LICL, LINCL, CLN2)	Jansky-Bielschowsky	2–3 years	Curvilinear, (in some cases also fingerprint), mitochondrial subunit c of ATP synthase	Tripeptidyl peptidase 1 (TPP1)
Juvenile (JNCL, CLN3)	Batten-Speilmeyer-Vogt	4–9 years	Fingerprint, mitochondrial subunit c of ATP synthase	Battenin (a lysosomal transmembrane protein)
Adult (ANCL, CLN4)	Kufs, Parry	30 years	Granular osmiophilic, finger print bodies,[b] mitochondrial subunit c of ATP synthase	Unknown

[a]There is overlap in character of storage among these disorders.
[b]Storage may be sparse outside the CNS.

Autofluorescent PAS-positive glycolipid accumulates in lysosomes in lymphocytes, cells in skin (particularly pericytes, endothelial, smooth muscle, and sweat gland epithelial cells), conjunctiva, skeletal muscle, and rectal mucosal neurons (322). As many as 10% to 20% of lymphocytes may have storage in late infantile NCL, but these cells are generally normal in adult NCL (Figure 5-3A) (322). Although the stored lipopigment is ultrastructurally different in each NCL type, there is morphological overlap (Figure 5-3B to H).

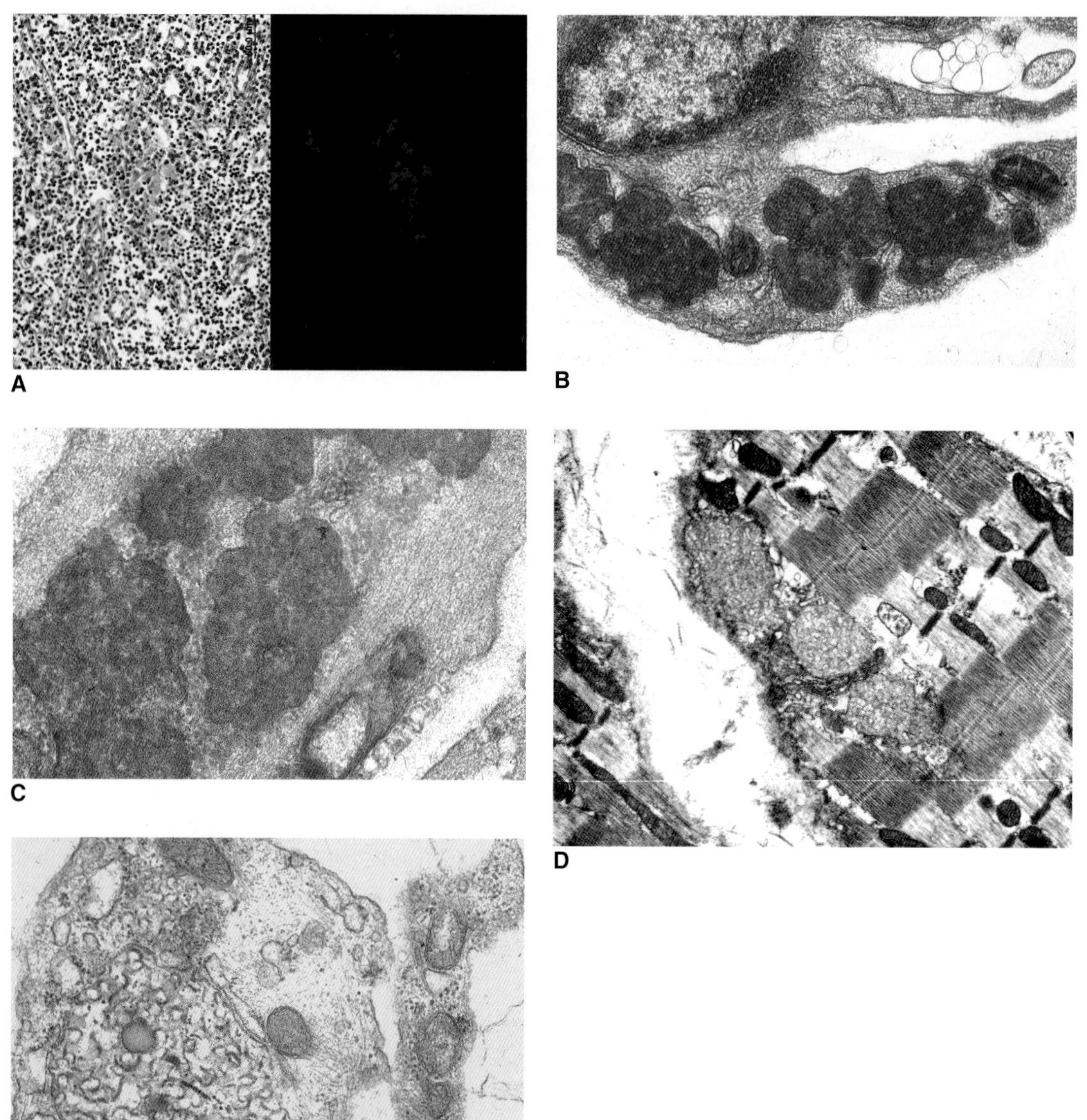

FIGURE 5-3 ■ **Neuronal ceroid lipofuscinosis. A:** Enlarged cells in a lymph node of a patient with neuronal ceroid lipofuscinosis have cytoplasmic glycolipid storage within a background of normal-appearing lymphocytes. A cluster of cells with prominent eosinophilic cytoplasm is easily identified in the center of the field (**left image**). Epifluorescence of the same microscopic field (**right image**) highlights the glycolipid storage, with a central cluster of storage cells as well as additional, scattered storage cells (H&E, autofluorescence). **B,C:** In infantile neuronal ceroid lipofuscinosis, lysosomal storage is typified by osmiophilic granular bodies. **D,E:** In late infantile neuronal ceroid lipofuscinosis, lysosomal storage is typified by osmiophilic curvilinear material.

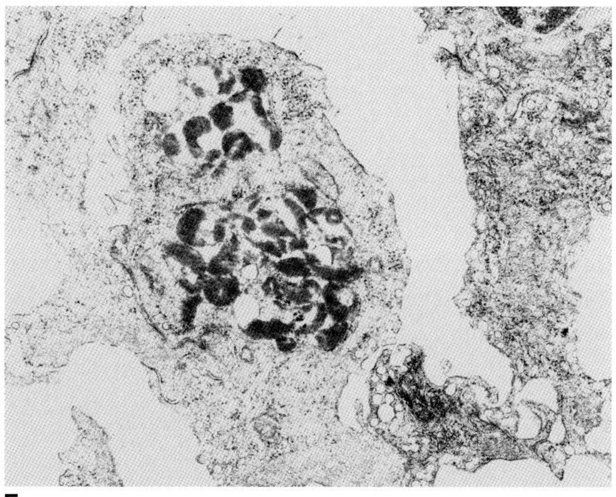

F

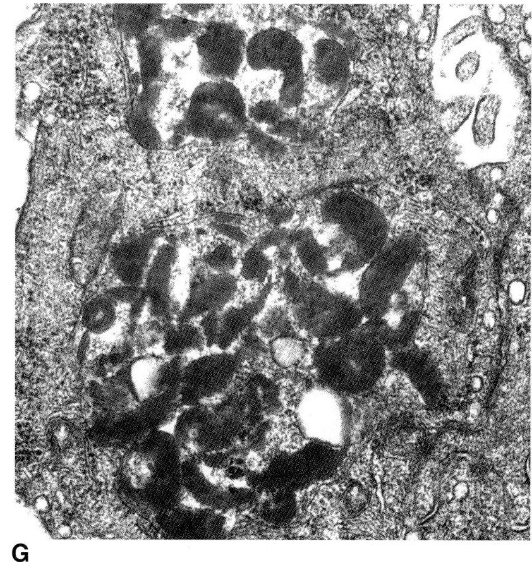

G

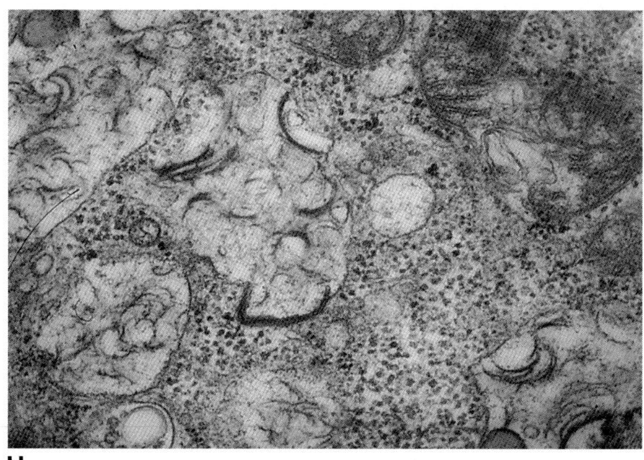

H

FIGURE 5-3▪ *(continued)* **F,G:** In juvenile neuronal ceroid lipofuscinosis, storage material is typified by osmiophilic "fingerprint bodies." **H:** Despite the association of granular bodies with infantile neuronal ceroid lipofuscinosis, curvilinear bodies with late infantile neuronal ceroid lipofuscinosis, and fingerprint bodies with juvenile neuronal ceroid lipofuscinosis, there is overlap in the morphologic appearance of storage material. In this image, the bulk of the storage material has the curvilinear appearance typical of late infantile neuronal ceroid lipofuscinosis; however, some of the darker material approaches the morphology of fingerprint bodies typical of juvenile neuronal ceroid lipofuscinosis (**B–H** Uranyl acetate, lead citrate).

Cerebral and cerebellar atrophy with neuronal loss, apoptosis, and gliosis occurs in the central nervous system with neural and extraneural lysosomal storage (116,274). Neuronal storage and loss is severe in the CA2 sector of the hippocampus (109). The heart has myocardial, valvular, and conduction system storage (116). Diagnosis can be made using DNA analysis.

Pompe Disease (Glycogen Storage Disease Type II, GSD-II)

A range of phenotypes occurs in GSD II patients, reflecting the variety of mutations in the alpha-glucosidase (acid maltase) gene, residual enzyme activity, and tissue-specific isoenzymes (80) (Table 5-10). All are autosomal recessive. Patients have hypotonia and cardiomegaly but differ in age of onset, extent of organ involvement, and rate of progression (84,115,222,300). Infants with classical Pompe disease die of cardiac or respiratory failure in the first several years of life. The "muscular variants" are generally less severe (80).

PAS-positive, diastase-digestible glycogen lysosomal storage is generalized but most severe in the skeletal muscle, heart, liver, and brain. Increased acid phosphatase activity indicates lysosomal distention and secondary elevation of other lysosomal enzymes (Figure 5-4A). A vacuolar myopathy with disruption of cytoplasmic structure affects skeletal,

Table 5-10 ▪ CLINICAL FORMS OF GLYCOGEN STORAGE DISEASE II

Type	Symptoms
Infantile (Pompe disease)	Hypotonia, cardiomegaly, macroglossia; Hepatomegaly is mild or absent; hypoglycemia and acidosis are uncommon; death from respiratory or cardiac failure in 1st years of life
Childhood, juvenile, or muscular	Onset after early infancy, predominant skeletal muscle involvement, usually without heart involvement, slowly progressive course, exercise intolerance, myalgia, weakness (in some cases rhabdomyolysis), impaired respiratory function; death usually from respiratory failure
Adult	Slowly progressive proximal myopathy, respiratory insufficiency

cardiac, and smooth muscle (Figure 5-4B,C). Cardiac hypertrophy (Figure 5-4D) and endocardial fibroelastosis occur, and the conduction system may be involved (40).

Glycogen is increased in Schwann cells, anterior horn cells, brain stem motor nuclei and spinal ganglia, myenteric plexus, astrocytes, oligodendroglia, endothelial cells, and pericytes with relative sparing of cortical neurons (115). Hepatocytes are only slightly enlarged with delicate glycogen-containing vacuoles. Liver lacks the mosaic pattern and nuclear glycogenation seen in other GSD (Figure 5-4E) (80). In kidney, glycogen accumulates in epithelium of loops of Henle and collecting tubules (221,300), and the adrenal zona fasciculata has prominent storage (80).

Skin, conjunctiva, liver, muscle, lymphocytes, and placenta can show diagnostic lysosomal glycogen accumulation by EM (Figure 5-4F to I). Glycogen in muscle is both lysosomal and cytoplasmic. Diagnosis is confirmed by demonstrating absent enzyme in dried blood spots, leukocytes, muscle, liver, or fibroblasts.

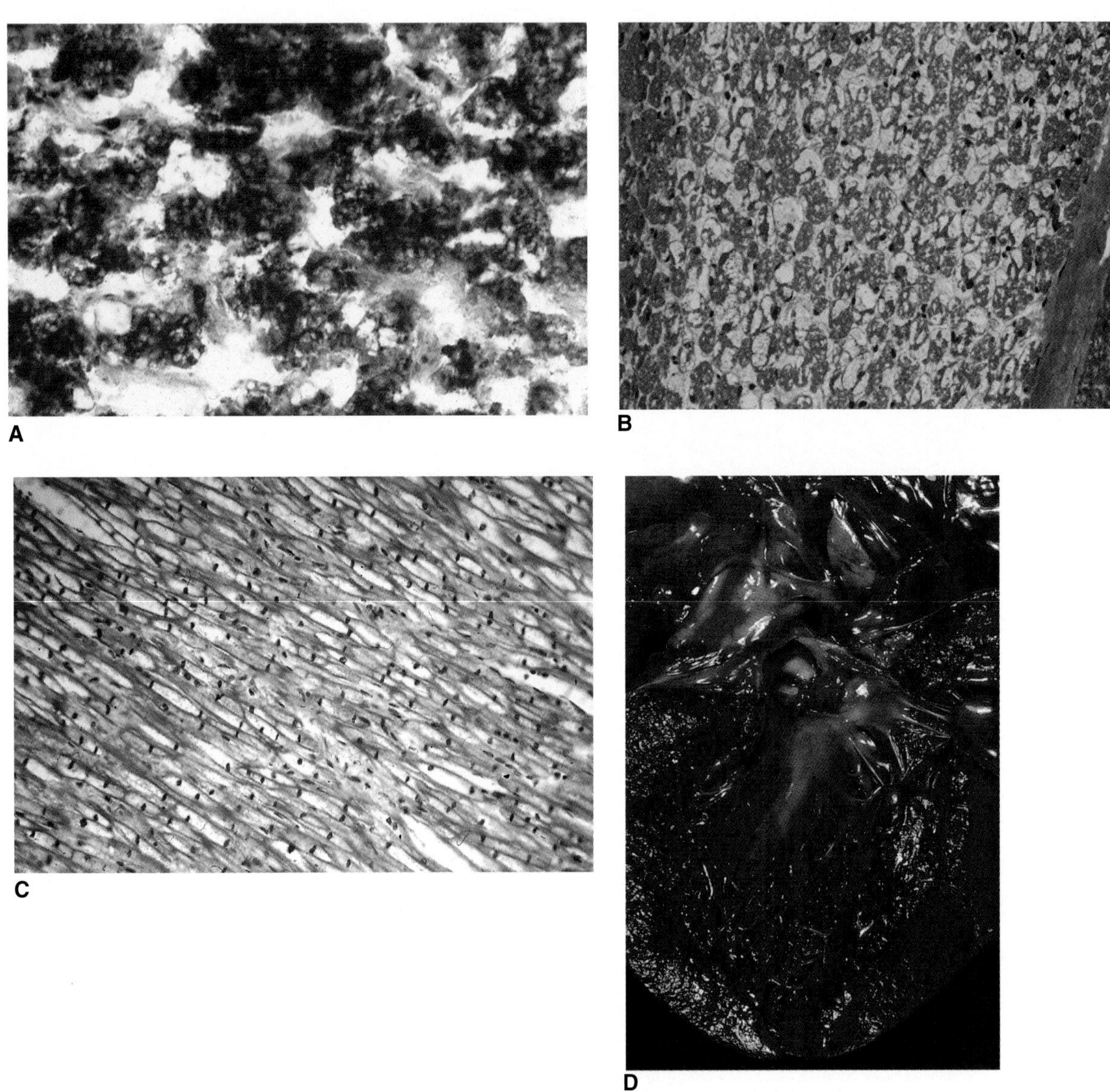

FIGURE 5-4 ■ **Pompe disease (type II glycogen storage disease). A:** Glycogen storage in Pompe disease is lysosomal (in contrast to glycogen storage in the other types of glycogen storage disease). The distended lysosomes also contain abundant acid phosphatase activity, which can be demonstrated histochemically, here in skeletal muscle by acid phosphatase staining (acid phosphatase stain). **B:** Vacuolar myopathy, though not specific for Pompe disease, is nonetheless characteristic and often striking in this LSD. The pale vacuoles in skeletal muscle fibers (representing glycogen storage) seen with H&E stain can be highlighted by PAS stain (not shown) (H&E). **C:** Histologically, cardiac myocytes are enlarged due to sarcoplasmic expansion by pale, often vacuolar material (H&E). **D:** Cardiac myocyte enlargement can lead to a hypertrophic gross appearance of myocardium, as seen in this image of the left ventricle from an infant who died with Pompe disease.

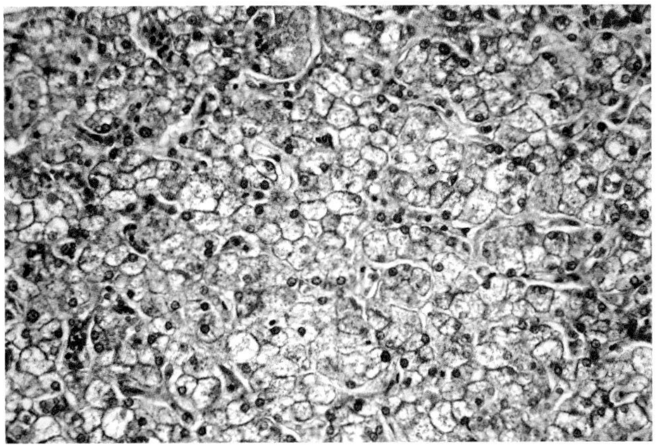

E

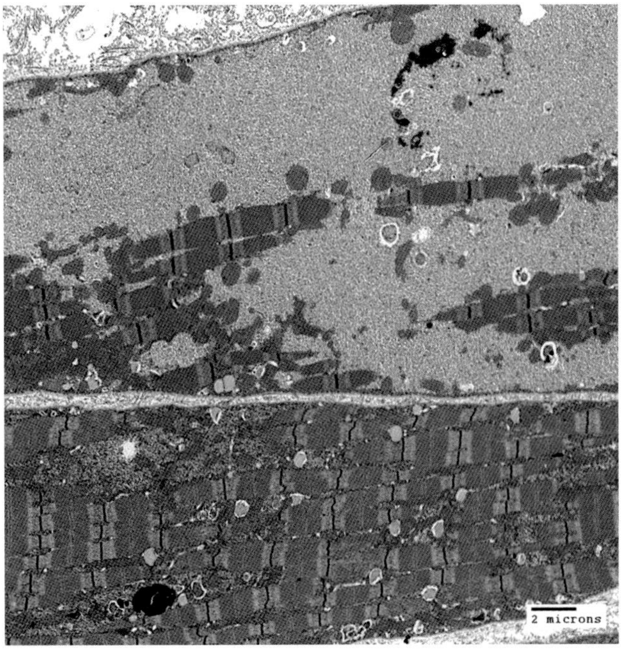

F

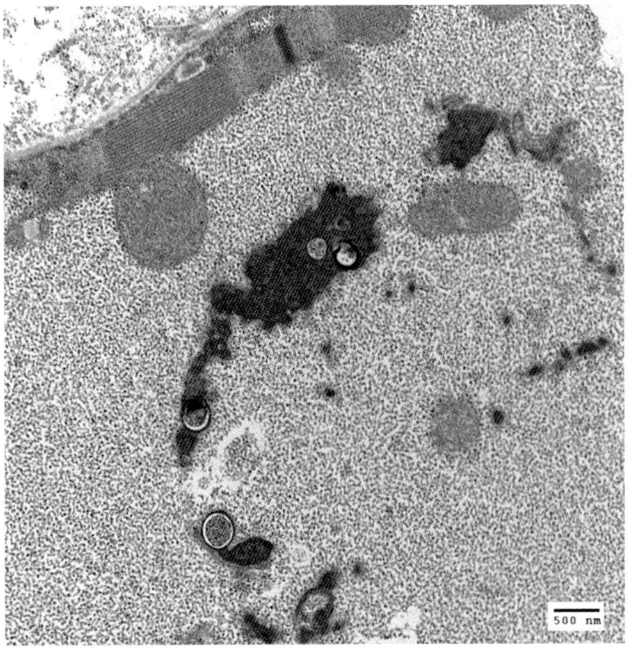

G

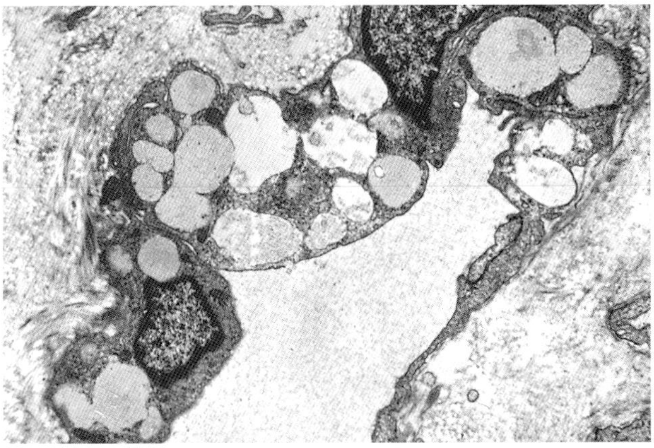

H

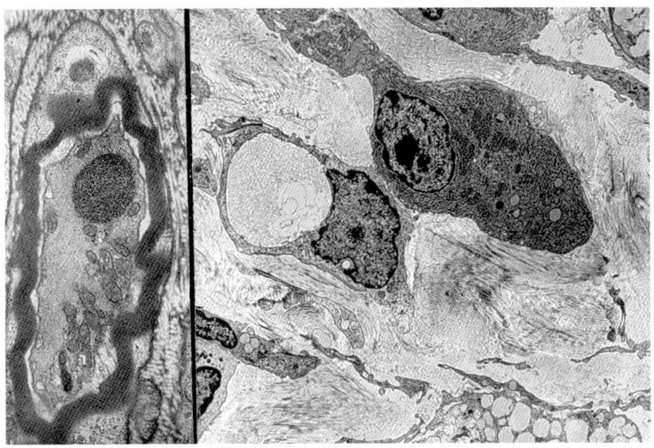

I

FIGURE 5-4■ *(continued)* **E:** The histologic appearance of hepatocytes in Pompe disease is usually less striking than that of skeletal muscle. Hepatocytes are slightly enlarged with somewhat rarefied, vacuolar cytoplasm. Note the absence of glycogenated nuclei, which are typically not seen in the liver in Pompe disease but are observed in several other types of glycogen storage disease (H&E). **F,G:** Though glycogen storage in Pompe disease (and morphologically indistinguishable Danon disease) is lysosomal (in contrast to other glycogen storage diseases), ultrastructural analysis of skeletal muscle often shows both widespread extra-lysosomal and lysosomal glycogen accumulation. **H:** Endomysial capillaries in skeletal muscle biopsy material as well as in other tissues, such as skin and conjunctiva, typically reveal membrane-bound glycogen. **I:** Most cells in conjunctival biopsy show lysosomal storage. In the left image, an axon contains a distended lysosome filled with glycogen granules. The right image shows prominent membrane-bound glycogen storage within a myelinated axon (**F–I** Uranyl acetate, lead citrate). (Image **I:** Used from, *American Journal of Medical Genetics*, with permission.)

Danon Disease, X-Linked Vacuolar Cardiomyopathy and Myopathy

Originally described as *lysosomal glycogen storage disease with normal acid maltase* (90), this disorder is characterized by mental retardation, hypertrophic cardiomyopathy, skeletal myopathy, and death due to heart failure in the third decade (89,275). X-linked dominant mutation in the *LAMP-2* gene encoding lysosome-associated membrane protein-2 leads to failure of fusion of endosome and lysosome (13). Some children with hypertrophic cardiomyopathy (especially if skeletal myopathy is also present) have been found to have LAMP-2 deficiency (377).

Muscle fibers have degeneration, size variation, and PAS-positive vacuoles that contain glycogen and autophagic material; the amount of vacuolization correlates with clinical disease. LAMP-2 is not identifiable immunohistochemically in leukocytes, skeletal muscle, and myocardium in affected patients (84,88,376), and definitive diagnosis is based on DNA testing for the mutation (8).

Mucopolysaccharidoses

The mucopolysaccharidoses (MPSs) are systemic diseases due to deficiency of an enzyme needed for catabolism of glycosaminoglycans (GAG) including dermatan, heparan, chondroitin, and keratan sulfate, with resultant storage of undegraded GAG in lysosomes in a variety of cell types (279). The clinical course is variable; MPS patients may have progressive psychomotor delay, coarse facial features, short stature, and bone and joint abnormalities (dysostosis multiplex), hepatosplenomegaly, corneal clouding, macroglossia, and airway narrowing (Figure 5-5A to C) (Table 5-11). All MPS are autosomal recessive traits except X-linked Hunter syndrome; Hurler (Type I) and Hunter (Type II) syndromes are the most common types. Scheie and Hurler-Scheie syndromes are subtypes of MPS I with a milder disease. Some infants, particularly with MPS VII, present with hydrops (Table 5-5).

In MPS, many organs have lysosomal storage. Grossly, the liver is enlarged and firm. Vacuolization is more prominent in Kupffer cells than hepatocytes. Fibrosis of Disse's

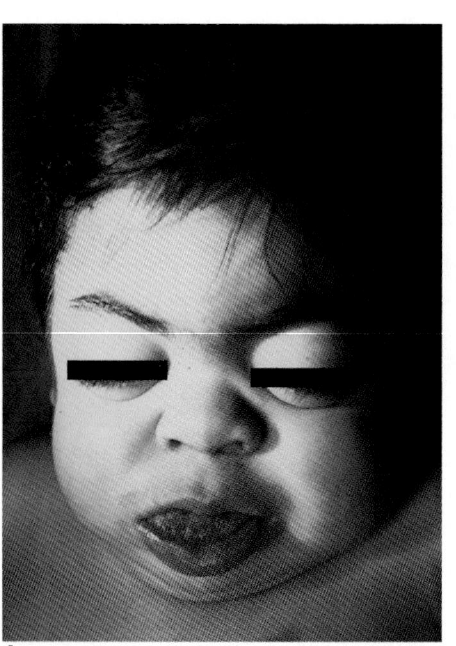
A

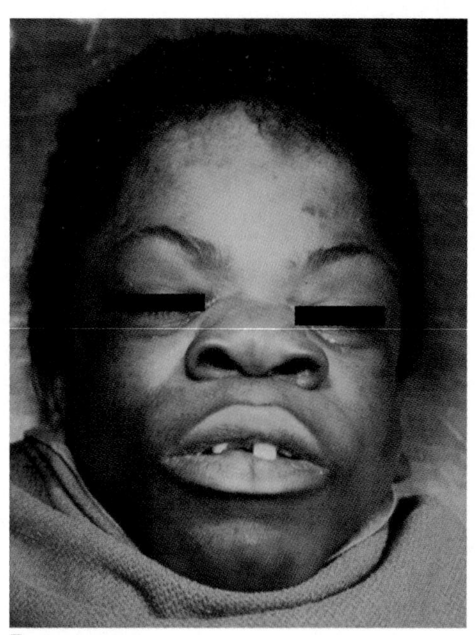
B

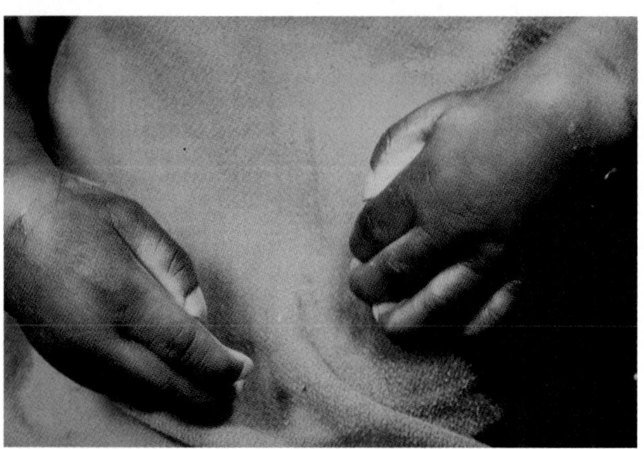
C

FIGURE 5-5 ■ **Mucopolysaccharidosis. A,B:** MPS patients have a characteristic facial appearance with coarse facial appearance, thick doughy skin, coarse hair, flattened midface, wide nasal bridge, and macroglossia, here seen in two children who died with MPS. **C:** The hands in MPS patients have joint stiffness and are held in a flexed position, a function of periarticular altered connective tissue and altered bone formation.

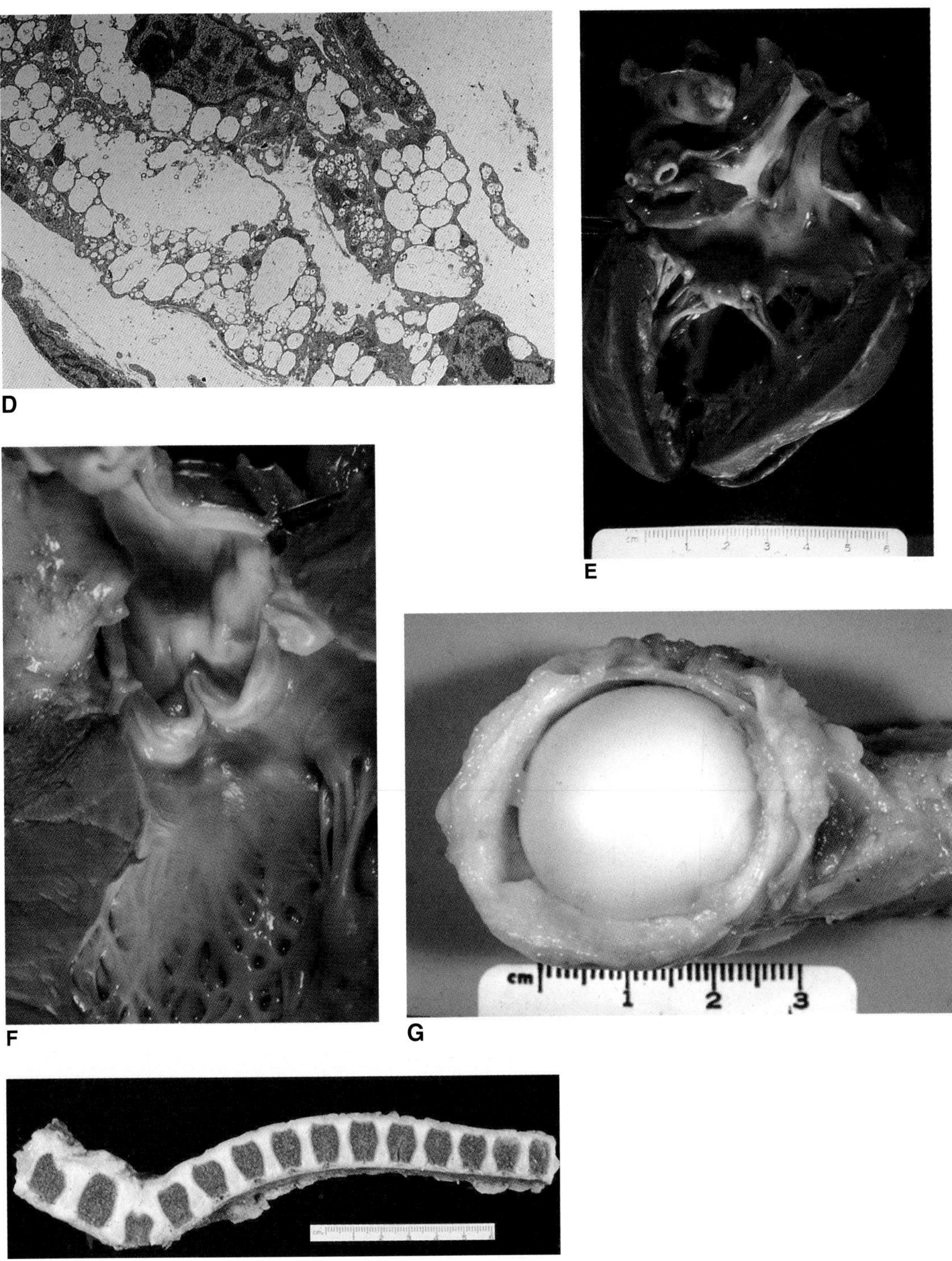

FIGURE 5-5 *(continued)* **D:** In mucopolysaccharidosis, stored GAGs (previously called *mucopolysaccharides*) have the ultrastructural appearance of fine fibrillogranular material and clear membrane-bound vacuoles. Distinguishing different types of mucopolysaccharidosis based on ultrastructural morphologic characteristics is not possible. **E,F:** The heart in patients with MPS typically has thickened sclerotic valves, due to GAG storage in heart valve stromal cells and altered extracellular connective tissue in the valve. Endocardial thickening is also frequent. **G,H:** The femoral head of a patient from MPS shows articular synechiae and thick, poorly pliable periarticular connective tissue. These joint changes cause marked joint stiffness and make normal movement impossible. The vertebral column from an MPS patient shows characteristic anterior inferior beaking of the lower thoracic and upper lumbar areas caused by hypoplasia of the anterior superior aspect. This change results in the dorsal kyphosis or gibbus deformation often seen in MPS patients and it is part of the widespread dysostosis multiplex.

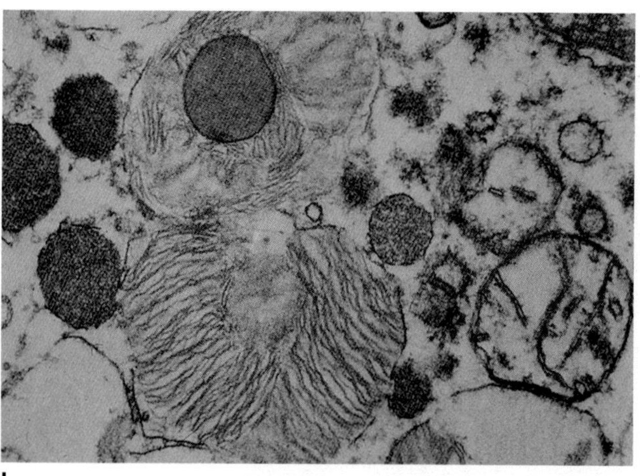

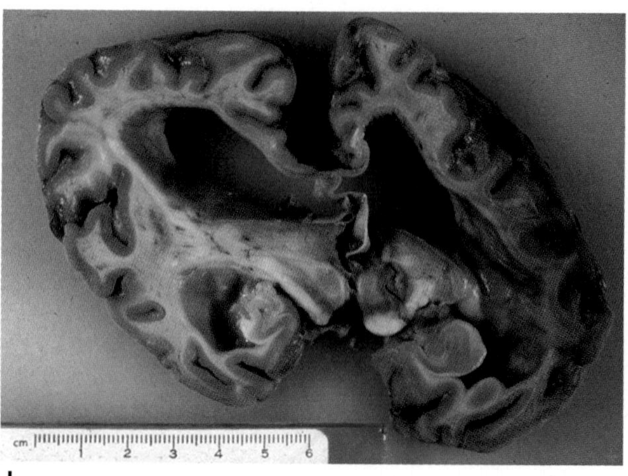

FIGURE 5-5 ■ *(continued)* **I:** Though storage material in neurons can resemble that seen in other organs, it can also take the form of "zebra bodies," as shown in this case of Hurler syndrome (**D,I**: Uranyl acetate, lead citrate). **J:** Note the presence of cortical atrophy, loss of white matter and hydrocephalus.

space occurs late in disease; rarely, more severe fibrosis can develop in older patients (73,188,300). The stored GAG can be highlighted with colloidal iron and Alcian blue stains and are digested by hyaluronidase. Adding 10% acetyltrimethylammonium bromide to formalin may help preserve tissue GAG (300). By EM, visceral lysosomal storage is fine fibrillogranular material (Figure 5-5D). Vessel walls and heart valves are often affected with storage with resultant sclerosis (Figure 5-5E,F) and endocardial fibroelastosis may occur (80). In bone, in most patients, storage in osteocytes and chondrocytes alters bone growth (Figure 5-5G,H). Neurons store both GAG and gangliosides, with membranous cytoplasmic bodies, zebra bodies, and fibrillogranular storage (Figure 5-5I). Neuronal loss and gliosis are seen in some patients, and meningeal storage may contribute to hydrocephalus (Figure 5-5J).

Diagnosis is suggested by increased urine GAG and the presence of vacuoles and metachromatic Adler-Reilly granules in peripheral blood leukocytes. EM of skin, conjunctiva, buffy coat, or liver can show characteristic fibrillogranular lysosomal storage. LM of thick sections of tissue prepared for EM are useful for identifying the multiple clear cytoplasmic vacuoles indicative of lysosomal storage. Enzyme assay of serum, leukocytes, or fibroblast culture provides definitive diagnosis, and carrier testing using DNA analysis is practical (80,100).

Mucolipidoses

I-cell disease (ML II) and pseudo-Hurler polydystrophy (ML III) are autosomal recessive traits due to altered lysosomal enzyme phosphorylation and localization (252).

Table 5-11 ■ MUCOPOLYSACCHARIDOSIS

MPS	Eponym	Enzyme Deficient	Clinical and Pathology Findings
I	Hurler, Scheie, Hurler-Scheie	Alpha-L-iduronidase	Corneal clouding, dysostosis multiplex, hepatosplenomegaly, cardiac valve sclerosis, mental retardation, premature death (Scheie has milder phenotype without mental retardation), rarely hydrops fetalis
II	Hunter	Iduronate sulfatase	Dysostosis multiplex, hepatosplenomegaly, cardiac valve sclerosis, mental retardation, X-linked
IIIA	Sanfilippo A	Heparan *N*-sulfatase (sulfamidase)	Mental retardation, mild somatic disease
IIIB	Sanfilippo B	*N*-acetyl-alpha-D-glucosaminidase	Similar to IIIA
IIIC	Sanfilippo C	Acetyl-CoA:alpha-glucosaminidase *N*-acetyl transferase	Similar to IIIA
IIID	Sanfilippo D	*N*-acetylglucosamine-6-sulfatase	Similar to IIIA
IVA	Morquio A	Galactosamine-6-sulfatase	Skeletal abnormalities, corneal clouding, odontoid hypoplasia, hydrops fetalis
IVB	Morquio B	Beta-galactosidase	Similar to IVA
VI	Maroteaux-Lamy	*N*-acetylgalactosamine 4-sulphatase (arylsulfatase B)	Dysostosis multiplex, corneal clouding, normal intelligence
VII	Sly	Beta-glucuronidase	Dysostosis multiplex, hepatosplenomegaly, mental retardation, hydrops fetalis

Both have disordered lysosomal enzyme targeting to lysosomes due to defective *N*-acetylglucosamine 1-phosphotransferase activity in Golgi. In normal cells, lysosomal targeting of enzymes is mediated by receptors that bind mannose 6-phosphate recognition markers on the enzymes. The recognition marker is synthesized in the Golgi, catalyzed by the phosphotransferase (252). Phosphotransferase deficiency results in abnormal lysosomal enzyme transport with synthesized enzyme being secreted out of the cell instead of being targeted to lysosomes. Elevated plasma lysosomal enzymes result.

Affected patients have features of both MPS and sphingolipidoses, hence the designation *mucolipidoses*. Clinical and radiologic findings (coarse facial features, psychomotor retardation, failure to thrive, hepatomegaly, dysostosis multiplex) are similar to those seen in MPS I, but earlier onset, a more rapid course, marked gingival hyperplasia, and absence of mucopolysacchariduria help distinguish ML II and III clinically from MPS I (252).

The term *I-cell disease* was coined because cultured fibroblasts from affected patients contain dense inclusions (252,300). PAS-positive and Hale's-colloidal-iron-positive vacuoles are prominent in endothelial cells and fibroblasts and occur in lymphocytes, Kupffer cells, glomerular visceral epithelial cells, satellite cells in muscle, myocardium, and pancreatic acinar cells (37,300,305). Storage in stromal fibroblasts in heart is associated with valve thickening. Granulomas with finely vacuolated histocytes may occur in lung and portal areas as well as portal tract fibroblasts. Hepatocytes are normal or only mildly altered and contain triglyceride droplets (300).

The CNS may be normal morphologically, except for lamellar bodies in spinal ganglia neurons and anterior horn cells, or may have cerebral cortical atrophy with neuronal loss (100,252). Storage may be apparent in affected fetuses and their placentas (252). I-cell disease can present as nonimmune hydrops (Table 5-5) (327). By EM, storage is electron lucent or fibrillogranular and includes oligosaccharides, mucopolysaccharides, and lipids (252); EM of skin or conjunctiva can be used for diagnostic evaluation (Figure 5-6). Increased serum lysosomal enzymes and decreased *N*-acetylglucosamine 1-phosphotransferase provide biochemical confirmation (100).

ML III (pseudo-Hurler polydystrophy) symptoms are similar to ML II but milder with growth retardation, coarse facial features, cardiac valve disease, dysostosis multiplex with stiff joints, and corneal clouding (80). ML II and III are distinguished on clinical findings and progression of disease (252). The pathology of ML III is not as well documented as that of ML II patients (80,100,252). Storage is identified in skin fibroblasts, but lymphocytes are normal (82).

Mucolipidosis Type IV

Mucolipidosis type IV (ML IV, sialolipidosis, ganglioside-sialidase deficiency) results from mutations in the gene *MCOLN1*, which codes for the TRP family ion membrane channel, mucolipidin 1, a transient receptor potential protein important in endocytosis (323). As a result, there is abnormal intracellular membrane trafficking (12,104). This disorder is classified as a mucolipidosis because of the storage of both lipids and mucopolysaccharides (36). Although panethnic, ML IV is more common among Ashkenazi Jewish individuals (104,111). Patients have severe psychomotor retardation, ophthalmologic abnormalities with corneal clouding, retinal degeneration, and optic nerve atrophy, but they do not have dysostosis multiplex (80).

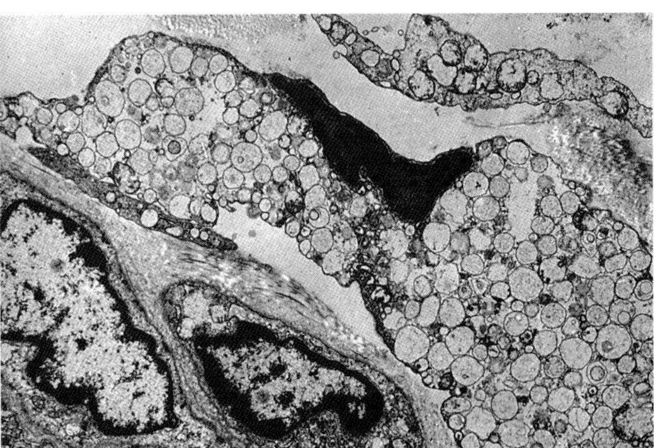

FIGURE 5-6 ■ **I-cell disease.** In I-cell disease, fibroblast cytoplasm is expanded by numerous membrane-bound vacuoles containing electron-lucent to fibrillogranular material (Uranyl acetate, lead citrate).

Widespread storage affects brain and viscera including liver, pancreas, kidney, marrow, conjunctiva, cornea, skin, muscle, peripheral nerve, rectum, and placenta (300). In neurons and glia, ganglioside, phospholipid, and GAG accumulation is variably PAS-positive and Sudanophilic and is associated with neuronal loss and astrocytosis (100). By EM, lysosomes contain heterogeneous material with fibrillogranular and concentric membranous bodies.

Hypergastrinemia and achlorhydria are described (264). Chronic atrophic gastritis and enterochromaffin-like cell hyperplasia are seen along with cytoplasmic vacuolization of parietal cells due to lysosomal storage (104,265). Confirmatory diagnosis of ML IV should include screening for mutations in *MCOLN1* (104).

Disorders of Glycoprotein Degradation (Oligosaccharidoses/Glycoproteinoses)

These autosomal recessive disorders are due to deficiency of a lysosomal enzyme that degrades glycoprotein oligosaccharide side chains of glycoproteins (173,300,334). The phenotype resembles that of MPS, and tissues accumulate glycoproteins and oligosaccharides (Table 5-12).

Alpha-mannosidosis. Affected patients have deficient alpha-mannosidase and increased plasma levels and excretion of small mannose-rich oligosaccharides (334). Phenotype is variable (Table 5-12). Frequent infections may relate to a defect in leukocyte chemotaxis (334), decreased serum IgG, or an impaired leukocyte membrane recognition

Table 5-12 ■ DISORDERS OF GLYCOPROTEIN DEGRADATION (OLIGOSACCHARIDOSES/ GLYCOPROTEINOSES)

Disorder	Enzyme Deficiency	Clinical Findings
Alpha-Mannosidosis	Alpha-mannosidase	Mental retardation, coarse facies, dysostosis multiplex, hepatosplenomegaly frequent infections
Beta-Mannosidosis	Beta-mannosidase	Angiokeratomas, mental retardation, hearing loss, respiratory infections, seizures, quadriplegia, death in early childhood
Fucosidosis	Alpha-L-fucosidases	Mental retardation, hepatosplenomegaly, angiokeratomas, thick skin, cardiomegaly, respiratory infections, dysostosis multiplex, mental retardation, increased sweat sodium chloride
Sialidosis (Mucolipidosis I)	Neuraminidase	Cherry-red spot-myoclonus syndrome, decreased visual acuity, corneal clouding, seizures, hyper-reflexia, ataxia, dysostosis multiplex, hepatosplenomegaly, nephrotic syndrome, infantile form may have hydrops fetalis
Aspartylglycosaminuria	Aspartylglucosaminidase	Onset by 1 year, hypotonia, coarse facies, thick calvarium, osteoporosis, seizures, abnormal gray and white matter differentiation, delayed myelination.

process that results from defective catabolism of substrates with alpha-D-mannose residues. Hepatocytes have granular or foamy cytoplasm, and Kupffer cells and hepatocytes contain reticulogranular, amorphous, or membranous storage by EM (300). In brain, neurons have marked and widespread ballooning with membrane-bound vacuoles containing reticulogranular material (334). Diagnosis can be based on ultrastructural morphology of skin, conjunctiva, or peripheral blood lymphocytes; demonstration of oligosacchariuria; and measurement of tissue alpha-mannosidase activity (57,334).

Beta-mannosidosis. This LSD, due to deficiency of beta-mannosidase, has a variable phenotype (Table 5-12). Cytoplasmic vacuoles are described in skin and bone marrow in isolated patients, and the diagnosis rests on measurement of beta-mannosidase in leukocytes or fibroblasts (334).

Fucosidosis. This LSD, due to deficient alpha-L-fucosidase, causes accumulation of fucoside moiety-containing glycolipids, glycoproteins, and oligosaccharides (Table 5-12). Most patients are of Italian or Spanish descent or from the southwestern United States (100,334). Some patients have a rapidly progressive course with death in the first decade, while others have a milder course with survival into the teen years and beyond. Angiokeratoma corporis diffusum occurs with fucosidosis and is essentially identical in appearance and distribution to that seen in Fabry disease (334). Hepatocytes, Kupffer cells, and bile duct epithelial cells are vacuolated. The CNS also may have lysosomal storage (334). Conjunctiva, muscle, skin sweat gland epithelium, and peripheral blood lymphocytes all show granular lysosomal storage by EM (Figure 5-7). Diagnosis is based on demonstrating deficient alpha-L-fucosidase in leukocytes and fibroblasts. Some clinically normal individuals have low alpha-L-fucosidase levels in plasma (334).

Sialidosis. This LSD, previously called *Mucolipidosis I*, results from a recessively inherited deficiency of neuraminidase, an enzyme that cleaves terminal sialic acid residues from oligosaccharides and glycoproteins. The deficiency results in lysosomal accumulation of sialylated glycoproteins and oligosaccharides (Table 5-12) (80,327). Patients may present with hydrops, facial dysmorphism, psychomotor retardation, dysostosis multiplex, hepatosplenomegaly, and cardiomegaly (100). Hepatomegaly and portal fibrosis may be present. Kupffer cells, endothelial and stellate cells, lymphocytes, glomerular visceral epithelial cells, neurons in myenteric plexus and brain, fixed tissue macrophages in marrow and lung, biliary epithelium, chondrocytes, and placental stromal and trophoblast cells have cytoplasmic vacuolization (Figure 5-8A,B) (80,229). By EM, lysosomes contain osmiophilic droplets and lamellar and fibrillogranular material (Figure 5-8C) (300,334). Vacuolated lymphocytes and

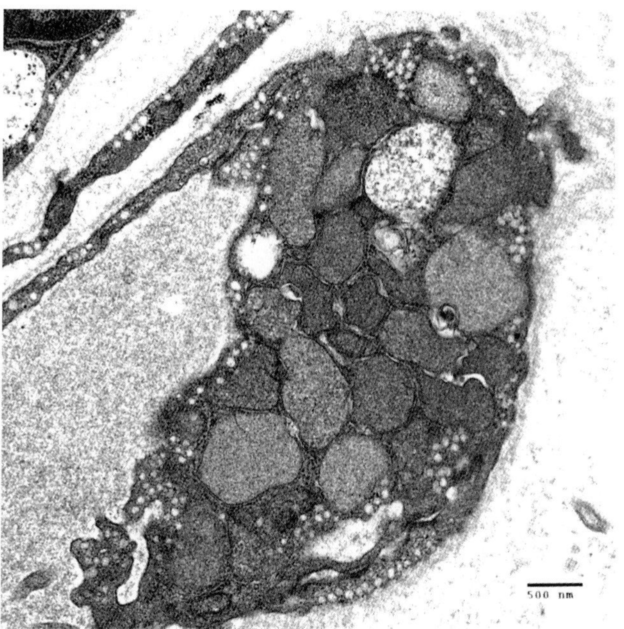

FIGURE 5-7 ■ **Fucosidosis.** Granular storage material distends the cytoplasm of this endomysial endothelial cell from a muscle biopsy of a 2-year-old girl with fucosidosis (Uranyl acetate, lead citrate).

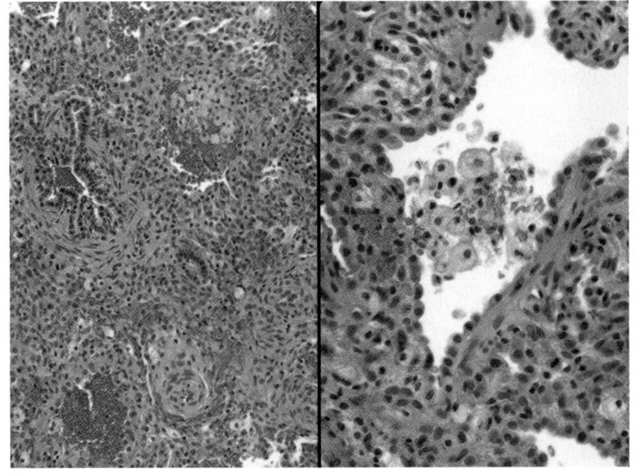

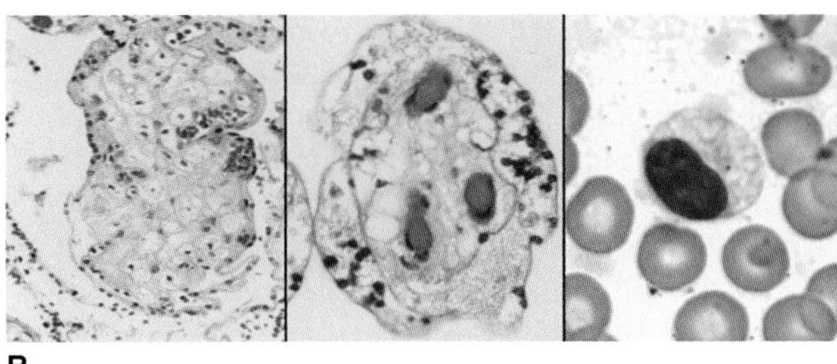

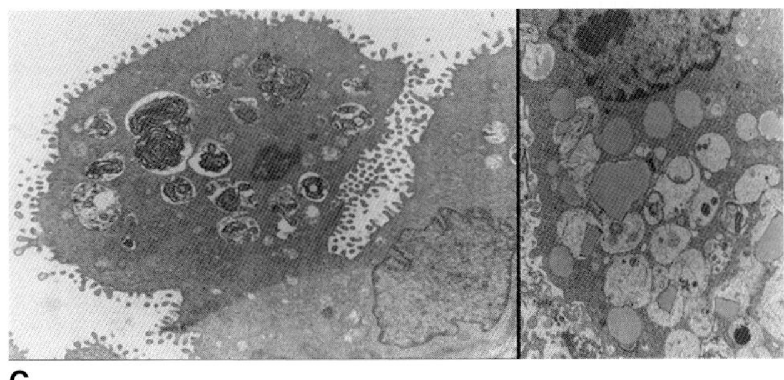

FIGURE 5-8 ▪ **Sialidosis (mucolipidosis I). A:** Foamy macrophages in lung tissue are present in this case of sialidosis (H&E). **B:** Cells of the reticuloendothelial system in sialidosis are vacuolated, as seen in chorionic villi (**left and middle images**) and a peripheral blood monocyte (**right image**) (H&E and Wright's). **C:** Ultrastructurally, storage material in sialidosis can manifest as lamellar inclusions (**left image**) or fibrillogranular material (**right image**) (Uranyl acetate, lead citrate).

increased urine sialyloligosaccharides can suggest the need for enzymatic evaluation (80). Definitive diagnosis is based on measurement of neuraminidase activity in cultivated fibroblasts or leukocytes. If tissue is used for analysis, it cannot have been frozen or exposed to prolonged sonication (334).

Aspartylglycosaminuria. This autosomal recessive glycoprotein degradation defect occurs predominantly in Finland (100) and is due to lack of aspartylglucosaminidase, an enzyme important in liver and brain (Table 5-12). Enlarged lysosomes contain aspartylglucosamine that appears as fibrillogranular storage in skin, conjunctiva, rectal mucosa, peripheral blood lymphocytes, and viscera including liver (34,118). Despite normal liver function, hepatocytes and Kupffer cells have abundant storage (34,117,297,300). In the CNS, delayed myelination, white matter gliosis, and gray matter atrophy are seen; storage affects cortical and deep gray matter neurons and is variably lucent, dense granular, or lipofuscin (35). Fetuses can have storage in liver, kidney, skin, and placenta as early as 20 weeks' gestation (34). Diagnosis is based on enzyme assay or DNA molecular analysis (34).

Gangliosidoses

These autosomal recessive disorders all have lysosomal accumulation of glycosphingolipids (gangliosides).

G_{M1} gangliosidosis. Beta-galactosidase is deficient with accumulation of gangliosides in CNS, and galactosyl oligosaccharides and keratan sulfate in viscera (5). Beta-galactosidase is also deficient in MPS IVB but presumably with some residual enzyme activity allowing sparing of the CNS (80,327,328). Patients resemble those with MPS with coarse facies, dysostosis multiplex, hepatosplenomegaly, rapid neurological deterioration, and seizures; infants may have hydrops fetalis, and the disease is fatal generally by 2 years of age. A late infantile/juvenile G_{M1} gangliosidosis presents at 1 year of age, is clinically similar to the early-onset form but with milder dysostosis, and leads to death by 5 years of age.

Sudanophilic gangliosides accumulate in CNS neurons with ballooning, neuronal loss, gliosis, and atrophy; by EM the storage includes membranous cytoplasmic bodies. Peripheral nerve is also affected (80). PAS-positive GAG accumulation causes vacuolization of Kupffer cells, hepatocytes, glomerular visceral epithelial cells and endothelial cells, placental syncytiotrophoblasts, marrow histiocytes, lymphocytes and cells in spleen, nodes, thymus, lung, intestine, pancreas, pituitary, thyroid, salivary gland, skin (including sweat glands), and conjunctiva (119,180,328). By EM, visceral storage is fibrillogranular. Definitive diagnosis rests on demonstrating beta-galactosidase deficiency in leukocytes, fibroblasts, or amniocytes or on DNA analysis (80,328).

G_{M2} gangliosidosis. These gangliosidoses are due to autosomal recessive defects in lysosomal hexosaminidase with resultant accumulation of G_{M2} gangliosides mainly in neurons.

G_{M2} Type 1, Tay-Sachs disease, B variant. This form of G_{M2} gangliosidosis is due to hexosaminidase A deficiency; G_{M2}-containing gangliosides accumulate particularly in the CNS. The incidence is increased in Jewish populations (105,179). Psychomotor deterioration, seizures, blindness, and death by 3 to 5 years of age characterize most patients, although milder juvenile and adult forms are recognized. The liver appears normal by LM, but, by EM, there is granular and zebra body storage (178,300). The brain is atrophic with neuronal loss and secondary gliosis; cholesterol, phospholipid, and G_{M2} ganglioside accumulate as sudanophilic storage in essentially all neurons (80,105). The stored material is PAS-positive in frozen but not in paraffin sections (105). By EM, stored material in the CNS is concentrically lamellated, membranous, and granular (80). More pleomorphic inclusions are present in glia. Diagnosis is based on hexosaminidase A (decreased) and B (normal) assay in leukocytes or fibroblasts (4).

G_{M2} Type II, Sandhoff disease, O variant patients have no hexosaminidase A or B activity (hence "O" variant) and are clinically indistinguishable from Tay-Sachs disease patients. The cerebral cortex is atrophic and yellowed by accumulated asialoganglioside. PAS-positive sphingolipids and glycoprotein accumulate in liver, both in hepatocytes and Kupffer cells; in histiocytes of the spleen, lymph nodes, and bone marrow; and in lymphocytes and pancreatic acinar cells (80,105,300). By EM, storage is similar to that of Tay Sachs disease with prominent membranous cytoplasmic bodies in brain and heterogeneous material in viscera (80,105). Diagnosis can be determined by enzyme assay or DNA analysis (3,105).

G_{M2} activator protein deficiency, AB variant (indicating normal hexosaminidase A and B activity) is due to a mutation in the *GM2A* gene. Patients cannot form a functional ganglioside G_{M2}/G_{M2} activator complex to interact with hexosaminidase A and G_{M2} ganglioside to facilitate the hydrolysis of G_{M2} ganglioside (105,353). Clinically, they resemble infantile Tay-Sachs and Sandhoff diseases but with normal total hexosaminidase A and B levels. By LM, neuropathologic findings are identical to those of other G_{M2} gangliosidosis. Visceral organs are not involved. Zebra and membranous cytoplasmic bodies accumulate (Figure 5-9A,B), and heterogeneous storage affects glial cells (105). Diagnosis is based on increased G_{M2} ganglioside in cerebrospinal fluid and reduced activator protein level in fibroblasts (356).

Niemann-Pick Disease (sphingolipidoses, sphingomyelin lipidosis, sphingomyelin-cholesterol lipidosis, NPD). There are at least 6 types (A to F) of NPD; all are autosomal recessive. NPD A and B, both due to sphingomyelinase deficiency, have lysosomal sphingomyelin, cholesterol, glycolipid, and acylglyceropyrophosphate. Residual sphingomyelinase level is less and the phenotype more severe in Type A than Type B patients. Type A is the most common (85% of cases) and most severe, infantile, neuronopathic form of NPD. Hydrops fetalis, failure to thrive, hepatosplenomegaly, hypotonia, and progressive neurological deterioration end with death by 3 to 4 years of age (312). Ashkenazi Jewish populations have a higher incidence: 1:80 in this population are carriers. Heterozygote detection, unreliable by enzyme assay, requires molecular studies (312). Type B is phenotypically variable, more chronic, and nonneuronopathic; the disease presents

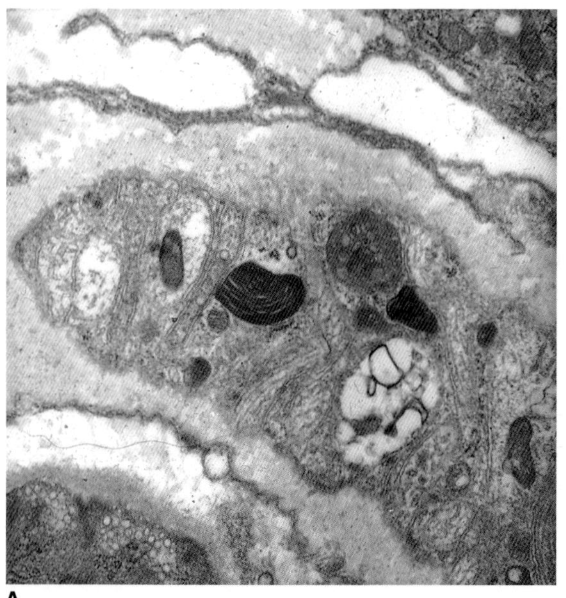
A

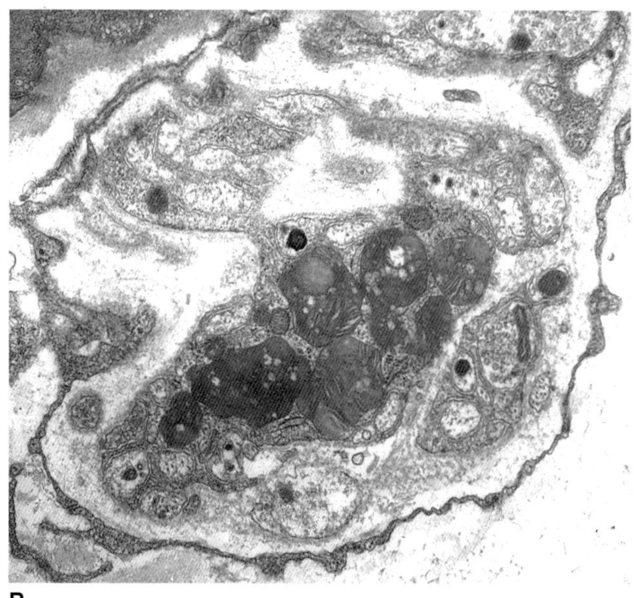
B

FIGURE 5-9■**Gangliosidosis. A,B:** Membranous cytoplasmic bodies in G_{M2} (AB variant) gangliosidosis are heterogeneous and can show concentric or parallel structure, here in peripheral nerve axons. Though the morphology of the stored gangliosides is often not helpful in distinguishing the gangliosidoses, location of the storage material can be helpful (Uranyl acetate, lead citrate. (Image **B** used from, *American Journal of Medical Genetics*, with permission.)

in older infants with hepatosplenomegaly, and progressive pulmonary disease may become a major complication. This form does not show an increased prevalence in Jewish patients (312).

The pathologic hallmark of NPD is the Niemann Pick (NP) cell (Figure 5-10A), though NP cells may be infrequent in the very young child (133,181). These 25 to 75 μm in diameter foamy lipid-laden histocytes have pale yellow or tan cytoplasmic pigmentation with H&E stain, the result of lipofuscin, sphingomyelin, ganglioside, and cholesterol storage. The vacuoles are birefringent with polarized light and stain with Sudan black B, oil red O (ORO), and Schultz reaction (312) but stain poorly with PAS and for acid phosphatase (312). The blue green cytoplasm of histiocytes with storage stained with Wright-Giemsa stain led to the term *sea-blue histiocytes*.

Kupffer cells (Figure 5-10B) (and, in some cases, hepatocytes) have progressive increase in foamy cytoplasm, and portal fibrosis and cholestasis are observed, but cirrhosis is rare (177). Infants with NPD A may have cholestasis, bile duct paucity, pseudoglandular formation, and giant cell transformation with a neonatal hepatitis pattern (100,300). The spleen may be as much as ten times normal size with extensive infiltrate and replacement of red pulp by NP cells, some of which show erythrophagocytosis. By EM, liver, spleen, lung, marrow, kidney, and lymph node storage is lipid with membranous lamellar or concentrically laminated myelin-like and lipofuscin storage (Figure 5-10C to F). Brain is atrophic with neuron loss, gliosis, and demyelination. Vacuolated neurons have sudanophilic, ORO-positive, and Luxol-fast-blue-positive storage (80), and foam cells and lipid-laden glia are in brain parenchyma and Virchow-Robin space.

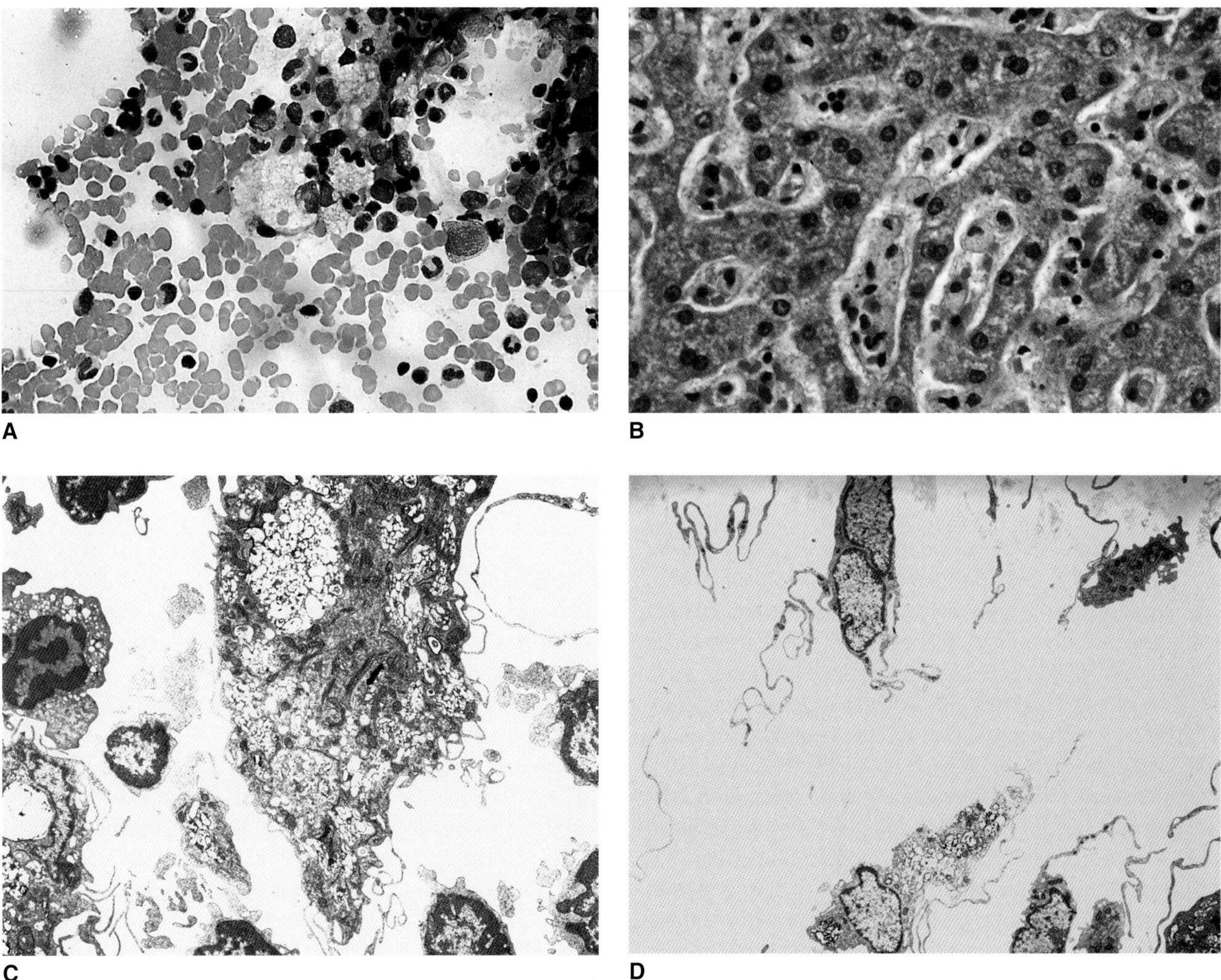

FIGURE 5-10 **Niemann-Pick disease. A:** Several vacuolated "Niemann-Pick" cells, the pathologic hallmark of types A and B Niemann-Pick disease, are present and show "sea blue" coloration by Wright-Giemsa stain in this smear of a bone marrow aspirate. Niemann-Pick cells are capable of erythrophagocytosis and emperipolesis. **B:** Enlarged, foamy Kupffer cells in Niemann-Pick disease, as shown here, may be absent in very young children but become more prominent with time (H&E). **C–F:** Ultrastructurally, storage material in Niemann-Pick disease is a heterogeneous mix of membranous lamellar material, concentrically lamellated myelin-like material, and lipofuscin (**C–F** Uranyl acetate, lead citrate).

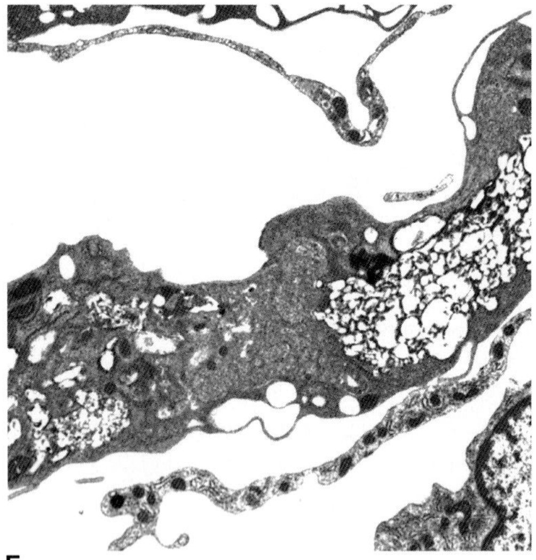
E

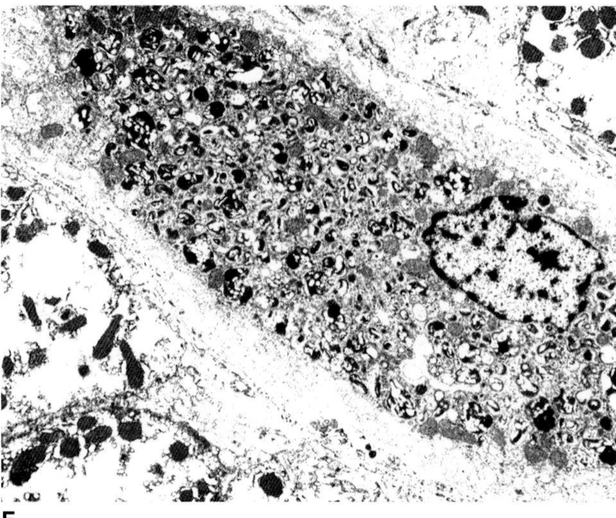
F

FIGURE 5-10■ *(continued).*

Diagnosis rests with identifying sphingomyelinase deficiency in leukocytes or fibroblasts. In families with a known molecular lesion, heterozygote status can be determined by DNA analysis (312).

NPD C, a cholesterol esterification and intracellular trafficking defect, leads to lysosomal accumulation of sphingomyelin and unesterified cholesterol and secondary reduction in sphingomyelinase activity (298,312). NPD C and D are allelic and are due to mutations in the *NPC-1* and *NPC-2* genes; NPD D is thus a variant phenotype of NPD C rather than a separate entity (298,312). NPD C is most commonly caused by mutations in the *NPC-I* gene. The protein product of *NPC-1* is thought to facilitate the egress of cholesterol and other lipids from the late endosomes and lysosomes to other cellular compartments. Protean manifestations can begin any time from intrauterine life to adulthood. Patients may present with fetal ascites or with transient neonatal jaundice and hepatitis. Hepatosplenomegaly may occur in some patients but usually regresses over time, and in general, is less severe than that seen with NPD A or B. Neurologic disease is progressive with spasticity and seizures (80). NPD D occurs in Nova Scotian Acadians with neurological disease beginning in childhood, generally later than in NPD C (80,298,312,327).

Neurovisceral storage is prominent with vacuolated cells in viscera and storage in neurons and glia (298). Vacuolated cells stain with Luxol fast blue, PAS, and Sudan black B and are positive for cholesterol with the Schultz reaction and for acid phosphatase. EM identifies membrane-bound whorled and dense osmiophilic lysosomal storage in skin and conjunctival cells, endothelial and perithelial cells, keratinocytes, retinal ganglion cells, retinal pigment epithelium, Schwann cells, smooth muscle cells, and fibroblasts (298).

NPD C and D may cause a neonatal hepatitis-like histology with giant cell transformation, fibrosis, or cirrhosis (80,176). The pathogenesis of this injury is unknown (175). Storage in liver is inconspicuous and easily overlooked, particularly in the setting of hepatitis. With time, whorled and irregular lamellar inclusions, clefts, and lipid storage accumulate in macrophages and Kupffer cells and to a lesser extent in hepatocytes (174). Neuronal storage occurs throughout the nervous system with neurofibrillary tangles, meganeurites, and axonal spheroids (298). Cerebral atrophy is generally severe, and neuronal loss may occur by apoptosis (298). A screening test involves staining cultivated cells with filipin to detect free cholesterol (359). Diagnosis is based on measurement of cholesterol esterification in fibroblasts during LDL uptake (15) and molecular analysis of the *NPC-1* or *NPC-2* genes.

Metachromatic Leukodystrophy (Sulfatide Lipidosis, MLD)

Autosomal recessive deficiency of arylsulfatatse A, which hydrolyzes galactocerebroside sulfate to galactocerebroside, leads to accumulation of sulfated glycolipids primarily in the CNS but also in extraneural sites. There are several clinical forms with infantile, juvenile, and adult types recognized; multiple mutations have been described, and patients have a variable course with progressive neurological disease. The central and peripheral nervous system have demyelination, and the cerebellum is atrophic with Purkinje and granule cell loss. Accumulation of 15 to 20 μm in diameter spherical masses of metachromatic material occurs in oligodendrocytes and macrophages in Virchow-Robin space and Schwann cells. This material comprises sulfatide, cholesterol, and phosphatides, and in frozen sections it stains positive with PAS, Alcian blue, and colloidal iron, is brown metachromatic (with 1% cresyl violet at low pH), and stains purple with toluidine blue (341). By EM, storage in oligodendrocytes, astrocytes, Schwann cells, and endoneurial cells in peripheral nerve is closely packed, lamellar, amorphous, or prismatic material with alternately leaflets and tubules giving it a "herringbone" or "tuffstone" pattern (Figure 5-11A,B) (80).

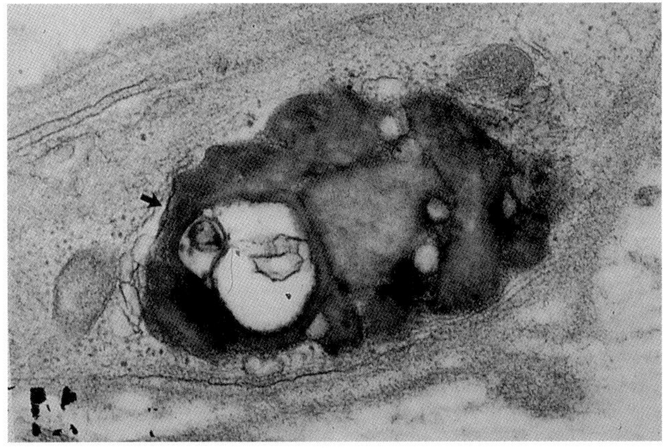
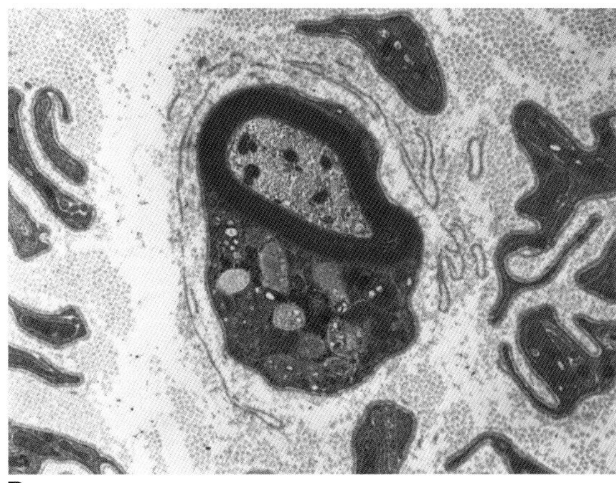

A B

FIGURE 5-11 ■ **Metachromatic leukodystrophy. A:** This unmyelinated nerve from a conjunctival biopsy contains an inclusion of variable electron density. In some foci (*arrow*), closely approximated osmiophilic lamellae contribute to a subtle herringbone pattern. **B:** Myelinated nerve with pleomorphic lysosomes of variable density, "tuffstone" inclusions from a sural nerve of a patient with metachromatic leukodystrophy. (**A, B:** Uranyl acetate, lead citrate, **A:** Used from *American Journal of Medical Genetics*, with permission.)

The gallbladder may be small and fibrotic with multiple mucosal papillomas and radiolucent choleliths; lamina propria macrophages, gall bladder epithelial cells, and intrahepatic bile ducts have storage. However, patients only rarely present with cholecystitis or pancreatitis (341). Liver macrophages, Kupffer cells, hepatocytes, and renal tubular epithelial cells also contain metachromatic storage (58,182).

Diagnosis is based on measuring arylsulfatase A activity. However, a low level does not prove MLD nor does a normal level exclude the diagnosis (341,355). A deficiency of the sphingolipid activator protein saposin B (80) can result in a normal or heterozygous range arylsulfatase A level in an affected patient. Pseudo-arylsulfatase A deficiency occurs when an abnormal allele that encodes only 5% to 15% of residual activity leads to low arylsulfatase A activity in a person who does not have MLD (341). Excessive urine sulfatides can confirm the diagnosis of MLD (358); a sulfatide-loading test allows distinction between patients homozygous for the pseudodeficiency allele and MLD patients (341).

Wolman Disease and Cholesterol Ester Storage Disease (CESD)

These autosomal recessive phenotypic variants, due to absence or reduction in acid lipase, have accumulation of cholesterol esters and triglyceride. Wolman disease patients have complete deficiency of acid lipase. Death often occurs in infancy, preceded by hydrops, steatorrhea, hepatosplenomegaly, jaundice, abnormal neurological development, and failure to thrive. The enlarged liver is a distinctive bright orange-yellow with a greasy consistency. Bile duct proliferation and cholestasis are described, and periportal fibrosis with portal bridging may progress to cirrhosis (183). In viscera—including liver, spleen, adrenal, lymph nodes, lymphocytes, marrow, and intestine—cholesterol esters and triglycerides accumulate as cholesterol crystals in foamy histiocytes (Figure 5-12A to C) (184). This storage can be identified by viewing sections of unfixed frozen tissue with polarized light (Figure 5-12D). Cholesterol and triglycerides in these cells can also be highlighted histochemically with the Schultz modification of the Lieberman-Burchard reaction (59,300). EM shows lipid droplets and membrane-bound angular cholesterol clefts in hepatocytes, Kupffer cells, fibroblasts, and macrophages (Figure 5-12E) (14,185). The mucosa of the small intestine, particularly duodenum and ileum, is velvety yellow (300) due to lamina propria storage. Adrenal glands are large, hard, and bright yellow, with dystrophic calcification and necrosis of the inner fasciculata and residual fetal cortex (80,300). Oligodendroglia, ganglia neurons of the CNS, and Schwann cells of the peripheral nervous system contain lipid. Placental syncytiotrophoblasts may be affected. Demonstration of acid lipase deficiency in tissue, cultivated fibroblasts, or leukocytes confirms the diagnosis (33).

Since CESD patients have 3% to 8% residual acid lipase activity, their phenotype is similar but more benign than that seen in Wolman disease, and diagnosis may not be made until childhood or early adulthood (33). Hyperbetalipoproteinemia and premature atherosclerosis may complicate CESD (60,80). The liver morphology is indistinguishable from that of Wolman disease. Hepatomegaly may be the sole clinical feature; cirrhosis is unusual, although periportal fibrosis may be present (186,300). Storage affects hepatocytes, bile duct epithelium, and endothelium (61). Unlike in Wolman disease, adrenals may not be calcified, but lymphocytes and histiocytes in intestinal lamina propria and marrow contain storage (38,80).

Farber Disease (Disseminated Lipogranulomatosis)

A rare autosomal recessive deficiency of acid ceramidase leads to accumulation of ceramide, which is formed from turnover

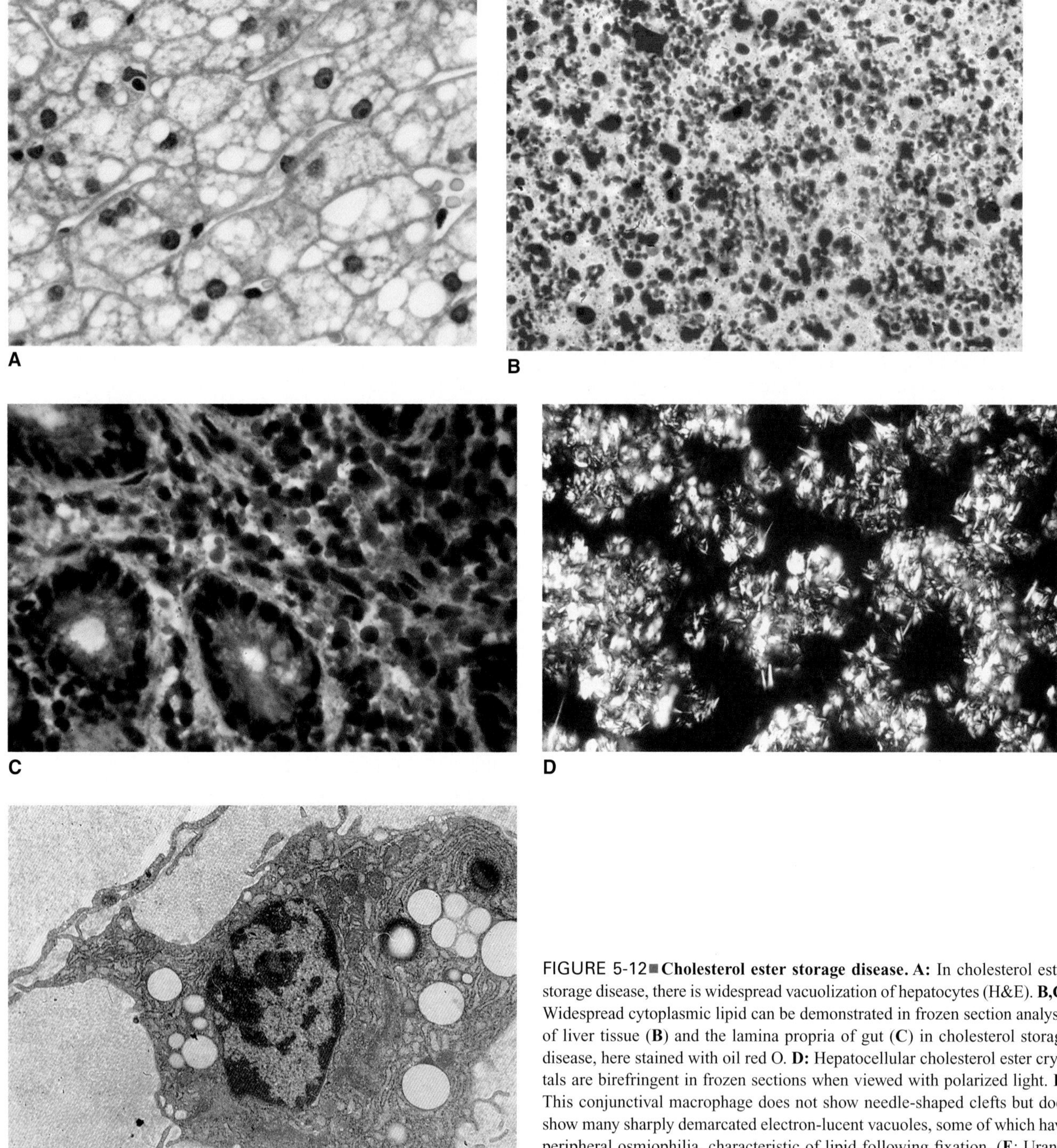

FIGURE 5-12 **Cholesterol ester storage disease. A:** In cholesterol ester storage disease, there is widespread vacuolization of hepatocytes (H&E). **B,C:** Widespread cytoplasmic lipid can be demonstrated in frozen section analysis of liver tissue (**B**) and the lamina propria of gut (**C**) in cholesterol storage disease, here stained with oil red O. **D:** Hepatocellular cholesterol ester crystals are birefringent in frozen sections when viewed with polarized light. **E:** This conjunctival macrophage does not show needle-shaped clefts but does show many sharply demarcated electron-lucent vacuoles, some of which have peripheral osmiophilia, characteristic of lipid following fixation. (**E**: Uranyl acetate, lead citrate, Used from *American Journal of Medical Genetics*, with permission)

of sphingolipids in lymph nodes, liver, kidney, and lung. Mucopolysaccharides and gangliosides also accumulate (80,276). Symptoms begin in infancy and include failure to thrive; vomiting; painful, progressively deformed joints; subcutaneous nodules, particularly near joints; and laryngeal involvement with hoarseness and respiratory insufficiency (276). Clinically, histocytosis is often in the differential diagnosis (80). Farber disease may present *in utero* with hydrops fetalis (187,327).

Lymph node, lung, larynx, spleen, liver, heart, subcutaneous, and periarticular nodular lipogranulomas contain PAS-positive storage in foam cells and multinucleated giant cells. Storage is also present in endothelial cells, pericytes, Schwann cells, hepatocytes, renal tubular epithelium, and glomerular visceral epithelial cells. Brain and spinal cord neurons are distended with PAS-positive ceramides and gangliosides (276). By EM, storage is membrane-bound, comma-shaped curvilinear tubular profiles, termed *banana-bodies* or *Farber bodies*, along with concentric lamellar, zebra-body, and fibrillogranular material (62). Diagnosis is confirmed by demonstration of decreased acid ceramidase activity in leukocytes, fibroblasts, or amniocytes (276).

Krabbe Disease (Galactosylceramide Lipidosis, Globoid Cell Leukodystrophy)

Autosomal recessive deficiency of galactocerebroside beta-galactosidase activity results in rapidly progressive neurological deterioration in affected infants (360). The pathology is limited largely to the nervous system (360): The brain has atrophy, myelin loss, neuronal degeneration, and gliosis. Distinctive "globoid cells" derived from monocyte-macrophage marrow stem cells are distended by PAS-positive and acid phosphatase-positive undigested psychosine (galactosylsphingosine), and galactosylceramide and accumulate in white matter and perivascular spaces; gray matter is generally less affected (360). Psychosine accumulation causes oligodendroglia destruction (80). By EM, storage comprises electron-dense, straight or curved, hollow tubular profiles in longitudinal section with crystalloid profiles in cross section (Figure 5-13A,B) (360). Peripheral nerves have endoneural fibrosis, demyelination, and infiltration of PAS-positive macrophages, similar to CNS globoid cells (360). Storage also occurs in sweat gland epithelium (360). Diagnosis is based on identifying galactocerebroside beta-galactosidase deficiency in leukocytes, fibroblasts, amniotic, or chorionic villous cells.

Cystinosis

In cystinosis, cystine accumulates because of defective transport of cystine out of lysosomes into the cytoplasm. This transport defect is due to an autosomal recessively inherited deficiency of cystinosin, a lysosomal membrane protein (97,228). Of the several forms of cystinosis, the most severe, nephropathic cystinosis, presents in the 1st year of life with Fanconi syndrome, rickets, photophobia, and short stature and can result in renal failure if untreated (80).

Rectangular, rhomboid, or polymorphic cystine crystals accumulate in lysosomes in most tissues, particularly in the fixed tissue macrophage system in liver, marrow, kidney, liver, lung, pancreas, intestine, appendix, spleen, conjunctiva, cornea, retina, lymph nodes, thyroid, thymus, muscle, brain, gingiva, and placenta (Figure 5-14) (9,80,97). The crystals are apparent in unfixed frozen or alcohol-fixed tissue examined with polarized light (80), which gives them a brilliant silvery birefringence (300). Kidney is the most severely affected organ, and cystine crystals may be present in interstitial, glomerular, and tubular cells (80). A "swan neck" deformity with atrophy of proximal tubule segments adjacent to cystine-containing interstitial cells is seen early in the disease. Progressive interstitial fibrosis and inflammation with tubular atrophy is associated with end-stage renal failure. Other organs also are affected, particularly after renal transplantation. Hepatomegaly is not associated with significant liver dysfunction. Perivenular Kupffer cells accumulate refractile crystals in clusters, and spaces left by crystals can be seen by EM. Pancreatic endocrine and exocrine insufficiency is due to long-standing cystine accumulation. Skeletal muscle fiber atrophy, ring fibers, and cystine crystals in endomysial cells lead to a myopathy (97). CNS involvement may cause nonobstructive hydrocephalus, demyelination, and cystic necrosis with calcification and spongy change (97). Diagnosis is based on the presence of ophthalmologic demonstration of cystine crystals; identification of cystine crystals in bone marrow, cornea, fixed tissue macrophages, or amniocytes; and measurement of leukocyte or fibroblast cystine content (97).

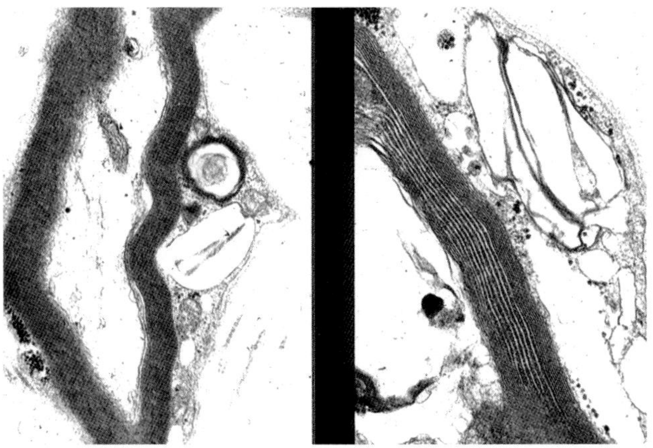
A

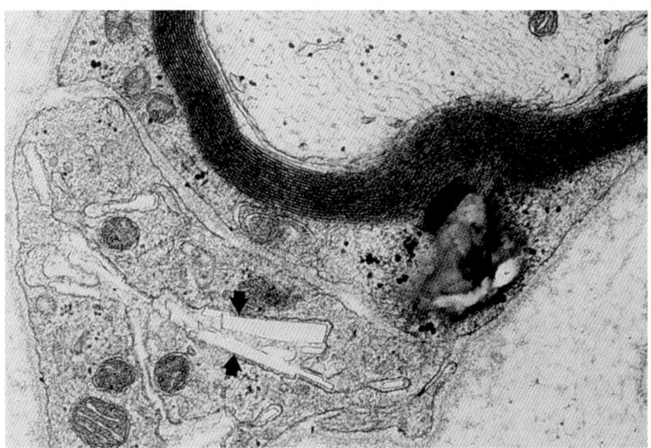
B

FIGURE 5-13■ **Krabbe disease. A,B:** Electron-lucent, angulated, and needle-shaped inclusions in conjunctival myelinated nerve Schwann cells, characteristic of Krabbe disease. (**A,B:** Uranyl acetate, lead citrate; **B:** Used from *American Journal of Medical Genetics*, with permission.)

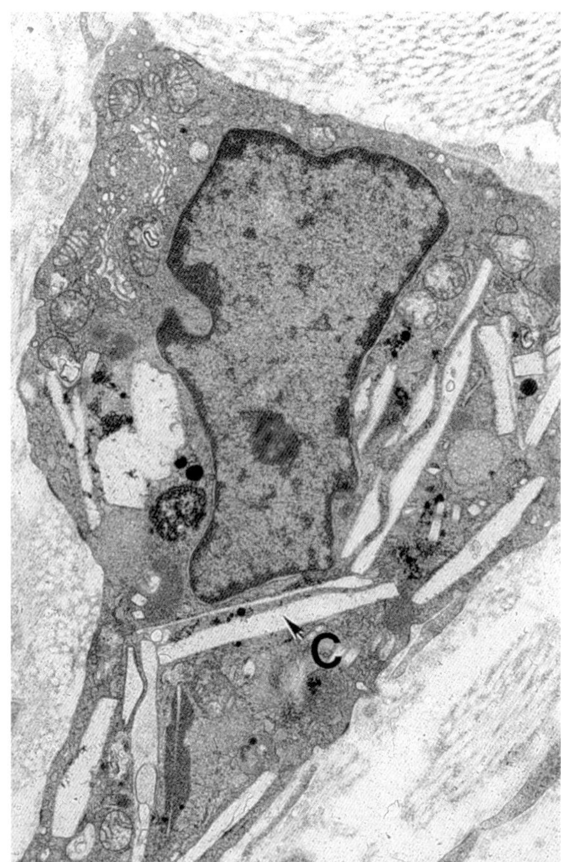

FIGURE 5-14 ▪ **Cystinosis.** Electron-lucent, pleomorphic, polygonal, and rectilinear cystine crystals (C) in dermal macrophage from a 22-year-old with cystinosis. (Uranyl acetate, lead citrate; Usedfrom *American Journal of Medical Genetics*, with permission.)

AMINOACIDOPATHIES

In these disorders, amino acid catabolism is blocked because of an enzyme deficiency with resultant accumulation of a specific amino acid (80).

Phenylketonuria (PKU, hyperphenylalaninemia) is usually due to a mutation in the gene encoding for hepatic phenylalanine hydroxylase (PAH), which converts phenylalanine to tyrosine. Both deficient PAH and exposure to dietary phenylalanine are necessary for expression of the phenotype (313). The biochemical consequence is accumulation of phenylalanine and its metabolites and a relative deficiency of tyrosine, which becomes an essential amino acid in PKU patients (112,231). Clinical features are the result of tyrosine deficiency and elevated phenylalanine (313). The main clinical effect is in the brain with microcephaly, severe mental retardation, seizures, and progressive motor dysfunction. Affected patients have a mousy odor, eczema, and light skin and hair due to deficiency of tyrosine, a precursor of melanin. A strictly reduced phenylalanine diet begun in infancy can prevent severe neurological damage, although treated patients may have a lower IQ, neuropsychological or neurological abnormalities, and abnormal cerebral white matter; adults who relax their diet may have motor or cognitive decline (112). Some patients respond to treatment with BH_4, the cofactor for PAH, with reduction of phenylalanine levels, allowing a less restricted diet.

Pregnant women with PKU must keep phenylalanine concentrations low to prevent toxic embryopathy/fetopathy. Microcephaly, callosal hypoplasia, mental retardation, growth restriction, and heart malformations (aortic coarctation with hypoplastic left heart syndrome, tetralogy of Fallot, patent ductus arteriosus) are seen in heterozygous infants of PKU mothers with hyperphenylalaninemia during pregnancy (313).

Some patients with hyperphenylalaninemia have a milder form of PKU with residual PAH activity; they may not require dietary therapy or may only need general protein restriction. However, even women with mild PKU need to keep phenylalanine levels in a safe range for the fetus during pregnancy.

The brain injury in untreated PKU patients is secondary to phenylalanine accumulation in blood (which increases brain phenylalanine), combined with deficiency of other large neutral amino acids (especially tyrosine and methionine). This results in abnormal brain protein synthesis, myelin turnover, and biogenic amine neurotransmission (112). Untreated patients have variable white matter alterations with spongiosis, delayed myelination or demyelination, focal myelin pallor, or breakdown with deposition of neutral fat, gliosis, and neuronal loss. Diagnosis is based on blood phenylalanine level. MS/MS has recently become the main method of screening for PKU (80).

PKU variants are caused by deficiency of the PAH cofactor tetrahydrobiopterin (BH4), due to one of several defects in the biosynthesis or recycling of BH4. These patients respond to oral BH4 treatment with normalization of serum phenylalanine. BH4 is also a cofactor for tyrosine and tryptophan hydroxylases and nitric oxide synthase (112), and BH4 deficiency results in neurotransmitter deficiencies, in addition to hyperphenylalaninemia. These patients also need treatment for their CNS dopamine and serotonin deficiencies, with L-dopa and 5-hydroxytryptophan, respectively, as well as carbidopa, since BH4 does not adequately cross the blood-brain barrier. Deficiencies of GTP cyclohydrolase I (GTPCH), 6-pyruvoyltetrahydropterin synthase (PTPS), dihydropteridine reductase (DHPR), and pterin-4a-carbinolamine dehydratase (PCD) have been described. GTPCH and PTPS are involved in synthesis of BH4 from GTP, and DHPR and PCD are involved in recycling BH4. Patients with DHPR deficiency also need folinic acid supplementation. All newborns with hyperphenylalaninemia should be screened for these less common disorders by testing for abnormal urine pterins and DHPR enzyme activity on a dried blood spot.

Tyrosinemia Type I (Hepatorenal Tyrosinemia, Congenital Tyrosinosis)

This autosomal recessive trait due to deficient or defective fumarylacetoacetate hydrolase (FAH), the last enzyme of tyrosine degradation, is due to one of a number of mutations at 15q23-q25. Tyrosine degradation by FAH normally primarily occurs in hepatocytes and renal tubular epithelium (132,273). Tyrosinemia I has an incidence of approximately 1/100,000 with an increased prevalence in French Canadians. Symptoms vary, but, in general, the earlier the presentation, the worse the prognosis (336). Patients may have failure to thrive; a distinctive boiled cabbage or fishy odor; hepatomegaly, and acute liver failure, cirrhosis, renal Fanconi syndrome, rickets, proteinuria, and peripheral neuropathy; hepatocellular carcinoma may develop as early as 15 months of age (145,273).

Liver, kidney, and peripheral nerve damage result from tyrosine degradation products fumarylacetoacetate and maleylacetoacetate that may act as alkylating agents, disrupt sulfhydryl metabolism, and inhibit transport function (146,273). In the chronic form of tyrosinemia I, symptoms develop later and are less severe but include mental retardation, rickets, and hepatocellular carcinoma.

Liver lesions can begin *in utero*. The liver is generally enlarged with sharply demarcated regenerative nodules with variegated colors, ranging from yellow to deep green. Microscopically, zones of hepatocellular collapse, cirrhosis, steatosis, intracanalicular and ductal cholestasis, cholangiolar proliferation, pseudoacinar transformation, and giant cell change are seen. Alpha fetoprotein is demonstrable in hepatocytes in cirrhotic areas. Sinusoidal collagen deposition is often present and may be prominent (228). Dysplasia, adenomas, and hepatocellular carcinoma can be seen (Figure 5-15) (80,121,228,273,300). Hepatocellular carcinoma occurs in a third of patients who survive beyond 2 years of age, may occur as early as the 1st year of life, and may be accompanied by normal or increased alpha fetoprotein level (100,300). Transplantation by 2 years of age is recommended by some to prevent carcinoma (147). Iron accumulates in hepatocytes and Kupffer cells and other organs including spleen, pancreas, thyroid, and peritracheal mucous glands. Kidneys are enlarged, with cortical tubular ectasia, tubular calcification, glomerulosclerosis, interstitial nephritis, and fibrosis. Half of affected patients have islet hyperplasia, but hypoglycemia is unusual. Hypertrophic obstructive cardiomyopathy is also described (230). Axonal degeneration with demyelination similar to that seen in porphyrias occurs, and a third of patients have white matter spongiosis (80,228,273,300,310).

Diagnosis is based on increased levels of succinylacetone in dried blood samples, plasma, or urine (148,228,273). FAH can be assayed in lymphocytes, fibroblasts, or liver. Demonstration of two mutant alleles known to cause FAH deficiency confirms the diagnosis.

Treatment includes phenylalanine and tyrosine dietary restriction and liver transplantation. Treatment with the herbicide 2-(2-nitro-4-trifluoromethylbenzoyl)-1,3 cyclohexanedione (NTBC), which blocks tyrosine's degradative pathway and prevents accumulation of maleylacetoacetate and fumarylacetoacetate, may improve liver and renal function and reduce mortality from liver failure.

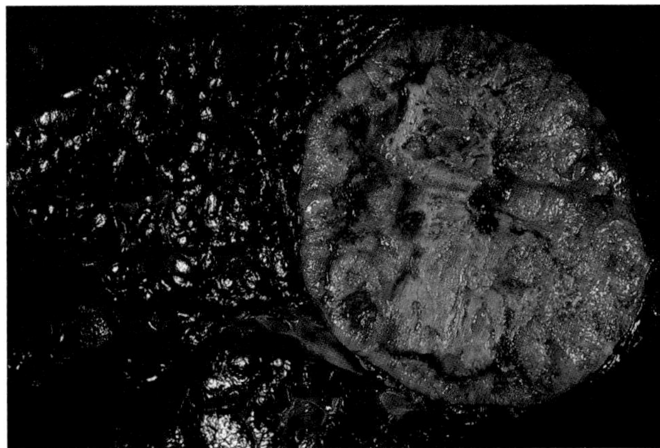

FIGURE 5-15 **Tyrosinemia.** Hepatocellular carcinoma in liver from a young child with tyrosinemia.

Its impact on the risk of hepatocellular carcinoma is uncertain (80,120,149,273).

Tyrosinemia Type II (Oculocutaneous Tyrosinemia, Richner-Hanhart Syndrome)

Oculocutaneous tyrosinemia is due to deficient cytoplasmic tyrosine aminotransferase (237,273). Patients have palmoplantar keratosis, corneal erosions, photophobia, and variable mental retardation but no liver dysfunction. Skin shows hyperkeratosis, acanthosis, and parakeratosis (236). Conjunctival and skin biopsies may have large lipid-like inclusion bodies with filaments and myelin-like figures in epithelium, fibrocytes, and endothelium (273).

Homocystinuria

Classical homocystinuria is due to cystathionine beta-synthetase (CBS) deficiency, inherited as an autosomal recessive disorder. Affected patients have increased urine and serum homocysteine and methionine (235,277). This multisystem disorder affects eye, skeleton, liver, vessels, and CNS. Extra-CNS complications of CBS deficiency are secondary to accumulation of homocysteine (277). CNS complications may be due to the metabolic defect as well as cerebrovascular disease (112). The risk of venous (and less likely arterial) thromboembolism increases with age. Thromboemboli can occur in children, particularly with dehydration, and can be multiple and recurrent (112,234).

Ischemic lesions due to occlusive thromboemboli in veins, arteries, and the dural sinus can cause multifocal CNS infarction. Approximately 50% of untreated patients die as young adults, often due to a thromboembolic event (233). Leukoencephalopathy with focal perivascular demyelination may also occur. The liver shows zone 3 steatosis, mild to moderate periportal fibrosis, and portal arteriole thickening with intimal hyperplasia. By EM, liver mitochondria are pleomorphic, and there are increased smooth endoplasmic reticulum and pericanalicular lysosomes (112). Newborn screening by MS/MS for hypermethioninemia is useful in identifying patients with CBS deficiency (232).

Nonketotic Hyperglycinemia (NKH)

This is an autosomal recessive error of glycine degradation by an intramitochondrial enzyme complex. Patients have undetectable or low glycine cleavage system activity (110,112). Affected children have a broad range of phenotypes. Hypotonia, lethargy, abnormal eye movements, mental retardation, seizures, and death in the first 6 months of life occur in more severely affected patients (80,112,114). There is no ketosis or organic acid excretion, unlike with the hyperglycinemia that occurs in methylmalonic aciduria or propionic acidemia (80). Glycine accumulates in all body fluids and all tissues, including brain; it is preferentially elevated in the cerebrospinal fluid (112).

In the CNS, abnormal myelination, callosal agenesis or thinning, cerebellar hypoplasia, and gyral defects, related to abnormal neuronal migration, and spongiform myelopathy (particularly of cerebellar white matter, corticospinal and optic tracts) are described (110). These CNS abnormalities are thought to reflect brain amino acid imbalance (which interferes with myelin synthesis) or increased spinal fluid glycine (which may impair neuronal function) (113). Liver may be steatotic, and skeletal muscle may have intranuclear filamentous inclusions and abnormal mitochondria (2).

The diagnosis is suggested by a cerebrospinal fluid/plasma glycine concentration ratio of greater than 0.08 (55). Confirmation is based on measurement of glycine cleavage system activity in liver (53). The normal hyperglycinuria in newborns makes measurement of the urine glycine not useful for diagnosis (55).

Maple Syrup Urine Disease (MSUD, Branched-Chain Ketoaciduria)

This autosomal recessive disorder is due to a mutation in a gene encoding any subunit of the α-ketoacid dehydrogenase complex (69). Branched-chain amino acids (leucine, isoleucine, and valine) accumulate in plasma. MSUD is the most common inborn error of metabolism among Mennonites; in some communities, MSUD occurs in approximately 1 in 176 newborns. In non-Mennonites, the incidence is 1 in 185,000 (20,69). In the classical phenotype, neonates present in the 1st days of life with poor feeding, alternating hyper- and hypotonia, ketoacidosis, seizures, and sudden unexpected death. Less severe, later-onset forms also occur (55).

Sotolone imparts a maple syrup, burnt sugar, or curry odor to urine, sweat, and saliva (20,29,55). Brain abnormalities include edema, astrocytosis, and delayed myelination without myelin destruction. Gray matter is unaffected. Loss of cerebellar granule cell layer has been described (20,55). The liver contains increased glycogen (43). Evaluation of plasma amino acids with MS/MS, urine organic acids measurement, and leukocyte or fibroblast branched-chain ketoacid decarboxylase measurement can provide the diagnosis.

CARBOHYDRATE METABOLISM ABNORMALITIES

Galactosemia

Affected patients have deficiency of one of three enzymes that convert galactose to glucose (99,130). Deficiency of erythrocyte galactose-1-phosphate uridyl transferase (GALT), galactokinase (GALK), or uridine diphosphate galactose-4-epimerase (GALE) can cause galactosemia. Newborn screening is usually aimed at identifying the classical form, due to decreased GALT, and characterized by toxic accumulation of galactose, galactose-1-phosphate, and galactitol that damage liver, kidneys, and lungs. A number of mutations have been identified; incidence is 1/35,000; and the disease shows autosomal recessive inheritance (29). Severe disease clinically mimics hereditary fructose intolerance but follows galactose feeding, usually after milk, and is characterized by feeding intolerance, failure to thrive, vomiting, diarrhea, lethargy, hypotonia, jaundice, and hypoglycemia (64). Galactosemia can present with sepsis (often with *E. coli*) due to depressed neutrophil function (64,99).

Cataracts, caused by galactitol accumulation in the lens, are typical at presentation but are mild and may be detected only by slit lamp examination in the first few weeks of life (29,69,121,130). Hemolysis, coagulopathy, aminoaciduria, proteinuria, and renal failure occur (43). Extensive liver damage may be prevented or reversed by a galactose-free diet, though CNS complications may not be avoided by dietary restriction (65,99). Patients may have serious long-term neurological complications such as tremor and ataxia, possibly due to endogenous galactose production (130). Hypergonadotrophic hypogonadism and ovarian failure with amenorrhea and delayed puberty occur in females.

In infants with galactosemia, the liver is enlarged and yellow with panlobular macrovesicular steatosis, followed by periportal ductular reaction with bile-plugged cholangioles surrounded by acute inflammation. The early liver lesions resemble those of hereditary fructose intolerance (29). By 1 to 1½ months of age, pseudoacinar transformation of hepatic plates occurs, and hepatocytes surround dilated canaliculi that may contain bile. Extramedullary hematopoiesis and iron deposition may be prominent. Fibrosis, apparent as early as 2 weeks of age, progresses to cirrhosis by 3 to 6 months. In some cases, giant cell transformation and regenerative or dysplastic nodules occur (63,99). The most severe hepatic abnormalities occur during episodes of sepsis; endotoxin may contribute to liver injury (121). Pancreatic islets are hyperplastic, and vacuolization of renal tubular epithelium (similar to that seen in hereditary fructose intolerance and tyrosinemia) is accompanied by tubular dilatation and necrosis. Ovarian histology in ovarian failure is variable: oocytes may be absent or reduced in number (42,130).

Diagnosis may be suspected if non–glucose-reducing substances are present in urine, although this test is neither sensitive nor specific (69). Diagnosis of classical galactosemia is based on red cell GALT assay (65) and can only be done if red cells have not been transfused in the last 3 months. GALK and GALE deficiencies can be identified by newborn screening if galactose is measured on a blood spot, and specific enzyme assays then confirm the diagnosis (69).

Hereditary Fructose Intolerance (HFI)

Deficiency of fructose-1-phosphate aldolase (fructoaldolase B), inherited as an autosomal recessive disorder, leads to fructose-1-phosphate accumulation. This toxic substrate damages liver, kidney, and brain, and inhibits glycogenolysis and gluconeogenesis, resulting in hypoglycemia, phosphate sequestration, and ATP depletion (65). It has been proposed that acute lesions in HFI are due to ATP depletion and osmotic effects of fructose-1-phosphate accumulation (60). Fructose-1,6-diphosphatase deficiency can cause a similar inhibition of gluconeogenesis with fructose- and fasting-induced hypoglycemia (65).

Symptoms develop when fructose in fruits and some vegetables or sucrose in candy is introduced into the diet, and clinical improvement occurs if fructose, sorbitol, and sucrose are withdrawn from the diet (65,99). Older children with HFI may avoid sweet foods (65,99). Liver, kidney, and intestine are affected; symptoms vary but include failure to thrive, vomiting, hepatomegaly, coagulopathy, and renal failure with renal tubular acidosis, aminoaciduria, and proteinuria. Acute liver failure may occur if fructose or sucrose is ingested in the newborn period.

Liver lesions resemble those of neonatal hepatitis and galactosemia with giant cell transformation, steatosis (Figure 5-16), ductular proliferation, cholestasis, and portal fibrosis. Acute hepatic necrosis with little inflammation may be seen in the acute phase (63). Progression to cirrhosis with portal hypertension, ascites, and splenomegaly occurs but is rare (60,65,99). Older infants may have less severe liver damage with variable steatosis and portal fibrosis (63). By EM, characteristic but not pathognomonic changes include "fructose holes" in hepatocytes: lucent spaces with sparse glycogen and membranous arrays surrounded by a single membrane. These lesions may result from dilated degranulated rough endoplasmic reticulum and relate to intracellular accumulation of enzyme substrate or ATP depletion (65). Pancreatic islet hyperplasia is seen, and, in kidney, proximal tubule epithelium is granular and vacuolated with slight tubule dilatation (116).

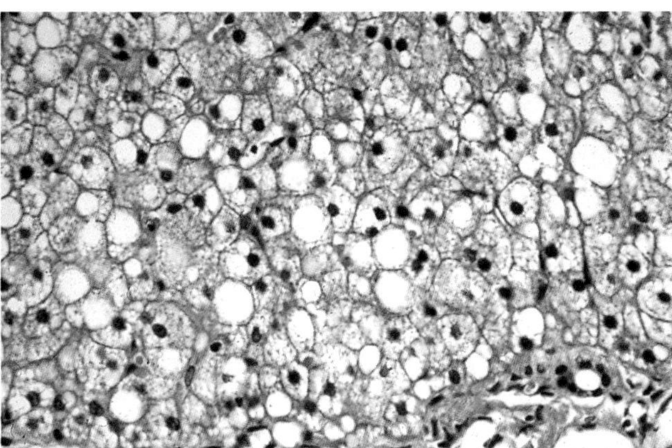

FIGURE 5-16 **Hereditary fructose intolerance.** In hereditary fructose intolerance, the liver shows microvesicular and macrovesicular steatosis. The histologic appearance of the liver can also resemble neonatal hepatitis with giant cell transformation, ductular proliferation, cholestasis, fibrosis, and necrosis (not shown here) (H&E).

Hypophosphatemia, metabolic acidosis, and elevated transaminases are typical but not diagnostic (99). Fructose tolerance test is not recommended for diagnosis because of potential danger to the patient. Analysis of leukocyte DNA for the aldolase B gene is generally performed first, and, if DNA is normal, measurement of aldolase B activity in liver or intestinal tissue can be done (99,116).

Glycogen Storage Diseases (GSD)

Glycogen catabolism is an important energy source. The many forms of GSD are generally associated with glycogen accumulation and deficiency of an enzyme important in glycogen synthesis or degradation (Table 5-13) (18,64,67). Many organs, including liver, heart and skeletal muscle, kidney, erythrocytes, and intestine, are affected by GSD (67). GSD can cause muscle fatigue, cramps, progressive weakness, rhabdomyolysis, hypoglycemia, acidosis, failure to thrive, or hepatomegaly. Overall incidence is approximately 1/20,000 (18). The various GSD have specific treatments, so early identification of an enzyme defect is important (67,99).

Subtle differences in liver morphology in GSD have been described (82) but, in general, pathological features are clearly distinctive in only a few GSD, such as the light microscopic findings in GSD IV and the ultrastructural appearance of hepatocytes in GSD II and IV (64,99). In general, hepatocytes are enlarged with clear or vacuolated cytoplasm (67) and resemble plant cells in that cell membranes appear thick, due to peripheral displacement of organelles by glycogen. Cytoplasm is PAS-positive and diastase digestible. Some glycogen is lost due to its water solubility with formalin fixation; optimal glycogen preservation can be achieved by alcohol fixation or by using fresh frozen tissue. Nuclei may be glycogenated, particularly in types I and III; types VI and IX typically do not have glycogenated nuclei (64). Increased collagen in Disse's space occurs in GSD I, III, IV, VI, and IX. By EM, cytoplasmic glycogen pools in hepatocytes, and variably sized lipid droplets occur in most GSD but are particularly abundant in GSD I, II, and VI (60,99).

GSD 0 is not true a GSD but is an autosomal recessive deficiency of glycogen synthase that results in ketotic hypoglycemia without hepatomegaly or muscle symptoms (132). Steatosis and a slight decrease in liver glycogen content with normal glycogen structure are seen (29,94,99,132).

GSD I, von Gierke disease. In classical GSD I, GSD Ia, glucose-6-phosphatase enzyme complex in endoplasmic reticulum is defective, and diagnosis is based on glycogen

Table 5-13 ■ GLYCOGEN STORAGE DISEASES

Type	Eponym	Clinical	Tissues Affected	Enzyme Deficient
O		Fasting ketotic hypoglycemia, short stature, osteopenia, without hepatomegaly or weakness	Liver	Glycogen synthase
I	von Gierke 1a and 1b (non-a)	Ia-most severe of GSD, recurrent hypoglycemia, hepatomegaly, nephromegaly, proteinuria, muscle atrophy, failure to thrive, xanthomas, 1b also has recurrent bacterial infections	Liver, kidney, hepatic adenoma, hepatocellular carcinoma (1b: neutropenia, inflammatory bowel disease)	1a-glucose-6-phosphatase 1b-glucose-6-phosphatase translocase
II	Pompe	Hypotonia, cardiomyopathy, hepatomegaly	Muscle, heart, CNS, lymphocytes, liver, kidney, adrenal	Alpha-1,4-glucosidase (acid maltase)
III	Forbe, Cori, limit dextrinosis	Hypotonia, hypoglycemia, ketosis, growth failure, infections, hepatosplenomegaly, cardiomyopathy	Muscle, heart, liver, WBC	Amylo-1,6-glucosidase, 4-alpha-glucanotransferase (debrancher enzyme)
IV	Amylopectinosis, Andersen	Hepatosplenomegaly, cirrhosis, muscle wasting, gastroenteritis, osteoporosis, cardiomyopathy, hydrops	Liver, heart, muscle, CNS, PNS	Amylo (1,4-1,6) transglucosidase (brancher enzyme)
V	McArdle	Exercise intolerance, cramps, fatigue, myoglobinuria	Muscle	Muscle myophosphorylase
VI	Hers	Growth retardation, hepatomegaly, hypoglycemia	Liver	Hepatic phosphorylase
VII	Tarui	Exercise intolerance, cramps, fatigue myoglobinuria	Muscle, hemolytic anemia	Phosphofructokinase
IX		Exercise intolerance, stiffness, weakness, includes GSD VIII and X	Liver, heart, blood cells, muscle	Phosphorylase kinase complex
XI	Fanconi-Bickel	Hepatorenal glycogen accumulation,	Liver and kidney	Glucose transporter 2 (GLUT2)

CNS, central nervous system; PNS, peripheral nervous system; WBC, white blood cell.

quantitation and glucose-6-phosphatase analysis. In GSD Ib, glucose-6-phosphatase is normal, but a defect in glucose-6-phosphatase translocase transporter protein results in failure of enzyme transport (29). Patients with GSD Ia present in infancy with hepatomegaly, recurrent ketotic hypoglycemia with acidosis, hyperuricemia, hyperlipidemia, seizures, liver failure, and failure to thrive. Truncal obesity, short stature, aminoaciduria, phosphaturia, muscle atrophy, and a bleeding tendency due to hypoglycemia-induced platelet dysfunction are also described (29,99). Patients with Type 1b additionally have neutropenia and impaired neutrophil function, with recurrent bacterial infections and oral and intestinal mucosal ulcerations indistinguishable from Crohn disease (18,64,99,133).

In GSD Ia, liver involvement is prominent with uniformly increased hepatocellular glycogen, nuclear glycogenation, and steatosis with small and medium-sized lipid droplets (Figure 5-17A to D). In the GSD 1b liver, minimal or no nuclear glycogenation is seen, unlike in GSD Ia (Figure 5-17E,F) (29). Sinusoids are compressed by distended hepatocytes (60,64). Mallory bodies and zone 3 and periportal fibrosis have been reported (Figure 5-17C) (60). Focal nodular hyperplasia, adenomas (often multiple with atypical cytologic features including dysplasia and hepatocellular carcinoma), may occur in patients with GSD 1a, particularly with the G727T mutation (Figure 5-17G,H). Adenomas may arise because of glucagon stimulation and can regress if hypoglycemia is reduced with diet (29). They are more common in boys than girls and are seen as early as 3 years of age (99). Hepatoblastomas have also been described in GSD I (29).

Nephromegaly, increased glycogen in tubular epithelium, focal segmental glomerulosclerosis, and interstitial fibrosis occur in GSD 1. Nephrocalcinosis relates to hypercalcuria due to tubular acidosis (29). Xanthomas and chronic pancreatitis may reflect hyperlipidemia (29).

GSD II is included above in the section on LSD.

GSD III (Cori-Forbe disease, Forbe disease, limit dextrinosis) patients have amylo-1,6-glucosidase,4-alpha-glucanotransferase (debrancher enzyme) deficiency, which can be measured in liver, fibroblasts, skin, or lymphocytes (29,111). This clinically and genetically heterogeneous disorder has symptoms similar but less severe than those seen in GSD I. Progressive weakness may be the predominant

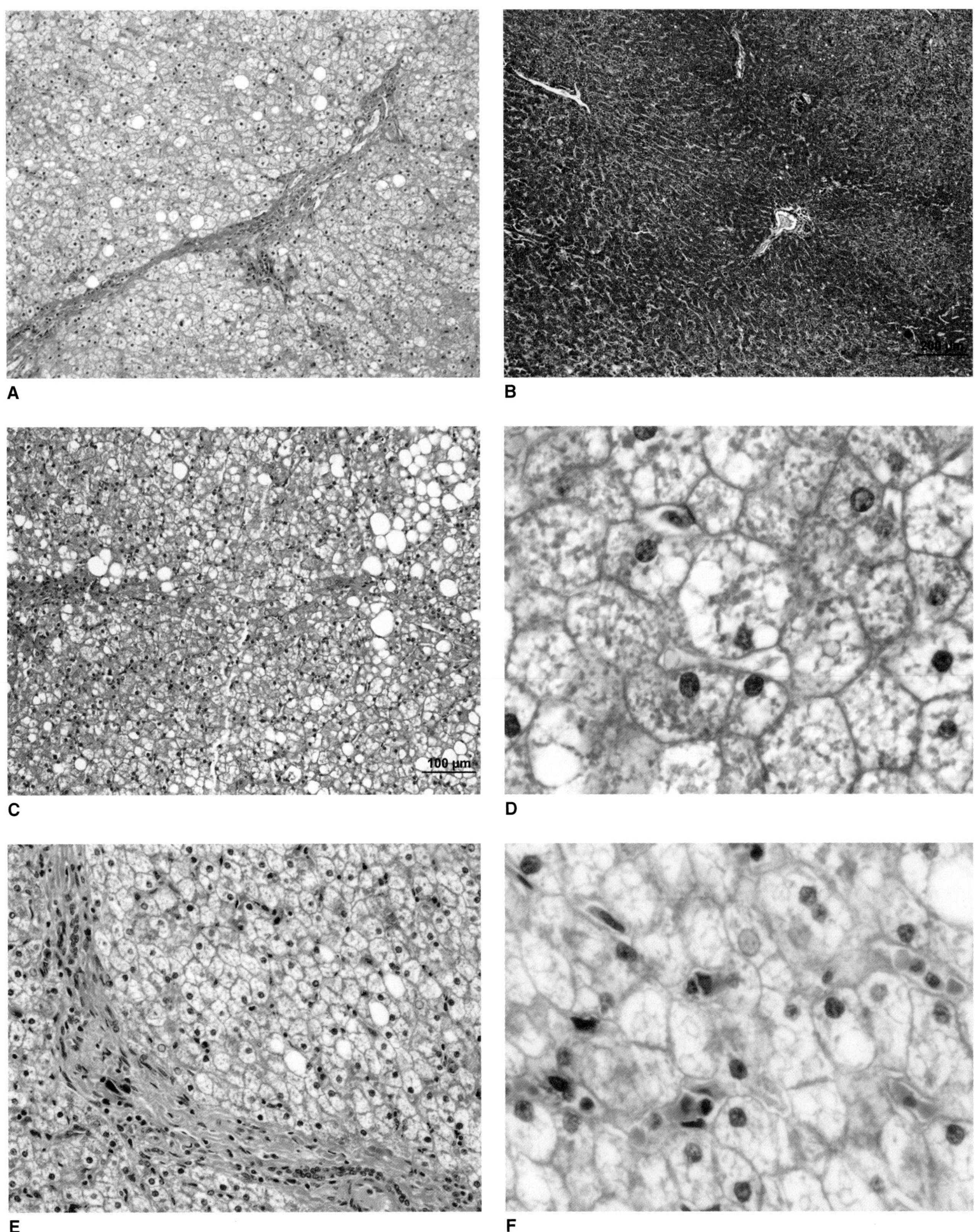

FIGURE 5-17 ■ **Glycogen storage disease, type I. A:** The liver in type I glycogen storage disease shows diffuse steatosis with hepatocyte distension obscuring sinusoids (H&E). **B:** Despite diffuse hepatocellular involvement, the liver in type I disease shows little (if any) fibrosis (trichrome). **C,D:** In type Ia disease, the liver shows steatosis (**C**) and hepatocellular Mallory's hyaline (**D**); note the presence of glycogenated nuclei (**C**), typical of type Ia disease (H&E). **E,F:** This example of type Ib disease shows steatosis and occasional pigment-laden macrophages (H&E).

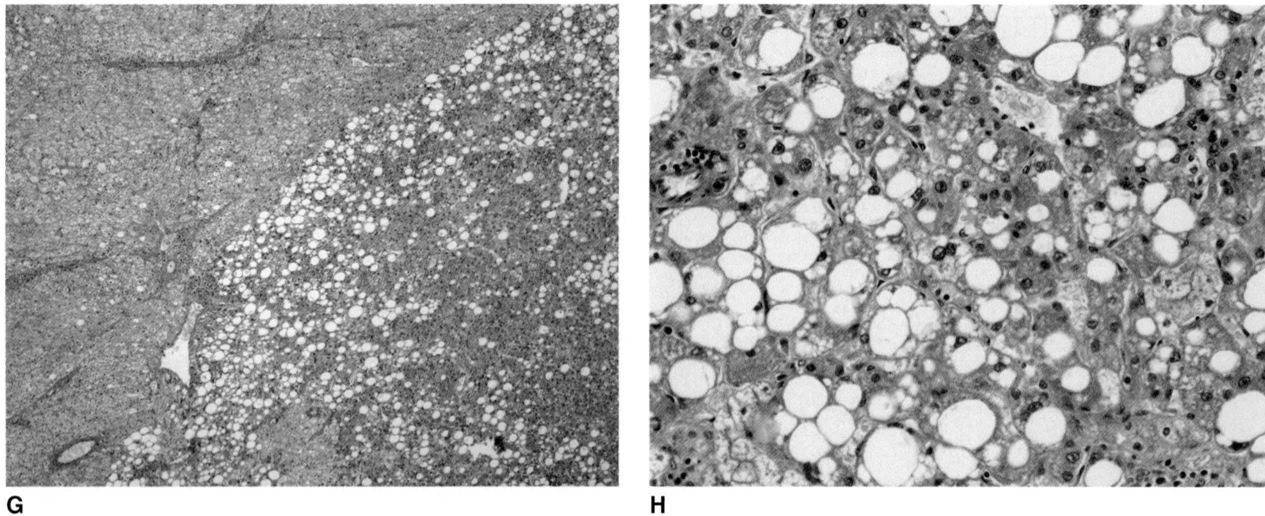

FIGURE 5-17 ■ *(continued)* **G,H:** Patients with type I GSD are at increased risk for the development of hepatocellular adenoma (with varying degrees of dysplasia), which can evolve into hepatocellular carcinoma. In (**G**), the interface between the hepatocellular adenoma (**lower right**) and nonneoplastic liver (**upper left**) is shown; in (**H**), the cells of the adenoma show dysplastic cytologic features (H&E).

feature in adults, and cardiomyopathy occurs in some patients (29). Liver failure can occur, though liver function often improves with age (18,29). GSD IIIa has liver and muscle involvement; GSD IIIb has liver involvement only; and GSD IIIc is an isolated muscle disease (111).

If restricted to muscle, enzyme assay of muscle is required for diagnosis. Muscle biopsy may show slight fiber size variation with little vacuolization or increased glycogen. Some patients have vacuolar myopathy with glycogen accumulation at the periphery of fibers (31). Liver has delicate reticular septal fibrosis or, less commonly, micronodular or mixed cirrhosis, and glycogenated nuclei can occur (67). Hepatic adenomas occur in up to 25% of GSD III patients, but hepatocellular carcinoma is rare (60,65,99).

GSD IV (Andersen disease, branching enzyme deficiency, amylopectinosis). Amylo (1,4-1,6) transglucosidase (brancher enzyme) deficiency can be identified in liver, muscle, leukocytes, and fibroblasts (29). Abnormally long, relatively insoluble amylopectin-like glycogen chains with reduced branch points accumulate in all tissues, particularly liver, skeletal muscle, and heart (46,64). GSD IV is autosomal recessive, and there are multiple mutations causing the enzyme deficiency, reflected in clinical variability (99). Infants may appear normal or have nonimmune hydrops and failure to thrive. In classical GSD IV, hepatomegaly occurs in the first months of life and progresses to cirrhosis and liver failure without hypoglycemia by 2 to 5 years (46,61,72). A neonatal neuromuscular form has been identified, and some infants present with dilated cardiomyopathy and arthrogryposis. Later-onset nonprogressive hepatic disease with hypotonia and cardiomyopathy may also occur (110).

The liver is tan with a waxy or a tough leathery consistency and tiny nodules that may aggregate into larger nodules (61). The liver resembles that seen in Lafora disease but with progression to fibrosis and cirrhosis. Only rarely do hepatic neoplasms occur with GSD IV (65). Pericellular fibrosis encircles clusters of hepatocytes with round or oval ground-glass intracytoplasmic inclusions primarily in periportal hepatocytes (Figure 5-18A). These PAS-positive, diastase-resistant inclusions stain green with colloidal iron; stain either brown, blue, or not at all with Lugol's iodine; are removed by pectinase or alpha-amylase; and have an artifactual space around them (60,65,99). By EM, inclusions are non–membrane-bound with undulating random delicate fibrils up to 5 nm in diameter surrounded by glycogen rosettes (65). Similar inclusions are seen in heart, skeletal muscle, skin, CNS neurons, and lymph node macrophages (Figure 5-18B) (29,46,61,65).

GSD V, McArdle disease is due to autosomal recessive inherited myophosphorylase deficiency. Children with GSD V typically have exercise intolerance, and this disease rarely presents as respiratory failure in infancy (29,111). Patients have no rise in lactic acid after ischemic exercise. By LM, muscle may appear normal or may have mild alterations, with occasional degenerating fibers and subsarcolemmal glycogen-containing vacuoles. EM highlights subsarcolemmal and sarcoplasmic glycogen, and histochemically demonstrable myophosphorylase activity is absent (31).

GSD VI, Hers disease due to hepatic phosphorylase deficiency is a relatively benign autosomal recessive disorder that causes hypoglycemia and growth failure. The disease improves with age: hepatomegaly decreases after puberty, and adults are typically asymptomatic (99). A nonuniform mosaic pattern of distended hepatocytes without nuclear glycogenation is accompanied by mild fibrosis and steatosis (Figure 5-19). Heart and skeletal muscle are not altered.

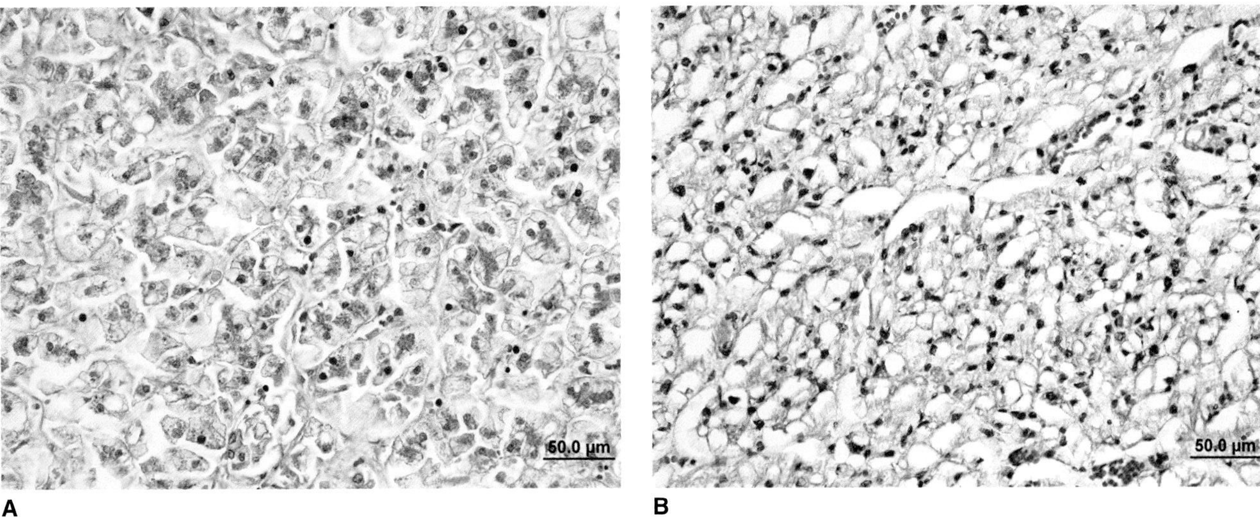

FIGURE 5-18 ■ **Glycogen storage disease, type IV. A:** In type IV disease, hepatocytes are enlarged with ground glass cytoplasmic inclusions (H&E). **B:** Skeletal muscle involvement in type IV disease, with rarefaction of myofibers due to non–membrane-bound glycogen accumulation (H&E).

GSD VII, Tarui disease is characterized by absent phosphofructokinase activity, easy fatigability, and exercise intolerance in children. Severe infantile cases with respiratory failure also occur (18,31,49,111). Patients have hemolytic anemia due to absence of a muscle isoenzyme in red blood cells, hyperuricemia, and myoglobinuria (111). Muscle has extensive subsarcolemmal and sarcoplasmic glycogen, and a few fibers contain hyaline, PAS-positive, diastase-resistant inclusions with a filamentous fine structure resembling amylopectin. Histochemical staining suggests these are an insoluble form of glycogen (1).

GSD VIII and GSD IX have been grouped together (18), both with mutations in genes that encode subunits of phosphorylase kinase; a defect in one of the four subunits of phosphorylase kinase result in a variable clinical presentation with hepatomegaly and growth failure (18). GSD IXa is X-linked, and the autosomal recessive forms (IXb, IXc) have more severe liver disease that can progress to cirrhosis (99).

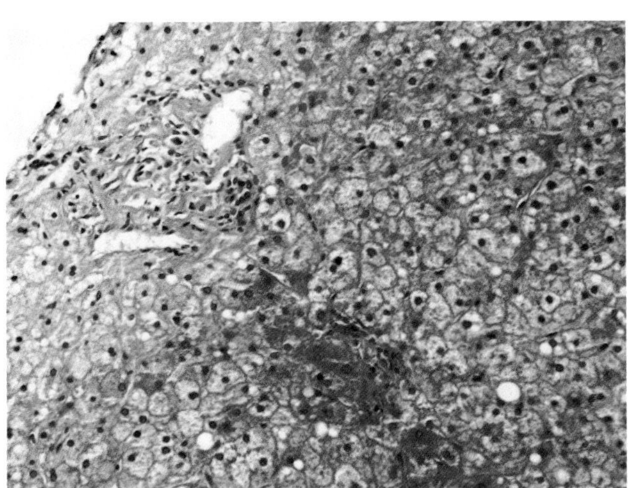

FIGURE 5-19 ■ **Glycogen storage disease, type VI.** Mosaic pattern of nondistended (lower middle) and distended hepatocytes, characteristic of type VI disease, with mild steatosis and absence of glycogenated nuclei (H&E).

GSD XI, Fanconi-Bickel patients have failure to thrive, rickets, hepatomegaly, nephromegaly, hyperglycemia when not fasting, glucosuria, and aminoaciduria. Hepatorenal glycogen accumulation is secondary to nonfunctional glucose transport due to a mutation in the *GLUT2* gene.

FATTY ACID OXIDATION DEFECTS

A number of enzymes and transporters are involved in intramitochondrial fatty acid oxidation (FAO), and defects in these pathways lead to a heterogeneous group of disorders (32). Inherited disorders of fatty acid transport and mitochondrial oxidation can present with acute liver failure and sudden unexpected death in children (Tables 5-14 and 5-15) (64).

Acyl-CoA Dehydrogenase Deficiencies

Before beta-oxidation of fatty acids occurs, fatty acids must be converted first to their coenzyme A (CoA) thioesters. This conversion is catalyzed by acyl-CoA dehydrogenases, of which there are at least four types—classified based on chain lengths as short-, medium-, long-, and very-long-chain synthetases. Any of these four forms of acyl-CoA dehydrogenases can be deficient, and these deficiencies are the most frequently identified abnormalities of FAO (32). Where known, inheritance is autosomal recessive.

In general, patients with acyl-CoA dehydrogenase deficiency have hypoketotic hypoglycemia, liver and skeletal muscle abnormalities, cardiomyopathy, and sudden unexpected death in childhood (63). Patients with short-chain

Table 5-14 ■ FATTY ACID OXIDATION DEFECTS

Acyl-CoA dehydrogenase deficiencies
- Medium-chain acyl-CoA dehydrogenase deficiency (MCADD, MCAD)
- Short-chain acyl-CoA dehydrogenase deficiency (SCAD)
- Long-chain hydroxylacyl-CoA dehydrogenase deficiency (LCHAD)/Trifunctional protein deficiency (TFP)
- Very-long-chain acyl-CoA dehydrogenase (VLCAD)
- Glutaric acidemia type II (Multiple acyl-CoA dehydrogenase deficiency, MADD)

Substrate Transport Defects
- Carnitine palmitoyltransferase (CPT) deficiency
  - CPT I and CPT II deficiency
- Primary systemic carnitine deficiency (carnitine transporter deficiency)
- Carnitine acylcarnitine translocase deficiency

defects may have ketotic hypoglycemia. Panlobular microvesicular or macrovesicular steatosis may disappear between crises when the patient is well (63). Fat accumulation may also be seen in the myocardium and skeletal muscle. EM shows enlarged mitochondria with increased matrical density, crystals, and widened intercristal space (64). Establishing a diagnosis may allow for successful treatment, and these disorders are included in newborn screening programs (Table 5-6) (137).

Medium-chain acyl-CoA dehydrogenase deficiency (MCADD, MCAD). Affected patients are often homozygous for the A985G mutation, and carriers are particularly common in northwest Europe (29). This is one of the most common IEM, with an incidence of 1/5–8,000; it is the most common FAO defect in central Europe (69,104). Patients present between 3 and 15 months of age with hypoketotic hypoglycemia after fasting, lethargy, vomiting, and sudden unexpected death (69). Fatal cases may resemble SIDS or Reye syndrome (69). They can also present in later life with exercise-induced muscle pain, and rhabdomyolysis, and there is marked clinical variability even in the same family.

Liver may be normal grossly or have minimal steatosis, and the heart may show lipid accumulation (16,63). Mitochondria may be enlarged with crystals, increased matrix density, and dilated cristae (63). Encephalopathy and cerebral edema are due to accumulation of fatty acids in the CNS (69). Octanoylcarnitine is elevated on plasma acylcarnitine analysis, and further confirmatory testing may include urine acylglycine analysis and molecular testing (69).

Short-chain acyl-CoA dehydrogenase deficiency (SCADD, SCAD). There are two clinical forms: (a) a myopathic form limited to muscle (with progressive weakness and exercise-induced pain) and (b) a systemic form with neonatal onset of vomiting, lethargy, acidosis, ketotic hypoglycemia, hepatomegaly, hypotonia, seizures, and microcephaly. However, the vast majority of patients with SCAD deficiency detected through newborn screening programs do not demonstrate any symptoms. There are two common mutations in the SCAD gene that are associated

Table 5-15 ■ METABOLIC CAUSES OF SUDDEN UNEXPECTED DEATH IN INFANCY

Inherited defects of fatty acid oxidation (FAO)
- Medium-chain acyl-CoA dehydrogenase deficiency (MCAD)
- Very-long-chain acyl-CoA dehydrogenase deficiency (VLCAD)
- Long-chain 3-hydroxy acyl-CoA dehydrogenase deficiency (LCHAD)/Trifunctional protein deficiency
- Glutaric acidemia type 2 (multiple acyl-CoA dehydrogenase deficiency (MADD)
- Carnitine palmitoyltransferase II deficiency (CPT II)
- Primary carnitine deficiency (carnitine transporter deficiency)
- Carnitine acylcarnitine translocase deficiency (CAT)

Hyperammonemia/urea cycle disorders
- Ornithine transcarbamylase (OTC) deficiency
- Argininosuccinate synthetase deficiency (citrullinemia)
- Argininosuccinate lyase deficiency (argininosuccinic aciduria)
- Carbamoylphosphate synthetase deficiency
- Lysinuric protein intolerance

Organic acidemias
- Methylmalonic acidemia
- Propionic acidemia
- Isovaleric acidemia
- Glutaric acidemia type 1
- 3-hydroxy-3-methyl-glutaryl-CoA lyase deficiency
- 3-methylcrotonyl-CoA carboxylase deficiency

Congenital lactic acidosis
- Pyruvate dehydrogenase deficiency
- Pyruvate carboxylase deficiency
- Phosphoenolpyruvate carboxykinase (PEPCK) deficiency

Amino acid disorders
- Maple syrup urine disease
- Tyrosinemia type 1

Carbohydrate disorders
- Galactosemia
- Glycogen storage disease type I
- Hereditary fructose intolerance
  - Fructose-1,6-bisphosphate deficiency

with mild disease. Increased lipid in muscle and liver are described (43).

Long-chain hydroxylacyl-CoA dehydrogenase deficiency (LCHADD, LCHAD) and trifunctional protein deficiency. LCHAD is part of the trifunctional protein (TFP) complex, comprising LCHAD, long-chain enoyl-CoA hydratase and long-chain beta-ketoacyl-CoA thiolase activities. Most patients have isolated LCHAD deficiency, but some are also deficient in the other two enzymes and have generalized TFP deficiency. Similar clinical and biochemical manifestations occur in affected individuals.

About 75% of LCHAD-deficient patients carry a G-to-C mutation at nucleotide position 1528 (Glu474Gln, E474Q) on both chromosomes, while up to 25% are compound heterozygotes for E474Q on one allele and a second different LCHAD mutation on the other allele. LCHAD patients have episodic nonketotic hypoglycemia, cardiomyopathy, and liver dysfunction (29,64). Infants can present with hydrops (72), cardiac involvement, coma associated with fasting, and death; a later-onset form causes myalgias with myoglobinuria.

The HELLP syndrome (hemolysis, elevated liver enzymes, and low platelet count) with hypertension can occur in mothers of fetuses with LCHAD and at least one E474Q allele. Why HELLP occurs with this mutation is not known (37). TFP deficiency is also associated with maternal HELLP syndrome. Acute fatty liver of pregnancy and prolonged hyperemesis can also occur in mothers of affected fetuses (78). The liver in LCHAD patients has bile duct proliferation, cholestasis, steatosis, fibrosis, and cirrhosis, and fat accumulates in skeletal and cardiac muscle (29,65,104).

Very-long-chain acyl-CoA dehydrogenase (VLCADD, VLCAD). Affected patients may have a lethal childhood form with early-onset, hypertrophic or dilated cardiomyopathy, and hypoglycemia (32,16). A milder childhood form with hypoglycemia and dicarboxylic aciduria is less common, and some patients resemble those with CPT II deficiency with rhabdomyolysis and myoglobinuria (32). Muscle pathology is generally mild with increased variation in fiber size and a mild increase in muscle fiber lipid (32). Bile duct proliferation, hepatic fibrosis, and cirrhosis can occur (65).

Glutaric acidemia type II (Multiple acyl-CoA dehydrogenase deficiency, MADD). Glutaric acidemia type II is caused by deficiency of the electron-accepting protein electron transfer flavoprotein (ETF) or ETF-ubiquinone oxidoreductase (ETF-QO). Patients may present in early infancy with hypotonia, hepatomegaly, sweaty feet odor, acidosis, and nonketotic hypoglycemia; death may occur in the first few weeks of life in the most severe form. Congenital anomalies include cerebral cortical dysgenesis with abnormal neuronal migration, facial dysmorphism, genital defects, and renal cystic dysplasia (Figure 5-20A) as well as irregular glomerular basement membrane can be seen (43). Later-onset disease is variable. It can present in infants with episodic vomiting, acidosis, and hypoglycemia or in adults with similar biochemical findings, hepatomegaly, and proximal myopathy. Hepatic steatosis, intracytoplasmic cholestasis, paucity of intrahepatic bile ducts, mild portal fibrosis, and hepatocellular necrosis are described (Figure 5-20B), and some patients respond to riboflavin (32,63).

Substrate Transport Defects

Carnitine palmitoyltransferase (CPT) is an enzyme that catalyzes the reaction of carnitine and long-chain fatty acyl groups for transport into mitochondria. There are two forms of this enzyme, CPT I and CPT II, associated with the outer and inner mitochondrial membranes, respectively. Either can be deficient leading to a myopathy. Most patients are males, although the defective CPT genes are on autosomes (32). Beginning in childhood, patients have recurrent myoglobinuria, often after exercise or fasting, and recurrent myalgia but no muscle cramps or intolerance to short spells of exercise. Respiratory muscles may be affected (32). Between attacks, patients are normal without weakness. CPT II deficiency can result in sudden unexpected death (16).

Muscle biopsy obtained when the patient is without symptoms may be normal or have only mild lipid accumulation. Biopsies obtained after an episode of myoglobinuria have fiber necrosis. At autopsy, fatty infiltration of myocardium, liver, kidneys, and muscle has been described (16).

Carnitine deficiency. Carnitine is an essential cofactor for transport of medium- and long-chain fatty acids across the inner mitochondrial membranes, where they undergo beta-oxidation (32). Carnitine is derived either from the diet or via biosynthesis; it is made in liver and transported to other tissues, including muscle, which has the highest concentration of free carnitine, followed by liver and heart.

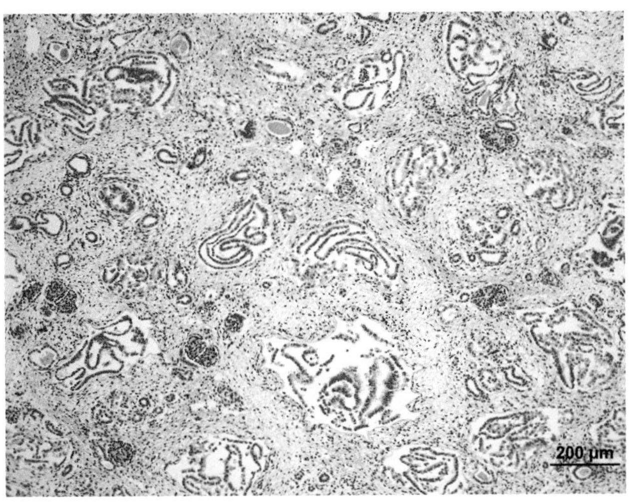

A

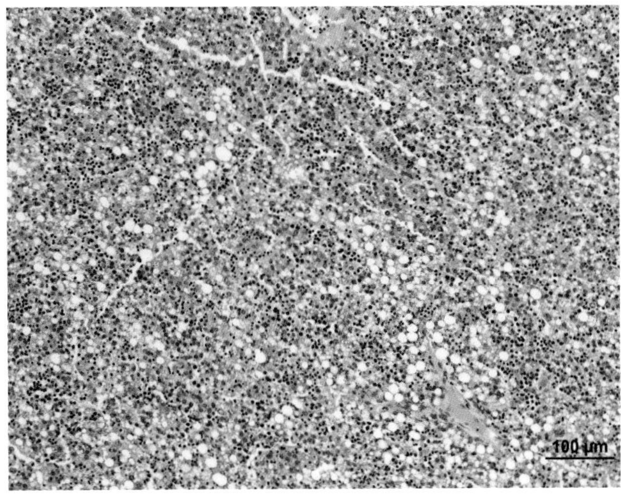

B

FIGURE 5-20 ■ **Glutaric acidemia, type II. A:** Renal dysplasia in an infant with glutaric acidemia, type II (H&E). **B:** Hepatic steatosis in glutaric acidemia, type II (as well as widespread extramedullary hematopoiesis, reflective of the patient's neonatal state) (H&E).

Decreased concentration of carnitine in skeletal muscle occurs in two biochemically and clinically distinct syndromes (32). Primary systemic carnitine deficiency (OMIM 212140), or carnitine uptake deficiency, is an autosomal recessive disorder caused by a defect in a sodium-dependent transporter protein OCTN2, which is encoded by the gene *SLC22A5*. In systemic carnitine deficiency, liver, muscle, and serum carnitine concentrations are all reduced. This disorder can present with hydrops fetalis and has been linked to sudden unexpected infant death (29). Generally, beginning in childhood, patients have muscle weakness, progressive cardiomyopathy, and recurrent acute hepatic encephalopathy with hypoglycemia, hyperammonemia, nausea, emesis, confusion, or coma. In some cases, hypoglycemia occurs with metabolic acidosis with increased lactate and ketoacids (32). Death due to cardiorespiratory failure occurs in many before 20 years of age. The muscle has severe lipid storage and panacinar microvesicular steatosis in the liver mimicking that seen in Reye syndrome. Fat may not be seen during asymptomatic periods or may be present in sinusoidal lining cells. Mild periportal fibrosis can occur (60). In some patients, there is cardiomegaly and endocardial fibroelastosis (16,32), and myocardium and renal tubular epithelium can contain increased lipid. This disorder responds very well to treatment with carnitine supplementation.

Myopathic carnitine deficiency (OMIM 212160) is an autosomal recessive disorder, associated with progressive weakness beginning in childhood. Cardiac involvement can occur (32). Carnitine is decreased in muscle but is normal or only slightly decreased in serum and liver. Lipid storage myopathy is seen with increased lipid, often adjacent to mitochondria (32).

MITOCHONDRIAL DISORDERS

The mitochondriopathies are a heterogeneous group of neuromuscular and multisystemic disorders due to altered mitochondrial metabolic function. This altered function is the result of an abnormal enzyme complex involved in energy production; patients have impaired respiratory chain function or oxidative phosphorylation. Some mitochondriopathies are inherited as autosomal dominant or recessive traits and others are maternally inherited due to mutations in mitochondrial DNA. The same molecular abnormality can cause very different clinical presentation, and even in a single family there may be a wide range of phenotypes (Table 5-16) (32). Some mitochondrial disorders affect only a single organ, while others involve multiple organ systems and have complex clinical features. Likewise, some individuals will have a distinct cluster of symptoms that fall into a specific clinical syndrome, such as Kearns-Sayre syndrome, while others will have a variety of problems that are more difficult to categorize. Nuclear gene defects are more likely to present in infancy or early childhood, while mitochondrial DNA defects often become symptomatic later in childhood or in adult life, although there are exceptions.

There are over 70 different polypeptides on the inner mitochondrial membrane that form the enzyme complexes I, II, III, IV, and V of the respiratory chain. Thirteen of these subunits are encoded by the mitochondrial DNA, but all of the rest are encoded by nuclear genes. In addition, the mitochondrial DNA encodes 22 transfer RNAs (tRNAs) and 2 ribosomal RNAs (rRNAs) that are essential for normal intramitochondrial protein synthesis. Of the 13 mitochondrial DNA-encoded polypeptides involved in the formation of the enzyme complexes, 7 are in complex I, 1 is in complex III, 3 are in complex IV, and 2 are in complex V. All of the complex II polypeptides and the remaining mitochondrial proteins are encoded by nuclear genes.

Patients with mitochondriopathies may present with ptosis, ophthalmoplegia, exercise intolerance, increased lactate level, or abnormal brain MRI. Onset may be from birth to adulthood and may be rapidly progressive or static; weakness may be generalized or proximal. There may be associated mitochondrial alterations including abnormal number or altered cristal structure (32). Secondary multiorgan damage occurs, with steatosis, cardiomyopathy, and, in the CNS, spongiosis, neuronal loss, gliosis, and demyelinization.

Subacute necrotizing encephalopathy (Leigh syndrome) can occur as a result of multiple different molecular defects (Tables 5-16 and 5-17). Brain lesions in Leigh syndrome include focal, symmetric necrotizing lesions in the brainstem and thalamus, basal ganglia, cerebellum and spinal cord with associated demyelination, astrocytosis, and vascular proliferation. Hypertrophic cardiomyopathy with concentric left ventricular hypertrophy is also associated with Leigh syndrome, and abnormal mitochondria have been described in lymphocytes in children with Leigh syndrome (43,62).

Ragged-red fibers (Figure 5-21A) may be seen with the Gomori trichrome stain in mitochondriopathies. With H&E, these fibers are basophilic and granular (Figure 5-21B); they react with NADH and may lack cytochrome oxidase activity (32). The presence of ragged-red fibers indicates ultrastructural abnormalities in mitochondria or increased number of morphologically normal mitochondria (32). Ragged-red fibers are more common in patients with mitochondrial gene mutations than nuclear gene mutations, but the number of these fibers is variable and does not correlate with phenotype (32). In some cases, ragged-red fibers are not apparent by LM (Figure 5-21C) and EM is required to see mitochondrial alterations: abnormalities in number, size, or shape; giant or bizarre mitochondria: altered cristae; or crystalline or osmiophilic intramitochondrial inclusions (Figure 5-21D to G). Such structurally abnormal mitochondria are not specific for a single clinical syndrome or molecular defect (32).

The liver in Complex IV and I deficiencies (the most common generalized enzyme deficiencies) has microvesicular and macrovesicular steatosis, cholestasis, and giant cell transformation. Portal fibrosis and cirrhosis are common. The number of hepatocyte mitochondria may be increased, and they may be pleomorphic with abnormal cristae and intramitochondrial inclusions (63,65).

Table 5-16 ■ MITOCHONDRIAL DEFECTS (MITOCHONDRIOPATHIES)

Primary Mitochondrial DNA Disorders		Clinical Features	Inheritance Pattern
Rearrangements (large-scale partial deletions and duplications)	Chronic progressive external ophthalmoplegia (CPEO)	External ophthalmoplegia Ptosis	Sporadic or mitochondrial
	Kearns-Sayre syndrome (KSS)	PEO before age 20 years Pigmentary retinopathy Heart block Cerebellar ataxia Deafness Myopathy Dysphagia Diabetes mellitus Hypoparathyroidism Dementia	Sporadic or mitochondrial
	Pearson marrow-pancreas syndrome	Sideroblastic anemia Exocrine pancreatic dysfunction Neonatal or infantile onset Survivors may develop KSS symptoms later in life	Sporadic or mitochondrial
	Diabetes mellitus and deafness		Sporadic
Point mutations	**Genes encoding structural proteins**		
	Leber hereditary optic neuropathy	Sudden loss of vision, usually bilateral, onset 18 to 30 years	Mitochondrial
	LHON (G11778A, T14484C, G3460A)	Males: females 4:1	
	NARP (T8993G/C)(ATPase6 gene)	Neuropathy, late childhood or adult onset Ataxia Retinitis pigmentosa	Mitochondrial
	Leigh syndrome (T8993G/C)(ATPase6 gene)	Onset of symptoms in 1st year of life Hypotonia and motor retardation Seizures Lactic acidosis Pigmentary retinopathy Necrotizing encephalomyopathy	Mitochondrial
	Genes encoding transfer RNAs		
	MELAS (A3243G, T3271C, A3251G)	Seizures and/or dementia Lactic acidosis Stroke-like events Ragged red fiber myopathy	Mitochondrial
	MERRF (A8344G, T8356C)	Myoclonic epilepsy Ragged red fiber myopathy	Mitochondrial
	CPEO (A3243G, T4274C)	Chronic progressive external ophthalmoplegia	Mitochondrial
	Myopathy (T14709C, A12320G)		Mitochondrial
	Hypertrophic cardiomyopathy (A3243G, A4269G, A4300G)		Mitochondrial
	Diabetes and deafness (A3243G, C12258A)		Mitochondrial
	Encephalomyopathy (G1606A, T10010C)		Mitochondrial
	Genes encoding ribosomal RNAs		
	Nonsyndromic sensorineural deafness (A7445G)		Mitochondrial
	Aminoglycoside induced nonsyndromic deafness (A1555G)		Mitochondrial

(Continued)

Table 5-16 ■ MITOCHONDRIAL DEFECTS (MITOCHONDRIOPATHIES) *(Continued)*

Primary Mitochondrial DNA Disorders		Clinical Features	Inheritance Pattern
Nuclear Gene Disorders			
Disorders of mtDNA maintenance	Autosomal dominant progressive external ophthalmoplegia		
	Mutations in adenine nucleotide translocator *(ANT1)*	PEO, muscle weakness, bipolar disease	AD
	Mutations in DNA polymerase *(POLG1)*	PEO, muscle weakness, psychiatric disease, neuropathy, ataxia	AD or AR
	Mutations in Twinkle helicase *(C10ORF2)*	PEO, myalgia, exercise intolerance, peripheral neuropathy, psychiatric disease	AD
	Mitochondrial neurogastrointestinal encephalomyopathy (MNGIE)(2° multiple mtDNA deletions): Mutations in thymidine phosphorylase *(ECGF1)*	Onset in infant to adult ages Gastrointestinal dysmotility (pseudo-obstruction) Leukoencephalopathy Neuropathy Ophthalmoplegia Myopathy	AR
	Myopathy with mtDNA depletion: Mutations in thymidine kinase *(TK2)*		AR
	Encephalopathy with liver failure and mitochondrial DNA depletion: Mutations in deoxyguanosine kinase *(DGUOK), MPV17* or *POLG1*	Neonatal or infantile onset Progressive liver disease	AR
	Mitochondrial DNA depletion due to ATP-forming beta subunit of the Krebs cycle enzyme succinyl-CoA ligase (SLUCA2)	Hypotonia Muscle atrophy Hyperkinesia Severe hearing impairment Postnatal growth retardation Methylmalonic acidemia	AR
Primary disorders of the respiratory chain	Leigh syndrome (Subacute necrotizing encephalomyopathy)		
	Complex I deficiency—mutations in complex I subunits *(NDUFS2,4,7,8* and *NDUFV1)*		AR
	Complex II deficiency—mutations in complex II flavoprotein subunit *(SDHA)*		AR
	Leukodystrophy and myoclonic epilepsy: Complex I deficiency - mutations in complex I subunit *(NDUFV1)*		AR
	Cardioencephalomyopathy: Complex I deficiency—mutations in complex I subunit *(NDUFS2)*		AR
	Optic atrophy and ataxia: Complex II deficiency - mutations in complex II flavoprotein subunit *(SDHA)*		AD
Disorders of mitochondrial protein import	Dystonia-deafness: Mutations in deafness-dystonia protein DDP1 *(TIMM8)*		XLR
Disorders of assembly of the respiratory chain	Leigh syndrome (Subacute necrotizing encephalomyopathy)		
	Complex IV deficiency—mutations in COX assembly protein *(SURFI)*	Most common cause of Leigh syndrome	AR
	Complex IV deficiency—mutations in COX assembly protein *(COX10)*		AR

(Continued)

Table 5-16 ■ MITOCHONDRIAL DEFECTS (MITOCHONDRIOPATHIES) *(Continued)*

Primary Mitochondrial DNA Disorders		Clinical Features	Inheritance Pattern
	Cardioencephalomyopathy: Complex IV deficiency—mutations in COX assembly protein *(SCO2)*		AR
	Hepatic failure and encephalopathy: Complex IV deficiency—mutations in COX assembly protein *(SCO1)*		AR
	Complex IV deficiency—mutations in protein affecting COX mRNA stability (Leucine rich pentatricopeptide repeat cassette, *LRPPRC)*		AR
	Tubulopathy, encephalopathy, and liver failure: Complex III deficiency—mutations in complex III assembly *(BSC1L)*		AR
	Encephalopathy: Complex I deficiency—mutations in the complex I assembly protein *(B17.2L)*		AR
Disorders of RNA metabolism	Leigh syndrome (Subacute necrotizing encephalomyopathy)		
	Complex IV deficiency *(LRPPRC)*		AR
	Multiple complex defects with mutations in mitochondrial elongation factor G1 *(EFG1)*		AR
Disorders of the lipid membrane	Coenzyme Q10 deficiency *(COQ2)*	Ataxia, seizures, encephalomyopathy Cerebellar atrophy Renal dysfunction Treatable with coenzyme Q10	AR
	Barth syndrome (Tafazzin)	Cardiomyopathy Noncompaction of left ventricle Neutropenia 3-methylglutaconic aciduria Skeletal muscle myopathy	XLR

PEO, progressive external ophthalmoplegia; AD, autosomal dominant; AR, autosomal recessive; XLR, X-linked recessive.

Mitochondrial DNA (mtDNA) Abnormalities

In these disorders, heteroplasmy is common, with a mixture of mutant and normal mtDNAs in the same patient, varying from mitochondrion to mitochondrion, cell to cell, and tissue to tissue, rather than the normal identical mtDNA (homoplasmy) in all cells and tissues (29). Heteroplasmy impacts clinical symptoms and organ dysfunction. Diagnosis may be made with histochemistry, EM, respiratory chain enzyme analysis, or mtDNA mutation analysis using muscle tissue. In families with mtDNA mutations, there is marked phenotype variability (Table 5-16) (29).

Mitochondrial DNA Rearrangements

Chronic progressive external ophthalmoplegia (CPEO) with ragged-red fibers is generally a benign disorder with slowly progressive ophthalmoplegia, ptosis, and proximal limb weakness beginning in adolescence. Most cases are sporadic and have deletions or duplications of mtDNA (29). Muscle biopsy shows ragged-red and cytochrome oxidase (COX)-negative fibers.

Kearns-Sayre syndrome (KSS) patients have a severe mitochondriopathy and may have retinitis pigmentosa, progressive external ophthalmoplegia, and heart block beginning before 20 years of age. Ptosis, cerebellar involvement, ataxia, and endocrinopathies (diabetes mellitus,

Table 5-17 ■ METABOLIC CAUSES OF LEIGH SYNDROME (SUBACUTE NECROTIZING ENCEPHALOMYELOPATHY)

Pyruvate dehydrogenase deficiency
Pyruvate carboxylase deficiency
Complex I
  Mutations in *NDUFS 1,2,3, 4,7,8, NDUFV1, MTND2,3,5,6*
Complex II
  Mutations in *SDHA*
Complex III
  Mutations in *BCS1L*
Complex IV
  Mutations in *SURFI, COX10, COX15, LRPPRC, MTCO3, SCO2*
Complex V
  Mutation of *MTATP6* (T8993G/C)
Mitochondrial tRNA protein mutations
  MTTV, MTTK, MTTW, MTTL1(A3243G)
Coenzyme Q10 deficiency *(COQ2)*
Mitochondrial elongation factor G1 *(EGF1)*

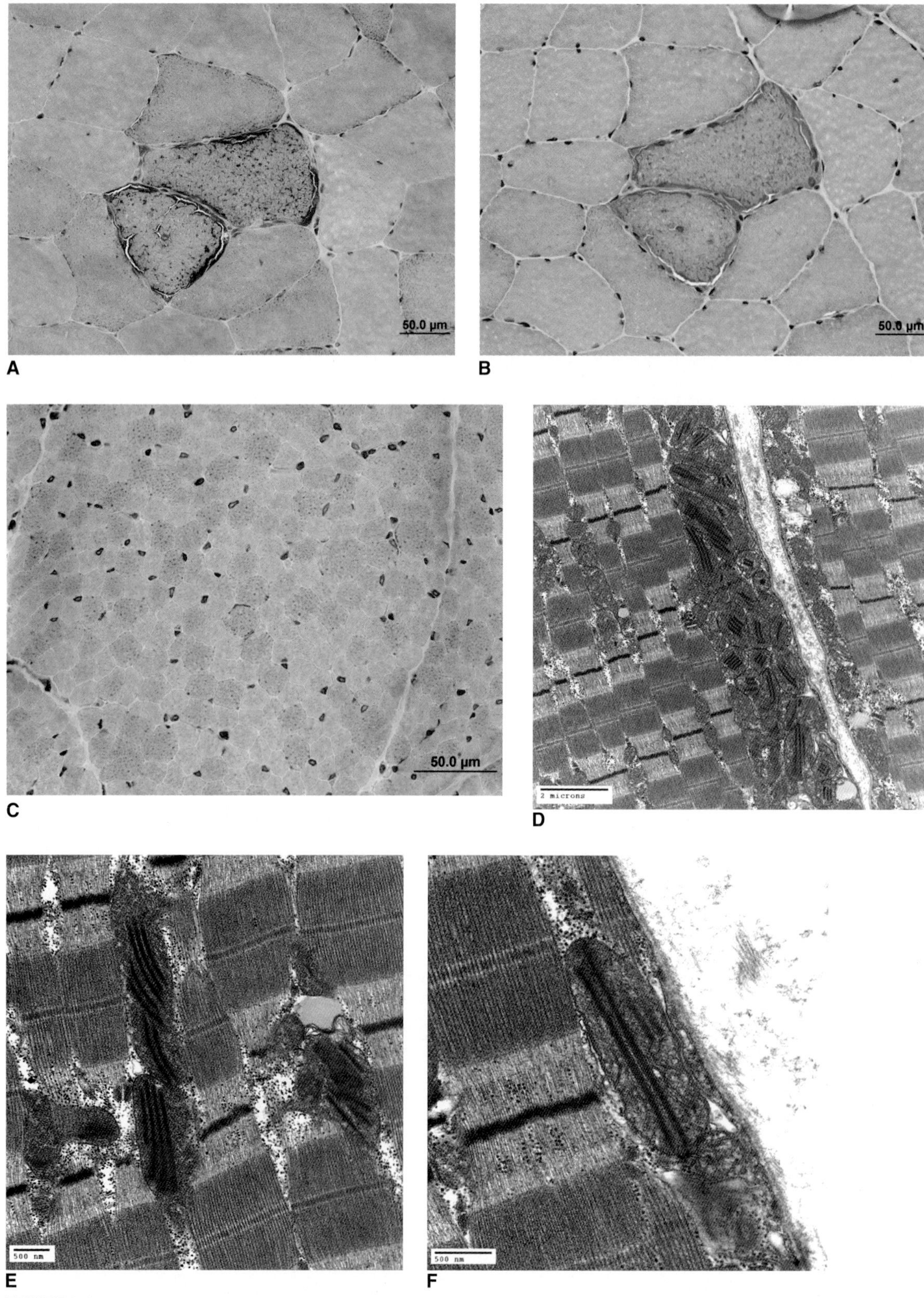

FIGURE 5-21 ■ **Mitochondrial disorders. A,B:** Many mitochondrial disorders are characterized by peripheral red granularity on Gomori trichrome stain, frequently described as *ragged red fibers* (**A**); by H&E (**B**) a similar pattern of basophilic granularity is present in myofibers [Gomori trichrome (**A**) and H&E (**B**)]. **C:** The absence of "ragged red fibers" does not exclude mitochondrial disease. In this case of Complex 1 deficiency, there is a subtle increase in red granularity of myofibers (i.e., mitochondrial prominence) but no frank "ragged red fibers" (Gomori trichrome). **D–G:** Though mitochondria can assume a variety of, often striking, morphological abnormalities—including crystalline/paracrystalline inclusions (**D–G:** uncharacterized mitochondrial disease;

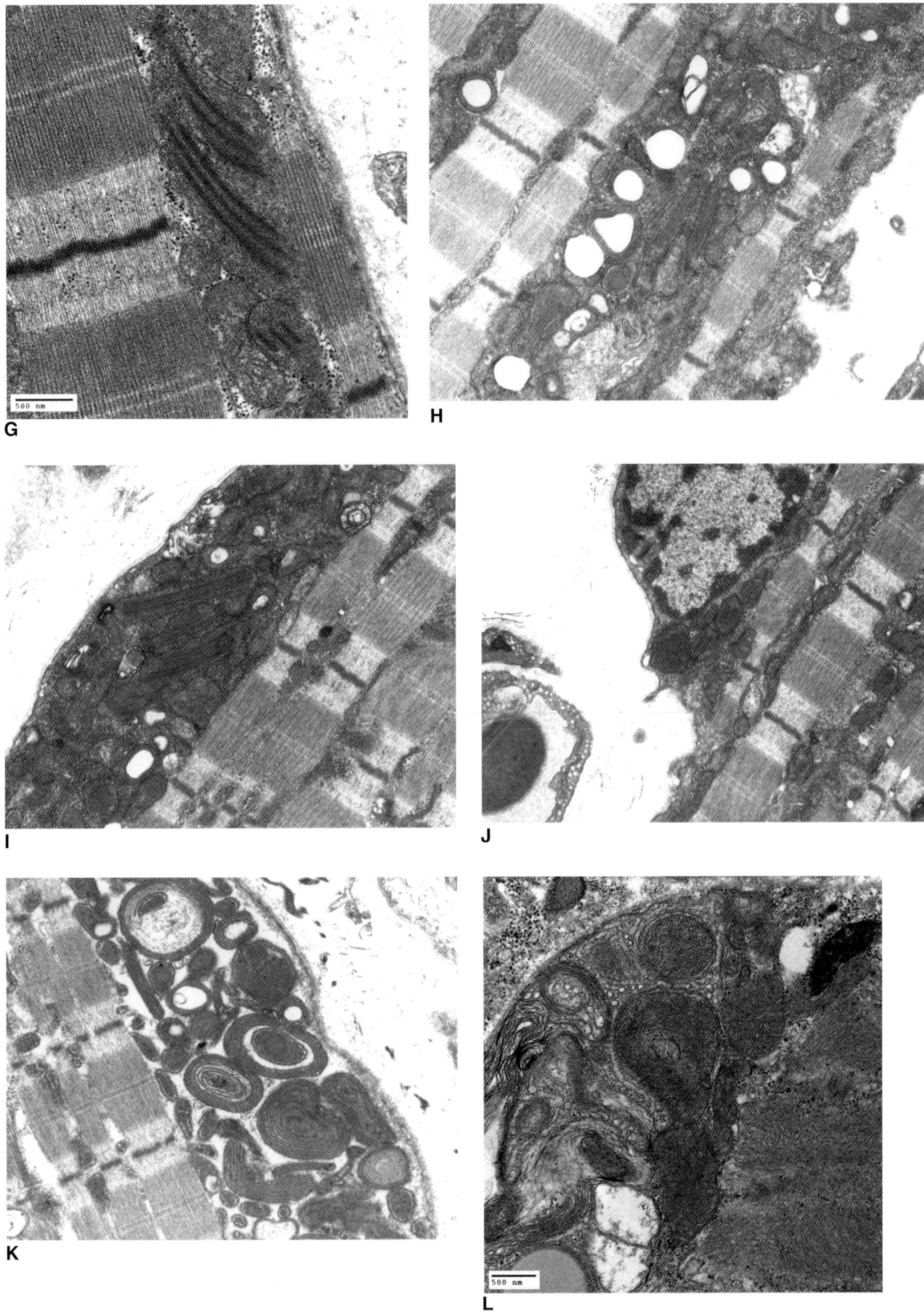

FIGURE 5-21 ■ *(continued)* **H–J**: MELAS) sometimes with a "parking lot appearance (**J:** MELAS), concentric cristae (**K:** MELAS), and other variable abnormalities in size and arrangement of cristae (**L–O**: Complex 1 Deficiency)—the specific morphologic features of abnormal mitochondria cannot reliably determine which mitochondrial disease is present (**D–O:** Uranyl acetate, lead citrate).

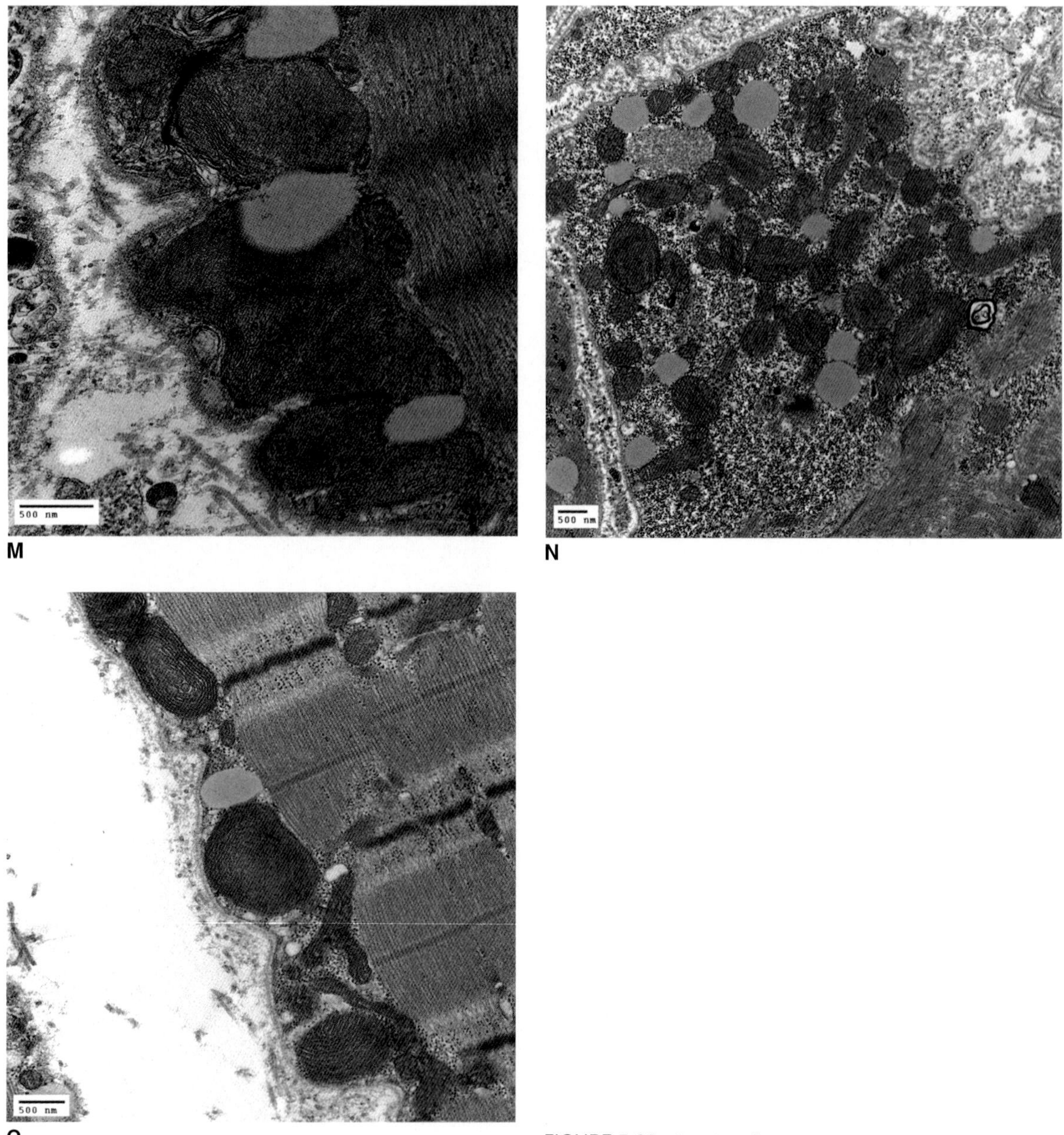

FIGURE 5-21 ■ *(continued).*

hypoparathyroidism, growth hormone deficiency, Addison disease, and hypogonadism) also occur. The brain may have basal ganglia calcification. Muscle biopsy shows numerous or infrequent ragged-red fibers and COX-negative fibers. Structurally abnormal mitochondria are apparent by EM (32).

Pearson marrow-pancreas syndrome is a sporadic disorder that is generally fatal in early childhood due to sepsis with bone marrow failure with pancytopenia, exocrine pancreatic failure, and refractory sideroblastic anemia (105). This disorder may cause hydrops fetalis (78), renal tubular disease, diarrhea, and liver failure. Neuromuscular symptoms resembling those seen in KSS may develop in older children. The marrow shows vacuolization of marrow precursors (29).

Point Mutations in Genes Encoding Mitochondrial Structural Proteins

Leber hereditary optic neuropathy (LHON) patients have painless vision loss as teens or young adults. Only a few have neurological symptoms or dystonia and lactic acidosis is absent. Mutations in ND4 complex I are associated with this disorder. Optic nerve pathology with ganglion cell atrophy and loss and retina nerve fiber atrophy may be seen, but ragged-red fibers are not present (29,31).

Neuropathy, ataxia, and retinitis pigmentosa (NARP) and Leigh syndrome (subacute necrotizing encephalomyopathy) are two syndromes that are phenotypic variants due to variation in the ratio of wild type to abnormal mitochondrial

DNA. They are both associated with T8993G/C mutations in the ATPase6 gene that causes a deficiency in complex V (32). The Leigh syndrome clinical presentation with this mutation is severe (91). Ragged-red fibers are not typically seen on muscle biopsy (32).

Point Mutations in Genes Encoding Mitochondrial Transfer RNA (tRNA)

Mitochondrial encephalopathy, lactic acidosis, and stroke-like episodes (MELAS) is one of the most common respiratory chain disorders. Patients have sudden onset of stroke-like episodes, usually in adulthood, along with myopathy, ataxia, headaches, deafness, cardiomyopathy, and diabetes mellitus (29). Ragged-red fibers are seen in muscle biopsy, but these fibers have cytochrome oxidase activity unlike in most other cases of mitochondrial myopathy with ragged-red fibers (32).

Myoclonic epilepsy with ragged-red fibers (MERRF) patients have myoclonic epilepsy, cerebellar ataxia, dementia, myopathy, deafness, short stature, and increased lactate and pyruvate levels (32). Ragged-red fibers are present in muscle biopsy along with numerous COX-negative fibers.

Disorders of Mitochondrial DNA Maintenance

These disorders are caused by defects in nuclear-encoded factors required for maintenance of mtDNA stability and replication. Mutations in these genes result in depletion of mtDNA and/or multiple mtDNA deletions.

Multiple mitochondrial DNA deletions. Mutations in adenine nucleotide translocator-1 (*ANT-1*) and the mitochondrial helicase Twinkle (*C10ORF2*) can lead to autosomal dominant or recessive progressive ophthalmoplegia and in some cases multisystemic symptoms.

Mitochondrial neurogastrointestinal encephalopathy (MNGIE) disease. This autosomal recessive condition usually presents before age 20 years and is characterized by severe gastrointestinal dysmotility (pseudo-obstruction), poor weight gain, gastroesophageal reflux, vomiting, diarrhea, abdominal pain, and abdominal distension. Patients may also have hearing loss, ptosis, external ophthalmoplegia, sensorimotor neuropathy, and leukoencephalopathy on brain MRI scan. Demyelinating peripheral neuropathy is associated with paresthesias and distal limb weakness. The gene encoding thymidine phosphorylase, *ECGF1*, is the only known gene associated with MNGIE disease. Both mitochondrial DNA depletion and multiple mitochondrial DNA deletions are found in patients with MNGIE disease.

Muscle biopsy shows ragged-red fibers; eosinophilic cytoplasmic inclusions, representing enlarged mitochondria, occur in rectal submucosal ganglia and smooth muscle cells (97). The duodenum may demonstrate focal atrophy or absence of the muscularis propria with increased number of nerves and focal loss of Auerbach's plexus with fibrosis (122).

Diagnosis may be made by demonstrating elevated plasma thymidine and deoxyuridine or by demonstrating less than 10% of the control mean thymidine phosphorylase activity in buffy coat leukocytes. Respiratory chain enzyme assays on tissues demonstrate defects in single or multiple complexes. The most common defect is in cytochrome c oxidase (complex IV). Molecular genetic testing of the *ECGF1* gene detects essentially 100% of affected individuals.

Mitochondrial DNA depletion syndrome patients have disease onset in the early months of life with progressive liver failure and encephalopathy. Three nuclear-encoded mitochondrial genes associated with hepatocerebral syndrome have been identified: deoxyguanosine kinase (*DGUOK*), *MPV17*, and DNA polymerase gamma (*POLG1*).

Mutations in the *POLG1* gene have been associated with autosomal recessive Alpers syndrome characterized by progressive encephalopathy, ataxia, and liver failure; intractable seizures may be the predominant clinical feature. Liver histopathology in patients with *POLG1* mutations is variable, ranging from steatosis and mild fibrosis to marked fibrosis and cirrhosis, hepatocyte degeneration, and bile duct proliferation. Muscle biopsy shows COX-deficient fibers and ragged-red fibers (71).

Liver failure is the major presenting symptom in patients with *DGUOK* or *MPV17* mutations, although there is overlap in these defects. In DGUOK deficiency, progressive liver disease leads to steatosis, siderosis, canalicular and hepatocellular cholestasis, multinucleated giant cells, cirrhosis, and, in some patients, hepatocellular carcinoma; fatal infantile liver disease may occur with or without encephalopathy (39). By EM, there is accumulation of mitochondria with reduced cristae. Mutations in *MPV17*, encoding an inner mitochondrial membrane protein, have been reported in patients with infantile hepatic mtDNA depletion.

Diagnosis may be made by demonstration of depletion of mitochondrial DNA by real-time PCR analysis on liver or muscle tissue. Also, DNA analysis of the *POLG1, DGUOK*, and *MPV17* genes is available.

Other mitochondrial DNA depletion disorders include a myopathy associated with thymidine kinase (TK2) deficiency and encephalomyopathy and anemia associated with mutations in *SUCLA2* encoding the beta subunit of the ADP-forming succinyl-CoA synthetase ligase.

Nuclear DNA Mutations That Cause Primary Disorders or Disorders of Assembly of the Respiratory Chain

These disorders are generally inherited as autosomal recessive traits (91).

Complex I deficiency. NADH-coenzyme Q (CoQ, ubiquinone) reductase is the largest complex of the respiratory chain and includes many polypeptides and several nonprotein components. Patients with abnormalities of complex I can present with an infantile multisystem disease with lactic acidosis, psychomotor delay, hypotonia, exercise intolerance, and weakness. Cardiomyopathy occurs with childhood or adult-onset forms. Others have encephalomyopathy beginning in childhood or adulthood, accompanied by ophthalmoplegia, seizures, dementia, ataxia, deafness, and sensory neuropathy.

Complex II deficiency. Patients with succinate CoQ reductase defect have encephalomyopathy with exercise-induced myoglobinuria and lack of SDH activity in muscle biopsy. Some patients with complex II defects may present with the more severe Leigh syndrome phenotype of subacute necrotizing encephalomyopathy.

Complex III deficiency. Defects in succinate cytochrome *c* reductase and NADH cytochrome *c* reductase (reduced CoQ-cytochrome *c* reductase) present clinically with encephalomyopathy and myopathy or with cardiomyopathy (91). There is also an autosomal recessive defect in complex III assembly caused by mutations in the *BSC1L* gene that presents with renal tubulopathy, encephalopathy, and liver disease.

Complex IV (cytochrome c oxidase, COX) deficiency. Patients may present with myopathy or encephalopathy. The encephalopathic form of cytochrome oxidase deficiency is the most common biochemical abnormality in Leigh syndrome (32), and a number of mutations in genes encoding proteins with a role in cytochrome oxidase assembly have been identified (Table 5-16).

Defects of the Inner Mitochondrial Membrane

Coenzyme Q_{10} (CoQ_{10}, ubiquinone) deficiency. CoQ_{10} is a lipid-soluble component of essentially all cell membranes and functions as an electron and proton carrier. CoQ_{10} deficiency is caused by mutations in the *COQ2* gene and is inherited as an autosomal recessive disorder. CoQ_{10} deficiency can present in infancy with encephalomyopathy and renal dysfunction; later in life as a myopathic form with myoglobinuria, exercise intolerance, and weakness; or may be associated with cerebellar atrophy, ataxia, and seizures. It is treatable with CoQ_{10} supplementation. Muscle biopsy shows increased lipid and ragged-red fibers (32).

Barth syndrome is due to defects in the *TAZ* gene that encodes the protein tafazzin, which influences incorporation of cardiolipin, an essential part of the inner mitochondrial membrane. This X-linked disorder causes mitochondrial myopathy with ragged-red fibers, dilated cardiomyopathy with abnormal left ventricular compaction, and neutropenia (32).

HYPERAMMONEMIAS/UREA CYCLE DISORDERS

The urea cycle, important in liver and intestine, converts toxic nitrogenous waste into water-soluble urea. Blocks in this pathway lead to hyperammonemia with neurotoxicity and cerebral edema. Presentation is variable: neonates can have hypotonia, seizures, respiratory alkalosis, hyperammonemia, coma, and death (65). Cerebral or pulmonary hemorrhage may be the terminal event (78). Alternatively, children or even adults with urea cycle defects can present when high-protein diet or infection precipitates symptoms.

Liver biopsy may be normal or show mild steatosis, glycogenated nuclei, occasional necrotic hepatocytes, or interface hepatitis, and mild portal or bridging fibrosis. Mitochondria may be normal or have nonspecific pleomorphism and swollen or shortened cristae (63,65). Diagnosis is based on plasma or urine amino acid analysis.

Ornithine Transcarbamylase (OTC) Deficiency

This is the most common urea cycle disorder. It is inherited as an X-linked dominant disease with variably symptomatic heterozygotes (55). A large number of mutations at Xp21 have been described. In the neonatal form, patients have emesis, hyperammonemia, progressive encephalopathy, and focal neurological defects. Hemizygous boys typically present in the first days of life, but heterozygous girls may be intermittently symptomatic. All patients with OTC deficiency patients are vulnerable to valproate-associated hepatotoxicity (61), and OTC-deficient heterozygote mothers may have postpartum hyperammonemic encephalopathy (65).

Liver may be normal even in fatal disease. Microscopically, islands of pale, water-clear hepatocytes, with lipid accumulation, are characteristic but not unique (being seen in a variety of urea cycle defects) (61). Centrilobular microvesicular steatosis, glycogenated nuclei, mild hepatitis, focal necrosis, cholestasis, mild periportal fibrosis, and, in severe cases, interface hepatitis and bridging fibrosis have been described (65). Heterozygote girls may have portal fibrosis or a hepatitic pattern with inflammation and piecemeal necrosis, steatosis, and fibrosis (64). By EM, lipid and pleomorphic, elongated, enlarged, or branching mitochondria (some with paracrystalline inclusions and peroxisomal swelling and matrix rarefaction) are seen (29,60,61).

The brain is edematous with Alzheimer type II astrocytosis. Spongiosis with hypomyelination or cystic destruction of the cerebellar hemispheres and mineralization of deep gray matter neurons occur in severely affected girls (29,55). Others have described ulegyria and atrophy of the cerebellar granular layer (73). Diagnosis is confirmed by mutation analysis, urine amino acid analyses to identify increased orotic acid, and low leukocyte, fibroblast, or liver OTC.

Carbamoyl Phosphate Synthetase I Deficiency

Carbamoyl phosphate synthase is a mitochondrial enzyme responsible for the first part of urea synthesis (61). Deficiency is inherited as an autosomal recessive disorder, and there are a lethal neonatal onset form and a delayed onset milder form with episodic hyperammonemia (61). The liver is normal or has mild steatosis with focal necrosis and slight portal fibrosis (29). Mitochondria may be normal or dilated and pleomorphic with increased matrix density (29,61). The brain shows Alzheimer type II astrocytosis and spongiosis (29). Diagnosis is confirmed by enzyme assay on liver tissue (29).

Citrullinemia

This disorder, due to autosomal recessive deficiency of argininosuccinic acid synthetase, leads to steatosis, focal hepatocellular necrosis, and patchy cholestasis. By EM, numerous small mitochondria with increased matrix density and paracrystalline and electron-dense bodies may be due to increased citrulline. Rough endoplasmic reticulum has a concentric profile and peroxisomes may be increased (29,140). Diagnosis is based on enzyme assay of fibroblasts or amniocyte cultures (29).

Argininosuccinic Aciduria

This autosomal recessive defect in argininosuccinate lyase (argininosuccinase) is associated with a nodular liver with severe septal portal fibrosis or cirrhosis, steatosis, and focal hepatocellular necrosis. Ultrastructural mitochondrial abnormalities are not seen (29). Older infants may have brittle hair with trichorrhexis nodosa, particularly if protein in the diet is low (29).

Argininemia

This autosomal recessive disease, due to arginase deficiency, presents later than other urea cycle disorders with spastic paraplegia, dementia, dystonia, ataxia, and mental retardation (55). Hepatomegaly with steatosis and periportal fibrosis but with normal mitochondria may be seen (43).

Hyperornithinemia, Hyperammonemia, Homocitrullinuria (HHH Disease)

This rare autosomal recessive disorder, due to mutations in the *SLC25A15* gene, is characterized by impaired transfer of ornithine from cytoplasm to mitochondria where it is normally converted to citrulline (29). Affected patients have increased plasma ornithine concentration, homocitrullinuria, and hyperammonemia (124). Increased mitochondrial number and giant pleomorphic hepatocyte mitochondria contain crystalline inclusions (29,124). Abnormal mitochondria may also be found in muscle and leukocytes (43).

Lysinuric Protein Intolerance (LPI)

This disorder, due to a mutation in amino acid transporter gene *SLC7A7*, is inherited as an autosomal recessive trait (112). The mutation results in lack of normal absorption and excessive loss of the cationic amino acids lysine, ornithine, and arginine with resultant low plasma levels of these amino acids and increased urine lysine. Affected patients may have failure to thrive, feeding difficulty, hepatomegaly, mental retardation, sparse hair, osteoporosis, hypotonia, and, in some cases, sudden unexpected death in infancy (24). Episodic hyperammonemia is due to deficient ornithine.

Pathologic alterations include interstitial pneumonia, alveolar proteinosis, and pulmonary hemorrhage, and immune complex–mediated IgA mesangial proliferative or membranous glomerulonephritis. In liver, periportal steatosis, fibrosis, and micronodular cirrhosis, with decreased glycogen and nuclei with PAS-positive inclusions are described (83,112). These changes may reflect protein malnutrition (112). Pancreatic atrophy and fibrosis and hemophagocytic lymphohistiocytosis with macrophage activation also occur (33,112).

ORGANIC ACIDEMIAS

In these disorders, catabolism of amino acids, carbohydrates, or fatty acids is blocked due to an enzyme or cofactor deficiency with resultant accumulation of organic acids, which can be identified by MS of urine (29). Clinically, the organic acidemias are characterized by severe, progressive encephalopathy with coma, seizures, and death (Table 5-18). Liver changes are nonspecific and include hepatomegaly and mild steatosis (65).

Propionic Acidemia

Actual or functional deficiency of the biotin-dependent enzyme propionyl-CoA carboxylase, inherited as an autosomal recessive disorder, leads to tissue propionic acid accumulation. Patients can present with ketotic hyperglycinemia, and most have neonatal progressive encephalopathy with coma, myoclonus, and early death. Later-onset forms have acute encephalopathy, anorexia, failure to thrive, and developmental delay (55). Neutropenia, thrombocytopenia, acidosis, hyperammonemia, decreased free carnitine, increased propionyl carnitine, and increased urine excretion of propionyl glycine and methylcitrate characterize this disorder (55).

Hepatomegaly and steatosis are seen. By EM, liver mitochondria are enlarged with decreased cristae and amorphous matrix material (43). In early-onset forms, spongy white matter degeneration occurs, particularly in the globus pallidus (55). In later-onset patients, the basal ganglia have perivascular rarefaction in caudate with bilateral symmetrical encephalomalacia in the lentiform nucleus, along with neuronal loss (55).

Methylmalonic Acidemia

Accumulation of methylmalonic acid in body fluids and urine is due to actual or functional deficiency of methylmalonyl-CoA mutase activity. Clinically, patients are similar to those with propionic acidemia, and the pathology is nonspecific. Diffuse white matter gliosis with Alzheimer type II astrocytosis has been described (43).

Table 5-18 ■ ORGANIC ACIDEMIAS

Name	Common Clinical Presentation	Enzyme Deficiency	Substrate Accumulation	Laboratory Evaluation	Pathology
Propionic acidemia	Neonate, vomiting, respiratory distress, hypotonia, seizures, death	Actual or functional biotin-dependent propionyl-CoA carboxylase	Propionic acid (U, B)	Ketoacidosis, Hyperammonemia, Hypoglycemia or Hyperglycinemia	Hepatomegaly, steatosis, spongy white matter degeneration, particularly of globus pallidus
			Methylcitrate (U) Tiglylglycine (U) 3-hydroxypropionate (U)	Neutropenia Thrombocytopenia	
Methylmalonic acidemia	Similar to propionic acidemia	Actual or functional methylmalonyl-CoA mutase	Methylmalonic acid (U, B)	Ketoacidosis, Hyperammonemia, Hypoglycemia	Spongy white matter degeneration
			Methylcitrate (U) Tiglylglycine (U) 3-hydroxypropionate (U)	Hyperglycinemia Neutropenia Thrombocytopenia	
Isovaleric acidemia	Similar to propionic acidemia; May have later age of onset	Isovaleryl-CoA dehydrogenase	Isovaleric acid (B)	Acidosis,	Spongy white matter degeneration, steatosis
			Isovalerylglycine (U)	Sweaty feet odor Pancytopenia	
Glutaric acidemia type 1	Developmental delay, macrocephaly, choreoathetosis, dystonia	Glutaryl-CoA dehydrogenase	Glutaric acid (U)	Acidosis	Frontotemporal atrophy, striatal degeneration, white matter spongiosis, subdural hematoma, steatosis, myocardial and smooth muscle and renal tubular epithelium fat deposition
			3-OH-glutaric acid (U)		

U, urine; B, blood.

Isovaleric Acidemia

Deficiency of isovaleryl-CoA dehydrogenase is inherited as an autosomal recessive disorder and causes patients to be acidotic and have a sweaty feet odor (43). Patients may have pancytopenia, white matter spongiosis, and hepatic steatosis (43).

Glutaric Acidemia Type I

Glutaryl-CoA dehydrogenase (GCDH) deficiency is inherited as an autosomal recessive trait and results in choreoathetosis and a severe dystonic-dyskinetic syndrome. Rarely, this organic acidemia can present with subdural hematoma and bilateral retinal hemorrhage that mimic shaken baby syndrome (55,93). The CNS is remarkable for frontotemporal atrophy, striatal degeneration, and white matter spongiosis (55). Steatosis and lipid deposition in myocardium and renal tubular epithelium are seen. Diagnosis is based on increased glutaric and hydroxyglutaric acid in urine and decreased GCDH in fibroblasts; molecular diagnosis is possible (43).

HYPERLACTATEMIA, LACTIC ACIDEMIA

The normal lactate:pyruvate ratio in human plasma is 10:1 to 25:1. Increased lactate can be due to nongenetic disease (including tissue necrosis and sepsis), but there are also primary genetic disorders of lactate metabolism.

Pyruvate dehydrogenase (PDH) deficiency. The clinical spectrum of PDH deficiency ranges from fatal lactic acidosis in the newborn to chronic neurologic dysfunction with structural abnormalities of the brain without systemic acidosis. The most common defect affects the X-linked E1-alpha subunit of the PDH complex. Affected males may have a thin callosum or callosal agenesis, polymicrogyria, and facial dysmorphism resembling fetal alcohol syndrome. Liver shows diffuse microvesicular steatosis, and the brain may show Leigh encephalopathy (43). Female heterozygotes may have as severe a presentation as affected males (Figure 5-22A to C) or may be normal. The E1-beta, E2, and E3 subunits of the complex are encoded by autosomal genes, and deficiencies are inherited as autosomal recessive traits. If low PDH activity is found in leukocytes or fibroblasts, the activities of the individual PDH components—E1, E2, and E3—can be assayed for further classification, and DNA analysis is available for the E1-alpha gene.

Pyruvate carboxylase deficiency. This autosomal recessive disorder results in persistent lactic acidosis and hepatomegaly. There is hepatocyte swelling with prominent nucleoli, steatosis, cholestasis, ductular proliferation, and mild portal fibrosis with acinar transformation (43,63). Other clinical features can include mental retardation, developmental delay, hypotonia, and seizures. Some patients present with cystic lesions of the brain consistent with Leigh syndrome, along with neuronal loss in the cerebral cortex, poor myelination, astrocytosis, thin callosum, and periventricular leukomalacia (43).

PEROXISOMAL DISORDERS

Although peroxisomes were named for their peroxide-based reactions, they have many other important metabolic biosynthetic and degradative functions (131). Peroxisomes are spherical with a diameter of 0.1 to 1 μm, bound by a single lipid bilayer. They are larger and more abundant in liver and kidney than in other tissues. In general, peroxisomal disorders can be identified by increased tissue and body fluid very-long-chain fatty acids (VLCFA), decreased plasmalogen, and increased phytanic acid levels (43). EM may be useful in defining the number and size of peroxisomes and in identifying trilaminate inclusions thought to be related to VLCFA deposition (29). Peroxisomal disorders can be divided into two groups (Table 5-19) (131).

Peroxisomal Biogenesis Disorders

In patients with abnormal peroxisomal biogenesis, there is a reduced number of peroxisomes because of defective peroxisomal assembly, and there is defective function of multiple peroxisomal enzymes (43,65). The Zellweger

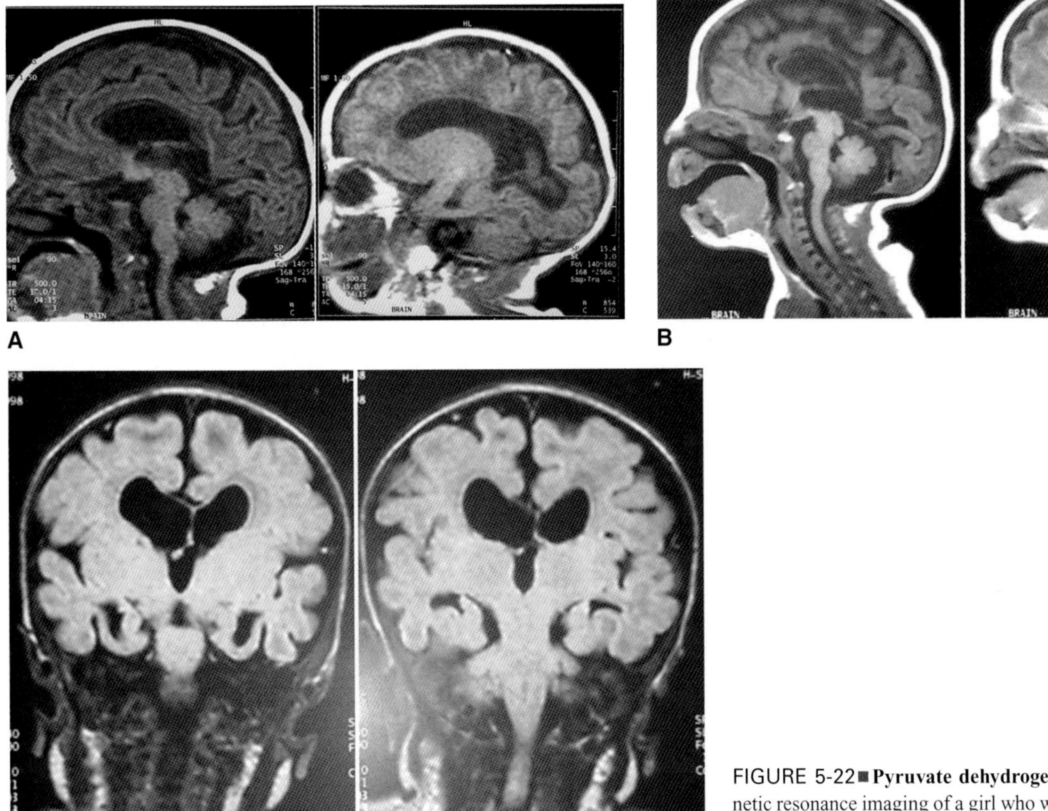

FIGURE 5-22 ■ **Pyruvate dehydrogenase deficiency. A–C:** Magnetic resonance imaging of a girl who was heterozygous for pyruvate dehydrogenase deficiency. Note atrophy, abnormal gyral formation, and absence of the corpus callosum.

Table 5-19 ■ PEROXISOMAL DISORDERS

Peroxisomal biogenesis disorders
- Zellweger syndrome (cerebrohepatorenal syndrome)
- Neonatal adrenoleukodystrophy
- Infantile Refsum disease
- Rhizomelic chondrodysplasia punctata type 1

Single peroxisomal enzyme deficiencies
- X-linked adrenoleukodystrophy
- Acyl-CoA oxidase deficiency (pseudo-neonatal adrenoleukodystrophy)
- Rhizomelic chondrodysplasia punctata type 2
- Rhizomelic chondrodysplasia punctata type 3
- D-bifunctional protein deficiency
- 2-Methylacyl-CoA racemase deficiency
- Sterol carrier protein X deficiency
- Refsum disease
- Hyperoxaluria type I (oxalosis 1).

syndrome spectrum is caused by defects in any of the *PEX* genes required for normal peroxisome assembly (15,99,131) and includes the first three diseases listed below. These disorders have similar biochemical findings. At least 10 genetic defects may be responsible for these disorders.

Zellweger (cerebrohepatorenal) syndrome is the most severe of the biogenesis disorders. An autosomal recessive disease, it presents in neonates with metabolic abnormalities; distinctive facial dysmorphology; severe hypotonia; failure to thrive; mental retardation; seizures; ocular, genital, and cardiovascular malformations; renal glomerular cysts; and calcific stippling of the patellae.

In the brain, premature arrest of migrating neuroblasts during development results in site-specific cerebral microgyria and pachygyria with neuronal heterotopia, an abnormal convolution pattern and olivary dysplasia. Liver initially shows a hepatitic pattern, with hepatocellular unrest, focal necrosis, steatosis, and canalicular and cytoplasmic cholestasis with pseudoacinar and giant cell transformation. Lymphocytes and macrophages accumulate in sinusoids and portal spaces. Intrahepatic bile ducts may be normal, decreased, or hyperplastic. With time, the liver becomes firm and fibrotic with micronodular cirrhosis (65). By EM, peroxisomes are absent or rare in liver and kidney (60,65). The pathogenesis of the liver injury is unknown but may relate to injury by abnormal bile acids (65).

Neonatal adrenoleukodystrophy is an autosomal recessive disorder that is less severe than Zellweger syndrome and is characterized by hypotonia, craniofacial dysmorphism, adrenocortical atrophy, and psychomotor deterioration. The brain shows progressive dysmyelination/demyelination of cerebral and cerebellar white matter, and polymicrogyria. Hepatic peroxisomes are reduced in number and size (43,60). PAS-positive macrophages with angulate lysosomes are present in viscera and brain.

Infantile Refsum disease patients resemble those with Zellweger syndrome with hypotonia, seizures, mental retardation, hearing loss, and dysmorphic facies. Their course is milder than seen in Zellweger syndrome or neonatal adrenoleukodystrophy (84). Hepatomegaly with fibrosis and portal-to-portal bridging is seen and, by EM, peroxisomes are deficient or very small (60). Lysosomal PAS-positive trilaminate inclusions with two dense outer and an inner lucent lamellae and an outer thickness of 6 to 14 μm accumulate first in macrophages and then in hepatocytes and suggest VLCFA storage (63,84). An elevated phytanic acid, trihydroxycoprostanoic acid, pipecolic acid, and VLCFA and decreased phytanic acid oxidase are laboratory abnormalities (60).

Rhizomelic chondrodysplasia punctata type 1 is a peroxisomal disorder that is genetically and biochemically distinct from Zellweger syndrome and is due to a defect in a peroxisomal targeting gene that affects importation of enzymes into peroxisomes (29). Patients have impaired plasmalogen synthesis and phytanic acid oxidation, severe proximal limb shortening, calcific stippling in hyaline cartilage, cataracts, renal dysfunction, facial dysmorphism, ichthyosis, and death in childhood. Hepatocytes may have absent or large irregularly shaped peroxisomes (43). Plasma phytanic acid is increased, and RBC and tissue plasmalogen are decreased (29) (see Chapter 27).

Single Peroxisomal Enzyme Deficiency

In these disorders, peroxisome structure is intact (43).

X-linked adrenoleukodystrophy. Very-long-chain fatty acyl-CoA synthetase is impaired and plasma and fibroblast VLCFA are increased due to impaired capacity to degrade these molecules (43). Progressive behavioral, cognitive, and neurologic deterioration occurs with a 1/21,000 incidence in boys. Adrenal glands are small, and zona fasciculata cells contain cytoplasmic lipid inclusions with a lamellar pattern (44). Lipid accumulation in CNS causes demyelination with a perivascular lymphocytic infiltrate that resembles that seen in multiple sclerosis (131). Rarely, sheaves of thin hollow needles in Schwann cells in skin are seen (30).

Acyl-CoA oxidase deficiency (pseudo-neonatal adrenoleukodystrophy) presents clinically with hypotonia, psychomotor retardation, sensory deafness, hepatomegaly, retinopathy and with or without mild craniofacial dysmorphism. Atrophy of skeletal muscle, brain stem ganglia, and cranial nerves along with hepatic fibrosis and large PAS-positive, sudanophilic adrenal macrophages, and brain astrocytes are described in this disorder (131). Hepatic peroxisomes are heterogeneous in size and increased in number.

Rhizomelic chondrodysplasia punctata type 2, due to dihydroxyacetonephosphate acyltransferase deficiency, presents with craniofacial abnormalities, hypotonia, cataracts, mental retardation, eczema, cerebral atrophy, and dwarfism with rhizomelic shortening of the upper arms but no stippled patellar calcifications.

Rhizomelic chondrodysplasia punctata type 3, due to alkyl dihydroxyacetonephosphate synthase deficiency, is clinically similar to rhizomelic chondrodysplasia punctata type 1.

D-bifunctional protein deficiency presents with neonatal hypotonia, seizures, failure to thrive, visual abnormalities, psychomotor delay, and dysmorphism that resembles that seen in Zellweger syndrome (131).

2-Methylacyl-CoA racemase deficiency has a variable clinical course, with adult-onset sensory motor neuropathy and fulminant liver disease described (131).

Sterol carrier protein X (SCPx) deficiency. Dystonic tremor, hypergonadotropic hypogonadism, and sensory motor neuropathy are seen in this rare disorder (131).

Refsum disease is due to autosomal recessively inherited phytanoyl-CoA hydroxylase deficiency. Patients have deterioration of night vision, retinitis pigmentosa, anosmia, deafness, ataxia, and arrhythmias.

Hyperoxaluria type I (oxalosis 1). Hepatic peroxisomal alanine:glyoxylate aminotransferase is deficient (61). High urine oxalate, progressive oxalate nephrocalcinosis, and oxalate urolithiasis are seen, and calcium oxalates deposit in many sites including bone, soft tissue, eye, and cardiac conduction system (61). The patients may have renal failure, recurrent fractures, and cardiac arrhythmias, and die before 20 years of age (43). The liver is grossly normal, but oxalate crystals may be present in the hepatic arterioles and gallbladder (60,61). The crystals have a rosette pattern with radial striations and a star-burst appearance seen with polarized light (43).

METAL METABOLISM ABNORMALITIES

Neonatal Hemochromatosis (Neonatal Iron Storage Disease)

This is one of the most commonly recognized causes of liver failure in the neonate. The disease is inherited as an autosomal recessive or codominant trait. Liver injury begins *in utero* and can result in stillbirth, hydrops, or severe neonatal liver disease, and extrahepatic siderosis. Infants can have intrauterine growth restriction, polyhydramnios, or oligohydramnios and prognosis is poor (43,61,63). The underlying metabolic defect is unknown, but some cases may be an alloimmune gestational disease (136). Alternatively, iron may be a marker for massive intrauterine liver destruction and iron redistribution (61).

The liver morphology is that of extensive hepatocellular loss. Cirrhosis occurs in a small bile-stained liver (136). Central veins may have obliterative fibrosis extending into sinusoids (61,136). Regenerative nodules may be present and, in other cases, almost no hepatocytes remain. Residual hepatocytes show giant cell or pseudoacinar transformation with canalicular bile plugs and acute and chronic inflammation. Hepatocytes may have coarsely granular siderosis (Figure 5-23A,B), but Kupffer cells do not accumulate iron (136). By EM, hemosiderin is present in hepatocyte lysosomes.

Extrahepatic iron storage is not associated with organ dysfunction, and the fixed tissue macrophage system is spared (61,136). Hypertrophy and hyperplasia of the islets of Langerhans accompanies pancreatic acinar and islet cell iron accumulation. Iron also accumulates in myocardium, oropharyngeal and respiratory submucosal glands, renal tubule epithelium, adrenal cortex, thyroid follicular epithelium, and other sites (136). Biopsy of oral submucosal glands can be used to demonstrate siderosis.

Wilson Disease (Hepatolenticular Degeneration, ATP7B Disease)

This autosomal recessive inherited mutations of the *ATP7B* gene result in copper retention in liver and other organs. Incidence is approximately 1:30,000, and 1:90 are heterozygous carriers. Over 200 mutations in the *ATP7B* gene have been identified. Most Wilson disease patients are compound heterozygotes (5). Copper homeostasis is controlled by the gene product ATP7B-ATPase, expressed in the canalicular membrane and involved in incorporation of copper into apoceruloplasm to form ceruloplasmin with subsequent biliary excretion (65). Absent or reduced ATP7B-ATPase function leads to hepatic copper retention by interfering with biliary copper excretion and incorporation into ceruloplasmin (5).

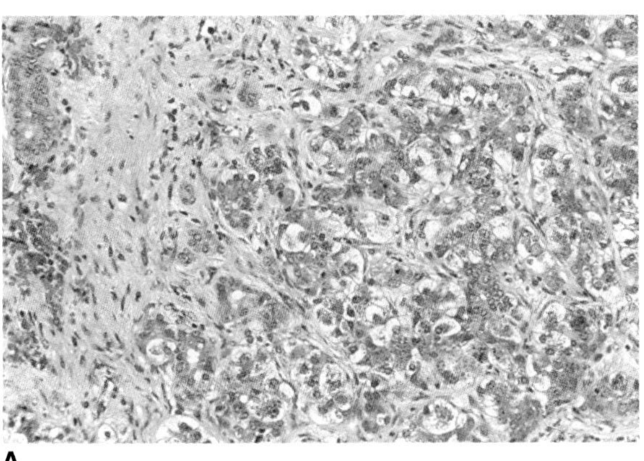

A

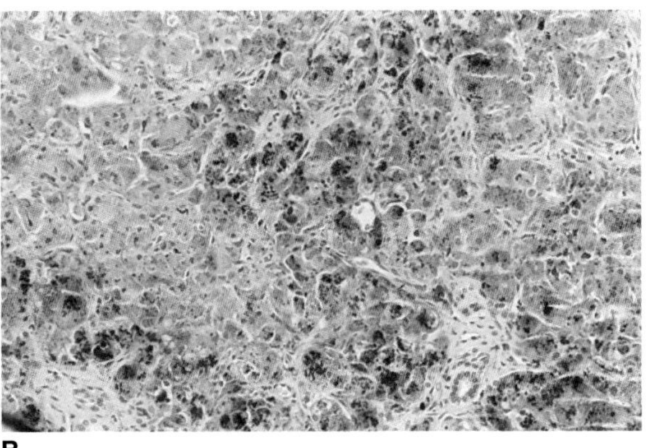

B

FIGURE 5-23 **Neonatal hemochromatosis. A,B:** Widespread hemosiderin accumulation in hepatocytes as shown by H&E (**A**) and Prussian blue (**B**) stains in neonatal hemochromatosis. (Images' courtesy of Elizabeth Brunt, M.D., Washington University, Department of Pathology and Immunology, St. Louis, Missouri).

Progressive copper ion accumulation is hepatotoxic and also injures kidneys, brain, and cornea. The unbound copper ion may act as a free radical, damaging cell and organelle membranes, causing oxidative injury to membranes, depletion of mitochondrial glutathione, and DNA-copper, and DNA-protein complexes that may result in DNA mutations (65).

Patients present in the 1st or 2nd decade with hepatomegaly, acute or chronic hepatitis, cirrhosis, or acute fulminant liver failure often accompanied by hemolytic anemia; hepatic symptoms are more common in children (5). Copper measurement confirms the diagnosis – the copper content is greater than 250 μg/g dry weight (normal <50 μg/g). It is important to select for analysis tissue not affected by fibroconnective tissue scar (65). Tissue copper quantitation can be done on 1 to 2 mg of fresh or frozen tissue (about 0.5 cm of a liver biopsy obtained with a 14-gauge needle or 1 cm of a biopsy obtained with an 18-gauge needle) or on tissue excised from the paraffin block (5,81). Copper levels may be normal in advanced Wilson disease due to variability in copper distribution in fibrotic liver or due to release of copper from necrotic hepatocytes in fulminant hepatic failure (5,61). Serum ceruloplasmin levels should be measured if Wilson disease is suspected. The level is less than 20 mg/dL in most affected patients. However, ceruloplasmin is an acute phase reactant, and an elevated or normal level does not rule out Wilson disease (5).

The liver initially shows glycogenated nuclei (in periportal hepatocytes) and steatosis, followed by periportal mononuclear inflammation with focal hepatocyte necrosis, fibrosis, hepatocyte swelling, and cholestasis. Chronic active hepatitis with marked portal inflammation and interface hepatitis may occur with progression to cirrhosis with cholestasis and small neocholangiole proliferation around the nodules (Figure 5-24A). Mallory bodies may be present in periportal hepatocytes (5,61,65). In some children, fulminant acute hepatitis with submassive or massive hepatocellular necrosis can occur (61). Kupffer cells may contain hemosiderin, particularly if there is a hemolytic crisis.

Cytoplasmic copper is soluble and does not stain with copper and copper-associated protein stains (Table 5-2). Thus, special stains may be negative for copper in the early precirrhotic stage of disease, becoming positive when lysosomal copper accumulates (5,65). When identified by stains, copper is generally in periportal hepatocytes in children and in panlobular hepatocytes in patients with more advanced disease (Figure 5-24B,C) (5,65). Copper accumulates in Kupffer cells as it is released from hepatocytes and nodules may have a variable amount of copper (64).

By EM, mitochondria are enlarged, pleomorphic, with increased matrix density, separation of inner and outer membranes, and widened intracristal spaces with dilatation and microcyst formations at the tips of cristae (Figure 5-24D). Electron-dense granular copper accumulates in mitochondria and lysosomes (65). Nonimmune hemolytic anemia is associated with macrophage erythrophagocytosis and fulminant liver failure (5). Copper deposition in the brain leads to neuropsychiatric symptoms, and corneal Kayser-Fleischer rings are characteristic. Neurologic symptoms are more common in adults and reflect basal ganglia cavitary degeneration, gliosis, neuronal loss, and copper accumulation. The mechanisms causing basal ganglia damage with relative sparing of the cortex in Wilson disease, despite the diffuse increase in copper throughout the CNS, are unknown (22).

Menkes Disease (Menkes Kinky Hair Syndrome)

This X-linked recessive disorder of copper transport is caused by mutations in the *ATP7A* gene at Xq13.3. It is rare, with an estimated incidence of 1:250,000, and is characterized by profound neurodevelopmental deterioration, seizures, poor growth, hypothermia, brittle and kinky hair, hypopigmentation, and connective tissue abnormalities. Most affected boys die within the first 3 years of life with

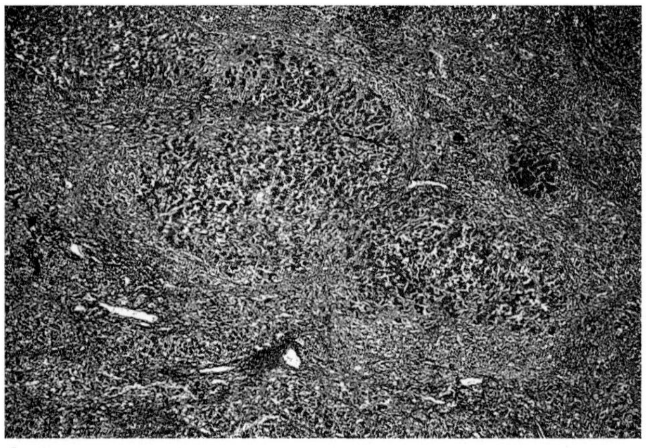

A

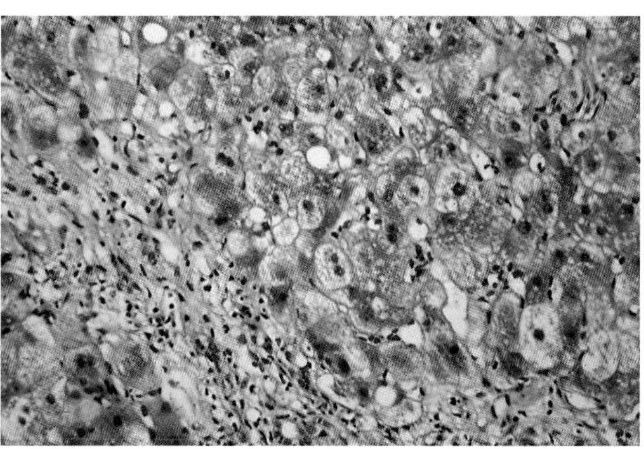

B

FIGURE 5-24 **Wilson disease. A:** Micronodular cirrhosis in late-stage Wilson disease: regenerative hepatocellular nodules (*red*) contrast with diffuse bridging fibrosis (*blue*) (trichrome). **B:** In late-stage Wilson disease, copper accumulation is apparent as cytoplasmic pigment within periportal hepatocytes (H&E).

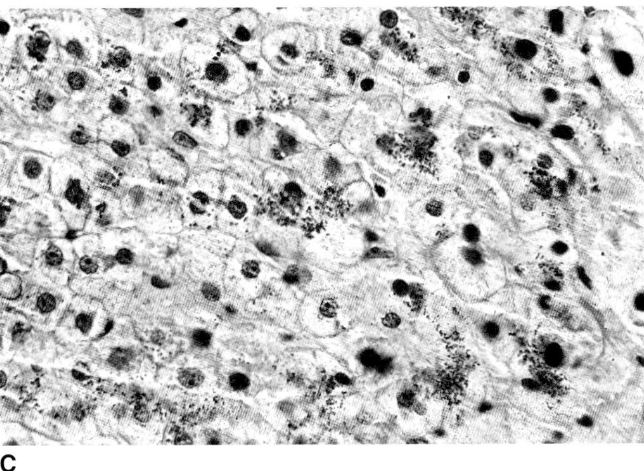
C

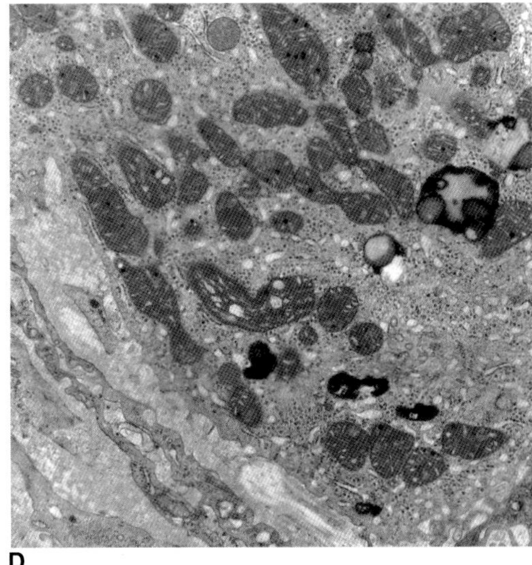
D

FIGURE 5-24■ *(continued)* **C:** Copper stain showing abundant hepatocellular copper accumulation in late-stage Wilson disease (Rhodanine). **D:** Ultrastructurally, Wilson disease shows mitochondrial abnormalities including widening of space between cristae and dilatation with microcystic expansion of the tips of cristae (**D**: Uranyl acetate, lead citrate).

progressive neurological deterioration. Carrier females may have abnormal hair. *ATP7A* encodes an intracellular copper-transporting ATPase, and patients have defective intestinal copper absorption, leading to copper deficiency.

Multiple copper-dependent enzymes become secondarily deficient, resulting in the multiple phenotypic features. One of the deficient copper-dependent enzymes, lysyl oxidase, is involved in collagen and elastin crosslinking; the multiple connective tissue defects in Menkes disease presumably are due to deficiency of lysyl oxidase and include loose and redundant skin, hyperextensible joints, vessel (including intracranial vessel) tortuosity and ectasia, emphysema, hypoplasia of arteries (including aorta and pulmonary arteries), bladder and bowel diverticula, gastric polyps, and bone fragility (with recurrent fractures and osteopenia) (22). The skeletal changes have been confused with those seen in child abuse.

Hair is normal at birth but is replaced by about 6 weeks of age with sparse, hypopigmented, brittle, twisted hair. Microscopic hair examination shows pili torti. Hypopigmentation is related to deficiency of tyrosinase, with decreased melanin production. Deficiency of the copper-dependent enzymes cytochrome c oxidase, dopamine β-hydroxylase, and peptidyl α-monoxygenase is thought to be responsible for the neurodevelopmental problems in Menkes disease.

The cerebral cortex and the cerebellum have abnormal myelination, progressive gliosis, and atrophy. Blood vessels have disruption of elastic lamina. Brain at autopsy may show subdural hematomas and diffuse atrophy, focal gray matter degeneration, and cerebellar neuronal loss. The Purkinje cells show abnormal dendrite arborization and axonal swelling.

Both serum copper and ceruloplasmin levels are low in Menkes disease. Deficiency of dopamine-β-hydroxylase leads to increased plasma dihydroxyphenylalanine (DOPA), dihydroxyphenylacetic acid (DOPAC), and dopamine, and to reduced norepinephrine and dihydroxyphenylglycol (DGPG). Since copper and ceruloplasmin are relatively low in normal newborns and young infants, measurement of these plasma catecholamines can provide an earlier definitive diagnosis of Menkes disease.

Treatment with subcutaneous copper histidine injections and other forms of copper replacement have been attempted with limited success. Serum copper and ceruloplasmin levels are corrected, but unless started very early in life, copper supplementation has not been able to prevent progressive neurological complications.

DISORDERS OF THE ENDOPLASMIC RETICULUM

These disorders include alpha-1-antitypsin deficiency, congenital disorders of glycosylation, and GSD I (29).

Alpha-1-antitypsin (A1AT) Deficiency

A1AT, synthesized primarily by hepatocytes, is an acute phase reactant glycoprotein that accounts for most alpha-1-globulins in serum. Its principal function is inhibition of proteases in lung. In A1AT-deficient patients, proteolytic enzymes released during inflammation are not inhibited normally, leading to lung damage (67,117). A1AT deficiency is the most common pediatric genetic liver disease with an incidence of 1/600 to 1/2,000 (5,67,99). More than 100 alleles of the A1AT gene have been identified, each inherited as an autosomal codominant (5,99).

Serum A1AT level should be determined in children with neonatal hepatitis or undefined liver disease. Levels in A1AT

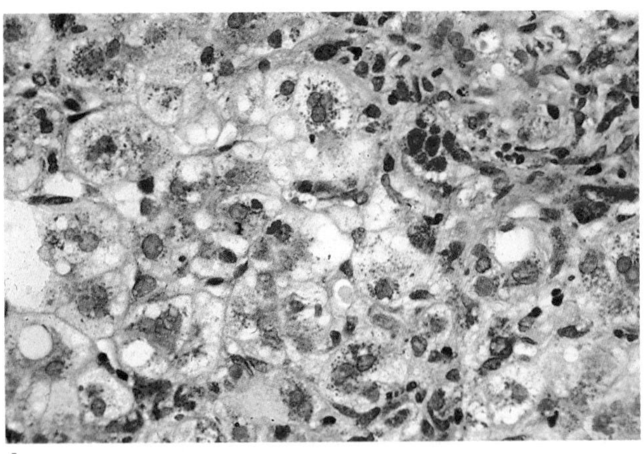
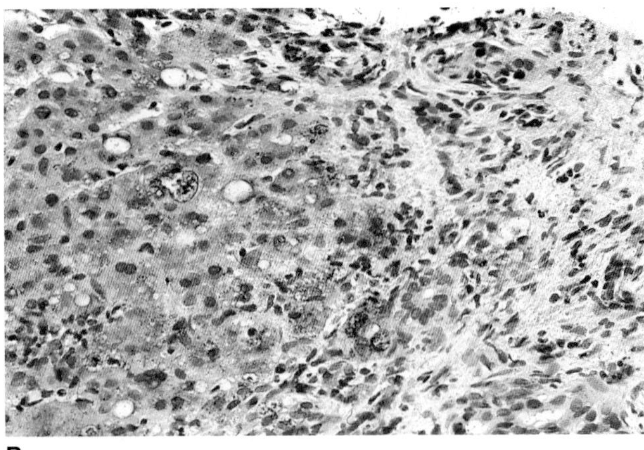

A B

FIGURE 5-25 **Alpha-1-antitrypsin deficiency. A:** PAS-positive, diastase-resistant globules of alpha-1-antitrypsin expand the cytoplasm of periportal hepatocytes in a patient with alpha-1-antitrypsin deficiency (PAS-diastase). **B:** Immunoperoxidase staining for alpha-1-antitrypsin highlights enzyme accumulation (*red-brown*) in periportal hepatocytes in a patient with alpha-1-antitrypsin deficiency (alpha-1-antitrypsin immunoperoxidase).

deficient children are usually 10% to 40% of normal (65). Diagnosis and genotype are confirmed by protease *i*nhibitor (Pi) phenotyping. The abnormal proteins are designated alphabetically, based on isoelectric focusing electrophoresis relative to the normal protein, PiM. The two most common deficiency variants are the S and Z alleles (5). PiZZ genotype patients have liver and lung disease with serum A1AT levels less than 20% of normal. The Z allele is present in 1% to 2% of Caucasians of northern European ancestry and is virtually absent in African-Americans and Asians (99).

In patients with ZZ phenotype, a point mutation in the *SERPINA 1* gene leads to aggregation and polymerization of the abnormal protein (5). The misfolded protein cannot be secreted normally, and A1AT accumulates in the endoplasmic reticulum, leading to serum A1AT deficiency with resultant lung damage. Liver accumulation and delayed degradation of misfolded A1AT leads to hepatocyte injury, and, in some patients, hepatocellular carcinoma; the mechanism of hepatotoxicity is unknown (65). The lack of antiprotease function of bile in A1AT deficiency may make patients prone to epithelial injury during ascending infection (29).

Several patterns of liver injury are seen in A1AT-deficient infants (5). Only 10% to 20% of PiZZ infants develop cholestatic liver disease, and the prognosis is variable (61,121). Intense lymphocytic portal and lobular inflammation with bile plugs, acinar formation, and mild giant cell transformation resembles neonatal hepatitis. Giant cell transformation is generally not as prominent in A1AT deficiency as in viral-related neonatal hepatitis or biliary atresia (67). Extensive bile duct proliferation, bile plugs, and varying fibrosis may suggest biliary atresia. A less common ductopenic pattern has paucity of bile ducts (5). With progression, inflammation may resolve, periportal steatosis is common, and cirrhosis develops with large hyperplastic regenerative nodules (61).

Numerous eosinophilic, 1 to 40 μm PAS-positive, diastase-resistant round hyaline-like globules with peripheral clearing in periportal hepatocytes, hepatocytes adjacent to fibrous septa, and bile duct epithelium are seen, generally after 3 to 4 months of age, although they can be identified immunohistochemically earlier (but hepatocytes in unaffected infants may also stain similarly) (Figure 5-25A,B) (5,65,67). These globules are abnormal A1AT retained in rough endoplasmic reticulum. In young infants, diffuse staining without distinct globules occurs in periportal hepatocytes (67). The globules can also occur in heterozygotes (e.g., PiMZ) with no liver disease and are not specific for the diagnosis of A1AT deficiency (5,67). By EM, electron-dense finely granular material distends endoplasmic reticulum even in infants.

Several forms of glomerulonephritis occur in patients with A1AT deficiency–associated liver disease. Immunoglobulin, complement, and A1AT accumulate in a subendothelial location in glomeruli, and IgA deposition is also seen (23,99,120).

Replacement therapy with purified human A1AT is helpful for progressive lung disease but is ineffective in treatment of liver disease (which is due to accumulation of A1AT rather than its deficiency). Liver transplantation cures the liver disease and corrects the deficiency (5).

Congenital Disorders of Glycosylation (CDG) (Formerly Known as Carbohydrate-Deficient Glycoprotein Syndromes)

Congenital disorders of glycosylation (CDG) are a heterogeneous group of multisystem disorders caused by abnormal glycosylation of *N*-linked oligosaccharides. The wide range of phenotypes associated with CDGs has resulted in underrecognition of these disorders. All known CDGs are inherited as autosomal recessive traits and are due to enzymatic defects. Because of the abnormal assembly or processing of carbohydrate moieties of glycoconjugates, there is abnormal glycosylation of glycoproteins (25,29,38). Diagnosis is usually made by analyzing the glycosylation status of transferrin, most commonly by isoelectric focusing, chromatography, or capillary electrophoresis. Newer methodology using mass spectrometry is likely to be more informative.

Subsequent confirmatory testing by enzyme assay, DNA analysis, glycan analysis on fibroblasts, or complementation assays is required if the screening test is abnormal. At least 25 subtypes due to deficiencies in enzymes that function in the endoplasmic reticulum and Golgi have been identified (Table 5-20) (25,55). The CDGs are classified into two major groups, CDG-I and CDG-II.

CDG-I patients have a defect in assembly of *N*-glycan moieties in the cytosol and endoplasmic reticulum. CDG-Ia is the most common CDG and is caused by deficient phosphomannomutase (25,55). Patients have a variable phenotype with developmental delay, hypotonia, ataxia, stroke-like episodes, seizures, and facial dysmorphism (Table 5-20). Nonimmune hydrops has also been described in CDG-Ia (25). In CDG-Ib, the liver is affected; CDG-Ib patients may have cyclic vomiting, hypoglycemia, failure to thrive, liver fibrosis, and protein-losing enteropathy, without brain involvement (Table 5-20). This form responds to oral mannose supplement and is the only currently successfully treatable type of CDG.

CDG-II patients have a defect in processing of *N*-glycan moieties of glycoconjugate in the Golgi (38,55). Clinical findings are variable depending upon the type and include dysmorphism, microcephaly, liver dysfunction, hypotonia, severe mental retardation, seizures, lipodystrophy, hypertrophic cardiomyopathy, peripheral neuropathy, and hydrops fetalis (Table 5-20) (38). CDG-IIb, IIc, and IIf have normal transferrin glycosylation and thus are more difficult to diagnose.

In CDG patients, there is often severe neonatal onset olivopontocerebellar atrophy with Purkinje and granule cell depletion; atrophy of cerebellar white matter; loss of pontine nuclei, inferior olives, and middle and inferior cerebellar peduncles with relative sparing of dentate neurons (55). Outside the CNS, pleural and pericardial effusions, hypertrophic obstructive cardiomyopathy, cystic dilatation of renal tubules and collecting ducts, steatosis, ductal plate abnormalities, portal fibrosis, cirrhosis, and retinal dystrophy with pigment epithelium degeneration are seen (21,55). Many patients have a coagulopathy due to low levels of clotting factors, although it is usually not clinically significant except during surgery or following trauma.

LIPID METABOLISM DISORDERS

Smith-Lemli-Opitz Syndrome

This autosomal recessive disorder of cholesterol biosynthesis is due to deficiency in 7-dehydrocholesterol reductase. The defect in cholesterol synthesis leads to abnormal development with a variable phenotype that can include microcephaly, mental retardation, hypotonia, dysmorphic facies, cleft palate, ambiguous genitalia, and congenital heart disease (44). Plasma cholesterol is reduced; patients with very low cholesterol levels have a more severe phenotype, and cholesterol deficiency may have a role in dysmorphogenesis (29).

Morphological findings include reduced myelination of the cerebral hemispheres and cranial and peripheral nerves, absent corpus callosum, cerebellar hypoplasia, abnormal gyral pattern, and altered neuronal migration. There is pancreatic enlargement and islet cell nuclear hyperchromasia (44), and liver has nonspecific changes (Figure 5-26A,B) with cholestasis.

Conradi-Hunermann Syndrome (CDPX2)

This X-linked dominant disorder of sterol metabolism is caused by a deficiency of sterol-Δ^8-isomerase that converts 8-dehydrocholesterol to 7-dehydrocholesterol, one step before the enzymatic step that is abnormal in Smith-Lemli-Opitz syndrome. Typical features include chondrodysplasia punctata, bilateral and asymmetrical limb anomalies, joint contractures, ichthyosiform skin lesions, patchy alopecia, and short stature. The skin lesions are most severe at birth and histologically show hyperkeratosis, parakeratosis, and marked acanthosis. They improve with age, leaving behind follicular atrophoderma ("orange peel" lesions) and hypopigmented streaks that follow Blaschko's lines. It was originally thought that this defect would be lethal in males; however, there have been two affected males reported (one of whom was a somatic mosaic for the genetic defect, and the other of whom had a very severe phenotype). Plasma sterol analysis shows elevated 8-dehydrocholesterol and 8(9)-cholestenol. Blood cholesterol levels are typically normal (see Chapter 27).

CHILD Syndrome (*C*ongenital *H*emidysplasia, *I*chthyosis, and *L*imb *D*efects)

This is another rare X-linked dominant disorder of sterol metabolism characterized by unilateral ichthyosiform skin lesions, often sharply demarcated at the midline of the trunk; limb deficiencies; and punctate calcifications of the epiphyses and other cartilaginous structures. In addition, ipsilateral visceral anomalies can be present, including brain, renal, lung, and cardiac defects. While some of the skin lesions follow Blaschko lines, many patients have more extensive patches of abnormal skin. It is presumed generally lethal males. In most patients, it is caused by a defect in the *NSDHL* [*N*AD(P)H *s*teroid *deh*ydrogenase-*l*ike] gene, which encodes the 3ß-hydroxysteroid dehydrogenase component of the sterol-4-demethylase protein, one step above the defect for CDPX2 in the cholesterol biosynthesis pathway. A few patients with the CHILD phenotype have been found to have a defect in sterol-Δ^8-isomerase as in CDPX2.

The skin abnormality in the *NSDHL* defect is typically a persistent scaly, raised, and sometimes verrucous lesion. Skin biopsy in the *NSDHL* defect shows marked ichthyosiform epidermal hyperplasia, inflammation, and sometimes foamy histiocytes within the dermal papillae (referred to as *verruciform xanthoma*). The lesions may regress with age. Sterol analysis of plasma, lymphocytes, and fibroblasts shows abnormally increased levels of 4-methylsterols.

Table 5-20 ■ CARBOHYDRATE-DEFICIENT GLYCOPROTEIN DISORDERS

CDG Subtype	Gene	Protein	Major Clinical Features	Comments
CDG-Ia	*PMM2*	Phosphomannomutase II	Mental retardation (MR) Seizures Hypotonia Strabismus Abnormal fat distribution Inverted nipples Coagulopathy Cerebellar hypoplasia/ atrophy Ataxia Hydrops	Most common form of CDG Incidence may be 1:20,000 Enzyme and mutation analysis clinically available No treatment available Occasionally normal transferrin electrophoresis
CDG-Ib	*MPI*	Phosphomannose isomerase	Hepatic fibrosis Coagulopathy Protein-losing enteropathy Hypoglycemia Cyclic vomiting	Treatment with oral mannose resolves symptoms No brain involvement; normal development
CDG-Ic	*ALG6*	Glucosyltransferase I Dol-p-Glc: Man(9)GlcNAc(2)-PP-dolichyl glucosyltransferase	MR Seizures Hypotonia Strabismus	Second most common form of CDG
CDG-Id	*ALG3*	Dolichyl-P-Man:Man(5)GlcNAc(2)-PP- dolichyl mannosyltransferase	Severe MR Seizures; hypsarrhythmia Optic nerve atrophy Iris colobomas	
CDG-Ie	*DPM1*	Dolichol-phosphate mannose synthetase I	Severe MR Seizures Hypotonia Coagulopathy	
CDG-If	*MPDU1*	Mannose-P-dolichol utilization defect 1/Lec 35	MR Pigmentary retinopathy Short stature Ichthyosis	Episodes of hypertonia
CDG-Ig	*ALG12*	Dolichyl-P-Man:Man(7)GlcNAc(2)-PP-dolichyl mannosyltransferase	MR Hypotonia Microcephaly Frequent infections	
CDG-Ih	*ALG8*	Glucosyltransferase II Dolichyl-P-Glc: Glc(1)Man(9)GlcNAc(2)-P-P-Dol glucosyltransferase	Hepatomegaly Protein losing enteropathy Coagulopathy Renal failure	
CDG-Ii	*ALG2*	Mannosyltransferase II GDP-Man:Man(1)GlcNAc(2)-P-P-Dol mannosyltransferase	MR Severe seizures Coloboma of eye Coagulopathy	
CDG-Ij	*DPAGT1*	UDP-GlcNAc: Dolichol phosphate *N*-acetylglucosamine-1 phosphate transferase	Severe MR Seizures Hypotonia Microcephaly	
CDG-Ik	*ALG1*	Mannosyltransferase I GDP-Man: GlcNAc(2)-PP-Dol mannosyltransferase	Severe MR Hypotonia Microcephaly Coagulopathy Nephrotic syndrome	
CDG-Il	*ALG9*	Mannosyltransferase Dol-P-Man: Man(6)- and Man(8)-GlcNAc(2)-P-P-Dol mannosyltransferase	Severe microcephaly Seizures Hypotonia Hepatomegaly	
CDG-IIa	*MGAT2*	GlcNAc transferase II	MR Seizures Dysmorphic facies	Normal cerebellum

(Continued)

Table 5-20 ■ CARBOHYDRATE-DEFICIENT GLYCOPROTEIN DISORDERS *(Continued)*

CDG Subtype	Gene	Protein	Major Clinical Features	Comments
CDG-IIb	*GCS1*	Glucosidase I	Hepatomegaly; hepatic fibrosis Seizures Hypotonia Dysmorphic facies	Normal transferrin isoelectric focusing
CDG-IIc	*SLC35C1*	GDP-fucose transporter 1	MR Hypotonia Microcephaly Frequent infections; persistently elevated peripheral leukocyte count	Normal transferrin isoelectric focusing May be treatable with fucose supplementation
CDG-IId	*B4GALT1*	Beta-1,4-galactosyltransferase 1	Hypotonia due to myopathy Spontaneous hemorrhage Dandy-Walker malformation with hydrocephalus	
CDG-IIe	*COG7*	Conserved oligomeric Golgi complex subunit 7	Severe seizures Hepatomegaly Progressive jaundice Frequent infections Cardiac failure Dysmorphic facies	Fatal in infancy
CDG-IIf	*SLC35A1*	CMP-sialic acid transporter	Thrombocytopenia Abnormal platelet glycoproteins	Normal transferrin isoelectric focusing No neurological abnormality

Sudden Death in Infants with Inborn Errors of Metabolism

Sudden unexpected death in infancy (SUDI) is defined as sudden unexpected death occurring before the age of 12 months (137). Many metabolic disorders can cause SUDI or acute metabolic crisis in infants, in some cases without preceding clinical symptoms (Table 5-15) (93). Key to the clinical history of a metabolic error presenting in the young infant is deterioration in clinical status after a symptom-free interval of hours to days (29). Findings that may indicate an IEM include family history of a similar sudden death, particularly in a sibling; dysmorphic features; enlarged liver, spleen, or heart; fatty or pale liver, heart, muscle, or kidney; or cerebral edema (16).

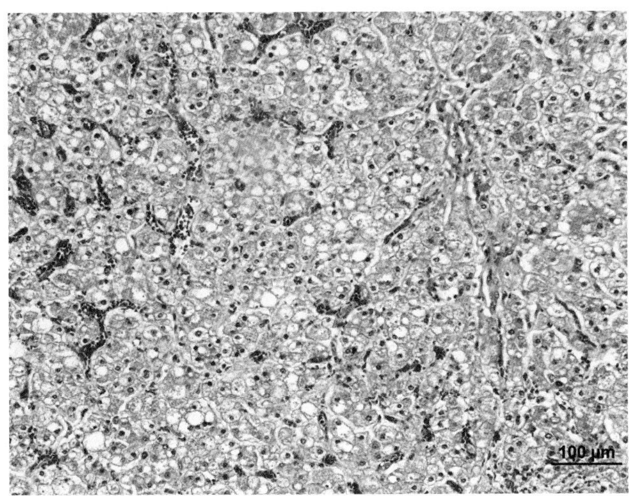

A

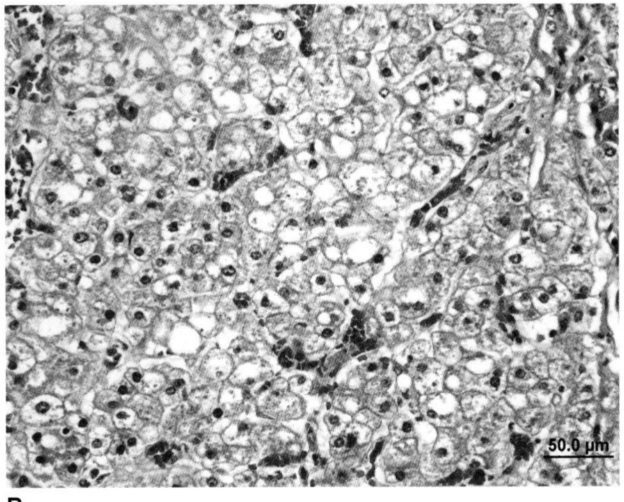

B

FIGURE 5-26 ■ **Smith-Lemli-Opitz syndrome. A,B:** Hepatocellular disarray in Smith-Lemli-Opitz syndrome (H&E).

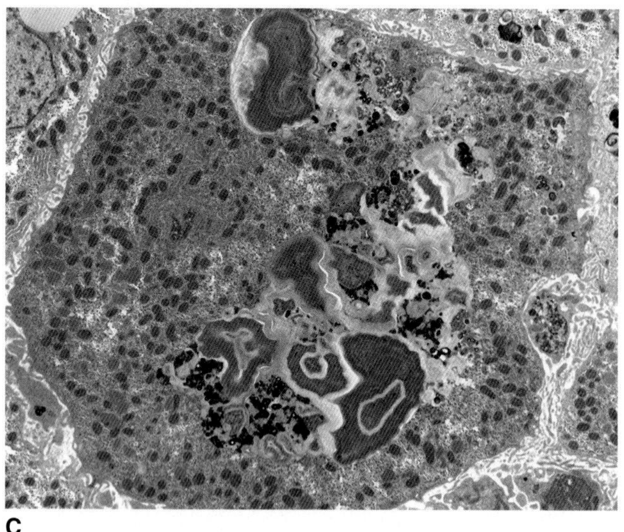
C

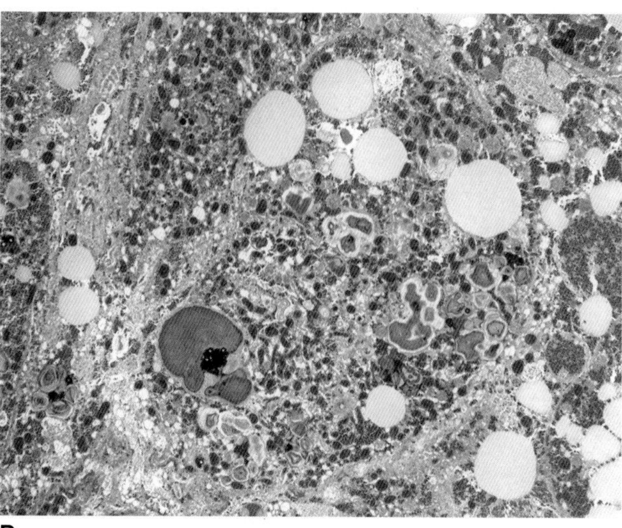
D

FIGURE 5-26 ■ *(continued)* **C,D:** Hepatocytes with multiple cytoplasmic whorled structures, lamellar structures, lipid droplets, and lipofuscin in Smith-Lemli-Opitz syndrome (**C,D**: Uranyl acetate, lead citrate).

Inherited defects of FAO have been shown to cause 4% to 5% of SUDI cases, and these are the most common disorders presenting as SUDI (93,137). Of these, medium-chain acyl-CoA dehydrogenase deficiency (MCAD) is the most common IEM that causes SUDI. As many as a third of affected infants die during the initial presentation, often without previous clinical evidence of a FAO defect (137). Hypoglycemia following birth or hypoketotic hypoglycemia suggests the diagnostic possibility of MCAD.

Autopsy of Child with Suspected Inborn Errors of Metabolism

The autopsy may include photography, radiography, histology, histochemistry, ultrastructure, fibroblast culture, biochemical analysis, and DNA analysis. It is important to do the autopsy as soon as possible after death, preferably within 2 hours. Photographs and whole-body radiographs will document dysmorphology that can be seen in a number of IEM. Hydrops suggests another group of disorders (Tables 5-5 and 5-21). There are several suggested protocols for sample collection in cases of unexpected metabolic death (16,77,93).

Biochemical studies will be directed based on the autopsy findings, but it is important to collect tissue and fluids that may be useful for further evaluation (Table 5-22). Since sepsis and intoxication can mimic IEM, cultures and toxicology may be necessary. Urine should be collected by catheterization or suprapubic tap, placed in a preservative-free container and frozen at −20°C for amino and organic acid analysis (37,93). Blood, serum, and plasma are useful for whole-blood acylcarnitine analysis by MS/MS, which is compared to postmortem sample reference ranges (93). Spotting a few drops of whole blood obtained by cardiac puncture onto filter paper (i.e., Guthrie card) is the most efficient collection method and suitable for many analyses (77,93,137). If more blood is available, collect heparinized blood, separate, and store plasma at −20°C (16,37,77). Red blood cells can be stored at +4°C (93).

If DNA is to be analyzed, collect whole blood in EDTA and keep at room temperature or +4°C until DNA can be extracted (37). Genomic DNA (25 to 60 μg) can be obtained from 1 to 2 mL of blood, and 5 to 10 μg of DNA is sufficient for a single analysis.

CSF can be obtained by cisternal puncture by hyperflexing the neck and inserting a needle between the atlas and the axis vertebrae. CSF may only provide reliable information if collected before death, but it is useful in certain

Table 5-21 ■ INBORN ERRORS OF METABOLISM THAT CAUSE HYDROPS FETALIS

Lysosomal storage disease
Mucopolysaccharidosis types I, IVA and VII
I-cell disease (mucolipidosis II)
Mucolipidosis IV
G_{M1} gangliosidosis
Wolman disease
Fabry disease
Farber disease
Gaucher disease type II
Sialidosis
Galactosialidosis
Niemann Pick disease type A, C
Glycogen storage disease type IV
Long-chain hydroxylacyl-CoA dehydrogenase deficiency
Primary carnitine deficiency
Pearson marrow-pancreas syndrome
Congenital disorders of glycosylation (CDG)
Neonatal hemochromatosis

Table 5-22 ■ SPECIMENS TO BE TAKEN IN AUTOPSY OF AN INFANT WITH POSSIBLE INBORN ERROR IN METABOLISM

Specimen	Store
Urine	−20°C
CSF	−70°C
Whole blood in EDTA for DNA	Room temperature or +4°C
Serum	−20°C
Vitreous	−20°C
Erythrocytes	+4°C
Bile	−20°C
Skin for fibroblast culture	Room temperature or +4°C
Brain, heart, kidney, liver, skeletal muscle, adrenal	−70°C
Brain, heart, kidney, liver, skeletal muscle	In 2% glutaraldehyde

Sources: Byard RW. *Sudden death in infancy, childhood and adolescence.* Cambridge, UK: Cambridge University Press, 2004; Fitzpatrick D. Genetic metabolic disease. In: Keeling JW, ed. *Fetal and neonatal pathology.* London, UK; New York, NY: Springer, 2001:153–174.

circumstances, especially for mitochondrial respiratory chain diseases and organic acid and acylcarnitine analyses (93). Collect two 1-mL samples, one in a plain tube and one in fluoride oxalate, and store at −70°C (93). Vitreous humor can be collected into a fluoride tube and stored at −20°C for glucose and electrolyte analysis.

Bile may be the only analyzable fluid in cases where the interval between death and autopsy is long. In all cases where there is a possibility of underlying metabolic disease, a sample of bile should be obtained (93). Bile can be collected on filter paper or a Guthrie card for acylcarnitine testing or collected in a plain tube for storage at −20°C.

Tissues must be taken promptly if accurate results are to be obtained. One cubic centimeter of tissue from brain, kidney, muscle, liver, and other viscera can be snap frozen in liquid nitrogen, wrapped in foil, and stored at −70°C. Liver and skeletal muscle can be obtained at the bedside after death (93). Fresh-frozen muscle is the tissue of choice for diagnosis of mitochondrial respiratory chain disorders. Complexes I, II, III, and IV of the respiratory chain can be measured (93). Some enzymes of intermediary metabolism are more stable, and tissue analysis may provide essential diagnostic information, even when obtained at the time of a routine autopsy (93). Both MCAD and LCAD in liver may be stable up to 100 hours after death if the body is refrigerated and for 5 years if tissue is kept at −70°C (16).

Fibroblast culture is essential for evaluation of many IEM, and obtaining skin for fibroblasts should be part of any autopsy on an infant or child who dies from unknown cause; this may be the only tissue on which a suspected diagnosis can be confirmed (93). Fibroblasts can be used for studies of DNA, enzymes, and metabolites and for karyotype and can be saved for future studies (29). Achilles tendon, kidney, pericardium, and fascia may also be used for a source of fibroblasts (29). Skin is not a good choice for cell culture for a macerated fetus; in that case, placental villi, kidney, lung, or heart could be used for culture. Take two pieces of tissue from different sites, using sterile technique, place in separate sterile vials containing culture transport medium (Ham's F10, Eagle's MEM, Dulbecco's medium, or sterile normal saline if the only solution available). Taking samples at the beginning of the autopsy is recommended because of the lower risk of bacterial contamination (93). Skin fibroblasts remain viable for up to 9 days after death, but they should be obtained as soon as possible as this increases chance of successful culture (16). Store specimen at 4°C (not below 0°C) until it can be delivered to the cell culture lab. Cultivated fibroblasts can be cryopreserved for indefinite period for future studies.

Histologic, histochemical, and ultrastructural findings can be a guide to diagnosis but are unfortunately often nonspecific. Liver and kidney frozen can be used to look for lipid. Although not specific for and not always present in FAO defects, steatosis can occur in SUID due to these disorders (137). Increased glycogen suggests altered glycogen metabolism. If membrane bound, it suggests GSD Type II.

Unless tissue is obtained minutes after death, ultrastructure is seldom well preserved; however, storage may remain identifiable even in autolyzed tissue (Figure 5-1D,E) (29). EM requires mincing tissues into 1-mm^3 pieces and fixation in 2% glutaraldehyde. LM and histochemistry can be performed on skeletal muscle up to 24 hours after death in children using a 1 to 2 mm in diameter, 1-cm long strip of muscle frozen in mountant in isopentane cooled to −170°C in liquid nitrogen. An infant with unexplained nonimmune hydrops may show characteristic lysosomal material suggesting a storage disease in viscera, brain, placental villi, or amnion cells (103).

REFERENCES

1. Agamanolis DP, Askari AD, Di MS, et al. Muscle phosphofructokinase deficiency: two cases with unusual polysaccharide accumulation and immunologically active enzyme protein. *Muscle Nerve* 1980;3:456–467.
2. Agamanolis DP, Potter JL, Herrick MK, et al. The neuropathology of glycine encephalopathy: a report of five cases with immunohistochemical and ultrastructural observations. *Neurology* 1982;32:975–985.
3. Alroy J, Ucci AA. Skin biopsy: a useful tool in the diagnosis of lysosomal storage diseases. *Ultrastruct Pathol* 2006;30:489–503.
4. Applegarth DA, Toone JR, Wilson RD, et al. Morquio disease presenting as hydrops fetalis and enzyme analysis of chorionic villus tissue in a subsequent pregnancy. *Pediatr Pathol* 1987;7:593–599.
5. Arroyo M, Crawford JM. Hepatitic inherited metabolic disorders. *Semin Diagn Pathol* 2006;23:182–189.
6. Assman G, Seedorf U. Acid lipase deficiency: Wolman disease and cholesteryl ester storage disease. In: Scriver CR, Beaudet AL, Sly WS, et al., eds. *The metabolic & molecular bases of inherited disease.* St. Louis, MO: McGraw-Hill Medical Publishing Division, 2001:3551–3572.
7. Aula P, Jalanko A, Peltonen L. Aspartylglucosaminuria. In: Scriver CR, Beaudet AL, Sly WS, et al., eds. *The metabolic & molecular*

bases of inherited disease. St. Louis, MO: McGraw-Hill Medical Publishing Division, 2001:3535–3550.

8. Autti T, Raininko R, Haltia M, et al. Aspartylglucosaminuria: radiologic course of the disease with histopathologic correlation. *J Child Neurol* 1997;12:369–375.
9. Bach G. Mucolipidosis type IV. *Mol Genet Metab* 2001;73:197–203.
10. Benirschke K, Kaufmann P, Baergen R. *Pathology of the human placenta*. New York, NY: Springer-Verlag, 2006.
11. Besley GT, Broadhead DM, Lawlor E, et al. Cholesterol ester storage disease in an adult presenting with sea-blue histiocytosis. *Clin Genet* 1984;26:195–203.
12. Beutler E, Grabowski GA. Gaucher disease. In: Scriver CR, Beaudet AL, Sly WS, et al., eds. *The metabolic & molecular bases of inherited disease*. St. Louis, MO: McGraw-Hill Medical Publishing Division, 2001:3635–3668.
13. Bharati S, Serratto M, DuBrow I, et al. The conduction system in Pompe's disease. *Pediatr Cardiol* 1982;2:25–32.
14. Bonduelle M, Lissens W, Goossens A, et al. Lysosomal storage diseases presenting as transient or persistent hydrops fetalis. *Genet Couns* 1991;2:227–232.
15. Brosius U, Gartner J. Cellular and molecular aspects of Zellweger syndrome and other peroxisome biogenesis disorders. *Cell Mol Life Sci* 2002;59:1058–1069.
16. Byard RW. *Sudden death in infancy, childhood and adolescence*. Cambridge, UK: Cambridge University Press, 2004.
17. Ceuterick-deGroote C, Martin JJ. Extracerebral biopsy in lysosomal and peroxisomal disorders. Ultrastructural findings. *Brain Pathol* 1998;8:121–132.
18. Chen Y-T. Glycogen storage diseases. In: Scriver CR, Beaudet AL, Sly WS, et al., eds. *The metabolic & molecular bases of inherited disease*. St. Louis, MO: McGraw-Hill Medical Publishing Division, 2001:1521–1551.
19. Cheng Y, Verp MS, Knutel T, et al. Mucopolysaccharidosis type VII as a cause of recurrent non-immune hydrops fetalis. *J Perinat Med* 2003;31:535–537.
20. Chuang DT, Shih VE. Maple syrup urine disease (branched-chain ketoaciduria). In: Scriver CR, Beaudet AL, Sly WS, et al., eds. *The metabolic & molecular bases of inherited disease*. St. Louis, MO: McGraw-Hill Medical Publishing Division, 2001:1971–2005.
21. Clayton PT, Winchester BG, Keir G. Hypertrophic obstructive cardiomyopathy in a neonate with the carbohydrate-deficient glycoprotein syndrome. *J Inherit Metab Dis* 1992;15:857–861.
22. Culotta VC, Gitlin JD. Disorders of copper transport. In: Scriver CR, Beaudet AL, Sly WS, et al., eds. *Metabolic & molecular bases of inherited disease*. St. Louis, MO: McGraw-Hill Medical Publishing Division, 2001:3105–3126.
23. Davis ID, Burke B, Freese D, et al. The pathologic spectrum of the nephropathy associated with α-antitrypsin deficiency. *Hum Pathol* 1992;23:57–62.
24. de Klerk JB, Duran M, Huijmans JG, et al. Sudden infant death and lysinuric protein intolerance. *Eur J Pediatr* 1996;155:256–257.
25. de Koning TJ, Toet M, Dorland L, et al. Recurrent nonimmune hydrops fetalis associated with carbohydrate-deficient glycoprotein syndrome. *J Inherit Metab Dis* 1998;21:681–682.
26. Desnick RJ, Ioannou YA, Eng CM. α-Galactosidase A deficiency: Fabry disease. In: Scriver CR, Beaudet AL, Sly WS, et al., eds. *The metabolic & molecular bases of inherited disease*. St. Louis, MO: McGraw-Hill Medical Publishing Division, 2001:3733–3774.
27. Desnick RJ, Sharp HL, Grabowski GA, et al. Mannosidosis: clinical, morphologic, immunologic, and biochemical studies. *Pediatr Res* 1976;10:985–996.
28. Di Bisceglie AM, Ishak KG, Rabin L, et al. Cholesteryl ester storage disease: hepatopathology and effects of therapy with lovastatin. *Hepatology* 1990;11:764–772.
29. Dimmick JE, Vallance HD. Inborn errors of metabolism. In: Stocker JT, Dehner LP, eds. *Pediatric Pathology*. Philadelphia, PA: Lippincott Williams & Wilkins, 2001:159–196.
30. Dolman CL. Diagnosis of neurometabolic disorders by examination of skin biopsies and lymphocytes. *Semin Diagn Pathol* 1984;1:82–97.
31. Dubowitz V, Sewry C. Metabolic myopathies I: Glycogenoses. *Muscle biopsy—a practical approach*. Philadelphia, PA: Saunders/Elsevier, 2007:453–468.
32. Dubowitz V, Sewry C. Metabolic myopathies II: Lipid related disorders and mitochondrial myopathies. *Muscle biopsy - a practical approach*. Philadelphia, PA: Saunders/Elsevier, 2007:469–492.
33. Duval M, Fenneteau O, Doireau V, et al. Intermittent hemophagocytic lymphohistiocytosis is a regular feature of lysinuric protein intolerance. *J Pediatr* 1999;134:236–239.
34. Elleder M. Sequelae of storage in Fabry disease—pathology and comparison with other lysosomal storage diseases. *Acta Paediatr Suppl* 2003;92:46–53.
35. Fanin M, Nascimbeni AC, Fulizio L, et al. Generalized lysosome-associated membrane protein-2 defect explains multisystem clinical involvement and allows leukocyte diagnostic screening in Danon disease. *Am J Pathol* 2006;168:1309–1320.
36. Fischer EG, Moore MJ, Lager DJ. Fabry disease: a morphologic study of 11 cases. *Mod Pathol* 2006;19:1295–1301.
37. Fitzpatrick D. Genetic metabolic disease. In: Keeling JW, ed. *Fetal and neonatal pathology*. London, UK; New York, NY: Springer, 2001:153–174.
38. Freeze HH. Genetic defects in the human glycome. *Nat Rev Genet* 2006;7:537–551.
39. Freisinger P, Futterer N, Lankes E, et al. Hepatocerebral mitochondrial DNA depletion syndrome caused by deoxyguanosine kinase (DGUOK) mutations. *Arch Neurol* 2006;63:1129–1134.
40. Gahl WA, Thoene JG, Schneider JA. Cystinosis: a disorder of lysosomal membrane transport. In: Scriver CR, Beaudet AL, Sly WS, et al., eds. *The metabolic & molecular bases of inherited disease*. St. Louis, MO: McGraw-Hill Medical Publishing Division, 2001: 5085–5108.
41. Garrod AE. *Inborn errors of metabolism*. London, UK: The Oxford University Press, 1923.
42. Gibson JB. Gonadal function in galactosemics and in galactose-intoxicated animals. *Eur J Pediatr* 1995;154:S14–S20.
43. Gilbert-Barness E, Barness LA. Metabolic diseases. In: Gilbert-Barness E, Kapur RP, Oligny LL, et al., eds. *Potter's pathology of the fetus, infant and child*. Philadelphia, PA: Mosby Elsevier, 2007: 463–572.
44. Gilbert-Barness E, Debich-Spicer D. Metabolic diseases. *Handbook of pediatric autopsy pathology*. Totowa, NJ: Humana Press, 2005:415–447.
45. Gilbert-Barness E, Debich-Spicer D. Metabolic diseases. *Embryo and fetal pathology: color atlas with ultrasound correlation*. Cambridge, UK; New York, NY: Cambridge University Press, 2004: 635–656.
46. Giuffre B, Parinii R, Rizzuti T, et al. Severe neonatal onset of glycogenosis type IV: clinical and laboratory findings leading to diagnosis in two siblings. *J Inherit Metab Dis* 2004;27:609–619.
47. Goldin E, Slaugenhaupt SA, Smith JA, et al. Mucolipidoses type IV. In: Scriver CR, Beaudet AL, Sly WS, et al., eds. *Metabolic & molecular bases of inherited disease*. St. Louis, MO: McGraw-Hill Medical Publishing Division, 2001.
48. Gravel RA, Kaback MM, Proia RL, et al. The G_{M2} gangliosidoses. In: Scriver CR, Beaudet AL, Sly WS, et al., eds. *The metabolic & molecular bases of inherited disease*. St. Louis, MO: McGraw-Hill Medical Publishing Division, 2001:3827–3876.
49. Guibaud P, Carrier H, Mathieu M, et al. Familial congenital muscular dystrophy caused by phosphofructokinase deficiency. *Arch Fr Pediatr*. 1978;35:1105–1115.
50. Hale LP, van deVen C, Wenger DA, et al. Infantile sialic acid storage disease: a rare cause of cytoplasmic vacuolation in pediatric patients. *Pediatr Pathol Lab Med*. 1995;15:443–453.
51. Haltia M. The neuronal ceroid-lipofuscinoses: from past to present. *Biochim Biophys Acta*. 2006;1762:850–856.

52. Haltia M, Herva R, Suopanki J, et al. Hippocampal lesions in the neuronal ceroid lipofuscinoses. *Eur J Paediatr Neurol.* 2001;5(Suppl A): 209–211.
53. Hamosh A, Johnston MV. Nonketotic hyperglycinemia. In: Scriver CR, Beaudet AL, Sly WS, et al., eds. *The metabolic & molecular bases of inherited disease*. St. Louis, MO: McGraw-Hill Medical Publishing Division, 2001:2065–2078.
54. Hantash FM, Olson SC, Anderson B, et al. Rapid one-step carrier detection assay of mucolipidosis IV mutations in the Ashkenazi Jewish population. *J Mol Diagn* 2006;8:282–287.
55. Harding B, Surtees R. Metabolic and neurodegenerative diseases of childhood. In: Graham DILPL, ed. *Greenfield's neuropathology*. London, UK: Arnold, a member of the Hodder Headline Group, 2002:485–517.
56. Hayasaka K, Tada K, Fueki N, et al. Nonketotic hyperglycinemia: analyses of glycine cleavage system in typical and atypical cases. *J Pediatr*. 1987;110:873–877.
57. Hirschhorn R, Reuser AJJ. Glycogen storage disease type II: Acid α-glucosidase (acid maltase) deficiency. In: Scriver CR, Beaudet AL, Sly WS, et al., eds. *The metabolic & molecular bases of inherited disease*. St. Louis, MO: McGraw-Hill Medical Publishing Division, 2001:3389–3420.
58. Hofmann SL, Peltonen L. The neuronal ceroid lipofuscinoses. In: Scriver CR, Beaudet AL, Sly WS, et al., eds. *The metabolic & molecular bases of inherited disease*. St. Louis, MO: McGraw-Hill Medical Publishing Division, 2001:3877–3894.
59. Isenberg JN, Sharp HL. Aspartylglucosaminuria: unique biochemical and ultrastructural characteristics. *Hum Pathol* 1976;7:469–481.
60. Ishak KG. Pathology of inherited metabolic disorders. In: Balisteri WF, Stocker JT, eds. *Pediatric hepatology*. New York, NY: Hemisphere Publishing Corporation, 1990:77–158.
61. Jaffe R. Liver transplant pathology in pediatric metabolic disorders. *Pediatr Dev Pathol* 1998;1:102–117.
62. Jamroz E, Marszal E, Glinka Z, et al. Ultrastructure of peripheral blood lymphocytes in some degenerative central nervous system disease. *Folia Neuropathol* 1994;32:81–86.
63. Jevon GP, Dimmick JE. Histopathologic approach to metabolic liver disease: Part 2. *Pediatr Dev Pathol* 1998;1:261–269.
64. Jevon GP, Dimmick JE. Histopathologic approach to metabolic liver disease: Part 1. *Pediatr Dev Pathol* 1998;1:179–199.
65. Jevon G, Dimmick J. Metabolic disorders in childhood. In: Russo P, Ruchelli E, Piccoli D, eds. *Pathology of pediatric gastrointestinal and liver disease*. New York, NY: Springer-Verlag New York, Inc., 2004:270–299.
66. Jones CJ, Lendon M, Chawner LE, et al. Ultrastructure of the human placenta in metabolic storage disease. *Placenta* 1990;11:395–411.
67. Kanel G, Korula J. Developmental, familial, and metabolic disorders. *Atlas of liver pathology*. Philadelphia, PA: Elsevier/Saunders, 2005:173–209.
68. Kashtan CE, Nevins TE, Posalaky Z, et al. Proteinuria in a child with sialidosis: case report and histological studies. *Pediatr Nephrol* 1989;3:166–174.
69. Kaye CI, Accurso F, La FS, et al. Newborn screening fact sheets. *Pediatrics* 2006;118:e934–e963.
70. Kieseier BC, Wisniewski KE, Goebel HH. The monocyte-macrophage system is affected in lysosomal storage diseases: an immunoelectron microscopic study. *Acta Neuropathol (Berl)* 1997;94:359–362.
71. Kollberg G, Moslemi AR, Darin N, et al. POLG1 mutations associated with progressive encephalopathy in childhood. *J Neuropathol Exp Neurol* 2006;65:758–768.
72. Kooper AJA, Janssens PMW, de Groot ANJA, et al. Lysosomal storage diseases in non-immune hydrops fetalis pregnancies. *Clinica Chimica Acta* 2006;371:176–182.
73. Kornfeld M, Woodfin BM, Papile L, et al. Neuropathology of ornithine carbamyl transferase deficiency. *Acta Neuropathol (Berl)* 1985;65:261–264.
74. Kornfeld S, Sly WS. I-cell disease and pseudo-Hurler polydystrophy: disorders of lysosomal enzyme phosphorylation and localization. In: Scriver CR, Beaudet AL, Sly WS, et al., eds. *The metabolic & molecular bases of inherited disease*. St. Louis, MO: McGraw-Hill Medical Publishing Division, 2001:3469–3482.
75. Kraus FT, Redline RW, Gersell DJ, et al. *Placental pathology (atlas of nontumor pathology)*. Washington, DC: American Registry of Pathology, 2004.
76. Lefkowitch JH. Special stains in diagnostic liver pathology. *Semin Diagn Pathol* 2006;23:190–198.
77. Leonard JV, Morris AA. Inborn errors of metabolism around time of birth. *Lancet* 2000;356:583–587.
78. Leonard JV, Morris AA. Diagnosis and early management of inborn errors of metabolism presenting around the time of birth. *Acta Paediatr* 2006;95:6–14.
79. Libert J. Diagnosis of lysosomal storage diseases by the ultrastructural study of conjunctival biopsies. *Pathol Annu* 1980;15:37–66.
80. Lubensky IA, Schiffmann R, Goldin E, et al. Lysosomal inclusions in gastric parietal cells in mucolipidosis type IV: a novel cause of achlorhydria and hypergastrinemia. *Am J Surg Pathol* 1999;23:1527–1531.
81. Ludwig J, Moyer TP, Rakela J. The liver biopsy diagnosis of Wilson's disease. Methods in pathology. *Am J Clin Pathol* 1994;102:443–446.
82. McAdams AJ, Hug G, Bove KE. Glycogen storage disease, types I to X: criteria for morphologic diagnosis. *Hum Pathol* 1974;5: 463–487.
83. McManus DT, Moore R, Hill CM, et al. Necropsy findings in lysinuric protein intolerance. *J Clin Pathol* 1996;49:345–347.
84. Mierau GW, Weeks DA. Role of electron microscopy in the diagnosis of metabolic storage diseases affecting the nervous system of children. *Ultrastruct Pathol* 1997;21:345–354.
85. Mitchell GA, Grompe M, Lambert M, et al. Hypertyrosinemia. In: Scriver CR, Beaudet AL, Sly WS, et al., eds. *The metabolic & molecular bases of inherited disease*. St. Louis, MO: McGraw-Hill Medical Publishing Division, 2001:1777–1805.
86. Mitchison HM, Mole SE. Neurodegenerative disease: the neuronal ceroid lipofuscinoses (Batten disease). *Curr Opin Neurol* 2001;14:795–803.
87. Molyneux AJ, Blair E, Coleman N, et al. Mucopolysaccharidosis type VII associated with hydrops fetalis: histopathological and ultrastructural features with genetic implications. *J Clin Pathol* 1997;50: 252–254.
88. Morisawa Y, Fujieda M, Murakami N, et al. Lysosomal glycogen storage disease with normal acid maltase with early fatal outcome. *J Neurol Sci* 1998;160:175–179.
89. Moser HW, Linke T, Fensom AH, et al. Acid ceramidase deficiency: Farber lipogranulomatosis. In: Scriver CR, Beaudet AL, Sly WS, et al., eds. *The metabolic & molecular bases of inherited disease*. St. Louis, MO: McGraw-Hill Medical Publishing Division, 2001:3573–3588.
90. Mudd SH, Levy HL, Kraus JP. Disorders of transsulfuration. In: Scriver CR, Beaudet AL, Sly WS, et al., eds. *The metabolic & molecular bases of inherited disease*. St. Louis, MO: McGraw-Hill Medical Publishing Division, 2001:2007–2056.
91. Munnich A, Rotig A, Cormier-Daire V, et al. Clinical presentation of respiratory chain deficiency. In: Scriver CR, Beaudet AL, Sly WS, et al., eds. *The metabolic & molecular bases of inherited disease*. St. Louis, MO: McGraw-Hill Medical Publishing Division, 2001: 2261–2274.
92. Neufeld EF, Muenzer J. The mucopolysaccharidoses. In: Scriver CR, Beaudet AL, Sly WS, et al., eds. *The metabolic & molecular bases of inherited disease*. St. Louis, MO: McGraw-Hill Medical Publishing Division, 2001:3421–3452.
93. Olpin SE. The metabolic investigation of sudden infant death. *Ann Clin Biochem* 2004;41:282–293.
94. Orho M, Bosshard NU, Buist NR, et al. Mutations in the liver glycogen synthase gene in children with hypoglycemia due to glycogen storage disease type 0. *J Clin Invest* 1998;102:507–515.

95. Palo J, Riekkinen P, Arstila A, et al. Biochemical and fine structural studies on brain and liver biopsies in aspartylglucosaminuria. *Neurology* 1971;21:1198–1204.
96. Patterson MC, Vanier MT, Suzuki K, et al. Niemann-Pick disease Type C: a lipid trafficking disorder. In: Scriver CR, Beaudet AL, Sly WS, et al., eds. *The metabolic & molecular bases of inherited disease*. St. Louis, MO: McGraw-Hill Medical Publishing Division, 2001:3611–3633.
97. Perez-Atayde AR, Fox V, Teitelbaum JE, et al. Mitochondrial neurogastrointestinal encephalomyopathy: diagnosis by rectal biopsy. *Am J Surg Pathol* 1998;22:1141–1147.
98. Poorthuis BJ, Wevers RA, Kleijer WJ, et al. The frequency of lysosomal storage diseases in The Netherlands. *Hum Genet* 1999;105:151–156.
99. Portmann B, Thompson R, Roberts E, et al. Genetic and metabolic liver disease. In: Burt A, Portman B, Ferrell L, eds. *MacSween's pathology of the liver*. Philadelphia, PA: Churchill Livingstone/Elsevier, 2007:199–326.
100. Prasad A, Kaye EM, Alroy J. Electron microscopic examination of skin biopsy as a cost-effective tool in the diagnosis of lysosomal storage diseases. *J Child Neurol* 1996;11:301–308.
101. Raghuveer TS, Garg U, Graf WD. Inborn errors of metabolism in infancy and early childhood: an update. *Am Fam Physician* 2006;73:1981–1990.
102. Renwick N, Nasr SH, Chung WK, et al. Foamy podocytes. *Am J Kidney Dis* 2003;41:891–896.
103. Roberts DJ, Ampola MG, Lage JM. Diagnosis of unsuspected fetal metabolic storage disease by routine placental examination. *Pediatr Pathol* 1991;11:647–656.
104. Roe CR, Ding J. Mitochondrial fatty acid oxidation disorders. In: Scriver CR, Beaudet AL, Sly WS, et al., eds. *The metabolic & molecular bases of inherited disease*. St. Louis, MO: McGraw-Hill Medical Publishing Division, 2001:2297–2326.
105. Rotig A, Cormier V, Blanche S, et al. Pearson's marrow-pancreas syndrome. A multisystem mitochondrial disorder in infancy. *J Clin Invest* 1990;86:1601–1608.
106. Russo P, O'Regan S. Visceral pathology of hereditary tyrosinemia type I. *Am J Hum Genet* 1990;47:317–324.
107. Sarfati R, Hubert A, Dugue-Marechaud M, et al. Prenatal diagnosis of Gaucher's disease type 2. Ultrasonographic, biochemical and histological aspects. *Prenat Diagn* 2000;20:340–343.
108. Schuchman EH, Desnick RJ. Niemann-Pick disease types A and B: acid sphingomyelinase deficiencies. In: Scriver CR, Beaudet AL, Sly WS, et al., eds. *The metabolic & molecular bases of inherited disease*. St. Louis, MO: McGraw-Hill Medical Publishing Division, 2001:3589–3610.
109. Scriver CR, Kaufman S. Hyperphenylalaninemia: phenylalanine hydroxylase deficiency. In: Scriver CR, Beaudet AL, Sly WS, et al., eds. *The metabolic & molecular bases of inherited disease*. St. Louis, MO: McGraw-Hill Medical Publishing Division, 2001:1667–1724.
110. Servidei S, Riepe RE, Langston C, et al. Severe cardiopathy in branching enzyme deficiency. *J Pediatr* 1987;111:51–56.
111. Shin YS. Glycogen storage disease: clinical, biochemical, and molecular heterogeneity. *Semin Pediatr Neurol* 2006;13:115–120.
112. Simell O. Lysinuric protein intolerance and other cationic aminoacidurias. In: Scriver C, Beaudet A, Sly W, et al., eds. *The metabolic & molecular bases of inherited disease*. St. Louis, MO: McGraw-Hill Medical Publishing Division, 2001:4933–4956.
113. Simonati A, Rizzuto N. Neuronal ceroid lipofuscinoses: pathological features of bioptic specimens from 28 patients. *Neurol Sci* 2000;21:S63–S70.
114. Slaugenhaupt SA. The molecular basis of mucolipidosis type IV. *Curr Mol Med* 2002;2:445–450.
115. Soma H, Yamada K, Osawa H, et al. Identification of Gaucher cells in the chorionic villi associated with recurrent hydrops fetalis. *Placenta* 2000;21:412–416.
116. Steinmann B, Gitzelmann R, Van den Berghe G. Disorders of fructose metabolism. In: Scriver CR, Beaudet A, Sly W, et al. eds. *The Metabolic & molecular bases of inherited disease*. St. Louis, MO: McGraw Hill Medical Publishing Division, 2001:1489–1520.
117. Stoller JK, Aboussouan LS. Alpha1-antitrypsin deficiency. *Lancet* 2005;365:2225–2236.
118. Stone DL, Sidransky E. Hydrops fetalis: lysosomal storage disorders in extremis. *Adv Pediatr* 1999;46:409–440.
119. Suzuki Y, Oshima A, Nanba E. β-galactosidase deficiency (β-galactosidosis): G_{M1} gangliosidosis and Morquio B disease. In: Scriver CR, Beaudet AL, Sly WS, et al., eds. *The metabolic & molecular bases of inherited disease*. St. Louis, MO: McGraw-Hill Medical Publishing Division, 2001:3775–3809.
120. Szonyi L, Dobos M, Vasarhelyi B, et al. Prevalence of α1-antitrypsin phenotypes in patients with IgA nephropathy. *Clin Nephrol* 2004;62: 418–422.
121. Tanner MS. Mechanisms of liver injury relevant to pediatric hepatology. *Crit Rev Clin Lab Sci* 2002;39:1–61.
122. Teitelbaum JE, Berde CB, Nurko S, et al. Diagnosis and management of MNGIE syndrome in children: case report and review of the literature. *J Pediatr Gastroenterol Nutr* 2002;35:377–383.
123. Thomas GH. Disorders of glycoprotein degradation: α-mannosidoses, β-mannosidosis, fucosidoses, and sialidosis. In: Scriver CR, Beaudet AL, Sly WS, et al., eds. *The metabolic & molecular bases of inherited disease*. St. Louis, MO: McGraw-Hill Medical Publishing Division, 2001:3507–3533.
124. Valle D, Simell O. The hyperornithinemias. In: Scriver CR, Beaudet AL, Sly WS, et al., eds. *The metabolic & molecular bases of inherited disease*. St. Louis, MO: McGraw-Hill Medical Publishing Division, 2001:1857–1895.
125. van Spronsen FJ, Bijleveld CM, van Maldegem BT, et al. Hepatocellular carcinoma in hereditary tyrosinemia type I despite 2-(2 nitro-4–3 trifluoro- methylbenzoyl)-1, 3-cyclohexanedione treatment. *J Pediatr Gastroenterol Nutr* 2005;40:90–93.
126. Vedder AC, Strijland A, vd Bergh Weerman MA, et al. Manifestations of Fabry disease in placental tissue. *J Inherit Metab Dis* 2006;29:106–111.
127. Vellodi A. Lysosomal storage disorders. *Br J Haematol* 2005;128: 413–431.
128. Vogler C, Rosenberg HS, Williams JC, et al. Electron microscopy in the diagnosis of lysosomal storage diseases. *Am J Med Genet Suppl* 1987;3:243–255.
129. von Figura K, Gieselmann V, Jaeken J. Metachromatic leukodystrophy. In: Scriver CR, Beaudet AL, Sly WS, et al., eds. *The metabolic & molecular bases of inherited disease* St. Louis, MO: McGraw-Hill Medical Publishing Division, 2001:3695–3724.
130. Walter JH, Tyfield LA. Galactosemia. In: Scriver CR, Beaudet A, Sly W, et al. eds. *The Metabolic & molecular bases of inherited disease*. St. Louis, MO: McGraw Hill Medical Publishing Division, 2001:1553–1587.
131. Wanders RJ, Waterham HR. Peroxisomal disorders: the single peroxisomal enzyme deficiencies. *Biochim Biophys Acta* 2006;1763: 1707–1720.
132. Weinstein DA, Correia CE, Saunders AC, et al. Hepatic glycogen synthase deficiency: an infrequently recognized cause of ketotic hypoglycemia. *Mol Genet Metab* 2006;87:284–288.
133. Wendel U, Schroten H, Burdach S, et al. Glycogen storage disease type Ib: infectious complications and measures for prevention. *Eur J Pediatr* 1993;152(Suppl 1):S49–S51.
134. Wenger DA, Coppola S, Liu SL. Lysosomal storage disorders: diagnostic dilemmas and prospects for therapy. *Genet Med* 2002;4: 412–419.
135. Wenger DA, Suzuki K, Suzuki Y, et al. Galactosylceramide lipidosis: globoid cell leukodystrophy (Krabbe disease). In: Scriver CR, Beaudet AL, Sly WS, et al., eds. *The metabolic & molecular bases of inherited disease* St. Louis, MO: McGraw-Hill Medical Publishing Division, 2001:3669–3694.

136. Whitington PF. Fetal and infantile hemochromatosis. *Hepatology* 2006;43:654–660.
137. Wilcox RL, Nelson CC, Stenzel P, et al. Postmortem screening for fatty acid oxidation disorders by analysis of Guthrie cards with tandem mass spectrometry in sudden unexpected death in infancy. *J Pediatr* 2002;141:833–836.
138. Wraith JE. Lysosomal disorders. *Semin Neonatol* 2002;7:75–83.
139. Yang Z, McMahon CJ, Smith LR, et al. Danon disease as an underrecognized cause of hypertrophic cardiomyopathy in children. *Circulation* 2005;112:1612–1617.
140. Zamora SA, Pinto A, Scott RB, et al. Mitochondrial abnormalities of liver in two children with citrullinaemia. *J Inherit Metab Dis* 1997;20:509–516.

CHAPTER 6

Congenital and Acquired Systemic Infectious Diseases

HARESH MANI
J. THOMAS STOCKER

> As it takes two to make a quarrel,
> so it takes two to make a disease,
> the microbe and its host.
>
> —Charles V. Chapin, 1856–1941

Infections are the leading cause of death in the pediatric population (e333). The optimism that accompanied the advent of antibiotics in the mid-20th century was premature, and even advances such as immunization and improved sanitation have not stopped microbial reemergence time and again. The importance of infectious diseases is underscored by the ever-increasing antimicrobial resistance and the resurgence of infections such as tuberculosis (TB), malaria, and syphilis; once thought eradicated from developed countries. Further, international travel has removed boundaries from the spread of infection, as exemplified by the rapid spread of infections such as severe acute respiratory syndrome (SARS) across countries. There is voluminous literature on this subject, with numerous heavy tomes devoted to individual infections. In this chapter, we aim to provide an overview of systemic infections that the pediatric pathologist is likely to encounter. Infections that are predominantly confined to a single organ system, (e.g., poliomyelitis, hepatitis) are not considered in this chapter, even though they may occasionally cause systemic manifestations. The reader is directed to chapters dealing with specific organ systems for information on such infections. Further, since it is impossible to comprehensively detail all facets of various systemic infections in a single chapter, we have generously referenced resources for the reader with specific interests. Detailed information is also available in standard textbooks including Feigin and Cherry's *Textbook of Pediatric Infectious Diseases* (56), Connor and Chandler's *Pathology of Infectious Diseases* (32) and the *American Academy of Pediatrics Red Book* (www.aapredbook.com).

THE PATHOGENESIS OF INFECTIOUS DISEASES

An infection is the result of an encounter between an infectious agent and a susceptible host. The microorganism is the *sine qua non*, but the occurrence of the disease, its pathophysiology, and its outcome are determined by host and environmental factors. A discussion of microbial virulence factors is beyond the scope of this chapter; various reviews cover the topic in considerable depth (130,184) (e37,e107).

HOST FACTORS

Host genetic factors, immune status, age, and geographic location determine exposure to and invasion by microorganisms. The apparent heritability of infectious disease susceptibility is determined by developmental and maturational changes in host defense, from embryo through adolescence, with resultant differences in response to infection (e65). The contribution of host genetics to infection susceptibility is complex (179) (e340). Genes responsible for simple or complex control of susceptibility to infection with different pathogens have been recently identified and characterized. Polymorphisms in genes coding for proteins that recognize bacterial pathogens [such as toll-like receptor 4, CD14, Fc(gamma) RIIa, and mannose-binding lectin] and the response to bacterial pathogens [with elaboration of cytokines such as tumor necrosis factor-α, interleukin (IL)-1α, IL-1β, IL-1 receptor agonist, IL-6, IL-10, heat shock proteins, angiotensin I converting enzyme, plasminogen activator inhibitor-1] can influence response to bacterial stimuli (33).

Immunologic maturity and immunodeficiencies (quantitative and qualitative) also determine susceptibility to invasive microbial infections. Neonates and infants are at a relative immunologic disadvantage since they have developmentally immature immune systems. The immaturity of the fetal immune system helps prevent "premature rejection" by the host (the mother). Paradoxically, this potential benefit also increases the risk of infections for the fetus and the prematurely born neonate. Term newborns have a higher frequency of microbial infections than older children and adults; extremely premature newborns (<28 weeks of gestation) have a five to tenfold higher frequency than even term newborns (e179). Immunological immaturity also obscures clinical symptoms in neonatal sepsis. Recent advancements in developmental immunology provide a framework for understanding the mechanisms underlying the propensity of infections in the preterm, near-term, and term newborn (28). The immune environment during early life favors innate over acquired immunity. Innate immunity against pathogens represents the critical first-line barrier of host defenses, as newborns have a naïve adaptive immune system. However, innate immune mechanisms are also relatively impaired in neonates as compared to older children and adults, thereby increasing neonatal susceptibility to infections (94) (e211). Further, the neonate is unable to produce antibody to thymus-independent antigens such as bacterial polysaccharides owing to multiple factors, although transplacentally acquired maternal antibodies confer some protection for the first few months of life. Neonatal B-cells are of an immature phenotype, the neonatal spleen has a different cellular composition and neonatal accessory cells (macrophages and dendritic cells) appear to produce lesser amounts of stimulatory cytokines and an overabundance of inhibitory cytokines (101).

Children with immunodeficiencies (primary or acquired) have an increased risk of infections (Tables 6-1 and 6-2). Impaired splenic function (due to asplenia, disease, or splenectomy) significantly increases the risk of life-threatening bacterial sepsis, especially with capsulated organisms, necessitating pneumococcal and meningococcal immunizations. Secondary factors such as comorbidities, medications, and nutritional status also dictate clinical course (Table 6-3). Organisms causing disease in a setting of immunodeficiency are, for the most part, "opportunists"; they are already on the scene, either as normal flora of skin, upper respiratory tract, or gastrointestinal tract (GIT), or they are ubiquitous in the environment where they ordinarily do no harm.

ENVIRONMENTAL FACTORS

Over 50 years ago, Haldane proposed that the prevalence of thalassemia in malaria-endemic areas was due to the heterozygotic advantage it conferred against malaria, despite its otherwise deleterious effects. Table 6-4 outlines examples of the influence of geographic, political, and socioeconomic factors on infectious diseases that account for a major part of the world's infant morbidity and mortality. Infectious disease risks associated with international travel are diverse and depend on the destination, planned activities, and baseline medical history. Children have special needs and vulnerabilities that should be addressed when preparing for travel abroad (109).

On a less global scale, certain local environments must frequently be considered as contributors to disease. Such nosocomial environments as intensive care units, neonatal nurseries, day care centers, schools, and summer camps play a role either by serving as reservoirs for pathogenic microbes or by facilitating their spread in a susceptible population. Finally, hospitalized or chronically ill children are exposed additionally to equipment and pharmaceutical agents that may be the source of iatrogenic infections.

Infections and Teratogenesis

In order to act as a teratogen, an agent must be capable of crossing the placenta at an early stage of embryogenesis or organogenesis and either inhibit cell growth and differentiation, or produce destructive fetal lesions. The spectrum of

Table 6-1 ■ INFECTIONS AND PRIMARY IMMUNODEFICIENCIES

General associations	
Recurrent respiratory and pyogenic infections by extracellular bacteria: *Streptococcus pneumoniae, Haemophilus influenzae, Staphylococcus aureus*	Antibody deficiencies
Chronic or severe infections with intracellular pathogens: viruses, mycobacteria, *Pneumocystis carinii, Toxoplasma gondii*, and others	Deficiencies of T lymphocytes
Specific associations	
Chronic viral encephalitis	X-linked agammaglobulinemla
Echo virus dermatomyositis	
Polio vaccine–induced paralysis	
Severe parainfluenza infection	Severe combined immunodeficiency
Severe varicella	Cartilage-hair hypoplasia
Severe Epstein-Barr virus infection	X-linked lymphoproliferative syndrome
Recurrent meningococcal sepsis	Complement deficiencies
Disseminated gonococcal infection	
Staphylococcal skin infections	Neutrophil abnormalities
Mucosal and periodontal infections	
Infections with *Aspergillus* sp., *S. aureus, Pseudomonas cepacia, Chromobacterium violaceum*	Chronic granulomatous disease
BCGosis and atypical myocobacteria	NF-γ and IL-12 deficiencies
Persistent mucocutaneous candidiasis	Chronic mucocutaneous candidiasis
Chronic/recurrent giardiasis	IgA deficiency

BCG, bacille Calmette-Guérin; INF, interferon; IL, interleukin; IgA, immunoglobulin A.

Table 6-2 ■ CONGENITAL IMMUNODEFICIENCIES WITH AN INCREASED RISK OF SEPSIS[a]

Immunodeficiency	Characteristic Susceptibility[b]	Estimated Sepsis Occurrence, %[c]
Innate immune defects		
Complement deficiency	*Neisseria*	28
Mannose binding lectin	*Neisseria*	
NEMO deficiency	*Klebsiella, S. pneumoniae*, mycobacteria	86
IRAK4 deficiency	Gram-positive bacteria	75
TLR-4	Gram-negative bacteria	
Caspase-12 defect		
CGD	*Salmonella, Burkholderia, Candida*	21 (X-linked) 10 (autosomal)
Leukocyte adhesion deficiency	*Pseudomonas aeruginosa*	28
Specific granule deficiency		
Severe chronic neutropenia		3[d]
Type-1 cytokine axis defects	Mycobacteria, *Salmonella*	
Adaptive immune defects		
SCID		5[e]
Agammaglobulinemia	*Pseudomonas*	10[f]
Hyper-IgM	*Pseudomonas*, pneumococcus, *Escherichia*	13
CVID		1[g]
Transient hypogammaglobulinemia of infancy		
IgG subclass deficiency		
Ataxia telangiectasia	Gram-positive bacteria	5
IPEX	Enteric bacteria	
Wiskott-Aldrich syndrome		36

[a]Sepsis, caused by bacteremia, fungemia, or viremia.
[b]Characteristic infectious susceptibility that can be useful in considering a particular diagnosis.
[c]Occurrence of sepsis within a particular population.
[d]Bacteremia in additional 15%.
[e]As high as 30% in reticular dysgenesis and 16% in Omenn syndrome.
[f]As a presenting manifestation before immunoglobulin replacement therapy.
[g]Higher in the Good syndrome variant (16%).
NEMO, nuclear factor_B; TLR, toll-like receptor; CGD, chronic granulomatous disease; SCID, severe combined immunodeficiency; Ig, immunoglobulin; CVID, common variable immunodeficiency; IPEX, immunodysregulation, polyendocrinopathy, enteropathy, X-linked.
Source: Orange JS. Congenital immunodeficiencies and sepsis. *Pediatr Crit Care Med* 2005;6(Suppl.):S99–S107.

Table 6-3 ■ PRIMARILY NONIMMUNE DISORDERS INFLUENCING INCIDENCE AND SEVERITY OF INFECTION

	Site	Predominant Organisms	Proposed Mechanism	References
Metabolic disorders				
Diabetes mellitus	Skin, GU tract	*S. aureus, E. coli*, yeasts, *Zygomycetes*	Impaired phagocytosis, neutrophilic chemotaxis, and opsonization	17
Galactosemia	Bacteremia, meningitis	*E. coli*, group D streptococci	Impaired phagocytosis due to hypoglycemia	117, 281
Uremia	Pneumonia, septicemia	Unspecified	Impaired macrophage function	314
Iron deficiency	Unspecified	Unspecified	Impaired bacterial killing	8, 356, 482
Nephrotic syndrome	Peritonitis	*S. pneumoniae*, enteric bacilli	Unknown, protein loss (?)	499
Intravenous lipid	Pulmonary arteritis, fungemia	*Malassezia furfur*	Lipophilic organism	369, 370, 384
Circulatory alterations				
Congenital/ rheumatic heart disease	Endocarditis, pericarditis	Viridans streptococci, *S. aureus*	Endocardial damage due to jet effects, turbulence	231, 308
Sickle cell disease	Meningitis, systemic osteomyelitis	*S. pneumoniae, Salmonella* sp.	Ischemia, functional asplenia, defective opsonization	25, 123, 211, 346, 357, 492, 504
Exudative enteropathy	Pneumonia, gastroenteritis	*S. pneumoniae*, enteric bacilli, *Giardia*	Intestinal loss of immunoglobulins and lymphocytes	156, 157

(continued)

Table 6-3 ■ PRIMARILY NONIMMUNE DISORDERS INFLUENCING INCIDENCE AND SEVERITY OF INFECTION *(Continued)*

	Site	Predominant Organisms	Proposed Mechanism	References
Obstructive phenomena				
Cystic fibrosis	Bronchitis, bronchiectasis, pneumonia	*S. aureus, Pseudomonas*	Defective ciliary movement, mechanical obstruction due to hyperviscosity of mucus	272, 298, 341, 446, 460
Immobile cilia syndromes	Otitis, sinusitis, bronchitis, bronchiectasis	*H. influenzae, Neisseria,* staphylococci, streptococci, *Pseudomonas*	Defective ciliary motility	376, 461
GU obstruction/ malfunction	Pyelonephritis, cystitis	*E. coli, Proteus, Enterobacteria*	Urinary stasis, instrumentation, trauma	93, 256, 266 267, 382, 427
Barrier defects				
Eczema, exfoliative dermatitis	Impetigo, sepsis	Staphylococci, β-hemolytic streptococci	Mechanical loss of skin barrier	156, 157
Burns	Skin, sepsis	*Pseudomonas, S. aureus, S. Epidermidis,* fungi, varicella, herpes simplex	Changes in flora, physiochemical properties of the skin	156, 157
Skull fractures	Meningitis	*S. pneumoniae*	Direct access to CSF via respiratory passages and sinuses	34, 55
Neural tube defects	Meningitis	*S. pneumoniae,* Gram-negative enterics, staphylococci	Direct access to CSF from skin	34, 156, 157
Foreign bodies				
Arterial and venous catheters	Phlebitis, omphalitis, endocarditis, arteritis, liver abscess	*S. epidermidis, Pseudomonas,* yeasts	Barrier bypass, nidus for infection	51, 277, 300
CSF shunts	Meningitis, peritonitis, septicemia, endocarditis, phlebitis	*S. epidermidis, S. aureus,* enteric organisms	Barrier bypass, nidus for infection	336, 415
Prostheses	Endocarditis	*S. aureus, S. epidermidis*	Nidus for infection	251, 448
Aspiration	Pneumonia, lung abscess	Anaerobes	Aspiration of infected material, bronchial obstruction by foreign bodies, necrosis of airway epithelium	47, 326
Splenectomy	Fulminant septicemia	*S. pneumoniae, Salmonella*	Defects in opsonization and clearing	146, 436
Malnutrition	Pneumonia	Measles, herpes simplex, staphylococci, enteric Gram-negatives, *Pneumocystis*	Depression of complement, cell-mediated immunity, and phagocytosis	215, 253

CSF, cerebrospinal fluid; GU, genitourinary.
? = Pathogenesis suspected, but largely unknown at present.

resulting defects depends both on the timing and the severity of the insult. The dysmorphogenetic syndromes produced by fetal infection are remarkable in their clinical and morphologic variability. The first such association was the recognition of congenital rubella by Sir Norman Gregg in 1941 (e126). Of the large number of agents causing fetal infection, only rubella, cytomegalovirus (CMV), varicella-zoster virus (VZV), herpes simplex virus (HSV), toxoplasma, and syphilis are firmly established as human teratogens. Early reports of a dysmorphic syndrome associated with human immunodeficiency virus (HIV) infection, distinguishable from the effects of drug/alcohol abuse or concomitant opportunistic infection (e156), have not been confirmed (e263). The evidence linking coxsackie viruses and mumps to congenital heart defects and endocardial fibroelastosis, respectively, is also inconclusive.

In-utero infections can result in a variety of adverse fetal outcomes. Microorganisms damage fetal cells or tissues (either directly or indirectly by elaborating toxic substances), interrupt cell division or migration, and/or evoke (or depress) host inflammatory and repair responses. Depending on the organism and the timing of the insult, intrauterine infection may result in no detectable damage, resorption of the embryo, spontaneous abortion, prematurity, stillbirth, intrauterine growth restriction, congenital malformation, acute or chronic neonatal infection, or clinically inapparent ongoing or static disease with late sequelae. Intrauterine rubella infection represents a paradigm of fetal infection because it

Table 6-4 ■ INFLUENCE OF ENVIRONMENTAL FACTORS ON INFECTIOUS DISEASES

	Example	Comment	References
Geographic			
Climate	Falciparum malaria	Requires summer average over 21°C	44, 381
Geologic characteristics	Onchocerciasis	Insect vector develops in fast-flowing rivers	381
Animal reservoirs	Toxoplasmosis	Oocysts produced in cats	166
Vector availability	Chagas disease	Transmitted by triatomid insects	500
Political and economic			
Population density/ overcrowding	Tuberculosis	Complex relationship, including ease of droplet transmission, malnutrition, presence of other chronic diseases	270, 278, 386, 388
Political structure and stability	Measles, polio	Can be eradicated by effective and sustained public health and immunization programs	163, 207
War, refugee status	Malaria	Refugee borne global spread of disease	355
Socioeconomic status	Tetanus	Most common cause of neonatal death in countries with lowest per capita income	455
Cultural/behavioral patterns	AIDS	Sexual and parenteral transmission of disease in homosexuals and drug addicts	167, 175, 398
Nosocomial sources of infection			
Pediatric ICU	*S. aureus, E. coli, Klebsiella, Enterobacter, Serratia*	Pediatric ICU–acquired infections less common than adult ICU–acquired	24, 37, 389
Neonatal ICU	Staphylococci, *E. coli*	Susceptibility Increased because of absence of normal flora	177, 217
Day care	Diarrheal illnesses, hepatitis A, *Haemophilus influenzae*, upper respiratory viruses	Close person-to-person contact in a highly susceptible population with behavior patterns facilitating transmission	26, 118, 483, 502
Contaminated ventilabory equipment	*Pseudomonas, Serratia*	Aerosols and nebulizers are reservoirs; cystic fibrosis patients especially affected	156, 157 363
Contaminated IV fluids	*E. coli, Erwinia, Pseudomonas*	Contamination of containers	156, 157
Contaminated water/air supplies	*Legionella*	Reservoirs in drinking water supply, air conditioning equipment. Rarely seen in normal children	139

ICU, intensive care unit; IV, intravenous.

operates by all of these mechanisms to affect virtually all of the possible outcomes. Table 6-5 lists various viral infections associated with adverse fetal outcomes. (146).

Intrapartum or neonatal infections are more limited in scope than those occurring *in utero* because of the relatively more advanced developmental state of the infant. Nonetheless, they may produce acute and possibly fatal disease (e.g., neonatal herpes virus infection), persistent infection with ongoing tissue or organ dysfunction (e.g., postnatal CMV infection), or late complications of the infection and its subsequent repair process (e.g., obstructive hydrocephalus resulting from neonatal meningitis).

TRANSMISSION

Materno-fetal transmission is specific to the pediatric population and may occur *in utero* ("vertical transmission") or during breast feeding. Other routes of transmission including inhalation, ingestion, and inoculation are similar in adults and children. Routes of fetal and neonatal infection have been thoroughly reviewed by Blanc (14). His findings are illustrated in Figure 6-1 and summarized in Table 6-6.

VERTICAL TRANSMISSION

Pathways of vertical transmission include *in utero* (transplacental and ascending), intrapartum (in the birth canal, from maternal genital and GITs), or immediately postnatally (although, strictly speaking, this is not vertical transmission). Although *in-utero* infection can occur in any trimester of pregnancy, the timing of infection significantly affects its clinical course resulting in asymptomatic infection, fetal demise, teratogenicity, prematurity, clinical disease present at birth, or later presentation. There are two major routes of intrauterine fetal infection. Organisms may ascend from the maternal genital tract through the cervix to the amniotic sac through either intact or ruptured membranes. This ascending route is the preferred one for HSV, most bacteria, and Candida. Hematogenous spread of maternal blood-borne organisms across the placenta is the pathway used by most

Table 6-5 ■ VIRAL INFECTIONS ASSOCIATED WITH ADVERSE FETAL OUTCOMES

	Transmission						
Virus	***In Utero***	**During Delivery**	**Breast Milk**	**Incidence per 1,000 Live Births**	**Present in AF/Fetus in Unaffected Cases**	**Clinical Consequences at Birth**	**Postnatal**
HSV	+	+++	++	0.04	Yes	IUGR, death, multiorgan disease	Recurrence
CMV	+++	+++	+++	5–22	Yes	IUGR, CNS disease, CID	Developmental delay, deafness
Adenovirus	+++	–	++	Unknown	Yes	IUGR, fetal hydrops	Unknown
AAV	+	+	++	Unknown	Unknown	Prematurity	—
EV	+	–	+++	Unknown	Unknown	Myocarditis	Neurodevelopmental delay, diabetes
HHV6	+	+	+	Unknown	Yes	Encephalitis	Unknown
LCMV	+	–	+	Unknown	Unknown	CNS disease, eye disease, death	Blindness
Parvovirus	++	+	+	Unknown	Unknown	Fetal hydrops	Anemia
Rubella	++	–	+	0.01	Unknown	CNS disease, eye disease	Deafness, exanthem
VZV	+	++	++	0.01	Yes	Limb disease, CNS disease	Disseminated VZV

+, rare; ++, frequent; +++, common.
AAV, adenovirus associated virus; AF, amniotic fluid; CID, chronic inflammatory disease; CMV, cytomegalovirus; CNS, central nervous system; EV, enterovirus; HHV, human herpes virus; HSV, herpes simplex virus; IUGR, intrauterine growth restriction; LCMV, lymphocytic choriomeningitis virus; VZV, varicella zoster virus.
Modified from Rawlinson WD, et al. Viruses and other infections in stillbirth: what is the evidence and what should we be doing? *Pathology* 2008;40(2):149–160.

viruses and protozoa such as plasmodia and toxoplasma. Intrauterine fetal manipulation, amniocentesis, and chorionic villus sampling represent potential risks for infection, but this appears to be a very rare event (e145,e219,e223).

Perinatal infections commonly occur from exposure to blood or body fluids and contact with pathogens from the maternal genitourinary and GITs. The likelihood that the exposed infant will be infected varies significantly with the specific organism and various host factors (e.g., passively acquired antibody levels in the infant). Intrapartum transmission is more efficient in a setting of prolonged labor combined with an infected maternal birth canal. Premature inspiratory movements on the part of the fetus may result in pneumonia occurring soon after birth, with high mortality. Postnatally acquired infections are transmitted most commonly through contact with caregivers (parents, relatives, visitors, and health care providers), the environment (medical equipment, other fomites), or breast milk, depending on the organism (97). In most situations of perinatal mother to child transmission, the infant is exposed before the illness is diagnosed in the mother (e.g., measles, Coxsackievirus infection) and frequently occurs even before the mother becomes ill (e.g., chickenpox, hepatitis).

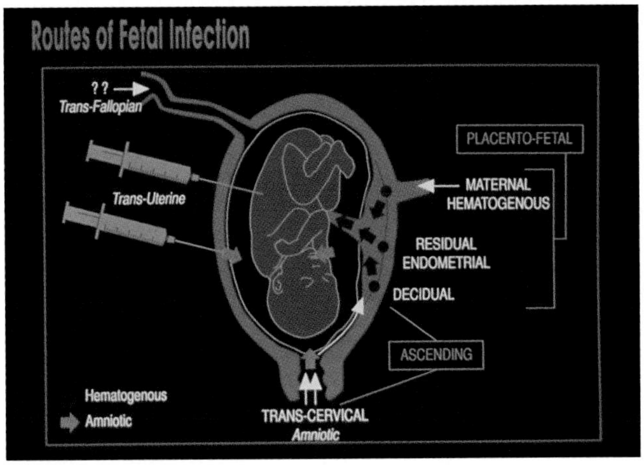

Routes of Fetal Infection

?? Trans-Fallopian
Trans-Uterine
PLACENTO-FETAL
MATERNAL HEMATOGENOUS
RESIDUAL ENDOMETRIAL
DECIDUAL
ASCENDING
Hematogenous
Amniotic
TRANS-CERVICAL Amniotic

FIGURE 6-1 ■ Routes of fetal infection.

BREAST MILK TRANSMISSION

Human milk protects against specific pathogens as well as separate clinical illnesses (e.g., necrotizing enterocolitis, bacteremia, meningitis, respiratory tract illness, diarrheal disease, and otitis media). Protective mechanisms of breast milk include improved growth of nonpathogenic flora, decreased colonization with enteropathogens, enhanced development of the respiratory and intestinal mucosal barriers, providing secretory IgA and functioning immune cells (neutrophils, macrophages, T and B lymphocytes), preventing gut inflammation and immunomodulation (51,104) (e123). Although breast milk may be a route for transmission of infection, organisms that are a concern for transmission through breastfeeding are transmitted more commonly through other mechanisms. Clinically significant infectious agents that are transmitted through breast milk include HIV-1, human

Table 6-6 ■ PREDOMINANT PATHWAYS OF THE MAJOR FETAL AND NEONATAL INFECTION

Transplacental	Ascending	Postpartum
Bacteria		
Listeria[a]	Group B streptococci	Staphylococci[a]
Treponema pallidum	Enteric bacilli[b]	*Pseudomonas*[a]
Mycobacterum tuberculosis	*Hemophilus influenzae*	Nongroup B streptococci[b]
Borrelia	*Neisseria gonorrhea*	
Campylobacter fetus (?)	Anaerobes	
	Actinomyces	
	Fusobacteria	
Viruses		
Cytomegalovirus[c]	Herpes simplex[c]	Respiratory syncytial virus
Human immunodeficiency virus		Coxsackie B[a]
Rubella		
Mumps		
Measles		
Variola		
Vaccinia		
Poliovirus		
ECHO		
Hepatitis B[c]		
Western equine encephalitis		
Human parvovirus		
Varicella zoster[a]		
Epstein-Barr virus		
Protozoa		
Toxoplasma		
Plasmodium		
Trypanosoma		
Babesia		
Fungi		
Coccidioides	*Candida*[c]	
	Aspergillus	
	Torulopsis	
Mycoplasmas		
	Mycoplasma hominis	
	Ureaplasma urealyticum	

[a]Also utilize ascending route.
[b]Also utilize hematogenous route.
[c]Also acquired postnatally.
From a summary of references 46, 130, 167, 184, 196, 306, 345, 400, 414, 437, and 441.

T-lymphocytotropic virus-1 (HTLV-1), CMV, measles virus, and streptococcus (104) (e290). Bacterial infections are rarely, if ever, transmitted to infants through breast milk. However, temporary cessation of breastfeeding has been recommended in certain maternal bacterial infections (*Neisseria gonorrhoeae*, *Haemophilus influenzae*, Group B streptococci (GBS), and staphylococci; longer period of cessation for others including *Borrelia burgdorferi*, *Treponema pallidum*, and *Mycobacterium tuberculosis*).

EVALUATION OF SUSPECTED FETAL INFECTION

Given the incredibly wide spectrum of disease produced by fetal infection, the pathologist must be prepared properly to evaluate fetal and neonatal deaths in order to arrive at a correct diagnosis. Infection should be suspected in newborns exhibiting any or all of the following: intrauterine growth restriction or failure to thrive, hydrops, jaundice or hepatosplenomegaly, skin rashes (especially vesicular or purpuric), hydrocephalus or microcephaly, and eye lesions such as microphthalmia, chorioretinitis, and cataract. Wigglesworth has outlined a procedure for autopsy evaluation of such infants using serologic studies, radiology, careful and complete bacteriologic studies including darkfield examination, viral diagnostic studies including culture, and electron microscopy (e365,e366). Nucleic acid amplification techniques, many applicable to formalin-fixed tissues, have made possible the identification of infectious agents hitherto difficult or impossible to detect (62) (e279). It cannot be overemphasized that histopathologic examination, however indispensable, constitutes only one facet of adequate autopsy examination in suspected prenatal or perinatal infection.

VIRAL INFECTIONS

Most significant viral infections in neonates or infants occur through transplacental or intrapartum transmission. The risk of transmission is dependant on whether the maternal infection is primary (e.g., HSV, HIV-1), secondary (reactivation) (e.g., HSV, CMV) or chronic (e.g., hepatitis B, HIV-1, HTLV-1). Fetal and neonatal viral infections are multifaceted. Many of these agents are teratogens, and most can affect the fetus or infant at any stage of development to produce fetal death or malformation, acute self-limited infection, ongoing infection, and late sequelae due to destructive, repair, or immune responses. Table 6-7 summarizes the main features of fetal and neonatal viral infections, while Table 6-8 outlines the major pathologic features of commonly seen viral infections in infants and older children. The number and diversity of the viruses affecting the human host have assumed substantial proportions. Of the more commonly encountered viral illnesses of children, many involve almost exclusively the nervous system (e.g., poliomyelitis, rabies) and are discussed in Chapter 10. The respiratory tract pathogens are included in Chapter 12, and the hepatitis viruses in Chapter 15. Of the remainder, relatively few are encountered with any frequency by the pathologist; many are opportunists in immunocompromised children. In general, these disseminated opportunistic viral infections resemble their perinatal counterparts. For comprehensive information, the reader is referred to Feigin and Cherry's textbook (56); only selected infections will be discussed here.

CYTOMEGALOVIRUS

Cytomegalovirus, the largest member of the family Herpesviridae, is encountered in all populations. CMV is ubiquitous and its seroprevalence in adult populations ranges from 50% to 90%. It is the most common cause of congenital infection in the United States, with frequency ranging from 0.2% to 2.2% of live-born babies in the United States (e76); 30% to 60% of fetuses of mothers with primary CMV infection during pregnancy are congenitally infected. However, unlike congenital infections with rubella and toxoplasma, intrauterine transmission of CMV can occur in women who are CMV-seroimmune before pregnancy, albeit at a much lower frequency. Approximately 1% of all infants excrete CMV in their urine at or within 3 weeks after birth; about 5% of congenitally infected infants manifest disease at birth and 15% develop late sequelae (137). More children may be affected by congenital CMV than by other, better known childhood conditions, such as Down syndrome, fetal alcohol syndrome, and spina bifida. CMV is, therefore, one of the most common causes of birth defects and childhood disability.

Transmission

Infection may be transplacental, perinatal, or postnatal. Early, hematogenous gestational infections are the most devastating. Primary maternal infection is much more likely to result in fetal infection than is recurrent maternal disease, but rarely congenital CMV infection "repeats" in subsequent pregnancies. Perinatal infection through body fluid contact at delivery and postnatal infection through breast milk do occur, but are rarely associated with clinical illness in full-term infants (160) (e132,212). Transplacental acquisition of maternal antibodies against CMV protects full-term infants of CMV-seropositive mothers. Rarely, primary CMV infection occurs in the mother around delivery or during lactation, increasing the risk for illness in the infant because of a lack of available anti-CMV antibodies. Postnatal exposure of susceptible infants (i.e., premature infants, infants of CMV-seronegative mothers, and immunodeficient infants) can lead to severe disease. CMV is also commonly reactivated in a setting of immunodeficiency, either congenital or acquired. Childcare centers are another significant source of transmission of CMV, propagated by frequent mouthing of hands and toys. Approximately 20% to 40% of toddlers in day care shed the virus for years. These children function as an important infectious source for other children, parents, and daycare workers (e151). Beyond puberty, infection is mainly sexually transmitted. Virus is present in urine, oropharyngeal, cervical and vaginal secretions, breast milk, semen, and tears and can be shed intermittently for years.

Clinical Features

Transplacental transmission can result in congenital infection and neurological sequelae. Perinatal and postnatal transmission does not usually manifest with clinical disease except in extremely preterm infants (157). Most (~90%) infants born with congenital CMV infection do not exhibit clinical abnormalities at birth (so-called asymptomatic congenital CMV infection). Of the 40,000 children born with congenital CMV infection each year, approximately 10% to 15% exhibit clinical abnormalities (symptomatic congenital infection). Infection involves multiple organ systems, with particular predilection for the reticuloendothelial and central nervous systems (CNS). The most commonly observed physical signs are petechiae, jaundice, and hepatosplenomegaly (Figure 6-2). Neurologic abnormalities such as microcephaly and lethargy affect a significant proportion of symptomatic children. Intrauterine growth restriction, chorioretinitis, optic atrophy, and seizures are other physical signs (157). Postnatal infection in the neonatal period results in an acute sepsis-like picture with apnea, bradycardia, hepatitis, leucopenia, and prolonged thrombocytopenia. In older children, severe infection occurs in a setting of immunodeficiency. Features of active disseminated CMV infection include fever, leucopenia, thrombocytopenia, pneumonia, hepatitis, chorioretinitis, adrenalitis, and encephalitis. Infected infants may have the characteristic "blueberry muffin lesions," a hemorrhagic purpura with mobile gray-blue skin lesions, which histologically show dermal extramedullary hematopoiesis. CNS lesions are irreversible and affect prognosis. There is a high incidence

Table 6-7 ■ VIRAL INFECTION IN THE FETUS AND NEONATE

	Abortion	Stillbirth	Intrauterine Growth Restriction	Congenital Defects	Acute Perinatal Infection	Late Effects	References
Rubella	+	+	+	Cataract, retinopathy sensorineural deafness, patent ductus arteriosus, pulmonary stenosis, VSD, microcephaly, mental retardation	Interstitial pneumonitis, cholestatic hepatitis with giant cell transformation, anemia, thrombocytopenia, myocarditis, immunopathy, osteoporosis, pancreatitis	Interstitial pulmonary fibrosis, hepatic fibrosis/cirrhosis, biliary atresia, arteriopathy with infarction, diabetes mellitus, chronic lymphocytic thyroiditis, panencephalitis, autism (?)	182, 183, 321 401, 441, 476
Cytomegalovirus	?	+	+	Microcephaly, hydrocephaly, microphthalmia	Necrotizing meningoencephalitis with arterial and periventricular calcification, hepatitis with giant cell transformation, cholangitis, inclusions in lung, renal tubules, rare pneumonitis and interstitial nephritis	Deafness, neurologic deficits, optic atrophy, noncirrhotic portal hypertension, and vascular and periventricular calcifications (brain) Hypoganglionosis of bowel (see *Pediatr Pathol* 1984;2:*85*–102)	32, 124, 129, 172
Herpes simplex	+	+	+	Microcephaly, hydranencephaly, microphthalmia	Hepatoadrenal necrosis, vesicular skin rash, vesicular/ulcerated stomatitis, esophagitis, necrotizing pneumonitis, chorioretinitis	Psychomotor retardation	36, 218, 390, 391, 437
Varicella zoster	?	?	+	Limb hypoplasia, rudimentary digits, cutaneous scars in dermatome distribution, chorioretinitis, microphthalmia	Typical varicella, acute disseminated varicella with necrotizing cutaneous and visceral lesions	Blindness, psychomotor retardation	4, 447

(*continued*)

Table 6-7 ■ VIRAL INFECTION IN THE FETUS AND NEONATE *(Continued)*

	Abortion	Stillbirth	Intrauterine Growth Restriction	Congenital Defects	Acute Perinatal Infection	Late Effects	References
HIV	+	+	+	None	See Table 6-9A	See Table 6-9B	See Table 7.7
Parvovirus	+	+	–	Ocular defects	Anemia, hydrops, hepatic fibrosis, siderosis	?	10, 52, 164, 202, 261, 432, 477
Hepatitis B	–	–	–	–	Acute hepatitis, giant cell transformation, chronic active hepatitis, fulminant hepatitis	Cirrhosis, carrier state Hepatocellular carcinoma	135, 283, 420, 435, 443
Hepatitis A	+	–	+	–	Rare	–	122
Mumps	+	+	–	Not proved	Perinatal parotitis (extremely rare)	Endocardial fibroclastosis (?)	234
Influenza	+	+	–	Unlikely	Rare influenza pneumonia, apnea	–	200
Vaccinia	+	+	+	–	Generalized vaccinia	–	
Variola	+	+	?	?	Smallpox	–	299
Measles	+	+	–	?	Measles pneumonia	–	
Polio	+	+	+	–	Paralytic polio	Paralysis	27, 28
Echo	–	–	–	–	Meningitis, DIC	–	
Coxsackie B	?	?	–	–	Disseminated disease, meningoencephalitis, myocarditis	–	258, 438
Adenovirus	–	–	–	–	Pneumonia	–	462
RSV	–	–	–	–	Apnea, bronchiolitis, pneumonia	Asthma (?), COPD	22, 192, 325, 434

DIC, disseminated intravascular coagulation; VSD, ventricular septal defect. +, occurs; –, does not occur.
From references 196, 345, 400, with permission.

Table 6-8 ■ COMMON SYSTEMIC VIRAL INFECTIONS IN INFANTS AND CHILDREN

Virus	Localized or Self-Limited Disease	Disseminated or Serious Disease	Specific Inclusions	Comments	References
Adenoviruses	Acute respiratory illness (Types 1, 2, 3, 4, 7, 21) Laryngotracheitis, pneumonia	Types 1, 2, 4, 5, 7, 11 Hepatitis, massive hepatic necrosis Pneumonia, Hemorrhagic cystitis, Gastroenteritis, Meningoencephalitis	1. Large basophilic indistinctly demarcated intranuclear inclusion (smudge cells) 2. Smaller eosinophilic intranuclear with incomplete halo	Easily confused with disseminated HSV infection	269, 402, 510
Cytomegalovirus	Mononucleosis	Interstitial pneumonia Gastroenteritis Retinitis, encephalitis, glomerulonephrits	1. Large amphophilic or basophilic nuclear inclusions with distinct halo 2. Smaller basophilic PAS positive indistinct cytoplasmic inclusions	Disease in immunocompromised host is similar to neonatal pattern	196, 239, 320
Herpes simplex	Localized oral, skin, or genital vesicular or ulcerated eruption, may be extensive	Hepatitis, hepatoadrenal necrosis, stomatitis, esophagitis, encephalitis, pneumonia	1. Type A-eosinophilic nuclear inclusions with halo 2. Type B-basophilic or amphophilic nuclear inclusions filling nucleus with peripheral chromatin rim, often multinucleate cells	Either type I or type II may disseminate: disseminated form resembles neonatal disease	151, 228, 263, 312, 408, 456
Varicella-Zoster	Localized herpes zoster, acute varicella, generalized vesicular eruption	Disseminated zoster Progressive disseminated varicella, pneumonia, meningo encephalitis, hepatitis	Multinuclear or mononuclear cells with nuclear type A inclusions, indistinguishable from HSV inclusions	Associated with Reye syndrome	158, 334
Epstein-Barr virus	Mononucleosis	Fatal mononucleosis, hepatitis, myocarditis, immunodeficiency various hematologic phenotypes in X-linked lymphoproliferative syndrome	None	Implicated in oncogenesis, especially in X-linked lymphoproliferative syndrome, posttransplant lymphoproliferative syndrome	77, 205, 285, 374, 422
Rubeola	Uncomplicated primary measles, skin, conjunctiva, respiratory tract	Progressive measles	Cytoplasmic and nuclear inclusions in epithelial and Warthin-Finkeldey giant cells	Subacute sclerosing panencephalitis, late	83, 380, 392
Mumps	Parotitis	Orchitis/oophoritis Meningitis pancreatitis Mastitis, nephritis, Arthritis	None	Late sequelae include deafness, diabetes mellitus	84
Coxsackie Virus	Coxsackie viruses A; benign, self-limited febrile illness with respiratory disease	Coxsackie viruses B; myocarditis meningoencephalitis	None		154
Echoviruses	Mild nonspecific febrile illness with respiratory disease	Hepatitis, hepatic necrosis, meningitis, adrenal and renal hemorrhage	None		265, 319
Variola (smallpox)	Disease declared eradicated by WHO in 1980		Cytoplasmic Guamieri bodies. Nuclear changes inconsistent		44
Vaccinia	Eczema vaccinatum	Disseminated vaccinia	Indistinguishable from smallpox		44
Hantavirus	?	Hantavirus pulmonary syndrome in adolescents	None	Noncarciogenic pulmonary edema	32, 243, 332, 511

HSV, herpes simplex virus; PAS, periodic acid-Schiff; WHO, World Health Organization.

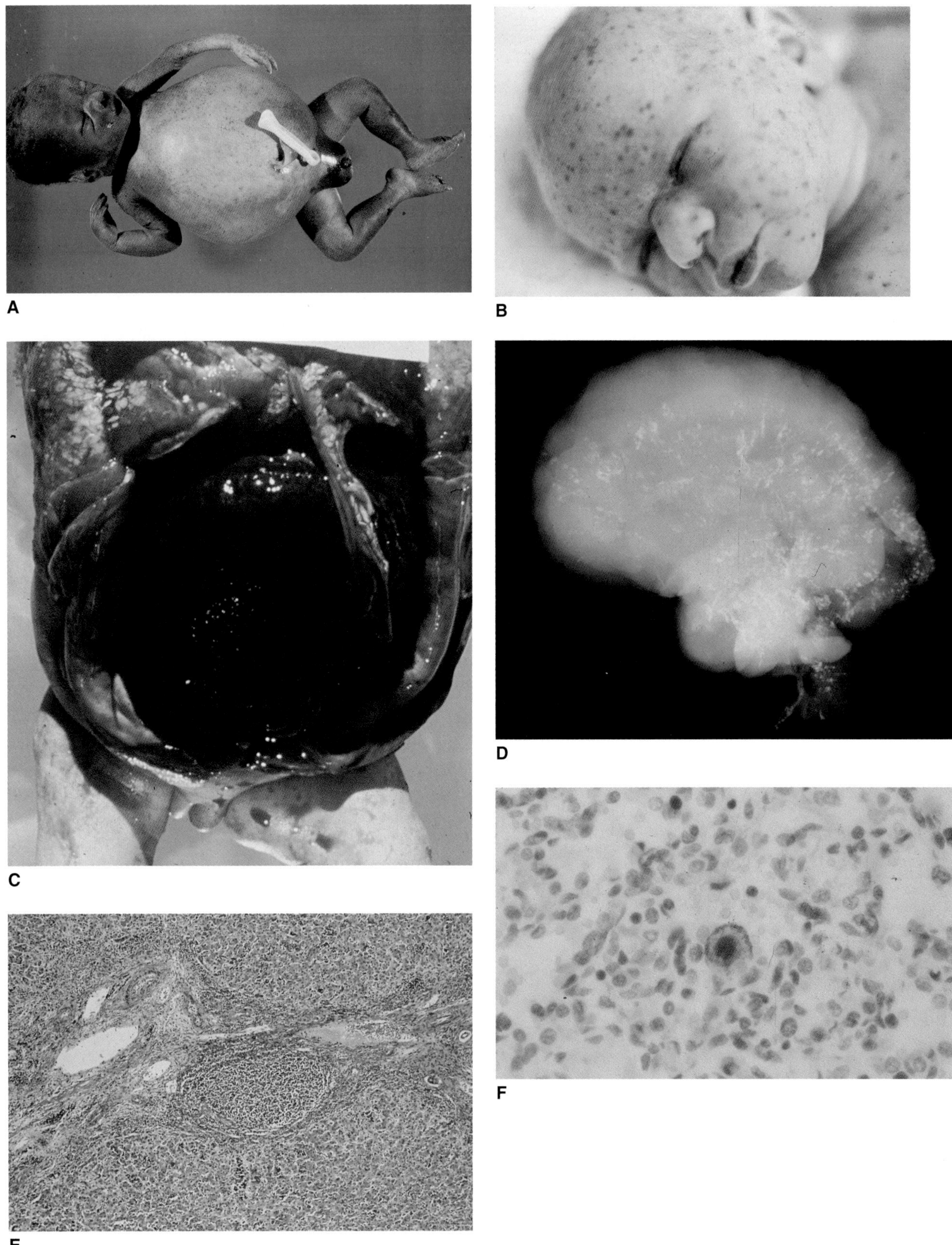

FIGURE 6-2 ■ Congenital CMV infection. **A**: Body with marked ascites. **B**: Face with petechiae as well as elsewhere. **C**: Abdominal cavity at autopsy showing hepatosplenomegaly. **D**: Skull x-ray with diffuse calcification secondary to necrosis. (See Malinger G, Lev D, Zahalka N, et al. *Am J Neuroradiol* 2003;24:28–32) **E**: CMV hepatitis with inflammation around a bile duct and within the lobules. **F**: Lung: CMV immunostain with large nuclear inclusion.

of symptomatic liver disease, ranging from mild cholangitis (with inclusions) to severe cholestatic hepatitis (Figure 6-2). Noncirrhotic portal fibrosis with portal hypertension is a rare but potentially lethal late sequela (e83,e120). Glomerulonephritis, ascites, and pulmonary hypoplasia are also described (e21,e317). A syndrome of hepatosplenomegaly, respiratory distress, a peculiar gray pallor, and atypical lymphocytosis occurs in multiple transfused low birth weight infants. Interstitial pneumonitis with inclusions (Figure 6-2) is the main pathologic feature and is likely responsible for the high (24%) mortality rate in this setting.

Pathology

The morphologic hallmark of CMV infection is cytomegaly with extremely large (25 to 40 μm) inclusion-bearing cells with both nuclear and cytoplasmic inclusions; often the nucleolus is retained within the inclusion, appearing as an "accessory body." A clear zone around the inclusion with chromatin margination gives an owl-eye appearance. The inclusion is eosinophilic in some stages of development but the fully developed inclusion is amphophilic to deeply basophilic. The inclusions are PAS and GMS positive, although immunostains are commonly used to specifically identify the virus. CMV is found in endothelial cells, epithelial cells (notably the biliary tree, pneumocytes, many exocrine cells, and renal tubular cells), fibroblasts, and histiocytes. Tissue damage is characterized by patchy and focal necrosis with mononuclear, and occasionally neutrophilic, inflammatory response, with vascular and parenchymal calcifications, the latter feature is seen especially in the brain. Giant cell transformation of hepatocytes is not a frequent feature. A complete picture of the morphologic spectrum appears in Becroft's review (10).

Congenital infection causes neurologic and hematologic damage and developmental defects which are evident at birth in 10% of infected babies. During infancy, sequelae such as sensorineural deafness, psychomotor retardation, and cerebral palsy develop, even in babies who are asymptomatic at birth. As a result about 20% of all infected neonates suffer sequelae of a congenital CMV infection (e76).

Laboratory Diagnosis

When the large inclusion-bearing cells are present, morphologic diagnosis is straight forward. Sensitivity of histopathologic methods can be improved with immunocytochemical and molecular virologic techniques. The reference method for diagnosing congenital CMV infection involves isolating the virus in cell culture from urine collected within 3 weeks of birth. A positive CMV result in urine collected after the third week might well be the consequence of exposure to infected vaginal secretions at delivery, through breast feeding, or untested transfusions (e76). Detection of CMV in the saliva and urine of infants is accomplished easily because newborns with congenital CMV shed large amounts of virus into these body fluids. Blood is also a useful specimen to identify viral DNA in serum or pp65 antigen in peripheral blood leukocytes (e334), but this method has not been evaluated for diagnosing congenital CMV infection. Tests for viral DNA have proved a valid means of diagnosing congenital CMV infection in neonatal blood dried on paper (DBS). The DBS test is simpler, faster, and less costly than viral isolation; in addition the samples can be safely stored for long periods, so diagnosis can be made even after several years. The DBS method is reported to have high sensitivity (71% to 100%) and specificity (99% to 100%) (7).

Laboratory findings in infected children include conjugated hyperbilirubinemia, thrombocytopenia, and elevations of hepatic transaminases in more than half of the symptomatic newborns, reflecting the involvement of the hepatobiliary and reticuloendothelial systems (157). Prenatal diagnosis of congenital CMV infection is feasible when maternal CMV infection occurs during pregnancy. Viral culture of amniotic fluid can identify fetal infection but has a high false-negative result (e198,e227). Molecular [polymerase chain reaction (PCR)] assays on amniotic fluid may have better sensitivity and specificity. However, PCR for CMV DNA requires the presence of viremia in the peripheral blood and may not identify every infant with congenital CMV infection (e232).

Prognosis and Outcome

Mortality rate among symptomatic children is now probably less than 5%. Of the symptomatic children who survive infancy, most will suffer mild to severe psychomotor and perceptual handicaps and approximately half will develop sensorineural hearing loss, mental retardation, and microcephaly (157). Predictors of adverse neurological outcome include microcephaly, chorioretinitis, presence of other neurologic abnormalities at birth or in early infancy, and presence of cranial abnormalities on CT scans within the first month of life. Petechiae and intrauterine growth restriction are independently predictive of hearing loss (157). Although, in general, children asymptomatic at birth have a better long-term prognosis, approximately 10% will develop sensorineural hearing loss (half of these have bilateral deficit). Other neurological complications can also occur in asymptomatic congenital CMV infection but at a much lower frequency than in symptomatic infection. The pathogenesis and mechanisms of hearing loss and other neurologic sequelae in children with congenital CMV infection, especially in those with asymptomatic infection, are not well understood. Furthermore, predictors of adverse outcomes in asymptomatic children have not been defined. This inability to identify infants at risk for the development of hearing loss and other sequelae necessitates monitoring and follow-up of all children with congenital CMV infection (154).

HERPES SIMPLEX VIRUS

First described as hepatoadrenal necrosis by Haas in 1935 (e135), HSV types 1 and 2 cause severe perinatal infections and, less frequently, prenatal and postnatal infections, with HSV-2 predominating; about 20% are caused by HSV-1 (e309). The risk to the infant is highest in mothers with primary genital herpes at the time of delivery (e33), but fetal infection may occur in the absence of visible maternal lesions.

Transmission

Most HSV infections in infants are acquired during passage through an infected birth canal. Maternal skin and nipple lesions, as well as paternal lesions pose a threat to the infant. Intrauterine infection can also occur as a consequence of either primary or recurrent maternal infection, with severe fetal consequences (e20,e151a,e276,e277). The pathogenesis is not well elucidated, but HSV antigen is demonstrable in endometrium, decidua, and placenta, suggesting that transplacental passage is possible. Case reports have demonstrated HSV infections in infants related to maternal HSV-positive breast lesions and inoculation of virus from primary gingivostomatitis in the infant to the mother's breast during breastfeeding (e90,e264,e323).

Clinical Features

Neonatal infections manifest in the first week of life. Although the neonatal form of the disease may be relatively benign, the majority of cases result in death from disseminated disease with meningoencephalitis (50%), or serious neurologic impairment (30%). Although no specific sign or symptom is diagnostic, the diagnosis should be strongly considered in the presence of HSV risk factors, atypical sepsis, unexplained acute hepatitis, or focal seizure activity. Neonatal HSV infection may be either disseminated or relatively localized; in general the younger the patient at presentation, the more disseminated the lesions, and even infants with encephalitis usually have at least skin and mucous membrane lesions (Figure 6-3A). Conversely, however, at least a third of newborns with disseminated HSV do not have detectable skin or mucous membrane lesions at the time of presentation (e309). The clinical presentation is variable and diagnosis may be extremely difficult; seizures, cyanosis, shock, and bleeding diathesis are common manifestations.

Pathology

The pathologic hallmark of disseminated HSV are patchy and focal well-demarcated punctuate areas of yellow-tan to hemorrhagic coagulative necrosis with little cellular inflammatory reaction at the periphery of irregular zones of necrosis (Figure 6-3B and C). The characteristic inclusions are beautifully illustrated in Singer's paper (e309) (Figure 6-3D) and are of two types. The early infectious inclusions (Cowdry type B) are variably staining (usually amphophilic, sometimes basophilic), homogeneous and glassy, occupying the entire nucleus, and pushing the chromatin to the nuclear membrane. The second type (Cowdry type A) is smaller, deeply eosinophilic, round or polygonal and separated from the nuclear membrane by a clear halo. Multinucleated cells are more likely to contain Cowdry type B inclusions. Type A inclusions occur later in the infection and reflect excess viral capsid material following extrusion of encapsidated viral DNA. In 75% to 80% of cases of disseminated HSV, the liver (Figure 6-3B and C) and adrenal glands are involved. Lesions may also be seen in the lung, brain, spleen, bone marrow, and GIT. Care must be exercised in the evaluation of necrotizing and ulcerated skin or mucous membrane lesions; HSV inclusions can usually be found at the periphery of such lesions, but secondary bacterial or yeast infection may obscure the underlying viral lesion.

Laboratory Diagnosis

If vesicular or ulcerated lesions are present, a firm diagnosis is usually possible using smears of vesical fluid or scrapings of the base of the lesion. In properly stained smears, identification of the characteristic, often multiple inclusions is straightforward; epithelial cells contain one or more large intranuclear inclusions, described with three Ms as multinucleate, with nuclear molding and chromatin margination (Figure 6-3D). Morphologic distinction from varicella-zoster inclusions is not possible, but in the usual clinical setting this is not a problem. Both immunohistochemical and molecular biologic techniques are available and are useful in distinguishing HSV from other viruses (e239).

Prognosis and Outcome

Neonatal herpes is a potentially devastating illness with 80% mortality without treatment. The mortality rate for disseminated disease remains very high at over 50%, even with therapy (e160). About 25% of survivors may have neurologic defects and/or blindness. Maternal treatment or prophylactic treatment of the infant may be reasonable in certain situations to decrease shedding, hasten clinical resolution of the lesions, and protect the infant.

The consequences of neonatal HSV infection can be severe (e175). Disease can be localized to skin, eye, and mouth (SEM disease), involve the CNS or manifest as disseminated infection involving multiple organs. Most surviving infants in the latter two categories have neurological sequelae. Neonatal herpes may occur in the absence of skin lesions; if infection is suspected, swabs of the oropharynx, conjunctiva, rectum, skin lesions, mucosal lesions, urine, and cerebrospinal fluid (CSF) should be promptly submitted for laboratory studies (96).

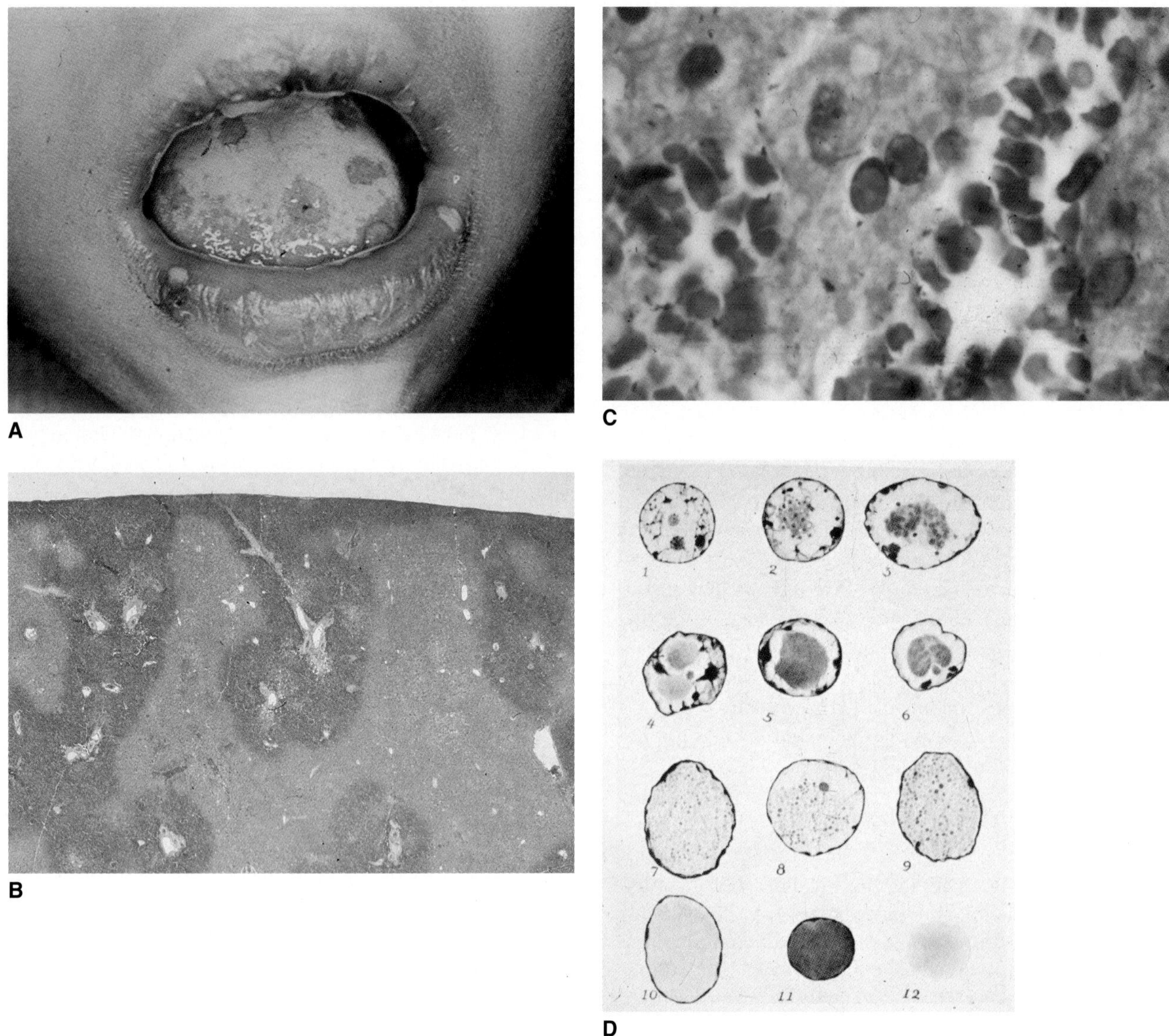

FIGURE 6-3 ■ Herpes simplex infection. **A**: Herpetic stomatitis. **B**: Liver (low power) with multifocal areas of coagulative necrosis. **C**: Liver (high power) with smooth nuclear inclusions usually at the interface between the necrotic and viable parenchyma. **D**: Pictorial representation of inclusions—camera lucida drawings by E. Piotti; each nucleus corresponds to the types of inclusions seen in the first reported case of HSV infection (With permission from Singer DB. Pathology of neonatal Herpes simplex virus infection. *Perspect pediatr pathol* 1981;6:243–278.)

HUMAN PARVOVIRUS INFECTION

The B19 parvovirus, although better known as a cause of erythema infectiosum (fifth disease), is a relatively recent entrant to the list of fetal pathogens (e8,e32). This single stranded DNA virus of the Erythrovirus genus primarily targets erythroid precursors in the bone marrow. Because the erythrocyte P antigen is the cellular receptor for the virus, individuals lacking this antigen are resistant to infection (e31).

Transmission

Transmission is through contact with respiratory secretions (droplets, saliva) and, less commonly, other body fluids (blood and urine). Seroprevalence data show peak parvovirus infection occurring in school-age children. Mode of entry into bloodstream and placental invasion is not clearly known.

Clinical Features

Intrauterine infection results in fetal anemia with a pronounced leukoerythroblastic reaction and hepatitis, with excessive iron deposition in the liver. Parvovirus is a major cause of nonimmune hydrops, possibly accounting for up to 16% of cases of "idiopathic" nonimmune hydrops (54). In Anand's series (e8), two of six affected pregnancies resulted in fetal hydrops and death; the other four infants were normal. Studies of fetuses and newborns infected with parvovirus have also described presentations other than fetal hydrops. Ocular lesions include microphthalmia, aphakia, and dysplasia of sclera, anterior segment, and retina (e134). In live-born infants, a lethal constellation of anemia, petechial rash, purpuric "blueberry muffin" appearance and severe liver disease with hepatic fibrosis and siderosis mimics the syndrome of neonatal hemochromatosis (188) (e218,e306,e364). (see Chapter 15).

Although postnatal infection is frequently asymptomatic, the best known clinical illness is the immune-mediated erythema infectiosum or fifth disease. Fifth disease is a highly contagious illness with a slapped cheek lacy erythematous exanthem on the face, trunk, and proximal limbs in children; adults manifest arthralgias and arthritis. Severe disease is seen most often in individuals with hemoglobinopathy, red blood cell abnormalities, and immune deficiency. Erythroid abnormalities include pure red cell aplasia and aplastic anemia (especially aplastic crisis in a setting of chronic hemolytic anemia). Vasculitis and hemophagocytic syndrome can also occur.

Pathology

The bone marrow may show erythroid hypoplasia of variable severity. Morphologic abnormalities in red cell precursors include giant pronormoblasts with vacuoles and multiple nucleoli. Distinctive eosinophilic intranuclear inclusions may be seen in erythroid lineage cells. The inclusions have been shown by DNA hybridization and electron microscopy (e8,e42,e181) to contain B19 virus, and the virus is readily detected in tissue with immunohistochemical and PCR techniques (54) (e209). Histologic studies on very young fetuses show ocular malformations and intense inflammatory reactions in all tissues (e348). The first clue to the infection may be the presence of infected red cells in the fetal capillaries of the placenta (see Chapter 9).

RUBELLA

Rubella is caused by a single stranded RNA virus. Originally described by Gregg as a classic triad of cataracts, deafness, and congenital heart disease (e126), the "expanded rubella syndrome," as it is sometimes referred to, is rare in countries where rubella vaccination is the norm. However, the congenital rubella syndrome (CRS) is unfortunately not just an item of historical interest due to the continued existence of both a nonimmune population of women of childbearing age and the many survivors of the 1964 to 1965 epidemic. Investigation of these individuals, now adults, has made possible the delineation of the late effects of congenital infection (156).

Transmission

The rubella virus is capable of infecting the fetus at any time during gestation. The virus reaches the fetus in emboli of necrotic placental tissue and affects the fetus by at least three mechanisms: (a) inhibition of cell growth, (b) cytolysis, and (c) compromise of blood supply (156). These, in turn, incite necrosis, inflammation, and scarring in virtually limitless combinations and permutations. Unlike in CMV infection, maternal antibodies to rubella virus protect the fetus from infection. Postnatal and childhood infections are transmitted through inhalation of droplets of nasopharyngeal secretions.

Clinical Features

The incidence and pattern of fetal disease vary strikingly with gestational age at the time of maternal viremia (e126,342). Congenital heart defects result from infection in the first trimester of gestation, deafness, and neurologic deficits from infection through the 4th gestational month, and retinopathy through the 5th gestational month. Infection late in gestation is more likely to produce inflammatory and destructive lesions, without evidence of malformation. The probability of the fetus suffering significant damage reduces from 80% to 90% in first trimester to negligible beyond 20-week gestation. In either case, the virus is recoverable for months to years after birth. With the possible exception of microcephaly, most of the CNS abnormalities are the result of meningoencephalitis and/or necrosis. Necrosis is presumably ischemic and related to the vascular lesions seen in a majority of cases. True developmental malformation is rare (156). A late-onset chronic progressive panencephalitis is seen in the second decade of life in some survivors of CRS; the neuropathologic changes are similar to those of subacute sclerosing panencephalitis (SSPE) including meningeal and perivascular infiltrates of lymphocytes and plasma cells with glial nodules, predominantly in the white matter (e338). Rubella virus has been recovered from these late lesions. Deafness in CRS is related to both CNS damage resulting in central auditory imperception and also to inflammation and scarring in the cochlea. The disseminated effects of infection may be related to vascular spread and cytopathic effects on endothelial cells. Interestingly, deafness, cardiovascular and neurological damage, and retinopathy are rare if infection occurs beyond the second trimester, raising the possibility of a protective role of maternal antibodies in the second trimester. Webster has reviewed these facets of rubella teratogenesis (192).

Rubella in postnatal life presents as a prodrome followed by a characteristic postauricular lymphadenopathy; a fine maculopapular rash appears 1 to 5 days later, starting in the face and spreading to limbs and face that lasts for about 3 days. Complications are infrequent and include immune manifestations such as arthritis, encephalitis, Guillian-Barre syndrome, and thrombocytopenia. Surveillance of postnatally and congenitally acquired infection is an essential component of CRS prevention since rubella is difficult to diagnose on clinical grounds alone. Laboratory differentiation of rubella from other rash-causing infections, such as measles, parvovirus B19, human herpes virus 6, enteroviruses in developed countries, and various endemic arboviruses is essential. Reverse transcriptase PCR and sequencing for diagnosis and molecular epidemiological investigation and detection of rubella-specific IgG and IgM salivary antibody responses in oral fluid are now available (6).

Pathology

A wide spectrum of cardiovascular disease is seen in CRS. In addition to the characteristic patent ductus arteriosus, the most common lesions are pulmonary artery branch stenosis, myocarditis, and systemic arterial hypoplasia and stenosis. Valvular sclerosis has been frequent in some series (156). The arterial lesion of CRS is distinctive and possibly unique: fibromuscular intimal proliferation, devoid of inflammatory change, leads to patchy and focal vascular stenosis. The media and adventitia are usually not disrupted, and there is no calcification (except in the brain). Chronic meningeal inflammation, perivascular lymphocytic infiltrates, gliosis, and mineralization of cerebral arterioles may occur. Bone lesions are transient and consist of focal osteopenia and growth inhibition. Metaphyseal changes reminiscent of syphilis, in the form of longitudinal radiologic striations are seen in half the patients. Interstitial pneumonitis is seen in up to 75% of CRS infants and may persist for up to a year after birth. Alterations of the lymphoreticular system are variable; both precocious germinal centers (from viral antigenic stimulus) and lymphoid depletion are encountered. Histiocytic proliferation and erythrophagocytosis may be seen. Hepatic changes include cholestatic hepatitis, giant cell transformation, necrosis, extramedullary hematopoiesis, and fibrosis; cirrhosis may ensue. On occasion, bile duct proliferation mimics extrahepatic biliary atresia; true biliary atresia has been reported anecdotally (e97). Eye changes include cataracts, lens necrosis, ciliary body inflammation, iridocyclitis, and retinitis. Interstitial nephritis and chronic lymphocytic thyroiditis have also been described. The placenta may show villitis, villous stromal necrosis, villous stromal sclerosis, and vascular endothelial lesions (92). No specific histopathologic studies are available of postnatal rubella infection, due to its short and benign course.

Prognosis and Outcome

Characteristically, complications affect the eyes (cataracts or retinopathy) and hearing (sensorineural deafness). Patients may have multiorgan involvement including myocarditis, hepatitis, cytopenia, meningoencephalitis, and visceromegaly. Cardiac teratogenic effects include patent ductus arteriosus, pulmonary artery stenosis, and supra-aortic stenosis. Long-term effects of intrauterine rubella infection have been studied in the original cohort of patients studied by Sir Norman Gregg and include an increase in the prevalence of diabetes, thyroid disorders, early menopause, and osteoporosis, as also an increased frequency of HLA haplotypes that are associated with autoimmune disorders (60). Approximately 20% of CRS survivors develop diabetes mellitus, usually in the second or third decade. The pathogenesis is not understood, but persistent viral infection is implicated; the virus may be recovered from the pancreas and lymphocytic infiltration of the pancreas has been seen at postmortem. Growth retardation continues postnatally probably because the virus remains active, as evidenced by its prolonged shedding in nasopharyngeal secretions.

VARICELLA ZOSTER VIRUS

The VZV is a double stranded DNA virus (human herpes virus 3). The existence of a fetal varicella syndrome was suggested in 1974 (e311), although the first case had been reported years earlier. Several studies have described the defects (e34,e140) associated with fetal varicella infection, and a specific neonatal syndrome is associated with maternal varicella (but not by maternal zoster) in the first half of pregnancy (e7).

Transmission

Congenital infections are transmitted transplacentally. The risk of embryopathy with maternal infection in the first 20 weeks of gestation is estimated at 0.4% to 2% (e25,252). Intrauterine insult occurs between 8 and 20 weeks of gestation resulting in a fetal disease with distinctive herpes zoster-like distribution. Although the virus has not been isolated from affected fetuses or newborns, virus specific IgM has been demonstrated in affected fetus (e68) and VZV DNA sequences have been recovered from the placenta (e157). Neonatal varicella infection is acquired *in utero* near term, or postnatally from the mother or other (household or nursery) contacts. Infants delivered of mothers who were infected more than 5 days before delivery were the best, presumably because there is time for production and transfer of maternal antibody. Perinatal infection can be severe when the mother presents with the rash of chickenpox from 5 days before to 2 days after delivery, since the virus is transmitted during maternal viremia and there is not sufficient time for transfer of antibodies to the infant in this narrow window. Postnatal transmission occurs through respiratory droplets and contact or aerosolization of virus from the skin lesions of either varicella or zoster. Infection peaks in winter and spring.

Clinical Features

Fetal varicella results in multiple defects of skin, limbs, eyes, and brain (e7,e326), giving an impression of a sudden devastating, but self-limited, herpes zoster-like illness occurring *in utero*. The most constant (100% of cases) are cicatricial skin lesions corresponding to the distribution of the affected dermatome. These are associated frequently with hypoplasia of the underlying bone and soft tissue. Hypoplastic limbs, many seriously deformed by scarring, are seen in 80% of cases. Calcification of the liver has been reported, suggesting dissemination, and viral-like inclusions have been reported in the lung (e278). CNS involvement may take the form of necrotizing encephalitis with calcification (e326). Microphthalmia, severe chorioretinitis with scarring and cataract lead to blindness. Neurologic abnormalities frequently correspond anatomically to the afflicted dermatome including limb paresis, microcephaly, Horner syndrome, cranial nerve palsies, and cortical atrophy.

Varicella in the newborn may be limited to the skin (Figure 6-4) or disseminate widely; disseminated disease carries a very high mortality rate, largely due to varicella pneumonia. Older children develop a prodrome for 2 to 3 days

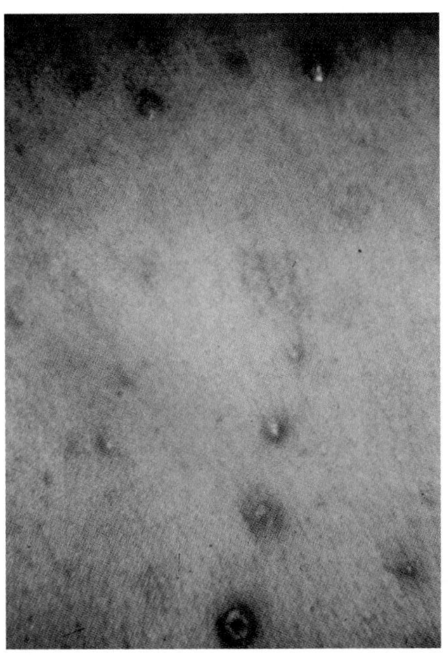

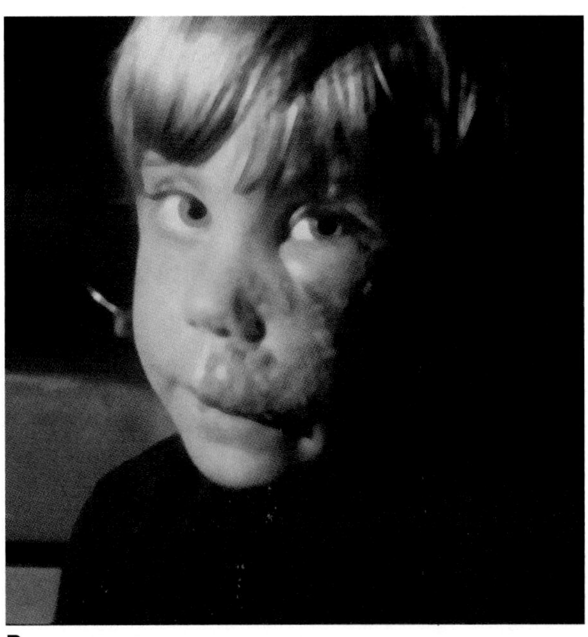

A B

FIGURE 6-4 ■ Varicella zoster virus infection. **A**: Neonatal varicella with skin lesions. **B**: Herpes zoster in an older child.

followed by a transient scarlatiniform rash that may precede or accompany the characteristic varicelliform rash that appears on the trunk and spreads out as crops of 1 to 4 mm maculopapular lesions that progress to clear fluid-filled vesicles ("dew drop on a rose petal") and pustules, with accompanying distressing pruritis. Lesions of various stages are seen in a given patient and the patient remains infectious till all the lesions have crusted. Excoriation may leave shallow pink depressions that get scarred if complicated by secondary bacterial infection. Vesicles may also develop on mucous membranes leaving multiple small ulcers. Rarely there may be septic shock, hemolytic-uremic syndrome, necrotizing pneumonia, encephalitis, hepatitis, and/or Reye's syndrome (e111).

VZV infects sensory nerves and migrates to sensory ganglia during acute infections and remains latent there to later cause herpes zoster (Figure 6-4). Involvement of nonneuronal satellite cells, which interface with multiple neurons, might allow the virus to involve large geographic areas (e.g., an entire dermatome) during reactivation (e66). A prodrome of pain, itching, burning, and paresthesia may precede the characteristic zosteriform eruption by 4 to 5 days, as may constitutional symptoms such as headache, fever, and malaise. Lesions may continue to develop within the dermatome over a week and last for 2 to 3 weeks, but may last longer in debilitated and immunodeficient patients. Ulcers, scaling, hyperpigmentation, and secondary bacterial infection with resultant scarring may complicate the clinical picture. Herpes zoster is uncommon in childhood.

Pathology

Chicken pox is a clinical diagnosis. However, Tzanck smears of vesicular or pustular fluid (of varicella or zoster) allows rapid identification of infected cells by demonstrating intranuclear inclusions and giant cells, similar to those seen in HSV infection. Skin biopsies also show features similar to HSV with ballooning degeneration progressing to acantholytic intraepidermal vesicles; adnexal structures may be involved. Unlike in HSV infection, however, a leukocytoclastic vasculitis with occasional hemorrhage may be seen in the dermis. Inclusions start as faint basophilic intranuclear bodies with peripheral chromatin condensation, later becoming eosinophilic with a surrounding halo. An immunostain is available for specific identification. Disseminated VZV may involve a variety of organs with hemorrhagic necrosis, little or no inflammation and eosinophilic intranuclear inclusions. Pulmonary lesions consist of an interstitial mononuclear infiltrate with edema, hemorrhage, and hyaline membranes with focal, sharply defined centrilobular areas of necrosis (e111).

Prognosis and Outcome

Chicken pox is almost always self-limited. Death from chickenpox is distinctly unusual (12 deaths/100,000 cases), except in immunodeficient patients in whom pneumonia, meningoencephalitis, and hepatitis may develop (141) (e258). Less frequently, other systemic infections may occur, including nephritis, myocarditis, arthritis, myositis, uveitis, orchitis, and idiopathic thrombocytopenic purpura (177). Reye syndrome has been described following chickenpox that was treated with salicylate administration, and aspirin is contraindicated in patients who have chickenpox (e324).

HUMAN IMMUNODEFICIENCY VIRUS

The first cases of pediatric AIDS were reported in 1982 to 1983, soon after recognition of this entity in adults (e240,e285,e343). Over 90% of cases of childhood HIV infection are acquired by vertical transmission. HIV/AIDS in children is similar in many respects to adult disease in both the primary viral cytopathic effects of HIV on the lymphoid and nervous systems, and the secondary effects of immunodeficiency including opportunistic infections and neoplasia. However, beyond the very different mode of transmission, there are important differences in diagnostic methods, response capability of the developing immune system, etiology of secondary infection, and type and distribution of pathologic lesions. HIV-2 causes clinical disease similar to HIV-1, but with a significantly slower progression to immune suppression. Ekpini and colleagues documented infrequent HIV-2 vertical transmission, but no cases of late postnatal seroconversion in a cohort of West African mothers and infants (e93). HIV-2 transmission through breast milk is less common than for HIV-1, but the risk and possible factors contributing to transmission have not been quantified adequately. Recent volumes have detailed the epidemiology, immunopathogenesis, molecular biology, and clinicopathologic aspects of pediatric AIDS (87,118,134). The Center for Disease Control has recently released revised surveillance case definitions for HIV and AIDS (Table 6-9) (161). However, the

Table 6-9A ■ 2008 SURVEILLANCE CASE DEFINITION FOR HIV INFECTION AMONG CHILDREN AGED <18 MONTHS[a]

Criteria for definitive or presumptive HIV infection

Child born to an HIV-infected mother and laboratory criterion or at least one other criteria met

Laboratory criterion for definitive HIV infection

Positive results on two separate specimens (not including cord blood) using HIV virologic (nonantibody) tests (HIV nucleic acid detection is method of choice):

Laboratory criterion for presumptive HIV infection

Criterion for definitively HIV infected not met, and

Positive result on one specimen (not including cord blood) using HIV virologic tests AND no subsequent negative results from HIV virologic or antibody tests

Other criteria (for cases that do not meet above laboratory criteria)

HIV infection diagnosed by a physician or qualified medical-care provider based on the laboratory criteria and documented in a medical record. Oral reports of prior laboratory test results are not acceptable.

or

When test results regarding HIV infection status are not available, documentation of a condition that meets the criteria in the 1987 pediatric surveillance case definition for AIDS

Criteria for uninfected with HIV, definitive or presumptive

Child born to an HIV-infected mother is either definitively or presumptively uninfected with HIV if (1) the criteria for definitive or presumptive HIV infection are not met and (2) at least one of the following laboratory criteria or other criteria are met.

Laboratory criteria for uninfected with HIV, definitive

At least two negative HIV DNA or RNA virologic tests from separate specimens, both of which were obtained at age ≥1 months and one of which was obtained at age ≥4 months.

or

At least two negative HIV antibody tests from separate specimens obtained at age ≥6 months.

and

No other laboratory or clinical evidence of HIV infection[b]

Laboratory criteria for uninfected with HIV, presumptive

Two negative RNA or DNA virologic tests, from separate specimens, both of which were obtained at age ≥2 wk and one of which was obtained at age ≥4 weeks

or

One negative RNA or a DNA virologic test from a specimen obtained at age ≥8 weeks.

or

One negative HIV antibody test from a specimen obtained at age ≥6 months.

or

One positive HIV virologic test followed by at least two negative tests from separate specimens, one of which is a virologic test from a specimen obtained at age ≥8 wk or an HIV antibody test from a specimen obtained at age ≥6 months.

and

No other laboratory or clinical evidence of HIV infection[b]

Other criteria (for cases that do not meet above laboratory criteria)

Determination of uninfected with HIV by a physician or qualified medical-care provider based on the laboratory criteria and who has noted the HIV diagnostic test results in the medical record. Oral reports of prior laboratory test results are not acceptable.

and

No other laboratory or clinical evidence of HIV infection[b]

Criteria for indeterminate HIV infection

Child born to an HIV-infected mother if the criteria for infected with HIV and uninfected with HIV are not met.

[a]These guidelines are intended for public health surveillance only and are not a guide for clinical diagnosis.
[b]No positive results from virologic tests (if tests were performed) and no AIDS-defining condition for which no other underlying condition indicative of immunosuppression exists (see Table 6-10).
Modified from Schneider E, Whitmore S, Glynn KM, et al. Centers for Disease Control and Prevention (CDC). Revised surveillance case definitions for HIV infection among adults, adolescents, and children aged <18 months and for HIV infection and AIDS among children aged 18 months to <13 years—United States, 2008. *MMWR Recomm Rep* 2008;57(RR-10):1–12.

Table 6-9B ■ 2008 SURVEILLANCE CASE DEFINITION FOR HIV INFECTION AMONG CHILDREN AGED 18 MONTHS TO <13 YEARS[a]

Criteria for HIV infection

At least one of laboratory criteria or the other criterion should be met

Laboratory criteria

Positive result from a screening test for HIV antibody (e.g., reactive EIA), confirmed by a positive result from a supplemental test for HIV antibody (e.g., Western blot or indirect immunofluorescence assay)

or

Positive result or a detectable quantity by a HIV virologic (nonantibody) tests[b]

Other criterion (for cases that do not meet laboratory criteria)

HIV infection diagnosed by a physician or qualified medical-care provider based on the laboratory criteria and documented in a medical record. Oral reports of prior laboratory test results are not acceptable.

Criteria for AIDS

Children aged 18 months to <13 years are categorized for surveillance purposes as having AIDS if the criteria for HIV infection are met and at least one of the AIDS-defining conditions has been documented.

[a]These guidelines are intended for public health surveillance only and are not a guide for clinical diagnosis. The 2008 laboratory criteria for reportable HIV infection among persons aged 18 mo to <13 y exclude confirmation of HIV infection through the diagnosis of AIDS-defining conditions alone (see Table 6-10). Laboratory-confirmed evidence of HIV infection is now required for all reported cases of HIV infection among children aged 18 mo to <13 y.

[b]For HIV screening among children aged 18 mo to <13 y infected through exposure other than perinatal exposure, HIV virologic (nonantibody) tests should not be used in lieu of approved HIV antibody screening tests. A negative result (i.e., undetectable or nonreactive) by an HIV virologic test (e.g., viral RNA nucleic acid test) does not rule out the diagnosis of HIV infection.

classification system for HIV infection among children aged 18 months to 13 years has not changed and the 1994 guidelines for AIDS-defining conditions remain valid (Table 6-10) (1).

Transmission

Vertical transmission is the most common mode of acquisition of pediatric HIV. Transmission of virus by breast feeding, sexual abuse, and heterosexual or homosexual relationships accounts for most of the remaining infection. The risk of transmission through transfusion of blood or blood products has been almost eliminated. The timing and mechanisms of mother-to-infant virus transmission are imprecisely understood. Vertical transmission can take place antepartum *in utero*, intrapartum, or postpartum, through breast feeding. To some extent, these are distinguishable on the basis of culturable virus or HIV genome in cord and infant blood. The best predictor of transmission risk is maternal viral burden, as measured by maternal plasma HIV-1 RNA level. Levels under 500 copies per milliliter are associated with minimal risk of perinatal transmission (116). Treatment of HIV-infected mothers with effective antiviral agents has significantly decreased the rate of vertical transmission (e64). Studies demonstrating lower transmission rates with caesarean section and with shortened interval between rupture of membranes and delivery indicate that obstetric interventions may also decrease the rate of perinatal infection (102) (e185,e280).

Breastfeeding by an HIV-1-positive mother increases transmission risk through breast milk by 4% to 22%, in addition to the risk for prenatal and perinatal transmission (e26,e72,e91). However, the lack of acceptable, feasible, affordable, sustainable, and safe (AFASS) water for breast milk alternatives has complicated infant feeding practices in less developed nations. Current WHO/UNICEF guidelines recommend exclusive breastfeeding for all infants for at least the first 6 months (unless AFASS criteria are satisfied) because of reduced infant mortality among exclusively breastfed, HIV-exposed infants (194). There are many issues related to breast milk HIV-1 transmission including the increased risk for transmission with primary HIV-1 infection in the mother during lactation, the health of the HIV-1-infected, breastfeeding mother, the presence of the virus and potentially immunologically protective factors in colostrum and breast milk, factors that contribute to HIV-1 transmission in breast milk, and possible interventions to prevent or limit HIV-1 transmission through breast milk (149). The avoidance of breastfeeding in maternal HIV-1 infection is an important component of preventing mother-to-child transmission in the United States and other countries. In resource-poor situations, where the complete avoidance of breast milk can increase morbidity and mortality because of poor nutrition or other infections, potential interventions can limit HIV-1 mother-to-child transmission, including exclusive breastfeeding, early weaning, education, and support to decrease the occurrence of mastitis or nipple lesions, antiretroviral therapy for the mother or infant, treating the human milk to decrease the viral burden (ultraviolet light, freezing, and thawing), and stimulating the infant's immune defenses with active or passive immunization.

Clinical Features

Clinical manifestations include hepatosplenomegaly, lymphadenopathy, failure to thrive, fever of unknown origin (FUO), chronic diarrhea, various infections, parotitis, chronic otitis media, lymphoid interstitial pneumonitis (LIP), HIV nephropathy, HIV encephalopathy, HIV cardiomyopathy, idiopathic thrombocytopenia purpura, and lymphoma. Age-specific data suggest that HIV manifestation changes with the child's age, and these may further vary based on geographic location (103,166,172). HIV encephalopathy,

Table 6-10 ■ AIDS DEFINING ILLNESSES IN THE PEDIATRIC AGE GROUP

Bacterial infections, multiple or recurrent[a]
Candidiasis of bronchi, trachea, or lungs
Candidiasis of esophagus[b]
Cervical cancer, invasive[c]
Coccidioidomycosis, disseminated or extrapulmonary
Cryptococcosis, extrapulmonary
Cryptosporidiosis, chronic intestinal (>1 month's duration)
Cytomegalovirus disease (other than liver, spleen, or nodes), onset at age >1 mo
Cytomegalovirus retinitis (with loss of vision)[b]
Encephalopathy, HIV related
Herpes simplex: chronic ulcers (>1 month's duration) or bronchitis, pneumonitis, or esophagitis (onset at age >1 mo)
Histoplasmosis, disseminated or extrapulmonary
Isosporiasis, chronic intestinal (>1 month's duration)
Kaposi sarcoma[b]
Lymphoid interstitial pneumonia or pulmonary lymphoid hyperplasia complex[a, b]
Lymphoma, Burkitt (or equivalent term)
Lymphoma, immunoblastic (or equivalent term)
Lymphoma, primary, of brain
Mycobacterium avium complex or *M. kansasii*, disseminated or extrapulmonary[b]
M. tuberculosis of any site, pulmonary,[b,c] disseminated,[b] or extrapulmonary[b]
Mycobacterium, other species or unidentified species, disseminated[b] or extrapulmonary[b]
Pneumocystis jirovecii pneumonia[b]
Pneumonia, recurrent[b,c]
Progressive multifocal leukoencephalopathy
Salmonella septicemia, recurrent
Toxoplasmosis of brain, onset at age >1 month[b]
Wasting syndrome attributed to HIV

[a]Only among children aged <13 years. (CDC. 1994 Revised classification system for human immunodeficiency virus infection in children <13 years of age. *MMWR* 1994;43[No. RR-12].)
[b]Condition that might be diagnosed presumptively.
[c]Only among adults and adloescents aged ≥13 years. (CDC. 1993 Revised classification system for HIV infection and expanded surveillance case definition for AIDS among adolescents and adults. *MMWR* 1992;41[No. RR-17].)
Source: Schneider E, Whitmore S, Glynn KM, et al. Centers for Disease Control and Prevention (CDC). Revised surveillance case definitions for HIV infection among adults, adolescents, and children aged <18 mo and for HIV infection and AIDS among children aged 18 mo to <13 y—United States, 2008. *MMWR Recomm Rep* 2008;57(RR-10):1-12.

HIV cardiomyopathy, idiopathic thrombocytopenia purpura, and lymphoma may occur later than other manifestations.

There is great variation in rapidity of onset, age of onset, and rate of progression in pediatric AIDS. In perinatally infected infants, the onset of symptomatic disease occurs at 6 to 8 months of age, as compared with a mean of about 18 months in transfusion acquired pediatric AIDS (and years in adults). This extremely rapid progression undoubtedly reflects early disruption of differentiation in the developing cellular immune system that results from HIV-induced destruction of CD4 lymphocytes before the establishment of a fully developed immunologic response. There is also marked variation in the rate of progression of HIV in pediatric patients once they are symptomatic. Some perinatally infected children have onset of disease in the first year of life characteristically with *Pneumocystis jiroveci* pneumonia (PCP), HIV encephalopathy, and recurrent severe bacterial infections. Another group is characterized by onset after the first year and a more indolent and chronic course of mucosal candidiasis, LIP, and cardiovascular disease. The reason(s) for these differences are, as yet, unclear. Children with AIDS do not show the marked degree of lymphopenia seen in adults but are more likely to have hyperglobulinemia. Cutaneous anergy is seen in infants. Severe bacterial infections are extremely common in pediatric AIDS, occurring in over 80% of affected children. Among pediatric opportunistic infections, candidiasis is the most frequent (Figure 6-5), beginning as oral thrush and affecting the entire GIT; PCP is the most frequent fatal infection in infancy (Figure 6-5). Other common opportunistic pathogens include CMV (Figure 6-5), MAIC, TB, aspergillosis, cryptococcosis, cryptosporidiosis, histoplasmosis, HSV, adenoviral pneumonia, measles, and RSV depending on the frequency of occurrence of the organism in a given geographic area and/or population. About 25% of children with AIDS develop a lymphoproliferative syndrome with generalized lymphadenopathy and splenomegaly.

Children with HIV demonstrate lower motor, cognitive, and adaptive functioning compared to uninfected children. Risk factors that may negatively affect the development of infected children include neurological abnormalities, progression of the disease, and poor environmental factors (15). Anemia is also a very common complication of pediatric HIV infection, associated with a poor prognosis. Failure of erythropoiesis may be the most important mechanism for anemia (18). Survival in children with AIDS is in general shorter than survival in HIV-infected adults.

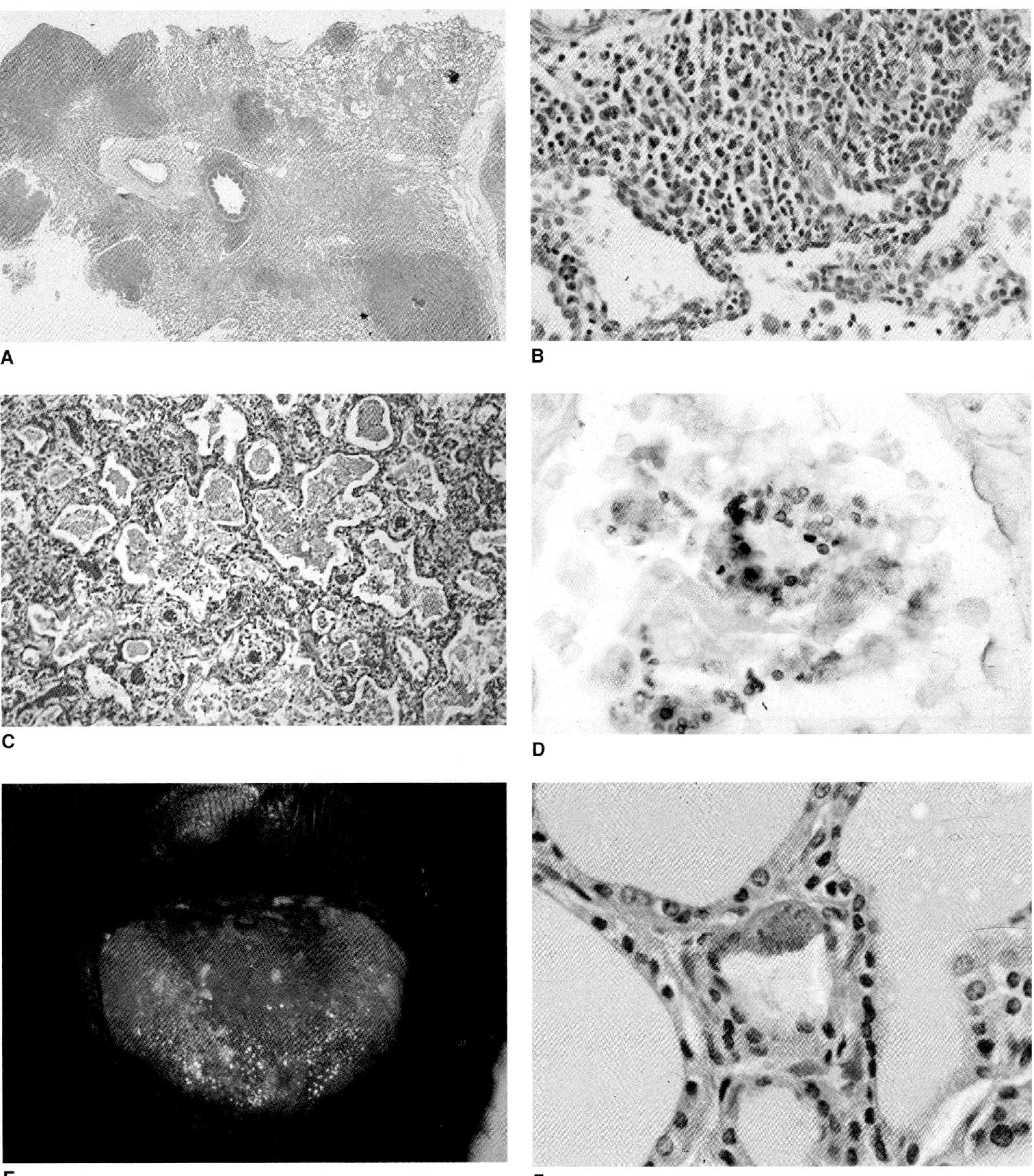

FIGURE 6-5 ■ HIV infection. **A,B**: Lymphoid interstitial pneumonia (low power and high power) with follicular bronchiolitis and diffuse interstitial lymphoplasmacytic inflammation. **C,D**: *Pneumocystis jiroveci* pneumonia—foamy alveolar material with saucer or cup-shaped organisms that stain heavily with silver (GMS stain). **E**: Oral thrush (candidal glossitis). **F**: Incidental HSV inclusions in thyroid follicular cells.

Pathology

All of the pathologic lesions that occur in adults with HIV infection are seen in children, but there are significant differences in frequency and distribution (87). Pathologies identified more frequently in children include thymic lesions, pulmonary lymphoid and lymphoproliferative disorders (LPDs), and arteriopathy. Polyclonal B-cell lymphoproliferative disorders (PBLD) and malignant lymphoma, especially of brain, are the common neoplasms in children; Kaposi sarcoma is rarely encountered (e63). Table 6-11 outlines the systemic pathology of pediatric HIV infection.

Table 6-11 ■ SYSTEMIC PATHOLOGY OF PEDIATRIC HIV INFECTION

Organ/System	References
Placenta Increased weight Chorioamnionitis Funisitis/fetal vasculitis Villitis	80, 174, 180, 227, 364, 418
Growth and development Increased fetal wastage, intrauterine demise Failure to thrive/wasting No increase in malformations	143, 197, 275, 377, 423
Thymus Small size, cortical atrophy Lymphoid depletion Warthin-Finkeldy-type giant cells Accelerated involution Fibrosis, plasmacytosis Calcified, cystic, or small Hassall corpuscles	18, 180, 235
Spleen Splenomegaly Immunoblastic proliferation Lymphoid depletion Histiocytosis Hemophagocytosis Opportunistic infection "Kaposiform" spindle cell proliferation	235, 469, 470
Lymph nodes Follicular hyperplasia, histiocytosis Plasmacytosis Multinucleate giant cells Hemophagocytosis Lymphoid depletion, fibrosis Lymphoproliferative disorders "Kaposiform" spindle cell proliferation Opportunistic infection	62, 235, 351, 411, 451
Bone marrow Hypoplasia or hyperplasia Myelodysplasia Plasmacytosis, histiocytosis Eosinophilia, lymphoid aggregates Hemosiderosis, fibrosis, granulomas Serous fat atrophy	180, 451
Cardiovascular system Dilated cardiomyopathy Myocarditis, pericarditis Vasculitis, vascular calcification Coronary and cerebral aneurysm Inflammation and fibrosis of conducting system	180, 236, 255, 286
Lung Opportunistic infection, especially PCP, CMV, RSV Lymphoproliferative disorders (PLH, LIP, PBLD) Malignant lymphoma Giant cell pneumonia Smooth muscle neoplasms	14, 49, 237, 238, 239, 463
Gastrointestinal tract Opportunistic infection, especially *Candida*, CMV, MAI, Cryptosporidium, Isospora, Salmonella, Shigella Lymphoid depletion of MALT Lymphoproliferative disorders Neoplasms (lymphoma, smooth muscle tumors, Kaposi sarcoma) Ulcers of undetermined etiology Pneumatosis, pseudomembranous enteritis	13, 180, 244
Liver Chronic active hepatitis, including HBV and HCV, giant cell hepatitis Opportunistic infection, especially CMV, adenovirus, MAI	233, 244, 246, 247, 359, 410
Pancreas Acute and chronic pancreatitis, some associated with pentamidine or dideoxyinosine Opportunistic infection (CMV, MAI, *Candida*) Steatonecrosis Islet hypertrophy and fibrosis Dilatation of ducts and acini Nodular lymphoid infiltrates	65, 245, 248
Kidney HIV-associated nephropathy: focal and segmental glomerulosclerosis, mesangial hyperplasia, immune complex glomerulonephritis, and minimal change disease Opportunistic infection (CMV, *Candida*, MAI) Nephromegaly Nephrocalcinosis	68, 107, 180, 235
Skin Opportunistic infection (*Candida*, HSV, VZ, HPV) Molluscum contagiosum Scabies Seborrheic dermatitis Kaposi sarcoma	180, 235, 282, 458
Nervous system Cerebral atrophy, multinucleate giant cells, microglial nodules, vascular mineralization Lymphoma Opportunistic infection (*Candida*, CMV, MAI, progressive mulfocal leukoencephalopathy) Nonspecific white matter pallor or gliosis	40, 121, 144, 145, 180, 427

Lymphoid Organs

The thymic lesions of childhood HIV infection include precocious or marked involution, marked reduction or absence of Hassall corpuscles, and thymitis (e165). Thymitis may take the form of follicular, mononuclear, or plasma cell infiltrates. Thymic dysfunction and thymic involution occur during HIV disease and have been associated with rapid progression in infants infected perinatally with HIV. Perivascular sclerosis is common. Thymic involvement may be due to direct infection or may represent an autoimmune process. Thymic recovery may be achieved in some patients as a result of potent antiretroviral therapy. Extensive thymic damage may, however, hamper immune reconstitution, particularly in pediatric patients (198).

Although splenomegaly is commonly seen in HIV-infected children, there is lymphoid depletion, architectural disarray, increased macrophages and functional hyposplenia. Cytologically, lymphoid organs show many large lymphocytes, immunoblasts, and also giant cells (polykaryocytes). Progression to lymphoma and Castleman disease may occur in nodal and extranodal sites. Quijano has detailed histopathologic findings in lymph nodes (144).

Lungs

HIV-related pulmonary lymphoid and lymphoproliferative lesions including pulmonary lymphoid hyperplasia (PLH), LIP, and PLBD (86) are more common in children than in adults. PLH is a peribronchial infiltrate of benign lymphoid follicles, often with germinal centers. LIP is characterized by a significant infiltrate of lymphocytes, plasmacytoid cells, plasma cells, and the occasional large immunoblastic cell that expand the interstitial septa (Figure 6-5). There is much overlap between PLH and LIP; they often coexist, hence the designation PLH-LIP complex. These disorders constitute a spectrum of disease related to Epstein-Barr virus (EBV) infection and may eventuate in PLBD or in malignant lymphoma (e164,e331).

Central Nervous System

Neurologic manifestations are frequent in children with AIDS (42) (e95); HIV-related encephalopathy is characterized by low IQ, loss of developmental milestones, microcephaly, progressive weakness, and seizures. Morphologic features include gross brain atrophy, hydrocephalus, diffuse gliosis, multinucleated giant cells, microglial nodules, basal ganglia mineralization, HIV encephalitis, corticospinal tract degeneration, and siderocalcinosis of blood vessels. Common lesions not directly related to HIV infection are lymphomas and cerebrovascular accidents. Opportunistic CNS infections are relatively uncommon, limited predominantly to monilial and cytomegaloviral encephalitides. CNS lymphoma, although less common in children than in adults, is the most common malignancy in pediatric AIDS and is usually EBV-associated. Myelin abnormalities occur both in the brain and the spinal cord and are attributed to delayed myelination, myelin injury, and/or Wallerian degeneration. Progressive multifocal leukoencephalopathy (PML) is rare in children. It has been suggested that most of the CNS effects of HIV infection cannot be attributed to detectable levels of viral antigen, but may be due to circulating cytokines and other soluble factors. The prevalence of HIV encephalopathy has not decreased despite use of HAART; as patients live longer, the prevalence of CNS manifestations may actually increase (e118).

Other Viscera

Liver disease manifests as hepatomegaly with altered enzymes, cholestasis, and/or hepatitis. Cholestatic hepatitis may be the first clue to a pediatric HIV infection. Giant cell transformation of hepatocytes is associated with poor outcomes in these children and is often associated with inflammation and diffuse fibrosis. Viral hepatitis (HBV, HCV, and EBV-hepatitis) and HAART-induced liver effects may contribute to liver injury (63,164,185) (e300). Morphologically, these may show chronic hepatitis with varying activity and/or cholestatic hepatitis. GI manifestations are similar to that in adults, the pathology including HIV enteropathy, opportunistic infections, and EBV-associated smooth muscle tumors (185) (e43,e155,e166). Renal lesions include focal segmental glomerulosclerosis, mesangial hypercellularity, microcystic transformation of renal tubules, immune complex glomerulonephritis, minimal change disease, and nephromegaly (due to glomerulomegaly, tubular dilatation, and interstitial inflammation) (114,147) (e5,e268). Secondary changes include drug-related nephrotoxicity and opportunistic infections. Salivary glands are often affected early giving an appearance of chronic mumps. In HIV-associated arteriopathy, small and medium-sized vessels in many organs (heart, lung, spleen, kidney, intestine, and brain) show fibrous intimal thickening, fragmentation or loss of elastica, and calcification. This results in luminal narrowing, aneurysmal dilatation, and distal ischemic lesions (e169). HIV infects the fetus through the placenta. Although chorioamnionitis, cytotrophoblastic hyperplasia, and other pathology have been identified in placentas of HIV-infected women, no lesion is specific for HIV infection (37) (e46). HIV antigens have been found in placental Hofbauer cells, trophoblasts, and villous endothelial cells (e16). Infected placental macrophages may infect fetal circulating cells or fetal endothelial cells.

Laboratory Diagnosis

As in adults, HIV-1 causes the majority of cases of childhood AIDS, but the diagnosis is more difficult in infants. In infants under the age of 18 months, HIV antibody tests such as the ELISA, western blot, and recently approved rapid tests are not used, since maternal HIV antibodies may persist in the child until 6 to 18 months (e281). In this age group, definitive diagnosis of HIV infection requires two positive viral detection assays on separate specimens, or documentation of an AIDS-defining illness (148,161) (e215). For children

Table 6-12 ■ COMPARISON OF WHO AND CDC STAGES OF HIV INFECTION[a]

WHO Stage[b]	WHO T-lymphocyte Count and Percentage[c]	CDC Stage[d]	CDC T-lymphocyte Count and Percentage
Stage 1 (HIV infection)	CD4⁺ T-lymphocyte count of ≥500 cells/μL	Stage 1 (HIV infection)	CD4⁺ T-lymphocyte count of ≥500 cells/μL or CD4⁺ T-lymphocyte percentage of ≥29
Stage 2 (HIV infection)	CD4⁺ T-lymphocyte count of 350–499 cells/μL	Stage 2 (HIV infection)	CD4⁺ T-lymphocyte count of 200–499 cells/μL or CD4⁺ T-lymphocyte percentage of 14–28
Stage 3 (advanced HIV disease [AHD])	CD4⁺ T-lymphocyte count of 200–349 cells/μL	Stage 2 (HIV infection)	CD4⁺ T-lymphocyte count of 200–499 cells/μL or CD4⁺ T-lymphocyte percentage of 14–28
Stage 4 (acquired immunodeficiency syndrome [AIDS])	CD4⁺ T-lymphocyte count of <200 cells/μL or CD4⁺ T-lymphocyte percentage of <15	Stage 3 (AIDS)	CD4⁺ T-lymphocyte count of <200 cells/μL or CD4⁺ T-lymphocyte percentage of <14

[a]For reporting purposes only.
[b]Among adults and children aged ≥5 years.
[c]Percentage applicable for stage 4 only.
[d]Among adults and adolescents (aged ≥13 years). CDC also includes a fourth stage, stage unknown: laboratory confirmation of HIV infection but no information on CD4⁺ T-lymphocyte count or percentage *and* no information on AIDS-defining conditions.
From Schneider E, Whitmore S, Glynn KM, et al. Centers for Disease Control and Prevention (CDC). Revised surveillance case definitions for HIV infection among adults, adolescents, and children aged <18 months and for HIV infection and AIDS among children aged 18 months to <13 years—United States, 2008. *MMWR Recomm Rep* 2008;57(RR-10):1-12.

aged 18 months to 13 years, laboratory-confirmed evidence of HIV infection is required in addition to the presence of one or more AIDS-defining conditions, to meet the surveillance case definition for AIDS (161). The salient differences between the 2007 World Health Organization (WHO) and 2008 CDC revised surveillance definitions are outlined in Table 6-12 (161).

MEASLES

The causative agent of measles (rubeola) is a single stranded RNA paramyxovirus virus of the genus morbillivirus. Suboptimum vaccination coverage raises serious doubts that the goal of elimination by 2010 can be attained (120) (e213,e228). Although global deaths from measles have decreased notably in past decades, due to both increases in immunization rates and decreases in measles case fatality ratios (CFRs), the values for measles CFR remain imprecise, resulting in continued uncertainty about the actual toll that measles exacts (195).

Transmission

Measles is highly contagious and is spread by aerosols and droplets of respiratory secretions. The viral receptor is CD46 for viral H and F glycoproteins and viremia is mediated through infection of lymphoid and endothelial cells. Host innate immune responses are effective in promptly eliminating the virus (70).

Clinical Features

After a 1- to 2-week(s) incubation period, there is a prodrome (of fever, cough, rhinorrhea, and/or conjunctivitis) with the development of Koplik spots characteristically seen in the oral mucosa. This is followed by an erythematous maculopapular (morbilliform) rash that begins on the face, spreads to the trunks and limbs (Figure 6-6), and fades about 6 days later in the same order in which it had appeared.

Complications are a result of progressive viral replication, secondary bacterial or viral infections, and/or an abnormal host-immune response. The most common complications are bacterial pneumonia or otitis media, the former being the most frequent cause of death. Other complications are febrile convulsions, encephalitis, chronic diarrhea, and liver function abnormalities. Pulmonary complications (secondary pneumonia, giant cell pneumonia, and atypical measles pneumonia) are the most feared. Prophylactic antibiotics may help prevent respiratory complications (88), although this has been refuted. While rare, the measles virus can infect the CNS and trigger fatal CNS diseases weeks to years after exposure (200). CNS complications include acute postinfectious allergic encephalitis, acute progressive measles (inclusion body) encephalitis, pseudotumor cerebri (e328), and SSPE. SSPE has an average 6-year latent period after infection/vaccination and is manifested as progressive mental retardation, motor dysfunction, seizures, coma, and death in 1 to 2 years.

Pathology

The pathology of measles infection is characterized by two types of multinucleated giant cells. Warthin Finkeldey giant cells are seen in lymphoid tissues throughout the body during the incubation period; while epithelial giant cells occur in the epithelia of all major organs (Figure 6-6). The giant cells may contain nuclear and/or cytoplasmic inclusions. Interstitial pneumonitis is characteristic, with or without a granulomatous response. Allergic phenomena (atypical measles

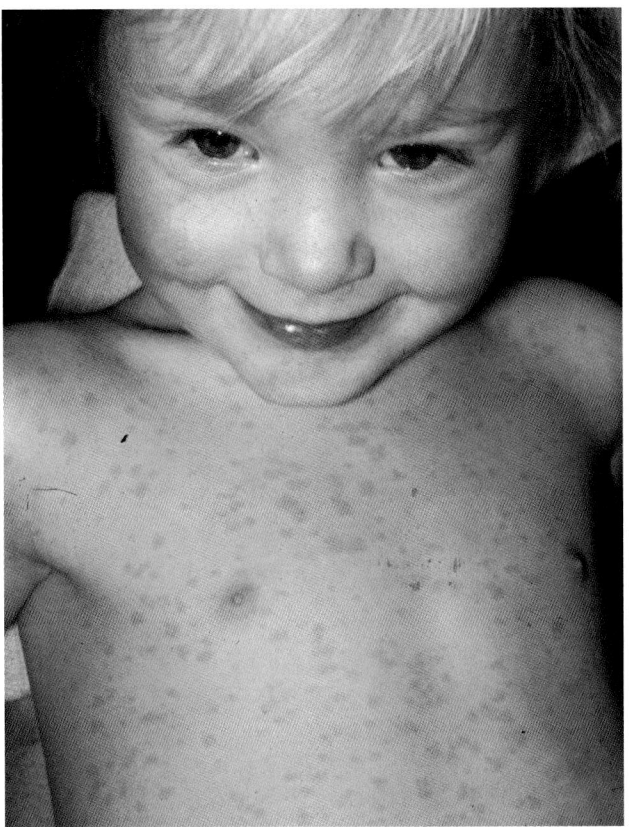

A

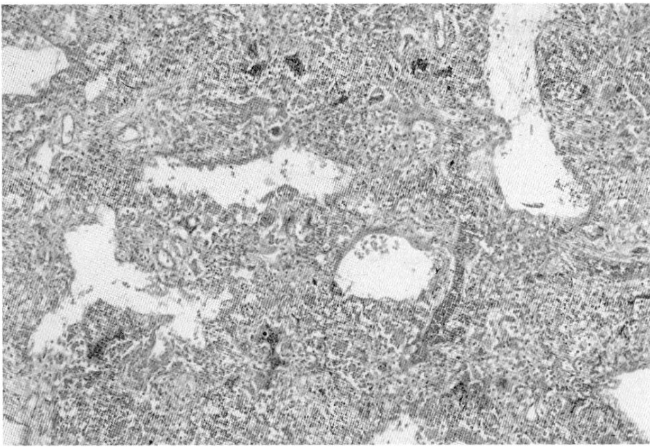

B

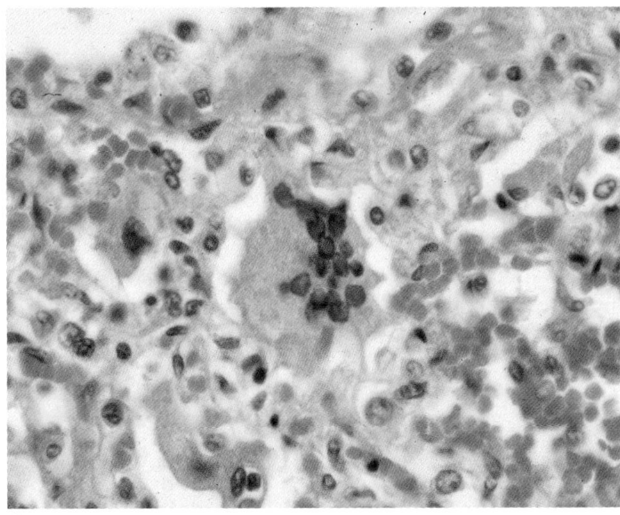

C

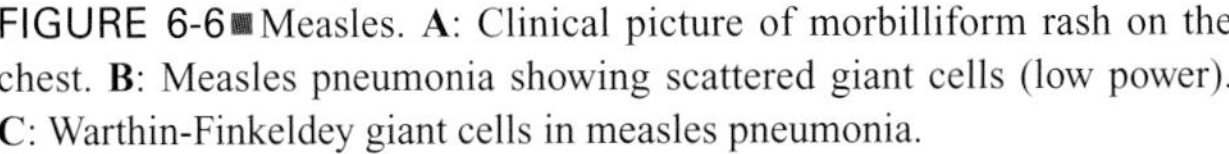

FIGURE 6-6■Measles. **A**: Clinical picture of morbilliform rash on the chest. **B**: Measles pneumonia showing scattered giant cells (low power). **C**: Warthin-Finkeldey giant cells in measles pneumonia.

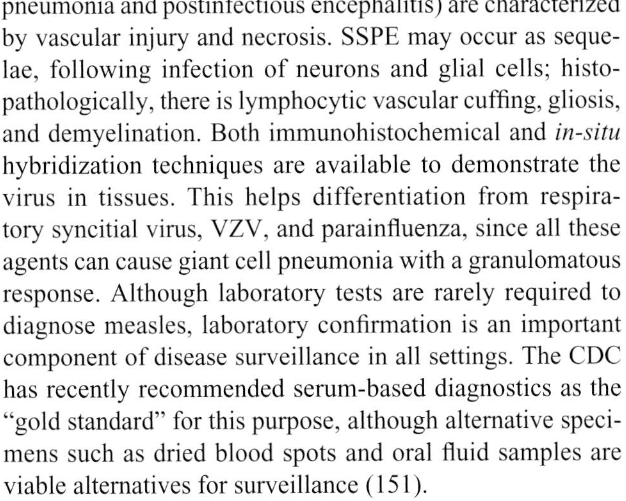

pneumonia and postinfectious encephalitis) are characterized by vascular injury and necrosis. SSPE may occur as sequelae, following infection of neurons and glial cells; histopathologically, there is lymphocytic vascular cuffing, gliosis, and demyelination. Both immunohistochemical and *in-situ* hybridization techniques are available to demonstrate the virus in tissues. This helps differentiation from respiratory syncitial virus, VZV, and parainfluenza, since all these agents can cause giant cell pneumonia with a granulomatous response. Although laboratory tests are rarely required to diagnose measles, laboratory confirmation is an important component of disease surveillance in all settings. The CDC has recently recommended serum-based diagnostics as the "gold standard" for this purpose, although alternative specimens such as dried blood spots and oral fluid samples are viable alternatives for surveillance (151).

EPSTEIN-BARR VIRUS

The EBV is a gamma-human herpes virus that infects B-lymphocytes and epithelial cells of the pharyngeal mucosa, salivary gland ducts, and uterine cervix. It has the unique distinction of being the first human tumor virus to be discovered, and has a diverse clinical disease spectrum including infectious mononucleosis (IM), LPDs, lymphoepithelioma-like (nasopharyngeal) carcinomas, and rare mesenchymal neoplasms. Infection of epithelial cells is lytic (productive), with resultant full cycle of viral replication and release of infectious virus particles into secretions. On the other hand, infection of B-lymphocytes is predominantly latent (nonproductive), with the potential for immortalization and activation of infected cells (e293). Only a limited set of genes are expressed during latent cycle infection [EBV nuclear antigens (EBNAs) and three latent membrane proteins (LMPs)]; these define different latency patterns (30) (e351).

The virus is ubiquitous and is transmitted primarily by saliva, although transmission by blood transfusion and allogeneic bone marrow transplantation is also documented. Recently, sexual transmission has also been proposed as a route of infection (75) (e371). Very little is known about the risk of congenital EBV infections, with only one well-documented case in the literature (e122). Since most adult women have become seropositive during childhood, primary

EBV infection during pregnancy is rare, whereas reactivation of a latent EBV infection seems to occur more often in seropositive pregnant women as compared to control subjects (e110). However, only primary infection (and not reactivation) may be harmful to the embryo or fetus. Worldwide, primary infection occurs within the first few years of life and is usually subclinical; symptomatic IM occurs when infection is delayed to adolescence or beyond.

Infectious Mononucleosis

IM, first detailed by Sprunt and Evans in 1920 (e310), is a self-limiting lymphoproliferative disease with a benign course. The highest rates of IM occurs between 10 and 19 years of age (6 to 8 cases per 1,000 persons per year) (e115,e138), although mild infections in younger children may often be undiagnosed. Rates of infection are highest in closeted populations of young adults such as active-duty military personnel and college students (11 to 48 cases per 1,000 persons per year) (19) (e346).

Most clinical symptoms are due to the host's immune response. The incubation period is estimated to be 5 to 7 weeks, followed by a prodrome of 3 to 5 days (with headache, malaise, and fever) and the characteristic triad of fever, sore throat, and extensive cervical lymphadenopathy/tonsillar enlargement. Pharyngeal inflammation and transient palatal petechiae are also common. Other frequent clinical manifestations include splenomegaly (identified in all patients by ultrasonography) and hepatomegaly with transient hepatic dysfunction. EBV infection must be considered in children with FUO (e251). Younger children may show less typical and less severe clinical disease. The well-known atypical lymphocytes (first described by Downing and McKinley) appear in circulation from 1 to 4 weeks after disease onset (e82). These atypical cells are mainly activated oligoclonal CD8-positive cytotoxic T-cells, with only a small proportion representing EBV-infected B-cells; in fact the CD8-proliferation may result in a reduction of the CD4/CD8 ratio (e337). The uncomplicated illness usually lasts for 2 to 4 weeks. Complications of IM involve the hematopoietic system (anemia, thrombocytopenia, neutropenia), heart (pericarditis, myocarditis), nervous system (meningo-encephalitis, cerebellitis, Guillain-Barre syndrome, Bell palsy, transverse myelitis, autoimmune neuropathies), skin (ampicillin-associated rash, Gianotti-Crosti syndrome), kidneys (nephritis, glomerulopathies), immune system (hypo-, hypergammaglobulinemia, auto-antibodies), and psychiatric diseases (85) (e293). Although most patients are advised to avoid contact sports to prevent potentitially serious splenic rupture, this is a rare complication (~0.1%) (e101). "Virus-associated hemophagocytic syndrome" is an unusual consequence of unknown pathogenesis, characterized by a benign generalized histiocytic proliferation with marked hemophagocytosis in bone marrow and lymph nodes (e275). Usually, IM is an acute, self-limiting disease that occurs only once in the host's lifetime. However, some patients suffer from recurrent fever, persistent hepatosplenomegaly, hematological abnormalities, neuromyasthenia, and the so-called chronic fatigue syndrome (e321). Many of these patients reveal immunological abnormalities such as deficient natural killer cell activity, and abnormal antibody responses to the different EBV antigens. Prolonged illness after IM may be due to altered immunity rather than increased viral load (e39).

The differential diagnoses for suspected IM include streptococcal pharyngitis, toxoplasmosis, CMV pharyngitis, acute HIV infection, and other viral pharyngitis (50). The presence of splenomegaly, posterior cervical adenopathy, axillary adenopathy, and inguinal adenopathy is most useful in considering the possibility of IM, while the absence of cervical adenopathy and fatigue is most helpful in dismissing the diagnosis. Hoagland's criteria (e142) for the diagnosis of IM are widely cited: at least 50% lymphocytes and at least 10% atypical lymphocytes in the presence of fever, pharyngitis, and adenopathy, and confirmed by a positive serologic test. Although specific, these criteria are not highly sensitive; only about one-half of symptomatic patients with a positive heterophile antibody test meet all the criteria.

Diagnosis rests on viral serology and the detection of the EBV genome, viral antigens, or infectious virus in saliva or lymphoid tissues. The accidental discovery of elevated heterophile antibody by Paul and Bunnell in 1932 (e253) forms the basis for the heterophile agglutination reaction. Although they are relatively specific, IgM heterophile antibody tests are somewhat insensitive, particularly in the first weeks of illness. Heterophile antibody tests are less sensitive in patients younger than 12 years, detecting only 25% to 50% of infections in this group, compared with 71% to 91% in older patients (e195). Antibodies to viral capsid antigen (i.e., VCA-IgG and VCA-IgM) are produced slightly earlier than the heterophile antibody and are more specific for EBV infection (e35); in acute infection IgM anti-VCA antibodies are present and anti-EBNA antibodies are absent. The VCA-IgG antibody persists past the stage of acute infection and signals the development of immunity (e9). A past infection is identified by the absence of IgM antibodies and the presence of IgG antibodies against VCA and EBNA. However, anti-EBNA antibodies may not be detected in immunodeficient children. Patients with latent infection have elevated antibodies against early antigen (EA). Although no evidence-based or consensus guidelines have been proposed to guide the evaluation of patients with suspected IM, Ebell has proposed an algorithmic approach based on the percentage of atypical lymphocytes and absence of streptococcal pharyngitis (50). At present, nucleic acid hybridization (by Southern blot, *in-situ* hybridization or PCR) is the most specific method for the detection of EBV in clinical material. The laboratory diagnosis of IM has been recently reviewed (69) (e150).

Histologically, enlarged lymph nodes show a predominant paracortical expansion, with atypical cells that are predominantly cytotoxic T-cells (CD8 and TIA-1 positive). EBV infected cells are best identified by *in-situ* hybridization for EBV-encoded small RNA (EBER) (Figure 6-7). Histologic

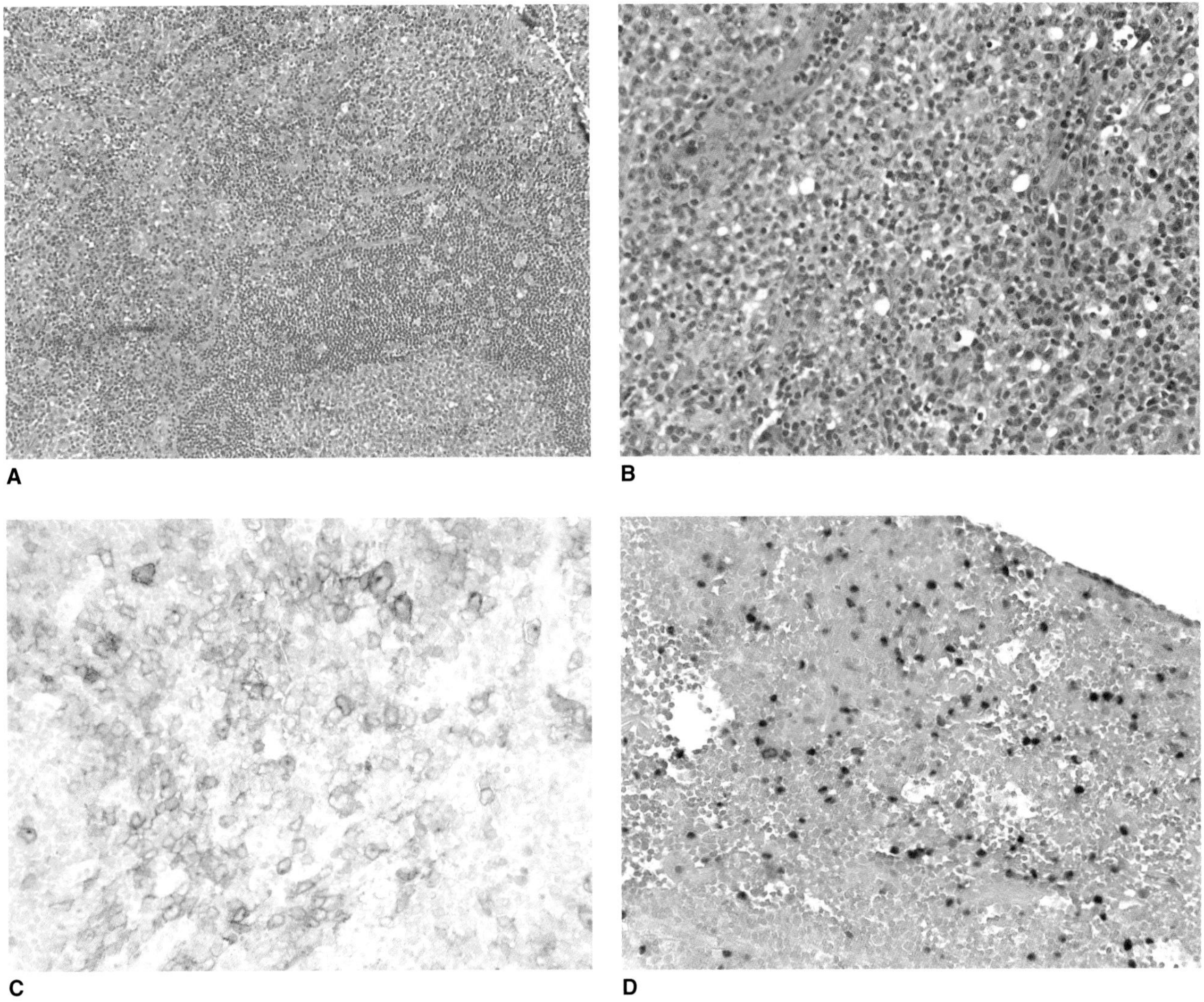

FIGURE 6-7 ■ Infectious mononucleosis. **AB:** Lymph node biopsy shows paracortical expansion and an atypical lymphoid infiltrate with numerous immunoblasts. **C:** These activated lymphoid cells are highlighted by CD30 immunostain. **D:** In-situ hybridization for EBV (EBER probe) shows strong, diffuse nuclear positivity.

findings of EBV-associated hepatitis include minimal swelling and vacuolization of the hepatocytes, and a peculiar sinusoidal infiltration of T-cells in an "Indian Bead" pattern, in addition to periportal inflammation. (see Chapter 15).

EBV-Associated Neoplasms

Neoplasms associated with latent EBV infection include lymphomas, nasopharyngeal carcinoma, lymphoepithelial carcinomas in various viscera, smooth muscle tumors, and inflammatory pseudotumor-like follicular dendritic cell tumor (30,38,40,153) (e12,e51). Different latency patterns are associated with different neoplasms (e.g., type I with Burkitt lymphoma, type II with Hodgkin lymphoma and nasopharyngeal carcinoma, and type III with posttransplant LPDs), with type III latency expressing more EBV proteins and being more immunogenic and type I being the least immunogenic (30). In lymphomagenesis, EBV either plays a direct role (such as in posttransplant LPDs and HIV-associated immunoblastic lymphoma occurring in immunodeficient individuals) or as a cofactor (such as in Burkitt lymphoma and some T/NK-cell malignancies occurring in immunocompetent individuals). EBV-associated T/natural killer (NK)-cell LPD (EBV-T/NK LPD) of children and young adults is generally referred to with the blanket nosological term of severe chronic active EBV infection (CAEBV) and overlaps with a unique disease previously described as infantile fulminant EBV-associated T-LPD. This disease is rare, is associated with high morbidity and mortality, and appears to be more prevalent in East Asian countries. The major signs and symptoms include fever, hepatomegaly, splenomegaly, liver dysfunction, thrombocytopenia, anemia, lymphadenopathy, hypersensitivity to mosquito bites, skin rash, hydroa vacciniforme, diarrhea, and uveitis. A classification system for EBV-T/NK LPD of children and young adults has been recently proposed based on morphology (polymorphic or monomorphic) and clonality (polyclonal or monoclonal NK or cytotoxic T-cells) (131).

VIRAL HEMORRHAGIC FEVERS

The combination of fever and hemorrhage can be caused by viruses, rickettsiae, bacteria, protozoa, and fungi. However, conventionally, the term "hemorrhagic fever" refers to fever and hemorrhage caused by viruses transmitted by arthropods ("arboviruses") and rodents. Viruses implicated in this syndrome are diverse and include arenaviridae (e.g., lassa virus), bunyaviridae (e.g., Hanta virus, Rift valley fever), flaviviridae (e.g., yellow fever, dengue), chikungunya, and filoviridae (Ebola, Marburg) (21,67) (e105,e139,e234,e327). The detailed description of each of these conditions is beyond the scope of this chapter. Certain general features common to these syndromes will be outlined, using dengue as a prototype (143) (e77,e298). The clinical differential diagnoses include leptospirosis, rickettsial fevers (e.g., typhus), complicated malaria, and disseminated intravascular coagulopathy (DIC) following severe sepsis of any etiology. Viral hemorrhagic fevers have become a major concern in the recent past. Agents such as Dengue virus have caused many recent epidemics; more than 1.2 million cases of dengue fever and dengue hemorrhagic fever (DHF) were reported to the WHO from 56 countries in the 1998 pandemic (106).

Transmission

Many of these arboviral fevers are transmitted to humans by mosquito bites (dengue is transmitted by the female Aedes mosquito) and several ecologic factors have contributed to a significant increase in the incidence of dengue fever and the emergence of DHF as a major public health problem in America and Asia. Prenatal or perinatal transmission has been reported in rare instances (e30). There is no evidence for transmission of dengue virus in breast milk, nor more severe disease in breast-fed infants compared with formula-fed infants. There has been no documented person-to-person transmission of dengue virus without a mosquito vector.

Clinical Features

Dengue viruses cause dengue fever, DHF, and dengue shock syndrome (DSS) in infants less than 1 year of age, but rarely in those younger than 3 months (e129). The disease spectrum ranges from a mild flu-like illness to life threatening manifestations with severe hypotension (due to vascular dysregulation), vascular abnormalities (manifested as conjunctival suffusion, flushing, and exanthem), capillary instability (manifested as edema), and hemorrhage (due to a combination of thrombocytopenia and microvascular damage with DIC). Visceral involvement manifests variably as renal, pulmonary, hepatic, and neurological dysfunction, and as a result of lymphoid necrosis and depletion. Infection of mononuclear cells leads to cytokine activation and plays a central role in the pathogenesis of DHF. Antibody-dependent enhancement due to preexisting antidengue IgG against the infecting strain causes more severe disease.

Infants and young children with dengue usually have only a nonspecific febrile illness, with a rash that is hard to distinguish from other viral illnesses. The more severe cases usually occur in older children and adults, characterized by a rapidly rising temperature and severe headache, myalgia and arthralgia that last for 5 to 6 days. Many patients have an initial macular to maculopapular rash that later becomes diffusely erythematous. Minor hemorrhagic manifestations such as petechiae, epistaxis, and gingival bleeding occur. Although dengue fever may be incapacitating, its prognosis is favorable and most patients generally recover after 7 to 10 days of illness. DHF, on the other hand, is an acute febrile illness with hemorrhagic manifestations, thrombocytopenia, and evidence of increased vascular permeability resulting in loss of plasma from the vascular compartment. Hypoproteinemia, an elevated hematocrit and serous effusion are indicators of plasma leakage, which may progress to circulatory failure, so-called dengue shock syndrome (DSS). The patient may die within 24 hours, or may recover quickly following appropriate volume replacement and supportive therapy. Neurological manifestations may occur in the absence of shock (90). Complications such as hepatic dysfunction and fluid overload are more commonly found in infants and the case fatality rate is also higher in this age group (89).

Pathology

Morphologically there is variably prominent capillary dilatation, endothelial swelling, edema, and/or vasculitis with fibrin thrombi. Target organs are different in different syndromes; for example, in Hantavirus syndromes the major target organ may be the lung or the kidney with brain, liver, and spleen being secondary target organs. Each involved organ may show features of severe injury such as diffuse alveolar damage, renal tubular necrosis, medullary hemorrhage, and features of DIC may be present.

OTHER SYSTEMIC VIRAL INFECTIONS

Disseminated *adenoviral* disease usually occurs in immunocompromised hosts, posttransplantation or in neonates, and manifests with clinically significant destructive hepatitis (e349). Rarely, infection may occur in healthy children (e98). The hepatitis is characterized by variable necrosis with intranuclear amphophilic or basophilic viral inclusions with peri-inclusional clearing or, in late stages, smudge cells. Adenovirus may also cause enterocolitis and pneumonia.

Echovirus can cause flu-like symptoms in any age group. However, fatal and severe infections are almost exclusively reported in neonates and infants. The spectrum of illness includes encephalitis, meningitis, hepatitis, and other unusual manifestations such as myocarditis, orchitis, postviral fatigue syndrome, and transient erythroblastopenia of childhood (e94).

Infection-associated hemophagocytic syndrome presents as a severe acute systemic illness with prolonged fever, constitutional symptoms, hepatosplenomegaly, cytopenias, and hepatic dysfunction. Conventionally thought to affect immunocompromised patients, in a relatively large study of 18 pediatric cases, almost 90% of patients were previously healthy; the case fatality rate was 61% with all fatal cases dying within 2 months of disease onset (23). Formerly thought to be a sequel to a viral infection (especially EBV), it is now known to be also associated with a wide variety of agents including Gram negative bacilli, mycobacteria, protozoa, and fungi. In the above study, children less than 3 years of age were more vulnerable to neutropenia-associated bacteremia. The histologic hallmark is widespread proliferation of cytologically benign histiocytes with erythrophagocytosis and lymphophagocytosis.

HTLV infection is endemic in southwest Japan, the Caribbean, South America, and sub-Saharan Africa (66) (e116). Transmission is through sexual contact, intravenous drug abuse, infected blood and blood products, and breast milk. The frequency of transmission and the contributing factors to sexual and mother-to-child transmission remain uncertain (e253). HTLV transmission is more frequent in breast-fed than formula-fed infants (e137,e183,e347). Duration of breastfeeding correlates with transmission rate (e10,e11,e236,e367). Transmission is also associated with higher maternal provirus levels and HTLV-1 antibody titers (76) (e345). The median time of transmission has been estimated at 11 to 12 months of age (e117). Complete avoidance of breastfeeding is reportedly effective in preventing mother-to-child transmission (e141). HTLV-1 causes adult

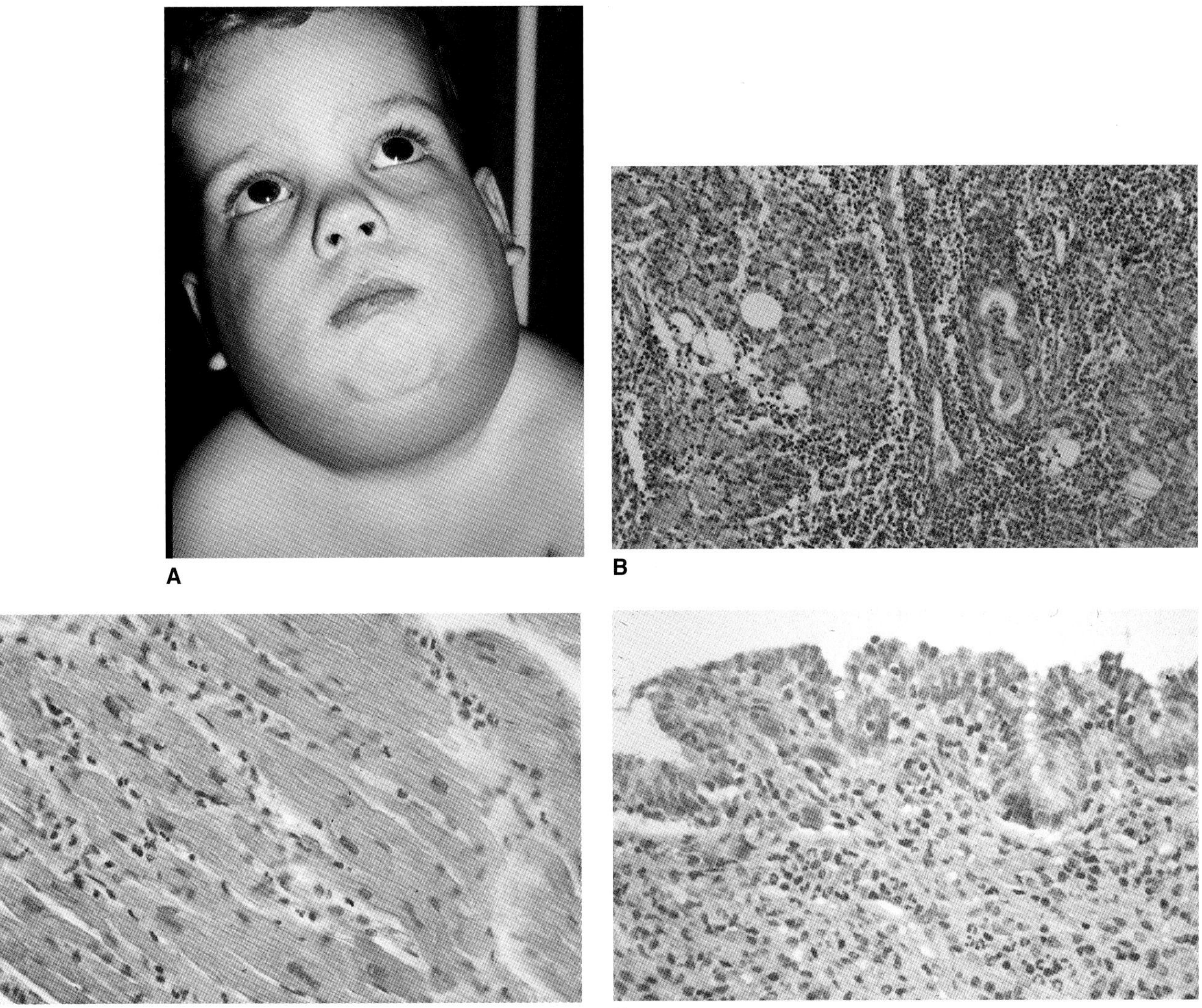

FIGURE 6-8 ■ Mumps. **A**: Bilateral parotitis is seen in this clinical photograph. **B**: Histological appearance of parotitis is shown with a diffuse lymphocytic infiltrate. **C**: Mumps myocarditis is characterized by the presence of a lymphocytic infiltrate and focal myonecrosis. **D**: Acute epididymoorchitis in mumps is seen as an active lymphocytic infiltrate in the interstitium.

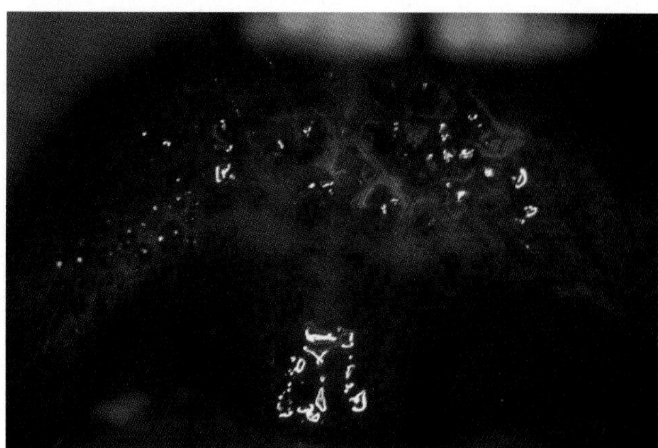

FIGURE 6-9 ■ Coxsackie infection with vesicular oral mucosal lesions.

T-cell leukemia/lymphoma (ATLL), a chronic, progressive neuropathy called HTLV-1 associated myelopathy, and tropical spastic paraparesis associated with various other chronic conditions (uveitis, arthritis, Sjogren syndrome, infective dermatitis, and a persistent lymphadenitis in children). Early life infection carries the greatest risk for later development of ATLL (e205). In areas of low prevalence, the likelihood of a false positive HTLV-1 test is high; therefore repeat testing is often indicated. In a pregnant woman, antibody titer testing and proviral load quantification are appropriate to estimate the risk for transmission to the infant. HTLV-2 causes at least two forms of chronic ataxia (spastic or tropical) (e199).

Mumps has been reported to be resurgent in the United States; over 2,500 cases were reported in 2006 alone (Figure 6-8). The majority of these cases occurred in college students aged 18 to 25 years, even though most had been vaccinated with two doses of measles, mumps, and rubella-containing vaccines. Kancherla has reviewed mumps and discussed potential mechanisms for vaccine failure (91).

Coxsackie viruses are implicated in hand, foot and mouth disease (Figure 6-9), myocarditis, and aseptic meningitis.

EMERGING VIRAL INFECTIONS

Every year seems to bring a new "emerging infectious disease" (20,25,26,27,44,71,107) (e58,59e,e106), the H1N1 "swine" influenza being the latest addition at the time of writing this section (83,128,175) (e108,e208,e254,e288). The influenza virus remains an important challenge, given its ability to mutate at a very high level. Although the common circulating influenza virus strains (H1N1 and H3N2) are not virulent enough to cause mortality, mutated strains may be lethal, especially in children (95). Apart from these circulating human strains, the avian influenza H5N1, H7, and H9 virus strains have also been reported to cause human disease. The major threats of emerging infections worldwide are from zoonotic diseases, foodborne diseases, waterborne diseases, and diseases caused by multiresistant organisms, and challenge clinical acumen, diagnostic armamentaria, and public health systems. Two are briefly discussed here including SARS and West Nile virus (WNV) infections.

SARS is caused by a coronavirus different from previously studied coronavirus groups (e283). Because the SARS-associated coronavirus was identified relatively recently, much about it is unknown. The SARS virus is transmitted primarily by respiratory droplets. In the pediatric cases reported in the literature, children had mild respiratory illness, although the severity of the disease in adolescents seemed more similar to that in adults (13,80). Infants born to mothers with confirmed SARS were born prematurely, presumably because of maternal illness. Two of the five infants described developed severe abdominal disease (coronavirus has been linked to necrotizing enterocolitis), although coronavirus was not identified in any of the infants (169).

WNV infection leads to approximately one case of severe neurologic disease for every 20 cases of nonspecific febrile illness and every 150 to 300 cases of asymptomatic infection (seroconversion). Clinical illness is rare in infants and children (140). Transmission occurs primarily through the bite of Culex mosquitoes, but may also occur during pregnancy (82), through organ transplants, following percutaneous exposure in laboratory workers, and possibly transfusion of blood products. One case of possible WNV transmission through breastfeeding has been reported (e256). However, the absence of illness in this infant (and most infants/children), the transient nature of maternal viremia with WNV infection, and the rarity of such a transmission event suggest that there is no reason to avoid breastfeeding or breast milk when a mother is infected with WNV (104).

BACTERIAL INFECTIONS

We will give an overview of neonatal sepsis followed by a discussion of the more common infections caused by individual groups of bacteria.

NEONATAL SEPSIS

Sepsis is a leading cause of death in infants and children, with over 42,000 cases of severe sepsis reported annually in the United States and millions worldwide. Sepsis is especially devastating in the neonatal population. Neonates significantly differ from adults in multiple respects including their naïve immune system, pathophysiologic response to sepsis, and response to treatment (108). Half of the children with severe sepsis in the United States are infants, and half of these are low- or very low–birth-weight babies. Incidence and mortality rates vary by age and the presence of underlying disease, if any (e360). Attack rates for infants of colonized mothers also vary with the organisms (e40), their serotype (e18), and the presence or absence of maternal antibody (e17). Sepsis neonatorum denotes fulminant bacterial sepsis occurring in the first 30 days of life, characterized clinically by abrupt onset, rapid progression, often without demonstrable anatomic localization, and very high morbidity and mortality rates even in the face of appropriate antibiotic therapy. The clinical manifestations are protean and include hypothermia, hyperthermia, respiratory distress, and feeding disturbances. Clinical distinction from noninfectious disease, especially hyaline membrane disease, is frequently impossible, and thorough microbiologic evaluation is mandatory in all cases of neonatal death. Unfortunately, sepsis is a term that has been, and continues to be, used very loosely in clinical practice, limiting comparison of studies from around the globe. Although bacteremia, systemic inflammatory response syndrome (SIRS), and septicemia have been defined for the adult population, these cannot be directly extrapolated to the pediatric population. Definitions for the pediatric population have only recently been agreed upon in consensus (Table 6-13) (65,165). SIRS is the body's response to an infectious or noninfectious insult. The name is only partially accurate since patients who develop SIRS have both an initial proinflammatory state (i.e., initially hyperimmune) and a later antiinflammatory state (i.e., hypoimmune). The pathophysiology of SIRS is complex and has been recently reviewed (155).

Neonatal sepsis is subclassified based on the timing of infection as early-onset (in the first week of life and especially within the first 24 hours), late-onset (7 to 30 days of age), and very late-onset (beyond 30 days). Early-onset disease is associated with obstetric complications including fever, prolonged labor, prolonged membrane rupture, and premature delivery. The predominant organisms causing early-onset infections are GBS and enteric bacilli, especially *Escherichia coli*. Less common early-onset pathogens include other streptococci, enterococci, *Listeria*, *H. influenzae*, *Streptococcus pneumoniae*, *Chlamydia*, and other organisms in the maternal genital flora. However, these organisms can also cause late- or very late-onset bacterial infections. Antibiotic-resistant strains of Gram negative bacilli and Staphylococci are important nosocomial pathogens in hospital settings. Anaerobic bacteria, *Serratia* and *N. meningitidis* are rare causes of neonatal sepsis. Timely detection and identification of offending organisms are among the most important functions of the microbiology laboratory. From a diagnostic standpoint, positive blood cultures can establish an infectious etiology for a patient's illness and provide a microorganism for susceptibility testing and optimization of antimicrobial therapy. Detection of positive blood cultures also has prognostic importance, providing evidence that the host defenses have failed to contain the infection locally and/or that the physician has failed to remove, drain, or otherwise eradicate the infection at its primary site. The key principles in obtaining blood cultures include choosing the best available site for culture, paying attention to aseptic technique, culturing an adequate volume of blood, and obtaining a sufficient number of blood culture sets. Technical variables that can affect results include culture medium, the ratio of blood to broth, additives to inactivate antimicrobial agents in the blood, and the duration of incubation and testing

Table 6-13 ■ DEFINITIONS OF SYSTEMIC INFLAMMATORY RESPONSE SYNDROME (SIRS), INFECTION, SEPSIS, SEVERE SEPSIS, AND SEPTIC SHOCK

SIRS

The presence of at least two of the following four criteria, one of which must be abnormal temperature or leukocyte count:

- Core temperature of >38.5°C or <36°C.
- Tachycardia, defined as a mean heart rate >2 SD above normal for age in the absence of external stimulus, chronic drugs, or painful stimuli; or otherwise unexplained persistent elevation over a 0.5- to 4-hour time period OR for children <1 year old: bradycardia, defined as a mean heart rate <10th percentile for age in the absence of external vagal stimulus, β-blocker drugs, or congenital heart disease; or otherwise unexplained persistent depression over a 0.5-hour time period.
- Mean respiratory rate >2 SD above normal for age or mechanical ventilation for an acute process not related to underlying neuromuscular disease or the receipt of general anesthesia.
- Leukocyte count elevated or depressed for age (not secondary to chemotherapy-induced leukopenia) or >10% immature neutrophils.

Infection

A suspected or proven (by positive culture, tissue stain, or polymerase chain reaction test) infection caused by any pathogen OR a clinical syndrome associated with a high probability of infection. Evidence of infection includes positive findings on clinical exam, imaging, or laboratory tests (e.g., white blood cells in a normally sterile body fluid, perforated viscus, chest radiograph consistent with pneumonia, petechial or purpuric rash, or purpura fulminans).

Sepsis

SIRS in the presence of or as a result of suspected or proven infection.

Severe sepsis

Sepsis plus one of the following: cardiovascular organ dysfunction OR acute respiratory distress syndrome OR two or more other organ dysfunctions.

Septic shock

Sepsis and cardiovascular organ dysfunction.

From Goldstein B, Giroir B, Randolph A. International Consensus Conference on Pediatric Sepsis. International pediatric sepsis consensus conference: definitions for sepsis and organ dysfunction in pediatrics. *Pediatr Crit Care Med* 2005; 6(1):2–8.

in the laboratory. Special considerations are required for organisms such as mycobacteria, *Bartonella*, anaerobes, and fungi (e203). Measures of acute phase proteins, cytokines, cell surface antigens, and bacterial genomes have been used alone or in combination to improve diagnosis of neonatal sepsis, but are not standardized and many are not available routinely (4,100). Real-time PCR methods that can simultaneously detect the 25 most important bacterial and fungal species which cause approximately 90% of all blood stream infections have been proposed for routine assessment of neonatal sepsis (122).

Pathologic changes in infants with neonatal sepsis vary little regardless of the agent responsible. Since the organism is commonly acquired from the mother's genital tract either directly, or through swallowing or aspiration of infected amniotic fluid, the main pathologic finding in early-onset disease is widespread pneumonia. The lungs are heavy, red, and airless. Histologically there is a widespread, relatively uniformly distributed, intraalveolar polymorphonuclear exudate. In infants dying within the first few hours of life, there may be little polymorphonuclear infiltrate, with collapse and congestion predominating. Hyaline membranes may be present, often containing large numbers of bacteria. Interstitial infiltrate may be prominent in GBS sepsis. Pulmonary hemorrhage is frequently seen. Amniotic squames are present in the alveoli, as they are in virtually all infants dying under 1 month of age. Systemic lesions are decidedly uncommon; splenitis is seen in 30% of cases, and meningitis is rare.

Late-onset neonatal sepsis, in contrast, has no association with obstetric complications, and the route of acquisition of the organism may be uncertain. Vertical transmission can be documented in most GBS disease (most commonly subtype III) and in some cases of *E. coli* infections (e177). Other Gram negative bacilli and, more recently, nosocomial *Acinetobacter* infections have also been implicated in late onset neonatal sepsis (e220,e332). Horizontal transmission from home or nursery contacts is presumed to account for the remainder. The onset is either insidious or fulminant, and mortality is less than that seen in early-onset disease. Bacteremia results in meningeal seeding in virtually all cases; ventriculitis is the rule and, together with arachnoidal fibrosis, accounts for the high incidence of hydrocephalus in survivors (e24,e255). The pathologic changes and sequelae are those of neonatal meningitis in general. Extrameningeal infectious foci were demonstrable in the majority of patients in Berman and Banker's series (e24). Various scoring systems are available to estimate the severity of illness and organ dysfunction (99).

Sepsis may have distinct characteristics in patients with congenital immunodeficiencies. Congenitally impaired immunity could paradoxically lead to a milder course of sepsis due to an incomplete inflammatory response, or result in a more severe course, due to a lack of regulatory responses and a higher pathogen burden. An association is seen between types of immune deficiencies and the class of infecting organisms (Tables 6-1 and 6-2) (132).

STAPHYLOCOCCAL INFECTIONS

Both coagulase-positive and coagulase-negative staphylococci are frequently encountered pathogens in the young. Staphylococcal infection usually occurs late in the neonatal period; 40% to 90% of infants in the nursery at 5 days of age are colonized with *Staphylococcus aureus*, skin and nares being the predominant sites of colonization (e99). The morphologic hallmark of infections by coagulase positive staphylococci is suppurative inflammation with necrosis (abscess formation) (Figure 6-10), with or without systemic manifestations of inflammation; any organ or organ-system may be involved. Cutaneous and subcutaneous infections can progress to necrotizing fasciitis, which may become fulminant. Methicillin-resistant *S. aureus* (MRSA) is now an established community pathogen with significant morbidity and mortality, and has changed the epidemiology, clinical manifestations, laboratory approach, antibiotic management, and prevention of staphylococcal infections in children (93). Spread of MRSA has also been documented in the school and daycare settings (e4). Community acquired MRSA isolates are now also associated with nosocomial infections in neonatal intensive care units (e178). Nursery outbreaks of *S. aureus* infections have been traced to postnatal contact with mothers, health care workers, and contaminated, unpasteurized, banked breast milk (e249). Differentiating between isolates that have the *pvl* genes and those that are negative for *pvl* has major therapeutic implications (93).

The most common bloodstream infection encountered in neonatal and pediatric intensive care units is coagulase-negative *Staphylococcus* (CONS) (186) (e231,e318,e319). CONS infections are almost always associated with intravenous catheters or invasive procedures. Since the organism is a normal skin commensal, differentiating infection from colonization and contamination can be difficult. These infections also pose serious concerns because of their high mortality rates and the frequent presence of the *mecA* gene, which is associated with β-lactam antibiotic resistance. Colonization rates are as high as 60% to 90% for infants hospitalized at 2 weeks of age.

Staphylococci can also cause diseases due to elaboration of soluble toxins, including food poisoning, the so-called staphylococcal scalded skin syndrome (SSSS), and toxic shock syndrome (TSS). SSSS (so-called Ritter disease in neonates and staphylococcal toxic epidermal necrolysis in older children) is caused by an epidermolytic exotoxin produced by phage group II staphylococcus. It is characterized by large intraepidermal bullae that rupture and lead to exfoliation (Figure 6-10); resultant fluid loss, and/or secondary infection may be fatal. Toxic shock syndrome is rare under age 10, with peak incidence in teenagers. Predisposing factors include tampon use, surgical procedures, skin infections, and abortions. The toxin (toxic shock syndrome toxin I, or TSST-I) causes massive intravascular fluid loss leading to edema, diarrhea, and hypotensive shock. Mucous membranes

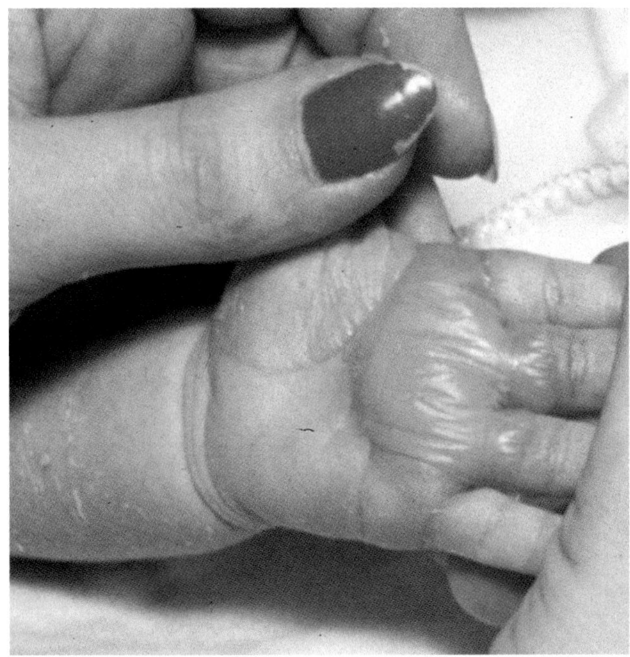

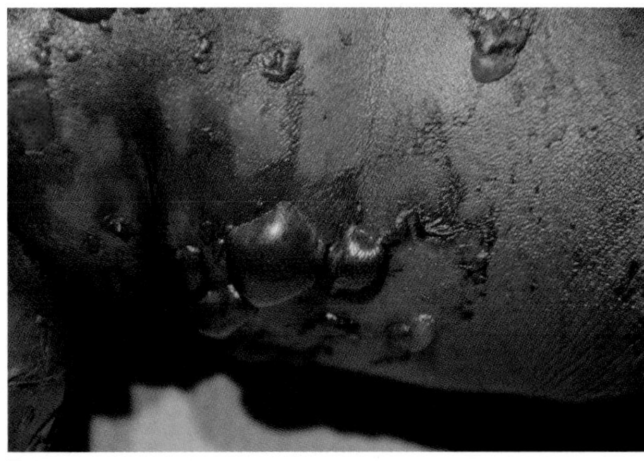

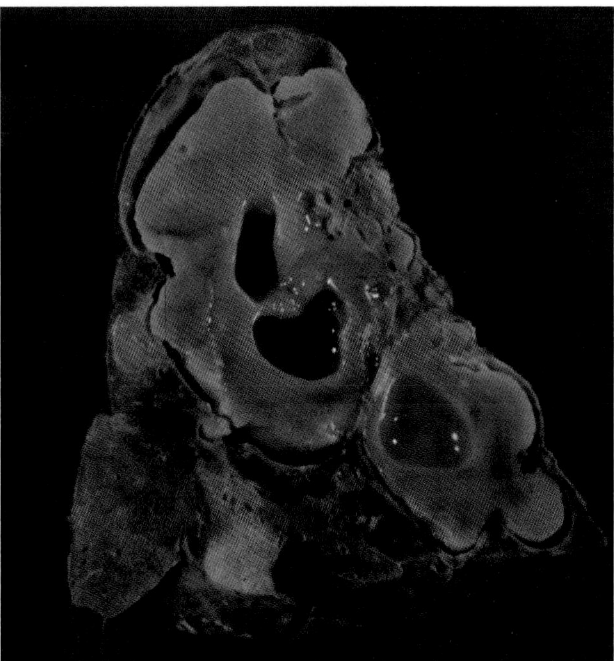

FIGURE 6-10 ■ Staphylococcal infections. **A**: Impetigo with bullous features. **B**: Staphylococcal scalded skin syndrome (toxic epidermal necrolysis) following MRSA infection. **C**: Partially "healed" or resolving staphylococcal lung abscess.

are red and edematous; in menstrual cases, erythema, edema, and ulceration involve the cervix, vagina, and perineum. Several autopsy studies reveal little in the way of specific findings; there is no evidence of bacterial invasion of tissues, and inflammatory reaction is negligible, supporting a toxin-mediated change. Reported findings include genitourinary tract ulceration, mild lymphoid depletion, a skin lesion remarkably similar to SSSS, and mild and nonspecific inflammation in kidney, liver, heart, and muscle (e186,e247).

STREPTOCOCCAL INFECTIONS

Pathogenic group A streptococci (GAS) are comprised of a number of serotypes based on the M protein, *S. pyogenes* being the most important. GAS produce disease by at least three mechanisms: (a) direct tissue invasion of skin and upper airways (impetigo, erysipelas, cellulitis, pharyngitis, tonsillitis, necrotizing fasciitis, necrotizing pneumonia), (b) toxin elaboration (scarlet fever), and (c) immune-mediated mechanisms (acute glomerulonephritis and rheumatic fever) (Figure 6-11). The prevalence of invasive GAS disease with resultant bacteremia and/or streptococcal toxic shock syndrome is on the rise (113) (e80,e224). Nonsuppurative immunologic complications can occur even in the neonate (e222). Maternal carriage is an important factor in neonatal GAS disease. Early onset disease is associated with concurrent maternal infection and manifests as respiratory distress, pneumonia, and toxic shock-like syndrome, while late onset disease is associated with soft tissue infections and meningitis.

The nonGAS are mainly encountered in the newborn. *S. pneumoniae* is a common cause of pneumonia, meningitis,

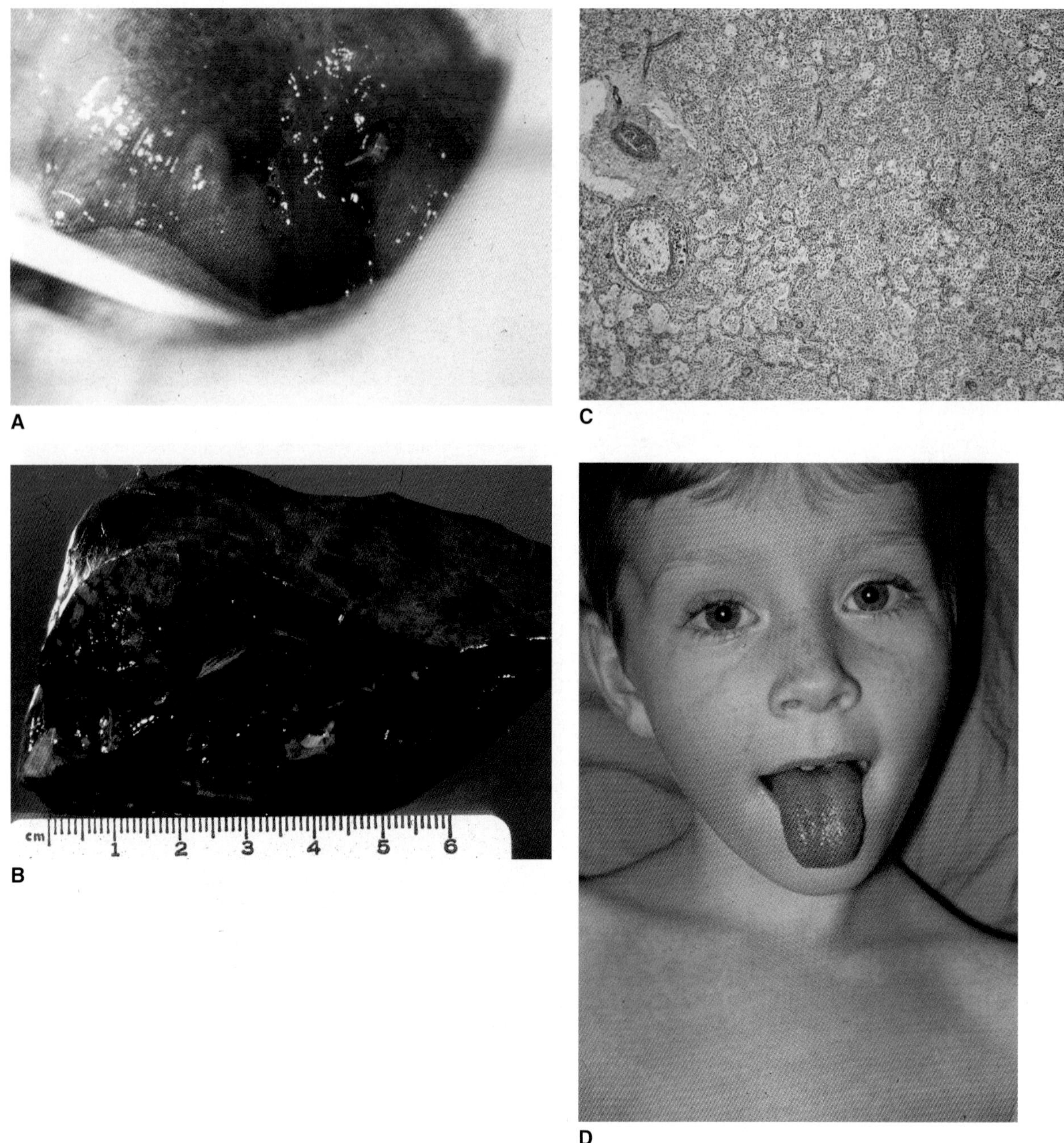

FIGURE 6-11 ■ Streptococcal infections. **A**: Streptococcal pharyngitis with erythematous, congested mucosa. **B**: Congenital streptococcal pneumonia with diffuse involvement. **C**: Diffuse alveolar exudates of neutrophils and fibrin in congenital streptococcal pneumonia. **D**: Scarlet fever with erythematous mucous membranes and tongue.

and otitis media (77). In asplenic patients, it is the single most common cause of sepsis, accounting for almost 50% of cases. *S. pneumoniae* has also been recognized as a cause of invasive soft tissue disease and a toxic shock-like syndrome in previously healthy children (e136). Group B streptococcus (GBS, e.g., *S. agalactiae*) is transmitted primarily *in utero* and during delivery, and is an important cause of early onset neonatal sepsis, meningitis, and pneumonia (182). Guidelines proposed by the American Academy of Pediatrics Committees on Infectious Diseases and the Fetus and Newborn use several variables to identify increased risk for GBS infection in the neonate and recommend intrapartum antimicrobial prophylaxis for infants at high risk (152). Other streptococcal infections, although much less common than GBS, are occasionally encountered; groups D and G have been reported to cause disease similar to GBS (49,84,170,171). Viridans group streptococci (VGS) are of particular concern in neutropenic children and can result in septic shock with median mortality of 10% (e301). VGS infection may be accompanied by neurological complications, myocarditis, and acute respiratory distress syndrome (e272). As is the case with other pathogens, their incidence and severity have increased during the past 15 years, and antibiotic resistance is commonplace. *S. viridans* infection may cause amniotic fluid infection in midgestation with resultant fetal-neonatal sepsis (e13).

ENTEROCOCCI

Enterococci are among the top four causes of nosocomial bacteremia in the United States (17) since they are bacteria that survive for brief periods on hands and inanimate surfaces. Risk factors for enterococcal bacteremia include prolonged hospital stay, exposure to antibiotics, central venous catheter use, and necrotizing enterocolitis (e217). They cause urinary tract infections, bloodstream infections (including neonatal sepsis and infections in older children), catheter-associated bacteremia, endocarditis, intra-abdominal infection, and meningitis. Enterococci are normal inhabitants of the human GIT and infection may ensue either from the patient's own indigenous flora or dissemination of acquired virulent clones. Virulence is dictated by genes that are clustered on the genome in distinct regions termed pathogenicity islands (PAIs), transfer and deletion of which are frequent. The management of patients with enterococcal infections is complex because it requires identifying the susceptibility of the isolate and the site of infection, both of which are key factors in providing optimal therapy. Glycopeptide-resistant/vancomycin-resistant enterococci (VRE) are increasing in prevalence and guidelines have been released for their control (150).

NEISSERIA INFECTIONS

N. gonorrhoeae can be transmitted *in utero*, intrapartum, or postpartum. Although gonococcal conjunctivitis is the most frequent clinical manifestation of neonatal infection (Figure 6-12), septicemia and arthritis can also develop (e6,e154). Gonococcal infections outside of the perinatal period are increasingly common and are associated with sexual abuse/sexual activity in children and adolescents; their clinical and pathologic features are similar to those in adults.

N. meningitidis is a major cause of childhood morbidity and mortality, causing meningococcal meningitis and meningococcemia. Fulminant meningococcemia ("purpura fulminans") is the form most likely to be encountered by the pathologist and is a catastrophic condition with hemorrhagic skin lesions that progress to gangrene (e56) (Figure 6-13). Lethargy or irritability, petechiae, and purpura are followed by circulatory collapse, shock, and death. The time from first symptom to death may be only a few hours. The combination of circulatory collapse, purpura, and bilateral adrenal cortical hemorrhage constitutes the Waterhouse-Friderichsen syndrome. The petechial skin lesions consist of extravasated red cells from small vessels in the absence of vasculitis; fibrin thrombi may be prominent, and the organism can be identified within endothelial cells or in smears from the lesions. Purpuric lesions show hemorrhagic infarction of skin and subcutis with vascular thrombi (e133). The pathogenesis of these lesions and the extreme variability of the clinical course are not well understood. The pathologic picture is reminiscent of generalized Schwartzman reaction and implicates an endotoxin-mediated process. Adrenal hemorrhage (Figure 6-13B and C), although striking, is unlikely to cause acute adrenal insufficiency and, by itself, does not cause death, given the great reserves of the adrenal. Acquired deficiencies of proteins C and S are probably more important players in fulminant meningococcemia (e259,e260). The propensity for severe disease in infants and very young children may be due to the fact that the protein C system is incompletely developed at this age. Early specific diagnosis is essential for optimal management and is based on CSF microscopy, culture, latex agglutination, and molecular (PCR-based) techniques. Latex agglutination allows serotyping while molecular methods are rapid and helpful in patients who have already received antibiotics. Traditional clinical prognostic signs include duration of petechiae, hypotension, presence of meningitis, leucopenia, and lack of elevation of erythrocyte sedimentation rate (e316). Mortality can be predicted by the pediatric risk of mortality (PRISM) score (e257,370). One must remember that the clinical syndrome of purpura fulminans may also be caused by infections with other bacteria (e.g., *E. coli, S. pneumoniae, P. mirabilis*) and viruses (varicella, rubella) (e56).

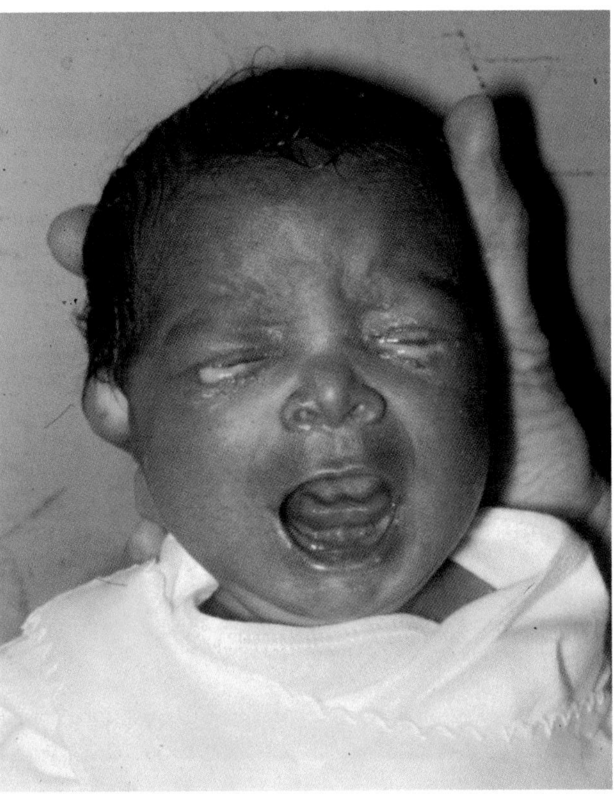

FIGURE 6-12 ■ Severe purulent gonococcal conjunctivitis is present in this infant.

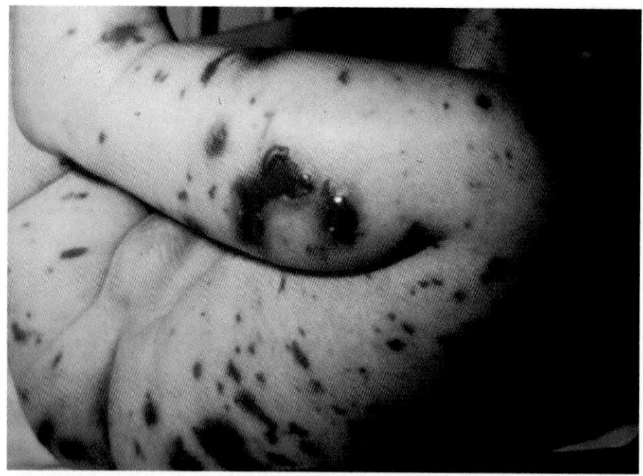
A

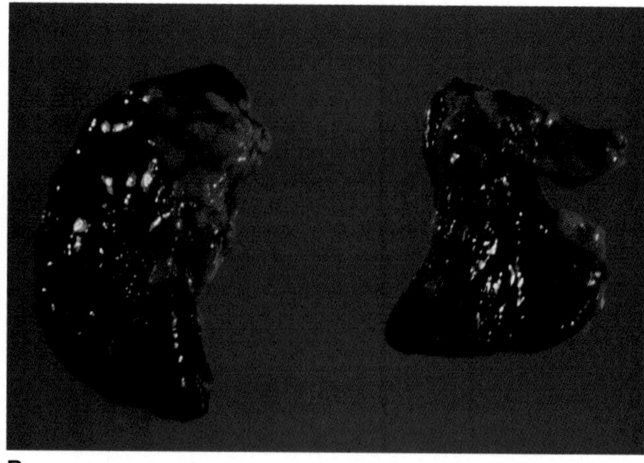
B

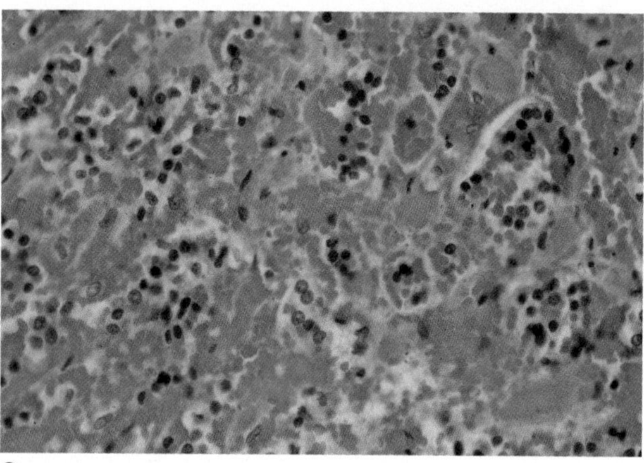
C

FIGURE 6-13 ■ Fulminant meningococcemia. **A:** Numerous petechial and ecchymotic foci with features of purpura fulminans of a consumptive coagulopathy. **B:** Bilateral adrenal hemorrhages of the Waterhouse-Friderichsen syndrome. **C:** The adrenal shows the presence of hemorrhagic necrosis.

ENTEROBACTERIACEAE

Except in the neonate, the enteric bacilli are either GI pathogens (see Chapter 14) or systemic opportunists in the compromised host (e102,e103,e104). As systemic opportunists they cause pneumonia, septicemia, and localized suppurative reactions depending on the nature of the underlying disease (Figure 6-14). Although the cellular reaction, when present, is entirely nonspecific, it must be emphasized that in the profoundly leukocytopenic host, the inflammatory reaction may consist solely of edema, vascular engorgement, hemorrhage, and fibrin deposition without much, if any, cellular

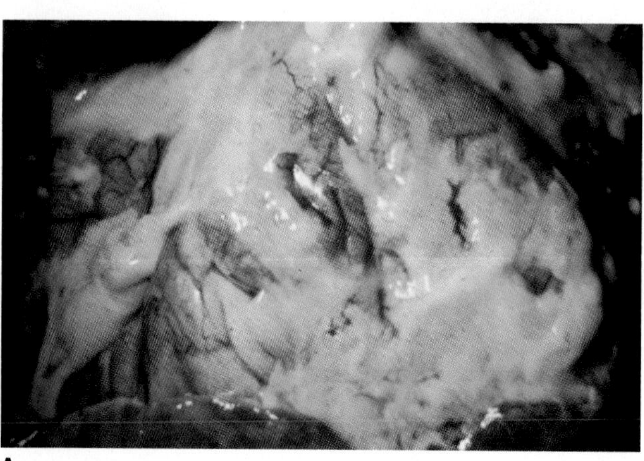
A

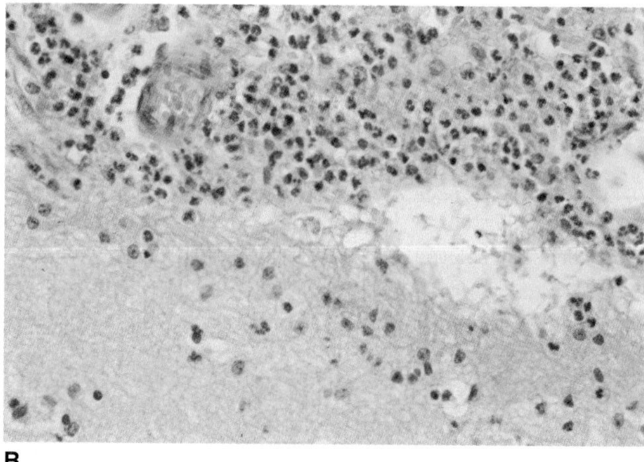
B

FIGURE 6-14 ■ **A:** Acute E.coli meningitis with purulent exudate covering convexities. **B:** Neutrophils filling the subarachoid space.

reaction. Enteric, usually food-borne, infections with verotoxin-producing strains of *E. coli* (O517: H7) are responsible for hemolytic uremic syndrome, which is discussed in Chapter 17.

SALMONELLA INFECTION (TYPHOID)

These Gram negative bacilli can cause localized infection (e.g., gastroenteritis by *S. typhimurium*) or systemic infection (e.g., typhoid by *S. typhi*). Typhoid and paratyphoid are relatively common infections in developing countries. Transmission is feco-oral and is the result of poor sanitation and fecal contamination of water and dairy products which is also seen in the United States. In the untreated patient, after an incubation period of 5 to 30 days, a febrile phase develops with stepwise daily elevations in temperature that may be associated with rose spots on the trunk, bradycardia, and leucopenia. Fever can be high grade and continuous, lasting up to 3 weeks, followed by a stage of decline and convalescence. In the present antibiotic era, patients may present with fever, diarrhea, abdominal pain, and hepatosplenomegaly (e204,e221). Specific symptoms and signs may be inapparent in children (e55,e125,e336). The bacteria gain access to the bowel wall and disseminate via lymphatics to lymph nodes, spleen, and liver. Salmonella proliferate in bile and amplify by a bacterial enterohepatic circulation. Intestinal typhoid ulcers are a result of necrosis of hyperplastic Peyer patches and are therefore arrayed in the long axis of the small bowel. Histology reveals numerous macrophages (so-called "typhoid cells" or "Mallory cells") forming "soft granulomas" with erythro- and lymphophagocytosis, plasma cells, and activated lymphocytes. Macrophage aggregates (so-called typhoid nodules) may be seen in the spleen, liver, bone marrow, kidneys, salivary glands, and testes. A fibrinous exudate may be seen on the splenic capsule that later becomes organized to produce the "sugar-coated" ("zuckergleiss") spleen. Laboratory diagnosis is by culture (from blood or bone marrow in the first week and stool by the third week) or by serology (Widal test) (e144) and more specific assays (e54,e161). Complications are numerous and include ileus, acute renal failure, cardiac arrhythmia (with sudden death), massive intestinal hemorrhage (following Peyer patch necrosis), pancreatic dysfunction, intestinal perforation, peritonitis, Zenker degeneration of abdominal skeletal muscles, liver necrosis, splenic rupture, and DIC (31) (e28,e73,e168,e174,e243). Atypical manifestations include pneumonitis, pericarditis, osteomyelitis (especially in sickle cell anemia patients), dactylitis, pericarditis, arthritis, meningitis, cerebellar ataxia, myelonecrosis, and a generalized hemophagocytic syndrome (78) (e192). A carrier stage may develop and carriers excrete the bacteria in their bile (stool) and urine, posing a health hazard to society, as exemplified by the infamous Typhoid Mary.

HEMOPHILUS INFLUENZA

This small Gram negative coccobacillus is a commensal of the upper respiratory tract and a major cause of morbidity and mortality in infants and young children. Colonization by capsular *H. influenza* type B is uncommon in a healthy

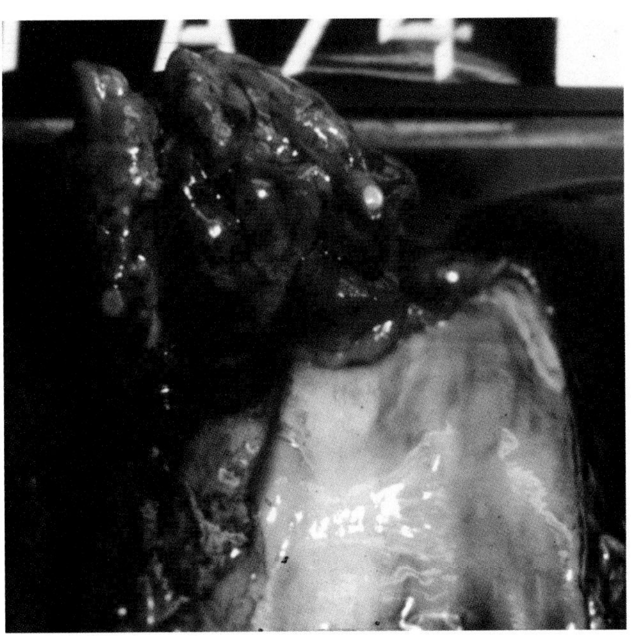

A

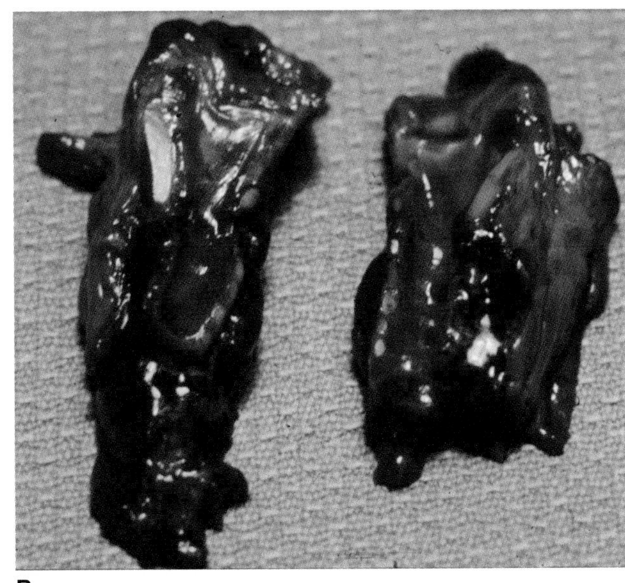

B

FIGURE 6-15■Hemophilus influenzae epiglottitis. **A**: Marked induration and enlargement of the epiglottis are features in this autopsy case. **B**: Involvement of the entire epiglottis and larynx by *H. influenzae*. results in these gross findings.

individual, but can cause severe disease in patients with respiratory compromise or immunodeficiency. Transmission is through direct contact and by respiratory droplets; there is no evidence for its transmission through breast milk. In fact, breast milk seems to limit colonization of *H. influenzae* in the infant's throat (e146). Most invasive disease outside the neonatal age group results from infection by encapsulated type B organisms. Infections range from mild (e.g., conjunctivitis and otitis media) to life threatening (epiglottitis, meningitis, pericarditis, pneumonia, septic arthritis, and facial cellulitis) (e71). Until recently, *H. influenzae* was the major cause of meningitis in infants accounting for 80% of cases under the age of 2 years and for at least one-third of bacterial pneumonia in this age group. This has, however, decreased significantly in countries where the use of the *H. influenzae* conjugate vaccines is the norm (12). In the upper airway, *H. influenzae* causes life-threatening acute epiglottitis (Figure 6-15). The larynx and especially the epiglottis are the site of marked congestion, edema, and leukocytic infiltration, which may completely occlude the small infant airway. The cherry red appearance is helpful in distinguishing this condition from severe viral laryngotracheitis (croup), which is occasionally severe enough to cause airway obstruction in this age group. Nontypeable strains commonly cause lower respiratory infections. In children, they are also the most common cause of bacterial conjunctivitis and the second most common cause (after *S. pneumoniae*) of otitis media (e121). *H. influenzae* also causes acute chorioamnionitis. Histopathologic features of *H. influenzae* infection are those of any other bacterial infection and are not distinctive.

DIPHTHERIA

Diphtheria is caused by a toxin produced by *Corynebacterium diphtheriae* carrying a particular lysogenic bacteriophage; all of the gross and microscopic features of the disease can be produced by purified toxin (e246). The toxin can affect all cells of the body, but is most potent on nerves, kidneys, and heart, and halts addition of amino acids to elongating polypeptide chains. Humans are the only identified reservoirs and symptom-free carriers. The major sources of infection are patients in the incubation stage of disease and fomites. The initial reaction appears to be toxin-induced necrosis of upper airway epithelium with abundant fibrin exudation, leading to the typical fibrinous pseudomembrane overlying mildly inflamed submucosa, accompanied by tremendous edema of the soft tissues of the neck. Death is related to airway obstruction, to toxin-mediated cardiomyopathy/myocarditis, and to diphtheritic peripheral and cranial neuropathy (e143).

Despite large scale and, on the whole, successful immunization, rare cases of diphtheria continue to occur in nonimmunized children and in young adults with nonprotective levels of antitoxin (e171). A massive epidemic in the independent states of the former USSR during the 1990s is a reminder of the breakdown of public health infrastructure in periods of socioeconomic and political upheaval (e352).

INFECTIONS BY OTHER GRAM-NEGATIVE BACILLI

Pseudomonas aeruginosa is ubiquitous in soil and water, and is seen almost exclusively as an opportunistic pathogen. Infection is frequently associated with cystic fibrosis. It also causes gangrenous lesions in the skin (pyoderma gangrenosum) and GIT of patients with malignancy. Pseudomonas sepsis is primarily a nosocomial infection that is seen as a late onset disease in very low birth weight infants and carries a 50% mortality rate (e189). Occasional cases may be associated with chorioamnionitis (e237). Pseudomonas sepsis is characterized by necrotizing vasculitis (e329), involving both arteries and veins; the vessel wall is replaced by collections of organisms, often with very little cellular infiltrate, and hemorrhagic infarction of the affected site. Particularly affected are the skin and mucous membranes (especially of the intestinal tract), manifesting as deep red or violaceous raised plaques, which rapidly undergo necrosis. Patients may also have a hemorrhagic necrotizing bronchopneumonia (Figure 6-16).

Serratia marcescens is an infrequent pathogen in the newborn and is usually nosocomially acquired through foreign bodies and instrumentation. Serratia sepsis is late-onset disease with severe meningitis and a high mortality rate (e230).

Citrobacter species (enteric Gram-negative bacilli) are an increasingly recognized cause of neonatal sepsis, meningitis, hemorrhagic encephalitis, and brain abscess. The majority of cases present in the first 10 days of life (e124). Most cases are apparently nosocomial following surgical manipulation of umbilical cord stumps (e250), although the existence of early onset sepsis suggests that vertical transmission may also occur (e339).

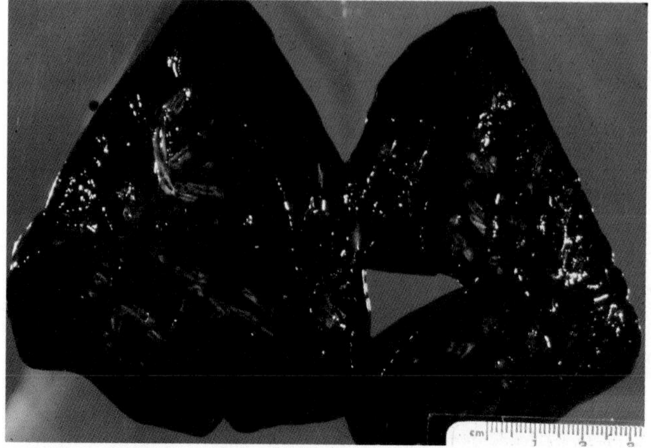

FIGURE 6-16 Necrotizing hemorrhagic pneumonia caused by *Pseudomonas aeruginosa.*

LISTERIOSIS

Listeria monocytogenes is a small, gram-positive bacillus that acts as a facultative intracellular parasite. The organism is a common intestinal and vaginal commensal. Human listeriosis presents as one of three clinical forms including febrile gastroenteritis, maternal-fetal/neonatal listeriosis, or bacteremia with or without CNS involvement. Infections are uncommon with the estimated incidence of listeriosis during pregnancy being 12 cases per 10^5 (124). Listeriosis during pregnancy is associated with second-trimester abortion (e184) and infrequently causes premature delivery or stillbirth. Up to two-thirds of surviving neonates born to infected mothers develop overt neonatal infection due to either transplacental or intrapartum transmission (124). Perinatal infection is an uncommon cause of severe disease in the neonate.

Neonatal listeriosis is classified as either early (occurring in the first 5 to 7 days following delivery) or late infection (123) (e187). Early-onset infection is due to types Ia, Ib, and IVb, while type IVb predominates in late-onset infection. Early disease is associated with maternal infection, is often overt at the time of delivery, and is associated with meconium staining of the amniotic fluid. Clinical presentation resembles neonatal sepsis with pneumonia, bacteremia, and/or meningitis (124) (e216). In some neonates, the infection manifests as "granulomatosis infantiseptica" with a salmon pink rash (papules surrounded by red margins) and mucosal nodules; there are widespread microabscesses and granulomata especially in the liver, spleen, and lungs (Figure 6-17). In contrast, late onset infection usually occurs in full term neonates delivered from uncomplicated pregnancies and presents as meningitis between the second and eighth week of life. The infection is presumed to be acquired from the maternal vaginal tract, at the time of delivery. Listerial meningoencephalitis cannot be distinguished from other systemic bacterial or viral infections. In Vawter's series, the organs most frequently involved were the adrenals, liver, GIT, skin, and tracheobronchial tree (e350). Mortality of untreated early-onset infection is 100%; survivors have CNS sequelae including hydrocephalus and mental retardation. Factors determining *L. monocytogenes* virulence have been recently reviewed (48).

Systemic infection is marked by bacterial replication in mononuclear cells in the liver, spleen, and bone marrow (e74,e84,e163). Parasitized monocytes play an important role in CNS invasion (46). The histopathologic features depend largely on the duration of the disease. Inflammatory foci may consist solely of necrosis with little cellular reaction (although fibrin thrombi and hemorrhage may be prominent) or miliary abscesses may be seen, particularly in liver and adrenal glands. Gram, Warthin-Starry, and immunohistochemical stains help identify organisms in tissues (e248). In patients who mount a specific immune response, the lesions, after several days, assume a granulomatous appearance as mononuclear cells replace polymorphonuclear leukocytes in the abscesses. Placental infection is common and manifests as intervillous and intravillous microabscesses with necrotizing villitis and chorioamnionitis, irrespective of route (transplacental or ascending) of infection (e23,e233). A definitive diagnosis of listeriosis is made by culturing *L. monocytogenes*. Blood and CSF are the most useful specimens; serologic assays are not useful. (see Chapter 9).

SYPHILIS

Treponemes are microaerophilic spiral gram-negative bacteria that are 6 to 20 μm long and 0.1 to 0.5 μm in diameter. Although this thickness is less than the resolution limits of conventional light microscopy, the microbe can be visualized by dark-field or phase-contrast microscopy. *T. pal-*

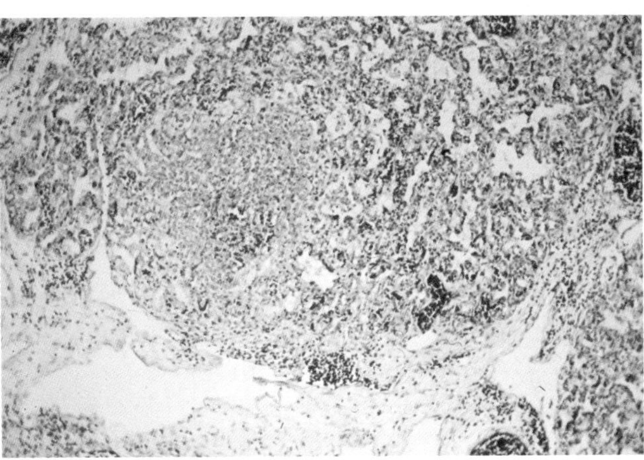

A

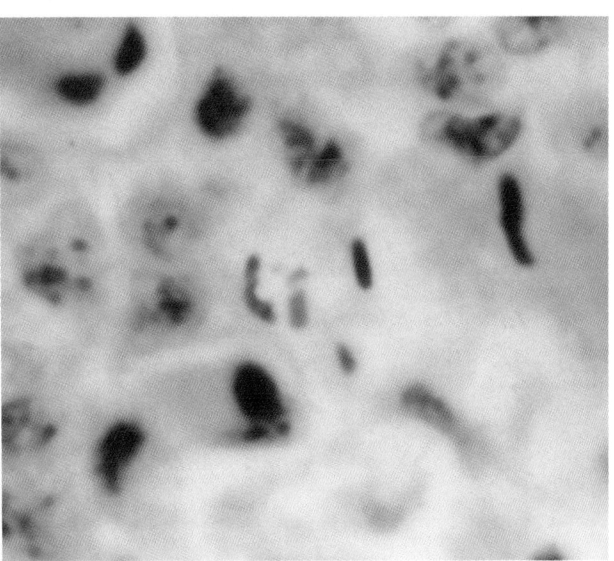

B

FIGURE 6-17 ■ Listeriosis. **A**: Lung abscess is seen in this infant with numerous such lesions with minimal inflammation. **B**: Brown-Hopps stain displays the rod-shaped bacteria.

lidum causes multisystem disease in stages similar to Lyme disease. Humans are the sole natural host of syphilis. The WHO estimates that maternal syphilis leads to 460,000 abortions/stillbirths and 270,000 live-born infants with congenital syphilis yearly (e106). The frequency of congenital syphilis in a specific locale is determined ultimately by both the prevalence of syphilis among adults and the effectiveness of prenatal screening and treatment programs. HIV-infected pregnant women are at high risk for having active syphilis. Pediatric syphilis has been the subject of many recent reviews (79,196).

Transmission

Transmission is through direct sexual contact and contact with open lesions or secretions from the lesions in the skin and mucous membranes. Congenital syphilis occurs in the fetus through placentitis, while perinatal infection occurs in the neonate through contact with the spirochete during passage through the birth canal. *T. pallidum* can cross the placenta and infect the developing fetus throughout pregnancy, from as early as 9 to 10 weeks of gestation. Vertical transmission during pregnancy occurs more frequently in primary or secondary syphilis than with latent maternal disease. Fetal infection is most efficient during the early stages of maternal infection when the transmission rate approaches 100%. The risk of transmission diminishes after 4 years of infection, even when the mother is untreated. Postnatal infection can occur in the infant through contact with open lesions or secretions in the infected mother or another adult. If syphilitic lesions involve the breast or nipples, then breastfeeding or using expressed breast milk should be avoided until the mother has completed treatment and the lesions have healed. There is no evidence for transmission of *T. pallidum* in breast milk without a breast or nipple lesion.

Clinical Features

Fetal infection can result in spontaneous abortion, stillbirth, early congenital syphilis, and late congenital syphilis (Figure 6-18). Congenital syphilis does not have a primary stage and may result in perinatal death in more than 40% of affected, untreated pregnancies. Among survivors, manifestations traditionally have been divided into early and late-onset types with early manifestations appearing in the first 2 years of life. With early-onset disease, manifestations result from transplacental spirochetemia and are analogous to the secondary stage of acquired syphilis. Late-onset disease is seen in children older than 2 years and is not considered contagious.

Although many features are nonspecific, certain lesions, when present, are pathognomonic, and the disease is recognizable even in severely macerated stillborns, who represent one-third to one-half of congenital syphilis cases (e167,e242,e372). Infection occurring prior to the fifth month

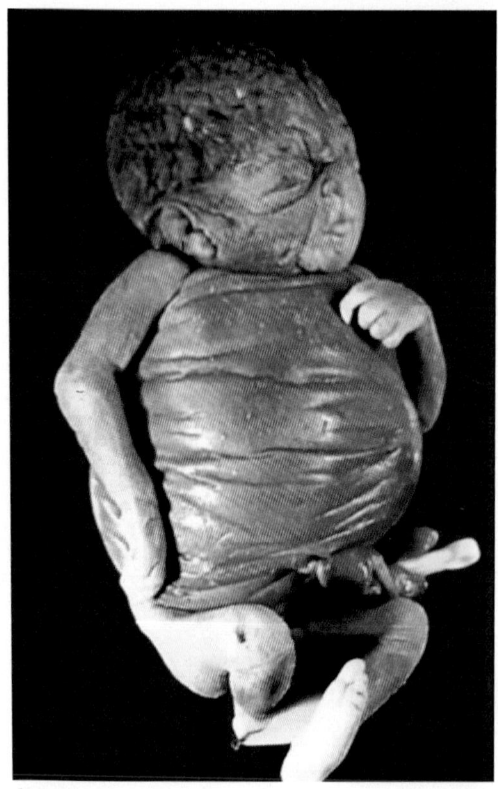
A

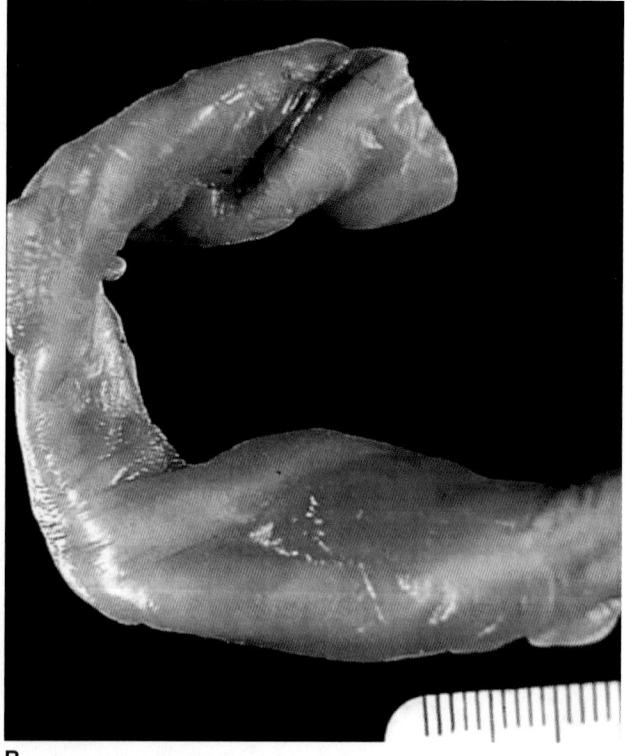
B

FIGURE 6-18 ■ Congenital syphilis with its various features. **A**: Congenital syphilis with hydrops fetalis. **B**: Congenital syphilis with "barber pole" funisitis.

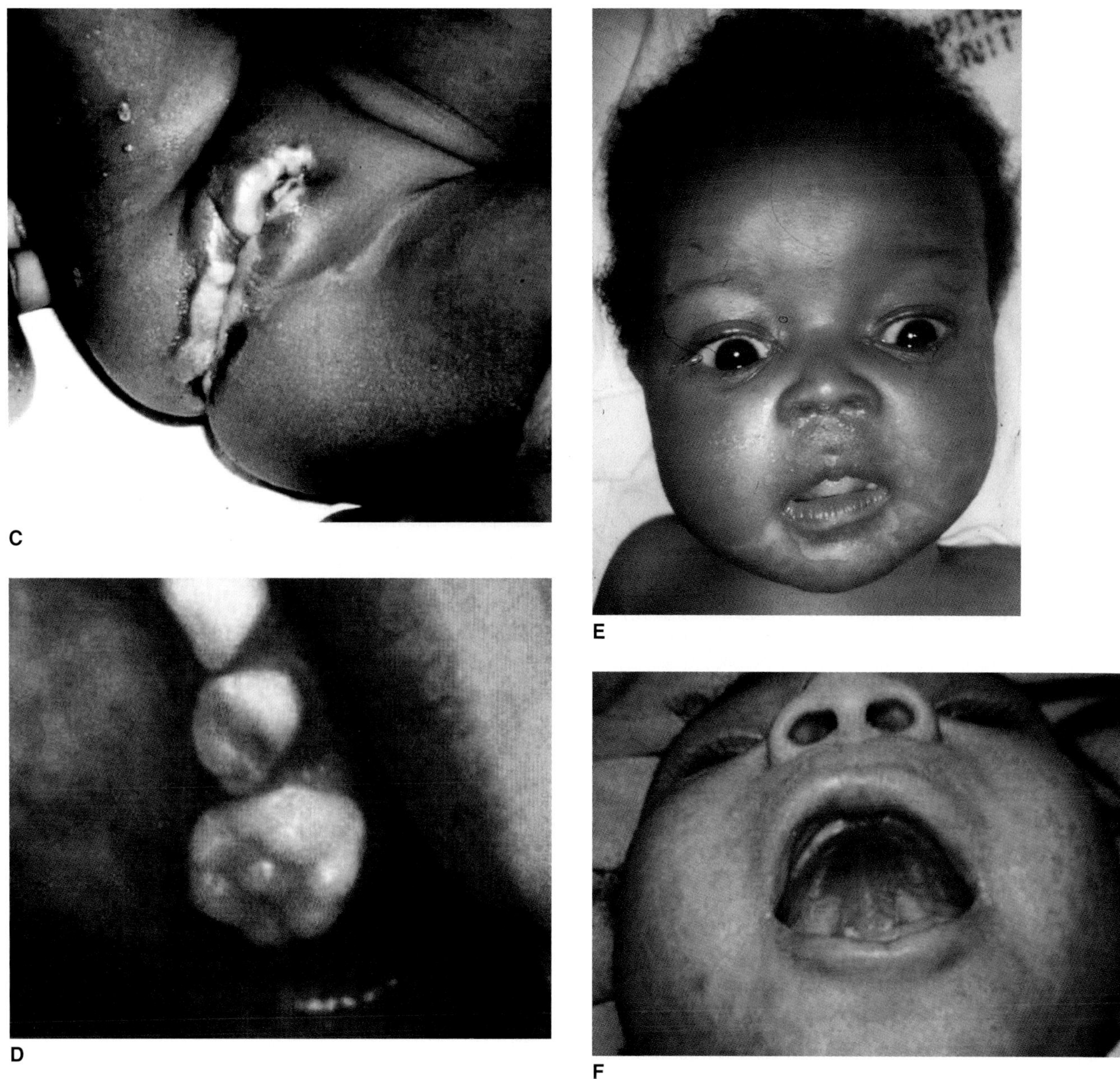

FIGURE 6-18▪ *(continued)* **C**: Labial lesions in neonatal syphilis forming condylomata lata. **D**: Bifid molar as a malformative manifestation in tooth development. **E**: Snuffles as a nasal discharge secondary to obstructive nasopharyngitis. The mucopurulent discharge contains viable organisms. **F**: Mucous patches representing an ulcerative mucositis.

of intrauterine life does not cause destructive changes and organogenesis is unaffected, although spirochetes are readily demonstrable in all fetal tissues. In the macerated second and third trimester stillborn infant, hepatomegaly, and/or hydrops may be the only gross evidence of disease (Figure 6-18A). Organisms are, however, abundant in all organs, including placenta, even when the internal organs have undergone extensive autolysis. Congenital syphilis can clinically mimic a number of neonatal conditions including other congenital infections (CMV, HSV, rubella, and toxoplasma), bacterial sepsis and blood group incompatibility, to name a few. A negative Coombs test in the setting of hydrops is suggestive of congenital syphilis (e36), although parvovirus infection should also be considered. In early-onset congenital syphilis, most affected infants are asymptomatic at birth and are identified only by routine prenatal screening. If untreated, symptoms develop within weeks or months. The typical stillborn or highly symptomatic newborn is born prematurely with an enlarged liver and spleen, skeletal involvement, and often pneumonia and bullous skin lesions. In others, the earliest signs of congenital syphilis may be poor feeding and snuffles (syphilitic rhinitis; Figure 6-18E). Early manifestations of congenital infection are varied and involve multiple organ systems. Hepatomegaly is reported in almost 100% of cases, and biochemical evidence of liver dysfunction is usually observed. The most striking lesions affect the mucocutaneous tissues and bones. Mucous patches, rhinitis, and condylomatous lesions are highly characteristic features of mucous membrane involvement in congenital syphilis (Figure 6-18F). Nasal fluid is highly infectious. Snuffles are followed quickly by a diffuse maculopapular desquamative rash that involves extensive sloughing of the epithelium, particularly on the palms and soles and about the mouth and anus. In contrast to acquired syphilis, a vesicular rash and bullae may develop in these areas that may weep and desquamate. These lesions teem with spirochetes and are highly infectious. Bone involvement in the form of multiple symmetric periostitis and joint osteochondritis occur in 60% to 80% of untreated early congenital cases. Bone involvement can be very painful, causing the infant to refuse to move the involved extremity (pseudoparalysis of Parrot). Tibial metaphyseal demineralization is seen radiologically (Wimberger sign). Bone involvement usually resolves spontaneously within 6 months. Neurosyphilis may be present even with normal CSF findings. Alternatively, it may present as acute meningitis (in the first 6 months) or a chronic meningovascular neurosyphilis (at the end of the first year of life) with progressive hydrocephalus, cranial nerve palsies, seizures, and neurodevelopmental regression. Cerebral infarction from syphilitic endarteritis may occur in the second year of life. Anemia, thrombocytopenia, leukopenia, and leukocytosis are common findings. The late manifestations of congenital syphilis are a consequence of scarring from the early systemic disease and involve teeth (Figure 6-18D), bones, eyes, the eighth cranial nerve, and CNS.

In older children and adolescents, syphilis is sexually transmitted and may be the result of sexual abuse. Manifestations and diagnosis are similar to that in adults. Neurosyphilis occurs in approximately 30% of patients with secondary syphilis; CSF pleocytosis and proteinosis are typical findings. Neurosyphilis may be clinically silent or present with meningeal, cranial nerve, or spinal nerve involvement. In addition to mucocutaneous involvement, secondary syphilis can also manifest with iritis, anterior uveitis, arthritis, and nephrotic syndrome, probably caused by deposition of immune complexes composed of treponemal antigens, fibronectin, antibodies, and complement. Secondary syphilis lesions resolve without treatment in 1 to 2 months. The infection then enters a latent period, without overt evidence of disease. The signs of secondary syphilis can recur during the first year (early latency) but not thereafter (late latency). Relative immunity to reinfection exists during latency, and approximately 60% of untreated patients will not progress from latency to tertiary syphilis, the remaining progressing after latent periods of 3 to 10 years. This time frame renders acquired tertiary syphilis a very rare occurrence during childhood and adolescence.

Pathology

In his seminal article Silverstein (e307) suggested that histopathologic changes of syphilis await the development of fetal immune competence. Humoral immunity is insufficient to control the infection. Cell-mediated immunity is suppressed during the primary and secondary stages of infection. Ultimate eradication of infection occurs when T-cells infiltrate syphilitic lesions. *T. pallidum* may escape immune surveillance by antigenic variation. Further, although a Th1 immune response is elicited in primary syphilis, progression to the secondary stage is accompanied by a shift to a Th2 response, allowing for incomplete clearance of the pathogen. In pregnancy, intense inflammatory responses and prostaglandins induced by fetal infection may be responsible for the various manifestations of congenital syphilis (139).

The main pathologic changes are seen in pancreas, liver, GIT, bones and nasal mucosa, and manifest as inflammation, scarring and developmental retardation (e241). The liver shows diffuse inflammation and fibrosis separating the liver into coarse nodules (hepar lobatum). Osteochondritis and periostitis of joints, long bones, palate, and nasal cartilage lead to skeletal deformities. Lung involvement leads to pale airless, heavy and fibrotic lungs (pneumonia alba). The viscera in general appear inappropriately immature for gestational age; there is prominent extramedullary hematopoiesis, persistence of fetal adrenal cortex, active glomerulogenesis, and persistence of fetal stroma in many organs, notably the pancreas and the pulmonary interstitium. The inflammatory response is mainly mononuclear and may be difficult to distinguish from extramedullary hematopoiesis. Polymorphonuclear leukocytes occur in response to tissue necrosis, producing the typical Dubois abscess. Gummata are rare in newborns. Oppenheimer and Dahms provide a complete description of the pathologic changes of congenital syphilis and describe a pathognomonic triad comprised of interstitial inflammation or fibrosis of the pancreas with pressure atrophy of the parenchyma, pneumonia alba (sharply defined fibrosing pneumonitis), and thickening of the bowel wall by submucosal infiltrates and fibrosis (e241). An obliterative endarteritis, consisting of concentric endothelial and fibroblastic proliferative thickening with plasma cell infiltration, should suggest syphilis. This endarteritis is also found in all stages of acquired syphilis (in the primary chancre, polymorphonuclear leukocytes, and macrophages often can be seen ingesting treponemes).

Placental examination is mandatory in suspected cases to allow for an early diagnosis. Grossly, the placenta is large and heavy. Syphilitic placentitis is histologically characterized by histiocytic-predominant villitis, proliferative endovasculitis of the stem villi (perivasculitis with concentric mural vascular sclerosis) and necrotizing umbilical periphlebitis. The umbilical periphlebitis is pathognomonic and comprises of abscess-like necrotic foci in the Wharton jelly, with eosinophilic precipitates around the umbilical vein. Other histopathologic findings may include villous dysmaturity, hypercellular villi with variable acute and chronic inflammation, numerous Hofbauer cells, endarteritis, perivascular fibrosis, numerous nucleated red cells in fetal vasculature, proliferative fetal vascular changes, chorioamnionitis, necrotizing funisitis, and/or plasma cell deciduitis. Spirochetes may be difficult to demonstrate in the placenta and their absence does not exclude the diagnosis. Spirochetes are easier to demonstrate in the umbilical cord, even if the cord does not show evidence of funisitis (168) (e294). (see Chapter 9).

Acquired syphilis is almost always by sexual contact. *T. pallidum* penetrates the skin or mucous membrane at a site of exposure, multiplies locally and spreads through the perivascular lymphatic system to the systemic circulation, which disseminates infection widely before the primary lesion(s) becomes evident. During the usual 3-week incubation period (range 10 to 90 days), an intense local inflammatory response develops, consisting of plasma cells, macrophages, and lymphocytes. This produces the red, indurated, ulcerative, spirochete-filled chancre. The host response likely is initiated by chemotactic effects of treponemal lipopeptide antigens (e296), but it seems to require proliferation of relatively large numbers of treponemes. Associated cellular proliferation in regional lymph nodes produces adenopathy. If the immune response is unable to fully eradicate the infection, replication at the site of early infection leads to dissemination and development of the lesions of secondary syphilis, over the course of 2 to 10 weeks. These lesions occur most commonly in ectodermal tissues (skin, mucous membranes) and the CNS. The tissue response is similar to that of primary lesions. Condylomata lata (venereal warts) are characterized by epithelial hyperplasia, hyperkeratosis, and plasma cell infiltrates. Even if untreated, the clinical manifestations of secondary syphilis resolve, and the disease process enters a period of relative immunologic control; viable organisms remain but in low numbers. Tertiary syphilis can involve any organ system and typically manifest as gummata, which are focal areas of nonsuppurative inflammatory necrosis surrounded by fibrotic scarring. These represent a granulomatous hypersensitivity reaction and viable organisms are rare or absent. Tertiary lesions also can take the form of a diffuse, chronic, noncaseating infiltrate of plasma cells and lymphocytes.

Laboratory Diagnosis

Definitive diagnosis requires demonstration of the spirochete; *T. pallidum* is a long (15-µm) slender organism that is optimally identified by darkfield examination, although, if fresh preparations are not available, the Levaditi, Steiner, and Warthin-Starry stains are helpful. An immunohistochemical procedure has been described, and PCR diagnosis has been useful in selected cases (e235). In the appropriate clinical setting, a diagnosis may also be made if serum quantitative antibody titer is at least four times greater than the maternal titer. CSF VDRL (Venereal Disease Research Laboratory) test is reactive and/or the IgM FTA-ABS is positive.

Prognosis and Outcome

If the newborn survives, progressive inflammation and fibrosis lead to the stigmata of late congenital syphilis: gummatous facial deformities (perforated palate and saddle nose), skeletal defects [frontal bossing, short maxillae, mandibular protruberance, high palatal arch, scaphoid scapulae, saber shins, Clutton joints, sternoclavicular thickening (Higoumenakis sign)], dental abnormalities (Hutchinson incisors, mulberry molars), rhagades, meningovasculitis leading to eighth nerve damage and optic atrophy, interstitial keratitis, and neurosyphilis (e109).

LEPTOSPIROSIS

Leptospirosis is a zoonotic disease caused by a single nontreponemal spirochete species (*Leptospira interrogans*) with several subgroups. The disease occurs in epidemic forms in tropical countries of especially South and Southeast Asia, with seasonal trends, and has recently been classified as an emerging global disease. Although primarily a zoonosis, humans are infected by exposure to water or soil contaminated with animal urine, or by the bite of a rat flea. Transplacental infection has been documented, as has fetal death due to maternal leptospirosis (e57,e61). Although the majority of leptospiral infections are either subclinical or result in very mild illness, a proportion of patients develop various complications due to multiorgan system involvement, with CFRs of over 40% (187). After an incubation period of 2 to 30 days, a flu-like septicemic phase ensues, followed by an immune phase (with involvement of kidneys, liver, meninges, eyes, skin, pancreas, heart spleen, and lymph nodes). Clinical presentation depends upon the predominant organs involved. Because of its protean manifestations, leptospirosis it is often misdiagnosed and under-reported. The more severe form (Weil disease) is characterized by jaundice, coagulopathy, and hematuria (hence the term "icterohemorrhagica"). When fatal, death is usually due to renal failure (22), although pulmonary involvement has recently emerged as a serious life threat (43). Identification methods include direct (darkfield) microscopy, culture, and the most widely used reference standard method—the microscopic agglutination test (3). In the first week, blood and CSF cultures are positive, while in the immune phase, leptospires may be recoverable only from the urine. Pathology reflects organ dysfunction and features of coagulopathy. Mortality is high in fulminant cases. Antibiotic therapy may cause a Jarisch-Herxheimer type reaction with clinical worsening.

LYME DISEASE

Lyme disease is the most common tickborne infection in both North America and Europe. In the United States, Lyme disease is caused by the spirochete *Borrelia burgdorferi*, transmitted by the bite of the deer tick species *Ixodes scapularis* and *I. pacificus*.

Transmission

Transplacental spread to the fetus is reported (e344); first-trimester infection may be followed by premature delivery with demonstrable spirochetes in many viscera and severe congenital cardiovascular abnormalities, including hypoplasia of the aorta and endocardial fibroelastosis (e291,e362). However, whether or not *B. burgdorferi* directly causes illness in the fetus or congenital abnormalities is debated (e322,e369). Prenatal transmission is uncommon, even in endemic areas (e305). The case against congenital infection is strong. No inflammation is seen in the placentas or tissues from children where spirochetes have been identified (e291,e201,e362). Further, longitudinal population studies and serosurveys have not shown any consistent evidence of adverse fetal effects of Lyme disease during pregnancy (178) (e210,e229,e368), and even when the placenta is infected (e359). Although *B. burgdorferi* DNA has been found in breast milk (e292), there is no evidence for transmission of illness through breast milk (167).

Clinical Features

Lyme disease is characterized by multiorgan system involvement (skin, heart, joints, and nervous system) and can occur in three stages (early localized, early disseminated, and late disease). Following the tick bite, the acute phase is characterized by the erythema migrans rash with or without systemic manifestations such as fever, headache, photophobia, myalgias, generalized lymphadenopathy and severe fatigue, without localizing signs. Erythema migrans is a round or oval, expanding erythematous skin lesion that develops at the site of deposition of *B. burgdorferi*, that typically become apparent approximately 7 to 14 days after the tick has detached and should be at least 5 cm in largest diameter for a secure diagnosis. The lesion may vary from erythematous to targetoid to vesicular, and are usually nonscaly and nonpruritic. Secondary skin lesions may arise by hematogenous dissemination from the site of primary infection. A tick bite hypersensitivity reaction is favored over erythema migrans if the erythematous skin lesion appears while an *Ixodes* tick is still attached to the skin, develops within 48 hours of detachment, is urticarial, is less than 5 cm and reduces in size over the 24 to 48 hours following its appearance. In addition, early Lyme disease manifestations include neurologic [triad of cranial neuropathy, especially Bell's palsy (e299), meningoradiculitis and encephalitis (e244), carditis (heart block or myopericarditis), and Borrelial lymphocytoma]. Late manifestations include recurrent large joint (typically knee) arthritis (e313), late neurologic Lyme disease (encephalopathy, encephalomyelitis, and peripheral neuropathy), and acrodermatitis chronica atrophicans (197). Acrodermatitis chronica atrophicans starts as a doughy bluish-red swelling on the extensor surfaces of the hands and feet and resolves over months to years with atrophy ("cigarette paper skin"). Most clinical features are immune mediated and are due to elaboration of various cytokines. There is no well-accepted definition of post-Lyme disease syndrome. Erythema migrans is the only manifestation of Lyme disease in the United States that is sufficiently distinctive to allow clinical diagnosis in the absence of laboratory confirmation; nearly 90% of children with Lyme disease have erythema migrans (167). In a community-based prospective study of 201 children with Lyme disease, the average age was 7 years and the initial manifestation was single erythema migrans (66%), multiple erythema migrans (23%), arthritis (7%), facial palsy (3%), aseptic meningitis (1%), and carditis (0.5%) (167).

Pathology

Histopathologically there is a perivascular and interstitial infiltration of lymphocytes, plasma cells, and histiocytes in involved organs. Borrelia may be demonstrated in the acute lesions of erythema migrans in hemorrhagic foci. Inflammatory changes are minimal to absent in neonates and, for that reason, spirochetes may be more numerous (e200). Placental changes range from none to a chorionic villitis with histiocytes, plasma cells, and increased Hofbauer cells, with intervillous and intravillous spirochetes. Borrelial lymphocytoma is a rare cutaneous manifestation of Lyme disease, which presents as a solitary bluish-red swelling with a diameter of up to a few centimeters, most commonly on the ear lobe in children and the breast, on or near the nipple, in adults. It may occasionally be the only sign of Lyme disease and may persist for months. As the name suggests, it is comprised of a dense lymphoid infiltrate in the cutis and subcutis with or without germinal centers and may suggest the diagnosis of a lymphoma to the unaware; the infiltrate, however, is polyclonal. Lesions of acrodermatitis chronica atrophicans show a pronounced lymphoplasmacellular infiltration of the skin and sometimes also of the subcutis, with or without atrophy (121).

Laboratory Diagnosis

Diagnosis is based on serology, and diagnostic testing performed in laboratories with excellent quality-control procedures is required for confirmation of extracutaneous Lyme disease (197). First-tier testing is most often performed using a polyvalent ELISA. If the first-tier assay result is positive or equivocal, then the same serum specimen is retested by separate IgM and IgG immunoblots. For patients with symptoms in excess of 4 weeks, reactivity must be present on the IgG immunoblot, to be considered seropositive. In interpreting the results of serologic tests, it is also important to remember that the background rates of seropositivity in areas with high endemicity may exceed 4%. False positive results on serology may be due to cross-reaction with other spirochetes, viruses and autoimmune diseases (e119). Although useful for documentation of *B. burgdorferi* infection in research studies, amplification of *B. burgdorferi* DNA by PCR or culture of specimens of skin or blood for *Borrelia* species is not recommended for diagnosis of erythema migrans in routine clinical care (197).

Prognosis and Outcomes

Long-term prognosis is excellent following treatment, irrespective of whether the children present with erythema migrans alone, early disseminated disease, or late Lyme disease (e3,e286,e325). Recurrence of arthritis may occur among patients with HLA-DR2, DR3, or DR4 phenotypes (e325). More recently, children with Lyme neuroborreliosis have been reported to have persistent facial nerve palsy (173). It has been suggested that therapy of pregnant women with syphilis and lyme borreliosis should follow the same strategy, since both diseases have similar etiologic, clinical, and epidemiologic characteristics (74).

"Piggyback" Infections Associated with Lyme Disease

The tick *I. scapularis* that transmits *B. burgdorferi* may also be infected with and transmit *Anaplasma phagocytophilum* (previously referred to as *Ehrlichia phagocytophila*) and/or *Babesia microti*, the primary cause of babesiosis. Thus, a bite from an *I. scapularis* tick may lead to the development of Lyme disease, human granulocytic anaplasmosis (HGA, formerly known as human granulocytic ehrlichiosis), or babesiosis as a single infection or, less frequently, as a coinfection (197). Coinfection should be considered in patients who present with more-severe initial symptoms than are commonly observed with Lyme disease alone, especially in those who have high-grade fever for over 48 hours despite receiving antibiotic therapy appropriate for Lyme disease, unexplained leukopenia, thrombocytopenia, or anemia. Coinfection may also be indicated by persistence of systemic viremic symptoms even after resolution of the erythema migrans skin lesion (197). *B. microti* is an erythrocyte parasitic infection, endemic to coastal New England, which causes a usually mild hemolytic disease with fever; transplacental babesiosis has been implicated in one perinatal case (e96). On peripheral smears, they may be mistaken for malarial parasites. HGA is discussed under "Ehrlichiosis."

Tick-borne lymphadenopathy has been recently described as a new childhood infectious disease. It is probably caused by *Rickettsia conorii* and *R. slovaca*, transmitted by the tick *Dermacentor marginatus* (142). The tick bite is usually on the scalp and a necrotic eschar surrounded by a perilesional erythematous halo is reported at the site of bite; there is painful regional lymphadenopathy, as the name suggests.

OTHER SPIROCHETAL INFECTIONS

Nonvenereal treponematoses (and their causative agents) include yaws (*T. pertenue*), pinta (*T. carateum*), and bejel (*T. endemicum*) (55,136). They are restricted to the tropics and subtropics, affect children and young adults, and are transmitted by direct personal contact, fomites (bejel), or arthropod vectors (yaws and pinta). Spirochetes multiply at site of primary infection and disseminate to regional lymph nodes, the adenopathy-mimicking syphilis. Although bejel and yaws have a systemic spirochetemia with tertiary lesions (in bones and joints), unlike in syphilis, transplacental infection, aortic, and neurologic involvement do not usually occur. Yaws affects the skin as fissured, verrucous, or oozing lesions; bejel causes mucocutaneous lesions of the mouth and nasopharynx; and pinta occurs as serpiginous plaques on the foot, hand, or arm.

Abramowsky et al. have described a novel nontreponemal spirochetosis eliciting a pronounced lymphoplasmacytic response in fetal intestine, lung, and meninges in second-trimester fetuses that is associated with chorioamnionitis and villitis. The organism is morphologically distinct from that causing syphilis, leptospirosis, and borreliosis (e2).

CLOSTRIDIAL INFECTIONS

Clostridia are ubiquitous, gram-positive, anaerobic, spore-forming organisms present in the environment, soil, and the GITs of humans, animals, and insects. Most clostridial syndromes are caused by toxins elaborated by the bacteria and include botulism, tetanus, myonecrosis (gas gangrene), and pseudomembranous colitis. Clostridial toxins are strongly antigenic and can be neutralized by antisera, a fact that is often used in therapy.

Botulism, an acute neuromuscular paralysis, is an acute systemic toxemia and not strictly an infection (59). It is caused by absorption of preformed botulinum toxin produced by *Clostridium botulinum*, usually from the GIT, although the toxin may rarely also be absorbed from infected wounds. The most common sources of food-borne botulism are home-canned fruits, vegetables, fish, honey, corn syrup, and the skin of fresh fruits such as grapes. It presents as a descending paralysis (cranial nerves, limbs, and trunk) about 12 to 36 hours after ingestion of toxin. Infant botulism presents with constipation, difficulty in feeding, weak cry, hypotonia, and drooling, progressing to cranial neuropathy and ventilatory failure. There are no specific morphologic findings. An association with sudden infant death syndrome has been postulated, but the data are inconclusive. Botulism most frequently occurs between 6 weeks and 6 months of age, with the youngest reported patient being 6 days of age (e15). Breast milk may protect against botulism by causing more acid stools and increasing the presence of *Bifidobacterium* species, thereby limiting the intestinal presence of *C. botulinum* or its spores (e14).

Tetanus, caused by the toxin tetanospasmin produced by *C. tetani*, is a major cause of neonatal infant mortality in many developing countries (e320). Neonatal tetanus follows contamination of the umbilical stump due to poor hygiene and certain traditional practices, especially when mothers are not adequately immunized. Tetanus neonatorum presents as generalized weakness and failure to nurse, progressing to muscular rigidity, spasms, and death (in over 90% of affected infants). There are no characteristic morphologic features. Older nonimmunized children can develop tetanus following trauma; often the colonized wound may be trivial.

Gas gangrene or clostridial myonecrosis caused by clostridial exotoxins (especially lecithinase) follows penetrating or crush injuries contaminated with soil or feces. Infection may also be nontraumatic in patients with reduced resistance to infections, following an insult to the intestines permitting transmucosal migration of intestinal clostridia into the blood. The myonecrosis is characterized by severe tissue damage associated with gas and fluid-filled bullae in necrotic skeletal muscle and surrounding soft tissues. Inflammation in the gangrenous muscle is scant to absent. *C. perfringens* causes about 80% of these infections followed by *C. septicum* and other clostridia (e315). Infection progresses very rapidly in the absence of prompt diagnosis and treatment; higher mortality rates are seen with *C. septicum* infections. Neutrophil dysfunction, bowel ischemia, and trauma predispose to *C. septicum* infection in children (174).

Pseudomembranous colitis (see Chapter 14) is a toxin-mediated condition produced by overgrowth of *C. difficile* in the large intestine; it may occur in the newborn (e308).

ZOONOSES

Space does not permit discussion of a large group of bacterial diseases that exist largely in domestic and wild animals; they are acquired only secondarily, and rarely, by humans. Examples include brucellosis, anthrax, tularemia, and plague. Although the clinical and epidemiologic aspects of these conditions may be distinctive in the pediatric age group, their pathologic manifestations are not different from those in adults. Recent reviews are comprehensive (24,119,129,176) (e38,e245,e287,e330). Anthrax, plague, and tularemia are potential agents of bioterrorism and are discussed in a later section. Brucellosis is briefly outlined below.

Brucellosis

Humans are accidental hosts to brucellosis and acquire the disease by direct contact with infected animals (cattle, pigs, or sheep) or by ingesting contaminated milk/milk products. The bacteria gain entry through skin abrasions, GIT, respiratory tract, or conjunctiva and then localize to the reticuloendothelial system (lymph node, spleen, liver, and bone marrow). After an incubation period of 3 to 4 weeks the patient has nonspecific symptoms including fever, chills, profuse sweats, body aches, mental inattention, and depression. Pathologic changes in involved organs include nonspecific inflammation, lymphoid hyperplasia, and (nonnecrotizing or necrotizing) granulomas. The coccobacillary organisms are rarely, if ever, demonstrable and culture isolation is also difficult. A presumptive diagnosis is made by demonstrating rising antibody titers in the serum. Complications include sacroiliitis, osteomyelitis (especially vertebral), neurobrucellosis (meningitis, encephalitis, radiculopathy, myelitis, and peripheral neuropathy), infective endocarditis, and mycotic aneurysms. (61) (e206, 287).

TUBERCULOSIS

Mycobacterial disease in children is encountered by the pathologist in three clinical forms: TB, pulmonary; disseminated *M. avium* infection in pediatric HIV infection; and lymphadenopathy caused by infection with atypical mycobacteria (usually *M. fortuitum*, *M. scrofulaceum*, or *M. avium-intracellulare*).

An estimated one-third of the world's population (2 billion people) is infected with the tubercle bacilli and the WHO estimates that more than 8 million new cases of TB occur each year, with 3 million persons dying from the disease. Childhood TB, defined as TB in patients less than 15 years of age, accounts for 2% to 40% of all cases (111) (e81). The current WHO practice of reporting only acid-fast bacillus (AFB) smear–positive cases would certainly underestimate global incidence and prevalence, since 95% of infected children may be AFB smear–negative (126). Difficulties in diagnosis stem from the low yield of mycobacteriologic cultures and the subsequent reliance on clinical case definitions (57). The epidemiology of pediatric TB continues to be shaped by risk factors such as age, race, immigration, poverty, overcrowding, and HIV/AIDS. The pathogenesis of disease differs from that in adults, because primary disease and its complications are more common in children, leading to differences in clinical and radiographic manifestations in pediatric TB. In some regions, TB accounts for 10% to 15% of all pediatric deaths (e225,226).

Transmission

Pediatric TB occurs in congenital and postnatal acquired forms; congenital TB is rare. Infection of the fetus may be transplacental (50% of cases) or by aspiration or ingestion of infected amniotic fluid (in maternal tuberculous endometritis or villitis). Transplacental infection leads to primary complex formation in the liver or lungs, whereas the latter leads to primary disease in the lungs or GIT (e41). Radiologic (CT scan) findings and the time course of the development of lesions may distinguish the two modes of transmission (e48). Perinatal TB is acquired from postnatal transmission from the mother, adult caregiver, health care worker, or other infectious source (e.g., *M. bovis* in cow's milk).

Acquired TB is transmitted by inhalation of infective airborne mucous droplets that are generated by an infected individual or produced by therapeutic manipulation (aerosol treatments, sputum induction, and through manipulation of lesions). The bacteria may also gain access by ingestion, or through the skin, mucous membranes, and conjunctiva. The risk of acquiring disease is greatest shortly after initial infection develops and is associated inversely with age, from birth to 8 years of age. For unknown reasons, a second peak in the risk of developing disease occurs during late adolescence and early adult life (111). Pediatric patients with TB are usually not infectious; they lack cavities with a large number of bacilli, and the relatively weak cough of young children is not conducive to the airborne transmission of organisms.

Clinical Features

Congenital TB presents with nonspecific symptoms during the second or third week of life (poor feeding, poor weight gain, cough, lethargy, irritability, fever) and may mimic other congenital infections such as syphilis, CMV, or neonatal sepsis. To make a diagnosis of congenital TB, the infant should have proven TB lesions, exclusion of postnatal transmission by thorough contact investigation of close contacts including health care workers and at least one of the following: papular or petechial lesions in the first week of life, documentation of TB infection of the placenta or the maternal genital tract, or a primary complex in the liver (caseating hepatic granulomas) (e41). Hepatosplenomegaly, respiratory distress, fever, lymphadenopathy, and abdominal distention are the most common signs and symptoms (2) (e41). Most infants have abnormal chest radiographs, usually showing a miliary pattern, hilar and mediastinal lymphadenopathy, or parenchymal infiltrates and, less commonly, multiple rim-enhancing pulmonary nodules with central hypodense areas (133) (e41). Fetal involvement is much less common than placental TB. The primary focus may be either in liver or in lung, depending on the route of access, and widespread miliary disease ensues. Perinatal TB presents at a later time than congenital TB; however, clinical manifestations may be similar to those of congenital TB (e289).

Clinical features of acquired TB depend on the evolution of disease. In contrast to adults and older adolescents, the clinical manifestations of TB in children are usually related to primary TB. Inhaled bacilli induce a localized pneumonia at a terminal airway (the Ghon focus), which, with resultant local tuberculous lymphangitis and hilar adenopathy forms the primary complex. An occult lymphohematogenous spread may disseminate bacilli to a variety of target organs, where the bacilli may survive for decades (e358). Most children do not develop further disease but instead develop "latent tubercular infection" (LTBI) with a positive tuberculin skin test result and no clinical or radiographic evidence of TB. Others (especially younger children) develop progressive primary TB, where the primary focus generally continues to grow even after the development of cellular immunity and may caseate centrally, liquefy, and empty into the bronchi resulting in further spread (Figure 6-19) (e193). Pleural involvement may result from direct spread of caseous material from a subpleural parenchymal or lymph node focus, or from hematogenous spread, and may present as pleural effusions or tuberculous empyema. Pleural TB is uncommon in children younger than 6 years of age and rare before 2 years of age. Mycobacteria disseminated by the bloodstream can cause extrapulmonary disease, including cervical lymphadenopathy (scrofula) and meningitis. Less common forms of extrathoracic disease are osteoarticular, abdominal, GI, genitourinary, and/or cutaneous disease. Extrapulmonary TB must be considered when evaluating children with a history of persistent fevers. Meningitis develops when caseating lesions in the cerebral cortex invade the meninges and disseminate into the subarachnoid space (e274). Children less than 2 years of age are more likely to experience a rapid progression of meningitis to hydrocephalus, seizures, and cerebral edema, whereas older children have a basal meningitis that slowly progresses over weeks (41) (e355). Tuberculomas, a less frequent manifestation of CNS disease, form when caseous foci within the brain enlarge and become encapsulated. Miliary TB occurs when large numbers of bacilli disseminate through the bloodstream and cause simultaneous disease in two or more organs, typically with millet-sized lesions (Figure 6-19). Miliary disease frequently has an insidious presentation with fever, lymphadenopathy, and hepatosplenomegaly developing before radiographic abnormalities. As many as 50% of children with military TB have a negative tuberculin skin test at presentation (e194). Extrapulmonary TB occurs in 9% to 23% of pediatric cases (110,127). Marais' review of information available from the prechemotherapy era provides a rich understanding of the natural evolution of childhood TB (112).

Infected children have a comparatively higher risk of progression to active disease than adults: 43% of infants, 24% of 1- to 5-year olds, and 15% of 11- to 15-year olds develop disease if not treated for latent TB (e312). In immune-competent children, the risk of developing TB and the clinical presentation are highly age-dependent, with younger children being at greatest risk of developing severe manifestations. After reaching the age of 10 years, children are much more likely to manifest adult-type disease that is primarily pulmonary in focus. Factors that increase the risk of progression from infection to disease include immunosuppressive therapy, HIV coinfection, malnutrition, medical conditions (e.g., renal and liver failure, diabetes mellitus, or cancer), and intercurrent viral infections such as measles (e312). Children have a relative deficiency of macrophage and dendritic cell function, and, in contrast to adults, tend to develop Th2-type T-cell responses to mycobacterial infection characterized by lack of CD8-positive cell response and interleukin (IL)-4 and IL-5 production by CD4-positive cells (105). Although BCG vaccination may not prevent infection (e214), it reduces the hematogenous complications of primary infection (183) and is reportedly efficacious in preventing tuberculous meningitis (e27, e335).

Pathology

The histopathologic features of TB are similar in children and adults. The classic morphologic feature of TB is the caseating granuloma (Figure 6-19). Immunocompromised children may have lesions that teem with acid-fast bacilli in macrophages and extracellularly, without granuloma formation.

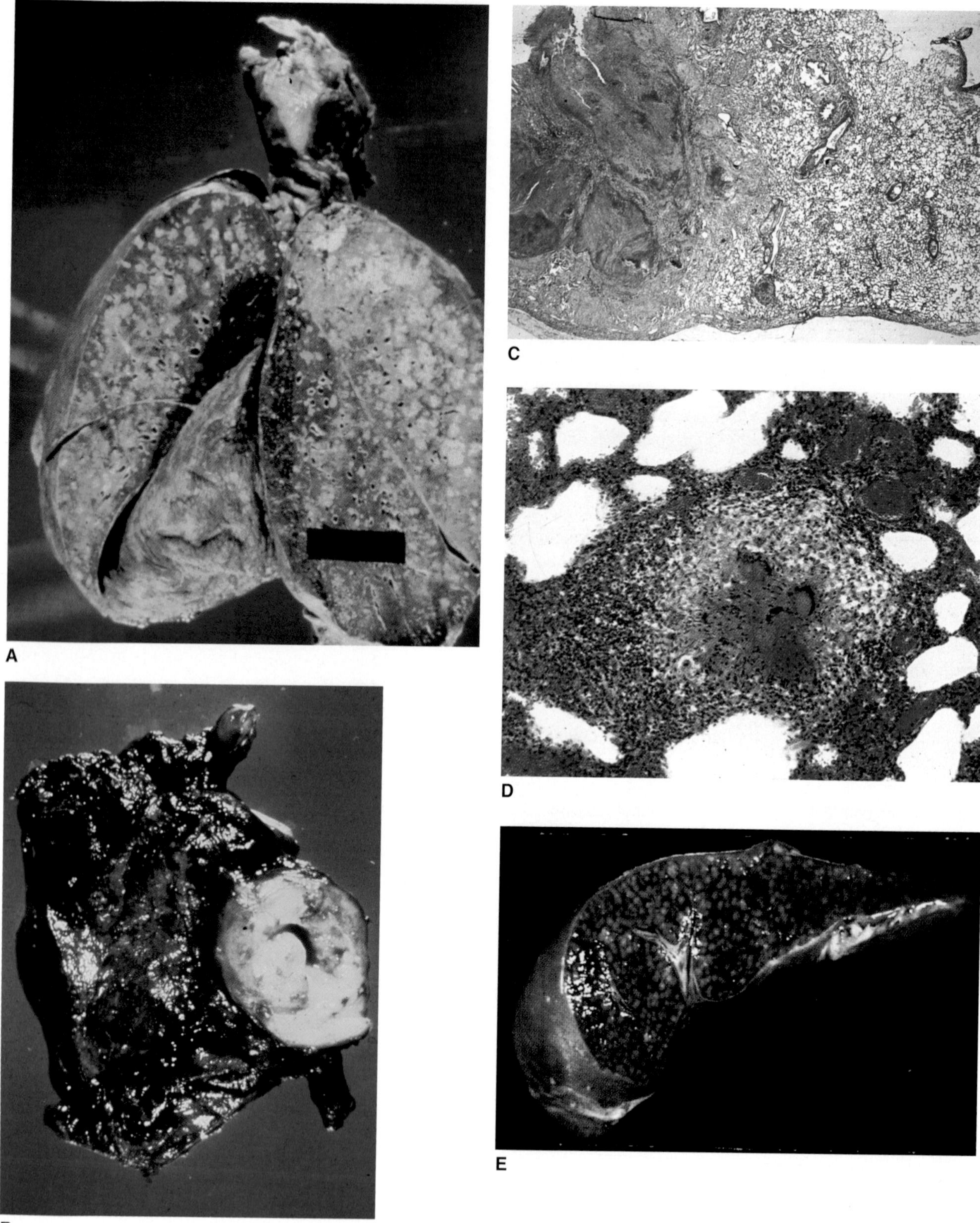

FIGURE 6-19 ■ Tuberculosis. **A**: Miliary pulmonary disease. **B**: Fibrocaseous cavitary lesion of secondary/progressive tuberculosis. **C:** Caseating granulomas in the lung (low power). **D**: Tuberculous granuloma, lung with central necrosis and Langhans type giant cells. **E**: Spleen with military tuberculosis.

Laboratory Diagnosis

Diagnostic challenges arise because children have less specific signs and symptoms of disease, have fewer positive mycobacterial cultures and, once infected, are at increased risk for progression to disseminated disease (57). Traditional techniques like microscopy (acid-fast stains, auramine-rhodamine fluorescence), and culture techniques (solid, liquid, radiometric, and nonradiometric systems) still remain the mainstay of diagnosis. Molecular amplification systems (PCR, NASBA, TMA, and LCR) can identify *M. tuberculosis* as well as nontuberculous mycobacteria and can also identify rifampin (rpoB gene)/isoniazide (katG gene) resistance. Although molecular assays have high sensitivity and specificity in smear positive sputum, they have variable sensitivity for sputum negative and extrapulmonary specimens (e361). Unfortunately, congenital and perinatal TB often eludes diagnosis until autopsy.

RICKETTSIAL INFECTIONS

Rickettsiae are arthropod-borne intracellular bacteria (small coccobacillary forms), which cause spotted fevers, typhus, and scrub typhus. A related organism, *Coxiella burnetii*, causes Q fever. The clinical and pathologic spectrum of rickettsial disease is discussed thoroughly by Walker et al. (190). The epidemiologic features of the diseases are listed in Table 6-14. Rickettsial diseases are all characterized by fever, headache, and (except for Q fever) rash. The pathologic substrate is inflammation of small blood vessels. Rocky Mountain spotted fever (RMSF) is endemic in the southeastern and south-central United States and in coastal New England, although it is reported from every state. Rickettsiae enter the blood during a tick bite and penetrate blood vessels. They multiply in endothelial cells and vascular smooth muscle, resulting in a systemic vasculitis, which is the basis for the rash (Figure 6-20), interstitial pneumonia, myocarditis, hepatic portal triaditis, meningoencephalomyelitis, and interstitial nephritis. Leakage of fluid from the injured vessels leads to edema and hypovolemia; vascular necrosis and inflammation can initiate consumption coagulopathy (e158,e356). The vasculitis of RMSF involves capillaries, venules, and arterioles; the cellular inflammatory reaction comprised of mainly macrophages and lymphocytes, with few polymorphonuclear leukocytes. Eccentric microthrombosis and microinfarction frequently result. Rickettsial organisms are visible, albeit very small (<2 μm), and may be demonstrated with difficulty using Giemsa or immunostains (e88,e357). Diagnosis, however, is usually accomplished serologically by the Weil-Felix test or by specific complement fixation. PCR-based methods are also available (e297,e341).

Ehrlichiosis

Ehrlichiae are small pleomorphic coccobacilli in the family Anaplasmataceae; they are tick-borne obligate intracellular parasites and are currently grouped with the rickettsiae. Human ehrlichiosis is a reportable disease in the United States and its incidence is on the rise. Ehrlichiae infect phagocytes (macrophages/monocytes and neutrophils). The three genera and the related infections include human monocytic ehrlichiosis (HME), caused by *E. chaffeensis*; HGA, caused by *A. phagocytophilum*; and human ewingii ehrlichiosis, caused by *E. ewingii* (47) (e159). Patients present with fever and myalgias, with or without rash and other systemic manifestations, and have leucopenia, thrombocytopenia, and raised transaminases (e114). Complications are uncommon and include meningitis, pneumonitis, renal failure, and septic shock. Diagnosis is established by blood smear examination for intracytoplasmic morulae or PCR in the first week

Table 6-14 ▪ RICKETTSIAL DISEASES

Disease	Agent	Transmission	Geographic Distribution
Spotted fever group			
RMSF	*R. rickettsii*	Tick bite	Western hemisphere
Rickettsial pox	*R. akari*	Tick bite	USA, Russia, Korea
Boutonneuse fever	*R. conorii*	Tick bite	Mediterranean, Africa, India
Tick typhus	Several	Tick bite	Asia, Australia, central Europe
Typhus group			
Epidemic typhus	*R. prowazekii*	Louse feces	Worldwide
Brill-Zinsser disease	*R. prowazekii*	Recrudescent form of epidemic typhus	Worldwide
Murine typhus	*R. mooseri (R. typin)*	Rat flea feces	Worldwide
Scrub typhus	*R. tsutsugamushi*	Mite bite	Japan, Southeast Asia, Pacific
Q fever	*Caxiella burnetii*	Aerosol	Worldwide
Ehrlichiosis			
Sennetsu fever	*E. sennetsu*	Tick bite	Japan, Malaysia
Monocytic ehrlichiosis	*E. chaffeensis*	Tick bite	United States, Portugal, Mali
Granulocytic ehrlichiosis	Unnamed species	Tick bite	United States: Midwest, northeast

RMSF, Rocky Mountain spotted fever.
Summarized and modified from references 134, 141, 178, 484, and 486.

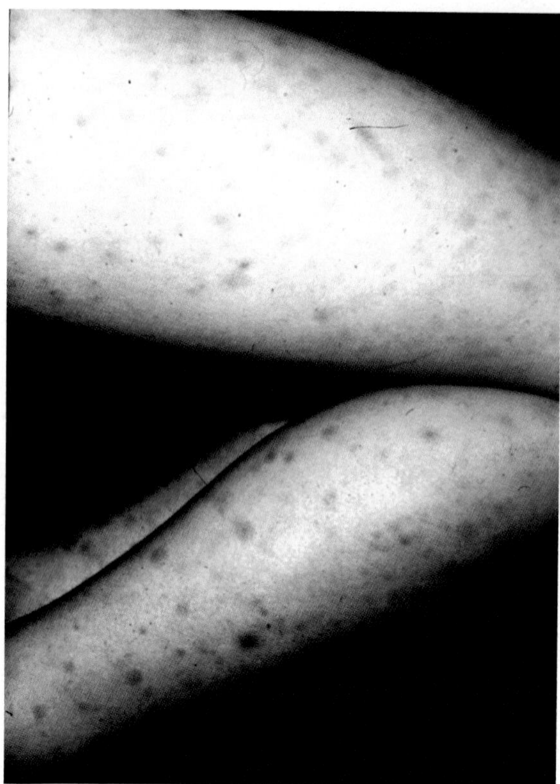

FIGURE 6-20 ▪ Rocky mountain spotted fever—lesions on the legs.

of infection, with serology being more sensitive beyond 2 weeks (47). Cultures are available in specialized centers. A high index of suspicion is required for diagnosis, especially in tick-endemic regions. The bone marrow is usually panhypercellular and shows increased histiocytes with granulomas, ring granulomas, erythrophagocytosis, plasmacytosis, and lymphoid aggregates (e89). The liver shows sinusoidal and portal lymphohistiocytic infiltrates and hepatocyte necrosis, and the spleen shows focal necrosis on a background of mild histiocytosis (e87). Interstitial pneumonitis and pulmonary hemorrhage have also been reported (e159). Other organs may show nonspecific perivascular lymphohistiocytic infiltrates. Immunohistochemical stains are available for diagnosis. Unfortunately, most of the literature pertains to adult infections and the true burden of pediatric infections and the natural course in children is unclear (162).

HGA, as the name suggests, is a rickettsial infection of neutrophils (e86). Clinical manifestations are nonspecific and may include fever, chills, headache, and myalgias. The incubation period is 5 to 21 days. In most cases, HGA is a mild, self-limited illness, even without antibiotic therapy. However, serious manifestations of infection, including a fatal outcome, have been reported in immunocompromised patients. Chronic infection due to *A. phagocytophilum* has not been described in humans. Laboratory features may include leukopenia, lymphopenia, thrombocytopenia, and mild elevation of liver enzyme levels. HGA can be detected in blood samples by smear examination, PCR, or culture using HL60 cells. Identification of the characteristic intragranulocytic inclusions on blood smear is the most rapid diagnostic method, but such inclusions are often scant in number or sometimes absent; in addition, overlying platelets or other types of inclusions unrelated to HGA can be misinterpreted by inexperienced observers. The most sensitive diagnostic method is paired (acute-phase and convalescent-phase) serologic testing using an indirect fluorescent antibody assay (acute-phase testing alone is not sufficiently sensitive). Serologic testing is often the only way to diagnose a patient who has already begun to receive antibiotic treatment. HGA is rare in children, but perinatal transmission from mother to child has been reported and is suspected to be transplacental (e147).

MYCOPLASMA INFECTIONS

Mycoplasma and ureaplasma are the smallest free living microorganisms, lacking cell wall peptidoglycans. *Mycoplasma hominus* and *Ureaplasma urealyticum* are frequent inhabitants of the maternal genital tract. They are associated with placental and perinatal pathology including chorioamnionitis (73) (e302, e314), funisitis (52), diffuse decidual leukocytoclastic necrosis (64), fetal vasculitis (34), fetal demise (e314), prematurity (64), premature rupture of membranes (e182), chronic lung disease of the newborn (81), and cerebral white matter echolucency (34). However, because both these organisms may be recovered from perfectly normal infants, a causal relationship to disease may be difficult to establish and requires vigorous exclusion of other pathogens. Histopathology of infected tissues varies from no pathologic changes to necrosis with or without an associated inflammatory reaction.

In older children, while pneumonia may be the most severe type of *M. pneumoniae* infection, the most typical syndrome is tracheobronchitis, accompanied by a variety of upper respiratory tract manifestations (53). The pneumonia is insidious in onset and chest radiographs show bronchopneumonia (often involving a single lower lobe), plate-like atelectasis, nodular infiltration, and hilar adenopathy (e60). As many as 25% of persons infected with *M. pneumoniae* may experience extrapulmonary complications at variable time periods after onset of, or even in the absence of, respiratory illness (158,180,189). Extrapulmonary pathology may be due to actual infection of other organs and/or host immune response to infection, and include neurologic (meningoencephalitis, encephalomyelitis, aseptic meningitis, cerebellar ataxia, isolated abducens palsy, ocular myasthenia, SIADH, transverse myelopathy, and Guillain-Barre syndrome) (199), dermatologic (maculopapular eruptions, erythema nodosum, erythema multiforme, and Stevens-Johnson syndrome), musculoskeletal (myalgias, arthritis, and rhabdomyolysis), GI (diarrhea, pancreatitis, cholestatic hepatitis), hematologic (hemolysis, DIC, thrombocytopenia, thrombocytosis) (135), cardiovascular (vasculitis, pericarditis, and myocarditis),

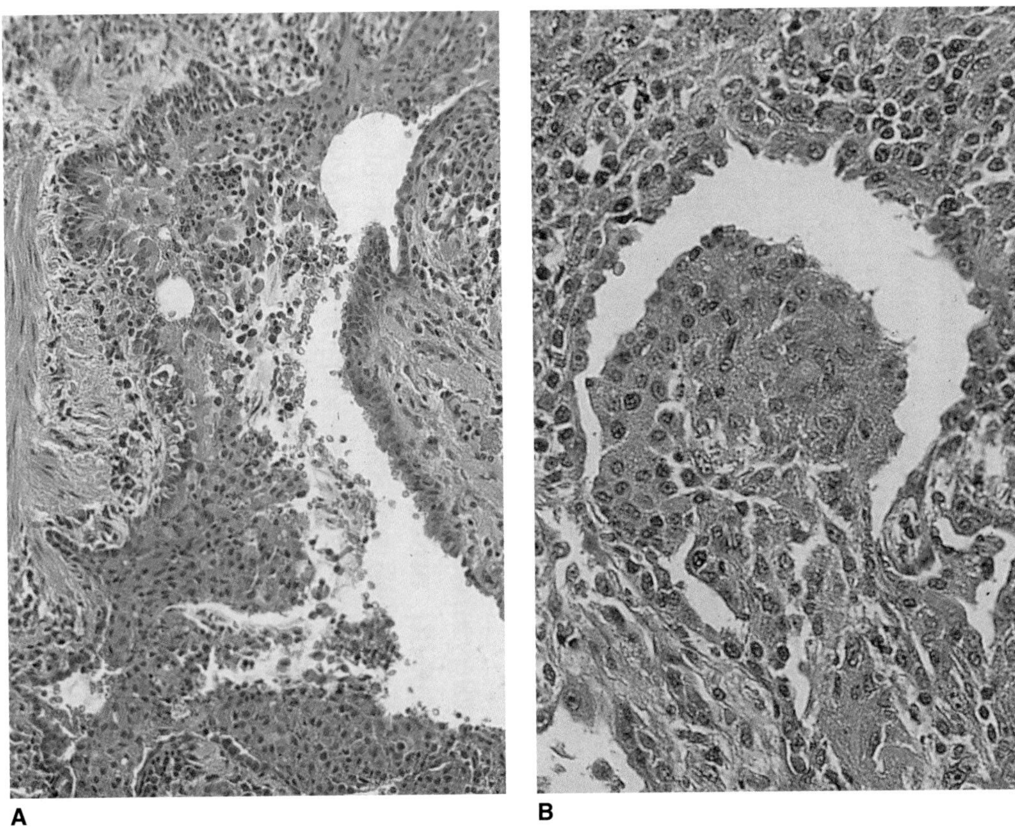

FIGURE 6-21 ■ Mycoplasma pneumonia. **A**: Inflamed bronchiole with epithelial metaplasia hyperplasia with surface necrosis. **B**: Partial occlusion of bronchiole.

renal (glomerulonephritis, renal failure, interstitial nephritis, and IgA nephropathy) (158), and lower genital tract (39) manifestations. Histopathological findings include bronchial epithelial ulceration with peribronchial and interstitial inflammation (e282) (Figure 6-21). Bronchiolitis obliterans (e190), type II pneumocyte hyperplasia, diffuse alveolar damage, lung abscess, and fibrinous pleuritis have also been reported, as have long-term sequelae including pleural scarring, bronchiectasis, and pulmonary fibrosis (e45,e75,e172,e266,e303,e354). Chen et al. have reported active lymphocytic myocarditis in *M. pneumoniae* infection (e49). The infection is routinely diagnosed by serological methods, although PCR and culture-based techniques are also available. Serology is more likely to be positive in children with pneumonia rather than in upper respiratory tract infection or asthma (135).

CHLAMYDIAL INFECTIONS

Chlamydiae are obligate intracellular pathogens; *Chlamydia trachomatis* and *C. pneumoniae* are important human pathogens, while *C. psittaci* is an important cause of zoonosis. Chlamydial infections in children have been comprehensively reviewed (36,72) (e131). *C. psittaci* and *C. trachomatis*, of which there are many subtypes, cause several distinct conditions in children (Table 6-15).

C. pneumoniae infects children of all ages. It is a common human respiratory pathogen with asymptomatic nasopharyngeal carriage occurring in up to 5% of the population. The nasopharynx is probably the most frequent site of perinatally-acquired chlamydial infection, with approximately 70% of infected infants having positive cultures at that site. Most infections are asymptomatic and may persist for over 2 years. The clinical presentation ranges from mild atypical pneumonia (similar to that seen with Mycoplasma) to severe disease. Their role in upper respiratory, sinus and middle ear infections is unclear. Infants with chlamydial pneumonia will usually be symptomatic before the eighth week of life with the insidious development of nasal obstruction and/or discharge, tachypnea, and a repetitive staccato cough. In very young infants, infection may be more severe and be associated with apnea. Possible laboratory findings include a distinctive peripheral eosinophilia, mild arterial hypoxemia, and elevated serum immunoglobulins. Untreated disease can linger or recur. Pulmonary disease takes the form of an interstitial pneumonitis with rare instances of necrotizing bronchiolitis and consolidation (e127). Because the pneumonia is rarely fatal, pathologic descriptions are few, and no characteristic features have been described. Definitive diagnosis is by cultures in cell lines, but is labor-intensive and needs special media for collection and transportation. Although serology is commonly used for diagnosis, infection may occur without seroconversion (45).

Table 6-15 ■ CHLAMYDIAL DISEASE IN CHILDHOOD

Organism	Disease	Pathologic Features	Transmission
C. psiltaci	Ornilhosis (Psittacosis)	Interstitial lobular or lobar pneumonia	Aerosol from infected birds
C. trachomatis			
Type A, B, C	Trachoma	Chronic progressive conjunctivitis with scarring leading to blindness. Cytoplasmic inclusions in early stage.	Contact
Type D–M	Inclusion conjunctivitis	Acute follicular conjunctivitis with cytoplasmic inclusions	Contact
	Nongonoccal urethritis, proctitis, salpingitis, cervicitis	Nonspecific, but prominent plasma cells and lymphoid nodules	Veneral; rare in prepubertal children and suggest sexual abuse
	Neonatal pneumonia and conjunctivitis	Interstitial pneumonitis with rare inclusions	Transit through birth canal
Type L_1, L_2, L_3	Lymphogranuloma venereum	Cutaneous ulcer, granulomatous lymphadenitis with stellate abscesses	Venereal

Modified and summarized from references 44, 189, 194.

C. trachomatis infection is arguably the most prevalent sexually transmitted infection in the United States, with prevalence rates exceeding 10% among sexually active adolescents (e53). Infection tends to be asymptomatic and of long duration. The rectum and vagina may also be infected at birth; however the presence of organisms in these sites in older children raises the possibility of sexual abuse (e130, e153). If a pregnant woman has active infection, the infant may acquire the infection during vaginal delivery, developing either inclusion conjunctivitis (e196) or pneumonitis (e19); the CDC recommends routine screening of all pregnant women during their first prenatal visit and again during the third trimester if they are at high risk (25 years of age or other risk factors such as new or multiple sexual partners) (e269). The evidence linking *C. trachomatis* to premature delivery and fetal loss is inconclusive. Further, transmission of the organism to other infants in nurseries or intensive care units has not been reported and there is no evidence to suggest that infants with chlamydial infections should be isolated.

Up to 50% of infants exposed to chlamydiae during vaginal delivery develop conjunctivitis (72). The incubation period for chlamydial conjunctivitis is 5 to 14 days after delivery or earlier if membranes have ruptured prematurely. The severity is variable, ranging from mild injection to purulent discharge with pseudomembrane formation. Clinical differentiation from gonococcal ophthalmia may be difficult. Inclusion conjunctivitis is characterized by clearly defined cytoplasmic microcolonies or inclusions in conjunctival epithelial cells. These contain large amounts of glycogen and are readily demonstrated with iodine or PAS stains. Although the conjunctivitis mostly resolves spontaneously during the first few months even in untreated patients, occasional infants maintain persistent inflammation with the formation of a micropannus (neovascularization of the cornea) and scarring typical of trachoma. Approximately 70% of infants who have perinatal chlamydial infection develop asymptomatic nasopharyngeal infection and about 30% of these develop pneumonia (72), usually presenting between 4 and 12 weeks of age with cough and tachypnea, but no fever. Radiographs do not show any consolidation; laboratory tests reveal eosinophilia and elevated immunoglobulin levels. Infected adolescents may develop urethritis, epididymitis, bartholinitis, endometritis, subclinical salpingitis, and perihepatitis (Fitz-Hugh-Curtis syndrome), as in adults.

Except for inclusion body conjunctivitis, early trachoma, and rare cases of neonatal pneumonia with inclusions, the clinical and pathologic features of chlamydial infections are not specific. Although cell culture techniques are the gold standard for laboratory diagnosis, enzyme immunoassays, direct fluorescent antibody assays, nucleic acid amplification tests, and microimmunofluorescence serology are more commonly used. However, nonculture techniques may yield false positive results (72).

ACTINOMYCOTIC INFECTIONS

Actinomycosis is a chronic suppurative inflammatory process caused by an anaerobic gram-positive bacterium, *Actinomyces israelii*, usually acting in concert with other bacteria. The organism is a part of the normal flora of the mouth. Actinomycosis is rare in children in the absence of underlying risk factors (8) (e112). The cervicofacial form of the disease is more likely to be encountered than abdominal and thoracopulmonary disease, and may be seen following trauma, surgery, or even tooth extraction (especially in a setting of caries). Diagnosis requires a high degree of suspicion (e112). In all locations, the lesion is an indolent, burrowing suppurative process with large aggregates of organisms forming "sulfur granules" with distinctive peripheral clubbing. The organism is rather pleomorphic, and diagnosis should ideally be confirmed by culture. Nocardiosis is caused by branching gram-positive coccobacilli; two species, *Nocardia asteroides* and *N. braziliensis*, cause most human diseases. Both are obligate aerobes and are weakly acid fast, the latter helping differentiate these from Actinomyces species. They are soil inhabitants and act, for the most part, as opportunistic pathogens. Primary infection is pulmonary (e188) and may take many forms including abscesses (often multiple and coalescent), pneumonia, or coin lesions. Extrapulmonary spread occurs most often to brain and kidney. In any location, the histologic hallmark is liquefaction necrosis and suppuration. The organisms, although small, are readily identifiable on Gram, acid fast or silver methenamine stains. Nocardiosis is also unusual in children, in the absence of immunosuppression.

FUNGAL INFECTIONS

In-utero fungal infections are decidedly rare. Only Candidiasis occurs with any frequency, the first case having been described in 1958 (e22). *Candida glabrata* (previously called *Torulopsis glabrata*) and Aspergillus have been shown to reach the fetus by the ascending transcervical route, while Coccidioides spreads by a hematogenous route (14).

Candidiasis ascends from the maternal genital tract and causes chorioamnionitis, from where it can gain access to the fetal skin, upper respiratory and intestinal tracts. Thus, it causes a generalized cutaneous rash, aspiration pneumonia (Figure 6-22), and intestinal mucositis (35) (e92). Affected infants are frequently growth restricted, and many are stillborn or abortuses. In recent years, candidiasis has been recognized as a complication of the intensive care of low birth weight infants; risk factors include parenteral nutrition, central arterial or venous catheters, and a history of broad-spectrum antibiotic therapy. These infants are older than the true congenital cases (e100,e173,e284) and tend to have more visceral dissemination with renal involvement, carditis, endophthalmitis, arthritis, osteomyelitis, and meningitis. Large aggregates of pseudohyphae may form endocardial vegetations and urinary tract fungus balls (e70). The lesions bear a striking resemblance grossly to whitish-yellow miliary abscesses of listeriosis and may even be confused with HSV on occasion. The cellular reaction is suppurative and budding yeast and pseudohyphae are easily demonstrated in the lesions with routine periodic acid-Schiff (PAS), methenamine silver, or even gram stains. *C. glabrata* is an occasional cause of neonatal sepsis in premature infants (e271).

Candida infections in later childhood range from relatively mundane cutaneous and mucous membrane infections (diaper rash, thrush, glossitis) to fatal septicemic illness with widespread miliary abscesses (191). Chronic mucocutaneous candidiasis is a cellular immunodeficiency with defective T-cell response to Candida antigens (e52). In the immune-deficient or multiple antibiotic-treated patients, the organism enters through intestinal or respiratory tract mucosa, producing local ulceration and necrosis and hematogenous spread to any organ. The usual suppurative reaction may be modified in the leukopenic host. The usual tissue form of the organism is a small unencapsulated budding yeast; occasionally blastospores with elongated germ tubes are seen. Confusion with Aspergillus arises when serially budding organisms are attached end-to-end to form pseudohyphae. A slight "pinching in" of *Candida* at the site of attachment is a helpful diagnostic feature. *C. glabrata*, does not form pseudohyphae. Further confusion with Aspergillus arises when masses of pseudohyphae cause vascular occlusion, thrombosis, and infarction.

Other fungi are occasionally encountered in the neonatal age group, chiefly as complications of intensive measures in seriously compromised infants. *Malassezia furfur* colonization and sepsis in neonates is related to indwelling Broviac catheters and long-term parenteral alimentation using lipid emulsion (e262). The organism is a lipophilic yeast that localizes in pulmonary vessels, which are the site of lipid deposits associated with parenteral lipid administration, and causes a pulmonary arteritis (e270). The organism is a tiny (2 to 4-μm) budding yeast with a distinctive "heel and sole" outline seen well on silver stains. Rare GI zygomycetes infection mimics necrotizing enterocolitis clinically; there is diffuse invasion of bowel wall, with necrosis and fungal invasion of vessels (e273).

Fungal diseases of older infants and children fall into two categories: the endemic mycoses, characterized by sharply defined geographic boundaries and occurrence in normal (nonimmunosuppressed) hosts, and the opportunistic mycoses, which are ubiquitous in the environment but do not ordinarily cause disease in healthy persons (191).

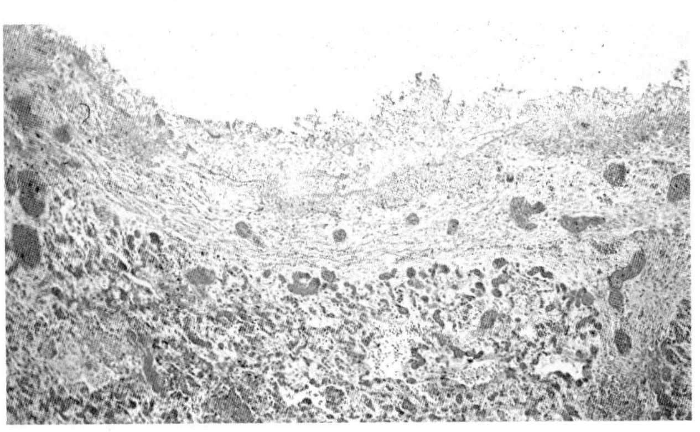

A

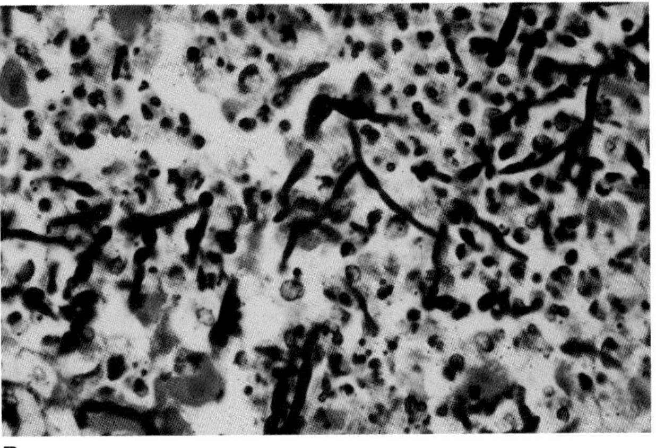

B

FIGURE 6-22 ■ **A**: Candidal pleuritis. **B**: Candidal pneumonia with yeast and pseudohyphal phase organisms. (PAS stain).

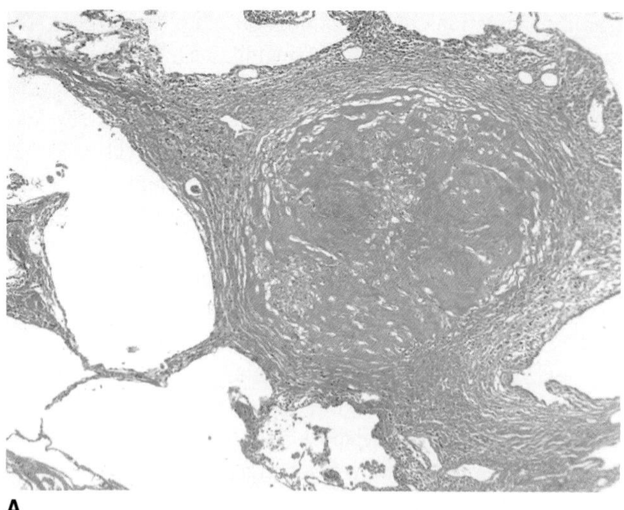

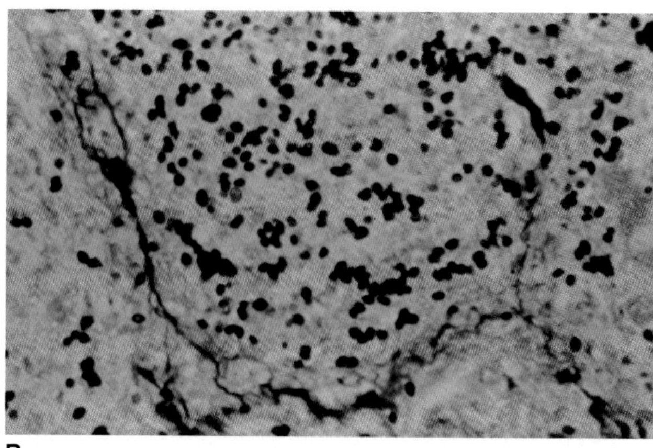

A B

FIGURE 6-23 ■ **A**: Histoplasma nodule, lung. **B**: Organisms highlighted by a GMS stain.

In North America, the endemic mycoses include blastomycosis, endemic in the eastern states, histoplasmosis in the Mississippi and Ohio River valleys, and coccidioidomycosis in the southwest. They have several features in common:

1. The organisms are dimorphic fungi; with rare exception, the yeast form is the one seen in tissue.
2. All three are primarily pulmonary diseases with clinical and morphologic features similar to TB.
3. Disseminated disease is the exception and tends to occur in very young children or in immunocompromised patients.
4. All evoke a host response which is primarily granulomatous, but mixed granulomatous and suppurative reactions are seen.
5. All are likely to be misdiagnosed, especially when encountered outside of their usual locale.

Blastomycosis in children ranges from asymptomatic to disseminated forms; most symptomatic disease consists of pneumonic infiltration or consolidation with or without cavitation (163) (e50,e261). Microscopically, there is a mixed granulomatous and suppurative reaction. *Blastomyces dermatitidis* is a large thick-walled yeast easily visible in sections or smears. A characteristic flat-based bud is helpful in distinguishing this organism from other yeasts. The organism is a rare cause of osteomyelitis (e44,e128). Delayed diagnosis may result in dissemination even in immunocompetent hosts (e67).

Histoplasmosis is asymptomatic in the majority of infected children. Acute pulmonary or disseminated disease may be seen in young infants or immunocompromised children (16) (e148,e238,e363). Dissemination occurs in pediatric HIV infections, as does cryptococcosis (e85). In the lung, histoplasmosis provokes a caseating, granulomatous reaction indistinguishable from TB; organisms may be very few (Figure 6-23). In the disseminated form of histoplasmosis, the organisms are found within macrophages in virtually any site but particularly in the reticuloendothelial system. Sclerosing mediastinitis is a rare form of thoracic disease. In endemic areas, histoplasmosis is a common cause of hepatic granulomas (e62). *Histoplasma capsulatum* is a tiny budding yeast best demonstrated with silver stains. An immunoperoxidase method has been described (e176), and PCR techniques are useful in archival tissues (e62).

Coccidioides immitis is a soil inhabitant that causes self-limited, often asymptomatic pulmonary disease in well children. Dissemination is unusual and seems to occur in the very young (e170,e197,e202). The pulmonary disease has many clinical and morphologic similarities to histoplasmosis, but *C. immitis* exists in tissues as large double-walled spherules (sporangia), 20 to 100 m in diameter, containing myriads of tiny endospores that are released by rupture of the spherule (Figure 6-24).

The main opportunists are four: two yeasts (*Candida* and *Cryptococcus*) and two mycelial forms (Aspergillus and zygomycetes). All have, in common, an ability to cause invasive and life-threatening infections in patients who are immunosuppressed or whose normal flora is altered by antibiotic therapy.

Cryptococcus neoformans infection is rarely encountered in immunocompetent children (e304); meningitis, pneumonia, cutaneous lesions (e267), and disseminated disease have been reported, usually in the compromised host. Two forms of inflammatory reaction are recognized: granulomatous inflammation and a gelatinous mass composed of large numbers of organisms almost devoid of cellular reaction. The organism is a multiple-budding yeast with a thick mucoid capsule that in most histologic preparations appears as a clear space. It may be visualized with mucicarmine stain and sometimes shows radial striations.

Aspergillosis is caused by several species, of which *Aspergillus fumigatus* is the most common. Four types of disease occur in children: hypersensitivity pneumonitis, saprophytic colonization of preexisting pulmonary cavities, invasive

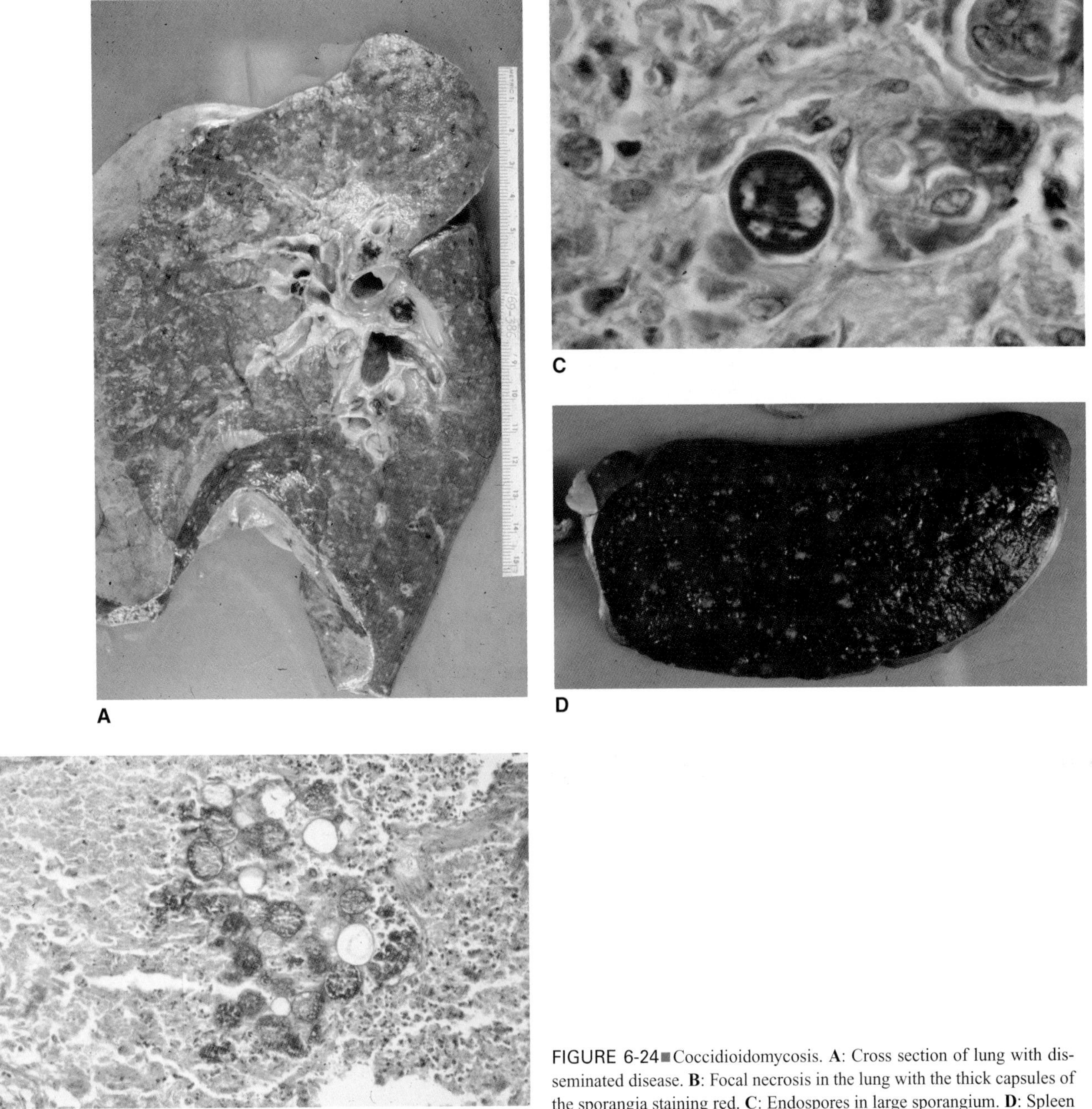

FIGURE 6-24 ■ Coccidioidomycosis. **A**: Cross section of lung with disseminated disease. **B**: Focal necrosis in the lung with the thick capsules of the sporangia staining red. **C**: Endospores in large sporangium. **D**: Spleen in a case of disseminated infection.

pulmonary aspergillosis, and disseminated aspergillosis (191). Invasive pulmonary and disseminated aspergillosis occurs almost exclusively in immunocompromised children. Aspergillus is easily identified in tissues as dichotomously branching septate hyphae uniformly 7 to 8 m in diameter. Radial or sunburst arrangement and a wavelike configuration are characteristic. The inflammatory reaction is suppurative and necrotizing. Aspergillus shares with zygomycetes (and to a lesser extent, *Candida*) a propensity for vascular invasion leading to infarction. Aspergillus is present in the sputum in a minority of patients, and the diagnosis is frequently established by lung biopsy; it is important that the surgeon understand that areas of infarction and necrosis distal to a fungal thrombus may not contain demonstrable fungi and that care should be used in selecting areas for biopsy.

Zygomycosis (or mucormycosis) is caused by several fungi (*Rhizopus* species, *Mucor* species, and *Absidia* species.) All are indistinguishable from each other in tissues (e207). These organisms are opportunists and are rarely, if ever, seen in normal children. Rhinocerebral and endobronchial zygormycosis occurs almost invariably in diabetic children (e162). Pulmonary GI and disseminated disease is seen in children with malignancy (e180). The typical pattern of tissue involvement includes granulomatous or suppurative inflammation, vascular invasion and thrombosis, and infarction. The fungi are coenocytic hyphae of rather variable diameter (5 to 20 μm) that branch at right angles. Folds and wrinkles may mimic septation.

Although histopathology is a major diagnostic tool in diagnosing fungal infections, diagnostic errors may result from morphologic mimics, use of inappropriate terminology, and incomplete knowledge in mycology (159). Template diagnosis formats have been suggested to minimize errors; species identification requires microbiology cultures.

PARASITIC DISEASES

The common protozoal and helminthic diseases are listed in Tables 6-16 and 6-17. Although parasitic infections have become more frequent even in the developed world, space does not permit a detailed review of each entity. Many of these organisms cause disease more or less confined to one organ system, and are discussed in the appropriate sections. Valuable sources for further details include *Pathology of Infectious Diseases* by Connor et al. (32), *Atlas of Human Parasitology* by Ash and Orihel (5), and Feigen and Cherry's encyclopedic *Textbook of Pediatric Infectious Diseases* (56). Protozoal infections of the fetus and neonate will be briefly discussed below.

TOXOPLASMOSIS

Toxoplasma gondii is a protozoan of the family Coccidia. The organism is a parasite of worldwide distribution; its definitive host is the cat. Clinical, epidemiologic, and pathologic features are the subject of recent reviews (9,117) (e79). Congenital toxoplasmosis, with very rare exceptions, occurs only with primary maternal infection; the exact route of transmission to the fetus is unknown, but clearly the placenta is involved. The risk to the fetus varies significantly with gestational age, increasing from 25% in the first trimester to 65% in the third for untreated maternal illness. Prenatal diagnosis is now feasible and maternal therapy during gestation appears to lessen the ill effects on the fetus (125) (e69,78,113). Among congenitally-infected infants, there is a wide spectrum of severity; most are asymptomatic, but 10% to 12% have severe morbidity and a few infants die. The characteristic clinical picture consists of fever, hydrocephalus or microcephaly, hepatosplenomegaly, jaundice, chorioretinitis, seizures, cerebral calcifications, and CSF pleocytosis. Newborns that die with toxoplasmosis generally have disseminated disease, even when clinical signs are confined to brain and eyes. Organisms may be identified in brain, eye, middle ear, blood vessels, heart, testes, adrenal,

Table 6-16 ■ PROTOZOAL INFECTIONS

Category	Organism	Disease	Transmission	References
Intestinal protozoa				
Amebae	*Entamoeba histolytica*	Amebiasis liver abscess	Fecal-oral	54
Flagellates	*Giardia lamblia*	Giardiasis	Fecal-oral	474, 505
Ciliates	*Balantidium coli*	Ciliary dysentery	Fecal-oral	
Coccidia	*Cryptosporidium*	Gastroenteritis	Meat, fecal-oral	5, 502
Extra-intestinal protozoa				
Amebae	*Naegleria fowleri*	Meningoencephalitis	Warm water	
	Acanthamoeba culbertsoni	Meningoencephalitis	Warm water	
Flagellates	*Trichomonas vaginalis*	Genitourinary infections	Venereal	104
Coccidia	*Toxoplasma gondii*	Mononucleosis like syndrome, lymphadenitis, disseminated	Infected meat oocysts in soil, sand, cat litter	166, 238, 239
Sporozoa	*Pneumocystis carinii*	Pneumonia, rarely disseminated	Droplet	215, 238, 239
Blood borne protozoa				
Sporozoa	*Plasmodium vivax*	Malaria	Arthropod born (mosquito)	381
	P. ovale	Malaria	Mosquito	
	P. malariae	Malaria	Mosquito	
	P. falciparum	Malaria	Mosquito	
	Babesia microti	Babesiosis	Tick bite	
Flagellates	*Leishmania tropica*	Cutaneous leshmaniasis	Arthropod borne (sandflies)	110, 204, 303
	L. mexicana	Cutaneous leshmaniasis	Sandflies	
	L. braziliensis	Mucotaneous leishmaniasis	Sandflies	
	L. donovani	Visceral leishmaniasis (Kala-Azar)	Sandflies	
	Trypanosoma cruzi	Chagas disease	Tristomid (reduvid) bugs	
	T. gambiense	African sleeping sickness	Tsetse flies	360
	T. rhodesiense	African sleeping sickness	Tsetse flies	

From references 44, 155, 297, and 320, in addition to those listed, with permission.

Table 6-17 ■ HELMINTHIC DISEASES

Category	Organisms	Disease	Transmission	References
Nematodes				
Intestinal	*Ascaris lumbricoides*	Ascariasis	Egg ingestion	114, 296, 488
	Enterobius vermicularis	Pinworm	Egg ingestion	79
	Ancylostoma duodenale	Old world hookworm	Skin penetration	
	Necator americanus	New world hookworm	Skin penetration	302
	Strongyloides stercoralis	Intestinal and disseminated strongyloidiasis	Skin penetration	375, 421
	Trichuris trichiura	Whip worm	Egg ingestion	296
Tissue	*Tricbineila spiratis*	Trichinosis	Ingestion of larvae	179, 226
	Toxicara canis, T. cati	Visceral larva migrans	Egg ingestion	111
	Ancylostoma brasiliense A. caninum	Cutaneous larva migrans	Skin penetration	
Filarial worms	*Wuchereria bancrofti*	Lymphangitis, elephantiasis	Mosquitos	
	Brugia malazi	Lymphangitis, elephantiasis	Mosquitos	
	Loa loa	Subcutaneous nodules, conjunctivitis	Chrysops flies	
	Onchocerca volvulus	River blindness, subcutaneous nodules, dermatitis	Black flies	96, 173
	Dirofilaria immitis	Pulmonary disease (coin lesions)	Mosquitos	70
	Dirofilaria sp.	Subcutaneous nodules, ocular lesions	Mosquitos	70
Cestodes				
Intestinal	*Diphyllobothrium latum*	Fish tapeworms	Ingestion of raw fish	
	Hymenolepsis nana	Dwarf tapeworms	Fecal-oral egg ingestion	
	Taenia solium	Pork tapeworm	Ingestion of rare pork	
	Taenia saginatum	Beef tapeworm	Ingestion of rare beef	
Larval	*Taenia solium*	Cysticercosis	Fecal-oral	58, 323
	Echinococcus	Hydatid disease	Egg ingestion	72
	Diphyllobothrium sp.	Sparganosis	Copepod ingestion	
Trematodes				
Intestinal	*Fasciolopsis buski*	Giant intestinal fluke	Larva ingestion (aquatic plants)	
Liver and lung	*Opisthorchis sinensis*	Oriental liver fluke	Ingestion of raw or undercooked fish	373
	Fasciola hepatica	Sheep liver fluke	Larva ingestion (aquatic plants)	
	Paragonimus westermani	Lung fluke	Larva ingestion (undercooked crabs and crayfish)	63, 213
Blood	*Schistosoma mansoni*	Schistosomiasis (intestinal)	Skin penetration	318
	S. haematobium	Schistosomiasis (urinary tract)	Skin penetration	442
	S. japonicum	Schistosomiasis (intestinal)	Skin penetration	493

Modified and summarized from 44, 155, 297, and 320.

lung, kidney, muscle, and occasionally, liver, spleen, and lymph nodes (Figure 6-25). The organisms appear in tissues both encysted and free. The cysts are round or oval bodies 10 to 30 m in diameter with a thick wall that is certainly visible on hematoxylin and eosin sections but better demonstrated with PAS, silver, or immunoperoxidase stains. Within the cyst are densely packed tiny trophozoites, 2 μm in diameter. The intact cysts are either intracellular or extracellular and rarely excite an inflammatory response. They rupture to liberate free trophozoites into the tissues. The host reaction is quite heterogenous and depends somewhat on the stage of disease (e79). Acute lesions are characterized by suppurative reaction, some eosinophilic infiltrate, and liquefactive necrosis, which may be extensive and confluent, particularly in the brain. Dystrophic calcification is most conspicuous in the brain. Trophozoites are numerous in these lesions. At a slightly later stage, the suppurative lesion gives way to a granulomatous one without significant necrosis; the cyst form is more frequently encountered in and around granulomatous lesions. Healing stages are highly variable in morphology with granulation tissue, gliosis, and fibrosis. Encysted organisms may persist in many tissues.

OTHER PROTOZOAL INFECTIONS

In endemic areas, malaria and trypanosomiasis constitute a threat to the fetus during episodes of maternal parasitemia. Congenital malaria, however, appears to be relatively rare (e265). Both *Plasmodium vivax* and *P. falciparum* are encountered. The infants develop fever, irritability, jaundice, and hepatosplenomegaly; the disease is usually not

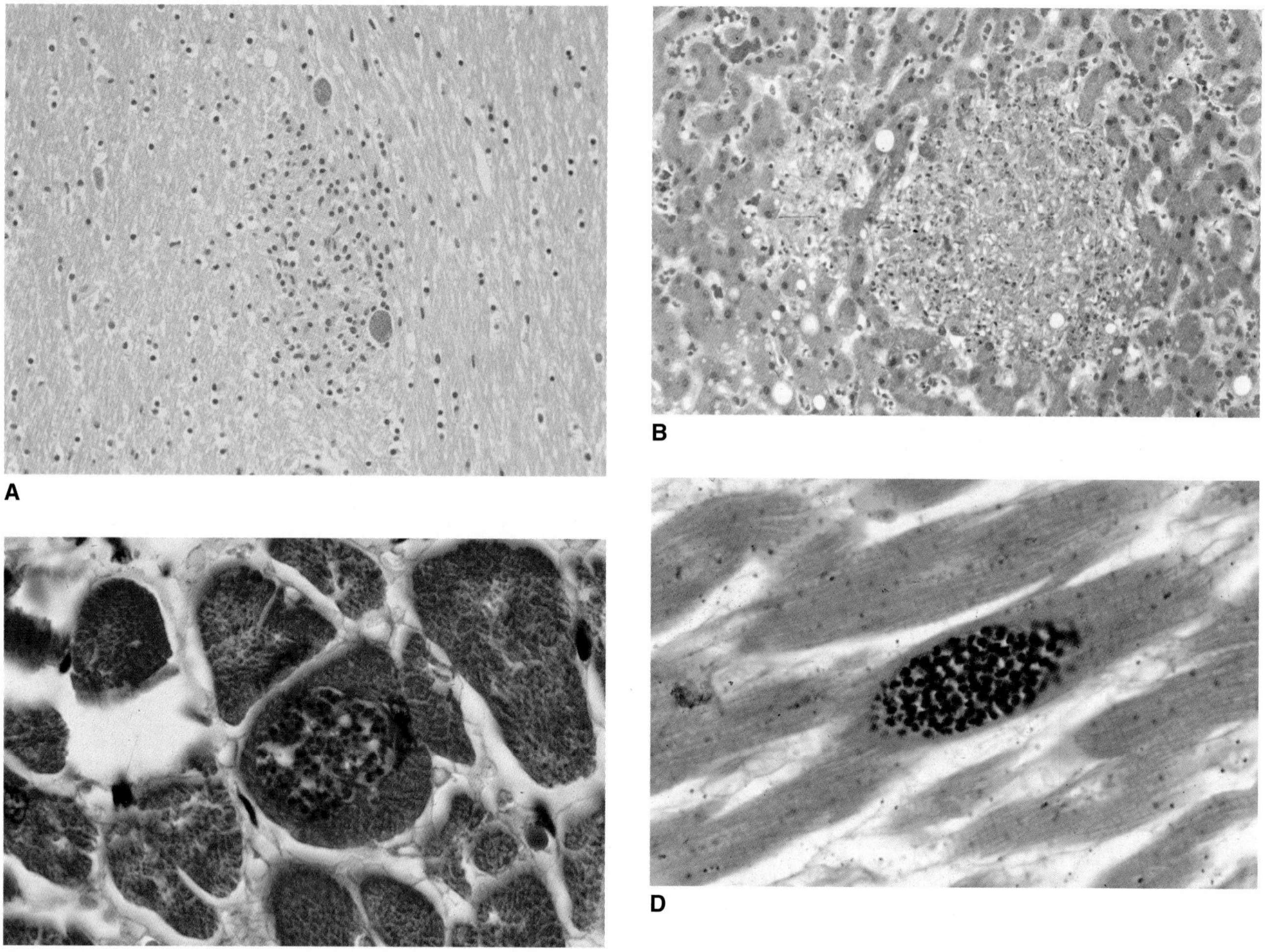

FIGURE 6-25 ■ Toxoplasmosis. **A**: Brain with microglial nodule and encysted organisms. **B**: Toxoplasmosis involving the liver with a granuloma-like lesion. **C**: Myocarditis with cyst forms within the muscle cells. **D**: Organisms highlighted by GMS stain.

suspected, and the diagnosis is almost invariably made by peripheral blood smear. Most reported fetal deaths due to malaria are associated with maternal falciparum malaria. It is not clear whether maternal anemia or fetal infection plays the most important role in fetal demise, but the parasites and malarial pigment may be identified in affected fetuses.

In Central and South America and Mexico, congenital Chagas disease results from transplacental spread of *Trypanosoma cruzi* to the fetus (11) (e29). In endemic areas, *T. cruzi* is a major cause of abortion and prematurity. Approximately 1% to 10% of pregnancies in women with chronic *T. cruzi* infection result in infants born with congenital infection (181). Most infected newborns are asymptomatic or have nonspecific findings such as low birth weight, prematurity, or low Apgar scores. Other signs include hepatosplenomegaly, anemia, and thrombocytopenia. When the disease follows an acute form in the neonate, organisms are found in many organs. The acute lesions are mixed granulomatous and suppurative, and *T. cruzi* is found within histiocytes in the leishmanial form. Meningoencephalitis, myocarditis, and respiratory distress have a high association with mortality (181).

Entamoeba histolytica is an important cause of morbidity in the developing countries, and causes amoebic colitis, hepatitis, liver abscess (Figure 6-26), and related complications. Leishmania species cause cutaneous (Figure 6-27) or systemic disease, with significant morbidity.

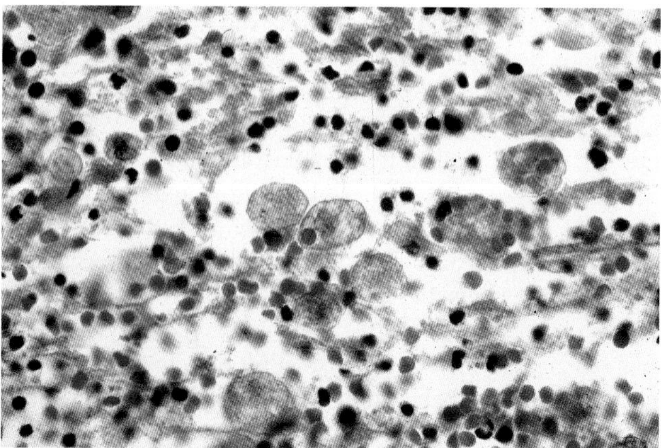

FIGURE 6-26 ■ *E. histolytica*—organisms showing erythrophagocytosis.

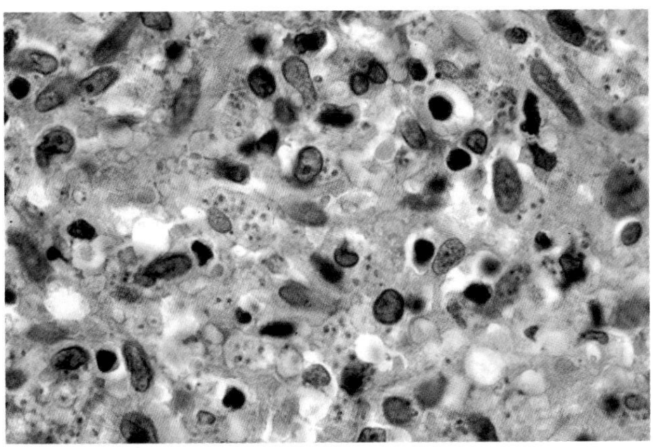

A

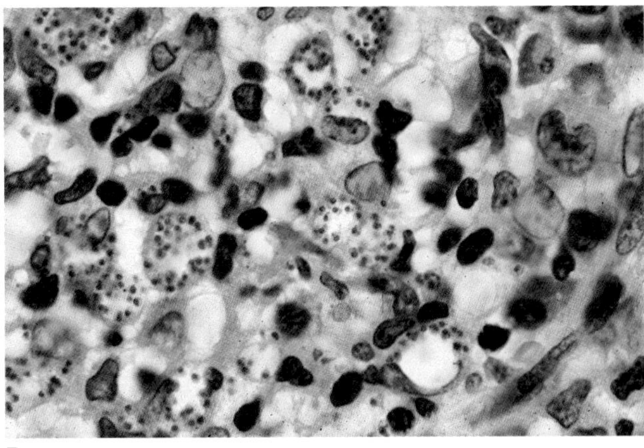

B

FIGURE 6-27 ■ Cutaneous leishmaniasis. **A**: Intracellular organisms (within histiocytes) (H&E). **B**: Brown-Hopps stain highlights organisms with their nucleus and kinetoplast.

SYSTEMIC INFECTIOUS AGENTS WITH BIOTERRORISM POTENTIAL

Fears of bioterrorism have exaggerated the importance of various infectious agents to the point of being considered in the routine differential diagnosis of many human illnesses. These agents have been categorized based, among other things, on their ease of dissemination or transmission, high mortality, degree of social disruption, and need for special preparation (58). Although any or all of the highest risk biological agents (including inhalation anthrax, pneumonic plague, smallpox, tularemia, botulism, and viral hemorrhagic fevers) can be seen in the pediatric patient, several agents might closely resemble some of the more common childhood illnesses (Table 6-18) (138,177). Selected infections are briefly outlined hereunder.

Smallpox is a highly contagious infection, caused by the variola virus, which is a strict human pathogen with no carrier state. Although smallpox was the first human epidemic disease to be eradicated, its high infectivity, ease of person-

Table 6-18 ■ DIFFERENTIAL DIAGNOSIS OF INFECTIONS BY AGENTS WITH BIOTERRORISM POTENTIAL

Agent	Differential Diagnosis
Smallpox: variola major	Chickenpox–herpes zoster
	Herpes
	Measles
	Mumps
	Vaccinia
	Epidermolysis bullosa
	Impetigo from *Staphylococcus aureus*, coagulase positive, group 2
Anthrax: *Bacillus anthracis*	Inhalation type: respiratory syncytial virus–"flu/cold"
	Cutaneous type: insect bites, cat scratch disease
	Gastrointestinal type: rotavirus, Norwalk virus, etc.
Plague: *Yersinia pestis*	Cat-scratch disease: *Bartonella henselae*
	Insect bites
	Necrotizing fasciitis: peripheral infarction
	Toxic shock syndrome
	Stevens-Johnson syndrome
Tularemia: *Francisella tularensis*	"Flu cold"
	Hemophilis influenza
	Primary pulmonary hemosiderosis
	Inhalation toxin with adult respiratory distress syndrome
Botulism: *Clostridium botulinum*	Viral gastroenteritis
	Inflammatory bowel disease
	Autoimmune disorder: dysarthria, generalized weakness
	Drug reaction
	Polio: paralysis
	Myesthenia gravis

Source: Stocker JT. Clinical and pathologic differential diagnosis of selected potential bioterrorism agents of interest to pediatric health care providers. *Clin Lab Med* 2006;26(2):329–344.

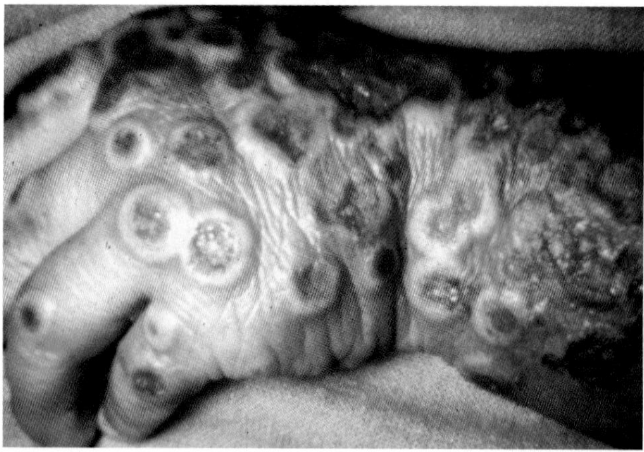

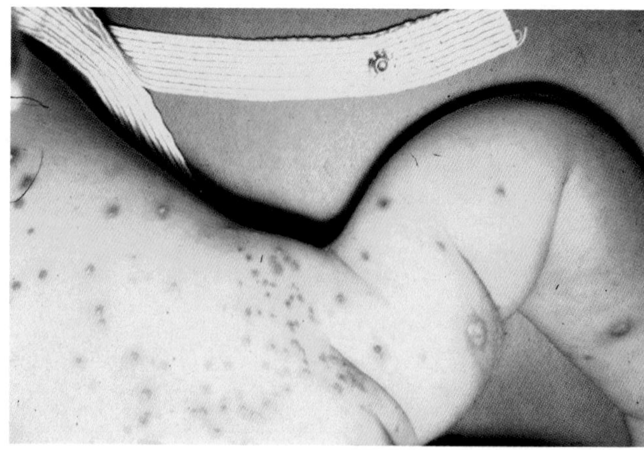

A B

FIGURE 6-28 ■ Vaccinia. **A**: Well developed lesions on the hand. **B**: Disseminated early lesions.

to-person transmission, high mortality, and lack of specific chemotherapeutic agents makes the virus an important biological weapon, especially since the majority of the world population would be susceptible to infection. Following aerial transmission, the virus spreads and multiplies in the reticuloendothelial system during the incubation period. A second phase of viremia ensues, associated with prodromal nonspecific symptoms, followed by the characteristic skin lesions. The differential diagnosis of smallpox includes infection by VZV, HSV, measles, vaccinia, impetigo from *S. aureus*, and epidermolysis bullosa (177). Unlike in chicken pox, however, fever precedes the rash by 2 to 3 days, the palms and soles are commonly involved and the vesicles are all in the same stage. Histologically, in smallpox, the papillary dermis shows signs of inflammation and capillary endothelial swelling, followed by reticulating degeneration of the overlying epidermis with the presence of basophilic inclusions (Guarneri bodies). Lysis of the infected cells leads to vesiculation; after 4 to 7 days, the clear vesicles become filled with neutrophils. The pustular fluid is usually bacteriologically sterile, unless secondarily infected. The umbilication characteristic of the mature smallpox vesicle is due to persistent septa and fixed dermal adnexa. Once the host immune response controls the infection, the vesicular fluid is resorbed and a scab is formed 10 to 15 days after the appearance of the rash. The scabs fall off by 3 weeks once the basal epithelium is replaced, leaving scars proportional to the depth of dermal involvement. Mucosal lesions are similar, except that they are covered by slough. The road to smallpox eradication, the weapon potential of the variola virus, and possible remedies has been reviewed by Raghunath (145). The Advisory Committee on Immunization Practices recommends not vaccinating pregnant or breastfeeding women or children less than 18 years old in preevent smallpox vaccination programs (193) Secondary contact vaccinia from smallpox vaccine is rare (Figure 6-28), estimated to occur at a rate of 5 to 7 cases per 100,000 vaccines (e295).

Anthrax, caused by *Bacillus anthracis*, is a worldwide zoonotic disease. Transmission in humans occurs through contact with animals or animal products (e.g., wool) and from person to person by way of cutaneous lesions. Anthrax occurs in three forms: cutaneous, GI, and inhalational. The cutaneous form accounts for nearly 95% of cases in children and adults. Pulmonary and GI infections may be complicated by sepsis and meningitis. In the initial stages, the cutaneous form may be mistaken for insect bites or cat scratch disease, the GI type for viral gastroenteritis, and the pulmonary type for respiratory syncytial viral or similar infections, leading to delay in instituting specific therapy (177). The hallmark lesions are edema and hemorrhage, including hemorrhagic thoracic lymphadenitis, hemorrhagic mediastinitis with radiographic mediastinal space expansion, meningeal hemorrhage/edema (so-called cardinal's cap), GI submucosa (in over 90% cases) hemorrhagic mesenteric lymphadenitis (in 20% cases) (68,115) (e1). The causative Gram positive bacilli may be identified in smear-preparations of lymph node, spleen, or blood. After presumed exposure, antimicrobial prophylaxis is recommended for up to 60 days. Adverse effects of prolonged antimicrobial use may cause added pathology, although little information is available on effects of such prolonged use.

PLAGUE

Plague is a bacterial zoonosis caused by *Yersinia pestis*, acquired through infected flea bites, and manifests as bubonic, septicemic, or pneumonic forms (98). The bubonic form is the most common and presents with one or more enlarged, tender, regional lymph nodes, so-called bubo, as a result of migration of bacteria from the bite site to the regional lymph nodes. A local skin lesion (papule, vesicle, ulcer, or eschar) may be seen at the bite site. There is marked neutrophilia (40,000 to 100,000 cells/μL); blood cultures are often positive (50%) and the organism may be identified readily in aspirates of the buboes. Morphologically, lymph nodes show congestion and edema progressing to hemorrhage and necrosis that spreads outside the nodes. The bacteria resist phagocytosis to cause lymph node necrosis, and may be seen as extracellular aggregates within necrotic foci. Ulceration and cutaneous fistulae may occur. The bacteria may be recognized in sections and smears by their bipolar "safety pin" morphology or by the identification of monoclonal antibodies to the F1 antigen of *Y. pestis* (e47). Destruction of the lymph nodes is followed by bacteremia, septicemia, and endotoxemia. Pneumonic plague, as the name suggests, have dyspnea, chest pain, and a cough with hemoptysis, while patients with septicemic plague often have prominent GI symptoms and abdominal pain. Gangrene of the fingers, toes, or the tip of the nose caused by small vessel thrombosis has led to the disease being referred to as the "black death." All three forms may have systemic manifestations of gram-negative sepsis. Septicemic and pneumonic plague progress rapidly and are usually fatal without prompt treatment; bubonic plague has a mortality rate of 50% to 60% (e149). Plague has historically been used as a biological warfare weapon, dating back to at least the early 14th century, when the Tartar army hurled its plague-infected corpses over the walls of the city during the siege of Caffa. In fact, the United States and the former Soviet Union were both involved in developing aerosolized *Y. pestis* before the 1972 convention on prohibition of biologic and toxin weapons (e152).

REFERENCES

1. Centers for Disease Control and Prevention. 1994 revised guidelines for the performance of CD4+ T-cell determinations in persons with human immunodeficiency virus (HIV) infections. *MMWR Recomm Rep* 1994;43(RR-3):1–21.
2. Adhikari M, Pillay T, Pillay DG. Tuberculosis in the newborn: an emerging disease. *Pediatr Infect Dis J* 1997;16(12):1108–1112.
3. Ahmad SN, Shah S, Ahmad FM. Laboratory diagnosis of leptospirosis. *J Postgrad Med* 2005;51(3):195–200.
4. Arnon S, Litmanovitz I. Diagnostic tests in neonatal sepsis. *Curr Opin Infect Dis* 2008;21(3):223–227.
5. Ash LR, Orihel TC. *Atlas of human parasitology*. Chicago: ASCP Press, 2007.
6. Banatvala JE, Brown DW. Rubella. *Lancet* 2004;363(9415):1127–1137.
7. Barbi M, Binda S, Caroppo S. Diagnosis of congenital CMV infection via dried blood spots. *Rev Med Virol* 2006;16(6):385–392.
8. Bartlett AH, et al. Thoracic actinomycosis in children: case report and review of the literature. *Pediatr Infect Dis J* 2008;27(2):165–169.
9. Beazley DM, Egerman RS. Toxoplasmosis. *Semin Perinatol* 1998;22(4):332–338.
10. Becroft DM. Prenatal cytomegalovirus infection: epidemiology, pathology and pathogenesis. *Perspect Pediatr Pathol* 1981;6:203–241.
11. Bern C, et al. Evaluation and treatment of chagas disease in the United States: a systematic review. *JAMA* 2007;298(18):2171–2181.
12. Bisgard KM, et al. Haemophilus influenzae invasive disease in the United States, 1994–1995: near disappearance of a vaccine-preventable-childhood disease. *Emerg Infect Dis* 1998;4(2):229–237.
13. Bitnun A, et al. Children hospitalized with severe acute respiratory syndrome-related illness in Toronto. *Pediatrics* 2003;112(4):e261.
14. Blanc W. Pathology of the placenta, membranes and umbilical cord. In: Kissane J, Naeye RL, Kaufman W, eds. *Perinatal diseases*. Baltimore: Williams & Wilkins, 1981:67–132.
15. Burns S, Hernandez-Reif M, Jessee P. A review of pediatric HIV effects on neurocognitive development. *Issues Compr Pediatr Nurs* 2008;31(3):107–121.
16. Butler JC, Heller R, Wright PF. Histoplasmosis during childhood. *South Med J* 1994;87(4):476–480.
17. Butler KM. Enterococcal infection in children. *Semin Pediatr Infect Dis* 2006;17(3):128–139.
18. Calis JC, et al. HIV-associated anemia in children: a systematic review from a global perspective. *AIDS* 2008;22(10):1099–1112.
19. Candy B, et al. Recovery from infectious mononucleosis: a case for more than symptomatic therapy? A systematic review. *Br J Gen Pract* 2002;52(483):844–851.
20. Cardoso TA, Navarro MB. Emerging and reemerging diseases in Brazil: data of a recent history of risks and uncertainties. *Braz J Infect Dis* 2007;11(4):430–434.
21. Carneiro SC, et al. Viral exanthems in the tropics. *Clin Dermatol* 2007;25(2):212–220.
22. Cerqueira TB, et al. Renal involvement in leptospirosis—new insights into pathophysiology and treatment. *Braz J Infect Dis* 2008;12(3):248–252.
23. Chen CJ, et al. Hemophagocytic syndrome: a review of 18 pediatric cases. *J Microbiol Immunol Infect* 2004;37(3):157–163.
24. Chomel BB. Zoonoses of house pets other than dogs, cats and birds. *Pediatr Infect Dis J* 1992;11(6):479–487.
25. Chugh TD. Emerging and re-emerging bacterial diseases in India. *J Biosci* 2008;33(4):549–555.
26. Cinatl J Jr, Michaelis M, Doerr HW. The threat of avian influenza A (H5N1). Part I: epidemiologic concerns and virulence determinants. *Med Microbiol Immunol* 2007;196(4):181–190.
27. Cinatl J Jr, Michaelis M, Doerr HW. The threat of avian influenza a (H5N1): part II: Clues to pathogenicity and pathology. *Med Microbiol Immunol* 2007;196(4):191–201.
28. Clapp DW. Developmental regulation of the immune system. *Semin Perinatol* 2006;30(2):69–72.
29. Cohen JI, et al. Current understanding of the role of Epstein-Barr virus in lymphomagenesis and therapeutic approaches to EBV-associated lymphomas. *Leuk Lymphoma* 2008;49(suppl 1):27–34.
30. Cohen JI, et al. Epstein-Barr virus-associated lymphoproliferative disease in non-immunocompromised hosts: a status report and summary of an international meeting, 8–9 September 2008. *Ann Oncol* 2009;20:1472–1482.
31. Connor BA, Schwartz E. Typhoid and paratyphoid fever in travellers. *Lancet Infect Dis* 2005;5(10):623–628.
32. Connor D, Chandler F, Manz H, eds. et al. *Pathology of infectious diseases*. Stamford, CT: Appleton and Lange, 1997.
33. Dahmer MK, et al. Genetic polymorphisms in sepsis. *Pediatr Crit Care Med* 2005;6(3 suppl):S61–S73.
34. Dammann O, et al. Antenatal mycoplasma infection, the fetal inflammatory response and cerebral white matter damage in very-low-birthweight infants. *Paediatr Perinat Epidemiol* 2003;17(1):49–57.
35. Darmstadt GL, Dinulos JG, Miller Z. Congenital cutaneous candidiasis: clinical presentation, pathogenesis, and management guidelines. *Pediatrics* 2000;105(2):438–444.
36. Darville T. Chlamydia trachomatis infections in neonates and young children. *Semin Pediatr Infect Dis* 2005;16(4):235–244.
37. D'Costa GF, Khadke K, Patil YV. Pathology of placenta in HIV infection. *Indian J Pathol Microbiol* 2007;50(3):515–519.
38. Delecluse HJ, et al. Epstein Barr virus-associated tumours: an update for the attention of the working pathologist. *J Clin Pathol* 2007;60(12):1358–1364.
39. Deligeoroglou E, et al. Infections of the lower female genital tract during childhood and adolescence. *Clin Exp Obstet Gynecol* 2004;31(3):175–178.
40. Deyrup AT. Epstein-Barr virus-associated epithelial and mesenchymal neoplasms. *Hum Pathol* 2008;39(4):473–483.
41. Diagnostic Standards and Classification of Tuberculosis in Adults and Children. This official statement of the American Thoracic Society and the Centers for Disease Control and Prevention was adopted by the ATS Board of Directors, July 1999. This statement

was endorsed by the Council of the Infectious Disease Society of America, September 1999. *Am J Respir Crit Care Med* 2000;161 (4 Pt 1):1376–1395.

42. Dickson DW, et al. Central nervous system pathology in pediatric AIDS. *Ann N Y Acad Sci* 1993;693:93–106.
43. Dolhnikoff M, et al. Pathology and pathophysiology of pulmonary manifestations in leptospirosis. *Braz J Infect Dis* 2007;11(1): 142–148.
44. Dong J, et al. Emerging pathogens: challenges and successes of molecular diagnostics. *J Mol Diagn* 2008;10(3):185–197.
45. Dowell SF, et al. Standardizing Chlamydia pneumoniae assays: recommendations from the Centers for Disease Control and Prevention (USA) and the Laboratory Centre for Disease Control (Canada). *Clin Infect Dis* 2001;33(4):492–503.
46. Drevets DA, Bronze MS. Listeria monocytogenes: epidemiology, human disease, and mechanisms of brain invasion. *FEMS Immunol Med Microbiol* 2008;53(2):151–165.
47. Dumler JS, et al. Ehrlichioses in humans: epidemiology, clinical presentation, diagnosis, and treatment. *Clin Infect Dis* 2007;45(suppl 1):S45–S51.
48. Dussurget O. New insights into determinants of Listeria monocytogenes virulence. *Int Rev Cell Mol Biol* 2008;270:1–38.
49. Dyson AE, Read SE. Group G streptococcal colonization and sepsis in neonates. *J Pediatr* 1981;99(6):944–947.
50. Ebell MH. Epstein-Barr virus infectious mononucleosis. *Am Fam Physician* 2004;70(7):1279–1287.
51. WHO Collaborative Study Team on the Role of Breastfeeding on the Prevention of Infant Mortality. Effect of breastfeeding on infant and child mortality due to infectious diseases in less developed countries: a pooled analysis. *Lancet* 2000;355(9202):451–455.
52. Egawa T, et al. Ureaplasma urealyticum and Mycoplasma hominis presence in umbilical cord is associated with pathogenesis of funisitis. *Kobe J Med Sci* 2007;53(5):241–249.
53. Esposito S, et al. Emerging role of Mycoplasma pneumoniae in children with acute pharyngitis. *Eur J Clin Microbiol Infect Dis* 2002;21(8):607–610.
54. Essary LR, et al. Frequency of parvovirus B19 infection in nonimmune hydrops fetalis and utility of three diagnostic methods. *Hum Pathol* 1998;29(7):696–701.
55. Farnsworth N, Rosen T. Endemic treponematosis: review and update. *Clin Dermatol* 2006;24(3):181–190.
56. Feigin RD, Cherry J, Demmler-Harrison GJ, eds, et al. *Feigen and Cherry's textbook of pediatric infectious diseases*, 6th ed. Philadelphia, PA: Saunders, 2009.
57. Feja K, Saiman L. Tuberculosis in children. *Clin Chest Med* 2005;26(2):295–312, vii.
58. Ferguson NE, et al. Bioterrorism web site resources for infectious disease clinicians and epidemiologists. *Clin Infect Dis* 2003;36(11): 1458–1473.
59. Ferrari ND III, Weisse ME. Botulism. *Adv Pediatr Infect Dis* 1995;10:81–91.
60. Forrest JM, et al. Gregg's congenital rubella patients 60 years later. *Med J Aust* 2002;177(11–12):664–667.
61. Franco MP, et al. Human brucellosis. *Lancet Infect Dis* 2007;7(12):775–786.
62. Garcia-de-Lomas J, Navarro D. New directions in diagnostics. *Pediatr Infect Dis J* 1997;16(3 suppl):S43–S48.
63. Gil AC, et al. Hepatotoxicity in HIV-infected children and adolescents on antiretroviral therapy. *Sao Paulo Med J* 2007;125(4): 205–209.
64. Goldenberg RL, et al. The Alabama Preterm Birth Study: diffuse decidual leukocytoclastic necrosis of the decidua basalis, a placental lesion associated with preeclampsia, indicated preterm birth and decreased fetal growth. *J Matern Fetal Neonatal Med* 2007;20(5):391–395.
65. Goldstein B, Giroir B, Randolph A. International pediatric sepsis consensus conference: definitions for sepsis and organ dysfunction in pediatrics. *Pediatr Crit Care Med* 2005;6(1):2–8.
66. Gotuzzo E, et al. Frequent HTLV-1 infection in the offspring of Peruvian women with HTLV-1-associated myelopathy/tropical spastic paraparesis or strongyloidiasis. *Rev Panam Salud Publica* 2007;22(4):223–230.
67. Gould EA, Solomon T. Pathogenic flaviviruses. *Lancet* 2008;371(9611):500–509.
68. Guarner J, et al. Pathology and pathogenesis of bioterrorism-related inhalational anthrax. *Am J Pathol* 2003;163(2):701–709.
69. Gulley ML, Tang W. Laboratory assays for Epstein-Barr virus-related disease. *J Mol Diagn* 2008;10(4):279–292.
70. Hahm B. Hostile communication of measles virus with host innate immunity and dendritic cells. *Curr Top Microbiol Immunol* 2009;330:271–287.
71. Halpin K, et al. Emerging viruses: coming in on a wrinkled wing and a prayer. *Clin Infect Dis* 2007;44(5):711–717.
72. Hammerschlag MR. *Chlamydia trachomatis* and *Chlamydia pneumoniae* infections in children and adolescents. *Pediatr Rev* 2004;25(2):43–51.
73. Hecht JL, et al. Characterization of chorioamnionitis in 2nd-trimester C-section placentas and correlation with microorganism recovery from subamniotic tissues. *Pediatr Dev Pathol* 2008;11(1):15–22.
74. Hercogova J, Vanousova D. Syphilis and borreliosis during pregnancy. *Dermatol Ther* 2008;21(3):205–209.
75. Higgins CD, et al. A study of risk factors for acquisition of Epstein-Barr virus and its subtypes. *J Infect Dis* 2007;195(4):474–82.
76. Hisada M, et al. Virus markers associated with vertical transmission of human T lymphotropic virus type 1 in Jamaica. *Clin Infect Dis* 2002;34(12):1551–1557.
77. Hoffman JA, et al. Streptococcus pneumoniae infections in the neonate. *Pediatrics* 2003;112(5):1095–1102.
78. Hoffner RJ, et al. Emergency department presentations of typhoid fever. *J Emerg Med* 2000;19(4):317–321.
79. Hollier LM, et al. Fetal syphilis: clinical and laboratory characteristics. *Obstet Gynecol* 2001;97(6):947–953.
80. Hon KL, et al. Clinical presentations and outcome of severe acute respiratory syndrome in children. *Lancet* 2003;361(9370):1701–1703.
81. Honma Y, et al. Certain type of chronic lung disease of newborns is associated with Ureaplasma urealyticum infection in utero. *Pediatr Int* 2007;49(4):479–484.
82. Intrauterine West Nile virus infection—New York, 2002. *MMWR Morb Mortal Wkly Rep* 2002;51(50):1135–1136.
83. Jain R, Goldman RD. Novel influenza A(H1N1): clinical presentation, diagnosis, and management. *Pediatr Emerg Care* 2009;25(11): 791–796.
84. Jeffery H, et al. Early neonatal bacteraemia: comparison of group B streptococcal, other Gram-positive and Gram-negative infections. *Arch Dis Child* 1977;52(9):683–686.
85. Jenson HB. Acute complications of Epstein-Barr virus infectious mononucleosis. *Curr Opin Pediatr* 2000;12(3):263–268.
86. Joshi VV, Oleske JM. Pulmonary lesions in children with the acquired immunodeficiency syndrome: a reappraisal based on data in additional cases and follow-up study of previously reported cases. *Hum Pathol* 1986;17(6):641–642.
87. Joshi VV, ed. *Pathology of AIDS and other manifestations of HIV infection*. New York: Igaku-Shoin, 1990:384.
88. Kabra SK, Lodha R, Hilton DJ. Antibiotics for preventing complications in children with measles. *Cochrane Database Syst Rev* 2008(3):CD001477.
89. Kalayanarooj S, Nimmannitya S. Clinical presentations of dengue hemorrhagic fever in infants compared to children. *J Med Assoc Thai* 2003;86(suppl 3):S673–S680.
90. Kamath SR, Ranjit S. Clinical features, complications and atypical manifestations of children with severe forms of dengue hemorrhagic fever in South India. *Indian J Pediatr* 2006;73(10):889–895.
91. Kancherla VS, Hanson IC. Mumps resurgence in the United States. *J Allergy Clin Immunol* 2006;118(4):938–941.
92. Kaplan C. The placenta and viral infections. *Semin Diagn Pathol* 1993;10(3):232–250.

93. Kaplan SL. Community-acquired methicillin-resistant *Staphylococcus aureus* infections in children. *Semin Pediatr Infect Dis* 2006;17(3):113–119.
94. Kenzel S, Henneke P. The innate immune system and its relevance to neonatal sepsis. *Curr Opin Infect Dis* 2006;19(3):264–270.
95. Khanna M, et al. Emerging influenza virus: a global threat. *J Biosci* 2008;33(4):475–482.
96. Kimberlin DW. Neonatal herpes simplex infection. *Clin Microbiol Rev* 2004;17(1):1–13.
97. Klein JO, Remington JS. Current concepts of infections of the fetus and newborn infant. In: Remington JS, Klein, JO, eds. *Infectious diseases of the fetus and newborn infant.* Philadelphia, PA: W.B. Saunders, 2001:1–24.
98. Koirala J. Plague: disease, management, and recognition of act of terrorism. *Infect Dis Clin North Am* 2006;20(2):273–287, viii.
99. Lacroix J, Cotting J. Severity of illness and organ dysfunction scoring in children. *Pediatr Crit Care Med* 2005;6(3 suppl):S126–S134.
100. Lam HS, Ng PC. Biochemical markers of neonatal sepsis. *Pathology* 2008;40(2):141–148.
101. Landers CD, Chelvarajan RL, Bondada S. The role of B cells and accessory cells in the neonatal response to TI-2 antigens. *Immunol Res* 2005;31(1):25–36.
102. Landesman SH, et al. The Women and Infants Transmission Study. Obstetrical factors and the transmission of human immunodeficiency virus type 1 from mother to child. *N Engl J Med* 1996;334(25): 1617–1623.
103. Laufer MK, et al. Observational cohort study of HIV-infected African children. *Pediatr Infect Dis J* 2006;25(7):623–627.
104. Lawrence RM, Lawrence RA. Breast milk and infection. *Clin Perinatol* 2004;31(3):501–528.
105. Lewinsohn DA, et al. Tuberculosis immunology in children: diagnostic and therapeutic challenges and opportunities. *Int J Tuberc Lung Dis* 2004;8(5):658–674.
106. Ligon BL. Dengue fever and dengue hemorrhagic fever: a review of the history, transmission, treatment, and prevention. *Semin Pediatr Infect Dis* 2005;16(1):60–65.
107. Ligon BL. Infectious diseases that pose specific challenges after natural disasters: a review. *Semin Pediatr Infect Dis* 2006;17(1):36–45.
108. Luce WA, Hoffman TM, Bauer JA. Bench-to-bedside review: developmental influences on the mechanisms, treatment and outcomes of cardiovascular dysfunction in neonatal versus adult sepsis. *Crit Care* 2007;11(5):228.
109. Maloney SA, Weinberg M. Prevention of infectious diseases among international pediatric travelers: considerations for clinicians. *Semin Pediatr Infect Dis* 2004;15(3):137–149.
110. Maltezou HC, Spyridis P, Kafetzis DA. Extra-pulmonary tuberculosis in children. *Arch Dis Child* 2000;83(4):342–346.
111. Mandalakas AM, Starke JR. Current concepts of childhood tuberculosis. *Semin Pediatr Infect Dis* 2005;16(2):93–104.
112. Marais BJ, et al. The natural history of childhood intra-thoracic tuberculosis: a critical review of literature from the pre-chemotherapy era. *Int J Tuberc Lung Dis* 2004;8(4):392–402.
113. Martin JM, Green M. Group A streptococcus. *Semin Pediatr Infect Dis* 2006;17(3):140–148.
114. McCulloch MI, Ray PE. Kidney disease in HIV-positive children. *Semin Nephrol* 2008;28(6):585–594.
115. Meyer MA. Neurologic complications of anthrax: a review of the literature. *Arch Neurol* 2003;60(4):483–488.
116. Mofenson LM, et al. Pediatric AIDS Clinical Trials Group Study 185 Team. Risk factors for perinatal transmission of human immunodeficiency virus type 1 in women treated with zidovudine. *N Engl J Med* 1999;341(6):385–393.
117. Montoya JG, Liesenfeld O. Toxoplasmosis. *Lancet* 2004;363 (9425):1965–1976.
118. Moran C, Mullick FG, ed. *Systemic pathology of HIV infection and AIDS in children.* Washington, D.C.: Armed Forces Institute of Pathology, 1997:325.
119. Morrison G. Zoonotic infections from pets: understanding the risks and treatment. *Postgrad Med* 2001;110(1):24–26, 29–30, 35–36 passim.
120. Moss WJ, Griffin DE. Global measles elimination. *Nat Rev Microbiol* 2006;4(12):900–908.
121. Mullegger RR. Dermatological manifestations of Lyme borreliosis. *Eur J Dermatol* 2004;14(5):296–309.
122. Mussap M, Molinari MP, Senno E, et al. New diagnostic tools for neonatal sepsis: the role of a real-time polymerase chain reaction for the early detection and identification of bacterial and fungal species in blood samples. *J Chemother* 2007;19(suppl 2):31–34.
123. Mylonakis E, Hohmann EL, Calderwood SB. Central nervous system infection with Listeria monocytogenes. 33 years' experience at a general hospital and review of 776 episodes from the literature. *Medicine (Baltimore)* 1998;77(5):313–336.
124. Mylonakis E, et al. Listeriosis during pregnancy: a case series and review of 222 cases. *Medicine (Baltimore)* 2002;81(4):260–269.
125. Naessens A, et al. Diagnosis of congenital toxoplasmosis in the neonatal period: A multicenter evaluation. *J Pediatr* 1999;135(6): 714–719.
126. Nelson LJ, Wells CD. Global epidemiology of childhood tuberculosis. *Int J Tuberc Lung Dis* 2004;8(5):636–647.
127. Nelson LJ, et al. Epidemiology of childhood tuberculosis in the United States, 1993–2001: the need for continued vigilance. *Pediatrics* 2004;114(2):333–341.
128. Neumann G, Noda T, Kawaoka Y. Emergence and pandemic potential of swine-origin H1N1 influenza virus. *Nature* 2009;459(7249):931–939.
129. Nicoll A. Children: avian influenza H5N1 and preparing for the next pandemic. *Arch Dis Child* 2008;93(5):433–438.
130. Nizet V. Understanding how leading bacterial pathogens subvert innate immunity to reveal novel therapeutic targets. *J Allergy Clin Immunol* 2007;120(1):13–22.
131. Ohshima K, et al. Proposed categorization of pathological states of EBV-associated T/natural killer-cell lymphoproliferative disorder (LPD) in children and young adults: overlap with chronic active EBV infection and infantile fulminant EBV T-LPD. *Pathol Int* 2008;58(4):209–217.
132. Orange JS. Congenital immunodeficiencies and sepsis. *Pediatr Crit Care Med* 2005;6(3 suppl):S99–S107.
133. Ormerod P. Tuberculosis in pregnancy and the puerperium. *Thorax* 2001;56(6):494–499.
134. Ortiz AM, Silvestri G. Immunopathogenesis of AIDS. *Curr Infect Dis Rep* 2009;11(3):239–245.
135. Othman N, et al. Mycoplasma pneumoniae infection in a clinical setting. *Pediatr Int* 2008;50(5):662–666.
136. Parish JL. Treponemal infections in the pediatric population. *Clin Dermatol* 2000;18(6):687–700.
137. Pass RF. Cytomegalovirus infection. *Pediatr Rev* 2002;23(5):163–170.
138. Patt HA, Feigin RD. Diagnosis and management of suspected cases of bioterrorism: a pediatric perspective. *Pediatrics* 2002;109(4):685–692.
139. Peeling RW, Hook EW III. The pathogenesis of syphilis: the Great Mimicker, revisited. *J Pathol* 2006;208(2):224–232.
140. Petersen LR, Marfin AA. West Nile virus: a primer for the clinician. *Ann Intern Med* 2002;137(3):173–179.
141. Pfeiffer H, Varchmin-Schultheiss K, Brinkmann B. Sudden death in childhood due to varicella pneumonia: a forensic case report with clinical implications. *Int J Legal Med* 2006;120(1):33–35.
142. Porta FS, et al. Tick-borne lymphadenopathy: a new infectious disease in children. *Pediatr Infect Dis J* 2008;27(7):618–622.
143. Potts JA, Rothman AL. Clinical and laboratory features that distinguish dengue from other febrile illnesses in endemic populations. *Trop Med Int Health* 2008;13(11):1328–1340.
144. Quijano G, Siminovich M, Drut R. Histopathologic findings in the lymphoid and reticuloendothelial system in pediatric HIV infection: a postmortem study. *Pediatr Pathol Lab Med* 1997;17(6):845–856.

145. Raghunath D. Smallpox revisited. *Curr Sci* 2002;83(5):566–576.
146. Rawlinson WD, et al. Viruses and other infections in stillbirth: what is the evidence and what should we be doing? *Pathology* 2008;40(2):149–160.
147. Ray PE. Taking a hard look at the pathogenesis of childhood HIV-associated nephropathy. *Pediatr Nephrol* 2009;24(11):2109–2119.
148. Read JS. Diagnosis of HIV-1 infection in children younger than 18 months in the United States. *Pediatrics* 2007;120(6):e1547–e1562.
149. Read JS. American Academy of Pediatrics Committee on Pediatric AIDS. Human milk, breastfeeding, and transmission of human immunodeficiency virus type 1 in the United States. *Pediatrics* 2003;112(5):1196–1205.
150. Recommendations of the Hospital Infection Control Practices Advisory Committee (HICPAC). Recommendations for preventing the spread of vancomycin resistance. *MMWR Recomm Rep* 1995;44(RR-12):1–13.
151. Recommendations from an ad hoc Meeting of the WHO Measles and Rubella Laboratory Network (LabNet) on use of alternative diagnostic samples for measles and rubella surveillance. *MMWR Morb Mortal Wkly Rep* 2008;57(24):657–660.
152. American Academy of Pediatrics Committee on Infectious Diseases and Committee on Fetus and Newborn. Revised guidelines for prevention of early-onset group B streptococcal (GBS) infection. *Pediatrics* 1997;99(3):489–496.
153. Rezk SA, Weiss LM. Epstein-Barr virus-associated lymphoproliferative disorders. *Hum Pathol* 2007;38(9):1293–1304.
154. Rivera LB, et al. Predictors of hearing loss in children with symptomatic congenital cytomegalovirus infection. *Pediatrics* 2002;110(4):762–767.
155. Robertson CM, Coopersmith CM. The systemic inflammatory response syndrome. *Microbes Infect* 2006;8(5):1382–1389.
156. Rosenberg HS, Oppenheimer EH, Esterly JR. Congenital rubella syndrome: the late effects and their relation to early lesions. *Perspect Pediatr Pathol* 1981;6:183–202.
157. Ross SA, Boppana SB. Congenital cytomegalovirus infection: outcome and diagnosis. *Semin Pediatr Infect Dis* 2005;16(1):44–49.
158. Sanchez-Vargas FM, Gomez-Duarte OG. Mycoplasma pneumoniae-an emerging extra-pulmonary pathogen. *Clin Microbiol Infect* 2008;14(2):105–117.
159. Sangoi AR, et al. Challenges and pitfalls of morphologic identification of fungal infections in histologic and cytologic specimens: a ten-year retrospective review at a single institution. *Am J Clin Pathol* 2009;131(3):364–375.
160. Schleiss MR. Acquisition of human cytomegalovirus infection in infants via breast milk: natural immunization or cause for concern? *Rev Med Virol* 2006;16(2):73–82.
161. Schneider E, et al. Revised surveillance case definitions for HIV infection among adults, adolescents, and children aged <18 months and for HIV infection and AIDS among children aged 18 months to <13 years—United States, 2008. *MMWR Recomm Rep* 2008;57 (RR-10):1–12.
162. Schutze GE, Buckingham SC, Marshall GS, et al. Tick-borne Infections in Children Study (TICS) Group. Human monocytic ehrlichiosis in children. *Pediatr Infect Dis J* 2007;26(6):475–479.
163. Schutze GE, et al. Blastomycosis in children. *Clin Infect Dis* 1996;22(3):496–502.
164. Schuval S, et al. Hepatitis C prevalence in children with perinatal human immunodeficiency virus infection enrolled in a long-term follow-up protocol. *Arch Pediatr Adolesc Med* 2004;158(10):1007–1013.
165. See LL. Bloodstream infection in children. *Pediatr Crit Care Med* 2005;6(3 suppl):S42–S44.
166. Shah I. Age related clinical manifestations of HIV infection in Indian children. *J Trop Pediatr* 2005;51(5):300–303.
167. Shapiro ED. Lyme disease in children. *Am J Med* 1995;98(4A):69S–73S.
168. Sheffield JS, et al. Placental histopathology of congenital syphilis. *Obstet Gynecol* 2002;100(1):126–133.
169. Shek CC, et al. Infants born to mothers with severe acute respiratory syndrome. *Pediatrics* 2003;112(4):e254.
170. Siegel JD, McCracken GH Jr. Group D streptococcal infections. *J Pediatr* 1978;93(3):542–543.
171. Siegel JD, McCracken GH Jr. Sepsis neonatorum. *N Engl J Med* 1981;304(11):642–647.
172. Singh HK, et al. The Indian pediatric HIV epidemic: a systematic review. *Curr HIV Res* 2008;6(5):419–432.
173. Skogman BH, et al. Lyme neuroborreliosis in children: a prospective study of clinical features, prognosis, and outcome. *Pediatr Infect Dis J* 2008;27(12):1089–1094.
174. Smith-Slatas CL, Bourque M, Salazar JC. Clostridium septicum infections in children: a case report and review of the literature. *Pediatrics* 2006;117(4):e796–e805.
175. Stein RA. Lessons from outbreaks of H1N1 influenza. *Ann Intern Med* 2009;151(1)59–62.
176. Stirling J, et al. Zoonoses associated with petting farms and open zoos. *Vector Borne Zoonotic Dis* 2008;8(1):85–92.
177. Stocker JT. Clinical and pathologic differential diagnosis of selected potential bioterrorism agents of interest to pediatric health care providers. *Clin Lab Med* 2006;26(2):329–344, viii.
178. Strobino BA, et al. Lyme disease and pregnancy outcome: a prospective study of two thousand prenatal patients. *Am J Obstet Gynecol* 1993;169(2 Pt 1):367–374.
179. Strunk T, Burgner D. Genetic susceptibility to neonatal infection. *Curr Opin Infect Dis* 2006;19(3):259–263.
180. Timitilli A, et al. Unusual manifestations of infections due to Mycoplasma pneumoniae in children. *Infez Med* 2004;12(2):113–117.
181. Torrico F, et al. Maternal *Trypanosoma cruzi* infection, pregnancy outcome, morbidity, and mortality of congenitally infected and non-infected newborns in Bolivia. *Am J Trop Med Hyg* 2004;70(2):201–209.
182. Trends in perinatal group B streptococcal disease—United States, 2000–2006. *MMWR Morb Mortal Wkly Rep* 2009;58(5):109–112.
183. Udani PM. BCG vaccination in India and tuberculosis in children: newer facets. *Indian J Pediatr* 1994;61(5):451–462.
184. van der Poll T, Opal SM. Host-pathogen interactions in sepsis. *Lancet Infect Dis* 2008;8(1):32–43.
185. Velasco-Benitez CA. Digestive, hepatic, and nutritional manifestations in Latin American children with HIV/AIDS. *J Pediatr Gastroenterol Nutr* 2008;47(suppl 1):S24–S26.
186. Venkatesh MP, Placencia F, Weisman LE. Coagulase-negative staphylococcal infections in the neonate and child: an update. *Semin Pediatr Infect Dis* 2006;17(3):120–127.
187. Vijayachari P, Sugunan AP, Shriram AN. Leptospirosis: an emerging global public health problem. *J Biosci* 2008;33(4):557–569.
188. Vogel H, et al. Congenital parvovirus infection. *Pediatr Pathol Lab Med* 1997;17(6):903–912.
189. Waites KB, Talkington DF. Mycoplasma pneumoniae and its role as a human pathogen. *Clin Microbiol Rev* 2004;17(4):697–728.
190. Walker DH, Paddock CD, Dumler JS. Emerging and re-emerging tick-transmitted rickettsial and ehrlichial infections. *Med Clin North Am* 2008;92(6):1345–1361, x.
191. Walsh TJ, et al. Invasive fungal infections in children: recent advances in diagnosis and treatment. *Adv Pediatr Infect Dis* 1996;11:187–290.
192. Webster WS. Teratogen update: congenital rubella. *Teratology* 1998;58(1):13–23.
193. Wharton M, et al. Supplemental recommendations of the Advisory Committee on Immunization Practices (ACIP) and the Healthcare Infection Control Practices Advisory Committee (HICPAC). Recommendations for using smallpox vaccine in a pre-event vaccination program. *MMWR Recomm Rep* 2003;52(RR-7):1–16.
194. *WHO HIV and infant feeding technical consultation—consensus statement, 2007*. Geneva: World Health Organization, 2007:5.
195. Wolfson LJ, et al. Estimates of measles case fatality ratios: a comprehensive review of community-based studies. *Int J Epidemiol* 2009;38(1):192–205.

196. Woods CR. Syphilis in children: congenital and acquired. *Semin Pediatr Infect Dis* 2005;16(4):245–257.
197. Wormser GP, et al. The clinical assessment, treatment, and prevention of lyme disease, human granulocytic anaplasmosis, and babesiosis: clinical practice guidelines by the Infectious Diseases Society of America. *Clin Infect Dis* 2006;43(9):1089–1134.
198. Ye P, Kirschner DE, Kourtis AP. The thymus during HIV disease: role in pathogenesis and in immune recovery. *Curr HIV Res* 2004;2(2): 177–183.
199. Yis U, et al. Mycoplasma pneumoniae: nervous system complications in childhood and review of the literature. *Eur J Pediatr* 2008;167(9):973–978.
200. Young VA, Rall GF. Making it to the synapse: measles virus spread in and among neurons. *Curr Top Microbiol Immunol* 2009; 330:3–30.

CHAPTER 7

Pediatric Forensic Pathology

TRACEY S. COREY
KIM A. COLLINS

Jurisdictions for forensic deaths vary between states, and often between counties within each state. In the medical examiner systems of some states, pathologists investigate deaths. In others, the investigator of deaths is the coroner, an elected lay official who often has no medical background. Some states have dual systems. Regardless of the particular system, modern death investigation involves forensic science, which is the application of physical sciences to legal matters. The numerous facets of forensic science include trace evidence, ballistics, forensic anthropology, forensic odontology, DNA analysis and serology, toxicology and drug identification, and forensic pathology. Depending on the case, different aspects of forensic science are employed. Forensic pathology is the study and investigation of bodily disease, injury, and death. The majority of cases referred to a forensic pathologist are postmortems. In these cases, the cause and manner of death are the usual focus. The cause of death is the disease or injury that initiates the sequence of events resulting in death. The manner of death refers to the circumstances under which the disease or injury occurred. Death can be categorized into five manners: natural, homicidal, suicidal, accidental, and undetermined. Natural deaths are solely the result of disease. Accidental deaths result from an unforeseen event or action with no harm intended. Homicides are deaths in which one person takes the life of another with an intended action, even though the intended result may not be death. Suicide is the taking of one's own life through a deliberate, self-inflicted action. A death is classified as undetermined when the evidence is insufficient for a manner to be assigned. Pediatric deaths can fall into any of the five categories. Usually, pediatric deaths are natural, especially during the first year of life, but a significant percentage is due to accidents or, unfortunately, homicides (63). Accidental deaths are more prevalent once children reach the toddler stage, and accidents continue to be the leading manner of death in persons up to the age of 18 (18). Causes of accidental death include asphyxia, as in drowning and choking, motor vehicle crashes, and recreational drug toxicity. At around the age of fourteen, we see the percentage of natural deaths decreases with accident, homicide, and suicide as the common manner of death in descending order (18,63). Many do not perceive that suicide occurs in this young age group. However, pediatric suicide rates have been increasing during the past two decades (185). Violent deaths (accident, homicide, and suicide) are challenging, and their classification requires expertise in the area of forensic pathology.

The investigation of the death scene is an important component of forensic pathology. Usually, such an investigation is conducted with law enforcement officials and, when applicable, the coroner or medical examiner. The death scene investigation provides an opportunity for the pathologist to view the incident site undisturbed, examine the body in its terminal state, and note its position and postmortem changes. This is also the preferred time to obtain an accurate history and interview family members or caretakers. At the death scene, the surroundings can be assessed [e.g., cleanliness, food, appearance of other family members, presence of animals or infestation, toys, furniture and surfaces (important in cases of falls), sleep location of the child and other family members, ambient temperature, water supply (in cases of scalds), dangerous objects, chemicals/drugs/medications]. Photographs should be taken of the immediate surroundings and of the body in its terminal location. Any items at the scene constituting potential evidence should be procured. Many times, the body is not at the scene because of prior transportation to a hospital. The scene has been disturbed and possibly altered, but valuable information may still be obtained by investigation. If present, the body is photographed and examined. The body position and postmortem changes (described later), any blood or froth, evidence of the body having been moved, clothing and bedding, nearby objects, and any medical intervention by emergency medical teams should be documented. Trace evidence, such as blood spots, hair, fibers, particulate matter, and semen, may be on the body and should be procured before the body is transported for autopsy. All information gained from the scene investigation will be correlated with the autopsy findings to assign the cause and manner of death accurately.

The primary investigative tool of the forensic pathologist is the autopsy. The best forensic autopsy is a complete autopsy, which includes examination of the brain. The external assessment begins with photographs and measurement of the growth indices. Special studies such as radiology and ultraviolet photography may be utilized. Postmortem changes are documented and interpreted at this time. These include rigor mortis, livor mortis, algor mortis, and changes of decomposition. Rigor mortis is the stiffening of the muscles after death secondary to the crosslinking of actin and myosin to form actomyosin as the ATP levels fall. The process begins soon after death (~2 hours); however, most studies of rigor and postmortem intervals have been performed on adults. Livor mortis is the pooling of blood with gravity when the circulation ceases. The lividity pattern depends on the position of the body after death. In adults, lividity appears within half an hour after death and becomes "fixed" after approximately 12 hours. Before this time, if the body is moved, the livor pattern can change as the blood redistributes according to gravity and points of pressure. Algor mortis is the cooling of the body. Determining the postmortem interval by means of the postmortem temperature is inaccurate. The rate of body cooling is affected by numerous variables, both between individuals and within the environment. Decomposition is a combination of autolysis and putrefaction—autolysis from internal cell breakdown and putrefaction from the action of bacteria and fungi. The rate and appearance of decomposition vary between environments. *In utero* within the amniotic sac, aseptic autolysis, or maceration, can occur (274). In cases of maceration, the fetus exhibits erythematous skin, sloughing epidermis, and overriding skull bones as the brain becomes liquefied. Fetal putrefaction may also be seen if the amniotic fluid or fetus is no longer sterile (274). Another postmortem change is adipocere, the formation of a waxy substance of fatty acids derived from the hydrolysis and hydrogenation of body fat. This process is largely attributed to *Clostridium perfringens* and most often occurs when a body is immersed. Other postmortem changes may include insect activity, marine activity, and animal activity (anthropophagy). Postmortem changes, external and internal gross findings, and the results of histopathology, laboratory, and ancillary studies are integrated into the final forensic autopsy report (48,59,62). The forensic autopsy provides answers to questions concerning the cause and manner of death, and it also provides an opportunity to determine the time of death and the body position, gather evidence, procure specimens for toxicology/chemistry/DNA analysis/metabolic testing, and correlate findings with the history (48,59,171,200). The pediatric autopsy, discussed below, is a specialized form of the forensic autopsy that is modified for each individual case.

THE PEDIATRIC FORENSIC AUTOPSY: HOW IT DIFFERS FROM THE HOSPITAL AUTOPSY

The pediatric forensic autopsy may involve procedures that are not performed by most hospital-based pathologists. One must remember that the focus and purpose of such an autopsy are very different from those of an autopsy performed after an attended, in-house, natural death. The forensic autopsy is conducted in an attempt to answer legal as well as medical questions. The main goals of the pediatric forensic autopsy are to establish the cause and manner of the death and, in certain instances, the identity of the child. Other goals are to document and interpret traumatic injuries, procure specimens for ancillary studies, and collect trace evidence (48,59,62,171).

Documentation and Collection of Trace Evidence and Clothing

Unlike the standard in-house autopsy, the forensic autopsy should include a detailed description of the clothing and personal effects of the decedent. A description of the clothing and its disposition is included in the autopsy protocol. Any external trace evidence, such as fibers and hairs adherent to the body, should be collected before the body is transferred to the autopsy table. It is recommended that a sample of scalp hair be removed and retained because in fatal cases of abuse with head trauma, an impact site containing scalp hair may be subsequently identified at the scene of injury. A record of chain of custody of any evidence must be maintained, and persons receiving evidence from the pathologist should sign a receipt for such evidence.

One must keep in mind that trace evidence may take many forms and can even include the presence of maggots. Good estimates of the time of death of a decomposed body may be obtained from the forensic entomologist who studies the insects that normally feed on human remains. From the succession of insects (maggots and beetles) infesting a body, the forensic entomologist can estimate the amount of time that a body has been infested under specific conditions. The estimate is based on the type and stage of maturity of the insects present. An accurate estimate requires the proper collection and preservation of evidence. Maggot infestation of a diaper and perineal region has been successfully used to estimate the time of abandonment of a living child (117).

Documentation of External Evidence of Injury

The forensic autopsy must include a detailed narrative account of any injuries present on the external body surface. Cutaneous manifestations of abuse may be the most striking visual evidence presented. If documented properly, such evidence may be used in a court of law and presented to a jury. If improperly documented, the evidence may be lost forever or considered "too inflammatory" for jury viewing. Therefore, a clear understanding of the proper documentation of cutaneous evidence of physical abuse is a prerequisite for any medical personnel who investigate death and injury in children.

Injuries in children that are suggestive or diagnostic of physical abuse should be documented in multiple forms—narrative, photographic, and diagrammatic. When injuries are described in written form, precise terminology should be employed. Terms that are used colloquially in an emergency care setting should be avoided.

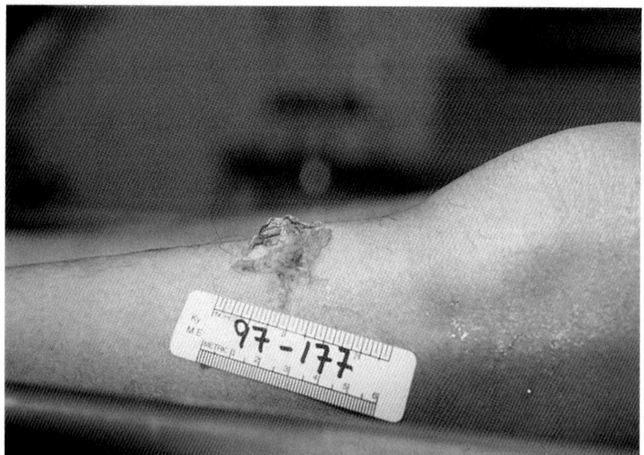

FIGURE 7-1 ■ Abrasion. A blunt force injury on the anterolateral leg. In this example, the direction of force can be determined from observation of the intact, rolled skin edge anteriorly. The force progressed posteriorly to anteriorly.

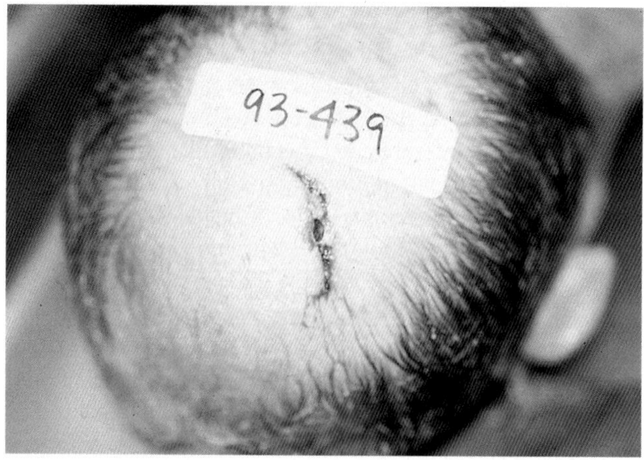

FIGURE 7-3 ■ Laceration, a blunt force injury.

Examples of blunt force injury include abrasion, contusion, and laceration. An abrasion (Figure 7-1) is the blunt removal of the upper layers of skin. Simply put, it is a scrape. The direction of force of an abrasion may sometimes be determined by observing a "rolled edge" of intact but displaced epidermis at the far end of the abrasion. A contusion, or bruise, is bleeding beneath intact skin at the site of a blunt impact. This differs from an ecchymosis, in which blood dissects through tissue planes to a site distant from the origin of the bleeding. An ecchymosis commonly occurs in the periorbital area in association with a basilar skull fracture (Figure 7-2). A laceration (Figure 7-3) is a specific term used to denote a tissue defect created by blunt force. A laceration can be differentiated from a sharp force injury by the presence of abraded wound margins or tissue bridging within the wound bed.

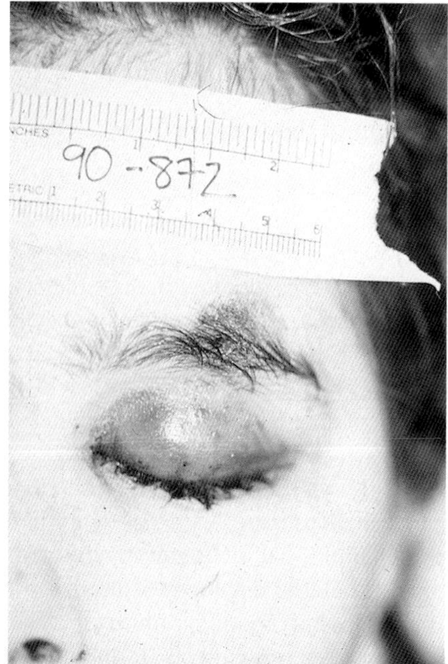

FIGURE 7-2 ■ Periorbital ecchymosis secondary to a fracture of the orbital roof caused by a gunshot wound to the eyebrow region.

Special mention should be made of the documentation of bite marks. The surface of a bite mark should be swabbed immediately with a sterile cotton applicator moistened with sterile water or saline solution to collect any saliva that may be on the skin surface. A control swab from another area of the body should be prepared at the same time. Bite marks generally appear as pattern contusions, often with multifocal overlying superficial abrasions (Figure 7-4). Some bite marks are of sufficient detail that, with proper documentation and subsequent examination and dental impressions of a suspect, a forensic odontologist may be able to identify a perpetrator or eliminate a suspect. These injuries must be carefully documented. If possible, the forensic odontologist should be called to the autopsy suite to view the injury firsthand and document it. If the forensic odontologist cannot attend the autopsy, the prosecting pathologist should discuss proper and preferred documentation of the injury with the forensic odontologist. The bite mark should be photographed at 90 degrees, with a linear scale included in the picture.

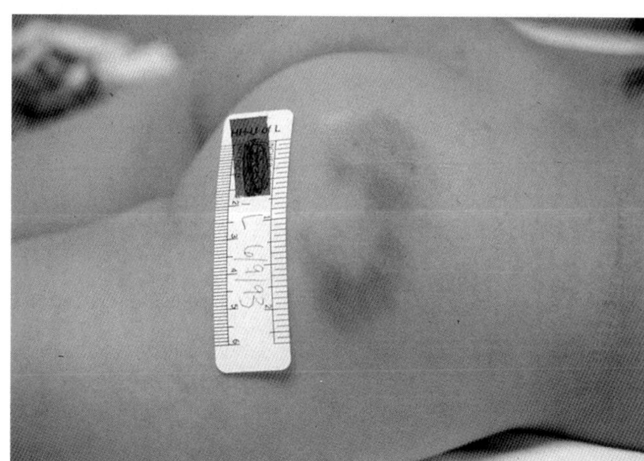

FIGURE 7-4 ■ Human bite mark on the buttock of a toddler.

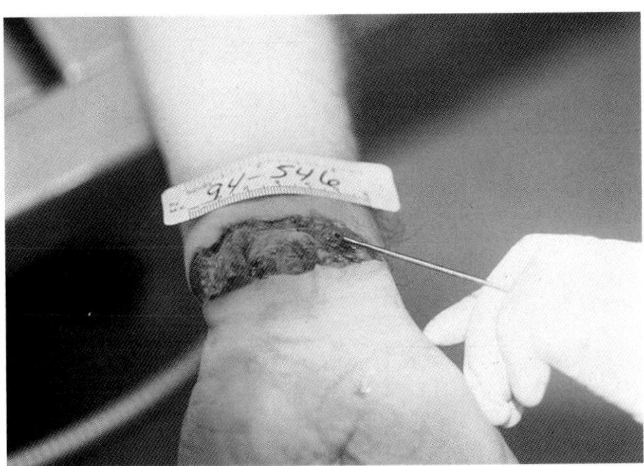

FIGURE 7-5 ▪ Incision of the wrist, a sharp force injury that is longer than it is deep.

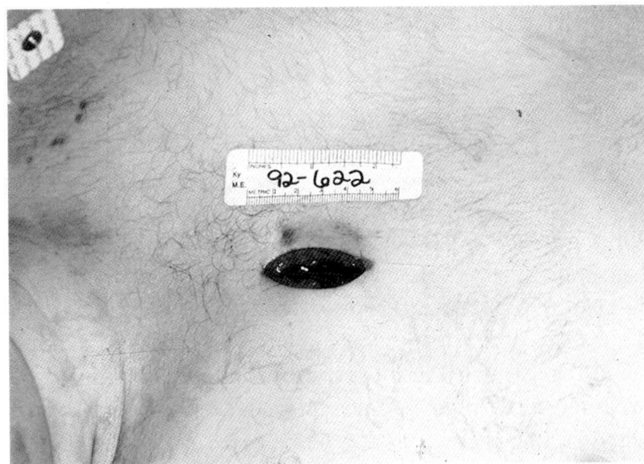

FIGURE 7-6 ▪ Stab wound of the chest, a sharp force injury that is deeper than it is long. The contusion adjacent to the stab wound is consistent with blunt force injury created by the knife handle.

A sharp force injury is created by a cutting instrument, such as a knife, scissors, or a piece of glass. The two main types of sharp force injury are the incision, a sharp force injury that is longer than it is deep, and the stab wound, which is deeper than it is long (Figures 7-5 and 7-6). In general, sharp force injuries have "clean" wound edges, without abrasions. On inspection, the wound bed displays a uniform, sharp demarcation of injured tissue on one side or the other, without the bridges of tissue of varying strength that are present in the wound depths of a laceration. It is important to adhere to a strict and precise use of terminology so that any reader at any time can recognize immediately the forces that created various described injuries. Such "universality" of terms facilitates meaningful discussions.

The injury location should be described in relation to a stable anatomic landmark. Examples of stable anatomic landmarks on the head include the external auditory canal, bridge of the nose, and occipital protuberance. Examples of stable anatomic landmarks on other areas of the body include the sternal notch, midline of the body, and heel. The general region of the body should also be noted (e.g., "the left frontal hair-bearing scalp"). When injuries over the extremities are documented, the body surfaces should be described with the body in the standard anatomic position. Each injury or injury cluster should be measured, and the number, shape, and color should be noted. General, nonspecific statements (e.g., "there are bruises on the face") are unacceptable and should be avoided.

If possible, the injuries should be documented photographically. Some type of linear scale and case identifier should be included in the photographs. An identifier may consist of a case number or initials with a date; use of a full name is discouraged. If available, a color standard may be useful when an attempt is made to delineate contusion colors at a later date. Areas notable for an absence of injury (e.g., the atraumatic shins of a preschooler) should also be photographically documented.

In living children, because variations in color and pattern may be observed as injuries heal, the use of sequential photography over several days should be considered. This may allow the emergence of faint or subtle patterns to be identified. Sequential documentation also allows the examiner to observe variations in healing patterns.

When injuries are photographed, attempts should be made to remove or cover extraneous and distracting objects or body parts (e.g., intravenous tubing, genitalia) from the photographic field. Usually, simple draping of the surrounding areas with surgical towels or sheets will suffice (Figure 7-7). A ring flash is useful in the documentation of small areas of injury and provides uniform lighting.

A collection of standard diagrams of the total body and specific anatomic regions should be kept on hand (Appendices 7 to 10). Quick sketching and notes on these diagrams provide a handy reference when a case is reviewed. If photographic documentation is not available or fails, these diagrams will be the only visual documentation of injury. Such diagrams may be useful in an attempt to explain the overall distribution of injury.

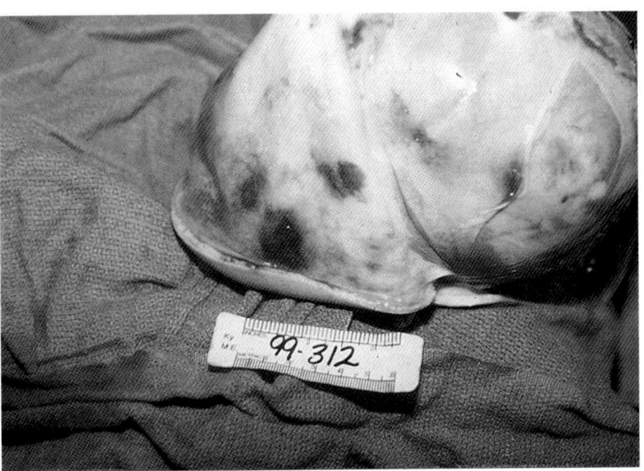

FIGURE 7-7 ▪ Multiple blunt impact sites of the scalp. The surrounding body parts are draped with surgical towels.

Autopsy Techniques and Procedures

The forensic autopsy begins with a thorough inspection of the external body surface. The body is examined from head to toe three separate times. First, traumatic injuries are described and documented from head to foot. It is helpful to describe injuries in separate paragraphs based on the anatomic regions of the body (e.g., injuries of the head listed first in one paragraph, then injuries of the anterior torso in a separate paragraph); such organization facilitates quick review and understanding at a later date. It must be remembered that all body surfaces must be viewed, including the intraoral mucosa, axillae, genitalia, posterior aspect of the body, and anus (Figure 7-8). Next, all evidence of medical treatment is documented. Lastly, a general external description is recorded.

In a forensic autopsy, it is often necessary to perform dissections and incisions other than the standard "Y incision" and scalp reflection. The soft tissues are reflected on the dorsal surface of the body, and incisions are made along the long axes of the extremities. Otherwise, the extent of soft tissue trauma in areas like the buttocks may not be visible, particularly in children with dark pigmentation (Figure 7-9). Such a dissection does not interfere with the undertaker's preparations; the incisions are on the posterior aspect of the body and can be closed at the completion of the autopsy. The dissection may be continued as a posterior neck dissection. The methodology of such a procedure has been detailed in the forensic literature (3). A posterior neck dissection may elucidate otherwise occult trauma in victims of abuse, especially those with inflicted head trauma (33,50).

In suspected abuse cases, a multiple-film "skeletal survey" before the postmortem dissection is strongly recommended. A standard, single-film "baby-gram" is insufficient and will not elucidate injuries common in cases of abuse, such as metaphyseal fractures (129,186,187,200). In fact, a skeletal survey should be conducted on all suspected victims of abuse under the age of 2 years. In older children, "spot films" dictated by history, signs, or symptoms may be sufficient. If feasible, postmortem neuroradiologic imaging with computed tomography or magnetic resonance imaging may also be useful (133,143). During the autopsy, the fractures in question may be excised for further radiologic and histologic examination (168,328).

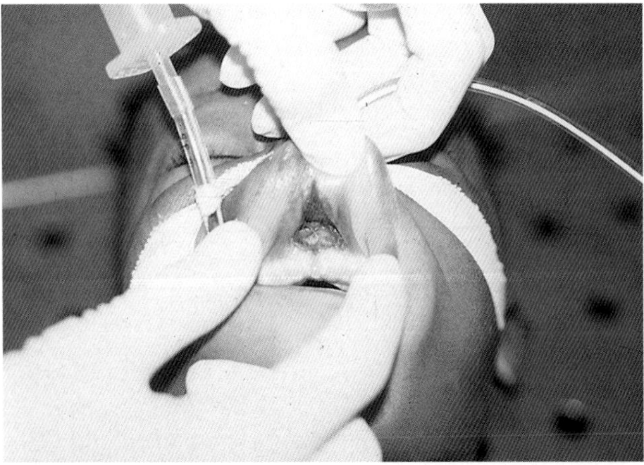

FIGURE 7-8 ■ Laceration of the intraoral mucosa and frenulum. The external surface of the philtrum region displayed no evidence of injury.

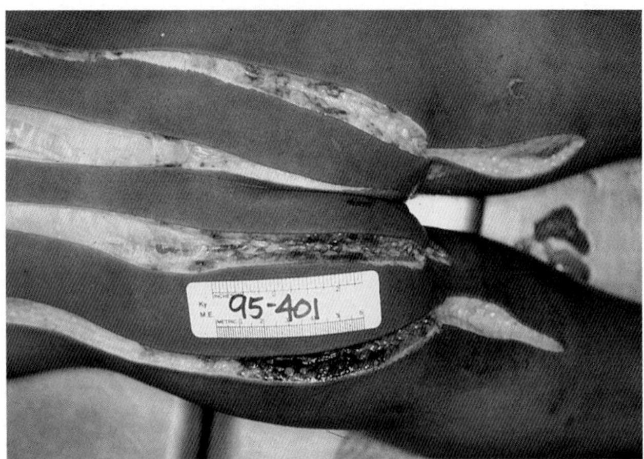

FIGURE 7-9 ■ Additional incisions along the dorsal aspect of the body of a child abuse homicide victim are evidence of blunt trauma to the buttocks, greater on the left than on the right.

The age of contusions is best estimated by histologic examination rather than by gross color determination (177,266,281,318). Therefore, when possible, cutaneous contusions should be sampled for microscopic examination. Obviously, this is not a feasible procedure for facial contusions. Even with histologic sampling, the dating of contusions remains an estimation (see "Cutaneous Evidence of Physical Abuse").

Diffuse, severe hemorrhages of the retina and along the optic nerve sheaths may be found in victims of inflicted head injury (25,89,115,127,176,194,226). For this reason, the globes of these victims are removed. The procedure, which is relatively simple, requires freeing of the extraocular muscles from an anterior approach, followed by globe removal from a superior approach. It is facilitated by removal of a window of bone from the orbital plate of the basilar skull. If the prosector is not familiar with this procedure and the subsequent fixation and sectioning of the globes, consultation with an ophthalmologic pathologist is strongly recommended. In cases of a postinjury survival interval, examination by a pediatric ophthalmologist is helpful. The pediatric ophthalmologist may be able to document retinal findings photographically.

When the hydration status of the child is in question, vitreous fluid may be aspirated for chemical analysis (59,62,171). Although the various electrolytes in the blood undergo rapid changes in the early postmortem interval, it has been shown that the vitreous compartment is relatively isolated and thus more stable. The chemistry values of the postmortem vitreous fluid mirror those of the antemortem blood in the early postmortem interval (55,78,130,171). With time, the vitreous potassium level rises in linear fashion and so is used by some forensic pathologists to estimate the postmortem interval. However, this linear increase is affected by factors such as ambient temperature and antemortem potassium concentration. The relative stability of sodium, urea nitrogen, and creatinine in the early postmortem interval allows the postmortem identification of antemortem pathologic processes such as dehydration, hypernatremia, and hyponatremia in low-salt syndrome (55,171). Vitreous fluid may be aspirated from the globe with a 20-gauge needle and a 10-mL syringe. The needle is inserted into the globe from the lateral aspect at an angle of approximately 45 degrees. When the needle is inserted into the center of the globe, the needle tip is visible through the pupil. Care should be taken to prevent the needle from being inserted too far and coming into contact with the retina. The fluid should be gently aspirated and placed into a small sterile red-top vacutainer. The aspirated fluid is clear and colorless. It may be stored in the refrigerator until it is transported to the chemistry laboratory. Because the fluid may be relatively viscous, it is helpful to centrifuge the fluid and use the supernatant for testing purposes (55).

In forensic pathology, we are often looking for subtle signs of injury that may have little clinical but considerable forensic significance. Some of these injury patterns may not be easily visualized when the body is first received. After the autopsy, intravascular blood has drained away from most cutaneous surfaces, so that faint injuries and contusions are more easily visualized. Furthermore, as the surface of an abrasion dries, it becomes more apparent (281). Therefore, in certain cases, it may be helpful to retain the body overnight and reinspect it the next morning (160–318).

SUDDEN INFANT DEATH SYNDROME

Sudden infant death syndrome (SIDS), a diagnosis of exclusion, is the sudden and unexpected death of a child under the age of 1 year that remains unexplained after a complete autopsy that includes toxicology studies, scene investigation, and review of the medical records. Although the exact cause of SIDS is unknown, the manner of death is presumed to be natural. SIDS accounts for 1 to 6 deaths per 1,000 live births per year, so that it is the leading cause of postneonatal mortality in the United States (38,61,62,223,316). Many risk factors have been reported for SIDS. These include male sex, black race, premature birth or low birth weight, and age between 2 and 4 months with approximately 80% less than 6 months (61,153,223,316). Most deaths occur during the winter months and during night sleep (138). The victims often have young parents of low socioeconomic status (138,180,315). Many mothers have used drugs, including tobacco, during pregnancy (128,142). Smoking is also associated with low birth weight, so that it compounds the risk for SIDS (170). Smoking in the household after birth results in passive inhalation by the infant and is also considered a risk factor (170,216). Research has shown that many of the victims were not breast fed (103,180). This finding has led to the hypothesis of a protective IgA factor in breast milk that bottle-fed infants lack. Overheating and overwrapping have also been well-documented frequent findings in these deaths and correlate with the increased occurrence during winter months (15,101,215,223,228,286,303). It is further proposed that overheating is more likely when a child sleeps in the prone position. Because the face is the main route for heat loss, thermoregulatory control is likely compromised in the prone position (228,326). With regard to risk factors, the greatest focus has been on sleep position and environment of the infant (140,215,223,246,295,326). Epidemiologic studies have shown that infants sleeping on their abdomen (prone) are at a greatly increased risk for SIDS (91,140,215,223,246, 295,316,326). When back or side sleep was promoted overseas, the incidence dropped by 50% to 70% (91,314,316). In 1992, the American Academy of Pediatrics recommended that infants sleep on their back or side, and in 1994 it supported the "back to sleep" campaign. This was and remains a successful effort to reduce the number of deaths. In reviews of the side-sleeping position, it has been reported that as prone-sleeping death rates have declined following reduction campaigns, side sleeping has become viewed by some as a risk factor and is not recommended (61,140). Along with the sleep position, the sleep environment, in particular fellow sleepers and abundant bedding, is a risk factor that is described below along with the scene investigation.

To classify a death as SIDS, a scene investigation must be conducted (292). In particular, this is an opportunity to examine the child's living and sleeping environment. The child's sleep position, location, bedding, room temperature, fellow sleepers (bedsharing), and clothing are documented at this time. The bedding should be well described because abundant, fluffy bedding and pillows are often implicated in SIDS (153,246). Water beds and adult beds are also a risk for infants (60,61,246). Broken cribs, areas of potential wedging, and nearby plastic should be sought (60). The temperature of the room should be noted, in addition to smoking in the household. The caretaker should be interviewed at this time to ascertain any recent illness and feeding and to record sleep patterns, time last seen alive, position the infant was put down to sleep, and time found dead. The infant's medical records should be reviewed.

The autopsy of a presumptive SIDS victim is essentially negative. Grossly, froth may be seen in the mouth and nares and is occasionally tinged with blood. The lungs may be congested and edematous. The notable finding in SIDS is the presence of intrathoracic petechiae (21). These are located on the serosal surfaces of the thymus, lungs, and heart. Such petechiae are nonspecific and can be seen in other conditions, including asphyxia, overlaying, and wedging (21,60,73). However, the quantity has been noted to be greater in SIDS than in cases of overlying, wedging, smothering, or other forms of asphyxia (23,73). Furthermore, resuscitation does not affect the number of petechiae (21). It has been theorized that intrathoracic petechiae are caused by changes in intrathoracic pressure resulting from forceful respiratory efforts against a mechanically occluded airway (73). Although many support an asphyxial mechanism for SIDS, most researchers do not believe that SIDS involves a forceful effort to breathe. Instead, hypoxia in and of itself has been regarded as the major systemic influence predisposing to the formation of petechiae in SIDS (21,61,215,326).

Microscopically, the intrathoracic serosal petechiae can be confirmed. One can see pulmonary edema with some extravasated red blood cells in the alveolar spaces, correlating with the froth seen grossly. Occasionally, chronic inflammatory cells are seen around the airways (bronchiolitis), but not to a sufficient extent to cause death. Hepatic steatosis, a nonspecific finding, has also been noted.

Toxicology must be performed in all cases (48,59,62). Vitreous electrolytes should be analyzed to rule out disturbances such as dehydration. The vitreous hypoxanthine level has been found to be elevated in cases of SIDS, but no specific causal or diagnostic conclusions can be drawn. Metabolic testing should also be performed, although not in the formal definition of SIDS. Likewise, microbiologic studies are advised; some researchers believe the investigation is incomplete without such studies (35).

Numerous theories have been proposed regarding the etiology of SIDS. Asphyxia resulting from partial or complete airway obstruction is supported by the studies of sleep position (prone) and sleep environment and by the physical findings of intrathoracic petechiae (153). The associated theory of rebreathing as the face is down toward the mattress or pressed into the bedding is plausible (140,153,326). Supporting this theory is the fact that the neck muscles of infants are weak, especially in the prone position, so that they are unable to turn and raise their head in response to hypoxia. Passive smoke inhalation reduces oxygen in the microenvironment and has been associated with SIDS (128,138,170,216,265). Apnea and apparent life-threatening events (ALTEs) have been proposed to result in SIDS. ALTEs, referred to as "near-miss" SIDS, occur when an infant has episodes of irregular breathing and is aroused. However, only a small number of these infants eventually die of SIDS, and the majority of SIDS victims never actually experienced a known ALTE (181). Some have proposed an anatomic variation in the airway of SIDS victims that results in obstruction, but findings have not been consistent (203). Cardiovascular theories have been proposed, including arrhythmias and a prolonged QT interval (267,324). However, the studies of prolonged QT interval have yielded conflicting results (125,309). Gastroesophageal reflux in infants has received attention (11,296). Stimulation of the esophageal and laryngeal receptors in cases of reflux results in apnea, bradycardia, and presumably death (11). However, many SIDS victims did not have reflux, and many children with reflux survive infancy. Gliosis of the brain stem, in particular the medulla tegmentum, has been documented in some SIDS victims (294). Gliosis, a reaction to previous necrosis, is presumed to inhibit vital centers. The immature brain control of cardiorespiratory function is also under study (66,181). This particularly correlates with the large number of SIDS victims born prematurely. Nutritional factors that appear to be associated with SIDS include deficiencies of trace metals (e.g., magnesium, selenium) and vitamins (e.g., C, D, E, biotin, and thiamine) (206,323). Infectious agents such as respiratory syncytial virus, cytomegalovirus, and toxin-producing bacteria have also been investigated without consistent findings (102,111,239). Others believe that SIDS is multifactorial, occurring in an infant at a critical period of development who is exogenously stressed. Thus, the exact cause of SIDS remains unknown, but through current research, we have been able to identify risk factors that may be "stressors" to the vulnerable infant.

The diagnosis of SIDS is one of exclusion; however, two other entities can present as SIDS and have similar autopsy findings: overlying and smothering (60). Intrathoracic petechiae are present in all three entities, although they are more numerous in SIDS (38). Overlying is an accidental cause of death in which mechanical asphyxia occurs when a larger person sleeps on top of an infant. At autopsy, one may see pressure marks from the bedding or the other person's clothing, but otherwise the autopsy findings are negative. The diagnosis of SIDS should not be designated in a situation that could be overlying. These cases are better designated as undetermined (i.e., SIDS versus overlying) or Sudden Unexplained Death in Infancy (SUDI). Smothering is a homicidal death in which the airway is intentionally occluded. If a child has teeth or is of an age to struggle, one may see lip abrasions, intraoral lesions, or a torn frenulum. Recently, Oehmichen et al. (235) reported the finding of skin petechiae in victims of smothering, and Meadow (209,210) reported the presence of respiratory tract bleeding in cases of smothering. Hemosiderin-laden macrophages in the alveolar spaces have been studied as a possible indicator of previous hemorrhage secondary to unnatural, inflicted asphyxia (19,22,41,173,174,264,290). Otherwise, the autopsy findings of a smothering victim are negative, and a case of smothering can present as SIDS.

Multiple SIDS deaths in a single family rarely occur. SIDS does not appear to have a genetic etiology, but certain situations, such as child abuse, inherited diseases, and unsafe sleeping environments, "run in families" (61). When a second child dies of SIDS, investigators are often suspicious of infanticide. Some researchers believe that the occurrence of three SIDS deaths in one family is so unlikely that the manner of death is considered homicide until proven otherwise (81).

Sudden infant death syndrome is a diagnosis of exclusion with an unknown cause. It is the number one cause of death in children of this age group. The findings are not specific, so that a thorough autopsy and investigation must be conducted.

MUNCHAUSEN SYNDROME BY PROXY

The term *Munchausen syndrome by proxy* (MSBP) was coined in 1977 by Meadow to describe illnesses in children produced by their caregivers (207). The syndrome was named as an extension of the disorder known as *Munchausen syndrome*, in which a patient "creates" an illness to obtain the attention afforded persons playing a "sick role." MSBP was defined as a cluster of four elements:

1. A child's illness is simulated (faked) or produced by a parent or someone who is in loco parentis.
2. The child is presented for medical assessment and care, usually persistently, and medical procedures are often performed.
3. The perpetrator denies knowledge of the cause of the child's illness.
4. Acute symptoms and signs of the illness abate when the child is separated from the perpetrator (260).

It must be stressed that the above definition excludes physical abuse only, sexual abuse only, and nonorganic failure to thrive only. In this particular disorder, the perpetrator (most often the mother) creates or feigns illness in the child to gain attention from the medical community. The methods by which disorders are created in the victims are often elaborate and almost beyond belief. In the series of 117 cases, common presentations included bleeding, seizures, central nervous system depression, apnea, diarrhea, vomiting, fever, and rash (260). Methods of production of various illnesses include forced oral ingestion of drugs or other substances (including salt), intentional manual suffocation, and intentional injection of nonprescribed substances and bacteria (255).

More recently, because of widespread inappropriate application of the term, Meadow (208) has suggested further specifications for its use. These include the following actions by and characteristics of the perpetrator:

1. A person intentionally produces or feigns physical or psychological signs or symptoms in someone under his or her care.
2. The motivation for the perpetrator's behavior is to assume the sick role by proxy.
3. External incentives for the behavior (such as economic gain) are absent.
4. The behavior is not better accounted for by another mental disorder.

Meadow stresses that the key discriminator in the above criteria is the second one—"in relation to the children, the mother would be harming the child (making the child ill) in order herself to assume the sick role and all its benefits" (208). It should be stressed that this disorder is not merely a "game" or an act of histrionics on the part of the mother. It constitutes true physical abuse and may be fatal if not detected by the medical community. Indeed, Rosenberg's series displayed a mortality rate of 9% (260). All the children who died were under the age of 3 years; the most common symptoms in these children were apnea and decreased levels of consciousness (260).

In recent years, covert video surveillance in the rooms of suspected victims of MSBP has proved useful in detecting and documenting this form of abuse. In such a procedure, the patient is admitted to a hospital room equipped with a hidden video monitor. Close by is an observation area where designated persons (law enforcement officers, hospital personnel) monitor the parental activities in the child's room. It is important that observation be continuous in these cases, so that intervention occurs in a timely fashion if the child is abused or assaulted. In a series published by Southall et al. in 1997, the use of covert video monitoring led to the identification and documentation of abuse in 33 of 39 suspected cases (278). Although vocal critics of such surveillance have emerged, it is certain that many of the cases presented in the article would not have been confirmed without such evidence, and the children would have remained "in harm's way" with the abusive caregiver.

When a case of possible MSBP is evaluated, all records should be completely and thoroughly reviewed. It is important to check multiple sources, including health insurance companies, to make sure that all medical evaluations have been discovered. It is helpful to construct a time line, as these are usually complicated, protracted cases. Such a time line is helpful in "keeping the facts straight" and is useful in explaining the condition and history to law enforcement officers, attorneys, and other lay persons. Information gleaned from extensive review of the often voluminous medical records should include documentation of admissions, outpatient and emergency department visits, calls to the physician, consultations, invasive procedures, and prescribed medications. An issue that should be considered during a review of medical records is the number of times visits were initiated by the caregiver, as opposed to the number of visits representing physician-ordered rechecks and specialty consultations. When a suspected victim of MSBP presents to the emergency department, blood and urine should be obtained for toxicologic analysis because multiple cases of forced ingestion of medication have been documented in MSBP (97,106,260). When a diagnosis of MSBP is considered, one should always keep in mind that the most common reason why a parent persistently seeks medical attention for a child is genuine illness of the child.

NEONATICIDE

Before the investigation of neonaticide is discussed, it is helpful to define the term. Neonatal may be defined as "newborn; relating to the period immediately succeeding birth and continuing through the first 28 days of life" (288). Based on this definition, neonaticide could be defined as the killing of any baby in the first 28 days of life. In reality, the term is usually reserved for homicides committed shortly after birth; it is this type of case that will be discussed here.

Around the country, state laws vary regarding the circumstances and time at which a fetus becomes a "person" in the context of criminal homicide statutes. In many states, several facts must be proven before such a death may be considered a homicide. First, the decedent must be shown to have been "viable"—that is, to have reached a gestational age at which independent, extrauterine survival is possible. This gestational age is generally legally considered to be around 24 to 28 weeks, but it varies from state to state. Second, it must be determined that the fetus was born alive and sustained an existence separate from the mother. Thus, in general, an intrauterine or intrapartum death of a baby or fetus arising as the result of a criminal act would not be considered a homicide. Further, the delivery and the subsequent demise of a previable fetus arising as a consequence of a criminal act also would not be considered a homicide in most courts of law.

When a possible neonaticide is investigated, the autopsy should not be conducted as a "black box" exercise (217). A complete postmortem investigation includes at least the three following components:

1. Examination of the scene of death and/or body discovery
2. Review of the case history
3. A complete autopsy

The precise incidence of neonaticide cannot be determined because some concealed babies are found decades after death, and undoubtedly some are never found. However, it appears that neonaticide is more prevalent in certain areas of the world. The reasons for this are probably multiple and include social customs, economic factors, and the availability of elective abortions. From the published literature, it appears that Japan has a higher incidence of neonaticide than the United States; neonaticide accounted for 10% to 24% of medicolegal autopsies performed in 1 series (272), and 12 cases of 3 or more consecutive neonaticides were described in another series (105).

Investigation of the Scene

Provided one keeps in mind that it is possible to suffocate an infant intentionally and leave no signs of trauma, the scene investigation may provide important information for a cause-of-death determination. If the pathologist does not examine the scene of death or body discovery, then it is important that scene information gathered by law enforcement officers or lay death investigators be communicated to the prosecting pathologist. Causes of death that leave little or no evidence on the body of an infant include the common methods of neonaticide—suffocation, drowning, and exposure (253). Without knowledge of the findings at the scene of death or body discovery, errors may occur in the determination of the cause and manner of death. If blood stain patterns are present at the scene, it is wise to have someone experienced in bloodstain pattern analysis examine the scene. Bloodstain pattern analysis is a scientific area of study based on the physical properties of liquids and the substances they affect; training seminars are conducted, and a scientific society (the International Association of Bloodstain Pattern Analysts) has been established. Courts around the country have qualified expert witnesses in the area of bloodstain pattern analysis based on their education, training, and experience. Among other things, bloodstain pattern analysis may reveal attempts to clean or conceal the delivery site, or even postpartum independent movement of the baby.

Case History Review

Historical information concerning the actions and statements of the mother in the months and weeks preceding the delivery and the actions and statements of the mother following the delivery may provide other "pieces of the puzzle" in the determination of the cause and manner of death. Ophoven noted "striking similarities in features of mothers committing infanticide" (238). These may include the following:

- Average intelligence
- Living at home with parents at the time of delivery
- Attempted concealment of pregnancy
- Statements on questioning that the child was born dead
- Lack of plans for delivery or for care of the infant thereafter
- Delivery alone in a high-risk location or circumstance
- Concealment of the delivery
- Concealment of the infant and placenta

Cases of neonaticide often come to the attention of medicolegal investigators when the mother presents for medical treatment of birth-related injuries or postpartum bleeding.

Autopsy

The pathologist performing the autopsy on an apparently newborn infant is confronted with three possibilities:

- Death *in utero*
- Intrapartum death
- Death after delivery

Depending on the time interval between death *in utero* and delivery, the stillborn infant will show varying degrees of maceration (274). Maceration is the progressive breakdown of tissues by sterile autolysis. Two of the earliest macerative changes include red-brown discoloration of the umbilical cord stump and skin slippage (109). The earliest reliable histologic feature of death *in utero* is the loss of nuclear basophilia in renal cortical tubular cells (109). The causes of death *in utero* are diverse and include maternal diseases, placental disorders, congenital anomalies, and infection.

Intrapartum death, defined as death occurring during labor and delivery, arises primarily from asphyxia or trauma (271,312). The prosecting pathologist must be cautious when attempting to differentiate between postpartum and intrapartum injuries. The pathologist should attempt to determine the presentation position by physical evidence. For instance, caput succedaneum identifies the area of the head that presented, whereas a large fluctuant hematoma over the

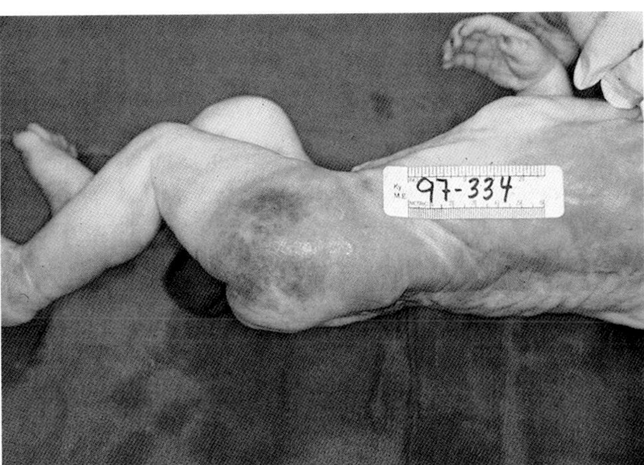

FIGURE 7-10 ■ Breech presentation with intrapartum death. Identification of the presentation position. Fluctuant hematoma of the buttock with associated swelling and congestion of the scrotal sac.

buttock may be seen in breech presentations (Figure 7-10). Other birth injuries include cephalhematoma, forceps abrasions, and shoulder dystocia.

The lungs of an infant succumbing *in utero* or during delivery generally display primary atelectasis—they are red-purple, rubbery, and airless. On *in situ* gross inspection, the lungs do not completely fill the pleural spaces. Some investigators report that partial pulmonary inflation can occur as a result of attempted resuscitation or intravaginal breathing. Full-body radiographs taken before the internal examination will document evidence of aeration within the lungs and gastrointestinal tract. However, it must be remembered that in decomposed bodies, putrefactive gases may be present (Figure 7-11). The distal edge of the umbilical stump should be examined to differentiate separation from the placenta by cutting versus tearing. It may be examined microscopically for histologic evidence of a vital tissue reaction.

After death *in utero* and intrapartum death have been ruled out, the pathologist is left with but one alternative: postpartum death. The questions then become: What is the cause of death? What is the manner of death? Natural causes must be eliminated. The lungs of an infant who has breathed after delivery are well aerated and light salmon pink in color, and they fill the pleural spaces. To assess aeration of the lungs further, a "flotation" test, first described in the 1600s, may be performed (238). The lungs, individual lobes, or tissue samples from each lobe are placed in water or formalin. Simply put, flotation is evidence of aeration once the presence of putrefactive gases has been ruled out. Evidence of aeration of the gastrointestinal tract should be documented because, in general, air within the gastrointestinal tract indicates extrauterine swallowing of air and thus extrauterine existence. Any stomach contents may be retained for possible analysis. The presence of indigestible vegetable matter representing feces may indicate swallowing of toilet water in cases of toilet water drowning.

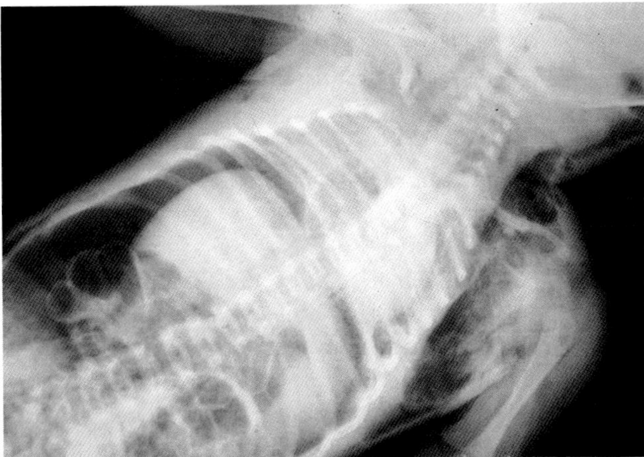

FIGURE 7-11 ■ Putrefactive gases in the soft tissues of an abandoned, decomposed term infant.

If available, the placenta should be thoroughly examined both grossly and microscopically. Examination of the placenta may shed light on both the cause and the time of death and may confirm or eliminate various factors contributing to death, such as infection and uterine-placental insufficiency.

No single objective laboratory test allows a diagnosis of neonaticide. Rather, the pathologist must compile and assess multiple findings before arriving at a conclusion regarding the cause and manner of death. These multiple findings include, but are not limited to, historical information, evidence from the scene examination, and the results of a complete autopsy. The pathologist should expect to encounter equivocal cases in which an opinion, to a reasonable degree of medical certainty, cannot be rendered. Cases may be equivocal for a variety of reasons, including decomposition of the body, severe natural disease, and indeterminate physical findings.

NEGLECT

Child maltreatment is an intentional act or omission by someone in the role of caretaker that endangers or impairs a child's physical, mental, or emotional health and development (54,62,171). The child from birth to age 18 who suffers maltreatment by parents, guardians, or other caretakers can broadly be defined as a victim of abuse (299). The four major categories of child maltreatment are physical abuse, sexual abuse, emotional abuse, and neglect (211). Neglect is the most common form of child maltreatment, three times more common than physical abuse (54,62,93,104,171,211,242). Neglect accounts for approximately two-thirds of maltreatment cases (85). Pediatric neglect is defined as the failure of a child's caregiver to provide adequate safety, food, clothing, shelter, education, protection, medical/dental care, and supervision. Multiple forms of neglect exist. Physical neglect refers to withholding nutrition, drink, hygiene, clothing, or shelter from a child (152). Emotional neglect occurs when nurturing or psychological needs are not met or are ignored. A child who is not immunized, does not attend school regularly, or is allowed to do dangerous things should alert one to a problem of neglect (242).

Neglect can be either active or passive. Active neglect involves a deliberate lack of care or the withholding of necessary components of a child's care. Passive neglect occurs when caretakers inadvertently do not provide for a child because their focus is elsewhere. The results of neglect range from slight morbidity to death and are the result of either short- or long-term failure to provide for a child. Lethal neglect usually denotes starvation or dehydration. Most victims of lethal neglect are under the age of 1 year. Once children are mobile, they are generally able to obtain drink and food, although the nutritional value is usually suboptimal.

A scene investigation is warranted in all cases of suspected lethal neglect. The caretaker should be interviewed and interrogated regarding the medical and feeding history. The medical history should include birth and medical records with chronologic recorded weights and measurements. The feeding history includes schedule and quantity of feedings. With starvation and dehydration, the history is inconsistent with the physical findings. If available, any formula given to the child should be procured. The consistency and concentration of the formula can be compared with the manufacturer's instructions to see if it was diluted and therefore inadequate for proper nourishment.

At autopsy, full-body radiographs (skeletal survey) should be obtained and interpreted by a pediatric radiologist. Usually, physical abuse/battering is not present in cases of physical neglect; however, it is not universally absent. Radiographs will reveal injuries in addition to signs of malnutrition, such as skeletal demineralization and rachitic changes. Proper external measurements of crown-heel and crown-rump length, head circumference, and body weight are extremely important, and these must be compared with standard measurements. If a child has been born prematurely, one can compare its measurements with the expected growth measurements. It is very useful to examine the aforementioned medical records to observe the chronologic pattern of growth and development. This can help narrow the time frame of neglect and often aids in ruling out organic disease. The child should be photographed in color from several views. A color card is useful in highlighting unusual pigmentation, hypopigmentation, or "blue pallor." Always back up photography with full-body infant/pediatric diagrams.

The gross findings at autopsy represent a decreased caloric intake over time and a decrease in total body adipose tissue, both deep and subcutaneous. The body is underweight for its length. The weight is usually around or below the fifth or third percentile (depending on the growth chart plotted) (158,171,322). The neck is narrow secondary to the loss of fat, so that the head has a deceptively large appearance. The occiput appears to protrude because of the decrease in neck adipose tissue and possible atrophy of the neck musculature. The eyes are sunken within the orbits from a loss of orbital fat and often from associated dehydration. The cheeks are sunken secondary to loss of the buccal fat pad. The ribs are prominent to the extent that the intercostal musculature is depressed (concave). The iliac crests are prominent and the abdomen is scaphoid. The skeletal muscles of the arms and legs are atrophied and the fat decreased, so that the appearance is skeletonized. The skin about the knees and ankles is wrinkled, and the knees appear "knobby." Posteriorly, the vertebral spinous processes are prominent. The scapulae are protuberant because the medial borders are accentuated secondary to a loss of muscle and adipose tissue. The buttocks are very wrinkled because of the near absence of gluteal fat. Pressure sores may accompany such a loss of fat over prominent bony planes. The skin is thin and dry and has a blue pallor. When pinched, the skin remains "tented," which indicates a loss of turgor resulting from a decrease of subcutaneous fat and fluid. The hair may be dry, pale, and brittle, with areas of alopecia. The fontanelles are often depressed as the cerebrospinal fluid pressure drops and the brain shrinks with dehydration of brain cells (123). Reflection of the scalp demonstrates more clearly the fontanelle depression. Internally, one sees the decrease in subcutaneous fat and the deeper fat around the gastrointestinal areas (omentum and mesentery) and kidneys. The serosal surfaces are "sticky." The organ weights, including those of the lymphoid organs, are decreased except for the brain, which may be smaller with dehydration, although not substantially. The organ weights are compared with the expected weights for the body length. The stomach and intestines have thinned walls, are empty of food material, and are often distended with gas. Any food material present should be quantified and qualified in regard to location in the tract. Fecoliths may be present secondary to dehydration. The gallbladder is distended with bile secondary to lack of secretion. Microscopically, the adipose tissue that remains is atrophied and transformed to brown fat. Brown fat is composed of adipocytes that are multivacuolated and univacuolated (171). The cytoplasm of the multivacuolated cells appears granular because of the presence of numerous mitochondria, and the nucleus is centrally located. The brown fat transformation is a protective mechanism; this type of fat has a higher energy- and heat-producing capacity. Hepatic microvesicular steatosis may be present, reflecting protein deficiency (62,171). Thymic involution is common. Hassall corpuscles undergo degeneration and calcification. The cuff of cortical lymphocytes becomes depleted, leaving a "starry sky" appearance. Eventually, the gland is replaced by fibroadipose tissue. The adrenal glands may be atrophic with a thin cortices, lipid depletion, and cortical pseudotubule formation.

To determine a component of dehydration, it is very useful to obtain an electrolyte analysis of the vitreous humor (57,59,171). Dehydration is a loss of fluid from vital tissues, with the potential for circulatory collapse. Infants are at increased risk for dehydration because their losses are higher (310). Their metabolic rates and surface-to-volume ratios are higher, and they are more prone to febrile illnesses (310). The three types of dehydration are isotonic, hypotonic, and hypertonic. Isotonic dehydration is the most common form in children and is usually a consequence of viral diarrhea (123). It is a loss of water coupled with a proportional loss of sodium. Hypotonic dehydration (sodium < 130 mmol/L) follows excessive fluid losses through gastrointestinal tubing and in cystic fibrosis, adrenal insufficiency, and bacillary dysentery. In hypotonic dehydration, the vitreous levels of sodium and chloride are low, as is the level of potassium, in contrast to the usual postmortem elevation of potassium (123). Hypertonic dehydration (sodium ≥ 155 mmol/L) is seen in salt (sodium) excess, diabetes mellitus, diabetes insipidus, mental retardation, high environmental temperature, and water deficit/withholding. This type of dehydration is associated with the highest mortality rate. Dehydration by neglect is usually hypertonic, with an increase in sodium, potassium (>135 mmol/L), and urea nitrogen (>40 mmol/L). The exact numeric levels of the electrolytes vary with the analytic method. In hypernatremic dehydration, the brain cells become dehydrated, the parenchyma shrinks, and tearing of cerebral vessels with hemorrhage may result (123). In hypertonic dehydration, the mechanism of death is probably arrhythmia resulting from circulatory collapse and hyperkalemia or, less commonly, cerebral hemorrhage.

Often, because malnutrition and dehydration depress the immune system, physical neglect is associated with certain diseases. These include bronchopneumonia, tuberculosis, urinary tract infections, skin infections, cellulitis, otitis media, meningitis, and intracranial abscesses. The immediate cause of death may be one of the above, but the underlying cause of death remains physical neglect.

Before a death is classified as having been caused by neglect, one must rule out organic diseases that produce a wasted appearance (70). Such diseases include partial cleft palate and other oral motor abnormalities, intestinal malabsorption, cystic fibrosis, protein-losing enteropathies, abetalipoproteinemia, pyloric stenosis, celiac disease, malignancies, and congenital metabolic disorders (e.g., congenital adrenal hyperplasia and glycogen storage diseases). In these organic diseases, absorption of the nutrients and calories necessary for development and the expenditure of energy are inadequate. Other conditions associated with such findings include congenital heart disease, cerebral palsy, and chromosomal abnormalities. Diseases such as cystic fibrosis, medium-chain acyl–CoA dehydrogenase deficiency (MCAD), diabetes mellitus, mental retardation/chromosomal abnormalities, congenital adrenal hyperplasia, and viral gastroenteritis can cause dehydration (122,310). Mentally retarded children are at increased risk for dehydration because their intake may be inadequate as a result of swallowing difficulties associated with neuromuscular incoordination (310). All such entities must be included in the differential diagnosis for pediatric neglect before such a serious conclusion can be made.

Other forms of physical neglect besides starvation and dehydration may be seen in forensic pathology. Hyperthermic and hypothermic deaths in cases of abandonment or exposure are seen in young children unable to protect themselves from the environment (171). Improper supervision or a lack of supervision combined with a dangerous environment can result in the death of a child. With the use of recreational drugs in our society, children are exposed to and may accidentally consume drugs. Another form of neglect is the failure to provide adequate dental and medical care. Dental caries, periodontal diseases, and other oral conditions, if left untreated, can lead to pain, infection, and loss of function (240,261). Infections may lead to meningitis or sepsis, an inflamed appendix may rupture, or a child may not receive immunizations. Certain cultural and religious practices that prohibit some types of medical treatment occasionally result in the death of a child. Care must be taken in the evaluation of such controversial situations. Respect for another person's beliefs must not be allowed to interfere with the welfare of a child.

Even though neglect is the most common form of child maltreatment, it remains a challenge to investigate and prove. A careful scene investigation, a review of the medical and feeding histories, a complete autopsy with radiographic, toxicologic, chemical, and metabolic studies, and a careful elimination of possible organic causes are all necessary before a death can be classified as resulting from neglect (59).

ACCIDENTAL CAUSES OF DEATH IN CHILDREN

Although this chapter focuses primarily on SIDS and inflicted injuries in children, it is important to remember that deaths from unintentional injury far outnumber abusive deaths in children. In most abusive deaths, a history of a minor household accident is often provided as the alleged history of injury. Some types of accidental deaths are indistinguishable from SIDS by autopsy alone, as are some types of homicide. Asphyxia is one of the more common causes of death in cases that may be mistaken for SIDS in the absence of a complete investigation. Thus, these cases require a thorough scene investigation and history review. Finally, it is important to recognize accidental deaths from a public health standpoint, so that the public may be made aware of such risks and changes in product design may be undertaken when appropriate. For these reasons, a brief discussion of accidental deaths in children is warranted. Perhaps the most important fact to remember is that children of different age groups are vulnerable to different hazards within their environments. Therefore, "childproofing" the home and discussing safety with parents and other caregivers must be age specific (47,64).

Infants less than 1 year old represent a unique age group with regard to death from unintentional injury. Unlike older children, infants are particularly vulnerable to hazards within their sleeping quarters. This is because infants are unable to extricate themselves from potentially dangerous positions and situations. Indeed, in an 11-year autopsy series by one of the authors (TSC), asphyxia after placement in unsafe sleeping quarters was the leading cause of accidental death in infants up to 1 year of age (56,60). Byard et al. reported similar findings in a 28-year retrospective review of sleeping environment deaths, and they reported wedging/entrapment, hanging, nose and mouth occlusion, and external chest compression as common situations conducive to asphyxia (39). In a follow-up study, Byard stressed the need for scene investigation in cases with relatively nonspecific autopsy findings (40). Other authors have stressed similar hazardous conditions in the sleeping quarters of infants (60,112,155).

Motor vehicle–related injuries remain the leading cause of death for persons of ages 1 to 24 years in the United States (18,95,126). In a study published in late 1997, it was noted that approximately one-fourth of all collisions in which children under 15 years of one-fourth age died involved a driver with a blood alcohol concentration above 0.10%. Furthermore, 60% died while riding with the drunk driver, and only 16% of the children were restrained. Studies have shown that fatalities among children ages 0 to 4 years have declined with the passage of child restraint laws (119,230). Even when caregivers are not driving while drunk and are placing children in safety restraint seats, the seats themselves are often improperly secured in the vehicle (71). New rules by the National Highway Traffic Safety Administration became effective November of 2009 that require that all safety seats be anchored to cars in a uniform way with a single type of anchoring system (250).

Other common causes of accidental death in early childhood include drowning and house fires (150,171,218, 219,234,243,327). Contrary to "information" portrayed on television and in the movies, no definitive postmortem test or finding indicates a drowning death. Drowning is determined by exclusion, based on scene circumstances and history and the lack of an overt cause of death at autopsy. Drowning is one of the leading causes of unintentional injury and death in children in the United States; although the circumstances are different among the various age groups, toddlers and adolescents are at high risk (29). Young infants are at risk for drowning during bath time if left unattended, either alone or with an older sibling (171,243). More than 50% of infant drowning deaths occur in bathtubs. One study found that infants placed in tub rings may be at a greater risk for drowning because of the caregiver's false sense of security and resultant increased likelihood that an infant will be left alone. As an infant grows and begins to interact more independently with the environment, new risks emerge. It is among toddlers that various household hazards such as 5-gallon buckets contribute to drowning deaths (150,198). Toddlers are also the age group in which swimming pools become a major circumstance in drowning deaths. During adolescence, boys are at a higher risk for unintentional drowning than girls. These drowning deaths often occur in natural bodies of fresh water (29). Thus, as in other categories of accidental death, prevention measures must be age specific. Caregivers of infants should be reminded of the dangers of leaving an infant unattended in the tub, "even for a minute." The dangers associated with tub rings should also be discussed. For caregivers of toddlers, safeguarding against "attractive nuisances" such as toilets, buckets, and pools should be emphasized. Adolescents benefit from campaigns alerting the public to common drowning scenarios. Further public awareness may help to reduce fatalities from these preventable accidents.

Like drowning, accidental strangulation characteristically involves distinct age groups of children. Preschool children may be strangled when they become entangled in common household items from which they are unable to extricate themselves. In part because of the actions of the Consumer Product Safety Commission and other organizations, accidental strangulations in structurally unsafe cribs are becoming less common (98). Some hazards are rather well-known, such as pacifier strings and cords on venetian blinds, but others are less well-known, such as cords to electric devices in a toddler's room (Figure 7-12). Adolescents may succumb to ligature hanging, either as a suicide or as an accident in association with autoerotic asphyxia (18,262). Victims of strangulation generally die of an interruption of blood flow to the brain rather than actual occlusion of the airway. Significantly less pressure is required to occlude the blood vessels than the airway (79). With the exception of judicial executions, injury to the cervical spine is very uncommon. Often, the physical findings in deaths from ligature hanging are few, especially if the victim was extricated from the asphyxiating device within a short period of time. When physical signs are present, they are generally the consequence of congestion distal to the ligature site. Such findings may include cephalic congestion, tongue protrusion with discoloration, and petechial hemorrhage. If the victim has been suspended for a postmortem interval measured in minutes to hours at a minimum, a ligature furrow may be seen about the neck. This furrow will have a yellow-brown, waxy base and display a suspension point based on the relative positions of the decedent and the ligature.

House fire deaths remain a significant source of pediatric morbidity and mortality. In fact, in one study of fatal residential fires, children less than 5 years of age were classified as one of several "high vulnerability" groups (327). Other highly vulnerable groups included persons aged 64 years

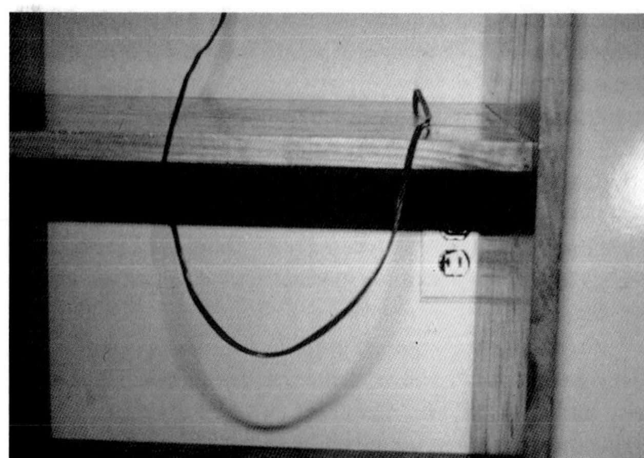

FIGURE 7-12 ■ Accidental ligature asphyxia. A toddler was found hanging by his neck from an electric cord. The cord connected to a clock radio on the shelf above.

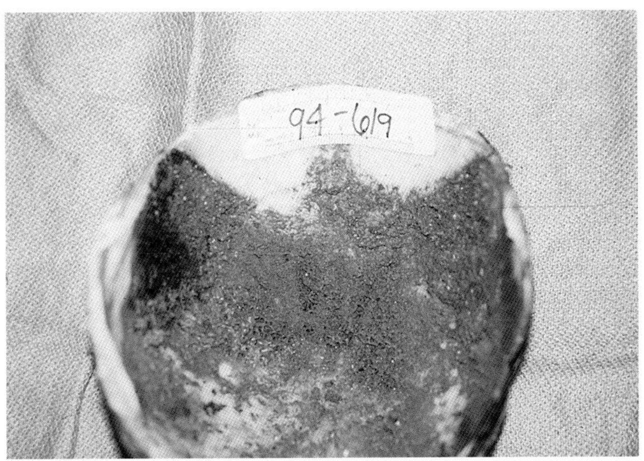

FIGURE 7-13 ■ Epidural heat hematoma along the inner table of the skull, a fire-related artifact that should not be confused with antemortem trauma.

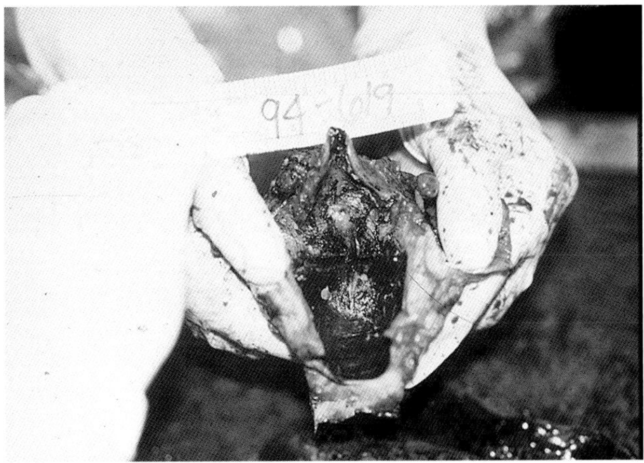

FIGURE 7-15 ■ Smoke inhalation. Black carbonaceous material adherent to the laryngeal mucosa.

or older, those with a physical or cognitive disability, and persons impaired by alcohol or other drugs (202). In most residential fire deaths, the actual cause of death is smoke inhalation. In such cases, the thermal injury to the body may be described as perimortem. Various fire-related artifacts may be mistaken for trauma by the uninitiated. Such artifacts include epidural heat hematomas, skin splitting, and heat fractures and disarticulations (83) (Figures 7-13 and 7-14). In most instances, even when a massive conflagration of the body has occurred, the various internal organ systems remain well preserved and sufficient blood remains for toxicologic study. Fire victims may demonstrate carboxyhemoglobin saturations less than the values encountered in pure carbon monoxide intoxications, but they are still high enough to allow the conclusion to be drawn that death was caused by smoke inhalation. A carboxyhemoglobin saturation above 10% is highly suggestive of life at the beginning of the fire. Gross findings in victims of smoke inhalation include black carbonaceous debris adherent to the respiratory mucosal surfaces and cherry red discoloration of the visceral surfaces, reflecting the carboxyhemoglobin saturation (Figure 7-15). From various published studies, it appears that prevention efforts regarding smoke detectors and egress routes should be directed at families of low socioeconomic status with children less than 5 years of age, as these families represent a high-risk group (202,234,327).

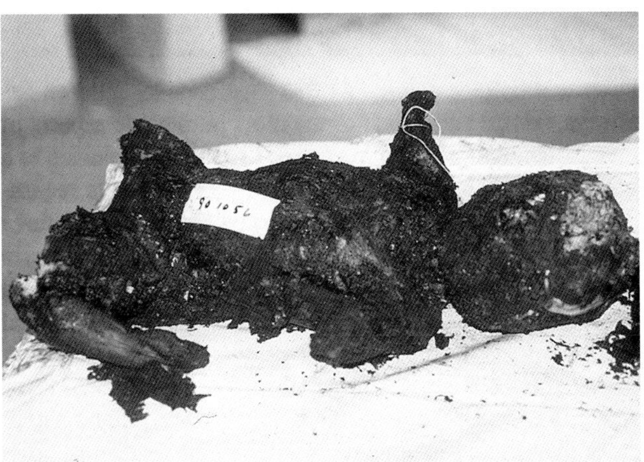

FIGURE 7-14 ■ Fire-related artifacts, including fractures and disarticulations, in a child who died of smoke inhalation in a house fire.

ASPHYXIA

Asphyxia may lead to death in young children in a variety of circumstances and may represent either an accident or a homicide. As discussed in the previous section, infants are particularly vulnerable to hazards in their sleeping quarters that can cause asphyxia (e.g., wedging, which obstructs the nose and mouth or compresses the chest; strangulation, which occludes the great vessels of the neck) (38,42,60,220,275). Infants placed on adult beds may slip between the headboard and the mattress, or between the mattress and the adjacent wall (Figure 7-16). Infants placed in cribs or bassinets with ill-fitting mattresses may become wedged in a similar fashion. Infants sleeping together with others may be killed by overlaying (16,60,65). Strangulation deaths may occur when a young child is left unattended in a day cradle, car seat, or swing and becomes entangled in the safety straps or some other portion of the device (2) (Figure 7-17). Another hazard in sleeping quarters may be soft bedding and a prone position of the infant, which leads to asphyxia from rebreathing (47,60,113,140,215,223,246, 263,295,316,326). A common feature to all the above causes of death is the fact that they often leave little, if any, physical evidence of trauma on the body. Strangulation and chest compression may leave scattered cutaneous petechiae distal to the site of occlusion/compression, but oronasal occlusion by soft substances and rebreathing may cause death without any evidence of injury. Without proper scene documentation and gathering of historical information, these cases may be erroneously ascribed to SIDS.

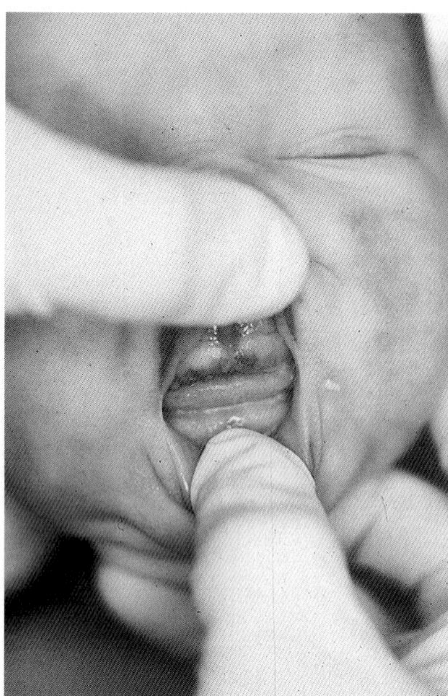

FIGURE 7-16 ■ Gingival abrasion in a 1-month-old child who became entrapped between the headboard and mattress of a standard adult bed.

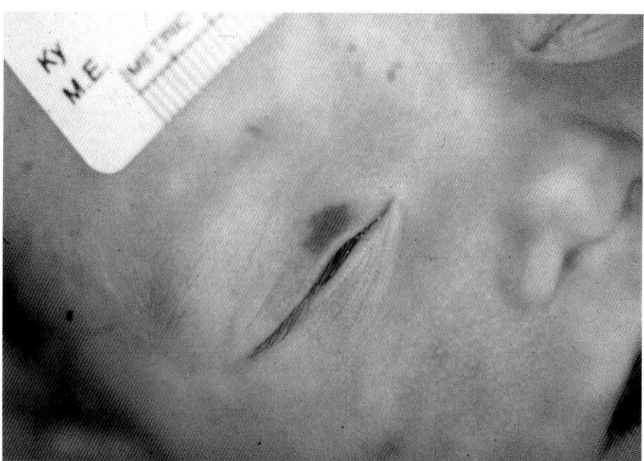

FIGURE 7-18 ■ Homicidal suffocation in a 6-week-old fraternal twin presenting as simultaneous sudden infant death syndrome. This baby had a small, superficial abrasion on the right upper lid. The other infant displayed no evidence of trauma.

Even more difficult to detect are cases of homicidal suffocation of an infant or a young child. Even with a careful scene examination, complete autopsy, and case history review, these cases may be erroneously ascribed to SIDS. Multiple cases of serial infanticides committed by parents or caregivers over a period of years before detection are now known (92,100). Many of these cases were initially erroneously ascribed to SIDS, and they illustrate the critical importance of strictly adhering to the definition of SIDS and obtaining a complete family history when investigating an apparent case of SIDS. In the absence of an identifiable metabolic or genetic defect, some forensic pathologists feel that that a second apparent "SIDS" case within a family should be classified as "undetermined," and that a third case should be classified as a homicide. The same thinking is relevant in alleged cases of "simultaneous SIDS" in twins. Although cases have been reported in the medical literature, many physicians are skeptical and feel that they represent undetected homicidal or accidental deaths (17,276). In the experience of one of the authors (T.S.C.), twins intentionally suffocated on the same night presented as simultaneous SIDS. One of the babies displayed no evidence of injury whatsoever, and the other baby displayed small, faint periorbital superficial abrasions about one eye (Figure 7-18). Although the parents denied use of the apnea monitors present in the home on the night of the infants' demise, the monitors were collected by the police. Downloading of the monitors provided documentation of the entire double homicide. When confronted with this evidence, the parents confessed. This case clearly illustrates that it is entirely possible to suffocate an infant intentionally and leave no evidence of injury whatsoever. Although some feel that intentional suffocation may account for up to 10% of cases classified as SIDS, most forensic pathologists believe that homicidal suffocation accounts for only a very small percentage of SIDS cases (80,94,233).

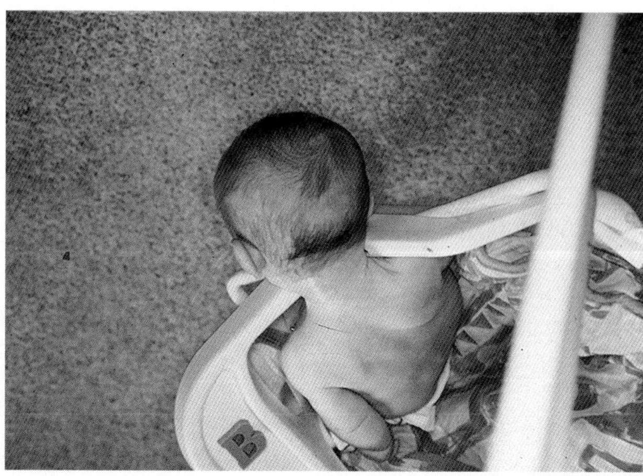

FIGURE 7-17 ■ Strangulation of a 2-month-old infant left unattended and unsecured in an infant swing.

CHARACTERISTICS OF VICTIMS AND PERPETRATORS OF PHYSICAL ABUSE

Despite the indisputable fact that "violence to children has always existed and is one of the most intractable aspects of human behavior," child abuse as a medical diagnosis is a relatively new phenomenon (26). Most of the data regarding physical abuse have been collected within the last three decades, since the publication of the landmark articles "Slaughter of the Innocents" in 1961 and "The Battered Child Syndrome" in 1962 (5,156). First and foremost, fatal child abuse is an intimate crime—the child is injured by the person or persons to whom society has entrusted it for care and nurturing. In one study, Starling et al. found that in cases of abusive head trauma, the perpetrator was most often the biologic father; the mother's boyfriend (unrelated to the child) was the second most common abuser (287). This same prevalence of biologic fathers as perpetrators was found in a study by one of the authors (T.S.C.) of fatally abused infants, in which the biologic father was identified as the perpetrator in 50% of cases undergoing autopsy during an 11-year period (65). Other researchers have reported that stepparents are statistically more likely to abuse children in their care fatally than are biologic or adoptive parents (301). Child abuse crosses all racial and socioeconomic lines, but common factors in most abusive households include an acceptance of physical punishment, social isolation, and stress (291). Most victims of fatal abuse are under 2 years of age, and homicide is the leading cause of traumatic infant death in the United States. Identified risk factors include childbearing at an early age, second or subsequent infants born to mothers less than 17 years of age, and lack of prenatal care (241). Common triggering mechanisms include crying, feeding difficulties, and toilet-training accidents (320). About 50% of fatally abused children display evidence of previous abuse at autopsy; this evidence may take the form of healing soft tissue injuries or skeletal injuries. In the families of living victims of maltreatment, maltreatment has been found to recur in more than 50% of families followed for more than 5 years (72).

Common presenting histories in physical abuse cases involve an account of a minor household fall, such as a tumble down the stairs or off a bed or couch (161). Other common histories in fatal abuse cases include sudden respiratory arrest, sudden onset of seizure activity with no previous history of seizure disorder, and simply finding the baby dead. These last histories are probably partial truths; the caregiver is simply omitting the assaultive act that precipitated the onset of symptoms described. Inflicted head injury is by far the most common cause of death in fatal abuse, especially in infants. Abdominal injury is the second most common fatal abusive injury encountered and is seen more often in toddlers than in infants.

CUTANEOUS EVIDENCE OF PHYSICAL ABUSE

First, it must be understood that a fatally abused child may display no external evidence of injury. The lack of cutaneous injuries such as abrasions and contusions does not eliminate homicide. Often, children with no external evidence of injury have massive internal injuries, including fatal head injuries and multiple skeletal fractures. Conversely, external evidence of contusion or abrasion does not necessarily indicate an abusive death. Adequate documentation and strict adherence to proper use of terminology in forensic reports is important.

When the external injuries of a suspected victim of physical abuse are examined, it is important to keep several points in mind:

- Evaluate the distribution of injury.
- Evaluate the pattern of injury.
- Evaluate the severity of injury.
- Compare the injury with the history provided.

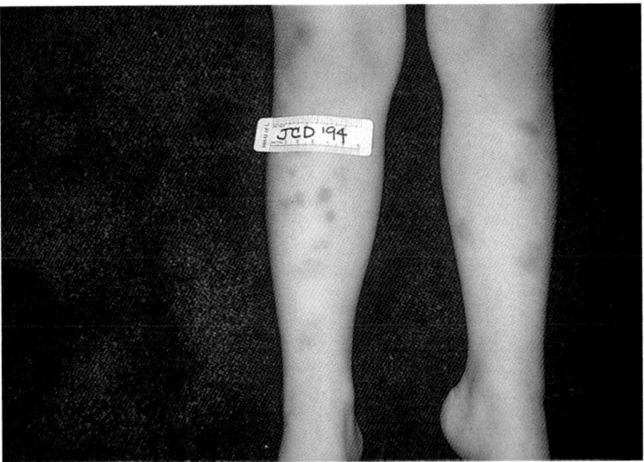

FIGURE 7-19 ▪ Toddler "wear-and-tear" injuries over the lower extremities of an active, healthy preschooler.

Evaluating Blunt Trauma

When the distribution of blunt force injuries is evaluated, it is important to recognize common sites of accidental injuries and the age groups in which these occur. Very young infants are relatively immobile and so do not commonly have contusions. Unexplained facial contusions in this age group may indicate physical abuse (224). As babies become more mobile, the likelihood of incurring accidental injury increases. Common sites of accidental injuries in infants learning to "pull up" and walk include the bony convexities of the anterior head, such as the forehead and the skin overlying the zygoma. Active, healthy toddlers engaging in play and exploration will incur a variety of (usually) superficial injuries. These normal toddler "wear-and-tear" injuries are distributed in a characteristic fashion. In toddlers and older children, accidental injuries are commonly encountered over the elbows, knees, shins, and forearms (308) (Figure 7-19). Isolated injuries in recessed or "protected" areas raise the index of suspicion of abuse. Accidental injuries may occur in these regions, but usually a correlating history can be elicited. Examples of recessed or protected areas that may be injured are the philtrum, submental space, midline of the abdomen, and low back and buttocks (Figures 7-20 and 7-21).

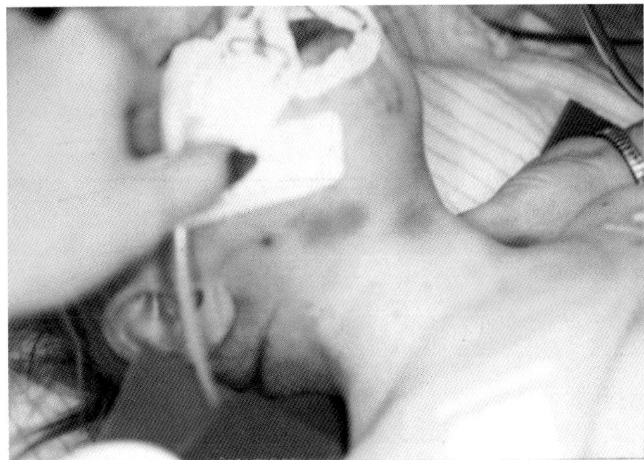

FIGURE 7-20 ▪ Contusions of a recessed area: the submental space in a 17-month-old victim of child abuse.

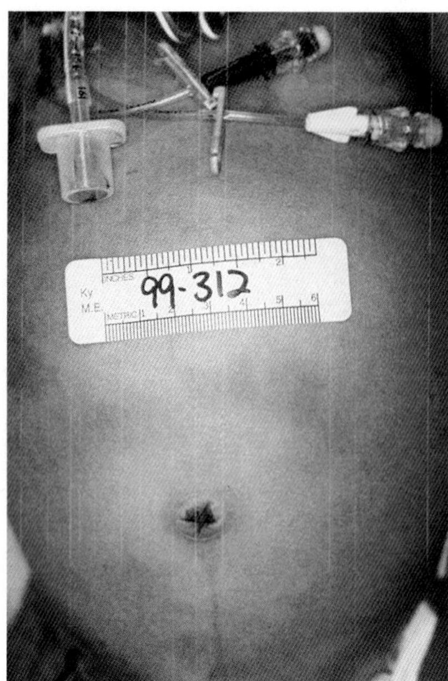

FIGURE 7-21 ■ Abdominal contusions in a 5-month-old victim of child abuse.

A pattern injury may be defined as an injury that mirrors at least a portion of the object that caused it, or an injury that is characteristic of a certain scenario. In cases of physical abuse of a child, most pattern injuries are created with either the hands of the perpetrator or common household items. The pattern varies depending on the velocity with which the object strikes the skin. In high-velocity events, such as whippings and slaps, the pattern often is a linear array of petechiae outlining the dimensions of the object, with a central, unbruised "negative image" of the object. In such cases, the tissues along the edge have been maximally distorted, with subsequent rupture of the capillaries in that region. With increasing force, the tissue immediately beneath the impact site is crushed and also displays bruising. If great forces are applied more slowly, the tissue at the margins of the impact site may conform and stretch without damage. In this scenario, the force ruptures the vessels directly impacted and leaves a "positive image" contusion at the site (99). When a strange or an unusual pattern is encountered, one is encouraged to think about common household items with similar dimensions and shapes. It is advisable to discuss the pattern and the items that possibly caused it with the investigators, so that the scene of injury can be examined for such items. A single object may leave many different patterns, depending on which of its many surfaces impacts the skin. Items often used as "weapons" in physical abuse include belts, electric cords, coat hangers, and curling irons (Figure 7-22). One may also encounter objects such as brooms, fly swatters, and kitchen utensils (Figures 7-23 and 7-24). Flexible objects such as belts or cords leave patterns that vary in length and arc, whereas rigid objects such as broomsticks leave relatively uniform patterns (Figure 7-25). However, the most common "instrument of injury" remains the human hand, with which the child may be slapped, punched, pinched, shaken, slammed, or thrown (Figure 7-26).

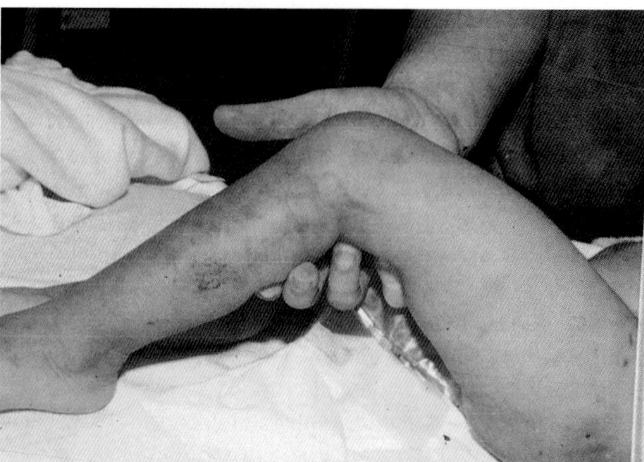

FIGURE 7-23 ■ Multiple diamond-shaped pattern injuries on the leg of a 3-year-old child inflicted by a fly swatter (see Figure 7-24).

Some patterns are characteristic of a particular method of injury. For example, a "brush-burn abrasion" occurs when a pedestrian is struck and has tangential contact with

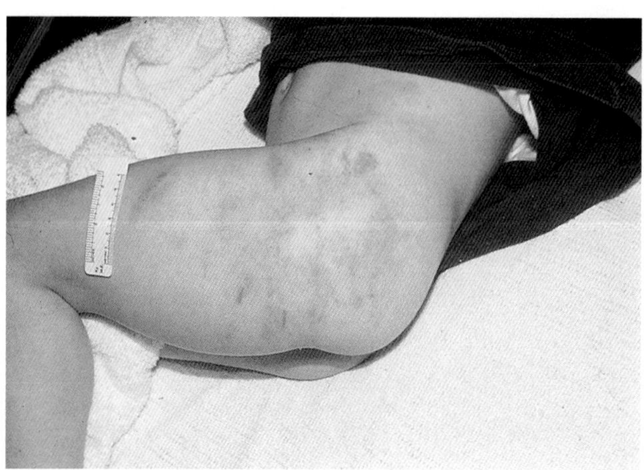

FIGURE 7-22 ■ Pattern injuries inflicted with a belt.

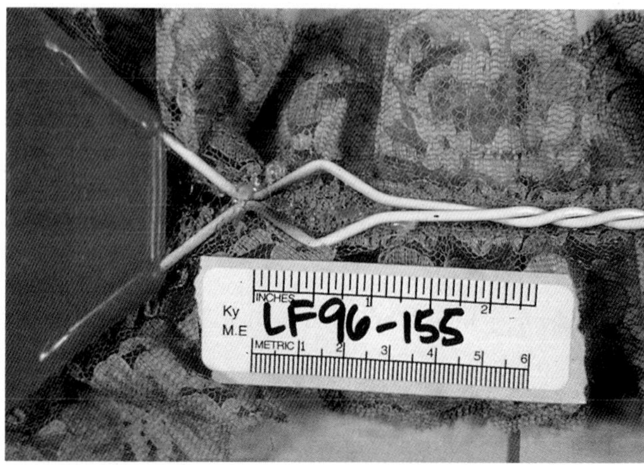

FIGURE 7-24 ■ Portion of the fly swatter corresponding to the pattern injuries depicted in Figure 7-23.

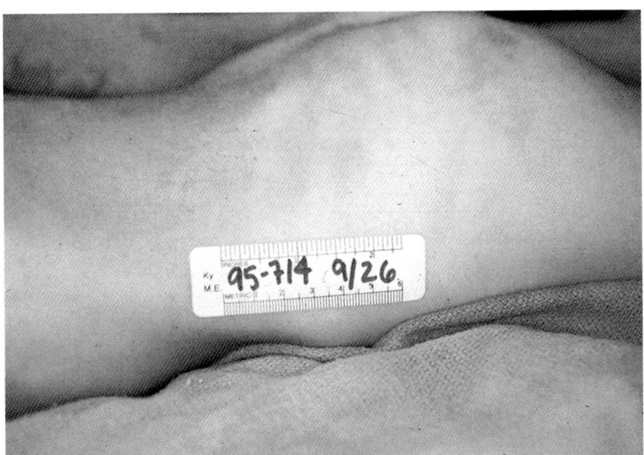

FIGURE 7-25■ Pattern injuries inflicted by beating with a broomstick.

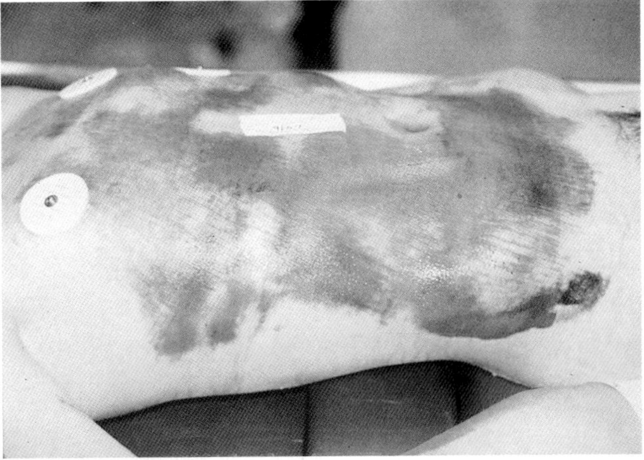

FIGURE 7-27■ Brush-burn abrasion. This injury is commonly seen in pedestrians struck by motor vehicles or occupants ejected during motor vehicle collisions.

the pavement (Figure 7-27). A vertical gluteal cleft injury occurs when a child is beaten over the buttocks; the convex surface flattens, and the regions immediately lateral to the vertical gluteal cleft, which are the interface between impacted and nonimpacted tissue, are subjected to shearing injury. The resulting pattern consists of vertically oriented, parallel linear contusions located on either side of the midline (Figure 7-28). A rim of petechiae may develop along the apex of the ear following direct blunt impact for the same reason. In these two examples, the pattern is dictated by the shape of the body and the anatomic lines of stress rather than by the shape of the object (99). When an injury over a joint is examined, it is helpful to move the joint into various positions. An injury viewed as irregular in the anatomic position may emerge as a pattern injury as the extremity is flexed or rotated (Figure 7-29).

When an external examination is conducted, all cutaneous and mucocutaneous surfaces should be inspected. Specific areas that may be overlooked include the skin surface in and behind the ear (Figure 7-30) and the axillae, intraoral mucosa, palpebral conjunctivae, buttocks, external genitalia, and anus (Figure 7-31).

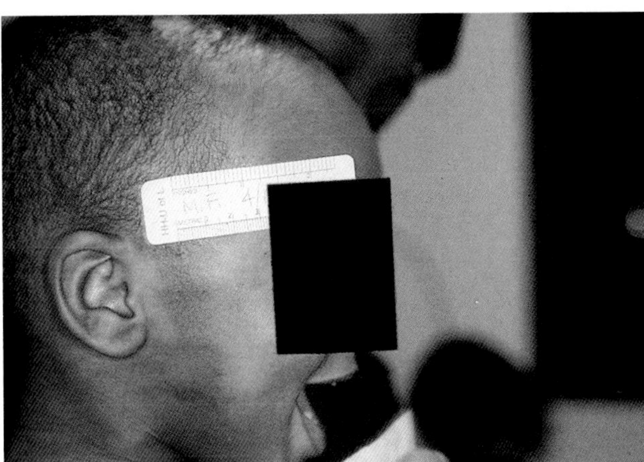

FIGURE 7-26■ Open-handed slap mark inflicted by a male adult.

The severity of the injury must be compared with the historical information. Often in cases of abusive injury and death, a history of a minor household accident, such as a fall from a bed, is given as an explanation (24,135). Other common histories include a sudden onset of seizures, choking, or simply discovering the baby dead. A history that does not agree with the physical findings is a hallmark of child abuse (148). The developmental skills of the child should be compared with the history to see if the alleged scenario is plausible. Therefore, the examiner should have at least a rough understanding of the basic developmental milestones, such as rolling over, crawling, and "cruising" (walking along a piece of furniture while using the hands to maintain balance and upright position).

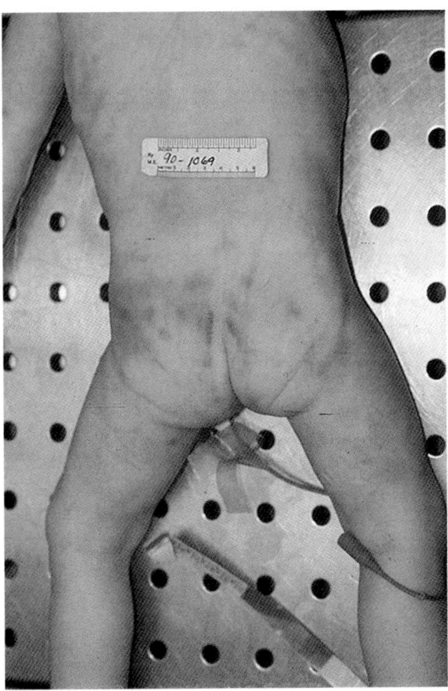

FIGURE 7-28■ Vertical gluteal cleft contusions and multiple additional contusions of varying colors and shapes.

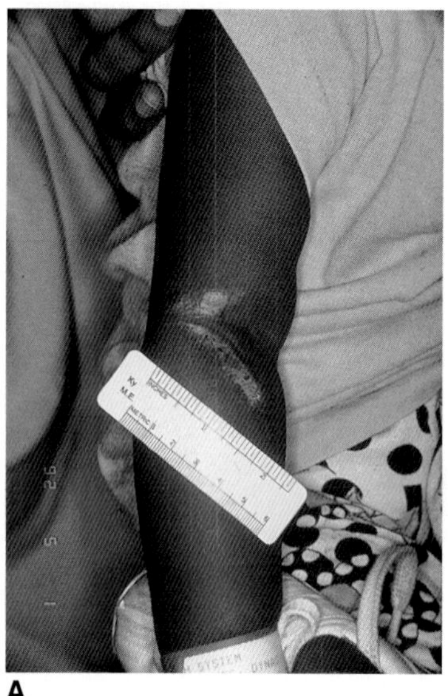

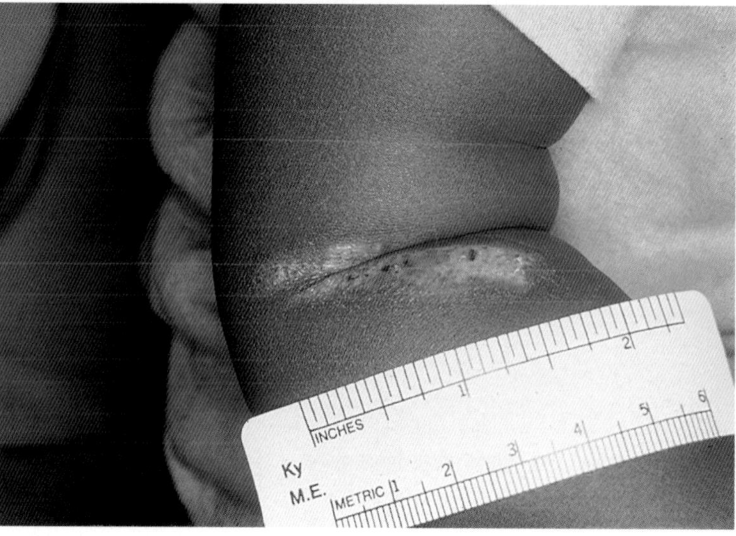

A B

FIGURE 7-29 ■ **AB:** Thermal injury over a joint. The injury pattern initially appears irregular, but when the elbow is flexed, one sees a patterned burn consistent with a curling iron (**B**). (Courtesy of William Smock, M.D., Department of Emergency Medicine, University of Louisville, Kentucky.)

Dating of Contusions

Many texts display charts and illustrations detailing the method of dating contusions by color. However, dating contusions by color is imprecise. Color may provide a rough estimate of age, but this should not be "set in stone." Many factors may affect the color of a contusion on the skin surface. These include the following:

- Depth of the contusion within the soft tissue
- Location on the body
- Amount of bleeding within the tissue
- Environmental lighting
- Overlying skin color of the patient

Although many texts detail an age range based on color, the descriptions often vary from one text to the next (318). Studies have shown that contusions do not progress through a predictable color change based on time (266,289). In fact, it has been shown that the color of bruises in one person at the same location, with the same cause, and of the same age may not change color at the same rate. It appears that the most one can say about the age of a contusion based on color is that a yellow coloration indicates that the bruise is at least 18 hours old (177). In deceased persons, samples of cutaneous contusions may be excised for microscopic examination, which allows a more precise estimation of the age of the injury; however, the dating of the injury remains general. Studies in sheep, calves, and guinea pigs have illustrated that microscopy aids in differentiating acute contusions from those more than 24 hours old (177,204,252). Thornton and Jolly examined 178 experimental bruises inflicted on sheep and aged from 1 to 72 hours; they found that the model was able to age bruises with an acceptable degree of accuracy only as 1 to 20 hours old or 24 to 72 hours old (298). In general, perivascular

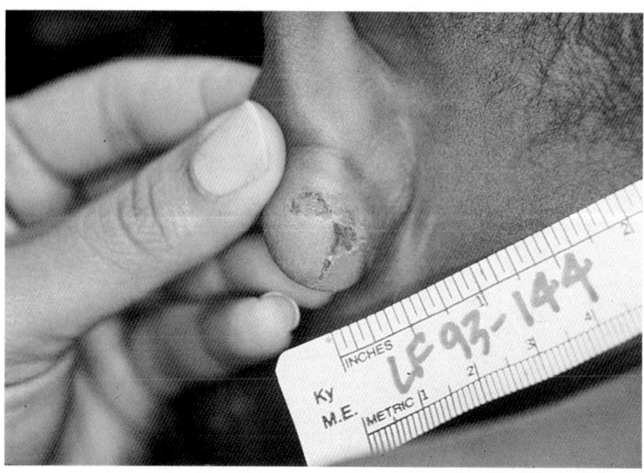

FIGURE 7-30 ■ Inflicted injury behind the ear.

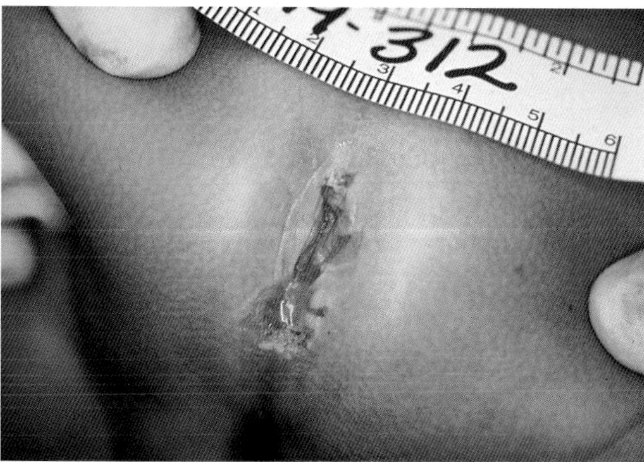

FIGURE 7-31 ■ Anal lacerations in a victim of fatal child abuse. Extensive associated subcutaneous hemorrhage was present.

polymorphonuclear leukocytes may be visible around 4 hours after injury, with a peripheral infiltration by around 12 hours. Macrophages peak around 16 to 24 hours and may contain hemosiderin by 72 hours. Fibroblasts may appear at 2 to 4 days (244). Unfortunately, even with the use of microscopy, "pathologic processes seldom cooperate fully with attempts to date or age them with precise reliability" (136).

Scald Burns and Contact Burns

Among tap water scald burn victims, 46% are under 5 years of age (8,69,84,214,236). When examining a scald burn victim, the pathologist should obtain and document a detailed, specific history of the scalding incident. As in the examination of contusions, observation, documentation, and correlation of the distribution of the injury are paramount (8,69,84,214,236). It is insufficient simply to estimate the total body surface area involved in the burn.

In incidents allegedly involving scalds from household tap water, scene investigation must be undertaken. Specifically, the hot water heater should be examined to document the temperature setting. The actual temperature of the hot water at the tap in question should be measured and recorded over time. Depending on the alleged history, it may be necessary to measure the tap water temperature with the hot and cold water running simultaneously, and also the temperature of the standing water in the tub. It may be helpful to utilize an immersion burn scene investigation worksheet. It is not necessary to purchase expensive medical equipment for these measurements—a candy thermometer from a retail store will suffice in most instances. When the data are presented to nonmedical persons, it is recommended that they be expressed in degrees Fahrenheit, as this will allow a more meaningful interpretation.

In general, accidental scald burns are seen in toddlers—children who are somewhat mobile and thus able to interact independently with their environment (8,69,84,214,236,327). Accidental scalds often involve the upper extremities and anterior surface of the head, neck, or upper chest. When a scald has been sustained by pulling a pan of liquid from the stove, the pattern may involve the axilla or submental space in addition to the face, neck, and upper chest (154). Accidental burns are often asymmetric in distribution and of varying severity and depth. At times, "flow patterns" may be observed, with the burn lessening in severity as the pattern progresses inferiorly, or with gravity. Overlying clothing, which holds the hot liquid next to the skin surface, may alter this pattern (Figure 7-32). In cases of accidental burns, small satellite "splash burns" are often apparent (Figure 7-33).

In contrast, victims of inflicted burns are generally younger, most being less than 2 years old (8,69,84,236,258,327). Inflicted burns are often symmetric and may be characterized by distinct immersion lines without evidence of splash burns. A glove or stocking distribution is a frequent finding. If a small child has been dipped into hot liquid, the skin folds of the popliteal fossae and inguinal regions will usually be spared, but the soles of the feet will not. These areas of sparing occur in regions of skin-to-skin contact, where hot liquid cannot penetrate (Figure 7-34). The depth of inflicted burns is usually relatively uniform. Occasionally, one may observe a "doughnut ring" area of sparing over the midportion of the

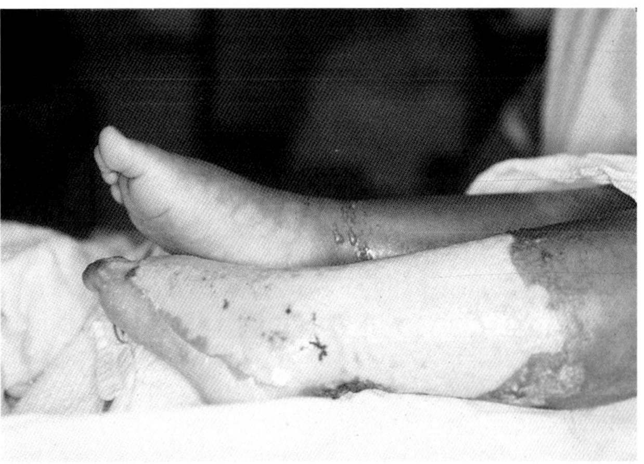

FIGURE 7-33 ■ Satellite splash burns on the medial aspect of the right ankle in an asymmetric scald burn.

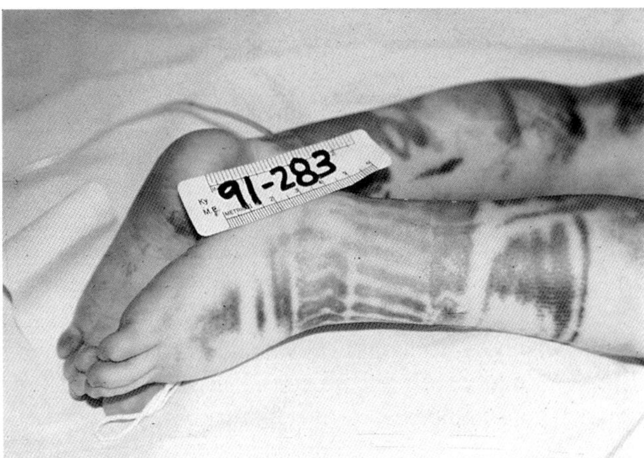

FIGURE 7-32 ■ Scald burns altered by clothing. The patterns of this child's socks and sweat pants are clearly visible.

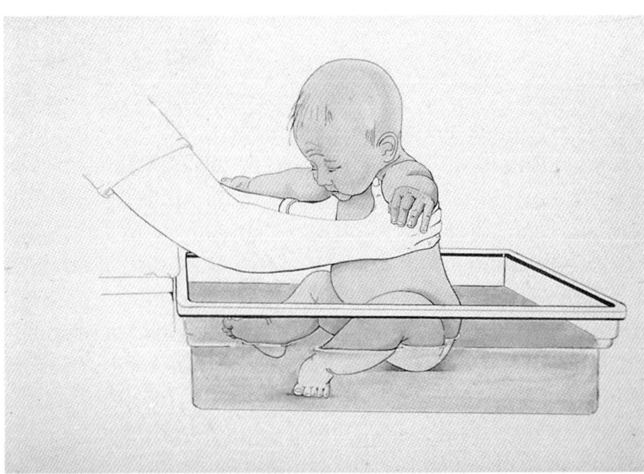

FIGURE 7-34 ■ Immersion pattern.

buttocks. This is created when that portion of the child's skin surface is in contact with the relatively cooler tub or basin surface and thus not directly exposed to the hot liquid.

The American Academy of Pediatrics recommends a "safe setting" of hot water heaters at 125°F or less. At 125°F, contact with water for 2 minutes is required to produce a full-thickness burn. At 130°F and higher, full-thickness burns can result with exposure times of 30 seconds or less (74,225). Of utmost importance in the investigation of scalds is the correlation of the history with the distribution of the scald burn. Simply put, "Does the injury pattern fit the history given?"

Contact burns are rarely fatal. Abusive contact burns are usually caused by common household appliances. Examples include clothing irons, curling irons, hair dryers, and cigarettes (249). Abusive contact burns are often uniform in depth in all directions. The shape of the burn may delineate the causative object. In accidental contact burns, the pattern is more irregular and does not mirror the object as faithfully. The burn is uneven, usually more severe on one side than the other (188). Although rare, abusive microwave burns have been reported (6). Microwave burns differ from scald or contact burns in that they produce an uneven burn pattern through the layers of tissue. Tissue with a high water content, such as muscle, heats to a greater degree than tissue with a relatively low water content, such as subcutaneous fat (255).

HEAD INJURIES

When one attempts to evaluate a head injury in a suspected victim of physical abuse, it may be helpful to refer to a paradigm such as that described by Hymel et al. (141). In this paradigm, injuries are classified as primary or secondary, and focal or diffuse. Cranial injuries are divided into three groups—contact injuries, acceleration injuries, and injuries resulting from hypoxia-ischemia. When a head-injured child is evaluated, the specific cranial injuries are classified, and then the required causal mechanism for each is defined. Finally, the biomechanical circumstances required to produce the injury are compared with the history given. Using such a paradigm allows one to analyze an injury in a systematic, logical, and reproducible way.

Falls

Often, an initial history of a fall is given to account for a young child's head injury. Review of the literature on witnessed, corroborated falls reveals that children generally tolerate such forces well—better than adults, in fact! This has been explained by factors unique to children, such as a smaller mass, which reduces the deceleration force on impact, and a higher proportion of cartilage and subcutaneous fat (307). Several authors have documented series of children sustaining minor household falls. In 1977, Helfer et al. reviewed a series of 246 children with a history of falling out of bed; 85 of the children were hospitalized at the time of their fall (135). No child in the study sustained central nervous system damage. The benign nature of falling out of bed was confirmed by two additional studies of falls in hospitals, one involving 76 children and another involving 207 children falling from beds, cribs, or chairs (196,231). No serious injuries occurred in either study. Stairway falls have also been examined and characterized as an initial "moderate impact" fall, followed by a series of minor impacts. Joffe and Ludwig documented 363 cases of falls down stairs seen in a pediatric emergency department (145). The majority of the children had only superficial injuries, and no child sustained life-threatening injuries or required intensive care (145).

Several series of witnessed, corroborated free falls in children have also been published. Barlow and colleagues examined 61 children during a 10-year period who were admitted to the hospital after falling from a height of one or more stories (13). Of the children who fell three stories or less, 100% survived. Mortality in those falling from the fifth and sixth floors was 50%. In one study of 106 witnessed, corroborated free falls in children less than 3 years old, only one death occurred—in a child who fell from 60 ft. The author concluded that falls of less than 10 ft are unlikely to produce serious or life-threatening injury (313). In yet another series, 70 children with a mean age of 5 years fell from heights ranging from one to 17 stories, and all survived (227). A study of fatal head injury with a history of a fall revealed only three fatalities from witnessed falls—all from heights greater than 10 ft and none with evidence of retinal hemorrhage or axonal injury. And yet in this same study, 19 fatalities occurred in children whose initial history was of a fall of 5 to 6 ft or less; investigation revealed that most of these cases were actually inflicted trauma with an initially false history (256). A study of 317 children brought to a children's trauma center with a history of a fall revealed only one death in 117 children falling from 10 to 45 ft, and seven deaths in children allegedly falling 4 ft or less. In all seven of the fatalities after a short fall, other factors suggested a false history (51). Compiling the multiple available studies, Chadwick concludes, "Death from a fall is now considered very unlikely when the fall is less than 20 feet" (52).

Inflicted Head Injuries

Inflicted head injury is the most common cause of traumatic death in infancy (24,86). Since Caffey first coined the term "whiplash shaken infant syndrome" in 1974, the medical community has used a variety of terms or phrases to describe the classic injury pattern. Terms include shaken baby syndrome, shaken/slammed baby syndrome, shaken impact syndrome, abusive head trauma, inflicted cerebral trauma, and inflicted closed head injury (43,49,86,144). All these terms describe a constellation of injuries seen with regularity in infants who have been physically abused; these include diffuse brain injury with altered consciousness, subdural and subarachnoid hemorrhages over the cerebral convexities, retinal hemorrhages, and scalp contusions. Many authors also include metaphyseal avulsions in this constellation, as Caffey did (43). It has been debated over the years whether

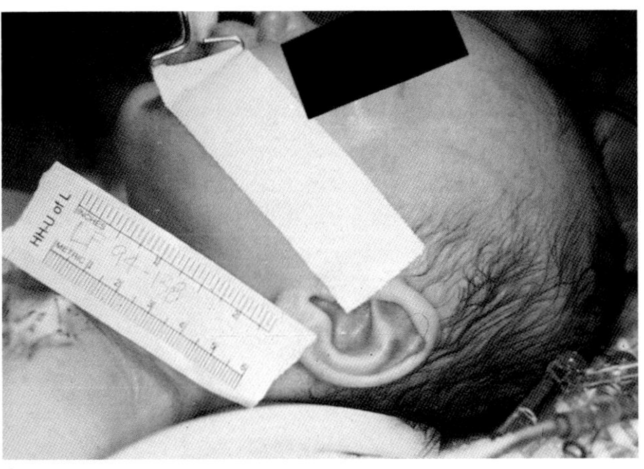

A

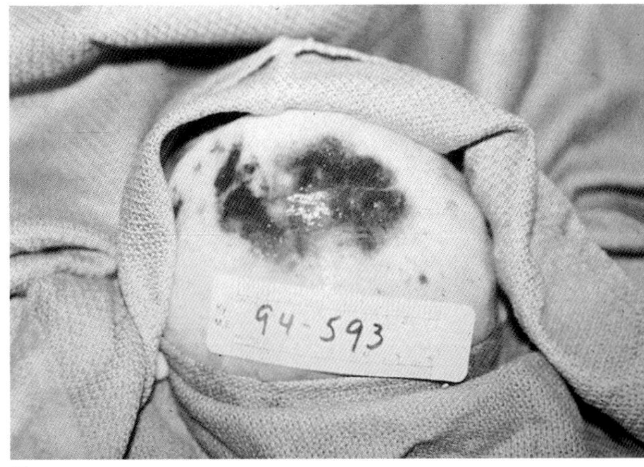

B

FIGURE 7-35 **AB**▪No external injury could be seen in this 2-month-old victim of fatal abusive head trauma (**A**). However, evidence of blunt trauma was identified on reflection of the scalp (**B**).

violent shaking alone is sufficient to cause diffuse, severe brain injury, or whether impact must occur (78,86,175). Many would now agree that pure shaking injury deaths do occur from time to time. Shaking as a mechanism of traumatic death has even been documented in an adult (247). However, in a far more common scenario, evidence of blunt impact to the head is also present (6,182). Many times, evidence of impact is not visible externally and is visualized only after reflection of the scalp at autopsy (Figure 7-35). Even at autopsy, the absence of evidence of cranial blunt trauma does not eliminate the possibility of an impact (283). If the impact occurs on a soft surface, such as a mattress, then the surface area of the impact could be large enough not to produce a scalp contusion. The use of terms such as shaken baby syndrome without adding an explanation that an impact cannot be excluded imparts incorrect information to investigators, who may not consider the possibility of an impact when examining the scene of injury and interviewing witnesses.

Infants and young children have unique characteristics that come into play in central nervous system trauma. The skull is pliable and unilaminar, with unfused sutures, open fontanelles, and a flat, shallow base. The brain constitutes a significantly larger percentage of the total body weight in children than in adults (10% to 15% in children versus 2% to 3% in adults). And this large, heavy head rests on a relatively weak neck. The infant's brain is less myelinated, has smaller axons, and has a higher water content (49).

Primate studies have shown that rotational acceleration of the head, with the low cervical region as the center of rotation, causes acute subdural hematomas (110). When the head is subjected to rotational acceleration, diffuse subdural hemorrhages may be produced over the convexities as a consequence of stretching and tearing of the bridging veins. These bridging veins travel from the brain surface to the dura. Subdural hemorrhages may be confined to the parafalcine area or may layer out over the convexities. Rarely are they space-occupying lesions (Figure 7-36). Rather, subdural hemorrhage is important as a marker of rotational acceleration of the head (141). Angular or rotational acceleration is poorly tolerated by the central nervous system, and shearing strains cause primary diffuse brain injury (86,141,283). Head acceleration with diffuse brain injury results in widespread brain dysfunction, which may range from concussion to traumatic coma with or without permanent neurologic sequelae to sudden death. The unifying feature across the spectrum from concussion to sudden death is the immediate loss of consciousness (110,237,317). In concussion, no pathology is visible; as the severity of the injury increases, pathologic changes become more apparent. These include subdural and subarachnoid hemorrhage as markers of the rotational forces that have occurred. Parenchymal pathologic changes may include contusional tears (slitlike tears at gray-white interfaces) and evidence of diffuse axonal injury, seen as actual axonal disruption (44) (Figure 7-37). In older children and

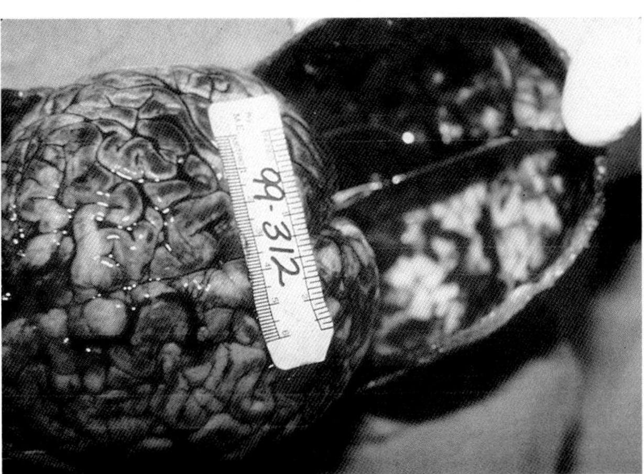

FIGURE 7-36▪Acute subdural hemorrhages over the cerebral convexities in a victim of fatal abusive head trauma. These subdural hemorrhages are very thin and are not space-occupying lesions.

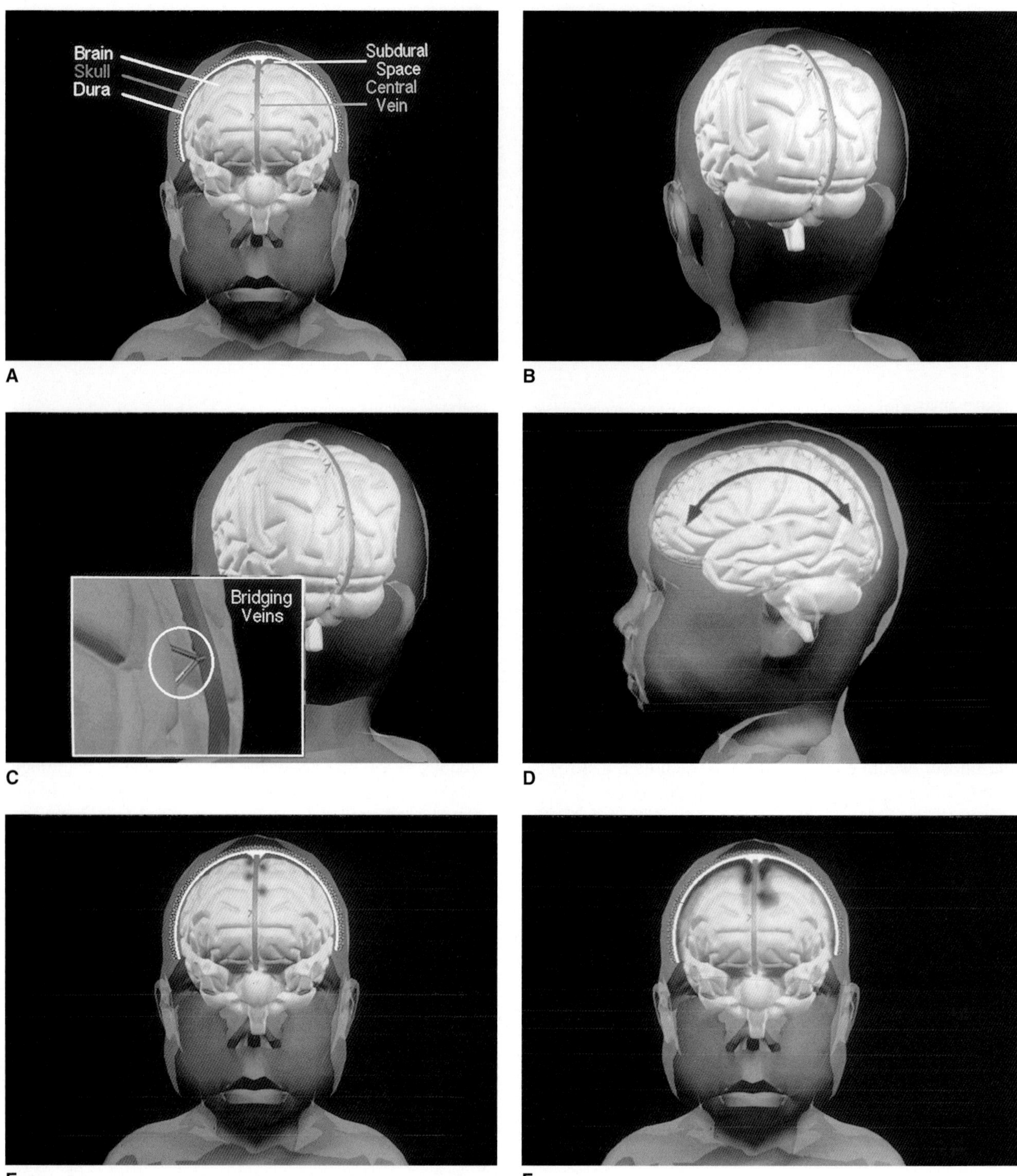

FIGURE 7-37 ■ Schematic representation of abusive head trauma. **A:** The various structures are defined. **B:** The central vein in the sagittal midline. **C:** Small bridging veins traversing the subdural space. **D:** Rotation of the central nervous system in angular acceleration. **E:** Parafalcine subdural hemorrhage. **F:** Subdural hemorrhage over the convexities.

adults, punctate hemorrhages throughout the white matter may accompany axonal disruption.

Because of the unique features of the infant brain, it has been difficult to demonstrate actual axonal disruption in victims of inflicted closed head injury, especially if the infant dies quickly. Even in adults, with good myelination, larger axons, and a higher fat content, histologic evidence of actual axon disruption in the form of retraction balls may

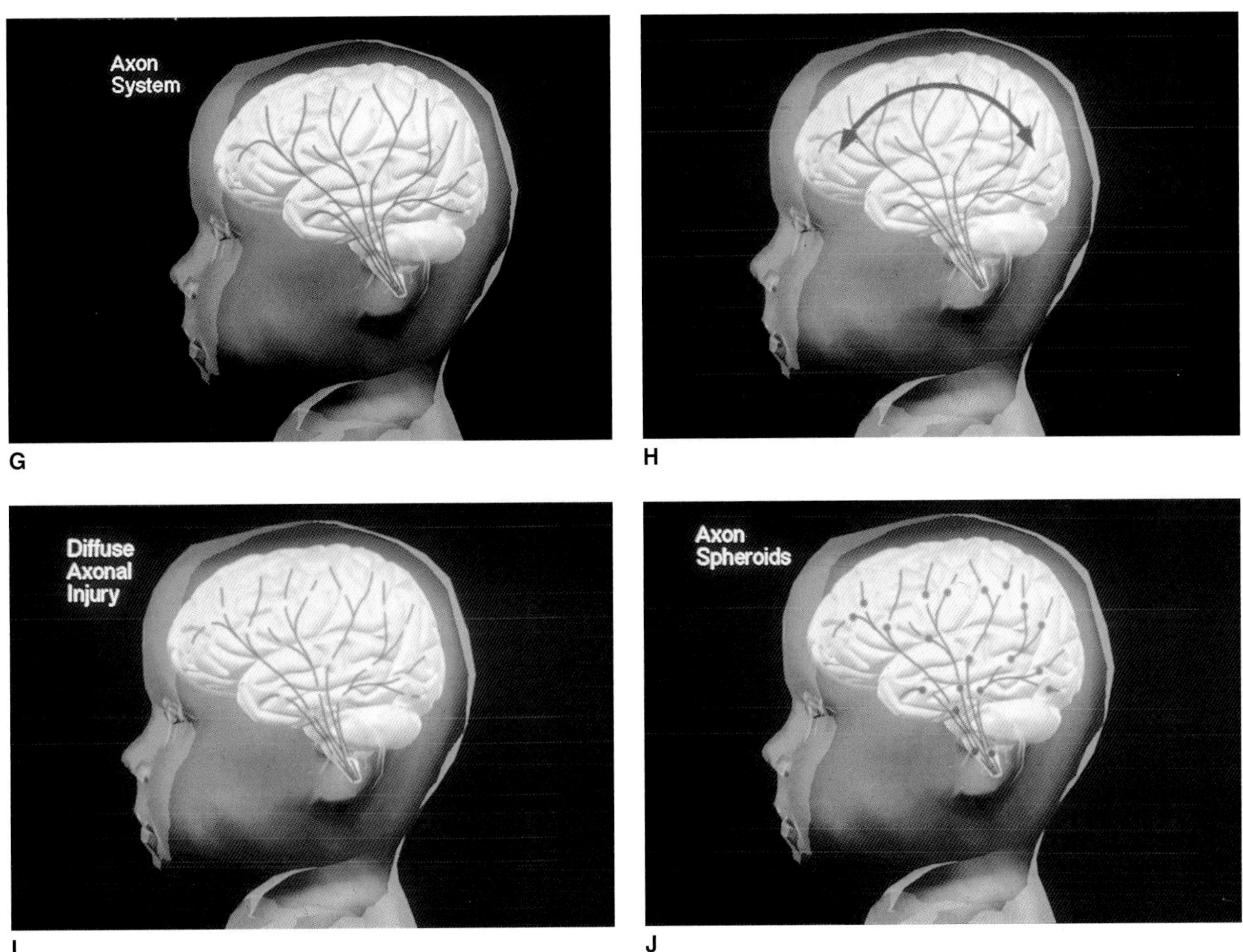

FIGURE 7-37 ▪ *(continued)* **G:** Depiction of the axon system. **H:** Rotation of the central nervous system with shearing. **I:** Resultant diffuse axonal injury. **J:** Eventual appearance of axon spheroids. (Courtesy of Dan Davis, M.D., Hennepin County Medical Examiner's Office, Minneapolis, Minnesota.)

not be apparent without a postinjury survival of at least several hours (4,50) (Figures 7-38 and 7-39). After several weeks, light microscopy reveals microglial nodules. Eventually, wallerian degeneration results in a loss of white matter. The areas most affected include the corpus callosum, fornix, corona radiata, and rostrolateral quadrants of the brain stem. Beta-amyloid precursor protein (b-APP) has been used to detect diffuse axonal injury in the early postinjury period. b-APP accumulates in the axon at or near the site of injury. Some researchers have found b-APP useful to demonstrate diffuse axonal injury in infants with inflicted head injury. Limitations to this method include the requirement for a postinjury survival of about 2 hours to allow the protein to accumulate, and for adequate cerebral vascular perfusion during this time (116). Additional limitations for coroner/medical examiner offices may include the cost and difficulty of routinely performing immunohistochemical studies.

"Tin ear syndrome" is a term used to denote a subset of rotational acceleration. It is a triad of unilateral ear bruising, ipsilateral cerebral edema, and hemorrhagic retinopathy. Each patient in the initial series was a toddler with thin subdural hemorrhages over the convexities (131).

A history of prehospitalization apnea is common in victims of abusive head trauma and is often the first symptom reported to emergency services. Apnea arising from angular acceleration may contribute to morbidity and mortality in these victims through the deleterious effects of ischemia and hypoxia (146). The true morbidity of abusive head trauma is not known because many children with survivable injuries are misdiagnosed or simply never present for medical evaluation. Infants with sublethal inflicted head injury may present for medical evaluation with nonspecific symptoms, including vomiting, fever, irritability, and lethargy. However, these are common symptoms in a variety of conditions. Because a forthcoming history of trauma is usually absent, the infant's traumatic injury may be misdiagnosed as a natural disease process, and the misdiagnosis may lead to further abusive injury and death (144,279). Some studies have

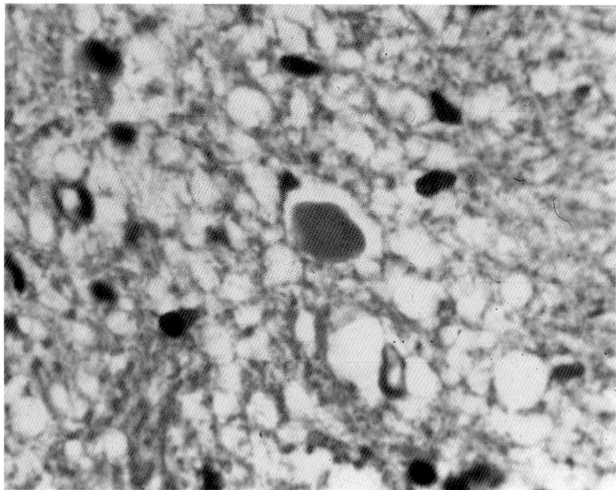

FIGURE 7-38 ■ An axon spheroid (also known as a retraction ball) appearing as an eosinophilic globule. (Hematoxylin and eosin ×400; courtesy of Mitch Morey, M.D., Hennepin County Medical Examiner's Office, Minneapolis, Minnesota.)

shown a "recovery rate" of victims of abusive head trauma of between 20% and 50%, but in one long-term study of victims of "whiplash shaken infant syndrome," many infants with what initially appeared to be a "full recovery" suffered medical, behavioral, and neuropsychological damage 2 to 6 years after the abusive event (27).

Contact Injuries

Head injuries resulting from direct blunt trauma include skull fractures, epidural hematomas, and, in severe cases, crush injuries. A focal area of subdural or subarachnoid hemorrhage may be localized under a contact injury, such as an epidural hematoma. In this case, the focal subdural hemorrhage represents a contact injury. In contrast, the classic findings in abusive head trauma (parafalcine subdural hemorrhage or thin bilateral subdural hemorrhages over the convexities) are produced by rotational forces and thus represent diffuse injury. In adults, epidural hematomas are usually found in association with a fracture of the ipsilateral temporal bone; the epidural hemorrhage arises from a tear in the middle meningeal artery immediately deep to this bone. In children, because of the pliant nature of the skull, the temporal bone may not actually be fractured. The bone may be able to bend in enough to prevent fracture, but the underlying artery may still be lacerated. Epidural hematomas result from brief, linear contact forces. These injuries can be caused by unintentional falls, especially onto pointed or protruding surfaces (273). Isolated epidural hemorrhages are not associated with an immediate loss of consciousness—a finding that makes sense because epidural hemorrhages do not represent primary diffuse brain injuries. Consciousness may be lost some time after the impact as the epidural hemorrhage becomes a space-occupying lesion that produces a mass effect.

Crushing head injury may be associated with incidents in the home environment, such as driveway runovers and toppled heavy objects. Such injuries are caused predominantly by static forces rather than the dynamic forces seen in rotational injuries. In one study of seven cases, including four cases in which the heads of children were run over by vehicles (usually on concrete or asphalt), only one fatality occurred. All the surviving children made a good cognitive recovery (88). In contrast, children with inflicted head injuries often have a poor neurologic outcome (118). Crushing head injuries consist of multiple fractures with deformity of the cranium and cutaneous pattern injuries that can be correlated with the impacting object (Figure 7-40).

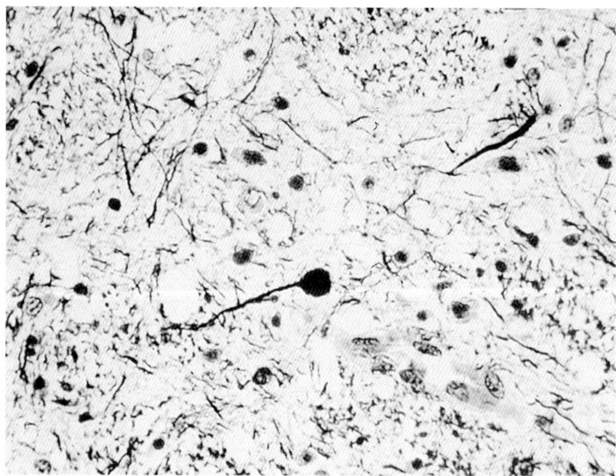

FIGURE 7-39 ■ An axon spheroid visualized with a silver stain. (Silver stain, ×250; courtesy of Mitch Moray, M.D., Hennepin County Medical Examiner's Office, Minneapolis, Minnesota.)

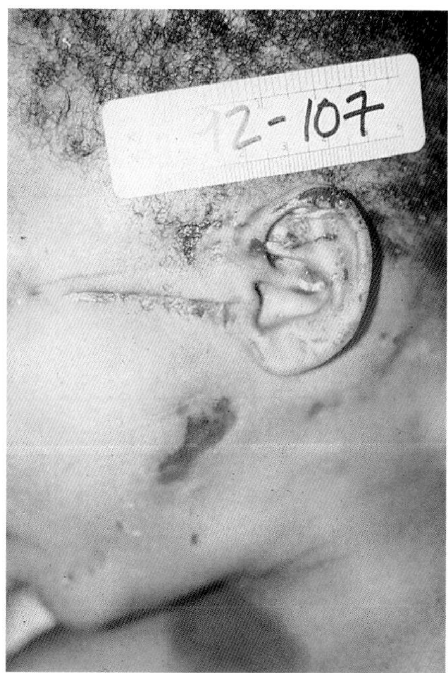

FIGURE 7-40 ■ Crushing head injury. Pattern injury corresponds to impacting object.

Retinal Hemorrhage

Retinal hemorrhages have been associated with abusive head trauma since Caffey included them in the constellation of injuries of the whiplash shaken infant syndrome (43). Although not always present in cases of abusive head trauma, retinal hemorrhages are disproportionately represented in inflicted head trauma, as opposed to head trauma caused by other mechanisms of force (50,88). The mechanism by which retinal hemorrhages are produced in pediatric inflicted head injury is not fully understood. Proposed mechanisms include vitreous traction on the retina during angular acceleration and elevated intracranial pressure (36,114). Studies indicate that retinal hemorrhages are found in from 50% to 100% of children with abusive head trauma (24,36).

Other causes of retinal hemorrhages include sepsis with coagulopathy and vaginal delivery in the newborn. Retinal hemorrhages have been reported in up to 20% of newborns, especially those with primiparous mothers or delivered vaginally. Most of the hemorrhages dissipate by the end of the first week of life. Virtually all resolve without incident by the end of the first month of life (269,271).

Although retinal hemorrhages may be found in a small percentage of children with accidental injuries, the injuries have generally been caused by extraordinary force, as in motor vehicle collisions (147). Although many articles do not describe in detail the pattern of retinal hemorrhages seen in accident victims, it is often different from that seen in shaken impact syndrome. In cases of accidental trauma, the hemorrhages may be less numerous and less severe than in abusive head trauma. In shaken impact syndrome, the hemorrhages are often diffuse, massive, and bilateral. Hemorrhage into the vitreous and traumatic retinoschisis may be seen in inflicted head trauma (120). Therefore, the often-heard statement that "retinal hemorrhages are nonspecific" is technically correct but no more meaningful than a statement such as "fractures are nonspecific." When retinal hemorrhages are characterized according to type, location, degree, and pattern of associated injuries, the specificity increases. Cardiopulmonary resuscitation has been offered as an explanation for retinal hemorrhages, but this hypothesis is not supported in several studies (114,147).

When the globes of a shaken impact syndrome victim are harvested at autopsy, various changes may be noted. Grossly, hemorrhage along the optic nerve sheath may be seen. It is relatively standard practice to prepare a pupillary-optic nerve section for microscopic examination. However, it should be remembered that this represents only a small surface area of the retina and that the overall pattern of retinal hemorrhage cannot be appreciated in such a section. Microscopically, hemorrhages frequently are seen in the nerve fiber and ganglion cell layers of the retina (226,254). Purtscher retinopathy is another distinct pattern of retinal hemorrhage associated with a distinct traumatic etiology. Purtscher retinopathy, which is seen following traumatic chest compression asphyxia, is characterized by large white patches on the retina in the macular and peripupillary areas (24,36). It has been reported in association with battered child syndrome (300).

SKELETAL EVIDENCE OF PHYSICAL ABUSE

As stated earlier, a skeletal survey should be conducted on victims of suspected physical abuse who are under the age of 2 years (212). In living children, it is recommended that a skeletal survey be repeated 2 weeks later, or, if this is unlikely to occur, a bone scan may be performed on the same day as the initial skeletal survey. Obviously, these are not options in deceased children. When abnormalities are suspected on skeletal survey, the bony area in question may be excised. Excision makes it possible to document associated soft tissue injuries, obtain more detailed radiographic images, and perform a direct visual and histologic examination. It is wise to review radiographs with a pediatric radiologist, who will recognize subtle but specific signs of inflicted injury. Kleinman has grouped skeletal injuries according to their relative specificity for abuse (162). Those with a high specificity for abuse, particularly in infants, include classic metaphyseal lesions, posterior rib fractures, scapular fractures, spinous process fractures, and sternal fractures.

Skull fractures in infancy may be associated with falls and also with inflicted blunt trauma. Most accidental skull fractures sustained in minor household falls are single, linear, nondisplaced fractures of unilateral parietal bones, with no associated underlying intracranial injury (137,270). Fractures that cross suture lines, multiple fractures, and bilateral fractures are associated with inflicted injury more than with minor accidents (213). Kleinman describes linear fractures as fractures with a low specificity for abuse, whereas complex skull fractures are regarded as moderately specific (162).

Classic metaphyseal lesions are distinctive injuries of infancy and are highly specific for inflicted injury—perhaps more so than any other skeletal or visceral abnormality. The lesion consists of a planar disruption through the primary spongiosa. Hemorrhage is usually inconspicuous. The distal femur and proximal tibia are the most common sites of these fractures, which are often bilateral. The lesions are thought to be produced by torsional and tractional forces generated when the infant is twisted or pulled by an extremity, or when the extremities are subjected to shear strains during violent shaking. Although extremely telling of abuse, these lesions are difficult to date because the usual markers, such as subperiosteal formation of new bone, are often lacking (162,163). Because of the subtlety and specificity of these lesions, some have suggested that even metaphyses that appear normal by radiographic examination be removed in postmortem cases in which abuse is strongly suspected (164). Fractures of the shaft of a long bone are four times more frequent than epiphyseal-metaphyseal injuries and are the most common fracture seen in child abuse (159,189,190,195). However, these fractures are of low specificity in ambulatory children (25,212). Indeed, nondisplaced oblique or spiral fractures of the tibia are so frequently caused by accidental falls in ambulating youngsters that they are referred to as "toddler's fractures" (90,162). The specificity for abuse increases as the age of the child decreases—spiral diaphyseal fractures of nonambulatory infants are highly suspect. However, a recent report of two unintentional spiral-oblique humeral fractures in preambulatory infants illustrates the importance of a investigating the case history thoroughly before formulating a final opinion (142). Although abusive fractures can occur anywhere along the ribs, they are often distributed in a posterior location. Anteroposterior compression of the thorax, as in squeezing by an adult, produces excess leverage over the fulcrum of the transverse processes at the costovertebral junction (169). This in turn creates tension along the inner aspects of the rib head and neck that leads to fractures. Abusive rib fractures may also be located laterally because the lateral aspects of the ribs represent areas of outbending and tension during squeezing (Figure 7-41). Acute rib fractures may not be visible radiographically. During healing, as calluses form, the fracture becomes visible radiographically (162) (Figure 7-42). Attempts at cardiopulmonary resuscitation may be offered as an explanation for rib fractures. However, in previous studies, routine skeletal survey or autopsy was unable to demonstrate rib fractures in infants following cardiopulmonary resuscitation (82,96,124,139,280,319,321).

Like the dating of soft tissue trauma, the dating of skeletal trauma is imprecise (328). In an attempt to age or date a skeletal injury, three separate factors must be taken into consideration. First, the age of the infant affects the healing process. Callus develops in neonates sooner than in older infants. Dynamic changes occur in the skeleton itself as an infant matures, and compact bone increases. Second, the history of the injury must be considered, although many times in abusive injuries accurate histories are not forthcoming. Third, many abusive skeletal fractures are subjected to repetitive trauma. Either the abusive act is repeated in the same location and affects the same bone, or a failure to seek medical attention results in lack of treatment and immobilization, so that the fracture is constantly disturbed (232). Histologic studies of the timing of abusive injuries are difficult to undertake. Multiple episodes of trauma have often occurred, accurate histories are rarely provided, and histology provides only a single window of time in a dynamic process. Consultation with a pediatric radiologist and correlation of the histopathologic findings with the radiologic appearance are strongly encouraged.

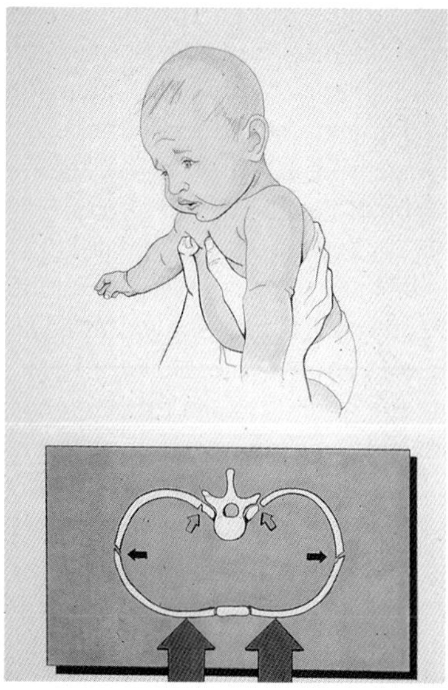

FIGURE 7-41 ■ Schematic representation of the production of abusive rib fractures. Anteroposterior squeezing results in posterior or lateral fractures.

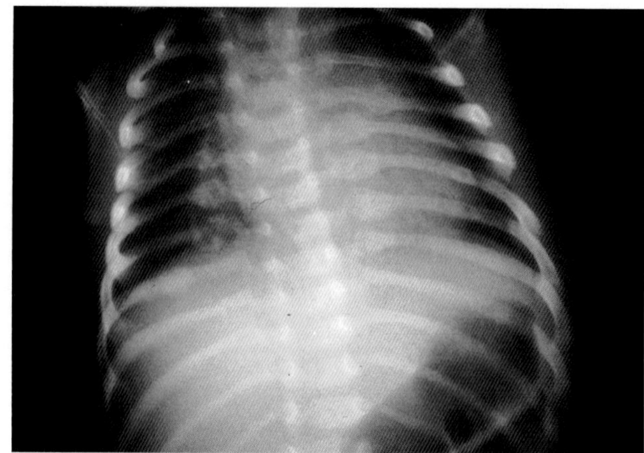

FIGURE 7-42 ■ Multiple posterior rib fractures with callus formation.

On occasion, caregivers attempt to conceal fatal child abuse by discarding the child's body and claiming that the child is missing. If the child is later discovered, the remains may be skeletonized. Ascertaining the cause and manner of death becomes more difficult when soft tissue is absent. Consultation with a forensic anthropologist may be extremely helpful in such cases. The forensic anthropologist can assist in determining the age, sex, and postmortem interval. The sex of a prepubertal child is extremely difficult to assess (157). The anthropologist may be able to detect subperiosteal new bone formation in association with healed fractures (305).

BLUNT TRAUMA OF THE ABDOMEN AND THORAX

Blunt abdominal trauma is the second leading cause of death in fatal child abuse (53). The victims are generally toddlers. The inflicted injury may represent the delivery of a large force, such as a punch or a kick, to a small surface area. The involved organs are trapped between the incoming force over the soft anterior abdominal wall and the rigid spine or thoracic cage along the posterior aspect of the body (Figure 7-43). Evidence of blunt trauma to the anterior abdominal wall is not a reliable marker for inflicted blunt abdominal trauma; in a study of 184 abusive child homicides in New York City, 43% of the children dying of blunt abdominal trauma displayed no external evidence of trauma along the anterior abdominal wall (75).

Several studies indicate that hollow viscera in the midline upper abdomen, such as the duodenum and jejunum, are the organs most commonly injured in abusive blunt abdominal trauma (184,245). The two most common causes of duodenal injury in children are abuse and motor vehicle collisions in which the lap belt has been placed over the abdomen rather

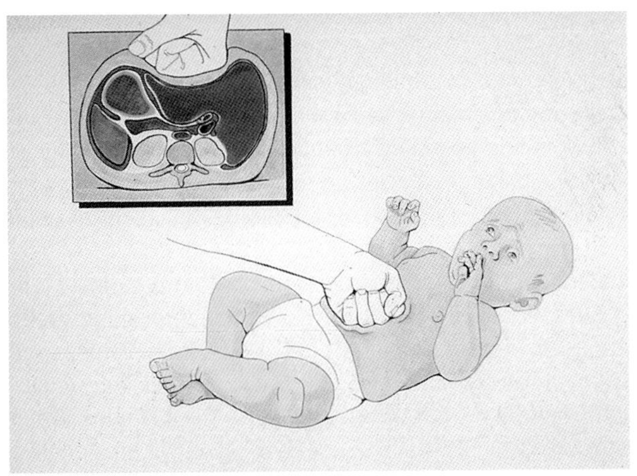

FIGURE 7-43 ▪ Schematic representation of abusive abdominal trauma.

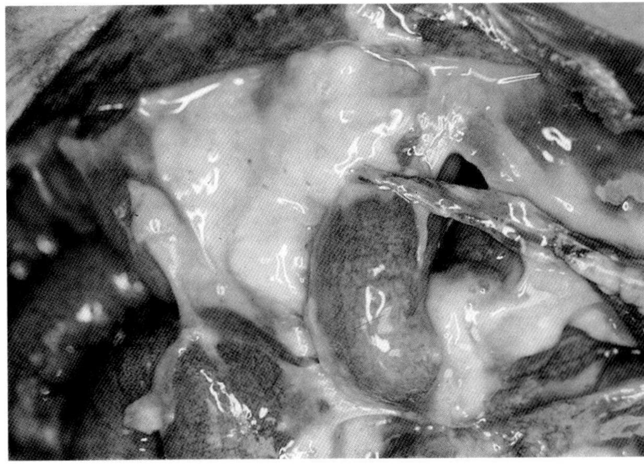

FIGURE 7-45 ▪ Acute peritonitis resulting from the small-bowel perforation shown in Figure 7-44.

than the pelvic region and iliac crests (28). The duodenum and jejunum are thought to be more vulnerable to blunt force injury in young children because of the unique characteristics of a toddler's abdomen—wide and comparatively flared costal margins and a short anteroposterior distance (31,245). Injuries to these organs include duodenal hematomas, serosal avulsions, and full-thickness perforations with resultant peritonitis. Because of its viscoelastic nature, human tissue responds in a rigid fashion when forces are rapidly applied. In contrast, the tissue is more deformable when forces are slowly applied (284). When subjected to a rapid force, such as a punch or kick, a hollow organ may perforate.

The mortality rate in victims with abusive hollow viscus perforations is very high [71% in a study by Ledbetter (184)], and they often present for medical care in extremis or are dead at the scene. Historical information usually reveals that the child has been ill, with nausea and vomiting, for a time period ranging from hours to days. At autopsy, the prosecting pathologist must examine the bowel carefully to identify the perforation—a task made more challenging by the accompanying peritonitis. The perforation itself is usually quite small. Such an injury is highly amenable to surgical intervention if medical treatment is obtained in a timely fashion (Figures 7-44 and 7-45). Injuries to the mesenteric root may be associated with the bowel perforation. All evidence of abdominal injury—abdominal wall contusion, small-bowel perforation, mesenteric root injury—should be histologically sampled to estimate the interval from "injury to death" and document any evidence of old injury. Vitreous electrolyte studies may reveal dehydration in these cases, which coincides with postinjury nausea and vomiting (59,62,171).

The solid organ most commonly injured in child abuse is the liver (75,184). Lacerations of the liver result in hemoperitoneum; the mechanism of death in these cases is internal exsanguination. In contrast to small-bowel perforation, injury to the liver is relatively quickly followed by profound symptoms of shock. The liver may display massive, stellate lacerations—more severe than those generally seen in high-velocity motor vehicle collisions (Figures 7-46 and 7-47). In cases of blunt force trauma, cardiopulmonary resuscitation may be offered as an explanation. However, studies have shown that injuries caused by cardiopulmonary resuscitation

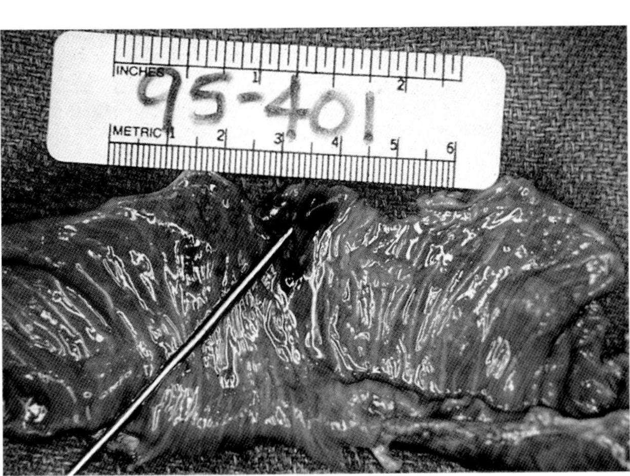

FIGURE 7-44 ▪ Small-bowel perforation with surrounding submucosal hemorrhage that resulted in death.

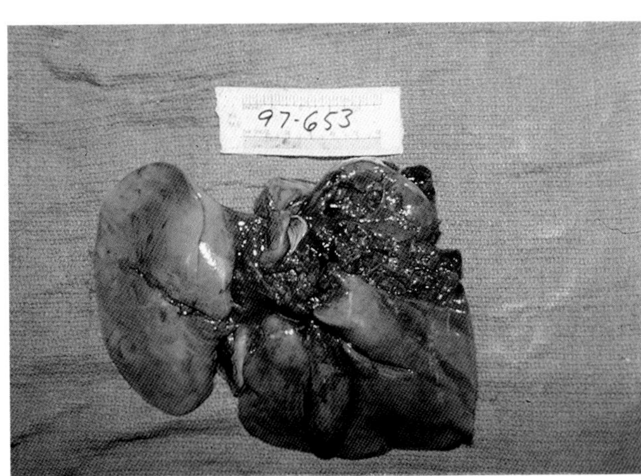

FIGURE 7-46 ▪ Extensive stellate liver lacerations resulting from fatal abusive abdominal trauma in a 3-year-old child.

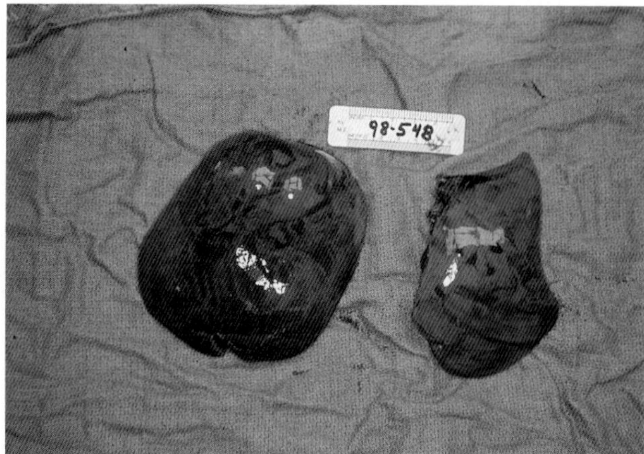

FIGURE 7-47 ■ Transection of the liver resulting from fatal abusive abdominal trauma in a 20-month-old child.

are rare in children and not as severe as abusive injuries (34,68,96,172,222,251,257,280,285,304). When such an explanation of massive abdominal injuries is offered, the question arises: "Why did the child require cardiopulmonary resuscitation in the first place?"

Another frequently affected solid organ is the pancreas. Injury to the pancreas may be associated with a small-bowel perforation or liver laceration which is the cause of death, but the pancreatic injury is further evidence of blunt force trauma (46). If the child survives the initial insult, pancreatitis and pseudocysts are the most common complications (9). As previously discussed (see "Skeletal Evidence of Physical Abuse"), rib fractures are often caused by anteroposterior squeezing. This represents a force applied slowly over a large surface area, rather than a large force delivered rapidly to a small surface area, as in a direct blow. The typical pattern is bilateral in approximately the same location (posterior or lateral). Abusive blunt force injury of the thoracic visceral organs from blows is relatively rare in comparison with head injuries and abdominal trauma. Homicidal cardiac lacerations often consist of rupture of the right atrium at its junction with the great veins. This rupture is caused by either of two possible mechanisms. In direct trauma to the precordial chest, the heart is compressed between the incoming sternum anteriorly and the rigid thoracic cage and vertebral column posteriorly (58). In trauma via a blow to the epigastric region of the abdomen, the force may be transmitted to the atrium via the inferior vena cava (67). In both scenarios, the forces are applied rapidly, so that energy cannot be absorbed through deformation of the viscoelastic tissue (302).

MIMICRY

Although some disorders can be mistaken for pediatric inflicted injury, courtroom claims are much more frequent than actual occurrences. Impostors of inflicted childhood injury may be divided into three main categories: cutaneous findings, bony abnormalities, and metabolic conditions.

Cutaneous Findings

Causes of cutaneous findings that can be mistaken for signs of abuse include natural diseases, congenital markings, cultural folk medicine practices, and decompositional changes.

Impetigo contagiosa is one of the more common cutaneous childhood infectious diseases that can be mistaken for child abuse. Impetigo contagiosa is most often a disease of preschoolers and may occur in epidemics. The two most common etiologic agents are Staphylococcus aureus and group A streptococci. The lesions, which usually occur in exposed areas, begin as relatively circular vesicopustules that rupture quickly and can be mistaken for cigarette burns (Figure 7-48). After rupture, the lesions become covered with a thick yellow crust. Histologically, the vesicopustule is located in the upper layers of the epidermis and contains numerous neutrophils. It also may contain Gram-positive cocci (191) (Figure 7-49).

Staphylococcal scalded skin syndrome, as the name implies, may be mistaken for scald burns. It is characterized by large, flaccid bullae that rupture almost immediately. In this syndrome, the staphylococcal infection is usually extracutaneous, such as pharyngitis or conjunctivitis. The bullae are caused by a toxin produced by the staphylococci (191). Streptococcal toxic shock syndrome may present in much the same way (229).

Cutaneous contact with calcium chloride may cause skin necrosis to an extent requiring debridement. Such a lesion may raise concerns about child abuse (329).

Ehlers-Danlos syndrome is an inherited connective tissue disorder with ten different subtypes. Some subtypes are characterized by poor wound healing with extremely thin skin, prolonged bleeding, and subsequent scarring (306). Because a severe injury accompanies a history of minor trauma, such lesions have been confused with abusive injuries.

Some hematologic disorders may cause a cutaneous manifestation of "unexplained bruising." This may lead to a suspicion of abuse. Disorders that have presented in this fashion include acute lymphoblastic leukemia and von Willebrand disease (205,306).

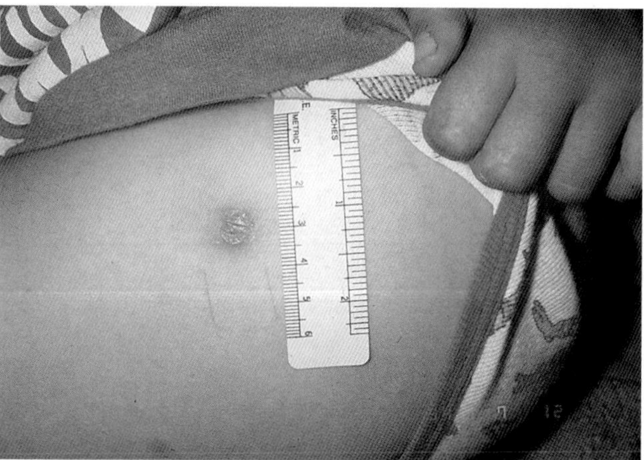

FIGURE 7-48 ■ Impetigo contagiosa, initially alleged to be a cigarette burn. Note additional lesion at the inferior margin of the photograph. (Courtesy of Bill Smock, M.D., Department of Emergency Medicine, University of Louisville, Kentucky.)

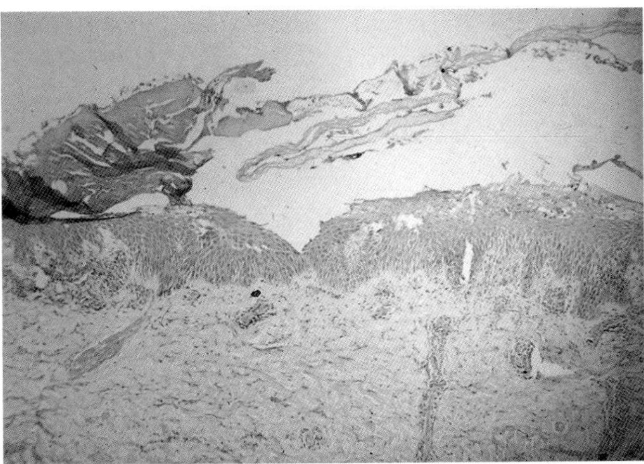

FIGURE 7-49 ▪ Impetigo contagiosa. Vesicle in the upper layers of the epidermis.

A common nonpathologic finding that may be mistaken for a contusion is a Mongolian spot. Mongolian spots are generally located over the lumbosacral region and are present at birth (Figure 7-50). They usually fade during the early years but may be retained into adulthood. They are seen in a high percentage of African-American, Hispanic, and Asian babies. They also occur in Caucasian babies. Mongolian spots occasionally develop outside the lumbosacral region (192). A congenital hemangioma known as nevus flammeus may be mistaken for a red contusion. Two types exist. The medially located nevus flammeus is commonly located in the occipital region or the center of the face. The laterally located nevus flammeus is found on the face or extremities. The laterally located lesion may become darker and raised with age, whereas the medially located lesion remains flat and may fade with age (193). These congenital hemangiomas are colloquially known as "stork bites" (Figure 7-51).

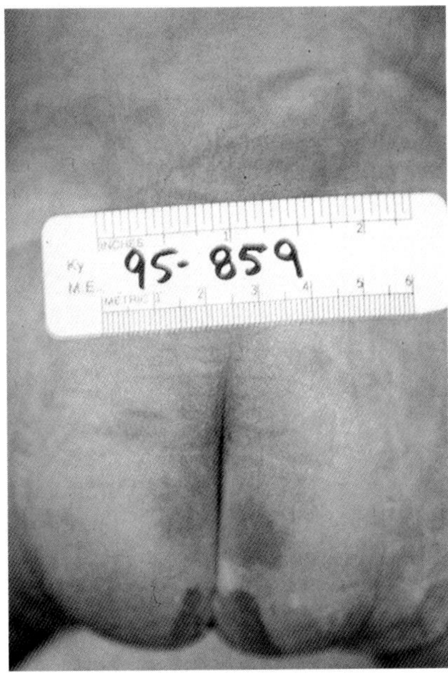

FIGURE 7-50 ▪ Mongolian spot over the midline buttocks of an infant.

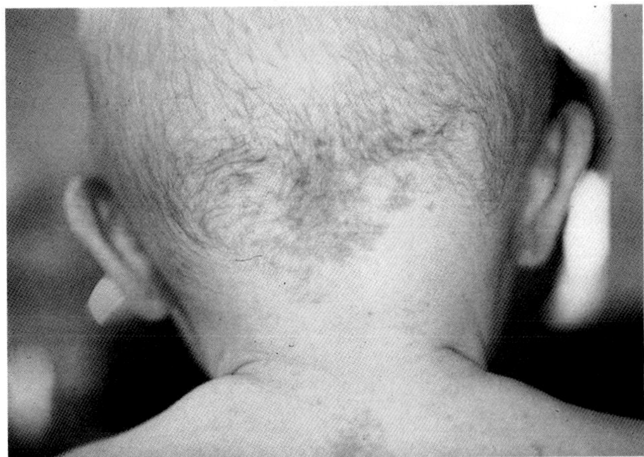

FIGURE 7-51 ▪ Congenital hemangioma over the midline occipital region. An additional hemangioma is visible at the bottom of the picture in the midline high thoracic region.

Various cultural folk medicine customs cause cutaneous lesions that can be confused with abuse if the examiner is unaware of them. One of the most common is a practice of Vietnamese immigrants. Cao gio ("coin rubbing") is used to alleviate common illnesses. The lesions are produced by rubbing the skin with a coin. Common sites include the back, neck, head, shoulders, and chest. Other practices include bat gio ("skin").

Postmortem changes that may be confused with traumatic injuries by nonpathologists include lividity and maceration. Victims of SIDS often are transported to the hospital with well-developed rigor mortis. Such infants show a well-developed lividity pattern. Those unfamiliar with lividity may confuse it with antemortem bruising. Lividity can be differentiated from contusion as follows: lividity occurs in dependent areas of the body as it rests in the postmortem state, and pressure points are spared. Prominent lividity is seen in association with well-developed rigor mortis. Livor mortis blanches under pressure for about the first 24 hours. It should be remembered that both rigor and livor are greatly influenced by environmental factors (including temperature and wind current) and by individual factors such as clothing and size of the decedent. Death *in utero* is followed by macerative changes in relatively short order (274). Skin slipping, separation of the epidermis from the underlying dermis, may be present as soon as 6 hours after death and is expected if the infant has been dead for 12 hours or longer (311). Because the epidermis easily peels away and the underlying dermis displays a generalized red color, skin slipping may be mistaken for scald burns.

Other Findings

Soon after death, the infant brain, with its very high water content, begins to liquefy. The bones of the cranium then override one another, so that deformity of the cranium results. Such deformity may be mistaken for head trauma.

Inherited metabolic conditions may cause signs and symptoms that can be confused with abuse (59,171,200).

Methylmalonic aciduria may present as failure to thrive (306). Glutaric aciduria type I is an inherited metabolic disorder that can be confused initially with head trauma. Children with glutaric aciduria type I may present at age 6 to 18 months with encephalopathic crisis following a minor illness. This encephalopathic crisis may lead to destruction of the basal ganglia. Children with glutaric aciduria type I characteristically display a head circumference above the 95th percentile at birth. Continued rapid growth of the head circumference after birth leads to macrocephaly with frontal bossing (12). Glutaric aciduria type I may be diagnosed by a metabolic screen of blood (see Chapter 5).

Osteogenesis imperfecta is a rare disorder of type I collagen that results in abnormal bone fragility. Type I collagen is the major structural protein of the extracellular matrix of bone, skin, and tendon (201). Four main types of osteogenesis imperfecta are known. Type I is the most common. It is characterized by abnormal fragility with osteoporosis, blue sclerae, defective dentition (dentinogenesis imperfecta), and presenile hearing impairment. Other features common in osteogenesis imperfecta type I include wormian bones of the skull and short stature. Osteogenesis imperfecta type I accounts for approximately 80% of all cases of osteogenesis imperfecta. It is inherited in an autosomal dominant fashion. The family history is extremely useful in evaluating children for osteogenesis imperfecta type I.

Osteogenesis imperfecta type II is known as the fetal or perinatal form. Severe osteoporosis is generally apparent at birth, and intrauterine growth retardation is present. The majority of children with osteogenesis imperfecta type II succumb within the first few weeks of life. These infants display deep blue-black sclerae, a characteristic facies, severe skeletal deformities, and multiple fractures and osteopenia at birth. Because of the obvious bony deformities, this form is unlikely to be mistaken for child abuse (107). Type III is thought to be caused by a sporadic mutation. The majority of patients with type III display characteristic triangular faces. These infants may have fractures at birth. The color of the sclerae may appear normal. Children with type III often display shortening, bowing, and angulation of the long bones in addition to growth retardation. Type IV, the rarest form, is most often confused with abuse. Osteoporosis and deformity are present but may be mild. Type IV children usually have wormian bones, and abnormal dentition is common. Metaphyseal fractures in osteogenesis imperfecta are different from the metaphyseal corner fractures and bucket handle fractures seen classically in child abuse (1). Although the potential for misdiagnosis exists, the probability is very small given the relative prevalences of type IV osteogenesis imperfecta and abusive fractures (167). Microscopically, the osseous tissue of a child with osteogenesis imperfecta demonstrates a relative abundance of osteocytes. The extracellular matrix is reduced, and so the cells are much closer together than is normal (32). The diagnosis of osteogenesis imperfecta remains a clinical one, based on the patient and family history and on the findings of diagnostic imaging and physical examination. A skin biopsy may be used as a confirmatory test (see Chapter 27).

CARDIOPULMONARY RESUSCITATION INJURIES

Often, a child is brought to the attention of a health care professional or death investigator and the etiology of injuries, in particular injuries secondary to cardiopulmonary resuscitation (CPR) versus inflicted blunt force trauma, becomes a crucial issue (20,124,132,134,149,172,183,222,248,251,297, 319,321). Perpetrators will claim that a child's injuries were caused by CPR, either by the child him/herself or by a first responder. Injuries secondary to CPR may be external and internal, usually involving the head/neck and rarely trunk (abdomen/thorax). These injuries are due to the compressions and to ventilation/intubation. Several studies report no injuries to children secondary to CPR. Others report that, if present, these CPR-related injuries are not significant or life threatening. Investigators should be aware of the resuscitative technique used on children, if abdominal compressions were performed, and note if the resuscitator is experienced in the technique(s) (222,304). The EMS personnel or emergency department physician can easily demonstrate how he/she performs CPR. The investigator can correlate injuries with points of contact during compressions and ventilation, type of mask, and type of airway. The mask should be retained for comparison to the facial injuries. A doll can be used as well as the type/size of mask. Note any adhesive used on the face to aid in ventilation/intubation.

Conventional CPR with chest compressions produces blood flow that is approximately 30% of normal. Interposed abdominal compressions (IAC) augmenting resuscitation may be performed resulting in improved hemodynamics without intra-abdominal injury (10,304). IAC can increase the blood flow twofold, and when performed by trained individuals, the midabdominal compressions increase organ perfusion without organ injury. Studies in canines show that IAC improves arterial pressure, central venous pressure, oxygen consumption, and cardiac output without causing trauma.

In children, unlike adults, rib and sternal fractures rarely if ever occur; this has even proven true in children with an underlying bone disease (124,134,139,172,199,268,319, 321). Ribs in children are flexible and more resilient against fracture. In the absence of radiographic evidence of bone disease, unexplained rib fractures are indicative of abuse. Often, such rib fractures are associated with other signs of abuse and/or different stages of rib healing. Recent radiographical studies have examined subtle CPR-related rib fractures (82). When present, these rib fractures are not usually associated with hemorrhage and are extremely difficult to notice without removal of the parietal pleura.

Abdominal injury is uncommon (14,68,178,197,248, 277,285,297). Rarely, gastric perforation (lesser curvature), epicardial hematoma, pulmonary interstitial hemorrhage, hepatic/splenic contusion or laceration, and pancreatic injury have been reported as secondary to CPR. Abdominal compressions in children may result in pancreatic hemorrhage as well as injury to the liver and spleen. Such abdominal compressions should be documented (304). However, it must be noted that some studies of many resuscitated children report no injuries. In one study, injuries were noted, but none were abdominal.

More of the CPR-related injuries in children are soft tissue injuries of the head and neck from ventilatory efforts (108,121,132,152). These include facial abrasions (nasal bridge, undersurface of the nose, anterior chin) from the air-bag-valve mask that are usually symmetrical. As the resuscitator positions his/her hand on the child, fingertip contusions beneath the chin and on the side of the head may be produced. If a mask is not used but instead mouth-to-mouth breathing is performed, one may see scrapes/fingernail scratches over the perinasal area. If intubated, adhesive tape marks may be present on the lateral aspects of the mouth and cheeks. The child's oropharynx is more susceptible to damage by forceful digital clearing and suction as well as by endoscopic instruments. Traumatic mucosal tears and hypopharyngeal perforation have occurred with digital clearing of the airway (108). The adult-type oral injuries secondary to teeth are not seen in the edentulous child (172). With regard to CPR causing retinal hemorrhages, studies and collaborative research conclude that CPR does not result in retinal hemorrhages.

Various forms of barotrauma have been described in adults and children (259). These include tympanic membrane injury, pneumothorax, pneumoperitoneum, pneumoscrotum, and air embolism (especially in the premature newborn). With ventilation, injuries such as pneumothorax (due to positive pressure ventilation) and gastric rupture (due to overdistension during ventilation; usually the lesser curvature) may result (257). Also, though rare, complications of mechanical positive pressure ventilation can occur related to faulty bag ventilation devices and the valve.

Findings secondary to CPR other than from compressions and ventilation include defibrillator marks over the thorax, venipuncture and intraosseous line access marks, bruising about the neck from attempted vascular access, adhesive marks from taping the endotracheal tube, and vomitus in the airway secondary to agonal regurgitation and subsequent compressions. One can also see cardiac contraction band necrosis and focal hemorrhage with the administration of catecholamines during prolonged resuscitation. Defibrillation can produce subepicardial myofibril disintegration. Gastric rupture secondary to nasogastric tube placement has also occurred.

GUNSHOT WOUNDS

Gunshot wounds are relatively uncommon in young children but account for significant morbidity and mortality in adolescents. It has been shown that the availability of guns in the home increases the risk for suicide among adolescents (18,30). Furthermore, many adolescent students report easy access to handguns (47% of boys and 22% of girls in one study) (18,45).

Information that may be derived from the examination of a gunshot wound includes an estimate of the range of fire and path of the projectile. Soot and gunpowder particles emerge from the muzzle of a fired gun along with the bullet. Depending on the distance of the target surface from the muzzle of the gun, these substances may be deposited in or on the target surface and may be used to estimate the range of fire. In contact wounds, all gas, soot, and gunpowder particles are blown into the wound bed along with the bullet. In wounds of the head, where relatively thin tissue is stretched over a rigid bony skull, gas is trapped between the outer table of the skull and the soft tissue. This causes a marked expansion of the soft tissue, which may exceed the elastic capability of the skin. When the elastic capability of the skin is exceeded, stellate lacerations radiate from the margins of the gunshot wound of entrance. Furthermore, as the skin is forced outward from the body by entrapped gas, a "muzzle stamp abrasion" may be produced (Figure 7-52). In wounds produced at close range, soot and burning gunpowder particles are deposited on the skin surrounding the gunshot wound of entrance. Soot is transient evidence because it may be wiped away during medical treatment. Therefore, it is imperative that this evidence be documented early or preserved in some fashion. As the distance between the muzzle and skin surface increases, soot can no longer reach the body surface. However, the burned and burning gunpowder particles continue to travel and become embedded in the skin. These are represented by small, reddish brown, punctate lesions surrounding the gunshot wound of entrance. The pattern is referred to as "stippling" or "tattooing" (Figure 7-53). The examiner should measure the dimensions of the stippling and describe

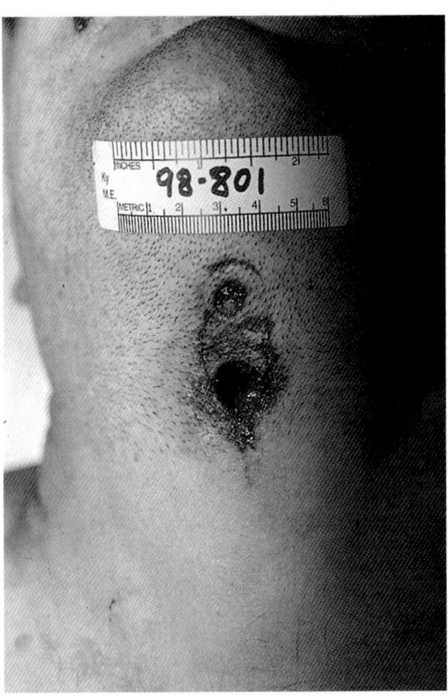

FIGURE 7-52 ■ Contact gunshot wound with muzzle stamp.

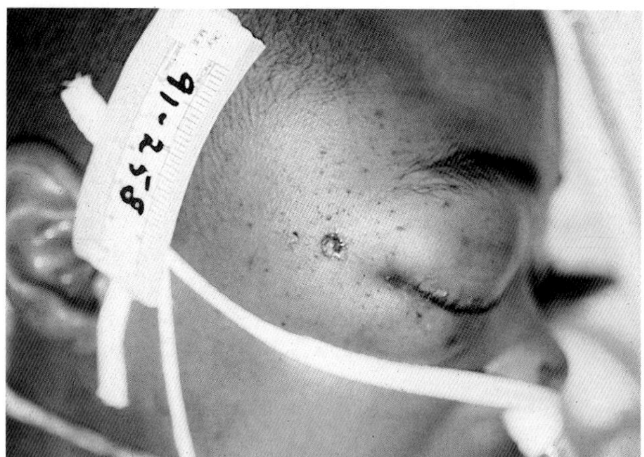

FIGURE 7-53 ■ Intermediate-range gunshot wound with surrounding tattooing.

its overall pattern. Also helpful is a notation concerning the location of the gunshot wound of entrance within the stippling (eccentric or central). In general, stippling is seen in handgun wounds inflicted within approximately 2 ft (76). However, actual numbers should be provided to investigators with caution.

It is better to use descriptive terms, such as "close range" or "intermediate range." When wounds have been inflicted from distances greater than about 2 ft (with standard handguns), the skin surrounding the gunshot of entrance does not display soot or stippling. The gunshot wound of entrance is represented by a defect with a small "abrasion collar." The abrasion collar is produced when the bullet initially encounters the skin and indents it, thereby stretching and rubbing the skin around the gunshot wound of entrance.

Gunshot wounds of exit are often irregular and stellate, and abrasions are absent (Figure 7-54). Contrary to a popular myth, the gunshot wound of exit is not always larger than the wound of entrance.

The path of the projectile through the body may be of forensic importance in proving or disproving a witness's account of the event. The path of the bullet should be described in three planes: anteroposterior, superoinferior, and lateral. Gunshot wounds should be classified as either penetrating or perforating. In a penetrating gunshot wound, the bullet is retained within the body. In a perforating gunshot wound, the bullet enters the body, proceeds through, and exits (77).

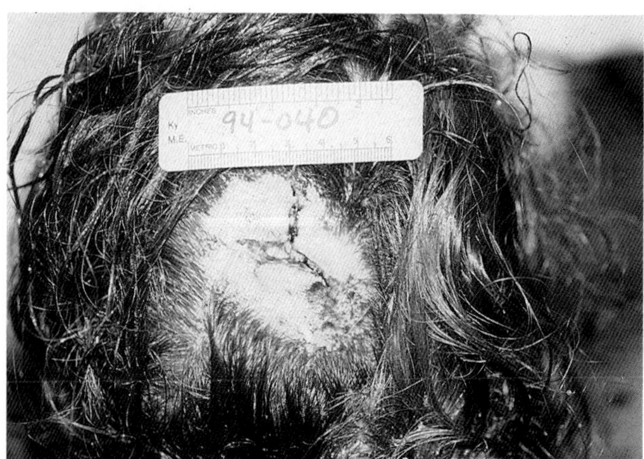

FIGURE 7-54 ■ Gunshot exit wound.

CONCLUSION

The diagnosis of physical abuse should be approached as a team effort because many disciplines are involved, including radiology, ophthalmology, surgery, pathology, social services, and law enforcement. It is useful to establish a child fatality review team within a community to review sudden unexpected and traumatic deaths of children. Such a team facilitates close working relationships and the exchange of information among multiple agencies. Furthermore, it allows for the discovery of trends and hazards concerning childhood deaths. The identification of common causes of accidental death may facilitate public awareness campaigns to lower the incidence of such tragedies in the future. Increased collaboration between pediatric pathologists, forensic pathologists, and pediatricians should be aggressively pursued. Collaborative efforts should involve research, scientific discussions, and publications, so that each specialty can benefit from the knowledge base of the others.

Of utmost importance in the evaluation of childhood injury is the correlation of the history with the physical findings. The pathologist must be familiar with various developmental milestones of infants and young children in order to properly evaluate the provided history. The severity, site, and distribution of the injury must also be correlated. Pattern injuries should be evaluated and properly documented. Ancillary studies should be utilized. The history should be adequately documented as well. Persons evaluating childhood injuries for forensic purposes are encouraged to keep an open mind when forming a differential diagnosis and employ common sense at all times.

REFERENCES

1. Ablin DS, Greenspan A, Reinhart M, et al. Differentiation of child abuse from osteogenesis imperfecta [see Comments]. *AJR Am J Roentgenol* 1990;154:1035–1046.
2. Ackerman J, Gilbert-Barness E. Suspended rocking cradles, positional asphyxia, and sudden infant death. *Arch Pediatr Adolesc Med* 1997;151:573–575.
3. Adams VI. Autopsy technique for neck examination. *Pathol Annu* 1991;26(Pt 1):211–225.
4. Adams JH, Doyle D, Ford I, Gennarelli TA, Graham DI, McLellan DR. Diffuse axonal injury in head injury: definition, diagnosis and grading. *Histopathology* 1989;15:49–59.
5. Adelson L. Pedicide revisited—the slaughter continues. *Am J Forensic Med Pathol* 1991;12:16–26.
6. Alexander RC, Surrell JA, Cohle SD. Microwave oven burns to children: an unusual manifestation of child abuse. *Pediatrics* 1987;79:255–260.
7. Alexander R, Sato Y, Smith W, Bennett T. Incidence of impact trauma with cranial injuries ascribed to shaking. *Am J Dis Child* 1990;144;724–726.

8. Allasio D, Fischer H. Immersion scald burns and the ability of young children to climb into a bathtub. *Pediatrics* 2005;115:1419–1421.
9. Arkovitz MS, John N, Garcia VF. Pancreatic trauma in children: mechanisms of injury. *J Trauma: Injury Infect Crit Care* 1997;42:49–53.
10. Babbs CF. Interposed abdominal compression CPR: a comprehensive evidence based review. *Resuscitation* 2003;59(1):71–82.
11. Baccino E, Le Goff D, Lancien G, Le Guillou M, Alix D, Mottier D, et al. Exploration of acid gastroesophageal reflux by 24-hour pH metry in infants at risk of sudden infant death syndrome: a study of 50 cases. *Forensic Sci Int* 1988;36:255–260.
12. Baric I, Zschoche J, Christensen E, Duran M, Goodman SI, Leonard JV, et al. Diagnosis and management of glutaric aciduria type I. *J Inherit Metab Dis* 1998;21:326–340.
13. Barlow B, Niemirska M, Gandhi RP, Leblanc W. Ten years of experience with falls from a height in children. *J Pediatr Surg* 1983;18: 509–511.
14. Barrowcliffe MP. Visceral injuries following external cardiac massage. *Anesthesia* 1984;39:347–350.
15. Bass M. The fallacy of the simultaneous sudden infant death syndrome in twins. *Am J Forensic Med Pathol* 1989;10:200–205.
16. Bass M, Kravath RE, Glass L. Death-scene investigation in sudden infant death. *N Engl J Med* 1986;315:100–105.
17. Bass M. The fallacy of the simultaneous sudden infant death syndrome in twins. *Am J Forensic Med Pathol* 1989;10:200–205.
18. Batalis NI, Collins, KA. Adolescent death: a 15-year retrospective study. *J Forensic Sci* 2005;50:1444–1449.
19. Batman P. Intra-alveolar hemorrhage in sudden infant death syndrome: a cause for concern? [Letter]. *J Clin Pathol* 2000;53:484.
20. Bedell AE, Fulton EJ. Unexpected findings and complications at autopsy after cardiopulmonary resuscitation (CPR). *Arch Intern Med* 1986;146:1725–1728.
21. Becroft DMO, Thompson JMD, Mitchell EA. Epidemiology of intrathoracic petechial hemorrhages in sudden infant death syndrome. *Pediatr Dev Pathol* 1998;1:200–209.
22. Becroft DMO, Lockett BK. Intra-alveolar pulmonary siderophages in sudden infant death: a marker for previous imposed suffocation. *Pathology* 1997;28:60–63.
23. Berry PJ. Pathological findings in SIDS. *J Clin Pathol* 1992;45:11–16.
24. Billmire ME, Myers PA. Serious head injury in infants: accident or abuse? *Pediatrics* 1985;75:340–342.
25. Blakemore LC, Loder RT, Hensinger RN. Role of intentional abuse in children 1 to 5 years old with isolated femoral shaft fractures. *J Pediatr Orthop* 1996;16:585–588.
26. Bloch H. Abandonment, infanticide, and filicide. *Am J Dis Child* 1988;142:1058–1060.
27. Bonnier C, Nassogne MC, Evrard P. Outcome and prognosis of whiplash shaken infant syndrome: late consequences after a symptom-free interval. *Dev Med Child Neurol* 1995;37:943–956.
28. Bowkett B, Kolbe A. Traumatic duodenal perforations in children: child abuse a frequent cause. *Aust N Z J Surg* 1998;68:380–382.
29. Brenner RA, Smith G, Overpeck M. Divergent trends in childhood drowning rates, 1971 through 1988. *JAMA* 1994;271:1606–1608.
30. Brent DA, Perper JA, Allman EJ, Moritz GM, Wartella ME, Zelenak JP. The presence and accessibility of firearms in the homes of adolescent suicides. *JAMA* 1991;266:2989–2995.
31. Buchino JJ. Recognition and management of child abuse by the surgical pathologist. *Arch Pathol Lab Med* 1983;107:204–205.
32. Bullough PG, Davidson DD, Lorenzo JC. The morbid anatomy of the skeleton in osteogenesis imperfecta. *Clin Orthop* 1982;59:42–57.
33. Burton B, Rooks VJ, Sisler C. Cervical spine injury in child abuse: report of two cases. *Pediatr Radiol* 1998;28:193–195.
34. Bush CM, Jones JS, Cohle SD, Johnson H. Pediatric injuries from cardiopulmonary resuscitation. *Ann Emerg Med* 1996;28:40–44.
35. Busuttil A, Burchell A. The SIDS phenomenon: an update. *J Clin Pathol* 1992;45:1–2.
36. Buys YM, Levin AV, Enzenauer RW, Elder JE, Letourneau MA, Humphreys RP, et al. Retinal findings after head trauma in infants and young children. *Ophthalmology* 1992;99:1718–1723.
37. Buys YM, et al. Retinal findings after head trauma in infants and young children. *Ophthalmology* 1992;99:1718–1723.
38. Byard RW, Becker LE, Berry PJ, Campbell PE, Fitzgerald K, Hilton JM, et al. The pathological approach to sudden infant death—consensus or confusion? *Am J Forensic Med Pathol* 1996;17:103–105.
39. Byard RW, Beal S, Bourne AJ. Potentially dangerous sleeping environments and accidental asphyxia in infancy and early childhood [see Comments]. *Arch Dis Child* 1994;71:497–500.
40. Byard RW. Hazardous infant and early childhood sleeping environments and death scene examination. *J Forensic Med* 1996;3:115–122.
41. Byard RW, Stewart WA, Telfer S, Beal SM. Assessment of pulmonary and intrathymic hemosiderin deposition in sudden infant death syndrome. *Pediatr Pathol Lab Med* 1997;17:275–282.
42. Byard RW, Kennedy JD. Diagnostic difficulties in cases of sudden death in infants with mandibular hypoplasia. *Am J Forensic Med Pathol* 1996;17:255–259.
43. Caffey J. The whiplash shaken infant syndrome: manual shaking by the extremities with whiplash-induced intracranial and intraocular bleedings, linked with residual permanent brain damage and mental retardation. *Pediatrics* 1974;54:396–403.
44. Calder IM, Hill I, Scholtz SL. Primary brain trauma in non-accidental injury. *J Clin Pathol* 1984;37:1095–1100.
45. Callahan CM, Rivara FP. Urban high school youth and handguns. *JAMA* 1992;267:3038–3042.
46. Cameron CM, Lazoritz S, Calhoun AD. Blunt abdominal injury: simultaneously occurring liver and pancreatic injury in child abuse. *Pediatr Emerg Care* 1997;13:334–336.
47. Campbell AJ, Taylor BJ, Bolton DP. Comparison of two methods of determining asphyxial potential of infant bedding. *J Pediatr* 1997;130:245–249.
48. Campbell TA, Collins KA. Pediatric toxicologic deaths: A ten year retrospective study. *Am J Forensic Med Pathol* 2001;22(2):184–187.
49. Case M. Head injury in a child. ASCP check sample. *Forensic Pathol* 1997;FP97–6.
50. Case MES. Head injury in child abuse. In: Monteleone JA, Brodeur AE, eds. *Child maltreatment: a clinical guide and reference*. St. Louis: GW Medical Publishing, 1998:87–101.
51. Chadwick DL. Falls and childhood deaths: sorting real falls from inflicted injuries. *APSAC Advisor* 1994;7:24–25.
52. Chadwick DL, Chin S, Salerno C, Landsverk J, Kitchen L. Deaths from falls in children: how far is fatal? *J Trauma* 1991;31:1353–1355.
53. Chadwick DL, Merten DF, Reece RM. Thoracic and abdominal injuries associated with child abuse. 1994:54–56.
54. Cheung KK. Identifying and documenting findings of physical child abuse and neglect. *J Pediatr Healthcare* 1999;13:142–143.
55. Coe JI. Postmortem chemistry update. Emphasis on forensic application. *Am J Forensic Med Pathol* 1993;14:91–117.
56. Coe JE, Dirlik P, Ommaya AK. An instrument for brain biopsy utilizing a new extraction principle. *J Neurosurg* 1965;23:217–218.
57. Coe JI. Postmortem chemistry update. *Am J Forensic Med Pathol* 1993;14:91–117.
58. Cohle SD, Hawley DA, Berg KK, Kiesel EL, Pless JE. Homicidal cardiac lacerations in children. *J Forensic Sci* 1995;40:212–218.
59. Collins KA, Nichols CA. A decade of pediatric homicide: a retrospective study at the Medical University of South Carolina. *Am J Forensic Med Pathol* 1999;20:169–172.
60. Collins KA. Ancillary studies in pediatric forensic pathology. Advance (August) 2001:14.
61. Collins KA. Death by overlaying and wedging: a 15-year retrospective study. *Am J Forensic Med Pathol* 2001;22(2):155–159.
62. Collins KA. Sudden infant death syndrome (Chapter 11). In: *Handbook of forensic pathology*, 2nd ed. Northfield: College of American Pathologists; 2003:105–110.

63. Collins KA, Knight LD. Pediatric Forensic Pathology (Chapter 17). In: *Basic competencies in forensic pathology*. Northfield: College of American Pathologists Press; 2006:135–156.
64. Corey TS, McCloud LC, Nichols GR 2nd, Buchino JJ. Infant deaths due to unintentional injury—an 11-year autopsy review. *Am J Dis Child* 1992;146:968–971.
65. Corey TS, et al. Infant deaths due to unintentional injury—an 11-year autopsy review. *Am J Dis Child* 1992;146:968–971.
66. Cruz-Sanchez FF, Lucena J, Ascaso C, Tolosa E, Quinto L, Rossi ML. Cerebellar cortex delayed maturation in sudden infant death syndrome. *J Neuropathol Exp Neurol* 1997;56:340–346.
67. Cumberland GD, Riddick L, McConnell CF. Intimal tears of the right atrium of the heart due to blunt force injuries to the abdomen. *Am J Forensic Med Pathol* 1991;12:102–104.
68. Custer JR, Polley TZ, Moler F. Gastric perforation following cardiopulmonary resuscitation in a child: Report of a case and review of the literature. *Pediatr Emerg Care* 1987;3(1):24–27.
69. Daria S, Sugar NF, Feldman KW, Boos SC, Benton SA, Ornstein A. Into hot water head first: distribution of intentional and unintentional immersion burns. *Pediatr Emerg Care* 2004;20:302–310.
70. Davis JH, Rao VJ, Valdes-Dapena M. A forensic approach to a starved child. *J Forensic Sci* 1984;29:663–669.
71. Decina LE, Temple MG, Dorer HS. Increasing child safety-seat use and proper use among toddlers—evaluation of an enforcement and education program. *Accid Anal Prev* 1994;26:667–673.
72. DePanfilis D, Zuravin S. Rates, patterns, and frequency of child maltreatment recurrences among families known to CPS. *Child Maltreatment* 1998;3:27–42.
73. DiMaio DJ, Di Maio VJM. *Forensic pathology*. New York: Elsevier, 1989.
74. DiMaio DJ, DiMaio VJM. *Forensic pathology*. Boca Raton: CRC Press, 1993:314.
75. DiMaio DJ. Neonaticide, infanticide, and child homicide. In: DiMaio DJ, DiMaio DVM. *Forensic pathology*. Boca Raton: CRC Press, 1993;299–326.
76. DiMaio VJM. *Gunshot wounds*. New York: Elsevier, 1985:113–125.
77. DiMaio VJM. An introduction to the classification of gunshot wounds. In: Geberth VJ, ed. *Gunshot wounds—practical aspects of firearms, ballistics and forensic techniques*. New York: Elsevier, 1985:51–98.
78. DiMaio VJM. The "shaken-baby syndrome." *N Engl J Med* 1998;338:1822–1829.
79. DiMaio VJ. Asphyxia. In: DiMaio VJ, DiMaio D. *Forensic Pathology*. 2nd ed. New York: CRC Press, 2001:230–262.
80. DiMaio VJ, DiMaio D. *Forensic pathology*. 2nd ed. New York: CRC Press, 2001:330–332.
81. DiMaio VJ, DiMaio D. *Forensic pathology*. 2nd ed. New York: CRC Press, 2001:327–329.
82. Dolinak D. Rib fractures in infants due to cardiopulmonary resuscitation efforts. *Am J Forensic Med Pathol* 2007;28:107–110.
83. Donoghue ER, Lifschultz BD. Investigation of fire-related deaths. *ASCP* 1991.
84. Drago DA. Kitchen scalds and thermal burns in children five years and younger. *Pediatrics* 2005;115:10–16.
85. Dubowitz H, Black MM, Kerr MA, Starr RH Jr, Harrington D. Fathers and child neglect. *Arch Pediatr Adolesc Med* 2000;154:135–141.
86. Duhaime AC, Christian LW, Rorke LB, Zimmerman RA, et al. Nonaccidental head injury in infants—the "shaken-baby syndrome" [see Comments]. *N Engl J Med* 1998;338:1822–1829.
87. Duhaime AC, Eppley M, Margulies S, Heher KL, Bartlett SP, et al. Crush injuries to the head in children. *Neurosurgery* 1995;35: 401–407.
88. Duhaime AC, Alario AJ, Lewander WJ, Schut L, Sutton LN, Séidl TS, et al. Head injury in very young children: mechanisms, injury types, and ophthalmologic findings in 100 hospitalized patients younger than 2 years of age. *Pediatrics* 1992;90(2 Pt 1):179–185.
89. Duhaime AC, Gennarelli TA, Thibault LE, Bruce DA, Margulies SS, Wiser R, et al. The shaken baby syndrome. A clinical, pathological, and biomechanical study. *J Neurosurg* 1987;66:409–415.
90. Dunbar JS, et al. Obscure tibial fracture of infants—the toddler's fracture. *J Can Assoc Radiol* 1964;15:136–144.
91. Dwyer T, Ponsonby AL, Blizzard L, Newman NM, Cochrane JA. The contribution of changes in the prevalence of prone sleeping position to the decline in sudden infant death syndrome in Tasmania. *JAMA* 1995;273:783–789.
92. Egginton J. *From cradle to grave*. New York: Jove Books, 1990.
93. Ellis PSJ. Review—the pathology of fatal child abuse. *Pathology* 1997;29:113–121.
94. Emery JL. Child abuse, sudden infant death syndrome, and unexpected infant death [see Comments]. *Am J Dis Child* 1993;147:1097–1100.
95. Fallat ME, Svenson JE, Roussell SS, Hardwick VG. Hazards to children riding in the back of pickup trucks. *J Ky Med Assoc* 1995;93:515–518.
96. Feldman KW, Brewer DK. Child abuse, cardiopulmonary resuscitation, and rib fractures. *Pediatrics* 1984;73:339–342.
97. Feldman KW, Christopher CM, Opheim KB. Munchausen syndrome/bulimia by proxy: ipecac as a toxin in child abuse. *Child Abuse Negl* 1989;13:257–261.
98. Feldman KW, Simms RJ. Strangulation in childhood: epidemiology and clinical course. *Pediatrics* 1980;65:1079–1085.
99. Feldman KW. Patterned abusive bruises of the buttocks and the pinnae. *Pediatrics* 1992;90:633–636.
100. Firstman R, Talan J. *The death of innocents*. New York: Bantam, 1997.
101. Fleming PJ, Gilbert R, Azaz Y, Berry PJ, Rudd PT, Stewart A, et al. Interaction between bedding and sleeping position in the sudden infant death syndrome: a population based case-control study. *BMJ* 1990;301:85–89.
102. Flemming KA. Viral respiratory infection and SIDS. *J Clin Pathol* 1992;45:29–32.
103. Ford RP, Taylor BJ, Mitchell EA, Enright SA, Stewart AW, Becroft DM, et al. Breastfeeding and the risk of sudden infant death syndrome. *Int J Epidemiol* 1993;22:366–375.
104. Frederickson D. Maltreatment of children. *J Child Fam Nurs* 1999;2:393–401.
105. Funayama M, Sagisaka K. Consecutive infanticides in Japan. *Am J Forensic Med Pathol* 1988;9:9–11.
106. Gaebel J. Cardiomyopathy from ipecac administration in MSBP. *Pediatrics* 1993;92:601–603.
107. Gahagan S, Rimsza ME. Child abuse or osteogenesis imperfecta: how can we tell? *Pediatrics* 1991;88:987–992.
108. Galvis AG, Kelley CF. Hypopharynx perforation during infant's resuscitation. *JAMA* 1979;242(14):1526–1527.
109. Genest DR. Estimating the time of death in stillborn fetuses: II: histologic evaluation of the placenta: a study of 71 stillborns. *Obstet Gynecol* 1991;80:585–592.
110. Gennarelli TA, Thibault LE, Adams JH, Graham DI, Thompson CJ, Marcincin RP. Diffuse axonal injury and traumatic coma in the primate. *Ann Neurol* 1982;12:564–574.
111. Gilbert R, Rudd P, Berry PJ, Fleming PJ, Hall E, White DG, et al. Combined effect of infection and heavy wrapping on the risk of sudden infant death. *Arch Dis Child* 1992;67:171–177.
112. Gilbert-Barness EF, Kenison K, Giuliam G, Chandra S. Extramedullary hematopoiesis in the liver in sudden infant death syndrome. *Arch Pathol Lab Med* 1991;115:226–229.
113. Gilbert-Barness E, Emery JL. Deaths of infants on polystyrene-filled beanbags. *Am J Forensic Med Pathol* 1995;17:202–206.
114. Gilliland MG, Luckenbach MW. Are retinal hemorrhages found after resuscitation attempts? A study of the eyes of 169 children. *Am J Forensic Med Pathol* 1993;14:187–192.
115. Gilliland MG, Luckenbach MW, Chenier TC. Systemic and ocular findings in 169 prospectively studied child deaths:

retinal hemorrhages usually mean child abuse. *Forensic Sci Int* 1994;68:117–132.

116. Gleckman AM, Bell MD, Evans RJ, Smith TW. Diffuse axonal injury in infants with nonaccidental craniocerebral trauma: enhanced detection by beta-amyloid precursor protein immunohistochemical staining. *Arch Pathol Lab Med* 1999;123:146–151.
117. Goff ML, Charbonneau S, Sullivan W. Presence of fecal material in diapers as a potential source of error in estimations of postmortem interval using arthropod development rates. *J Forensic Sci* 1991;36:1603–1606.
118. Goldstein B, Kelly MM, Bruton D, Cox C. Inflicted versus accidental head injury in critically injured children. *Crit Care Med* 1993;21:1328–1332.
119. Goldstein LA, Spurlock CW. Kentucky's child restraint law has saved lives: a 20-year review of fatalities among children (ages 0–4) as motor vehicle occupants. *Ky Med Assoc J* 1998;96:97–100.
120. Greenwald MJ, Weiss A, Oesterle CS, Friendly DS. Traumatic retinoschisis in battered babies. *Ophthalmology* 1986;93:618–625.
121. Gregersen M, Vesterby A. Iatrogenic fractures of the hyoid bond and the thyroid cartilage. A case report. *For Sci Inter* 1981;17:41–43.
122. Greig F, Schoeneman M, Kandall SR, Benforte RJ. Neonatal hyponatremic dehydration as an initial presentation of cystic fibrosis. *Clin Pediatr (Phila)* 1993;548–551.
123. Grisanti KA, Jaffe DM. Dehydration syndromes. Oral rehydration and fluid replacement. *Emerg Med Clin North Am* 1991;9:565–588.
124. Gunther WM, Symes SA, Berryman HE. Characteristics of child abuse by anteroposterior manual compression versus cardiopulmonary resuscitation. *Am J Forensic Med Pathol* 2000;21(1):5–10.
125. Guntheroth WG, Spiers PS. Prolongation of the QT interval and the sudden infant death syndrome. *Pediatrics* 1999;103:813.
126. Guyer MJ. Child psychiatry and legal liability: implications of recent case law [see Comments]. *J Am Acad Child Adolesc Psychiatry* 1990;29:958–962.
127. Hadley MN, Sonntag VK, Rekate HL, Murphy A. The infant whiplash-shake injury syndrome: a clinical and pathological study. *Neurosurgery* 1989;24:536–540.
128. Haglund B, Cnattingius S. Cigarette smoking as a risk factor for sudden infant death syndrome. *Am J Public Health* 1990;80:29–32.
129. Haller J, et al. Diagnostic imaging of child abuse. *Pediatrics* 1991;87:262–264.
130. Handy TC, Hanzlick R, Shields LB, Reichard R, Goudy S. Hypernatremia and subdural hematoma in the pediatric age group: is there a causal relationship? *J Forensic Sci* 1999;44:1114–8.
131. Hanigan WC, Peterson RA, Njus G. Tin ear syndrome: rotational acceleration in pediatric head injuries. *Pediatrics* 1987;80:618–622.
132. Harm T, Rajs J. Face and neck injuries due to resuscitation versus throttling. *For Sci Inter* 1983;23:109–116.
133. Hart BL, Dudley MH, Zumwalt RE. Postmortem cranial MRI and autopsy correlation in suspected child abuse. *Am J Forensic Med Pathol* 1996;17:217–224.
134. Hashimoto Y, Moriva F, Furumiya J. Forensic aspects of complications resulting from cardiopulmonary resuscitation. *Leg Med (Tokyo)* 2007;9:94–9.
135. Helfer RE, Slovis TL, Black M. Injuries resulting when small children fall out of bed. *Pediatrics* 1977;60:533–535.
136. Hirsch CS. Scientific death investigation. Presented at the 47th Annual Anatomic Pathology Slide Seminar of the American Society of Clinical Pathologists, Las Vegas, 1981.
137. Hobbs CJ. Skull fracture and the diagnosis of abuse. *Arch Dis Child* 1984;59:246–252.
138. Hoffman HJ, Hillman LS. Epidemiology of the sudden infant death syndrome: maternal, neonatal, and postneonatal risk factors. *Clin Perinatol* 1992;19:717–737.
139. Hoke RS, Chamberlain D. Skeletal chest injuries secondary to cardiopulmonary resuscitation. *Resuscitation* 2004;63:327–238.
140. Hutchison L, Stewart A, Mitchell E. Infant sleep position, head shape concerns, and sleep positioning devices. *J Paediatr Child Health* 2007;43:243–248.
141. Hymel KP, Jenny C, Block RW. Intracranial hemorrhage and rebleeding in suspected victims of abusive head trauma: addressing the forensic controversies. *Child Maltreat* 2002;7(4):329–348.
142. Hymel KP, Jenny C. Child sexual abuse. *Pediatr Rev* 1996;17:236–249; quiz 249–250.
143. Hymel KP, Rumack CM, Hay TC, Strain JD, Jenny C. Comparison of intracranial computed tomographic (CT) findings in pediatric abusive and accidental head trauma. *Pediatric Radiol* 1997;27:743–747.
144. Jenny C, Hymel KP, Ritzen A, Reinert SE, Hay TC. Analysis of missed cases of abusive head trauma [see Comments]. *JAMA* 1999;281:621–626.
145. Joffe M, Ludwig S. Stairway injuries to children. *Pediatrics* 1988;82:457–463.
146. Johnson DL, Boal D, Baule R. Role of apnea in nonaccidental head injury. *Pediatr Neurosurg* 1995;23:305–310.
147. Johnson DL, Braun D, Friendly D. Accidental head trauma and retinal hemorrhage. *Neurosurgery* 1993;33:231–234; discussion 234–235.
148. Johnson CF. Inflicted injury versus accidental injury. *Pediatr Clin North Am* 1990;37:791–814.
149. Jones J, Fletter B. Complication after cardiopulmonary resuscitation. *Am J Emerg Med* 1994;12(6):479–480.
150. Jumbelic MI, Chambliss M. Accidental toddler drowning in 5-gallon buckets. *JAMA* 1990;263.
151. Kaplan JA, Fossum RM. Patterns of facial resuscitation injury in infancy. *Am J Forensic Med Pathol* 1994;15(3):187–191.
152. Kaplan SJ, Pelcovitz D, Labruna V. Child and adolescent abuse and neglect research: a review of the past 10 years. Part 1: physical and emotional abuse and neglect. *J Am Acad Child Adolesc Psychiatry* 1999;38:1214–1222.
153. Kattwinkel J, Brooks JG, Keenan ME, et al. Task Force on Infant Positioning and SIDS of the American Academy of Pediatrics. Changing concepts of sudden infant death syndrome: implications for infant sleep environment and sleep position. *Pediatrics* 2000;105:650–656.
154. Keen JH, Lendrum J, Wolman B. Inflicted burns and scalds in children. *Br Med J* 1975;4(5991):268–269.
155. Kemp JS, Thach BT. Sudden death in infants sleeping on polystyrene-filled cushions [see Comments]. *N Engl J Med* 1991;324:1858–1864.
156. Kemp CH, Silverman FN, Steele BF, Droegemueller W, Silver HK. The battered-child syndrome. *JAMA* 1962;181:17–24.
157. Kerley ER. The identification of battered-infant skeletons. *J Forensic Sci* 1978;23:163–168.
158. Kerr MA, Black MM, Krishnakumar A. Failure-to-thrive, maltreatment and the behavior and development of 6-year-old children from low-income urban families: a cumulative risk model. *Child Abuse Negl* 2000;24:587–598.
159. King J, Diefendorf D, Apthorp J, Negrete VF, Carlson M. Analysis of 429 fractures in 189 battered children. *J Pediatr Orthop* 1988;8;585–589.
160. Kirschner RH, Wilson HL. Fatal child abuse: the pathologist's perspective. In: Reece R, ed. *Child abuse*. Philadelphia: Lea & Febiger, 1994:337.
161. Kirschner RH, Wilson HL. Fatal child abuse: the pathologist's perspective. In: Reece RM, ed. *Child abuse: medical diagnosis and management*. Philadelphia: Lea & Febiger, 1994:349.
162. Kleinman PK. Skeletal trauma: general considerations. In: Kleinman PK, ed. *Diagnostic imaging of child abuse*, 2nd ed. St. Louis: Mosby, 1998:12–22.
163. Kleinman PK, Spevak MR. Variations in acromial ossification simulating infant abuse in victims of sudden infant death syndrome. *Radiology* 1991;180:185–187.
164. Kleinman PK, Marks SC Jr, Spevak MR, Belancer PL, Richmond JM. Extension of growth-plate cartilage into the metaphysis: a sign of healing fracture in abused infants. *AJR Am J Roentgenol* 1991;156(4);775–779.
165. Kleinman PK. The lower extremity. In: Kleinman PK, ed. *Diagnostic imaging of child abuse*. St. Louis: Mosby, 1998:45.

166. Kleinman PK. Bony thoracic trauma. In: Kleinman PK, ed. *Diagnostic imaging of child abuse*. St. Louis: Mosby, 1998:110–148.
167. Kleinman PK. Diagnostic imaging in infant abuse. *Am J Radiol* 1990;155:703–710.
168. Kleinman PK. Chapter 13. In: Kleinman PK, ed. *Diagnostic imaging of child abuse*, 2nd ed. St. Louis: Mosby, 1998:244.
169. Kleinman PK, Shelton YA. Hangman's fracture in an abused infant: imaging features. *Pediatr Radiol* 1997;27:776–777.
170. Klonoff-Cohen HS, Edelstein SL, Lefkowitz ES, Srinivasan IP, Kaegi D, Chang JC, et al. The effect of passive smoking and tobacco exposure through breast milk on sudden infant death syndrome. *JAMA* 1995;273:795–798.
171. Knight L, Collins KA. A 25 Year Retrospective Review of Deaths Due to Child Neglect. *Am J Forensic Med Pathol* 2005;26(3):221–228.
172. Krischer JP, Fine EG, Davis, Nagel EL. Complications of cardiac resuscitation. *Chest* 1987;92(2):287–291.
173. Krous HF, Chadwick AE, Haas EA, Stanley C. Pulmonary intra-alveolar hemorrhage in SIDS and suffocation. *J Forensic Legal Med* 2007; 14(8):461–470.
174. Krous HF, Haas EA, Masoumi H, Chadwick AE, Stanley C. A comparison of pulmonary intra-alveolar hemorrhage in cases of sudden infant death due to SIDS in a safe sleep environment or to suffocation. *Forensic Sci Int* 2007;172(1):56–62.
175. Krugman RD, et al. Shaken baby syndrome: inflicted cerebral trauma. *Pediatrics* 1993;92:872–875.
176. Lambert SR, Johnson TE, Hoyt CS. Optic nerve sheath and retinal hemorrhages associated with the shaken baby syndrome. *Arch Ophthalmol* 1986;104:1509–1512.
177. Langlois NE, Gresham GA. The aging of bruises: a review and study of the colour changes with time. *Forensic Sci Int* 1991;50:227–238.
178. Larzon T, Jansson H, Holmstrom B, Lund P, Norgren L, Arfvidsson B, et al. Salvage of an acutely ruptured thoracic aortic aneurysm during CPR. *J Endovasc Ther* 2002;9(Suppl 2):1167–1171.
179. Lawes EG, Baskett PJ. Pulmonary aspiration during unsuccessful cardiopulmonary resuscitation. *Intensive Care Med* 1987;13:379–382.
180. Lazoff M, Kauffman F. Sudden infant death syndrome—part I: general features. *Acad Emerg Med* 1995;2:936–933.
181. Lazoff M, Kauffman F. Sudden infant death syndrome—part II: etiologic theories. *Acad Emerg Med* 1995;2:996–1000.
182. Lazoritz S, Baldwin S, Kini N. The whiplash shaken infant syndrome: has Caffey's syndrome changed or have we changed his syndrome? [see Comments]. *Child Abuse Negl* 1997;21:1009–1014.
183. Leadbeatter S, Knight B. Resuscitation artifact. *Med Sci Law* 1988;28(3):200–204.
184. Ledbetter DJ, Hatch EI Jr, Feldman KW, Fligner CL, Tapper D. Diagnostic and surgical implications of child abuse. *Arch Surg* 1988;123:1101–1105.
185. Lee JC, Collins KA, Burgess SE. Suicide under the age of eighteen: a 10-year retrospective study. *Am J Forensic Med Pathol* 1999;20:27–30.
186. Lenoski EF, Hunter KA. Specific patterns of inflicted burn injuries. *J Trauma* 1977;17:842–846.
187. Leionidas JC. Skeletal trauma in the child abuse syndrome. *Pediatr Ann* 1983;12:875–881.
188. Leonidas JC. The abused child: reappraisal. *Radiology* 1983;146: 377–381.
189. Leonidas JC. Skeletal trauma in the child abuse syndrome. *Pediatr Ann* 1983;12:875–881.
190. Leventhal JM, Thomas SA, Rosenfield NS, Markowite RI. Fractures in young children. Distinguishing child abuse from unintentional injuries. *Am J Dis Child* 1993;147:87–92.
191. Lever WF. Bacterial disease. In: Lever WF, ed. *Histopathology of the skin*. Philadelphia: JB Lippincott Co., 1990:318–319.
192. Lever WF. Benign melanocytic tumors and malignant melanoma. In: Lever WF, ed. *Histopathology of the skin*, 7th ed. Philadelphia: JB Lippincott Co, 1990:776.
193. Lever WF. Tumors of vascular disease. In: Lever WF, ed. *Histopathology of the skin*, 7th ed. Philadelphia: JB Lippincott Co, 1990:689–690.
194. Levin AV, Magnusson MR, Rafto SE, Zimmerman RA. Shaken baby syndrome diagnosed by magnetic resonance imaging. *Pediatr Emerg Care* 1989;5:181–186.
195. Loder RT, Bookout C. Fracture patterns in battered children. *J Orthop Trauma* 1991;5:428–433.
196. Lyons TJ, Oates RK. Falling out of bed: a relatively benign occurrence. *Pediatrics* 1993;92:125–127.
197. Machii M, Inaba H, Nakae H, Suzuki I, Tanaka H. Cardiac rupture by penetration of fractured sternum: A rare complication of cardiopulmonary resuscitation. *Resuscitation* 2000;43(2):151–153.
198. Mann NC, Weller SC, Rauchschwalbe R. Bucket-related drownings in the United States, 1984 through 1990. *Pediatrics* 1992;89:1.
199. Maguire S, Mann M, John N, Ellaway B, Sibert JR, Kemp AM, et al. Does cardiopulmonary resuscitation cause rib fractures in children? A systematic review. *Child Abuse Neglect* 2006;30:739–751.
200. Marcus BJ, Collins KA. Childhood panhypopituitarism presenting as child abuse: a case report and review of the literature. *Am J Forensic Med Pathol* 2004;25:265–269.
201. Marini JC, Gerber NL. Osteogenesis imperfecta. *JAMA* 1997;277:746–750.
202. Marshall SW, Runyan CW, Bangdiwala SI, Linzer MA, Sacks JJ, Butts JD. Fatal residential fires. *JAMA* 1998;279:1633–1637.
203. Martinez FD. Sudden infant death syndrome and small airway occlusion: facts and a hypothesis. *Pediatrics* 1991;87:190–198.
204. McCauseland IP, Dougherty RH. Histologic ageing of bruises in lambs and calves. *Aust Vet J* 1978;54:525–528.
205. McClain JL, Clark MA, Sandusky GE. Undiagnosed, untreated acute lymphoblastic leukemia presenting as suspected child abuse. *J Forensic Sci* 1990;35:735–739.
206. McGlashan ND. Low selenium status and cot deaths. *Med Hypotheses* 1991;35:311–314.
207. Meadow R. Munchausen syndrome by proxy. The hinterland of child abuse. *Lancet* 1977;2(8033):343–345.
208. Meadow R. What is, and what is not, "Munchausen syndrome by proxy"? [see Comments]. *Arch Dis Child* 1995;72:534–538.
209. Meadow R. Unnatural sudden infant death. *Arch Dis Child* 1999;80:7–14.
210. Meadow R. Suffocation, recurrent apnea, and sudden infant death. *J Pediatr* 1990;117:351–357.
211. Meadow R. Epidemiology. In: *ABC of child abuse*, 2nd ed. London, UK: BMJ Publishing, 1993.
212. Merten DF, Carpenter BL. Radiologic imaging of inflicted injury in the child abuse syndrome. *Pediatr Clin North Am* 1990;37: 815–837.
213. Meservy CJ, Towbin R, McLaurin RL, Myers PA, Ball W. Radiographic characteristics of skull fractures resulting from child abuse. *AJR Am J Roentgenol* 1987;149:173–175.
214. Mirowski GW, Frieden IJ, Miller C. Iatrogenic scald burn: a consequence of institutional infection control measures. *Pediatrics* 1996;98(5):963–965.
215. Mitchell EA, Thompson JM, Becroft DM, Bajanowski T, Brinkmann B, Happe A, et al. Head covering and the risk for SIDS: findings from the New Zealand and German SIDS case-control studies. *Pediatrics* 2008;121:e1478–e1483.
216. Mitchell EA, Ford RP, Stewart AW, Taylor BJ, Becroft DM, Thompson JM, et al. Smoking and the sudden infant death syndrome. *Pediatrics* 1993;91:893–896.
217. Mitchell G, et al. Congenital anomalies in glutaric aciduria type 2 [Letter]. *J Pediatr* 1984;104:961–962.
218. *MMWR Morb Mortal Wkly Rep* 1990;:442–451.
219. *MMWR Morb Mortal Wkly Rep* 1998;:803–809.
220. *MMWR Morb Mortal Wkly Rep* 1992;:271–272.
221. Mofenson HC, Wheatley GMP. Prevention of childhood injuries: morbidity and mortality-an overview. *Pediatr Ann* 1983:12;716–719.
222. Monsuez JJ, Charniot JC, Veilhan LA, Mougue F, Bellin MF, Boissonnas A. Subcapsular liver haematoma after cardiopulmonary resuscitation by untrained personnel. *Resuscitation* 2007;73:314–317.

223. Moon RY, Norne RS, Hauck FR. Sudden infant death syndrome. *Lancet* 2007;370:1578–1587.
224. Mortimer PE, Freeman M. Are facial bruises in babies ever accidental? [Letter]. *Arch Dis Child* 1983;58:75–76.
225. Moritz AR, Henriques FC. Studies of thermal injuries: II. The relative importance of time and surface temperature in the causation of cutaneous burns. *Am J Pathol* 1947;23:695–720.
226. Munger CE, Peiffer RL, Bouldin TW, Kylstra JA, Thompson RL. Ocular and associated neuropathologic observations in suspected whiplash shaken infant syndrome. A retrospective study of 12 cases. *Am J Forensic Med Pathol* 1993;14:193–200.
227. Musemeche CA, Barthel M, Cosentino C. Pediatric falls from heights. *J Trauma* 1991;31:1347–1349.
228. Nelson EAS, Taylor BJ, Wetherall IL. Sleeping position and infant bedding may predispose to hyperthermia and the sudden infant death syndrome. *Lancet* 1989;1:199–201.
229. Nields H, Kessler SC, Boisot S, Evans R. Streptococcal toxic shock syndrome presenting as suspected child abuse. *Am J Forensic Med Pathol* 1998;19:93–97.
230. Niemcryk SJ, Kaufmann CR. Motor vehicle crashes, restraint use, and severity of injury in children in Nevada. *Am J Prev Med* 1997;13:109–114.
231. Nimityongskul P, Anderson LD. The likelihood of injuries when children fall out of bed. *J Pediatr Orthop* 1987;7:184–186.
232. O'Connor JF, Cohen J. Dating fractures. In: Kleinman PK, ed. *Diagnostic imaging of child abuse*. St. Louis: Mosby, 1998:168–177.
233. O'Halloran RL, Ferratta F, Harris M, Ilbeigi P, Rom CD. Child abuse reports in families with sudden infant death syndrome. *Am J Forensic Med Pathol* 1998;19:57–62.
234. O'Shea J. House-fire and drowning deaths among children and young adults. *Am J Forensic Med Pathol* 1991;12:33–35.
235. Oehmichen M, Gerling I, MeiBner C. Petechiae of the baby's skin as differentiation symptom of infanticide versus SIDS. *J Forensic Sci* 2000;45:602–607.
236. Ojo P, Palmer J, Garvey R, Atweh N, Fidler P. Pattern of burns in child abuse. *Am Surg* 2007;73:253–255.
237. Ommaya AK, Gennarelli TA. Cerebral concussion and traumatic unconsciousness. Correlation of experimental and clinical observations of blunt head injuries. *Brain* 1974;97:633–654.
238. Ophoven J. Forensic pathology. In: Stocker JT, Dehner LP, eds. *Pediatric pathology*. Philadelphia: JB Lippincott Co., 1992.
239. Oppenheim BA, Barclay GR, Morris J, Knox F, Barson A, Drucker DB, et al. Antibodies to endotoxin core in sudden infant death syndrome. *Arch Dis Child* 1994;70:95–98.
240. Oral and dental aspects of child abuse and neglect. Joint statement of the American Academy of Pediatrics and the American Academy of Pediatric Dentistry. *Pediatrics* 1999;104:348–350.
241. Overpeck MD, Brenner RA,Trumble AC, Trifiletti LB, Berendes HW. Risk factors for infant homicide in the United States. *N Engl J Med* 1998;339:1211–1216.
242. Patterson MM. Child abuse: assessment and intervention. *Orthop Nurs* 1998;17:49–54.
243. Pearn JH, Brown J 3rd, Bart R. Bathtub drownings: report of seven cases. *Pediatrics* 1979;64:68–70.
244. Perper JA. Microscopic forensic pathology. In: Spitz W, ed. *Medicolegal investigation of death*. Springfield, IL: Charles C Thomas Publisher, 1993:660–661.
245. Philippart AI. Blunt abdominal trauma in childhood. *Surg Clin North Am* 1977:57;151–163.
246. Pike J, Moon RY. Bassinet use and sudden unexpected death in infancy. *J Pediatr* 2008;153(4):509–512.
247. Pounder DJ. Shaken adult syndrome. *Am J Forensic Med Pathol* 1997;18:321–324.
248. Powner DJ, Holcombe PA, Mello LA. Cardiopulmonary resuscitation-related injuries. *Crit Care Med* 1984;12(1):54–55.
249. Prescott PR. Hair dryer burns in children. *Pediatrics* 1990;86: 692–697.
250. Transport Accident Commission. www.tacsafety.com 2010
251. Price EA, Rush LR, Perper JA, Bell MD. Cardiopulmonary resuscitation-related injuries and homicidal blunt abdominal trauma in children. *Am J Forensic Med Pathol* 2000;21(4):307–310.
252. Raekallio J. Determination of the age of wounds by histochemical and biochemical methods. *Forensic Science* 1972:1;1–16.
253. Raff HN. Concealed pregnancies, clandestine births. ASCP check sample. *Forensic Pathol* 1995;FP95–7(FP208):11–123.
254. Rao N, Smith RE, Choi JH, Xu XH, Kornblum RN. Autopsy findings in the eyes of fourteen fatally abused children. *Forensic Sci Int* 1988;39:293–299.
255. Reece RM. Unusual manifestations of child abuse. *Pediatr Clin North Am* 1990;37:905–921.
256. Reiber GD. Fatal falls in childhood. How far must children fall to sustain fatal head injury? Report of cases and review of the literature. *Am J Forensic Med Pathol* 1993;14:201–207.
257. Reichardt JA, Casey GD, Krywko D. Gastric rupture from cardiopulmonary resuscitation or seizure activity? A case report. *J Emerg Med* 2008.
258. Reid-Nicholson MD, Escoffery CT. Severe pulmonary barotraumas. *West Indian Med J* 2000;49(4):344–346.
259. Renz BM, Sherman R. Abusive scald burns in infants and children: A prospective study. *Am Surg* 1993;59(5):329–334.
260. Rosenberg DA. Web of deceit: a literature review of Munchausen syndrome by proxy. *Child Abuse Negl* 1987;11:547–563.
261. Rupp R. Child abuse and neglect: a review of the literature. *J Kans Dent Assoc* 1996;81:20–24.
262. Sabo RA, Hankan WC, Flessner K, Rose J, Aaland M. Strangulation injuries in children. Part I. Clinical analysis. *J Trauma* 1996;40:68–72.
263. Scheers NJ, Dayton CM, Kemp JS. Sudden infant death with external airways covered: case–comparison study of 206 deaths in the United States. *Arch Pediatr Adolesc Med* 1998:152;540–547.
264. Schluckebier DA, Cool DC, Henry TE, Martin A, Wahe JW. Pulmonary siderophages and unexpected infant death. *Am J Forensic Med Pathol* 2002;23:360–363.
265. Schoendorf K, Kiely J. Relationship of sudden infant death syndrome to maternal smoking during and after pregnancy. *Pediatrics* 1992;90:905–908.
266. Schwartz AJ, Ricci LR. How accurately can bruises be aged in abused children? Literature review and synthesis. *Pediatrics* 1996;97: 254–257.
267. Schwartz PJ, Stramba-Badiale M, Segantini A, Austoni P, Bosi G, Giorgetti R, et al. Prolongation of the QT interval and the sudden infant death syndrome. *N Engl J Med* 1998;338:1709–1714.
268. Sewell RD, Steinberg MA. Chest compressions in an infant with osteogenesis imperfecta type II: No new rib fractures. *Pediatrics* 2000;106(5):E71.
269. Sezen F. Retinal haemorrhages in newborn infants. *Br J Ophthalmol* 1970;55:248–253.
270. Shane SA and SM Fuchs. Skull fractures in infants and predictors of associated intracranial injury. *Pediatr Emerg Care* 1997:13; 198–203.
271. Sheil AT, Collins KA. Fatal birth trauma due to an undiagnosed abdominal teratoma: case report and review of the literature. *Am J Forensic Med Pathol* 2007;28(2):121–127.
272. Shiono H, Maya A, Tabata N, Fujiwara M, Azumi J, Morita M. Medicolegal aspects of infanticide in Hokkaido District, Japan. *Am J Forensic Med Pathol* 1986;7:104–106.
273. Shugerman RP, Paez A, Grossman DC, Feldman KW, Grady MS. Epidural hemorrhage: is it abuse? *Pediatrics* 1996;97:664–668.
274. Sims MA, Collins KA. Fetal death: a 10 year retrospective study. *Am J Forensic Med Pathol* 2001;22(3):261–265.
275. Smialek JE, Smialek PZ, Spitz WU. Accidental bed deaths in infants due to unsafe sleeping situations. *Clin Pediatr* 1977;16:1031–1036.
276. Smialek JE. Simultaneous sudden infant death syndrome in twins. *Pediatrics* 1986;77:816–821.

277. Sokolove PE, Willis-Shore J, Panacek EA. Exsanguination due to right ventricular rupture during closed-chest cardiopulmonary resuscitation. *J Emerg Med* 2002;23(2):161–164.
278. Southall DP, Plunkett MC, Banks MW, Falkov AF, Samuels MP, et al. Covert video recordings of life-threatening child abuse: lessons for child protection. *Pediatrics* 1997;100:735–760.
279. Spear RM, Chadwick D, Peterson BM. Fatalities associated with misinterpretation of bloody cerebrospinal fluid in the "shaken baby syndrome" [Letter]. *Am J Dis Child* 1992;146:1415–1417.
280. Spevak MR, Kleinman PK, Belanger PL, Primack C, Richmond JM. Cardiopulmonary resuscitation and rib fractures in infants. A post-mortem radiologic-pathologic study. *JAMA* 1994;272:617–618.
281. Spitz W. Investigation of deaths in childhood. In: Spitz W, ed. *Medicolegal investigation of death*. Springfield, IL: Charles C Thomas Publisher, 1993:703.
282. Spitz W. Asphyxia, in medicolegal investigation of death. In: Spitz W, ed. *Medicolegal investigation of death*. Springfield, IL: Charles C. Thomas Publisher, 1993:467.
283. Spivack BS. Statistics and death certificates [Letter]. *Pediatrics* 1998;102(4 Pt 1):1000–1001.
284. Spivack B. Biomechanics of nonaccidental trauma. In: Ludwig S, Kornberg AE, eds. *Child abuse: a medical reference* 2nd ed. New York: Churchill Livingstone, 1992.
285. Stallard N, Findlay G, Smithies M. Splenic rupture following cardiopulmonary resuscitation. *Resuscitation* 1997;35:171–173.
286. Stanton AN. Overheating and cot death. *Lancet* 1984;2:1199–1201.
287. Starling SP, Holden JR, Jenny C. Abusive head trauma: the relationship of perpetrators to their victims. *Pediatrics* 1995;95:259–262.
288. *Stedman's medical dictionary*, 24th ed. Baltimore: Williams & Wilkins, 1983:931.
289. Stephenson T, Bialas Y. Estimation of the age of bruising. *Arch Dis Child* 1996;74:53–55.
290. Stewart S, Fawcett J, Jacobson W. Interstitial haemosiderin in the lungs of sudden infant death syndrome: a histological hallmark of "near-miss" episodes? *J Pathol* 985;145:53–58.
291. Straus MA, Kantor GK. Stress and child abuse. In: Helfer RE, Kemp RS, eds. *The battered child*, 4th ed. Chicago: University of Chicago Press, 1987:42–59.
292. Sturner WQ. SIDS redux: is it or isn't it? *Am J Forensic Med Pathol* 1998;19:107–108.
293. Subramani K, Thomas AN, Reeve RS. Occult splenic rupture with cardiovascular collapse: a report of three cases in critically ill patients. *Intensive Care Med* 2002;28(12):1819–1821.
294. Summers CG, Parker JC Jr. The brain stem in sudden infant death syndrome. A postmortem survey. *Am J Forensic Med Pathol* 1981;2:121–127.
295. Tablizo MA, Jacinto P, Parsley D, Chen ML, Ramanathan R, Keens TG. Supine sleeping position does not cause clinical aspiration in neonates in hospital newborn nurseries. *Arch Pediat Adolesc Med* 2007;161:507–510.
296. Thach BT. Sudden infant death syndrome: can gastroesophageal reflux cause sudden infant death? *Am J Med* 2000;108(4A):144S–148S.
297. Thaler MM, Krause VW. Serious trauma in children after external cardiac massage. *N Engl J Med* 1962;207:500–501.
298. Thornton RN, Jolly RD. The objective interpretation of histopathological data: an application to the aging of ovine bruises. *Forensic Sci Int* 1986;31:225–239.
299. Tober RB, Marting RE. Child abuse. *J Fla Med Assoc* 1995;82:679–683.
300. Tomasi LG, Rosman NP. Purtscher retinopathy in the battered child syndrome. *Am J Dis Child* 1975;129:1335–1337.
301. Tudge C. Relative danger. *Nat History J* 1997;9:28–31.
302. Viano DC, King AI, Melvin JW, et al. Injury biomechanics research: an essential element in the prevention of trauma. *J Biomechanics* 1989;22:403–417.
303. Wailoo MO, Petersen SA, Whittaker H, et al. The thermal environment in which 3- to 4-month-old infants sleep at home. *Arch Dis Childhood* 1989;64:600–604.
304. Waldman PJ, Walters BL, Grunau CF. Pancreatic injury associated with interposed abdominal compression in pediatric cardiopulmonary resuscitation. *Am J Emerg Med* 1984;2(6):510–512.
305. Walker PL, Cook DC, Lambert PM. Skeletal evidence for child abuse: a physical anthropological perspective. *J Forensic Sci* 1997;42:196–207.
306. Wardinsky TD. Genetic and congenital defect conditions that mimic child abuse. *J Fam Pract* 1995;41:377–383.
307. Warner KG, Deming RH. The pathophysiology of free-fall injury. *Ann Emerg Med* 1986;15:141–146.
308. Wedgewood J. Childhood bruising. *Practitioner* 1990;234:598–601.
309. Weinstein SL, Steinschneider A. Qtc and R-R intervals in victims of the sudden infant death syndrome. *Am J Dis Child* 1985;139:987–990.
310. Whitehead FJ, Couper RT, Moore L, Bourne AJ, Byard RW. Dehydration deaths in infants and young children. *Am J Forensic Med Pathol* 1996;17:73–78.
311. Wigglesworth JS. The macerated stillborn fetus. In: Livosi VA, ed. *Perinatal pathology*. Philadelphia: WB Saunders, 1996:78–80.
312. Wigglesworth A, Agnew J, Campbell H, Jones IG. The centre for the vulnerable child: a new model for the therapeutic provision for abused children and their families. *Public Health* 1996;110:373–377.
313. Williams RA. Injuries in infants and small children resulting from witnessed and corroborated free falls. *J Trauma* 1991;31:1350–1352.
314. Willinger M, Hoffman HJ, Hartford RB. Infant sleep position and risk for sudden infant death syndrome. National Institutes of Health report. *Pediatrics* 1994;93:814–819.
315. Willinger M. SIDS prevention. *Pediatr Ann* 1995;24:358–364.
316. Willinger M. Sleep position and sudden infant death syndrome. *JAMA* 1995;273:818–819.
317. Willman KY, Bank DE, Senac M, et al. Restricting the time of injury in fatal inflicted head injuries. *Child Abuse Negl* 1997;21:929–940.
318. Wilson EF. Estimation of the age of cutaneous contusions in child abuse. *Pediatrics* 1977;60:750–752.
319. Wininger KL. Chest compressions: biomechanics and injury. *Radiol Technol* 2007;78:269–274.
320. Wissow LS. Infanticide. *N Engl J Med* 1998;339:1239–1241.
321. Worn MJ, Jones MD. Rib fractures in infancy: establishing the mechanisms of cause from the injuries—a literature review. *Med Sci Law* 2007;47:200–212.
322. Wright CM. Identification and management of failure to thrive: a community perspective. *Arch Dis Child* 2000;82:5–9.
323. Wyatt DT, Erickson MM, Hillman RE, Hillman LS. Elevated thiamine levels in SIDS, non-SIDS, and adults: postmortem artifact. *J Pediatr* 1984;104:585–588.
324. Wynn VT, Southall DP. Normal relation between heart rate and cardiac repolarisation in sudden infant death syndrome. *Br Heart J* 1992;67:84–88.
325. Yeatman GW, Shaw C, Barlow MJ, Bartlett G. Pseudobattering in Vietnamese children. *Pediatrics* 1976;58:616–618.
326. Yiallourou SR, Walker AM, Horne RS. Prone sleeping impairs circulatory control during sleep in healthy term infants: implications for SIDS. *Sleep* 2008;31:1139–1146.
327. Zaloga WF, Collins KA. Pediatric homicides related to burn injury: a retrospective review at the Medical University of South Carolina. *J Forensic Sci* 2006;51:396–399.
328. Zumwalt RE, Fanizza-Orphanos AM. Dating of healing rib fractures in fatal child abuse. In: Fenoglio-Preiser CM, ed. *Advances in pathology*. St. Louis: Mosby, 1990:193–205.
329. Zurbuchen P, Le Coultre C, Caiza AM. Cutaneous necrosis after contact with calcium chloride: a mistaken diagnosis of child abuse. *Pediatrics* 1996;97:257–258.

CHAPTER 8

Transplant Pathology

RISH PAI
THEODORE J. PYSHER
ALIYA N. HUSAIN

Solid organ transplantation has become an accepted mode of therapy for a variety of end-stage diseases, with somewhat variable long-term outcome depending on the organ, as is discussed in this chapter (small bowel, liver, pancreas, kidney, heart, and lung). Kidney and liver transplant are relatively more common; thus, these are presented in greater detail. Although there are many organ-specific features in posttransplantation pathology, there are many similarities also. Postsurgical complications have markedly decreased due to better techniques and donor and recipient management. Immunosuppressive regimens, including multiple drug combinations, are standard of care. Antibody-mediated rejection is uncommon, while acute cellular rejection occurs in a majority of recipients and can usually be treated effectively. Chronic rejection is a fibrosing process that continues to be the major limiting factor to long-term survival, being more frequent in lung than in kidney, heart, and liver recipients. These immunocompromised patients are susceptible to both the usual bacterial as well as opportunistic infections, which often involve the lung. Posttransplant lymphoproliferative disease (PTLD), reported to occur in 3% to 5%, appears to be decreasing even further. It can involve the transplanted organ (rare in heart) as well as extranodal sites such as the gastrointestinal tract.

TRANSPLANT IMMUNOLOGY

Overview

The success of transplantation depends, in large part, on the immune response of the recipient to the donor tissue. The phenomenon of graft rejection was first identified by Peter Medawar in the early 1940s (71,111). Medawar and others demonstrated that allogeneic skin grafts (graft from a genetically distinct individual of the same species) would undergo rapid necrosis; however, syngeneic skin grafts (graft from a genetically identical individual) would survive. As almost all solid organ transplants occur between two genetically different individuals (allogeneic graft), many potential foreign or nonself molecules (alloantigens) are available to elicit an immune response and lead to graft failure. Most of these alloantigens are derived from polymorphic genes inherited from both parents and expressed codominantly. One of the most important alloantigens responsible for rejection is encoded by the major histocompatibility complex (MHC). There are three different histopathologic categories of rejection: hyperacute rejection, acute rejection, and chronic rejection, each of which can also be characterized by immunologic effector mechanisms (humoral versus cell-mediated). As transplant immunology is a complex field, only a limited discussion of this broad topic is presented here, and interested readers are referred to many excellent reviews for further reading (90,110,118).

Hyperacute Allograft Rejection

Hyperacute rejection is characterized by thrombotic occlusion of the graft vasculature that begins within minutes to hours after blood vessel anastomosis. The mechanism involves preformed antibodies present in the recipient that bind donor endothelial cells and elicit an immune response characterized by complement activation. Complement proteins are powerful serum proteins that are able to damage cells through either cell lysis or recruitment of inflammatory cells such as neutrophils and macrophages. Classical complement activation occurs when an antibody of the IgM or IgG subclass binds to its cognate antigen and activates C1q. The activation of complement leads to the destruction of donor endothelial cells, resulting in thrombosis. The IgM antibodies responsible for hyperacute rejection are mainly those against the carbohydrate ABO blood group antigen expressed primarily on red blood cells but also on vascular endothelial cells. As most donors and recipients are matched with respect to their ABO subtypes, hyperacute rejection due to anti-ABO antibodies is rare (118).

Acute Allograft Rejection

Acute allograft rejection is commonly encountered in solid organ transplants and has been an area of extensive research. Classically, acute rejection is characterized by the presence of infiltrating lymphocytes that mediate direct killing, macrophage activation, and tissue damage. The lymphocytes involved in this process include CD4$^+$ T-cells, CD8$^+$ T-cells, natural killer (NK) cells, and B-cells. Much of transplant immunology has been focused on the role of T-cells in rejection, as they are the principal mediators of acute rejection. Indeed, much of the immunosuppressive therapies in use today are directed toward interfering with T-cell function. The mechanism underlying T-cell activation is complex and involves two mechanisms: direct presentation of alloantigens (nonself MHC molecules) to recipient T-cells by donor-derived leukocytes and indirect presentation of alloantigens to recipient T-cells by recipient leukocytes (90). The process by which recipient T-cells can be directly activated by nonself MHC molecules on donor cells is still a mystery to most immunologists. During T-cell development in the thymus, those cells, with T-cell receptors, with high affinity for self-MHC molecules are deleted and only those with low affinity for self-MHC survive, thus preventing nonspecific T-cell activation (negative selection) (108). However, in the transplant setting, recipient peripheral T-cells are exposed to *nonself* MHC. Immunologists hypothesize that since T-cells with high affinity for these MHC-molecules were not deleted by negative selection, there will be a significant proportion (up to 1%) of circulating recipient T-cells with high affinity for nonself MHC (80). These T-cells could become activated and mediate allograft rejection. Both CD8$^+$ and CD4$^+$ T-cells become activated by allorecognition in response to class I and class II MHC molecules, respectively. The subsequent secretion of cytokines leads to macrophage, neutrophil, and natural killer cell recruitment (through chemokine and adhesion molecule expression) and tissue destruction (through reactive oxygen species, arachidonic acid metabolites, thrombosis, etc.). In addition, through direct allorecognition, donor CD8$^+$ T-cells can mediate killing. Direct allorecognition is thought to be the principle mechanism by which cellular rejection is mediated.

Indirect recognition of alloantigens is much better understood immunologically as it mirrors what occurs during infections. In this pathway, recipient antigen-presenting cells (dendritic cells and macrophages) phagocytose donor antigens and process them into peptides for presentation on class I and class II MHC. T-cells specific for these peptide:MHC complexes then can become activated and mediate rejection. The proportion of T-cells that would be activated in such a manner is much smaller than in direct allorecognition, and for many years, the significance of this pathway of T-cell activation has been unclear. Recently, indirect presentation has gained the interest of transplant immunologists as it can on its own mediate rejection (30). Moreover, indirect presentation is essential in producing highly specific antidonor antibodies (16). The donor-specific antibodies are mainly directed against donor MHC, both class I and class II. Once formed, these antibodies can bind to donor leukocytes and activated endothelial cells (anti-MHC class II) or all donor cells (anti-MHC class I) resulting in tissue damage through activation of complement and recruitment of inflammatory cells. Indeed, the use of C4d, a product of the complement cascade, as a surrogate of antibody-mediated complement activation has helped pathologists recognize acute humoral rejection (14,66).

Chronic Allograft Rejection

Histologically, chronic rejection in most organs is characterized by fibrosis and vascular damage, and immunologically this process most likely represents repeated bouts of acute rejection (sometimes subclinical). Thus, both cell-mediated and humoral mechanisms most likely contribute to chronic rejection. Upon activation, some T-cells can differentiate into effector cells that produce fibrosing cytokines (65) resulting in collagen deposition and parenchymal extinction. In addition, other cytokines such as platelet-derived growth factor and basic fibroblast growth factor can induce proliferation of smooth muscle cells leading to narrowing of the graft vessels. Moreover, antidonor antibodies have been shown to activate endothelial proliferation and vascular remodeling in animal models (16). The resulting ischemia further leads to parenchymal loss and graft dysfunction. Other causes of late graft dysfunction might not necessarily be related to immune-mediated rejection. Indeed, systemic disease such as diabetes, hyperlipidemia, viral infections, etc. can all contribute to late graft dysfunction and should be differentiated from chronic rejection.

Allograft Tolerance

Understanding the immunologic mechanisms of allograft rejection has been essential in developing new therapies as well as defining new histopathologic entities (acute humoral rejection); however, many questions remain. One of the most exciting fields in transplant immunology is uncovering the mechanisms behind allograft tolerance. The goal of such research is to determine which patients can be removed from immunosuppressive therapy due to tolerance toward the donor allograft. This is particularly important in the pediatric population as immunosuppressive therapy (particularly corticosteroids) is a major cause of morbidity and mortality. To date, no serologic or histopathologic data can accurately predict graft survival upon withdrawal of medications; however, evidence points to a role of donor-derived leukocytes in mediating allograft tolerance (110,111). It is hypothesized that patients who become microchimeras are more likely to become tolerant to their allografts (124). This finding is supported by the early observations that solid organ allografts are accepted to a great extent in individuals who are also receiving partial bone marrow transplants (63). In addition, the greater acceptance of liver allografts is thought to be due to the large number of donor-derived leukocytes present in this organ, some of which may be pluripotent stem cells that can migrate to recipient bone marrow and persist. The recent appreciation of regulatory T-cells has also shed light on allograft tolerance. Regulatory T-cells have been shown to suppress the function of effector T-cells, and active research is underway to enhance the activity of regulatory T-cells in order to achieve allograft tolerance (120).

TRANSPLANT PATHOLOGY OF THE INTESTINE

Overview

The introduction of improved immunosuppression (notably FK506) has led to a rise in small intestinal transplantation that is of particular importance to the pediatric pathologist as many of the disorders requiring transplantation occur in the pediatric population: necrotizing enterocolitis, intestinal volvulus, gastroschisis, massive resections, Hirschsprung disease, neuronal intestinal dysplasia, neuropathic and myopathic pseudo-obstruction, protein-losing enteropathy, and microvillous inclusion disease (29,51,89). The most frequent indication for intestinal transplantation in these patients is total parenteral nutrition–associated liver disease (52). When the liver disease is mild, the intestine can be transplanted in isolation. Signs of portal hypertension and cirrhosis mandate intestinal transplantation in combination with the liver, or as part of a multivisceral organ transplant. Indeed, patients receiving combined intestinal/liver transplantation or a multivisceral organ transplant experience fewer episodes of acute rejection and improved overall survival at 5 years (48). Currently, the major obstacle to intestinal transplantation is the availability of appropriate grafts. In particular, size matching is of extreme importance as many pediatric patients have contracted abdominal cavities as a result of previous surgeries.

The pathologist's role in intestinal transplantation is to evaluate mucosal biopsies in patients with graft dysfunction or as part of a surveillance program. Most institutions routinely take protocol biopsies for the first four to six weeks and when clinically indicated thereafter. In evaluating mucosal biopsies, the pathologist must correlate histologic findings with the clinical and endoscopic findings. As with most transplant specimens, a systematic approach evaluating the overall architecture, surface and crypt epithelium, inflammatory infiltrate, and vasculature can prevent pitfalls in diagnosis.

Preservation Injury and Hyperacute Rejection

Due to the intestinal villous circulation, the regenerative compartment of the epithelium is protected from ischemia; thus, preservation injury is less worrisome than in other solid organs. Biopsies taken prior to transplantation demonstrate lamina propria edema and separation of the epithelium from the basement membrane. Shortly after reperfusion, numerous mitoses can be seen within the regenerative compartment along with capillary congestion, villous blunting, and a mild neutrophilic infiltrate (58). Biopsies taken a week after transplantation usually show normal histology even when epithelial damage was quite severe. Hyperacute rejection in small bowel transplants has recently been described, and there is some overlap with preservation injury; however, distinction between the two is usually not difficult. In instances of hyperacute rejection, there is a positive cross-match indicating preformed donor-specific antibodies. These antibodies damage the endothelium leading to fibrin thrombi within the lamina propria vasculature resulting in severe congestion and focal hemorrhage. Neutrophils can be seen marginating within the congested vessels. The presence of fibrin thrombi and severe congestion distinguishes hyperacute rejection from preservation injury (125).

Acute Rejection

Unlike liver allografts, acute rejection is extremely common (up to 90% of patient's will experience at least one episode) and remains a major cause of intestinal graft failure (up to 50%). Acute rejection is clinically characterized by nonspecific symptoms such as fever, nausea, vomiting, increased stomal output, abdominal pain, and distention. In severe acute rejection, hemodynamic instability may occur leading to shock. Endoscopically, acute rejection is characterized by granularity, diminished peristalsis and, in some cases, mucosal ulceration. Acute rejection can occur at any time in the posttransplant period; however, the first episode of rejection usually occurs within 100 days (51,89). The landmark paper by Lee et al. (58) analyzed the first 62 intestinal transplants performed at the University of Pittsburgh and was the first study to develop histologic criteria for the diagnosis of acute rejection. Subsequent modifications have led to a well-developed histologic grading system for acute rejection that provides a reliable assessment of severity (126).

The histologic manifestations of acute rejection include crypt apoptosis, lamina propria inflammatory cell infiltrate, and crypt architectural distortion. During most episodes of acute rejection, all biopsies taken from multiple sites will show histologic features of rejection; however, in approximately 20% of cases, only the ileum will be involved. Crypt apoptosis is the earliest histologic sign of rejection, and apoptotic counts should be routinely performed on mucosal biopsy specimens. Rejection is characterized by greater than six apoptotic bodies per ten crypts, and in mild acute rejection, crypt apoptosis is the dominant histologic feature (Figure 8-1). In addition, mild localized collections of inflammatory cells (predominately activated/blastic lymphocytes with lesser numbers of eosinophils and neutrophils) are present around small venules and capillaries in the deep mucosa. Peyer patches become enlarged and contain large numbers of activated lymphocytes. The crypt epithelium commonly shows features of regeneration including mucin depletion, nuclear enlargement, and hyperchromasia. A mild increase in intraepithelial lymphocytes and occasional neutrophils is

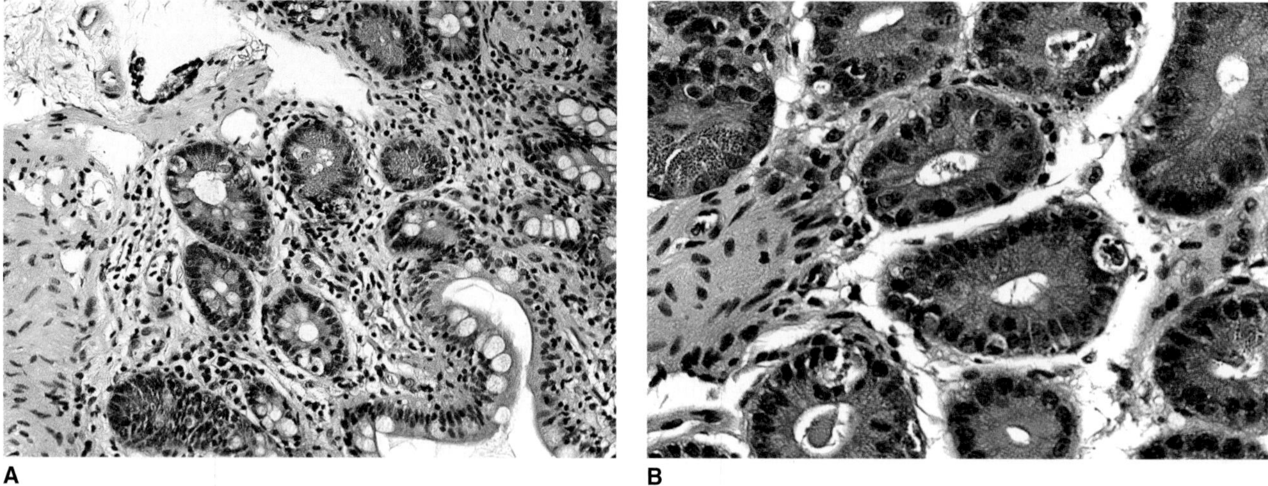

FIGURE 8-1 ■ Mild acute rejection of small bowel allografts. **A:** The villous architecture is usually preserved, and there is only a mild increase in lamina propria inflammation. **B:** Prominent apoptotic bodies are the most prominent feature. (Photos courtesy of Dr. Reetesh Pai, Stanford University.)

typically seen. The villi are shortened, and the crypts tend to be distorted due to lamina propria expansion.

Moderate rejection is characterized by increased crypt apoptotic bodies and a diffuse inflammatory cell infiltrate characterized by activated lymphocytes. Crypt apoptotic bodies are increased and begin to appear in the midportions of the crypt. The villi are flattened to a greater extent; however, extensive ulceration is not common. In severe acute rejection, crypt apoptotic body counts are further increased (up to 20) and become confluent (Figure 8-2). Mucosal ulcerations are common and, in its place, are fibrinous neutrophilic exudates mimicking pseudomembranous colitis. Care should be taken when evaluating biopsies for acute rejection 100 days posttransplant as the inflammatory infiltrate is generally mild and crypt apoptosis is the only dominant histologic feature (58).

Chronic Rejection

Chronic rejection in the intestine is less common than in heart, kidney, and lung; however, 8% of allografts at 5 years post-transplantation develop chronic rejection (79). Patients with chronic rejection have persistent diarrhea despite increased immunosuppressive therapy. Endoscopic and radiographic findings of chronic rejection include loss of mucosal folds, mural thickening, focal ulcers, and decreased arborization of the mesenteric vasculature. Clinically, chronic rejection is encountered late in the posttransplant period, with most cases occurring months after transplantation. There are many factors associated with the development of chronic rejection. Those individuals with acute rejection within 30 days of transplantation and those with severe acute rejection are more likely to develop chronic rejection. Other risk factors

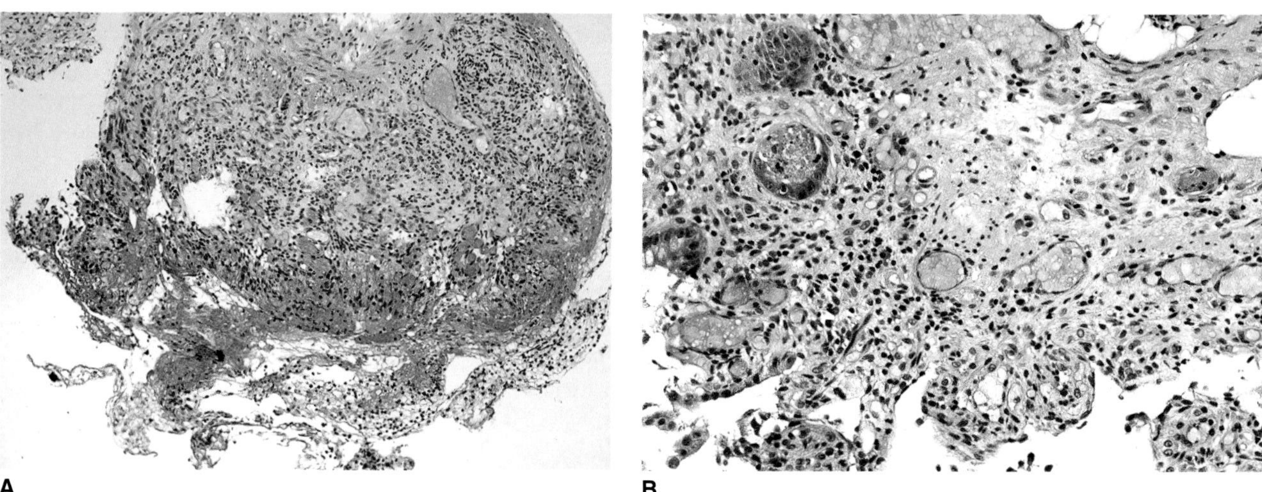

FIGURE 8-2 ■ Severe acute rejection of small bowel allografts. **A:** Surface ulceration with a prominent lymphocytic infiltrate is common. **B:** Crypts are typically lost, and the surviving crypts are severely damaged. This differential diagnosis includes ischemia and infection. (Photos courtesy of Dr. Reetesh Pai, Stanford University.)

include prolonged cold ischemic time, old donor age, and episodes of CMV infection (79). Simultaneous liver transplantation greatly protects from chronic rejection most likely by decreasing the number of acute rejection episodes. The pathologic process that results in chronic rejection involves arterial obliteration; however, arteries are rarely sampled in endoscopic biopsies. Thus, on mucosal biopsies, one can only suggest possible chronic rejection based on downstream features of chronic ischemia. Early histologic changes that suggest possible chronic rejection include patchy mild fibrosis and focal crypt loss. These nonspecific changes can persist for months. With worsening ischemia due to progression of chronic rejection, there is extensive loss of the intestinal crypts, villous atrophy, mucosal ulceration, and increased lamina propria inflammation and fibrosis. The surviving crypts show evidence of chronic damage including pyloric gland metaplasia and regenerative features (58,79). Once chronic rejection proceeds to the severe stage, the graft is very likely to fail. At resection, the vasculature should be adequately sampled to find the characteristic changes of chronic rejection. In addition, extensive neural hyperplasia is a common finding at resection (76).

Complications of Transplantation

Infection remains a very common complication of transplantation, whether in the postoperative setting or due to immunosuppressive therapies. The vast majority of infections are bacterial infections although fungal infections are also routinely encountered (89). Of more importance to the pathologist is recognizing viral infections, in particular cytomegalovirus (CMV), Epstein-Barr virus (EBV), and adenovirus. CMV infection is encountered in 5% to 29% of intestinal allograft specimens and can clinically mimic acute rejection (31,89). Negative CMV serology in the pediatric recipient is associated with increased CMV infection when transplanted with a serologic positive donor (60% will develop CMV enteritis) (64). In the majority of specimens, a moderate neutrophilic and mononuclear cell infiltrate is seen in the lamina propria as well as in the crypts. Ulceration with abundant granulation tissue can be seen in severe cases. In severely immunocompromised individuals, inflammation may be mild. In addition, crypt atrophy, cell drop out, and apoptotic bodies may be present, mimicking rejection. The characteristic CMV inclusions are mainly confined to the endothelial and stromal cells (Figure 8-3); however, epithelial cells can be infected in severe cases.

Adenovirus is a very common cause of pediatric gastroenteritis; however, until recently, infection of allografts has not been routinely recognized. Pinchoff et al. (81) found a high prevalence of adenoviral infection in pediatric small bowel allografts. Adenoviral enteritis most commonly affects the ileum and is characterized by smudgy epithelial cell nuclear inclusions, epithelial hyperplasia with disarray, and a prominent lymphoplasmacytic infiltrate. While adenoviral infection limited to the intestinal allograft is not in itself a matter of concern, disseminated adenoviral infection can be fatal. Moreover, those patients with a liver allograft are at risk of developing adenoviral hepatitis and fulminant hepatic failure.

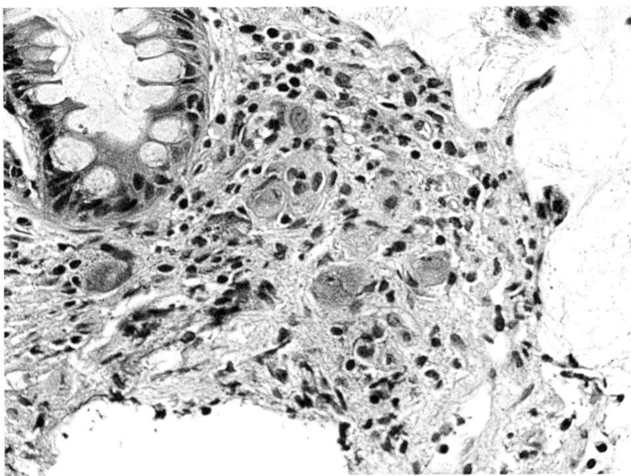

FIGURE 8-3 ■ Cytomegalovirus infection of small bowel allografts. In CMV infection, an inflammatory infiltrate with ulceration, crypt atrophy, and apoptotic bodies can be seen; however, the characteristic cytoplasmic and nuclear inclusions are key in differentiating CMV infection from rejection. (Photo courtesy of Dr. Reetesh Pai, Stanford University.)

Epstein-Barr virus (EBV) infection is another serious complication in the posttransplant period as it can lead to PTLD. Biopsy-proven EBV infection is fairly common and occurs in up to 50% of intestinal allograft specimens, higher than in many solid organs (27). EBV infection is associated with a wide histologic spectrum, from simple lymphoid hyperplasia to non-Hodgkin lymphoma. When evaluating a specimen, particular attention should be paid to the type of lymphoid infiltrate (Figure 8-4). If small lymphocytes predominate, one can be reassured; however, the presence of large atypical lymphoid cells should prompt concern for PTLD and *in situ* hybridization for EBV early RNA (EBER)

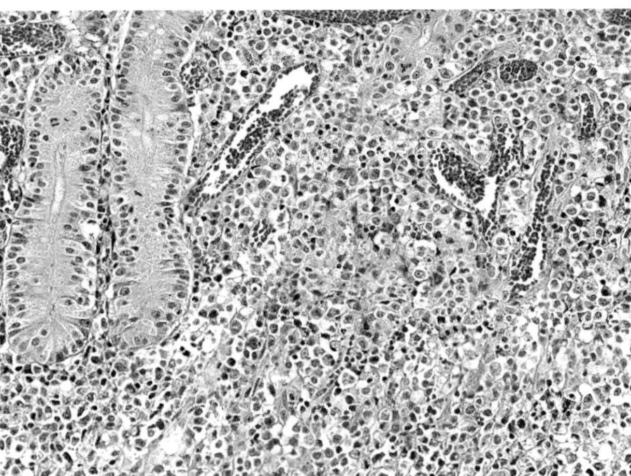

FIGURE 8-4 ■ Posttransplant lymphoproliferative disorder of small bowel allografts. PTLD is commonly characterized by an atypical inflammatory infiltrate, which can be mixed (polymorphous) as in this case or monomorphic. *In situ* hybridization for EBER can be helpful in confirming the diagnosis. (Photo courtesy of Dr. Reetesh Pai, Stanford University.)

should be performed. A large number of EBER positive cells (>15 per high power field) with a heterogeneous population of lymphoid cells, including immunoblasts, plasma cells, and large cleaved cells, are characteristic of polymorphous PTLD (Figure 8-4) (27). If the lymphoid population is homogenous, the designation of monomorphic PTLD is made and further classification is made according to established criteria (27). The vast majority of monomorphic PTLDs are B-cell in origin; however, T-cell PTLDs have been described.

The Gastrointestinal Tract in Graft-Versus-Host Disease

The intestinal tract is one of the three major target organs in graft-versus-host disease (GVHD) (69,70). The skin and the liver are the other two organs affected when donor lymphoid cells are transfused into immunosuppressed host. GVHD usually occurs in the setting of bone marrow transplantation but may also rarely occur following the transfusion of nonirradiated blood into patients with primary or secondary immunodeficiency disorders (75). Conceptually, GVHD mirrors allograft rejection as donor leukocytes recognize recipient tissues as "foreign" and attempt to "reject" them. Thus, the immunologic effector mechanisms are similar. GVHD develops in two phases: acute, which begins 1 week to 4 months after transplantation, and chronic, which begins approximately 4 months or more after transplantation. The clinical and pathologic features of the two phases are distinctly different.

The gastrointestinal tract is affected in at least half of patients with acute GVHD (69). Intestinal GVHD is usually heralded by profuse watery diarrhea, which indicates involvement of the small intestine and colon. Occasionally, the upper gastrointestinal tract will be involved first or exclusively; the symptoms are nausea, vomiting, and anorexia. Acute intestinal GVHD is usually diagnosed by colonoscopic biopsy or endoscopic biopsy of the upper gastrointestinal tract. The earliest histologic changes occur deep in the crypts (the regenerative compartment) with epithelial infiltration by lymphocytes and subsequent apoptosis of individual glandular cells, vacuolization of cytoplasm, and nuclear karyorrhexis (105,122), mimicking the changes seen in acute rejection (Figure 8-5). If appropriate therapy is not instituted, neutrophilic inflammation, glandular destruction, crypt abscesses, and ulceration are seen. Complete crypt loss, villous atrophy, and extensive mucosal denudation occur in advanced acute GVHD. In the esophagus, vacuolization and inflammation of the epithelial basal layer and eventual desquamation and ulceration are seen (103).

Chronic GVHD is a more insidious process that primarily affects the skin and liver. The intestinal tract is largely spared; however, features of chronic injury can be seen (2). In the esophagus, a scleroderma-like fibrosis and dysmotility may develop (72). In the evaluation of all the phases of intestinal GVHD, opportunistic infections must be ruled out (103) Interestingly, mycophenolate mofetil, a commonly used immunosuppressive drug in solid organ transplantation, can give rise to histologic findings similar to acute GVHD (78).

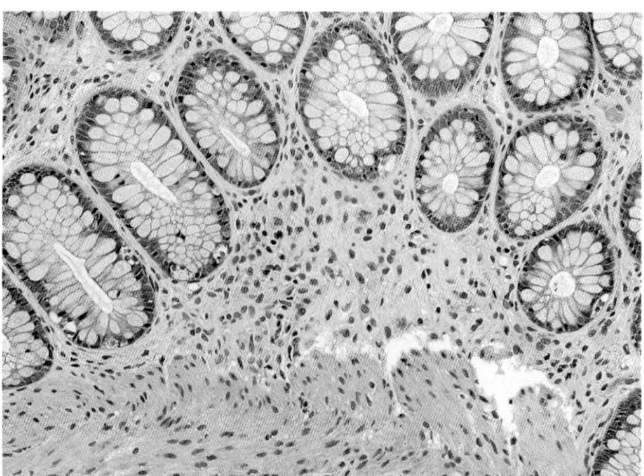

FIGURE 8-5 ■ Graft-versus-host disease of the small bowel. GVHD is characterized by apoptosis of individual epithelial cells lining the crypts similar to acute rejection seen in small bowel transplants. If severe, complete villous loss and surface ulceration can be seen.

TRANSPLANT PATHOLOGY OF THE LIVER

Overview

In the United States, between 1998 and 2007, 1,589 liver transplants were performed in patients under the age of 17 accounting for approximately 7% of the total number of liver transplants. Currently, there are approximately 800 pediatric patients on the transplant list (77). The indications for liver transplant are diverse (Table 8-1) (77); the most common continues to be extrahepatic biliary atresia.

Early in pediatric transplantation, the survival rates were dismal as only 30% of patients survived greater than 1 year (29). With improved surgical techniques, patient screening, and immunosuppression, the current 1-year patient survival is 90% and the 5-year survival is 80%. Graft survival is 85% at 1 year and 67% at 5 years (77). The early days of pediatric liver transplantation were also complicated by a shortage of appropriate-sized liver allografts. With the advent of reduced-sized liver transplantation, living-related transplantation and, most importantly, split-liver transplantation, the shortage of pediatric liver allografts has been somewhat alleviated (29,38,55). In split-liver transplants, the whole adult cadaveric liver is divided into two functional segments: one for adults (right trisegment) and one for children (left lateral segment). Recent studies have shown that split-liver recipients have comparable survival to whole liver recipients (4,49). Despite these improvements, surgical complications continue to be more common when compared with adults (29,38,68). In particular, the use of partial liver allografts predisposes to biliary complications (98). In addition, hepatic artery thrombosis is more common in pediatric patients owing to the technically difficult surgery. However, the improvement in surgical techniques and postoperative management has improved, allowing many of these grafts to be saved. Portal vein thrombosis is occasionally encountered, which, in most cases, resolves without need for intervention (68). Hepatic vein thrombosis is rarely encountered except in patients

Table 8-1 ▪ INDICATIONS FOR PEDIATRIC LIVER TRANSPLANTATION

Noncholestatic cirrhosis
- Autoimmune hepatitis
- Chronic viral hepatitis

Cholestatic liver disease/cirrhosis
- Caroli disease
- Choledochol cyst
- Primary sclerosing cholangitis

Biliary atresia
- Extrahepatic
- Alagille syndrome
- Hypoplasia

Acute hepatic necrosis
- Acute viral hepatitis
- Drugs

Metabolic diseases
- Alpha-1-antitrypsin deficiency
- Wilson disease
- Hemochromatosis
- Tyrosinemia
- Primary oxalosis
- Glycogen storage disease types Ia, Ib, III and IV
- Hyperlipidemia
- Urea cycle disorders
- Crigler-Najjar syndrome

Malignant neoplasms
- Hepatoblastoma
- Hepatocellular carcinoma

Other
- Cystic fibrosis
- Budd-Chiari syndrome
- Congenital hepatic fibrosis
- TPN/hyperalimentation
- Familial cholestasis
- Hepatic adenomatosis

undergoing liver transplantation for Budd-Chiari syndrome. Bowel perforation is common in the pediatric population as most of these patients have had previous abdominal surgery and suffer from poor nutrition. Other complications of liver transplant can be roughly grouped into the time periods in which they are most likely to occur (Table 8-2) (121).

The initial outcome of the liver allograft depends on the health of the donor liver, the amount of ischemic time the allograft suffered, the presence of preformed antiallograft antibodies, and complications encountered during surgery and the perioperative period. Acute rejection and viral infections tend to occur between 1 week and 2 months posttransplantation, whereas chronic rejection and recurrent disease are late manifestations. However, the timing can vary significantly (e.g., late-onset acute rejection) and biopsy interpretation remains essential.

Preservation Injury

Preservation (harvesting) injury results from donor and tissue procurement factors that contribute to poor allograft function in the perioperative period. In order to diagnose preservation injury, one must exclude injury due to surgical complications, immunologic reactions, and drug toxicity. Warm and cold ischemia preferentially damage hepatocytes and endothelial cells, respectively. Endothelial cell damage leads to interference with vascular blood flow and subsequent allograft injury. Many donor factors can increase the susceptibility of the allograft to ischemic time. One of the most studied is the presence of donor macrovesicular steatosis. Transplantation of liver allografts with greater than 50% macrovesicular steatosis, on frozen section analysis results in poor graft function as steatotic hepatocytes are

Table 8-2 ▪ APPROXIMATE TIMELINE OF BIOPSY FINDINGS IN LIVER TRANSPLANTATION

Posttransplant Interval	Complications	Histologic Features
Early (0–7 days)	Preservation/harvesting injury	Centrilobular pallor, ballooning degeneration, cholestasis
	Humoral rejection	Extensive necrosis and perivenular hemorrhage; positive C4d
	Early hepatic artery thrombosis	Zonal hepatocyte and bile duct necrosis
Middle (7–30 days)	Acute cellular rejection	Mixed portal infiltrate, bile duct damage, and endothelialitis
	CMV hepatitis	Microabscesses and viral inclusions
Late (>30 days)	Recurrent disease	Features of original disease
	Chronic rejection	Bile duct and arteriolar loss, foam cell arteriopathy
	Late-onset acute rejection	Perivenular inflammation; interface and lobular activity; less endothelialitis and portal inflammation than classic acute rejection
	PTLD	Atypical lymphoid infiltrate, EBER+
	Late hepatic artery thrombosis	Centrilobular hepatocyte dropout; biliary obstruction
	De novo autoimmune hepatitis	Lymphoplasmacytic infiltrate with interface activity

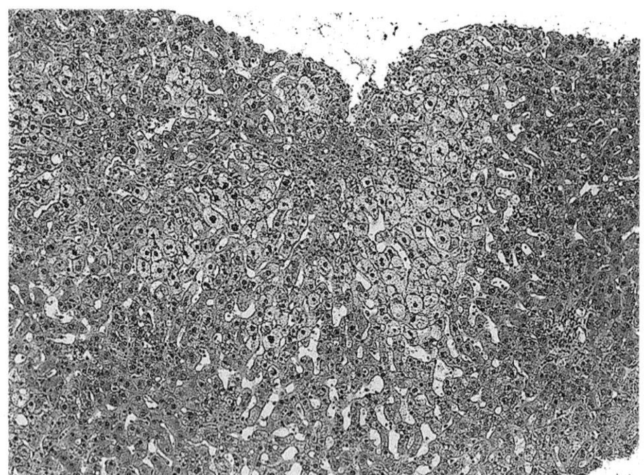

FIGURE 8-6 ■ Preservation injury of liver allografts. Pallor in the centrilobular areas with hepatocyte ballooning occurring shortly after transplantation is characteristic of mild preservation injury. Hepatocyte and canalicular cholestasis can also be quite prominent in some cases.

sensitive to ischemic damage. Other donor factors that influence graft function include fibrosis, chronic liver disease, hemodynamic instability, infections, donor atherosclerosis, and donor age (82,91).

Clinically, preservation injury is characterized by poor bile production and persistent elevations of serum ALT and AST. The histologic features of preservation injury are usually apparent within 1 to 2 days after revascularization. In mild preservation injury, mild centrilobular hepatocyte ballooning and canalicular cholestasis are commonly seen. Occasionally, neutrophils may be present. On low-power microscopic evaluation, preservation injury can be suggested by pallor in the centrilobular areas. The hepatocyte injury is rapidly reversible; however, the cholestasis may persist for several weeks (Figure 8-6). In more severe injury, zonal necrosis and severe neutrophilia may be seen. In these biopsies, bile ductular proliferation as well as cholestasis may be prominent. In patients receiving a steatotic liver, reperfusion results in lysis of the steatotic hepatocytes with formation of sinusoidal fat droplets that disrupt hepatic blood flow. The extracellular fat may persist for weeks after initial injury. Resolution of hepatic injury is the hallmark of preservation injury, but if severe, the allograft may fail resulting in primary nonfunction. If hepatocyte injury persists beyond one week, other diagnoses such as rejection and obstructive cholangitis should be considered.

It is our practice to report the percentage of macrovesicular steatotic hepatocytes, the amount of fibrosis, the presence of perivenular necrosis, and neutrophilic infiltration (excluding surgical hepatitis) (28) to our transplant surgeons who ultimately determine allograft use.

Hepatic Artery Thrombosis

As previously mentioned, hepatic artery thrombosis (HAT) remains a significant problem in pediatric liver transplantation and is a complication in 5% to 10% of pediatric liver allografts (68). The incidence of HAT increases with decreasing age due to the smaller size of the arterial anastomosis. As the hepatic artery is the sole blood supply to the biliary tree, HAT should be sought whenever a biliary leak is found. HAT can occur early in the posttransplant period or late (occurring >30 days posttransplant). Early HAT is associated with severe graft dysfunction and high mortality rate. In early HAT, rapid diagnosis and repair of the vascular tree are essential in reversing biliary damage and prevention of allograft failure. Even with aggressive treatment, retransplantation may be necessary; however, in one study, 40% of children with HAT survived without retransplantation (114).

In late HAT, the allograft is less susceptible to damage as collaterals have formed. Indeed, many patients are asymptomatic. Symptomatic patients commonly present with recurrent cholangitis, biliary tract strictures (due to prolonged ischemic damage), abscess, and fever. Biopsy findings in HAT are nonspecific, variable, and irregularly distributed within the graft (121). In early HAT, coagulative necrosis of the centrilobular hepatocytes is frequently encountered along with bile duct necrosis. In late HAT, features of biliary obstruction are encountered, including canalicular cholestasis, cholate stasis, and bile ductular proliferation. In addition, centrilobular hepatocyte ballooning and dropout are commonly seen. Although these findings suggest HAT, definitive diagnosis requires clinical correlation.

Biliary Complications

In children, biliary tract complications are more numerous due to surgical difficulties and the use of split-liver allografts (38,67,68). Clinically, biliary complications should be suspected when preferential increases in alkaline phosphatase and gamma-glutamyl transferase occur. Minor strictures may be asymptomatic with only minor elevations in biliary enzymes, whereas complete obstruction, cholangitic abscess, and ascending cholangitis result in fever, jaundice, right upper quadrant pain, and bacteremia. Liver biopsies typically show features of biliary obstruction. In the acute phase, portal edema, canalicular cholestasis, and portal inflammation (mostly neutrophils) are commonly seen. Chronic obstruction leads to cholate stasis, chronic portal inflammation, focal bile duct loss, and portal fibrosis. Progression to biliary cirrhosis can occur if the obstruction is not relieved. Biliary-vascular fistula is a serious complication that warrants prompt surgical correction. Histologically, bile is found in blood vessels often with a giant cell reaction, and red blood cells are found within bile ducts.

Hyperacute (Humoral) Rejection

Humoral rejection is a rare cause of early liver allograft failure and should be distinguished from primary nonfunction. Hyperacute rejection occurs in the setting of preformed cytotoxic antibodies directed mainly against ABO blood group antigens, but also against class I and II MHC antigens. The liver is relatively resistant to injury by these antibodies for multiple reasons including clearance of antibodies by resident Kupffer cells, dual blood supply, and absence of conventional basement membrane (which is prothrombotic) (21).

Hyperacute rejection is suspected first in the operating room when the liver becomes swollen and hard and bile is not produced, soon after revascularization. Hemostasis may be difficult to achieve in these patients. Histologically, hyperacute rejection may be difficult to distinguish from primary nonfunction. In severe cases (mostly those due to ABO-incompatibility), there tend to be large areas of infarction, portal vein thrombi, and necrotizing arteritis. In mild cases (ABO-compatible), centrilobular hepatocyte ballooning, canalicular cholestasis, acidophil bodies, and bile ductular proliferation may be seen (features almost indistinguishable from preservation injury). With appropriate clinical history, such as positive cross-match and short ischemic time, hyperacute rejection may be suggested. Detection of C4d (by immunohistochemistry or immunofluorescence) may be helpful as a recent study found 91% (10 of 11) of hyperacute rejection cases had positive staining for C4d in the hepatic vasculature (35).

Acute Rejection

Acute rejection is fairly common in pediatric liver allografts, affecting up to 60% of transplant recipients (67). Most episodes occur within the first few months after transplantation and can easily be controlled by traditional immunosuppressive therapy. However, a somewhat distinct form of acute rejection can occur late in the post transplant period, aptly termed late acute rejection. These rejection episodes tend to be more resistant to standard immunosuppressive therapy and have unique histologic features. Most cases of late acute rejection in children are due to inadequate immunosuppression (18). Clinically, acute rejection can be asymptomatic when mild. More severe cases present with fever, decreased bile flow, and elevations in liver chemistry tests. The gold standard for confirming the diagnosis remains liver biopsy; however, communication between the pathologists and clinician is essential in determining which patients with rejection require increased immunosuppression.

In 1997, the Banff working group convened to develop histologic criteria outlining three core histological features: (a) portal inflammation, (b) subendothelial inflammation, and (c) bile duct damage (5) (Figure 8-7). The portal inflammation is mixed. Activated (blastic) lymphocytes and small mononuclear cells tend to predominate; however, eosinophils, macrophages, and neutrophils can be prominent. Posttransplant lymphoproliferative disorder should be kept in mind when a monotonous portal infiltrate consisting of blastic lymphocytes is present without other features of rejection. The presence of mononuclear inflammatory cells between the endothelial cells of the portal or central vein and the underlying basement membrane, referred to as endothelialitis, is another common feature of rejection. Occasionally, central vein endothelialitis may be the only prominent feature of acute rejection. Bile duct damage is manifested by the presence of mononuclear cells inside the basement membrane and between cholangiocytes. In addition, the bile duct epithelium shows loss of apical cytoplasm (increased nuclear/cytoplasmic ratio), paranuclear vacuolization, nucleoli,

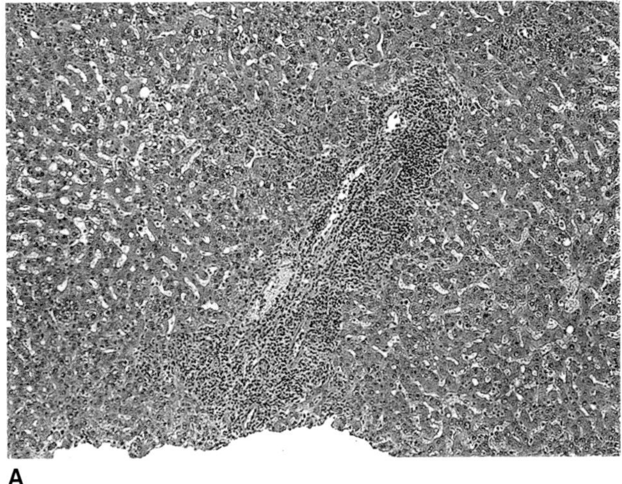

A

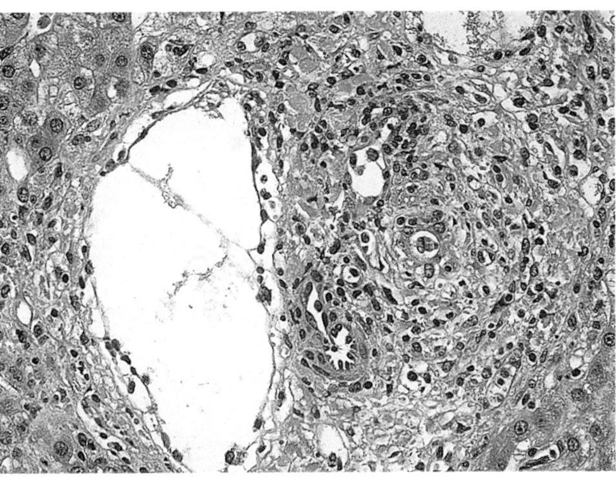

B

FIGURE 8-7 ▪ Acute rejection of liver allografts. **A:** The portal tracts in acute rejection are expanded by a dense mixed inflammatory infiltrate. **B:** Definitive evidence of endothelialitis along with bile duct damage confirms the diagnosis.

nuclear overlap, mitosis, apoptotic bodies, and cytoplasmic eosinophilia. To make a diagnosis of acute rejection, two of three of the above histologic features must be present. The diagnosis is further strengthened if greater than 50% of bile ducts are damaged or if unequivocal endothelialitis is present. Other findings such as necrotizing arteritis (rarely seen in needle biopsies), interface hepatitis, lobular inflammation, and eosinophilia are also seen in acute rejection but are not necessary for the diagnosis. Early in the postoperative period, acute rejection may resemble preservation injury; however, the presence of portal inflammation should distinguish between these two entities.

Once the diagnosis of acute rejection is made based on the above criteria, an indication of the global severity should be given. In mild acute rejection, portal inflammation is mild. In moderate rejection, most or all of the portal tracts are expanded by an inflammatory infiltrate. In severe rejection, there is spillover into the hepatic parenchyma with hepatocyte necrosis, both periportal and perivenular. At our institution, only a global assessment of rejection is given;

however, a rejection activity index has been developed to further characterize the severity of rejection and is routinely reported at some institutions (5,59).

As mentioned, late-onset acute rejection has some unique morphologic features when compared with acute rejection occurring early in the posttransplant period (18,20). Late acute rejection tends to have less portal inflammation, increased interface activity, less endothelialitis, and more lobular activity; however, traditional features of acute rejection should still be present. In some cases, only centrilobular pathology exists with perivenular inflammation and zone 3 hepatocyte dropout.

Chronic Rejection

Chronic rejection has become relatively rare with current immunosuppressive therapy and affects only 3% to 5% of total liver allografts (67). Some studies report almost no cases of chronic rejection in pediatric patients (46); however, chronic rejection does occur and is an important cause of late graft failure. Factors associated with chronic rejection include a primary diagnosis of autoimmune liver disease, late-onset acute rejection, nonwhite race, baseline immunosuppression, certain tumor necrosis factor-2 alleles, and CMV infection (controversial) (24,34,117). Despite the name, many cases of chronic rejection occur within months of transplant (2 to 6 months) and lead to graft failure within 2 years. Indeed, unlike other solid organ allografts, chronic rejection in the liver decreases with time, except for a small group of patients with late-onset chronic rejection. The classic presentation of chronic rejection is that of a patient with multiple episodes of acute rejection who develops progressive cholestasis and elevations in alkaline phosphatase, bilirubin, and gamma-glutamyl transferase, and is unresponsive to immunosuppressive therapy. Rarely patients present with chronic rejection in the absence of any documented history of acute rejection.

As chronic rejection most commonly results from repeated bouts of acute rejection, there will be a period of overlap. Conceptually, acute rejection refers to reversible and active lesions in which there is hepatocyte apoptosis and blastic portal inflammation, whereas chronic rejection is generally nonreversible and refers to loss of key structures. If both features are present, both acute and chronic rejection should be diagnosed based on their respective criteria. Late clinical findings of chronic rejection include hepatic infarction and loss of synthetic function. Clinically, chronic rejection can resemble biliary obstruction, and cholangiography is sometimes necessary to distinguish them.

Like acute rejection, there are three histopathologic features of chronic rejection: (a) bile duct atrophy, (b) foam cell arteriopathy, and (c) bile duct loss, at least one of which should be present (19,59). The diagnosis of chronic rejection mainly depends upon bile duct features as the characteristic foam cell arterial changes are rarely encountered on routine liver biopsies. Thus, it is important to exclude other causes of duct injury or loss such as hepatic artery thrombosis, obstructive biliary disease, recurrent chronic hepatitis, drug reactions, and cytomegalovirus infections. The bile duct damage is thought to be ischemic in nature due to damage to the peribiliary arterial plexus. The earliest manifestations of bile duct injury include eosinophilic transformation of the biliary cytoplasm, uneven nuclear spacing, syncytia formation, nuclear enlargement and hyperchromasia, and ducts with focal epithelial cell loss. At this early stage of chronic rejection, it is thought that these changes might be reversible with immunosuppression. In late chronic rejection, bile ducts and, to a lesser extent, terminal hepatic arterioles are lost. When quantifying bile duct and arterial loss, it is essential to remember that in a normal liver, not all portal tracts contain these structures. In fact, between 5% and 10% of portal tracts do not contain bile ducts or hepatic artery branches (17). Thus, bile duct loss is only significant if greater than

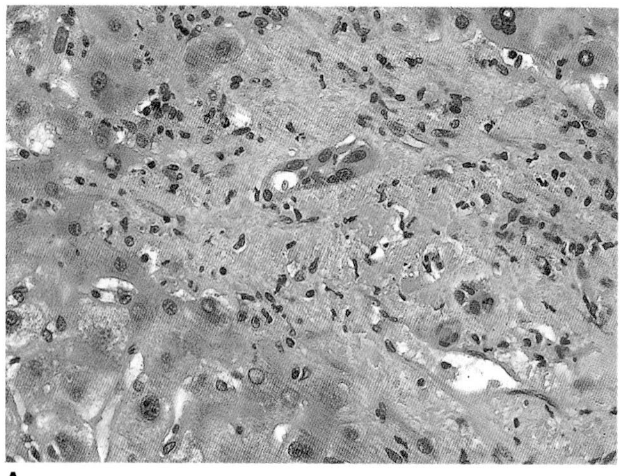
A

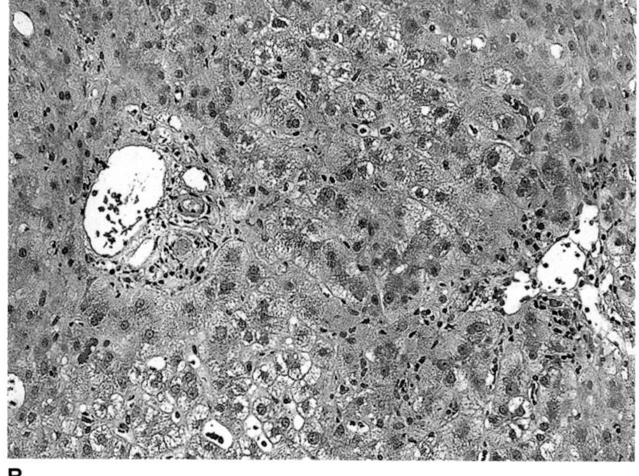
B

FIGURE 8-8 ■ Chronic rejection of liver allografts. **A:** In early chronic rejection, the biliary nuclear/cytoplasmic ratio is increased, and the cytoplasm shows prominent eosinophilia. **B:** In late chronic rejection, the bile ducts are lost and only portal veins and, to a lesser extent, terminal hepatic arterioles remain to identify portal tracts. There is an "empty" appearance to the often diminutive portal tracts.

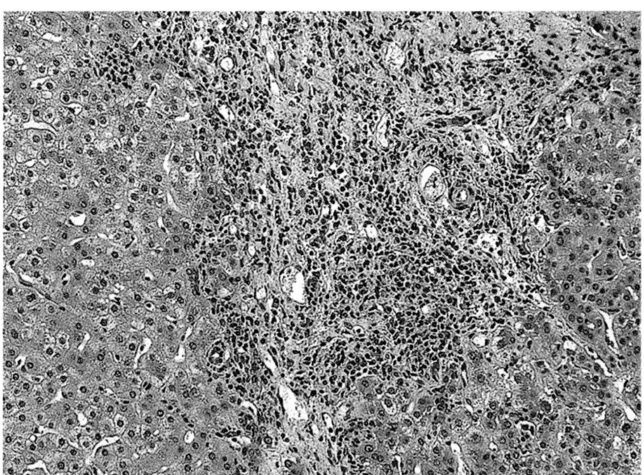

FIGURE 8-9 ▪ *De novo* autoimmune hepatitis. The portal tract is expanded by a dense lymphoplasmacytic infiltrate with prominent interface and lobular activity. Along with elevated ANA titers, these findings are consistent with a *de novo* autoimmune hepatitis.

20% of the portal tracts do not have bile ducts. However, quantification of bile duct and arterial loss can be complicated in late chronic rejection as portal tracts can be difficult to visualize. In these cases, portal tracts should be inferred from location within the lobule, presence of connective tissue, and shape. Additionally, inflammatory cells may obscure bile ducts. In such cases, immunohistochemistry for cytokeratin 7 may be useful in determining bile duct number; however, care must be taken to count only true bile ducts and not ductules (36).

Foam cell arteriopathy is another hallmark of chronic rejection; however, it is best appreciated in large-sized and medium-sized hepatic artery branches that can only be sampled on hepatectomy specimens. Early chronic rejection is characterized by accumulation of foam cells within the intima without luminal compromise. In late rejection, foam cell accumulation with luminal compromise predominates. Changes in large bile ducts can also be appreciated in hepatectomy specimens, including fibrosis of the wall, epithelial sloughing, and papillary hyperplasia. In most cases of chronic rejection, both bile duct loss and foam cell arterial changes co-exist; however, up to 15% of cases may have only one feature.

Centrilobular changes can also be seen in chronic rejection and may be a prominent feature. In early chronic rejection, perivenular mononuclear inflammation, hepatocyte dropout, acidophil bodies, pigmented macrophages, and mild fibrosis are commonly seen. Late chronic rejection is characterized by perivenular fibrosis that can be extensive, resulting in bridging fibrosis. Vascular damage due to chronic rejection may be a cause of these centrilobular changes; however, immunologic factors might also contribute to these findings. Centrilobular cholestasis can also be prominent, especially when bile duct loss becomes severe. Many factors not related to chronic rejection may also lead to similar centrilobular changes such as viral hepatitis, venous outflow obstruction, and hepatic artery thrombosis. Thus, definitive diagnosis of chronic rejection must rely on bile duct and arterial changes.

De novo and Recurrent Autoimmune Hepatitis

Patients who are transplanted due to autoimmune hepatitis (AIH) can develop recurrent disease (30% by 5 years); however, some patients without any prior history develop a syndrome remarkably similar to classic AIH termed *de novo* AIH. The diagnosis of *de novo* or recurrent AIH requires the presence of autoantibodies, lymphoplasmacytic portal inflammation with prominent interface and lobular activity, serologic evidence of liver injury, hypergammaglobulinemia, and no evidence of viral hepatitis, drug-related hepatitis, or rejection (Figure 8-9) (20).

Other Recurrent Diseases

In children, recurrent hepatitis C or B is generally not routinely encountered as chronic viral hepatitis is an uncommon indication of liver transplantation. In addition, intrinsic metabolic or synthetic liver disease does not recur in the allograft. However, metabolic diseases that secondarily affect the liver can recur in the allograft. These diseases include Niemann-Pick disease, Gaucher disease, cystinosis, and erythropoietic protoporphyria (45).

Recent evidence has confirmed that primary sclerosing cholangitis (PSC) can recur in approximately 5% to 20% of patients with most recurrences diagnosed more than 1 year posttransplant (32). Moreover, PSC patients are at a higher risk of developing rejection and worsening inflammatory bowel disease after transplantation. Because in the posttransplant setting there are many causes of biliary disease, the diagnosis of recurrent PSC is often difficult, and no gold standard exists. Thus, close clinical, radiologic, and histopathologic correlation is required to make this diagnosis. The presence of nonanastomotic biliary strictures is suggestive of recurrent PSC but only if occurring late in the posttransplant period. In addition, other causes of late-onset biliary strictures, such as chronic rejection and biliary infections must be excluded. Early stricturing is more likely due to complications of preservation injury and hepatic artery thrombosis. Biopsies showing characteristic "onion-skinning" cholangitis or fibro-obliterative changes have been shown to occur only in allografts from PSC patients, but these features are seen only in a small percentage of patients. Thus while specific, absence of these features does not rule out recurrent PSC. Features of biliary obstruction are more commonly seen in recurrent PSC; however, these features are nonspecific. Currently, guidelines suggest that recurrent PSC should be suggested in cases with a confirmed diagnosis of PSC before transplant; if there is cholangiographic evidence of extrahepatic biliary obstruction, beading, and irregularities at least greater then 90 days after transplantation; or if there is histologic evidence of fibrous cholangitis and/or fibro-obliterative lesions with or without ductopenia, biliary fibrosis, or biliary cirrhosis.

Idiopathic Posttransplantation Chronic Hepatitis

Recently, a group of patients without any previous history or serologic evidence of viral hepatitis or drug reaction has been shown to develop a picture resembling chronic hepatitis late in the posttransplant period (23). Remarkably, in one pediatric study, 64% of allograft biopsies at 10 years post-transplant had histopathologic features of chronic hepatitis including portal inflammation, necroinflammatory activity, and fibrosis. Less than 5% of these cases met the criteria of *de novo* autoimmune hepatitis; only 2 of 113 were positive for hepatitis C, whereas no cause was found in the vast majority of cases. Although only a subset met the criteria for *de novo* autoimmune hepatitis, many patients had increased ANA and SMA titers, some above 1:100. It is possible that these clinical and histopathologic abnormalities represent a subclinical form of *de novo* autoimmune hepatitis or atypical chronic rejection. These authors suggest that reinstitution of steroid therapy may be beneficial to these patients. As most institutions do not routinely obtain protocol liver biopsies late in the posttransplant course, these findings have yet to be corroborated at other institutions.

Posttransplant Opportunistic Infections

As the pediatric transplant recipient may be naïve for many viral infections and many would not have completed their vaccinations, viral infections of the allograft tend to be more severe. Indeed, even live attenuated viral vaccines are contraindicated in transplant patients due to the possibility of graft infections. Viral infections occur most commonly between 1 week to 2 months after transplantation and tend to follow episodes of acute rejection due to increased immunosuppression (121). Thus, distinction between ongoing acute rejection and new-onset viral infection may be difficult clinically and histologically. The most common viral infections leading to graft dysfunction are CMV and EBV. However, other, more rare viral infections such as adenovirus, varicella virus, and herpes simplex virus can lead to graft failure.

CMV hepatitis is fairly common in pediatric liver transplantation, affecting up to 10% of allografts. However, with the advent of prophylactic CMV therapy, the incidence and severity of disease have been reduced. Close monitoring of patients receiving an allograft from a CMV positive donor, is essential as CMV hepatitis tends to be more common and more severe. CMV infection of the allograft can lead to a variety of histologic manifestations, some of which overlap with acute rejection. As classic eosinophilic nuclear inclusions are rare and may be absent, reliance on multiple histologic features is necessary. Mild-to-moderate lymphocytic portal inflammation is found in almost all cases of CMV hepatitis. In addition, one of the most sensitive, but not specific, findings in CMV hepatitis is the presence of scattered clusters of necrotic hepatocytes surrounded by a neutrophilic infiltrate forming microabscesses (Figure 8-10A). However, microabscesses can be found in a wide variety of conditions such as biliary obstruction, ischemia, other infections, and sepsis (57), and, therefore, CMV immunohistochemistry is indicated when microabscesses are present. Kupffer cell hyperplasia, hepatocyte ballooning, and parenchymal inflammation are other common findings. Slight lymphocytic cholangitis may be seen and should not be mistaken for acute rejection.

Pediatric transplant recipients commonly develop manifestations of EBV infection that can ultimately lead to PTLD (67). Naïve recipients of EBV-positive allografts are at a much higher risk of developing infection in the posttransplant period. Interestingly, transplantation for Langerhans cell histiocytosis also predisposes to EBV-associated PTLD (98). Clinically, EBV infection first manifests as fever, pharyngitis, lymphadenitis, and jaundice. Liver enzymes are typically elevated. EBV infection results in a wide variety of histologic manifestations in the liver allograft. Nonspecific findings such as portal inflammation and sinusoidal mononuclear infiltrates, often forming linear aggregates, are common. Scattered acidophil bodies, hepatocyte ballooning, and mild lobular disarray with pseudoacinar formation and plate hypertrophy are commonly seen. If EBV infection is not controlled, progression to PTLD may occur. Early lesions consist of atypical lymphocytes in the portal inflammatory cell infiltrate. Endothelialitis may be present, closely mimicking acute rejection. Differentiation relies on the presence of a monotonous portal infiltrate with few atypical lymphocytes rather than the mixed infiltrate seen in acute rejection (Figure 8-10C). Frank PTLD can range from diffuse large B-cell lymphoma to Hodgkin-like lymphoma. Extrahepatic involvement is common. EBER as well as immunohistochemistry for CD20, kappa, and lambda is useful to confirm the diagnosis (Figure 8-10D).

Adenovirus, though rare, is more common in pediatric transplant recipients than in adults who are more likely to have protective immunity (42). Clinically, patients present with fever, difficulty breathing, diarrhea, and liver dysfunction. Usually infection occurs in the first 3 months, and serotype 5 is the most common. Large granulomas along with random areas of necrosis are characteristic of adenoviral hepatitis (Figure 8-10B). Smudgy and granular viral nuclear inclusions can be found at the edge of the necrotic zones and can be documented by immunohistochemistry. HSV and VZ are other rare causes of posttransplant viral hepatitis and can lead to fulminant hepatic failure if infection goes unrecognized. Once again, infection is more common and more severe in pediatric patients as they are more likely to lack protective immunity. HSV and VZ cause similar histopathologic findings, and because it is difficult to separate these two infections based on H&E alone, immunohistochemistry is required. As in adenoviral hepatitis, random confluent areas of coagulative-type necrosis are common. In the center of the necrotic areas, ghost hepatocytes and neutrophils are seen. At the edge of these zones, virally infected hepatocytes with characteristic ground-glass intranuclear inclusions may be present. Multinucleated infected hepatocytes are sometime seen.

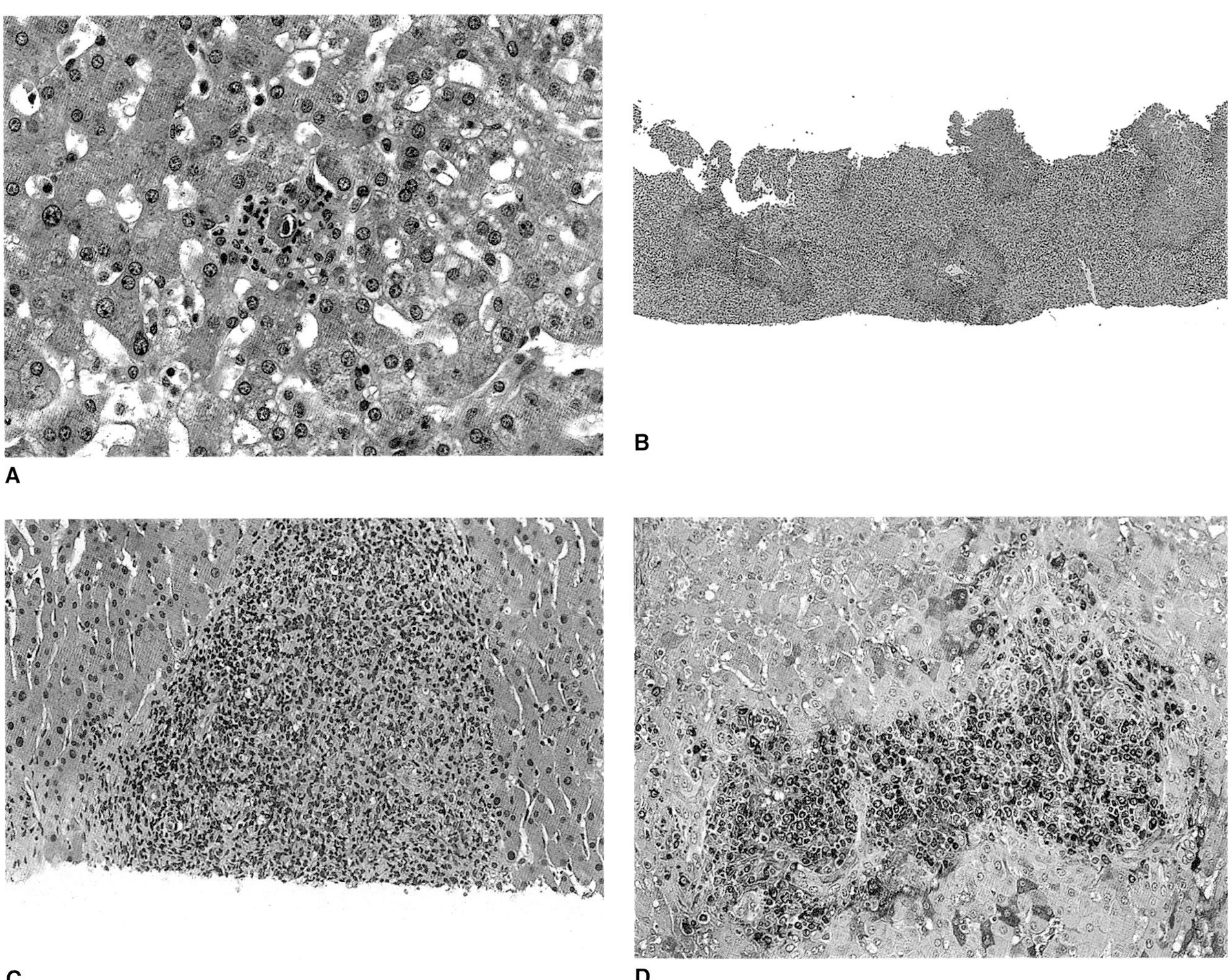

FIGURE 8-10 ■ Posttransplant infections of the liver allograft. **A:** Cytomegalovirus is a common infection in the posttransplant setting. Characteristic findings include microabscesses near infected cells. **B:** Adenovirus infection, although rare, is a serious complication in the pediatric setting. Zonal necrosis along with smudgy nuclear inclusions is characteristic. **C:** The histologic findings in PTLD are varied. In severe cases, the portal tracts are greatly expanded by a dense, atypical lymphoid infiltrate. **D:** *In situ* hybridization for EBER may be essential in confirming the diagnosis of PTLD.

If VZ or HSV is suspected, rapid communication to the clinicians is essential. Immediate antiviral therapy and cessation of immunosuppression may reduce graft dysfunction and prevent graft failure.

The Liver in Bone Marrow Transplantation

Bone marrow transplantation is used in the management of a wide variety of diseases, including aplastic anemia, leukemia, and immune disorders (70). Hepatic changes seen in these patients may be related to chemotherapy and total-body irradiation in preparation for transplantation, graft-versus-host disease (GVHD), or the infections to which these immunocompromised individuals are susceptible. Veno-occlusive disease (VOD) or sinusoidal occlusive syndrome (SOS) is a complication of chemotherapy (particularly cyclophosphamide-based regimens) and may be mild, with full recovery, or severe and lead to death (119). VOD usually occurs within the first 30 days after transplantation; however, late-onset VOD has been reported with newer chemotherapeutic regimens. Chemotherapeutic agents damage the sinusoidal endothelial cell layer, resulting in deposition of extracellular matrix in the sinusoids and terminal hepatic veins occluding blood flow. This results in ascites, weight gain, painful hepatomegaly, and jaundice. In the early phase, centrilobular hemorrhage is associated with damaged venules and sinusoids (Figure 8-11). There is narrowing of the lumina and widening of the subendothelial zone, which may contain collagen fibers, siderophages, and cell fragments. Progression is manifested by partial to complete occlusion of the venules and sinusoids and centrizonal hepatocellular atrophy. The reticulin stain is particularly helpful in identifying the occlusive sinusoidal and venular lesions (Figure 8-11). Cholestasis and distortion of the lobular architecture may occur (97).

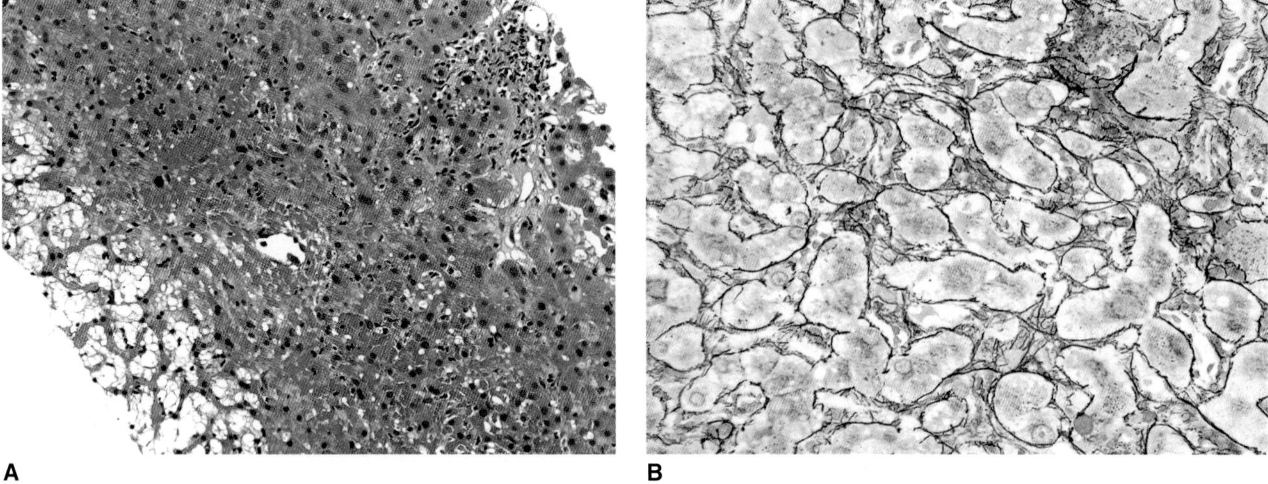

FIGURE 8-11 ■ Veno-occlusive syndrome/sinusoidal obstructive syndrome. **A:** VOD/SOS is characterized by centrilobular hemorrhage and necrosis. **B:** A reticulin stain is helpful in highlighting the sinusoidal and venular deposition of extracellular matrix.

Mild disease is followed by recovery by day 20, but death from fulminant hepatic failure occurs in some cases.

Immunologic mechanisms of rejection in liver allograft recipients and GVHD in bone marrow transplant patients are similar. They manifest many of the same histopathologic changes in the liver. Both are characterized by portal inflammation and bile duct injury in the acute phase, and severe duct damage and duct loss in the chronic stages (109). The acute form of GVHD manifests 3 to 4 weeks after transplantation with a skin rash, diarrhea, and jaundice. The early changes consist of mild, nonspecific lobular hepatitis. Liver biopsy specimens evaluated 1 to 2 weeks after the onset of the disease, show characteristic bile duct abnormalities. The bile ducts show epithelial degeneration and necrosis and lymphocytic infiltration (Figure 8-12). Destruction of ducts and ductular proliferation occurs with progressive disease. There is a lymphocytic portal inflammation, but spillover is usually minimal. Mild hepatocellular changes, occasional acidophil bodies, and cholestasis are seen in the lobule. Endothelialitis of the portal and central veins may be seen (104).

Chronic GVHD, seen 100 to 400 days after bone marrow transplantation, affects 30% of long-term survivors. It may be preceded by acute GVHD or develop in patients without prior episodes of disease. Chronic liver disease is seen in most patients with chronic GVHD with multisystem involvement or as a limited disorder with cutaneous and hepatic involvement, which has a more favorable prognosis. Although cirrhosis and its complications are unusual, micronodular cirrhosis leading to death from hepatic failure has been reported (69,70). The liver in chronic GVHD may show a histologic appearance of chronic hepatitis with portal infiltration by mononuclear cells. Long-standing GVHD results in bile duct loss (Figure 8-12). Additional findings include portal infiltration by plasma cells and cholestasis

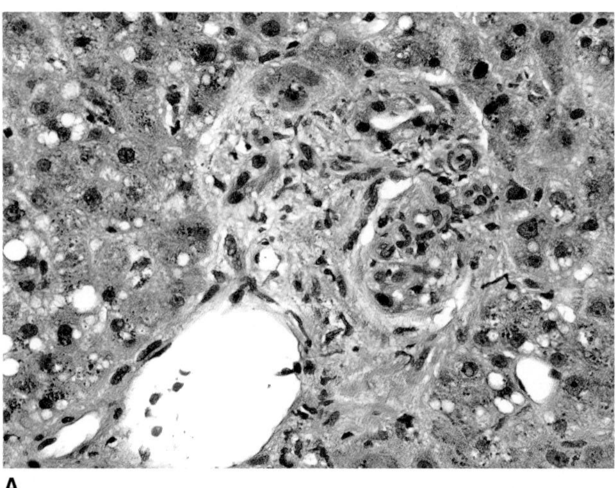

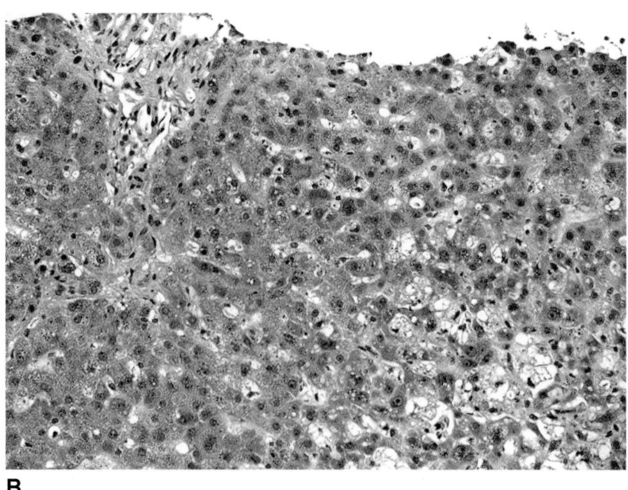

FIGURE 8-12 ■ Graft-versus-host disease of the liver. **A:** GVHD is characterized by destruction of the bile ducts with lymphocytic infiltration. Extensive iron deposition is commonly seen in these bone marrow transplant patients. **B:** In chronic GVHD, bile ducts are lost and cholestasis is evident. (Photos courtesy of Dr. John Hart, University of Chicago.)

with pseudoxanthomatous changes. Endothelialitis is not a feature of chronic GVHD (104).

TRANSPLANT PATHOLOGY OF THE PANCREAS

Overview and the Role of Histopathology

Pancreatic transplantation is becoming increasingly utilized for type I diabetes mellitus and is most commonly performed in conjunction with a kidney allograft due to end-stage renal failure. As end-stage renal failure in type I diabetes occurs mainly in adulthood, the pediatric pathologist is rarely asked to evaluate pancreatic biopsies in this setting. Moreover, histopathologic evaluation of pancreatic graft biopsies is rarely indicated in current practice for a variety of reasons. First, the pancreas is a very active exocrine and endocrine organ; thus, levels of synthetic products produced by the pancreas can accurately gauge graft function. Second, biopsies from the kidney have proven to be a fairly accurate surrogate in evaluating pancreatic rejection in patients who receive kidney/pancreas transplants (87). Third, in some instances, biopsies can be difficult to obtain and could cause severe injury to the pancreatic duct and vessels. Despite these caveats, biopsies obtained from the pancreatic grafts can occasionally provide useful information to the clinician, and at some large centers, biopsies are routinely performed (54).

Histopathology of Acute and Chronic Rejection

In 1997, a histologic grading scheme was proposed for acute rejection that divided acute rejection into six grades based on the degree of septal, acinar, ductal, and vascular inflammation (22). Inflammation in the islets of Langerhans is rarely encountered and is not a feature of acute rejection. This grading scheme showed good reproducibility, prognostic significance, correlation with laboratory data, and response to immunosuppressive treatment. Chronic rejection is characterized by fibrous expansion of the septal areas and loss of acinar parenchyma. Islets initially are not affected; however, extensive fibrosis can lead to loss of glycemic control. The vascular changes are similar to those seen in other solid organs with intimal and medial fibrosis and narrowing of the lumen. Critical to the evaluation of allograft pancreatic biopsies is assessment for other causes of graft dysfunction such as bacterial, fungal, or viral infections, especially CMV infection (53). Clinically and histologically, CMV pancreatitis can mimic acute rejection; however, the presence of the characteristic nuclear inclusions in endothelial or stromal cells is diagnostic.

RENAL TRANSPLANT PATHOLOGY

Overview

Approximately 600 renal transplants are performed on patients less than 18 years old each year in the United States. Based upon the 9,837 renal transplants performed in 8,990 patients from 1987 through 2005 in the North American Pediatric Renal Trials and Collaborative Studies (NAPRTCS) database, the primary diagnoses leading to renal transplantation in children are developmental abnormalities (renal aplasia/hypoplasia/dysplasia (15.9% of total), obstructive uropathy (15.8%), reflux nephropathy (5.2%), polycystic kidney disease (2.9%), medullary cystic disease (2.8%), and agenesis of abdominal musculature (2.7%), followed by focal segmental glomerulosclerosis (FSGS) (11.7%), specific glomerulonephritis (9.9%) in aggregate, chronic glomerulonephritis (3.4%), and hereditary nephritis (2.2%). Over this same period, the proportion of living donor (LD) renal allografts has increased from 43% to 60%, 81% of which were from a parent, and the proportion of cadaveric donor (CD) allografts has declined from 57% to 40% (101). From 1987 to 2000, the proportion of deceased donors less than 10 years of age declined from 35% to 10% due to the inferior outcomes of small CD kidneys given to small recipients (8). Approximately 25% of pediatric patients require removal of their native kidneys to alleviate problems related to polyuria, proteinuria (including hyperlipidemia and thrombophilia), recurrent pyelonephritis, and hypertension; and a similar percentage of pediatric renal transplants are performed preemptively, before reaching dialysis-dependent ESRD (7). One-year allograft survival improved from 91% in 1987–1995 to 94% in 1996–2000 for LD and 81% to 93% for CD, and the projected allograft half-life (the time at which one-half of allografts will be lost) improved from 15.4 (LD) and 9.5 (CD) years in the 1987–1989 cohort to 25.4 and 16.4 years for the 1996–1998 cohort (8). The causes of graft failure in pediatric renal transplants are chronic rejection (41.3%), vascular thrombosis (8.1%), recurrence of the original disease (7.9%), and acute rejection (6.3%) (101). Important morbidities in pediatric renal transplant recipients are growth failure, cardiovascular disease, and infectious diseases (7), and infectious diseases now exceed rejection as the most common reason for hospitalization of pediatric renal transplant recipients (84).

The pathologist may encounter autopsy, nephrectomy, biopsy, or cytologic specimens from pediatric renal transplant patients. Approximately 20% of our pediatric renal biopsy specimens are from renal allografts, all of which were performed to determine the cause of graft dysfunction. The differential diagnosis in that situation includes acute or chronic rejection, infection, drug toxicity, ischemic injury, urinary obstruction, recurrence of the original disease, *de novo* primary renal disease, posttransplant lymphoproliferative disorder, and chronic allograft nephropathy. The widely used Banff Classification of Renal Allograft Pathology defines a "minimal" sample for interpretation as seven glomeruli and one artery and an "adequate" sample as at least ten glomeruli and two arteries, and recommends that there be two cores or at least two separate cortical areas for examination (86,106). Multiple levels should be examined with hematoxylin and eosin (H&E), trichrome, periodic acid-Schiff (PAS), and Jones silver stains; and immunofluorescent or immunohistochemical stains for C4d and BK polyomavirus should be performed. Immunofluorescent stains for other immunoglobulin and complement components to look for recurrent or *de novo* disease or immunohistochemical stains for T-and B-lymphocytes and *in situ* hybridization for Epstein Barr virus to rule out posttransplant lymphoproliferative disease are performed without hesitation when these conditions are suspected clinically or pathologically.

Frozen section prior to implantation of kidneys from older donors has been recommended as a means of eliminating organs likely to experience delayed graft function or decreased survival, but glomerulosclerosis, interstitial fibrosis, and vascular disease may be difficult to recognize in frozen sections, and no absolute threshold has been established beyond which a donor kidney should not be used (15). Similarly, although Sarwal et al. (92) noted that the presence of acute tubular necrosis in the graft largely obviated the advantage of transplanting adult-sized kidneys to infants and small children, it is difficult to diagnose acute tubular necrosis in a frozen section. Permanent sections of biopsies obtained at the time of reperfusion (0-hour) or 1 hour later may show lesions predictive of hyperacute (neutrophils in glomeruli and peritubular capillaries) or acute rejection (neutrophils, macrophages or platelets in peritubular capillaries) and can provide a baseline for the interpretation of subsequent biopsies (15).

Protocol or surveillance biopsies taken at predetermined times irrespective of graft function may show evidence of acute rejection in the absence of clinical signs of graft dysfunction, allow earlier recognition of chronic lesions, and reveal unsuspected (and potentially treatable) infectious or inflammatory conditions. Postulating that the "renal reserve" created by transplantation of an adult-sized kidney to a small child may delay the clinical recognition of acute or chronic injury, Birk et al. (11) performed regular protocol biopsies on 21 pediatric renal allograft recipients and found subclinical acute rejection in four patients (19%). This group also performed routine follow-up biopsies 1 month after the diagnosis of acute rejection and showed that improvement of serum creatinine did not reliably predict resolution of rejection (10). In another descriptive study of protocol biopsies in children, Shishido et al. (96) found that subclinical acute rejection superimposed on chronic allograft nephropathy (CAN) had more graft dysfunction and diminished graft survival compared to patients with CAN alone. Protocol biopsies have also been used in studies of steroid-free immunosuppressive drug regimens in pediatric renal allograft recipients (1,93).

Hyperacute and Accelerated Acute Rejection and Delayed Graft Function

These early events represent variations on the theme of acute humoral rejection due to preformed antidonor antibodies and ischemic acute tubular necrosis. Hyperacute rejection is characterized by graft swelling and tenderness, and anuria almost immediately or within the first few days after transplantation. Glomerular capillaries are distended with platelets, erythrocytes, and fibrin thrombi, and there is necrosis of glomerular endothelium and tubular epithelium. Neutrophils marginate in small vessels and peritubular capillaries (an important finding that helps to distinguish humoral rejection from perfusional injury, arterial or venous thrombosis, or cyclosporine toxicity). Interstitial edema and hemorrhage progress to coagulative necrosis. Although the process is mediated by antibodies, immunofluorescent staining of vessels may be negative. C4d staining along peritubular capillaries similar to that seen in acute and chronic humoral rejection, as discussed below, is often seen in hyperacute rejection (15). The disease formerly known as accelerated acute rejection is also caused by preformed antibodies that may not be detectable until the plasma cell clone has been stimulated by the graft. It typically occurs 1 to 12 weeks after transplantation and is manifested by necrotizing arteritis or a thrombotic microangiopathy. Delayed graft function may be caused by a variety of donor factors, peritransplant ischemic injury, or drug toxicity. Typical histologic findings are reminiscent of acute tubular necrosis and include dilation of tubular lumens, loss of the brush border in proximal tubules, epithelial cell necrosis and apoptosis, and cellular casts (102).

Acute Rejection

Historically, renal allografts in children had higher rates and earlier and more refractory episodes of acute rejection than allografts in adults (7), but, with improved immunosuppressive therapy, the 12-month probability of acute rejection in children in the NAPRTCS series decreased from 54% to 13% in LD recipients and 69% to 16% in CD recipients between 1987–1990 and 2003–2005. 53% of LD recipients and 47% of CD recipients achieved complete reversal of rejection (return to baseline creatinine values), and only 4% and 6%, respectively, lost their grafts or died as a result of acute rejection (101). For LD recipients, the relative risk of developing acute rejection is increased in African-Americans, history of prior transplant or more than five blood transfusions, HLA mismatch, lack of induction therapy, and female gender; and for CD recipients, additional risk factors include recipient age less than 1 year, prior dialysis, and cold ischemic time greater than 24 hours (101). Tables 8-3 and 8-4 summarize the criteria for the scoring of lesions and classification of patterns of rejection in the Banff Classification of Renal Allograft Pathology.

Acute T-cell–mediated rejection: The minimum criteria for acute T-cell–mediated rejection in the Banff Classification (Type IA) are the following: mononuclear cell infiltrates involving more than 25% of the parenchyma (≥i2) and at least two foci with five to ten intraepithelial mononuclear cells in a tubular cross section or five to ten mononuclear cells per ten tubular epithelial cells in a longitudinal section (≥t2) (Figure 8-13A). Interstitial inflammation without tubulitis is not diagnostic of rejection, and lesser degrees of interstitial inflammation and tubulitis are considered borderline or "suspicious" for acute rejection, although immunosuppressive therapy

Table 8-3 ▪ BANFF CLASSIFICATION OF RENAL ALLOGRAFT PATHOLOGY (86,106)– I. LESION SCORING[a]

Lesion	Code	Grade 0	Grade 1	Grade 2	Grade 3	Comment
Findings associated with cell-mediated rejection						
Tubulitis	t	None	≥2 foci with 1–4 intraepithelial lymphocytes per tubular cross section or per 10 epithelial cells	≥2 foci with 5–10 intraepithelial lymphocytes per tubular cross section or per 10 epithelial cells	≥2 foci with >10 intraepithelial lymphocytes per tubular cross section or per 10 epithelial cells	Do not count atrophic tubules <50% normal size
Interstitial inflammation	i	<10% of unscarred parenchyma	10%–25% of unscarred parenchyma	26%–50% of unscarred parenchyma	>50% of unscarred parenchyma	Indicate >5%–10% eosinophils, neutrophils, or plasma cells and B-cell nodules with an
Total interstitial inflammation[b]	ti	<10% of total parenchyma	10%–25% of total parenchyma	26%–50% of total parenchyma	>50% of total parenchyma	
Arteritis	v	No intimal arteritis	≥1 artery with intimal arteritis and <25% luminal occlusion	≥1 artery with intimal arteritis and ≥ 25% luminal occlusion	≥1 artery with fibrinoid change and transmural arteritis with medial smooth muscle necrosis	Indicate infarction and/or interstitial hemorrhage with an
Findings associated with antibody-mediated rejection						
C4d staining	C4d	Negative (0%)	Minimal (1%–<10% of area with ≥2+ linear staining along peritubular capillaries)	Focal positive (10%–50% of area with ≥2+ linear staining along peritubular capillaries)	Diffuse positive (> 50% of area with ≥2+ linear staining along peritubular capillaries)	Immunohistochemistry may be one grade less sensitive than immunofluorescence
Glomerulitis	g	None	Glomerulitis in a minority of glomeruli	Segmental or global glomerulitis in 25%–75% of glomeruli	Glomerulitis (mostly global) in all or almost all glomeruli	Specify types of inflammatory cells
Peritubular capillaritis	ptc	No luminal inflammatory cells in cortical peritubular capillaries	Cortical peritubular capillary with 3–4 luminal inflammatory cells	Cortical peritubular capillary with 5–10 luminal inflammatory cells	Cortical peritubular capillary with >10 luminal inflammatory cells	Do not score if <10% of cortical capillaries involved. Specify type(s) of luminal cells.
Glomerular double contour	cg	Double contours in <10% of peripheral capillary loops in most severely affected nonsclerotic glomerulus	Double contours in 10%–25% of peripheral capillary loops in the most severely affected nonsclerotic glomerulus	Double contours in 26%–50% of capillary loops in the most severely affected nonsclerotic glomerulus	Double contours in >50% of peripheral capillary loops in the most severely affected nonsclerotic glomerulus	
Chronic changes						
Tubular atrophy	ct	No tubular atrophy	Tubular atrophy in ≥25% of the area of cortical tubules	Tubular atrophy in 26%–50% of the area of cortical tubules	Tubular atrophy in >50% of the area of cortical tubules	
Interstitial fibrosis	ci	Fibrosis of ≥5%of cortical area	Fibrosis of 6%–25% of cortical area	Fibrosis of 26%–50% of cortical area	Fibrosis of >50% of cortical area	Do not score subcapsular fibrosis

(Continued)

Table 8-3 ■ BANFF CLASSIFICATION OF RENAL ALLOGRAFT PATHOLOGY (86,106)– I. LESION SCORING[a] *(Continued)*

Lesion	Code	Grade 0	Grade 1	Grade 2	Grade 3	Comment
Subintimal fibrosis in arteries	cv	No chronic vascular changes	≥25% luminal narrowing by fibrointimal thickening	26%–50% luminal narrowing	>50% luminal narrowing	Elastica breaks, inflammatory cells in fibrosis suggest chronic rejection
Findings associated with calcineurin-inhibitor toxicity						
Arteriolar hyalinization	ah	No PAS-positive hyaline thickening	Mild-to-moderate PAS-positive hyaline thickening in at least one arteriole	Moderate-to-severe PAS-positive hyaline thickening in more than one arteriole	Severe PAS-positive hyaline thickening in many arterioles	
Alternate arteriolar hyalinization[b]	aah	No typical lesions of CNI arteriolopathy	Nodular hyaline deposits in only one arteriole and no circumferential involvement	Nodular hyaline deposits in more than one arteriole, but no circumferential involvement	Circumferential hyaline involvement; independent of the number of arterioles involved	

[a]Note the number of glomeruli and arteries present and number of sclerotic glomeruli.
[b]Total interstitial inflammation and alternate arteriolar hyalinization are undergoing evaluation.

Table 8-4 ■ BANFF CLASSIFICATION OF RENAL ALLOGRAFT PATHOLOGY (106)–II. DIAGNOSTIC CATEGORIES

T-cell–mediated rejection	
Suspicious	(v = 0 and (i = 0 or 1 and t = 1, 2 or 3)) OR (v = 0 and (i = 2 or 3 and t = 1))
IA	V = 0 and (i = 2 or 3 and t = 2)
IB	V = 0 and (i = 2 or 3 and t = 3)
IIA	v1
IIB	v2
III	v3
Chronic active	cv > 0 with mononuclear cells in subintimal fibrosis
Antibody-mediated rejection	
C4d+	C4d = 3, antidonor antibody detected, and no morphologic evidence of rejection
I	C4d = 3, antidonor antibody detected, and ATN-like change
II	C4d = 3, antidonor antibody detected, and (ptc > 0 and/or g > 0 and/or thromboses)
III	C4d = 3, antidonor antibody detected, and v = 3
Chronic active	C4d = 3, antidonor antibody detected, (cg > 0 and/or ct > 0 and/or ci > 0 and or cv > 0)
Interstitial fibrosis and tubular atrophy without evidence of any specific etiology	
I	ct = 1 and ci = 0 or 1
II	ct = 2 and ci = 2
III	ct = 3 and ci = 3

prior to biopsy may have reduced the interstitial inflammatory response, and in that context, i1t2 lesions may indicate rejection (86). Interstitial inflammation is not graded in areas of fibrosis, the immediate subcapsular cortex, and the adventitia around large veins, but this is being reevaluated. The interstitial infiltrate in acute rejection is often mixed, but if there are more than 5% to 10% eosinophils, neutrophils, or plasma cells, an asterisk is added to the "i" score and other diagnoses should be considered (hypersensitivity reaction, acute bacterial infection or infarction, and infection or posttransplant lymphoproliferative disorder, respectively). Similarly, while tubulitis should be assessed in the most severely involved area, there should be more than one focus with the highest grade of involvement, and since tubulitis in atrophic tubules may be seen in the absence of rejection, it should not be graded in tubules that show a 50% or greater reduction in caliber. Most of the infiltrating lymphocytes in acute rejection will be T-cells, and a predominantly B-cell infiltrate raises the question of a posttransplant lymphoproliferative disorder (86), while nodular aggregates of B-cell aggregates in a predominantly T-cell infiltrate may identify allografts that will be refractory to standard antirejection therapy but responsive to anti-B-cell immunotherapy (60).

Intimal arteritis, seen as lymphocytic infiltration beneath the endothelium of arteries (Figure 8-13B), is the criterion by which Type II acute T-cell–mediated rejection is defined. Type IIA shows mild-to-moderate endarteritis in at least one arterial cross section (v1), and Type IIB shows severe intimal arteritis with at least a 25% reduction of the luminal area in at least one arterial cross-section (v2) (86). Because of the potential for sampling error, the most severely involved

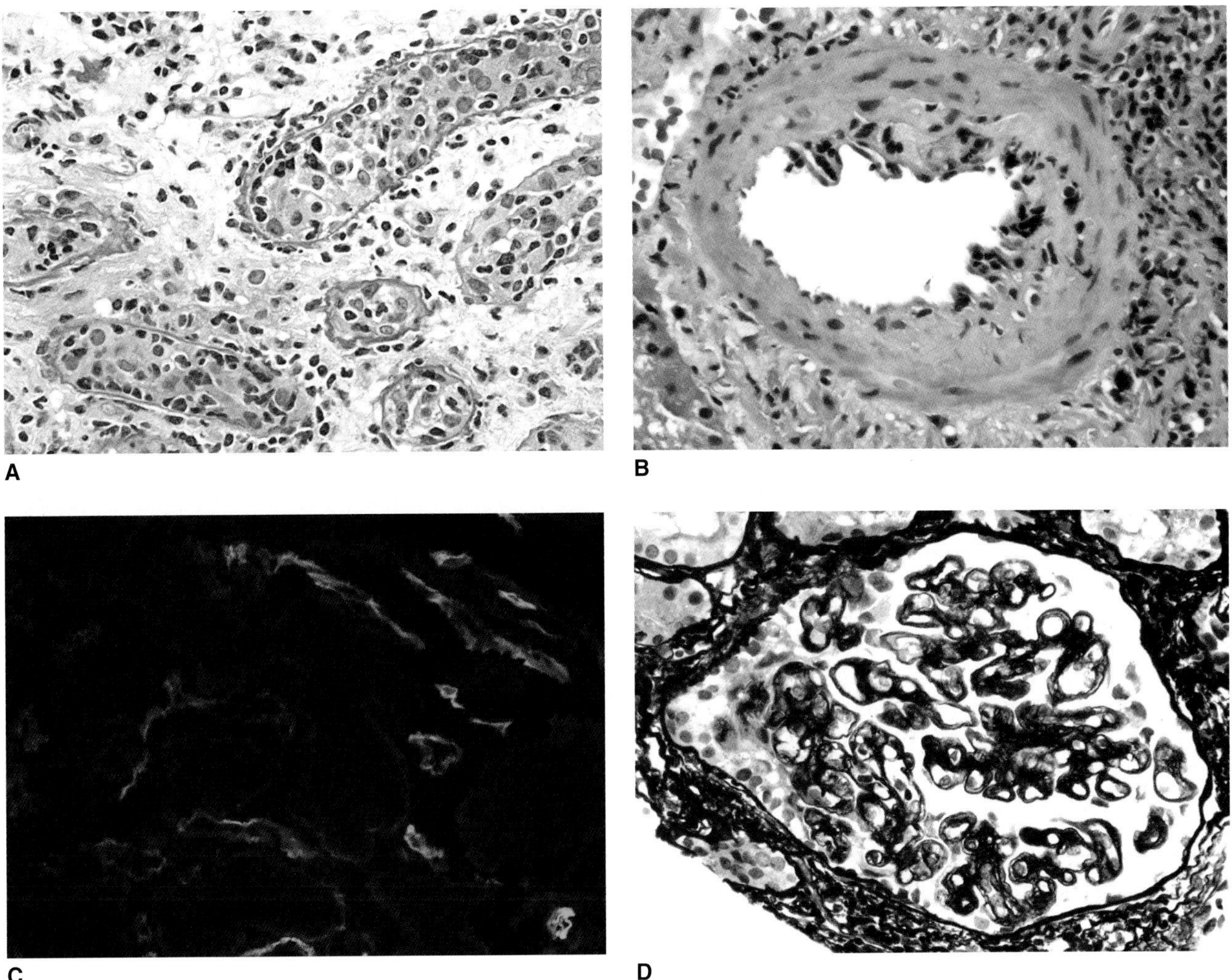

FIGURES 8-13 Acute and chronic rejection. **A:** Tubulitis is a feature of acute T-cell–mediated rejection, and the >10 intraepithelial lymphocytes per 10 epithelial cells in nonatrophic or only partially atrophic tubules seen here is a t3 lesion (PAS 40×). **B:** Intimal arteritis is indicative of grade II acute rejection, and the 25% to 30% luminal narrowing seen here is a borderline v2 lesion (H&E 40×). **C:** Bright ribbon-like staining for C4d along peritubular capillaries between tubules is the hallmark of antibody-mediated rejection (Fluorescein-conjugated anti-C4d 40×). **D:** Double contours along glomerular capillary loops are a sign of chronic antibody-mediated rejection (Jones methenamine silver 40×).

artery should be graded, and neither lymphocytes attached to (but not beneath) arterial endothelium nor lymphocytes in venous walls should be graded. Transmural arteritis or fibrinoid mural necrosis with lymphocytic inflammation is the criterion by which Type III acute rejection is defined. Interstitial hemorrhage and infarction are not sufficient for a diagnosis of Type III rejection but are designated with an asterisk after the "v" score (86).

Acute antibody-mediated rejection (AMR): Demonstration of diffuse linear staining for C4d along peritubular capillaries (C4d3) (Figure 8-13C) has become the hallmark of AMR (86) and is seen in 20% to 30% of biopsies for acute rejection. C4d is an inactive fragment of complement component C4 that binds covalently to adjacent structures, thereby avoiding the modulation that makes the immunoglobulins responsible for initiating the attack undetectable. In normal kidneys, immunofluorescent staining for C4d is found in the mesangium and at the vascular pole of glomeruli, presumably a consequence of the physiologic turnover of immune complexes, and may be seen along glomerular capillaries in immune complex disorders, but peritubular capillary staining is characteristic of AMR (26). Other histopathologic features of AMR include neutrophils in peritubular and glomerular capillaries and neutrophilic tubulitis, but these lesions are seen infrequently in some series, and the Banff Classification has categories of AMR in which there is C4d staining without these features, alone and with changes consistent with acute tubular necrosis (Table 8-4). AMR typically has its onset one to three weeks after transplantation but may arise after several months or years, especially if immunosuppression is decreased. There is no correlation with HLA match, ischemic time, or donor age. During episodes of rejection,

C4d-positive cases show higher serum creatinine levels and are less responsive to steroid and anti-T-cell immunotherapy compared to C4d-negative cases (66), and long-term graft survival is significantly reduced (40). Most patients with positive C4d staining have HLA class I or II donor-specific antibodies, but ABO and non-HLA antiendothelial antibodies have been demonstrated in a few patients (66).

Chronic Allograft Nephropathy (CAN)

Chronic Allograft Nephropathy (CAN), the leading cause of renal allograft failure in children, is due to a combination of immunologic and nonimmunologic mechanisms, ischemia, hypertension, infection, immunosuppressive drug toxicity and noncompliance, and recurrent disease. In the original Banff 97 classification, CAN was graded on the extent of tubular atrophy and interstitial fibrosis, but recently there has been an increased emphasis on identifying the underlying cause. Chronic transplant glomerulopathy, characterized by the presence of double contours along glomerular capillary walls on silver stains (Figure 8-13D), fibrous intimal thickening without duplication of the internal elastica in arteries, and diffuse C4d staining along peritubular capillaries, are suggestive of late or chronic AMR; and mononuclear cells in peritubular capillaries or glomeruli and interstitial plasma cell infiltrates may also be seen in this condition (107). In a pediatric series, 50% of biopsies that showed features of CAN were C4d-positive; these biopsies showed more transplant glomerulopathy and increased mesangial matrix, and patients with C4d-positive CAN had a higher rate of graft loss (39). Immunofluorescent microscopy of chronic transplant glomerulopathy may show nonspecific segmental granular deposits of IgG or IgM and C3 in the capillary wall and mesangium, and electron microscopy shows widening of the subendothelial space due to accumulation of electron lucent flocculent material, but no electron-dense deposits. Reduplication of the external lamina of peritubular capillaries is associated with positive C4d staining (44,66,74). Fibrointimal thickening with reduplication of the internal elastica (cv) and arteriolar hyaline change (ah) may be related to hypertension; peripheral hyaline nodules in arterioles suggest chronic calcineurin-inhibitor (cyclosporine, tacrolimus) toxicity as discussed below; marked tubular ectasia with Tamm-Horsfall casts raises the question of chronic obstruction; and intratubular neutrophils, lymphoid follicles, and viral inclusions are seen in infections (107).

Vascular Thrombosis

Vascular thrombosis accounts for 8.1% of graft failures and is the second leading cause of allograft loss in the NAPRTCS series (101). Risk factors for vascular thrombosis include peritoneal dialysis prior to transplantation, cadaver kidneys from donors less than 6 years old or with more than 24 hours cold ischemic time, recipients less than 2 years old, and a history of prior transplant (8).

Recurrent Disease

Recurrence of the original disease that necessitated renal transplantation accounts for 7.9% of allograft loss in children (101). In addition, any acquired renal disease may develop *de novo* in renal allografts. The most common recurrent disease in pediatric renal allograft recipients is focal segmental glomerulosclerosis (FSGS), which accounts for 12% of ESRD leading to transplantation in all children and adolescents in the United States and 23% among African-American patients, and recurs in the allograft in 20% to 50% of patients. Rapid progression from onset to ESRD, younger age, white race, mesangial proliferation on biopsy, and recurrent disease in one allograft are associated with a higher risk of recurrence (7). Autosomal recessive FSGS due to NPHS2 mutations appear to have a much lower risk of recurrence after transplantation (95). Recurrences occur early, 78% within the first posttransplant month (95), and patients with primary FSGS also experience twice the rate of early graft nonfunction/acute tubular necrosis, requiring dialysis compared to all other groups, raising the question of subclinical recurrence (7).

Membranoproliferative glomerulonephritis (MPGN) Type I accounts for 2.1% of ESRD leading to transplantation in children (101) and recurs in 30% to 77% of allografts, resulting in loss of the graft in approximately one-fourth to one-third of patients with recurrent disease (95). MPGN Type II (dense deposit disease) accounts for 0.9% of pediatric renal transplants (101), and recurs in nearly all allografts, but this results in graft loss in only 10% to 20% of patients (95). Lupus nephritis accounts for 1.6% of ESRD leading to transplantation in children (101) and may recur in 30% of allografts, but the incidence of graft failure due to recurrent disease is low (95). IgA nephropathy accounts for 1.3% of pediatric renal transplants (101) and has been reported to recur in 65% of adults who had a graft biopsy for any reason (83). However, graft loss from recurrence was only 7% in one pediatric series and 3% in adults (95). Henoch-Shoenlein purpura nephritis accounts for 1.4% of ESRD leading to transplantation in children (101), and recurrence has been reported in 53% of allografts, all from living related donors, and 22% of grafts were lost (95). Congenital nephrotic syndrome accounts for 2.6% of pediatric renal transplants (101), and though proteinuria recurs in 25% of patients with the Finnish type of congenital nephrotic syndrome (CNF) who receive transplants, these patients do not appear to have recurrent CNF (56). Membranous glomerulonephritis (MGN) accounts for 0.5% of ESRD leading to transplantation in children (101), and recurrence has been reported in adults but not in children. However, *de novo* MGN was reported in initial allografts of seven children, four of whom developed MGN in subsequent allografts (37). Familial nephritis accounts for 2.2% of pediatric renal transplants (101), but half of males with X-linked Alport syndrome will require transplantation by age 25. This genetic disease does not recur in the allograft, but crescentic glomerulonephritis due to antiglomerular basement membrane antibodies develops in 3% to 5% of transplanted Alport males, and nearly 90% of these grafts will fail (50).

Hemolytic uremic syndrome (HUS) is the most common cause of acute renal failure in children in developed countries and accounts for 2.7% of pediatric renal transplants (101). HUS recurred in only 1 of 118 (0.8%) transplanted children with classic postdiarrheal HUS, but in 13 of 63 (21%) of those with atypical HUS, and 5 of 11 (45%) of those with HUS due to Factor H deficiency (62). The rate of graft failure in a smaller series of recurrent HUS was 83% (85), and one would suspect that the rate of recurrence in subsequent grafts would also be high. A thrombotic microangiopathy indistinguishable from HUS may develop in transplants as a result of humoral rejection, drug toxicity (oral contraceptives, cyclosporine and, rarely, OKT3), pregnancy, or other infection.

Cystinosis accounts for 2.1% of ESRD leading to transplantation in children (101), and cystine deposits commonly occur in renal allografts of patients with cystinosis. This does not appear to affect graft function, but neither does the renal allograft prevent the systemic complications of cystinosis. In contrast, recurrence of oxalate deposits in oxalosis, which accounts for 0.5% of pediatric renal transplants (101), does impair graft function, and combined liver and kidney transplantation is the preferred treatment. Graft survival in children transplanted for ESRD due to urologic abnormalities is comparable to children with normal urinary tracts if the abnormalities can be corrected and careful attention is paid to possible sources of infection (9). Wilms tumor (WT) and Denys-Drash syndrome (DDS) each account for 0.5% of pediatric renal transplants (101), and transplantation should be delayed for 1 to 2 years after completion of chemotherapy.

Immunosuppressive Drug Toxicity

Of the immunosuppressive agents currently used in solid organ transplantation, the calcineurin inhibitors, cyclosporine and tacrolimus, have the most significant renal toxicity. The monoclonal and polyclonal antibodies that deplete the T-cell pool (OKT3 and antilymphocyte and antithymocyte globulins) or inhibit interleukin-2 (Basiliximab and Daclizumab) rarely cause renal disease (100). However, there have been case reports of glomerular and larger renal vessel thrombosis with OKT3 (15). Steroids and antiproliferative agents have numerous adverse effects but generally do not cause renal lesions. However, sirolimus has been reported to delay recovery from acute renal failure in cultured mouse proximal tubular epithelium (61) and to result in delayed graft function, which resulted in a myeloma-like cast nephropathy when sirolimus was used in combination with tacrolimus, possibly because these two drugs are metabolized by the same pathway (102). Sirolimus has also been reported to rarely cause reversible proteinuria and thrombotic microangiopathy (15).

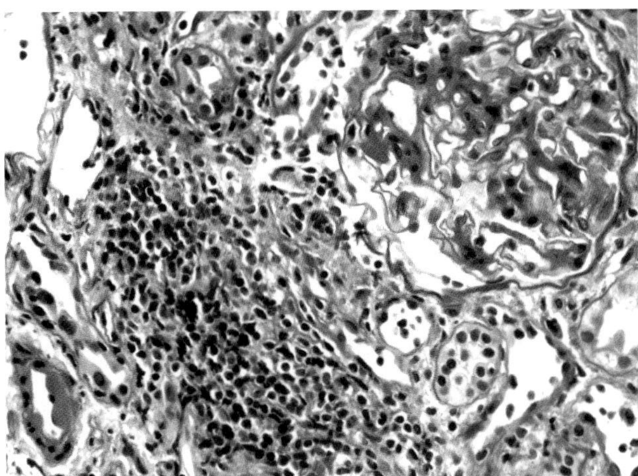

FIGURE 8-14■The PAS-positive nodules in the wall of the arteriole at the lower left are seen in calcineurin-inhibitor toxicity (PAS 40×).

Calcineurin inhibitors (CNI) can cause characteristic lesions in glomeruli, tubules, the interstitium, and vessels. Glomerular thrombotic microangiopathy (TMA) and isometric vacuolization of proximal tubular epithelial cells indicate acute or ongoing toxic injury, while chronic toxicity results in hyaline changes in arterioles and striped interstitial fibrosis (107). The differential diagnosis of glomerular TMA includes antibody-mediated rejection, but CNI-induced TMA does not show C4d staining along peritubular capillaries. The cytoplasmic vacuoles in CNI tubulopathy are small and uniform, in contrast to the large irregular vacuoles seen with ischemic tubular injury, and they do not stain with H&E or PAS stains. The differential diagnosis includes an osmotic nephrosis due to agents such as mannitol and intravenous immunoglobulin. Arteriolar lesions include ballooning of smooth muscle cells, probably an early and reversible lesion like isometric vacuolization in tubules, and PAS-positive mural hyaline nodules along the adventitial aspect of the vessel (Figure 8-14). The differential diagnosis of the hyalinosis includes diabetes mellitus and hypertension, but the subadventitial nodules are relatively specific for CNI toxicity (15).

Polyomavirus Type BK (BKV) Infection

Cytomegalovirus and adenovirus are important causes of infection in renal transplant patients and can be diagnosed in biopsies on the basis of characteristic inclusions or positive immunohistochemical stains. Epstein-Barr virus infection may lead to posttransplant lymphoproliferative disorders and is best diagnosed by *in situ* hybridization. However, over the past decade, polyomavirus type BK (BKV) has become the most important infection in kidney transplant patients. BKV infection develops in 1% to 5% of renal transplant recipients, and one-half of these patients lose graft function. Up to 90% of the population worldwide is BKV-seropositive, and the virus is known to persist in renal allografts (41). Histologically confirmed BKV nephropathy developed in six of 173 (3.5%) of pediatric renal transplant recipients 4 to 47 months

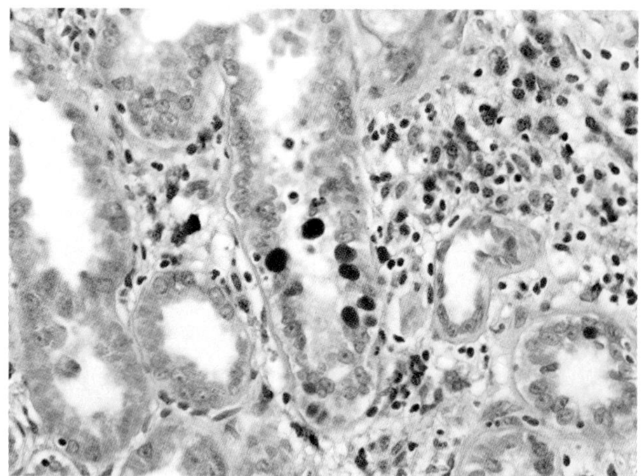

FIGURE 8-15 ■ BK virus infection is evidenced by the staining of enlarged nuclei in these tubular epithelial cells. Mouse anti-BK virus large T antibody 40×.

after transplant (median 15 months), which led to reduced long-term graft function, and BKV nephropathy was significantly associated with recipient seronegativity (99). Allograft biopsies with BKV nephropathy characteristically show large basophilic nuclear inclusions in tubular epithelial cells (Figure 8-15) that stain strongly with antibodies to the SV-40 T antigen, but central pale inclusions surrounded by dark chromatin and vesicular nuclei have been described. In early stages of viral replication, the immunohistochemical stain may be positive in normal-appearing nuclei and in late stages inclusion-bearing cells may be negative (15). Interstitial inflammation and tubulitis may be present in more advanced BKV nephropathy, and biopsies may show both acute rejection and BKV infection. Inclusion-bearing cells, known as "decoy" cells, can be identified in the urine, and in a prospective study of 78 adult renal allograft recipients, decoy cell shedding was seen in 30%, viremia assessed by nested PCR in 13%, and biopsy-proven nephropathy in 8%. With biopsy as the diagnostic standard, decoy cells had a sensitivity of 100% and specificity of 71%, and BKV viremia had a sensitivity of 100% and specificity of 88%, but the viral load in patients with BKV nephropathy was significantly higher than in those without nephropathy (41).

Posttransplant Lymphoproliferative Disorders

Posttransplant lymphoproliferative disorders (PTLDs) occur in 1% or less of pediatric renal transplant recipients, although there may be considerable variations in case definition between centers since EBV infection may present along a continuum of clinical features (33). There is also a continuum of pathologic lesions ranging from benign lymphoid hyperplasia to polymorphic PTLD to monomorphic PTLD, and tissue from suspected cases should be handled in the same manner as a suspected non-Hodgkin lymphoma, with samples sequestered for possible flow cytometry, immunohistochemical studies for T-cells and B-cells, *in situ* hybridization for EBV, and B-cell gene rearrangement studies. While the native kidney may be involved in PTLD arising in the setting of transplantation of other organs, the differentiation of PTLD from acute cellular rejection is a problem unique to the renal allograft. Typically, the interstitial infiltrate is very dense and is either monomorphic or contains a range of lymphoid cells, but no neutrophils or eosinophils, and tubulitis and endarteritis are usually absent. Since most PTLDs are B-cell proliferations, in contrast to the predominantly T-cell proliferation seen in acute cellular rejection, and more than 90% harbor the EBV genome, a combination of immunohistochemistry for T-cells and B-cells and *in situ* hybridization for EBV-encoded nuclear RNAs (EBERs) can sort out most cases (116).

PATHOLOGY OF HEART TRANSPLANTATION

Overview

In 1967, the first successful human heart transplant was achieved but survival was limited by infection, graft failure/hemodynamic collapse, and rejection. Important milestones include introduction of biopsy forceps for percutaneous endomyocardial biopsies in 1973, the development of calcineurin inhibitors and the introduction of Cyclosporine A in the heart transplant population in 1980, and the introduction of antithymocyte globulin (ATG) in 1990 for both induction and treatment of rejection.

Volumes and Indications

The total number of pediatric heart transplant procedures reported to the Registry of the International Society of Heart Lung Transplantation (ISHLT) has remained stable for the past 15 years at approximately 400 procedures per year (12). The 1st year of life is the single most common year for a heart transplant procedure in patients aged 18 years and younger. The indications for transplantation include congenital cardiac malformations in the infant [most often after surgery(ies)], and in the older child cardiomyopathy (dilated), congenital malformation [also after surgery(ies)], endocardial fibroelastosis, adriamycin toxicity, and retransplantation for chronic rejection. Dilated cardiomyopathy does not recur in the transplanted heart; however, the patient is at higher risk for developing chronic rejection again after retransplantation for it.

Surgical Complications

In the current setting, surgical complications are exceedingly rare and include hemorrhage and wound infections.

Rejection

Endomyocardial biopsy (EMB) remains the gold standard for rejection surveillance. It has a high sensitivity and specificity for the diagnosis of acute cellular rejection. There are currently no cardiac imaging modalities or serum markers that can replace it. Typically, surveillance biopsies are performed

Table 8-5 ■ OLD AND REVISED GRADING SYSTEMS OF THE ISHLT FOR ACUTE CELLULAR REJECTION

1990	2005
No rejection (grade 0)	No rejection (grade 0R)
Focal, mild acute rejection (grade 1A) Diffuse, mild acute rejection (grade 1B) Focal, moderate acute rejection (grade 2)	Mild, low-grade, rejection: interstitial and/or perivascular cellular infiltrate with up to one focus of myocyte damage (grade 1R)
Multifocal moderate rejection (grade 3A)	Moderate, intermediate-grade, rejection: two or more foci of cellular infiltrate with associated myocyte damage (grade 2R)
Diffuse, moderate rejection (grade 3B) Severe acute rejection (grade 4)	Severe, high-grade rejection: diffuse cellular infiltrate with multifocal myocyte damage ± edema, ± hemorrhage ± vasculitis (grade 3R)

once weekly for the 1st month, every 2 weeks for the 2nd month, and every 6 to 8 weeks between the 3rd and 12th months. After the 1st year, the frequency can be decreased to quarterly, biannually, or annually. The current working formulation suggests a minimum of three step levels for microscopic examination. No special stains are routinely required. Unstained slides can be saved for immunohistochemical staining if needed. One to two pieces of biopsy should be obtained in addition and frozen for immunofluorescence staining, if clinically indicated (115).

Hyperacute rejection is graft injury triggered by preformed antibodies and occurs rapidly after implantation of the graft, usually within minutes to hours. This type of rejection is now extremely rare.

Acute cellular rejection consists of an inflammatory infiltrate that is predominantly a T-cell–mediated response directed against the cardiac allograft. A substantial increase in activated B-lymphocytes and natural killer cells is seen in moderate rejection, suggesting their important role as promoters and effectors of cellular rejection. Eosinophils and neutrophils are also present in severe rejection. The grading system for acute cellular rejection has been revised by the ISHLT such that the old system can easily be translated into the new one, which is simpler and more reproducible (Table 8-5; Figures 8-16–8-21; eFigures 8-1 and 8-2) (113). In most transplant centers, mild as well as focal moderate rejection (grades 1A, 1B, 2/1R) is not treated if patient is asymptomatic and there is no clinical indication of rejection.

Antibody-mediated rejection (AMR): AMR is an immunopathologic process associated with the production of antidonor-reactive antibodies in which injury to the graft is, in part, the result of activation of the complement system. It is poorly responsive to conventional immunosuppression, which targets the cellular arm of the immune response. Risk

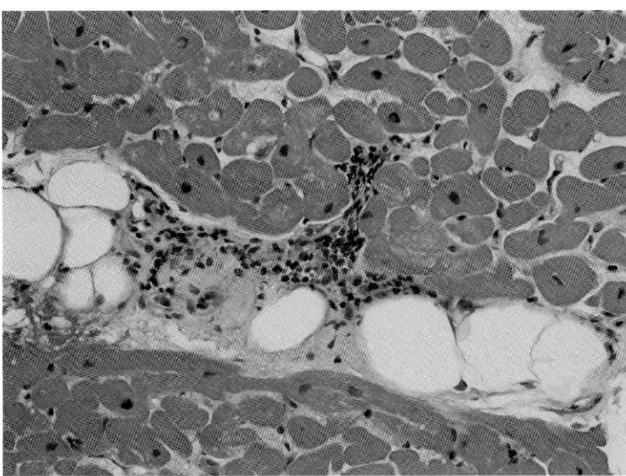

FIGURE 8-17 ■ Focal mild acute cellular rejection (grade 1A/1R). There is a focal infiltrate of lymphocytes between the myocytes and involving fat, which is often present in posttransplant biopsies (H&E, 200×).

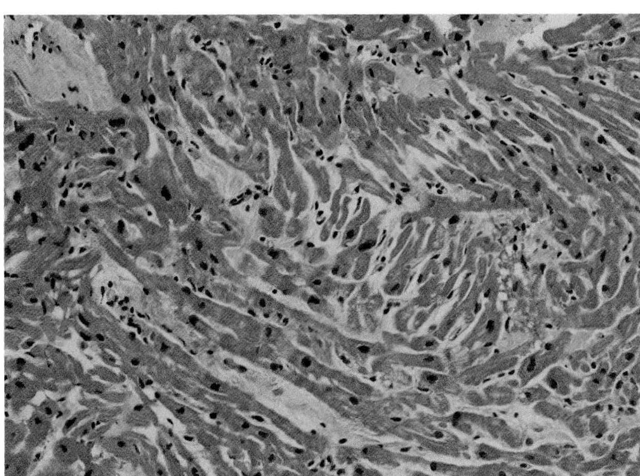

FIGURE 8-16 ■ Negative for acute cellular rejection (grade 0/0R). Pediatric heart biopsies appear more cellular than adults do since the myocytes are smaller. Also, capillary endothelium can be quite prominent in posttransplant biopsies (H&E, 200×).

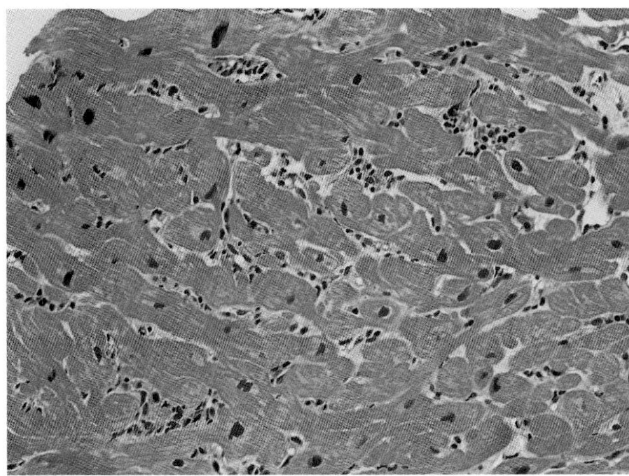

FIGURE 8-18 ■ Mild acute cellular rejection (grade 1B/1R). There is a sparse but diffuse lymphocytic infiltrate between myocytes, without any myocyte damage (H&E, 200×).

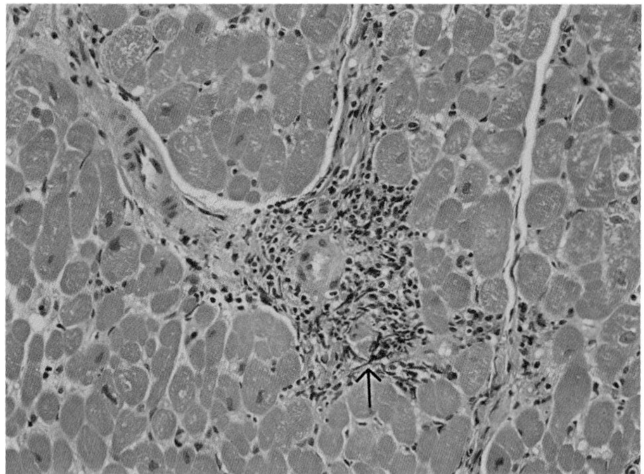

FIGURE 8-19 ■ Focal moderate acute cellular rejection (grade 2/1R). There is one focus of activated lymphocytes associated with myocyte damage (*arrow*) (H&E, 200×).

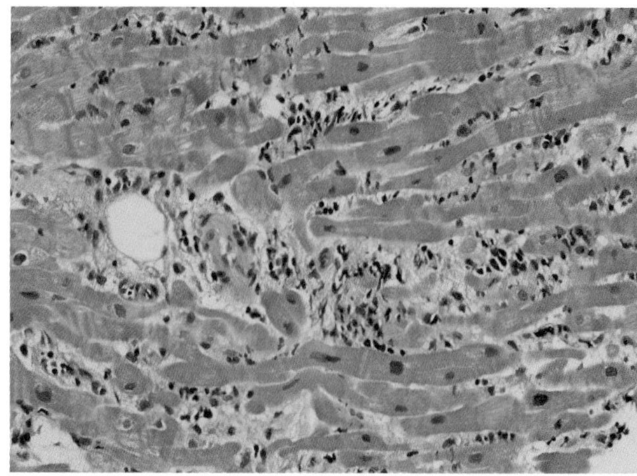

FIGURE 8-21 ■ Diffuse moderate acute cellular rejection (grade 3B/3R). There is a marked infiltrate associated with myocyte damage and few eosinophils and neutrophils (H&E, 200×).

factors for developing AMR include blood transfusions, previous transplantation, use of ventricular assist devices, presence of positive B-cell flow cytometry cross-match, and elevated panel-reactive antibodies. AMR has been associated with the development of cardiac allograft vasculopathy (CAV) and decreased survival (88).

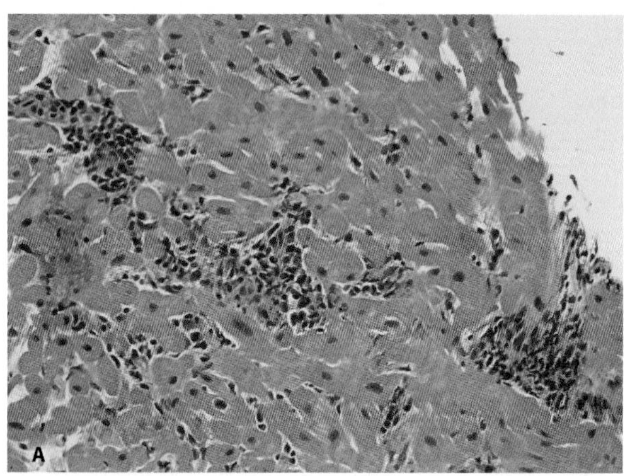

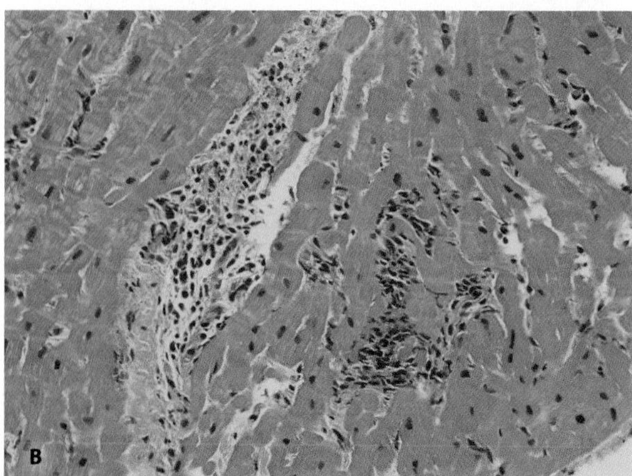

FIGURE 8-20 ■ Multifocal moderate acute cellular rejection (grade 3A/2R). The biopsy has two separate foci of moderate rejection seen in **A** and **B** (H&E, 200×).

Histological features are capillary endothelial changes (swelling or denudation with congestion), macrophages and neutrophils in capillaries, interstitial edema, and/or hemorrhage and fibrin in vessels. Immunopathologic evidence of AMR includes

- Immunoglobulin (IgG, IgM, and/or IgA) plus complement deposition (C3d, C4d, and/or C1q) in capillaries by immunofluorescence on frozen sections (Figure 8-22); and/or
- CD68 staining of macrophages within capillaries (CD31-positive or CD34-positive) by immunohistochemistry; and
- C4d staining of capillaries by paraffin immunohistochemistry (Figure 8-23) (25).

Chronic rejection (CAV) involves both epicardial and intramural coronary arteries. The whole length of the coronary vessels is usually affected. There is diffuse concentric

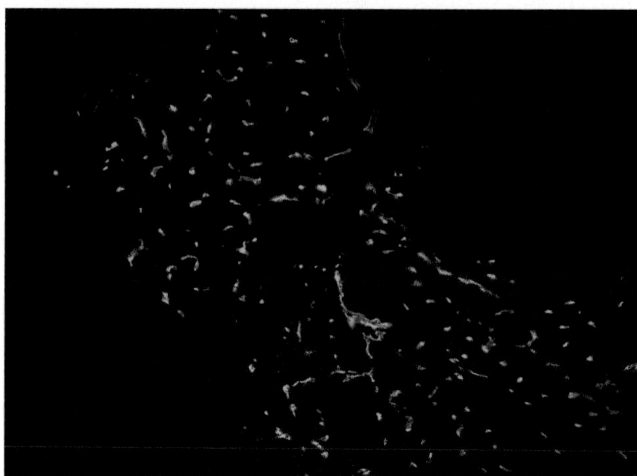

FIGURE 8-22 ■ Positive C4d staining is seen in all the vessels in this heart biopsy (Courtesy of Dr. Anthony Chang, University of Chicago Medical Center, indirect immunofluorescence, 40×).

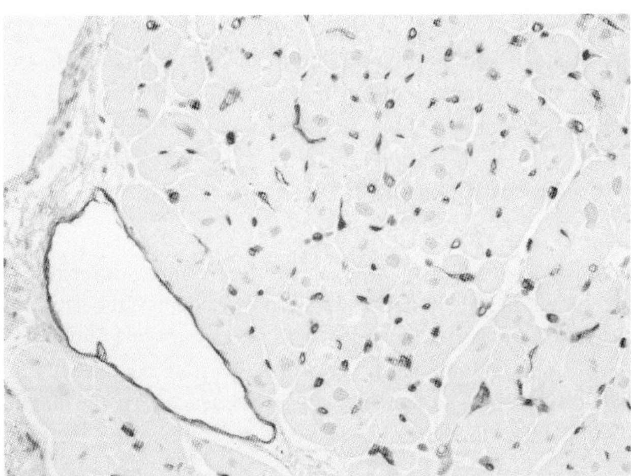

FIGURE 8-23 ▪ Positive C4d staining is seen in all the vessels in this heart biopsy with strong endothelial staining (immunohistochemical stain, 200×).

narrowing with luminal stenosis due to intimal fibrosis (eFigures 8-3 and 8-4) with long-term lesions resembling conventional atherosclerosis (Figure 8-24). The incidence of CAV in children is 2.5% at 1 year, 11% at 5 years, and 16.7% at 10 years after transplantation, which is much lower than that reported for adults. Infant recipients had the lowest risk of CAV, likely due to their lower incidence of acute cellular rejection.

Infection

These chronically immunosuppressed patients are prone to bacterial and opportunistic infections mostly in the lungs, GI tract, skin, and nervous system. Infection of the heart itself is rare; toxoplasmosis and CMV are seen most often.

The incidence of PTLD seems to be decreasing from the 3% to 5% reported in the past, perhaps due to better immunosuppressive regimens. The proliferation is EBV driven and can be polyclonal lymphoplasmacytoid or monoclonal. It most often involves extracardiac sites such as lymph nodes, gastrointestinal tract, lung, and skin.

Other Complications

Hypertension is reported in 47% at 1 year, 63% at 5 years, and 72% of pediatric recipients at 10 years after transplantation. Renal dysfunction occurs in 6% at 1 year, 9% at 5 years, and 17% at 10 years. Hyperlipidemia also increases steadily to 38% at 10 years after pediatric transplantation (12).

Other Biopsy Findings

Quilty lesion: This is an endocardial lymphocytic lesion composed of mature lymphocytes with a central dendritic cell network upon which the B- and T-cells are organized (neolymphogenesis) (94). The infiltrate often extends into the underlying myocardium where it may be associated with myocyte damage and fibrosis (Figure 8-25). It is not known to be related to acute or chronic rejection, infection, ischemic time, or poor outcome. The main issue is to differentiate it from cellular rejection and avoid over-treatment (eFigures 8-5 to 8-8)

Adipose tissue: Over time, more and more fat accumulates in the transplanted heart and can be seen in the endomyocardial biopsies (eFigure 8-9). Only when epicardial mesothelium is identified, should one alert the cardiologist as to the possibility of perforation.

Site of previous biopsy: Due to the structure of the heart, the bioptome tends to be guided to the same location for each biopsy. Thus, it is very common to see organizing biopsy site with fibrin, mild inflammation, granulation tissue, and fibrosis (eFigure 8-10).

Calcifications: Occasionally, dystrophic microcalcifications are seen on biopsy. These can be located in the myocyte or in areas of scarring.

Fibrosis: Focal fibrosis is often seen on biopsy, especially after the 1st year posttransplantation. It may represent old biopsy site, healed infarct, or drug-induced fibrosis.

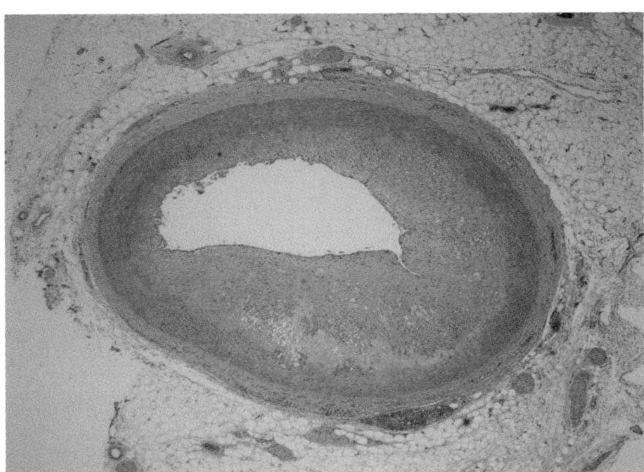

FIGURE 8-24 ▪ Chronic rejection (cardiac allograft vasculopathy) is seen in this epicardial coronary artery, which has eccentric intimal fibrosis (H&E, 20×).

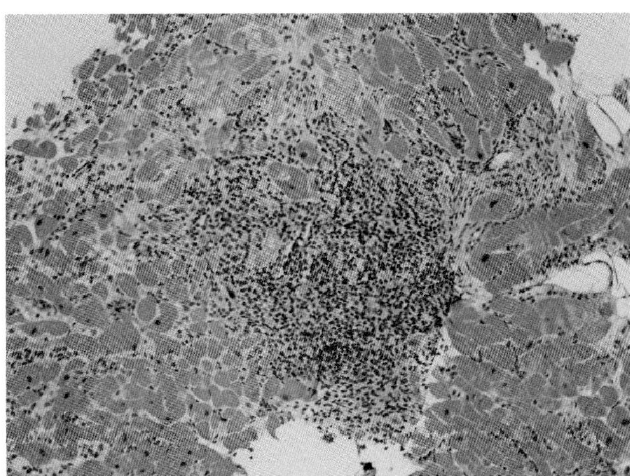

FIGURE 8-25 ▪ Quilty lesion. This endomyocardial biopsy shows a large infiltrate between myocytes, composed of mature lymphocytes with multiple capillaries (H&E, 100×).

Outcome

Overall survival is approximately 40% for patients up to 20 years after transplantation. The median survival is 15.8 years for infant recipients, 14.2 years for childhood-age recipients, and 11.4 years for adolescents. Late survivors have continued to show excellent rehabilitation in terms of functional status. The two main posttransplant morbidities that have steadily increased are CAV and renal failure. Malignancy has remained an important but low-frequency event (12).

PATHOLOGY OF LUNG TRANSPLANTATION

Lung transplantation, single, bilateral, or, less often, heart-lung, has been an accepted mode of therapy for a variety of end-stage lung diseases for about 20 years. Methods of evaluation of allograft dysfunction are variable and, depending on the clinical differential diagnosis, can include transbronchial biopsy (TBB), bronchoalveolar lavage (BAL) with culture, endobronchial biopsy (EBB), and, least often, wedge biopsy and fine needle aspiration biopsy (FNAB).

Volumes and Indications

Since 1995, the numbers of procedures worldwide that are reported to the ISHLT have been fairly constant, with 76 lung transplants in 2006. The majority of recipients are between 12 and 17 years of age with less than five procedures per year in infants (3). The most common indications for children are cystic fibrosis (CF) and primary pulmonary arterial hypertension (PPAH), in contrast to adults who are transplanted for emphysema, CF, idiopathic pulmonary fibrosis, and PPAH. Heritable surfactant deficiency and alveolar capillary dysplasia are indications in neonates. There is no recurrence of original disease in children except for the rare patient who gets retransplanted for chronic rejection and is at higher risk for developing chronic rejection again.

Vascular Complications

Postsurgical obstruction/thrombosis of the arterial or venous anastomosis, although rare, is a surgical emergency. Inflammatory cells, endothelial disruption, and recent thrombus are seen in the early posttransplant period, while organizing/organized thrombus, stenosis, and fibrosis with foreign body giant cells are present in the intermediate to late period.

Airway Anastomotic Complications

The anastomosis heals by formation of granulation tissue, the surface of which reepithelializes in a few days. Occasionally, exuberant polypoid granulation tissue forms, which may need to be removed. Varying degrees of ischemic injury, manifested as coagulative necrosis of airway wall components, are commonly present. Superimposed infection may interrupt and complicate the healing process. Common organisms found on culture, endobronchial biopsy, and special stains include fungi (*Candida* and *Aspergillus* sp.) and bacteria. Fungi tend to invade necrotic cartilage. Dehiscence of the anastomosis can allow infection to spread into the mediastinum. Healing may result in fibrosis and stenosis of the airway, treatment for which includes stent placement.

Primary Graft Dysfunction

Primary graft dysfunction occurs in 22% of pediatric lung recipients (similar to adults) in the first 30 days after transplantation due to some combination of ischemia, reperfusion, surgical trauma, denervation, and interruption of lymphatics, resulting in endothelial injury and pulmonary edema with or without diffuse alveolar damage. Recovery occurs in the majority of patients in a few days to weeks with supportive therapy, although the mortality and morbidity rates are high (73).

Rejection

Definite diagnosis and grading of rejection (especially acute rejection) are based on light microscopic examination of tissue obtained by TBB, which may be performed based on the clinical symptoms or based on a surveillance protocol. Since rejection is a patchy process, it is recommended that five fragments of alveolated lung tissue be examined at three different levels stained with hematoxylin and eosin. A working formulation for the grading of pulmonary allograft rejection, initially developed in 1990 and revised in 1996 (Table 8-6) and 2007, is widely used (112).

Hyperacute Rejection

Only a few well-documented cases of hyperacute (humoral or antibody-mediated) rejection of the lung (all in adults) have been reported in the literature (47). Preformed antibodies bind to the endothelium and epithelium of the donor lung and activate inflammatory, complement, and coagulation

Table 8-6 ■ WORKING FORMULATION FOR THE CLASSIFICATION AND GRADING OF PULMONARY ALLOGRAFT REJECTION

A. Acute rejection (perivascular)
   - Grade 0—none
   - Grade 1—minimal
   - Grade 2—mild
   - Grade 3—moderate
   - Grade 4—severe

B. Airway inflammation—lymphocytic bronchitis/bronchiolitis
   - Grade 0—none
   - Grade 1—minimal
   - Grade 2—mild
   - Grade 3—moderate
   - Grade 4—severe

C. Chronic airway rejection—bronchiolitis obliterans
   - Ca. Active
   - Cb. Inactive

D. Chronic vascular rejection—accelerated graft vascular sclerosis

Modified from Yousem SA, Berry GJ, Cagle PT, et al. Revision of the 1990 working formulation for the classification of pulmonary allograft rejection. Lung Rejection Study Group. *J Heart Lung Transplant* 1996;15:1–15.

cascades. Within minutes to hours after transplantation, there is progressive respiratory failure, pulmonary edema, and pleural effusion, with complete opacification of the allograft seen on radiologic examination. The histologic features of hyperacute rejection include diffuse alveolar damage (DAD), alveolar hemorrhage, interstitial neutrophilia, fibrin thrombi and vasculitis.

There is deposition of IgG and complement in the alveolar septa. Complement fragments C3d and C4d may also be detected. If fresh frozen tissue is not available for immunofluorescence studies, C4d deposition can be demonstrated in the vascular endothelium and/or the interstitium by IHC. Only strong staining without background should be interpreted as positive. However, staining is patchy and the sensitivity and specificity of C4d staining are low.

Acute Rejection

Acute rejection is a cell-mediated process during which there is progressive infiltration of the graft by host mononuclear cells. Immune cell activation causes release of inflammatory chemokines and upregulation of adhesion molecules. Major cellular targets include endothelial and epithelial cells. With current immunosuppressive therapy, it is rare for a lung transplant recipient to die of acute cellular rejection.

Although acute rejection can develop as early as 3 days to many years posttransplant, most patients experience some rejection commonly around 3 months, with most episodes occurring between 2 and 9 months (43). Noncompliance with immunosuppressive medications is a significant cause of late episodes of acute rejection.

Acute rejection is characterized by a predominantly lymphocytic infiltrate with scattered eosinophils, neutrophils, and plasma cells. The infiltrate begins in the perivascular areas and variably extends into the airways and lung parenchyma. In minimal acute rejection (grade A1/B1), there are scattered infrequent perivascular and airway mononuclear infiltrates forming two to three layers that are not obvious at low magnification (Figure 8-26). Mild acute rejection (grade A2/B2) consists of greater than three layers of activated lymphocytes,

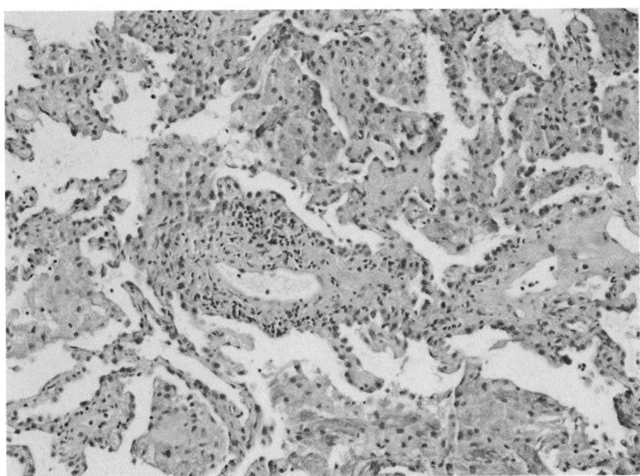

FIGURE 8-26 ■ Minimal acute cellular rejection of lung (A1). There is an incomplete perivascular cuff of lymphocytes (H&E, 100×).

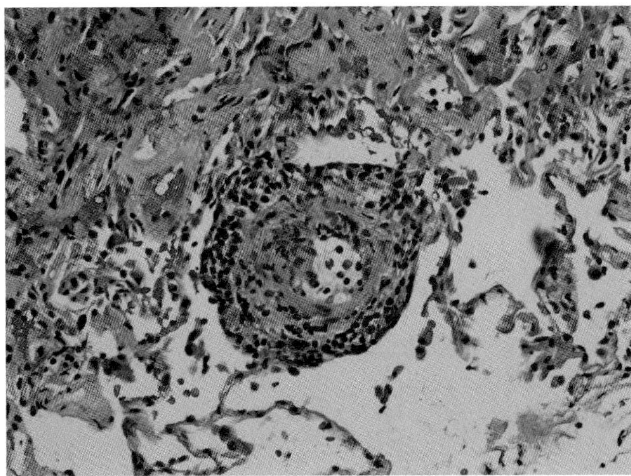

FIGURE 8-27 ■ Mild acute cellular rejection of lung (A2). There is a complete perivascular cuff, more than three layers thick, which is readily apparent at low power (H&E, 40×).

eosinophils, and neutrophils around small blood vessels (Figure 8-27) or a band-like infiltrate in the airway submucosa (eFigure 8-11). Moderate acute rejection (A3/B3) is characterized by an extension of the inflammation into alveolar septa with or without vasculitis or a band-like infiltrate in the submucosa extending into the airway epithelium with focal epithelial necrosis. In severe acute rejection (grade A4/B4), diffuse perivascular, interstitial, and air space infiltrates associated with pneumocyte damage, macrophages, hyaline membranes, hemorrhage and neutrophils or epithelial ulceration with fibrinopurulent exudates are seen.

In the 2007 revision, the grading of perivascular and interstitial infiltrates remains the same (i.e., A0 to A4); however, the airway inflammation is changed to B0 (none), B1R (low-grade, 1996 B1 and B2), Grade B2R (high-grade, 1996 B3 and B4) (112). The latter poses a problem for those centers that treat grade B2 rejection in a manner similar to grade A2. Asymptomatic minimal rejection is clinically insignificant and not treated. Mild (grade A2/B2) and higher grades are treated irrespective of symptoms.

The main differential diagnosis is infection, and microbiologic cultures and TBB are most useful to distinguish this (eFigure 8-11). Aspiration is a common event, which is gaining more significance since it may trigger episodes of acute rejection and increase the risk of patients to develop chronic rejection (eFigures 8-13 to 8-15) Bronchial-associated lymphoid tissue (BACT) is often prominent to lung transplant recipients, and care should be taken not to overcall it as rejection (eFigure 8-16).

Chronic Rejection

In the lung, chronic rejection is primarily manifested as bronchiolitis obliterans (BO). Despite improved baseline immunosuppression and treatment of acute rejection, BO remains the most important cause of late graft failure. Although its etiology and pathogenesis are still not completely understood, acute rejection is certainly one of the most important risk factors. In general, the process of chronic rejection is believed to occur in stages. The initial wave of antibody-mediated response is paralleled by a cellular infiltrate in which the monocyte/macrophage compartment plays a central role as the critical effector cells. The high antigenicity of airway epithelial cells through the upregulated expression of MHC, adhesion and co-stimulatory molecules, together with the abundance of antigen-presenting cells and circulating lymphocytes, provide an increased propensity to damage of these structures, similar to epithelial-lined conduits in other solid allografts (e.g., bile ducts, pancreatic ducts, and renal tubules). The production of inflammatory mediators and growth factors contribute to the fibroproliferative response of the damaged graft leading to BO.

Although the term chronic implies a late temporal process, BO can be seen as early as three to six weeks after transplantation, but primarily occurs 1 or more years later. The onset of chronic rejection is insidious with vague general symptoms and nonproductive cough. There is progressive dyspnea on exertion and irreversible decline in pulmonary function tests, not explained by other causes such as infection. When the decline is greater than 10% of baseline, a clinical diagnosis of bronchiolitis obliterans syndrome (BOS) is made, which does not need pathologic confirmation. BOS is graded from 1 to 3 based on the degree of loss of lung function (13). When the clinical diagnosis is not clear, a wedge biopsy is often needed since BO is a patchy process and diagnostic yield of TBB is low.

BO is patchy both in distribution and severity in individual lobes and in the same airway. There is submucosal fibrosis, which either bulges asymmetrically into the lumen and causes partial obstruction or is concentric and causes total obstruction (Figure 8-28; eFigure 8-17). Chronic vascular rejection occurs much less frequently and is histologically similar to the transplant vasculopathy seen in other solid organ allografts (intimal fibrosis and vascular thickening); however, in the lung, it does not usually cause significant allograft dysfunction.

The main histologic differential diagnosis is organizing pneumonia (formerly known as bronchiolitis obliterans organizing pneumonia or BOOP), which is a healing response to various forms of lung injury and manifests as loose fibromyxoid plugs of connective tissue within alveoli and bronchioles. On the other hand, BO is a dense scar tissue (mature collagen) within small airways.

Once there has been a decrease in lung function due to BO, it cannot be reversed, but aggressive immunosuppression can stabilize the disease for variable periods of time. Some patients can live with BO for a few years, but others have progressive dysfunction and complications and die unless retransplanted.

Infections

Like any immunocompromised patient, lung transplant recipients are at high risk of developing infections, which can be bacterial, viral, or fungal, and may cause tracheobronchitis, localized infection of the airway anastomosis or pneumonia. Most bacterial infections occur in the first posttransplant month, whereas viral and fungal infections tend to be seen in the 3- to 6-month period since they are on immunosuppressive drugs. Lung transplant patients remain susceptible to infections for the rest of their lives especially in that substantial population of children transplanted because of cystic fibrosis (50% of cases in most pediatric lung transplant programs).

Microscopic findings depend on the etiology of the infection and the host response, which may be minimal. Bacterial infections usually elicit neutrophilic infiltration of airway, interstitium, and alveolar spaces. Occasionally, there is only bacterial growth and infarction with no inflammation. The most common viral infection is caused by CMV, which often infects endothelial cells. This may lead to bleeding complications after diagnostic TBB. CMV is diagnosed by finding the classical single intranuclear and multiple small cytoplasmic inclusions in an enlarged cell (eFigure 8-21). Treated patients often have smudged, eosinophilic inclusions, which may be difficult to identify as CMV (Figure 8-29). Adenovirus infection is more common in children, and scattered adult and pediatric patients develop serious pneumonias due to the other

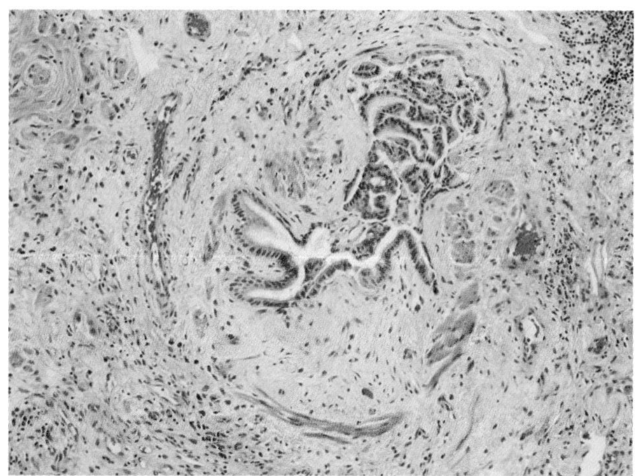

FIGURE 8-28 ■ Chronic rejection (bronchiolitis obliterans). Eccentric submucosal fibrosis partially occludes the lumen of this bronchiole (H&E, 100×).

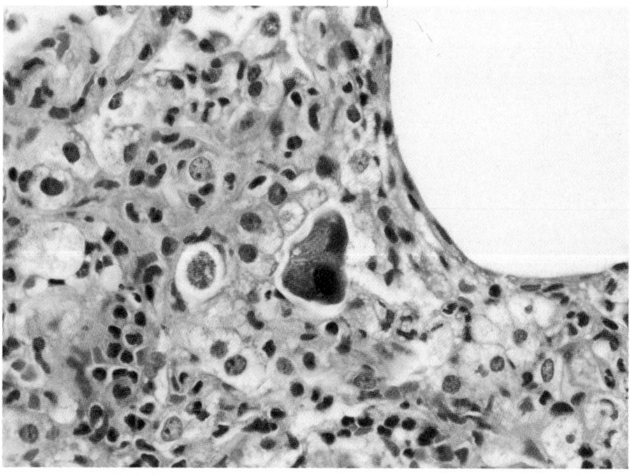

FIGURE 8-29 ■ Treated CMV. Soon after treatment, CMV inclusions become eosinophilic and smudged as seen in this photomicrograph (H&E, 200×).

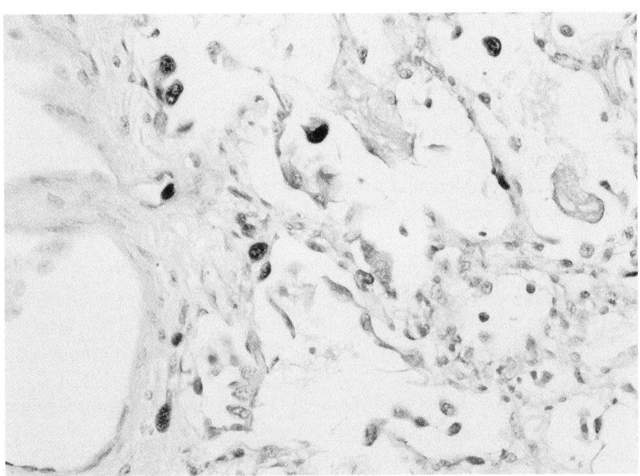

FIGURE 8-30▪Early CMV pneumonitis. In the lung transplant recipient, detection of any nuclear stain even without classic intranuclear inclusions is indicative of CMV infection (immunohistochemical stain, 200×).

respiratory viruses (respiratory syncytial virus, parainfluenza, influenza). Fungal infections are often caused by *Aspergillus* or *Candida* sp. especially in children with cystic fibrosis. Pneumocystis pneumonia is rare due to routine prophylaxis.

In the very early stage of CMV infection, IHC staining against immediate-early antigen may demonstrate nuclear positivity in cells lacking diagnostic cytopathic changes (Figure 8-30). IHC is also very useful for confirming the diagnosis in patients already on treatment for CMV.

The main differential diagnosis is from acute rejection, since the symptoms are similar. Infection may precipitate rejection and vice versa. Infections can be very difficult to treat, with new resistant strains emerging in some patients. Prophylaxis plays an important role in preventing PCP and CMV pneumonia.

OTHER FORMS OF LUNG INJURY

DAD, organizing pneumonia, acute interstitial pneumonia, and interstitial fibrosis may all be seen as nonspecific responses to lung injury in the posttransplant patient. The etiology of these responses is diverse and is not specifically related to either acute or chronic rejection.

Posttransplant Lymphoproliferative Disorder

PTLD occurs in 3% to 5% of lung transplant recipients with frequent involvement of the allograft, often as one or multiple nodules. A high index of suspicion should be maintained, and the diagnosis can be suggested on FNAB and TBB. Particularly with low-grade lesions, the need to obtain adequate tissue for complete workup may require a wedge biopsy. The histologic and molecular features are similar to those seen in any other transplant patient (Chapter 22).

Outcome

Advances in donor management, surgical techniques, and immunosuppressive drugs have led to improvement in the short-term survival of patients. However, in contrast to other solid organ transplants, over half of the lung transplant recipients (pediatric and adult) continue to suffer and die of chronic rejection (bronchiolitis obliterans) 3 to 10 years posttransplantation. Although surveillance biopsies can detect infection in asymptomatic children, the early detection of AR (seen in 4%) is unlikely to have a major impact on long-term survival (6).

Pulmonary Complications After Hematopoietic Stem Cell Transplant

With the use of effective infection prophylaxis, noninfectious causes of pulmonary dysfunction after stem cell transplant are the major pulmonary causes of morbidity and mortality. These include acute and chronic graft-versus-host-disease, idiopathic pneumonia syndrome, diffuse alveolar hemorrhage, pulmonary veno-occlusive disease, and organizing pneumonia (123).

REFERENCES

1. Aikawa A, Miyagi M, Motoyama O, et al. Pathological evaluation of steroid withdrawal in pediatric renal transplant recipients. *Pediatr Transplant* 1999;3(2):131–138.
2. Asplund S, Gramlich TL. Chronic mucosal changes of the colon in graft-versus-host disease. *Mod Pathol* 1998;11(6):513–515.
3. Aurora P, Edwards LB, Christie J, et al. Registry of the International Society for Heart and Lung Transplantation: eleventh official pediatric lung and heart/lung transplantation report—2008. *J Heart Lung Transplant* 2008;27(9):978–983.
4. Azoulay D, Astarcioglu I, Bismuth H, et al. Split-liver transplantation. The Paul Brousse policy. *Ann Surg* 1996;224(6):737–746; discussion 746–738.
5. Banff schema for grading liver allograft rejection: an international consensus document. *Hepatology* 1997;25(3):658–663.
6. Benden C, Boehler A, Faro A. Pediatric lung transplantation: literature review 2006–2007. *Pediatr Transplant* 2008;12(3):266–273.
7. Benfield MR. Current status of kidney transplant: update 2003. *Pediatr Clin North Am* 2003;50(6):1301–1334.
8. Benfield MR, McDonald RA, Bartosh S, et al. Changing trends in pediatric transplantation: 2001 Annual Report of the North American Pediatric Renal Transplant Cooperative Study. *Pediatr Transplant* 2003;7(4):321–335.
9. Bereket G, Fine RN. Pediatric renal transplantation. *Pediatr Clin North Am* 1995;42(6):1603–1628.
10. Birk PE, Rush DN. Protocol biopsies should be standard of care for pediatric renal allograft recipients! *Pediatr Transplant* 2006;10(7):760–765.
11. Birk PE, Stannard KM, Konrad HB, et al. Surveillance biopsies are superior to functional studies for the diagnosis of acute and chronic renal allograft pathology in children. *Pediatr Transplant* 2004;8(1):29–38.
12. Boucek MM, Aurora P, Edwards LB, et al. Registry of the International Society for Heart and Lung Transplantation: tenth official pediatric heart transplantation report—2007. *J Heart Lung Transplant* 2007;26(8):796–807.
13. Burton CM, Carlsen J, Mortensen J, et al. Long-term survival after lung transplantation depends on development and severity of bronchiolitis obliterans syndrome. *J Heart Lung Transplant* 2007;26(7):681–686.
14. Collins AB, Schneeberger EE, Pascual MA, et al. Complement activation in acute humoral renal allograft rejection: diagnostic

significance of C4d deposits in peritubular capillaries. *J Am Soc Nephrol* 1999;10(10):2208–2214.

15. Colvin RB, Nickeleit V. Renal transplant pathology (Chapter 28). In: Jennette JC, Olson JL, Schwartz MM, et al., eds. *Heptinstall's pathology of the kidney*, 6th ed. Philadelphia: Lippincott Williams & Wilkins. 2007;1349–1447.
16. Colvin RB, Smith RN. Antibody-mediated organ-allograft rejection. *Nat Rev Immunol* 2005;5(10):807–817.
17. Crawford AR, Lin XZ, Crawford JM. The normal adult human liver biopsy: a quantitative reference standard. *Hepatology* 1998;28(2):323–331.
18. D'Antiga L, Dhawan A, Portmann B, et al. Late cellular rejection in paediatric liver transplantation: aetiology and outcome. *Transplantation* 2002;73(1):80–84.
19. Demetris A, Adams D, Bellamy C, et al. Update of the International Banff Schema for Liver Allograft Rejection: working recommendations for the histopathologic staging and reporting of chronic rejection. An International Panel. *Hepatology* 2000;31(3):792–799.
20. Demetris AJ, Adeyi O, Bellamy CO, et al. Liver biopsy interpretation for causes of late liver allograft dysfunction. *Hepatology* 2006;44(2):489–501.
21. Demetris AJ, Markus BH. Immunopathology of liver transplantation. *Crit Rev Immunol* 1989;9(2):67–92.
22. Drachenberg CB, Papadimitriou JC, Klassen DK, et al. Evaluation of pancreas transplant needle biopsy: reproducibility and revision of histologic grading system. *Transplantation* 1997;63(11):1579–1586.
23. Evans HM, Kelly DA, McKiernan PJ, et al. Progressive histological damage in liver allografts following pediatric liver transplantation. *Hepatology* 2006;43(5):1109–1117.
24. Evans PC, Smith S, Hirschfield G, et al. Recipient HLA-DR3, tumour necrosis factor-alpha promoter allele-2 (tumour necrosis factor-2) and cytomegalovirus infection are interrelated risk factors for chronic rejection of liver grafts. *J Hepatol* 2001;34(5):711–715.
25. Fedson SE, Daniel SS, Husain AN. Immunohistochemistry staining of C4d to diagnose antibody-mediated rejection in cardiac transplantation. *J Heart Lung Transplant* 2008;27(4):372–379.
26. Feucht HE. Complement C4d in graft capillaries—the missing link in the recognition of humoral alloreactivity. *Am J Transplant* 2003;3(6):646–652.
27. Finn L, Reyes J, Bueno J, et al. Epstein-Barr virus infections in children after transplantation of the small intestine. *Am J Surg Pathol* 1998;22(3):299–309.
28. Gaffey MJ, Boyd JC, Traweek ST, et al. Predictive value of intraoperative biopsies and liver function tests for preservation injury in orthotopic liver transplantation. *Hepatology* 1997;25(1):184–189.
29. Ghobrial RM, Farmer DG, Amersi F, et al. Advances in pediatric liver and intestinal transplantation. *Am J Surg* 2000;180(5): 328–334.
30. Gould DS, Auchincloss H Jr. Direct and indirect recognition: the role of MHC antigens in graft rejection. *Immunol Today* 1999;20(2):77–82.
31. Goulet O. Complications after intestinal transplantation: traditional and new. *Pediatr Transplant* 1999;3(2):89–91.
32. Graziadei IW. Recurrence of primary sclerosing cholangitis after liver transplantation. *Liver Transpl* 2002;8(7):575–581.
33. Green M, Webber S. Posttransplantation lymphoproliferative disorders. *Pediatr Clin North Am* 2003;50(6):1471–1491.
34. Gupta P, Hart J, Cronin D, et al. Risk factors for chronic rejection after pediatric liver transplantation. *Transplantation* 2001;72(6):1098–1102.
35. Haga H, Egawa H, Fujimoto Y, et al. Acute humoral rejection and C4d immunostaining in ABO blood type-incompatible liver transplantation. *Liver Transpl* 2006;12(3):457–464.
36. Harrison RF, Patsiaoura K, Hubscher SG. Cytokeratin immunostaining for detection of biliary epithelium: its use in counting bile ducts in cases of liver allograft rejection. *J Clin Pathol* 1994;47(4):303–308.
37. Heidet L, Gagnadoux ME, Beziau A, et al. Recurrence of de novo membranous glomerulonephritis on renal grafts. *Clin Nephrol* 1994;41(5):314–318.
38. Hendrickson RJ, Karrer FM, Wachs ME, et al. Pediatric liver transplantation. *Curr Opin Pediatr* 2004;16(3):309–313.
39. Herman J, Lerut E, Van Damme-Lombaerts R, et al. Capillary deposition of complement C4d and C3d in pediatric renal allograft biopsies. *Transplantation* 2005;79(10):1435–1440.
40. Herzenberg AM, Gill JS, Djurdjev O, et al. C4d deposition in acute rejection: an independent long-term prognostic factor. *J Am Soc Nephrol* 2002;13(1):234–241.
41. Hirsch HH, Knowles W, Dickenmann M, et al. Prospective study of polyomavirus type BK replication and nephropathy in renal-transplant recipients. *N Engl J Med* 2002;347(7):488–496.
42. Hoffman JA. Adenoviral disease in pediatric solid organ transplant recipients. *Pediatr Transplant* 2006;10(1):17–25.
43. Husain AN. Transplantation related lung pathology (Chapter 24). In: Zander DS, Farver C, eds. *Pulmonary pathology*. Philadelphia: Elsevier; 2008.
44. Ivanyi B, Fahmy H, Brown H, et al. Peritubular capillaries in chronic renal allograft rejection: a quantitative ultrastructural study. *Hum Pathol* 2000;31(9):1129–1138.
45. Jaffe R. Liver transplant pathology in pediatric metabolic disorders. *Pediatr Dev Pathol* 1998;1(2):102–117.
46. Jain A, Mazariegos G, Pokharna R, et al. Almost total absence of chronic rejection in primary pediatric liver transplantation under tacrolimus. *Transplant Proc* 2002;34(5):1968–1969.
47. de Jesus Peixoto Camargo J, Marcantonio Camargo S, Marcelo Schio S, et al. Hyperacute rejection after single lung transplantation: a case report. *Transplant Proc* 2008;40(3):867–869.
48. Jugie M, Canioni D, Le Bihan C, et al. Study of the impact of liver transplantation on the outcome of intestinal grafts in children. *Transplantation* 2006;81(7):992–997.
49. Kalayoglu M, D'Alessandro AM, Knechtle SJ, et al. Preliminary experience with split liver transplantation. *J Am Coll Surg* 1996;182(5):381–387.
50. Kashtan CE. Renal transplantation in patients with Alport syndrome. *Pediatr Transplant* 2006;10(6):651–657.
51. Kato T, Tzakis AG, Selvaggi G, et al. Intestinal and multivisceral transplantation in children. *Ann Surg* 2006;243(6):756–764; discussion 764–756.
52. Kaufman SS. Small bowel transplantation: selection criteria, operative techniques, advances in specific immunosuppression, prognosis. *Curr Opin Pediatr* 2001;13(5):425–428.
53. Klassen DK, Drachenberg CB, Papadimitriou JC, et al. CMV allograft pancreatitis: diagnosis, treatment, and histological features. *Transplantation* 2000;69(9):1968–1971.
54. Klassen DK, Weir MR, Cangro CB, et al. Pancreas allograft biopsy: safety of percutaneous biopsy-results of a large experience. *Transplantation* 2002;73(4):553–555.
55. Kulkarni S, Malago M, Cronin DC II. Living donor liver transplantation for pediatric and adult recipients. *Nat Clin Pract Gastroenterol Hepatol* 2006;3(3):149–157.
56. Laine J, Jalanko H, Holthofer H, et al. Post-transplantation nephrosis in congenital nephrotic syndrome of the Finnish type. *Kidney Int* 1993;44(4):867–874.
57. Lamps LW, Pinson CW, Raiford DS, et al. The significance of microabscesses in liver transplant biopsies: a clinicopathological study. *Hepatology* 1998;28(6):1532–1537.
58. Lee RG, Nakamura K, Tsamandas AC, et al. Pathology of human intestinal transplantation. *Gastroenterology* 1996;110(6): 1820–1834.
59. Lefkowitch JH. Diagnostic issues in liver transplantation pathology. *Clin Liver Dis* 2002;6(2):555–570.
60. Lehnhardt A, Mengel M, Pape L, et al. Nodular B-cell aggregates associated with treatment refractory renal transplant rejection resolved by rituximab. *Am J Transplant* 2006;6(4):847–851.

61. Lieberthal W, Fuhro R, Andry CC, et al. Rapamycin impairs recovery from acute renal failure: role of cell-cycle arrest and apoptosis of tubular cells. *Am J Physiol Renal Physiol* 2001;281(4):F693–F706.
62. Loirat C, Niaudet P. The risk of recurrence of hemolytic uremic syndrome after renal transplantation in children. *Pediatr Nephrol* 2003;18(11):1095–1101.
63. Main JM, Prehn RT. Successful skin homografts after the administration of high dosage X radiation and homologous bone marrow. *J Natl Cancer Inst* 1955;15(4):1023–1029.
64. Manez R, Kusne S, Green M, et al. Incidence and risk factors associated with the development of cytomegalovirus disease after intestinal transplantation. *Transplantation* 1995;59(7):1010–1014.
65. Mannon RB. Therapeutic targets in the treatment of allograft fibrosis. *Am J Transplant* 2006;6(5 Pt 1):867–875.
66. Mauiyyedi S, Colvin RB. Humoral rejection in kidney transplantation: new concepts in diagnosis and treatment. *Curr Opin Nephrol Hypertens* 2002;11(6):609–618.
67. McDiarmid SV. Current status of liver transplantation in children. *Pediatr Clin North Am* 2003;50(6):1335–374.
68. McDiarmid SV. Management of the pediatric liver transplant patient. *Liver Transpl* 2001;7(11 Suppl 1):S77–S86.
69. McDonald GB, Shulman HM, Sullivan KM, et al. Intestinal and hepatic complications of human bone marrow transplantation. Part I. *Gastroenterology* 1986;90(2):460–477.
70. McDonald GB, Shulman HM, Sullivan KM, et al. Intestinal and hepatic complications of human bone marrow transplantation. Part II. *Gastroenterology* 1986;90(3):770–784.
71. Medawar PB. The behaviour and fate of skin autografts and skin homografts in rabbits: a report to the War Wounds Committee of the Medical Research Council. *J Anat* 1944. 78(Pt 5):176–199.
72. Mekori YA, Claman HN. Is graft-versus-host disease a reliable model for scleroderma? *Ric Clin Lab* 1986;16(4):509–513.
73. Meyers BF, de la Morena M, Sweet SC, et al. Primary graft dysfunction and other selected complications of lung transplantation: a single-center experience of 983 patients. *J Thorac Cardiovasc Surg* 2005;129(6):1421–1429.
74. Monga G, Mazzucco G, Novara R, et al. Intertubular capillary changes in kidney allografts: an ultrastructural study in patients with transplant glomerulopathy. *Ultrastruct Pathol* 1990;14(3):201–209.
75. Moroff G, Luban NL. The irradiation of blood and blood components to prevent graft-versus-host disease: technical issues and guidelines. *Transfus Med Rev* 1997;11(1):15–26.
76. Noguchi Si S, Reyes J, Mazariegos GV, et al. Pediatric intestinal transplantation: the resected allograft. *Pediatr Dev Pathol* 2002;5(1):3–21.
77. The Organ Procurement and Transplantation Network. [Internet] 2007 [cited; Available from: http://www.optn.org.]
78. Papadimitriou JC, Cangro CB, Lustberg A, et al. Histologic features of mycophenolate mofetil-related colitis: a graft-versus-host disease-like pattern. *Int J Surg Pathol* 2003;11(4):295–302.
79. Parizhskaya M, Redondo C, Demetris A, et al. Chronic rejection of small bowel grafts: pediatric and adult study of risk factors and morphologic progression. *Pediatr Dev Pathol* 2003;6(3):240–250.
80. Pietra BA. Transplantation immunology 2003: simplified approach. *Pediatr Clin North Am* 2003;50(6):1233–1259.
81. Pinchoff RJ, Kaufman SS, Magid MS, et al. Adenovirus infection in pediatric small bowel transplantation recipients. *Transplantation* 2003;76(1):183–189.
82. Ploeg RJ, D'Alessandro AM, Knechtle SJ, et al. Risk factors for primary dysfunction after liver transplantation—a multivariate analysis. *Transplantation* 1993;55(4):807–813.
83. Ponticelli C, Traversi L, Banfi G. Renal transplantation in patients with IgA mesangial glomerulonephritis. *Pediatr Transplant* 2004;8(4):334–338.
84. Puliyanda DP, Stablein DM, Dharnidharka VR. Younger age and antibody induction increase the risk for infection in pediatric renal transplantation: a NAPRTCS report. *Am J Transplant* 2007;7(3):662–666.
85. Quan A, Sullivan EK, Alexander SR. Recurrence of hemolytic uremic syndrome after renal transplantation in children: a report of the North American Pediatric Renal Transplant Cooperative Study. *Transplantation* 2001;72(4):742–745.
86. Racusen LC, Solez K, Colvin RB, et al., The Banff 97 working classification of renal allograft pathology. *Kidney Int* 1999;55(2): 713–723.
87. Randhawa P. Allograft biopsies in management of pancreas transplant recipients. *J Postgrad Med* 2002;48(1):56–63.
88. Reed EF, Demetris AJ, Hammond E, et al. Acute antibody-mediated rejection of cardiac transplants. *J Heart Lung Transplant* 2006;25(2): 153–159.
89. Reyes J, Bueno J, Kocoshis S, et al. Current status of intestinal transplantation in children. *J Pediatr Surg* 1998;33(2):243–254.
90. Rocha PN, Plumb TJ, Crowley SD, et al. Effector mechanisms in transplant rejection. *Immunol Rev* 2003;196:51–64.
91. Rull R, Vidal O, Momblan D, et al. Evaluation of potential liver donors: limits imposed by donor variables in liver transplantation. *Liver Transpl* 2003;9(4):389–393.
92. Sarwal MM, Cecka JM, Millan MT, et al. Adult-size kidneys without acute tubular necrosis provide exceedingly superior long-term graft outcomes for infants and small children: a single center and UNOS analysis. United Network for Organ Sharing. *Transplantation* 2000;70(12):1728–1736.
93. Sarwal MM, Yorgin PD, Alexander S, et al. Promising early outcomes with a novel, complete steroid avoidance immunosuppression protocol in pediatric renal transplantation. *Transplantation* 2001;72(1):13–21.
94. Sattar HA, Husain AN, Kim AY, et al. The presence of a CD21+ follicular dendritic cell network distinguishes invasive Quilty lesions from cardiac acute cellular rejection. *Am J Surg Pathol* 2006;30(8):1008–1013.
95. Seikaly MG. Recurrence of primary disease in children after renal transplantation: an evidence-based update. *Pediatr Transplant* 2004;8(2):113–119.
96. Shishido S, Asanuma H, Nakai H, et al. The impact of repeated subclinical acute rejection on the progression of chronic allograft nephropathy. *J Am Soc Nephrol* 2003;14(4):1046–1052.
97. Shulman HM, Fisher LB, Schoch HG, et al. Veno-occlusive disease of the liver after marrow transplantation: histological correlates of clinical signs and symptoms. *Hepatology* 1994;19(5): 1171–1181.
98. Sieders E, Peeters PM, TenVergert EM, et al. Analysis of survival and morbidity after pediatric liver transplantation with full-size and technical-variant grafts. *Transplantation* 1999;68(4):540–545.
99. Smith JM, McDonald RA, Finn LS, et al. Polyomavirus nephropathy in pediatric kidney transplant recipients. *Am J Transplant* 2004;4(12):2109–2117.
100. Smith JM, Nemeth TL, McDonald RA. Current immunosuppressive agents: efficacy, side effects, and utilization. *Pediatr Clin North Am* 2003;50(6):1283–1300.
101. Smith JM, Stablein DM, Munoz R, et al. Contributions of the Transplant Registry: The 2006 Annual Report of the North American Pediatric Renal Trials and Collaborative Studies (NAPRTCS). *Pediatr Transplant* 2007;11(4):366–373.
102. Smith KD, Wrenshall LE, Nicosia RF, et al. Delayed graft function and cast nephropathy associated with tacrolimus plus rapamycin use. *J Am Soc Nephrol* 2003;14(4):1037–1045.
103. Snover DC. Graft-versus-host disease of the gastrointestinal tract. *Am J Surg Pathol* 1990;14(Suppl 1):101–108.
104. Snover DC, Weisdorf SA, Ramsay NK, et al. Hepatic graft versus host disease: a study of the predictive value of liver biopsy in diagnosis. *Hepatology* 1984;4(1):123–130.
105. Snover DC, Weisdorf SA, Vercellotti GM, et al. A histopathologic study of gastric and small intestinal graft-versus-host disease following allogeneic bone marrow transplantation. *Hum Pathol* 1985;16(4):387–392.

106. Solez K, Colvin RB, Racusen LC, et al. Banff 07 classification of renal allograft pathology: updates and future directions. *Am J Transplant* 2008;8(4):753–760.
107. Solez K, Colvin RB, Racusen LC, et al. Banff '05 Meeting Report: differential diagnosis of chronic allograft injury and elimination of chronic allograft nephropathy ('CAN'). *Am J Transplant* 2007;7(3):518–526.
108. Starr TK, Jameson SC, Hogquist KA. Positive and negative selection of T cells. *Annu Rev Immunol* 2003;21:139–176.
109. Starzl TE, Demetris AJ. Transplantation milestones. Viewed with one- and two-way paradigms of tolerance. *JAMA* 1995;273(11): 876–879.
110. Starzl TE, Zinkernagel RM. Antigen localization and migration in immunity and tolerance. *N Engl J Med* 1998;339(26):1905–1913.
111. Starzl TE, Zinkernagel RM. Transplantation tolerance from a historical perspective. *Nat Rev Immunol* 2001;1(3):233–239.
112. Stewart S, Fishbein MC, Snell GI, et al. Revision of the 1996 working formulation for the standardization of nomenclature in the diagnosis of lung rejection. *J Heart Lung Transplant* 2007;26(12): 1229–1242.
113. Stewart S, Winters GL, Fishbein MC, et al. Revision of the 1990 working formulation for the standardization of nomenclature in the diagnosis of heart rejection. *J Heart Lung Transplant* 2005;24(11):1710–1720.
114. Stringer MD, Marshall MM, Muiesan P, et al. Survival and outcome after hepatic artery thrombosis complicating pediatric liver transplantation. *J Pediatr Surg* 2001;36(6):888–891.
115. Tan CD, Baldwin WM III, Rodriguez ER. Update on cardiac transplantation pathology. *Arch Pathol Lab Med* 2007;131(8):1169–1191.
116. Trpkov K, Marcussen N, Rayner D, et al. Kidney allograft with a lymphocytic infiltrate: acute rejection, posttransplantation lymphoproliferative disorder, neither, or both entities? *Am J Kidney Dis* 1997;30(3):449–454.
117. van den Berg AP, Klompmaker IJ, Hepkema BG, et al. Cytomegalovirus infection does not increase the risk of vanishing bile duct syndrome after liver transplantation. *Transpl Int* 1996;9(Suppl 1):S171–S173.
118. VanBuskirk AM, Pidwell DJ, Adams PW, et al. Transplantation immunology. *JAMA* 1997;278(22):1993–1999.
119. Wadleigh M, Ho V, Momtaz P, et al. Hepatic veno-occlusive disease: pathogenesis, diagnosis and treatment. *Curr Opin Hematol* 2003;10(6):451–462.
120. Waldmann H, Chen TC, Graca L, et al. Regulatory T cells in transplantation. *Semin Immunol* 2006;18(2):111–119.
121. Washington K. Update on post-liver transplantation infections, malignancies, and surgical complications. *Adv Anat Pathol* 2005;12(4):221–226.
122. Washington K, Bentley RC, Green A, et al. Gastric graft-versus-host disease: a blinded histologic study. *Am J Surg Pathol* 1997;21(9): 1037–1046.
123. Watkins TR, Chien JW, Crawford SW. Graft versus host-associated pulmonary disease and other idiopathic pulmonary complications after hematopoietic stem cell transplant. *Semin Respir Crit Care Med* 2005;26(5):482–489.
124. Wekerle T, Sykes M. Mixed chimerism and transplantation tolerance. *Annu Rev Med* 2001;52:353–370.
125. Wu T, Abu-Elmagd K, Bond G, et al. A clinicopathologic study of isolated intestinal allografts with preformed IgG lymphocytotoxic antibodies. *Hum Pathol* 2004;35(11):1332–1339.
126. Wu T, Abu-Elmagd K, Bond G, et al. A schema for histologic grading of small intestine allograft acute rejection. *Transplantation* 2003;75(8):1241–1248.

SECTION II
Organ System Pathology

CHAPTER 9

The Placenta

RAYMOND W. REDLINE

INTRODUCTION

Perinatal pathology, the subdiscipline of pediatric pathology devoted to the study of abnormal pregnancy outcomes, is a rapidly developing field interfacing with obstetrician-gynecologists, neonatologists, and clinical geneticists. A central tenet of this field is that analysis of adverse pregnancy outcome begins with study of the placenta and its adnexa. The fetus is entirely dependent on the placenta for sustenance and protection throughout gestation. Indeed the placenta has been called a "diary of intrauterine life." Artificial barriers are often placed between the study of so-called products of conception resulting from early pregnancy loss and placentas submitted to pathology following complications of later pregnancy. Such a separation has no anatomic or functional basis and has probably hindered a complete and holistic understanding of the underlying biologic factors responsible for adverse outcomes in couples with sporadic or recurrent pregnancy loss. The first part of this chapter briefly summarizes key stages of placental development as a basis for understanding the problems of the first and early second trimester. The second part outlines the structure of the mature placenta to provide an anatomic framework for disease processes occurring in the late second and third trimester of pregnancy.

EARLY PREGNANCY

Development

The fertilized zygote undergoes a series of cleavage divisions to form a solid 16-cell morula by 5 days following ovulation (123). Between 5 and 8 days, a number of important events occur: the loose aggregate of cells becomes compacted, cells at the periphery develop tight junctions and begin transporting fluid into the center of the morula (blastocyst formation), and the surrounding zona pellucida is shed as the blastocyst attaches to, crosses, and invades the endometrium (Figure 9-1). The formation of tight cell-cell junctions at the periphery of the blastocyst marks the emergence of the trophectoderm lineage (trophoblast), which is the principal component of the placenta. Transport of fluid into the blastocyst and invasion of the gestational endometrium (decidua) foreshadow the two most important functions of trophoblast throughout gestation: transport of maternal substrates to the fetus and tissue remodeling of the maternal uterus to ensure adequate delivery of these substrates. Cells within the blastocyst (inner cell mass) separate into two lineages: epiblast, which gives rise to the epithelium surrounding the amnionic cavity (day 8) and the embryonic germ layers (days 15 to 28), and hypoblast, which forms the connective tissue of the placenta (extraembryonic mesoderm) and the primary yolk sac (23).

Development of the maternal and fetal placental circulations occurs in parallel. The maternal circulation begins when capillaries are eroded by an outer layer of primitive syncytial trophoblasts (131). Blood subsequently flows into lacunar spaces within the syncytium. These lacunae gradually enlarge eventually forming the intervillous space. Trophoblasts also migrate centripetally within the arterial circulation, forming cellular plugs that retard blood flow into the intervillous space until approximately 10 weeks of gestation (Figure 9-2A) (69). The basis for arterial versus venous invasion is unknown but may involve differential expression of angiogenic signaling molecules (190). During this period of retarded blood flow, the walls of the spiral arteries are remodeled in a series of events that includes dissolution of the muscular media, dilatation of

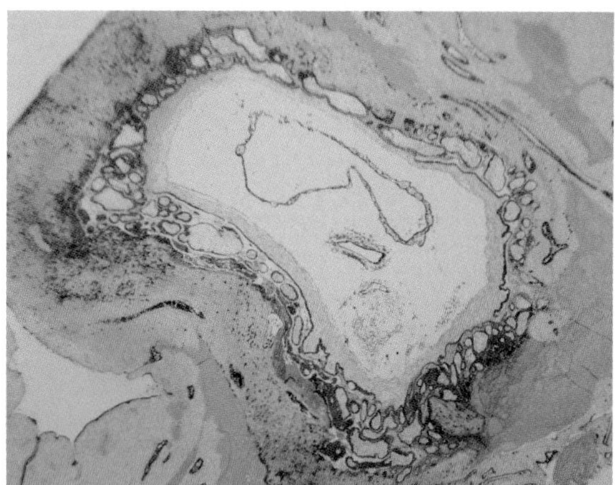

FIGURE 9-1 ■ Early implanting gestational sac (cytokeratin stain): Portions of embryo and unattached amnionic sac are surrounded by circumferential primary villi anchored in the peripheral cytotrophoblast shell with early intermediate trophoblasts infiltrating the adjacent endometrium.

the lumen, and reconstitution of the vessel wall by extracellular matrix secreted by endovascular trophoblasts. By the time that the plugs disappear, the cells of the developing placenta and the underlying structural integrity of the intervillous space are sufficient to withstand the oxygen tension and pressure of arterial blood flow. Subsequent remodeling of deeper arteries in the inner third of the myometrium continues until 18 weeks of pregnancy (the so-called secondary wave of implantation) (127). During this process, the placenta also expands laterally by attachment to and cooptation of large veins at the margins of the conceptus (so-called marginal sinus formation) (39). By the end of pregnancy, approximately 80 to 100 spiral arteries open into the mature intervillous space (28).

The fetal circulation of the placenta develops in two distinct phases (44). Extraembryonic mesoderm from the hypoblasts migrate peripherally into the primitive biphasic trophoblasts (cytotrophoblast stem cells and syncytial trophoblast) between the developing lacuna to form the so-called primary villi. A villous capillary circulation subsequently forms via local inductive interactions between cytotrophoblasts and extraembryonic mesoderm (Figure 9-2B). Later, this villous capillary net becomes connected to the embryonic circulation via anastomoses with large vessels growing out into extraembryonic connective tissue covering the trophoblastic portion of the placenta (chorionic plate). These large vessels reach the placenta via the body stalk, later to become the umbilical cord. Paired arteries develop along the allantoic duct and a vein develops along the omphalomesenteric duct. The vascularized extraembryonic mesoderm undergoes branching morphogenesis to form villous trees. As these trees increase in complexity and the placenta enlarges, the more proximal intraplacental vessels develop a muscular media and form the so-called stem villous arteries and veins.

The final stage of early placental development is formation of the membranes (185). The initial phase occurring at about 9 to 11 weeks of gestation is disappearance of the extraembryonic coelom and primitive yolk sac, resulting in attachment of the amnionic cavity surrounding the fetus to the chorionic connective tissue covering the trophoblastic portion of the placenta. This is followed at 11 to 17 weeks by the gradual atrophy and collapse of the intervillous space in all portions of the placenta not directly overlying the implantation site. It has been suggested that higher oxygen tension due to the lack of endovascular trophoblasts plugging away from the implantation site is responsible for this pattern of peripheral collapse (70). Finally, at about 17 to 20 weeks, the enlarging chorionic sac makes contact with and fuses to opposite side of the uterus, forming the mature multilayered placental membrane composed of vascularized decidua vera, avascular decidua capsularis, chorionic trophoblasts (chorion laeve), chorionic connective tissue, amnionic connective tissue, and amnionic epithelium.

Multiple Pregnancy

Background

Twinning (and higher order multiple pregnancies) can occur from either fertilization of multiple eggs (dizygotic) or fission of a single fertilized egg (monozygotic) (136).

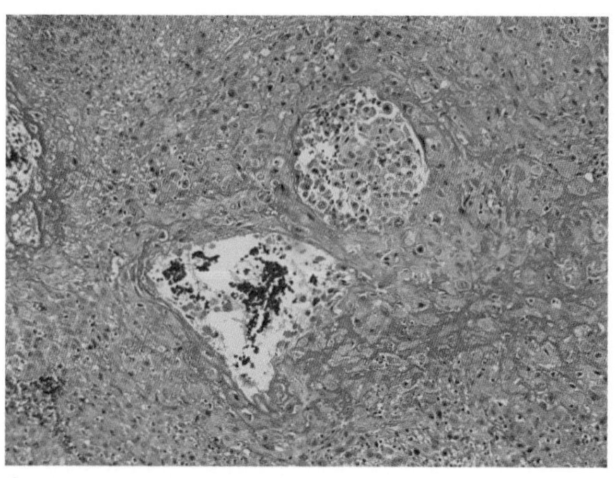

A

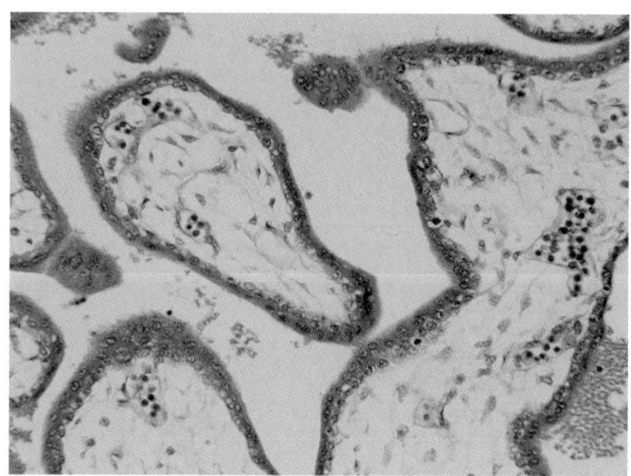

B

FIGURE 9-2 ■ Early pregnancy vascular development: **A:** Spiral arteries surrounded by intermediate trophoblasts with luminal plugs of endovascular trophoblasts and remodeling of the vessel wall. **B:** Fetal capillaries arising from pluripotent villous stromal cells induced by villous trophoblasts.

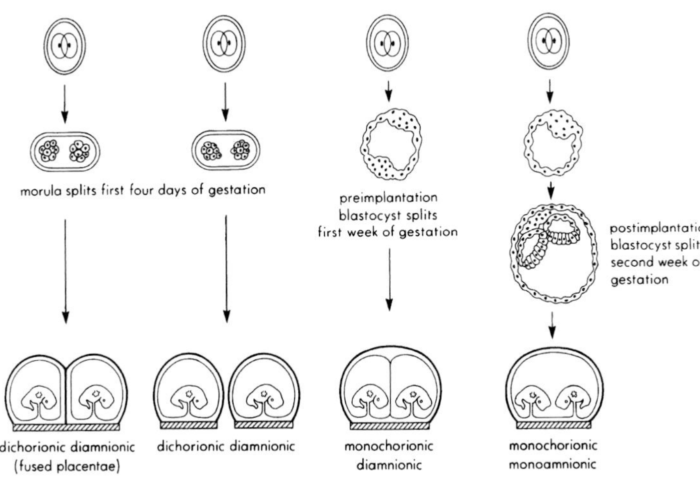

FIGURE 9-3 ■ Diagrammatic representation of placentation in monochorionic twinning. (From Gersell DJ, Kraus FT. Diseases of the placenta. In: Kurman RJ, ed. *Blausteins pathology of the female genital tract*. New York: Springer Verlag, 1998:986, with permission.)

Monozygotic twinning occurs at a constant rate in most populations and can be associated with a variety of different placental types (Figure 9-3). Separation prior to blastocyst formation leads to separate placentas (dichorionic diamnionic). Separation between blastocyst formation and amniogenesis leads to a single placenta but separate amnionic sacs (monochorionic diamnionic) while separation after amniogenesis results in a single placenta and amnionic sac (monochorionic monoamnionic). The incidence of dizygotic twinning is variable in different populations and depends on the frequency of polyovulation, either natural related to endogenous FSH levels or artificial related to ovulation-inducing drugs used in association with assisted reproductive technology. It had been thought that dizygotic twins always have separate (dichorionic) placentas, but a recent report has confirmed that on rare occasions, probably at the late morula stage, dizygotic twins can fuse to form a monochorionic placenta (172).

More important than zygosity per se from a clinical standpoint are connections in the placental vasculature (17,93). Surface anastomoses between chorionic arteries or veins (artery to artery and vein to vein) are common in monochorionic twins. These connections can lead to sharing of blood (chimerism) but do not generally cause circulatory imbalance. An exception may occur when major arteries immediately adjacent to their umbilical cord insertion sites are connected. In this situation, an artery from one twin may develop sufficient pressure to reverse the circulatory flow in the second twin, leading to secondary atrophy of the heart and other rostral structures (acardiac fetus) (21). Aberrant connections in the period when the villous circulation anastomoses with the embryonic circulation, on the other hand, may lead to areas of the placenta that are perfused by the arterial circulation of one twin and drained by the venous system of the other. The resulting twin-twin transfusion syndrome is discussed below.

Pathology

The most important role of the pathologist in multiple pregnancy is to determine the number of chorions and amnions in each placenta, usually by direct inspection followed by confirmatory histologic sections from the dividing membrane between the two placentas. Such examination is not required when the placental discs are completely separate. If a single placenta is noted and the dividing membrane is opaque, two amnions flanking a fused central chorion are most likely (dichorionic diamnionic). This can be confirmed at gross examination by peeling the three layers, and the placentas can then be separated for weighing and processing. If the dividing membrane is translucent, only two amnions are expected (monochorionic diamnionic). The chorion is absent because it surrounds but does not divide the two fetal sacs. This is again confirmed by peeling the two layers. A monochorionic placenta is, as the name indicates, one placenta and should be weighed without division. Inspection of the chorionic plate for surface anastomoses should be performed. Air injection studies are a quick and easy method for detecting clinically significant deep arteriovenous anastomoses (87). More complete injections with colored or radiopaque dyes are usually conducted only in a research context. Pathologic lesions, most frequently found with discordant twin growth (see below) in both monochorionic and dichorionic twins, include peripheral cord insertion, avascular villi, and indicators of maternal vascular under perfusion (60,154).

Clinical Correlation

Twin gestations of all types are at an increased risk for premature delivery, fetal growth restriction, preeclampsia, and cerebral palsy (129). Many of these complications are increased in the presence of discordant twin growth, usually defined as a greater than 25% difference in body weights. Adverse outcome is generally more frequent in the smaller and/or the nonpresenting (second) twin. Chronic twin-twin transfusion syndrome is a specific form of discordant growth related to deep arteriovenous anastomoses in monochorionic twins (183). The syndrome is characterized by marked growth restriction and anemia in the donor twin and macrosomia, polycythemia, and congestive heart failure in the recipient. Acute twin-twin transfusion without growth discordance can occasionally occur when previously balanced anastomoses become unbalanced due to either changes in fetal blood pressures or secondary occlusion of bridging fetal vessels. The most dramatic example of acute transfusion syndrome occurs after fetal demise of one twin. In this case, sudden blood shifts from the survivor to the decedent are associated with a very high risk of perinatal brain damage (126).

Gestational Trophoblastic Disease

Background

Trophoblast has two major functions: tissue invasion and substrate transfer. As described above, invasion occurs early in gestation as the primitive mononuclear and syncytial trophoblasts invade the superficial endometrium, and later in gestation, when intermediate trophoblasts implant more deeply in the myometrium. Neoplastic transformation of primitive mononuclear and syncytial trophoblasts result in choriocarcinoma while that of intermediate trophoblasts result in placental site trophoblastic tumor (PSTT). A third more recently described subtype of trophoblastic neoplasm, the epithelioid trophoblastic tumor (ETT), is derived from cells phenotypically similar to the trophoblasts of the membranes (chorion laeve trophoblasts) (166). While choriocarcinoma can develop *de novo* from apparently normal early and late placentas, more than half of cases are preceded by molar pregnancies. Trophoblastic proliferation is largely dependent on growth-promoting factors, transcribed only from paternally inherited genes (14). Control of proliferation and differentiation, on the other hand, depends on antiproliferative genes of maternal inheritance. Molar pregnancies have an overrepresentation of paternal chromosomes (141). Complete moles are derived from fertilization of an empty ovum and contain only paternal chromosomes, while partial moles are triploid gestations resulting from dispermy and have a 2:1 ratio of paternal to maternal chromosomes. The increased frequency of molar pregnancies accounts for the relatively high incidence of choriocarcinoma in Asian populations. PSTT and ETT, most commonly, develop after term pregnancies, often years after delivery. It is well known that some intermediate trophoblasts are left behind after delivery and can persist for many years. Although not proven, these persistent rests of trophoblasts, known as placental site nodules, may well be precursors for these rare tumors (189).

Pathology

Molar pregnancies are characterized by villous edema and trophoblastic hyperplasia. Edema is often extreme leading to cavitation of the villous stroma. In complete moles, the edema and hyperplasia affect the entire conceptus, while in partial moles, they affect only a subgroup of villi (Figure 9-4A). Partial moles also show irregularly shaped villi, as may be seen in

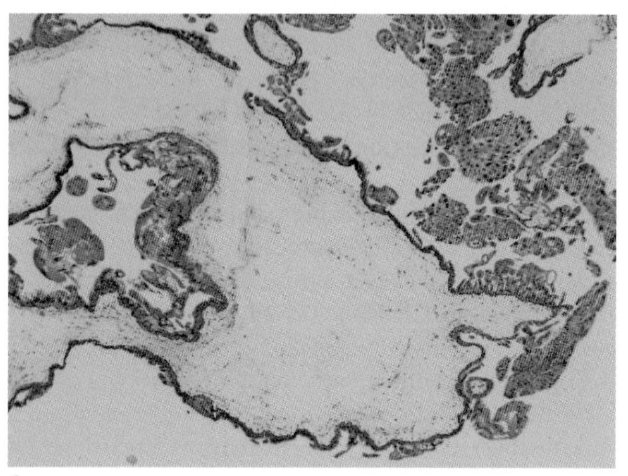

A

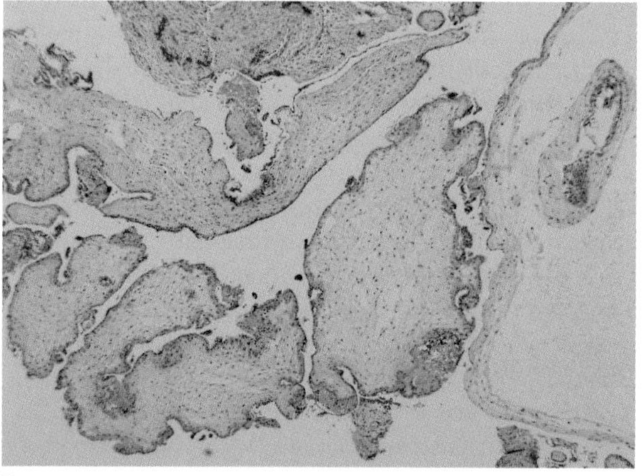

B

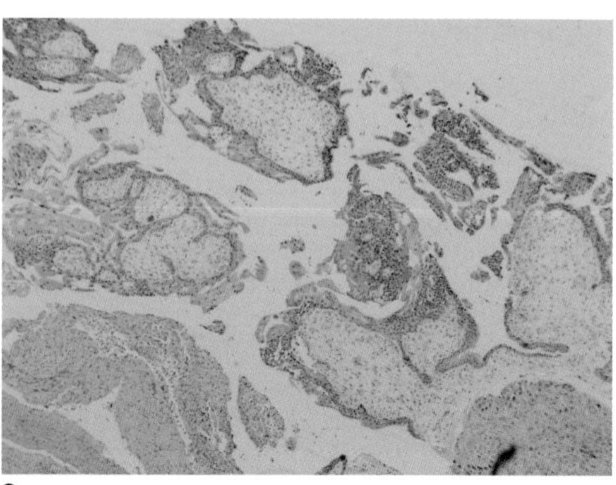

C

FIGURE 9-4 ■ Molar pregnancy: **A:** Complete hydatidiform mole—uniformly hydropic villi with central cisterns and circumferential trophoblastic hyperplasia. **B:** Partial hydatidiform mole—molar villi (**left**) and irregularly shaped fibrotic villi (**right**) showing mild circumferential syncytiotrophoblastic hyperplasia. **C:** Early complete hydatidiform mole—bulbous villous branching, densely cellular myxoid stroma, and trophoblastic hyperplasia.

other chromosomal abnormalities (Figure 9-4B) (147). Classic complete moles are easily diagnosed based on clusters of fluid-filled vesicles (hydatidiform or "grape-like" change) and marked trophoblastic hyperplasia. With current use of early ultrasound, approximately one-third of complete moles are curetted at a stage before development of edema or diffuse trophoblastic hyperplasia. These early complete moles can be difficult to recognize but manifest a number of helpful diagnostic features including a cauliflower-like growth pattern, densely cellular myxoid villous stroma, focal trophoblastic hyperplasia, and atypia of implantation site trophoblasts (Figure 9-4C) (80). Occasional early pregnancy specimens show nonspecific trophoblastic hyperplasia without edematous or molar villi. Cytogenetic study of these specimens has shown a high prevalence of the two relatively uncommon trisomies, 7 and 15 (146). Whether these cases have an increased risk of later choriocarcinoma is not known.

Choriocarcinomas are often characterized grossly by large areas of hemorrhage and necrosis. They are composed of two cellular populations—clusters of 10 to 50 mononuclear cytotrophoblasts surrounded by a wreath-like garland of syncytial trophoblasts (Figure 9-5A). The mononuclear trophoblast shows mild-moderate nuclear atypia and watery clear cytoplasm. Syncytial trophoblast contains multiple enlarged hyperchromatic nuclei and deep eosinophilic cytoplasm. The latter stains intensely for human chorionic gonadotropin and human placental lactogen, while the former lack both hormones. Both cell types are cytokeratin positive. Unlike normal trophoblasts, individual clusters of malignant cells in choriocarcinoma perpendicularly invade smooth muscle fascicles in the myometrium. PSTT is composed of larger mononuclear cells with more nuclear atypia and an intensely eosinophilic cytoplasm (Figure 9-5B) (167). Binucleation is occasionally seen, but greater numbers of nuclei are rare. Unlike normal intermediate trophoblasts, tumor cells invade in large cohesive sheets and are associated with tissue necrosis. Some large arteries show remodeling by tumor cells, but large nontransformed arteries are also seen and are diagnostically helpful. Tumor cells stain positively for cytokeratin and human placental lactogen but are usually only weakly and focally positive for human chorionic gonadotropin (hCG). ETT contains vacuolated cells often in a hyaline matrix, bearing a striking resemblance, by both light microscopy and immunostaining, to the cells of the membranous chorion laeve (Figure 9-5C). They tend to grow in a nodular expansile pattern in the lower uterine segment or cervix where

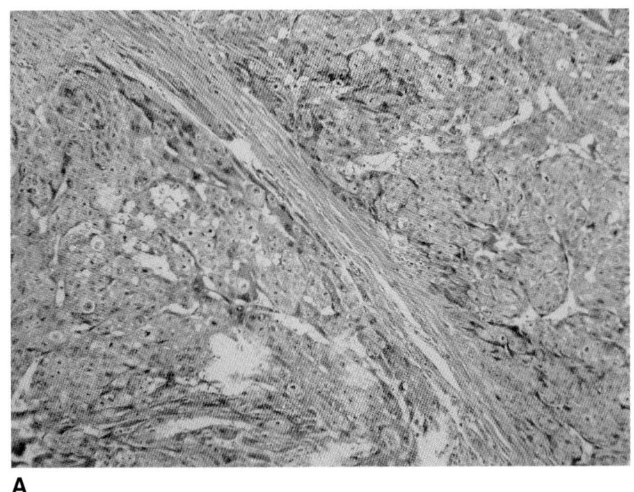

A

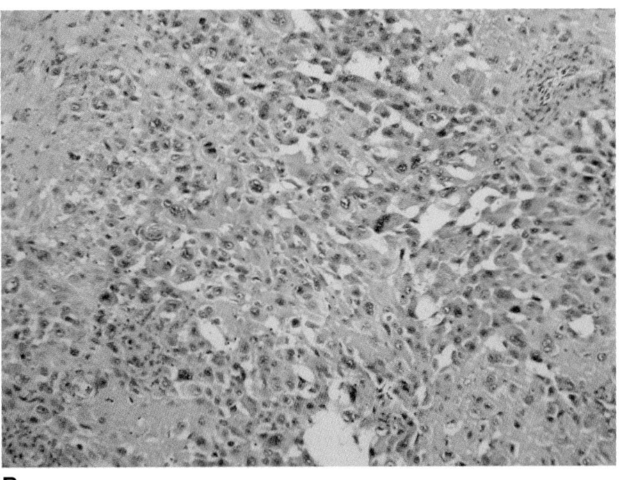

B

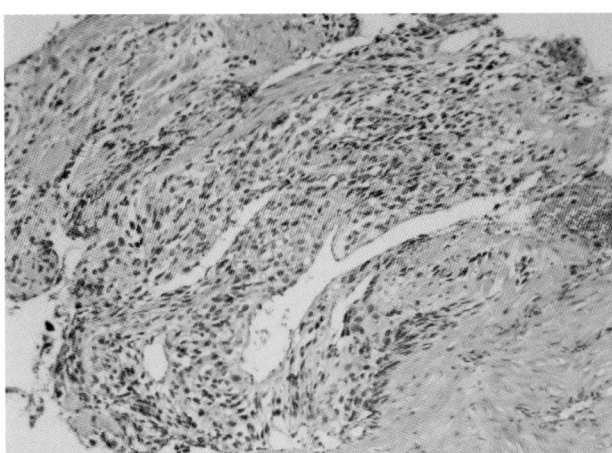

C

FIGURE 9-5 ■ Trophoblastic tumors: **A:** Choriocarcinoma—clusters of mononuclear cytotrophoblasts surrounded by a wreath-like garland of poorly differentiated syncytial trophoblasts. **B:** Placental site trophoblastic tumor—loosely cohesive sheets of atypical intermediate trophoblasts with strongly eosinophilic cytoplasm. **C:** Epithelioid trophoblastic tumor—sheets of vacuolated extravillous trophoblasts invading myometrium.

they can mimic squamous carcinomas. Their antigen profile includes diffuse expression of keratin, alpha inhibin and p63 plus focal/variable hCG, hPL, MelCAM (CD148), and placental alkaline phosphatase (168).

Clinical Correlation

All preneoplastic and neoplastic lesions of trophoblasts are combined under the rubric gestational trophoblastic disease (92). While molar pregnancies are usually confirmed by tissue diagnosis, subsequently developing choriocarcinomas are generally not. Clinical management relies on serum monitoring of the tumor marker, hCG, and radiographic imaging. Persistence or elevation of hCG levels, after evacuation of a molar pregnancy, is treated empirically with single agent chemotherapy. Tumors with extremely high hCG levels, metastasis to organs other than the lung, and other high-risk factors are treated with multiple agent chemotherapy. On rare occasions, chemotherapeutically resistant tumors manifest a distinct pathologic phenotype known as atypical choriocarcinoma (100). PSTT and ETT usually present with vaginal bleeding. Curettage is suspicious for a neoplasm and hCG levels are usually positive, but often at low levels. Radiographic studies confirm a mass lesion, and hysterectomy is performed. Unlike choriocarcinoma, PSTT and ETT are relatively indolent and only rarely metastasize. However, they respond poorly to chemotherapy so local control is paramount. Clinical management of the occasional early pregnancy specimens with nonspecific or unclassifiable trophoblastic hyperplasia referred to above should include a single hCG titer to ensure return to baseline.

Anembryonic Pregnancy

Background

Missed abortion refers to a pregnancy in which a nonviable chorionic sac is retained in the uterus requiring curettage for evacuation. An early gestational sac lacking sonographic and histologic evidence of embryonic development (anembryonic pregnancy) is the most common form of missed abortion. A large percentage of these specimens have embryonic lethal chromosomal abnormalities (158). The remaining chromosomally normal specimens most likely represent random major disruptions of early embryogenesis resulting in complete or partial resorption of the inner cell mass derivatives. The proportion with sporadic mutations in major developmental genes is unknown (see Chapters 2 and 3).

Pathology

Anembryonic pregnancies show a typical pathologic profile. They consist of a relatively thin chorionic membrane, uniformly edematous (hydropic) villi, and well-preserved gestational endometrium and implantation site (Figure 9-6A). Amnion, yolk sac, umbilical cord, and embryonic tissue are usually absent, and no fetal blood vessels are apparent. The uniformly hydropic nature of the villi is caused by continuing trophoblastic transport function leading to fluid buildup in villi with no egress to the fetal circulation. With prolonged retention, the hydropic villi can undergo secondary fibrosis (hyalinization). Gestational endometrium and an implantation site in these cases are usually unremarkable.

Clinical Correlation

The management of women with first trimester losses, particularly when recurrent, is highly dependent on the nature of the loss. A careful pathologic examination can often guide clinical management in cases where cytogenetic analysis has either not been obtained or is unsuccessful (158). Recognition of an anembryonic gestation (also referred to as blighted ovum or hydropic abortus) by early ultrasound or pathologic examination is clinically useful in that it identifies a cohort with a low recurrence rate. Early and late miscarriages with thromboinflammatory lesions or endometrial pathology and no apparent defects in fetal development are much more likely to recur in subsequent pregnancies.

Miscarriage

Background

The term miscarriage refers to early pregnancy specimens in the process of being expelled from the mother (threatened, incomplete, and complete abortions). Most common are specimens with evidence of remote fetal death (hyalinized villi, obliterated fetal vasculature) (Figure 9-6B). These cases are a heterogeneous mixture of chromosomally normal and abnormal gestations with intrauterine fetal demise due to malformation, deformation, or disruption. A second group is characterized by well-preserved and normally vascularized chorionic villi with copious intervillous hemorrhage (Breus mole) (Figure 9-6C). Specimens in this second group are often chromosomally normal. Several underlying maternal abnormalities may contribute to miscarriage. Antiphospholipid syndrome leads to maternal vascular maldevelopment, thrombosis, and hemorrhage via antibody plus complement-mediated interactions with maternal endothelial cells and trophoblasts (30,164). Other less specific maternal vascular abnormalities may interfere with the endovascular trophoblastic plugs that normally retard blood flow into the intervillous space in early pregnancy. This can lead to oxidative damage to the developing placenta and high-pressure flow into the early intervillous space (73). Finally, there is a group of poorly understood thromboinflammatory processes (see below) characterized by evidence of maternal immune responses in fetal tissues. Some evidence links these uncommon lesions to abnormal maternal immune responses to foreign fetal antigen in the placenta (158).

Pathology

The general phenotype of most miscarriages is a well-developed chorionic sac with adherent amnion, collagenized (hyalinized) villi, and hemorrhagic necrosis of the implantation site and gestational endometrium. More specific findings are sometimes

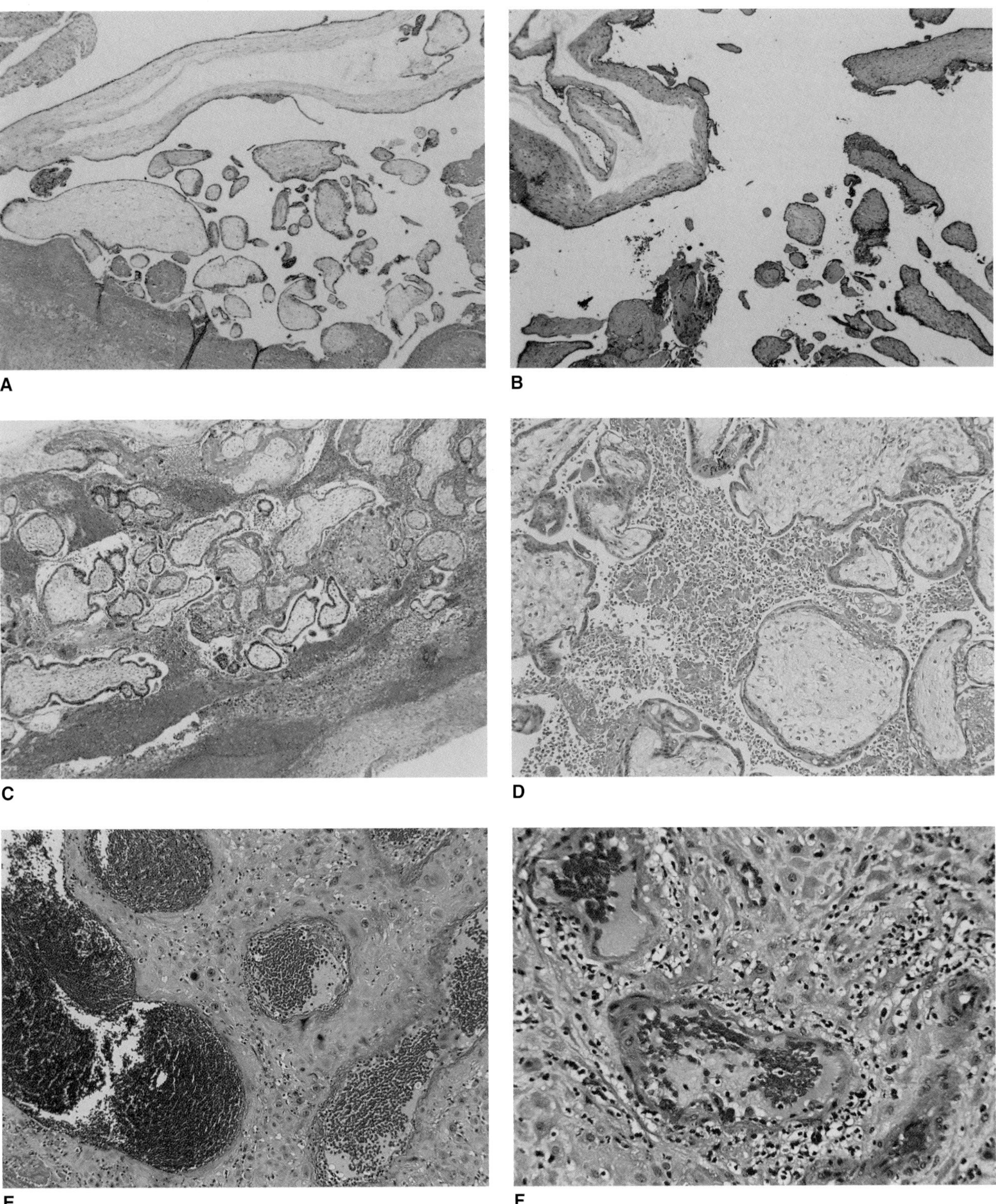

FIGURE 9-6■ Spontaneous abortion: **A:** Anembryonic pregnancy—uniformly hydropic villi adjacent to chorion without an adherent amnion. **B:** Hyalinized villi with adjacent fused chorioamnion, consistent with remote fetal death. **C:** Breus mole—well-preserved villi with marked intervillous hemorrhage. **D:** Chronic histiocytic intervillositis—early chorionic villi surrounded by sheets of immature monocytes-macrophages. **E:** Pathologic congested spiral arteries lacking endovascular trophoblast plugs. **F:** Spiral arterioles with marked chronic perivasculitis in maternal autoimmune disease.

identified in specimens from patients with multiple consecutive miscarriages. Massive perivillous fibrin deposition ("maternal floor infarction") can present at any gestational age and is discussed later. Chronic histiocytic intervillositis is characterized by extensive infiltration of the intervillous space by a monomorphic infiltrate of monocytes-macrophages (Figure 9-6D) (29). This lesion can also present at later stages but is most frequently observed in the first trimester. Breus mole, in addition to marked hemorrhage in the intervillous space, may show pathologic thrombosis or congestion of spiral arteries and an absence of endovascular trophoblastic plugs (Figure 9-6E). Finally, the spiral arteries of some patients with antiphospholipid syndrome or other autoimmune diseases may show vasculitis, mural hypertrophy, perivascular decidual fibrin deposition, and/or plasma cell infiltration (Figure 9-6F) (116).

Clinical Correlation

Patients with antiphospholipid syndrome are currently treated with low-dose heparin therapy often accompanied by low-dose aspirin. Approximately 70% to 80% of women treated with this regimen achieve successful pregnancy outcome in subsequent pregnancies (30). Those failing this regimen may be treated with full anticoagulation, intravenous gamma globulin, or corticosteroids with unclear efficacy. Patients with vascular pathology lacking antiphospholipid antibodies are often treated similarly. Chronic histiocytic intervillositis is more frequent in women with underlying immunologic abnormalities and abnormal alloimmune responses to fetal (paternal) antigens (29,47). They frequently have an abnormal cytokine response to pregnancy, as manifest by increased TNF-α (embryotoxic factor) (63). Women with abnormal alloimmune responses have been extensively studied often without any pathologic correlation. Although no randomized controlled trials demonstrating efficacy have been published, these patients are sometimes treated empirically with progesterone, immunosuppressive drugs, intravenous immunoglobulin, and immunization with paternal leukocytes (37).

Congenital Infection

Background

Although ascending infections caused by organisms from the cervicovaginal tract can occur in the second trimester, most congenital infections in the first half of pregnancy are acquired hematogenously (24,87). The majority are the result of primary infection, since previous exposure usually elicits protective antibodies in the mother. Bacterial and fungal infections are rare. Spirochetes (*T. pallidum, B. burgdorfei*), *parasites* (*T. gondii, T. cruzi, P. falciparum, S. hematobium*), and viruses (cytomegalovirus, varicella zoster virus, herpes simplex virus, rubellavirus, poxviruses, parvovirus B19, enteroviruses, HIV, hepatitis B and C) are the major causative agents. Organisms may localize to and elicit inflammation exclusively in the intervillous space (*P. falciparum, B. burgdorfei, S. hematobium*) or they may cross the placenta without eliciting an inflammatory response (parvovirus B19, HIV, hepatitis B and C, most enteroviruses), but more commonly they infect both placenta and fetus. Most fetal infections occur in the second trimester. Spread to the fetus in the first trimester is less common, but the infections are generally more severe. Maternal infections in very early pregnancy often spare the products of conception (see Chapter 6).

Pathology

Organisms limited to the intervillous space lead to accumulations of fibrin and chronic inflammatory cells at that location. The remaining infections lead to a diffuse chronic placentitis with chronic inflammatory cells in the chorion, decidua, and villous stroma (6). Unlike villitis of unknown etiology (also discussed below), infectious villitis tends to involve most or all villi. Two overlapping patterns are seen. The first, edematous villi with increased Hofbauer cells, is typical of syphilis (Figure 9-7A). The second, fibrotic villi with evidence of remote hemorrhage and, occasionally, villous plasma cells is typical of CMV (Figure 9-7B). Many infections have unique

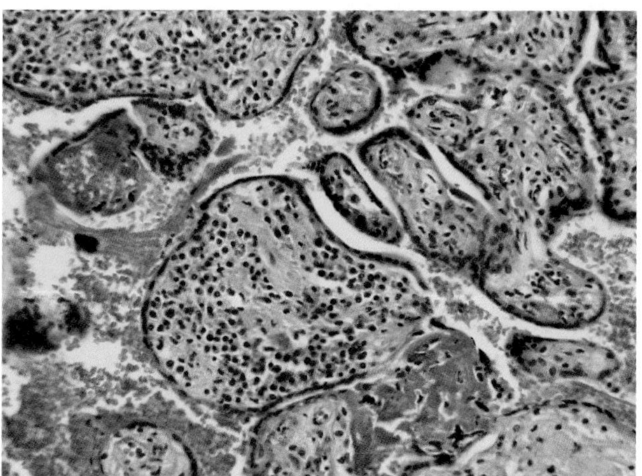

FIGURE 9-7 ■ TORCH infections: **A:** Syphilis—histiocytic villitis with villous edema. **B:** CMV-plasma cell villitis with villous fibrosis.

features allowing a specific histopathologic diagnosis. These include the presence of organisms or viral inclusions in the villous stroma (CMV, herpes simplex virus, varicella zoster virus, parvovirus B19, *T. cruzi*), umbilical cord (*T. pallidum, T. gondii*), or intervillous space (*P. falciparum, S. hematobium*).

Clinical Correlation

A common clinical mnemonic for congenital infection is the acronym TORCH standing for toxoplasmosis, (others), rubella virus, cytomegalovirus, and herpes simplex (58). In the United States, two infections, CMV and syphilis, account for more than 90% of congenital infections. Infants with any of the TORCH infections have a number of common features including intrauterine growth restriction (IUGR), pancytopenia, hepatosplenomegaly, and coagulopathy. Each infection also has specific features, a description of which is beyond the scope of this chapter. A standard serologic screen known as the "TORCH titer" tests for maternal IgG specific for the common TORCH agents and is part of the routine workup for IUGR or suspected antenatal maternal infection. Specific testing for IgM is required to distinguish recent from remote infection. Many infections can also be diagnosed by PCR testing of fetal blood or amniotic cells obtained by amniocentesis.

LATE PREGNANCY

Anatomy

The mature placenta is composed of four distinct units of structure-function:

1. Chorionic plate and its contiguous vascularized fetal connective tissue
2. Interhemal villous trophoblasts and the adjacent intervillous space
3. Basal plate and underlying maternal uterine vasculature
4. Tripartite placental membranes, consisting of amnion, chorion, and decidua.

The chorionic plate (or fetal surface) consists of the fibrous connective tissue supporting the large muscular arteries and veins that distribute fetal blood flow from the umbilical cord to the family of 20 to 30 large villous trees (20,28). The umbilical cord is a squamous epithelial-lined conduit normally measuring between 40 to 80 cm in length at term that conducts fetal blood from the umbilicus to some location on the chorionic plate (or occasionally the adjacent placental membranes). It contains paired arteries that spiral around a central vein, all surrounded by a hyaluronate-rich matrix (Wharton jelly), which provides considerable protection from external compression. The two arteries are connected, at or just before their insertion site, into the chorionic plate by an anastomosis (Hyrtyl anastomosis). Villous trees, emanating from the underside of the chorionic plate, branch multiple times as they conduct fetal blood through a succession of smaller arteries and veins until they reach capillaries that abut the trophoblastic interhemal membrane in the terminal villi. These conducting villi are referred to as stem and intermediate villi, with the latter representing the arteriolar level at which blood flow to the gas-exchanging terminal villi is ultimately regulated (54). The two critical anatomic features that must be maintained in this compartment are patency of the large villous vessels and short diffusion distance between fetal capillaries and interhemal villous trophoblasts. Maturation of the villous tree with advancing gestational age in the third trimester is characterized by an increase in the number of terminal villi relative to intermediate villi and a decrease in the amount of villous connective tissue associated with the peripheralization of capillaries and the formation of specialized vasculosyncytial membranes. However, there is considerable regional variation in villous maturity. Well-perfused villi, overlying the opening of the maternal spiral artery (central cotyledon), appear considerably less mature than those at the "watershed" between arteries (peripheral cotyledon) (Figure 9-8A and B).

Interhemal villous trophoblasts consist of a single multinucleated layer of differentiated syncytiotrophoblasts with underlying basement membrane and occasional basally located cytotrophoblastic stem cells. Each stem cell is the progenitor for 80 to 100 fused syncytiotrophoblastic cells, and these large syncytial sheets form a mosaic covering the entirety of the villous tree (169). Turnover of syncytiotrophoblasts occur via clustering of nuclei in syncytial knots followed by apoptosis and shedding into the maternal circulation (98). Critical features for the interhemal membrane are cellular viability, appropriate maturation in terms of endocrine, transport, anticoagulant, and immunoprotective functions, and accessibility to maternal blood flow—meaning absence of adherent fibrin or inflammatory exudate.

The basal plate consists of 80 to 100 anchoring villi inserted into the endometrium plus a similar number of perpendicularly oriented perforating maternal arteries and tangentially oriented draining maternal veins. Intermediate trophoblasts, arising from cytotrophoblasts on the underside of the anchoring villi, diffusely infiltrate the basal plate and elaborate large amounts of a fibronectin-rich extracellular matrix that provides structural integrity and unites these elements into a coherent anatomic structure (Nitabuch layer). Closely related endovascular trophoblasts are normally present in the wall of basal plate arteries. Important features of the normal basal plate are adequate remodeling of maternal arteries to ensure adequate blood flow into the intervillous space and sufficient depth and extent of trophoblastic implantation to prevent premature separation. The margins of the placenta require additional consideration. The process of continuing lateral placental growth involves growth of villous trees into maternal veins at the periphery of the disc (39,115). This process results in the formation of distinct large sinusoidally dilated veins surrounding the placenta, structures previously misinterpreted as a discrete marginal venous sinus (Figure 9-8C).

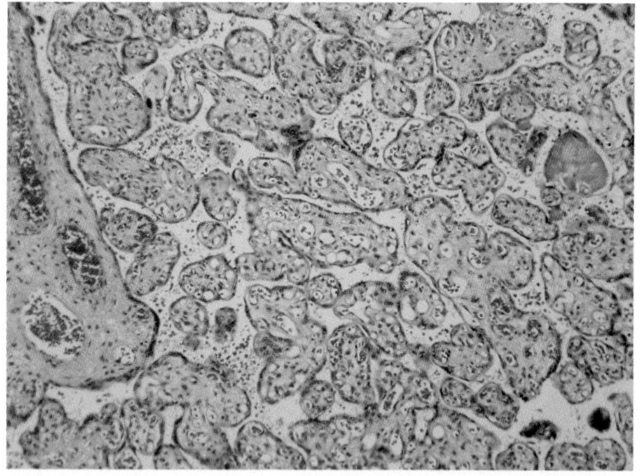
A

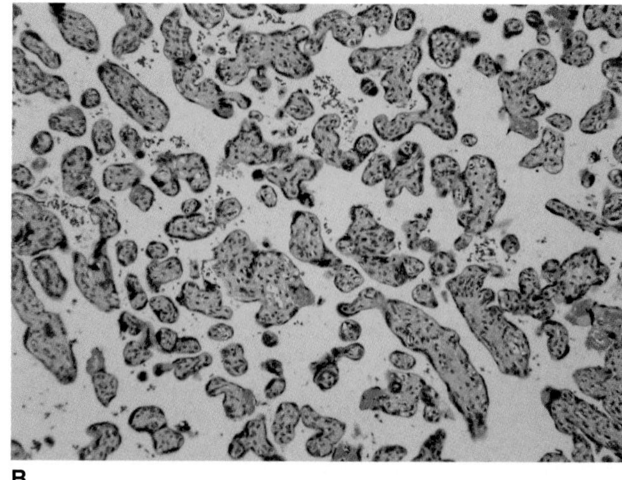
B

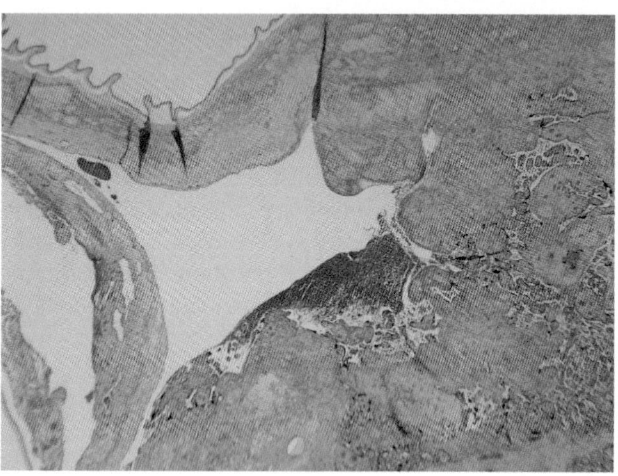
C

FIGURE 9-8 ■ Normal placental anatomy at term: **A:** Central lobule—distal villi are enlarged with abundant stroma, numerous capillaries, and uniform layer of villous trophoblasts. **B:** Peripheral lobule—distal villi are much smaller with scant peripheral capillaries and prominent syncytial knots. **C:** Margin/membrane—peripheral villi extend into a large venous space within the basal plate that is covered by fused amniochorion and decidua.

The placental membranes, at first glance, appear distinct from the first three compartments. While this is certainly true in terms of function, the anatomic differences are minor. The membranes form by involution of the placenta and retain all of its layers. The fetal surface of the membranes is covered by amnion and consists of chorionic connective tissue and occasional chorionic villi, albeit without fetal blood vessels. The villous trophoblasts coalesce as the intervillous space is obliterated to form a third distinct morphologic variant of trophoblast known as chorion laeve or epithelioid trophoblast. This noninvasive trophoblastic layer is supported by underlying maternal decidua. Critical requirements for this compartment include the integrity and contiguity of all layers. In particular, chorionic prostaglandin dehydrogenase in chorion laeve trophoblasts must be functionally active and spatially positioned to inactivate labor-inducing prostaglandins elaborated by the amnion, decidua, and myometrium (34,179).

Chronic Disease Processes

Disease processes affecting the placenta can be classified in a variety of ways including anatomic location, mechanism of injury, or clinical outcome. Another way that is particularly useful for understanding the causal sequence of events leading to adverse pregnancy outcome is time of onset (149). The rationale for such a separation is that earlier events and placental lesions may significantly decrease placental reserve lowering the threshold for fetal injury and resulting in an enhanced effect of comparatively minor stresses at the time of parturition. In the following scheme the term chronic refers to lesions evolving over weeks, subacute to those evolving over many hours to days, and acute to those evolving over just a few hours.

Maternal Vascular Under Perfusion

Background

Chronic maternal underperfusion of the intervillous space can result from a variety of causes including underlying cardiac insufficiency, failure to expand intravascular volume during pregnancy, or structural abnormalities in arteries supplying the uterus. It is currently believed that the major process leading to underperfusion is failure of trophoblasts to appropriately invade and remodel the uterine spiral arteries. While the exact sequence or sequences of events leading to this outcome have not yet been worked out, a number of contributing factors have been identified. These include initial exposure to fetoplacental antigens in first pregnancies, inherited polymorphisms in genes of the renin-angiotensin system, antiendothelial cell antibodies, and underlying uterine small vessel disease (15,105,161,181). The common denominator for all of these factors seems to be decreased oxygen delivery to the implantation site resulting in dysregulation of growth factor and protease expression, impaired trophoblastic differentiation, and inadequate placentation (32). In the absence of arterial remodeling, the placenta is chronically underperfused leading to decreased fetoplacental growth and, in some cases, the release of vasoactive mediators in late pregnancy leading to the clinical syndrome of preeclampsia. Several of these mediators have been identified in the last few years including soluble form of vascular endothelial growth factor (VEGF) receptor 1 (sflt-1), soluble endoglin, and circulating AT1 receptor antibodies (67,90,99,165).

Pathology

Placentas affected by maternal underperfusion generally show two or more of a constellation of features that together allow a specific diagnosis to be rendered (144). One important and often overlooked feature is decreased weight for gestational age and decreased placental weight relative to that of the infant (increased fetoplacental weight ratio) (109,187). In severe cases, this correlates with late impairment of placental growth (distal villous hypoplasia) as the fetus sacrifices placental perfusion in order to supply critical vascular beds such as the central nervous and cardiovascular systems (Figure 9-9A) (68,88). Also, common in severe cases is a thin umbilical cord resulting from extracellular volume depletion and decreased hydration of Wharton jelly. Complete maternal vascular obstruction secondary to spiral artery thrombi leads to villous infarcts (Figure 9-9B) (31,180). Partial maternal vascular obstruction can lead to stasis with intervillous fibrin deposition (Figure 9-9C), hypoxia with accelerated syncytiotrophoblast turnover and increased syncytial knots (Figure 9-9D), and localized ischemia with villous agglutination (Figure 9-9E) (7,65,132). Two other types of placental abnormalities may also be seen. First, persistent muscularization of basal plate arteries and aggregates of placental site giant cells or epithelioid (chorion laeve type) trophoblasts in the basal plate) correlate with superficial implantation (153). Second, maternal arteriopathies, medial hypertrophy (Figure 9-9F) and fibrinoid necrosis (acute atherosis) (Figure 9-9G), may be linked to inheritance of a variant

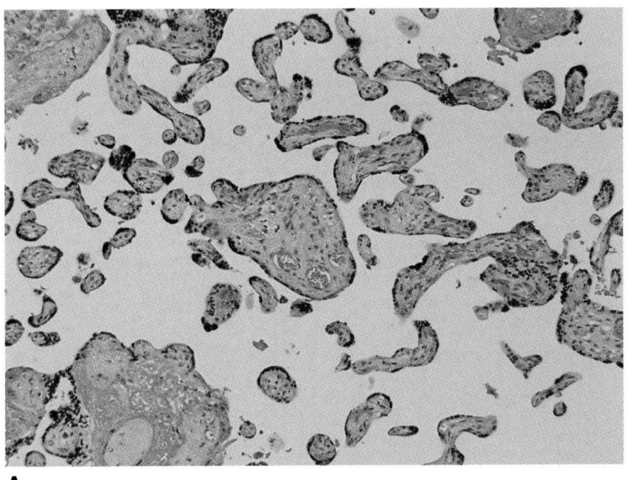

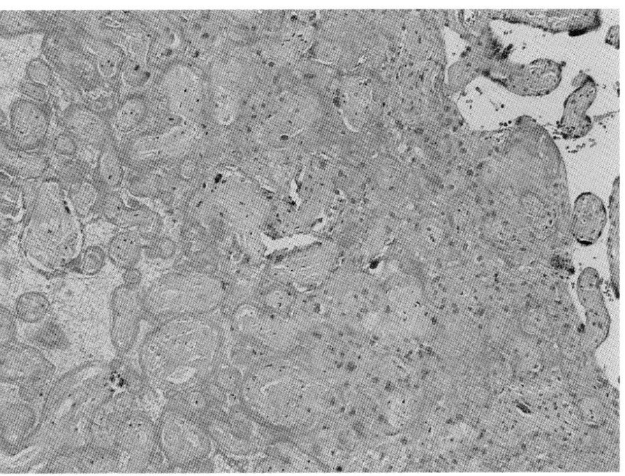

FIGURE 9-9 ■ Maternal underperfusion: **A:** Distal villous hypoplasia—decreased number of long thin poorly branching distal villi. **B:** Villous infarction—large aggregate of nonviable villi with collapse of the intervillous space and remote ischemic necrosis of the villous trophoblast. **C:** Increased intervillous fibrin—irregular aggregates of fibrin coating large proximal villi and protruding from denuded portions of the distal villous tree.

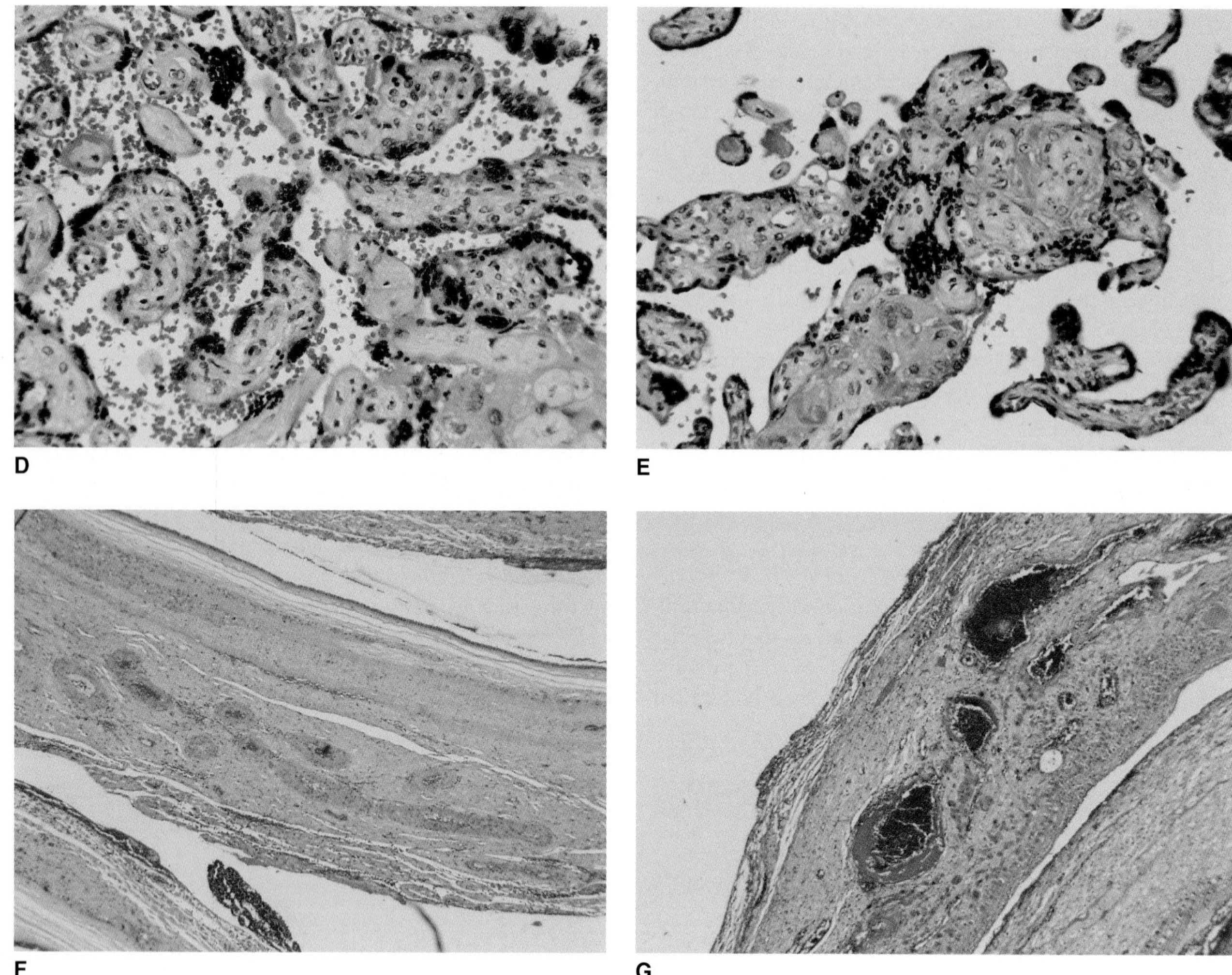

FIGURE 9-9 ■ **D:** (*continued*) Increased syncytial knots—numerous aggregates of large numbers of syncytiotrophoblastic nuclei within the villous trophoblast layer. **E:** Villous agglutination—small areas of aggregated villi with syncytial knots and intervillous fibrin (microinfarct). **F:** Mural hypertrophy of decidual arterioles–hypertrophy of the vascular smooth muscle wall (arteriolosclerosis). **G:** Acute atherosis of decidual arterioles—fibrinoid necrosis of the vascular smooth muscle wall with scattered aggregates of embedded lipid-laden macrophages.

angiotensinogen allele and/or the vasoactive mediators discussed above (82,90,105,182).

Clinical Correlation

Chronically underperfused placentas are associated with fetal growth restriction, premature birth owing to either premature labor or premature rupture of membranes, premature placental separation (abruptio placenta), and an increased risk for the development of preeclampsia (10,43,110,186). Clinical conditions predisposing to maternal underperfusion include type I diabetes mellitus, connective tissue disease, chronic renal insufficiency, essential hypertension, and underlying maternal coagulopathies including thrombophilic mutations and antiphospholipid syndrome (119). Familial aggregation of preeclampsia and underlying maternal vascular disease may at least in part be due to inheritance of the so-called metabolic syndrome characterized by abnormal serum lipid levels, enhanced production of acute phase inflammatory mediators, and a predisposition to vascular damage related to oxidative stress. These patients are often overweight and predisposed to developing cardiovascular disease, type II diabetes, and sleep-disordered breathing in later life.

Chronic Abruption

Background

As discussed above, lateral growth of the placenta involves remodeling of large uterine veins (39). These large obliquely oriented structures may rupture prematurely if poorly supported by the surrounding endometrium or subjected to elevated intramural pressure due to obstruction of larger upstream maternal veins (38,130). Unlike arterial rupture resulting in abruptio placenta, venous hemorrhages tend to occur at the placental margins and at relatively lower pressure (61). For these reasons, marginal separation may not cause immediate delivery but may instead present as threatened

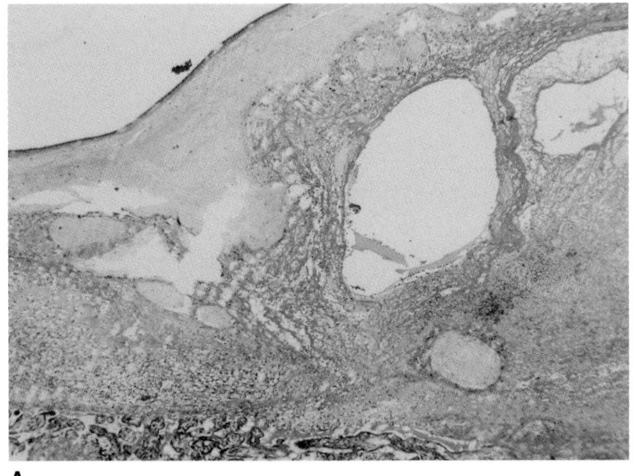

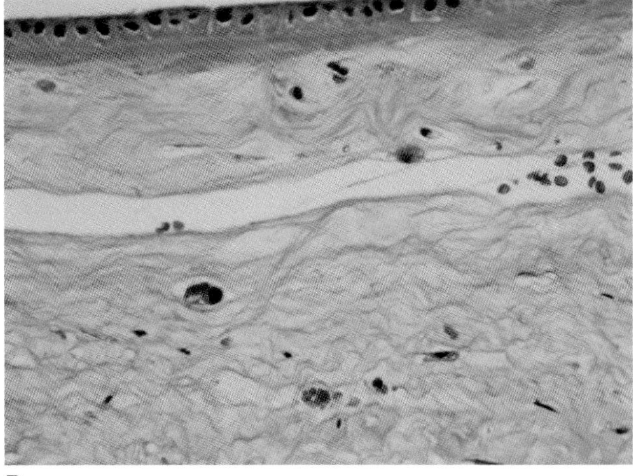

A B

FIGURE 9-10 ■ Chronic abruption: **A:** Circumvallation—nonperipheral membrane insertion with underlying organizing blood clot. **B:** Membrane hemosiderin—cytoplasmic golden-brown refractile pigment within macrophages in the chorioamnion.

abortion in early pregnancy or vaginal bleeding in later pregnancy. Factors that have been associated with chronic abruption include multiparity, smoking, oligohydramnios, and excessively deep uterine implantation (114,177).

Pathology

Chronic abruption, like maternal underperfusion, is associated with a constellation of placental findings. These include old marginal blood clot, circumvallate membrane insertion, chorioamnionic hemosiderin deposition, and green (biliverdin) staining of the fetal surface (Figure 9-10) (155). Circumvallation develops as a consequence of blood accumulating in the space between the decidua and chorion, leading to undermining or folding of the marginal chorionic plate. When circumvallation is attributable to chronic marginal separation, old blood clot and local hemosiderin deposition are seen on histologic sections. Hemosiderin stains blue by iron stain, but other hemoglobin-related pigments do not. Any pigment seen in a premature placenta favors chronic abruption rather than meconium release, which is uncommon before 37 weeks.

Clinical Correlation

Chronic abruption is often clinically associated with oligohydramnios, a syndrome known as the chronic abruption-oligohydramnios sequence (48). Chronic marginal hemorrhages may be detected by ultrasound as so-called subchorionic hemorrhages (74). Serial ultrasound studies have documented the development of circumvallation following repeated subchorionic hemorrhages (22). Chronic abruption is an important cause of preterm delivery and may be associated with an atypical form of neonatal lung disease (188). It is also a significant risk factor for cerebral palsy and other forms of neurologic impairment in term infants (118,149). Finally, acute marginal hemorrhages that result in immediate delivery (marginal abruptions) are important causes of preterm delivery and should be distinguished from abruptio placenta (see below) by pathologic examination.

Villitis of Unknown Etiology

Background

Diffuse chronic villous inflammation with fibrosis and mineralization is typical of relatively rare TORCH-type congenital infections (see above). Localized lymphohistiocytic villous inflammation is far more common and is seen in approximately 5% to 10% of term pregnancies (84). While these localized infiltrates could reflect unrecognized infections, extensive investigation over many years has failed to reveal organisms and neither the mothers nor the infants of these pregnancies have shown any consistent clinical or laboratory evidence of an infectious process. It has been shown that the villous infiltrates are largely composed of maternal T-lymphocytes (151). It is currently believed that this lesion, known by convention as villitis of unknown etiology (VUE), is the result of maternofetal cell trafficking with a localized host-versus-graft reaction in the villous tree. Maternofetal cell trafficking is a well-known phenomena in animal and human pregnancies and can rarely result in neonatal graft-versus-host disease and connective tissue diseases of childhood (16,117).

Pathology

The majority of cases of VUE are characterized by small groups of less than 10 affected villi in either a random or predominantly basal distribution (Figure 9-11A,B). Less commonly, larger groups of villi are involved (patchy or diffuse VUE) (Figure 9-11C). Stem villous vasculitis and perivasculitis are a special subcategory of VUE, where lymphocytic infiltration is not confined to the distal villous tree (Figure 9-11D). This pattern is often associated with extensive downstream avascular villi and has been termed obliterative fetal vasculopathy (139,143). All types of VUE are commonly accompanied by a lymphoplasmacytic infiltrate in the basal plate (chronic deciduitis). Diffuse perivillous fibrin deposition and intervillositis with a polymorphous inflammatory infiltrate including neutrophils (active chronic

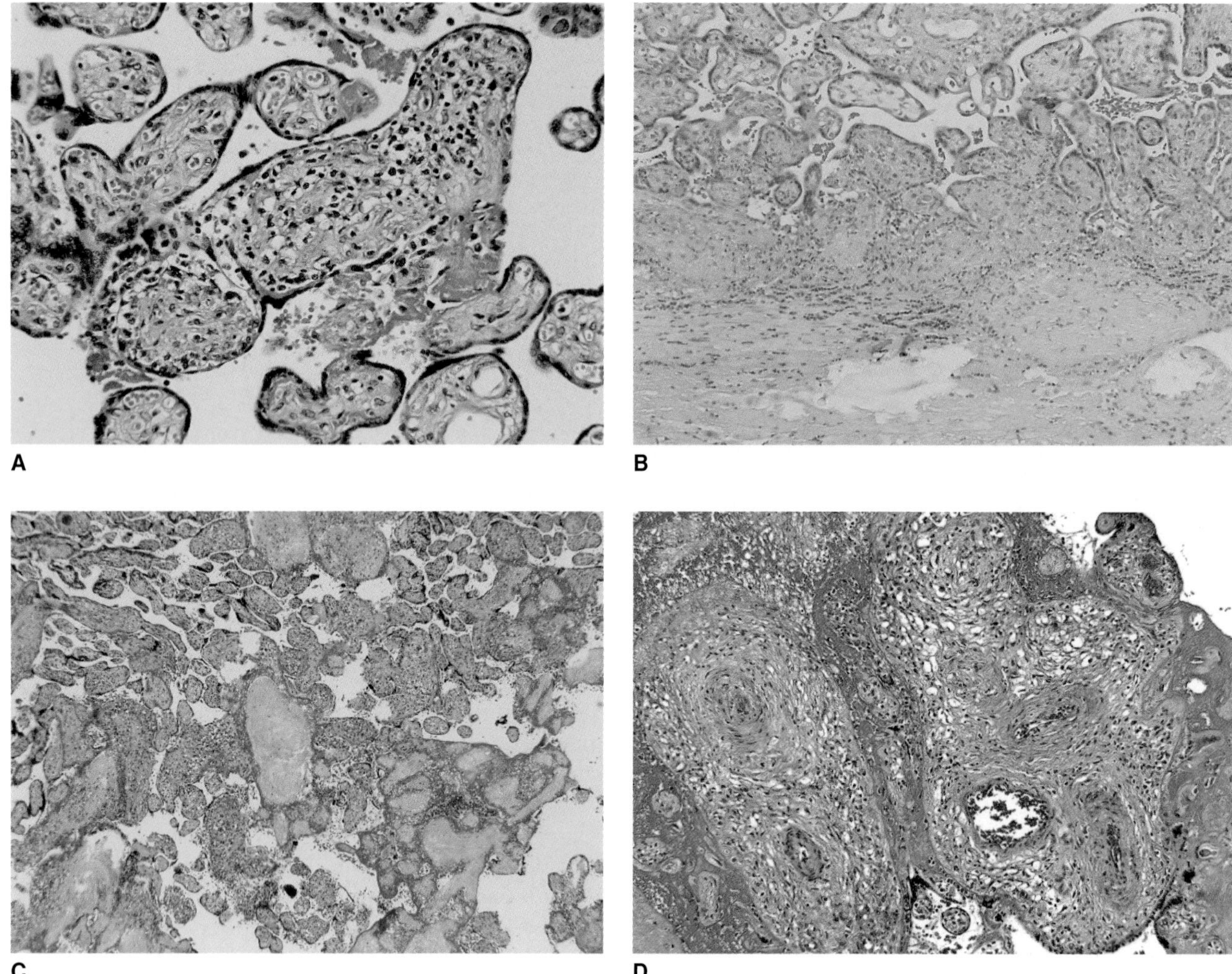

FIGURE 9-11 ■ Chronic villitis: **A:** Focal—clusters of less than ten villi with a nonuniform lymphohistiocytic infiltrate in the villous stroma. **B:** Basal—lymphohistiocytic infiltrate involving anchoring stem and adjacent villi accompanied by a lymphoplasmacytic infiltrate in the decidua basalis. **C:** Patchy/diffuse—aggregates of ten or more chronically inflamed villi. **D:** Obliterative fetal vasculopathy—marked perivascular chronic inflammation involving stem villi leading to vascular occlusion.

villitis) are other variations most commonly seen with patchy or diffuse VUE. The presence of neutrophils, plasma cells, or eosinophils increases the possibility of an underlying infection, which can be further evaluated by special stains and clinical correlation. Histiocytic giant cells, on the other hand, are common and do not suggest an infectious etiology.

Clinical Correlation

Focal and basal villitis are generally not associated with adverse outcomes (149). Basal villitis is more common with underlying uterine abnormalities such as malformations, leiomyomas, previous curettage, chronic endometritis, low implantation, and adherent placenta (142). Patchy and diffuse villitis is associated with IUGR, particularly when it occurs at term in the absence of hypertension (152). Stem villous vasculitis and perivasculitis with avascular villi (VUE with obliterative fetal vasculopathy) are associated with an increased risk of cerebral palsy and other forms of neurologic impairment. Recurrence of VUE occurs in approximately 10% to 25% of cases (142,160). This is particularly common with more severe involvement. A small subgroup of women experience recurrent fetal losses at all gestational ages secondary to diffuse chronic villitis. Also of interest is the association of VUE with ovum donation pregnancies where the fetus shares no antigens with the mother (125,175).

Fetal Vascular Thrombo-occlusive Disease

Background

Thrombo-occlusive lesions of large fetal vessels in the placenta and umbilical cord occur in the context of one or more of the classic triad of risk factors: vascular stasis, loss of endothelial resistance to coagulation, and circulatory hypercoagulability (143). Possible causes of fetal vascular stasis include prolonged umbilical cord obstruction, increased central venous pressure, and elevated hematocrit. Loss of endothelial resistance to coagulation may occur with severe fetal inflammation, antiphospholipid syndrome, and other forms of vessel wall damage. Circulatory hypercoagulability may be present with platelet disorders, maternal diabetes, or thrombophilic mutations involving protein C, protein S, antithrombin II, factor V, prothrombin 2010, and methyltetrahydrofolate reductase. Other causes of inherited and acquired thrombophilia are emerging with increasing recognition.

Pathology

Sustained proximal vascular occlusion leads to degenerative changes in the distal villous tree. Because of the extensive branching of the villous tree, changes in distal villi are a more sensitive indicator of disease than the obstructive lesions themselves. Long-standing occlusion of large fetal vessels leads to hyalinized avascular villi (Figure 9-12A) (150). Earlier stages lead to circulatory stasis with degeneration of red blood cells, endothelial cells, and villous stromal fibroblasts (Figure 9-12B). This pattern of change occurs diffusely in the placentas of stillbirths (52). When seen in a focal distribution in either livebirths or stillborns, it has been termed hemorrhagic endovasculitis (162) or more recently villous stromal-vascular karyorrhexis (143). Both types of degenerative villous change can affect large or small groups of villi and can either be localized or distributed throughout the placental parenchyma. When the number of affected villi exceeds an average of ≥15 villi/slide, the term fetal thrombotic vasculopathy is used. Thrombi in large fetal vessels are identified in approximately one-third of such cases (Figure 9-12C). Other lesions associated with fetal thrombo-occlusive disease include intimal fibrin cushions and fibromuscular sclerosis of stem arteries (45). Intimal fibrin cushions are intramural aggregates of fibrin or fibrinoid in proximal fetal veins that may be attributable to increased intramural pressure (Figure 9-12D). At late stages, they may undergo mineralization. Fibromuscular sclerosis represents concentric narrowing of the vascular lumen by proliferating smooth muscle cells and subendothelial fibroblasts, typically occurring in placental vessels lying between the point of occlusion and the distal villi secondary to lack of flow (Figure 9-12E).

Clinical Correlation

Fetal thrombotic vasculopathy is a significant risk factor for cerebral palsy and other forms of neurologic impairment in term infants (86,137,149). It may also be associated with other manifestations of thromboembolic disease in the fetus

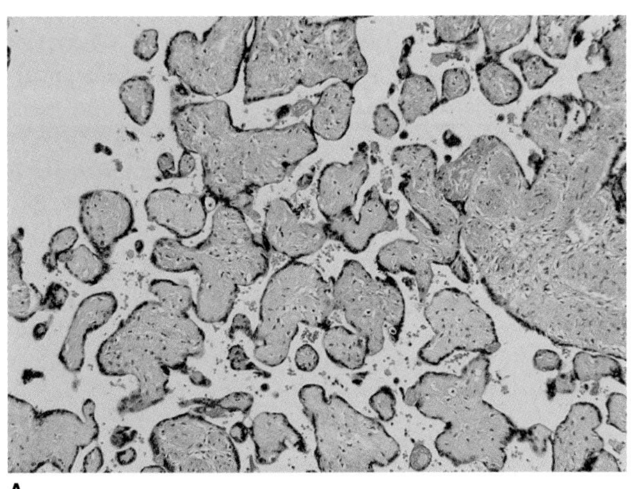

A

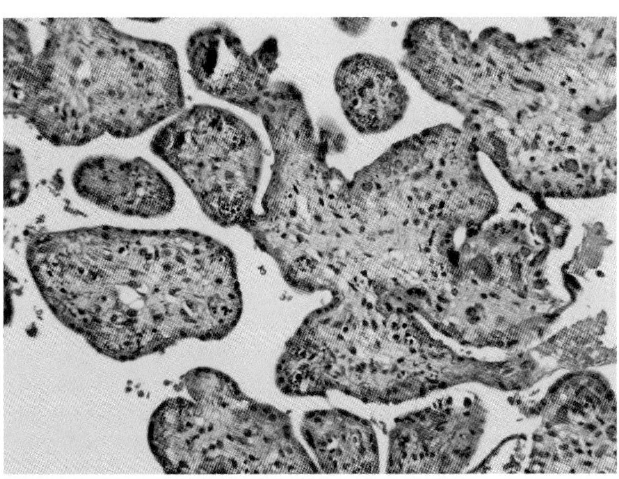

B

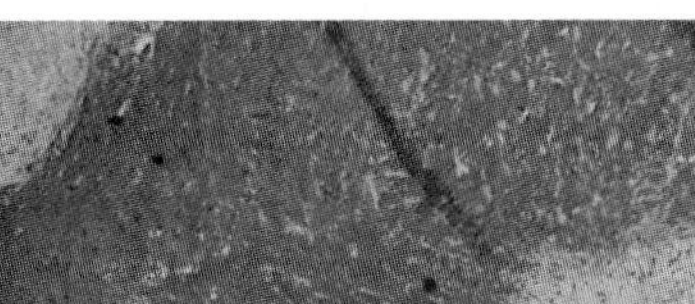

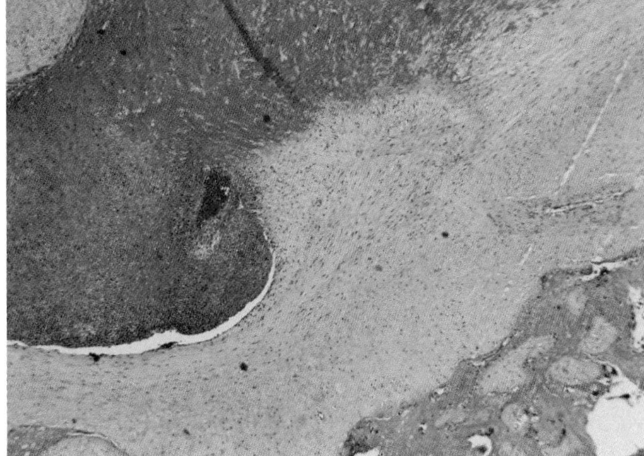

C

FIGURE 9-12 ▪ Fetal thrombo-occlusive lesions: **A:** Extensive hyalinized avascular distal villi. **B:** Distal villi with degenerative stromal-vascular karyorrhexis. **C:** Occlusive stem villous thrombus.

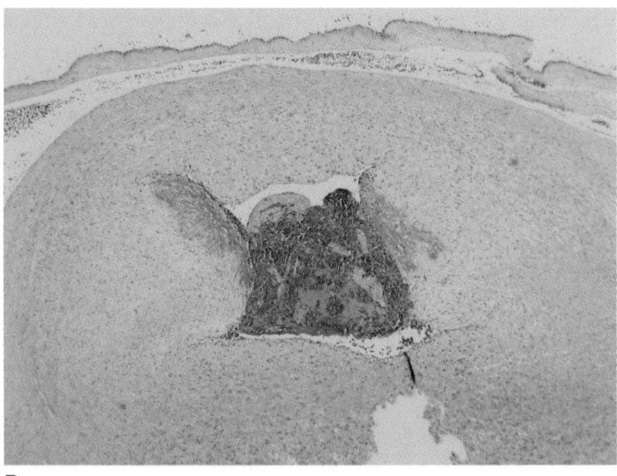

D

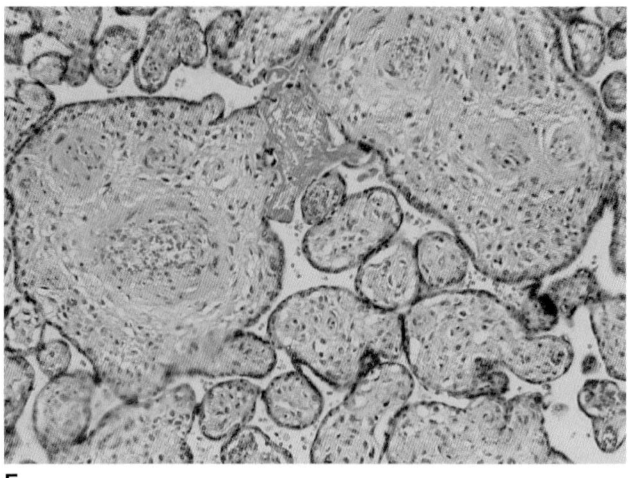

E

FIGURE 9-12 ■ (*continued*) **D:** Recent intimal fibrin cushions—layered subendothelial eosinophilic fibrin/matrix deposits in the walls of large stem villous or chorionic veins. **E:** Fibromuscular sclerosis—concentric fibrosis of large fetal vessels with entrapment of degenerating red blood cells.

including renal vein thrombosis, perinatal liver disease, and limb infarction (41,122). Avascular villi are also associated with IUGR, chronic monitoring abnormalities, and discordant twin growth (134,152). Nonocclusive thrombi in severely inflamed chorionic vessels are occasionally seen with severe acute chorioamnionitis in very low–birth-weight infants and represent a risk factor for neurologic impairment in this subgroup (156).

Massive Perivillous Fibrin Deposition ("Maternal Floor Infarction")

Background

Massive perivillous fibrin deposition is characterized by the accumulation of excessive amounts of fibrin and extracellular matrix-rich fibrinoid around gas-exchanging distal villi in the lower two-thirds of the placenta (9,35,108). It should be distinguished from increased intervillous fibrin owing to maternal underperfusion, which usually begins around proximal villi in the upper portions of the placenta (7). Deposition of fibrin and/or other matrix components could be the primary abnormality providing a substrate that may promote differentiation of villous to intermediate trophoblasts followed by migration into the intervillous space. Alternatively, the lesion may represent an aberrant response to trophoblastic injury in which cytotrophoblasts generate intermediate trophoblasts, rather than syncytiotrophoblasts (trophoblastic metaplasia). These intermediate trophoblasts would then, in turn, secrete large quantities of extracellular matrix proteins that surround the distal villous tree (42,50). Massive perivillous fibrin deposition is idiopathic and often recurrent in subsequent pregnancies. Maternal autoimmune disease, preeclampsia, and thrombophilic states have all been implicated in its pathogenesis (18,78,163). Case reports of discordancy in twins and an association with fetal long-chain acyl CoA dehydrogenase deficiency suggest a fetal genetic component as well (97,148).

Pathology

Massive perivillous fibrin deposition occurs in two distinct patterns: basal-predominant with a rind-like gross thickening of the basal plate and diffuse with fine lacy strands of firm with fibrin marbling the entire cut surface of the placenta. Microscopically, distal villi are surrounded by a matrix of fibrin and fibrinoid elements intermixed with large numbers of intermediate trophoblasts (Figure 9-13). In some cases, degenerative changes such as eosinophilia or karyorrhexis of villous trophoblasts and stroma may be seen. The lesion is distinguished from villous infarction by lack of villous agglutination and the absence of degenerating cellular debris in the intervillous space. Localized plaques of perivillous fibrin and increased intervillous fibrin in areas of marginal placental atrophy may be seen at all gestational ages (51). These localized lesions should not be mistaken for massive perivillous fibrin deposition.

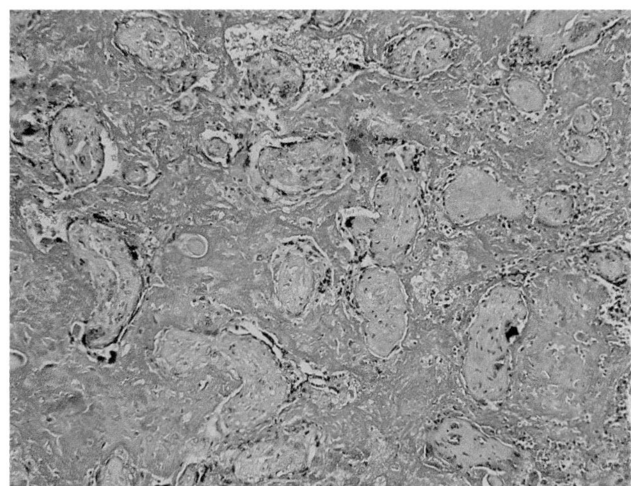

FIGURE 9-13 ■ Massive perivillous fibrin deposition/maternal floor infarction: eosinophilic fibrin/ matrix material with embedded intermediate trophoblasts completely surrounding large portions of the distal villous tree.

Clinical Correlation

Massive perivillous fibrin deposition ("maternal floor infarction") is a rare but important placental lesion associated with spontaneous abortion, stillbirth, severe IUGR, and neurologic impairment (2,9,108). It is a recognized cause of recurrent reproductive failure (13). It most commonly begins in the late second and early third trimester and can develop quite rapidly. It has been associated with a typical sonographic picture, which some have termed a "jelly-like" placenta (72). Severe IUGR, decreased pulsed flow Doppler studies, and abnormal biophysical profile are common, and delivery at the earliest possible opportunity is recommended (95). No controlled trials of therapy have been conducted. Empiric use of heparin, aspirin, or immunomodulatory agents has been attempted in some cases.

Villous Capillary Proliferations (Chorangioma/Chorangiomatosis/ Chorangiosis)

Background

As described above, early vascularization of the first trimester placenta occurs by vasculogenesis. Mesenchymal precursor cells form vessels de novo under the inductive influence of adjacent villous trophoblasts. At later stages of pregnancy, new vessels form by angiogenesis in which new vessels arise via budding and sprouting from existing vessels. Angiogenic growth factors such as VEGF released under the influence of hypoxia, growth factors, or inflammatory cytokines can stimulate reactive villous capillary proliferative lesions at several sites in the mature placenta (121).

Pathology

Chorangiomas are spherical expansile lesions usually found arising from major stem villi under the chorionic plate or at the placental margins (Figure 9-14A). Histologically, they resemble capillary hemangiomas and are composed of a mixture of endothelial cells, pericytes, and myofibroblastic stromal cells. Associated nonspecific surface trophoblastic proliferation is seen in up to 40% of cases and is benign (81). Chorangiomatosis can arise in the loose reticular connective tissue of either stem or intermediate villi. The lesion is composed of small vessels with endothelial cells and pericytes surrounding an intact central villous core (Figure 9-14B). Rather than expanding eccentrically to form a mass as in chorangioma, the vessels in localized chorangiomatosis extend proximally, distally, and around their site of origin. Diffuse multifocal involvement of immature intermediate villi appears to be a distinct pattern. Chorangiosis is confined to distal villi, and the vessels are lined by endothelium alone (Figure 9-14C). The threshold for making a diagnosis of chorangiosis is the presence of ten or more capillary cross sections in ten or more villi in several areas of the placenta (3). Occasional villi with 15 to 20 or more capillaries are usually identified (174).

Clinical Correlation

Chorangiomas are most frequent at sites such as the placental margin and with scenarios such as preeclampsia and multiple gestations that are associated with relative hypoxia (19,121). They may be multifocal in rare cases and are occasionally associated with hemangiomas in the fetus. When large, they can serve as niduses for fetal consumptive coagulopathy or may act as arteriovenous shunts leading to heart failure and hydrops fetalis (75,176). Localized chorangiomatosis and chorangioma have similar associations, while diffuse multifocal chorangiomatosis is more common in preterm placentas and has been associated with IUGR (121). Chorangiosis is most common in large diabetic placentas but often accompanies placentas with other chronic and subacute pathologic processes (3,170). It is also seen in placentas delivered at high altitude and may be a compensatory physiologic adaptation to reduced oxygen tension without maternal underperfusion of the intervillous space. Villous capillary vascular lesions of all three types are increased in Beckwith-Wiedemann syndrome as is mesenchymal dysplasia, a more pervasive abnormality presenting with abnormal large and small fetal vessels, increased villous connective tissue, and villous cavitation (Figure 9-14D) (71). Mesenchymal dysplasia has also been associated with several types of confined placental mosaicism (11,64) (see Chapter 3).

Subacute Disease Processes

Amniotic Fluid Infection/Chorioamnionitis

Background

The products of conception develop in the normally sterile uterine cavity. Parturition, however, requires an outlet to the external environment. This outlet, the cervicovaginal tract, like most other body orifices has a rich and complex microbial flora that can include aerobic and anaerobic bacteria, mycoplasma, and fungi. This environment can also transiently harbor organisms with a particular capacity to infect the products of conception. These include group B streptococci, *Listeria monocytogenes*, and the predominantly anaerobic flora associated with bacterial vaginosis. A connection between the gestational sac and the cervicovaginal tract does not occur until about 18 to 19 weeks of gestation (55). After that time, the secretory immune system, structural integrity of the cervix, and the placental membranes serve to protect the fetoplacental unit from ascending infection. Failure of one or more of these mechanisms may allow organisms to enter the endometrium or amniotic fluid. Local immunosuppressive mechanisms, fetal immunologic immaturity, and the anatomic enclosure of the fetoplacental unit all inhibit effective immune responses at these sites. The early inflammatory response to ascending infection is composed of maternal neutrophils emanating from the intervillous circulation and small venules in the membranous decidua (26,27). Later this maternal response may be supplemented by a fetal response composed of neutrophils emanating from large vessels of the umbilical cord and chorionic plate. The localization of the inflammatory response reflects the site of infection in the amniotic cavity and the placental layers through which maternal and fetal neutrophils migrate (chorion and amnion).

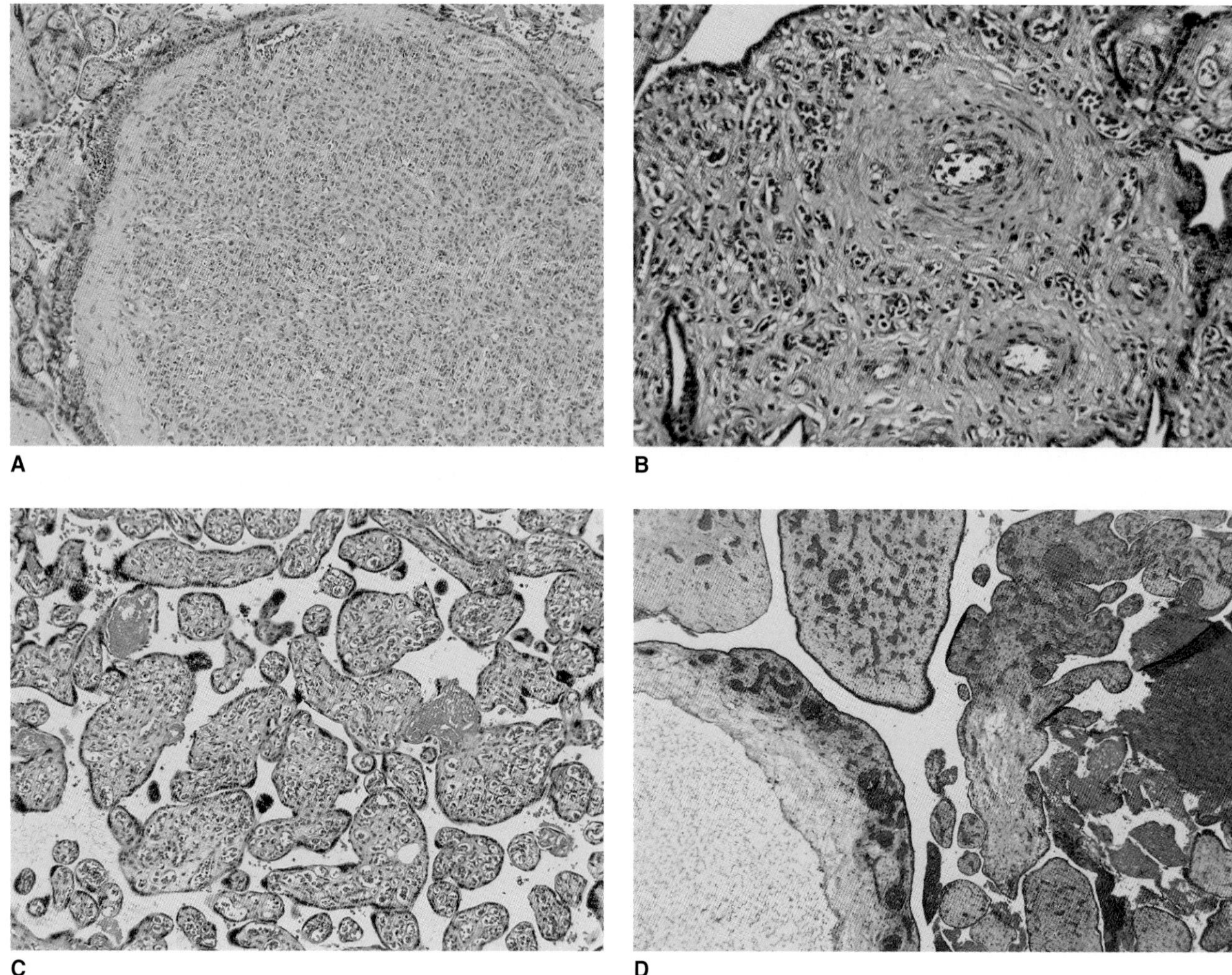

FIGURE 9-14 Villous capillary lesions: **A:** Chorangioma—nodular vascular tumor composed of capillaries, surrounding pericytes, and adjacent fibrous stroma. **B:** Chorangiomatosis—proliferating capillaries with surrounding pericytes in the outer reticular zone of an immature intermediate villus. **C:** Chorangiosis—increased (>10) number of capillary cross sections in the terminal villi. **D:** Mesenchymal dysplasia—varying combinations of increased small and large fetal vessels, excessive villous stroma, and cavitated edematous cisterns affecting large segments of the villous tree.

While the majority of amniotic fluid infections occur via the ascending route, other mechanisms including hematogenous spread from distant sites, contiguous spread from other pelvic organs, and direct inoculation of organisms during diagnostic procedures such as amniocentesis also occur.

Pathology

The pathologic description of chorioamnionitis must be separated into its two components: the maternal and fetal responses. Each of these in turn should be subcategorized in terms of spatiotemporal progression (stage) and severity (grade) (145). The stages of maternal infection are (a) acute subchorionitis (neutrophils restricted to subchorionic fibrin and the membranous decidual-chorionic interface) (Figure 9-15A), (b) acute chorioamnionitis (neutrophils in chorion and amnion), and (c) necrotizing chorioamnionitis (signs of amnion necrosis) (Figure 9-15B). These signs include karyorrhexis of neutrophils, desquamation of amnionic epithelial cells, and intense eosinophilia of the amnionic basement membrane. The stages of fetal infection are (a) neutrophils in chorionic vessels (chorionic vasculitis) and/or umbilical vein (umbilical phlebitis), (b) neutrophils in one or both umbilical arteries (umbilical arteritis), and (c) neutrophils and neutrophilic debris forming arcs around umbilical vessels in the Wharton jelly (necrotizing funisitis) (Figure 9-15C). Severe maternal responses are characterized by large accumulations of neutrophils (microabscesses) under the chorion (79). Severe fetal responses are characterized by near confluent neutrophilic infiltrates in the amnionic side of chorionic vessels with attenuation and degenerative changes of the vessel wall (intense chorionic vasculitis) (Figure 9-15D). Severe fetal responses may in some cases lead to the formation of mural thrombi in affected vessels.

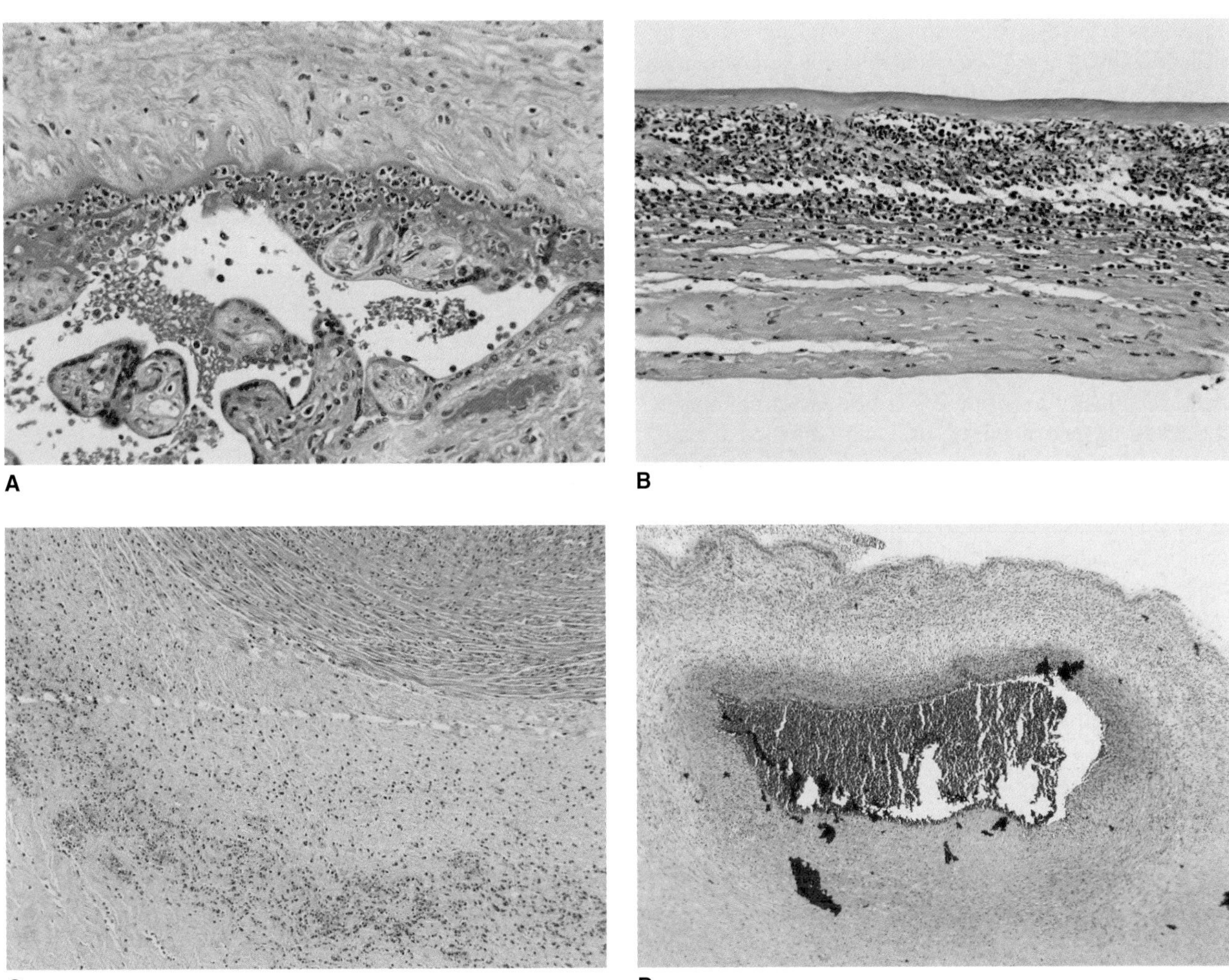

FIGURE 9-15 ■ Chorioamnionitis: **A:** Early subchorionitis—diffuse neutrophilic infiltration of the subchorionic fibrin. **B:** Necrotizing chorioamnionitis—necrosis and sloughage of amniocytes combined with a thickened eosinophilic basement membrane and karyorrhexis of adjacent neutrophils. **C:** Necrotizing funisitis—loosely organized perivascular arcs of eosinophilic precipitate and degenerating neutrophilic debris in the umbilical Wharton jelly. **D:** Intense chorionic vasculitis—near confluent neutrophilic infiltration of the amnionic side of major chorionic vessels accompanied by myocyte disarray and/or endothelial activation.

Clinical Correlation

The prevalence of histologic chorioamnionitis is inversely proportional to gestational age reaching over 50% below 28 weeks (33,106). It is believed that placental infection is the leading cause of premature delivery at less than 32 weeks. In some cases, chorioamnionitis may be preceded by premature membrane rupture. Bacterial vaginosis is another risk factor for infection (53). In general, the ability to effectively eradicate intrauterine infections with antibiotics is limited and preterm delivery is inevitable. Spread of organisms from the infected placenta to the fetus (early onset sepsis) is much less common, and chorioamnionitis is rarely the direct cause of intrauterine fetal death. An exception is untreated group B streptococcal infection, which is associated with a higher but still limited risk of fetal infection. Recently, the fetal response to amniotic fluid infection has received special attention (fetal inflammatory response syndrome). It is currently believed that various aspects of this response including circulating cytokines, bacterial toxins, and activation of the coagulation cascade predispose to cerebral palsy and other forms of neurologic impairment (56,91,135). A role for fetal inflammatory response syndrome in the development of chronic lung disease has also been proposed with conflicting evidence (57,157,178).

Amniotic Fluid Meconium

Background

Acute episodes of *in utero* hypoxia, regardless of duration, can trigger redistribution of blood flow resulting in the release of fetal stool (meconium) into the amniotic fluid (101). This vagally mediated reflex is believed to represent an adaptation preserving adequate perfusion to more critical vascular beds such as the central nervous and cardiovascular systems.

In most cases, the hypoxic episodes are brief and caused by transient umbilical cord occlusion, which is common after 39 weeks as the fetus continues to grow and move in the face of decrease in the amount of protective amniotic fluid and umbilical cord Wharton jelly. Meconium is composed of large amounts of bile acid and phospholipases that have direct caustic effects on fetal and placental tissues. Particularly important are effects on umbilical and chorionic blood vessels (5). The amount of meconium passed and the volume of fluid available to suspend it are important variables in determining its effects on the placenta and fetal lungs. Since meconium diffuses relatively slowly through fetoplacental tissues, duration of exposure is a critical factor in terms of toxic effects on fetal blood vessels. Longer duration of exposure is also significant insofar as it is an indicator of hypoxia occurring more remote from the time of labor and delivery. Meconium increases the risk for chorioamnionitis by several mechanisms including neutralization of bacterial inhibitory factors in amniotic fluid and direct chemotactic properties (128). In some cases, prolonged meconium exposure and severe fetal chorioamnionitis may synergize to cause chorionic vessel injury.

Pathology

The pathologist's role is to determine the chronicity and secondary effects of meconium exposure. Meconium is a fine particulate red-brown pigment generally found within the vacuolated cytoplasm of tissue macrophages. Other membrane pigments such as hemosiderin and lipofuscin are morphologically distinct, are not associated with a clinical history of meconium-stained fluid, and do not cause degenerative changes in the amnion such as dehiscence from the chorion, necrosis of amniocytes, and connective tissue edema (Figure 9-16A). Estimating the duration of meconium exposure is inexact (102). It is believed that meconium pigment–laden macrophages appear in amnion approximately 1 hour after release. Spread to the membranous decidua takes at least 3 hours. Significant accumulations of pigment-laden macrophages in the deeper layers of the chorionic plate and Wharton jelly, and green staining of the umbilical cord probably take at least 6 to 12 hours (Figure 9-16B). A rare and clinically significant lesion associated with prolonged meconium exposure is meconium-associated vascular necrosis (4). This lesion is characterized by apoptotic cell death of peripheral myocytes in the umbilical and chorionic vessels (Figure 9-16C).

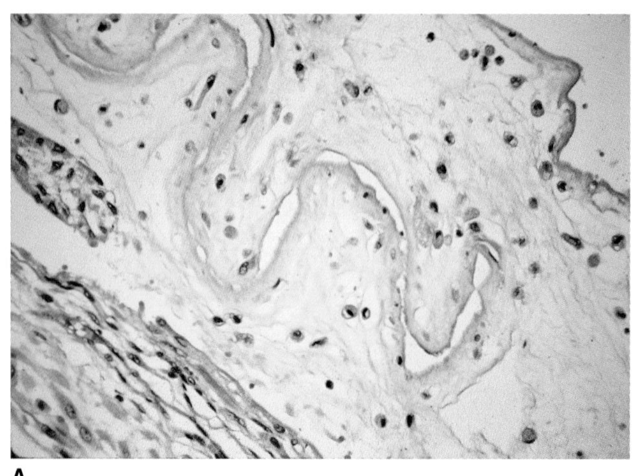
A

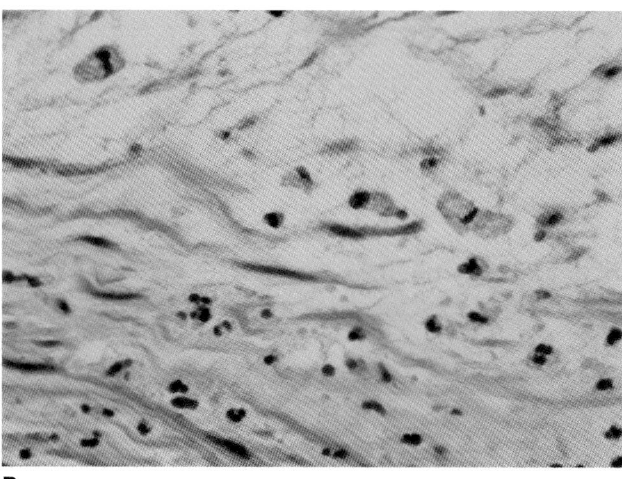
B

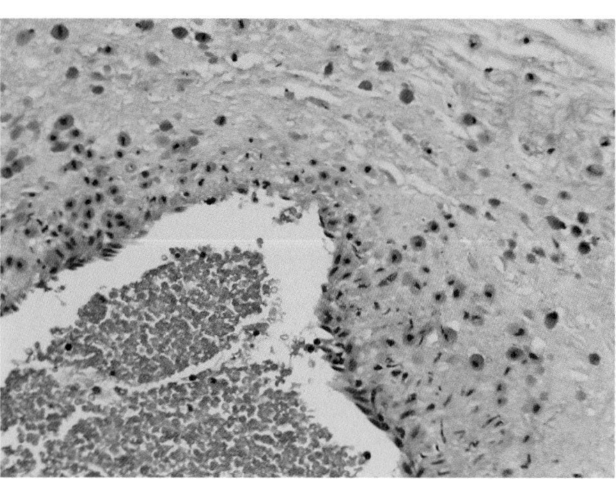
C

FIGURE 9-16 Meconium: **A:** Numerous vacuolated pigment-laden macrophages and amnionic edema with necrosis of amniocytes. **B:** Numerous vacuolated pigment-laden macrophages deep in the connective tissue of the chorionic plate. **C:** Meconium-associated vascular necrosis—diffuse eosinophilic cytoplasmic degeneration and nuclear pyknosis (apoptosis) of peripheral vascular smooth muscle cells in the vessels of the chorionic plate and/or umbilical cord.

Clinical Correlation

Meconium passage occurs in approximately 14% of all deliveries but rarely occurs before 34 weeks of gestation. While statistically associated with obstetric and neonatal complications, it is neither a specific nor a sensitive indicator for them. Meconium-associated vascular necrosis has been strongly associated with cerebral palsy and other adverse neurologic outcomes (149). The presence of abundant pigment-laden macrophages in the chorionic plate also has a borderline significant association with adverse outcome (138). The meconium aspiration syndrome is defined as respiratory distress requiring oxygen therapy associated with meconium release and an abnormal chest x-ray (159). It is associated with serious respiratory and neurologic complications and a significant mortality rate. It occurs in 11% of meconium-stained infants and has been correlated with the presence of meconium below the vocal cords. However, prompt suctioning of meconium from the airways after delivery has not made a major impact on morbidity and mortality (77). Current thinking suggests that meconium aspiration syndrome is largely due to significant perinatal stresses that lead to the deep aspiration of the meconium prior to birth.

Fetomaternal Hemorrhage

Background

One of the consequences of the close proximity of maternal and fetal circulations in the placenta is that small disruptions in the integrity of the villous tree can lead to fetal hemorrhage into the intervillous space. Some degree of fetomaternal hemorrhage has been estimated to occur in at least 50% of all pregnancies, and fetal cells may persist in the mother for many years leading to modulation of the immune response and in some cases maternal autoimmune diseases such as scleroderma (117). More substantial hemorrhages of 0.5 to 40 mL occur in 8% of pregnancies and hemorrhages of greater than 40 mL in 0.3% to 1% of pregnancies (49). Diagnosis of fetomaternal hemorrhages depends on either flow cytometry or the Kleihauer-Betke test. These tests are performed on a peripheral blood sample from the mother, and the volume of hemorrhage is calculated from the percentage of fetal cells relative to the maternal blood volume.

Pathology

Definitive diagnosis of massive fetomaternal hemorrhage can be confirmed only by direct measurement of fetal red blood cells in the maternal circulation. Placental findings, which suggest the diagnosis in the proper clinical context are intervillous thrombi (Figure 9-17A), markedly increased circulating nucleated red blood cells (NRBC) (Figure 9-17B), or signs of developing hydrops fetalis (placentomegaly, villous immaturity, diffuse villous edema) (Figure 9-17C). NRBCs are discussed below. Intervillous thrombi are spherical collections of clotted blood that are completely surrounded by villous tissue. They have been shown to represent sites of fetomaternal hemorrhage (76). However, they are extremely common and are not, in most cases, associated with large volume bleeds. The finding of multiple or large intervillous thrombi increases the probability of a clinically significant hemorrhage.

Clinical Correlation

Predisposing factors for massive fetomaternal hemorrhage include severe maternal underperfusion of the placenta; large edematous placentas associated with fetal congestive heart failure; and traumatic insults including abruptio placenta, amniocentesis, maternal trauma, or external cephalic version. Most cases have none of these predisposing factors (49). Cases may present *in utero* with decreased fetal movements, nonreactive fetal monitoring, or a distinct sinusoidal fetal heart rate pattern. Affected fetuses and neonates can develop circulatory collapse, CNS damage, hydrops fetalis, or stillbirth due to a combination of hypovolemia and chronic high output congestive heart failure due to profound fetal anemia (89).

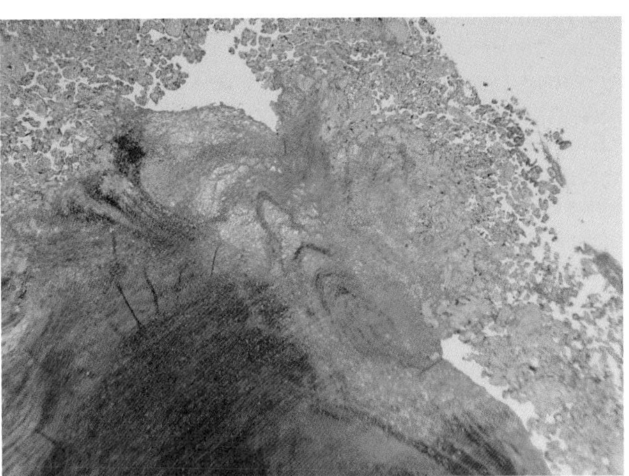

A

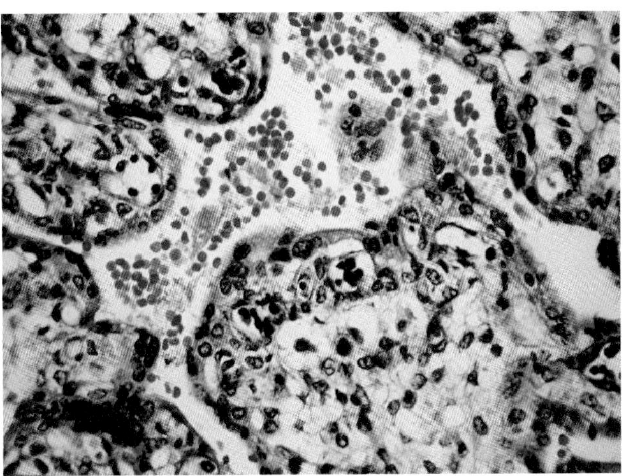

B

FIGURE 9-17 ■ Fetomaternal hemorrhage/increased NRBC. **A:** Intervillous thrombus—fresh laminated hematoma completely surrounded by distal villi. **B:** Marked increase in circulating NRBC—clusters of immature nucleated red blood cells including erythroblasts in villous capillaries.

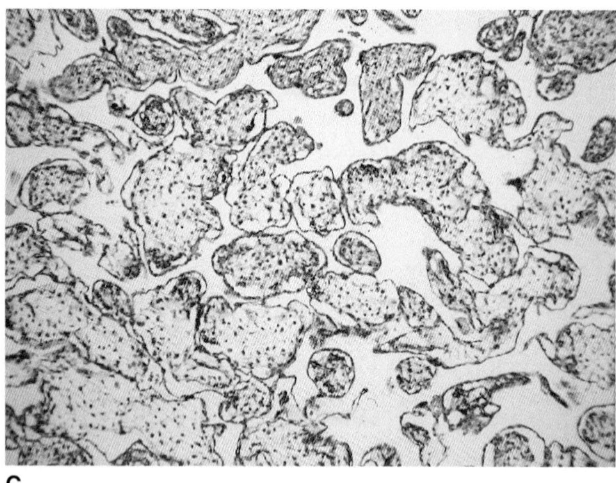

C

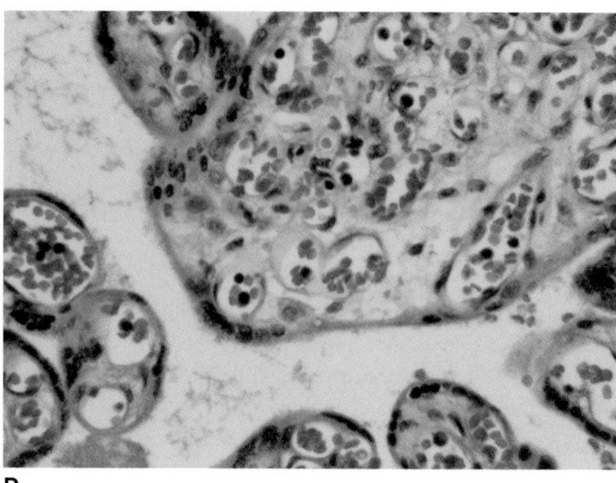

D

FIGURE 9-17 (*continued*) **C:** Villous hydrops-marked stromal edema with artifactual dehiscence of the villous trophoblastic layer. **D:** Mild-to-moderate increase in circulating NRBC—scattered normoblasts in terminal villous capillaries

Prolonged/Repetitive Antenatal Hypoxia

Background

Prolonged or repetitive shorter periods of antenatal fetal hypoxia are well-documented causes of CNS damage in experimental pregnancy models and selected clinical cases (107). While the underlying cause of hypoxia is sometimes indicated by one or more of the pathologic lesions discussed above, in other cases, the insults are not accompanied by recognizable tissue changes. One useful indicator of sustained significant hypoxia is the finding of an increased number of circulating NRBC in the placental circulation (113,171). This physiologic response is the result of both premature release of red blood cell precursors into the systemic circulation and, later, increased fetal erythropoiesis. It is, at least in part, mediated by hypoxia-inducible elements in the promoter regions of erythropoietin.

Pathology

The identification of increased NRBCs in the placental circulation is most important in cases such as stillbirths where early neonatal blood counts are not available. While erythroblastosis is readily identified (Figure 9-17B), the recognition of lesser numbers of circulating normoblasts requires a conscious effort to inspect several fields of distal villi at 40× magnification in every case (Figure 9-17D). A relatively simple semiquantitative method for the estimation of increased NRBCs in the placenta has been described (140). Others have actually counted NRBCs in cross sections of large umbilical or chorionic vessels (40).

Clinical Correlation

Increased NRBCs reflect decreased oxygen availability in the fetal hematopoietic microenvironment. This can occur secondary to maternal hypoxemia, decreased placental oxygen transfer, or insufficient fetal oxygen-carrying capacity (anemia). Accumulation of red blood cell precursors in hematopoietic tissues and their subsequent release in large numbers in the fetal circulation require a time interval measured in hours. Variable estimates of the time required vary from 2 to 24 hours and are controversial (62,112). Our patient data and the available animal studies suggest that a marked significant elevation in a previously normal host probably requires at least 6 to 12 hours to develop (25,103,140). Persistence of elevated NRBCs for several days postnatally may indicate a longer period of antenatal hypoxia associated with markedly increased fetal erythropoiesis.

Acute Disease Processes

Abruptio Placenta

Background

Abruptio placenta (placental abruption), the sudden separation of a significant portion of the placenta from its underlying maternal blood supply prior to delivery, is one important cause of acute hypoxic injury. While separation can occur at any location, clinically significant abruptions tend to occur in the central part of the disc and tend to involve the rupture of maternal spiral arteries rather than veins. Three major factors are associated with arterial rupture: (a) an abnormal vessel wall (e.g., acute atherosis in preeclampsia), (b) physical force (e.g., increased luminal pressure secondary to severe hypertension or shear force associated with maternal trauma), and (c) ischemia-reperfusion injury (e.g., vasospasm associated with substance abuse involving cocaine or nicotine) (1,120,186). Other processes leading to sudden catastrophic uteroplacental separation include cervical dilatation with placenta previa and uterine rupture with attempted vaginal delivery following a previous C-section.

Pathology

It is often stated that the correlation between pathologic and clinical abruption is poor (59). Indeed vaginal bleeding followed by immediate delivery can occur in the absence of placental lesions. Likewise, clinical signs and symptoms of abruption may also prove unreliable. The gold standard for diagnosis of abruptio placenta is direct visualization of retroplacental hemorrhage at the time of C-section. Nevertheless, most placentas in cases of abruptio placenta show one or more of a constellation of findings that allow a diagnosis of findings consistent with abruption to be made with some confidence. The best pathologic evidence is a finding of a retroplacental hematoma with either placental indentation or intraplacental extension (Figure 9-18A). In the absence of these findings, microscopic evidence of interstitial hemorrhage in the basal plate or diffuse retromembranous hemorrhage is helpful. Ischemic changes in the overlying placenta such as recent villous infarction (Figure 9-18B) or villous stromal hemorrhage (Figure 9-18C) are also highly suggestive of abruption (104). Finally, lesions associated with chronic maternal underperfusion, as listed above, are often associated with abruption and can help strengthen a strong clinical suspicion of the diagnosis (46).

Clinical Correlation

The classical clinical signs of abruptio placenta include vaginal bleeding, abdominal pain, and uterine rigidity. Abruption is associated with a number of adverse outcomes including preterm delivery, fetal growth restriction, stillbirth, and hypoxic ischemic encephalopathy (8,111). Hypertension, maternal substance abuse, advanced maternal age, low pregnancy weight gain, grand multiparity, and strenuous physical labor are known predisposing risk factors. A subgroup of patients have repetitive abruptions and both inherited and acquired maternal coagulation disorders may play a role in some of these patients (66,83,184).

Umbilical Cord Occlusion

Background

A second common cause of acute hypoxic injury is complete obstruction to umbilical blood flow (cord occlusion). Obstruction to flow can occur via a variety of mechanisms including occlusive umbilical venous thrombi, tight true knots, compression of the cord between the fetus and the bony pelvis, hypercoiling, torsion of bridging vessels associated with anomalous cord insertions (marginal, membranous, furcate) and cord entanglements around fetal body parts (12,36,85,94,173). Several scenarios increase the risk of cord occlusion including decreased Wharton jelly, increased cord length, decreased amniotic fluid volume, sudden changes in

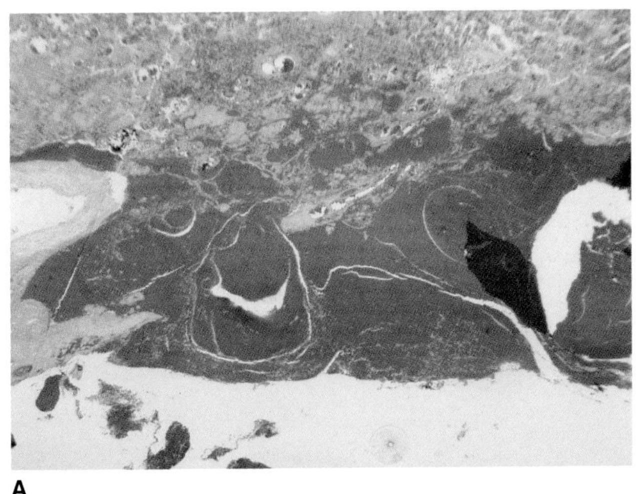

A

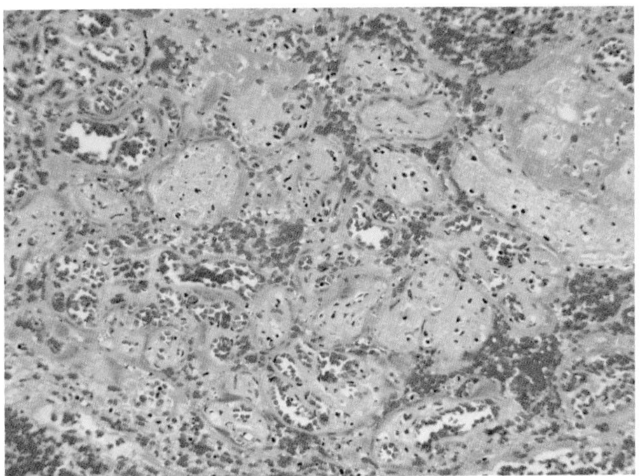

B

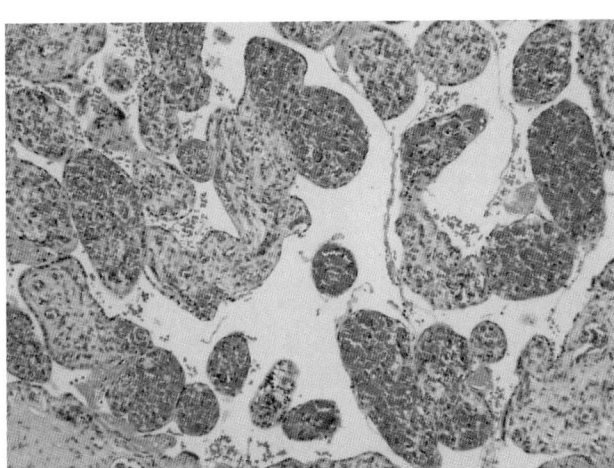

C

FIGURE 9-18 ■ Recent abruption: **A:** Laminated blood clot spreading within, indenting, and focally perforating the basal plate. **B:** Recent villous infarction—eosinophilic degeneration and karyorrhexis of villous trophoblast with partial collapse of the intervillous space. **C:** Villous stromal hemorrhage—diffuse fresh hemorrhage filling the stroma of immature distal villi.

fetal position, and fetal thrombophilic states. The umbilical vein is the more easily compressed structure by virtue of its thin wall and its nonduplicated status compared to the umbilical arteries. Cord occlusion prevents oxygenated placental venous blood from returning to the fetus and may be associated with dramatic differences between umbilical arterial and venous pH and base excess values (96).

Pathology

The umbilical cord itself may show a distinct abnormality such as a tight overhand knot (Figure 9-19A). Sometimes, the only gross clue is a difference in diameter and/or color on opposite sides of a putative site of obstruction (Figure 9-19B). In other cases, obstruction can be inferred by changes within the placenta such as intimal fibrin cushions (increased venous pressure) or villous stromal karyorrhexis (circulatory stasis). More recently, the degree of dilatation in chorionic stem villous veins has been used to help make the diagnosis of cord obstruction as a cause of stillbirth (Figure 9-19C) (124). Also important is documentation of pathologic abnormalities that may predispose to cord obstruction such as long, thin, hypercoiled, and/or marginally inserted umbilical cords (Figure 9-19D).

Clinical Correlation

A recent study found either clinical or pathologic abnormalities of the umbilical cord in 63% of term infants with cerebral palsy (133). Cord occlusion is also a well-recognized, although occasionally controversial, cause of intrauterine fetal demise (124). Prolapse of the cord with compression between the fetus and pelvic brim is most commonly seen in premature or breech deliveries and can be a cause of intrapartum death. Transient umbilical cord occlusion during labor is believed to be responsible for the fetal heart rate abnormality known as variable decelerations. Variable decelerations can develop a "late" component, a pattern indicative of acidosis and suggestive of more prolonged and severe occlusion. The correlation between clinical cord entanglements and outcome is weak and controversial. This reflects the fact that the severity and duration of cord occlusion are poorly estimated by the observed state of the cord at the time of delivery.

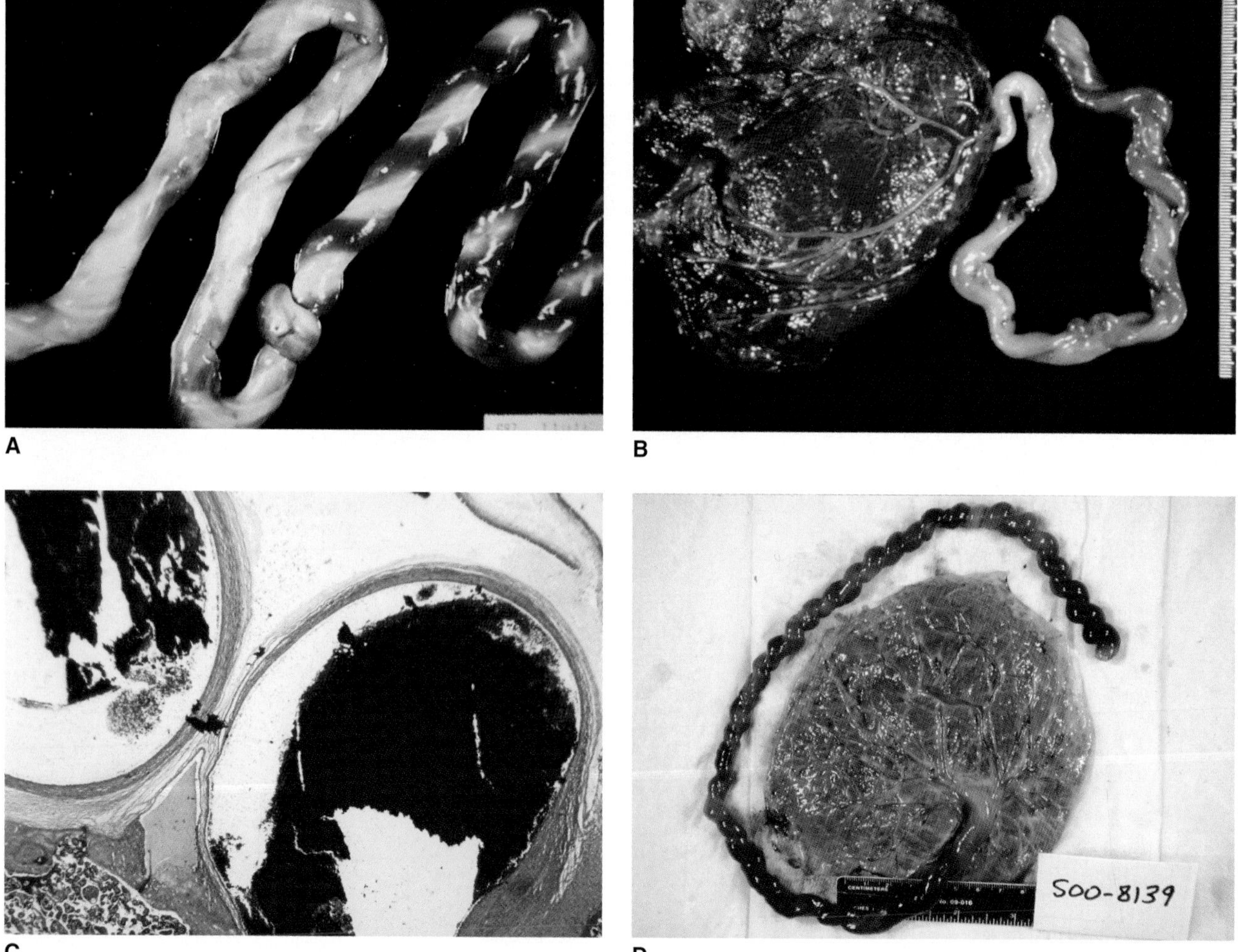

FIGURE 9-19 ■ Umbilical cord obstruction: **A:** Tight overhand umbilical cord knot with marked morphologic changes in vessels on one side of the obstruction. **B:** Acute cord prolapse—transverse indentation of the umbilical cord with congestion on the fetal side. **C:** Markedly dilated chorionic plate veins. **D:** Excessive long, diffusely hypercoiled, and macerated umbilical cord associated with an intrauterine fetal demise.

Fetal Hemorrhage

Background

Finally, the least common mechanism of acute hypoxic injury is fetal hemorrhage. One cause of acute fetal hemorrhage is massive fetomaternal hemorrhage (discussed above) occurring during labor. Other causes include transection of umbilical vessels in the placental membranes at the time of membrane rupture; perforation of umbilical or chorionic vessels at the time of amniocentesis; and sequestration of extravasated blood in the placenta (subamnionic or subchorionic hemorrhage), umbilical cord (umbilical hematoma), or fetus (liver, lung, GI tract, central nervous system, caput succedaneum).

Pathology and Clinical Correlation

The relationship between intervillous thrombi and fetomaternal hemorrhage is discussed above and the pathology of hemorrhages in the fetus is outside of the scope of this chapter. Other placental hemorrhages must be carefully considered in terms of the clinical history. Fetal vessels traveling in the fetal membranes associated with peripheral cord insertion are quite common, and these vessels are frequently torn after delivery of the infant in the third stage of labor. Only tears showing significant amounts of adjacent hemorrhage, distortion of neighboring tissues, or organization of the hematoma in the setting of fetal distress should be diagnosed. Likewise, subamnionic and intraumbilical hemorrhages commonly occur with traction on the umbilical cord after delivery of the infant. Hemorrhages at these sites should be diagnosed only in the presence of predisposing events such as *in utero* instrumentation or cord traction (e.g., external version, short umbilical cord) followed by fetal distress with neonatal anemia and/or hypovolemia.

REFERENCES

1. Acker D, Sachs BP, Tracey KJ, et al. Abruptio placentae associated with cocaine use. *Am J Obstet Gynecol* 1983;146:218–219.
2. Adams-Chapman I, Vaucher YE, Bejar RF, et al. Maternal floor infarction of the placenta: association with central nervous system injury and adverse neurodevelopmental outcome. *J Perinatol* 2002;22:236–241.
3. Altshuler G. Chorangiosis: an important placental sign of neonatal morbidity and mortality. *Arch Pathol Lab Med* 1984;108:71–74.
4. Altshuler G, Arizawa M, Molnar-Nadasdy G. Meconium-induced umbilical cord vascular necrosis and ulceration: a potential link between the placenta and poor pregnancy outcome. *Obstet Gynecol* 1992;79:760–766.
5. Altshuler G, Hyde S. Meconium-induced vasocontraction: a potential cause of cerebral and other fetal hypoperfusion and of poor pregnancy outcome. *J Child Neurol* 1989;4:137–142.
6. Altshuler G, Russell P. The human placental villitides: a review of chronic intrauterine infection. *Curr Topics Pathol* 1975;60:63–112.
7. Altshuler G, Russell P, Ermocilla R. The placental pathology of small-for-gestational age infants. *Am J Obstet Gynecol* 1975;121: 351–359.
8. Ananth CV, Wilcox AJ. Placental abruption and perinatal mortality in the United States. *Am J Epidemiol* 2001;153:332–337.
9. Andres RL, Kuyper W, Resnik R, et al. The association of maternal floor infarction of the placenta with adverse perinatal outcome. *Am J Obstet Gynecol* 1990;163:935–938.
10. Arias F, Victorio A, Cho K, et al. Placental histology and clinical characteristics of patients with preterm premature rupture of membranes. *Obstet Gynecol* 1997;89:265–271.
11. Aviram R, Kidron D, Silverstein S, et al. Placental mesenchymal dysplasia associated with transient neonatal diabetes mellitus and paternal UPD6. *Placenta* 2008;29:646–649.
12. Baergen RN, Malicki D, Behling C, et al. Morbidity, mortality, and placental pathology in excessively long umbilical cords: retrospective study. *Pediatr Dev Pathol* 2001;4:144–153.
13. Bane AL, Gillan JE. Massive perivillous fibrinoid causing recurrent placental failure. *Br J Obstet Gynaecol* 2003;110:292–295.
14. Barton SC, Surani MA, Norris ML. Role of paternal and maternal genomes in mouse development. *Nature* 1984;311:374–376.
15. Basso O, Christensen K, Olsen J. Higher risk of pre-eclampsia after change of partner. An effect of longer interpregnancy intervals? *Epidemiology* 2001;12:624–629.
16. Beer AE, Billingham RE. Maternally acquired runt disease. *Science* 1973;179:240–243.
17. Bendon RW. Twin transfusion: pathologic studies of the monochorionic placenta in liveborn twins and of the perinatal autopsy in monochorionic twin pairs. *Pediatr Pathol Lab Med* 1995;15:363–376.
18. Bendon RW, Hommel AB. Maternal floor infarction in autoimmune disease: two cases. *Pediatr Pathol Lab Med* 1996;16:293–297.
19. Benirschke K. Recent trends in chorangiomas, especially those of multiple and recurrent chorangiomas. *Pediatr Dev Pathol* 1999;2:264–269.
20. Benirschke K, Kaufmann P, Baergen RN, eds. *Pathology of the human placenta*, 5th ed. New York, NY: Springer, 2006.
21. Benson CB, Bieber FR, Genest DR, et al. Doppler demonstration of reversed umbilical blood flow in an acardiac twin. *J Clin Ultrasound* 1989;17:291–295.
22. Bey M, Dott A, Miller JM. The sonographic diagnosis of circumvallate placenta. *Obstet Gynecol* 1991;78:515–517.
23. Bianchi DW, Wilkins-Haug LE, Enders AC, et al. Origin of extraembryonic mesoderm in experimental animals: relevance to chorionic mosaicism in humans. *Am J Med Genet* 1993;46:542–550.
24. Bittencourt AL, Garcia AG. The placenta in hematogenous infections. *Pediatr Pathol Mol Med* 2002;21:401–432.
25. Blackwell SC, Hallak M, Hotra JW, et al. Timing of fetal nucleated red blood cell count elevation in response to acute hypoxia. *Biol Neonate* 2004;85:217–220.
26. Blanc W. Amniotic infection syndrome: pathogenesis, morphology, and significance in circumnatal mortality. *Clin Obstet Gynecol* 1959;2:705–734.
27. Blanc W. Pathology of the placenta and cord in ascending and hematogenous infections. In: Marshall W, ed. *Perinatal infections, CIBA Foundation Symposium 77*. London, UK: Excerpta Medica, 1980:17–38.
28. Boyd JD, Hamilton WJ. *The human placenta*. Cambridge, UK: W Heffer & Sons, 1970.
29. Boyd TK, Redline RW. Chronic histiocytic intervillositis: a placental lesion associated with recurrent reproductive loss. *Hum Pathol* 2000;31:1389–1392.
30. Branch DW, Khamashta MA. Antiphospholipid syndrome: obstetric diagnosis, management, and controversies. *Obstet Gynecol* 2003;101:1333–1344.
31. Bruch JF, Sibony O, Benali K, et al. Computerized microscope morphometry of umbilical vessels from pregnancies with intrauterine growth retardation and abnormal umbilical artery Doppler. *Hum Pathol* 1997;28:1139–1145.
32. Caniggia I, Winter J, Lye SJ, et al. Oxygen and placental development during the first trimester: implications for the pathophysiology of pre-eclampsia. *Placenta* 2000;21(suppl. A):S25–S30.
33. Chellam VG, Rushton DI. Chorioamnionitis and funiculitis in the placentas of 200 births weighing less than 2.5 kg. *Br J Obstet Gynaecol* 1985;92:808–814.
34. Cheung PY, Walton JC, Tai HH, et al. Immunocytochemical distribution and localization of 15-hydroxyprostaglandin dehydrogenase in

human fetal membranes, decidua, and placenta. *Am J Obstet Gynecol* 1990;163:1445–1449.
35. Clewell WH, Manchester DK. Recurrent maternal floor infarction: a preventable cause of fetal death. *Am J Obstet Gynecol* 1983;147:346–347.
36. Collins JH. Nuchal cord type A and type B. *Am J Obstet Gynecol* 1997;177:94.
37. Coulam CB, Stephenson M, Stern JJ, et al. Immunotherapy for recurrent pregnancy loss: analysis of results from clinical trials. *Am J Reprod Immunol* 1996;35:352–359.
38. Craven CM, Chedwick LR, Ward K. Placental basal plate formation is associated with fibrin deposition in decidual veins at sites of trophoblast cell invasion. *Am J Obstet Gynecol* 2002;186:291–296.
39. Craven CM, Zhao L, Ward K. Lateral placental growth occurs by trophoblast cell invasion of decidual veins. *Placenta* 2000;21:160–169.
40. Curtin WM, Shehata BM, Khuder SA, et al. The feasibility of using histologic placental sections to predict newborn nucleated red blood cell counts. *Obstet Gynecol* 2002;100:305–310.
41. Dahms BB, Boyd T, Redline RW. Severe perinatal liver disease associated with fetal thrombotic vasculopathy. *Pediatr Dev Pathol* 2002;5:80–85.
42. Damsky CH, Fitzgerald ML, Fisher SJ. Distribution patterns of extracellular matrix components and adhesion receptors are intricately modulated during first trimester cytotrophoblast differentiation along the invasive pathway, in vivo. *J Clin Invest* 1992;89:210–222.
43. De Wolf F, Brosens I, Renaer M. Fetal growth retardation and the maternal arterial supply of the human placenta in the absence of sustained hypertension. *Br J Obstet Gynaecol* 1980;87:678–684.
44. Demir R, Kaufmann P, Castellucci M, et al. Fetal vasculogenesis and angiogenesis in human placental villi. *Acta Anat* 1989;136: 190–203.
45. DeSa DJ. Intimal cushions in foetal placental veins. *J Pathol* 1973;110:347–352.
46. Dommisse J, Tiltman AJ. Placental bed biopsies in placental abruption. *Br J Obstet Gynaecol* 1992;99:651–654.
47. Doss BJ, Greene MF, Hill J, et al. Massive chronic intervillositis associated with recurrent abortions. *Hum Pathol* 1995;26:1245–1251.
48. Elliott JP, Gilpin B, Strong TH Jr, et al. Chronic abruption-oligohydramnios sequence. *J Reprod Med* 1998;43:418–422.
49. Faxelius G, Raye J, Gutberlet R, et al. Red cell volume measurements and acute blood loss in high-risk newborn infants. *J Pediatr* 1977;90:273–281.
50. Feinberg RF, Kliman HJ, Lockwood CJ. Is oncofetal fibronectin a trophoblast glue for human implantation? *Am J Pathol* 1991;138:537–543.
51. Fox H. Perivillous fibrin deposition in the human placenta. *Am J Obstet Gynecol* 1967;98:245–250.
52. Genest DR. Estimating the time of death in stillborn fetuses. 2. Histologic evaluation of the placenta—a study of 71 stillborns. *Obstet Gynecol* 1992;80:585–592.
53. Gibbs RS. Chorioamnionitis and bacterial vaginosis. *Am J Obstet Gynecol* 1993;169:460–462.
54. Giles WB, Trudinger BJ, Baird PJ. Fetal umbilical artery flow velocity waveforms and placental resistance: pathological correlation. *Br J Obstet Gynaecol* 1985;92:490–497.
55. Goldenberg R, Hauth J, Andrews W. Intrauterine infection and preterm delivery. *N Engl J Med* 2000;342:1500–1507.
56. Gomez B, Romero R, Ghezzi F, et al. The fetal inflammatory response syndrome. *Am J Obstet Gynecol* 1998;179:194–202.
57. Gonzalez A, Sosenko IR, Chandar J, et al. Influence of infection on patent ductus arteriosus and chronic lung disease in premature infants weighing 1000 grams or less. *J Pediatr* 1996;128:470–478.
58. Greenough A. The TORCH screen and intrauterine infections. *Arch Dis Child* 1994;70:F163–F165.
59. Gruenwald P, Levin H, Yousem H. Abruption and premature separation of the placenta. The clinical and pathologic entity. *Am J Obstet Gynecol* 1968;102:604–610.
60. Hanley ML, Shen-Schwartz S, Anath CV, et al. Birthweight discordancy in twin gestation-Is it related to discordancy of placental mass or histopathologic lesions. *Am J Obstet Gynecol* 2000;178:S83.
61. Harris BA. Peripheral placental separation: a review. *Obstet Gynecol Surv* 1988;43:577–581.
62. Hermansen MC. Nucleated red blood cells in the Fetus and newborn. *Arch Dis Child Fetal Neonatal Ed* 2001;84:F211–F215.
63. Hill JA, Polgar K, Anderson DJ. T-helper 1-type immunity to trophoblast in women with recurrent spontaneous abortion. *JAMA* 1995;273:1933–1936.
64. Hoffner L, Dunn J, Esposito N, et al. P57KIP2 immunostaining and molecular cytogenetics: combined approach aids in diagnosis of morphologically challenging cases with molar phenotype and in detecting androgenetic cell lines in mosaic/chimeric conceptions. *Hum Pathol* 2008;39:63–72.
65. Huppertz B, Kingdom J, Caniggia I, et al. Hypoxia favours necrotic versus apoptotic shedding of placental syncytiotrophoblast into the maternal circulation. *Placenta* 2003;24:181–190.
66. Inbal A, Muszbek L. Coagulation factor deficiencies and pregnancy loss. *Semin Thromb Hemost* 2003;29:171–174.
67. Irani RA, Xia Y. The functional role of the Renin-Angiotensin system in pregnancy and preeclampsia. *Placenta* 2008;29:763–771.
68. Jackson MR, Walsh AJ, Morrow RJ, et al. Reduced placental villous tree elaboration in small-for-gestational-age pregnancies: relationship with umbilical artery Doppler waveforms. *Am J Obstet Gynecol* 1995;172:518–525.
69. Jauniaux E, Gulbis B, Burton GJ. The first trimester gestational sac limits rather than facilitates oxygen transfer to the foetus—a review. *Placenta* 2003;24(suppl A):S86–S93.
70. Jauniaux E, Hempstock J, Greenwold N, et al. Trophoblastic oxidative stress in relation to temporal and regional differences in maternal placental blood flow in normal and abnormal early pregnancies. *Am J Pathol* 2003;162:115–125.
71. Jauniaux E, Nicolaides KH, Hustin J. Perinatal features associated with placental mesenchymal dysplasia. *Placenta* 1997;18:701–706.
72. Jauniaux E, Ramsay B, Campbell S. Ultrasonographic investigation of placental morphologic characteristics and size during the second trimester of pregnancy. *Am J Obstet Gynecol* 1994;170:130–137.
73. Jauniaux E, Watson AL, Hempstock J, et al. Onset of maternal arterial blood flow and placental oxidative stress—a possible factor in human early pregnancy failure. *Am J Pathol* 2000;157:2111–2122.
74. Johns J, Hyett J, Jauniaux E. Obstetric outcome after threatened miscarriage with and without a hematoma on ultrasound. *Obstet Gynecol* 2003;102:483–487.
75. Jones EEM, Rivers RPA, Taghizadeh A. Disseminated intravascular coagulation and fetal hydrops in a newborn infant in association with a chorangioma of placenta. *Pediatrics* 1972;50:901–905.
76. Kaplan C, Blanc WA, Elias J. Identification of erythrocytes in intervillous thrombi: a study using immunoperoxidase identification of hemoglobins. *Hum Pathol* 1982;13:554–557.
77. Katz VL, Bowes WA. Meconium aspiration syndrome: reflections on a murky subject. *Am J Obstet Gynecol* 1992;166:171–183.
78. Katz VL, DiTomasso J, Farmer R, et al. Activated protein C resistance associated with maternal floor infarction treated with low-molecular-weight heparin. *Am J Perinatol* 2002;19:273–277.
79. Keenan WJ, Steichen JJ, Mahmood K, et al. Placental pathology compared with clinical outcome. *Am J Dis Child* 1977;131: 1224–1227.
80. Keep D, Zaragoza M, Hassold T, et al. Very early complete hydatidiform mole. *Hum Pathol* 1996;27:708–713.
81. Khong TY. Chorangioma with trophoblastic proliferation. *Virchows Arch* 2000;436:167–171.
82. Khong TY, De Wolf F, Robertson WB, et al. Inadequate maternal vascular response to placentation in pregnancies complicated by pre-eclampsia and by small-for-gestational age infants. *Br J Obstet Gynaecol* 1986;93:1049–1059.

83. Khong TY, Hague WM. The placenta in maternal hyperhomocysteinaemia. *Br J Obstet Gynaecol* 1999;106:273–278.
84. Knox WF, Fox H. Villitis of unknown aetiology: its incidence and significance in placentae from a British population. *Placenta* 1984;5:395–402.
85. Kouyoumdijian A. Velamentous insertion of the umbilical cord. *Obstet Gynecol* 1980;56:737–742.
86. Kraus FT, Acheen VI. Fetal thrombotic vasculopathy in the placenta: cerebral thrombi and infarcts, coagulopathies, and cerebral palsy. *Hum Pathol* 1999;30:759–769.
87. Kraus FT, Redline R, Gersell DJ, et al. *Placental pathology*. Washington, DC: American Registry of Pathology, 2004.
88. Krebs C, Macara LM, Leiser R, et al. Intrauterine growth restriction with absent end-diastolic flow velocity in the umbilical artery is associated with maldevelopment of the placental terminal villous tree. *Am J Obstet Gynecol* 1996;175:1534–1542.
89. Laube DW, Schauberger CW. Fetomaternal bleeding as a cause for 'unexplained' fetal death. *Obstet Gynecol* 1982;60:649–651.
90. Levine RJ, Lam C, Qian C, et al. Soluble endoglin and other circulating antiangiogenic factors in preeclampsia. *N Engl J Med* 2006;355:992–1005.
91. Leviton A, Paneth N, Reuss ML, et al. Maternal infection, fetal inflammatory response, and brain damage in very low birth weight infants. Developmental Epidemiology Network Investigators. *Pediatr Res* 1999;46:566–575.
92. Lewin SL, Herzog TJ. Current perspectives on gestational trophoblastic disease. *Women's Oncol Rev* 2003;3:109–116.
93. Machin G, Still K, Lalani T. Correlations of placental vascular anatomy and clinical outcomes in 69 monochorionic twin pregnancies. *Am J Med Genet* 1996;61:229–236.
94. Machin GA, Ackerman J, Gilbert-Barness E. Abnormal umbilical cord coiling is associated with adverse perinatal outcomes. *Pediatr Dev Pathol* 2000;3:462–471.
95. Mandsager NT, Bendon RW, Mostello D, et al. Maternal floor infarction of placenta: prenatal diagnosis and clinical significance. *Obstet Gynecol* 1994;83:750–754.
96. Martin GC, Green RS, Holzman IR. Acidosis in newborns with nuchal cords and normal Apgar scores. *J Perinatol* 2005;25:162–165.
97. Matern D, Schehata BM, Shekhawa P, et al. Placental floor infarction complicating the pregnancy of a fetus with long-chain 3-hydroxyacyl-CoA dehydrogenase (LCHAD) deficiency. *Mol Genet Metab* 2001;72:265–268.
98. Mayhew TM, Barker BL. Villous trophoblast: morphometric perspectives on growth, differentiation, turnover and deposition of fibrin-type fibrinoid during gestation. *Placenta* 2001;22:628–638.
99. Maynard SE, Min JY, Merchan J, et al. Excess placental soluble fms-like tyrosine kinase 1 (sFlt1) may contribute to endothelial dysfunction, hypertension, and proteinuria in preeclampsia. *J Clin Invest* 2003;111:649–658.
100. Mazur MT, Lurain JR, Brewer JI. Fatal gestational choriocarcinoma. Clinicopathologic study of patients treated at a trophoblastic disease center. *Cancer* 1982;50:1833–1846.
101. Miller FC, Sacks DA, Yeh SY, et al. Significance of meconium during labor. *Am J Obstet Gynecol* 1975;122:573–579.
102. Miller PW, Coen RW, Benirschke K. Dating the time interval from meconium passage to birth. *Obstet Gynecol* 1985;66:459–462.
103. Minior V, Levine B, Guller S, et al. Antenatal fetal hypoxemia gradually increases fetal nucleated red blood cells in a rat model. *Am J Obstet Gynecol* 2004;191:S168.
104. Mooney EE, al Shunnar A, O'Regan M, et al. Chorionic villous haemorrhage is associated with retroplacental haemorrhage. *Br J Obstet Gynaecol* 1994;101:965–969.
105. Morgan T, Craven C, Lalouel JM, et al. Angiotensinogen Thr235 variant is associated with abnormal physiologic change of the uterine spiral arteries in first-trimester decidua. *Am J Obstet Gynecol* 1999;180:95–102.
106. Mueller-Heubach E, Rubinstein DN, Schwarz SS. Histologic chorioamnionitis and preterm delivery in different patient populations. *Obstet Gynecol* 1990;75:622–626.
107. Myers RE. Four patterns of perinatal brain damage and their conditions of occurrence in primates. *Adv Neurol* 1975;10:223–234.
108. Naeye RL. Maternal floor infarction. *Hum Pathol* 1985;16:823–828.
109. Naeye RL. Do placental weights have clinical significance? *Hum Pathol* 1987;18:387–391.
110. Naeye RL. Pregnancy hypertension, placental evidences of low utero-placental blood flow and spontaneous premature delivery. *Hum Pathol* 1989;20:441–444.
111. Naeye RL, Harkness WL, Utls J. Abruptio placentae and perinatal death. A prospective study. *Am J Obstet Gynecol* 1977;128: 740–748.
112. Naeye RL, Lin HM. Determination of the timing of fetal brain damage from hypoxemia-ischemia. *Am J Obstet Gynecol* 2001;184: 217–224.
113. Naeye RL, Localio AR. Determining the time before birth when ischemia and hypoxemia initiated cerebral palsy. *Obstet Gynecol* 1995;86:713–719.
114. Naftolin F, Khudr G, Benirschke K, et al. The syndrome of chronic abruptio placentae, hydrorrhea, and circumallate placenta. *Am J Obstet Gynecol* 1973;116:347–350.
115. Nanaev AK, Kosanke G, Kemp B, et al. The human placenta is encircled by a ring of smooth muscle cells. *Placenta* 2000;21:122–125.
116. Nayar R, Lage JM. Placental changes in a first trimester missed abortion in maternal systemic lupus erythematosus with antiphospholipid syndrome: a case report and review of the literature. *Hum Pathol* 1996;27:201–206.
117. Nelson JL. Pregnancy, persistent microchimerism, and autoimmune disease. *J Am Med Womens Assoc* 1998;53:31–32, 47.
118. Nelson KB, Ellenberg JH. Antecedents of cerebral palsy: multivariate analysis of risk. *N Engl J Med* 1986;315:81–86.
119. Ness RB, Roberts JM. Heterogeneous causes constituting the single syndrome of preeclampsia: a hypothesis and its implications. *Am J Obstet Gynecol* 1996;175:1365–1370.
120. Odegard RA, Vatten LJ, Nilsen ST, et al. Risk factors and clinical manifestations of pre-eclampsia. *Br J Obstet Gynaecol* 2000;107:1410–1416
121. Ogino S, Redline RW. Villous capillary lesions of the placenta: Distinctions between chorangioma, chorangiomatosis, and chorangiosis. *Hum Pathol* 2000;31:945–954
122. Oppenheimer EH, Esterly JR. Thrombosis in the newborn: comparison between infants of diabetic and nondiabetic mothers. *J Pediatr* 1965;67:549–556.
123. O'Rahilly R, Muller F. *Developmental stages in human embryos*. Washington D.C.: Carnegie Institute of Washington, 1987.
124. Parast MM, Crum CP, Boyd TK. Placental histologic criteria for umbilical blood flow restriction in unexplained stillbirth. *Hum Pathol* 2008;39:948–953.
125. Perni SC, Cho JE, Baergen RN. Placental pathology and pregnancy outcomes in donor and non-donor oocyte in vitro fertilization pregnancies. *Am J Obstet Gynecol* 2003;189:S122.
126. Pharoah PO, Adi Y. Consequences of in-utero death in a twin pregnancy. *Lancet* 2000;355:1597–1602.
127. Pijnenborg R, Dixon G, Robertson WB, et al. Trophoblastic invasion of human decidua from 8 to 18 weeks of pregnancy. *Placenta* 1980;1:3–19.
128. Piper J, Newton E, Berkus M, et al. Meconium: a marker of peripartum infection. *Obstet Gynecol* 1998;91:741–745.
129. Powers WF, Kiely JL. The risks confronting twins: a national perspective. *Am J Obstet Gynecol* 1994;170:456–461.
130. Pritchard JA, Mason R, Corley M, et al. Genesis of severe placental abruption. *Am J Obstet Gynecol* 1970;108:22–27.
131. Ramsey EM, Donner MW. *Placental Vasculature and Circulation*. Philadelphia, PA: W. B. Saunders Co., 1980.

132. Redline R. Disorders of the placental parenchyma. In: Lewis SH, Perrin E, eds. *Pathology of the Placenta*. Philadelphia, PA: Churchill Livingstone, 1999:161–184.
133. Redline R. Cerebral palsy in term infants: a clinicopathologic analysis of 158 medicolegal case reviews. *Pediatr Dev Pathol* 2008;11: 456–464.
134. Redline R, Shah D, Sakar H, et al. Placental lesions associated with abnormal growth in twins. *Pediatr Dev Pathol* 2001;4:473–481.
135. Redline R, Wilson-Costello D, Borawski E, et al. The relationship between placental and other perinatal risk factors for neurologic impairment in very low birth weith children. *Pediatr Res* 2000;47:721–726.
136. Redline RW. Nonidentical twins with a single placenta–disproving dogma in perinatal pathology. *N Engl J Med* 2003;349:111–114.
137. Redline RW. Severe fetal placental vascular lesions in term infants with neurologic impairment. *Am J Obstet Gynecol* 2005;192: 452–457.
138. Redline RW. Placental lesions and neurologic outcome. In: Baker P, Sibley C, eds. *The placenta and neurodisability*. London, UK: MacKeith Press, 2006:pp. 58–69.
139. Redline RW. Villitis of unknown etiology: noninfectious chronic villitis in the placenta. *Hum Pathol* 2007;38:1439–1446.
140. Redline RW. Elevated circulating fetal nucleated red blood cells and placental pathology in term infants who develop cerebral palsy. *Hum Pathol* 2008;39:1378–1384.
141. Redline RW, Abdul-Karim FW. Pathology of gestational trophoblastic disease. *Semin Oncol* 1995;22:96–108.
142. Redline RW, Abramowsky CR. Clinical and pathologic aspects of recurrent placental villitis. *Hum Pathol* 1985;16:727–731.
143. Redline RW, Ariel I, Baergen RN, et al. Fetal vascular obstructive lesions: nosology and reproducibility of placental reaction patterns. *Pediatr Dev Pathol* 2004;7:443–452.
144. Redline RW, Boyd T, Campbell V, et al. Maternal vascular underperfusion: nosology and reproducibility of placental reaction patterns. *Pediatr Dev Pathol* 2004;7:237–249.
145. Redline RW, Faye-Petersen O, Heller D, et al. Amniotic infection syndrome: nosology and reproducibility of placental reaction patterns. *Pediatr Dev Pathol* 2003;6:435–448.
146. Redline RW, Hassold T, Zaragoza MV. Determinants of trophoblast hyperplasia in spontaneous abortions. *Mod Pathol* 1998;11: 762–768.
147. Redline RW, Hassold T, Zaragoza MV. Prevalence of the partial molar phenotype in triploidy of maternal and paternal origin. *Hum Pathol* 1998;28:505–511.
148. Redline RW, Jiang JG, Shah D. Discordancy for maternal floor infarction in dizygotic twin placentas. *Hum Pathol* 2003;34:822–824.
149. Redline RW, O'Riordan MA. Placental lesions associated with cerebral palsy and neurologic impairment following term birth. *Arch Pathol Lab Med* 2000;124:1785–1791.
150. Redline RW, Pappin A. Fetal thrombotic vasculopathy: The clinical significance of extensive avascular villi. *Hum Pathol* 1995;26: 80–85.
151. Redline RW, Patterson P. Villitis of unknown etiology is associated with major infiltration of fetal tissue by maternal inflammatory cells. *Am J Pathol* 1993;143:473–479.
152. Redline RW, Patterson P. Patterns of placental injury: correlations with gestational age, placental weight, and clinical diagnosis. *Arch Pathol Lab Med* 1994;118:698–701.
153. Redline RW, Patterson P. Preeclampsia is associated with an excess of proliferative immature intermediate trophoblast. *Hum Pathol* 1995;26:594–600.
154. Redline RW, Shah D, Sakar H, et al. Placental lesions associated with abnormal growth in twins. *Pediatr Dev Pathol* 2001;4:473–481.
155. Redline RW, Wilson-Costello D. Chronic peripheral separation of placenta: The significance of diffuse chorioamnionic hemosiderosis. *Am J Clin Pathol* 1999;111:804–810.
156. Redline RW, Wilson-Costello D, Borawski E, et al. Placental lesions associated with neurologic impairment and cerebral palsy in very low birth weight infants. *Arch Pathol Lab Med* 1998;122:1091–1098.
157. Redline RW, Wilson-Costello D, Hack M. Placental and other perinatal risk factors for chronic lung disease in very low birth weight infants. *Pediatr Res* 2002;52:713–719.
158. Redline RW, Zaragoza MV, Hassold T. Prevalence of developmental and inflammatory lesions in non-molar first trimester spontaneous abortions. *Hum Pathol* 1999;30:93–100.
159. Rossi EM, Philipson EH, Williams TG, et al. Meconium aspiration syndrome: Intrapartum and neonatal attributes. *Am J Obstet Gynecol* 1989;161:106–110.
160. Russell P, Atkinson K, Krishnan L. Recurrent reproductive failure due to severe villitis of unknown etiology. *J Reprod Med* 1980; 24:93–98.
161. Saftlas AF, Olson DR, Franks AL, et al. Epidemiology of preeclampsia and eclampsia in the United States, 1979–1986. *Am J Obstet Gynecol* 1990;163:460–465.
162. Sander CH. Hemorrhagic endovasculitis and hemorrhagic villitis of the placenta. *Arch Pathol Lab Med* 1980;104:371–373.
163. Sebire NJ, Backos M, Goldin RD, et al. Placental massive perivillous fibrin deposition associated with antiphospholipid antibody syndrome. *Br J Obstet Gynaecol* 2002;109:570–573.
164. Sebire NJ, Fox H, Backos M, et al. Defective endovascular trophoblast invasion in primary antiphospholipid antibody syndrome-associated early pregnancy failure. *Hum Reprod* 2002;17:1067–1071.
165. Sela S, Itin A, Natanson-Yaron S, et al. A novel human-specific soluble vascular endothelial growth factor receptor 1: cell-type-specific splicing and implications to vascular endothelial growth factor homeostasis and preeclampsia. *Circ Res* 2008;102:1566–1574.
166. Shih IM, Kurman RJ. Epithelioid trophoblastic tumor: a neoplasm distinct from choriocarcinoma and placental site trophoblastic tumor simulating carcinoma. *Am J Surg Pathol* 1998;22:1393–1403.
167. Shih IM, Kurman RJ. The pathology of intermediate trophoblastic tumors and tumor-like lesions. *Int J Gynecol Pathol* 2001; 20:31–47.
168. Shih IM, Kurman RJ. p63 expression is useful in the distinction of epithelioid trophoblastic and placental site trophoblastic tumors by profiling trophoblastic subpopulations. *Am J Surg Pathol* 2004;28:1177–1183.
169. Simpson RA, Mayhew TM, Barnes PR. From 13 weeks to term, the trophoblast of human placenta grows by the continuous recruitment of new proliferative units: a study of nuclear number using the dissector. *Placenta* 1992;13:501–512.
170. Soma H, Watanabe Y, Hata T. Chorangiosis and chorangioma in three cohorts of placentas from Nepal, Tibet and Japan. *Reprod Fertil Devel* 1996;7:1533–1538.
171. Soothill PW, Nicolaides KH, Campbell S. Prenatal asphyxia, hyperlacticaemia, hypoglycaemia, and erythroblastosis in growth retarded fetuses. *Br Med J* 1987;294:1051–1053.
172. Souter VL, Kapur RP, Nyholt DR, et al. A report of dizygous monochorionic twins. *N Engl J Med* 2003;349:154–158.
173. Spellacy WN, Graven H, Fisch RO. The umbilical cord complications of true knots, nuchal coils and cords around the body. *Am J Obstet Gynecol* 1966;94:1136–1142.
174. Stanek J. Numerical criteria for the diagnosis of placental chorangiosis using CD34 immunostaining. *Trophoblast Res* 1999;13: 443–452.
175. Styer AK, Parker HJ, Roberts DJ, et al. Placental villitis of unclear etiology during ovum donor in vitro fertilization pregnancy. *Am J Obstet Gynecol* 2003;189:1184–1186.
176. Tonkin IL, Setzer ES, Ermocilla R. Placental chorangioma: a rare cause of congestive heart failure and hydrops fetalis in the newborn. *Am J Roentgenol* 1980;134:181–183.
177. Torpin R. Evolution of a placenta circumvallata. *Obstet Gynecol*. 1966;27:98–101.

178. Van Marter LJ, Dammann O, Allred EN, et al. Chorioamnionitis, mechanical ventilation, and postnatal sepsis as modulators of chronic lung disease in preterm infants. *J Pediatr* 2002;140:171–176.
179. van Meir CA, Matthews SG, Keirse MJ, et al. 15-hydroxyprostaglandin dehydrogenase: implications in preterm labor with and without ascending infection. *J Clin Endocrinol Metab* 1997;82:969–976.
180. Wallenburg HCS, Stolte LAM, Jannsens J. The pathogenesis of placental infarction. I. A morphologic study in the human placenta. *Am J Obstet Gynecol* 1973;116:835–846.
181. Wallukat G, Homuth V, Fischer T, et al. Patients with preeclampsia develop agonistic autoantibodies against the angiotensin AT1 receptor. *J Clin Invest* 1999;103:945–952.
182. Wallukat G, Neichel D, Nissen E, et al. Agonistic autoantibodies directed against the angiotensin II AT1 receptor in patients with preeclampsia. *Can J Physiol Pharmacol* 2003;81:79–83.
183. Wee LY, Fisk NM. The twin-twin transfusion syndrome. *Semin Neonatol* 2002;7:187–202.
184. Wiener-Megnagi Z, Ben-Shlomo I, Goldberg Y, et al. Resistance to activated protein C and the leiden mutation: high prevalence in patients with abruptio placentae. *Am J Obstet Gynecol* 1998;179:1565–1567.
185. Wigglesworth JS, Singer DB, eds. *Textbook of fetal and perinatal pathology*. Boston, MA: Blackwell Scientific Publications, 1991.
186. Williams MA, Lieberman E, Mittendorf R, et al. Risk factors for abruptio placentae. *Am J Epidemiol* 1991;134:965–972.
187. Williams MC, O'Brien WF. Elevated placenta/birthweight ratio as a marker for increased risk of perinatal morbidity and mortality in growth restricted infants. *Am J Obstet Gynecol* 2000;182:S73.
188. Yoshida S, Kikuchi A, Sunagawa S et al. Pregnancy complicated by diffuse chorioamniotic hemosiderosis: obstetric features and influence on respiratory diseases of the infant. *J Obstet Gynaecol Res* 2007;33:788–792.
189. Young RH, Kurman RJ, Scully RE. Placental site nodules and plaques. A clinicopathologic analysis of 20 cases. *Am J Surg Pathol* 1990;14:1001–1009.
190. Zhang J, Dong H, Wang B, et al. Dynamic changes occur in patterns of endometrial EFNB2/EPHB4 expression during the period of spiral arterial modification in mice. *Biol Reprod* 2008;79:450–458.

CHAPTER 10

The Nervous System

CHRISTOPHER DUNHAM
ARIE PERRY

GENERAL NEUROPATHOLOGIC PROCESSES AND PRINCIPLES

The practice of neuropathology demands an extensive knowledge of normal central nervous system (CNS) cytology and architecture, in addition to common artifacts. During development, the CNS (from fetal life and beyond) changes dramatically, especially in terms of histology, making pathologic assessments even more challenging. A full discussion of normal CNS histology and common artifacts is beyond the scope of this text. Some of the more common neuropathologic changes and pathophysiologic processes are introduced below.

The CNS contains a variety of neurons, which vary in size from the small neocortical granular (stellate) neurons (<15 μm) to the large neocortical pyramidal neurons (measuring from 10 to 100 μm for the Betz cells of the primary motor cortex). Pyramidal neurons are often considered the morphologic prototype that bears ample lightly basophilic cytoplasm, darker clumpy Nissl substance, a large central nucleus, a prominent nucleolus (the "Owl's eye"), and coarse cytoplasmic processes. Neocortical neurons exhibit a prominent apical dendrite oriented perpendicular to the cortical surface. Neurons may display several different cytologic abnormalities, some of which are specific, but many of which are nonspecific and must thus be interpreted in the correct clinico-pathologic context. Acutely necrotic (or "dead") neurons are a form of nonspecific change that contain two essential components: (a) shrunken pyknotic angular nuclei and (b) cytoplasmic eosinophilia ("red is dead") (Figure 10-1A). Although commonly caused by ischemia (and hence often referred to as ischemic neurons), any process that causes acute neuronal death may lead to the formation of red neurons (e.g., hypoxia, hypoglycemia, carbon monoxide, epilepsy, HSV encephalitis). Acute neuronal death is much more difficult to appreciate in fetal brains that contain a predominance of primitive neurons (small dark nuclei with little cytoplasm); in such cases, nuclear fragmentation or karyorrhexis (at times in keeping with apoptosis) can be appreciated on high magnification (Figure 10-1B). A large variety of neuronal inclusions may be seen, including both intranuclear and intracytoplasmic types. These inclusions vary tremendously in color, size, and shape, from essentially rounded and eosinophilic/basophilic to more fibrillar (e.g., neurofibrillary tangle). These inclusions are commonly seen in viral and neurodegenerative/metabolic diseases. Abnormal vacuolization of the cytoplasm can be seen and may correlate with swelling of ultrastructural elements (e.g., mitochondria). Vacuolization that seemingly occurs within the neuropil (the meshwork of neuronal processes among which all the cell bodies of the neocortex reside) may be a result of neuronal loss or the expansion of neuronal processes (which occurs with the prion diseases or "spongiform" encephalopathies). Some damaged neurons, for instance those near infarction, may undergo mineralization (i.e., ferruginization). Damage to the axon can lead to several cytologic alterations. Disruption of the axon may result in chromatolytic changes that include swelling of the soma, dispersion of the Nissl substance, eccentric displacement of the nucleus, and accumulation of cytoskeletal filaments. This latter event results in axonal spheroids (i.e., swellings) that can be highlighted with immunohistochemical (IHC) stains [e.g., β-amyloid precursor protein (β-APP)] (Figure 10-2). The distally transected portion of the axon degenerates and initially forms ovoids that are later taken up by macrophages, which serve to localize areas of degeneration (26). Somewhat more fusiform axonal spheroids known as "torpedoes" are commonly found in the upper cerebellar cortex and reflect Purkinje cell damage.

Normal astrocytes are situated throughout the gray (protoplasmic astrocytes) and white (fibrillary astrocytes) matter. For the most part, these astrocytes partake in their physiologic duties rather inconspicuously. However, in response to almost any insult, these cells undergo proliferation (i.e., hyperplasia) and enlargement (i.e., hypertrophy) termed reactive astrocytosis or gliosis, which has been equated to the "scar tissue" of the CNS. Their normally inapparent cytoplasmic processes (by routine H&E staining) accumulate intermediate GFAP filaments after stimulation, and thus take on a starburst-like pattern (Figure 10-3). In contrast to astrocytic neoplasms, these reactive astrocytes are

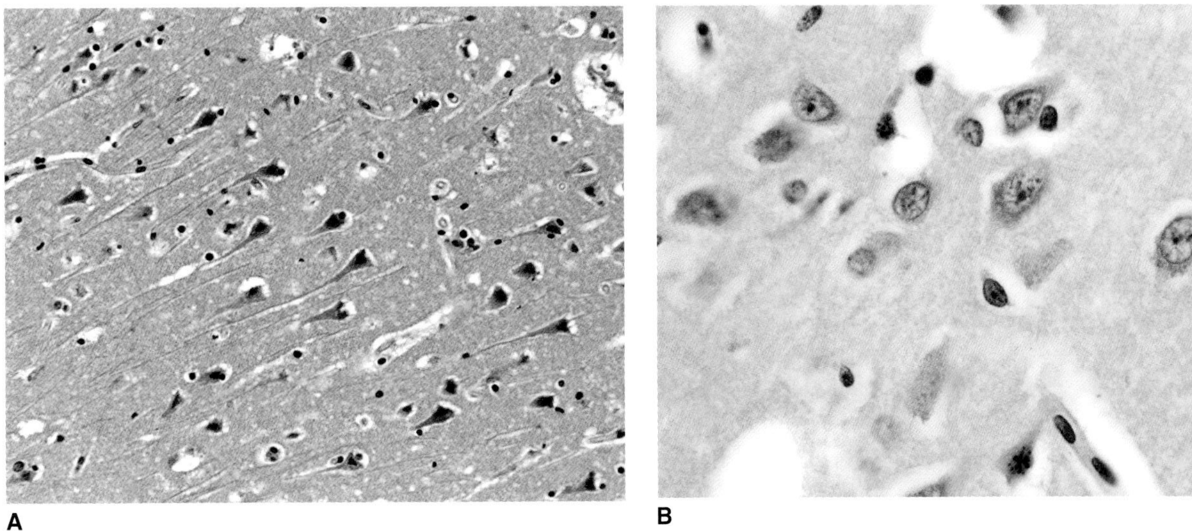

FIGURE 10-1▪Acutely "necrotic" or dead neurons. **A:** Adult. **B:** Premature infant. Note the nuclear fragmentation (i.e., karyorrhexis) and eosinophilic cytoplasm in two shrunken subicular neurons.

typically distributed evenly throughout the parenchyma. Myelination glia are a notable pitfall to the determination of gliosis in the newborn; these glia also display relatively abundant eosinophilic cytoplasm, but they are a normal finding in the young myelinating nervous system. Although their distinction from gliosis is often difficult, myelination glia often display hyperchromatic small round nuclei associated with cytoplasm that is shaped like a comet. In the more chronic stages of gliosis, the cytoplasmic processes of astrocytes retract and become less obvious on routine staining, although their nuclei remain in increased number and continue to mark areas of prior damage. Gliosis occurring in the cerebellar cortex in response to Purkinje cell loss is termed Bergmann gliosis, which is characterized by parallel fibrillary processes radiating through the molecular layer toward the pial surface and the accumulation of astrocytic nuclei within the Purkinje layer. The somewhat nonspecific form of gliosis that occurs immediately under the pia mater in the neocortex is called Chaslin gliosis, a reaction that is often attributed to previous seizure activity. Occasionally found within these areas of longstanding gliosis are the brightly eosinophilic structures termed Rosenthal fibers (RFs) and less often eosinophilic granular bodies (EGBs); however, these structures are also seen in a variety of neoplastic [e.g., pilocytic astrocytoma (PA)] and nonneoplastic (i.e., Alexander disease) conditions (Figure 10-4). RFs have a characteristic EM appearance, manifesting as an electron-dense core surrounded by fibrillary material. An entirely nonspecific but characteristic astrocytic reaction occurs in abnormal physiologic states often associated with hyperammonemia; under these conditions, Alzheimer type II astrocytes (of no relation to Alzheimer disease) accumulate, particularly in the basal ganglia and deep layers of the neocortex. These astrocytes,

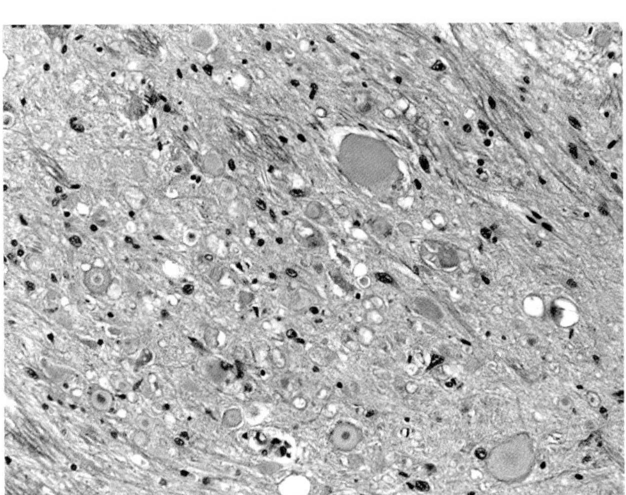

FIGURE 10-2▪Axonal spheroids from a case of infantile neuroaxonal dystrophy (i.e., Seitelberger disease).

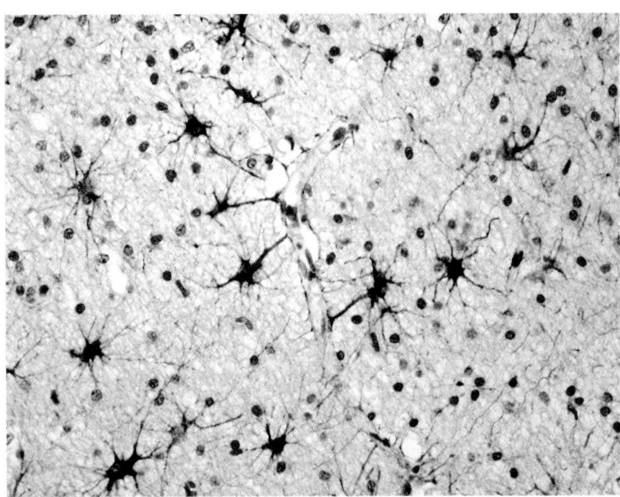

FIGURE 10-3▪Reactive gliosis (Glial fibrillary acidic protein immunohistochemistry (IHC)).

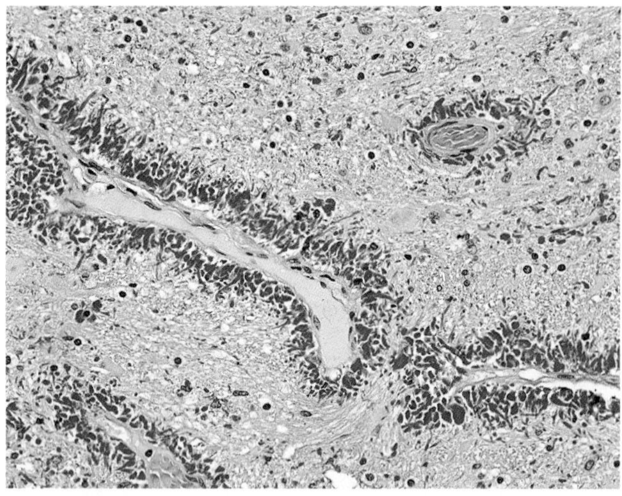

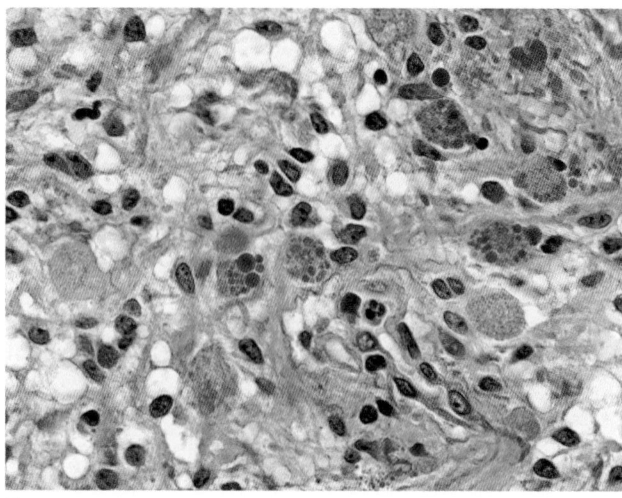

A B

FIGURE 10-4 ■ Rosenthal fibers and eosinophilic granular bodies are nonspecific eosinophilic structures that are most commonly seen in the context of long-standing gliosis or within low-grade primary brain neoplasms. **A:** Perivascular accumulation of RFs in this case of Alexander disease. **B:** EGBs within the microcystic component of a pilocytic astrocytoma.

often seen in pairs, exhibit inconspicuous cytoplasm, enlarged pale nuclei, and often a prominent nucleolus. Astrocytes may bear inclusions, both cytoplasmic and nuclear, although these are often difficult to appreciate on routine stains, necessitating the use of special stains and immunohistochemistry for their detection.

Normal oligodendroglia fulfill their metabolic roles (most importantly myelination) rather inconspicuously from a histologic point of view. As opposed to astrocytes, the spectrum of pathology occurring in oligodendroglia is much more restricted. By routine staining, normal oligodendroglia exhibit inconspicuous cytoplasmic processes and hyperchromatic, round regular nuclei. As may be predicted, insults affecting oligodendroglia result in demyelination (i.e., myelin destruction), which can be elucidated with myelin special stains [e.g., Luxol fast blue (LFB)]. Usually, there is concomitant oligodendroglial dropout and astrocytic gliosis. Some pathologic processes cause myelin to separate between its layers, resulting in intramyelinic splitting, which manifests as vacuolar change in the white matter on light microscopy. Like astrocytes, oligodendroglia may bear abnormal nuclear [e.g., progressive multifocal leukoencephalopathy (PML)] or cytoplasmic inclusions [e.g., multiple systems atrophy (MSA)], the latter of which usually require special/IHC stains for their detection. The normally inconspicuous cytoplasm of oligodendroglia may become slightly more conspicuous when they suffer cytotoxic insults (e.g., ischemia).

Pathologic reactions of the ventricular lining cells, or ependyma, are generally very limited and nonspecific. These normally columnar to cuboidal cells form a simple (i.e., single layered) epithelium. With hydrocephalus (HCP) or cerebral atrophy, the epithelium stretches and becomes atrophic, or even discontinuous. Soon after acute injury, subependymal astrocytes proliferate and produce nodular excrescences, which protrude into the ventricular cavity. Although previously termed granular ependymitis, this nonspecific pathologic reaction is not always related to an underlying inflammatory process; as such, the terms subventricular gliosis or ependymal granulations are preferable. If exuberant, this gliosis may entrap portions of ependyma resulting in subependymal rosettes/tubules. As with the other cellular elements of the CNS, residual ependymal cells may bear inclusions, usually of viral etiology.

Microglial reactions are unique to the CNS. Microglia are inflammatory and antigen-presenting cells derived from bone marrow monocytes. The nuclei and cytoplasmic processes of these parenchymal cells are very inconspicuous within normal CNS tissue. Generally, they are of two types: (a) resident microglia are those that reside within the neuropil (and also the perivascular space) and do not undergo significant turnover with hematogenous monocytes and (b) perivascular microglia, whose population is continually renewed via hematogenous monocytes (26). Microglia have also been termed rod cells since, after parenchymal insult, their presence is heralded by a proliferation of small elongate naked nuclei. After CNS damage, perivascular microglia phagocytose necrotic debris and accordingly accumulate lipid material, which distends their cytoplasm yielding a foamy appearance. When resident microglia are stimulated, two basic pathologic patterns may be seen. First, there may be a diffuse microglial activation, wherein rod cells are evenly distributed throughout the diseased tissue; some have termed this uniquely CNS reaction "neuroinflammation" (21) (Figure 10-5A). Second, and often associated with viral encephalitides, are microglial nodules, which are roughly spherical aggregates of microglia (Figure 10-5B). Microglia may also surround and digest dying neurons, a process termed neuronophagia.

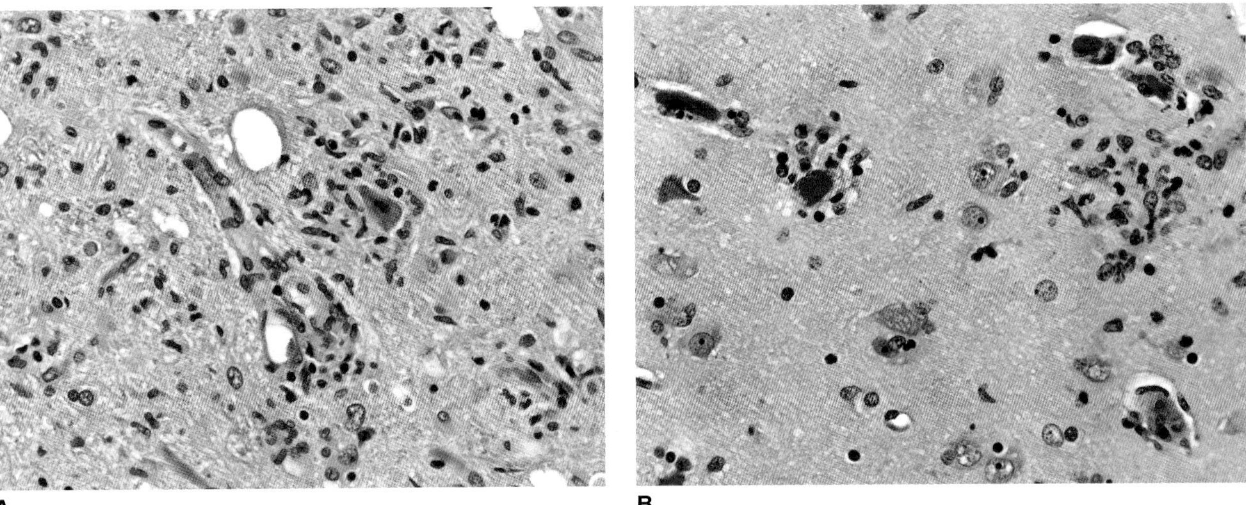

FIGURE 10-5 ▪ Activated microglia. **A:** Neuronophagia is seen within this diffuse microgliosis. **B:** In addition to some perivascular lymphocytes, a microglial nodule is seen toward the left side of the figure.

Increased Intracranial Pressure, Edema, and Hydrocephalus (HCP)

Once the cranial sutures fuse early on in postnatal life, the skull essentially acts as a rigid closed box, the contents of which include brain parenchyma, blood, and cerebrospinal fluid (CSF). A mature- sized brain (~1,400 g) contains 75 mL each of blood and CSF (*Note*: a term brain weighs ~300 to 350 g). This CSF results in a normal intracranial pressure (ICP) of 15 mm Hg. The cerebral perfusion pressure (CPP) equals the mean arterial pressure minus the ICP. Cerebral blood flow (CBF), which for the brain as a whole is 50 mL/100 g/minute, is calculated by dividing CPP by resistance (i.e., the vasculature). Through autoregulation, the CBF is kept constant despite changes in the systemic blood pressure. Notably, the autoregulatory capabilities of the prenatal cerebral vasculature are poor, making the brain vulnerable to fluctuations in blood pressure. When a mass-forming disease process increases the intracranial contents and elevates ICP (e.g., brain tumor), the brain compensates by expelling contents from the "closed box" so as to maintain the CBF at near normal levels. CSF leaves the cranial cavity first, and once autoregulatory mechanisms fail, blood is expelled (i.e., global ischemia), and then finally brain tissue (i.e., cerebral herniation). Several dural folds exist in the cranial cavity (e.g., cerebral falx, tentorium) and effectively serve to compartmentalize the brain. However, these extremely tough pieces of connective tissue are unyielding in the setting of increased ICP. In response to a mass lesion, brain tissue will shift or herniate from one compartment to the next, resulting in tissue damage (including contusion). Subfalcine, transtentorial (i.e., uncal), and tonsillar herniations are the most important forms, with the latter often being fatal due to compression of nearby cardiorespiratory centers in the medulla (26).

Cerebral edema is a local or generalized accumulation of fluid within the brain parenchyma that can result in increased ICP. If severe, cerebral edema may result in herniation. There are three main types of cerebral edema: (a) vasogenic, (b) cytotoxic, and (c) hydrocephalic. The blood-brain-barrier (BBB) results from the specialized properties of the endothelial cells, their intercellular junctions, and a relative lack of vesicular transport (51). Breakdown of the BBB results in vasogenic cerebral edema. This type of cerebral edema is often seen in the context of CNS neoplasia and is responsive to steroid therapy. Cytotoxic cerebral edema refers to the intracellular swelling that occurs in neurons, glia, and endothelial cells. This results from failure of the ATP-dependent Na^+/K^+ pump, and subsequent osmotic accumulation of intracellular fluids. Cytotoxic cerebral edema occurs after hypoxia, or more commonly with global ischemia due to cardiac arrest. Hydrocephalic cerebral edema is the result of transependymal CSF accumulation. Both vasogenic and hydrocephalic cerebral edema are elucidated by hyperintense signals seen on T2-weighted MRI and fluid-attenuated inversion recovery (FLAIR) sequences. Notably, these forms of cerebral edema are not mutually exclusive, and often occur simultaneously. Grossly, the edematous brain exhibits congestion, with flattening of gyri and narrowing of sulci. There may be evidence of cerebral herniation (see above) manifesting as areas of necrosis and hemorrhage. Certain types of herniation routinely cause compression of large arteries and hence infarction (e.g., uncal herniation with posterior cerebral artery compression and primary occipital lobe infarction). On coronal sectioning, the ventricles are collapsed from surrounding pressure and appear slit-like. By histology, the parenchyma is pale and vacuolated.

HCP refers to the accumulation of excess CSF and concurrent expansion of the cerebral ventricles (Figure 10-6). CSF can accumulate under normal ICP, usually in the context of cerebral atrophy; this is called HCP *ex vacuo*. Conventional HCP occurs under the pressure of excess CSF, usually resulting from a paucity of CSF absorption but also more

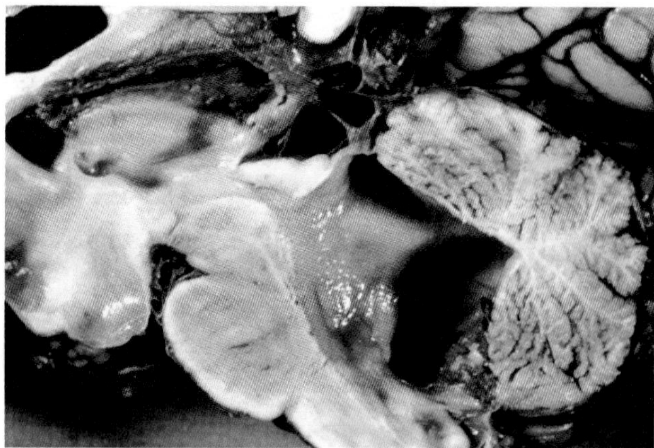

FIGURE 10-6 ■ Hydrocephalus. There is marked dilatation proximal to and including the fourth ventricle in this sagittally sectioned autopsy brain, which also exhibited evidence of meningitis.

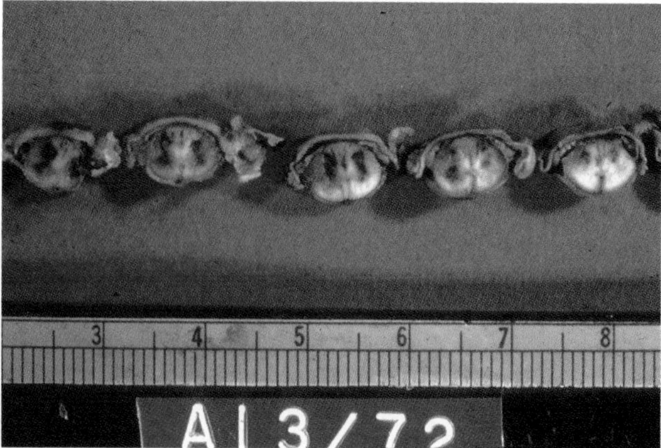

FIGURE 10-7 ■ Laceration and intraparenchymal hemorrhage within the spinal cord secondary to a complicated breech delivery seen here in cross sections of the spinal cord.

uncommonly from abnormal CSF production [e.g., from a choroid plexus papilloma (CPP)]. HCP due to impaired resorption can be communicating or noncommunicating, with the former resulting from a lack of arachnoid granulation–mediated CSF uptake, and the latter being caused by an obstruction in the ventricular system. Communicating HCP is often a result of meningitis or subarachnoid hemorrhage (SAH), while more rare causes include arachnoid villi aplasia or dural venous sinus obstruction. Noncommunicating HCP may be primary (i.e., congenital) or secondary (i.e., acquired). Primary causes include the enigmatic aqueductal obstruction (e.g., related to gliosis, stenosis, atresia/forking, or an obstructing septum) and X-linked HCP (caused by mutations in the L1CAM gene on Xq28). Secondary causes include tumor, hemorrhage, or infection. Several structural CNS abnormalities may exhibit concurrent HCP (e.g., holoprosencephaly) of unknown pathogenesis, and some suggest that the nonspecific term ventriculomegaly may be more appropriate in these cases.

TRAUMA

Birth

Various craniospinal injuries may be mechanically incurred at birth. A number of extracranial hemorrhages may occur within the scalp whose layers can be remembered via the mnemonic "scalp" (Skin, Connective tissue, Aponeurosis epicranialis or galea, Loose connective tissue, Periosteum). Hemorrhage into the subcutaneous connective tissue is called caput succedaneum. There may be subgaleal bleeding and subperiosteal hemorrhage (i.e., cephalohematoma) that often occur over the parietal bone, which may be attributable to forceps delivery. Usually these hemorrhages resolve after a few weeks or months. Perinatal skull fractures are also frequently parietal in location, and often linear in quality. Depressed skull fractures tend to be more common in children over 2 years of age. Separation of the squamous and lateral aspects of the occipital bone is called occipital osteodiastasis, and this may result in contusion of the cerebellum and posterior fossa subdural hemorrhage (SDH). Epidural hemorrhage is less common than SDH and SAH. A cerebral contusion with subsequent evolution to intracerebral/intraventricular hemorrhage (IVH) is rare. However, white matter tears, that are potentially hemorrhagic (i.e., gliding or internal contusions), may be seen in young infants and are thought to arise from shearing forces between the gray and white matter.

The spinal cord may absorb tractional or rotational forces at the time of birth. Breech and cephalic deliveries typically result in upper thoracic/low cervical and midcervical damage, respectively. Large forces can result in laceration (i.e., tearing) of the parenchyma (Figure 10-7). Petechial hemorrhages and axonal spheroids may be seen microscopically. Clinical outcome is variable; there may be acute respiratory failure and death or, in those survivors who are initially hypotonic, spasticity. The brachial plexus may be injured via tractional forces at the time of delivery. Damage to the C5-6 roots results in shoulder deficits (i.e., Erb paralysis), whereas the wrist and digits are affected with C8-T1 insult (Klumpke paralysis). Simplistically, surgical repair involves resection of the resultant traumatic neuroma with anastomosis of more normal proximal and distal nerve stumps; frozen section assessment of the degree of nerve stump viability may be requested intraoperatively.

Infancy and Childhood

Pediatric patients may suffer from both accidental and nonaccidental (i.e., inflicted or abusive) injury. Motor vehicle accidents (MVAs), falls, and assaults are the leading causes of pediatric neurotrauma. The neuropathology of severe or fatal head injury in children older than 1 year is very similar to that seen in adults (26). Infants less than 1 year old suffer a different pattern of injuries, which is thought to be related to the unique anatomic features of this age (39). These include a highly deformable skull, unfused cranial sutures, a high head:body ratio, an elastic spinal column with immature joints, reduced neck muscle tone, and a relatively unmyelinated brain. Accordingly, the cause of death in fatal infant craniospinal injury is often related to cerebral edema, secondary to hypoxia-ischemia. The craniocervical junction is particularly vulnerable and damage to vital brainstem cardiorespiratory centers may account for the frequent clinical presentation of apnea (39). SDH may be seen and is typically thin and bilateral (see below).

Inflicted Injury in Infants

The pathogenesis of fatally inflicted CNS injury among infants is controversial. Several terms have been used to describe the classic pattern injuries and circumstances, the most common of which is likely "shaken baby syndrome." Many disfavor the use of this term since it implies knowledge of the mechanisms surrounding injury; hence we use the term "inflicted injury." Infants suffering inflicted injury often present clinically in a moribund state with respiratory distress or apnea. There may be lethargy, irritation, poor feeding, vomiting, and seizures. Fundoscopy may reveal retinal hemorrhages and CT/MRI often reveals cerebral swelling and a diffuse thin layer of subarachnoid blood. In addition to inflicted mechanisms, this clinical feature may be mimicked by other etiologic entities, including MVAs, vasculopathies/coagulopathies, infection, dehydration, and metabolic abnormalities; hence a thorough forensic-based investigation of these cases may be required (see Chapter 7).

Autopsy of an infant with inflicted injury needs to be meticulous since many findings may be subtle. Extracranial injuries may include rib and long bone fractures, which may be more conspicuous in older children. A variety of cranial fractures and hemorrhages is somewhat characteristic but nevertheless nonspecific in isolation. Skull fractures are relatively common in infants despite the inherent deformability of these bones at this age. Fractures tend to be linear and may result in dural tears and hence CSF leaks (e.g., rhinorrhea, otorrhea). Growing fractures occur when a portion of the leptomeninges herniate through the dural defect and intercede between the two sides of a bony interruption; with time, CSF accumulates in a cyst-like space and erodes bone, thus preventing proper healing. In general, skull fractures are most often parieto-occipital in location. Several different types of hemorrhage may be incurred. Epidural hemorrhage occurs between the outer surface of the dura and the adjacent skull. It is uncommon in infants, possibly because the dura is tightly adherent to the skull, and since the middle meningeal artery is more easily displaced than torn (39). SDHs are common yet different than the space-occupying variety seen in older children and adults. They are thin and bilateral and are often described as "trivial." Accordingly, infant SDHs are not thought to be due to the tearing of bridging veins, and they tend to be accompanied by retinal hemorrhages (which are somewhat nonspecific). SAH and IVHs are generally negligible. Cerebral contusions are essentially "brain bruises," which manifest as areas of parenchymal hemorrhage and necrosis among the crests of gyri. Acutely, the hemorrhage of contusions is perivascular and oriented perpendicular to the cortical surface. Although they may be seen beneath skull fractures, contusions are generally uncommon. Cerebral edema is often the immediate cause of death, and is related to global hypoxic-ischemic injury. As mentioned above, the craniocervical junction is particularly susceptible to injury, especially that which is related to stretch. Careful dissection of the cervical paraspinal muscles may reveal soft-tissue hemorrhage. Spinal epidural hemorrhage may be seen but must be cautiously interpreted since this can be artifactually induced. When the craniocervical region suffers from severe hyperextension injury, pontomedullary rents (or tears) may be identified. If the injured infant survives but dies later on, signs of cerebral atrophy in keeping with hypoxic-ischemic encephalopathy (HIE) may be seen.

Although previously claimed to be indicative of diffuse axonal injury (DAI) by some, the microscopic feature of infant-inflicted injury is not in keeping with such. DAI is due to profound acceleration/deceleration and rotational forces placed upon the head, and results in widespread axonal damage. As opposed to the axonal damage of DAI, infant-inflicted injury is localized often to the lower pons and upper medulla, and particularly to descending corticospinal tracts (32). In addition, axonal damage may be apparent in the cervical and other spinal roots (95). Axonal spheroids can be seen on routine stains about 24 hours after injury, but IHC staining for β-APP can highlight microscopic axonal damage after as little as 2 hours. The lysosomal marker, CD68, is often used to label microglia, and may be used to highlight the acute and more remote cellular reactions to axonal damage. HIE is frequent and is seen more diffusely throughout the brain. Early features include acute neuronal necrosis (i.e., red neurons), parenchymal vacuolation, microglial activation, and myelin pallor, whereas in chronic stages, parenchymal rarefaction predominates with neuronal loss and gliosis.

SUDDEN INFANT DEATH SYNDROME

Sudden infant death syndrome (SIDS) is a complex multifactorial disorder characterized by the sudden clinico-pathologically unexplained death of an infant (<1 year old). Numerous factors are associated with SIDS, but the role to which each impacts this disorder remains elusive. Many of these factors are hypothesized in terms of their effect on the infant's innate autonomic physiologic response to normal homeostatic stressors (e.g., apnea, hypercarbia/blood pH, hypotension, etc.). These infant responses are largely mediated by brainstem nuclei. Maternal factors increasing the risk of SIDS include low socioeconomic status, low maternal education, cigarette smoking, and alcohol consumption. These maternal factors may play a role in predisposing the embryo/infant to hypoxic-ischemic damage [e.g., periventricular leukomalacia (PVL)] or brainstem abnormalities, which can be seen pathologically in a subset of SIDS cases (67); notably, the histopathologic changes seen in SIDS cases are often inconspicuous.

Cerebellar and more so medullary abnormalities have been hypothesized. Derivatives of the rhombic lip [e.g., external granule layer (EGL) of the cerebellum, inferior olive, and the arcuate nucleus] have been implicated in SIDS. Abnormalities in medullary serotonergic (5HT) nuclei have been postulated (74). These nuclei have been suggested to normally modulate and integrate autonomic, respiratory, and somatomotor responses to homeostatic stressors; in particular, lowered 5HT receptor binding has been demonstrated in the arcuate nucleus (56). Susceptibility genes have been proposed, as evidenced by the detection of polymorphisms in the promoter regions/coding sequences; candidate genes include the 5HT transporter, IL-10, and heat shock protein 60 (39). Rare SIDS-like cases have even been associated with cardiac sodium channel mutations (causing arrhythmias) and inborn errors of metabolism (especially medium chain acetyl-CoA dehydrogenase deficiency). Death often occurs during sleep and is associated with the prone position. Integration and synthesis of these factors have led to the triple risk model of SIDS (27). This model proposes that there are three key factors leading to infant death when present simultaneously: (a) a vulnerable infant (i.e., those with pathophysiologic abnormalities), (b) a critical period of development (the peak incidence of SIDS cases occurs at 2 to 4 months and may be related to brain maturation), and (c) an exogenous stressor (e.g., prone sleeping). As researchers continue to unravel the mysteries of this disorder, management and minimization of these recognizable risk factors are the best means of preventing this devastating syndrome (see Chapter 7).

STRUCTURAL MALFORMATIONS OF THE CNS

Neural Tube Defects, Axial Mesodermal Defects, and Tail Bud Defects

Classic embryologic describes three primitive germ layers: endoderm, mesoderm, and ectoderm. Near 16 days postovulation, the mesodermally derived notochord induces the development of CNS tissue from the overlying ectoderm; the signaling molecule sonic hedgehog (Shh) is important to this process. This newly formed neuroectoderm first thickens into the neural plate. A longitudinal neural groove then develops, and subsequently at 18 to 20 days postovulation, neural folds arise from the lateral aspects of the plate. The neural crest (the forerunner of the spinal, cranial nerve and autonomic ganglia, leptomeninges, Schwann cells, melanocytes, and other tissues) originates from the apices of these folds, which eventually meet at distinct closure sites in the midline to form the neural tube. In humans, two initial closure sites are well recognized, one (Site 1) at the cervical-occipital boundary (on day 22 postfertilization), and a second (Site 2) at the extreme rostral end of the neural plate. A third closure site at the forebrain-midbrain boundary may also exist. Fusion of the neural fold proceeds bidirectionally from Site 1 and caudally from Site 2. Fusion of the cranial portion of the neural tube is completed at the anterior neuropore (24 days postfertilization), which subsequently develops into the lamina terminalis. The caudal aspect of the neural tube finishes closure at the posterior neuropore (28 days postfertilization). In general, the process of neural tube formation is called neurulation and is divided into two aspects: (a) primary neurulation describes the fusion of neural folds, which form the rostral aspects of the CNS and (b) secondary neurulation describes the formation of the caudal-most neural tube (i.e., lumbosacral spinal cord) that occurs through canalization of a solid mass of cells. Primary and secondary neurulated tissues eventually join to form the complete neural tube. After neural tube formation, the axial skeleton begins its development and eventually encases the maturing CNS. The skull has a dual origin: the cranial vault and occiput develop from axial mesoderm (endochondral bone formation), while the skull base and facial bones arise from cranial neural crest (membranous bone). The vertebrae also arise from axial mesoderm.

Neural Tube Defects

Neural tube defects (NTDs) are the result of defective neural tube closure during the third to fourth week of gestational age (GA). The true incidence of NTD is difficult to determine since severe forms lead to spontaneous abortion. Birth prevalence has been estimated to be between 3 and 7/1,000 depending on several factors, including geography (e.g., high prevalence in Northern Ireland) (30). There is a spectrum of CNS involvement, from widespread (e.g., complete craniorachischisis) to more focal (e.g., lumbosacral myelomeningocele). Patients with focal spinal forms may survive with motor and sensory deficits below the level of nonclosure, which include rectal and urinary sphincter involvement (e.g., incontinence, urinary tract infections). Additional problems may include HCP, Chiari II malformation, and kyphosis. Although the use of folic acid supplements has reduced the frequency of NTDs, the mechanism by which they act is unclear. Craniorachischisis is the most severe form of NTD wherein there is complete failure of neural tube closure such that the brain and spinal cord are exposed to the amniotic fluid. There may be some forebrain development rostrally, but neural tube closure is usually deficient distal to the midbrain. In anencephaly, the NTD is generally limited to the cranial and cervical regions (Figure 10-8). The skull vault is absent, the skull base is malformed (thick and flat anomalous sphenoid bones), and the orbits are shallow. The majority of the brain (minus portions of the anterior pituitary, cranial nerves, medulla, and some cerebellar folia) is replaced by the area cerebrovasculosa. This CSF-filled cystic angiomatous area contains neuroepithelial remnants (including ependyma, neurons, neuroblasts, and choroid plexus) and numerous thin-walled blood vessels. Keratinizing squamous epithelium, that is continuous with normal skin, covers the defect. Due to the deficiency of cerebral tissue, there is a paucity of descending spinal cord tracts.

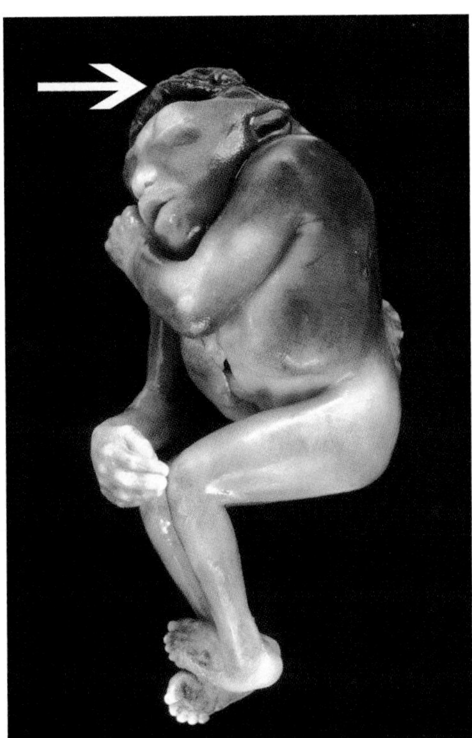

FIGURE 10-8 ■ Anencephaly. Because of the absent calvarium (or "skull cap"), malformed vascularized neuroglial tissue (i.e., area cerebrovasculosa) can be directly visualized (see *arrow*).

Overlying spinal leptomeninges are vascular and may contain glioneuronal heterotopias (39). Associated abnormalities include hypoplastic adrenals and lungs, plus an enlarged thymus. Myelomeningoceles can occur throughout the spinal cord, but lumbosacral lesions are the most frequent (Figure 10-9). An association with the Chiari II malformation may be noted. The spinal cord may be "closed" (i.e., no NTD *per se*) or "open" posteriorly as a flattened lesion. Closed lesions are cystic and covered by a delicate membrane/skin that contains a hydromyelic cord (Figure 10-9 A,B). Open lesions contain a vascularized mass of disorganized neuroepithelial tissue, the area medullovasculosa that is covered by atrophic cutaneous tissue. In either case, the spinal cord and meninges herniate through an associated vertebral defect. There may be spinal cord abnormalities above the NTD (e.g., hydromyelia, syringomyelia, and diplomyelia).

Herniation Through Axial Mesodermal Defects

Portions of CNS tissue (with proper neural tube closure) may herniate through axial mesodermal (i.e., bony) defects. These include encephaloceles and meningoceles. Encephaloceles may be anteriorly located (fronto-ethmoidal cases are common in Southeast Asia), but occipital cases are the most frequent (Figure 10-10). Occipital encephaloceles can involve the foramen magnum and include portions of cerebellum, brainstem, and occipital lobe (e.g., Chiari III malformation). Meckel-Gruber syndrome is a lethal autosomal recessive disorder that is characterized by the triad of CNS malformations (especially occipital encephalocele), cystic dysplasia of the kidneys, and ductal plate malformations of the liver (3). It can be detected by ultrasound prior to 14 weeks gestation. There is genetic linkage to three loci: 17q21-24 (MKS1), 11q13 (MKS2), and 8q24 (MKS3). Meningoceles are typically lumbosacral in location. All three layers of meninges herniate through the bony vertebral defect, while the spinal cord remains in a normal position. Accompanying

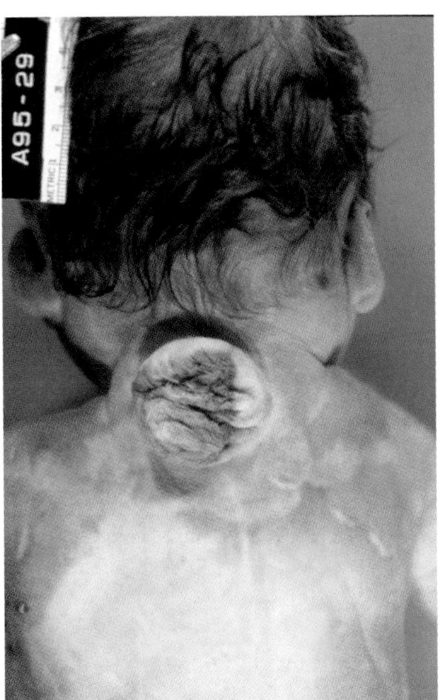

A

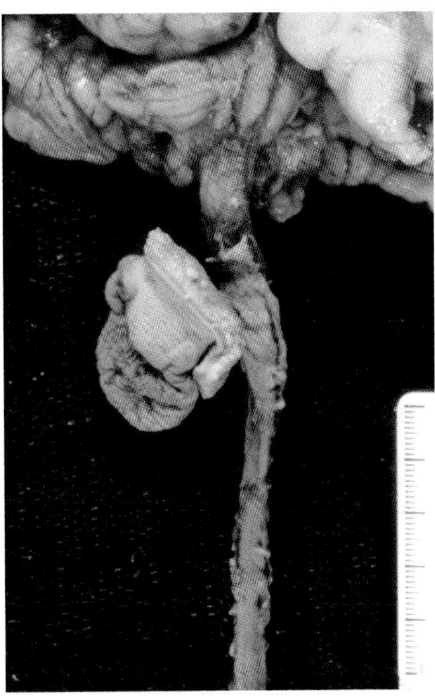

B

FIGURE 10-9 ■ Cervical myelomeningocele (**A and B**). Gross dissection revealed contiguity of the midline cervical mass and the cervical spinal cord. (Images courtesy of Dr. Beth Levy, Department of Pathology, St. Louis University School of Medicine, St. Louis, MO.)

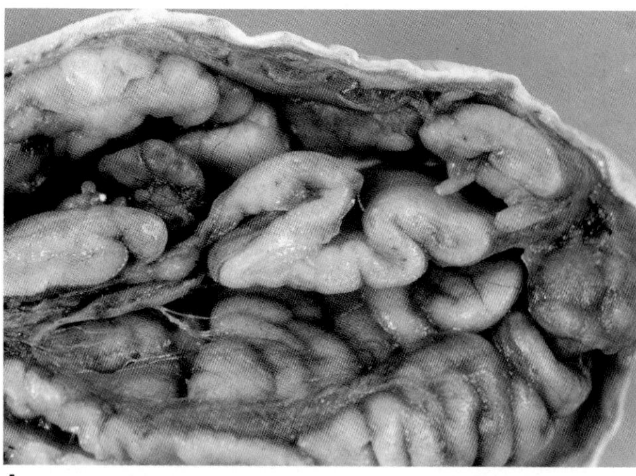
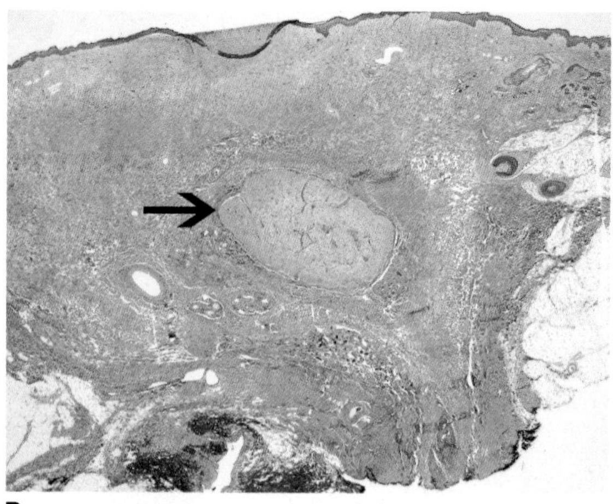

A B

FIGURE 10-10 ■ Encephalocele. **A:** Atrophic cutaneous tissue overlies brain parenchyma in this surgical specimen. (Image courtesy of Dr. Beth Levy, St. Louis University.) **B:** Histologically, neuroglial tissue (*arrow*) is embedded within the deep subcutaneous connective tissue from a more subtly involved example.

spinal cord defects may be seen and include hydromyelia, syringomyelia, diastematomyelia, and cord tethering.

Tailbud Defects

Tailbud defects are thought to involve abnormalities of secondary neurulation. Cord abnormalities are lumbosacral and include hydromyelia (dilatation of the central canal), diastematomyelia (splitting of the cord into hemisections and often due to a bony spur), diplomyelia (duplication), and cord tethering. The tethered cord syndrome *per se* involves lower limb motor and sensory deficits, pain, and neuropathic bladder, all of which presumably result from traction on distal cord elements. There may be a thickened filum terminale, low or dilated conus medullaris, spinal lipoma, or other abnormalities in the lumbosacral cord or sacral region in general (39). Detethering frequently leads to clinical improvement, although surgical specimens are not common (61).

Disorders of Forebrain Development

The early development of the forebrain and midline structures, as it pertains to the neuropathology of structural malformations, is described in greater detail by Ellison (26). Three primary brain vesicles are present by the fourth week of gestational age (GA): (a) prosencephalon (forebrain), (b) mesencephalon (midbrain), and (c) rhombencephalon (hindbrain). Forebrain induction is thought to be governed by the prechordal plate, the ventralizing molecule Shh, and the dorsalizing molecule bone morphogenic protein 7. By constraining growth in the ventral midline of the forebrain primordium, the relatively rapid dorsolateral growth leads to the formation of paired telencephalic secondary vesicles by the sixth week GA. There are five secondary brain vesicles: (a) the telencephalon (cerebral hemispheres and basal ganglia) and (b) diencephalon (thalamic substructures), both arise from the prosencephalon; (c) mesencephalon; (d) the metencephalon (pons and cerebellum) and (e) myelencephalon (medulla), both arise from the rhombencephalon. Shh also induces the optic primordium to divide and grow out from the diencephalon at 4 to 5 weeks GA. The paired olfactory vesicles are induced by the olfactory placodes and their ingrowing olfactory nerves at 6 weeks GA. The anterior commissure begins its development at 10 weeks GA, arising from or adjacent to the lamina terminalis. At this same time, the fornices and hippocampal primordia arise nearby and grow in a reverse C-shaped manner en route to their destination in the temporal lobe. The corpus callosum arises at 12 weeks GA from the massa commissuralis, which is slightly rostral and superior to the anterior commissure. It grows in a rostro-caudal manner, and in doing so results in the formation of the septum pellucidum at 20 weeks GA.

Holoprosencephaly and Agenesis of the Corpus Callosum

Holoprosencephaly is a disorder of induction and patterning of the rostral neural tube occurring at 4 to 5 weeks GA. This may be the result of a faulty prechordal plate (17). The majority of cases are sporadic, and the incidence is approximately 5 to 9/100,000 live births. Risk factors for holoprosencephaly include maternal diabetes and possibly alcohol consumption. Chromosomal abnormalities are commonly seen, the most frequent of which is trisomy 13 (Patau syndrome). Molecular genetic investigations have revealed seven genes that are associated with holoprosencephaly, including SIX3 (HPE2), SHH (HPE3), TGIF (HPE4), ZIC2 (HPE5), and PTCH (HPE7). Mutation of the sonic hedgehog gene (SHH) is especially intriguing in light of its role in neuroectodermal induction. Holoprosencephaly may be seen in the context of a well-recognized syndrome, such as Smith-Lemli-Opitz syndrome (due to a defect in cholesterol biosynthesis). Notably, the Shh molecule must undergo autoproteolytic cleavage for proper functioning, which in turn is dependent on cholesterol attachment to its carboxy-terminus. Holoprosencephaly has a variable clinical picture; severe forms result in death early in life, while more mild forms allow survival into adulthood. Craniofacial and ocular abnormalities that can be present have been hypothesized to be a result of defective mesencephalic neural crest (94) (Figure 10-11A). Microcephaly (i.e., small head) is common; brains are correspondingly micrencephalic (i.e., low weight) and often less than 100 g at term. There may be hypotonia, seizures, developmental delay, and mental retardation. Hypofunctioning of the pituitary gland results in pan-endocrinopathies.

There are three main clinico-pathologic categories of holoprosencephaly that together likely represent a spectrum of disease severity. Lobar, semilobar, and alobar forms correspond to increasingly severe structural and clinical diseases, which is generally defined by the extent of the midline longitudinal fissure. In less severe forms, the fissure can be seen "cleaving" the cerebrum into two cerebral hemispheres more caudally. In alobar holoprosencephaly, this midline fissure is absent, resulting in a single cerebral mass or holosphere. The Sylvian fissure, gyrus rectus, and the olfactory structures are also absent. This anomalous gyral pattern prohibits the delineation of cerebral lobes. The holosphere is horseshoe shaped and contains a single ventricle that opens postero-dorsally (Figure 10-11B). The opening of this ventricle is covered by a delicate membranous roof that attaches to the tentorium; this membrane may balloon to form a dorsal cyst. The lateral aspects of this membrane are bounded by a single arch-shaped hippocampus. The floor of the single ventricle is formed by the fused deep gray nuclei. Although the corpus callosum is absent, there is no bundle of Probst (see below). The anterior commissure and the septum pellucidum are also absent. Both the brainstem and the cerebellum are grossly normal (with the exception of hypoplastic corticospinal tracts). The skull base is malformed. The anterior aspects of the circle of Willis are anomalous, and both the anterior and middle cerebral arteries are replaced by a disorganized collection of vessels called the rete mirable. Microscopically, the cortical gray matter is dysplastic (93). It is excessively thick and dyslaminated, and may demonstrate a progressively abnormal latero-medial gradient of architectural disturbance (94). The sparsely cellular external layer is segmented and arranged into irregular clusters, which may form thick cords of neurons that can traverse the entire pallium (i.e., developing cortical gray matter). There may be acellular deep zones or "glomeruli." The deeper neocortical neurons are often maloriented. The leptomeninges of the holosphere can be laden with glioneuronal rests and form a superficial "crust" over the brain. The architecture of the hippocampi, deep gray nuclei, and cerebellum is also often abnormal, with the latter exhibiting dysplasia, heterotopia, and an association with trisomy 13.

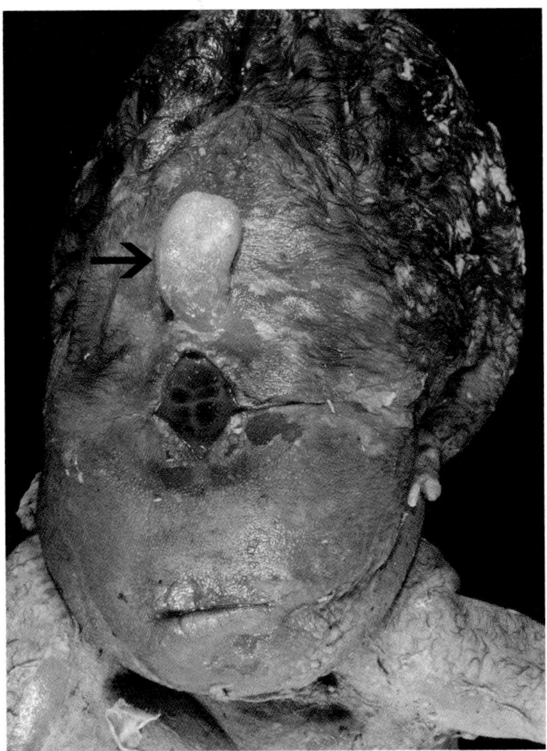

A

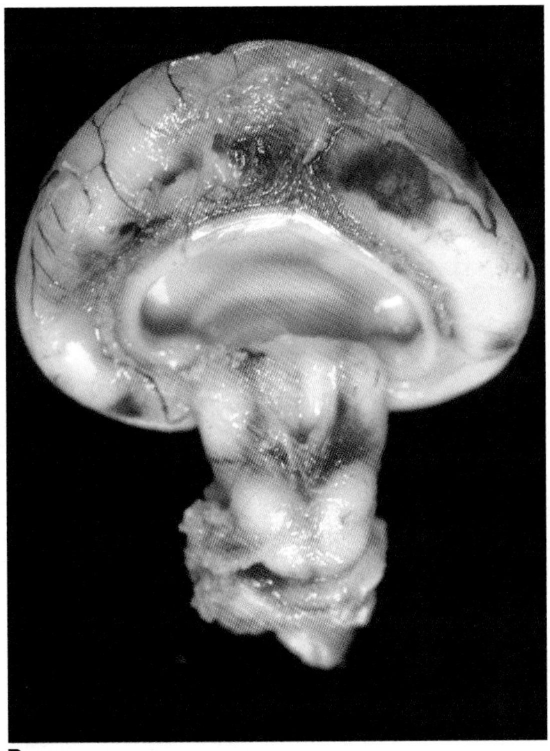

B

FIGURE 10-11 ▪ Alobar holoprosencephaly. **A:** Examination of the face reveals a proboscis (*arrow*), which is superior to a single orbit bearing two fused globes. **B:** Superior and caudal views of the brain reveal the horseshoe-shaped holosphere containing a single ventricle that opens postero-dorsally. (Images courtesy of Dr. Robert Schmidt, Department of Pathology and Immunology, Washington University School of Medicine, St. Louis, MO.)

The least severe lobar form of holoprosencephaly, despite its resemblance to normal brain, still contains cerebral cortex that is continuous across the midline (at the frontal pole, in the orbital region or above the corpus callosum causing cingulosynapsis). Portions of the olfactory structures and posterior corpus callosum may be present. Semilobar holoprosencephaly is intermediate in appearance. In the recently described middle hemispheric variant of holoprosencephaly, portions of the deep gray nuclei and fronto-parietal lobe are fused across the midline, with relative rostral, caudal, and ventral brain sparing.

Agenesis of the corpus callosum (ACC) may be isolated or seen in combination with other CNS abnormalities. These associations (e.g., a neuronal migration disorder) make it difficult to assess the clinical impact of agenesis of the corpus callosum *per se*. However, isolated agenesis of the corpus callosum is most often asymptomatic and found incidentally on imaging. Potential signs and symptoms may include seizures, mental retardation, subtle perceptual deficits, or a disconnection-like syndrome. ACC may be associated with a well-recognized syndrome (e.g., Aicardi) or an inborn error of metabolism (e.g., nonketotic hyperglycinemia). Pathologically, the characteristic findings of ACC are seen grossly on coronal sectioning of the brain. Agenesis may be complete or partial, with latter forms being found more caudally (i.e., splenium) in keeping with the corpus callosum's rostro-caudal embryologic development. Laterally situated and longitudinally directed bundles of white matter are usually identified immediately superior to the lateral ventricles; these are called the bundles of Probst, and are thought to represent misdirected callosal fibers (Figure 10-12). The normal dorso-lateral angles of the lateral ventricles take on an abnormal superior orientation (i.e., "bat-wing ventricles").

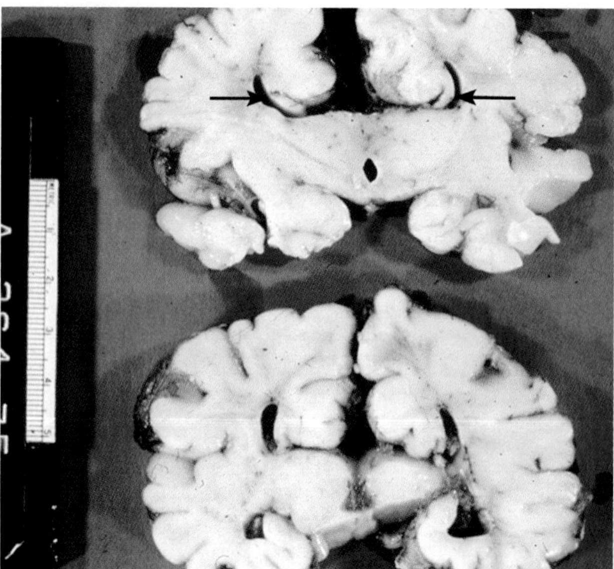

FIGURE 10-12 ■ Agenesis of the corpus callosum. Coronal sections of the brain do not reveal a normal corpus callosum; in its absence, dorso-laterally directed "bundles of Probst" (*arrows*) are noted. (Image courtesy of Dr. Barry Rewcastle.)

The distended membranous roof of the 3rd ventricle displaces the fornices and leaves of the septum pellucidum laterally. The cingulate gyrus is replaced by several short radiating gyri, and the anterior commissure may also be absent. Other structural abnormalities that may accompany agenesis of the corpus callosum include HCP, olfactory hypoplasia and neuronal migration deficits (see below). A subset of ACC may be the result of mechanically impeding mass lesion (e.g., lipoma), but the pathogenesis of most other cases is unclear. Some have speculated that abnormalities in the "glial sling," which normally guides commissural fibers across the midline, may be a potential cause of ACC (20).

Other disorders of forebrain induction include olfactory aplasia, atelencephaly, aprosencephaly, and abnormalities involving the septum pellucidum (26). Just as the development of the cingulate gyrus and that of corpus callosum are linked, so are those of the olfactory bulbs and the gyrus rectus; true olfactory aplasia is usually accompanied by absence of the gyrus rectus.

Cell Migration and Specification Disorders

The embryology of early neocortical development is reviewed in greater detail by Golden (39). The wall of the early neural tube is composed of a pseudostratified neuroepithelial layer. By 4 weeks GA, the outer preplate zone has emerged from the inner ventricular zone of neuroepithelium. The preplate is composed of two layers: an outer layer of Cajal Retzius cells (CRCs) (i.e., neurons) and an inner layer of subplate neurons. These transient subplate neurons play an important role in the early organization of neocortical connectivity. CRCs secrete reelin, an important extracellular matrix protein that assists migrating neuroblasts in finding their correct neocortical laminar destination. By 6 weeks GA, radial glia processes have essentially spanned the cortical mantle and aligned themselves perpendicular to the brain surface. These radial glia processes serve as physical guides for the migrating neuroblasts, which will form the cortical plate and eventual neocortex. The process of radial migration is complex and involves numerous molecules, including neuregulin, ErbB4, cell adhesion molecules, astrotactin, extracellular matrix molecules, and their receptors (39). A two-part physical barrier to overmigration lies in the marginal zone (i.e., laminae I) of the pallium and is composed of (a) the glia limitans, which is formed by the expanded end feet of the radial glia and the basal lamina of pial blood vessels, and (b) the horizontal processes and synapses of CRCs. Neuroblasts leave the ventricular zone to populate the cortical plate "split the preplate" and form the future neocortical laminae in an inside-to-outside sequence, with the deepest layers forming prior to more superficial layers (i.e., laminae VI prior to V, etc.). These neuroblasts migrate in waves between 6 and 20 weeks GA. There is also tangential migration in the developing neocortex, wherein migrating neuroblasts (future inhibitory neurons) are guided by neuronal processes (rather than radial glia) to their destination. The primitive neocortex is initially overpopulated by neurons, and their numbers are normally culled by apoptosis. The remaining neurons terminally differentiate and establish the connectivity pattern indicative of the developed neocortex.

Lissencephaly, Types I and II

Lissencephaly type I (i.e., classical type) is a diffuse and abnormally "smooth" (i.e., agyric) cerebral surface, whereas pachygyria represents a more focal agyric abnormality among more normally gyrated cortex. Lissencephaly type I is caused by disrupted neocortical cell migration. A number of additional CNS malformations may be associated with lissencephaly type I, and imaging that reveals such features can guide genetic testing. Four main genes have been linked to lissencephaly type I and some appear associated with distinct histopathology (39). LIS1 (17p13.3) encodes the LIS1 protein [aka platelet-activating factor acetyl hydrolase 1 subunit β1 (PAFAH1β1)] that is involved in a complex cellular cascade, which influences dynein (and hence cell movement) and possibly cell proliferation. LIS1 is associated with Miller-Dieker syndrome. XLIS (Xq22.3-23) (or DCX) encodes doublecortin, which is a microtubule-associated protein; while affected males have lissencephaly type I, females exhibit subcortical band heterotopia (SBH; see "Cerebral Heterotopia" below). The reelin gene's (RELN; 7q22) product (i.e., reelin) is the extracellular ligand that influences intracellular downstream targets (e.g., LIS1 protein). Clinically, mutation in RELN causes lissencephaly type I associated with cerebellar malformations. Finally, ARX (Xp21) encodes a transcription factor important in CNS/PNS development; mutations result in lissencephaly type I and ambiguous genitalia. The general clinical features of lissencephaly type I include developmental delay, mental retardation, seizures (including infantile spasms), and microcephaly.

Pathologically, lissencephaly type I is characterized by thickened neocortical gray matter and a paucity of white matter (Figure 10-13). The aygric cortex may be preferentially seen more rostrally (XLIS or RELN mutation) or caudally (LIS1 mutation). Foci of pachygyria tend to have an ill-defined border with more normal brain. Heterotopic gray matter may be seen in the periventricular and deep white matter, and if associated with an XLIS mutation, a subcortical band of gray matter may be seen. There may be HCP. The cerebellum is typically hypoplastic in cases associated with RELN mutations. The inferior olives may be dysplastic, and the cortico-spinal tracts may be abnormal. Classically, the histology of lissencephaly type I is described as a malformed four-layer cortex: (a) the outer first layer (i.e., molecular layer) is fairly normal and contains CRCs, (b) the second layer contains large maloriented pyramidal neuron, (c) the cell poor third layer may be myelinated in older children, and (d) the fourth layer is a thick and contains disorganized small to medium pyramidal and granular neurons. This classic four-layer pattern corresponds to the LIS1 mutation and

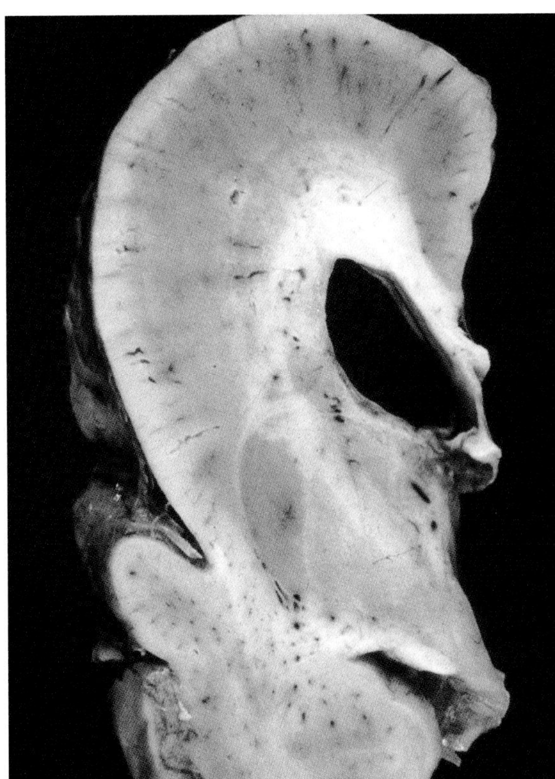

FIGURE 10-13 ■ Lissencephaly type I. The markedly thickened cerebral gray matter displays an absence of gyration. There is a concomitant paucity of cerebral white matter (coronal section). (Image courtesy of Dr. Beth Levy, St. Louis University.)

is more prominent in the posterior cerebral aspects. Recent investigations have suggested additional histologic variants, including four-layer anteriorly predominant (DCX mutation), three-layer (ARX mutation), and two-layer forms (29).

The cell migratory defect in lissencephaly type II (i.e., cobblestone type) appears to be one of overmigration. A defective glia limitans allows radial glial processes to extend beyond the normal limits of the neocortex, facilitating the excessive migration of neuroglial precursors. Lissencephaly type II shares a thickened neocortical gray ribbon and at times an agyric surface with lissencephaly type I. However, the five main autosomal recessive syndromes associated with lissencephaly type II exhibit a characteristic triad of cerebral, ocular, and muscle diseases that are not seen in type I disease. These syndromes include Walker-Warburg syndrome, Fukuyama congenital muscular dystrophy (FCMD), Muscle-Eye-Brain disease, congenital muscular dystrophy type 1D (MDC1D), and, MDC1C, a disorder associated with fukutin-related protein (FKRP). FCMD is the most common (incidence of 3/100,000/year) and characteristically occurs in Japan. The abnormalities in these syndromes (and hence lissencephaly type II) are thought to be due to defective glycosylation, in particular O-mannosylation. Glycosylation is a common posttranslational protein modification and, in general, is important to normal development. O-glycosylation of α-dystroglycan appears particularly important to the etiology of these conditions (65). Pathologically, these micrencephalic brains have a lissencephalic cortex that may have a "bumpy" quality (i.e., cobblestone). The gray-white junction tends to be distinct below the thickened gray matter. White matter is deficient, and there may be HCP. The brainstem is small, in part due to hypoplastic corticospinal tracts. The cerebellum in these cases is characteristically small, especially in the vermal region, and cases of Walker-Warburg syndrome may exhibit features of a Dandy-Walker malformation (DWM) and an occipital encephalocele. Microscopically, the cortex is very disorganized and unlaminated. Superficial aspects tend to be more abnormal and may resemble polymicrogyria. The gray-white junction may exhibit a nodular appearance. The deep and superficial areas are separated by large internalized and hyalinized blood vessels that likely represent the original overrun leptomeningeal vasculature. Less severely affected areas may contain a leptomeningeal "crust" of glioneuronal ectopia. The cerebellum is disorganized, and although the internal granular and Purkinje neurons retain their somewhat normal relations, the normal architecture is disrupted. Bands of white matter are seen over the cerebellar surface. The overall appearance of the cerebellum may also resemble polymicrogyria.

Polymicrogyria

Polymicrogyria is a cortical malformation where the neocortical gray matter ribbon is microscopically thin, excessively folded, and fused. Intrinsic and acquired origins for this lesion have been proposed (39). The risk factors for polymicrogyria include (a) intrauterine infection (e.g., "TORCH"), (b) intrauterine ischemia, (c) metabolic diseases (e.g., Zellweger syndrome), and (d) a family history. Polymicrogyria may also be associated with well-recognized syndromes. Karyotypic abnormalities have been noted (e.g., −1p36, −22q11), but with the exception of FGRR3 mutations in thanatophoric dwarfism, specific mutational information is limited (44). Clinically, localized polymicrogyria may be asymptomatic, but more often it is associated with developmental delay, psychomotor retardation, spastic diplegia, pseudobulbar palsy, and seizures. MRI highlights this abnormal cortex and may reveal additional structural abnormalities (e.g., decreased white matter or other white matter changes, calcification, schizencephaly, porencephaly, etc.). Grossly, the cerebral surface in polymicrogyria is irregular and bumpy. Coronal sections reveal thickened neocortical gray matter composed of serpiginous, heaped-up thin layers. Polymicrogyria may be widespread and symmetric, or focal and asymmetric. Cingulate and striate cortices are often spared. Polymicrogyria may be seen in the relatively spared temporal lobe of hydranencephaly, or adjacent to porencephalic defects. Microscopically, the cortex is composed of numerous attenuated, excessively folded, and fused layers (Figure 10-14). Fusion of adjacent molecular layers results in a branching pattern of paucicellular tissue, which often bears a central blood vessel. The cortex is usually unlayered but may be four layered (similar to lissencephaly type I). Leptomeningeal glioneuronal and nodular heterotopias may also be seen.

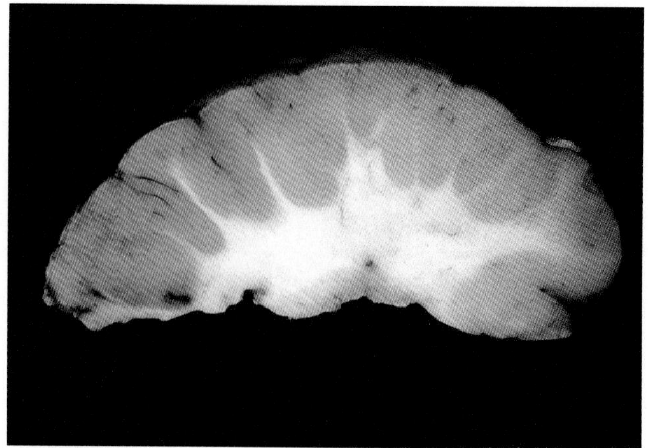

FIGURE 10-14 ■ Polymicrogyria. Transverse sectioning of this surgical brain specimen reveals abnormal undulation of the cortical ribbon.

Cerebral Heterotopia

Cerebral heterotopia refers to malformative lesions wherein groups of cytologically normal brain cells (i.e., neurons and glia) do not reach their neocortical destination. Three main categories are discussed here: leptomeningeal heterotopia (LH), periventricular heterotopia (PH), and SBH. LH and PH are often associated with other CNS malformations, while SBH is usually seen in isolation. LH is likely the most common of these three forms and is usually focal. Genetic and epigenetic risk factors are associated with each form of cerebral heterotopia. Genetic syndromes linked to LH include trisomy 13, holoprosencephaly, and lissencephaly type II. The genetics of PH are complex, but one X-linked form involves mutations of the FLNA gene (Xq28) (99). SBH is usually due to mutations in the X-LIS gene (i.e., doublecortin, DCX) (see above). Epigenetic risk factors likely represent the most common mechanisms underlying LH/PH and include HIE, PVL, and germinal matrix/subpial hemorrhage. Damage to the glia limitans and radial glia likely underlies the pathogenesis of LH and PH, respectively. It is difficult to assess the clinical impact of these heterotopias since LH and PH are frequently associated with other CNS malformations. However, mental retardation and seizures often accompany all three forms of cerebral heterotopia. Grossly, LH is often inapparent unless seen in the context of lissencephaly type II. SBH appears as a band of gray matter (outside of the intragyral white matter) that is flanked on either side by white matter. On close inspection, the gray matter of the SBH may be broken up into nodules, which are split by white matter bundles. PH may also be confluent (i.e., band-like) or nodular. Like LH, PH is associated with abnormal adjacent neocortex (cortical dysplasia with LH, and polymicrogyria with PH). Microscopically, all three forms of cerebral heterotopia appear similar.

Pyramidal and granular neurons are associated with glia and other normal neocortical elements, but there is no lamination and the neurons are maloriented. In LH, there is usually some connection to the underlying cortex.

"Malformations of Cortical Development," Including Focal Cortical Dysplasia

This group of epileptogenic CNS malformations regrettably has been plagued by a plethora of confusing terminology. A recent multidisciplinary consensus has been achieved regarding the terminology of these cortical lesions (72). Malformations of cortical development (MCD) is the umbrella term and encompasses several entities such as the neuronal migration disorders (NMD; see above), focal cortical dysplasia (FCD), and microdysgenesis. Previously, the term "cortical dysplasia" was often used nonspecifically to describe many different abnormal cortical histologies. Microdysgenesis has similarly been utilized in the past to describe more mild abnormalities in cortical architecture (e.g., excess white matter neurons, excess perivascular oligodendroglia in the white matter, "glioneuronal hamartia," abnormal neuronal clustering, dyslamination, cortical columnarization) (52); however, the term mild MCD is now favored over microdysgenesis (see below).

FCDs are a relatively common surgical specimen. The seizures associated with FCD usually manifest in the first decade. A variety of genetic predispositions and environmental insults have been hypothesized to play a role in the pathogenesis of FCD. At what time FCD arise during embryology is unclear (i.e., insult occurring before, during, or after neuroglial migration). Genetic studies have suggested general roles for the PI3K/mTOR and reelin pathways in FCD. In addition, polymorphisms of the TSC1 gene have been associated with FCD type IIb, while polymorphisms of the TSC2 gene have been seen with ganglioglioma (GG) and FCD type IIa (5). Identification of these lesions has been facilitated by MRI (90). Pathologically, lesions may be grossly inapparent or seen as a focal thickening of gray matter with blurring of the underlying gray-white matter junction. The main histologic features of FCD were recently reviewed and used to devise a new classification scheme (72). Dyslamination and columnar disorganization are common findings among most FCDs, and are usually associated with other

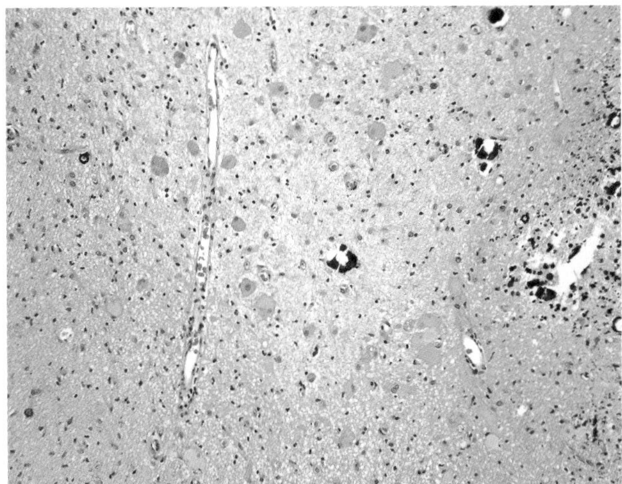

FIGURE 10-15 ■ FCD type IIb. Balloon cells are seen within the gliotic and calcified white matter immediately subjacent to malformed cortical gray matter.

"mild" abnormalities (in particular, ectopic neurons in the subarachnoid space or within layer I of the cortex); these findings have been termed mild MCD. FCD has been divided into types I and II (i.e., Taylor type), with only the latter containing overtly dysmorphic neurons and balloon cells (Figure 10-15). Dysmorphic neurons are neurofilament (NFP)-rich, maloriented, and/or abnormally large neurons with atypical coarse Nissl substance and thick dendritic processes. Balloon cells are abnormal cells with abundant glassy eosinophilic cytoplasm and eccentrically placed vesicular nuclei, often with prominent nucleoli; larger than gemistocytes, these cells may demonstrate neuronal, glial, or hybrid features by routine staining and by immunohistochemistry (e.g., coexpressing GFAP and neuronal markers). Neuronal abnormalities are limited to immature (round/oval cells with an enlarged nucleus and a thin rim of cytoplasm) and or giant (normal but enlarged, 50 to 80 μm pyramidal) neurons in FCD type I (see Table 10-1). Other changes may be numerous but often include gliosis, hypomyelinated zones, an abnormally myelinated layer I, and calcification (39). FCD type IIb is often indistinguishable from the tubers of tuberous sclerosis (TS), and as such may represent a forme fruste of this condition, a hypothesis which is somewhat strengthened by genetic studies (see above). The histologic changes of FCD

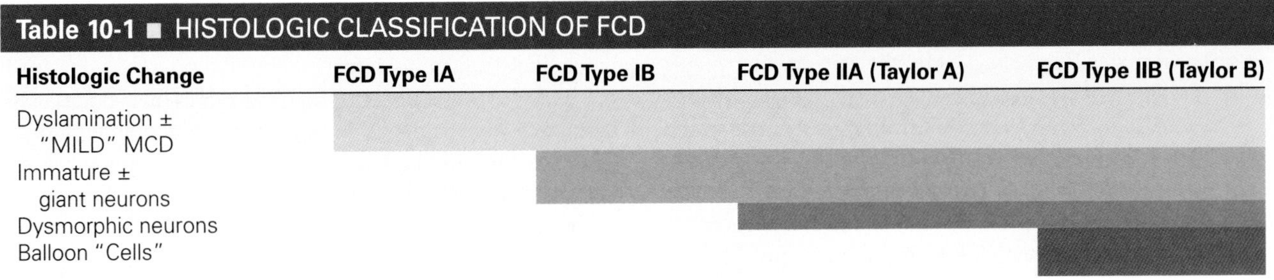

Table 10-1 ■ HISTOLOGIC CLASSIFICATION OF FCD

Histologic Change	FCD Type IA	FCD Type IB	FCD Type IIA (Taylor A)	FCD Type IIB (Taylor B)
Dyslamination ± "MILD" MCD				
Immature ± giant neurons				
Dysmorphic neurons				
Balloon "Cells"				

FCD, focal cortical dysplasia; MCD, malformation of cortical development (see text for details).
Adapted from Palmini A, Najm I, Avanzini G, et al. Terminology and classification of the FCDs. *Neurology* 2004;62(Suppl. 3):S2–S8.

may also be similar to those seen in hemimegalencephaly, an epileptogenic disorder that describes the syndromic or isolated occurrence of an enlarged abnormal hemisphere associated with hemiparesis and developmental delay (39).

Antenatal Disruptive Lesions

Although in a sense this group of lesions could be considered malformative, they are felt to be largely due to the impact of a hypoxic-ischemic insult on the developing brain. These insults are acquired *in utero*. Intrauterine infections may play a role in the etiology of some of these lesions. Hydranencephaly is the severe and diffuse necrosis of the cerebral mantle and deep gray (and concomitant HCP *ex vacuo*) due to perfusion failure of the internal carotid territory at 15 to 16 weeks gestation. The residual mantle is markedly thinned, and there is evidence of secondary brainstem and spinal cord atrophy. There may be sparing of parenchyma supplied by the posterior cerebral artery. Porencephaly describes the focal transmantle necrosis of cerebrum (most often in the middle cerebral artery territory) wherein the ventricle communicates with the subarachnoid space. Polymicrogyria, gliosis, and calcification often rim the porencephalic defect. If there is bilateral MCA damage that spares the cingulate gyri (i.e., leaving a "handle"), the resulting defect is called basket brain. Schizencephaly describes a nontransmantle cleft in the cerebrum. Multicystic encephalopathy is the result of a diffuse white/gray matter insult to the cerebrum, causing widespread necrosis and cystic change. The insult in MCE is presumed to occur late in gestation.

Microcephaly and Micrencephaly

Microcephaly refers to a small head, whereas micrencephaly refers to a small brain. Some authors have used the term microcephaly interchangeably to refer to both of these abnormalities.

Hindbrain Malformations

As described above, by the sixth week of GA, the secondary brain vesicles that give rise to the cerebellum and pons (metencephalon), in addition to the medulla (myelencephalon), have begun their development. There are similarities in the development of the hindbrain and the spinal cord. The alar and basal plates give rise to the dorsal sensory and ventral motor spinal cord horns, respectively. With respect to hindbrain, its dorsal aspect is essentially splayed out such that the motor basal plates lie medial, while the sensory alar plates lie lateral. The metencephalic alar plates fuse and give rise to the cerebellum. The Purkinje and deep gray neurons of the cerebellum arise from the ventricular zone of the alar plate, while the eventual internal granule neurons arise from the upper aspect of an alar plate derivative called the rhombic lip (109). A lateral to medial outward migration of granule neuron precursors has populated the EGL by 14 weeks, and persists until 1 year of age. Neurons from the EGL migrate inward to their eventual destination in the internal granule layer. The flocculonodular, anterior and posterior lobes are already identifiable by 12 weeks GA. Cerebellar folia can be seen by 20 weeks. Precerebellar nuclei (i.e., the pontine and inferior olivary nuclei) arise from the lower rhombic lip.

Chiari and Dandy-Walker Malformations

Although the Chiari malformations are discussed in the context of the hindbrain, their actual pathogenesis is unclear (see below). Three forms are well recognized. Chiari I malformations are characterized by the caudal displacement (not true herniation) of the cerebellar tonsils through the foramen magnum and into the upper cervical spinal canal. Chiari I malformations are often associated with syringomyelia. The clinical picture includes neck pain and signs/symptoms associated with syringomyelia (i.e., "cape-like" or "hanging" dissociated sensory loss in the shoulders and arms) that develops in older teenagers and young adults. Pathologically, surgical resection specimens reveal sclerotic and gliotic degenerated tonsillar tissue. Pathogenesis of the Chiari I malformation is unclear. Chiari II malformations (previously known as the Arnold-Chiari malformation) occur in young children and describe the caudal displacement of cerebellar vermis into the upper cervical spinal canal plus added hindbrain abnormalities. Ninety-five percent of Chiari II malformations are associated with a lumbosacral myelomeninocele (39). Maternal vitamin A deficiency is a risk factor for Chiari II. The clinical picture of Chiari II is dominated by HCP and the myelomeningocele. Pathologically, the fourth ventricle, midbrain, pons, and medulla are all elongated and caudally displaced. There may be "tectal beaking" and an S-shaped "kinking" of the medulla onto the dorsal spinal cord (Figure 10-16). The posterior fossa is small, and there may be abnormalities of the cranial nerves. Additional CNS malformations may include PH, polymicrogyria, and pachygyria. Pathogenesis of the Chiari II malformation is unknown. Hypotheses include (a) hydrodynamic (related to mechanic pressure from HCP or excess CSF egress from the myelomeningocele), (b) cord tethering, (c) a defect in neurulation, or (d) a defect in the posterior fossa mesenchyme leading to restricted cerebellar growth. Chiari III malformations are rare and are defined by an occipito-cervical encephalocele (that includes cerebellar tissue) that is accompanied by a distorted brainstem and local anatomy. The clinical picture is similar to Chiari II but is more severe and the prognosis is poor. Pathologic changes may include cerebellar dysplasia. Pathogenesis is also unclear but is likely related to defective neurulation.

The DWM (or syndrome) typically presents sporadically in infancy as an isolated finding or in association with other CNS malformations. It contains five main features. First, there is cystic dilatation of the fourth ventricle. Second, the cerebellar vermis is hypoplastic or absent. Third, as opposed to the Chiari II malformation, DWM is characterized by a large posterior fossa. Fourth, and likely related to the large posterior fossa, is the elevation of the tentorium and related

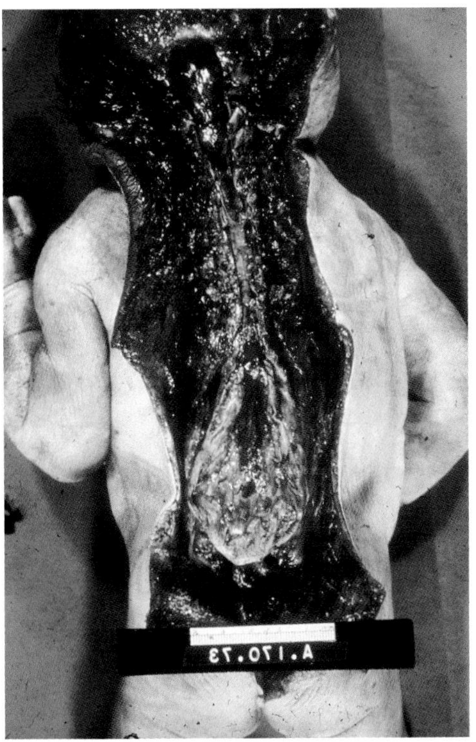

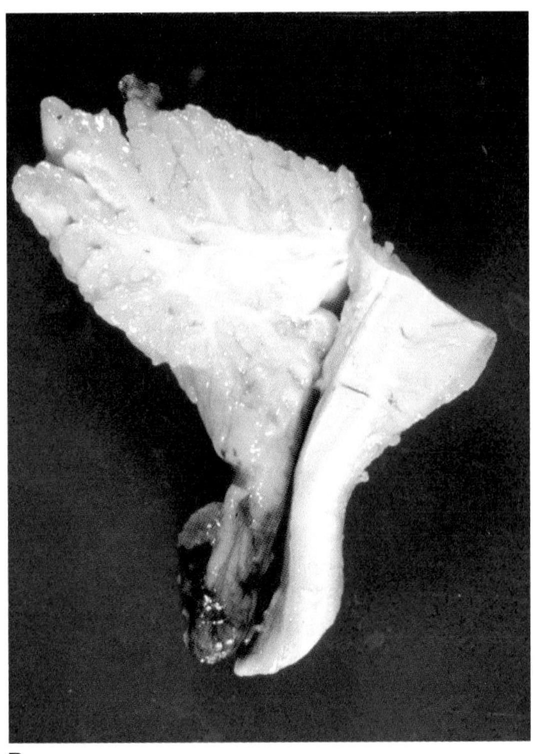

A B

FIGURE 10-16 Chiari II malformation. **A:** This posterior dissection reveals cerebellar vermis that has herniated through the foramen magnum and an associated lumbar myelomeningocele. (Image courtesy of Dr. Barry Rewcastle.) **B:** Sagittal section of the brain highlights herniated and discolored cerebellar vermis along the posterior aspect of the spinal cord. (Image courtesy of Dr. Robert Schmidt, Washington University School of Medicine, St. Louis, MO.)

dural sinuses. Finally, there is HCP. The Dandy-Walker variant has only some of the features of the DWM, which include an anteriorly rotated vermis ± fourth ventricular dilatation. The pathogenesis of the DWM is unknown, but the development of the fourth ventricular roof and its outlet foramina (especially Magendie) is thought to be important. Maternal isoretinoin use is a risk factor. Clinically, features related to HCP and increased ICP are common. Surprisingly, cerebellar signs/symptoms are less common. There may be concomitant mental retardation. Pathologically, the main findings are those seen grossly (see above). The fourth ventricular cyst wall is composed of an outer pial and inner ependymal layers, with residual cerebellar parenchymal in between.

A variety of additional cerebellar malformations has been characterized. Cerebellar heterotopia and dysplasia are reviewed by Golden (39). Rarer malformations include cerebellar agenesis, Joubert syndrome, pontoneocerebellar hypoplasia, and granular cell aplasia.

Malformations of the brainstem are numerous but rare. Some are described elsewhere in this chapter (i.e., Moebius syndrome, X-linked HCP with congenital absence of the pyramids). Olivary heterotopia and dentate/olivary dysplasias may occur in association with a number of different CNS malformations or syndromes, and in light of their origin from the metencephalic alar plate, it is not surprising that these may occur in conjunction with cerebellar abnormalities.

Cystic Lesions of the CNS

"Cysts" within the CNS are biologically benign and nonneoplastic. Their characteristic sites and pathology are summarized in Table 10-2. During embryologic development, ectopic placement of germ layer tissue may account for the formation of many of these lesions.

METABOLIC, NEURODEGENERATIVE, AND MISCELLANEOUS DISORDERS

Lysosomal Storage Disorders

Lysosomes are the digestive organelles of the cell. They contain numerous hydrolytic enzymes (e.g., phosphatases, nucleases, glycosidases, proteases, sulfatases, phospholipases, etc.) that assist in normal cellular metabolism. These enzymes are often directed to cleave off the sugar chains from larger macromolecules. A deficiency in one or more of the glycoprotein enzymes results in a lysosomal storage disorder (LSD). The LSDs are relatively uncommon disorders that often result in progressive and multisystemic disease that is fatal in childhood. LSD can be subdivided into categories, which are roughly based on the class of macromolecule that is not correctly metabolized; these include (a) sphingolipidoses (lipids), (b) mucopolysaccharidoses (MPS)

Table 10-2 ■ CNS CYSTS

Cyst Type	Common Sites	Pathology
Neurenteric (i.e., endodermal)	Intradural, extramedullary, and ventral to the cervical spinal cord	Cuboidal to columnar respiratory-type or GI-type epithelium covering a connective tissue stroma. Possible goblet cells and cilia. Immunohistochemistry[a] (IHC)
Colloid	Antero-superior third ventricle near the Foramen of Monroe	Simple columnar epithelium. Possible cilia. Cyst contents PAS-positive. IHC[a]
Rathke cleft	Sella	Similar to neurenteric. Degenerate forms with atrophic epithelium and xanthogranulomatous inflammation. IHC[a]
Dermoid	Midline: fontanelle, fourth ventricle, cauda equina.	Stratified squamous epithelium with dermal adnexal appendages. Cyst contents (grossly "cheesy"): degenerate keratinocytes, sebaceous material, hair, etc.
Epidermoid	Cerebello-pontine angle (CPA), parasellar, diploe of skull	Similar to dermoid epithelium but without dermal appendages. Keratinizing epithelium. Cyst contents: "dry" keratin. Gross "pearly" appearance
Ependymal	Intraventricular, leptomeningeal, intraparenchymal	Columnar epithelium similar to ependyma. Possible cilia. No goblet cells. IHC: GFAP-positive and S-100 protein-positive.
Choroid plexus	Lateral ventricles	Simple cuboidal to columnar epithelium. Cytokeratin-positive and S-100-positive.
Pineal	Pineal parenchyma	Three layers: (a) internal fibrillar layer with RFs. IHC: GFAP-positive. (b) Pineal parenchymal "middle" layer. IHC: Synaptophysin-positive. (c) Outer connective tissue layer.
Arachnoid	CPA, Sylvian fissure	CSF filled. Inner arachnoid (EMA-positive) and outer connective tissue layers.

[a]Cytokeratin and EMA-positive, with collagen IV immunoreactive subepithelial basement membrane. Usually CK7-positive, CK20-negative.

[disaccharide molecules of glycosaminoglycans (GAGs)], (c) glycoproteinoses (glycoproteins), and (d) a number of miscellaneous LSDs, which include the neuronal ceroid lipofuscinoses (NCL) and Pompe disease (type II glycogenosis).

The LSDs are generally autosomal recessive disorders that are usually the result of a mutation in the gene that encodes a particular lysosomal enzyme. There is extensive clinicopathologic overlap among the LSDs as a whole, many of which are individually indistinguishable without ancillary biochemical and genetic testing.

Conceptually, the LSDs can be divided into four basic clinico-pathologic phenotypes: (a) neuronal lipidoses, (b) leukodystrophies, (c) storage histiocytoses, and (d) MPS (or the Hurler phenotype) (81). Most LSD storage products are water soluble and thus are washed out during routine histologic processing, leaving behind only the clear, vacuolated, and distended cytoplasm of the cells they have affected. This accumulated material mechanically disrupts cellular processes and eventually leads to cell death. The neuronal lipidoses are characterized by substrate storage in cytoplasm of neurons, leading to the gross finding of megalencephaly early in the disease course (Figure 10-17). Subsequent neuronal death and gliosis eventually result in cerebral atrophy. Involvement of the retina may lead to the characteristic "cherry red spot," while other clinical manifestations of the neuronal lipidosis (NL) phenotype include psychomotor retardation and dementia, loss of acquired motor and perceptual skills, epilepsy, and myoclonus. The leukodystrophies, which are part of the LSDs [e.g., metachromatic leukodystrophy (MLD) and Krabbe leukodystrophy (KLD)], are the result of substrate accumulation in oligodendrocytes and Schwann cells, causing a loss of myelin and myelinating cells. Clinical manifestations include psychomotor retardation, spasticity, ataxia, visual abnormalities, and a demyelinative peripheral neuropathy. Substrate accumulation in mesenchymal and epithelial cells, in addition to the extracellular matrix, results in the Hurler phenotype. Clinically, these patients have core features, which include coarse facies, skeletal and joint abnormalities (i.e., dysostosis multiplex and arthropathies), organomegaly, cloudy corneas, cardiovascular disease, and CNS disease (entrapment neuropathies, HCP, and NL). Finally, substrate storage in monocytes/macrophages causes

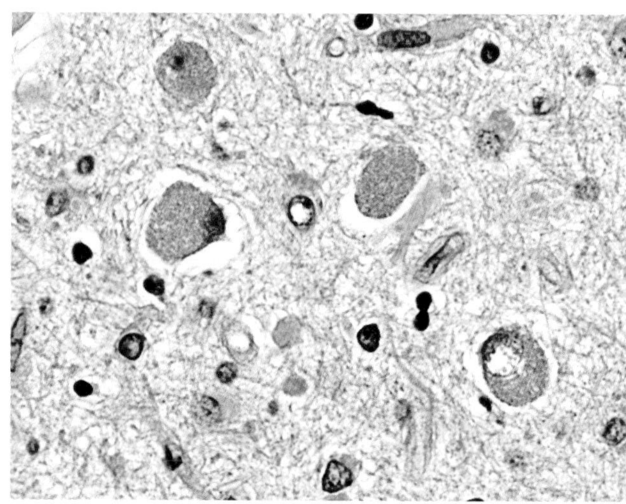

FIGURE 10-17 ■ Neuronal lipidosis (NL). The cytoplasm of these neurons is markedly distended by lipofuscin-like storage products in this example of neuronal ceroid lipofuscinosis (NCL).

the storage histiocytosis (SH) phenotype, which clinically manifests in hepatosplenomegaly, hematologic, and skeletal abnormalities. Table 10-3 lists a subset of the LSD, their specific enzymatic defects, and some of their characteristic clinico-pathologic features (note: MLD and KLD are further described below) (see Chapter 5).

Leukodystrophies

The leukodystrophies are a group of genetically based progressive disorders that share common abnormalities in myelin formation and metabolism. These disorders have hence been referred to as dysmyelinating, to distinguish them from demyelinating disorders (e.g., multiple sclerosis) where myelin is thought to form normally but is later destroyed. Pathogenetically, the leukodystrophies are a heterogeneous group of disorders, which, for example, include some of the lysosomal and peroxisomal storage disorders. These disorders often have onset during childhood, but adults can also be affected. Clinically, these disorders can affect numerous neurologic modalities and hence result in a myriad of signs and symptoms, which may include psychomotor retardation and dementia, pyramidal and extrapyramidal manifestations including spastic paraparesis, ataxia, visual and hearing abnormalities, as well as signs of bulbar involvement. Characteristic clinical manifestations (i.e., age of onset, signs/symptoms) may accompany specific forms of leukodystrophy. The white matter of not only the CNS but also the PNS [e.g., MLD, KLD, and less so adrenoleukodystrophy (ALD)] may be affected. Some leukodystrophies are more systemic in nature and thus bear extra-CNS/PNS disease manifestations (e.g., adrenal and testicular involvement with ALD; biliary and renal involvement with MLD). Genetically, many of these disorders are inherited in

Table 10-3 ■ LYSOSOMAL STORAGE DISEASES

LSD	Enzymatic/Protein Deficiency	Stored Material	Characteristic Clinico-Pathologic Features
GM1 gangliosidosis	β-Galactosidase	GM1 ganglioside, Keratan sulfate	NL, MPS, cherry red spot[a]
GM2 gangliosidosis (Tay-Sachs and Sandhoffs)	Hexosaminidase A and/or B	GM2 gangliosides	NL, SH (Sandhoff), cherry red spot[a]
Niemann-Pick A/B	Sphingomyelinase	Sphingomyelin	NL, SH (Niemann-Pick cells), cherry red spot[a]
Niemann-Pick C	ER membrane protein with role in intracellular cholesterol transport	Phospholipids and glycolipids	NL, SH (Niemann-Pick cells), axonal swellings, and neurofibrillary tangles[a]
Gaucher disease	Glucocerebrosidase	Glucocerebroside	SH with Gaucher cells ("wrinkled tissue paper")[a]
Fabry disease	α-Galactosidase	Trihexosylceramide	Painful peripheral neuropathy; ischemic CNS and heart disease; bathing trunk telangectasias, renal, and eye disease[a]
Farber granulomatosis	Ceramidase	Ceramide	NL, LD, cherry red spot; painful arthropathy, subcutaneous nodules, and hoarseness related to lipid granulomas[a]
MPS type I: Hurler disease	α-L-Iduronidase	Dermatan and heparan sulfate	MPS, mental retardation, dysostosis multiplex, cloudy corneas, heart disease. EM: reticulogranular inclusions
NCL 1–4	Palmitoyl protein thioesterase (NCL1), Tripeptidyl peptidase (NCL2)	Saposin A&D (NCL1), SCMAS (subunit C of mitochondrial ATPase synthase), (NCL2–4)	NL. EM: granular osmiophilic deposit (NCL1), curvilinear bodies (NCL2), fingerprint bodies (NCL3), or "mixed" with lipofuscin-like (NCL4)
Pompe disease (glycogenosis type 2)	α-Glucosidase (acid maltase)	Glycogen (membrane bound and free by EM)	Vacuolar myopathy, cardiomegaly, macroglossia

EM: in general, many of these disorders contain membranous cytoplasmic or zebra body inclusions within lysosomes; GM1 may contain added reticulogranular material; Gaucher disease exhibits tubular inclusions; Farber granulomatosis features "banana bodies."
[a]Sphingolipidoses.
LSD, lysosomal storage disease; NL, neuronal lipidosis; MPS, mucopolysaccharidosis; SH, storage histiocytosis; ER, endoplasmic reticulum; NCL, neuronal ceroid lipofuscinosis.

an autosomal recessive manner; however, some follow an X-linked or sporadic pattern.

Pathologically, the leukodystrophies characteristically cause bilaterally symmetric white matter–predominant disease that can involve the cerebrum, brainstem, cerebellum, and even the spinal cord. Usually, subcortical U-fibers are spared from myelin destruction (Figure 10-18A). There may be a rostral (Alexander disease, MLD) or caudal (ALD; KLD) predominance of cerebral white matter disease. In general, early stages of disease are characterized by widespread myelin destruction with relative axonal preservation; macrophages are often present and distended by bubbly PAS-positive cytoplasmic material. Later stages often demonstrate axonal and oligodendrocyte destruction plus reactive gliosis. Characteristic pathologic changes often accompany individual leukodystrophies and hence assist in diagnosis (Table 10-4; Figure 10-18B). A subset of leukodystrophies are considered "sudanophilic" since macrophages and other cells that accumulate indigestible substrates stain positive with Sudan B or Oil Red O fat stains. Included in these sudanophilic leukodystrophies are ALD, Pelizaeus-Merzbacher disease (PMD), and a host of less well-described entities that may contain characteristic histopathology including calcification, pigmentation, meningeal angiomatosis, and cavitation with oligodendrocyte proliferation or vanishing white matter disease, which recently has been linked to mutations in any of the genes encoding subunits of the eukaryotic translation factor eIF2B (87,115).

Peroxisomal Disorders

Peroxisomes are cellular organelles that have a single membrane, which encloses a matrix wherein numerous important biochemical reactions take place. Peroxisomes generate hydrogen peroxide (H_2O_2), a molecule that assists in oxidizing several cellular toxins. However, H_2O_2 can itself be toxic; hence peroxisomes contain catalase, an enzyme that serves to break down H_2O_2 into water and oxygen. Peroxisomes also play an important role in the β-oxidation of very long chain fatty acids (VLCFAs), plasmalogen biosynthesis (an important cell membrane and myelin component), cholesterol biosynthesis, and the metabolism of amino acids, bile acids, and purine nucleotides. Knowledge of these basic biologic functions is clinically useful since the routine laboratory workup of the peroxisomal disorders often involves initial assessment of VLCFAs, hepatic peroxisomes, and RBC plasmalogens.

There are three main categories of peroxisomal disorders: (a) the peroxisomal biogenesis disorders (e.g., Zellweger spectrum, and rhizomelic chondrodysplasia punctata type 1), (b) the single enzyme deficiencies (e.g., D-bifunctional protein deficiency and adult Refsum disease), and (c) X-linked ALD. In general, these disorders are neuropathologically characterized by neuronal migration defects, leukodystrophy-like white matter abnormalities, CNS lipid deposition, and systemic abnormalities (including the adrenal cortex and liver). Both the biogenesis disorders and the single enzymes deficiencies include autosomal recessive inheritance. The former involve mutations in the PEX genes; these encode the peroxin proteins that are important to peroxisomal functioning. Zellweger spectrum includes three disorders, which are considered to form a spectrum of diseases related to mutations in PEX1. These include (from most to least severe) the following: Zellweger syndrome, neonatal ALD, and infantile Refsum disease. Zellweger syndrome (aka, cerebrohepatorenal syndrome) is a systemic disorder primarily affecting the liver (cirrhosis) and brain. Patients have dysmorphic facies and neurologic manifestations that include psychomotor retardation, hypotonia, depressed deep tendon and Moro reflexes, seizures and nystagmus. These infants die within the 1st year of life. Neuropathologic findings include NMD

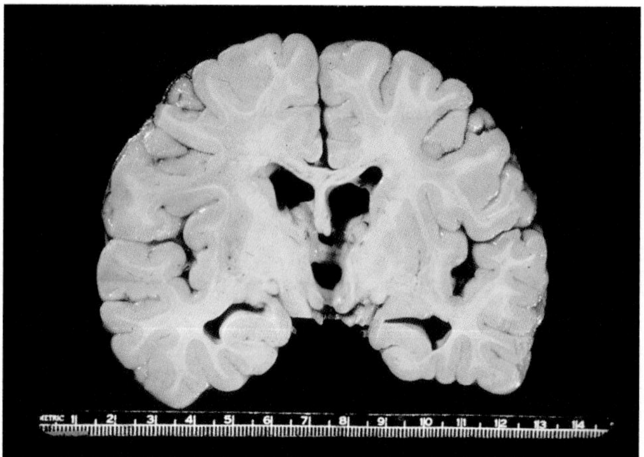

A

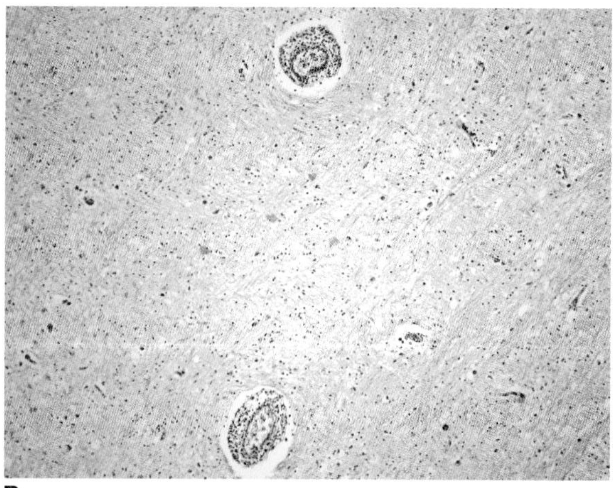

B

FIGURE 10-18 ■ Leukodystrophy. **A:** Coronally sectioned case of Krabbe disease demonstrates symmetric dysmyelination of cerebral white matter with relative sparing of the subcortical U-fibers. (Image courtesy of Dr. Barry Rewcastle.) **B:** LFB-PAS–stained case of ALD demonstrates pale white matter and characteristic perivascular lymphocytic cuffing.

Table 10-4 ■ THE LEUKODYSTROPHIES

Leukodystrophy	Biochemical/Genetic Abnormality (Chromosomal Locus)	Characteristic Pathology
Adrenoleukodystrophy (ALD)	Deficiency of a peroxisomal ATP-binding cassette transporter, resulting in accumulation of VLCFAs. X-linked (Xq28)	Perivascular lymphocytic inflammation. EM: trilaminar inclusions. Striated lamellar cytoplasm inclusions in CNS and select systemic organs
Metachromatic leukodystrophy (MLD)	Aryl-sulfatase A deficiency. Accumulate sulfatide (22q13)	Metachromatic material (using acidic cresyl violet or toluidine blue) in the brain (macrophages), PNS (Schwann cells), and viscera (biliary epithelium and renal tubules). EM: herringbone, prismatic, and tuftstone inclusions.
Krabbe leukodystrophy (KLD)	Galactocerebroside β-galactosidase deficiency. Accumulate psychosine (14q25-31)	Globoid cells, often perivascular. PNS: hypertrophic neuropathy with fibrosis and "onion-bulbs." EM: tubular inclusions
Alexander disease	Sporadic mutation of the GFAP gene (17q21)	RF accumulation, especially in perivascular and subpial locations. Grossly cavitated white matter. EM: amorphous electron-dense material surrounded by 10-nm intermediate filaments
Canavan disease	Aspartoacylase deficiency. Accumulate *N*-acetylaspartate (17p13-ter)	More central aspects of central myelin lost with relative oligodendroglial and axonal sparing. Vacuolation at neocortical gray-white junction. No macrophages and little gliosis (versus other LSDs). EM: myelin splitting at intraperiod line plus elongate mitochondrial with "ladder-like" cristae
Pelizaeus-Merzbacher disease (PMD)	Deficiency of normal proteolipid protein (PLP). Accumulate abnormally folded PLP in the ER. X-linked (Xq22)	Perivascular patchy dysmyelination (i.e., tigroid).

(pachygyria, polymicrogyria), leukodystrophy-like white matter abnormalities, abnormalities of rhombic lip–derived structures (dentate nucleus/inferior olivary dysplasias, cerebellar heterotopias), and prominent deposition of sudanophilic lipid in the CNS (primarily within macrophages and showing trilaminar appearance on EM) (Chapters 5 and 15).

Mitochondrial Disorders

The mitochondria are the "powerhouse" of the cell. They produce the energy needed for life in the form of ATP via aerobic respiration. The final stages of aerobic respiration are mediated by the electron transport chain, which comprises five protein complexes that are embedded within the inner mitochondrial membrane. Each of these five complexes is composed of multiple protein subunits (86 in total), most of which are encoded by nuclear DNA. The mtDNA genome is circular, double stranded, and includes 16,569 base pairs. Up to ten copies of the mtDNA genome may be seen within a cell. This genome encodes for 22 tRNAs, 2 rRNAs, and 13 subunits of the electron transport chain. Genetically induced defects in the assembly or formation of the electron transport chain, or in the maintenance of the mitochondrial DNA, result in mitochondrial disorders. Dysfunction of the electron transport chain presumably results in cell death via numerous mechanisms, including energy deprivation, free radical toxicity, and apoptosis. Since electron transport chain functioning relies on proteins encoded by both mitochondrial and nuclear DNA, mitochondrial disorders may be inherited via either maternal or classic Mendelian patterns.

Mitochondrial disorders, such as the LSDs, may display significant clinico-pathologic overlap. Many of these disorders, when viewed in isolation, may be caused by more than one mutation, and in turn, any given mutation may lead to more than one mitochondrial disorder. This biologic complexity makes the diagnosis of mitochondrial disorders challenging. These disorders are often described as encephalomyopathies, since muscle (cardiac and skeletal) and brain tissues are usually affected due to their heavy reliance on mitochondrial energy production. Clinically, the presence of a mitochondrial disorder may be suspected via characteristic lab abnormalities, which often include an elevation in blood/CSF lactate and the lactate-to-pyruvate ratio. Ragged red fibers (RRF) are a common manifestation of muscle disease and represent a localized proliferation of abnormal mitochondria. RRFs are detected histochemically on frozen sections via modified Gomori trichrome (dark red) or succinic dehydrogenase (dark blue) stains (Figure 10-19A). The cytochrome oxidase C (COX) stain often fails to stain such affected fibers (i.e., "pale fibers"). By EM, the abnormal mitochondria of RRFs may take several unusual configurations including concentric spirals and rectangular paracrystalline arrays that resemble "parking lots" (Figure 10-19B). It is important to note that RRFs are not entirely specific for the mitochondrial disorders, and that not all mitochondrial disorders bear RRFs. Other common neuropathologic findings seen among the mitochondrial disorders include hypoxic-ischemic-like and infarct-like changes, intramyelinic edema/spongy myelinopathy, tract/system

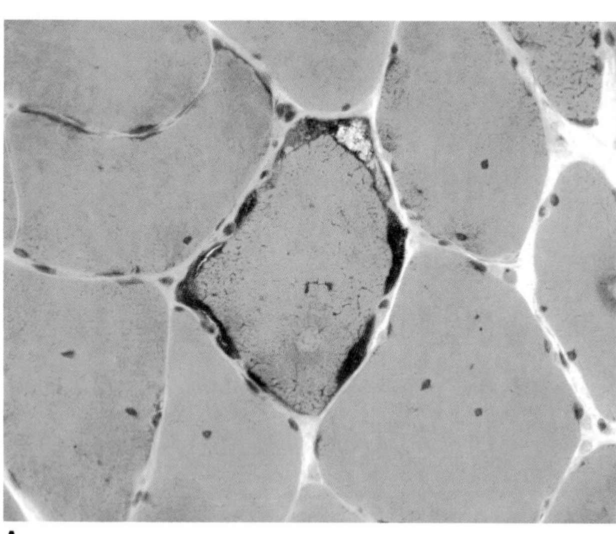
A

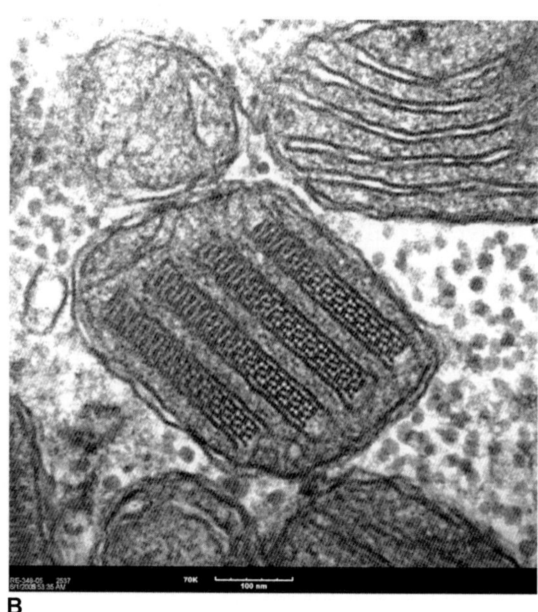
B

FIGURE 10-19 ■ Mitochondrial myopathy. **A:** RRF. (Modified Gomori trichrome.) **B:** EM reveals abnormal mitochondria with paracrystalline ("parking lot") inclusions.

degenerations, and vascular mineralization (deep gray and adjacent white matter, dentate nucleus and the brain stem). Only a few of the more common mitochondrial disorders are briefly discussed below.

Mitochondrial encephalopathy with lactic acidosis and strokes (MELAS) is a maternally inherited disorder that most often results from an adenine to guanine point mutation at nucleotide 3,243 of mtDNA. This mutation is within the gene that encodes the tRNA for leucine. Those afflicted are usually young, although both the age of onset and initial presentation may be quite variable. Sudden focal neurologic signs (e.g., hemiplegia, hemianopsia, seizures, etc.), migraine-like attacks, or more nonspecific symptoms (such as vomiting or a change in mental status) may be seen. Myopathic features include proximal limb weakness, fatigability, and deficits in eye movements. Episodes of such neurologic dysfunction tend to be recurrent. Pathologically, foci of necrotic brain damage resemble true infarcts; however, these lesions do not follow standard vascular distributions. The occipital lobes, deep gray matter (which also may demonstrate vascular mineralization), and cerebellum are often affected. RRFs are present.

Myoclonic epilepsy with ragged red fibers (MERRF) is another maternally inherited disorder. MERRF most often results from an adenine to guanine point mutation at nucleotide 8,344 of mtDNA. This mutation is within the gene that encodes the tRNA for lysine. Like MELAS, those afflicted are often young. Clinical features include a proximal myopathy, myoclonic epilepsy, sensorineural hearing loss, cognitive deficits, short stature, and ataxia. Pathologic changes involve neuronal loss and gliosis among the dentato-rubro-olivary system, substantia nigra, dorsal column nuclei (gracile and cuneate), and Clarke column. Vascular mineralization may be noted in the deep gray matter, and muscle pathology includes RRFs.

Leigh disease (subacute necrotizing encephalopathy) is most frequently caused by nuclear DNA mutations, and hence usually inherited in an autosomal recessive pattern. Genes encoding subunits of the electron transport chain complexes I, II, IV, and V may be mutated, or alternatively there may be a deficiency of pyruvate dehydrogenase. Disease onset often manifests prior to 2 years of age and includes weight loss, vomiting, psychomotor retardation, and weakness. Movement disorders, ataxia, eye abnormalities (optic atrophy, ophthalmoplegia, nystagmus), respiratory difficulties, hypotonia, and epilepsy are also often characteristic. Pathologically, the deep gray and brainstem are primarily affected by vasculo-necrotic lesions. The brainstem tegmentum, inferior colliculi, and substantia nigra are characteristically affected. Grossly, these lesions are atrophic, soft, and symmetrically distributed. Microscopically, the findings resemble those seen in Wernicke-Korsakoff syndrome (although hemorrhagic features are absent and the mamillary bodies are normal). Typical lesions bear rarefaction of the neuropil with spongiosis and relative neuron preservation, foamy macrophages, and gliosis and an increased density of capillaries that is thought to result from vascular proliferation and/or neuropil collapse.

Kearns-Sayre syndrome (KSS) is a sporadic disorder that is most frequently due to a deletion in the mtDNA genome (~5 kb). KSS is usually of pediatric onset and is neurologically characterized by eye findings (ophthalmoplegia, ptosis, retinitis pigmentosa, and vision loss), hearing deficits, weakness, ataxia, proximal myopathy, cognitive impairment, and seizures. Extra-CNS abnormalities include short stature, often fatal cardiac pathology (cardiomyopathy and conduction problems), plus additional GI, renal and endocrine perturbations. Chronic progressive external ophthalmoplegia (CPEO) may be seen as a component of KSS, or alternatively can be the sole manifestation of a mitochondrial disorder. Neuropathologic abnormalities classically include RRFs on muscle biopsy and a diffuse spongy myelinopathy. This white matter pathology is not accompanied by prominent gliosis or macrophagic infiltrates. As can be seen in many of the disorders characterized by spongy myelinopathy, splitting of myelin lamellae at the intraperiod line results in vacuole formation. Like many mitochondrial diseases, deep gray matter may bear vascular mineralization. Correlating with clinical ataxia, cerebellar pathology includes Purkinje neuron dendritic deformities plus eventual neuronal dropout.

Amino Acid Disorders

Amino acid disorders are inherited (mostly autosomal recessive) deficits in the enzymatic degradation of amino acids. This group includes the urea cycle disorders, phenylketonuria (PKU), nonketotic hyperglycinemia, homocystinuria, maple syrup urine disease (MSUD), and some of the organic acidemias (e.g., proprionic and methylmalonic acidemia). Although some of these diseases have an insidious onset and pursue a chronic course, most follow a severe and fatal clinical picture in early childhood. Encephalopathy/psychomotor retardation, seizures and motor findings (spasticity, tetraplegia) are seen. Neurologic dysfunction is thought to be related to a combination of toxic biochemical accumulations (e.g., amino acid intermediaries, hyperammonemia), deficits in the biosynthesis of key metabolic compounds, and energy dysfunction. Neuropathologic alterations commonly include a spongy myelinopathy (like that seen in KSS) that tends to affect infratentorial structures, Alzheimer type II astrocytes (see below), and neocortical/deep gray hypoxic-ischemic lesions. Vascular pathology (i.e., infarction) is characteristic of homocystinuria.

Congenital Disorders of Glycosylation

The congenital disorders of glycosylation (CDGs) are an uncommon but evolving group of relatively recently described inborn errors of metabolism. *N*- and *O*-linked glycan synthesis/processing are affected and ultimately result in hypoglycosylated glycoproteins; hence, these disorders are often multisystemic in nature. These disorders are inherited in an autosomal recessive manner, and the genetic basis underlying many of the CDGs is a missense mutation. Isoelectric focusing of transferritin is the common test used in the diagnosis of CDGs. CDG type Ia is the most common and best described entity. The R141H missense mutation in the PMM2 gene on 16p13.3-13.2 is the most frequent mutation in CDG Ia. Infants are affected, in the early stages, by prominent psychomotor retardation, ataxia, and alternating strabismus. This early phase of disease is often fatal. If the patient survives, later neurologic manifestations include retinitis pigmentosa, seizures, and stroke-like episodes. Other clinical aspects of CDG Ia may include hypotonia, feeding problems, liver disease (fatty infiltration and cirrhosis, leading to coagulopathies), pericardial effusions, dysmorphic features (inverted nipples, subcutaneous buttock fat pads, and contractures), and musculoskeletal abnormalities. Neuropathologic features are dominated by olivopontocerebellar atrophy (OPCA); EM may reveal myelin-like lysosomal inclusions.

Acquired Metabolic Disorders and Vitamin Deficiencies

Acquired metabolic diseases affecting the nervous system are numerous. They are encountered more frequently in adults, although pediatric examples are clinically and pathologically similar. Some of these include hypoglycemia, electrolyte disorders [e.g., central pontine myelinolysis (CPM), disorders of calcium hemostasis], hepatic encephalopathy, porphyria, uremic, and dialysis-related encephalopathy. Several vitamin deficiencies may also characteristically lead to neurologic disease. These include thiamine (B1) and Wernicke-Korsakoff syndrome, pyridoxine (B6), B12 (subacute combined degeneration), nicotinic acid (pellagra), folic acid, vitamin A (including intoxication), and vitamin E.

Neurodegenerative and Miscellaneous Disorders

There are a number of neurodegenerative and more nondescript neurologic disorders that characteristically affect the pediatric population. A subset of these entities are discussed below.

Alpers-Huttenlocher syndrome [progressive neurodegeneration of childhood (PNDC)] is now considered by many to reside among the mitochondrial disorders (40). This disease manifests in infancy and is characterized by the acute onset of intractable seizures, developmental delay, hypotonia, ataxia, cortical blindness, failure to thrive, and liver disease (which pathologically reveals bile duct proliferation and cirrhosis). Death frequently occurs by 3 years of age. Molecular genetic studies have revealed mtDNA depletion and mutations in the polymerase gamma gene (POLG). Genetic transmission has been suggested to be autosomal recessive. Gross pathologic findings reveal a patchy neocortical atrophy that has a predilection for the visual cortex. Along with thalamic and focal hippocampal atrophy, there may be concomitant HCP *ex vacuo*. Microscopically, the neocortex is especially affected by a spongy rarefaction, with superimposed neuronal loss and gliosis; severe cases are transcortical, while less involved cortex shows these abnormalities more superficially. These spongy changes are reminiscent of those seen in Creutzfeld-Jacob disease (CJD). Neuronal loss is often prominent in the inferior olives. Neutral fat deposition in diseased parenchyma is highlighted with oil red O staining.

Axonal spheroids are a microscopic accompaniment of many diseases that affect the nervous system. When numerous, these axonal spheroids may signify the presence of a *neuroaxonal dystrophy (NAD)*. Axonal spheroids are rounded eosinophilic structures ranging in size from 20 to 120 μm. They are highlighted with silver stains or by various IHC stains (e.g., NFP and ubiquitin). EM reveals mitochondria, membrane-bound electron-dense granules, tubulomembranous structures all among an amorphous matrix; NFPs are surprising sparse but if seen are often displaced toward the periphery. Two NADs are discussed further: infantile neuroaxonal dystrophy (INAD, or Seitelberger disease) and neurodegeneration with brain iron accumulation type 1 [NBIA; pantothenate kinase–associated neurodegeneration (PANK), or Hallervorden-Spatz disease (HSD)]. Both are rare progressive neurologic diseases.

INAD typically has an onset just after 1 year of age. Sporadic and familial forms (with an autosomal recessive inheritance pattern) may be seen. A definitive pathogenesis has not been defined. Normal development may be seen early on, but psychomotor retardation eventually develops. Weakness, hypotonia, depressed deep tendon reflexes, visual difficulties, and cerebellar deficits (ataxia, pendular nystagmus) may also be seen clinically. Terminal stages of disease (between 6 and 15 years of age) include tetraplegia/spasticity with decerebrate posturing, bulbar palsies, and bowel/bladder incontinence. Gross pathologic changes reveal cerebral and cerebellar atrophy with HCP *ex vacuo*. Optic nerves may be atrophic as well. The globus pallidus is large and pale early on but later takes on a rusty discoloration. Microscopically, the deep gray, brainstem (including the substantia nigra), cerebellar cortex, and spinal cord are especially affected; abnormalities include axonal spheroids (central, peripheral, and in the autonomic nervous systems), spongy degeneration, gliosis, and lipid/iron pigment accumulation (especially within the globus pallidus and the substantia nigra reticulata). These regions as well as a few white matter tracts (e.g., corticospinal, spinobulbar, optic, olfactory) may display demyelinating-like pathology.

NBIA occurs in both sporadic and familial (autosomal recessive) forms and may have an onset at any age. Infantile (<1 years old), late infantile (2 to 5 years old), juvenile ("classic;" 7 to 15 years old), and rarely adult onset cases have been described. Infantile/late infantile cases are often fatal before 10 years of age and are more often associated with mutations in the PANK2 gene. An insidious gait disorder with hypotonia often heralds the onset of disease, although psychomotor deficits may predate such manifestations. Hyperkinetic movement disorders are a key clinical feature and are seen in approximately 50%; these include choreoathetosis, dystonia, and tremors, which may result in dysarthria, dysphagia, and abnormal extraocular movements. Additional neurologic deficits include ataxia and nystagmus, visual abnormalities, hyper-reflexia with a Babinski response, and leg amyotrophy. Cognitive impairment leads to dementia. HARP syndrome (hypo-β-lipoproteinemia, acanthocytosis, retinitis pigmentosa, and pallidal degeneration) is considered to reside within the NBIA clinico-pathologic spectrum (15). MRI findings characteristically reveal the "eye of the tiger" sign where a ring-like region of T2 hypointensity is seen in the globus pallidus externa and the substantia nigra, while T2 hyperintensity is seen in the globus pallidus interna. Gross pathology reveals atrophy within the cerebrum and cerebellum; this atrophy has a rusty hue in the globus pallidus interna and substantia nigra (Figure 10-20). Microscopically, the pallidonigral system is characteristically affected by iron pigment deposition, neuronal loss, gliosis, and spheroid formation. Granular pigment containing iron, lipofuscin, and neuromelanin may be intracellular (neuronal somata and axons, astrocytes, and microglia) or extracellular. Spheroids may also be seen in other deep gray nuclei, as well as the neocortex, brainstem tegmentum, and the spinal cord. Notably, the peripheral nervous system is not affected.

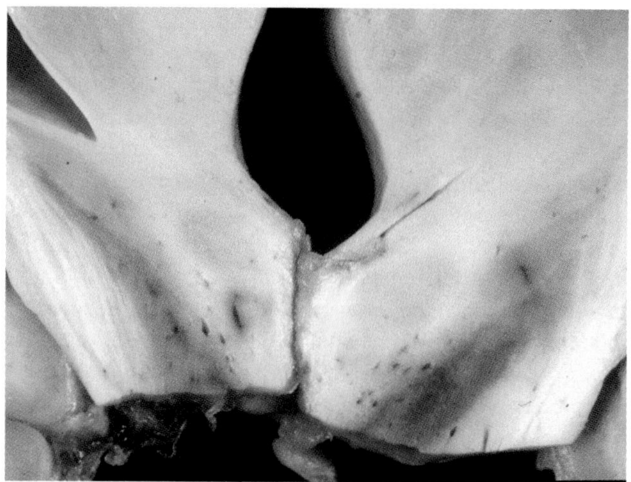

FIGURE 10-20 ■ NIBA (PANK or HSD). This coronal brain section reveals a rusty discoloration of the substantia nigra.

Epilepsy may be a manifestation of a number of different disorders that cause dysfunctioning of the neocortex. Vascular, infectious, traumatic, autoimmune, neoplastic, metabolic, malformative, and neurodegenerative are some of the etiologic classes that may be involved in the pathogenesis of epilepsy. Pasquier et al. (73) discussed their surgical pathology experience with 327 cases of drug-resistant epilepsy and highlighted the spectrum of disease that may be seen in this context. Included within these specimens was a large number displaying a common form of idiopathic pathology to which we will limit our discussion: mesial temporal sclerosis (MTS). MTS (also known as Ammon horn sclerosis or hippocampal sclerosis) is not usually associated with a clear genetic abnormality and does not have a clear pathogenesis. However, some cases are associated with a history of prolonged febrile seizures during infancy, and moreover, the pathology is similar if not identical to that seen within the context of hypoxic-ischemic injury. MTS may be seen in isolation or in conjunction with a second form of temporal lobe pathology (e.g., neoplasm, vascular formation, cortical dysplasia, etc.). Gross pathology reveals atrophy of the hippocampal formation with concomitant dilatation of the adjacent inferior temporal horn of the lateral ventricle (Figure 10-21A). Microscopically, neuronal loss and gliosis are most striking in

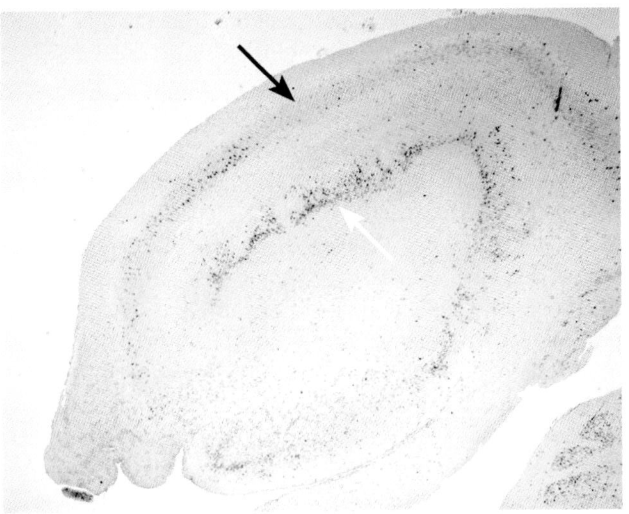

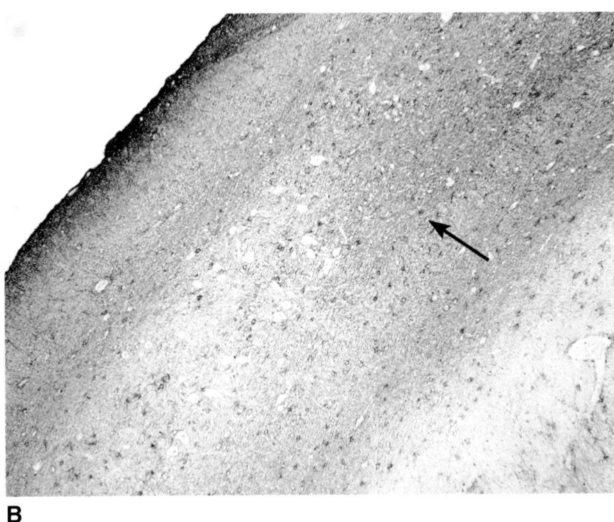

FIGURE 10-21 ■ Mesial temporal sclerosis (MTS). **A:** Using NeuN immunohistochemistry, this low-power magnification image reveals a dropout of neurons in the hippocampal CA1 subregion (*black arrow*), as well as neuronal dispersion within the dentate granule layer of the hippocampal formation (*white arrow*). **B:** GFAP-stained section reveals marked gliosis of CA1. Note: unstained neurons (**left**) taper off into a region of more intense gliosis (*arrow*).

the CA1 and CA4 (i.e., endfolium) hippocampal subregions (Figure 10-21B). Neuronal loss, dispersion, and/or duplication may also be seen within the dentate granular layer. Dysmorphic neurons may occasionally be seen in the endfolium and, like some of the dentate granule neuron alterations, may be a reactive, rather than primary component of MTS.

Neurodegenerative disorders that prominently affect the cerebellum are numerous but uncommon. Secondary forms of cerebellar disease (i.e., paraneoplastic, toxic/nutritional, vascular, infectious/inflammatory, prion related, and metabolic) will not be discussed here. Primary forms of cerebellar disease may be inherited or sporadic (e.g., multiple system atrophy, idiopathic degeneration) in nature. Familial cerebellar ataxia may follow an autosomal recessive or dominant pattern of inheritance. Some of the more common forms of autosomal recessive [*Friedreich ataxia (FA)*; ataxia telangectasia (AT)] and autosomal dominant diseases [the "spinocerebellar ataxias"; dentatorubropallidoluysial atrophy (DRPLA); and the episodic ataxias (EA1 and EA2)] are discussed below.

FA is a progressive multisystem disorder that typically has an onset prior to 15 years of age and results in death by the end of the fourth decade. This disorder involves an abnormally expanded intronic GAA trinucleotide repeat within the frataxin gene located on 9q13-21.1. The gene product frataxin encodes for a mitochondrial protein involved in iron transport; dysfunction of this protein with disease is thought to lead to iron accumulation and oxidative neuronal damage. Ataxia (of gait, limb and voice, or dysarthria) is the result of cerebellar and sensory degeneration. There is a loss of position and vibratory sense, along with areflexia. A pyramidal pattern of leg weakness is accompanied by a Babinski response. Extra-CNS manifestations include pes cavus, scoliosis, cardiomyopathy, and diabetes mellitus. Gross pathologic CNS findings are generally limited to atrophic dorsal roots of the spinal cord; ischemic CNS disease may be seen and may be attributed to cardiac disease. Microscopic changes are prominent within the spinal cord and include tract degenerations (spinocerebellar, corticospinal, and dorsal columns) plus degeneration of Clarke columns (Figure 10-22). The dorsal root ganglion shows neuronal depletion and concomitant nodule of Nageotte formation (a proliferation of satellite cells that normally rim sensory neurons of the dorsal root ganglia). Large myelinated sensory fibers are lost in peripheral nerves. Neuronal loss in the accessory cuneate and gracile nuclei reflects transsynaptic degeneration. Neuronal loss and gliosis are seen in the vestibular, cochlear, and superior olivary nuclei. Cerebellar abnormalities include white matter gliosis plus neuronal loss in the dentate nuclei with concomitant superior cerebellar peduncle atrophy. Hypoxic-ischemic changes may be seen in the cerebellum and neocortex.

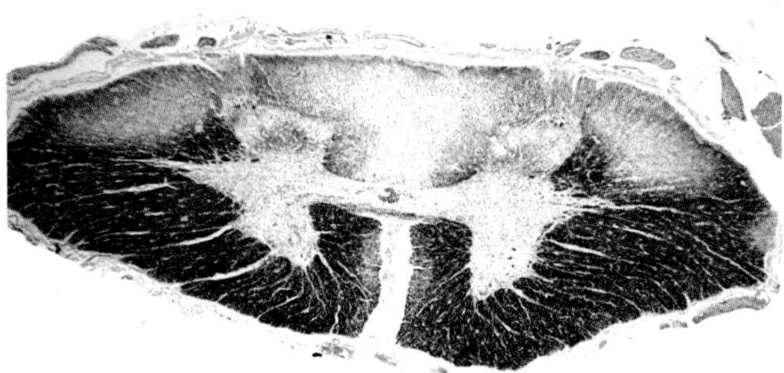

FIGURE 10-22 ■ Friedreich ataxia (FA). In this myelin-stained histologic preparation of the spinal cord in transverse section, there is a symmetric lack of staining in the dorsal columns, corticospinal tracts, and less so in the spinocerebellar tracts.

Strictly speaking, spinocerebellar atrophy (SCA) is a heterogeneous group of autosomal dominant neurodegenerative disorders affecting the cerebellum and additional CNS structures. The reciprocal circuitry between the cerebellar cortex, dentate nucleus, and the inferior olive (the "cerebellar module") is thought to be particularly important to the pathogenesis of ataxia (57). The number of disorders included under the rubric of SCA continues to grow at a rapid pace, and types 1 to 25 have recently been described (note: there is no SCA 9) (114). Many of the SCAs are trinucleotide repeat disorders, of which six forms (SCA 1 to 3, 6, 7, and 17) bear expanded CAG coding repeats along with clinical evidence of "anticipation," wherein the repeat becomes progressively longer, and disease onset is progressively earlier with increasing disease severity for each subsequent generation of patients. SCA 10 is exceptional in that it exhibits an ATTCT pentanucleotide noncoding repeat. Despite their recognition, the mechanism by which these repeats cause disease is unclear.

Although the atypical age of onset is usually after the fifth decade, pediatric forms of SCA may be seen. The spectrum of neurologic deficits includes cerebellar dysfunction (truncal and limb ataxia, dysarthria, nystagmus), abnormal gait, spasticity, weakness, parkinsonism and other extrapyramidal movement disorders, pyramidal signs, autonomic dysfunction, sensory abnormalities (including visual difficulties), and cognitive impairment. Some SCAs cause a multitude of neurologic deficits, while others are considered "purely" cerebellar. SCA 3 (or Machado Joseph disease) is the most common form among this group of diseases. Pathologic descriptions are available for only a subset of these disorders. SCA 2 affects many neurologic systems. The gross brain weight is reduced, and there is OPCA. Although there may be gross cerebellar atrophy in SCA 6, considered one of the "purely" cerebellar forms, such atrophy is not conspicuous in SCA 3. Microscopically, both SCA 2 and SCA 6 demonstrate cerebellar cortical atrophy with Purkinje cell dropout, while SCA 3 cerebellar disease is centered upon the dentate nucleus (with neuron loss and "grumose degeneration"). SCA 2 demonstrates dropout of neurons from the basis pontis and inferior olive. The spinal cord is abnormal in both SCA 2 and 3; while both demonstrate fiber loss in the posterior columns and neuronal loss in Clarkes nucleus, SCA 3 exhibits additional lateral column degeneration reminiscent of FA (but without dorsal spinal root involvement). Immunohistochemistry may reveal diagnostically useful intranuclear inclusions or more diffuse staining in the SCAs with expanded CAG repeats (SCA 6 bears abnormal cytoplasmic staining only). These inclusions may stain with antibodies targeted against the abnormal gene product involved, ubiquitin, expanded polyglutamine residues (e.g., IC2), or against other "chaperone" proteins.

Spinal muscular atrophy (SMA) is an autosomal recessive neuromuscular disorder resulting from the homozygous mutation or deletion of the SMN1 gene on 5q13. Three forms are generally recognized. SMA 1 (or Werdnig-Hoffmann disease) has an onset early in infancy. Proximal muscle weakness in the limbs progresses to involve the axial and diaphragmatic muscles; there may be bulbar involvement with respiratory insufficiency related to intercurrent infection and aspiration. Death is often seen prior to 1 year of age. In SMA 2, early motor development may be normal, but weakness prevails by 3 months of age. There may be tongue atrophy and hand tremor. Fasciculations and depressed deep tendon reflexes are also seen. Eventually, contractures and kyphoscoliosis develop. Most die by 25 years of age. SMA 3 is a more chronic form of disease but still may have a young onset. A functional motor deficit is appreciated and includes clinical weakness. Knee jerk reflexes are depressed and there may also be hand tremor. This gradual form of disease does not affect respiratory musculature or lead to a shortened life span. Pathologically, SMA 3 exhibits an adult pattern of denervation within muscles. In contrast, SMA 1 and 2 show large groups/fascicles of small rounded (not angular like that seen in adults) type I and II fibers intermixed with hypertrophic type I fibers, the latter possibly reflecting a compensatory response (Figure 10-23). In the end stage, endomysial

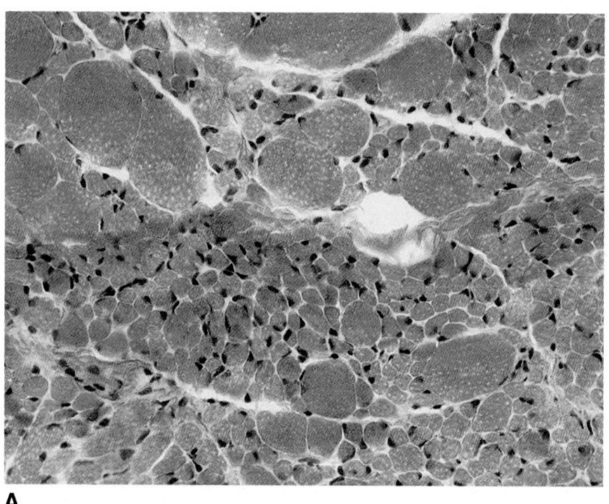
A

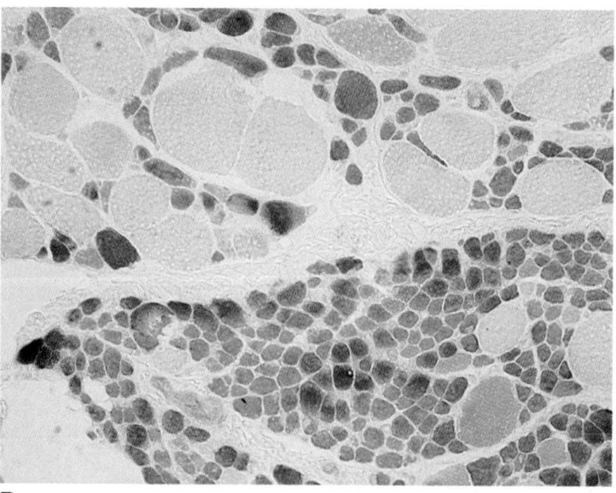
B

FIGURE 10-23 ■ Spinal muscular atrophy (SMA). **A:** H&E-stained frozen section of skeletal muscle reveals the typical distribution of rounded atrophic and enlarged fibers. **B:** Many of the latter prove to be type I (ATPase pH 10.4).

connective tissue and fat replacement may mimic a muscular dystrophy. Within the CNS, all forms of disease demonstrate anterior spinal root atrophy grossly, with anterior horn cell loss and concomitant gliosis microscopically. Earlier stages may feature neuronophagia and ballooned (NFP) neurons. A useful diagnostic feature in the thalamus is the presence of chromatolytic neurons. Bulbar motor neurons may also be affected.

Autism is an enigmatic neurologic disorder characterized by three key features: impaired social interaction, communication deficits (both verbal and nonverbal), and restricted/stereotyped behavior. Onset is before 3 years of age, and there is a 4:1 male-to-female sex distribution. Prevalence has most recently been estimated at 1/150 live births, making autism a rather common disorder. Genetic factors are clearly critical, but rather than a simple Mendelian pattern of inheritance, multiple genes are likely to be involved in the predisposition to this disease. In particular, duplication of chromosome 15q11-q13 is observed in a subset, and there appears to be a strong linkage between this GABA β3 subunit–encoding locus and the clinical feature of "insistence on sameness" (96). Neurotransmitter studies have suggested deficits in GABA-A receptors (hippocampal formation), ACh receptors (frontal and parietal lobes plus the cerebellar cortex), and decreased 5-HT synthesis (dentothalamocortical pathway) (7,16,78). Although the prevalence of autism is clearly higher in monozygotic (60% to 90% concordance) versus dizygotic (5% to 10% concordance) twins, environmental factors likely play a significant etiologic role as well. Neuropathologic descriptions remain limited, although the most common gross finding, especially in young patients, is a nonspecific megalencephaly. Purkinje cell dropout is the most common histologic finding. Limbic structures (including the amygdala, hippocampus, and entorrhinal cortex) exhibit small and closely packed neurons. Neocortical malformations may be seen and include a thickened neocortex, focal increased neuronal density, dyslamination, pyramidal neuronal malorientation, an increase in white matter, and molecular layer neurons (4). Cortical microcolumns, thought to be the smallest functional unit of the neocortex, have also been studied and found to be abnormally developed (13). Several brain regions, including the vertical limb of the nucleus of the diagonal band of Broca, the dentate nucleus, and the inferior olive, demonstrate neuronomegaly in younger patients with autism, followed by atrophy in older patients; there may be superimposed neuronal loss in some of these regions.

Neoplasia

Primary CNS tumors are common in pediatrics and only superseded by lymphoid-hematopoietic disorders in terms of frequency (86). Although adults and children may incur similar tumors, their individual incidence varies significantly with age. Prominent in adults are the following: diffusely infiltrating astrocytomas (DAs), metastases (primarily carcinoma), meningioma, and nerve sheath tumors (especially schwannoma). In pediatrics, PAs are the most frequent. Other common pediatric CNS tumors include DA, medulloblastoma, ependymoma, and craniopharyngioma (CPG) (Table 10-5). The current epidemiologic data are due in part to the ongoing refinements of our classification schemes, of which the WHO Classification of Tumors of the Nervous System (2007) is considered the standard (Table 10-6) (63). Despite these advances, several pediatric neoplasms remain difficult to classify.

Clinical Considerations

The presenting signs and symptoms of pediatric brain tumors are largely similar to those described in adults (Table 10-7). However, tumors occurring in infancy often display more insidious features. The myriad of focal neurologic abnormalities are more easily appreciated in older children who are better able to articulate their deficits. For example, tumors of the pineal gland characteristically result in Parinaud syndrome, typified by upgaze paralysis and convergence

Table 10-5 ■ THE MAIN HISTOLOGIC TYPES OF PRIMARY CNS TUMORS IN CHILDREN AND THEIR RELATIVE FREQUENCIES

Tumor Type, WHO Grade	Percentage
Pilocytic astrocytoma (PA), I	23.5
Diffuse astrocytoma, II	5
Anaplastic astrocytoma, III	7.2
Glioblastoma (GBM), IV	7.2
Pleomorphic xanthoastrocytoma (PXA), II–III[a]	1.9
Subependymal giant cell astrocytoma (SEGA), I	2.5
Medulloblastoma, IV	16.3
Ependymoma, II–III[a]	10.1
Craniopharyngioma (CPG), I	5.6
Germ cell tumors	2.5
Ganglioglioma (GG), I–III[a]	2.5
Meningioma, I–III[a]	2.5
Supratentorial primitive neuroectodermal tumor (sPNET), IV	1.9
Pineal parenchymal tumors (PPTs) (pineocytoma; pineoblastoma), II–IV	1.9
Atypical teratoid rhabdoid tumor (ATRT), IV	1.3
Choroid plexus tumors (CPTs) (papilloma; carcinoma), I and III	0.9
Desmoplastic infantile ganglioglioma (DIG)/astrocytoma (DIA), I	0.6
Dysembryoplastic neuroepithelial tumor (DNT), I	0.6
Pituitary adenoma	0.9
Schwannoma	1.3
Neurofibroma	0.3
Langerhans' cell histiocytosis	0.6

[a]Tumors where a range of grades are listed, the highest grade is generally called "anaplastic."
Data from Rickert CH, Paulus W. Epidemiology of central nervous system tumors in childhood and adolescence based on the new WHO classification. *Childs Nerv System* 2001;17:503–511.

Table 10-6 ■ WHO CLASSIFICATION OF TUMORS OF THE NERVOUS SYSTEM

Tumors of Neuroepithelial Tissue

Astrocytic tumors
- Pilocytic astrocytoma (PA)
- Pilomyxoid astrocytoma
- Subependymal giant cell astrocytoma (SEGA)
- Pleomorphic xanthoastrocytoma (PXA)
- Diffuse astrocytoma
- Fibrillary astrocytoma
- Protoplasmic astrocytoma
- Gemistocytic astrocytoma
- Anaplastic astrocytoma
- Glioblastoma (GBM)
- Giant cell GBM
- Gliosarcoma
- Gliomatosis cerebri

Oligodendroglial tumors
- Oligodendroglioma
- Anaplastic oligodendroglioma

Oligoastrocytic tumors
- Oligoastrocytoma
- Anaplastic oligoastrocytoma

Ependymal tumors
- Subependymoma
- Myxopapillary ependymoma
- Ependymoma
- Cellular
- Papillary
- Clear cell
- Tanycytic
- Anaplastic ependymoma

Choroid plexus tumors (CPTs)
- Choroid plexus papilloma (CPP)
- Atypical CPP
- Choroid plexus carcinoma (CPC)

Other neuroepithelial tumors
- Astroblastoma
- Chordoid glioma of the third ventricle
- Angiocentric glioma

Neuronal and mixed glioneuronal tumors
- Dysplastic gangliocytoma of cerebellum (Lhermitte-Duclos)
- Desmoplastic infantile astrocytoma/ganglioglioma
- Dysembryoplastic neuroepithelial tumor (DNT)
- Gangliocytoma
- Ganglioglioma (GG)
- Anaplastic ganglioglioma
- Papillary glioneuronal tumor
- Rosette-forming glioneuronal tumor of the fourth ventricle
- Central neurocytoma
- Extraventricular neurocytoma
- Cerebellar liponeurocytoma
- Paraganglioma of the filum terminale

Tumors of the pineal region
- Pineal parenchymal tumors (PPTs)
- Pineocytoma
- PPT of intermediate differentiation
- Pineoblastoma
- Papillary tumor of the pineal region

Embryonal tumors
- Medulloblastoma
- Desmoplastic/nodular medulloblastoma
- Medulloblastoma with extensive nodularity
- Anaplastic medulloblastoma
- Large cell medulloblastoma
- CNS primitive neuroectodermal tumors (PNETs)
- CNS PNET, NOS
- CNS neuroblastoma
- CNS ganglioneuroblastoma
- Medulloepithelioma
- Ependymoblastoma
- Atypical teratoid/rhabdoid tumor

Tumors of Cranial and Paraspinal Nerves

Schwannoma (Neurilemmoma, Neurinoma)
- Cellular
- Plexiform
- Melanotic

Neurofibroma
- Plexiform

Perineurioma
- Intraneural perineurioma
- Soft-tissue perineurioma

Malignant peripheral nerve sheath tumor (MPNST)
- Epithelioid
- MPNST with divergent mesenchymal and/or epithelial differentiation
- Melanotic

Tumors of the Meninges

Tumors of meningothelial cells
- Meningioma
- Meningothelial
- Fibrous (fibroblastic)
- Transitional (mixed)
- Psammomatous
- Angiomatous
- Microcystic
- Secretory
- Lymphoplasmacyte-rich
- Metaplastic
- Chordoid
- Clear cell
- Atypical
- Papillary
- Rhabdoid
- Anaplastic (malignant)

Mesenchymal tumors
- Lipoma
- Angiolipoma
- Hibernoma
- Liposarcoma (intracranial)
- Solitary fibrous tumor
- Fibrosarcoma
- Malignant fibrous histiocytoma
- Leiomyoma
- Leiomyosarcoma
- Rhabdomyoma
- Rhabdomyosarcoma
- Chondroma
- Chondrosarcoma
- Osteoma
- Osteosarcoma
- Osteochondroma
- Hemangioma
- Epithelioid hemangioendothelioma

(Continued)

Table 10-6 ▪ WHO CLASSIFICATION OF TUMORS OF THE NERVOUS SYSTEM *(Continued)*

Hemangiopericytoma
- Angiosarcoma
- Kaposi sarcoma

Primary melanocytic lesions
- Diffuse melanocytosis
- Melanocytoma
- Malignant melanoma
- Meningeal melanomatosis

Other neoplasms related to the meninges
- Hemangioblastoma

Lymphomas and Hematopoietic Neoplasms
- Malignant lymphomas
- Plasmacytoma
- Granulocytic sarcoma

Germ Cell Tumors
- Germinoma
- Embryonal carcinoma
- Yolk sac tumor
- Choriocarcinoma
- Teratoma
- Mature
- Immature
- Teratoma with malignant transformation
- Mixed germ cell tumors

Tumors of the Sellar Region
- Craniopharyngioma (CPG)
  - Adamantinomatous
  - Papillary
- Granular cell tumor
- Pituicytoma
- Spindle cell oncocytoma of the adenohypophysis

Metastatic Tumors

Modified from the WHO 2007 classification scheme (63).

nystagmus due to compression of dorsal midbrain visual centers. Seizure activity is an especially frequent presenting feature; not only do they suggest cortical involvement, but they also commonly accompany temporal lobe tumors. Posterior fossa tumors are anatomically speaking in a "high-traffic area" and result in a number of cerebellar, brainstem, and "long tract" abnormalities.

Neuroradiologic studies are an important tool of the neuropathologist. In particular, T1-weighted MR images with gadolinium enhancement and T2-weighted/FLAIR (fluid-attenuated inversion recovery) studies allow (somewhat simplistically) assessment of the vascularity and edema associated with a tumor, respectively. These radiologic studies help tremendously in the formation of differential diagnoses. Cystic lesions bearing a mural nodule [e.g., PA, pleomorphic xanthoastrocytoma (PXA) and GG], intracortical lesions [e.g., dysembryoplastic neuroepithelial tumor (DNT)], and other tumors that remodel the inner table of the skull (presumably through mechanical compression) all suggest a slowly growing low-grade lesion. An exophytic lesion of the dorsal brainstem is usually PA, while an intrinsic pontine or white matter–based cerebral lesion (especially enhancing cases) points to a more ominous tumor, such as a DA (28). Newer imaging modalities may also prove useful in the future. For example, using magnetic resonance spectroscopy (MRS), Tamiya et al. (106) found positive correlations between choline to creatinine ratios and the proliferative IHC marker Ki-67, suggesting that this modality may assist in tumor grading.

Table 10-7 ▪ PRESENTING SIGNS AND SYMPTOMS OF PEDIATRIC BRAIN TUMORS

Symptom/Sign Category	Specific Feature
General illness	Irritability, listlessness, failure to thrive, loss of developmental milestones, behavioral disturbance, poor feeding
Increased ICP or HCP	Headache, nausea, vomiting, macrocephaly, "sun-setting eyes," papilledema
Focal neurological disturbances ("focality")	Seizures Motor deficits (e.g., weakness) Visual field loss/deficit (e.g., Parinauds') Neuroendocrine dysfunction Cranial neuropathies Cerebellar dysfunction (nystagmus, ataxia, Romberg sign, abnormal tone, tremor, vertigo, etc.) Long tract signs (paraparesis, hyperreflexia, Babinski sign)

Treatment strategies generally involve three modalities: surgery, radiotherapy, and chemotherapy. Low-grade tumors are generally treated with surgery alone since this circumvents potential negative sequelae of chemotherapy and radiotherapy (113). High-grade neoplasms (i.e., WHO grade III–IV) usually receive adjuvant radiation and chemotherapy. Stereotactic biopsy may be performed in cases where the tumor lies within delicate anatomy (e.g., brainstem, pineal, and spinal cord); however, this yields very small biopsies, and therefore sampling adequacy is often a concern. A more thorough assessment of the current state of therapeutic neuro-oncology is available elsewhere (113).

General Pathologic Considerations

The workup of pediatric CNS tumors often employs both routine and adjuvant pathologic studies. As classification schemes are regularly updated, it is important to review prior surgical specimens at the time of recurrence or progression, as previous diagnoses occasionally need revision.

The frozen section provides a preliminary diagnosis and enables tissue allocation algorithms, the latter of which are increasingly being utilized for tumor banking, local research, ancillary molecular testing, and participation in clinical protocols. However, diagnostic accuracy ultimately remains most critical, and ensuring histologically superior permanent sections [i.e., formalin-fixed and paraffin-embedded (FFPE) sections] should always be the first priority. Retention and processing of the cavitronic ultrasound aspirator (CUSA) material may be somewhat less preserved than resected tissue due to partial autolysis and other artifacts but can nonetheless be essential to the final diagnosis, especially in the context of small tumors. Fixing a small portion of the tumor (i.e., 1 mm^3) in glutaraldehyde for ultrastructural analysis is recommended when the initial diagnosis is in question. If sufficient tissue is provided, a fragment should be snap frozen and stored for future studies. If only a small portion of tumor remains for FFPE, requesting a number of unstained sections upfront will avoid wasting any tissue at the time of slide preparation.

Evaluation of the FFPE material allows the first precise characterization of tumor. Primary CNS tumors may simplistically be considered as either "well circumscribed" or "diffusely infiltrating," and this dichotomization often assists in narrowing the differential diagnosis. Glial, neuronal, embryonal, and a number of other cytologic features can usually be appreciated on routine stains. Detail should be directed at the nuclear features since these are often key to many diagnoses (especially gliomas). Degenerative-type atypia (large hyperchromatic nuclei, often bearing pseudoinclusions of cytoplasm) is a common feature to many low-grade primary brain tumors and should not be over-interpreted as a concerning finding in the absence of other malignant features. Mitotic activity is critical to the grading of many CNS primary tumors, and specific cutoff numbers [generally expressed as #/10 high-powered fields (HPF)] exist for some tumor types. Grading is generally based not on the entirety of the specimen but on the most malignant portion identified (i.e., one rotten apple spoils the bunch). Microvascular proliferation (MVP), also referred to as endothelial proliferation or endothelial hyperplasia, represents foci of multilayering in blood vessel; several cellular elements (including smooth muscle cells, pericytes, and endothelial cells) are identified in these hyperplastic walls despite the focus on endothelia in the name. It is an important finding in the diffuse gliomas, as is necrosis (which may be pseudopalisading), where both of these features raise the WHO grade; notably both of these features may be seen in PA but do not impact prognosis and, thus, do not elevate the tumor grade. EGBs and RFs, while nonspecific, usually imply the presence of a slow-growing neoplasm, as does calcification to a lesser extent.

IHC analysis plays an important ancillary role in the diagnosis of brain tumors. The more commonly utilized stains are listed in Table 10-8. Special histochemical stains and electron microscopy (EM) modalities have been supplanted by IHC; but the former still have great utility in some scenarios. Reticulin is frequently used to identify extracellular matrix deposition in several tumors (e.g., PXA, gliosarcoma, GG, desmoplastic medulloblastoma, etc.) and in some tumors may stain in a pericellular pattern (e.g., schwannoma), indicative of basal lamina (The immunostain collagen IV is a more specific marker of such.). Periodic acid Schiff (PAS) and PAS-with-diastase confirm the presence of glycogen within the

Table 10-8 ■ IHC STAINS COMMONLY USED IN THE INVESTIGATION OF PEDIATRIC CNS TUMORS

Stain	Utility
GFAP	Glial differentiation, primarily in gliomas, reactive gliosis
S-100 protein	Nonspecific neuroectodermal marker, gliomas, DNT (OLCs), CPT, nerve sheath tumors, melanocytic tumors, histiocytic tumors
Neuronal markers[a]	Facilitate identification of a "neuronal component" in a tumor. Synaptophysin and chromogranin also for neuroendocrine differentiation; NFP labels normal axons and hence infiltration
Cytokeratin[b]	Epithelial differentiation in CPTs, ATRT, metastatic carcinoma
EMA	Ependymoma[c], meningioma, ATRT, metastatic carcinoma
CD34	Epileptogenic tumors: GG and PXA
INI1/BAF47	ATRT[d]
c-kit	Germinomatous differentiation in germ cell tumors
Ki-67	Proliferative marker
CD68	Lysosomal marker; used to identify reactive elements, including macrophages and microglia; histiocytic tumors
p53	Labels many tumors including astrocytic tumors, high-grade CPTs and MPNSTs. Particularly useful to identify "naked nuclei" of an infiltrating astrocytoma when strongly positive
HMB-45 and Melan-A	Melanocytic markers
CD45, CD20 and 79a, CD3	Markers of white blood cells (CD45 is general, CD20 and 79a for B-cells, and CD3 for T-cells) in reactive conditions and lymphoma
Muscle markers[e]	Muscle type differentiation in rhabdomyosarcoma, ATRT, medullomyoblastoma, etc.

[a]Neuronal markers: synaptophysin, Neu-N, NFP, MAP-2, chromogranin.
[b]CAM 5.2 (low molecular weight cytokeratin most commonly used).
[c]Ependymomas also stain with CD99 in a membranous and dot-like pattern.
[d]For ATRT, a triad of vimentin, EMA and SMA positivity also useful.
[e]Includes SMA, MSA, desmin, myogenin, myoglobin, and caldesmon.
DNT, dysembryoplastic neuroepithelial tumor; OLC, oligodendroglial-like cells; CPT, choroid plexus tumors; NFP, neurofilament; ATRT, atypical teratoid rhabdoid tumor; GG, ganglioglioma; PXA, pleomorphic xanthoastrocytoma; MPNST, malignant peripheral nerve sheath tumor.

cytoplasm of tumor cells (diastase sensitive), while the latter also highlights EGBs. Trichrome stains highlight RFs in addition to collagen. Bielschowsky silver stain labels axons (like NFP by IHC) and often the ganglion cell component of glio-neuronal tumors. LFB, counterstained with H&E or PAS, can be used to stain myelin and, hence, highlight tumor infiltration of white matter, or active demyelination (note: myelin breakdown products within macrophages is first blue, then changes to magenta or PAS-positive with time and concomitant degradation.), as seen in tumefactive (or tumor-like) multiple sclerosis. Ultrastructural analysis remains the gold standard for a few tumor types, such as ependymoma. The cilia, basal bodies, and intercellular "zipper-like" junctions of ependymoma are often well preserved and may even be identified in tissue that was previously subject to FFPE. EM can also help support the presence of a neuronal differentiation when dense-core granules, clear vesicles, microtubule-filled processes, and synapse formation are seen.

Genetic studies are becoming more frequent in the daily practice of neuropathology. Karyotyping remains an excellent method of globally screening rare pediatric brain tumors for cytogenetic abnormalities. Several pediatric brain tumors are amenable to testing, and some may exhibit signature molecular alterations. Fluorescence in situ hybridization (FISH) is occasionally used in the workup of several tumor types, including astrocytomas, oligodendrogliomas, medulloblastomas, atypical teratoid rhabdoid tumors (ATRTs), and meningiomas. Polymerase chain reaction (PCR)–based loss of heterozygosity (LOH) analysis is also used by some, as is chromogenic in situ hybridization (CISH). As newer genetic techniques continue to elucidate the molecular underpinnings of these tumors [e.g., gene expression profiling, array comparative genomic hybridization (aCGH), and single nucleotide polymorphism (SNP) arrays or "chips"], it is anticipated that additional routine genetic testing will be employed for diagnostic, prognostic, and predictive purposes.

What follows here is a brief account of the pertinent pathologic and molecular genetics of the most common pediatric brain neoplasms. A more exhaustive description exists elsewhere (10,63,68).

Gliomas

Pilocytic Astrocytomas

PAs, WHO grade I, are slowly growing tumors that most commonly occur in the cerebellum, hypothalamus, and in relation to the optic pathway (especially in relation to NF1), although cerebral, brainstem, and spinal cord cases also occur. Imaging often reveals a cystic lesion bearing an enhancing mural nodule.

Histologically, PAs are fairly discrete GFAP-positive tumors that exhibit only limited infiltration of adjacent native parenchyma. They are classically described as biphasic with (a) compact areas that contain spindled cells with long thin fibrillary processes (i.e., "piloid" or hair-like) emanating from opposite ends of the cell (i.e., bipolar); and (b) more loosely textured microcystic areas populated by small cells with round-oval nuclei bearing short cytoplasmic processes (Figure 10-24); RFs are seen in the former areas, while EGBs are seen in the latter. Degenerative atypia (see above) and vascular hyalinization are both common. Several histologic features, taken out of this typical context, can raise suspicion of a more ominous neoplasm, in particular a diffusely infiltrating type glioma. Areas of a PA may closely resemble DA or oligodendroglioma. MVP, often termed "glomeruloid-type," can closely mimic that found in high-grade gliomas, and may be accompanied by a bland "infarct-like" necrosis. Mitotic activity can be seen but is generally low. Extension involving the local subarachnoid space is fairly common, but does not adversely impact prognosis. Cases of anaplastic PA (WHO grade III), which secondarily develop the typical features of a high-grade DA (see below), have been reported but are exceedingly rare and remain poorly characterized to date. Pilomyxoid astrocytomas (PMA), considered by some to be an infantile-variant of PA, typically occur in the hypothalamus and are characterized by a monotonous population of small oval-to-elongate cells; these cells are embedded in mucoid background and form occasional perivascular pseudorosettes similar to those seen in ependymoma along with mitoses, necrosis, and variable infiltration. This proposed variant has been suggested to recur and seed the CSF spaces more frequently than typical PA (111). As such, it has been designated as WHO grade II in the 2007 WHO classification scheme. With exception of these latter two variants, WHO grade I PAs behave in a prognostically favorable manner.

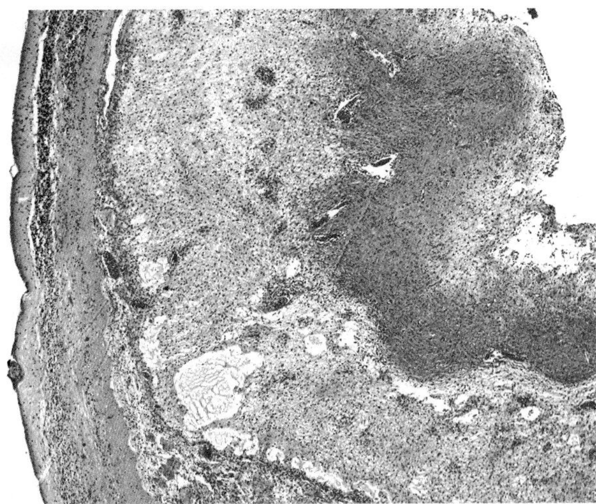

FIGURE 10-24 ■ Pilocytic astrocytoma (PA). Low-power magnification demonstrating a sharp tumor-brain interface (**left**), and a typical biphasic solid/microcystic architecture.

Genetic studies of PA have failed to identify a consistent signature abnormality. Cytogenetic abnormalities are often limited to gains of only a single chromosome (92). Gene expression profiling of 21 PAs suggested deregulation of several groups of genes in PA, including those involved in neurogenesis, cell adhesion, synaptic transmission, and CNS development in cellular differentiation (119). In addition to demonstrating that PAs could be separated into two groups based upon differences in gene expression, this latter study also showed that PAs immunonegative for myelin basic protein were more likely to progress. Although loss of the tumor suppressor gene, neurofibromin, appears to play a role in NF1-related PAs, its role in sporadic PAs is less clear (112). More recent studies suggest roles for Sox-10-regulated overexpression of ErbB3 (as part of a tyrosine kinase receptor–mediated pathway) (2), and overexpression of mRNA related to matrilin-2 (an extracellular matrix protein) in sporadic PA (98).

Diffusely Infiltrating Astrocytomas

As a group, DAs, WHO grade II-IV, represent the second most common pediatric tumor type. These grossly gray-tan-to-gelatinous tumors obscure the native gray-white boundaries, with higher grade examples often containing additional hemorrhage and necrosis. Microscopically, tumor cells invade adjacent brain structures in a single cell manner and have a tendency to aggregate around preexisting structural elements (neurons, blood vessels, underneath pial, and ependymal surfaces); these are called secondary structures of Scherer. Irregularly arranged infiltrating astrocytic tumor cells' morphology range from uniform, and minimally atypical, to highly pleomorphic in terms of both their cytoplasmic and nuclear features (Figure 10-25). Eosinophilic cytoplasm is fibrillary to gemistocytic ("belly-like"), and processes are often few and coarse; this cytoplasm is often immunoreactive for GFAP. In contrast, reactive astrocytes are evenly spaced and have a "starburst" appearance with several thin processes. "Naked nuclei" (i.e., nuclei without discernable cytoplasm on routine staining) may be common or predominant in fibrillary astrocytomas, making their identification difficult in cases with only mild hypercellularity and atypia. Nuclear features often reflect tumor grade. In general, the lowest grade tumors (i.e., WHO II) display less pleomorphism; they are moderately hyperchromatic, oval to slightly angulated, and bear indistinct nuclear membranes/nucleoli. In higher grade examples (i.e., WHO III-IV), nuclei often become increasingly pleomorphic and hyperchromatic.

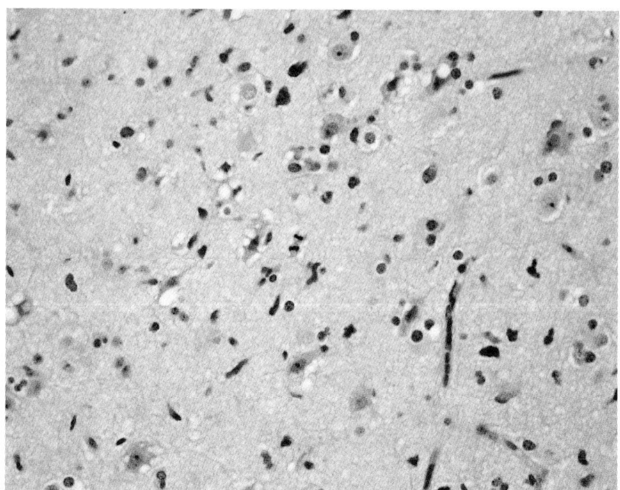

FIGURE 10-25 ■ Anaplastic astrocytoma, WHO grade III. Enlarged, hyperchromatic, and irregular tumor nuclei are associated with little cytoplasm and are seen diffusely invading neocortical gray matter.

DA grading criteria are currently fairly well defined. The four key features are encompassed by the mnemonic "AMEN": nuclear atypia, mitoses, endothelial proliferation, and necrosis. WHO grade II tumors show nuclear atypia alone. One mitotic figure is generally not considered sufficient to warrant an anaplastic designation, especially in large resections (35). WHO grade III tumors (i.e., anaplastic astrocytoma) generally exhibit mitotic activity (at least 2 to 3 mitoses within the entire surgical material). Suspicion of a higher grade neoplasm is also often deduced from radiologic enhancement, which often (but not always) correlates with the presence of MVP. Either MVP or necrosis (in particular pseudopalisading necrosis, wherein tumor cells cluster or palisade around an area of central necrosis) elevates the grade to IV [i.e., glioblastoma (GBM)].

The inherently infiltrative nature of diffuse astrocytomas precludes surgical resection, and recurrences are inevitable despite current adjuvant therapy. Although some studies suggest better outcomes for childhood versus adult DAs, the prognosis remains poor (9). A recent epidemiological study of 987 children and adults estimated the median survival times for grade II, III and IV DAs at 5.6, 1.6, and 0.4 years, respectively (71).

The traditional EGFR (seen in primary or de novo GBM) versus p53 (secondary GBMs developing from a lower grade precursor) molecular pathogenic dichotomy, which characterizes adult DAs does not appear to be entirely applicable to pediatric DAs: EGFR and p53 mutations are relatively infrequent (83,112). However, Phosphatase and Tensin homolog (PTEN) mutations, which characterize both primary and secondary adult GBMs, may be seen in children and appear to portend a poor prognosis (83); therefore, pediatric DAs may involve similar but also potentially different components of these complicated pathways. In general, mouse modeling of gliomas has suggested molecular abnormalities in three basic cellular processes: (a) external signaling (e.g., involving receptor tyrosine kinases EGFR and PDGFR), (b) signal transduction (SRC, AKT, PTEN, RAS, RHO), and (c) cell cycling (INK4a/CDK4/RB/E2F and ARF/MDM2/p53 pathways) (68). Notably, one recent pediatric microarray study found differential expression of the EGFR/FKBP12/HIF2-alpha growth and angiogenesis-promoting pathway in higher grade DAs (54). In addition, microsatellite instability, considered a marker of defective DNA repair, has been noted by some researchers to be more common in pediatric versus adult high-grade DAs (103), although a recent study has failed to find such an association (25).

Ependymomas

Ependymomas, WHO grade II–III, are discrete radiologically enhancing gliomas, which in children most often occur

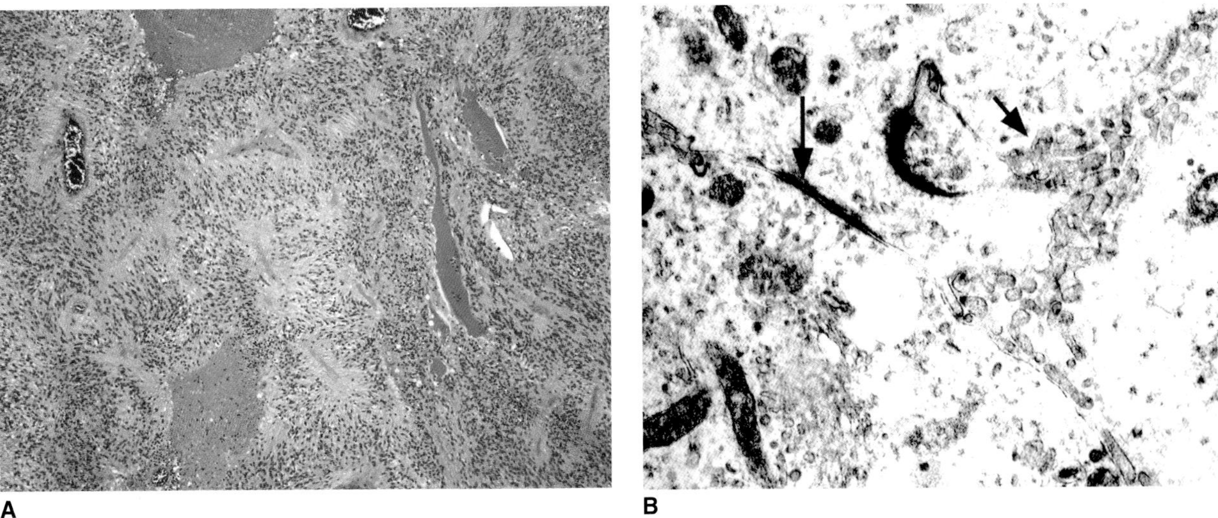

FIGURE 10-26 ▪ Ependymoma. **A:** Perivascular pseudorosettes. **B:** EM demonstrating "zipper-like" intercellular junctions (*long arrow*) and microvilli (*short arrow*).

in relation to the fourth ventricle. Supratentorial and spinal cord cases also occur, the latter of which are more common in adults. Of several microscopic variants (classic, cellular, papillary, clear cell, tanycytic, and myxopapillary), the classic and cellular types are the most common. The interface with adjacent brain is sharp. Tumor cells are more often fibrillar, but epithelial morphologies can be seen; the former result in characteristic perivascular pseudorosettes and the less common true rosettes, while the latter form epithelial canals and surfaces (Figure 10-26A). Long GFAP-positive fibrillary processes radiate toward a central blood vessel, creating perivascular nuclear free zones and hence pseudorosettes. The epithelial quality of many ependymomas is reflected in IHC cytoplasmic dot-like positivity seen for epithelial membrane antigen (EMA) and CD99. EM can facilitate the diagnosis by demonstrating long zipper-like intercellular junctions, microvilli, cilia, and intracytoplasmic lumina (Figure 10-26B).

Numerous grading systems have been proposed for ependymomas. Regrettably, no consensus has been achieved as to the criteria that best typify anaplastic (WHO grade III) examples. Ho et al. (45) suggested that two of the following four criteria were indicative of anaplasia: mitoses ≥4/10 hpf, hypercellularity, MVP, and necrosis. Other studies have found atypia, hypercellularity, and MVP to be reliable prognosticators (58,70). One recent study suggested that indicators of cellular proliferation, in particular cell density–adjusted mitotic rate and ki-67, are especially important (60). Another new study claims that telomerase activity is reflective of anaplasia, with IHC positivity for h-TERT seen in those cases (104).

Ependymomas are usually treated with surgery and, in many cases, radiation. Gross total resection has been proven a key prognostic indicator. Radiotherapy is often withheld in children under 3 years of age because of the heightened risk of CNS damage in this cohort. Five-year progression free survival (PFS) and overall survival (OS) for grade II and grade III ependymomas were 90 and 93 months versus 27 and 61 months, respectively (58).

To date, no single genetic feature characterizes the majority of pediatric ependymomas. While overall, loss of chromosome 22q is the most commonly seen abnormality, this usually occurs in the context of adult spinal cases and in NF2 patients. Loss of the tumor suppressor gene 4.1B (DAL-1 on 18p11.3) has been noted to be more common in intracranial examples (especially in the "clear cell variant"), and abnormalities of the 4.1R gene (on 1p32-33) may also be important (85,100). Various CGH studies on pediatric intracranial ependymoma have revealed gain on 1q (spinal cases may show gain of chromosome 7) and losses on chromosomes 6q, 9, 13, and 17p in subsets of tumors (79). Poorer clinical outcomes have been suggested in cases with (a) partial chromosomal losses (or structural alterations) and gain of 1q (23) and (b) elevated ErbB2/4 receptor coexpression levels, which is especially predictive when combined with the IHC Ki67 index and the extent of resection (37). More recently, microarray and Q-PCR data have suggested several potential genes of interest in the pathogenesis of pediatric ependymoma (102), with patterns supporting a possible histogenetic link to radial glia (108).

Less Common Gliomas

Additional relatively discrete and generally low-grade gliomas include PXAs, SEGAs, and DIAs. These neoplasms are usually associated with a favorable prognosis post resection and are briefly discussed below. Both astroblastoma (with low-grade and high-grade forms proposed) and gliomatosis cerebri (generally considered WHO grade III) are rare tumors that are essentially considered forms of glioma (the former sharing some ependymal features, while the latter demonstrates astrocytic or rarely oligodendrocytic cytology). Astroblastomas are discrete and contain epithelioid-to-fibrillary GFAP positive cells arranged in distinctive astroblastomatous-type rosettes (i.e., perivascular pseudorosettes containing cellular processes with broad-based vascular attachments). Vascular hyalinization is characteristic. Gliomatosis cerebri is defined as a widely infiltrative glioma involving more than two lobes and potentially infratentorial structures. Types I and II are recognized, with the latter being associated with a distinct mass. Prognosis is poor for these patients; the majority of whom die within 12 months (63). Angiocentric glioma is a recently described epileptogenic primary neoplasm that displays ependymal-like differentiation, characteristic nuclear cytology, and a perivascular/subpial infiltrative growth pattern (118).

In comparison with adults, oligodendrogliomas (WHO grade II and III) are much less common. These tumors are generally white matter–based lesions of the cerebrum that have a tropism for the neocortical gray matter. Secondary structures of Scherer and calcification tend to be more prominent in oligodendrogliomas as opposed to DAs. The typical "fried-egg" appearance of tumor cells is a helpful, although not entirely consistent, tissue-processing artifact wherein round/regular tumor nuclei are surrounded by a clear halo of cytoplasm. Delicate chicken-wire-type vasculature courses between the tumor cells. Scattered mitotic activity is tolerated within grade II forms. In general, mitotic activity greater than 6/10 HPF and/or MVP is necessary for a designation of anaplastic oligodendroglioma (WHO grade III) (36). Oligodendrogliomas are probably best known for their favorable prognosis and chemotherapeutic responsiveness when accompanied by codeletion of the 1p and 19q chromosomal arms (12). Unfortunately, this favorable genetic signature is more commonly encountered in adult oligodendrogliomas and is uncommon in pediatric cases (59,84). Moreover, when present in children, the prognostic significance of this deletional pattern is not as clearly established. Mixed oligoastrocytomas (MOA) contain both oligodendroglial and astrocytic tumor components, manifesting either as geographically separate forms or more often intermingled forms.

PXAs, WHO grade II and III, are epileptogenic and usually occur as cortically superficial lesions of the temporal lobe. Histologic features are quite characteristic, but prior to its recognition as a distinct entity, PXA was commonly misdiagnosed as GBM. Large pleomorphic cells are variably GFAP-positive, and often contain substantial eosinophilic to lipidized clear cytoplasm. Spindle-shaped cells are arranged in interweaving fascicles that often engender a mesenchymal quality, which is accompanied by pericellular reticulin deposition. EGBs and perivascular lymphocytes are typical. Both subarachnoid space involvement and a limited infiltrative component can be seen and are not indicative of a poor outcome. Grading criteria have been proposed to mark a subset of PXAs that are associated with a poor prognosis; five mitoses/10 HPF has been suggested as a criterion for anaplastic PXA (WHO grade III) (34). Genetic studies are limited and initially suggested alterations that differ from DAs (53). More recently, some of the abnormalities previously described in DA have also been identified in PXAs, namely changes in chromosome 9p (53) and the MDM2 gene (66).

SEGA, WHO grade I, is almost entirely restricted to patients with TS (see later discussion). They usually occur near the foramen of Monro, and accordingly result in obstructive HCP. Whether this entity is neoplastic or hamartomatous remains unclear. Imaging reveals contrast enhancement and often calcification. Tumor cells contain abundant glassy eosinophilic cytoplasm and, despite their name, are more aptly considered larger than "giant" (giant cells of a giant cell GBM are much larger, bizarre, and are often multinucleate.). Both spindled cells and epithelioid to gemistocyte-like forms are seen, typically forming sweeping fascicles and occasional perivascular pseudorosettes. Nuclei often bear prominent nucleoli, resulting in comparisons to ganglion-like cells. These hybrid astrocytic/neuronal features are reiterated in the IHC results in these cases that sometimes reveals both GFAP and neuronal marker positivity. Accordingly, some experts have favored the alternative term subependymal giant cell tumor. Mitoses, MVP, and necrosis are usually absent.

Embryonal Tumors

This group of tumors comprises approximately 20% of pediatric tumors. Histologically, they are united by their small round blue cell cytology: primitive appearing cells exhibiting a high nuclear-to-cytoplasmic ratio and hyperchromatic nuclei. All are WHO grade IV.

Medulloblastoma

Medulloblastomas are tumors of the cerebellum, and generally originate from the vermis. They are contrast-enhancing tumors that may contain necrosis, although MVP is somewhat uncommon. These tumors have a tendency to seed the CSF pathways and may result in "drop metastases" to the spinal cord. Distant metastases may also rarely occur (most frequently bone and lymph nodes).

Numerous histologic subtypes of medulloblastoma exist, the most common of which include classic (i.e., undifferentiated); desmoplastic-nodular (D-N); medulloblastomas with extensive nodularity (MBEN); and large cell-anaplastic (LC-A). Less commonly, medulloblastomas may exhibit glial, skeletal muscle, and/or melanotic types of differentiation. Classic medulloblastomas contain patternless sheets of "small round blue cells," with or without Homer Wright rosettes, wherein primitive tumor cells surround a central island of delicate fibrillary material (i.e., neuropil) (Figure 10-27A). These Homer Wright rosettes are also sometimes referred to as neuroblastic rosettes since they are identical to those encountered in neuroblastomas of the peripheral nervous system. Ganglioid (intermediate in size between neurocytes and ganglion cells) and ganglion cells are less common manifestations of neuronal differentiation and maturation. When significant nuclear atypia accumulates, this variant essentially blends into the more aggressive LC-A variant.

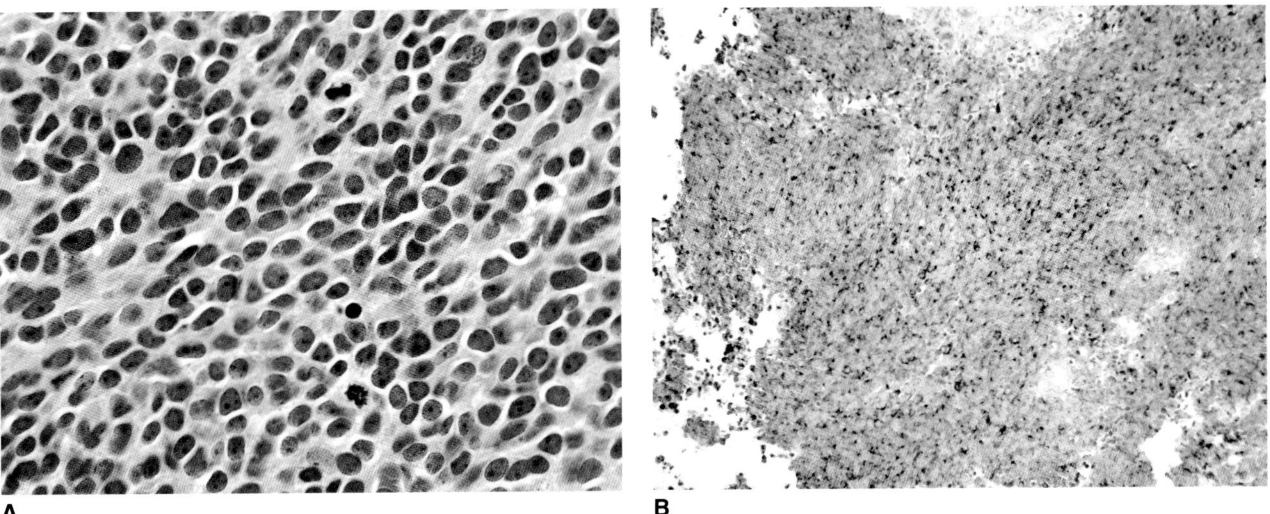

FIGURE 10-27 ▪ Medulloblastoma, "classic" subtype. **A:** H&E 1,000× magnification. **B:** Synaptophysin immunohistochemistry.

LC-As medulloblastomas are characterized by two types of tumor cells, either of which may predominate: (a) large cells are rounded and contain enlarged vesicular nuclei, prominent nucleoli, and variable amounts of cytoplasm and (b) anaplastic cells are similarly enlarged, but show significant nuclear atypia and hyperchromasia. These anaplastic regions often display "nuclear molding" and "cell wrapping" (Figure 10-28).

D-N medulloblastomas have a characteristic low-power appearance of rounded pale islands of tumor, separated by darker internodular tumor. The pale islands are less cell dense and composed of uniform round-oval, less mitotically active and cells embedded within a fine fibrillary/neuropil-like reticulin-poor background. These slightly more mature neuronal-appearing cells sometimes resemble neurocytes. The internodular tumor is more cell dense and primitive appearing, with mitotically active cells embedded within reticulin-rich tissue. Sometimes parallel rows of single tumor cells are identified (cellular streaming). D-N medulloblastomas comprise a genetically distinct subset of medulloblastomas that behave in a prognostically favorable manner (69). Tumors bearing a predominance of large pale islands (which are often grossly or radiologically visible) and minimal internodular areas have been termed MBENs; these rare medulloblastomas seen in very young children are also considered to form a prognostically more favorable subgroup. Such tumors have been referred to as cerebellar neuroblastoma in the past.

IHC staining of tumor cells in medulloblastoma is most reliably done with synaptophysin, consistent with at least a limited degree of neuronal differentiation in the vast majority of medulloblastomas (Figure 10-27B). More variable and often limited degrees of GFAP positivity may also be seen. In the D-N medulloblastomas, the greatest degree of synaptophysin and GFAP positivity is usually seen in the intranodular regions, consistent with the notion that these represent islands of maturation. Occasionally, Neu-N nuclear positivity may be seen within the neurocytic-like tumor cells of these intranodular areas. As expected, ultrastructural evidence of neuronal differentiation is also common.

Recent attempts at grading medulloblastomas have concluded that greater degrees of anaplasia (as defined by nuclear enlargement, mitoses, apoptosis, large cells, angulation/pleomorphism, cell crowding, and cell wrapping) are associated with worse clinical outcomes (Fig. 10-28) (24,33).

Several biologic pathways have been implicated in medulloblastoma pathogenesis: (a) sonic hedgehog (SHH), (b) wingless (WNT), and (c) ERBB receptor tyrosine kinase I family. SHH is important to cerebellar granular cell development and mutations in the SHH pathway (most notably the PTCH gene associated with Gorlin syndrome) have been linked to D-N medulloblastoma (80). Approximately, 15% of sporadic medulloblastomas involve mutations in the WNT pathway, which includes contributions from APC (related to Turcot syndrome), axin, GSK-3beta, beta-catenin, and the

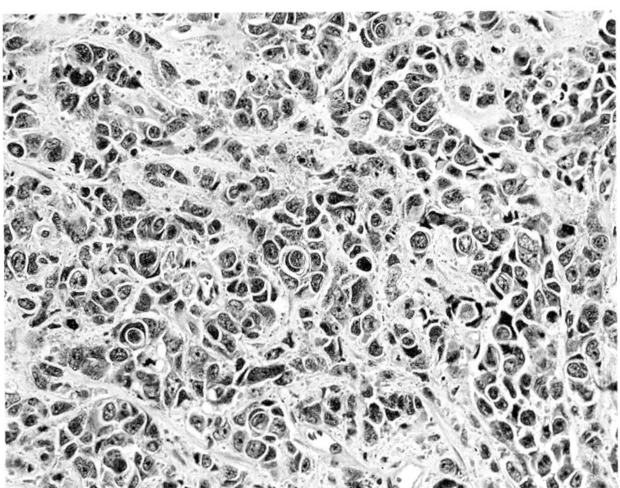

FIGURE 10-28 ▪ Large cell—anaplastic medulloblastoma. "Cell wrapping" is prominent in this example.

transcription factor complex TCF/LEF (105). Overexpression of the ERBB2 receptor has been associated with poor clinical outcome, while elevated Trk-C expression has been linked to a more favorable behavior and the D-N medulloblastoma variant (42,112). The most common cytogenetic alteration in medulloblastomas involves loss of chromosome 17p, most often resulting from the formation of an isochromosome 17q [i(17q)] with an associated duplication of the long arm; i17q is encountered in about 30% of cases (79). Isolated losses of 17p have been associated with aggressive behavior, as have amplifications in the MYC oncogenes, either c-MYC or N-MYC; such amplifications are seen in approximately 10% of cases (105,112). More recent data have drawn attention to epigenetic phenomena, in particular hypermethylation of key DNA segments involved in transcriptional regulation, including the tumor suppressor genes RASSF1A and HIC-1 (64,117).

Five-year survival rates for medulloblastomas have continually improved over the last 25 years, rising from 36% in 1980 to approximately 70% to 80% now. However, this has come with a significant price in terms of long-term side effects, since craniospinal radiation is particularly toxic to the developing CNS, especially in those children less than 5 years old.

Supratentorial Primitive Neuroectodermal Tumor

A previously held conceptualization suggested that all CNS embryonal neoplasms were of a similar origin. For example, supratentorial primitive neuroectodermal tumor (sPNET) was considered to simply represent the supratentorial form of medulloblastoma. However, the prognosis for sPNET has been demonstrated to be significantly worse than for its postulated cerebellar counterpart; moreover, recent studies have revealed separate genetic alterations (see below). sPNETs are contrast enhancing and may exhibit calcification, hemorrhage, and/or necrosis. Histologically, these densely cellular tumors are reminiscent of classic medulloblastomas, but sometimes with greater evidence of divergent differentiation, both on routine stains (Homer-Wright rosettes, perivascular pseudorosettes, ependymal canals, pigmented cells, neurons) and immunohistochemically (positivity with neuronal markers including synaptophysin, GFAP, muscle markers, epithelial markers). Tumors with evidence of extensive neuronal differentiation have been alternately termed cerebral neuroblastoma.

Gene expression profiling (80) and CGH data (46) support the separation of medulloblastoma from sPNETs. In particular, CGH has revealed that sPNET, as compared to medulloblastoma, do not demonstrate i(17q) or −10q but do exhibit +1q, −16p and −19p. This latter study also revealed a significantly worse prognosis for sPNET. One recent review suggested a role for the pRB/Ink4/p53 and DNA repair pathways in the development of sPNETs (62). With such a paucity of data accumulated to date, additional molecular genetic investigations of sPNET are clearly needed.

Atypical Teratoid/Rhabdoid Tumor (ATRT)

ATRT is an uncommon, but distinctive tumor of infants and young children (generally <5 years old). These often large, cystic, hemorrhagic, and enhancing tumors may be seen supratentorially, in the posterior fossa or rarely in the spinal cord. Routine and IHC stains yield a polyphenotypic pattern (i.e., presence of multiple lineage-associated markers that are usually not coexpressed). Characteristic to ATRT are rhabdoid cells, which exhibit eccentrically placed vesicular nuclei, prominent nucleoli, and a globular or fibrillar eosinophilic paranuclear inclusion corresponding to whorled bundles of intermediate filaments ultrastructurally (Figure 10-29A). Areas of both mesenchymal and epithelial differentiation may be noted. Primitive appearing cells may predominate in some, causing diagnostic confusion with sPNET or medulloblastoma (43). The IHC profile is highly variable but typically includes a triad of positivity for EMA, smooth muscle actin (SMA), and vimentin. ATRTs result from biallelic inactivation of the INI1/BAF47/hSNF5 gene tumor suppressor gene (located at 22q11) via either large-scale deletion (which may be identified with FISH) or smaller single base pair mutation (detected through gene sequencing). A highly sensitive and specific IHC stain for this gene's protein product (called INI1/BAF47) has recently become commercially available; non-neoplastic nuclei retain nuclear staining of this ubiquitously expressed protein, whereas there is loss of expression in tumor nuclei (43) (Figure 10-29B). These extremely aggressive tumors often cause death within 1 year.

Other rare embryonal neoplasms are listed in Table 10-9. Pineoblastomas are also a form of embryonal tumor but are discussed under the pineal parenchymal tumors (PPTs) section below.

Tumors Related to the Third Ventricle/ Suprasellar Space

Craniopharyngioma (CPGs), WHO grade I, are squamous epithelial neoplasms that are thought to be derived from remnants of Rathke pouch. They are typically suprasellar and result in dysfunction of the hypothalamic-pituitary axis, visual difficulties, obstructive HCP, and increased ICP. These contrast-enhancing, cystic and calcified tumors contain a characteristic dark sparkled fluid similar to "machinery oil" (when spilled *in vivo* may result in chemical meningitis). Papillary and adamantinomatous are the two main subtypes.

Adamantinomatous CPGs are typically present in children, although there is also a second smaller peak in adults. Epithelial cells are arranged in sheets, whorls, and trabeculae, and may line cyst spaces. Solid foci bear orderly islands of epithelia with (a) peripheral or basal palisades, (b) adjacent polygonal cells, and (c) a loose meshwork of epithelial cells termed stellate reticulum resulting from intercellular fluid accumulation (Figure 10-30). Cellular outlines (or "ghosts") of squamoid tumor cells with brightly eosinophilic cytoplasm and indistinct nuclei constitute wet-keratin, a diagnostic feature even in the absence of viable epithelium. A xanthogranulomatous inflammatory

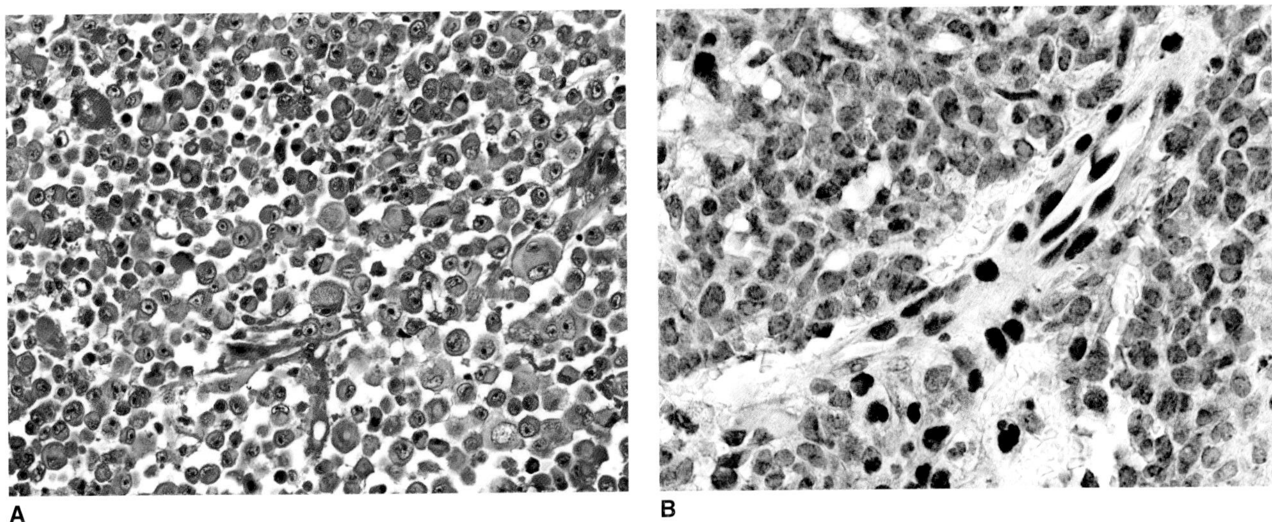

FIGURE 10-29 ■ Atypical teratoid rhabdoid tumor (ATRT). **A:** Rhabdoid cells. **B:** INI-1/BAF-47 immunohistochemistry demonstrating a lack of staining in tumor nuclei, while nonneoplastic lymphocytes and endothelial cells retain nuclear positivity.

reaction is typical and accompanied by needle-shaped clear cholesterol clefts and necrosis. The ragged interface with adjacent brain is typified by dense piloid gliosis (including RFs), which may resemble PA in the absence of adjacent epithelium. Immunohistochemistry is positive for cytokeratins and EMA. The outcome is dependent on the extent of surgical resection and tumor size, with 10-year survivals ranging from 64% to 96% (63). Recent mutational and IHC analyses have suggested a role for abnormal WNT pathway signaling in adamantinomatous CPGs; exon 3 of beta-catenin was mutated in 77% of these tumors, with corresponding nuclear accumulation of beta-catenin in 94% (11).

Papillary CPGs are relatively discrete papillary tumors that primarily affect adults. These tumors are composed of stratified, nonkeratinizing squamous epithelium situated on a fibrovascular stroma that lacks the characteristic histology of the adamantinomatous variant. Scattered goblet cells may be highlighted with mucin stains. Papillary CPGs are more commonly intraventricular (third ventricular), and although some studies have suggested that this variant displays a better prognosis than the adamantinomatous variety (107), other studies have failed to demonstrate such an association (22).

Germ cell tumors are thought to be derived from ectopically placed germ cells during gestation. Included in this group are germinoma, yolk sac tumor, choriocarcinoma, embryonal carcinoma, teratoma (mature and immature variants), and mixed neoplasms (comprised of two or more of the preceding types). Pineal and suprasellar regions are especially favored; at times, synchronous (and separate) lesions may be detected in each of these two areas. Suprasellar lesions typically result in dysfunction of the hypothalamic-pituitary axis and abnormal vision, whereas pineal lesions result in Parinaud syndrome and HCP. Clinical outcomes correlate with certain subtypes and segregate into favorable (e.g., germinoma, teratoma) and unfavorable groups (e.g., yolk sac tumor, choriocarcinoma, embryonal carcinoma), the latter of which are often suspected via imaging/gross features of necrosis and hemorrhage. Histologic features of CNS germ cell tumors are essentially identical to their extra-CNS counterparts (nongerminomatous examples are discussed in Chapters 18 and 19).

CNS germinomas have a characteristic histology composed of two cell types. The neoplastic component has large round-to-oval epithelioid cells that are glycogen rich and have a clear-to-eosinophilic cytoplasm; the associated

Table 10-9 ■ RARE EMBRYONAL TUMORS

Tumor Type (ref)	Key Histologic Features	IHC/EM
Medulloepithelioma (Molloy et al., 1996)*	Neoplastic epithelium bearing an external limiting membrane; divergent differentiation.	Vimentin and nestin
Ependymoblastoma (Cruz-Sanchez et al., 1988)**	Multilayered true rosettes (ependymoblastic)	Vimentin, S-100; "abortive" ependymoma-like ultrastructure
ETANTR (Eberhart et al., 2000)***	Ependymoblastoma-like rosettes, neuropil and variable neuronal differentiation	Synaptophysin, NFP,GFAP; EM as above

ETANTR, embryonal tumor with abundant neuropil and true rosettes.
*_J Neurosurg_ 1996;84:430–436.
**_Histopathology_ 1988;12:17–27.
***_Pediatr Dev Pathol_ 2000;3:346–352.

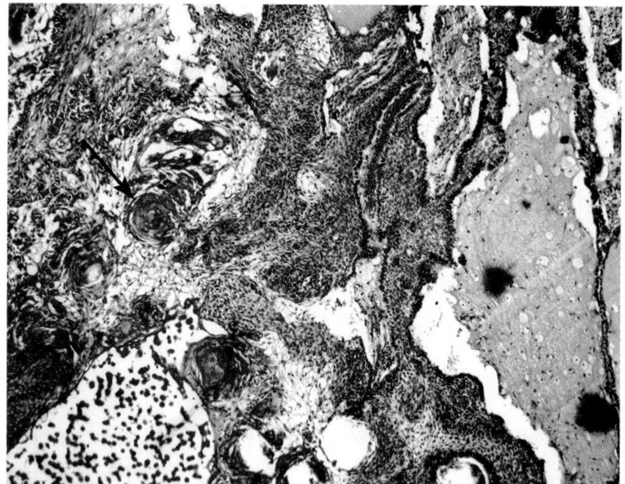

FIGURE 10-30 ■ Adamantinomatous CPG. In addition to its characteristic epithelium, "wet keratin" (*arrow*) can be seen and often bears "ghosts" of degenerate tumor cells.

nucleus is large, vesicular and bears a prominent nucleus (Figure 10-31A). The second cell type comprises a variably prominent reactive lymphocytic infiltrate, which is dispersed within an architectural lobularity created by delicate fibrovascular septae. This inflammation can also be granulomatous and may overshadow the tumor cells, occasionally leading to a misdiagnosis of inflammatory disorders; this pitfall is particularly important to consider when dealing with small biopsy specimens. Immunohistochemically, the large tumor cells stain positively for placental alkaline phosphatase (PLAP) and c-kit (CD117) in a membranous pattern, of which the latter is now preferred (49) (Figure 10-31B). Recent genetic studies have yielded similar cytogenetic alterations within CNS and extra-CNS germinomas: isochromosome 12p [i(12p)] which should not come as a surprise. Germinomas are extremely radiosensitive and chemosensitive and therefore are among the prognostically favorable group of CNS germ cell tumors, with 5-year survival varying from 80% to 96% (10).

PPTs are thought to be derived from the native pineocyte, a neuron-like cell with photoreceptor and neuroendocrine characteristics. These contrast-enhancing tumors obstruct CSF flow and compress adjacent structures with Parinaud syndrome being typical. The WHO 2000 classification system recognizes three main PPTs: Pineoblastoma, WHO grade IV, primarily affects children, while pineocytoma, WHO grade II, usually occurs in adults. PPT of intermediate grade is "intermediate" in terms of grade and clinical features and is considered WHO grade III. Jouvet et al. (48) have proposed an alternative four-tier grading scheme for PPTs, where pineocytomas are grade I, PPT of intermediate grade are grade II and III, and pineoblastomas are grade IV; the degrees of mitotic activity and NFP staining in tandem serve to differentiate these groups into prognostically meaningful categories. Pineoblastomas are somewhat poorly demarcated and may contain hemorrhage and or necrosis. Histologically, these embryonal tumors are populated by primitive mitotically active cells. Hypercellular sheets of tumor cells may contain Homer-Wright rosettes or Flexner-Wintersteiner rosettes, but none of the pineocytic rosettes are characteristic of pineocytoma. Pineocytomas bear uniform small mature cells with round-oval bland nuclei and moderate amounts of eosinophilic cytoplasm. These cells closely resemble the neurocytes encountered in central neurocytoma. Mitoses and necrosis are infrequent. Pineocytic rosettes resemble Homer-Wright rosettes but are larger and are not formed by primitive cells (Figure 10-32). Degenerative atypia and ganglionic differentiation may also be seen. Immunohistochemistry reveals staining for neuronal markers, especially synaptophysin, but also for the more nonspecific neural/neuroendocrine marker neuron specific enolase (NSE). In general, the grading of PPTs utilizes cytology, mitotic activity, necrosis,

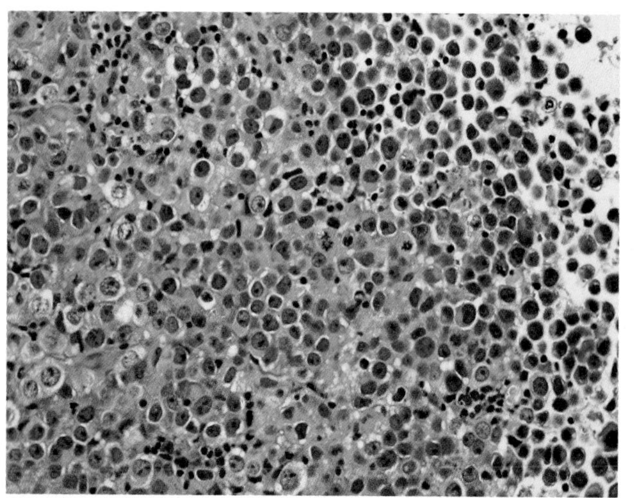

A

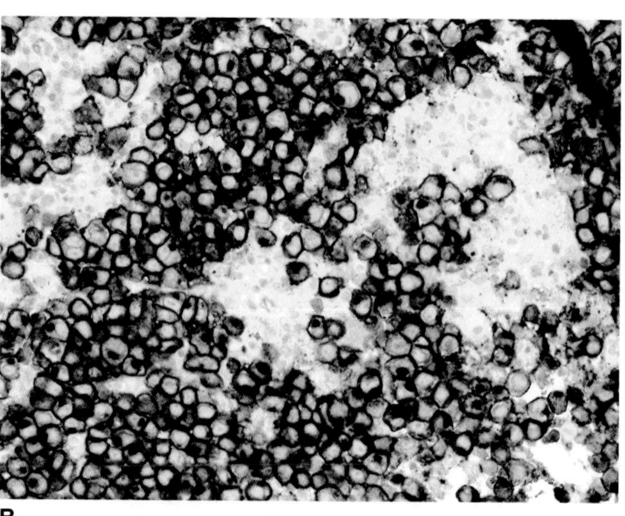

B

FIGURE 10-31 ■ Intracranial germinoma. **A:** Typical biphasic histology including large mitotically active cells and reactive lymphocytes. **B:** CD117 (c-kit) immunohistochemistry demonstrating membranous positivity in the large tumor cells.

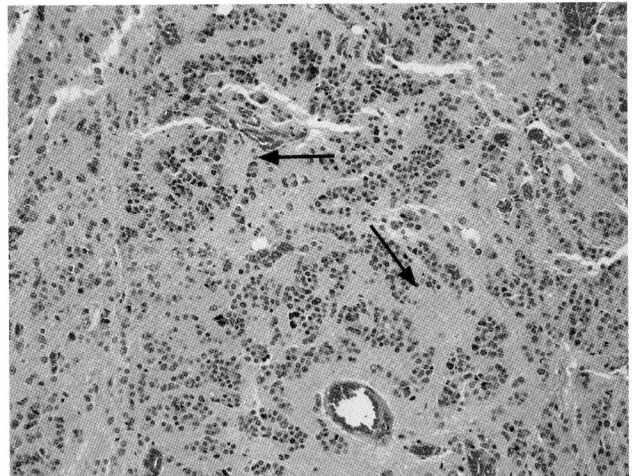

FIGURE 10-32 ■ Pineocytoma. Pineocytic rosettes (*arrows*), which are larger than Homer Wright rosettes, are scattered throughout this example.

the present or absence of pineocytic/Homer-Wright/Flexner-Wintersteiner rosettes, and a decrease in NFP staining (10) (see also above). Five-year survival rates for pineocytoma and pineoblastoma have been estimated at 86% and 58%, respectively (63). Genetic information on PPTs is very limited and reviewed elsewhere (62).

Neuronal and Mixed Glioneuronal Tumors

Ganglioglioma (GG)

GGs (usually WHO grade I) are epileptogenic tumors that preferentially occur in the temporal lobe. The defining feature of GGs is dysmorphic neurons. Their morphology deviates from normal neurons (large vesicular nucleus, prominent nucleolus, basophilic cytoplasm bearing Nissl substance) in exhibiting binucleation or multinucleation, vacuolated cytoplasm, and clumpy irregularly formed Nissl substance (Figure 10-33A). Coarse irregular processes and Alzheimer type degenerative changes (including neurofibrillary tangles and granulovacuolar degeneration) may be seen. Architecturally, the ganglion cells are often clumped or haphazardly arranged in comparison to the laminar, well-ordered arrangement of normal cortex. However, in areas where the glial component predominates, GGs may resemble DA, oligodendroglioma, and even PA. Gangliocytomas are essentially GGs without the glial component; in cases where a glial component is more equivocal, a diagnosis of "ganglion cell tumor" may be more appropriate. Connective tissue–rich areas and calcification may also be seen. Although generally considered noninfiltrating and discrete neoplasms, neuropil-like areas (including axons) indistinguishable from native parenchyma are frequent and make the designation of infiltration versus neoplastic neuropil (i.e., tumor cell process constitute the meshwork of process, which to some degree mimics the appearance of normal neuropil) difficult. EGBs are very common, as are perivascular lymphocytes. Features characteristic of high-grade gliomas (mitoses and necrosis) are usually absent, although MVP is fairly common. High-grade glial transformation (i.e., anaplastic GG, WHO grade III, and rarely IV) is exceedingly rare and difficult to define (10). The glial and neuronal components can be highlighted immunohistochemically with GFAP and neuronal markers (most commonly synaptophysin), respectively. More recently, scattered CD34 positivity has been suggested to be characteristic of GG, both within tumor cells and in the adjacent dysplastic cortex (8) (Figure 10-33B). EM can also be used to support the finding of neuronal differentiation. Prognosis is favorable with surgical resection.

Dysembryoplastic Neuroepithelial Tumor (DNT)

DNT, WHO grade I, is a controversial lesion that was first described in 1988 (18). Although currently considered a mixed glioneuronal tumor by the WHO, many consider it

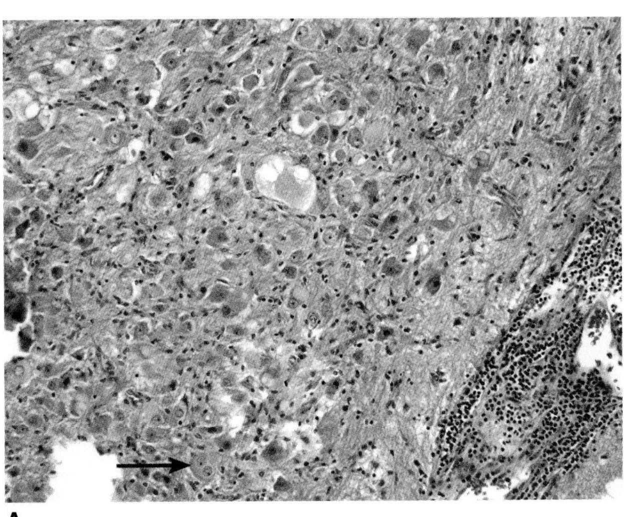

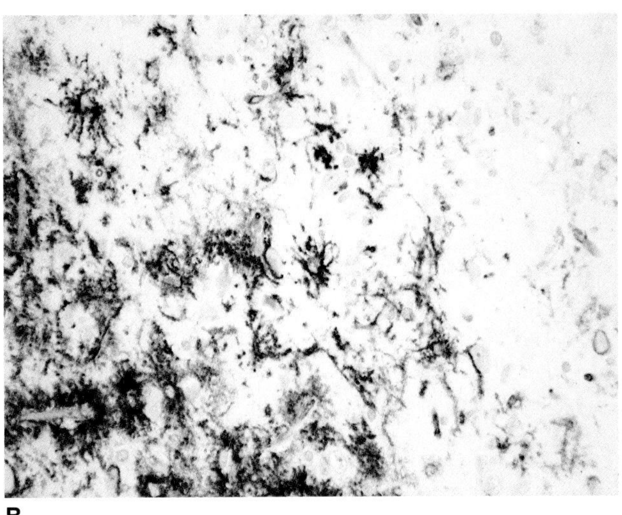

A B

FIGURE 10-33 ■ Ganglioglioma (GG). **A:** H&E section reveals numerous neoplastic neurons, including vacuolated and binucleate (*arrow*) forms. **B:** CD34 immunohistochemistry highlights tumor cells with highly ramifying cytoplasmic processes.

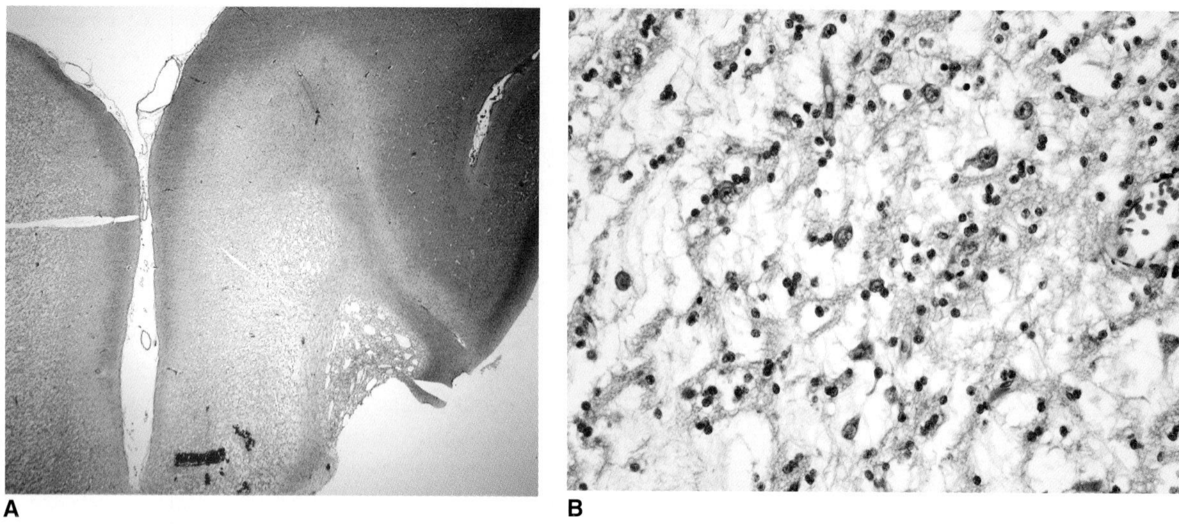

FIGURE 10-34 ■ Dysembryoplastic neuroepithelial tumor (DNT). **A:** Low-power microscopy reveals a cortically based neoplasm. **B:** High-power microscopy demonstrates "floating neurons" and "oligodendroglial-like cells."

a hamartomatous mass. These epileptogenic lesions are cortically based, with a marked predilection for the temporal lobe. Imaging may reveal calcifications, cyst formation, and enhancement. The histologic hallmark of classic DNT is the specific glioneuronal element, which is composed of columns of bundled axons/capillaries (arranged perpendicular to the cortical surface) that are lined by oligodendroglial-like cells (OLCs). The exact histogenesis of OLCs is debated; they stain for S-100 and are negative for both GFAP and neuronal markers, suggesting a nondescript neuroepithelial origin. The columns of the specific glioneuronal element are separated by pale basophilic mucin, within which are nondysmorphic floating neurons (Figure 10-34 A, B). Stellate astrocytes may be seen among the specific glioneuronal element. Complex and simple forms of DNT are the most commonly recognized. Complex DNTs contain patterned glial nodules (mucin ±) and a multinodular architecture associated with the specific glioneuronal element and/or foci of cortical dysplasia. The glial component, although typically nodular, may resemble conventional diffuse glioma or low-grade glioma. In addition, this glial component may exhibit rare mitoses, nuclear atypia, necrosis, and even MVP, but these features are not common. Areas of cortical dysplasia, characterized mainly by disorganized and dyslaminated cortex, may lie adjacent to DNTs. Even more controversial is the proposed nonspecific variant of DNT; this variant is not widely accepted (19). Chief in differential diagnosis of DNT is oligodendroglioma; features used to differentiate these tumors are described by Burger et al. (10). DNTs have a favorable prognosis, even after subtotal resection. Genetic studies of DNT are rare, but unlike oligodendrogliomas, they lack 1p and 19q codeletions (31,76,82).

Other Neuronal/Glioneuronal Tumors

Desmoplastic infantile ganglioglioma (DIG), WHO grade I, is a distinctive tumor usually occurring in the 1st year of life. These large superficial lesions often have dural attachment, cyst formation, and contrast enhancement. Macrocephaly and increased ICP herald its presence. Histologically, reticulin-rich desmoplastic areas contain spindled cells with a fascicular or storiform arrangement; these areas often obscure the astrocytic component that often requires GFAP IHC to fully appreciate. The latter resemble slender fibrillary astrocytes embedded within the densely desmoplastic stroma; scattered small gemistocytes may be seen. The neuronal component is often equally subtle since they are often considerably smaller than the neurons of conventional GG. Less common are more classic ganglioglioma-like foci complete with EGBs. As with the glial element, IHC or EM may be needed to detect this neuronal component. If neuronal elements are still lacking after special studies, the term "dyplastic infantile astrocytomas" (DIA) is appropriate. However, both DIA and DIG are now thought to represent opposite ends of a single entity (i.e., dysplastic infantile tumors). Worrisome and mitotically active primitive neuroectodermal tumor (PNET)-like foci bearing MVP and necrosis may be seen but fortunately do not impact prognosis since these patients have favorable outcomes after surgery.

Dysplastic gangliocytoma of the cerebellum (Lhermitte Duclos disease) (DGCC), WHO grade I, is a unique cerebellar neoplasm often associated with Cowden syndrome. Predictably, these patients present with signs and symptoms of cerebellar dysfunction and CSF obstruction. These solid tumors are characteristically striped on T2-weighted MRI due to in part to thickened folia. Microscopically, a distinctive abnormal architecture is seen and has been likened to cortex "flipped inside-out." More normal cerebellar cortex is progressively replaced by two layers. The outer layer consists of parallel arrays of myelinated axons, whereas the inner layer is composed of abnormal smaller and larger neurons (ganglioid and ganglion-like, respectively), which replace the internal granule cells. These ganglion cells may resemble Purkinje cells but are far too numerous, disordered, and pleomorphic. Abnormal vascular proliferation may be noted in the subarachnoid space and white matter (which may be vacuolated). Since patients with Cowden syndrome bear germline mutations in the PTEN tumor suppressor gene on chromosome 10q23, genetic studies (including sporadic cases) have investigated the PTEN/Akt/mTOR pathway. IHC and mutational analysis have confirmed frequent PTEN mutations (15/18, 83%) and secondary activation of mTOR (1,120). A workup for other features of Cowden syndrome may also be warranted since such patients are at risk for numerous systemic manifestations, including breast and gastrointestinal (GI) carcinomas.

Choroid Plexus Tumors

Choroid plexus tumors (CPTs) are intraventricular papillary epithelial tumors that are derived from the choroid plexus. These are intensely enhancing lesions that often present with increased ICP and HCP. Although CPTs may affect any site where native choroid plexus resides, the lateral ventricle is the most frequent location in children.

CPP, WHO grade I, closely resembles normal choroid plexus in that papillae contain a fibrovascular core, a simple to cuboidal epithelium with minimal to mild atypia, and little mitotic activity. However, this neoplastic epithelium differs from normal choroid plexus in being more cell dense and lacking the normal surface hobnailing (i.e., bumpy) architecture (Figure 10-35A). Mesenchymal type metaplasia, pigmented epithelium, and focal ependymal differentiation may all be seen rarely, the latter manifesting GFAP immunoreactivity.

Choroid plexus carcinoma (CPC), WHO grade III, usually presents before 3 years of age. Papillary architecture is variably replaced by areas of solid tumor growth (Figure 10-35B). Epithelium is clearly anaplastic in most examples, although transitions with better-differentiated areas are occasionally seen and may suggest a role for progressive malignant transformation in some. Pseudostratified epithelium is markedly cell dense and tumor cells exhibit a high nuclear-to-cytoplasmic ratio. Nuclei are hyperchromatic and mitotic activity is generally prominent (>5 per 10 HPF). Foci of necrosis are characteristic, and MVP may be seen. CPCs often invade adjacent brain parenchyma.

Atypical CPP is considered an intermediate WHO grade II tumor. Atypical CPP has recently been defined by a minimum of two mitoses per 10 HPF, while often containing at least two of the following as well: hypercellularity, pleomorphism, foci of solid growth, and necrosis (47).

In general, CPT immunohistochemistry reveals positivity for cytokeratins and S-100 protein, with the latter often being more limited in CPCs. Unlike most carcinomas, EMA is usually negative and focal GFAP expression is relatively common. Transthyretin and synaptophysin staining have been touted as markers of CPTs, but these are generally unreliable due to poor specificities. The genetics of CPTs are reviewed by Kamaly-Asl et al. (50). TP53 mutations may be frequent in CPC (especially those related to Li-Fraumeni syndrome) but are rare in CPP. Kamaly et al. further suggest that rare cases of CPC with INI1 mutation are truly ATRTs, an important differential diagnostic consideration, since this tumor afflicts the same age group, can be intraventricular, and may show papillary features. CPPs are often cured with surgery (5-year survival 100%), while CPCs often grow rapidly and have an unfavorable prognosis (5-year survival 40%) (63).

Miscellaneous CNS Tumors

A variety of less common tumors arise in the CNS of pediatric patients. As opposed to adult patients, Meningeal-based tumors, in particular meningioma, are uncommon (75). Pituitary adenoma is also much more common in adults. Nerve sheath tumors (including schwannoma and neurofibroma) are covered in the soft tissue chapter (Chapter 24), whereas bony skull–based tumors (including chordoma, Langerhans cell histiocytosis) are covered in the chapter on the skeletal system (Chapter 27). Primary melanocytic lesions (melanomas,

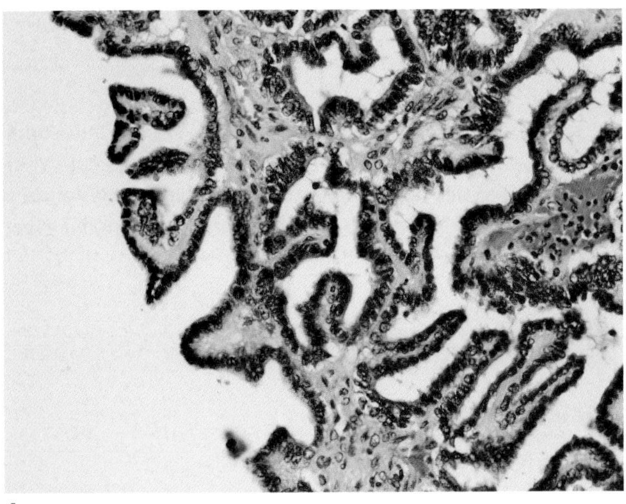

A

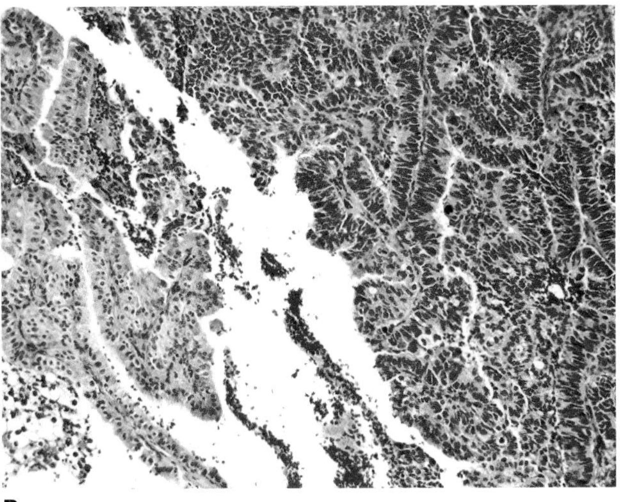

B

FIGURE 10-35■ Choroid plexus tumors (CPTs). **A:** Choroid plexus papilloma (CPP). **B:** CPC; note the better differentiated area left versus the more poorly differentiated tumor right.

Table 10-10 ■ CANCER PREDISPOSITION (NEUROCUTANEOUS) SYNDROMES

Syndrome	Gene (Locus)	Nervous System Pathology	Extraneural Manifestations
Neurofibromatosis type 1	NF1 (17q11)	Neurofibromas (diffuse, nodular, plexiform); MPNSTs; optic/ hypothalamic gliomas; diffuse astrocytomas; "UBOs"	Skin (café au lait spots, axillary freckling); Lisch nodules; pheochromocytoma; carcinoid tumors; rhabdomyosarcoma; CML; bone lesions
Neurofibromatosis type 2	NF2 (22q12)	Bilateral vestibular schwannomas; schwannosis; multiple meningiomas; MA; spinal cord ependymomas; glial microhamartoma	Minimal skin stigmata (rare plexiform schwannomas); cataracts.
Ataxia telangectasia (AT)	ATM (11q22–23)	Cerebellar degeneration; intracranial hemorrhage; cytomegaly and nuclear atypia (CNS and extra-CNS tissues)	Mucocutaneous and conjunctival telangectasias; immunodeficiency and related respiratory infections; tumor predilection and radiation sensitivity
Neurocutaneous melanosis syndrome	sporadic	Diffuse melanocytosis, melanocytoma, or primary malignant melanoma of the leptomeninges	Cutaneous nevi (giant and or multiple, including the congenital nevus of Ota)
Nevoid basal cell carcinoma (Gorlin) syndrome	PTCH (9q22.3)	Desmoplastic medulloblastomas; meningioma; CNS malformations (agenesis of the corpus callosum, cerebral falcine calcifications; HCP)	Odontogenic keratocysts; palmar/ plantar dyskeratoses; skeletal malformations; ovarian fibromas; melanoma; leukemia/lymphoma; breast/lung carcinoma
Von Hippel-Lindau (VHL)	VHL (3p25–26)	Hemangioblastomas (cerebellum, retina); papillary endolymphatic sac tumor (PELST)	Renal cell carcinoma; pheochromocytoma; pancreatic tumors; polycythemia
Cowden	PTEN/MMA C1 (10q23)	DGCC (Lhermitte Duclos disease)	Verrucous skin; cobblestone oral papules; trichilemmomas; colonic polyps; thyroid nodules; breast carcinoma
Li-Fraumeni	TP53 (17p13.3)	Gliomas (astrocytoma, ependymoma; ± multicentric); cerebral PNETs; CPTs; meningioma; schwannoma	Bone and soft-tissue sarcomas; leukemia; adrenocortical/breast carcinoma; visceral epithelial malignancies
Turcot	Type 1: hMLH1 (3p21); hMSH2 (2p22–21); hPMS2 (7p22) Type 2: APC (5q21)	Type 1: GBM (younger onset versus sporadic) Type 2: medulloblastoma	Type 1: ± hereditary nonpolyposis colorectal carcinoma Type 2: familial adenomatous polyposis
Familial retinoblastoma	RB (13q14)	Retinoblastoma; pineoblastoma	Osteosarcoma

MPNST, malignant peripheral nerve sheath tumor; UBOs, unidentified bright object on T2-weighted or FLAIR MR images; MA, Meningioangiomatosis.

melanocytoma) are rare and thought to be derived from leptomeningeal melanocytes, hence their typical extra-axial location. Vascular tumors are similarly rare, with hemangioblastomas being common only in adults. Their presence in children strongly raises the possibility of von Hippel-Lindau (VHL) disease.

Cancer Predispostion (Neurocutaneous) Syndromes

These syndromes are summarized in Table 10-10. Patients with one of these syndromes may incur both neoplastic and nonneoplastic forms of pathology and hence are often multisystemic in nature. Onset of these syndromes is often during the pediatric years. While many of these syndromes are inherited in an AD pattern, some (e.g., AT) are autosomal recessive in nature, while others (e.g., neurocutaneous melanosis syndrome) appear sporadically. The specific clinical diagnostic criteria for each of these syndromes are not given here; for such, the reader is directed to other texts (81).

INFECTIOUS DISEASE

Bacterial Infections

Acute Meningitis

Neonatal acute bacterial meningitis is most frequently due to group B streptococcus (*Streptococcus agalactiae*) and *Escherichia coli*. Several other Gram-positive

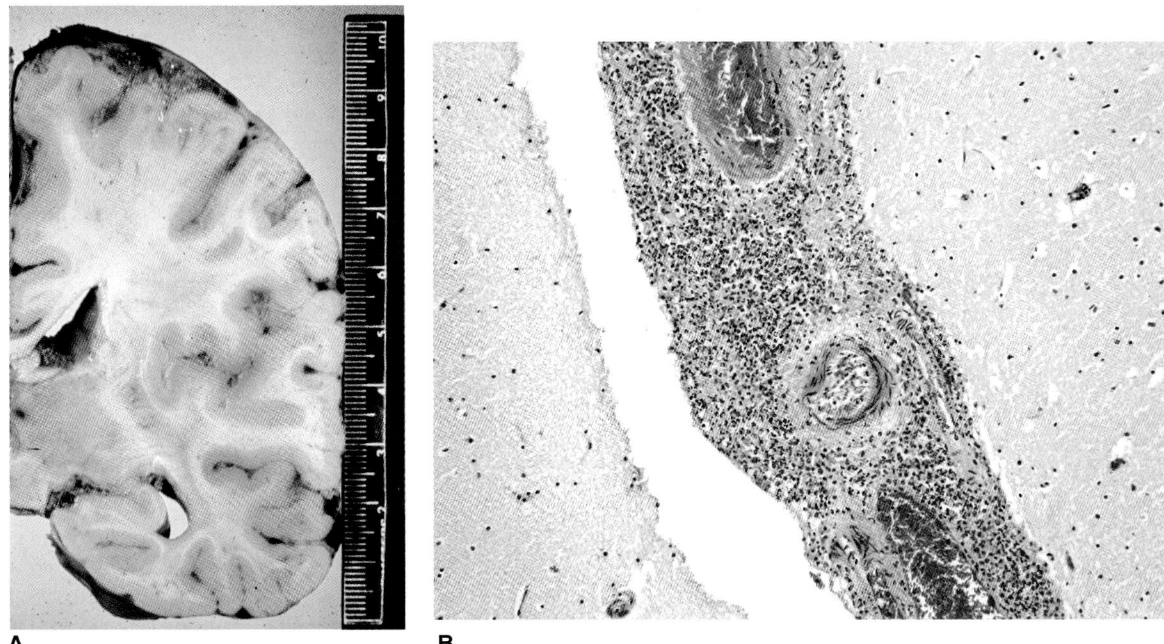

FIGURE 10-36 ▪ Acute bacterial meningitis. **A:** Coronal section of the cerebrum reveals abundant purulent material within the leptomeninges. **B:** Microscopy highlights a neutrophil-rich leptomeningeal infiltrate.

(*Listeria monocytogenes* and *Staphylococcus aureus*) and Gram-negative (*Citrobacter*, *Klebsiella*, *Enterobacter*, *Proteus*, and *Salmonella* species, as well as *Pseudomonas aeruginosa*) bacteria may also be causative. Infants and young children are affected primarily by *S. pneumoniae*, *Neiserria meningitides*, and *Haemophilus influenzae* type b (Hib), while children older than five (like adults) are infected most frequently with the former two pathogens. Notably, immunization with the Haemophilus, pneumococcal, and meningococcal conjugate vaccines has significantly reduced the incidence of previously devastating infections (14).

Bacteria reach the CNS via hematogenous spread, often from an upper respiratory focus, or direct spread from a contiguous site of disease (i.e., mastoids, inner ear, nasal sinus, mouth). Neonates often acquire organisms via passage through an infected birth canal. Once arriving at the CNS, breech of the blood-brain barrier is facilitated by bacterial surface proteins. Although host immune defenses and antimicrobial therapy may effectively neutralize the pathogen at hand, bacterial products can persist in stimulating the inflammatory response (14).

Focal neurologic deficits, changes in mental status, fever, rash, seizures, and signs of meningeal irritation herald the presence of acute meningitis. Nonspecific changes such as irritability, lethargy, poor feeding, apneic spells, and a bulging fontanelle may be seen in infants. CSF examination is key to the diagnosis, and findings include granulocytic pleocytosis, elevated protein, decreased CSF to serum glucose ratio, and identification of organisms on Gram stain. Definitive diagnosis is made with culture, organism specific PCR, and latex agglutination tests.

Gross examination of the brain reveals diffuse edema and possibly cerebral herniation. Surface vasculature is congested. A light-colored thick leptomeningeal exudate may be seen grossly but may be less prominent in partially treated cases. Focal areas of parenchymal softening are suggestive of infarction (Figure 10-36A). Microscopic sections reveal a neutrophil-predominant exudate (lymphocytes and macrophages are seen in later stages.) that often extends down the Virchow-Robin spaces (Figure 10-36B). This inflammation can result in a vasculitis with secondary thrombosis (and hence infarction). Inflammation may also be seen in the choroid plexus and along the ventricular lining. Organisms are highlighted with the Gram stain. Complications among survivors predictably follow the areas of pathologic damage. Cortical infarcts lead to focal neurologic deficits (e.g., spasticity, dysphasia) and seizures and, when widespread, may result in mental retardation (or when less pronounced, learning disabilities and behavioral disturbances). Resolution of leptomeningeal inflammation with concomitant fibrosis overlying cranial nerves may result in cranial nerve palsies (e.g., hearing loss). Scarring (i.e., gliosis and fibrosis) of the ependyma and leptomeninges can obstruct the flow of CSF causing HCP (see Chapter 6).

Cerebral Abscess

Bacteria, which cause abscesses, like those causing meningitis, also arrive at the CNS via hematogenous or direct contiguous spread. Children with congenital heart disease are particularly predisposed to hematogenous dissemination of bacteria, resulting in abscesses within brain regions receiving a high blood flow (e.g., middle cerebral artery territory). Dental infections (i.e., abscesses), mastoiditis, paranasal sinusitis, or otitis media may traverse local anatomic boundaries and lead to abscess formation in adjacent brain parenchyma.

The spectrum of microorganisms causing abscesses has changed with time (91). While the incidence of *S. aureus* has been decreasing, the identification of anaerobes has increased. *Streptococcus milleri* and *S. viridans* are frequently associated with direct brain inoculation and hematogenous spread, respectively, and as a group, aerobic and anaerobic forms of streptococcus cause 60% to 70% of cerebral abscesses (26). Other causative aerobic and microaerophilic bacteria may include *Haemophilus*, Gram-negative enteric bacilli, and *Pseudomonas aeruginosa*. Common anaerobes include Bacteroides, Peptostreptococcus, Fusobacterium, Propionbacterium, Prevotella, and Actinomyces. Penetrating head injuries, neurosurgical procedures, and immunocompromised states all predispose to abscess formation, with the latter invoking less common bacterial (e.g., *Nocardia*, *Listeria*, *Mycobacterial* species), fungal (e.g., *Candida*, *Aspergillus*, *Cryptococcus*, *Histoplasma*, *Coccidioides*, and *Mucor*), and parasitic (e.g., *Toxoplasmosis*) pathogens. MR imaging reveals a mass with a thin smooth rim of enhancement. The resulting gross and microscopic appearance of cerebral abscesses evolves through stages. Early stages (<4 days) begin with a cerebritis that grossly appears as an ill-defined area of hyperemia and edema; microscopically endothelial swelling is accompanied by perivascular and parenchymal neutrophils. After 4 days, areas of confluent necrosis emerge, as both macrophage and mononuclear infiltrates become more conspicuous. An early granulation tissue reaction at the margin of necrosis heralds the initiation of capsule formation at approximately 10 days; chronic inflammatory cells are noted within the capsule, which is in turn surrounded by edema and reactive astrocytosis in the adjacent brain. A well-formed reticulin-rich capsule is noted at 2 weeks, at which time the classic multilayered abscess wall is best appreciated. Organisms (most highlighted with the Gram stain) are seen at all stages of evolution, particularly at the capsule-necrosis boundary.

Subdural empyema and epidural abscesses are uncommon and not discussed further here.

Chronic Bacterial Infections

Mycobacteria uncommonly cause infection in North American children. Most cases are seen in the immunocompromised (in particular, AIDS patients) and importantly in the developing world. *Mycobacterium tuberculosis* (TB) causes meningitis (the most common form of disease), tuberculous masses (i.e., tuberculomas), and spinal epidural abscesses. Initial infection results from inhalation of bacteria-laden droplets; subsequent CNS spread is related to hematogenous dissemination. Reactivation of a focus of latent CNS infection (i.e., a "tubercle" or "Rich focus") is also a source of active disease. Symptoms in children are subacute (occur over 2 to 3 weeks) and may include fever, meningismus, signs of increased ICP (headache, nausea, and vomiting), seizures, cranial nerve palsies, and epilepsy, with changes in mental status seen later on. Examination may reveal a sixth cranial nerve palsy. Diagnosis may be made on CSF specimens via culture (often slow growing) and PCR, or via direct visualization using Ziehl-Nielsen or auramine rhodamine fluorescence staining (see below).

Gross pathologic findings include a gelatinous and, at times, nodular leptomeningeal exudate that is often most prominent along the Sylvian fissure and base of the brain. The choroid plexus and ventricular lining may be similarly affected, and result in HCP. Areas of parenchymal softening are suggestive of superimposed infarcts related to endarteritis obliterans with vascular thrombosis. Necrotizing granulomas are typical. Chronic type inflammatory cells, variable fibrosis, and multinucleated (Langhans type) giant cells may be accompanied, albeit rarely in most cases, by acid-fast bacilli on Ziehl-Nelsen staining (i.e., "red snappers"). Inflammation may spill over into the adjacent brain, causing microglial activation and gliosis. Tubercles are the nodular macroscopic confluence of these granulomas, while the histologically similar tuberculomas are grossly "mass forming."

Other bacteria causing chronic CNS disease are uncommon but include Lyme disease (*Borrelia burgdorferi*) and syphilis (*Treponema pallidum*).

Viral Infections

Viral meningitis is defined as a febrile illness associated with clinical signs of meningeal irritation but lacking neurologic dysfunction and positive cultures. These often banal cases occur with seasonal and geographic variations; rarely do they come to the attention of the pathologist. The most common causative entities include the enteroviruses (echoviruses, Coxsackie A and B, and enterovirus *per se*) and HSV-2 (i.e., Mollaret meningitis). Histology reveals, at best, a scanty lymphocytic predominant perivascular and leptomeningeal infiltrate, which may affect the choroid plexus and creep into the superficial aspects of the brain parenchyma.

Viral encephalitis also causes fever but is additionally characterized by brain parenchymal dysfunction manifesting as an altered state of consciousness and/or objective signs of neurologic dysfunction (i.e., seizures, focal neurologic deficits); the equivalent pathologic process occurring in the spinal cord is called myelitis. Mixed forms (i.e., meningoencephalitis or encephalomyelitis) also occur. Each of these main pathologic processes can result in either acute or chronic disease depending on the particular type of viral pathogen involved. The clinical severity of disease induced by these viruses ranges from minimal to fatal. Antivirals exist for some pathogens (e.g., HSV and acyclovir), but care is limited to supportive therapy for others. Diagnoses are made by serology, culture (in the past from CNS biopsy specimens), and more recently via PCR-based assays (especially of CSF), which uncover specific viral nucleic acids.

Herpes simplex virus (HSV) is one of the most common members of the Herpesviridae family, a group of generally necrotizing double-stranded DNA viruses that also include varicella-zoster (VZV), cytomegalovirus (CMV), and Epstein-Barr virus (EBV). Viral DNA is enclosed in a nucleocapsid and surrounded by a viral envelope. Neonatal disease is most often caused by the HSV type 2, while the less frequent childhood form of infection is caused by HSV type 1. Neonatal disease is usually acquired in the perinatal period from an infected mother bearing recurrent but often asymptomatic genital disease (55). Neonates present within the first 4 weeks of life with one of three main forms of disease: (a) localized skin, eyes, or mouth (SEM) disease including vesicles and/or keratoconjunctivitis; (b) encephalitis ± SEM; or (3) diffuse or disseminated HSV with SEM, encephalitis, and multiple visceral organ disease. These affected infants may be lethargic, irritable, feed poorly, and suffer from seizures. Pathology reveals a diffusely swollen and congested brain. Hemorrhagic and necrotic lesions of the gray and white matter are accompanied by macrophages and lymphocytes. Intranuclear viral inclusions may be seen within neurons, glia, and/or endothelia. Survivors are left with a parenchymal loss and gliosis (i.e., cystic encephalomalacia).

Childhood disease is much less common and presents in a similar fashion to that in adults. Primary HSV infection is often asymptomatic, although some may develop oropharyngeal ulcers. Once the virus is absorbed, it replicates and subsequently travels in a retrograde fashion along sensory axons (e.g., olfactory or trigeminal) toward the respective ganglion where a latent infection ensues. Reactivation of viral disease is accompanied by replication and anterograde travel down sensory axons toward the periphery whereupon mucocutaneous vesicles erupt. HSV encephalitis is thought to arise either with primary infection or after reactivation of latent trigeminal ganglia disease. Common clinical presenting features include fever, headache, altered mental status, and seizures. The classic distribution of disease (see below) may be seen via imaging, and definitive diagnosis using PCR to find viral DNA in the CSF has largely supplanted brain biopsy. Swelling, congestion, hemorrhage, and necrosis are typically localized initially (often asymmetrically) to the posterior orbitofrontal, temporal lobes, cingulate gyrus, and insulae (Figure 10-37A). Acutely necrotic (i.e., "red") neurons are accompanied by parenchymal/perivascular lymphocytes and macrophages, plus the nonspecific but characteristic viral encephalitic features of perivascular lymphocytes, microglial activation, microglial nodule formation, and neuronophagia. Neuronal, glial, and/or endothelial intranuclear viral inclusions (Figure 10-37B) may be difficult to appreciate in some cases, wherein IHC staining for HSV can be very helpful. Endothelial and hence vascular involvement may result in thrombosis and infarction. A necrotizing myelopathy may be seen but is rare. In survivors, the extensive residual damage usually manifests in the form of cystic encephalomalacia.

CMV is the most common intrauterine viral infection. Congenital CMV is usually acquired transplacentally from a newly infected mother, and while acquisition is most successful in third trimester gestations, first trimester infections lead to the most severe (often systemic and fatal) disease. Survivors are left with sequelae that include hearing loss, language disorders, microcephaly (the most common neurologic presentation), mental retardation, seizures, chorioretinitis, and motor deficits. Imaging reveals micrencephaly, cerebral microcalcifications (often periventricular), HCP, and gyral abnormalities. Diagnosis of fetal infection can be made via viral culture or PCR of amniotic fluid, or by fetal IgM serology. Gross pathology confirms the imaging impressions, and

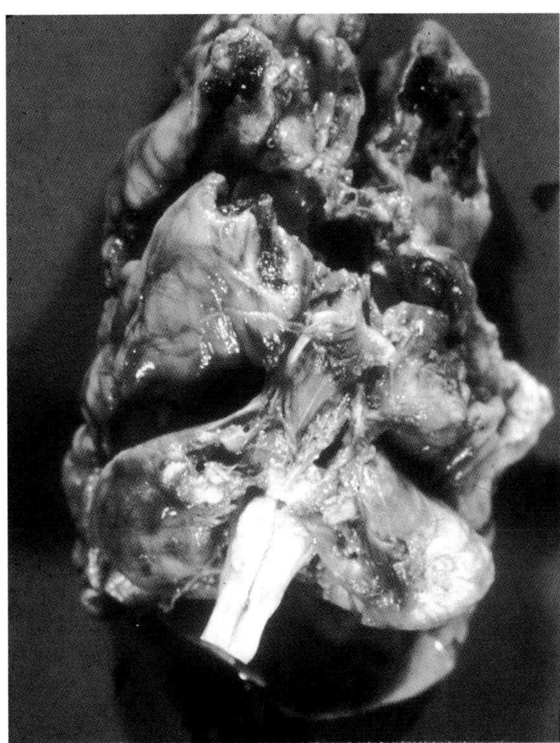

A

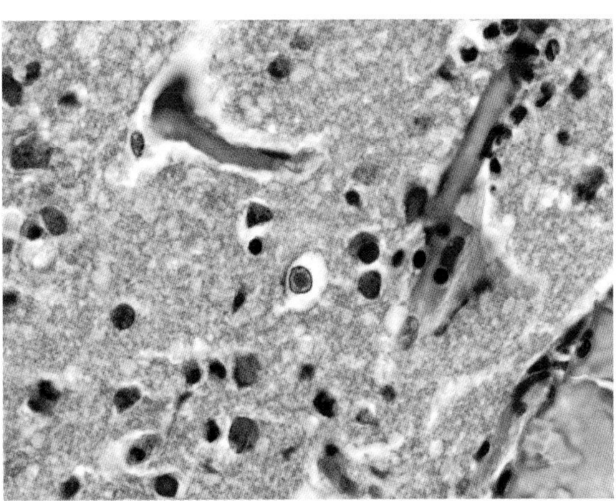

B

FIGURE 10-37 ▪ Herpes simplex encephalitis. **A:** Ventral view of the brain demonstrating marked hemorrhagic necrosis in a congenital case caused by HSV 2 (image courtesy of Dr. Barry Rewcastle). **B:** High-power histology showing an eosinophilic intranuclear inclusion, likely within a glial cell.

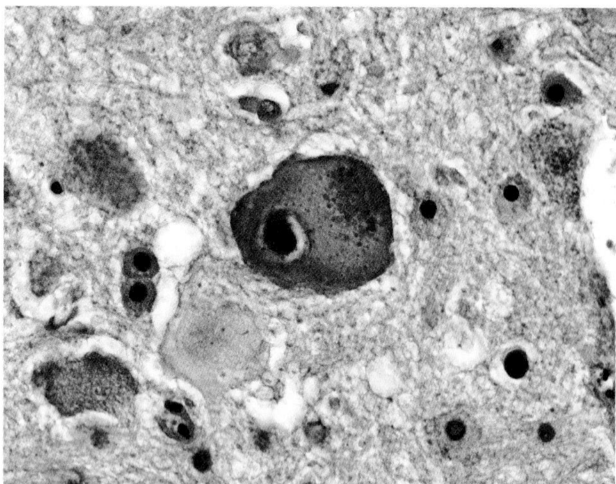

FIGURE 10-38 ■ CMV encephalitis. Cytomegalic cell containing a large intranuclear inclusion.

may reveal porencephaly and polymicrogyria. Microscopy reveals a necrotizing ventriculoencephalits, with areas of calcification and gliosis. Perivascular lymphocytes are accompanied by macrophages and activated microglia (± nodules). Cytomegalic cells bear a single haloed intranuclear inclusion whose abundant cytoplasm also contains multiple small inclusions (Figure 10-38); immunohistochemistry often highlights more widespread involvement than is appreciated by routine stains. Subependymal gliosis may result in HCP. CMV infections are less common in older children and are largely restricted to immunosuppressed patients (e.g., those with HIV) with systemic disease, which may be related to reactivation of latent bone marrow virus. Symptoms may include changes in mental status, nystagmus, and cranial nerve palsies, all of which are often indicative of a poor prognosis. Pathologically, several forms of disease may be seen including encephalitis of varying severity, ventriculitis, and lumbosacral myeloradiculitis (see Chapter 6).

Primary infection with VZV results in chicken pox (varicella), whereas reactivation of latent sensory ganglia disease causes shingles (zoster). Either form of VZV may result in CNS disease, which is typically necrotizing and accompanied by intranuclear inclusions. Varicella may cause an embryopathy, transient cerebellitis, meningoencephalitis (that can resemble Acute Disseminated Encephalomyelitis (ADEM), and has been associated with Reye syndrome (an encephalopathic illness that has been correlated with salicylate ingestion). Zoster has been associated with encephalitis, myeloradiculitis, and a vasculopathy/vasculitis. Varicella embryopathy is acquired transplacentally and results in the most severe disease when acquired in the first half of gestation. Cutaneous scarring, limb hypoplasia, chorioretinitis, cataracts, and mental retardation are seen. Pathologically, scarring and gliosis are seen within the meninges and parenchyma, respectively, with the latter showing evidence of degeneration but rarely an active necrotizing infection with demonstrable virus. A chronic inflammatory infiltrate is accompanied by microglial activation. There may be neuronal loss and degeneration within the dorsal root ganglia, anterior horns, and posterior/lateral funiculi, along with denervation muscular atrophy. Vasculitis (± granulomatous) with infarction is seen in AIDS patients. The recent development of a live attenuated vaccine will likely decrease the future incidence of VZV-related CNS disease.

The *arboviruses* are a group of mostly single-stranded RNA viruses that are usually transmitted to humans via mosquitos. Infections are seasonally distributed and generally occur in the summer and fall. While West Nile virus has garnered much of recent spotlight, it only rarely results in symptomatic CNS disease in pediatric patients. More common in children, yet still rare, are Western and Eastern equine encephalitides and La Crosse encephalitis (88). Incubation periods are less than 3 weeks and presenting symptoms include fever, malaise, and myalgias. Neurologic disease is diverse and includes aseptic meningitis, increased ICP, altered level of consciousness (which can lead to coma), motor deficits, and seizures. Diagnosis is made via serology or via PCR-specific RNA assay of the CSF. Gross pathology may reveal swelling, congestion, hemorrhage, and, if severe, necrosis. Some arboviruses tend to affect certain areas of the brain and spinal cord (26), but despite these predilections, the microscopic features are nonspecific. Chronic leptomeningeal inflammation is accompanied by the typical features of encephalitis (microglial activation, microglial nodules, perivascular lymphocytes) and occasionally perivascular hemorrhage/myelin destruction. Vessels may be thrombosed, but only rare and severe cases demonstrate significant necrosis. Notably, although viral inclusions are absent on routine staining, IHC staining (available for some arboviruses) can help to highlight neuronal and glial infection.

Although more commonly associated with meningitis, the enteroviruses (see above) may all rarely cause a poliomyelitis. These small single-stranded RNA viruses (including the formerly more common Poliovirus) cause a lytic infection of motor neurons in the anterior horn of the spinal cord and in the brainstem. Initial infection is via the fecal-oral route, and after hematogenous dissemination, the virus enters the CNS. Roughly 10 days after the resolution of a nonspecific flu-like illness, a prodrome of fever, headache, vomiting, meningismus, irritability, and myalgia ensues. Paralytic encephalomyelitis follows this prodrome and is often asymmetric and lower extremity predominant. Gross pathologic findings are uncommon, but severe cases include congestion, hemorrhage, and necrosis of motor nuclei within the brainstem and spinal cord anterior gray matter. Microscopically, affected areas are intensely inflamed. Parenchyma and leptomeninges first contain neutrophils and later lymphocytes plus activated microglia (with microglial nodules and neuronophagia). Chronic forms of disease manifest as areas of neuronal loss, gliosis, and scanty inflammatory infiltrates.

The *measles virus* is a single-stranded RNA pathogen from the paramyxoviridae family. Measles is highly contagious virus that is acquired through inhalation. Primary infection is systemic and results in fever, a maculopapular rash, and rarely CNS disease, which can include aseptic meningitis or ADEM. Measles mediates two less common chronic CNS diseases that are now rare since the institution of the MMR vaccine: measles inclusion body encephalitis (MIBE) (which occurs in the immunocompromised a few months after primary infection) and the more acclaimed subacute sclerosing panencephalitis (SSPE). SSPE results in CNS disease approximately 5 to 10 years after primary infection, with some occurring after vaccination (which normally reduces the risk of disease dramatically). In SSPE, the viral genome is mutated such that the virus is unable to assemble or bud from infected cells. Clinical disease progresses through the early stages of cognitive and behavioral dysfunction; through motor deficits, seizures, and ataxia; and finally autonomic dysfunction, altered mental status, and finally death. Median survival is less than 2 years. Diagnosis can be made via antibody titers or PCR of fresh frozen brain. Pathologically, the gross brain may show signs of atrophy and leukodystrophy-like changes. A meningoencephalitis is seen microscopically, with lymphocytic infiltrates (including perivascular) and parenchymal microglial activation. The neocortex, deep cerebral gray, and white matter regions are especially involved. There may be neuronal loss, and Alzheimer-like neurofibrillary tangles may be identified in residual neurons. Extensive white matter gliosis (i.e., "sclerosing") may be accompanied by demyelinated patches. Intranuclear eosinophilic and haloed viral inclusions may be seen in neurons and oligodendroglia, but these are often sparse, necessitating immunohistochemistry for their detection.

Human immunodeficiency virus (HIV) is a single-stranded RNA retrovirus that causes AIDS. HIV infection is acquired by numerous routes, including sexual, hematologic, iatrogenic (e.g., contaminated instruments), and perinatal. This latter mode of infection is the most common in children. Primary infection may result in aseptic meningitis, after which a reservoir of virus is established in CD4-positive T-cells, macrophages, and microglia. With viral-mediated destruction, CD4-positive T-cells plummet to numbers less than 200/μL; thereafter, the systemic and CNS features of AIDS ensue. CNS disease related to AIDS includes (a) direct HIV infection, (b) opportunistic infections, (c) nonspecific CNS damage (related to ischemia, metabolic insults, etc.), and (d) treatment-related disease (e.g., AZT myopathy). Although pathologic reports are early, highly active antiretroviral therapy (HAART) appears to have significantly impacted the patterns (i.e., incidence, prevalence) of AIDS-related disease in developed nations, especially in terms of reducing opportunistic infections (41). However, these opportunistic infections are much less common in children as compared to adults regardless. Moreover, socioeconomic barriers have impeded the implementation of HAART therapy in many developing nations. HIV encephalitis/encephalopathy (HIVE) and vacuolar myelopathy are disorders that are thought to be directly related to CNS HIV infection. Almost 40% of HIV-positive children develop HIVE, which is the most frequent HIV-specific disease and tends to occur in the later stages of immune suppression (6). Clinically, HIVE is characterized by developmental delay, apathy, seizures, and spastic quadriparesis (39). Grossly, HIVE brains may be atrophic. Microscopically, the multinucleated giant cell is characteristic; it is thought to be of phagocytic lineage, expresses HIV antigens, and harbors virus (97). Loosely aggregated microglia and glial cells (similar to microglial nodules) and perivascular (at times vasculitic) inflammatory infiltrates may be seen and predominate in the deep cerebral white, basal ganglia, and brainstem. Leukoencephalopathic features can be present and include white matter myelin pallor and gliosis; there also may be degeneration of the corticospinal tracts. Somewhat characteristic of pediatric AIDS brains are the angiocentric calcifications seen within basal ganglia and frontal white matter.

Fungal Infections

Fungal infections are largely restricted to those pediatric patients who are immunocompromised. Typically, these pathogens gain access to the CNS through hematogenous dissemination, often via lung infection. CNS invasion may be accompanied by only a sparse inflammatory reaction, which in part may be related to the patient's immunosuppression. The clinico-pathologic features of the most commonly encountered fungal pathogens are summarized in Table 10-11. Other CNS fungal infections include Mucormycosis, Coccidiomycosis, Blastomycosis, Histoplasmosis, and Chromoblastomycosis.

Parasitic Infections

Parasitic infections of the pediatric CNS are uncommon. Two of the most common, toxoplasmosis and neurocysticercosis (NEC) are briefly described below. Other parasitic infections include cerebral malaria, amoebic infections (e.g., *Entamoeba histolytica*, *Nagleria fowleri*, *Acanthamoeba* species), neuroschistosomiasis, trypanosomiasis, and helminthic infections (e.g., *Ecchinococcus granulosis*).

Toxoplasmosis is caused by *Toxoplasma gondii*, an obligate intracellular protozoan. Cats are the definitive host, and human infection is acquired via inadvertent ingestion of parasitic oocysts passed through feline feces. Primary infection is essentially asymptomatic in the immunocompetent; although the immune system may prevent the development of disease, the parasite is not eradicated, and lies dormant in muscle/brain cysts. Of particular interest is the CNS toxoplasmal disease, which is congenital or occurs in the immunosuppressed. Congenital toxoplasmosis results from transplacental spread of organisms primarily during initial maternal infection and parasitemia. Like CMV, transmission of disease is most efficient during late gestation but more severe earlier on (highest risk for severe disease is 10 to 24 weeks). Following birth, affected infants classically present with Sabin tetrad, which includes seizures, chorioretinitis, cerebral calcifications, and HCP. The pathology of congenital toxoplasmosis differs from the disease seen in

Table 10-11 ■ SUMMARY OF COMMON FUNGAL INFECTIONS

Organism	Fungal Morphology	Source	Clinical Presentation	Pathology
Cryptococcus neoformans	Narrow budding yeast; polysaccharide capsule	Pigeon excreta Inhaled	Subacute to chronic meningitis	Thick gelatinous meninges and soap bubble' deep gray matter lesions. Perivascular yeast accumulation. PAS-positive and mucicarmine-positive
Candida albicans	Pseudohyphae and yeast	Endogenous (e.g., GI, GU, skin, etc.)	Low-grade meningitis	Cerebritis and microabscesses in an ACA/MCA distribution. PAS and Grocott methenamine Silver (GMS)-positive
Aspergillus species (*fumigatus* and *flavus*)	Acutely branching septated hyphae	Soil Inhaled	Hemorrhagic infarction and abscess formation	Hyphal angioinvasion ± granulomatous reaction. PAS-positive and GMS-positive

older immunosuppressed individuals. Parasites proliferate in ependymal and periventricular regions, disseminating widely from there. Ependymal destruction and gliosis result in obstructive HCP. There is leptomeningeal, parenchymal, and perivascular inflammation, in addition to vascular thrombosis with secondary coagulative necrosis with mineralization. Inflammation is chronic, and there is often microglial activation. Encysted bradyzoites are more easily appreciated, whereas extracellular tachyzoites may be difficult to distinguish from karyorrhectic nuclear debris; in these cases, IHC stains and EM help to highlight the parasites (Figure 10-39). Toxoplasmosis disease related to immunosupression is associated with reactivation of a dormant infection. Clinical presentation is variable but can include changes in mental status, features of increased ICP, and focal neurologic deficits. Imaging usually reveals multiple ring enhancing lesions. Pathologically, areas of hemorrhage and necrosis are often centered upon the basal ganglia. Microscopically, foci of coagulative necrosis are surrounded by mononuclear and neutrophilic inflammation plus granulation tissue and gliosis/microgliosis. Inflammation may also be perivascular. These pathologic changes depend in part on the immune status of the host: greater degrees of suppression are associated with less inflammation and scarring. Vascular damage with superimposed thrombosis is often present. Older lesions can become cystic.

NEC is likely the most common parasitic CNS infection worldwide. Humans are the definitive host in the non-CNS form of disease wherein larval forms residing in poorly cooked pork are ingested; thereafter, the larvae mature into the adult tapeworms (*Taenia solium*), which reside in the GI tract. CNS disease occurs when humans become the intermediate host after eating food contaminated with tapeworm eggs (or oocytes). Once ingested, the eggs develop into larvae, which burrow through the GI tract wall and disseminate hematogenously throughout the body (including the CNS

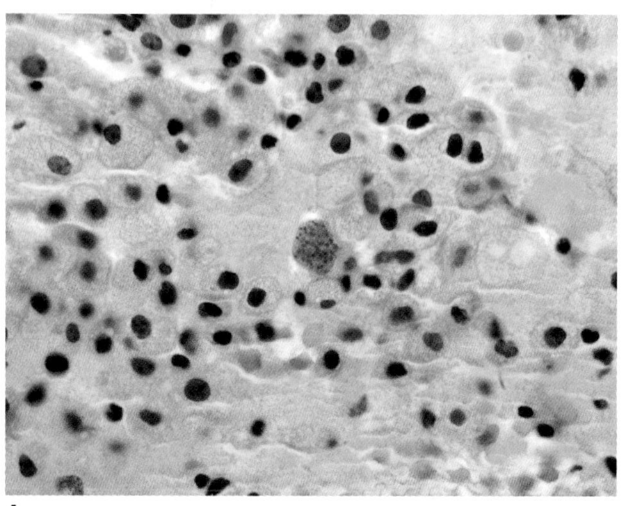

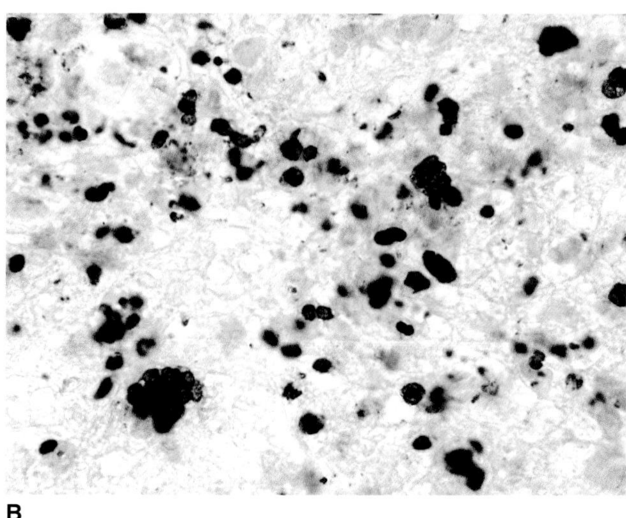

FIGURE 10-39 ■ Toxoplasmosis. **A:** An encysted organism (bradyzoites) is accompanied by foamy macrophages and coagulative necrosis. **B:** Immunohistochemistry against toxoplasmosis helps to highlight free-living tachyzoite forms that mimic karyorrhectic debris on routine staining.

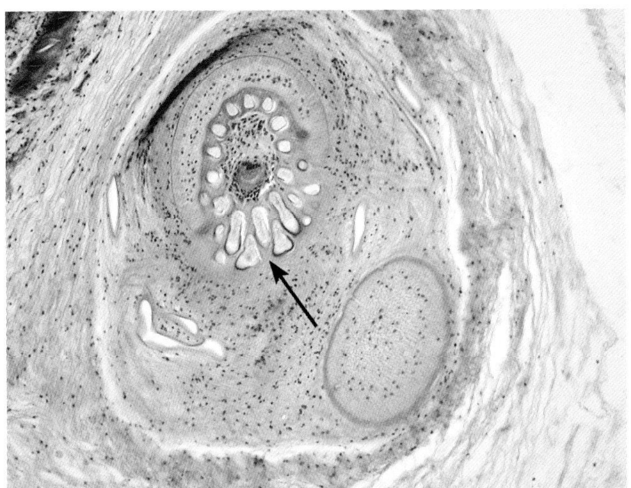

FIGURE 10-40 ■ Neurocysticercosis (NEC). This viable larval form has been favorably sectioned and reveals the characteristic hooklets of the scolex (*arrow*).

and muscle). Numerous larval cysts may develop within the brain and often remain asymptomatic for years. However, if the larvae are in eloquent brain or die, an intense inflammatory reaction may occur and herald the parasites' presence via a myriad of often location-dependent specific neurologic signs and symptoms. Imaging reveals 1 to 2 cm ring enhancing cystic lesions that may bear a calcified scolex. Microscopically, the larval cyst wall contains three layers: outer/cuticular, middle/cellular, and inner/reticular/fibrillary components. Favorable sections of the scolex may reveal parts of the four muscular suckers and or the double row of 22 to 32 hooklets (i.e., teeth) (Figure 10-40). Once the larvae dies and begins to degenerate, a chronic inflammatory response (including multinucleate giant cells, eosinophils, and neutrophils) ensues and a zone of granulation tissue may eventually wall off the deceased larva, which in turn undergoes fibrosis and mineralization.

VASCULAR DISORDERS

Several pediatric CNS disorders are best considered within the vascular category. These include both congenital and acquired disorders, and they may affect all pediatric age groups. In general, these cause an interruption of blood supply (either global or localized), which results in ischemia and/or hemorrhage. The incidence of pediatric CNS vascular disorders varies tremendously; likely the most commonly encountered entities are those affecting premature infants [e.g., HIE and germinal matrix hemorrhage (GMH)]. The gray or white matter may be preferential targets of damage.

Hypoxic-ischemic encephalopathy (HIE) is a common form of injury, especially in premature infants. HIE causes a global insult (e.g., with septic shock or cardiac arrest). The clinical impact may be minimal or may lead to profound neurologic impairment and even death. The areas of the brain that are susceptible to damage are age dependent; premature infants suffer damage primarily in the deep gray matter (i.e., basal ganglia and thalamus), while term infants and older children exhibit hippocampal and neocortical damage preferentially. However, these general patterns are only guidelines and damage can be more widespread in all ages. Regional factors associated with increased vulnerability include (a) high metabolic activity; (b) vascular watershed zones; and (c) specific neurotransmitter receptor distributions (especially glutaminergic). These factors contribute to the general concept of selective vulnerability, which dictates that certain areas of the CNS are preferentially susceptible to certain injurious processes, such as hypoxia and ischemia. Grossly, there may be cerebral swelling, dusky gray matter, and loss of normal gray-white junctions that eventually result in cerebral atrophy.

The microscopic CNS pathologic changes of HIE are age and region dependent. Neocortical damage may occur in a variety of patterns. As with any HIE, the initial phase is one of cerebral swelling and edema that manifests as parenchymal pallor and vacuolation. Acute neuronal death occurs within the first 24 hours. If mature neurons contain ample cytoplasm (i.e., large pyramidal neurons), the latter will become brightly eosinophilic (Figure 10-1A). The neuronal nucleus becomes pyknotic and angulated. However, if cells are small and immature (i.e., little cytoplasm), evidence of HIE will be limited to nuclear fragmentation (i.e., karyorrhexis) (Figure 10-1B). If the nucleus fragments into multiple rounded bodies, cell death may be considered apoptotic rather than necrotic. Microglial activation is a common early occurrence, while foamy macrophages appear after a few days. Vascular changes include early swelling of endothelia, while capillary proliferation occurs after a week. Reactive gliosis is generally not apparent until 1 week after injury. Some have suggested that the premature brain cannot demonstrate gliosis in the first half of gestational development; as such, this would facilitate the rough dating of an *in utero* insult; however, exceptions to this rule clearly exist (101). Mineralization within neurons and macrophages may be seen after 10 to 14 days. Notably, these changes are very similar to those of frank infarction, although the latter typically involves all cell types within a vascular region, rather than individual neurons. For example, vascular watershed zones are particularly susceptible to HIE, resulting in selective neuronal necrosis, but if injury is more severe, complete parenchymal involvement occurs (i.e., watershed infarction). Near-term infants may display a peri-Rolandic or rarely a columnar distribution of cortical damage. The sulcal cortical depths are particularly susceptible to HIE, leading over time to deep sulcal atrophy and superficial sparing; grossly, this pathology is termed ulegyria because of the "mushroom-like" appearance of the affected gyrus.

The hippocampus is somewhat more resistant to the effects of HIE in premature infants, as compared to its more classic involvement in older patients. If involved, however, acute neuronal cell death (i.e., red neurons) is most often seen in Sommer sector (CA1) and the end folium (i.e., CA4), while CA2 (the "dorsal resistant zone") is largely spared. Later stages are characterized by neuronal loss and gliosis (i.e., hippocampal sclerosis). Infants less than 8 to 9 months may display a microglial reaction beneath the dentate gyrus as a marker of HIE. The hippocampal subiculum is more commonly affected in premature infants with HIE; although initially called pontosubicular necrosis (PSN) when seen in association with pontine damage, it has been shown that the neuronal cell death is actually apoptotic and not necrotic (89).

HIE may preferentially affect the deep gray nuclei (including the basal ganglia and thalami), primarily in preterm but also term infants. These nuclei display a high metabolic activity near term, which might underlie their susceptibility to insult (110). Histologic changes are similar to those in the neocortex. As a response to injury, the deep gray nuclei may display abnormal myelination, wherein oligodendroglia mistakenly invest reactive astrocytic, rather than axonal processes. Grossly, these deep gray nuclei adopt a marbled appearance called status marmoratus. Survivors with this type of damage may suffer from cerebral palsy.

The cerebellum is also commonly affected by HIE. Both the cortex and dentate nuclei are often damaged. While Purkinje and dentate neurons die via necrosis, internal granule neurons are lost by apoptosis (39).

Overall, the brainstem is uncommonly affected by HIE (with the exception of the aforementioned PSN). While the inferior olives may incur neuronal death, other changes are generally rare. Severe HIE may result in bilaterally symmetric dorsal lower brainstem necrosis, which may explain the pathogenesis behind a subset of Moebius syndrome cases (facial diplegia and bilateral abducens palsies). Only severe cases of HIE tend to affect the entirety of the brainstem, and for that matter the spinal cord.

If HIE occurs during prenatal life, the pathways and cytoarchitecture of the developing brain may be significantly disturbed. Accordingly, this may lead to secondary malformations (i.e., acquired and not congenital). The type of malformation that results is GA dependent. It would be predicted that earlier insults result in more profound malformations. Polymicrogyria and schizencephaly are thought to be the result of early damage, while some forms of cortical dysplasia and hippocampal sclerosis are considered to be of late onset (39).

The white matter may be preferentially damaged in premature (and less so term) infants. The most acclaimed member of this group of lesions is *periventricular leukomalacia (PVL)*.

PVL is less frequently encountered than it was in the past, likely because of advances in prenatal care. Premature infants between GAs of 24 and 35 weeks (peak age is 28 weeks) are most frequently affected. Besides age, two of the most important risk factors include feto-maternal cardiorespiratory instability (e.g., fetal cerebral hypoperfusion and immature cerebral autoregulatory mechanisms) and intrauterine infection (e.g., chorioamnionitis). These two factors may act synergistically to trigger an inflammatory response (in part mediated by reactive astrocytes and activated microglia) that primarily targets the premyelinating oligodendrocytes of the fetal brain via excitotoxic amino acid–based mechanisms, oxidative stress, and cytokine cascades (116). Clinically these premature infants are generally "sick" (i.e., septic with unstable cardiac and respiratory function), and neurologically, they may have weak legs and seizures. The more uncommonly affected term infant often suffers from congestive heart disease or a congenital diaphragmatic hernia. Long-term sequelae include cerebral palsy, cognitive deficits (mental retardation, learning deficits), behavioral abnormalities, and epilepsy. Twenty-five percent of SIDS cases display evidence of PVL at autopsy. Genetic features of PVL are not well understood.

Pathologically, PVL is defined by two features: (a) periventricular necrosis that may be cystic and mineralized and (b) evidence for a more diffuse white matter gliosis (Figure 10-41). Some have conceptualized these two lesional components as the vascular "core" and the "penumbra," respectively. Adding further to the vascular hypothesis is the suggestion that the periventricular areas of predilection likely represent a region of vascular watershed during this age (26). Microscopically, periventricular white matter damage begins with the development of coagulative necrosis of all cell types within the first 24 hours of the insult (all cells develop nuclear pyknosis and eosinophilic cytoplasm). Axonal spheroids are seen on routine staining but can be further highlighted with β-APP IHC. Activated microglia, elucidated with CD68 immunohistochemistry, are prominent in early stages. Within the first week, macrophages infiltrate the areas of necrosis and are surrounded by early reactive gliosis. Gross cavitation and mineralization (of axons) can be seen after a few weeks. Cystic spaces collapse to form glial scars or areas of encephalomalacia. Destruction of these axonal processes undoubtedly affects the development of the overlying neocortical gray matter and likely accounts for subsequent cytoarchitectural abnormalities. Surrounding these areas of periventricular

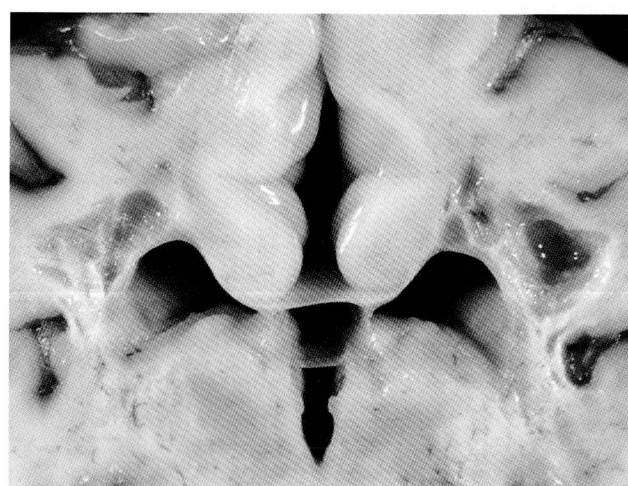

FIGURE 10-41 ■ Periventricular leukomalacia (PVL). Coronal section of the brain demonstrating cystic abnormalities in the white matter; note the markedly thinned corpus callosum.

necrosis is a more subtle diffuse white matter gliosis that is relatively devoid of axonal pathology. However, prominent loss of premyelinating oligodendrocytes from these areas leads to delayed and impaired myelination. Since premature infants are mainly at risk, it is not uncommon to see coexistent *germinal matrix hemorrhage (GMH)* (see below) and HIE.

GMH is also characteristic of premature infants. Given its subependymal location, IVH is present in most examples. Although in rare examples term infant may also experience GMH and IVH, the latter is more often a result of choroid plexus hemorrhage, possibly related to congenital vascular malformation (see below). Young GA is the most important risk factor; the incidence of GMH is inversely proportional to GA. Those infants less than 28 weeks are at the greatest risk for severe GMH (38). Other risk factor may include respiratory compromise (which is interrelated with age), intrauterine growth retardation (IUGR), feto-maternal sepsis (e.g., related to chorioamnionitis), hypothermia, intubation, and transportation between hospitals. Although the large veins of the germinal matrix are the likely source of the hemorrhage, the exact pathogenesis of GMH remains unclear. The germinal matrix is a major source of neuroglial precursors and persists until 34 weeks gestation (involution occurs by 38 to 40 weeks gestation). Enhanced fibrinolytic activity is characteristic of the involuting matrix making it susceptible to hemorrhage, in part due to the lack of sufficient parenchymal support of the matrix vasculature and poor hemostasis. Hypoxic-ischemic injury of the germinal matrix may further impair the already primitive autoregulatory capabilities of these vessels, making them vulnerable to fluctuations in CPP.

Clinically, GMH usually presents within the first 24 to 48 hours after birth. There may be a decreased level of consciousness or irritability, a tense fontanelle, and seizure activity. Severe GMH is often fatal (38). Occult cases of GMH are presumably of less clinical severity. Grading of the extent of GMH has been widely applied to ultrasonography. Grade I is confined to the germinal matrix; grade II additionally includes IVH that in grade III causes HCP; and finally, grade IV adds intraparenchymal extension of hemorrhage beyond the germinal matrix. Higher grades of GMH correlate with greater degrees of long-term neurological disability (39). Grossly, the appearance of GMH is in keeping with the aforementioned grading scheme (Figure 10-42). Extension of ventricular blood out of the foramina of the fourth ventricle into the basal cisterns yields a subarachnoid component that likely plays a role in chronic HCP. Areas of parenchyma adjacent to GMH may be necrotic (with microscopic mineralization) and often show concomitant PVL. Microscopically, there are relatively few reactive changes in the parenchyma.

A variety of acquired vascular disorders may be seen in children, many of which are rarely encountered by the neuropathologist. Essentially, all of these disorders result in "stroke" (i.e., infarction). Risk factors for pediatric stroke include diabetes, cardiac abnormalities (e.g., congenital and rheumatic heart disease, arrhythmias), thrombophilias, hyperhomocysteinemia, hematologic conditions, trauma, drug use (e.g., smoking, amphetamines, etc.), hypertension, obesity, and oral contraceptive use. Meningitis often leads to infarction via inflammation, damage, and thrombosis of leptomeningeal vessels (i.e., secondary vasculitis). Clinically, pediatric and adult stroke may present similarly (i.e., focal signs/symptoms and or more global neurologic impairment). Angiography and diffusion/perfusion weight MRI are frequently used in the patient's workup. Microscopically, edema and congestion precede acute neuronal cell death that is most readily visible by 24 hours. At 1 to 2 days, there is infiltration of neutrophils (PMNs) and endothelial swelling. Within the first week, PMNs make way for macrophages. Angiogenesis and reactive gliosis are seen by 2 weeks. Later stages are characterized by neuronal loss, gliosis, and cystic degeneration. Well-recognized clinico-pathologic entities that have a relative predilection for the CNS vasculature include Moyamoya disease, fibromuscular dysplasia, venous sinus thrombosis, arterial dissection, vasculitides (e.g., Takayasu arteritis, primary angiitis of the CNS), and vasculopathies (e.g., HIV vasculopathy). Many systemic disorders characteristically affect the large and small blood vessels of the CNS including systemic lupus erythematosis, other collagen vascular disorders, sickle cell disease, antiphospholipid antibody syndrome, fat emboli, thrombotic thrombocytopenic purpura, and hemolytic uremic syndrome.

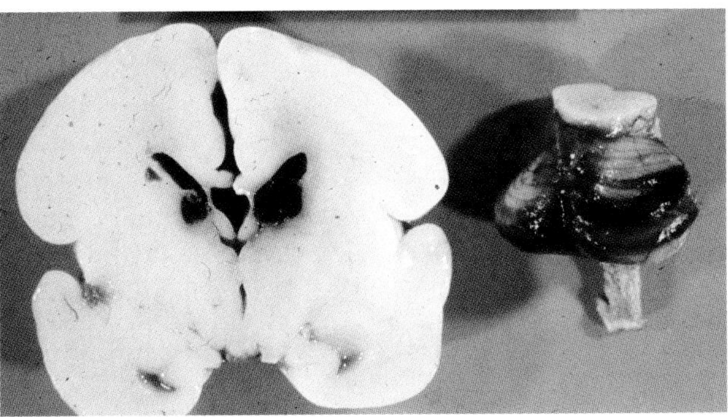

FIGURE 10-42 ■ Bilateral GMH. Hemorrhage on left side has extended into the adjacent ventricular system and out into the subarachnoid space (cisterna magna) overlying the cerebellum through the foramina of the fourth ventricle (coronal section). (Image courtesy of Dr. Barry Rewcastle.)

Many of the congenital CNS vascular anomalies are also uncommonly seen. Berry (i.e., saccular) aneurysms are extremely rare in young children. A defective internal elastic lamina may predispose to their formation over time and thus accounts for the low prevalence in this population. These often present with massive and fatal SAH. The key to their discovery is a careful dissection of blood and the circle of Willis in the fresh state when structures are more manipulatable. Microscopically, the aneurysm wall is focally attenuated; the internal elastic lamina and media are replaced by fibrous connective tissue, and possibly atherosclerosis plus hemosiderin.

Vascular malformations include arterio-venous malformations (AVMs), cavernous hemangiomas (i.e., cavernous angiomas or "cavernomas"), venous angiomas, and capillary telangectasias, the former two of which are more commonly symptomatic. AVMs may present with hemorrhage or with ischemic signs and symptoms that relate to arterio-venous shunting and vascular steal. Arterial feeders and draining veins are usually well appreciated angiographically. Microscopically, there are arteries, veins, and "arterialized veins" of varying mural thickness and caliber, often with entrapped fragments of gliotic brain between these abnormal vessels. Hybrid vessels appear partly arterial and partly venous in favorable histologic sections. Staining of the internal elastic lamina (e.g., Musto Moat, Verhoff van Gieson) assists in highlighting the arterial components. Recent and remote hemorrhage may be seen in the abnormal vessels, as well as gliotic brain. Evidence of embolization may be seen in the form of foreign material within the vascular lumina of the malformation. Cavernous angiomas are essentially venous structures that present as mass lesions, which may cause hemorrhage, focal neurologic deficits, or seizures. Gradient echo MRI sequences highlight these malformations. Microscopically, hyalinized veins of various caliber are packed together in a back-to-back fashion, generally excluding intervening parenchyma in most examples. Gliosis and signs of prior hemorrhage surround these abnormal blood vessels.

Vein of Galen aneurysms are actually arterio-venous fistulas that are associated with aneurysmal dilatation of the vein of Galen. These are thought to arise early in gestation (between 6 and 11 weeks) (39). The posterior cerebral artery is a frequent "feeder artery." The most common clinical presentation is high output congestive heart failure in a young child. Vascular steal may lead to atrophy and parenchymal necrosis (with dystrophic calcification). Microscopically, feeder vessels are dilated and hypertrophic, while the "aneurysmal" vein similarly displays a thickened wall. Vessels in the adjacent brain parenchyma may also be hyperplastic in response to high pressure shunting.

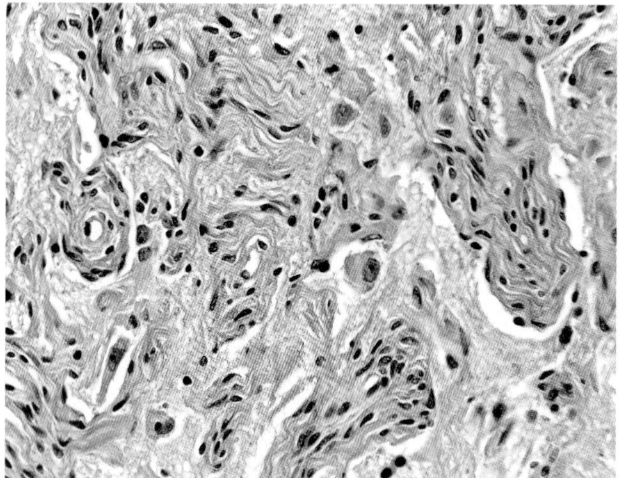

FIGURE 10-43 ■ MA characterized by a variably hyalinized, fibroblast-like perivascular spindle cell proliferation, adjacent to normal-appearing or mildly dysmorphic cortical neurons.

Meningioangiomatosis (MA) is a form of meningovascular malformation or hamartoma occurring either in the setting of NF2 or sporadically (77). The former is typically asymptomatic, whereas the latter usually presents before adulthood with seizures and/or headache. This often plaque-like proliferation of meningothelial, smooth muscle, and fibroblast-like spindled cells appears to extend down the Virchow-Robin spaces into the superficial brain and invest blood vessels (Figure 10-43). The surrounding brain is gliotic and often displays dysmorphic neurons, dystrophic calcification, and fibrosis. In contrast to pure MA, cases associated with an overlying meningioma likely represent an unusual mimic with perivascular tumoral spread, rather than a true malformation. Other CNS vascular anomalies include Fowler syndrome, meningocerebral angiodysplasia/renal agenesis, and Sturge-Weber-Dimitri disease (i.e., encephalotrigeminal angiomatosis) (39).

REFERENCES

1. Abel TW, Baker SJ, Fraser MM, et al. Lhermitte-Duclos disease: a report of 31 cases with immunohistochemical analysis of the PTEN/AKT/mTOR pathway. *J Neuropathol Exp Neurol* 2005;64:341–349.
2. Addo-Yobo SO, Straessle J, Anwar A, et al. Paired overexpression of ErbB3 and Sox10 in pilocytic astrocytoma. *J Neuropathol Exp Neurol* 2006;65:769–775.
3. Alexiev BA, Lin X, Sun CC, et al. Meckel-Gruber syndrome: pathologic manifestations, minimal diagnostic criteria, and differential diagnosis. *Arch Pathol Lab Med* 2006;130:1236–1238.
4. Bailey A, Luthert P, Dean A, et al. A clinicopathological study of autism. *Brain* 1998;121(Pt 5):889–905.
5. Becker AJ, Blumcke I, Urbach H, et al. Molecular neuropathology of epilepsy-associated glioneuronal malformations. *J Neuropathol Exp Neurol* 2006;65:99–108.
6. Bell JE, Lowrie S, Koffi K, et al. The neuropathology of HIV-infected African children in Abidjan, Cote d'Ivoire. *J Neuropathol Exp Neurol* 1997;56:686–692.
7. Blatt GJ, Fitzgerald CM, Guptill JT, et al. Density and distribution of hippocampal neurotransmitter receptors in autism: an autoradiographic study. *J Autism Dev Disord* 2001;31:537–543.
8. Blumcke I, Wiestler OD. Gangliogliomas: an intriguing tumor entity associated with focal epilepsies. *J Neuropathol Exp Neurol* 2002;61:575–584.
9. Broniscer A, Gajjar A. Supratentorial high-grade astrocytoma and diffuse brainstem glioma: two challenges for the pediatric oncologist. *Oncologist* 2004;9:197–206.
10. Burger PC, Scheithauer BW, Vogel FS. *Surgical pathology of the nervous system and its coverings*. New York: Churchill Livingstone, 2002.
11. Buslei R, Nolde M, Hofmann B, et al. Common mutations of beta-catenin in adamantinomatous craniopharyngiomas but not in other tumours originating from the sellar region. *Acta Neuropathol* 2005;109:589–597.
12. Cairncross JG, Ueki K, Zlatescu MC, et al. Specific genetic predictors of chemotherapeutic response and survival in patients with anaplastic oligodendrogliomas. *J Natl Cancer Inst* 1998;90:1473–1479.
13. Casanova MF, Buxhoeveden DP, Switala AE, et al. Minicolumnar pathology in autism. *Neurology* 2002;58:428–432.
14. Chavez-Bueno S, McCracken GH Jr. Bacterial meningitis in children. *Pediatr Clin North Am* 2005;52:795–810, vii.

15. Ching KH, Westaway SK, Gitschier J, et al. HARP syndrome is allelic with pantothenate kinase-associated neurodegeneration. *Neurology* 2002;58:1673–1674.
16. Chugani DC, Muzik O, Rothermel R, et al. Altered serotonin synthesis in the dentatothalamocortical pathway in autistic boys. *Ann Neurol* 1997;42:666–669.
17. Dale JK, Vesque C, Lints TJ, et al. Cooperation of BMP7 and SHH in the induction of forebrain ventral midline cells by prechordal mesoderm. *Cell* 1997;90:257–269.
18. Daumas-Duport C, Scheithauer BW, Chodkiewicz JP, et al. Dysembryoplastic neuroepithelial tumor: a surgically curable tumor of young patients with intractable partial seizures. Report of thirty-nine cases. *Neurosurgery* 1988;23:545–556.
19. Daumas-Duport C, Varlet P, Bacha S, et al. Dysembryoplastic neuroepithelial tumors: nonspecific histological forms—a study of 40 cases. *J Neurooncol* 1999;41:267–280.
20. Davila-Gutierrez G. Agenesis and dysgenesis of the corpus callosum. *Semin Pediatr Neurol* 2002;9:292–301.
21. Dickson D. *Neurodegeneration: the molecular pathology of dementia and movement disorders*. Basel, Switzerland: International Society of Neuropathology, 2003.
22. Duff J, Meyer FB, Ilstrup DM, et al. Long-term outcomes for surgically resected craniopharyngiomas. *Neurosurgery* 2000;46:291–302; discussion 302–295.
23. Dyer S, Prebble E, Davison V, et al. Genomic imbalances in pediatric intracranial ependymomas define clinically relevant groups. *Am J Pathol* 2002;161:2133–2141.
24. Eberhart CG, Kepner JL, Goldthwaite PT, et al. Histopathologic grading of medulloblastomas: a Pediatric Oncology Group study. *Cancer* 2002;94:552–560.
25. Eckert A, Kloor M, Giersch A, et al. Microsatellite instability in pediatric and adult high-grade gliomas. *Brain Pathol* 2007;17:146–150.
26. Ellison D, Love S, Chimelli L, et al. *Neuropathology: a reference text of CNS pathology*. Edinburgh; New York: Mosby, 2004.
27. Filiano JJ, Kinney HC. A perspective on neuropathologic findings in victims of the sudden infant death syndrome: the triple-risk model. *Biol Neonate* 1994;65:194–197.
28. Fisher PG, Breiter SN, Carson BS, et al. A clinicopathologic reappraisal of brain stem tumor classification. Identification of pilocystic astrocytoma and fibrillary astrocytoma as distinct entities. *Cancer* 2000;89:1569–1576.
29. Forman MS, Squier W, Dobyns WB, et al. Genotypically defined lissencephalies show distinct pathologies. *J Neuropathol Exp Neurol* 2005;64:847–857.
30. Frey L, Hauser WA. Epidemiology of neural tube defects. *Epilepsia* 2003;44(Suppl 3):4–13.
31. Fujisawa H, Marukawa K, Hasegawa M, et al. Genetic differences between neurocytoma and dysembryoplastic neuroepithelial tumor and oligodendroglial tumors. *J Neurosurg* 2002;97:1350–1355.
32. Geddes JF, Hackshaw AK, Vowles GH, et al. Neuropathology of inflicted head injury in children. I. Patterns of brain damage. *Brain* 2001;124:1290–1298.
33. Giangaspero F, Wellek S, Masuoka J, et al. Stratification of medulloblastoma on the basis of histopathological grading. *Acta Neuropathol* 2006;112:5–12.
34. Giannini C, Scheithauer BW, Burger PC, et al. Pleomorphic xanthoastrocytoma: what do we really know about it? *Cancer* 1999;85:2033–2045.
35. Giannini C, Scheithauer BW, Burger PC, et al. Cellular proliferation in pilocytic and diffuse astrocytomas. *J Neuropathol Exp Neurol* 1999;58:46–53.
36. Giannini C, Scheithauer BW, Weaver AL, et al. Oligodendrogliomas: reproducibility and prognostic value of histologic diagnosis and grading. *J Neuropathol Exp Neurol* 2001;60:248–262.
37. Gilbertson RJ, Bentley L, Hernan R, et al. ERBB receptor signaling promotes ependymoma cell proliferation and represents a potential novel therapeutic target for this disease. *Clin Cancer Res* 2002;8:3054–3064.
38. Gleissner M, Jorch G, Avenarius S. Risk factors for intraventricular hemorrhage in a birth cohort of 3721 premature infants. *J Perinat Med* 2000;28:104–110.
39. Golden JA, Harding BN, International Society of Neuropathology. *Developmental neuropathology*. Basel, Switzerland: International Society of Neuropathology, 2004.
40. Gordon N. Alpers syndrome: progressive neuronal degeneration of children with liver disease. *Dev Med Child Neurol* 2006;48:1001–1003.
41. Gray F, Chretien F, Vallat-Decouvelaere AV, et al. The changing pattern of HIV neuropathology in the HAART era. *J Neuropathol Exp Neurol* 2003;62:429–440.
42. Grotzer MA, Janss AJ, Phillips PC, et al. Neurotrophin receptor TrkC predicts good clinical outcome in medulloblastoma and other primitive neuroectodermal brain tumors. *Klin Padiatr* 2000;212:196–199.
43. Haberler C, Laggner U, Slavc I, et al. Immunohistochemical analysis of INI1 protein in malignant pediatric CNS tumors: lack of INI1 in atypical teratoid/rhabdoid tumors and in a fraction of primitive neuroectodermal tumors without rhabdoid phenotype. *Am J Surg Pathol* 2006;30:1462–1468.
44. Hevner RF. The cerebral cortex malformation in thanatophoric dysplasia: neuropathology and pathogenesis. *Acta Neuropathol* 2005;110:208–221.
45. Ho DM, Hsu CY, Wong TT, et al. A clinicopathologic study of 81 patients with ependymomas and proposal of diagnostic criteria for anaplastic ependymoma. *J Neurooncol* 2001;54:77–85.
46. Inda MM, Perot C, Guillaud-Bataille M, et al. Genetic heterogeneity in supratentorial and infratentorial primitive neuroectodermal tumours of the central nervous system. *Histopathology* 2005;47:631–637.
47. Jeibmann A, Hasselblatt M, Gerss J, et al. Prognostic implications of atypical histologic features in choroid plexus papilloma. *J Neuropathol Exp Neurol* 2006;65:1069–1073.
48. Jouvet A, Saint-Pierre G, Fauchon F, et al. Pineal parenchymal tumors: a correlation of histological features with prognosis in 66 cases. *Brain Pathol* 2000;10:49–60.
49. Kamakura Y, Hasegawa M, Minamoto T, et al. C-kit gene mutation: common and widely distributed in intracranial germinomas. *J Neurosurg* 2006;104:173–180.
50. Kamaly-Asl ID, Shams N, Taylor MD. Genetics of choroid plexus tumors. *Neurosurg Focus* 2006;20:E10.
51. Kandel ER, Schwartz JH, Jessell TM. *Principles of neural science*. New York: McGraw-Hill, Health Professions Division, 2000.
52. Kasper BS, Stefan H, Buchfelder M, et al. Temporal lobe microdysgenesis in epilepsy versus control brains. *J Neuropathol Exp Neurol* 1999;58:22–28.
53. Kaulich K, Blaschke B, Numann A, et al. Genetic alterations commonly found in diffusely infiltrating cerebral gliomas are rare or absent in pleomorphic xanthoastrocytomas. *J Neuropathol Exp Neurol* 2002;61:1092–1099.
54. Khatua S, Peterson KM, Brown KM, et al. Overexpression of the EGFR/FKBP12/HIF-2alpha pathway identified in childhood astrocytomas by angiogenesis gene profiling. *Cancer Res* 2003;63:1865–1870.
55. Kimberlin DW. Herpes simplex virus infections of the central nervous system. *Semin Pediatr Infect Dis* 2003;14:83–89.
56. Kinney HC, Randall LL, Sleeper LA, et al. Serotonergic brainstem abnormalities in Northern Plains Indians with the sudden infant death syndrome. *J Neuropathol Exp Neurol* 2003;62:1178–1191.
57. Koeppen AH. The pathogenesis of spinocerebellar ataxia. *Cerebellum* 2005;4:62–73.
58. Korshunov A, Golanov A, Sycheva R, et al. The histologic grade is a main prognostic factor for patients with intracranial ependymomas treated in the microneurosurgical era: an analysis of 258 patients. *Cancer* 2004;100:1230–1237.

59. Kreiger PA, Okada Y, Simon S, et al. Losses of chromosomes 1p and 19q are rare in pediatric oligodendrogliomas. *Acta Neuropathol* 2005;109:387–392.
60. Kurt E, Zheng PP, Hop WC, et al. Identification of relevant prognostic histopathologic features in 69 intracranial ependymomas, excluding myxopapillary ependymomas and subependymomas. *Cancer* 2006;106:388–395.
61. Lee GY, Paradiso G, Tator CH, et al. Surgical management of tethered cord syndrome in adults: indications, techniques, and long-term outcomes in 60 patients. *J Neurosurg Spine* 2006;4:123–131.
62. Li MH, Bouffet E, Hawkins CE, et al. Molecular genetics of supratentorial primitive neuroectodermal tumors and pineoblastoma. *Neurosurg Focus* 2005;19:E3.
63. Louis DN, Ohgaki H, Wiestler OD, et al., eds. *WHO classification of tumours of the central nervous system*, 4th ed. Lyon, France: IARC, 2007.
64. Lusher ME, Lindsey JC, Latif F, et al. Biallelic epigenetic inactivation of the RASSF1A tumor suppressor gene in medulloblastoma development. *Cancer Res* 2002;62:5906–5911.
65. Martin-Rendon E, Blake DJ. Protein glycosylation in disease: new insights into the congenital muscular dystrophies. *Trends Pharmacol Sci* 2003;24:178–183.
66. Matsumoto K, Suzuki SO, Fukui M, et al. Accumulation of MDM2 in pleomorphic xanthoastrocytomas. *Pathol Int* 2004;54:387–391.
67. Matturri L, Ottaviani G, Lavezzi AM. Maternal smoking and sudden infant death syndrome: epidemiological study related to pathology. *Virchows Arch* 2006;449:697–706.
68. McLendon RE, Rosenblum MK, Bigner DD. *Russell & Rubinstein's pathology of tumors of the nervous system*. London, UK: Hodder Arnold, 2006.
69. McManamy CS, Pears J, Weston CL, et al. Nodule formation and desmoplasia in medulloblastomas-defining the nodular/desmoplastic variant and its biological behavior. *Brain Pathol* 2007;17:151–164.
70. Merchant TE, Jenkins JJ, Burger PC, et al. Influence of tumor grade on time to progression after irradiation for localized ependymoma in children. *Int J Radiat Oncol Biol Phys* 2002;53:52–57.
71. Ohgaki H, Kleihues P. Population-based studies on incidence, survival rates, and genetic alterations in astrocytic and oligodendroglial gliomas. *J Neuropathol Exp Neurol* 2005;64:479–489.
72. Palmini A, Najm I, Avanzini G, et al. Terminology and classification of the cortical dysplasias. *Neurology* 2004;62:S2–S8.
73. Pasquier B, Peoc HM, Fabre-Bocquentin B, et al. Surgical pathology of drug-resistant partial epilepsy. A 10-year-experience with a series of 327 consecutive resections. *Epileptic Disord* 2002;4:99–119.
74. Paterson DS, Trachtenberg FL, Thompson EG, et al. Multiple serotonergic brainstem abnormalities in sudden infant death syndrome. *JAMA* 2006;296:2124–2132.
75. Perry A, Dehner LP. Meningeal tumors of childhood and infancy. An update and literature review. *Brain Pathol* 2003;13:386–408.
76. Perry A, Fuller CE, Banerjee R, et al. Ancillary FISH analysis for 1p and 19q status: preliminary observations in 287 gliomas and oligodendroglioma mimics. *Front Biosci* 2003;8:a1–a9.
77. Perry A, Kurtkaya-Yapicier O, Scheithauer BW, et al. Insights into meningioangiomatosis with and without meningioma: a clinicopathologic and genetic series of 24 cases with review of the literature. *Brain Pathol* 2005;15:55–65.
78. Perry EK, Lee ML, Martin-Ruiz CM, et al. Cholinergic activity in autism: abnormalities in the cerebral cortex and basal forebrain. *Am J Psychiatry* 2001;158:1058–1066.
79. Pfeifer JD. *Molecular genetic testing in surgical pathology*. Philadelphia: Lippincott Williams & Wilkins, 2006.
80. Pomeroy SL, Tamayo P, Gaasenbeek M, et al. Prediction of central nervous system embryonal tumour outcome based on gene expression. *Nature* 2002;415:436–442.
81. Prayson RA. *Neuropathology*. Philadelphia: Churchill-Livingstone, 2005.
82. Prayson RA, Castilla EA, Hartke M, et al. Chromosome 1p allelic loss by fluorescence in situ hybridization is not observed in dysembryoplastic neuroepithelial tumors. *Am J Clin Pathol* 2002;118:512–517.
83. Raffel C, Frederick L, O'Fallon JR, et al. Analysis of oncogene and tumor suppressor gene alterations in pediatric malignant astrocytomas reveals reduced survival for patients with PTEN mutations. *Clin Cancer Res* 1999;5:4085–4090.
84. Raghavan R, Balani J, Perry A, et al. Pediatric oligodendrogliomas: a study of molecular alterations on 1p and 19q using fluorescence in situ hybridization. *J Neuropathol Exp Neurol* 2003;62: 530–537.
85. Rajaram V, Gutmann DH, Prasad SK, et al. Alterations of protein 4.1 family members in ependymomas: a study of 84 cases. *Mod Pathol* 2005;18:991–997.
86. Rickert CH, Paulus W. Epidemiology of central nervous system tumors in childhood and adolescence based on the new WHO classification. *Childs Nerv Syst* 2001;17:503–511.
87. Rodriguez D, Gelot A, della Gaspera B, et al. Increased density of oligodendrocytes in childhood ataxia with diffuse central hypomyelination (CACH) syndrome: neuropathological and biochemical study of two cases. *Acta Neuropathol* 1999;97:469–480.
88. Romero JR, Newland JG. Viral meningitis and encephalitis: traditional and emerging viral agents. *Semin Pediatr Infect Dis* 2003;14:72–82.
89. Rossiter JP, Anderson LL, Yang F, et al. Caspase-3 activation and caspase-like proteolytic activity in human perinatal hypoxic-ischemic brain injury. *Acta Neuropathol* 2002;103:66–73.
90. Ruggieri PM, Najm I, Bronen R, et al. Neuroimaging of the cortical dysplasias. *Neurology* 2004;62:S27–S29.
91. Saez-Llorens X. Brain abscess in children. *Semin Pediatr Infect Dis* 2003;14:108–114.
92. Sanoudou D, Tingby O, Ferguson-Smith MA, et al. Analysis of pilocytic astrocytoma by comparative genomic hybridization. *Br J Cancer* 2000;82:1218–1222.
93. Sarnat HB. *Cerebral dysgenesis: embryology and clinical expression*. New York: Oxford University Press, 1992.
94. Sarnat HB, Flores-Sarnat L. Neuropathologic research strategies in holoprosencephaly. *J Child Neurol* 2001;16:918–931.
95. Shannon P, Smith CR, Deck J, et al. Axonal injury and the neuropathology of shaken baby syndrome. *Acta Neuropathol* 1998;95:625–631.
96. Shao Y, Cuccaro ML, Hauser ER, et al. Fine mapping of autistic disorder to chromosome 15q11-q13 by use of phenotypic subtypes. *Am J Hum Genet* 2003;72:539–548.
97. Sharer LR. Pathology of HIV-1 infection of the central nervous system. A review. *J Neuropathol Exp Neurol* 1992;51:3–11.
98. Sharma MK, Watson MA, Lyman M, et al. Matrilin-2 expression distinguishes clinically relevant subsets of pilocytic astrocytoma. *Neurology* 2006;66:127–130.
99. Sheen VL, Dixon PH, Fox JW, et al. Mutations in the X-linked filamin 1 gene cause periventricular nodular heterotopia in males as well as in females. *Hum Mol Genet* 2001;10:1775–1783.
100. Singh PK, Gutmann DH, Fuller CE, et al. Differential involvement of protein 4.1 family members DAL-1 and NF2 in intracranial and intraspinal ependymomas. *Mod Pathol* 2002;15:526–531.
101. Squier M, Chamberlain P, Zaiwalla Z, et al. Five cases of brain injury following amniocentesis in mid-term pregnancy. *Develop Med Child Neurol* 2000;42:554–560.
102. Suarez-Merino B, Hubank M, Revesz T, et al. Microarray analysis of pediatric ependymoma identifies a cluster of 112 candidate genes including four transcripts at 22q12.1-q13.3. *Neurooncol* 2005;7:20–31.
103. Szybka M, Bartkowiak J, Zakrzewski K, et al. Microsatellite instability and expression of DNA mismatch repair genes in malignant astrocytic tumors from adult and pediatric patients. *Clin Neuropathol* 2003;22:180–186.

104. Tabori U, Ma J, Carter M, et al. Human telomere reverse transcriptase expression predicts progression and survival in pediatric intracranial ependymoma. *J Clin Oncol* 2006;24:1522–1528.
105. Tamber MS, Bansal K, Liang ML, et al. Current concepts in the molecular genetics of pediatric brain tumors: implications for emerging therapies. *Childs Nerv Syst* 2006;22:1379–1394.
106. Tamiya T, Kinoshita K, Ono Y, et al. Proton magnetic resonance spectroscopy reflects cellular proliferative activity in astrocytomas. *Neuroradiology* 2000;42:333–338.
107. Tavangar SM, Larijani B, Mahta A, et al. Craniopharyngioma: a clinicopathological study of 141 cases. *Endocr Pathol* 2004;15:339–344.
108. Taylor MD, Poppleton H, Fuller C, et al. Radial glia cells are candidate stem cells of ependymoma. *Cancer Cell* 2005;8:323–335.
109. ten Donkelaar HJ, Lammens M, Wesseling P, et al. Development and developmental disorders of the human cerebellum. *J Neurol* 2003;250:1025–1036.
110. Thorngren-Jerneck K, Ohlsson T, Sandell A, et al. Cerebral glucose metabolism measured by positron emission tomography in term newborn infants with hypoxic ischemic encephalopathy. *Pediatr Res* 2001;49:495–501.
111. Tihan T, Fisher PG, Kepner JL, et al. Pediatric astrocytomas with monomorphous pilomyxoid features and a less favorable outcome. *J Neuropathol Exp Neurol* 1999;58:1061–1068.
112. Ullrich NJ, Pomeroy SL. Molecular genetics of pediatric central nervous system tumors. *Curr Oncol Rep* 2006;8:423–429.
113. Ullrich NJ, Pomeroy SL. Pediatric brain tumors. *Neurol Clin* 2003;21:897–913.
114. van de Warrenburg BP, Sinke RJ, Kremer B. Recent advances in hereditary spinocerebellar ataxias. *J Neuropathol Exp Neurol* 2005;64:171–180.
115. van der Knaap MS, Leegwater PA, Konst AA, et al. Mutations in each of the five subunits of translation initiation factor eIF2B can cause leukoencephalopathy with vanishing white matter. *Ann Neurol* 2002;51:264–270.
116. Volpe JJ. Cerebral white matter injury of the premature infant-more common than you think. *Pediatrics* 2003;112:176–180.
117. Waha A, Waha A, Koch A, et al. Epigenetic silencing of the HIC-1 gene in human medulloblastomas. *J Neuropathol Exp Neurol* 2003;62:1192–1201.
118. Wang M, Tihan T, Rojiani AM, et al. Monomorphous angiocentric glioma: a distinctive epileptogenic neoplasm with features of infiltrating astrocytoma and ependymoma. *J Neuropathol Exp Neurol* 2005;64:875–881.
119. Wong KK, Chang YM, Tsang YT, et al. Expression analysis of juvenile pilocytic astrocytomas by oligonucleotide microarray reveals two potential subgroups. *Cancer Res* 2005;65:76–84.
120. Zhou XP, Marsh DJ, Morrison CD, et al. Germline inactivation of PTEN and dysregulation of the phosphoinositol-3-kinase/Akt pathway cause human Lhermitte-Duclos disease in adults. *Am J Hum Genet* 2003;73:1191–1198.

CHAPTER 11

Pediatric Ophthalmic Pathology

J. DOUGLAS CAMERON

INTRODUCTION

The observations and opinions of surgical pathologists are critical in managing many pediatric ocular conditions including potentially fatal entities such as retinoblastoma and suspected nonaccidental trauma.

Because pediatric ophthalmic surgical specimens tend to be infrequent, this chapter includes a discussion of pertinent ocular anatomy and pivotal events in embryologic development of the eye; the intention is to provide a context for pathologic features. In addition, the type of surgical procedure used to obtain the tissue specimen is described to assist in understanding the origin of the specimen and orientation of gross specimens.

This chapter is organized by the types of tissue most frequently received in the laboratory; eyelid tissue, conjunctiva, cornea, vitreous, orbital soft tissues, whole globes removed surgically, and globes removed at autopsy. Crystalline lens tissue removed because of congenital cataracts and extraocular muscle tissues removed during some types of strabismus procedures are infrequently processed because histological observations of this type of specimen are not relevant to management of the ocular abnormality.

THE NORMAL EYELID

Structure of the Eyelid

The eyelid is covered by stratified squamous epithelium associated with a thin keratin layer. The surface merges with the mucous membrane at the mucocutaneous junction located on the eyelid margin (Figure 11-1). The epidermis is associated with pilosebaceous units, eccrine glands, and apocrine glands. The apocrine glands have no recognized function in the eyelid tissues. The cilia are the product of a modified pilosebaceous unit in that there are no associated piloerector muscles and there is a prominent sebaceous component (glands of Zeis). The tarsal plate is a dense collagenous structure that supports the delicate eyelid and houses a large volume of sebaceous glands (the Meibomion glands). No cartilage is present in the eyelid. The holocrine secretion of the Meibomion gland is applied to the tear film surface from pores located along the eyelid margin anterior to the mucocutaneous junction and posterior to the eyelid cilia (38,61).

SURGICAL PROCEDURES OF THE EYELID

An eyelid biopsy may be a simple removal of an ellipse of skin because of the suspicion of cutaneous neoplasm. These specimens are handled as are cutaneous biopsies elsewhere. When a lesion involves the eyelid margin, particularly near the punctum, the surgery becomes more complicated because scarring in the region of punctum may cause lacrimal drainage abnormalities (chronic tearing, epiphora) and because scarring of the eyelid margin may damage the cornea. Some type of superficial lamellar dissection in the region of the punctum may be done to spare punctal function. For lid margin lesions a full-thickness wedge of eyelid is removed because restoration of lid margin function is facilitated. A lid-splitting procedure removes the tissue either anterior or posterior to the anterior border of the tarsal plate. Full-thickness and partial-thickness lid margin specimens are generally oriented perpendicular to the lid margin (or row of cilia) with nasal and lateral surgical margins.

VASCULAR ABNORMALITIES OF THE EYELID

Capillary hemangioma is a benign proliferation of blood vessels of the soft tissue of the face that may involve both eyelids and the orbit (57). The proliferation does not usually involve the contents of the globe. The cutaneous lesions are red and lobulated, and may markedly distort the contours of the face (Figure 11-2). The lesions are rarely biopsied but occasionally may be surgically debulked. Initially, there is capillary lesion in a lobular pattern characterized by proliferation of endothelial cells around a small caliber vascular channel. The lesion is not encapsulated and lobules of the hemangioma extend into the surrounding soft tissue. With time the endothelial profile flattens and the lumen becomes

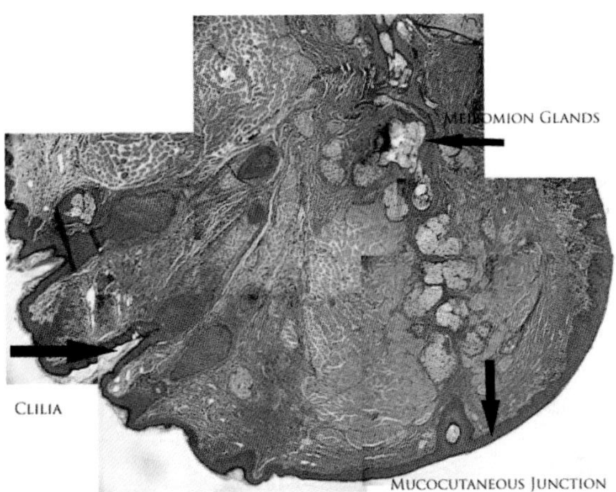

FIGURE 11-1 ▪ Structure of the eyelid: The anterior surface of the eyelid is composed of stratified squamous epithelium with a thin keratin layer. The keratinized surface merges with mucous membrane lining the posterior surface of the eyelid at the mucocutaneous junction (*arrow*). Large pilosebaceous units represent the eyelashes that lack a piloerector muscle. Meibomion gland secretion covers the surface of the tear film at the mucocutaneous junction. (Hematoxylin-eosin stain, original magnification ×40).

more prominent as interstitial tissue develops. Intralesional steroids are sometimes injected to shrink the mass and may be seen as amorphous material in the vascular lumen or in the interstitial space (128). The lesions appear clinically at birth or 2 to 4 weeks after birth and may progress rapidly to produce soft-tissue enlargement and mechanical ptosis of the eyelid. Obstruction of vision by mechanical ptosis may interfere with the development of visual function (amblyopia) (77). The hemangioma may enlarge over the following several years. The lesions tend to spontaneously involute generally by age 7 years. There may be vascular abnormalities elsewhere in the body.

Nevus flammeus is congenital vascular lesion in the distribution of the first and second divisions of the trigeminal nerve (42). The vascular abnormality is present at birth and does not progress or regress. The cutaneous lesion may be treated with laser but is generally not biopsied (117). It is clinically important because this vascular malformation is associated with ipsilateral glaucoma and ipsilateral choroidal hemangioma. Glaucoma, when present, is treated as are cases of glaucoma from other causes. The choroidal hemangioma is very difficult to treat and may progress to serious retinal detachment, a potential cause of loss of vision (98,133).

INFLAMMATORY ABNORMALITIES OF THE EYELID

Pyogenic granuloma refers to a polypoid lobular capillary hemangioma of the skin in the discipline of dermatopathology. This term is used by clinical ophthalmologists to describe a granulation tissue reaction usually located in the tarsal conjunctiva, which is a response to mechanical trauma or to the presence of a chalazion (Figure 11-3) (37). A reddish lobulated mass develops on the conjunctival surface that may be large enough to protrude through the interpalpebral fissure. The area is excised if the mass interferes with the surface lubrication of the eye from malpositioning of the eyelid margin. The overlying mucous membrane may show effects of drying and reactive proliferation. In the subepithelial tissue there are acute and chronic inflammatory reactions associated with multiple delicate vascular channels and an edematous stroma (granulation tissue). Conjunctival pyogenic granuloma usually will spontaneously involute over days to weeks.

Chalazion is a granulomatous reaction to sebaceous products of the Meibomion gland of the eyelid. The gland becomes occluded and ruptures into the surrounding soft tissue. The affected area is initially tender but evolves into a firm nontender nodule. In cases of exceptional size, an incision and curettage is performed. The tissue is usually friable

FIGURE 11-2 ▪ Capillary hemangiomas in the periorbital soft tissue of the face cause dysfunction of the eyelid because of mechanical ptosis. If the eye is not stimulated by formed images the retinal function will not develop (amblyopia).

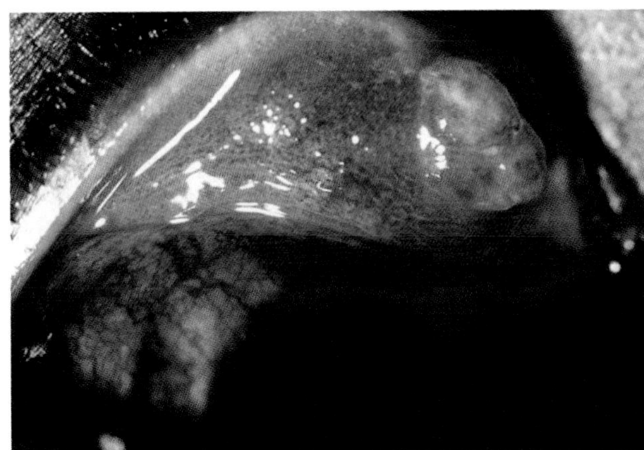

FIGURE 11-3 ▪ Pyogenic granuloma is a clinical term used by ophthalmologists to refer to a transient fibrovascular response in a mucous membrane (the conjunctiva). With remodeling normally found in the repair process the lesion will spontaneously diminish over time. The lesion is occasionally removed if it causes symptoms related to eyelid dysfunction.

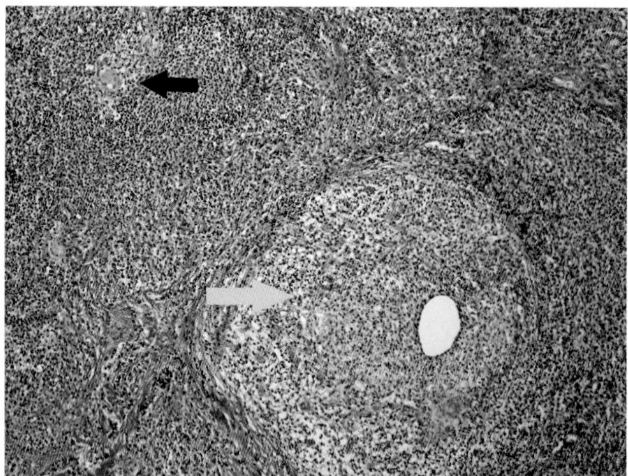

FIGURE 11-4 ▪ Chalazion is a lipogranulomatous reaction to a lipid globule (*white arrow*) representing sebaceous secretion from a ruptured Meibomion gland of the eyelid (*black arrow*). The rupture is thought to be the result of blockage of the outlet mechanism of the gland. The tissue submitted will often be limited to the contents of the chalazion (Hematoxylin-eosin stain, original magnification ×100).

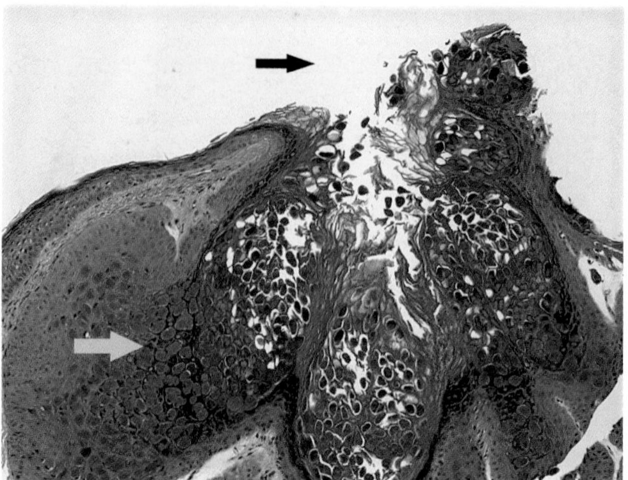

FIGURE 11-5 ▪ Molluscum contageosum consists of virus-infected cells (*white arrow*) of the eyelid margin that may cause regional conjunctivitis because of exfoliation of infected cells and debris (*black arrow*) (Hematoxylin-eosin stain, original magnification ×20).

amorphous gray tissue composed of a lipogranulomatous reaction with foreign body and occasional Langhans-type giant cells (Figure 11-4). The surrounding normal tissue is usually not represented in the specimen, however, infiltration among the fibers of the orbicularis muscle may be observed occasionally.

Generally, the nodule resolves over weeks or months. In some individuals, there may be multiple episodes in different locations in the eyelid. In children, chalazion may cause refractive error and pose a risk of amblyopia if persistent (4). In adults, a coexisting sebaceous carcinoma may be present.

Juvenile xanthogranuloma (nevoxanthoendothelioma) is a non-Langerhans' cell histiocytosis. Well-defined purple to red nodules appear on the skin and the anterior surface of the eye (24,135). The reaction may also appear in the orbit and in the uveal tract within the eye. Lesions in the iris may cause spontaneous hyphema, which may be bilateral (22). The cutaneous lesions are characterized by a mononuclear lipidized or non-lipidized cells and Touton giant cells. The lesions tend to involute spontaneously. Occasionally, intraocular lesions cause intractable glaucoma requiring enucleation. The mononuclear cells are usually limited to the uveal tract but may involve adjacent structures as well. This type of proliferation may occur in adults as well as in children.

Molluscum contageosum is a poxvirus infection of the epithelium of the skin. Multiple, well-demarcated, elevated, umbilicated, nontender nodules develop on the skin. Shedding of viral particles from infected epithelial cells near the lid margin may produce a localized, persistent, follicular conjunctivitis, which brings the patient to medical attention (113). This infection is often found associated with immune deficiency (23). The lesion consists of acanthotic stratified squamous epithelial cells with prominent intracytoplasmic inclusions (Figure 11-5). The contents of infected cells desquamate into the environment from the umbilicated region. Conjunctival follicular reaction from *Molluscum contageosum* is difficult to treat medically. Lid margin lesions often require surgical excision.

A *sty or hordeolum* is an abscess of one of the adnexal units of the eyelid skin. This condition is very infrequent and is generally not biopsied. An external hordeolum is superficial and an internal hordeolum is located deeper in the eyelid skin. In most cases, a lesion described clinically as a sty may actually be a chalazion (see above) (108).

Preseptal cellulitis is a bacterial infection of the subcutaneous tissue of the eyelid anterior to the orbital septum. The orbital septum is a fibrous diaphragm extending from the periosteum of the orbital rim to the eyelid margin. Its major function is to compartmentalize and protect orbital fat from external influences. Preseptal cellulitis may present with a marked increase in soft-tissue volume. If the inflammatory reaction or infection extends posterior to the orbital septum (orbital cellulitis), there is swelling of intraorbial tissue forcing the globe to move anteriorly (proptosis or exophthalmoses). The malposition of the globe as well as direct inflammation of the extraocular muscle may cause limitation of excursion of the globe (ophthalmoparesis) resulting in double vision (diplopia). The infected tissue is rarely biopsied, although fine needle aspirations may be used for culturing microorganisms. The most common organisms found are *Haemophilus influenza* and *Streptococcus* species (31,76). Treatment is with systemic antibiotics.

NEOPLASTIC LESIONS OF THE EYELID SKIN

Melanocytic nevus is a proliferation of abnormal melanocytes at the dermal-epidermal junction. Clinically, the lesions appear as hyperpigmented areas of the skin that vary in degree and extent of pigmentation (see Chapter 25).

Spindle cell and epithelioid nevus (Spitz nevus) is a proliferation of melanocytes that has many histological features of melanoma even though the clinical course is usually benign. The lesion may present as a rapidly enlarging, well-demarcated nodule of the eyelid skin (60). Histological patterns include spindle and epithelioid cell as well as mixed types. The mitotic rate is usually low, and actively dividing cells are generally located near the superficial dermis. The size of the melanocytes usually diminishes toward the base of the lesion. Regional lymph node metastasis has been reported; however, even in those cases the long-term course remains favorable. Cutaneous malignant melanoma of the skin may arise in childhood (18).

Oculodermal melanocytosis is congenital hyperpigmentation of the skin associated with hyperpigmentation of the ipsilateral episcleral tissue located deep to the conjunctiva. Hyperpigmentation is present at birth and generally remains stationary in intensity and extent throughout the life of the individual. The lesions may become more prominent during puberty (120). An increased concentration of typical melanocytes is located at the dermal-epidermal junction and in the episcleral tissue. There is minimal risk of malignant transformation of cutaneous and episcleral melanocytes. There is an increased risk for ipsilateral uveal melanoma, particularly for Caucasians affected with the problem. Malignant transformation may also occur in the nevus itself as well as orbit, optic nerve, and brain (97).

Xeroderma pigmentosa is an autosomal recessive defect in the DNA repair systems of the body. Exposure to ultraviolet light induces the formation of basal cell carcinoma, squamous cell carcinoma, and malignant melanoma in the facial skin of even young children. The number of lesions is characteristically large. Children may also develop squamous cell carcinoma of the conjunctiva as well as pterygia. Ocular surface scarring from these lesions may significantly affect visual function (51,85). There is no treatment to replace the deficient DNAase that normally repairs ultraviolet-damaged DNA. Treatment of individual lesions is accomplished by standard surgical therapy. Prevention is attempted by limiting exposure of the facial skin to sun light.

Basal cell nevus syndrome (Gorlin-Goltz) is an autosomal dominant condition associated with the development of basal cell carcinoma at multiple sites. Basal cell carcinoma of the eyelid has been observed in a 16-year old. The eyelid lesions tend to be aggressive and may involve the orbit (63). In addition to cutaneous malignancies there are associated skeletal abnormalities such as odontogenic cysts of the jaw and bifid ribs. Palmar and plantar pits as well as mental retardation and intracranial calcifications may be present. As with other ectodermal dysplasia syndromes, the ocular surface may be abnormal due to meibomion gland dysfunction. Degenerative pannus may be associated with loss of vision (68).

Neurofibromatosis type I (NF-1) is an autosomal dominant condition in which various types of abnormally produced cytokines lead to the development of neoplasia of various types. The syndrome is recognized by the presence of hyperpigmented cutaneous regions with a smooth contour (Café-au-lait) spots and proliferation of elements of peripheral nerve (neurofibroma) within the eyelid skin. The neurofibromas are acquired and consist of nodular or plexiform patterns. The nodular form generally does not affect eyelid function. The plexiform variety may produce massive enlargement of the soft tissues of the face including the eyelid, causing major deformations of the eyelid margin (ectropion or entropion). The cornea depends on normal eyelid function to maintain corneal clarity. Corneal scarring can result from eyelid distortions. Surgical debulking of lesions is occasionally performed to improve eyelid function, which is often only partially successful (34). The lesion consists of proliferation of all cellular elements of the peripheral nerve including axons, Schwann cells, and perineural cells. Occasionally, the native peripheral nerve trunk can be identified. The lesions of plexiform deformity are often progressive. In this tissue as well as elsewhere, there is a risk of developing malignant peripheral nerve sheath tumors.

Optic pathway glioma may be found in 15% to 20% of individuals with NF-1 and may account for significant morbidity in young children. Symptoms include vision loss, proptosis, and precocious puberty (34,79). Globe enlargement and glaucoma have been reported on the ipsilateral side of orbito-facial NF-1 (95). The association of NF-1 and uveal melanoma appears to be coincidental (64) (see Chapter 10).

THE PEDIATRIC CONJUNCTIVA

Structure of the Conjunctiva

The conjunctiva extends from the eyelid margin to the junction of the cornea and sclera (the limbus). The conjunctiva is a mucous membrane with many specialized regions. Along the internal lining of the eyelid (the tarsal conjunctiva) the surface is tightly adherent to the tarsal plate. There is redundant conjunctiva at the forniceal regions of the eyelid to allow full mobility of the globe. The conjunctiva over the globe (bulbar conjunctiva) is loosely applied. The associated accessory lacrimal tissue is regional and clinically inconspicuous. There is associated nonnodal lymphoid tissue in the subepithelial space, particularly in the region of the fornix. The conjunctival surface is composed of stratified, nonkeratinizing epithelium containing a variable number of intraepithelial goblet cells found most prominently in the bulbar conjunctiva (Figure 11-6A,B). Dendritic melanocytes and antigen-processing cells (Langerhans cells) are present throughout the surface epithelium. The underlying tissue is nonspecific, delicate fibrovascular tissue (substancia propria). The substancia propria of the conjunctiva fuses with the fibrovascular tissue of the globe (episcleral tissue and Tenon capsule) at the limbus but is otherwise distinct and separate. Lymphatic channels are present throughout the substancia propria of the conjunctiva to the limbus where they form arcades. The limbus is one of the locations of stem cells

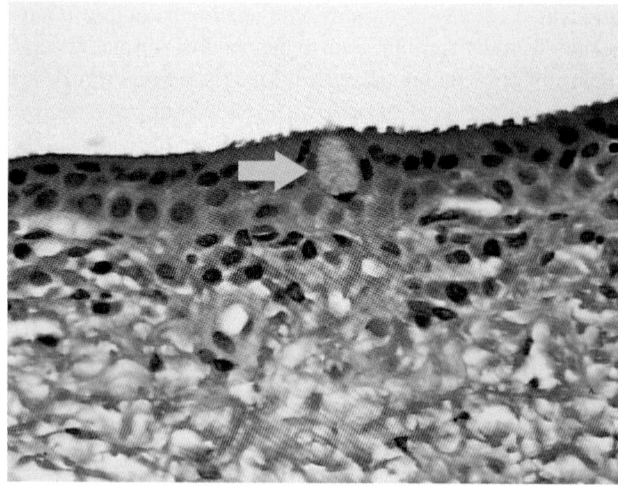
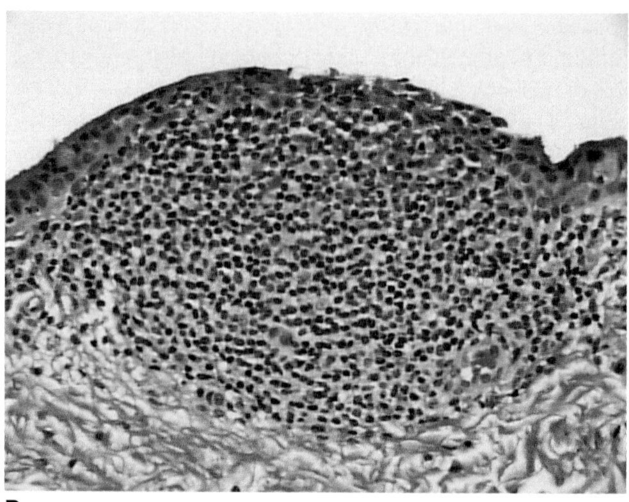

A B

FIGURE 11-6■ **A:** The normal conjunctiva is composed of nonkeratinizing squamous epithelium containing goblet cells (*arrow*). Goblet cells are concentrated in the bulbar conjunctiva (Hematoxylin-eosin stain, original magnification ×100). **B:** There is normally a nonnodal collection of lymphocytes within the stroma of the conjunctiva, particularly in the far periphery (conjunctival fornix) (Hematoxylin-eosin stain, original magnification ×100).

and is a common site for the development of both squamous cell carcinoma and malignant melanoma. Lymphatic channels of the conjunctiva drain to the preauricular, parotid, and submental nodes (38,61).

SURGICAL PROCEDURES OF THE CONJUNCTIVA

The repair process of the conjunctiva results in scarring that may restrict movement of the globe and may result in a cosmetically unacceptable appearance. Therefore, biopsies of the conjunctiva are generally limited in extent even in the presence of a suspected malignancy. Most biopsy sites of the conjunctiva are described in reference to the limbus (e.g., the specimen is from the 3 o'clock position of the right eye and extended nasally). Biopsies for the diagnosis of systemic disease (e.g., sarcoidosis) are often performed in the inferior fornix where there is a normal high density of resting lymphocytes. Surgical access to the eye (cataract incision, orbital biopsy) and for strabismus procedures is through the conjunctiva. Inclusion cysts may arise at a suture line if the wound margins are not precisely apposed. Inclusion cysts may be removed by a second procedure to improve cosmetic appearance. Conjunctival tissue is essentially a nonrenewable resource, making the surgeon hesitant to remove any more tissue than is absolutely necessary. Histopathologic interpretation of biopsy is often difficult because this tissue, which may harbor potentially serious disease (melanoma, lymphoma, rhabdomyosarcoma), is delicate and can easily be crushed with the forceps; furthermore the samples are usually small. Adding to the processing problem is the tendency of the conjunctival tissue to curl or deform, if immersion fixed in formalin. The optimal method of submission is to fix the conjunctiva after the tissue has been flattened on support media such as filter paper. Many tumors of significance arise at the limbus (the junction of cornea and sclera). Therefore, the tissue sections are usually oriented perpendicular to the limbus. Close communication with the surgeon is necessary to establish tissue margins of significance.

INFLAMMATORY CONDITIONS OF THE CONJUNCTIVA

Microbial infections of the conjunctiva due to bacteria, viruses, and fungi occur commonly but are rarely biopsied. Trachoma remains a worldwide cause of significant blindness that results from infection with *Chlamydia trachomatis*. Early stages of the disease are characterized by an indolent follicular conjunctivitis. Late in the evolution of the disease, superficial scarring of the tarsal conjunctiva deforms the eyelid orientation (entropion) to allow eyelashes (cilia) to come in contact with and damage the superficial structure of the cornea. Blindness from trachoma results from the corneal scarring and not from the conjunctival infection. Treatment of established cases is surgical (132).

Ligneous conjunctivitis is an accumulation of fibrin in the subepithelial space of mucous membranes throughout the body, caused by a systemic reduction in the levels of plasminogen (90,136). The condition usually presents in young females due to conjunctival symptoms (itching, burning, decreased vision) because of the presence of subconjunctival nodules composed of a woody-like accumulation of fibrin (114). The overlying epithelium is usually unremarkable, although signs of drying (epithelial thinning, reactive keratinization) may be present. Amorphous fibrin sometimes associated with an acute or chronic nongranulomatous inflammatory infiltrate may be present. Topical plasminogen concentrate has been used for treatment (90). Ligneous conjunctivitis may be associated with congenital occlusive hydrocephalus and juvenile colloid milium (114).

DEVELOPMENTAL ABNORMALITIES OF THE CONJUNCTIVA

Developmental abnormalities of the conjunctiva are infrequent. Occasionally, redundant, tortuous, dilated lymphatic vessels (lymphangiectasia) are present that may lead to symptoms because of dryness of elevated portions of the tissue or because of hemorrhage into the lymphatic spaces.

Episcleral osseous choristoma is due to embryonic rests of bone in the episcleral tissue, which may present as a stationary nodule often in the upper temporal quadrant of the conjunctiva or of the lower eyelid (50). The lesion generally consists of mature bone surrounded by mature fibrous tissue.

Limbal dermoid of the conjunctiva is a choristomatous nodule of dermal tissue, usually located at the limbus. The nodule may also be situated on the central corneal surface with only a minimal connection with the vascular system of the conjunctiva. The mass is an obstruction to vision light and alters the contour of the cornea. Without treatment, the lack of symmetric vision in a child can lead to amblyopia (failure of physiologic development of vision, "lazy eye") (12). The surface is nonkeratinizing squamous epithelium overlying dermal elements including mature fat. The lesion may involve the full thickness of the cornea and sclera but does not involve intraocular structures (93) (Figure 11-7). The lesion is usually solid without cystic elements as are found in cystic dermoid of the orbit (see below). Surgical removal may not result in normalization of corneal curvature.

Neuronal ceroid lipofuscinosis is a group of neurodegenerative diseases inherited in an autosomal recessive pattern that results in accumulation of lipopigments within cells and consequently with disruption of cellular function (94). The conjunctiva is considered a convenient site for diagnostic biopsy. Intracellular "curvilinear bodies and fingerprint bodies" are found by examination with transmission electron microscopy (126) (Figure 11-8A,B) (see Chapters 5 and 10).

MELANOCYTIC ABNORMALITIES OF THE CONJUNCTIVA

Melanosis of the conjunctiva is recognized clinically as hyperpigmentation of the conjunctiva without alteration of the surface contour of the conjunctiva. The lesion is present at birth or develops in early childhood as a yellow-brown to brownish black discoloration. There is a larger than average number of typical melanocytes and a higher than average accumulation of melanin in the conjunctival epithelium basal layers. This lesion is not a precursor for melanoma.

Melanosis of the episclera and scleral tissue is visible melanosis of the tissues deep to the conjunctiva, although the normal, transparent conjunctiva is visible as an area of slate gray discoloration. Heterochromia iridis and hyperpigmentation of the uveal tract may be present. Hyperpigmentation may extend to the meninges of the optic nerve and the brain. The contour of the overlying conjunctiva is not altered. The lesion may also present at birth and is generally stationary. A larger than average number of melanocytes is present as individual cells or small clusters interspersed in connective tissue. There is an increase in the number of melanocytes in the uveal tract; these melanocytes are larger than the indigenous melanocytes. The melanocytes are relatively hyperpigmented (Figure 11-9A,B). This lesion is a risk factor for melanoma, but the melanoma arises in the ipsilateral uveal tract or deep orbital tissues but not in the conjunctiva.

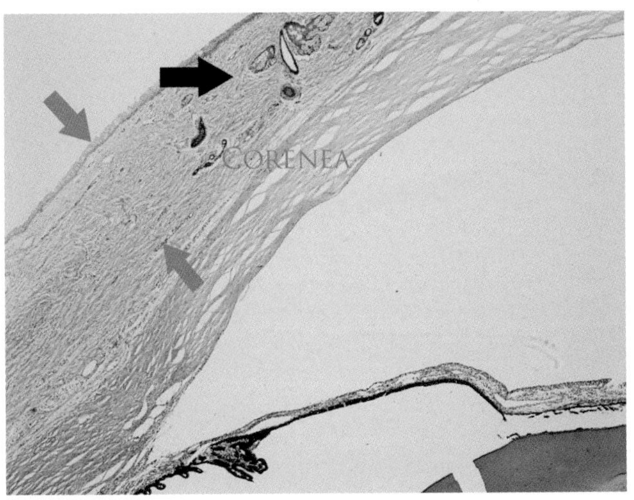

A

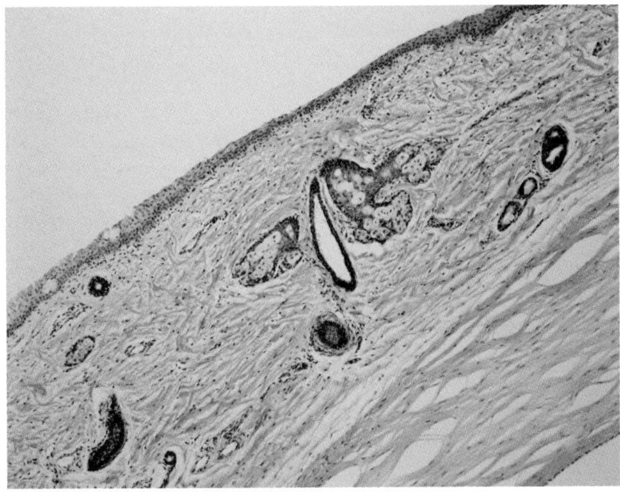

B

FIGURE 11-7 ■ Limbal dermoid, light micrograph. **A:** Solid dermoid is present at the limbus (junction of cornea and sclera) involving the eye of a child, which was enucleated for other reasons. The conjunctiva is markedly thickened (between two *gray arrows*) (Hematoxylin-eosin stain, original magnification ×20). **B:** Mature pilosebaceous units as well as eccrine and apocrine glands (*black arrow*) are present. The lesion tends to remain stationary in size and location. If the opacity involves the central visual axis retinal function may not develop in a normal manner (amblyopia) (Hematoxylin-eosin stain, ×40 original magnification).

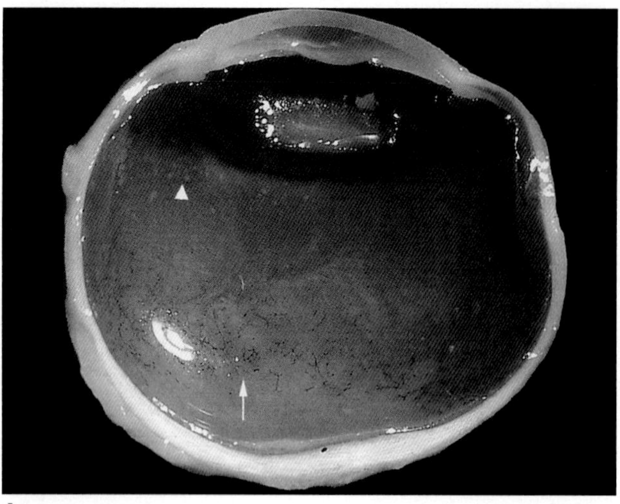

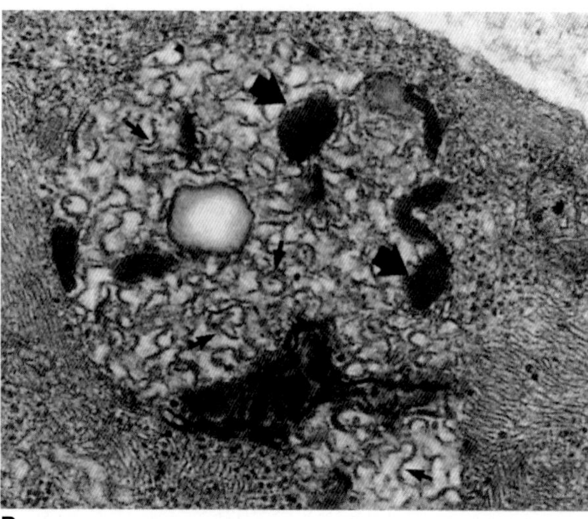

A B

FIGURE 11-8■ **A:** Neuronal lipofuscinosis is a neurodegenerative disease resulting in pigment degeneration of the retina (*arrow* and *arrow head*). **B:** The conjunctiva may be used as a biopsy site to confirm the diagnosis by transmission electron microscopy. Within affected cells curvilinear and fingerprint bodies are recognized (*arrows*).

Nevus of Ota is a risk factor for ipsilateral uveal and orbital melanoma, particularly if it occurs in Caucasians. In addition to the hyperpigmentation of the eye (melanosis oculi) and orbit, there is hyperpigmentation of the skin of the eyelids and periorbital facial skin. Meningeal melanocytoma has also been associated with the nevus of Ota (104).

Acquired melanosis of the conjunctiva may be a characteristic of aging in races with high-density melanin pigmentation of the skin. Onset is well beyond the pediatric age and is generally bilateral and indolent. Primary acquired melanosis (PAM) of the conjunctiva primarily involves women. PAM in races with low-density melanin pigmentation is a risk factor for conjunctival melanoma, if the condition is unilateral with the onset in middle age. The risk is greatest if atypia of the abnormal melanocytes is present. This condition has not been reported to involve the pediatric age group (39).

Melanocytic nevus of the conjunctiva is an accumulation of abnormal nevus cells in the region of the conjunctival epithelium. Early in life, in the junctional nevus stage, the nevus is a relatively well-demarcated area of the conjunctiva, which may not alter the surface contour and may be amelanotic or lightly pigmented. Conjunctival nevi are often

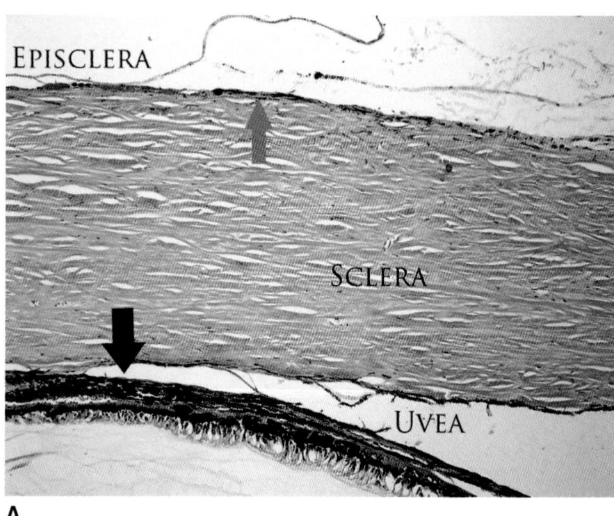

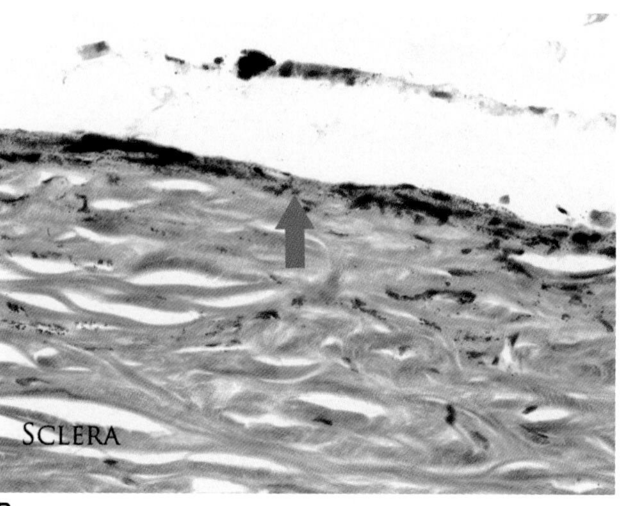

A B

FIGURE 11-9■ **A:** Melanosis oculi may be associated with hyperpigmentation of the uveal tract (*black arrow*) as well the episcleral surface (*gray arrow*). The uveal pigmentation is a clinical risk factor for the development of uveal melanoma (Hematoxylin-eosin A ×40 original magnification). **B:** The hyperpigmentation of the episcleral fibrous tissue is clearly visible clinically but subtle histopathologically (*gray arrow*) (Hematoxylin-eosin stain, original magnification ×200).

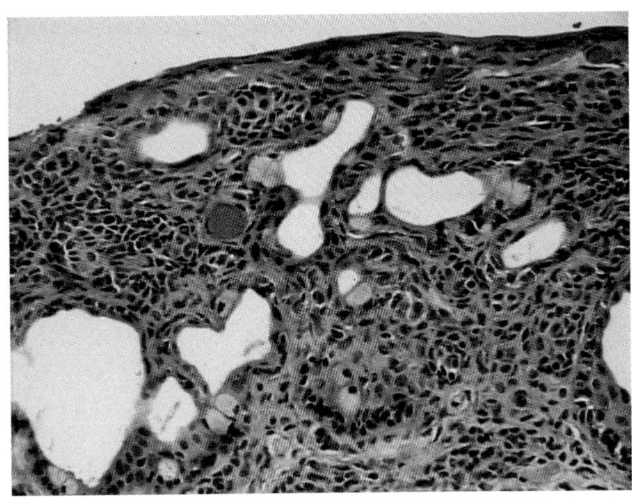

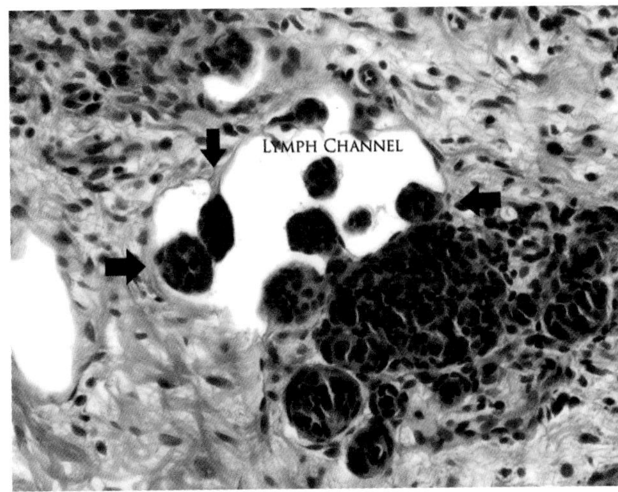

A B

FIGURE 11-10 ■ **A:** Conjunctival nevus. The surface stratified squamous cells are somewhat flattened. Multiple cysts lined by squamous epithelial cells are located among nests of nevus cells in the subepithelial tissue. Material accumulating in the cystic spaces may simulate growth by clinical appearance (Hematoxylin-eosin stain, original magnification ×100). **B:** Aggregates of melanocytic nevus cells may indent the lining of lymphocytic channels in the conjunctival stroma suggesting lymphatic invasion and possible metastasis. The appearance of the cells is bland and the aggregates are covered by lymphatic endothelial cells (Hematoxylin-eosin, original magnification ×400).

associated with an anomalous development of the conjunctival epithelium, where the conjunctival epithelium is drawn into the substancia propria of the conjunctiva to form solid nests of squamous epithelium or cysts lined by squamous epithelium (Figure 11-10). The cysts may alter the surface contour of the conjunctiva, particularly if the cystic lining contains goblet cells or accessory lacrimal tissue that secretes into the lumen of the cysts. The melanocytes may be extensively pleomorphic, ranging from spindle-shaped cells to epithelioid cells. These atypical melanocytes may occur in the epithelium of the inclusion cysts giving the false impression of lymphatic spread of a melanoma. Clusters of melanocytic nevus cells may indent the lining of lymphatic channels also giving the appearance of possible distant spread (41).

Later in the natural history of a conjunctival melanocytic nevus, a dermal component develops (compound nevus). At puberty, there may be proliferation of melanocytes and increased density of pigmentation creating concern about the presence of a conjunctival melanoma. The nevus may appear to enlarge because of simultaneous proliferation of the squamous epithelial component of the inclusion cysts and increasing volume of the contents of the cyst (137). Irritation from drying of the elevated surface of the conjunctiva may also add to the impression of growth due to reactive inflammation and vascularization.

Melanoma of the conjunctiva is the possibility of melanoma arising in a preexisting nevus or *de novo* even though PAM with atypia does not generally occur in the pediatric age group. A review of the international literature by Taban found 28 reported cases in individuals under the age of 15 years (125,137).

A conjunctival melanoma is an atypical proliferation of conjunctival melanocytes that has the potential of wide spread metastasis and death. In the presence of a preexisting nevus or in the absence of histological signs of a preexisting nevus there is invasion of the substancia propria of the conjunctiva by atypical melanocytes. Features of malignancy include the presence of mitotic figures, atypical melanocytes in clusters, lack of the expected maturation with depth, and infiltrative growth at the deep margin. Cytological features such as a spindle-shaped appearance of the cells is of no prognostic significance (87).

Squamous carcinoma of the conjunctiva is usually associated with exposure to ultraviolet light in middle-aged or elderly persons (99). The lesion may present as a papilloma, a gelatinous lesion, or as a leukoplakic mass of the conjunctiva. The initial histopathologic findings are atypia progressing to carcinoma *in situ*. The lesions are invasive if the underlying basement membrane is breached. Squamous cell carcinoma of the conjunctiva is usually indolent but may spread to regional nodes. Spindle cell and mucoepidermoid variants tend to be more aggressive and may invade the eye itself. Squamous cell carcinoma of the conjunctiva rarely involves the pediatric age group, and is seen in xeroderma pigmentosum.

THE PEDIATRIC CORNEA

Structure of the Cornea

The cornea is the dominant element of optical system of the eye, providing up to 80% of its refracting power. The power of the cornea is determined by its curvature, a feature that is highly conserved throughout life. The cornea is composed primarily of extracellular matrix (the corneal stroma). The principal component of the corneal stroma

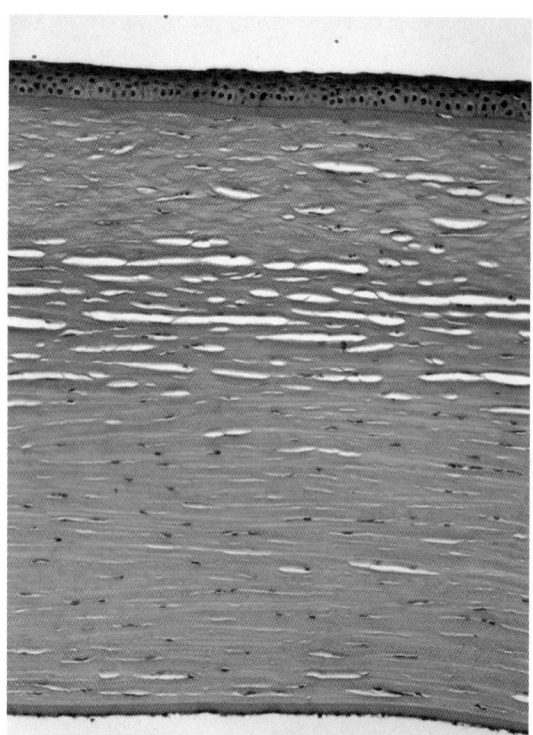

FIGURE 11-11 ■ Normal cornea. The surface epithelium is stratified, nonkeratinized squamous epithelium that does not contain goblet cells. The epithelial basement membrane is not visible by light microscopy when the epithelium is normal. The corneal stroma is composed of uniform collagenous fibers regularly separated by proteoglycans. The splitting artifact of the stroma between collagenous lamellae is a normal finding. Lack of the splitting artifact correlates with clinical corneal edema. Descemet membrane continues to thicken throughout life. There are no firm architectural attachments between Descemet membrane and corneal stroma and Descemet membrane and corneal endothelial cells. Corneal endothelial cells are similar to mesothelial cells of the pleura and maintain corneal hydration (Periodic acid/Schiff stain; original magnifications ×20).

is uniform type I collagen bundles separated at a precise distance by highly specialized and uniform proteoglycans. The interfiber distance is determined by the degree of hydration of the proteoglycans (Figure 11-11). The anterior surface of the cornea is composed of extraordinarily homogeneous nonkeratinizing squamous epithelium. The corneal epithelium does not contain goblet cells or antigen-processing cells. The normal basement membrane of the corneal epithelium is not visible by light microcopy. It rests on an acellular band of dense type I collagen (Bowman membrane) that is found only in primates and birds. Bowman membrane probably functions in maintaining corneal curvature, does not thicken with age, and is not restored if damaged by pathologic processes (Figure 11-12). The corneal endothelium is derived from neural crest and not mesoderm and therefore, is not stained by vascular endothelial markers (e.g., factor VIII). The corneal endothelium produces a thick basement membrane (Descemet membrane) that is not physically attached to the corneal stroma and thickens continuously throughout life (38,61).

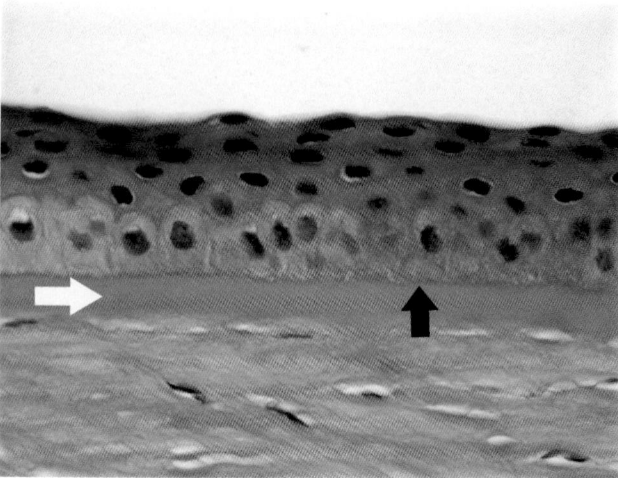

FIGURE 11-12 ■ Normal corneal anterior surface. The corneal surface is nonkeratinized and is composed of extremely uniform cells. The epithelial basement membrane is not visible by light microscopy when the epithelium is normal (*black arrow*). Bowman layer is acellular type I collagen that is not replaced if damaged (*white arrow*) (Periodic acid/Schiff stain, original magnification ×200).

SURGICAL PROCEDURES OF THE CORNEA

Biopsy of the cornea is performed infrequently except in the case of infection (fungus and acanthamoeba) that is resistant to therapy. Repair processes of the cornea result in loss of transparency and therefore, biopsies are extremely small and originate as far away from the visual axis (center of the cornea) as possible. Most of the biopsy specimens, in the case of suspected fungus, will be submitted for culture; however, histopathologic evaluation in cases of suspected acanthamoeba is more likely to be diagnostic than microbiologic studies.

Classically full-thickness penetrating keratoplasty has been the most common method of treating disease-damaged corneas. A trephine, usually 7.5 mm in diameter, is used to create an incision through 90% of the thickness of the cornea. The incision is completed with scissors. The entire specimen is submitted only after the donor graft is in place and secured. Drying artifacts of the host cornea may accumulate during the interval. The most common indications for penetrating keratoplasty in the pediatric age group are keratoconus and opacity from corneal trauma. More recently surgical techniques have been developed in which only the specific layer of the cornea, which has been altered by disease, is removed [deep lamellar keratoplasty (DLK)]. Currently, the most common use of this procedure is for the removal of the diseased posterior corneal stroma (e.g., Descemet membrane and endothelium in Fuchs endothelial dystrophy). The diseased host tissue is replaced by a similar donor graft tissue. Surgical treatment of Fuchs endothelial dystrophy is not usually performed in the pediatric age group. Surface damage of the cornea at any age may be treated with anterior lamellar keratoplasty. The surgical procedure and problems associated with visual recovery limit the use of this procedure in children.

The object of refractive corneal surgery is to change the optical qualities of the cornea. Initially, the strategy was to flatten the central cornea by weakening the peripheral cornea (radial keratotomy). Currently various methods are used to decrease corneal thickness [photorefractive keratectomy (PRK) and laser *in situ* keratomileusis (LASIK)] and thus, reduce the refractive error of myopia (nearsightedness, the eye is too long). Because the optical system of the eye is not stable until age 18 to 22 years, these procedures are generally not performed in children.

DEVELOPMENTAL ABNORMALITIES OF THE CORNEA

There is a small range of tolerance of corneal diameter in which the normal optical properties of the cornea function. Similarly, the radius of curvature must be precise in order to focus light on the retina.

Microcornea is a condition in which the cornea is less than 9 mm in diameter (horizontal limbus to limbus) at 1 year of age. Other anatomic abnormalities such as microphthalmos with cyst or persistent hyperplastic primary vitreous (PHPV) often coexist. Even nonsyndromic-associated abnormalities of the trabecular meshwork are likely to cause glaucoma. The cornea tissue generally has a normal histological appearance except in the case of Peters syndrome (see following).

Megalocornea is a condition in which the cornea is greater than 11.5 mm in diameter (horizontal limbus to limbus) at 1 year of age. If the megalocornea is acquired and unilateral, then distortion by intraocular pressure (buphthalmos of congenital glaucoma) may be the cause of enlargement rather than developmental process. Developmental abnormalities are generally stationary and tend to be bilateral. Megalocornea may be associated with ectopia lentis and other abnormalities of the anterior segment. The structure of the cornea in megalocornea is generally normal.

Cornea plana refers to a flattened corneal contour (decreased radius of curvature). The associated decrease in axial length often results in severe degrees of hyperopia (farsightedness) (44). The corneal structure may have characteristics of nonuniform sclera rather than uniform cornea and be opaque (129).

Sclerocornea is the result of failure in the development of the unique homogeneous architecture of the cornea. The corneal tissue resembles sclera both in radius of curvature (cornea plana) and in characteristics of extracellular matrix.

Peters anomaly most likely results from failure of separation of the cornea from the crystalline lens during embryonic development. In most cases the central posterior corneal stroma, Descemet membrane and central corneal endothelium are absent. Rupture of Descemet membrane (Haab stria), during forceps delivery or with corneal enlargement from glaucoma (buphthalmos), may have a similar histological appearance.

INFLAMMATORY CONDITIONS OF THE CORNEA

Herpes Simplex Keratitis

The herpes simplex virus initially affects the body as a systemic infectious disease with the cutaneous expression being a vesicular dermatitis. Live virus is retained in the Gasserian ganglion and, for undetermined reasons, will periodically travel via sensory peripheral nerve to infect the corneal epithelium. Cytopathologic effects of the infected cells are seen as a linear, branching ulcer of the corneal epithelium (dendritic figure). With repeated episodes of infection, the corneal stroma becomes involved, not with direct viral infection but with lymphocytic infiltration, peripheral vascularization, and proteolysis of the extracellular matrix (discoid herpes keratitis, herpes metaherpetica). The cornea can thin to the point of rupture. There may or may not be an intact epithelial covering. Bowman membrane ulcerates and Descemet membrane ruptures resulting in perforation of the cornea. A foreign body granulomatous response to the severed ends of either or both Bowman membrane and Descemet membrane is a unique response in herpes simplex keratitis. There may be an extensive lymphocytic infiltrate in the keratoplasty specimen that may not be appreciated clinically. The degree of vascularization of the cornea is a risk factor for immunologic corneal rejection (119) (see Chapter 6).

Acanthamoeba Keratitis

Acanthamoeba is a protozoa commonly found in soil and water. The organism can gain access to the cornea via microabrasions often associated with wearing contact lenses (17). The organism is neurotropic accounting for the extreme pain associated with infection. Organisms can be identified clinically by using confocal microscopy (35). The trophozoite form is motile and is able to spread extensively throughout the corneal stroma creating necrotizing keratitis and scarring. The encysted form can be identified throughout the cornea with most commonly used stains (Figure 11-13). There

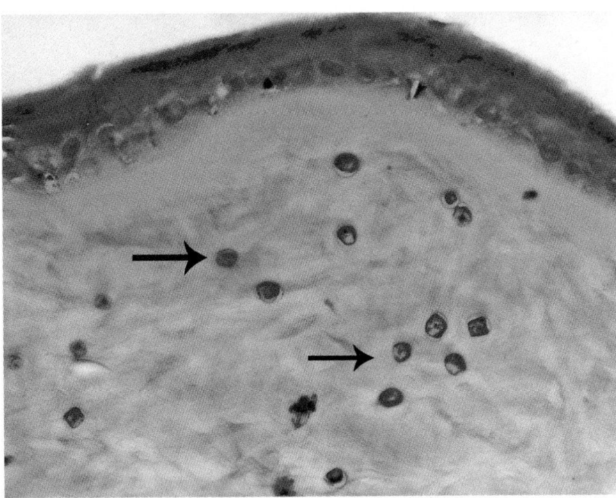

FIGURE 11-13■Acanthamoeba keratitis. Multiple encysted acanthamoeba organisms are present throughout the corneal stroma (Periodic acid/Schiff, original magnification ×200).

may be a limited inflammatory response because of topical treatment. Acanthamoeba is resistant to most forms of therapy (29). Occasionally, biopsy for diagnosis or penetrating keratoplasty for advanced stages of the infection is performed.

DYSTROPHIC CONDITIONS OF THE CORNEA

Corneal dystrophies are metabolic abnormalities of the cornea that cause clinically detectable opacities. The prevalence of corneal dystrophy is extremely low. Dystrophies are mostly inherited (usually in an autosomal dominant pattern, except for macular corneal dystrophy), bilateral, usually symmetric, progressive (at markedly variable rates), and recur in corneal grafted tissue. Recently, multiple clinical entities that were thought to be distinct from each other have been found to have a common genetic defect located at 5q31 (62,71,74,124). The discovery has totally changed the classification of corneal stromal dystrophies. The dystrophies reclassified include Reis-*Bücklers* dystrophy, lattice corneal dystrophy type I, granular corneal dystrophy, and Avellino corneal dystrophy (103). Even though the conditions are inherited, they generally do not progress sufficiently to be treated with penetrating keratoplasty in the pediatric age group except for congenital hereditary corneal dystrophy (CHED). (See cornea 2008;27(Suppl 2:S1–S42)).

CHED is a congenital structural abnormality of the corneal stroma and endothelium that is inherited both in autosomal recessive (2,116) and autosomal dominant forms (70). The two forms are genetically distinct but both involve a region of chromosome 20 (13) with the recessive form mapping to 20p13 (92). At birth both corneas of an affected individual are thickened and opaque. The corneal collagen fiber diameter is nearly twice the normal diameter and is haphazardly arranged in a manner that limits transmission of light. Descemet membrane is often thin and the endothelium is abnormal. There is associated secondary bullous keratopathy and degeneration of Bowman membrane. Subepithelial amyloid accumulation has been observed in some cases (81). Treatment is penetrating keratoplasty.

Map-dot-fingerprint dystrophy, also known as anterior basement membrane or Logan-Guerry dystrophy, is characterized by excessive production of basement membrane material by the corneal epithelial cells (105). The epithelium is loosely adherent because of abnormal adhesive properties of the redundant basement membrane. Corneal abrasions tend to occur more frequently (recurrent erosion) (Figure 11-14). Secondary reactive degeneration of the Bowman membrane and anterior corneal stroma may occur if the abrasions are extensive, leading to superficial corneal opacification that is permanent. The condition rarely affects the pediatric age group and is treated topically.

Meesmann corneal dystrophy is a degeneration of the corneal epithelial cell cytoskeleton. Because the corneal epithelial cells are replaced in a 10-day cycle this condition is rarely symptomatic and does not require treatment.

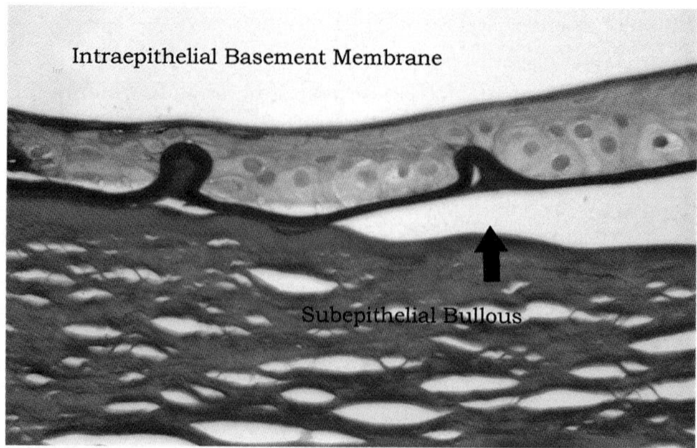

FIGURE 11-14 ▪ Map-dot-fingerprint dystrophy. Epithelial cells have produced a defective basement membrane with abnormal adhesive characteristics. The epithelium has separated from Bowman membrane to form a subepithelial bulla. The bullae are fragile and may rupture causing exposure of nerve endings and pain. The absence of epithelial cover is a risk factor for corneal infection (Periodic acid/Schiff stain, original magnification ×100).

Dystrophies of Bowman membrane (Reis-*Bücklers* and Thiel-Behnke dystrophies) occur extremely rarely. There is destruction of Bowman membrane possibly due to a protease produced in the corneal epithelium. Recent evidence suggests a relationship to a mutation of the TGFBI gene (21).

Macular corneal dystrophy is an abnormality of mucopolysaccharide production by corneal keratocytes (1). The condition is inherited in an autosomal recessive pattern (16q22). Unlike the other corneal dystrophies, there is a systemic abnormality in a subset of persons with macular corneal dystrophy.

Granular corneal dystrophy is an abnormality of protein metabolism of the corneal epithelial cells associated with the genetic defect at 5q31. Well-demarcated deposits occur initially in the anterior corneal stroma and progress to accumulate in deeper stromal layers. The intervening collagen is normal.

Lattice corneal dystrophy type I is an accumulation of amyloid in the corneal stroma often in a linear pattern associated with the genetic abnormality at 5q31. Other subgroups of lattice corneal dystrophy involve other processes leading to amyloid deposition and are extremely rare (123).

Avellino corneal dystrophy is caused by the genetic defect at 5q31 that presents initially with features of granular corneal dystrophy and then progresses to develop features of lattice corneal dystrophy in addition to the features of granular corneal dystrophy. Persons living in Avellino, Italy were the initial group studied that led to the discovery of the common genetic defect at 5q31 being associated with multiple phenotypic expressions (40).

Fuchs endothelial dystrophy is a common corneal dystrophy that is expressed generally in the older age groups. The corneal endothelium is not able to dehydrate the cornea and the corneal stroma becomes thickened and opaque. Descemet membrane becomes thickened focally (corneal guttata) or generally (multilaminar Descemet membrane). There is a significant loss of corneal endothelial cells far beyond what

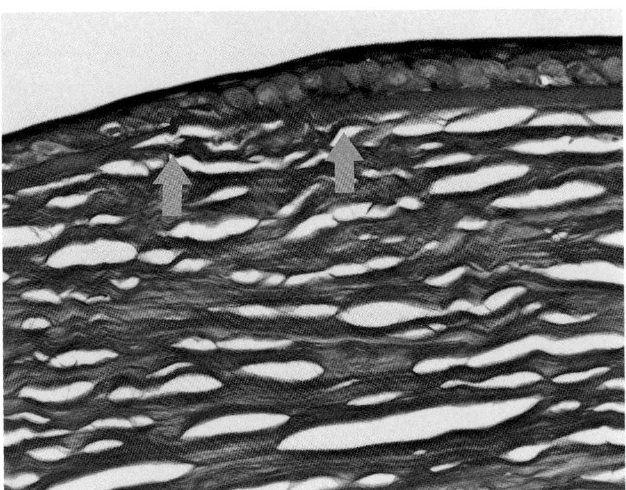

FIGURE 11-15 ■ Keratoconus. There is a break in Bowman membrane (*arrows*) that is associated with alteration of the anterior contour of the cornea (formation of a "cone") (Periodic acid/Schiff stain, original magnification ×200).

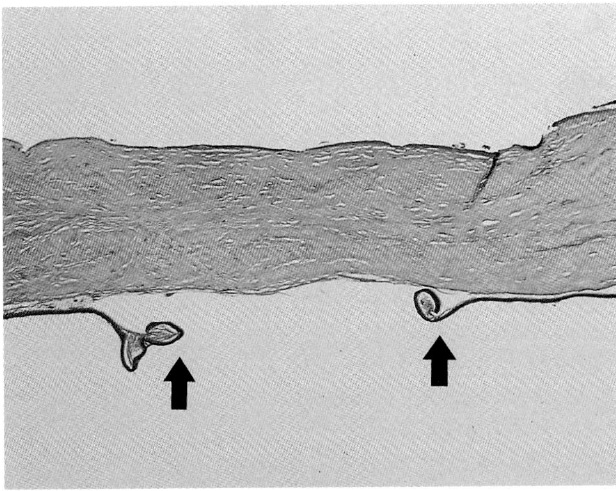

FIGURE 11-16 ■ Corneal hydrops. The lack of tensile strength of the cornea has progressed to the point of rupture of Descemet membrane, exposing the relatively dehydrated corneal stroma to be exposed to aqueous humor (*arrows*). Hydration of the corneal stroma results in opacity in the region of rupture. With time, the posterior cornea may repair causing at least partial clearing of the stroma and improved vision. (Periodic acid/Schiff, original magnification ×40).

is observed during normal age-related attrition. There are secondary degenerative changes of the corneal epithelium, bullous keratopathy, including intraepithelial basement membrane formation, subepithelial bullae, degenerative pannus, and reactive destruction of Bowman membrane. This condition is one of the most common indications for penetrating keratoplasty particularly following cataract extraction in older age groups (131).

Posterior polymorphous dystrophy consists of endothelial cells with epithelial cell characteristics (59). The epithelial cell metaplasia can be detected clinically but is generally stationary and does not affect visual function. Generally, no treatment is required.

Keratoconus is an acquired localized stromal thinning of the cornea, usually located in the inferior nasal quadrant (Figure 11-15). The thin area is displaced anteriorly by normal levels of intraocular pressure altering the anterior corneal curvature. Keratoconus is not considered to be a corneal dystrophy. Its etiology has not been established but appears to relate to abnormal activity of the matrix metalloproteases normally produced by corneal keratinocytes. The natural history is one of progressive myopia and irregular astigmatism that can be corrected initially with contact lenses. In time, some cases progress to corneal stromal scarring in the region of the cone (the area of maximal distortion). The stroma becomes thin to the point where corneal rupture is possible. Rupture of Descemet membrane in the region of the cone may allow aqueous from the anterior chamber to instantaneously hydrate the normally dehydrated corneal stroma (corneal hydrops). There is sudden appearance of corneal opacity that may slowly clear over weeks or months as the corneal endothelium repairs. Complete clarity is rarely accomplished. Distinct, focal breaks of Bowman membrane characterize keratoconus. Scarring of variable degrees is associated with the breaks in Bowman membrane. In the event of corneal hydrops, there is rupture of Descemet membrane. The severed ends of Descemet membrane generally curl inward. Endothelial cells may migrate over exposed posterior corneal stroma to establish a new, but considerably thinner Descemet membrane. Keratoconus is one of the most common indications for penetrating keratoplasty in children (36) (Figure 11-16).

DEGENERATIONS OF THE CORNEA

Band keratopathy is a degeneration of the anterior cornea often associated with chronic anterior uveitis or chronic keratitis. It appears as superficial opacification of the anterior cornea with focal oval well-demarcated areas of translucency that causes marked loss of vision. Calcium is deposited in Bowman membrane and corneal stroma by dystrophic calcification (Figure 11-17). The calcified Bowman membrane is as fragile as an egg shell and may fracture and extrude onto the anterior corneal surface. There is no effective treatment for band keratopathy (20).

THE CRYSTALLINE LENS

Structure of the Crystalline Lens

The crystalline biconvex lens is located in the visual axis posterior to the iris diaphragm and contributes about 10% of the refractive power of the eye. Until approximately age 40 years, the lens is pliable enough to allow variable focus from distance to near. After age 40, the lens loses its pliability and bifocals or reading spectacles are necessary for near

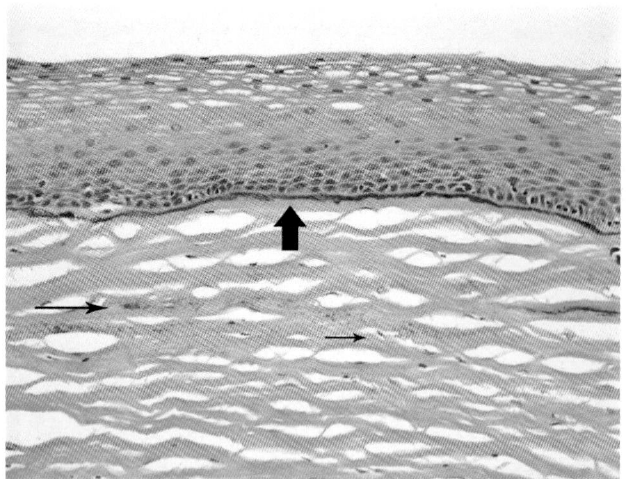

FIGURE 11-17 ■ Band keratopathy is dystrophic calcification of Bowman membrane (*large arrow*) and corneal stroma (*small arrows*) following chronic keratitis or uveitis. In advanced cases, calcified Bowman membrane may fracture and be displaced onto the corneal surface causing a foreign body sensation (Hematoxylin-eosin stain, original magnification ×40).

tasks. After age 70 years, the lens loses its transparency to the point where cataract surgery may be necessary.

The crystalline lens is surrounded by a dense type IV collagen capsule that is variable in thickness. The thickest portion of the capsule is at the point of insertion of the supportive lens zonule system of fibers and is thinnest at the posterior pole, adjacent to the vitreous in the visual axis. The lens cortex and nucleus are initially entirely cellular. In the anterior hemisphere there is a single layer of cuboidal "epithelial cells" that terminate at the lens equator by forming a curvilinear "lens bow" (the stem cells of the lens). The remainder of the lens cells lose their nuclei and become anucleate lens fibers. The lens fibers have a very regular structure associated with few organelles but have an intricate system of ball-and-socket connections between lens fibers. Lens fibers are continuously added to the surface of the cortex beneath the lens. The older fibers are compacted in central lens and tend to become opaque (nuclear cataract). Lens zonules originate from the surface cells of the pars plana, anterior to the vitreous base, and extend through the posterior chamber to the equator of the lens. Zonules are composed of fibrillin, maintain lens position, and change lens shape (and optical power) during accommodation (38,61).

SURGICAL PROCEDURES OF THE CRYSTALLINE LENS

Cataract extraction is one of the most common surgical procedures performed on the elderly in the United States. Cataract surgery is infrequently performed in the pediatric age group except for congenital cataract or inflammation-related cataract (e.g., uveitis associated with juvenile rheumatoid arthritis and trauma). Surgery is usually performed through a small corneal incision. The opaque material of the lens is removed by mechanical aspiration through a sophisticated auger-like device. The lens is replaced by a synthetic (usually plastic) lens constructed of various types of biostable polymers. In children, glasses for near tasks will be necessary because the current intraocular lenses correct only for distance. The intact lens is usually not removed, and the aspirated lens cortical material is usually not submitted for histopathologic examination. The lens capsule remains to support the intraocular lens. The posterior lens capsule often becomes opaque due to fibrous metaplasia of the remaining lens epithelial cells. A YAG laser is used as a postoperative office procedure to create a clear axial opening through this type of reactive membrane.

DEVELOPMENTAL ABNORMALITIES OF THE CRYSTALLINE LENS

The crystalline lens develops from an invagination of the surface ectoderm to form the lens vesicle. The developing lens interacts with the retina derived from the neuroectoderm to form the functional aspects of the eye. Neural crest cells form the supportive tissue of the eye and orbit. Fibers of the lens cortex form a visible suture in the shape of an inverted Y anteriorly and an inverted Y posteriorly. Subtle changes in lens biochemistry may lead to opacification of lens fibers as punctate or diffuse opacities or opacification of the Y sutures. A rich, temporary, vascular plexus (tunica vasculosa lentis) supports the lens during embryonic development, which will undergo apoptosis approximately at birth. At that time, nutritional support for the lens changes to the aqueous produced by the cilia epithelium. The tunica vasculosa lentis may be retained in various degrees to form fibrovascular membranes in the papillary space (persistent fetal vasculature.) The lens is supported by a system of zonules composed primarily of fibrillin. Variations in zonular structure may allow various degrees of lens dislocation (15).

Primary aphakia is an exceedingly rare event because of the contribution of the lens to ocular development; if the lens is not present the remainder of the globe is unable to develop.

Microphakia may occur in generalized ocular abnormalities such as *PHPV*. In this situation abnormalities of the vitreous will limit development of the lens. Eyes affected by PHPV are usually small with limited visual potential. Many complex factors determine lens size, most of which are not yet fully characterized. The microphakic lens is usually also spherical. The abnormal shape may be caused by deficiencies in the quality or quantity of lens zonules (19,56).

In *Lowe syndrome* the lens is small and has a discoid shape with no clear demarcation between fetal nucleus and cortex. There is apparent lack of formation or, alternatively, a degeneration of primary lens fibers at the lens equator. The profile of the equatorial lens is sharply angled and the anterior-posterior dimension of the lens is reduced. The lens is densely opaque.

A *pyramidal cataract* is a dense elevation on the anterior surface of the lens usually in the visual axis. In addition there may be absence of axial posterior corneal stroma and Descemet membrane and endothelium (Peters syndrome).

A *lens notch* may be observed in an inferior nasal hiatus of the iris diaphragm of an iris coloboma. Faulty closure of the fetal fissure during development leads to failure of formation of lens zonules in the area of the coloboma. The absence of lens zonules allows the natural pliability of the lens to form a notch at the lens equator. A lens notch is usually not associated with opacification of the lens.

Phakomatous choristoma is the presence of ectopic lens tissue in the cutaneous structures of the anterior orbital soft tissue, usually in the inferior nasal quadrant. The abnormal lens is characterized by basement membrane–producing epithelial cells and primitive lens fibers. The condition is usually stationary and not associated with other ocular abnormalities (88,140).

In *Alports syndrome*, most often inherited in an X-lined pattern, abnormal basement membrane may lead to alteration in lens contours; increase in anterior lens curvature, *anterior lenticonus*, or increase in posterior lens curvature, *posterior lenticonus*. The anterior lens capsule is thin and is characterized ultrastructurally by numerous full-thickness cracks associated with degeneration of regional epithelial cells. The capsule appears thin enough and weak enough to explain reported spontaneous lenticular ruptures. Posterior lenticonus, independent of Alport syndrome, has also been reported (102). A dot-and-fleck retinopathy also occurs in a high percentage of affected individuals (28).

CONGENITAL LENS OPACITIES

Congenital cataracts are the final expression of many types of developmental and metabolic defects and are relatively rare (52). Autosomal dominant transmission with high penetrance is most common, but autosomal recessive and X-linked transmissions also occur. It is not surprising that several cataract types have been linked to regions that regulate crystallin genes, the major proteins of the lens fibers (100). The pathologic features of congenital cataracts are classified by geographic localization of the clinical opacity.

Anterior polar cataracts arise in the papillary space as an elevated plaque that may be the result of faulty separation of the lens vesicle from the surface ectoderm or may be the result of a momentary toxic environment (e.g., inflammation) during gestation. *Posterior polar cataracts* are more likely related to failure of involution of components of the tunica vasculosa lentis (*Mittendorf dot*). Opacification in the region of the Y sutures is common and is estimated to occur in at least 20% of the population. Congenital cataract may affect any region of the lens with markedly variable degrees and patterns of relative opacity. A *cerulean cataract* is a club-shaped opacity with a blue tinge. A *zonular congenital cataract* has opacification in zones around a clear nucleus. In contrast, the fetal nucleus may be translucent or totally opaque as found in the *rubella syndrome*. There is potential risk indicated by cataract as there is intracellular sequestration of live virus within the central fiber cells of the lens, which may persist long after birth and may cause viral endophthalmitis if released during cataract surgery.

LENS OPACITIES IN DISEASES OF GENETIC ORIGIN

There are dozens of other syndromes of known or suspected genetic cause in which some form of cataract has been described; however, seldom are the clinical characteristics of the lens opacity specific for that syndrome. Extensive bibliographies of these associations are available (45), and new examples are reported yearly. The most common lens opacity in these often autosomal dominant diseases is the posterior subcapsular cataract (PSC). What may be difficult to determine is whether the cataract is directly due to the genetic defect or is a secondary effect of the disease process. Discoveries such as expression of crystallins in nonlenticular cells promise new avenues for understanding these associations (100).

In *galactosemia*, polysaccharides may accumulate in the lens, changing the state of hydration and the clarity of the lens. If the biochemical abnormality is corrected through dietary measures early in the course of the disease, the lens may return to its normal state of transparency. If the condition persists, secondary structural changes in the lens will cause permanent opacity (see Chapter 5).

Lysosomal storage diseases result from deficiency of the lysosomal enzymes necessary for cellular metabolic functions and are transmitted as autosomal or X-linked recessive traits. They show lysosomal inclusions that occur in lens epithelial cells, causing subtle anterior lens opacification.

In ***Fabry disease***, there is an intracellular accumulation of neutral glycosphingolipids, especially trihexosylceramide, in many ocular and systemic epithelial and endothelial cells (43). *Niemann-Pick disease* is characterized by accumulation of laminated membranous inclusions in many cells including the lens epithelial cells although causing minimal opacification (110).

Cataract formation is an important feature in *myotonic dystrophy*, the clinical characteristics of which include muscle weakness, cardiac muscle conduction defects, and a slowness of contracted muscles to relax. Cataracts occur in almost all adults, with myotonic dystrophy, as iridescent polychromatic crystals in a zone deep to the anterior and posterior capsules, exhibiting especially green and red colors. A posterior subcapsular stellate cataract may then develop, followed by cortical vacuoles and clefts of a nonspecific type that are not distinguishable from an aging cataract.

THE ZONULAR APPARATUS AND LENS DISLOCATION (ECTOPIA LENTIS)

The lens zonules are composed of a cystine-rich glycoprotein fibrillin, which is encoded on chromosome 15q21.1 (80).

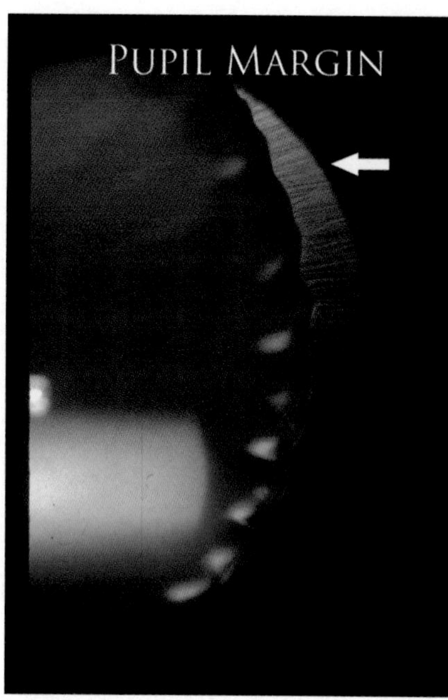

FIGURE 11-18 ■ Crystalline lens dislocation. The center of the lens is displaced (subluxated) from the pupillary margin (*white arrow*) but is not completely dislocated (luxated). Stretched zonules can be seen extending from the margin of the lens posteriorly to their insertion. The majority of lens zonules attached to the elevated portions of the lens margin.

A lens is *luxated* when it is completely dislocated from its normal position and the zonular support is nearly or completely absent. *Subluxated* lenses are partially removed from their normal position with variable degrees of zonular support remaining (Figure 11-18).

The most common cause of lens subluxation-luxation in most large series has been trauma (96). It usually follows penetrating injury or severe contusive injury and is often associated with cataract and rhegmatogenous retinal detachment.

Marfan syndrome is the most common heritable cause of crystalline lens dislocation; it is caused by mutations in the fibrillin-1 gene (*FBN1*) on chromosome 15q21.1 (30). The most important systemic abnormality of Marfan syndrome is the high risk of dissecting aneurysm of the aorta. Lens subluxation may be present at birth or may appear after birth, and may be stationary or progressive (84). The zonules can be easily seen stretching from the periphery of the lens across the peripheral pupillary space. The subluxated lens may be normal in size or small, with a flatter curvature of the lower half and a posterior bulge as a result of weakness or absence of the inferior zonules. The zonular bundles may be thin, thick, or of normal caliber but in most cases show thin and poorly aggregated zonules (106) (see Chapter 13).

Homocystinuria is an autosomal recessive disease based on a virtual absence of cystathionine β-synthase (58). Lens dislocation is not present at birth but is usually present by age 30 years. The lens is often spherical to the point where it may dislocate into the anterior chamber producing pupillary block glaucoma. The globe tends to be elongated, increasing the risk of retinal detachment and the ciliary musculature tends to be hypodeveloped. The zonular bundles inserting on the lens show an abnormal porous sponge-like appearance (107), probably as a result of the short, disoriented fibrils of which they are composed. The zonules tend to rupture midway between origin and insertion.

The biochemical defects of *Weill-Marchesani syndrome* and *sulfite oxidase deficiency* are also associated with abnormalities of zonular structure that may lead to ectopia lentis.

CONGENITAL CATARACT FROM ENVIRONMENTAL FACTORS

The developing lens is extremely sensitive to changes in its biochemical microenvironment. Even transient changes may lead to localized opacities in specific regions of the lens cortex. The closer the opacity to the epicenter of the lens the more likely the event was early in development. Lens opacities formed in this manner generally do not progress after birth and may not affect visual function.

Rubella: The rubella virus may gain access to the developing lens and infect the cells of the lens cortex during pregnancy. Infection in this manner produces a dense white (pearl-like) cataract that may be limited to the embryonic nucleus. The cataract is distinguished by retention of lens cells with nuclei in the center of the lens, which, in normal development, would have involuted and disappeared except at the equatorial lens bow (Figure 11-19). Rubella virus remains viable in the lens for years after birth (130,139). Early surgical procedures designed to remove congenital cataracts piecemeal may have contributed to virus release into the eye and subsequent viral panophthalmitis.

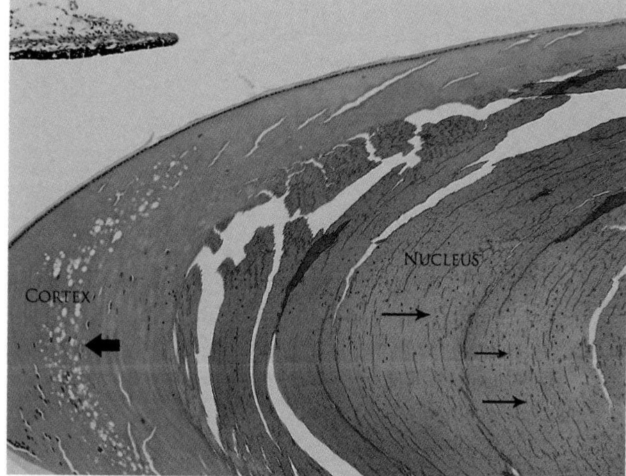

FIGURE 11-19 ■ Rubella cataract. Normally, there are no nucleated crystalline lens cells in the center of the lens, the lens nucleus. With rubella infection early in gestation the central lens cells are infected with the rubella virus, retain their nuclei (*small arrows*), and are densely opaque. There is also some degeneration of the lens cortex (*large arrow*) which also causes peripheral translucent opacity (Hematoxylin-eosin stain, original magnification ×20).

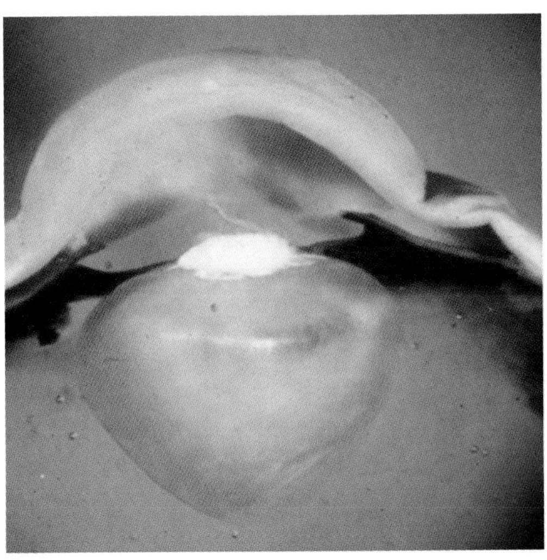

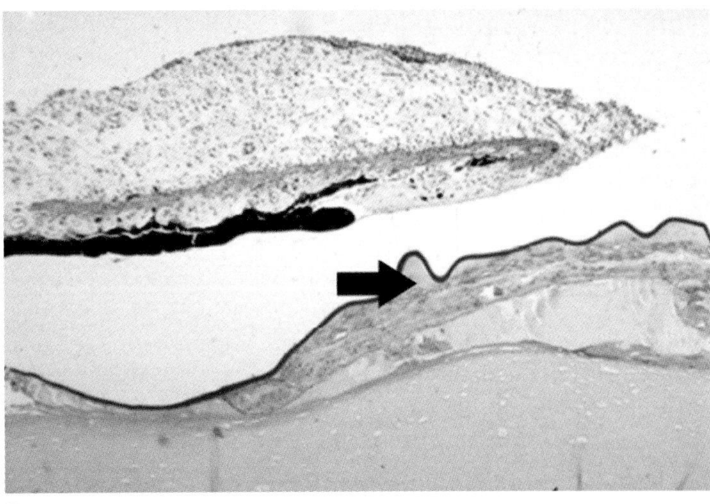

A B

FIGURE 11-20 ■ Anterior subcapsular cataract. **A:** The cornea is opaque from long-standing anterior uveitis and keratitis creating a toxic environment in the anterior chamber. **B:** Crystalline lens repair processes have caused a dense anterior subcapsular cataract (*arrow*) by fibrous metaplasia of the crystalline lens epithelium. The lens capsule undulates because of contracture of the fibrous scar (Periodic acid/Schiff stain, original magnification ×40).

Toxic cataract: With chronic damage from anterior uveitis, the anterior lens epithelial cells will be stimulated to undergo fibrous metaplasia resulting in dense anterior subcapsular cataract (Figure 11-20). Following trauma, intraocular inflammation, or vitrectomy, crystalline lens cells may migrate from the lens equator to the posterior pole of the lens to create a "ground-glass" opacification of the posterior lens cortex. The migrating cells retain their nuclei but are very polymorphic. The posterior subcapsular cells are said to resemble urothelial cells of the bladder and have been called "bladder cells (15) (Figure 11-21).

Traumatic cataract: The crystalline lens will instantly become opaque if the lens capsule is disrupted allowing fluid to disturb the homogeneity of the lens cortex as in a penetrating injury of the cornea or sclera. A shock wave associated with blunt trauma may also cause the formation of a cataract; however, the clinical onset of the opacity may be days or years following the injury. This type of cataract may be characterized by posterior migration of the lens epithelium from the equator along the internal surface of the posterior capsule to the posterior pole of the lens. This type of PSC is also associated with advanced diabetes mellitus, chronic treatment with corticosteroids and with inflammation (14).

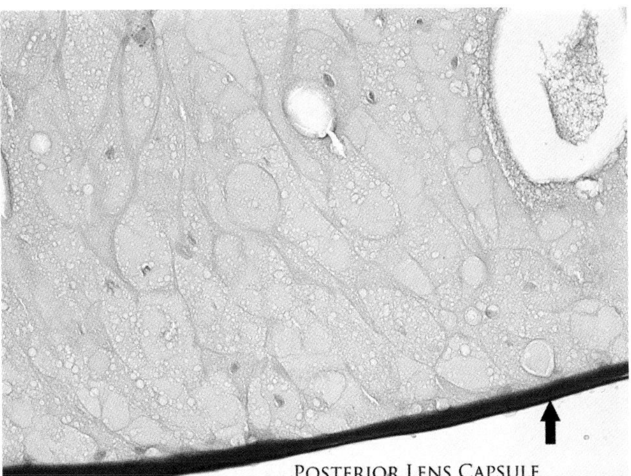

FIGURE 11-21 ■ Posterior subcapsular cataract (PSC). Lens epithelial cells have migrated from the lens equator to the posterior cortex of the lens in the visual axis. The cells have retained their nuclei and are irregular in shape and size manifesting as a "ground glass" appearance of the posterior lens cortex clinically (Periodic acid/Schiff stain, original magnification ×40).

THE VITREOUS

Structure of the Vitreous

The vitreous is composed of a type II collagen matrix containing hyaluronic acid. The majority of the vitreous is composed of water and may attain a volume of 4 cc weighing 4 g. The vitreous is formed near the junction adherent to the internal surface of the retina at the optic disc, in the region of the peripheral macula, along the course of retinal blood vessels and at the posterior surface of the crystalline lens. The matrix of the vitreous degenerates over time (usually beyond the pediatric age) and separates from the surface of the posterior retina forming "floaters," which cast a symptomatic shadow on the retina. The vitreous is a biochemical sink and also functions in maintaining retinal attachment (38,61).

Surgical Procedures of the Vitreous

The entire vitreous can be surgically removed (vitrectomy) without immediate effect on the structure of the eye. In most cases, a cataract will develop due to subtle biochemical alteration. Vitrectomy is most often used to remove acquired mechanical factors affecting the retina (e.g., epiretinal membrane formation associated with macular hole and subretinal neovascularization from a variety of causes). Vitrectomy is also used to correct fibrovascular membranes (traction retinal detachment) that are found in advanced stages of diabetic retinopathy. Occasionally, vitrectomy is used in pediatric cases for diagnostic purposes (diffuse infiltrating retinoblastoma, medulloepithelioma). The specimen often contains only a small number of cells, as is found in fine needle aspirations used at other sites. Usually, the histopathologic diagnosis is established by examining a cellblock. Fine needle aspiration is rarely done intraocularly because the mechanical forces generated during aspiration are much more difficult to control than the aspiration forces generated by the highly sophisticated vitrectomy instrument.

Intermediate uveitis or pars planitis is a localized inflammation probably of autoimmune origin that involves the vitreous base and peripheral retina (8). Children and young adults are primarily affected. The majority of affected patients are asymptomatic and become symptomatic only with secondary changes such as cystoid macular edema (reactive swelling of the retina), cataract, or glaucoma. In the region of the peripheral retina there is phlebitis and retinal edema. The vitreous structure collapses and becomes opaque over the area of proliferation of the nonpigmented epithelium of the ciliary body. Granulomatous inflammation is present in the region of reactive proliferation (53). Medulloepithelioma of the ciliary body and diffuse infiltrating retinoblastoma may present in a similar manner (122).

Familial exudative vitreoretinopathy is a congenital abnormality of the peripheral retinal circulation resulting in secondary extracellular matrix abnormalities throughout the vitreous in the form of organized membranes and focal opacities (snowflake-like) (7). Autosomal dominant, recessive, and X-lined inheritance patterns have been identified. At least five mutations associated with familial exudative vitreoretinopathy have been identified on the long arm of chromosome 11 (67). Along with the basic vascular abnormality the membranes are responsible for causing retinal detachment, displacement of the macula, cataract, and anterior chamber angle closure (6).

THE OPTIC NERVE

Structure of the Optic Nerve

The optic nerve is the aggregation of retinal ganglion cell axons that exit the eye through the scleral canal in the posterior medial portion of the sclera. The hydraulic integrity of the globe is maintained by a sieve-like structure (the lamina cribrosa) at the plane of the sclera through which the optic nerve axons pass. Just beyond the lamina cribrosa, oligodendroglia form a myelin sheath around each axon. This addition increases the diameter of the optic nerve from 1.5 mm at the scleral canal to 3.0 mm in the myelinated portion. The axons of the optic nerve are supplied by branches of the ophthalmic artery in the arachnoid, extending across the subarachnoid space to the pia. The central retinal artery crosses the dura and arachnoid 12 mm posterior to the lamina to assume a central position in the proximal optic nerve but does not supply the optic nerve itself. The dura of the optic nerve is contiguous with the periostium of the orbital apex and with the sclera. The subdural space is truncated or closed through the optic canal of the sphenoid bone. The subarachnoid space of the optic nerve is contiguous with the subarachnoid space of the central nervous system (38,61).

Surgical Procedures of the Optic Nerve

The optic nerve is a sensitive structure that is in a relatively surgically inaccessible position. The anterior approach usually requires removal of a portion of the orbital rim. The best exposure is via a frontal craniotomy. On occasion biopsy of the optic nerve may be necessary in cases where a diagnosis cannot be established by other means and usually where there is no or limited visual potential for the eye. Fistualization of the meninges (optic nerve fenestration) has been attempted in certain limited medical conditions that do not usually affect the pediatric age group.

Optic nerve gliomas are juvenile pilocytic astrocytomas that cause fusiform enlargement of the optic nerve. In many cases the tumor limits visual potential but is not a threat to the life of the child. Approximately 15% of persons with NF-1 will have optic nerve gliomas. In this setting, the clinical course may be more aggressive but the tumor rarely, if ever, undergoes malignant transformation (78,112). Only rarely will an optic nerve glioma extend into the eye. Two cytological patterns are found in pilocytic astrocytomas: areas of fibrillar matrix with oval to round nuclei and a more mucoid matrix that may contain microcysts. Rosenthal fibers (intracellular electron-dense material surrounded by glial elements), eosinophilic granular bodies (membrane-bound intracellular osmophilic material), and microcalcifications also characterize the lesion. Neither Rosenthal fibers nor granular bodies are unique to pilocytic astrocytoma. Surgical resection of the optic nerve or enucleation may be necessary if there is sufficient proptosis to cause degeneration of the cornea or abnormal development of the orbit. Risk factors for a poor therapeutic outcome include the association with NF1 or involvement of sensitive structures such as the optic chiasm (3,65) (see Chapter 10).

Meningioma of the optic nerve may arise in the arachnoid sheath of the optic nerve (primary optic nerve meningioma) or may involve the orbit from an intracranial meningioma, usually one situated along the sphenoid ridge. Optic nerve meningioma is uncommon. Most are of the transitional and meningotheliomatous types. They usually do not invade the eye itself but may cause proptosis and ophthalmoplegia due to mass effect of the tumor. Treatment is usually surgical. Treatment with external beam radiation is being evaluated (75).

THE ORBIT

Structure of the Orbit

The globe is housed in a 30 cc orbit bordered by bone that provides physical protection for the globe, primarily by the presence of the orbital rim. The interior orbit is separated from the soft tissues of the face by the orbital septum, a fibrous membrane that originates from the periostium of the facial bones at the orbital rim. The rectus and oblique muscles have their origin at the periosteum of the orbital apex and function to align the two globes, allowing the brain to receive two slightly dissimilar images providing for perception of depth. The veins traversing the orbit have no valves. Direction of blood flow is determined by differential pressure gradients between the internal and external carotid systems. The only epithelial structure in the orbit is the lacrimal gland, a portion of which is located anterior to the orbital septum (the palpebral lobe) and a portion is posterior to the septum (the orbital lobe). The ducts from the orbital lobe extend through the palpebral lobe to reach ostia in forniceal region of the conjunctiva. There are no lymphatic channels or lymph nodes in the orbit except the lymphoid tissue associated directly with the lacrimal gland. The only cartilaginous structure in the orbit is the trochlea in the superior nasal orbit that serves as a pulley to direct orientation of the superior oblique tendon. Orbital soft tissue is divided into multiple intercommunicating compartments by delicate fibrous septa. The area between the rectus muscles has been referred to as the intraconal space, but that space has no unique functional or prognostic significance for tumors. Preseptal soft tissue forms the eyelids, the conjunctiva, and the lacrimal drainage apparatus. The eyelids protect the eye from the external environment and close when stimulated by visual threats, movement of the eyelashes, or disturbance of corneal sensation. The orbicularis oculi closes the eyelids, and the levator palpebrae open the eyelids. The eyelid is also responsible for forming and maintaining the tear film. The tear film has at least three functional layers: an aqueous portion that contains oxygen and other nutrients, a mucous portion that allows smooth layering of the aqueous portion, and a lipid portion that retards evaporation of the aqueous portion. The major volume of aqueous is not formed by the lacrimal gland in the orbit but is formed by accessory lacrimal gland acini located in the upper eyelid, the upper conjunctival fold (the fornix), and the conjunctiva directly covering the globe (bulbar conjunctiva). The lacrimal gland itself plays only a minor reflex role of tear film function. Tear film components exit via puncta located at the superior and inferior nasal eyelid margins. Tears and surface debris flow through the canaliculus to the nasal lacrimal duct and finally to the lateral wall of the nasal mucosa under the inferior turbinate. A pumping mechanism for aqueous is thought to function via contraction of the orbicularis oculi. The caruncle is a sequestered portion of the lower eyelid margin and contains all of the dermal elements of the eyelid but is covered by mucous membrane contiguous with the conjunctiva (38,61).

Surgical Procedures of the Orbit

As indicated with the optic nerve, surgical approaches to the orbit are technically difficult and undertaken only with strong clinical indications. Lacrimal gland tissue is usually removed anteriorly through the skin and orbital septum. Particularly when adenoid cystic carcinoma is encountered, bone in the region of the lacrimal fossa is often removed. Because of the evolution of treatment of rhabdomyosarcoma only a biopsy sampling of the tumor is required prior to chemotherapy and radiation (although debulking procedures may be performed). In the past the entire contents of the orbit including all eyelid tissue to the orbital rim (exenteration) were required. Tumors located in the posterior orbit are best approached via a frontal craniotomy. Occasionally expanded orbital contents are decompressed into an adjacent sinus cavity such as in aggressive Graves disease. Release of trapped orbital contents in an orbital floor fracture is indicated only if the entrapped tissue causes major abnormalities of movement of the globe.

A *dermoid cyst* of orbital tissue is a cystic choristoma usually containing benign dermal elements that tend to progressively enlarge because of internal desquamation of the surface epithelium and adnexal units. The cyst arises from embryonic rests of mesenchyme that tend to be adjacent to membranous bones particularly in the region of facial fusion lines (46). A classification by location has been proposed. Juxtasutural cysts are often found along the orbital rim and are attached to bone by fibrous septa that do not distort the bone. Sutural dermoid cysts (including giant dermoid cysts) originate in the synostosis of orbital bones and may extend within cancellous bone or may extend either into the orbital cavity or into the intracranial cavity. This type of cyst is associated with defects of bone and may develop the appearance of a draining sinus. A soft-tissue dermoid cyst develops within soft tissue and is not associated with bone.

Orbital dermoid cysts may develop either anterior or posterior to the orbital septum. Cysts present anterior to the orbital septum tend to occur at an earlier age (usually before age 5 years) and are often found at orbital rim suture lines. The cyst is usually a smooth, firm, nontender, oval mass along the superior orbital rim and is less than 2 cm in diameter. Cysts posterior to the orbital septum tend to be associated with intraorbital suture lines and present at a later age. Anteriorly positioned cysts may herniate through the orbital septum. Posterior lesions may extend through the superior orbital fissure or into the temporal fossa. Medial lesions generally do not extend into the ethmoid air cells, but superior cysts may extend into the frontal sinus. Most lesions present in the first two decades, although presentation in advanced age is also possible. There is no gender specificity.

There has been a distinction between epidermoid cysts that do not contain adnexal elements and dermoid cysts that do contain adnexal elements. However, the histological distinction does not guide management and the general term dermoid cyst is most often used. The lining of the cyst is

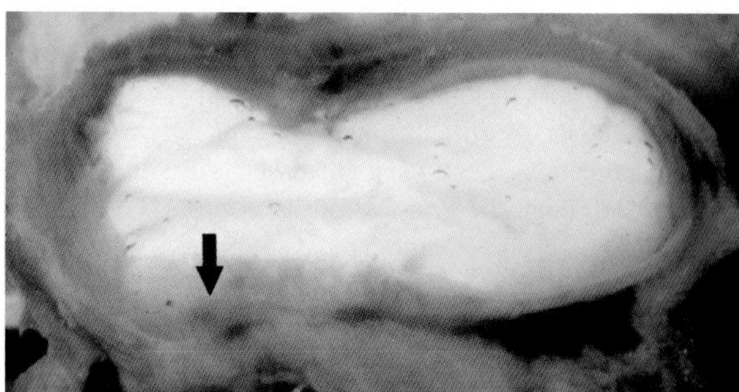

FIGURE 11-22 ■ Dermoid cyst. This cyst was removed from a 3-year old who developed superior temporal orbital rim pain and tenderness. The symptoms may have been due to rupture of the cyst wall (*arrow*), allowing a foreign body granulomatous reaction to the keratin contents of the cyst.

stratified, keratinizing squamous epithelium with or without adnexal units. When adnexal units are present, the cyst wall is usually more robust than in those lesions without adnexal units. The cyst may contain desquamated squamous epithelium, cholesterol, hemorrhage (hemosiderin), hair, or calcium. The contents may subdivide into various fluid levels. In regions were the cyst wall has ruptured, there is a granulomatous foreign body reaction and fibrous reaction that may be extensive (Figure 11-22).

Generally there is progressive enlargement of the lesion because of expanding volume of the intraluminal contents. Continuous pressure may cause erosion through bone into contiguous tissues and spaces. There is no malignant transformation. Treatment is surgical excision.

Langerhans cell histiocytosis (LCH) (formerly known as histiocytosis X) is a proliferative disorder with multiple clinically distinct forms (Hand-Schuller-Christian disease, Letterer-Siwe disease, and eosinophilic granuloma). The pathophysiology of LCH is not understood; however, there is no evidence of metabolic abnormality or infection (83). The Langerhans cell is an immune-processing cell of the monocyte-macrophage system found among the squamous epithelial cells in the skin, in bone marrow, and in the paracortical region of lymph nodes as well as multiple other sites. Despite the clinical dissimilarity, all these diseases have a histological pattern that suggests a granulomatous inflammatory infiltrate containing pathologic Langerhans cells. The normal Langerhans cell has dendritic processes, an eccentric folded nucleus, small nucleolus, and a cytoplasmic structure, the Birbeck granules, that has a central striation and a "tennis racket" profile. The function of the Birbeck granule is unknown, but it appears to be composed of plasma membrane components. Pathologic Langerhans cells lack dendritic processes but retain Birbeck granules. CD1a positivity differentiates Langerhans cells from other macrophages.

The prevalence of LCH in children under age 15 years ranges between 4.6 (55) and 8.9 (121) per 100,000. There have been no reported instances of familial, time, or geographic location clustering (83). There appears to be no gender specificity.

LCH may present as a single system disease with a lesion in a single tissue type or a multisystem disease including disseminated forms. Orbital involvement most often presents as a single system disease of orbital bone. The onset of proptosis is acute, and there are associated signs of inflammation. The degree of involvement is highly variable. When the lesion is located in orbital bones there has been concern that there would be progression to central nervous system involvement and such lesions have been treated with chemotherapy with conflicting opinions about long-term benefit. Extraocular lesions of sufficient size may cause intraocular findings of compression (choroidal folds, optic disc swelling) and compressive optic neuropathy. Rarely, LCH may present as uveitis where a vitreous biopsy could be interpreted as containing only macrophages and other benign inflammatory cells (unless stained for CD1a) (127). Secondary glaucoma may develop if the trabecular meshwork is affected. The eyelid skin is unusually not involved. Late recurrences have been reported (134) (see Chapters 22 and 27).

The light microscopic pattern is that of chronic granulomatous inflammation characterized by an infiltrate of histiocytes, lymphocytes, giant cells, and eosinophils. The presence of eosinophils is not essential for the diagnosis of LCH. Birbeck granules can be detected only by transmission electron microscopy and are found in only 20% of the cases studied (91). Langerhans cells can be identified by the CD1a stain. The number of CD1a-stained cells generally decreases as the lesion matures or regresses.

Single system disease survival is nearly 100%. Multisystem disease survival is associated with an 80% survival. Age at presentation of less than 1 year is a risk factor for a poor prognosis. LCH itself is a risk factor for secondary malignancy including Hodgkin lymphoma and acute leukemia. Treatment includes surgical debulking, chemotherapy, and simple observation.

Lymphangioma is a developmental abnormality of lymphatic vessels and their precursor cells and lymphoid tissue in the soft issue of the orbit. Normally no lymphatic channels or populations of lymphocytes are found in the orbit, thus this lesion is a choristoma and presents at birth, although the condition may not present clinically until advanced age. One clinical classification is by the character of hemodynamics in the lesion (no flow, venous flow, or arterial flow) that guides surgical and other means of therapy (49). There is no gender specificity with the majority of lesions presenting in the first decade.

Lesions of various sizes and degrees of functional significance may be found in the eyelid, the conjunctiva, anterior (preseptal) orbital soft tissue, and posterior (postseptal) orbital soft tissue. The eye itself is not involved. Noncontinuous vascular lesions may be present in patients with intracranial vascular lesions (69). The size of the lymphangioma may vary with posture, straining, or inflammation of the upper respiratory tract. There is usually less effect during indolent periods on the optical system than that found with hemangioma of similar volume. There is minimal pain unless acute hemorrhage suddenly expands the volume of the lesion. In this circumstance, there may be various degrees of loss of vision, development of an afferent pupillary defect, choroidal folds, optic disc swelling, and compressive optic neuropathy (potentially to the point of complete and permanent loss of vision). Hemorrhage may be spontaneous or associated with trauma and is more likely to occur in a child or adolescent than in older persons. This event is also more likely in the postoperative period after debulking procedures. Long-standing lesions beginning in childhood may result in expansion of the orbital contours.

The gross appearance is that of diffuse lesion with no external capsule. The cut surface is composed of vascular channels of various sizes that may contain translucent fluid or hemorrhage or both. The vascular channels are separated by fibrous septa that also may contain areas of fresh to old brownish hemorrhage. The vascular channels are lined by low-profile vascular endothelial cells with little apparent support by pericytes or extracellular matrix. Within the fibrous septa there are variable amounts of lymphoid tissue, some of which may contain germinal centers. By transmission electron microscopy endothelial cell gaps and fragmented basement membrane may be seen.

Treatment is limited to embolization and surgical debulking (27). Multiple procedures are often necessary. In extreme cases, due to corneal exposure and ulceration, enucleation of the eye may be necessary.

Idiopathic inflammatory disease of the orbit (also known as inflammatory pseudotumor of the orbit) is a syndrome of inflammation of the soft tissues of the orbit of undetermined cause. The condition may arise at any age (range 2 to 89 years) with no gender predilection (47). Approximately, 5% of cases arise in the 2 to 18 years age-group. The usual presentation is orbital pain. The onset is often explosive and may be either unilateral or bilateral. The bilateral cases may be simultaneous or sequential. The presentation tends to be bilateral in children (44%) (47). Other common findings are ophthalmoparesis, proptosis, and a palpable mass. Cerebrospinal fluid pleocytosis may be present in cases of extraobital inflammation (82). Imaging findings include thickening of extraocular muscles including the tendon insertion to the sclera (in contrast with thyroid ophthalmopathy where the tendon is spared), lacrimal gland enlargement, contrast enhancement of the sclera, and inflammation of orbital fat. Histological findings include pleomorphic inflammation, fibrovascular tissue proliferation, and fat necrosis (granulomatous inflammation to fat necrosis). There is no clonal restriction. The plasma cells may be IgG4-positive (89). Early in the course of the disease, there is a fine collagenous stroma and a rich cellular infiltrate consisting of plasma cells, eosinophils, and lymphocytes. Later in the course of disease there is often a dense deposition of extracellular matrix and a granulomatous pattern in the region of fat necrosis. The rate of progression is variable from case to case and within a given case. The response to treatment is variable. Bilaterality is a risk factor for poor therapeutic response. The histological character of the lesion may not be predictive of therapeutic success.

Rhabdomyosarcoma is the most common sarcoma in children as a proliferation of primitive rhabdomyoblasts. There are two distinct clinical presentations. The most characteristic is the sudden, unexplained onset of signs of inflammation in a child suggestive of preseptal or orbital cellulitis, except that there is no response to conventional treatment, indicating that a biopsy is necessary. In the embryonal variant, there may be marked pleomorphism of cells, which are often spindled, with prominent nucleoli and a variable degree of cytoplasmic eosinophila. Rarely, actin and myosin filaments may be identified by PTAH staining. Myosin filaments and sarcomeric units with Z-banding are evident in the tumor cells by transmission electron microscopy. The immunohistochemical profile is positive for desmin, smooth muscle actin, and focally for myogenin. A rare subtype is the botryoid rhabdomyosarcoma that may present in the subconjunctival space or anterior orbital soft tissues, suggestive of a lymphoma. It is most often seen in older children and its prognosis is more favorable than with other types of rhabdomyosarcoma (10,101).

In older children, the alveolar variant may present in paraorbital sinuses and secondarily may involve the tissues of the orbit. Clinical signs are those of a soft-tissue mass in the orbit or more likely in the ethmoid sinuses with temporal displacement of the globe. The tumor is composed of aggregation of primitive round cells with an acellular center vaguely suggestive of alveoli of a normal lung. Positive immunohistochemical markers include those for muscle with strong reactivity for myogenin.

Treatment of orbital rhabdomyosarcoma is no longer surgical but a combination of chemotherapy and radiation (25).

Tumors of the lacrimal gland, which is the only epithelial structure of the orbit, most often tend to be the result of inflammation or lymphoma, generally in the adult age groups. The most common epithelial tumor of the lacrimal gland is pleomorphic adenoma (benign mixed tumor), which is generally found in adults. The most common malignant tumor of the lacrimal gland is *adenoid cystic carcinoma*, which can occur in the pediatric age group. Early clinical signs and tumification of this neoplasm may be subtle. The most common histological pattern is that of proliferation of small cells with hyperchromatic nuclei in a "Swiss cheese" pattern. Solid, basaloid, and sclerosis patterns are also possible. The tumor tends to spread early due to its propensity to involve perineural spaces, to adjacent orbital bone. Evaluation of surgical margins in this situation is at best problematic. The long-term outcome for all cases is generally poor (48).

THE EYE

Structure of the Eye

The eye (globus oculi) is an extension of the brain that collects and transmits images gathered from the environment. Two elements are essential: a method of focusing light with tissue

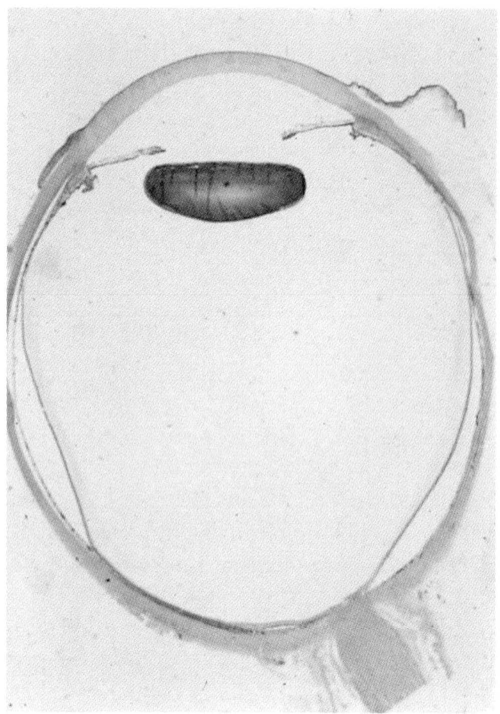

FIGURE 11-23■The normal eye. The anterior segment is composed of the cornea, anterior chamber and the posteior chamber, and cyrstalline lens. The posterior segment is composed of the vitreous, retina, choroid, and optic nerve.

lenses (the anterior segment) and a method of converting energy from a restricted portion of the electromagnetic spectrum via a photochemical process into impulses that can be integrated with the remaining processes of the brain (the posterior segment) (38,61).

The anterior segment is composed of the cornea, the anterior chamber, the iris, the posterior chamber, and the crystalline lens (Figure 11-23). The main function of the anterior segment is to transmit and refract light (reorient parallel rays of light to a focal point). The anterior chamber is bordered anteriorly by the cornea, peripherally by the anterior chamber aqueous filtering apparatus (the trabecular meshwork), and posteriorly by the iris stroma and the anterior crystalline lens capsule at the pupil. Aqueous is produced by the nonpigmented epithelium of the ciliary processes and flows through the pupil into the anterior chamber. The aqueous nourishes the anterior hemisphere of the crystalline lens and all of the tissues bordering the anterior chamber. Spent aqueous is filtered into the systemic vascular system, at the periphery of the anterior chamber initially, through a porous trabecular meshwork and then through a protein membrane [the juxtacanalicular connective tissue (JXT)]. Beyond the JXT the aqueous is discharged through the canal of Schlemm, through emissary veins, and finally into veins of the general circulatory system. Abnormalities of drainage (glaucoma) usually occur in the JXT. Tumor cells in the anterior chamber may exit the eye via the aqueous drainage channels.

The trabecular meshwork collagen cores are covered by an endothelium contiguous with the corneal epithelium. There is no epithelial or endothelial lining of the anterior surface of the iris. The iris stroma is variably pigmented by dendritic melanocytes allowing for iris "color." The degree of iris epithelial pigmentation is uniformly dense despite the degree of iris stromal pigmentation. The vessels of the iris stroma are unique because of a very thick adventitial lining. The blood column cannot be seen during clinical evaluation. The thick adventitia is probably necessary because of the continuous movement of the iris associated with changes in pupil diameter. The sphincter muscle at the pupil is located in the iris stroma. The dilator muscle fibers are located in the cytoplasm of the anterior iris pigment epithelium.

The posterior chamber is bordered by the posterior surface of the iris, the equatorial crystalline lens, the ciliary body, and the anterior border of the vitreous (the vitreous face). The posterior chamber contains aqueous. The lens zonules extend through the posterior chamber from posterior ciliary body to the lens equator and are freely mobile in that space.

The posterior segment is composed of the vitreous, the retina, the optic disc, the uveal tract, and the sclera. The main function of the posterior segment is to detect and transfer images from the external environment to the brain.

The main architectural structure of the retina is provided by the Müller cells. Incident light travels through the full-thickness of the retina before it is absorbed by visual pigments in the photoreceptor outer segments and is converted into electrical signals for the brain. The outer limiting membrane of the retina is not a true retina but a series of attachments between Müller cells and photoreceptors. The visual pigments of the rods are embedded in the plasma membrane of separate disc-shaped structures of the photoreceptor outer segments. The visual pigments of the cones are located in a folded but continuous plasma membrane of the outer segments. In both the rods and cones, the signal is transported from the photoreceptor outer segments via cilia to the photoreceptor inner segments. The photoreceptor inner segments contain abundant mitochondria. The visual signal is then passed to the horizontal, bipolar, and amacrine signal-processing cells in the middle retina across connections in the outer plexiform layer. A series of synapses in this layer forms the middle limiting membrane. The modified signal is then passed to the ganglion cells across connections of the inner plexiform layer and passed to the lateral geniculate via long axonal processes that make up the optic nerve (Figure 11-24).

Muller cells, modified astrocytes, support the retina by extending from the internal limiting membrane (a true basement membrane that it produces) across the full-thickness of the neurosensory retina to the external limiting membrane that is actually a series of connections between the apical portion of the Muller cell and the photoreceptor cells. The nuclei of the Muller cells are located in the same region as the nuclei of the photoreceptors. The retina also contains microglia and oligodendroglia. The central retinal artery supplies the internal retina to the level of the middle limiting membrane. There are three layers of capillaries posteriorly

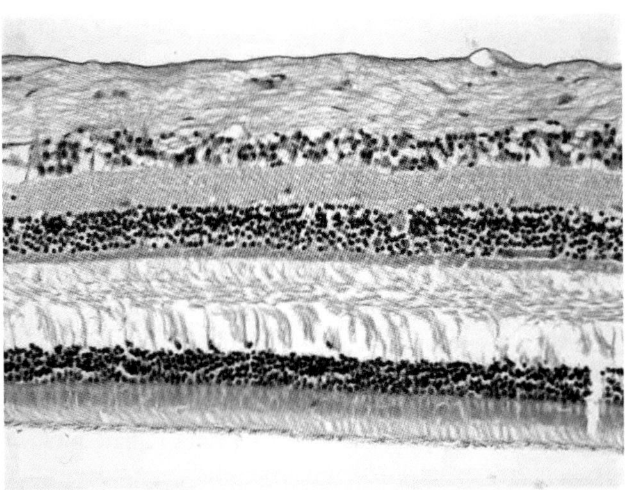

FIGURE 11-24 ▪ The normal retina: The retina contains photoreception system, an image processing system, and image transmission system. The retina is rarely biopsied (Hematoxylin-eosin stain, original magnification ×20).

and two layers in the equatorial retina. Beyond the equator there is a single capillary layer and at the periphery the retina is solely supplied by external sources in the uveal tract.

The retinal pigment epithelium (RPE) is derived from neuroectodermal cells of the outer layer of the optic cup. The RPE cell is among the first in the body to produce melanin a molecule that is necessary for the development of the neurosensory retina. The retina does not fully develop in ocular albinism. The melanin granules, which are large and oval, are easily distinguished as individual granules by light microcopy. Collections of extracellular RPE melanin in the vitreous may be mistaken for bacteria. In contrast, individual melanin granules in the dendritic melanocytes of the uveal tract have a small diameter that is not easily resolvable by light microscopy. The RPE is a monolayer of cells residing on its basement membrane with an undulating basal surface and long apical processes. The apical processes interdigitate among the photoreceptor outer segments and help to physically isolate individual photoreceptor outer segments. Interphotoreceptor mucoid substance is also present among the photoreceptor outer segments. Among the functions of the RPE is metabolism of spent photoreceptor outer segment lipoproteins and visual pigment molecules. The RPE has no physical connection with the overlying neurosensory retina but is held in place by physiologic forces generated between the vitreous and the choroid. If these factors are altered, or if the physical integrity of the neurosensory retina is violated by the formation of a physical hole, the retina will detach from the RPE (retinal detachment).

The fovea centralis is the most highly specialized region of the retina. It is a thin area of the retina located directly in the visual axis in the center of a portion of the retina designated as the macula. The macula is a region of the retina generally lying between the temporal inferior and superior vascular arcades. All factors that might interfere with the transmission of light are eliminated. The internal limiting membrane is thin; the internal retina including ganglion cells and nerve fiber layer are absent; the internal retinal circulation is absent; and the external plexiform layer is oriented obliquely to reach peripherally located ganglion cells. Only cones are present and are in such a high concentration that their profiles are cylindrical rather than cone-shaped. The RPE is thicker in this region and there is a higher concentration of melanin granules. In the center there is a avascular zone of diameter 500 μm where nutrition is solely supplied by the uveal tract vessels (choriocapillaris). There is compensatory thickening of the ganglion cell and nerve fiber layer in the retina immediately peripheral to the fovea centralis.

The uveal tract receives its blood supply from the short and long posterior ciliary system. The larger vessels are located external and progressively diminish in caliber to finally form the choriocapillaris, which is a large volume chamber lined by fenestrated vascular endothelial cells. The basement membrane of the vascular endothelium, a layer of extracellular matrix containing elastin and the basement membrane of the RPE cells together make up Bruch membrane. In the region between lumens of the choriocapillaris vessels, Bruch membrane is composed of only two layers. Venous blood is drained via vortex veins located in each quadrant through a long intrascleral channel to mix with systemic venous blood on the episcleral surface. Among the vascular channels there is a dense concentration of dendritic melanocytes characterized by retention of intracellular small caliber melanin granules. The uveal tract also contains the long posterior ciliary nerve, a branch of the trigeminal, and may contain collections of peripheral nervous system ganglion cells.

The retina is protected from vascular insults by a blood-retinal barrier similar in function and form to the blood-brain barrier. The vessels of the choriocapillaris are porous but any extravascular fluid is blocked from retinal penetration by intercellular tight junctions near the apical portions of the RPE cell. Similarly, the vascular endothelial cells of the intraretinal vascular system are connected by tight junctions to form the intraretinal portion of the blood-retinal barrier. This barrier may be breached by either inflammation or degeneration.

The optic disc is formed by the confluence of ganglion cell axons exiting through the scleral canal to form the optic nerve. The hydraulic integrity of the globe is maintained at the level of a specialized relatively porous zone of the sclera, the lamina cribrosa. The majority of the fibers exit via large pores in the superior and inferior lamina. The region is not supplied by the central retinal artery but by end arteries of the short posterior ciliary system, which is a branch of the ophthalmic artery. The exiting fibers form a central concavity, the optic cup, which is not covered by the internal limiting membrane of the retina but does contain glial tissue.

The sclera is formed by randomly oriented collagenous fibers that are more hydrated than the cornea and are therefore opaque. The sclera contains elastin fibers to accommodate changes in intravascular blood volume during systole and diastole. The sclera is relatively thin at the insertions of the four rectus muscles and the insertion of the superior oblique. The insertion of the inferior oblique is muscular rather than tendinous, and therefore, there is no compensatory thinning. The sclera is breached by multiple ostia for the short and long posterior ciliary arteries posteriorly, the vortex veins near the equator, sensory nerves anteriorly, and multiple emissary channels carrying aqueous to the venous system near the limbus.

Surgical Procedures of the Eye

In addition to cataract extraction and penetrating keratoplasty, glaucoma-filtering procedures are performed on the anterior segment. In order to reduce intraocular pressure a fistula is created at the limbus (trabeculectomy). In certain difficult cases (neovascular glaucoma) a silicone tube is placed in the anterior chamber to route aqueous posteriorly to a filtration chamber placed at the equator of the eye. Strabismus procedures consist of surgically transposing the insertion of a rectus muscle or oblique muscle or surgically shortening a muscle by excising a portion of the muscle. At the site of insertion the sclera is reduced to half thickness to allow attachment of the rectus muscle. Penetration of the globe is possible when resuturing rectus muscles. In cases of intraocular tumor or advanced degeneration of the eye from trauma or other insults (atrophia bulbae, phthisis bulbi), the entire eye is removed (enucleation). The volume of the eye is replaced with a plastic sphere and covered with conjunctiva. A contact lens-like prosthesis ("glass eye") is then placed behind the eyelids but anterior to the conjunctiva. The prosthesis should be removed and cleaned similar to cleaning a contact lens. In some circumstances, particularly with advanced endophthalmitis, and when there is no evidence of intraocular malignancy, the cornea and ocular contents are removed leaving the rectus muscles attached to the sclera, which is left in place (evisceration). Processed coral material (hydroxyl apatite) is placed in the scleral shell. Fibrous tissue will grow into and stabilize the coral relative to the sclera. A prosthesis is attached to the coral by a peg, which extends thorough a fistula in the conjunctiva. Increased mobility of the prosthesis is the clinical advantage to evisceration versus enucleation.

Abnormalities of the Eye

Retinoblastoma is a malignant tumor of the retina, resulting from an uncontrolled proliferation of retinoblasts. The malignancy is capable of widespread metastasis leading to death. The retinoblast is a pleuripotential neuroectodermal cell that will differentiate into the various components of mature retina. This tumor has become a model for heritable malignant tumors based on a genetic deletion of the Rb (retinoblastoma) gene. The tumor initially proliferates in the plane of the retina but is capable of involving all structures within the eye. The tumor may spread to the central nervous system via the optic nerve and through lymphatics and blood vessels to tissues at distant sites. In the past 10 years retinoblastoma has changed from an almost uniformly fatal disease to one in which 95% of the patients are stabilized using methods that preserve the eye and vision.

The genetic defect at chromosome 13q14 is associated with retinoblastoma in early childhood and is also associated with malignant tumors in other tissues (e.g., pinealoblastoma, osteosarcoma) at later stages of life. Thus, there is a risk of death not only from the initial retinoblastoma but from other second primary malignancies as well.

The Knudson two-hit hypothesis states that retinoblastoma arises as a result of two mutational events (72,73). If both chromosomal 13q14 regions are normal, no retinoblastoma develops; if one of the two 13q14 regions is abnormal, no retinoblastoma results. If both chromosomes 13 have a 13q14 deletion or functional abnormality, retinoblastoma results. When both mutations occur in the same somatic postzygotic cell, a single unilateral retinoblastoma results. Because the mutations occur in a somatic cell, this condition is, therefore, not inherited. In the hereditary form, the first mutation occurs in a germinal prezygotic cell, which means that this mutation is present in all resulting somatic cells and a second mutation occurs in the somatic postzygotic cells, resulting in multiple retinal tumors as well as nonretinal tumors in other sites at different times of life, such as sarcomas. In the inherited form with a germ-line mutation (i.e., a carrier of the retinoblastoma genetic abnormality), the probability of developing the tumor is 95 in 100 (32).

The tumor arises when the retinoblastoma gene is absent (point deletion) or nonfunctional in affected cells. The protein produced by the gene (RB1) is a phosphoprotein that inhibits progression through the cell cycle by binding to DNA. The RB1 protein functions as a tumor suppressor in the retina by inhibiting proliferation and promoting differentiation of retinal progenitor cells. In the absence of this protein there is an accumulation of proliferating embryonic retinal cells (9,138). In the eye the tumor arises in differentiated retina, may arise in multiple sites of the same eye and may develop in both eyes.

Retinoblastoma is inherited in an autosomal dominant pattern with incomplete penetrance even though at a cellular level the disease is autosomal recessive. In heritable retinoblastoma all of the 200 million cells of the developing retina of an individual are susceptible to acquiring a second mutation. Even though the probability of any one cell being damaged is low, the chance of one hit in 200 million is high.

Small subsets of cases of retinoblastoma arise in children with extensive deletions in chromosome 13. These children in addition may exhibit holoprosencephaly, midface dysmorphism including cleft lip and palate, and mental and growth retardation. This is the least frequent form of retinoblastoma (115).

Retinoblastoma is the most common intraocular neoplasm in children with a frequency of 1 in 16,000 to 1 in 20,000 live births in the United States (86,111). The incidence of retinoblastoma decreases with age. There is no significant sex or race predilection, and 20% to 35% of the cases are bilateral (resulting from germ-line mutations), although only

5% of all children with retinoblastomas have a family history of retinoblastoma (111). The tumor occurs in both sexes and is found in all cultures and all geographic areas. The incidence of heritable retinoblastoma appears stable. There is a recent suggestion that the incidence of nonheritable, unilateral retinoblastoma is increasing in certain groups due to environmental influences (nutritional deficiencies and human papilloma virus infection).

The heritable form is likely when another family member has been identified with retinoblastoma. Approximately 40% of cases of retinoblastoma are heritable. This form is generally diagnosed before age 12 months, much earlier than the nonheritable form. In 80% of cases of heritable retinoblastoma, retinal tumors are multiple in each eye and are found in both eyes. An associated intracranial tumor (primitive neuroectodermal tumor or trilateral retinoblastoma) is found in 2% to 3% of cases. The children who survive heritable retinoblastoma are at risk of developing osteosarcoma, soft-tissue sarcoma, and other mesenchymal tumors during the first two decades of life or later. In adulthood there is a significant risk of developing malignant melanoma and central nervous system tumors. In the elderly there is an increased incidence of cancer of the bladder. The 30-year cumulative incidence rate for second, nonocular, primary tumors is approximately 26%. The risk may be increased with radiation and chemotherapy (109).

The nonheritable form arises spontaneously and comprises about 60% of cases. The average age at presentation is 24 months. There is generally a single tumor in one eye. There is no detectable chromosomal abnormality and, therefore, much less risk of developing retinoblastoma in succeeding generations. These children have the same risk for second primary tumors, as does the general population.

Historically, retinoblastoma has presented as a fungating mass emanating from a ruptured globe. There was often associated facial soft-tissue invasion and involvement of the central nervous system. Death usually followed in the subsequent weeks or months.

Currently retinoblastoma is often discovered by parents or relatives who notice a difference between the quality of the light reflex in one eye relative to the other either in person or on viewing family photographs (118) (Figure 11-25). At this relatively early stage, usually at age less than 3 years, the eye does not appear to be inflamed and the child does not appear to be aware of loss of vision. The tumor, whether limited to the posterior retina, in the vitreous or in the subretinal space associated with retinal detachment, will reflect the light that is normally absorbed by blood pigments and melanin in the RPE and choroid. Children with retinoblastoma also may present with strabismus (misalignment of the visual axes of the two eyes), iris neovascularization (response to retinal ischemia leading to heterochromia, dilated fixed pupil, secondary glaucoma), or tumor accumulation in the anterior chamber (neoplastic hypopyon). More advanced cases may present with signs of intraocular inflammation (panophthalmitis), or ruptured globe with orbital extension. In some of cases of regressed retinoblastoma, the sole clinical sign may be a small calcified tumor in the plane of the retina with surrounding retinal pigment epithelial scarring.

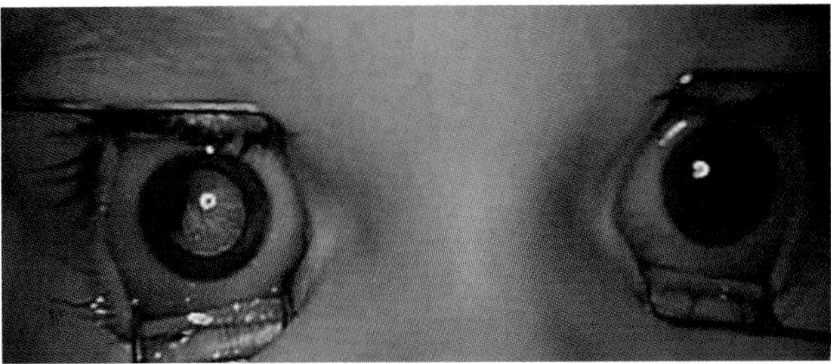

FIGURE 11-25 ■ Retinoblastoma. The right pupil appears white (*leukocoria*) because of light reflecting off a large intraocular tumor (retinoblastoma) through a clear lens and cornea. Cataract and corneal opacification are features of only an advanced retinoblastoma that fills the entire eye.

Leukocoria (white pupil) is not an exclusive sign of retinoblastoma. Any condition that changes absorption of ambient light to reflection of ambient light through the pupil may cause this sign. Some of the more common nonretinoblastoma conditions presenting with leukocoria include PHPV (a developmental anomaly of the vitreous resulting in intraocular fibrosis and retinal detachment), Coats disease (a developmental vascular malformation of the retina leading to retinal detachment) and presumed ocular toxacariasis (a parasitic intraocular infection leading to intraocular scarring and retinal detachment).

Clinical findings may be unilateral or bilateral. Bilateral cases are often asymmetric. Retinoblastoma appears initially as an isolated or multicentric translucent-to-opaque thickening or globular expansion of the retina in any quadrant of the eye (Figure 11-26). Larger tumors become vascularized with a feeding artery and a draining vein. Focal opacities within larger masses correspond to areas of dystrophic calcification. The mass progressively enlarges and expands into the vitreous where it may simulate vitreous inflammation or

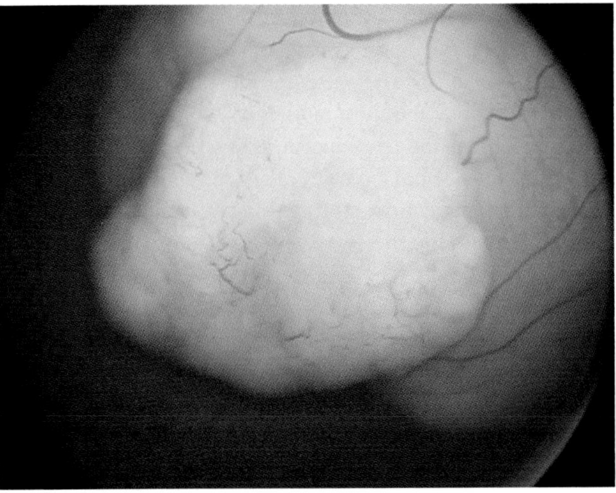

FIGURE 11-26 ■ Retinoblastoma. The intraocular tumor causing the leukocoria in Figure 11-25 extends into the vitreous space from the retina. Areas of calcification and irregular vascularization are evident.

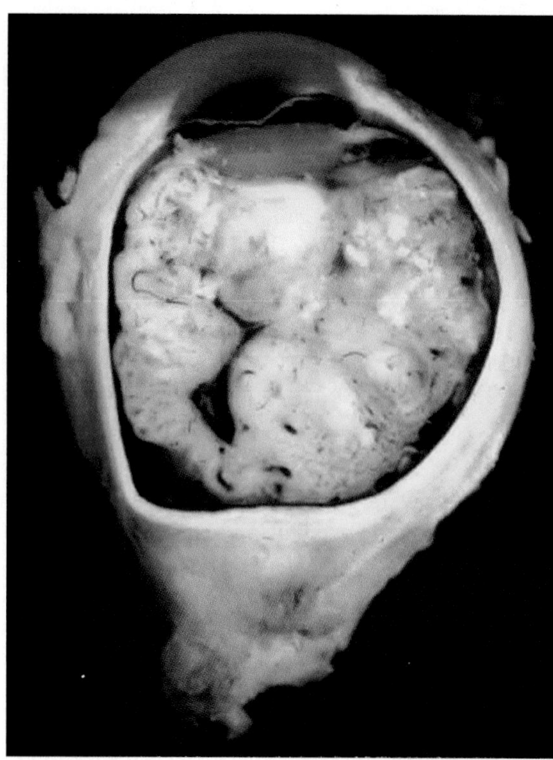

FIGURE 11-27 ■ Retinoblastoma. The tumor has filled the entire volume of the posterior segment and is displacing the lens-iris diaphragm anteriorly. The cut surface of the tumor has a "brain-like" quality. Multiple calcific highlights are present.

into the subretinal space causing a serous retinal detachment. The mass continues to enlarge to fill the entire posterior compartment and displaces the lens-iris diaphragm anteriorly (Figure 11-27). Retinal ischemia associated with tumor growth will promote neovascularization of the anterior iris surface. The anterior contour of the iris flattens and the pupil may become distorted, enlarged, and nonreactive. The delicate neovascular vessels may hemorrhage and deposit hemosiderin within the iris stroma that darkens the iris color (heterochromia iridis). Neovascularization of the trabecular meshwork interferes with the egress of aqueous and causes the intraocular pressure to rise (neovascular glaucoma). The sclera of a child is pliable and may markedly expand in an anterior-posterior dimension resulting in a large eye (buphthalmos). Increased intraocular pressure also causes corneal decompensation, opacification, and scarring. With additional tumor growth, the tumor will seek sites of weakness in the eyewall (cornea and sclera). The largest opening is the scleral canal containing the optic nerve, the most likely and earliest site of extraocular extension. The tumor may also extend through any of the numerous scleral ostia; however, this stage in the evolution of the tumor is not visible clinically. When extraocular, the tumor may extend through the lymphatics of the conjunctiva and infiltrate the soft preseptal tissues of the orbit and facial lymph nodes. Direct expansion to the posterior septal orbital tissues is usually across the posterior sclera, presenting as proptosis. The cornea is the most likely site of frank rupture of the eye when the tumor completely fills the eye. Extension through the blood vessels of the choroid, orbit, and face allows the tumor to spread to distant sites.

Fluorescein angiography of the retinoblastoma is characterized by early filling and late hyperfluorescense associated with leakage of fluorescein into the vitreous. Echographic features of retinoblastoma include general low internal reflectivity alternating with intense hyper-reflectivity in regions of dystrophic calcification. There is a shadow effect posterior to thick areas of the tumor.

Standard radiography has been important in identifying intraocular opacities (dystrophic calcification) and outlining signs of extraocular extension. Dystrophic calcification, however, can occur in nonneoplastic conditions, particularly those associated with degeneration (e.g., following trauma). Computed tomography (CT) and magnetic resonance imaging (MRI) allow more precise recognition of extraocular extension. These techniques are particularly important in the detection of mass lesions in the pineal and suprasellar regions of the brain (trilateral retinoblastoma). By CT imaging, retinoblastoma has approximately the same density as brain. By MRI T1-weighted imaging, the tumor is hyperdense relative to the vitreous, and by T2-weighted imaging, the tumor is hypodense relative to the vitreous. There is minimal-to-marked enhancement on contrast-enhanced T1-weighted images with fat suppression techniques.

In most cases of retinoblastoma, the external dimensions of the eye are normal for the patient's age. The exceptions are rare and are associated with developmental abnormalities affecting the size of the globe (e.g., microphthalmos) and advanced cases with buphthalmos or frank rupture of the globe. On gross sectioning the tumor has a brain-like consistency associated with focal areas of dystrophic calcification. The tumor may arise in any region of the retina. The location of greatest clinical significance is near the optic disc.

There are several growth patterns. The tumor may remain confined to the plane of the retina usually at the retinal periphery in a rare variant of retinoblastoma, diffuse infiltrating retinoblastoma. The usual tumor is densely white or gray with an irregular outline that is sharply demarcated from surrounding differentiated, uninvolved retina. In most cases the tumor invades the vitreous (endophytic growth pattern), into the subretinal space (exophytic growth pattern) or both. Tumor within the vitreous is poorly supported by blood vessels and develops extensive areas of necrosis giving it a friable character that appears similar to inflammation within the vitreous. This form of tumor extension may also be associated with metastatic seeding to the surface of the retina or optic disc making the distinction between multiple primary sites and multiple metastatic sites difficult. The posterior chamber, the anterior chamber, and the surface of the optic disc may similarly be seeded by tumor from the vitreous. Tumor in the subretinal space is associated with serous fluid accumulating in the subretinal space and detaching the overlying retina. Advanced tumors may invade the choroidal tissues (26).

The final growth pattern is regression. Retinoblastoma may progress in one eye and regress in the other. The remaining tumor tissue is often extensively calcified and surrounded by retinal pigment epithelial reaction for a variable distance from the main tumor.

The cross-sectional diameter of the optic disc in most patients is 1.5 mm. Immediately posterior to the lamina cribrosa, the ganglion cell axons acquire a myelin coat increasing the cross-sectional diameter of the optic nerve (dural sheaths and neural axis) to 3.0 mm. Any optic nerve cross-sectional diameter, greater than 3.0 mm, harbors extraocular retinoblastoma until proven otherwise. The desired length of the optic nerve specimen is a minimum of 10 mm. Removal of 20 mm of optic nerve is technically possible, even in a child. A short optic nerve specimen is a prognostic risk factor.

It is unusual for a cataract to form, except in the most advanced tumors characterized by extensive necrosis. In these cases iris neovascularization and anterior chamber hemorrhage (hyphema) may be a presenting clinical feature.

The majority of the tumor cells are characterized by a large vesicular nucleus with homogeneously dispersed chromatin of variable shape and size without a nucleolus. There is only a small amount of visible cytoplasm. Retinoblastoma cells are positive with S100 but are usually negative with glial fibrillary acidic protein. Ultrastructurally, the cells contain few internal organelles. In some regions there may be triplication of the nuclear membrane. Numerous mitotic figures are present throughout the tumor. There may be some background cells with features of glial cells; however, it is difficult to distinguish neoplastic glial cells from reactive glial cells originating in surrounding normally differentiated retina. Outside the confines of the retina (e.g., in the subretinal space) retinoblastoma cells tend to adhere to each other in small clusters. Multiple bizarre cells may be present. Inflammatory cells and macrophages may be present in vitreous samples.

There are several types of more differentiated cells generally grouping in the form of rosettes. Rosettes are composed of one or two layers of nuclei encircling a central space. Mitotic figures may be seen in the cells making up the rosettes. Some rosettes are incompletely formed and blend with the surrounding undifferentiated cells. Rosettes are usually found in random areas of greater differentiation rather than within areas of totally undifferentiated retinoblasts.

The most primitive and least specific of the forms is the Homer-Wright rosette. It is composed of poorly differentiated cells with definite epithelial characteristics. The central portion of the rosette does not form a definitive lumen but contains neurofibrillary processes and is thought to be composed of cells with ganglion cell characteristics. This type of configuration is found in neuroblastoma of the adrenal gland and cerebellar medulloblastoma among others. The Homer-Wright rosette appears much less frequently in retinoblastoma than the Flexner-Wintersteiner rosette.

The Flexner-Wintersteiner rosette is more differentiated and more specific for retinoblastoma as compared with the Homer-Wright rosette (Figure 11-28). The layer of cuboidal cells is taller and has a more definite epithelial character. The apical portion of the cell forms an inner limiting structure of terminal bars, delimiting the cells from a central lumen. The central lumen contains acid mucopolysaccharide that is similar to the acid mucopolysaccharide found in the interphotoreceptor mucoid substance. Some cells may have characteristics of inner photoreceptor elements such as abundant nuclei, cytoplasmic microtubules, and 9 + 0 cilia. Occasionally laminated membranous structures resembling the discs of rod outer segments have been identified.

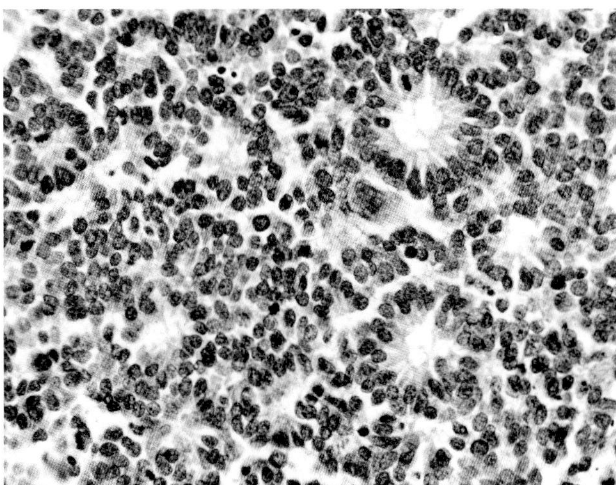

FIGURE 11-28 ▪ Retinoblastoma. Flexner-Wintersteiner rosettes are an indication of tumor differentiation.

The fluerette is the most differentiated and is the most specific for retinoblastoma but is identified in only 6% of cases of retinoblastoma. This type of rosette is more linear than round and is composed of more differentiated cells with small less basophilic nuclei and prominent eosinophilic cytoplasm. Cytoplasmic processes extend through a fenestrated membrane in a cluster-like configuration suggesting a bouquet of flowers (i.e., a "fleurette"). There may be associated areas of deposited calcium, but mitotic figures are rare in fleurettes and there is no necrosis. The cells have ultrastructural characteristics of cone photoreceptors.

Retinoblasts spread initially in the plane of the retina. There does not seem to be any architectural resistance of either the inner or outer retina to the advance of the tumor cells. The tumor spreads across the inner limiting membrane into the substance of the vitreous. In the vitreous, proliferation of blood vessels appears to be limited. Tumor cells are arranged in sleeves around dilated blood vessels originating in the retina. Approximately 50 to 200 cells are seen surrounding the lumen of blood vessels in contrast with the one to two cell layers that make up a true rosette. The thickness of the sleeve depends on the metabolic activity of the cells of the tumor. If twenty to one-hundred and ten micrometer from the vessel lumen there is ischemic necrosis and dystrophic calcification but little or no inflammatory infiltrate. Extensive cellular necrosis leads to liberation of substantial amounts of DNA that can deposit and be identified by light microscopy

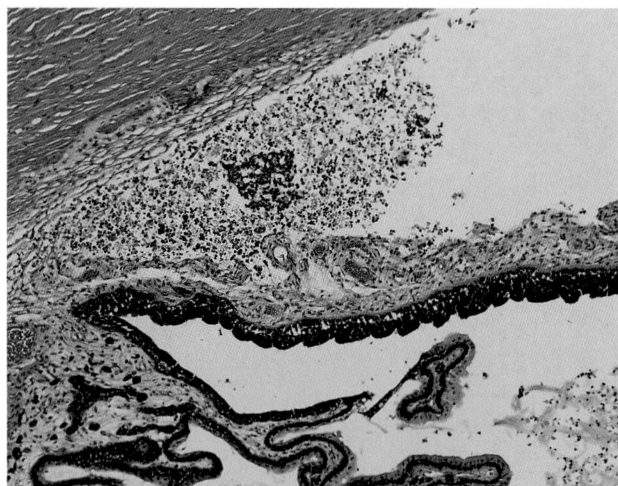

FIGURE 11-29 ■ Retinoblastoma. Both viable and necrotic tumor has extended into the anterior chamber in a case of advanced retinoblastoma (Hematoxylin-eosin stain, original magnification ×40).

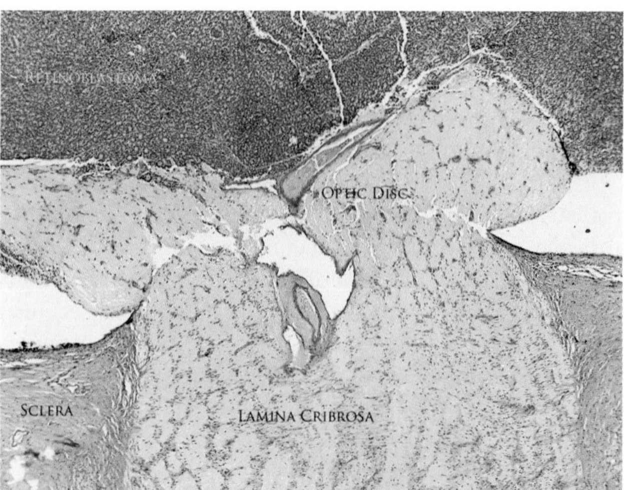

FIGURE 11-31 ■ Retinoblastoma. The intraocular retinoblastoma has extended to the superficial tissues of the optic disc but not through the lamina cribrosa (Hematoxylin-eosin stain, original magnification ×20).

along the internal limiting membrane of the retina, along blood vessel walls, and along the posterior crystalline lens capsule.

The mode of spread for retinoblastoma includes local extension, extension into the optic nerve and intracranial spread, and distant metastases. Spherules of tumor cells separate from the primary tumor in the vitreous and deposit on the inner limiting membrane and secondarily reinvade the retina at a site distant from the original tumor. Spherules also gain access to the posterior chamber where aqueous convection currents carry the cells to the iris surface and trabecular meshwork of the anterior chamber (Figure 11-29). Aqueous seeding may simulate a hypopyon.

Tumor cells readily cross the external limiting membrane of the retina and enter into the subretinal space (Figure 11-30). Disturbance of retinal pigment epithelial function due to the presence of tumor cells breaks down the blood retinal barrier and allows fluid to accumulate in the subretinal space (serous retinal detachment). There is no secondary neovascularization to support tumor cells in the subretinal space. Nutrition appears to be derived from the serous fluid itself. Tumor cells become configured into spherules as in the vitreous cavity; however, the inner most cells of the spherules tend to be necrotic rather than the externally situated cells in the vitreous. Cells may obtain access to the space under the RPE and across Bruch membrane and choriocapillaris to the vessel-rich choroidal layer.

Retinoblastoma spreads in the plane of the retina, to the optic disc, through the lamina cribrosa into the substance of the optic nerve (Figure 11-31). Once beyond the lamina cribrosa, extraocular extension has occurred (Figure 11-32). The tumor in the optic nerve axis has access to the subarachnoid space through which it is able to spread throughout the central nervous system (Figure 11-33).

In the uveal tract, tumor cells have access to the intravascular compartment and may spread extensively to the liver,

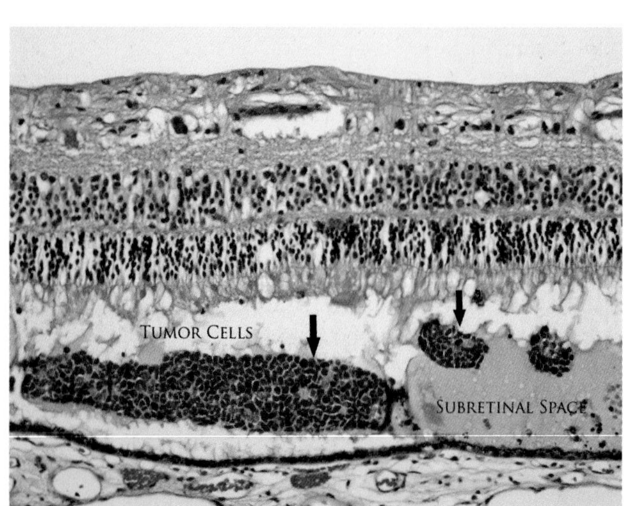

FIGURE 11-30 ■ Tumor cells (*arrows*) have extended from the plane of the retina into the subretinal space (Hematoxylin-eosin, original magnification ×20).

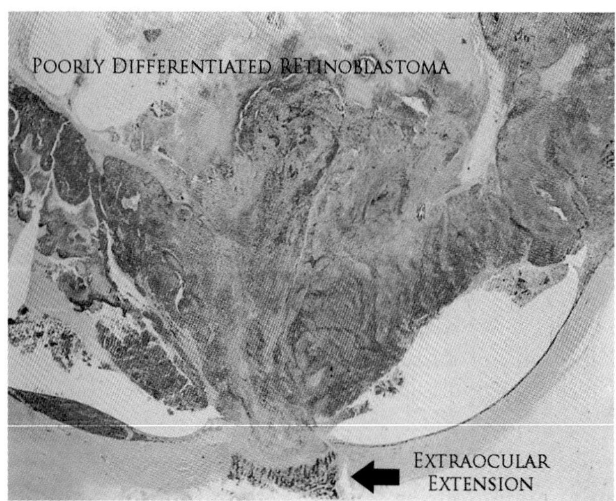

FIGURE 11-32 ■ Retinoblastoma. The tumor has spread beyound the lamina cribrosa to the optic nerve (Hematoxylin-eosin stain, original magnification ×20).

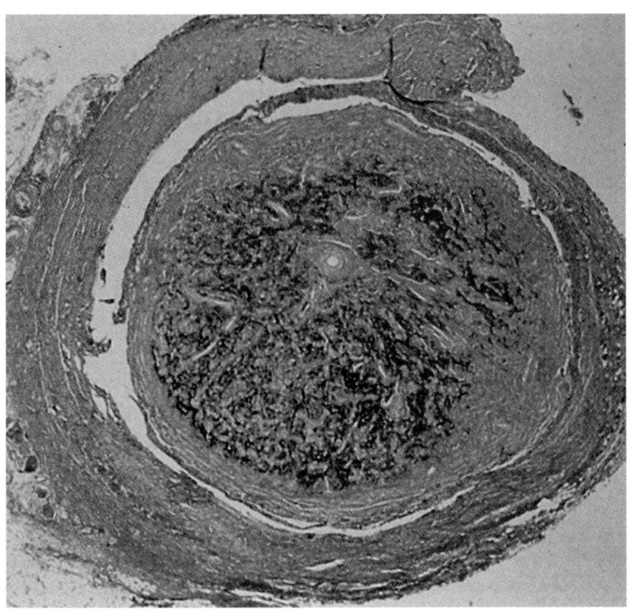

FIGURE 11-33 ▪ Retinoblastoma tumor cells have completely replaced the axons of the optic nerve (Hematoxylin-eosin stain, original magnification ×20).

bones, and lungs. In the anterior chamber, tumor cells may traverse the trabecular meshwork to gain access to episcleral tissue including the lymphatics of the conjunctival stroma. The lymphatic channels collect at the preauricular nodes and submental nodes of the soft tissues of the face.

Tumor cells may escape the eye along surgical wounds in those unfortunate cases where retinoblastoma has been misinterpreted as a congenital cataract and the cataract has been surgically removed.

In terms of prognostic factors, besides tumor size and location, a differentiated tumor with abundant Flexner-Wintersteiner rosettes has a better prognosis than one without rosettes. Similarly, a tumor composed entirely of fleurettes (retinocytoma) has a much better prognosis (73). Although many factors affect the prognosis, the most important is the extent of invasion by the retinoblastoma, with extension into the optic nerve and ocular coats being the two most important predictors of outcome (77) and extraocular invasion being the most important predictor of death. Massive choroidal invasion and extension into the sclera are associated with a high incidence of systemic metastases. With respect to assessing extraocular extension, it is important to note that isolated episcleral "free-floating" tumor cells may sometimes represent artifact of dislodged tumor cells during opening of the globe. Full-thickness choroidal involvement is associated with 60% mortality. Subretinal pigment epithelial or superficial choroidal extension is frequent and is not very significant. Uveal inflammation in the presence of choroidal invasion is associated with a poor prognosis. Thus, massive choroidal involvement, deep choroidal involvement with emissarial extension short of the surface of the eye, concomitant choroidal inflammation, and a large tumor are associated with an adverse outcome (102). With respect to invasion of the optic nerve, invasion up to but not beyond the lamina cribrosa has relatively little prognostic significance, but invasion up to the line of transection carries a poor prognosis. Tumor beyond the lamina cribrosa and involving the pia arachnoid also is associated with a poor prognosis (111). Presence of iris neovascularization is a poor prognostic sign and may relate to the quantitative volume of tumor and to significant choroidal invasion (102). Besides local extension and intracranial involvement, distant metastases may involve long bones and skull, viscera (most often the liver), and lymph nodes.

Medulloepithelioma is a rare tumor originating from the medullary epithelial cells of the optic vesicle that have differentiated toward the epithelium of the ciliary body. There is a bimodal distribution of tumors presenting as congenital lesions in children and acquired lesions in adults. In both instances, the clinical and histopathologic distinction between benign and malignant lesions may be difficult in the early stages of tumor progression. The single best differentiating feature is invasion of adjacent tissues and even that finding can be found in tumors with an indolent course.

Congenital medulloepitheliomas tend to arise in the first decade of life presenting with pain, decreased vision, a sectoral cataract (leukocoria), or increased intraocular pressure (11). The tumors are not heritable. A ciliary body mass is found by clinical examination. The tumors tend to be white or gray with an irregular, sometimes cystic surface. The cystic components of the tumor may separate from the primary mass and may float freely in the anterior chamber or even in the vitreous. Infrequently the tumor may arise in the plane of the RPE or along the course of the optic nerve. The tumor is composed of primitive neuroblastic cells arranged in chords or sheets of cells associated with an extracellular matrix containing hyaluronic acid. Flexner-Wintersteiner (photoreceptor differentiation) and Homer-Wright rosettes (ganglion cell differentiation) lined by a single layer of cells may be present. In addition, primitive rosettes (ciliary epithelial differentiation) may be present; however, this type of rosette is lined by several layers of undifferentiated neuroepithelial cells. Reactive proliferation and formation of a cellular membrane may also occur and extend across the vitreous face. Because there is often an inconsistent degree of pleomorphism and variable mitotic activity, the natural history may be difficult to predict by cytological features. Invasion of adjacent uveal structures, especially extension to and through the sclera, is a distinct risk factor for additional local invasion, although the tumor only rarely produces distant metastasis (54). Tumors significantly affecting ocular function are often treated with enucleation because of the uncertainty of the natural history of any individual tumor and the difficulty in determining the significance of involvement of adjacent structures, particularly the vitreous (33).

A subgroup of medulloepitheliomas (*teratoid medulloepithelioma*) contain heterotopic elements, particularly cartilage, however brain and muscle tissue may also be present. Again, histological clues to a malignant course are not distinctive enough for certain categorization. Tumors with heterotopic elements tend to have a more aggressive course. Treatment criteria for the two groups are similar because the heterotopic elements cannot be distinguished clinically with any degree of certainty. The overall mortality in one series was reported in the range of 10% (11).

Benign and malignant acquired medulloepitheliomas also occur, but arise most often in adults. Again, the distinction between benign and malignant lesions may be difficult. Treatment is usually surgical depending on symptoms and volume of tumor (33,54).

Fuchs adenoma is a benign proliferation of fully differentiated ciliary epithelium of adults that is found in up to 30% of autopsy series (5,66). The lesion is of no clinical significance.

PEDIATRIC GLAUCOMA

Glaucoma is an imbalance between production of aqueous and drainage of aqueous into the systemic circulation. Any developmental abnormality of the anterior segment may lead to glaucoma; the more extensive the architectural abnormality the more likely is glaucoma to develop. In the vast majority of cases, the imbalance is caused by abnormalities of filtration rather than overproduction of aqueous. Increased intraocular pressure will not decrease aqueous production until the intraocular pressure is in the range of the diastolic blood pressure. In the pediatric age group the tissues of the eye remain pliable to the point where increased intraocular pressure may actually expand the dimensions of the eye leading to apparent enlargement of the cornea and anterior-posterior dimensions of the globe (buphthalmos). The expansion is not uniform enlargement of the globe, rather it is stretching of the thinnest portion of the eyewall at the junction of the cornea and sclera (the intercalary zone)). In advanced cases of glaucoma from any cause, the anterior chamber may collapse allowing the anterior surface of the iris to come in contact with the posterior surface of the cornea (total anterior synechiae), further limiting the ability of aqueous to exit the eye. The front of the eye may bulge forward (ectasia) and the ectatic area may become lined by iris (anterior staphyloma).

In many cases of congenital glaucoma there is no histological sign of architectural abnormality of the anterior chamber angle including the delicate trabecular meshwork. However, there is a range of anatomic abnormalities in developmental disturbances from total immaturity of the draining structures to regional minimal structural changes. Except in extreme cases, the intraocular pressure cannot be predicted from the nature of the architectural changes.

In the pediatric age group, one of the most common forms of secondary glaucoma is neovascular glaucoma. In this situation ischemia of the retina induces formation of local angiogenic factors [e.g., vascular endothelial growth factor (VEGF)]. The process stimulates angiogenesis of the anterior surface of the iris. This fibrovascular growth flattens the contour of the anterior iris (clearly seen by light microscopy) and also causes adhesions between the anterior surface of the iris and the posterior surface of the peripheral cornea [peripheral anterior synechia (PAS)]. The PAS limit aqueous access to the trabecular meshwork and cause increased intraocular pressure. This mechanism is found in retinopathy of prematurity, advanced retinoblastoma, and uncontrolled diabetic retinopathy, among others.

Sustained increased intraocular pressure causes degeneration of the ganglion cell and nerve fiber layer of the retina. The exact cause for internal retinal atrophy has not been definitely determined for all types of glaucoma. In addition, there is retrodisplacement of the structural support of the optic disc (the lamina cribrosa), which is a finding unique to increased intraocular pressure. In other forms of atrophic optic neuropathy the position of the lamina cribrosa relative to the surrounding sclera is not affected. Progressive loss of retinal ganglion cell axons progressively increases the cup-to-disc ratio to the point of "total cupping" of the optic disc. This clinical finding can be confirmed by anterior-posterior histological sections of the eye if the plane of section is through the optic disc. Total optic cupping correlates with total loss of optic nerve axons, widening of pial septa, and enlargement of the subretinal space. The character of the dura is not changed by increased intraocular pressure.

OCULAR TRAUMA

The most common indication for the surgical removal of an eye in the pediatric age group is trauma. Loss of visual function of the eye is usually due to a combination of hemorrhage, inflammation, and ultimately glaucoma.

Accidental trauma to the eye is generally categorized into nonpenetrating or penetrating trauma. The distinction is important in guiding the initial therapy of the injured eye. Generally, a nonpenetrating injury does not require surgical repair, although the degree of injury in many cases exceeds that found in penetrating injury. Surgical repair is usually necessary in cases of penetrating trauma (open globe injury).

In most cases of severe trauma treated with enucleation there is a rupture or laceration of the corneal-scleral coat, the "eye wall". Most ruptures are found in the region of the corneal sclera limbus, which is a normally thin region of the eye wall. Lacerations are also most commonly found in the anterior eye wall but may also be located posteriorly. By the time of enucleation there usually has been fibrovascular repair of the eye wall wound that can be identified by discontinuity of the collagen pattern, rupture of Bowman or Descemet membrane, or interruption of one of the pigmented coats of the eye. The anterior chamber is usually disorganized and PAS are present. The lens may be totally absent, be represented by crystalline lens remnants (best identified by Periodic acid/Schiff staining), or show changes of anterior or posterior fibrous metaplasia of the crystalline lens epithelial cells. The retina is most often detached with blood or serous fluid in the subretinal space. The surface of the retina may undulate due to the formation of a contracted membrane on its surface (epiretinal membrane). The vitreous may be contracted and filled with inflammatory cells or with proliferating fibrovascular tissue (proliferative vitreoretinopathy). There may be hemorrhage within, superficial to, or deep to any of the coats of the eye. The choroid may be infiltrated by nongranulomatous or granulomatous inflammatory cells either diffusely (see below) or focally. The optic nerve frequently has signs of early or advanced atrophy (14).

The eye may be collapsed, if there has been loss of intraocular contents, including the lens, vitreous, and retina. Intraocular foreign material may be present, depending on the nature of the original injury. Identifying foreign material is aided by the use of polarized light.

The eye is removed within 2 weeks, if there is no clinical indication of retention of useful vision (no light perception) in order to reduce the risk of losing vision in the contralateral eye because of sympathetic ophthalmia (14).

Sympathetic ophthalmia is a bilateral granulomatous inflammation of the uveal tract appearing 5 days to many years following trauma to one of the two eyes. The inflammation is thought to be due to an autoimmune response to an unknown type of antigen that is expressed during trauma. The first clinical indication of the presence of sympathetic ophthalmia is a loss of the ability to focus at near objects (accommodation) followed by a generalized uveitis. Untreated, the uveitis in the initially uninvolved eye may be more severe than in the injured eye. The major histological sign is a granulomatous inflammatory response in any portion of the uveal tract characterized by epithelioid histiocytes and giant cells. The giant cells may contain melanin pigment, but this finding is not specific to sympathetic ophthalmia. There is generally an intense infiltrate of lymphocytes but not plasma cells or eosinophils in the surrounding tissue. Epithelioid histiocytes also accumulate between the RPE and Bruch membrane (Dahlen-Fuchs nodules) (Figure 11-34). Dahlen-Fuchs nodules may also be found in sarcoid uveitis. There may be some sparing of the choriocapillaris in the noninjured (sympathizing) eye, but the finding is also not specific for sympathetic ophthalmia. An inflammatory reaction to exposed lens protein (lens-induced uveitis or phacoanaphylactic endophthalmitis) is also found in some cases. All of the histological findings are nonspecific. To establish the diagnosis of sympathetic ophthalmia there must be a history of some type of ocular trauma, which may include such surgical procedures such as cyclocryotherapy (freezing of the ciliary body to treat intractable glaucoma) or pars plana vitrectomy (see above).

Eyes removed within the 2-week risk period for sympathetic ophthalmia may still have suture material at sites of penetration of the sclera and may also have surgical appliances used in retinal detachment repair (scleral buckles) and treatment of glaucoma (glaucoma filtration devices) on the episcleral surface. There may be considerable fibrosis from the episcleral tissue at sites of injury and at surgical sites even a few days after the original injury.

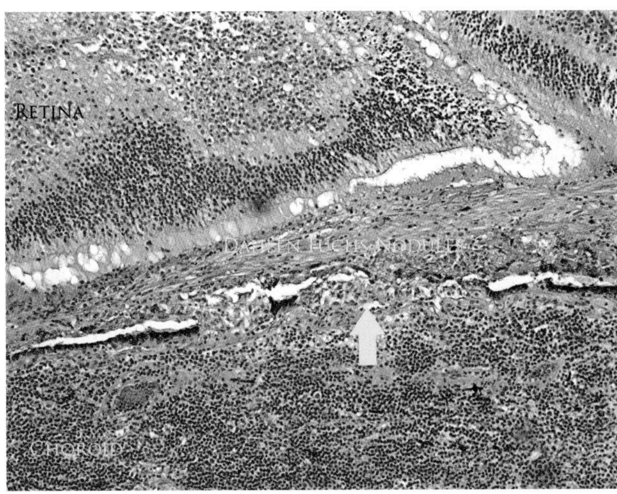

FIGURE 11-34 ▪ Sympathetic ophthalmia. There is a massive chronic granulomatous inflammatory infiltration of the uveal tract. Epithelioid histiocytes have accumulated between the RPE and Bruch membrane (*arrow*). The features of the retina are distorted by trauma, inflammation, and sectioning artifacts (Hematoxylin-eosin stain, original magnification ×40).

Eyes removed months or years following trauma are generally small, shrunken, and have assumed a cuboidal shape (phthisis) (Figure 11-35). The ocular degeneration may be so advanced as to make identification of laterality difficult. The most reliable landmarks are the insertion of the superior and inferior oblique muscles. On sectioning, there may be extreme resistance because of dystrophic calcification both in the remaining lens tissue and in the plane of the RPE. Decalcification for several days is often necessary. Histologically, there is often scarring and vascularization of the cornea, complete fibrosis of the anterior chamber, atrophy of the iris, cataract (potions of which may be calcified), total retinal detachment with atrophy and gliosis, fibrosis of the vitreous, and, most often, profound optic atrophy. The most important observations are those of the uveal tract to determine the presence or absence of sympathetic ophthalmia.

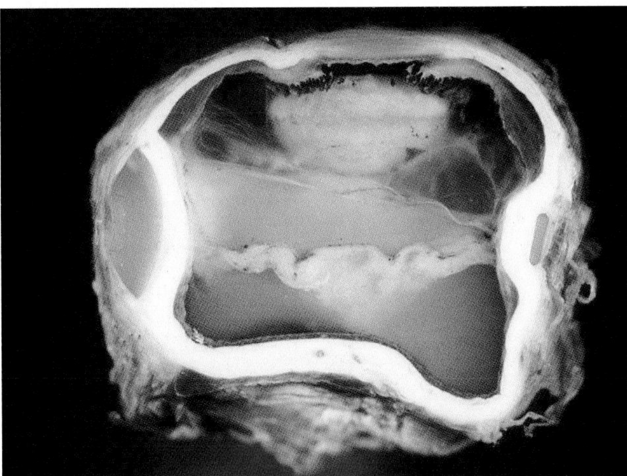

FIGURE 11-35 ▪ Phthisis. This eye has degenerated following surgical repair for a detached retina. The eye is small and cuboidal in shape.

In adults, it is also important to determine if this "blind painful eye" has been harboring a neoplasm such as malignant melanoma (14).

AUTOPSY SPECIMEN

Removing the eyes of a child at autopsy is a very uncommon event, except when there is suspicion of child abuse homicide (16). Globes may be removed via an anterior approach as with surgical enucleation or may be removed through a window created in orbital roof. Whichever approach is used, it is important to obtain as much optic nerve as possible and to obtain a sample of orbital fat.

In most cases of death due to shaking or simple blunt force injury in which death occurred shortly following the injury there is little external sign of trauma. There is also usually no abnormality of the cornea, anterior chamber, or external surface of the globe. It is important to note any signs of scleral thinning indicated by a blue tinge of the sclera, which may be found in very young infants or in individuals affected by osteogenesis imperfecta. Subdural and subarachnoid hemorrhage of the optic nerve is indicated also by a blue-to-gray discoloration of the dura. Cross sections of the optic nerve itself are normal in diameter and character, however, there may be marked expansion of the dural and subdural spaces by hemorrhage (Figure 11-36). On sectioning of the eye the cornea, lens, and anterior chamber generally are normal. Retinal hemorrhages may be present. The location and extent of the intraretinal hemorrhage, particularly if the hemorrhage extends to the ora serrata, is an important observation (Figure 11-37). The retina in the region of the macula may also be elevated. Hemorrhage may extend into the vitreous itself. Histologically, the hemorrhages may be located completely within the architecture of the retina (intraretinal), between the neurosensory retina and the RPE (subretinal), between the retina and the cortex of the vitreous (subhyaloid), or within the vitreous (intravitreal). There may also be signs of disruption of the internal limiting membrane in the region of the macula. Hemorrhage may also be noted in the sclera at the insertion of the dura of the optic nerve (the circle of Zinn-Haller). Hemorrhage may be found in the surrounding orbital fat (see Chapter 7).

In cases where the child died after a longer interval from abuse, the hemorrhages may be less apparent. There may be atrophy and gliosis in the region of resolved retinal hemorrhage. There may or may not be hemosiderin staining in the area of suspected former hemorrhage. There may be considerable optic atrophy.

SUMMARY

The most common eyelid specimens in the pediatric age group usually consist of inflammatory lesions: Molluscum contageosum and chalazion. Most important lesions would be those of metastatic neuroblastoma in very young children and rhabdomyosarcoma in slightly older children. There is a variant of rhabdomyosarcoma with a subconjunctival presentation, the botryoid variant. Basal cell carcinoma and squamous cell carcinoma can occur with xeroderma pigmentosa but are otherwise uncommon. Sebaceous cell carcinoma can occur but again is extremely rare.

Conjunctival nevus may be an important clinical problem in the pediatric age group. Malignant melanoma can occur in very young children but most of the pigmented lesions will be nevi. Concern is generated because of enlarging size due to expansion of subepithelial squamous cysts, increased pigmentation found during adolescence, and inflammation of the nevus from a combination of factors. Pterygium and squamous cell carcinoma are found generally in a much older age group.

Corneal tissue is most often evaluated because of surgical treatment of keratoconus. Confirmatory findings include focal ruptures of Bowman membrane and occasionally rupture of Descemet membrane (corneal hydrops). Other corneal

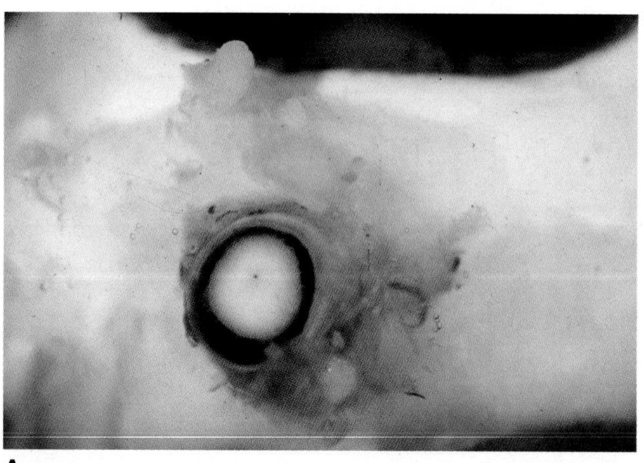

A

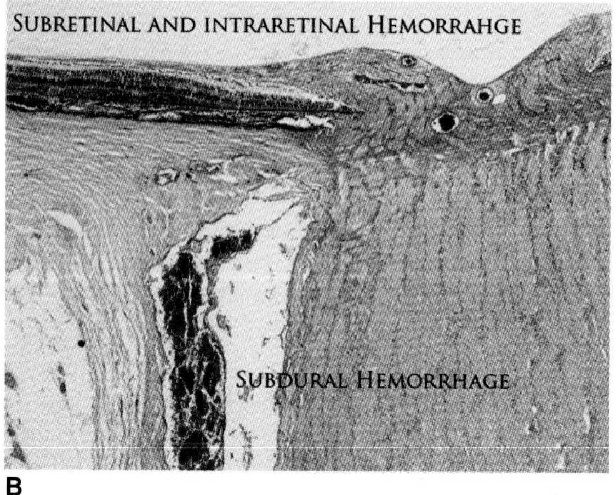

B

FIGURE 11-36■ Nonaccidental trauma. **A:** The cross section of the optic nerve is normal at 3.0 mm. There is extensive hemorrhage in the subdural and subarachnoid spaces. **B:** Subdural and subretinal hemorrhages are present in this low magnification view.

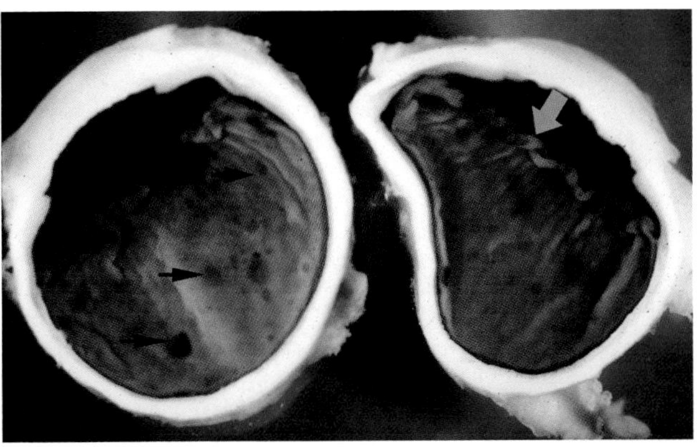

A

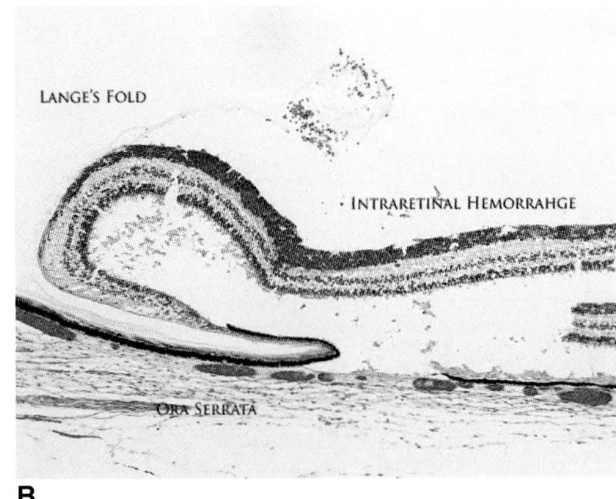

B

FIGURE 11-37 ▪ Nonaccidental trauma. **A:** Hemorrhages are found throughout the retina (*black arrows*) and extend as far anteriorly as the ora serrata (*yellow arrow*). **B:** Intraretinal hemorrhage is shown extending to the ora serrata.

specimens will be submitted following accidental trauma and will show evidence of repair with fibrous proliferation. Corneal dystrophies, except for CHED in some restricted geographic areas, are not commonly treated with surgery in this age group. An important biopsy evaluation would be for acanthamoeba keratitis, particularly if there is a history of correction of refractive error with soft contact lenses.

Cataracts in this age group are treated surgically, but the tissue is generally not examined histologically.

Retina, vitreous, and uveal tract are very infrequently evaluated by fine needle aspiration biopsy. The major exception would be anterior chamber paracentesis for diffuse infiltrating retinoblastoma as a differential diagnosis in the evaluation of protracted intermediate uveitis, both found in the older child-younger teenage group. Congenital melanoma of the uveal tract has been reported but uveal melanoma generally occurs in the fifth to sixth decade.

The most common orbital lesions in children include ruptured dermoid cyst and various vascular developmental abnormalities such as lymphangioma. Idiopathic orbital inflammation (orbital inflammatory pseudotumor) can occur in children where the presentation is often bilateral and the progression more aggressive. Rhabdomyosarcoma has a predilection for orbital tissue in children. Surgical treatment for rhabdomyosarcoma is now not as common as formerly, being replaced currently by combinations of chemotherapy and occasionally radiation. The biopsy of orbital tumor tissue is often essential in managing treatment strategies for rhabdomyosarcoma. Adenoid cystic carcinoma of the lacrimal gland can occur in children. Its treatment at any age is difficult as the outcome tends to be poor.

The treatment of retinoblastoma is in rapid evolution. Enucleation, once the standard of care for all cases of retinoblastoma, is now done selectively and often after prior treatment with chemotherapy, cryotherapy, photocoagulation, transpupillary thermotherapy, and, occasionally, radiation. All therapeutic efforts will change the histological appearance of the primary tumor. Definite histologically defined risk factors, especially optic nerve involvement by the retinoblastoma tumor, continue to guide therapy when enucleation is performed. The most important part of gross examination of a retinoblastoma eye is extremely careful evaluation of the surgical margin at the site of transaction of the optic nerve. Sections of the retinoblastoma eye must include levels through the optic disc.

Most eyes enucleated in children are the result of irreparable trauma to the eye. The most important histological observations include those for diffuse granulomatous inflammation of the uveal tract with or without signs of Dalen-Fuchs nodules (i.e., sympathetic ophthalmia). Sarcoidosis and other inflammatory lesions may have exactly the same histological appearance as sympathetic ophthalmia. Correlation of histopathologic findings of the pathologist with clinical findings of the ophthalmologist is essential in establishing the diagnosis of sympathetic ophthalmia. Eyes removed many years following the original trauma may even become small externally and distorted internally (phthisis bulbi). The evaluation for sympathetic ophthalmia remains an important function of the pathologist even if the interval between the injury and enucleation has been decades.

Autopsy eye specimens are usually collected for assessment of ocular developmental abnormalities as part of evaluation for congenital syndromes (e.g., trisomy 13 or 18) or as a part of a homicide investigation for child abuse. In cases of suspected nonaccidental injury, important observations include external signs of ocular injury; the apparent thinness of the sclera (osteogenesis imperfecta); sign of cataract formation; the presence, location, and extent of retinal hemorrhage; the presence and extent of vitreous hemorrhage; the presence and extent of subretinal hemorrhage; signs of traction retinal detachment; signs of intrascleral hemorrhage at the sclera insertion of the dura of the optic nerve (Circle of Zinn-Haller); the presence of hemorrhage in the soft tissues of the orbit; presence and extent of subdural and subarachnoid hemorrhage; and finally the presence and degree of optic atrophy.

REFERENCES

1. Abbruzzese C, Kuhn U, Molina F, et al. Novel mutations in the CHST6 gene causing macular corneal dystrophy. *Clin Genet* 2004;65(2):120–125.
2. Aldahmesh M, Khan A, Meyer B, et al. Mutational spectrum of SLC4A11 in autosomal recessive CHED in Saudi Arabia. *Invest Ophthal Vis Sci* 2009;50(9):4142–4145.
3. Alvord EJ, Lofton S. Gliomas of the optic nerve or chiasm. Outcome by patient's age, tumor site, and treatment. *J Neurosurg* 1988;68:85–98.
4. Bagheri A, Hasani H, Karimaian F, et al. Effect of chalazion excision on refractive error and corneal topography. *Eur J Ophthalmol* 2009;19(4):521–526.
5. Bateman J, Foos R. Coronal adenomas. *Arch Ophthalmol* 1979;97:2379–2384.
6. Benson W. Familial exudative vitreoretinopathy. *Trans Am Ophthalmol Soc* 1995;93:473–521.
7. Boldrey E, Egbert P, Gass JF. The histopathology of familial exudative vitreoretinopathy. A report of two cases. *Arch Ophthalmol* 1985;103(2):238–241.
8. Boyd S, Young S, Lightman S. Immunopathology of the noninfectious posterior and intermediate uveitides. *Surv Ophthalmol* 2001;46(3):209–233.
9. Brantley MJ, Harbour JW. The molecular biology of retinoblastoma. *Ocul Immunol Inflam* 2001;9(1):1–8.
10. Brichard B, De Potter P, Godfraind C, et al. Embryonal rhabdomyosarcoma presenting as a conjunctival tumor. *J Pediatr Hematol Oncol* 2003;25(8):651–652.
11. Broughton W, Zimmerman L. A clinicopathologic study of 56 cases of intraocular medulloepithelioma. *Am J Ophthalmol* 1978;84:407–418.
12. Burillon C, Durand L. Solid dermoids of the limbus and cornea. *Ophthalmologica* 1997;211(6):367–372.
13. Callaghan M, Hand C, Kennedy S, et al. Homozygosity mapping and linkage analysis demonstrate that autosomal recessive congenital hereditary endothelial dystrophy (CHED) and autosomally dominant CHED are genetically distinct. *Br J Ophthalmol* 1999;83(1):115–119.
14. Cameron J. Ocular trauma (Chapter 13). In: Klintworth GK, Garner A, eds. *Gardner and Klintworth's pathobiology of ocular disease*. New York: Informa Healthcare, 2008:333–360.
15. Cameron J, Streeten BW. Pathology of the lens (Chapter 272). In: Albert DM, Miller, eds. *Albert and Jakobiec's principles and practice of ophthalmology*. Philadelphia: Saunders Elsevier, 2008:3653–3678.
16. Cameron JD, Emerson MV. Ophthalmic pathologic findings in infantile traumatic brain injury. In: Troncoso JC, Rubio A, Fowler DR, eds. *Essential forensic neuropathology*. Philadelphia: Wolters Kluwer/Lippincott Williams & Wilkins, 2010:203.
17. Carvalho F, Foronda A, Mannis M, et al. Twenty years of acanthamoeba keratitis. *Cornea* 2009;28(5):516–519.
18. Ceballos P, Ruiz-Maldonado R, Mihm MJ. Melaoma in children. *N Engl J Med* 1995;332(10):656–662.
19. Ceron O, Lou P, Walton D. The vitreo-retinal manifestations of persistent hyperplastic primary vitreous (PHPV) and their management. *Int Ophthalmol Clin* 2008;48(2):53–62.
20. Chang L, Ching SS. Corneal and conjunctival degenerations. In: Krachmer J, Mannis M, Holland E, eds. *Cornea*. Philadelphia: Elsevier Mosby, 2008:987–1004.
21. Chang L, Zhigum W, Shijing D, et al. Arg124Cys mutation of the TGFBI gene in 2 Chinese families with Thiel-Behnke corneal dystrophy. *Arch Ophthalmol* 2009;127(5):641–644.
22. Chang M, Frieden I, Good W. The risk of intraocular juvenile xanthogranuloma: survey of current practices and assessment of risk. *J Am Acad Dermatol* 1996;34(3):445–449.
23. Charles N, Friedberg D. Epibulbar molluscum contagiosum in acquired immune deficiency syndrome. Case report and review of the literature. *Ophthalmology* 1992;99(7):1123–1126.
24. Chaudhry I, Al-Jishi Z, Samsi F, et al. Juvenile xanthogranuloma of the corneoscleral limbus: case report and review of the literature. *Surv Ophthalmol* 2004;49(6):608–614.
25. Chen B, Perry JD. Rhabdomyosarcoma. In: Singh A, Damato BE, Pe'er J, et al., eds. *Clinical ophthalmic oncology*. Philadelphia: Saunders Elsevier, 2007:581–585.
26. Chevez-Barrios P, Eagle RJ, Marback EF. Histopathologic features and prognostic factors. In: Singh AD, Damato BE, Pe'er J, et al., eds. *Clinical ophthalmic oncology*. Philadelphia: Saunders Elsevier, 2007:468–483.
27. Couch S, Garrity J, Cameron JD, et al. Embolizatin of orbital varicies with n-butyl cyanoacrylate as an aid in surgical excision: results of four cases with histopathologic examination. *Am J Ophthalmol* 2009;148(4):614–616.
28. Coville D, Savige J. Alport's syndrome. A review of the ocular manifestations. *Ophthalmic Genet* 1997;18(4):161–173.
29. Dart JK, Saw VP, Kilvington S. Acanthamoeba keratitis: diagnosis and treatment update 2009. *Am J Ophthalmol* 2009;148(4):487–499.
30. Dietz HC, Cutting GR, Pyeritz RE, et al. Marfan syndrome caused by a recurrent de novo missense mutation in the fibrillin gene. *Nature* 1991;352(6333):337–339.
31. Donahue S, Schwartz G. Preseptal and orbital cellulitis in childhood. A changing microbiologic spectrum. *Ophthalmology* 1998;105(10):1902–1905.
32. Dyer MA, Harbour JW. Cellular and genetic events in retinoblastoma tumorgenesis. In: Singh AD, Damato BE, Pe'er, et al., eds. *Clinical ophthalmic oncology*. Philadelphia: Saunders Elsevier, 2007:405–409.
33. Elizalde J, de la Paz M, Barraquer RI. Tumors of the ciliary pigment epithelium. In: Singh AD, Damato BE, Pe'er, et al., eds. *Clinical ophthalmic oncology*. Philadelphia: Saunders Elsevier, 2007:366–371.
34. Erb M, Uzcategui N, Burnstine M. Orbitotemporal neurofibromatosis: classification and treatment. *Orbit* 2007;26(4):223–228.
35. Erie JC, McLaren JW, Patel SV. Confocal microscopy in ophthalmology. *Am J Ophthalmol* 2009;148(5):639–646.
36. Feder R, Kshettry P. Noninflammatory ectatic disorders. In: Krachmer J, Mannis M, Holland E, eds. *Cornea*. Philadelphia: Elsevier Mosby, 2005:955–966.
37. Ferry A. Pyogenic granulomas of the eye and ocular adnexa: a study of 100 cases. *Trans Am Ophthalmol Soc* 1989;87:327–343.
38. Fine BS, Yanoff M. *Ocular histology. A text and atlas*, 2nd ed. Hagerstown, Maryland: Harper & Row, 1979.
39. Folberg R, Jakobiec F, Bernardino V, et al. Benign conjunctival melanocytic lesions. Clinicopathologic features. *Ophthalmology* 1989;96(4):436–461.
40. Folberg R, Stone E, Sheffield V, et al. The relationship between granular, lattice type 1, and Avellino corneal dystrophies. A histopathologic study. *Arch Ophthalmol* 1994;112(8):1080–1085.
41. Font R, Croxatto JO, Rao NA. *Tumors of the eye and adnexa*, Vol. Fourth Series: Fascicle 5. Washington, DC: American Registry of Pathology, 2006.
42. Font R, Ferry A. The phakomatoses. *Int Ophthal Clin* 1972;12(1):1–50.
43. Font R, Fine B. Ocular findings in Fabry disease. Histochemical and electron microscopic observations. *Am J Ophthalmol* 1972;73: 410–430.
44. Forsius H, Damsten M, Eriksson A, et al. Autosomal recessive cornea plana. A clinical and genetic study of 78 cases in Finland. *Acta Ophthalmol Scand* 1998;76(2):196–203.
45. Garner A, Klintworth G. The causes and morphology of cataracts. In: Garner A, Klintworth G, eds. *Pathobiology of ocular disease: a dynamic approach*. New York: Marcel Dekker, 1994:481.
46. Garrity J, Henderson JW, Cameron JD. Cysts and celes. In: Garrity J, Henderson JW, Cameron JD, eds. *Henderson's orbital tumors*. Philadelphia: Lippincott Williams & Wilkins, 2007:33–39.
47. Garrity J, Henderson JW, Cameron JD. Inflammatory orbital pseudotumors. In: Garrity J, Henderson JW, Cameron JD, eds. *Henderson's orbital tumors*. Philadelphia: Lippincott Williams & Wilkins, 2007:343–351.

48. Garrity J, Henderson JW, Cameron JD. Primary epithelial neoplasms. In: Garrity J, Henderson JW, Cameron JD, eds. *Henderson's orbital tumors*. Philadelphia: Lippincott Williams & Wilkins, 2007:33–39.
49. Garrity J, Henderson JW, Cameron JD. Vascular hamartomas, hyperplasia and neoplasms. In: Garrity J, Henderson JW, Cameron JD, eds. *Henderson's orbital tumors*. Philadelphia: Lippincott Williams & Wilkins, 2007:210–215.
50. Gayre G, Prola A, Dutton J. Epibulbar osseous choristoma: case report and review of the literature. *Ophthalmic Surg Laser* 2002;33(5):410–415.
51. Goval J, Rao V, Srinlvasan R, et al. Oculocutaneous manifestations in xeroderma pigmentosa. *Br J Ophthalmol* 1994;78(4):295–297.
52. Graw J. Congenital hereditary cataracts. *Int J Dev Biol* 2004;48(8–9): 1031–1044.
53. Green W, Kincaid M, Michaels R, et al. Pars planitis. *Trans Ophthalmol Soc U K* 1981;101:361–367.
54. Green WR, McLean IW. Neuroepithelial tumors of the ciliary body. In: Spencer W, ed. *Ophthalmic pathology. A text and atlas*. Philadelphia: W.B. Saunders Co, 1996:1316–1324.
55. Guyot-Goubin A, Donadieu J, Barkaoui M, et al. Descriptive epidemiology of childhood Langerhans cell histiocytosis in France, 2000–2004. *Pediatr Blood Cancer* 2008;51(1):3–4.
56. Haddad R, Font R, Reeser F. Persistent hyperplastic primary vitreous. A clinicopathologic study of 62 cases and review of the literature. *Surv Ophthalmol* 1978;23(2):123–134.
57. Haik B, Karcioglu Z, Gordon R, et al. Capillary hemangioma (infantile periocular hemangioma). *Surv Ophthalmol* 1994;38(5): 399–426.
58. Henkind P, Ashton N. Ocular pathology in homocystinuria. *Trans Ophthalmol Soc U K* 1965;85:21.
59. Henriquez A, Kenyon K, Dohlman C, et al. Morphologic characteristics of posterior polymorphous dystrophy. A study of nine corneas and review of the literature. *Surv Ophthalmol* 1984;29(2):139–147.
60. Hiscott P, Seitz B, Naumann G. Epithelioid cell Spitz nevus of the eyelid. *Am J Ophthalmol* 1998;126(5):735–737.
61. Hogan MJ, Alvarado JA, Weddell JE. *Histology of the human eye*. Philadelphia: W.B. Saunders Company, 1971.
62. Holland E, Daya S, Stone E, et al. Avellino corneal dystrophy. Clinical manifestations and natural history. *Ophthalmology* 1992;99(10):1564–1568.
63. Honavar S, Shields J, Shields C, et al. Basal cell carcinoma of the eyelid associated with Gorlin-Goltz syndrome. *Ophthalmology* 2001;108(6):1115–1123.
64. Honavar S, Singh A, Shields C, et al. Iris melanoma in a patient with neurofibromatosis. *Semin Ophthalmol* 2000;45(3):231–236.
65. Ilgren E, Kinnier-Wilson L, Stiller C. Gliomas in neurofibromatosis. A series of 89 cases with evidence for enhanced malignancy in associated cerebellar astroctyomas. *Pathol Annu* 1985;20(Pt 1): 331–358.
66. Iliff W, Green WR. The incidence and histology of Fuchs' adenoma. *Arch Ophthalmol* 1972;88:249–254.
67. Jiao X, Ventruto V, Trese M, et al. Autosomal recessive familial exudative vitreoretiopathy is associated with mutations in LRP5. *Am J Human Genet* 2004;75:878–884.
68. Kaercher T. Ocular symptoms and signs in patients with ectodermal dysplasia syndromes. *Graefes Arch Clin Exp Ophthalmol* 2004;242(6):495–500.
69. Katz S, Rootman J, Vangveeravong S, et al. Combined venous lymphatic malformations of the orbit (so-called lymphangiomas). Association with noncontiguous intracranial vascular anomalies. *Ophthalmology* 1998;105(1):176–184.
70. Kenyon K, Maumenee A. The histological and ultrastructural pathology of congenital hereditary corneal dystrophy: a case report. *Invest Ophthalmol Vis Sci* 1968;7(5):475–500.
71. Klintworth G. The molecular genetics of the corneal dystrophies—current status. *Front Biosci* 2003;1(8):687–713.
72. Knudson A. Mutation and cancer: a statistical study of retinoblastoma. *Proc Natl Acad Sci USA* 1971;68:820–828.
73. Knudson AJ. Retinoblastoma and cancer genetics. In: Singh AD, Damato BE, Pe'er, et al., eds. *Clinical ophthalmic oncology*. Philadelphia: Saunders Elsevier, 2007:403–404.
74. Korvatska E, Munier F, Kjemai A, et al. Kerato-epithelin mutations in four 5q31-linked corneal dystrophies. *Am J Human Genet* 1998;15(3):247–251.
75. Lee H, Garrity J, Cameron J, et al. Primary optic nerve sheath meningioma in children. *Surv Ophthalmol* 2008;53(6):543–558.
76. Lessner A, Stern G. Preseptal and orbital cellulitis. *Infect Dis Clin North Am* 1992;6(4):933–952.
77. Levi M, Schwartz S, Blei F, et al. Surgical treatment of capillary hemangioma causing amblyopia. *J Am Assoc Pediatr Ophthalmol Strabismus* 2007;11(3):230–234.
78. Lewis R, Gerson L, Axelson K, et al. von Recklinghausen neurofibromatosis. II. Incidence of optic gliomata. *Ophthalmology* 1984;91:929–935.
79. Listernick R, Ferner R, Liu G, et al. Optic pathway gliomas in neurofibromatosis-1: controversies and recommendations. *Ann Neurol* 2007;61(3):189–198.
80. Magenis RE, Maslen CL, Smith L, et al. Localization of the fibrillin (FBN) gene to chromosome 15, band q21.1. *Genomics* 1991;11(2):346–351.
81. Mahmood E, Teichmann K. Corneal amyloidosis associated with congenital hereditary endothelial dystrophy. *Cornea* 2000;19(4): 570–573.
82. Mahr M, Salomao D, Garrity J. Inflammatory orbital pseudotumor with extension beyond the orbit. *Am J Ophthalmol* 2004;138(3): 396–400.
83. Margo C, Goldman D. Langerhans cell histiocytosis. *Surv Ophthalmol* 2008; 53(4):332–358.
84. Maumenee IH. The eye in the Marfan syndrome. *Trans Am Ophthalmol Soc* 1981;79:684–733.
85. McKelvie P, Daniell M, McNab A, et al. Squamous cell carcinoma of the conjunctiva: a series of 26 cases. *Br J Ophthalmol* 2002; 86(2):18–173.
86. McLean I. Retinoblastoma, retinocytomas, and pseudoretinoblastomas. In: Spencer W, ed. *Ophthalmic pathology*. Philadelphia: W.B. Saunders Company, 1996:1332–1438.
87. McLean I, Burnier M, Zimmerman L, et al. *Tumors of the eye and ocular adnexa*. Washington, DC: Armed Forces Institute of Pathology, 1994.
88. McMahon R, Font R, McLean I. Phakomatous choristoma of eyelid: electron microscopical confirmation of lenticular derivation. *Arch Ophthalmol* 1976;94:1778–1781.
89. Mehta M, Jakobiec F, Fay A. Idiopathic fibroinflammatory disease of the face, eyelids, and periorbital membranes with immunoglobulin G4-positive plasma cells. *Arch Pathol Lab Med* 2009;133(8):1251–1255.
90. Mehta R, Shapiro A. Plasminogen deficiency. *Haemophilia* 2008;14(6):1261–1268.
91. Mierau G. Intranuclear Birbeck granules in Langerhans cell histiocytosis. *Pediatr Pathol* 1994;14(6):1051–1054.
92. Mohamed M, McKibbin M, Jafri H, et al. A new pedigree with recessive mapping to CHED2 locus on 20p13. *Br J Ophthalmol* 2001;85(6):758–759.
93. Mohammad A, Kroosh S. Huge corneal dermoid in a well-formed eye: a case report and review of the literature. *Orbit* 2002;21(4): 295–299.
94. Mole S, Gardiner M. Molecular genetic analysis of neuronal lipofuscinosis. *Int J Neurol* 1991–1992;25–26:52–59.
95. Morales J, Chaudhry I, Bosley T. Glaucoma and globe enlargement associated with neurofibromatosis type I. *Ophthalmology* 2009;116(9):1725–1730.
96. Nirankari MS, Chaddah MR. Displaced lens. *Am J Ophthalmol* 1967;63(6):1719–1723.

97. Patel B, Egan C, Luclus R, et al. Cutaneous malignant melaonoma and oculodermal melanocytosis (nevus of Ota): report of a case and review of the literature. *Am J Dermatol* 1998;35(5):862–865.
98. Paulus Y, Jain A, Moshfeghi D. Resolution of persistent exudative retinal detachment in a case of Sturge-Weber syndrome with anti-VEGF administration. *Ocul Immunol Inflam* 2009;17(4):292–294.
99. Pe'er J. Ocular surface squamous neoplasia. *Ophthalmol Clin North Am* 2005;18(1):1–13.
100. Piatigorski J. Molecular biology: recent studies on the enzyme/crystallins and alpha-crystallin gene expression. *Exp Eye Res* 1990;50:725–727.
101. Polito E, Pichierri P, Loffredo A, et al. A case of primary botryoid conjunctival rhabdomyosarcoma. *Graefes Arch Clin Exp Ophthalmol* 2006;244(4):517–519.
102. Pollard ZF. Familial bilateral posterior lenticonus. *Arch Ophthalmol* 1983;101(8):1238–1240.
103. Poulaki V, Colby K. Genetics of anterior and stromal corneal dystrophies. *Semin Ophthalmol* 2008;23(1):9–17.
104. Rahimi-Movagahr V, Karimi M. Meningeal melaonocytoma of the brain and oculodermal melanocytosis (nevus of Ota): case report and review of the literature. *Surg Neurol* 2003;59(3):200–210.
105. Ramamurthi S, Rahman M, Dutton G, et al. Pathogenesis, clinical features and management of recurrent corneal erosions. *Eye* 2006;20(6):635–644.
106. Ramsey M, Fine B, Shields J, et al. The Marfan syndrome. A histopathologic study of ocular findings. *Am J Ophthalmol* 1973;76: 102–116.
107. Ramsey MS, Yanoff M, Fine BS, The ocular histopathology of homocystinuria. A light and electron microscopic study. *Am J Ophthalmol* 1972;74(3):377–385.
108. Raskin E, Speaker M, Laibson P. Blepharitis. *Infect Dis Clin North Am* 1992;6(4):777–787.
109. Roarty J, McLean IW, Zimmerman L. Incidence of seond neoplasms in patients with bilateral retinoblastoma. *Ophthalmology* 1988;95:1583–1587.
110. Robb R, Kuwabara T. The ocular pathology of type A Niemann-Pick disease: a light and electron microscopic study. *Invest Ophthalmol Vis Sci* 1973;12:366.
111. Rootman J, Carruthers J, Miller R. Retinoblastoma. *Perspect Pediatr Pathol* 1987;10:208–258.
112. Rosenblum MK, Bilbao JM, Ang L-C. Neuromuscular system. In: Rosai J, ed. *Rosai and Ackerman's surgical pathology*. Edinburgh, UK: Mosby, 1996:2515–2517.
113. Schornack M, Siemsen D, Bradley C, et al. Ocular manifestations of molluscum contagiosum. *Clin Exp Optom* 2006;89(6):390–393.
114. Schuster B, Seregard S. Ligneous conjunctivitis. *Surv Ophthalmol* 2003;48(4):369–388.
115. Seidman D, Shields J, Augsburger J, et al. Early diagnosis of retinoblastoma on dysmorphic features and karyotype analysis. *Ophthalmology* 1987;94(6):663–666.
116. Shah S, Al-Rajhi A, Brandt J, et al. Mutation in the SLC4A11 gene associated with autosomal recessive congenital hereditary endothelial dystrophy in a large Saudi family. *Ophthalmic Genet* 2008;29(1):41–45.
117. Sharan S, Swamy B, Taranath D, et al. Port-wine vascular malformation and glucoma risk in Sturge-Weber syndrome. *J Am Assoc Pediatr Ophthalmol Strabismus* 2009;13(4):374–378.
118. Shields J, Parsons H, Shields C, et al. Lesions simulating retinoblastoma. *J Am Assoc Pediatr Ophthalmol Strabismus* 1991;1991(6): 338–340.
119. Shtein R, Garcia D, Musch D, et al. Herpes simplex virus keratitis: histopathologic neovascularization and corneal allograft failure. *Ophthalmology* 2009;116(7):1301–1305.
120. Sinha S, Cohen P, Schwartz R. Nevus of Ota in children. *Cutis* 2008;82(1):25–29.
121. Stalemark H, Laurencikas E, Karis J, et al. Incidence of Langerhans cell histiocytosis in children: a population based study. *Pediatr Blood Cancer* 2008;51(1):76–81.
122. Stavrou P, Balatzis S, Letko E, et al. Pars plana vitrectomy in patients with intermediate uveitis. *Ocul Immunol Inflam* 2001;9(3):141–151.
123. Stock E, Feder R, O'Grady R, et al. Lattice corneal dystrophy type IIIA. Clinical and histopathologic correlations. *Arch Ophthalmol* 1991;109(3):354–358.
124. Stone E, Mathers W, Rosenwasser G, et al. Three autosomal dominant corneal dystrophies map to chromosome 5q. *Nat Genet* 1994;6(1):47–51.
125. Taban M, Traboulsi E. Malignant melanoma of the conjunctiva in children. *J Am Assoc Pediatr Ophthalmol Strabismus* 2007;44(5): 277–282.
126. Traboulsi E, Maumenee I. Peters' anomaly and assorted congenital malformations. *Arch Ophthalmol* 1992;110:1739–1742.
127. Tsai J, Galaydh F, Ching S. Anterior uveitis and iris nodules that are associated with Langerhans cell histiocytosis. *Am J Ophthalmol* 2005;140(6):1143–1145.
128. Verity D, Restori M, Rose G. Natural history of periocular capillary haemangiomas: changes in internal blood velocity and lesion volume. *Eye* 2006;20(10):1228–1237.
129. Vesaluoma M, Sankila E, Gallar J, et al. Autosomal recessive cornea plana: in vivo corneal morphology and corneal sensitivity. *Invest Ophthalmol Vis Sci* 2000;41(8):2120–2126.
130. de Visser L, Braakenburg A, Rothova A, et al. Rubella virus-associated uveitis: clinical manifestations and visual prognosis. *Am J Ophthalmol* 2008;146:292–297.
131. Weisenthal RW, Streeten BW. Posterior membrane dystrophies. In: Krachmer J, Mannis M, Holland E, eds. *Cornea*. Philadelphia: Elsevier Mosby, 2005:938–948.
132. West S, Taylor H. Bilamellar tarsal rotation is the preferred treatment for trachomatous trichiasis. *Surv Ophthalmol* 1999;43(5):468.
133. Witchel H, Font R. Hemangioma of the choroid. A clinicopathologic study of 71 cases and a review of the literature. *Surv Ophthalmol* 1976;20(6):415–431.
134. Wladis E, Tomaszewski J, Gausas R. Langerhans histiocytosis of the orbit 10 years after involvement at other sites. *Ophthalmic Plast Reconstruct Surg* 2008;24(2):142–143.
135. Yanoff M, Perry H. Juvenile xanthogranuloma of the corneoscleral limbus. *Arch Ophthalmol* 1995;113(7):915–917.
136. Yohe S, Reyes M, Johnson D, et al. Plaminogen deficiency as a rare cause of conjunctivitis and lymphadenopathy. *Am J Surg Pathol* 2009;33(2):313–319.
137. Zamir E, Mechoulam H, Micera A, et al. Inflamed juvenile conjunctival nevus: clinicopathologic correlations. *Br J Ophthalmol* 2002;86(1):28–30.
138. Zhang J, Gray J, Wu L, et al. Rb regulates proliferation and rod photoreceptor development in the mouse retina. *Nat Genet* 2004;36(4):351–360.
139. Zimmerman L. Histopathologic basis for ocular manifestations of congenital rubella syndrome (the eighth William Hamilin Wilder Memorial Lecture). *Am J Ophthalmol* 1968;65:837–862.
140. Zimmerman L. Phakomatous choristoma of the eyelid. A tumor of lenticular origin. *Am J Ophthalmol* 1971;71:169–171.

CHAPTER 12

The Respiratory Tract

J. THOMAS STOCKER
HARESH MANI
ALIYA N. HUSAIN

DEVELOPMENT OF THE LUNG

The lung begins as a pouch or groove originating from the primitive foregut in week 3 of embryologic development, when the embryo is 3 mm long. As the groove enlarges caudally, a tubular lung bud is formed; the upper portion develops into the epithelium of the larynx, and the caudal portion into the epithelium of the tracheobronchial tree (1).

The embryonic period of lung development (Table 12-1) begins in week 4 of gestation as the single lung bud from the foregut divides into two primary bronchial buds, the forerunners of the right and left lungs (Figure 12-1A to C). During week 5 of gestation, the primary bronchi divide. Each forms three lobar buds that, by the end of week 6 of gestation, divide again to form 10 segmental bronchi on the right and eight to nine on the left. These potential airways consist of a central core of epithelial cells surrounded by loose primitive mesenchyme that contains widely separated capillaries. The primitive pulmonary arteries begin to form from the sixth aortic arch, near the end of the embryonic period (2). The pulmonary veins begin as evaginations of the left atrium during week 4 of gestation and coalesce with the mesenchymal capillary plexus early in week 5 (3).

The pseudoglandular period (weeks 6 to 16 of gestation) begins with the completion of the proximal airways and encompasses the development of the conducting airway system to the level of the terminal bronchioles (Figure 12-2A,B). The pseudostratified columnar epithelium of the proximal airway displays cilia at week 10 of gestation. The appearance of cilia extends to the epithelial cells of the peripheral airways by week 13. Goblet cells appear in the bronchial epithelium at weeks 13 to 14 of gestation, and submucosal glands begin as solid buds originating from the basal layers of the epithelium by weeks 15 to 16. Smooth muscle cells develop around airways by the end of gestational week 7 and organize to form an identifiable wall to the larger bronchi by week 12. Lymphatics appear first in the hilar region of the lung in gestational week 8 and in the lung itself by week 10 (4). Cartilage is first seen in week 4 of gestation and forms distinct rings along the trachea and main bronchi by the end of week 10.

The acinar or canalicular period extends from weeks 17 to 28 of gestation and is characterized by the development of the basic structure of the gas-exchanging portion of the lung (Figure 12-3A,B). Smooth-walled respiratory bronchioles, lined by cuboidal epithelium, subdivide into multiple, irregular alveolar ducts. By week 20 of gestation, the cells lining the ducts develop into type II alveolar lining cells with lamellar and multivesicular bodies associated with surfactant synthesis. Type I alveolar lining cells then differentiate from type II cells to form the thin air-blood interface required for gas exchange. As the interstitium thins in the latter portion of the acinar period, the capillaries of the interstitium proliferate and come to lie beneath the type I cells. Submucosal glands in the trachea and bronchi progress from tubules to mucus-containing acini. By week 24, the cartilage has extended to the most distal bronchi.

Table 12-1 ■ PHASES OF INTRAUTERINE LUNG DEVELOPMENT

Phase	Gestation Period	Major Event
Embryonic	26 days to 6 weeks	Development of major airways
Pseudoglandular	6–16 weeks	Development of airways to terminal bronchioles
Acinar or canalicular	16–28 weeks	Development of acinus and its vascularization
Saccular	28–34 weeks	Subdivision of saccules by secondary crests to term
Alveolar	34 weeks (and beyond)	Alveolar acquisition

Adapted from Langston C. Prenatal lung growth and pulmonary hypoplasia. In: Stocker JT, ed. *Pediatric pulmonary disease.* Washington, DC: Hemisphere, 1989:2, with permission.

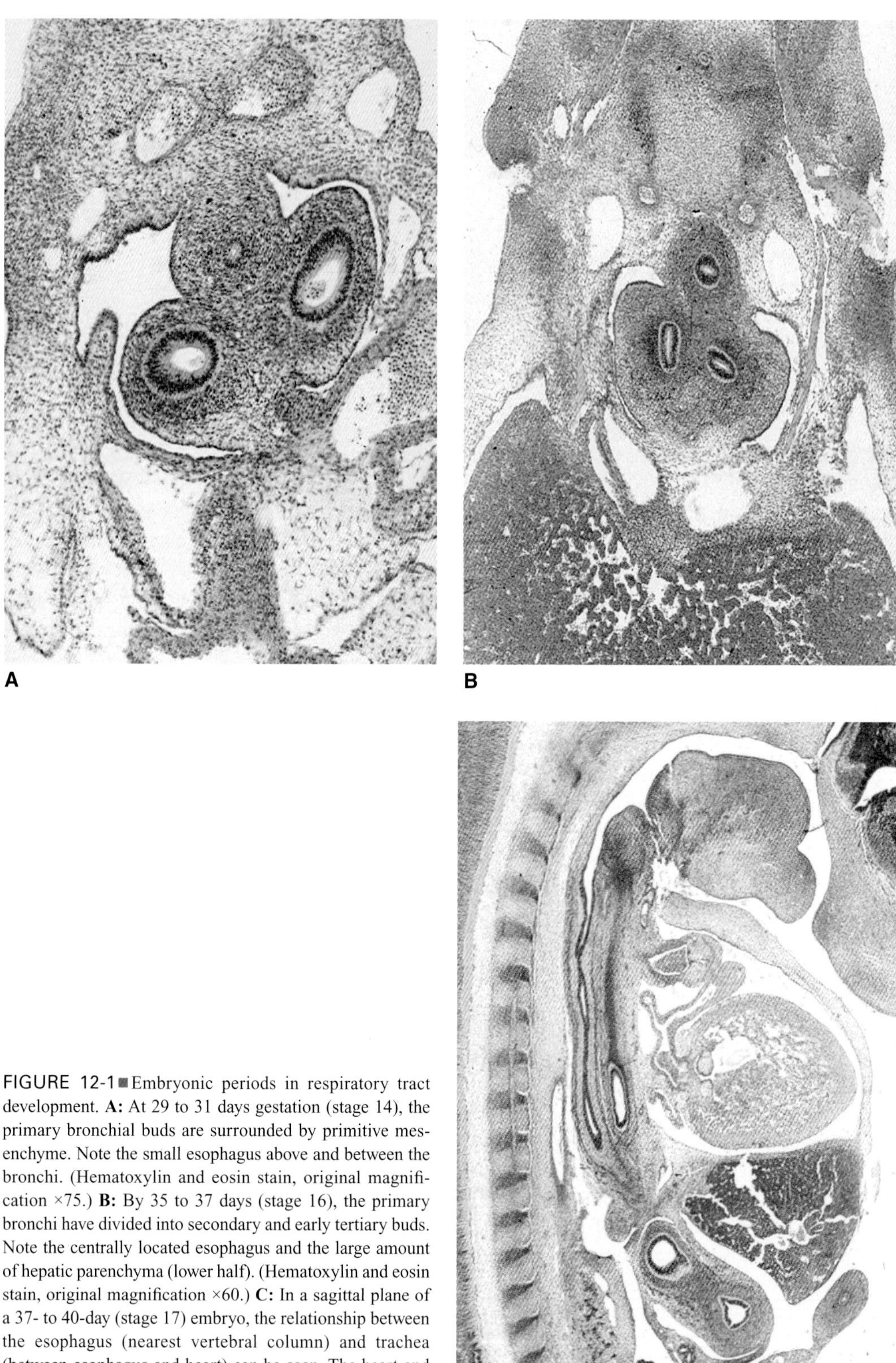

FIGURE 12-1 ■ Embryonic periods in respiratory tract development. **A:** At 29 to 31 days gestation (stage 14), the primary bronchial buds are surrounded by primitive mesenchyme. Note the small esophagus above and between the bronchi. (Hematoxylin and eosin stain, original magnification ×75.) **B:** By 35 to 37 days (stage 16), the primary bronchi have divided into secondary and early tertiary buds. Note the centrally located esophagus and the large amount of hepatic parenchyma (lower half). (Hematoxylin and eosin stain, original magnification ×60.) **C:** In a sagittal plane of a 37- to 40-day (stage 17) embryo, the relationship between the esophagus (nearest vertebral column) and trachea (between esophagus and heart) can be seen. The heart and liver are ventral to the foregut structures. (Hematoxylin and eosin stain, original magnification ×20.)

The saccular period begins at week 28 of gestation with the development of secondary crests, which are formed as distal airspaces divide into smaller units (Figure 12-4A,B). With an accompanying marked decrease in the interstitial tissue and further increase in the capillary bed, a complex, interwoven capillary network develops in the wall of the saccules. This provides for effective gas exchange as alveoli begin to develop at the end of the period (32 to 36 weeks of gestation).

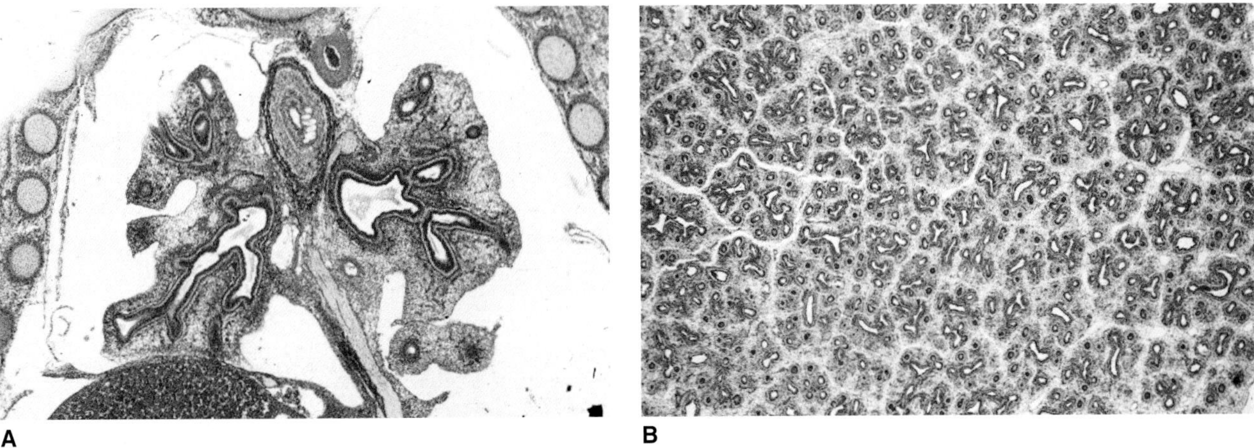

FIGURE 12-2 Pseudoglandular period. **A:** At 9 weeks gestation, the proximal airways are present throughout the right and left lobes. (Hematoxylin and eosin stain, original magnification ×30.) **B:** By 13 weeks, bronchiolar development is well under way and early division into lobules and clusters of acini is apparent. (Hematoxylin and eosin stain, original magnification ×40.)

The final period of development, the alveolar period, begins *in utero* at 32 to 36 weeks of gestation and extends until 18 to 24 months after birth. Alveoli develop as flask-shaped structures with thin walls whose double capillary network meshes to appear as a single capillary bed (Figure 12-5). At term, type I alveolar cells are extremely thin, resulting in an air-blood barrier of only 0.2 μm including the type I cell, the underlying basement membrane, and the cytoplasm of the capillary endothelial cell. Lymphatic channels are distributed around pulmonary arteries, bronchi, and bronchioles

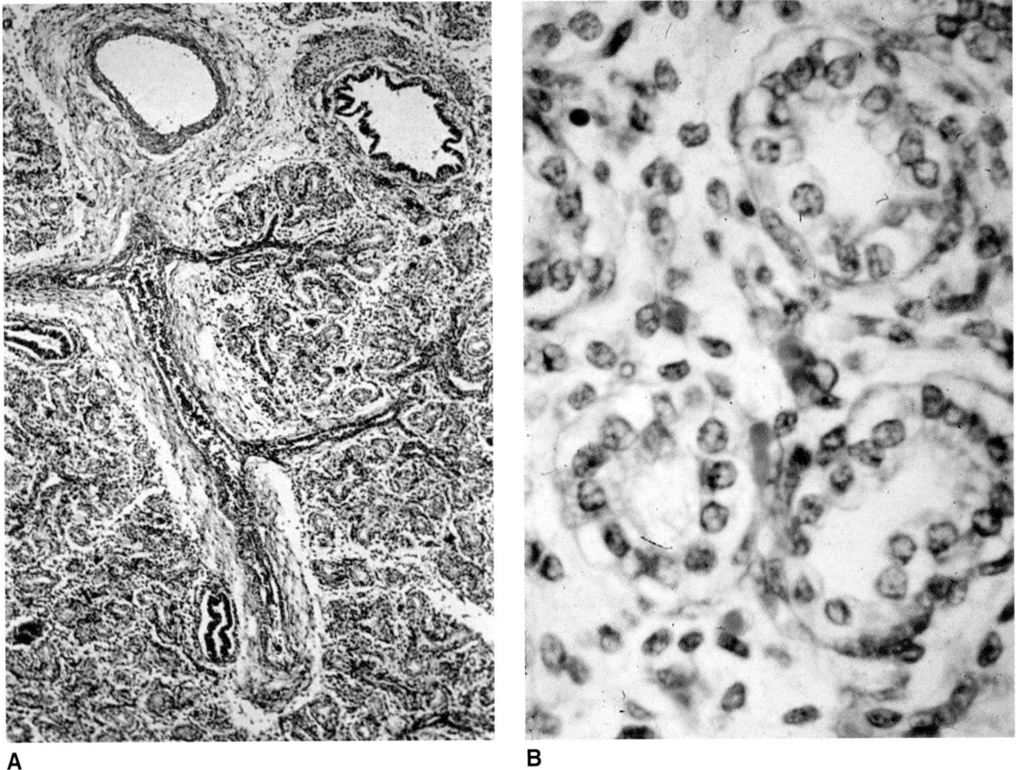

FIGURE 12-3 Acinar period. **A:** In a 370-g fetus, acinar development is characterized by pulmonary arteries and proximal bronchioles surrounded by alveolar ducts still widely separated by mesenchymal tissue. (Hematoxylin and eosin stain, original magnification ×40.) **B:** The alveolar duct structures are lined by cuboidal epithelium (early type II cells), but blood-filled capillaries are present just beneath the cells. (Hematoxylin and eosin stain, original magnification ×425.)

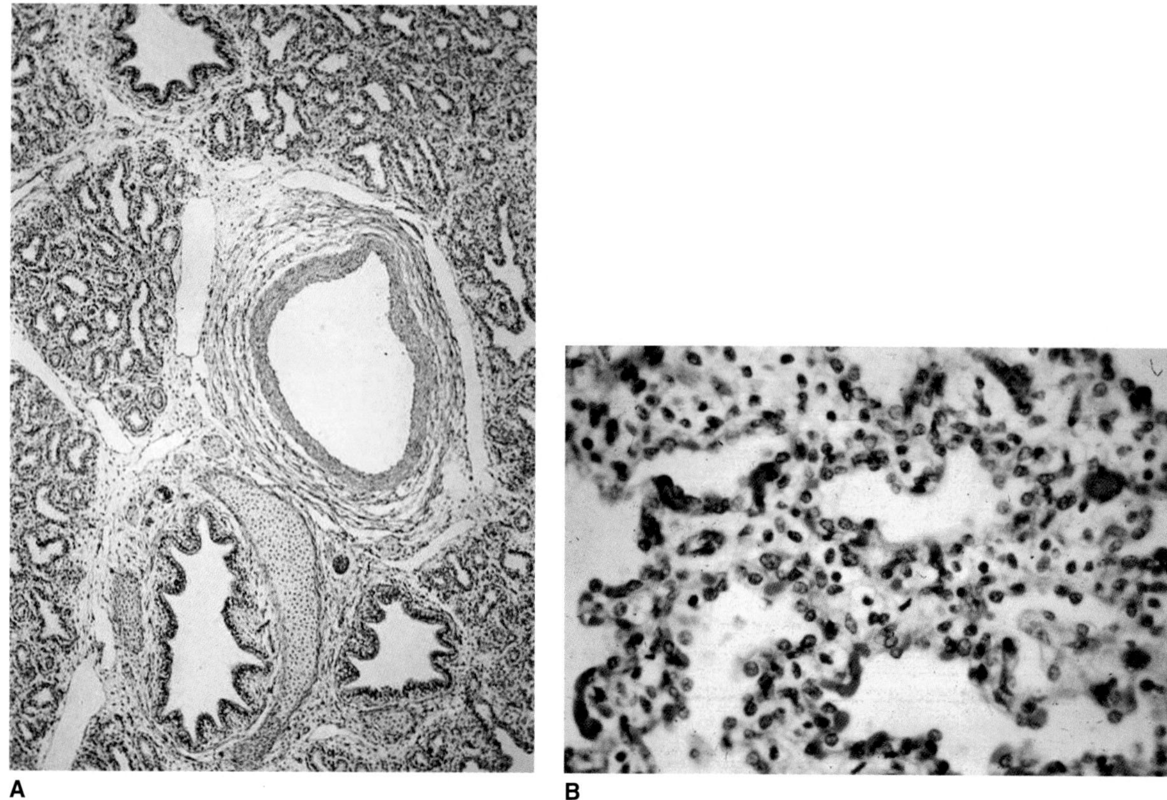

FIGURE 12-4■Saccular period. **A:** In a 650-g fetus, discrete acini are identifiable within a lobule. (Hematoxylin and eosin stain, original magnification ×50.) **B:** Secondary crests are covered by thinning type I cells, which expose capillary beds immediately beneath the cells. (Hematoxylin and eosin stain, original magnification ×350.)

and extend along interlobular septa to anastomose with a plexus beneath the pleura. Lymphatic spaces do not exist between alveoli (4).

The vascular supply of the lung changes appreciably in late gestation and infancy. The bronchial arterial circulation, originating from the aortic arch, supplies the bronchi, bronchioles, and interlobular septa in older children and adults; however, the bronchial artery contributes substantially to the circulation of the alveolar ducts and alveoli in the central portions of the lungs through bronchopulmonary artery anastomoses *in utero* and in early infancy (5).

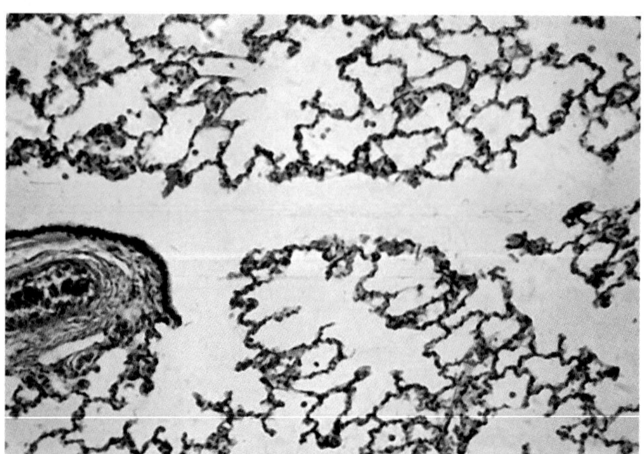

FIGURE 12-5■Alveolar period. At 2 months of age, a respiratory bronchiole (left) gives rise to alveolar ducts, alveolar saccules, and thin-walled alveoli. (Hematoxylin and eosin stain, original magnification ×50.)

At birth, the surface area of the lung is about 4 m^2, with the number of alveoli ranging from 10 to 150 million (mean of 53 million) (6). Alveoli increase in number after birth, reaching the adult range of 300 to 600 million alveoli by 2 years of age. Thereafter, lung growth occurs in terms of volume and alveolar size, with no further increase in alveolar numbers (7).

NASOPHARYNX

Choanal Atresia

Choanal atresia occurs in about 1 in 5 to 8,000 livebirths and consists of unilateral or bilateral occlusion of the airway between the posterior nasal passage and the nasopharynx (8,9). The entity has been seen in monozygotic twins (10) and has also been noted following radiotherapy for nasopharyngeal carcinoma (11,12). The septum blocking the airway is usually composed of bone or cartilage, but in as many as 20% to 50% of cases, it may be composed of mucous membrane alone (13). Choanal atresia may exist as an isolated sporadic lesion, in an autosomal dominant form, or possibly in an autosomal recessive form. It has been associated with palatal defects, tracheoesophageal fistula (TEF), congenital heart malformations (14), trisomy 6 (15), Pfeiffer syndrome (16), Treacher Collins syndrome (17), the fetal carbimazole syndrome (18), and the CHARGE (Coloboma, Heart defect, choanal Atresia, Retardation, Genital, Ear anomaly) association (CHD7 mutation on 8q12.2) (19,20), of which it is a major component.

Cleft Lip and/or Palate

Cleft lip, with or without unilateral and bilateral involvement of the hard palate, the soft palate, or both, is the most common malformation of the respiratory tract (21,22). It occurs once in 750 live births as an isolated anomaly or as part of a wide variety of chromosomal, inherited, and noninherited syndromes, of which over 250 have been described (23) (Table 12-2). Cleft palate is associated with other anomalies in 47% of cases, cleft lip and palate in 37%, and cleft lip alone in 14%. Anomalies most frequently seen are those in the central nervous system (CNS) and skeletal system, followed by urogenital and cardiovascular anomalies. Maternal cigarette smoking and alcohol use are associated with a 1.6- to 2.0-fold increase in isolated cleft lip, cleft palate, or both (24). The incidence of cleft lip and palate is dose-related, increasing with increased cigarette smoking (25).

Laryngocele

Laryngoceles occur rarely in childhood but may present as airway obstruction or as a neck mass in a neonate or an older child (26,27). The lesion, seen predominantly in boys and containing air or fluid, or both, may be within the larynx behind the thyroid cartilage (33%), external to the larynx (25%), or involving both locations (28). Infection of the lesion may occur (pyolaryngocele), leading to acute respiratory distress (29). Laryngoceles have been described in association with laryngeal papillomatosis (30) and in later life with laryngeal carcinoma (31).

Laryngomalacia

Stridor and feeding difficulties in the newborn may be caused by laryngomalacia due to flaccidity of a long epiglottis, short arytenoepiglottic folds, or bulky arytenoid swellings, resulting in partial obstruction of the larynx. Kay and Goldsmith (32) have developed a classification based on the underlying pathophysiologic processes with type 1 characterized by a

Table 12-2 ■ EXAMPLES OF SYNDROMES ASSOCIATED WITH ISOLATED CLEFT PALATE-PRESUMED INHERITANCE

Autosomal Dominant	Autosomal Recessive	X-Linked	Sporadic Occurrence
Stickler syndrome	Diastrophic dwarfism	Oculopalatodigital syndrome	Hanhart or aglossia-adactyl complex
Apert syndrome	Smith-Lemli-Opitz syndrome	Bruan-type nephrosis	Congenital oral teratoma
Marfan syndrome	Multiple pterygium syndrome	Gorlin skeletovascular syndrome	Buccopharyngeal membrane
Mandibulofacial dysotosis	Stapes fixation and oligodontia	Bilateral renal agenesis	Oral duplication
Spondyloepiphyseal dysplasia congenita	Cerebro-costo-mandibular syndrome		Caudal regression anomaly
Camptodactyly and clubfoot	Chondrodystrophia calcificans congenital		Klippel-Feil anomaly
Larsen syndrome	Dubowitz syndrome		Oligohydramnios sequence
Beckwith-Wiedemann syndrome	Campomelic syndrome		Bilateral renal agenesis
Wildervanck syndrome	Tel Hasomer camptodactyly syndrome		Various chromosomal syndromes
Chotzen syndrome	Juberg-Haywood syndrome		
CPLS syndrome			
Achondroplasia			
Cleidocranial dysplasia			
Brachmann-de Lange syndrome			
Hereditary renal adysplasia			
Maternally transmitted myotonic dystrophy			
Ectodactly, ectodermal dysplasia syndrome			
Popliteal pterygium syndrome			
Rapp-Hodgkin syndrome			
Shprintzen syndrome			
Treacher Collins syndrome			

CPLS, cleft palate-lateral synechia.
Adapted from Gilbert EF. Respiratory system. In: Gilbert-Barness E, ed. *Potter pathology of the fetus and infant.* St. Louis: Mosby, 1997:721, with permission.

foreshortened or tight aryepiglottic fold, type 2 defined by the presence of redundant soft tissue in the supraglottis, and type 3 applying to cases caused by other etiologies. Potentially serious complications of the obstruction include pulmonary hypertension and cor pulmonale, sudden death during respiratory tract infections, failure to thrive, and possible impaired intellectual development secondary to episodes of hypoxia and hypercapnia. Twenty percent of these infants have severe neurologic compromise or multiple congenital anomalies (33). Surgical procedures including supraglottoplasty have been used in severe cases (about 10% to 15% of cases) and have been successful in relieving respiratory symptoms in 80% of those cases (33,34). Laryngomalacia-induced stridor has been reported in patients with Pierre Robin (35), acrocallosal, Marshall-Smith (36), cri du chat, fetal warfarin (37), Down (38), Freeman-Sheldon (39), and Mohr syndromes. Chen et al. (40) have described a familial form of laryngomalacia.

Laryngeal Stenosis and Atresia

Supraglottic, glottic, and subglottic developmental webs may produce varying degrees of laryngeal stenosis and have been described in families with an autosomal dominant inheritance pattern.

Subglottic stenosis, as an acquired lesion, has been seen secondary to short-term and long-term intubation in the neonatal intensive care nursery with increased incidence when the infant is intubated for longer periods (41). With acquired stenosis, dense submucosal fibrous connective tissue is present circumferentially in the subglottic area and may narrow the lumen significantly. Submucosal glands are usually absent, and the cricoid cartilage may display evidence of erosion.

Congenital laryngeal atresia occurs in three patterns:

1. Type 1, atresia of both supraglottic and infraglottic portions of the larynx
2. Type 2, atresia of the infraglottic region (Figure 12-6A,B)
3. Type 3, glottic atresia (42)

Associated conditions include esophageal atresia (EA), TEF, "total sequestration" of the lungs in the absence of TEF, anal anomalies, urinary tract malformations, skeletal anomalies, and heart malformations (43). Many of the conditions are part of the vertebral, anal atresia, cardiac, TEF, renal, and limb (VATER or VACTERL) association. Other associations include partial diaphragmatic obliteration (44), Frasier

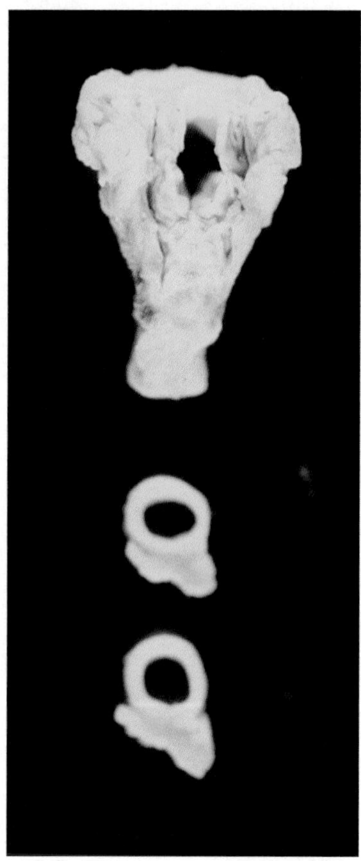
A

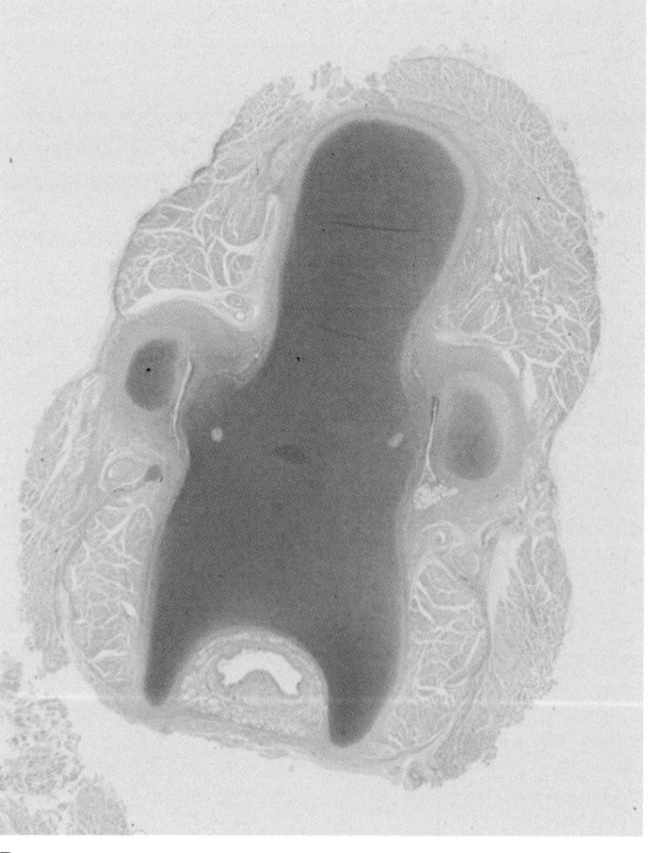
B

FIGURE 12-6 ■ Laryngeal atresia. **A:** The larynx reveals a patent upper opening (upper piece) and a patent trachea (lower two cross sections). **B:** A histologic section from the area in the region of the cricoid cartilage reveals only a pinpoint lumen (bottom center). (Hematoxylin and eosin stain, original magnification ×4.)

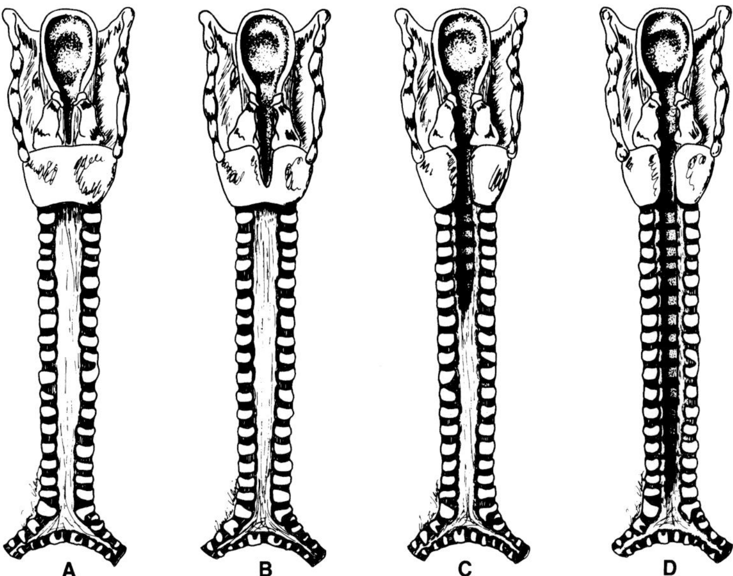

FIGURE 12-7 ■ Types of laryngotracheoesophageal cleft. **A:** Supraglottic interarytenoid cleft. **B:** Partial cricoids cleft. **C:** Total cricoid cleft. **D:** Complete cleft to level of carina.

syndrome, DiGeorge developmental field defect, and partial trisomy 9 (45–47). Pulmonary hyperplasia has been noted in infants who have laryngeal atresia with lung weights ranging from 150% to 300% of normal (48).

Laryngotracheoesophageal Cleft

Failure in formation of the tracheoesophageal septum, normally complete by day 35 of gestation, leads to the development of one of four forms of laryngotracheoesophageal cleft (Figure 12-7A to D):

1. Supraglottic interarytenoid cleft (50% of cases)
2. Partial cricoid cleft
3. Total cricoid cleft
4. Complete cleft of the trachea to the level of the carina (42,116)

Maternal polyhydramnios is seen in many cases, and a familial occurrence has been reported with relative frequency. Associated conditions include TEF and other elements of the VATER association—pulmonary hypoplasia, exstrophy of the bladder, polysplenia, double outlet right ventricle, and the G syndrome (49).

TRACHEA

Tracheal Agenesis

Tracheal agenesis is a rarely occurring, uniformly fatal malformation that is usually associated with tracheoesophageal or bronchoesophageal fistula. Various classifications divide the entity into three to seven types (Figure 12-8A to G); however, nearly 70% of cases consist of agenesis of the entire trachea with a small fistulous connection between the esophagus and the carina (Figure 12-8C to E) (50,51). The lungs may be normally developed or totally absent (pulmonary agenesis). In the rare cases of tracheal agenesis with no fistulous connection to the esophagus (i.e., total sequestration of the lungs), the lungs are uniformly distended, histologically resembling extralobar sequestration (48). There is a male predominance of approximately 2:1 and an association with maternal polyhydramnios in tracheal agenesis. In addition to the anomalies of the VATER association, tracheal agenesis has been seen in association with duodenal atresia, annular pancreas, syndactyly, and CNS malformations (52). Evans et al. (51) describe four groups based on the type of anomalies associated with the tracheal agenesis: group 1, anomalies restricted to the trachea, larynx, and cardiovascular system; group 2, severe cardiovascular anomalies and abnormal lung lobulation; group 3, a caudal component in addition to thoracic abnormalities, with anal and renal anomalies being common; and group 4, multisystem involvement with a high incidence of aberrant vessels, complex cardiac malformations, lung lobation defects, and anomalies of other foregut derivatives.

Tracheal Stenosis

Although laryngeal, or tracheal, stenosis is usually seen as an acquired lesion related to intubation or to the presence of a foreign body, congenital stenosis of the trachea is rare (53–55). Congenital stenosis may be diffuse, funnel-like, or segmental. Diffuse, generalized hypoplasia accounts for about 30% of cases, funnel-shaped or "carrot-shaped" stenosis for 20%, and segmental stenosis for the remaining 50%. Segmental stenosis may be due to complete tracheal cartilage

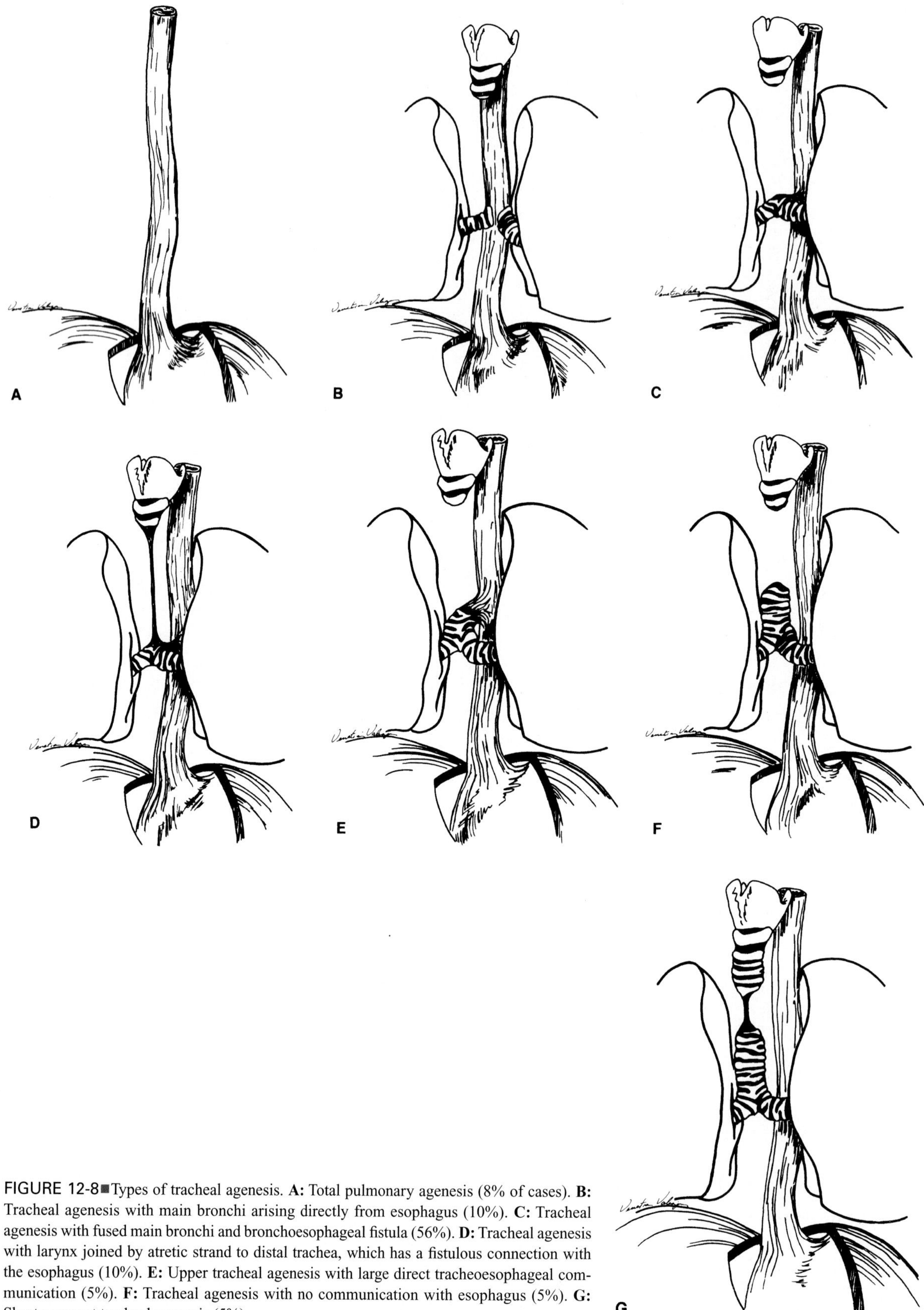

FIGURE 12-8 Types of tracheal agenesis. **A:** Total pulmonary agenesis (8% of cases). **B:** Tracheal agenesis with main bronchi arising directly from esophagus (10%). **C:** Tracheal agenesis with fused main bronchi and bronchoesophageal fistula (56%). **D:** Tracheal agenesis with larynx joined by atretic strand to distal trachea, which has a fistulous connection with the esophagus (10%). **E:** Upper tracheal agenesis with large direct tracheoesophageal communication (5%). **F:** Tracheal agenesis with no communication with esophagus (5%). **G:** Short-segment tracheal agenesis (5%).

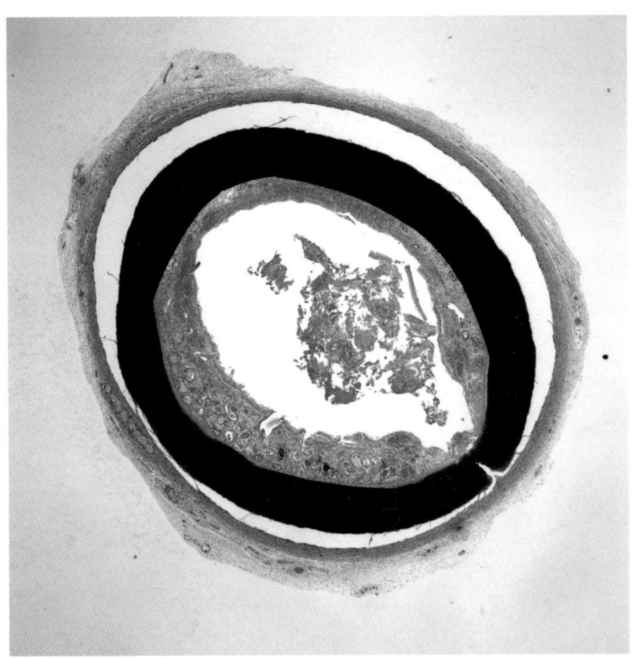

FIGURE 12-9 ■ Tracheal stenosis. A cross section from the mid trachea shows a complete cartilage ring beneath the mucosa, significantly narrowing the tracheal lumen. (H&E, ×2.)

rings, "napkin-ring" stenosis, or too small but normally shaped rings with a narrow pars membranosa (Figure 12-9) (56). Associated anomalies include anomalous bronchi, TEF, unilateral pulmonary agenesis, Crouzon syndrome, Larsen syndrome, Down syndrome (57), Alagille syndrome, and ventricular septal defect (58). Wong et al. (59) describe tracheobronchial stenosis in monozygotic twins.

Tracheal stenosis, or narrowing, may also be produced by extrinsic pressure, most commonly by abnormally placed or abnormally large blood vessels including

- Vascular ring due to double aortic arch
- Vascular ring due to right aortic arch
- Aberrant right subclavian artery
- Anomalous innominate artery
- Anomalous left carotid artery—aneurysmal left and right pulmonary arteries
- "Sling" retrotracheal left pulmonary artery

Advances in surgical management of congenital tracheal stenosis have improved survival, especially since the advent of extracorporeal membrane oxygenation (ECMO) (60,61).

Tracheomalacia

Congenital tracheomalacia (i.e., soft or collapsing trachea) is exceedingly rare and overlaps with tracheal stenosis secondary to cartilage plate deficiency (62). Isolated cases have, however, been reported in association with Down syndrome (63), EA, CHARGE association, Larsen syndrome (64), pulmonary vascular sling (65), polychondritis, and various chondrodystrophies including Ellis–van Creveld syndrome, Langer-type mesomelic dwarfism, and diastrophic dwarfism (66). Aortopexy has been successfully employed in the treatment of tracheomalacia in infants (67). Acquired tracheomalacia may be seen in infants and young children who have been intubated for prolonged periods or as a result of trauma, radiation, or a neoplasm (68,69).

Tracheobronchiomegaly

Tracheobronchiomegaly, or the Mounier-Kuhn syndrome, usually involves men 20 to 40 years of age but has been reported in children of both sexes and has a familial occurrence, suggesting an autosomal recessive type of inheritance (70). The tracheal diameter exceeds the normal by three standard deviations. Saccular bulging of the intercartilaginous membranes is frequent. The disorder has been noted in a child with cutis laxa and in an adult with Ehlers-Danlos syndrome (71).

Tracheoesophageal Fistula and Esophageal Atresia

EA, with or without TEF, occurs sporadically with an incidence of 1 in 3,500 live births (72,73). Maternal polyhydramnios is present in more than 30% of cases, and nearly 35% of the infants are premature (56). The anomaly can be divided into five (or more) types (Figure 12-10A to E). More than 95% of the patients have EA with the clinical findings of excessive oral and pharyngeal secretions or choking, cyanosis, or coughing during first attempts at feeding. A least three separate genetic factors have been identified for esophageal atresia (74).

TEF and EA can be most easily demonstrated at autopsy by removing the esophagus and trachea en bloc (see Chapter 1), and then opening the esophagus lengthwise along its posterior or dorsal margin. EA is readily apparent as a blind pouch (Figure 12-11A,B), but a small fistula between the anterior or ventral portion of the esophagus and the trachea can also be visualized, as can the rare esophagobronchial fistula. Histologically, squamous metaplasia of the trachea and bronchi may be seen in 80% of patients, primarily along the posterior wall of the trachea but frequently extending around the entire internal surface of the trachea and into the bronchi. The segment of esophagus may show tracheobronchial remnants in the form of abnormal mucous glands and ducts, abnormal mucin secretion, the presence of cartilage, and a disorganized muscle coat (75). Aspiration of gastric contents may be present in the lung, producing pneumonia with foreign body giant cell reaction.

Associated anomalies are seen in 49% to 72% of infants with EA and TEF, with multiple anomalies frequently present (Table 12-3) (76). A nonrandom association of TEF with other malformations has been recognized in about 45% of cases and given the acronyms of VATER, VACTER, or VACTERL (vertebral, anal, cardiac, tracheoesophageal, renal, or radial and limb anomalies) (77–79).

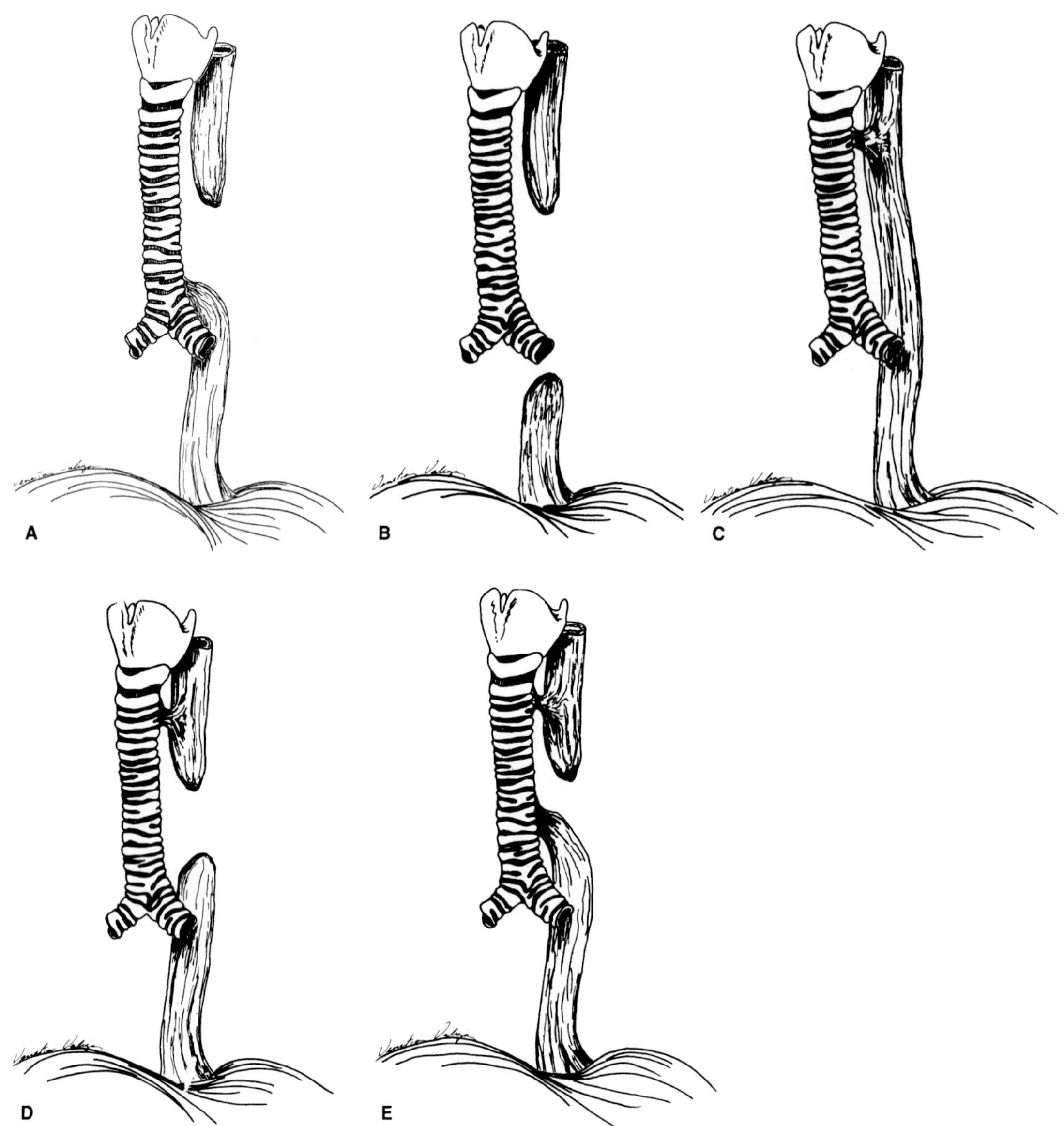

FIGURE 12-10 ■ Types of TEF and esophageal atresia (EA). **A:** EA with TEF to the distal esophageal segment (>85% of cases in various series). **B:** EA without TEF (8%). **C:** TEF without EA (4%). **D:** EA with TEF to the proximal esophageal segment (1%). **E:** EA with TEF to both proximal and distal esophageal segments (1%).

Other less frequently associated anomalies include congenital pulmonary airway malformation (CPAM) (80), diaphragmatic hernia, duodenal atresia, biliary atresia, sirenomelia, trisomy 18, and intracardiac epithelial cyst (81).

Postsurgical survival of patients with EA and TEF has increased steadily over the last 50 years, presently ranging from 75% to over 90% (43,77). The highest mortality rate occurs in infants with low birth weight or with coexisting cardiac malformations. TEF may recur after surgical repair in nearly 10% of cases (82). Tracheal narrowing may persist for years in nearly one-third of the patients, along with respiratory infections and gastroesophageal reflux. Histologically, esophageal inflammation may be seen in 51% of cases, Barrett esophagus in 6%, and Helicobacter pylori infection in 21% of cases (83). TEFs may develop in burn patients, with foreign body impaction, such as a disc battery (84), and following radiation and chemotherapy for mediastinal malignancies, including lymphoma (85). An increased incidence of esophageal adenocarcinoma in adulthood in patients with TEF has been suggested (86).

BRONCHUS

Bronchial Atresia

Bronchial atresia is an entity seen almost exclusively in infants and is most frequently associated with infantile (congenital) lobar emphysema (87). Cases of bronchial atresia with mild emphysema, however, have been reported in children from 1 day to 13 years (median, 4 years) with

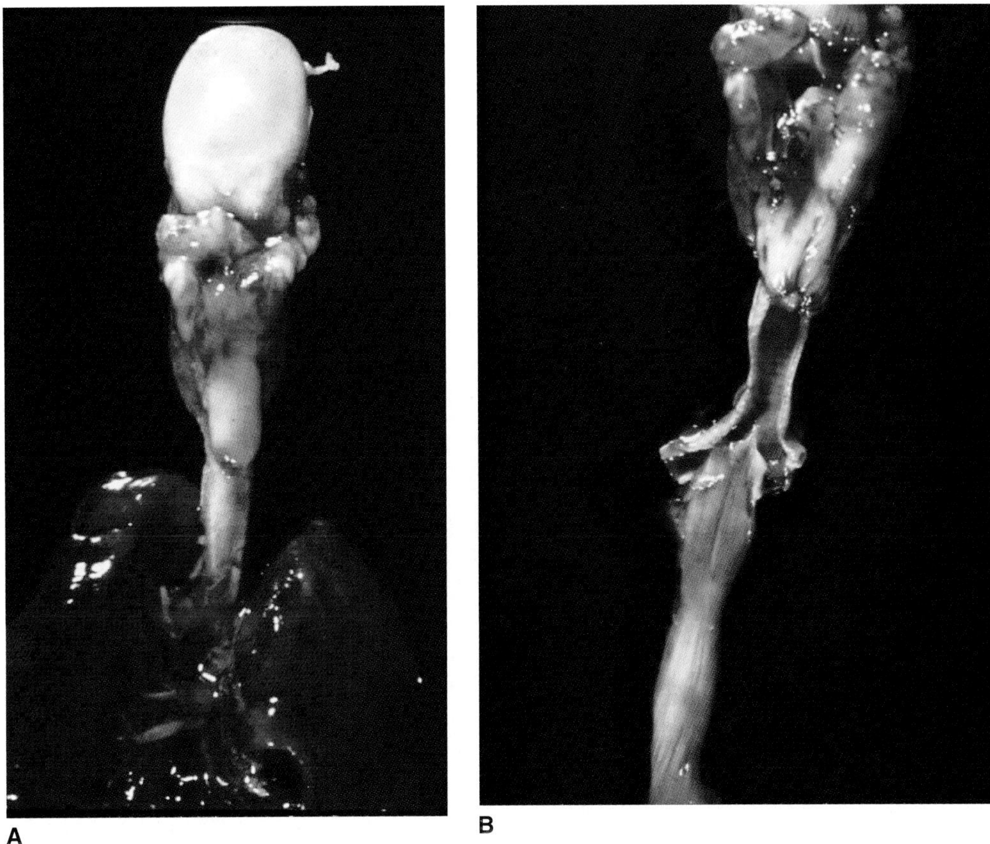

FIGURE 12-11 ■ TEF and esophageal atresia. **A:** In a posterior view of the tongue **(top)**, trachea, and lung, the esophagus is seen to end in a blind pouch **(center)**. **B:** With the trachea and esophagus open posteriorly, a fistula can be seen connecting the carina with the distal end of the esophagus. (Courtesy of David Kelly, M.D., University of Alabama, Birmingham, Alabama.)

symptoms of chronic cough and fever in nearly all of the cases, often related to the recurrent pneumonia noted in more than 90% of cases. The atretic bronchus is connected to the right lower lobe, left upper lobe, and right upper lobe in decreasing order of frequency. Histologically, the affected bronchus may be obstructed by circumferential or eccentric luminal fibrosis with or without abnormalities of the cartilage plates. The fibrosis may be the result of *in utero* inflammation in the neonate or possibly postpartum inflammation in the case of children and adults. The similarity between the lungs of congenital bronchial atresia and infantile lobar emphysema (ILE), both radiographically and pathologically, is striking, and suggests that they may be a single entity.

Bronchial stenosis may also be associated with ILE. The lumen of the bronchus may be intrinsically narrowed by postinflammatory fibrosis or by an intraluminal mass such as aspirated meconium or other foreign material, bronchial adenoma, ectopic thyroid tissue, or bronchial mucosal web. Extrinsic causes of bronchial stenosis include parabronchial masses such as teratoma and bronchogenic cyst, enlarged or abnormally located pulmonary arteries, and cardiac or

Table 12-3 ■ ANOMALIES ASSOCIATED WITH ESOPHAGEAL ATRESIA AND TEF

Organ System	Incidence (%)	Most Frequent Examples
Musculoskeletal	14.7–24	Vertebral defects, rib defects, radial amelia, caudal dysgenesis
Cardiovascular	11.0–49	Ventricular septal defect, patent ductus arteriosus, right aortic arch
Gastrointestinal	20.3	Imperforate anus, malrotation, duodenal atresia
Genitourinary agenesis	12.2–50	Renal malposition, renal cysts or hypospadias, horseshoe kidney
Craniofacial	9.7	Choanal stenosis, ear malformations, micrognathia
Central nervous system	7.2	Hydrocephalus
Pulmonary	2.1	CPAM pulmonary hypoplasia

Adapted from Stocker JT. Congenital and development diseases. In: Dail DH, Hammer SP, eds. *Pulmonary pathology*. 2nd ed. Heidelberg: Springer-Verlag, 1994:163, with permission.

left atrial enlargement (88,89). Bronchial stenosis has also been associated with EA and TEF. More recently, studies have also suggested that bronchial stenosis and/or atresia are common features of CPAM, extralobar sequestration, and intralobar sequestration (ILS) as well as ILE (90,91).

Bronchomalacia

Bronchomalacia and tracheobronchomalacia are seen most frequently in premature infants treated for prolonged periods with mechanical ventilation (92). Congenital bronchomalacia, however, is a rarely occurring disorder in which there is abnormal development of bronchial cartilage, leading to collapse of the lumen and possible development of secondary pneumonia. Bronchomalacia has also been suggested as a cause of sudden death, especially in those infants with respiratory distress (93). Deficiency of subsegmental bronchial cartilage with bronchial collapse is also a feature of Williams-Campbell syndrome and has been noted in children with Larsen syndrome (64,94). Children with Down syndrome have a high incidence (to 50%) of laryngomalacia, tracheomalacia, and bronchomalacia (63).

Histologically, the affected bronchus is decreased in size, with the usual cartilage plates replaced by scattered small islands of immature-appearing cartilage. The lung, distal to the collapsed bronchus, may show pneumonia or is distended in a pattern typical of ILE. Bronchial stents are used in the treatment of this abnormality but have been associated with complications including an aortobronchial fistula (95).

Bronchial Isomerism Syndromes

Bronchial isomerism results in "mirror–image" lungs (i.e., bilateral right or left lung), and is associated with five types of "polysplenia/asplenia" or heterotaxy syndromes (96).

Type 1, Ivemark asplenia syndrome, is a nonfamilial malformation complex involving bilateral right-sidedness, including absence of the spleen, intestinal malrotation, symmetric liver, and bilateral three-lobed "right" lungs with bronchi for both lungs. A variety of cardiac malformations are also associated with this type, including right aortic arch, symmetric venae cavae, transposition of the great vessels, and total anomalous pulmonary venous return.

Type 2, M-anisosplenia, involves boys who have one or more larger and one or more smaller spleens, along with congenital heart malformations, bilateral three-lobed "right" lungs, and relatively normal visceral situs.

Type 3, the polysplenia syndrome, is characterized by a bilateral two-lobed "left" lung bronchial pattern with intestinal malrotation, symmetric liver, congenital heart malformations, and 4 to 14 uniform small spleens.

Type 4, *F*-anisosplenia, involves females who have bilateral two-lobed "left" lungs, congenital heart malformation (usually double-outlet right ventricle), and anisosplenia.

Type 5, *O*-anisosplenia, is characterized by bilateral two-lobed "left" lungs, an approximately 50% incidence of intestinal malrotation, multiple spleens, an equal sex ratio, and congenital heart malformations, particularly double-outlet right ventricle, ostium atrioventriculare commune, or both (see Chapter 13).

Abnormal Bronchial Branching and Origin

Abnormal branching patterns, mostly minor anomalies such as double stem superior segments of lower lobe bronchi and trifurcation of the left upper lobe bronchus, are seen in nearly 10% of bronchograms (97). However, major anomalies are also seen, including double right lobe bronchus, accessory cardiac bronchus, tracheal origin of the right upper lobe bronchus (also called pre-eparterial bronchus), and bridging bronchus (Figure 12-12) (98,99).

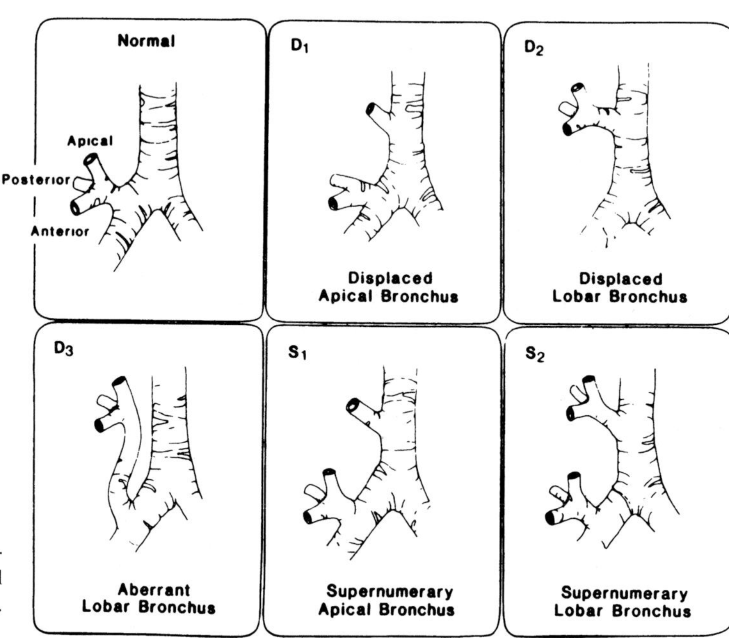

FIGURE 12-12 ■ Anatomic variations of right upper lobe bronchus. (From McLaughlin FJ, Strieder DJ, Harris GB, et al. Tracheal bronchus: association with respiratory morbidity in childhood. *J Pediatr* 1985;106:751, with permission.)

McLaughlin et al. (100) noted a tracheal origin of a bronchus in 2% of 412 symptomatic patients younger than 5 years of age who were undergoing bronchoscopy. The various forms of tracheal bronchus (Figure 12-12) may lead to recurrent episodes of pneumonia requiring resection of the bronchus and lobe. Other anomalies are noted in more than 75% of patients with tracheal bronchus. Wells et al. suggest that in patients with sling left pulmonary artery, the tracheal bronchus often associated with the right upper lobe may represent the "normal" origin of the bronchus, and the bronchi supplying the right middle and lower lobes are branches of the left main bronchus that are crossing or "bridging" the mediastinum (Figure 12-13). They note that the origin of the tracheal bronchus is at the normal level of tracheal bifurcation (T4-5) and the bifurcation of the bronchi supplying the left lung and right middle and lower lobes is at the T6-7 level.

Bronchobiliary and Bronchoesophageal Fistulae

Bronchoesophageal fistula probably represents a variation of TEF (101) but may also be seen with infectious diseases such as tuberculosis (102) and has been reported in association with Crohn disease (103).

Congenital bronchobiliary fistula rarely occurs (104); however, when it does, it is usually located between the right mainstem bronchus and the left hepatic duct (105). The bronchobiliary fistula is thought to represent a duplication of the upper gastrointestinal tract from its junction with the airway to the level of the ampulla of Vater. The fistula arises from the proximal portion of the right main bronchus, accompanies the esophagus through the diaphragm, and joins the biliary tree at the left hepatic duct. In its proximal portion, the tract resembles a bronchus with cartilage rings and respiratory epithelium, and in its distal portion, the tract resembles a bile duct or esophagus. Bronchobiliary fistulas may be seen in older children and adults in association with biliary obstruction or infections (such as echinococcosis) involving the liver (106). It has also been noted as a postsurgical complication in a child with undifferentiated embryonal sarcoma of the liver (107).

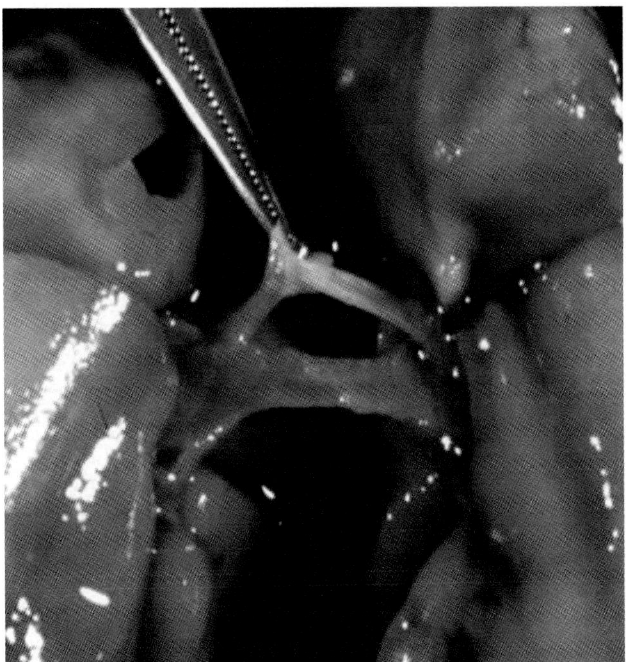

FIGURE 12-13■A bronchus "bridges" the mediastinum in the case of tracheal agenesis.

Bronchiectasis

Bronchiectasis was once a common acquired disorder seen in a variety of infectious diseases associated with chronic inflammation of the bronchi (e.g., tuberculosis and pertussis). It is now primarily associated with a number of congenital and familial conditions including immunodeficiency states (e.g., IgG, IgA, α-1-antitrypsin, neutrophil, or complement deficiency), the immotile cilia syndrome, cystic fibrosis (CF), and the Williams-Campbell syndrome.

Primary ciliary dyskinesis or the immotile cilia syndrome, also called Kartagener syndrome when associated with situs inversus (50% of cases), is characterized by immobility of the cilia of mucosal cells in the upper and lower airways, in the ependymal lining of the ventricular system, and in the various cells of the reproductive tract (including tails of spermatozoa) (108). The incidence of the disease is 1 in 20,000 to 30,000. The abnormalities of these cells lead to the clinical manifestations of chronic rhinitis, sinusitis, otitis, bronchitis, diffuse or localized bronchiectasis, headaches, and male subfertility. A variety of ultrastructural abnormalities, many nonspecific, have been described. These abnormalities include the absence of both inner and outer dynein arms, radial spoke defects, missing nexin links, microtubular transpositions, and compound cilia (109). An autosomal recessive mode of inheritance is suspected with extensive locus heterogeneity primarily on chromosome 19q and 10% of patients having a mutation in DNAI1or DNAH5 (110). An association with rheumatoid arthritis has recently been noticed (111). Treatment may require bilateral lung transplantation.

The Williams-Campbell syndrome, or familial congenital bronchiectasis, is a disorder characterized by a deficiency of bronchial cartilage distal to the main segmental bronchi, usually of the fourth to sixth order (112). Cartilage is absent, markedly diminished, or soft. The syndrome usually is seen in the neonatal period or early infancy, and familial cases have been reported. The disease may proceed rapidly or have a more benign course compatible with prolonged survival. Lung transplantation may be unsuccessful because of cartilage problems in the recipients' residual right and left mainstem bronchi (94).

CF (see below) is probably the most common cause of bronchiectasis, accounting for about 50% of all cases. No airway lesion specific for CF has been discovered, although mucus stasis in bronchi and pseudomonas pneumonia are frequently seen.

Bronchogenic Cyst

The bronchogenic cyst is a discrete, extrapulmonary mass filled with fluid and composed of a wall lined by respiratory epithelium overlying fibromuscular connective tissue that contains seromucinous glands and cartilage plates. It is noted most frequently in the hilar or middle-mediastinal area, but it may be present in a midline location from the subcutaneous region of the suprasternal area to beneath the diaphragm (113,114). Esophageal and enteric duplication cysts and pericardial cysts may also be present in the mediastinal region. Bronchogenic cysts are rarely connected to the tracheobronchial tree or involve the pulmonary parenchyma. Case reports of "intrapulmonary bronchogenic cysts" probably represent instances of type 1 CPAM [formerly congenital cystic adenomatoid malformation (CCAM)] (115).

Bronchogenic cysts are seen most frequently in children and young adults as incidental findings on chest radiographs, at surgery, or at autopsy, but they may present with symptoms related to secondary infection of the cyst, including fever, hemorrhage, or perforation. In infants, bronchogenic cysts located near the trachea, especially the carina, may produce obstruction and respiratory distress (116).

In infants, the gross appearance of the cysts consists of a 1- to 4-cm, smooth-to-irregular, spheroid mass attached to, but not in communication with the tracheobronchial tree (Figure 12-14A–C). The cysts may contain clear serous fluid, but if they are infected, the fluid may be turbid or hemorrhagic. In older patients, the cysts may reach a diameter of 8 to 10 cm and may be found throughout the mediastinum as well as in or beneath the diaphragm. Extrathoracic cysts are usually confined to the subcutaneous region in the suprasternal area (117).

Microscopically, the lining of the cyst is composed of ciliated, cuboidal to pseudostratified columnar epithelium. Cartilage plates and seromucinous glands are present in the wall, as is fibromuscular connective tissue (Figure 12-14C). The presence of striated muscle and stratified squamous or columnar epithelium is consistent with an esophageal cyst (Figure 12-15). Enteric cysts are lined by mucus-secreting columnar epithelium and contain gastric glands with parietal cells in the wall. All three types of cysts may display squamous metaplasia, mucosal ulceration, inflammation, extensive necrosis, or a combination of these, making an exact diagnosis difficult.

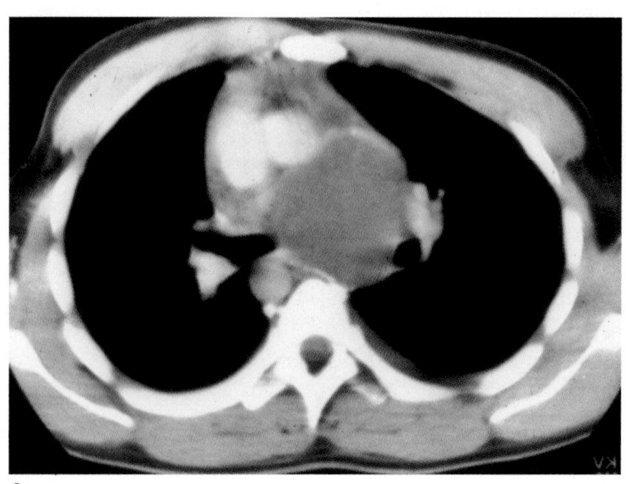

A

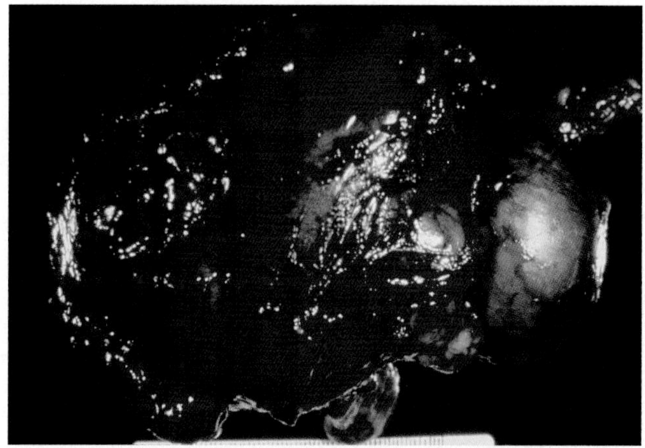

B

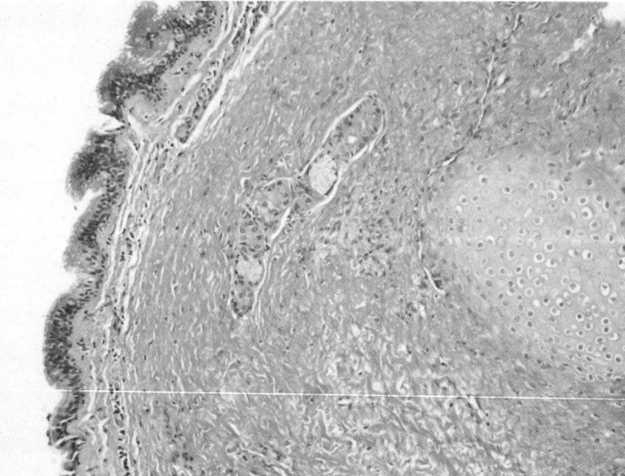

C

FIGURE 12-14 ■ Bronchogenic cyst. **A:** A CT of the chest displays a large mass in the middle mediastinum. **B:** A resected bronchogenic cyst, which was separate from the lung, is covered by connective tissue. **C:** Ciliated pseudostratifi ed columnar epithelium overlies a wall composed of fibrous connective tissue, glands, and a cartilage plate in a bronchogenic cyst. (H&E, ×100.)

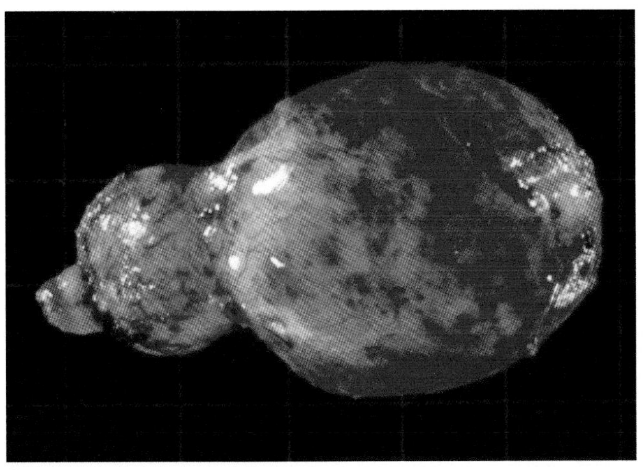

A

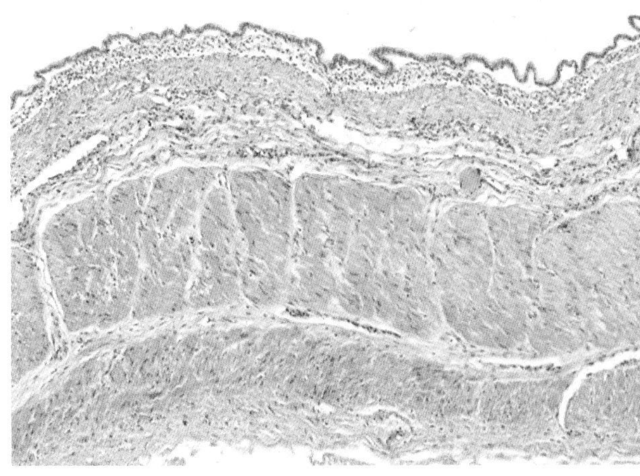

B

FIGURE 12-15▪Esophageal cyst. **A:** A cystic structure was resected from the middle mediastinum adjacent to the esophagus. **B:** Columnar epithelium overlies a wall composed of thick muscular bands in this esophageal cyst from the mediastinum. (Hematoxylin and eosin stain, original magnification ×75.)

Bronchogenic cysts have been noted between the sequestration and the midline in association with extralobar sequestrations in older children. This suggests that the cysts have arisen from "rests" of bronchogenic cells along the abortive foregut tract that gave rise to the sequestration (118).

Plastic Bronchitis

Children with cardiac defects (119) or an underlying pulmonary disease (asthma or allergic disease) may develop obstructive bronchial casts (120). There are two types of casts: type I, cellular cast made up of inflammatory cells with fibrin, and type II, acellular casts composed mainly of mucin (121). Other underlying causes include CF, neoplasia (122), thalassemia α (123), and acute chest syndrome of sickle-cell disease (124).

Grossly the cast may display a partial or complete outline of the bronchial tree with either tube-like features or partial or completely solid cores. Those composed of acellular mucin may be partially clear to opaque. Microscopically, the structures, as indicated by the types, are composed of an inflammatory cellular infiltrate embedded in fibrin (type I) or mucin-like material with scattered cellular debris (type II) (120).

LUNG

Pulmonary Agenesis

Complete absence of both lungs is extremely unusual and incompatible with life. However, unilateral agenesis, involving one or more lobes, has been seen in 1 in 10,000 to 20,000 autopsies and, in the absence of other severe anomalies, is compatible with long-term survival (113,125). There is a 1.3:1 female predominance with unilateral agenesis; the right and left lungs are absent with equal frequency. Associated anomalies are noted in about 75% of cases and include, in decreasing order of frequency, cardiovascular, gastrointestinal, skeletal, and urogenital systems (126). Cardiovascular malformations include dextrocardia, septal defects, patent ductus arteriosus, and total anomalous pulmonary venous return (127). Skeletal anomalies include hemivertebrae and a high frequency of thumb malformations, especially triphalangeal thumb (128). Along with the radial and vertebral anomalies, imperforate anus and TEF have been described, suggesting an association of pulmonary agenesis with the VATER or VACTERL association (129). Osborne et al. (126) propose that a neural crest injury may account for both the skeletal and pulmonary abnormalities because both are supplied by the second, third, and fourth thoracic nerves.

The larynx and upper trachea are usually well formed in unilateral pulmonary agenesis, although with bilateral agenesis the total trachea may be absent. The lower trachea in unilateral agenesis may continue directly into the existing lung as a tracheobronchus or bifurcate at the carina, giving rise to a rudimentary, blind-ending bronchus on the side of the agenesis. The pulmonary artery and vein to the side of the agenesis are absent or hypoplastic and may have an unusual course to the lung, often forming a pulmonary sling (130). Shift of the mediastinum to the side of the agenesis is usually present, often giving the appearance of dextrocardia in right-sided agenesis. Studies in older infants have demonstrated an absolute increase in the number of alveoli in the existing lung despite a reduced number of bronchial generations and pulmonary artery branches.

Abnormal Lobation, Location, and Shape

Abnormalities of lobation of the lung are usually of little clinical significance unless they are associated with other anomalies such as the asplenia or polysplenia syndrome (discussed earlier in chapter). Lobes may be fused to give the appearance of a single lobe on the right or left, or pleural fissures may produce the appearance of multiple lobes.

The appearance of multiple lobes may be seen in infants with long-standing healed bronchopulmonary dysplasia (LSHBPD) (131). Fusion of the lungs in the midline behind the heart produces a conjoined, or "horseshoe," lung analogous to the horseshoe kidney (132). Additional anomalies are often present, including those of the VATER association and the PAGOD syndrome (Pulmonary hypoplasia, Agonadism, Omphalocele, Dextrocardia and Diaphragmatic defect), among others (133,134). Bronchial supply to both lungs may be anatomically normal, but there is usually an anomalous pulmonary artery supply and venous drainage resembling that seen in scimitar syndrome (135).

Herniation of the lung across the mediastinum into the opposite hemithorax, associated with ILE, CPAM, extralobar sequestration, and other conditions, occurs relatively frequently (1). The lung can also herniate outside the thoracic cavity, usually into the neck. Cervical herniation or "protrusion" is most frequently reported as a "normal variant" in some infants and children (136). It may also be seen, however, as a result of trauma or surgery, and in association with iniencephalus, the Klippel-Feil syndrome, and the cri du chat syndrome (137). A familial occurrence has been noted, and the condition is thought to be an autosomal dominant hereditary disease (138). Herniation through the diaphragm and intercostal spaces may also occur (139).

Sequestrations

Extralobar

Extralobar sequestrations of the lung are discrete masses of pulmonary parenchyma outside the normal pleural investment of the lung and are not connected to the tracheobronchial tree. They apparently originate from an outpouching of the foregut, separate from the normally developing lung (Figure 12-16A). This outpouching then loses its connection with the foregut, isolating the parenchyma from the tracheobronchial tree (118). Extralobar sequestrations are diagnosed prenatally in about 25% of cases, and about 60% of patients present with it by 3 months of age (140). Presenting symptoms, often noted on the first day of life, include cyanosis, dyspnea, and difficulty in feeding. Approximately 10% of patients are asymptomatic. Fetal nonimmune hydrops, anasarca, pleural effusion, or localized edema may be present along with maternal polyhydramnios. Extralobar sequestrations may be seen in older children, occasionally in association with a bronchogenic cyst, and they have been reported in adults as old as 81 years of age (141). There is a slight female predominance.

Associated anomalies are present in more than 65% of cases of extralobar sequestration, with 50% of lesions containing CPAM type 2 within the sequestration or, less frequently, in a lobe of the "normal" lung. The ELS/CPAM cases are seen more frequently in the first 3 months of life and on the left side (140). Other anomalies include bronchogenic cyst, cardiovascular malformations, bronchopulmonary-foregut connection, pectus excavation, absence of pericardium, and diaphragmatic hernia with concomitant pulmonary hypoplasia (142,143). High levels of CA19–19 have been reported in a few cases of extralobar sequestration (142,144).

Extralobar sequestration is usually a single round to ovoid lesion ranging from 0.5 to 15 cm in diameter (Figure 12-16B). In a report of 50 cases, 48% of the lesions were located in the left hemithorax, 20% in the right hemithorax, 8% in the anterior mediastinum, 6% in the posterior mediastinum, and 18% beneath the diaphragm (140). The blood supply to the extralobar sequestration is through a direct branch of the thoracic or abdominal aorta in over 75% of cases. The remaining receive their blood supply from smaller systemic arteries, the pulmonary artery, or rarely, from the pulmonary artery and a systemic artery (48). Venous drainage is through the systemic circulation in over 80% of cases; the remaining 20% of cases are drained either partially or completely by the pulmonary veins, or rarely, by the portal vein (145).

Grossly, the lesion is covered by a smooth to wrinkled pleura overlying a fine, reticular network of lymphatics. These lymphatics may be prominent in 30% or more of cases. Cut sections of the lesion display homogenous, pink-to-tan tissue resembling normal pulmonary parenchyma, or clusters of small cysts. Prominent subpleural lymphatics may also be seen.

Microscopically, extralobar sequestrations consist of uniformly dilated bronchioles, alveolar ducts, and alveoli in a normal acinar pattern (Figure 12-16C). Bronchioles are usually tortuous with undulating, cuboidal to columnar epithelium. In 50% of cases, the lesion may consist partially or entirely of back-to-back, dilated, bronchiole-like structures typical of CPAM type 2 (Figure 12-16D). Lymphatics are unremarkable in the majority of cases but may be dilated and increased in number beneath the pleura and around bronchovascular bundles, occasionally resembling congenital pulmonary lymphangiectasia (CPL) (Figure 12-16C). Although they are rare, infarction, arteritis, and inflammation may be present in an extralobar sequestration. In the absence of severe anomalies, survival is good, although with large intrathoracic lesions, the associated pulmonary hypoplasia may be severe enough to cause death. Rhabdomyomatous dysplasia is seen 25%–30% of cases (Figure 12-16D).

"Total" Sequestration with Pulmonary Hyperplasia

Infants with laryngeal or tracheal atresia without TEF have, in effect, "total" sequestration of the lungs and display a histologic appearance virtually identical with that seen in extralobar sequestration. The lungs are often two to four times the expected weight and crowd the chest cavity, flattening the diaphragm and leaving an impression of the ribs on the visceral pleural surface (Figure 12-17) (48). Similar pulmonary changes may be seen with *in utero* hyperextension of the neck that appears to compress and obstruct the larynx. Scurry et al. (146) have noted normal sized or hyperplastic lungs in infants with varying degrees of upper airway obstruction despite the presence of renal dysgenesis

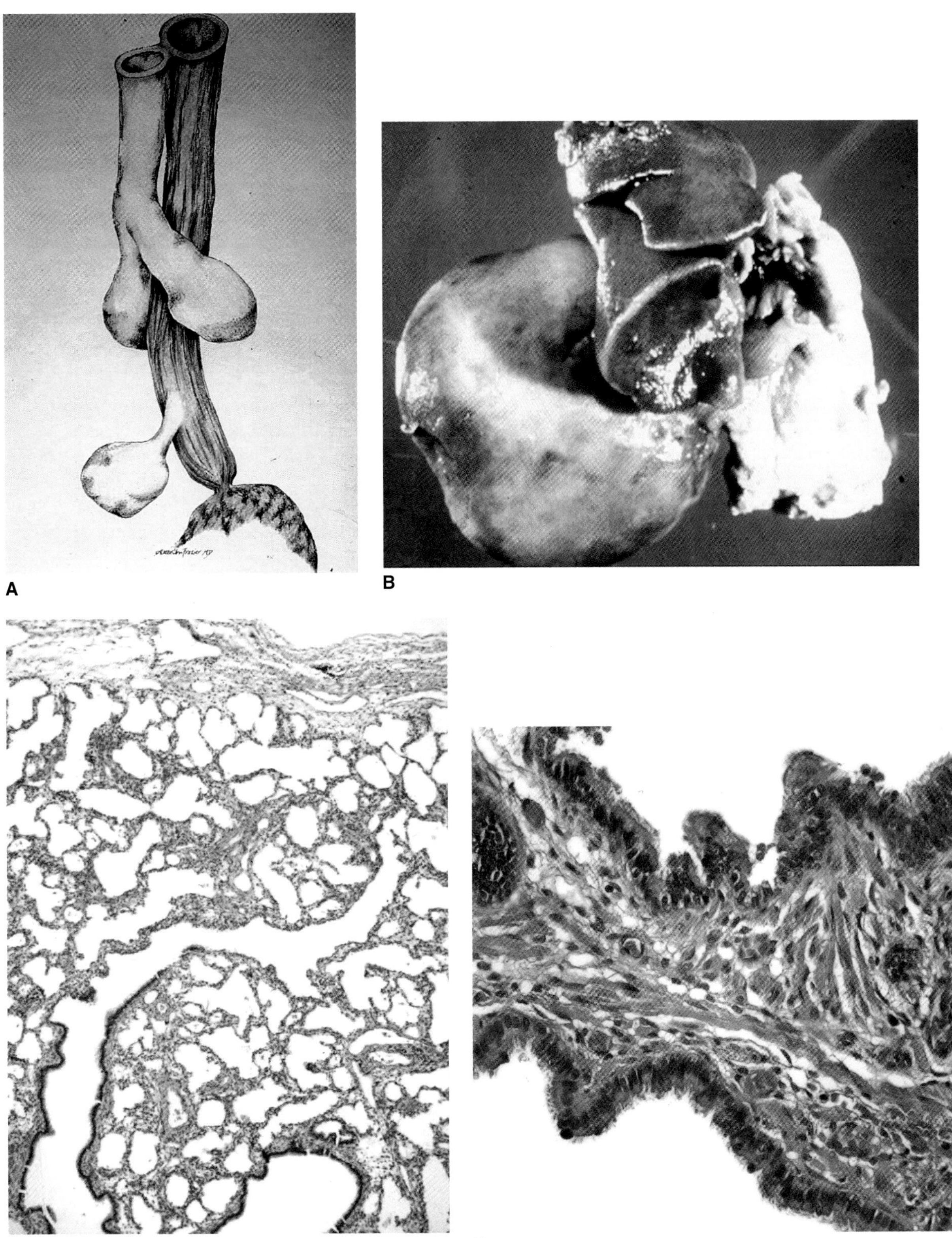

FIGURE 12-16 Extralobar sequestration. **A:** The normal lung develops as an evagination from the foregut (**top half**). A second evagination (**bottom**) from the foregut gives rise to lung tissue not attached to the normally developing lung. **B:** A large right-sided thoracic mass is attached to the mediastinum by a thin vascular pedicle. Note the hypoplasia of the right lung. **C:** The pulmonary parenchyma is uniformly dilated from the bronchioles to the most distal alveoli. (Hematoxylin and eosin stain, original magnification ×25.) **D:** Back-to-back bronchiole-like structures typical of CPAM type 2 are seen in 50% of extralobar sequestrations. Note also the rhabdomyomatous dysplasia. (Hematoxylin and eosin stain, original magnification ×75.)

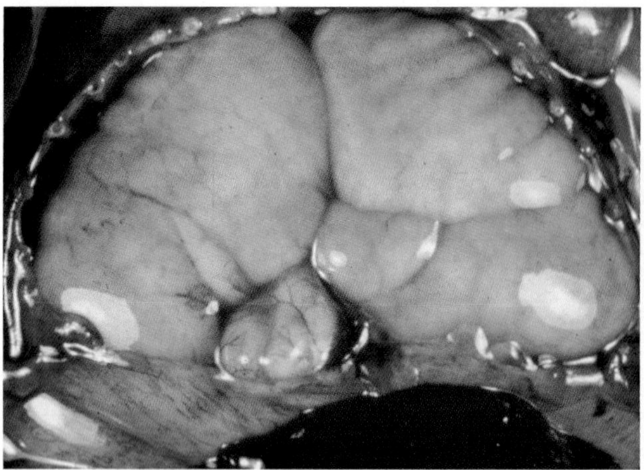

FIGURE 12-17■Hyperplastic lungs in the case of laryngeal atresia are massively enlarged, displaying the markings of the ribs on their surface.

and oligohydramnios, conditions more frequently associated with pulmonary hypoplasia. Lymphatics are unremarkable. Atresia or obstruction of a single bronchus to a lobe may lead to hyperplasia of that lobe and the development of one form of ILE (see below) (147).

Intralobar

ILS, by definition, consists of a portion of lung within the normal pleural investment that is isolated (sequestered) from the tracheobronchial tree and is supplied by a systemic artery (Figure 12-18) (148). Although a small percentage of ILSs are clearly congenital in origin and might more correctly be called arteriovenous malformations (149,150), the vast majority of ILSs are probably acquired lesions formed through repeated episodes of pneumonia. During the course of these episodes, normal pulmonary ligament arteries become hypertrophic to provide the systemic artery supply (Figure 12-18A–C) (48,151,152). Some examples of ILS may develop from a previously existing malformation (e.g., CPAM) (142,153). The following evidence suggests the acquired nature of ILS:

- ILS is rarely seen in the newborn (<15 cases described in children younger than 5 years of age).
- ILS is infrequently associated with other congenital malformations.
- ILS is limited to the lower lobes in 98% of cases, allowing access to normally occurring pulmonary ligament arteries.

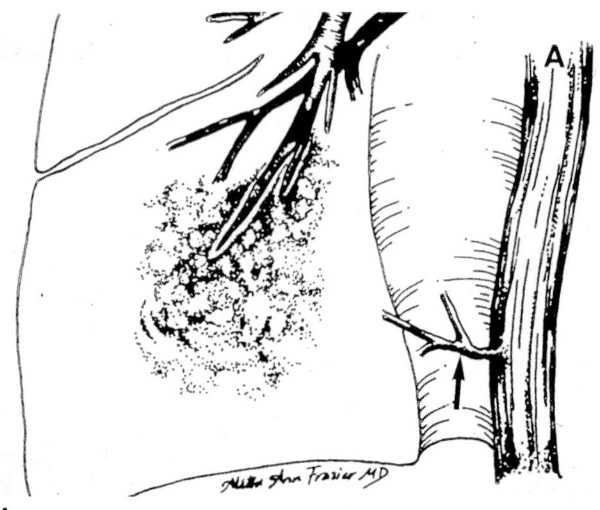

A

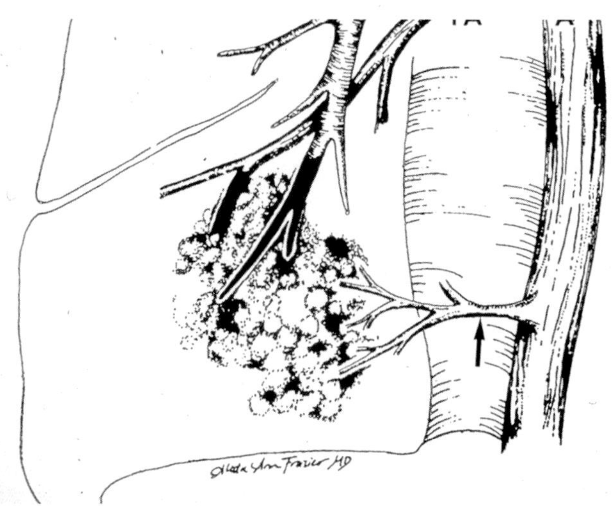

B

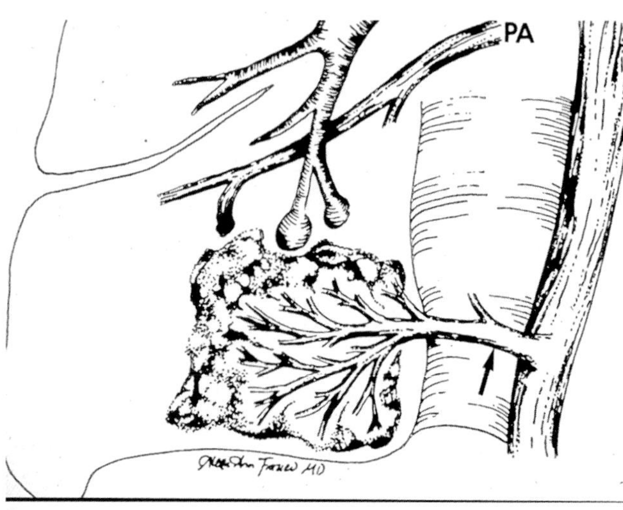

C

FIGURE 12-18■Sequence of events in the formation of intralobar pulmonary sequestration. **A:** Occlusion of a bronchial branch by means such as aspirated material or inflammatory debris can lead to the development of pneumonia distal to the occlusion. **B:** As the pneumonia persists or progresses, the lung seeks oxygenated blood to aid in resolution and repair. If pulmonary artery flow is inadequate, systemic blood supplying pleural granulation tissue through the pulmonary ligament arteries may be "parasitized." **C:** As the pneumonia resolves (or progresses or recurs), the major arterial supply to the sequestered portion of lung is derived from the hypertrophied pulmonary ligament artery (or arteries). (From Stocker JT, Malczak HT. A study of pulmonary ligament arteries: relationship to intralobar pulmonary sequestration. *Chest* 1984;86:611, with permission.)

ILS-affected patients have a frequent history of repeated pulmonary infections (154,155).

ILS presents with a clinical picture of chronic or recurrent pneumonia (e.g., cough, sputum production) in over 85% of cases (148).

ILSs involve the lower lobe in 98% of cases with this probably reflecting the availability, within pleural granulation tissues, of branches of normally occurring pulmonary ligament arteries or arteries within the diaphragm that are parasitized for access to oxygen-rich systemic blood. The pulmonary ligament arteries originate from the thoracic aorta and extend through the pulmonary ligament between the mediastinum and the lower lobes of the lung (152). No comparable arteries except the bronchial arteries are present for potential use by the upper lobes in cases of chronic or recurrent pneumonia.

Radiographic findings include cystic areas, some with fluid levels, along with homogenous and inhomogeneous shadows. Lack of communication with the tracheobronchial tree is demonstrable by bronchography in about 85% of cases; the other 15% of cases show some communication between the bronchial tree and the sequestration. Arteriography demonstrates single (84%) or multiple (10%) systemic arteries (Figure 12-19A,B). The majority of the arteries (73%) originate from the thoracic aorta, but about 21% originate from the abdominal aorta or celiac axis and another 4% from the intercostal arteries (156). In rare instances, arteries may originate from the coronary, subclavian, innominate, internal thoracic, or pericardiophrenic arteries (156). Venous drainage occurs through the pulmonary veins in 95% of cases, and the remaining 5% of cases drain into the systemic circulation. Increased serum levels of CA19-19 and CA125 have been noted in patients with ILS (157).

ILS is located on the left side in 55% of cases and on the right in 45% of cases; bilateral involvement is rare (48). Grossly, the sequestered segment of lung displays variable pleural thickening with adhesions between mediastinal structures, the diaphragm, and the parietal pleura. Variably sized (1 mm to 5.0 cm) cysts filled with thin to viscid fluid are noted amid a dense fibrous parenchyma on cut section (Figure 12-19). Microscopically, the pulmonary parenchyma is distorted by chronic inflammation and fibrosis (Figure 12-19C). The cysts are lined with cuboidal or columnar epithelium and are filled with amorphous eosinophilic material, foamy macrophages, or both (Figure 12-19D). Elastic and muscular arteries are present within the interstitium and may show medial hypertrophy, thrombosis, and arteritis.

Hypoplasia

Pulmonary hypoplasia is the incomplete or defective development of the lung resulting in overall reduced size due to reduced numbers or size of acini (Figure 12-20A). Lung weight and lung weight–to–body weight ratio are the simplest means of determining whether hypoplasia exists. The normal lung weight–to–body weight ratio for term and near-term infants is 0.222 ± 0.002 (158). Emery and Methal (159) describe a radial alveolar count using a line intersect method in which a line is drawn from a terminal bronchiole perpendicular to the nearest septal division or pleura surface (Figure 12-20B). The number of alveoli intersected by the line determines the count with the mean for term infants of 4.4 ± 0.9 (160). Alveolar counting and lung volume measurements may also be used (161). MRI, and two-dimensional or three-dimensional ultrasound have also been used in determining whether the lungs of an *in utero* fetus or newborn infant may be hypoplastic (162,163).

Pulmonary hypoplasia is noted in more than 10% of neonatal autopsies and occurs in association with another malformation (or malformations) in more than 85% of cases (164). The most frequently occurring anomalies are diaphragmatic defects and renal malformations (Table 12-4), but a wide variety of anomalies have been described (1). The common feature of most of these anomalies is that they directly or indirectly compromise the thoracic space available for lung growth. The cause of the decreased thoracic space may be intrathoracic (e.g., abdominal contents herniated through a defect in the diaphragm) or extrathoracic (e.g., oligohydramnios with uterine fetal compression). The thorax itself may be abnormal as in Jeune asphyxiating thoracic dystrophy, spondyloepiphyseal dysplasia congenita, and achondroplasia (165). *In utero* accumulation of fluid within the thorax as pleural effusion or chylothorax has also been implicated in the production of pulmonary hypoplasia.

Pulmonary hypoplasia may also occur in the absence of other anomalies or in cases of preterm premature rupture of amniotic membranes (162,166–169). As with infants with hypoplasia secondary to other anomalies, these infants present with respiratory distress, are difficult to ventilate, and frequently have episodes of pneumothorax (PT) and interstitial pulmonary emphysema (IPE). Potter sequence with sloping forehead, flattened face and nose, receding chin, large ears, broad spade-like hands, and deformations of the limbs secondary to compression by the uterus in the absence of adequate amniotic fluid is a consistent finding in cases associated with oligohydramnios from any cause. Pulmonary hypoplasia has been noted in children with Down syndrome, but it is thought to result from failure of the lung to develop properly in the postnatal period (170).

At autopsy, the lungs may be either uniformly reduced in size or markedly asymmetric (e.g., with diaphragmatic hernia). In cases in which the pulmonary hypoplasia is the direct cause of death, the lung weight usually is less than 40% of expected and is often as low as 20% to 30%. Histologically, the acini are small for the infant's gestational age, but alveolar and capillary development is usually consistent with the gestational age.

Infantile (Congenital) Lobar Emphysema

ILE is the overdistension or hyperplasia of a pulmonary lobe as the result of a partial or complete obstruction of the bronchus to the lobe by intrinsic or extrinsic factors (171–173) (Table 12-5). Boys are more frequently affected than girls

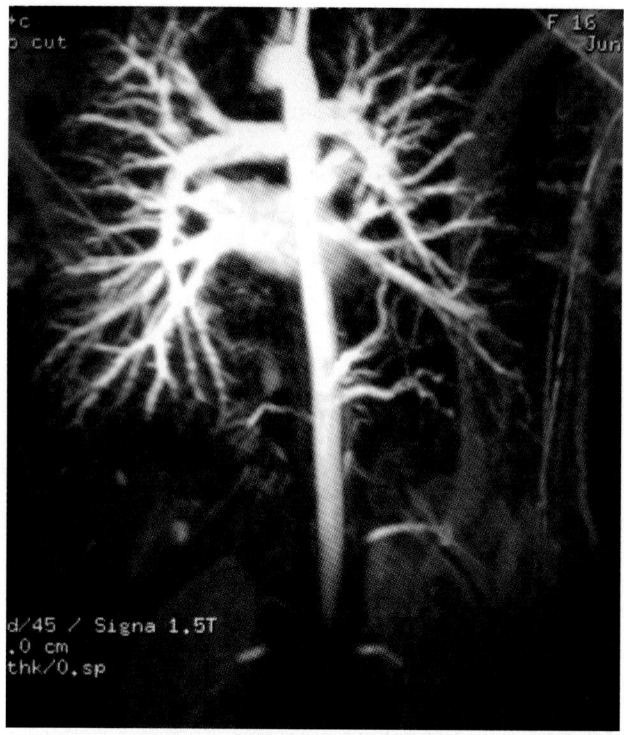

A

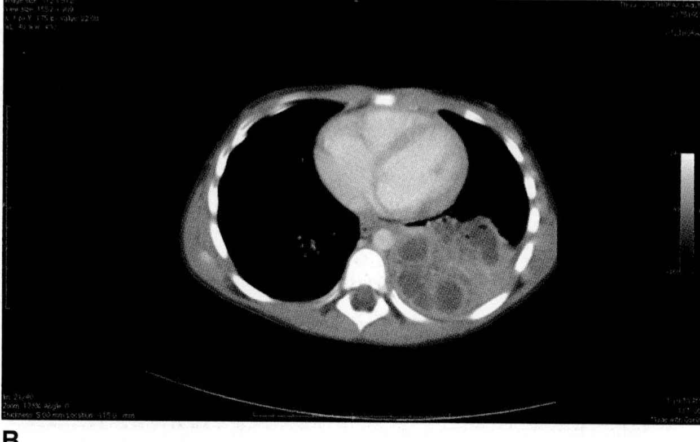

B

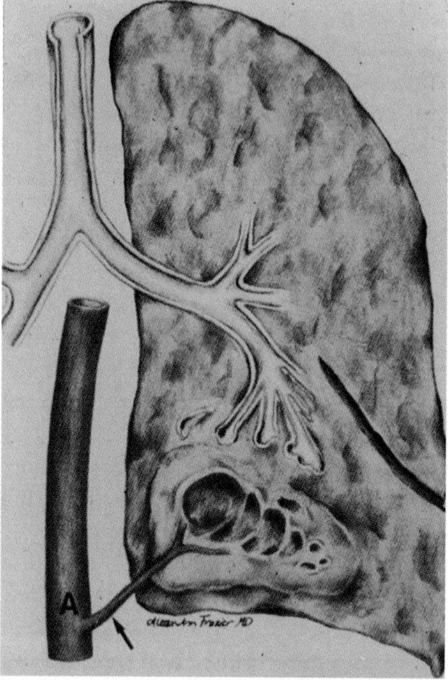

C

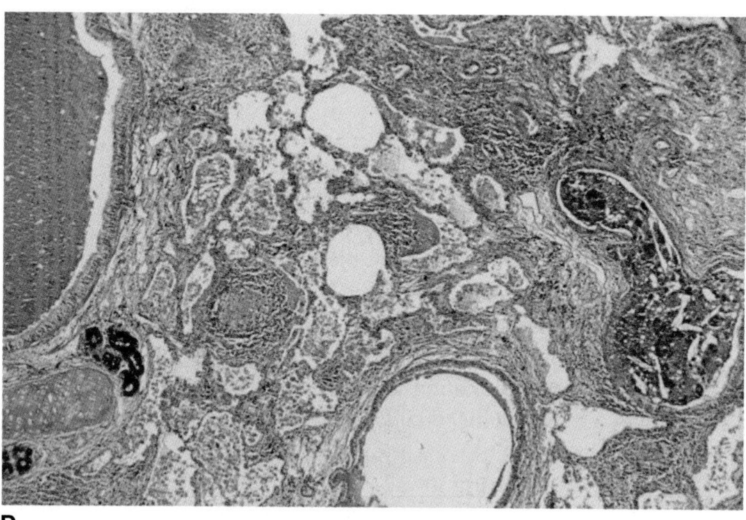

D

FIGURE 12-19 ■ Intralobar sequestration. **A:** An arteriogram demonstrated arteries arising from the descending aorta (**mid right**) supplying a portion of pulmonary parenchyma. **B:** A CT demonstrates a mass in the posterior area of the right hemithorax. **C:** An artery arising from the descending aorta and passing through the pulmonary ligament supplies a cystic portion of lung in the left lower lobe. **D:** Dense fibrous connective tissue containing lymphoid aggregates surrounds irregular cysts filled with debris and macrophages. (Hematoxylin and eosin stain, original magnification ×25.)

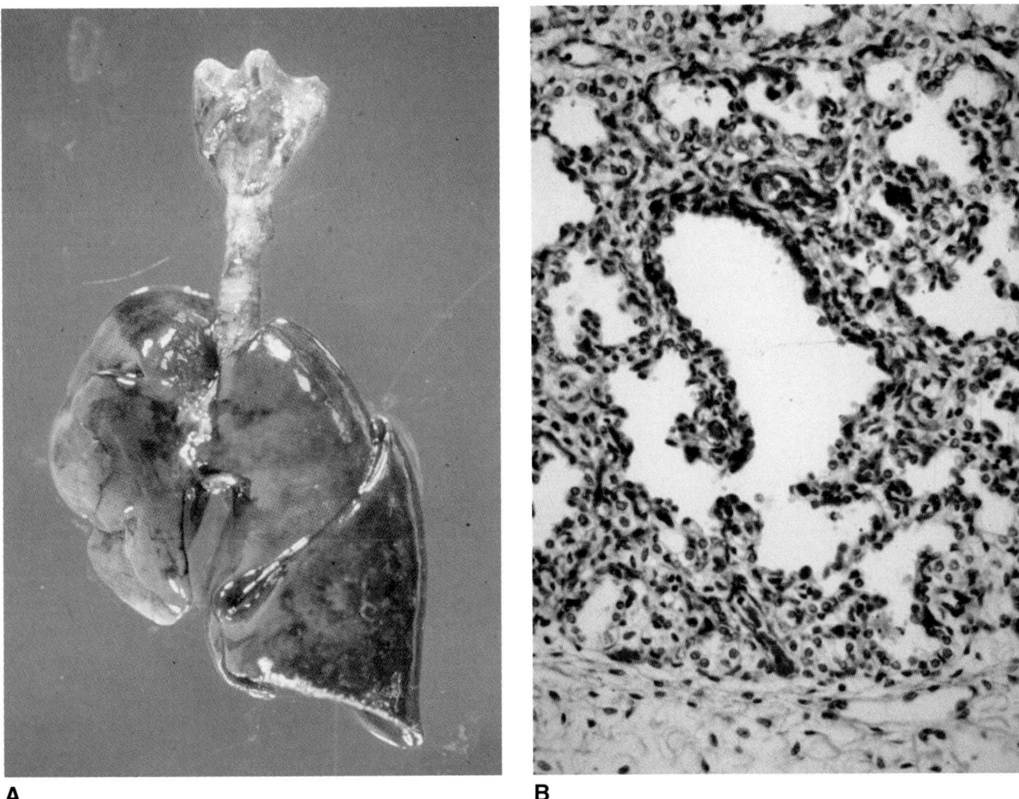

FIGURE 12-20 ▪ Pulmonary hypoplasia. **A:** The right lobes of the lung are markedly diminished in size, secondary to herniated abdominal organs through a right-sided diaphragmatic hernia. By weight, the left lung is also hypoplastic. **B:** At the periphery of an acinus in this hypoplastic lung, a radial alveolar count (RAC) is far below the normal of 4 to 6 for a term infant, confirming the diagnosis of hypoplasia. (H&E, ×50.)

Table 12-4 ▪ ANOMALIES ASSOCIATED WITH PULMONARY HYPOPLASIA

Common

- Diaphragmatic hernia
- Renal agenesis, bilateral
- Renal dysgenesis, bilateral
- Obstructive uropathy
- Polycystic renal disease (autosomal recessive)
- Large abdominal wall defects

Infrequent

- Diaphragmatic hypoplasia or eventration
- Anophthalmia/microphthalmia—usually in association with diaphragmatic hernia
- Hemolytic disease of the newborn
- Pleural effusion, as with nonimmune fetal hydrops
- Musculoskeletal abnormalities, such as thoracic dystrophies
- Anencephaly
- Scimitar syndrome
- Chromosomal anomalies, including trisomy 13, 18, and 21

Rare

- Abdominal pregnancy
- Ascites secondary to congenital cytomegalovirus infection
- Cloacal dysgenesis
- Congenital hydropericardium
- Down syndrome (probably postnatal "hypoplasia")
- Eagle-Barret syndrome
- Giant cervical teratoma
- Glutaric acidemia, type II
- Homozygous α-thalassemia
- Horseshoe lung
- Hypoplasia of the arcuate nucleus
- Laryngotracheoesophageal cleft
- Neonatal hypophosphatasia
- Pena-Shokeir syndrome, type I
- Phrenic nerve agenesis
- Right-sided cardiovascular malformation, as with hypoplastic right side of heart and pulmonary valve or artery atresia
- Rhabdomyoma in tuberous sclerosis
- Thoracic neuroblastoma
- Upper cervical spinal cord
- Extralobar sequestration

Table 12-5 ■ CAUSES OF ILE

Bronchial abnormality
Bronchial stenosis
Bronchial atresia
Abnormal origin of bronchus
Extrinsic obstruction of bronchus
Vascular anomaly
Pulmonary artery sling
Anomalous pulmonary venous return
Left-to-right shunting with dilated pulmonary arteries
External mass
Bronchogenic cyst
Intrinsic obstruction of bronchus
Aspirated meconium
Mucous plug
Granulation tissue
Bronchial mucosal folds
Torsion of bronchus
Foreign body

Adapted from Stocker JT. Congenital and developmental diseases. In: Dail DH, Hammer SP, eds. *Pulmonary pathology*. Heidelberg: Springer-Verlag, 1989:55, with permission.

(1.5:1) (147). ILE presents in the first week of life in about 50% of cases (with about 40% presenting in the first day of life) and in the first 6 months of life in over 80%, but ILE can occasionally be seen in children and young adults from 7 months to 20 years of age. Wall et al. (174) described ILE in a mother and daughter each presenting in their first month of life and Roberts et al. (175) noted the lesion in a father and son, both with cartilage deficiency of the bronchus. Symptoms are those of mild respiratory distress increasing over a period of hours to days to weeks; cyanosis, respiratory infections, vomiting, choking, and feeding difficulties may also be seen. Rarely, the lesion may present as a sudden pneumothorax (147). Imaging studies reveal, in the classic form (see below), a characteristic hyperlucent, overdistended lobe producing mediastinal shift and compression of the uninvolved lobes (176) (Figure 12-21A). In the polyalveolar lobe form (see below), imaging may display a lobe of normal lucency but one that occupies a disproportionate part of the hemithorax with mediastinal shift. Less frequently, retained lung fluid may be seen in the involved hyperexpanded lobe (usually the polyalveolar lobe type) on initial examination but which may clear over subsequent days. Associated anomalies are present in from 5% to 40% of patients, and 70% of these anomalies are cardiovascular (177–179). The upper lobes are involved in over 95% of cases—the left slightly more often than the right. Multiple lobe involvement occurs in about 15% of cases, usually with at least one lobe being an upper lobe. Bilateral involvement has been reported in one case with the left upper and right middle lobes displaying ILE (180). Lower lobe involvement is rarely seen except in the "acquired" form of ILE, as in premature infants receiving mechanical ventilation who develop granulation tissue obstruction of a lower lobe bronchus, probably as a result of endotracheal tube suctioning (181).

Grossly, the lobe *in vivo* and after resection is hyperexpanded with individual alveoli, which may be readily visualized (Figure 12-21B). Microscopically, two patterns (classic and polyalveolar) are identified. Nearly, 70% (the classic pattern) display a uniform overdistension of apparently normally developed acini with alveolar saccules and alveoli three to ten times the normal size but with radial alveolar counts (RAC) similar to those of age-matched controls (Figure 12-21C) (147). There may be focal disruption of alveolar walls. The other 30% (the polyalveolar pattern) show only little overdistension of what appear to be "complex" acini of

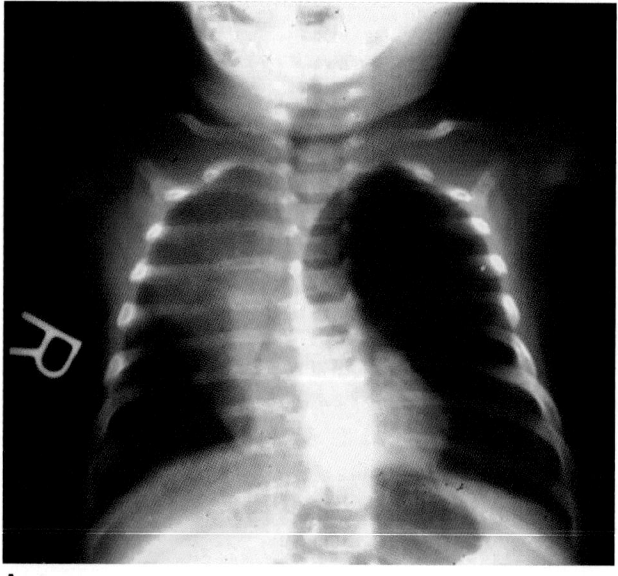

A

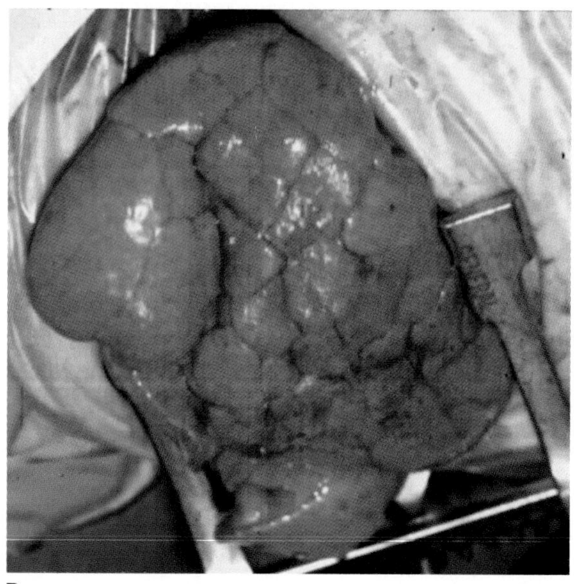

B

FIGURE 12-21 ■ Infantile lobar emphysema. **A:** A hyperinflated left lung shifts the mediastinum to the right. **B:** At surgery, the hyperinflated lung bulges from the opening in the thorax.

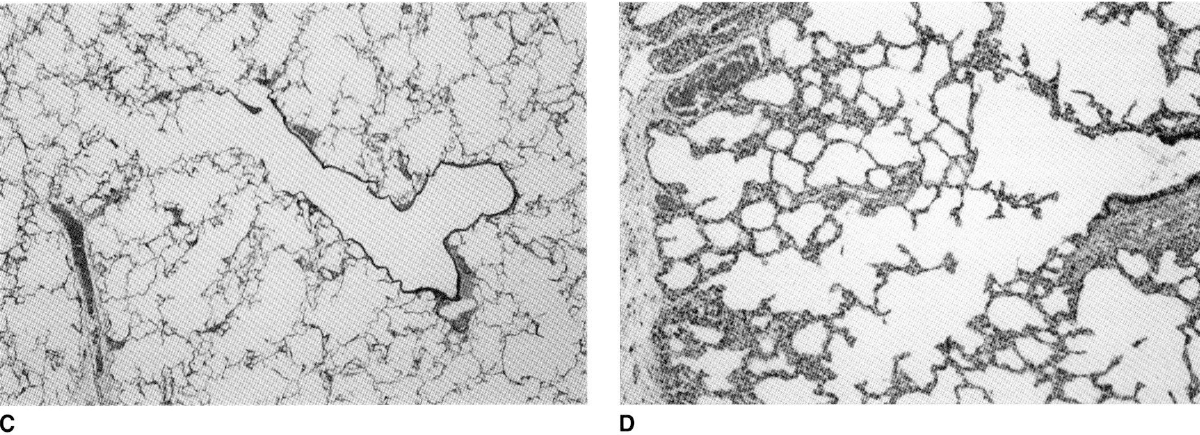

FIGURE 12-21 ▪ *(continued)* **C:** "Classic" form of ILE. The alveolar duct and alveoli are dilated to 3 to 10 times the normal size but are otherwise unremarkable. (Hematoxylin and eosin stain, original magnification ×60.) **D:** "Hyperplastic" form of ILE. While not overinflated, this lung displays a complex acinar formation with a larger number of alveoli (and consequently a large radial alveolar count) than would be expected at this age. (Hematoxylin and eosin stain, original magnification ×25.)

the type seen in polyalveolar lobes and hyperplastic lungs (Figure 12-21D) (Munnell, 1973), and these have RACs that are two standard deviations beyond the mean of age-matched controls. Seventy-five percent of these infants with polyalveolar lobe present clinically within the first day or two of life and are likely to show radiologic features of retained lung fluid (182,183). Examination of the bronchus to the lobe may reveal stenosis, atresia, or intrinsic obstruction (Table 12-5), or the bronchus may be unremarkable if extrinsic compression was present. Cartilage abnormalities of the bronchial wall have been described, but special techniques must be employed to demonstrate these changes convincingly. Surgical resection of the involved lobe is curative, although nonsurgical management has been successful in unusual cases (176).

Congenital Pulmonary Lymphangiectasis

CPL is a rare, usually fatal disorder that presents in the first hours to days of life (184). It is characterized by the presence of dilated thin-walled to thick-walled lymphatics within the interlobular septa and beneath the pleura of the lung. CPL may be seen as a primary disorder or as secondary to obstructive cardiovascular lesions, particularly total anomalous pulmonary venous return, but it may occur as part of a generalized lymphangiectasis or as an isolated pulmonary lesion (185,186). There is a distinct male predominance in occurrence of CPL of over 2.5:1, and 5% to 10% of affected infants are stillborn. Symptoms include cyanosis and acute respiratory distress. Fluid abnormalities including chylothorax, pleural effusion, fetal hydrops, and maternal polyhydramnios have been described *in utero* and postpartum (187). In addition to the 60% of cases with cardiovascular anomalies, CPL is associated with renal malformations, generalized lymphangiectasis, and other anomalies in another 20% of cases (1). The confusion between CPL and interstitial pulmonary emphysema (IPE) has led to the misdiagnosis of CPL in many cases, including the purported occurrence of CPL in two related female infants (188). Illustrations of one of these

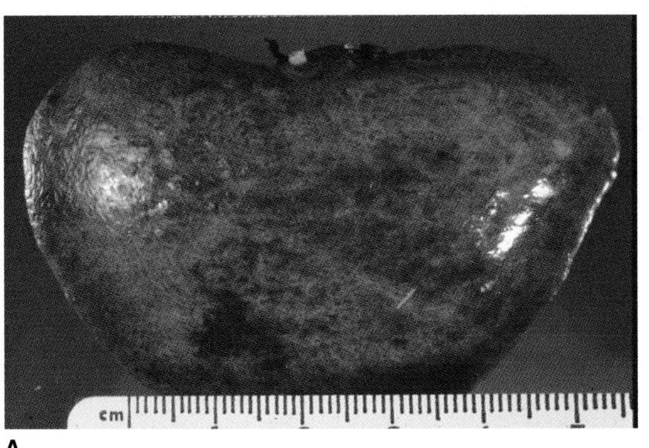

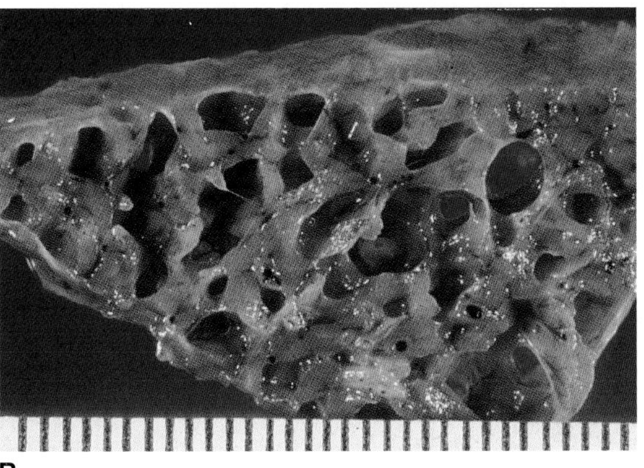

FIGURE 12-22 ▪ Congenital pulmonary lymphangiectasis. **A:** A fine network of dilated lymphatics is present beneath the pleura, most notably where interlobular septa intersect the pleura. **B:** Cut section of the lung from an infant with total anomalous pulmonary return reveals enormously dilated lymphatics.

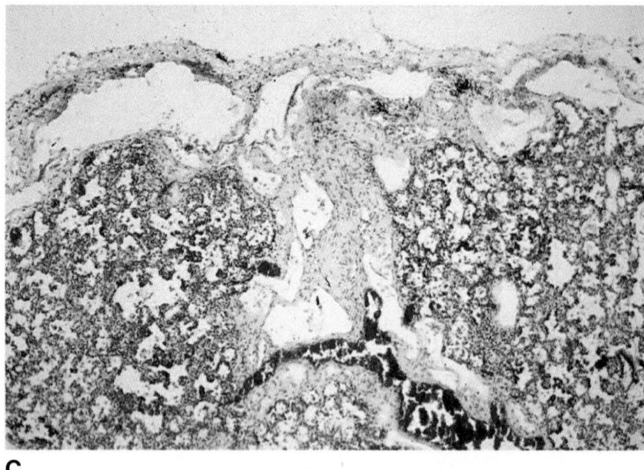

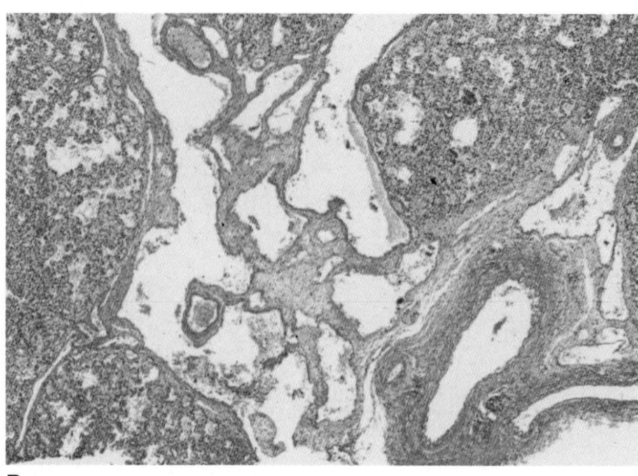

C D

FIGURE 12-22■ *(continued)* **C:** Dilated lymphatics extend laterally beneath the pleura (**top**) and centrally along an interlobular septum (**center**). Note the slight increase in connective tissue between the channels. (Hematoxylin and eosin stain, original magnification ×60.) **D:** Numerous dilated lymphatics extend along interlobular septa surrounding bronchovascular bundles. (Hematoxylin and eosin stain, original magnification ×20.)

cases strongly suggest that IPE was the pulmonary lesion. The diagnosis of CPL in the absence of cardiovascular or other anomalies should be strongly suspect.

The lungs in CPL are bulky, firm, noncompressible, and covered by a milky network of dilated subpleural lymphatics (Figure 12-22A). Rarely, a single lobe is involved by this process (189). On cut section, the lymphatics are fluid filled and extend from the interconnecting subpleural network into the interlobular septa and around the bronchovascular bundles (Figure 12-22B). Microscopically, the lymphatics are diffusely and uniformly dilated, and may appear to be increased in number. Identification of lymphatics can be aided by the CD31 and D2-40 immunohistochemical marking of endothelial cells (186). These small, irregular cysts are lined with a thin layer of endothelial cells and surrounded by a loose myxoid to occasionally dense connective tissue that often contains foci of extramedullary hematopoiesis. Clusters of lymphatics surround bronchovascular bundles within the interlobular septa and may separate acini beneath the pleura (Figure 12-22C,D). This is in contrast to the air-filled, larger, "unlined" cysts of IPE that are limited to the interlobular septa and do not extend laterally beneath the pleura.

Congenital Pulmonary Airway Malformation (CPAM)

CPAM is a hamartomatous lesion of the lung, with an incidence of about 1 in 5,000 live births, that can be separated into five major types based on clinical and pathologic features (Figure 12-23) (190). We proposed that the former designation of this lesion as "CCAM" be changed to "CPAM" to reflect the fact that the lesions as described below are "cystic" in only three of the five types and "adenomatoid" in only one type (type 3). CPAM more accurately encompasses all five types in this classification.

CPAM, type 0, also known as acinar dysplasia or agenesis, is a rarely occurring, infrequently described malformation that is largely incompatible with life (191). It is seen in term and premature infants who are cyanotic at birth and survive only a few hours and is associated with cardiovascular abnormalities and dermal hypoplasia. Grossly, the lungs are small and firm and have a diffusely granular surface (Figure 12-24A). Microscopically, tissue consists of bronchus-like structures with muscle, glands, and numerous cartilage plates

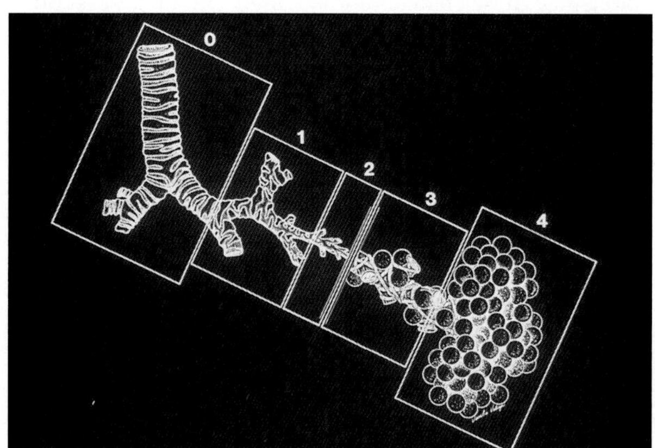

FIGURE 12-23■ Classification of CPAM. The classification is based on the similarity in appearance of the hamartomatous components of the lesion with the various areas of the normal tracheobronchial tree. Type 0, composed of bronchus-like structures, appears to be a malformation of the most proximal tracheobronchial tree. Type 1, containing bronchus-like and proximal bronchiole-like structures, mimics the distal bronchial tree and proximal acinus. Type 2, composed of bronchiole-like structures, resembles the bronchiolar segment of the acinus. Type 3, composed of bronchiole-like structures and alveolar ducts and saccules lined by cuboidal epithelium, resembles the midacinar region. Type 4, with thin-walled structures lined by type 1 alveolar lining cells, suggests a malformation of the distal acinar components. (From Stocker JT. Congenital and developmental diseases. In: Dail HD, Hammer SP, eds. *Pulmonary pathology*. 2nd ed. New York: Springer-Verlag, 1994:182, with permission.)

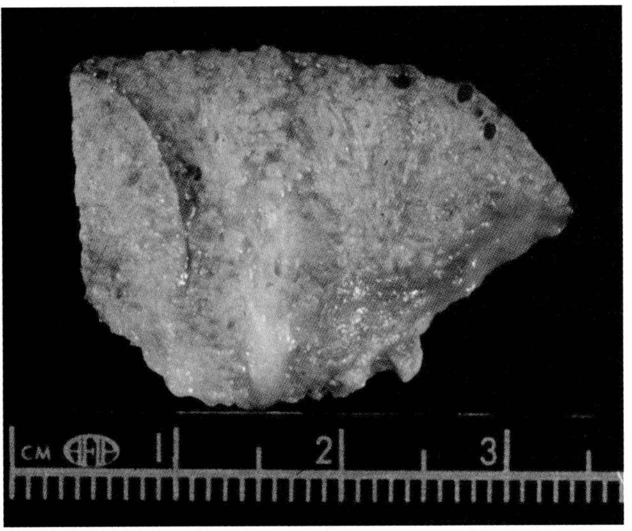

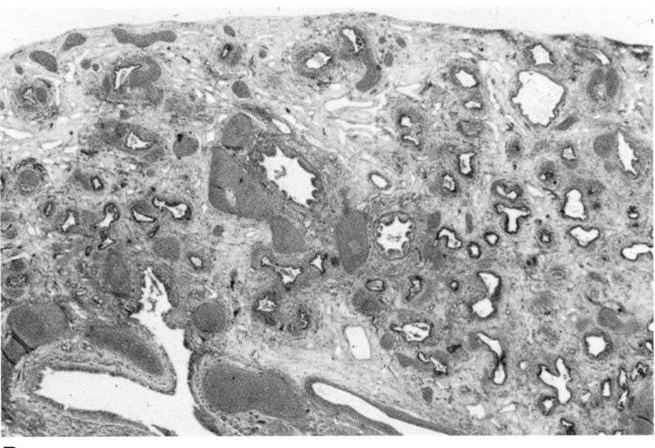

A B

FIGURE 12-24 ■ CPAM, type 0. **A:** A small nodular mass representing the right lung is largely devoid of air. A similar lung was present on the left side. **B:** Bronchial-like structures are surrounded by irregular cartilage plates and loose mesenchyme-containing thin-walled vascular structures. (Hematoxylin and eosin stain, original magnification ×25.)

(Figure 12-24B). Prominent mesenchymal tissue separates these structures and contains extramedullary hematopoiesis, large thin-walled vascular channels, and collections of amorphic basophilic debris. Rarely, structures resembling proximal bronchioles are present, along with a few scattered acini at the periphery of the lesion.

CPAM, type 1, the large or predominant cyst type, presents primarily within the first week to month of life but can be seen in older children and even young adults (Figure 12-25A) (192). It accounts for nearly 65% of cases and is usually readily amenable to surgery with a good prognosis. Grossly, the type 1 lesion is characterized by single or multiple large cysts (3 to 10 cm in diameter) surrounded by smaller cysts and compressed normal parenchyma (Figure 12-25B,C). Microscopically, the larger cysts are lined with ciliated, pseudostratified columnar epithelium and the smaller ones by cuboidal to columnar epithelium (Figure 12-25D,E). More than 45% of the cases display segments of mucus-producing cells among the epithelial

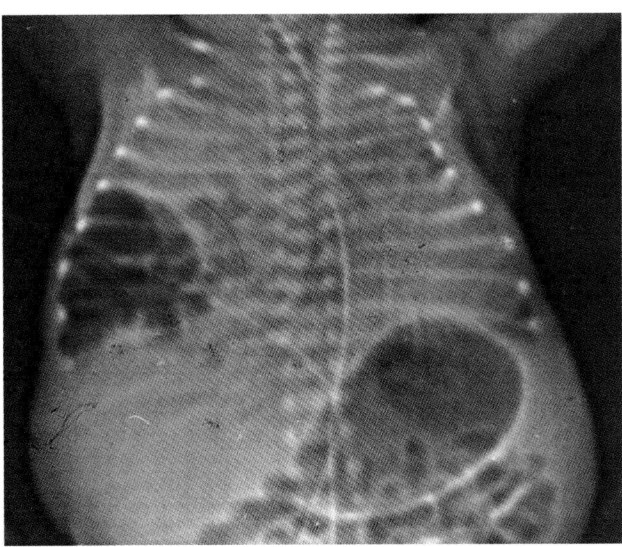

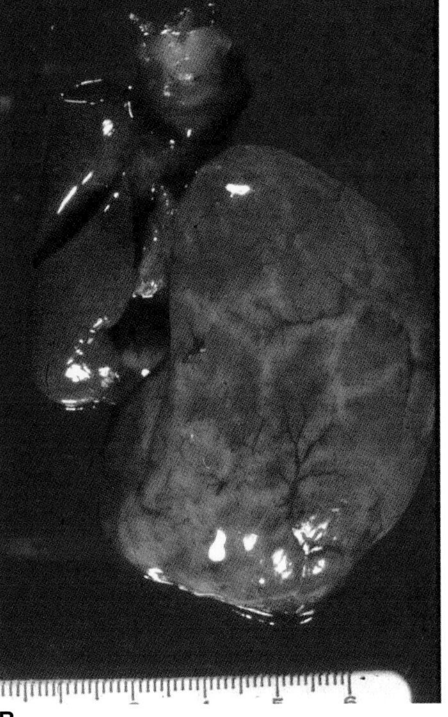

A B

FIGURE 12-25 ■ CPAM, type 1. **A:** A cystic mass is present in the lower right hemithorax in a newborn with respiratory distress. **B:** Multiple large, fluid-filled cysts distend the left lobe from a fetus in the second trimester.

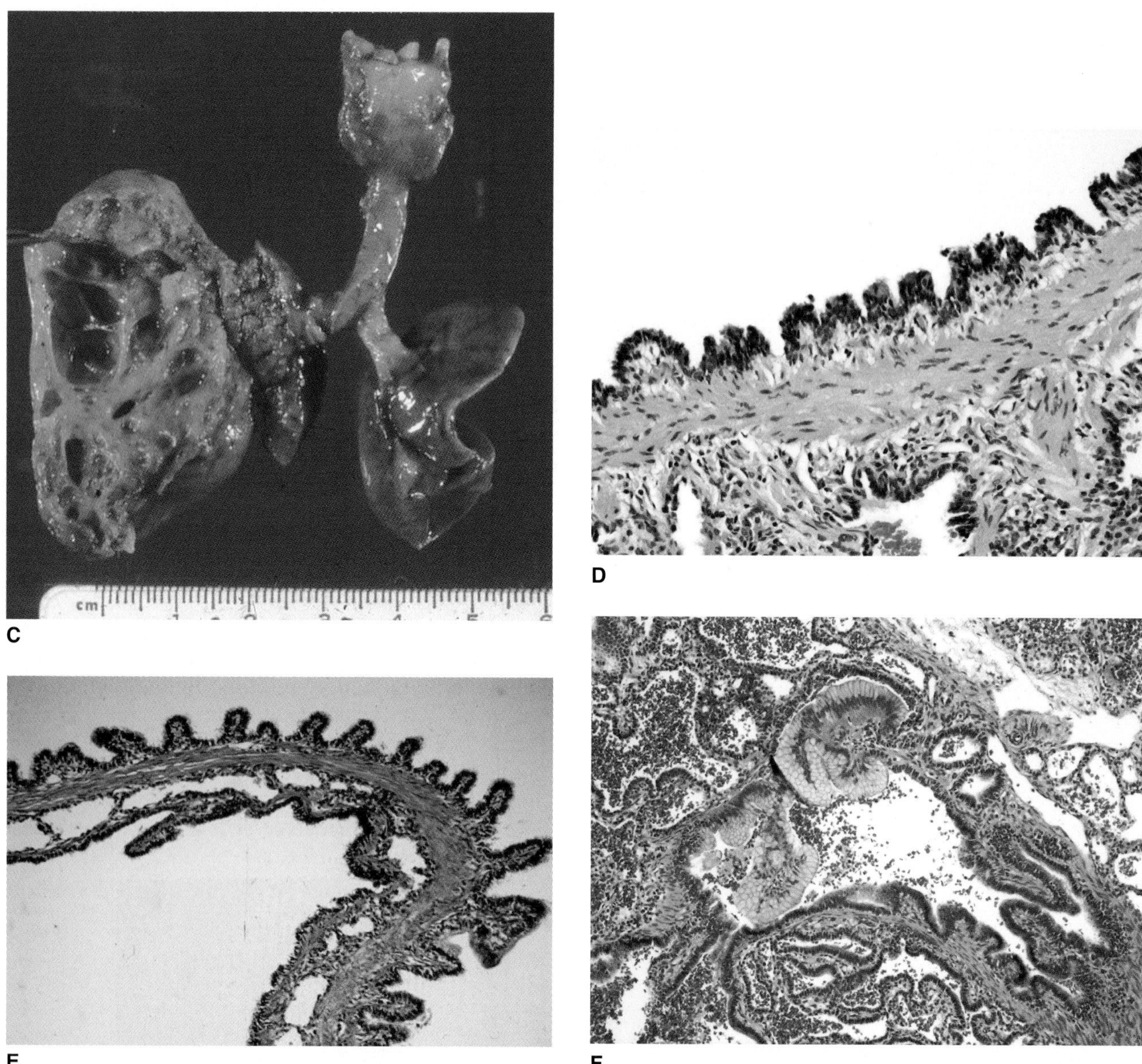

FIGURE 12-25■ *(continued)* **C:** When opened, the mass consists of intercommunication cysts. **D:** Cysts of type 1 CPAM are chararacteristically lined by ciliated columnar epithelium in a sawtooth configuration with underlying fibromuscular connective tissue. (H&E, ×200). **E:** A larger cyst wall (top) is covered by columnar epithelium in a papillary configuration. Note the columnar epithelial lining of the smaller cysts as well. (Hematoxylin and eosin stain, original magnification ×20.) **F:** Clusters of mucogenic cells line are present within the cyst lining. (H&E, ×200.)

lining of the larger cysts or in bronchioles and alveolar duct–like structures adjacent to the larger cysts (Figure 12-25F). These mucous cells have similar characteristics to those of pyloric mucosa (193). Wang et al. (194,195) suggest that these mucous cells may have the potential for malignant transformation to bronchioloalveolar carcinoma. Several reports of the occurrence of CPAM and bronchioloalveolar carcinoma have been published, and a convincing argument can be made in establishing an association between the two diseases (196–200). The walls of the CPAM, type 1 cysts are composed of elastic tissue overlying fibromuscular connective tissue, and in 5% to 10% of cases, cartilage plates.

CPAM, type 2, the medium cyst type, accounts for 10% to 15% of cases, is seen exclusively within the first year of life, and has a poorer outcome owing to its more frequent association with other anomalies (140), some of which are incompatible with life (e.g., renal agenesis). The type 2 lesion is composed of cysts 0.5 to 2.0 cm in diameter (rarely larger) that are evenly distributed and blend with the adjacent normal parenchyma (Figure 12-26A). The cysts occasionally surround normal appearing bronchi. The typical back-to-back bronchiole-like structures are lined by cuboidal to columnar epithelial cells with a thin, underlying, fibromuscular layer (Figure 12-26B). Mucous cells and cartilage plates are absent

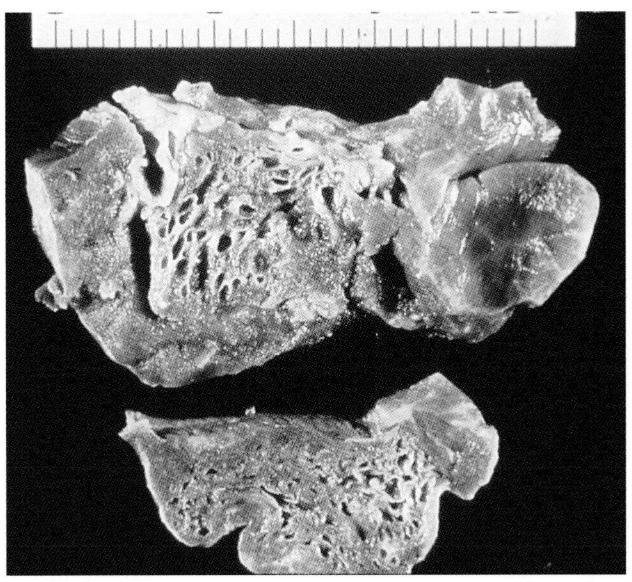

A

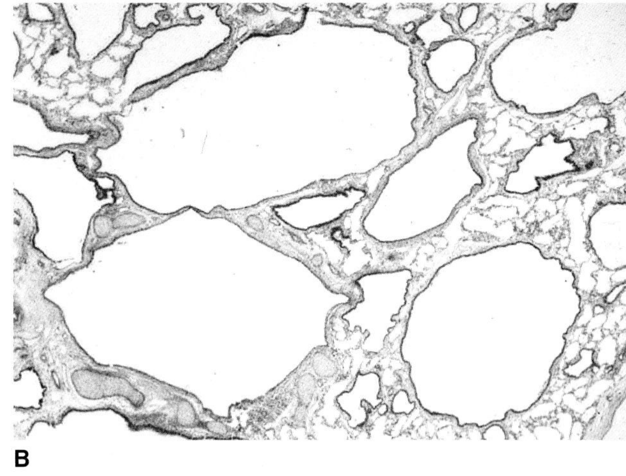

B

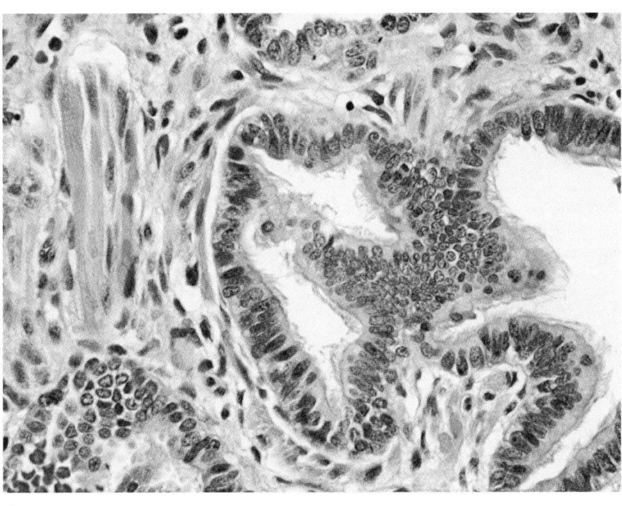

C

FIGURE 12-26■CPAM, type 2. **A:** Small cysts (0.2 to 0.5 cm) are scattered throughout the lobe and blend with normal parenchyma. **B:** The back-to-back bronchiole-like structures are separated by structures resembling alveolar ducts. (Hematoxylin and eosin stain, original magnification ×40.) **C:** In a variant of type 2, striated muscle fibers are present in the connective tissue between and around cysts. (H&E, ×200.)

except as components of "entrapped" normal bronchi. A variant or subgroup of the type 2 lesion, termed rhabdomyomatous dysplasia (201–203), contains ribbons of striated muscle fibers throughout the lesion, both in association with the cysts and between alveolar ducts and around blood vessels (Figure 12-26C). The cysts of this rhabdomyomatous variant may be less prominent than other type 2 lesions. Rhabdomyosarcoma has been reported to originate from CPAM, but this represents a pleuropulmonary blastoma (PPB) rather than CPAM. CPAM, type 2-like features are present in 50% of extralobar sequestrations (140).

CPAM, type 3, the small cystic or solid type, occurs infrequently (5% of cases), is seen exclusively in the first days to month of life, has a notable male predominance, and owing to its large size and association with maternal polyhydramnios and fetal anasarca, has a high mortality rate (204). Increased maternal levels of serum α-fetoprotein have been noted in the second trimester of two cases of type 3 CPAM (205,206). CPAM, type 3, the original lesion described by Ch'in and Tang (207), consists of a large, bulky, parenchymal mass involving an entire lobe or even an entire lung (Figure 12-27A,B). The mass effect of the lesion consistently produces mediastinal shift and often results in hypoplasia of the uninvolved lung. Cysts are rarely larger than 0.2 cm in diameter, with the exception of scattered, larger, bronchiole-like structures. Microscopically, the lesion resembles an immature lung devoid of bronchi. Irregular, stellate-shaped, bronchiole-like structures lined with cuboidal epithelial cells are surrounded by alveolar ductules and saccules that are also lined by cuboidal cells, imparting the "adenomatoid" appearance for which this lesion was originally named (Figure 12-27C). Mucous cells, cartilage, and rhabdomyomatous cells are not present, and there is a paucity of vessels within the lesion.

CPAM, type 4, the peripheral acinar cyst type, appears to be a hamartomatous malformation of the distal acinus. This variant is seen equally in boys and girls, with an age range of newborn to 4 years and accounts for 10% to 15%

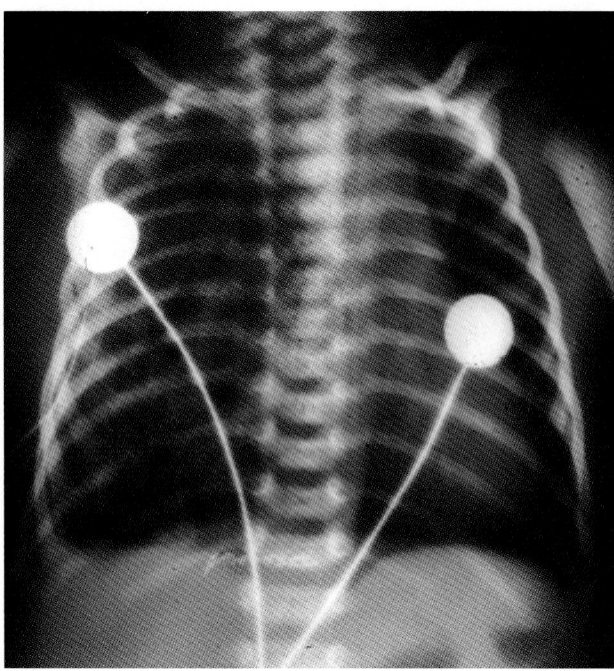

A

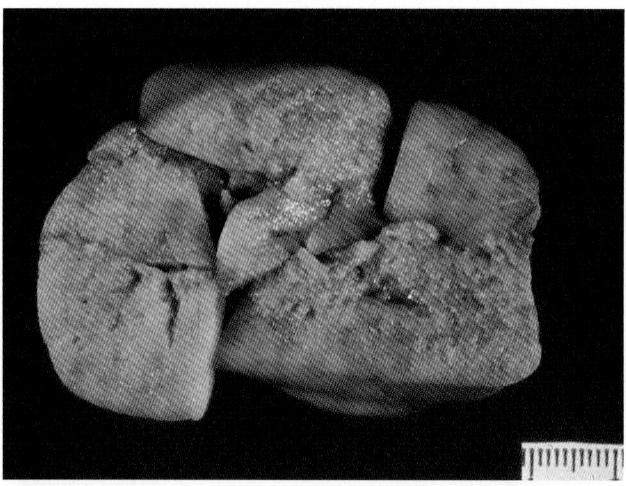

B

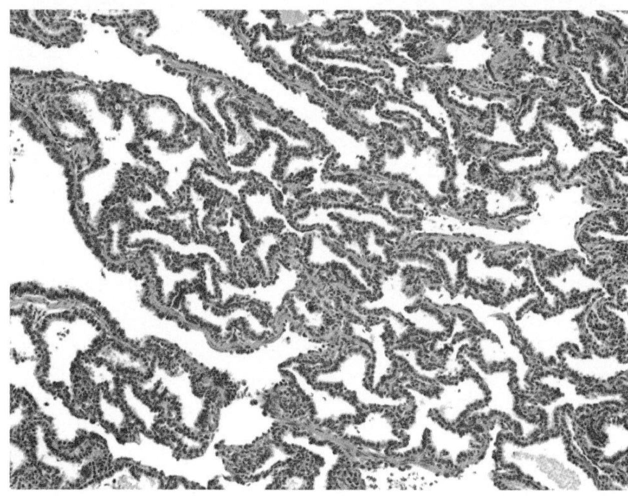

C

FIGURE 12-27 ■ CPAM, type 3. **A:** A large air-containing mass in the right hemithorax pushes the mediastinum to the left. **B:** The resected lesion is nearly solid with only a few slit-like openings. **C:** Randomly distributed irregular bronchiole-like structures are separated by dilated alveolus-like structures all of which are lined by cuboidal epithelial cell imparting an adenomatoid (or gland-like) appearance. (H&E, ×100.)

of cases. Until recently, most of these cases were included in the type 1 category. Clinically, the type 4 lesions may present with mild respiratory distress, sudden respiratory distress from tension PT, pneumonia, or on occasion, as an incidental finding with no symptoms (190,192). Radiographically, the lesion displays large air-filled cysts with mediastinal shift and, occasionally, is associated with a PT. The lesion involves a single lobe in about 80% of cases and rarely may be bilateral. Grossly, large thin-walled cysts are present at the "periphery" of the lobe and appear to be lined by a smooth membrane (Figure 12-28A). Microscopically, the cysts are lined by flattened epithelial cells (type I and II alveolar lining cells) over most of wall, with occasional low cuboidal epithelium seen (Figure 12-28B to D). The wall of the cyst is composed of loose mesenchymal tissue with prominent arteries and arterioles. Loose mesenchyme must not be confused with similar features seen in the cystic type of PPB (see later). Dense connective tissue may be present in some cases in older patients. Survival is excellent with resection.

Ultrasonography has been demonstrated to be a highly useful modality in the *in utero* diagnosis of CPAM (208). *In utero* serial sonography has demonstrated the gradual reduction in the size of CPAM, type 1 and 2, with subsequent normal development of the uninvolved lung (209).

There are several examples of anomalies seen in association with CPAM, mostly with type 2:

- Bilateral renal agenesis/dysgenesis
- Extralobar pulmonary sequestration
- Cardiovascular malformation
- Diaphragmatic hernia
- Hydrocephalus and macrocephaly
- Myelomeningocele
- Jejunal atresia
- Prune-belly syndrome
- Sirenomelia
- Bilateral nephromegaly
- Pierre Robin syndrome
- Pulmonary hypoplasia
- Skeletal malformation
- Bile duct hypoplasia
- Left heart hypoplasia
- Polycytosis of a solitary medial kidney

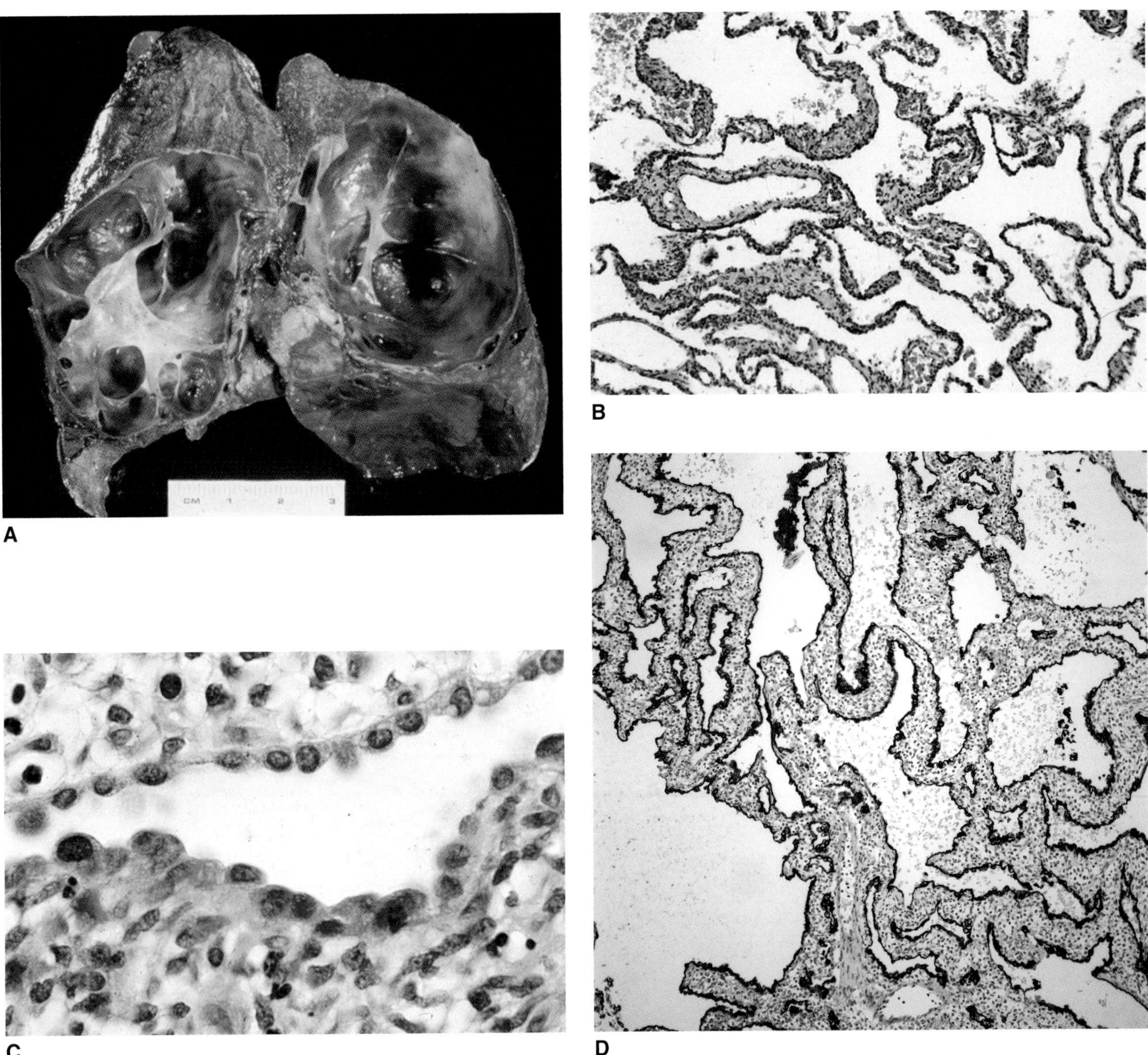

FIGURE 12-28 CPAM, type 4. **A:** The lung is distended by thin, almost translucent cyst walls. **B:** The walls of the cysts are composed of loose mesenchyme covered by an indistinct epithelial lining not apparent at this magnification (Hematoxylin and eosin stain, original magnification ×25) **C:** The cyst walls are variously covered by an attenuated epithelium of alveolar lining cells. (Hematoxylin and eosin stain, original magnification ×150). **D:** The epithelium stains positively for cytokeratin (H&E, ×50).

Anomalies are noted in 15% to 20% of all cases of CPAM, particularly in association with the type 2 lesion (210). CPAM is a unilateral lesion in about 95% of cases and involves a single lobe in 80% to 90% of cases. The right and left sides of the lung are nearly equally involved, with the lower lobes affected in about 60% of cases. Type 2 CPAM has been noted in nearly 50% of cases of extralobar sequestrations. An association of CPAM with the later development of a bronchioloalveolar carcinoma has been established (211,212).

Variants of CPAM exist as unique entities or are the result of alteration by associated anomalies. Fisher et al. (213) described a type 1 CPAM with large cysts filled with large papillary projections that consisted of delicately branching fibrovascular stalks covered with cuboidal to columnar epithelial cells.

Congenital Alveolar Capillary Dysplasia

Congenital alveolar capillary dysplasia with or without misalignment of pulmonary veins is a rare entity that presents as progressive hypoxemia in the newborn and is uniformly fatal (214,215). Familial occurrence has been noted (216). A number of cases have been shown to be associated with mutations in STRA6 on chromosome 15q24.1 (217). Associated anomalies (Table 12-6) are seen in over 50% of cases and include duodenal atresia, congenital heart disease, asplenia, phocomelia, and ureteric and urethral obstruction, among others (218). It is characterized by the failure of formation and ingrowth of alveolar capillaries. Broad alveolar septa with large alveolar capillaries within the septal wall are the hallmark of this disorder (Figure 12-29A to D) (219). Capillaries

Table 12-6 ■ ANOMALIES ASSOCIATED WITH ALVEOLAR CAPILLARY DYSPLASIA

Anophthalmia and distinct eyebrows (217)
Familiary microphthalmia (460)
Degeneration of the anterior segment of the eye (461)
Atrioventricular septal defect and quadricuspid pulmonary valve (462)
Down syndrome (463)
Gastrointestinal (464)
  Duodenal atresia and anorectal anomaly
  Intestinal malrotation
  Total colonic Hirschsprung disease.
  Duodenal atresia (216,465)
Left-right asymmetry (466)
Arteriovenous malformation of the liver
Bilateral ureteropelvic junction obstruction
Atrioseptal defect
Abnormally lobated lungs
Hydronephrosis
Urethral atresia (467)
Atrioventricular canal
Absence of gall bladder
Absence of left umbilical artery
Pulmonary lymphangiectasia
Hypoplastic left heart (468)
Sturge-Weber syndrome
Anomalous pulmonary veins (466)
Diaphragmatic hernia (469)
Bilateral tibial agenesis/ectrodactyly dysostosis (470)

are centrally placed well beneath the basement membrane of the alveolar lining cells and surrounded by loose mesenchyme (Figure 12-29C). Ectatic veins are present within bronchovascular bundles, occasionally within the adventitia of the pulmonary arteries, and may form an intermittent ring around the bronchiole (Figure 12-29B). Small muscularized arteries are also present within the acini, extending to the precapillary area (Figure 12-29D). Treatment with inhaled nitric oxide and ECMO has prolonged life but has been uniformly unsuccessful in changing the fatal outcome of this disorder without lung transplantation (220).

Peripheral Cysts of the Lung

Peripheral, air-containing cysts of the lung can be seen in neonates, infants, and young children; it occurs in association with Down syndrome as a result of pulmonary infarction, or in association with idiopathic spontaneous PT (5). Occlusion of the pulmonary artery in infants can result in peripheral infarction of the lung, which, with necrosis and organization, can produce subpleural cysts of varying size. Gonzalez et al. (221) reported peripheral cysts in 18 of 98 patients with Down syndrome and suggested that the cysts are an intrinsic feature of the disease that may result from reduced postnatal production of peripheral small air passages and alveoli. The 0.2- to 1.0-cm air-filled cysts are located beneath the pleura and are formed of vascular fibrous connective tissue walls lined by alveolar lining cells (Figure 12-30A,B). The cysts communicate with more centrally located bronchioles and alveolar ducts. The cysts resemble those seen in the upper lobes of adult males with idiopathic spontaneous PT and have also been noted in a case of ILE (147).

Hyaline Membrane Disease (HMD)

HMD is the pathologic counterpart of neonatal or idiopathic respiratory distress syndrome (RDS). It is characterized by firm, atelectatic lungs with an uneven air-expansion pattern, focal hemorrhage, edema fluid in alveoli, and hyaline membranes along terminal and respiratory bronchioles and alveolar ducts (222).

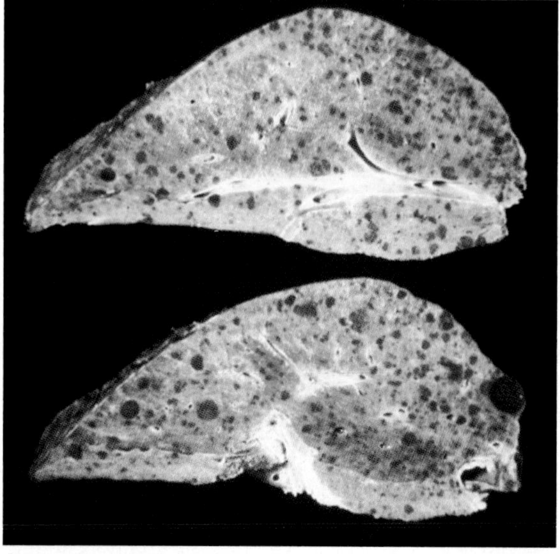

A

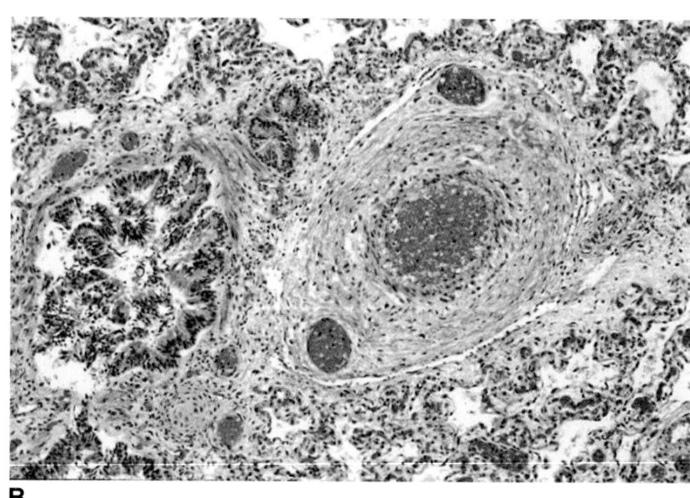

B

FIGURE 12-29 ■ Congenital alveolar capillary dysplasia. **A:** Bulky stiff lungs display focal hemorrhage and prominent interlobular septa. **B:** Dilated veins are present adjacent to and within the adventita of a pulmonary artery (**center-right**). (Hematoxylin and eosin stain, original magnification ×40.)

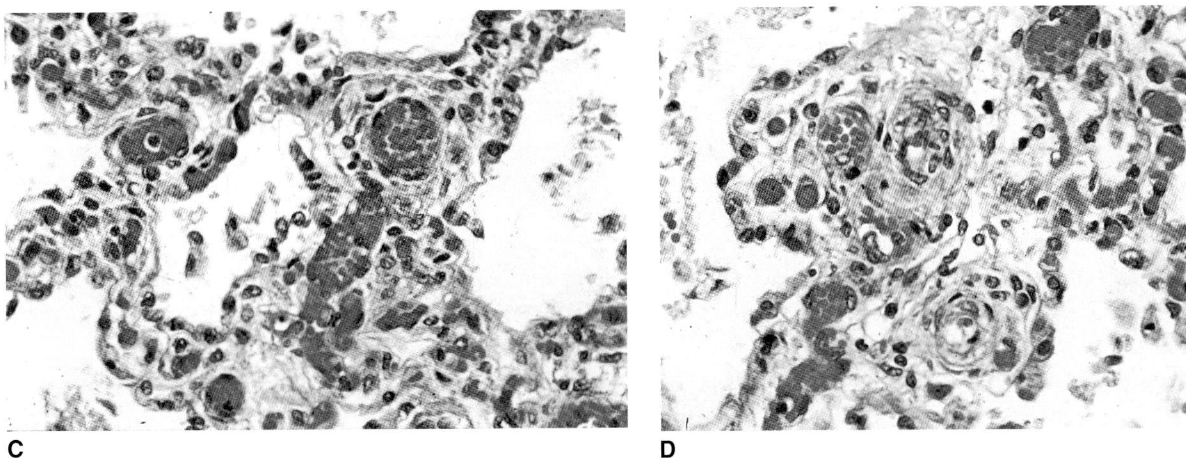

FIGURE 12-29 (*continued*) **C:** Broad alveolar septa contain many centrally located capillaries with only a few of them approaching the alveolar epithelium. (Hematoxylin and eosin stain, original magnification ×75.) **D:** Muscularized arteries are present within alveolar septa well away from bronchioles. (Hematoxylin and eosin stain, original magnification ×75.)

Although infrequently seen in its "pure" form since the advent of surfactant replacement, sophisticated mechanical ventilation and oxygen supplementation, HMD occurs primarily in premature infants with pulmonary surfactant deficiency due to a variety of conditions. There is also, however, an increased incidence of HMD in postterm infants (223). Infants present with tachypnea, intercostal retractions, and hypoxemia and display a typical x-ray image of ground-glass alterations of the lungs with an air bronchogram and diffusely scattered reticulogranular opacities (Figure 12-31A) (1).

Grossly, the lungs are firm and resemble liver more than lung. Microscopically, there is an uneven air-expansion pattern with atelectatic acini and dilated bronchioles and alveolar ducts (Figure 12-31B). Scattered foci of alveolar hemorrhage and edema are present, but most striking is the presence of smooth, homogeneous, pink membranes lining

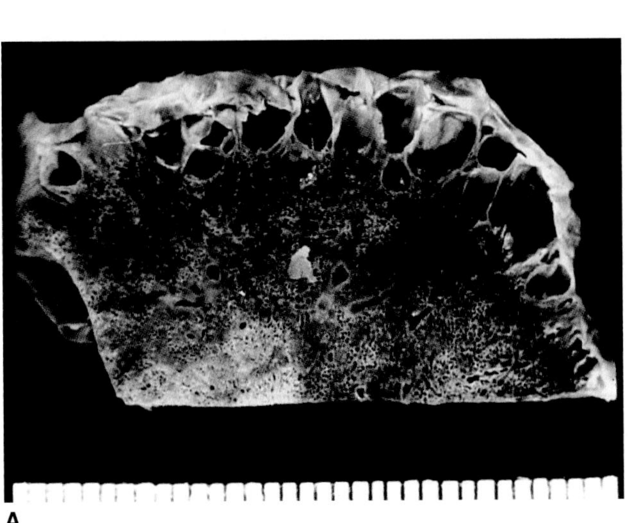

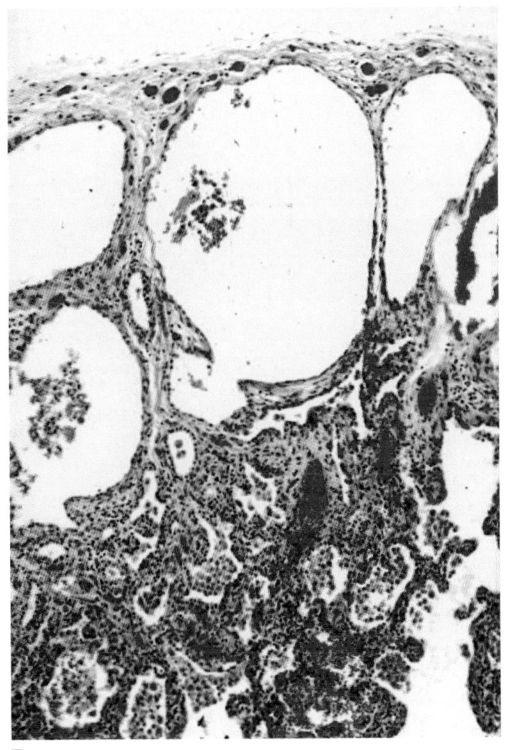

FIGURE 12-30 Peripheral cysts of the lung. **A:** Small intercommunicating cysts lie between the pleura and normal pulmonary parenchyma. **B:** The fibrovascular cyst walls are continuous with the interlobular septa of the underlying lung. (Hematoxylin and eosin stain, original magnification ×15.)

terminal and respiratory bronchioles and alveolar ducts, particularly at points of division or branching (Figure 12-31C). These hyaline membranes are composed of necrotic alveolar lining cells, plasma transudate, inhaled amniotic fluid including squames, and fibrin, if hemorrhage is present. Hyaline membranes may be seen in infants who die as early as 3 to 4 hours after birth and are uniformly present as well-formed structures by 12 to 24 hours in infants with RDS. In the absence of severe disease requiring high oxygen tensions and ventilatory pressures, at 36 to 48 hours the membranes begin to organize and separate from the underlying wall to be replaced by alveolar lining cells or bronchiolar cuboidal or columnar epithelium (Figure 12-31D) (131).

Bacteria may alter the appearance of the membranes by producing fragmented, faintly basophilic structures, with organisms often readily demonstrable by Gram stain on or within the membranes. Conditions associated with hyperbilirubinemia (e.g., kernicterus, intraventricular hemorrhage,

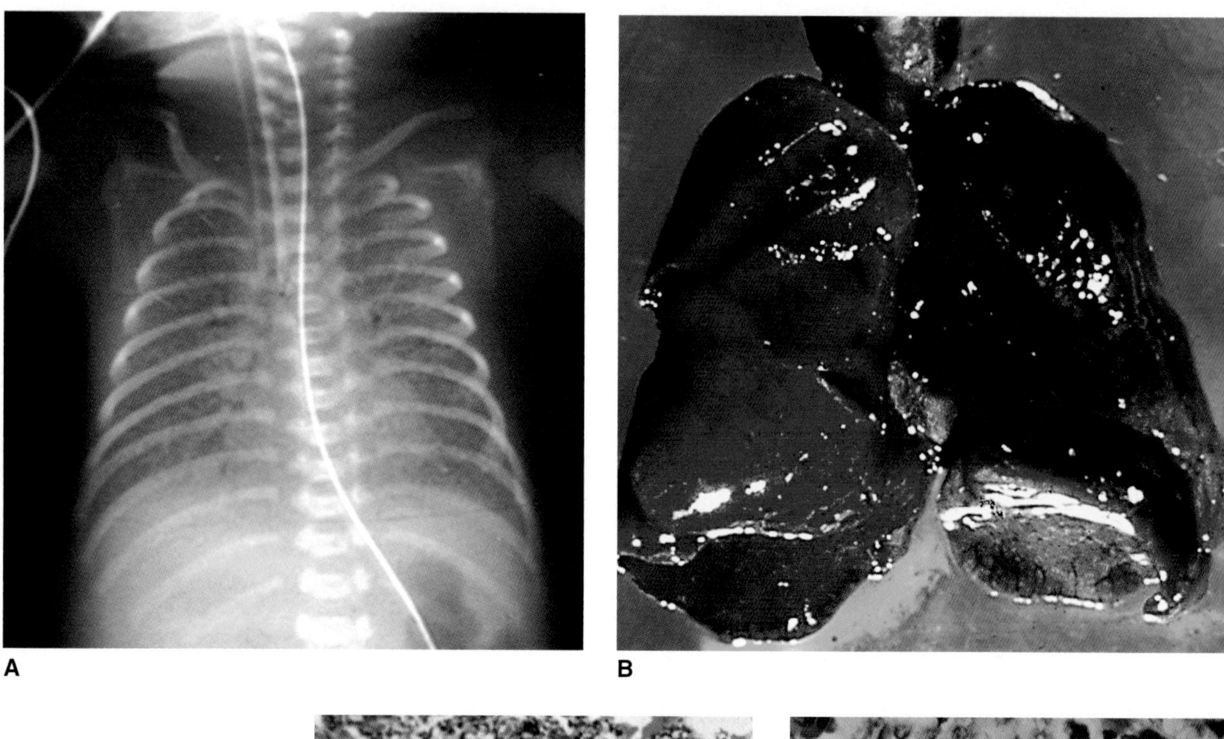

A B

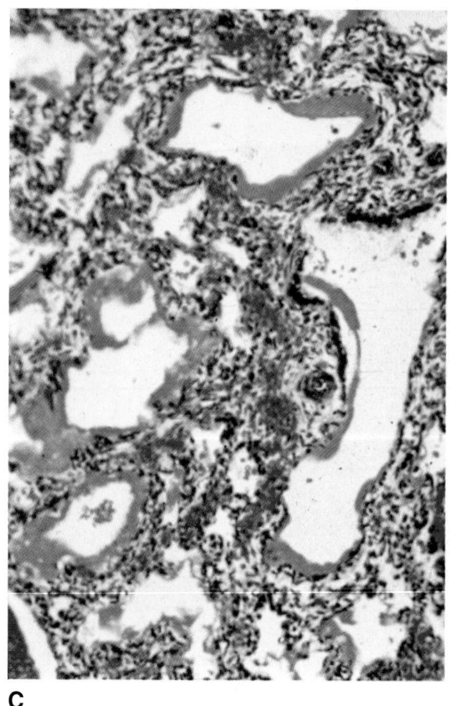

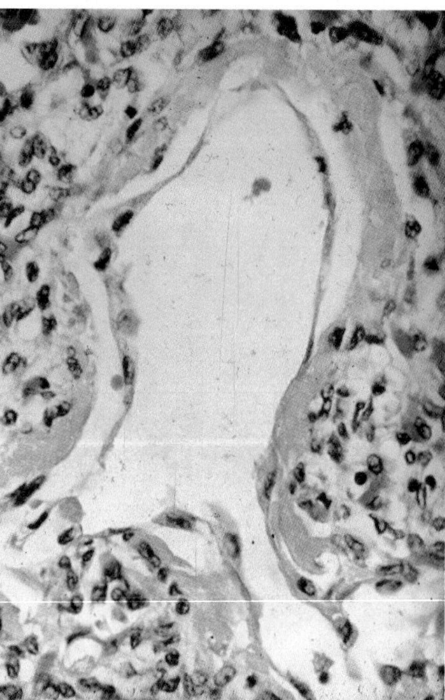

C D

FIGURE 12-31 ■ Hyaline membrane disease. **A:** In this 24-hour-old, 1,050-g infant with respiratory distress, the lungs display a classic "ground glass" opacity. **B:** The lungs in HMD are often atelectatic and display focal hemorrhage. **C:** Dilated bronchioles and alveolar ducts are lined by thick hyaline membranes. (Hematoxylin and eosin stain, original magnification ×25.) **D:** At 72 hours of age, the membranes are being covered by regenerating alveolar lining cells. (Hematoxylin and eosin stain, original magnification ×100.)

intrahepatic bile stasis, disseminated intravascular coagulation) may produce, in infants surviving 3 or more days, yellow hyaline membranes as a result of the presence of unconjugated bilirubin (151).

Surfactant replacement therapy, although radically decreasing the incidence of HMD in premature infants and its morbidity and mortality in these infants, does not appear to alter the pathologic features of HMD in infants dying of RDS, although clinically there may be a slightly higher incidence of pulmonary hemorrhage and a lower incidence of IPE, PT, and retinopathy of prematurity (224,225). Surfactant therapy appears to accelerate the rate of epithelial cell regeneration (226).

Bronchopulmonary Dysplasia (Chronic Lung Disease of Prematurity)

Bronchopulmonary dysplasia was first described in 1967 by Northway et al. (227). In a retrospective study, they describe the clinical and pathologic features of 19 infants dying following mechanical ventilation with high concentrations of oxygen for severe HMD (RDS). The pathology was correlated with clinical and radiographic findings and included a 2- to 3-day period of acute RDS, followed by a weeklong period of "regeneration," another 10-day period of transition to chronic disease, and a final period of chronic disease extending beyond 1 month of life. The pathologic features in the first stage included the typical findings of HMD (e.g., atelectasis, uneven air expansion pattern, hemorrhage, and hyaline membranes). During the second stage, there was necrosis of bronchiolar and alveolar epithelium with persistence of hyaline membranes (Figure 12-32A to C). In the transition to chronic disease, injury to alveolar epithelium continued, along with widespread bronchial and bronchiolar mucosal metaplasia and marked mucus secretion. Clusters of hyperexpanded alveoli alternated with areas of atelectasis. In the chronic stage, bronchioles displayed marked peribronchiolar smooth muscle hypertrophy associated with clusters of "emphysematous alveoli." The birth weights of the 19 infants dying of bronchopulmonary dysplasia varied from 900 to 2,466 g, with two-thirds of them weighing more than 1,300 g. Northway et al. (227) suggested that bronchopulmonary dysplasia was due to the toxic effects of oxygen, poor bronchial drainage, and the effects of mechanical ventilation.

In the 10 years following that initial brief description of the pathology of BPD, a number of other studies described in more detail the pathologic features including the changes noted in alveoli, airways, lymphatics, vessels, and connective tissue as criteria for the staging of bronchopulmonary dysplasia. In 1976, Bonikos et al. (228) described a severe necrotizing bronchiolitis in the acute stages of BPD and

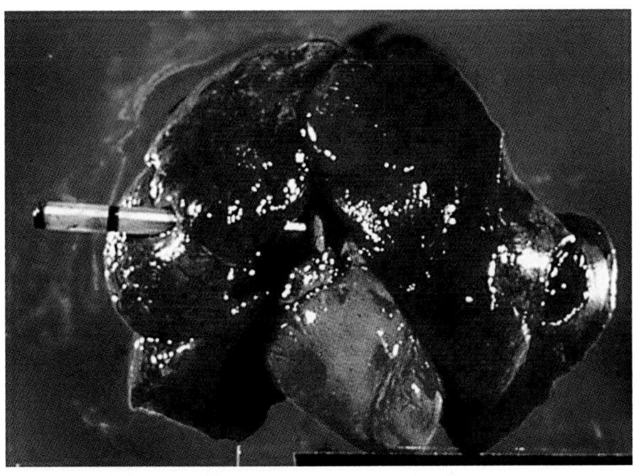
A

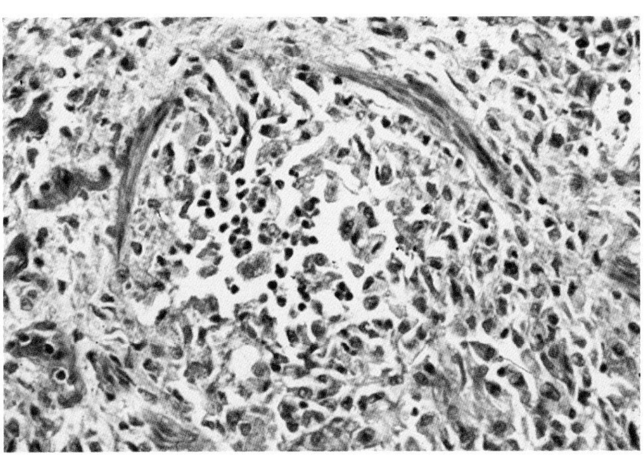
B

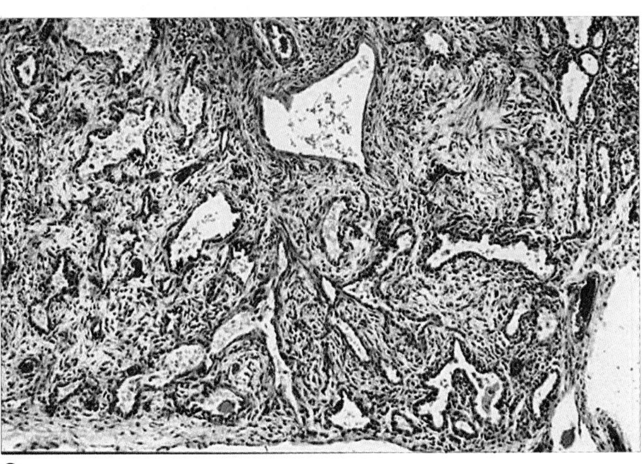
C

FIGURE 12-32 ■ Bronchopulmonary dysplasia (BPD), acute and severe. **A:** The lungs are bulky and firm. Note the tube perforating the upper lobe. **B:** Necrotizing bronchiolitis is a key feature of acute BPD and with occlusion such as this precludes the acinus distal to it from being available for air exchange (H&E, ×125). **C:** In acini whose bronchioles are not occluded by necrotizing bronchiolitis, the distal portion is exposed to the full barotrauma and oxygen toxicity used in the treatment of HMD. As a result, there is alveolar cell hyperplasia/dysplasia and alveolar septal fibroplasia (H&E, ×25).

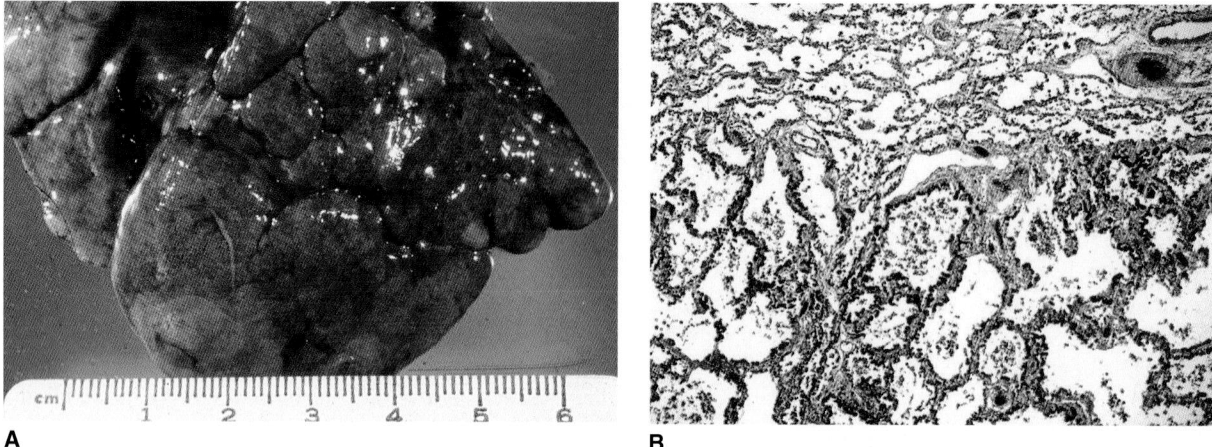

FIGURE 12-33 Long-standing healed bronchopulmonary dysplasia. **A:** Irregular clefting and fissuring of pulmonary lobes probably represent the loss of acini during the acute phases of BPD. **B:** The acinus at top represents the one "protected" by occluded bronchioles from the damage of barotrauma and high oxygen pressures. At the bottom, this acinus displays the diffuse alveolar septal fibrosis caused by previous exposure to barotrauma and high oxygen pressures (Masson trichrome, ×25).

implicated prolonged exposure to high levels of oxygen as a major feature in the cause of bronchiolitis. Since that time, a number of additional factors, including infection, inflammation, poor nutrition, dehydration, and others, have been implicated in the pathogenesis of BPD (229). In addition to the bronchiolitis, Bonikos et al. (230) described a prominent alveolar septal fibrosis in the healed stages along with an increased incidence of cardiac hypertrophy.

The sequelae of this necrotizing bronchiolitis was described by Stocker in 1986 in a series of 28 patients with long-standing "healed" bronchopulmonary dysplasia, who died at 3 to 40 months of age (131). Noting the presence of deep pleural fissures and acini with varying degrees of alveolar septal fibrosis (Figure 12-33), It was suggested that the necrotizing bronchiolitis seen in the acute phases, while prohibiting adequate ventilation, often served to "protect" acini from damage by mechanical ventilation or high levels of oxygen (Figure 12-34A–C). Stocker also suggested that the alveolar fissures might represent areas of complete loss of acini corresponding to the marked decrease in internal surface area and number alveoli noted by Sobonya et al. (231). The 6- to 10-fold reduction in number of alveoli suggested not only an absolute loss of some acini but a generalized reduction in lung growth. In 1991, Margraf et al. (232) confirmed the reduction in lung volume and small airway density noted by Sobonya.

In recent years, with the advent of surfactant replacement therapy and increased sophistication in the use of mechanical ventilation (including high frequency jet ventilation) and oxygen supplementation, another stage in the evolution of

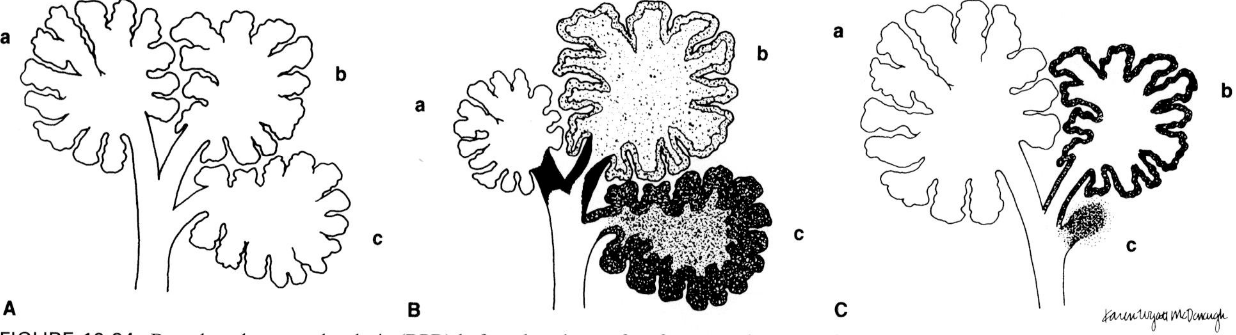

FIGURE 12-34 Bronchopulmonary dysplasia (BPD) before the advent of surfactant replacement therapy. **A:** Schematic representation of three uniformly distended acini (a to c) with associated bronchiole, alveolar ducts, and alveoli. **B:** In the early stages of BPD, hyaline membranes or necrotic debris may totally occlude a bronchiole (a) protecting the distal acinus. Bronchioles that remain partially or completely open (b, c) allow the distal acinus to be exposed to varying degrees of injury from barotrauma and high oxygen tension. **C:** In the healed stages of BPD with resolution of the bronchiolar obstruction in (**A**), the "protected" distal acinus expands and continues to develop new alveoli. Depending on the degree of injury, acini may atrophy and disappear (c), producing pleural fissures (see Figure 12-33A), or display varying degrees of alveolar septal fibrosis (b) and be inhibited from further alveolar development. (From Stocker JT. Pathologic features of long-standing "healed" bronchopulmonary dysplasia: a study of 28 3- to 40-month-old infants. *Hum Pathol* 1986;17:943, with permission.)

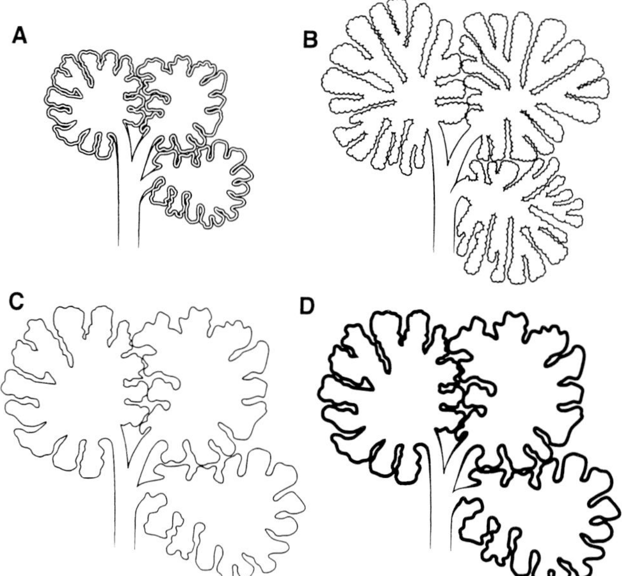

FIGURE 12-35■ Bronchopulmonary dysplasia or chronic lung disease of the premature since the advent of surfactant replacement therapy. **A:** Schematic representation of three normally expanded and aerated pulmonary acini in an immature infant. Note the appropriately thick septa of the developing lung. **B:** With normal growth and development, the acini not only increase in size [relative to (**A**)] but also in complexity, with the appearance of "new" alveolar saccules and alveoli. **C** and **D:** In infants receiving surfactant replacement therapy who develop moderate-to-severe BPD, the acini increase in size [relative to (**A**)] but show little, if any, increase in the number of alveolar saccules or alveoli. The alveolar septa in (**C**) appear normal in thickness compared with the less injured or uninjured lung (**B**), or they may display a uniform mild alveolar septal fibrosis as in (**D**).

the pathology of bronchopulmonary dysplasia has been seen. Although the occasional case of "classic" acute bronchopulmonary dysplasia with necrotizing bronchiolitis, alveolar cell hyperplasia, and peribronchiolar and alveolar septal fibroplasia is still seen along with focal alveolar septal fibrosis in the older patient (Figure 12-35A to D), the few infants who now die from bronchopulmonary dysplasia display what might best be described as "acinar simplification." These simplified acini are characterized by uniformly dilated alveoli whose walls consist of thin alveolar septa with little or no interstitial fibrosis (233).

The bronchioles are similarly unremarkable, with only an occasional mild increase in peribronchiolar musculature. These changes seem to represent an "arrest" of development of the acini, with a resulting markedly decreased number of alveoli within each acinus (Figure 12-36A to C). As a result, the surface area of the lung is significantly decreased even in the absence of significant pathology (e.g., alveolar septal fibrosis).

Although high concentrations of oxygen over prolonged periods of time are known to cause alveolar cell hyperplasia and necrotizing bronchiolitis with resulting alveolar septal fibrosis, it is possible that low levels of oxygen (25% to 35%), while not producing significant alteration in the epithelial lining of the lung or not causing damage sufficient to cause septal fibrosis, may, in very immature infants, inhibit growth of the lung, that is, the development of new alveolar ducts and alveoli. Although the lung appears to "mature" and alveolar septa appear to thin and expand to resemble the septa of term infants, there is no accompanying significant increase in the surface area of the lung through an increase in number of alveoli. Thus, although recent advances in mechanical ventilation have limited the amount of injury to the bronchiole (i.e., no necrotizing bronchiolitis), the continued patency of all bronchioles throughout the course of therapy allows equal injury or inhibition of growth to all acini from even low levels of oxygen therapy.

Husain et al. (233) examined the lungs at autopsy of 22 patients with BPD, of whom 14 had received surfactant therapy and compared them with 15 age-matched controls. Using readily available morphometric techniques [RAC and mean linear intercept (MLI)], they displayed a virtual arrest of alveolar development in both the surfactant-treated and nonsurfactant-treated infants whether or not the typical feature of LSHBPD (i.e., alveolar septal fibrosis) was present. Incidentally, septal fibrosis was infrequently seen in surfactant-treated BPD patients even though their disease was severe enough to contribute significantly to their death. The RAC/MLI ratio (an indicator of the number of alveoli) in the BPD patients who lived weeks to months was virtually unchanged from that expected at the infant's birth weight. In other words, an infant born at 28 weeks' gestation, who developed HMD and BPD and lived for 12 weeks, had the same number of alveoli as the one born at 28 weeks' gestation who died in a few days.

As a result of surfactant replacement therapy and sophisticated methods of ventilation, we now see a much smaller percentage of immature and premature infants with chronic lung disease, and when this chronic lung disease does occur, it does not at all resemble the BPD described in the 1970s and 1980s. The classic features of BPD (necrotizing bronchiolitis, epithelial cell hyperplasia, bronchiolar muscular hyperplasia, and alveolar septal fibrosis) are, in fact, rarely seen today. The chronic lung disease of prematurity of today is an extremely subtle disease (at least from a pathologic perspective) that manifests itself primarily as an inhibited or arrested growth and development of the lung. The etiology of this type of failure of development is unclear. Long-term sequelae of BPD include late sudden unexpected death, lobar overinflation, and right, left, or biventricular myocardial hypertrophy (234).

Congenital Surfactant Deficiency

Inherited deficiency of one or more surfactant proteins (most frequently surfactant protein B) is often a fatal autosomal recessive disorder of lung cell metabolism and is characterized by rapidly progressive respiratory failure immediately after birth (235). The disease is caused by a deficiency of adenosine triphosphate–binding cassette (ABC) protein (236), most frequently ABCA3 (237). Chorionic villous sampling can be used to identify the homozygous state *in utero* (238). Less frequently, abnormalities of surfactant protein-A

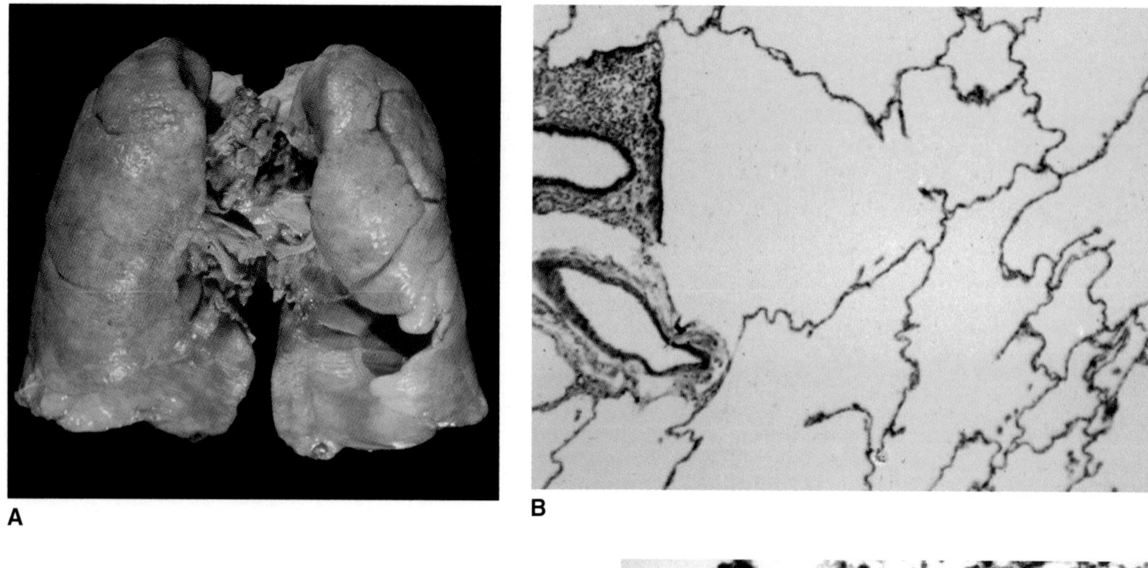

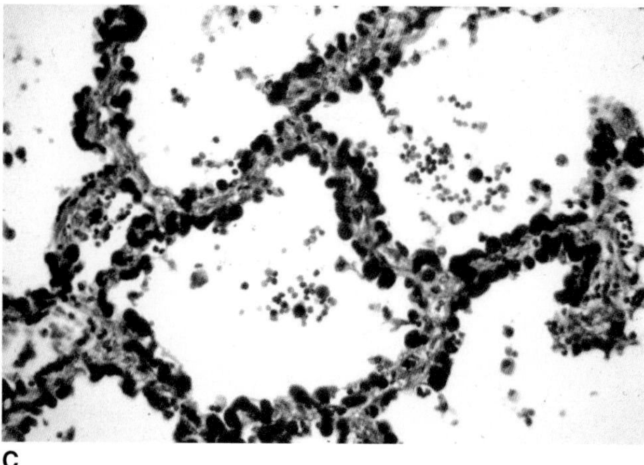

FIGURE 12-36■Chronic lung disease of the premature. **A:** The lung appears largely unremarkable (compare with Figure 12-33B) with an evenly aerated parenchyma. **B:** In this section of lung from a 4-month-old infant born at 26 week's gestation who developed moderate respiratory distress and clinical BPD, the acinus is simplified with dilated alveolar ducts and saccules and with very few alveoli arising from them (see Figure 12-35C) (Hematoxylin and eosin stain, original magnification ×60.). **C:** In this section of lung from a 2-month-old infant born at 28 week's gestation who developed severe prolonged respiratory distress and clinical BPD, the alveolar septa of all acini show mild though uniformly interstitial fibrous thickening. (Masson trichrome stain, ×40.)

and surfactant protein-C may occur. Lung transplantation has been successful, although patients may develop anti–surfactant protein-B antibody (239). Gene therapy utilizing adenoviral vectors has been studied for surfactant protein B deficiency (240).

Grossly, the lungs in congenital surfactant deficiency are heavy and appear consolidated. Microscopically, in the early stages, alveoli are lined by a continuous layer of cuboidal alveolar lining cells (Figure 12-37A). As the disease progresses, alveoli may be filled with eosinophilic granular material admixed with desquamated alveolar cells and macrophages resembling congenital alveolar proteinosis (241) (Figure 12-37B). In the later stages, alveolar septa are widened by fibroblasts producing alveolar septal fibrosis, although the alveolar cell hyperplasia persists (Figure 12-37C). Immunohistochemical stains of the typical SP-B-deficient lung demonstrate decreased to absent SP-B and normal to increased amounts of A and C in alveolar lining cells (Figure 12-37D,E). Electron microscopy displays alveolar type II cells with irregular electron-dense bodies, which also may be present in alveolar spaces and macrophages (242).

Interstitial Pulmonary Emphysema

IPE is the dissection by air around bronchovascular bundles and along intralobular septa as the result of rupture of alveoli, usually in association with mechanical ventilation (Figure 12-38). Dissection of air peripherally through the pleura produces PT, whereas medial dissection can lead to pneumomediastinum, pneumopericardium, and, rarely, pneumomyocardium (Figure 12-39A to C) (192). Although these air leaks can occasionally be observed in normal infants and may spontaneously occur in about 5% of infants with RDS, the highest incidence is seen in infants with RDS who are receiving mechanical ventilation. Although the incidence of IPE and its complications in neonatal intensive care nurseries (NICU) was as high as 40% or more among all NICU patients 30 years ago, early administration of surfactant and increasingly sophisticated means of ventilation have reduced the incidence to 20% to 35% in only the sickest infants. Those particularly at risk include infants with lower 1 and 5 minute APGAR scores, increased surfactant utilization, and higher inspired oxygen concentration (243). IPE has also been reported in 20% of patients dying of acute asthma, as

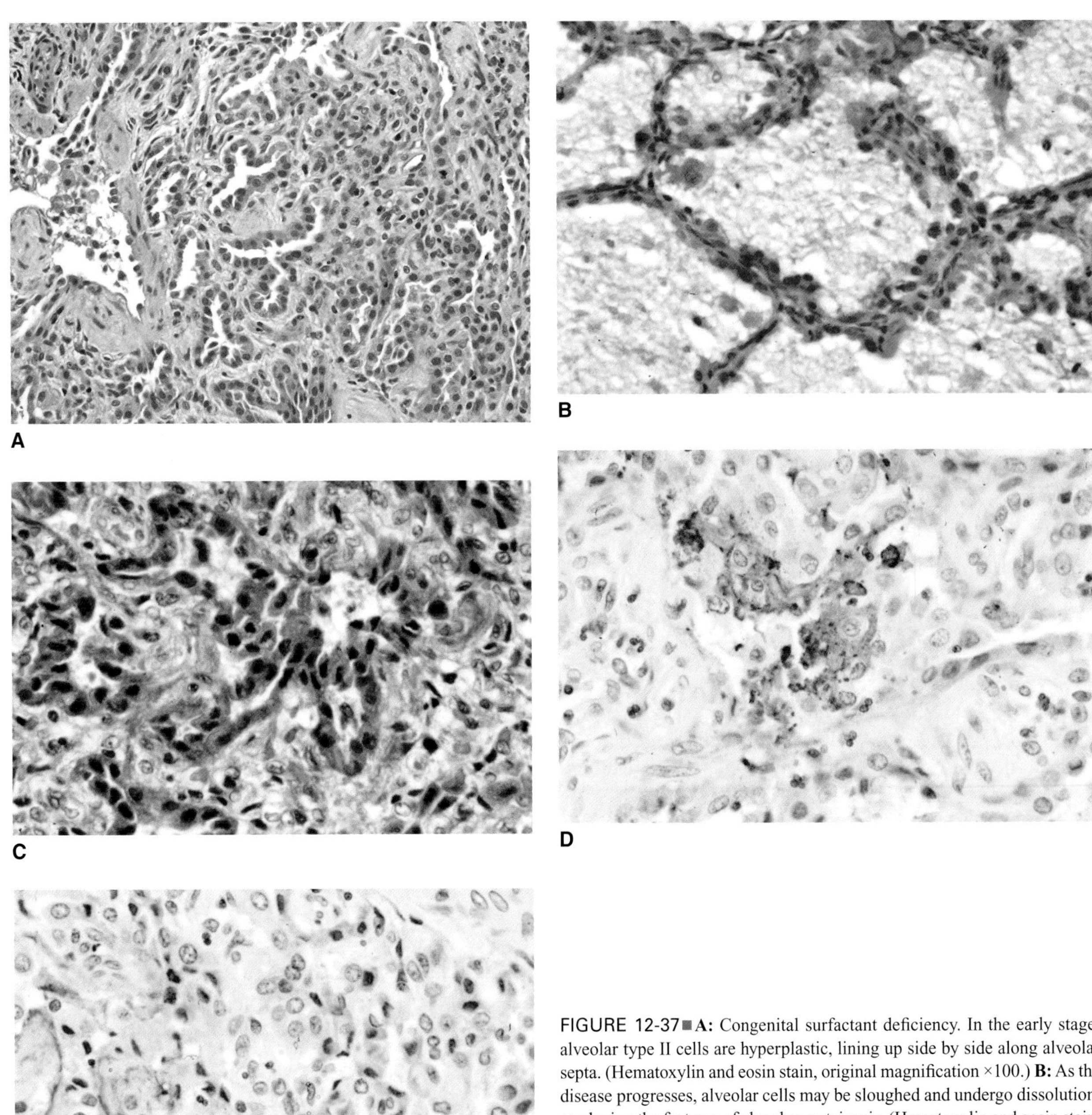

FIGURE 12-37 ■ **A:** Congenital surfactant deficiency. In the early stage, alveolar type II cells are hyperplastic, lining up side by side along alveolar septa. (Hematoxylin and eosin stain, original magnification ×100.) **B:** As the disease progresses, alveolar cells may be sloughed and undergo dissolution, producing the features of alveolar proteinosis. (Hematoxylin and eosin stain, original magnification ×100.) **C:** With further progression, alveolar septa become widened with fibrous connective tissue. Note the continued alveolar cell hyperplasia. (Masson trichrome stain, original magnification ×100. **D** and **E:** Stains for surfactant in this surfactant-deficient lung are positive for surfactant A (**D**) and negative for surfactant B (**E**). (Immunoperoxidase stains ×125.)

a result of cardiopulmonary resuscitation, and in association with a variety of infectious diseases (244).

IPE can be acute (<7 days' duration) or persistent and may be localized to a single lobe or distributed diffusely through all lobes (245). Acute IPE (AIPE) presents grossly as 0.1- to 0.5-cm air blebs located beneath the pleura along junctions between the interlobular septa and the pleura (Figure 12-40A). On cut section, round to oval air spaces may be seen around bronchovascular bundles and along the interlobular septa (Figure 12-40B). Only rarely do the air-filled cysts dissect laterally from the septa beneath the pleura, which aids in the differentiation of IPE from CPL. Microscopically, the cysts of AIPE are confined to the interlobular septal and peribronchial region, compressing the adjacent blood vessels and acini (Figure 12-40C). The walls consist primarily of loose connective tissue and compressed parenchyma. AIPE may incorporate some of the lymphatics of the interlobular septa, but the vast majority of cysts appear to be formed from air-dissected connective tissue. Subpleural lymphatics are rarely involved and appear unremarkable.

Persistent interstitial pulmonary emphysema (PIPE) occurs in infants with AIPE that lasts more than 1 week. The cysts of

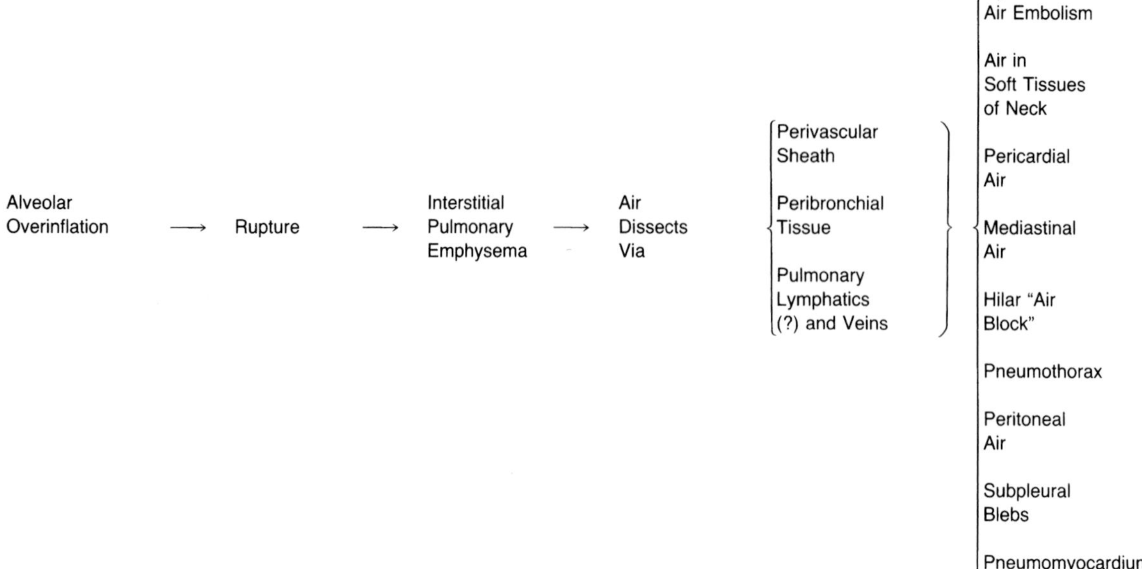

FIGURE 12-38 ■ Potential complications related to mechanical ventilation and pulmonary interstitial air. (From Askin FB. Pulmonary interstitial air and pneumothorax in the neonate. In: Stocker JT, ed. *Pediatric pulmonary disease*. Washington, DC: Hemisphere, 1989:166, with permission.)

PIPE may be localized to a single lobe or, when seen in association with BPD, diffusely radiate throughout most or all of the lobes (245). PIPE is grossly characterized by multiple 0.1- to 0.3-cm cysts localized to the interlobular septa and extending radially from the hilum to the pleura (Figure 12-41A,B). Cysts in the localized form of PIPE tend to be larger than those in lungs that are diffusely involved, occasionally as large as 5 cm (246,247). The intercommunicating, irregularly shaped cysts are air-filled and lined with a smooth, glistening membrane. A communication between the airway system and the interstitium may be demonstrable (245). Microscopically, the cysts are composed of a thin to thick fibrous connective tissue wall intermittently "lined" with multinucleated foreign body giant cells, the pathognomonic feature of PIPE

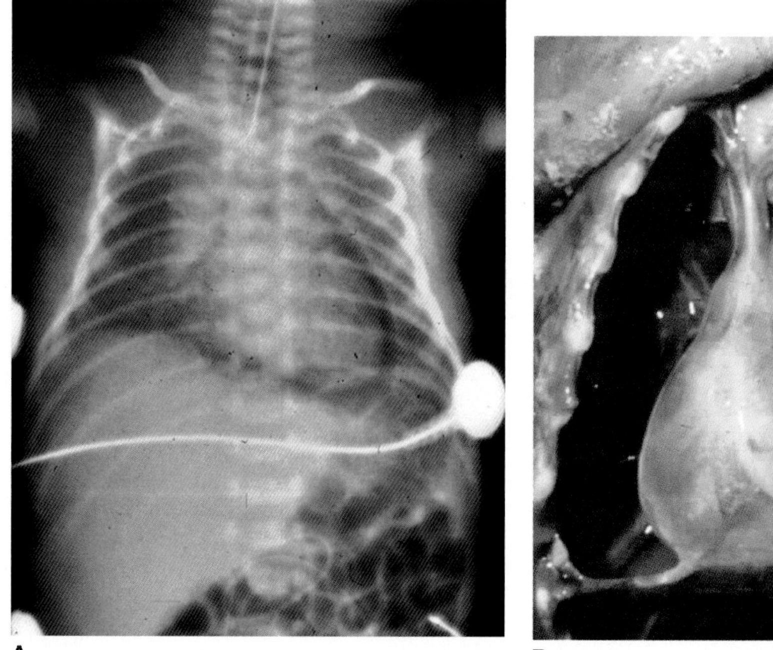

FIGURE 12-39 ■ Pneumopericardium, PT, and pneumomediastinum. **A:** In this chest x-ray, air can be seen within the pericardial sac surrounding the heart (pneumopericardium), and in the right hemithorax (PT). **B:** At autopsy, the air distended the pericardial sac. (Courtesy of Ralph E. Franciosi, M.D., Children's Hospital of Wisconsin, Milwaukee, Wisconsin.)

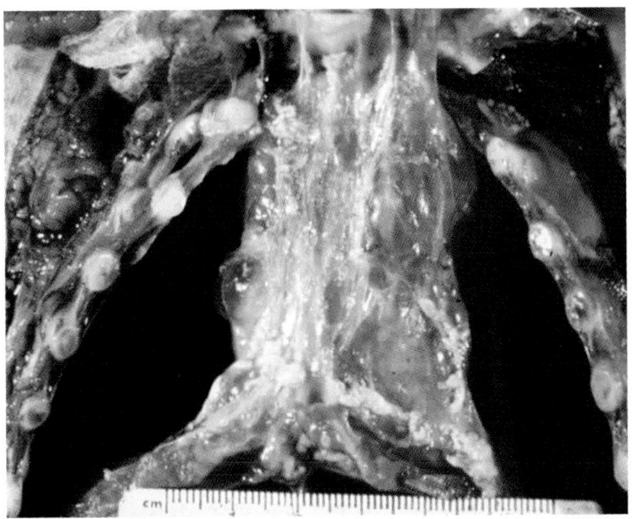

C

FIGURE 12-39■*(continued)* **C:** Blebs of air dissect the tissues of the mediastinum (pneumomediastinum).

(Figure 12-41C,D). The adjacent parenchyma is usually compressed and, in the diffuse form, frequently displays the features of BPD. Treatment of localized PIPE consists of surgical resection or a variety of forms of selective intubation, mechanical ventilation, or both (248).

Aspiration

Aspiration of material into the tracheobronchial tree can occur *in utero*, during delivery, or in the neonate or young child (Table 12-7). The material aspirated may obstruct the major airways and produce sudden respiratory distress and even death (e.g., tracheal obstruction from aspiration of a peanut), or the distribution of the material may be more diffuse, leading to a "chemical" pneumonitis (e.g., aspiration of meconium or gastric contents). Aspiration of amniotic fluid *in utero* is a normal physiologic process, and a few sloughed squamous epithelial cells ("squames") can be seen in the lungs of virtually every term or near-term infant, but massive aspiration of amniotic debris may be seen in postterm infants or in infants with oligohydramnios.

Grossly, the lungs are expanded and firm. Microscopically, squames distend alveolar ducts and alveoli. As noted above, however, small number of squames can be seen in the lungs of virtually all infants born after 34 to 36 weeks of gestation (249).

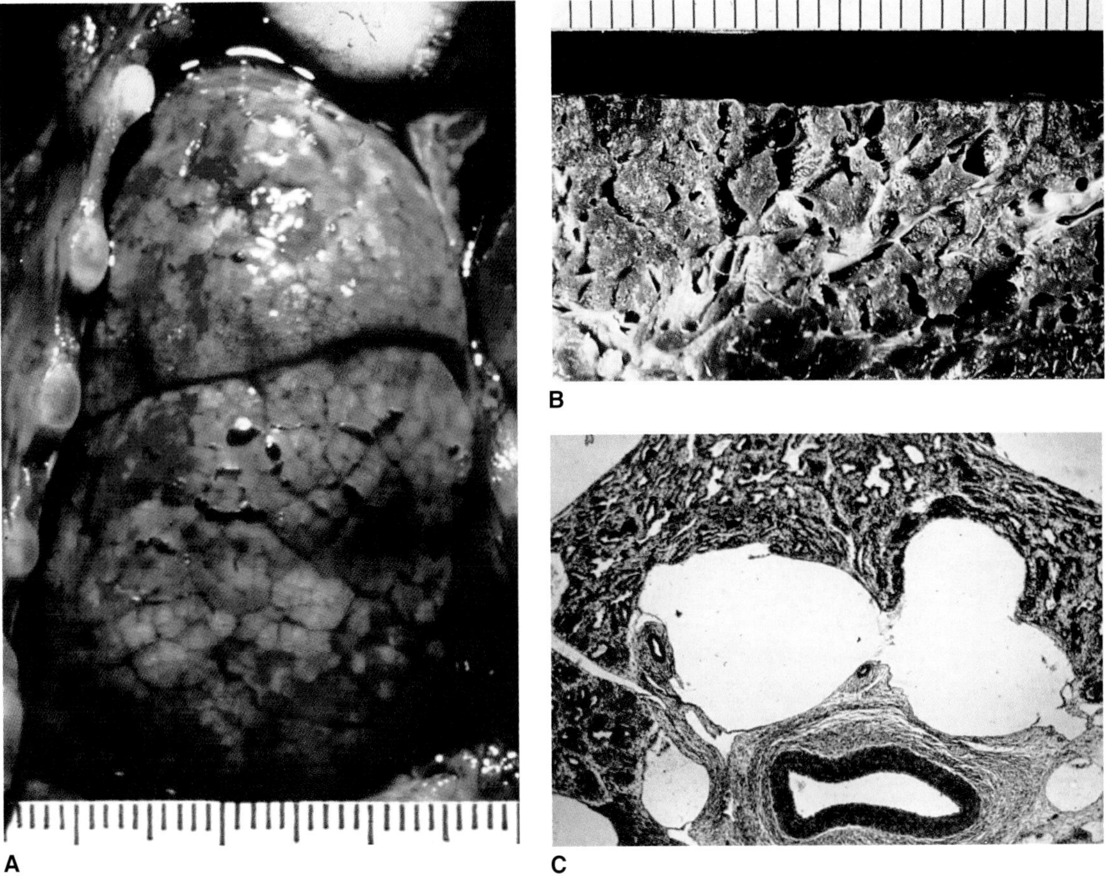

A B C

FIGURE 12-40■Acute PIPE. **A:** Air can be seen beneath the pleura at the junction of interlobular septa and pleura. **B:** Round to oval, air-containing cysts are present within interlobular septa. The cysts extend radially from the hilum to the pleura. **C:** The pulmonary artery (**bottom**) is surrounded and partially compressed by air-filled spaces. (Masson trichrome, ×50.)

Meconium staining of amniotic fluid is seen in up to 29% of all pregnancies and was noted in 12.15% of 176,790 neonates reported by Wiswell et al. (250). Approximately, 5.5% of meconium-stained neonates (0.66% of all neonates) develop the meconium aspiration syndrome (MAS). Boys are more frequently affected than girls. MAS may cause death in approximately 4% of affected neonates.

MAS presents as respiratory distress in the meconium-stained neonate and requires mechanical ventilation in about 30% of cases (251). Pneumothoraces are noted in more than 11% of MAS infants. ECMO and surfactant lavage have contributed to the increasing survival of neonates with MAS (252).

Meconium, the residual of gastrointestinal secretions accumulated in the lower gastrointestinal tract of the fetus, can, when aspirated, obstruct the trachea, bronchi, and bronchioles. The tenacious green–yellow material can frequently be seen grossly as plugs within bronchi and bronchioles on cut section of the lung. Microscopically, the material is composed of amorphous, acellular, faintly basophilic debris (Figure 12-42A). In infants surviving more than a few hours, a chemical pneumonitis develops with alveoli filled with neutrophils and basophilic debris. Chronic intrauterine meconium aspiration may cause pulmonary infarction, rupture, and meconium embolism.

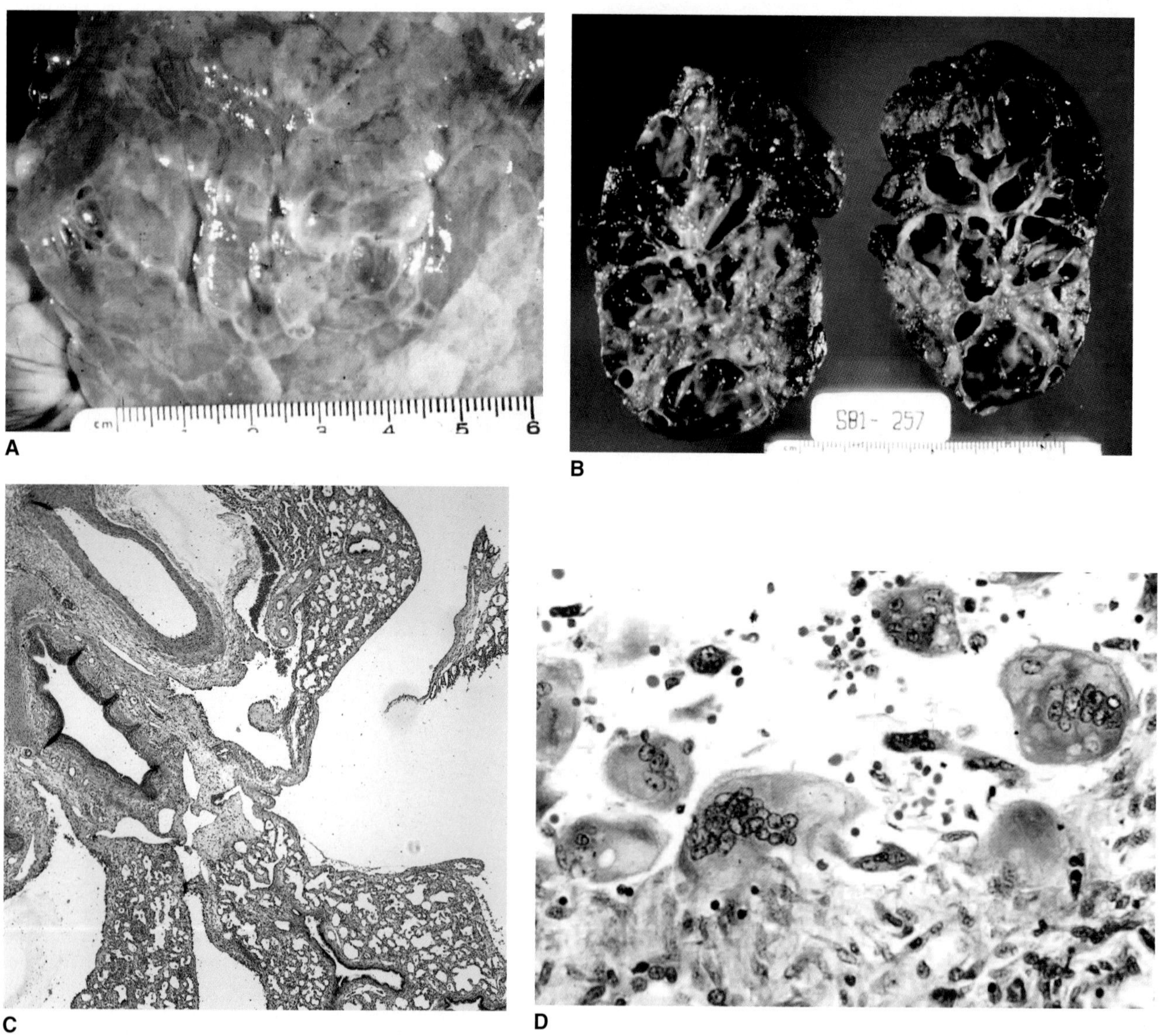

FIGURE 12-41 ■ Persistent PIPE. **A:** Air blebs are noted beneath a partially "clouded" pleura. **B:** Intercommunicating, irregular, air-filled cysts lined by a smooth membrane compress the pulmonary parenchyma. **C:** The irregular cysts extend along interlobular septa. The cyst walls are composed of fibrous connective tissue of varying thickness, irregularly covered by foreign body giant cells. Note the bronchus (**left**). (Hematoxylin and eosin stain, original magnification ×4.) **D:** The foreign body giant cells contain multiple, eccentrically placed nuclei amid a smooth to granular cytoplasm. (Hematoxylin and eosin stain, original magnification ×210.)

Table 12-7 ■ SOURCES OF ASPIRATED MATERIAL
Amniotic debris
Meconium
Blood
Milk
Gastric contents
Foreign bodies
Plants
Pins
Pieces of toys
Small batteries
Toxic fluids
Kerosene
Furniture polish
Mineral oil

Aspiration of maternal blood during delivery may produce clinical features that mimics pulmonary hemorrhage. In infants, milk may be aspirated during feeding or regurgitation. Older infants with esophageal reflux or neurologic disorders (e.g., cerebral palsy) are also prone to aspiration. Gastric contents may obstruct bronchi or bronchioles and produce a chemical pneumonitis in which meat and vegetable fibers may be identified in association with granulomata and foreign body giant cells. (Figure 12-42B to D)

Aspirated foreign bodies are responsible for about 2,000 deaths a year in children, usually lodge in the upper airway or bronchi, and include virtually any object that will pass through the glottis into the larynx (253,254). Bronchial obstruction may lead to acute or chronic pneumonia including the development of an ILS (48).

Aspirated fluid such as kerosene, mineral oil, and furniture polish may result in severe pulmonary damage including diffuse alveolar damage, lipoid pneumonia, and diffuse necrosis. ECMO has been helpful in treating these patients, as well as patients with meconium aspiration (see below).

Extracorporeal Membrane Oxygenation

The development of ECMO and its use in the treatment of meconium aspiration, alveolar capillary dysplasia, diaphragmatic hernia (among other causes of pulmonary hypoplasia), *Listeria monocytogenes* infection, and congenital heart malformations have produced a variety of pathologic changes involving the lung and other organs (220,255).

Chou et al. (256) have described the autopsy findings in 23 infants receiving ECMO therapy and noted the presence of interstitial and intra-alveolar hemorrhage along with hyaline membrane formation during the first few days of therapy. They described the hyperplasia of type II alveolar cells and bronchial epithelial cells after 2 days of ECMO therapy in some patients and, by 7 days, in all patients. Interstitial fibrosis was also noted beginning at 7 days. After 15 days of treatment, there was replacement of the terminal airways and alveoli by tall columnar and mucin-producing epithelium (Figure 12-43). Squamous metaplasia of bronchial epithelium was also seen in the majority of patients, and one patient developed mucinous metaplasia as well. Clusters of calcified material were present in the alveoli of 7 of 23 cases (255). Long-term survivors of ECMO show a high frequency of hyperinflation and airway obstruction (257).

Extrapulmonary changes include ischemic neuronal necrosis, focal cerebral infarcts, intracerebral hemorrhages, periventricular leukomalacia, pericardial hemorrhage, carotid artery injury, and retinal vasculopathy (258,259).

Pulmonary Hemorrhage

Hemorrhage into the alveoli or interstitium of the lung is a frequent finding in tissue removed at surgery at all ages. In the neonatal period, however, pulmonary hemorrhage is frequently associated with HMD and BPD but may also occur in association with patent ductus arteriosus (260), erythroblastosis, congestive heart failure, disseminated intravascular coagulation, congenital malformations, acute pneumonia,

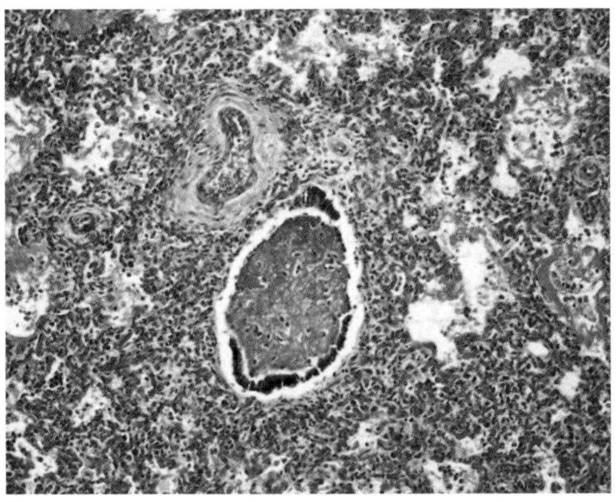
A

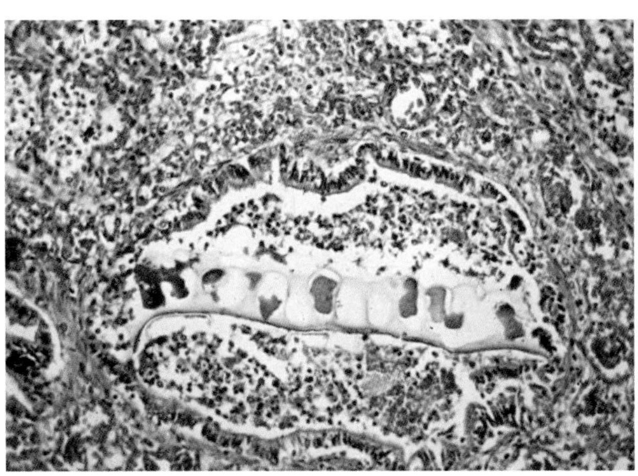
B

FIGURE 12-42 ■ Aspiration. **A:** Meconium. Amorphous debris containing scattered neutrophils occludes a bronchiole in this term infant who was intensely meconium stained. (H&E, ×50) **B:** Vegetable fibers are accompanied by acute bronchiolitis (H&E, ×50).

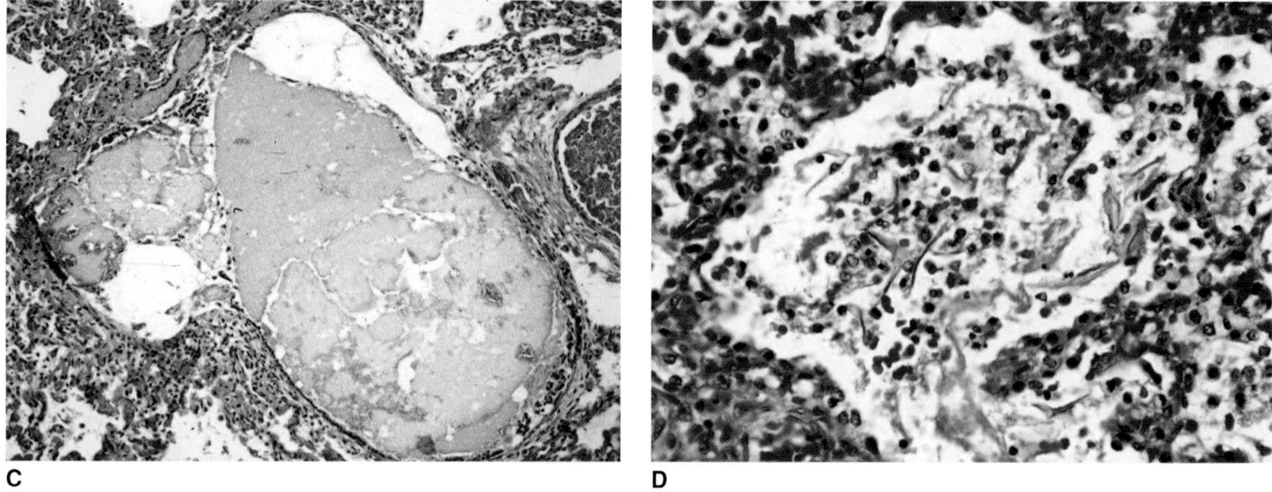

FIGURE 12-42 ■ *(continued)* **C:** Gastric contents—milk. (H&E, ×40) **D:** Amniotic debris. (H&E, ×50).

systemic lupus erythematosus (261), Goodpasture syndrome (262), and rarely, as an isolated finding (263, 264). The incidence of neonatal massive pulmonary hemorrhage, defined as hemorrhage involving more than two-thirds of the lung, is seen in up to 40% of neonatal autopsies. The appearance of hemorrhage may also be produced by the intrapartum aspiration of maternal blood, which may mimic both the clinical and pathologic features of massive pulmonary hemorrhage. Identification of the type of alveolar red blood cells (maternal versus fetal) allows for separation of the two entities.

Pulmonary Veno-occlusive Disease

Pulmonary venous obstruction may be secondary to congenital cardiac malformations such as mitral stenosis or cor triatriatum, or it may be due to an intrinsic disease of the pulmonary veins, that is, pulmonary veno-occlusive disease (PVOD). PVOD is a rare cause of pulmonary hypertension that mainly affects children and young adults (265). Patients with PVOD present with symptoms of right-sided heart failure. Radiologic examination shows prominent pulmonary arteries with Kerley B lines, interlobular septal thickening, pleural effusion, and mediastinal adenopathy (266). Microscopically, pulmonary veins and venules show eccentric intimal fibrosis or are occluded by thrombi, which may be partially recanalized and are best seen with an elastic or connective tissue stain. Evidence of pulmonary hypertension is seen in arterialized veins and medial hypertrophy of arteries.

Its cause is unknown, although viral infections (including HIV), antiphospholipid antibody, and drugs have been implicated (267,268). PVOD has also been seen to develop in patients following bone marrow transplantation (269) and as a component of pulmonary capillary hemangiomatosis (268,270). No effective treatment is available; lung transplantation has been tried. The prognosis associated with PVOD is poor.

Pulmonary Alveolar Microlithiasis

Pulmonary alveolar microlithiasis is a rare and unusual disorder reported worldwide as single cases or in siblings or other family members (271). Patients often are asymptomatic with a diffuse miliary pattern concentrated along bronchovascular bundles, interlobular septa, and beneath the pleura on routine chest x-ray study (272). Diagnosis is made by demonstrating calcium phosphate microconcretions on bronchoalveolar lavage or lung biopsy. An autosomal recessive inheritance pattern has been proposed, and one case has been associated with the Waardenburg-anophthalmia syndrome (273). The disease progresses with eventual pulmonary hypertension, cor pulmonale, and respiratory failure.

Pulmonary Hemosiderosis

Hemosiderin in the lung usually indicates previous hemorrhage or aspiration of blood and is thus relatively nonspecific

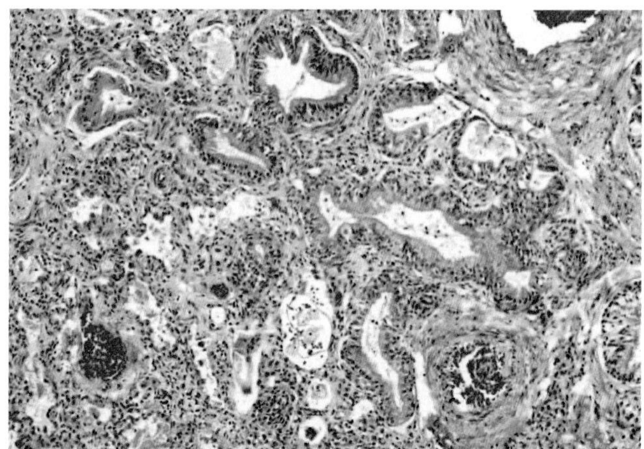

FIGURE 12-43 ■ Extracorporeal membrane oxygenation. This term infant with a large left-sided diaphragmatic hernia and severe pulmonary hypoplasia was on ECMO for 16 days before dying. Note the alveolar septal fibrosis and the replacement of the terminal airways and alveoli (**right**) by cuboidal to columnar epithelium. (Hematoxylin and eosin stain, original magnification ×40.)

Table 12-8 ▪ DISORDERS ASSOCIATED WITH DIFFUSE PULMONARY HEMORRHAGE AND HEMOSIDEROSIS IN INFANCY AND CHILDHOOD

Idiopathic pulmonary hemosiderosis (isolated)
Pulmonary hemosiderosis associated with sensitivity to cow's milk
Pulmonary hemosiderosis and glomerulonephritis
  With antibodies to GBM (Goodpasture syndrome)
  Without antibodies to GBM (usually immune-complex glomerulonephritis)
Pulmonary hemosiderosis associated with collagen-vascular or purpuric disease
  Systemic lupus erythematosus
  Wegener granulomatosis
  Polyarteritis nodosa
  Rheumatoid arthritis
  Schönlein-Henoch purpura
  Idiopathic thrombocytopenic purpura
Pulmonary hemosiderosis secondary to cardiac disease, Intrapulmonary vascular lesions, or malformations
  Chronic left-sided or right-sided heart failure (e.g., mitral stenosis)
  Pulmonary hypertension
  Pulmonary veno-occlusive disease
  Pulmonary lymphangiomyomatosis
  Arteriovenous fistulas and other congenital vascular malformations
  Vascular thrombosis with infarction

GBM, glomerular basement membrane.
From Cutz E. Idiopathic pulmonary hemosiderosis and related disorders in infancy and childhood. *Perspect Pediatr Pathol* 1987;11:49, with permission.

(Table 12-8). Macrophages containing hemosiderin can be found in alveolar or interstitial regions in association with conditions such as infection, blood dyscrasia, chronic heart failure, pulmonary hypertension, and neoplasia. There exists a group of rare disorders that are characterized by single or repeated episodes of bleeding that can lead to massive hemorrhage or progress to chronic pulmonary disease. Based on the clinical, laboratory, and immunopathologic findings, they are divided into two categories:

1. Idiopathic pulmonary hemosiderosis (IPH), with pulmonary hemorrhage as an isolated process
2. Secondary pulmonary hemorrhage associated with immunologically mediated renal or vascular disease.

Idiopathic Pulmonary Hemosiderosis

IPH presents with symptoms including anemia, hypoxemia (85%), dyspnea, and hemoptysis (65%). It occurs primarily in children 3 to 6 years of age but can be seen in children as young as 4 to 6 months of age. Consanguinity and environmental factors may be involved in the development of IPH (274). Sex incidence is equal, and 15% to 20% of cases occur in adolescents and young adults. Less specific non-pulmonary symptoms include fever (in as many as 79% of cases), lymphadenopathy, hepatomegaly, and splenomegaly. Radiographically, early stages are characterized by patchy or diffuse pulmonary infiltrates or massive confluent shadows that may rapidly clear. In later stages of the disease, there is a perihilar reticulation or a pattern of diffuse interstitial disease. The clinical triad of hemoptysis, iron deficiency anemia, and diffuse parenchymal infiltrates is strongly suggestive of IPH (274). The presence of hemosiderin-laden macrophages on bronchoalveolar lavage is also highly correlated with IPH, with the presence of 35% or more hemosiderin-laden macrophages associated with a sensitivity of 1% and a specificity of 96% (275).

Hypochromic microcytic anemia is seen in virtually all cases of IPH, and eosinophilia is present in 12% to 15% of patients (276). Bone marrow examination shows reactive erythroid hyperplasia and depleted iron stores. Levels of serum iron are low, and total iron binding capacity is increased. Most patients with IPH have normal renal function without circulating autoantibodies (compare with Goodpasture syndrome; see Chapter 17). An association with celiac disease has also been reported (277,278) and, rarely, juvenile dermatomyositis (279). Although some children with IPH may die of massive hemorrhage shortly after presentation, other patients have a history of progressive respiratory insufficiency leading to death 2 to 5 years after diagnosis, although a 5-year survival of 86% was reported in 17 patients receiving corticosteroids (280) and other immunosuppressant agents (281,282).

Bronchoalveolar lavage demonstrates hemosiderin-laden alveolar macrophages in large numbers (283). Lung biopsy and autopsy specimens show varied involvement. Focal areas of consolidation are common owing to massive accumulations of hemosiderin-laden macrophages, which obliterate alveolar spaces and are associated with interstitial fibrosis. Corrin et al. (284) describe capillary endothelial swelling and focal thickening of the basement membrane. Stainable iron is present in alveolar and tissue macrophages, free in connective tissues, and encrusting elastic fibers of small blood vessels and alveolar septa (Figure 12-44A to C). There is mild-to-moderate alveolar cell hyperplasia, peribronchial lymphoid hyperplasia, and alveolar septal mastocytosis (75). Immunofluorescence is negative for immunoglobulin, complement and antibasement membrane antibodies (285).

Infectious Diseases

Infectious diseases affecting the lungs (among other organs) are described in detail in Chapter 6. Organisms specifically or primarily affecting the lungs bear special mention.

Respiratory Syncytial Virus

Respiratory syncytial virus (RSV) is the most important respiratory pathogen of infancy and childhood, and creates sizable outbreaks of infection each year. An RNA virus, RSV occurs in regularly recurring epidemics in midwinter and early spring. It has been identified as causing 5% to 40% of pneumonias (50% of viral pneumonias), from 50% to 90% of cases of bronchiolitis, and from 10% to 30% of cases of persistant bronchitis in young children (286). RSV presents clinically with fever, cough, rhinitis, pharyngitis, and dyspnea and can

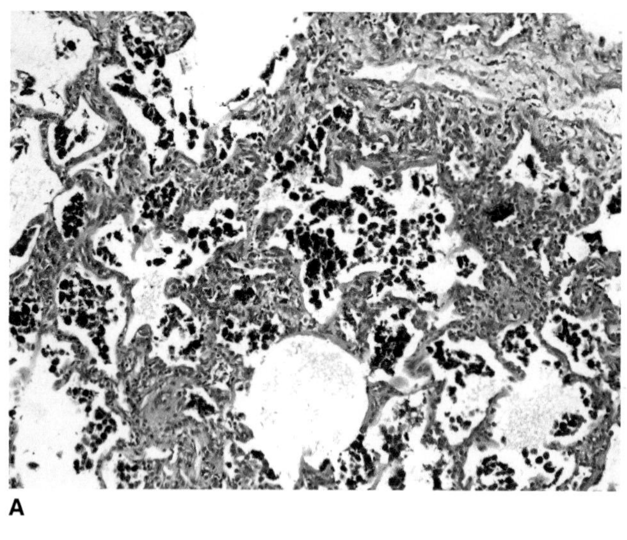

A

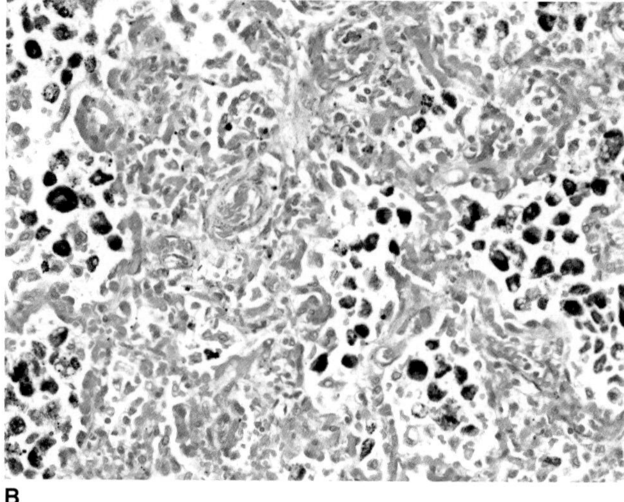

B

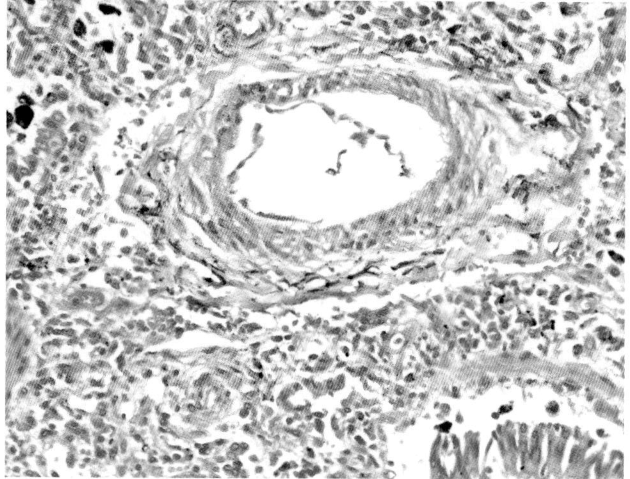

C

FIGURE 12-44 ■ Idiopathic pulmonary hemosiderosis. **A:** Hemosiderin is present in clusters of alveolar and septal macrophages. **B:** An iron stain demonstrates masses of iron in alveolar macrophages and in connective tissue. (Prussian iron stain, ×40.) **C:** Iron is also present in the media as well as encrusting elastic fibers adjacent to a pulmonary artery. (Prussian iron stain, ×70.)

produce severe enough bronchiolitis to require hospitalization in 1% to 2% of cases, primarily in children 2 to 5 months of age, accounting for 90,000 hospital admissions annually in the United States (286). The mortality rate in these hospitalized patients is 1% to 3%, causing 4,500 deaths in infants and children in the United States annually. RSV may, however, be associated with a higher mortality rate in children infected with pathogens such as adenovirus, pneumococcus, cytomegalovirus, and *Pneumocystis jiroveci* (287). Of patients with RSV requiring mechanical ventilation, the majority have at least one additional risk factor for a severe course of infection (prematurity 50%, chronic lung disease 20%, congenital heart disease 35%, immunodeficiency 20%) (288). Of those dying of RSV, Thorburn noted one of the following preexisting medical conditions in every patient–chromosomal abnormalities 29%, cardiac lesions 27%, neuromuscular disorder 15%, chronic lung disease 12%, large airway abnormality 9%, and immunodeficiency 9% (289).

In fatal cases, RSV produces extensive alveolar and terminal bronchiolar plugging by granular eosinophilic debris accompanied by peribronchiolar lymphocytic inflammation and edema (290). Eosinophils may be an integral part of the inflammatory process (291). In less severely involved areas, bronchiolar epithelium displays uneven proliferation with a polypoid appearance, squamous metaplasia, and desquamation. Syncytial giant cells may be present along alveolar walls and may contain granular, mildly basophilic cytoplasmic inclusions, which may also be seen in bronchial, bronchiolar, and alveolar epithelia (Figure 12-45A to C). Dense cytoplasmic inclusions can be demonstrated by electron microscopy (286). RSV antigen can be demonstrated in formalin-fixed, paraffin-embedded autopsy tissue by immunohistochemical techniques (Figure 12-45C).

Human Metapneumovirus

Human metapneumovirus (MNPV) accounts for nearly 10% of community-acquired alveolar pneumonia, but, when compared with infants with RSV pneumonia, are older and have a more common history of acute otitis media requiring tympanocentesis, wheezing and gastrointestinal symptoms, and a lower hospitalization rate (292). MNVP is also seen more frequently

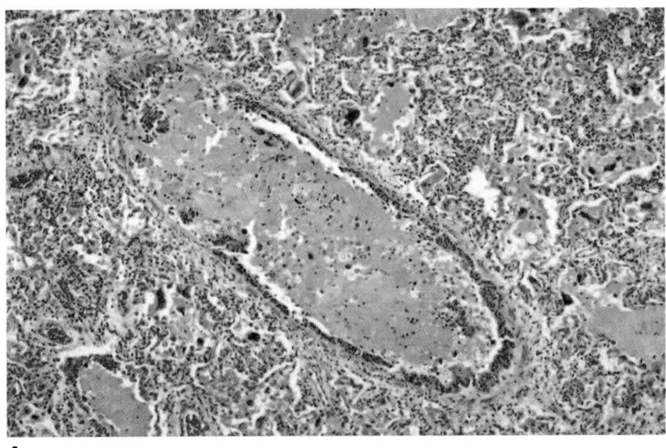

A

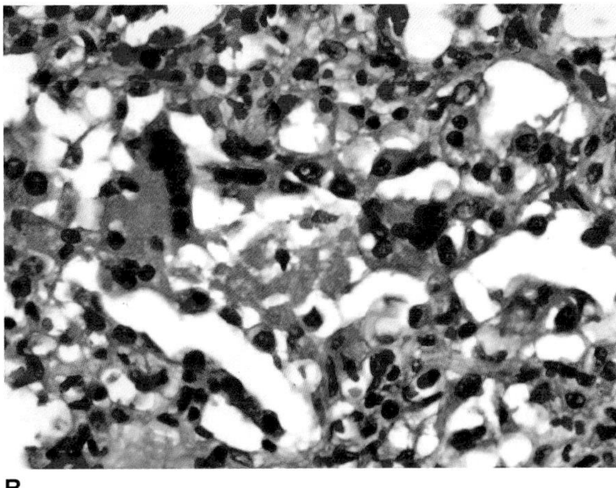

B

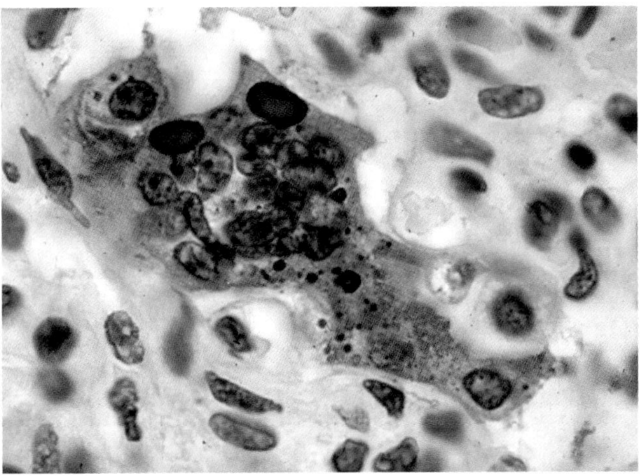

C

FIGURE 12-45 Respiratory syncytial virus. **A:** Amorphous inflammatory debris fills a bronchiole and surrounding alveoli. Note the syncytial giant cells throughout the section. (H&E, ×75.) **B:** Hyperplastic alveolar cells line the surface of this alveolus, which contains numerous syncytial giant cells. (H&E, ×200; courtesy of Eduardo J. Yunis, M.D., Children's Hospital, Pittsburgh, Pennsylvania.). **C:** The cytoplasmic viral inclusions stain intensely positive for RSV. (RSV immunoperoxidase stain, ×400.)

than RSV in children with congenital abnormalities, particularly those with cardio-pulmonary problems and when associated with an increased ventilatory requirement (293).

The pathology of HMPV has only recently been described (294). Bronchoalveolar lavage shows epithelial degenerative changes and eosinophilic cytoplasmic inclusions within epithelial cells, multinucleate giant cells, and histiocytes. Lung biopsy shows chronic airway inflammation and intra-alveolar foamy and hemosiderin-laden macrophages.

Adenovirus

Adenovirus, a DNA virus, is frequently associated with gastroenteritis in infants and young children but also accounts for 5% to 11% of cases of bronchitis, 2% to 10% of bronchiolitis, and 4% to 10% of pneumonia in children (295). Adenovirus infections are seen most frequently in children younger than 5 years of age who spend portions of their days in child care centers or other closed environments. Infections are also common in grade and junior high school children during winter, spring, and early summer.

Severe cases of pneumonia are most common in children 3 to 18 months of age and are associated with adenovirus types 3, 7, and 21. The onset is acute, and the child presents with high fever, persistent cough, lethargy, diarrhea, vomiting, and pharyngitis. Adenovirus infection with or without interstitial pneumonia has been implicated in up to 25% of sudden deaths in infants. Extrapulmonary complications (e.g., meningitis, myocarditis) are common, and serious pulmonary sequelae (e.g., bronchiectasis, bronchiolitis obliterans (296), unilateral hyperlucent lung) are seen in 14% to 60% of cases with documented lower respiratory tract disease (297).

The pneumonia is characterized by severe necrotizing bronchitis, bronchiolitis, and alveolitis (298). Adjacent to areas of necrosis, the alveolar and bronchiolar epithelial cells are enlarged and contain small eosinophilic and larger basophilic intranuclear inclusions. These inclusions have a characteristic amphophilic (smudged) appearance. When viewed by electron microscopy, it can be seen that these inclusions contain viral particles that measure 70 to 80 nm and are arrayed in a tight periodic pattern along diagonals, which create hexagonal unit groups.

Legionella Pneumonia

Legionella pneumonia is seen infrequently in infants and children, but may be one of the many infections seen in immunocompromised patients (299).

Chlamydia Trachomatis

Chlamydia trachomatis, an obligate intracellular bacterial parasite, is a well-known oculogenital pathogen that can also produce pneumonia in infants. Respiratory distress is noted in premature infants, and a progressive staccato cough is seen in older infants. The disease is readily treatable with antibiotics, and the mortality rate is low. Lung biopsy specimens display interstitial and intra-alveolar infiltrates of lymphocytes, plasma cells, histiocytes, eosinophils, and neutrophils (300). Necrotizing bronchiolitis may be present, along with emphysema, airway plugging, and atelectasis. Intracytoplasmic inclusions of *Chlamydia trachomatis* are only rarely seen in the lung.

Eosinophilic Pneumonia

Acute eosinophilic pneumonia (AEP), while rare in the pediatric age group, can be seen in older children and is characterized by acute onset, respiratory distress, eosinophilic infiltration in the lung, resolution of symptoms with corticosteroids, and the absence of relapse (301,302). An increase in peripheral blood hypersegmented eosinophils may precede the onset of symptoms (303). Bronchoalveolar lavage also demonstrates the presence of many eosinophils. Although the etiology of AEP is often unknown, it has been associated with a wide variety of drugs, parasites, and other infectious agents (304). The lungs are consolidated with alveoli filled with eosinophils and macrophages, accompanied in about 50% of the cases with an eosinophilic proteinaceous exudate. The interstitium may be widened by a mixture of inflammatory cells rich in eosinophils but also containing plasma cells and lymphocytes. Alveolar cells may be hyperplastic. Chronic eosinophilic pneumonia is rarely seen in children (305).

Interstitial Lung Diseases

As the name implies, these are diseases, which primarily affect the interstitium (alveolar walls, interlobular septae, and connective tissue surrounding bronchovascular bundles) of the lung. They are bilateral with multilobar involvement. Terminology and definitions of acute and chronic interstitial lung diseases (ILDs) have evolved over the last few years, both in children and adults. Use of uniform criteria has helped characterize clinico-pathological entities whose course, response to treatment, and prognosis are better understood, although there are still many patients whose diseases cannot be classified. It has also become evident that responses to lung injuries occur in certain pathologic patterns that can be recognized on light microscopy, such as organizing pneumonia, which point to a differential diagnosis but are not specific for a disease.

The spectrum of diseases seen in the pediatric population is almost completely different from that in adults. Idiopathic pulmonary fibrosis/usual interstitial pneumonia and smoking-related disorders [desquamative interstitial pneumonia (DIP) and respiratory bronchiolitis-interstitial lung disease] are never seen in children. Nonspecific interstitial pneumonia (NSIP), which is usually associated with connective tissue diseases, can rarely be seen in older children. The terms DIP and NSIP have been used in children, but these are not specific diagnoses, rather the intent is to be descriptive. Thus, it is better to avoid terminology, which leads to confusion; rather one should be as specific as possible.

A multidisciplinary working group reviewed 165 lung biopsies from children less than 2 years of age who had diffuse lung disease and grouped them according to clinical and pathologic features (306). These groups are given below, with the first four being more prevalent in infancy:

1. Diffuse developmental disorders
   a. Acinar dysplasia
   b. Congenital alveolar dysplasia
   c. Alveolar capillary dysplasia with misalignment of pulmonary veins
2. Growth abnormalities reflecting deficient alveolarization
   a. Pulmonary hypoplasia
   b. Chronic neonatal lung disease
   c. Related to chromosomal disorders
   d. Related to congenital heart disease
3. Specific conditions of undefined etiology
   a. Neuroendocrine cell hyperplasia of infancy
   b. Pulmonary interstitial glycogenosis
4. Surfactant dysfunction disorders
   a. Surfactant protein B mutations
   b. Surfactant protein C mutations
   c. ABCA3 mutations
   d. Histology consistent with surfactant dysfunction disorder
      i. Pulmonary alveolar proteinosis
      ii. Chronic pneumonitis of infancy
      iii. Desquamative interstitial pneumonia
      iv. Nonspecific interstitial pneumonia
5. Disorders related to systemic disease processes
   a. Immune-mediated collagen vascular disorders
   b. Storage disease
   c. Sarcoidosis
   d. Langerhans cell histiocytosis
   e. Malignant infiltrates
6. Disorders of the normal host-presumed immune intact
   a. Infectious/post–infectious processes
   b. Related to environmental agents
      i. Hypersensitivity pneumonitis
      ii. Toxic inhalation
   c. Aspiration syndrome
   d. Eosinophilic pneumonia
7. Disorders of the immunocompromised host
   a. Opportunistic infections
   b. Related to therapeutic interventions
   c. Related to transplantation and rejection
   d. Diffuse alveolar damage, unknown etiology

8. Disorders masquerading as ILD
   a. Arterial hypertensive vasculopathy
   b. Congestive changes related to cardiac dysfunction
   c. Veno-occlusive disease
   d. Lymphatic disorders

As evident from the above groups, these include all diffuse lung diseases including developmental disorders, not just interstitial diseases. However, this is workable framework in which to develop a differential diagnosis when looking at a lung biopsy. Many of these conditions are discussed in other sections of this chapter.

Chronic Lung Disease of Infancy

After excluding known causes of ILDs, such as surfactant disorders and complications of prematurity (bronchopulmonary dysplasia), there remains a group of infants who were born at term or near-term and developed slowly progressive respiratory insufficiency several days or weeks after birth. On biopsy, there is a mild chronic interstitial inflammation with minimal-to-mild fibrosis, reactive type 2 pneumocytes, and some simplification of alveolar architecture. Possible etiologies are postinfectious changes, nutritional deficiencies, and circulatory imbalances such as edema.

Neuroendocrine Cell Hyperplasia of Infancy

This is a relatively recently described rare disorder of unknown etiology seen in infants and young children. It is characterized by significant tachypnea, hypoxia, and failure to thrive. Radiographs demonstrate hyperinflation, interstitial markings, and ground glass densities. Lung biopsies show minimal changes on routine H&E stain. By immunohistochemistry (bombesin and serotonin) significant increase in neuroendocrine cells is seen. All patients in the initial series improved and survived for a mean of 5 years (307).

Pulmonary Interstitial Glycogenosis

This entity was first described in 2002 (308) based on seven infants who presented with tachypnea, hypoxemia, and diffuse interstitial infiltrates with overinflated lungs on chest radiographs in the first month of life. Lung biopsies from all cases showed expansion of the interstitium by spindle-shaped and polygonal cells containing periodic acid–Schiff-positive, diastase-labile material consistent with glycogen (Figure 12-46A,B). Immunohistochemical staining showed these cells to be vimentin-positive but negative for leukocyte common antigen, lysozyme, and other macrophage markers. Electron microscopy revealed primitive interstitial mesenchymal cells with few cytoplasmic organelles and abundant monoparticulate glycogen. Minimal or no glycogen was seen in the alveolar lining cells. Since then a few more case reports have been reported. It appears that this is most likely a relatively benign disease with resolution of signs and symptoms over the course of a few months, with or without treatment (309).

LUNG TUMORS

Tumors of the lung, both benign and malignant, are decidedly unusual in the pediatric age group (310). In a review of the files of the Armed Forces Institute of Pathology (AFIP) over a 40-year period, 166 pulmonary tumors (including "pseudotumors") were noted in patients 21 years of age and younger (Table 12-9). The ratio of benign to malignant tumors in this series, 1:1.68, is similar to that appearing in the English literature, as described by Hartman and Schochat, who identified 230 examples of primary neoplasms, 79 benign and 151 malignant (311), whereas Hancock et al. (312) reported a ratio of 1:3.16 in a more recent literature review. However, metastatic tumors are much more common than primary lung tumors in children (313). Fever, cough, and pneumonitis are the most frequent presenting symptoms; respiratory distress

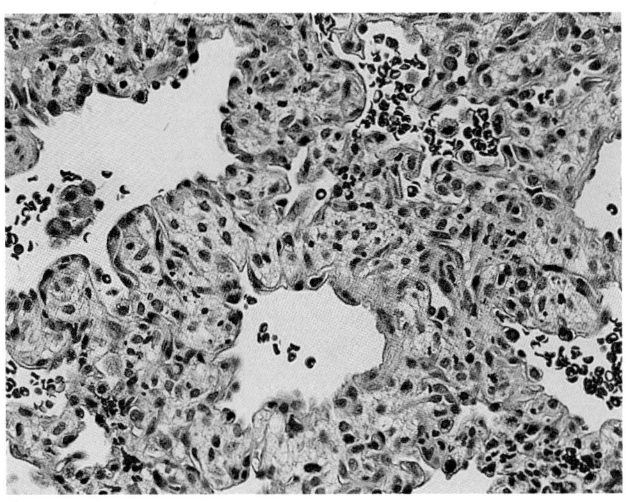
A

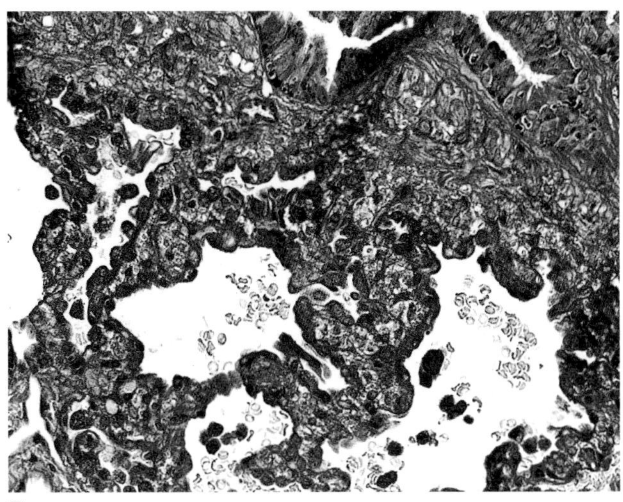
B

FIGURE 12-46 **A:** Pulmonary interstitial glycogenosis is illustrated in this lung biopsy from a young infant, showing widened alveolar septa. **B:** These cells contain glycogen. (**A:** H&E stain, ×200, **B:** PAS stain, ×200.)

Table 12-9 ■ PRIMARY PULMONARY TUMORS IN CHILDREN

Benign		**62 total**
Inflammatory pseudotumor	52	
Chondromatous hamartoma	3	
Granular cell myoblastoma	3	
Leiomyoma	2	
Bronchial chondroma	1	
Teratoma	1	
Malignant		**104 total**
Bronchial adenoma		46 subtotal
Carcinoid	35	
Mucoepidermoid	9	
Adenoid cystic	2	
Bronchogenic carcinoma		27 subtotal
Adenocarcinoma	14	
Squamous cell carcinoma	7	
Small-cell carcinoma	3	
Large-cell carcinoma	3	
Sarcoma		25 subtotal
Fibrosarcoma	8	
Rhabdomyosarcoma	7	
Leiomyosarcoma	6	
Undifferentiated	4	
Pulmonary blastoma	6	

Compiled from cases seen at the Armed Forces Institute of Pathology from 1950 to 1989 (166 cases).

and hemoptysis are more often seen with malignant tumors. About a quarter of children with benign neoplasms are asymptomatic. These earlier series were compiled before the advent of pleuropulmonary blastoma (PPB).

Benign Tumors

Inflammatory Pseudotumor/Inflammatory Myofibroblastic Tumor

Inflammatory pseudotumor of the lung (IPL) is by far the most common "benign tumor" of the lung in children, accounting for up to 84% of cases; these tumors are more common in older children, and only anecdotal in infancy (Table 12-10) (314). Unfortunately, the term "inflammatory pseudotumor" has been rather loosely used in older literature to encompass different lesions including organizing pneumonia, so-called pseudolymphoma and inflammatory myofibroblastic tumor (IMT). In the current literature, the term inflammatory pseudotumor is largely restricted to IMT and its variant, the so-called plasma cell granuloma (315).

Table 12-10 ■ INFLAMMATORY PSEUDOTUMOR IN CHILDREN (MYOFIBROBLASTIC TUMOR)

Age (years)	No. of Cases
<1	1
1–4	3
5–9	5
10–14	8
15–21	17

Male:female ratio, 15:19 (34 cases).
Compiled from cases seen at the Armed Forces Institute of Pathology.
Adapted from Stocker JT. Congenital and developmental diseases. In: Dail DH, Hammer SP, eds. *Pulmonary athology.* Heidelberg: Springer-Verlag, 1988:53, with permission.

Children with IPL present with fever (22%), cough (20%), chest pain (11%), hemoptysis (9%), or pneumonia (8%). Although IPL is thought by many to begin as a reactive process, a history of preceding pulmonary disease is noted in only 20% to 33% of cases, and about 30% of cases (70% in some series) are asymptomatic when discovered (314). The presence of clonal chromosomal aberrations also suggests that these lesions may be neoplastic proliferations (316), and IMT is considered to be of intermediate biologic potential neoplasm. Although the WHO classification of lung tumors (317) has defined IMT as being characterized by a molecular rearrangement on chromosome 2p23 involving the tyrosine kinase receptor anaplastic lymphoma kinase (ALK) (318), this genetic association is seen in less than 50% of all cases (319, 320). HHV-8 sequences with IL-6 overexpression have been described in pulmonary IMT/IPL (321), although this has not been substantiated by other authors (322). Arber et al. (323) have reported frequent presence of Epstein-Barr virus (EBV) in IPL. Pulmonary IMT may also represent metastasis from an extrapulmonary site (324,325). In a study of 59 IMTs, Coffin et al. (325) observed a mean age of 13.2 years, mean tumor size of 7.8 cm, and involvement of the lung in 22% of cases. Imaging studies usually show a single round, well-defined, peripheral mass with visible calcium deposits in 25% to 35% of cases (Figure 12-47A) (314). Grossly, the lesion is usually seen as a firm, circumscribed, 3- to 10-cm, grayish white mass, peripherally or centrally (Figure 12-47B), although they may also involve the major bronchi and trachea (326,327). Even peripheral lesions have been suggested to be closely related to airways, as peribronchial, submucosal, or endobronchial nodules (328).

Microscopically, the tumor infiltrates adjacent lung, even though it may appear grossly well defined. There are different histologic patterns, probably representing a morphologic continuum (329). The so-called plasma cell granuloma pattern comprises of a fasciitis-like spindle cell proliferation with a vascular stroma rich in lymphocytes, plasma cells, histiocytes, and mast cells (Figure 12-47C). Large lymphoid aggregates with or without germinal centers may be seen, along with multinucleated giant cells, xanthoma cells, and/or abscess formation. Some cases show a sclerosed hypocellular desmoid-like stroma, probably representing a burnt-out stage. In other cases, the spindle cell proliferation may mimic a sarcoma but retains a prominent inflammatory component; these cellular lesions may recur as inflammatory fibrosarcomas and have metastatic potential. Atypical histologic features included hypercellularity, a prominent fascicular architecture, a focal herringbone pattern, necrosis, abundant large ganglion-like cells, multinucleated or anaplastic giant cells, cellular and nuclear pleomorphism,

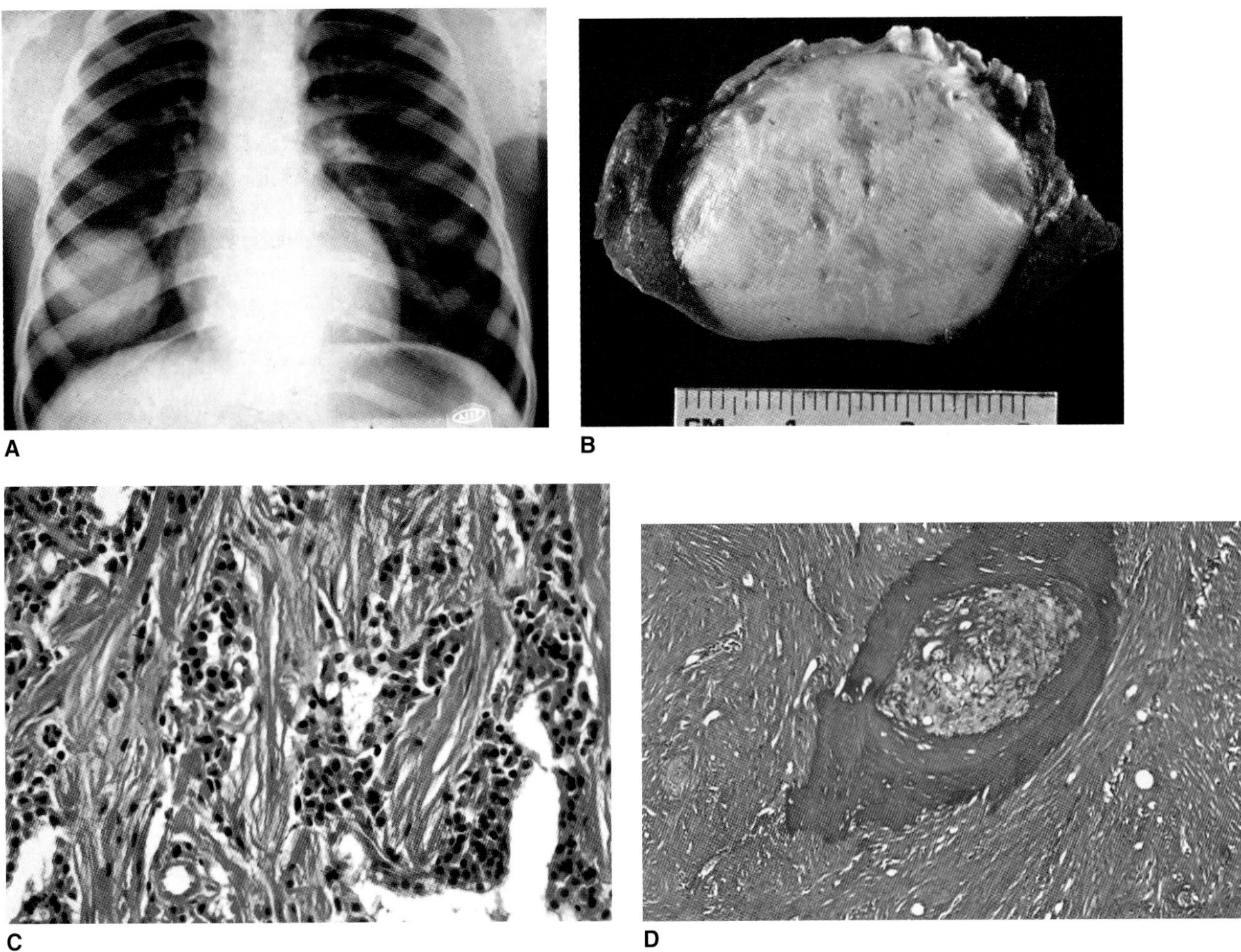

FIGURE 12-47 Inflammatory pseudotumor. **A:** A discrete round mass is present in the right lower lobe of this 4-year-old boy. **B:** A circumscribed nodule bulges from the cut surface of a resected section of lung. **C:** Interlacing fascicles of myofibroblasts are separated by an infiltrate of lymphocytes and plasma cells. (Masson trichrome stain, ×50.) **D:** A densely sclerotic area contains a focus of osteoid material. (H&E, ×75.)

atypical mitoses, a round or polygonal cell component, and necrosis (325). Areas of organizing pneumonia may be present at the margin of the lesion. Foci of calcification, osteoid metaplasia, and myxomatous changes may be present (Figure 12-47D). Immunohistochemistry for smooth muscle actin and/or desmin may be helpful in demonstrating the myofibroblastic nature of these cells. ALK positivity may or may not correlate with more aggressive histology and behavior (330,331). Electron microscopy indicates that the spindle cells are fibroblasts or myofibroblasts. Treatment of IPL is by excision of the mass. The lesion tends to grow slowly and is locally invasive and recurs in up to 24% of cases (332,333). Recurrence correlates with local invasion and is rare following complete excision but is more likely after simple enucleation (334). In Coffins series, three of 13 pulmonary IMTs metastasized. Metastasis was confined to ALK-negative lesions, although ALK reactivity was associated with local recurrence (325). Secondary nephrotic syndrome has been reported in association with pulmonary IMT (335). At present, there is no specific accepted adjuvant therapy for aggressive lesions.

Chondroma and Chondromatous Hamartoma

Although pulmonary chondroid hamartoma is the most common benign neoplasm of the lung in adulthood, they are rare in children (312). They occur as isolated lesions and show a pathognomonic stippled, "popcorn" calcification on chest radiographs, although this finding is present in less than 25% of cases. They are usually single and variable in size; a giant (18 cm) cystic chondroid hamartoma has been reported in an asymptomatic 11-year-old boy (336). When discovered in adolescent girls, they may be associated with the Carney triad (pulmonary chondroma, gastric epithelioid gastrointestinal stromal tumor, and functioning extra-adrenal paraganglioma) (337). In this situation, the lung tumors, which may be multiple, are soft to firm bosselated masses composed of a mixture of mature cartilage, bone, vascular adipose tissue, and stellate cells in a myxoid stroma (Figure 12-48). Chondroid matrix may also be seen in pulmonary epithelioid hemangioendothelioma (338) and pleomorphic adenoma (339); the latter tends to occur in association with large airways, whereas the former is more likely to be peripheral and pleural based.

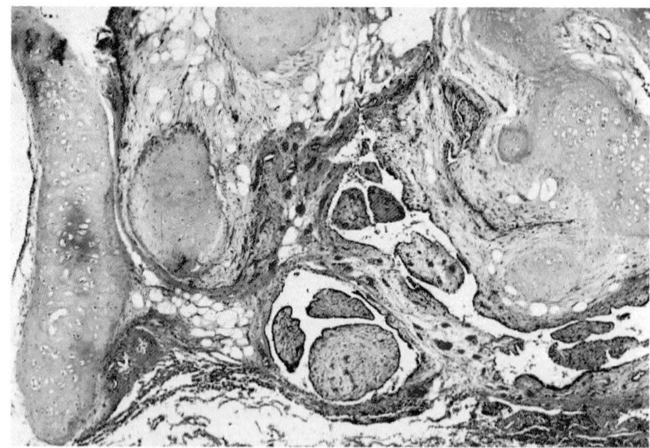

FIGURE 12-48 ■ Chondromatous hamartoma. Irregular lobules of cartilage are separated by vascular adipose tissue and fibrous connective tissue. (H&E, ×30.)

Juvenile Laryngotracheal Papillomatosis

Juvenile squamous papillomas are benign neoplasms that occur most commonly in the larynx but in 5% of patients extend into the trachea and, rarely, into the pulmonary parenchyma. The papillomas occur in 1,500 to 2,000 infants and children in the United States each year and are caused by a human papillomavirus (HPV) 6 and 11, which may be transmitted to the child from the mother during parturition (340,341). The papillary growths in the larynx produce hoarseness and inspiratory stridor, which may progress to acute respiratory distress. Treatment includes standard surgical resection, cryosurgery, and laser therapy (342,343). Within the larynx and trachea, the lesion grows as papillary or sessile structures along the mucosal surface (Figure 12-49A) and shows the morphology of a benign squamous papilloma with orderly stratified squamous epithelium covering a vascular connective tissue core or stalk (340). Koilocytes are seen as evidence of HPV infection. Recurrences are noted in many patients requiring multiple resections and even tracheostomy. However, spontaneous regression may occur in older children. With repeated manipulation (e.g., surgery, intubation) fragments of the papillomas may spread down the trachea into the bronchi and pulmonary parenchyma and produce solid and cavitary lesions composed of sheets of squamous epithelial cells (Figure 12-49B to D) (344). The incidence of lung involvement in recurrent papillomatosis has been estimated at 3.3% (345). Dissemination and subsequent growth of the benign squamous epithelium may be extensive enough to produce respiratory insufficiency and, rarely, death. Squamous cell carcinoma of the lung has been reported in patients with recurrent juvenile laryngotracheal papillomatosis (346,347), with a 16% incidence of cancer in cases with lung involvement (345). HPV 11 transforms in these cases of malignancy.

Other Benign Tumors

Leiomyomas of the lung are seen in children, but leiomyosarcomas are more frequent (348,349). In addition to cartilage-containing hamartomata of the lung, a wide variety of benign lesions composed of varying amounts of fibrous tissue, smooth muscle, adipose tissue, and vascular tissue are occasionally seen in children. Hull et al. (350) described multiple pulmonary fibroleiomyomatous hamartomata in a 9-year-old girl. EBV-associated smooth muscle tumors may occur in immunocompromised children (351).

Mesenchymal cystic hamartomas of the lung, first reported in 1986 (352), are rare tumors originating from nodules of primitive mesenchymal cells, that gradually increase in size and then become cystic. They may occur multifocally and should be distinguished from both pulmonary metastasis of endometrial stromal sarcoma and lymphangioleiomyomatosis (353). Complications include hemorrhage from systemic arteries within the cyst wall, PT, and hemothorax (354, 355). Mesenchymal cystic hamartoma is usually considered to carry a good prognosis. However, malignant transformation has been reported (356). These are suspected PPBs.

Benign vascular tumors of the lung in children are rare and include *lymphangiomatosis*, *lymphangiomyomatosis*, and *pulmonary capillary hemangiomatosis*. Diffuse pulmonary lymphangiomatosis is a rare disorder that presents as wheezing or dyspnea over a period of months. Patients are from 1 month to 35 years of age at presentation, with a mean age of 10 to 15 years. There is a male predominance (357). Chest images display bilateral interstitial infiltrates, which are often greatest in the lower lobes associated with smooth thickening of the interlobular septa and bronchovascular bundles (358). Microscopically, anastomosing endothelium-lined spaces are present beneath the pleura and along interlobular septa, accompanied by irregular collections of spindle cells containing hemosiderin and reactive for vimentin, desmin, actin, and progesterone receptor (357). The endothelial lining cells are positive for factor VIII and ulex europaeus. The disease is progressive, especially in younger children. Small pulmonary nodules, possibly representing early vascular malformations, may be seen in patients with hereditary hemorrhagic telangiectasia (359).

The so-called *sugar tumor* of the lung is a tumor of the perivascular epithelioid cells (PEComa) and presents as a circumscribed mass that is histologically composed of cells with clear cytoplasm rich in glycogen and immunoreactivity for HMB45 and Melan-A, but negative for cytokeratin (360). These tumors may reach large sizes, up to 12 cm (361). *Lymphangioleiomyomatosis*, a related lesion, has been reported in prepubertal girls in association with renal and hepatic angiomyolipomas with or without tuberous sclerosis (362).

Sclerosing hemangioma (although not a vascular tumor), seen most frequently in adult women (363), also occurs in the 15- to 21-year age group and is usually asymptomatic (364). The solitary, well-circumscribed peripheral lesion measures 0.4 to 8 cm in diameter and shows a constellation of microscopic findings with two cell types (surface and round cells) in a mixture of solid, hemorrhagic, papillary, and sclerotic patterns.. The distinct round cells have abundant, pale, eosinophilic cytoplasm. Immunohistochemically, both surface and round

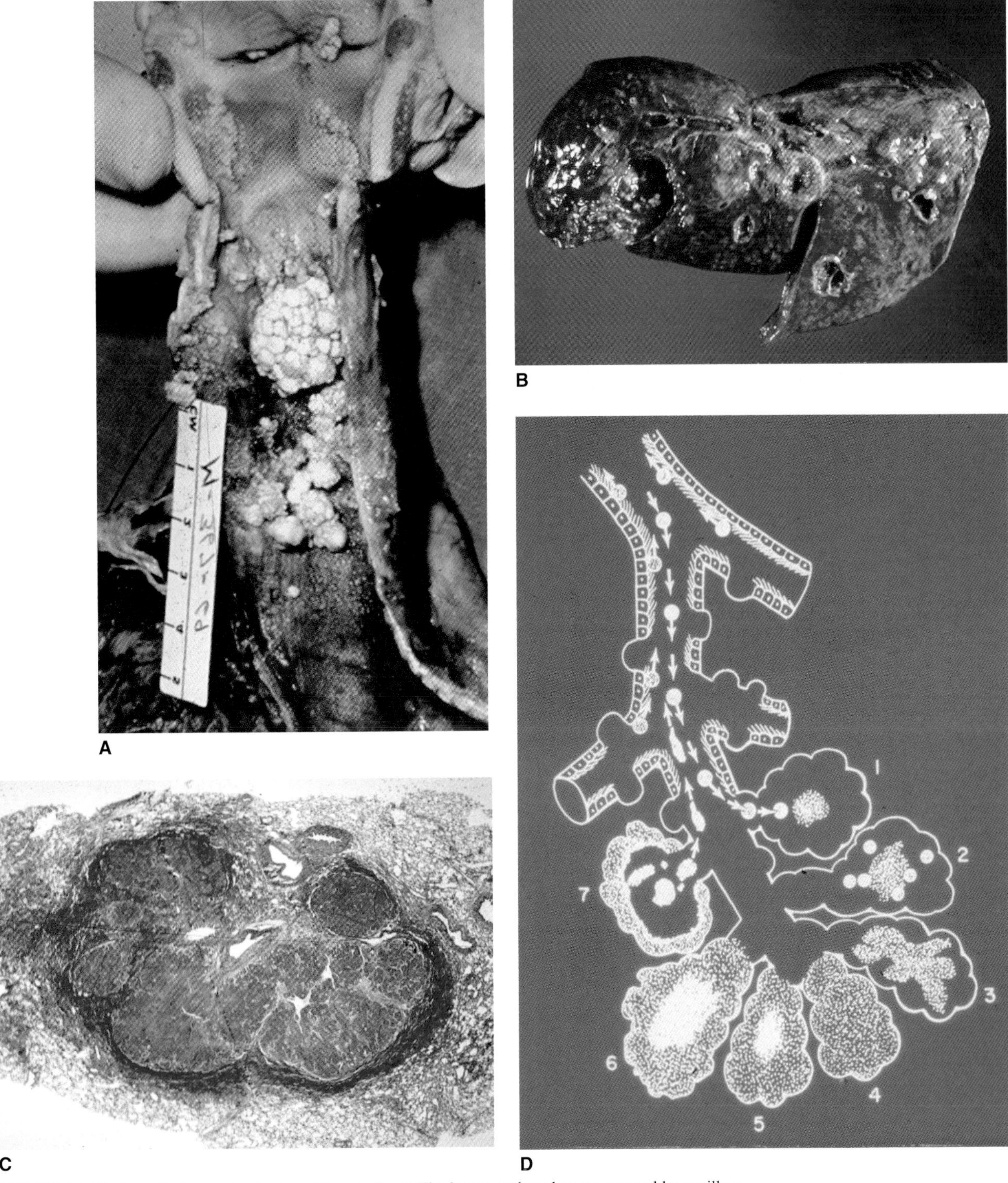

FIGURE 12-49■Juvenile laryngotracheal papillomatosis. **A:** The larynx and trachea are covered by papillary growths of firm, tan tissue. **B:** The lung contains cystic areas where fragments of tissue broken off from the trachea and larynx have settled into the distal airways. **C:** Fragments of squamous papillomas that disseminated to the lung have proliferated to fill alveoli (H&E, ×60). **D:** Fragments of papillomas from the larynx and trachea can move down the trachea to lodge in alveolar ducts and alveoli (*1, 2*), where they can proliferate and extend throughout adjacent acini (*3, 4*). Central cavitation of large lesions may take place (*5 to 7*) with further spread of the tissue fragments. (From Kramer SS, Wehunt WD, Stocker JT, Kashema H. Pulmonary manifestations of juvenile laryngotracheal papillomatosis. *AJR Am J Roentgenol* 1985;144:687, with permission.)

cells stain with epithelial membrane antigen (EMA) and thyroid transcription factor-1 (TTF-1), while the round cells are uniformly negative for pancytokeratin, surfactant proteins (A and B), and Clara cell antigens, suggesting that they are derived from primitive respiratory epithelium (365). Rare cases are reported to have regional lymph node metastases, which does not appear to affect the excellent prognosis.

Although tumors of neural origin are relatively common in the mediastinum, they are rarely seen in the bronchi or lung parenchyma. *Neurofibromas* and *neurilemomas*, however, have been reported and successfully treated with conservative resection (311). *Granular cell tumor* is a disproportionately frequent endobronchial tumor in children, considering its rarity in all sites (Figure 12-50A,B) (366). Multifocal intrapulmonary and hilar *infantile myofibromatosis* has been described in a neonate (367). The lung may be secondarily involved in thoracic fibromatosis. Similarly, teratomas are seen much more frequently in the mediastinum, and are exceedingly rare as primary lesions of the lung (368).

Malignant Tumors

The most common malignant tumors in the lung are metastatic lesions (313). Although the lungs are frequently involved in children dying from a variety of malignancies, in surgical pathology practice, the most frequently encountered resections are metastatic osteosarcoma (348,369,370). Other common childhood tumors that metastasize to the lung include Ewing sarcoma, rhabdomyosarcoma, Wilms tumor, hepatoblastoma, and germ cell tumors. It must be remembered, however, that in patients with multiple lung lesions, all lesions may not represent metastases and the possibility of a primary lung cancer following treatment of sarcoma must also be considered in the differential diagnosis (371).

The most common malignant primary pediatric pulmonary tumors are the so-called "bronchial adenomas," which include carcinoid, mucoepidermoid carcinoma, adenoid cystic carcinoma, and the benign mucous gland adenoma, in view of their intra-endobronchial nature. Carcinoids arise from bronchial neuroendocrine cells, whereas the other two tumors arise from bronchial minor salivary glands.

Carcinoid

Carcinoid is the single most common primary malignant tumor of the lung in children and adolescents, accounting for about 35% of all cases and nearly 50% of all malignant epithelial tumors. Presenting symptoms are cough (80%), pneumonitis (60%), and hemoptysis (33%). Although the condition is occasionally seen in younger children, more than 75% of pediatric carcinoids occur in patients older than 15 years of age (372). Carcinoid syndrome is rarely seen in children although Cushing syndrome has been reported (372,373). The tumors usually arise in a bronchus (Figure 12-51A) as a fleshy, smooth, polypoid mass covered by intact mucosa but may extend through the bronchial wall to invade the adjacent parenchyma. Peripheral carcinoids are rare in children.

Microscopically, the lesion presents a mosaic pattern of solid ducts, cords, nests, trabeculae, and ribbons of uniform cells with abundant clear or lightly eosinophilic cytoplasm and regular, centrally placed nuclei (Figure 12-51B). Numerous capillaries are present in the delicate fibrous septa separating the cells. Rarely, spindle cell or other atypical patterns may be seen. Argyrophilic granules may be demonstrated by Grimelius or Churukian Schenk stains, but the tumors are usually argentaffin-negative, consistent with their foregut derivation. Immunohistochemically, the tumors are positive for cytokeratin, synaptophysin, chromogranin, Leu-7 (CD56), and variably positive for a variety of other neuroendocrine products including bombesin, serotonin, vasoactive intestinal peptide, somatostatin, calcitonin, and/or adrenocorticotrophic hormone. Treatment of pulmonary carcinoid is by conservative resection with removal of involved lymph nodes. Prognosis is excellent (374), with about 90% survival.

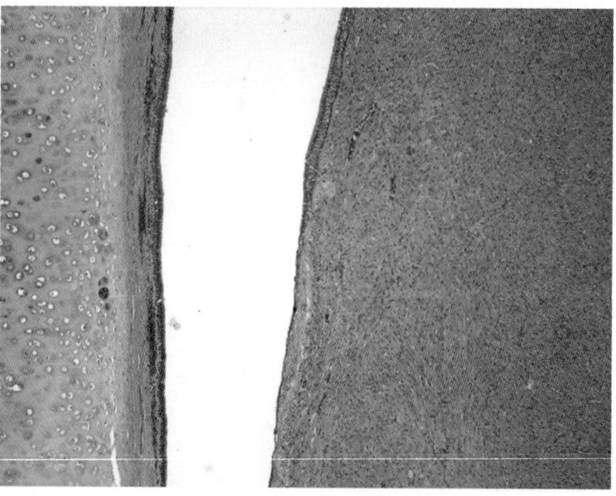
A

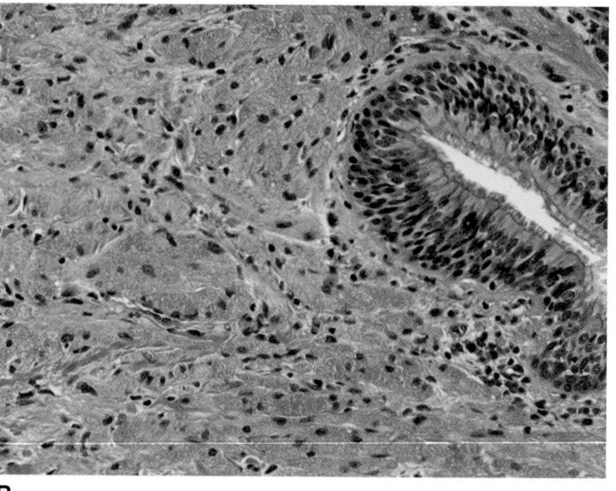
B

FIGURE 12-50 Granular cell tumor. **A:** A densely cellular tumor nodule abuts a bronchus (H&E, ×100). **B:** The tumor nodule is composed of large uniform cells with abundant granular cytoplasm. (H&E, ×200.)

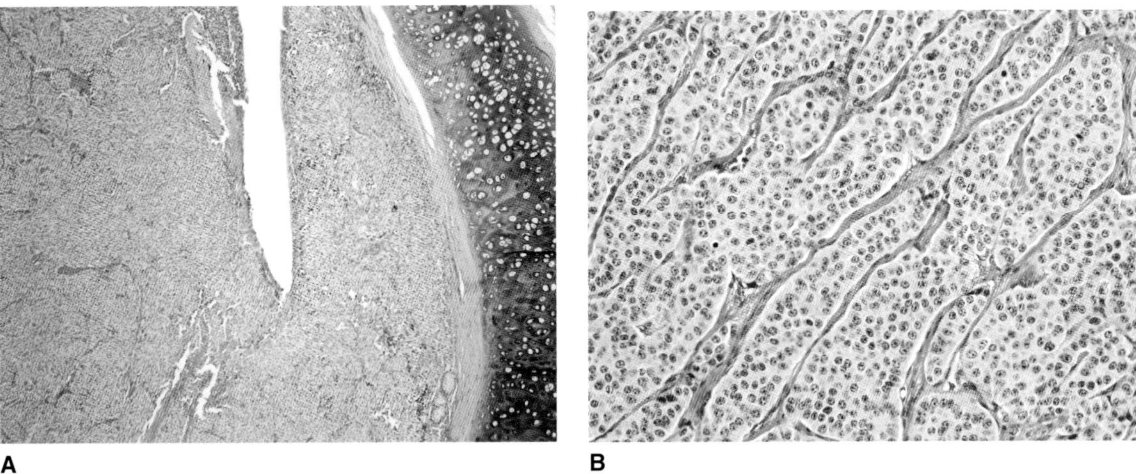

FIGURE 12-51 Bronchial carcinoid. **A:** A bronchus is occluded by a densely cellular tumor mass. (H&E, ×100.) **B:** Uniform cells with round nuclei and finely granular cytoplasm are separated into discrete bundles by delicate vascular septa. (H&E, ×200.)

However, long-term follow-up is mandated since metastases occur in 10% to 25% of cases (366).

Mucoepidermoid Carcinoma

Mucoepidermoid carcinoma accounts for up to 20% of bronchial adenomas and, like carcinoids, presents with cough, fever, hemoptysis, recurrent pneumonia, or a combination of these symptoms (366). The lesion usually occurs in a main bronchus as an obstructing, soft, polypoid mass. Microscopically, the tumor presents a solid and cystic appearance with an admixture of mucus-secreting, intermediate, and epidermoid cells arranged in sheets and glands (Figure 12-52), and may be associated with a dense lymphoplasmacytic infiltrate (375). Tumors with higher proportions of squamoid cells tend to be of higher grade and higher stage, and have worse outcomes (376). Translocation *t*(11;19) has been reported to be the primary chromosomal aberration for pulmonary MEC in children, and the MECT1-MAML2 fusion transcript may be associated with better prognosis in these tumors (377). Prognosis is favorable after conservative resection (374), although lymph node metastases may rarely be present.

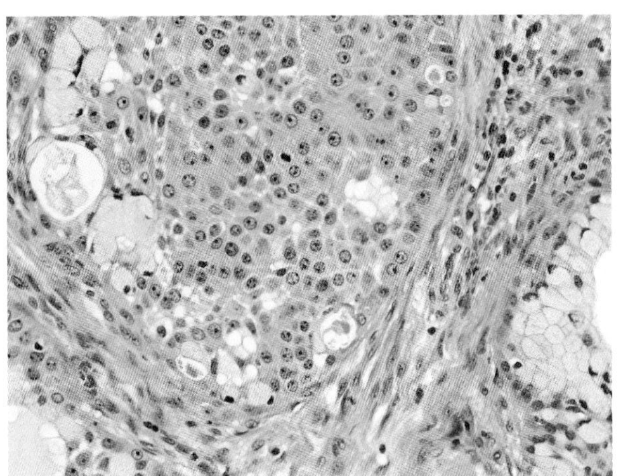

FIGURE 12-52 Bronchial mucoepidermoid carcinoma. Epidermoid and intermediate cells are admixed with mucinous cells in the same tumor cluster (H&E, ×200.)

Adenoid Cystic Carcinoma

Adenoid cystic carcinoma accounts for less than 5% of bronchial adenomas in children, and presents in a manner similar to other bronchial adenomas. The tumor resembles that seen in the salivary gland with groups of cells arranged in cords or nests. Accumulation of mucin or hyaline material within the clusters imparts a characteristic cribriform pattern. Treatment is by resection, and although metastases may occur, prognosis is relatively favorable (311).

Other salivary-gland type malignancies are rare in children, with only anecdotal reports of acinic cell carcinoma of the bronchus (378,379) and epithelial-myoepithelial carcinoma (380).

Bronchogenic Carcinoma

Bronchogenic carcinoma accounts for up to 25% of primary malignant tumors of the lung and was the second most common primary malignant pediatric pulmonary neoplasm until PPB. The majority of lesions are adenocarcinomas or undifferentiated carcinomas (311,312). Patients present with cough, pneumonitis, and chest pain but may be asymptomatic if the tumor is peripheral. Over 60% of children and adolescents with primary lung carcinoma experience a delay in diagnosis, leading to an advanced stage at diagnosis and poor outcome. However, patients with localized resectable disease have a more favorable prognosis (312,381,382). Over 60% of children and adolescents with primary lung carcinoma experience a delay in diagnosis, with advanced stage at diagnosis and poor outcomes. However, patients with localized resectable disease have favorable prognosis (312,381,382).

Adenocarcinomas in children may be primary or may occur as a second malignancy following treatment for Hodgkin lymphoma, Ewing sarcoma, and testicular germ cell tumor (383,384). Adenocarcinoma may also arise in a setting of type 1 CPAM and is thought to derive from the mucogenic cells seen in this entity (194,200). Parenthetically, mucinous areas in type 1 CPAM are reported to lack EGFR expression, whereas adjacent epithelial cystic linings are strongly positive, suggesting that EGFR may play an important role in the pathogenesis of CPAM but not in the associated malignant transformation (198). *Bronchioloalveolar carcinoma* has also been reported in a child with hepatoblastoma (385). Radiographically, the mass is usually localized to the midlung or peripheral lung fields. Grossly, the tumor is a moderately firm mucoid mass, which may display central necrosis. Microscopically, the tumor presents a characteristic lepidic growth pattern with columnar cells extending along alveolar walls, with little apparent destruction of the walls (Figure12-53A,B). Mucinous cells may line alveoli, replacing normal alveolar lining cells and filling the lumen with mucin, which may extend into and fill adjacent normal alveoli. Aerogenic spread (with resultant secondary lesions) may occur to other lobes of both lungs. Treatment is by resection, and prognosis is favorable if resection is complete and no metastatic disease is present at the time of diagnosis (386). Invasion of alveolar septa, pleura, or vascular spaces precludes a diagnosis of bronchioloalveolar carcinoma and should be considered as an invasive adenocarcinoma even in the presence of a predominant bronchioloalveolar component (384). Pulmonary adenocarcinoma has also been reported in a child with prior tuberculosis (387).

Squamous cell carcinoma has been reported in children from 2 to 21 years of age with a nearly equal male-female incidence (348,388). Presenting symptoms include cough, hemoptysis, chest pain, or indication of extrapulmonary metastatic disease (Figure 12-54A). Radiographically, the lesion may be central or peripheral, occasionally involving an entire lobe or lung. Microscopically, sheets of cells range from small to large undifferentiated cells to keratinizing squamous epithelial cells (Figure 12-54B). Areas of necrosis may be extensive. Squamous cell carcinoma must be differentiated from disseminated laryngeal papillomatosis, which may "seed" squamous cells throughout the lobes, which then grow into nodules. Malignant transformation of papillomatosis has been reported in children (347). Squamous cell carcinomas of the lung may also arise in a setting of bronchogenic cyst or teratoma. Treatment of squamous cell carcinoma is by resection, chemotherapy, and radiation; prognosis is poor (348).

Pulmonary blastoma, as first described (and named embryoma of lung) by Barnard in 1952 and subsequently redefined by Spencer in 1961, is a primary lung tumor consisting of a mixture of immature, embryonic-like mesenchymal and epithelial components (389). These tumors are typically seen in adults, are usually solid, and morphologically show either a well-differentiated fetal adenocarcinoma pattern or a biphasic

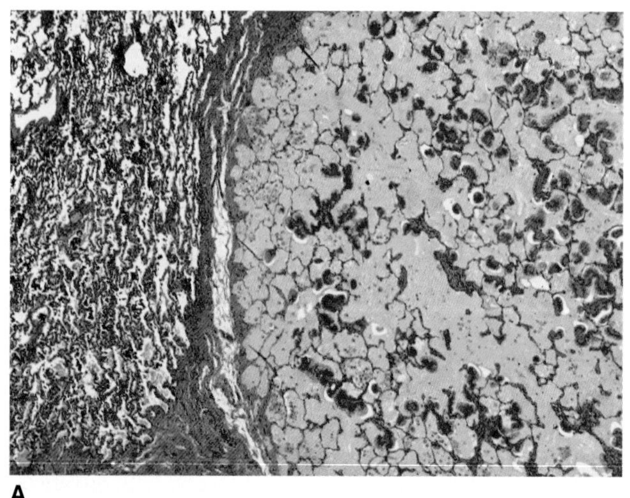

A

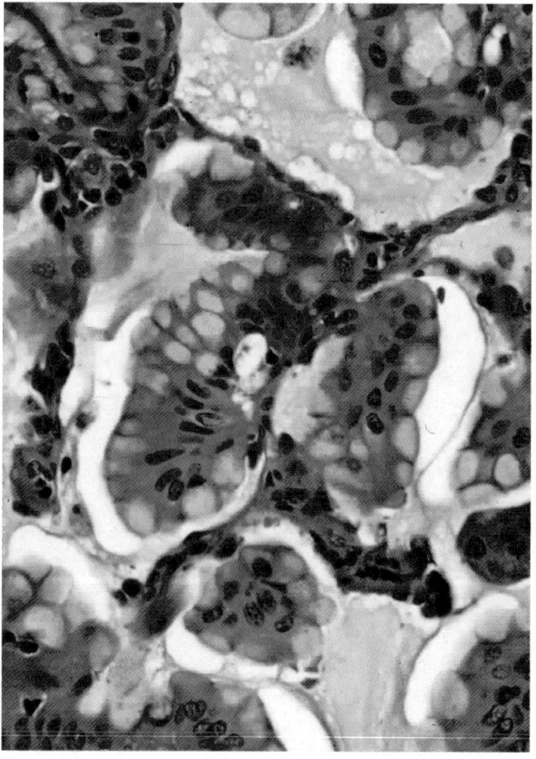

B

FIGURE 12-53 ■ Bronchioloalveolar carcinoma. **A:** A large, peripherally placed tumor nodule is composed of dilated alveoli filled with mucin and clusters of tumor cells. (H&E, ×30.) **B:** Alveolar septa are lined by papillary growths of columnar epithelial cells with irregular basal nuclei and apical mucin. Note the mucin lying free in the alveoli. (H&E, ×300.)

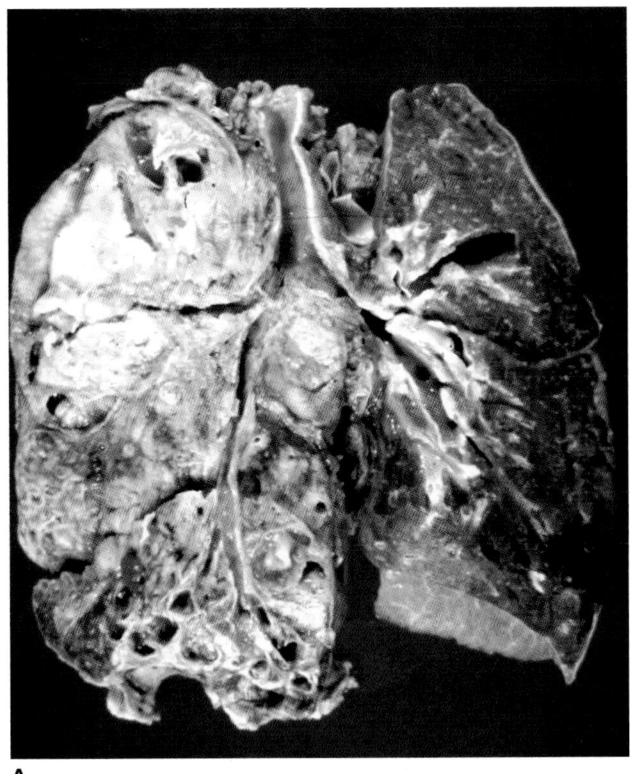

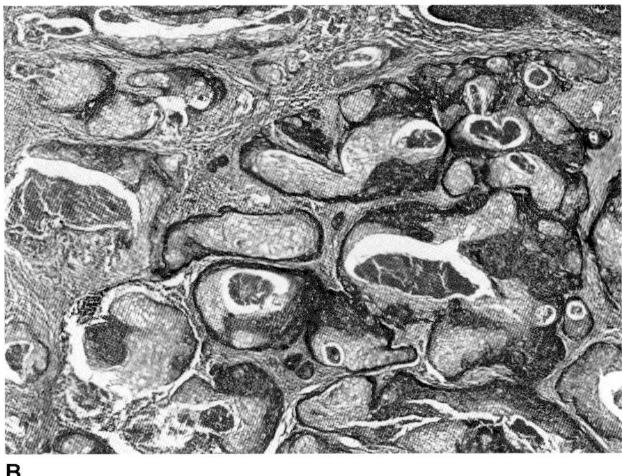

A B

FIGURE 12-54 ■ Squamous cell carcinoma. **A:** The entire right lung of this 10-year-old boy is infiltrated by dense tan-white tumor. **B:** Clusters of well-differentiated stratified squamous epithelial cells invade the parenchyma. (H&E, ×30.)

epithelial and mesenchymal pattern. Although, the older literature describes similar tumors in children (usually over 10 years of age), most tumors diagnosed as pulmonary blastomas in children are now classified as PPBs (see below) in view of their variable anatomic location, primitive embryonic-like blastema and stroma, absence of a carcinomatous component, and potential for sarcomatous differentiation (390).

Sarcomas

Sarcomas of the lung account for a small but significant number of primary malignant tumors, and include malignant fibrous histiocytoma, monophasic and biphasic synovial sarcoma, malignant peripheral nerve sheath tumor, leiomyosarcoma, angiosarcoma, pulmonary vascular intimal sarcoma, fibrosarcoma, and epithelial hemangioendothelioma (349).

Malignant fibrous histiocytoma accounted for seven (27%) of 26 primary pulmonary sarcomas in children in Keel's series (349). All but one of the cases were of the storiform-pleomorphic subtype with spindle-shaped cells arranged in fascicles that intersected in a cartwheel-like fashion. Mitoses ranged from 6 to 10 per 10 high-power fields, with some atypical forms. Areas of necrosis were consistently seen, occasionally comprising up to 90% of the mass. Treatment consisted of resection (and chemotherapy in one case) and, of six with follow-up, all were alive at 8 to 94 months, although one continued to have demonstrable disease at 53 months.

Primary pulmonary synovial sarcomas may be either monophasic or biphasic, and may be confused with fibrosarcoma and other lesions. Monophasic synovial sarcomas are composed of hypercellular fascicles of spindle cells that intersect randomly or are arranged in a herringbone pattern separated by collagen bundles. Diagnosis often requires confirmation by electron microscopy (cells with cytoplasmic projections and intercellular spaces that contain amorphous extracellular matrix) or immunohistochemistry (positive for keratins, EMA, CD99, BCL2, and CD34) (391). The presence of the *t*(X;18) translocation is confirmatory. Compared with soft-tissue synovial sarcoma, primary pulmonary and mediastinal synovial sarcoma has less calcification, less obvious mast cell influx, less radiologic vascularity but similar magnetic resonance imaging features, percentage of poorly differentiated tumors, and number of *t*(X;18)-positive tumors (391). Survival with resection is relatively good, although late metastases may occur.

Malignant peripheral nerve sheath tumors are uncommon in children and almost 50% of the cases occur in patients with neurofibromatosis 1 (392). These tumors are composed of spindle cells with wavy hyperchromatic nuclei arranged randomly, in fascicles or in a storiform pattern. Areas representing more conventional neurofibroma may be seen at the periphery. Immunostains may not be helpful in diagnosis; electron microscopy shows prominent basal lamina. Despite resection and chemotherapy, death usually occurs in 6 to 20 months (349) (see Chapter 24).

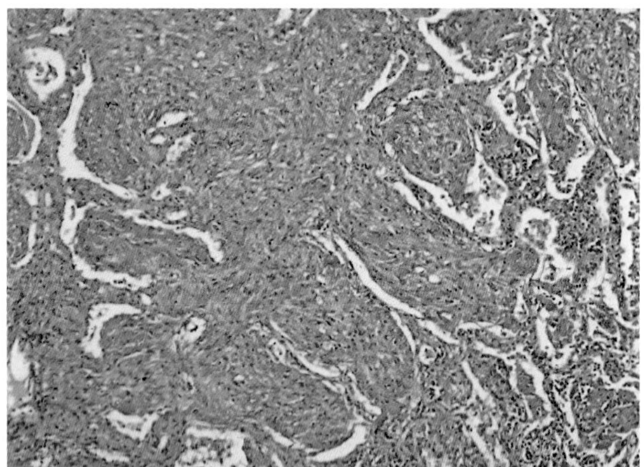

FIGURE 12-55 ■ Leiomyosarcoma. Interlacing bundles of fusiform cells extend along alveolar septa. (H&E, ×75.)

Leiomyosarcoma occurs primarily in young children (5 to 10 years of age) but may also be seen in the newborn period. Infants may present with respiratory distress, whereas older children display cough, anorexia, weight loss, hemoptysis, pneumonia, or a combination of symptoms. The lesion may develop in a bronchus or in the pulmonary parenchyma, frequently attaining a size of 7 cm or greater (393). Tumors arising in immunosuppressed individuals (394), may be related to EBV infection (313,351). Microscopically, the firm, gray-yellow mass is composed of interlacing bundles of fusiform cells with oval vesicular nuclei, scanty cytoplasm, and ill-defined cellular borders (Figure 12-55). Collagen is abundant, and actin-like filaments with focal condensations (i.e., dense bodies) can be seen by electron microscopy (349). With total resection, prognosis is very good.

Primary pulmonary fibrosarcoma is a very low-grade malignancy seen in newborns presenting with respiratory distress or in older children presenting with cough, fever, and chest pain (395). The lesions may be endobronchial or parenchymal and vary in size from 1.0 to 7.5 cm. The firm gray, yellow, or white lesions may display areas of hemorrhage or cyst formation. Microscopically, the tumors are highly cellular with sheets and interlacing bundles of densely packed spindle cells arranged in a herringbone-like pattern (Figure 12-56A,B). Mitotic activity is lower in endobronchial lesions (0 to 3/10 hpf) than in parenchymal lesions (8 to 12/10 hpf). The tumor cells display strong, diffuse cytoplasmic staining for vimentin but are nonreactive for muscle-specific actin, desmin, Ulex europaeus, NSE, S-100 protein, Leu-7, EMA, or factor VIII–related antigen. Prognosis with complete resection is excellent (395). Those in infants may represent congenital peribronchial myofibroblastic tumor.

In a study of six HIV-positive children (aged 18 months to 10 years) with pulmonary Kaposi sarcoma, Theron et al. (396) found predominantly perihilar and lower lobe involvement, and reported that pleural effusion, air space involvement, and lymphadenopathy (mediastinal and axillary) were much more common in children than in adults with pulmonary Kaposi sarcoma.

Primary intrathoracic rhabdomyosarcoma occurs rarely as mediastinal, pleural, pulmonary, or endobronchial solid tumors with typical embryonal or alveolar patterns (397). More frequently, rhabdomyosarcoma-like foci are noted in association with PPB (see below).

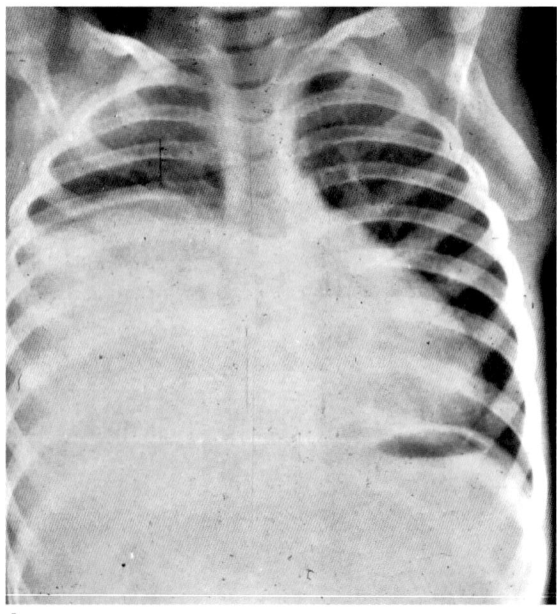

A

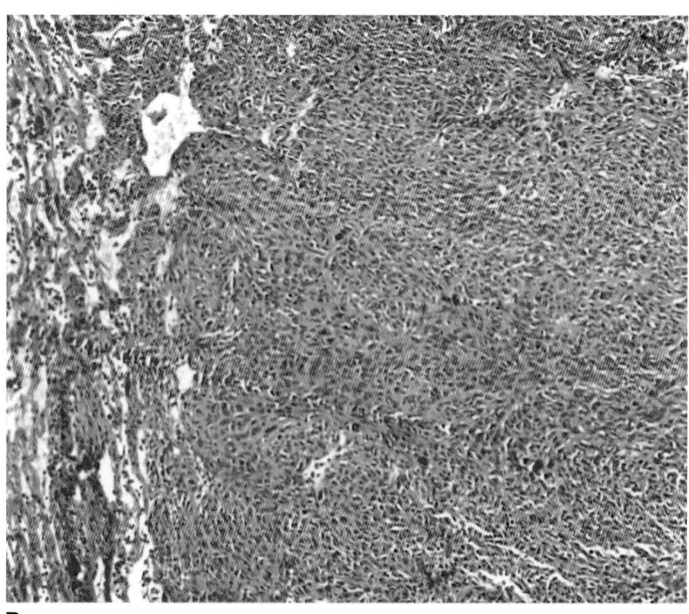

B

FIGURE 12-56 ■ Fibrosarcoma. **A:** The entire lower right hemithorax is filled with a homogenous mass. **B:** The tumor infiltrating the normal lung (**at left**) is composed of individual spindle cells in a somewhat woven pattern. (H&E, ×30.)

Pleuropulmonary Blastoma

PPB is a rare distinct embryonic primary pulmonary tumor in children, with over 220 confirmed cases in the International PPB registry (www.ppbregistry.org). There is an equal gender incidence, and the vast majority (94%) present in the first 6 years of life (398), although cases have been reported in older children and even in adulthood (399). Presenting symptoms include respiratory distress, nonproductive cough, fever, chest pain, or a combination of symptoms of days to weeks duration (398). The lesion is considered to be part of a hereditary tumor predisposition syndrome, and there is often a positive family history of childhood neoplasms, including PPBs in siblings, cousins, and other close relatives. Other associations in PPB patients include familial cystic nephroma and other renal tumors, medulloblastoma, ovarian tumors (germ cell tumor and sex cord stromal tumor), seminoma, Hodgkin lymphoma, leukemia, thyroid neoplasia, and intestinal polyps (400–406). Imaging studies may show a solid and/or cystic lesion that may be intrapulmonary, pleural based, or mediastinal; a cystic component is more prominent in younger children consistent with the supposed progression of lesions with increasing age. Tumors are classified as type I (cystic, 14% of cases, median age 9 months), type II (cystic and solid, 48% of cases, median age 36 months), and type III (solid, 38% of cases, median age 42 months (398,407). The multilobated masses measure 8 to 23 cm in diameter and weigh up to 1,100 g.

Type I PPB (Figure 57A to D) occurs as a delicate multilocular cyst with variable numbers of primitive mesenchymal cells beneath a benign respiratory (bronchial or alveolar) epithelium, with the presence of rhabdomyoblasts (49% of cases) and cartilage nodules (40% of cases) (407). Rhabdomyoblasts may be seen as a subepithelial cambium layer (403). Tumors in patients less than 2 months of age are more uniform in composition and cellularity compared with those in older groups, and have a subtle transition between normal developing lung and tumor, showing bland interstitial mesenchymal cells uniformly expanding the alveolar septa. Presumed regressive changes including cyst wall necrosis are common, and may explain the variable and sometimes sparse tumor cellularity seen in some type I PPBs. Factors that control the balance between progression and regression may be important in predicting tumor behavior and determining which patients will benefit from adjuvant chemotherapy (407). The solid areas of type II (Figure 12-58A to C) and III PPB (Figure 12-59A to D) consist of blastomatous islands of loose mesenchyme blending into fibrosarcoma-like foci; nodules of benign-appearing to overtly malignant cartilage; rhabdomyosarcomatous component; and areas of large, bizarre, pleomorphic, multinucleated mesenchymal cells (408). Immunohistochemical staining is variable from one tissue type to another (390,409). Cytogenetic analyses have revealed complex abnormalities with gain in chromosome 8q being the most frequent single abnormality (410). PPB families harbor heterozygous germ-line mutations in DICER1, a gene encoding an endoribonuclease critical to the generation of small noncoding regulatory RNAs; loss of DICER1 in the epithelium of the developing lung may alter the regulation of diffusible factors that promote mesenchymal proliferation and sarcomatous transformation (411).

Local recurrence may developed in fewer than 15% of type I PPBs but is seen in over 45% of type II and III PPBs. Metastatic disease occurs in about 25% of patients (all with type II or III PPB), chiefly in the brain, spinal cord, or bone. Cerebral metastasis is more frequent in PPB than in other childhood sarcomas (412). The 5-year survival rate in a series of 50 cases reported by Priest et al. (398) was 83% for type I and 42% for types II and III. Gender, side, tumor size, preexisting lung cysts, and extent of surgical resection at diagnosis do not impact prognosis, whereas incomplete resection and extrapulmonary involvement at diagnosis result in a significantly worse prognosis (413). As a final note, it is necessary to rule out type I PPB before a diagnosis of CPAM IV is made.

Miscellaneous Tumors of Pleura and Thorax

Calcifying fibrous pseudotumor is a rare benign tumor of the pleura, characterized by a dense hyalinized collagenous tissue interspersed with benign spindle cells, lymphoplasmacytic infiltrate, and, particularly, psammomatous and/or dystrophic calcifications (414,415). *Mesenchymal hamartoma of the chest wall* usually arises from the posterior or lateral portions of the rib and usually involves many ribs. Chest wall mesenchymal hamartoma associated with a massive fetal pleural effusion has been detected antenatally by ultrasound (416). Multifocal bilateral mesenchymal hamartomas of the chest wall have been reported in a neonate (417) (see Chapter 27). *Pleuropulmonary desmoid* tumor is rare, shows nuclear positivity for β-catenin, and may resemble solitary fibrous tumors. However, unlike the latter, desmoids are negative for CD34 (418).

Malignant small cell tumor of thoracopulmonary region (Askin tumor) is a tumor with a neural phenotype and is presently included in the Ewing sarcoma family (see Chapter 24). *Malignant mesothelioma* of the pleura is seen in children as young as 5 years of age and accounts for about 10% of childhood mesotheliomas (419).

Miscellaneous Other Disorders of Lung

Sarcoidosis

Sarcoidosis is a chronic multisystem disorder characterized by the formation of noncaseating granulomata (420). Although the condition is uncommon in children, when mass screening is performed, the incidence of the disease approaches that of adults with similar demographics. The peak occurrence of the disease is between 20 and 40 years of age, but in children, most cases occur between 9 and 15 years of age, with a separate cluster seen in children younger than 4 years of age in whom a distinct clinical triad of rash, uveitis, and arthritis is seen (421–423). It is occasionally seen in children as young as 2 months of age. Childhood sarcoidosis is seen with near-equal frequency in boys and

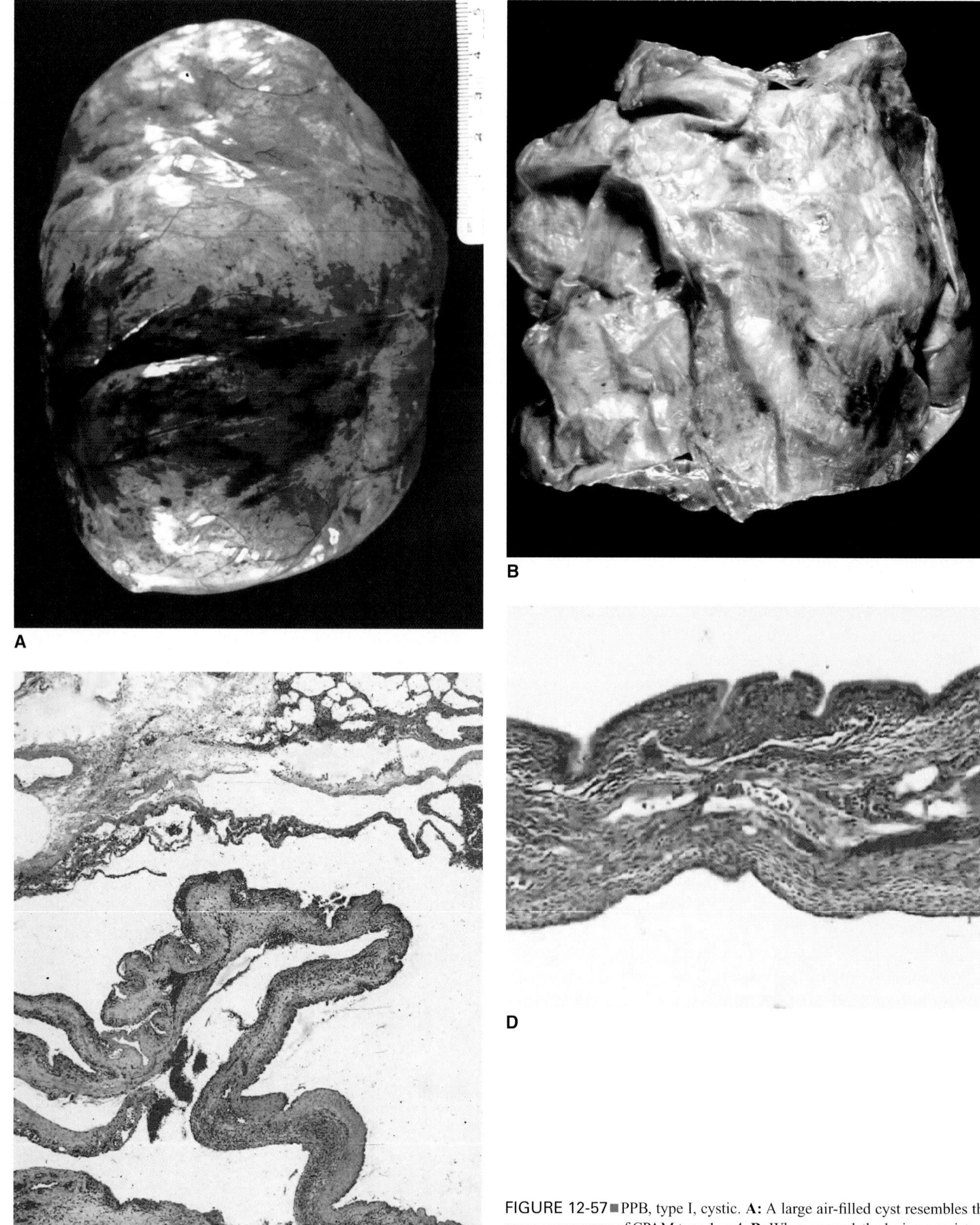

FIGURE 12-57 ■ PPB, type I, cystic. **A:** A large air-filled cyst resembles the gross appearance of CPAM type 1 or 4. **B:** When opened, the lesion consists of a large, very thin-walled cystic with a small area of hemorrhage. **C:** The cyst walls are lined by interrupted lines of cuboidal/columnar epithelial cells that overlie a fibromuscular stroma that displays/contains vessels of varying sizes. (H&E, ×40) **D:** The cells beneath the epithelium form a dense cambium layer of a rhabdomyosarcoma, displaying staining characteristics of rhabdomyoblasts. (H&E, ×80.)

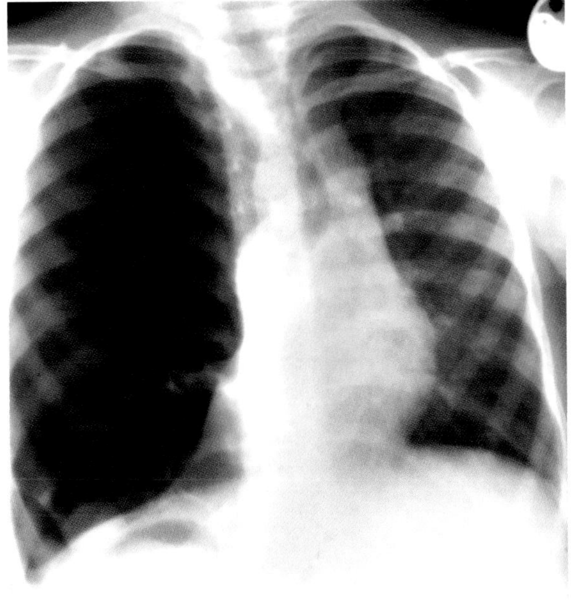

A

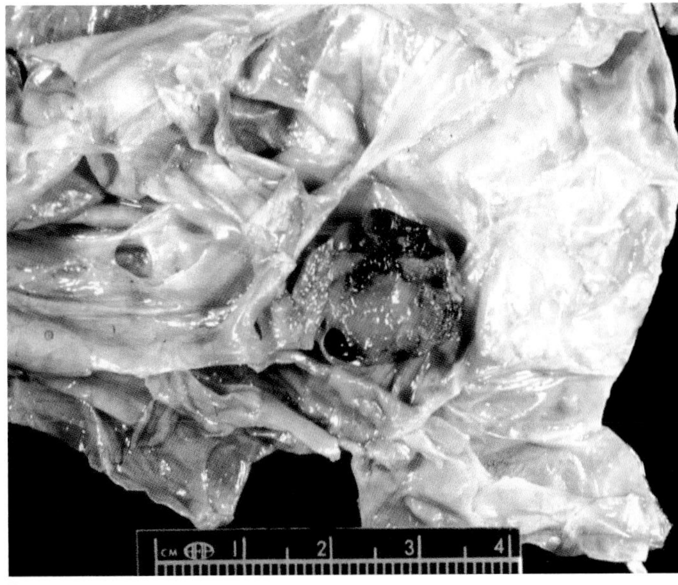

B

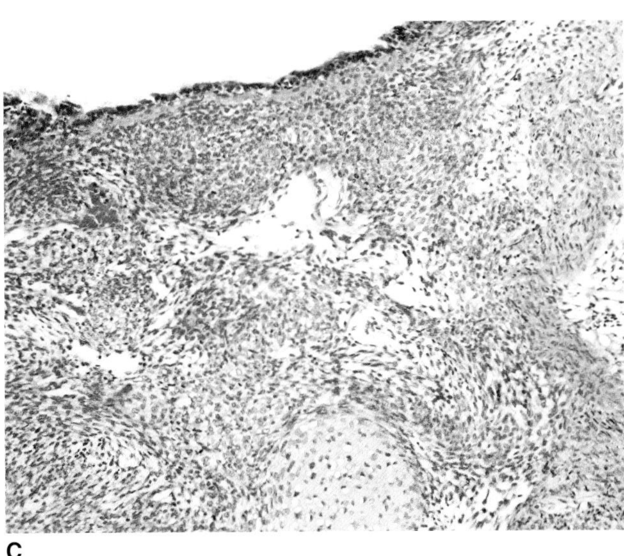

C

FIGURE 12-58 PPB, type II, cystic/solid. **A:** A large cystic lesion occupies the entire right hemithorax. Note the opacity just above the right leaflet of the diaphragm. **B:** The opened resected specimen is composed of multiple cysts and a small, irregular partially solid nodule. **C:** The nodule is covered by cuboidal epithelium and is composed of rhabdomyosarcoma, chondrosarcoma and other areas of undifferentiated sarcoma. (H&E, ×20.)

girls and is significantly more common in blacks (55% to 80% of cases) and American Indians (5%) (424,425).

Although the condition is asymptomatic in 5% to 16% of cases, older children frequently present with cough, dyspnea, weight loss, lethargy, adenopathy, and headache. At presentation, 50% of children have characteristic functional changes of restrictive lung disease. Nearly all patients, on radiographic observation, have bilateral hilar lymphadenopathy, which is frequently associated with bilateral paratracheal adenopathy (Figure 12-60A). Pulmonary parenchymal involvement is noted radiographically in about 50% of cases, but extrapulmonary lesions (e.g., skeletal, CNS, skin, GI) are seen in 10% to 15% of cases, a number more frequent than in adults (426,427). Sarcoidosis may be confused with tuberculosis in its early stages (428).

Clinically, lymphadenopathy is the most common sign, with firm, movable, nontender nodes palpable in over 60% of cases. Skin and eye changes are also noted in 40% to 50% of patients, and hepatosplenomegaly is found in about 35%. Findings noted in less than 20% of patients include fever, pulmonary signs (e.g., rales, rhonchi), joint effusions, muscle masses, meningitis, and seizures.

Laboratory findings are nonspecific but include hypercalcemia, hypercalciuria, high serum immunoglobulins, leukopenia, eosinophilia, and proteinuria. Angiotensin-converting enzyme elevation is noted in approximately 50% of childhood cases, and although not specific for sarcoidosis, its presence does correlate with disease activity (420,429). Bronchoalveolar lavage displays a threefold to fivefold increase in the number of

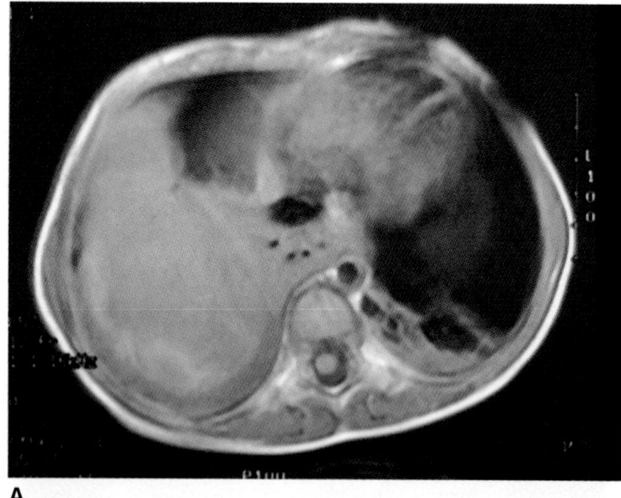
A

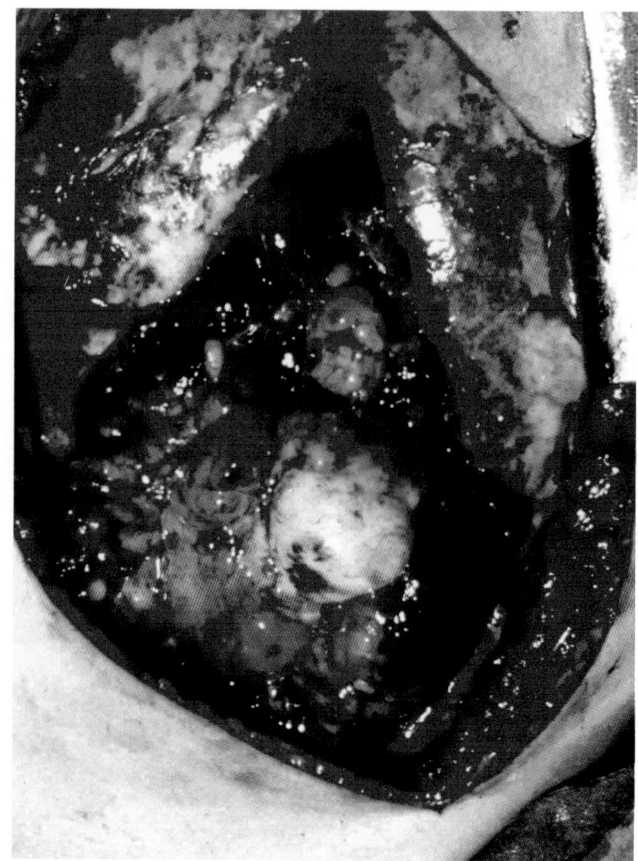
B

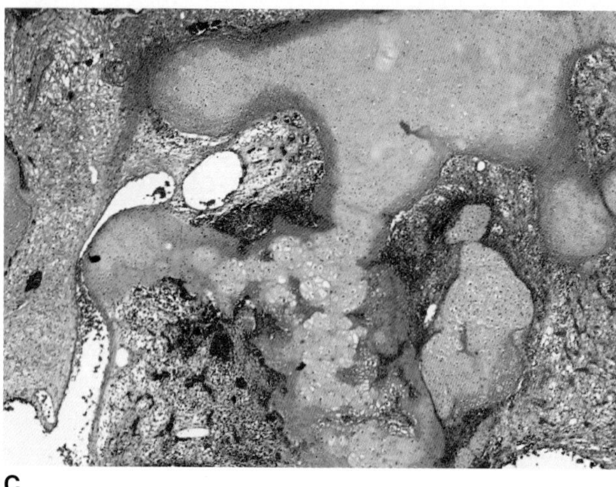
C

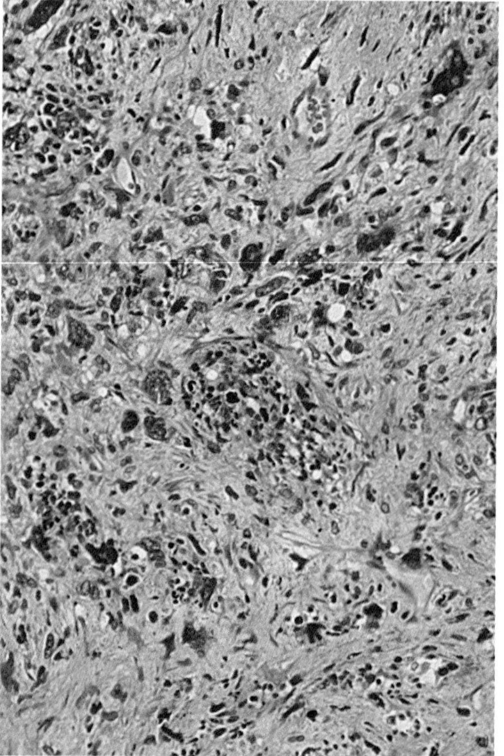
D

FIGURE 12-59 PPB, type III, solid. **A:** A large mass fills the anterior portion of the right hemithorax of a one-year-old boy. **B:** A multilobulated mass of hemorrhagic and focally necrotic tissue is seen *in situ* attached to the pleura. (Courtesy of Louis P. Dehner, M.D., St. Louis Children's Hospital, St. Louis, Missouri.) **C:** Immature cartilage blends with blastemal and mesenchymal components. (H&E, ×75.) **D:** Clusters of anaplastic blastemal cells displaying marked mitotic activity are separated by fibrovascular septa. (H&E, ×150.)

lymphocytes, disproportionately represented by helper T-cells and causing the helper-suppressor ratio to be as high as 10:1 (normally <1:1.8) (430). Bronchoalveolar lavage cytokine expression patterns may be helpful in evaluating disease activity and planning treatment (431).

Although it is observed in less than 25% of children younger than 4 years of age, pulmonary involvement is a consistent finding in older children. It begins as alveolitis consisting of inflammatory cells and immune effector cells in the interstitium and alveolar areas of the lung. As the alveolitis progresses, epithelioid cells develop, and the typical noncaseating granuloma is formed. Necrotizing granulomas may rarely be seen. The more typical noncaseating granulomas are sharply circumscribed and composed of a focal collection of radially arranged epithelioid cells and multinucleated giant cells surrounded by a rim of lymphocytes (Figure 12-60B,C). The large epithelioid cells have pale, eosinophilic cytoplasm with round or oval nuclei. The giant cells, 150 to 300 g in diameter, are of the Langhans cellular type formed from the coalescence of epithelioid cells. These cells may contain large, nonspecific, concentrically laminated, basophilic inclusion bodies (Schaumann bodies) or small star-shaped inclusion bodies with a central core of multiple radiating curved spines (asteroid bodies) (432). The granulomata contain fibroblasts and varying amounts of amorphous hyaline or reticular material, which increases with the age and maturation of the granulomata.

Although seen primarily in the interstitium of the lung, the granulomata may also be peribronchial or perivascular. Granulomata may completely resolve to leave normal lung parenchyma or, with hyalinization and fibrosis, give rise to nonspecific interstitial pulmonary fibrosis and, rarely in children, end-stage honeycomb lung. Involvement of the upper airway is unusual. Granulomata also develop in lymph nodes, liver, spleen, eye, skin, parotid gland, brain, heart, skeletal muscle, kidney, and bone (433).

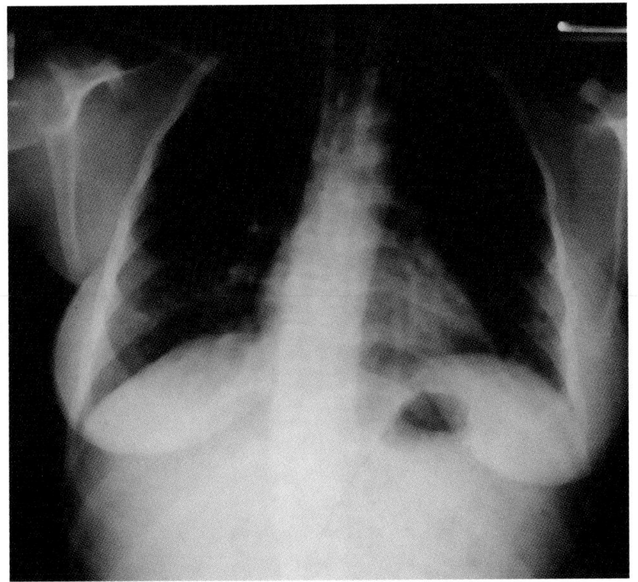

A

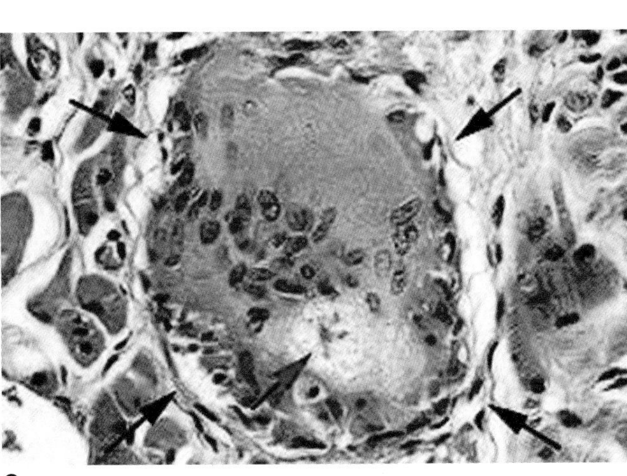

C

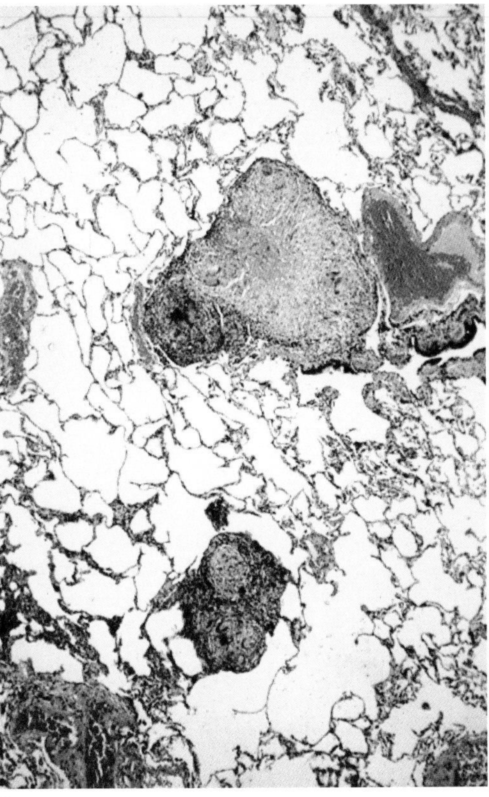

B

FIGURE 12-60■ Sarcoidosis. **A:** Bilateral hilar lymphadenopathy is noted in the 14-year-old black female. **B:** In these classic sarcoid granulomas, the central core of epithelioid cells and multinucleated giant cells is surrounded by a rim of lymphocytes. (H&E, ×40.) **C:** The granulomas contain multinucleated giant cells (*black arrows*), some of which may display asteroid bodies (*blue arrow*). (H&E, ×125.)

With early recognition and treatment with corticosteroids, complications such as blindness, pulmonary insufficiency, and renal impairment can be diminished. Although long-term sequelae occur in 10% to 20% of childhood cases, the mortality rate is only about 5% (434). Transplantation is a treatment option in severe cases, but recurrence in the transplanted lung may occur (435).

Cystic Fibrosis

CF is a multisystem disorder of children and adults, the most common lethal genetic disease of the white population, and the major cause of severe chronic lung disease of children (see Chapters 5 and 6). CF is inherited as an autosomal recessive disorder, with 70% of cases caused by mutations in the CF transmembrane conductance regulator gene located on chromosome 7 at ΔF508 (436–438). The other 30% of the mutations number over 1,000 (439–441).

CF is characterized by high viscosity of the mucoid secretion products in the lungs, pancreas, liver, and gastrointestinal tract, which causes plugging and secondary damage to these organs (see Chapters 14 to 16). Nasal and sinus polyposis are commonly seen in patients with CF, and pulmonary infection has long been recognized to be the most common cause of morbidity and mortality in these patients (442). The respiratory flora of patients with CF include *Staphylococcus aureus* and *Haemophilus influenzae* in the early stages of the disease, but repeated and chronic infections with *Pseudomonas aeruginosa* frequently occur (443). Eradication of *P. aeruginosa* is extremely difficult in CF patients, and the organism may be the dominant respiratory pathogen for years even after lung transplantation.

Fungal infections are present in over 20% of CF patients as a result of extensive lung damage, long-term antibiotic therapy, and repeated exposure to pathogenic microorganisms. The most frequently encountered organisms include members of the *Aspergillus* and *Candida* species, with allergic bronchopulmonary aspergillosis reported in up to 11% of patients (444).

Bronchiectasis is the predominant lesion of CF and begins in infancy as mucous plugging of bronchi, followed by infection, inflammation, mucosal necrosis and ulceration, and ectasia (Figure 12-61A–C). The chronic bronchitis may be associated with bronchiolitis obliterans and pneumonia. Bronchiectatic changes can alter the bronchial volume (normally 4% of a lobe's volume in healthy lungs) by increasing it to 10% to 20% of the total lung volume and occasionally as high as 50%.

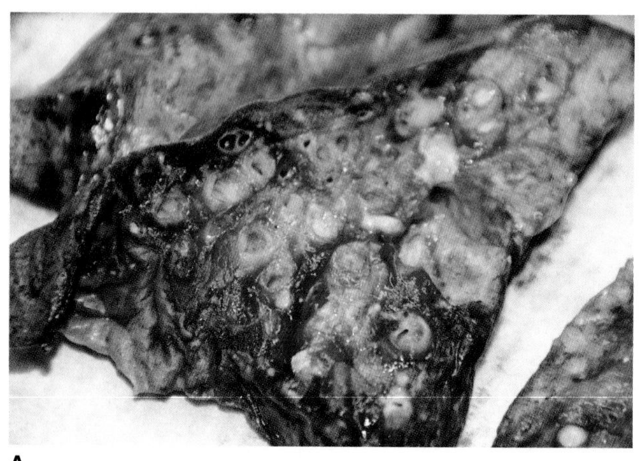

A

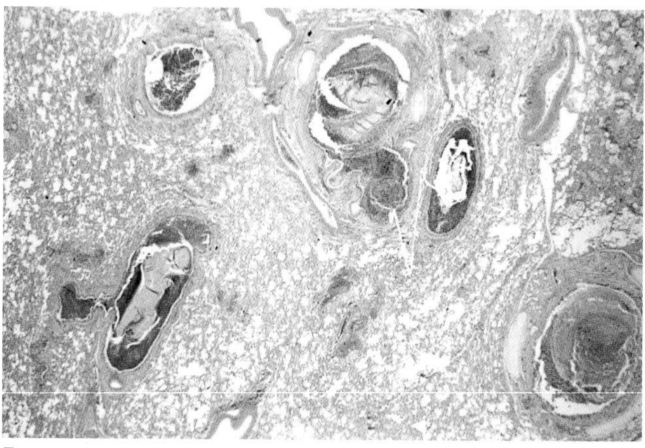

B

C

FIGURE 12-61 ■ Cystic fibrosis. **A:** Massively ectatic bronchi are filled with viscid mucus in the explanted lung of a 22-year-old woman. **B:** Bronchi are obstructed by a mixture of mucus and inflammatory debris that expands the airway and occasionally extends into the adjacent parenchyma (H&E, ×15). **C:** Hyperplastic submucosal glands exude a tenacious mucus that fills and adheres to the bronchial mucosa. (H&E, ×25.)

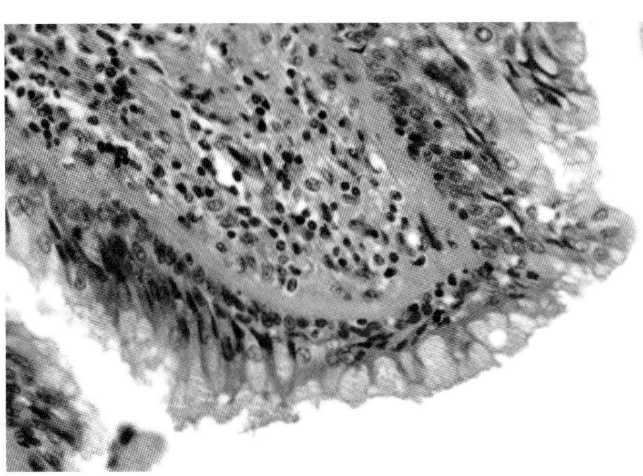
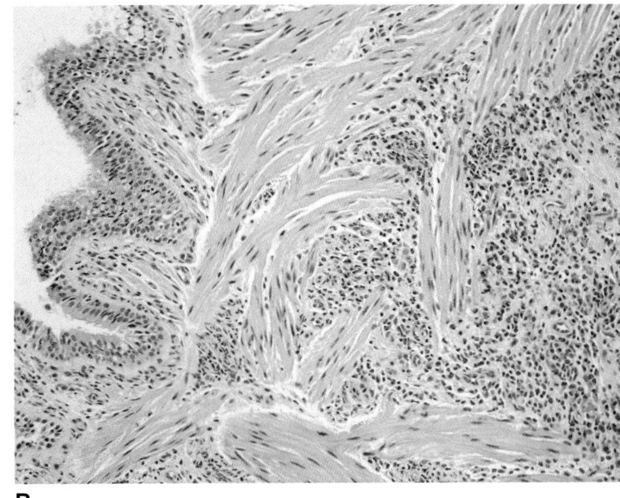

FIGURE 12-62 ▪ Asthma. **A:** A markedly thickened undulating basement membrane separates the lumen of a bronchus from the muscular wall that is heavily infiltrated with eosinophils, lymphocytes, and plasma cells (H&E, ×100). **B:** The wall of the bronchus displays markedly thickened muscle layers (H&E, ×20).

Changes in bronchi are most prominent in the upper lobes and may be accompanied by the development of large subpleural cysts that communicate with bronchi (bronchiectatic cysts), are confined to the interstitium, or distend the visceral pleura and merge with emphysematous pneumothoraces in CF patients. Transplantation of one or both lungs is increasingly successful in the treatment of chronic pulmonary CF (445,446).

Asthma

Asthma is an acute, usually reversible airway disease that results in spasmodic, diffuse airway narrowing, with persistent airway hyperreactivity (447,448). It affects 3% to 8% of the population and accounts for 2,000 to 3,000 deaths each year in the United States. In autopsy specimens of patients dying during an acute attack, the lungs show alternating areas of atelectasis and hyperexpansion. Mucus plugs composed of soft, gelatinous, or rubbery grey material fill medium-to-small bronchi. The smooth muscle of bronchi is markedly thickened, often 2.5-fold or more than normal (Figure 12-62A,B) (449). There is also a prominent thickening of the basal lamina of the mucosa, and the submucosa shows edema, vessel dilatation, and an inflammatory infiltrate of eosinophils, plasma cells, lymphocytes, and neutrophils (304,450). The bronchial mucosal lining and the submucosal glands display an increased number of goblet cells. Microscopically, the mucus plugs in bronchioles and smaller bron-

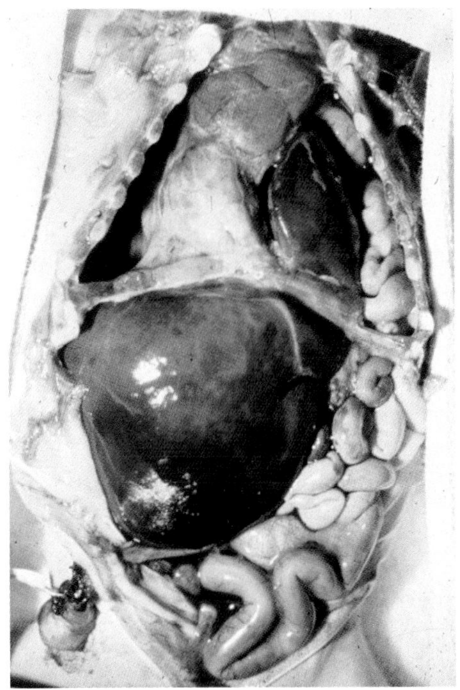
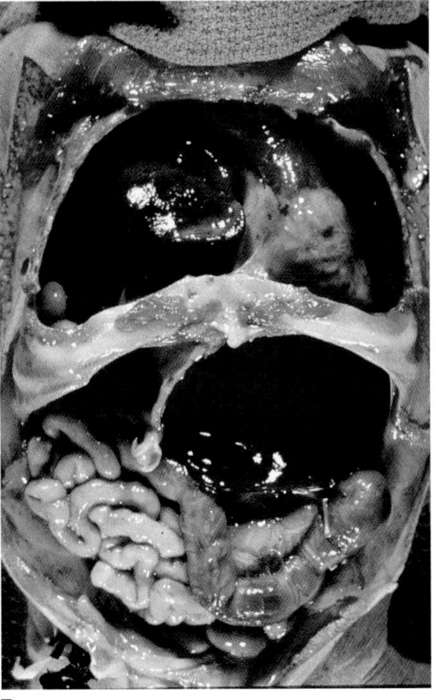

FIGURE 12-63 ▪ Diaphragmatic hernia. **A:** A large defect in the left leaflet of the diaphragm allows herniation of the liver and portions of gastrointestinal tract into the right hemithorax. **B:** A similar defect of the right leaflet allowed the liver to herniate and shifted the mediastinum to the left side. When the liver is returned through the diaphragm to the abdomen at the time of autopsy, the profound hypoplasia of the right lung can be seen.

chi may contain small linear whorled strands of material that are twisted in a common direction with a central highly refractile densely coiled or braided coil, called a Curshmann spiral. Inflammatory cells are admixed with the material in the lumen, and degranulated eosinophils may form crystals, called Charcot-Leyden crystals. Sloughed segments of respiratory epithelium may also be present as Creola bodies. These structures—Curshmann spirals, Charcot-Leyden crystals and Creola bodies—may also be found in sputum specimens of asthmatic patients (304). Similar findings are seen in allergic bronchopulmonary aspergillosis.

Transplantation

Lung transplantation in children is becoming increasingly common for treatment of a variety of pulmonary diseases, especially CF, but also PVOD, congenital surfactant deficiency, BPD, and other forms of interstitial lung disease with fibrosis, pulmonary vein stenosis (often in association with congenital heart disease), and pulmonary hypertension (446,451–454) (see Chapter 8).

DIAPHRAGM

Abnormalities of the diaphragm are both congenital and acquired. Developmental anomalies include accessory diaphragm, agenesis of one or both leaflets, defective formation with herniation, and aplasia or hypoplasia of muscle with eventration. Acquired diseases such as traumatic rupture, denervation, and muscular atrophy are also seen.

The diaphragm develops from the septum transversum, pleuroperitoneal membranes, and dorsal mesentery during the first 6 to 8 weeks of gestation. Under normal circumstances,

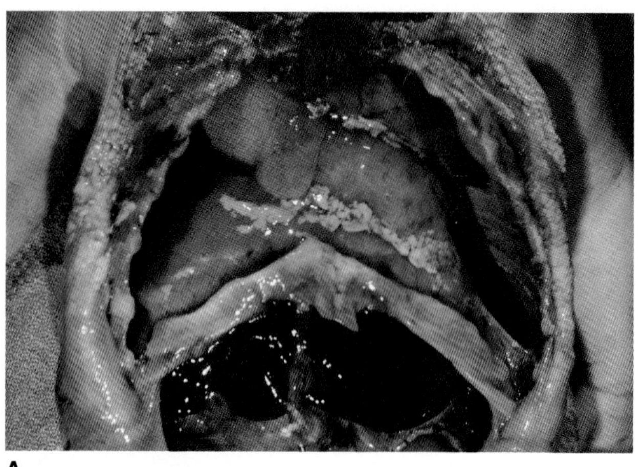

A

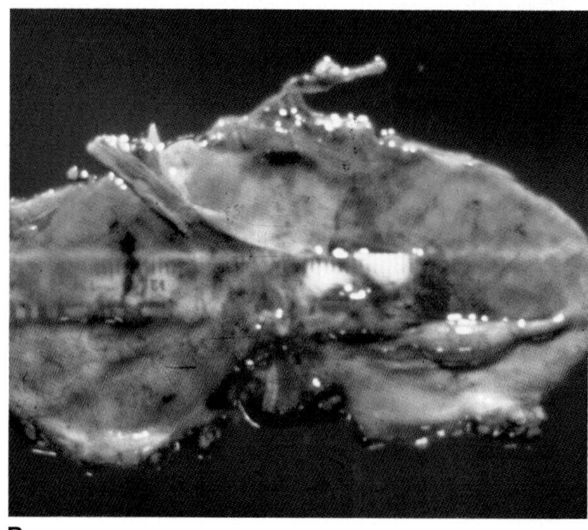

B

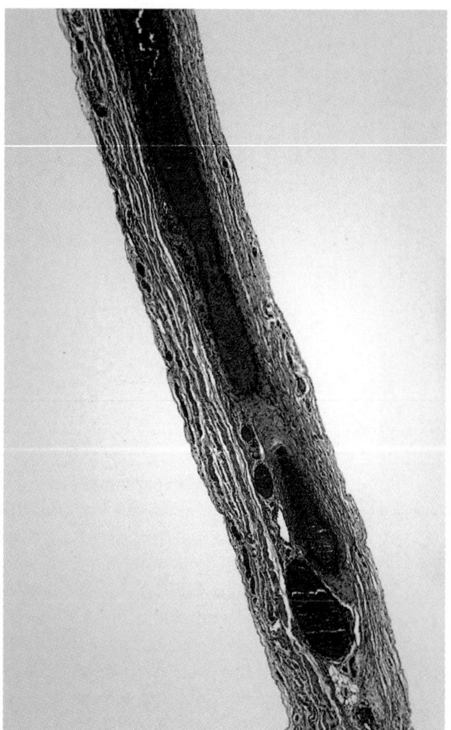

C

FIGURE 12-64 ■ Diaphragmatic eventration. **A:** The thorax in this newborn is markedly reduced in size by the elevation of the diaphragm and protrusion upward of the abdominal organs. **B:** At autopsy, the diaphragm consisted only of a thin and largely translucent membrane. **C:** A section of the diaphragm displays only vessels and a few strands of muscle between the thoracic and abdominal membranes. (H&E, ×50.)

Table 12-11 ■ ANOMALIES ASSOCIATED WITH DIAPHRAGMATIC HERNIA

Pulmonary
- Hypoplasia
- Extralobar sequestration
- Tracheoesophageal fistula
- Congenital pulmonary airway malformation

Cardiovascular
- Tetralogy of Fallot
- Endocardial cushion defect
- Atrial and ventricular septal defects
- Ectopia cordis
- Coarctation of the aorta
- Pulmonic stenosis

Gastrointestinal
- Imperforate anus
- Omphalocele
- Pyloric stenosis
- Stomach duplication
- Malrotation of bowel

Genitourinary
- Hydronephrosis
- Multicystic kidney
- Duplicated collecting system

Chromosomal
- Trisomy 18 and 21

Other
- Arthrogryposis
- Cleft lip and palate
- Meningomyelocele
- Hemivertebrae
- Fetal alcohol syndrome
- Cornelia de Lange syndrome
- Syndactyly
- Ullrich-Turner syndrome

Modified from Stocker JT. Congenital and developmental diseases. In: Dail DH, Hammer SP, eds. *Pulmonary pathology*. Heidelberg: Springer-Verlag, 1994, with permission.

the diaphragm separates the thoracic and abdominal contents completely by weeks 8 to 9 of gestation. Rarely, the septum transversum fails to descend completely, and an accessory diaphragm divides the hemithorax into upper and lower compartments. Always unilateral, and right-sided in more than 90% of cases, the accessory diaphragm can produce respiratory distress in infants but may be asymptomatic and seen only incidentally (192). Associated cardiovascular anomalies are seen in more than 40% of cases, and the entrapped portion of lung may be hypoplastic.

Complete absence of the diaphragm has been reported in a family, and agenesis of a hemidiaphragm is occasionally seen (455).

Diaphragmatic hernia is one of the most frequently occurring anomalies of the lungs and thorax, seen once in every 2,000 to 5,000 births. Herniation of abdominal contents into the thoracic cavity through a defect in the diaphragm occurs early in gestation and results in varying degrees of pulmonary hypoplasia. The defect is usually in the posterolateral (i.e., foramen of Bochdalek) aspect of the diaphragm. The size of the defect and location on the right (20% to 35% of cases) or left (65% to 80% of cases) side influence the degree of pulmonary hypoplasia and the clinical presentation.

Right-sided diaphragmatic hernias are often partially or completely occluded by the liver, and the degree of pulmonary compromise is mild. Delayed presentation has been reported in infants with right-sided diaphragmatic hernia whose symptoms are masked by a group B streptococcal sepsis (456).

Infants with the more typical large, left-sided hernia may present in the first minutes to hours of life with severe respiratory distress. Herniation of abdominal contents including liver, spleen, and loops of intestine may result in severe pulmonary hypoplasia (Figure 12-63A,B). Survival rates for infants with congenital diaphragmatic hernia (CDH) have increased dramatically with the increased availability of surgical repair of the hernia (both *in utero* and after birth) and the development of ECMO to support infants with mild-to-moderate pulmonary hypoplasia. Current survival rates are up to 75% to 95% of liveborn infants with CDH (457). Those with the poorest prognosis have the most severe pulmonary hypoplasia and are unable to maintain adequate oxygenation after repair of the hernia. Pulmonary hypoplasia is life threatening when the lung weights are less than 30% to 40% of expected weight. Infants with more than 45% to 50% of expected weight, including those whose entire right or left lung has been removed because of a congenital malformation (e.g., CPAM), often survive with little respiratory difficulty. Associated anomalies are noted in approximately 25% of cases of CDH and include a variety of pulmonary, cardiovascular, gastrointestinal, and genitourinary malformations (Table 12-10). In addition, tracheobronchomalacia may be seen in 5% to 10% of infants with CDH. CDH is also part of the phenotype of Fryns syndrome.

Aplasia or hypoplasia of musculature within the leaflets of the diaphragm, either partial or complete, produces *eventration of the diaphragm* (Figure 12-64A to C). Congenital eventration, usually seen in boys (62%), is unilateral in 85% of cases, with the right side involved in 67% and the left in 33% (458). Phrenic nerve palsy from birth injury or iatrogenic damage can lead to diaphragmatic elevation mimicking eventration (459)]. Associated anomalies, present in over 30% of cases, are similar to those seen with diaphragmatic hernia (Table 12-11) but also include cases of arthrogryposis. The involved segments of the diaphragm display normal parietal thoracic and abdominal mesothelium separated by delicate fibrovascular connective tissue either devoid of muscle or with only a few skeletal muscle fibers present.

REFERENCES

1. Stocker JT. Congenital and developmental diseases. In: Dail DH, Hammer SP, eds. *Pulmonary Pathology*, 2nd ed. New York: Springer-Verlag, 1994:155–190.
2. Hislop A, Reid L. Pulmonary arterial development during childhood: branching pattern and structure. *Thorax* 1973;28(2):129–135.
3. Hislop A, Reid L. Fetal and childhood development of the intrapulmonary veins in man—branching pattern and structure. *Thorax* 1973;28(3):313–319.
4. Lauweryns JM. The blood and lymphatic microcirculation of the lung. *Pathol Annu* 1971;6:365–415.

5. Stocker JT, McGill LC, Orsini EN. Post-infarction peripheral cysts of the lung in pediatric patients: a possible cause of idiopathic spontaneous pneumothorax. *Pediatr Pulmonol* 1985;1(1):7–18.
6. Langston C, Thurlbeck WM. Lung growth and development in late gestation and early postnatal life. *Perspect Pediatr Pathol* 1982;7:203–235.
7. Langston C. Prenatal lung growth and pulmonary hypoplasia. In: Stocker JT, ed. *Pediatric Pulmonary Disease*. Washington, D.C.: Hemisphere, 1989:1–27.
8. Issekutz KA, Graham JM, Jr., Prasad C, et al. An epidemiological analysis of CHARGE syndrome: preliminary results from a Canadian study. *Am J Med Genet A* 2005;133(3):309–317.
9. da Fontoura Rey Bergonse G, Carneiro AF, Vassoler TM. Choanal atresia: analysis of 16 cases–the experience of HRAC-USP from 2000 to 2004. *Rev Bras Otorrinolaringol (Engl Ed)* 2005;71(6):730–733.
10. Vatansever U, Duran R, Acunas B, et al. Bilateral choanal atresia in premature monozygotic twins. *J Perinatol* 2005;25(12):800–802.
11. Shepard PM, Houser SM. Choanal stenosis: an unusual late complication of radiation therapy for nasopharyngeal carcinoma. *Am J Rhinol* 2005;19(1):105–108.
12. Marina MB, Gendeh BS. Acquired nasal posterior choanal atresia: postradiotherapy. *Med J Malaysia* 2006;61(1):94–96.
13. Hsu CY, Li YW, Hsu JC. Congenital choanal atresia: computed tomographic and clinical findings. *Chung Hua Min Kuo Hsiao Erh Ko I Hsueh Hui Tsa Chih* 1999;40(1):13–17.
14. Devine WA, Webber SA, Anderson RH. Congenitally malformed hearts from a population of children undergoing cardiac transplantation: comments on sequential segmental analysis and dissection. *Pediatr Dev Pathol* 2000;3(2):140–154.
15. Jacob R, Priolo C, Farina D, et al. Trisomy 6 with choanal atresia. The first Italian case. *Minerva Pediatr* 1999;51(6):213–215.
16. Park MS, Yoo JE, Chung J, et al. A case of Pfeiffer syndrome. *J Korean Med Sci* 2006;21(2):374–378.
17. Andrade EC, Junior VS, Didoni AL, et al. Treacher Collins Syndrome with choanal atresia: a case report and review of disease features. *Rev Bras Otorrinolaringol (Engl Ed)* 2005;71(1):107–110.
18. Myers AK, Reardon W. Choanal atresia—a recurrent feature of foetal carbimazole syndrome. *Clin Otolaryngol* 2005;30(4):375–377.
19. Aramaki M, Udaka T, Kosaki R, et al. Phenotypic spectrum of CHARGE syndrome with CHD7 mutations. *J Pediatr* 2006;148(3):410–414.
20. Lalani SR, Safiullah AM, Fernbach SD, et al. Spectrum of CHD7 Mutations in 110 Individuals with CHARGE Syndrome and Genotype-Phenotype Correlation. *Am J Hum Genet* 2006;78(2):303–314.
21. Bill J, Proff P, Bayerlein T, et al. Treatment of patients with cleft lip, alveolus and palate—a short outline of history and current interdisciplinary treatment approaches. *J Craniomaxillofac Surg* 2006;34(Suppl 2):17–21.
22. Canfield MA, Honein MA, Yuskiv N, et al. National estimates and race/ethnic-specific variation of selected birth defects in the United States, 1999-2001. *Birth Defects Res A Clin Mol Teratol* 2006;76(11):747–756.
23. Warrington A, Vieira AR, Christensen K, et al. Genetic evidence for the role of loci at 19q13 in cleft lip and palate. *J Med Genet* 2006;43(6):e26.
24. Lorente C, Cordier S, Goujard J, et al. Tobacco and alcohol use during pregnancy and risk of oral clefts. Occupational Exposure and Congenital Malformation Working Group. *Am J Public Health* 2000;90(3):415–419.
25. Chung KC, Kowalski CP, Kim HM, et al. Maternal cigarette smoking during pregnancy and the risk of having a child with cleft lip/palate. *Plast Reconstr Surg* 2000;105(2):485–491.
26. Pennings RJ, van den Hoogen FJ, Marres HA. Giant laryngoceles: a cause of upper airway obstruction. *Eur Arch Otorhinolaryngol* 2001;258(3):137–140.
27. Chu L, Gussack GS, Orr JB, et al. Neonatal laryngoceles. a cause for airway obstruction. *Arch Otolaryngol Head Neck Surg* 1994;120(4):454–458.
28. Zelman WH, Burke LI. External laryngocele: an unusual cause of respiratory distress in a newborn. *Ear Nose Throat J* 1994;73(1):19–22.
29. Cassano L, Lombardo P, Marchese-Ragona R, et al. Laryngopyocele: three new clinical cases and review of the literature. *Eur Arch Otorhinolaryngol* 2000;257(9):507–511.
30. Altamar-Rios J, Morales Rozo O. Laryngocele and pyolaryngocele. *An Otorrinolaringol Ibero Am* 1992;19(4):393–399.
31. Righini C, Mouret P, Reyt E. Pyolaryngocele: case report of an uncommon laryngeal disease. *Ann Otolaryngol Chir Cervicofac* 2001;118(4):261–264.
32. Kay DJ, Goldsmith AJ. Laryngomalacia: a classification system and surgical treatment strategy. *Ear Nose Throat J* 2006;85(5):328–331, 336.
33. Olney DR, Greinwald JH, Jr., Smith RJ, et al. Laryngomalacia and its treatment. *Laryngoscope* 1999;109(11):1770–1775.
34. Sichel JY, Dangoor E, Eliashar R, et al. Management of congenital laryngeal malformations. *Am J Otolaryngol* 2000;21(1):22–30.
35. Waters ET, Oberman JP, Biswas AK. Pierre Robin sequence and double aortic arch: a case report. *Int J Pediatr Otorhinolaryngol* 2005;69(1):105–110.
36. Hou JW. Long-term follow-up of Marshall-Smith syndrome: report of one case. *Acta Paediatr Taiwan* 2004;45(4):232–235.
37. Hou JW. Fetal warfarin syndrome. *Chang Gung Med J* 2004;27(9):691–695.
38. Shing Yan Robert L, Daniel Kwok-Keung N, Pok Yu C, et al. Obstructive sleep apnea syndrome secondary to pharyngolaryngomalacia in a neonate with Down syndrome. *Int J Pediatr Otorhinolaryngol* 2005;69(7):919–921.
39. Tastekin A, Ikbal M, Ors R. Laryngomalacia, choanal atresia and renal anomaly in a newborn with Freeman-Sheldon syndrome phenotype. *Genet Couns* 2004;15(3):383–386.
40. Chen JL, Messner AH, Chang KW. Familial laryngomalacia in two siblings with syndromic features. *Int J Pediatr Otorhinolaryngol* 2006;70(9):1651–1655.
41. Choi SS, Zalzal GH. Changing trends in neonatal subglottic stenosis. *Otolaryngol Head Neck Surg* 2000;122(1):61–63.
42. Gatti WM, MacDonald E, Orfei E. Congenital laryngeal atresia. *Laryngoscope* 1987;97(8 Pt 1):966–969.
43. Okuyama H, Kubota A, Kawahara H, et al. Congenital laryngeal atresia associated with esophageal atresia and tracheoesophageal fistula: a case of long-term survival. *J Pediatr Surg* 2006;41(11):e29–e32.
44. Minior VK, Gagner JP, Landi K, et al. Congenital laryngeal atresia associated with partial diaphragmatic obliteration. *J Ultrasound Med* 2004;23(2):291–296.
45. Balci S, Altinok G, Ozaltin F, et al. Laryngeal atresia presenting as fetal ascites, oligohydramnios and lung appearance mimicking cystic adenomatoid malformation in a 25-week-old fetus with Fraser syndrome. *Prenat Diagn* 1999;19(9):856–858.
46. Moerman P, de Zegher F, Vandenberghe K, et al. Laryngeal atresia sequence as part of the DiGeorge developmental field defect. *Genet Couns* 1992;3(3):133–137.
47. Van den Boogaard MJ, De Pater J, Hennekam RC. A case with laryngeal atresia and partial trisomy 9 due to maternal 9; 16 translocation. *Genet Couns* 1991;2(2):83–91.
48. Stocker JT. Sequestrations of the lung. *Semin Diagn Pathol* 1986;3(2):106–121.
49. Alabdulgader A, Patten D, Harder J, et al. Laryngotracheoesophageal cleft type 3 and double outlet right ventricle: unique combination. *Ann Diagn Pathol* 2005;9(6):323–326.
50. Heimann K, Bartz C, Naami A, et al. Three new cases of congenital agenesis of the trachea. *Eur J Pediatr* 2007;166(1):79–82.
51. Evans JA, Greenberg CR, Erdile L. Tracheal agenesis revisited: analysis of associated anomalies. *Am J Med Genet* 1999;82(5):415–422.
52. van Veenendaal MB, Liem KD, Marres HA. Congenital absence of the trachea. *Eur J Pediatr* 2000;159(1–2):8–13.
53. Altman KW, Wetmore RF, Marsh RR. Congenital airway abnormalities requiring tracheotomy: a profile of 56 patients and their diagnoses over a 9 year period [see comments]. *Int J Pediatr Otorhinolaryngol* 1997;41(2):199–206.

54. Altman KW, Wetmore RF, Marsh RR. Congenital airway abnormalities in patients requiring hospitalization. *Arch Otolaryngol Head Neck Surg* 1999;125(5):525–528.
55. Tsugawa J, Satoh S, Nishijima E, et al. Development of acquired tracheal stenosis in premature infants due to prolonged endotracheal ventilation: etiological considerations and surgical management. *Pediatr Surg Int* 2006;22(11):887–890.
56. Faust RA, Stroh B, Rimell F. The near complete tracheal ring deformity. *Int J Pediatr Otorhinolaryngol* 1998;45(2):171–176.
57. Bravo MN, Kaul A, Rutter MJ, et al. Down syndrome and complete tracheal rings. *J Pediatr* 2006;148(3):392–395.
58. Quiros-Tejeira RE, Ament ME, Heyman MB, et al. Variable morbidity in alagille syndrome: a review of 43 cases. *J Pediatr Gastroenterol Nutr* 1999;29(4):431–437.
59. Wong KS, Lien R, Lin TY. Clinical and computed tomographic features of tracheal bronchus in children. *J Formos Med Assoc* 1999;98(9): 646–648.
60. Cordovilla Zurdo G, Cabo Salvador J, Sanz Galeote E, et al. Congenital heart defects with tracheal and bronchial stenoses: surgical treatment with extracorporeal circulation. *An Esp Pediatr* 1999;51(2): 149–153.
61. Lang FJ, Hurni M, Monnier P. Long-segment congenital tracheal stenosis: treatment by slide- tracheoplasty. *J Pediatr Surg* 1999;34(8): 1216–1222.
62. Berrocal T, Madrid C, Novo S, et al. Congenital anomalies of the tracheobronchial tree, lung, and mediastinum: embryology, radiology, and pathology. *Radiographics* 2004;24(1):e17.
63. Bertrand P, Navarro H, Caussade S, et al. Airway anomalies in children with Down syndrome: endoscopic findings. *Pediatr Pulmonol* 2003;36(2):137–141.
64. Rock MJ, Green CG, Pauli RM, et al. Tracheomalacia and bronchomalacia associated with Larsen syndrome. *Pediatr Pulmonol* 1988;5(1):55–59.
65. Triglia JM, Nicollas R, Roman S, et al. Tracheomalacia associated with compressive cardiovascular anomalies in children. *Pediatr Pulmonol* 2001;23(Suppl):8–9.
66. Masters IB, Chang AB, Patterson L, et al. Series of laryngomalacia, tracheomalacia, and bronchomalacia disorders and their associations with other conditions in children. *Pediatr Pulmonol* 2002;34(3):189–195.
67. Kamata S, Usui N, Sawai T, et al. Pexis of the great vessels for patients with tracheobronchomalacia in infancy. *J Pediatr Surg* 2000;35(3): 454–457.
68. Carden KA, Boiselle PM, Waltz DA, et al. Tracheomalacia and tracheobronchomalacia in children and adults: an in-depth review. *Chest* 2005;127(3):984–1005.
69. Kang FC, Tsai YC, Jiang CY, et al. Acquired tracheomalacia–a case report. *Acta Anaesthesiol Sin* 1996;34(4):239–242.
70. Sane AC, Effmann EL, Brown SD. Tracheobronchiomegaly. The Mounier-Kuhn syndrome in a patient with the Kenny-Caffey syndrome. *Chest* 1992;102(2):618–619.
71. Wanderer AA, Ellis EF, Goltz RW, et al. Tracheobronchiomegaly and acquired cutis laxa in a child. Physiologic and immunologic studies. *Pediatrics* 1969;44(5):709–715.
72. Shaw A, Ko C, Tomlinson J. A 2-year-old boy, born with polysplenia syndrome, esophageal atresia, and tracheoesophageal fistula (TEF). *J Pediatr Surg* 2004;39(6):1002.
73. Genty E, Attal P, Nicollas R, et al. Congenital tracheoesophageal fistula without esophageal atresia. *Int J Pediatr Otorhinolaryngol* 1999;48(3):231–238.
74. Shaw-Smith C. Oesophageal atresia, tracheo-oesophageal fistula, and the VACTERL association: review of genetics and epidemiology. *J Med Genet* 2006;43(7):545–554.
75. Dutta HK, Mathur M, Bhatnagar V. A histopathological study of esophageal atresia and tracheoesophageal fistula. *J Pediatr Surg* 2000;35(3):438–441.
76. Al-Salem AH, Tayeb M, Khogair S, et al. Esophageal atresia with or without tracheoesophageal fistula: success and failure in 94 cases. *Ann Saudi Med* 2006;26(2):116–119.
77. Diaz LK, Akpek EA, Dinavahi R, et al. Tracheoesophageal fistula and associated congenital heart disease: implications for anesthetic management and survival. *Paediatr Anaesth* 2005;15(10):862–869.
78. Ratan SK, Grover SB. Lung agenesis in a neonate presenting with contralateral mediastinal shift. *Am J Perinatol* 2001;18(8):441–446.
79. Ratan SK, Rattan KN, Pandey RM, et al. Associated congenital anomalies in patients with anorectal malformations—a need for developing a uniform practical approach. *J Pediatr Surg* 2004;39(11):1706–1711.
80. De Felice C, Di Maggio G, Messina M, et al. Congenital cystic adenomatoid malformation of the lung associated with esophageal atresia and tracheoesophageal fistula. *Pediatr Surg Int* 1999;15(3–4): 260–263.
81. Onyeije CI, Sherer DM, Handwerker S, et al. Prenatal diagnosis of sirenomelia with bilateral hydrocephalus: report of a previously undocumented form of VACTERL-H association. *Am J Perinatol* 1998;15(3):193–197.
82. Tsai JY, Berkery L, Wesson DE, et al. Esophageal atresia and tracheoesophageal fistula: surgical experience over two decades. *Ann Thorac Surg* 1997;64(3):778–783; discussion 783–774.
83. Somppi E, Tammela O, Ruuska T, et al. Outcome of patients operated on for esophageal atresia: 30 years' experience. *J Pediatr Surg* 1998;33(9):1341–1346.
84. Alkan M, Buyukyavuz I, Dogru D, et al. Tracheoesophageal fistula due to disc-battery ingestion. *Eur J Pediatr Surg* 2004;14(4):274–278.
85. Birman C, Beckenham E. Acquired tracheo-esophageal fistula in the pediatric population. *Int J Pediatr Otorhinolaryngol* 1998;44(2): 109–113.
86. Alfaro L, Bermas H, Fenoglio M, et al. Are patients who have had a tracheoesophageal fistula repair during infancy at risk for esophageal adenocarcinoma during adulthood? *J Pediatr Surg* 2005;40(4):719–720.
87. Ward S, Morcos SK. Congenital bronchial atresia–presentation of three cases and a pictorial review. *Clin Radiol* 1999;54(3):144–148.
88. Zylak CJ, Eyler WR, Spizarny DL, et al. Developmental lung anomalies in the adult: radiologic-pathologic correlation. *Radiographics* 2002;22 Spec No:S25–S43.
89. Landing B, Wells T. Tracheobronchial anomalies in children. *Perspect Pediatr Pathol* 1973;1:1–32.
90. Riedlinger WF, Vargas SO, Jennings RW, et al. Bronchial atresia is common to extralobar sequestration, intralobar sequestration, congenital cystic adenomatoid malformation, and lobar emphysema. *Pediatr Dev Pathol* 2006;9(5):361–373.
91. Kunisaki SM, Fauza DO, Nemes LP, et al. Bronchial atresia: the hidden pathology within a spectrum of prenatally diagnosed lung masses. *J Pediatr Surg* 2006;41(1):61–65; discussion 61–65.
92. Murray C, Pilling DW, Shaw NJ. Persistent acquired lobar overinflation complicating bronchopulmonary dysplasia. *Eur J Pediatr* 2000;159(1-2):14–17.
93. Rohde M, Banner J. Respiratory tract malacia: possible cause of sudden death in infancy and early childhood. *Acta Paediatr* 2006;95(7):867–870.
94. Palmer SM, Jr., Layish DT, Kussin PS, et al. Lung transplantation for Williams-Campbell syndrome. *Chest* 1998;113(2):534–537.
95. Ide Y, Nemoto S, Ikeda T, et al. Successful implantation of a metal coronary angioplasty stent for bronchomalacia of the right tracheal bronchus associated with right isomerism complex in an early infant. *Kyobu Geka* 2005;58(7):537–541.
96. Landing BH. Five syndromes (malformation complexes) of pulmonary symmetry, congenital heart disease, and multiple spleens. *Pediatr Pathol* 1984;2(2):148–151.
97. Atwell SW. Major anomalies of the tracheobronchial tree: with a list of the minor anomalies. *Dis Chest* 1967;52(5):611–615.
98. Stokes JR, Heatley DG, Lusk RP, et al. The bridging bronchus. Successful diagnosis and repair. *Arch Otolaryngol Head Neck Surg* 1997;123(12):1344–1347.
99. Wheeler DS, Poss WB, Cocalis M, et al. Braided bronchus: a previously undescribed airway anomaly. *Pediatr Pulmonol* 1998;25(5):348–351.
100. McLaughlin FJ, Strieder DJ, Harris GB, Vawter GP, Eraklis AJ. Tracheal bronchus: association with respiratory morbidity in childhood. *J Pediatr* 1985;106(5):751–755.

101. Linnane BM, Canny G. Congenital broncho-esophageal fistula: a case report. *Respir Med* 2006;100(10):1855–1857.
102. Chiu HH, Chen CM, Mo LR, et al. Gastrointestinal: tuberculous bronchoesophageal fistula. *J Gastroenterol Hepatol* 2006;21(6):1074.
103. Devbhandari MP, Raco L, Hendrickse MT, et al. Congenital bronchoesophageal fistula in a patient with Crohn's disease: a cautionary tale. *Ann Thorac Surg* 2005;79(5):1776–1777.
104. Aguilar C, Cano R, Camasca A, et al. Congenital bronchobiliary fistula detected by cholescintigraphy. *Rev Gastroenterol Peru* 2005;25(2):216–218.
105. Hourigan JS, Carr MG, Burton EM, et al. Congenital bronchobiliary fistula: MRI appearance. *Pediatr Radiol* 2004;34(4):348–350.
106. Uchikov AP, Safev GP, Stefanov CS, et al. Surgical treatment of bronchobiliary fistulas due to complicated echinococcosis of the liver: case report and literature review. *Folia Med (Plovdiv)* 2003;45(4):22–24.
107. Corapcioglu F, Sarper N, Demir H, et al. A child with undifferentiated sarcoma of the liver complicated with bronchobiliary fistula and detected by hepatobiliary scintigraphy. *Pediatr Hematol Oncol* 2004;21(5):427–433.
108. Carlen B, Stenram U. Primary ciliary dyskinesia: a review. *Ultrastruct Pathol* 2005;29(3–4):217–220.
109. Roomans GM, Ivanovs A, Shebani EB, et al. Transmission electron microscopy in the diagnosis of primary ciliary dyskinesia. *Ups J Med Sci* 2006;111(1):155–168.
110. Hornef N, Olbrich H, Horvath J, et al. DNAH5 mutations are a common cause of primary ciliary dyskinesia with outer dynein arm defects. *Am J Respir Crit Care Med* 2006;174(2):120–126.
111. Rebora ME, Cuneo JA, Marcos J, et al. Kartagener syndrome and rheumatoid arthritis. *J Clin Rheumatol* 2006;12(1):26–29.
112. George J, Jain R, Tariq SM. CT bronchoscopy in the diagnosis of Williams-Campbell syndrome. *Respirology* 2006;11(1):117–119.
113. Sauvat F, Fusaro F, Jaubert F, et al. Paraesophageal bronchogenic cyst: first case reports in pediatric. *Pediatr Surg Int* 2006;22(10):849–851.
114. Mehta RP, Faquin WC, Cunningham MJ. Cervical bronchogenic cysts: a consideration in the differential diagnosis of pediatric cervical cystic masses. *Int J Pediatr Otorhinolaryngol* 2004;68(5):563–568.
115. Tireli GA, Ozbey H, Temiz A, et al. Bronchogenic cysts: a rare congenital cystic malformation of the lung. *Surg Today* 2004;34(7):573–576.
116. Baets FD, Daele SV, Schelstraete P, et al. Asphyxiating tracheal bronchogenic cyst. *Pediatr Pulmonol* 2004;38(6):488–490.
117. Zvulunov A, Amichai B, Grunwald MH, et al. Cutaneous bronchogenic cyst: delineation of a poorly recognized lesion. *Pediatr Dermatol* 1998;15(4):277–281.
118. Stocker JT, Kagan-Hallet K. Extralobar pulmonary sequestration: analysis of 15 cases. *Am J Clin Pathol* 1979;72(6):917–925.
119. Tzifa A, Robards M, Simpson JM. Plastic bronchitis; a serious complication of the Fontan operation. *Int J Cardiol* 2005;101(3):513–514.
120. Madsen P, Shah SA, Rubin BK. Plastic bronchitis: new insights and a classification scheme. *Paediatr Respir Rev* 2005;6(4):292–300.
121. Brogan TV, Finn LS, Pyskaty DJ, Jr., et al. Plastic bronchitis in children: a case series and review of the medical literature. *Pediatr Pulmonol* 2002;34(6):482–487.
122. Kuperman T, Wexler ID, Shoseyov D, et al. Plastic bronchitis caused by neoplastic infiltrates in a child. *Pediatr Pulmonol* 2006;41(9):893–896.
123. Veras TN, Lannes GM, Piva JP, et al. Plastic bronchitis in a child with thalassemia alpha. *J Pediatr (Rio J)* 2005;81(6):499–502.
124. Manna SS, Shaw J, Tibby SM, et al. Treatment of plastic bronchitis in acute chest syndrome of sickle cell disease with intratracheal rhDNase. *Arch Dis Child* 2003;88(7):626–627.
125. Sharma S, Kumar S, Yaduvanshi D, et al. Isolated unilateral pulmonary agenesis. *Indian Pediatr* 2005;42(2):170–172.
126. Osborne J, Masel J, McCredie J. A spectrum of skeletal anomalies associated with pulmonary agenesis: possible neural crest injuries. *Pediatr Radiol* 1989;19(6–7):425–432.
127. Eroglu A, Alper F, Turkyilmaz A, et al. Pulmonary agenesis associated with dextrocardia, sternal defects, and ectopic kidney. *Pediatr Pulmonol* 2005;40(6):547–549.
128. Cunningham ML, Mann N. Pulmonary agenesis: a predictor of ipsilateral malformations. *Am J Med Genet* 1997;70(4):391–398.
129. Knowles S, Thomas RM, Lindenbaum RH, et al. Pulmonary agenesis as part of the VACTERL sequence. *Arch Dis Child* 1988;63(7 Spec No):723–726.
130. Lin JH, Chen SJ, Wu MH, et al. Right lung agenesis with left pulmonary artery sling. *Pediatr Pulmonol* 2000;29(3):239–241.
131. Stocker JT. Pathologic features of long-standing "healed" bronchopulmonary dysplasia: a study of 28 3- to 40-month-old infants. *Hum Pathol* 1986;17(9):943–961.
132. Goldberg S, Ringertz H, Barth RA. Prenatal diagnosis of horseshoe lung and esophageal atresia. *Pediatr Radiol* 2006;36(9):983–986.
133. Lutterman J, Jedeikin R, Cleveland DC. Horseshoe lung with left lung hypoplasia and critical pulmonary venous stenosis. *Ann Thorac Surg* 2004;77(3):1085–1087.
134. Kim JB, Park JJ, Ko JK, et al. A case of PAGOD syndrome with hypoplastic left heart syndrome. *Int J Cardiol* 2007;114(2):270–271.
135. Dikensoy O, Kervancioglu R, Bayram NG, et al. Horseshoe lung associated with scimitar syndrome and pleural lipoma. *J Thorac Imaging* 2006;21(1):73–75.
136. Currarino G. Cervical lung protrusions in children [see comments]. *Pediatr Radiol* 1998;28(7):533–538.
137. Cunningham D, Peters ER. Cervical hernia of the lung associated with the cri du chat syndrome. *Am J Dis Child* 1969;118(5):769–771.
138. Chen RD, Liu XD, Liu LX. Familial cervical lung hernia: a report of 4 cases in a family. *Chung Hua Chieh Ho Ho Hu Hsi Tsa Chih* 1994;17(4):230–231, 255.
139. Moncada R, Vade A, Gimenez C, et al. Congenital and acquired lung hernias. *J Thorac Imaging* 1996;11(1):75–82.
140. Conran RM, Stocker JT. Extralobar sequestration with frequently associated congenital cystic adenomatoid malformation, type 2: report of 50 cases. *Pediatr Dev Pathol* 1999;2(5):454–463.
141. Arslanian A, Leflour N, Hernigou A, et al. Complex extralobar sequestration in a 24-year-old woman. *Ann Thorac Surg* 2003;76(6):2077–2078.
142. Datta G, Tambiah J, Rankin S, et al. Atypical presentation of extralobar sequestration with absence of pericardium in an adult. *J Thorac Cardiovasc Surg* 2006;132(5):1239–1240.
143. Lucaya J, Garel L, Martin C. Clinical quiz. Extralobar sequestration, esophageal bronchus (bronchopulmonary foregut malformation). *Pediatr Radiol* 2003;33(9):665–666.
144. Kugai T, Kinjyo M. Extralobar sequestration presenting increased serum CA19-9 and associated with lung aspergillosis–an unusual case. *Nippon Kyobu Geka Gakkai Zasshi* 1996;44(4):565–569.
145. Kamata S, Sawai T, Nose K, et al. Extralobar pulmonary sequestration with venous drainage to the portal vein: a case report. *Pediatr Radiol* 2000;30(7):492–494.
146. Scurry JP, Adamson TM, Cussen LJ. Fetal lung growth in laryngeal atresia and tracheal agenesis. *Aust Paediatr J* 1989;25(1):47–51.
147. Mani H, Suarez E, Stocker JT. The morphologic spectrum of infantile lobar emphysema: a study of 33 cases. *Paediatr Respir Rev* 2004;5(Suppl A):S313–S320.
148. Frazier AA, Rosado de Christenson ML, Stocker JT, et al. Intralobar sequestration: radiologic-pathologic correlation. *Radiographics* 1997;17(3):725–745.
149. Yamanaka A, Hirai T, Fujimoto T, et al. Anomalous systemic arterial supply to normal basal segments of the left lower lobe. *Ann Thorac Surg* 1999;68(2):332–338.
150. Walford N, Htun K, Chen J, et al. Intralobar sequestration of the lung is a congenital anomaly: anatomopathological analysis of four cases diagnosed in fetal life. *Pediatr Dev Pathol* 2003;6(4):314–321.
151. Stocker JT, Dehner LP. Acquired neonatal and pediatric diseases. In: Dail DH, Hammer SP, eds. *Pulmonary Pathology*, 2nd ed. New York: Springer-Verlag, 1994:191–254.
152. Stocker JT, Malczak HT. A study of pulmonary ligament arteries. Relationship to intralobar pulmonary sequestration. *Chest* 1984;86(4):611–615.

153. Holder PD, Langston C. Intralobar pulmonary sequestration (a nonentity?). *Pediatr Pulmonol* 1986;2(3):147–153.
154. Yatera K, Izumi M, Imai M, et al. A case report of intralobar sequestration with a Mycobacterium tuberculosis infection limited to the sequestrated lung. *Respiratory* 2005;10(5):684–688.
155. Shanmugam G, MacArthur K, et al. Congenital lung malformations–antenatal and postnatal evaluation and management. *Eur J Cardiothorac Surg* 2005;27(1):45–52.
156. Hayasaka K, Saitoh T, Tanaka Y. Intralobar pulmonary sequestration receiving arterial supply from the superior mesenteric artery: a case report. *Comput Med Imaging Graph* 2006;30(2):135–137.
157. Yagyu H, Adachi H, Furukawa K, et al. Intralobar pulmonary sequestration presenting increased serum CA19-9 and CA125. *Intern Med* 2002;41(10):875–878.
158. Reale FR, Esterly JR. Pulmonary hypoplasia: a morphometric study of the lungs of infants with diaphragmatic hernia, anencephaly, and renal malformations. *Pediatrics* 1973;51(1):91–96.
159. Emery JL, Mithal A. The number of alveoli in the terminal respiratory unit of man during late intrauterine life and childhood. *Arch Dis Child* 1960;35:544–549.
160. Askenazi SS, Perlman M. Pulmonary hypoplasia: lung weight and radial alveolar count as criteria of diagnosis. *Arch Dis Child* 1979;54(8): 614–618.
161. Thurlbeck WM. Post-mortem lung volumes. *Thorax* 1979;34(6): 735–739.
162. Gerards FA, Twisk JW, Fetter WP, et al. Two- or three-dimensional ultrasonography to predict pulmonary hypoplasia in pregnancies complicated by preterm premature rupture of the membranes. *Prenat Diagn* 2007;27(3):216–221.
163. Ruano R, Martinovic J, Aubry MC, et al. Predicting pulmonary hypoplasia using the sonographic fetal lung volume to body weight ratio–how precise and accurate is it? *Ultrasound Obstet Gynecol* 2006;28(7):958–962.
164. Page DV, Stocker JT. Anomalies associated with pulmonary hypoplasia. *Am Rev Respir Dis* 1982;125(2):216–221.
165. Rodriguez LM, Garcia-Garcia I, Correa-Rivas MS, et al. Pulmonary hypoplasia in Jarcho-Levin syndrome. *P R Health Sci J* 2004;23(1): 65–67.
166. Odd DE, Battin MR, Hallam L, et al. Primary pulmonary hypoplasia: a case report and review of the literature. *J Paediatr Child Health* 2003;39(6):467–469.
167. Cregg N, Casey W. Primary congenital pulmonary hypoplasia–genetic component to aetiology. *Paediatr Anaesth* 1997;7(4):329–333.
168. Vergani P, Locatelli A, Strobelt N, et al. Amnioinfusion for prevention of pulmonary hypoplasia in second- trimester rupture of membranes. *Am J Perinatol* 1997;14(6):325–329.
169. Green RA, Shaw DG, Haworth SG. Familial pulmonary hypoplasia: plain film appearances with histopathological correlation. *Pediatr Radiol* 1999;29(6):455–458.
170. Cooney TP, Thurlbeck WM. The radial alveolar count method of Emery and Mithal: a reappraisal 2–intrauterine and early postnatal lung growth. *Thorax* 1982;37(8):580–583.
171. Aslan AT, Yalcin E, Ozcelik U, et al. Foreign-body aspiration mimicking congenital lobar emphysema in a forty-eight-day-old girl. *Pediatr Pulmonol* 2005;39(2):189–191.
172. Clubley E, England RJ, Cullinane C, et al. Ball valve obstruction of a bronchus causing lobar emphysema in a neonate. *Pediatr Surg Int* 2007;23(7):699–702.
173. Seo T, Ando H, Kaneko K, et al. Two cases of prenatally diagnosed congenital lobar emphysema caused by lobar bronchial atresia. *J Pediatr Surg* 2006;41(11):e17–e20.
174. Wall MA, Eisenberg JD, Campbell JR. Congenital lobar emphysema in a mother and daughter. *Pediatrics* 1982;70(1):131–133.
175. Roberts PA, Holland AJ, Halliday RJ, et al. Congenital lobar emphysema: Like father, like son. *J Pediatr Surg* 2002;37(5):799–801.
176. Karnak I, Senocak ME, Ciftci AO, et al. Congenital lobar emphysema: diagnostic and therapeutic considerations. *J Pediatr Surg* 1999;34(9):1347–1351.
177. Moideen I, Nair SG, Cherian A, et al. Congenital lobar emphysema associated with congenital heart disease. *J Cardiothorac Vasc Anesth* 2006;20(2):239–241.
178. Gordon I, Dempsey JE. Infantile lobar emphysema in association with congenital heart disease. *Clin Radiol* 1990;41(1):48–52.
179. Ozcelik U, Gocmen A, Kiper N, et al. Congenital lobar emphysema: evaluation and long-term follow-up of thirty cases at a single center. *Pediatr Pulmonol* 2003;35(5):384–391.
180. Ekkelkamp S, Vos A. Successful surgical treatment of a newborn with bilateral congenital lobar emphysema. *J Pediatr Surg* 1987;22(11):1001–1002.
181. Miller KE, Edwards DK, Hilton S, et al. Acquired lobar emphysema in premature infants with bronchopulmonary dysplasia: an iatrogenic disease? *Radiology* 1981;138(3):589–592.
182. Giudici R, Leao LE, Moura LA, et al. Polyalveolosis: pathogenesis of congenital lobar emphysema?. *Rev Assoc Med Bras* 1998;44(2):99–105.
183. Cleveland RH, Weber B. Retained fetal lung liquid in congenital lobar emphysema: a possible predictor of polyalveolar lobe. *Pediatr Radiol* 1993;23(4):291–295.
184. Bellini C, Boccardo F, Campisi C, et al. Congenital pulmonary lymphangiectasia. *Orphanet J Rare Dis* 2006;1:43.
185. Bellini C, Mazzella M, Arioni C, et al. Hennekam syndrome presenting as nonimmune hydrops fetalis, congenital chylothorax, and congenital pulmonary lymphangiectasia. *Am J Med Genet* 2003;120A(1):92–96.
186. Nobre LF, Muller NL, de Souza Junior AS, et al. Congenital pulmonary lymphangiectasia: CT and pathologic findings. *J Thorac Imaging* 2004;19(1):56–59.
187. Dempsey EM, Sant'Anna GM, Williams RL, et al. Congenital pulmonary lymphangiectasia presenting as nonimmune fetal hydrops and severe respiratory distress at birth: not uniformly fatal. *Pediatr Pulmonol* 2005;40(3):270–274.
188. Scott-Emuakpor AB, Warren ST, Kapur S, et al. Familial occurrence of congenital pulmonary lymphangiectasis. Genetic implications. *Am J Dis Child* 1981;135(6):532–534.
189. Rettwitz-Volk W, Schlosser R, Ahrens P, et al. Congenital unilobar pulmonary lymphangiectasis. *Pediatr Pulmonol* 1999;27(4): 290–292.
190. Stocker JT. Congenital pulmonary airway malformation—a new name for and an expanded classification of congenital cystic adenomatoid malformation of the lung. *Histopathology* 2002;41(suppl. 2): 424–430.
191. Rutledge JC, Jensen P. Acinar dysplasia: a new form of pulmonary maldevelopment. *Hum Pathol* 1986;17(12):1290–1293.
192. Stocker JT. Congenital and developmental diseases. In: Tomashefski JF, Jr, ed. *Dail and Hammer's Pulmonary Pathology*, 3rd ed. New York: Springer, 2008:132–175.
193. Ota H, Langston C, Honda T, et al. Histochemical analysis of mucous cells of congenital adenomatoid malformation of the lung: insights into the carcinogenesis of pulmonary adenocarcinoma expressing gastric mucins. *Am J Clin Pathol* 1998;110(4):450–455.
194. Wang NS, Chen MF, Chen FF. The glandular component in congenital cystic adenomatoid malformation of the lung. *Respirology* 1999;4(2):147–153.
195. Benjamin DR, Cahill JL. Bronchioloalveolar carcinoma of the lung and congenital cystic adenomatoid malformation. *Am J Clin Pathol* 1991;95(6):889–892.
196. Abecasis F, Gomes Ferreira M, Oliveira A, et al. Bronchioloalveolar carcinoma associated with congenital pulmonary airway malformation in an asymptomatic adolescent. *Rev Port Pneumol* 2008;14(2):285–290.
197. Barlesi F, Doddoli C, Gimenez C, et al. Bronchioloalveolar carcinoma: myths and realities in the surgical management. *Eur J Cardiothorac Surg* 2003;24(1):159–164.
198. Guo H, Cajaiba MM, Borys D, et al. Expression of epidermal growth factor receptor, but not K-RAS mutations, is present in congenital cystic airway malformation/congenital pulmonary airway malformation. *Hum Pathol* 2007;38(12):1772–1778.

199. Ioachimescu OC, Mehta AC. From cystic pulmonary airway malformation, to bronchioloalveolar carcinoma and adenocarcinoma of the lung. *Eur Respir J* 2005;26(6):1181–1187.
200. Mani H, Shilo K, Galvin JR, et al. Spectrum of precursor and invasive neoplastic lesions in type 1 congenital pulmonary airway malformation: case report and review of the literature. *Histopathology* 2007;51(4):561–565.
201. Orpen N, Goodman R, Bowker C, et al. Intralobar pulmonary sequestration with congenital cystic adematous malformation and rhabdomyomatous dysplasia. *Pediatr Surg Int* 2003;19(8):610–611.
202. Lienicke U, Hammer H, Schneider M, et al. Rhabdomyomatous dysplasia of the newborn lung associated with multiple congenital malformations of the heart and great vessels. *Pediatr Pulmonol* 2002;34(3):222–225.
203. Drut RM, Quijano G, Drut R, et al. Rhabdomyomatous dysplasia of the lung. *Pediatr Pathol* 1988;8(4):385–390.
204. Sherer DM, Abramowicz JS, Metlay LA, et al. Nonimmune fetal hydrops caused by bilateral type III congenital cystic adenomatoid malformation of the lung at 17 weeks' gestation. *Am J Obstet Gynecol* 1992;167(2):503–505.
205. Journel H, Le Guern H, Le Goff JL. Congenital cystic adenomatoid malformation of the lung and alpha fetoprotein. *Clin Genet* 1988;34(5):344.
206. Calderwood G, Nguyen DL, Leonard JC. Hepatoblastoma. *Clin Nucl Med* 1986;11(12):880–881.
207. Ch'in KY, Tang MY. Congenital adenomatoid malformation of one lobe of a lung with general anasarca. *Arch Path* 1949;48:221–225.
208. Azizkhan RG, Crombleholme TM. Congenital cystic lung disease: contemporary antenatal and postnatal management. *Pediatr Surg Int* 2008;24(6):643–657.
209. Fine C, Adzick NS, Doubilet PM. Decreasing size of a congenital cystic adenomatoid malformation in utero. *J Ultrasound Med* 1988;7(7):405–408.
210. Stocker JT, Madewell JE, Drake RM. Congenital cystic adenomatoid malformation of the lung. Classification and morphologic spectrum. *Hum Pathol* 1977;8(2):155–171.
211. West D, Nicholson AG, Colquhoun I, et al. Bronchioloalveolar carcinoma in congenital cystic adenomatoid malformation of lung. *Ann Thorac Surg* 2007;83(2):687–689.
212. Ramos SG, Barbosa GH, Tavora FR, et al. Bronchioloalveolar carcinoma arising in a congenital pulmonary airway malformation in a child: case report with an update of this association. *J Pediatr Surg* 2007;42(5):E1–E4.
213. Fisher JE, Nelson SJ, Allen JE, et al. Congenital cystic adenomatoid malformation of the lung. A unique variant. *Am J Dis Child* 1982;136(12):1071–1074.
214. Janney CG, Askin FB, Kuhn C, III. Congenital alveolar capillary dysplasia–an unusual cause of respiratory distress in the newborn. *Am J Clin Pathol* 1981;76(5):722–727.
215. Eulmesekian P, Cutz E, Parvez B, et al. Alveolar capillary dysplasia: a six-year single center experience. *J Perinat Med* 2005;33(4): 347–352.
216. Gutierrez C, Rodriguez A, Palenzuela S, et al. Congenital misalignment of pulmonary veins with alveolar capillary dysplasia causing persistent neonatal pulmonary hypertension: report of two affected siblings [In Process Citation]. *Pediatr Dev Pathol* 2000;3(3):271–276.
217. Pasutto F, Sticht H, Hammersen G, et al. Mutations in STRA6 cause a broad spectrum of malformations including anophthalmia, congenital heart defects, diaphragmatic hernia, alveolar capillary dysplasia, lung hypoplasia, and mental retardation. *Am J Hum Genet.* 2007;80(3): 550–560.
218. Chalabreysse L, Allias F, Bourgeois J, et al. Alveolar capillary dysplasia with misalignment of pulmonary vessels. *Ann Pathol* 2004; 24(4):349–355.
219. Pucci A, Zanini C, Ferrero F, et al. Misalignment of lung vessels: diagnostic role of conventional histology and immunohistochemistry. *Virchows Arch* 2003;442(6):597–600.
220. Farrow KN, Fliman P, Steinhorn RH. The diseases treated with ECMO: focus on PPHN. *Semin Perinatol* 2005;29(1):8–14.
221. Gonzalez OR, Gomez IG, Recalde AL, et al. Postnatal development of the cystic lung lesion of Down syndrome: suggestion that the cause is reduced formation of peripheral air spaces. *Pediatr Pathol* 1991;11(4):623–633.
222. Pinar H, Makarova N, Rubin LP, et al. Pathology of the lung in surfactant-treated neonates. *Pediatr Pathol* 1994;14(4):627–636.
223. Seo IS, Gillim SE, Mirkin LD. Hyaline membranes in postmature infants. *Pediatr Pathol* 1990;10(4):539–548.
224. Shaw NJ, Kotecha S. Management of infants with chronic lung disease of prematurity in the United Kingdom. *Early Hum Dev* 2005;81(2):165–170.
225. Toti P, Buonocore G, Rinaldi G, et al. Pulmonary pathology in surfactant-treated preterm infants with respiratory distress syndrome: an autopsy study. *Biol Neonate* 1996;70(1):21–28.
226. Gonda TA, Hutchins GM. Surfactant treatment may accelerate epithelial cell regeneration in hyaline membrane disease of the newborn. *Am J Perinatol* 1998;15(9):539–544.
227. Northway WH, Jr., Rosan RC, Porter DY. Pulmonary disease following respirator therapy of hyaline-membrane disease. Bronchopulmonary dysplasia. *N Engl J Med* 1967;276(7):357–368.
228. Bonikos D, Bensch K, Northway WJ. Oxygen toxicity in the newborn. The effect of chronic continuous 100 percent oxygen exposure on the lungs of newborn mice. *Am J Pathol* 1976;85:623–650.
229. Hislop AA. Bronchopulmonary dysplasia: pre- and postnatal influences and outcome. *Pediatr Pulmonol* 1997;23(2):71–75.
230. Bonikos DS, Bensch KG, Northway WH, Jr., et al. Bronchopulmonary dysplasia: the pulmonary pathologic sequel of necrotizing bronchiolitis and pulmonary fibrosis. *Hum Pathol* 1976;7(6):643–666.
231. Sobonya RE, Logvinoff MM, Taussig LM, et al. Morphometric analysis of the lung in prolonged bronchopulmonary dysplasia. *Pediatr Res* 1982;16(11):969–972.
232. Margraf LR, Tomashefski JF, Jr., Bruce MC, et al. Morphometric analysis of the lung in bronchopulmonary dysplasia. *Am Rev Respir Dis* 1991;143(2):391–400.
233. Husain AN, Siddiqui NH, Stocker JT. Pathology of arrested acinar development in postsurfactant bronchopulmonary dysplasia. *Hum Pathol* 1998;29(7):710–717.
234. Walsh MC, Yao Q, Horbar JD, et al. Changes in the use of postnatal steroids for bronchopulmonary dysplasia in 3 large neonatal networks. *Pediatrics* 2006;118(5):e1328–e1335.
235. Wegner DJ, Hertzberg T, Heins HB, et al. A major deletion in the surfactant protein-B gene causing lethal respiratory distress. *Acta Paediatr* 2007;96(4):516–520.
236. Somaschini M, Nogee LM, Sassi I, et al. Unexplained neonatal respiratory distress due to congenital surfactant deficiency. *J Pediatr* 2007;150(6):649–653, 653 e641.
237. Brasch F, Schimanski S, Muhlfeld C, et al. Alteration of the pulmonary surfactant system in full-term infants with hereditary ABCA3 deficiency. *Am J Respir Crit Care Med* 2006;174(5):571–580.
238. Stuhrmann M, Bohnhorst B, Peters U, et al. Prenatal diagnosis of congenital alveolar proteinosis (surfactant protein B deficiency). *Prenat Diagn* 1998;18(9):953–955.
239. Hamvas A, Nogee LM, Mallory GB, Jr., et al. Lung transplantation for treatment of infants with surfactant protein B deficiency. *J Pediatr* 1997;130(2):231–239.
240. Aneja MK, Rudolph C. Gene therapy of surfactant protein B deficiency. *Curr Opin Mol Ther* 2006;8(5):432–438.
241. Kattan AK, Bulagannawar PS, Malik IH. Congenital alveolar proteinosis. *Saudi Med J* 2004;25(10):1474–1477.
242. Tryka AF, Wert SE, Mazursky JE, et al. Absence of lamellar bodies with accumulation of dense bodies characterizes a novel form of congenital surfactant defect. *Pediatr Dev Pathol* 2000;3(4):335–345.
243. McAdams RM. Risk factors and clinical outcomes of pulmonary interstitial emphysema in extremely low birth weight infants. *J Perinatol* 2006;26(8):521–522; author reply 522–523.

244. O'Donovan D, Wearden M, Adams J. Unilateral pulmonary interstitial emphysema following pneumonia in a preterm infant successfully treated with prolonged selective bronchial intubation. *Am J Perinatol* 1999;16(7):327–331.
245. Stocker JT, Madewell JE. Persistent interstitial pulmonary emphysema: another complication of the respiratory distress syndrome. *Pediatrics* 1977;59(6):847–857.
246. Rastogi S, Gupta A, Wung JT, et al. Treatment of giant pulmonary interstitial emphysema by ipsilateral bronchial occlusion with a Swan-Ganz catheter. *Pediatr Radiol* 2007;37(11):1130–1134.
247. Demura Y, Ishizaki T, Nakanishi M, et al. Persistent diffuse pulmonary interstitial emphysema mimicking pulmonary emphysema. *Thorax* 2007;62(7):652.
248. Chalak LF, Kaiser JR, Arrington RW. Resolution of pulmonary interstitial emphysema following selective left main stem intubation in a premature newborn: an old procedure revisited. *Paediatr Anaesth* 2007;17(2):183–186.
249. Wigglesworth JS, Desai R, Hislop AA. Fetal lung growth in congenital laryngeal atresia. *Pediatr Pathol* 1987;7(5–6):515–525.
250. Wiswell TE, Tuggle JM, Turner BS. Meconium aspiration syndrome: have we made a difference? [see comments]. *Pediatrics* 1990;85(5):715–721.
251. Wiswell TE, Gannon CM, Jacob J, et al. Delivery room management of the apparently vigorous meconium-stained neonate: results of the multicenter, international collaborative trial. *Pediatrics* 2000;105(1 Pt 1):1–7.
252. Lam BC, Yeung CY. Surfactant lavage for meconium aspiration syndrome: a pilot study. *Pediatrics* 1999;103(5 Pt 1):1014–1018.
253. Oguz F, Citak A, Unuvar E, et al. Airway foreign bodies in childhood. *Int J Pediatr Otorhinolaryngol* 2000;52(1):11–16.
254. Baharloo F, Veyckemans F, Francis C, et al. Tracheobronchial foreign bodies: presentation and management in children and adults. *Chest* 1999;115(5):1357–1362.
255. Sebire NJ, Ramsay AD, Malone M. Histopathological features of open lung biopsies in children treated with extracorporeal membrane oxygenation (ECMO). *Early Hum Dev* 2005;81(5):455–460.
256. Chou P, Blei ED, Shen-Schwarz S, et al. Pulmonary changes following extracorporeal membrane oxygenation: autopsy study of 23 cases. *Hum Pathol* 1993;24(4):405–412.
257. Hamutcu R, Nield TA, Garg M, et al. Long-term pulmonary sequelae in children who were treated with extracorporeal membrane oxygenation for neonatal respiratory failure. *Pediatrics* 2004;114(5):1292–1296.
258. Young TL, Quinn GE, Baumgart S, et al. Extracorporeal membrane oxygenation causing asymmetric vasculopathy in neonatal infants. *J AAPOS* 1997;1(4):235–240.
259. Jarjour IT, Ahdab-Barmada M. Cerebrovascular lesions in infants and children dying after extracorporeal membrane oxygenation. *Pediatr Neurol* 1994;10(1):13–19.
260. Lewis MJ, McKeever PK, Rutty GN. Patent ductus arteriosus as a natural cause of pulmonary hemorrhage in infants: a medicolegal dilemma. *Am J Forensic Med Pathol* 2004;25(3):200–204.
261. Kreindler J, Ellis D, Vats A, et al. Infantile systemic lupus erythematosus presenting with pulmonary hemorrhage. *Pediatr Nephrol* 2005;20(4):522–525.
262. Godfrey S. Pulmonary hemorrhage/hemoptysis in children. *Pediatr Pulmonol* 2004;37(6):476–484.
263. Coffin CM, Schechtman K, Cole FS, et al. Neonatal and infantile pulmonary hemorrhage: an autopsy study with clinical correlation. *Pediatr Pathol* 1993;13(5):583–589.
264. Cetin H, Yalaz M, Akisu M, et al. The use of recombinant activated factor VII in the treatment of massive pulmonary hemorrhage in a preterm infant. *Blood Coagul Fibrinolysis* 2006;17(3):213–216.
265. Veeraraghavan S, Koss MN, Sharma OP. Pulmonary veno-occlusive disease. *Curr Opin Pulm Med* 1999;5(5):310–313.
266. Swensen SJ, Tashjian JH, Myers JL, et al. Pulmonary venoocclusive disease: CT findings in eight patients. *AJR Am J Roentgenol* 1996;167(4):937–940.
267. Chazova I, Robbins I, Loyd J, et al. Venous and arterial changes in pulmonary veno-occlusive disease, mitral stenosis and fibrosing mediastinitis. *Eur Respir J* 2000;15(1):116–122.
268. Frazier AA, Franks TJ, Mohammed TL, et al. From the Archives of the AFIP: pulmonary veno-occlusive disease and pulmonary capillary hemangiomatosis. *Radiographics* 2007;27(3):867–882.
269. Alam S, Chan KM. Noninfectious pulmonary complications after organ transplantation. *Curr Opin Pulm Med* 1996;2(5):412–418.
270. Lantuejoul S, Sheppard MN, Corrin B, et al. Pulmonary veno-occlusive disease and pulmonary capillary hemangiomatosis: a clinicopathologic study of 35 cases. *Am J Surg Pathol* 2006;30(7):850–857.
271. Thapa R, Ganguly D, Ghosh A. Pulmonary alveolar microlithiasis in siblings. *Indian Pediatr* 2008;45(2):154–156.
272. Marchiori E, Goncalves CM, Escuissato DL, et al. Pulmonary alveolar microlithiasis: high-resolution computed tomography findings in 10 patients. *J Bras Pneumol* 2007;33(5):552–557.
273. Al-Alawi AS. Familial occurrence of pulmonary alveolar microlithiasis in 3 siblings. *Saudi Med J* 2006;27(2):238–240.
274. Kiper N, Gocmen A, Ozcelik U, et al. Long-term clinical course of patients with idiopathic pulmonary hemosiderosis (1979-1994): prolonged survival with low-dose corticosteroid therapy. *Pediatr Pulmonol* 1999;27(3):180–184.
275. Salih ZN, Akhter A, Akhter J. Specificity and sensitivity of hemosiderin-laden macrophages in routine bronchoalveolar lavage in children. *Arch Pathol Lab Med* 2006;130(11):1684–1686.
276. Cohen S. Idiopathic pulmonary hemosiderosis. *Am J Med Sci* 1999; 317(1):67–74.
277. Khemiri M, Ouederni M, Khaldi F, et al. Screening for celiac disease in idiopathic pulmonary hemosiderosis. *Gastroenterol Clin Biol* 2008;32(8–9):745–748.
278. Hammami S, Ghedira Besbes L, Hadded S, et al. Co-occurrence pulmonary haemosiderosis with coeliac disease in child. *Respir Med* 2008;102(6):935–936.
279. Omori CH, Jesus AA, Sallum AM, et al. Association between pulmonary hemosiderosis and juvenile dermatomyositis. *Acta Reumatol Port* 2009;34(2A):271–275.
280. Saeed MM, Woo MS, MacLaughlin EF, et al. Prognosis in pediatric idiopathic pulmonary hemosiderosis. *Chest* 1999;116(3):721–725.
281. Luo XQ, Ke ZY, Huang LB, et al. Maintenance therapy with dose-adjusted 6-mercaptopurine in idiopathic pulmonary hemosiderosis. *Pediatr Pulmonol* 2008;43(11):1067–1071.
282. Chen CH, Yang HB, Chiang SR, et al. Idiopathic pulmonary hemosiderosis: favorable response to corticosteroids. *J Chin Med Assoc* 2008;71(8):421–424.
283. Milman N, Pedersen FM. Idiopathic pulmonary haemosiderosis. Epidemiology, pathogenic aspects and diagnosis. *Respir Med* 1998;92(7):902–907.
284. Corrin B, Jagusch M, Dewar A, et al. Fine structural changes in idiopathic pulmonary haemosiderosis. *J Pathol* 1987;153(3):249–256.
285. Cutz E. Idiopathic pulmonary hemosiderosis and related disorders in infancy and childhood. *Perspect Pediatr Pathol* 1987;11:47–81.
286. Stocker JT, Conran RM, Fishback N. Respiratory syncytial virus. In: Conner DH, Chandler FW, eds. *Pathology of Infectious Diseases,* vol 1. Stanford, CT: Appleton & Lange, 1997:287–295.
287. Jeena PM, Bobat B, Thula SA, et al. Children with Pneumocystis jiroveci pneumonia and acute hypoxaemic respiratory failure admitted to a PICU, Durban, South Africa. *Arch Dis Child* 2008;93(6):545.
288. von Renesse A, Schildgen O, Klinkenberg D, et al. Respiratory syncytial virus infection in children admitted to hospital but ventilated mechanically for other reasons. *J Med Virol* 2009;81(1):160–166.
289. Thorburn K. Pre-existing disease is associated with a significantly higher risk of death in severe respiratory syncytial virus infection. *Arch Dis Child* 2009;94(2):99–103.
290. Neilson KA, Yunis EJ. Demonstration of respiratory syncytial virus in an autopsy series. *Pediatr Pathol* 1990;10(4):491–502.
291. Rosenberg HF, Dyer KD, Domachowske JB. Respiratory viruses and eosinophils: exploring the connections. *Antiviral Res* 2009;83(1):1–9.

292. Wolf BC, Lavezzi WA. Pulmonary interstitial emphysema and live birth. *Am J Forensic Med Pathol* 2008;29(4):382.
293. Zhang SX, Tellier R, Zafar R, et al. Comparison of human metapneumovirus infection with respiratory syncytial virus infection in children. *Pediatr Infect Dis J* 2009;28(11):1022–1024.
294. Vargas SO, Kozakewich HP, Perez-Atayde AR, et al. Pathology of human metapneumovirus infection: insights into the pathogenesis of a newly identified respiratory virus. *Pediatr Dev Pathol* 2004;7(5):478–486; discussion 421.
295. Spencer MJ, Cherry JD. Adenoviral infections. In: Feigin RD, Cherry JD, eds. *Textbook of Pediatric Infectious Diseases*, 2nd ed. Philadelphia: WB Saunders, 1987:1688.
296. Mauad T, Dolhnikoff M. Histology of childhood bronchiolitis obliterans. *Pediatr Pulmonol* 2002;33(6):466–474.
297. Murtagh P, Kajon A. Chronic pulmonary sequelae of adenovirus infection. *Pediatr Pulmonol Suppl* 1997;16:150–151.
298. Vaideeswar P, Bavdekar SB, Jadhav SM, et al. Necrotizing adenoviral pneumonia: manifestation of nosocomial infection in pediatric intensive care unit. *Indian J Pediatr* 2008;75(11):1171–1174.
299. Hughes WT. Pneumonia in the immunocompromised child. *Semin Respir Infect* 1987;2(3):177–183.
300. Griffin M, Pushpanathan C, Andrews W. Chlamydia trachomatis pneumonitis: a case study and literature review. *Pediatr Pathol* 1990;10(5):843–852.
301. Godding V, Bodart E, Delos M, et al. Mechanisms of acute eosinophilic inflammation in a case of acute eosinophilic pneumonia in a 14-year-old girl. *Clin Exp Allergy* 1998;28(4):504–509.
302. Khemiri M, Ouederni M, Ben Mansour F, et al. Acute respiratory failure revealing an idiopathic acute eosinophilic pneumonia: report of a pediatric case. *Ann Fr Anesth Reanim* 2008;27(6):502–504.
303. Maeno T, Maeno Y, Sando Y, et al. Nuclear hypersegmentation precedes the increase in blood eosinophils in acute eosinophilic pneumonia. *Intern Med* 2000;39(2):157–159.
304. Dail DH. Eosinophilic infiltrates. In: Dail DH, Hammer SP, eds. *Pulmonary Pathology,* 2nd ed. New York: Springer-Verlag, 1994: 537–566.
305. Wubbel C, Fulmer D, Sherman J. Chronic eosinophilic pneumonia: a case report and national survey. *Chest* 2003;123(5):1763–1766.
306. Deutsch GH, Young LR, Deterding RR, et al. Diffuse lung disease in young children: application of a novel classification scheme. *Am J Respir Crit Care Med* 2007;176(11):1120–1128.
307. Deterding RR, Pye C, Fan LL, et al. Persistent tachypnea of infancy is associated with neuroendocrine cell hyperplasia. *Pediatr Pulmonol* 2005;40(2):157–165.
308. Canakis AM, Cutz E, Manson D, et al. Pulmonary interstitial glycogenosis: a new variant of neonatal interstitial lung disease. *Am J Respir Crit Care Med* 2002;165(11):1557–1565.
309. Deutsch GH, Young LR. Histologic Resolution of Pulmonary Interstitial Glycogenosis. *Pediatr Dev Pathol* 2009;12(6):475–480.
310. Stocker JT, Husain AN, Dehner LP. Pediatric tumors. In: Tomashefski JF, Jr, ed. *Dail and Hammer's Pulmonary Pathology*, vol II, 3rd ed. New York: Springer, 2008:542–557.
311. Hartman GE, Schochat SJ. Primary pulmonary neoplasms of childhood: A review. *Ann Thorac Surg* 1983;1983:108.
312. Hancock BJ, Di Lorenzo M, Youssef S, et al. Childhood primary pulmonary neoplasms. *J Pediatr Surg* 1993;28(9):1133–1136.
313. Dishop MK, Kuruvilla S. Primary and metastatic lung tumors in the pediatric population: a review and 25-year experience at a large children's hospital. *Arch Pathol Lab Med* 2008;132(7):1079–1103.
314. Agrons GA, Rosado-de-Christenson ML, Kirejczyk WM, et al. Pulmonary inflammatory pseudotumor: radiologic features. *Radiology* 1998;206(2):511–518.
315. Monzon CM, Gilchrist GS, Burgert EO, Jr., et al. Plasma cell granuloma of the lung in children. *Pediatrics* 1982;70(2):268–274.
316. Su LD, Atayde-Perez A, Sheldon S, et al. Inflammatory myofibroblastic tumor: cytogenetic evidence supporting clonal origin. *Mod Pathol* 1998;11(4):364–368.
317. Travis W, Dehner L, Manabe T, et al. Congenital peribronchial myofibroblastic tumour. In: Travis W, Brambilla E, Muller-Hermelink H, et al., eds. *Pathology and Genetics of the Lung, Pleura, Thymus and Heart. World Health Classification of Tumours*. Lyon: IARC Press, 2004:102–103.
318. Griffin CA, Hawkins AL, Dvorak C, et al. Recurrent involvement of 2p23 in inflammatory myofibroblastic tumors. *Cancer Res* 1999;59(12): 2776–2780.
319. Cook JR, Dehner LP, Collins MH, et al. Anaplastic lymphoma kinase (ALK) expression in the inflammatory myofibroblastic tumor: a comparative immunohistochemical study. *Am J Surg Pathol* 2001;25(11): 1364–1371.
320. Chan JK, Cheuk W, Shimizu M. Anaplastic lymphoma kinase expression in inflammatory pseudotumors. *Am J Surg Pathol* 2001;25(6): 761–768.
321. Gomez-Roman JJ, Sanchez-Velasco P, Ocejo-Vinyals G, et al. Human herpesvirus-8 genes are expressed in pulmonary inflammatory myofibroblastic tumor (inflammatory pseudotumor). *Am J Surg Pathol* 2001;25(5):624–629.
322. Tavora F, Shilo K, Ozbudak IH, et al. Absence of human herpesvirus-8 in pulmonary inflammatory myofibroblastic tumor: immunohistochemical and molecular analysis of 20 cases. *Mod Pathol* 2007;20(9):995–999.
323. Arber DA, Kamel OW, van de Rijn M, et al. Frequent presence of the Epstein-Barr virus in inflammatory pseudotumor. *Hum Pathol* 1995;26(10):1093–1098.
324. Morotti RA, Legman MD, Kerkar N, et al. Pediatric inflammatory myofibroblastic tumor with late metastasis to the lung: case report and review of the literature. *Pediatr Dev Pathol* 2005;8(2):224–229.
325. Coffin CM, Hornick JL, Fletcher CD. Inflammatory myofibroblastic tumor: comparison of clinicopathologic, histologic, and immunohistochemical features including ALK expression in atypical and aggressive cases. *Am J Surg Pathol* 2007;31(4):509–520.
326. Storck M, Liewald F, Heymer B, et al. Inflammatory pseudotumors of the lung and trachea. *Zentralbl Chir* 1995;120(8):650–656.
327. Sivanandan S, Lodha R, Agarwala S, et al. Inflammatory myofibroblastic tumor of the trachea. *Pediatr Pulmonol* 2007;42(9): 847–850.
328. Kim TS, Han J, Kim GY, et al. Pulmonary inflammatory pseudotumor (inflammatory myofibroblastic tumor): CT features with pathologic correlation. *J Comput Assist Tomogr* 2005;29(5):633–639.
329. Dehner L. Inflammatory myofibroblastic tumor: the continued definition of one type of so-called inflammatory pseudotumor. *Am J Surg Pathol* 2004;28:1652–1654.
330. Mergan F, Jaubert F, Sauvat F, et al. Inflammatory myofibroblastic tumor in children: clinical review with anaplastic lymphoma kinase, Epstein-Barr virus, and human herpesvirus 8 detection analysis. *J Pediatr Surg* 2005;40(10):1581–1586.
331. Chun YS, Wang L, Nascimento AG, et al. Pediatric inflammatory myofibroblastic tumor: Anaplastic lymphoma kinase (ALK) expression and prognosis. *Pediatr Blood Cancer* 2005;45(6):796–801.
332. Chan YF, White J, Brash H. Metachronous pulmonary and cerebral inflammatory pseudotumor in a child. *Pediatr Pathol* 1994;14(5): 805–815.
333. Janik JS, Janik JP, Lovell MA, et al. Recurrent inflammatory pseudotumors in children. *J Pediatr Surg* 2003;38(10):1491–1495.
334. Hedlund GL, Navoy JF, Galliani CA, et al. Aggressive manifestations of inflammatory pulmonary pseudotumor in children. *Pediatr Radiol* 1999;29(2):112–116.
335. Kruscic D, Peco-Antic A, Spasojevic-Dimitrijeva B, et al. Pulmonary inflammatory myofibroblastic tumor associated with nephrotic syndrome. *Pediatr Nephrol* 2007;22(10):1785–1786.
336. Ozbudak IH, Dertsiz L, Bassorgun CI, et al. Giant cystic chondroid hamartoma of the lung. *J Pediatr Surg* 2008;43(10):1909–1911.
337. Carney JA. Gastric stromal sarcoma, pulmonary chondroma, and extra-adrenal paraganglioma (Carney Triad): natural history, adrenocortical component, and possible familial occurrence [see comments]. *Mayo Clin Proc* 1999;74(6):543–552.

338. Bagan P, Hassan M, Le Pimpec Barthes F, et al. Prognostic factors and surgical indications of pulmonary epithelioid hemangioendothelioma: a review of the literature. *Ann Thorac Surg* 2006;82(6):2010–2013.
339. Baghai-Wadji M, Sianati M, Nikpour H, et al. Pleomorphic adenoma of the trachea in an 8-year-old boy: a case report. *J Pediatr Surg* 2006;41(8):e23–e26.
340. Somers GR, Tabrizi SN, Borg AJ, et al. Juvenile laryngeal papillomatosis in a pediatric population: a clinicopathologic study. *Pediatr Pathol Lab Med* 1997;17(1):53–64.
341. Wiatrak BJ, Wiatrak DW, Broker TR, et al. Recurrent respiratory papillomatosis: a longitudinal study comparing severity associated with human papilloma viral types 6 and 11 and other risk factors in a large pediatric population. *Laryngoscope* 2004;114(11 Pt 2 Suppl 104):1–23.
342. Andrews SE. Laser ablation of recurrent laryngeal papillomas in children. *Aorn J* 1995;61(3):532–540, 543–534.
343. Chmielik M, Piekarniak P, Snieg B. Microsurgical treatment of laryngeal papillomatosis. *Otolaryngol Pol* 1997;51(1):26–30.
344. Kramer SS, Wehunt WD, Stocker JT, et al. Pulmonary manifestations of juvenile laryngotracheal papillomatosis. *AJR Am J Roentgenol* 1985;144(4):687–694.
345. Gelinas JF, Manoukian J, Cote A. Lung involvement in juvenile onset recurrent respiratory papillomatosis: a systematic review of the literature. *Int J Pediatr Otorhinolaryngol* 2008;72(4):433–452.
346. Lie ES, Engh V, Boysen M, et al. Squamous cell carcinoma of the respiratory tract following laryngeal papillomatosis. *Acta Otolaryngol* 1994;114(2):209–212.
347. Simma B, Burger R, Uehlinger J, et al. Squamous-cell carcinoma arising in a non-irradiated child with recurrent respiratory papillomatosis. *Eur J Pediatr* 1993;152(9):776–778.
348. Dehner LP. Tumors and tumor-like lesion of the lung and chest wall in childhood:clinical and pathologic review. In: Stocker JT, ed. *Pediatric Pulmonary Disease*. Washington, D.C.: Hemisphere, 1989:207–267.
349. Keel SB, Bacha E, Mark EJ, et al. Primary pulmonary sarcoma: a clinicopathologic study of 26 cases. *Mod Pathol* 1999;12(12):1124–1131.
350. Hull MT, Gonzalez-Crussi F, Grosfeld JL. Multiple pulmonary fibroleiomyomatous hamartomata in childhood. *J Pediatr Surg* 1979;14(4):428–431.
351. Atluri S, Neville K, Davis M, et al. Epstein-Barr-associated leiomyomatosis and T-cell chimerism after haploidentical bone marrow transplantation for severe combined immunodeficiency disease. *J Pediatr Hematol Oncol* 2007;29(3):166–172.
352. Mark EJ. Mesenchymal cystic hamartoma of the lung. *N Engl J Med* 1986;315(20):1255–1259.
353. Leroyer C, Quiot JJ, Dewitte JD, et al. Mesenchymal cystic hamartoma of the lung. *Respiration* 1993;60(5):305–306.
354. Chadwick SL, Corrin B, Hansell DM, et al. Fatal haemorrhage from mesenchymal cystic hamartoma of the lung. *Eur Respir J* 1995;8(12):2182–2184.
355. Chida M, Minowa M, Eba S, et al. Mesenchymal cystic hamartoma of the lung: a rare cause of pneumothorax. *Gen Thorac Cardiovasc Surg* 2009;57(3):166–168.
356. Hedlund GL, Bisset GS, III, Bove KE. Malignant neoplasms arising in cystic hamartomas of the lung in childhood. *Radiology* 1989;173(1):77–79.
357. Tazelaar HD, Kerr D, Yousem SA, et al. Diffuse pulmonary lymphangiomatosis. *Hum Pathol* 1993;24(12):1313–1322.
358. Swensen SJ, Hartman TE, Mayo JR, et al. Diffuse pulmonary lymphangiomatosis: CT findings. *J Comput Assist Tomogr* 1995;19(3):348–352.
359. Manson D, Traubici J, Mei-Zahav M, et al. Pulmonary nodular opacities in children with hereditary hemorrhagic telangiectasia. *Pediatr Radiol* 2007;37(3):264–268.
360. Gora-Gebka M, Liberek A, Bako W, et al. The "sugar" clear cell tumor of the lung-clinical presentation and diagnostic difficulties of an unusual lung tumor in youth. *J Pediatr Surg* 2006;41(6):e27–e29.
361. Kavunkal AM, Pandiyan MS, Philip MA, et al. Large clear cell tumor of the lung mimicking malignant behavior. *Ann Thorac Surg* 2007;83(1):310–312.
362. Ciftci AO, Sanlialp I, Tanyel FC, et al. The association of pulmonary lymphangioleiomyomatosis with renal and hepatic angiomyolipomas in a prepubertal girl: a previously unreported entity. *Respiration* 2007;74(3):335–337.
363. Keylock JB, Galvin JR, Franks TJ. Sclerosing hemangioma of the lung. *Arch Pathol Lab Med* 2009;133(5):820–825.
364. Rodriguez-Soto J, Colby TV, Rouse RV. A critical examination of the immunophenotype of pulmonary sclerosing hemangioma. *Am J Surg Pathol* 2000;24(3):442–450.
365. Devouassoux-Shisheboran M, Hayashi T, Linnoila RI, et al. A clinicopathologic study of 100 cases of pulmonary sclerosing hemangioma with immunohistochemical studies: TTF-1 is expressed in both round and surface cells, suggesting an origin from primitive respiratory epithelium. *Am J Surg Pathol* 2000;24(7):906–916.
366. Lack EE, Harris GB, Eraklis AJ, et al. Primary bronchial tumors in childhood. A clinicopathologic study of six cases. *Cancer* 1983;51(3):492–497.
367. Short M, Dramis A, Ramani P, et al. Mediastinal and pulmonary infantile myofibromatosis: an unusual surgical presentation. *J Pediatr Surg* 2008;43(11):e29–e31.
368. Greif J, Schwarz Y, Sperber F, et al. Benign cystic teratoma simulating organized empyema. *Pediatr Pulmonol* 1997;23(4):310–313.
369. Tronc F, Conter C, Marec-Berard P, et al. Prognostic factors and long-term results of pulmonary metastasectomy for pediatric histologies. *Eur J Cardiothorac Surg* 2008;34(6):1240–1246.
370. Absalon MJ, McCarville MB, Liu T, et al. Pulmonary nodules discovered during the initial evaluation of pediatric patients with bone and soft-tissue sarcoma. *Pediatr Blood Cancer* 2008;50(6):1147–1153.
371. Longhi A, Bertoni F, Bacchini P, et al. Simultaneous osteosarcoma lung metastasis and second primary lung cancer. *J Pediatr Hematol Oncol* 2004;26(7):457–461.
372. Wang LT, Wilkins EW, Jr., Bode HH. Bronchial carcinoid tumors in pediatric patients. *Chest* 1993;103(5):1426–1428.
373. de Matos LL, Trufelli DC, das Neves-Pereira JC, et al. Cushing's syndrome secondary to bronchopulmonary carcinoid tumor: report of two cases and literature review. *Lung Cancer* 2006;53(3):381–386.
374. Fauroux B, Aynie V, Larroquet M, et al. Carcinoid and mucoepidermoid bronchial tumours in children. *Eur J Pediatr* 2005;164(12):748–752.
375. Shilo K, Foss RD, Franks TJ, et al. Pulmonary mucoepidermoid carcinoma with prominent tumor-associated lymphoid proliferation. *Am J Surg Pathol* 2005;29(3):407–411.
376. Chin CH, Huang CC, Lin MC, et al. Prognostic factors of tracheobronchial mucoepidermoid carcinoma–15 years experience. *Respirology* 2008;13(2):275–280.
377. Serra A, Schackert HK, Mohr B, et al. t(11;19)(q21;p12 p13.11) and MECT1-MAML2 fusion transcript expression as a prognostic marker in infantile lung mucoepidermoid carcinoma. *J Pediatr Surg* 2007;42(7):E23–E29.
378. Katz DR, Bubis JJ. Acinic cell tumor of the bronchus. *Cancer* 1976;38(2):830–832.
379. Sabaratnam R, Anunathan R, Govender D. Acinic cell carcinoma: an unusual case of bronchial obstruction in an child. *Pediatr Dev Pathol* 2004;7:521–526.
380. Rosenfeld A, Schwartz D, Garzon S, et al. Epithelial-myoepithelial carcinoma of the lung: a case report and review of the literature. *J Pediatr Hematol Oncol* 2009;31(3):206–208.
381. Laberge JM, Bratu I, Flageole H. The management of asymptomatic congenital lung malformations. *Paediatr Respir Rev* 2004;5 (Suppl A):S305–S312.
382. Lal D, Clark I, Shalkow J, et al. Primary epithelial lung malignancies in the pediatric population. *Pediatr Blood Cancer* 2005;44:1–4.

383. Kowalski P, Rodziewicz B, Pejcz J. Bilateral bronchioloalveolar carcinoma of the lungs in a 7 year old girl treated for Hodgkin's disease. *Tumori* 1989;75(5):449–451.
384. Travis WD, Linnoila RI, Horowitz M, et al. Pulmonary nodules resembling bronchioloalveolar carcinoma in adolescent cancer patients. *Mod Pathol* 1988;1(5):372–377.
385. Spaner SJ, Raymond G, Puttagunta L, et al. Bronchioloalveolar cell carcinoma in a child with hepatoblastoma: case report. *Can Assoc Radiol J* 1999;50(5):343–345.
386. Ohye RG, Cohen DM, Caldwell S, et al. Pediatric bronchioloalveolar carcinoma: a favorable pediatric malignancy? *J Pediatr Surg* 1998;33(5):730–732.
387. Park JA, Park HJ, Lee JS, et al. Adenocarcinoma of lung in never smoked children. *Lung Cancer* 2008;61(2):266–269.
388. Abuzetun JY, Hazin R, Suker M, et al. Primary squamous cell carcinoma of the lung with bony metastasis in a 13-year-old boy: case report and review of literature. *J Pediatr Hematol Oncol* 2008;30(8): 635–637.
389. Koss MN. Pulmonary blastomas. *Cancer Treat Res* 1995;72:349–362.
390. Manivel JC, Priest JR, Watterson J, et al. Pleuropulmonary blastoma. The so-called pulmonary blastoma of childhood. *Cancer* 1988;62(8):1516–1526.
391. Hartel PH, Fanburg-Smith JC, Frazier AA, et al. Primary pulmonary and mediastinal synovial sarcoma: a clinicopathologic study of 60 cases and comparison with five prior series. *Mod Pathol* 2007;20(7):760–769.
392. Muwakkit SA, Rodriguez-Galindo C, El Samra AI, et al. Primary malignant peripheral nerve sheath tumor of the lung in a young child without neurofibromatosis type 1. *Pediatr Blood Cancer* 2006;47(5):636–638.
393. McLeod AJ, Zornoza J, Shirkhoda A. Leiomyosarcoma: computed tomographic findings. *Radiology* 1984;152(1):133–136.
394. Sabatino D, Martinez S, Young R, et al. Simultaneous pulmonary leiomyosarcoma and leiomyoma in pediatric HIV infection. *Pediatr Hematol Oncol* 1991;8(4):355–359.
395. Pettinato G, Manivel JC, Saldana MJ, et al. Primary bronchopulmonary fibrosarcoma of childhood and adolescence: reassessment of a low-grade malignancy. Clinicopathologic study of five cases and review of the literature. *Hum Pathol* 1989;20(5):463–471.
396. Theron S, Andronikou S, Du Plessis J, et al. Pulmonary Kaposi sarcoma in six children. *Pediatr Radiol* 2007;37(12):1224–1229.
397. Schiavetti A, Dominici C, Matrunola M, et al. Primary pulmonary rhabdomyosarcoma in childhood: clinico-biologic features in two cases with review of the literature. *Med Pediatr Oncol* 1996;26(3): 201–207.
398. Priest JR, McDermott MB, Bhatia S, et al. Pleuropulmonary blastoma: a clinicopathologic study of 50 cases. *Cancer* 1997;80(1):147–161.
399. Hill DA, Sadeghi S, Schultz MZ, et al. Pleuropulmonary blastoma in an adult: an initial case report. *Cancer* 1999;85(11):2368–2374.
400. Priest JR, Watterson J, Strong L, et al. Pleuropulmonary blastoma: a marker for familial disease. *J Pediatr* 1996;128(2):220–224.
401. Delahunt B, Thomson KJ, Ferguson AF, et al. Familial cystic nephroma and pleuropulmonary blastoma [see comments]. *Cancer* 1993;71(4):1338–1342.
402. Kiziltepe TT, Patrick E, Alvarado C, et al. Pleuropulmonary blastoma and ovarian teratoma. *Pediatr Radiol* 1999;29(12):901–903.
403. Dehner LP, Watterson J, Priest JR. Pleuropulmonary blastoma. *Perspect Pediatr Pathol* 1995;18:214–226.
404. Rome A, Gentet JC, Coze C, et al. Pediatric thyroid cancer arising as a fourth cancer in a child with pleuropulmonary blastoma. *Pediatr Blood Cancer* 2008;50(5):1081.
405. Boman F, Hill DA, Williams GM, et al. Familial association of pleuropulmonary blastoma with cystic nephroma and other renal tumors: a report from the International Pleuropulmonary Blastoma Registry. *J Pediatr* 2006;149(6):850–854.
406. Priest JR, Williams GM, Hill DA, et al. Pulmonary cysts in early childhood and the risk of malignancy. *Pediatr Pulmonol* 2009;44(1):14–30.
407. Hill DA, Jarzembowski JA, Priest JR, et al. Type I pleuropulmonary blastoma: pathology and biology study of 51 cases from the international pleuropulmonary blastoma registry. *Am J Surg Pathol* 2008;32(2):282–295.
408. Nicol KK, Geisinger KR. The cytomorphology of pleuropulmonary blastoma. *Arch Pathol Lab Med* 2000;124(3):416–418.
409. Sciot R, Dal Cin P, Brock P, et al. Pleuropulmonary blastoma (pulmonary blastoma of childhood): genetic link with other embryonal malignancies? *Histopathology* 1994;24(6):559–563.
410. de Krijger RR, Claessen SM, van der Ham F, et al. Gain of chromosome 8q is a frequent finding in pleuropulmonary blastoma. *Mod Pathol* 2007;20(11):1191–1199.
411. Hill DA, Ivanovich J, Priest JR, et al. DICER1 mutations in familial pleuropulmonary blastoma. *Science* 2009;325(5943):965.
412. Priest JR, Magnuson J, Williams GM, et al. Cerebral metastasis and other central nervous system complications of pleuropulmonary blastoma. *Pediatr Blood Cancer* 2007;49(3):266–273.
413. Indolfi P, Bisogno G, Casale F, et al. Prognostic factors in pleuropulmonary blastoma. *Pediatr Blood Cancer* 2007;48(3):318–323.
414. Reed MK, Margraf LR, Nikaidoh H, et al. Calcifying fibrous pseudotumor of the chest wall. *Ann Thorac Surg* 1996;62(3):873–874.
415. Soyer T, Ciftci AO, Gucer S, et al. Calcifying fibrous pseudotumor of lung: a previously unreported entity. *J Pediatr Surg* 2004;39(11):1729–1730.
416. Odaka A, Takahashi S, Tanimizu T, et al. Chest wall mesenchymal hamartoma associated with a massive fetal pleural effusion: a case report. *J Pediatr Surg* 2005;40(5):e5–e7.
417. Hemsrichart V, Charoenkwan P. Fatal bilateral congenital mesenchymal hamartoma of the chest wall. *J Med Assoc Thai* 2007;90(11): 2519–2523.
418. Andino L, Cagle PT, Murer B, et al. Pleuropulmonary desmoid tumors: immunohistochemical comparison with solitary fibrous tumors and assessment of beta-catenin and cyclin D1 expression. *Arch Pathol Lab Med* 2006;130(10):1503–1509.
419. Fraire AE, Cooper S, Greenberg SD, et al. Mesothelioma of childhood. *Cancer* 1988;62(4):838–847.
420. Loddenkemper R, Kloppenborg A, Schoenfeld N, et al. Clinical findings in 715 patients with newly detected pulmonary sarcoidosis–results of a cooperative study in former West Germany and Switzerland. WATL Study Group. Wissenschaftliche Arbeitsgemeinschaft fur die Therapie von Lungenkrankheitan. *Sarcoidosis Vasc Diffuse Lung Dis* 1998;15(2):178–182.
421. Fauroux B, Clement A. Paediatric sarcoidosis. *Paediatr Respir Rev* 2005;6(2):128–133.
422. Shetty AK, Gedalia A. Sarcoidosis: a pediatric perspective. *Clin Pediatr (Phila)* 1998;37(12):707–717.
423. Fink CW, Cimaz R. Early onset sarcoidosis: not a benign disease [see comments]. *J Rheumatol* 1997;24(1):174–177.
424. Reich JM, Johnson RE. Incidence of clinically identified sarcoidosis in a northwest United States population. *Sarcoidosis Vasc Diffuse Lung Dis* 1996;13(2):173–177.
425. Torrington KG, Shorr AF, Parker JW. Endobronchial disease and racial differences in pulmonary sarcoidosis [see comments]. *Chest* 1997;111(3):619–622.
426. Yanardag H, Pamuk ON, Uygun S, et al. Sarcoidosis: child vs adult. *Indian J Pediatr* 2006;73(2):143–145.
427. Kwon EJ, Hivnor CM, Yan AC, et al. Interstitial granulomatous lesions as part of the spectrum of presenting cutaneous signs in pediatric sarcoidosis. *Pediatr Dermatol* 2007;24(5):517–524.
428. Singh M, Kothur K. Pulmonary sarcoidosis masquerading as tuberculosis. *Indian Pediatr* 2007;44(8):615–617.
429. Cimaz R, Ansell BM. Sarcoidosis in the pediatric age. *Clin Exp Rheumatol* 2002;20(2):231–237.
430. Chadelat K, Baculard A, Grimfeld A, et al. Pulmonary sarcoidosis in children: serial evaluation of bronchoalveolar lavage cells during corticosteroid treatment. *Pediatr Pulmonol* 1993;16(1):41–47.
431. Tessier V, Chadelat K, Baculard A, et al. BAL in children: a controlled study of differential cytology and cytokine expression profiles by alveolar cells in pediatric sarcoidosis. *Chest* 1996;109(6):1430–1438.

432. Hsu RM, Connors AF, Jr., Tomashefski JF, Jr. Histologic, microbiologic, and clinical correlates of the diagnosis of sarcoidosis by transbronchial biopsy. *Arch Pathol Lab Med* 1996;120(4):364–368.
433. Dimitriades C, Shetty AK, Vehaskari M, et al. Membranous nephropathy associated with childhood sarcoidosis. *Pediatr Nephrol* 1999;13(5):444–447.
434. Clark SK. Sarcoidosis in children. *Pediatr Dermatol* 1987;4(4):291–299.
435. Kazerooni EA, Jackson C, Cascade PN. Sarcoidosis: recurrence of primary disease in transplanted lungs. *Radiology* 1994;192(2):461–464.
436. Dinwiddie R. Pathogenesis of lung disease in cystic fibrosis. *Respiration* 2000;67(1):3–8.
437. Trapnell BC, Chu CS, Paakko PK, et al. Expression of the cystic fibrosis transmembrane conductance regulator gene in the respiratory tract of normal individuals and individuals with cystic fibrosis. *Proc Natl Acad Sci U S A* 1991;88(15):6565–6569.
438. Ott CJ, Suszko M, Blackledge NP, et al. A complex intronic enhancer regulates expression of the CFTR gene by direct interaction with the promoter. *J Cell Mol Med* 2009;13(4):680–692.
439. Planells-Cases R, Jentsch TJ. Chloride channelopathies. *Biochim Biophys Acta* 2009;1792(3):173–189.
440. Pierce BL, Carlson CS, Kuszler PC, et al. The impact of patents on the development of genome-based clinical diagnostics: an analysis of case studies. *Genet Med* 2009;11(3):202–209.
441. de Faria EJ, de Faria IC, Ribeiro JD, et al. Association of MBL2, TGF-beta1 and CD14 gene polymorphisms with lung disease severity in cystic fibrosis. *J Bras Pneumol* 2009;35(4):334–342.
442. De Gaudemar I, Contencin P, Van den Abbeele T, et al. Is nasal polyposis in cystic fibrosis a direct manifestation of genetic mutation or a complication of chronic infection? *Rhinology* 1996;34(4):194–197.
443. Qiu X, Kulasekara BR, Lory S. Role of horizontal gene transfer in the evolution of pseudomonas aeruginosa virulence. *Genome Dyn* 2009;6:126–139.
444. Aquino SL, Kee ST, Warnock ML, et al. Pulmonary aspergillosis: imaging findings with pathologic correlation. *AJR Am J Roentgenol* 1994;163(4):811–815.
445. Aurora P, Whitehead B, Wade A, et al. Lung transplantation and life extension in children with cystic fibrosis. *Lancet* 1999;354(9190):1591–1593.
446. Morton J, Glanville AR. Lung transplantation in patients with cystic fibrosis. *Semin Respir Crit Care Med* 2009;30(5):559–568.
447. Cutz E, Yeger H, Pan J. Pulmonary neuroendocrine cell system in pediatric lung disease-recent advances. *Pediatr Dev Pathol* 2007;10(6):419–435.
448. Carver TW, Jr. Pediatric athletic asthmatics. *Curr Allergy Asthma Rep* 2008;8(6):500–504.
449. Gomperts BN, Strieter RM. Fibrocytes in lung disease. *J Leukoc Biol* 2007;82(3):449–456.
450. Wagelie-Steffen A, Aceves SS. Eosinophilic disorders in children. *Curr Allergy Asthma Rep* 2006;6(6):475–482.
451. Gaynor JW, Bridges ND, Clark BJ, et al. Update on lung transplantation in children. *Curr Opin Pediatr* 1998;10(3):256–261.
452. Sweet SC. Pediatric lung transplantation. *Proc Am Thorac Soc* 2009;6(1):122–127.
453. Aurora P, Edwards LB, Christie JD, et al. Registry of the international society for heart and lung transplantation: twelfth official pediatric lung and heart/lung transplantation report-2009. *J Heart Lung Transplant* 2009;28(10):1023–1030.
454. Elizur A, Faro A, Huddleston CB, et al. Lung transplantation in infants and toddlers from 1990 to 2004 at St. Louis Children's Hospital. *Am J Transplant* 2009;9(4):719–726.
455. Singh SJ, Cummins GE, Cohen RC, et al. Adverse outcome of congenital diaphragmatic hernia is determined by diaphragmatic agenesis, not by antenatal diagnosis. *J Pediatr Surg* 1999;34(11):1740–1742.
456. Rescorla FJ, Yoder MC, West KW, et al. Delayed presentation of a right-sided diaphragmatic hernia and group B streptococcal sepsis. Two case reports and a review of the literature. *Arch Surg* 1989;124(9):1083–1086.
457. Stevens TP, van Wijngaarden E, Ackerman KG, et al. Timing of delivery and survival rates for infants with prenatal diagnoses of congenital diaphragmatic hernia. *Pediatrics* 2009;123(2):494–502.
458. Deslauriers J. Eventration of the diaphragm. *Chest Surg Clin N Am* 1998;8(2):315–330.
459. de Vries TS, Koens BL, Vos A. Surgical treatment of diaphragmatic eventration caused by phrenic nerve injury in the newborn. *J Pediatr Surg* 1998;33(4):602–605.
460. Schirmer-Zimmerman H, Hammersen G, Scheuerlen W, et al. CR3/108–Congenital alveolar capillary dysplasia with familiary microphthalmia. *Paediatr Respir Rev* 2006;7(Suppl 1):S326.
461. Merchak A, Lueder GT, White FV, et al. Alveolar capillary dysplasia with misalignment of pulmonary veins and anterior segment dysgenesis of the eye: a report of a new association and review of the literature. *J Perinatol* 2001;21(5):327–330.
462. Roth W, Bucsenez D, Blaker H, et al. Misalignment of pulmonary vessels with alveolar capillary dysplasia: association with atrioventricular septal defect and quadricuspid pulmonary valve. *Virchows Arch* 2006;448(3):375–378.
463. Galambos C. Alveolar capillary dysplasia in a patient with Down's syndrome. *Pediatr Dev Pathol* 2006;9(3):254–255; author reply 256.
464. Antao B, Samuel M, Kiely E, et al. Congenital alveolar capillary dysplasia and associated gastrointestinal anomalies. *Fetal Pediatr Pathol* 2006;25(3):137–145.
465. Usui N, Kamiyama M, Kamata S, et al. A novel association of alveolar capillary dysplasia and duodenal atresia with paradoxical dilatation of the duodenum. *J Pediatr Surg* 2004;39(12):1808–1811.
466. Sen P, Thakur N, Stockton DW, et al. Expanding the phenotype of alveolar capillary dysplasia (ACD). *J Pediatr* 2004;145(5):646–651.
467. Vick RN, Owens T, Moise KJ, et al. Urethral atresia in a neonate with alveolar capillary dysplasia and pulmonary venous misalignment. *Urology* 2000;55(5):774.
468. Rabah R, Poulik JM. Congenital alveolar capillary dysplasia with misalignment of pulmonary veins associated with hypoplastic left heart syndrome. *Pediatr Dev Pathol* 2001;4(2):167–174.
469. Adolph V, Flageole H, Perreault T, et al. Repair of congenital diaphragmatic hernia after weaning from extracorporeal membrane oxygenation. *J Pediatr Surg* 1995;30(2):349–352.
470. Witters I, Devriendt K, Moerman P, et al. Bilateral tibial agenesis with ectrodactyly (OMIM 119100): further evidence for autosomal recessive inheritance. *Am J Med Genet* 2001;104(3):209–213.

CHAPTER 13

The Cardiovascular System

KATHLEEN PATTERSON

CONGENITAL MALFORMATIONS OF THE CARDIOVASCULAR SYSTEM

Incidence

The heart, first recognizable at 15 days of gestation, develops from a single tube into a four-chambered structure via an extraordinary series of loopings and septations (e1–e3). Given the complexity of cardiac development, it is not surprising that congenital cardiac defects account for the vast majority of cases of cardiac disease in childhood. The reported incidence of congenital heart disease (CHD) varies widely, ranging from 2.4/1,000 to 8.8/1,000 live births (1) (e4–e12). The incidence statistics vary depending on the age of the patient population, the criteria used for diagnosis and inclusion in a study, and the length of study group follow-up. Inconsistency in the methods of classifying hearts, especially when the lesions are multiple or complex, introduces an additional level of variability to the reported relative frequency of individual defects (Table 13-1).

Etiology

The etiology of congenital heart malformations is multifactorial, with both genetic and environmental factors playing a role (2) (e3). From 15% to 45% of patients with CHD have additional developmental anomalies, including chromosomal and nonchromosomal syndromes, malformation associations or sequences, and teratogen-associated defects (e13–e15). Genetic factors have long been recognized as a major player; approximately 10% of patients with CHD exhibit a trisomy, monosomy, duplication, or deletion on routine cytogenetic study, with trisomy 21 being the most common (e16,e14). Over the past 15 years, microdeletions and mutations of single genes have been identified in many of the developmental syndromes that include CHD as a major factor, with the 22q11 deletion, characteristic of the diGeorge/velocardiofacial syndrome, being the most prevalent (2) (e17,e18). The ever-increasing number of identified chromosomal abnormalities linked with heart malformations unfortunately does not mean that genetic screening can predict a specific form of CHD. Instead, it has become clear that mutations at multiple genetic loci can cause the same cardiac malformation, and that mutations at a single locus can cause multiple different malformations. Meanwhile, molecular and biochemical analysis of normal gene products from many of these CHD-associated genes is leading to increased understanding of the developmental mechanisms in the heart (e19).

Pathophysiology

Simplistically, two major factors, shunting and obstruction to flow, are central to an understanding of the pathophysiology of CHD. In the normal heart, the pulmonary and systemic vascular circuits are completely separate, functioning as two parallel circuits. Loss of this separation results in shunting of blood between the two circuits. The size and the predominant direction of the shunt (i.e., right to left or left to right) are dynamic and determined by a variety of factors, including the

Table 13-1 ■ PREVALENCE OF CONGENITAL HEART DEFECTS

Type	Range (%)[a]	M:F
VSD	30–52	1:1
PDA	2.5–8.5	1:2
TOF	3.5–10.5	1:1
COTA	4.5–6.5	3:2
TGA	2.5–6.5	2:1
ASD	6.0–8.0	1:2
PS-IVS	2.5–9.0	1:1
AVSD	1.5–9.5	2:3
HLHS	2.0–5.0	3:2
AS	3.0–6.0	2:1

[a]Percentage of total for ten most common defects; see references (e4–e8,e10–e12,e14).
VSD, ventricular septal defect; PDA, patent ductus arteriosus; TOF, tetralogy of Fallot; COTA, coarctation of the aorta; TGA, transposition of the great arteries; ASD, atrial septal defect; PS-IVS, pulmonary stenosis with intact ventricular septum; AVSD, atrioventricular septal defect; HLHS, hypoplastic left-heart syndrome; AS, aortic stenosis; TAPVC, total anomalous pulmonary venous connection; DORV, double-outlet right ventricle; PA-IVS, pulmonary atresia with intact ventricular septum; SV, single ventricle; TA, tricuspid atresia; TRUN, truncus arteriosus.

Table 13-2 ▪ CONGENITAL HEART DEFECTS: MAJOR CLINICAL FINDINGS

	SHUNT		PBF				
	L→R	R→L	INC	DEC	Cyanosis	Ductus Dependent	Complications
ASD	X	—	X	—	—	—	PVOD
ECD	X	—	X	—	—	—	PVOD
VSD	X	—	X	—	—	—	PVOD
TGV	—	—	X	—	X	X	PVOD
TRUN	X	—	X	—	—	—	PVOD
EBS	—	X	—	X	X	—	Arrhythmia
TOF	—	X	—	X	X	—	Polycythemia
HRHS	—	X	—	X	X	X	—
HLHS	—	—	—	—	—	X	Shock
PDA	X	—	X	—	—	—	PVOD

PBF, pulmonary blood flow; L→R, left to right; R→L, right to left; INC, increased; DEC, decreased; ASD, atrial septal defect; ECD, endocardial cushion defect; VSD, ventricular septal defect; TGV, transposition of the great vessels; TRUN, truncus arteriosus; EBS, Ebstein malformation; TOF, tetralogy of Fallot; HRHS, hypoplastic right-heart syndrome; HLHS, hypoplastic left-heart syndrome; PDA, patent ductus arteriosus; PVOD, pulmonary vascular obstructive disease.

relative resistance to flow in the two circuits and the presence or the absence of an associated obstructive lesion. Shunting lesions are often not apparent at birth, when resistance in the two circuits is similar, but become clinically evident over time with the normal decrease in pulmonary vascular resistance (PVR). In general, right-to-left shunts are associated with cyanosis, and left-to-right shunts with increased pulmonary blood flow, congestive heart failure, and a risk for the development of pulmonary artery hypertension.

Obstructive lesions can occur at almost any site in either of the circuits, with the cardiac chambers proximal to the site of obstruction showing marked hypertrophy in response to the increased work load. In general, right-sided obstruction produces decreased pulmonary blood flow and cyanosis; left-sided obstruction results in decreased systemic blood flow. In cases of severe obstruction, the obstructed circuit is often dependent on blood flow across the ductus arteriosus (i.e., ductus-dependent lesions), and symptoms characteristically appear at the time of ductus closure in the 1st day or two of life.

These generalizations presuppose normal connections between the respective cardiac chambers and the great vessels. When these connections are abnormal, as in transposition of the great vessels, additional pathophysiologic consequences develop, which are discussed in the context of the individual lesions. A summary of the clinicopathologic features in some of the more common congenital cardiac defects is presented in Table 13-2.

Classification

An accurate classification of congenital heart malformations requires knowledge of the normal anatomy of the heart and a careful systematic approach to the examination (e20,e21). Normal values for heart weight relative to age and body size are readily available (see Appendix); normal values for the ventricular wall thickness and valve sizes have been reported for fetuses and newborns by Oyer et al. (3) and for infants and children by Rowlett et al. (4) and Scholz et al. (5). Following a careful external examination of the shape and the position of the heart, relationships of the great vessels, and venous drainage pattern, a sequential evaluation of the three segments of the heart (atria, ventricles, and great vessels) is undertaken. The connections of the segments, the relationship between the chambers within a segment, and the morphology of the segments are all assessed (6) (e20,e22–e24) (Table 13-3). When this segmental approach is used for

Table 13-3 ▪ SEQUENTIAL EXAMINATION OF HEART SEGMENTS

Atrial situs: determined by position of morphologic RA
- Situs solitus: RA on right; LA on left
- Situs inversus: RA on left; LA on right
- Situs ambiguus: indeterminate atrial situs
  - Bilateral right-sided atria
  - Bilateral left-sided atria

Atrioventricular connections
- Atrioventricular concordance: RA → RV; LA → LV
- Atrioventricular discordance: RA → LV; LA → RV
- Ambiguous (indeterminate) connection
  - Double inlet ventricle: RA + LA → one ventricle
- Absence of one atrioventricular connection

Ventricular organization
- Normal or D-looped: morphologic RV to the right of the morphologic LV
- Inverted or L-looped: morphologic RV to the left of the morphologic LV

Ventricular morphology
- Three normal components: inlet = trabecular = and outlet
  - Trabecular component determines morphologic right and left ventricles
- Rudimentary chamber: absent inlet portion

Ventriculoarterial connections
- Ventriculoarterial concordance: RV → PA; LV → Ao
- Ventriculoarterial discordance: RV → Ao; LV → PA
- Double outlet ventricle: one ventricle → PA + Ao
- Single outlet of heart: includes truncus = pulmonary atresia = aortic atresia

RA, right atrium; RV, right ventricle; LA, left atrium; LV, left ventricle; PA, pulmonary artery; Ao, aorta.

classification, normal connections, relationships, and morphology are not incorporated into the diagnosis. In the majority of cases of CHD, a single defect is present [e.g., a ventricular septal defect (VSD)], and the heart is classified on the basis of that solitary anomaly. With the increasing use of cardiac transplantation for complex congenital heart defects, both before and after repair, accurate morphologic diagnosis of cardiac explants becomes a challenge. Although the atrial anatomy and vascular connections can no longer be evaluated, careful examination of atrioventricular (AV) connections, the ventricular anatomy, and the ventriculoarterial connections is still warranted (e25).

Septal Malformations

Malformations of the Atrial Septum

The atrial septum forms from three distinct embryonic structures: the septum primum, endocardial cushions, and septum secundum (e1,e2,e26). In the fetus, blood flows freely between the right and the left atria via the foramen ovale, bordered by the superior right-sided septum secundum (limbus of fossa ovalis) and the inferior left-sided septum primum (valve of fossa ovalis). This opening normally fuses during the 1st year of life. However, in 25% to 30% of people, this fusion never occurs, leaving a "probe–patent" or "valvular-competent" foramen ovale (e27).

Atrial Septal Defect

An atrial septal defect (ASD), the most common atrial septal malformation, can occur in one or more of four sites (Figure 13-1 and Table 13-4). A secundum ASD, the most common of the four types, manifests as multiple perforations of, a deficiency in, or absence of the fossa ovalis flap valve (eFigure 13-1) (7) (e26). In patients with a probe-patent fossa ovalis, a secondary functional secundum ASD may appear following atrial dilatation. An isolated secundum ASD usually remains asymptomatic through childhood with 80% to 90% closing spontaneously, especially when of a small size (≤4 mm diameter) (8) (e28,e29). Defects greater than 8 mm on the other hand rarely close spontaneously, requiring instead surgical closure (8) (e28,e29). Complicating pulmonary vascular hypertension, which develops in 10% of adult patients, occurs rarely in the pediatric population (e30–e32).

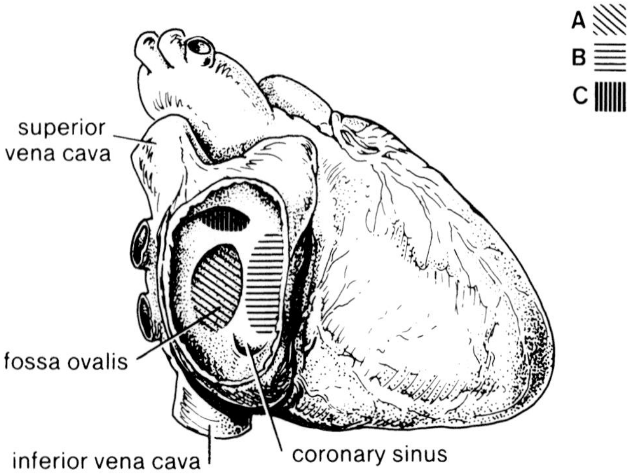

FIGURE 13-1 ■ The positions of various atrial septal defects from the perspective of the right atrium, which has been opened laterally. **A:** Secundum defect. **B:** Primum defect. **C:** Sinus venosus defect.

Table 13-4 ■ TYPES OF ATRIAL SEPTAL MALFORMATION

Septal defects
Secundum atrial septal defect
Primum atrial septal defect
Sinus venosus atrial septal defect
Coronary sinus atrial septal defect
Single atrium (cor triloculare biventricularis)
Premature closure of foramen ovale

Primum defects are discussed later with AV septal defects. Sinus venosus defects result from a deficiency of the posterior superior aspect of the atrial wall that normally separates the right pulmonary veins from the superior vena cava/right atrium junction. A defect in this area therefore almost always occurs in conjunction with partial anomalous pulmonary venous return (9) (e33,e34). Coronary sinus defects result from an unroofing or a fenestration of the coronary sinus on the posterior aspect of the left atrium and occur most often in association with a persistent left superior vena cava (LSVC) (10) (e35,e36). Although most isolated ASDs occur sporadically, they can occasionally be inherited as an autosomal dominant anomaly with or without associated conduction system abnormalities (e37). In a small subgroup of these patients with associated radial limb defects (Holt-Oram syndrome), the underlying genetic abnormality on chromosome 12q2 has been identified (e38,e39) (see Chapter 27).

Single Atrium

Complete absence of the atrial septum, a rare anomaly, results in a single atrial cavity, also termed *common atrium* or *cor triloculare biventricularis*. The single atrium usually accompanies other severe cardiac anomalies and is often associated with AV septal defects and situs ambiguous (7) (e40,e41).

Premature Closure of the Foramen Ovale

Premature closure of the foramen ovale manifests as a normally positioned but imperforate foramen ovale, an unidentifiable fossa ovalis, or an aneurysmal pouch bulging into the left atrium. The restricted mixing *in utero* can be complicated by hydrops fetalis and the hypoplastic left-heart syndrome (7) (e42–e44).

Malformations of the Ventricular Septum

The ventricular septum is a complex structure that can be divided into four components: inlet, trabecular, outlet, and membranous (e45–e47). From the right ventricular aspect, the inlet septum lies superiorly and posteriorly behind the septal

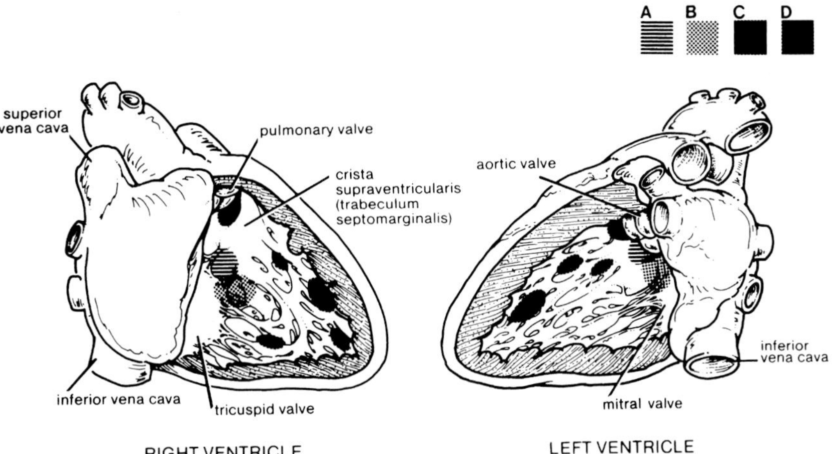

FIGURE 13-2 ▪ The positions of the ventricular septal components and the corresponding ventricular septal defects from the lateral perspectives of the opened right and left ventricles. **A:** Membranous septum and perimembranous defect. **B:** Inlet septum and defect. **C:** Trabecular septum and trabecular muscular defects. **D:** Outlet septum and defect.

tricuspid valve, the trabecular septum occupies the apex, the outlet septum sits between the crista supraventricularis and the pulmonary valve, and the membranous septum lies at the anteroseptal tricuspid commissure, where the tricuspid, mitral, and aortic valves converge (Figure 13-2). From the left ventricular aspect, the inlet septum lies posteriorly adjacent to the mitral valve, the trabecular septum occupies the apical region, the outlet septum sits beneath the right cusp of the aortic valve, and the membranous septum lies below the right and posterior aortic valve commissure (Figure 13-2).

VSDs, the most common type of congenital heart defect, can occur anywhere in the ventricular septum (11) (e47). VSDs are subclassified according to the nature of the defect rim and its anatomic position in the septum (Table 13-5).

Perimembranous (membranous, infracristal) defects account for up to 80% of VSDs (11) (e45,e47). These defects are most easily seen from the left side, where they lie in the left ventricular outflow tract just beneath the aortic valve (Figure 13-3). In the right ventricle, they reside beneath the crista supraventricularis and behind the papillary muscle of the conus, partially obscured by the septal leaflet of the tricuspid valve (12) (e46,e47) (Figure 13-4).

Outlet (infundibular) defects account for 5% to 7% of VSDs in the Western world but nearly 30% of VSDs in Japan and the East Asia (e45,e48,e49). These defects are often roofed by pulmonary and aortic valve tissue (i.e., doubly committed subarterial) (11,12) (e47) and can be complicated by prolapse of the right coronary cusp of the aortic valve into the defect; 40% to 60% are complicated by aortic regurgitation (e49,e48). Outlet and occasionally perimembranous trabecular defects may be associated with malalignment between the outlet and the trabecular portions of the ventricular septum. Anterior malalignment results in aortic override and posterior malalignment results in pulmonic override. Either can be complicated by subaortic stenosis, often with associated arch anomalies (13) (e45,e50–e52).

Inlet defects, which account for 5% to 8% of VSDs, reside beneath the septal leaflet of the tricuspid valve, but posterior and inferior to the position of perimembranous trabecular defects (e45). Although inlet defects are similar in location

Table 13-5 ▪ VENTRICULAR SEPTAL DEFECTS: CLASSIFICATION

Defect Rim	Defect Location	Historical
Perimembranous	Inlet	Posterior AV canal
	Outlet	Supracristal Infundibular
	Trabecular	Membranous Infracristal
Muscular	Inlet	AV canal
	Outlet	Infundibular Subpulmonic Supracristal
	Central Trabecular	Infracristal
	Remote Trabecular	Muscular
Doubly committed subarterial	Outlet	Infundibular Supracristal

AV, atrioventricular.

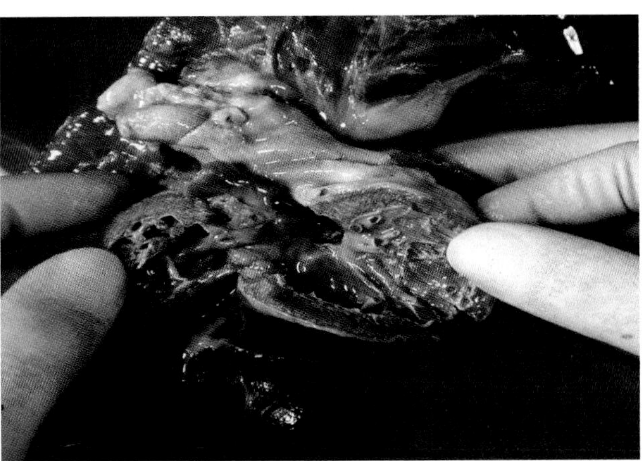

FIGURE 13-3 ▪ Ventricular septal defect. An opened left ventricle with the free wall reflected laterally contains a perimembranous defect, visible in the outflow tract inferior to the aortic valve. The probe visible in the right ventricle in figure 13-4 traverses the defect opening.

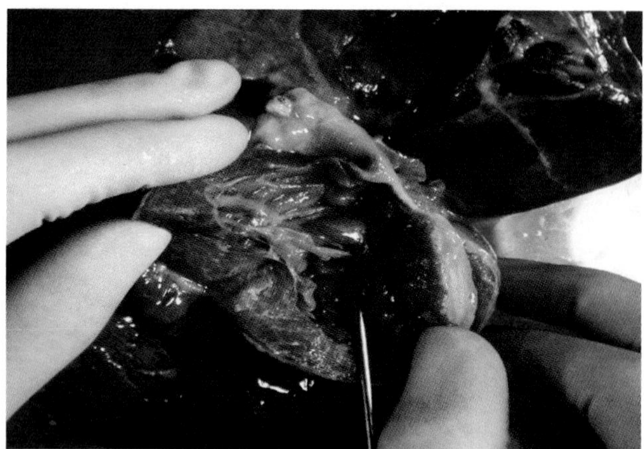

FIGURE 13-4 ■ Ventricular septal defect. An opened right ventricle with the free wall reflected superiorly contains a perimembranous defect hiding beneath the septal leaflet of the tricuspid valve. The probe traversing the defect is visible from the left ventricular aspect in Figure 13-3.

to the VSD component of AV septal defects, hearts with isolated inlet defects do not show the other characteristic features of AV septal defects (11) (e45).

Muscular trabecular defects, representing 5% to 20% of VSDs, often are multiple and may be difficult to see beneath the trabeculations on the right ventricular aspect of the ventricular septum (e45,e47,e53). What appear to be multiple muscular defects on the right ventricular side ("Swiss cheese" septum) may coalesce to form what appears to be a single defect in the left ventricular aspect of the septum (e53).

Clinical manifestations of a VSD usually first appear at the age of 2 to 6 weeks, when the normal drop in PVR results in the onset of a harsh holosystolic murmur at the left sternal border. The size of the defect and the state of the PVR rather than the anatomic location of the defect determine the nature of the symptoms (e54,e55) (Table 13-6). In VSDs with large shunts, congestive heart failure may be resistant to therapy, and the risk for pulmonary vascular obstructive disease is substantial (e54).

Spontaneous closure occurs in 25% to 40% of all VSDs and in up to 85% if the defect is small (e10,e54,e56,e57). Closure of membranous VSDs by overgrowth of fibrous connective tissue or adherence of the tricuspid valve septal leaflet can result in the formation of a ventricular septal "aneurysm" (e58,e59). Ventricular septal aneurysms, with or without complete defect closure, are seen in more than 40% of patients with VSD, usually appearing after 2 years of age (e59).

The penetrating and branching bundles of the conduction system traverse the membranous portion of the ventricular septum (12,14). This relationship is of particular concern during the surgical repair of perimembranous and inlet defects. Anomalies in the conduction system or an ill-placed suture can result in postoperative bundle branch block (12) (e60) or, rarely, sudden death (e61).

Malformations of the Atrioventricular Septum

The AV septum is a structure at the crux of the heart that separates the right atrium from the left ventricle (15) (e62). In the embryo, the AV septum forms at the site of fusion of the four endocardial cushions (16) (e2,e40). The spectrum of lesions resulting from defects of the AV septum has been traditionally called *endocardial cushion defects* (Figure 13-5). All forms of AV septal defect display the following features (15) (e41,e63,e64):

1. Disproportion between the inlet and the outlet dimensions of the interventricular septum, which gives the inlet septum a "scooped out" appearance
2. Elongation of the left ventricular outflow tract, which creates the "gooseneck" deformity
3. Abnormal formation of the AV valves, with a characteristic "cleft" in the left-sided anterior leaflet

AV septal defects are subdivided into partial and complete forms, depending on the morphology of the AV valve leaflets.

Partial Atrioventricular Septal Defect

Partial AV septal defect is defined by the presence of two discrete AV valve annuli. Partial AV septal defects account for approximately one-third of cases (17) (e65–e69).

Table 13-6 ■ VENTRICULAR SEPTAL DEFECTS: CLINICAL GROUPS

Group	Defect Size	Shunt	PVR	Complications	Prognosis/Therapy
1	Small	L→R	Nl	SBE	Spontaneous closure 75%–83%
2	Moderate	L→R	Nl	SBE CHF	Surgical closure required 15%–20%
3	Large	L→R	Nl Inc	SBE CHF	Surgical closure <2 years
4	Large	R→L	Inc	CHF Cyanosis	Inoperable

PVR, pulmonary vascular resistance; L→R, left to right; R→L, right to left; Nl, normal; Inc, increased; SBE, subacute bacterial endocarditis; CHF, congestive heart failure.

ENDOCARDIAL CUSHION DEFECTS

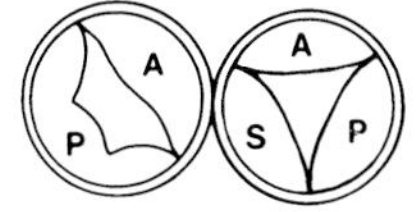

Normal Mitral & Tricuspid Valves

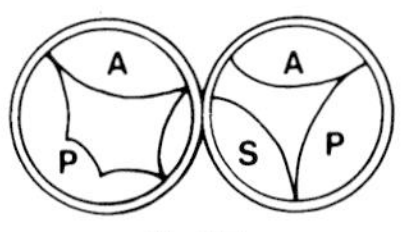

Partial Atrioventricular Canal

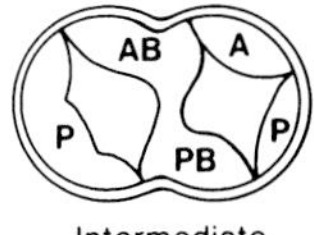

Intermediate Atrioventricular Canal

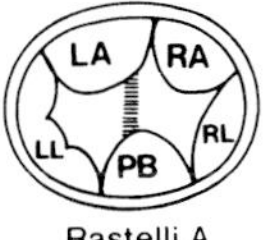

Rastelli A

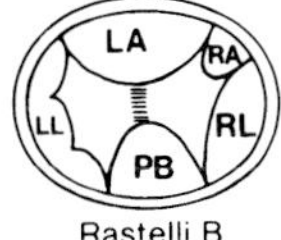

Rastelli B

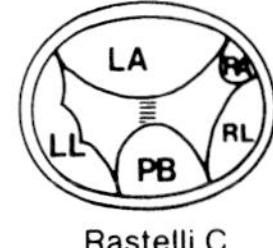

Rastelli C

Complete Atrioventricular Canal

FIGURE 13-5 ■ Diagrammatic representation of the atrioventricular valves as viewed from the atria in a normal heart and various atrioventricular septal defects. A, anterior leaflet; P, posterior leaflet; S, septal leaflet; AB, anterior bridging leaflet; PB, posterior bridging leaflet; LA, left anterior leaflet; RA, right anterior leaflet; RL, right lateral leaflet; LL, left lateral leaflet.

Most hearts in this group contain an ostium primum ASD (Figure 13-6) in conjunction with a cleft in the anterior mitral valve leaflet (15,17) (e64) (eFigure 13-2). Although these hearts have traditionally been considered to have ASDs, echocardiographic studies demonstrate that the atrial septum is, in fact, normal in size and that the defect is located in the ventricular septum, with inferior displacement of the AV valves causing interatrial shunting (e70). The cleft mitral leaflet inserts, commissure-like, on the ventricular septum. The septal leaflet of the tricuspid valve displays variable degrees

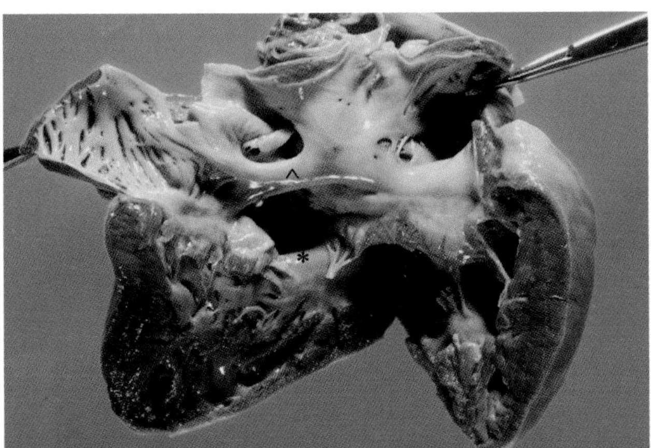

FIGURE 13-6 ■ Complete atrioventricular septal defect. A complete atrioventricular septal defect is readily visible centrally in this opened left atrium and ventricle. At the upper rim of the defect a band of atrial septal tissue marked by the ^ separates the upper secundum ASD from the lower ostium primum ASD. The lower rim of the defect marked by the * represents the upper rim of the ventricular septum. The anterior and the posterior bridging leaflets of the common AV valve extend over the defect without chordal insertion.

of deficiency. When both the mitral and the tricuspid valves are cleft, the valves insert, commissure-like, onto the rim of the ventricular septum; a connecting tongue of valve tissue covers the ventricular septum and closes the ring (e63,e41). The size of the defect in the ventricular septum also varies in these hearts, and in some cases the valve leaflets may be less firmly adherent to the ventricular septum so that some interventricular shunting occurs (17) (e63). Hearts with associated interventricular shunting are said to have "intermediate" AV septal defects in some reports (e71,e40).

Complete Atrioventricular Septal Defect

In the complete AV septal defect (*endocardial cushion defect, complete AV canal*) (Figure 13-6), the single AV orifice is guarded by five valve leaflets: posterior (inferior) bridging, right lateral, left lateral, right anterior, and left anterior (superior, bridging) (17) (e68,e72). The complete AV septal defect is further subclassified according to the extent of septal bridging of the left anterior leaflet and the site of medial insertion (e40, e41,e68,e72).

Rastelli A: minimal bridging, attachment to right rim of septum or medial papillary muscle
Rastelli B: moderate bridging, attachment to an aberrant right apical papillary muscle
Rastelli C: marked bridging, attachment to the anterolateral papillary muscle of the right ventricle

Rastelli types A and C account for the vast majority of cases.

Additional cardiovascular anomalies occur in up to 50% of hearts with either partial or complete AV septal defects (e67,e73–e76). The commonly associated anomalies vary in the different subtypes of AV septal defect, as outlined in Table 13-7. At least 50% of patients have trisomy 21 with a variety of other syndromes in another 25% including the heterotaxy syndromes in particular (e67,e73,e77). The ventricles are "unbalanced" in approximately 10% of AV septal defects, with dominant right and dominant left ventricles occurring in nearly equal numbers (17) (e69,e73).

Clinically, the large left-to-right shunt precipitates severe congestive heart failure. Pulmonary hypertensive vascular changes can appear in the 1st year of life, further complicating the clinical picture (18) (e77,e78). Without intervention, almost 50% of infants with a complete AV septal defect die by 6 months of age, and only 15% survive to 2 years (e79). Early surgical repair, usually in the 1st year of life, is recommended (e40,e77,e78,e80,e81).

Malformations of the Conus and Truncus

The conotruncal structures of the heart arise embryologically from the distal aspect of the heart tube and represent the outflow region of the developing heart (e1,e2,e82). Embryologic research demonstrates the importance of cells derived from the neural crest in normal conotruncal development (e75,e83–e85). This finding is reflected in humans by the close association between conotruncal malformations and

Table 13-7 ■ ATRIOVENTRICULAR SEPTAL DEFECTS: ASSOCIATED CARDIAC ANOMALIES AND SYNDROMES

Type AVSD	Relative Incidence %Total[c]	Associated Syndrome[a]	Associated CV Anomalies[b]
Partial	35%	33% with Trisomy 21	All AVSD:
Complete	65%	48% with Trisomy 21	Subaortic stenosis
Subtypes	% Complete[d]		Coarctation of the aorta
			Patent ductus arteriosus
			Double-orifice mitral valve
			Parachute mitral valve
			Tetralogy of Fallot
			Double outlet right ventricle
			Common atrium
Rastelli A	55%–70%	Trisomy 21	Subaortic stenosis
Rastelli B	<10%	—	Valvular aortic stenosis
			Coarctation of aorta
			Hypoplastic left ventricle
Rastelli C	25%–40%	Heterotaxy	Tetralogy of Fallot
			Double outlet right ventricle
			Common atrium

[a]See references (17) (e67,e69).
[b]See references (e40,e69,e73,e75,e76).
[c]See references (17) (e64–e69).
[d]See references (e66,e72,e75,e76).
AVSD, atrioventricular septal defect; CV, cardiovascular.

the diGeorge/velocardiofacial syndrome and its associated 22q11.2 chromosomal deletion (e86,e87). Table 13-8 outlines the spectrum of malformations that occur in the conotruncal region.

Transposition of the Great Vessels

In transposition of the great vessels, the aorta arises from the right ventricle and the pulmonary artery from the left ventricle (i.e., discordant ventriculoarterial connections). The transposed aorta thus originates in an anterior position, either to the right (dextrotransposition, or D-transposition) or the left (levotransposition, or L-transposition) of the pulmonary artery. Hearts with transposition are further classified according to their AV connection, as depicted in Figure 13-7.

Complete Transposition

Complete transposition, the most common form, accounts for 2.5% to 6.5% of all congenital heart malformations (see Table 13-1), with a 2:1 male predominance (e88). The D–transposed aorta ascends parallel and to the right of the pulmonary artery rather than following its normal, twisted course (Figure 13-8). Internal examination reveals AV concordance with ventriculoarterial discordance (19). The aorta originates from the normally positioned morphologic right ventricle, with a muscular band separating the aortic and the tricuspid valves; the pulmonary artery arises posteriorly from the normally positioned morphologic left ventricle and is in fibrous continuity with the anterior mitral valve leaflet. The coronary arteries originate from one or both of the "facing sinuses" of the aorta (i.e., the sinuses adjacent to the

Table 13-8 ■ TYPES OF CONOTRUNCAL MALFORMATIONS

Transposition of the great vessels
Complete transposition (D-transposition)
Corrected transposition (L-transposition)
Double outlet ventricles
Double outlet right ventricle
Double outlet left ventricle
Persistent truncus arteriosus
Aortopulmonary window (aortopulmonary septal defect)

D, dextro; L, levo.

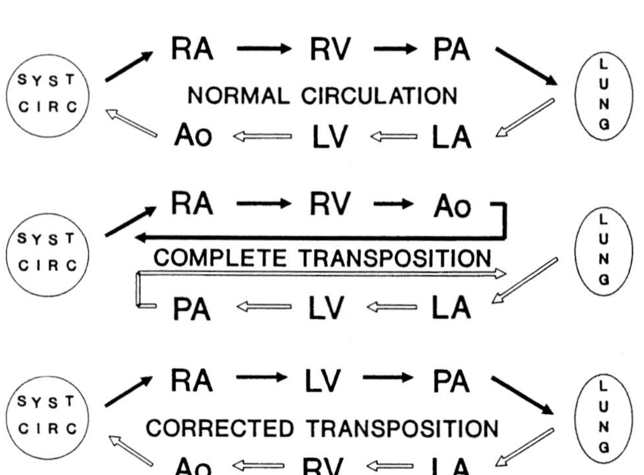

FIGURE 13-7 ■ Diagrammatic representation of normal blood flow (**top**), blood flow through complete transposition (**middle**), and blood flow through "corrected" transposition (**bottom**).

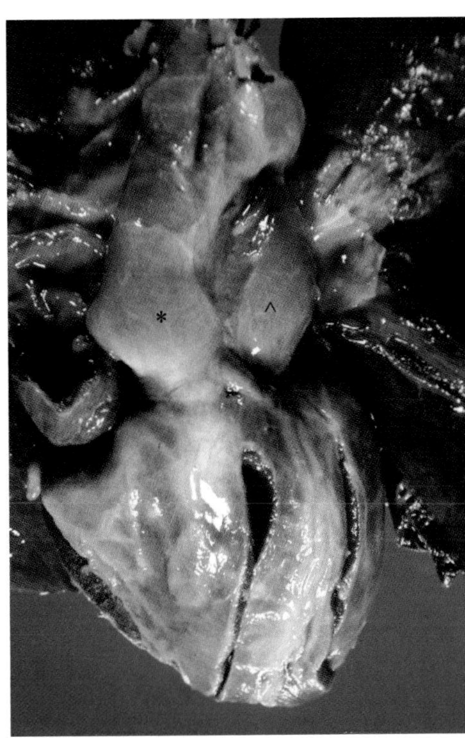

FIGURE 13-8 ▪ Complete transposition of the great vessels from the anterior aspect of the heart. The aorta, marked with *, is situated to the right and slightly anterior to the pulmonary artery, marked with ^. The two vessels ascend in a parallel course.

pulmonary artery) (19,20) (e89,e90). The anatomic course traversed by the coronary arteries varies considerably, a feature of significance when arterial switch surgery is planned (20,21) (e88,e89,e91).

A VSD accompanies the complete transposition in approximately 40% of cases, with 40% to 60% of the VSDs showing septal malalignment (22) (e92). Anterior (rightward) malalignment, present in 20% to 25% of cases with VSD, results in subaortic (right ventricular outflow tract) obstruction, often with associated coarctation (22) (e92–e94). Pulmonary (left ventricular outflow tract) obstruction occurs in 25% to 30% of hearts with or without VSD, secondary to a malaligned VSD or subvalvular fibrous or fibromuscular tissue bundles (21,22) (e88,e95).

Patients with complete transposition of the great vessels can be divided into three clinical groups based on the status of the ventricular septum and pulmonary outflow tract (Table 13-9). In groups 1 and 2, massive pulmonary blood flow is associated with a high rate of early and accelerated pulmonary hypertensive vascular disease (e96–e98). A variety of surgical repairs have been devised for transposition of the great vessels, depending in part on the group. Uncomplicated transposition was in the past most commonly repaired with an atrial baffle (Mustard or Senning) procedure, which shunted systemic venous return to the left ventricle and pulmonary venous return to the right ventricle. The atrial baffle repairs result in good long-term survival, but these hearts are prone to late right ventricular dysfunction and arrhythmias

Table 13-9 ▪ TRANSPOSITION OF THE GREAT VESSELS: CLINICAL GROUPS

	Group 1	Group 2	Group 3
Ventricular septum	Intact Small defect	Large defect	Defect
Outflow tract	Not obstructed	Not obstructed RVOT obstructed	LVOT Obstructed
Presentation	Cyanosis	Heart failure	Cyanosis
Surgical repair	Arterial switch	Arterial switch + VSD closure	Rastelli

LVOT, left ventricular outflow tract; RVOT, right ventricular outflow tract; VSD, ventricular septal defect.

(e99–e103). The more anatomically correct arterial switch procedure is therefore the currently favored repair for hearts in groups 1 and 2 (e100,e104). In hearts with VSD and significant left ventricular outflow tract obstruction (group 3), repair focuses on directing the left ventricular flow into the aorta and creating a shunt between the right ventricle and the pulmonary circulation (Rastelli procedure) (21) (e95,e105).

Corrected Transposition

In the much less common corrected transposition, also known as *L-transposition* or *ventricular inversion*, an L-transposed aorta ascends parallel to and to the left of the pulmonary artery. Internally, both AV and ventriculoarterial discordance are present. The right atrium is in continuity with a right-sided morphologic left ventricle from which the pulmonary artery arises; the left atrium is in continuity with a left-sided morphologic right ventricle from which the aorta originates; blood flow is thus anatomically "corrected" (e106,e107) (Figure 13-7). The defect is frequently associated with other congenital anomalies, including tricuspid valve dysplasia, pulmonary outflow tract obstruction, and VSDs (e106–e108). When corrected transposition is present as an isolated defect, patients are initially asymptomatic but prone to late right ventricular dysfunction and arrhythmias, which reflect the limited ability of the right ventricle to support the systemic circulation (e109). AV discordance can occur with other types of ventriculoarterial connections, including double outlet right ventricle and ventriculoarterial concordance (e110).

Double Outlet Ventricle

Double Outlet Right Ventricle

Of the two forms of double outlet ventricle (Table 13-8), double outlet right ventricle (DORV) is the more common, accounting for 1% to 1.5% of congenital heart defects (1) (e9,e10). The term *DORV* denotes a heart in which both great vessels originate from the right ventricle. This seemingly straightforward term incorporates a currently controversial range of morphologic entities. The strictest criterion requires that both great arteries arise exclusively from the right ventricle, with no fibrous continuity between the mitral and the outflow valves (23) (e111,e112). A somewhat less strict criterion requires only that both great vessels arise exclusively from the right ventricle; 50% to 60% of such hearts display at least focal fibrous continuity between the mitral and the outflow valves (24) (e113,e114). The broadest criterion requires only that more than 50% of one great vessel override the ventricular septum; when this criterion is used, DORV overlaps with tetralogy of Fallot (25) (e115–e117). A VSD almost always accompanies the double outlet right ventricle, serving as the only site for left ventricular outflow. The variable location of the VSD relative to the pulmonary and aortic valves serves to define pathologic subcategories (23,26) (e111,e118) (Figure 13-9). The anatomic relationship between the great arteries also varies, as outlined in Table 13-10. In earlier reports, the side-by-side relationship of the great arteries was described as the most frequent one, but more recent series describe the posterior normal pattern as the most common (23,24) (e114,e117). The wide variety of coronary artery anomalies that are associated with side-by-side or malposed great arteries affect surgical repair options and procedures (e117,e119–e121).

The Taussig-Bing malformation, first described in 1949 (e122), is an uncommon variant of double outlet right ventricle in which the VSD is subpulmonic; no pulmonary stenosis is present. When strict criteria are used, fewer than 10% of DORV are of the Taussig-Bing variant (23). When broader criteria are used ("a spectrum of anomalies unified by a juxtapulmonary VSD with malalignment of the infundibular septum"), some hearts can be classified both as the Taussig-Bing variant and as transposition of the great vessels with a malaligned VSD (25) (e123).

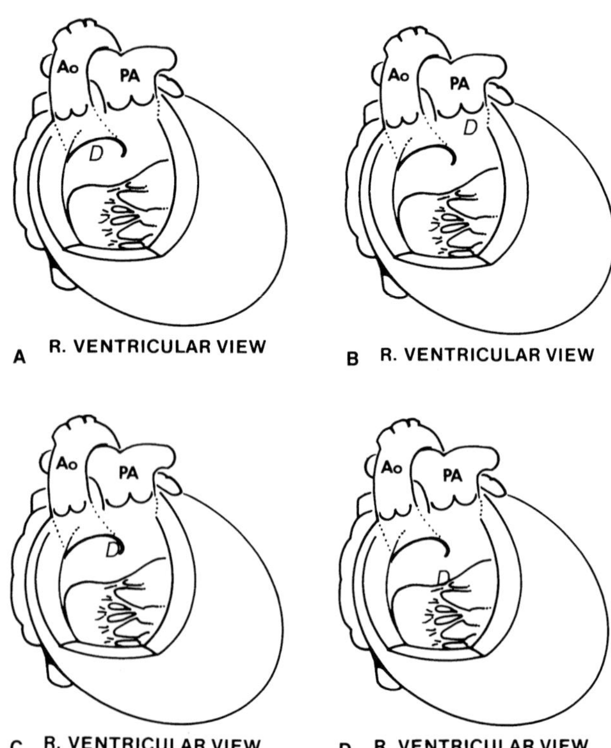

FIGURE 13-9 ■ The sites, *D*, of the ventricular septal defects in a double outlet right ventricle. **A:** Subaortic (60% to 65% of total cases). **B:** Subpulmonic (25% to 30%). **C:** Doubly committed (5% to 15%). **D:** Remote (10% to 15%). Ao, aorta; PA, pulmonary artery.

Table 13-10 ■ DOUBLE-OUTLET RIGHT VENTRICLE: RELATIONSHIP OF GREAT ARTERIES

Root of Ao Relative to Root of PA	Descriptive Terms	Ascending Ao and PA
Posterior and right	Normal or dextroposition	Spiral
Parallel and right	Side by side	Parallel
Anterior and right	D-malposition	Parallel
Anterior and left	L-malposition	Parallel

Ao, aorta; PA, pulmonary artery; D, dextro; L, levo.

Various other cardiac malformations accompany many double outlet right ventricles. Pulmonary infundibular stenosis with or without valvular stenosis occurs in 40% to 70% of hearts (23,24) (e112,e113,e116). ASDs are not uncommon; complete AV septal defects are less common (e112,e117,e124,e125). Left-sided inflow and outflow obstructive lesions may be accompanied by left ventricular hypoplasia (24) (e112,e113,e116,e117).

The clinical presentation of DORV depends on the location of the VSD and the presence of associated malformations, particularly pulmonary stenosis (e111,e126) (Table 13-11). Surgical correction varies depending on the anatomic configuration of the heart (e118,e121,e126,–e129) (Table 13-11).

Double Outlet Left Ventricle

Double outlet left ventricle (DOLV) is a rare malformation in which both great vessels arise predominantly from the morphologic left ventricle; a VSD accompanies the vast majority (27) (e130–e132). Similar to DORV, the DOLV is classified by the location of the VSD relative to the great vessels (27). The DOLV with subaortic VSD is frequently complicated by pulmonary outflow tract obstruction and DOLV with subpulmonic VSD by aortic outflow tract obstruction (27) (e132).

Persistent Truncus Arteriosus

Persistent truncus arteriosus is defined as a single arterial trunk that originates from a single semilunar valve and supplies the aorta, one or both pulmonary arteries, and the coronary arteries (Figure 13-10). The truncal valve is tricuspid in 50% to 70% of cases, quadricuspid in 25%, and bicuspid in most of the rest (e133–e137). The truncal vessel overlies and usually overrides an infundibular VSD, although occasionally it is predominantly committed to one ventricular chamber (e133, e137,e138). The truncal valve is always in fibrous continuity with the mitral valve; fibrous continuity may also be present between the truncal and tricuspid valves (e134,e137). The truncal valve leaflets are frequently thickened and myxomatous, with valvular insufficiency

Table 13-11 ■ DOUBLE-OUTLET RIGHT VENTRICLE: CLINICOPATHOLOGIC CATEGORIES

Clinical Type	VSD Location	RVOTO	LVOTO	Surgical Repair
VSD	Subaortic Doubly committed	Absent	Absent	Intraventricular tunnel
TOF	Subaortic Doubly committed	Present	Absent	TOF type
TGA	Subpulmonic (Taussig-Bing)	Absent	Often present	Arterial switch + VSD closure Intraventricular tunnel Damus-Kaye-Stansel
Remote VSD	Noncommitted	Absent	Often present	Intraventricular tunnel Single ventricle repair

VSD, ventricular septal defect; TOF, tetralogy of Fallot; TGV, transposition of the great vessels; RVOTO, right ventricular outflow tract obstruction; LVOTO, left ventricular outflow tract obstruction.

present in approximately 15% to 30% (e134,e138–e140). The coronary arteries originate from the sinuses of the truncal valve in a variable pattern, with a single coronary artery present in 15% to 20% (e133–e135,e137,e141).

Truncus arteriosus is subclassified according to the pattern of origin of the pulmonary arteries from the truncal root (Figure 13-11). However, this classification by Collet and Edwards (28) (e142) has two problems:

1. It classifies hearts in which both pulmonary arteries arise directly from the descending aorta as type 4 truncus. The "type 4 truncus" instead represents a variant of pulmonary atresia (PA) with VSD (e134).
2. It does not address the aberrant origin of one pulmonary artery from the ascending or descending aorta. In approximately 15% of cases, one pulmonary artery arises from the truncus and the other from the ductus or ascending aorta, so that a pulmonary artery is "absent" (e143).

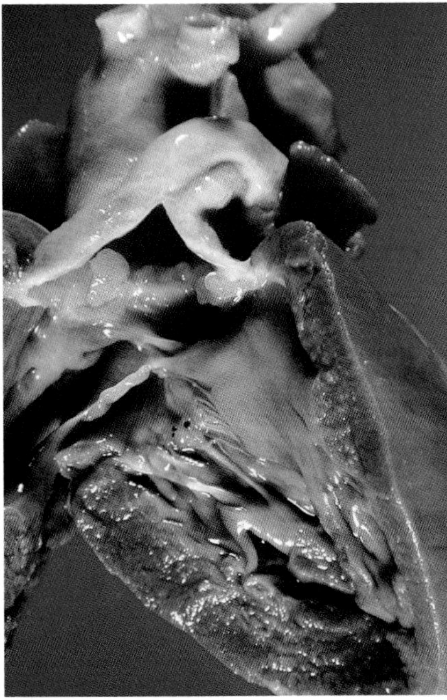

FIGURE 13-10 ■ Truncus arteriosus. The left ventricle free wall has been lifted to uncover the smooth surfaced left ventricular outflow tract with a VSD opening at the top. Above the VSD lies a somewhat nodular truncus arteriosus valve. The main pulmonary artery almost immediately branches to the left from the common trunk; the aorta continues ascending posteriorly.

A classification devised by van Praagh creates a separate subtype for this latter finding and also acknowledges the rare case in which there is no VSD (e144). The classification was subsequently revised by van Praagh to simplify the scheme in a surgically meaningful fashion (29) (Table 13-12).

Associated anomalies most frequently involve the aortic arch and include absent ductus arteriosus (>50%), right-sided aortic arch (20% to 35%), and interrupted aortic arch type B (10%) (e133,e134,e140). Extracardiac anomalies, especially those related to diGeorge syndrome, occur in 20% to 30% (e145,e146). The diGeorge syndrome-associated chromosome 22q11 deletion can be detected by fluorescence *in situ* hybridization (FISH) in 35% to 50% of infants with persistent truncus arteriosus (e87,e147,e148).

The early clinical manifestation of congestive heart failure results from intracardiac shunting and markedly excessive pulmonary blood flow. The excessive pulmonary blood flow also produces rapidly progressive pulmonary hypertensive vascular disease; early surgical repair is therefore recommended (e141,e149,e150).

Aortopulmonary Window

Aortopulmonary window, or *aortopulmonary septal defect*, is a rare malformation characterized by a defect in the vessel wall between the ascending aorta and the main pulmonary artery. The defect may lie proximally (just above the aortic and the pulmonary valves), distally (in the upper ascending aorta adjacent to the right pulmonary artery), or as a combined opening that involves the majority of the ascending aorta (7) (e151,e152). Associated anomalies, present in more than 50% of cases, commonly include a VSD, interrupted aortic arch type A, and anomalous origin of one pulmonary artery from the ascending aorta (30) (e153–e155). Although aortopulmonary window occurs in the same general region as persistent truncus arteriosus, it is not seen in the chromosome 22q11 deletion syndromes (30) (e156,e157).

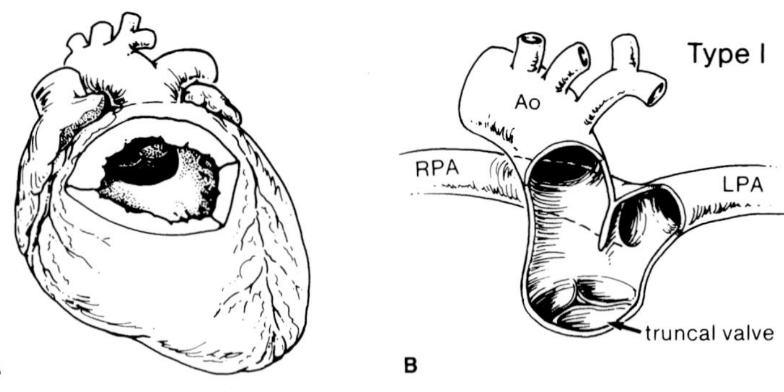

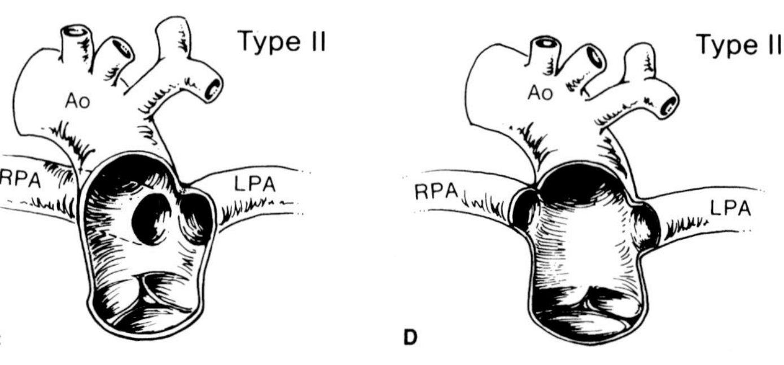

FIGURE 13-11 ■ Truncus arteriosus. **A:** A window in the right ventricle shows a tricuspid truncal valve through an infundibular ventricular septal defect, with an associated right aortic arch. There are three main truncus types. **B:** In type I, a single pulmonary trunk arises from the truncus and divides into two pulmonary arteries. **C:** In type II, two pulmonary arteries originate from closely apposed orifices in the common trunk. **D:** In type III, the two pulmonary arteries originate from widely separated orifices in the common trunk. Ao, aorta; LPA, left pulmonary artery; RPA, right pulmonary artery.

Malformations of the Ventricular Inflow Tracts

Tricuspid Valve Malformations

Tricuspid Atresia

Tricuspid atresia, in which the only outlet to the right atrium is via a patent fossa ovalis or an ASD, accounts for 1% to 1.5% of congenital heart malformations (e4–e6,e10,e15). The markedly hypoplastic right ventricle, positioned along the right anterosuperior border of the heart, has no inlet segment. The markedly dilated right atrium contains no grossly identifiable valvular tissue in more than 85% of cases (31,32) (e158). A dimple in the muscular atrial floor, presumably marking the site of the missing valve, may have a fibrous attachment to the right ventricle, but often is instead in continuity with the left ventricle by transillumination and pin prick studies (32) (e158,e159). The remaining 5% to 15% of hearts display a tricuspid valve remnant in the form of an imperforate fibrous membrane (e158,e160). A muscular VSD, termed the *outlet foramen*, allows communication between the dominant left ventricular chamber and the rudimentary right ventricle; however, the VSD or the infundibular outflow tract may be restrictive (31) (e161,e162).

Tricuspid atresia is subclassified according to the size of the VSD, concordance or discordance of the great vessels,

Table 13-12 ■ TRUNCUS ARTERIOSUS CLASSIFICATION

Collet and Edwards(e142)	Van Praagh (e144)	Modified van Praagh (29)
Type 1 PAs arise as a single main artery and then divide	*Type 1* PAs arise as a single main artery and then divide	*Large aorta type* TA with confluent or near confluent PAs
Type 2 PAs arise separate but next to each	*Type 2* PAs arise separately	
Type 3 PAs arise widely separated		
	Type 3 One PA branch "absent" Arises from ductus or aorta	TA (large aorta type) with absence of one PA
	Type 4 Aortic arch hypoplastic or interrupted	*Large pulmonary artery type* TA with IAA or severe COTA
	Type A = VSD present *Type B* = VSD absent	

PA, pulmonary artery; VSD, ventricular septal defect; TA, truncus arteriosus; IAA, interrupted aortic arch; COTA, coarctation of the aorta.

Table 13-13 ▪ TRICUSPID ATRESIA: CLINICAL CLASSIFICATION

I. Normally related great vessels (60%–70%)
   A. Intact ventricular septum with pulmonary atresia
   B. Small VSD with pulmonary stenosis
   C. Large VSD without pulmonary stenosis
II. D-transposition of the great arteries (25%–30%)
   A. VSD with pulmonary atresia
   B. VSD with pulmonary stenosis
   C. VSD without pulmonary stenosis
III. Malposition other than D-transposition of the great arteries (5%)

and the presence or absence of pulmonary stenosis/atresia (e163,e164) (Table 13-13). The clinical symptoms depend on these anatomic variables; more than 50% of cases present with cyanosis and murmur in the newborn period (e162,e164,e165). In the vast majority of hearts, the right ventricle is too small to function adequately as a pumping chamber (eFigure 13-3), and repair relies on the Fontan operation or one of it modifications (e162,e165,e166).

Ebstein Malformation

Ebstein malformation accounts for fewer than 1% of all cases of CHD, but is the most common cause of isolated tricuspid stenosis or insufficiency (1,33) (e11). It is characterized by adherence of variable portions of the septal and posterior tricuspid valve leaflets to the right ventricular wall, with "atrialization" (i.e., downward displacement of the functional annulus) of a portion of the right ventricle (Figure 13-12) (33,34) (e167). The anterior valve annulus

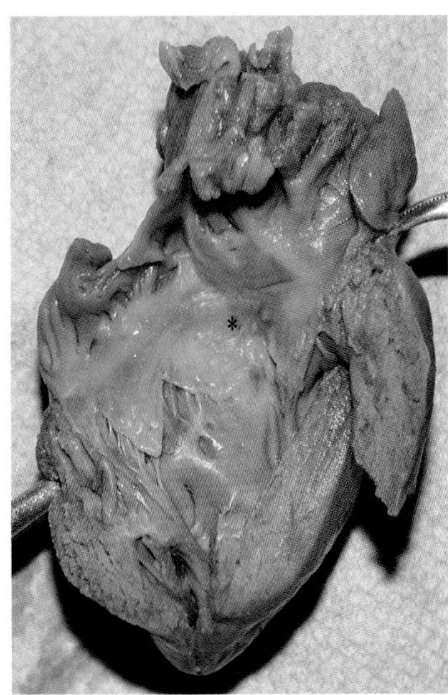

FIGURE 13-12 ▪ Mild form of Ebstein anomaly. The opened right atrium and right ventricle display a markedly thickened ventricular wall. The septal (*) and posterior leaflets of the tricuspid valve are fixed to the underlying ventricular wall.

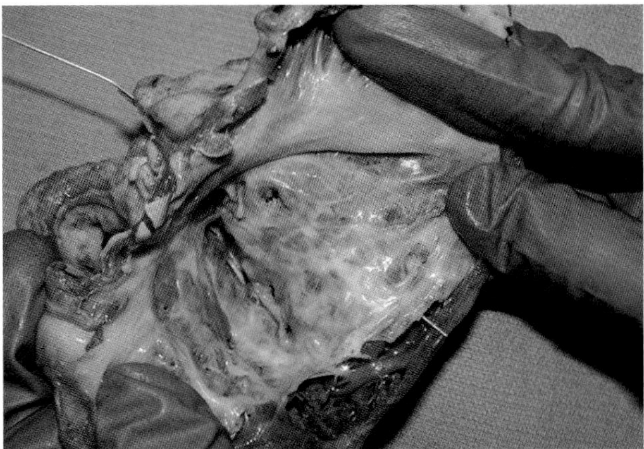

FIGURE 13-13 ▪ Severe form of Ebstein anomaly. The opened right atrium uncovers a markedly enlarged and dysplastic anterior tricuspid leaflet attached to the apical myocardium by tiny chordae. A probe placed in the pulmonary artery traverses the remaining right ventricular cavity and appears at the base of this dysplastic valve, illustrating the severe obstruction to pulmonary inflow and outflow created by this defect.

insertion is normally positioned, with a large, redundant, and often muscularized leaflet. The margin of the leaflet may be attached to the posteroinferior right ventricular wall and produce obstruction and in some cases complete occlusion of the AV orifice (Figure 13-13) (34) (e167,e168). Tricuspid regurgitation occurs across the dilated AV junction (true annulus). Right-to-left shunting across a patent fossa ovalis or ASD and supraventricular arrhythmias due to accessory conduction pathways frequently complicate Ebstein malformation (33) (e169,e170). A variety of other associated cardiovascular defects, most commonly pulmonary valvular stenosis, PA, or a VSD, occur in 30% to 40% of cases (33) (e169,e171e172). Abnormalities of the left ventricle include not only valvular dysplasia, but also noncompaction of the myocardium (e170).

Given the broad range of anatomic alterations encompassed by Ebstein malformation, it is not surprising to find a broad range of clinical manifestations for the disorder. One-third to one-half of patients present in the newborn period with cyanosis and a murmur; the mortality rate among such infants is high, particularly when the malformation is associated with additional cardiac anomalies (e171–e174). In many patients, however, the diagnosis is delayed until the second decade of life or later, when arrhythmias often represent the major clinical problem (33) (e169,e174). Surgical repair, required in approximately 40% of patients, includes either tricuspid valvuloplasty or valve replacement with concomitant repair of associated lesions, most commonly ASD closure (e175–e178).

Mitral Valve Malformations

Mitral Stenosis

The normal mitral valve apparatus is a complex structure with four primary components: annulus, anterior and posterior valve leaflets, chordae tendineae, and anterolateral and posteromedial papillary muscles. A variety of malformations

Table 13-14 ■ MITRAL VALVE MALFORMATIONS

Supravalvar lesions
Supramitral ring
Valvar lesions
Valve hypoplasia
Valve dysplasia
Commissural fusion
Valve leaflet excess or agenesis
Double orifice valve
Cleft mitral valve
Subvalvar lesions
Parachute deformity (Single papillary muscle)
Funnel deformity (shortened fused chordae)
Arcade deformity (Papillary muscle fused with valve)
Mixed
Shone syndrome

affecting any or all of the valve components result in congenital mitral stenosis and insufficiency (e179–e181) (Table 13-14). A supramitral ring, a ridge of connective tissue at the atrial surface of the mitral leaflets, usually occurs with deformities of the mitral valve apparatus (e180,e182–e184). Valve hypoplasia, in which the valve components are small but otherwise normally formed, most commonly associated with left ventricle hypoplasia, VSDs, and coarctation of the aorta (COTA) (7) (e180). The "typical" mitral stenosis manifests as lesions at both the valvar and the subvalvar areas including valve dysplasia with commissure fusion, obliteration of the intrachordal spaces, and shortening of the chordae tendineae and papillary muscles. Associated malformations include tetralogy of Fallot, COTA, and subaortic stenosis with a near-normal-sized left ventricle (7) (e180). The double orifice mitral valve results when excessive valve tissue bridges between the anterior and posterior valve leaflets to create two, usually unequally sized, orifices, both supported by chordal attachments that insert into often abnormally positioned papillary muscle (eFigure 13-4) (e185,e186). The double orifice valve almost always occurs in company with other cardiac malformations, especially AV septal defects (50% of cases) or left-sided obstructive lesions (40%) (e187,e186) Two forms of cleft mitral valve without associated primum ASD or VSD have been described (e188):

1. Associated with normally related great vessels and a shortened inlet septum (i.e., forme fruste of an AV septal defect)
2. Associated with TGA or DORV and a normal inlet septum.

Parachute deformity of the mitral valve, defined as insertion of all the chordae into a single papillary muscle group, also usually occurs with other malformations of the heart, particularly VSDs and obstructive lesions of the aortic valve and arch (7,35) (e180,e182,e189). The eponym *Shone syndrome* denotes the association of a parachute mitral valve with a supramitral ring, subaortic stenosis, and COTA (35) (e190). Repair strategies include balloon dilation and mitral valve reconstruction, mitral valve replacement surgery, and the more recent pulmonary valve autograft (Ross II) (e191–e193).

Mitral Atresia

Mitral atresia, defined as the absence of a left AV connection, is marked on the left atrial aspect by muscular atrial floor with or without a visible dimple or, less commonly, by an imperforate membrane (7,36,37) (e194). The microscopic examination of hearts with no grossly obvious membrane between the left atrium and the left ventricle uniformly reveals a fibrous connection at the presumed site of the absent valve (36). The outlet for pulmonary venous return is by way of a patent fossa ovalis or less commonly an ASD (7). Rarely, the fossa ovalis is prematurely closed, and pulmonary venous return is shunted to the right side of the heart by anomalous venous connections (7,38) (e195). When the great vessels are normally related, mitral atresia is most commonly associated with aortic atresia and, as such, is included in the hypoplastic left-heart syndrome. The left ventricle exists as a diminutive chamber lined by translucent endocardium, which in some cases is evident only on microscopic examination of the posterosuperior aspect of the hypertrophic right ventricle (7,37). Less often a VSD is present and a patent aortic valve arises from either the right (DORV) or left ventricular chamber (7,37) (e194). Repair strategies are similar to those employed for other hypoplastic left ventricles (see below).

Floppy Mitral Valve

Floppy mitral valve represents the central defect in the floppy mitral valve (FMV)/mitral valve prolapse (MVP)/ mitral valve regurgitation (MVR) triad. The primary defect in the "floppy" valve is deposition of acid mucopolysaccharides and dissolution of the collagen in the pars spongiosa and fibrosa of the valve (39) (e196,e197). The accumulation of myxoid material leads to thickened and enlarged valve leaflets often with increased chordal insertions on the ventricular surface, elongation of the chordae tendenae, and dilatation of the valve annulus (39). With prolapse, the valve becomes "hooded," defined as the presence of ballooning to a height of at least 4 mm and involving at least one-half of the anterior or two-thirds of the posterior mitral leaflets (40). The myxomatous degeneration in the valves leaflets is without inflammation and does not lead to fusion of the valve commissures, distinguishing these valvular changes from those of rheumatic fever. Similar myxomatous changes occur elsewhere in the heart, including the conduction system; a feature that likely explains the associated arrhythmias and the conduction defects (e198).

The reported incidence of FMV/MVP/MVR varies considerably, with less than 1% to 5% of children exhibiting clinical or echocardiographic features of MVP (41) (e199,e200). In the pediatric population, the incidence increases with age; MVP is extremely rare before 2 years of age (e201,e200). Most children are asymptomatic, presenting with the characteristic late systolic "click" on ascultation; an occasional child presents with chest pain of unclear etiology (41) (e201,e200). Skeletal anomalies, especially pectus excavatum, are common (42) (e196,e201). The 2:1 female predominance described in adults is also observed in some but not all groups of children studied (41) (e200,e201). Progressive MVR, a major problem in adults with FMV, occurs rarely during childhood. Other complications, including infectious endocarditis, thromboembolism, arrhythmias, and even sudden death, do occur occasionally in the pediatric population (e196,e200,e202).

The disorder frequently occurs in families, following either an autosomal dominant or X-linked inheritance pattern (e196). The linkage of MVP to loci on chromosomes 11, 13, and 16 has so far failed to yield an identifiable underlying genetic mutation (e203). A small subgroup of patients with FMV/MVP/MVR do have an associated connective tissue disorder such as Marfan or Ehler-Danlos syndrome (e196).

Univentricular Atrioventricular Connection

The term *univentricular AV connection* denotes the connection of the AV valves to a single ventricular cavity (37) (e204,e205). Table 13-15 lists at least some of the terms previously used for this condition and outlines the range of anomalies encompassed. The anatomy of such hearts can be highly complex and variable, so that sequential segmental analysis is an essential tool for accurate classification (37) (e206,e207).

Double Inlet Ventricle

In double inlet left ventricle, the most common of the double inlet malformations, both the left and right AV valves open into a dominant left ventricular cavity (e205,e208,e209). The rudimentary right ventricle occupies the right anterosuperior border of a normally related, D-looped left ventricle or the left anterosuperior border of an inverted, L-looped left ventricle. The rudimentary right ventricle communicates with the dominant left ventricle via a variably sized VSD. The great vessels are transposed in the vast majority of cases but may be normally related, atretic, or in a double outlet configuration.

Table 13-15 ■ UNIVENTRICULAR ATRIOVENTRICULAR CONNECTION

- Common synonyms
  - Single ventricle
  - Common ventricle
  - Holmes heart
  - Univentricular heart
  - Cor triloculare biatriatum
  - Primitive ventricle
- Anatomic subtypes
  - Double-inlet ventricle
    - Double-inlet left ventricle
    - Double-inlet right ventricle
    - Double-inlet ventricle of mixed morphology (absent ventricular septum)
    - Double-inlet ventricle of indeterminate morphology
  - Single-inlet ventricle
    - Mitral atresia
    - Tricuspid atresia
  - Common-inlet ventricle
  - Overriding atrioventricular valves

Common Inlet Ventricle

In common inlet ventricle, both atria communicate with a single ventricle via a common AV valve (e205,e210). Many of these hearts represent the extreme form of unbalanced AV septal defect and thus include a dominant right or left ventricular cavity and a rudimentary second ventricle. Less often, the common AV valve communicates with a single ventricular chamber of indeterminate type without an identifiable rudimentary ventricle. These hearts frequently have abnormal ventriculoarterial connections as well.

Straddling and Overriding Atrioventricular Valves

An AV valve annulus may override, or its chordal insertion may straddle, the ventricular septum (43) (e205). In hearts with valve annulus override, the AV connection is assigned to the ventricle to which more than 50% of the valve annulus is attached (e211). Straddling of the chordae without valve annulus override does not change the AV connection designation.

Malformations of the Ventricular Outflow Tracts

Pulmonary Outflow Tract and Valve Malformations

Tetralogy of Fallot

Four components comprise the tetralogy of Fallot (TOF): infundibular pulmonic stenosis, VSD, aortic valve dextroposition, and right ventricular hypertrophy (Figure 13-14). However, the morphologic detail surrounding these four components can vary considerably (7,44) (e212,e213). Infundibular pulmonic stenosis, the consequence of anterosuperior malalignment of the outlet septum, leads to decreased pulmonary blood flow with an associated small pulmonary artery (Figure 13-15). Over time, the stenosis becomes exacerbated by hypertrophy of the infundibular septum or cristal structures (e212,e213). The invariably large and nonrestrictive VSD is perimembranous in 75% of cases, located in the muscular outlet in 20%, and subarterial only rarely (44) (e212,e214). The degree of aortic override varies from 15% to 95%. In the extreme situation, the differentiation of TOF from double outlet right ventricle depends on the presence of the characteristic infundibular stenosis and fibrous continuity between the aortic and mitral valves; some investigators classify hearts with more than 50% aortic override as TOF with double outlet right ventricle (25).

The pulmonary valve is abnormal in 66% to 75% of cases. It is most often bicuspid but may be unicuspid or stenotic by virtue of thickened dysplastic valve leaflets (7,44) (e215). The 20% to 25% of cases with an imperforate pulmonary

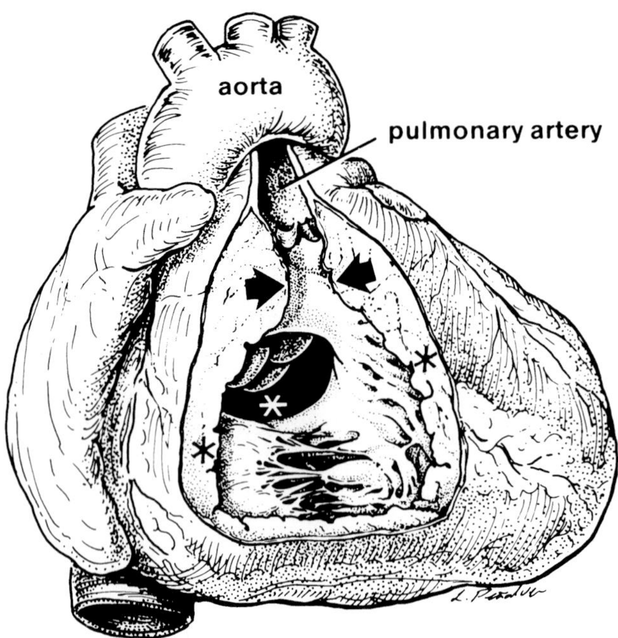

FIGURE 13-14 ■ An opened anterior right ventricle illustrates the four primary features of tetralogy of Fallot: marked narrowing of the pulmonary infundibulum (between *arrows*); a large perimembranous ventricular septal defect (*white asterisk*); dextroposed overriding aorta, visible through the ventricular septal defect; and hypertrophy of the right ventricular myocardium (*black asterisk*).

valve orifice are classified as PA with VSD, discussed in more detail later. The pulmonary arteries show a range of accompanying abnormalities that includes localized stenosis at the origin of the pulmonary artery branches, central pulmonary artery discontinuity, absent left pulmonary artery branch, and pulmonary hilar artery hypoplasia (45) (e216). When the pulmonary artery stenosis is severe, pulmonary artery hypertension may develop after surgical repair of the TOF (46) (e217). In 3% to 6% of cases, the pulmonary valve is absent (e216) and the pulmonary arteries are dilated; this dilatation may be massive.

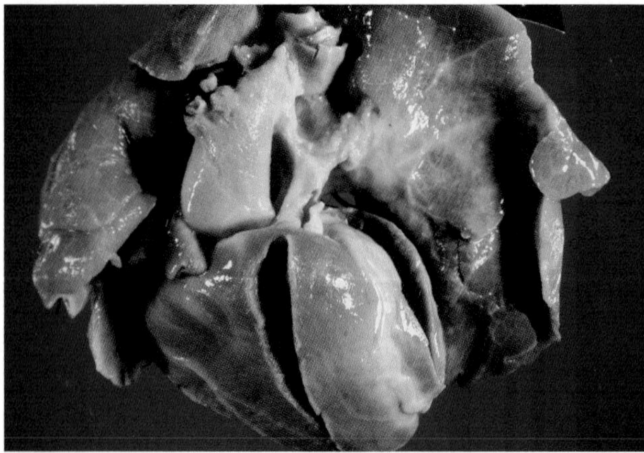

FIGURE 13-15 ■ Heart and lungs removed at autopsy with an unrepaired tetralogy of Fallot. An incision through the anterior right ventricle ends at the base of a small pulmonary artery. The markedly enlarged aorta arises behind and to the right of the pulmonary artery.

A variety of other cardiovascular defects occur with TOF. Commonly associated anomalies include right-sided aortic arch (20% to 30%) and absent ductus arteriosus (20% to 25%) (e216,e215). Although a patent fossa ovalis occurs commonly in infants with TOF, a true ASD is present in only 20% to 25% (e216,e215). A complete AV septal defect accompanies TOF in 1% to 2% of cases, most often in children with trisomy 21 (e218,e219).

TOF accounts for 3.5% to 10.5% of all CHD and represents the most common cyanotic CHD. In approximately 33% of cases, TOF occurs as part of a recognizable syndrome, most commonly DiGeorge syndrome or trisomy 21 (45).

Hypoxia and cyanosis are the principal symptoms of TOF; their severity varying with the degree of pulmonary obstruction (45). In the presence of marked stenosis or atresia, cyanosis is evident in the neonatal period. More commonly, cyanosis appears in the first 6 months of life, associated with increasing infundibular stenosis. Required treatment consists of widening of the outflow tract by surgical resection of outflow tract muscle and, in severe cases, insertion of a transannular patch (45) (e165).

Pulmonary Atresia with Ventricular Septal Defect

Although the designation PA with VSD (PA/VSD) is frequently used as a synonym for TOF with PA, not all hearts with PA/VSD display the hypoplastic right ventricular infundibulum characteristic of TOF (47) (e220). Most commonly, a dimple (more rarely recognizable fused bicuspid valve cusps) marks the site of the pulmonary valve (e221). Abnormalities of the pulmonary arteries include a connection of confluent, bilateral pulmonary arteries to the right ventricle by an atretic cord, absence of the left pulmonary artery, and absence of all intrapericardial pulmonary arteries (48) (e222–e224). This latter group was classified as truncus arteriosus type IV in the past. The ductus arteriosus supplies blood to one or both of the pulmonary arteries in 40% to 65% of cases. The lungs also receive blood via collateral arteries that originate from the descending aorta and supply the pulmonary arteries via intrapulmonary, hilar, or extrapulmonary anastomoses (48) (e225,e226). Recent studies demonstrate that the chromosome 22q11 deletion increases the likelihood of an absent ductus arteriosus and a major aortopulmonary collateral artery supply (e227,e228). With a major aortopulmonary collateral artery supply, hypoplasia and arborization of the pulmonary arteries make surgical management problematic (49) (e229,e222). Early unifocalization of the pulmonary blood supply seems to improve pulmonary circulation and makes later corrective surgery possible in some patients (e230–e233).

Absent Pulmonary Valve

Absent pulmonary valve is a rare anomaly usually associated with TOF (e234–e236). At the site of the expected valve, a narrow valve annulus is rimmed by rudimentary, nodular, gelatinous tissue with massive poststenotic dilation (e234). More complex pulmonary artery anomalies, including discontinuity of the main pulmonary arteries, anomalous origin of the pulmonary arteries, and absence of the left pulmonary artery, occur less often (50) (e235,e237). The ductus arteriosus is frequently absent (e238,e235). Dilated pulmonary arteries can compress the adjacent bronchi and cause respiratory compromise; abnormalities of the intrapulmonary arteries and bronchi may exacerbate these pulmonary problems (50) (e239).

Pulmonary Stenosis with Intact Ventricular Septum

Pulmonary stenosis with intact ventricular septum (IVS) accounts for 2.5% to 8.0% of all cases of CHD (Table 13-1). The obstruction is usually valvular, with secondary right ventricular hypertrophy and poststenotic dilation of the pulmonary trunk. The valve is most often dome shaped with fused cusps and a single central orifice, but it may be unicuspid, bicuspid, or tricuspid with partially fused commissures (51) (e240). Thickened dysplastic valve leaflets with nonfused cusps occur sporadically (e240,e241), and as one form of pulmonary stenosis in Noonan syndrome (e242). The pulmonary artery trunk usually exhibits poststenotic dilation; pulmonary artery hypoplasia is rare even with critical stenosis (e243,e244). Symptoms depend on the severity of the stenosis. Critical stenosis, presenting as cyanosis in infancy, requires early balloon angioplasty, surgical valvotomy, or transannular patch (e243–e246). More commonly, infants are asymptomatic; stenosis develops and worsens in early childhood in approximately 15%, and many remain asymptomatic into adulthood (52) (e247–e249). Secondary infundibular stenosis secondary to right ventricular hypertrophy can further complicate the course over time (e248).

Subvalvular Stenosis

Pulmonary subvalvular or infundibular stenosis, which accounts for fewer than 10% of cases of pulmonary stenosis with IVS, occurs when fibrous thickening at the junction of the trabecular and outlet segments divides the right ventricle into two chambers; it may also be caused by tubular hypoplasia of the infundibulum (7) (e244). Double chamber right ventricle is a closely related anomaly in which hypertrophied muscle bands cross the right ventricular cavity just proximal to the infundibulum and divide a high-pressure proximal chamber from a low-pressure infundibular chamber (53) (e250,e251). The majority of hearts with double chamber right ventricle exhibit other anomalies, most often (65% to 75%) a VSD (53) (e252,e253).

Supravalvular and Peripheral Pulmonary Artery Stenosis

Supravalvular or pulmonary artery stenosis occurs as a localized area of narrowing in the pulmonary trunk or branch or as multiple areas of narrowing throughout the pulmonary artery tree (54) (e254). The stenosis is subclassified into four types, based on the site of the obstruction, with type III accounting for approximately one-third of cases (e254) (Table 13-16). Associated cardiac malformations, present in approximately 66% of cases, include VSD, ASD, valvular pulmonary stenosis, and TOF (55) (e244). A variety of malformation syndromes include pulmonary artery stenosis (Table 13-17).

Pulmonary Atresia with Intact Ventricular Septum

PA with IVS accounts for 1% to 3% of all cases of CHD. The atresia is usually valvular, with a fibrous membrane containing commissural lines present at the expected site of the valve (7) (e221,e255,e256). The pulmonary artery is funnel shaped and usually only mildly to moderately hypoplastic (7) (e221,e256). The right ventricular myocardium is hypertrophied and the cavity of variable size, with the size of the tricuspid valve directly related to the size of the right ventricle (56) (e255–e257). The right ventricle and tricuspid valve are usually small, often with associated pulmonary infundibular stenosis or atresia (56) (e256,e258). Right ventricle-coronary artery fistulas develop in more than 50% of hearts with small ventricular cavities; in a subgroup of these hearts, the volume of flow through the fistula results in right ventricle-dependent coronary blood flow (57) (e259–e262). Accompanying coronary artery luminal stenosis and vessel atrophy proximal to the fistula site can result in myocardial ischemia and sudden death (57) (e10,e263). At the opposite extreme, the right ventricular cavity may be dilated, with the tricuspid valve showing dysplasia and often Ebsteinization (56) (e256,e257,e264).

Table 13-16 ■ SUPRAVALVAR AND PERIPHERAL PULMONARY ARTERY STENOSIS

Type I Single central stenosis of:
- A Main pulmonary artery
- B Right main pulmonary artery
- C Left main pulmonary artery

Type II Bifurcation stenosis
- A Short, localized stenosis
- B Long, narrow segments of stenosis

Type III Multiple stenoses of peripheral segmental arteries

Type IV Multiple stenoses of peripheral and central arteries

Table 13-17 ■ PULMONARY ARTERY STENOSIS-ASSOCIATED MALFORMATION SYNDROMES

Syndrome	Location of Stenosis	Reference
Rubella	Peripheral pulmonary arteries	e342
Williams	Peripheral pulmonary arteries	e308,e309
Alagille	Peripheral pulmonary arteries	e711
Noonan	Main pulmonary artery	e242

PA with IVS is a severe form of CHD in which pulmonary blood flow depends on a patent ductus arteriosus; initial palliative therapy therefore includes infusions of prostaglandin E2. The definitive surgical management varies according to the degree of right ventricular hypoplasia, the presence and severity of coronary artery fistula, and the status of the tricuspid valve with options including a variety of outflow tract ("biventricular") repairs, univentricular (Fontan) repair, or transplantation (58) (e259,e265–e267).

Aortic Outflow Tract and Valve Malformations

Aortic Valvular Stenosis

The left ventricular outflow tract may be obstructed at any level, but the most common form of obstruction is aortic valvular stenosis. The spectrum of abnormal valvular morphology is similar to that in pulmonary valvular stenosis, but a bicuspid valve is the most common form (7) (e268,e269). Bicuspid aortic valves are not congenitally stenotic and many remain asymptomatic throughout childhood, with a smaller subset progressing quickly to significant stenosis requiring intervention (e268–e271). Unicommissural and the less common tricuspid dysplastic and dome-shaped valves are stenotic from birth and therefore more likely to be symptomatic in early childhood (e272–e275). With congenitally stenotic valves, the left ventricle may be dilated, normal in size, or hypoplastic. In infants with severe stenosis, endocardial fibroelastosis and subendocardial ischemic damage often further complicate the picture (e275–e277). COTA commonly accompanies a congenitally malformed aortic valve in two clinical settings: critical aortic stenosis (59) (e278,e276) and bicuspid valves related to Turner syndrome (e279,e280).

Clinical features vary, depending largely on the severity of the stenosis. In "critical" stenosis, newborn infants present with heart failure and shock (e281–e283). Treatment then depends on the morphology of the left ventricle. With a normally sized ventricular cavity, surgical or balloon valvotomy relieves the obstruction (e282–e284). Infants with left ventricular hypoplasia or other confounding malformations require more complex surgical procedures (e285–e288). Outside the newborn period, aortic stenosis usually presents as an asymptomatic murmur (e289). Complications of the stenosis include bacterial endocarditis, myocardial ischemic damage, arrhythmias, and sudden death (e268,e289,e290). Initial treatment involves surgical or balloon valvotomy (e282,e291,e292), with up to 40% of patients requiring valve replacement later in life (60) (e290,e291). Given the growth requirement inherent in pediatric valve replacement surgery, the potential for continued somatic growth makes the pulmonary autograft (Ross) procedure particularly attractive (e293,e294).

Subvalvular Aortic Stenosis

Discrete subvalvular aortic stenosis most frequently takes the form of a fibroelastic diaphragm just beneath the base of the aortic valve; less common forms include a thickened diaphragm with a muscular base or a tunnel-like narrowing of the outflow tract (7) (e295–e297). Commonly associated heart defects, present in 50% to 75% of cases, include a maligned VSD, aortic valvular stenosis or regurgitation, aortic coarctation, and AV septal defects (59) (e273,e296–e298). These subaortic lesions rarely present in infancy, and current theories consider them to be acquired progressively, perhaps on the framework of an underlying subtle deformation of the outflow tract (61) (e295,e296,e299).

Supravalvular Aortic Stenosis

Supravalvular aortic stenosis occurs in three forms (62) (e300–e302):

1. An hourglass deformity caused by a constrictive annular ridge at the superior margin of the sinuses of Valsalva (66%)
2. A discrete fibromuscular membrane with a central opening in the lumen of the aorta (12%)
3. A diffuse hypoplasia of the ascending aorta with involvement of the arch and the branches (23%)

The coronary arteries may also be involved in the process, with ostial stenosis or luminal narrowing resulting in myocardial ischemia or even sudden death (62) (e303–e306). Supravalvar aortic stenosis occurs sporadically but may also be familial (e307) or part of the Williams syndrome (e308,e309). The latter two disorders have both been mapped to the elastin gene on chromosome 7 (e310,e311).

Aortic Atresia

Aortic atresia, the most common defect seen in the hypoplastic left-heart syndrome (e312–e314), shows a 2:1 to 3:1 male predominance (7,63) (e313,e315–e317). In isolated aortic atresia, the mitral valve and the left ventricular cavity are hypoplastic, with secondary left ventricular endocardial fibroelastosis and myocardial hypertrophy (eFigure 13-5) (e312,e313,e316). In the 30% to 50% of cases with associated mitral atresia, the left ventricle is diminutive (Figure 13-16) visible only on serial sections or definitively identified only on microscopic examination (63) (e313,e316,e318). VSDs, present in fewer than 10% of cases, may on the other hand be associated with a more normally sized ventricular cavity, with or without endocardial fibroelastosis (7,63) (e317,e319,e320). The site of the aortic valve may be invisible, or the valve may be represented by an imperforate membrane (e312,e313). The ascending aorta is represented by a narrow vessel functioning as a conduit to the coronary arteries, which arise normally. In 60% to 80% of cases, a discrete COTA is present (63) (e315,e316,e321). The descending aorta may then appear to arise from the ductus arteriosus, which is widely patent in most cases (63). Coronary artery changes and ventricle-coronary arterial connections, similar to those complicating PA, have been described in the left coronary artery and ventricle of hearts with aortic atresia and mitral stenosis (e320,e322,e323).

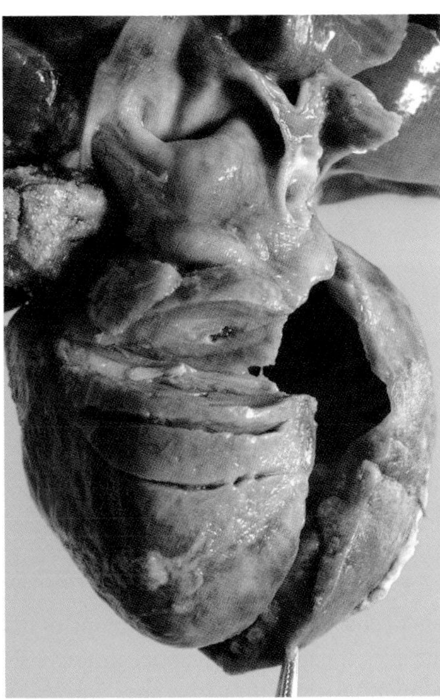

FIGURE 13-16 ▪ Posterior view of a heart removed at autopsy with mitral atresia and a hypoplastic left ventricle. At the left an incision opens into the large dilated right ventricle. Serial transverse sections across the thick posterior wall of the right atrium reveal a tiny opening just beneath an atretic mitral valve that represents the residuum of the left ventricle.

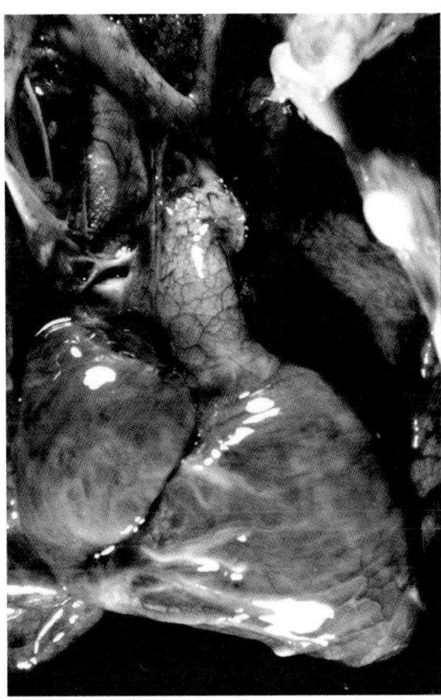

FIGURE 13-17 ▪ External view of a heart with hypoplastic left-heart syndrome, as seen from the anterior aspect. A dilated right atrial appendage hugs the large pulmonary artery and atrioventricular groove. A large right ventricle occupies the entire anterior ventricular surface.

Hypoplastic Left-Heart Syndrome

Hypoplastic left-heart syndrome is a clinicopathologic condition in which underdevelopment of the left side of the heart and the ascending aorta results in obstruction to the pulmonary venous outflow and dependence on a patent ductus arteriosus for adequate systemic blood flow (e324,e325). Without surgical intervention, severe congestive heart failure and death invariably ensue, usually in the first 2 months of life (1) (e281,e326). The uniform right atrial and ventricular enlargement combined with the small left ventricle, ascending aorta, and aortic arch give these hearts a characteristic external appearance (e313) (Figure 13-17). Pulmonary venous outflow depends on a left-to-right shunt across the atrial septum, usually via a patent fossa ovalis or secundum ASD (7) (e327). However, hypoplastic left-heart syndrome is associated with and possibly caused by premature closure of the foramen ovale in 5% to 10% of cases; in this situation, the pulmonary venous return must to be shunted to the right side of the heart via anomalous venous connections or intramyocardial sinusoids (38,63) (e43,e323,e328). The closed fossa ovalis worsens the already present pulmonary venous obstruction and predisposes an infant to significant pulmonary hypertension early in life (e328,e329). Stenotic or atretic mitral and aortic valves, with or without COTA, are the usual malformations resulting in hypoplastic left-heart syndrome (e312–e315,e327). Occasional reports describe instead left ventricular hypoplasia with a "contracted" form of endocardial fibroelastosis and hypoplastic but otherwise normally formed valves (e330,e331). In recent years, staged surgical correction of the hypoplastic left-heart syndrome (Table 13-18) and neonatal cardiac transplantation have dramatically improved the outlook for infants with this otherwise uniformly fatal disorder (64) (e318,e332–e336).

Malformations of the Aortic Arch System

Ductus Arteriosus

The ductus arteriosus differs from the aorta and pulmonary arteries in that its media is formed predominantly of smooth muscle layers (65) (e337). Control of ductus patency during fetal life relies on many factors, including relatively low oxygen tension and high circulating prostaglandins (65). In normal full-term infants, the rapidly rising oxygen and the falling prostaglandin levels result in functional ductus closure within 15 hours of birth. In premature infants, the immature state of the ductal response combined with relative hypoxia and prostaglandin excess lead to persistent ductal patency in 40% of infants weighing less than 2,000 g and up to 80% of infants weighing less than 1,200 g (e338). In premature infants with an inherently normal ductal structure, the administration of prostaglandin inhibitors such as indomethacin usually induces closure (e338).

Patent Ductus Arteriosus

A persistently patent ductus arteriosus (eFigure 13-6) beyond the first 2 or 3 weeks of life accounts for 2.5% to 8.5% of cases of CHD with a 2:1 female predominance (Table 13-1). In these older infants, the persistence of ductal patency is

Table 13-18 ■ HYPOPLASTIC LEFT HEART: MULTISTAGE "NORWOOD" REPAIR

Stage 1: Initial palliative surgery at age 1–3 weeks	
Purpose	Establish unobstructed systemic blood supply Limit pulmonary blood flow and pressure to normal levels
Procedures	Transect proximal main pulmonary artery Allograft reconstruction of ascending aorta (i.e., neoaorta) Pulmonary root-neoaorta anastomosis Atrial septectomy Blalock-Taussig shunt
Stage 2: Intermediate palliation at age 4–6 months	
Purpose	Decrease right ventricular load
Procedure	Superior vena cava-right pulmonary artery anastomosis (i.e., bidirectional Glenn procedure)
Stage 3: Definitive repair at age 18 months–2 years	
Purpose	Complete separation of pulmonary and systemic venous blood
Procedure	Tunnel anastomosis between inferior vena cava and right pulmonary artery (i.e., Fontan variant procedure)

probably caused by an inherent structural abnormality, and prostaglandin inhibitors rarely induce closure (e337,e339). Grossly, the patent ductus is usually thin-walled with a smooth intima, in contrast to the thick-walled irregular appearance of the normally closing ductus (7). Occasionally, the communication between the pulmonary artery and the aorta is in the form of a window at the expected site of the ductus (7). Microscopically, the internal elastic lamina is intact rather than fragmented, and a paucity of the intimal cushions present in the normal ductus can be seen (e339,e340).

In children outside the newborn period, a patent ductus arteriosus without other structural heart defects raises the possibility of an underlying infectious or genetic disorder. Patent ductus arteriosus is a frequent manifestation of the congenital rubella syndrome (e341,e342). Familial recurrence has been documented approximately in 3% of cases, and abnormal neural crest development may play a role (66) (e343,e344).

The clinical manifestations of patent ductus arteriosus relate to the size of the left-to-right shunt. Children with a small shunt are usually asymptomatic, coming to medical attention because of the characteristic continuous murmur. With increasing shunt size, congestive heart failure develops. Like patients with other right-to-left shunting lesions, these patients are at risk for the development of pulmonary obstructive vascular disease (7,65) (e337). Closure options include surgical ligation and nonsurgical insertion via a catheter of an occluding device or coils (65) (e345,e346).

Obstructive Anomalies of the Aortic Arch

The aortic arch can be divided into three segments: proximal transverse, distal transverse, and isthmus (67) (e347) (Table 13-19). Obstructive arch anomalies occur in any of the segments with varying frequency, depending on the type of obstruction.

Coarctation of the Aorta

COTA, defined as a discrete, shelflike area of narrowing in the descending aorta, accounts for 5% to 6.5% of congenital heart defects (Table 13-1). In the vast majority of instances, the coarctation is located in the upper thoracic aorta opposite the ductus arteriosus insertion site, and the previously used "preductal" and "postductal" designations have been replaced in the newer literature with the broader "juxtaductal" designation (e348). The site of narrowing is formed by a shelf of fibroelastic tissue and smooth muscle that is in continuity with similar tissue in the ductus (7) (e349,e350).

Associated cardiovascular anomalies, present in 50% to 60% of cases, include bicuspid aortic valve (40% to 50%), VSD (40% to 50%), and a variety of complex obstructive lesions of the left side of the heart (24%) (e351). The associated VSDs show malalignment and abnormalities of the left outflow tract that could reduce aortic arch blood flow *in utero* (e352). Decreased arch flow is postulated to play a role in the pathogenesis of the obstructive aortic arch lesions (e352–e354).

Clinical symptoms of coarctation are related to the severity of the obstruction. In infancy coarctation presents with heart failure; these infants often have associated tubular hypoplasia (7,68). Children less than 1year old at diagnosis are usually asymptomatic and present with upper extremity hypertension and decreased pulse and blood pressure. Surgical repair can be accomplished by resection of the coarctation ridge and end-to-end anastomosis of the aorta or by means of a subclavian flap or patch aortoplasty (e355,e356). Balloon aortoplasty and implantation of stents have also

Table 13-19 ■ AORTIC ARCH SEGMENTS

Arch Segment	Anatomic Location	Diameter[a]
A. Isthmus	Between L subclavian and ductus	≥40%
B. Distal transverse	Between L carotid and L subclavian	≥50%
C. Proximal transverse	Between R innominate and L carotid	≥60%

[a]% of diameter compared with ascending aorta.
L, left; R, right

Table 13-20 ■ COARCTATION OF THE AORTA: SURGICAL CLASSIFICATION[a]

Type I Primary coarctation
A. With ventricular septal defect
B. With other major cardiac defects

Type II Coarctation with isthmus hypoplasia
A. With ventricular septal defect
B. With other major cardiac defects

Type III Coarctation with tubular hypoplasia of isthmus and transverse arch
A. With ventricular septal defect
B. With other major cardiac defects

[a]All types with or without patent ductus arteriosus.

been used with some success in infants and older children, particularly those with discrete coarctation sites (e357–e359). Restenosis, aneurysm formation, or aortic dissection can occur as a complication in any of these procedures with the highest risk for complications in the very young infants (e349,e358,e360–e362).

Tubular Hypoplasia

The term *tubular hypoplasia* denotes an elongated (>5 mm) and hypoplastic segment of aortic arch, usually with an associated discrete coarctation site (7,68) (e363). In normal infants, the diameter of the aortic arch is smaller than that of the ascending aorta (67) (e347). The normal values used to determine whether true arch hypoplasia is present are outlined in Table 13-20. In the vast majority of instances, tubular hypoplasia is associated with other complex heart malformations, most often left ventricular hypoplasia or DOLV (67). Amato et al. (69) have proposed a classification system for coarctation that incorporates many of these anatomic variables (Table 13-20).

Interruption of the Aortic Arch

Complete obstruction of the aortic arch is subdivided into two lesions. In aortic arch atresia, an imperforate membrane or cord occludes the arch isthmus (7) (e347). Interruption of the aortic arch refers to a complete loss of aortic arch continuity, which is subclassified according to the interruption site (70) (e364–e367) (Table 13-21). Blood flow to the lower body depends on a patent ductus arteriosus; most hearts also contain a VSD (70) (e364,e366,e368,e369). In a smaller number (one-third to two-third), additional anomalies accompany the interrupted arch (70) (e369,e370). DiGeorge syndrome and its associated chromosome 22q11 deletion are identified in approximately 30% of cases with 90% of the cases of deletion occurring with the type B interruption (70) (e369–e371).

Table 13-21 ■ INTERRUPTED AORTIC ARCH SUBCLASSIFICATION

Type	Interruption Site	Relative Incidence
A	Isthmus	15%–30%
B	Distal transverse arch	70%–85%
C	Proximal transverse arch	0%–8%

Aortic Arch Branching Anomalies

The normal aortic arch, ductus arteriosus, and main pulmonary arteries develop from a sequence of six paired vessels, which then persist or disappear (71). The most significant of the myriad of anomalies that can result will be discussed briefly here.

Left Aortic Arch with Aberrant Right Subclavian Artery

The aberrant right subclavian artery originates distal to the left subclavian artery as a fourth branch of a left aortic arch, coursing behind the esophagus to the right arm. It occurs as an asymptomatic and usually isolated anomaly in 0.5% of the general population (72). It also accompanies other anomalies, appearing in 0.9% of children undergoing cardiac catheterization for other heart disease (72). During its retroesophageal course, the aberrant artery compresses the esophagus; it rarely causes symptoms, but the anomaly is visible on barium swallow. Rarely, a right-sided ductus arteriosus attaches to the anomalous right subclavian artery to form a vascular ring (71,72) (e372).

Right-sided Aortic Arch

A right-sided aortic arch, defined by a rightward sweep of the aorta as it arches into the posterior mediastinum, may display mirror-image branching or may be accompanied by a variety of additional branching anomalies (72). A right aortic arch with mirror image branching, the most common arch anomaly, is by itself of no clinical significance but almost always accompanies other cardiac malformations, especially TOF, which is present in 50% of cases (72) (e373). Hearts with mirror-image branching usually retain a left-sided ductus.

An aberrant left subclavian artery originating distal to the right subclavian artery as a fourth arch branch is the most frequent right-sided arch branching anomaly. The aberrant subclavian artery follows a retroesophageal course to enter the left side of the chest, where it usually attaches to a left-sided ductus arteriosus or ligamentum arteriosum to form a vascular ring. The origin of the aberrant subclavian artery from the aortic arch frequently appears dilated—hence the designation of *Kommerall diverticulum* (71,72). Additional cardiac malformations accompany the right-sided arch with aberrant left subclavian artery in less than 20% of cases (e372,e374,e375).

Vascular Rings

Vascular rings are malformations of the aortic arch structures that encircle and compress the trachea and the esophagus, causing respiratory symptoms and dysphagia (e374–e377). The most common vascular rings are formed by a double aortic arch, a right aortic arch with aberrant left subclavian artery and left ductus, or an anomalous left pulmonary artery (pulmonary sling) (71) (e374–e376,e378). The most common of these, the double aortic arch, occurs with associated cardiac anomalies in less than 20% of cases (e379). The anomalous left pulmonary artery (pulmonary sling) originates from the right pulmonary artery anterior to the right main bronchus and then passes between the trachea and the esophagus to enter the hilum of the left lung (73) (e380,e381). A variety of tracheobronchial and cardiovascular anomalies occur in at least 50% of these infants with tracheal cartilaginous rings or tracheal stenosis being the most common (73) (e382,e383).

Malformations of the Coronary Arteries

Anomalous Origin of the Left Coronary Artery

A variety of coronary artery anomalies have been described, but the only one of clinical significance is anomalous origin of the left coronary artery from the pulmonary trunk, a rare malformation (74) (e384). Beyond the newborn period, blood from the low-pressure pulmonary artery inadequately perfuses the high-pressure left ventricular myocardium. The resulting myocardial ischemia manifests clinically as congestive heart failure and pathologically as extensive subendocardial fibrosis or fibroelastosis and anterolateral wall infarction (74,75). The clinical course depends largely on the adequacy of the collateral flow that develops during the first weeks of life (75) (e385,e386). Most infants become symptomatic in the 1st months of life, and 65% to 85% die in early childhood if the anomaly is not corrected by surgery (7,74) (e386,e387). An anomalous origin of the right coronary artery is usually inconsequential because the low-pressure right ventricle is adequately perfused by blood from the low-pressure pulmonary artery (7,74).

Malformations of the Venous System

Systemic Venous Anomalies

Systemic venous blood returns to the heart via five sources: superior vena cava, coronary veins, hepatic veins, inferior vena cava, and azygos veins. With normally lateralized situs (situs solitus or situs inversus), anomalies of the systemic venous system are not uncommon but usually of little clinical significance. With situs ambiguus, complex systemic venous malformations are the rule.

Persistent Left Superior Vena Cava

A persistent LSVC is present in 0.3% to 0.5% of the general population and up to 10% of patients with other cardiovascular anomalies (7,76) (e388,e389). Absence of the innominate vein serves as a clue to the presence of a persistent LSVC in approximately 40% of cases (7) (e390). The LSCV traverses the posterior surface of the left atrium to enter the coronary sinus in the AV sulcus. Occasionally, the coronary sinus becomes dilated to the point of compressing the posterior wall of the left atrium, mimicking cor triatriatum (e391,e392). The wall between the coronary sinus and the left atrium becomes unroofed in approximately 8% of cases, resulting in drainage of the LSCV into the left atrium (76). This latter morphology occurs most frequently in the setting of the heterotaxy syndromes (10).

Coronary Sinus Ostium Atresia

With atresia of the coronary sinus ostium, a rare anomaly, cardiac venous drainage relies on a persistent LSVC with a patent innominate vein or other left-to-right connection (e393). The obstructed coronary sinus ostium by itself creates few clinical problems, but ligation of the persistent LSVC should be avoided during heart surgery (10) (e394).

Interruption of the Inferior Vena Cava with Azygos Continuation

Anomalies of the inferior vena cava are much less common. Infrahepatic interruption of the inferior vena cava with azygos continuation results in an absence of the inferior vena cava between the renal and hepatic veins (7,76). The inferior vena cava below the renal veins drains via an enlarged azygos vein, which enters the thorax through the aortic hiatus and joins the superior vena cava just superior to its junction with the right atrium. This anomaly is usually associated with other cardiovascular malformations and is frequently present in the polysplenia syndrome (7,77) (e395–e397).

Pulmonary Venous Anomalies

Pulmonary venous anomalies are listed in Table 13-22.

Partial Anomalous Pulmonary Venous Connection

Anomalous pulmonary venous connection refers to a group of conditions in which the pulmonary venous drainage is routed partially or totally to the right atrium. In the more common anomaly, partial anomalous pulmonary venous connection, blood from one or more, but not all, of the pulmonary veins drains into a systemic vein or right atrium. This anomalous drainage is right sided in more than 80% of cases and most frequently enters the superior vena cava or the right atrium (7) (e398–e400). More than 80% of cases occur in the setting of sinus venosus ASDs as described earlier (e33,e34,e398). The Scimitar syndrome represents a variant of partial anomalous pulmonary venous connection characterized by anomalous pulmonary venous drainage into the inferior vena cava with a variety of associated cardiopulmonary anomalies. The most frequent associations include right lung hypoplasia,

Table 13-22 ■ PULMONARY VENOUS MALFORMATIONS

- Partial anomalous pulmonary venous connection
  - Sinus venosus atrial septal defect
  - Scimitar syndrome
- Total anomalous pulmonary venous connection
  - Supradiaphragmatic
    - Supracardiac
    - Intracardiac
  - Infradiaphragmatic
- Pulmonary vein atresia
- Cor triatriatum

Table 13-23 ■ TOTAL ANOMALOUS PULMONARY VENOUS CONNECTION: CLASSIFICATION

Site of Connection	% Total	% Obstructed
Supracardiac	45%	45%
Left innominate vein	25%–35%	
Right SVC	10%–15%	
Cardiac	25%	0%–20%
Coronary sinus	15%–20%	
Right atrium	5%–15%	
Infracardiac	25%	80%–90%
Portal vein	15%–25%	
Mixed	5%–10%	35%–60%

dextrocardia, systemic arterial supply to the lung, and abnormal bronchial anatomy (78) (e401,e402).

Total Anomalous Pulmonary Venous Connection

Total anomalous pulmonary venous connection, in which all the pulmonary veins drain to the systemic circuit, is subclassified according to the route of the abnormal venous drainage and the presence or absence of obstruction to that drainage (79) (e403–e405) (Table 13-23). The most common route of drainage is through a vertical vein that arises from a confluence of the pulmonary veins posterior to the left atrium, traverses superiorly along the left side of the mediastinum, and drains into the innominate vein at its junction with the left subclavian vein (7) (e403,e404). Less frequently, the common trunk drains into the superior vena cava, right atrium, coronary sinus, or subdiaphragmatic portal venous system (Figure 13-18). In up to 10% of cases, the pulmonary veins drain to multiple different sites (80) (e406,e407). Drainage is obstructed in approximately 60% of cases of total anomalous pulmonary venous connection, with the cardiac sites having the lowest risk and the infracardiac the highest risk for obstruction (80) (e408) (Table 13-23). The venous drainage can be obstructed by intrinsically small vessels, external compression, or interposition of a capillary bed (7) (e403,e404). The pulmonary venous obstruction leads to early and often severe pulmonary hypertensive changes, manifested as medial hypertrophy of the pulmonary arteries and veins combined with intimal proliferation and eventually arterialization in the pulmonary veins (e409–e411). Total anomalous pulmonary venous connection is associated with other cardiac anomalies in approximately one-third of cases, particularly with the heterotaxy syndromes (7) (e403,e412). Occasionally, it occurs in families; the inherited form has been linked to chromosome 4p13 (e413,e414). The clinical manifestations of total anomalous pulmonary venous connection vary with the degree of obstruction and the resultant PVR (79) (e407,e415,e405). With significant obstruction and high levels of resistance, cyanosis, heart failure, and death occur in the 1st months of life (79). With low resistance, infants may be asymptomatic at birth,

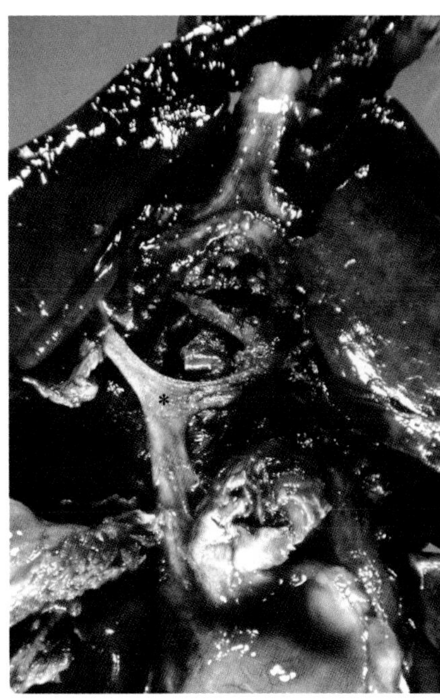

FIGURE 13-18■Total anomalous pulmonary venous connection, infradiapragmatic type seen from the posterior view. A confluence of the pulmonary veins (*) is isolated from the left atrium and drains into a vertical vein. This vein traverses the diaphragm to enter the portal venous system of the liver.

and right-sided heart failure is the predominant manifestation (79). Surgical correction in the modern era yields more than 90% short-term survival with only rare late deaths, usually caused by pulmonary venous stenosis (80) (e405,e407,e415). In large series, risk factors for death include young age at surgery, cardiac or infracardiac connection sites, and preoperative pulmonary venous obstruction (80) (e407).

Pulmonary Vein Atresia/Stenosis

In pulmonary vein atresia, the entire pulmonary venous system drains into a common chamber from which there is no site for egress (7,79). In pulmonary vein stenosis, which is less severe, luminal narrowing occurs at the venoatrial junction of one or more of the pulmonary veins (e416).

Cor Triatriatum

In cor triatriatum, the left atrium is partitioned by a fibromuscular shelf separating the pulmonary venous compartment from the atrial appendage and the mitral valve orifice compartment (eFigure 13-7) (7,79). The dividing membrane contains a variably sized opening, which results in most instances in pulmonary venous obstruction (7) (e417,e418). The foramen ovale may open into either compartment; when the opening is proximal to the obstruction, it can function as an escape valve for the pulmonary venous obstruction (7) (e417,e418).

Malformations of Position and Situs

Dextrocardia

Dextrocardia, in which the heart is located in the right side of the chest with a right-sided apex, occurs with situs inversus, situs ambiguous, and as an isolated finding (7) (e419,e420). Except when occurring with situs inversus, the incidence of associated intracardiac and extracardiac anomalies is high (1) (e420). Dextrocardia should be distinguished from dextroposition, in which the heart is displaced to the right side of the chest with a left-sided apex (7).

Ectopia Cordis

Ectopia cordis, a rare anomaly in which the heart is partially or totally outside the chest (Figure 13-19), is subclassified according to the location of the defect (7,81) (e421). Thoracic ectopia cordis, the most common type, is the result of a sternal cleft. The heart is usually located on the anterior surface of the chest without skin or a pericardial covering (81) (e421). Thoracoabdominal (abdominal) ectopia cordis is associated with a defect in the lower sternum, diaphragm, and abdominal wall; the heart is usually located with the abdominal viscera in a common omphalocele sac (81) (e421–e423). Intracardiac defects occur frequently but are not inevitable (81).

Situs Ambiguous

Situs ambiguous (heterotaxia) occurs when the usual markers of situs are disorganized or missing as a result of disruption of the left-right axis determination early in development (77) (e424–e426). The two best-described forms of situs ambiguous are asplenia (bilateral right sidedness) and polysplenia (bilateral left sidedness). The "sidedness" of the heart is determined by the atrial appendage morphology (82) (e427).

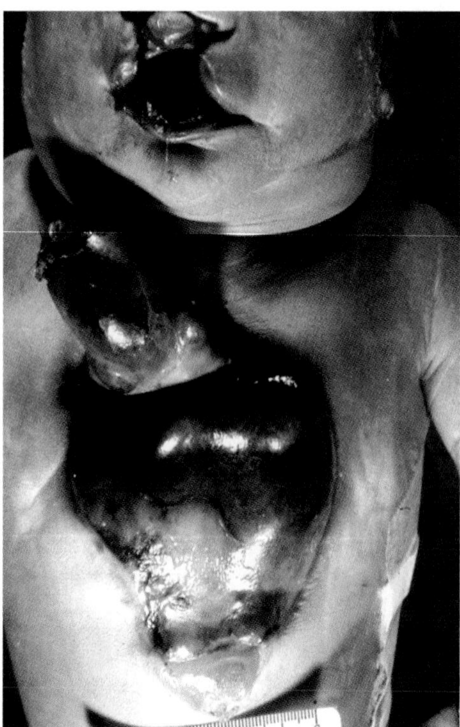

FIGURE 13-19 ■ Infant with multiple congenital anomalies including cleft lip seen at the top of the photograph and an anterior defect in the chest and abdomen through which the heart and liver protrude.

The heterotaxic syndromes are frequently associated with complex congenital heart and venous malformations and a variety of extracardiac defects (77) (e412,e424,e428,e429). Heterotaxic syndromes occasionally complicate maternal diabetes (e430), and the familial recurrence suggests a genetic factor (e431). Recent molecular studies have identified a variety of genes involved in left-right patterning during development (83) (e432). The heterotaxy syndromes are likely multifactorial in origin.

Juxtaposition of Atrial Appendages

Juxtaposition of the atrial appendages, diagnosed when both atrial appendages reside partially or completely on the same side of the great vessels, is a harbinger of underlying heart malformations (e433). Left-sided juxtaposition accounts for 86% of cases, with tricuspid atresia and transposition of the great vessels the most common associated malformations (e433). On the flip side, 11% of hearts with tricuspid atresia and 3% of hearts with D-transposition exhibit left-sided juxtaposition of the atrial appendages (32) (e434).

HEREDITARY AND NONHEREDITARY FUNCTIONAL CARDIOVASCULAR DISEASES

Myocardial Disease

Cardiomyopathies

The designation *cardiomyopathy* (CMP) encompasses a heterogeneous group of diseases with dysfunction of the myocardium, unaccompanied by structural malformations, as the defining pathophysiologic abnormality. Their classification, once largely descriptive, continues to evolve with the recent explosion in understanding of the underlying molecular aspects of these diseases and the ability to identify associated genetic mutations.

In 1980, the World Health Organization (WHO) presented a consensus definition of CMP as "heart muscle disease of unknown etiology," which was then divided into four subcategories (e435) (Table 13-24). Myocardial dysfunction of known etiology was considered a "specific disease of heart muscle" rather than a CMP (e435). In 1995, with improved understanding of disease pathogenesis, a revised WHO classification redefined CMP as "diseases of the myocardium associated with cardiac dysfunction" (e436). These diseases were then classified into five categories based largely on the dominant pathophysiologic abnormality. Myocardial diseases associated with specific cardiac or systemic disorders were reclassified as specific cardiomyopathies (Table 13-24). Over the ensuing 10 years, the explosion in molecular biology and genetic techniques resulted in dramatic advances in the knowledge of disease pathogenesis and ability to make more specific diagnoses. With this advance in understanding, the prior classification system has become increasingly incomplete and unwieldy. In response to this, the American Heart Association recently proposed a new classification scheme as outlined in Table 13-24 (84).

Table 13-24 ▪ CARDIOMYOPATHY: CLASSIFICATION

WHO 1980 (e435)	WHO 1995 (e436)	AHA 1006 (84)
Cardiomyopathy	Cardiomyopathy	Primary cardiomyopathy
Dilated	Dilated	Genetic
Hypertrophic	Hypertrophic	Hypertrophic
Restrictive	Restrictive	Arrhythmogenic RVC/D
Unclassified	Arrhythmogenic RV	LV noncompaction
Endocardial fibroelastosis	Unclassified	Conduction system disease
Histiocytoid	Fibroelastosis	Ion channelopathies
Fiedler myocarditis	Non compacted myocardium	Mixed (genetic and nongenetic)
Specific heart muscle disease	Mildly DCMP	Dilated
Infective	Mitochondrial CMP	Primary restrictive nonhypertrophied
Metabolic	Specific cardiomyopathy	Acquired
General system disease	Ischemic CMP	Myocarditis (inflammatory CMP)
Heredo-familial	Valvular CMP	Stress (Taku-Tsubo) CMP
Sensitivity and toxic reaction	Hypertensive CMP	Others
	Inflammatory CMP	Secondary cardiomyopathy
	Metabolic CMP	Infiltrative Storage
	Others	Endomyocardial Toxicity
		Endocrine Cardiofacial
		Inflammatory (granulomatous)
		Neuromuscular/neurological
		Nutritional deficiencies
		Autoimmune/collagen
		Electrolyte imbalance
		Consequence of cancer therapy

CMP occurs rarely in children, with 0.74 to 1.24 cases per 100,000 children in a year (e437–e439). In the pediatric population, dilated CMP (DCMP) accounts for 50% to 60% of cases and hypertrophic CMP (HCMP) another 25% to 40% (e437–e441). The clinical approach to a child presenting with CMP has been nicely summarized by Schwartz et al. (85).

Primary Cardiomyopathies

Hypertrophic Cardiomyopathy

HCMP is characterized by left ventricular hypertrophy, either symmetric or asymmetric, with a small ventricular cavity in a structurally normal heart (Figure 13-20). Idiopathic hypertrophic subaortic stenosis, hypertrophic obstructive CMP, and muscular subaortic stenosis are among the more than 50 synonyms used in the past (86).

At explant or autopsy, the heart is massively enlarged, weighing as much as two to three times the normal weight. The thickening of the left ventricular free wall and the interventricular septum may be either symmetric (concentric) or asymmetric. With asymmetric hypertrophy, which accounts for approximately two-thirds of cases, the thickness of the interventricular septum at its base measures greater than 1.3 times the thickness at the posterior left ventricular free wall (S/P ratio) (87) This asymmetric hypertrophy is often accompanied by an enlarged elongated mitral valve (86,87). The resulting abnormal mitral valve movement contributes to left ventricular outflow tract obstruction. This physiologic state may be marked by a fibrous imprint of the mitral valve septal leaflet on the apposing septal endocardium (87).

At the microscopic level, HCMP manifests a triad of features: myocyte hypertrophy, interstitial fibrosis, and myofiber disarray defined by whorled and intertwined clusters of myocytes surrounding a central fibrotic core (86,87). At the ultrastructural level, the myofilaments also display "disarray" (e442). Myofiber disarray is unfortunately not pathognomonic of HCMP, but can occur in secondary hypertrophy, or even normal hearts, and the finding of "extensive" (i.e., >10% and usually ≥30% of septum) disarray is therefore

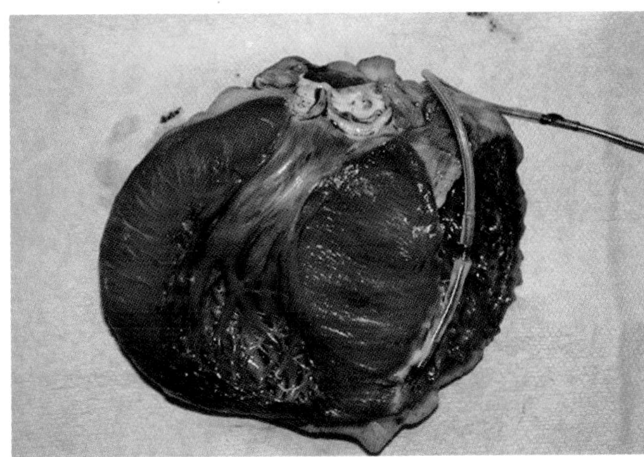

FIGURE 13-20 ▪ Coronal section through an explanted heart with hypertrophic cardiomyopathy as viewed from behind. A catheter marks the right atrium and right ventricle. Two cusps of the aortic valve are visible above the markedly thick walled left ventricle. The hypertrophic interventricular septum narrows and distorts the left ventricular outflow tract.

needed to make a diagnosis (87) (e443). The intramyocardial arteries in HCMP often display dysplastic changes similar to those seen in fibromuscular dysplasia (86,87). This small vessel disease may contribute to the myocardial ischemia, interstitial fibrosis, and development of a dilated phase late in the course of the disease (e443).

It should be noted that the S/P ratio of greater than 1.3 is not an appropriate criteria in stillborn or newborn infants. In the developing heart, the ventricular septum is disproportionately thick and an S/P ratio greater than 1.3 occurs in greater than 90% of embryos and young fetuses, in 65% of older fetuses, and in 25% of normal-term newborns (e444).

Primary HCMP represents a common autosomal dominant disorder with an estimated incidence of 1:500 in the general population (86). Causative mutations in at least ten different genes encoding sarcomere proteins have been identified in families with HCMP, with mutations in the myosin-binding protein C or β-myosin heavy chains accounting for 80% of cases (86) (e445). Mutations can also be identified in up to 60% of adults with sporadic HCMP (e445). In children under 10 years of age, underlying metabolic or syndromatic causes, including Noonan syndrome in particular, account for 20% to 35% of cases of HCMP (88) (e446). The spectrum of diseases that can present with HCMP is broad, as outlined in Table 13-25.

Table 13-25 ■ HYPERTROPHIC CARDIOMYOPATHY

Autosomal dominant inheritance		
Familial HCMP	Gene	
Defect in cardiac myosin-binding protein C	*MYBPC3*	11p11.2
Defect in cardiac β-myosin heavy chain	*MYH7*	14q12
Defect in cardiac troponin T	*TNNT2*	1q32
Defect in cardiac troponin 1	*TNNI3*	19q13.4
Defect in myosin light chain 2	*MYL2*	12q23-q24.3
Defect in myosin light chain 3	*MYL3*	3p
Defects in α-tropomyosin	*TPM1*	15q22.1
Defect in cardiac α-actin	*ACTC1*	15q14
Defect in titin	*TTN*	2q31
HCMP with Wolff-Parkinson-White syndrome	*PRKAG*	7q36
Noncompaction of the left ventricle[a]		
Syndromic disorders		
Noonan syndrome		
Friedreich ataxia		
Myotonic dystrophy		
Cardiofaciocutaneous syndrome		
Leopard syndrome/lentiginosis/multiple lentigines		
Neurofibromatosis		
Beckwith-Wiedemann syndrome		
Telecanthus, multiple congenital anomalies		
Deaf mutism		
Rubinstein-Taybi syndrome		
Autosomal recessive inheritance		
Total lipodystrophy, insulin resistance, leprechaunism		
Costello syndrome		
Sporadic		
Infant of diabetic mother[a]		
Infiltrative (storage) disorders		
Disorders of glycogen metabolism		
Glycogen storage disease type II (Pompe disease: acid maltase deficiency)		
Glycogen storage disease type IIb (Danon disease: lysosome-associated membrane protein-2)		
Glycogen storage disease type III (Cori disease: debranching enzyme)		
Glycogen storage disease type IX (cardiac phosphorylase kinase deficiency)		
Disorders of mucopolysaccharide degradation		
Mucopolysaccharidosis type I (Hurler syndrome)[a]		
Mucopolysaccharidosis type II (Hunter syndrome)		
Mucopolysaccharidosis type III (Sanfilippo syndrome)		
Mucopolysaccharidosis type IV (Morquio syndrome)		
Mucopolysaccharidosis type VII (Sly syndrome)		
Disorder of glycosphingolipid degradation (Fabry disease)		
Disorder of glycosylceramide degradation (Gaucher disease)		
Disorder of *N*-glycosylation		
Disorder of phytanic acid oxidation (Refsum disease)[a]		
Disorders of combined ganglioside/mucopolysaccharide and oligosaccharide degradation		
GM1 gangliosidosis[a]		
GM2 gangliosidosis (Sandhoff disease)[a]		

(Continued)

Table 13-25 ■ HYPERTROPHIC CARDIOMYOPATHY AUTOSOMAL DOMINANT INHERITANCE *(Continued)*

Diminished energy production (mitochondrial disorders)
- Disorders of pyruvate metabolism
  - Pyruvate dehydrogenase complex deficiency (Leigh disease)
- Disorders of oxidative phosphorylation
  - Complex I deficiency
  - Complex III deficiency (histiocytoid CM)
  - Complex IV deficiency (muscle and Leigh disease forms)
  - Complex V deficiency
  - Mitochondrial transfer RNA mutation
    - MERRF syndrome[a]
    - MELAS syndrome
- Mitochondrial DNA deletions and duplications
    - Kearns-Sayre syndrome
    - Barth syndrome (3-methylglucurconic aciduria type II)[a]
    - Senger syndrome

Disorders of fatty acid metabolism
- Primary carnitine deficiency[a]
- Very-long-chain acyl-CoA dehydrogenase deficiency
- Long-chain acyl-CoA dehydrogenase deficiency
- Long-chain 3-hydroxyacyl-CoA dehydrogenase deficiency[a]
- Multiple acyl-CoA dehydrogenase deficiency (glutaric acidemia type II)

Toxic intermediary metabolite
- Disorders of amino acid or organic acid metabolism
- Tyrosinemia

[a]Causes both HCMP and DCMP.
DCMP, dilated cardiomyopathy; HCMP, hypertrophic cardiomyopathy; AR, autosomal recessive; CM, cardiomyopathy.
Modified from Schwartz ML, Cox GF, Lin AE, et al. Clinical approach to genetic cardiomyopathy in children. *Circulation* 1996;94:2021–2038.
See also Callis TE, Jensen BC, Weck KE, et al. *Expert Rev Mol Diagn* 2010;10:329–351.

In primary HCMP, the symptoms of hypertrophy most commonly develop only after adolescent growth has been completed (86). However, up to one-third of cases can present in infancy (e447). In infants, the hypertrophy tends to cause restriction of right ventricular outflow in addition to obstruction of left ventricular outflow (86) (e446). When this occurs, HCMP may masquerade clinically as pulmonary valvular stenosis, congenital mitral insufficiency, VSD, endocardial fibroelastosis, or myocarditis. Sudden death may occur in 1% to 2% of affected children, whether they are symptomatic or not (86) (e447).

Arrhythmogenic Right Ventricular Dysplasia

Arrhythmogenic right ventricular dysplasia (ARVD) is characterized by partial or massive transmural fibrofatty replacement of the right ventricular myocardium with associated ventricular arrhythmias (89) (e448).

Hearts removed at transplant or autopsy are large with the right ventricle appearing yellow or white. The fatty replacement occurs initially in the anterior free wall of the right ventricle adjacent to the septum, with progressive involvement extending to the lateral ventricular wall (89) (e448) (Figure 13-21). In the most severe cases, the entire right ventricle may be involved. In areas of thinning, the ventricle wall may display focal aneurysm formation (89) (e448). At microscopic examination, fat mixed with variable amounts of fibrous tissue and inflammatory cells replaces the normal myocardium (89) (e448). The extension of fat and fibrosis into the conduction pathways correlates the histopathology with the clinical course (89). The left ventricle may be thickened in 15% of cases and shows histologic features of patchy fibrosis with or without subepicardial fat infiltration in up to 50% of cases (89) (e448). Distinguishing the normal fatty infiltration of the right ventricle, which occurs with increasing age and obesity, from ARVD can be difficult. Suggested criteria include the association of fat with disorganized myocardium and presence of fibrosis with the fat (90) (e449).

ARVD presents as a familial disease in 50% of cases with both autosomal dominant and autosomal recessive (Naxos

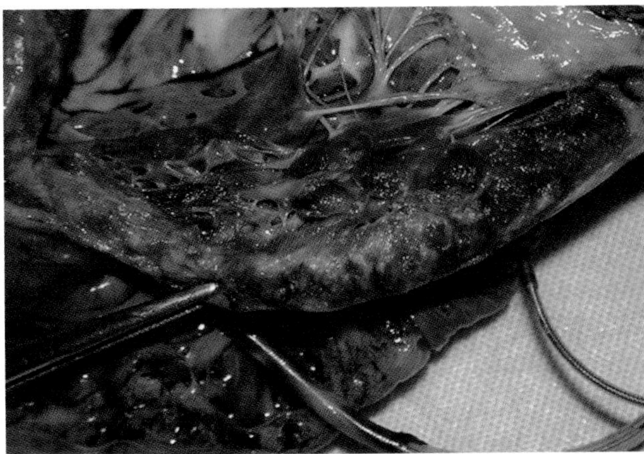

FIGURE 13-21 ■ A close-up view of the right ventricular wall cut surface showing near complete replacement of the normally deep red myocardium by pale yellow fibrofatty tissue.

disease) inheritance patterns (e450). Search for a gene has yielded a variety of mutations related to desmosomal junction proteins and calcium receptors without a well-defined unifying disease mechanism (91) (e450). Apoptosis in the condition suggests that the genes involved may play a role in programmed cell death and that apoptosis may precede the infiltration (e451).

ARVD clinically presents with an arrhythmia or sudden death in young adults, especially males (M:F, 2.7:1) and has been reported in children as young as 5 years (89,90). The overall disease prevalence is estimated at 1:5,000 with certain regions (e.g., Greek Island of Naxos) having an increased prevalence (90). ARVD accounts for up to 5% of sudden unexpected deaths in young adults. Patients with known disease experience an annual mortality rate of approximately 2% due to arrhythmia or right-heart failure (90). Therefore, treatment often requires aggressive measures such as radiofrequency ablation, implantable defibrillators, or transplantation (90).

Noncompaction of the Ventricular Myocardium

Noncompaction of the ventricular myocardium (NCVM), also called *persistence of spongy myocardium*, refers to a luminal meshwork of interlacing endomyocardial trabeculae intersected by irregular endocardial-lined sinusoids that communicate with the ventricular lumen (92) (e452,e453). A similar pattern of spongy myocardium occurs in the very early stages of heart embryogenesis (92) (e454,e455). During normal development, as the coronary arteries and veins develop, the sinusoids involute and the surrounding myocardium becomes compacted, proceeding from the epicardium to endocardium and base to apex (e452,e454,e455). The earliest description of noncompaction included hearts both with and without associated complex malformations (e456). The noncompacted sinusoids in hearts with severe malformations, PA with IVS in particular, connect with the subepicardial coronary arteries, whereas the sinusoids in hearts with isolated noncompaction communicate with the ventricular lumen (92). Isolated noncompaction, recognized with increasing frequency in recent years, occurs at all ages (92) (e452,e453). In recent studies, it accounts for up to 10% of heart lesions presenting to cardiology clinics (92).

The clinical diagnosis of NCVM hinges on echocardiographic findings with the diagnostic criteria varying between institutions (e457–e460). The echocardiagraphic features of dilated, restrictive, or HCMP may accompany the noncompaction (e460,e461). These echocardiographic findings correlate with the pathologic changes described in hearts examined at autopsy or following transplant (92,93). The left ventricular cavity contains poorly defined papillary muscles as an initial clue to the diagnosis. The excess trabeculation may or may not be grossly visible on the luminal surface. Full thickness sections from the ventricular apex and/or free wall will, however, yield the histologic picture of deep invaginations of endocardial-lined spaces with variable degrees of associated fibroelastosois. The normal luminal trabeculae are of variable thickness and a definitive pathologic diagnosis of noncompaction requires that the

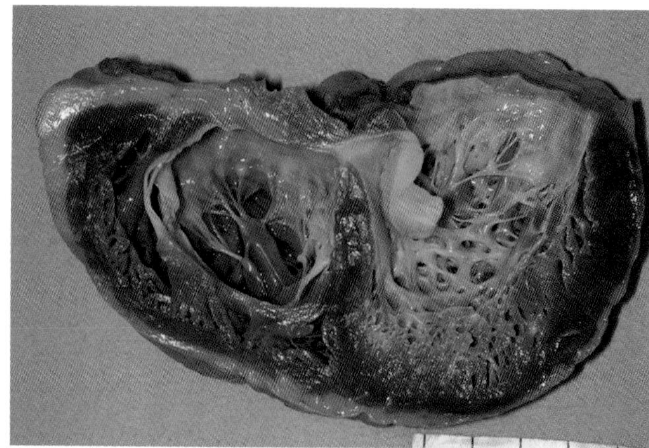

FIGURE 13-22 ■ Coronal section through an explanted heart with noncompaction as viewed from the front. Both the right and left ventricles of this globular heart appear thick walled and dilated. The endocardium appears whitened due to endocardial fibroelastosis, particularly in the left ventricle. At the apex of the left ventricle, only the external 25% of the wall has the appearance of normal deep red compact myocardium. The fine trabeculations characteristic of noncompaction occupy the majority of the wall.

trabeculae and intervening sinusoids account for at least 50% of the myocardial wall thickness (Figure 13-22) (93). Although left ventricular involvement represents the hallmark of this disease, the right ventricle is also involved in approximately 40% of cases (e460,e462).

Clinically, NCVM manifests as arrhythmias and congestive heart failure. In adults, thrombi within the sinusoids often lead to systemic emboli; this complication occurs less frequently in children (e460,e463,e464). Although in adults the disorder is reported more commonly in males, in the pediatric population the M:F ratio is near equal (e452,e458, e460,e462,e463,e465). A variety of extracardiac manifestations have been described, with neuromuscular disorders being the most frequent (92) (e466). Genetic studies of family cohorts have yielded several associated gene mutations, the most frequent being the tafazzin gene on chromosome Xp28, which is also associated with Barth syndrome (Table 13-26).

The underlying pathogenesis of NCVM remains unclear. Abnormal embryonic development currently represents the most popular theory (e454). However, this theory does not explain the full clinical spectrum of disease, and the noncompaction phenotype likely represents a final common pathway for a variety of etiologic factors.

Table 13-26 ■ LEFT VENTRICULAR NONCOMPACTION GENETIC MUTATIONS

Gene	Chromosome	Reference
Tafazzin	Xp28	(e712,e713)
α-dystrobrevin	18q12.1-q12.2	(e712)
CSX	5q del	(e714)
CypherZasp	10q22.2-q23.3	(e715)
Lamin A/C	1q12.1-q23 and 10	(e716)

Dilated Cardiomyopathy

DCMP represents a spectrum of disorders in which a dilated, poorly contracting, failing heart exhibits systolic and diastolic dysfunction. DCMP represents the common endpoint for multiple underlying conditions (Table 13-27).

Table 13-27 ■ DILATED CARDIOMYOPATHY

- **Nongenetic conditions**
  - Infectious or postinfectious condition
    - Enteroviruses
    - Mumps
    - *Corynebacterium diphtheroides*
  - Endocrine/vitamin/mineral disorders
    - Thyrotoxicosis
    - Hypothyroidism
    - Vitamin E and selenium deficiency
    - Infants of diabetic mothers[a]
  - Cellular toxicity
    - Anthracycline toxicity
    - Hemochromatosis
    - Alcohol
    - Cyclophosphamide
- **Genetic/familial conditions**
  - Infiltrative (storage) disorders
    - Glycogen storage disease type IV (Andersen disease: branching enzyme deficiency)
    - Mucopolysaccharidosis type I (Hurler syndrome)[a]
    - Mucopolysaccharidosis type VI (Maroteaux-Lamy syndrome)
  - Disorders of oxidative phosphorylation
    - Complex I deficiency
    - Mitochondrial transfer RNA mutations
      - MERRF syndrome[a]
    - Mitochondrial DNA deletions and duplications
      - Barth syndrome (3-methylglucuronic aciduria type II)[a]
  - Disorders of fatty acid metabolism
    - Primary or systemic carnitine uptake deficiency[a]
    - Long-chain 3-hydroxyacyl-CoA dehydrogenase deficiency[a]
  - Toxic intermediary metabolite disorders
    - Proprionic acidemia
    - Ketothiolase deficiency
  - Familial and neuromuscular conditions
    - Familial DCMP
    - Familial DCMP with conduction defects
    - Isolated ventricular noncompaction[a]
    - Muscular dystrophies
      - Duchenne and Becker muscular dystrophy
      - Emery-Dreifuss muscular dystrophy
      - Myotonic dystrophy[a]
      - Limb-girdle muscular dystrophy
      - Congenital muscular dystrophy
    - Congenital myopathies
      - Centronuclear (myotubular) myopathy
      - Nemaline rod myopathy[a]
      - Minicore-multicore myopathy
    - Friedreich ataxia[a]
    - Refsum disease[a]

[a]Cause both DCMP and HCMP
DCMP, dilated cardiomyopathy; HCMP, hypertrophic cardiomyopathy; AR, autosomal recessive; AD, autosomal dominant.
Modified from Schwartz ML, Cox GF, Lin AE, et al. Clinical approach to genetic cardiomyopathy in children. *Circulation* 1996;94:2021–2038.

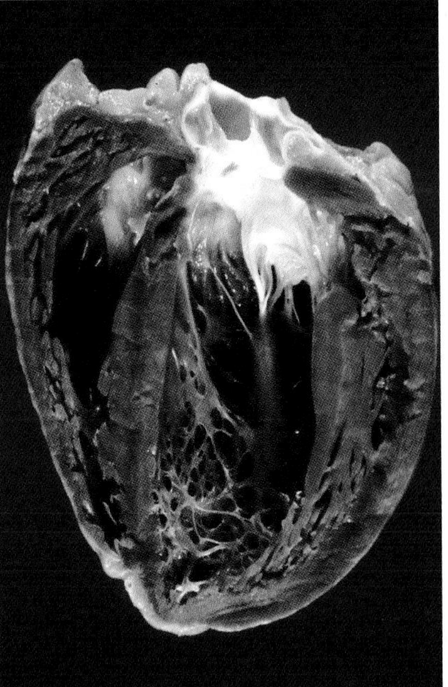

FIGURE 13-23 ■ Coronal section through an explanted heart with dilated cardiomyopathy. Both ventricles appear dilated with minimally thickened myocardium.

The gross appearance of a heart with DCMP is the same regardless of the cause (94). The key feature is biventricular dilation (Figure 13-23), and often all four cardiac chambers are dilated. The enlarged heart may weigh 25% to 50% more than normal and has a globular appearance. The dilated flabby, pale left ventricular wall is of normal thickness or appears thinned despite hypertrophy of the myofibers. Stasis in the large end-diastolic atrial and ventricular cavities results in the formation of mural thrombi. Interstitial myocardial fibrosis is the histologic feature common to all cases of DCMP, whatever the cause (94). Because these histologic features are generally nonspecific, the diagnosis of DCMP based on biopsy material is difficult.

In childhood, an underlying etiology can be identified in 33% to 60% of cases of DCMP with lymphocytic myocarditis accounting for 15% to 45% (95) (e441,e467,e468). Biopsy early in the course of disease leads to a higher number of myocarditis diagnoses (e467). Under the new classification scheme, these cases would be termed *inflammatory CMP* and are discussed further later.

Familial DCMP accounts for 10% to 45% of cases depending on the study methods used (95) (e467,e469,e470). Familial forms of DCMP cover a broad spectrum of disease processes (Table 13-27). The most common familial diseases are neuromuscular, with the majority having a known underlying muscular dystrophy. In a small subgroup of patients, however, the CMP represents the presenting feature of the underlying neuromuscular disorder (e471,e472). The identification of clinical features such as weakness, elevated creatine kinase, lactic acidosis, ptosis, granulocytopenia, and conduction abnormalities can help focus the search for the underlying genetic defect (85) (e473).

In a large combined prospective and retrospective review of DCMP in childhood, the majority of children (>70%) presented in congestive heart failure with the median age at diagnosis of 1.5 years; 42% were under 1 year. There was an M:F ratio of 3:2 and a 2 to 3× increased incidence in the black versus white populations (95). Fifty percent of children in this study died or required heart transplant.

Restrictive Cardiomyopathy

Restrictive CMP (RCMP) represents a heart in which the ventricular diastolic volume is decreased with near-normal systolic function and wall thickness. This wall "stiffness" results from infiltrative or fibrotic disorders that may be primary in the heart or secondary to a systemic disorder. RCMP occurs rarely in childhood accounting for less than 5% of all cardiomyopathies (e438–e440), with the majority of cases being familial isolated CMP (e441).

Hearts from patients with the echocardiographic features of RCMP include three pathologic forms (96) (e474). The "pure" restrictive form manifests a normal weight with small ventricular size and no hypertrophy; the hypertensive restrictive form manifests increased weight, with free wall and septal hypertrophy; the dilated restrictive form manifests increased weight without hypertrophy and with mild ventricular dilatation. Microscopic examination similarly displays overlapping features including fibrosis, hypertrophy, and even myofiber disarray (96). With the restricted ventricular filling, atrial dilatation is often striking (97) (e475,e476). The increased left ventricular filling pressure leads to pulmonary hypertension and associated right ventricular hypertrophy.

In children, RCMP most often occurs as a primary myocardial disease rather than secondary to infiltrative processes (97) (e477). Although the majority of primary and familial RCMP are idiopathic, some have now been linked to some of the same genetic mutations found in HCMP (e478). CMP associated with underlying genetic disorders, such as Noonan syndrome, can also present as RCMP rather than HCMP.

Although children with RCMP can present at any age, in most series the mean age is under 5 years (97) (e475,e476). Symptoms at presentation often reflect the increased PVR. The long-term prognosis in these children is poor, with up to 60% dying within 5 years of diagnosis (97) (e476). Cardiac transplantation early in the course of disease offers the best opportunity for long-term survival (97) (e475,e479).

Endocardial Fibroelastosis

Endocardial fibroelastosis (EFE) is a focal or a diffuse proliferation of fibroelastic tissue beneath the endocardium of any chamber of the heart, but predominantly the left ventricle. EFE occurs in both structurally normal and structurally malformed hearts. In the past, EFE in a structurally normal heart was considered a form of primary CMP. In recent years, with the overall improved understanding of the cardiomyopathies, EFE is no longer considered a primary form of CMP and has instead been relegated to the status "associated finding" in a wide variety of cardiomyopathic processes. In infants with primary EFE, mumps and/or adenovirus have been identified in 90% of cases by PCR, suggesting *in utero* viral infection as an etiology for this disorder (e480).

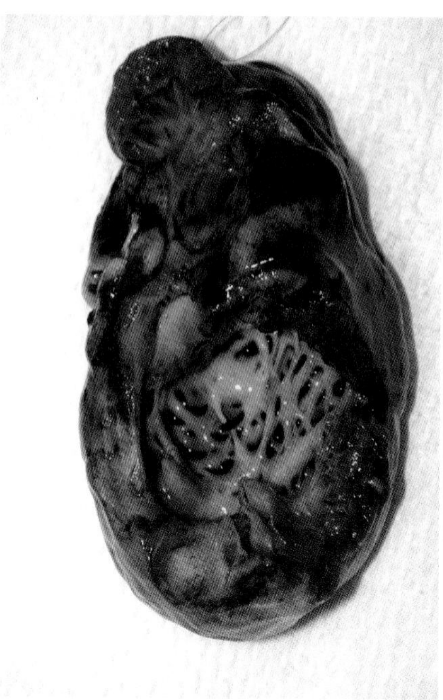

FIGURE 13-24 ■ Posterior view of an infant heart with windows opened into the left atrium and the left ventricle. The left ventricle endocardium appears white due to the diffuse endocardial fibroelastosis.

EFE gives the normally thin translucent endocardium a white opaque appearance (Figure 13-24). Microscopic examination reveals subendocardial layers of dense collagen and elastic fibers that extend into all the crevices of the chamber walls and even into the myocardium to surround vessels and groups of myocytes. Focal dystrophic calcification and necrosis may also occur. The elastic fibers in EFE often appear larger, more darkly staining, and more uniformly oriented than those found in the subendocardial fibrosis that follows ischemic heart disease (e481).

Myocarditis (Inflammatory Cardiomyopathy)

Although the term *myocarditis* denotes inflammation of the myocardium, experienced physicians and pathologists recognize that the clinical and morphologic diagnosis of myocarditis can be exceedingly difficult. The current widely accepted criteria for a morphologic diagnosis of myocarditis requires the presence of an inflammatory infiltrate directly associated with myocyte damage that occurs in the absence of ischemic changes associated with vascular disease (Figure 13-25) (98) (e482).

The macroscopic appearance of the heart, clinically or at autopsy, depends on the age of the patient, causative agent, time course of the infection, and associated complications. In acute fulminant myocarditis, the myocardium is often flabby; it may have a gray and glassy cast and be studded with scattered hemorrhagic foci. Although their overall shape may not be altered, the ventricular walls are usually much softer than expected (99) (e483). With more longstanding disease,

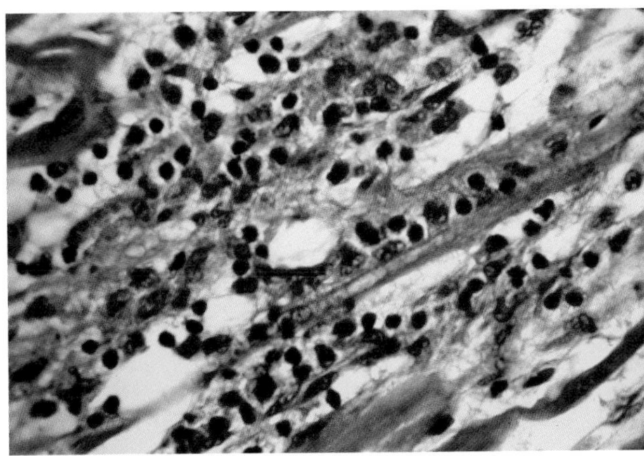

FIGURE 13-25 ■ Acute myocarditis. Mononuclear cells infiltrate frayed and damaged cardiac myocytes. (Hematoxylin and eosin stain, original magnification 400×.)

Table 13-28 ■ MYOCARDITIS

Dallas Criteria

Myocarditis—requires both inflammation and myocyte damage
Borderline myocarditis = Inflammation without myocyte damage
Inflammation = Lymphocytic ± neutrophils ± giant cells ± eosinophils
Myocyte damage = Frank fiber necrosis and/or intracellular lymphocytes and/or fiber vacuolization or disruption
First biopsy
  Myocarditis with/without fibrosis
  Borderline myocarditis
  No myocarditis
Subsequent biopsy (requires myocarditis dx on first biopsy)
  Ongoing (persistent) myocarditis with/without fibrosis
  Resolving (healing) myocarditis with/without fibrosis
    Inflammation still present; no myofiber necrosis; reparative changes present
  Resolved (healed) myocarditis with/without fibrosis
    No inflammation in myocardium (may be in center of scar)

German Criteria

Myocarditis = ≥ 14 leukocytes/mm^2 or clusters of ≥ 3 T-cells in myocardium; leukocytes quantitated using IHC
First biopsy
  Acute (active) myocarditis—≥ 14 leukocytes/mm^2 + myocyte damage ± fibrosis
  Chronic myocarditis—≥ 14 leukocytes/mm^2 without myocyte damage ± fibrosis
Subsequent biopsy
  Ongoing (persistent) myocarditis—may be acute or chronic
  Resolving (healing) myocarditis—acute or chronic but "sparser" than first biopsy
  Resolved (healed) myocarditis—no inflammation in myocardium

multifocal fibrosis of the ventricular wall and septum and endocardial thickening are common.

Microscopic features include inflammation and myocyte damage. Myocyte damage, best seen in longitudinal section, consists of necrosis and myocyte debris; degenerative changes and altered staining characteristics (especially with Masson trichrome); vacuolization, which causes a ragged, frayed appearance of the margins of the myocytes and cellular disruption with infiltration of inflammatory cells. The nature of inflammatory infiltrates varies with the time course and underlying etiology; infiltrates may be diffuse or focal and may include neutrophils, lymphocytes, macrophages, plasma cells, eosinophils, and/or giant cells (GCs) (98) (e482). The histologic appearance of the inflammatory infiltrate, coupled with the type and extent of the myocyte damage, may offer clues to the cause of myocarditis (99).

Endomyocardial biopsy currently serves as the major tool for diagnosing myocarditis based on the Dallas criteria (Table 13-28). These criteria are however fraught with problems of sampling and interobserver variability (e484,e485). In an attempt to address the biopsy interpretation difficulties, among other things, a new set of diagnostic criteria have recently been advanced (Table 13-28) (e486,e487).

Myocarditis presents clinically in one of three patterns: sudden unexpected death, acute heart failure, and more insidious heart disease that can mimic DCMP. In one large autopsy series, myocarditis accounted for 7% of sudden deaths (e488). Luckily, myocarditis presents more commonly as acute heart failure, manifesting as a wide spectrum of clinical symptoms. Diagnosis relies on EKG and echocardiographic features, with identification of the underlying organisms usually requiring serologic studies (e489). The incidence of acute myocarditis is best estimated from a large prospective study of myocarditis in Finnish military conscripts with a mean age of 20 years that yielded an incidence of 0.17/1,000 person-years (e490). With aggressive clinical support, the death rate in this group is less than 10% and the vast majority recover normal heart function (e489,e491). A young age of onset renders the best long-term prognosis. The one exception to this overall good outlook is idiopathic GC myocarditis, discussed later.

Myocarditis has been linked to most human pathogens and also to a variety of noninfectious conditions (88,100) (Table 13-29).

Bacterial myocarditis occurs rarely, usually as a complication of septicemia. Streptococci, staphylococci, and Neisseria result in suppurative myocarditis (7); in rickettsial infections organisms directly invade the endothelium of myocardial vessels (e492). Bacterial exotoxins have been implicated as the causative mechanism in diphtheria-(*Corynebacterium diphtheriae*) related myocarditis (7,100). The suggestion that a bacterial infection could elicit myocarditis through antigenic mimicry has received support from studies of *Chlamydia spp.* infections and heart disease (e493).

Protozoal myocardial infections, rare in North America and Europe, lead to significant diseases in many parts of the world. Chagas disease (*Trypanosoma cruzi*), an endemic infection in South and Central America, represents the most common form of myocarditis worldwide (88). Acute disseminated infection occurs predominantly in children following a focal lesion. Chronic Chagas disease is a leading

Table 13-29 ■ AGENTS AND CONDITIONS ASSOCIATED WITH MYOCARDITIS

I. Infections			
A. Viruses			
Enterovirus			
Coxsackie A	Coxsackie B	Echovirus	Poliovirus
Adenovirus			
Herpes virus			
Cytomegalovirus	Herpes simplex	Varicella	Ebstein-Barr virus
Influenza A or B			
Paramyxovirus			
Respiratory syncytial virus	Measles	Mumps	
Parvovirus			
Human immunodeficiency virus	Hepatitis B	Hepatitis C	
Rubella	Dengue virus	Yellow fever virus	
B. Bacteria			
Gram positive			
Streptococcus	*Staphylococcus*	*Corynebacterium diphtheriae*	
Clostridium			
Gram negative			
Meningococcus	*Brucella*	*Neisseria*	*Salmonella*
Hemophilus influenza		*Serratia marcescens*	
Acid-fast			
Myocobacteria tuberculosis			
Spirochetes			
Leptospira	*Treponema pallidum*		*Borrelia*
Rickettsia			
Rickettsia rickettsii	*Coxiella burnetii*	*Rickettsia prowazekii*	
Other			
Chlamydia	*Mycoplasma pneumoniae*		
Actinomycetes	Nocardia		
C. Fungi			
Candida	Histoplasma	*Aspergillus*	Coccidioides
Cryptococcus	Blastomyces	Mucormycoses	
D. Parasites			
Trypanosoma cruzi	*Toxoplasma gondii*	Amoebiasis	
Toxocara canis	*Schistosoma*	Visceral larva migrans	
Trichinella	*Echinococcus*	Cystocercosis	
II. Noninfectious			
A. Connective tissue disease			
Rheumatic heart diseases		Systemic lupus erythematosus	
Rheumatoid heart disease		Mixed connective tissue	
Ulcerative colitis		Scleroderma	
B. Drugs and toxins			
Anthracyclines	Acetazolamide	Antibiotics	
Cyclophosphamide	Amphotericin B	Indomethacin	
Phenytoin	Heavy metals	Cocaine	
C. Other			
Giant cell myocarditis		Kawasaki disease	
Sarcoidosis		Thyrotoxicosis	

cause of cardiac failure and sudden death in endemic areas (7). Toxoplasmosis (*Toxoplasma gondii*) is widespread and may be acquired or occur *in utero* (e494), but isolated myocardial disease is uncommon. Necrotizing inflammation with edema, lymphocytes, histiocytes, and plasma cells is typical (e495). Occasionally, one finds pseudocysts or sporozoites in the site. *Toxocara canis* causes severe granulomatous inflammation with an occasionally intense eosinophilic infiltrate (100) (e496). *Trichinella spiralis* infection may lead to cardiac failure with a focal or a diffuse infiltration by lymphocytes and eosinophils; the parasites are however rarely found in the sites of myocardial injury, having been either destroyed or passed directly into the circulation (7). Echinococcal heart disease is rare in North America but is common in countries with large sheep-grazing programs.

Viral infections account for most cases of infectious myocarditis, with a wide number of agents implicated (Table 13-29). Coxsackievirus B is the most commonly recognized cause in infants and children (e497). Although polymorphonuclear leukocytes may predominate initially, lymphocytes, plasma cells, and eosinophils soon replace them, followed by fibroblasts attempting repair (7) (e483).

The diagnosis of viral myocarditis can be established by (a) isolation and identification through cytopathic effects in culture, (b) identification of pathognomonic tissue changes with light or electron microscopy, (c) tissue identification of specific viral antigens with monoclonal antibodies, (d) recognition of a fourfold rise in specific antibodies in acute and convalescent serum samples, and (e) specific identification with molecular methods (100). Most acute cases are identified by serologic study. In recent years, molecular methods, in particular PCR, have become widely used to test for viral genome in inflamed myocardial tissue (e498,e499). Using these techniques, viral genome can be detected in 23% to 46% of cases (e499,e500).

The role viral infection plays in biopsy-proven chronic myocarditis remains unclear. Using PCR, viral nuclei acid can be detected in biopsy material from 10% to 60% of patients presenting with DCMP (e501). In infants with primary EFE, mumps virus and adenovirus have been identified by PCR, suggesting *in utero* viral infection as an etiology for this disorder (e480). Early studies suggested that treatment with steroids and other immunoregulatory drugs improved the clinical outcome; more recent studies call this into question (e502).

Idiopathic GC myocarditis represents a distinct clinical entity with a rapidly progressive course leading to death or cardiac transplant in 89% of patients (101) (e503). The pathologic features include three phases of disease, which may all be present simultaneously within the same heart (102). The acute phase includes extensive zones of myocardial necrosis with an associated mixed inflammatory infiltrate including CD8 T-lymphocytes, eosinophils, and macrophages including multinucleated GCs. Despite the GCs, granulomas are not seen, distinguishing this disorder from infectious and sarcoid-related GC disease. In the healing phase, granulation tissue containing inflammatory GCs mixed with myocardial GCs replaces the necrotic regions. Healed areas contain fibrous scar tissue without GCs. Although predominantly an adult disease, GC myocarditis does occur in the pediatric age range, predominantly the second decade. A variety of features have led to the speculation that GC myocarditis represents an autoimmune disorder: (a) About 20% of patients have an underlying autoimmune disease, especially inflammatory bowel disease (101) (e504). (b) GC myocarditis occurred in a child with common variable immunodeficiency, a disorder prone to the development of autoimmune disorders (e505); and (c) recurrent disease occurs in approximately 25% of transplanted hearts (101).

Secondary Cardiomyopathies

Glycogen Storage Disorders

The glycogen storage diseases (GSD) are predominantly autosomal recessive conditions characterized by a deficiency in one of the enzymes involved in the synthesis or degradation of glycogen. Significant cardiac involvement occurs in GSD types IIa (Pompe disease) and IIb (Danon disease).

Pompe disease (type IIa GSD) results from a deficiency in α-1,4-glucosidase (acid maltase) causing accumulation of lysosomal-bound glycogen in the heart and skeletal muscle. The disease manifests as infantile and late forms, depending on the severity of the enzyme deficiency (e506). With complete loss of enzyme (infantile Pompe), glycogen accumulates in the heart at a rapid rate, leading to onset of disease in the 1st month or two of life and death in the 1st year (e507). Involved infants invariably display cardiomegaly on chest x-ray and a hypertrophic left ventricle by EKG and echocardiogram (e507). At autopsy, the heart weighs three to ten times the expected weight for age and the walls of all the chambers appear thickened, giving the heart a globular appearance. Mild degrees of EFE may be present. At microscopic examination, the cardiac myocytes appear markedly distended by vacuolated and lacy cytoplasm due to the accumulation of PAS-positive digestible glycogen displacing the myofibrils (103). Ultrastructural exam shows the glycogen to be at least partially membrane bound, a feature that distinguishes Pompe disease from other forms of glycogen storage disease. The deficiency of α-1, 4-glucosidase (acid maltase) can be readily proved in muscle, fibroblasts, lymphocytes, or urine (see Chapter 5).

Danon disease (type IIb GSD) represents an X-linked disorder caused by primary deficiency of lysosome-associated membrane protein-2 (LAMP-2). Affected males present during childhood with muscle weakness, HCMP, and frequently (70%) mental retardation with death from cardiac failure in the second or the third decade (104) (e508). Affected females also almost invariably manifest disease, but at an older age. At the time of diagnosis, EKG displays features of both left ventricular hypertrophy and rhythm disturbance including Wolff-Parkinson-White syndrome and bundle branch block. The pathologic changes are best described in skeletal muscle biopsies (104). Muscle fibers contain PAS- and acid phosphatase–positive inclusions that exhibit dystrophin and sarcoglycan staining of their membranes. Ultrastructural study shows the intracytoplasmic membrane-bound vacuoles to contain glycogen mixed with cytoplasmic debris (104).

Mucopolysaccaridoses

Mucopolysaccharidoses (MPS) represent a group of lysosomal storage disorders caused by defects in the intralysosomal degradation of acid mucopolysaccharides (glycosaminoglycans). Seven forms of MPS have been identified, all but one of which are transmitted in an autosomal recessive fashion (e509,e510) (Table 13-30). Cardiovascular abnormalities occur in most forms of MPS, with the degree of involvement varying between forms and over time for any one form (105) (e511). During life valvular insufficiency due to thickening of the mitral, or less often aortic valve represents the most significant cardiovascular complication (105). At autopsy, more extensive involvement can be identified. These cardiovascular changes are best described in MPS I (Hurler syndrome). (106). The valves and the endocardium

Table 13-30 ■ MUCOPOLYSACCHARIDOSE

Type	Chromosome Locus	Stored Material	Deficient Enzyme
MPS IH Hurler	4p16.3	Dermatan sulfate Heparin sulfate	α-L-Iduronidase
MPS IS Scheie	4p16.3	Dermatan sulfate Heparin sulfate	α-L-Iduronidase
MPS IH/S Hurler-Scheie	4p16.3	Dermatan sulfate Heparin sulfate	α-L-Iduronidase
MPS II Hunter	Xq28	Dermatan sulfate Heparin sulfate	Iduronate sulfatase
MPS IIIA Sanfilippo A	17q25.3	Heparan sulfate	Heparan *N*-sulfatase
MPS IIIB Sanfilippo B	17q21	Heparan sulfate	α-*N*-Acetyl-glucosaminidase
MPS IIIC Sanfilippo C	NK	Heparan sulfate	Acetyl-CoA:α-glucosaminide acetyltransferase
MPS IIID Sanfilippo D	12q14	Heparan sulfate	*N*-Acetylglucosamine 6-sulfatase
MPS IVA Morquio A	16q24.3	Keratan sulfate chondroitin 6-sulfate	Galactose 6-sulfatase
MPS IVB Morquio B	3q21.33	Keratan sulfate	β-Galactosidase
MPS VI Maroteaux-Lamy	5q13-114	Dermatan sulfate	Arylsulfatase B
MPS VII Sly	7q21.1	Dermatan sulfate, Heparin sulfate Chondroitin 4-,6-sulfates	β-Glucuronidase
MPS IX	3p21.2–21.3	Hyaluronan	Hyaluronidase

See references (e509,e510).

of all four cardiac chambers are thickened, the mitral valve especially so, with irregular nodules along its free margin (Figure 13-26). The coronary arteries appear thickened with luminal narrowing; the aorta and systemic vessels exhibit substantial intimal plaque formation. Subendocardial fibrosis may be severe, especially in the left ventricle with occasional patients presenting as newborns with EFE (e512,e513). Histologically, the thickened connective tissues of the cardiovascular system and other sites are populated by vacuolated "Hurler" cells containing large vesicles of soluble acid mucopolysaccharides and glycolipids. Ultrastructurally, membrane-bound vacuoles contain concentric and parallel lamellae (106) (see Chapter 5).

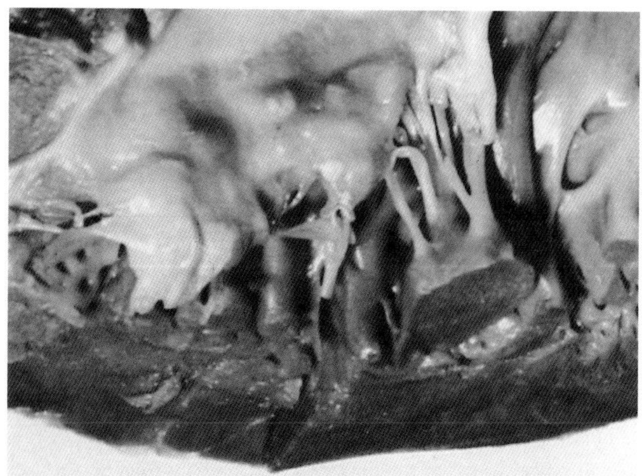

FIGURE 13-26 ■ Mucopolysaccharidosis type IV. A thickened, nodular mitral valve is characteristic of most mucopolysaccharidoses.

Mucolipidosis

Mucolipidosis II (I-cell disease) (gene map locus 4q21-23), an autosomal recessive disorder caused by a deficiency of multiple lysosomal hydrolases that degrade lipids and mucopolysaccharides, leads to a Hurler-like clinical presentation (e514). Fibroblasts accumulate storage material leading to thickened and nodular valvular leaflets and abnormal chordae (107). The coronary artery intima may contain foam cells (e515). Progressive left ventricular hypertrophy can contribute to the risk for sudden death in some patients (e514).

Gangliosidoses

The gangliosidoses are autosomal recessive enzymatic defects of glycosphingolipid metabolism. Although manifesting predominantly as disorders of neuronal tissues, accumulation of storage material in the myocardium mimicking that seen in the MPS may cause significant disease in at least two of these disorders (see Chapters 5 and 10).

GM1 gangliosidosis resulting from a deficiency in acid β-galactosidase causes storage of GM1 ganglioside material in neuronal tissue and glycosaminoglycans and glycopeptides in visceral organs (108). Cardiac involvement occurs in a subgroup of infants, manifesting as CMP or valve insufficiency (e516,e517). Foamy histiocytes containing periodic acid–Schiff and alcian blue–positive storage material accumulate in the heart valves, subendocardial regions, and vessel adventitia (108) (e518).

GM2 gangliosidosis type II (Sandhoff disease) results from deficiency of the hexosaminidase β-subunit (e519). Storage material, described in the connective tissue cells throughout the heart, consists of membrane-bound concentric bodies

(109) (e520). The resulting cardiac disease manifests clinically as HCMP and valvular insufficiency (109) (e519).

Fabry Disease

Fabry (Anderson-Fabry) disease, an X-linked recessive inborn error of glycosphingolipid metabolism (gene locus 3p21-23), results from a deficiency of lysosomal α-galactosidase A (ceramide trihexosidase). The neutral glycosphingolipids deposit in lysosomes of cells throughout the body, with the renal, cardiovascular, and peripheral nervous systems taking the largest "hit" (110). In cardiac muscle cells, the deposits occupy the central, perinuclear areas and displace the contractile elements toward the periphery. In frozen tissue, the storage material appears as PAS positive and birefringent. At electron microscopic study, the deposits form intralysosomal aggregates of concentric or parallel lamellae (110). Cardiac disease manifests most commonly as left ventricular hypertrophy, with less common clinically significant valve and conduction system alterations. The disease occurs with an incidence of 1/40,000 to 117,000 male live births and accounts for 3% to 4% of unexplained LVH in young adult males (110). Although commonly considered an adult disease, symptoms begin in childhood. The majority of patients manifest neurologic pain and/or skin angiokeratomas and nearly 40% have cardiac manifestation in the second decade (e521–e523). Female heterozygous patients are affected, though usually with a less severe and more delayed course compared with the male hemizygous patients. With the possibility of affective enzyme replacement therapy, early diagnosis has become more important (110) (e521).

N-Glycosylation Disorders

N-glycosylation disorders refer to a group of multisystem diseases caused by at least 12 different defects in the attachment of *N*-linked oligosaccharide chains to glycoproteins (e524). Hypertrophic or DCMP complicates at least a small subgroup of these patients (111). Cardiac manifestations including pericardial effusions and HCMP may be the presenting symptoms in some patients (111). Endomyocardial biopsy in one patient with DCMP revealed nonspecific findings of myocyte hypertrophy and interstitial fibrosis without inflammation (111).

Fatty Acid Oxidation Defects

Fatty acid oxidation is a complex metabolic pathway that can go awry at a variety of points leading to cardiac dysfunction (Table 13-31) (112) (e525). The majority of theses enzyme defects present in infancy, with abnormal free carnitine levels and acylcarnitine profiles serving as diagnostic clues (112). Primary carnitine deficiency presents with hypoglycemia and CMP (113) (e526–e528). The CMP may be either dilated or hypertrophic and there is often associated EFE (113) (e527). In both biopsy and autopsy material, the cytoplasm of skeletal muscle and cardiac myocytes contain accumulations of neutral lipid vacuoles with associated large aggregates of mitochondria (114) (e527). The CPT II and translocase deficiencies often present with an arrhythmia with or without associated CMP (e525,e529) (see Chapter 5).

Table 13-31 ■ FATTY ACID OXIDATION DISORDERS WITH CARDIOMYOPATHY

Enzyme	Gene
Carnitine transporter	OCTN2
Carnitine/acylcarnitine translocase	CACT
Carnitine palmitoyltransferase II	CPT-II
Very-long-chain acyl CoA dehydrogenase	VLCAD
Electron transfer flavoprotein dehydrogenase[a]	ETF-DH
Electron transfer flavoprotein-α[a]	α-ETF
Electron transfer flavoprotein-β[a]	β-ETF
Short-chain L-3-hydroxyacyl CoA dehydrogenase	SCHAD
Mitochondrial trifunctional protein	MTP
Long-chain 3-ketoacyl-CoA thiolase	LKAT

[a]These deficiencies also known as glutaric *aciduria type II.*
CoA, coenzyme A.

Mitochondrial Electron Transport Chain Disorders

The mitochondria, home of energy production via oxidative phosphorylation (OXPHOS), represent a unique structure within cells. The electron transport chain pathways involved in OXPHOS include five enzyme complexes, each including multiple proteins produced by a mix of mitochondrial DNA (mtDNA) and nuclear DNA (nDNA). Mitochondrial enzyme deficiencies can be derived from either mtDNA or nDNA mutations. This fact combined with the ability of mitochondria to divide independent of cell division (heteroplasmy) results in an exuberant array of phenotypic variations for the electron transport chain deficiencies (e530,e531). Out of this phenotypic array, a group of mitochondrial enzyme deficiency syndromes have been identified, some of which include cardiac manifestations, especially hypertrophic or DCMP and conduction defects, as an important element (e530,e531). Up to 40% of patients with mitochondrial cytopathy manifest cardiac disease, including both hypertrophic and DCMP with approximately 10% of patients presenting as an isolated CMP (115) (e532). Patients whose mitochondrial disorder includes CMP follow a more severe clinical course compared with patients without CMP (115,116) (see Chapter 5).

The pathologic features of mitochondrial disease in cardiac muscle include replacement of the cardiac myofibers by pools of mitochondria that ultrastructually may contain closely compacted stacks or circular arrays of cristae (116). In a subgroup of patients, negative COX staining of frozen tissue serves as a clue to the diagnosis (116). Making a definitive diagnosis of a mitochondrial cytopathy is, however, not straightforward requiring not only light and electron microscopic examination of the endomyocardial biopsy material, but also mtDNA and nDNA analysis of blood or tissue and frequently electron transport chain analysis of fresh/frozen skeletal muscle.

Iron Overload

The most common form of severe iron overload in childhood is transfusional siderosis, or secondary hemochromatosis, caused by the repeated transfusions (e533). The excess iron is primarily deposited in the mononuclear phagocyte system and by itself it does not cause significant cellular dysfunction or injury. During long-term transfusion therapy, cardiac iron deposits become readily demonstrable but usually cause no clinical problems.

Hereditary hemochromatosis occurs as a juvenile form due to mutations in hemojuvelin (*HJV*, 1q21) or hepcidin (*HAMP*, 19q13.1) genes, rather than the *HFE* gene common in adult hemochromatosis (e534,e535). Clinical features are similar to those in the adult disease but with earlier onset of cardiac symptoms and endocrine dysfunctions. Iron accumulation begins early in life and causes clinical symptoms including arrhythmias and DCMP before the age of 30 years. The heart may be two or three times the normal weight with a rusty brown discoloration (117). On microscopic exam, both biopsy and heart explant iron deposits, readily identified by histochemical staining, are visible in both myocardial connective tissue cells and in cardiac myocytes (117) (e533).

Neuromuscular Disorders

Given the similar myofibrillar structure in skeletal and cardiac muscle fibers, it is not surprising that cardiac involvement occurs as a part of many neuromuscular diseases (118). DCMP is the most common form. Conduction abnormalities and arrhythmias without apparent cardiac histopathology are also common (see Chapter 26).

Muscular Dystrophies

Both the Duchenne and the Becker forms of muscular dystrophy involve mutations in the dystrophin gene (Xp21.2). At autopsy, most patients with this X-linked recessive disorder have a DCMP with epicardial and extensive interstitial fibrosis (119) (e536). Dystrophic changes may also develop in the left ventricular papillary muscles with MVP or involve the conduction system (e537,e538). In a small subgroup of people with a dystrophin gene mutation, the DCMP may be the presenting feature of the disease (e472).

Emery-Dreifuss muscular dystrophy represents a slowly progressive form of muscular dystrophy that presents with contractures at the elbows and the ankles. This phenotype occurs in both X-linked (emerin gene Xq28) and autosomal dominant (lamin gene 1q21.2-q21.3) forms (118). Cardiac involvement manifests as conduction defects with DCMP occurring less frequently (e539). Mutations in the lamin gene also cause a DCMP with conduction defects without the skeletal muscle disease (e540).

Myotonic dystrophy, an autosomal dominant disorder characterized by muscle delayed muscle relaxation (myotonia), results from an abnormal expansion of a cytosine-thymine-guanine (CTG) trinucleotide repeat in chromosome 19 (120). The dystrophic changes in the heart manifest most frequently as conduction defects, though left ventricular hypertrophy, dilatation, and valve prolapse also occur (120) (e541). Ventricular noncompaction has also been described in occasional families (e542). The CTG repeat length is unstable with a trend toward increased length over time. This phenomenon is important as repeat length correlates with disease severity in the heart as well as the muscle (e543).

Congenital Myopathies

Myofibrillar myopathy presents in the second decade of life with muscle weakness, cramps, or exercise intolerance. The finding of abnormal accumulations of desmin material in the muscle fibers led to identifying mutations in the desmin gene in many of the patients (121). A DCMP frequently accompanies and may predate the myopathy in affected families (e544). The disorder is transmitted as an autosomal dominant trait with variable penetrance.

Central core disease represents a slowly progressive form of congenital myopathy diagnosed by the distinctive pathologic absence of central mitochondria in skeletal muscle. Most cases can be linked to a mutation in the ryanodine receptor (RYR1) gene on chromosome 19 and are without associated heart disease (e545). The central core phenotype has, however, also been identified in skeletal muscle from patients with HCMP and a mutation in the β-myosin heavy-chain (MYH7) gene on chromosome 14 (e546). Mutations in a different region of the MYH7 gene have been identified in the myosin storage myopathy in which myofibers contain aggregates of myosin myofilaments beneath the cell membrane (e547). Patients with myosin myopathy present in childhood with slowly progressive limb weakness; CMP is usually not a part of this disorder.

Friedreich Ataxia

Friedreich ataxia, the commonest form of inherited ataxia, results from an expansion of the GAA trinucleotide repeat in the frataxin gene on chromosome 9q13 (122) (e548–e550). The frataxin gene is involved with mitochondrial iron metabolism and mitochondrial dysfunction is believed to be the mechanism behind this disorder (e550). Cardiac disease, usually manifesting as HCMP, complicates the clinical course in 65% to 75% of patients (e548–e550) and occasionally young patients present with CMP (e551). The severity of the cardiac manifestations correlates with the number of GAA repeats (122). Examination of hearts at autopsy reveals myocyte hypertrophy and fibrosis with myocyte degeneration and iron deposition (123) (e552).

Inflammatory/Autoimmune Disorders

Systemic Lupus Erythematosus

Most of the classic autoimmune diffuse connective tissue diseases, including systemic lupus erythematosis (SLE), rheumatoid arthritis, scleroderma, polyarteritis, and dermatomyositis, occur in children and adolescents. These diseases manifest overlapping clinical features, with heart involvement occurring as a component in many. SLE, which includes a well-studied significant cardiac component, will be the focus of the discussion here.

In the pediatric population, SLE usually occurs after the age of 9 years with a striking (6:1) female predominance (124). The patients present with a bewildering febrile illnesses that over time involve the joints, skin, serosal membranes, and kidneys. There is a large clinical and serology overlap between the various autoimmune connective tissue disorders with a positive double-stranded DNA antibody helping to discriminate SLE from the other forms. A transient similar condition may occur in infants born to mothers with active SLE (see later). Cardiac disease, involving any and all portions of the heart, occurs commonly.

Pericardium: In collected autopsy series, pericarditis occurs in 65% of SLE cases (125). By echocardiography evidence, 35% to 40% of patients have evidence of pericardial effusions and/or pericardial thickening (e553). Clinical evidence of pericardial disease occurs in even fewer patients, up to 30% (124,125). The pericardial effusion is typically neutrophilic with a decreased glucose, mimicking bacterial pericarditis (124). The histopathologic changes in the pericardium include mesothelial proliferation and necrosis with a fibrinous exudate and underlying inflammation and granulation tissue formation. Fibrous obliteration of the pericardial space occurs infrequently.

Myocardium: Autopsy series identify myocarditis in up to 40% of hearts though clinical evidence of myocarditis occurs in 2% to 25% of patients (124,125) (e554). Echocardiographic studies identify left ventricular hypertrophy and/or abnormal wall motion in 20% (e553,e555). The pathologic features include small-vessel inflammation, interstitial inflammation with or without necrosis, and interstitial fibrosis (124). The demonstration of immune complex deposition in intramyocardial vessels indicates that the myocarditis can be attributed, at least in part, to the underlying autoimmune disorder (e555). The presence of hypertension and coronary vascular narrowing in many patients suggests however that at least some of the myocardial disease occurs as a secondary complication.

Endocardium and Valves: In his classic descriptions, Gross (126) described discrete vegetations of three types on the valves and endocardium in SLE: the "pyramidal ridge type," similar to that seen in rheumatic fever; the "massive thrombotic type" around commissures, similar to that seen in nonbacterial endocarditis; and the "flat spreading type," which he considered the most characteristic form. These latter lesions represent the most notable gross cardiac feature in SLE, "nonbacterial verrucous" or "Libman-Sacks" endocarditis. Libman-Sachs endocarditis manifest as smooth and friable vegetations, up to about 4 mm in greatest diameter, which can be flat and granular, warty, or nodular, resembling mulberries. These vegetations, found most often on mitral and aortic valves, are located on the valve surface impacted by blood away from the line of closure. Similar vegetations often spread along the chordae tendinae and onto the endocardium. Microscopic changes begin on the surface of the valve leaflets and include hematoxylin bodies, valvular necrosis without bacterial presence, widespread multinucleated eosinophilic coalescent bodies, and a characteristic valvulitis with plasma cells and thick granulation bud capillaries (126). The valve under the vegetations is minimally deformed and these small lesions may be difficult to identify by echocardiogram. A second type of valve abnormality in SLE, diffuse thickening without discrete vegetations, has been described with increasing frequency in recent years, predominantly in adults with longstanding disease (e556). Valvular disease is identified at autopsy in up to 65% of patients (124) and by echocardiography in 20% to 35%, including a group of patients with mitral and/or aortic regurgitation without visible structural defects (e553,e556,e557). The Libman-Sacks vegetations have been attributed, at least in some case to antiphospholipid antibody deposition (125) (e555).

Neonatal SLE

Neonatal SLE manifests as characteristic skin lesions and cardiac involvement, especially heart block, with other systemic organ involvement occurring only rarely. The skin rash may not be present at birth, appearing on the scalp and elsewhere by 2 months of age and disappearing by 6 months of age. The heart disease frequently manifests *in utero*, with bradycardia frequently detectable before 30 weeks of gestation (e558). Virtually all infants and their mothers have demonstrable 48-kD SSB/La, 52-kD SSA/Ro, and/or 60-kD SSA/Ro autoantibodies. Despite the serologic abnormalities, approximately 40% of the mothers are without autoimmune disease symptoms (e559). The antibodies apparently cross react with fetal cardiac tissue resulting in permanent damage to the conduction system. Histologic studies of the conduction system in these infants show the AV node and parts of the bundle branches to be replaced by fibrous scar tissue; a few lymphocytes may also be present as a residuum of prior inflammatory damage (127,128). When diagnosed *in utero*, complete heart block as a result of maternal autoantibodies leads to death in approximately 40% of cases (129), with fetal hydrops a particularly poor prognosis marker. When diagnosed in the neonatal period, morbidity is much lower (~5%), but nearly all infants who survive require placement of a pacemaker (129) (e560,e558). Secondary DCMP and EFE may further complicate the long-term cardiac function in these children (129) (e561).

Rheumatic Fever and Rheumatic Heart Disease

Rheumatic fever (RF), once the leading cause of death in young people age 5 to 20, has nearly disappeared from the developed world, but it remains the leading cause of acquired heart disease in the developing world (e562,e563). RF represents a delayed autoimmune reaction to group A β-hemolytic streptococcal pharyngitis. Whether strep throat leads to RF depends on several factors, including the M-protein type of the infecting bacteria, the genetic background of the infected individual, and the socioeconomic environment surrounding the infection (130). The appropriate infecting agent evokes a T- and B-cell response against the myosin-like M-protein, which then crossreacts with antigens in myocardium, endothelium, and neurons (130) (e564). The resulting acute RF is characterized by (a) migratory polyarthritis of large joints, (b) carditis, (c) erythema marginatum, a striking evanescent skin rash, (d) subcutaneous nodules, and (e) Sydenham chorea, a neurologic disorder with features of involuntary, purposeless, rapid movements (130,131) (e565). The presenting symptoms in an individual patient may vary greatly, making a definite diagnosis of RF difficult. In 1944, T. Duckett Jones published clinical criteria for making the diagnosis; the Jones criteria withstood the test of time and remain in use today with only minor modifications (Table 13-32) (131) (e565,e566).

The pathologic response to this autoimmune disorder results in formation of Aschoff nodules, comprising central fibrinoid necrosis surrounded by inflammatory cells. Included in the inflammation are lymphocytes, plasma cells, and a characteristic histiocytic cell with ragged edges, and vesicular nucleus containing a dense central spiculated bar of chromatin named the Anitschkow cell (Figure 13-27) (e565). The carditis, which occurs in roughly 50% of RF patients, involves all layers of the heart. Rheumatic endocarditis induces injury to the heart valves, representing the most clinically significant disease. The mitral valve is involved alone in 40% to 50% of cases, the aortic and the mitral valves together in 35% to 40%, the aortic valve alone in 15% to 20%, and the mitral, aortic, and tricuspid valves together in 2% to 3% (e567). On gross examination, the valves display a nearly continuous row of translucent verrucae near the closure margins of swollen, focally hemorrhagic valve leaflets. On the mitral and the tricuspid valves, the verrucae lie on the atrial surfaces, a few millimeters from the free edges; the attached

Table 13-32 ■ DIAGNOSIS OF RHEUMATIC FEVER AND HEART DISEASE 2002–2004 WHO CRITERIA (BASED ON REVISED JONES CRITERIA)

Major manifestations
- Carditis
- Polyarthritis
- Chorea
- Erythema marginatum
- Subcutaneous nodules

Minor manifestations
- Clinical: fever, polyarthralgia
- Laboratory: elevated acute phase reactants (ESR, WBC)

Supporting evidence of preceding streptoccocal infection within last 45 days
- Electrocardiogram: prolonged P-R interval
- Elevated or rising antistreptolysin-O or other streptococcal antibody

OR
Positive throat culture
OR
Rapid antigen test for group A streptococci
OR
Recent scarlet fever

Diagnostic categories	**Criteria**
Primary episode of RF	2 major **or** 1 major + 2 minor manifestations **Plus** Evidence of preceding group A streptococcal infection
Recurrent attack of RF in patient **without** established RHD	2 major **or** 1 major + 2 minor manifestations **Plus** Evidence of preceding group A streptococcal infection
Recurrent attack of RF in patient **with** established RHD	2 minor manifestations **Plus** Evidence of preceding group A streptococcal infection[a]
Rheumatic chorea Insidious onset rheumatic carditis	Other major manifestations or evidence of group A streptococcal infection not required
Chronic valve lesions of RHD (presenting with pure mitral stenosis or mixed mitral valve disease and/or aortic valve disease)	Do not require any other criteria to be diagnosed as RHD

RF, Rheumatic fever; RHD, Rheumatic heart disease.

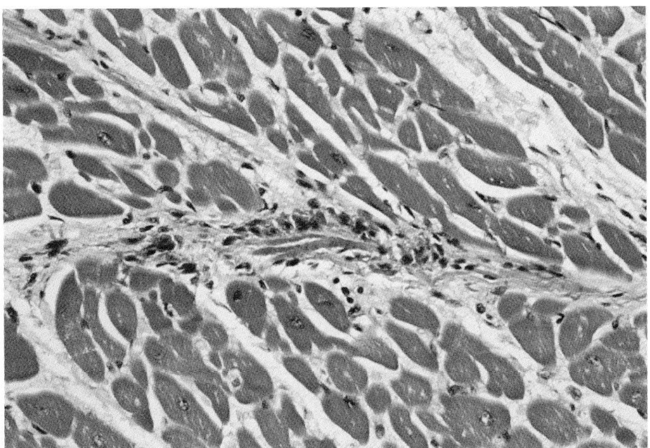

FIGURE 13-27 ▪ Acute rheumatic carditis. A characteristic Aschoff body is seen in this section of the left ventricle. There is a central degenerating fiber surrounded by large mononuclear cells (200×).

chordae may also be involved (Figure 13-28). Verrucae on the aortic and pulmonic valves involve the ventricular surface. Microscopically, the entire leaflet is usually inflamed and edematous with focal formation of Aschoff nodules; new vessels extend from the base of the valve into the leaflet. In about half of the patients, a series of thickened subendocardial ridges, the MacCallum patch, develops in the left atrium immediately above and perpendicular to the posterior leaflet of the mitral valve (7,131). The ventricular endocardium is rarely involved. Rheumatic myocarditis results in left-heart dilatation with minimal associated inflammation early in the course (131). With time, mononuclear cell infiltrates and characteristic Aschoff bodies are often found in the edematous perivascular or subendocardial interstitium of the interventricular septum and left ventricle. Rheumatic pericarditis develops only in people with underlying endocarditis and myocarditis (131). Characteristically, a fibrinous exudate thickens the pericardium, binding the visceral and parietal layers together and obliterating the pericardial space. Microscopically, fibrin layers containing scattered neutrophils cover the reactive mesothelial surfaces. Beneath this layer lie infiltrates of lymphocytes, plasma cells, macrophages, and polymorphonuclear leukocytes. With resolution of the acute phase, the exudate may resolve completely or leave variable patterns of adhesions.

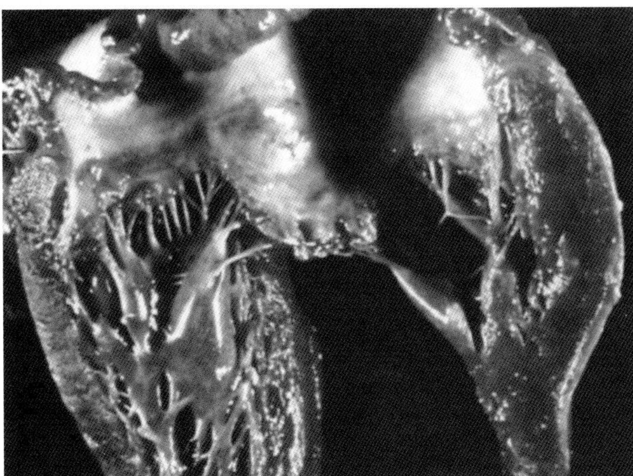

FIGURE 13-28 ▪ Acute rheumatic carditis. Characteristic dark, nodular excrescences line the margins of closure on the mitral valve leaflets. Rarely seen today, these sites often heal as fibrous nodules with associated valvular distortion. (Courtesy of Roma Chandra, M.D., National Children's Hospital, Washington, DC.)

Infant of Diabetic Mother Cardiomyopathy

Maternal diabetes places an infant at significantly increased risk of heart disease at birth, including both a 5 to 10× greater relative risk of having a malformed heart and a 15% to 40% risk of HCMP in an otherwise normally formed heart (132) (e568,e569). The HCMP remains asymptomatic in the majority of infants but may also present with congestive heart failure or even stillbirth (132) (e570). The HCMP is often asymmetric and in an occasional infant, this hypertrophied septum causes a transient left ventricular outflow obstruction. The ventricular hypertrophy usually resolves completely in 2 to 12 months (e570). Given the transient and rarely fatal nature of this disorder, histologic examination of involved myocardium is limited. In the few studied cases, the myocardium appears hypertrophic with EFE in some cases (132) (e571,e572). Myofiber disarray similar to that seen in familial HCMP, which occurs in some cases, is believed to be a normal feature of development.

Ischemic Myocardial Necrosis

Ischemic myocardial necrosis is relatively common in the normal and malformed hearts of infants and children, especially those in which profound hypoperfusion develops for any reason. Ischemia primarily damages the papillary muscles and ventricular subendocardium of either ventricle. Thus, sampling the infant heart requires examination of all the papillary muscles, the adjacent free ventricular and atrial walls, and ventricular septal myocardium near the membranous septum. Given that the myocardial fibers of the papillary muscles and much of the subendocardium are arrayed longitudinally, sections taken in the long axis of the heart give the best sampling yield (133) (e573). Small deep red or yellow ischemic foci near the apex of a papillary muscle represent the earliest and the mildest form of injury. The more severe the injury in papillary muscles, the greater the likelihood of subendocardial necrosis in the ventricular free walls (134). Longitudinal sections through the septum may expose unsuspected large infarcts near the AV ring that may involve the AV node or the bundle of His (134).

For the most part, the histopathology of ischemic myocardial injury in children resembles that in adult humans. However, in very young infants, the chronology of injury repair does not follow that of adults and is in fact not well defined. Using birth as the time of injury yields the following chronology of pathologic changes (134):

0 to 9 hours—histopathologic evidence of ischemic injury in the myocardium may be entirely lacking. The ninth component of complement (C9), part of the C5-9 membrane attack complex, has been used to identify sites of very early perinatal myocardial injury (e574).

24 to 48 hours—Myocyte necrosis manifests as cytoplasmic eosinophilia and nuclear pyknosis; cross-striations may persist in necrotic fibers; marginated cells in capillaries may be the only neutrophilic response.

72 to 96 hours—neutrophils infiltrate the margins of necrotic foci; the mononuclear, vascular, and fibroblastic responses may be slowed by associated systemic problems.

Dystrophic calcification is common in the most frequent sites of perinatal myocardial injury, such as the papillary muscles and ventricular subendocardial myocytes, and calcium may provide a sharp outline of the sarcolemmal membranes when no other signs are present (133) (e575). Massive myocardial calcification may occur in perinates subjected to various causes of hypoxic-ischemic injury (e576).

Endomyocardial Biopsy and Heart Transplant

Diagnostic Biopsy

The usefulness of myocardial biopsy in the evaluation of CMP remains controversial. The initial evaluation includes history, physical examination, electrocardiography, echocardiography, and metabolic/genetic screens (85) (e577). When these studies fail to identify an underlying etiology, especially in the setting of DCMP, cardiac catheterization with endomyocardial biopsy often becomes indicated (e578). Given the broad differential diagnoses encompassed, appropriate handling of the biopsy material requires (a) communication with the cardiologists regarding the patient's clinical picture; (b) information about specific disorders being addressed by the biopsy; and (c) adequate tissue samples. In our laboratory, all endomyocardial biopsies are received fresh accompanied by a standardized form (Table 13-33) outlining briefly the reason for the biopsy. The biopsy material is then divided with one piece snap frozen in OCT for viral PCR or special stains (including PAS, oil-red-O, NADH reductase, cytochrome C oxidase, succinate dehydrogenase, and immunohistochemical stains for dystrophin and sarcoglycans), one piece placed in glutaraldehyde for electron microscopy, and the remaining three to four pieces fixed in formalin for routine light microscopy.

Heart Explants

At the time of heart transplantation, examination of the explanted heart yields an opportunity to confirm, further delineate, or change the prior clinical diagnosis. In our laboratory, 40% of heart transplants are currently performed for a cardiomyopathic process and 60% for congenital malformations. Examination of the cardiomyopathic hearts has yielded previously unknown diagnoses of noncompaction and arrhythmogenic right ventricular CMP.

Table 13-33 ■ HEART BIOPSY

Clinical (to be completed by Cardiologist)
_____Diagnostic
Clinical Suspicion: _____
_____Transplant Biopsy
Date of transplant: _____
Indications for Transplant: _____
Current Rx: _____
Reason for Biopsy
_____Rejection Surveillance (cellular and humoral)
_____Clinical Rejection, cellular (describe indications: ______________________________)
_____Clinical Rejection, humoral (describe indications: ______________________________)
Results to: _____________ Pager _____________

Specimens submitted (to be completed by Cardiologist)
Right ventricular endomyocardial biopsies
large _____ # medium _____ # small _____
_____ Routine processing (results reported the next business day)
_____ Stat processing. NOTE—Stat processing requires the following:
1. The pathologist on call must be consulted at the time the biopsy is scheduled
2. The specimen must be in the histology laboratory by 10:00 AM for same day results
Special requests:

Transplant Biopsy

Transplant biopsies play an integral role in the management of cardiac transplant patients. To be considered adequate, the biopsy must include at least three fragments of myocardial tissue with the myocardium occupying greater than 50% of the tissue in the biopsy fragment (135). Rejection may be either cellular or humoral. Cellular rejection manifests as interstitial lymphocytic inflammation with or without myocyte necrosis. The extent of the inflammation and necrosis determines the grade of rejection. The grading schemes for rejection have changed over the years with often poor interobserver concordance (e579,e580). In response to this, the 2004 ISHLT working formulation (135) (e581) significantly modified the prior 1990 ISHLT/2001 Banff formulation (Table 13-34). Humoral rejection refers to antibody and complement mediated graft dysfunction. Humoral rejection most commonly occurs in the 1st month following transplant, but may persist for several months with an associated poor outcome (135,136). Diagnostic criteria for humoral rejection include evidence of endocapillary injury manifest as endothelial swelling, capillary neutrophil or macrophage infiltrates, and interstitial edema and/or hemorrhage (135). These morphologic changes can however be difficult to identify in biopsy material (e582). Positive immunocytochemical staining for C4d, when diffuse and intense, can serve as an aid in the evaluation for humoral rejection (136) (e583).

Transplant biopsies can also display nonrejection alterations. In the early post-transplant period, differentiating harvest injury from acute rejection may be problematic. Ischemic harvest injury results in contraction band or coagulative

Table 13-34 ■ 1990 WORKING FORMULATION FOR THE STANDARDIZATION OF NOMENCLATURE IN THE DIAGNOSIS OF HEART REJECTION

	2004 ISHLT	Banff (2001)/1990 ISHLT
No Rejection	**Grade 0**	**Grade 0**
Interstitial and/or perivascular infiltrate without myocyte damage	Grade 1 R, mild	Grade 1, mild A—Focal B—Multifocal or diffuse sparse
Single focus of dense infiltrate with myocyte injury	Grade 1 R, mild	Grade 2, moderate (focal)
Multifocal (≥2 foci) of dense infiltrate with myocyte injury	Grade 2 R, moderate	Grade 3, moderate A—Focal
Diffuse infiltrate with multifocal myocyte damage	Grade 3 R, severe	Grade 3, moderate B—Diffuse
Diffuse infiltrate with multifocal myocyte damage, ± edema, ± hemorrhage, ± vasculitis	Grade 3 R, severe	Grade 4, severe

myocyte necrosis with the inflammatory response relatively mild in comparison to the degree of injury, whereas in acute rejection the opposite relationship occurs (inflammation > necrosis) (135). The "Quilty" lesion, defined as nodular lymphocytic infiltrates in the endocardium with or without extension into the adjacent myocardium, occurs frequently in biopsies (e584). Recognizing the invasive form of a Quilty lesion where the myocardial lymphocytic inflammation is in direct continuity with the endocardial infiltrates often requires examination of serial sections. This distinction is however important, as "invasive" Quilty is not considered rejection and requires no treatment. The possibility of post-transplant lymphoproliferative disorder must also be kept in mind when examining the biopsy transplant material.

Conduction System Abnormalities

The conduction system represents a part of the heart that is functionally important but anatomically difficult to identify. The physiology of the conduction system and its broad range of abnormalities are beyond the scope of this chapter (e585). A basic understanding of the conduction system anatomy is however important for pathologists, especially if they examine the hearts of children at autopsy or abnormal native hearts removed during cardiac transplantation. This section will focus on the examination of the conduction system and its abnormalities that can lead to sudden death.

The cardiac conduction system includes the sinus (SA) node, AV node, bundle of His, and bundle branches (137,138) (e586). The sinus node lies in the right atrium at its junction with the superior vena cava. Electrical impulses from the sinus node are transmitted via the atrial myocardium to the AV node. The AV node lies just above the septal leaflet of the tricuspid valve in the apex of the "triangle of Koch." From the AV node, the electrical impulse is transmitted via the bundle of His through the central fibrous body and membranous system to the superior margin of the muscular interventricular septum. Here the conduction tract divides, forming bundle branches that extend along the right and the left sides of the septum. These bundle branches pass the impulse on to an interweaving network of subendocardial Purkinje fibers, which transmit the signal simultaneously to the entire right and left ventricular myocardium.

Histologic examination of the AV node and its connections to the ventricular myocardium represents the key to most pathologic examinations of the conduction system. The *Histology for Pathologists* text and a recent forensic paper nicely describe in detail methods for examination of conduction system (138,139). Under the microscope, the nodal tissue includes three zones: (a) an inner zone of pale staining specialized myocardial cells containing sparse myofibrils and inconspicuous striations embedded within a fibrous stroma, (b) an outer zone of normal atrial myocardium, and (c) an intermediate zone containing transitional cells with a mixed appearance. Both the SA and the AV nodes are innervated by sympathetic and parasympathetic nerve fibers. With formation of the penetrating bundle and bundle branches, the specialized cells become surrounded by a fibrous tissue coat.

Interfering with this normal conduction at any point along the pathway can result in arrhythmias. Current classification divides the arrhythmias into three basic types: supraventricular tachycardia, AV conduction disorders, and ventricular tachycardias (140) (Table 13-35).

The *supraventricular tachycardias* are predominantly medical disorders that rarely cause sudden death, with Wolff-Parkinson-White (WPW) being the main exception (e587,e588). WPW results from persistence of cardiac muscle strands connecting atrial and ventricular muscle. These accessory pathways cross the AV sulcus, bypassing the normal AV node (141) (e589). The pathologic evaluation for accessory pathways requires systematic study of both AV rings (139). The faster conduction through these accessory pathways leads to pre-excitation of the ventricular muscle and the diagnostic ECG findings of a short PR interval, delta wave, and widened QRS complex (e585). Pre-excitation due to accessory pathways occurs with a prevalence of 0.1 to 3.1/1,000 in the general population (e589).

Table 13-35 ■ ARRHYTHMIA CLASSIFICATION

	Neonate	Childhood
Supraventricular tachycardia		
Primary atrial tachycardia	10%–15%	10%–15%
Sinus tachycardia		
Atrial flutter		
Atrial fibrillation		
Atrial reentry		
AV nodal tachycardia	<5%	5%–30%
AV nodal reentry		
Junctional ectopia		
[a]Accessory connection mediated	>80%	>60%
Wolff-Parkinson-White		
[a]AV Conduction Disorders (AV block)		
Congenital		
Acquired		
Ventricular tachycardia		
Scar mediated		
Cardiomyopathy related		
[a]Long QT syndrome		
Idiopathic		

[a]Disorders discussed in text.
AV, atrioventricular.
Data from Calder L, Van Praagh R, Van Praagh S, et al. Truncus arteriosus communis: clinical, angiocardiographic, and pathologic findings in 100 patients. *Am Heart J* 1976;92:23–38.

These abnormal conduction circuits can result in supraventricular tachycardia that manifests in young infants as congestive heart failure or collapse and in older children as anxiety, chest discomfort, syncope, or cardiac arrest (e590). In symptomatic children, the lifetime risk for sudden death is estimated as 3% to 4% (e591). However, not all individuals with pre-excitation ECG changes develop symptomatic arrhythmias. Asymptomatic adults have a very low risk of cardiac arrest/sudden death (e592). In contrast, the risk for cardiac arrest or sudden death in asymptomatic children is currently not known. In one multicenter study, 48% of WPW deaths occurred in children without prior cardiac events (e593). In children with "high-risk" features (positive family history, multiple accessory pathways), ablation of the accessory pathways resulted in improved survival (e587,e588). The appropriate use of invasive treatment in asymptomatic children will depend on ascertaining appropriate risk stratification criteria.

Although usually sporadic, in 10% to 20% of instances WPW occurs in association with other congenital abnormalities (e589), especially Ebstein malformation. Its association with an unusual form of glycogen storage type HCMP led to the identification of a mutation in the *PRKAG2* (e594,e595). Less commonly, ventricular pre-excitation result from accelerated conduction through a hypoplastic AV node (e596,e597).

AV conduction disorders (AV block), due to interruption of impulse conduction from the atrium to the ventricle, are further characterized as to the degree (first, second, and third or complete) of block. Congenital AV block (CAVB) is associated with a variety of heart malformations, in particular AV septal defects and left atrial isomerism, and may also occur following surgical repair of heart defects or ablation of arrhythmogenic foci (142) (e585,e598,e599). In the fetus CAVB can lead to hydrops, with an associated high risk for fetal or neonatal death (129,142) (e560,e599).

When not associated with underlying heart disease, CAVB occurs most commonly (85%) in the setting of maternal autoimmune disease with anti-SSA/Ro and/or anti-SSB/La antibodies (e560,e600). Despite this high association between fetal CAVB and positive maternal antibodies, the reverse is not true. Fetal CAVB complicates pregnancy in only 2% of women with positive anti-SSA/Ro or SSB/La and the risk for recurrence following a pregnancy with CAVB is less than 20% (e558–e600). In fetuses and infants with antibody-induced CAVB, histopathologic examination reveals fibrosis and calcification with or without inflammation in the AV nodes as well as other sites along the conduction pathway (127,128) (e601). Given the severity of these pathologic changes, it is not surprising that antibody-induced CAVB is permanent with 60% to 90% of children requiring pacemaker implantation (129) (e558–e560).

Ventricular tachycardia can occur with a broad spectrum of precipitating causes of which the long QT syndrome (LQTS) is of particular interest. The LQTS, manifest as QT prolongation and slowed repolarization on ECG, encompasses a group of disorders affecting the cardiac muscle potassium, sodium, and calcium channels (channelopathies). Currently, LQTS can be subdivided into eight major genotypes (LQTS1–8) (143), with some of the genotypes also expressing extracardiac abnormalities (Table 13-36). Individuals with LQTS carry a significant risk of syncope and sudden death with the relative risk and event triggers (exercise, emotional stress, sleep) correlating with the genotype (e602–e604). Recent molecular studies have identified LQTS mutations in up to 9.5% of SIDS cases (144) (e605) and up to 20% of sudden cardiac deaths in older children (e606).

Catecholaminergic polymorphic ventricular tachycardia (CPVT), a form of ventricular tachycardia with a distinctive

Table 13-36 ■ LONG QT SYNDROME

	Gene	Locus	Phenotype
LQT1	KvLQT1, KCNQ1	11p15.5	RWS JLNS
LQT2	HERG, KCNH2	7q35–36	RWS
LQT3	SCN5A	3p21-24	RWS Brugada syndrome
LQT4	ANKB, ANK2	4q25-27	
LQT5	Mink, IsK, KCNE1	21q22.1-2	RWS JLNS
LQT6	MiRP1, KCNE2	21q22.1	RWS
LQT7	Kir2.1, KCNJ2	17q23	Anderson syndrome
LQT8	CACNA1C	12p13.3	Timothy syndrome

RWS, Roman-Ward syndrome (143): ECG changes only.
Brugada syndrome (143): ECG changes only.
JLNS, Jervell and Lange-Nielsen syndrome: ECT changes + sensorineural hearing loss.
Anderson syndrome (e717): Ventricular arrhythmia, periodic paralysis, dysmorphic facies, syndactyly, clinodactyly, cleft palate, scoliosis.
Timothy syndrome (e718): Ventricular arrhythmia, heart malformation, syndactyly, immune deficiency, dysmorphic facies, autism.

bidirectional polymorphic pattern on ECG, leads to recurrent episodes of stress-related syncope in childhood (e607). Following identification of mutations in the human cardiac ryanodine receptor gene (*hRyR2*) in CPVT, a molecular autopsy study identified the same mutations in 14% of sudden unexpected childhood deaths (145).

These recent molecular genetic findings in infant and childhood sudden deaths serve to emphasize the importance of a comprehensive autopsy examination including molecular and genetic testing in cases of unexpected sudden death (e608,e609).

Extracardiac Vascular Disease

Pulmonary Hypertension

Pulmonary hypertension, defined as a mean pulmonary artery pressure at rest of greater than 25 mm Hg, represents a common pathophysiologic state arrived at from a variety of etiologic pathways. Advances in understanding the underlying vascular biology, physiology, and genetics, combined with new treatment modalities led in 2003 to a proposed revision in the classification of these disorders (Table 13-37) (146) (e610,e611). In pediatrics, persistent pulmonary hypertension of the newborn (PPHN), and pulmonary hypertension complicating L→R shunts represent the most common etiologies with primary (idiopathic or familial) PHT accounting for many of the remaining cases. Before discussing the specifics of these conditions, it seems prudent to review (a) normal pulmonary vascular development and (b) the pathologic changes associated with pulmonary artery hypertension.

Table 13-37 ▪ PULMONARY HYPERTENSION—WHO CLASSIFICATION

- I. Pulmonary artery hypertension
  - A. **Idiopathic**
  - B. **Familial**
  - C. Associated with:
    - 1. Collagen vascular disease
    - 2. **Congenital heart disease with L→R shunt**
    - 3. Portal hypertension
    - 4. HIV disease
    - 5. Drugs and toxins
    - 6. Other
  - D. Associated with significant venous or capillary involvement
    - 1. Pulmonary veno-occlusive disease
    - 2. Pulmonary capillary hemangiomatosis
  - E. **Persistent pulmonary hypertension of the newborn**
- II. **Pulmonary hypertension with left-heart disease**
  - A. Left-sided atrial or ventricular disease
  - B. Left-sided heart valve disease
- III. Pulmonary hypertension associated with respiratory disorders or hypoxemia
- IV. Pulmonary hypertension caused by chronic thrombotic/embolic disease
- V. Miscellaneous (sarcoid, Langerhans cell histiocytosis, compression of pulmonary vessels, lymphangiomatosis)

Bold indicates disorders discussed in this section.

Normal Pulmonary Vascular Development

The vasculature in fully developed lung includes preacinar and intra-acinar arteries. The preacinar arteries travel in parallel with the pulmonary airways and contain a well-developed muscle wall. The preacinar pulmonary arterial tree develops in synchrony with the pulmonary airways becoming completely formed by 16 to 17 weeks of gestation (147) (e612). The intra-acinar arteries arise as a network of supernumerary vessels that supply the terminal airspaces, and in the adult carry up to 40% of the pulmonary blood flow (147). The development of the terminal airspaces and the intra-acinar arteries begins *in utero* but is incomplete at birth and continues for many months thereafter. The formation of a muscle layer around the intra-acinar arteries lags behind the development of the alveoli, and the medial muscle of these intra-acinar arteries normally extends into the alveoli only after 8 to 10 years of age (148) (e612).

The pathophysiology of the pulmonary vasculature clearly differs before and after birth. In the fetus, there is little pulmonary blood flow with the high PVR due to increased thickness of the artery walls. At birth, this high PVR rapidly falls due to release of nitric oxide and prostacyclin from the pulmonary artery endothelial cells, with resultant dilatation of the pulmonary arteries. Subsequent thinning of the muscular media requires time and is complete only at 4 months of age (147).

Pulmonary Artery Hypertensive Changes

Pulmonary artery hypertension results in a constellation of changes outlined in Table 13-38 (149). The pulmonary artery changes were traditionally graded by the Heath-Edwards scoring system (e613) (Table 13-38). However, with the advances in drug treatment modalities gained from improved understanding of the underlying pathophysiology of pulmonary hypertension, this scoring system has lost most of its value. The complex lesions are a marker of severe disease. The plexiform lesion is defined by "glomeruloid" endothelial proliferation that extends through an area of vessel wall destruction into perivascular tissue (eFigure 13-8). These lesions frequently occur adjacent to an area of concentric intimal fibrosis at an artery branch point. The plexiform lesions are not only specific to primary/idiopathic pulmonary hypertension but also occur in the setting of cardiac shunting lesions. They are however not a feature of PPHN (149). The dilation lesion refers to an area of artery wall thinning, often located distal to a plexiform lesion. These dilated areas can serve as a focal point of hemorrhage.

Persistent Pulmonary Hypertension of the Newborn

PPHN occurs when the fetal circulation fails to adapt normally at birth due to underdevelopment, maldevelopment, or maladaptation (148). The failed drop in PVR leads to right→left shunting at the foramen ovale and ductus

Table 13-38 ■ PULMONARY ARTERY HYPERTENSION PATHOLOGIC GRADING

Pulmonary Arteriopathy	Heath and Edwards Grade
Pulmonary arteriopathy with isolated medial hypertrophy	Grade 1
Pulmonary arteriopathy with medial hypertrophy + intimal thickening (cellular or fibrotic)	
Concentric laminar intimal fibrosis	Grade 2 or 3
Eccentric or concentric nonlaminar intimal fibrosis	
Pulmonary arteriopathy with complex lesion	
Plexiform lesion	Grade 5
Dilation lesion	Grade 4
Arteritis	Grade 6
Pulmonary arteriopathy with isolated arteritis	Grade 6

Compiled from references (149) (e613).

arteriosus with resultant central cyanosis. PPHN most often occurs as a hypoxia-related maladaptation secondary to underlying pneumonia, sepsis, or meconium aspiration. In infants with meconium aspiration, there is also abnormal extension of smooth muscle into the media of the more peripheral, normally nonmuscular intra-acinar arteries suggesting *in utero* onset of the vascular dysfunction (148). In approximately 20% of cases, peripheral muscle extension occurs without an obvious underlying etiology resulting in "idiopathic" PPHN (146). Epidemiologic studies suggest that nonsteroidal anti-inflammatory drugs taken by the mother may play a role in this vasculopathy. PPHN also occurs when the lungs fail to grow normally, resulting in a parallel underdevelopment of the pulmonary vasculature. This manifests most dramatically in infants with congenital diaphragmatic hernias who often develop severe respiratory insufficiency following repair (148). In recent years, the use of vasodilators, prostacyclin, and ECMO has dramatically improved the survival of these infants.

Congenital Heart Disease with Left→Right Shunt

A left→right shunt, particularly at the post-tricuspid valve level, results in increased volumes of blood flow at an increased pressure in the lungs. This stimulates smooth muscle hyperplasia along with the intimal changes of pulmonary hypertension. An additional feature seen in the left→right shunt scenario is the decrease in numbers of peripheral arteries (150) (e614). If the shunt can be repaired early enough, these pulmonary hypertensive changes are reversible (150). However, if the repair is delayed, the pulmonary vascular changes can become nonreversible and the pulmonary hypertension will continue to progress following surgery. Predicting in an individual patient how quickly pulmonary hypertensive changes will progress to a nonreversible stage remains problematic (e611). Age at surgery does play a role. In one study, in infants with a variety of shunting lesion operated upon before 9 months, the PVR uniformly returned to normal postoperatively, irrespective of pulmonary vascular histology. In older infants, medial wall thickening greater than 2× normal resulted in an increased risk of persistent PHT following surgery (150). In the worst-case scenario, the pulmonary hypertension progresses to a point where PVR exceeds systemic vascular resistance and the shunt becomes right→left with resultant cyanosis (Eisenmenger syndrome) (e611).

Familial and Idiopathic Pulmonary Artery Hypertension

Primary pulmonary hypertension (PPH) occurs as a familial disease in 6% to 12% of cases with the remainder occurring sporadically. The striking 1:2 female predominance observed in adults with PPH is less obvious in children where the M:F ratio is 1:1.3 to 1.5 (146,151). The familial disease follows an autosomal dominant inheritance pattern with incomplete penetrance and genetic anticipation (successive generations with worse disease) (151). In 50% of families, a mutation in the gene encoding bone morphogenetic protein receptor-2 (BMRP-2) can be identified; similar mutations occur in approximately 25% of sporadic cases (146,151) (e615). The involved pulmonary arteries display the range of pathologic changes described earlier. Improved understanding of the pathophysiology of pulmonary hypertension in recent years has led to significant improvements in treatment for patients with PPH. This disease, which once led to death within a year of diagnosis, can now be managed in most patients by initially using vasodilator therapy with lung transplantation as a final option (e610).

Pulmonary Hypertension with Obstructive Left-Heart Disease

In the face of obstruction to pulmonary venous return, the vascular changes in the lungs include not only arterial but also venous thickening. With extrapulmonary venous obstruction, the pulmonary arteries develop medial hypertrophy and intimal fibroplasia without the more complex lesions. The pulmonary veins also develop medial hyperplasia with "arterialization"; that is, formation of a discrete internal and external elastic lamina (e616). These venous changes, though striking, are reversible following repair of the obstructive defect. The long-term outcome of the pulmonary hypertension depends instead on the severity of the associated arterial disease.

Systemic Artery Disease

Arteriopathy

Idiopathic infantile arterial calcification (IIAC) represents a metabolic disorder of the arteries resulting in deposition of calcium hydroxyapatite in and around the internal elastic lamina and intimal fibrous proliferation (e617). The calcification occurs in any artery, with the coronary arteries involved in greater than 75% of cases and the cerebral arteries involved only rarely (e617). The calcification may elicit an inflammatory response including lymphocytes, eosinophils, and foreign body GCs. Ultrastructural exam identified hydroxyapatite deposition in the elastic laminae, collagen fibers, smooth muscle, and fibroblasts (e618). This rare condition most often presents as heart failure in early infancy, but may manifest prenatally as nonimmune hydrops. The artery luminal narrowing caused by the calcification and intimal proliferation can lead to ischemic injury in the involved organ, most commonly the heart, with 85% of infants dying in the first 6 months (e617). IIAC occurs in an autosomal recessive pattern in some families. The presence of associated periarticular calcification in a few instances led to the finding of low nucleotide pyrophosphatase (NPP) activity and inorganic pyrophosphate levels in some patients (e619). These observations in turn led to identification of loss-of-function mutations in *ENPP1*, a gene encoding for NPP protein, in 8 of 11 kindreds with IIAC (e620).

Fibromuscular dysplasia represents a noninflammatory disorganization and fibrosis of large muscular arteries leading to segmental luminal narrowing with the renal, internal carotid, coronary, celiac, hepatic, and mesenteric arteries most frequently involved. The pathologic changes can involve all layers of the vessel wall. Several forms have been described, including medial fibroplasia, perimedial fibroplasia, medial hyperplasia, and intimal fibroplasia (152) (e621). In medial fibroplasia, disorderly arrays of medial smooth muscle cells form luminal ridges that narrow the artery lumen. Between the ridges, the artery contains abnormally thin layers of otherwise normal smooth muscle cells. This alternating thick and thin luminal diameter gives an angiographic appearance of a "string of beads." Perimedial fibroplasia is characterized by layers of circumferential elastic-like tissue between the media and the adventitia. With intimal fibroplasia, the intima may be thickened and the internal elastic lamina duplicated and fragmented. Alternatively, the internal and the external elastic laminae may be disrupted and the intima and the media may merge. Fibromuscular dysplasia accounts for up to 45% of renal hypertension in childhood with multifocal vascular involvement present in many (e622–e624). A form of severe arterial dysplasia involving the aorta with its main branches has been described in both stillborn infants and infants with sudden death. The vessels in these infants display medial thickening due to hyperplasia of the elastic fibers (e625,e626).

Aneurysms

Aneurysmal dilatation of vessels, rare in childhood, occur both as primary defects in vessel wall structure and secondary to underlying inflammatory or infectious disease (153). Inherited/genetic causes of aortic aneurysm are the focus here.

Dilatation and dissection of the ascending aorta occurs most commonly in Marfan syndrome but may also complicate a spectrum of other disorders (Table 13-39). In all these disorders, microscopic examination reveals cystic medial degeneration with accumulation of mucopolysaccharides in the tunica media in the involved aorta (153) (e627–e629). At the ultrastructural level, the elastic lamella appears torn with loss of the connection between elastic lamella and smooth muscle cells (e630,e629).

Table 13-39 ■ ANEURYSMS OF AORTA

Syndrome	Gene	Reference
Marfan's	Fibrillin-1	(155)
Loeys-Dietz	TGFBR-1 TGFBR-2	(156)
Ehlers-Danlos	COL3A1	(158)
Turner	Monosomy X	(157)

Marfan syndrome represents an autosomal dominant disorder of connective tissue with high penetrance but variable phenotype due to the broad spectrum of organ involvement. A set of diagnostic criteria, combining clinical and genetic features, has been devised to aid in accurate diagnosis (Table 13-40) (154) (e627). Marfan syndrome occurs from mutations in the fibrillin-1 gene (*FBN1*, gene 15q21.1), with approximately 25% of cases representing new mutations. Signs of the disease can appear at any age but most patients come to diagnosis in the second or third decade. There is, however, a "neonatal" form of Marfan, associated with mutations in exons 24 to 32 of the fibrillin-1 gene (155) (e628) that presents in infancy with aortic dilatation accompanied by mitral and tricuspid regurgitation with death often occurring in the first 2 years (e631,e632).

Loeys-Dietz syndrome mimics many of the clinical features of Marfan syndrome, with craniofacial features of hypertelorism, low set ears, and bifid uvular or cleft palate serving to distinguish the two (154,156). Loeys-Dietz also represents an autosomal dominant disorder, due to mutations in transforming growth factor beta receptors 1 or 2 (*TGFBR1/2*). The aortic dilatation progresses to dissection at a younger age in these patients, with a mean age of death at 26 years (156).

Ascending aortic dilatation also occurs with increased frequency in Turner syndrome and in isolated bicuspid aortic valve patients (157) (e633,e634). The distribution of the aneurysms in the bicuspid aortic valve patients is however somewhat different from that of Marfan. In Marfan, the dilatation occurs predominantly at the level of the aortic valve cusps, whereas in the bicuspid aortic valve group the dilatation extends for longer distance up the aorta (e633).

Ehlers-Danlos syndrome is a heterogeneous group of at least ten generalized disorders of connective tissue synthesis, many involving different forms of collagen and their genes (158). Ehlers-Danlos type IV (vascular type) manifests thin-walled vessels and a diffuse decrease in elastic tissue in the media, deposition of acid mucopolysaccharide material between the medial elastic lamellae, and a decrease

Table 13-40 ■ MARFAN SYNDROME: GHENT DIAGNOSTIC CRITERIA[a]

System	Major Criteria	Minor Criteria
Family history	Diagnosis in first degree relative	None
Genetics	Mutation FBN1	None
Cardiovascular	Aortic root dilatation Dissection of ascending aorta	Mitral valve prolapse Mitral valve calcification (<40 years) Pulmonary artery dilatation Descending aorta dilatation/ dissection
Ocular	Ectopia lentis	2 of the 3 Flat cornea; elongate globe; myopia
Skeletal	At least 4 major: Pectus excavatum with surgery Pectus carinatum Pes planus Positive wrist or thumb sign Scoliosis >20° or spondylolithiasis Arm span/height ratio >1.05 Protrusio-acetabulae Elbow extension <170 degrees	2–3 major or 1 major + 2 minor Minor: Moderate pectus excavatum High arched palate Typical facial features Joint hypermobility
Pulmonary	None	Spontaneous pneumothorax Apical bulla
Skin	None	Stria Recurrent or incisional hernia
Central nervous system	Lumbosacral dural ectasia	

[a]Need major criteria in two organ systems + minor criteria in a third system.
See references (154) (e627).

in adventitial and medial collagen. Aortic dilatation with dissection and rupture, often intra-abdominal in location, can complicate clinical course and even cause death (158). This form of Ehlers-Danlos syndrome is caused by a mutation in the COL3A1 gene transmitted in an autosomal dominant fashion.

Menkes steely hair syndrome (gene Xq12-13) is an X-linked, recessively transmitted deficiency state associated with the defective intestinal absorption of copper. The disease manifestations result from reduced activities of the numerous copper-dependent enzymes. One such enzyme, lysyl oxidase, plays a role in formation and repair of extracellular matrix material. With impaired enzyme activity, vessel wall tensile strength is diminished leading to aneurysm formation in the high flow vessels (e635,e636). Arterial walls exhibit abnormalities of the internal elastic lamina at both the light and electron microscopic level (159) (see Chapter 5).

Atherosclerosis

A spectrum of inherited disorders cause congenital hypercholesterolemia; the complicating atherosclerotic cardiovascular disease occurs in childhood in a subgroup of these disorders (160) (Table 13-41). Atherosclerosis in childhood has been best described in familial hypercholesterolemia caused by a mutation in the gene encoding the receptor for low-density lipoprotein located on chromosome 19p13.2 (e637). Mutations in this gene occur frequently with heterozygotes identified at a 1:500 frequency (160) (e638). About one person in a million is a homozygote resulting in plasma cholesterol levels in excess of 650 mg/dL from infancy (e637). Study of an involved 20-week fetus revealed lipid deposits already present in the aorta intima (e639). Aortic atherosclerosis, although generalized, tends to be worse in the ascending aorta near the coronary arteries, and in the thoracic segment

Table 13-41 ■ INHERITED HYPERCHOLESTEROLEMIAS

Disorder	Inherit.	Gene Product	Gene	Childhood CVD
Homozygous familial hypercholesterolemia	AD	Low-density lipoprotein receptor	*LDLR*	Yes
Heterozygous familial hypercholesterolemia	AD	Low-density lipoprotein receptor	*LDLR*	No
Familial defective apolipoprotein B	AD	Apoplipoprotein B-100	*APOB*	No
PCSK9 gain- of function	AD	Proprotein convertase subtisilin/kexin 9	*PCSK9*	No
Autosomal recessive hypercholesterolemia	AR	ARH adaptor protein	*ARH*	Variable
Phytosterolemia	AR	ATP-binding cassette g5, g8	*ABCG5ABCG8*	Yes

Inherit., Inheritance pattern; CVD, cardiovascular disease; AD, autosomal dominant; AR, autosomal recessive.
From Rahalkar AR, Hegele RA. Monogenic pediatric dyslipidemias: classification, genetics and clinical spectrum. *Mol Genet Metab* 2008;93: 282–294.

and can result in supravalvular aortic stenosis as well as stenosis of the coronary artery ostia (161) (e640). Deposits of foam cells in the aortic and mitral valves with fibrosis and cholesterol clefts also cause valvular stenosis or insufficiency (161) (e640). Disease is widespread throughout the coronary arteries, and death from coronary artery disease can occur as early as 3 years of age (e641). Treatment modalities include plasmapheresis, high-dose statins, and bypass surgery to treat the coronary artery disease as well as the possibility of liver transplantation to reverse the metabolic defect (e8).

Vasculitis

Vasculitis by definition is an inflammatory, even destructive, process involving arteries and veins that can occur as one of many manifestations in a broad spectrum of infectious and inflammatory disorders. Involvement of the heart and great vessels occurs predominantly in two of these vasculitic disorders: Kawasaki disease and Takayasu arteritis.

Kawasaki Disease (Mucocutaneous Lymph Node Syndrome)

Kawasaki disease (KD), also called *mucocutaneous lymph node syndrome*, is an acute febrile exanthematous vasculitis that affects infants and young children. First reported in Japanese children in 1967 (e642), KD is now recognized worldwide. Although the initial febrile illness is self-limited, the vasculitic damage to the coronary arteries can lead to ischemic heart disease and occasionally death. In the developed world, KD now represents the most common cause of acquired heart disease in childhood (e643).

KD occurs almost exclusively in young children with the peak incidence at 6 months to 1 year, and greater than 75% of cases occurring before 5 years of life. There is a slight male predominance (M:F 1.5:1) and a prominent racial trend (Table 13-42) (162,163) (e643,e644). This racial trend is reflected in the reported incidence of KD in Japan of 137.7 cases per 100,000 children compared with that in the United States of 17.1 per 100,000 children (e645,e644).

Although the epidemiologic features of KD, including its acute febrile nature, seasonal occurrence, age of onset, and temporal and geographic clustering point to an infectious etiology, a causal agent continues to elude detection. The possibility that it represents a response to superantigens of group A *Streptococcus* or *Staphylococcus aureus* has attracted a lot of attention but has not been proven (e646). An alternative theory suggests an antigen-mediated immune response with IgA plasma cells playing a central role (e644). Epidemiologic data (Table 13-42) also suggest an underlying genetic predisposition to developing KD (e647).

The disease typically presents as a sudden febrile illness in young children between 6 months and 5 years of life. The fever, which lasts 5 days or more, is accompanied by the development of bilateral conjunctivitis, erythematous changes of the lips and oral cavity, a nonvesicular polymorphous rash of the trunk, erythematous desquamation of the palms and soles, and cervical lymphadenopathy (162,163). This constellation of features (Table 13-43) evolves over a 10-day period of time, often obscuring the diagnosis particularly in the early stages. Affected children often manifest a marked increase in acute-phase reactants and the erythrocyte sedimentation rate is generally elevated (162). This initial febrile illness is self-limited, but in 20% to 35% of patients the underlying vasculitis leads to coronary artery aneurysm formation (164,165) (e648). The risk of coronary artery disease is highest in young infants, a group in which the symptoms are also most likely to be incomplete (e649). The natural history of the aneurysms depends on their size and shape (164). Overall, 50% of the aneurysms resolve in the first 2 years; 20% become stenotic. Giant aneurysms (≥8 mm), which account for 20% of all aneurysms, do not resolve and 45% become stenotic. Although the death rate from Kawaski disease overall is much below 1%, up to 40% of children with stenotic vessels experience myocardial infarction, with death in 18% (164). The advent of intravenous immunoglobulin therapy has dramatically reduced the incidence of coronary artery aneurysms, particularly when given in the 10 days of illness (e650).

Table 13-42 ▪ KAWASAKI DISEASE EPIDEMIOLOGY: GENETIC FACTORS

Seasonal incidence
- Japan—biphasic winter and summer peak
- United States—winter/spring peak

Race-specific incidence (highest to lowest)
- Asia or Pacific Island
- African American
- Hispanic
- Caucasian

Sibling risk 2.1% = 10 × increase
Twin risk 13%

Data compiled from references (162,163) (e643,e644,e645,e647).

Table 13-43 ▪ CLINICAL CRITERIA FOR KAWASAKI DISEASE DIAGNOSIS

Fever persisting for ≥5 days
Presence of at least four of the following clinical features:
- Bilateral nonpurulent conjunctivitis
- Oral mucosal changes
  - Erythema, cracked lips, strawberry tongue or pharyngeal injection
- Polymorphous exanthemous skin rash
- Extremity changes
  - Acute = desquamative erythema of palms and soles; edema of hands and feet
  - Subacute = periungual peeling of digits
- Cervical lymphadenopathy (usually unilateral)

Patients with fever and less than four clinical features can be diagnosed with Kawasaki disease if coronary artery changes are identified with echocardiography or angiography

Compiled from references (162,163).

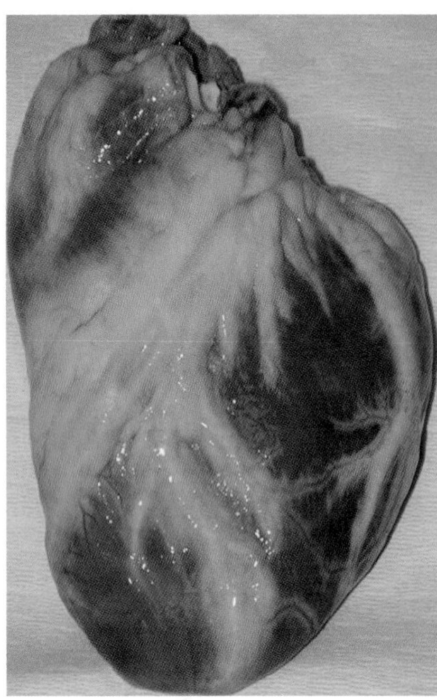

FIGURE 13-29 ■ Kawasaki disease. The heart from this 4-year-old is enlarged, has excessive fat deposition, and shows thick dilated coronary arteries.

The pathologic features of Kawaski disease are limited to autopsy studies and therefore represent the most severe pathologic changes. Within the first 10 days, vessel walls appear edematous with acute inflammation in the perivascular soft tissue and vasa vasorum without inflammation or necrosis in the media. From 12 to 25 days, the inflammation extends into the artery wall with a mixed inflammatory infiltrate including lymphocytes, plasma cells, and eosinophils accompanied by necrosis, thrombosis, and granulation tissue formation. Healing of the inflammation and organization of thrombi lead to aneurysm formation and luminal stenosis (166) (e651) (Figure 13-29). In the acute phase, pericarditis, myocarditis, and endocarditis are often present with involvement of the conduction system (166) (e652,e651). Overtime myocardial fibrosis and EFE appear. Endomyocardial biopsies from Kawasaki disease patients also reveal evidence of myocardial fibrosis with or without inflammation although progression to CMP is not a described feature (e653). In resected regressing aneurysms and coronary arteries from former Kawasaki patients dying of unrelated disease, intimal thickening with or without organizing thrombus material raises the speculation that KD may lead to early-onset coronary vascular disease (e654,e655).

Takayasu Arteritis

Takayasu arteritis (167) (e656) represents a form of large vessel vasculitis first described as "pulseless disease" because of subclavian artery occlusion. The vasculitis manifests in the aorta and its main branches initially as chronic granulomatous inflammation in the media and adventia of the vessel wall. Subsequent thrombosis and intimal and wall fibrosis may lead to vessel occlusion; alternatively, the damaged vessel may aneurysmally dilated. Symptoms of fever, malaise, arthralgias, and myalgias reflect the underlying inflammatory process. Occlusive symptoms, which vary depending on the anatomic location of the involved vessels, include seizures or stroke, renal hypertension, extremity claudication, aortic regurgitation, and pulmonary hypertension. Virtually all patients manifest multifocal bruits and/or absent pulses at presentation as a clue to the underlying disease. Takayasu arteritis has a striking 80% to 90% prevalence in young woman, and occurs most commonly in southeast Asia and Mexico (167) (e656). The underlying etiology for this rare disorder remains unknown.

Endocardial Diseases

The major pathologic process that affects the endocardium is endocarditis, defined by the presence of inflammatory cells within the endocardium. With few exceptions, the surface of an inflamed endocardium is marked by friable or partly healed excrescences termed *vegetations*. Although the heart valves are the most common sites, endocarditis also occurs on atrial walls, along the chamber trabeculae, and on the papillary muscles or chordae tendineae. Endocarditis due to microbial infection has classically been termed *bacterial endocarditis* and without infection nonbacterial endocarditis. With the increasing incidence of fungal endocarditis in recent years, the more general terms infective and noninfective endocarditis are replacing the classic language.

Noninfective Endocarditis

Noninfective endocarditis does not occur commonly in childhood. In a review of large published series of nonbacterial thrombotic endocarditis, only 3.2% of the reported cases occurred under 20 years of age (168). Noninfective endocarditis can be further subdivided into three groups (Table 13-44) with the rheumatic and Libman-Sacks forms discussed previously.

Nonbacterial thrombotic endocarditis is believed to occur in the setting of endothelial/endocardial injury serving as a nidus for platelet aggregation and thrombus formation. The associated vegetations, characterized by single or multiple, white-tan to pink, friable, verrucous projections of variable size, lie along the contact margins of the valve leaflets (Figure 13-19). Vegetations may occur as obvious warty, nodular or, sessile lesions occupying part or all of a valve leaflet, or they may be so small as to escape detection until coming to light under the microscope. They consist of fibrin strands among which lie trapped platelets, scattered erythrocytes, and occasional leukocytes. The underlying valves may appear normal or may be thickened and fibrotic (168) (e657). The actual valvular inflammatory reaction is minimal, in contrast to the pronounced reaction seen in infective endocarditis (IE). Visceral emboli are common, occurring in about 40% of cases, and resemble the parent lesions on the heart valve (168).

Table 13-44 ▪ FEATURES OF INFECTIVE AND NONINFECTIVE ENDOCARDITIS

Infective Endocarditis		Noninfective Endocarditis		
Bacterial	**Fungal**	**Rheumatic**	**Thrombotic**	**Libman-Sacks**
Underlying disease				
CHD	Surgically repaired CHD	Rheumatic fever	Indwelling arterial catheter	Systemic lupus erythematosis
Rheumatic heart disease	Prosthetic valve		Malignancy	
Prematurity	Immune deficit		Hypercoagulable states	
	IV drug abuse		Severe burns	
Valve before onset of endocarditis				
Normal	Normal Abnormal Prosthetic	Normal	Normal	Normal
Abnormal				
Appearance of vegetations				
Variable size	Large	Small (<4mm)	Small, uniform size	Variable size
Tan and friable	Friable	Row near cusp margin	Friable	Ventricular surface
			Patchy along cusp margin	
Valve ulceration and perforation				
Ulceration ±	Ulceration ±	No	No	No
Perforation ±	Rare perforation			
Mural involvement				
Rare	Rare	Rare	Rare	Common
Common sites				
Septal defects	Prosthetic valve	Mitral valve	Neonates—right-heart valves	Tricuspid valve
Suture lines	Suture lines	Aortic valve	Others—left-heart valves	Mitral valve
Damaged valve				
Peripheral embolization				
Common	Common	Rare	Occasional	Rare
Often large				

Neonates primarily have right-sided lesions associated with the use of intracardiac catheters, persistent fetal circulation, and disseminated intravascular coagulation (e658,e659). In older children and adults, the vegetations occur more often on the aortic and mitral valves and are associated with underlying malignancy, hypercoagulable states, septicemia, and extensive burns (168).

Infective Endocarditis

IE also occurs infrequently in children, making epidemiology data difficult to ascertain. The overall incidence of IE seems to be on the rise (e660) and the few pediatric studies available suggest a similar trend in children (e661). In the past, rheumatic fever served as the major underlying condition. Although this remains true in much of the developing world (169), in developed countries underlying congenital heart defects serve as the nidus for infection in the majority of pediatric patients (Table 13-45) (170) (e662–e664). The degree of risk for developing IE varies with the type of defect; the highest risk occurs in patients with complex cyanotic heart defects, prior episodes of endocarditis, or repairs that include placement of shunt or prosthetic valve material (171) (e665). Neonates with IE do not usually have underlying congenital heart defects; risk factors include prematurity and the presence of central vascular catheters (e666,e667).

The clinical presentation for children with IE includes fever and malaise with a new or changing heart murmur, when detectable, serving as a clue (e661,e665). Embolic phenomenon occurs in approximately 15% of patients (169,170) (e662). With longstanding disease, splenomegaly and immunologic stimulation leading to hypergammaglobulinemia, autoantibody formation, and immune complex deposition may further confuse the clinical picture (e661).

Table 13-45 ▪ PEDIATRIC INFECTIVE ENDOCARDITIS CARDIAC ANATOMY

New York City, USA (170)	
Complex cyanotic heart disease	35%
Normal anatomy	31%
Ventricular septal defect	15%
Other acyanotic heart disease	8%
Mitral valve prolapse	6%
Rheumatic heart disease	5%
Lahore, Pakistan (169)	
Rheumatic heart disease	53%
Ventricular septal defect	18%
Tetralogy of Fallot	9%
Patent ductus arteriosus	9%
Aortic stenosis	4%
Complex congenital heart disease	4%
Myocarditis	2%

Neonates more often present with a septic picture including thrombocytopenia, disseminated intravascular coagulation, and septic emboli (e661). Echocardiographic demonstration of vegetations aids in the diagnosis of IE, particularly in children without complex heart defects (170) (e661,e665). Diagnosis depends on clinical or pathologic findings (Table 13-46) that include positive blood cultures and echocardiographic identification of vegetations (e668).

The formation of infected vegetations begins with endothelial injury or erosion, often at a site of turbulent blood flow. The injury site serves as a nidus for fibrin clot formation. Gram-positive organisms, which account for 90% of identified organisms, have a propensity to adhere to fibronectin and lamin within the clot material and activate further clot formation (e661). In the past, *Streptococcus viridans* was the most common organisms causing IE; in more recent years, *S. aureus* has become nearly as common (170) (e661,e662). Gram-negative, fastidious, and fungal organisms are identified infrequently, occurring most often in the setting of prior heart surgery, underlying immune deficiency, or central line placement (Figure 13-30) (e661).

Table 13-46 ■ DIAGNOSIS OF INFECTIVE ENDOCARDITIS

Modified Duke Criteria for Pathologic or Clinical Diagnosis

Pathologic Criteria

Organisms identified in vegetation, embolized vegetation, or cardiac abscess by either culture or histology

OR

Pathologic lesions present (vegetation or cardiac abscess) + histologic confirmation of endocarditis

Clinical Criteria

Two major criteria

OR

1 major and 3 minor criteria

OR

5 minor criteria

Major Criteria

1. Positive blood culture
   —Typical IE microorganisms from ≥ 2 blood cultures
   OR
   —Microorganisms consistent with IE from blood cultures drawn ≥12 hours apart or all of 3 or majority of 4 or more blood cultures with first and last ≥1 hour apart
2. Evidence of endocardial involvement by
   —Positive echocardiogram of IE
   Oscillating intracardiac mass or
   abscess or
   New partial dehiscence of prosthetic valve
   OR
   —New valvular regurgitation

Minor Criteria

1. Predisposing heart condition or intravenous drug use
2. Fever ≤38°F
3. Vascular phenomena
   Major artery emboli, pulmonary infarct, intracranial hemorrhage
4. Immunologic phenomena
   Glomerulonephritis, Osler nodes, Roth spots, rheumatoid factor
5. Microbiologic evidence
   Positive blood culture not meeting major criteria or serologic evidence of active infection with consistent organism
6. Echocardiographic evidence
   consistent with IE but not meeting major criteria

IE, infective endocarditis.
See references (e661,e665,e668).

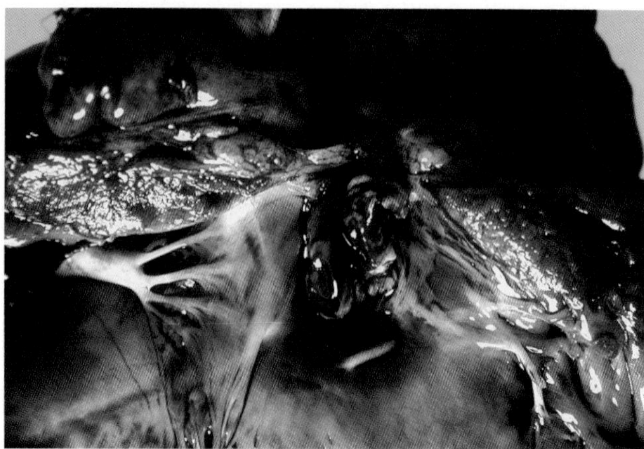

FIGURE 13-30 ■ Close-up view of the left ventricular outflow tract from a child with bicuspid aortic valve and *Streptococcus* endocarditis. Two large irregular vegetations obscure and partially destroy the aortic valve leaflets.

The infected vegetations tend to occur on the atrial surface of the AV valves and the ventricular surface of the outflow valves (172). In neonates without underlying heart malformations, the vegetations are often right sided (e666). With underlying heart malformations, the vegetations may occur at the edge of VSDs or at the site of flow turbulence on the ventricular or malformed valve surface (172). The infective organisms elicit an acute inflammatory response leading to destruction and perforation of the valve tissue. The infection may spread into the adjacent vessel or heart tissue leading to abscess or fistula formation. Microscopically, acute vegetations consist of granular, heaped-up layers of fibrin, platelets, necrotic materials, and polymorphonuclear leukocytes. Organisms may or may not be identified. Similar neutrophil-rich infiltrates with granulation tissue formation help distinguish infected from noninfected prosthetic valve specimens (e669). With time (and antibiotic treatment), organisms are lost and the damaged valve tissue undergoes calcification, chronic and at times granulomatous inflammation, and granulation tissue formation. Whether a native valve was initially normal or not, the subsequently damaged valve becomes a potential site for recurrent endocarditis.

Pericardial Diseases

Pericarditis

The two-layered pericardium forms a sac around the heart that normally contains less than 30 mL of serous fluid. However, when the pericardium becomes inflamed, the normally smooth mesothelium lining the sac becomes rough. A fibrinous exudate, rich in fibrinogen and other plasma proteins,

Table 13-47 ■ CAUSES OF PERICARDITIS

Infectious agents
Viral
Bacterial
Fungal
Parasitic
Immunologically mediated
Rheumatic fever
Systemic lupus erythematosus
Scleroderma
Postcardiotomy syndrome
Drug hypersensitivity
Other
Uremia
Postsurgical
Neoplasia
Trauma
Radiation

accumulates a dull-colored film over the pericardial surface. Friction between the two roughened surfaces results in the pericardial friction rub that serves as a clinical marker of pericarditis. In many instances, pericarditis also leads to increased fluid volume in the pericardial sac. The serous versus purulent versus hemorrhagic nature of this fluid varies with the underlying etiology.

Pericarditis occurs in a wide variety of clinical settings (Table 13-47) (173). When the etiology is viral or noninfectious, a serous effusion, rich in protein containing lymphocytes, accompanies a fibrinous exudate. Viral pericarditis typically follows a respiratory or gastrointestinal illness with enteroviruses the common responsible viral agent (173). Noninfectious pericarditis may complicate a variety of systemic illnesses, including rheumatic fever, systemic lupus erythematosis, juvenile rheumatoid arthritis, and KD (173,174). Postoperative pericardial effusions occur in approximately 15% to 25% of children undergoing open heart surgery (175) (e670). Approximately 25% of these postoperative effusions become symptomatic (postpericardiotomy syndrome) (175) (e670).

Purulent pericarditis is largely caused by pyogenic bacteria, with the most common cause in North American children being *S. aureus* (173,174) (e671). Purulent pericarditis usually results from a primary infection spreading to the pericardium either by direct extension from an adjacent purulent pneumonia, mediastinitis, or empyema, or by hematogenous seeding from pyelonephritis or osteomyelitis (174). Most patients are acutely ill with fever, tachypnea, and even chest pain. A shaggy, thick, yellow or gray exudate covers the pericardial surfaces (Figure 13-31). Organisms are numerous, and large numbers of neutrophils infiltrate the strands and local tissues.

Tuberculous pericarditis results as a direct extension of infection from tracheobronchial lymph nodes or from hematogenous spread. The clinical onset may be insidious with fever and chest pain. Pericardiocentesis returns often bloody fluid containing numerous lymphocytes and few neutrophils. Acid-fast bacilli can be identified in fluid smears from 15% to 40% of patients, and biopsy of the thickened pericardium often reveals caseating granulomas (173).

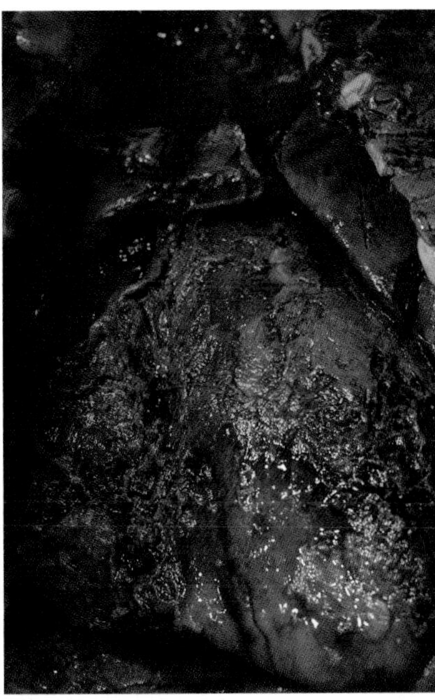

FIGURE 13-31 ■ The opened pericardium in an immune-compromised patient with disseminated Aspergillus infection. The pericardium appears thickened and shaggy due to the intense inflammatory response to the infection.

Chronic or healed pericarditis manifests in two major patterns, adhesive (obliterative) and constrictive. Adhesive pericarditis is characterized by the presence of small nodules of vascularized granulation tissue between fibrin aggregates and mesothelial cell proliferations leading eventually to partial or complete obliteration of the pericardial cavity. In the more clinically significant constrictive pericarditis, the heart becomes encased in a dense fibrous and even calcified shell, the rigidity of which may mechanically interfere with cardiac diastolic function and venous return to the atria (173).

Developmental Abnormalities

Congenital aplasia of the pericardium occurs either as complete or partial absence of the parietal pericardium. When complete, the defect is usually asymptomatic. Partial deficiency, which occurs mostly on the left side of the heart, may be complicated by herniation and strangulation of myocardium (176). Small defects may be associated with other congenital mediastinal lesions, such as bronchogenic cysts, pulmonary sequestration, and ectopia cordis. The defect is thought to result from a failure of the normal pleuropericardial foramen to close in the pleuropericardial membrane.

Pericardial cysts are thin-walled, generally unilocular structures filled with clear fluid that tend to be benign and asymptomatic. They are encountered in children only rarely at autopsy. The cysts are most often located at the costophrenic angles but may also appear higher in the mediastinum. The cysts vary markedly in size with mesothelium lining the thin walls of fibrous tissue. Though believed to be

Table 13-48 ■ TUMOR INCIDENCE BY AGE

Ref. No.	Age Range (No.)	Rhabdomyoma (%)	Fibroma (%)	Teratoma (%)	Myxoma (%)	Histiocytoid (%)	Other benign (%)	Malignant (%)
186	Fetal (89)	64	11	22	0	0	6	0
	Neonatal (135)	47	16	15	4	11	5	2
194	<1 year (35)	54	23	3	0	6	6	8
	1–16 year (21)	5	24	0	19	0	14	38
e719	≤1year (48)	58	13	19	0	0	6	4
	1–15 year (89)	39	14	12	14		12	9
177	0–17 year (56) (Benign only)	79	11	2	0	0	8	—

developmental, the embryonic origin of these cysts remains unclear (e672).

Cardiac Tumors

Primary cardiac tumors occur rarely in both adults and children. In a review of 22 large autopsy series, Reynen (e673) identified a frequency of 0.02%, or 200 primary tumors in 1 million autopsies in a general population. A large autopsy series of infants and children yielded an estimated frequency of 0.08% (e674). Even among infants presenting for evaluation of cardiac disease, tumors account for only 0.2% to 0.4% of lesions (1,177). New imaging techniques have led to increased numbers of tumors identified during life. Fetal echocardiographic studies report cardiac tumors in 0.11% to 0.14% of referred pregnancies (178) (e675) with prenatal ultrasound identifying 21% of congenital cardiac tumors in one study (177).

The type of primary cardiac tumor present varies considerably with age (Table 13-48). In fetuses and newborn infants, rhabdomyomas account for the vast majority followed by pericardial teratomas (178). During the first 2 years of life, rhabdomyomas continue to be the most common tumor, with fibromas representing the second most common (179) (e676). Myxomas, the most common tumor in adults, account for 6% of tumors in children, occurring almost exclusively in adolescents (179). In rare instances, a cardiac tumor (especially rhabdomyoma) occurs in association with a heart malformation (180) (e677,e678). The space-occupying aspect of these tumors suggests that they in fact may play a role in inducing the associated malformation.

Primary Tumors

Rhabdomyomas

The most common cardiac tumor in infants occurs as a solitary or, more often (77% to 90%) (181,182) (e679–e681) multiple, nodules anywhere in the heart (Figure 13-32). They are highly associated with tuberous sclerosis (TS), occurring in 40% to 60% of patients examined echocardiographically (180,181). Rhabdomyomas may be the first clue to the diagnosis of TS, with 70% to 80% of fetuses and infants carrying rhabdomyomas subsequently having a diagnosis of TS confirmed (181) (e679,e680,e682). Rhabdomyomas display a striking propensity to regress spontaneously. When identified in infancy, 50% to 70% will regress, especially when associated with TS (180) (e675,e679,e683). Tumors identified in older children are less likely to regress (180).

Clinically, many rhabdomyomas remain asymptomatic. Larger rhabdomyomas may project from the ventricular wall or septum into the cardiac cavity and obstruct cardiac flow or valvular motion (181) (e680,e681). Disruption of the conduction system with resultant arrhythmias also frequently occurs (180,181). The tumors come to light in fetuses due to nonimmune hydrops, arrhythmias, a mass noted on routine prenatal ultrasound, or a family history of TS (178) (e679). Postnatally, tumors may present clinically with a murmur, heart failure, arrhythmia, or sudden death. When symptomatic, partial resection to relieve symptoms may be required, but more aggressive surgical intervention is contraindicated (e684).

Grossly, rhabdomyomas appear as well-circumscribed, yellow-to-gray nodules that vary in size from microscopic to 10 cm in diameter (183). Usually multiple, they occur with about equal frequency in either ventricle. They also may occur in the atrial walls; they have not been described in cardiac valves (182). Microscopically, the typical rhabdomyoma cells are much larger (up to 80 mm) than those of normal myocardium, due to accumulation of glycogen within

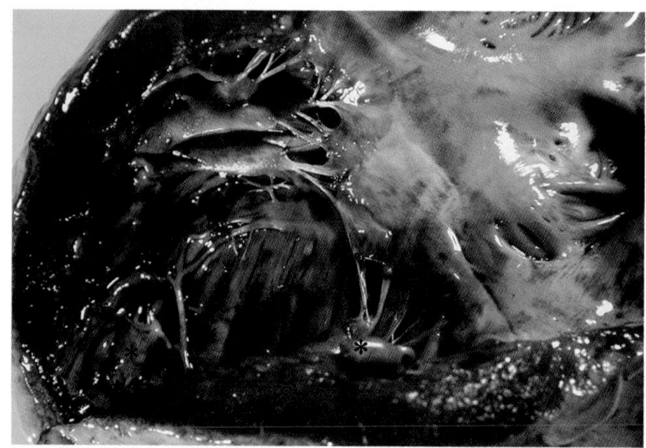

FIGURE 13-32 ■ Multiple small rhabdomyomas. In this opened left ventricular cavity, the trabeculae appear thickened and somewhat pale due to multiple small rhabdomyomas highlighted by asterisks. These rhabdomyomas were asymptomatic in this child with tuberous sclerosis.

the cell cytoplasm, resulting in the formation of "spider cells". By electron microscopy, the "spider cells" contain diffuse glycogen, few myofibrils, scattered leptofibrils, and poorly developed sarcoplasmic reticulum. Well-formed intercalated disc-like intercellular junctions surround the periphery of the cells, mimicking cardiac myoblasts (182) (e681,e685). The clinical pattern of multiple tumors that tend to regress, combined with the ultrastructural appearance of the tumor cells, led to the conclusion that cardiac rhabdomyomas represent a hamartomatous rather than a neoplastic process (182) (e681).

Cardiac Fibroma

The second most common tumor outside the fetal period presents most frequently (>1/3 of cases) in the 1st year of life with the remaining spread out over the following two decades (184). These fibromas characteristically arise as a single ventricular mass in an otherwise normal child, although a small subgroup occur with Gorlin syndrome (184) (e686,e687). They present with cardiomegaly, arrhythmias, and heart failure; sudden death occurs in one-third of cases, probably as the result of arrhythmias or outflow obstruction (182,184). The tumors arise most frequently in the left ventricle or intraventricular septum, but may also occur in the right ventricle and occasionally in the atria (183,184). They reach large size, occasionally exceeding 10 cm (182). On cut surface, these firm white trabeculated tumors grossly resemble a leiomyoma (Figure 13-33). Microscopically, the tumors display a monomorphic population of bland spindled cells embedded within a variably collagenized stroma that often appears infiltrative at the periphery (182). Tumors from young infants tend to appear more cellular and mitotically active, features that do not denote more aggressive behavior (183,184). In older children, calcification and focal cystic degeneration become more prevalent. Although benign, cardiac fibromas do not regress and in fact tend to slowly increase in size (183). Surgical excision is the treatment of choice (183) (e688); unresectable tumors may require transplantation (183) (e689).

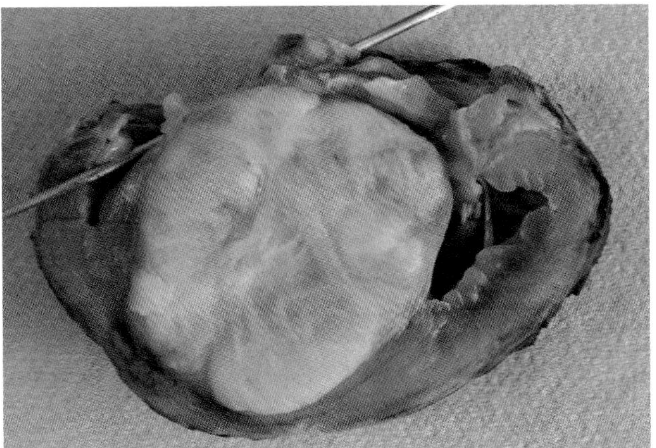

FIGURE 13-33▪Transverse section of an explanted heart as viewed from the back. A white firm trabeculated mass replaces the interventricular septum and protrudes into the left and right ventricular cavities. A probe inserted into the aortic valve exits into the left ventricular chamber under the mitral valve leaflet, highlighting the obstruction to the left ventricular outflow caused by this large cardiac fibroma.

Teratoma

Teratoma represents the second most common cardiac tumor in fetuses, with 50% of this rare tumor being diagnosed before or during the 1st month of life and two-thirds in the 1st year (185,186). In its more common intrapericardial location, the tumor originates from the external surface of the heart base and gives rise to an often marked pericardial effusion (185,187). Compression of the heart by the mass combined with the effusion leads to nonimmune hydrops in the fetus and cardiac tamponade in infants (186). Intrauterine pericardiocentesis is reported to effectively relieve the fetal distress (e690–e692). Surgical excision is curative (186) (e693). Rarely teratomas occur in the intraventricular septum where they clinically mimic cardiac rhabdomyomas and fibromas (185) (e693,e694). The pathologic features of the tumor, when reported, are similar to benign teratomas occurring elsewhere in the body (186) (e693,e695). Intrapericardial bronchogenic cysts overlap clinically with teratomas and may be included as teratomas in the older literature (185,187).

Myxomas

They present the most common (50% to 75%) cardiac tumor in adults (182) (e696,e694) but account for only 5% of tumors in infancy and 15% to 20% of tumors in older children and adolescents (179,182,186). They arise from endocardium, usually adjacent to the fossa ovalis, in the left (75%) or right (18%) atrium (182,188). Presenting symptoms include one or more components of a clinical triad (Table 13-49) (182,188,189). Although the vast majority of atrial myxomas occur sporadically, approximately 5% occur in families as part of the familial atrial myxoma syndrome (Carney complex) (Table 13-49) (190,191) (e697,e698). The Carney

Table 13-49 ▪ ATRIAL MYXOMAS—CLINICAL FEATURES

Clinical Triad (188,189)
- Valvular obstruction
- Tumor emboli
- Constitutional symptoms
  - Malaise, fever, weight loss, anemia, elevated ESR, hypergammaglobulinemia

Carney Complex (190,191) (e698)
- Skin lesions: Lentigines, blue nevi,
- Myxomas: cardiac, breast, skin, mucus membranes, bone
- Endocrine abnormalities:
  - Adrenal pigmented cortical hyperplasia
  - Pituitary adenoma
  - Thyroid nodules
  - Breast adenomas
  - Testicular large cell calcifying Sertoli cell tumors

complex, an autosomal dominant disorder, results from a mutation in the *PRKAR1A* gene on chromosome 17q2 in 90% of cases (190,191). The syndromic form of atrial myxoma tends to occur at a younger age, in atypical locations, and with a higher frequency of multiple recurrent tumors as compared with the sporadic form (192) (e699). Atrial myxomas occurring in children and adolescents should therefore elicit a search for other manifestations of this complex in both patients and other family members.

Identical pathologic features occur in syndromic and sporadic forms of atrial myxoma (182,183,188,193). Grossly, the tumors appear gelatinous with either a narrow or a broad base, and a frond-like or smooth surface. Cut surface appears variegated with scattered gritty calcification. Microscopically stellate or elongate cells with scant eosinophilic cytoplasm disperse singly or as small nests, trabeculae or perivascular rings in an acid mucopolysaccharide-rich myxoid matrix. With immunocytochemical stains, the cells mark reliably with vimentin and variably with endothelial, actin, and cytokeratin markers (189,193).

Histiocytoid Cardiomyopathy

This represents a rare myocardial disease of infancy and early childhood characterized by cardiomegaly, incessant ventricular tachycardia, and sudden death. More than 70 cases have been reported under a variety of synonyms, including isolated cardiac lipidosis, xanthomatous CMP, foamy myocardial transformation of infancy, oncocytic CMP, myocardial hamartoma, and Purkinje cell tumor (194,195) (e700–e702). The lesion presents almost exclusively in the first 2 years of life with a 75% predominance in girls (194). Both cardiac and noncardiac malformations occur in a subgroup of these patients including atrial and VSDs, EFE, hypoplastic left heart, corneal opacities, microphthalmia, cataracts, cleft palate, hydrocephalus, agenesis of the corpus callosum, and renal cysts (194) (e702).

At surgery or autopsy, the heart is often enlarged with the left ventricular surface studded by multiple flat to round, smooth, yellow to tan-white nodules that may or may not be visible to the naked eye. Similar nodules may also occur on the papillary muscles, right ventricle, atria, and all four heart valves (194,196) (e703). Histologically, the nodules contain cells that differ from the adjacent myocardial cells in both their larger size (20 to 40 mm diameter) and the pale foamy nature of their cytoplasm, which gives them their histiocytic appearance (Figure 13-34). Nodules of similar cells are also often present in the conduction system, the midmyocardium, and beneath the epicardium. Immunocytochemical stains identify the cells as myocardial in origin based on positive muscle-specific actin and myosin, and negative lysozyme and CD68 (197). These foamy cells contain only small amounts of glycogen, and lipid; the mitochondria-rich nature of the cytoplasm becoming evident only at the ultrastructural level. By electron microscopy, the large unusual cells have the configuration of swollen abnormal myocytes that contain

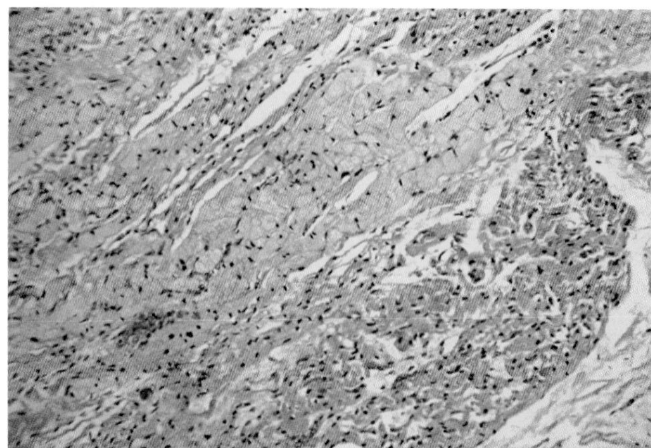

FIGURE 13-34 ■ Histiocytoid cardiomyopathy. Enlarged, granular-appearing myocytes on the upper left contrast with the normal compact myocytes on the lower right. (Hematoxylin and eosin stain, original magnification 100×.)

abundant mitochondria with only rare peripherally placed myofibrils, scattered leptofibrils, no T tubules, and decreased numbers of the usual desmosomes (196,197) (e702,e704).

The pathogenesis for this unusual pathologic condition remains controversial. The ultrastructural features suggest a relationship with primitive Purkinje cells (196) (e705) or primitive myocardial cells and support a hamartomatous process. Comparable cellular changes may occur in other organs of infants with the cardiac lesions (e704,e706). The possibility of an underlying mitochondrial disorder has been raised by the finding of respiratory chain enzyme deficiencies and mtDNA mutations in a few cases (195) (e701,e707). The possibility of an X-linked chromosomal abnormalities has been suggested in a few other cases (198) (e708).

Unfortunately, the diagnosis of histiocytoid CMP is most often made at autopsy. When the presenting ventricular arrhythmias can be initially controlled medically, subsequent electrophysiologic mapping and surgical ablation of the lesions can lead to long-term survival (e590,e709). Cardiac transplantation in a single case has also been reported (e700).

Other Benign Tumors

A variety of other benign tumors and malformations have been described in the heart (Table 13-50). The vascular tumors may occur in the setting of multiple cutaneous hemangiomas (186).

Table 13-50 ■ OTHER BENIGN CARDIAC TUMORS AND MALFORMATIONS

Hemangioma and vascular malformation	4%
Mesothelioma of AV node	3%
Neurofibroma	<1%
Bronchogenic cysts	
Lipoblastoma	
Inflammatory pseudotumor	
Lipoma	
Multicystic hamartoma	

See references (179,182,183) (e710,e720).

Table 13-51 ■ MALIGNANT CARDIAC TUMORS

Primary (e510,e721–e724)
Rhabdomyosarcoma
Fibrosarcoma
Undifferentiated sarcoma
Angiosarcoma
Malignant germ cell tumor
Leiomyosarcoma
Malignant nerve sheath tumor
Pleomorphic sarcoma
Synovial sarcoma
Myxosarcoma
Secondary (metastatic) (199) (e725,e726)
Non-Hodgkin lymphoma
Neuroblastoma
Wilms tumor
Hepatoblastoma
Hepatoma
Rhabdomyosarcoma
Undifferentiated sarcoma
Osteosarcoma
Adrenal carcinoma
Ewing sarcoma
Endodermal sinus tumor
Brain tumor
Hodgkin disease
Pleuropulmonary blastoma

Malignant Tumors

Malignant tumors account for less than 1% of the primary cardiac tumors in the fetus and newborn. In older infants and children, malignancies become more prevalent, accounting for 10% to 20% of primary cardiac tumors (179,182) (e710). A broad range of diagnoses encompass the remaining reported cases (Table 13-51).

In children, as in adults, metastatic tumors outnumber the primary cardiac malignancies. In a review of records from Hospital for Sick Children in Toronto over a 62-year period, Chan et al. (199) identified 16 primary cardiac tumors of which only one was malignant. Over the same time period, 59 secondary malignant tumors were identified in the heart, of which 45 were distant metastases and 14 resulted from direct extension (199). Table 13-51 outlines the range of metastatic tumor types identified.

REFERENCES

1. Fyler DC, Buckley LP, Hellenbrand WE, et al. Report of the New England Regional Infant Cardiac Program. *Pediatrics* 1980;65:377–461.
2. Brennan P, Young ID. Congenital heart malformations: aetiology and associations. *Semin Neonatol* 2001;6:17–25.
3. Oyer CE, Sung CJ, Friedman R, et al. Reference values for valve circumferences and ventricular wall thicknesses of fetal and neonatal hearts. *Pediatr Dev Pathol* 2004;7:499–505.
4. Rowlatt UF, Rimoldi HJA, Lev M. The quantitative anatomy of the normal child's heart. *Pediatr Clin North Am* 1963;10:499–588.
5. Scholz DG, Kitzman DW, Hagen PT, et al. Age-related changes in normal human hearts during the first 10 decades of life. Part I (Growth): a quantitative anatomic study of 200 specimens from subjects from birth to 19 years old. *Mayo Clin Proc* 1988;63:126–136.
6. Anderson RH. How should we optimally describe complex congenitally malformed hearts? *Ann Thorac Surg* 1996;62:710–716.
7. Arey JB. *Cardiovascular pathology in infants and children*. Philadelphia, PA: W.B. Saunders, Company, 1984.
8. Azhari N, Shihata MS, Al-Fatani A. Spontaneous closure of atrial septal defects within the oval fossa. *Cardiol Young* 2004;14:148–155.
9. al Zaghal AM, Li J, Anderson RH, et al. Anatomical criteria for the diagnosis of sinus venosus defects. *Heart* 1997;78:298–304.
10. Adatia I, Gittenberger-de Groot AC. Unroofed coronary sinus and coronary sinus orifice atresia: implications for management of complex congenital heart disease. *J Am Coll Cardiol* 1995;25:948–953.
11. Anderson RH, Lenox CC, Zuberbuhler JR. The morphology of ventricular septal defects. *Perspect Pediatr Pathol* 1984;8:235–268.
12. Milo S, Ho SY, Wilkinson JL, et al. Surgical anatomy and atrioventricular conduction tissues of hearts with isolated ventricular septal defects. *J Thorac Cardiovasc Surg* 1980;79:244–255.
13. Zielinsky P, Rossi M, Haertel JC, et al. Subaortic fibrous ridge and ventricular septal defect: role of septal malalignment. *Circulation* 1987;75:1124–1129.
14. Anderson RH, Ho SY, Becker AE. The surgical anatomy of the conduction tissues. *Thorax* 1983;38:408–420.
15. Becker AE, Anderson RH. Atrioventricular septal defects: what's in a name? *J Thorac Cardiovasc Surg* 1982;83:461–469.
16. Pierpont MEM, Markwald RR, Lin AE. Genetic aspects of atrioventricular septal defects. *Am J Med Genet* 2000;97:289–296.
17. Silverman NH, Zuberbuhler JR, Anderson RH. Atrioventricular septal defects: cross-sectional echocardiographic and morphologic comparisons. *Int J Cardiol* 1986;13:309–331.
18. Newfeld EA, Sher M, Paul MH, et al. Pulmonary vascular disease in complete atrioventricular canal defect. *Am J Cardiol* 1977;39: 721–726.
19. Anderson RH, Weinberg PM. The clinical anatomy of transposition. *Cardiol Young* 2005;15:76–87.
20. Smith A, Arnold R, Wilkinson JL, et al. An anatomical study of the patterns of the coronary arteries and sinus nodal artery in complete transposition. *Int J Cardiol* 1986;12:295–307.
21. Mavroudis C, Backer CL. Transposition of the great arteries. In: Mavroudis C, Baker CJ, eds. *Pediatric cardiac surgery*, 3rd ed. Philadelphia, PA: Mosby, 2003: 442–475.
22. Milanesi O, Ho SY, Thiene G, et al. The ventricular septal defect in complete transposition of the great arteries: pathologic anatomy in 57 cases with emphasis on subaortic, subpulmonary, and aortic arch obstruction. *Hum Pathol* 1987;18:392–396.
23. Sridaromont S, Feldt RH, Ritter DG, et al. Double outlet right ventricle: hemodynamic and anatomic correlations. *Am J Cardiol* 1976;38:85–94.
24. Lev M, Bharati S, Meng L, et al. A concept of double-outlet right ventricle. *J Thorac Cardiovasc Surg* 1972;64:271–281.
25. Ueda M, Becker AE. Classification of hearts with overriding aortic and pulmonary valves. *Int J Cardiol* 1985;9:357–369.
26. Anderson RH, Ho SY, Wilcox BR. The surgical anatomy of ventricular septal defect part IV: double outlet ventricle. *J Card Surg* 1996;11:2–11.
27. Tchervenkov CI, Walters HL, Chu VF. Congenital heart surgery nomenclature and database project: double outlet left ventricle. *Ann Thorac Surg* 2000;69:S264–S269.
28. Collett RW, Edwards JE. Persistent truncus arteriosus: a classification according to anatomic types. *Surg Clin North Am* 1949;29: 1245–1270.
29. Van Praagh R. Truncus arteriosus: what is it really and how should it be classified? *Eur J Cardiothorac Surg* 1987;1:65–70.
30. Kutsche LM, Van Mierop LH. Anatomy and pathogenesis of aorticopulmonary septal defect. *Am J Cardiol* 1987;59:443–447.
31. Scalia D, Russo P, Anderson RH, et al. The surgical anatomy of hearts with no direct communication between the right atrium and the ventricular mass–so-called tricuspid atresia. *J Thorac Cardiovasc Surg* 1984;87:743–755.

32. Thoele DG, Ursell PC, Ho SY. Atrial morphologic features in tricuspid atresia. *J Thorac Cardiovasc Surg* 1991;102:606–610.
33. Attenhofer Jost CH, Connolly HM, Dearani JA, et al. Ebstein's anomaly. *Circulation* 2007;115:277–285.
34. Schreiber C, Cook A, Ho SY, et al. Morphologic spectrum of Ebstein's malformation: revisitation relative to surgical repair. *J Thorac Cardiovasc Surg* 1999;117:148–155.
35. Tandon R, Moller JH, Edwards JE. Anomalies associated with the parachute mitral valve: a pathologic analysis of 52 cases. *Canad J Cardiol* 1986;2:278–281.
36. Gittenberger-de Groot AC, Wenink AC. Mitral atresia: morphological details. *Br Heart J* 1984;51:252–258.
37. Ho SY, Zuberbuhler JR, Anderson RH. Pathology of hearts with a univentricular atrioventricular connection. *Perspect Pediatr Pathol* 1988;12:69–99.
38. Beckman CB, Moller JH, Edwards JE. Alternate pathways to pulmonary venous flow in left-sided obstructive anomalies. *Circulation* 1975;52:509–516.
39. Virmani R, Atkinson JB, Forman NB, et al. Mitral valve prolapse. *Hum Pathol* 1987;18:596–602.
40. Edwards JE. Floppy mitral valve syndrome. *Cardiovasc Clin* 1988;18:249–271.
41. Greenwood RD. Mitral valve prolapse: incidence and clinical course in a pediatric population. *Clin Pediatr (Phila)* 1984;23:318–320.
42. Bissett GSI, Schwartz DC, Meyer RA, et al. Clinical spectrum and long term follow-up of isolated mitral valve prolapse in 119 children. *Circulation* 1980;62:423–429.
43. Milo S, Ho SY, Macartney FJ, et al. Straddling and overriding atrioventricular valves: morphology and classification. *Am J Cardiol* 1979;44:1122–1134.
44. Anderson RH, Allwork SP, Ho SY, et al. Surgical anatomy of tetralogy of Fallot. *J Thorac Cardiovasc Surg* 1981;81:887–896.
45. Siwik ES, Patel CR, Zahka KG, Goldmuntz E. Tetralogy of fallot. In: Allen HD, Gutgesell HP, Clark BJ, et al., eds. *Moss & Adams' heart disease in infants, children & adolescents: including the fetus and young adults*, 6th ed. Philadelphia, PA: Lippincott Williams & Wilkins, 2001:880–902.
46. Kinsley RH, McGoon DC, Danielson GK, et al. Pulmonary arterial hypertension after repair of tetralogy of Fallot. *J Thorac Cardiovasc Surg* 1974;67:111–120.
47. Tchervenkov CI, Roy N. Congenital heart surgery nomenclature and database project: pulmonary atresia–ventricular septal defect. *Ann Thorac Surg* 2000;69:S97–S105.
48. Hadjo A, Jimenez M, Baudet E, et al. Review of the long-term course of 52 patients with pulmonary atresia and ventricular septal defect: anatomical and surgical considerations. *Eur Heart J* 1995;16:1668–1674.
49. Johnson RJ, Sauer U, Buhlmeyer K, et al. Hypoplasia of the intrapulmonary arteries in children with right ventricular outflow tract obstruction, ventricular septal defect, and major aortopulmonary collateral arteries. *Pediatr Cardiol* 1985;6:137–143.
50. Buendia A, Attie F, Ovseyevitz J, et al. Congenital absence of pulmonary valve leaflets. *Br Heart J* 1983;50:31–41.
51. Stamm C, Anderson RH, Ho SY. Clinical anatomy of the normal pulmonary root compared with that in isolated pulmonary valvular stenosis. *J Am Coll Cardiol* 1998;31:1420–1425.
52. Gielen H, Daniels O, van Lier H. Natural history of congenital pulmonary valvar stenosis: an echo and Doppler cardiographic study. *Cardiol Young* 1999;9:129–135.
53. Cil E, Saraclar M, Ozkutlu S, et al. Double-chambered right ventricle: experience with 52 cases. *Int J Cardiol* 1995;50:19–29.
54. Franch RH, Gay BB, Jr. Congenital stenosis of the pulmonary artery branches: a classification, with post mortem findings in two cases. *Am J Cardiol* 1963;35:512.
55. Latson LA, Prieto LR. Pulmonary stenosis. In: Allen HD, Gutgesell HP, Clark EB, et al., eds. *Moss & Adams' heart disease in infants, children & adolescents: including the fetus and young adults*, 6th ed. Philadelphia, PA: Lippincott Williams & Wilkins, 2001:820–844.
56. Choi YH, Seo JW, Choi JY, et al. Morphology of tricuspid valve in pulmonary atresia with intact ventricular septum. *Pediatr Cardiol* 1998;19:381–389.
57. Hausdorf G, Gravinghoff L, Keck EW. Effects of persisting myocardial sinusoids on left ventricular performance in pulmonary atresia with intact ventricular septum. *Eur Heart J* 1987;8:291–296.
58. Vricella LA, Kanani M, Cook AC, et al. Problems with the right ventricular outflow tract: a review of morphologic features and current therapeutic options. *Cardiol Young* 2005;14:533–549.
59. Brown JW, Stevens LS, Holly S, et al. Surgical spectrum of aortic stenosis in children: a thirty-year experience with 257 children. *Ann Thorac Surg* 1988;45:393–403.
60. Hawkins JA, Minich LL, Tani LY, et al. Late results and reintervention after aortic valvotomy for critical aortic stenosis in neonates and infants. *Ann Thorac Surg* 1998;65:1758–1762.
61. Vogt J, Dische R, Rupprath G, et al. Fixed subaortic stenosis: an acquired secondary obstruction? A twenty- seven year experience with 168 patients. *Thorac Cardiovasc Surg* 1989;37:199–206.
62. Stamm C, Li J, Ho SY, et al. The aortic root in supravalvular aortic stenosis: the potential surgical relevance of morphologic findings. *J Thorac Cardiovasc Surg* 1997;114:16–24.
63. Mahowald JM, Lucas RV, Jr, Edwards JE. Aortic valvular atresia: associated cardiovascular anomalies. *Pediatr Cardiol* 1982;2: 99–105.
64. Hagemo PS, Skarbo A-B, Rasmussen M, et al. An extensive long term follow-up of a cohort of patients with hypoplasia of the left heart. *Cardiol Young* 2007;17:51–55.
65. Schneider DJ, Moore JW. Patent ductus arteriosus. *Circulation* 2006;114:1873–1882.
66. Satoda M, Zhao F, Diaz GA, et al. Mutations in TFAP2B cause Char syndrome, a familial form of patent ductus arteriosus. *Nat Genet* 2000;25:42–46.
67. Machii M, Becker AE. Hypoplastic aortic arch morphology pertinent to growth after surgical correction of aortic coarctation. *Ann Thorac Surg* 1997;64:516–520.
68. Pellegrino A, Deverall PB, Anderson RH, et al. Aortic coarctation in the first three months of life: an anatomopathological study with respect to treatment. *J Thorac Cardiovasc Surg* 1985;89: 121–127.
69. Amato JJ, Galdieri RJ, Cotroneo JV. Role of extended aortoplasty related to the definition of coarctation of the aorta. *Ann Thorac Surg* 1991;52:615–620.
70. Loffredo CA, Ferencz C, Wilson PD, et al. Interrupted aortic arch: an epidemiologic study. *Teratology* 2000;61:368–375.
71. Kussman BD, Geva T, McGowan FX, Jr. Cardiovascular causes of airway compression. *Pediatr Anesth* 2004;14:60–74.
72. Weinberg PM. Aortic arch anomalies. In: Allen HD, Gutgesell HP, Clark EB, et al., eds. *Moss & Adams' heart disease in infants, children & adolescents: including the fetus and young adults*, 6th ed. Philadelphia, PA: Lippincott Williams & Wilkins, 2001:707–772.
73. Gikonyo BM, Jue KL, Edwards JE. Pulmonary vascular sling: report of seven cases and review of the literature. *Pediatr Cardiol* 1989;10:81–89.
74. Matherne GP. Congenital anomalies of the coronary vessels and the aortic root. In: Allen HD, Gutgesell HP, Clark EB, et al., eds. *Moss & Adams' heart disease in infants, children & adolescents: including the fetus and young adults*, 6th ed. Philadelphia, PA: Lippincott Williams & Wilkins, 2001:675–688.
75. Smith A, Arnold R, Anderson RH, et al. Anomalous origin of the left coronary artery from the pulmonary trunk. Anatomic findings in relation to pathophysiology and surgical repair. *J Thorac Cardiovasc Surg* 1989;98:16–24.
76. Geva T, Van Praagh S. Abnormal systemic venous connections. In: Allen HD, Gutgesell HP, Clark EB, et al., eds. *Moss & Adams' Heart Disease in Infants, Children & Adolescents: Including the Fetus and Young Adults*, 6th ed. Philadelphia, PA: Lippincott Williams & Wilkins, 2001:773–798.

77. Moller JH, Nakib A, Eliot RS, et al. Congenital cardiac disease associated with polysplenia: a developmental complex of bilateral "left-sidedness". *Circulation* 1967;36:789–799.
78. Najm HK, Williams WG, Coles JG, et al. Scimitar syndrome: twenty years' experience and results of repair. *J Thorac Cardiovasc Surg* 1996;112:1161–1169.
79. Geva T, Van Praagh S. Anomalies of the pulmonary veins. In: Allen HD, Gutgesell HP, Clark EB et al., eds. *Moss & Adams' Heart Disease in Infants, Children & Adolescents: Including the Fetus and Young Adults*, 6th ed. Philadelphia, PA: Lippincott Williams & Wilkins, 2001:736–772.
80. Karamlou T, Gurofsky R, Al Sukhni E, et al. Factors associated with mortality and reoperation in 377 children with total anomalous pulmonary venous connection. *Circulation* 2007;115:1591–1598.
81. Leca F, Thibert M, Khoury W, et al. Extrathoracic heart (ectopia cordis). Report of two cases and review of the literature. *Int J Cardiol* 1989;22:221–228.
82. Sharma S, Devine WA, Anderson RH, et al. The determination of atrial arrangement by examination of appendage morphology in 1842 heart specimens. *Br Heart J* 1988;60:227–231.
83. Belmont JW, Mohapatra B, Towbin JA, et al. Molecular genetics of heterotaxy syndromes. *Curr Opin Cardiol* 2004;19:216–220.
84. Maron BJ, Towbin JA, Thiene G, et al. Contemporary definitions and classification of the cardiomyopathies: an American Heart Association Scientific Statement from the Council on Clinical Cardiology, Heart Failure and Transplantation Committee; Quality of Care and Outcomes Research and Functional Genomics and Translational Biology Interdisciplinary Working Groups; and Council on Epidemiology and Prevention. *Circulation* 2006;113:1807–1816.
85. Schwartz ML, Cox GF, Lin AE, et al. Clinical approach to genetic cardiomyopathy in children. *Circulation* 1996;94:2021–2038.
86. Maron BJ. Hypertrophic cardiomyopathy in childhood. *Pediatr Clin North Am* 2004;51:1305–1346.
87. Hughes SE. The pathology of hypertrophic cardiomyopathy. *Histopathology* 2004;44:412–427.
88. Feldman AM, McNamara D. Myocarditis. *N Engl J Med* 2000; 343:1388–1398.
89. Tabib A, Loire R, Chalabreysse L, et al. Circumstances of death and gross and microscopic observations in a series of 200 cases of sudden death associated with arrhythmogenic right ventricular cardiomyopathy and/or dysplasia. *Circulation* 2003;108:3000–3005.
90. Kies P, Bootsma M, Bax J, et al. Arrhythmogenic right ventricular dysplasia/cardiomyopathy: screening, diagnosis, and treatment. *Heart Rhythm* 2006;3:225–234.
91. Dokuparti M, Pamuru P, Thakkar B, et al. Etiopathogenesis of arrhythmogenic right ventricular cardiomyopathy. *J Hum Genet* 2005;50:375–381.
92. Freedom RM, Yoo SJ, Perrin D, et al. The morphological spectrum of ventricular noncompaction. *Cardiol Young* 2005;15:345–364.
93. Burke A, Mont E, Kutys R, et al. Left ventricular noncompaction: a pathological study of 14 cases. *Hum Pathol* 2005;36:403–411.
94. Edwards WD. Cardiomyopathies. *Hum Pathol* 1987;18:625–635.
95. Towbin JA, Lowe AM, Colan SD, et al. Incidence, causes, and outcomes of dilated cardiomyopathy in children. *JAMA* 2006;296: 1867–1876.
96. Angelini A, Calzolari V, Thiene G, et al. Morphologic spectrum of primary restrictive cardiomyopathy. *Am J Cardiol* 1997;80: 1046–1050.
97. Denfield SW, Rosenthal G, Gajarski RJ. Restrictive cardiomyopathies in childhood: etiologies and natural history. *Tex Heart Inst J* 1997;24:38–44.
98. Aretz HT, Billingham ME, Edwards WD, et al. Myocarditis. A histopathologic definition and classification. *Am J Cardiovasc Pathol* 1986;1:3–14.
99. Marboe CC, Fenoglio JJ. Pathology and natural history of human myocarditis. *Pathol Immunopathol Res* 1988;7:226–239.
100. Calabrese F, Thiene G. Myocarditis and inflammatory cardiomyopathy: microbiological and molecular biological aspects. *Cardiovasc Res* 2003;60:11–25.
101. Cooper LT, Berry GJ, Shabetai R, et al. Idiopathic giant-cell myocarditis – natural history and treatment. *N Engl J Med* 1997; 336:1860–1866.
102. Litvosky SH, Burke AP, Virmani R. Giant cell myocarditis: an entity distinct from sarcoidosis characterized by multiphasic myocyte destruction by cytotoxic T cells and histiocytic giant cells. *Mod Pathol* 1996;9:1126–1134.
103. Thurberg BL, Lynch Maloney C, Vaccaro C, et al. Characterization of pre- and post-treatment pathology after enzyme replacement therapy for Pompe disease. *Lab Invest* 2006;86:1208–1220.
104. Sugie K, Yamamoto A, Murayama K, et al. Clinicopathological features of genetically confirmed Danon disease. *Neurology* 2002;58:1773–1778.
105. Mohan UR, Hay AA, Cleary MA, et al. Cardiovascular changes in children with mucopolysaccharide disorders. *Acta Paediatr* 2002;91:799–804.
106. Renteria VG, Ferrans VJ, Roberts WC. The heart in the Hurler syndrome: gross, histologic and ultrastructural observations in five necropsy cases. *Am J Cardiol* 1976;38:487–501.
107. Gilbert EF, Dawson G, zu Rhein GM, et al. I-cell disease, mucolipidosis II. Pathological, histochemical, ultrastructural and biochemical observations in four cases. *Z Kinderheilkd* 1973;114:259–292.
108. Suzuki Y, Oshima A, Nanba E. β-Galactosidase deficiency (β-galactosidosis): GM1 gangliosidosis and Morquio B disease. In: Scriver CR, Beaudet AL, Sly WS et al., eds. *The Metabolic & Molecular Bases of Inherited Disease*, 8th ed. New York: McGraw-Hill, 2001:3775–3809.
109. Blieden LC, Desnick RJ, Carter JB, et al. Cardiac involvement in Sandhoff's disease. Inborn error of glycosphingolipid metabolism. *Am J Cardiol* 1974;34:83–88.
110. Linhart A, Elliott PM. The heart in Anderson-Fabry disease and other lysosomal storage disorders. *Heart* 2007;93:528–535.
111. Gehrmann J, Sohlbach K, Linnebank M, et al. Cardiomyopathy in congenital disorders of glycosylation. *Cardiol Young* 2003;13:345–351.
112. Shekhawat PS, Matem D, Strauss AW. Fetal fatty acid oxidation disorders, their effect on maternal health and neonatal outcome: impact of expanded newborn screening on their diagnosis and management. *Pediatr Res* 2005;57:78R-86R.
113. Pierpont ME, Breningstall GN, Stanley CA, et al. Familial carnitine transporter defect: a treatable cause of cardiomyopathy in children. *Am Heart J* 2000;139:s96-s106.
114. Tripp ME, Katcher ML, Peters HA, et al. Systemic carnitine deficiency presenting as familial endocardial fibroelastosis. A treatable cardiomyopathy. *N Engl J Med* 1981;305:385–390.
115. Scaglia F, Towbin JA, Craigen WJ, et al. Clinical spectrum, morbidity, and mortality in 113 pediatric patients with mitochondrial disease. *Pediatrics* 2004;114:925–931.
116. Holmgren D, Wahlander H, Eriksson BO, et al. Cardiomyopathy in children with mitochondrial disease: clinical course and cardiological findings. *Eur Heart J* 2003;24:280–288.
117. Kelly AL, Rhodes DA, Roland JM, et al. Hereditary juvenile haemochromatosis: a genetically heterogeneous life- threatening iron-storage disease. *QJMed* 1998;91:607–618.
118. Finsterer J, Stollberger C. Cardiac involvement in primary myopathies. *Cardiology* 2000;94:1–11.
119. Frankel KA, Rosser RJ. The pathology of the heart in progressive muscular dystrophy: epimyocardial fibrosis. *Hum Pathol* 1976;7:375–386.
120. Sovari AA, Bodine CK, Farokhi F. Cardiovascular manifestations of myotonic dystrophy-1. *Cardio Rev* 2007;15:191–194.
121. Dalakas MC, Park KY, Semino-Mora C, et al. Desmin myopathy, a skeletal myopathy with cardiomyopathy caused by mutations in the desmin gene. *N Engl J Med* 2000;342:770–780.

122. Bit-Avragim N, Perrot A, Schöls L, et al. The GAA repeat expansion in intron 1 of the frataxin gene is related to the severity of cardiac manifestation in patients with Friedreich's ataxia. *J Mol Med* 2001; 78:626–632.
123. Delatycki MB, Williamson R, Forrest SM. Friedreich ataxia: an overview. *J Med Genet* 2000;37:1–8.
124. Rennebohm RM. Inflammatory "noninfectious" cardiovascular diseases. In: Allen HD, Gutgesell HP, Clark EB et al., eds. *Moss and Adams' Heart Disease in Infants, Children, and Adolescents Including the Fetus and Young Adult*, 6th ed. Philadelphia, PA: Lippincott Williams & Wilkins, 2001:1242–1253.
125. Moder KG, Miller T, Tazelaar HD. Cardiac involvement in systemic lupus erythematosus. *Mayo Clin Proc* 1999;74:275–284.
126. Gross L. The cardiac lesions in Libman-Sacks disease. With a consideration of its relationship to acute diffuse lupus erythematosus. *Am J Pathol* 1940;16:375–407.
127. Ho SY, Esscher E, Anderson RH, et al. Anatomy of congenital complete heart block and relation to maternal anti-Ro antibodies. *Am J Cardiol* 1986;58:291–294.
128. Meckler KA, Kapur RP. Congenital heart block and associated cardiac pathology in neonatal lupus syndrome. *Pediatr Dev Pathol* 1998;1:136–142.
129. Jaeggi ET, Hamilton RM, Silverman ED, et al. Outcome of children with fetal, neonatal or childhood diagnosis of isolated congenital atrioventricular block: a single institution's experience of 30 years. *J Am Coll Cardiol* 2002;39:130–137.
130. da Silva NA, Pereira BA. Acute rheumatic fever. Still a challenge. *Rheum Dis Clin North Am* 1997;23:545–568.
131. Ayoub EM. Acute rheumatic fever. In: Allen BS, Gutgesell HP, Clark EB et al., eds. *Moss & Adams' heart disease in infants, children & adolescents: including the fetus and young adults*, 6th ed. Lippincott Williams & Wilkins, 2001:1226–1241.
132. Ullmo S, Vial Y, Di Bernardo S, et al. Pathologic ventricular hypertrophy in the offspring of diabetic mothers: a retrospective study. *Eur Heart J* 2007;28:1319–1325.
133. Donnelly WH, Hawkins H. Optimum examination of the normally formed perinatal heart. *Hum Pathol* 1987;18:55–60.
134. Donnelly WH. Ischemic myocardial necrosis and papillary muscle dysfunction in infants and children. *Am J Cardiovasc Pathol* 1987;1:173–188.
135. Stewart S, Winters GL, Fishbein MC, et al. Revision of the 1990 Working Formulation for the Standardization of Nomenclature in the Diagnosis of Heart Rejection. *J Heart Lung Transplant* 2005;24:1710–1720.
136. Crespo-Leiro MG, Veiga-Barreiro A, Doménech N, et al. Humoral heart rejection (severe allograft dysfunction with no signs of cellular rejection or ischemia): incidence, management, and the value of C4d for diagnosis. *Am J Transplant* 2005;5:2560–2564.
137. Anderson RH, Ho SY. The architecture of the sinus node, the atrioventricular conduction axis, and the internodal atrial myocardium. *J Cardiovasc Electrophysiol* 1998;9:1233–1248.
138. Berry GJ, Billingham ME. Normal heart. In: Mills SE, ed. *Histology for Pathologists*, 3rd ed. Philadelphia, PA: Lippincott Williams & Wilkins, 2007:527–545.
139. Gulino SPM. Examination of the cardiac conduction system: forensic application in cases of sudden cardiac death. *Am J Forensic Med Pathol* 2003;24:227–238.
140. Deal BJ, Jacobs JP, Mavroudis C. Congenital Heart Surgery Nomenclature and Database Project: arrhythmias. *Ann Thorac Surg* 2000;69(4 suppl):S319–S331.
141. Anderson RH, Ho SY. Anatomy of the atrioventricular junctions with regard to ventricular preexcitation. *Pacing Clin Electrophysiol* 1997;20:2072–2076.
142. Schmidt KG, Ulmer HE, Silverman NH, et al. Perinatal outcome of fetal complete atrioventricular block: a multicenter experience. *J Am Coll Cardiol* 1991;17:1360–1366.
143. Modell SM, Lehmann MH. The long QT syndrome family of cardiac ion channelopathies: a huGE review. *Genet Med* 2006;8:143–155.
144. Tester DJ, Ackerman MJ. Sudden infant death syndrome: how significant are the cardiac channelopathies? *Cardiovasc Res* 2005;67:388–396.
145. Tester DJ, Spoon DB, Valdiva HH, et al. Targeted mutational analysis of the RyR2-encoded cardiac ryanodine receptor in sudden unexplained death: a molecular autopsy of 49 medical examiner/coroner's cases. *Mayo Clin Proc* 2004;79:1380–1384.
146. Berger S, Konduri GG. Pulmonary hypertension in children: the twenty-first century. *Pediatr Clin North Am* 2006;53:961–987.
147. Hislop AA, Pierce E. Growth of the vascular tree. *Paediatr Resp Rev* 2000;1:321–327.
148. Geggel RL, Reid LM. The structural basis of PPHN. *Clin Perinatol* 1984;2:525–549.
149. Pietra GG, Capron F, Stewart S, et al. Pathologic assessment of vasculopathies in pulmonary hypertension. *J Am Coll Cardiol* 2004;43:S25-S32.
150. Rabinovitch M, Keane JF, Norwood WI, et al. Vascular structure in lung tissue obtained at biopsy correlated with pulmonary hemodynamic findings after repair of congenital heart defects. *Circulation* 1984;69:655–667.
151. Adatia I. Recent advances in pulmonary vascular disease. *Curr Opin Pediatr* 2002;14:292–297.
152. Slovut DP, Olin JW. Fibromuscular dysplasia. *N Engl J Med* 2004;350:1862–1871.
153. Sarkar R, Coran AG, Cilley RE, et al. Arterial aneurysms in children: clinicopathologic classification. *J Vasc Surg* 1991;13:47–56.
154. Stuart AG, Williams A. Marfan's syndrome and the heart. *Arch Dis Child* 2007;92:351–356.
155. Faivre L, Collod-Beround G, Loeys BL, et al. Effect of mutation type and location on clinical outcome in 1,013 probands with Marfan syndrome or related phenotypes and *FBN1* mutations: an international study. *Am J Hum Genet* 2007;81:454–466.
156. Loeys BL, Schwarze U, Holm T, et al. Aneurysm syndromes caused by mutations in the TGF-{beta} receptor. *N Engl J Med* 2006;355:788–798.
157. Carlson M, Silberbach M. Dissection of the aorta in Turner syndrome: two cases and review of 85 cases in the literature. *J Med Genet* 2007;44:745–749.
158. Byers PH. Disorders of collagen biosynthesis and structure. In: Scriver CR, Beaudet AL, Sly WS et al., eds. *The Metabolic & Molecular Bases of Inherited Disease*, 8th ed. New York: McGraw-Hill, 2001:5241–5285.
159. Murakami H, Kodama H, Nemoto N. Abnormality of vascular elastic fibers in the macular mouse and a patient with Menkes' disease: ultrastructural and immunohistochemical study. *Med Electron Microsc* 2002;35:24–30.
160. Rahalkar AR, Hegele RA. Monogenic pediatric dyslipidemias: classification, genetics and clinical spectrum. *Mol Genet Metab* 2008;93:282–294.
161. Kawaguchi A, Miyatake K, Yutani C, et al. Characteristic cardiovascular manifestation in homozygous and heterozygous familial hypercholesterolemia. *Am Heart J* 1999;137:410–418.
162. Satou GM, Giamelli J, Gewitz MH. Kawasaki disease: diagnosis, management, and long-term implications. *Cardio Rev* 2007;15: 163–169.
163. Burns JC, Glode MP. Kawasaki syndrome. *Lancet* 2004;364:533–544.
164. Kato H, Sugimura T, Akagi T, et al. Long-term consequences of Kawasaki disease: a 10- to 21-year follow-up study of 594 patients. *Circulation* 1996;94:1379–1385.
165. Suzuki A, Kamiya T, Kuwahara N, et al. Coronary arterial lesions of Kawasaki disease: cardiac catheterization findings of 1100 cases. *Pediatr Cardiol* 1986;7:3–9.
166. Fujiwara H, Hamashima Y. Pathology of the heart in Kawasaki disease. *Pediatrics* 1978;61:100–107.

167. Hall S, Barr W, Lie JT, et al. Takayasu arteritis. A study of 32 North American patients. *Medicine* (*Baltimore*) 1985;64:89–99.
168. Lopez JA, Ross RS, Fishbein MC, et al. Nonbacterial thrombotic endocarditis: a review. *Am Heart J* 1987;113:773–784.
169. Sadiq M, Nazir M, Sheikh SA. Infective endocarditis in children–incidence, pattern, diagnosis and management in a developing country. *Int J Cardiol* 2001;78:175–182.
170. Saimon L, Prince A, Gersong WM. Pediatric infective endocarditis in the modern era. *J Pediatr* 1993;122:847–853.
171. Dajani AS, Taubert KA. Infective endocarditis. In: Allen BS, Gutgesell HP, Clark EB et al., eds. *Moss & Adams' heart disease in infants, children & adolescents: including the fetus and young adults*, 6th ed. Lippincott Williams & Wilkins, 2001:1297–1308.
172. Thiene G, Basso C. Pathology and pathogenesis of infective endocarditis in native heart valves. *Cardiovasc Pathol* 2006;15:256–263.
173. Rheuban KS. Pericardial diseases. In: Allen BS, Gutgesell HP, Clark EB et al., eds. *Moss & Adams' heart disease in infants, children & adolescents: including the fetus and young adults*, 6th ed. Lippincott Williams & Wilkins, 2001:1287–1296.
174. Roodpeyma S, Sadeghian N. Acute pericarditis in childhood: a 10-year experience. *Pediatr Cardiol* 2000;21:363–367.
175. Cheung EW, Ho SA, Tang KK, et al. Pericardial effusion after open heart surgery for congenital heart disease. *Heart* 2003;89:780–783.
176. Montaudon M, Roubertie F, Bire F, et al. Congenital pericardial defect: report of two cases and literature review. *Surg Radiol Anat* 2007;29:195–200.
177. Beghetti M, Gow RM, Haney I, et al. Pediatric primary benign cardiac tumors: a 15-year review,. *Am Heart J* 1997;134:1107–1114.
178. Groves AM, Fagg NL, Cook A, et al. Cardiac tumours in intrauterine life. *Arch Dis Child* 1992;67:1189–1192.
179. Burke A, Virmani R. Classification and incidence of cardiac tumors. *Tumors of the Heart and Great Vessels*, 3rd Series. Washington, D.C.: Armed Forces Institute of Pathology 1996; 1–11.
180. Nir A, Tajik AJ, Freeman WK, et al. Tuberous sclerosis and cardiac rhabdomyoma. *Am J Cardiol* 1995;76:419–421.
181. Webb DW, Thomas RD, Osborne JP. Cardiac rhabdomyomas and their association with tuberous sclerosis. *Arch Dis Child* 1993;68:367–370.
182. McAllister HAJ, Hall RJ, Cooley DA. Tumors of the heart and pericardium. *Curr Probl Cardiol* 1999;24:57–116.
183. Freedom RM, Lee KJ, MacDonald C, et al. Selected aspects of cardiac tumors in infancy and childhood. *Pediatr Cardiol* 2000;21:299–316.
184. Burke A, Rosado-de-Christenson M, Templeton PA, et al. Cardiac fibroma: clinicopathologic correlates and surgical treatment. *J Thorac Cardiovasc Surg* 1994;108:862–870.
185. Marx GR, Moran AM. Cardiac tumors. In: Allen HD, Gutgesell HP, Clark EB et al., eds. *Moss & Adams' heart disease in infants, children & adolescents: including the fetus and young adults*, 6th ed. Lippincott Williams & Wilkins, 2001:1431–1445.
186. Isaacs H. Fetal and neonatal cardiac tumors. *Pediatr Cardiol* 2004;25:252–273.
187. Burke A, Virmani R. Heterotopias and tumors originating from ectopic tissues. In: Burke A, Virmani R, eds. *Tumors of the Heart and Great Vessels*, 3rd Series. Washington, D.C.: Armed Forces Institute of Pathology, 1996:111–125.
188. Burke A, Virmani R. Cardiac myxoma. *Tumors of the Heart and Great Vessels*, 3rd Series. Washington, D.C.: Armed Forces Institute of Pathology, 1996; 21–46.
189. Reynen K. Cardiac myxomas. *N Engl J Med* 1995;333:1610–1617.
190. Boikos SA, Stratakis CA. Carney complex: the first 20 years. *Curr Opin Oncol* 2007;19:24–29.
191. Wilkes D, McDermott DA, Basson CT. Clinical phenotypes and molecular genetic mechanisms of Carney complex. *Lancet Oncol* 2005;6:501–508.
192. McCarthy PM, Piehler JM, Schaff HV, et al. The significance of multiple, recurrent, and "complex" cardiac myxomas. *J Thorac Cardiovasc Surg* 1986;91:389–396.
193. Burke AP, Virmani R. Cardiac myxoma. A clinicopathologic study. *Am J Clin Pathol* 1993;100:671–680.
194. Shehata BM, Patterson K, Thomas JE, et al. Histiocytoid cardiomyopathy: three new cases and a review of the literature. *Pediatr Dev Pathol* 1998;1:56–69.
195. Vallance HD, Jeven G, Wallace DC, et al. A case of sporadic infantile histiocytoid cardiomyopathy caused by the A8344G (MERRF) mitochondrial DNA mutation. *Pediat Cardiol* 2004;25:538–540.
196. Kearney DL, Titus JL, Hawkins EP, et al. Pathologic features of myocardial hamartomas causing childhood tachyarrhythmias. *Circulation* 1987;75:705–710.
197. Gelb AB, Van Meter SH, Billingham ME, et al. Infantile histiocytoid cardiomyopathy– Myocardial or conduction system hamartoma: what is the cell type involved? *Hum Pathol* 1993;24:1226–1231.
198. Bird LM, Krous HF, Eichenfield LF, et al. Female infant with oncocytic cardiomyopathy and microphthalmia with linear skin defects (MLS): a clue to the pathogenesis of oncocytic cardiomyopathy? *Am J Med Genet* 1994;53:141–148.
199. Chan HSL, Sonley MJ, Moësmd CAF, et al. Primary and secondary tumors of childhood involving the heart, pericardium, and great vessels: a report of 75 cases and review of the literature. *Cancer* 200;56:825–836.

CHAPTER 14

The Gastrointestinal Tract

JOHN HART
REBECCA WILCOX
CHRISOPHER R. WEBER

EMBRYOLOGY

The gastrointestinal tract is derived largely from the endodermal germ layer. During the 3rd week of embryonic development, cephalocaudal and lateral folds of the trilaminar germ disk develop and progressively incorporate parts of the endoderm-lined yolk sac into the body cavity to form a tubelike gut. By the end of week 3 of gestation, an open connection between the anterior portion of this tube, the foregut, and the amniotic cavity is established at the site of the future mouth. During early embryonic life, the vitelline or omphalomesenteric duct provides an open connection between the midgut and the yolk sac (Figure 14-1). This connection becomes progressively longer and narrower as gestation proceeds and eventually forms part of the umbilical cord. By week 10, the communication between the lumen of the midgut and the umbilicus becomes obliterated and soon disappears (e328).

The laryngotracheal diverticulum develops from the ventral foregut during week 4 of gestation (Chapter 12). Gradual formation of an esophagotracheal septum along the length of the laryngotracheal diverticulum separates the ventral respiratory and the dorsal digestive tubes (Figure 14-2).

During the 2nd month of embryonic life, rapid cellular proliferation within the digestive tube causes a transient partial obliteration of the duodenal lumen, the so-called solid stage of development. Recanalization occurs by week 8 of gestation. Rapid midgut growth within the relatively small body cavity results in a temporary herniation of the lengthening midgut into the umbilical stalk during weeks 6 to 11 (Figure 14-3). During this physiologic herniation, the intestinal loops rotate counterclockwise, a process that continues as the intestinal loops return to the abdominal cavity during weeks 10 and 11, so that the cecum comes to lie in the right side of the abdomen. If this orderly process fails to occur or is anomalous, the locations of the small and large intestine, mesentery, and fixation points of the intestine to the body wall will be abnormal. The hindgut, or posterior portion of the primitive digestive tube, initially ends posteriorly in the

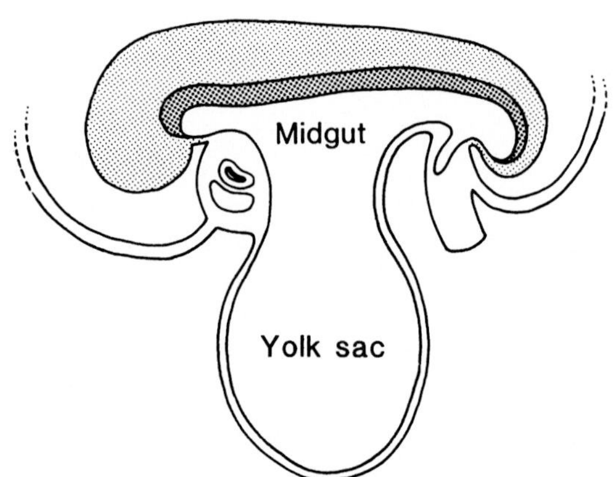

FIGURE 14-1 ■ During week 4 of gestation, head and tail folds of the embryo surround portions of the yolk sac. An open connection between the primitive midgut and the yolk sac exists. After this connection narrows, it is known as the vitelline or omphalomesenteric duct.

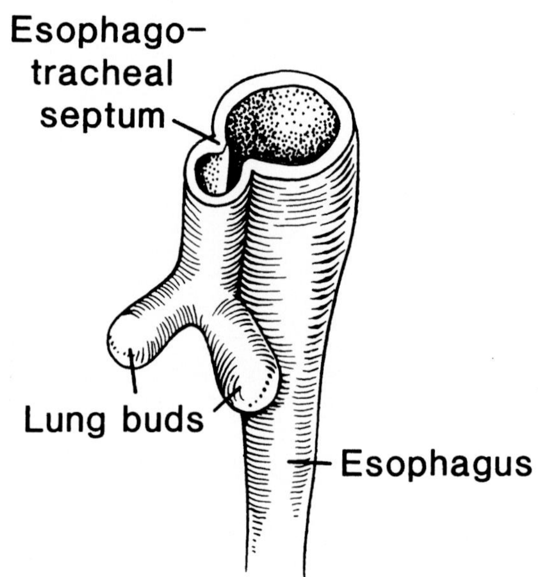

FIGURE 14-2 ■ Development of the respiratory system from the foregut at week 4 of gestation. The esophagotracheal septum develops from the two lateral folds that migrate toward the midline to separate the developing respiratory diverticulum from the primitive gut.

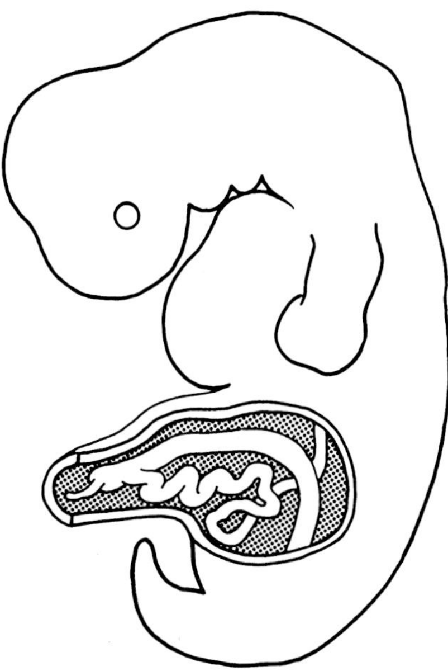

FIGURE 14-3■Physiologic gut herniation in an embryo at week 8 of gestation. Rapid elongation of the intestine in a relatively small abdominal cavity causes the gut to herniate into the umbilical cord. This herniation resolves at the end of the 3rd month of gestation. A failure in the normal events at this stage explains the omphalocele and malrotation.

cloaca, separated from superficial ectoderm by the cloacal membrane (Figure 14-4). A transverse ridge, the urorectal septum, grows posteriorly from the umbilical stalk and gradually divides the cloaca into a ventral portion, the urogenital sinus, and a dorsal portion, the future rectum, and anus. This division is normally complete at the end of week 6 of gestation. The membrane covering the anal canal disappears by week 9, so that communication between the digestive tract and the amniotic cavity is established caudally.

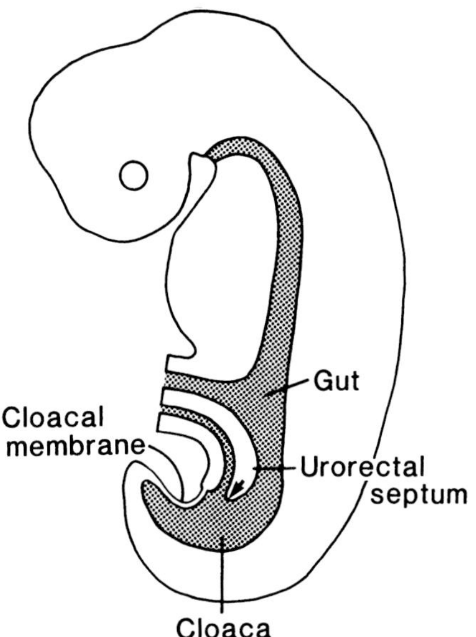

FIGURE 14-4■Primitive hindgut region in an embryo at 6 weeks of gestation. The urorectal septum grows posteriorly to divide the cloaca into a urogenital portion separate from the intestinal portion. Note the intact cloacal membrane.

DISORDERS OF THE ESOPHAGUS

Congenital Abnormalities

Persistent Embryonic Epithelium

The embryonic and early fetal esophagus is lined by ciliated stratified columnar epithelium. The transformation to stratified squamous epithelium is usually complete by week 25 of gestation, but occasionally a patch of superficial columnar epithelium persists at birth, especially in premature infants. Persistent embryonic epithelium is usually found incidentally at autopsy as microscopic foci in either the proximal or distal end of the esophagus and is of little clinical consequence. This change is limited to surface epithelium only; glandular mucosa, as in gastric heterotopia of the esophagus, is not present. Because it is not usually found after early infancy, persistent embryonic epithelium is presumed to be replaced by squamous epithelium.

Heterotopic Gastric Mucosa (Inlet Patch)

Single or multiple small patches (5 to 30 mm) of gastric cardiac or fundic type mucosa can sometimes be found incidentally in the cervical esophagus (eFigure 14-1). The incidence in patients undergoing esophagogastroduodenoscopy has been reported to be 3.6% (120). These patches of heterotopic gastric epithelium usually are not clinically important and are rarely biopsied since most endoscopists are familiar with them. They can be colonized by *Helicobacter pylori* organisms (120). Confusion with Barrett esophagus can occur if the endoscopic findings are not communicated to the surgical pathologist.

Esophageal Duplication

Duplication of the esophagus is rare. The duplicated segment may be a separate cylindrical tube alongside part of the normal esophagus with a complete mucosa, submucosa, and two-layered muscularis externa (double esophagus). Alternatively, a spherical, intramural esophageal cyst may form and share a portion of muscularis propria with the adjacent esophageal wall. Esophageal duplication occurs most often in the thorax adjacent to the distal two thirds of the esophagus, but it may also occur in the lateral cervical area. Esophageal duplication cysts may be asymptomatic and discovered incidentally, or they may cause tracheal or esophageal compression. The epithelium is either stratified squamous or columnar; the latter is derived from persistent embryonic esophageal ciliated columnar epithelium. Distinction between esophageal and bronchogenic cysts may be difficult because they occur at similar locations in the mediastinum and show similar ciliated columnar epithelium. The diagnosis of esophageal cyst is made if a two-layered muscularis externa is present. A bronchial origin is favored if cartilage or respiratory glands are identified (e396). The generic designation of "foregut cyst" is used in cases in which the lining epithelium is primitive columnar without the distinguishing features cited.

Enteric Cyst of the Mediastinum

Mediastinal enteric (gastroenteric) cyst is distinct from the esophagus; however, because of its location, it may be confused with esophageal duplication cyst. Mediastinal enteric cyst is found in the right posterior mediastinum in a retrocardiac position, often extending into the right thorax. Vertebral anomalies, especially cervical hemivertebra, are associated in a high percentage of cases (e33,e36). A small number of enteric cysts extend through an intervertebral space into the spinal canal, in which case the designation of neurenteric cyst is given. Enteric cysts are often lined partially or completely by gastric mucosa, and some present with peptic ulceration, perforation, and hemorrhage. Small-intestinal mucosa and primitive columnar epithelial lining have also been described.

Esophageal Atresia and Tracheoesophageal Fistula

Esophageal atresia and tracheoesophageal fistula occur together in most cases (e24,e438). The dual anomalies, which occur approximately once in 3,000 births, result from faulty division of the foregut into tracheal and esophageal channels during the 1st month of embryonic life. Additional congenital anomalies (usually midline) occur in 50% of these infants, directly affecting the prognosis. Congenital heart disease, especially ventricular septal defect, patent ductus arteriosus, and tetralogy of Fallot, are seen in 30% of cases of esophageal atresia, and imperforate anus occurs in approximately 10%. In babies with multiple malformations, the VATER (vertebrae, anal, tracheoesophageal, radial, and renal anomalies) association or the VATERL (vertebrae, anal, tracheoesophageal, renal, and limb) association should be considered (e374). Approximately one-third of the infants with esophageal atresia are born prematurely, so that morbidity is further increased.

Variations in the anatomy of esophageal atresia and tracheoesophageal fistula are diagrammed in Figure 12-10 (see Chapter 12). Esophageal atresia without tracheoesophageal fistula occurs rarely, and tracheoesophageal fistula without esophageal atresia (H-type fistula) is even more unusual. The most common type is esophageal atresia with distal tracheoesophageal fistula, which accounts for 85% of the cases (Figure 14-5). The esophagus ends in a blind pouch in the upper chest, and the lower portion of the esophagus is connected to the trachea at or near the carina by a tracheoesophageal fistula less than 0.5 cm in diameter (Figure 12-10A). During breathing, air enters the stomach through the fistula, and as the stomach becomes distended, gastric secretions pass through the fistula into the lungs, causing pneumonia. The infant cannot swallow oral secretions or food; attempts at feeding produce regurgitation and aspiration. The diagnosis is suggested by the inability to pass a tube from the mouth to the stomach and is confirmed by plain x-ray films of the chest and abdomen. Treatment is surgical and consists of extrapleural transection of the fistula and anastomosis of the two ends of the esophagus.

Isolated esophageal atresia without an associated fistula, found in 7% to 8% of cases, is usually characterized by blind proximal and distal esophageal pouches, often separated by a wide gap. Multiple surgical procedures are usually required for repair.

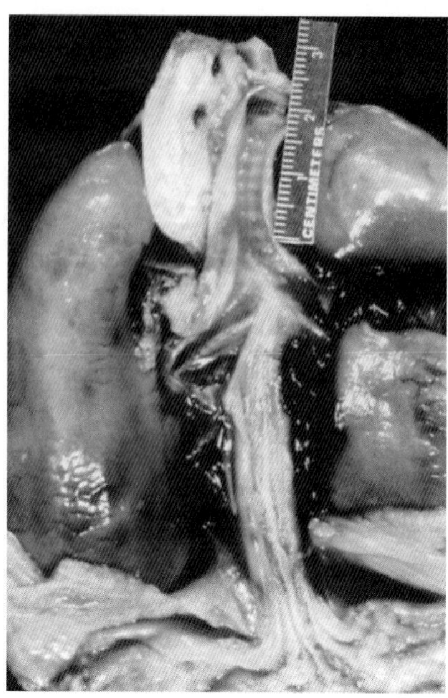

FIGURE 14-5 ■ Tracheoesophageal fistula at autopsy (posterior view of thoracic organ block). The blind esophageal pouch is at the upper left, and the tracheoesophageal fistula arises at the tracheal bifurcation.

In the relatively rare cases of isolated tracheoesophageal fistula without esophageal atresia (H-type fistula), the diagnosis is often delayed beyond the newborn period. Patients with this anomaly present with coughing or choking during feeding and with recurrent pneumonia. Histologic study of the tracheoesophageal fistula often reveals foci of primitive ciliated columnar epithelium, respiratory glands, and even cartilage. These tracheobronchial elements and abnormalities in smooth muscle may extend for some distance into the distal esophagus.

Esophageal Stenosis

In most cases, esophageal stenosis is an acquired lesion caused by gastroesophageal reflux with severe peptic esophagitis. However, rare forms of congenital esophageal stenosis have been described resulting from membranous mucosal rings and webs. Stenotic segments surrounded by respiratory epithelium, submucosal glands, and cartilage rings derived from remnants of the embryonic tracheoesophageal bud may occur rarely (e220). Sloughing of esophageal mucosa occurs in inherited epidermolysis bullosa, which is complicated by stenosis.

Acquired Diseases

Gastroesophageal Reflux and Reflux Esophagitis

Gastroesophageal reflux is common during the first few months of life, as evidenced by the frequent occurrence of effortless regurgitation at this age (e53,e205,e348).

It is considered a physiologic process secondary to immature esophageal peristaltic and lower esophageal sphincter function and gradually improves during the 1st year of life. If reflux is excessive during infancy or persists beyond that period, peptic esophagitis may ensue.

The symptoms of reflux esophagitis differ with the age of the patient. Infants show effortless regurgitation and sometimes forceful vomiting, excessive irritability, and failure to thrive as a consequence of caloric losses. Children present with vomiting and poorly characterized abdominal or chest pain. Patients of any age may exhibit gastrointestinal blood loss (from esophageal ulceration), failure to thrive, and recurrent pulmonary problems (e.g., asthma, pneumonia, and night cough). Most children with reflux esophagitis are otherwise normal, but certain groups of children are predisposed, including those with mental retardation, cystic fibrosis, and bronchopulmonary dysplasia, and those who have undergone repair of esophageal atresia and tracheoesophageal fistula in infancy (e53,e166,e218,e348). Esophageal pH monitoring, esophageal manometry, and barium esophagography may be used in patient evaluation. If a patient has signs of esophagitis, such as pain, gastrointestinal blood loss, or failure to thrive, esophagoscopy and esophageal biopsy are indicated. However, histologic changes are found in only 40% to 50% of symptomatic infants and children with clinical evidence of reflux esophagitis (e101,e501).

Histologic features in children with reflux esophagitis are similar to those widely described in adults with the same condition (e42,e89,e101,e154,e382,e421) (Figure 14-6). Diagnostic histologic findings include intraepithelial lymphocytes (IELs), neutrophils and eosinophils, basal cell hyperplasia (>15% to 20% of total epithelial thickness), papillary elongation (>50% to 66% of epithelial thickness), and dilated intraepithelial spaces (2,100). Basal cell hyperplasia and papillary elongation are the most sensitive histologic features of reflux, but unfortunately these features cannot be assessed accurately in poorly oriented specimens. They are also common in biopsies obtained from near the squamocolumnar junction (Z-line) in patients without reflux. Dilated intracellular spaces between the squamous cells (spongiosis) are also a sensitive marker of epithelial cell injury, usually best seen in the lower cell layers, and can be evaluated even in poorly oriented biopsies (110). Intraepithelial eosinophils and neutrophils are very specific features of esophagitis but are not sensitive indicators of reflux as they are usually present only at the more severe end of the spectrum, when erosions are evident endoscopically. Of course, eosinophils are also present in fungal and pill esophagitis and in eosinophilic esophagitis. There is considerable controversy regarding whether rare eosinophils are present in the esophageal squamous mucosa of normal individuals. A recent well-performed study that included 20 healthy adult controls with normal pH monitoring did find one to two eosinophils in two of them (110). Lymphocytes and Langerhans cells are normally present in the esophageal squamous mucosa, so the determination of an abnormal increase in these cells is subjective. Also, the presence of increased IELs alone is not diagnostic of esophagitis, since this finding has also been reported in patients with Crohn disease, celiac disease and other autoimmune disorders, and *H. pylori* infection (126). In a more recent study esophageal squamous intraepithelial lymphocytosis was not found to be associated with any particular pathologic condition, including reflux esophagitis (121).

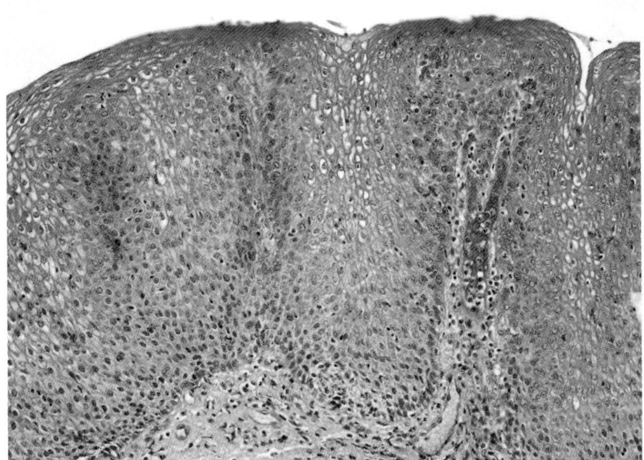

FIGURE 14-6 ▪ Reflux esophagitis. Note the presence of basal cell hyperplasia and lengthening of the papillae. There are also scattered intraepithelial eosinophils (Hematoxylin and eosin, 200×).

In otherwise healthy pediatric outpatients, occasional cases of infectious esophagitis, particularly herpes simplex esophagitis, present with signs and symptoms mimicking those of reflux esophagitis. Ingestion of caustic substances, Crohn disease, and dermatologic conditions, such as bullous pemphigoid and Stevens-Johnson syndrome, are rare possibilities, and other suggestive clinical findings are usually present. In children who are immunosuppressed or severely debilitated from another illness, infectious esophagitis is an important diagnostic consideration (Table 14-1).

Reflux esophagitis is managed with thickened, small feedings; maintenance of an upright posture after meals; and antacids, histamine H2-receptor antagonists (e.g., cimetidine and ranitidine), and proton pump inhibitors. In the few cases resistant to medical therapy, surgical fundoplication procedures are performed to increase the efficacy of the lower esophageal sphincter mechanism (e363). Sequelae of gastroesophageal reflux include ulcers (usually of the distal one third of the esophagus and often associated with blood loss), stricture, and Barrett esophagus.

Table 14-1 ▪ CAUSES OF ESOPHAGITIS IN CHILDREN
Reflux esophagitis
Eosinophilic esophagitis
Ingestion of drugs or caustic substances
Chemotherapy induced injury
Trauma (e.g., nasogastric tube)
Crohn disease
Dermatologic conditions
Graft-versus-host disease
Eosinophilic gastroenteritis
Infections (*Candida*, herpes simplex virus, and CMV)

Barrett Esophagus

Barrett esophagus, in which columnar epithelium replaces the normal squamous lining of the distal esophagus, is an acquired metaplastic condition caused by chronic gastroesophageal reflux. It is now established that even in children, Barrett esophagus is invariably found in association with severe reflux esophagitis; however, it is rare in children, occurring in only a small percentage who undergo biopsy for symptomatic gastroesophageal reflux (e96,e102,e201). Usually older children, not infants, are affected. Barrett esophagus cannot be predicted by the clinical presentation; the symptoms are those of the associated reflux esophagitis.

The changes in Barrett esophagus affect the lower portion of the esophagus (Figure 14-7A) and involvement may be either circumferential or patchy. The usual squamous lining is transformed to a columnar mucosa. Several types of columnar-lined mucosa have been described in Barrett esophagus (e354). These include intestinal type mucosa with absorptive cells and goblet cells (Figure 14-7B), gastric fundic type mucosa with parietal and chief cells, a junctional type resembling gastric cardia; and a mixed type with tall columnar surface cells and a mixture of fundic and mucous glands, but no goblet cells. In all types of Barrett mucosa, inflammation and glandular distortion and atrophy are often noted. The squamous mucosa proximal to the affected esophagus often shows changes of reflux esophagitis.

In the United States, a consensus panel of experts has required the presence of specialized columnar mucosa containing goblet cells in biopsies confirmed by the endoscopist to have been obtained from the tubular esophagus to make a diagnosis of Barrett esophagus (151). Thus, the location of the biopsy site in relation to the lower esophageal sphincter must be known by the pathologist before Barrett esophagus can be diagnosed. In Great Britain, columnar type mucosa without goblet cells is accepted as diagnostic of Barrett esophagus, provided the endoscopist is certain that the biopsies were obtained from the tubular esophagus and not the proximal stomach (20). However, because the endoscopic landmarks used to separate esophagus and stomach (primarily the upper extent of the gastric rugal folds) are not precise, particularly in the presence of a hiatal hernia, confusion between distal esophagus and gastric cardia is possible. The use of a CDX2 immunostain to confirm the presence of intestinal metaplasia even in the absence of goblet cells has been proposed but has not been widely adopted to date (118). In one study of pediatric Barrett esophagus CDX2 immunoreactivity was evident only when goblet cells were also present, and not in epithelium comprised entirely of gastric cardiac or cardio-oxyntic type epithelium (32).

Well-formed barrel-shaped goblet cells are usually easily recognizable with ordinary hematoxylin and eosin staining, but recognition can be enhanced and confirmed by staining with Alcian blue at pH 2.5, which imparts a blue color to

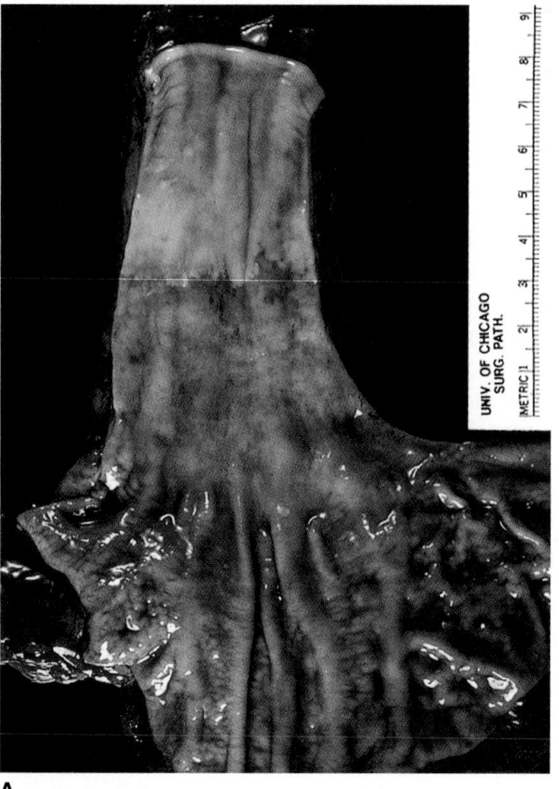

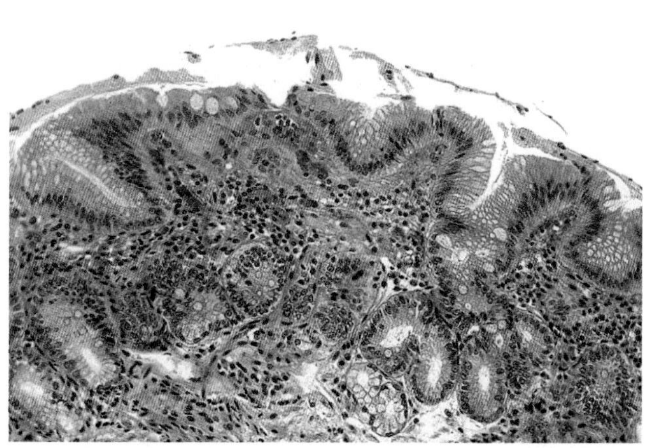

A B

FIGURE 14-7 ■ Barrett esophagus. **A:** Esophagectomy specimen exhibiting a 5-cm circumferential segment of Barrett mucosa. **B:** Barrett mucosa, characterized by specialized columnar mucosa with goblet cells (Hematoxylin and eosin, 200×).

intestinal-type acidic mucins (e173). This histologic type of Barrett mucosa has the potential to progress to dysplasia and, after many years, to adenocarcinoma in about 1% to 2% of cases (e191,e201,e382). Adenocarcinoma in Barrett esophagus in children is very rare but has been reported (e203,e209).

Eosinophilic Esophagitis

Recently, it was recognized that esophageal biopsies containing large numbers of intraepithelial eosinophils and exhibiting basal cell hyperplasia can represent an allergic reaction to dietary or inhaled allergens, rather than representing severe gastroesophageal reflux disease (88) (e488). This disorder, termed eosinophilic esophagitis, often presents in childhood, although diagnosis in adults is also possible (81). Children are usually unable to distinguish between heartburn due to reflux and dysphagia due to eosinophilic esophagitis. In young children presenting symptoms include difficulty feeding, prolonged irritability and crying, failure to thrive, and growth delay. Characteristic endoscopic findings include wrinkled or thickened esophageal squamous mucosa, sometimes with circumferential rings, linear furrows, or tiny vesicles. Although this disorder has only recently been recognized, retrospective studies have shown that in the past cases were interpreted as severe reflux esophagitis. Treatment with an elimination diet or topical or oral steroids is usually effective, but esophageal stricture can develop in refractory cases (30).

Endoscopic biopsies of the esophagus typically reveal a heavy but patchy infiltrate of eosinophils, including clusters of eosinophils (microabscesses), often near the luminal surface (Figure 14-8A to C). Basal cell hyperplasia is usually quite prominent. Originally a cutoff of 24 eosinophils per high power field was suggested as useful in distinguishing between eosinophilic esophagitis and reflux esophagitis, since in most cases of reflux esophagitis the density of intramucosal eosinophils is less than seven per high power field. More recently an expert panel suggested that 15 eosinophils in any single high power field (400×) should be regarded as consistent with eosinophilic esophagitis in the proper clinical context (46). However, it is likely that in some patients even fewer eosinophils are present, or at least that limited sampling will not identify areas of high eosinophil density. A trial of proton pump inhibitors as treatment for presumptive reflux esophagitis before endoscopy is usual clinical practice, something the surgical pathologist should keep in mind when evaluating esophageal biopsies. It must also be recognized that patients may have both gastroesophageal reflux and eosinophilic esophagitis. In fact, reflux could conceivably predispose to the development of eosinophilic esophagitis, and the presence of eosinophilic esophagitis may make the mucosa more susceptible to reflux injury (145).

The presence of inflammatory changes that are equally severe in biopsies from the midesophagus and distal

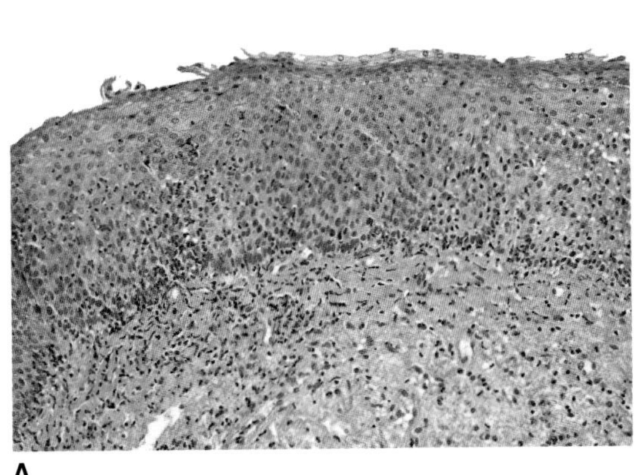

A

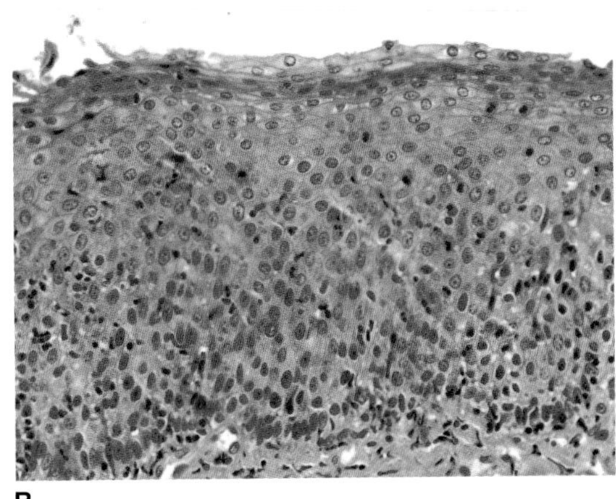

B

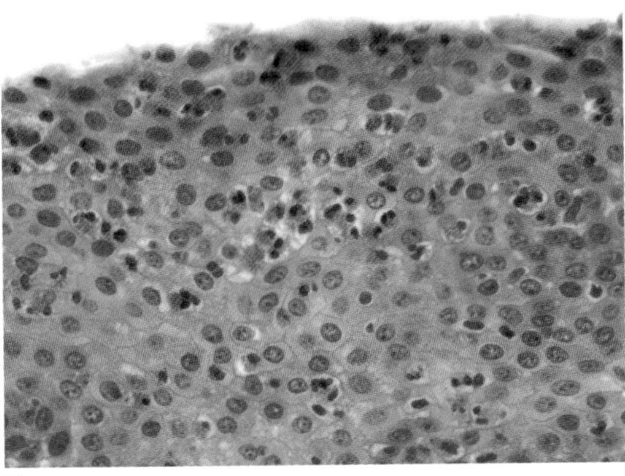

C

FIGURE 14-8■Eosinophilic esophagitis. **A:** Low power showing basal cell hyperplasia. Note the fibrosis of the subepithelial stroma. **B:** There are more than 40 eosinophils per high power field. **C:** An eosinophilic microabscess in the superficial epithelium (Hematoxylin and eosin, **A:** 100×, **B:** 200×, **C:** 400×).

esophagus is a useful finding in making the diagnosis of eosinophilic esophagitis (since reflux changes are typically more severe distally than proximally). The presence of admixed neutrophils, on the other hand, favors the presence of reflux esophagitis, since in general only eosinophils are present in eosinophilic esophagitis unless ulceration has occurred. Biopsies of the gastric cardia can also be useful in distinguishing between reflux esophagitis and eosinophilic esophagitis. In reflux esophagitis the cardia is uniformly inflamed (i.e., "carditis"), while in eosinophilic esophagitis the cardia is typically not inflamed. The presence or absence of increased eosinophils in any gastric or duodenal biopsies obtained during the endoscopy should also be mentioned in the surgical pathology report, to address the possibility of a more generalized eosinophilic gastrointestinal disorder.

In some cases it is not possible to make a firm histologic distinction between eosinophilic esophagitis and severe reflux esophagitis. Correlation with the clinical history and the endoscopic appearance is often sufficient to arrive at the proper diagnosis, but 24-hour esophageal pH monitoring may be necessary in some patients.

Infectious Esophagitis

Infectious esophagitis is rare except in hospitalized, immunosuppressed, and debilitated children, who are at significant risk for the development of esophagitis in association with infection by Candida species, herpes simplex virus, and cytomegalovirus (CMV). Bacterial infection is a practical consideration only as a superinfection.

Herpes Simplex Esophagitis

Herpes esophagitis presents as odynophagia and is often accompanied by gingivostomatitis (e313,e333). Multiple small, discrete ulcers separated by normal mucosa are distributed throughout the esophagus (Figure 14-9A). In severe cases, confluent ulceration can occur. Microscopically, severe necrotizing esophagitis, abundant neutrophils, and ulceration are found. Epithelial cells at ulcer margins often demonstrate discrete eosinophilic intranuclear inclusions (Cowdry type A) or ground-glass intranuclear inclusions (Cowdry type B) (Figure 14-9B,C). Only the squamous cell can be infected by the herpes simplex virus; so if the biopsy consists only of granulation tissue and necrotic debris, no comment can

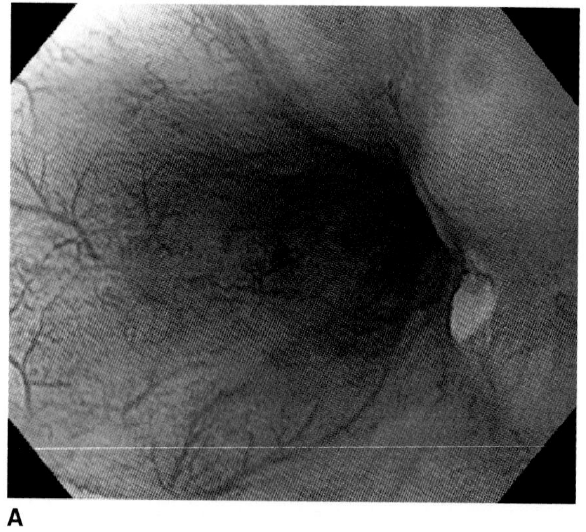

A

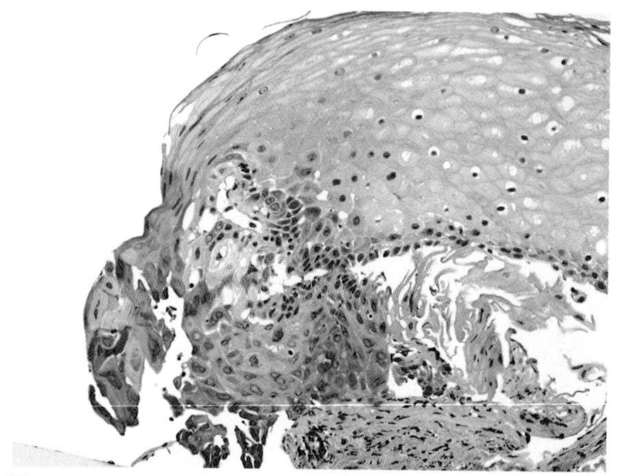

B

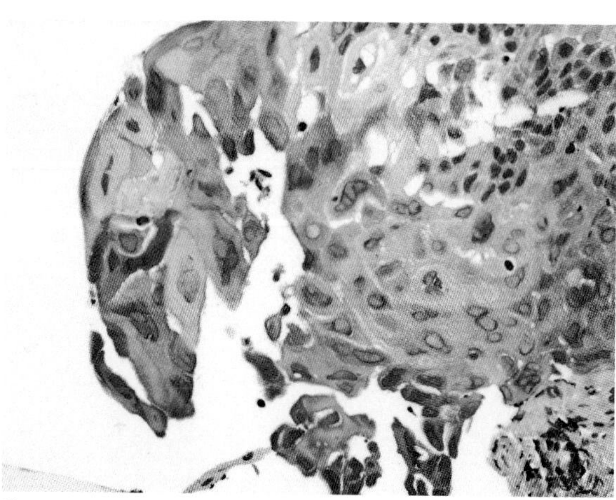

C

FIGURE 14-9 ■ Herpes simplex virus esophagitis. **A:** Endoscopic appearance of a midesophageal ulcer. **B:** Viral inclusions in squamous epithelium at the edge of the ulcer 200×. **C:** High power to demonstrate typical intranuclear inclusions and multinucleated cells 400×.

be made regarding the presence or absence of this infection. Although it occurs most often in immunosuppressed persons, herpetic esophagitis may occasionally be found in otherwise normal children.

Candida Esophagitis

Immunosuppression, premature birth, cancer chemotherapy, and AIDS are the most significant risk factors for the development of esophageal candidiasis in infants and children (e256,e409). Esophageal involvement is common in children with mucocutaneous candidiasis. In debilitated patients, esophageal infection may lead to systemic candidiasis. The gross appearance is usually a combination of white plaques and ulcerations. Histologically, the plaques consist of masses of pseudohyphae and yeast forms admixed with inflammatory debris and fibrin (eFigure 14-2A to C).

Cytomegalovirus Esophagitis

CMV esophagitis is uncommon and limited to immunosuppressed persons. It rarely occurs alone; it is usually part of a systemic CMV infection or an infection involving the whole gastrointestinal tract. In contrast to herpes simplex esophagitis, CMV cannot infect squamous epithelial cells; so if the biopsy consists only of squamous epithelium, no comment can be made regarding the presence or absence of this infection.

DISORDERS OF THE STOMACH

Congenital Anomalies

Hypertrophic Pyloric Stenosis

Although pyloric stenosis is diagnosed as early as 2 weeks of age, it is not a congenital anomaly in the usual sense because it has rarely been demonstrated at birth (e437). Pyloric stenosis is a common condition, seen in 1 of 200 infant boys. The male-to-female ratio is 5:1 or greater, and white, firstborn boys are at greatest risk. A definite familial incidence has been noted, but there is no definite inheritance pattern. Neurons supplying the circular muscle layer of the pylorus lack activity of the enzyme nitric oxide synthase (e476). The circular muscle layer undergoes hypertrophy and elongation, and gastric outlet obstruction ensues. Progressive nonbilious vomiting, the primary manifestation, commences at 2 to 6 weeks of age in an otherwise healthy infant. The diagnosis is suggested when the hypertrophic pyloric muscle mass, approximately the size of an olive, is palpated in the right upper quadrant after a feeding. Abdominal x-ray films show marked gaseous distension of the stomach, and barium studies demonstrate a narrow and elongated pyloric channel ("string sign"). Treatment is surgical. At operation, the hypertrophic pyloric muscle appears as an elongated sphere ("olive"), approximately 2.5 cm long and 1.5 cm in diameter. A longitudinal surgical incision of the hypertrophic muscle down to the submucosa (pyloromyotomy) immediately and efficaciously relieves the obstruction. Occasional postmortem observations indicate that the circular layer of muscularis propria is hypertrophic, hyperplastic, and disorganized in appearance. The outer, longitudinal muscle layer is attenuated and of variable thickness. The cause of infantile hypertrophic pyloric stenosis is unknown.

Antral Web

A very unusual cause of gastric outlet obstruction in young infants is an antral web (antral diaphragm) of fibrous tissue and gastric mucosa obstructing the antrum a few centimeters proximal to the pylorus (e34). A small, central aperture, usually no more than several millimeters in diameter, permits passage of some stomach contents; variability in the size of the opening explains the variability in age at presentation. The diagnosis is made by barium studies, and endoscopy is often difficult.

Duplication

Gastric duplication presents as a cystic mass on the greater curvature or at the pylorus and may present with bleeding, rupture, or obstruction. The pathologic features are similar to those of the more commonly encountered small-intestinal duplication. The mucosa of a gastric duplication resembles stomach mucosa most of the time, but primitive or simplified gut epithelium or intestinal mucosa is also encountered.

Pancreatic Heterotopia

An island of ectopic pancreas may occur as an intramural nodule or mass on the greater curvature near the antrum (e443). It is often detected incidentally on imaging studies or at autopsy. A central depression may be seen, corresponding to the opening of the pancreatic duct draining the heterotopic tissue. Occasionally, ulceration develops in the overlying mucosa and causes epigastric pain.

Acquired Diseases

Spontaneous Gastric Perforation in the Neonate

Spontaneous perforation of the body of the stomach occasionally develops in premature neonates, especially those under intensive care (e221). The cause of the perforation is inapparent, although it often occurs in an area of hemorrhagic or coagulative necrosis and may be ischemic or traumatic in origin. The usual presentation is sudden abdominal distension and pneumoperitoneum.

Gastritis

A list of the types of gastritis in children is much shorter than a similar list in adults because of the absence of many of the atrophic, metaplastic, and dysplastic conditions of the adult stomach. However, it is clear that gastritis occurs with considerable frequency in children and adolescents. Numerous classification schemes exist (e119), but for practical purposes, gastritis is categorized by etiology if apparent.

Hemorrhagic and Erosive Gastritis

The etiology of acute hemorrhagic gastritis is multifactorial, with ischemia, stress, and drug therapy playing contributory roles. Drugs known to damage the gastric mucosa include aspirin, corticosteroids, alcohol, and nonsteroidal anti-inflammatory drugs (NSAIDs), such as indomethacin. The ingestion of corrosive substances also causes a similar picture. At endoscopy, a diffusely injected and edematous mucosa, often with petechial hemorrhages and small erosions, is seen. In severe cases, which usually occur in very ill children hospitalized for sepsis, hemorrhagic shock, major surgery, burns, central nervous system disorders, or other severe illness, the changes are most severe in the gastric body and fundus.

Biopsies are usually not obtained in these severely ill patients, and therefore this condition is usually seen at the time of autopsy. The histologic changes essentially represent a chemical injury to the gastric mucosal caused by reduced host defense against the injurious action of gastric acid and digestive enzymes. Hemorrhage and mucosal edema dominate the histologic picture. Significant inflammation is not present except directly adjacent to areas of ulceration (eFigure 14-3A,B).

Helicobacter pylori Gastritis

Since the early 1980s, it has been recognized that diffuse antral gastritis is caused by infection with *H. pylori*, a small Gram-negative bacillus (e124,e202,e248,e300,e506). This organism, which is the pathogen responsible for the associated symptoms and pathologic changes, is not an opportunist or a commensal. Children with *H. pylori* infection usually present with nausea, vomiting, and epigastric pain. Endoscopy shows erythema, particularly in the antrum, and in the more severe cases erosion, antral nodularity, and thickened gastric folds. However, there is not a good correlation between the endoscopic and histologic findings of gastritis. That is, in many cases where endoscopic findings of gastric mucosal erythema, granularity, or erosion are described, biopsies are entirely unremarkable. Conversely, in many cases where the gastric mucosa is described as endoscopically normal, gastritis is actually evident histologically.

Currently, endoscopy and biopsy are the most widely used methods for the diagnosis of *H. pylori* infection. Culturing the endoscopy specimen directly for *H. pylori* is difficult and not performed routinely. A commercial test is available in which the presence of the organism in a fresh biopsy specimen causes a change in the color of a solution. This reaction is based on the production of urease enzyme by the organism. A number of commercially available enzyme-linked immunosorbent assay (ELISA) kits are also available for serologic testing, but they lack the sensitivity and specificity of biopsy. On biopsy, the organisms are most reliably found in the antrum, although the fundus and cardia of the stomach may also be affected. The bacilli can be seen faintly on ordinary preparations stained with hematoxylin and eosin, but they are more easily seen with Giemsa, Genta (e160), Warthin-Starry, or immunoperoxidase staining; they appear as small curved or slightly twisted rods, 4 to 5 μm in length, within the mucous coat overlying the surface or superficial foveolar epithelium (Figure 14-10). Organisms are usually most easily found in areas of active inflammation.

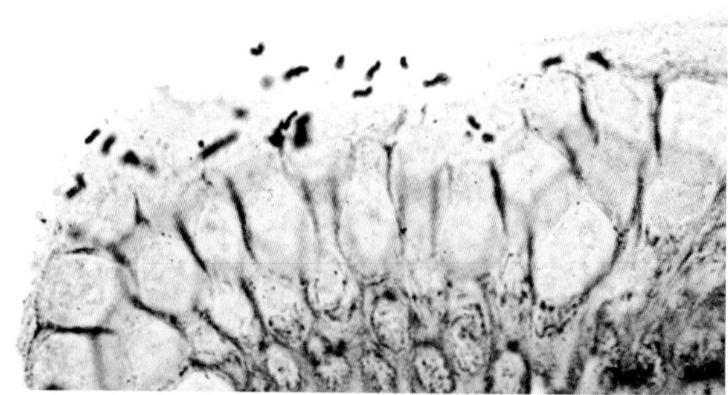

FIGURE 14-10 ▪ *Helicobacter pylori* organisms over antral mucosa (Warthin-Starry stain, 400×).

The antral mucosa exhibits a diffuse superficial infiltrate composed primarily of plasma cells and lymphocytes. Active foci of neutrophilic infiltration may be seen in the lamina propria or in glandular or surface epithelium. Although lymphoid aggregates are normal in the gastric mucosa, the presence of lymphoid follicles with germinal centers is highly suggestive of past or current *H. pylori* infection (e159). In patients on a proton pump inhibitor for dyspepsia or symptoms of gastroesophageal reflux, the *H. pylori* organism may migrate to cause active gastritis of the gastric body mucosa, resulting in an inactive appearance of the antral gastritis.

Treatment of *H. pylori* with antibiotics results in prompt disappearance of the organisms and the neutrophilic component of the mucosal inflammatory cell infiltrates. By contrast, it may take many months for the lymphocytic and plasma cell infiltrates to disappear. Biopsies obtained during this period may be diagnosed as inactive gastritis. The diagnosis of inactive gastritis can be difficult, as there are a small number of lamina propria lymphocytes and plasma cells in the gastric mucosa normally. As a general rule of thumb, when the density of plasma cells is such that they are clustered and touching each other, this can be regarded as indicative of inactive gastritis. In some patients with inactive antral gastritis there may not be an antecedent diagnosis of *H. pylori* gastritis, as the infection may have been treated incidentally during antibiotic treatment of infection elsewhere (e.g., otitis media).

Even though *H. pylori* causes duodenal ulcers, the organism is not found in duodenal mucosa except in instances of gastric metaplasia of the duodenum, which is rare in children. The mechanism of duodenal ulcer formation in *H. pylori* infection is thought to involve increased acid secretion as a response to the gastric infection, as well as direct damage by the organism in the areas of duodenal gastric foveolar metaplasia.

In addition to the immediate morbidity of gastritis and ulcer disease in children and adults, infection with *H. pylori* is known to carry a risk for future adenocarcinoma of the stomach (e16,e351) and gastric lymphoma arising in mucosa-associated lymphoid tissue (MALT) (e352). H. pylori infection can be difficult to eradicate. Bismuth preparations and multiple antibiotic regimens are effective, but relapses are common.

The histologic differential diagnosis of *H. pylori* gastritis includes a small number of unusual conditions of the stomach with distinctive clinical and histologic findings, including involvement by eosinophilic gastroenteritis, Crohn disease (e505), or, less frequently, Langerhans cell histiocytosis (e182,e243), chronic granulomatous disease (e9,e117), and Henoch-Schönlein purpura (e460). Lymphocytic gastritis, characterized by increased lymphocytes in the gastric foveolar and glandular epithelium, can occur in patients with celiac disease and has also been reported as a consequence of *H. pylori* infection. An increase in IELs above 1 per 25 gastric foveolar or glandular epithelial cells is generally regarded as abnormal and diagnostic of lymphocytic gastritis. (eFigure 14-4A to C) (e6,e112,e503).

Helicobacter heilmannii (Gastrospirillum hominis) Gastritis

Helicobacter heilmannii infection of the stomach is much more rare and not as serious or chronic a disease as *H. pylori* gastritis. The clinical presentation and histologic picture are similar except that *H. heilmannii* is a much larger organism than *H. pylori*, much more obviously spiraled, and more readily seen on slides stained with hematoxylin and eosin (Figure 14-11). It also resides on the gastric epithelial surface and does not invade tissue (e3,e111,e343).

Peptic Ulcer Disease

The widespread use of fiberoptic endoscopy has led to the realization that ulcer disease in children is not as rare as was formerly thought (e127,e224). Peptic ulcers are of two types: acute (stress) and chronic. Nearly all peptic ulcers occur in the stomach and duodenum, but they may occur in any location where acid- and pepsin-secreting gastric mucosa is found, including Meckel diverticulum.

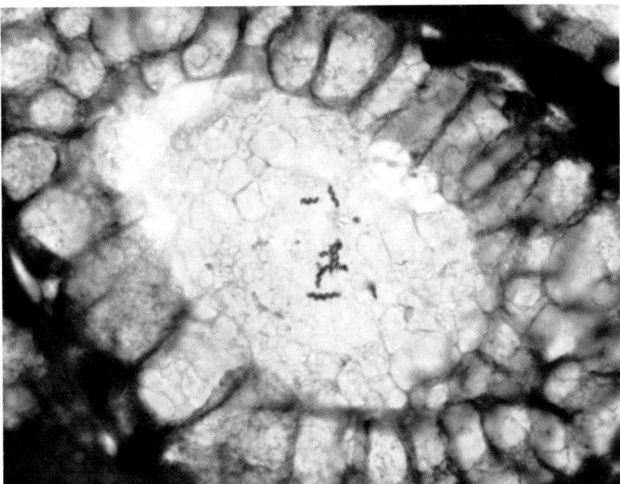

FIGURE 14-11 ■ *Helicobacter heilmannii* organisms over antral mucosa (Giemsa stain, 1,000×).

Nearly all cases of childhood and adult chronic ulcers have been shown to be caused by infection with *H. pylori* in the stomach (e15,e202,e224,e248,e300,e506). Chronic (or primary) peptic ulceration in children is the same acid-peptic disease that is so common in adults. This condition can develop in children as young as 4 or 5 years old, although it is more common in preadolescents and adolescents of either sex. It is most common in adolescent boys. Duodenal ulcer is much more common than gastric ulcer. Chronic abdominal pain is the most frequent presenting symptom. More than 50% of the patients have hematemesis, melena, or occult bleeding at the time of presentation. At endoscopy, chronic peptic ulcers are usually round to oval, less than 2 cm in diameter, well delineated from the surrounding mucosa by sharp margins, and covered by exudate at the base.

Microscopically, granulation and scar tissue form the ulcer base, which often extends deep into the muscularis propria. The stomach invariably shows active antral gastritis, and *H. pylori* is usually readily identified. If the ulcer is duodenal, active duodenitis is usually present in surrounding, nonulcerated mucosa. Chronic peptic ulcers usually heal with a medical regimen. Zollinger-Ellison syndrome, characterized by peptic ulceration resistant to therapy, giant gastric rugal folds, and increased serum levels of gastrin, is very rare in children; fewer than 30 cases have been reported in this age group. Ulceration due to mucosal injury caused by NSAIDs or other medications is also a diagnostic consideration in older children.

Ménétrier Disease

Ménétrier disease is found primarily in adults, but cases in children have been described (e79,e80,e371). The disease appears similar symptomatically and pathologically, but the clinical course and etiology are different. In adults, the cause is unknown and the disease is usually severe and often requires gastrectomy. Childhood cases are often self-limited, and most are caused by CMV infection. Classic Ménétrier disease presents with epigastric or abdominal pain, weight loss, and peripheral edema. The edema is caused by protein loss in the stomach with resultant hypoalbuminemia.

Radiographs and endoscopic examination reveal prominent or "giant" gastric folds of the corpus; the antrum is usually spared. Histologic features include mucous cell hyperplasia, pronounced elongation and tortuosity of the usually short gastric pits (foveolae), glandular atrophy, and reversal of the usual pit-to-gland ratio. Cysts lined by superficial mucous cells are found deep in the mucosa. Inflammation is more prominent in children than in adults, reflecting the infectious etiology in most children. CMV inclusions are often evident in biopsy material in children. If they are not seen, polymerase chain reaction testing may be positive for CMV (e80,e371). Not all pediatric cases of Ménétrier disease are caused by CMV. Formula protein intolerance has been suggested as an alternate cause in young infants (e145).

Ménétrier disease is difficult to diagnose in superficial mucosal biopsy specimens. The differential diagnosis includes other causes of large gastric folds: *H. pylori* gastritis, peptic ulcers, Crohn disease, eosinophilic gastroenteritis, and gastric lymphoma (e19). Foveolar hyperplasia of the antrum in neonates may be caused by prostaglandin therapy administered to maintain patency of the ductus arteriosus in certain forms of congenital heart disease (e356). Usually, the clinical setting, antral location, and presence of hypoalbuminemia make it possible to distinguish this group of neonates from those with Ménétrier disease.

Eosinophilic Gastroenteritis

Eosinophilic gastroenteritis can occur at any age but is rare in infants and children. It is characterized by striking eosinophilic infiltration of any part of the gastrointestinal wall (e44,e171,e278,e425,e453,e465,e495). A poorly understood allergic reaction is thought to be responsible for the disease because most patients have an allergic history and increased serum IgE levels. However, specific allergens have not been implicated in every case, and patients do not respond to food elimination diets. Symptoms vary depending on which part of the gastrointestinal tract is affected and on whether the disease is mucosal or transmural. The gastric antrum and proximal small intestine are affected in most cases; isolated small intestinal, colonic, or esophageal involvement accounts for the remainder. In the transmural form of the disease, submucosal edema and eosinophilic infiltration compromise the lumen and obstruct the intestine or gastric outflow tract. Abdominal pain, vomiting, and weight loss are frequently the presenting complaints in this form (e453). Disease limited to the mucosa may have a more insidious onset. Malabsorption and weight loss are found with small-intestinal mucosal disease. Radiologic studies are often helpful in the diagnosis by demonstrating either antral narrowing with a "mass" of inflammation and edema, or nodularity and thickening of the small-intestinal wall.

Histologically, the mucosal form of the disease is characterized by prominent and diffuse inflammatory infiltration in the lamina propria, with eosinophils accounting for the majority of the inflammatory cells. Eosinophils infiltrate and damage to the surface and glandular epithelium, and eosinophilic glandular abscesses are occasionally found. Infiltration of the muscularis mucosae is also a useful feature indicating true pathology (Figure 14-12A,B). The presence of increased numbers of eosinophils in the lamina propria alone is insufficient to make the diagnosis of eosinophilic gastroenteritis because the same phenomenon may occur in Crohn disease or infection, as a drug response, or as a normal finding in some persons. Normal mucosal architecture is preserved; ulceration is unusual. In transmural forms of the disease, eosinophil infiltration is often maximal in the submucosa, with lesser numbers seen in the muscularis externa and serosa. Rarely, eosinophilic ascites and eosinophilic infiltration of regional lymph nodes are found. Most patients with eosinophilic gastroenteritis have a chronic waxing and waning of symptoms. Steroids are often necessary to control the symptoms. Because the disease is quite patchy and may not affect the mucosa, full-thickness biopsy is sometimes necessary for diagnosis.

Crohn Disease of the Stomach

Involvement of the stomach by Crohn disease usually occurs in association with disease in the more usual locations—the distal ileum and colon (e192,e280,e302,e338,e392,e400, e505). On occasion, the initial presentation of Crohn disease

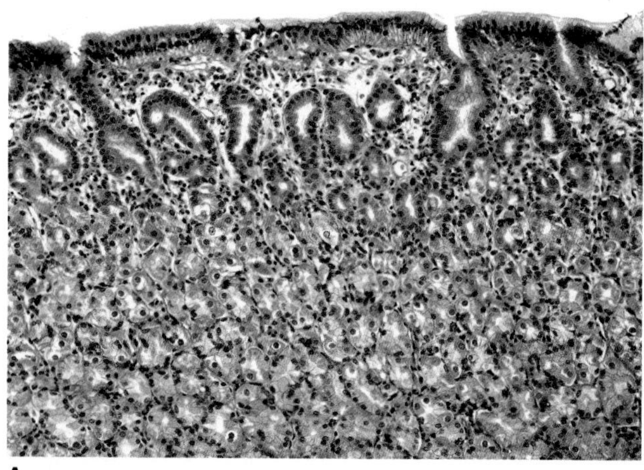

A

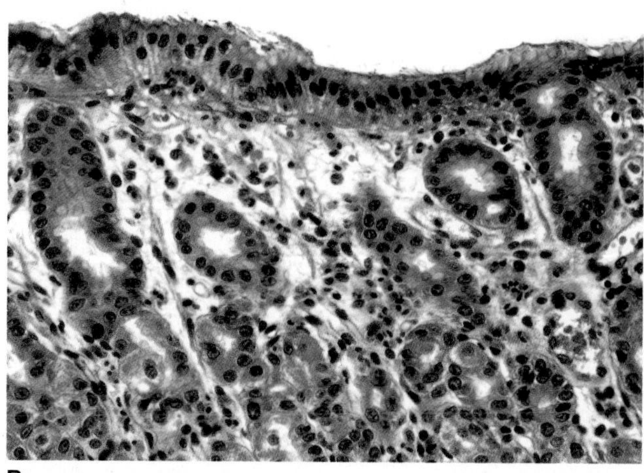

B

FIGURE 14-12 ■ Eosinophilic gastritis. **A:** A pure infiltrate of abundant eosinophils 200×. **B:** Eosinophils infiltrate the surface epithelium 400×.

is as a gastroduodenal process. In such cases, the antrum is usually involved, often in continuity with the proximal duodenum. Obstruction of the gastric outlet is a feature shared with eosinophilic gastroenteritis and some cases of *H. pylori* gastritis. The histology of gastric Crohn disease is similar to that in other sites. Particularly suggestive of gastroduodenal Crohn disease is the combination of distinctly focal acute inflammation causing destruction of glandular epithelium plus spotty chronic inflammation similar to the characteristic focal involvement of the distal gastrointestinal tract in Crohn disease. This focally enhanced pattern of active gastritis in Crohn disease is usually distinct from the more diffuse, superficial and plasma cell predominant pattern of gastritis due to *H. pylori* infection (e338,e505). The presence of granulomas is very helpful in addition to these nonspecific inflammatory features.

Granulomatous Gastritis

Granulomatous gastritis not associated with Crohn disease has rarely been described in adults. Tuberculosis, fungal infections, chronic granulomatous disease (e117), and sarcoidosis are other rare causes of gastric granulomas (e131). In biopsy specimens, most granulomas associated with chronic inflammation in the stomach of a child or adolescent prove to be Crohn disease.

Polyps and Tumors of the Stomach

Gastric polyps are rare in children. Juvenile polyps and Peutz-Jeghers polyps may occur in the stomach as part of a generalized polyposis syndrome. Gastric hyperplastic polyps are rare in children but can occur in the setting of *H. pylori* gastritis. Fundic gland polyps are a more common clinically insignificant consequence of chronic administration of proton pump inhibitors used to treat gastroesophageal reflux disease and dyspepsia (72,116). They are usually small and often multiple and are restricted to the oxyntic mucosa of the proximal stomach. Histologically they can be difficult to distinguish from normal gastric fundic mucosa as the histological features can be subtle, despite the endoscopic appearance of a polypoid lesion. The diagnostic histologic features include dilatation of the fundic glands and parietal cells with cytoplasmic protrusions extending into the glandular lumina. Cytoplasmic vacuolization of parietal cells is also common. The complete absence of lamina propria inflammation and edema is a striking feature of these polyps (eFigure 14-5). The surrounding flat fundic mucosa often exhibits histologic features similar to but not as pronounced as those evident in the polyps. Fundic gland polyps also develop commonly in patients with familial polyposis coli. Thus, if a fundic gland polyp is identified in a young patient not taking a proton pump inhibitor, colonoscopy to exclude colonic polyposis may be indicated. Dysplasia does occur in fundic gland polyps associated with familial polyposis coli but is exceedingly rare in the sporadic setting (142). For this reason it is not necessary to remove multiple sporadic fundic gland polyps.

Gastric teratomas are large, bulky multicystic masses that project into the gastric lumen or outward into the peritoneal space (35). Heterotopic pancreatic tissue should be considered in the differential diagnosis of gastric tumors. This is usually a sessile mass in the antrum and easily recognized histologically as acinar and endocrine pancreas (e443). The term adenomyoma has been applied to a variant characterized by a predominance of pancreatic duct structures interlaced with smooth muscle bundles but without pancreatic parenchyma (e157).

Malignant tumors of the stomach are quite rare in children. MALT lymphomas associated with *H. pylori* infection and Burkitt lymphomas are the most common types of lymphoma reported (35) (e53). Adenocarcinoma of the stomach is distinctly rare but has been reported in otherwise normal children (35) (e82,e294,e444). It is also known to occur in ataxia-telangiectasia and other primary immunodeficiency disorders (e190). Rare examples of inflammatory myofibroblastic tumor (e84) and rhabdomyosarcoma have also been reported (35) (e444).

Gastrointestinal Stromal Tumors

Gastrointestinal stromal tumors present occasionally in children, either as sporadic tumors or in the setting of a syndrome. The vast majority of, but not all, gastrointestinal stromal tumors in children occur in the stomach. Iron deficiency anemia is the most common presenting symptom in sporadic cases, while abdominal pain, a palpable mass, or vomiting occurs rarely (77). Carney triad is used to describe patients with paragangliomas, pulmonary chondromas, and gastric gastrointestinal stromal tumors (e69). About 85% of patients with Carney triad are female, and the gastrointestinal stromal tumors are often multifocal, which is unusual for sporadic tumors. Despite extensive molecular analysis, a specific underlying genetic defect has not been identified in patients with Carney triad (144). Carney-Stratakis syndrome designates a separate group of patients with gastric gastrointestinal stromal tumors and paragangliomas but no pulmonary chondromas. In these patients, autosomal dominant transmission has been demonstrated and germline mutations in any of three mitochondrial complex II succinate dehydrogenase (SDH) enzyme subunits (SDHB, SDHC or SDHD) have been documented (144). Gastrointestinal stromal tumors can also develop in individuals with neurofibromatosis type 1, although usually not in childhood. Lastly, individuals with germline mutations in the KIT or PDGFRA genes are at risk for the development of gastrointestinal stromal tumors, although again the tumors usually occur outside of the pediatric age range (114).

Gastrointestinal stromal tumors are presumed to develop from the interstitial cells of Cajal, which are thought to represent the pacemaker cells throughout the gastrointestinal tract. These cells are normally located within the myenteric plexus and the muscularis propria and have an important role in the regulation of peristalsis. A gain of function mutation in either the c-kit or platelet-derived growth factor receptor A gene can be detected in about 85% of gastrointestinal stromal tumors in adults (92). By contrast, mutations in these two genes are rare in pediatric tumors, with reported rates from 0% to 10%. Thus, the molecular pathogenesis of pediatric gastrointestinal stromal tumor is distinct from the adult counterparts, and the underlying mechanisms are currently undefined (1,114).

Pediatric gastrointestinal stromal tumors can be of spindle cell or epithelioid morphology, and mixed forms are also common. Among sporadic tumors, epithelioid tumors are more common overall, but spindle cell morphology is more common in boys (154). The epithelioid tumors are composed of round to polygonal cells, which may have little or abundant cytoplasm. Cytoplasmic vacuolization is common in these tumors and sometimes can be so prominent as to produce a signet-ring cell-like appearance (Figure 14-13A,B). The vacuoles do not stain for mucosubstances, glycogen, or fat and appear to represent an artifact of formalin fixation. The spindle cell variant of the tumor resembles smooth muscle tumors, but the cells are usually not as long and slender. Areas of hyaline fibrosis are common in both spindle cell and epithelioid variants of the tumor.

The diagnosis of gastrointestinal stromal tumor is confirmed by immunohistologic detection of cytoplasmic reactivity in tumor cells with the c-kit antibody. Even in pediatric tumors where 10% or less of the tumors have mutations in either the c-kit or PDGFRA genes, most of the tumors still express c-kit by immunohistochemistry. In adults immunohistologic detection utilizing a recently developed antibody designated DOG1 has been reported as highly sensitive and specific for the diagnosis of gastrointestinal stromal tumors, including those that are nonreactive with the c-kit antibody (104,154). The antigen detected by the DOG1 antibody is uniformly present in Cajal cells throughout the gastrointestinal tract, but not in mast cells, unlike the c-kit protein (104). In one study 9 of 11 pediatric gastrointestinal stromal tumors were reactive with the DOG1 antibody (91).

Various schemes have been utilized to stratify the risk of prognosis of gastrointestinal stromal tumors (76). Most systems, including a consensus scheme developed under the auspices of the National Institutes of Health, rely primarily on tumor size and mitotic rate (mitotic figures per 50 high power fields) (44). However, it has been known for some time that the site of tumor origin also has an important influence of the risk of poor outcome. Therefore, tumor site has been incorporated into several subsequent iterations of risk assessment schemes proposed by various groups (41,49,76). In addition, tumor rupture appears to be an important risk factor for tumor spread (68). These schemes have not been applied specifically to pediatric gastrointestinal tumors. Retrospective data suggests that the prognosis of these tumors in children is more difficult to predict (1,114).

DISORDERS OF THE SMALL AND LARGE INTESTINE

Congenital Abnormalities

Omphalocele

Omphalocele (exomphalos) is a developmental defect of the anterior abdominal wall in which the abdominal musculature, fascia, and skin are absent in the midline at the point of insertion of the umbilical cord (e301,e510). Abdominal organs extrude anteriorly through the defect and are covered by a saclike membrane consisting of amnion externally and parietal peritoneum internally (Figure 14-14). Omphalocele results from failure of the intestine to return to the body cavity after its normal herniation into the umbilical stalk during

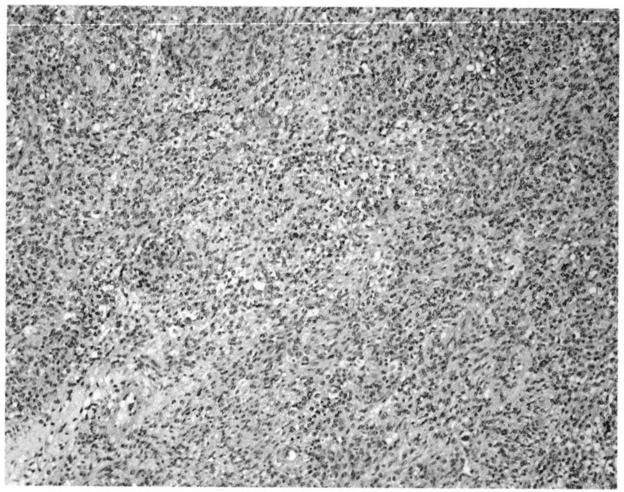
A

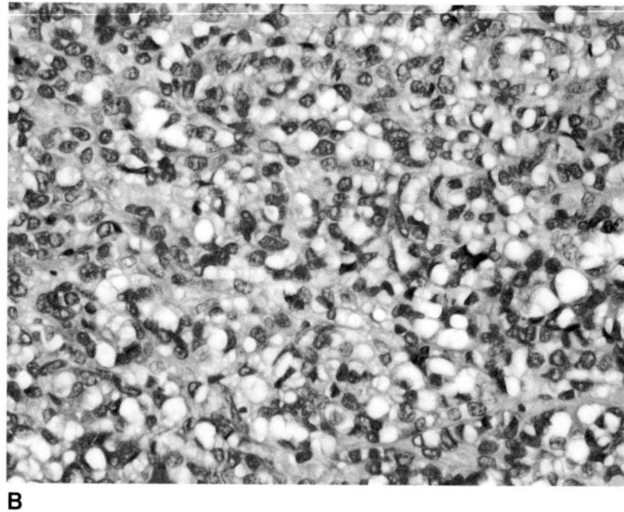
B

FIGURE 14-13 ■ Gastric gastrointestinal stromal tumor. **A:** This example demonstrates epithelioid histology, which is more common in the pediatric age group 100×. **B:** Cytoplasmic vacuoles are sometimes prominent, as seen here 200×.

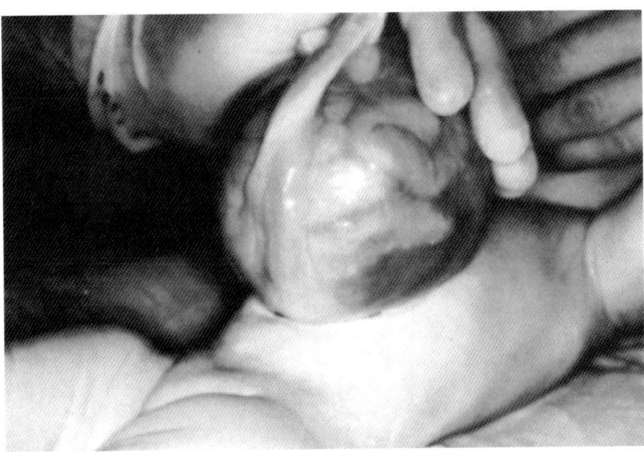

FIGURE 14-14 ▪ Omphalocele. A translucent membrane covers the abdominal organs, which are protruding through an abdominal wall defect in this newborn. Note the insertion of the umbilicus into the center of the omphalocele sac. (Courtesy of Robert J Izant Jr, M.D., Case Western Reserve University, Cleveland, Ohio.)

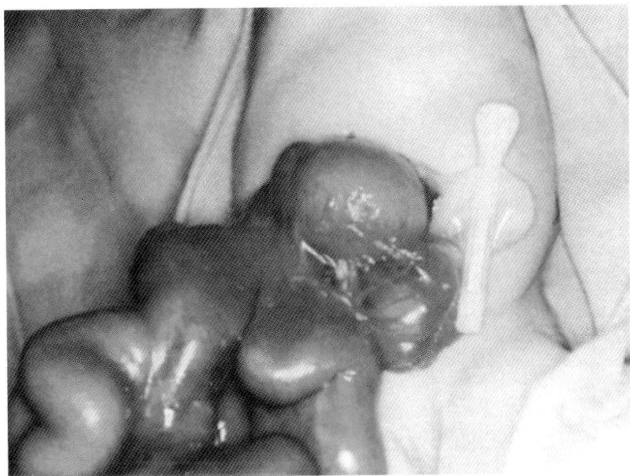

FIGURE 14-15 ▪ Gastroschisis. Loops of intestine extrude through an abdominal wall defect located to the right of the normally placed umbilicus. The intestines are not covered by a sac. (Courtesy of Robert J Izant Jr, M.D., Case Western Reserve University, Cleveland, Ohio.)

embryonic life (e301). Omphaloceles vary in size; the defect may be a few centimeters in diameter, or most of the anterior abdominal wall may be lacking. Depending on the size of the defect, small intestine, liver, spleen, and pancreas may be in the sac. The umbilicus usually inserts at the dome of the sac, and umbilical vessels ramify across the membrane. Intrauterine rupture of the sac may occur; exposure of the gut to amniotic fluid results in edema, bowel wall thickening, and matting of intestinal loops. Such cases must be distinguished from gastroschisis. The intestine is nearly always malrotated and shorter than normal.

Other congenital anomalies are found in at least one third of these infants, including gastrointestinal malformations, congenital heart disease, genitourinary anomalies, imperforate anus, and central nervous system defects. The incidence of omphalocele is increased in infants with trisomy 18, trisomy 13, and trisomy 21. Omphalocele is a key feature of Beckwith-Wiedemann syndrome (gigantism, macroglossia, hemihypertrophy, visceromegaly, and hypoglycemia) (33) (e164).

The prognosis in omphalocele is usually determined by the other anomalies and the size of the defect. The omphalocele sac is excised surgically just after birth, with closure of the defect primarily or with temporary prosthetic material.

Gastroschisis

Gastroschisis occurs much less frequently than omphalocele (e115,e301,e461). In gastroschisis, a relatively small paraumbilical abdominal wall defect (right side–to–left side ratio of 9:1) is distinctly separate from the normally placed umbilicus. Loops of bowel, not covered by a membrane, extrude through the opening (Figure 14-15). Because the extruded intestine has been bathed in amniotic fluid in utero, it appears abnormally thickened and edematous and may be coated with fibrin. The intestine is usually not rotated and is much shorter than normal. Jejunoileal atresia is another recognized association. In contrast to omphalocele, gastroschisis is rarely associated with concurrent major congenital anomalies (e115,e461).

Gastroschisis is believed to result from failure of the umbilical cord to form properly, so that the elongating midgut ruptures into the amniotic cavity during the first trimester (e301). Treatment consists of surgical closure of the defect at birth or staged procedures with the use of prosthetic material.

Malrotation

The term malrotation includes a group of congenital positional and associated abnormalities of the intestine and mesentery resulting from nonrotation or abnormal rotation and fixation of the developing embryonic gut (e150,e462). During the most rapid period of growth, the embryonic intestine extends outside the abdominal cavity (Figure 14-3). During weeks 10 and 11 of gestation, the intestine returns to the abdomen in sequential stages, the first of which is a 270-degree counterclockwise rotation of the midgut around the superior mesenteric artery until the duodenum comes to rest in its usual position posterior to the superior mesenteric artery. After that, the cecum and right colon rotate, first entering the abdomen on the left side, then crossing to the right and descending into the right lower quadrant anterior to the superior mesenteric artery. At week 11, fixation of the gut to the abdominal wall occurs. A broad-based mesentery extending from the ligament of Treitz to the ileocecal area attaches the intestine to the posterior abdominal wall and stabilizes it. The right and left portions of the colon become fixed retroperitoneally.

Failure of this sequence to take place at all (nonrotation) or failure at any step produces a spectrum of malrotation abnormalities. Any arrest in the process of rotation also tends to interfere with the normal mesenteric fixation of the bowel and results in a narrow mesenteric base and a mobile intestine that is predisposed to volvulus. A person with an incompletely rotated bowel is likely to have abnormal mesenteric fixations and associated extrinsic intestinal obstruction and volvulus. Malrotation often occurs together with other congenital anomalies, including duodenal atresia, omphalocele, gastroschisis, jejunoileal atresia, and Meckel diverticulum.

Variations of malrotation are diagrammed in Figure 14-16. In the case of nonrotation (Figure 14-16A), the duodenum is directed inferiorly and lacks the usual sweep to the left. The distal portion of the duodenum and the ascending colon lie together in the midabdomen and are attached to the abdominal wall posteriorly by a very short mesenteric root containing the superior mesenteric artery. The descending colon is not fixed. The narrow mesenteric root and nonfixed descending colon result in midgut volvulus and duodenal obstruction (Figure 14-16C). The rapid progression of volvulus causes the most dreaded and lethal complication of malrotation, which is cessation of mesenteric artery blood flow at the base of the twisted mesentery and infarction of the entire midgut. Midgut volvulus usually presents in the 1st month of life with intestinal obstruction. Normal rotation of the duodenal loop with nonrotation of the colon is associated with the same potential for midgut volvulus (Figure 14-16B).

In the variation of normal colonic rotation with nonrotation of the duodenum, abnormal mesenteric bands may intermittently obstruct the duodenum. In another variation, both the duodenum and the colon rotate normally, but the ascending colon does not become fixed. Abnormal peritoneal (Ladd) bands between the hepatic flexure and lateral abdominal wall overlie the duodenum and may obstruct it (Figure 14-16D).

Intestinal Atresia and Stenosis

Intestinal atresia is the complete absence of a segment of the intestine or complete occlusion of the intestinal lumen. Either situation is a common cause of neonatal intestinal obstruction, with a prevalence of 2 in 10,000 live births (1). The rates of atresia in the duodenum and in the more distal jejunum and ileum are approximately equal; colonic atresia is much less frequent. Multiple jejunoileal atresias are found in approximately 10% of cases.

Clinical, pathologic, histologic, and experimental observations indicate that most jejunoileal atresias and stenoses are secondary malformations. The disruptions are caused by intrauterine vascular accidents, with infarction and subsequent resorption or scarring of the affected segment (e114). The fact that bile and squamous epithelial cells are often found distal to the obstruction indicates that the lumen was patent early in gestation. The presence of serosal fibrosis and meconium indicates previous (intrauterine) intestinal perforation and peritonitis. Experimental occlusion of portions of the mesenteric circulation in fetal animals results in identical atretic lesions. Atresias are associated with known vascular insults, such as intrauterine malrotation with volvulus, intussusception, internal hernia, and constricting gastroschisis. Familial patterns in some cases of multiple jejunoileal atresias suggest that not all cases result from vascular accidents. Some arise from abnormal development of the mesenteric vasculature, probably genetically-based (134,138). A particularly distinctive form of multiple intestinal atresias occurs in French Canadians, although it is not limited to this ethnic group (e273,e415).

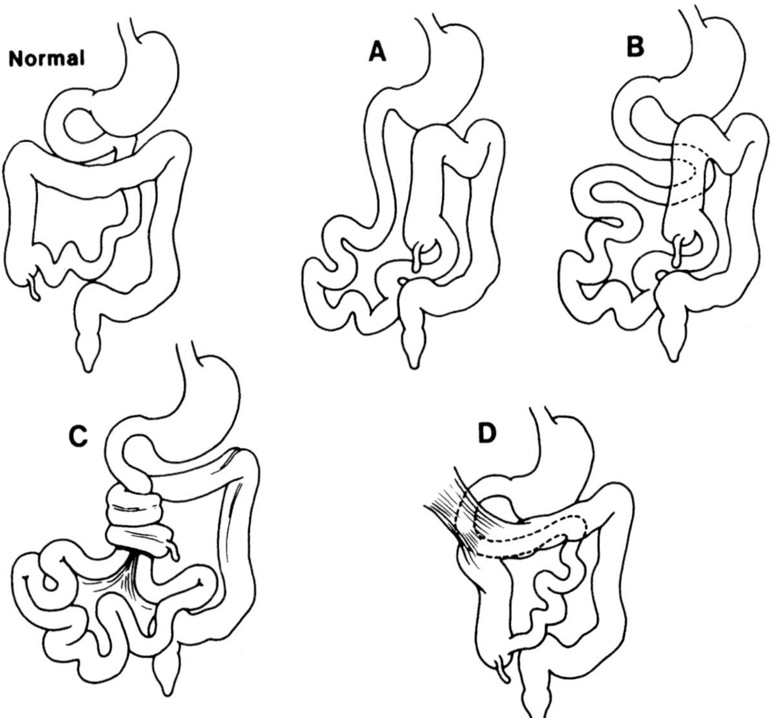

FIGURE 14-16■Normal rotation and variations in position of stomach and intestines due to malrotation. **A:** Nonrotation of duodenum and colon. **B:** Nonrotation of colon. **C:** Midgut volvulus resulting from a narrow mesenteric root and nonfixed descending colon in malrotation. Occlusion of mesenteric blood flow leads to midgut infarction. **D:** Ladd (peritoneal) fibrous bands (**upper left**) may extend from the lateral abdominal wall to the right colon, compressing and obstructing the duodenum.

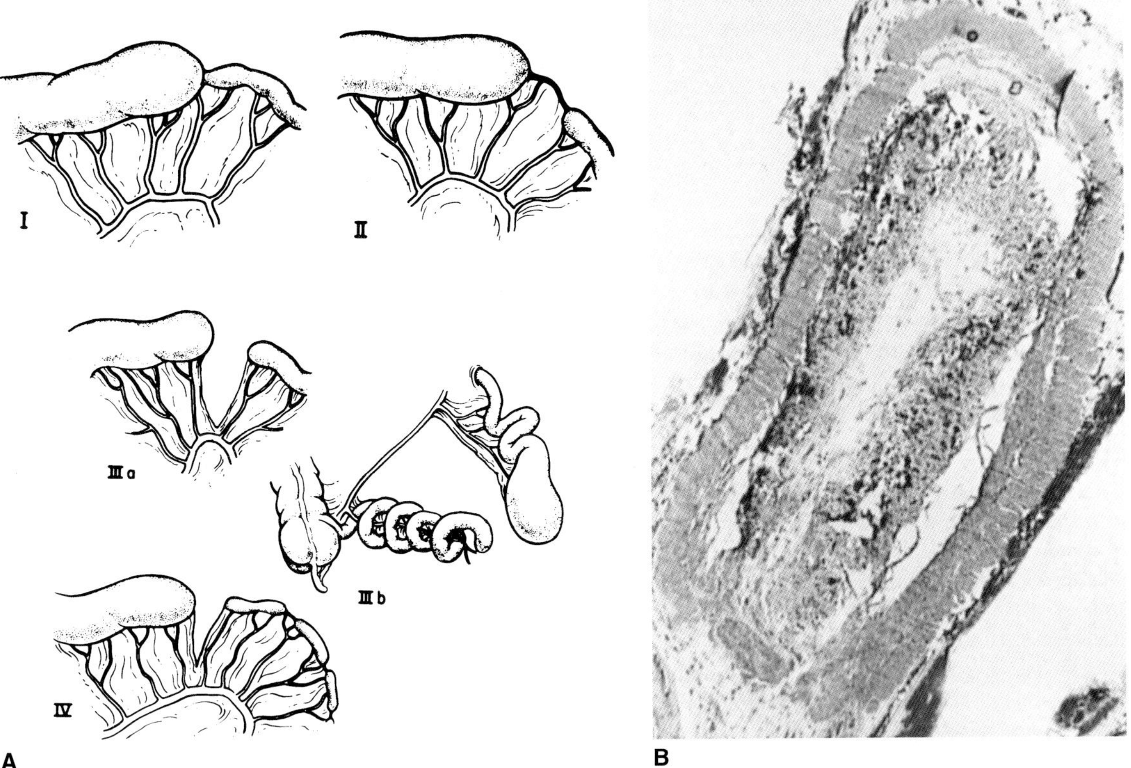

FIGURE 14-17■ **A:** Classification of intestinal atresia. I: mucosal (membranous) atresia with intact bowel wall and mesentery; II: blind intestinal ends attached by a fibrous cord; IIIA: blind intestinal ends separated by a V-shaped mesenteric defect without an intervening cord; IIIb: "apple-peel" atresia; and IV: multiple atresia. (From Grosfeld JL. Jejunoileal atresia and stenosis. In: Welch KJ, Randolph SG, Ravich MM et al., eds. *Pediatric surgery*. 4th ed. Chicago: Year Book, 1986:843, with permission.) **B:** Photomicrograph of a "fibrous cord" of intestinal atresia reveals an intact muscularis propria, but there is fibrous obliteration of the lumen and submucosal calcification, consistent with intrauterine ischemia and healing (H&E, original magnification 20×).

The embryologic basis of duodenal atresia probably differs from that of jejunoileal and colonic atresia. Because most cases of duodenal atresia are of the membranous type, they probably result from a lack of central vacuolization during the solid cord stage of duodenal development. The rate of associated anomalies in infants with duodenal atresia is high. One-fourth of infants with duodenal atresia have Down syndrome, an association not noted with atresia at other sites. Additional congenital anomalies associated with duodenal atresia include cardiac and renal malformations, esophageal atresia, imperforate anus, and vertebral anomalies. Annular pancreas and malrotation are each found in approximately one-fourth of infants with duodenal atresia (e103). Jejunoileal atresia is less likely to be associated with other anomalies, although an association between cystic fibrosis and jejunoileal atresia has been noted (e40).

The symptoms of intestinal atresia depend on the level of gastrointestinal tract affected. Duodenal and proximal jejunal atresia cause maternal polyhydramnios (secondary to reduced absorption of swallowed amniotic fluid), vomiting, and abdominal distension in the first 24 hours of life; these symptoms are delayed with more distal obstruction. Abdominal radiographs show gaseous distension of the stomach with duodenal atresia and, in lower intestinal atresias, air-fluid levels. Many cases of jejunoileal atresia are now detected by prenatal ultrasonography.

Intestinal atresias have been classified according to their gross appearance (e184) (Figure 14-17A). Type I has an intact intestinal wall and mesentery but a septal or membranous luminal obstruction. Because the proximal segment is obstructed, its diameter greatly exceeds that of the distal segment. In type II, two intestinal segments with blind ends are separated by a fibrous cord. In type III, the most common, two blind ends are present without an intervening cord; a wedge-shaped mesenteric defect is also present. In the "apple-peel" or "Christmas tree" variety of extensive jejunal atresia, the intestine is very short and the distal ileal segment is coiled around its arterial blood supply (the ileocecal artery). Type III may also be associated with a congenitally short small intestine.

Histologic examination of a type II atresia usually shows a recognizable intestinal wall with muscularis layers but fibrous obliteration of the mucosa and submucosa. The frequent presence of luminal granulation tissue, fibrosis, and calcification suggests previous ischemia and healing (Figure 14-17B).

Intestinal segments adjacent to regions of atresia or stenosis should be examined for changes suggestive of cystic fibrosis: dilated glands with eosinophilic inspissated secretions, unusually viscid secretions in the lumen, and hyperplasia of goblet cells (e121). In one study, 8% of neonates with jejunoileal atresia had cystic fibrosis (4).

Congenital intestinal stenosis is less common than intestinal atresia; it may be solitary or multiple and may affect a short or long segment. The bowel diameter is greatly reduced, although the lumen is patent throughout. Histologic examination of the intestinal wall often shows evidence of previous ischemia and healing, including mucosal atrophy, submucosal fibrosis, and scarring of smooth muscle. As in intestinal atresia, most cases are presumed to result from an intrauterine ischemic insult, although a history of an untoward event during pregnancy is often lacking (e114).

Duplications of the Gastrointestinal Tract

Gastrointestinal (enteric) duplications are tubular or cystic structures that lie alongside the intestinal tube. The duplication and the intestinal tube often share a muscular wall (intramural); less often, the duplication is separated from the intestine proper but in close proximity to it (extramural) (e51,e183). Duplications may occur anywhere near the gastrointestinal tract from the neck to rectum; the single most common site is the ileum (Figure 14-18A).

No single theory of embryogenesis satisfactorily explains the origin of all duplications. They are thought to result from aberrant diverticula in embryonic life (e469) or as a consequence of incomplete intestinal infarction in the fetus with isolation of a viable portion of intestine adjacent to the regenerated intestinal tube (e138).

Symptoms vary widely, depending on the location of the duplication. Thoracic enteric duplication cysts are usually extramural and found in the posterior mediastinum; they present with respiratory symptoms in infancy and may communicate across the diaphragm with the intraabdominal gastrointestinal tract. Abdominal duplications may present with pain, a palpable mass, intestinal obstruction, and, if peptic ulceration occurs in ectopic gastric mucosa, intestinal bleeding.

Multiple duplications are found in 5% of patients. The usual intestinal duplication is a cystic mass located on the mesenteric border. It ranges in size from 2 to 7 cm in diameter, although much larger ones may also be found (Figure 14-18B). The cyst lumen usually does not communicate with the intestinal lumen. Occasionally, tubular duplications paralleling a long segment of intestine are found; these form a blind pouch proximally but communicate with the intestinal lumen distally. Noncommunicating cysts are filled with mucoid material and histologically mimic normal gastrointestinal tract with enteric mucosa, submucosa, muscularis propria, and a myenteric plexus. Intramural duplications usually do not have a complete muscularis layer but rather share a muscularis layer with the adjacent intestine. The mucosa may resemble adjacent normal gastrointestinal mucosa, but it is often very simplified and difficult to categorize except that columnar epithelium bears a generic resemblance to intestinal surface epithelial cells. Cilia may be present, as in embryonic intestinal epithelium. Gastric mucosa is found in approximately 20% of duplications and may cause peptic ulceration in unlikely sites, such as the ileum and posterior mediastinum. Intestinal duplications in the abdomen must be distinguished from a Meckel diverticulum and other vitelline duct remnants, mesenteric cyst (which lacks intestinal wall morphology), and cystic lymphangioma.

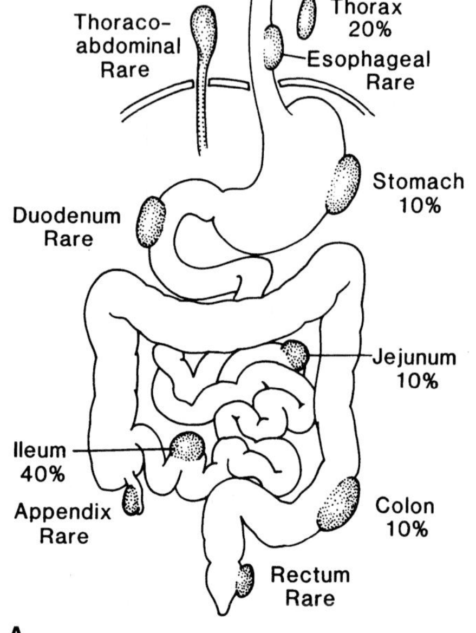

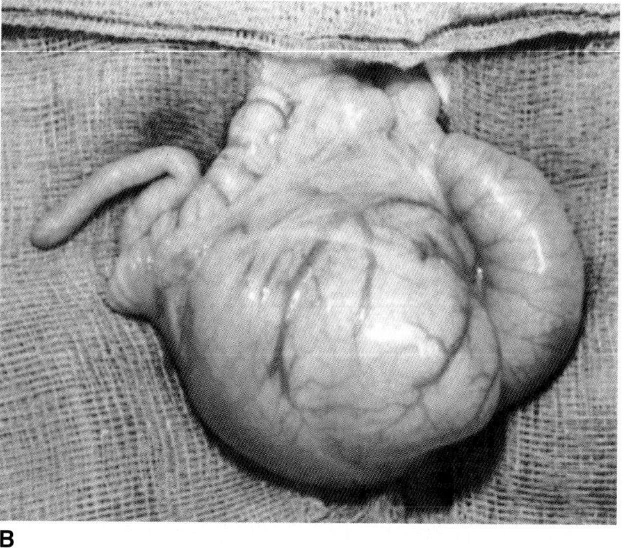

FIGURE 14-18■**A:** Locations and incidence of gastrointestinal duplication cysts. **B:** Ileal duplication cyst located near the ileocecal valve. The appendix and cecum are on the left, and the dilated obstructed ileum is on the right. (Courtesy of Robert J. Izant Jr, M.D., case-Western reserve University, Cleveland, Ohio.)

Meckel Diverticulum and Other Vitelline Duct Anomalies

The vitelline (omphalomesenteric) duct usually becomes obliterated by week 10 of embryonic life and subsequently disappears completely (e226,e477). In approximately 2% of the population, however, it remains in various forms (Figure 14-19A–E). These include Meckel diverticulum or, less commonly, a fibrous cord extending from ileum to umbilicus, a cyst, or an umbilical sinus. Many of these remnants are asymptomatic, but others cause symptoms that develop most frequently in the first few years of life.

Meckel diverticulum is the most common vitelline duct remnant and also the most common congenital anomaly of the gastrointestinal tract. It results from incomplete obliteration of the vitelline duct at the ileum and appears as a 1- to 5-cm fingerlike protrusion of the intestine on the antimesenteric surface of the middle ileum (Figure 14-19D). When found incidentally at autopsy or surgery, most Meckel diverticula are lined by small-intestinal epithelium. Those causing symptoms are likely to contain heterotopic gastric mucosa (Figure 14-20A,B), which secretes acid and leads to peptic ulceration of adjacent intestinal mucosa with subsequent abdominal pain, rectal bleeding, and occasionally intestinal perforation. Approximately 25% of all Meckel diverticula contain foci of gastric mucosa. Occasionally, a Meckel diverticulum may invert into the intestinal lumen and serve as the lead point of an ileal intussusception.

Other vitelline duct remnants are much less common than Meckel diverticulum. A vitelline cyst (Figure 14-19B) results from partial obliteration of the vitelline duct and presents as a mass subjacent to the umbilicus. Microscopically, the cyst wall resembles that of the intestine and is lined by mucus-secreting intestinal epithelium. A vitelline band is a fibrous cord that persists after obliteration of the vitelline duct (Figure 14-19E). These bands extend from umbilicus to ileum, a Meckel diverticulum, or a vitelline cyst and they may serve as a fulcrum for volvulus. Persistence of part of the vitelline duct at the umbilicus causes an umbilical sinus, which presents with mucous discharge from the umbilicus (Figure 14-19C). This must be distinguished from the very rare persistence of the entire vitelline duct (Figure 14-19A). Vitelline cysts and sinuses at the umbilicus are distinguished histologically from urachal remnants at the same site by the presence of intestinal or columnar epithelium. Urachal remnants have an urothelial lining.

Meconium and Meconium Abnormalities

Meconium is the dark green–to-black mucoid material that fills the neonatal colon and distal small intestine. It consists predominantly of water (75%) admixed with mucous glycoproteins, swallowed vernix caseosa, gastrointestinal secretions, bile, pancreatic enzymes, plasma proteins, minerals, and lipids. More than 90% of healthy term newborns pass a meconium stool averaging 200 mL within the first 24 hours of life, and nearly all have done so by 48 hours. Abnormalities of meconium (e.g., in cystic fibrosis) or of intestinal motility (e.g., in Hirschsprung disease) result in a delayed meconium passage (e18).

Meconium Ileus

Meconium ileus is neonatal obstruction of the ileal lumen by abnormally viscid and inspissated meconium containing an abnormally high level of albumin (e122,e211,e345,e513). Most but not all cases occur as the initial manifestation of

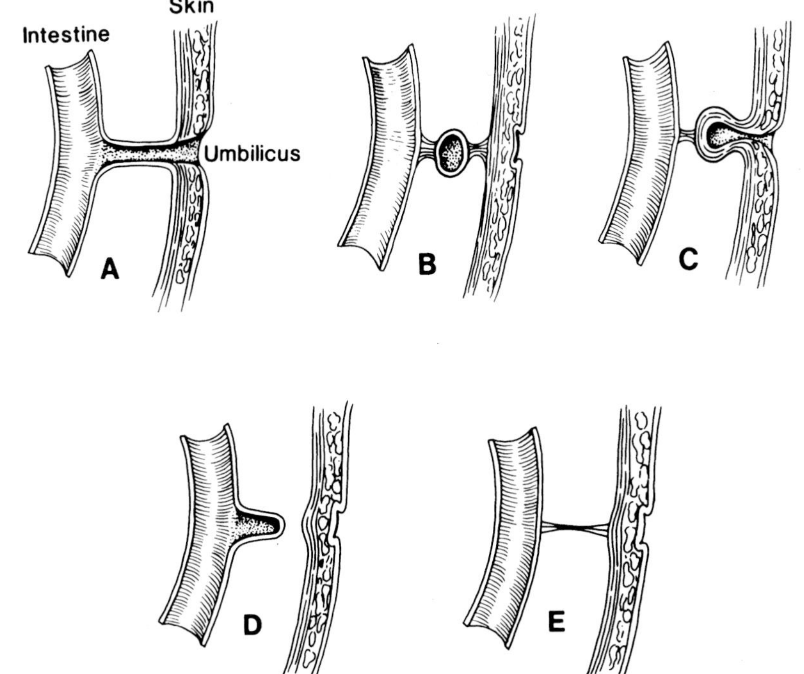

FIGURE 14-19 ▪ Vitelline (omphalomesenteric) duct anomalies. **A:** Persistence of the entire vitelline duct from the ileum to umbilicus. **B:** Vitelline duct cyst. **C:** Vitelline duct and umbilical sinus. **D:** Meckel diverticulum. **E:** Vitelline band.

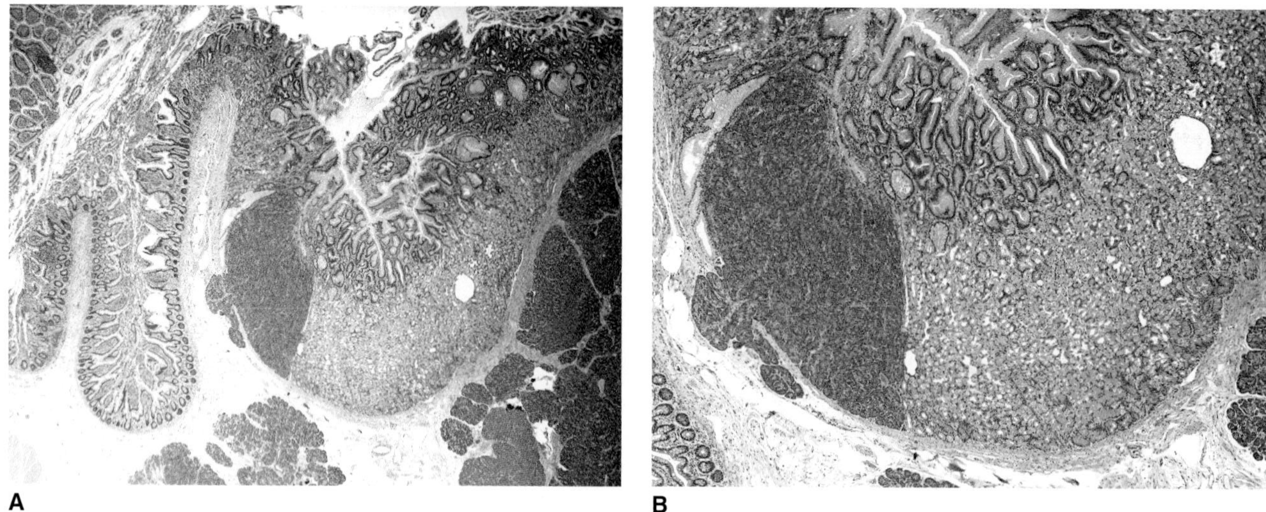

FIGURE 14-20■**AB:** Meckel diverticulum. Ectopic gastric fundic and pancreatic tissue in the mucosa lines the diverticulum. **A:** 40×. **B:** 100×.

cystic fibrosis; 10% to 15% of patients with cystic fibrosis are born with meconium ileus. Rarely, infants with congenital pancreatic or pancreatic duct abnormalities have meconium ileus without cystic fibrosis, but these account for fewer than 5% of cases. The diagnosis of cystic fibrosis should be pursued in every infant with meconium ileus. In the classic case, the distal one third of the ileum has a nearly normal diameter, but the lumen is filled with dense gray beadlike or solid meconium having the consistency and appearance of putty. The middle one third of the ileum, proximal to the obstructing meconium, is dilated and filled with dark gelatinous or tarlike meconium. Because the colon in meconium ileus is empty throughout the fetal life, its diameter is smaller than normal.

Microscopically, the distal ileal lumen is filled with hypereosinophilic, focally calcified meconium. Intestinal glands are dilated, often V-shaped, and plugged with hypereosinophilic secretions that are continuous with the luminal meconium. If intrauterine intestinal perforation has occurred, the infant will also have meconium peritonitis. Approximately 50% of the patients with meconium ileus have meconium peritonitis or other complications of meconium ileus, which include intestinal atresia (e40) and volvulus.

The overall survival rate of infants with meconium ileus exceeds 80%, although they often have a prolonged hospital course.

Meconium Peritonitis

Intestinal perforation *in utero* causes meconium to be released into the peritoneal space. The result is a distinctive chemical peritonitis, with sterile inflammation, fibrosis, and characteristic calcifications (e151,e287). Between 33% and 50% of patients with meconium peritonitis have meconium ileus and cystic fibrosis. In half of the remaining patients, perforation is the result of intrauterine intestinal obstruction resulting from atresia, malrotation with volvulus, mesenteric hernias, or congenital bands. In the others, the bowel perforation and its cause are no longer apparent at birth, but it is believed that intrauterine vascular insufficiency has caused the intestinal perforation (e459). Meconium peritonitis is usually seen just after birth and is temporally remote from the intrauterine intestinal perforation that caused it. At gross examination, the peritonitis is usually organized, with fibrosis, calcifications, and often dense intestinal adhesions. Occasionally encountered is a meconium pseudocyst, a collection of soft meconium walled off by peritoneal fibrosis.

Microscopically, collections of squames and bile pigment in the peritoneal space, florid fibrosis, and calcifications indicate the presence of meconium. Inflammation is usually chronic, and a well-developed foreign body response to squames and calcifications may be noted. Because the fetal gut is sterile, the degree of inflammation is much less than in the usual case of postnatal peritonitis. If meconium is released into the peritoneal space during intrauterine life, when the inguinal canal to the scrotum is patent, the migration of meconium into the paratesticular area results in a condition called meconium periorchitis (e113). Inguinal and even labial meconium masses may also occur, although more rarely, in girls (e251).

Meconium Plug

Meconium plug is a syndrome of neonatal colonic obstruction caused by a plug of desiccated meconium, usually in the ascending colon or, in infants with a very low birth weight, the ileum or proximal colon (e345,e484). It is a much less serious condition than meconium ileus, but it may present with a similar clinical picture. The plug is usually passed after a Gastrografin enema, and the infant has no further problems. Meconium plug syndrome may rarely occur in patients with cystic fibrosis. It is essential that Hirschsprung disease be excluded. However, most infants with a meconium plug have neither of these conditions.

Gastrointestinal Involvement in Cystic Fibrosis

Cystic fibrosis, the most common lethal genetic disease in white children, is an autosomal recessive condition with an incidence of 1 in 3,000 live births in the United States and Canada (e260,e422) (Chapters 5, 12, 15). The past decade has seen great advances in the understanding of its pathogenesis. It is now known that mutations in the gene that encodes the cystic fibrosis transmembrane conductance regulator result in faulty electrolyte transport across epithelial surfaces and subsequent dehydration of luminal contents, which in turn leads to obstruction of glands and ducts by thick, viscid secretions. The pancreas, intestines, and lungs are the chief organ systems affected. Gastrointestinal symptoms may be present at birth and almost invariably appear during the first few months of life. Malabsorption resulting from exocrine pancreatic insufficiency is a prominent manifestation in nearly all children and adults with cystic fibrosis. Many gastrointestinal tract abnormalities are also characteristic signs of cystic fibrosis (e260,e346,e350,e422) (Table 14-2).

Meconium ileus is the first sign of cystic fibrosis in approximately 10% to 15% of patients (e122,e211,e513). It usually presents as intestinal obstruction in the 1st hours or days of life but has also been diagnosed antenatally by obstetric ultrasonography. It should be considered a manifestation of cystic fibrosis until proven otherwise. Up to one-half of the infants with meconium ileus have concurrent gastrointestinal manifestations of cystic fibrosis, including meconium peritonitis, small-intestinal atresias and stenoses, duplication, volvulus, microcolon, and mesenteric bands or adhesions.

Distal intestinal obstruction syndrome, formerly called meconium ileus equivalent, is partial or total distal intestinal obstruction by inspissated fecal material occurring in older children and adults with cystic fibrosis. It has nothing to do with meconium. Viscid intestinal contents, a change in dietary habits, dehydration, and temporary disturbances in motility are all thought to be etiologic (e81,e198). Up to 33% of all patients with cystic fibrosis are affected at one time or another. The incidence of meconium plug syndrome is increased in neonates with cystic fibrosis, although most cases occur in infants without cystic fibrosis (e345,e388). Fibrosing colonopathy is a rare distinctive stricturing process of the colon first described in patients with cystic fibrosis in the 1990s, when it was linked to the ingestion of new preparations of high-dose pancreatic enzyme replacement capsules. The condition usually presents with partial or complete intestinal obstruction, and symptoms may mimic those of distal ileal obstruction syndrome (meconium ileus equivalent) or chronic inflammatory bowel disease (e254,e355,e408,e433). Fibrosing colonopathy usually affects a long segment of the ascending colon but may involve the entire colon. The lumen is compromised by circumferential submucosal fibrosis along the length of the strictured segment. Fibrosis of the lamina propria, mucosal ulceration, acute and chronic mucosal inflammation, and granulation tissue can also be seen. One series noted increased numbers of eosinophils in the mucosa (e355). Because of the strong association between fibrosing colonopathy and high-strength pancreatic enzyme supplements, it was recommended that the daily dose be reduced (e146).

Table 14-2 ■ GASTROINTESTINAL MANIFESTATIONS OF CYSTIC FIBROSIS

Gastroesophageal reflux and Barrett esophagus
Malabsorption and pancreatic insufficiency
Meconium ileus, peritonitis, and meconium plug syndrome
Microcolon
Small-intestinal obstruction and atresia
Intussusception
Volvulus
Rectal prolapse
Brunner gland hyperplasia
Fibrosing colonopathy (due to pancreatic enzyme replacement)
Pneumatosis intestinalis
Mucocele
Gallbadder disease

HIRSCHSPRUNG DISEASE

Hirschsprung disease is characterized by an absence of intramural parasympathetic ganglion cells in the distal gastrointestinal tract in association with a loss of tonic neural inhibition, persistent contraction of the affected segment, and subsequent colonic obstruction. The condition usually results from defective craniocaudal migration of vagal neural crest cells (the progenitors of ganglion cells) between gestational weeks 5 and 12. Interruption of craniocaudal migration of neural crest cells explains the distal aganglionosis in Hirschsprung disease, but development of the ganglia is also influenced by local factors in the intestinal wall (e234). The physiology of the disease is more complex than can be explained by colonic ganglion cell absence alone; abnormalities of both adrenergic and cholinergic fibers are demonstrable in the aganglionic bowel, and function of the internal anal sphincter is also abnormal.

Hirschsprung disease is a congenital disorder with an incidence of one per 5,000 live births and is much more common in male infants (85%) than in female infants (e48). Most cases are sporadic, although a familial component has been noted in approximately 10% of cases (13). Long-segment Hirschsprung disease and total colonic aganglionosis are the types most likely to be familial conditions. It has a complex genetic basis, involving defects in at least ten genes, with mutation in the RET gene playing a central role (4). In most cases, Hirschsprung disease is an isolated congenital anomaly, but associations have been noted with Down syndrome (10% of patients with Hirschsprung disease have Down syndrome), congenital heart disease, genitourinary anomalies, Waardenburg syndrome, congenital deafness, intestinal atresia, and Ondine curse.

More than 90% of patients with Hirschsprung disease are born at full term with a normal birth weight. Presenting symptoms in neonates include delayed passage of meconium, vomiting, abdominal distention, and enterocolitis. Hirschsprung enterocolitis, a grave complication that may develop rapidly, results from vascular compromise caused by the distal obstruction and superimposed bacterial infection. More than 90% of infants with Hirschsprung disease fail to pass meconium within 24 hours after birth (39).

The aganglionic segment in Hirschsprung disease begins at the anal sphincter and extends proximally (Figure 14-21A to E). In 80% of cases, aganglionosis is limited to the rectum and distal sigmoid colon; this situation is sometimes referred to as short-segment Hirschsprung disease. In the remaining patients, the aganglionic segment is longer (long-segment Hirschsprung disease) and extends as far proximally as the splenic flexure or transverse colon in 10% and the cecum in 5% (total colonic aganglionosis or Zuelzer-Wilson disease). In rare cases, aganglionosis extends into the small intestine and may reach as far as the proximal duodenum (e46). In the usual case, barium enema shows a narrow rectum and rectosigmoid colon with a proximal funneling transition to a very dilated sigmoid colon. Neonates and infants with long aganglionic segments do not have this diagnostic radiologic picture. Anal manometry is another valuable diagnostic tool used in certain clinical settings. Despite the relative rarity of Hirschsprung disease, it enters into the differential diagnosis of many other conditions because of its varied modes of presentation and the common occurrence of functional constipation in children.

Although radiographic and manometric studies are routine diagnostic screening procedures, microscopic evaluation of rectal biopsies is regarded as the gold standard for the diagnosis of this disorder. Suction biopsies are preferable over routine forceps biopsies in order that an adequate sample of submucosal tissue is obtained (e512). The biopsy should be performed at least 2 cm above the dentate line in order to avoid the normal zone of hypoganglionic distal rectum (e4,e490). Thus, the first task of the surgical pathologist is to assess the adequacy of the biopsy material. A biopsy that contains squamous or anal transitional epithelium should be reported as inadequate and the absence of ganglion cells in such a specimen is disregarded. The biopsy must also contain an adequate thickness of submucosa in order to evaluate for loss of ganglion cells. An accepted rule of thumb is that in a well-oriented biopsy the portion of submucosa sampled should be at least as thick as the overlying mucosa.

Ganglion cells in neonates can have an immature morphology that can be difficult to recognize in H&E sections, particularly in the submucosa (Meissner plexus) (e483). Confusion between endothelial cells and neuronal cells may lead to a false negative diagnosis (Figure 14-22A,B). Careful examination of a large number of serial sections of each biopsy is necessary before a diagnosis of Hirschsprung disease is made.

Normal A B

Squamo-columnar junction

C D E

FIGURE 14-21 ■ Distribution of affected colon in Hirschsprung disease (stippled area). **A:** Rectosigmoid aganglionosis. **B:** Ultrashort Hirschsprung disease affected the distal rectum near the anal sphincter. **C:** Long-segment Hirschsprung disease with involvement of the hepatic flexure. **D:** Total colonic aganglionosis. **E:** aganglionosis involving the entire colon and the distal small bowel (in exceptional cases the distal duodenum may be involved).

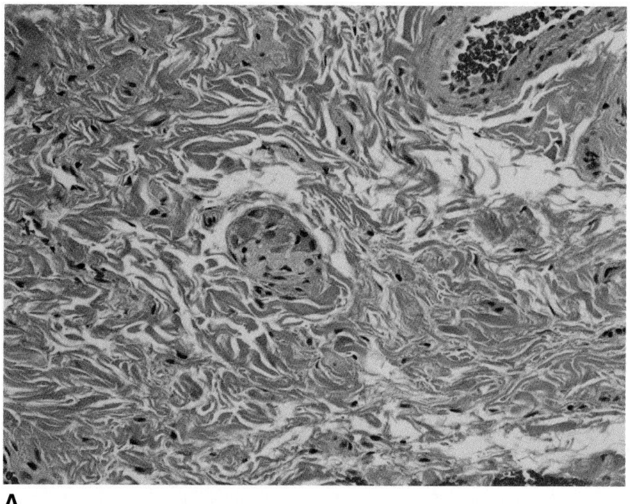

A

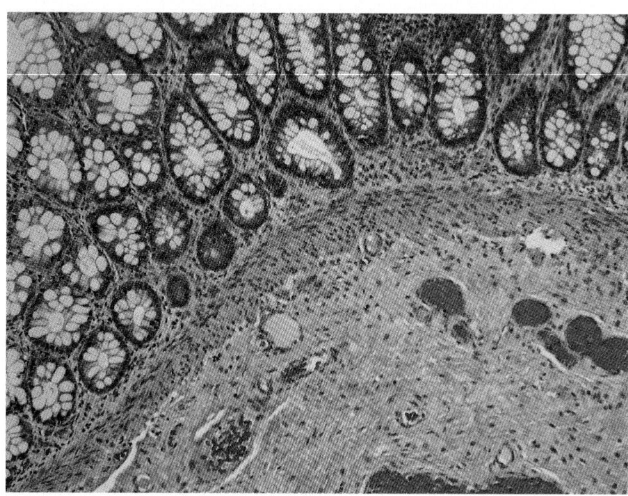

B

FIGURE 14-22 ■ Normal submucosal ganglion cells **A:** In this 7-month-old child ganglion cells are easy to identify 200×. **B:** In this 11-day-old infant the ganglion cells are immature appearing and therefore more difficult to identify 200×. (Courtesy of Dr. Aliya N. Husain, University of Chicago Medical Center.)

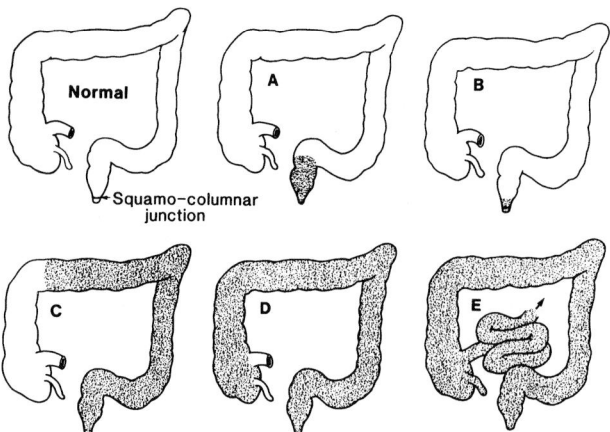

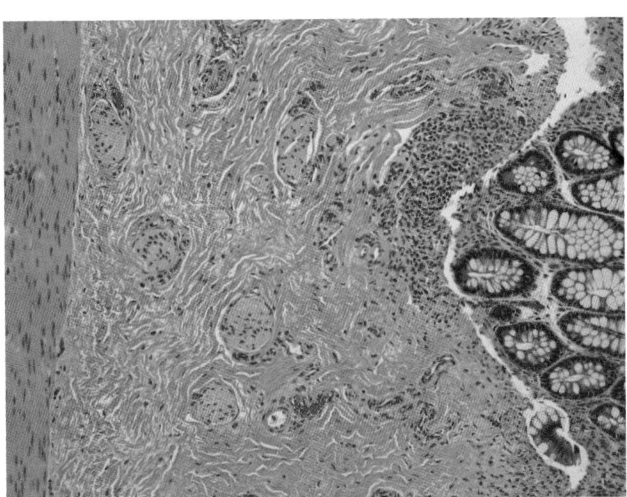

FIGURE 14-23▪Hypertrophic submucosal nerve fibers in a patient with Hirschsprung disease 200×. (Courtesy of Dr. Aliya N. Husain, University of Chicago Medical Center.)

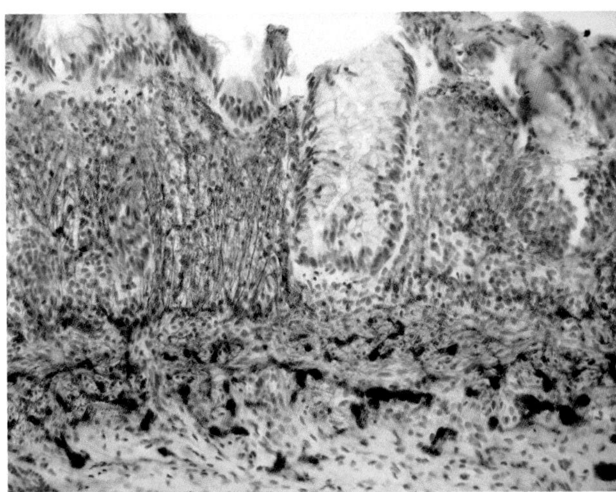

FIGURE 14-24▪Acetylcholinesterase stain of a rectal biopsy in a patient with Hirschsprung disease. Note the presence of abnormal ropey nerve fibers in the lamina propria 400×.

The absence of ganglion cells in an adequate biopsy is diagnostic of Hirschsprung disease, but the presence of multiple submucosal hypertrophic extrinsic nerve fibers is regarded as a helpful additional "positive" feature in making the diagnosis. These abnormally thick fibers should be at least 40 μm in diameter (Figure 14-23). This feature is present in more than 90% of the rectal suction biopsies of patients with Hirschsprung disease (e326). Thick submucosal nerve fibers are reportedly less common in short segment Hirschsprung disease and in total colonic aganglionosis (112). Immunohistologic stains to highlight these nerve fibers utilizing nerve growth factor receptor, glial fibrillary acidic protein, or glutose transporter-1 antibodies can be performed on paraffin embedded biopsies, but the sensitivity and specificity are not as good as that for acetylcholinesterase stains (79,82) (e235,e507).

Histochemical demonstration of acetylcholinesterase positive cholinergic nerve fibers within the lamina propria provides supportive evidence for the diagnosis of Hirschsprung disease, since they are not present in normal individuals (Figure 14-24). The presence of thick ropy fibers in the lamina propria between the crypts is regarded as highly specific for the diagnosis (99) (e75). However, this change may not be clearly evident in patients under the age of 6 months, particularly in short-segment Hirschsprung disease (112). In these patients the abnormal fibers may be present only in the submucosa and muscularis mucosae, and since some positively stained thinner fibers are also present in these locations in healthy infants, the diagnosis in this circumstance is problematic (99,112). In addition, this technique can only be performed on frozen sections, requiring the clinician to obtain extra biopsies, and the staining procedure must be followed meticulously using freshly prepared reagents (98) (e272). The frozen sections should be cut at 15 μm thickness so that the nerve fibers can be properly highlighted. Recently, a prepackaged kit for acetylcholinesterase staining has become available, and this may increase usage of this methodology (99).

There are also a variety of histochemical and immunohistologic stains that can be used to visualize submucosal ganglion cells in suction rectal biopsies. The histochemical stains, which must be performed on frozen sections, highlight enzymes present in ganglion cells, including lactic dehydrogenase, alpha-naphthyl esterase, and NADPH-diaphorase. These stains are not commonly performed in the United States, but the availability of a prepackaged kit may increase their usage in the future (99). Immunohistologic stains have the advantage of being performed on sections from paraffin embedded biopsies, obviating the need to obtain extra biopsies. However, they all suffer from the distinct disadvantage of having to be performed on multiple levels to ensure that no ganglion cells are present. Antibodies that have been utilized to highlight the presence of ganglion cells include NSE, bcl-2, bone morphogenic protein 1A, and RET (19,85) (e492). In addition, S-100 immunostains can highlight the presence of hypertrophic submucosal nerve fibers and highlight the presence of ganglion cell bodies by their lack of staining (e386,e451).

Recently, the observation was made that patients with Hirschsprung disease lacked calretinin immunoreactive submucosal nerve fibers in the aganglionic segment of colon (13). This observation has led to a proposal to use calretinin immunostains on rectal suction biopsies as a diagnostic test. In the single report to date, calretinin reactive nerve fibers were absent from all rectal biopsies from Hirschsprung patients and present in all patients where ganglion cells were present in the biopsy (Figure 14-25A,B). The authors stressed that for unclear reasons the density of calretinin reactive submucosal fibers varied greatly among the patients without Hirschsprung disease and that at the anorectal junction no reactive fibers are normally present (84). If the utility of this staining pattern can be confirmed by other authors, this technique may represent a valuable diagnostic adjunct in Hirschsprung disease.

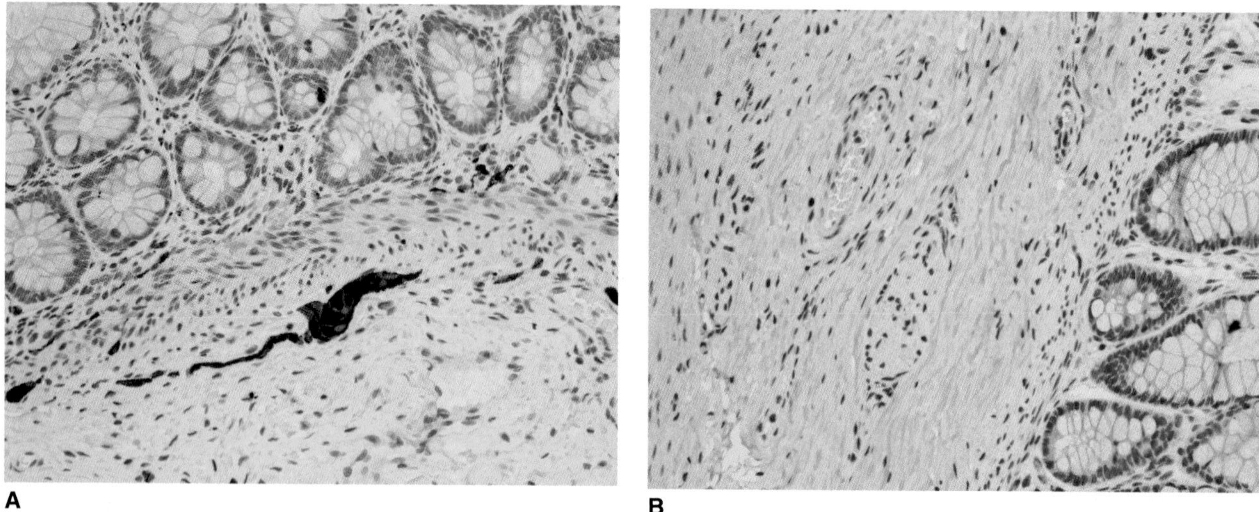

FIGURE 14-25■Calretinin immunostains performed on sections from suction rectal biopsies. **A:** In a normal infant, calretinin reactive submucosal nerve fibers are prominent 400×. **B:** In an infant with Hirschsprung disease, there is no reactivity in submucosal nerve fibers in the aganglionic segment 400×. (Courtesy of Dr. Aliya N. Husain, University of Chicago Medical Center.)

A histologic diagnosis of Hirschsprung disease made from examination of a suction rectal biopsy should be confirmed by frozen section at the time corrective surgery is performed. A seromuscular biopsy containing the full thickness of the muscularis propria from the abnormally narrowed aganglionic segment allows for examination to confirm the absence of ganglion cells within the myenteric (Auerbach) plexus. The myenteric (Auerbach) plexus and ganglion cells within it are much larger and easier to interpret than those in the submucosal (Meissner) plexus. Normal myenteric plexus, found between the inner circular and outer longitudinal layers of the muscularis externa, consists of unmyelinated nerve fibers and clusters of rounded Schwann cells and large ganglion cells around the perimeter of the nerve fibers. Myenteric ganglion cells can be recognized by their polygonal shape, abundant cytoplasm, round and eccentric nucleus, and prominent nucleolus. These features are apparent even on frozen section. In Hirschsprung disease, by contrast, nerves are present but ganglion cells are completely absent.

If a full-thickness biopsy is performed, the submucosa can be examined for the presence of ganglion cells in Auerbach plexus. The ganglion cells are contained within "neural units", first described by Yunis is a seminal 1976 publication, consisting of vaguely organoid structures containing two to ten nuclei in a horseshoe-shaped array surrounding a central core of pale, bubbly neural tissue. The ganglion cells are located at the periphery of these neural units (e512).

There is often a hypoganglionic colonic segment of variable length just proximal to the aganglionic segment (e162). Thus, frozen sections are also performed on muscularis propria from above the grossly narrowed segment to confirm that normal numbers of ganglion cells are present. This allows the surgeon to identify the proper level at which to transect the colon. However, it must be admitted that the confident recognition of immature ganglion cells in frozen sections is problematic, and both false positive and negative errors are possible (97).

In some patients the distal functional obstruction leads to the development of diversion-like colitis changes in the aganglionic segment and obstructive-like colitis in the segment just proximal to it (e372). Colitis is a major cause of morbidity and mortality in patients with untreated Hirschsprung disease (e456).

Chronic Intestinal Pseudo-Obstruction

The term intestinal pseudo-obstruction denotes greatly impaired or absent peristalsis without mechanical obstruction to luminal flow (e390,e480). Pseudo-obstruction is a clinical syndrome, not a pathologic diagnosis. A recent consensus workshop of pediatric gastroenterologists defined the clinical features of chronic intestinal pseudo-obstruction as intermittent or continuous bowel obstruction, including radiologic documentation of dilated bowel with air-fluid levels but without a lumen-occluding lesion. A wide clinical spectrum comprises more than 70 known entities, all of them rare. The diagnosis is often elusive and difficult for both gastroenterologists and pathologists (e167). Both congenital and acquired forms exist, and the pseudo-obstruction may occur in any region of the gastrointestinal tract. By the above definition, cases of Hirschsprung disease would be included, but by convention, they are excluded. However, Hirschsprung disease is considered in the differential diagnosis of colonic pseudo-obstruction presenting early in life.

The two major subclasses of pseudo-obstruction are myopathic and neurogenic, with primary and secondary subcategories in each (Table 14-3). In primary chronic intestinal pseudo-obstruction, manifestations of the disease are limited chiefly to the gastrointestinal tract; in the secondary form, the

Table 14-3 ■ CHRONIC INTESTINAL PSEUDO-OBSTRUCTION IN CHILDREN

Primary visceral myopathies
- Congenital megacystis-microcolon-hypoperistalsis
- Other familial visceral myopathies

Secondary visceral myopathies
- Muscular dystrophies
- Connective tissue disorders
- Ehlers-Danlos syndrome

Primary visceral neuropathies
- Familial visceral neuropathies
- Neuropathies associated with malrotation and gastroschisis
- Myenteric plexus neuropathies
- Intestinal neuronal dysplasia

Secondary visceral neuropathies
- Familial dysautonomia
- Myotonic dystrophy
- Postviral pseudo-obstruction

gastrointestinal manifestations are part of a systemic disease. A panel of immunohistologic stains can be used to systematically evaluate both the muscular and neural elements of the bowel wall in specimens submitted for diagnostic purposes (5).

Visceral myopathies can be appreciated by conventional microscopy, although full-thickness specimens of intestinal wall are necessary because the abnormalities are in the muscularis propria. Degeneration, atrophy, and sometimes fibrosis of intestinal smooth muscle are revealed by hematoxylin and eosin stain and enhanced by Masson trichrome stain. The outer, longitudinal layer of the muscularis propria is almost always more affected than the inner, circular layer. The most widely recognized of the visceral myopathies is congenital megacystis-microcolon-intestinal hypoperistalsis syndrome, also called hollow visceral myopathy (e13,e37,e405,e502). It is transmitted as an autosomal dominant trait and is diagnosed at birth or by prenatal ultrasonography. Many other familial visceral myopathies without megacystis also occur. The inheritance of these varies with type and from family to family (e267,e336,e405,e432). Smooth muscle degenerative changes also occur secondarily in the muscular dystrophies, particularly Duchenne muscular dystrophy (e281), and in connective tissue disorders, such as polymyositis, lupus erythematosus (e65), and scleroderma. Genetic defects of the mitochondrial oxidative phosphorylation pathway have been determined to be responsible for a small subset of the myopathic form of pseudo-obstruction (6). Structural malformation of the intestinal muscularis propria has also been reported as a rare cause of pseudo-obstruction (83).

Study of the visceral neuropathies is less easily accomplished because conventional light microscopy of paraffin-embedded sections of intestine stained with hematoxylin and eosin often does not demonstrate any changes. Special techniques such as electron microscopy and acetylcholinesterase staining of frozen sections may demonstrate abnormalities. Even more technically difficult and not often performed in routine practice is the sectioning and staining technique devised by Smith to demonstrate subtle changes in the myenteric plexus. With this method, a large surgical biopsy specimen of muscularis propria is embedded flat so that the myenteric plexus is sectioned longitudinally or obliquely rather than in the more conventional perpendicular plane. Much thicker sections are used than in conventional microscopy, and these are prepared with a special silver stain (e406,e431). By means of this technique, Schuffler and others have described a number of rare abnormalities of the myenteric plexus (e266,e334,e406). The submucosal plexus is usually normal. The onset of symptoms in the pediatric visceral neuropathies is usually between birth and the first few months of life. Depending on the location and length of the affected intestinal segment(s), symptoms include abdominal distension, vomiting, and constipation. Many of the visceral neuropathies in children show no familial pattern (e266), although familial forms are also known (e29,e68,e135,e267,e390). Familial forms of visceral myopathy involving the gastrointestinal tract have been reported (125).

Intestinal Neuronal Dysplasia

Isolated intestinal neuronal dysplasia has been described in the distal colon and rectum, and its clinical presentation, with constipation and intestinal obstruction, mimics that of Hirschsprung disease (e136,e399). Intestinal neuronal dysplasia type A is extremely rare, if it exists at all. The term has been used variously to describe either hypoganglionosis or complete aganglionosis, involving either the myenteric plexus alone or affecting both the myenteric and submucosal plexi (101) (e210,e255). Accepted diagnostic criteria have not been agreed upon. Neuronal intestinal dysplasia type B was first described and strictly defined by Meier-Ruge and Scharli (e399) in newborns with colonic obstruction, hyperplasia of the submucosal and myenteric plexuses, giant ganglia, and increased nerve fibers in acetylcholinesterase-stained frozen sections of bowel wall. The original definition required visualization of the myenteric plexus in a full-thickness biopsy specimen plus the demonstration of increased numbers of nerve fibers in acetylcholinesterase-stained frozen sections. Since the entity was first described, others proposed adjustments to the criteria so that the diagnosis could be made by rectal suction biopsy alone. This resulted in variable diagnostic criteria, continued controversy, and wide variations in the reported incidence of intestinal neuronal dysplasia (99) (e92). Some investigators believe that histologic features of intestinal neuronal dysplasia type B can be seen in suction biopsy specimens in a variety of clinical settings and that it is more a descriptive entity than a specific disease requiring surgical intervention (e90,e257,e322,e402,e403). Many patients in whom this condition was diagnosed by suction biopsy have improved over time with conservative measures exclusive of surgery (e90,e402,e427).

Diagnostic criteria developed by a consensus panel of European pathologists that were published in 1991 included obligatory features (hyperplasia of submucosal nerves, increased acetylcholinesterase activity in submucosal nerve fibers, and giant submucosal ganglia) as well as facilitative features (increased acetylcholinesterase activity in lamina propria nerve fibers and heterotopic ganglia in the lamina propria) (e50). At this time the disorder was recognized to affect only the submucosal nerve plexus, and thus diagnosis by sampling of the myenteric plexus is not possible. The criteria, which have been adopted by many clinical studies, have subsequently been revised and updated (140) (e317,e318). For instance, the number of ganglion cells defining a giant ganglion has varied from seven to nine (Figure 14-26). The subsequent recognition of age-dependent changes in the histologic features of the disease has led to further refinement of the diagnostic criteria. Specifically, the number of acetylcholinesterase-positive submucosal nerve fibers has been shown to decrease with age in affected patients (140).

Currently, some experts in the field have stated that the histologic diagnosis of intestinal neuronal dysplasia type B rests primarily upon the identification of giant submucosal ganglia, defined as a ganglion containing eight or more identifiable ganglion cells (102). If more than 20% of the submucosal ganglia in a rectal biopsy are giant ganglia, a diagnosis of intestinal neuronal hyperplasia is appropriate. However, since it is now recognized that giant ganglia are more numerous in premature infants and neonates, this diagnostic criterion is felt to be diagnostic only in patients more than 1 year of age. In addition, the criteria above were developed based on the examination of well-oriented frozen sections cut at 15 μm thickness and utilizing enzymatic histochemical stains for dehydrogenases to highlight ganglion cells. The applicability of these criteria to the evaluation of H&E stained 4 μm-thick paraffin sections is uncertain (102). The reproducibility of the histologic diagnosis of intestinal neuronal dysplasia type B remains poor (e258). It appears that even as currently defined the symptoms of patients with intestinal neuronal dysplasia type B improve with age and therefore conservative therapy is more appropriate that surgical treatment (131) (e257).

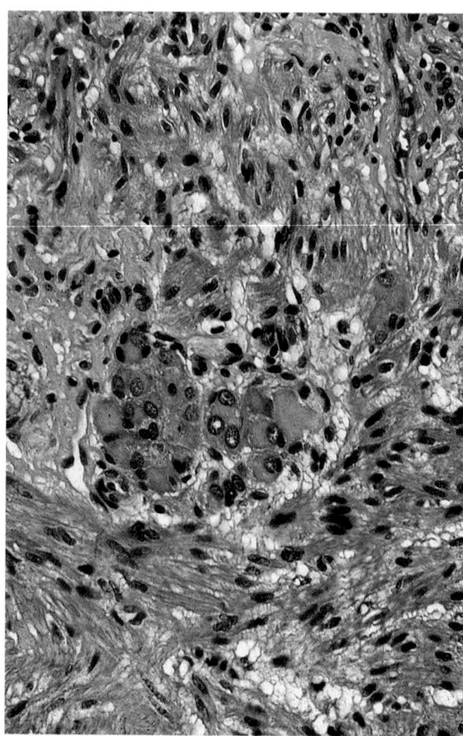

FIGURE 14-26 ■ Giant ganglion in a patient with intestinal neuronal dysplasia 400×.

Histological features overlapping with those of intestinal neuronal dysplasia type B have been reported in some patients with neurofibromatosis type I (von Recklinghausen disease) (e99,e140,e155,e414) and multiple endocrine neoplasia type IIB (e70,e99,e414). Intestinal neuronal dysplasia has also been described in association with Hirschsprung disease, at sites proximal to the classic aganglionic segment of Hirschsprung disease (e58,e369).

Acquired Diseases

Intussusception

Intussusception, or the invagination of a portion of the intestine into itself, is a relatively common pediatric surgical problem (e132). Infants, particularly those between 5 and 9 months of age, are most commonly affected. More than 90% of cases of childhood intussusception begin at the ileocecal valve, and the intussusceptum may reach as far as the descending colon or rectum. Progressive compression of the mesentery and blood supply of the invaginated bowel causes edema, hemorrhage, and ischemic necrosis. In the classic case, severe, intermittent, colicky pain begins suddenly in an infant, followed after a few hours by vomiting and the passage of blood and mucus from the rectum. Barium enema is both diagnostic and therapeutic. The obstructing mass of invaginated bowel can be recognized, and if the congestion and edema are not too advanced, the application of hydrostatic pressure by the radiologist reduces the intussusception. Operative reduction is required if barium enema reduction fails, as happens in 20% to 30% of cases (e511).

Gangrene of a portion of the intussusceptum necessitates segmental intestinal resection in approximately 10% of cases. These specimens exhibit edema, congestion, and coagulative and hemorrhagic necrosis indicative of combined ischemia and venous outflow obstruction.

In most cases, the cause is unknown. Large Peyer patches have been proposed as the possible lead point in many cases. Lymphoid hyperplasia due to adenovirus infection has been implicated in a subset of patients (Figure 14-27A to C) (16) (e327). Use of the first commercially available oral rotavirus vaccine was associated with an increased risk of intussusception in children, leading to withdrawal of the vaccine from the market (117). Newer generation vaccines do not appear to have this risk (34).

Approximately 10% of cases of childhood intussusception do not conform to the typical picture. In children past infancy and in atypically located intussusceptions (i.e., those not in

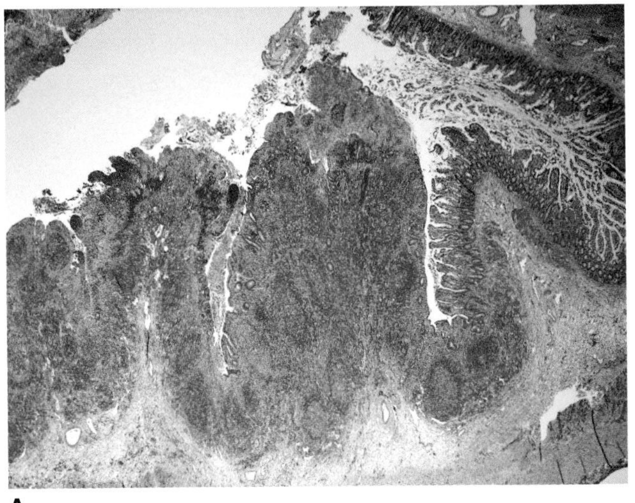

A

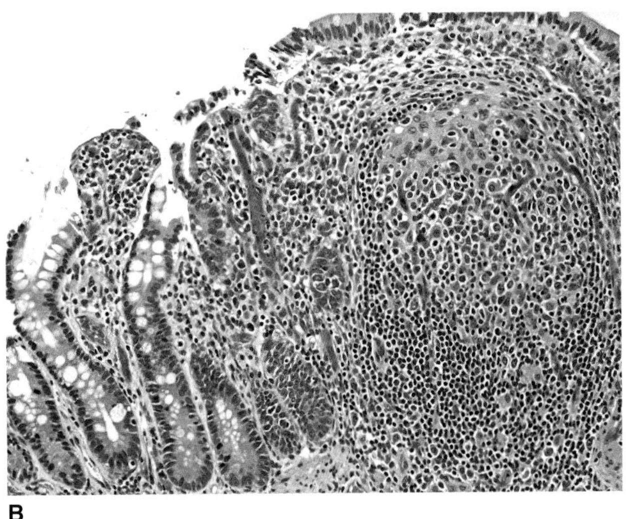

B

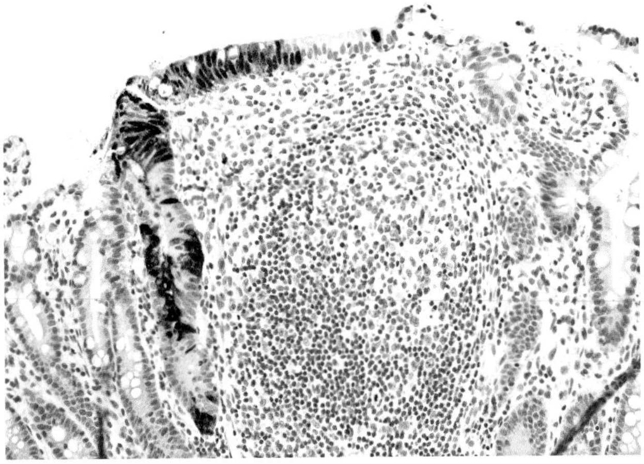

C

FIGURE 14-27 ▪ Small-bowel intussusception in an infant due to adenovirus infection. **A:** Histologic section from the lead point of the intussusception demonstrating lymphoid hyperplasia 20×. **B:** High power demonstrates smudgy intranuclear inclusion within enterocytes 200×. **C:** Immunostain utilizing an adenovirus antibody confirms the diagnosis 200×.

the ileocecal valve region), a discrete lead point is usually identified. Meckel diverticula, Peutz-Jeghers polyps, juvenile polyps, small-intestinal duplications, and Burkitt lymphoma have been implicated (70).

GASTROINTESTINAL INFECTIONS

Infections of the gastrointestinal tract are the leading cause of morbidity in infants and children in all parts of the world (e188) (Table 14-4). Mortality resulting from this group of illnesses is common in infants in underdeveloped countries where malnutrition contributes to the poor outcome. In developed countries, gastroenteritis and diarrhea are frequent causes of illness, but they seldom cause death because nutrition is better and medical care and intravenous fluids are available (e165).

In the 1970s, viruses, particularly rotavirus, were identified as the causal agents in more than half the cases of gastroenteritis and diarrhea worldwide. In developed countries, bacterial infections account for approximately 15% of hospitalized cases of diarrhea. Many of the causative strains have been identified only relatively recently; these include *Clostridium difficile*, *Campylobacter jejuni*, *H. pylori*, *Yersinia enterocolitica*, and the enteroinvasive, toxigenic, and hemorrhagic strains of *Escherichia coli*. The AIDS epidemic and advances in immunosuppressive chemotherapy have led to recognition of "new" organisms. At the same time, rapid advances in microbiologic, serologic, and molecular diagnosis have made it possible to identify them in patients.

Viral Diarrhea

Most cases of acute infection, gastroenteritis, and diarrhea in infants and children are caused by viruses (e43,e66). Typically, the viruses localize in the small intestine and cause a noninflammatory, watery diarrhea; neutrophils and red blood cells are not found in the stool. Patients usually have nausea, vomiting, and low-grade fever. Infants are often quite ill and may become severely dehydrated.

Rotaviruses

Rotaviruses have been extensively studied (e43, e148,e467). Group A rotaviruses are responsible for

Table 14-4 ■ PEDIATRIC GASTROINTESTINAL INFECTIONS

Organism	Location	Symptom/Syndrome	Histology	Means of Diagnosis
Bacteria				
Helicobacter pylori	Stomach, especially antrum	Epigastric abdominal pain in surface	Active chronic nonspecific gastritis; organisms visible muous coat	Histologic identification of bacilli on biopsy, culture of endoscopic biopsy
Salmonella (*S. enteritidis, S. typhi, S. cholerasuis*)	Distal SI, especially ileum, colon	Gastroenteritis, inflammatory bloody, mucoid stools; enteric (typhoid) fever	Acute enteritis with exudation, hemorrhage, focal ulceration; acute infective colitis; hypertrophy, necrosis and macrophage infiltration of Peyer patches, mesenteric LN	Stool culture, blood culture (*S. typhi*)
Shigella	Colon, distal SI	Bloody, mucoid stools, diarrhea, cramps, fever, convulsions	Acute infective colitis.	Stool culture
Vibrio cholerae	SI	Massive watery diarrhea and dehydration	Minimal change	Stool culture
Escherichia coli				
Enteropathogenic	SI	Diarrhea	Enteritis; may show villous atrophy	Stool culture and serotyping
Enterotoxigenic	SI	Watery diarrhea, traveler's diarrhea	Minimal change	Stool culture and serotyping
Enteroinvasive	Distal SI, colon	Bloody, mucoid diarrhea	Acute infective colitis	Stool culture and serotyping
Enterohemorrhagic	Colon, distal SI	Bloody diarrhea hemolytic uremic syndrome	Acute infective colitis	Stool culture on selective medium, serotyping, toxin assay
Campylobacter jejuni	SI, colon	Abdominal pain, diarrhea, bloody stools	Acute enteritis, acute infective colitis, acute appendicitis, mesenteric adenitis	Stool culture
Yersinia enterocolitica	Entire GI tract especially ileum, appendix, colon	Diarrhea, abdominal pain, fever	Enteritis with ulcerations and microabscesses; terminal ileitis mimicking Crohn disease; necrotizing appendicitis; acute infective colitis with apthoid ulceration; mesenteric adenitis	Stool culture
Clostridium difficile	Colon	Pseudomembranous colitis, antibiotic-associated diarrhea	Pseudomembranous colitis; acute colitis	Toxin assay on stools
Listeria monocytogenes	SI, colon; systemic spread in immuno-suppressed	Fever, gastroenteritis	ND for GI tract	Stool culture, rectal swab on selective media
Aeromonas	Colon, SI	Acute watery diarrhea; dysenteric-like illness, colitis	Acute colitis	Stool culture
Mycobacterium avium complex	SI, colon	Diarrhea, abdominal pain, malabsorption in AIDS	Acid-fast bacilli in macrophages throughout lamina propria	Identification of acid-fast bacilli in macrophages in lamina propria of intestinal biopsy
Fungi				
Candida	All GI tract	Depends on location	Pseudohyphae and yeast forms with acute inflammation	Fungal stain on biopsy
Protozoa				
Giardia lamblia	Proximal SI	Diarrhea, malabsorption; failure to thrive	Proximal SI changes range from minimal change to chronic inflammation and villous atrophy; organisms on H&E	Stool examination for cysts; mucus smears of intestinal biopsy; identification visible of trophozoites on proximal SI biopsy

(*Continued*)

Table 14-4 ■ PEDIATRIC GASTROINTESTINAL INFECTIONS *(Continued)*

Organism	Location	Symptom/Syndrome	Histology	Means of Diagnosis
Crytosporidium	Small intestine in normal hosts; stomach, SI and colon in AIDS patients	Watery diarrhea	Minimal change or mild, nonspecific enteritis; organisms visible on H and E	Stool examination for cysts; identification by histologic examination of proximal SI biopsy
Entamoeba histolytica	Colon	Hematochezia; diarrhea; bloody, mucoid diarrhea	Diffuse acute colitis, microulcerations; deep ulcers undermining mucosa, organism visible on H and E	Stool examination for trophozoites and cysts; identification of trophozoites on histologic examination of colonic biopsy; serology; identification of organism on biopsy
Viruses				
Rotavirus	SI	Watery diarrhea, vomiting	Enterocyte necrosis, partial villous atrophy, mononuclear inflammation	Stool ELISA
Norwalk virus	SI	Watery diarrhea, vomiting	See text	Stool ELISA, PCR on stool
Adenovirus	Colon, SI	Diarrhea	Inclusions in surface epithelium	Identification of inclusion on biopsy
Astrovirus	ND	Diarrhea	ND	ELISA on stool
Calicivirus	ND	Diarrhea	ND	
Cytomegalovirus	All parts of GI tract	GI bleeding; hemorrhagic colitis; esophagitis	Focal necrotizing colitis, esophagitis, gastritis; inclusions visible in endothelium and mesenchymal cells	Identification of inclusions on endoscopic biopsy, culture of biopsy or stool
Herpes simplex	Esophagus, colon	Esophagitis, colitis	Small focal (apthous) ulcerations, inclusion in epithelium	Identification of inclusions on biopsy, culture of biopsy

GI, gastrointestinal; H and E, hematoxylin and eosin; LN, lymph node; SI, small intestine; ND, not described; ELISA, enzyme-linked immunosorbent assay; RT-PCR, reverse transcriptase polymerase chain reaction.

approximately 50% of hospitalized cases of diarrhea in all parts of the world (e105,e148). Children younger than 2 years are most susceptible; they are usually ill for 4 to 7 days and are most likely to be admitted to a hospital for treatment of dehydration resulting from watery diarrhea and vomiting. Rotavirus was first identified by electron microscopy in small-intestinal epithelial cells and later in the stools of infants with diarrhea. Rotavirus infection was formerly diagnosed by the ultrastructural identification of virus particles in stools, but this method has been replaced by ELISA of stool samples. Biopsies are almost never performed during the acute illness, but several morphologic studies have shown proximal small-intestinal mucosal injury with surface enterocyte necrosis, partial villous atrophy, and chronic inflammation in the lamina propria (e27,e105,e501). The loss of enterocytes greatly reduces the capacity of the intestine to absorb fluid and electrolytes, and the effect is compounded when damage to brush border enzymes results in malabsorption. The mucosa takes 3 to 8 weeks to recover; during this time, malabsorption may persist (e105). Immunodeficient patients may take months to clear the virus and suffer a more chronic illness. Rotavirus vaccines are now available.

Norwalk Virus

Norwalk virus is the second most commonly encountered cause of viral gastroenteritis. Cases tend to occur in clusters, and epidemics are more frequent in children of school age than in infants. This is a briefer, less severe illness characterized by vomiting and watery diarrhea. No method to diagnose this infection is readily available, although immune electron microscopy and recently developed ELISAs to detect viral antigen and antibody responses are used in reference laboratories. Only samples taken from patients during diarrhea epidemics are likely to be studied by these means. Histologic studies are sparse, but villous blunting, infiltration of mononuclear cells and neutrophils into the lamina propria, and vacuolization of enterocytes have been described (e2,e404).

Electron microscopic studies of stool specimens during outbreaks of gastroenteritis and diarrhea have led to the identification of other viruses, although none of these is encountered as often as rotavirus and Norwalk virus.

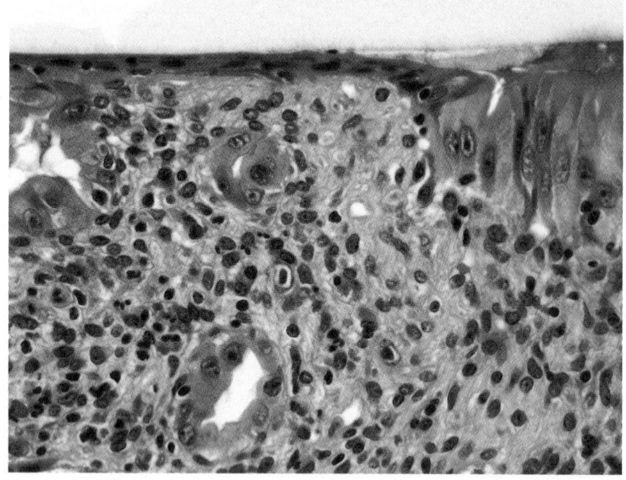
A

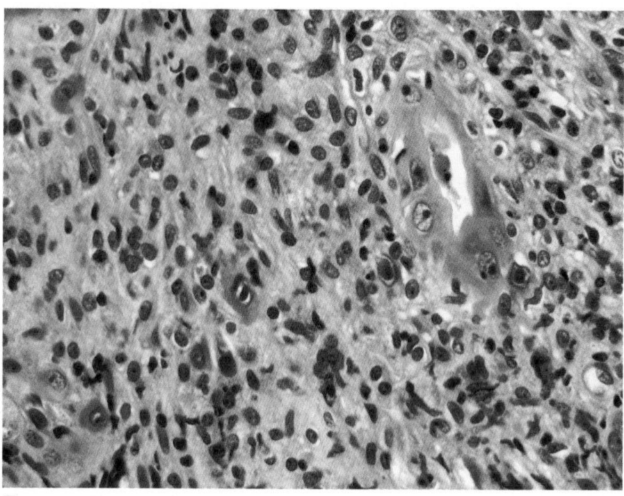
B

FIGURE 14-28■CMV colitis in a child status post stem cell transplantation. **A:** Mild colitis is evident in this biopsy 400×. **B:** Several classic intranuclear viral inclusions are present 400×.

Enteric Adenovirus

Enteric adenoviruses are serologically distinct from respiratory adenoviruses, and for a long time they eluded detection except by electron microscopy and difficult immunologic methods not widely available (e293). Several outbreaks of enteric adenovirus gastroenteritis have been described in normal infants, and this infection is probably a common cause of pediatric viral gastroenteritis. Immunocompromised patients, particularly those with AIDS, are highly susceptible to adenovirus infection (e264,e292,e508). Patients with solid organ and bone marrow transplants are also at risk (e147,e418,e442).

Nonspecific watery diarrhea with vomiting, dehydration, and abdominal pain characterizes the illness (e467). Lactose intolerance and other malabsorptive states may follow adenovirus enteritis and last for months. Adenovirus nuclear inclusions can be identified by light microscopy within infected surface epithelial cells, but the presence of adenovirus should be confirmed by immunohistochemical stains or electron microscopy (e508). Enteric adenovirus infection can result in small intestinal mucosal lymphoid hyperplasia, which can form the lead point of an intussusception (Figure 14-27A–C).

Cytomegalovirus

Gastrointestinal infection with CMV has become a significant clinical problem in persons with bone marrow or solid organ transplants and in patients with AIDS or other conditions associated with immune compromise (e368,e389). Occasional cases have been reported in patients with ulcerative colitis and Crohn disease. Any site in the gastrointestinal tract can be affected, from esophagus to colon. In the most severe cases, the patient often also has evidence of a systemic infection, with CMV pneumonia, hepatitis, and retinitis. Symptoms vary according to the affected site of the gastrointestinal tract. Particularly characteristic is a fulminant hemorrhagic colitis with multiple focal ulcerations resulting from CMV vasculitis and thrombosis; this sometimes leads to toxic megacolon, necrotizing colitis, and intestinal perforation (e14,e152,e319). Esophageal involvement is usually distal, with ulcerations and erythema. Gastric and small-intestinal involvement is also generally manifested as erosions and ulcerations. Because it tends to affect blood vessels, CMV infection often presents with gastrointestinal bleeding. The diagnosis is made by endoscopic biopsy, with typical inclusion bodies usually seen in vascular endothelium, mesenchymal cells of the lamina propria, and more rarely in glandular epithelial cells (Figure 14-28A,B). Inclusions are not seen in squamous cells (e389). Variable degrees of acute and chronic inflammation, vasculitis, thrombosis, and ulceration are present, depending on the extent of the infection and the degree of ulceration.

Herpes Simplex Virus

Gastrointestinal infection with this group of viruses is usually limited to immunosuppressed patients, although herpes esophagitis occasionally develops in normal children. In the gastrointestinal tract, herpesvirus most commonly causes esophagitis (see previous section) or proctocolitis. At both sites aphthous and more extensive ulceration is characteristic. Viral cytopathic changes and inclusions are most commonly seen in squamous epithelium, but glandular epithelium and mesenchymal cells may also be involved. The accompanying inflammation commonly contains neutrophils and histiocytes (e305,e389).

Other Viruses

Other recently described viruses associated with gastroenteritis include coronaviruses, astroviruses, (e206,e323) and caliciviruses (e28,e323).

Bacterial Diarrhea

Bacteria cause diarrhea through multiple pathophysiologic mechanisms that are categorized as inflammatory or noninflammatory (e176,e379). *Salmonella* species, *Shigella* species, and *Campylobacter jejuni* are the most common causes of inflammatory infectious diarrhea in children (e85), with *C. difficile*, *Y. enterocolitica*, enteroinvasive *E. coli,* and the protozoan *Entamoeba histolytica* causing a similar picture. Most of these organisms invade the mucosa, usually in the colon and distal small intestine, and cause epithelial necrosis and a neutrophilic response. The same inflammatory response may be elicited by the cytotoxins of some noninvasive pathogens, such as *C. difficile*, and some toxin-producing *E. coli*, including enterohemorrhagic *E. coli* 0157:H7 (e85). Dysentery is said to be present if inflammatory diarrhea is accompanied by systemic manifestations such as fever, abdominal pain, and prostration. The stool contains neutrophils, mucus, and blood. A mucosal biopsy is not usually obtained if the organism is identified by stool culture, but a biopsy may be performed in a patient with infectious colitis before the organism is cultured or if rectal bleeding persists. The pathologist may be asked to distinguish infection from ulcerative colitis or Crohn disease (e337,e448).

In contrast, organisms causing noninflammatory diarrhea exert their effect through a toxin or other mechanism without penetration of the intestinal mucosa. Watery diarrhea is characteristic, and neutrophils and blood are not found in the stool. The tissue response is less pronounced and usually localized to the small intestine. Examples of organisms causing noninflammatory infectious diarrhea include *Vibrio cholerae*, *C. jejuni*, enteropathogenic *E. coli*, enterotoxigenic *E. coli*, and some Salmonella organisms. *Giardia lamblia*, *Cryptosporidium*, and viruses, especially rotaviruses, are nonbacterial causes of noninflammatory diarrhea.

Salmonella

Salmonella-induced diarrhea is a worldwide food-borne and waterborne illness. In the United States and Canada, infants and children are most often affected. In a large series of infants with diarrhea at the Hospital for Sick Children, Toronto, *Salmonella* organisms were the most common bacterial pathogens isolated. Infants may present with the acute onset of watery diarrhea, abdominal pain, and fever, but a dysenteric presentation with mucus, pus, and blood in the stools is also encountered (e108,e311). *Salmonella* organisms penetrate the intestinal mucosa and invade the submucosa, stimulating a neutrophilic response, epithelial necrosis with focal ulceration, hyperemia, and sometimes hemorrhage. In typhoid fever (*Salmonella typhi* infection), the organisms are carried by macrophages to intestinal lymphoid tissues, particularly Peyer patches, which become hyperplastic and necrotic. From there, bacilli enter the bloodstream. Morbidity and mortality are high (e457). The more common childhood enteric infections with other strains of *Salmonella* (*S. enteritidis* and *S. typhimurium*) are usually acquired through the ingestion of contaminated eggs, poultry, and other animal products, and their course is more self-limited. The histology of the usually self-limited acute enteritis caused by *Salmonella* species is rarely observed in clinical practice. However, a colonic mucosal biopsy specimen is occasionally encountered and shows nonspecific edema, neutrophilic exudate in the lamina propria and epithelium, and crypt abscesses (e180). Rarely does a colonic biopsy in salmonellosis show the florid crypt abscess formation, goblet cell depletion, and chronic crypt alterations characteristic of ulcerative colitis. Patients with AIDS are especially susceptible to severe Salmonella infections, sometimes with enterocolitis and bacteremia that are resistant to therapy (e284).

Shigella

Shigella dysenteriae is the prototype organism producing dysentery (the frequent passage of bloody mucoid stools with fever and abdominal cramps) (e282). *Shigella dysenteriae* and *Shigella flexneri* are the species responsible for most infections in developing countries (e11), and *Shigella sonnei* is usually isolated in industrialized countries. Direct invasion of the colonic epithelium and lamina propria by the organism causes cell death, ulceration, and hemorrhage. *Shigella* also produces potent toxins, known as Shiga toxins, which compound the intestinal damage. *Shigella* colitis is characterized by superficial ulceration, purulent mucosal exudate, and, in severe cases, confluent hemorrhagic necrosis of large areas of mucosa with pseudomembrane formation. The microscopic picture is that of an acute colitis with ulceration, crypt abscess formation, and goblet cell depletion (eFigure 14–6). In fulminant cases distinction from ulcerative colitis can be difficult in the absence of culture results (e436).

The potent Shiga toxins produce watery diarrhea in some cases and also have far-reaching effects throughout the body (e242,e282). Hemolytic-uremic syndrome is known to occur after shigellosis in a small percentage of children (e263,e288). Thrombotic thrombocytopenic purpura, a similar illness with more central nervous system manifestations, is the adult counterpart of hemolytic-uremic syndrome. Both these conditions are caused by Shiga toxin and a group of similar toxins, Shiga-like toxins, produced by enterohemorrhagic strains of *E. coli*, particularly 0157:H7. Shiga toxin not only affects the gastrointestinal tract but also exerts a cytotoxic effect on endothelial cells throughout the body and is a neurotoxin. The toxin causes extensive platelet fibrin thrombi to form in small blood vessels, impairing perfusion to vital organs. Hemolytic-uremic syndrome, a microangiopathic hemolytic anemia, results from the effect of the toxin on the kidneys. In the most severe cases, acute renal failure may follow the thrombotic microangiopathic renal process (see Chapter 17).

Vibrio Cholerae

Cholera is rarely encountered in developed countries, but it is an important cause of morbidity and mortality in children worldwide. Cholera is a classic example of enterotoxigenic diarrhea, in which massive fecal fluid losses rapidly lead to dehydration in the absence of any tissue invasion by the organism, whose enterotoxin stimulates the secretion of water and electrolytes and inhibits absorption by epithelial cells (e375). Morphologic changes are minimal. Surface epithelium of the small intestine remains intact, and at most, a mild increase in cellularity of the lamina propria and vascular congestion are observed (e104).

Escherichia coli

Various strains of *E. coli* were first recognized as stool pathogens after the development of specific serotyping, which made it possible to differentiate them from normal gut flora. More recent molecular, genetic, and biochemical differences have led to the identification of many classes of *E. coli* that cause diarrhea, with a different pathogenesis and clinical picture for each (e176).

Enteropathogenic *E. coli* was the first of these to be identified in association with epidemics of diarrhea in infant hospital wards, nurseries, and day care centers. It is one of the major causes of bacterial diarrhea in infants worldwide and is also one cause of traveler's diarrhea in adults who visit underdeveloped countries. It produces a toxin that acts on the small-intestinal epithelium to produce profuse watery diarrhea. Numerous serotypes have been identified, but serologic testing is usually performed only in epidemic clusters and not in sporadic cases. Electron microscopy of infected small intestine shows adherence of the bacteria to the brush border of enterocytes, with dissolution of microvilli. Adherent *E. coli* can sometimes be identified on the intestinal epithelial surface, associated with villous atrophy and inflammation of the lamina propria. Enterotoxigenic strains of *E. coli* produce secretory enterotoxins and commonly cause watery diarrhea in children and adults in developing countries, in addition to traveler's diarrhea. Occasional outbreaks from contaminated food or water are reported in developed countries. A cholera-like illness characterized by noninflammatory watery diarrhea results from the effect of bacterial toxin on the small intestine. The illness is usually self-limited and resolves in a few days unless the child is malnourished or very young. Enteroinvasive *E. coli* affects the colon rather than the small intestine. It invades the mucosa, much like *Shigella*, and in severe cases produces a similar dysenteric disease, with bloody and mucoid diarrhea, neutrophils in the stool, and systemic symptoms, including fever, headache, myalgia, and abdominal pain.

Enterohemorrhagic *E. coli* was first identified in the early 1980s in association with outbreaks of hemorrhagic colitis in children and adults in North America (e52,e85,e180,e393). It is a commensal in a small percentage of beef cattle and is usually spread to humans through the ingestion of undercooked ground beef or contamination of fruits or vegetables. It produces a Shiga-like toxin (verotoxin) that shares many features with the Shiga toxin of *Shigella* (e237,e242,e393). The most notorious enterohemorrhagic serotype is *E. coli* 0157:H7, which has been responsible for numerous epidemics and sporadic cases of hemorrhagic colitis in the past decade (e52,e56,e85,e237,e335,e380). In contrast to most *E. coli* strains, *E. coli* 0157:H7 does not ferment sorbitol and can thus be recognized by a characteristic pattern on a selective growth medium, sorbitol-MacConkey agar. Since its recognition and the development of a relatively easy method of identification, E. coli 0157:H7 has been detected more frequently than *Shigella*, averaging approximately 21,000 infections and 240 deaths per year in the United States alone (e52). The Shiga-like toxin causes endothelial damage in the kidney, which results in hemolytic-uremic syndrome in 6% of infected persons, usually young children. It is the most common cause of hemolytic-uremic syndrome in North America (e52,e56,e237,e380). In older patients, the toxin may cause thrombotic thrombocytopenic purpura. In epidemics in the United States, approximately one-fourth of infected persons become ill enough to be hospitalized. The toxin produces watery stools at first, which progress to bloody diarrhea over several days. Abdominal pain, diarrhea, and rectal bleeding may mimic ulcerative colitis or appendicitis. Stool is negative for leukocytes in mild infections but positive in more severe cases. Endoscopy shows colonic edema, hyperemia, superficial ulcers, and, in the most severe cases, pseudomembranous colitis.

The early histopathology consists of focal hemorrhagic colitis with ischemic changes, edema, and acute inflammation in the superficial mucosa, which progress to confluent ulceration and pseudomembrane formation in the most severe cases (Figure 14-29). Small blood vessels in the lamina propria and submucosa may contain platelet-fibrin thrombi, and occasional vasculitis is responsible for the superficial ischemic changes and hemorrhage (108) (e180,e245,e380). Most of the fatalities are associated with the complications of hemolytic-uremic syndrome. Although *E. coli* 0157:H7 has achieved notoriety, at least 100 other serotypes of enterohemorrhagic *E. coli* have been reported to cause bloody diarrhea via Shiga toxin production, and several of these

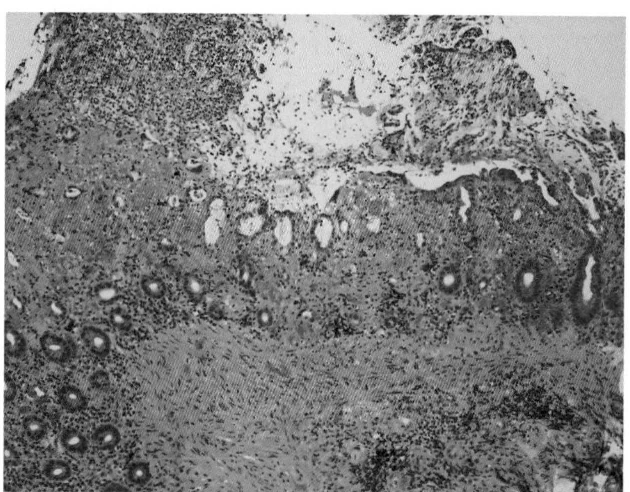

FIGURE 14-29 ■ Colitis due to *E. coli* O157:H7. The combination of histologic features of infectious colitis seen at each end of the biopsy and ischemic changes in the middle of the biopsy is typical of this infection 200×.

also cause hemolytic-uremic syndrome (e381). Many of the non-0157:H7 enterohemorrhagic *E. coli* strains are not detected on sorbitol-MacConkey agar but demonstrate production of Shiga-like toxin. Assay for Shiga toxin is indicated in the clinical situation of bloody diarrhea, especially if culture on sorbitol-MacConkey agar does not yield growth characteristic of *E. coli* 0157:H7.

Unfortunately, none of the pathogenic strains of *E. coli* can be identified on routine stool culture. Some microbiology laboratories routinely screen for *E. coli* 0157:H7 with selective media, but some do not. A sporadic case of enteropathogenic or enterohemorrhagic *E. coli* can easily elude diagnosis. *E. coli* is rarely serotyped in sporadic cases of noninflammatory diarrhea; only reference laboratories perform this procedure with any degree of regularity, and most detailed investigations are saved for outbreaks or clusters.

Campylobacter jejuni

Campylobacter jejuni is now the major cause of acute bacterial diarrhea in older infants and children in developed countries (e45,e236,e385,e430). Virtually unknown as recently as the early 1970s because of the unique conditions required for it to grow in culture, *C. jejuni* is now isolated as often as *Salmonella, Shigella,* and enteropathogenic strains of *E. coli* from children with diarrhea. Ordinary laboratory stool culture techniques are unsatisfactory to isolate this fastidious organism; a microaerophilic environment and selective media must be used. *Campylobacter* infection is acquired from animals in which the organism is a commensal, including pets and poultry, and from contaminated water or milk. The infection presents with abdominal pain, low-grade fever, and diarrhea that becomes bloody after a few days. Direct examination of the stool usually shows neutrophils. The illness is usually self-limited and lasts approximately one week, but it may linger for 5 or 6 weeks or relapse after initial improvement. Jejunum, ileum, colon, rectum, and appendix may all be affected. *Campylobacter* colitis may be sufficiently severe to mimic Crohn disease, with cobblestone mucosa and aphthous ulcers. Toxic megacolon has also been described. Rectal and colonic biopsy specimens show an infective proctocolitis with edema, neutrophils in the lamina propria, and crypt abscesses (eFigure 14-7) (e86,e367,e499).

Yersinia enterocolitica

Yersinia enterocolitica is a Gram-negative coccobacillus known to cause diarrhea, gastroenteritis, and mesenteric adenitis in older children; more rarely, it causes enterocolitis, appendicitis, arthritis, erythema nodosum, and sepsis (e54,e57). In children younger than 5 years of age, a mild, self-limiting, febrile gastroenteritis lasting 1 to 2 weeks is characteristic (e297). In more severe cases in older children, fever, leukocytosis, and abdominal symptoms may be mistaken for appendicitis and a laparotomy performed unnecessarily; in this situation, inflammation of the terminal ileum, cecum, appendix, and mesenteric lymph nodes is found, often with an inflammatory mass in the ileocecal region, mimicking Crohn disease (e54,e60,e91,e168,e478). In severe cases, extensive ulceration and inflammation of the small intestine and colon, sepsis, and extraintestinal abscesses may develop. Microabscesses and neutrophilic infiltrate characterize the tissue response in *Yersinia* infection; the sarcoidlike granulomas of Crohn disease do not occur (eFigure 14-8A,B). Gram-negative coccobacilli may be found in microabscesses and areas of mucosal necrosis and within the generally enlarged and sometimes necrotic lymphoid tissue (e54,e60).

Y. enterocolitica is usually identified by stool culture. The organism grows on standard selective stool culture media, such as MacConkey agar, but overgrowth of normal flora makes identification difficult unless specific subculturing and other identification techniques are used. The anatomic pathologist may encounter relatively severe or prolonged cases of *Yersinia* infection in a variety of circumstances: acute inflammation and mucosal ulceration of the colon, necrotizing appendicitis and periappendicitis, terminal ileitis thought to be Crohn disease, or even severe mesenteric lymphadenitis mistaken for intestinal lymphoma.

Clostridium difficile

Clostridium difficile is best known as a cause of pseudomembranous colitis, but it is also responsible for many cases of antibiotic-associated diarrhea without pseudomembranous colitis, in addition to occasional cases of diarrhea unrelated to antibiotic exposure (e30,e244). It is a common nosocomial pathogen that is notoriously difficult to eradicate once established (e244,e310). Most of the work implicating this organism as a human enteric pathogen dates from the late 1970s. Before this, *C. difficile* was extremely difficult to isolate and culture from fecal flora, hence its designation "difficile." Since then, it has been shown that this Gram-negative anaerobe can be recovered from the intestine of only 2% to 3% of normal adults. In adults and children over the age of 2 years, antibiotic treatment alters normal gut flora and allows intestinal overgrowth of *C. difficile* from endogenous and exogenous sources, which leads to diarrhea. In this age group and setting, *C. difficile* is a pathogen. More rarely, *C. difficile* causes diarrhea, with or without pseudomembranes, in an older child without antecedent antibiotic therapy. Neutropenic patients and those with inflammatory bowel disease are susceptible to such infections, although healthy children are also occasionally affected (31,115). The *C. difficile* strains that cause disease produce potent toxins that induce fluid secretion and colonic mucosal necrosis and inflammation. The diagnosis of *C. difficile* infection is usually established by demonstrating *C. difficile* toxins in stool with a commercially available enzyme immunoassay (e244). Stool culture for the organism is also performed in many centers.

The situation in infants is more complex. *C. difficile* is harbored in 30% to 70% of healthy neonates, in whom the organism may produce toxin without causing disease

(23,147) (e123). The carriage rate decreases abruptly in the first 5 months of life but does not decline to adult levels until approximately 2 years of age (e440,e491). However, *C. difficile* is known to cause severe disease in certain groups of young infants, particularly those with Hirschsprung disease and malignancies, in whom organisms can be demonstrated invading colonic mucosa (e373). Recently, a hypervirulent strain of *C. difficile* has emerged as an important cause of nosocomial colitis in hospitalized patients, including children (23,147).

C. difficile colitis ranges in severity from mild watery diarrhea noticed shortly after the initiation of antibiotic therapy, which can be controlled merely by discontinuing antibiotic therapy, to severe colitis with or without pseudomembranous colitis (see "Pseudomembranous Colitis"). A characteristic form of necrotizing enteropathy may also be seen, in which focal superficial or deep areas of coagulative necrosis and ulceration are surrounded by neutrophils, with sparing of intervening areas. Marked submucosal edema is also characteristic. The Gram-positive organisms can be seen invading tissue; the large size of the bacilli and spore formation are unique in this setting. Metronidazole and vancomycin are used to treat the more severe cases. Relapse of infection following therapy and the development of vancomycin-resistant strains are emerging problems. Surgical intervention may be required in extreme cases.

Aeromonas

In the 1990s, Aeromonas species were increasingly implicated in a variety of gastrointestinal illnesses, although they are still relatively uncommon isolates in the microbiology laboratory. In young children, acute watery diarrhea (e76) or gastroenteritis (e397) is the usual presentation. More rarely, especially in adults, an acute dysenteric illness is seen, sometimes with a severe colitis mimicking chronic inflammatory bowel disease (e137).

Protozoal Infections

Giardia lamblia (Intestinalis)

Giardia lamblia is a flagellated protozoan capable of causing diarrhea and malabsorption in human hosts (e128) (Table 14-4). In some parts of the world, cyst forms of the organism can be frequently identified in the stools of asymptomatic carriers, but in developed countries, ingestion of the organism usually leads to clinically apparent illness. Toddlers and children and persons with selective IgA deficiency and other primary immunodeficiencies are more susceptible to infection. Case clusters of giardiasis have been reported in day care centers and residential institutions. Travelers drinking untreated water in Rocky Mountain areas and in the Soviet Union are also at risk.

Affected children manifest diarrhea, nausea, weight loss, malabsorption, and failure to thrive. The host ingests the cyst form of the organism. In the proximal small intestine, the cyst wall dissolves and trophozoites are released; these adhere to the brush border of epithelial cells, damaging the microvilli. In small-intestinal biopsy specimens, trophozoites are 10 to 18 μm long, have an arched or curved appearance at high levels of magnification, and are visible at the surface of enterocytes or in the mucous coat (eFigure 14-9). They do not invade tissue. The trophozoites can be highlighted with a trichrome stain or CD117 immunostain.

In immunocompetent hosts, the degree of intestinal reaction varies from insignificant to severe. The villous architecture is usually normal, but increased numbers of chronic inflammatory cells and eosinophils in the lamina propria and increased numbers of IELs may be seen. Patients with severe diarrhea and malabsorption show variable degrees of villous atrophy and more severe chronic inflammation (e339). Patients with selective IgA deficiency or other immunodeficiency syndromes are highly susceptible to giardiasis, and villous atrophy and inflammation are usually more severe in these cases (e200). Identification of Giardia in the intestine should prompt consideration of an immunodeficiency, although normal infants and children can also become infected.

In approximately one-third of patients, giardiasis becomes chronic and causes secondary effects of malabsorption, including macrocytic anemia, lactose malabsorption with bloating, and growth impairment. The diagnosis is best accomplished by microscopic examination of stool specimens for Giardia cysts. Commercial ELISAs are available to detect Giardia antigens in stool. All too often, however, microscopic examination of a duodenal biopsy specimen will provide the first clue that a patient has giardiasis.

Cryptosporidium

Cryptosporidium was first identified as a human pathogen in 1976, as a rare cause of self-limited, watery diarrhea in immunocompetent persons (e95,e223,e279). Clusters of diarrhea in day care centers and families have been described. In the early 1980s, Cryptosporidium was identified with increasing frequency as a cause of severe chronic diarrhea in patients with AIDS, and cryptosporidiosis as one of the opportunistic infections that often heralds the onset of AIDS (e187). Once immunodeficient patients are infected, they are plagued with chronic diarrhea, which is often severe and difficult to eradicate. Cryptosporidium species are present in a large number of domestic and wild animals. Both zoonotic and person-to-person spread occurs. In 1993, a widely publicized outbreak in Milwaukee, Wisconsin, was traced to contamination of the municipal water supply (e290). Oocysts are ingested orally and progress through stages of the life cycle in the proximal small intestine where they are recognized on the surface of epithelial cells in mucosal biopsy specimens as a line of spherical basophilic structures 3 to 4 μm in diameter. They are recognizable with hematoxylin and eosin stains, but they also may be stained with Giemsa. They usually cause minimal morphologic changes in the intestine except for chronic inflammatory infiltration of the lamina propria

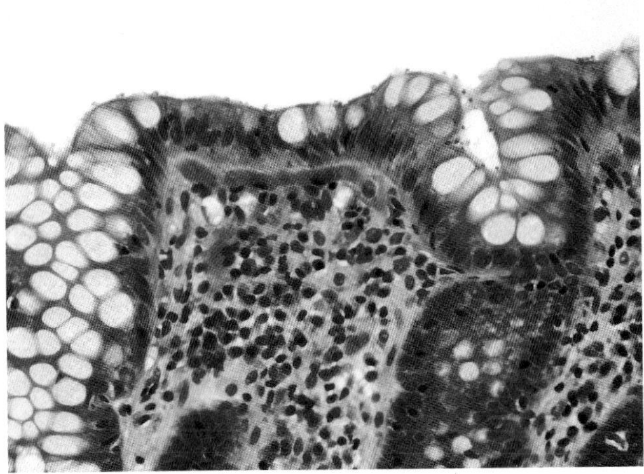

FIGURE 14-30▪Colonic cryptosporidium infection. Numerous small dot-like organisms line the crypt luminal surfaces 400×.

(Figure 14-30). Electron microscopy reveals destruction of enterocyte microvilli. Diagnosis is accomplished by microscopic examination of stool specimens for oocysts with an acid-fast stain. ELISA kits are commercially available to aid in the detection of oocysts. The infection is self-limited in normal hosts. No satisfactory treatment is available for chronic infection in immunosuppressed persons.

Entamoeba histolytica

Entamoeba histolytica infection (amebiasis) is a major cause of diarrhea in third world countries (e320,e361,e364). In the United States, it is diagnosed most often in southwestern states, especially in Hispanic patients and those who have recently traveled to Latin America. Infection may be asymptomatic (carrier state), or it may cause isolated hematochezia or a dysentery-like syndrome with diarrhea and blood and mucus in the stools. Children often acquire the organism by fecal-oral transmission from an asymptomatic adult and are more likely than adults to become ill when infected. The diagnosis is made by finding cysts or trophozoites in fresh stool smears or trophozoites in biopsy material. The diagnosis may also be made serologically by an elevated indirect hemaglutination titer.

In acute amebic infection, the organism invades the colon and causes a diffuse acute inflammation that may be difficult to distinguish from ulcerative colitis or Crohn disease, both endoscopically and pathologically. Rectal biopsy specimens often show no more than edema, scattered intraepithelial and lamina propria neutrophils, and a mild increase in lamina propria cellularity. Superficial microscopic ulcerations usually indicate invasion of the trophozoites into the lamina propria. Organisms resemble large, pale histiocytes, 15 to 30 μm in diameter, with a pale nucleus and ingested red blood cells in the cytoplasm. They may be found in the surface mucous coat or in the superficial lamina propria beneath a microscopic ulceration (Figure 14-31A to D). Organisms are not found in up to 50% of rectal biopsy specimens from patients with acute-onset amebiasis (e361). Examination of stool smears is a more sensitive method of diagnosis. In advanced cases, amebiasis causes multiple ulcerations, particularly in the cecum and ascending colon. Microscopically, these have a characteristic flask shape at low levels of magnification, a consequence of epithelial undermining. At this stage, abundant trophozoites are found in the intestinal wall. Sequelae include intestinal perforation, peritonitis, lymphatic and hematogenous dissemination, and systemic amebiasis.

Fungal Disease of the Gastrointestinal Tract

Candida is regarded as part of the normal flora in healthy persons. It becomes a pathogen only when immunodeficiency, immunosuppression, debilitation, or prolonged antibiotic therapy supervene. Since the onset of the AIDS epidemic, esophageal candidiasis has been recognized as an AIDS-defining condition in many patients. Candidiasis develops in most patients with AIDS sometime during their illness (e389). Zygomycosis and Aspergillus infection are also usually limited to debilitated and immunosuppressed patients (e321). The gastrointestinal tract is often the portal of entry for fungal septicemia in these people. Any portion of the gastrointestinal tract may be infected by these three groups of fungi. Multiple fungal microabscesses a few millimeters in diameter or focal ulcerations are grossly identifiable on mucosal surfaces. Histoplasma capsulatum may cause gastrointestinal disease in immunocompetent persons in endemic areas (e435).

MALABSORPTION

Malabsorption in children has many causes, only some of which have anatomic correlates of concern to the pathologist viewing an abnormal biopsy specimen. Conditions associated with a failure to absorb nutrients but without diagnosable histologic abnormalities include pancreatic and liver diseases, enterocyte enzyme deficiencies, alterations of normal bacterial flora, some infections, some immunodeficiency states, and decreases in intestinal surface area. These extraintestinal, enzymatic, metabolic, and other nonstructural causes of malabsorption in children are covered in standard textbooks and review articles (e384).

Children with malabsorption of any cause usually present with growth failure, bulky or diarrheal stools, and anemia. Edema and hypoalbuminemia occur if inadequate protein is absorbed or if enough serum protein is lost through the intestine. Steatorrhea results in a failure to absorb fat-soluble vitamins, associated with a prolonged prothrombin time and manifestations of bleeding (vitamin K deficiency), rickets and hypocalcemia (vitamin D deficiency), and night blindness (vitamin A deficiency). Zinc malabsorption produces a characteristic dermatitis. Anemia results from malabsorption of iron, folate, or vitamin B12. The laboratory diagnosis of malabsorption is complex but usually includes documentation of fat, carbohydrate, and protein loss in the stools.

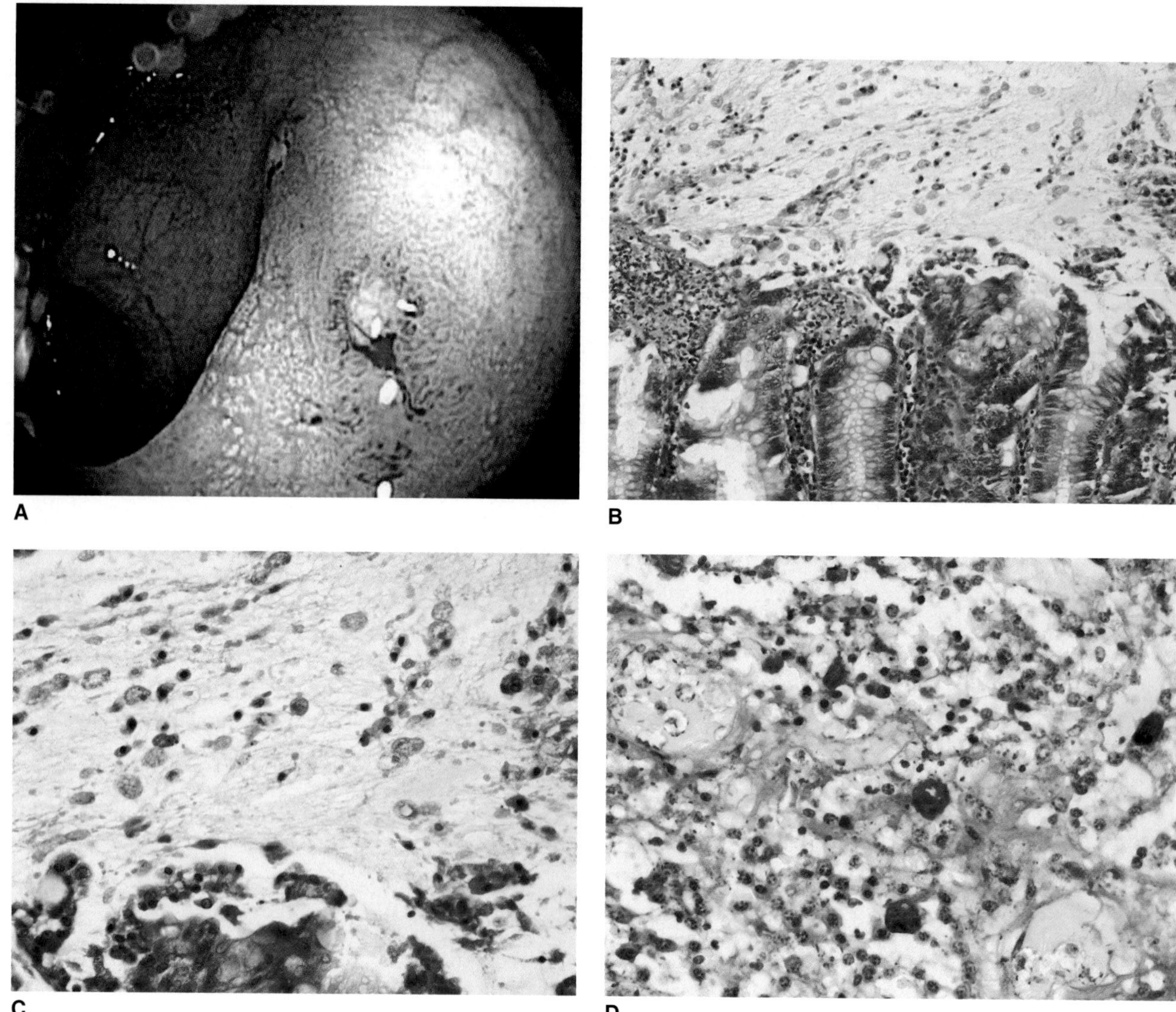

FIGURE 14-31 ■ *Entamoeba histolytica* colitis. **A:** Colonoscopy revealed scattered ulcers. **B:** Trophozoites can be seen within mucus and debris at the luminal surface 200×. **C:** The trophozoites are slightly bigger than histiocytes and contain a nucleus 400×. **D:** The organisms are highlighted in a PAS stain 400×.

A 72-hour quantitative stool fat excretion is used to quantify steatorrhea. Carbohydrate absorption is evaluated by means of the H2 breath test, fecal pH, and D-xylose absorption. Serum proteins, immunoglobulins, calcium, carotene, folic acid, and vitamin B12 are all subject to intestinal loss and can be measured directly. Stool is cultured and examined for ova and parasites, especially *G. lamblia*. Because cystic fibrosis is a common cause of malabsorption in children in North America and northern Europe, a sweat test is often performed. Antigliadin and antiendomysial antibodies are sought in serum to rule out celiac disease.

A small-intestinal biopsy specimen is evaluated for inflammation, plasma cells, and the ratio of villus height to crypt length (normal, 3:1 in infants; 4:1 in older children) (Figure 14-32). Duodenal biopsy specimens should be examined for *G. lamblia* and cryptosporidium within the surface mucous coat.

Causes of malabsorption in children with morphologic abnormalities of the small intestine are listed in Table 14-5. Several excellent review articles are available on the examination of small-intestinal mucosal biopsy specimens (e357,e481). Of the causes of intestinal malabsorption, the most commonly encountered in developed countries are celiac disease, temporary postgastroenteritis syndrome (postenteritis enteropathy), cow's milk protein intolerance, short-gut syndrome (postoperative), Crohn disease, and immunodeficiency states.

Celiac Disease

Celiac disease, or gluten-sensitivity enteropathy, is the most common small-intestinal mucosal disease causing malabsorption in white children. It can be diagnosed at any age after institution of gluten into the diet. One recent screening

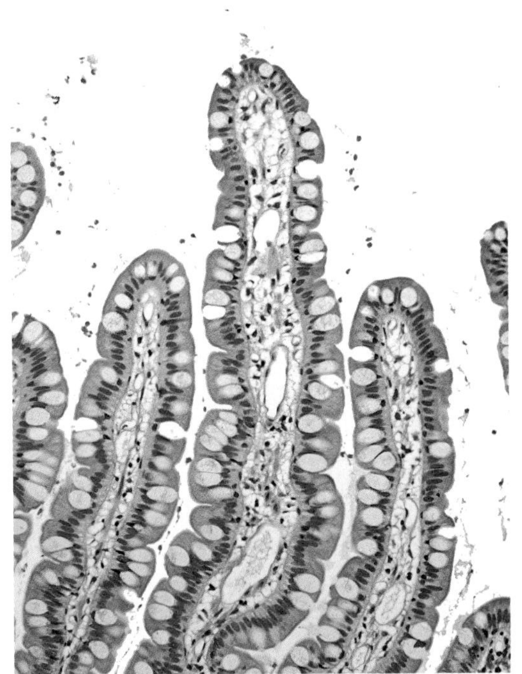

FIGURE 14-32 ■ Normal duodenal mucosa. Although scattered IELs are evident in the lower portions of the villi, they become progressively less numerous toward the tips of the villi. This normal "decrescendo" pattern is helpful to rule out a borderline increase as seen in various pathologic conditions 200×.

study of unselected healthy infants reported that 9 of 484 had a positive anti–tissue transglutaminase test at age 2½ years. In seven of these children duodenal biopsies confirmed the diagnosis of celiac disease (27). Presentation with the classic symptoms of malabsorption (diarrhea, steatorrhea, abdominal bloating and pain, weight loss, poor weight gain, failure to thrive, fatigue, and metabolic bone disease) is becoming less and less frequent. Instead, a wide (and ever expanding) range of "atypical" presenting symptoms is being reported, including low serum folate, calcium, magnesium or phosphorus levels, intracranial calcifications causing seizures, and growth retardation (94). Unexplained iron deficiency anemia is now one of the leading presenting signs of celiac disease, particularly among adolescent patients (e55,e247). One study proposes that gastrointestinal blood loss is partially responsible for the anemia, in addition to the obvious decrease in iron absorption (e143). There has also been a significant increase in diagnosis through screening of patients with Down syndrome, juvenile-onset diabetes mellitus, and other autoimmune disorders. Virtually every patient with dermatitis herpetiformis has or will develop celiac disease. About 90% of patients with celiac disease carry a HLA-DQ2 of HLA-DQ8 allele. There is a 70% concordance rate in identical twins (94).

Celiac disease occurs because of the ingestion of alpha-gliadin within gluten-containing foods by sensitive individuals. Gluten is present at high levels in wheat, rye, and barley but is absent in corn and rice. Oats (in moderate amounts) has been shown to be tolerated by some celiac patients without adverse effects (e225). Gliadin injures the enterocytes in celiac disease patients, causing them to aberrantly express HLA antigens and secrete IL-15. This in turn may lead to the intraepithelial infiltration of $CD8^+$ T-cells that is so characteristic of celiac disease. The gliadin is deaminated by tissue transglutaminase in the interstitium, resulting in a peptide that is recognized by an expanded population of $CD4^+$ T-cells (DQ2 and DQ8 restricted) in the lamina propria (56).

In the past elevation of serum antigliadin and antiendomysial antibody titers were required to establish a diagnosis of celiac disease. In patients with a high clinical suspicion of celiac disease (i.e., those with classic symptomatology) the sensitivity and specificity of these assays were in the range of 90%. However, as screening tests in asymptomatic adult blood donors, for example, the positive predictive value for a positive antigliadin antibody test was only 20% (e181). Moreover, the value of these serologic tests varied by geographic area and ethnicity, even among high-risk patient populations (e349,e470). It is important to remember, though, that the antiendomysial antibody test only detects IgA antibodies, while both IgA and IgG antigliadin antibody tests are available. This is important because the frequency of selective IgA deficiency is more than ten times higher in patients with celiac disease than in the general population (e94).

Recently, it was demonstrated that the primary antigen detected by the antiendomysial indirect immunofluorescent test is a peptide portion of tissue transglutaminase (tTG) (e118). Automated ELISA assays have become the primary test for celiac disease and have supplanted the more time-consuming and subjective antiendomysial antibody test (e445) (130). However, no single test is 100% sensitive and specific in all testing situations, and currently a panel

Table 14-5 ■ CAUSES OF MALABSORPTION IN CHILDREN
Celiac disease
Postviral enteropathy
Cow's milk and other dietary protein intolerance
Eosinophilic gastroenteritis
Immunodeficiency states (e.g., common variable immunodeficiency)
Bacterial overgrowth/stasis
Bacterial infection (e.g. mycobacterium avium intracellular)
Parasitic infections (Giardia and Cryptosporidium)
Crohn disease
Autoimmune enteritis
Microvillous inclusion disease
Tufting enteropathy
Intestinal lymphangiectasia
Abetalipoproteinemia
Cystic fibrosis
Langerhans cell histiocytosis
Chronic granulomatous disease

including anti-tTG, antiendomysial, and antigliadin antibody tests is usually performed (133).

The classic histologic features of celiac disease in patients ingesting gluten include villous blunting, crypt hyperplasia, an increased number of mitotic figures in the crypts, dense mixed inflammatory cell infiltration of the lamina propria, and an increased number of IELs. The lamina propria inflammatory cell infiltrates are composed mostly of plasma cells and lymphocytes, with scattered admixed eosinophils. Although not characteristic, a few scattered neutrophils may be present as well. Disorganization, flattening, and/or vacuolization of the surface epithelium are also evident in some cases of celiac disease (eFigure 14-10A,B). After withdrawal of gluten from the diet, there is slow resolution toward normal villous architecture. The mucosa of the most distal portion of the small bowel recovers most quickly, while the duodenum is the last to normalize. It may take several months or longer of a strict gluten-free diet before the biopsy appearance returns to normal. Ileal biopsies obtained during a colonoscopy may exhibit the same histologic features seen in duodenal biopsies, although significant villous blunting is very unusual.

The degree of villous blunting in celiac disease varies in individual patients and even among duodenal biopsies from a single patient. Multiple biopsies are recommended because the pathologic changes can be patchy, and because some of the biopsies may be poorly oriented or artifactually distorted, interfering with proper interpretation. The number of duodenal biopsies that are obtained have been shown to influence the likelihood of identifying flat mucosa (e359,e410). Since a flat mucosa with increased IELs is much more specific for celiac disease than an increase in IELs alone, the procurement of multiple biopsies is clearly desirable (e463). If the duodenal mucosa is completely flat the diagnosis of celiac disease is almost ensured, although rarely autoimmune enteropathy, viral enteritis, and tropical sprue can result in a flat mucosa. Villous architecture is difficult to accurately assess in the proximal duodenum because Brunner glands can cause mild villous architecture distortion and shortening. In addition, the inflammatory changes of peptic duodenitis are most severe in the proximal duodenum and when present, interfere with the recognition of the histologic features of celiac disease. For these reasons surgical pathologists should encourage gastroenterologists to obtain small bowel biopsies for the evaluation of malabsorption from as far distally in the duodenum as is practical.

As more patients with "atypical" symptoms underwent duodenal biopsy to rule out celiac disease, it became clear that a range of pathologic abnormalities could be expected. Marsh proposed a classification for the morphologic appearance of duodenal biopsies in celiac disease patients (e298,e299), which can be briefly summarized as follows:

Type 0—normal crypt and villous architecture with no increase in IELs

Type 1—normal crypt and villous architecture with greater than 40 IELs/100 enterocytes

Type 2—crypt hyperplasia but normal villous length; greater than 40 IELs/100 enterocytes

Type 3—crypt hyperplasia and villous blunting (mild to flat) with greater than 40 IEL/100 enterocytes

Type 1 morphology, also known as the "infiltrative lesion," which represents the earliest recognizable light microscopic change, was first documented in biopsies from first-degree relatives of celiac disease patients and in patients with dermatitis herpetiformis (Figure 14-33A to D). These patients had no gastrointestinal complaints and were considered to suffer from a *form fruste* of celiac disease (e298). It has been shown that the infiltrative lesion can be induced in full-fledged celiac disease patients who have been on a gluten-free diet (with a documented entirely normal duodenal mucosa) by administering a low dose of dietary gluten. Increasing the load of dietary gluten can produce evolution to a flat mucosa (e141,e153). It has recently been estimated that only 30% of "gluten-sensitive" patients exhibit a flat mucosa (e298). It appears that many of the "asymptomatic" first-degree relatives of celiac disease patients often do have subtle symptoms (e.g., iron deficiency anemia) related to abnormal small bowel morphology. It is important to realize that 10% of patients with dermatitis herpetiformis actually exhibit a flat mucosa on duodenal biopsy and still do not suffer diarrhea or significant malabsorption (e298). Obviously, the clinical presentation is dependent to some extent on the length of the small bowel mucosa that is severely affected.

It is currently unknown what percentage of patients with the "infiltrative lesion" will go on to develop flat mucosa and the full blown clinical syndrome of celiac disease. It is important to recognize this morphologic expression of gluten sensitivity because the atypical symptoms of these patients will respond to dietary gluten withdrawal. For that reason, and because of the greater long-term risk of lymphoma in untreated patients, a gluten-free diet is recommended by most gastroenterologists for all celiac patients, regardless of the presence or absence of villous blunting. On the other hand, it is clear that celiac disease is not the only cause of intraepithelial lymphocytosis. Other disease states in which an increased number of IELs may occur include tropical sprue, autoimmune enteropathy, cryptosporidiosis, giardiasis, microsporidiosis, bacterial overgrowth, other food allergies, viral enteritis, Crohn disease, Zollinger-Ellison syndrome, and systemic autoimmune states. It is also possible that NSAIDs can cause intraepithelial lymphocytosis (22,50,78). Severe *H. pylori* gastritis may also cause a mild increase in IELs in biopsies of the duodenal bulb, but usually not more distally (103).

Most cases of flat duodenal mucosa and increased intraepithelial lymphocytosis are due to celiac disease, but common variable immunodeficiency, autoimmune enteritis, and severe viral enteritis can also produce this pattern of injury. With lesser degrees of villous blunting, the differential diagnosis broadens considerably. Given the large number of disorders that can cause intraepithelial lymphocytosis and villous

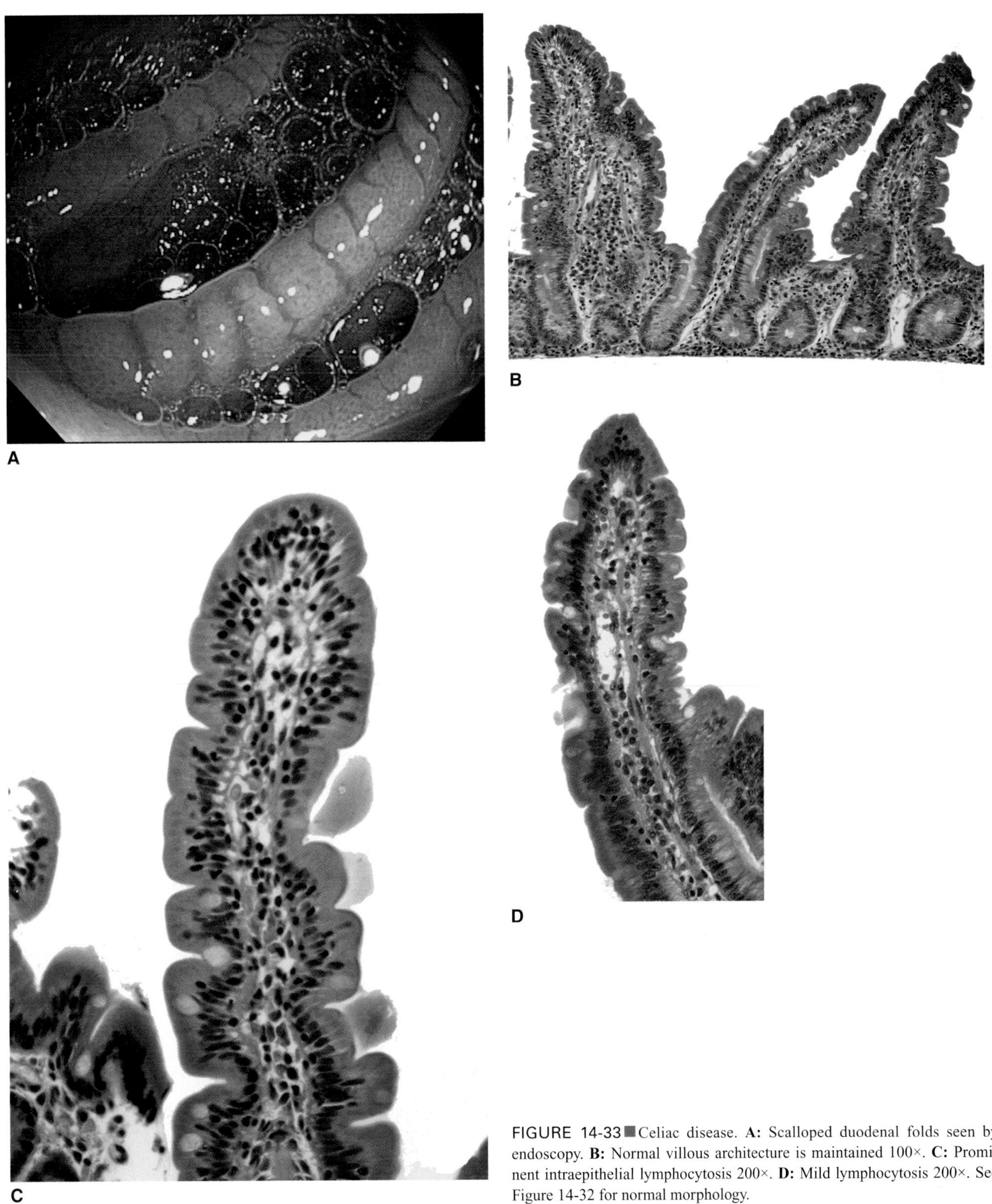

FIGURE 14-33 Celiac disease. **A:** Scalloped duodenal folds seen by endoscopy. **B:** Normal villous architecture is maintained 100×. **C:** Prominent intraepithelial lymphocytosis 200×. **D:** Mild lymphocytosis 200×. See Figure 14-32 for normal morphology.

blunting, it is clear that a diagnosis of celiac disease is not possible solely by histologic examination of duodenal biopsies. Instead, correlation of the serologic tests results and the biopsy findings is necessary to establish a firm diagnosis of celiac disease. Resolution of symptoms or abnormal laboratory tests after a gluten-free diet is an important confirmatory sign. Re-biopsy after a gluten-free diet is instituted or after gluten rechallenge is no longer standard clinical practice.

The number of IELs that separate normal individuals from those with small bowel disease have, surprisingly, not been studied extensively. Forty IELs per 100 enterocytes were adopted as the cutoff for the diagnosis of celiac disease by Furguson and Murray because the highest level in their control group of normal individuals was 40 and the mean value plus two standard deviations (SD) was 36.1 (e156). However, a recent larger study of a Swedish population concluded that a value of 20 IELs per 100 enterocytes was more appropriate (their mean plus 3 SD was 18.5). The authors calculated that using that cutoff no more that 1 in 1000 healthy persons would be falsely diagnosed with intraepithelial lymphocytosis (149). They also studied the use of CD3 immunostains to highlight IELs and calculated a cutoff of 30 per 100 enterocytes, with 25 to 29 IELs reported as "borderline" (149). The authors stress the importance of not performing counts of IELs in the epithelium anywhere in the vicinity of even small lamina propria lymphoid aggregates, since increased numbers of IELs are normal there. This is particularly critical in the evaluation of biopsies of the terminal ileum, since lymphoid aggregates and follicles often occupy large portions of such samples. Immunohistologic studies to highlight IELs utilizing a CD3 antibody may aid in the recognition of intraepithelial lymphocytosis in biopsies without villous blunting (105), but the use of this strategy is generally not required in daily practice.

Recently, it has been proposed that an abnormal distribution of IELs along the length of the villi, even if the overall number is not significantly increased, is suggestive of celiac disease (52). This proposal is based on the observation that in healthy individuals there is a progressive decrease in the density of IELs from the base of a villus to its tip. In contrast, in a subset of patients with celiac disease this normal "decrescendo pattern" of IEL distribution is lost, and instead, the number of IELs is similar along the entire length of the villus or is actually higher at the tip than at the base. However, the author emphasizes that this pattern of IEL distribution merely suggests the need for serologic testing to rule out celiac disease, as there are other causes of this histologic finding, and some patients may have no disease state at all (51).

Gastric antral biopsies from patients with celiac disease, particularly children exposed to gluten at a young age, may also exhibit an intraepithelial lymphocytosis, and the term "lymphocytic gastritis" has been applied in such cases. More than 25 IELs per 100 foveolar epithelial cells is considered abnormal. There is conflicting data on whether patients with lymphocytic gastritis experience upper gastrointestinal symptoms, such as nausea and vomiting or dyspepsia, more often than patients without this finding (e6,e112,e503).

Some celiac patients who are asymptomatic on a gluten-free diet sudden redevelop symptoms of malabsorption. Most of these patients are ultimately discovered to have discontinued the gluten-free diet, inadvertently or not. Some patients, however, relapse despite strict adherence to the proper diet and are said to suffer from refractory sprue. The most feared complication of celiac disease is the development of small bowel lymphoma, which is sometimes heralded by the redevelopment of malabsorption. These lymphomas are unusual in that they are almost always of T-cell phenotype (e329), while almost all sporadic gastrointestinal lymphomas are of B-cell origin. In many patients gene rearrangement studies are necessary to confirm the diagnosis of a clonal T-cell proliferation, since significant cytological atypia may not be present. The relative risk of small bowel lymphoma in celiac patients has been variously estimated at 40- to 100-fold greater than that for the general population (e134), but there is some evidence that strict adherence to a gluten-free diet may prevent the development of lymphoma (e88). The mucosa in celiac patients with lymphoma often appears atrophic, with both crypt hypoplasia and total villous blunting (Marsh type 4 morphology). The evolution to lymphoma was initially overlooked in some celiac patients who developed diffuse ulceration of the small bowel mucosa (the so-called ulcerative jejunoileitis), making it difficult to discern the underlying clonal lymphoid infiltrate, especially in biopsies (28) (e73). There has been some confusion in the literature, however, in that the term ulcerative jejunoileitis is also used to describe large areas of small bowel mucosal ulceration in nonceliac patients. In this population there is no association with lymphoma. A small number of patients also develop lymphocytic or collagenous colitis, which may manifest simultaneously, before or after the diagnosis of sprue (e504). In one study of 21 patients with "refractory sprue," collagenous colitis was responsible for the development of diarrhea in three patients on a strict gluten-free diet (e144).

Gastroenteritis and Postenteritis Enteropathy

Most cases of acute gastroenteritis in children are caused by viruses. Biopsies are usually not performed during the acute infection. Of more concern is the infant or child who apparently recovers from an episode of acute viral gastroenteritis but then lapses into a malabsorptive state lasting weeks to months. These children may undergo endoscopic examination and their biopsy findings must be distinguished from those of celiac disease. Cases of postenteritis enteropathy show villous atrophy and chronic inflammation, but the changes characteristically vary in severity from one piece of tissue to another (e458). Cow's milk protein intolerance is sometimes unmasked by acute gastroenteritis and should be considered.

Enteropathy Induced by Cow's Milk Proteins

Enteropathy associated with malabsorption is one of several gastrointestinal symptom complexes in infants caused by cow's milk proteins. The others are occult gastrointestinal blood loss and iron-deficiency anemia, protein-losing enteropathy, and allergic proctocolitis. Enteropathy, with or without protein loss, is well-known (e149,e269,e270,e295,e487). Other dietary proteins, including soy protein and even casein hydrolysate in formulas, may also cause the syndrome (e195,e475). Symptoms usually develop in the first 6 months of life in a bottle-fed baby. The onset may be sudden, with vomiting and diarrhea, or more gradual, with failure to thrive and chronic loose stools. In some cases, hypoproteinemia

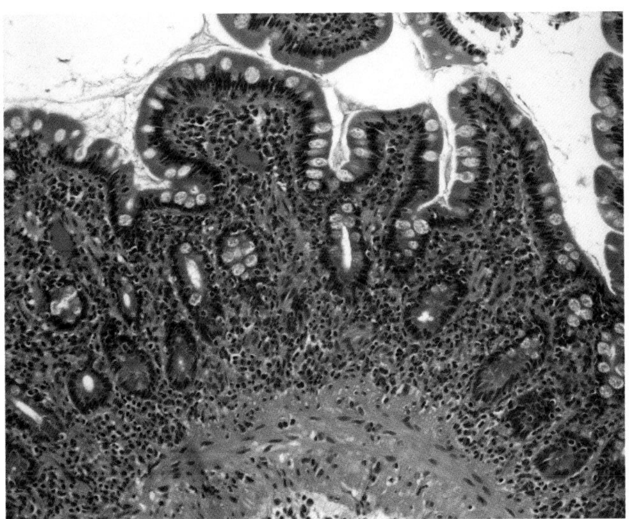

FIGURE 14-34 ■ Cow's milk protein intolerance. This duodenal biopsy demonstrates villous blunting (without crypt hyperplasia) and an intense infiltrate of eosinophils 200×.

and edema (protein-losing enteropathy) dominate the picture. Steatorrhea and carbohydrate malabsorption can be demonstrated, and some patients have a mild peripheral eosinophilia. Small-intestinal biopsy specimens (Figure 14-34) show villous blunting and inflammation of the lamina propria, which is often quite patchy, which necessitates procurement of multiple biopsies for diagnosis. Lamina propria cells are usually a mixture of mononuclear cells and eosinophils; polymorphonuclear leukocytes are rare. IELs are not increased in number. Sigmoidoscopic biopsies are easier to obtain in infants than duodenal biopsies and are therefore the most common specimens seen by surgical pathologists. Normal crypt architecture is well preserved in all cases. The inflammatory infiltrates are usually eosinophil predominant, always distinctly patchy, and sometimes also include neutrophilic infiltrates. In fact, some of the biopsies from a given case may be entirely normal. More than 60 eosinophils/10 hpf has been used as a diagnostic cutoff for colonic biopsies, while others have suggested 20 eosinophils/hpf. However, most biopsies (from any site) also exhibit focal eosinophilic cryptitis and/or infiltration of the muscularis mucosae, and these features are useful to make a firm diagnosis. It must be emphasized that increased eosinophils are not present in every case, and the presence of a neutrophilic predominant colitis is also consistent with the diagnosis. However, in that situation infectious colitis and Hirschsprung disease–associated colitis must also be ruled out clinically.

Infants with cow's milk protein-induced enteropathy usually respond to a diet free of cow's milk with resolution of symptoms and morphologic abnormalities. Identical symptoms of malabsorption and enteropathy often develop in infants who cannot tolerate cow's milk protein when they are switched to a soy protein formula or even a casein hydrolysate formula (e424,e475). Such patients respond to an elemental formula containing amino acids. In any case, milk-sensitive enteropathy is a temporary state. By the age of 1 year, most patients can ingest products containing cow's milk without difficulty.

Intestinal Lymphangiectasia

Intestinal lymphangiectasia is a disease category rather than a single entity. It is characterized by greatly dilated lymphatic vessels in the lamina propria of the small intestine with leakage of lymph into the intestine and consequent protein-losing enteropathy (e1,e479). Primary (congenital) forms often are associated with extraintestinal lymphatic abnormalities. Secondary forms are caused by lymphatic obstruction resulting from cardiac failure, pericarditis, abdominal tumors, inflammatory bowel disease, and other conditions. Patients with both primary and secondary forms present with diarrhea and protein-losing enteropathy (i.e., intestinal protein loss, hypoalbuminemia, and edema). Lymphocyte and immunoglobulin losses into the intestine through the lymphatics also produce lymphopenia and hypogammaglobulinemia. The dilated lymphatics can often be seen through the endoscope as multiple, white, pinhead-sized spots on the small-intestinal mucosa. On biopsy specimens, the abnormally dilated lymphatic vessels are often grouped at the tips of villi (Figure 14-35A,B) but may appear elsewhere in the lamina propria. A distinct endothelial lining helps differentiate lymphatic vessels from artificial tears caused by biopsy trauma. Because intestinal lymphangiectasia is a focal abnormality, multiple biopsies and serial sections are indicated if this diagnosis is suspected. Unaffected villi are normal or show a mildly increased cellularity in the lamina propria.

Immunodeficiency

Immunodeficiency diseases may present in infancy and childhood as malabsorption, diarrhea, and failure to thrive (e8,e10). The most common disorders are selective IgA deficiency, which may present at any age; common variable immunodeficiency, which usually presents in the older child or adult; and AIDS. In all three conditions, villous atrophy and inflammation mimicking celiac disease may occur. Plasma cells are conspicuously absent from the lamina propria, and the enteropathy is patchy in common variable immunodeficiency and severe combined immunodeficiency. Plasma cells are also absent in X-linked agammaglobulinemia. Exacerbation of malabsorption in many immunodeficient patients often indicates superimposed giardiasis.

IPEX (immune dysregulation, polyendocrinopathy, enteropathy, and X-linkage) syndrome is due to a mutation in the FOXP3 (scurfin) gene, which codes for a transcription factor involved in the development and proliferation of $CD4^+$ T-cells. Affected infants may develop severe enteropathy, diabetes mellitus, eczematous ichthyosis, hemolytic anemia, and thyroid and/or adrenal dysfunction. The duodenal morphology resembles autoimmune enteropathy. Although immunosuppressive therapy may ameliorate symptoms for a time, death will occur without stem cell transplantation (14).

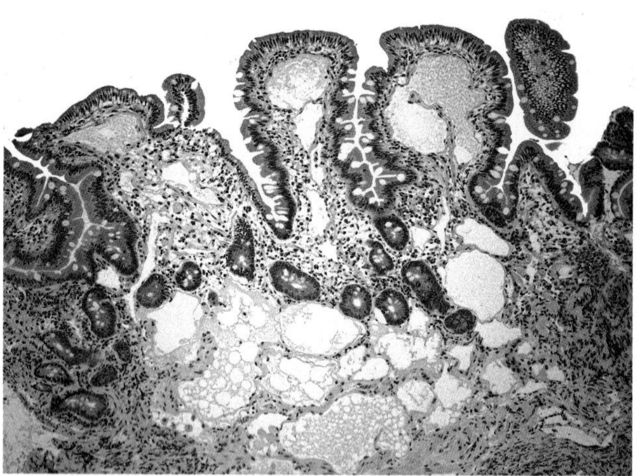

A

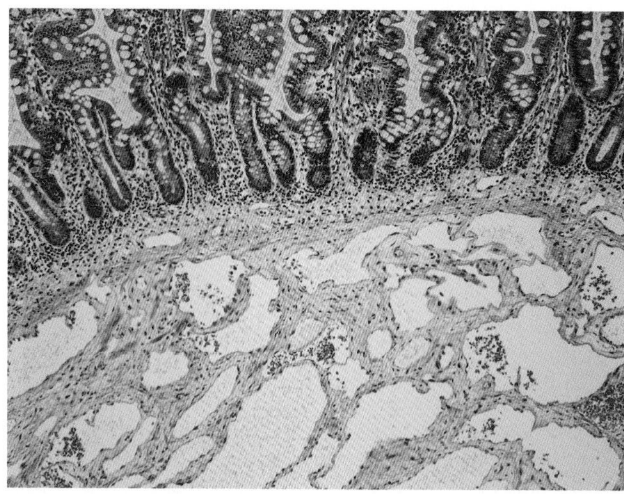

B

FIGURE 14-35 ■ Small-bowel lymphangiectasia. **A:** This duodenal biopsy demonstrates dilated lymphatic channels within the lamina propria 200×. **B:** In this resection specimen the dilated lymphatic vessels are within the superficial submucosa 100×.

Short-bowel Syndrome and Bacterial Overgrowth

Extensive surgical resection of the intestine is the usual cause of short-bowel syndrome, defined as malabsorption in the presence of reduced intestinal length, usually 50 cm or less of small intestine in a neonate. The normal small-intestinal length in the term neonate is 239 ± 67 cm (e426). Extensive intestinal resection is performed in patients with such conditions as neonatal necrotizing enterocolitis, malrotation with volvulus, multiple intestinal atresias, and, in older children, Crohn disease. Very rarely, the intestine is congenitally very short (e197,e454). In any case, diarrhea results from a shortened transit time, and malabsorption of nutrients results from an inadequate absorptive surface area. In some patients, a reduction in peristalsis leads to intestinal dilation. Bacterial overgrowth in the intestinal lumen contributes substantially to malabsorption in many cases of short-bowel syndrome (e241,e474). Small-intestinal biopsy specimens often show nonspecific partial villous atrophy, crypt hypertrophy, and inflammation with lymphocytes, plasma cells, and eosinophils. In severe cases of bacterial overgrowth, an acute enteritis with polymorphonuclear leukocytes in the lamina propria or crypts may be present. The colon is often also involved (e455). Bacterial overgrowth can be diagnosed by culture of proximal intestinal fluid; organisms are rarely seen on biopsy specimens. Intravenous alimentation with amino acid and lipid preparations has made long-term survival possible in these patients. Antibiotics often decrease the bacterial overgrowth. Newer bowel-lengthening procedures have been used to correct selected cases, and in the most severe cases, small-bowel transplantation is possible.

Bacterial overgrowth is most often seen in children with short-bowel syndrome (see above). However, the same bacterial overgrowth and subsequent enteropathy may also occur in children with a normal intestinal length if they have severe malnutrition, an alteration of peristalsis and stasis, as in one of the pseudo-obstruction syndromes, or a surgically created blind loop. The clinical picture is that of malabsorption (e241,e417).

Malnutrition

Kwashiorkor and marasmus may both produce villous atrophy and inflammation, although this is rare in developed countries. Patients with protein-calorie malnutrition and gastrointestinal symptoms often have a superimposed infection (e59).

Abetalipoproteinemia

Patients with this rare autosomal recessive metabolic disease are unable to synthesize and transport low-density lipoproteins (β-lipoproteins) and manifest numerous extraintestinal abnormalities, including red cell acanthocytosis, retinitis pigmentosa, and neuromuscular degeneration. Malabsorption and diarrhea are conspicuous within the 1st year of life and are often the earliest manifestations of the disease (152) (e494). On small-intestinal biopsy specimens, surface epithelial cells are markedly vacuolated by lipid that has been absorbed but cannot be normally transported out of the cells (Figure 14-36). Villous architecture is otherwise normal (e376).

Microvillus Inclusion Disease

Microvillus inclusion disease (congenital microvillous atrophy and familial enteropathy) is a rare, lethal, familial disease that presents at birth with relentless secretory diarrhea (e97,e98,e106,e358). Small-bowel transplantation is required in many cases (127). Small-intestinal biopsy specimens show villous atrophy, hypoplasia of crypts, an inappropriate lack of compensatory mitosis, and vacuolization of enterocyte apical

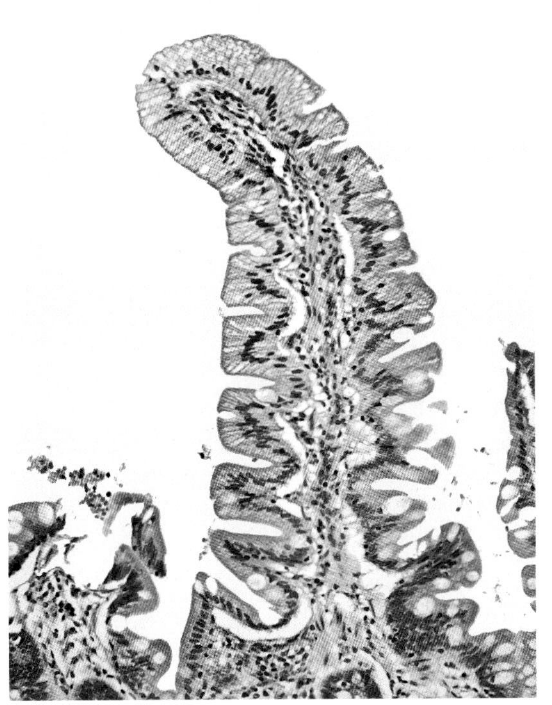

FIGURE 14-36 ▪ Abetalipoproteinemia. There is prominent accumulation of small droplets of lipid within the enterocytes from this duodenal biopsy 200×.

cytoplasm (Figure 14-37A,B). The lack of inflammation is striking in comparison with other enteropathies. Similar changes are also evident in colonic and gastric mucosa (e401).

Electron microscopy of surface enterocytes shows distinctive intracytoplasmic inclusions and absent or shortened microvilli (Figure 14-37C) (e35,e97,e98,e358). Although electron microscopic demonstration of the unique cytoplasmic inclusions confirms the diagnosis, paraffin-embedded sections can also be evaluated; affected enterocytes contain periodic acid-Schiff (PAS)–positive and diastase-resistant material (e98) and show distinctive inclusions utilizing a CD10 antibody by immunohistochemistry (58).

Autoimmune Enteropathy

To date, approximately 100 infants have been described in the world literature with a severe protein-losing enteropathy refractory to treatment except for potent immunosuppressive agents such as cyclosporine or FK506 (tacrolimus) or small-bowel transplantation (137) (e72). The onset of diarrhea and protein-losing enteropathy may be at any time between several weeks after birth to approximately 2 years of age. Many of the infants have had an associated autoimmune disease of some type, including diabetes, thyroid disease, atopic dermatitis, glomerulonephritis, autoimmune hemolytic anemia,

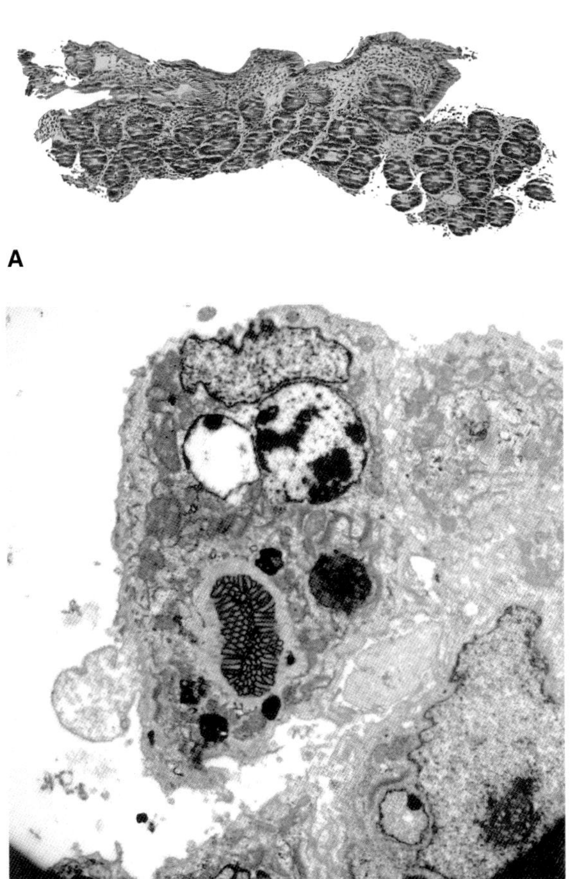

A

C

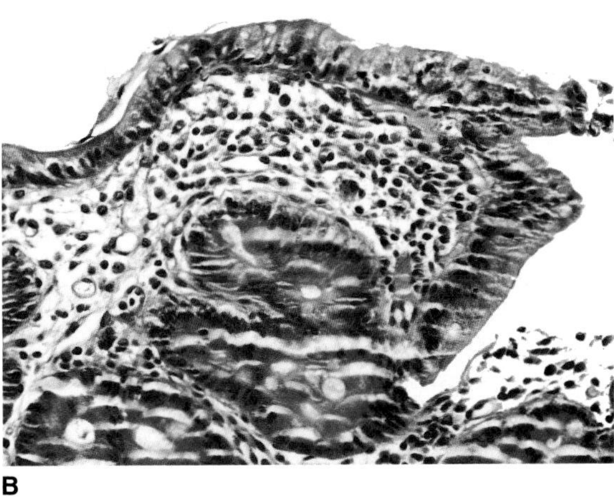

B

FIGURE 14-37 ▪ Microvillous inclusion disease. **A:** This duodenal biopsy exhibits both villous blunt and crypt hypoplasia, resulting in atrophic appearing mucosa 100×. **B:** A well-developed brush boarder is not visible 400×. **C:** Electron microscopy demonstrates a microvillous inclusion body in the cytoplasm of an enterocyte.

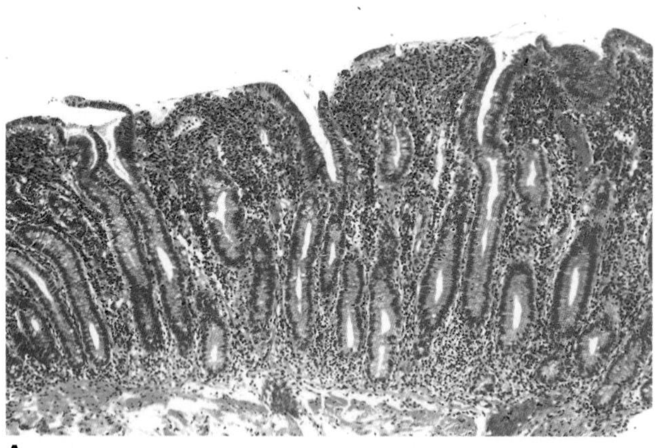
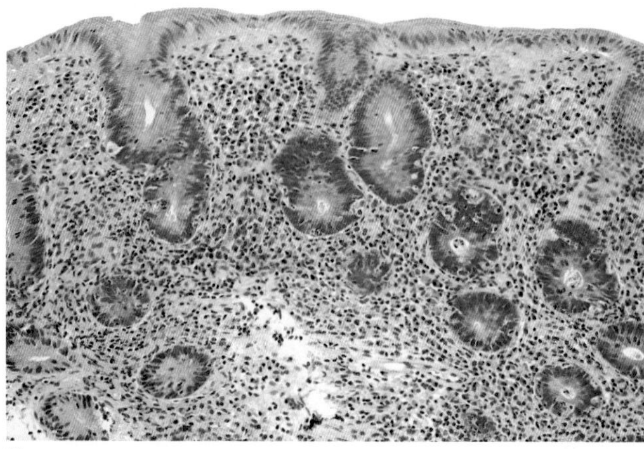

A B

FIGURE 14-38 ■ Autoimmune enterocolitis. **A:** This duodenal biopsy exhibits total villous blunting and mild intraepithelial lymphocytosis, but serologic tests for celiac disease were negative. A serum antienterocyte antibody titer was elevated 100×. **B:** This colonic biopsy from a different child exhibits mild colitis with prominent epithelial cell apoptosis and a complete absence of goblet cells. The serum antigoblet cell antibody titer was elevated 200×.

polyarthritis, and autoimmune hepatitis. Some of the cases are familial (e87,e93,e98,e175,e391). Some of the patients have serum antibodies against either enterocyte or goblet cell antigens, but these assays are available only in specialized centers. Small-intestinal biopsy changes are variable, ranging from partial to total villous atrophy with lymphoplasmacytic infiltration in the lamina propria and crypt elongation. IELs in surface enterocytes, similar to the characteristic finding in celiac disease, are also present in some cases. Absence of goblet cells is an easily overlooked feature in some cases (Figure 14-38A,B). Colonic and gastric mucosa may be involved (e98,e208).

Tufting Enteropathy

This rare genetic disorder is responsible for some cases of intractable congenital diarrhea (e98,e174,e378). Small-intestinal biopsy specimens show moderate to severe villous atrophy and crypt hyperplasia without significant inflammatory cell infiltrates (Figure 14-39A to C). The diagnostic histologic feature is the disorganization of the surface epithelium, with crowding, tufting, and shedding of enterocytes (54). Decreased epithelial cell adhesion molecule expression due to an underlying gene mutation has been found in some patients (139).

GASTROINTESTINAL MANIFESTATIONS OF IMMUNODEFICIENCY

Gastrointestinal symptoms, infections, and morphologic abnormalities figure prominently in many primary and secondary immunodeficiency syndromes (see Chapter 22). Excellent review articles on this subject are available (e9,e10,e120,e216,e389). Biopsy specimens from immunodeficient patients may come to the pathologist masquerading as malabsorption, inflammatory bowel disease, giardiasis, or lymphoid hyperplasia. The pathologist evaluating an intestinal mucosal biopsy specimen or resected tissue for any of these clinical indications may be the first to suspect AIDS, hypogammaglobulinemia, agammaglobulinemia, or, if plasma cells are absent in the lamina propria, severe combined immunodeficiency or X-linked agammaglobulinemia (e489).

At times, a primary gastrointestinal abnormality may result in a secondary immunodeficiency. Leakage from intestinal lymphatics, as in intestinal lymphangiectasia and Crohn disease, may lead to lymphopenia and functional T-cell deficiency (e120). Protein-losing enteropathy in cow's milk protein intolerance can produce hypogammaglobulinemia and lymphopenia. Structural defects, such as malrotation and cavernous hemangioma of the jejunum, have been associated with defects of both humoral and cellular immunity, postulated to result from intestinal losses of protein and lymphocytes (e139).

Immunosuppression caused by steroids and cytotoxic agents, especially in children with malignancies, increases the risk for fungal or viral infection of the gastrointestinal tract. Necrotizing inflammation of the cecum or typhlitis (neutropenic colitis) is likely to develop in children being treated for leukemia (e413,e482).

Primary Immunodeficiencies

Selective IgA deficiency is the most common primary immunodeficiency in the general population, with an incidence of 1 to 2 in 1,000. Diarrhea and steatorrhea may occur at any age and are often the initial manifestations of immunodeficiency. The incidence of celiac disease is increased in IgA-deficient patients, and the diagnosis may be more difficult than usual

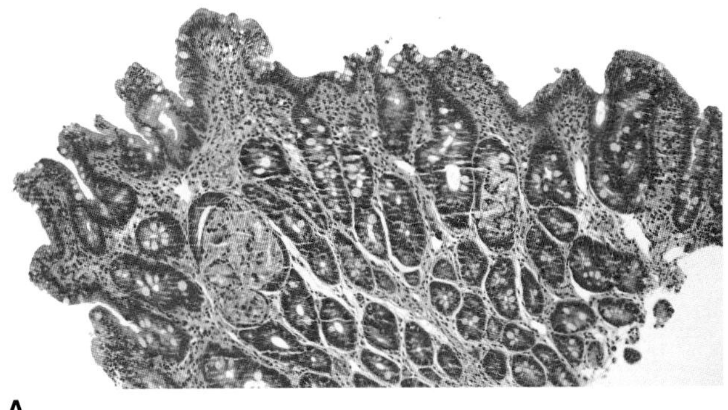
A

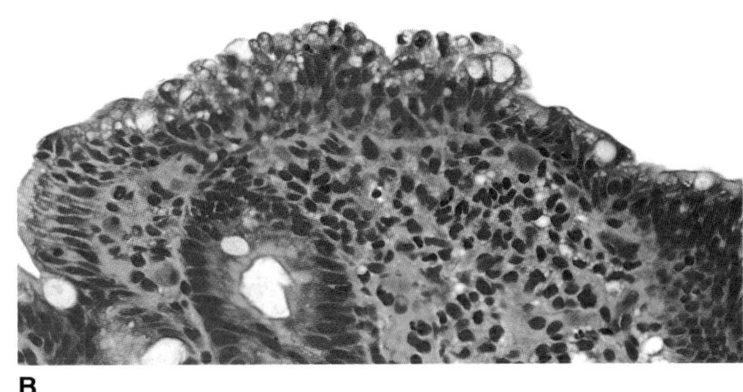
B

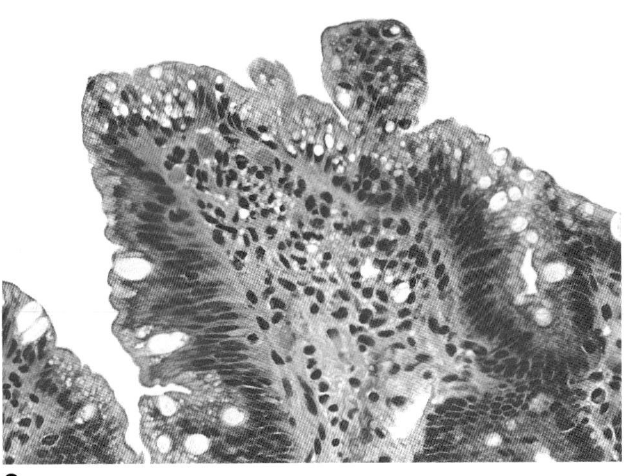
C

FIGURE 14-39■Congenital tufting enteropathy. **A:** Duodenal biopsy reveals villous and crypt hypoplasia 200×. **B:** Tufting of the surface epithelium 400×. **C:** Note the lack of intraepithelial lymphocytosis 400×.

because the serum levels of antigliadin and antiendomysial IgA antibodies are not elevated. Intestinal giardiasis may also cause malabsorption, but malabsorption persists in some IgA-deficient patients even after elimination of gluten from the diet and treatment of *Giardia* infestation. Various chronic inflammatory bowel diseases, morphologically identical to Crohn disease and ulcerative colitis, have also been reported in IgA-deficient patients. Nodular lymphoid hyperplasia of the small intestine occurs in both selective IgA deficiency and common variable hypogammaglobulinemia, but is rare in children.

Common variable immunodeficiency (common variable hypogammaglobulinemia) may also first come to clinical attention with gastrointestinal symptoms in older children (148). The diagnosis is often delayed because a pattern of recurrent infections involving multiple organs is not recognized (122). They are susceptible to a host of gastrointestinal complications, which often become the dominant clinical problem. Infections are common, with giardiasis, bacterial infections, and chronic viral infections reported. The diagnosis rests upon the findings of abnormally low serum immunoglobulin (IgA, IgM, and IgG) levels without another explanation. A poor or absent response to immunization is helpful to confirm the diagnosis (80). Malabsorption states, nonspecific colitis, gastritis, and chronic inflammatory bowel diseases resembling Crohn disease and ulcerative colitis are also found.

Gastrointestinal plasma cells are absent or markedly decreased in most but not all cases. Duodenal biopsies in patients with malabsorption may exhibit villous blunting, crypt hyperplasia, and intraepithelial lymphocytosis, closely resembling the histologic features of celiac disease (Figure 14-40A,B). The proper diagnosis rests on the recognition of the lack of a dense lamina propria infiltrate of lymphocytes and plasma cells, as expected in celiac disease. Since patients with common variable immunodeficiency are at particularly increased risk of Giardia infection, this possibility should be excluded by special stain (trichrome or CD117 immunostain). In some duodenal biopsies epithelial apoptosis is prominent, resulting in an appearance similar to severe graft-versus-host disease or autoimmune enteritis. Esophageal biopsies may reveal Candida esophagitis. Severe diffuse nonspecific gastritis may be seen in antral or gastric body biopsies. Colonic

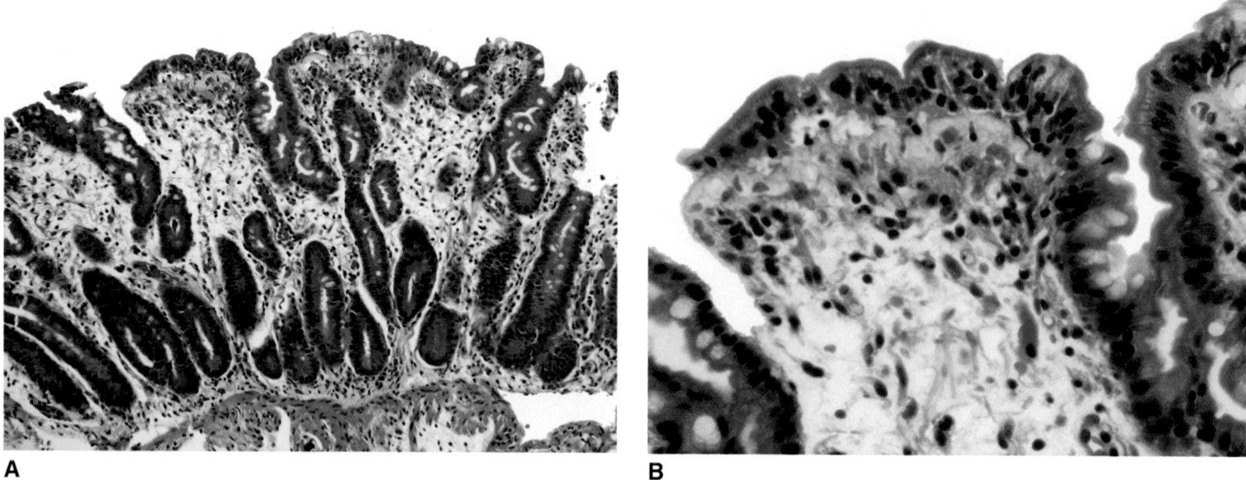

FIGURE 14-40 ■ Common variable immunodeficiency. **A:** This duodenal biopsy exhibits complete villous blunting and crypt hyperplasia 200×. **B:** There is also a mild intraepithelial lymphocytosis, similar to that seen in celiac disease. However, the complete absence of lamina propria plasma cells suggests the correct diagnosis 400×.

biopsies may reveal features consistent with lymphocytic or collagenous colitis or exhibit crypt architectural distortion and active inflammation resembling inflammatory bowel disease. Granulomas may also be present (37). Again, the absence of plasma cells is a clue to the proper diagnosis in most cases.

X-linked agammaglobulinemia presents in the first 6 months of life with severe respiratory infections and meningitis. Diarrhea, malabsorption, giardiasis, and colitis are frequent manifestations and may dominate in any given case (e489). Examination of the lamina propria reveals an absence of plasma cells.

Severe combined immunodeficiency is fatal in the first few months of life unless a bone marrow transplant is successful. Malabsorption, villous atrophy, diarrhea, and severe failure to thrive regularly develop in untreated patients. Gastrointestinal plasma cells are lacking.

Immunodeficient patients are predisposed to gastrointestinal infections by usual and unusual pathogens (e480). *G. lamblia* infection of the small intestine has been found in up to 50% of symptomatic patients with primary immunodeficiency syndromes and is responsible for many of the cases of chronic diarrhea and malabsorption in patients with common variable hypogammaglobulinemia, selective IgA deficiency, and X-linked agammaglobulinemia. Eradication of the parasite usually relieves the symptoms.

Gastrointestinal Involvement in Pediatric AIDS

Gastrointestinal disorders, especially infections, are the chief cause of morbidity and mortality worldwide in patients infected with HIV. Some of the conditions may occur anywhere in the digestive tract, including Candida, CMV, and *Mycobacterium avium complex* infections, smooth muscle tumors, and atypical lymphoid proliferations. Most of the infections listed are discussed in the section on gastrointestinal infections. Several excellent reviews on this topic are available (e232,e389).

Much of the chronic failure to thrive, diarrhea, and malabsorption seen in infants and children with AIDS result from a condition known as AIDS enteropathy, with or without infection(s). AIDS enteropathy is a poorly understood syndrome of chronic diarrhea and weight loss associated with small-intestinal changes of villous atrophy, mononuclear cell infiltration of the lamina propria, and crypt hyperplasia, all in the absence of a known pathogen. The etiology is currently unknown; theories include intestinal infection by the HIV virus or an agent not yet identified, an immune dysregulation, or a reaction to luminal antigens. A deficiency of brush border enzymes in AIDS enteropathy results in lactose and fat malabsorption (e32,e177,e232,e468). Infections develop in many children with AIDS that also occur in immunocompetent children, but they are more severe or sustained than in the normal host; agents include rotavirus, *Salmonella*, *Shigella*, *Campylobacter*, *Cryptosporidium*, and *Giardia*. In addition, AIDS patients are unusually susceptible to infections with certain opportunistic agents, including *Candida albicans*, CMV, *Mycobacterium avium* complex, and Microsporium. Candida infection of the mouth and esophagus is the most common opportunistic infection in children with AIDS. More than half of all children with AIDS carry CMV; in some, it causes a fulminant hemorrhagic, ulcerative, and necrotizing gastrointestinal illness to erupt suddenly that is often fatal.

A number of atypical proliferations may develop in gastrointestinal lymphoid tissue in AIDS patients, including the following: (a) endoscopically visible lymphoid aggregates of duodenal mucosa, (b) a polyclonal lymphoproliferative process resembling posttransplant lymphoproliferative

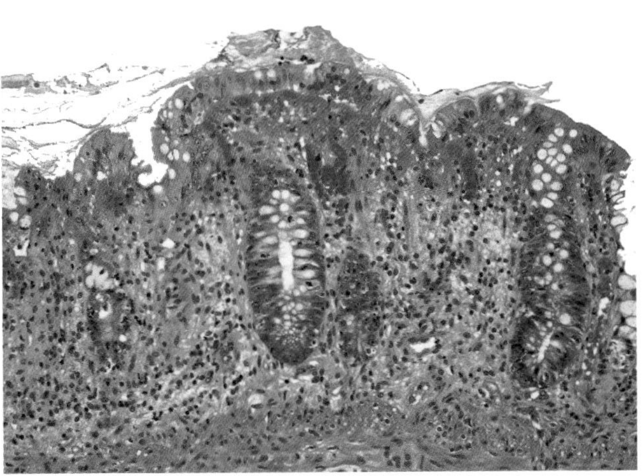

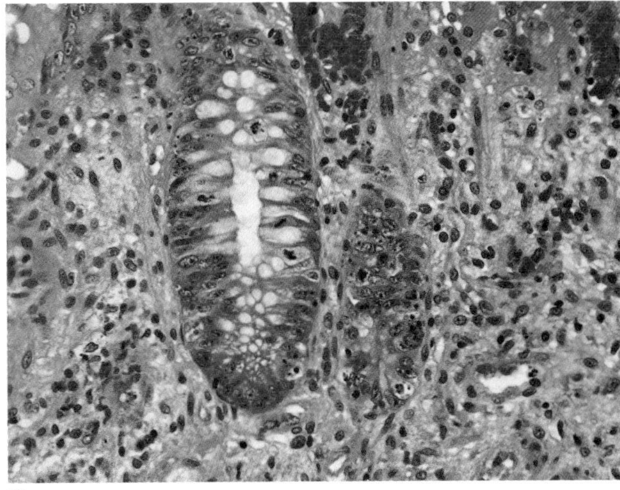

A B

FIGURE 14-41 ▪ Colonic acute graft-versus-host disease. **A:** Lamina propria cellularity is decreased from normal due to the effect of induction chemotherapy prior to the stem cell transplantation 200×. **B:** Note the characteristic epithelial cell apoptosis 400×.

syndrome (e230,e232,e394), and (c) AIDS-associated non-Hodgkin lymphoma (e222,e394). Children with AIDS have a disproportionate number of smooth muscle tumors in the gastrointestinal tract and extraintestinal sites. Most are leiomyomas, sometimes multiple; more rarely, leiomyosarcoma has been diagnosed. These tumors have been demonstrated to be Epstein-Barr virus (EBV)–related (e74,e307,e314).

Graft-versus-Host Disease (GVHD)

The intestinal tract is one of the three major target organs in graft-versus-host disease. The skin and the liver are the other two organs affected when donor lymphoid cells are transfused into an immunosuppressed host. Donor T-lymphocytes target epithelial cells in these organs and initiate an immune response that destroys them. GVHD is usually diagnosed following allogeneic bone marrow or stem cell transplant to treat leukemia and other malignant and nonmalignant diseases, but it may also rarely occur following the transfusion of nonirradiated blood into patients with primary or secondary immunodeficiency disorders (e411). GVHD develops in two phases: acute, which begins 1 week to 4 months after transplantation, and chronic, which begins approximately 4 months or more after the transplant. The clinical and pathologic features of the two phases are distinctly different.

The gastrointestinal tract is affected in at least half of the patients with acute GVHD. The skin and liver may be involved at the same time, at different times, or not at all. Intestinal GVHD is usually heralded by profuse watery diarrhea, which indicates involvement of the small intestine and colon. Occasionally, the upper gastrointestinal tract will be involved first or exclusively; the symptoms are nausea, vomiting, and anorexia (e434). Acute intestinal graft-versus-host disease is diagnosed by colonoscopic or upper endoscopic biopsies. The earliest histologic change is the development of apoptosis of individual epithelial cells in the regenerative (stem cell) compartment, characterized by vacuolization of the cytoplasm and nuclear karyorrhexis (Figure 14-41A,B). The stem cell population in the small bowel and colon resides in the lower portions of the crypts. In the esophageal squamous mucosa apoptosis is seen in the basal cell layer, similar to that seen in skin involvement. In the stomach the stem cell population is located in the neck zone of the mucosa. Inflammatory cell infiltrates are typically quite sparse, and lymphocytic infiltration of the epithelium in areas exhibiting apoptosis is usually not apparent. Scattered eosinophils are usually present. Diagnostic histologic features of graft-versus-host disease are often quite patchy, and many biopsies are necessary to exclude the diagnosis (21). Grading schemes for acute graft-versus-host disease have been proposed, usually based on features best seen in the colonic mucosa, but there is not a close relationship between clinical findings and grade. If the process is not arrested by appropriate medical therapy, it progresses to glandular attenuation, destruction, and dropout. Areas of complete glandular loss and extensive mucosal denudation occur in severe graft-versus-host disease (e308,e309,e395,e434).

Apoptosis can also occur as a consequence of the induction chemoradiation therapy regime used prior to stem cell transplantation. Thus, histologic distinction between therapy-related mucosal damage and graft-versus-host disease is usually not possible in the first 20 to 30 days after induction therapy is instituted. CMV infection can cause epithelial cell apoptosis and therefore the diagnosis of concurrent GVHD is problematic. In addition, mycophenolate mofetil can cause diarrhea and produce a graft-versus-host–like appearance in the gastrointestinal mucosa, and this agent is used in some stem cell transplant patients. After appropriate therapy the mucosa has a regenerative appearance with mucosal architectural distortion but absence of ongoing apoptosis (153).

Chronic graft-versus-host disease is a more insidious process that primarily affects skin and liver. The intestinal tract is largely spared except for the esophagus, in which a scleroderma-like fibrosis and dysmotility develop (e308,e309,e446). In the evaluation of all the phases of intestinal graft-versus-host disease, the differential diagnosis must include infection, particularly with opportunistic organisms.

Henoch-Schönlein Purpura and Other Systemic Vasculitides

Henoch-Schönlein purpura is a systemic vasculitis affecting mainly the skin, gastrointestinal tract, joints, and kidneys (e239,e387,e460). It is believed to be triggered by a humoral response to a variety of antigens, including viruses, bacteria, and some drugs. Gastrointestinal involvement is usually in the stomach or small intestine and presents with abdominal pain and bleeding. These may be the heralding symptoms or may follow the characteristic purpuric rash. The underlying gastrointestinal pathology is an acute leukocytoclastic vasculitis of small blood vessels in the submucosa or deep lamina propria (Figure 14-42). Only rarely is this sampled by endoscopic biopsy; instead, nonspecific focal mucosal hemorrhage, edema, erosions, and aphthous ulceration are seen, and endoscopic biopsy shows nonspecific inflammation. These nonspecific histologic features often lead to an erroneous diagnosis of inflammatory bowel disease or nonspecific colitis, resulting in a delay in proper diagnosis (21).

Other forms of vasculitis affecting the intestinal tract include systemic lupus erythematosus, Churg-Strauss syndrome, Wegener granulomatosis, and microscopic polyangiitis (e62). Some cases in the past classified as polyarteritis nodosa affecting the gastrointestinal tract actually represent microscopic polyangiitis using current diagnostic criteria. Some infectious agents, notably enterohemorrhagic strains of *E. coli*, including serotype 0157:H7, and CMV, may target blood vessels and cause small-vessel vasculitis, platelet-fibrin thrombi, and patchy hemorrhage and necrosis.

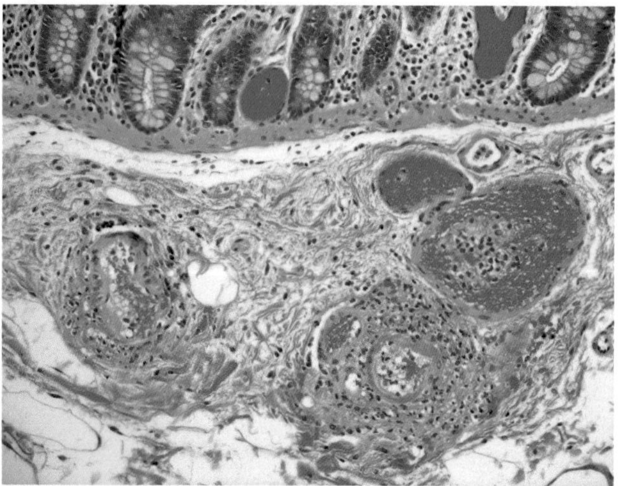

FIGURE 14-42 ■ Henoch-Schönlein purpura. Leukocytoclastic vasculitis involving small submucosal arterioles of the colon 200×.

Table 14-6 ■ CAUSES OF COLITIS IN PEDIATRIC PATIENTS

Idiopathic disorders
Ulcerative colitis
Crohn disease
Lymphocytic/collagenous colitis (rare)
Infections (see Table 14-4)
Viral (e.g., CMV, adenovirus, and enteric viruses)
Bacterial (e.g., *Shigella, Salmonella, E. coli, Clostridium difficile,* etc.)
Fungal (e.g., Zygomycoses)
Parasitic (e.g., Strongyloides)
Autoimmune and immunodeficiency
Autoimmune enterocolitis
Common variable immunodeficiency
Chronic granulomatous disease
Typhlitis (neutropenic enterocolitis)
Miscellaneous
Diversion colitis
Hirschsprung enterocolitis
Allergic colitis
Vasculitides

COLITIS

The numerous causes of colitis in infants and children are listed in Table 14-6. A comprehensive review of this topic is available (e17).

Inflammatory Bowel Disease (IBD)

The term inflammatory bowel disease, as it is commonly used, encompasses only the chronic idiopathic conditions of ulcerative colitis and Crohn disease. Specifically excluded are numerous other gastrointestinal inflammatory processes, including infections, antibiotic-associated colitis, ischemia, and allergic diseases (e78,e246,e250). Ulcerative colitis and Crohn disease have many similar features—enigmatic etiology, familial predisposition, clinical presentation, chronic course, extraintestinal manifestations, and response to treatment. However, important differences make it possible to differentiate between the two entities in most patients, and it is desirable for long-term prognostic and therapeutic purposes to make this distinction if possible. Differentiating Crohn disease from ulcerative colitis may be difficult if the disease is limited to the colon. The clinical findings, pattern of involvement in the gastrointestinal tract, radiologic studies, and histopathology must all be integrated for a diagnosis to be made. In some cases, the distinction is impossible, even after surgical resection and careful pathologic examination; in these cases, the designation inflammatory bowel disease, indeterminate type is used (see below.)

Crohn disease and ulcerative colitis are far from rare in children. Among all cases of inflammatory bowel disease,

20% to 30% are diagnosed before the age of 20 years. The incidence of Crohn disease and ulcerative colitis was approximately equal until the 1970s, but since then, the incidence of Crohn disease in children has risen steadily while the incidence of ulcerative colitis has remained relatively stable (e31,e185). Caucasians are at greatest risk, but other races are also affected. Although most cases in children are diagnosed in the second decade, toddlers and young children may also be affected (e100,e185,e186,e246). The symptoms of inflammatory bowel disease in children are similar to those in adults, but in addition, growth retardation and delayed puberty are commonly encountered, particularly in children with Crohn disease. Cessation of growth resulting from steroid therapy is also an important consideration in the treatment of Crohn disease and ulcerative colitis in children.

Before idiopathic inflammatory bowel disease is diagnosed, intestinal infections with organisms such as *Salmonella*, *Shigella*, *Campylobacter*, *Yersinia*, pathogenic strains of *E. coli*, and *E. histolytica* must be ruled out by appropriate cultures and stool examination. The pathology of inflammatory bowel disease in children is identical to that in adults in most respects (e17,e96,e228).

Ulcerative Colitis

Ulcerative colitis is an idiopathic chronic inflammatory disease that begins in the rectum and extends proximally and contiguously for a variable distance. In a given patient disease may be limited to the rectum, involve only the left colon, or involve the right colon as well. A fluctuating clinical course with exacerbations and remissions is typical. A fulminant presentation with toxic megacolon is also seen. Ulcerative colitis is limited to the colon, although in patients with active pancolitis mild inflammation may also involve the mucosa of the distal few centimeters of the terminal ileum (the so-called backwash ileitis).

Diarrhea and rectal bleeding are the presenting symptoms in nearly all cases, although abdominal pain, cramping, anorexia, and weight loss are also frequently seen. A small percentage of patients have a fulminant presentation, with acute abdominal signs and toxic megacolon. As many as 20% of children have extraintestinal manifestations, with arthritis of the large joints being the most common; uveitis, growth failure, skin involvement, and liver disease are more unusual. Infections (e.g., with *Shigella*, *Salmonella*, *C. difficile*, *Yersinia*, and *E. histolytica*) must be ruled out, and radiologic investigation, including barium enema and radiography of the upper gastrointestinal tract with small-bowel follow-through, is undertaken to determine the extent and type of disease. Endoscopic features of ulcerative colitis include mucosal hyperemia, friability, and ulceration beginning at the rectum and extending proximally. Biopsy specimens taken at multiple levels during colonoscopy are important in diagnosing the disease, monitoring its progress, and evaluating the response to therapy.

Ulcerative colitis can usually be well controlled medically, although powerful immunosuppressive drugs are sometimes necessary. Surgery, usually a total proctocolectomy, cures the disease. Surgery is performed in ulcerative colitis for both acute and chronic indications, including massive bleeding, acute fulminant colitis with megacolon, a chronic course with severe disability or complications of medical therapy, and retardation of growth and sexual maturation. Sphincter-sparing ileal reservoir (ileal "pouch") operations spare the patient a permanent ileostomy (e17,e129). Patients with ulcerative colitis of more than 10 years' duration are advised to undergo periodic surveillance colonoscopy with biopsies to monitor for the development of dysplasia. Cancer is usually preceded by histologic evidence of dysplasia in biopsy specimens (e383).

Pathologic findings in the first endoscopic biopsy specimens from a given patient may not be diagnostic by themselves, but they are extremely helpful in arriving at a diagnosis when integrated with clinical and radiologic findings. In most cases of untreated ulcerative colitis, the mucosal biopsy specimen shows diffusely increased numbers of chronic inflammatory cells (plasma cells and lymphocytes) and acute inflammatory cells (polymorphonuclear leukocytes and eosinophils) in the lamina propria. Plasma cells dominate the inflammatory response, often densely packing the lamina propria and extending beneath crypts (basal plasmacytosis). Crypt abscesses and intraepithelial neutrophils may be present at the initial diagnosis and during exacerbations (Figure 14-43). Superficial ulcerations may be seen, but even in their absence, damage to the surface epithelium is nearly always indicated by the presence of regenerating epithelial cells without goblet cells.

In normal colonic mucosa the crypts are arranged in straight and evenly spaced rows. Even at the time of the initial presentation of ulcerative colitis, with symptoms of short duration, biopsies of involved segments will usually exhibit distortion of this normal crypt architecture. This is typically

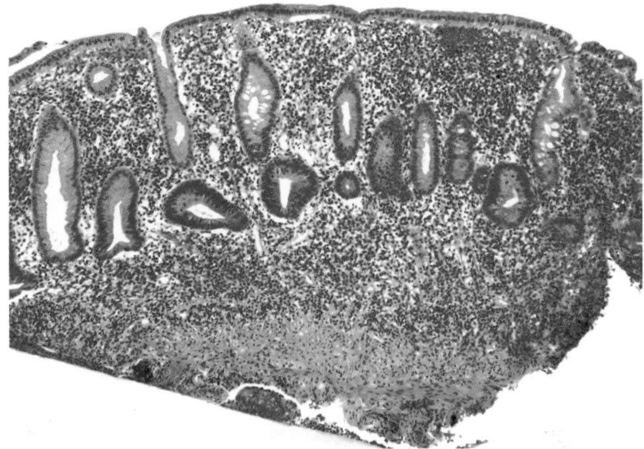

FIGURE 14-43 ▪ Colonic biopsy demonstrating active ulcerative colitis. Note the presence of crypt architectural distortion and a basal infiltrate of lymphocytes and plasma cells between the bases of the crypts and the muscularis mucosae 100×.

manifested by scattered branched and irregularly shaped crypts, as well as crypts that no longer extend all the way down to the muscularis mucosae. Assessment of crypt architecture is much easier in well-oriented biopsies. In poorly oriented biopsies the crypts are usually seen in cross section as doughnut-shaped profiles, which makes it difficult to evaluate branching and foreshortening. However, irregular spacing and variation in crypt diameter may still be observed in tangential sections. A feature often associated with crypt architectural distortion is the presence of Paneth cell metaplasia. Paneth cells are normally present in the mucosa throughout the small intestine but in the colon are limited to crypts of the cecum and ascending colon. In IBD Paneth cells may be present more distally, and their presence is a good marker of chronic colitis. In patients with inactive disease of very long duration crypt architectural distortion may become very subtle, to the point where the histologic (and endoscopic) appearance may be indistinguishable from normal. In this situation review of biopsies obtained during previous colonoscopic procedures may be necessary to confirm a diagnosis of IBD.

In the relatively recent era of routine colonoscopy and effective medical therapy for IBD it has become clear that healing ulcerative colitis can appear quite patchy endoscopically, simulating the appearance of Crohn colitis (e38,e39,e249). Fortunately, microscopic examination of these apparent "skip areas" of endoscopically normal mucosa in patients with treated ulcerative colitis usually reveals evidence of quiescent disease, as indicated by the presence of (sometimes subtle) crypt architectural distortion. However, patchy areas of completely normal mucosa have been documented in long-standing ulcerative colitis. Often this is a result of intensive long-term medical therapy, but it can also be seen before therapy is instituted. There are also cases in which skip areas of normal mucosa are definitely present from the onset (typically a segment in the transverse or descending colon), and yet all other clinical and histologic features are consistent with the diagnosis of ulcerative colitis. The clinical course in such a patient is almost always that of typical ulcerative colitis (e249,e252). Topical steroid therapy delivered via enema has been convincingly demonstrated to result in complete resolution of active inflammation and regression of crypt architectural distortion in rectal biopsies from ulcerative colitis patients (e283,e340).

Histologically, rectal sparing at the onset of symptoms has been documented to occur in a subset of pediatric patients with ulcerative colitis (48,123,152) (e296). These patients may also have histologically patchy disease at presentation (59,155). No clinical feature appears to separate children who present with rectal sparing from those who do not, although atypical histology may be more common in the youngest children (124).

The distinctive features of ulcerative colitis are better visualized in colonic resection specimens. Ulcerative colitis is most often characterized by uninterrupted mucosal involvement beginning at the rectum and extending proximally in a circumferential and contiguous manner.

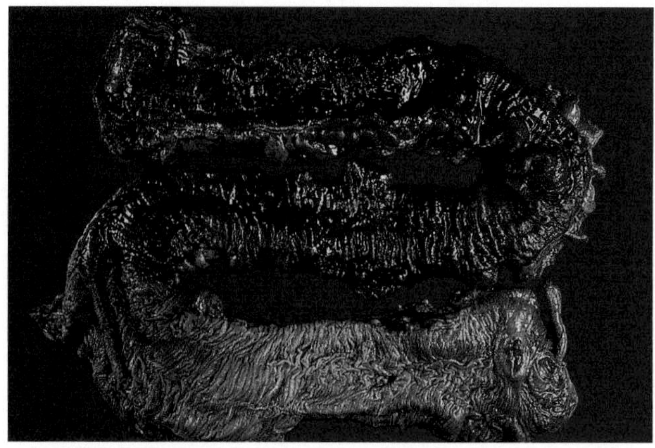

FIGURE 14-44 ■ Total abdominal colectomy specimen from a patient with ulcerative colitis involving the left colon.

The mucosa is usually diffusely hyperemic and granular, with areas of superficial or deep ulceration in patients under poor medical control at the time of colectomy (Figure 14-44). Inflammatory polyps may be present, and in some cases are numerous (Figure 14-45). The ileal mucosa is generally grossly unremarkable. The rectum and descending colon may show more chronic changes, such as loss of the haustral folds and a smooth or granular mucosal surface. Conspicuously absent are skip (uninvolved) areas, strictures, fistulas, and fibrotic thickening of the colonic wall, all of which are commonly seen in Crohn disease.

Histologic examination reveals inflammation that most severely affects the mucosa and submucosa, with lesser severity or sparing of the muscularis layers and serosa. Extensively ulcerated areas show mucosal and submucosal destruction, with replacement by granulation tissue. Inflammatory polyps are composed of islands of surviving mucosa with pronounced glandular distortion, inflammation, and capillary dilation. After the acute inflammation has subsided and healing has occurred, evidence of ulcerative colitis remains as a loss of crypt parallelism, crypt atrophy and shortening, hypertrophy of the muscularis mucosae, and metaplasia of Paneth cells. The appendix is commonly involved in resected specimens (e170,e233) even when the cecum is spared, an

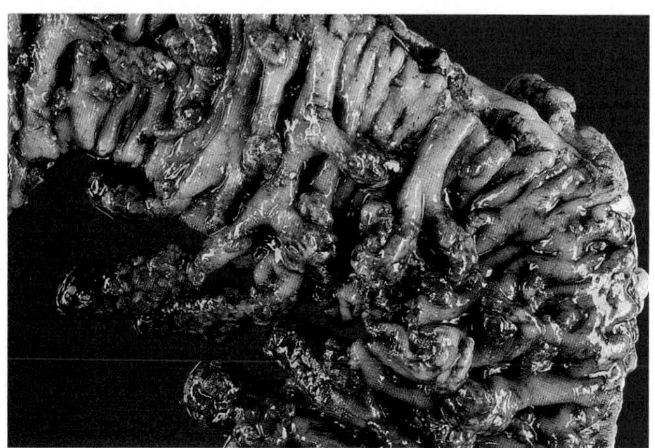

FIGURE 14-45 ■ Ulcerative colitis with inflammatory polyps.

exception to the diffuse contiguous involvement characteristic of ulcerative colitis (e107,e268).

Crohn Disease

In contrast to ulcerative colitis, Crohn disease may arise anywhere in the gastrointestinal tract, from mouth to anus. In approximately 50% of children with Crohn disease, the classic distal ileal and proximal colonic involvement is seen. Approximately 15% of children have only diffuse small-bowel disease, another 15% have only distal ileal involvement, and 10% have isolated colonic disease. The remaining 10% have disease in another site, as in gastroduodenal Crohn disease (e280,e302,e392,e505), or combination of sites.

Symptoms depend on the site of involvement, but in general the presentation of Crohn disease is more insidious than that of ulcerative colitis, so that the diagnosis is often delayed. Vague abdominal pain, diarrhea, growth failure, and anorexia are common. Small-bowel involvement may present as diarrhea and malabsorption. Colonic involvement may present as bloody diarrhea and mimic ulcerative colitis. Endoscopic and radiologic studies of the upper and lower gastrointestinal tract are important in determining the extent of involvement.

Unlike ulcerative colitis, Crohn disease is characterized by a segmental or skip pattern, in which involved areas of intestine are often separated by normal intestine. Another important distinguishing feature is that the inflammation in Crohn disease is transmural rather than mucosal, so that fissures, fistulas, intramural abscesses, strictures, and fibrous adhesions develop (Figure 14-46). Thickening of the bowel wall as a result of edema and fibrosis occurs at the expense of the lumen and causes intestinal obstruction. Inflammation, edema, and fibrosis of the bowel and regional lymph nodes may cause adjacent structures to mat together and form an ileocecal mass. Perianal fissures, skin tags, and rectal-perineal fistulas and abscesses are common in children with Crohn disease.

Endoscopic examination in Crohn disease often reveals patchy involvement and skip areas of normal mucosa. Ulcerations are often linear, with intervening preserved mucosal islands, resulting in a cobblestone appearance. Small (<5 mm), round, superficial "aphthoid" ulcerations are common in otherwise normal mucosa at the periphery of more severely involved segments. In Crohn colitis the right side of the colon is often more severely affected than the left, and the rectum may be completely spared.

The histologic hallmark of Crohn disease is the presence of noncaseating epithelioid granulomas (eFigure 14-11). Unfortunately, granulomas can be identified in biopsy specimens in less than 50% of Crohn disease patients, limiting the utility of this feature. The routine examination of serial sections increases the likelihood of the identification of granulomas (e271). Poorly formed granulomas can occur in association with ruptured crypt abscesses in ulcerative colitis, presumably in response to extravasated mucin. Examination of serial sections may be necessary to demonstrate the relationship between the damaged crypt and the granuloma (eFigure 14-12). Also, in a tangential section the pericryptal fibroblast sheath can resemble a small granuloma. Distinction between Crohn disease and intestinal tuberculosis can also be problematic (86).

Mucosal biopsy specimens in Crohn disease show increased numbers of chronic and acute inflammatory cells in the lamina propria, crypt abscesses, and superficial ulcerations, all of which are nondiagnostic in the absence of granulomas. In many cases the degree of crypt architectural distortion is less severe in Crohn disease than is typical of ulcerative colitis, but confident distinction between the two diseases cannot rest on the assessment of this feature. Relative preservation of the mucin content of goblet cells, even in cases of severe inflammation, is also more characteristic of Crohn colitis than ulcerative colitis (9).

The histologic features of Crohn ileitis are essentially identical to those evident in colonic biopsies. There is usually clear-cut distortion of normal villous architecture at least focally. Mucous (pyloric) gland metaplasia is a reliable marker of long-standing inflammation and is common in ileal biopsies from patients with Crohn disease (Figure 14-47). However, mucous gland metaplasia has also

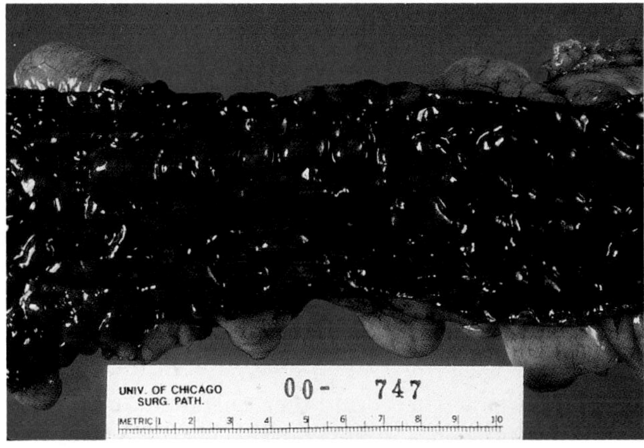

FIGURE 14-46 ▪ Crohn enteritis with cobblestoned mucosa.

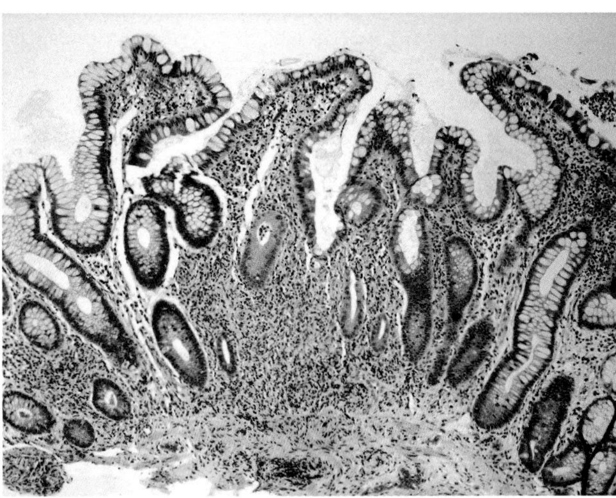

FIGURE 14-47 ▪ Crohn ileitis. The inflammatory cell infiltrates are distinctly focal and destructive of the crypt epithelium (100×).

been documented in biopsies of ileal ulcers from patients taking NSAIDs (90). Although ulcerative colitis is classically limited to the colon, some patients with pancolitis may exhibit the so-called "backwash ileitis." "Backwash ileitis" generally consists only of scattered neutrophils in the lamina propria and surface epithelium, with relative preservation of the mucosal architecture. However, the spectrum of ileal mucosal damage in backwash ileitis has not been well-defined in the current era of routine colonoscopic ileal biopsies (36).

Transmural chronic inflammation is the most helpful histologic feature in a resected intestinal specimen from a patient with Crohn disease. Deep knifelike fissures, fistulas lined by granulation tissue, and fibrous strictures are also characteristic. Submucosal fibrosis and the presence of many lymphoid aggregates or follicles also suggest Crohn disease rather than ulcerative colitis (e17,e228,e366).

One of the best ways to distinguish between ulcerative colitis and Crohn disease is by examination of biopsies from the upper gastrointestinal tract. The presence of significant patchy inflammatory changes of the esophageal, gastric, or duodenal mucosa, while usually not diagnostic in isolation, can be very helpful in confirming a diagnosis of Crohn disease (89) (e505).

The medical treatment of Crohn disease is similar to that of ulcerative colitis, although anti–tumor necrosis factor monoclonal antibody therapy plays a more central role in Crohn disease. Surgery is not curative in Crohn disease and is generally undertaken only when intestinal obstruction, fistulas, massive hemorrhage, or abscesses supervene. Growth failure while the patient is on medical therapy and failure of medical therapy may also be reasons for a limited surgical resection.

Indeterminate Colitis

The term indeterminate colitis is descriptive rather than diagnostic and is applied to cases of chronic inflammatory bowel disease in which ulcerative colitis cannot be distinguished from Crohn disease. The term was first used by Price (e365) in a description of fulminant pancolitis with overlapping pathologic findings, but it has gradually come to encompass other cases with a gradual onset. In up to one-fourth of patients with a colitic presentation of chronic inflammatory bowel disease, the distinction between Crohn disease and ulcerative colitis cannot be made, even when the endoscopic, imaging, and biopsy findings are known. The term indeterminate colitis is often used as a temporary designation until evolution of the disease provides further clues, such as the development of granulomas, fistulas, or gastroduodenal or perineal involvement in Crohn disease. In a small percentage of patients, the distinction between Crohn disease and ulcerative colitis is extremely difficult or impossible, even after a chronic course and colonic resection.

It is important to make the distinction between ulcerative colitis and Crohn disease if possible because the surgical treatment of ulcerative colitis is significantly different from that of Crohn colitis. Patients with severe ulcerative colitis who fail medical therapy undergo a total proctocolectomy with creation of an internal ileal reservoir (J-pouch) and ileal pouch–anal anastomosis, which allow defecation through the anus. Patients with Crohn colitis often do poorly after the creation of an ileal reservoir, and the procedure is contraindicated in them (e17).

Lymphocytic Colitis

Lymphocytic colitis was originally called microscopic colitis when it was first described in adults with chronic diarrhea and normal colonoscopy findings, but demonstrable mucosal inflammation on colonic biopsy specimens. In the past decade, the definition has been refined and the name changed to lymphocytic colitis with the recognition that patients often have other autoimmune diseases, such as diabetes and arthritis, and that the colonic inflammation is characterized by an increase in T-lymphocytes. On biopsy specimens, characteristic findings are increased numbers of IELs, surface epithelial damage, and dense mononuclear cell inflammation of the lamina propria in the absence of crypt architectural distortion and acute cryptitis (e49,e227,e276,e509). Similar findings are encountered in some patients with celiac disease (e504). Lymphocytic colitis is seldom diagnosed in children, although occasional cases have been described (e303).

Collagenous Colitis

Collagenous colitis has many of the same clinical and histologic characteristics as lymphocytic colitis (see above), with the additional histologic finding of a distinct subepithelial collagen band that is obvious with hematoxylin and eosin stain and highlighted by Masson trichrome stain. The collagen band represents a thickened basement membrane that is unevenly distributed in specimens from different areas of the colon and is probably thickest in the proximal colon. A basement membrane thickness of at least 10 μm is suggested for the diagnosis of collagenous colitis, measured in well-oriented sections in which crypts are longitudinally sectioned. In adults, the thickness of the basement membrane in collagenous colitis is variable up to 50 μm (e49,e227,e276,e509). The many similarities of lymphocytic and collagenous colitis suggest a similar pathogenesis. This condition is almost never diagnosed in children, but an occasional report is the exception (e179). Crypt architectural distortion and acute cryptitis are found in Crohn disease and ulcerative colitis, neither of which is seen in microscopic or collagenous colitis.

Acute Self-limited Colitis (Infectious Colitis)

Acute self-limited colitis is defined clinically as a condition in which diarrhea, often bloody and with a sudden onset, resolves spontaneously after several weeks. It is presumed to be bacterial in nature but since stool cultures are not routinely obtained in every case of diarrhea a specific causal organism is not identified in a given patient. The histologic features include neutrophils in the lamina propria, cryptitis, and, in the most severe cases, erosions and microscopic ulcerations, but normal crypt architecture is well maintained (e17,e178,e447,e448). In some cases the superficial portion of the mucosa is focally necrotic and hemorrhagic (eFigure 14-13). The lamina propria lacks the basal lymphoplasmacytosis seen in chronic inflammatory bowel disease (e126,e277,e337,e407,e447,e448). Despite these differences, in the absence of a stool culture positive for organisms, it is still sometimes difficult to assign an initial biopsy to the self-limited infectious category rather than to chronic inflammatory bowel disease. Further clinical studies and a follow-up period of observation usually clarify the situation.

Pseudomembranous Colitis

The term pseudomembranous colitis refers to a gross or endoscopic appearance of the colonic mucosa in which numerous discrete, irregular, yellow plaques, 0.2 to 2.0 cm in diameter, appear anywhere on the colonic mucosal surface. In the most severe cases, the membranes coalesce and become nearly confluent, and the process spreads to involve most of the colon. The membranes are tightly adherent to the mucosal surface; wiping does not remove them.

Formerly thought to represent *C. difficile* infection in nearly all cases, pseudomembranous colitis is now known to occur in infection with *E. coli* 0157:H7 (e380), other toxin-producing strains of *E. coli*, and *Shigella*, and in ischemia, ulcerative colitis and Crohn colitis, uremia, fungal infections, neonatal necrotizing enterocolitis, and Hirschsprung disease–associated enterocolitis (e373). However, antibiotic-associated *C. difficile* infection is still the most common cause. When *C. difficile* infection is responsible, pseudomembranous colitis typically develops during a course of antibiotic therapy or up to 6 weeks afterward (e30,e64,e244,e316,e485). *C. difficile* overgrows in the colon after antibiotic alteration of normal flora. Clindamycin, ampicillin, penicillin, cephalosporins, and many other antibiotics have been implicated. The onset of watery diarrhea is usually abrupt and accompanied by systemic signs, including fever, abdominal pain, and leukocytosis.

Histologically, pseudomembranes are composed of inflammatory cell exudate, necrotic debris, and desquamated and apoptotic epithelial cells, admixed with red blood cells and mucus. The pseudomembrane overlies acutely inflamed colonic mucosa. In cases of pseudomembranous colitis due to due to *C. difficile* infection there is a characteristic lesion that has been likened to a mushroom or volcano erupting from the crypts (Figure 14-48). The surface epithelium is often destroyed, and in severe cases, much of the mucosa is necrotic. The intervening areas of mucosa are normal or show nonspecific colitis while the submucosa is often edematous the deeper bowel layers are usually normal (e17,e64,e244,e316).

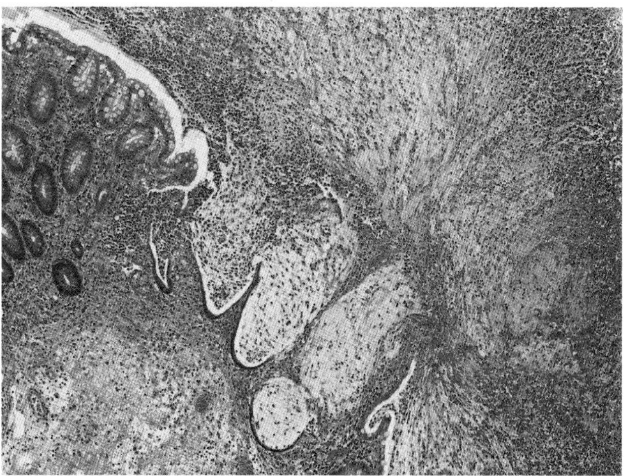

FIGURE 14-48 ■ *Clostridium difficile* infection. The classic "erupting volcano" appearance with a pseudomembrane composed of desquamated epithelial cells, inflammatory cells, and red blood cells admixed with mucus and fibrin 100×.

Colitis Associated with Antibiotics

By altering the normal gut flora, antibiotics can cause a wide variety of gastrointestinal symptoms; these range from innocuous diarrhea that ceases with the antibiotic therapy to fatal pseudomembranous colitis (see preceding section) (e244,e316,e485). Tissue alterations, when they occur at all, can be manifested as an enteritis or colitis. When the colon is affected, findings range from acute self-limited colitis to hemorrhagic colitis (e238) and pseudomembranous colitis. *C. difficile* infection is sought by either toxin assay or selective culture in the most severe cases because it is responsible much of the time.

Diversion Colitis

Diversion colitis is a chronic inflammatory process in an intestinal segment that has been bypassed by ileostomy or colostomy and left in place, as in Hirschsprung disease, Crohn disease, ulcerative colitis, or other conditions that are treated surgically. The cause is unknown but is thought to be an interplay between altered bacterial flora and a deficiency of short chain fatty acids in the bypassed segment (e17,e199). In milder cases, the findings are identified incidentally during pathologic examination of a bypassed segment removed during a "pull-through" procedure for Hirschsprung disease. Other patients may become symptomatic and demonstrate endoscopic mucosal abnormalities, including erythema, friability, and aphthous ulcerations. The most characteristic histologic finding is mucosal and submucosal follicular lymphoid hyperplasia. Chronic mucosal inflammation, acute cryptitis, crypt abscesses, and epithelial injury are seen in the most severe cases. The clinical setting usually suggests the diagnosis, but in patients with chronic inflammatory bowel disease, these findings in the rectosigmoid colon may pose a diagnostic dilemma when ulcerative colitis must be distinguished from Crohn disease (e17,e169,e194,e199,e259,e289).

Typhlitis (Neutropenic Enterocolitis)

The term typhilitis is derived from the Greek word meaning "blind sac" (referring to the cecum). It is a necrotizing enterocolitis typically centered around or limited to the cecum. It was first described in children with leukemia (e486), but other susceptible persons are patients undergoing cancer chemotherapy or being treated with immunosuppressive drugs following bone marrow or solid organ transplantation, children with AIDS, and those with neutropenia secondary to hematologic diseases. Symptoms include fever, diarrhea, and right lower quadrant pain. Bacterial sepsis with recovery of enteric bacteria is common, and polymicrobial sepsis is not unusual. The involved bowel is edematous, hemorrhagic, and ulcerated. Transmural necrosis not uncommonly leads to bowel perforation. Antibiotics are sometimes effective in arresting the infection, but intestinal resection is necessary in many cases (e240,e413,e482,e486).

Neonatal Necrotizing Enterocolitis

Neonatal necrotizing enterocolitis is a distinctive common disease of premature infants in the neonatal intensive care unit characterized by coagulative and hemorrhagic necrosis and inflammation of portions of the small and large intestine (e214,e253). Despite decades of research, the precise pathogenesis of this disease remains enigmatic (93,107,132). Important contributing factors include altered bowel motility and digestion, immature intestinal circulatory regulation, abnormal bacterial colonization, immature intestinal mucosal barrier, and enteral formula feedings. Intestinal ischemia results from reduced splanchnic perfusion, systemic hypoperfusion, systemic hypoxia, or local factors such as intestinal gaseous distension. Bacterial colonization is nearly always present, although neonatal necrotizing enterocolitis is not primarily an infectious process in the usual sense and no specific organisms or group of organisms have been implicated. Immature innate intestinal immune function likely contributes to the process of bacterial colonization. Inflammatory mediators, especially platelet-activating factor and tumor necrosis factor, are endogenously induced by the presence of bacterial toxins and play an important role in the pathophysiology of intestinal necrosis in neonatal necrotizing enterocolitis. The role of oral feeding strategies in the pathogenesis of neonatal necrotizing enterocolitis has been debated for years. There does appear to consensus that human breast milk feeds have a beneficial role, perhaps by aiding in establishing a healthy intestinal bacterial flora and by augmenting cellular and humoral immunity. The feeding of hyperosmolar formulas, in contrast, may result in the proliferation of abnormal gut flora and may adversely affect intestinal perfusion (93,107,132).

Neonatal necrotizing enterocolitis occurs primarily in premature infants with birth weights ranging from 1,000 to 1,500 g who are more than 2 weeks of age and who are severely ill with respiratory distress syndrome (Chapter 12). However, up to 10% of infants with neonatal necrotizing enterocolitis are born at term, and the disease may develop as early as the 1st day of life (143). Manifestations include abdominal distension, bloody stools, diarrhea, gastric retention of feedings, shock, and apnea. As many as one-third of the affected infants have a fulminant course with intestinal perforation, and a similar number have bacterial sepsis. The overall mortality is approximately 15% to 30%. The diagnosis of neonatal necrotizing enterocolitis requires a suggestive clinical picture and radiographic demonstration of pneumatosis intestinalis (i.e., gas within the bowel wall) or gas in the portal or hepatic veins. However, positive radiologic signs may be lacking in one-third of the patients in whom the diagnosis is confirmed at surgery or autopsy (93,107,132).

In most cases, the most severely affected portions of the gastrointestinal tract are the terminal ileum and cecum (80%) and the ascending colon, although either the small intestine or colon alone may be affected, or the entire small intestine and colon. The gross appearance of neonatal necrotizing enterocolitis in 50% of the cases is that of a patchy segmental necrosis with intervening spared areas; half of the cases show a continuous segment of intestine with circumferential necrosis, dilation, and friability. If perforation has occurred, peritonitis is present. The mucosa shows a combination of coagulative necrosis, inflammation, and hemorrhage. Focal necrotic pseudomembrane formation is seen in approximately 10% of cases. Overall microscopic features are similar in most cases of neonatal necrotizing enterocolitis, but the findings vary considerably from one microscopic field to another. Coagulative and hemorrhagic necrosis is always present; it is limited to the mucosa in the early stages but at least focally transmural in the surgical or autopsy cases (Figure 14-49). Acute and chronic inflammation is commonly

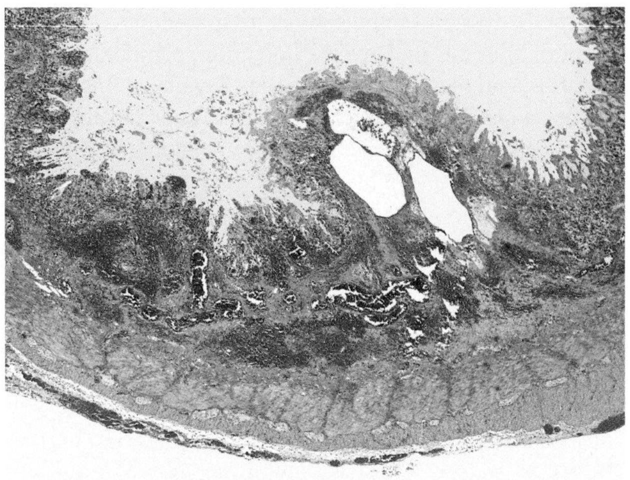

FIGURE 14-49 ■ Necrotizing enterocolitis. This section from a resected portion of small bowel reveals extensive mucosal necrosis and submucosal hemorrhage. Note the large air spaces in the submucosa consistent with pneumatosis cystoides 40×.

found, limited to the mucosa in some foci but transmural in others. Inflammation and coagulative necrosis often occur together in a given segment, but in some instances, one or the other may predominate (e26).

Mixed intestinal bacteria are often visible in the lumen or within the necrotic superficial mucosa. Fungal growth is unusual, occurring in 3.5% of cases in one large series (e26). Pneumatosis intestinalis is found in approximately one-half of surgical specimens with neonatal necrotizing enterocolitis, usually limited to the submucosa. These gas bubbles have been shown to contain hydrogen, a product of bacterial fermentation. More than 50% of the cases of neonatal necrotizing enterocolitis undergoing laparotomy show focal reparative epithelial changes and other evidence of healing, such as the formation of granulation tissue and crypt distortion. Villous atrophy may be observed (e26,e231). Such changes suggest that neonatal necrotizing enterocolitis evolves gradually before a catastrophic event, such as perforation, brings it to clinical attention.

Intestine compromised by neonatal necrotizing enterocolitis, but not resected during the acute phase of the disease, may develop progressive circumferential submucosal fibrosis during healing, causing intestinal stricture (e35,e262,e265). Strictures are found in 10% to 20% of infants between 3 and 10 or more weeks after neonatal necrotizing enterocolitis has been diagnosed. Before oral feedings are resumed, strictures are routinely sought by barium enema.

The treatment of neonatal necrotizing enterocolitis includes cessation of oral feedings, administration of antibiotics, and surgery or percutaneous peritoneal drainage for perforation or other evidence of severe bowel compromise. Lengthy intestinal resection may produce short-bowel syndrome. Other complications include peritonitis, sepsis and its complications, and compromised nutrition. Long-term parenteral nutrition is required in many cases (65).

Spontaneous Perforation of the Gastrointestinal Tract

Isolated spontaneous perforation of the gastrointestinal tract in premature and term neonates occurs occasionally as a clinical event distinct from neonatal necrotizing enterocolitis. It is usually an unexpected event in an infant not known to have any prior gastrointestinal compromise (e23). The perforation develops in a single location in almost any part of the stomach (e221), small intestine, or colon, and at laparotomy, the damage to surrounding tissue is inapparent or minimal. Some cases have been explained by prior exposure of the infant to indomethacin to close a patent ductus arteriosus or arrest maternal preterm labor (e5,e419). In other cases, localized segmental absence or thinning of the muscularis externa has been observed (e217,e286) and is thought to represent a congenital abnormality. This view is not universally accepted; however, an opposing view is that the thinning of muscle layers occurs secondary to excessive distension, tearing, and retraction of muscle fibers. A final common pathway in these cases is probably localized ischemia (e217), caused by a drug, a transient local decrease in splanchnic circulation, or a combination of these factors. One case report noted the simultaneous occurrence of intestinal atresia, known to be ischemic in origin in most cases, and a segmental absence of muscle coats (e7). Defects in muscle have also been described in strictures developing after neonatal necrotizing enterocolitis and after ischemic bowel disease in older patients.

Allergic Colitis (Allergic Proctocolitis)

Allergic proctocolitis is a common cause of rectal bleeding and diarrhea in infants younger than 6 months to 1 year of age. Most of those affected have been fed artificial formulas, usually based on cow's milk protein, or have recently been switched from breast- to bottle-feedings. However, any dietary protein can be responsible, and cases have been described in infants fed with soy milks, casein hydrolysate formulas, and even breast milk; in the latter cases, the offending protein is thought to originate in the mother's diet and be transmitted in breast milk (e171,e207,e229,e291,e341,e362, e475,e500).

The presenting symptom is usually blood streaks on the surface of stools or bloody diarrhea in an otherwise healthy infant. Constipation is a presenting symptom in some patients. Fever, leukocytosis, and other signs of infection are lacking. A peripheral blood eosinophilia is characteristic, but is not present in every patient (109) (e219,e291,e500). Colonoscopy may be normal, but most often there is mucosal erythema, erosions, and loss of the normal vascular pattern (e291).

Colonic biopsies usually reveal preservation of the normal crypt architecture. The most characteristic histologic feature is a patchy or diffuse increase in eosinophils. Various studies have used different cutoff values to separate normal controls from patients with allergic colitis (109) (e171,e500). A frequently cited rule of thumb regarding the number of eosinophils is that 60 eosinophils should be seen in 10 high power fields in the lamina propria plus eosinophils within the epithelium (e109). The presence of focal eosinophilic cryptitis with damage to crypt epithelium, eosinophilic crypt abscesses, or infiltration of fibers of the muscularis mucosa, are features helpful in confirming the diagnosis when sheets of lamina propria eosinophils are not present. (Figure 14-50A,B).

The differential diagnosis includes infectious colitis, which may present with similar symptoms but is characterized by polymorphonuclear leukocytes rather than eosinophils. Eosinophilic gastroenteritis should also be considered in the differential diagnosis if tissue eosinophils are very prominent, although this is much less likely to occur in infants.

The treatment of allergic proctitis consists of a dietary change to eliminate the offending protein. A large number of special formulas are commercially available. The diagnosis of allergic proctitis is not considered confirmed unless the symptoms and rectal eosinophilia resolve on the elimination diet and recur with challenge feedings of the offending protein.

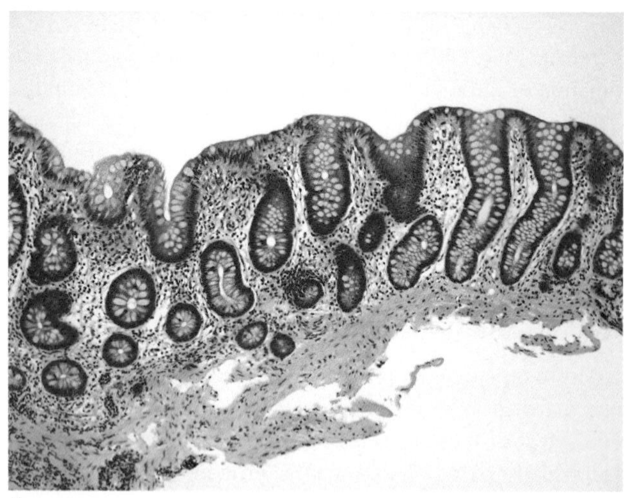

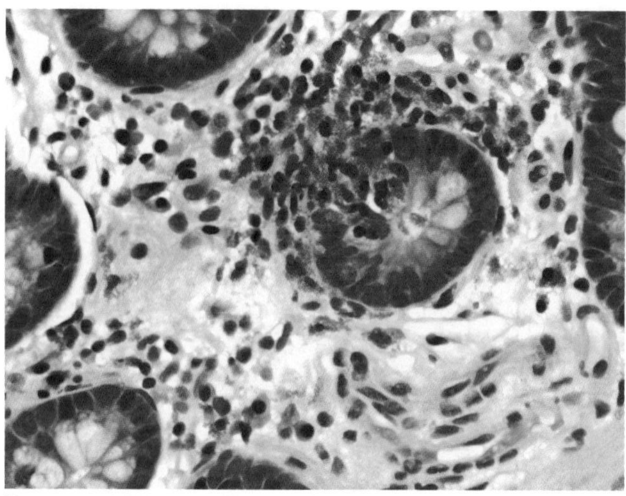

A B

FIGURE 14-50 ■ Eosinophilic colitis due to food allergy in an infant. **A:** Normal crypt architecture is maintained 100×. **B:** Eosinophilic infiltrates can be quite patchy 400×.

INTESTINAL NEOPLASMS

Intestinal tumors are uncommon in children, and most of them are not malignant. Many childhood intestinal masses prove not to be tumors at all but rather inflammatory processes, such as ileocecal Crohn disease, or developmental anomalies, such as duplication cyst or pancreatic heterotopia. Except for juvenile and Peutz-Jeghers polyps, epithelial lesions are unusual, in contrast to their frequent occurrence in the adult intestine. The most common category of intestinal malignancy in children is non-Hodgkin lymphoma, particularly Burkitt lymphoma. Hereditary syndromes should be kept in mind when certain types of gastrointestinal polyps and tumors appear in children. An excellent comprehensive review of pediatric gastrointestinal tract polyps and neoplasms is available (e82).

Polyps

Juvenile polyps of the rectosigmoid colon are the most commonly encountered gastrointestinal neoplasms in children. Other polyps of the gastrointestinal tract are rare in children, yet they merit precise identification because of potentially important long-term implications to both the children and their families. Most polyposis syndromes are hereditary and associated with an increased risk for gastrointestinal and other malignancies (e82,e193).

Juvenile Polyps and Juvenile Polyposis Syndrome

Juvenile polyposis is an autosomal dominant syndrome characterized by the development of multiple hamartomatous gastrointestinal hamartomatous polyps. The prevalence is approximately 1 in 100,000 (47,69,73). Germline mutations in either of two genes of the TGF-beta signaling pathway, the SMAD4 gene located on chromosome 18q21, or the BMPR1a gene on chromosome 10q23 are identified in about 45% of affected patients. Between 25% and 50% of cases there is no family history of the disorder (25,29).

Polyps usually develop during childhood and number between 5 and 100. Presenting symptoms and the gastrointestinal distribution of polyps have led to the clinical subclassification of juvenile polyposis. There is a rare infantile form in which severe polyposis of the entire gastrointestinal tract leads to clinically significant protein-losing enteropathy, rectal bleeding, intussusception or prolapse of polyps, and involvement of other organ systems. In some affected probands an autosomal recessive pattern of inheritance has been suggested. Another group of patients present later in childhood with a milder form of generalized gastrointestinal involvement. There is also a subset of patients who develop only colonic polyps. Finally, there is a small group of patients with both hereditary hemorrhagic telangiectasia and juvenile polyposis syndrome who develop vascular ectasias throughout the body, including the gastrointestinal tract, as well as gastrointestinal juvenile polyps (47,69).

Because isolated colonic juvenile type polyps occur in up to 2% of children who do not have juvenile polyposis syndrome, criteria for the diagnosis of the syndrome have been developed. The diagnosis requires either (a) documentation of five juvenile polyps, (b) the presence of juvenile polyps in the stomach or small bowel, or (c) the presence of any juvenile polyp and a positive family history of juvenile polyposis syndrome. Because there is some overlap of the histologic features of juvenile polyps and other types of gastrointestinal hamartomatous polyps [especially the phosphatase and tensin homolog (PTEN) hamartoma syndromes, discussed below], the diagnosis also requires the absence of extraintestinal manifestations of any other polyposis syndrome (47,69).

Juvenile polyps develop as a disordered overgrowth of mucosal elements. Colonic juvenile polyps consist of hyperplastic and cystically dilatated crypts set in an abundant

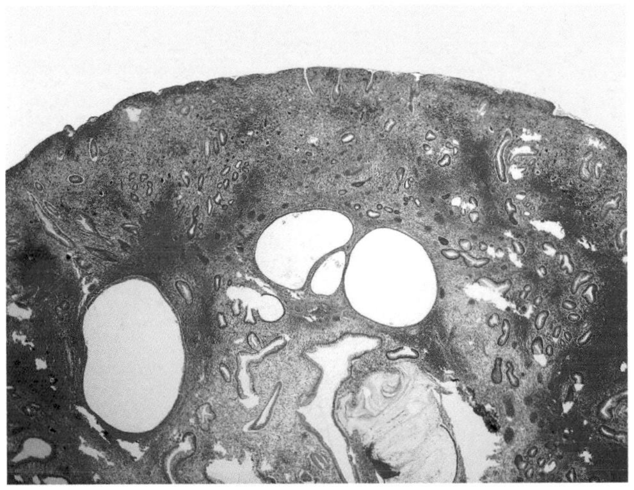

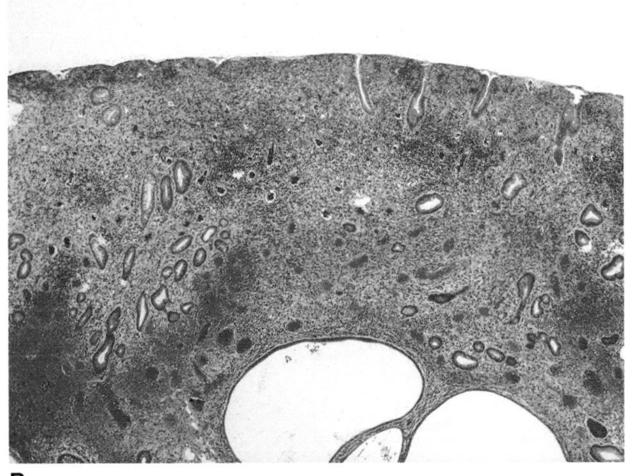

A B

FIGURE 14-51 ▪ **AB:** Sporadic juvenile polyps usually exhibit cystically dilated crypts, abundant edematous and inflamed stroma with numerous eosinophils, and surface erosion. **A:** 40×, **B:** 100×.

edematous and markedly inflamed stroma. Isolated juvenile polyps are usually sessile and extensively eroded, resulting in the development of abundant superficial granulation tissue (Figure 14-51A,B) (73). This produces a highly characteristic strawberry-like endoscopic appearance. The polyps in patients with the juvenile polyposis syndrome, in contrast, often lack this extensive surface erosion and may have a more pedunculated configuration. In addition, there is usually a greater amount of the epithelial component and less of the stromal elements in the syndromic polyps (Figure 14-52). In contrast to colonic Peutz-Jeghers polyps an arborizing core of smooth muscle is usually not present, although a few smooth muscle fibers may be evident if the polyp has been prolapsing. In small polyps the crypt hyperplasia and stromal edema and inflammation may be minimal, making accurate recognition difficult. Dysplasia does occur rarely in the polyps of patients with colonic juvenile polyposis polyps, but great care must be taken to avoid overcalling reactive changes related to the inflammatory background (Figure 14-53A,B).

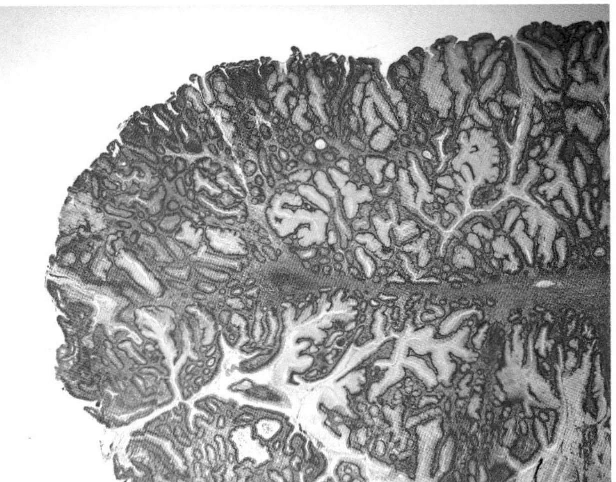

FIGURE 14-52 ▪ Juvenile polyposis syndrome in which the polyps typically exhibit greater epithelial proliferation, less stroma, and an intact surface epithelium 20×.

Gastric juvenile polyps are histologically similar to their colonic counterparts. There is disorganized hyperplasia and cystic dilatation of the gastric foveolar epithelium set in a background of inflamed and edematous stroma (Figure 14-54A,B). Unfortunately, these same features also characterize sporadic gastric hyperplastic polyps, and histologic distinction is generally not possible. Sporadic gastric hyperplastic polyps can be multiple and do not always occur in a background of diffuse gastritis, which makes separation from gastric involvement by juvenile polyposis even more problematic. Furthermore, gastric Peutz-Jeghers polyps often have a very poorly developed core of arborizing smooth muscle fibers and therefore can also closely resemble gastric juvenile polyps. These confounding factors suggest that histologic classification of hamartomatous polyps is best performed by analysis of small-bowel or colonic polyps. If gastric polyps are discovered first, the prudent course for the surgical pathologist is to suggest the possibility of a polyposis syndrome and to recommend examination for small-bowel or colonic polyps. Gastric juvenile polyps may also develop dysplastic changes, but once again care must be taken not to mistake reactive epithelial changes due to inflammation for dysplasia (73).

Involvement of the small bowel by juvenile polyposis is less common than colonic and gastric involvement, and the polyps are less often sampled endoscopically. Small intestinal juvenile polyps lack the well-developed core of smooth muscle of Peutz-Jeghers polyps and are generally much more inflamed, so accurate distinction is usually not problematic.

There is a significant lifetime risk of malignancy in patients with juvenile polyposis syndrome, including cancers of the pancreas, stomach, small bowel, and colon. One study of the risk of colorectal cancer yielded an absolute risk of 38.7 per

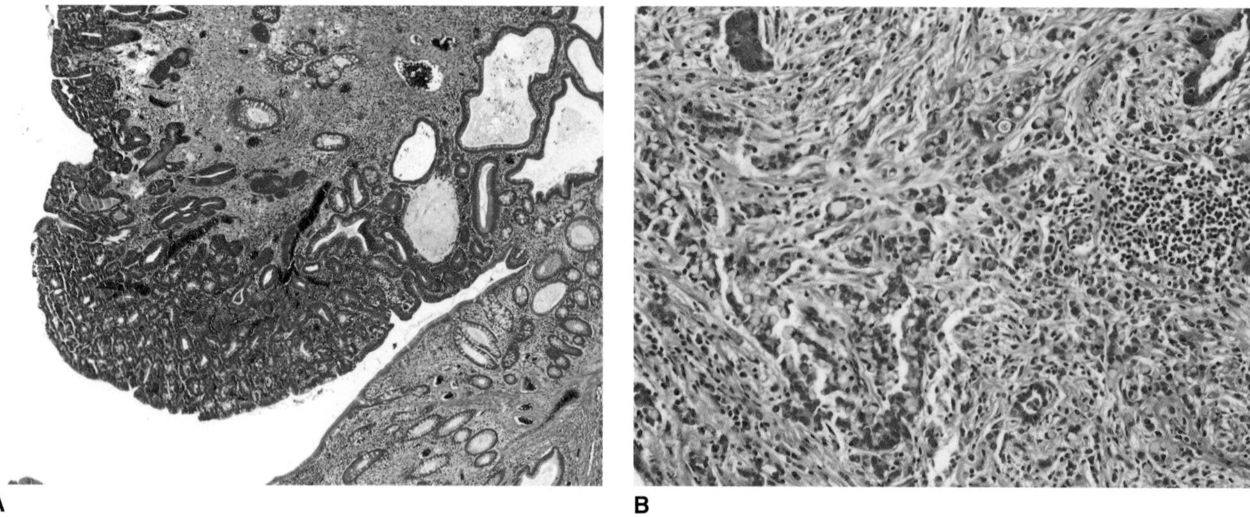

FIGURE 14-53 ■ Juvenile polyposis syndrome. **A:** Colonic polyp with a focus of high-grade dysplasia 40×. **B:** Focus of invasive signet ring adenocarcinoma in a colonic polyp from an adult patient 200×.

100 affected persons and a relative risk of 34 times compared to the general population (18).

PTEN Hamartoma Tumor Syndrome

A number of clinical syndromes including hamartomatous gastrointestinal polyps have been linked to mutations in the PTEN tumor suppressor gene on chromosome 10q23.3 (17,67). The best characterized of these disorders is Cowden syndrome, an autosomal dominant disorder with hamartomatous lesions involving multiple organ systems, as well as a substantially increased risk of thyroid, breast, and endometrial cancer. Mucocutaneous lesions, including multiple facial trichilemmomas, acral keratosis, and papillomas (particularly of the oral cavity) are pathognomic features of the syndrome. However, because these lesions can also occur sporadically in the general population, diagnosis requires finding multiple such lesions or additional features of the syndrome. Macrocephaly and a large variety of benign lesions of the breast, thyroid, and brain are also recognized as major manifestations of the syndrome. These lesions may begin to develop in childhood and are usually diagnosed by the third decade of life. A consensus panel of diagnostic criteria have been developed and more than 80% of individuals fulfilling these criteria harbor a mutation in the PTEN gene. Screening and surveillance strategies for early detection of the various types of tumors have been advocated (17,67,119).

Bannayan-Riley-Ruvalcaba syndrome is also caused by mutation in the PTEN gene. Cardinal clinical features include macrocephaly, pigmented penile macules, lipomas,

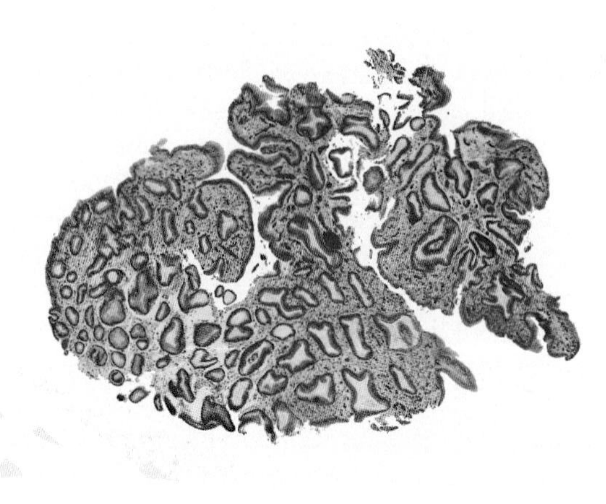

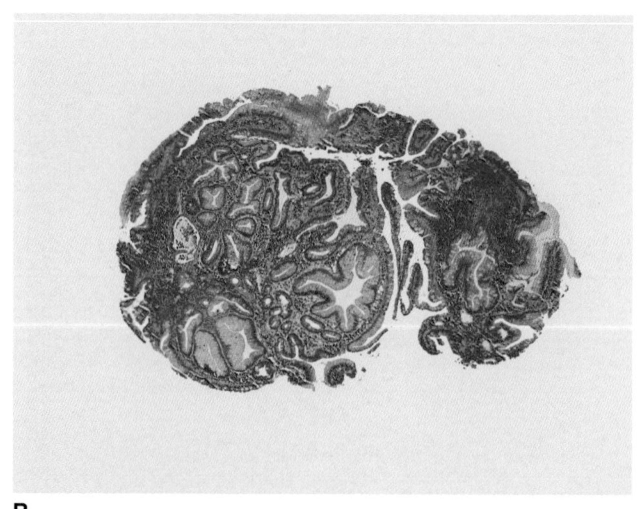

FIGURE 14-54 ■ Juvenile polyposis syndrome. **A:** The gastric polyps in this syndrome closely resemble sporadic gastric hyperplastic polyps 40×. **B:** This duodenal polyp lacks the central core of smooth muscle typical of small-bowel Peutz-Jeghers polyps 40×.

hemangiomas, and gastrointestinal hamartomas. Additional described features include developmental delay, thyroiditis, proximal muscle myopathy, and joint hyperextensibility. Consensus criteria for clinical diagnosis have not yet been formulated. About 70% of patients with this syndrome have mutations or large deletions in the PTEN gene. While an increased risk of malignancy has not been firmly documented in Bannayan-Riley-Ruvacaba syndrome, affected probands with overlap between this disorder and Cowden disease have been reported to have an increased risk of breast cancer, and therefore the same cancer screening and surveillance recommendations have been advocated for all affected individuals (17,67).

Because the gastrointestinal hamartomas are usually asymptomatic and documentation of their presence is not necessary to establish a diagnosis of either Cowden syndrome or Bannayan-Rubalcava-Riley syndrome, the incidence of polyps in these disorders is not known precisely. In one review of reports of patients with Cowden syndrome in the literature, gastrointestinal polyps were identified in 85% of patients who underwent endoscopic screening (67). The hamartomatous polyps in both syndromes resemble those present in juvenile polyposis syndrome, and therefore distinction between these disorders rests upon the presence of other diagnostic clinical features and genetic testing. The polyps in Cowden syndrome have been reported to exhibit more stromal myofibroblastic proliferation and less edema than juvenile polyps, and scattered lamina propria ganglion cells have also been described (73). Inflammatory type polyps and lipomas have also been reported. Dysplasia and malignant degeneration of the hamartomatous polyps do not appear to occur in these syndromes. Colonic adenomas have been reported in affected individuals, but currently it is thought that they are sporadic and do not occur at increased incidence compared to the general population (17,67) (see Chapter 24 for other PTEN findings).

Peutz-Jeghers Polyposis Syndrome

Peutz-Jeghers syndrome is an autosomal dominant disorder with an incidence of between 1:8,300 and 1:280,000 in the general population. It is characterized by the development of mucocutaneous hyperpigmentation, hamartomatous polyps throughout the gastrointestinal tract, and an increased risk of malignancy at many sites. The median age of onset of symptoms caused by the gastrointestinal polyps is 13 years of age. Presenting symptoms include bowel obstruction, intussusception, and gastrointestinal bleeding or anemia. Recognition of the characteristic hyperpigmented macules can also lead to proper diagnosis. They occur most often on the lips, buccal mucosa, or periorbital skin, but can also develop on the skin of the fingers, palms and soles, genitalia, and perianally. The macules may fade with age (47,67). Diagnosis and follow-up with new technologies such as video capsule endoscopy and double balloon enteroscopy likely will be beneficial to the clinical management of affected individuals (150).

More than 90% of patients have a detectable mutation in the SKT11 gene on chromosome 19p13.3. About 10% to 20% of patients present with *de novo* mutations. The protein product is a serine/threonine kinase that is expressed ubiquitously in human tissues. It regulated a number of downstream kinases and has important roles in the cellular response to energy stress and in the establishment of cell polarity (66,75,135).

The hamartomatous polyps occur primarily in the small bowel (92%) but can also develop in the colon (30%) and stomach (25%). Hamartomatous polyps may also occur in the nasal cavity, bladder, and lungs. The burden of gastrointestinal polyps is usually lower than in juvenile polyposis syndrome; often less than ten polyps are present. A clinical diagnosis of Peutz-Jeghers syndrome is made when two of the following three criteria are met: (a) two or more small bowel Peutz-Jeghers type polyps; (b) characteristic hyperpigmented macules of the nose, lips, nose eyes, genitalia, or fingers; and (c) a family history of Peutz-Jeghers syndrome (47,69,73). Peutz-Jeghers polyps are quite rare outside the setting of the syndrome, with less than 50 cases reported in the literature (146).

The characteristic histologic features are best developed in Peutz-Jeghers polyps of the small intestine. The arborizing central core of haphazardly arranged smooth muscle bundles is the most distinctive feature. The epithelial elements are hyperplastic and disorganized. The inflammatory component is sparse when compared to juvenile polyps, and stromal edema is not prominent (Figure 14-55). Displacement of the hyperplastic epithelial component into the deeper bowel layers is not uncommon, particularly in larger polyps that have caused bowel obstruction or intussusception (Figure 14-56). At frozen section the herniation of the epithelium into submucosa or muscularis propria can be confused with invasive adenocarcinoma by the unwary surgical pathologist (e416,e493).

Peutz-Jeghers polyps of the stomach and colon often do not exhibit a prominent central core of arborizing smooth

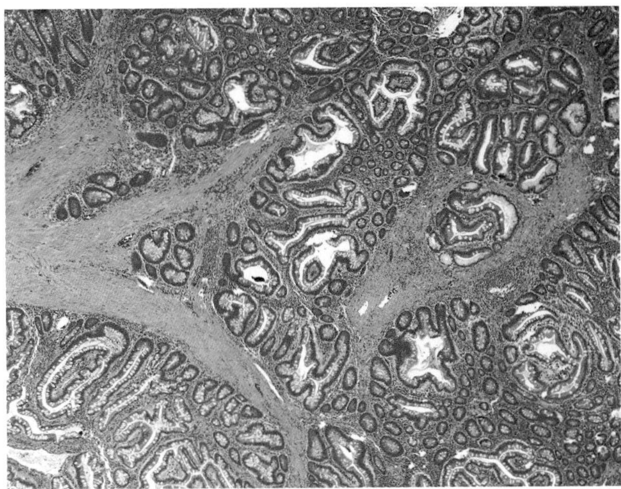

FIGURE 14-55 ■ Peutz-Jeghers polyp. Jejunal polyp with hyperplastic and disorganized mucosal elements and the characteristic central arborizing core of smooth muscle 40×.

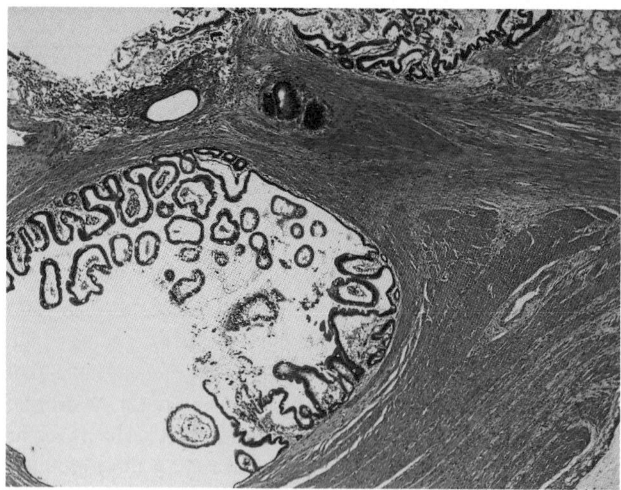

FIGURE 14-56 ■ Jejunal Peutz-Jeghers polyp. Displacement of epithelial elements into the muscularis can be confused with invasive adenocarcinoma, particularly in frozen sections, but the epithelium is clearly benign 40×.

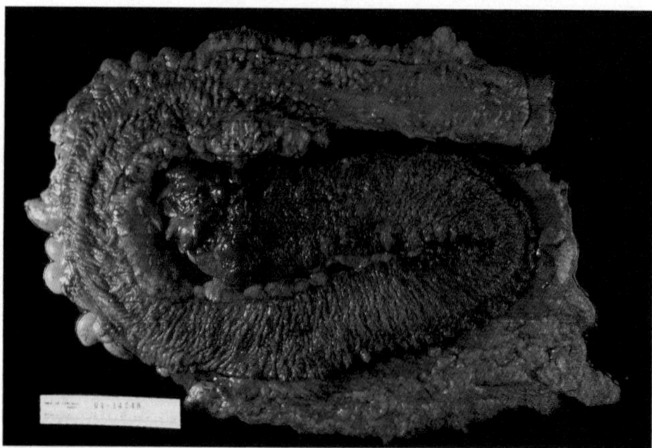

FIGURE 14-57 ■ Prophylactic colectomy specimen from a 27-year-old female with familial adenomatosis polyposis. No invasive adenocarcinoma was identified.

muscle and therefore can be confused with the more common juvenile polyps at these sites. They are less inflamed and edematous than juvenile polyps, but accurate diagnosis is problematic unless small-bowel polyps are also present. While there is a significant increased risk of gastrointestinal malignancy in patients with Peutz-Jeghers syndrome, dysplasia and cancer development within the polyps themselves is extraordinarily rare (38,43).

Individuals with Peutz-Jeghers syndrome have a significantly increased risk of malignancy compared to the general population (e163). Gastrointestinal, pulmonary, breast, gynecological, and pancreatic malignancies all occur with increased incidence. The cumulative incidence of malignancy is reported to reach 85% by the age of 70 years (63). A number of screening and surveillance programs have been advocated to monitor patients with Peutz-Jeghers syndrome (29,47,69).

Adenomatous Polyps and Adenocarcinoma

Adenomatous polyps are true neoplasms and are rare in children. When identified in a child, even a single adenomatous polyp should prompt consideration of familial adenomatous polyposis (96) (e82) and related polyposis syndromes. An adenomatous polyp may be grossly sessile or pedunculated and microscopically exhibit a tubular or villous growth pattern. Microscopically, it exhibits both architectural and cytologic features of dysplasia. Architectural features include crowded crypts or cribriforming. Cytologic features of dysplasia include elongation and stratification of nuclei, nuclear contour irregularity, and nuclear hyperchromasia. Adenomas lack the cystic dilatation of crypts and abundant inflammatory stroma of juvenile polyps and the arborizing core of smooth muscle of Peutz-Jeghers polyps.

Familial adenomatous polyposis (adenomatous polyposis coli), the most common of the polyposis syndromes, is an autosomal dominant disorder with an incidence of 1 in 8,000 persons. Approximately one-third of the cases are sporadic (96). In 1991, the defective gene in familial adenomatous polyposis was localized to chromosome 5, and shortly after, Gardner syndrome and Turcot syndrome were mapped to the same locus. In patients with familial adenomatous polyposis, hundreds of adenomatous polyps usually carpet the colonic mucosa (Figure 14-57). The disease may become symptomatic in adolescents, usually causing diarrhea and abdominal pain. The incidence of colonic adenocarcinoma is very high in patients with familial polyposis, approaching 100% by age 50. Malignancy may occur as early as the second decade. For this reason, colectomy is recommended whenever symptoms develop or in early adulthood (12,96). Multiple colonic adenomas also occur in the MUTYH polyposis syndrome, another autosomal recessive disorder with a significantly increased risk of colonic adenocarcinoma. In this condition, however, colonic adenomas almost never develop during childhood (128).

After colectomy continued surveillance is necessary since small intestinal adenomas will almost always develop, frequently in the area of the ampulla of Vater. Patients also commonly develop gastric fundic gland polyps. Dysplasia has been reported to develop in these polyps, but progression to invasive gastric adenocarcinoma is exceedingly rare (15,142).

Patients with familial polyposis coli may exhibit a variety of extraintestinal malignancies, including thyroid and pancreatic carcinomas, hepatoblastoma, and fibromatosis (desmoid tumor). There is also an increased incidence of a variety of benign lesions, including dermatofibroma, lipoma, and bone lesions (e.g., osteoma, exostosis, cortical thickening of long bones, and dental cysts). Congenital hypertrophy of the retinal pigment is the most common extracolonic manifestation of familial adenomatous polyposis and may be detected before the gastrointestinal polyps.

Gastrointestinal and extraintestinal components of the syndrome may appear in different members of a family.

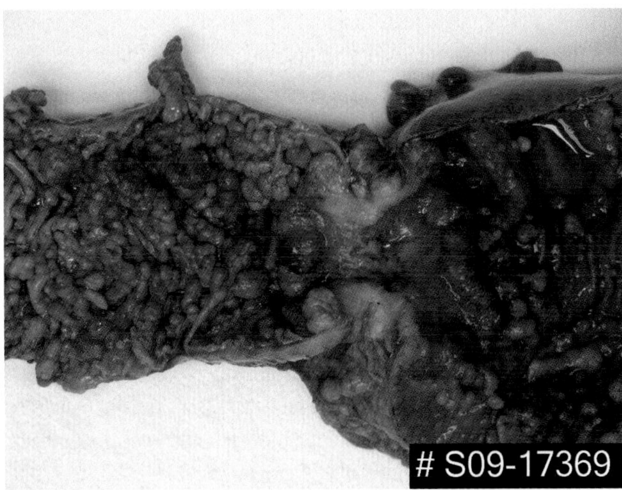

FIGURE 14-58▪Invasive colonic adenocarcinoma arising in an adult patient with familial adenomatosis polyposis. (Courtesy of Richard R. Anderson, M.D., Laboratory & Pathology Diagnostics, LLC.)

The designation of Turcot syndrome has been applied to patients with familial adenomatous polyposis who also develop malignant central nervous system tumor. Glioblastoma and medulloblastoma usually cause death, although ependymoma has also been reported (57) (e466).

Adenocarcinoma of the colon and rectum remains a rare diagnosis in children, with an incidence of only 1 in several million (e82). Recognized antecedent conditions, such as familial adenomatous polyposis, familial juvenile polyposis, and ulcerative colitis, account for a minority of the cases (Figure 14-58). Hereditary nonpolyposis colon cancer (Lynch syndrome) (95) and other syndromes account for a few more, but most childhood cases appear sporadically. Presenting symptoms of pain, vomiting, weight loss, and constipation are similar to those in adults. The diagnosis tends to be delayed in children and therefore many have advanced disease and a rapidly fatal course shortly after presentation. Involvement of the right colon where early disease is clinically silent is more frequent in children than in adults. Histologically, the tumor in children tends to show poor differentiation with abundant mucin and often "signet ring" features (e274,e377).

In addition to true polyps, other conditions may present as polypoid masses in the gastrointestinal tract. These include inflammatory pseudopolyp in inflammatory bowel disease, pancreatic or gastric heterotopia, and tumors such as leiomyoma, adenocarcinoma, lipoma, neurofibroma, and ganglioneuroma.

Nonepithelial Gastrointestinal Tumors

In children with congenital immunodeficiency or AIDS, smooth muscle tumors may develop in association with EBV infection in either gastrointestinal or extraintestinal sites (e74,e307,e314). The tumors are commonly multifocal and are uniformly reactive by in situ hybridization with probes to the EBV small noncoding RNAs (EBER) (40,42).

Spindle cell tumors of smooth muscle origin must be distinguished from others with similar histology, including inflammatory myofibroblastic tumor and fibromatosis (e82,e83).

Inflammatory fibroid polyp can occur at any age in the gastric or intestinal wall or adjacent mesentery and can become a large mass (e84). The histologic picture is variable but usually includes loose fascicles of bland spindle cells admixed with a mixed inflammatory cell infiltrate with a prominent component of eosinophils (111). The spindle cells often exhibit a perivascular whorling orientation that is characteristic. Because of its large size, a malignancy may be considered clinically, but the low cellularity of the lesion and lack of significant cytologic atypia usually lead to the correct diagnosis. Recently, gain of function mutations of the PDGFRA gene has been documented in a subset of small-bowel and gastric inflammatory fibroid polyps (87). Ganglioneuroma is yet another intestinal spindle cell tumor that is usually easily distinguished by a frequent polypoid configuration and a positive reaction with neural immunocytochemical markers (e99,e414).

Mesenteric or omental cysts, although not strictly gastrointestinal tumors, should be considered in the differential diagnosis of abdominal masses in children (e71,e204,e325). Ultrasonography reveals their typical unilocular or multilocular cystic nature. Most are located in the mesentery immediately adjacent to the small intestine. Mesenteric cyst is lined by a single layer of cells or consists only of fibrous septa. It may be confused with a similar cystic lesion, cystic lymphangioma, which has an endothelial lining in addition to lymphoid tissue and smooth muscle in its walls (e172,e261,e452). Cystic lymphangioma often spans both the bowel wall and adjacent mesentery, so that a segmental bowel resection is required; in contrast, mesenteric cyst is usually easily separated from the bowel wall.

Lymphoma

The intestine is the most common site of primary extranodal lymphoma (e41), and non-Hodgkin lymphoma is the most common malignant intestinal tumor in children. Boys from 5 to 10 years of age account for most of the affected children, and the usual clinical presentation is abdominal pain and a palpable right lower quadrant mass. Burkitt lymphoma is by far the most common gastrointestinal lymphoma of childhood. It usually arises in the submucosal lymphoid tissue of the ileocecal region and extends transmurally to involve local mesenteric lymph nodes and form a bulky tumor mass. Less advanced cases may present with intussusception or intestinal obstruction. Histologically, the mucosa and submucosa are replaced by sheets of uniform lymphoblastic cells with very regular, round, noncleaved nuclei, usually arranged in a "starry sky" pattern. Appropriate hematopathologic evaluation of Burkitt lymphoma reveals a B-cell lineage; a translocation, t(8;14), is characteristic.

The prognosis is related to the extent of abdominal or systemic tumor spread. If the intestinal and nodal masses are amenable to resection and appropriate chemotherapy is administered, approximately 80% of these children are cured. Other non-Hodgkin lymphomas, in addition to Burkitt lymphoma, have been reported in the gastrointestinal tract but are less frequent in otherwise healthy children (e82).

In immunodeficient patients, malignant lymphoma occurs anywhere in the intestinal tract and does not demonstrate a preference for the ileocecal area. Unusual large-cell lymphoproliferative disorders have been reported in the gastrointestinal tract in primary immunodeficiency diseases (e133). A number of lymphoproliferative processes in addition to AIDS-associated non-Hodgkin lymphoma develop in patients with AIDS (e222,e230,e232,e394). A spectrum of posttransplant lymphoproliferative disorders associated with EBV infection, which involves the gastrointestinal tract in many cases, may develop in recipients of solid organ and bone marrow transplants (e142,e332,e450). These include polyclonal and monomorphic B-lineage lymphomas at the most advanced end of the spectrum.

Langerhans cell histiocytosis (formerly called histiocytosis X) may affect any portion of the gastrointestinal tract to produce malabsorption, diarrhea, ulceration, or bleeding. Gastrointestinal involvement occurs as a component of widespread systemic infiltration. The infiltrate is usually mucosal and consists of the characteristic histiocyte-like cells with grooved nuclei admixed with a mixed inflammatory cell infiltrate including a prominent component of eosinophils (Figure 14-59A,B). Immunohistochemical reactivity for S-100 protein and CD1a confirms the diagnosis. Because of the presence of multinucleated giant cells in some cases, this condition may be mistaken for a granulomatous infectious process or Crohn disease (62) (e47,e158,e182,e243).

Systemic mastocytosis develops due to a specific activating mutation (codon 816) in the *c-kit* gene. Gastrointestinal involvement occurs in about 70% to 80% of patients with systemic mastocytosis. The stomach and duodenum are the most commonly involved. Common symptoms include abdominal pain, diarrhea, and bleeding. Peptic ulcer disease can develop due to hypergastrinemia stimulated by the release of histamine from the mast cells. Serum tryptase levels greater than 20 ng/mL are considered abnormal (74).

Mast cells are cytologically bland and are inconspicuous in H&E sections of normal mucosa. With the use of special stains, scattered mast cells can be seen in the lamina propria. In patients with systemic mastocytosis, endoscopy may be normal or reveal thickened mucosal folds and erosions. In most cases the infiltrate of mast cells is dense (eFigure 14-14A,B). Eosinophils are often also increased in number. Chloracetate esterase, toluidine blue, or Giemsa stains can be used to highlight the mast cells. Immunohistologic stains utilizing mast cell tryptase or CD117 antibodies are probably more sensitive and easier to perform (eFigure 14-14C) (74).

APPENDIX

Normal Anatomy and Histology

The appendix is present at the tip of the cecum at birth, but as the cecum grows the appendix moves to a position on the posteromedial wall below the ileocecal valve (e498). However, aberrant takeoff from the cecum is not unusual, and both anterior and retrocecal positions are particularly commonly encountered (e189). The average length of the adult appendix is 9 cm, with a reported range of 2 to 25 cm (e12,e498).

The overall gross anatomy of the appendix is most similar to the colon. There is a serosa, muscularis propria with an outer longitudinal and inner circular layer, submucosa,

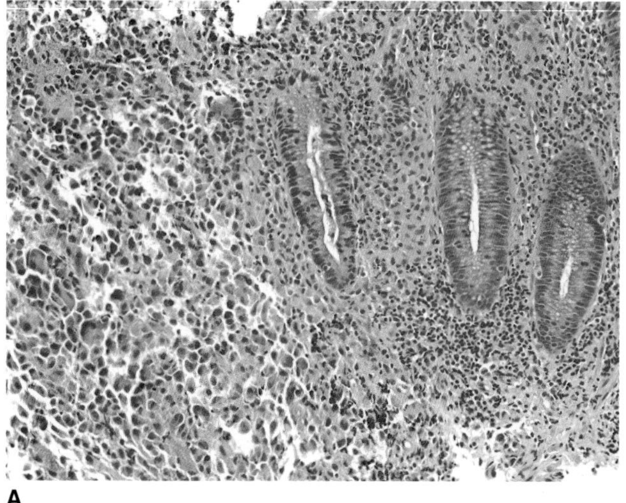
A

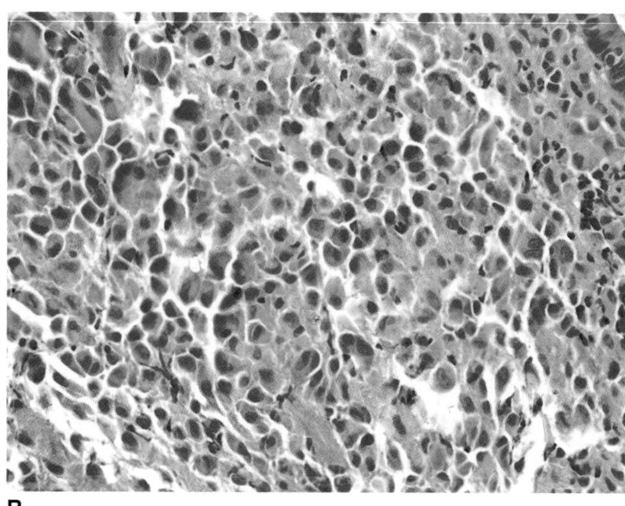
B

FIGURE 14-59 ■ Colonic involvement by Langerhans cell histiocytosis. **A:** Histiocytic infiltrate in the lamina propria 200×. **B:** Higher power reveals mixture of histiocytic cells with grooved nuclei, multinucleated giant cells, and a few admixed eosinophils 400×.

muscularis mucosae, and mucosa (e498). The mucosa closely resembles its colonic counterpart, although branched crypts are regarded as a normal finding in the appendix. Endocrine cells and Paneth cells are scattered throughout the mucosa. The lymphoid tissue component is also exaggerated in the appendix, more akin to that seen in the terminal ileum. In children lymphoid follicles may be confluent over large areas of the mucosa. Within the lamina propria there are numerous ganglion cells, Schwann cells, and nerve fibers, as well as endocrine cells, which may be the origin for carcinoid tumors (e116).

Congenital and Neuromuscular Disorders

Diverticula of the appendix may be congenital or acquired, with acquired lesions being ten times more common (e285,e464). Acquired diverticula may easily rupture during bouts of acute appendicitis. Inflammation of the diverticula (akin to sigmoid diverticulitis) may present as a mild form of appendicitis (e285). Appendiceal diverticula are particularly common in patients with cystic fibrosis (e161). Appendiceal intussusception is usually the result of a pathologic process involving the appendix itself, such as a tumor, endometriosis, cystic fibrosis, or virally induced lymphoid hyperplasia (e15,e312). Adenovirus infection has specifically been implicated in some cases.

Fibrous obliteration of the appendiceal tip, a common finding in adults, is uncommon in childhood and is of no clinical significance. In some cases a disorganized hyperplasia of neural elements is evident within the fibrous tissue, including nonmyelinated nerve fibers and Schwann cells, and in some cases endocrine cells (156) (e25,e344,e439). Some authors have applied the term "appendiceal neuroma" to this finding (e439). It is unclear whether the presence of these elements is indicative of prior acute appendicitis. A lesser degree of neural proliferation is sometimes present within the mucosa in appendices without luminal obliteration (e344).

Acute Appendicitis

Acute appendicitis is the most common indication for emergent surgery in the United States, with about 250,000 appendectomies performed each year (136). The epidemiology, pathogenesis, and clinical features of acute appendicitis have been extensively investigated for many decades, but certain aspects of this very common disorder remain controversial. The peak age of incidence is from 10 to 30 years of age, although cases in infants and the elderly do occur (26). The lifetime risk of the development of acute appendicitis is about 7% in the United States (136). About twice as many women as men undergo appendectomy, although the disorder has about an equal incidence in females and males. The overlap in symptomatology and laboratory findings between acute appendicitis and a variety reproductive tract diseases accounts for the high frequency of unnecessary appendectomy in women (7). The rate of appendectomy in which acute appendicitis is not confirmed pathologically is currently approximately 15% (45). The rate has not decreased significantly in the past 70 years, despite the use of even more sophisticated and expensive laboratory and imaging techniques (26).

The classic early symptoms of acute appendicitis include abdominal pain, anorexia, nausea, and vomiting. McBurney described progression from vague periumbilical pain to localized pain in the right lower quadrant more than 100 years ago (e306). Physical examination typically reveals mild tachycardia, low-grade fever, decreased bowel sounds, and tenderness to palpation in the right lower quadrant. Laboratory evaluation usually reveals a mildly elevated white blood cell count with a left shift (136). The use of abdominal ultrasound and helical computed tomography has been proposed to increase the sensitivity and specificity of the diagnosis of acute appendicitis (136). Appendectomy remains the mainstay of treatment for acute appendicitis. However, when perforation has already occurred at the time of diagnosis, some surgeons advocate delaying surgery until after a course of antibiotics.

The pathogenesis of acute appendicitis is still a matter of debate (e498). Many investigators are convinced that luminal obstruction (usually by a fecalith or lymphoid hyperplasia) leads to distension and ischemia followed by bacterial invasion (136) (e21,e22,e275). Ligation of the appendix in animals has consistently resulted in the development of acute appendicitis (e360). However, there are some data that suggest that this mechanism is not operative in the majority of human cases. Alternative hypotheses include primary viral infection or local ischemia producing microscopic ulcers, thus allowing for bacterial invasion (26).

Although ultimately bacterial invasion plays a central role in the pathogenesis of acute appendicitis, microbiologic studies have shown that any of a variety of enteric organisms could be responsible in an individual case. In a recent study involving peritoneal swabs performed at the time of appendectomy for perforated appendicitis, *E. coli* was cultured in about 75%, with *P. aeruginosa* and *Streptococcus* responsible for the majority of the remaining cases (141).

The gross appearance in acute appendicitis varies depending on the severity of the acute inflammatory process. In classic cases with transmural involvement the serosa appears dull, discolored, and shaggy. The wall is edematous and swollen and retracts when incised. Acute inflammatory cell exudate may be evident at the site of a perforation. If the appendix is removed before transmural inflammation has developed, the appendix may grossly appear normal or exhibit only mild serosal hyperemia.

The histologic features of acute appendicitis reflect the gross appearance. In severe acute appendicitis there may be transmural necrosis with perforation and acute peritonitis.

There is debate, however, regarding the minimal degree of neutrophilic inflammation that is required to render a diagnosis of acute appendicitis. Most authors will accept neutrophilic mucosal infiltrates if associated with at least focal ulceration as diagnostic (e77,e130,e498). However, others point to data suggesting that such changes can be present in incidental appendectomies performed in asymptomatic patients. These authors insist that for this reason a diagnosis of acute appendicitis is not warranted until neutrophilic inflammation extends into the muscularis propria (26). The point has been made that if multiple additional sections are obtained from an appendix that on initial examination exhibits only superficial inflammation, there is a high likelihood of finding involvement of the muscularis propria (e63,e429). There is uniform agreement that luminal neutrophils or focal infiltration of the surface epithelium alone is insufficient ground for a diagnosis of acute appendicitis (assuming that the entire appendix has been examined). The possibility of an enteric infection (such as *Campylobacter* ileocolitis) should be considered in such patients (26) (e498).

Interval Appendectomy

It has become accepted practice in many centers to delay appendectomy in patients in whom perforation and abscess formation have occurred. Instead, the patient is treated conservatively with supportive care and antibiotics, and appendectomy is thus delayed for 4 to 8 weeks, at which time the patient is clinically stable and the complication rate is therefore lower. In fact, some surgeons question the need for appendectomy at all if conservative management is successful (8).

Histologic examination of interval appendectomy specimens most often reveals mural thickening and fibrosis, transmural lymphoid aggregates, and mucosal architectural distortion (e304) (Figure 14-60A,B). Not infrequently granulomas are also evident, resulting in a histologic appearance that closely mimics Crohn disease. Occasionally, xanthogranulomatous inflammation is evident (61) (e304). In some cases the appendix is histologically normal or exhibits only mild serosal fibrosis.

Unusual Infections of the Appendix

A variety of viral pathogens can produce inflammation of the appendix and many produce clinical features similar to acute appendicitis. Measles virus infection involving the appendix is very rare but is well described. In most patients appendectomy is performed during the prodromal stage of the illness, before the diagnosis of measles is established. The histologic hallmark is the presence of Warthin-Finkeldey cells similar to those seen in the tonsillar tissue of infected patients. Lymphoid hyperplasia is also prominent, but there is little evidence of acute inflammation (113). However, if appendectomy is delayed superimposed bacterial appendicitis of the traditional type may develop (113). Adenovirus and rotavirus infection has already been mentioned as a cause of appendiceal intussusception. Smudgy appearing viral inclusions can be identified in epithelial cells, but rotavirus does not produce inclusions visible by light microscopy (60).

Yersinia, Campylobacter, or *Salmonella* infection can cause ilocecitis that results in symptoms, laboratory test abnormalities, and radiographic findings difficult to distinguish from acute appendicitis (e370,e472). Histologic examination in cases where an appendectomy is performed usually reveals only mild mucosal neutrophilic infiltrates, without involvement of the submucosa (e331,e420,e473). However, there are also cases of true acute appendicitis caused by *Yersinia* infection (e420). Histologic examination in these cases has revealed severe neutrophilic infiltrates extending into the muscularis, as well as prominent granulomatous inflammation. In these cases isolated Crohn appendicitis must also be considered, and distinction between these two disorders is usually not possible on histologic grounds alone.

Enterobius vermicularis (pinworm) is infrequently seen in the lumen of the appendix, but this parasite is not thought to cause acute appendicitis (e61,e428,e497). On occasion ova that become embedded in the mucosa may produce mild

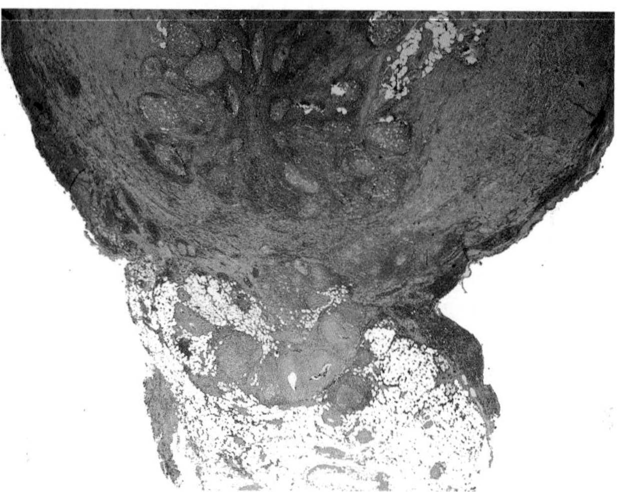

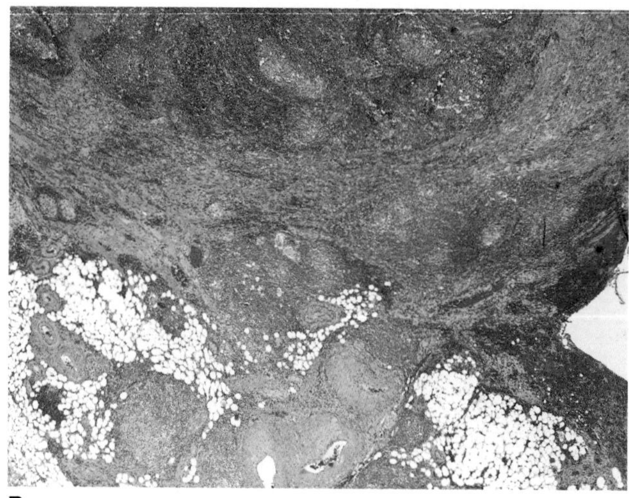

FIGURE 14-60 ■ Interval appendicitis. **A:** There is fibrosis of the serosa with lymphoid follicles, consistent with resolution of a prior episode of acute appendicitis with perforation 20×. **B:** The acute inflammation has completely resolved 40×.

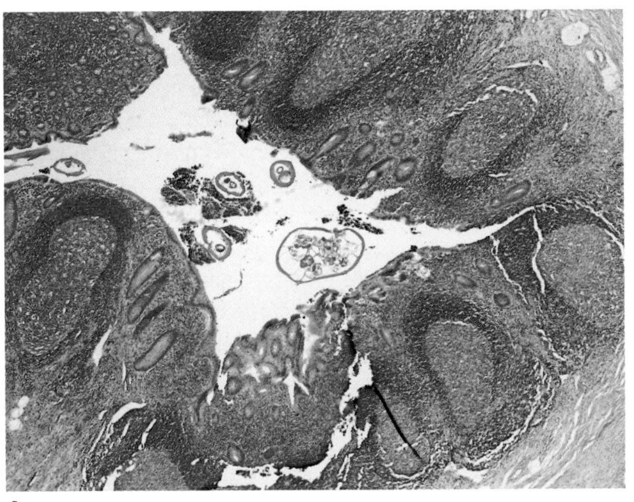

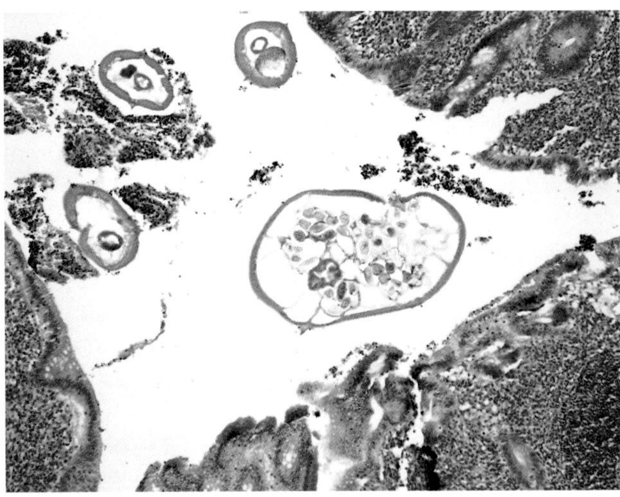

FIGURE 14-61 ■ **A** and **B:** Appendix with *Enterobius vermicularis*. The adult worms can be seen in cross section within the appendiceal lumen. **A:** 40×. **B:** 200×.

mucosal inflammation (e497) (Figure 14-61A,B). In some parts of the world, appendiceal infection by *E. histolytica*, schistosomiasis, tuberculosis, and Toxoplasma are not uncommon (53) (e342).

Miscellaneous Conditions

Mucosal melanosis has been documented in 46% of appendices removed from pediatric patients. It has no clinical significance and does not appear to be related to the use of laxatives (55). In pregnancy submesothelial deposits of decidualized cells may develop in the absence of endometriosis (e449). Confusion with metastatic tumor is avoided by use of immunohistologic stains, since the decidualized cells are uniformly negative with keratin antibodies. The relationship between deciduosis and symptoms of acute appendicitis is unclear, as no neutrophilic infiltrates are present (e449). Endometriosis of the appendix is not uncommon. The appearance is histologically similar to that seen with involvement in other pelvic sites. Although appendiceal endometriosis usually does not cause acute inflammation, it can produce cyclic abdominal pain (e67).

Cystic fibrosis has already been mentioned as a cause of appendiceal intussusception and diverticular disease. Gross examination usually reveals a dilated appendix that is filled with thick, tenacious mucus. Histologic examination reveals densely eosinophilic mucin filling the lumen and sometimes causing dilatation of the crypts (e330,e423) (Figure 14-62A,B).

Both Crohn disease and ulcerative colitis often involve the appendix (e233). In some cases of ulcerative colitis, the appendix is involved even when the proximal colon is not, an exception to the rule that ulcerative colitis does not "skip" segments (e268). Appendiceal inflammation clinically

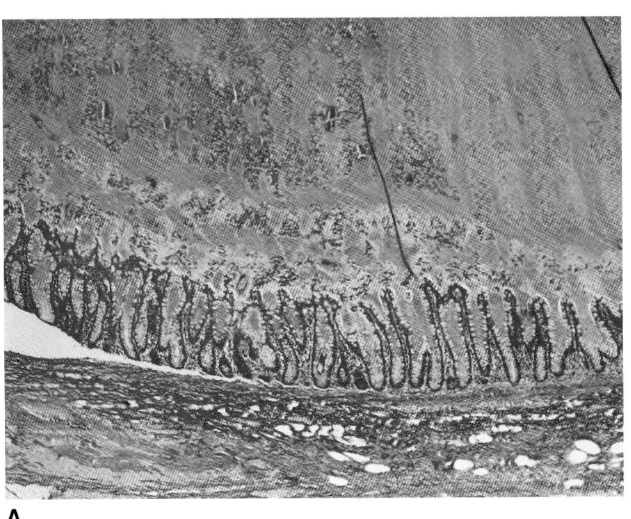

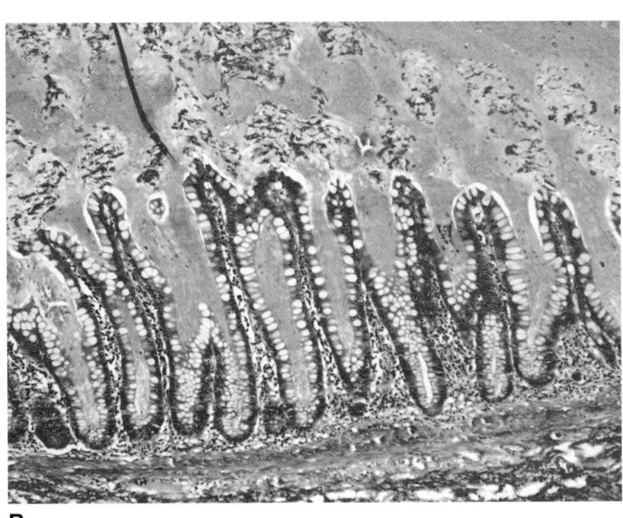

FIGURE 14-62 ■ Appendix in a patient with cystic fibrosis. **A:** Thick mucinous secretions fill the appendiceal lumen 40×. **B:** The crypts are distended by thick mucinous secretions 200×.

mimicking acute appendicitis may be the heralding event that leads to the diagnosis of Crohn disease. In the absence of known chronic inflammatory bowel disease, it is rarely possible to diagnose either Crohn disease or ulcerative colitis when an abnormal appendix is encountered. However, because appendicitis is ordinarily an acute suppurative process, the presence of unusual or chronic features, such as predominantly chronic inflammation, fibrosis, fissuring ulcers, or granulomas, should lead to a consideration of another diagnosis. Noncaseating granulomas, in addition to being characteristic of Crohn disease, are also found in idiopathic granulomatous appendicitis, an entity that is felt to be different from Crohn disease (e20,e125,e215). Granulomatous appendicitis presents with appendiceal symptoms, and the histology shows chronic appendicitis with granulomas. It is possible that most of these cases represent a chronic resolving phase of acute appendicitis, as the histologic features are identical to those seen at the time of interval appendectomy for resolved acute appendicitis with perforation.

Appendiceal Carcinoid Tumors

About 70% of carcinoids are located at the tip of the appendix, allowing for appendectomy with a negative surgical margin. Generally, a well-circumscribed firm yellowish nodule is evident. The tumor is centered in the submucosa but may extend into the overlying mucosa and into the underlying muscularis propria. A precise size should be recorded in the gross description (106). Histologic examination usually reveals an insular or trabecular arrangement of tumor cells. Depth of invasion and the presence or absence of angiolymphatic invasion are important prognostic factors.

Immunohistologic studies are usually not required for diagnosis. Classic carcinoid tumors are usually reactive with neuroendocrine markers such as synaptophysin, chromogranin A, neuron specific enolase, and CD56. About 15% of the tumors are reactive with the CK20 antibody, but they are consistently CK 7 nonreactive. About 85% of appendiceal carcinoids are reactive with the CDX2 antibody, even in metastatic sites. As expected, appendiceal carcinoids are nonreactive with the TTF-1 antibody, which is useful in the distinction in a metastatic site from pulmonary primaries, which are usually positive with this marker (3,11,24,71,129).

Carcinoids less than 1 cm in dimension are regarded as benign since lymph node metastasis and distant metastasis are vanishingly rare. Appendectomy with a negative margin is regarded as curative for these tumors. In contrast, lymph node or distant metastasis occurs in about 5% of carcinoids greater than 2 cm in size and therefore right hemicolectomy is recommended for these tumors. The proper management of carcinoids between 1 and 2 cm is unclear since prospective data regarding the natural history of these tumors is limited. Many authors recommend right hemicolectomy if tumor invades the mesoappendiceal fat or if angiolymphatic invasion is detected. However, it should be noted that some advocate simple appendectomy even for carcinoids larger than 2 cm, given the indolent natural history of even metastatic carcinoid tumor, and the lack of a proven survival advantage for right hemicolectomy (10) (e324). Goblet cell or adenocarcinoid is a more treacherous neoplasm.

DISORDERS OF THE ANUS

Congenital Abnormalities

Anorectal anomalies comprise a spectrum of malformations. These range from a thin membrane obstructing an otherwise normal rectum and anus (true imperforate anus) to atresia of the entire distal rectum, in which the proximal rectum ends as a blind pouch in the pelvis (e496). The term imperforate anus is a misnomer because the anomaly usually consists of considerably more than an imperforate anal membrane. The anal canal and rectum are usually both affected. The incidence of these malformations is approximately 1 in 5,000 births.

The classification of anorectal malformations has long been confusing and nonstandardized. The malformation is usually classified as high, intermediate, or low, depending on the location of the distal rectum in relation to the levator ani muscle, which can be demonstrated radiologically in relation to bony landmarks (e.g., the pubococcygeal line on a lateral radiograph) (e398). Fistulas between the rectal pouch and perineal skin or various locations in the urinary and genital systems are often found. The most common variations are

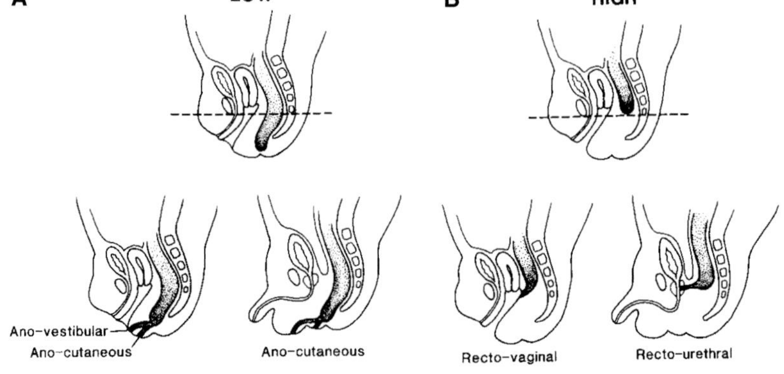

FIGURE 14-63 ■ Classification of anorectal malformations. Anomalies are classified as low or high depending on their relationship to the pubococcygeal line on x-ray film (*broken line*). Fistulas tracts between the rectum and other structures are indicated by stippling. **A:** low anomalies are usually associated with an external fistula to the vestibule (in girls) or the skin. **B:** In high anomalies, fistulas are internal, usually to the posterior vagina in girls or the proximal urethra in boys.

shown in Figure 14-63. Persons with a low imperforate anus have an intact anal sphincter and usually a fistula from the rectal pouch to the perineal skin anterior to a covered anal dimple, although in up to 25% of the cases, a fistula is not present. High malformations, formerly known as anorectal agenesis, are associated with absence of the anal sphincter and complex abnormal interval anomalies. A rectourethral fistula is present in most boys with this malformation; girls usually have a fistula between the rectal pouch and the vagina, bladder, or urethra. The term persistent cloaca describes the condition in which a girl has a single perineal opening draining an internal pouch comprised of the terminal portions of rectum, vagina, and urinary tract structures.

Other congenital anomalies are found in as many as 50% of infants with high anorectal malformations. The most frequent associations are genitourinary and skeletal abnormalities (especially of vertebrae and pelvis), congenital heart disease, and esophageal atresia with tracheoesophageal fistula. A diagnosis of VATER syndrome, VATERL syndrome, or caudal regression syndrome (e353,e441) should be considered in every infant with an anorectal anomaly.

Acquired Diseases

Condylomata Acuminata

Condylomata acuminata, or venereal warts, are being increasingly reported in prepubertal children (e110,e412,e471). In boys, they occur in the perianal region, and in girls, they are found in the perianal or genital regions. The etiologic agent is human papillomavirus of the same DNA sequence types that are responsible for condylomata acuminata in adults (e471). In many but not all cases, a history of sexual abuse of the affected child is obtained (e412) (see Chapter 7). Alternatively, the mother of an affected child may have transmitted the virus. Histologically, the lesions are identical to those seen in adults.

Perianal Abscess and Anal Fistula

Perianal abscesses, usually found in infants, result from breaks in the skin or anal mucosa or an infection in the anal glands. Treatment consists of surgical incision and drainage. Anal fistulas between the anal canal and skin may develop secondarily, requiring surgical excision of the fibrous and granulation tissue tract in perianal soft tissues and muscle. Older children with leukemia, Crohn disease, and immunodeficiency states are especially susceptible to perianal abscesses and fistulas (e411).

All References are listed on the Stocker Website.

CHAPTER 15

The Liver, Gallbladder, and Biliary Tract

JOHN HICKS
HARESH MANI
J. THOMAS STOCKER

DEVELOPMENT

Hepatobiliary morphogenesis occurs during the first 10 weeks of gestation (e473,e685,e686,e697). The liver primordium appears in week 3 as a tubular evagination of the future duodenal segment of the foregut endoderm. The hepatic diverticulum differentiates cranially into the proliferating hepatic cords and caudally into the extrahepatic bile ducts and the gallbladder. The hepatic diverticulum branches dichotomously, and thick anastomosing sheets of epithelial cells grow into the mesenchyme of the septum transversum, and the mesenchymal cells form the connective tissue elements of the hepatic stroma and capsule. As the hepatic sheets extend outward in the septum transversum, they are penetrated by the capillary plexus derived from the vitelline veins, which arise from the primitive hepatic sinusoids (e695).

In the 10-mm embryo, bile canaliculi appear as intercellular spaces between sheets of presumptive hepatocytes. The epithelial lining of the extrahepatic bile ducts is continuous with the primitive hepatic sheets that give rise to the epithelium of the intrahepatic bile ducts. The epithelium of the intrahepatic bile ducts is probably generated by interaction of the primitive hepatic epithelium and the mesenchyme surrounding the developing and branching portal vein. The epithelial layer, which is in direct contact with the mesenchyme around the portal vein, transforms into bile duct–like cells, after which a second layer transforms into bile duct epithelial cells (e694). At around 8 weeks' gestation, the ductal plate develops, appearing as a cleft in the shape of a cylinder around the mesenchyme of the progressively developing and branching portal vein (e741). The ductal plate (Figure 15-1) undergoes gradual remodeling to form the interlobular bile ducts in the portal tract, undergoing a balanced process of cell proliferation and apoptosis (e696). Intrahepatic bile ducts are recognized in the 20- to 30-mm embryo. The hepatocytes and bile duct epithelial cells are structurally and functionally distinct. The canals of Hering, which connect the canaliculi to the bile ducts, consist of both typical hepatocytes and bile duct epithelial cells (e742).

The development of the liver is associated with changes in the primordial vitelline veins, which give rise to the portal, hepatic, and umbilical veins. The definitive pattern of veins within the liver is established in the 10-mm embryo. The proximal end of the right vitelline vein forms the terminal part of the inferior vena cava. The portal vein arises from persistence of segments of both right and left vitelline veins and three anastomotic channels between the two. The right umbilical vein disappears, and all blood from the placenta enters the liver from the left umbilical vein. The coalescence of some of the hepatic sinusoids produces an oblique channel, the ductus venosus, which connects the left umbilical vein to the right vitelline vein, diverting some of the oxygenated blood directly to the heart.

The right side of the liver receives blood predominantly from the portal vein, and the left lobe is supplied mainly

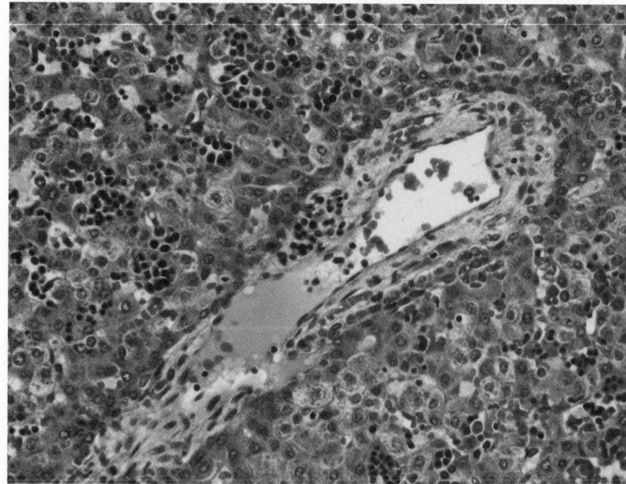

FIGURE 15-1 ■ Ductal plate in the fetal liver is formed by a collar of epithelial cells at the periphery of the portal tract and abuts against zone 1 hepatocytes. Note the presence of extramedullary hematopoiesis (H&E stain, 200×).

by oxygenated blood from the left umbilical vein. This may account for the difference in the appearance of the two lobes. At birth, the left lobe is larger relative to its size in later life. Moreover, the right lobe shows more hematopoiesis, and the hepatocytes contain more glycogen, lipid, and iron pigment than those in the left lobe. Fetal blood flow through the hepatic artery is insignificant compared with that delivered by the umbilical and portal veins.

The caudal part of the hollow diverticulum elongates and presumably becomes the common bile duct, hepatic duct, cystic duct, and the gallbladder between weeks 5 and 7.5. The liver is the site of hematopoiesis between weeks 6 and 7, and erythropoiesis dominates from week 12 until the beginning of the third trimester (e641). During the third trimester, the bone marrow is the dominant site of hematopoiesis, and hepatic erythropoiesis decreases, although it continues in the newborn period and may persist into the first few weeks of life.

HISTOLOGY

The conventional histologic unit of the liver is the hepatic lobule, which consists of a central efferent vein with cords of hepatocytes radiating to several peripheral portal tracts. The portal tract contains the interlobular bile ducts, branches of the portal vein, and hepatic artery and lymphatics. The functional unit of the liver is the hepatic acinus (Figure 15-2). The hepatic acinus is a three-dimensional structure with the portal tract as the central point (zone 1) where blood flows from terminal branches of the portal vein and hepatic arteries into the sinusoids and empties into the terminal hepatic venules at the periphery of the acinus (centrilobular/zone 3). Bile is secreted into the canaliculi and flows toward the portal areas into the interlobular bile ducts that are connected to the canaliculi by canals of Hering. The acinus thus includes parts of several adjacent lobules.

The hepatocytes in children older than 5 or 6 years of age are organized into single-cell plates. In younger children, the liver cells are arranged in two-cells–thick plates. In the preterm infant, the lobular structure of the liver is poorly defined and hepatic plates are more than one cell thick. Canaliculi lie between adjacent hepatocytes, and, ultrastructurally, tight junctions are present between the hepatocytes surrounding the canaliculus. Microvilli from the hepatocytes project into the canalicular lumen. The hepatocytes in childhood often have nuclear glycogen, and lipofuscin in the cytoplasm is usually scanty. The hepatic sinusoidal lining cells include endothelial and Kupffer cells. The endothelial cells are supported by reticulin fibers, and between the endothelial cells and hepatocytes is the space of Disse. Perisinusoidal cells (cells of Ito) are interstitial fat-storing cells and appear to play a significant role in hepatic fibrogenesis.

CONGENITAL ANOMALIES

Agenesis of the liver is incompatible with life and is usually associated with other severe congenital anomalies in stillborn fetuses. Agenesis of one lobe of the liver, usually the right, is seen infrequently and is rarely associated with clinical symptoms (e327,e412). In situs inversus totalis, the liver, its peritoneal and vascular connections, and the gallbladder and extrahepatic ducts have a mirror-image configuration to normal situs. In the asplenia-polysplenia syndromes, the liver may be midline and bilaterally symmetrical (e468).

The liver may herniate through defects in the diaphragm (Figure 15-3). Diaphragmatic defects are more common on the left side, and the liver often herniates into the left pleural

FIGURE 15-2 ■ Schematic view of hepatic lobule or acinus. The conventional view of the liver consisted of a hepatic lobule with a central vein (CV) surrounded by hepatocyte cords radiating to peripheral portal areas. The functional unit of the liver, the acinus, however, consists of a three-dimensional structure with a central portal tract surrounded by concentric zones of hepatocytes (I, II, and III), with the most peripheral zone (III) lying near the central vein.

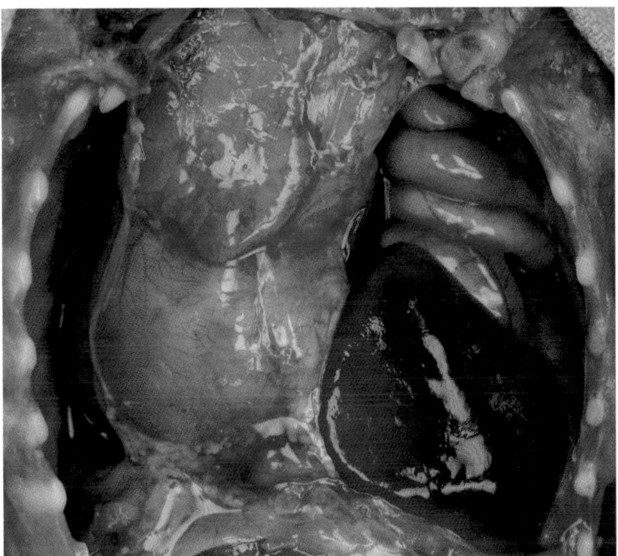

FIGURE 15-3 ■ Herniation of liver through diaphragmatic defect. A large defect in the left leaflet of the diaphragm has led to herniation of the left lobe of the liver and intestines into the left hemithorax, resulting in mediastinal shift to the right and severe pulmonary hypoplasia.

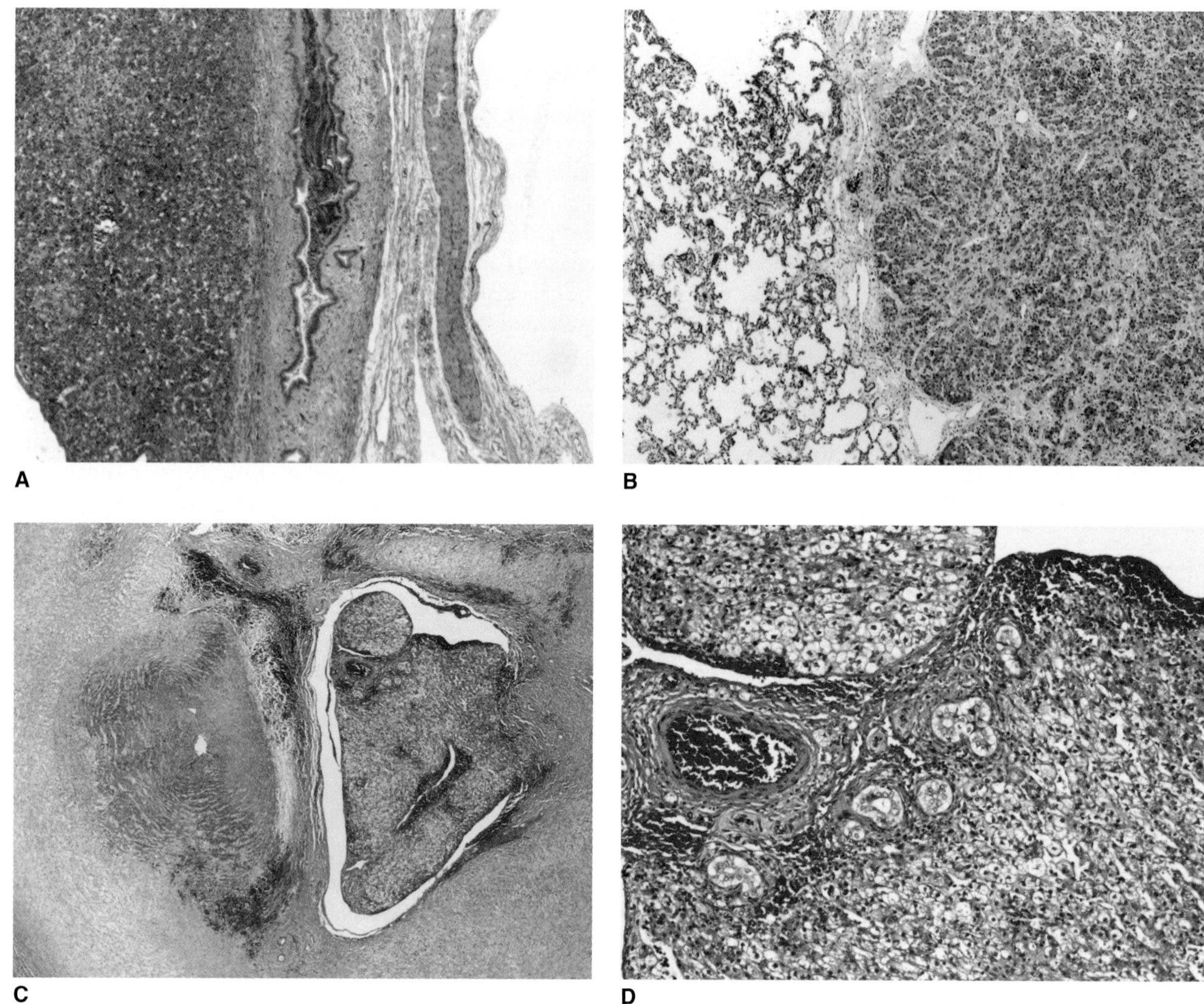

FIGURE 15-4 ■ **A:** Ectopic liver tissue within the diaphragm, **B:** lung, and **C:** umbilical cord (H&E, 40×). **D:** Ectopic liver tissue in the umbilical cord with bile ducts (H&E stain, 200×).

cavity (61) (e159,e161,e453,e568). The herniated portion of the liver may be dusky, and a groove often marks the site of compression by the margin of the diaphragm. The right lobe of the liver may bulge into the right pleural cavity in association with eventration of the right hemidiaphragm (e453). In cases of omphalocele, the liver is often herniated into the omphalocele sac. In large omphaloceles, there is often distortion of the liver and its vascular and biliary connections. The liver may have signs of marked congestion and even hemorrhagic necrosis. Intrapericardial herniation of the liver occurs rarely and may result in massive pericardial effusion in neonates (e159). Nearly all cases of the thoracopagus type of conjoined twins show connections between the two livers, ranging from a bridge to a common liver between the two twins (e652).

Hepatic ectopia or heterotopia is extremely unusual, with only rare reports of distinct lobules of hepatic tissue within the gallbladder wall, the substance of the diaphragm, lung, and umbilical cord (Figure 15-4) (101) (e83,e520,e611). Often times, this liver tissue is seen in conjunction with congenital diaphragmatic hernias and congenital heart disease. Ectopic pancreatic tissue within the liver or in the porta hepatis may also be seen, occasionally obstructing the common hepatic duct (e611). Adrenal heterotopias are usually the result of adrenal-hepatic adhesion or fusion depending on the presence (adhesion) or absence (fusion) of a capsule between the organs. Liver tissue at these variable sites is at the same risk for viral hepatitis and subsequent hepatocellular carcinoma (HCC) as an orthotopic liver tissue infected with hepatitis viruses.

TISSUE TRIAGING

The most important aspect of providing an accurate diagnosis is appropriate triaging of tissue to allow for optimal evaluation (Figure 15-5). It is imperative that adequate tissue is obtained to perform all necessary tests for an appropriate diagnosis to guide future therapy and to avoid repeat biopsy.

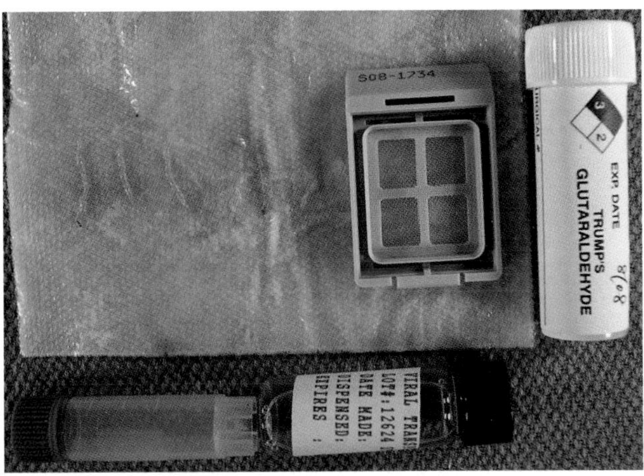

FIGURE 15-5■Liver biopsy triaging consists of tissue submitted for formalin-fixation and paraffin embedding, freezing tissue at −70°C, viral or microbiologic culture submission, and glutaraldehyde fixation for electron microscopy.

Fresh tissue can be obtained for microbiologic and viral cultures and polymerase chain reaction (PCR) testing. Tissue should be obtained for routine histology (formalin fixation), histochemical stains (frozen in optimal cryomatrix material [OCT] at −20°C and alcohol fixation), electron microscopy (glutaraldehyde), and genetic/molecular evaluation (frozen at −70°C). It is especially important with glycogen storage diseases (GSDs) to maintain optimal preservation of glycogen. With formalin fixation, up to 70% of glycogen is lost due to the soluble nature of the predominant form of glycogen in the cytoplasm. Glycogen can be preserved with freezing and/or alcohol fixation, allowing for quantitative evaluation by analytical techniques (frozen tissue) and qualitative assessment by histochemical staining (PAS, PAS-diastase). Quantitative analysis of enzyme(s) responsible for suspected metabolic and mitochondrial diseases must be done on frozen tissue. Assessment of gene mutation and sequencing of the gene responsible for the enzyme defect or mitochondrial disease also require frozen tissue. Preservation of the enzyme, enzyme activity, DNA, and RNA requires cryopreservation at −70°C and maintaining this temperature until the tissue reaches the appropriate reference laboratory. Depending on the testing required for a definitive diagnosis, tissue requirements may dictate an open biopsy of the liver or skeletal muscle. Obtaining fibroblast cultures from a skin biopsy may also be necessary for genetic and enzyme studies. Current trend in surgical and interventional radiology practice has been toward needle core biopsies for diagnosis. The pathologist should be aware of necessary tissue requirements (tissue weights and preservation methods) for appropriate testing to be completed. A single tissue core of 20 mm length from a 16-gauge needle with a 1.5 mm diameter yields about 15 mg of tissue. Several metabolic disease tests require a minimum of 20 mg of tissue. With GSDs, 100 mg or more of tissue will be needed. This may necessitate numerous tissue cores, or an open biopsy, to obtain adequate tissue for all tests. This emphasizes the importance of active communication between the healthcare team and the pathologist. Because tissue will be preserved in a steady state with cryopreservation (−70°C), comprehensive workup (histopathology, histochemistry, electron microscopy) by the pathologist to determine which additional testing is most appropriate can be completed prior to performing specialized testing on the frozen tissue.

PHYSIOLOGIC JAUNDICE

Hyperbilirubinemia in the neonatal period is one of the earliest postnatal events that requires clinical assessment to determine its clinical significance (83,147) (e158,e534). In the majority of cases, it is assessed to be physiologic jaundice with an elevated unconjugated bilirubin, which resolves within the first 2 weeks of life. However, in the presence of conjugated hyperbilirubinemia and other concurrent hepatic enzyme abnormalities, a clinically serious underlying disorder must be given consideration. With infants and older children, development of jaundice is a sign of hepatic or biliary tract disease of diverse etiologies, requires thorough clinical, imaging and laboratory evaluation, and may need liver biopsy to determine the exact nature of the underlying disease.

Physiologic jaundice is characterized by an increase in serum unconjugated bilirubin of 5 to 6 mg/dL by 2 to 4 days of age. This is a result of increased bilirubin production following breakdown of fetal red blood cells, combined with transient limitation in the conjugation of bilirubin by the liver. Levels of up to 12 mg/dL may be seen in Chinese, Japanese, Korean, or Native American infants. Other risk factors include maternal diabetes, prematurity, altitude, polycythemia, male sex, trisomy 21, cutaneous bleeding, cephalohematoma, oxytocin induction, and vitamin K use (e499). Other causes of unconjugated hyperbilirubinemia are listed in Table 15-1. Cholestasis is rarely present in the liver in the absence of other diseases.

HEREDITARY HYPERBILIRUBINEMIAS

Crigler-Najjar syndrome (CNS), an autosomal dominant disorder, results from a mutation in one of the five exons of the UGT1A1 gene coding for the enzyme bilirubin-UDP-glucuronosyltransferase (24) (e143,e323,e506,e590,e760). UGTIA1 mutation leads to elevated unconjugated bilirubin levels. In type 1 CNS, enzymatic activity is completely absent and the neonate presents with jaundice and frequently kernicterus with death by 1 year of age. Liver transplantation has been successfully used in management. The liver may show prominent canalicular bile or may appear normal. With type 2 CNS, there is only partial deficiency of glucuronyl transferase, and this has milder clinical course with most affected individuals being asymptomatic. Gilbert syndrome is a benign condition with minimal clinical manifestations, owing to greater preservation of enzyme activity. Although the condition is occasionally seen in children, the diagnosis is usually made incidentally in young adults or in later life (e242).

Dubin-Johnson syndrome, an autosomal recessive trait, may present in the neonatal period with conjugated and

Table 15-1 ■ JAUNDICE IN INFANTS DUE TO UNCONJUGATED HYPERBILIRUBINEMIA

Physiologic Features	Associated Conditions
Overproduction of bilirubin	Sepsis Rh/ABO incompatibility Erythrocyte defects Hemoglobinopathies Hematoma, birth trauma Polycythemia, maternal fetal or fetal maternal transfusion Drugs
Impaired transport of bilirubin	Hypoxia Acidosis Drugs Hypoalbuminemia Intralipid
Impaired hepatic uptake	Decreased sinusoidal perfusion Gilbert syndrome
Impaired conjugation	Breast milk jaundice Hypoglycemia Hypothyroidism High intestinal obstruction Glucoronyl transferase deficiency, types I and II Drugs
Impaired enterohepatic circulation	Low intestinal obstruction Meconium ileus

unconjugated hyperbilirubinemia and severe cholestasis (145,181) (e249,e630,e713). This syndrome has mutation in the ABCC2 gene that is responsible for synthesis of MRP2/cMOAT, an organic ion transporter. Zone 3 hepatocytes contain deposits of a granular golden-brown pigment, with staining characteristics of melanin. Ultrastructurally, however, these granules do not have the features of melanosomes, but are lysosomes with a distinctive appearance.

Rotor syndrome is characterized by persistent elevation of conjugated and unconjugated serum bilirubin and presents infrequently in children (181) (e132,e251,e329,e722). It differs from Dubin-Johnson syndrome clinically and morphologically and can be distinguished from Dubin-Johnson syndrome by elevated urinary coproporphyrin levels (2.5 to 5 times normal) (e132,e251,e722). The liver is normal histologically, but ultrastructurally immature bile canaliculi and osmiophilic lysosomal granules have been described.

CONGENITAL AND ACQUIRED CHOLESTATIC DISORDERS IN THE NEWBORN AND INFANT

Idiopathic Neonatal Hepatitis

Idiopathic neonatal hepatitis (INH) is largely a diagnosis of exclusion, because there are many infectious, metabolic, toxic, and anatomic etiologies to explain neonatal cholestasis (Table 15-2) (15,69,153). Once other disorders have been excluded, INH accounts for approximately 25% to 40% of

Table 15-2 ■ CHOLESTATIC DISEASE IN INFANCY

- Extrahepatic obstruction
  - Biliary atresia
  - Bile duct stenosis
  - Sclerosing cholangitis
  - Stone
  - Neoplasm
  - Mucus/bile plug
- Intrahepatic disorders
  - Giant cell hepatitis
  - Paucity of intrahepatic bile ducts
    - Syndromic (Alagille)
    - Nonsyndromic
  - Byler syndrome (progressive hepatocellular disease with persistent cholestasis)
  - Defects in bile acid metabolism (trihydroxycoprostanic acidemia)
- Congenital abnormalities
  - CHF
  - Caroli disease
- Toxic
  - TPN
  - Sepsis
    - Endotoxemia
- Chromosomal
  - Down syndrome
  - Trisomy 17,18
- Inborn errors of metabolism
  - Amino acid
    - Tyrosinemia
  - Carbohydrate
    - Galactosemia
    - Fructosemia
    - Glycogen storage disease, type IV
  - Lipid
    - Gaucher disease
    - Niemann-Pick disease
    - Wolman disease
  - Glycolipid
    - A1AT deficiency
  - Miscellaneous
    - CF
    - Neonatal iron storage
    - Copper overload Indian childhood cirrhosis
    - Cerebrohepatorenal syndrome of Zellweger
    - Hypopituitarism
    - Hypothyroidism
- Infections
  - Viral
    - Cytomegalovirus
    - Hepatitis B
    - Herpes simplex
    - Rubella
    - Reovirus
    - ECHO
    - Coxsackie
    - Varicella
  - Bacterial
    - Mycobacterium
    - Listeria
  - Syphilis
  - Toxoplasmosis
- Infiltrative disorders
  - Langerhans cell (histrocytosis X)
  - Familial erythrophagocytic lymphohistiocytosis
- Other
  - Shock
  - Cardiac failure

cases, with an incidence of 1 in 4,500 to 9,000 live births. Although two subsets are seen, sporadic INH (85% to 90%) and familial INH (10% to 15%), it is likely that INH will become a better defined diagnostic category with the elucidation of addition etiologies for cases considered to be INH. For example, alpha1-antitrypsin deficiency was included in the idiopathic category prior to discovery of the clinical and genetic features of this disease. It is now a separate and distinct entity, accounting for 25% to 30% of neonatal hepatitis cases (69). It should be noted that there are some familial INH cases without a defined genetic pattern.

Grossly, the liver in neonatal hepatitis may be enlarged, is usually smooth, and has a deep green bilious appearance. Microscopically, cholestasis is usually seen in zone 3 hepatocytes and canaliculi and rarely in the interlobular bile ducts. Giant cell transformation is usually prominent, but is a nonspecific finding, because it may be seen in many disorders involving the neonatal liver (Figure 15-6). Hepatocytes may show ballooning, acidophilic necrosis, and pseudoglandular or acinar formation. Lobular or portal mononuclear cells are generally sparse, but a prominent inflammatory component and extramedullary erythropoiesis should suggest an infectious etiology. The portal areas in INH are usually not expanded, and the bile ducts are normal or may be inconspicuous. Rarely, there may be mild proliferation of the interlobular bile ducts (69). Histologic features comparing INH with those of extrahepatic biliary atresia (EHBA) are listed in Table 15-3 (177).

The prognosis of sporadic cases of INH is generally favorable (74% complete recovery, 7% chronic liver disease, 19% death). Infants with the familial form (family history of neonatal cholestasis) have a considerably poorer prognosis (22% recovery, 16% chronic liver disease, and 63% death) (69).

Extrahepatic Biliary Atresia

EHBA is a disorder of infants that occurs worldwide with an incidence of 1 in 8,000 to 12,000 live births (14,66,80) (e45,e46,e163,e270). EHBA presents in two forms: an embryonic or fetal type (10% to 35%) and a perinatal form (65% to 90%). The embryonic or fetal form is characterized by early onset of neonatal cholestasis without a jaundice-free

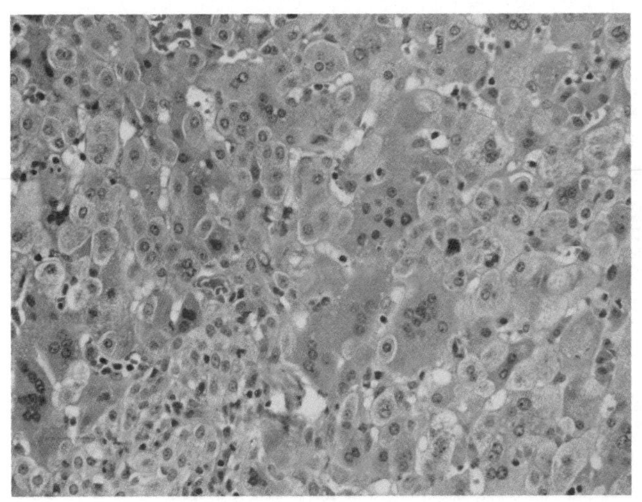

A

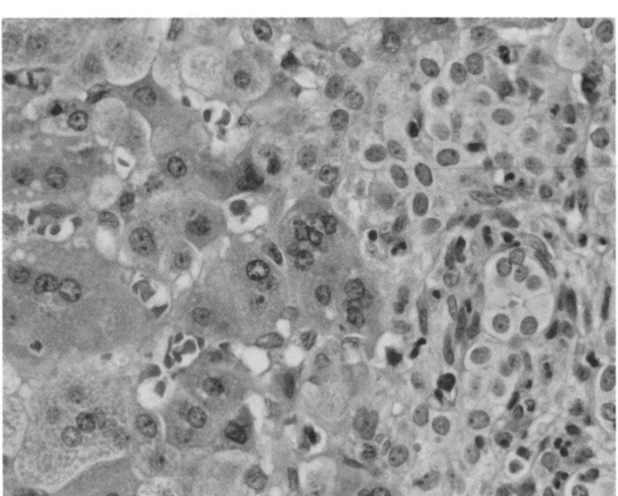

B

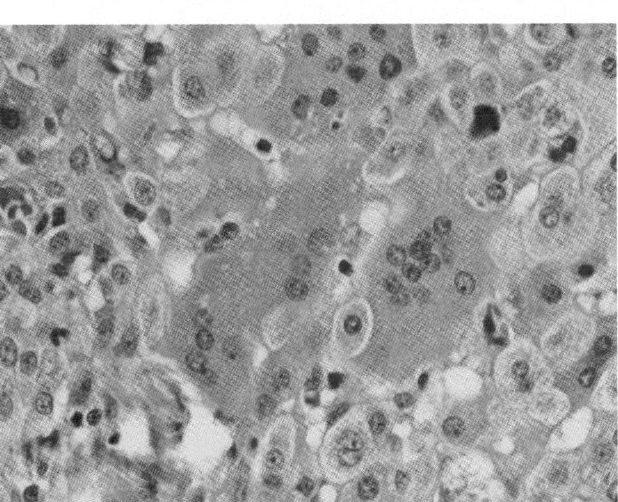

C

FIGURE 15-6 **A-C:** Idiopathic neonatal hepatitis. Giant cell transformation with expansion of the portal region by chronic inflammatory cells, prominent bile ducts, and readily identified cholestasis (**A** at 100×, **B** at 200×, **C** at 200×, H&E).

Table 15-3 ■ COMPARISON OF BILIARY ATRESIA AND NEONATAL HEPATITIS SYNDROME

Features	Biliary Atresia	Neonatal Hepatitis
Giant cell transformation	Usually focal	Diffuse; occasionally focal
Hepatocellular necrosis	Variable	Variable
Lobular disarray	Usually mild	May be marked
Cholestasis	Hepatocytes, canaliculi, and ducts	Hepatocytes and canaliculi; ducts (rare)
Portal fibrosis	In all portal areas	Absent early in the course
Bile ducts	Proliferation typically seen in all portal areas	Normal; rarely focal proliferation
Cellular infiltrate	Variable; mononuclear	Variable; mononuclear
Extramedullary hematopoiesis	Usually present	Usually present
Fat	Typically absent	Typically absent

period, unlike neonatal physiologic jaundice. This form is also associated with other anomalies, such as polysplenia and asplenia, cardiovascular defects, abdominal situs inversus, intestinal malrotation, and portal vein and hepatic artery anomalies. The perinatal form presents as late-onset neonatal cholestasis (4 to 8 weeks of age) following a jaundice-free period with passage of normally pigmented stools at birth. There is no associated anomaly with the perinatal form (14). Similar to neonatal hepatitis, EHBA is also considered to be a condition with more than one etiology. In fact, INH and EHBA have been seen as sequential processes in the same infant over a period of several weeks or months.

The liver biopsy remains an integral component in the diagnosis of a neonate or young infant with persistent conjugated hyperbilirubinemia and is a highly reliable means of establishing the diagnosis of EHBA in 85% to 97% of cases (14). Ductular proliferation is the most common finding and is considered a diagnostic feature of EHBA, although modest bile duct proliferation may be seen in neonatal hepatitis (Figures 15-7 to 15-9) (e381). The interlobular bile ducts are

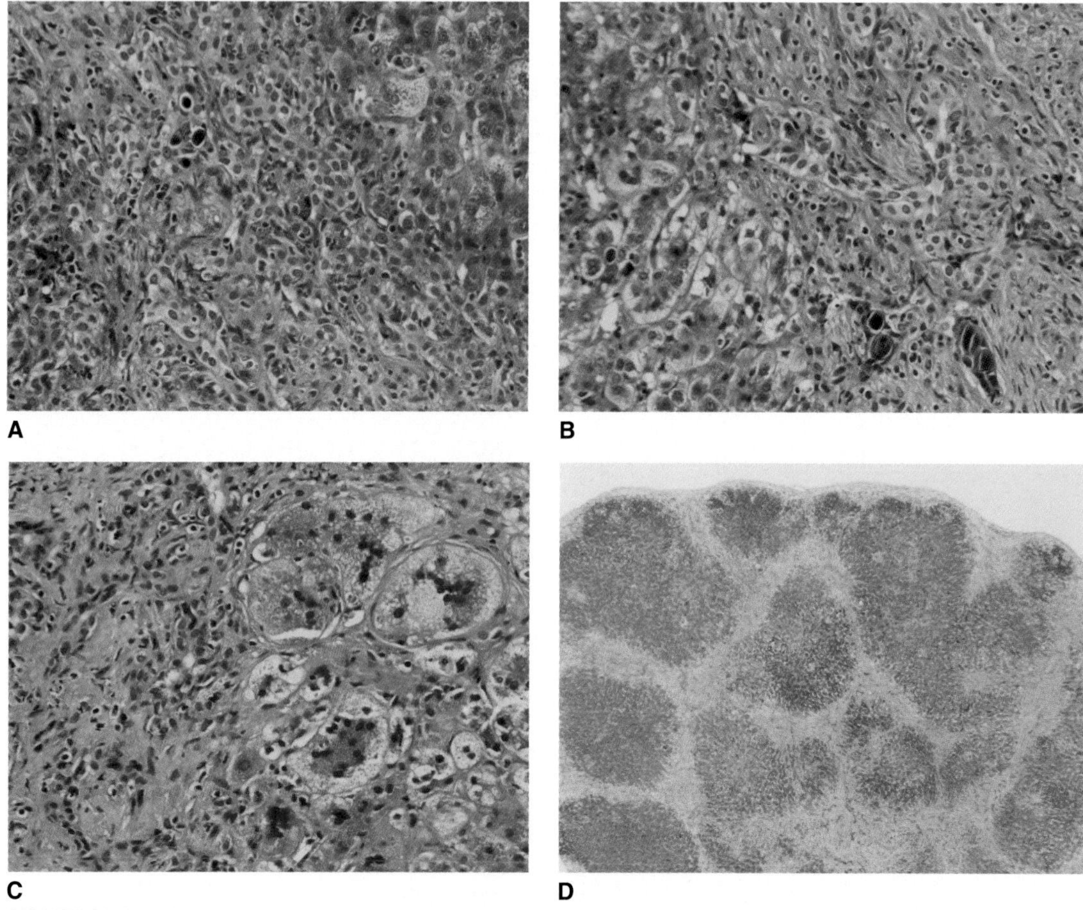

FIGURE 15-7 ■ **A:** Extrahepatic biliary atresia liver biopsy. Histopathologic features include diffuse bile duct proliferation in expanded portal region with canalicular cholestasis. **B:** Hepatocytes organized into pseudoacinar pattern, **C:** giant cell transformation adjacent to fibrotic portal region. **D:** Cirrhosis may occur rapidly without surgical intervention (H&E stains, A, B, C at 200×, D 40×).

tortuous and have distorted contours, readily demonstrated with pancytokeratin. The lining epithelium shows degenerative changes, and periductal reactive fibrosis may occur with plump fibroblasts surrounded by a loose edematous stroma. Lymphocytes and even neutrophils are found within the portal areas, with occasional infiltration of the bile duct epithelium. Portal lymphocytes, which are usually few in number, should not be confused with extramedullary hematopoiesis in younger infants. As the disease progresses in the first few weeks of life, nearly all portal areas are expanded by fibrosis, with type IV collagen deposition. Bridging fibrosis occurs, and early nodular transformation is evident as a prelude to the development of secondary biliary cirrhosis. The progression to cirrhosis varies considerably from one case to another, but there is some direct relationship with age.

Hepatocellular alterations include cholestasis (canalicular, hepatocellular, ductular), feathery (pseudoxanthomatous) degeneration, pseudoacinar transformation, and focal giant cell transformation. These features overlap with those of neonatal hepatitis. The cholestasis in EHBA is usually severe. The most prominent cholestasis is in zone 3, but is also present in the ductules and bile ducts at the zone 1 interface. Hepatocytes may form glandlike structures around bile plugs, imparting a "pseudoacinar" configuration, the so-called cholestatic rosettes. Bile "lakes" consisting of amorphous collections of bile surrounded by inflammatory cells and connective tissue are seen rarely in liver biopsies, unlike in adults with obstruction of the biliary tract. Hepatocytes may display mild enlargement and rarefaction of the cytoplasm (feathery degeneration), but fatty change is

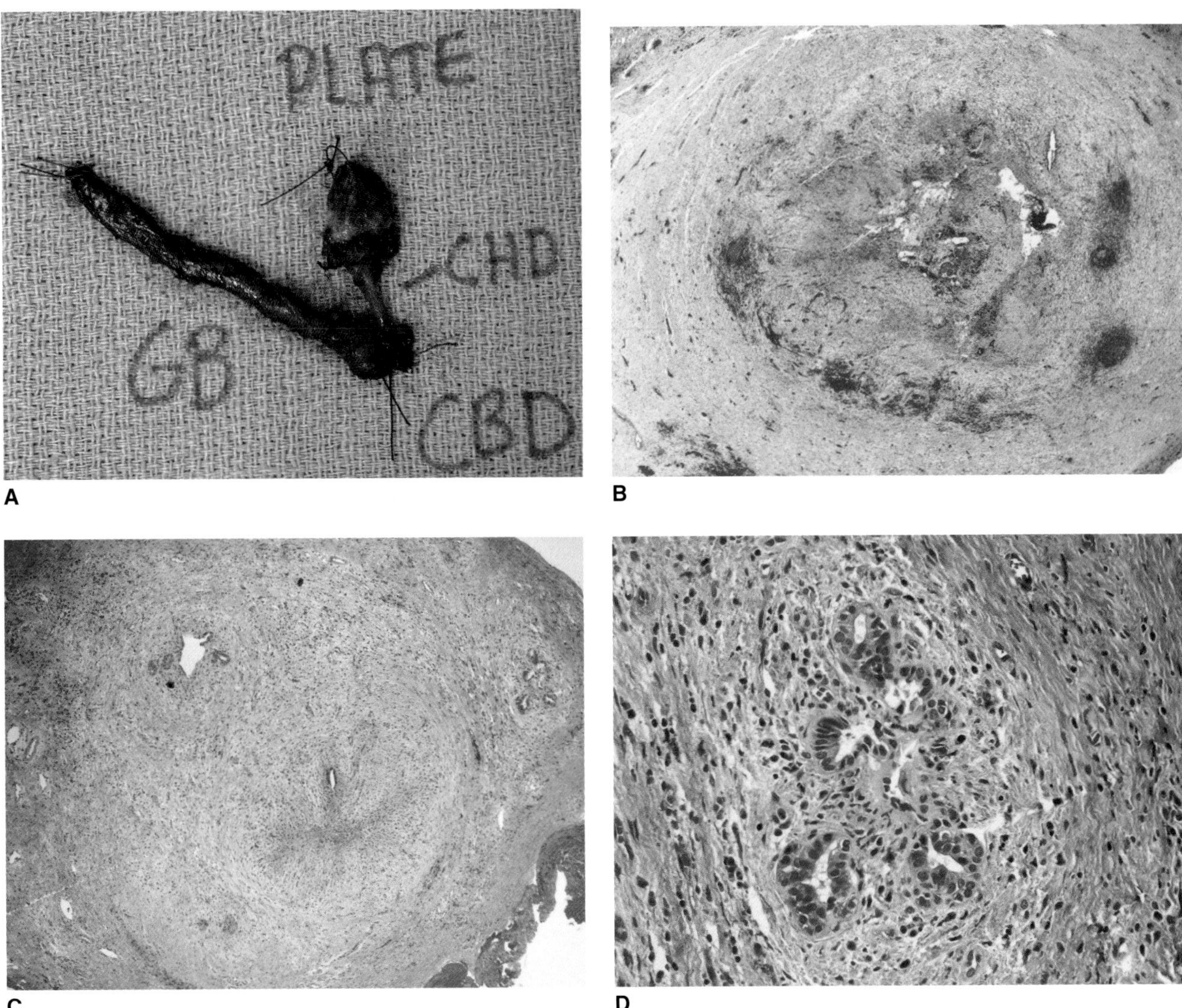

FIGURE 15-8 ■ Resection of residual common bile duct during Kasai procedure. **A:** Common bile duct remnant with orientation by surgeon. CHD, hepatic duct, GB; gallbladder, CBD; common bile duct; plate, liver plate. **B:** Near total obliteration of common bile duct lumen with no residual epithelial lining (H&E, 20×). **C:** Microscopic residual common bile duct lumen with epithelial lining (H&E, 20×). **D:** Nests of bile duct epithelium in common bile duct wall (H&E, 200×). The latter side chain structures should not be mistaken as evidence of a patent bile duct.

rarely seen. Giant cell transformation, if present, is generally restricted to zone 1 at the interface with the expanded portal tracts (Table 15-3).

The most frequently observed changes within the liver in EHBA are the cholestasis, portal fibrosis, and ductular proliferation. Other causes of obstruction (bile duct stenosis, choledochal cyst, mucous or bile plug) produce similar changes, as will disorders such as alpha-1-antitrypsin deficiency and total parenteral nutrition (TPN)–associated cholestasis. It is important to realize that other disorders can simulate patterns of liver injury similar to those for EHBA.

The extrahepatic ducts may display a wide variety of histopathologic changes, ranging from a mild degree of inflammation to complete obliteration (Figure 15-8). The epithelium

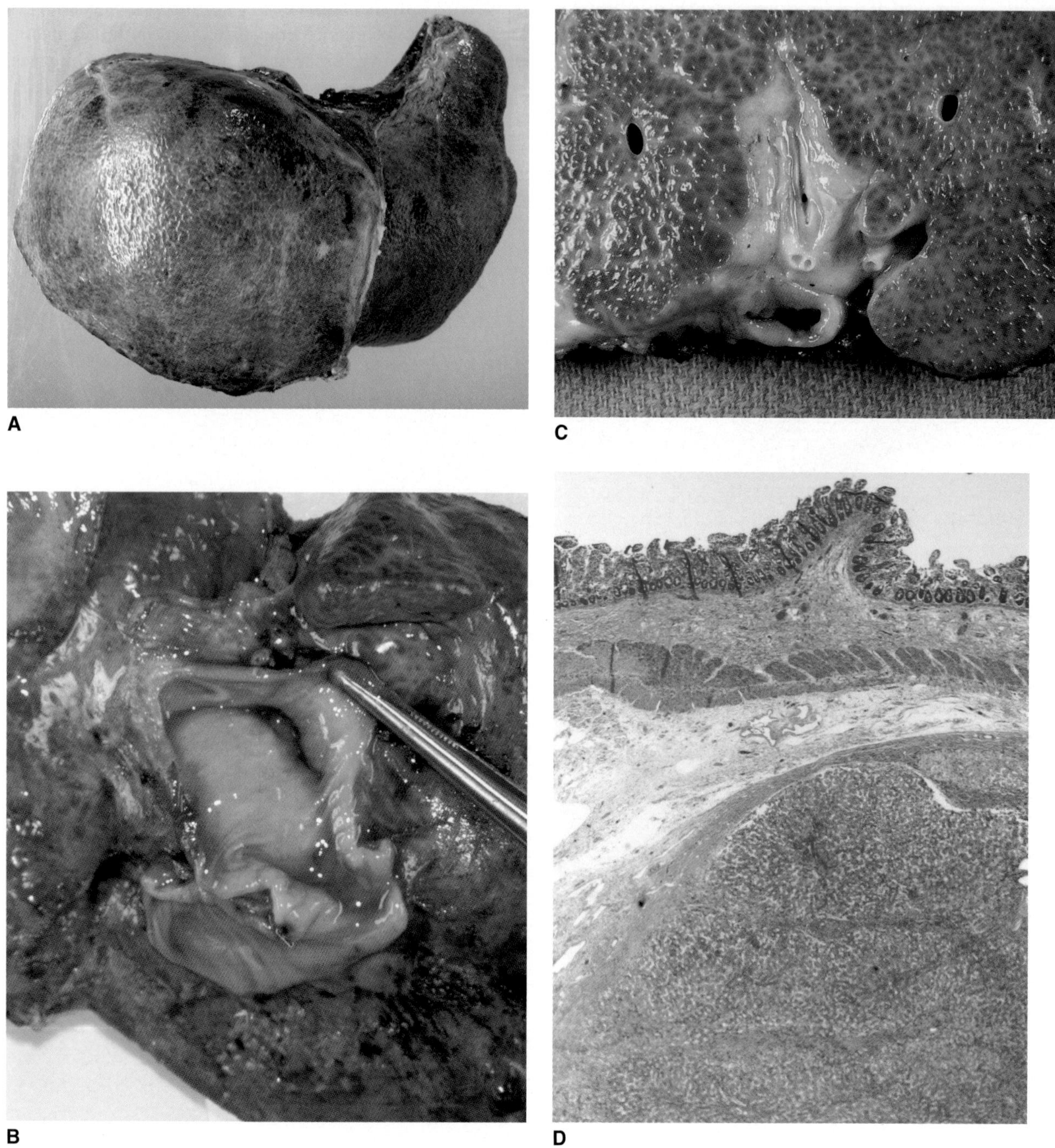

FIGURE 15-9 Explanted liver with prior Kasai procedure. **A:** Explanted liver with micronodular cirrhosis. **B:** Patent small bowel anastomosis site at liver hilum. **C:** Liver in cross section with close apposition of small bowel anastomosis to liver hilum and micronodular liver parenchyma with diffuse bile staining. **D:** Small bowel anastomosis separated by muscular wall of small bowel and fibrous tissue from the underlying liver parenchyma (H&E, 10×).

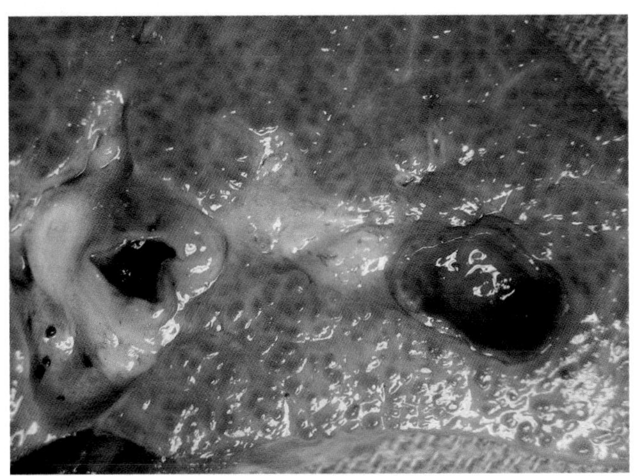

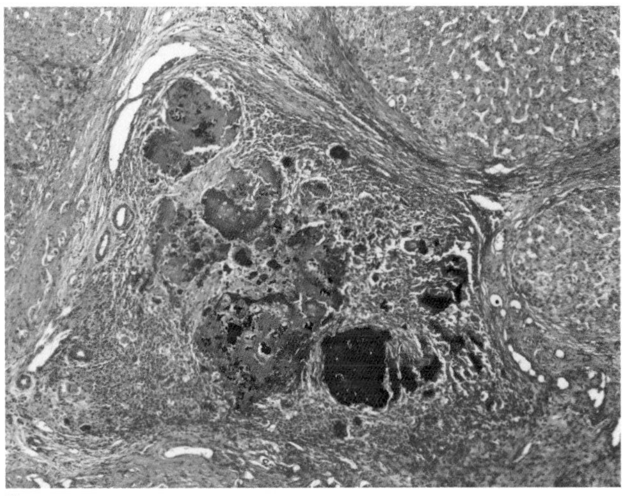

E F

FIGURE 15-9■ *(continued)* **E:** Large bile-filled lakes within the liver parenchyma and micronodular cirrhosis with diffuse bile staining, and **F:** bile plugs distending portal legion with adjacent micronodular liver parenchyma (H&E, 40×).

of large, medium, and small ducts shows nuclear irregularity and pyknosis with cellular degeneration and necrosis. Cellular debris and bile-stained macrophages may be present in the lumen. The duct lining is often infiltrated by neutrophils and is ulcerated, with intraluminal and extraluminal fibrosis distorting the lumen. As the epithelial inflammation and degeneration progresses, fibrosis increases and eventually obliterates the duct. With active ductular destruction, the stroma around and between ducts becomes infiltrated by neutrophils, lymphocytes, and macrophages, along with a prominent fibroblastic proliferation. As the ductular inflammation diminishes and the ducts are destroyed, the stromal activity is replaced by dense fibrosis, containing a few residual inflammatory cells and remnants of bile ducts. Choi et al. (e128) have used ultrasonography to define a "triangular cord" of fibrous connective tissue in the portal hepatis of infants with EHBA. Rarely, islands of hyaline cartilage may be found in the porta hepatis, suggesting a congenital malformation as the cause of the atresia in these selected cases (e447). The gallbladder may be diminutive and exhibit varying degrees of fibrosis, epithelial degeneration and destruction, and luminal compromise.

Biliary remnants have been classified by Gautier and Eliot (58) into three types:

1. Absence of any lumen lined by biliary epithelium, with little or no inflammatory cells in the connective tissue (Figure 15-8).
2. Presence of lumina lined by cuboidal epithelium. The remnants may be numerous, have a lumen less than 50 μm, and be surrounded by a neutrophilic infiltrate. Cellular debris and bile may be present in the lumen, and epithelial necrosis may be seen in ducts with a diameter exceeding 300 μm.
3. The presence of a central altered bile duct incompletely lined by columnar epithelium, in addition to smaller epithelial structures resembling those in the second type.

The size of the ducts tends to be larger in infants younger than 12 weeks of age, and beyond this age, total obliteration of ducts is the common finding. Tan et al. (e687) noted that few or absent ductal remnants at the porta hepatis and absence of portal inflammation were predictors of poor prognosis. However, this finding has not been confirmed in other clinical studies. Age at operation (improved outcome at <60 days of age), the surgical team's experience, and the degree of liver disease are factors associated with prognosis.

Persistent Intrahepatic Cholestasis

Once the presence of a normal biliary tract has been established through a variety of studies and procedures, the differential diagnosis of persistent conjugated hyperbilirubinemia shifts in the direction of inherited and infectious etiologies. The inherited disorders include those conditions of a primary nature affecting the structure of intrahepatic bile ducts or bile secretion with secondary effects on the intrahepatic ducts. The first category is represented primarily by the Alagille and Byler (progressive familial intrahepatic cholestasis [PFIC]) syndromes, and the second by a diverse group of infectious, metabolic, and inherited disorders.

Alagille Syndrome (Syndromic Paucity of Interlobular Bile Ducts, Arteriohepatic Dysplasia)

Alagille syndrome is an autosomal dominant disorder associated with abnormalities of the liver, heart, eye, skeleton, and a characteristic facial appearance (Table 15-4) (82) (e60,e320,e344,e360,e532,e584,e730). The genetic defect for this syndrome is the JAG1 gene locus on chromosome 20p12. JAG1 encodes a ligand for the Notch signaling

Table 15-4 ■ FAMILIAL CHOLESTATIC SYNDROMES

Syndrome	Age at Onset	Associated Anomalies	Inheritance	Outcome	Pathologic Features
Alagille	<3 months	Facies, heart, eye, bone, kidneys	Autosomal dominant	Mild disease, cirrhosis in 12%–14%	Paucity of ducts, cholestasis, giant cells; pigment in Golgi, ER, and lysosomes
Byler	3–12 months	None	Autosomal recessive	Fatal in childhood	Cholestasis, giant cells, fibrosis
Norwegian	<3 months	Lymphedema	Autosomal recessive	Mild disease	Cholestasis, portal fibrosis
Benign, recurrent	1–15 years	None	Unknown	No disease	Cholestasis
North American Indian	<3 months	None	Autosomal recessive	Fatal cirrhosis	Cholestasis, giant cells, actin filament hyperplasia

ER, endoplasmic reticulum.

pathway that is important in early cellular development, particularly in the liver, kidney, and heart. Alagille syndrome is the most frequent condition associated with paucity of intrahepatic bile ducts and has been referred to as syndromic paucity of interlobular bile ducts. The onset of cholestasis occurs in the first 3 months of life with unconjugated hyperbilirubinemia and an obstructive pattern on laboratory evaluation and hepatobiliary scintigraphy. Cutaneous manifestations occur later in the course and include pruritus (hyperbilirubinemia) and xanthomas (hypercholesterolemia). The typical facies includes a prominent forehead, hypertelorism, flattened malar eminence, and a pointed chin, although the specificity of the abnormal facies has been questioned. Characteristic eye findings include a posterior embryotoxon. The cardiovascular anomaly most often reported is pulmonic stenosis with a heart murmur (95%). Vertebral abnormalities (butterfly vertebrae, 60% to 70%) and foreshortened fingers are skeletal anomalies associated with the syndrome. Renal abnormalities leading to renal failure include interstitial nephritis and membranoproliferative glomerulonephritis with mesangial lipid deposits. Unilateral renal cystic dysplasia, renal hypoplasia, ureteropelvic obstruction, and renal artery stenosis may also be seen (e427). Other features include mental retardation, stunted growth, cerebrovascular accidents (15%), pancreatic insufficiency, moyamoya, and middle aortic syndrome. Incomplete forms of the syndrome have been described in which only some of the major features are present. The mortality rate is 17% to 28%, which is largely determined by the presence of cardiovascular disease or progressive liver disease (e195).

Liver disease is noted in almost 95% of cases within the 1st year of life, with progression to cirrhosis. HCC is an infrequent complication (e553). Transplantation has been performed in approximately 50% of patients in some series, with approximately a 75% survival rate (e103,e552).

The characteristic histopathologic feature of Alagille syndrome is absence or paucity of interlobular bile ducts (Figure 15-10). Because normal numbers of bile ducts may be present in early biopsies and even ductal proliferation, it is assumed that the syndrome is characterized by progressive damage and subsequent loss of intrahepatic ducts, as noted in liver biopsies from older children (e714). Loss of ducts through atrophy secondary to decreased bile flow is an alternative explanation for the paucity of bile ducts. An optimal diagnostic liver biopsy should contain 20 portal areas, which may require a wedge biopsy, but a needle biopsy containing at least six portal areas may be adequate. Portal triads may be diminished in size and number and show no or mild fibrosis. Cholestasis is usually present in zone 3, but may be seen in zone 1. Hepatocellular ballooning, pseudoacinar transformation, focal giant cell formation, and lobular disarray are other nonspecific features. A quantitative increase in hepatic copper may occur and is demonstrable by rhodamine or other copper stains in zone 1 hepatocytes, a finding also common in other obstructive or cholestatic hepatopathies. Ultrastructural changes are distinctive with bile pigment retention in the cytoplasm, especially in lysosomes and in vesicles in the outer convex region of the Golgi apparatus. Rarely, bile pigment is present in the bile canaliculi or immediate pericanalicular region, suggesting a block in the bile secretory apparatus (e730).

Progressive Familial Intrahepatic Cholestasis (Byler Disease and Byler Syndrome)

PFIC is a group of severe genetic cholestatic hepatopathies of early life, including the archetypical PFIC1 (Byler disease) first described in Amish children. This autosomal recessive disorder is heralded by infantile cholestasis, which leads to hepatic fibrosis and death (90) (e18,e160,e243,e275,e352). Children who have a clinically similar disorder, but are not members of the Amish kindred in which Byler disease was described, are said to have Byler syndrome. The gene for Byler disease is at 18q21 locus of the ATP8P1 gene, which synthesizes an aminophospholipid translocating ATPase on the bile duct epithelium. This same gene mutation is

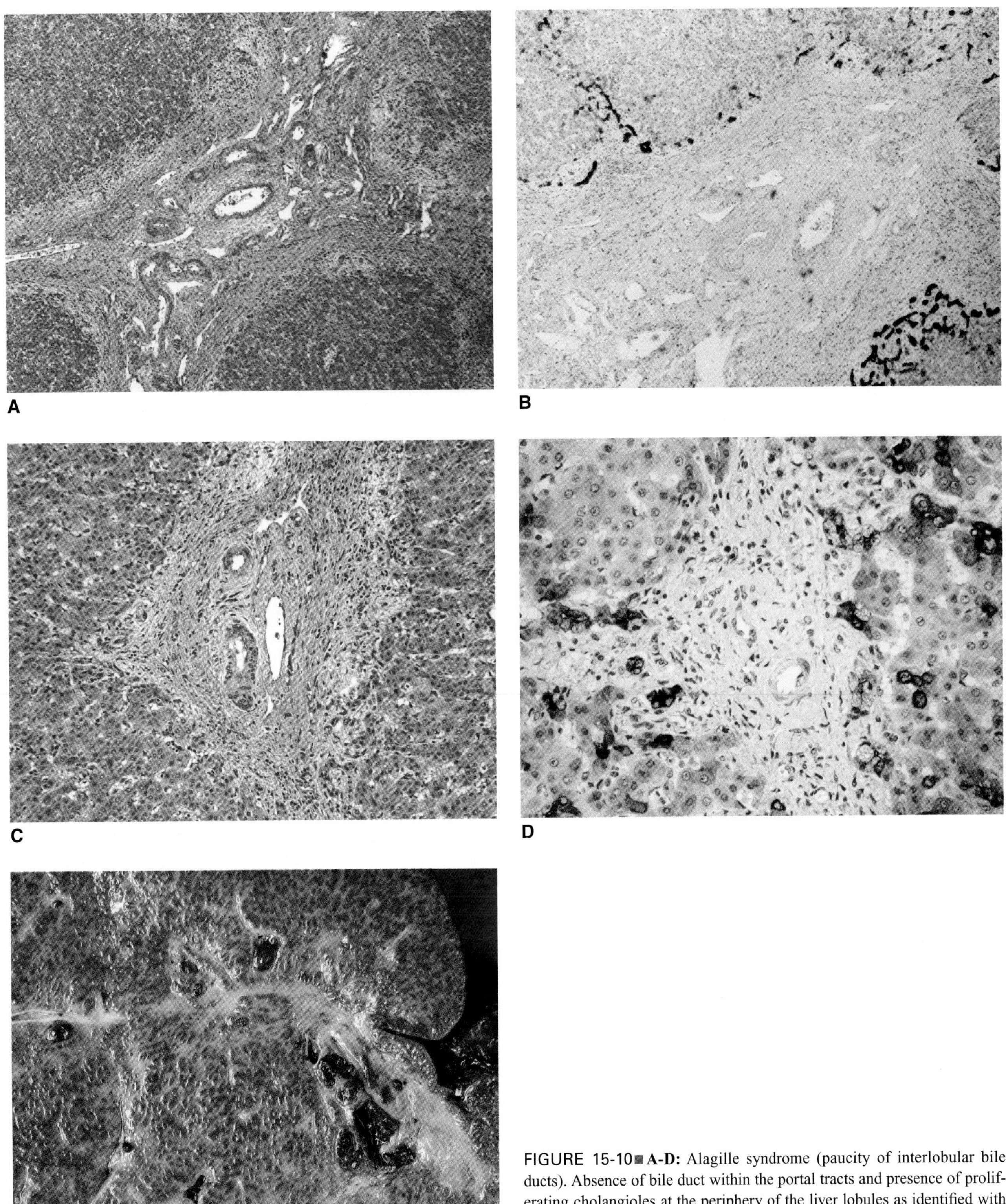

FIGURE 15-10 ■ **A-D:** Alagille syndrome (paucity of interlobular bile ducts). Absence of bile duct within the portal tracts and presence of proliferating cholangioles at the periphery of the liver lobules as identified with cytokeratin 7 immunostaining (H&E staining, **A,C:** 20×; Cytokeratin 7 immunostaining, **B,D:** 20×). **E:** Micronodular cirrhosis with bile plugs and diffuse bile staining.

implicated in benign recurrent intrahepatic cholestasis (BRIC), which is associated with recurrent cholestasis with pruritus. PFIC types 1 (ATP8B1 gene mutation at 18q21) and 2 (ABCB11 gene mutation at 2q24) (e311,e665) are characterized by cholestasis and low serum gamma-glutamyltransferase (GGT) activity. With PFIC type 3, serum GGT is elevated and is associated with mutation of the ABCB4 gene (7q21). This gene encodes the canalicular protein

MDR3 responsible for translocation phospholipids from hepatocytes to canalicular lumens. Intrahepatic cholestasis of pregnancy occurs in heterozygotes with an ABCB4 gene mutation and is associated with elevated aminotransferases, cholestasis with pruritus, and recurrent fetal losses.

Histologically, PFIC type 1 exhibits giant cell transformation and paucity of bile ducts, which progresses through a spidery fibrosis beginning in zone 3 and extending to zone 1, eventually leading to cirrhosis (Figure 15-11). The bile has a coarse granular appearance on electron microscopic examination. In contrast, non-Amish children have neonatal hepatitis, amorphous to finely filamentous bile, and a more benign course, but with recurrent cholestasis (33). PFIC type 2 is characterized by persistent neonatal cholestasis with features of neonatal hepatitis and later biliary cirrhosis. PFIC type 3 displays periportal inflammation, extensive bile duct proliferation, feathery hepatocyte degeneration, and fibrosis, which progresses to biliary cirrhosis (e664). Partial external biliary diversion and transplantation have been helpful in 80% of patients (e307). Liver biopsies in Amish and Mennonite children with familial hypercholesterolemia have bland intracanalicular cholestasis and low GGT and improve with ursodeoxycholic acid treatment. The genetic defects in these children are associated with aberrant tight junction proteins (claudin, TJP2 gene) and a defective bile acid conjugation enzyme (gene BAAT).

Other conditions may also present initially with cholestasis and end in cirrhosis. A disease that presents with neonatal cholestasis and may mimic EHBA is North American Indian cirrhosis. This disease has progressive fibrosis and usually culminates in cirrhosis early in life. The genetic defect has

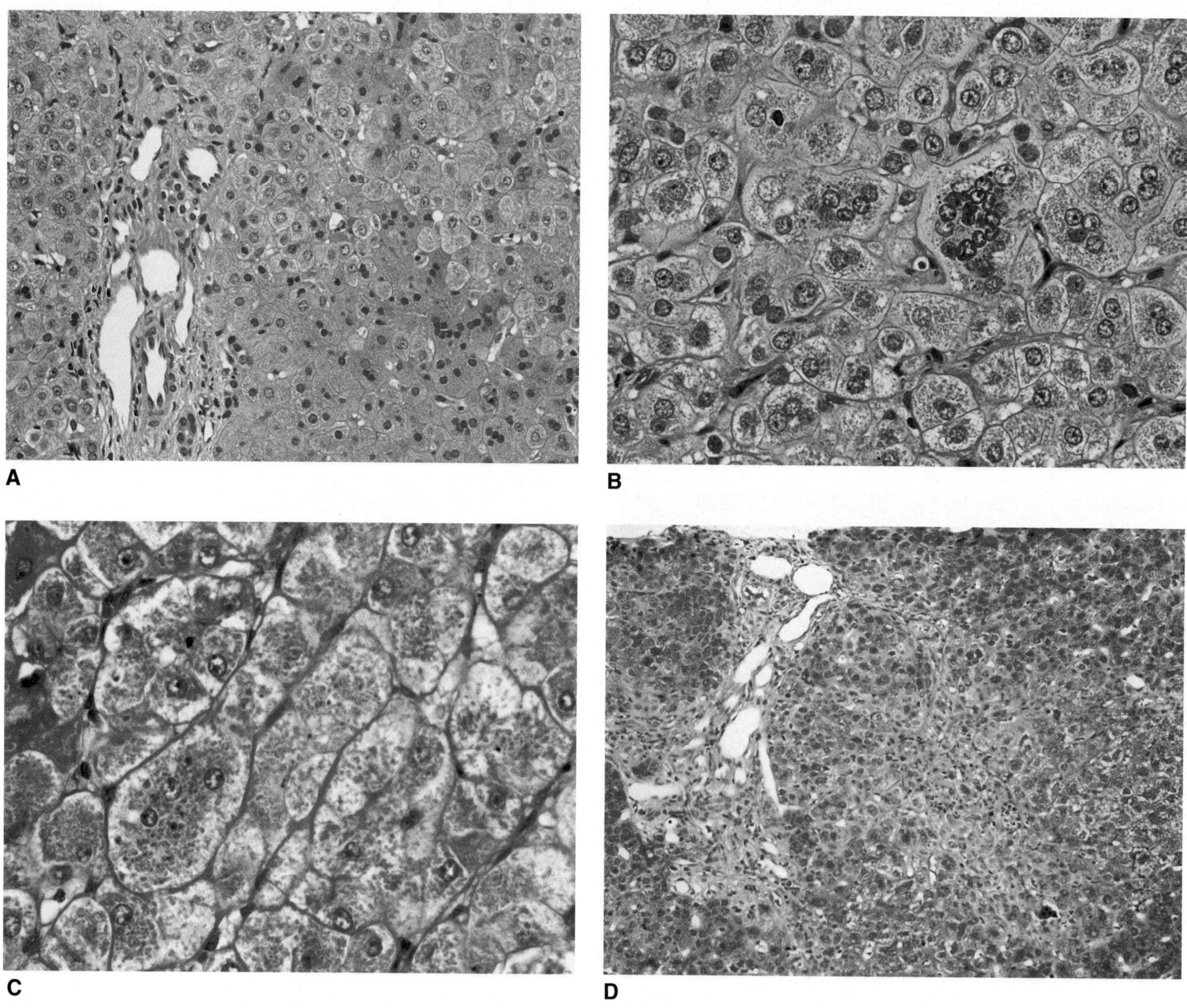

FIGURE 15-11 ■ **A-B:** Progressive familial intrahepatic cholestasis (PFIC). Hepatic lobular disarray with giant cell transformation and focal canalicular cholestasis (H&E, **A:** 100×, **B:** 400×). **C:** Diffuse cytoplasmic cholestasis of hepatocytes with granular bile (H&E, **C** 400×). **D:** Central lobular fibrosis with fine feathery extension into the peripheral zone toward the portal region (Trichrome, **D:** 100×).

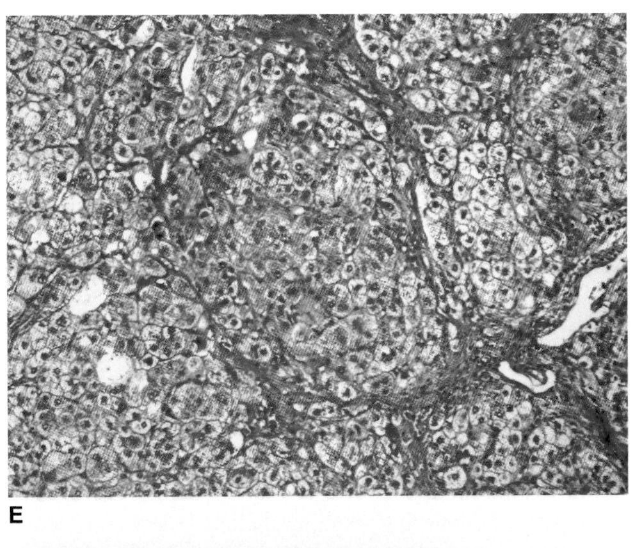
E

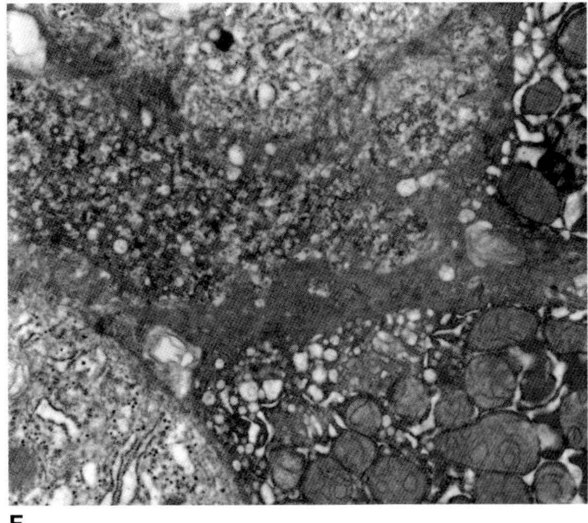
F

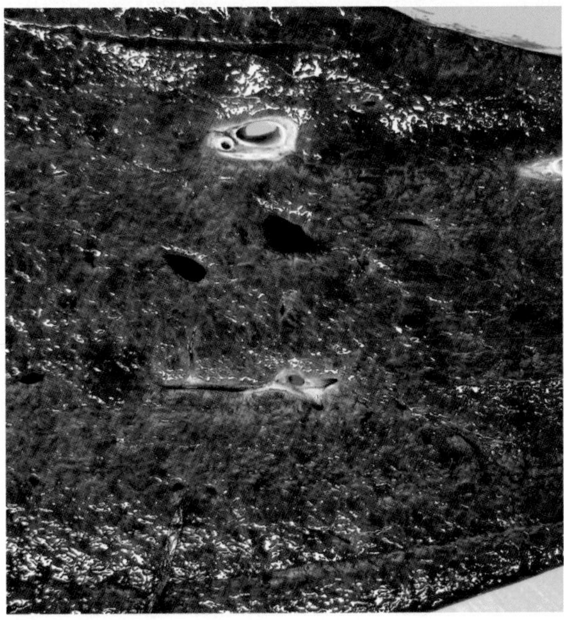
G

FIGURE 15-11 ■ *(continued)* **E:** Micronodular cirrhosis with portal to portal bridging fibrosis and loss of central veins (H&E, **E**, 100×; **G:** Gross appearance). **F:** Electron microscopic appearance of coarse granular bile markedly distending a canalicular space between hepatocytes (Electron microscopy, **F:** 20,000×).

been localized to a mitochondrial protein gene, CIRHIN. A syndrome that is comprised of arthrogryposis, renal tubular dysfunction, and cholestasis (ARC) may present initially as cholestasis with a low GGT, and is typically fatal in the first few years of life.

Nonsyndromic Paucity of Intrahepatic Ducts

Paucity of intrahepatic bile ducts have been reported in several sporadic cases of neonatal cholestasis with progressive liver disease, but rarely does the condition evolve into cirrhosis. Alpha-1-antitrypsin deficiency has been associated with paucity of intrahepatic bile ducts in a subgroup of patients. Other conditions include congenital syphilis, Turner syndrome, Down syndrome, cytomegaloviral infection, hepatitis B antigenemia, hypopituitarism, medications, infections, toxins, immune-mediated injury, and graft-versus-host disease (79,107,111) (e664,e672). Ultrastructural evidence of bile duct destruction in nonsyndromic paucity of bile ducts has been regarded as representing a primary ductal injury (79).

Recurrent Intrahepatic Cholestasis

Benign Recurrent Intrahepatic Cholestasis

BRIC and PFIC type 1 share the same locus on 18q21 (108) (e91,e92,e364). The gene PFIC1 has been identified in both groups of patients, but the relationship between these two entities is unclear (91). BRIC is characterized by recurrent episodes of cholestasis without permanent liver damage.

Hereditary Cholestasis with Lymphedema (Aagenaes Syndrome)

Hereditary intrahepatic cholestasis with lymphedema (Aagenaes syndrome) is an autosomal recessive, inherited syndrome with more than 75% of the cases occurring in Norwegians, and is associated with a genetic defect on chromosome 15q (2,184) (e225). Cholestasis with high serum GGT is present before or shortly after birth. With modern treatment, the cholestasis usually improves considerably during the first 2 years of life, but periods of recurrent cholestasis occur later. In some cases, lymphedema is present at birth, but this usually comes to light during childhood. The prognosis for the liver disease is good, but cirrhosis develops in about 15% of Norwegian cases (e2).

Anatomic Anomalies and Disorders of Biliary and Hepatic Ducts

Agenesis of the Common Bile or Hepatic Duct

Agenesis of the common bile duct or hepatic duct is extremely rare. With common duct atresia, the hepatic duct enters directly into the gallbladder, and a long cystic duct drains into the duodenum (e426).

Congenital Bronchobiliary Fistula

Congenital bronchobiliary fistula (CBBF) is a rare anomaly with varied presentations, including aspiration pneumonia and atelectasis, and may be associated with common bile duct abnormalities, including biliary atresia and diaphragmatic hernia (e110,e112,e179,e192,e261,e296). CBBF usually arises from the proximal part of the right main bronchus, a short distance below the carina, and joins the biliary system at the level of the left hepatic duct. The intrahepatic portion is usually lined by squamous or columnar epithelium, whereas the proximal section resembles a bronchus with respiratory epithelial lining and cartilage plates in the wall (e192).

Ciliated Foregut Cyst

Ciliated hepatic foregut cyst is usually seen in adults, but may rarely present in childhood with abdominal pain or portal hypertension (38,165) (e626,e668,e740,e787). The cyst is thought to arise from the migration of a bronchiolar bud of the foregut through the pleuroperitoneal canal. The cyst is subcapsular, measuring from 1 to 4 cm in diameter, and is composed of a lining of ciliated pseudostratified columnar epithelium overlying connective tissue, a layer of smooth muscle bundles, and a fibrous capsule.

Congenital Dilatation of the Bile Ducts

Choledochal cyst is a presumed congenital anomaly of the intrahepatic and extrahepatic ducts characterized by segmental ductal dilatation, bile stasis, and hyperbilirubinemia (167–169) (e338,e460). An association with malunion of the pancreatic and distal common bile ducts is a common finding. The prevalence of choledochal cysts is 1:15,000 live births and is higher in Asian populations. There is a female predilection. Secondary causes of bile duct dilatation include cholangitis, biliary perforation, biliary tract carcinoma, acute pancreatitis, and biliary cirrhosis (e704). The cysts are classified (Figure 15-12) as:

- Type Ia—large cystic or saccular dilatation of the choledochus
- Type Ib—segmental dilatation with no pancreaticobiliary malunion
- Type Ic—diffuse cylindrical or fusiform dilatation
- Type II—diverticulum of the common bile duct or gallbladder
- Type III—choledochocele of the distal common bile duct that usually extends into the wall of the duodenum
- Type IVA—multiple choledochal cysts with intrahepatic and extrahepatic involvement (Caroli disease)
- Type IVB—multiple extrahepatic cysts
- Type V—single or multiple intrahepatic dilatations (may belong to Caroli disease—see later)

Choledochal cysts present most often with nonspecific symptoms. In 40% of patients, most of whom are children, a classic clinical triad of pain, jaundice, and right upper quadrant mass is seen. Irritability, nausea, vomiting, and a palpable abdominal mass may also be present. Affected infants often have large choledochal cysts, presenting as abdominal

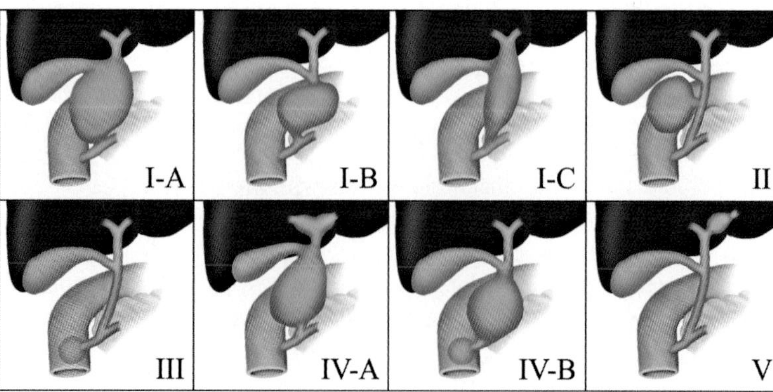

FIGURE 15-12 ■ Classification of congenital bile duct cysts.

masses (e759). Associated atresia or stenosis of the biliary tree is often present, and has a greater risk for cirrhosis in infants (e673). Diagnostic imaging studies, including isotope scan, ultrasonography, CT scan, and endoscopic or percutaneous cholangiography are useful in establishing a preoperative diagnosis (e345,e377). With some, prenatal ultrasound examination may identify dilatation of the bile ducts, suggesting choledochal cyst or extrahepatic biliary obstruction.

Intrahepatic histopathology is similar to that seen with EHBA. There is bile ductular proliferation and periportal fibrosis, which may progress to biliary cirrhosis. Regression of biliary cirrhosis has been documented after drainage of the choledochal cyst. Total excision of the cyst is recommended to avoid ascending cholangitis, choledocholithiasis, chronic liver disease, pancreatitis, and carcinoma of the bile ducts, liver, or pancreatic ducts that may be associated with internal drainage alone (e673). The excised cyst wall is usually 1 to 2 mm thick and bile stained (Figure 15-13). It consists of dense fibrous tissue containing a few to no inflammatory cells. Only a few smooth muscle fibers may be identifiable within the wall. An epithelium is generally lacking, but occasional foci of residual columnar epithelium may be identified and some cysts may even have a complex epithelial pattern.

Congenital polycystic dilatation of the larger intrahepatic bile ducts is known as Caroli disease and has a marked predisposition to cholangitis, liver abscess, and portal hypertension (109) (e28,e535,e627,e718,e784). Caroli disease occurs most frequently in adults, but may be seen in children and

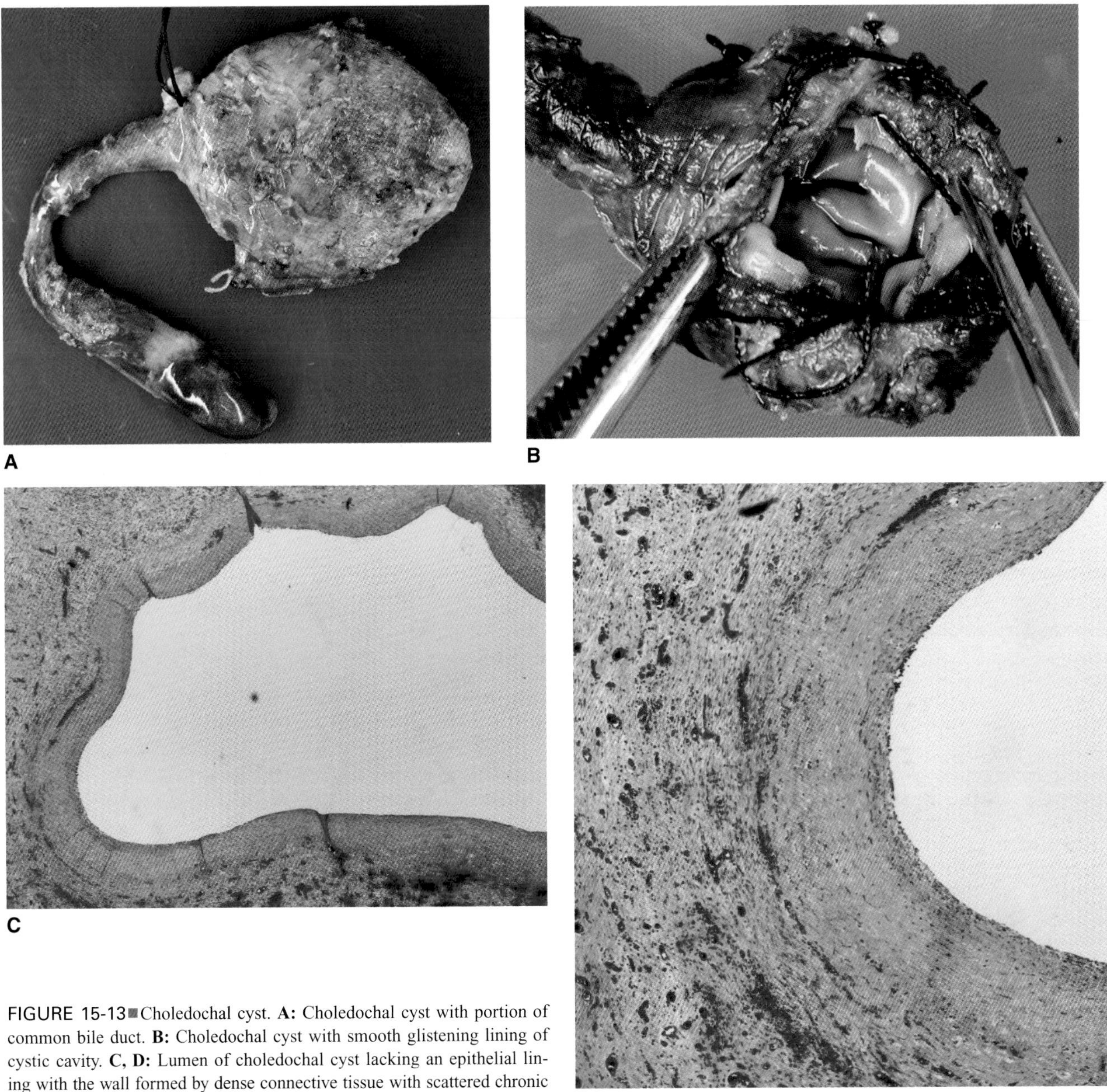

FIGURE 15-13 ■ Choledochal cyst. **A:** Choledochal cyst with portion of common bile duct. **B:** Choledochal cyst with smooth glistening lining of cystic cavity. **C, D:** Lumen of choledochal cyst lacking an epithelial lining with the wall formed by dense connective tissue with scattered chronic inflammatory cells and no residual smooth muscle (H&E, **C:** 20×, **D:** 40×).

infants if there are severe clinical symptoms (e335,e404). The diagnosis is based on cholangiographic findings of polycystic segmental dilatation of the intrahepatic biliary tree, including multiple small saccular dilatations of the peripheral segments of the intrahepatic biliary ductal system (e718). Histopathologically, a pattern of dysplastic portal ducts and fibrosis resemble congenital hepatic fibrosis (CHF) in 90% of cases, even though only 10% have clinical evidence of portal hypertension. The combination of intrahepatic bile duct cystic changes and CHF has been termed Caroli syndrome. Medullary sponge kidney or renal tubular ectasia may be present in approximately 50% of patients with Caroli disease (e718). Isolated hepatic polycystic liver disease may also occur that histopathologically appears similar to autosomal dominant polycystic kidney disease (ADPKD). The genetic defect lies at the 19p13.2 locus and is associated with mutation in the PRKCSH gene. This gene is responsible for synthesis of hepatocystin, which modulates fibroblast growth factor receptor functions. Predominantly, young adult females are affected.

Fibropolycystic Disease of the Liver Associated with Cystic Renal Disease

Ductal plate abnormalities of the liver and portal fibrosis may occur in the presence or absence of renal cysts in several inherited syndromes (Table 15-5) (47,49,63) (e58,e276,e514,e721). These syndromes include autosomal recessive polycystic kidney disease (ARPKD), ADPKD, hereditary renal dysplasia, and hereditary tubulointerstitial nephritis. Morphometric studies show that the hepatic lesions in the infantile, juvenile, and adult types of polycystic disease are identical initially as ductal plate malformations. Both liver and kidneys are involved, and patients present with hepatomegaly and enlarged kidneys at birth or in early infancy (see Chapter 17).

During the neonatal period, the liver has increased fibrous tissue in the portal areas and a striking increase in the number of bile ducts (Figure 15-14). The bile ducts are dilated and have cleftlike or irregular contours. The dilated bile ducts are most prominent at the periphery of the portal areas and may extend into the periportal lobule. The ductal epithelium is bland and lacks epithelial degenerative changes or mitoses, in contrast to the increased numbers of bile ducts associated with extrahepatic obstruction. Inflammation is usually not a feature. Hepatocytes appear normal. Occasionally, cholestasis may be seen.

Table 15-5 ■ CYSTIC LESIONS OF THE LIVER AND ASSOCIATED CONDITIONS

Infantile polycystic disease
Hereditary renal dysplasia
Meckel syndrome and congeners
Chondrodysplasia syndromes
Majewski and Saldino-Noonan short rib polydactyly syndromes
Jeune asphyxiating thoracic dystrophy syndrome
Ellis-van Creveld chondroectodermal dysplasia
Elejalde acrocephalopolydactylous dysplasia
Trisomy 9 syndrome
Trisomy 13 syndrome
Zellweger cerebrohepatorenal syndrome
Ivemark renal-hepatic-pancreatic dysplasia
Glutaric aciduria, type II
Hereditary tubulointerstitial nephritis
Juvenile nephronophthisis
Bardet-Biedl syndrome
Adult polycystic disease
Isolated nonsyndromatic disease

Congenital Hepatic Fibrosis

CHF presents in a seemingly healthy child or young adult with hematemesis from esophageal varices secondary to portal

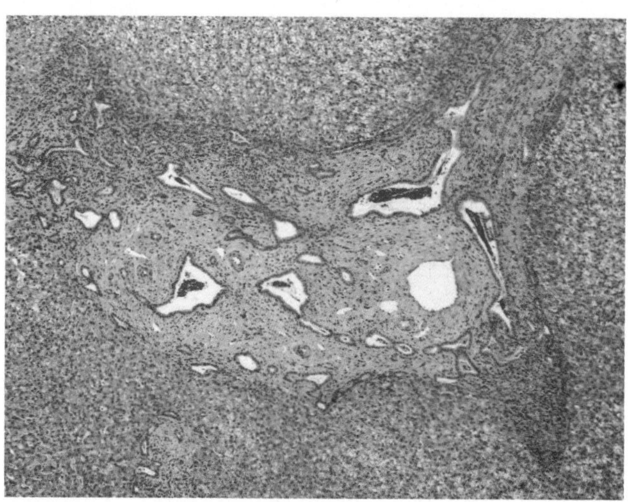

A

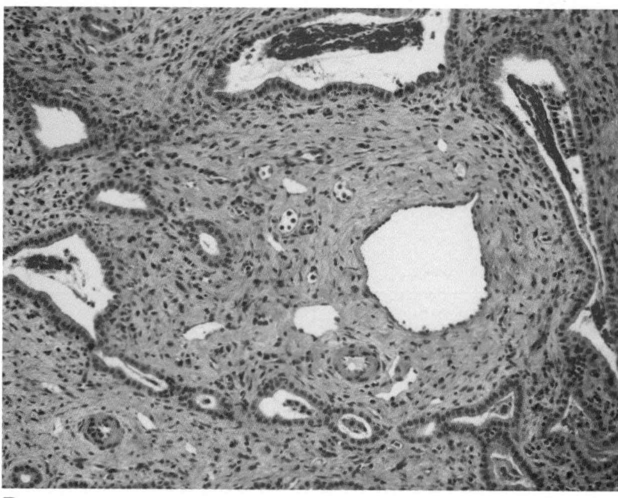

B

FIGURE 15-14 ■ Congenital hepatic fibrosis associated with autosomal recessive polycystic kidney disease. **A**, **B:** Ductal plate abnormality with dilated and concentric arrangement of bile ducts in expanded and fibrotic portal regions (H&E, **A:** 20×, **B:** 40×).

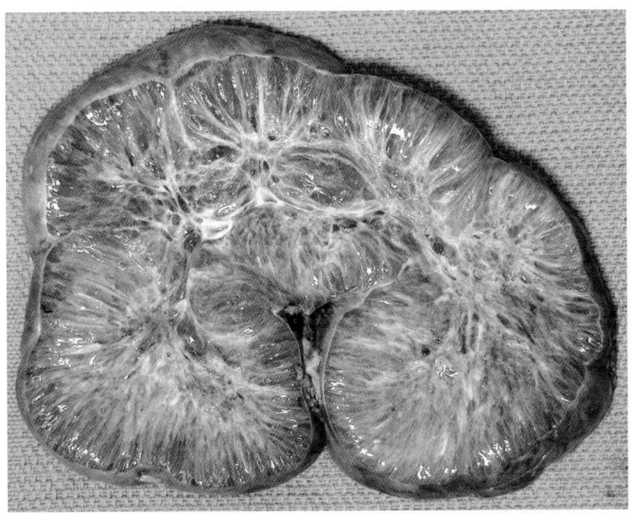

C

FIGURE 15-14 ■ *(continued)* C: Autosomal recessive polycystic kidney disease with markedly enlarged kidney due to numerous thin cystics extending from the cortical to medullary regions.

hypertension. Cholangitis may also be seen on occasion. CHF has been noted in association with a variety of renal lesions (Figure 15-14) (47,49,63) (e58,e276,e514,e721) including ARPKD (mutation of PKHD1-fibrocystin at 6p21 locus), ADPKD (mutation of PKD1-polycystin-1 or mutated PKD2-polycystin-2), and rarely in Meckel-Gruber syndrome (mutation of MKS1 at 17q, MKS2 at 1q, or MKS3 at 8q) and Jeune syndrome. Because Caroli disease and choledochal cyst are associated with CHF in a small proportion of cases, a common pathogenesis is worth consideration. CHF has also been seen in association with a variety of other syndromes including Joubert syndrome (agenesis or hypoplasia of the cerebellar vermis, retinal dystrophy, chorioretinal colobomata, oculomotor abnormalities, episodic hyperpnea, ataxia, mental retardation), Ivemark syndrome (renal, pancreatic, hepatic dysplasia), Down syndrome, Laurence-Moon-Biedl syndrome (mental retardation, retinitis pigmentosa, obesity), and COACH syndrome (hypoplasia of the cerebellar vermis, oligophrenia, congenital ataxia, coloboma, hepatic fibrosis) (47,49,63) (e58,e276,e365,e514,e721).

Desmet (49) suggested that CHF is caused by faulty development of the interlobular bile ducts with a disturbance in epithelial-mesenchymal inductive interactions. As a result, the ducts are subject to progressive destructive cholangiopathy of variable progression and duration that leads to biliary fibrosis. In addition, HCC has been reported to arise in a case of CHF (e48).

There is nearly a 1:1 correlation between the frequency of liver and kidney disease in ARPKD, although the degree of kidney involvement may vary considerably. The majority of ARPKD patients present *in utero* or shortly after birth with abdominal masses, anuria, and oligohydramnios and frequently die within days. With the milder (juvenile) ARPKD form in older children, the clinical picture may be dominated by cholestasis in the newborn period or symptoms related to CHF (portal hypertension, bleeding esophageal varices). A number of diagnostic imaging studies are available for the diagnosis of CHF.

The liver in ARPKD displays a gross pattern of interweaving white "streaks" beneath the capsule. The cut surface may also show small cysts of a few millimeters in diameter. Microscopically, the portal areas contain increased numbers of bile duct structures usually arranged in concentric rings around the portal area (Figure 15-14). The anastomosing and branching ducts are associated with an increase in connective tissue, which is minimal at first but expands to form broad fibrous bands over time. Unlike cirrhosis, the fibrosis does not have a bridging appearance, and there are no regenerative nodules. However, there is the potential for the misinterpretation of CHF for cirrhosis. The portal bile ducts in infants are lined by cuboidal to columnar epithelium, which may form small polypoid projections. Pink or orange secretions are often present in bile duct lumina.

Unlike in ARPKD, CHF is rare in ADPKD (e58). Hepatic involvement varies widely from one kindred to another, with CHF reportedly causing death shortly after birth in one ADPKD family. Other ADPKD families have shown little tendency for progression of the hepatic manifestations over long periods of clinical follow-up.

Several syndromes of inherited renal dysplasia are characteristically associated with hepatic changes that are identical to CHF and carry the designation of biliary dysgenesis (e58,e59). These include Meckel-Gruber syndrome, chondrodysplasia (short-rib polydactyly), Jeune asphyxiating thoracic dysplasia, trisomy 21, Bardet-Biedl syndrome, Ivemark syndrome (renal-hepatic-pancreatic dysplasia), Zellweger cerebrohepatorenal syndrome, and type II glutaric aciduria (e181,e509,e666). Central nervous system, ocular, and pancreatic abnormalities are additional components of these syndromes. Compared with CHF, the differences in the hepatic lesions in these syndromes are a matter of degree rather than type, with less severe fibrosis and bile duct abnormalities being a general observation. The essential saclike structure of the biliary passages is similar, and ductal dilatation resembling Caroli disease has been seen. Large intrahepatic cysts may be present. A similar hepatic lesion has been described in some cases of vaginal atresia syndrome and tuberous sclerosis (e371). Another condition that is associated with CHF is nephronophthisis (mutation in NPHP1 [nephrocystin], NPHP2 [inversin], NPHP3, or NPHP4). Ductal plate abnormalities in the liver and marked tubulointerstitial kidney disease are the features of this familial condition. Progressive renal failure occurs during the first two decades of life.

METABOLIC DISORDERS

A wide variety of metabolic disorders involve the liver, in addition to other organs, and a number of these disorders may present in the neonatal period as cholestasis and with

Table 15-6 ■ DISTINCTIVE FEATURES IN METABOLIC DISORDERS WITH NEONATAL HEPATITIS-LIKE CHANGES

Disorders	Histologic Features
Galactosemia	Moderate-to-severe fatty change, fibrosis, no other distinctive features
Fructosemia	Moderate-to-severe fatty change, fibrosis, EM shows characteristic "fructose holes"
Tyrosinemia	Moderate-to-severe fatty change and fibrosis; regenerative nodules and hepatocellular dysplasia are suggestive
A1AT deficiency	Stored A1AT in hepatocytes PAS-positive diastase-resistant globules; immunohistochemistry and EM are diagnostic aids, especially in the neonate
Glycogenosis (IV)	Early cirrhosis; stored structurally abnormal glycogen (diastase-resistant PAS-positive material with characteristic fibrillar nonmembrane-bound dense material by EM) in hepatocytes
CF (mucoviscidosis)	"Focal biliary cirrhosis" manifests as proliferated bile ducts with intraluminal inspissated material in expanded and fibrotic portal areas; rarely seen in the newborn
Niemann-Pick disease	Stored sphingolipids in Kupffer cells demonstrable histochemically; EM shows characteristic pleomorphic lamellar inclusions in lysosomes
Idiopathic iron storage	Hepatocellular necrosis with collapse; fibrosis; massive amounts of iron in hepatocytes and duct epithelial cells with negligible amounts in Kupffer cells

EM, electron microscopy.

neonatal hepatitis-like changes (Table 15-6). The overall incidence of metabolic disease is approximately 4 per 10,000 live births (e32). The following disorders are considered in some detail because of their association with significant liver disease (see Chapter 5).

Carbohydrate Metabolism Disorders

Galactosemia

Hereditary galactosemia, an autosomal recessive disorder, is most commonly due to deficiency of galactose-1-phosphate uridyl transferase, an enzyme encoded on the GALT gene on chromosome 9q13 (57) (e76,e77,e391,e488,e701). Genetic defects in the enzymes galactokinase and uridyl diphosphate galactose-4-epimerase are less common causes of galactosemia. These three enzymatic defects impair conversion of galactose to glucose. The incidence varies from approximately 1.5 to 4 per 100,000 whites to 1 per 400,000 in Chinese (e32,e39,e723,e751). The disorder exhibits considerable allelic heterogeneity, and more than 150 different mutations have been identified in 24 different populations and ethnic groups in 15 countries. The mutations most frequently cited are Q188R, K285N, S135L, and N314D. Q188R is the most common mutation in European populations or in those predominantly of European descent (e723). The clinical features in neonates includes hepatomegaly, jaundice, hypoglycemia, generalized aminoaciduria, presence of reducing substances in the urine, diarrhea, and vomiting. The differential diagnosis includes inborn errors of metabolism that manifest as neonatal hepatitis (Table 15-6). Histopathologically, canalicular and intracellular cholestasis, pseudoacinar transformation, bile ductular proliferation, focal giant cell transformation of hepatocytes, and presence of lipid are the notable features (Figure 15-15). These features in the

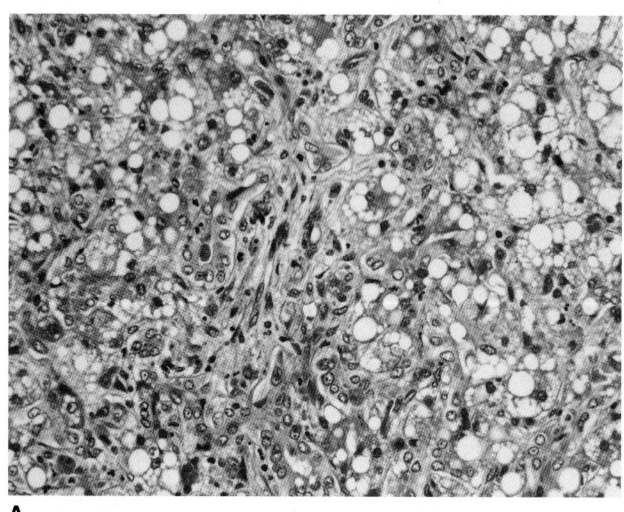

A

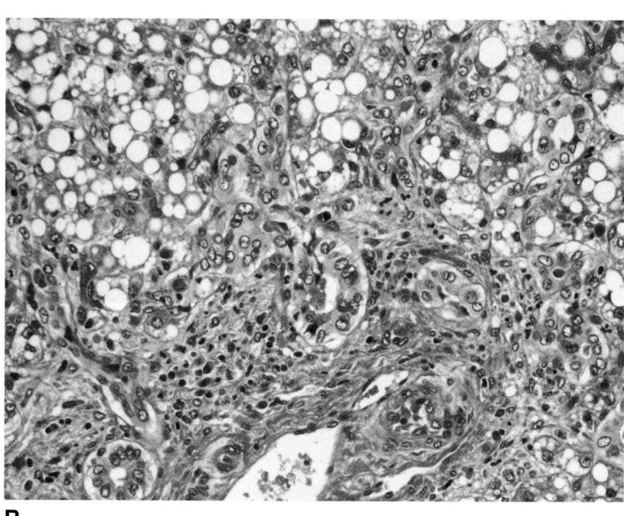

B

FIGURE 15-15 ■ Galactosemia. **A, B:** Hepatocytes display medium to large droplet fatty metamorphosis, along with pseudoglandular transformation (H&E, **A:** 100×, **B:** 200×).

Table 15-7 ■ HEPATIC FINDINGS IN GLYCOGEN STORAGE DISEASE

Disease	Light Microscopic Findings	Electron Microscopic Findings
Type I von Gierke disease	Excess glycogen in enlarged hepatocytes and in nuclei; uniform mosaic pattern; lipid droplets	Accumulation of cytoplasmic glycogen and lipid; nuclear glycogen
Type II Pompe disease	Nonuniform, mild distension, and vacuolation of hepatocytes	Lysosomal monoparticulate glycogen
Type III Cori glycogenosis	Uniform mosaic pattern, resembling type I; portal fibrosis	Similar to type I; lipid and nuclear glycogen less pronounced
Type IV Andersen disease	Inclusions in periportal hepatocytes; cirrhosis	Nonmembrane-bound inclusions of fibrillary material, glycogen, and tubules
Type VI Her disease	Nonuniform enlargement of hepatocytes; periportal fibrosis	Glycogen and finely granular material in cytoplasm
Type VIII	Glycogen deposition	Glycogenosis
Type IX	Glycogen deposition	Glycogen deposition with "starry-sky" pattern
Type X	Glycogenosis	Glycogenosis

neonatal period are similar to those seen in tyrosinemia and fructosemia. Fibrosis occurs early and progresses to cirrhosis if left untreated within the first 3 to 6 months of life (e765a). The ultrastructural features are diagnostic, although the individual features are not specific. The diagnosis is made by demonstration of enzyme deficiency in erythrocytes. Neonatal screening tests are available. Liver effects may be reversible with dietary galactose restriction.

Fructosemia

Hereditary fructose intolerance is caused by catalytic deficiency of aldolase B (fructose-1,6-bisphosphate aldolase) in the liver, intestines, and kidneys, and is a recessively inherited condition (193) (e16). Aldolase B deficiency inhibits gluconeogenesis and glycogenolysis. Two mutations on chromosome 9q (A149P and A174D) account for more than 70% of cases (193) (e372). The disease becomes manifest when fructose is introduced into the diet and presents with vomiting, diarrhea, failure to thrive, jaundice, renal failure, and hepatomegaly. Liver failure may be severe, with hepatic necrosis during the acute phase (e145). More commonly, there is variable fibrosis involving the portal and lobular regions, as well as microsteatosis and macrosteatosis. Chronic disease may be associated with severe fibrosis, potentially leading to cirrhosis. A neonatal hepatitis-like pattern may be seen with diffuse hepatocellular steatosis, a frequent feature. Electron microscopy of hepatocytes shows endoplasmic reticulum degranulation with membrane profiles. The response to dietary exclusion of fructose is rapid, and when so treated, the disease is compatible with a normal life span (e145).

Glycogen Storage Diseases

The GSDs are a group of metabolic disorders with specific enzyme defects resulting in accumulation of abnormal amounts of structurally normal or abnormal glycogen in the liver and other tissues (136,176) (e328,e632,e732,e770). The GSDs most frequently associated with hepatic manifestations include types I, II, III, IV, VI, and IX. The mode of inheritance is autosomal recessive in all the types described, with the exception of type IXb, which is inherited as a sex-linked recessive trait. Some forms of the disease present in infancy and others in early childhood, with failure to thrive, developmental delays, acidosis, hypoglycemia, and hepatomegaly. The morphologic changes have been reviewed by McAdams et al. (119), and the ultrastructural features have been illustrated by Phillips et al. (141). Features of those glycogenoses that significantly involve the liver are summarized in Table 15-7.

Type I Glycogenosis (von Gierke Disease)

GSD type I is the most common form of glycogenosis and potentially the most severe (77,136,176) (e129,e328,e459, e632,e732,e770). There is no gender predilection. Children with this disease present in infancy with hypoglycemia and hepatomegaly. There is lactic acidosis, seizures, and failure to thrive. The subsequent course is characterized by the development of hyperlipidemia, xanthomata, hyperuricemia, cyclic neutropenia with recurrent infections, nephropathy, and chronic bowel inflammation with type 1b GSD. Type 1a GSD is due to a deficiency in the enzyme glucose-6-phosphatase (17q21). Type 1b GSD has a deficiency in a transmembrane protein required for glucose-6-phosphate transport (11q23) into microsomes. Type 1c has a deficiency in a phosphatase transporter (11q23-24.2). These deficiencies result in the accumulation of large amounts of normal glycogen in the liver, kidney, and intestine.

Histopathologically, the liver shows marked distension of the hepatocytes with glycogen, resulting in a diffuse mosaic pattern with compression of the sinusoids (Figure 15-16). Intranuclear glycogen is a common feature (77,119). The glycogen is best demonstrated by periodic acid–Schiff (PAS) stains of unfixed frozen sections or alcohol-fixed tissue. Lipid is also present, while fibrosis is typically absent. Rarely, Mallory bodies may be seen (e309). Ultrastructurally, there are pools of monoparticulate glycogen in the cytoplasm and nuclei of hepatocytes. Lipid vacuoles are found in the cytoplasm. The organelles are displaced, and the size of the mitochondria may be increased. Hepatic adenomas have

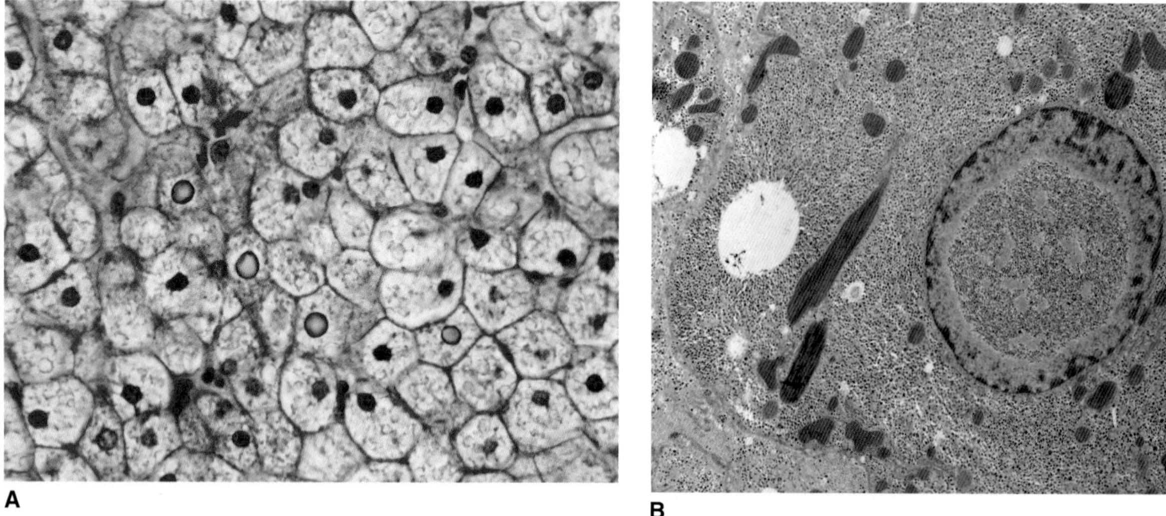

FIGURE 15-16 ■ Glycogen storage disease, Type I. **A:** Hepatocytes distended by glycogen with obliteration of the sinusoids, forming a mosaic pattern, and glycogenated nuclei. (H&E, 400×). **B:** Hepatocyte with glycogenated nuclei, cytoplasmic monoparticulate glycogen, large lipid droplet, and abnormally shaped mitochondria (Electron microscopy, 7,500×).

been reported with some frequency, and cases of HCC and hepatoblastoma have been described in type 1 glycogenosis (e67,e309,e318,e471). Hepatic transplantation has been used in the treatment of types I, III and IV GSD (e432).

Type II Glycogenosis (Pompe Disease, Generalized Glycogenosis, or Acid Maltase Deficiency)

GSD type II is classified as a lysosomal storage disorder in contrast to the cytoplasmic storage disorder that occurs in the other GSDs. It is the result of a deficiency in acid maltase caused by mutations in the alpha-1,4-glucosidase (GAA, 17q25.2-25.4) gene (77,136,176) (e177,e328,e355, e459,e632,e732,e770). The major manifestations are muscular and cardiac, and the liver shows changes as a component of the generalized involvement. Three clinical types have been described (e177,e438,e459,e732). Infantile or classic Pompe disease manifests in infancy with hypotonia and cardiomyopathy, leading to death in infancy. The second type presents in childhood with predominant involvement of the skeletal musculature, and a third type is described with an onset in the second to fourth decades. Cardiac involvement in these latter variants is minimal. Affected hepatocytes are mildly enlarged and have finely vacuolated cytoplasm (Figure 15-17). Ultrastructural features are characterized by the presence of monoparticulate glycogen within membrane-bound lysosomal vacuoles. Acid phosphatase activity is associated with the lysosomal vacuoles.

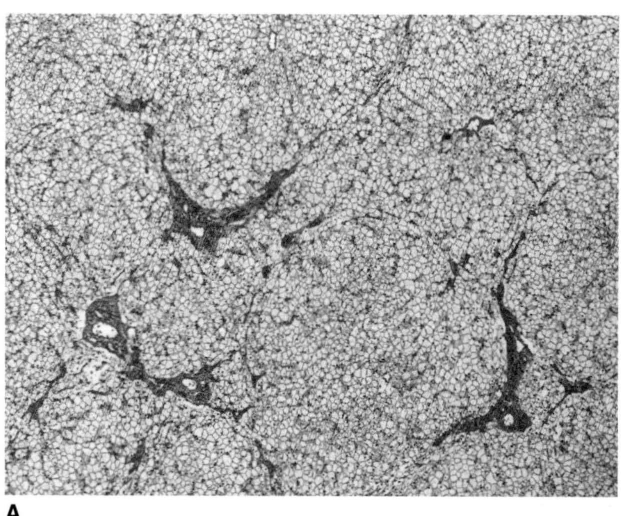

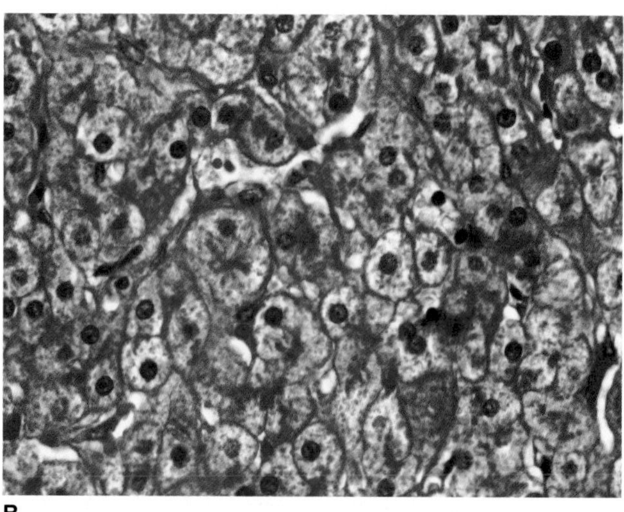

FIGURE 15-17 ■ Glycogen storage disease, type II. **A:** Hepatocytes demonstrating mosaic pattern with obliteration of sinusoids (H&E, 40×). **B:** Hepatocytes in close proximity to one another, with thickened cell membranes, fine cytoplasmic vacuolization, and indistinct sinusoids (H&E, 400×).

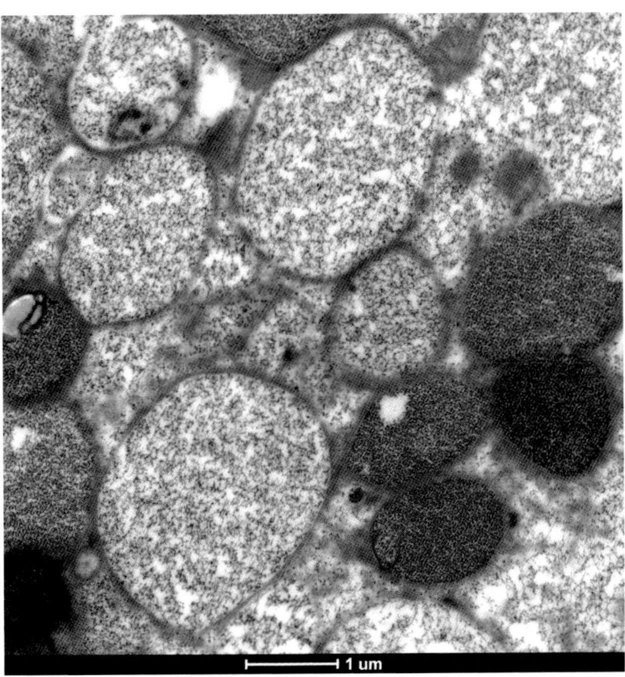

C

FIGURE 15-17 ■ *(continued)* **C:** Monoparticulate glycogen within membrane bound lysosomes (Electron microscopy, 20,000×).

Type III Glycogenosis (Cori Disease, Forbes Disease, Limit Dextrinosis, Debranching Enzyme Disease)

GSD type III is the result of a deficiency in the amylo-1, 6-glucosidase (debrancher enzyme, 1p21) activity (77,136,176) (e328,e459,e632,e732,e770). This deficiency leads to abnormal glycogen formation with increased branching points that accumulate in the liver and muscle. Hypoglycemia develops during stress or fasting due to lack of conversion of the abnormal glycogen to glucose. Hepatic morphologic features are very similar to those seen in type I GSD with panlobular cytoplasmic distension by glycogen and a uniform mosaic pattern. Accumulated glycogen is demonstrable by the presence of diastase-digestible PAS-positive material in the cytoplasm. Nuclear glycogen is not as prominent as in type I GSD, but is a distinguishing feature from other types of GSD, especially types VI and IX (77). Hepatomegaly with hepatic fibrosis may be prominent and may progress to cirrhosis by the third or fourth decade of life.

Type IV Glycogenosis (Andersen disease, Amylopectinosis; Glycogen Branching Enzyme Disease)

GSD type IV manifests at birth or in early infancy with failure to thrive and hepatosplenomegaly (77,136,176) (e323,e632,e732,e770). In the absence of transplantation, there is progression to cirrhosis and death in early childhood (e422). The brancher enzyme 1,4-1,6-glucon:1-4-glucan, 6-glycosyl transferase (3p12) is absent, resulting in abnormal glycogen with decreased branch points that resembles amylopectin or starch. Deposits of the abnormal glycogen are generalized with significant involvement of the liver, skeletal and cardiac muscles, and intestine. Microscopically, the hepatocytes in the periportal region (zone 1) contain pale eosinophilic hyaline inclusions surrounded by a clear halo, resembling Lafora bodies. These inclusions resist diastase digestion, but are digestible with pectinase treatment (Figure 15-18). Colloidal iron staining is also seen in the cytoplasmic inclusions. Ultrastructurally, the inclusions consist of central fibrillar glycogen surrounded by polyparticulate glycogen rosettes (e109). Prenatal diagnosis is possible (e628).

Type VI Glycogenosis (Hers disease)

GSD type VI, a deficiency in hepatic phosphorylase E activity (14q21-22), presents with hepatomegaly in the absence of the serious complications seen in other glycogenoses (77,136,176) (e115,e328,e459,e632,e732,e770). Histopathologically, there is a mosaic pattern of hepatocellular distension with glycogen in zone 1 hepatocytes. Mild portal fibrosis may be seen. Ultrastructurally, pools of monoparticulate glycogen with interspersed glycogen rosettes displace the cytoplasmic organelles. A finely granular material of low electron density that is devoid of organelles may be scattered in the glycogen aggregates, imparting a starry-sky appearance (77).

Type VIII Glycogenosis

GSD type VIII, a deficiency in phosphorylase kinase (16q12-13), is accompanied by progressive neurologic deterioration leading to death in early childhood secondary to glycogen accumulation within the central nervous system (136,176) (e328,e459,e632,e732,e770). Hepatic changes are those of glycogen accumulation with nonspecific features, although a rare case of cirrhosis and adenomatous hyperplasia has been reported (e633).

Type IX, X, and XI Glycogenoses

Other glycogenoses with hepatic manifestations are GSD types IX (phosphorylase b kinase deficiency, Xp22.2-22.1) and X (cyclic 3,5 AMP-dependent kinase deficiency, 17q23-24) (136,176) (e328,e459,e632,e732,e770). Hepatic glycogenosis with stunted growth (type XI, Fanconi-Bickel syndrome) is associated with renal glycogen deposition. Type XI glycogenosis is caused by mutations in the glucose transporter 2 (GLUT2, 3q26.1-26.3) gene (136,176) (e328,e459,e632,e732,e770). Generalized glycogen deposition is accompanied by cirrhosis, but with normal glycogen metabolism.

Other Glycogenoses

Hepatic involvement is not a feature of GSD types V (McArdle disease, muscle glycogen phosphorylase [myophosphorylase], 11q13) and VII (Tarui disease, phosphofructokinase enzyme deficiency, 12q13), in which skeletal muscle is primarily affected (136,176) (e29,e328,e470,e632,e710, e732,e770). GSD type 0 (aglycogenosis) is an autosomal recessive disease with a deficiency in glycogen synthase (chromosome 12p12.2) (136,176) (e328,e459,e632,e732, e770). Deficiency in glycogen synthase leads to a marked

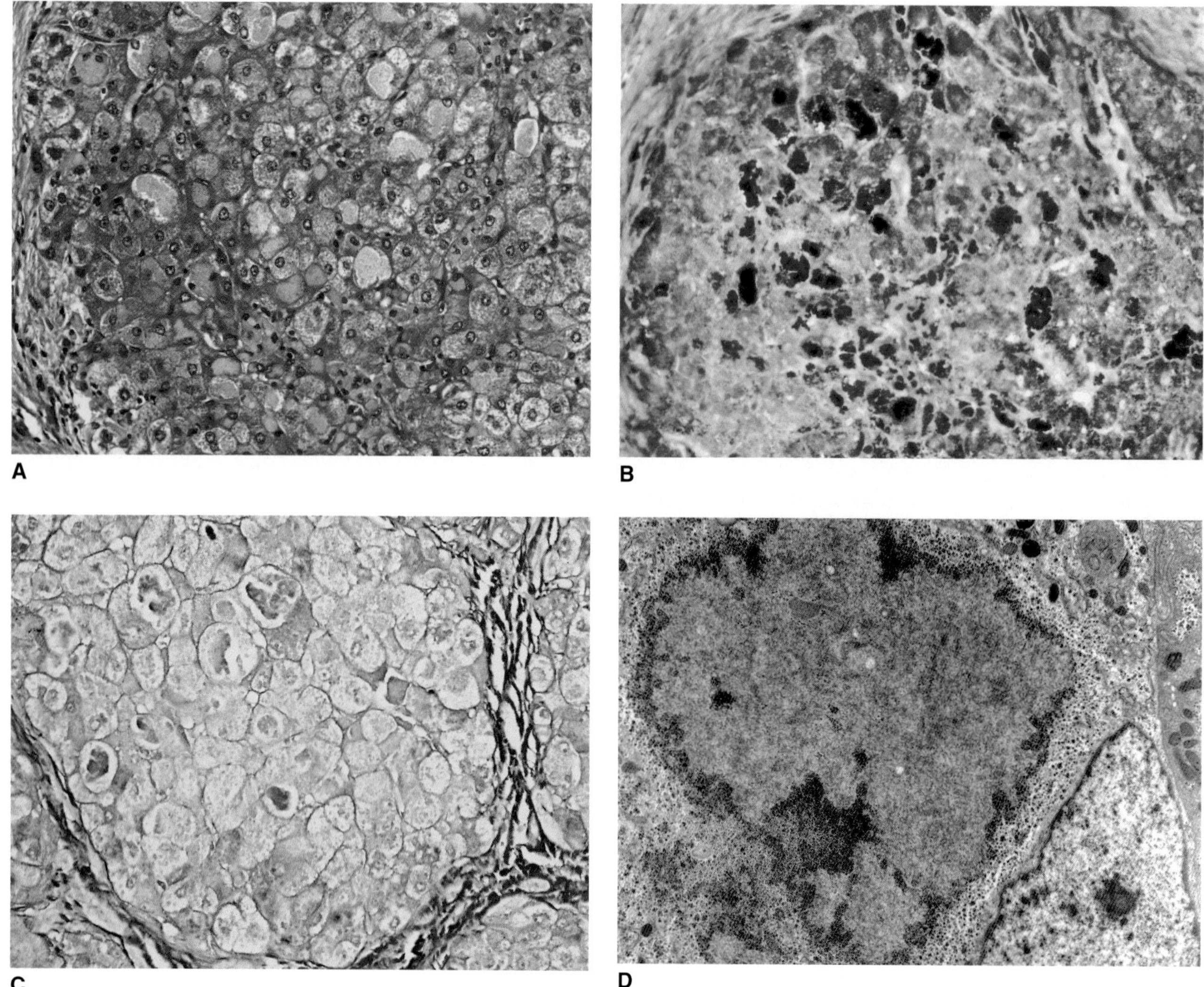

FIGURE 15-18 **A:** Glycogen storage disease, type IV. Hepatocytes with pale hyaline inclusions surrounded by indistinct halos, resembling LaFora bodies (H&E, 200×). **B, C:** The inclusions stain intensely with PAS (400×). and colloidal iron (400×). **D:** Hepatocyte with hyaline inclusion comprised of fibrillary glycogen (electron microscopy, 6,000×).

reduction in liver glycogen stores. The symptoms of GSD type 0 are those associated with hypoglycemia and include lethargy, pallor, nausea, vomiting and, rarely, seizures in the early morning before breakfast. Liver biopsy will demonstrate moderate steatosis and small amounts of glycogen (0.5% versus 1.6% for normal wet liver weight) on quantitative analysis. There have also been reports of liver fibrosis in some GSD type 0 cases.

Amino Acid Metabolism Disorders

Tyrosinemia

Tyrosinemia results from a deficiency of fumaryl acetoacetate hydrolase (FAH, 15q23-25) and presents as acute fulminant disease in infancy or as a chronic liver disease later in childhood (157,161) (e198,e257,e536). Diagnosis is based upon serologic or urinary determination of succinylacetone level and FAH assays. Liver biopsy in the acute form reveals cholestasis, pseudoacinar transformation of hepatocytes, fatty change, marked intralobular fibrosis, and variable giant cell transformation (Figure 15-19) (78). These features are indicative of a metabolic hepatopathy, but are not specific for tyrosinemia. Regenerative nodules may already be present in early liver biopsies. The chronic form is characterized by cirrhosis with variable-sized nodules separated by thick bands of fibrous connective tissue with little inflammation or bile duct proliferation. Hepatocytes may demonstrate nuclear hyperchromasia, dysplasia, or adenomatous hyperplasia. The incidence of HCC is quite high with tyrosinemia (e544). Liver transplantation is advisable soon after diagnosis and before 2 years of age, because of the high risk of HCC. Treatment with NTBC [2(-nitro-4-trifluoromethylbenzoyl)-1-3-cyclohexanedione] prevents accumulation of the toxic metabolites of FAH and the

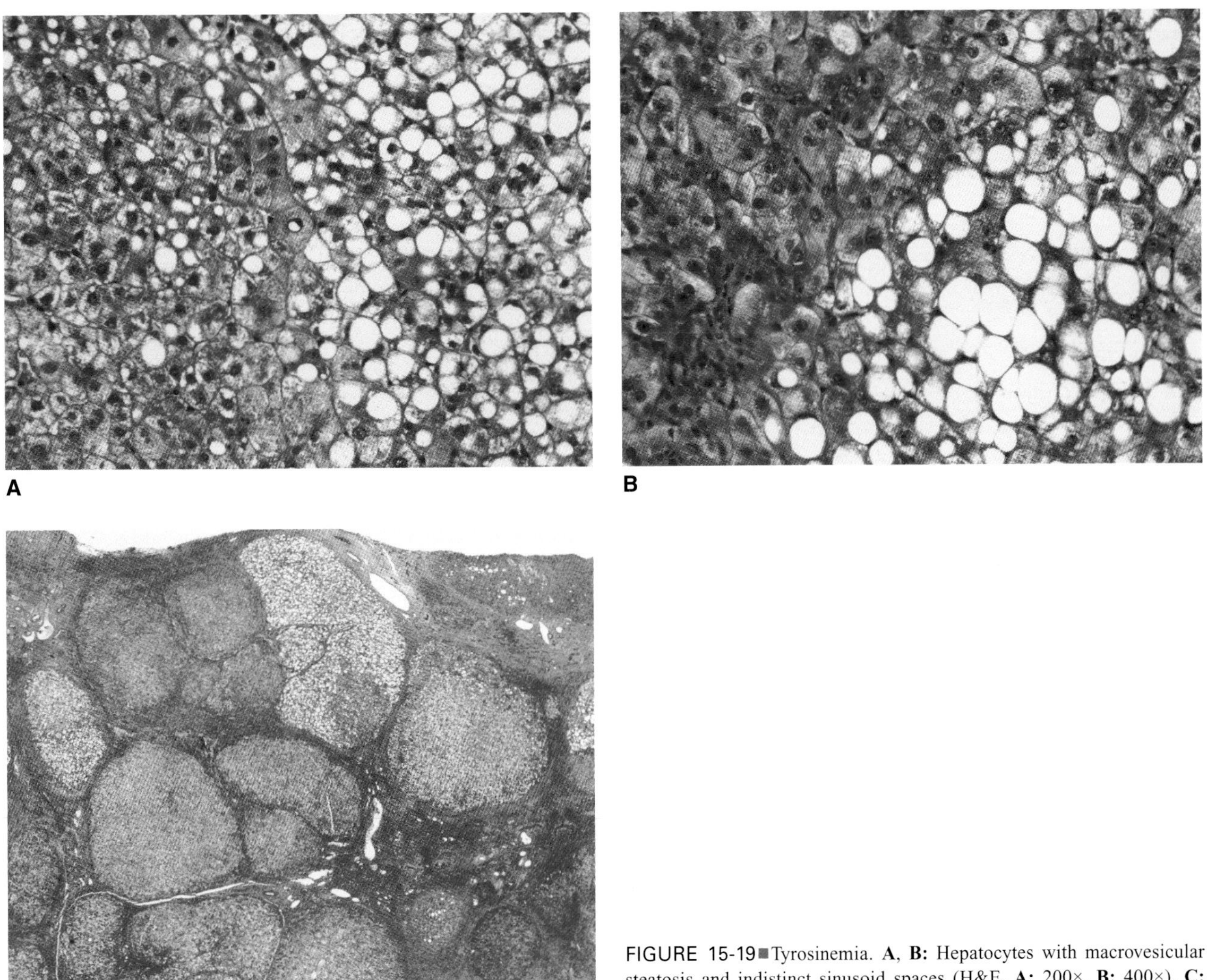

FIGURE 15-19 ■ Tyrosinemia. **A**, **B:** Hepatocytes with macrovesicular steatosis and indistinct sinusoid spaces (H&E, **A:** 200×, **B:** 400×). **C:** Micronodular cirrhosis in chronic form of tyrosinemia (H&E, 40×).

subsequent liver and neurologic effects, but does not entirely eliminate the risk of HCC.

Lysosomal Storage Diseases

Lipidoses

Wolman Disease

Wolman disease and cholesterol ester storage disease (CESD) are rare autosomal recessive lipoprotein-processing disorders caused by mutations in the gene encoding human lysosomal acid lipase (10q24-25; Table 15-8) (e185,e281,e399,e724, e727,e771). Wolman disease is fatal in early life, presents with failure to thrive and diarrhea, and is characterized by generalized accumulation of foam cells and adrenal calcifications. Because there is partial enzyme activity, CESD is a milder clinical form of the disorder, generally limited to the gastrointestinal tract and the liver. Liver pathology includes steatosis and numerous foamy macrophages that contain cholesterol and lipid (Figure 15-20) and are similar in both diseases, although cirrhosis may occur in CESD. Cholesterol accumulation is demonstrated with frozen sections using polarized light microscopy. Ultrastructurally, hepatocytes, Kupffer cells, and portal macrophages are engorged with membrane-bound lipid vacuoles with dense membranes. Cholesterol clefts are seen in the cytoplasm.

Mucolipidoses

The mucolipidoses are a group of disorders caused by defects of various lysosomal hydrolases and include sialidosis (ML I, neuraminidase gene at 6p21.3), I-cell disease (ML II, GNPTAB gene at 12q23.3), pseudo-Hurler disease (ML III, GNPTAB gene at 12q23.3), and sialolipidosis (ML IV, mucolipin-1 gene at 19p13.3) (60,116) (e37,e178,e548,e550,e667). Many of the clinical stigmata of mucopolysaccharidoses may be seen, but mucopolysaccharides are not excreted in the urine. I-cell disease and pseudo-Hurler polydystrophy are autosomal recessive disorders. Coarse facies, skeletal changes, hepatosplenomegaly, and delayed growth and

Table 15-8 ■ LYSOSOMAL DISORDERS

Disease	Enzyme Deficiency	Light Microscopic Findings	Electron Microscopic Findings
Gaucher	Glucocerebrosidase	Gaucher cells with striated cytoplasm; fibrosis	Membrane-bound inclusions with twisted tubules in Kupffer cells
Niemann-Pick	Sphingomyelinase	Finely vacuolated cytoplasm of Kupffer cells	Myelin figures in Kupffer cells and hepatocytes
Wolman and cholesterol ester storage	Acid lipase	Steatosis of hepatocytes and Kupffer cells; cholesterol clefts, fibrosis	Lipid droplets and lipolysosomes and cholesterol clefts in hepatocytes and histiocytes
Mucopolysaccharidoses, Hurler, Hunter, Scheie	Iduronidases sulfatases	Swollen clear cytoplasm of hepatocytes and Kupffer cells; fibrosis; cirrhosis	Membrane-bound, sharply delimited, electron-lucent inclusions with some granular material
Mucolipidoses, I-cell disease	Acid hydrolases	Vacuolated hepatocytes, Kupffer cells	Membrane-bound vacuoles with flocculent material
Oligosaccharidoses	Sialidase, mannosidase, fucosidase	Vacuolated hepatocytes and Kupffer cells	Membrane-bound vacuoles with finely granular material
Metachromatic leukodystrophy	Aryl sulfatase A	Metachromatic granules in portal macrophages	Lamellar prismatic inclusions within macrophages, hepatocytes, and Kupffer cells
Farber	Acid ceramidase	Lipogranulomatous infiltrates	Curvilinear lysosomal material
Gangliosidosis GM_1	β-galactosidase	Vacuolated hepatocytes and Kupffer cells	Membrane-bound vacuoles with granular material

development are some of the clinical features. The primary histopathologic and ultrastructural changes are cytoplasmic vacuolization of hepatocytes, Kupffer cells, and less frequently, biliary epithelial cells. Inclusions within clear vacuoles can be demonstrated within fibroblasts and peripheral nerves in skin and conjunctival biopsies (141). Glomeruli and renal tubular epithelium contain similar inclusions, and the inclusions are also present in the urine.

Oligosaccharidoses (Glycoproteinoses)

Disorders of glycoprotein degradation resulting from defects in specific lysosomal enzymes lead to the accumulation of oligosaccharides in tissues and urinary excretion of these substances. These are rare autosomal recessive conditions with a phenotypic similarity to the mucopolysaccharidoses (e359,e522,e541). These disorders include sialidosis (neuraminidase gene at 6p21.3), mannosidosis (mannosidase 2B1 gene at 19cen-q12), fucosidosis (FUCA1 gene at 1p34), and aspartylglycosaminuria (aspartylglucosaminidase gene at 4q32-33). The liver is involved in all forms and has enlarged vacuolated hepatocytes. Ultrastructurally, the foamy appearance is due to cytoplasmic membrane-bound clear vacuoles (141). The vacuoles are of variable sizes, may be molded by adjacent vacuoles, and fuse to form larger vacuoles. They are composed of finely granular to flocculent material intermingled with membrane material. Kupffer cells, biliary epithelial cells, and endothelial cells show similar vacuoles.

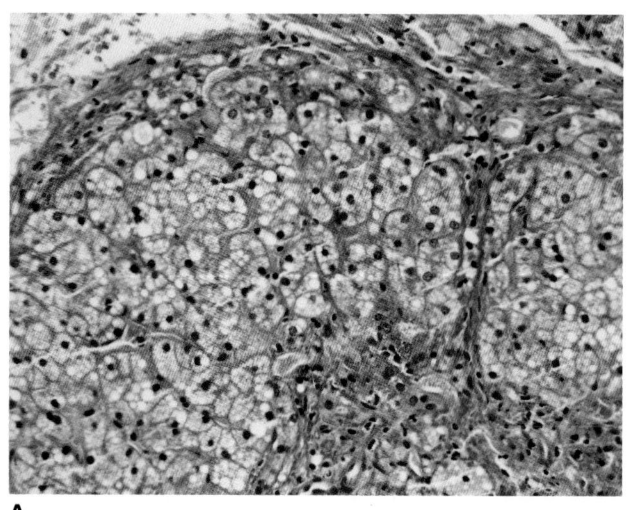
A

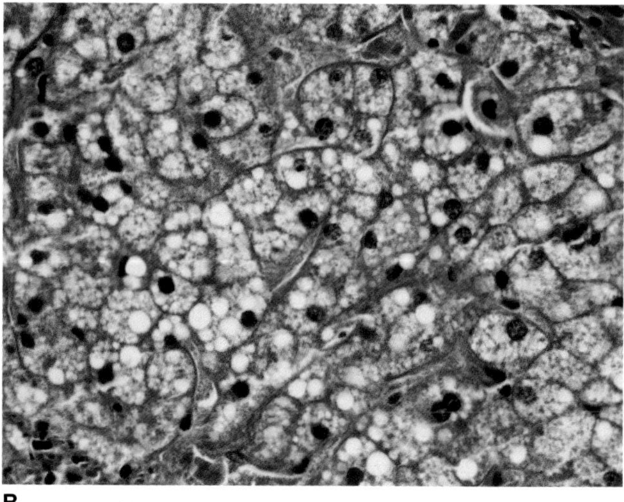
B

FIGURE 15-20■**A, B:** Cholesterol ester storage disease. Hepatocytes with diffuse microsteatosis (H&E, **A** 200×, **B** 400×).

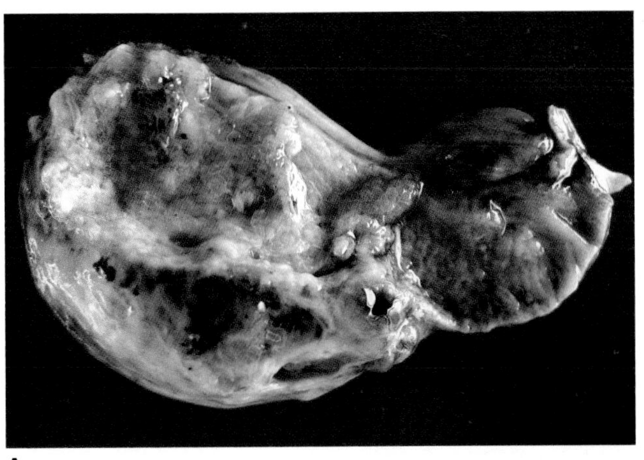

A

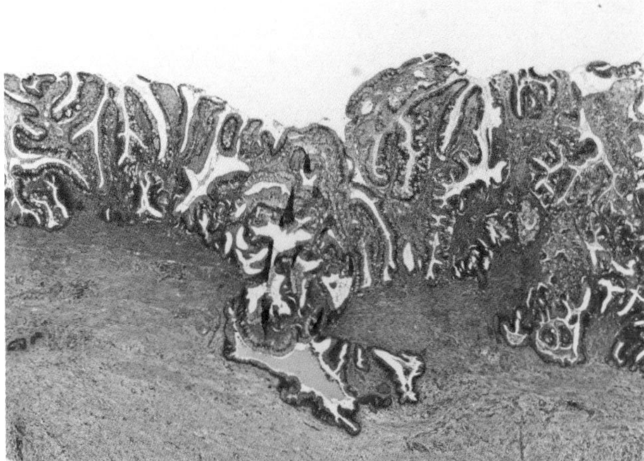

B

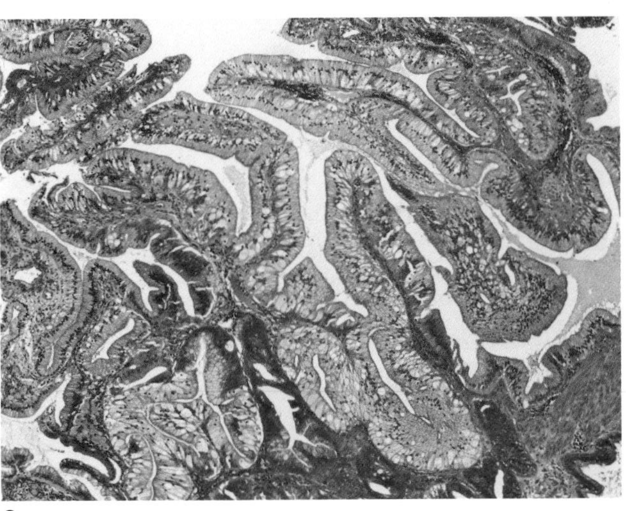

C

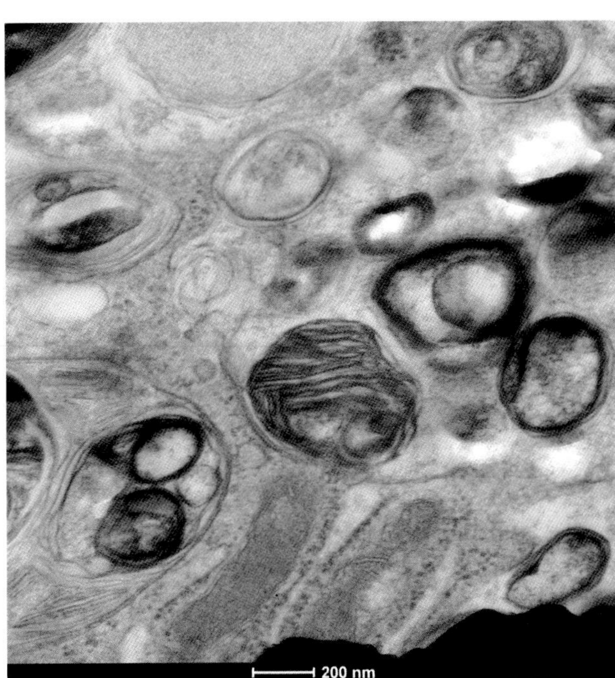

D

FIGURE 15-21 ■ Metachromatic leukodystrophy. **A:** Gallbladder with markedly thickened mucosa with fine cobblestone to papillary surface. **B, C:** Papillary fronds lined by columnar epithelial cells with amphophilic cytoplasm (H&E, **B:** 100×, **C:** 200×). **D:** Lysosomal inclusions with closely packed herringbone appearance (Electron microscopy, 25,000×).

Metachromatic Leukodystrophy

Metachromatic leukodystrophy is an autosomal recessive condition caused by a deficiency in lysosomal aryl sulfatase activity (arylsulfatase A gene at 22q13.31-qter) (59) (e54,e68,e238,e239,e314,e428). This results in accumulation of galactosyl sulfatide in the tissues and excessive urinary excretion of the metachromatic material (e314). Demyelination occurs with excess storage of the substrate in the central and peripheral nervous system (59) (e428). The storage material is metachromatic and shows brown granules with a characteristic birefringence in cresyl-violet-stained, unfixed frozen sections. By light microscopy, foam cells are seen in the nervous system, liver, kidneys, pancreas, adrenal cortex, and gallbladder. The gallbladder may show papillary fronds lined by epithelial cells and with foam cells in the subepithelial stroma (Figure 15-21) (5). Ultrastructurally, the lysosomal inclusions consist of prismatic structures with closely packed periodic leaflets that display a herringbone pattern. In the liver, the inclusions are found in portal macrophages, fibroblasts, and Kupffer cells.

Farber Disease (Farber Lipogranulomatosis)

Farber disease is an autosomal recessive condition in which ceramide, a sphingolipid, accumulates in the tissues due to a deficiency of the lysosomal enzyme acid ceramidase (N-acylsphingosine amidohydrolase gene at 8p22-21.3) (e227,e392,e516,e735). Disseminated lipogranulomata are the morphologic findings. The liver is mildly affected, with clear

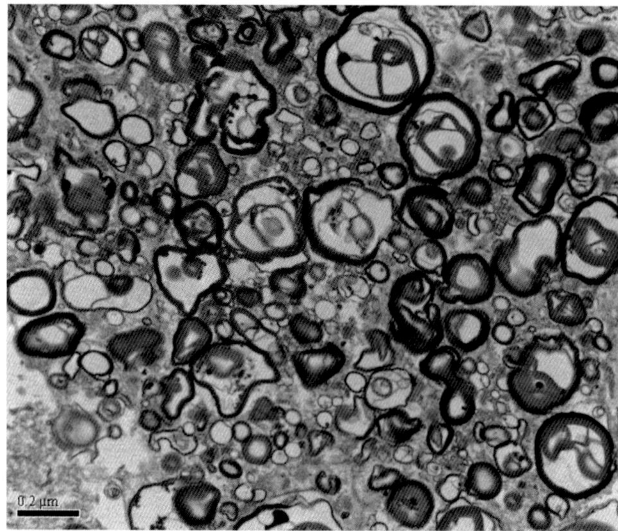

FIGURE 15-22 ■ Fabry disease. Membrane-bound lysosomal inclusions with lamellar and concentric pattern (Electron microscopy, 12,000×).

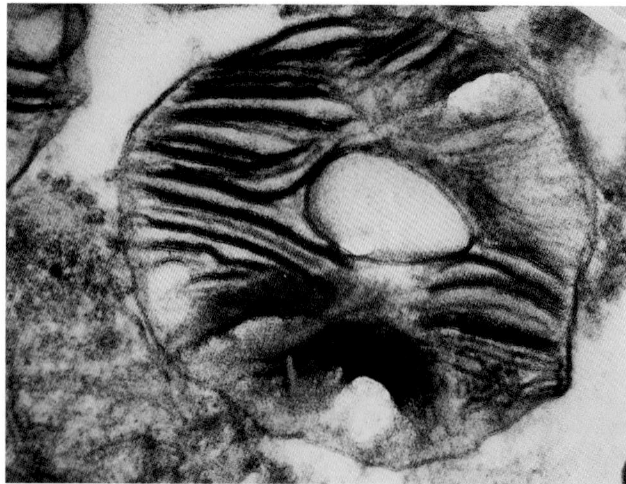

FIGURE 15-23 ■ Tay-Sachs disease. "Zebra bodies" comprised of concentric membrane-bound lysosomal inclusions (Electron microscopy, 20,000×).

vacuoles in the hepatocytes similar to the membrane-bound vacuoles in mucopolysaccharidoses. The Kupffer cells and portal macrophages have lysosomal comma-shaped, banana-shaped, and curvilinear inclusions in common with other tissues. Death occurs in adolescence or early adulthood.

Fabry Disease

Fabry disease is an X-linked recessive disorder caused by mutations in the alpha-galactosidase A gene (GLA gene, Xp22) and results in globotriaosylceramide accumulation in the liver and other organs (70) (e134,e194,e292,e786). Endothelial cells are the most commonly affected cell type. Ultrastructural findings are characterized by pleomorphic, membrane-bound, osmiophilic lamellar and concentric inclusions (Figure 15-22).

Gangliosidoses

The gangliosidoses are a group of autosomal recessive disorders with impairment of ganglioside metabolism (28,59,110) (e207,e288). GM1 and GM2 gangliosidoses have several clinical variants in each group. Five types of GM1 gangliosidosis have been described. The infantile type presents in infancy with coarse facies, skeletal abnormalities, retinal cherry-red spot, hepatosplenomegaly, and progressive deterioration (beta-galactosidase-1 at 3p21.33). Lysosomal beta-galactosidase is deficient, and the substrate accumulates in the brain and the viscera. Hepatocytes and Kupffer cells are foamy and vacuolated. Ultrastructurally, the cells are distended with large lysosomes that appear as electron lucent vacuoles filled with reticular granular (141). Lamellar, concentric, membrane-bound bodies may also be seen. GM2 gangliosidosis is a group of heterogeneous disorders that includes Tay-Sachs disease (hexosaminidase A gene at 15q23-24) with a hexosaminidase A deficiency, and Sandhoff disease with hexosaminidase A and B deficiencies (beta subunit hexosaminidase at 5q13). In Tay-Sachs disease, the central nervous system is primarily affected. The liver appears normal by light microscopy, but concentric membrane-bound inclusions ("zebra bodies") may be seen on electron microscopic examination (Figure 15-23).

Mucopolysaccharidoses

The mucopolysaccharidoses are a group of distinct genetic disorders with accumulation of acid mucopolysaccharides (glycosaminoglycans), dermatan sulfate, heparan sulfate, chondroitin sulfate, and keratin sulfate in the tissues with excretion of these substances in the urine (59,129) (e135,e224,e562). Multiple clinical types have been described, each associated with a specific enzyme defect. With the exception of Hunter disease (type II), which is an X-linked recessive condition (Xq28), mucopolysaccharidoses are inherited in an autosomal recessive pattern. The major clinical manifestations are caused by involvement of the brain, skeletal system, liver, cornea, and other organ systems. Because the histopathologic and ultrastructural features are identical, the various syndromes cannot be differentiated on morphologic grounds alone.

The liver is involved in all types with marked cytoplasmic vacuolization of the hepatocytes, Kupffer cells, and Ito cells. Stored acid mucopolysaccharide can be demonstrated with colloidal iron staining, but requires frozen sections or nonaqueous fixatives. Numerous electron lucent membrane-bound vacuoles are seen with electron microscopic examination, corresponding to acid mucopolysaccharides that are extracted with routine tissue processing. Finely granular to flocculent material may be seen in some of the vacuoles arranged in concentric whorls. Hepatic fibrosis may occur.

Sphingolipidoses

Niemann-Pick Disease

Niemann-Pick disease is an autosomal recessive lysosomal disorder associated with a deficiency of sphingomyelinase (type IA and 1B [type A and B], sphingomyelin phosphodiesterase-1 gene at 11p15.4-15.1) or a defect in cholesterol esterification (type II or type C, NPC gene at 18q11-12) (59,77,195) (e178,e301,e503,e507,e508,e616, e671,e738,e774). This disease is characterized by sphingomyelin storage in various organs (59,77). Sphingomyelin accumulation varies in extent, but it is most pronounced in type A (type 1A), the acute neuropathic form, and in type B (type 1B), the chronic nonneuropathic form. Sea blue histiocytes are seen in the bone marrow. The liver is enlarged and pale on gross examination. The lobular structure of the liver is not disorganized, and fibrosis is generally not a feature. However, cirrhosis may rarely occur.

Type C (type II) disease usually presents with neurologic symptoms between 2 and 4 years of age (59,77,195) (e178,e301,e503,e507,e508,e616,e671,e738,e774). However, it may present in the neonatal period with jaundice, hepatosplenomegaly, and failure to thrive and progress to death in months. Foamy macrophages and Kupffer cells may be infrequent initially, but there is progression to the more classic swollen, foamy vacuolated appearance of the cytoplasm (Figure 15-24). Hepatocytes show similar alterations. Ceroid pigment, cholesterol, and phospholipids accumulate in the cells. The stored material is best demonstrated by the Baker hematin reaction for phospholipids. Histochemical staining for acid phosphatase activity reveals a reticular pattern. Ultrastructurally, the appearance is distinctive (141). Large, pleomorphic, membrane-bound inclusions composed of concentric or parallel osmiophilic lamellae are seen in the Kupffer cells and to a lesser extent in the hepatocytes. Bone marrow transplantation has been reported to reverse the amount of storage material in the liver, spleen, lung, and bone marrow, but it does not prevent progression of the neurologic changes.

Gaucher Disease

Gaucher disease is caused by glucocerebrosidase deficiency (acid beta-glucosidase gene at1q21) and leads to glucosyl ceramide accumulation in various organs (39) (e63,e64,e97, e274,e319,e484,e635,e788). The disorder is inherited in an autosomal recessive manner, and three clinical types have been described. Type I, the most common, is the adult or chronic nonneuropathic form; type II is the acute neuropathic or infantile form; type III is the juvenile or subacute neuropathic form. The liver has a similar appearance in all three clinical types. There is massive hepatosplenomegaly with portal hypertension. Gaucher cells are the hallmark. These cells are distended and have a characteristic striated, "wrinkled tissue paper" appearance of the cytoplasm (Figure 15-25). The striations are accentuated with the PAS stain, and acid phosphatase activity can be demonstrated histochemically (39) (e6). Hemosiderin and lipofuscin are frequently present. These macrophages are also seen within the spleen and bone marrow. Clusters of Gaucher cells in the lobule and in portal areas may be associated with fibrosis and cirrhosis in some cases (e519). The ultrastructural features are distinctive with closely apposed, irregular lysosomal inclusions, which correspond to the wrinkled tissue paper light microscopic appearance of Gaucher cells. The inclusions are composed of innumerable tubules with circular profiles on cross section. "Pseudo-Gaucher" cells have been described in association with benign and malignant hematologic diseases and HIV and mycobacterial infections (e657).

Bile Acid Metabolism Disorders

Bile acid synthesis defects are inherited in an autosomal recessive manner, have low to normal GGT, present in infancy, and are progressive (e675). These diseases typically

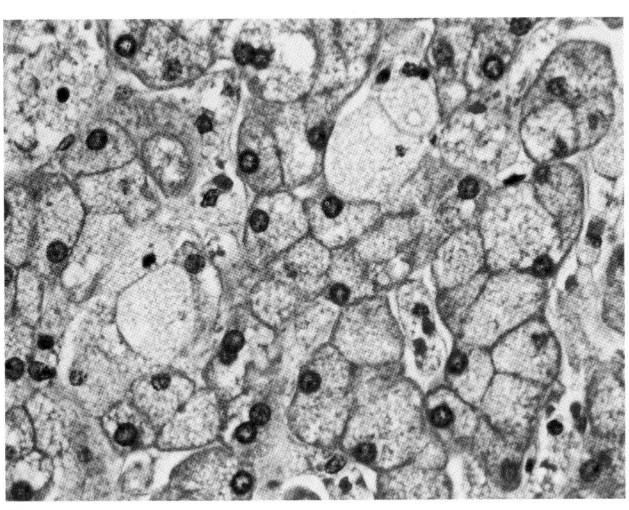

A

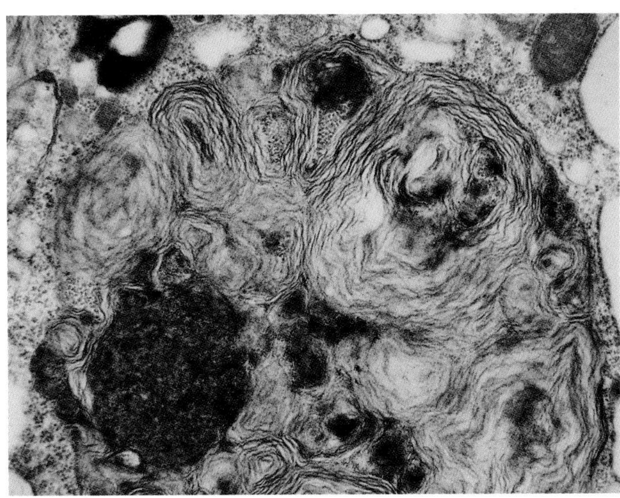

B

FIGURE 15-24 ■ Niemann-Pick disease, Type C. **A:** Hepatocytes and Kupffer cells with swollen, granular to foamly vacuolated cytoplasm (H&E, 400×). **B:** Large pleomorphic membrane-bound lysosomal inclusions with concentric to parallel lamellae (Electron microscopy, 15,000×).

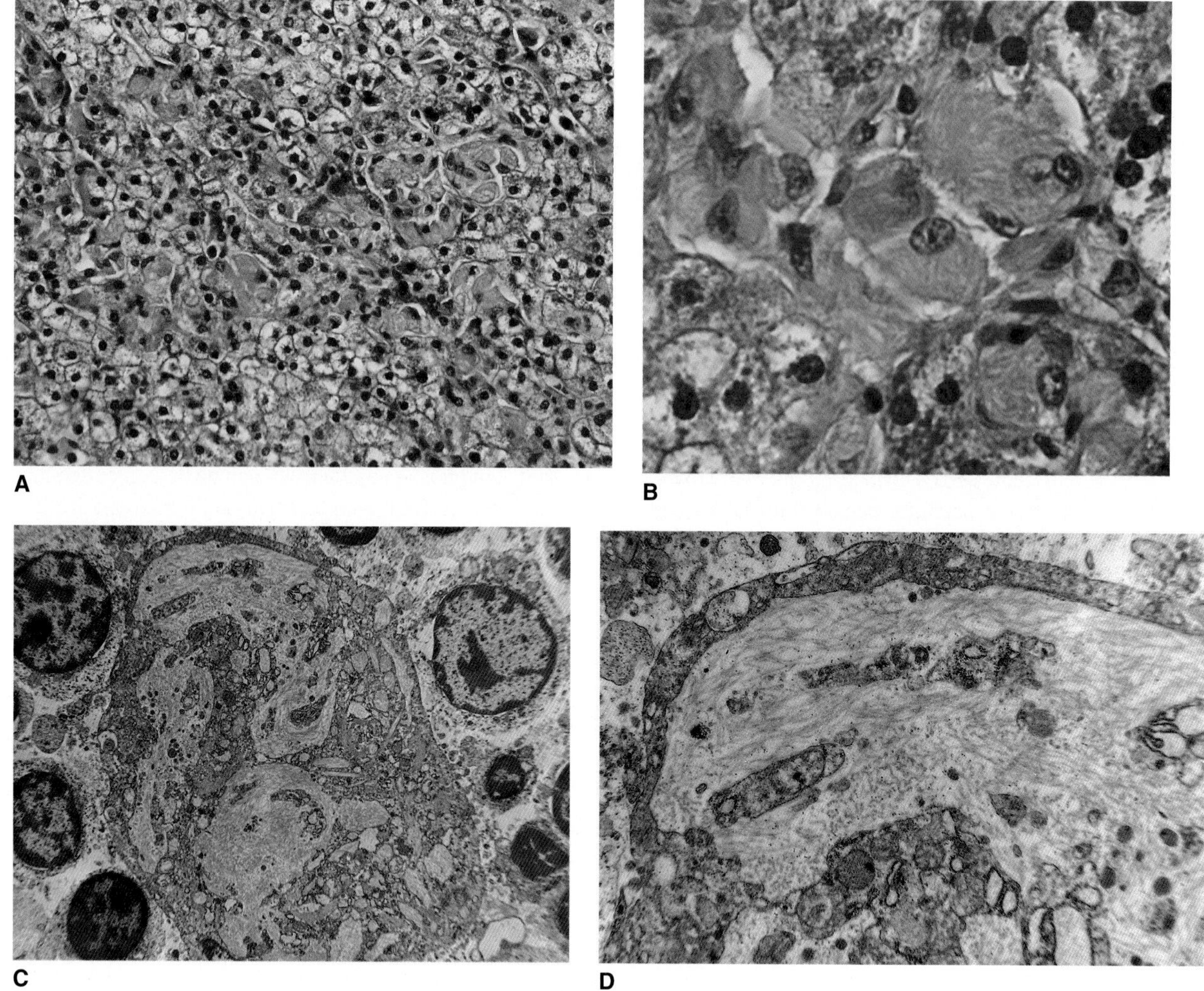

FIGURE 15-25 Gaucher disease. **A, B:** Markedly enlarged Kupffer cells with cytoplasm with a striated, wrinkled tissue paper appearance (H&E, **A:** 100×, **B:** 800×). **C,D:** Kupffer cells with cytoplasmic tubular inclusions with a circular profile on cross section (Electron microscopy, **C:** 6,000×, **D:** 24,000×).

present with neonatal hepatitis and mimic other etiologies for this nonspecific disease process. In older children, there is a more chronic hepatitis-like picture. Clinical signs and symptoms include pruritus with hyperbilirubinemia, difficulty with lipid absorption, and failure to thrive. With some conditions, bile acid substitution will reverse the clinical and histopathologic effects of the bile synthesis deficiencies.

Zellweger Syndrome (Cerebrohepatorenal Syndrome)

Zellweger syndrome (cerebrohepatorenal syndrome) is an autosomal recessive disorder characterized clinically by multiple congenital abnormalities, including craniofacial abnormalities, hypotonia, and psychomotor retardation. Renal cortical cysts, cerebral dysgenesis, and hepatic abnormalities are present (188) (e49,e176,e233,e417,e655,e678). Several different genes involved in peroxisome biogenesis occur in different forms of Zellweger syndrome, including peroxin-1 (PEX1 at 7q21-q22), peroxin-2 (PEX2, 8q21.1), peroxin-3 (PEX3 6q23-q24), peroxin-5 (PEX5 12p13.3), peroxin-6 (PEX6 6p21.1), peroxin-12 (PEX12 on chromosome 17), peroxin-14 (PEX14 1p36.2), and peroxin-26 (PEX26 22q11.21). Absence of peroxisomes in hepatocytes and renal tubular cells is a distinctive feature (77,156) (e325,e571). Death occurs in early infancy. The liver shows hepatocellular disarray, biliary dysgenesis, portal inflammation, and striking iron deposition in Kupffer cells and hepatocytes. Giant cell transformation, steatosis, and hepatic fibrosis or cirrhosis may be seen.

Other Bile Acid Synthesis Defects

Many genetic defects of bile acid synthesis are known (25) (e763). The most common defect among these is 3-beta-hydroxy dehydrogenase deficiency caused by mutation in the gene encoding 3-beta-hydroxy-delta-5-C27-steroid oxidoreductase (16p12-p11.2). This entity is referred to as

Congenital Bile Acid Synthesis Defect Type 1. This leads to neonatal hepatitis and will progress to chronic liver disease without appropriate diagnosis and bile acid substitution. Another form of a congenital defect in bile acid synthesis is due to delta(4)-3-oxosteroid 5-beta-reductase deficiency (Congenital Bile Acid Synthesis Defect Type 2). This is caused by mutation in the AKR1D1 gene (7q32-33). Congenital Bile Acid Synthesis Defect Type 4 is caused by mutation in the alpha-methylacyl-CoA racemase gene located at 5p13.2-q11.1. Neonatal hepatitis with bile duct proliferation is associated with a bile synthesis defect in oxysterol 7-alpha-hydroxylase (gene at 6p21.1-p11.2). Cholesterol is converted into one of several oxysterols prior to being 7-alpha-hydroxylated by an oxysterol 7-alpha-hydroxylase (gene at 6p21.1-p11.2). Lack of this enzyme leads to neonatal hepatitis and the potential for progressive liver disease. A deficiency in 25-hyroxylase (gene at 10q23) results in a bile acid synthesis defect. This is due to the role of this enzyme in expression of genes involved in cholesterol and lipid metabolism. Liver fibrosis is somewhat variable, with a more prolonged course of fibrosis in affected neonates and children. Familial hypercholanemia is characterized by elevated serum bile acid concentrations, itching, and fat malabsorption (BAAT gene at 9q22.3). The defect in this condition is associated with the enzyme bile acid CoA amino acid *N*-acyltransferase (BAAT). This enzyme produces *N*-acyl conjugates of cholanoates (C24 bile acids) with glycine or taurine. The resulting bile acid–amino acid conjugates serve as detergents in the gastrointestinal tract. Those affected with bile acid conjugation defects may present as neonatal hepatitis with fibrosis or as mild chronic liver disease. There are several other conditions that may also have bile acid synthesis defects, such as peroxisome diseases (Zellweger syndrome, Refsum disease, hyperpipecolic anemia, adrenolipodystrophies) and cerebrotendinous xanthomatosis (CYP27A1 gene encoding sterol 27-hydroxylase at 2q33-qter).

Alpha-1-Antitrypsin Deficiency

Liver disease associated with alpha-1-antitrypsin deficiency (A1AT) was initially described by Sharp et al. and has been extensively reviewed (140,166,176) (e201,e222,e350,e357, e529,e528,e624,e662). This is an autosomal recessive disease caused by mutations in the protease inhibitor gene (Pi) on chromosome 14. Both liver and lung diseases (emphysema) occur due to lack of neutralization of neutrophil elastase secondary to absent or decreased protease inhibitor activity. Liver disease without pulmonary emphysema occurs when a mutant but functional form of protease inhibitor is present that inhibits neutrophil elastase activity. This mutant form of AIAT has a defect that does not allow for proper folding, resulting in failure of the material to be translocated from the endoplasmic reticulum to the Golgi for further processing before release from the hepatocyte. The AIAT continues to accumulate in the rough endoplasmic reticulum, leading to hepatocyte injury and liver disease. Clinical presentations vary from neonatal hepatitis with cholestatic jaundice, to young adults with recurrent hepatitis that may lead to chronic hepatitis and cirrhosis, and to older adults with a silent clinical course and cirrhosis development.

A close association of A1AT deficiency has been noted with neonatal cholestasis, accounting for over 10% of cases of neonatal cholestasis, making it the most common genetic cause of neonatal liver disease (78) (e527). Bleeding diathesis, including intracranial hemorrhage, may be the presenting manifestation in the newborn, probably related to an associated vitamin K deficiency (e308).

A1AT is a glycoprotein that is synthesized in the liver and secreted into the serum. Its biosynthesis is controlled by a pair of genes at the protease inhibitor (Pi) locus (140,166,176) (e 202,e222,e350,e357,e528,e529,e662). More than 25 alleles have been described and are responsible for A1AT variant molecules. The normal genotype is PiMM. PiZZ is the most clinically significant genotype with respect to liver disease, and is due to a point mutation with substitution of Lys for Glu. PiMZ genotype patients have 50% normal A1AT and 50% mutant A1AT. Other mutant gene alleles include PiS with reduced A1AT level and no clinical disease, and PiNull with no detectable A1AT. With electrophoresis, PiZ is the slowest of the A1AT variants. In the homozygous (PiZZ) state, there is a marked reduction in the serum A1AT levels. Homozygous PiZZ A1AT has an incidence of 1 in 1,600 to 2,000 live births, making it nearly as frequent as cystic fibrosis (CF) (e527). A few cases of liver disease have been reported in association with PiSZ (e679). Neonatal liver injury has occurred with the PiZ null phenotype (e551). The risk of HCC is increased, especially in homozygous patients, with most cases being reported in adults.

Liver morphology varies in the early phase of the disease. Hepatocellular injury is manifested principally as cholestasis, pseudoacinar transformation, and giant cell transformation, similar to other metabolic hepatopathies (Figure 15-26). Extramedullary hematopoiesis is usually seen. Cholestasis is hepatocellular and present in the form of plugs within the canaliculi. Three morphologic patterns with prognostic significance have been described for the early cholestatic phase. In group 1, portal areas show mild portal fibrosis and no bile duct proliferation, which has a neonatal hepatitis-like appearance (Figure 15-26). In group 2, the portal triads are fibrotic and expanded and contain proliferating bile ducts in which bile may be present. This pattern may be mistaken for the obstructive changes seen in EHBA, and is associated with persistent hepatic disease leading to cirrhosis with a higher frequency. With group 3, there is a paucity of extrahepatic ducts. The prognosis of this group is uncertain. Extensive hepatocellular necrosis may also occur and lead to fulminant hepatic failure.

The morphologic hallmark of the disease is the presence of A1AT in the hepatocytes, predominantly in zone 1 and occasionally in bile duct epithelium. The stored material appears in the form of eosinophilic hyaline globules that are PAS-positive and resist diastase digestion. The globules

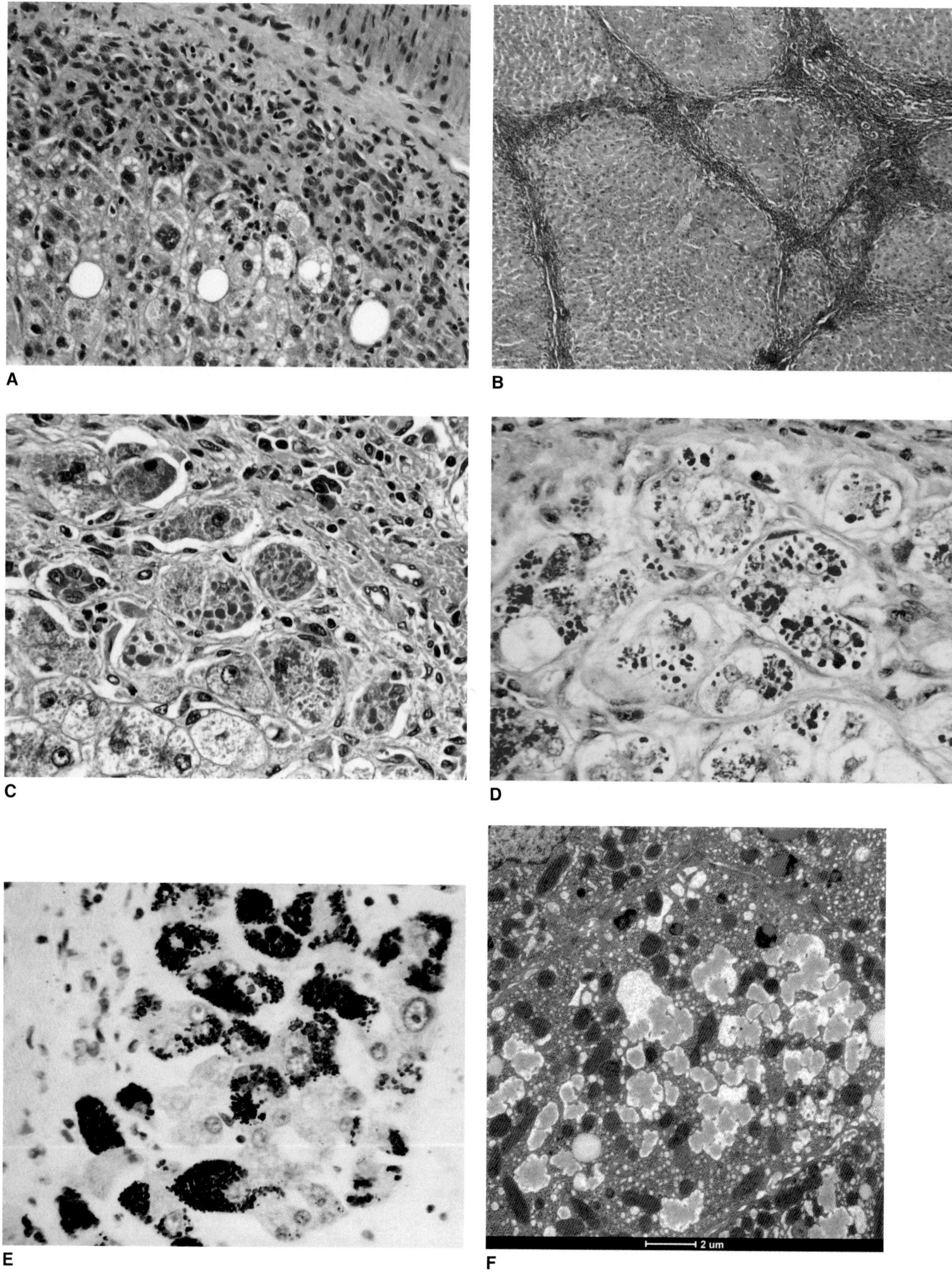

FIGURE 15-26 **A:** Alpha-1-antitrypsin deficiency. Zone 1 hepatocytes with reactive changes and portal areas with chronic inflammation and mild bile duct proliferation (**A:** H&E, 200×). **B:** Cirrhosis in late stage of disease detection (**B:** H&E, 40×). **C, D:** Zone 1 hepatocytes with PAS-positive (**C:** 400×) cytoplasmic globules that are diastase resistant (**D:** 400×). **E:** Immunostaining for alpha-1-antitrypsin reacts with the cytoplasmic globules (**E:** 400×). **F:** Granular, flocculent material distends cisternae of the rough endoplasmic reticulum (**F:** Electron microscopy, 10,000×).

progressively increase in number and may not be visible by hematoxylin and eosin sections in biopsy specimens obtained in the first 3 months of life (e527). The stored material may be demonstrable by immunohistochemistry, even in the absence of appreciable globules. Ultrastructurally, the stored material appears as flocculent, moderately electron-dense material within dilated cisternae of rough endoplasmic reticulum.

The frequency of progression to cirrhosis after neonatal presentation with prolonged cholestasis is variable. Only about 15% of the PiZZ population develop liver disease in the first 20 years of life. If A1AT deficiency is manifested in the neonatal period, as many as 50% of cases progress to cirrhosis, typically micronodular (Figure 15-26) (78). The presence of PAS-positive diastase-resistant globules is the pathologic hallmark, differentiating the micronodular cirrhosis associated with A1AT deficiency from micronodular cirrhosis associated with other disorders. The extrahepatic bile ducts are usually normal. A few cases of hypoplasia of the extrahepatic bile ducts with A1AT deficiency have been described, and the hypoplasia has been ascribed to a low-flow state.

Cystic Fibrosis

CF is caused by mutations in the CFTR gene (CF transmembrane conductance regulator, 7q31.2) that regulates a cyclic AMP-dependent chloride channel (55) (e401,e492,e589). CFTR gene mutation results in decreased sodium and water content of bile with an increase in bile viscosity and reduction in bile low, leading to intrahepatic bile duct obstruction and injury. The incidence of hepatic involvement in CF has increased over the past several decades with increased life expectancy of CF patients. Although pulmonary complications are the predominant clinical manifestations, up to 5% of CF patients may have substantial hepatic dysfunction and an even larger proportion have the typical histologic lesions of CF in the liver without abnormal liver function tests (41,103,128) (e138,e152,e180,e639). The liver may have multiple capsular depressed scars, with a resemblance to hepar lobatum. Histopathologically, there are focal irregular areas of fibrosis with bile duct proliferation and intraluminal inspissated eosinophilic or pale orange secretions (Figure 15-27). This pathognomonic hepatic lesion is the so-called focal biliary cirrhosis. Mononuclear cell infiltration may be seen.

A

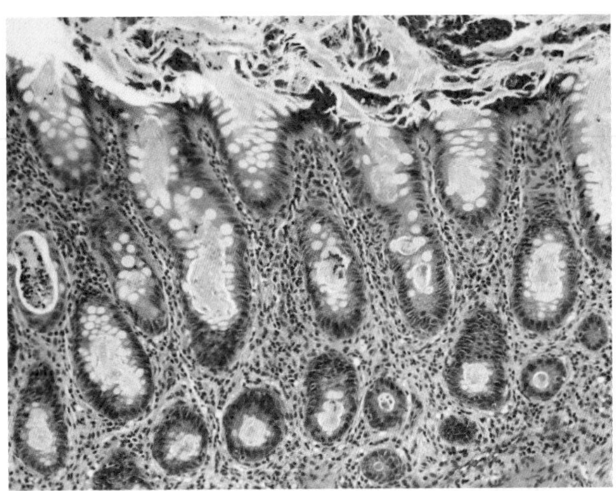

B

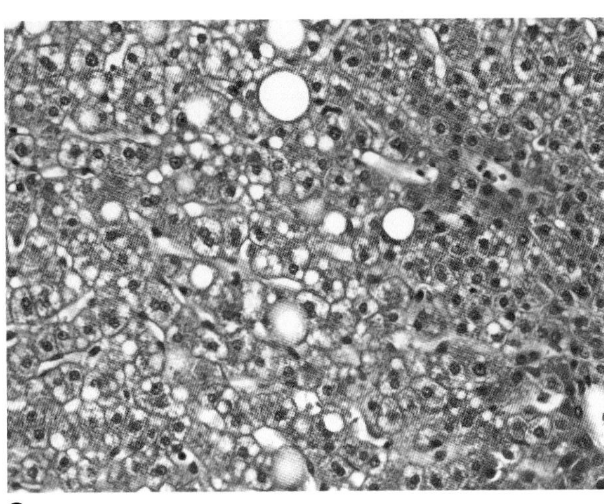

C

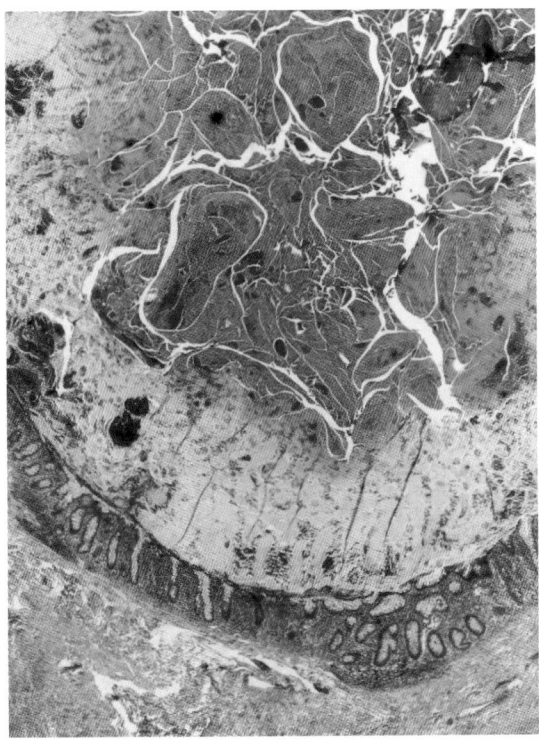

FIGURE 15-27 ■ Cystic fibrosis. **A:** Appendix with dilated lumen and dense eosinophilic mucin in lumen (H&E, 20×). **B:** Appendiceal glands with insipissated densely eosinophilic mucin (H&E, 200×). **C:** Hepatocytes with diffuse microsteatosis and focal macrosteatosis (H&E, 200×).

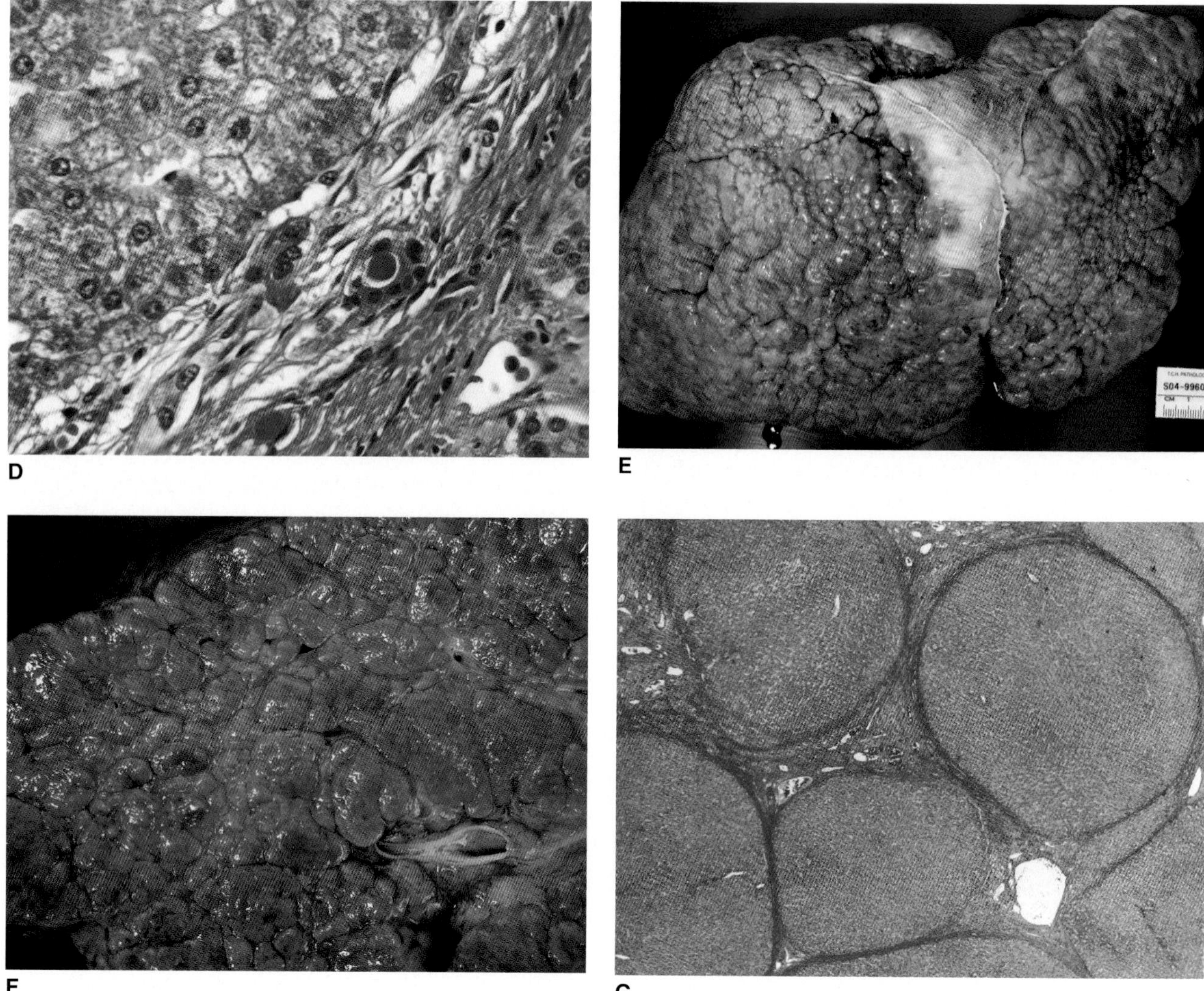

FIGURE 27-7 ■ *(continued)* **D:** Bile ducts in fibrotic portal region with lumenal insipissated densely eosinophilic secretions (H&E, 400×). **E–G:** Explanted liver with macronodular and micronodular cirrhosis (H&E, G 40×).

Steatosis is confined to zone 3 or shows a panacinar distribution, especially in infants with newly diagnosed CF whose pancreatic enzyme replacement has not yet been initiated.

The disease may present in the neonate with cholestatic changes with giant cell transformation and steatosis as the feature of a metabolic hepatopathy. A liver biopsy in an infant with CF may not show the distinctive bile duct lesion (focal biliary cirrhosis). The progression from neonatal cholestasis to focal biliary cirrhosis is not clear.

A coarsely nodular cirrhosis is present in 4% to 10% of cases, with the prevalence increasing through childhood (41,103,128) (e138,e152,e180,e639). Interestingly, there is a diminished prevalence of cirrhosis in those surviving to young adulthood, suggesting that liver disease may influence premature respiratory death in teenagers. At the cirrhotic stage, the liver shows multiple, large nodules, with areas between the nodules appearing depressed and presenting a finely nodular appearance. Portal hypertension and its complications may occur and, rarely, death may ensue acute bleeding from esophageal varices. Combined liver and lung transplantation are necessary in a minority of cases.

The gallbladder is frequently abnormal. The prevalence of gallbladder abnormalities increases with age (103,128) (e152,e180). The gallbladder may be small, with the epithelium frequently having mucinous metaplasia. Diagnostic imaging may show a diminutive or nonfunctioning gallbladder. Cholesterol gallstones are seen in 6% to 12% of patients over 12 years of age, with the risk of developing calculi increasing with age.

Iron Storage Disease

Primary and secondary disorders of iron metabolism are characterized by excessive iron accumulation in the liver (Figure 15-28) as a component of increased total body iron stores (16,59,77,192) (e15,e86,e216,e315,e481,e613,e750). Secondary iron overload may be the result of multiple transfusions for hemoglobin disorders such as thalassemia and

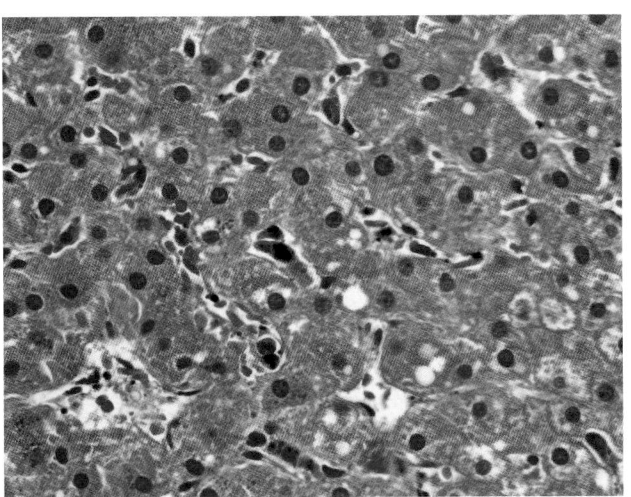

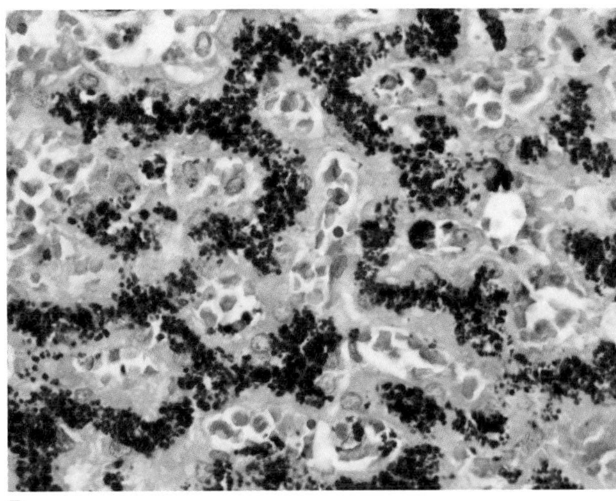

FIGURE 15-28 ▪ Secondary hemosiderosis due to chronic transfusion therapy. **A:** Occasional Kupffer cells with iron pigment in their cytoplasm (H&E, 400×). **B:** Abundant iron storage in Kupffer cells revealed with Prussian blue histochemical stain for iron (400×).

sickle cell disease, or may be due to excessive iron intake. Inherited iron storage disease or hemochromatosis is most often an autosomal recessive condition characterized by a defect in the regulation of iron absorption in the intestine and may present in childhood. There are several inherited forms of hemochromatosis caused by different gene mutations. The clinical features of hemochromatosis include cirrhosis of the liver, diabetes, hypermelanotic pigmentation of the skin, and heart failure. Pancreatic deposition of iron leads to diabetes, and congestive cardiomyopathy is the result of iron deposition in the myocardium. Primary HCC, complicating cirrhosis, is responsible for about one-third of deaths in affected homozygotes. Because hemochromatosis is a relatively easily treated disorder if diagnosed early, this is a form of preventable cancer. At least five iron-overload disorders labeled hemochromatosis have been identified on the basis of clinical, biochemical, and genetic characteristics (6). Classic hemochromatosis (HFE), an autosomal recessive disorder, is most often caused by mutation in a gene designated HFE on chromosome 6p21.3. It has also been found to be caused by mutation in the gene encoding hemojuvelin (HJV), which maps to 1q21. Juvenile hemochromatosis or hemochromatosis type 2 (HFE2) is also autosomal recessive. One form, designated HFE2A, is caused by mutation in the HJV gene (1q21). A second form, designated HFE2B, is caused by mutation in the gene encoding hepcidin antimicrobial peptide, which maps to 19q13. Hemochromatosis type 3, also an autosomal recessive disorder, is caused by mutation in the gene encoding transferrin receptor-2 (TFR2), which maps to 7q22. Hemochromatosis type 4, an autosomal dominant disorder, is caused by mutation in the SLC40A1 gene, which encodes ferroprotein and maps to 2q32. Most affected children and adolescents are asymptomatic with periportal iron accumulations extending toward the central lobule during adolescents. With juvenile hemochromatosis, organ failure with severe iron overload presents before age 30. Both the inherited (hemochromatosis) and secondary (transfusion) forms of iron storage differ from hemosiderosis in that the iron, in addition to being deposited in mononuclear phagocytic cells, is also deposited in the parenchymal cells. Iron deposition in biliary epithelial cells is seen more often in inherited iron storage disease.

Neonatal Iron Storage Disease

Neonatal iron storage disease (NISD), a fatal neonatal disorder, is characterized by massive iron overload (192) (e146, e353,e463,e743,e764,e765). The liver is the predominant organ affected, but iron is also deposited in the pancreas, thyroid, adrenals, pituitary, heart, intestinal mucosa, salivary glands, and sweat glands. The basic defect has not been defined, but most reports suggest that it is a metabolic error, unrelated to classic iron storage disease or hemochromatosis. The condition should be differentiated from other disorders such as tyrosinemia, galactosemia, and Zellweger syndrome, in which excess iron is usually present. More recently, NISD has been considered a gestational disease in which fetal liver injury leads to the phenotype in the neonate. NISD recurrence rate in siblings after the index case is 60% to 80%, implicating maternal alloimmune damage to fetal liver. Pregnant mice injected with human IgG from women with NISD offspring had pups with extensive hepatic injury and liver necrosis. Clinical investigations have evaluated treatment of pregnant women with a prior NISD neonate with intravenous immunoglobulin (IV Ig). In these clinical studies, prior gestational histories indicated a high risk for NISD occurrence, with 92% of at-risk pregnancies resulting in intrauterine fetal demise, neonatal death, or liver failure necessitating transplant. With IV Ig gestational therapy during pregnancy, there were only three failures, while 52 infants did not experience NISD (192).

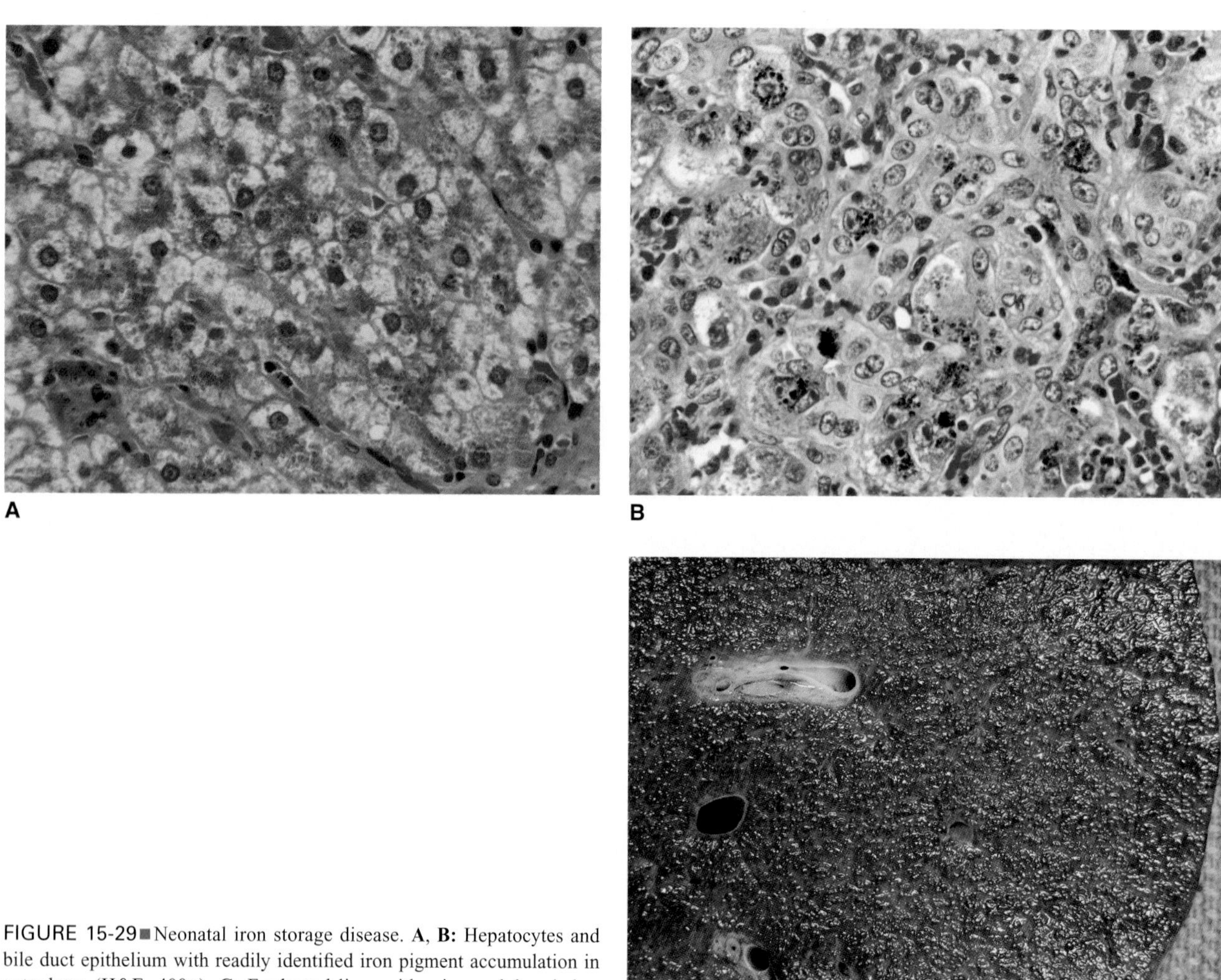

FIGURE 15-29 Neonatal iron storage disease. **A**, **B:** Hepatocytes and bile duct epithelium with readily identified iron pigment accumulation in cytoplasm (H&E, 400×). **C:** Explanted liver with micronodular cirrhosis and green and brown pigmentation from bile and iron accumulation, respectively.

In NISD, the hepatic architecture is markedly disorganized with lobular collapse and early fibrosis (Figure 15-29). Scattered nests of hepatocytes with heavy iron deposits, pseudoacinar profiles, and multinucleated hepatocytes are other microscopic features. Iron may also be demonstrable in biliary epithelial cells. With other organ systems, the iron deposits tend to be within the reticuloendothelial system, with sparing of the parenchymal cells. Minor salivary glands in the oral mucosa show iron deposition in NISD and may be biopsied for diagnosis in suspected cases while awaiting genetic testing results for hemochromatosis.

Wilson Disease

Wilson disease is an inborn error of copper metabolism with an autosomal recessive pattern of inheritance. A genetic defect in ATP7B on chromosome 13q14-21 has been described. This gene encodes a transmembrane copper-transporting adenosine triphosphatase (ATPase) that is located on the canalicular membrane of hepatocytes, and is also homologous with Menkes disease gene. The genetic defect results in reduced copper excretion in the bile and decreased copper incorporation into ceruloplasmin. There are many different mutations in ATP7B, which account for the variable clinical phenotypes.

In normal metabolism, copper is taken up by the stomach and duodenum, weakly bound to albumin, and transferred to hepatocytes (113) (e12,e206,e213,e298,e437,e603). Within the hepatocytes, copper is incorporated into the alpha-2-globulin of ceruloplasmin and released into the bloodstream. Senescent ceruloplasmin is reabsorbed by the hepatocytes and undergoes lysosomal degradation and excreted into the bile. In Wilson disease, copper accumulation occurs in the liver, brain, eyes, and other organs. Elevated levels of serum and hepatic copper, increased urinary copper excretion, and diminished levels of serum ceruloplasmin are the common laboratory abnormalities. In some cases, serum ceruloplasmin values may be within normal limits. A normal serum level of copper excludes Wilson disease, but an elevated level is not always diagnostic, because elevations in copper may be seen in other forms of liver disease, especially of cholestatic type, and in chronic hepatitis. Genetic analysis is available for the diagnosis of Wilson disease in patients and their families.

The clinical presentation varies according to the age of the patient and the stage of the disease (113) (e12,e206,e213,e298,e437,e603). The most frequent symptoms are related to hepatic involvement. Liver disease may be chronic, and cirrhosis or chronic hepatitis may be evident at clinical presentation. Acute hepatitis and fulminant hepatic failure may be the presenting features in a minority of cases, especially in the first two decades of life. Hemolytic anemia is frequent. Central nervous system signs, neuropsychiatric symptoms associated with basal ganglia involvement, and Kayser-Fleischer rings develop in the course of the disease. The latter are characterized by green-brown deposits of copper in Descemet membranes of the corneal limbus.

Penicillamine therapy has been reported to alter the natural course of the disease, and, when instituted early, can prevent progression of liver disease (113) (e12,e206,e213, e298,e437,e603). Controversy, however, exists as to the timing of the use of penicillamine in treatment. Treatment using zinc and trientine has also been studied. Transplantation may be necessary in some cases.

Histopathologic features in the liver vary from mild to moderate fatty changes, focal cytoplasmic swelling, glycogenated nuclei, and occasional acidophilic bodies in the early stages (Figure 15-30). Generally, portal tract inflammation, lobular chronic inflammation, and fibrosis are not seen at this stage. Copper is diffusely dispersed in the cytoplasm and usually cannot be demonstrated histochemically. In the symptomatic stage, the liver may have features of chronic hepatitis (interface hepatitis, portal inflammation, fibrosis, and spotty acidophilic necrosis of hepatocytes). Mallory bodies may be seen, especially in the zone 1 hepatocytes. Glycogenated nuclei are a frequent, but nonspecific, feature. A mixed micronodular-macronodular cirrhosis is the consequence of the chronic hepatitis. Rarely, massive liver necrosis is seen.

Copper can be demonstrated histochemically and is most pronounced in the periportal hepatocytes. The rhodamine

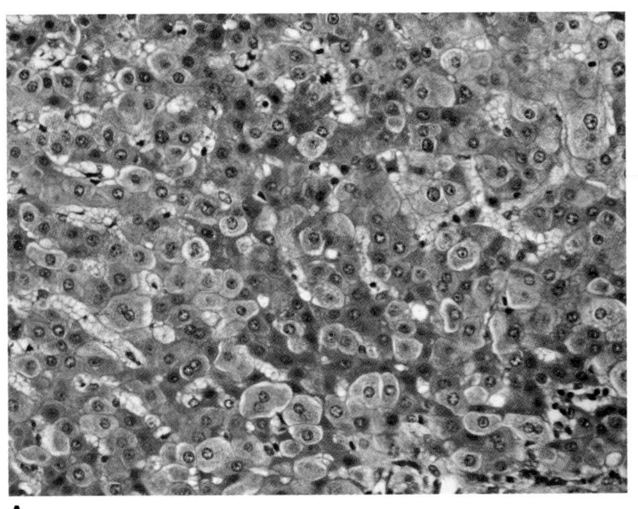

A

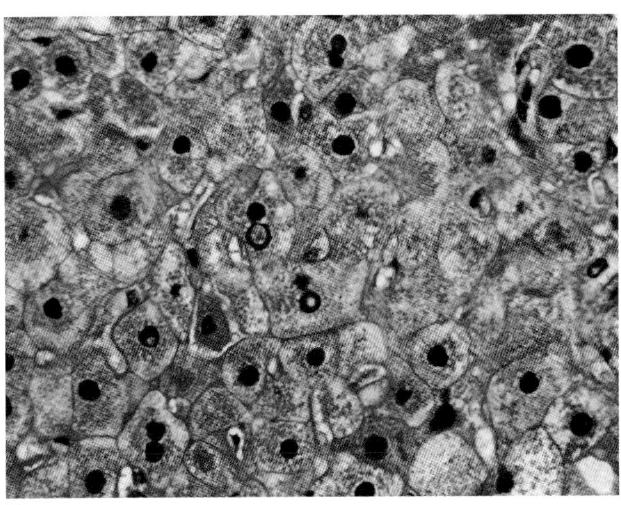

B

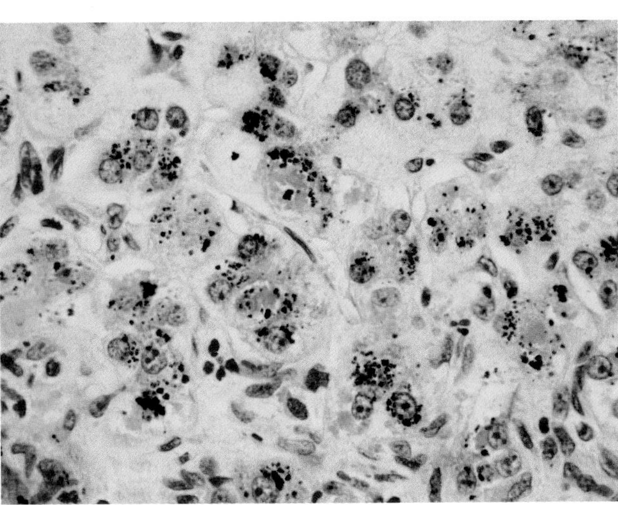

C

FIGURE 15-30 ■ Wilson disease. **A:** Hepatocytes with variable cytoplasmic swelling and decreased cytoplasmic eosinophilia (H&E, 200×). **B:** Infrequent hepatocytes with glycogenated nuclei, apoptotic (acidophil) bodies, and fine granular cytoplasm with a certain degree of cytoplasmic swelling (H&E, 400×). **C:** Cytoplasmic copper detection in periportal hepatocytes (Rhodamine stain, 400×).

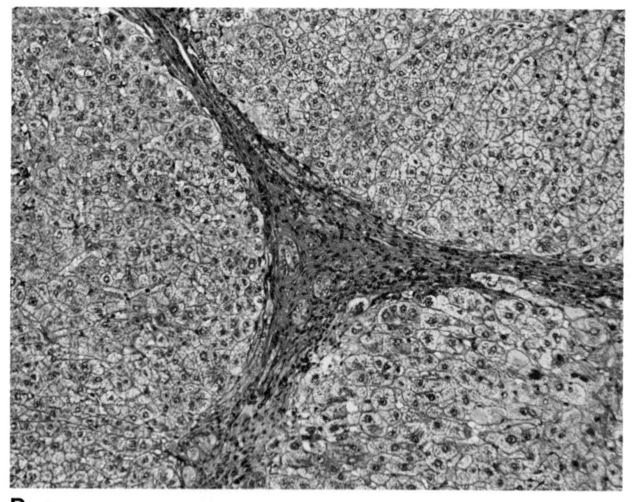

D

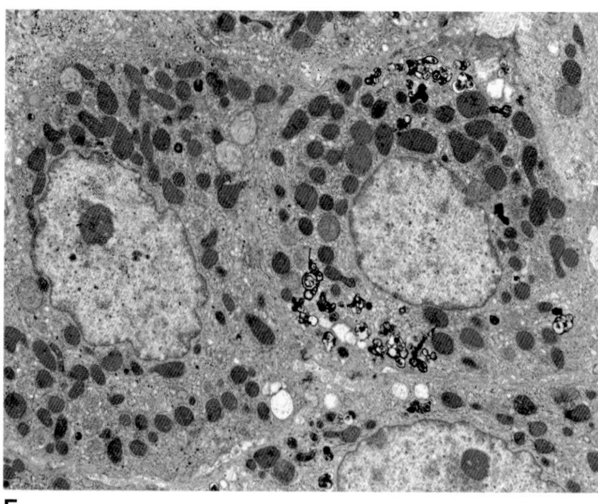

E

FIGURE 15-30 ■ *(continued)* **D:** Wilson disease with cirrhosis of liver (H&E, 100×). **E:** Variably sized and relatively pleomorphic mitochondria and dense lysosomal deposits in Wilson disease (Electron microscopy, 3,000×).

stain gives a brick red reaction product, while rubeanic acid stains the copper gray-black. The Shikata orcein stain demonstrates associated copper-binding protein. Copper may be irregularly distributed in the hepatocyte nodules and may be absent in the regenerative nodules by histochemical methods. Biochemical quantitation of hepatic copper typically demonstrates marked elevations (>250 ug/g dry weight). This can be performed on fresh tissue or a paraffin block. Ultrastructurally, the mitochondria show characteristic alterations appearing enlarged and pleomorphic. Separation of the inner membranes, widening of the intracristal space with microcystic formations at the tips of the cristae, crystalloid inclusions, disoriented cristae, and increased granules in the matrix of the mitochondria are regarded as diagnostic of the disorder (77). Copper deposits are seen in the lysosomes of zone 1 hepatocytes and appear extremely electron-dense. Peroxisomal deposition of copper has also been described.

Porphyrias

Porphyrias are a group of disorders of porphyrin and heme biosynthesis (16,59) (e30,e73,e370). Porphyria may be inherited or acquired and is characterized by increased excretion of porphyrins and storage of abnormal types of porphyrin pigments within tissues. Hepatic abnormalities may be seen in acute intermittent porphyria (hydroxymethylbilane synthase 11q23.3), porphyria cutanea tarda (hemochromatosis gene at 6p21.3, uroporphyrinogen decarboxylase gene at 1p34), and congenital erythropoietic protoporphyria (uroporphyrinogen III synthase gene at 10q25.2-q26.3). The changes in acute intermittent porphyria and porphyria cutanea tarda are similar, although the severity of hepatic injury is greater in porphyria cutanea tarda. Fatty changes and iron overload are evident. Cirrhosis and hepatic failure may occur in porphyria patients, and HCC has been described as a complication in later life. The uroporphyrin crystals are water-soluble, needle-shaped, and have a red fluorescence on examination under ultraviolet light. The needle-shaped inclusions are seen in the hepatic cells by electron microscopy. Additional ultrastructural features include abnormal mitochondria, autophagic vacuoles, and myelin figures. In congenital erythropoietic protoporphyria, the hepatic findings consist of focal accumulation of dark brown pigment in the canaliculi, bile duct epithelium, Kupffer cells, and connective tissue. The pigment is birefringent with bright granules and central Maltese crosses. An intense red fluorescence is seen in frozen sections examined under ultraviolet light. Ultrastructurally, the crystals are electron-dense, straight or curved, and arranged singly or in a radiating star-burst pattern.

Urea Cycle Disorders

Hyperammonemia is characteristic of this group of disorders and should be differentiated from other conditions with elevated ammonia levels (59) (e95,e150,e199,e200,e247, e386,e406,e441,e600,e644). In the newborn, hyperammonemia may be found in premature infants or infants with birth asphyxia. *In utero* hepatic necrosis of undetermined cause has been found to be associated with hyperammonemia (59). Defects of the urea cycle include deficiency of ornithine transcarbamylase (Xp21.1), deficiency of carbamyl synthetase (2q35), citrullinemia associated with deficiency of argininosuccinic acid synthetase (9q34.1), argininosuccinic aciduria due to deficiency of argininosuccinase lyase (7cen-q11.2), argininemia associated with arginase deficiency (6q23), and deficiency of N-acetyl-glutamate synthetase (17q21.31) (e95, e150,e199,e200,e247,e386,e406,e441,e600,e644). With the exception of ornithine transcarbamylase deficiency, which is inherited as an X-linked dominant condition, the other conditions have an autosomal recessive pattern of inheritance.

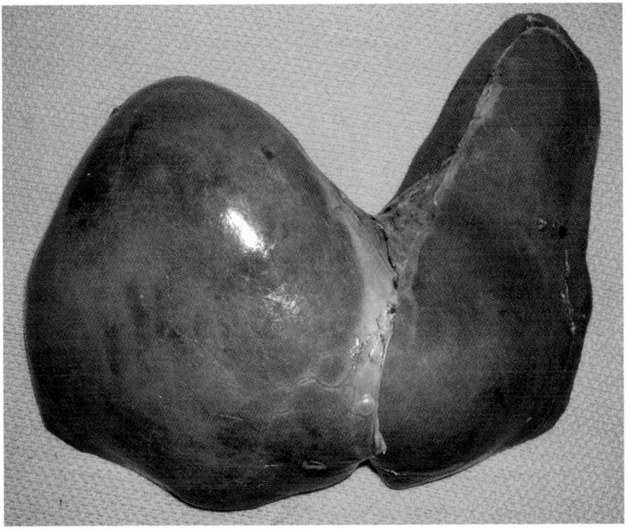

A

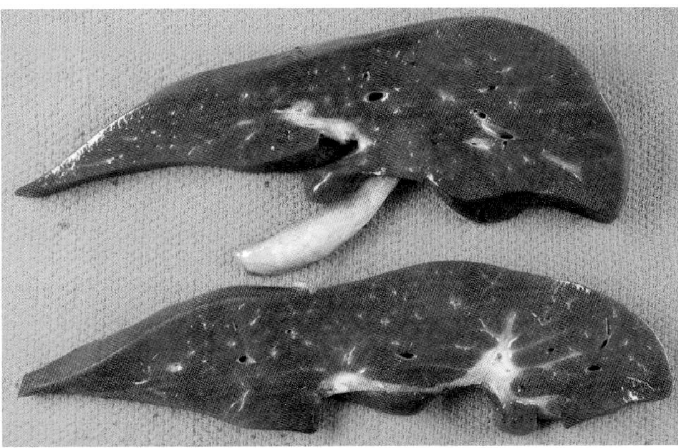

B

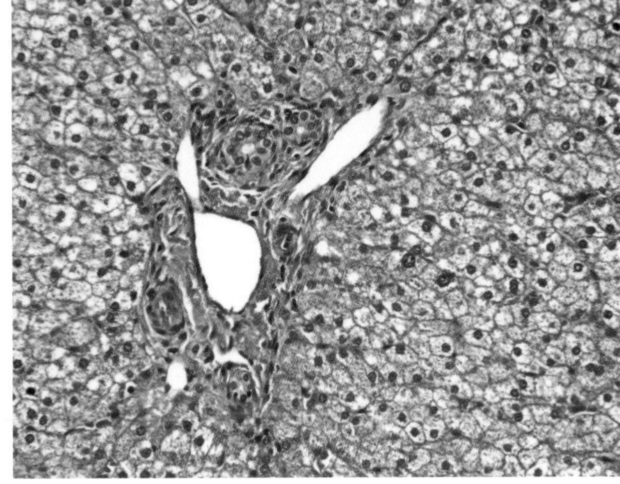

C

FIGURE 15-31 ■ Urea cycle disorder—ornithine transcarbamylase deficiency. **A**, **B:** Explanted liver with no gross abnormalities in ornithine transcarbamylase deficiency. **C:** Portal triad and zone 1 and 2 hepatocytes with no histopathologic abnormalities (H&E, 200×).

Prenatal diagnosis is possible. Liver biopsy in urea cycle defects may be normal or may have only mild nonspecific changes including steatosis, cholestasis, individual cell necrosis, and early fibrosis (Figure 15-31). Liver transplantation may be necessary depending upon the specific urea cycle defect disorder.

Hepatic Steatosis and Steatohepatitis

Fatty change of the liver is a frequent, nonspecific finding associated with a variety of metabolic and nutritional disorders (29,104) (e17,e89,e118,e390,e416,e521,e565,e566, e674,e779). Diagnosis of the specific metabolic disorder associated with this change requires the demonstration of pathognomonic biochemical and morphologic features of that disease. Disorders of lipid and lipoprotein metabolism include abetalipoproteinemia, hypercholesterolemia, congenital lipodystrophy, and fatty acid oxidation defects. The ultrastructural features of these diseases have been described elsewhere (141). Various chemical agents, drugs (valproate, asparaginase, steroids, amiodarone), and toxins (alcohol) are known to induce hepatosteatosis. Other causes of hepatosteatosis in childhood include protein malnutrition, kwashiorkor, obesity, chronic illnesses, type I diabetes, hepatitis C, TPN, mitochondrial disease, inborn errors of metabolism, and severe infection. In the case of obesity, fatty change may be accompanied by inflammation in the lobules and portal tracts as features of steatohepatitis.

This is a reversible form of cellular injury. The lipid may accumulate in the form of small droplets of microvesicular fat, or in the form of large (macrovesicular) droplets that occupy most of the cytoplasm and displace the nucleus to the periphery (Figure 15-32). Microvesicular fat leads to a foamy or clear appearance of the hepatocyte cytoplasm, without displacement of the nucleus, and may not be obvious as fat in the usual preparation. Fat stains on frozen sections and electron microscopy conclusively demonstrate the fat.

The marked increase in childhood obesity and type II diabetes has significantly increased the prevalence of nonalcoholic fatty liver disease (NAFLD) in the pediatric population (29,104) (e17,e89,e118,e390,e416,e521,e565,e566,e674, e779). In fact, NAFLD has emerged as the leading cause of chronic liver disease in children and adolescents in the United States. Elevated insulin, ALT levels, and hyperlipidemia (increased cholesterol and triglyceride) are commonly present in these children. Further, cardiovascular risk and

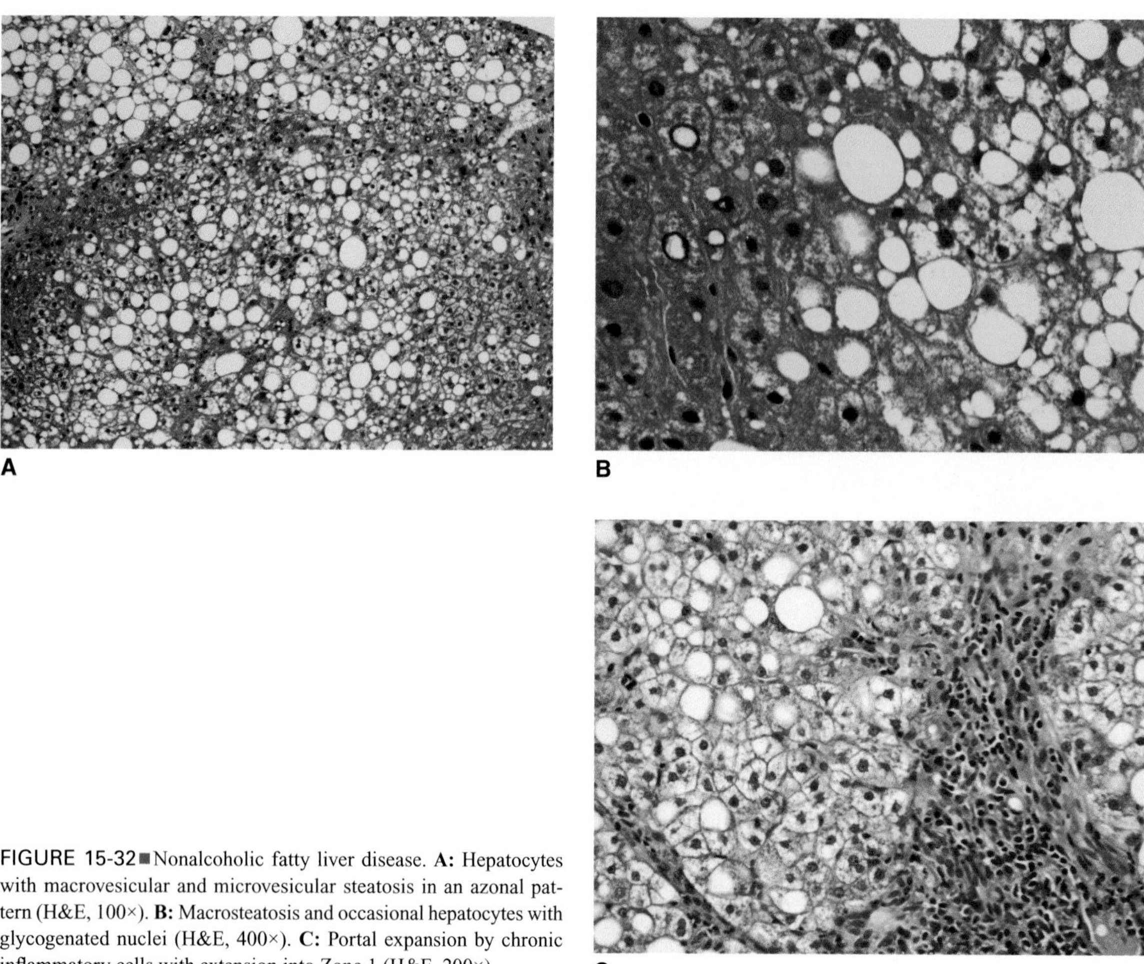

FIGURE 15-32 ■ Nonalcoholic fatty liver disease. **A:** Hepatocytes with macrovesicular and microvesicular steatosis in an azonal pattern (H&E, 100×). **B:** Macrosteatosis and occasional hepatocytes with glycogenated nuclei (H&E, 400×). **C:** Portal expansion by chronic inflammatory cells with extension into Zone 1 (H&E, 200×).

morbidity in children and adolescents are associated with fatty liver.

The characteristic histological features of NAFLD range from steatosis alone to steatohepatitis (NASH) with or without fibrosis to cirrhosis (Figure 15-32). Liver biopsy remains the gold standard for the diagnosis of NASH. NAFLD grading systems are based upon the proportion of hepatocytes demonstrating macrovesicular steatosis, hepatocyte injury (ballooning degeneration), lobular inflammation, and stage of fibrosis (29) (e89,e779). In adults, the histological features of NAFLD have been well-described and include macrovesicular steatosis, perisinusoidal or pericellular fibrosis, foci of lobular inflammation, lipid granulomas, Mallory hyaline, and megamitochondria (29). The combination of macrovesicular steatosis with ballooning change of hepatocytes and/or perisinusoidal fibrosis constitutes a pattern of histology considered diagnostic of NASH in an appropriate clinical context. However, pediatric fatty liver disease often displays a histologic pattern distinct from that found in adults (104,160). In a large study of 100 children with biopsy-proven NAFLD, Schwimmer et al. demonstrated two different forms of steatohepatitis. While both types showed steatosis, "type 1" was characterized by ballooning degeneration, and perisinusoidal fibrosis (as in adults) affecting 17% of subjects while "type 2" was more common (affecting 51% of subjects) and was characterized by portal inflammation and portal fibrosis. Boys were significantly more likely to have type 2 NASH than girls. Further, type 1 NASH was more common in white children, whereas type 2 NASH was more common in children of Asian, Native American, and Hispanic ethnicity. In cases of advanced fibrosis, the pattern was generally that of type 2 NASH (160).

Reye Syndrome

Reye syndrome (acute encephalopathy with hepatic fatty degeneration) is an acute disease of childhood that presents as an encephalopathy, which may progress rapidly to irreversible coma and death (35) (e240,e326,e549,e610). The disease has decreased dramatically since its association with salicylate use was described and warnings issued about the use of salicylates in febrile children. The disease has a biphasic clinical course with an initial febrile illness, usually associated with an upper respiratory viral infection, followed by apparent recovery and the abrupt onset of protracted vomiting, delirium, and stupor. The basic damage appears to be a widespread mitochondrial injury, especially in the liver, brain, and muscle, leading to abnormal metabolism of lipids. Children with symptoms mimicking Reye syndrome may have metabolic disorders, such as organic acid and beta-oxidation defects, and urea cycle disorders. This emphasizes the need to evaluate these children thoroughly, setting aside tissue appropriate for metabolic disorder investigations and molecular genetic studies.

Liver dysfunction is manifested by elevations in transaminases, hypoprothrombinemia, and hyperammonemia (35) (e240,e326,e549,e610). Hypoglycemia may be present. Serum amino acid and free fatty acid levels may be elevated. Grossly, the liver is enlarged and is yellow to pale due to increased parenchymal lipid. Microscopically, the hepatocytes appear either normal or contain finely vacuolated microvesicular steatosis, which does not displace the nucleus. Oil-red-O stains on frozen sections reveal the panlobular distribution of lipid, and virtually all hepatocytes contain small droplets of lipid (34). Characteristically, there is no hepatocellular necrosis or inflammation. Severe decrease or absence of succinate dehydrogenase enzyme activity is demonstrable histochemically.

The ultrastructural features of microvesicular lipid droplets and typical mitochondrial abnormalities are considered virtually diagnostic of the syndrome (141). The changes are reversible, and in children who recover, the liver may show normal morphology, except for the presence of lipid in some hepatocytes and Kupffer cells, and occasional large mitochondria.

Lipid accumulation is also seen in other organs, notably renal tubular epithelium, myocardial and skeletal muscles, lungs, and pancreatic islets. The brain is edematous and mitochondrial changes similar to those in the liver have been described.

Defects in Fatty Acid Oxidation

Defects in fatty acid oxidation, such as carnitine deficiency (SLC22A5 gene at 5q31.1) and acyl-CoA-dehydrogenase deficiency (gene locus at 12q22-qter), may be associated with clinical features resembling Reye syndrome (e356–e361). Episodes of a recurrent Reye-like illness or siblings similarly affected should raise the distinct possibility of fatty acid oxidative disorder.

Carnitine has a role in the beta-oxidation of fatty acids by aiding in their transport across the inner mitochondrial membranes (e75,e87,e402,e403,e449,e577,e599). Three clinical types of carnitine deficiency (SLC22A5 gene at 5q31.1) have been described: myopathic, systemic, and mixed. In the systemic form, carnitine levels are reduced in the serum, liver, and muscle. During the acute episode, often initiated by a relative minor clinical event such as gastroenteritis, the liver shows microvesicular steatosis with panacinar distribution (Figure 15-33) (e102). Ultrastructurally, there is nonmembrane-bound lipid and proliferation of smooth endoplasmic reticulum, increased numbers of lysosomes and accumulation of lipofuscin. Mitochondria may be abnormal in a nonspecific manner. Between clinical episodes, the liver may appear normal. It is important to keep this group of metabolic disorders in mind when a child dies rather abruptly during a seemingly innocuous febrile illness. Tissue and fluids should be obtained at the time of autopsy and be appropriately preserved for possible biochemical and genetic analysis.

Glutaric aciduria type II (type IIA, ETFA gene at15q23-25; type II B, ETFB gene at 4q32-qter; type IIC ETFDH gene at 19q13.3) is associated with deficiency of several mitochondrial acyl-CoA-dehydrogenases and is characterized by acidosis, nonketotic hypoglycemia, organic aciduria, hyperammonemia, and accumulation of lipid in the liver, myocardium, and renal tubular epithelium (59) (e248,e449). One of the unique aspects of this inherited metabolic disorder is the presence of several congenital malformations, including renal cortical and medullary cysts, cerebral pachygyria, pulmonary hypoplasia, and facial dysmorphism. A familial

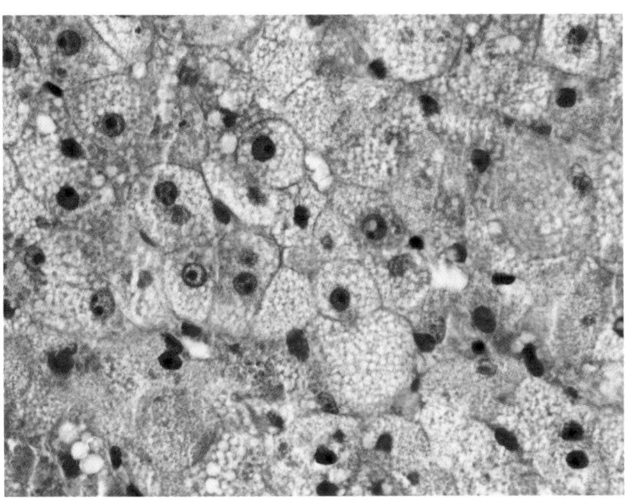

A

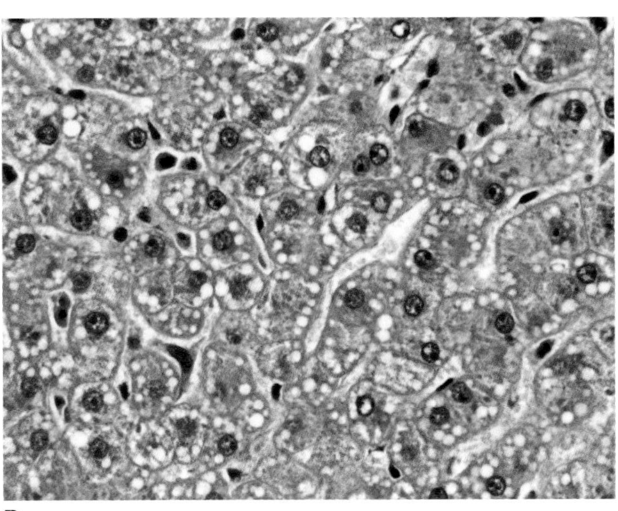

B

FIGURE 15-33 ■ Fatty acid oxidation defect—carnitine deficiency. **A–C:** Variable lipid deposition from fine cytoplasmic vacuolization (**A**) to microsteatosis (**B**) to macrosteatosis (**C**)

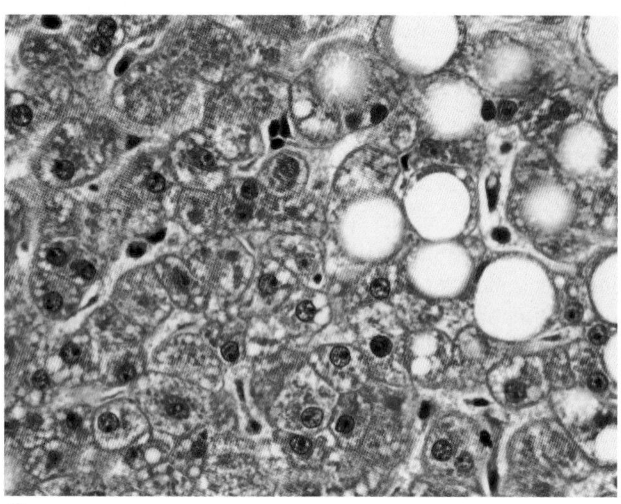

C

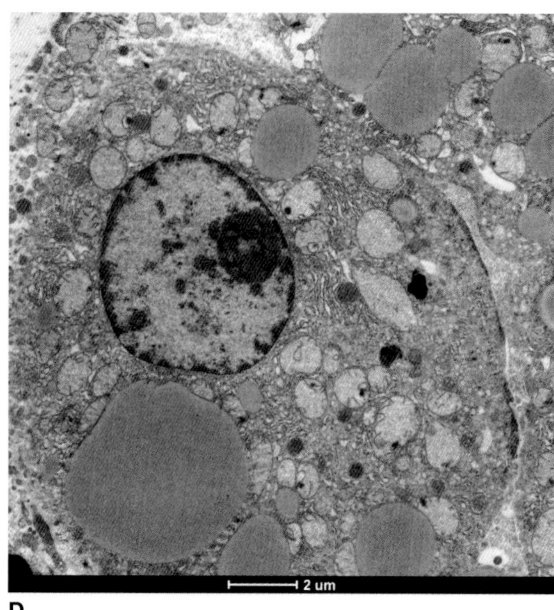

D

FIGURE 15-33■ *(continued)* within hepatocytes (H&E, **A:** 400×, **B:** 200×, **C:** 400×). **D:** Nonmembrane-bound lipid droplets within the hepatocyte cytoplasm (Electron microscopy, 4,000×).

syndrome of hepatosteatosis, jaundice, and kernicterus has been described (e560,e595,e676). Death occurs in the first 3 months of life. Histologically, the liver shows panlobular steatosis with variable cholestasis and portal fibrosis. Lipid is also demonstrable in the renal tubular epithelium and myocardium. The basic mechanism of this disease has not been defined, and there is a possibility that the disease may not be a distinct entity.

VIRAL HEPATITIS

Viral hepatitis is the result of primary infection of the liver by specific hepatotropic viruses. These include hepatitis A, B, C, D, E and possibly G (GB virus C) viruses. Many studies and reviews of clinical findings, the nature of the viruses, morphologic findings, and immunopathology are available that discuss the disease as it affects adult and pediatric age groups (e168,e476,e688,e768). Some characteristics of these viruses and the associated hepatic diseases are shown in Table 15-9.

Hepatitis A

Infectious hepatitis, or hepatitis A, accounts for one-third of reported pediatric cases. This virus is a single-stranded RNA virus (picornavirus). Transmission is by the fecal-oral route because the virus is resistant to low gastric pH (e609). Sexual transmission is prominent among homosexual men. Epidemics of the disease occur, and there are endemic areas, especially in the tropics, with a high rate of infection. Institutionalized children are at risk owing to poor hygienic conditions. In countries with poor sanitary conditions, most children are infected at an early age. Seroepidemiologic studies have routinely shown that up to 100% of preschool children have detectable anti–hepatitis A virus (HAV) antibodies, presumably reflecting previous subclinical infection (e265). The average age of infection is rapidly increasing to 5 years and older, when symptomatic infection is more likely (e304). In industrialized countries, there is a low prevalence of HAV infection among children and young adults. Thus, in the United States, the prevalence of anti–HAV antibodies is approximately 10% in children and 37% in adults (e1).

HAV causes acute inflammation of the liver, which resolves without chronic carrier status, chronic hepatitis, or HCC in infected patients. The incubation period is 2 to 4 weeks, rarely up to 6 weeks. Histologically, acute hepatitis manifests as lobular disarray with ballooned hepatocytes, apoptotic (Councilman) bodies, lymphomononuclear inflammation, and zone 3 cholestasis. However, the diagnosis is established on serology and biopsy is not required. Mortality rate is low in previously healthy individuals. The real impact of the disease is in the morbidity it causes, usually a significant problem only in adults and older children. Approximately 11% to 22% of patients with acute HAV require hospitalization (e271). Young children (below 2 years of age) are usually asymptomatic with only 20% developing jaundice, whereas most 5-year-old children (80%) develop symptoms. Management includes only general supportive measures. A highly effective vaccine is available; however, it is not recommended for children younger than 2 years of age.

Hepatitis B

The hepatitis B virus (HBV), a partially circular double-stranded DNA virus (hepadnavirus), is usually transmitted perinatally, sexually, and parenterally by means of blood or

Table 15-9 ▪ HEPATITIS VIRUSES AND LIVER DISEASE

				Tissue Markers	
Virus	**Characteristics**	**Antigen**	**Disease**	**Nucleus**	**Cytoplasm**
HAV	27-nm RNA virus found in stool, blood, and liver	Hepatitis A (HAAg)	Acute viral hepatitis	None	+
HBV	42-nm DNA virus with envelope, 27-nm core in nucleus and 22-nm coat found in blood and hepatocyte cytoplasm	Hepatitis B surface (HBsAG)	Acute viral hepatitis	None	None
		Hepatitis B core (HBcAg)	Acute hepatitis with bridging	1+ HBcAg	1+ HBsAg
		Hepatitis E (HBeAg)	Carrier state, no liver disease	None	4+ HBsAg
			CAH	1+ HBcAg	1+ HBsAg
			Chronic hepatitis, immune suppressed	4+ HBcAg	1+ HBsAg
			Carrier state, mild hepatitis	4+ HBcAg	1+ HBsAg
Hepatitis C (non-A, non-B)	Single RNA strand 6 genotypes, 80 subtypes	Hepatitis C	Acute viral hepatitis CAH	None	None
Hepatitis D virus (HDV) delta agent	RNA defective virus; 35–37-nm incomplete virion, requires HBsAg to be infective	Delta	In the presence of coinfection with HBV, implicated in massive hepatic necrosis; and higher frequency of chronic disease	4+ delta	1+ delta
Hepatitis E virus (HEV)	27–30-nm nonenveloped RNA virus	Hepatitis E	Acute self-limiting hepatitis	Immunofluorescence positive in frozen tissue	

other body fluids including semen, saliva, and breast milk (183) (e642). HBV has an incubation period of 6 to 8 weeks. Among children, those at increased risk include hemophiliacs and others who require frequent transfusions, adolescent intravenous drug abusers, institutionalized children, and infants of mothers with chronic HBV infection.

The prevalence of HBV infection varies in different geographic areas (e424). In most high-prevalence areas such as Hong Kong and China, perinatal transmission is the major mode of spread, accounting for 40% to 50% of chronic HBV infection (e400). However, horizontal spread during the first 2 years of life is the major mode of transmission in other endemic areas including Africa and the Middle East (e340,e711). In intermediate-prevalence areas, transmission occurs in all age groups, but early childhood infection accounts for most cases of chronic infection (defined as persistent serum HBsAg for 6 or more months after initial diagnosis). In low-prevalence areas, such as the United States, Western Europe, and Australia, most infections are acquired in early adult life through unprotected sexual intercourse or intravenous drug abuse. Age at infection has a significant impact on the clinical outcome, because chronic infection occurs in approximately 90% of infants infected at birth, in 25% to 50% of children infected between the ages of 1 and 5 years, and in less than 5% of those infected during adult life (183) (e51,e114,e144,e642,e656,e690).

Acute HBV infection has been estimated to account for 10% to 25% of all cases of childhood acute hepatitis (183) (e113,e642). Acute hepatitis B can cause fulminant hepatitis. Acute and chronic hepatitis B morphologically may resemble hepatitis of other etiologies and requires serology for definitive diagnosis. Chronically infected patients may have acute hepatitis B flares; superinfection with hepatitis D virus (HDV) should be considered in this setting. Chronic hepatitis B is an important risk factor for cirrhosis, dysplasia, and HCC.

Anti-HB confers long-term immunity. An effective and safe vaccine has been available since the early 1980s and is now included in the routine pediatric immunization schedule. Following infection, treatment should be instituted as early as possible, before there is irreversible liver damage. Extrahepatic manifestations including arthralgia, arthritis, skin rash, and Gianotti-Crosti syndrome (papular acrodermatitis) are common (in 25% of patients). Many new antiviral and immunomodulatory therapies have become available in recent years; however, these therapies are efficacious in less than 50% of patients. Liver biopsy is also useful in confirming virologic clearance or persistence; a part of the specimen should be routinely preserved for viral DNA quantitation.

Hepatitis C

The hepatitis C virus (HCV) infects over 100 million people worldwide, mostly adults, and is perhaps the most common cause of chronic hepatitis (126). Hepatitis C is a single-stranded RNA virus (flavivirus-like). The development of serologic tests has led to donor screening and its decrease in transfusion recipients. A population at risk is injection drug abusers. The most common transmittal route is parenteral, with an incubation period of 6 to 12 weeks. Although transfusions were the most common mode of spread, nucleic acid–based screening of blood and blood products has almost eliminated this route of spread. Intravenous drug abuse is presently the most common route of transmission. Perinatal transmission is known to occur, but the predominant route (transplacental or perinatal) and incidence of transmission are not known (183) (e214,e303,e496,e642). Perinatal transmission has been documented only from anti-HCV women who are HCV-RNA positive. Transmission is more efficient if mothers have acute HCV infection during pregnancy, high circulating HCV-RNA levels, and/or HIV coinfection. HCV is not transmitted by breast-feeding. Since maternal HCV antibodies are passively transferred to the neonate, diagnosis requires RNA-based tests.

Eighty percent of patients develop chronic hepatitis, with 20% developing cirrhosis and 20% developing HCC. Histopathologically, chronic hepatitis C is characterized by predominant portal lymphomononuclear inflammation with or without lymphoid aggregates and bile duct (Poulsen) lesions, lobular inflammation, and varying degrees of fibrosis. The standard grading and staging systems in use for the histopathologic assessment of most chronic hepatitis were originally developed for evaluating chronic hepatitis C and as such are best standardized in this setting. Transplantation is not curative, and recurrent infection is universal. No vaccine is available, and antiviral therapy is effective in only 25% to 40% of patients. Anti-HCV antibody does not confer immunity. Serum transaminases fluctuate markedly and cannot be used as surrogate markers of infection or the degree of hepatic injury (126,183).

Hepatitis D

The HDV (or delta agent) is a unique defective passenger RNA virus requiring helper functions provided by the HBV, including provision of the hepatitis B surface antigen coat for virion assembly and penetration into hepatocytes (151) (e262). Transmission is via a parenteral route. In about 80% of those affected, chronic hepatitis D progresses to cirrhosis. These individuals are also at risk for HCC. Survival after transplantation is better than for other types of viral hepatitis, and reinfection is rare.

Hepatitis E

The hepatitis E virus (HEV; enterically transmitted non-A, non-B hepatitis) was identified in 1983 and cloned in 1990 (3) (e9,e111,e157,e342,e464). HEV is a single-stranded RNA virus that is water-borne and has an incubation period of 6 weeks. It is responsible for large epidemics of acute hepatitis in parts of Asia, Middle East, Africa, and Mexico. Transmission is fecal-oral, through contaminated water secondary to virion shedding in stools. Young adults are most commonly infected. The illness is usually self-limiting, except in pregnant women who tend to have severe disease and a high mortality rate (up to 25%). Chronic infection is unknown. Diagnosis is based on serologic detection of anti-HEV antibodies. Liver biopsy is not usually performed for diagnosis. Biopsy morphology is of acute hepatitis; fatal cases may show submassive to massive necrosis. No specific treatment or vaccine is available.

Hepatitis G

The Hepatitis G virus (HGV or GB virus-C) is a flavivirus with global distribution that is transmitted primarily by parental routes, but can also be transmitted sexually and perinatally (149) (e40,e61,e411). There is no convincing evidence that HGV is a primary hepatotropic virus, and it has not been known to cause acute or chronic hepatitis. There is controversy as to whether HGV should be included among the well-established hepatitis viruses A through E; however, there is coinfection with HCV in up to 20% of patients with hepatitis E and coinfection in patients with HIV infection.

Pathology of the Viral Hepatitides

Microscopic features of acute viral hepatitis, regardless of specific viral etiology, are characterized by lobular disarray and inflammation (Figure 15-34). Liver injury is manifest by ballooning degeneration, individual cell necrosis with dropout of hepatocytes, and acidophilic (Councilman) bodies. Concomitant regenerative activity is evidenced by mitoses and binucleate or multinucleate cells. The cellular infiltrate is predominantly mononuclear and has a lobular and portal distribution. Portal areas are uniformly infiltrated with lymphocytes. Plasma cells, neutrophils, and eosinophils may be present. The infiltrate may extend into the periportal lobule, but in contrast to chronic hepatitis with marked activity, periportal necrosis is not usual, and all portal areas are uniformly involved. There is hyperplasia of the sinusoidal lining cells, and Kupffer cells may contain lipofuscin pigment. Cholestasis is variable and usually mild, seen most often in zone 3. In the cholestatic form of hepatitis, prominent cholestasis simulating extrahepatic obstruction may be seen. In subsiding hepatitis, the changes become less prominent and may resemble chronic hepatitis with mild to moderate activity. Clusters of macrophages (PAS-positive, diastase-resistant) may suggest a recent acute hepatitis in these cases. In more severe forms of acute hepatitis, bridging necrosis with loss of hepatocytes may be accompanied by reticulin collapse and the formation of passive septa between central veins and between central veins and portal areas. The presence of bridging necrosis is an adverse prognostic factor that may be associated with a fatal outcome or progression to cirrhosis (118) (e82). In a few cases, the course may be fulminant with a high mortality rate; at autopsy, submassive necrosis with few surviving hepatocytes is seen in the

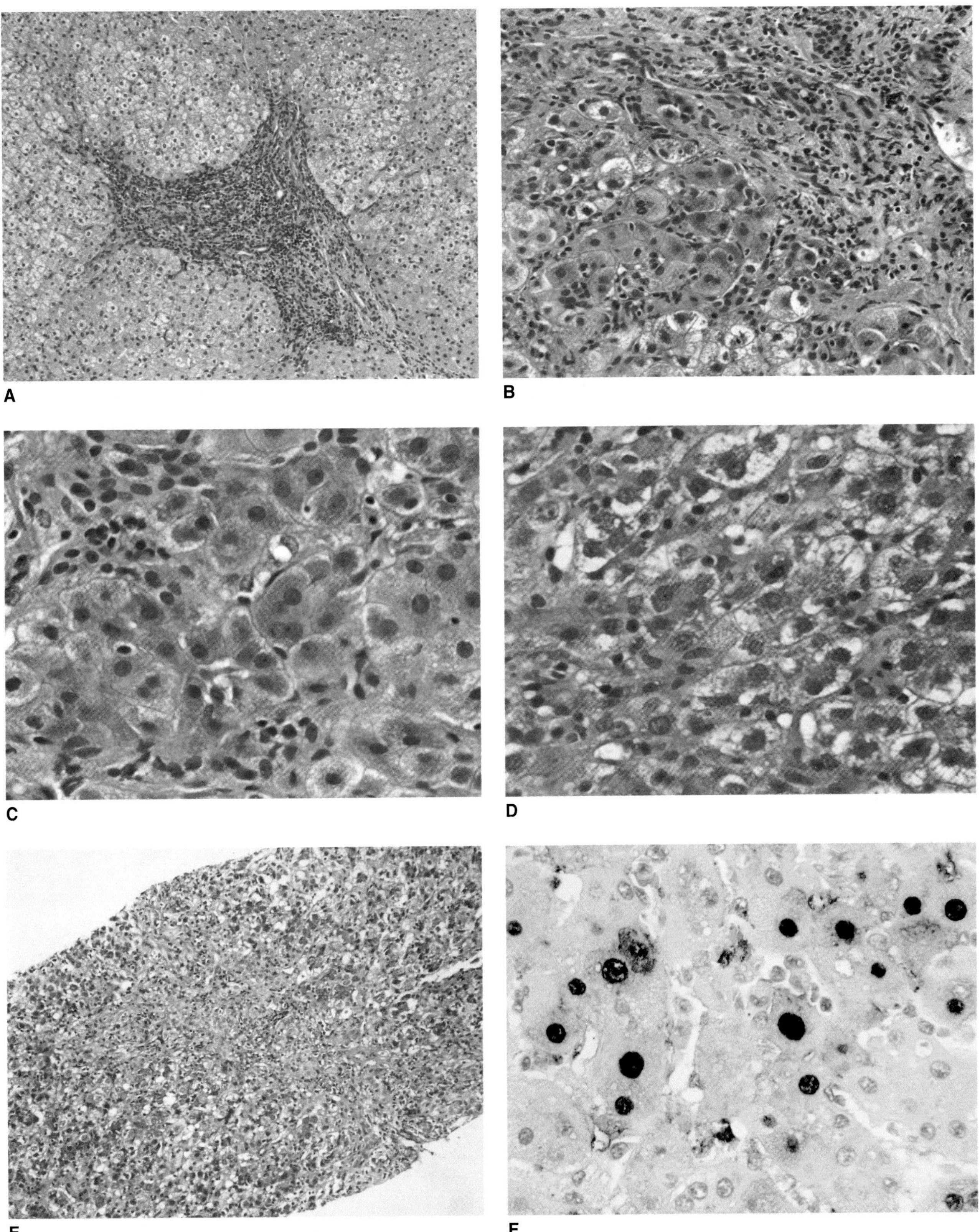

FIGURE 15-34 ■ Viral hepatitis—Hepatitis B. **A:** Expansion of portal region by chronic inflammatory cells with extension into zone 1 by piecemeal necrosis (H&E, 100×). **B**, **C:** Zone 1 hepatocytes with deeply eosinophilic, glassine cytoplasm, and chronic inflammatory cells extending into Zone 1 (H&E, **B:** 200×, **C:** 400×). **D:** Necrotic hepatocytes (apoptotic/acidophil bodies) with pyknotic nuclei and densely eosinophilic cytoplasm (H&E, 400×). **E:** Diffuse fibrosis extending from the portal region into the hepatic lobule (Trichrome, 40×).

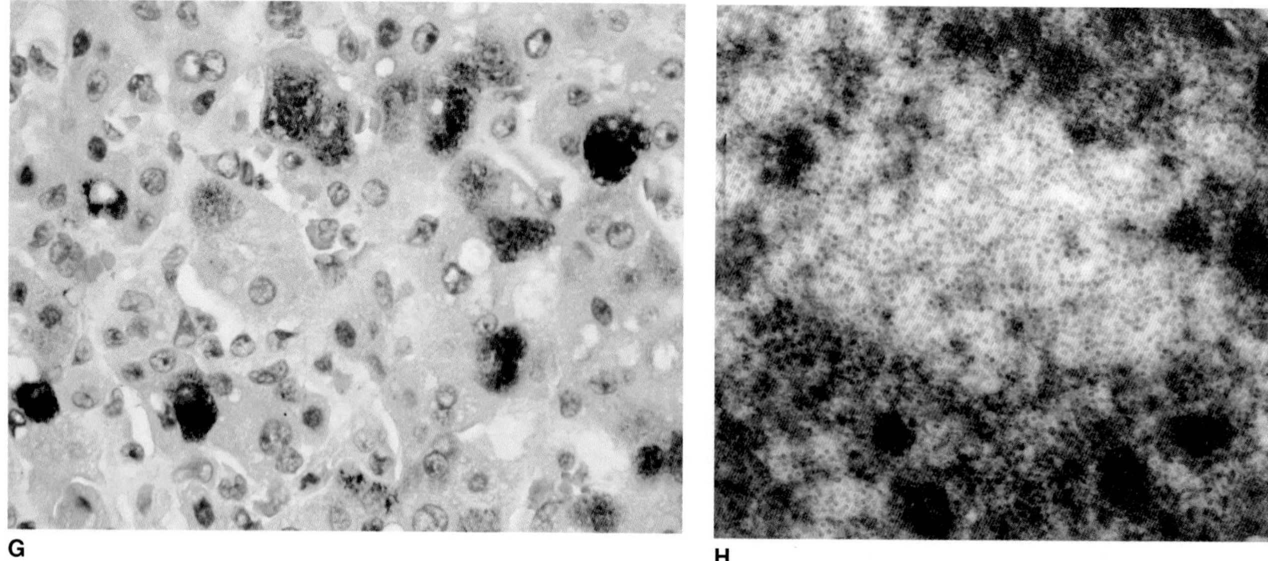

FIGURE 15-34■ *(continued)* **F, G:** Hepatocytes immunoreact with Hepatitis B core antigen in nuclear pattern (**F:** 400×) and with Hepatitis B surface antigen in cytoplasmic pattern (**G:** 400×). **H:** Hepatocyte with intranuclear hepatitis B virus inclusions (Electron microscopy, 75,000×).

periportal zones. The major portion of the lobule shows diffuse loss of hepatocytes accompanied by collapse and approximation of the portal areas. Some degree of regenerative activity of the surviving periportal hepatocytes may be evident in the form of pseudoductular or neocholangiolar proliferation (e531). Lymphocytes, plasma cells, neutrophils, and eosinophils are seen in the sinusoids and space of Disse, and an endophlebitis may be seen, particularly if more than 10 days have elapsed since the onset of the process. Inflammation is seen in the portal areas. Kupffer cells contain cell debris and lipofuscin pigment. An etiologic distinction between the acute hepatitis caused by hepatitis A, B, C, D, and E viruses is not possible on morphologic grounds alone, although reports of acute hepatitis caused by hepatitis C describe the presence of lipid in the hepatocytes and a prominent sinusoidal mononuclear cell infiltrate with marked hypertrophy of the sinusoidal lining cells (Figure 15-35). The differences between hepatitis A and B infection are not readily appreciated. Perivenular cholestasis, interface hepatitis with a dense portal infiltrate with frequent plasma cells, and extensive microvesicular steatosis are considered to be more characteristic for HAV-associated acute viral hepatitis. With HBV acute viral infection, hepatocytes with ground-glass cytoplasm is associated with abundant HBsAg production and may be somewhat helpful in differentiating HBV from HAV.

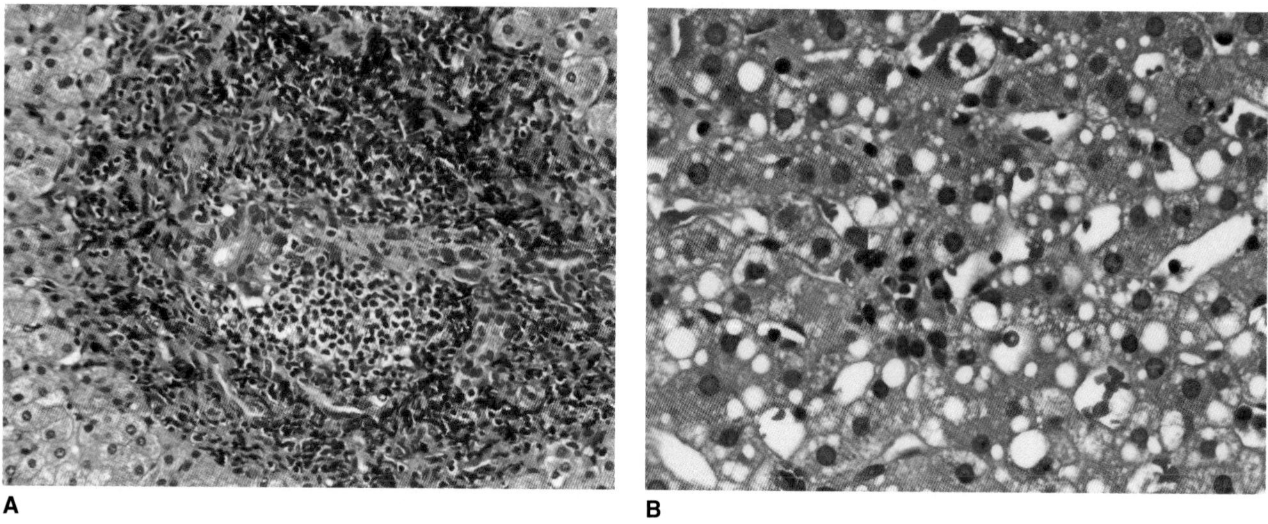

FIGURE 15-35■ Viral hepatitis—Hepatitis C. **A:** Portal chronic inflammation with lymphoid aggregate with germinal center (H&E, 200×). **B:** Hepatocytes with microsteatosis and occasional chronic inflammatory cells in sinusoids (H&E, 400×).

HBV and HCV infection may lead to chronic liver disease. Histopathologic features that predict progression to chronicity include bridging necrosis, prominent portal infiltrate with periportal extension, and distortion of the lamina limitans, lymphoid follicles, and early fibrosis. The concomitant demonstration of the surface and core antigen of HBV by immunohistochemistry has been associated with progression to chronic liver disease. The histopathology of hepatitis B infection has been recently comprehensively reviewed (118).

Chronic hepatitis is not a single disease, but rather a clinicopathologic syndrome that may have a variety of causes (48,126) (e166,e466,e677,e756). Traditionally, chronicity has been defined clinically as continuing disease for at least 6 months. This definition still has some practical utility, but asymptomatic disease must also be taken into account; for example, both HCV and autoimmune hepatitis (AIH) may remain asymptomatic for long periods. The terms chronic active hepatitis (CAH), chronic persistent hepatitis (CPH), and chronic lobular hepatitis (CLH) have become obsolete and should not be used.

The chronic hepatitides consist of chronic necroinflammatory diseases in which hepatocytes rather than biliary structures appear to be the main target of attack. Chronic cholestatic diseases, such as primary biliary cirrhosis (PBC) and primary sclerosing cholangitis (PSC), and metabolic disorders, such as Wilson disease and A1AT deficiency, are not always included under the headings of chronic hepatitis (48). However, they may show similar morphologic features, and there is thus practical merit in considering them in the broader spectrum of chronic hepatitis (2).

Various etiologic types of chronic hepatitis share a number of histopathologic characteristics that may vary over time in an affected individual. Most of these common morphologic features allow the pathologist to assess the grade (severity of inflammatory activity) and stage (degree of fibrosis) of the disease process, but do not always allow a definitive distinction between the various etiologies. In general, lobular inflammation predominates in acute forms of hepatitis, and portal and periportal inflammation predominates in chronic hepatitis. Chronic hepatitis with flares of disease activity commonly shows lobular hepatitis, together with portal and periportal inflammation and fibrosis (48,118) (e94).

Portal inflammation (Figures 15-34 and 15-35) is common to all forms of chronic hepatitis and is composed mainly of a mixture of lymphocytes, plasma cells, and macrophages. Lymphoid aggregates with or without germinal centers are more often seen in HCV-associated chronic viral hepatitis (Figure 15-35). Periportal inflammation commonly accompanies local hepatocyte damage. This necroinflammatory process is referred to as lymphocytic piecemeal necrosis or interface hepatitis. The composition of these inflammatory infiltrates is identical to those in the portal tracts. As a consequence of the necroinflammatory process, collagen and elastin is deposited. In contrast to portal and periportal inflammation, lobular inflammation usually consists of single small clusters of mononuclear cells rather than confluent sheets. Lobular inflammation is usually accompanied by hepatocellular damage. Hepatocellular damage is generally manifested by scattered necrotic hepatocytes (acidophilic, apoptotic, or Councilman bodies), hepatocellular nuclear disarray (anisonucleosis), mitotic activity, and hepatocellular swelling (ballooning degeneration). Apoptotic hepatocytes are characterized by pyknotic nuclear remnants and dense retracted cytoplasm. Degenerative and regenerative hepatocellular changes are frequently more impressive than the number of inflammatory cells.

Over time, chronic hepatitis leads to progressive fibrosis, which begins in portal areas, extends to periportal zones, and eventually links portal tracts to other portal tracts and to terminal hepatic venules. After fibrous septa have formed, regenerative nodules, indicative of cirrhosis, may appear. With the exception of HCV, in which approximately 70% of cases show fatty change (12), steatosis is uncommon in chronic hepatitis. Steatosis in a liver biopsy may be unrelated to viral hepatitis and may purely reflect of background fatty change. Chronic viral hepatitis is rarely cholestatic.

Pathologic reporting of liver biopsies should include the etiology, grade, and stage of the chronic hepatitis in the final diagnosis (Tables 15-10 and 15-11). Development of cirrhosis may be related to the duration of CAH.

In the asymptomatic patient with chronic hepatitis B, the liver may show no abnormality except for the ground-glass hepatocytes, which represent cells containing HBsAg (Figure 15-34). The ground-glass hepatocyte is larger than

Table 15-10 ■ GRADING OF DISEASE ACTIVITY IN CHRONIC HEPATITIS[a]

Grading Terminology		Criteria	
Semiquantitative	**Descriptive**	**Lymphocytic Piecemeal Necrosis**	**Lobular Inflammation and Necrosis**
0	Portal inflammation only; no activity	None	None
1	Minimal	Minimal, patchy	Minimal; occasional spotty necrosis
2	Mild	Mild; involving some or all portal tracts	Mild; little hepatocellular damage
3	Moderate	Moderate; involving all portal tracts	Moderate; with noticeable hepatocellular change
4	Severe	Severe; may have bridging fibrosis	Severe; with prominent diffuse hepatocellular damage

[a]When a discrepancy exists between criteria, the more severe lesion should determine the grade.

Table 15-11 ■ STAGING OF CHRONIC HEPATITIS

Staging Terminology		
Semiquantitative	**Descriptive**	**Criteria**
0	No fibrosis	Normal connective tissue
1	Portal fibrosis	Fibrous portal expansion
2	Periportal fibrosis	Periportal or rare portal-portal septa
3	Septal fibrosis	Fibrous septa with architectural distortion; no obvious cirrhosis
4	Cirrhosis	Cirrhosis

the normal hepatocyte and has a smooth, uniform, pale, eosinophilic cytoplasm, often with a clear halo. The nucleus may be displaced to the periphery. These cells show a positive staining reaction with orcein and aldehyde fuchsin. Immunohistochemical staining is more sensitive and specific. The hepatitis B core antigen (HBcAg) is identified predominantly in the nuclei (Figure 15-34), and may correspond with the so-called sanded nuclei seen on hematoxylin and eosin stains. The distribution pattern of the tissue markers varies with the type of hepatic disease and is related to the host's immune response. Immunocytochemical staining for HBsAg and hepatitis B early antigen is also available. Electron microscopic examination may reveal HBsAg in the cytoplasm of hepatocytes, as 22 nm spheres and rods (Figure 15-34).

Nonhepatotropic viruses that may involve the liver as part of a systemic infection include herpes simplex, human herpesvirus-6, varicella, adenovirus, ECHO virus, Epstein-Barr virus (EBV), parvovirus, and cytomegalovirus (CMV). The liver may also be affected in acquired immune deficiency syndrome (AIDS), and a chronic hepatitis-like disorder has been described in children with AIDS. Hepatic involvement can occur in rickettsial diseases. The hepatic lesion in childhood cases of Rocky Mountain spotted fever has been described elsewhere.

FULMINANT HEPATIC FAILURE

Fulminant hepatic failure is characterized clinically by altered mental status and coagulopathy of rapid onset (<8 weeks after jaundice) (88,99) (e136,e203,e379,e380,e410). Its etiology is variable around the world and includes viruses (most commonly HBV, EBV, herpes simplex viruses, CMV) (Figure 15-36), drugs (most commonly acetaminophen, other drugs with idiosyncratic reactions), pregnancy-induced, metabolic (inborn errors of metabolism), malignancy, and other rare causes. Ten to twenty percent of cases remain cryptogenic. Prognosis depends on age, etiology, and rapidity of onset of disease. A liver biopsy reveals zones of hepatocellular loss, a variable inflammatory reaction, and residual foci of hepatocytes (Figure 15-37). Residual hepatocytes have abnormalities ranging from steatosis to ballooning degeneration. Small regenerative nodules of hepatocytes may be seen at a somewhat later stage in the evolution of the process. In most cases, there are few clues about the etiology in the biopsy findings. Liver transplantation is often successful. New experimental treatments include use of extracorporeal liver assist devices and hepatocyte transplantation.

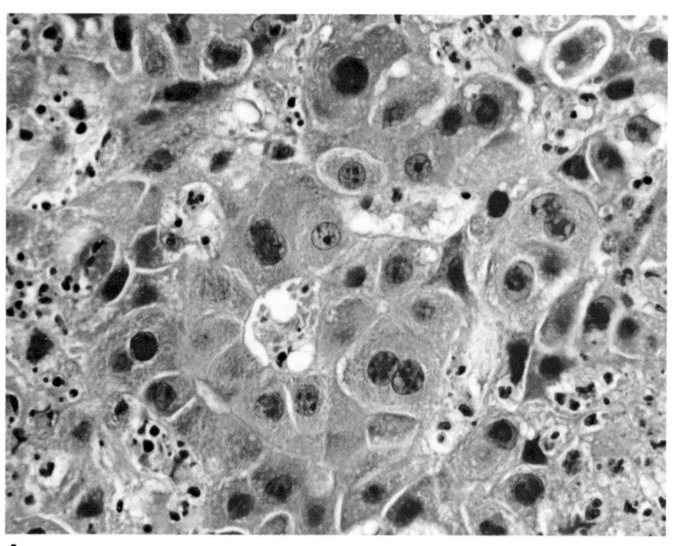
A

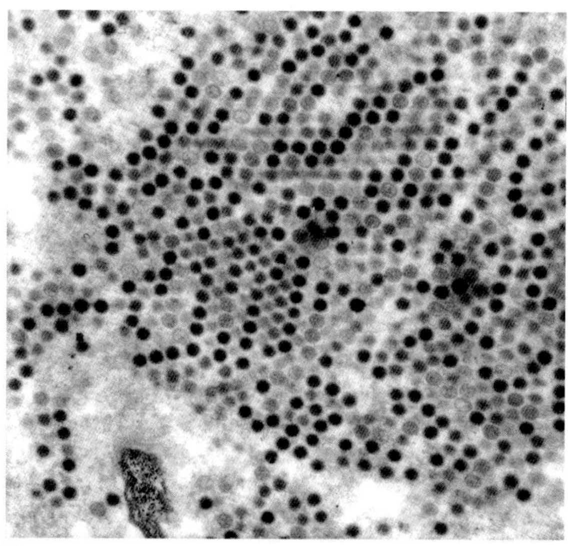
B

FIGURE 15-36 ■ Viral agents in fulminant hepatic failure. **A, B:** Adenovirus hepatitis with deeply eosinophilic cherry-red homogenous smudgy inclusions with hepatocytes (H&E, **A:** 400×), and adenovirus particles in nuclei by electron microscopy (**B:** 75,000×).

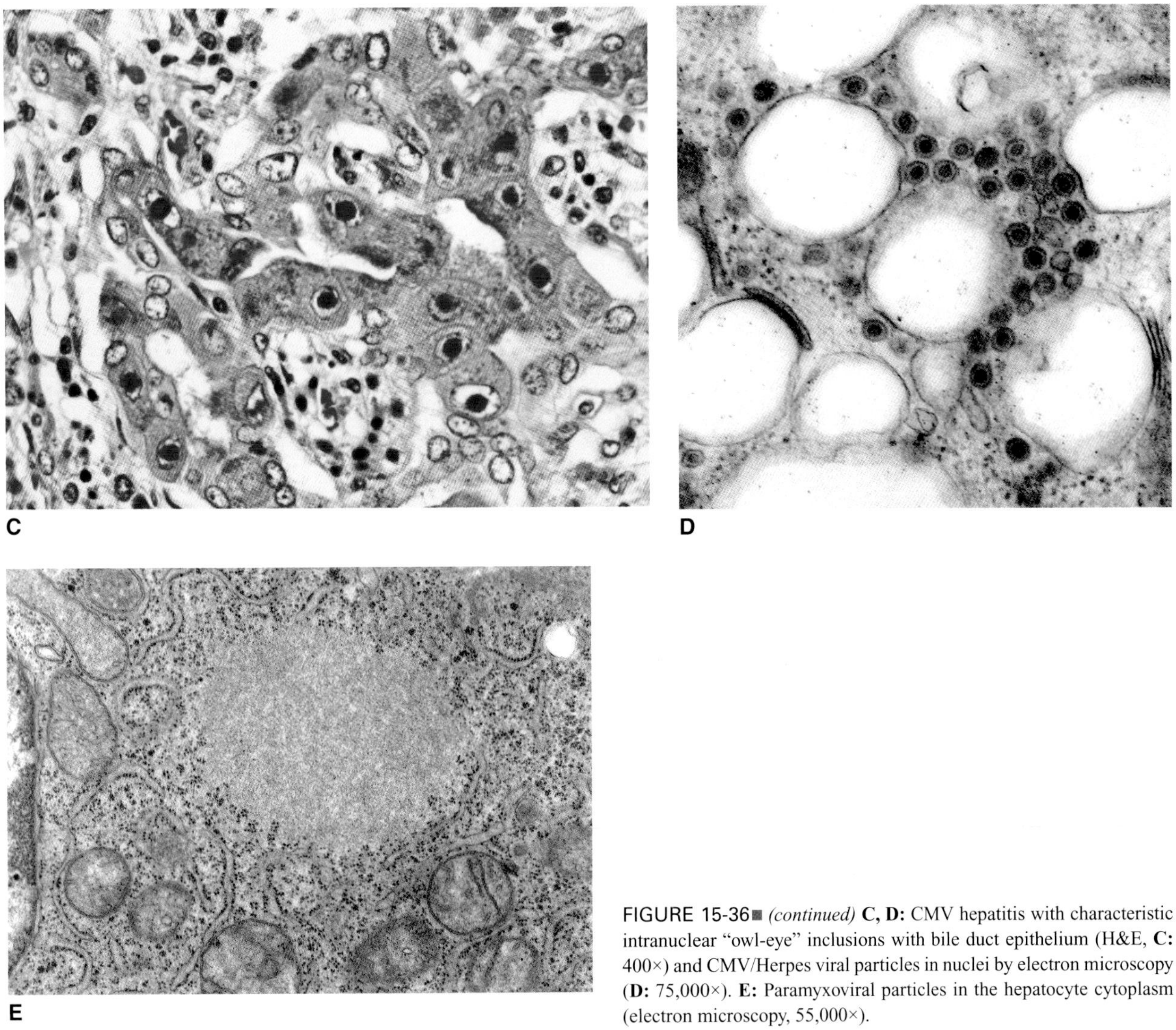

C

D

E

FIGURE 15-36 ■ *(continued)* **C, D:** CMV hepatitis with characteristic intranuclear "owl-eye" inclusions with bile duct epithelium (H&E, **C:** 400×) and CMV/Herpes viral particles in nuclei by electron microscopy (**D:** 75,000×). **E:** Paramyxoviral particles in the hepatocyte cytoplasm (electron microscopy, 55,000×).

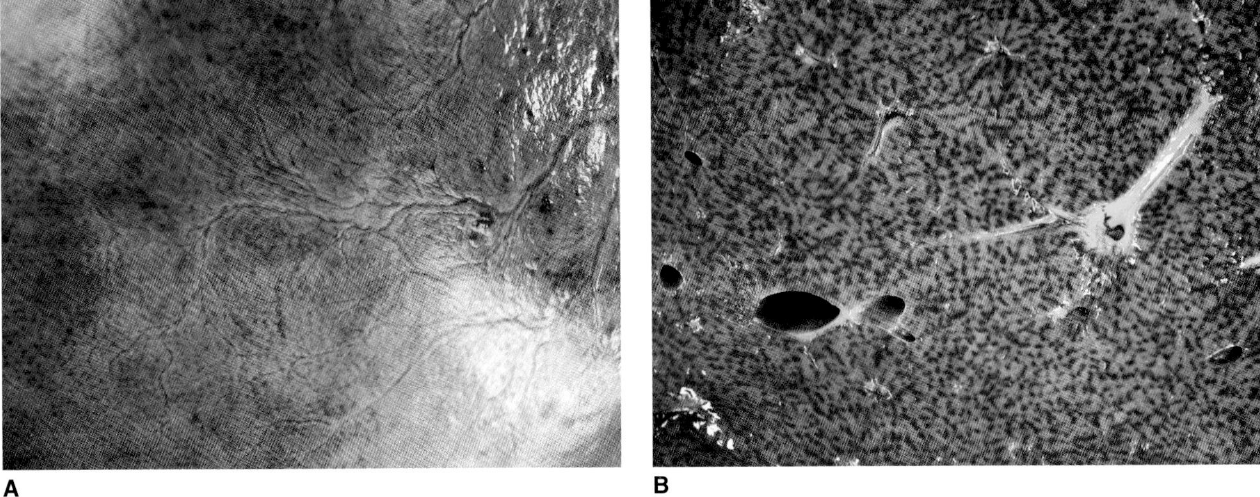

FIGURE 15-37 ■ Fulminant hepatic failure. **A:** Liver explant with tense, distended liver capsule. **B:** Liver explant cross section demonstrating diffuse liver necrosis with red-brown fine punctate areas representing viable liver parenchyma.

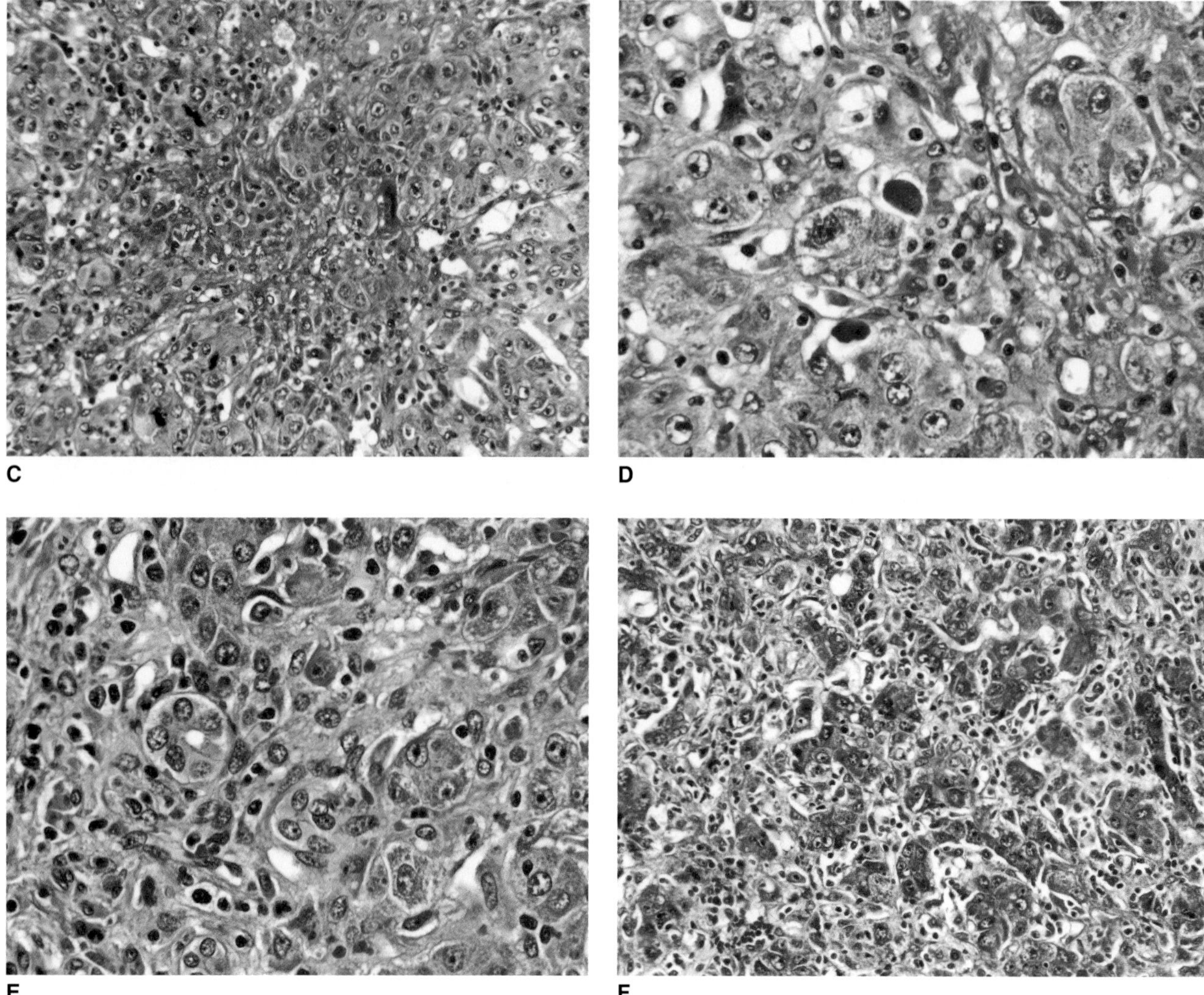

FIGURE 15-37 ■ *(continued)* **C:** Central area of hepatocyte necrosis with dense eosinophilia, hemorrhage in the background and necrotic hepatocytes (H&E, 200×). **D:** Residual bile ducts, hepatocytes organized into pseudoacini and necrotic hepatocytes (H&E, 400×). **E:** Residual bile ducts with rare hepatocytes and background of chronic inflammatory cells (H&E, 400×). **F:** Trichrome stain highlights residual bile ducts, loss of hepatocytes, and replacement by fibrotic tissue (200×).

PRIMARY SCLEROSING CHOLANGITIS AND AUTOIMMUNE HEPATITIS

PSC is a progressive hepatobiliary disease characterized by a cholestatic syndrome (98) (e21,e35,e116,e246,e351,e375, e394,e407,e408,e491,e636,e637,e703). Diagnostic imaging abnormalities consist of segmental narrowing and dilatation of intrahepatic and extrahepatic ducts. The disease is seen primarily in young men in the third to fifth decades of life, but it also seen in the pediatric population including neonates.

The pathogenesis is unknown, but a strong association with ulcerative colitis (UC) has been documented in most cases. Inflammatory bowel disease (UC) has been associated with sclerosing cholangitis in 70% of cases (98) (e21,e351,e394,e408). However, PSC is seen in only about 5% of patients with UC. Langerhans cell histiocytosis occurs in 15% of cases, and immunodeficiency is associated with another 10% of children. No apparent underlying disease is present in 24%, including cases of neonatal onset. The clinical presentation of childhood PSC is highly variable and frequently without features of cholestasis. Typically, elevated alkaline phosphatase (ALP) and bilirubin are noted. In addition, hypergammaglobulinemia, DRw52a (HLA subtype), perinuclear-antineutrophil cytoplasmic antibody (p-ANCA), and IgM elevation may be identified by serologic tests. Clinical similarity to AIH is common (152). Contrast digital imaging of the intrahepatic biliary tree by retrograde endoscopy shows a characteristic beaded appearance. This is due to strictures and secondary dilation of the affected bile ducts.

The histopathologic changes in the liver are not diagnostic in most cases (Figure 15-38). Portal fibrosis, pericholangitis, fibrous obliterative cholangitis, and cirrhosis are the range of microscopic features. Fibrous obliterative cholangitis consisting of concentric whorls of dense collagen, with an onion

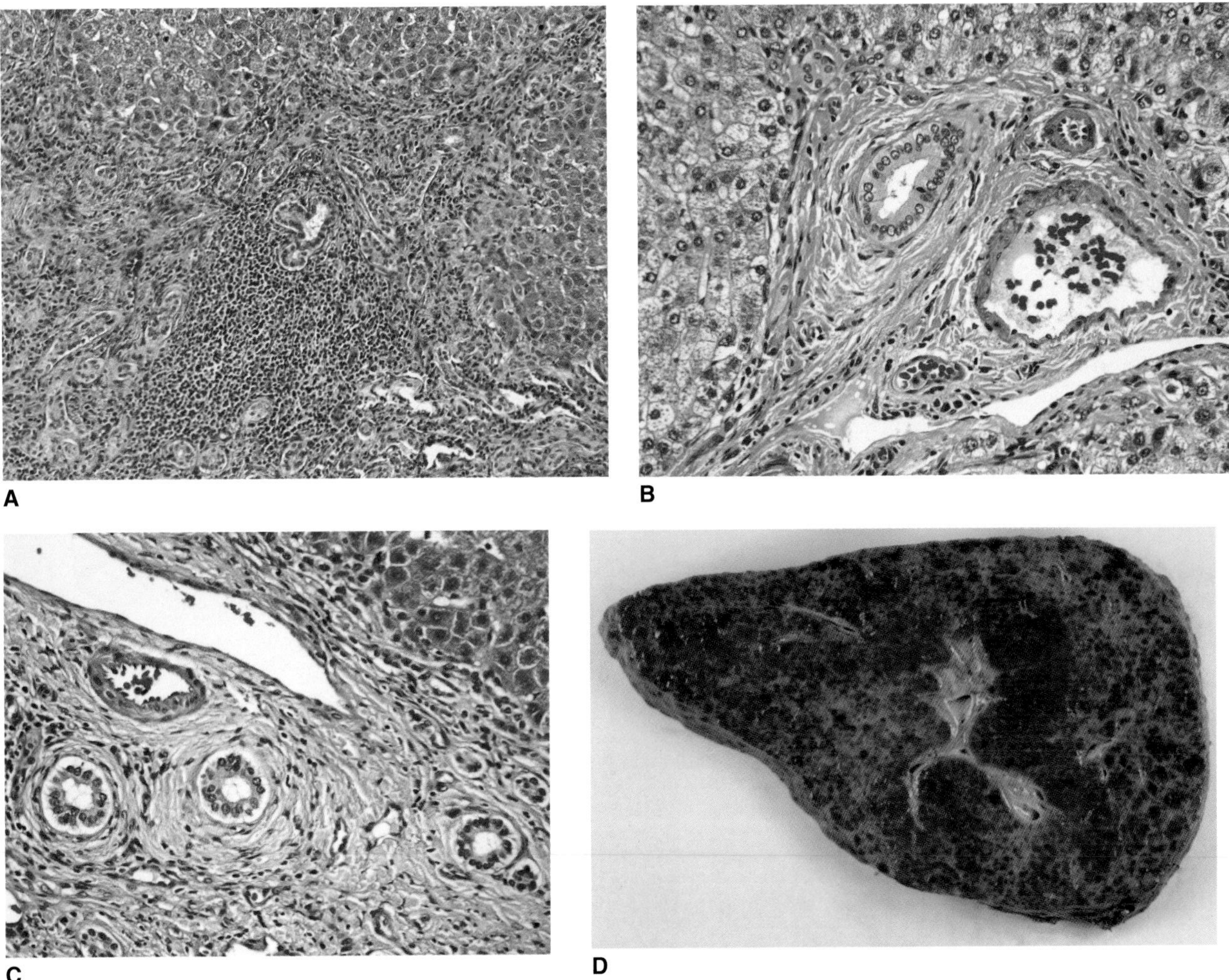

FIGURE 15-38 ■ Primary sclerosing cholangitis. **A:** Severe portal chronic inflammation with bile duct proliferation, fibrosis, and interface hepatitis (H&E, 100×). **B, C:** Concentric fibrosis around bile ducts (onion-skinning) and portal fibrosis (H&E, 200×). **D:** Liver explant for primary sclerosing cholangitis with diffuse bile pigmentation and biliary cirrhotic pattern.

skin appearance, surrounding the bile ducts is regarded as a characteristic lesion. This is seen only early in the evolution of the disease. Fibroinflammatory stricture of bile ducts may be seen at various sites from the ampulla of Vater to the interlobular bile ducts. Histopathologic staging of PSC is based upon degree of involvement (Stage I—portal; Stage II—periportal; Stage III—septal; Stage IV—cirrhosis). Stage I (portal) has concentric periductal fibrosis with a lymphocytic infiltrate around bile ducts. Stage II (periportal) has fibrosis extending in the periportal tissues with interface hepatitis and reactive bile ducts. Stage III (septal) has obliterated bile ducts and bridging fibrosis. Stage IV (cirrhosis) has biliary type cirrhosis.

Cholangiography is essential for diagnosis to evaluate medium to large intrahepatic ducts, since 40% of children lack extrahepatic duct involvement (152). The most serious complication is adenocarcinoma of the bile duct and colon in patients with concurrent PSC and UC (e376). The prognosis appears to be more favorable in children than in adults. Liver transplantation is required for children who progress to biliary cirrhosis and hepatic decompensation. Recurrence of PSC may occur in the transplanted liver.

AIH may be present in children with signs and symptoms of acute hepatitis (50% to 60%), fulminant liver failure (10%), or a more chronic, insidious onset (30% to 40%) (111,123) (e26,e74,e153,e256,e443,e444,e663,e699,e739). This disease is more typically seen in young and middle age women. Two types of AIH are recognized: type 1 with antinuclear antibodies (ANA), antismooth muscle antibodies (SMA), antiactin antibodies, soluble liver antigen, and acute asialoglycoprotein receptor; and type 2 with anti-LKM1. Younger children present with anti-LKM1 with or without ANA or SMA antibodies. There is no difference in clinical outcome between the types of AIH. Family history of autoimmune disorder is noted in 40% of cases. Affected children may have other autoimmune disorders including lymphocytic (Hashimoto) thyroiditis, rheumatoid arthritis, Sjögren syndrome, and UC. Hyperglobulinemia is a common feature. It is important to ensure that viral serologic markers are negative. Liver biopsy demonstrates plasma

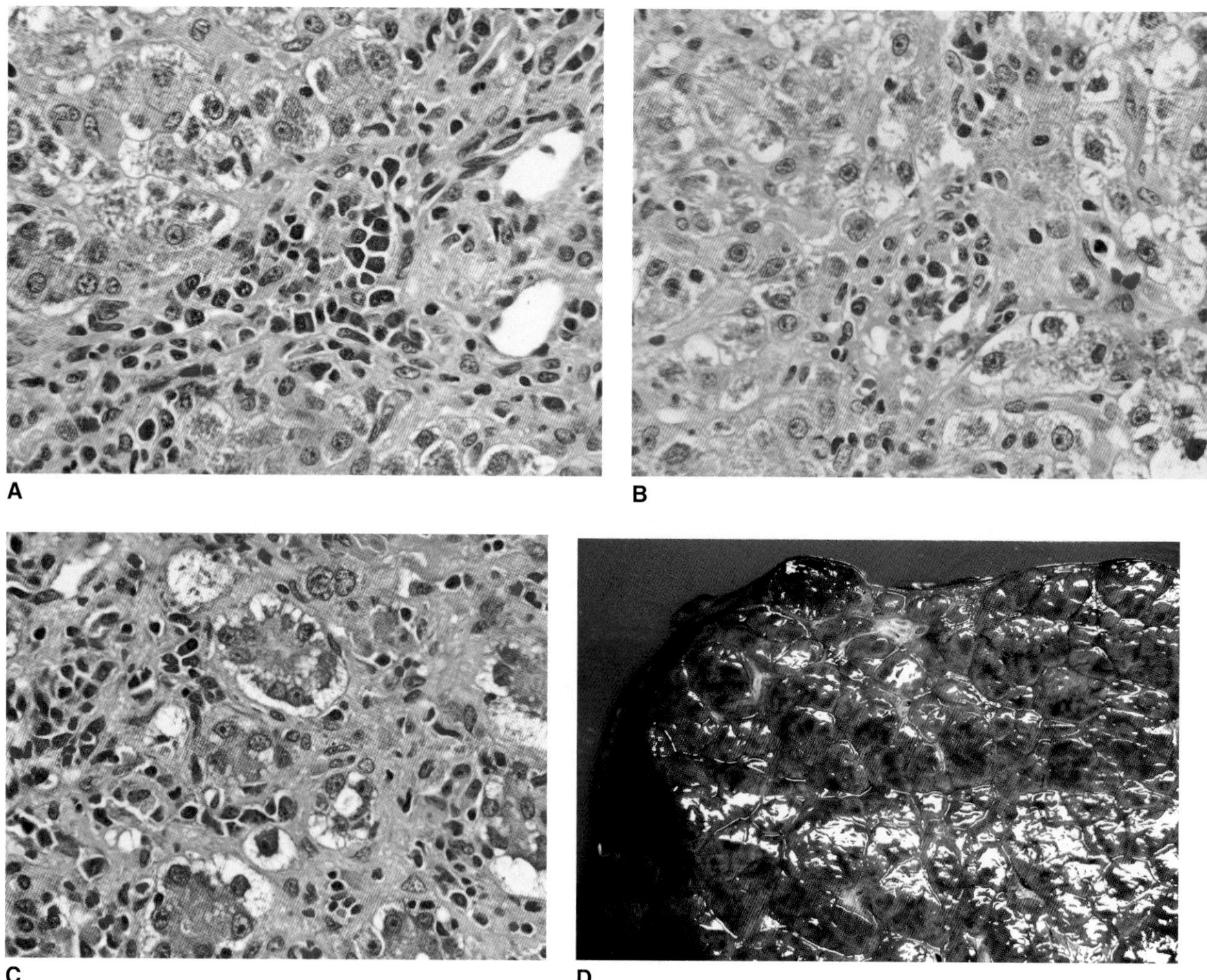

FIGURE 15-39 ■ Autoimmune hepatitis. **A, B:** Plasma cells within portal regions and within the hepatic lobules (H&E, 400×). **C:** Hepatocytes arranged in pseudoacinar pattern with occasional plasma cells and increased fibrous tissue (H&E, 400×). **D:** Explanted liver for autoimmune hepatitis with macronodular pattern of cirrhosis and bile staining.

cells within the chronic inflammatory infiltrate in the portal tracts and an aggressive interface hepatitis, which may lead to collapse (Figure 15-39). Marked lobular chronic inflammatory infiltrates with plasma cells may be seen. Hepatocellular injury with acinar (rosette) formation and syncytial giant hepatocytes can be features as well. Plasma cells with or without hepatocyte rosette formation are considered to be highly suggestive of AIH. However, one should remember that plasma cells can be seen in other chronic hepatitides as well. Because lymphoid aggregates may be seen in HCV, it is important to eliminate this from consideration. Cirrhosis develops in 90% of cases. In a certain proportion of children, serologic and histologic evidence is supportive of AIH at initial diagnostic evaluation. However, diagnostic imaging and liver biopsy have features that support PSC. When this occurs, the term autoimmune sclerosing cholangitis overlap syndrome is employed. These patients appear to respond to immune suppression therapy.

ABSCESSES

Pyogenic abscesses are uncommon in the liver in the pediatric patient and, when they occur, may be single or multiple (76,91) (e615,e623,e638). The infection may be hematogenous or ascend via the biliary tract. In the neonate, umbilical vein catheterization complicated by septic omphalitis poses an additional hazard. Ascending cholangitis may be associated with intrahepatic abscesses, especially after a portoenterostomy procedure for EHBA. Hepatic abscess may occur in the setting of a systemic disorder. In patients with congenital or acquired neutropenia or aplastic anemia, hepatic abscesses may show a paucity of neutrophils, and coagulative necrosis without liquefaction may be seen. Hepatic abscesses may be the initial presentation of chronic granulomatous disease (CGD) (91); as many as one-third of hepatic abscesses in children are a complication of CGD (72). These abscesses show a central area of suppuration, often with a surrounding palisade of macrophages. Pigmented lipid-laden histiocytes in the portal tracts and sinusoidal lining cells are characteristic of this process. Blunt trauma associated with hepatic necrosis may be complicated by abscess formation. Occasional reports have documented hepatic abscess without a predisposing condition. Amebic liver abscess may be seen in areas endemic for amebiasis.

Grossly, the abscesses may be multiple and range from small yellow foci scattered throughout the liver to large cavitary lesions with purulent debris. Microabscesses consist of focal collections of neutrophils with no zonal distribution. Larger abscesses show a central area of liquefaction necrosis in which degenerating neutrophils are seen. At the periphery, there is characteristically a mixed cellular infiltrate consisting of neutrophils and mononuclear cells and a variable fibroblastic proliferation.

Polymicrobial infection is present in about 80% of cases (2.4 isolates per specimen), with anaerobes and microaerophilic streptococci being more common (76) (e42,e88,e638). The predominant anaerobes implicated are Peptostreptococcus, *Bacteroides* sp., *Fusobacterium* sp., and *Clostridium* sp., whereas common aerobes implicated are *Escherichia coli*, Streptococcus group D, *Klebsiella pneumoniae*, and *Staphylococcus aureus*. Diminutive abscesses consisting of no more that a few neutrophils are seen in CMV hepatitis in immunosuppressed children and adults. The mortality rate for pyogenic liver abscesses has decreased to less than 10% with improved diagnostic imaging, percutaneous draining techniques, and antibiotics (e42).

PARASITIC DISEASES

A variety of parasitic diseases can involve the liver (144) (e250,e348,e395,e422,e588). Among the protozoal infections are toxoplasmosis, malaria, leishmaniasis, and amebiasis. Toxoplasma infections have a worldwide distribution. Infection may be transmitted through contact with house pets, such as cats. Congenital infections are an important cause of illness with prominent hepatic manifestations. Giant cell transformation of hepatocytes may be seen. Occasionally, the parasite may be demonstrable.

Acute *Plasmodium falciparum* malaria may be fatal. At autopsy, the liver is enlarged and tense with a dark red or slate gray color. There is marked engorgement of the sinusoids and central veins, and erythrocytes may contain parasites. There is Kupffer cell hyperplasia and phagocytosis of ruptured erythrocytes. Within Kupffer cells, the dark brown malarial pigment is a characteristic cytoplasmic feature. This hemazoin pigment is formed by the trophozoite from the breakdown of hemoglobin and does not give a positive Prussian blue reaction.

In leishmaniasis (kala-azar), hyperplastic Kupffer cells contain the parasites (Leishman-Donovan bodies). Infiltration with lymphocytes, plasma cells, and histiocytes may be seen in portal areas and lobules, and granulomas may form.

Amebic infection of the liver is the most frequent extraintestinal complication of the disease and it manifests usually as a single abscess, most often involving the right lobe. The abscess cavity contains red-brown, thick ("anchovy sauce-like") material. The abscess wall consists of a layer of necrotic parenchyma, external to which a mixed inflammatory cell infiltrate is seen. A fibrous capsule may be present, and the adjacent liver is compressed. Amebae may be demonstrable in the necrotic zone or in the compressed parenchyma as PAS-positive round or oval bodies about the size of macrophages.

Liver involvement may also occur in infestation by a variety of helminths. In schistosomiasis, liver injury results through migration of ova in the portal venous system. The ova elicit a granulomatous response, and in severe infection with *Schistosoma japonicum*, diffuse fibrosis and portal hypertension may result. Liver flukes (*Clonorchis sinensis*, *Fasciola hepatica*) inhabit major intrahepatic ducts and cause inflammation and epithelial injury. Biliary hyperplasia, cholangitis, and periductal fibrosis are common findings with liver flukes. Hydatid cyst is caused by infestation with the larval stage of the cestodes *Echinococcus granulosus* and *E. multilocularis*. The right lobe is more frequently involved. The cyst has a thick, white wall and a cavity in which the fluid contains fine granular sediment ("hydatid sand"). The cyst may be unilocular or multilocular. The cyst has a characteristic laminated outer layer and an inner layer containing multiple nuclei. Brood capsules are formed from numerous scolices and arise from the inner germinal layer. Invaginations of the cyst give rise to daughter cysts. Secondary cholangitis may result from intrahepatic bile duct obstruction. Toxocariasis (visceral larva migrans) results from migration of the larvae of *Toxocara canis* or *T. cati* (144) (e395). Granulomas containing larval fragments may be seen in the liver. Ascariasis infestation is associated with numerous foul-smelling cavities in the liver upon gross examination. The liver tissue demonstrates necrotic debris with a granulomatous and eosinophil inflammatory response to degenerated parasites.

GRANULOMATOUS HEPATITIS

Granulomas in the liver are associated with the same etiologic agents as granulomas at other sites (97) (e65,e189, e330,e358,e748). The frequency of granulomas in the liver varies with geographic location, due to variation in causative agents in different populations. The etiologic associations are shown in Table 15-12. Nevertheless, tuberculosis and sarcoidosis account for the majority of cases.

Histopathologic evaluation includes a search for an etiologic agent with appropriate special stains, especially for acid-fast bacilli and fungi. The auramine O stain for fluorescent microscopy is more sensitive in demonstrating acid-fast bacilli than standard stains. PCR for mycobacteria is also possible from formalin-fixed and paraffin-embedded tissue.

Table 15-12 ■ HEPATIC GRANULOMAS

Bacterial
Tuberculosis
Atypical mycobacteria
Listeriosis
Tularemia
Brucellosis
Rochalimaea henselae (cat scratch disease)
Mycotic
Candida
Histoplasmosis
Cryptococcosis
Blastomycosis
Coccidioidomycosis
Rickettsial and spirochetal
Q fever
Syphilis
Viral
Infectious mononucleosis
Cytomegalovirus
Parasitic and protozoal
Schistosomiasis
Visceral larva migrans
Ascariasis
Toxoplasmosis
Leishmaniasis (kala-azar)
Drug-related
Sulfonamides
Diphenylhydantoin
Sulfonyl urea compounds
Allopurinol
Miscellaneous
CGD of childhood
Sarcoidosis
Hodgkin lymphoma
Crohn disease
Foreign body
Undetermined etiology

VASCULAR DISORDERS

Cavernous Transformation of the Portal Vein

The most important entity in this group of disorders is portal vein obstruction due to thrombosis and cavernous transformation resulting from recanalization of the thrombus (e25,e290,e299,e333,e783). This is the most frequent cause of noncirrhotic portal hypertension in children. Extrahepatic causes of portal hypertension, including portal vein obstruction, are reported in approximately 50% of cases (e25). Umbilical vein catheterization and omphalitis have been incriminated most frequently, with other mechanisms including local infections, portoenterostomy, sepsis, and chemotherapy (e299,e333). Hypercoagulopathy secondary to protein C, protein S, and antithrombin III deficiencies are frequently found in children with portal vein obstruction (e186). The liver is histologically normal in most cases of portal vein thrombosis or cavernous transformation of the portal vein.

Budd-Chiari Syndrome

Obstruction of the hepatic veins may occur in the main branches or ostia leading to Budd-Chiari syndrome (198) (e38,e188,e264,e294,e537,e731). The lesion occurs most frequently in women in the third and fourth decades of life and is uncommon in childhood. In young women, there is an association with contraceptive medications and pregnancy. Paroxysmal nocturnal hemoglobinuria, sickle cell disease, nephrotic syndrome, TPN, blunt trauma, myeloproliferative disorders, and coagulation abnormalities may also be associated with Budd-Chiari syndrome. Venous occlusion by tumor occurs less frequently in childhood than in adults. Congenital webs and obliteration of the suprahepatic inferior vena cava are seen in children. Budd-Chiari syndrome may occur after giant omphalocele repair. Thrombosis of hepatic veins and retrohepatic inferior vena cava may result from direct pressure on the hepatic venous outlet after visceral reduction and final abdominal wall closure. Gaucher disease has also been implicated in rare instances.

Clinical features associated with Budd-Chiari syndrome include ascites and hepatomegaly (198) (e38,e188, e264,e294,e537,e731). The liver, in early stages, shows severe centrilobular congestion, hepatocyte degeneration and loss, and erythrocytes in the space previously occupied by the liver cells in zone 3 (Figure 15-40). Central veins are not affected, but sublobular veins may contain thrombi. Pericentral fibrosis with extension into adjacent parenchyma causes distortion of the architecture and may progress to cirrhosis.

Venoocclusive Disease

Venoocclusive disease (VOD) (18) (e50,e104,e142,e173, e287,e393) was initially described in Jamaican children and ascribed to pyrrolizidine alkaloids in Senecio tea. Other etiologic associations are cytotoxic agents used

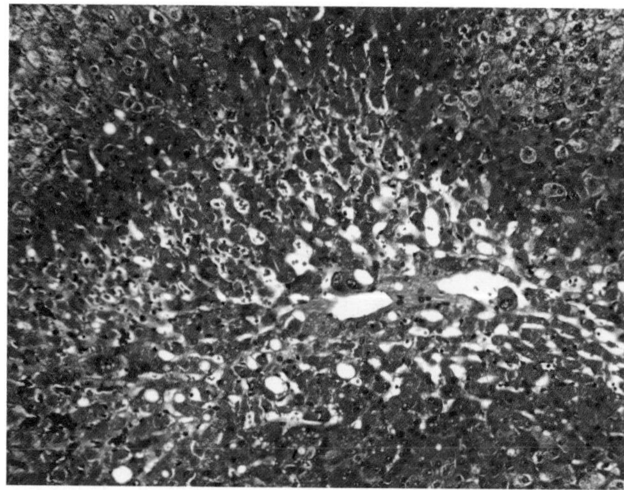

FIGURE 15-40■ Budd Chiari syndrome. Centrilobular ischemia and hepatocyte degeneration with less affected hepatocytes away from Zone 3 (H&E, 200×).

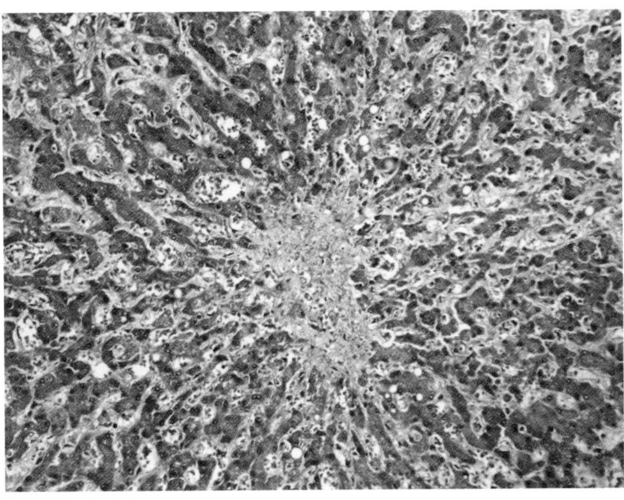

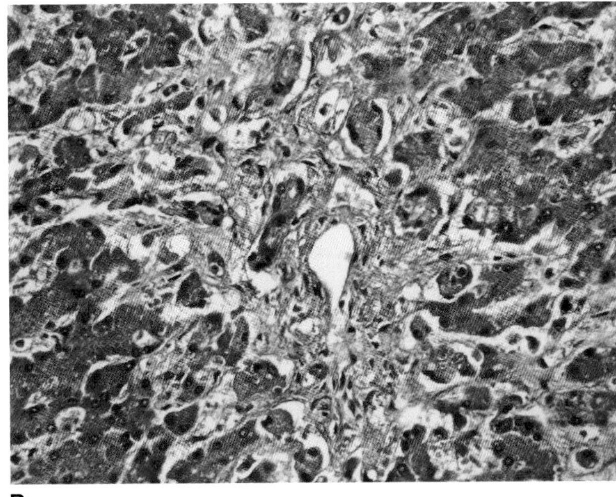

A B

FIGURE 15-41 ▪ Venoocclusive disease. **A, B:** Partial to nearly complete obliteration of central veins with pericentral vein fibrosis (H&E, 400×).

for malignant disease therapy and in preparation for bone marrow transplantation, hereditary tyrosinemia, familial immune deficiency disorders, and irradiation (e500,e509). The condition has also been described in newborn infants (e80,e167,e313).

Early in the course of the disease, there is massive centrilobular hemorrhage with hepatocyte degeneration or loss. The abnormal central veins have narrowed lumina and widened subendothelial spaces, containing collagen fibers, fragmented cells, cell debris, and hemosiderin-laden macrophages. At this stage, central vein abnormalities are subtle and require special stains to demonstrate collagen deposition. Later in the course of the disease, there is intimal thickening due to reticulin and collagen deposition, and presence of foam cells, causing partial or complete obliteration of vessel lumens (Figure 15-41). Central hepatocytes (zone 3) are atrophic, and cholestasis may be seen. Pericentral fibrosis with extension into the adjacent parenchyma distorts the architecture, but true cirrhosis is infrequent. Allograft rejection may resemble VOD, and this needs to be taken into consideration prior to making a diagnosis of VOD.

Peliosis Hepatis

Peliosis hepatis was initially described in adults with chronic debilitating diseases, steroid medications, HIV, mycobacterial infection, and wasting conditions (186) (e173,e174,e334,e592,e729). This condition was described in a child with CF who died at the age of 11 years, after which additional reports documented peliosis hepatis in the pediatric age group, including the neonatal period. Two previously healthy young children in whom peliosis hepatis presented as acute hepatic failure associated with *E. coli* pyelonephritis have also been reported. Both patients had active intraperitoneal hemorrhage from the peliotic liver lesions (e312). Focal peliosis hepatis has been found incidentally in five children succumbing to an asphyxiating death (e614). Androgenic anabolic steroids, oral contraceptives, thiopurines, and danazol play a role in development of this lesion. Resolution of the lesion tends to occur after discontinuing such medications. Liver infection by *Bartonella henselae* in HIV-infected patients is known to lead to peliosis hepatis (186). Also, peliosis hepatis occurs with increased frequency in renal transplant recipients (e107). The liver contains grossly identifiable multiple blood-filled spaces, which, on microscopic examination, consist of pools of erythrocytes in the hepatic lobule with no zonal predilection (Figure 15-42). A definitive endothelial lining is not identified. The early lesion consists of localized areas of sinusoidal dilatation, likely due to disruption and injury to the sinusoidal endothelial cells. Disruption of sinusoidal reticulin fibers may be demonstrated using typical reticulin stains. In HIV-infected patients with Bartonella-associated lesions, there may be myxoid perisinusoidal stroma with granular clumped material. Within the granular material, organisms may be detected with Warthin-Starry staining and PCR. Rupture and hemoperitoneum are potential complications.

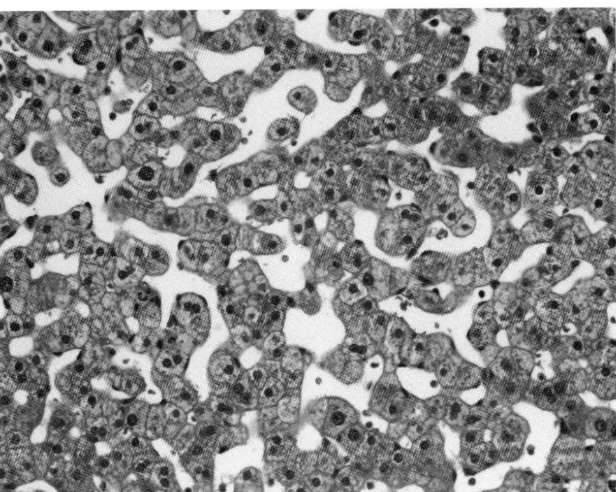

FIGURE 15-42 ▪ Peliosis hepatis. Early lesion of peliosis with widely dilated sinusoids, which tends to be localized due to sinusoidal endothelial injury (H&E, 400×).

Hepatic Hemorrhage

Hepatic hemorrhage may occur as a result of blunt or sharp trauma (e215,e223,e625). Spontaneous subcapsular hemorrhage in the newborn occurs most frequently in premature infants and may be a cause of morbidity. A review of infant autopsies showed a 15% incidence of subcapsular hemorrhage. At-risk infants tend to be premature male infants with chronic problems during gestation and complications during labor and delivery, as well as sepsis. Hemoperitoneum due to liver rupture may lead to hypovolemic shock.

TOTAL PARENTERAL NUTRITION RELATED INJURY

Hepatic abnormalities secondary to TPN were first described in a premature infant. The infant died after 71 days, and the liver at postmortem examination showed cirrhosis, bile duct proliferation, and cholestasis. Subsequent reports have confirmed the association of hepatobiliary dysfunction with TPN (62) (e90,e259,e337,e451,e556,e706). The associated cholestasis is seen most frequently in the premature infant, with low birth weight and low gestational age being the greatest risk factors. The incidence and severity of the disease are greater in infants with gastrointestinal disease or intestinal resection.

Cholestasis increases with prolonged TPN infusion (62). Most infants with TPN-associated cholestasis and subsequent cirrhosis have severe gastrointestinal disease, such as necrotizing enterocolitis, gastroschisis, and volvulus, or have undergone intestinal resection. These infants are also subject to infection, cardiopulmonary dysfunction, shock, and hypoxia. Toxicity of the infusate, especially amino acid composition and lipid content, has been considered a factor in liver dysfunction associated with TPN.

The onset of jaundice is insidious, and the infant may manifest no other evidence of hepatic disease. The earliest biochemical abnormality is the elevation of serum bile acid concentration, as early as 5 days after beginning TPN, and routine study of serum bile acids may help in diagnosis. Hyperbilirubinemia is usually seen 3 to 4 weeks after TPN initiation.

Histopathologic changes noted in TPN-associated disease are nonspecific and quite variable (Figure 15-43). Because

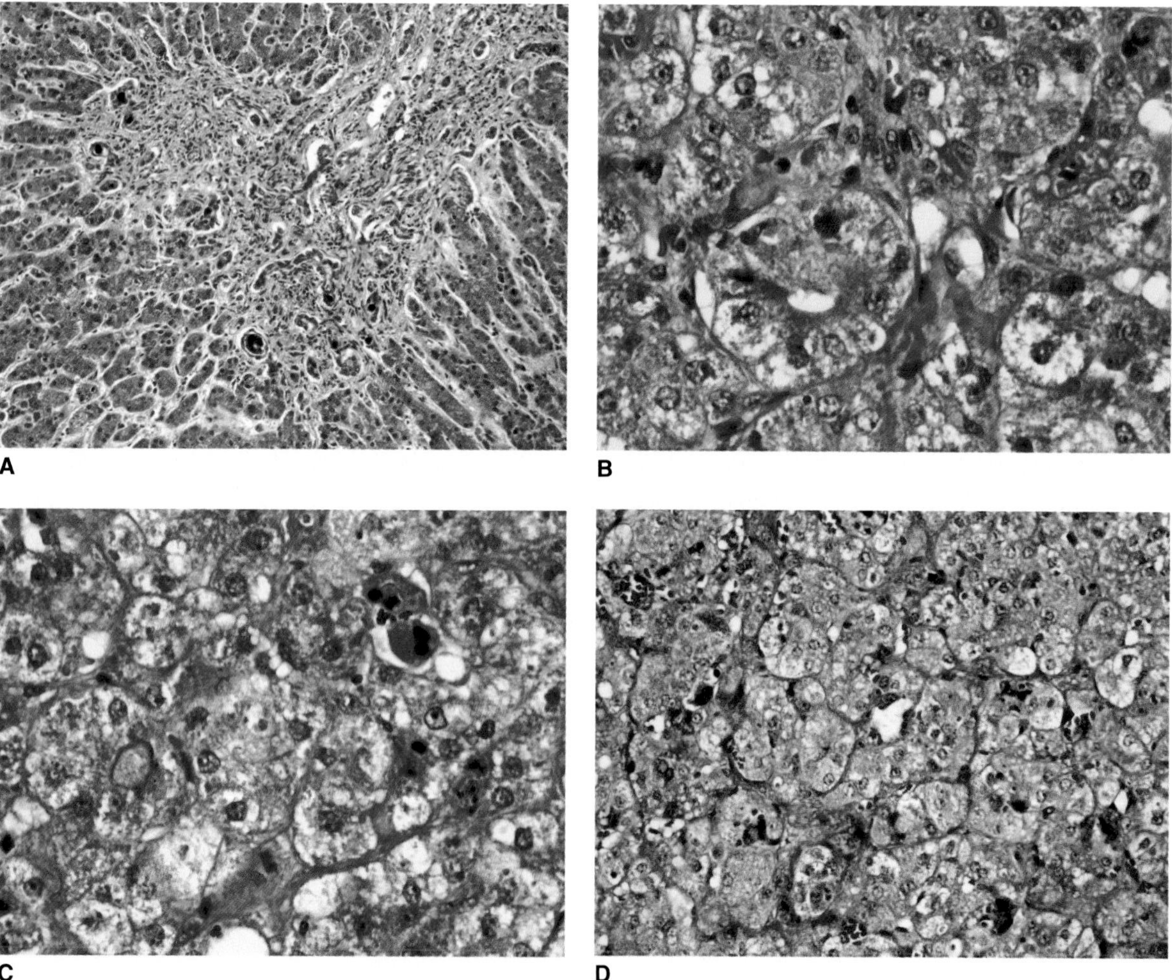

FIGURE 15-43 ■ Total parenteral nutrition. **A:** Portal tract expansion by fibrous tissue with bile duct proliferation and cholestasis (H&E, 100×). **B, C:** Pseudoacinar arrangement of hepatocytes with obvious cytoplasmic cholestasis, apoptotic hepatocytes (**C**), and increased sinusoidal fibrous tissue (H&E, 400×). **D:** Trichrome staining highlights pseudoacinar pattern and lobular fibrosis (H&E, 200×).

there is no specific clinical, biochemical, or histopathologic marker, the diagnosis remains one of exclusion. Canalicular and hepatocellular cholestasis, most pronounced in zone 3, is the initial finding and a constant feature of TPN. There is lobular disarray with ballooned hepatocytes. Kupffer cell hyperplasia is present, with the Kupffer cells containing lipofuscin pigment. Iron pigment is demonstrable within hepatocytes. Giant cell transformation, pseudoacinar formation, and scattered foci of hepatocyte necrosis may be present. Extramedullary hematopoiesis may be prominent. Focal inflammation is usually seen and may vary from mild to severe. The cellular infiltrate is predominantly lymphocytic, but neutrophils and eosinophils may also be present. A pericholangitis may be seen, along with focal fibrosis of variable degree. The vast majority of patients recover with clearing of the jaundice after cessation of TPN, and commencement of enteral feedings. In repeat liver biopsies, cholestasis usually clears. Hepatocyte ballooning, lobular disarray, and occasional cholestasis and portal fibrosis may persist. However, cirrhosis and hepatic failure have been noted in infants receiving TPN.

CIRRHOSIS

Cirrhosis has been defined by the Working Group of the World Health Organization as a diffuse process characterized by fibrosis and conversion of normal liver architecture into structurally abnormal nodules (9). Cirrhosis is the end result of hepatic cell necrosis caused by a variety of injurious agents (9,100) (e602). Necrosis is associated with collapse, fibrosis, and regeneration, resulting in the formation of nodules.

The classification of cirrhosis may be etiologic or morphologic. Cirrhosis has many etiologies. Many metabolic disorders are associated with cirrhosis and have been reviewed elsewhere (65). Alper disease, a putative mitochondrial disorder, is characterized by progressive neuronal degeneration and cirrhosis in childhood (e8,e191,e273). Alcoholic cirrhosis, a common cause of liver injury in adults, may rarely be seen in adolescents. Hepatic changes resembling adult alcohol-associated injury has been described in the fetal alcohol syndrome (e382). Cardiac cirrhosis in the pediatric population occurs most commonly in association with congenital heart disease (e383). Hematologic conditions, such as hemophilia, can be associated with progressive liver disease (e282). The role of trace metals in childhood cirrhosis has been detailed elsewhere (e241). Gallbladder duplication has been described in association with childhood obstructive biliary disease and biliary cirrhosis (e253). Etiologic associations with cirrhosis in childhood are presented in Table 15-13. Establishing the etiology requires demonstration of the specific histopathologic characteristics of a disease, such as AIAT stored in hepatocytes, ground-glass hepatocytes in HBV, or biochemical evaluation in metabolic disorders. As in the adult, cirrhosis in childhood may be cryptogenic, with failure to identify an etiologic agent in the explanted liver.

Table 15-13 ■ CIRRHOSIS IN INFANCY AND CHILDHOOD

Causes of Cirrhosis	Related Disorder
Infections	Neonatal viral infection
	Neonatal hepatitis
	Viral hepatitis
	CAH
	Syphilis
Biliary obstruction	EHBA
	Choledochal cyst
	Familial cholestatic syndromes
	Paucity of intrahepatic bile ducts
	Cholangitis
Vascular disease	Hepatic vein occlusion
	VOD
	Constrictive pericarditis
	Chronic congestive cardiac failure
	Rendu-Osler-Weber disease
Hereditary syndromes	Cerebrohepatorenal (Zellweger syndrome)
	CF
	Indian childhood cirrhosis
	CHF
Metabolic abnormalities	Galactosemia
	Fructosemia
	Tyrosinemia
	Glycogenoses, types III and IV
	A1AT deficiency
	Gaucher disease
	Niemann-Pack disease
	Wolman disease
	Cholesterol ester storage disease
	Mucopolysaccharidoses
	Wilson disease
	Hemochromatoses
	Arginosuccinic aciduria
	Cystinosis
	Porphyria
Miscellaneous	TPN
	Malnutrition
	Obesity
	Alcohol
	Sclerosing cholangitis
	Histiocytosis X
	Drugs

Morphologic classification is based on nodule size. In micronodular cirrhosis, nodules measure less than 3 mm in diameter and are relatively uniform throughout the liver. Fibrous septa are delicate and extend from portal to central areas or encircle the lobule. Macronodular cirrhosis is characterized by nodules larger than 3 mm, usually with broad bands of fibrous tissue (Figure 15-44). Large nodules contain several lobules in which portal areas and central veins are identifiable. In mixed type cirrhosis, the liver contains an approximately equal proportion of small and large nodules. Transformation of one type to another can occur with continuing necrosis, collapse, and fibrosis. In some conditions,

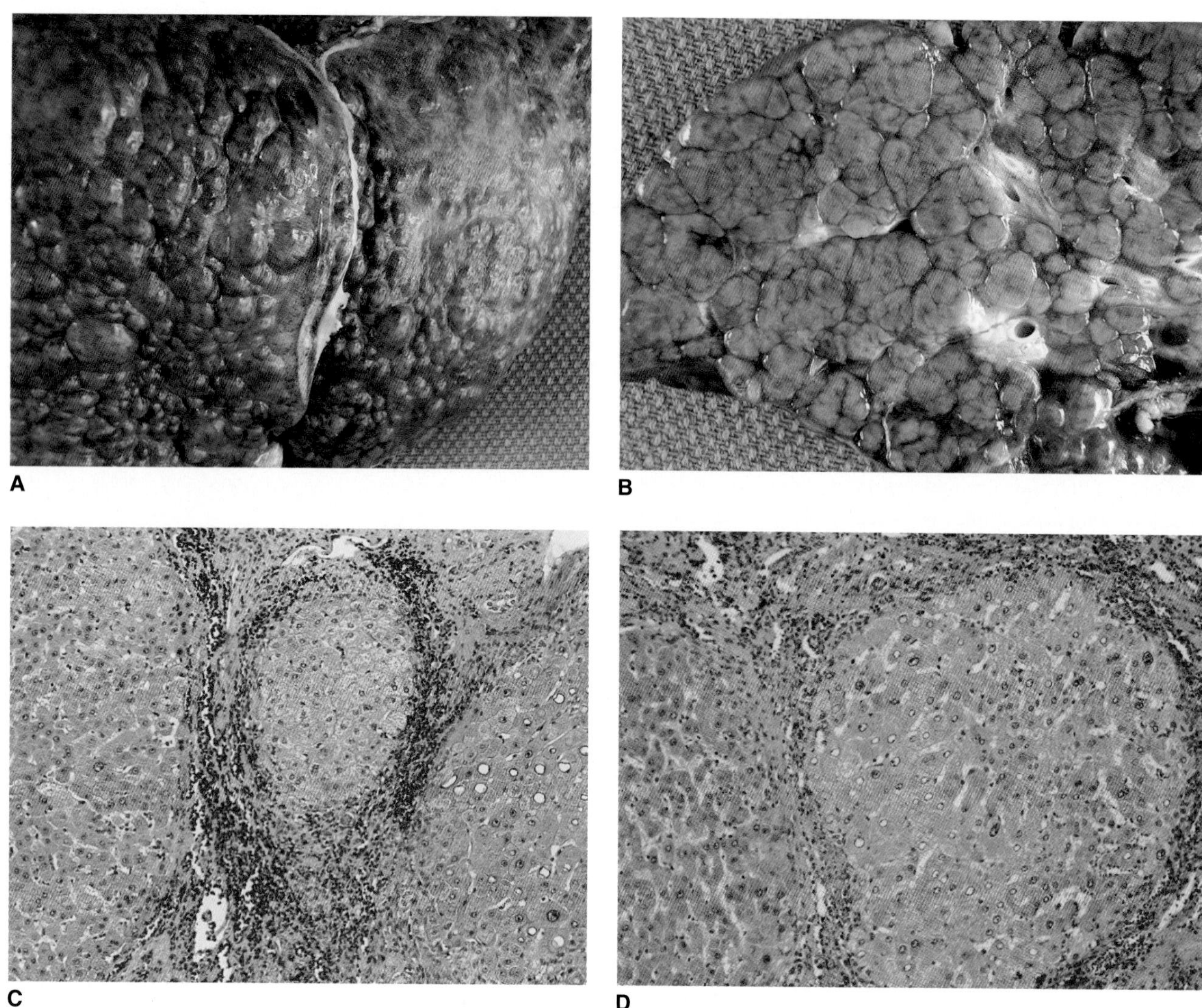

FIGURE 15-44 ■ Cirrhosis. **A, B:** Liver explant with a cirrhotic surface and cross section demonstrating numerous macronodules and micronodules. **C, D:** Fibrous tissue separates nodules of hepatocytes lacking central veins from each other. Note the variable size to the nodules (H&E, 200×).

cirrhosis is predominantly macronodular, such as after submassive bridging hepatic necrosis due to hepatitis or toxic agents. A predominantly micronodular cirrhosis is associated with biliary atresia and cholestatic syndromes. However, considerable overlaps exist owing to the transformation that may occur between the various morphologic types of cirrhosis, and the etiology of cirrhosis cannot be ascertained from the morphologic type of cirrhosis in all cases. This morphologic classification has therefore fallen out of favor.

Activity of cirrhosis is evaluated by identifying continuing hepatocellular necrosis and the degree of septal inflammation. Portal hypertension with all its sequelae is a frequent complication (e405), although portal hypertension may also be noncirrhotic in origin. Noncirrhotic portal hypertension may be suspected when the patient presents with portal hypertension without parenchymal dysfunction (as reflected by maintained albumin level and prothrombin time indicating preserved synthetic function) (e594).

Putative preneoplastic hepatic lesions may be found in cirrhotic livers. Liver cell dysplasia (large cell dysplasia) is characterized by nuclear and cytoplasmic enlargement, nuclear hyperchromasia, prominent nucleoli, and occasionally, multinucleation (8). Adenomatous hyperplasia (macroregenerative nodule) is a nodular lesion that occurs in cirrhosis and is thought to progress to HCC through an intermediate lesion termed atypical adenomatous hyperplasia (small cell dysplasia) (130). Atypical adenomatous hyperplasia occurs as an ill-defined nodule within a cirrhotic nodule (the so-called nodule-in-nodule formation), identified by compression of surrounding reticulin fibers and a different orientation of the liver plates. The evidence suggests that this lesion, rather than liver cell dysplasia, is more likely the precursor of HCC in a cirrhotic liver. Although it typically takes many years for HCC to develop, HCC may be associated with cirrhosis even in a neonate (e434).

Table 15-14 ■ HEPATICTUMORS IN PEDIATRIC PATIENTS, BIRTHTO 20YEARS (AFIP 1970–1999)

Type of Tumor	N	%
Hepatoblastoma	198	27.6
Hepatocellular carcinoma	135	18.9
Infantile hemangioendothelioma	119	16.5
Focal nodular hyperplasia	72	10.1
Mesenchymal hamartoma	57	8.0
Undifferentiated "embryonal" sarcoma	52	7.2
Nodular regenerative hyperplasia	32	4.5
Hepatocellular adenoma	27	3.8
Angiosarcoma	17	2.4
Embryonal rhabdomyosarcoma	7	1.0
TOTAL	716	100.0

HEPATIC TUMORS

Primary hepatic neoplasms account for 0.5% to 2.0% of all pediatric neoplasms and comprise a variety of benign and malignant epithelial and mesodermal tumors. Incidences of these tumors change significantly from birth to 20 years of age (Tables 15-14 to 15-16). Of 716 cases of the 10 most commonly occurring hepatic neoplasms seen at the Armed Forces Institute of Pathology between 1970 and 1999, hepatoblastoma, HCC, and hemangioendothelioma accounted for almost 65% (see Table 15-14).

FOCAL NODULAR HYPERPLASIA

Focal nodular hyperplasia (FNH) is a benign tumorlike lesion of the liver. Rather than a true neoplasm, it is considered to be the result of a hyperplastic response to hemodynamic disturbance related to vascular abnormalities. Although it most commonly occurs in women of childbearing and middle age, nearly 8% of cases present in the first 15 years of life, with a slightly increased frequency in those 6 to 10 years of age (39%) and a distinct female predominance of more than 3:1 (171) (Figure 15-45A).

Table 15-15 ■ HEPATICTUMORS IN PEDIATRIC PATIENTS, BIRTHTO 2YEARS (AFIP 1970–1999)

Type of Tumor	N	%
Hepatoblastoma	124	43.5
Infantile hemangioendothelioma	103	36.1
Mesenchymal hamartoma	38	13.3
Nodular regenerative hyperplasia	6	2.1
Hepatocellular carcinoma	4	1.4
Angiosarcoma	4	1.4
Focal nodular hyperplasia	3	1.1
Undifferentiated "embryonal" sarcoma	3	1.1
Hepatocellular adenoma	0	0
Embryonal/rhabdomyosarcoma	0	0
TOTAL	285	100.0

Table 15-16 ■ HEPATICTUMORS IN PEDIATRIC PATIENTS, 5–20YEARS (AFIP 1970–1999)

Type of Tumor	N	%
Hepatocellular carcinoma	96	36.6
Focal nodular hyperplasia	40	15.3
Undifferentiated "embryonal" sarcoma	39	14.9
Nodular regenerative hyperplasia	26	9.9
Hepatocellular adenoma	22	8.4
Hepatoblastoma	22	8.4
Angiosarcoma	6	2.3
Mesenchymal hamartoma	5	1.9
Infantile hemangioendothelioma	4	1.5
Embryonal rhabdomyosarcoma	2	.8
TOTAL	262	100.0

[a]Portions of this section were adapted from Stocker, JT. Hepatic tumors in children. In: Suchy FJ, *Liver disease in children*. 2nd ed. Philadelphia: Lippincott Williams and Wilkins. In press.

Pathogenesis

In 1985, Wanless and collaborators proposed that FNH is a hyperplastic response of the hepatic parenchyma to a preexisting local arterial spiderlike malformation, likely with a developmentally abnormal origin (e752). FNH is also related to well-known vascular diseases, such as hereditary hemorrhagic telangiectasia or congenital portal vein absence (e24,e96,e165). Hepatocellular hyperplasia in FNH is thought to be secondary to increased arterial flow and hyperperfusion of localized parenchyma (e228,e229,e752). An association between the use of oral contraceptives in older children and adults and the development of FNH is still under debate. However, some studies suggest that the use of contraceptive pills may increase the size of the nodules (e433,e601) or may predispose to bleeding (e634).

A variety of associations have been anecdotally noted in children with FNH (Table 15-17) (e497,e586). FNH is associated with vascular abnormalities, including hepatic hemangiomas, which supports the concept of a vascular component in the pathogenesis of this lesion. FNH has also been reported in patients with a variety of nonhepatic tumors and tumorlike conditions (21).

Clinical Features

The vast majority of lesions (90%) are asymptomatic, presenting as a mass on routine physical examination or as an incidental finding at surgery or autopsy. Symptomatic cases may present with abdominal pain, weight loss, vomiting, or diarrhea. Laboratory parameters in patients with FNH are rarely abnormal, and alpha-fetoprotein (AFP) is not elevated.

Imaging studies can be extremely helpful in differentiating FNH from other benign or malignant hepatic lesions (e20,e295), especially hypervascular lesions such as hepatocellular adenoma (HCA), HCC, and hypervascular metastases. Color power Doppler allows, in most cases, its distinction from other focal liver lesions (e648). In contrast

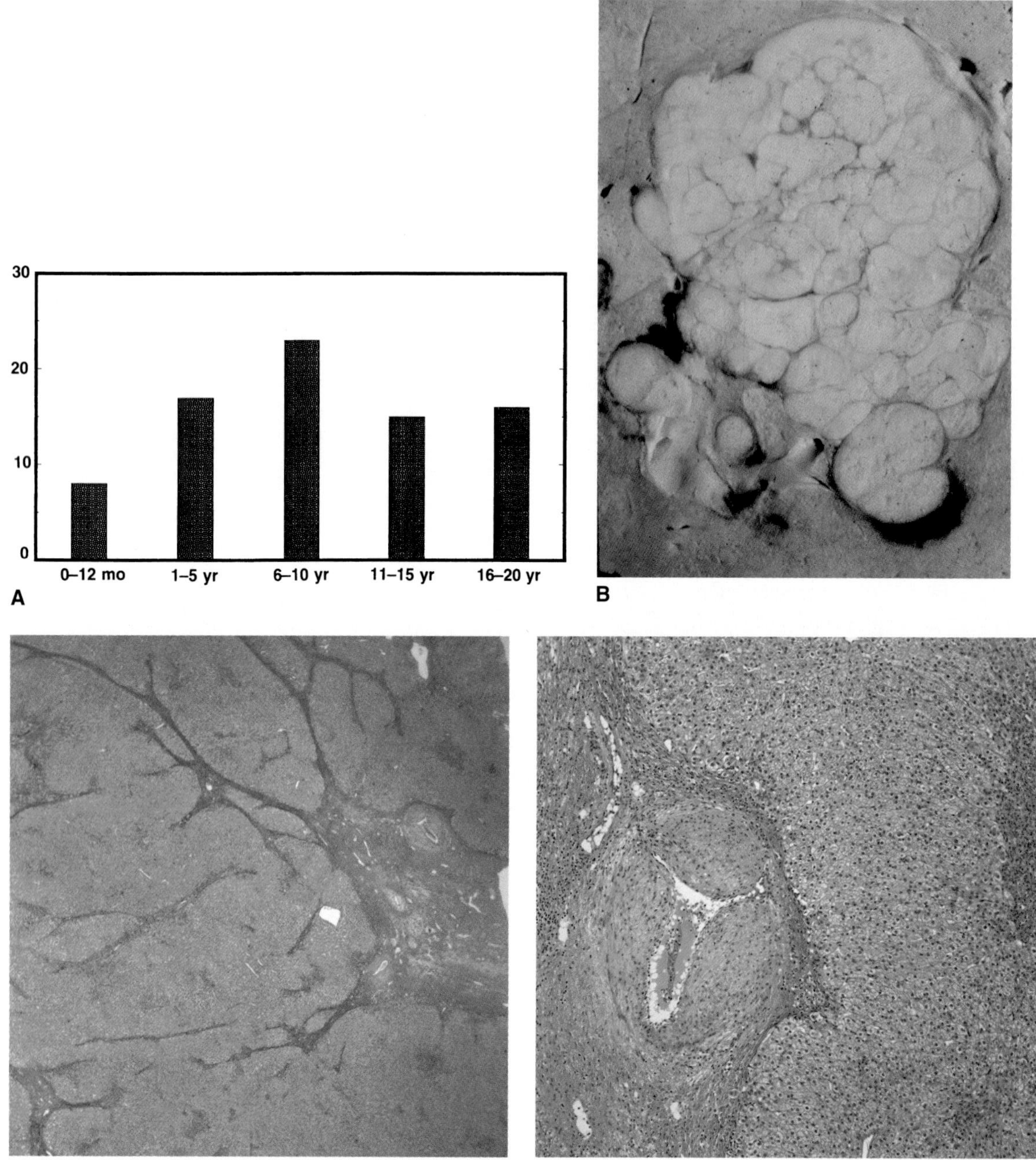

FIGURE 15-45 ■ Focal nodular hyperplasia. **A:** Age distribution in 79 cases. **B:** A well-circumscribed lesion is subdivided into smaller nodules by bands of connective tissue. **C:** Arborizing septa of fibrous connective tissue surround and subdivide nodules of hepatocytes (Reticulin stain, original magnification 15×). **D:** The edges of the fibrous septa contain scattered small ducts along with small to large vessels, some displaying eccentric subintimal thickening (H&E stain, original magnification 60×).

to adenomas, imaging techniques are sufficient for diagnosis in 70% of cases. Magnetic resonance imaging (MRI) has higher sensitivity and specificity for FNH than does ultrasonography or computed tomography. Typically, FNH is isointense or hypointense on T1-weighted images, is slightly hyperintense or isointense on T2-weighted images, and has a hyperintense central scar on T2-weighted images. FNH demonstrates intense homogeneous enhancement during the arterial phase of gadolinium-enhanced imaging and enhancement of the central scar during later phases (71). Arteriography often displays the prominent single or multiple feeder arteries associated with FNH. Centrifugal filling from the feeder artery to the periphery of the lesion may be seen. Ultrasonography may demonstrate a feeding artery with a radial vascular architecture, which, however, may not be present in a lesion smaller than 3 cm in size. Cheon et al.

Table 15-17 ■ ASSOCIATED ANOMALIES IN CHILDREN WITH FOCAL NODULAR HYPERPLASIA

Glycogen storage disease
Gastroschisis, absent gallbladder
Cardiac hypertrophy, nodular hyperplasia of thyroid and adrenal cortex
Ovarian dysgerminoma
Persistent hypoglycemia
Multiple telangiectasia on arms and legs
Hypospadias, bilateral syndactyly of toes, bilateral hydrocele
Left-sided hemihypertrophy, syndactyly, absent distal phalanges of second and third fingers on left hand, multiple telangiectasia over face and lips, umbilical hernia
Sickle cell disease
Biliary atresia with portoenterostomy
Fibrolamellar hepatocellular carcinoma
Adrenocortical tumor

Modified from Stocker JT, Ishak KG: Focal nodular hyperplasia of the liver: a study of 21 pediatric cases. *Cancer* 1918;48:336–345, with permission.

(e125), however, noted that children often display a wide spectrum of imaging findings on various radiologic examinations and that the typical centrally placed scar is not always seen. Superparamagnetic iron oxide (SPIO)–enhanced MRI has been shown to be useful in differentiating benign lesions such as FNH and hepatic adenoma from malignant hepatocellular lesions (e53).

Treatment

Symptomatic children are treated with resection of the lesion. However, since morbidity and death have been associated with attempts at resection, Pain et al. (e510) suggested that asymptomatic lesions be observed with regular ultrasonography and treated only if they enlarge or become symptomatic. Young girls with FNH should be cautioned on the use of oral contraceptives, because bleeding may occur within the lesion (e204). FNH does not undergo malignant transformation. Although Saul et al. (e596) described the association of FNH with fibrolamellar HCC (FL-HCC), they also suggested that the FNH, usually found either in or adjacent to the FL-HCC, is a phenomenon secondary to the highly vascular nature of FL-HCC. There is currently no proof of FL-HCC arising in a preexisting FNH. However, the radiologist should be cautious about the similar radiographic appearance of FL-HCC and FNH, both of which may contain central scars (e436).

Gross Appearance

FNH occurs most frequently (90%) as a single mass within the right or left lobe (Figure 15-45B). Bilateral involvement by a large lesion may be present in 10% of cases. Multiple lesions within both lobes are seen in 10% of cases and often have a histologic appearance different from that in cases with a single lesion (see later). The single lesions are firm, irregular in outline, and range from 1 to 17 cm in greatest diameter with weights as high as 1,500 g (171) (e659). The lesions often bulge from the surface of the liver and may be pedunculated. On cut section, the lesion is sharply demarcated from the surrounding liver and displays a nodular tan-brown parenchyma subdivided by gray-white septa radiating from a central area of fibrosis. Prominent vessels may be seen near the edge of the lesion arising within the normal liver parenchyma and ramifying within the lesion. Areas of hemorrhage or necrosis may rarely be seen.

Histopathology

The typical histopathological features of classical FNH include a firm, well-delimited but not encapsulated lesion composed of hepatocellular nodules with normal hepatocytes, a central scar, and radiating fibrous septa. The central scars of the single lesions display broad bands of fibrous connective tissue typically containing large dystrophic arteries (ectatic vessels with eccentric intimal thickening and medial hyperplasia) (Figure 15-45C, D). Frequently, there is a lymphocytic infiltrate. The fibrous septa subdivide, partially or completely enclosing lobules of parenchymal cells arranged in cords, almost imparting an appearance of a focal biliary cirrhosis. Numerous small bile ducts, arterioles, and venules are present within the septa, along with varying numbers of lymphocytes and neutrophils. Bile ductules are usually found at the interface between hepatocytes and fibrous regions. VanEyken et al. (e733) demonstrated that hepatocytes within the liver express cytokeratins of bile duct type, suggesting that the ductular proliferation of FNH is derived from ductular metaplasia of hepatocytes. Interlobular bile ducts are usually absent. The cords within the nodules contain hepatocytes in 1- to 2-cell–thick plates that may be slightly larger than those of the normal liver and may contain intracellular fat and variable amounts of glycogen (22,114). The cells within the FNH show no evidence of dysplasia (e596). The lesion often compresses the adjacent parenchyma but is separated from it only by a discontinuous fibrous capsule. A large feeder artery is frequently present within this capsule. Wanless et al. (190) demonstrated a connection between this feeder artery and a spiderlike structure of smaller vessels supplying 1-mm nodules within the lesion.

The diagnosis of FNH is usually evident in a liver biopsy specimen. However, some cases of FNH may show atypical clinical and/or histopathologic features and the diagnosis is difficult in these even in the resected specimen, let alone on a biopsy (114) (e387,e483). In atypical FNH, the above key diagnostic features are either lacking or inconspicuous. Differential diagnosis with adenomas may be difficult in these cases, especially when the nodules are small (<10 mm) or associated with significant steatosis. Fabre et al. (52) have proposed a scoring system for the reliable diagnosis of FNH with atypical features. In their study, most radiologically atypical tumors also showed nonclassic histopathology.

Some lesions have histological features of both adenoma and FNH. These variant lesions have often been classified as the telangiectatic type of FNH (1) (e754). These tumors are often multiple and the cut surface displays a spongy telangiectatic appearance with numerous small, blood-filled cavities. In these multifocal telangiectatic lesions, connection(s) between the vessels within the connective tissue and dilated sinusoids within the parenchymal nodules can be readily demonstrated. As a result of this connection, the telangiectatic lesion displays markedly dilated sinusoids filled with red blood cells clearly separating the hepatic cords (190). Foci of more firm tissue resembling the single FNH lesions may be present in the multiple telangiectatic lesions. It is not clear if all nodules originally called telangiectatic FNH (e388,e483) and progressive FNH (e585) are histologically the same lesions as those subsequently included in the studies that demonstrated monoclonality (e70,e512) and/or were associated with syndromes such as meningioma, astrocytoma, telangiectasia of the brain, and berry aneurysm (e754). Clinical and molecular evidence indicates that telangiectatic FNH should be reclassified as adenomas (e70,e791).

Molecular Pathology

The molecular pathogenesis of FNH was recently reviewed by Rebouissou et al. (146). Of 33 FNH lesions evaluated by the HUMARA assay in the literature, 9 (27%) showed a uniform pattern of X chromosome inactivation consistent with clonality. Other studies analyzing chromosome gains and losses by comparative genomic hybridization (CGH), allelotyping, or karyotype have identified chromosome alterations indicating a clonal origin in 14% to 50% of cases (e70,e123,e336,e554) Although somatic gene mutations in β-catenin gene (*CTNNB1*), *TP53*, *APC* or HNF1α (e70,e72,e124) have not been identified in FNH, mRNA expression levels of the angiopoietin genes (ANGPT1 and ANGPT2) involved in vessel maturation are altered, with increased ANGPT1/ANGPT2 ratio (e70).

Immunohistochemical assays of extracellular matrix proteins also support the hypothesis that FNH is merely a hyperplastic response of liver parenchyma to local vascular abnormalities and have shown that the lesions of perisinusoidal fibrosis associated with FNH are accompanied by the induction of integrin receptors on hepatocytes and sinusoidal endothelial cells (e612).

NODULAR REGENERATIVE HYPERPLASIA

Nodular regenerative hyperplasia (NRH) of the liver is an uncommon condition characterized by the presence of widely distributed to diffuse parenchymal nodules with little or no fibrosis. The condition is more common in adults than in children and increases with age. In a study of 2,500 consecutive autopsies, Wanless (190) found a prevalence of 2.6%, rising to 5.3% above 80 years of age at death. Over 30 cases of NRH have been reported in children, including two cases in fetal livers (127) (e230,e715). In the pediatric age group, NRH has been demonstrated in 4.5% of a large series of 716 pediatric liver tumors, but only in 2.1% of liver tumors from birth to 2 years of age. However, since liver tumors are in general rare, NRH remains the fourth most common "liver tumor" from 5 to 20 years of age (Figure 15-46A), after HCC, FNH, and undifferentiated embryonal sarcoma (UES) (174).

Pathogenesis

Originally described as "miliary hepatocellular adenomatosis" in a patient with Felty syndrome (e558), NRH is seen in association with other rheumatologic and autoimmune diseases, hematological disorders, drug therapy, PBC, congestive heart failure, other hepatic circulatory disorders, metastases, tuberculosis, and CGD (112,148) (e413,e542) (Table 15-18). Three familial cases of NRH have been reported in literature (e187). In a series of 16 children with NRH, clinical associations included a history of anticonvulsant drug therapy (four patients), Donohue syndrome, disseminated intravascular coagulation, renal angiomyolipoma, other intraabdominal tumors, thrombocytopenia, and pancytopenia (127). Other pediatric reports have been associated with congenital heart disease (e715,e719), Krabbe disease (e450), Still disease (e465), chronic inflammation (e530), sacrococcygeal teratoma (e155), autoimmune disorders (112) (e22), and multiple organ malformation in fetuses (e230).

The etiopathogenesis of NRH is not fully understood. NRH may be a hyperproliferative response to an obstructive portal venopathy resulting in an uneven perfusion of the hepatic parenchyma (148) (e137,e472,e753). It is hypothesized that the portal venopathy leads to centrilobular (acinar zone 3) ischemic atrophy with compensatory proliferation of zone 1 hepatocytes. The resultant "regenerative nodules" compress the atrophic hepatocytes, yielding the characteristic pattern highlighted by reticulin stains. This hypothesis is supported by the association of NRH with diseases that are known to cause vascular injury and the frequent histologic finding of portal venous abnormalities in NRH. Vascular abnormalities such as atrial septal defects, ventricular septal defects, abnormal junction of pulmonary veins, congenital absence of portal vein, and other congenital anomalies are reported in children diagnosed with NRH, strengthening the argument that NRH may result from microcirculatory derangements (e254,e756). However, other investigators have not confirmed these findings (e670) and suggest that NRH is a primary generalized proliferative disorder of the liver (112). In cases associated with drug therapy, it has been suggested that polymorphisms in genes encoding thiopurine methyltransferase may be linked to development of NRH probably through altered drug metabolism (e85). Some NRH cases have been suggested to result from chronic, cytotoxic CD8+ T-lymphocyte targeting of sinusoidal endothelial cells (e790), and NRH has also been postulated to be an organ-specific form of antiphospholipid syndrome (e349).

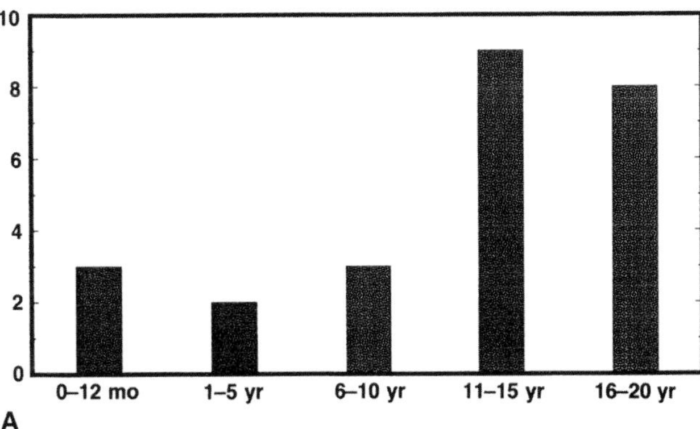

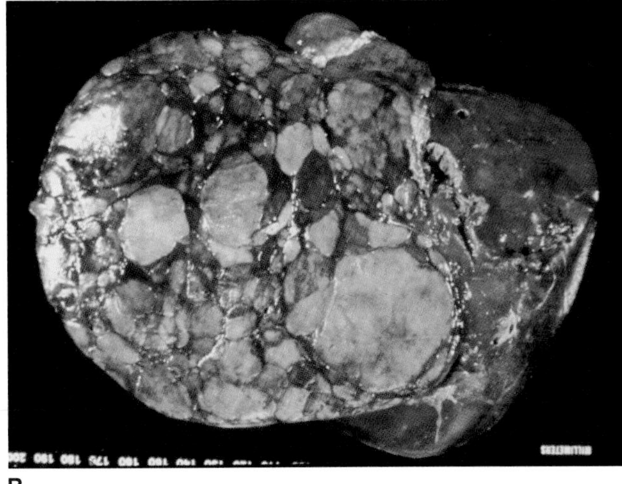

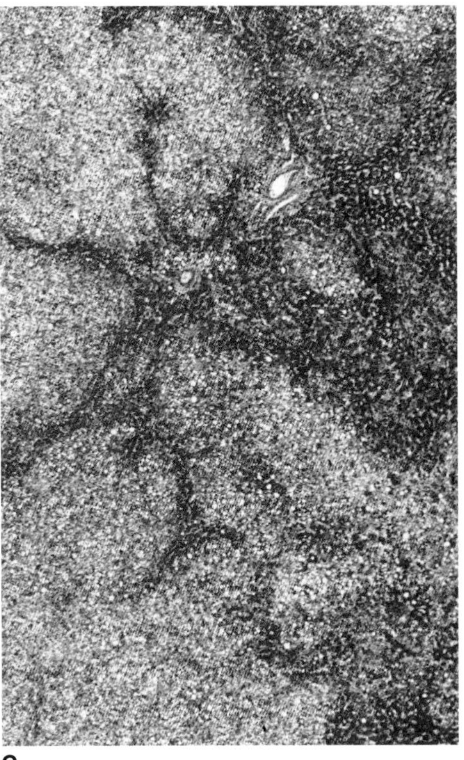

FIGURE 15-46 ■ Nodular regenerative hyperplasia. **A:** Age distribution in 25 cases. **B:** A large mass of different-sized nodules occupies most of the liver. **C:** The nodules are composed of hyperplasic "regenerative" hepatocytes, which are light staining and compress remnants of atrophic lobules into thin bands. (H&E stain, original magnification 30×).

Clinical Features, Diagnosis, and Management

Most patients with NRH may remain asymptomatic for years before coming to clinical attention. The diagnosis of NRH requires a high index of suspicion and awareness of its associations detailed above; NRH should be considered in the differential diagnosis of patients who present with unexplained portal hypertension. NRH may also clinically simulate metastates and should be considered in patients with history of malignancy treated with chemotherapy and/or radiotherapy who develop single or multiple hepatic masses (e133).

Table 15-18 ■ CONDITIONS ASSOCIATED WITH NODULAR REGENERATIVE HYPERPLASIA IN CHILDREN

Donohue syndrome
Mental retardation
Anticonvulsant therapy
Vater syndrome
Renal angiomyolipoma
Disseminated intravascular coagulopathy
Krabbe disease
Portal hypertension
Wilms tumor
Down syndrome
Still disease

In symptomatic patients, portal hypertension and its complications dominate. However, ascites is relatively uncommon since patients typically have normal hepatic synthetic function with normal albumin levels. Although based on the vascular compromise hypothesis, portal hypertension should be presinusoidal in nature (190), portal pressure measurements in a small number of patients have been more consistent with a sinusoidal portal hypertension, possibly due to sinusoidal compression by the regenerating nodules in later stages of the disease (148).

The radiological findings of NRH reflect clinical observations (e154,e670,e715). Liver size can be normal, reduced, or increased; immense hepatomegaly leading to abdominal deformity is very rare. Nodules range in size from 0.1 to 10 cm in diameter and are often hyperechoic on ultrasound, although they may be even undetectable by this modality. CT scans generally show hypodense nodules with respect to the adjacent liver parenchyma, without significant contrast enhancement (e27). On MRI, lesions are described as isointense to normal liver on T2-weighted images and contain foci of high signal intensity on T1-weighted scans (e106). Kobayashi et al. report typical imaging findings to include hyperintensity on T1-weighted MRI, hyperdensity on CT during arterial portography (CTAP), and isointensity to hypointensity onSPIO–enhanced T2-weighted MRI (e356).

Laboratory parameters of liver function are also usually normal in NRH, although approximately 25% of cases reported in the literature note an elevated ALP (148). Liver biopsy is essential for diagnosis. It has been emphasized that the histologic findings of NRH may not be detected by a needle biopsy of the liver and a wedge biopsy may be required (112) (e716). In the case of needle biopsy, the gauge of the needle is an important consideration. Regenerative nodules may be missed if the needle is too narrow, as is often the case with transjugular liver biopsy, thus making the diagnosis of NRH difficult.

The mainstay of treatment is to manage the underlying disease, remove offending drugs, if any, and control portal hypertension. Given the uncommon nature of NRH, there is scant literature on the natural history of this disease and treatment strategies are based on experience with other more common causes of portal hypertension (148). It is not known whether NRH is a reversible process once the presumed cause is removed, such as might occur with stopping a drug. Since the synthetic function of the liver is generally intact in NRH, despite the potential for the development of significant portal hypertension, liver transplantation is not a conventional therapy. The outcome of NRH depends on the presence of portal hypertension, associated systemic disease, and the risk of rupture of a large hyperplastic nodule. Some investigators claim that NRH is a premalignant condition, which may progress to hepatocyte dysplasia and HCC. Nzeako et al. (e489) demonstrated that 23 of 342 patients without cirrhosis who had HCC also had NRH and also found that 73.9% of their patients with NRH and HCC had liver cell dysplasia. Liver cell dysplasia is a common finding in NRH and has been noted in 20% to 42% of cases (e489,e670).

The largest pediatric series of NRH (127) comprised 16 patients (10 girls and 6 boys) with a median age of 6 years (range 7 months to 13 years). Nine presented with hepatomegaly or splenomegaly, with and without signs of portal hypertension. Follow-up was available for eight patients; six patients died of causes unrelated to the nodular hyperplasia. Two patients were asymptomatic when last seen 5 and 18 years after the initial diagnosis of nodular hyperplasia.

Pathology

Based on autopsy studies, the liver with NRH shows a diffuse transformation into nodules of 1 to 3 mm in size (Figure 15-46). Unlike cirrhosis, there is no fibrosis separating nodules; each nodule presses directly against its neighbor. Although nodules greater than 15 mm have been described grossly, these are frequently revealed to be composed of smaller nodules when examined microscopically (190).

Histopathology is the only means of definitive diagnosis and is also required to rule out cirrhosis and HCC. By definition, the nodules are less than 3 mm in thickness and perisinosoidal fibrosis is absent to minimal (1,148). At a minimum, to make the diagnosis of NRH, one should see the characteristic nodular zones of widened hepatocyte plates bounded by narrowed and compressed plates. Parenchymal nodularity can be appreciated on scanning magnification with a characteristic pattern of light and dark areas (127). The light areas are comprised of swollen liver cells with empty to clear cytoplasm, whereas the dark areas correspond to compressed liver cell plates between the nodules. The hepatocytes within the nodule may be arranged in plates that are more than one cell thick. The individual hepatocytes may be enlarged and have hypertrophic nuclei. Between individual nodules, the hepatocytes are small and atrophic and are pressed together into thin, parallel plates. This compression is best visualized using a reticulin stain and may be associated with slitlike central veins and sinusoidal dilation (in areas of hepatocellular atrophy). Immunohistochemical granular staining for alpha-1-antitrypsin is reportedly increased in the regenerating (periportal) compartment and this may help in the histological evaluation of difficult cases (e474). Whereas the larger portal veins may be widely patent, portal venous structures in smaller radicals may be absent or occluded. Central veins may show venoocclusive changes or may be compressed into narrowed slits. However, no vascular abnormalities were noted in Moran's series (127). Fibrosis typical of chronic liver disease is usually not present, although there may be some degree of periportal fibrosis or perisinusoidal fibrosis, the latter frequently associated with the atrophic areas. There is usually little or no inflammation or cholestasis, and normal bile ducts and arteries can be easily identified. In needle biopsies of the liver, the changes of regeneration and atrophy may be very subtle on routine hematoxylin-eosin stains. Therefore, any "normal" liver biopsy specimens, particularly those from patients with portal hypertension, should be investigated further using reticulin stains (148).

The differential diagnosis of NRH includes hepatic adenoma, FNH, partial nodular transformation, large regenerative nodule, CHF, incomplete cirrhosis, cirrhosis, and HCC. The International Working Party has published guidelines and definitions for these nodular hepatic lesions (1). It is important to remember that more than one type of nodular lesion can coexist in the same liver since clinical portal hypertension may result from NRH, whereas disabling pain or hemorrhage may be due to other pathology such as hepatic adenoma, with different treatment options for each situation. Histologically, patients with portal hypertension not associated with cirrhosis may present with NRH, hepatoportal sclerosis (portal venopathy), central venous obliteration, sinusoidal dilatation, or some combination of these lesions (131). Histologic findings in these settings may be subtle and awareness of these will prevent underdiagnosis.

HEPATOCELLULAR ADENOMA

HCA is a rare benign tumor of the liver. In the pediatric age group, it is seen most frequently in teenage girls (Figure 15-47A) but has also been described in younger children with GSD and galactosemia, in infants, and even *in utero* (150) (e33,e477,e561,e762). Most patients, however, are older than 10 years of age and, like adults, have a history of oral contraceptive use (e659).

Pathogenesis

In addition to oral contraceptive use, HCA has been described in a variety of conditions in children, including GSD types I, III, and IV; galactosemia; Hurler syndrome; severe combined immunodeficiency; diabetes mellitus; and androgen therapy for Fanconi anemia (150) (e23). Osteoporosis has been noted in some children with HCA (e762).

Clinical, Laboratory, and Imaging Features

The lesion may be asymptomatic, produce mild episodic abdominal pain, or present as acute abdominal pain due to hemorrhage into the tumor or peritoneal cavity. Laboratory studies are usually not helpful with normal or only mildly elevated serum aminotransferases, ALP, and bilirubin values (150).

Although imaging studies are helpful in demonstrating the large single mass usually seen in this disorder, at present, HCA cannot be conclusively identified by any currently available imaging technique. Arteriography displays hypervascular masses that in some areas are hypovascular, presumably because of intratumor bleeding or necrosis (e339). Ultrasound has detected the lesions *in utero* (150) (e33). Imaging findings of HCA and adenomatosis are similar and vary according to the particular characteristics of the lesional tissue: there are fatty patterns, peliotic patterns, and heterogeneous patterns with necrotic and hemorrhagic foci (e458). Currently, imaging techniques are unable to detect early malignant transformation in HCA.

Treatment and Outcomes

HCAs require excision, in view of their propensity to bleed or rupture, association with osteoporosis, and the inability to predict malignant transformation (e762). HCAs in girls using

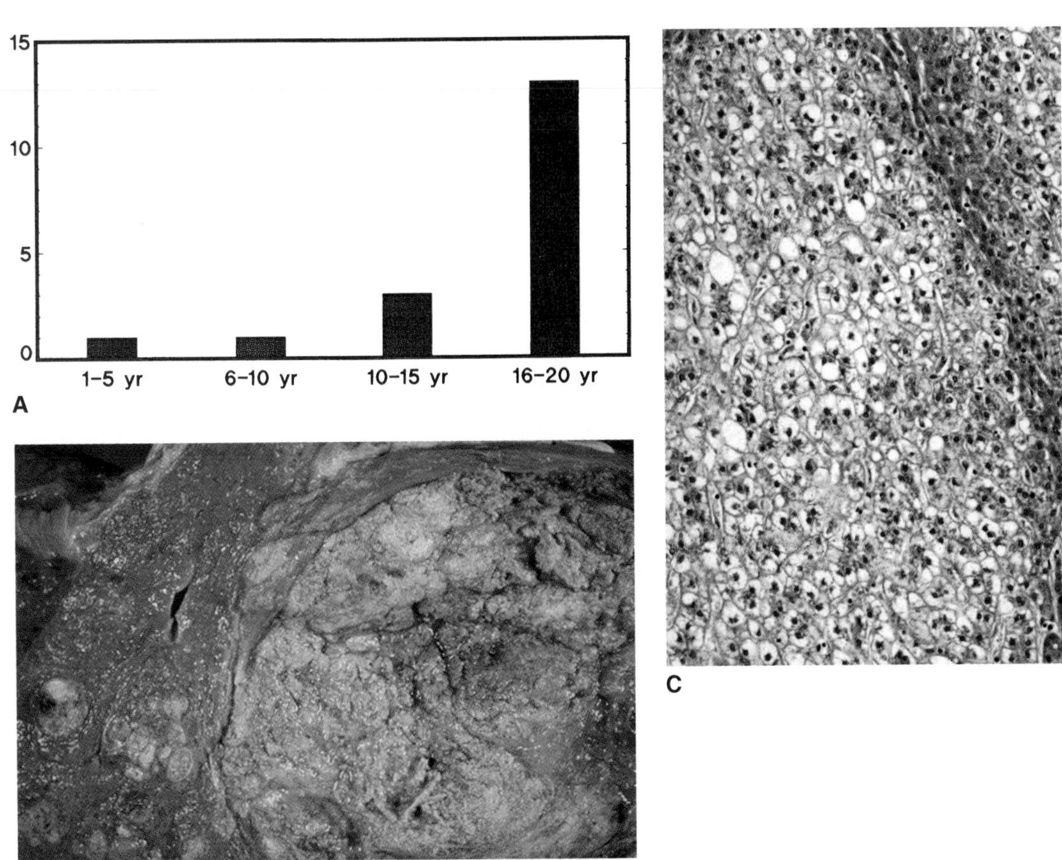

FIGURE 15-47 ■ Hepatocellular adenoma. **A:** Age distribution in 18 cases. **B:** A poorly circumscribed light yellow-tan mass occupies a large portion of the liver. Note the smaller nodules of similar colored tissue in the adjacent normal liver parenchyma. **C:** The lesion is composed of trabeculae of uniform hepatocytes, some surrounding canaliculi. Note the absence of portal areas and bile ducts. (H&E stain, original magnification 100×).

contraceptive steroids may regress after discontinuation of their use (e23).

There is, at present, inadequate data regarding the growth and involution of HCAs. Also, the risk of hemorrhage in an HCA is not restricted to larger lesions and is unpredictable. There are no longitudinal studies evaluating transformation of HCA to HCC, although a recent study found malignancy only in adenomas larger than 4 cm and more often in men than in women (20).

Gross Pathology

HCA is usually a solitary, well-demarcated, globular to ovoid lesion measuring 0.1 to 15 cm in diameter, often with large vessels coursing over its surface (150). The lesion is soft to firm in consistency and has a variegated appearance ranging from light brown to tan, with or without areas of yellow necrosis or reddish-brown hemorrhage. Multiple lesions may be present (Figure 15-47B). By definition, "adenomatosis" requires the presence of at least ten adenomas in the liver (e126,e217). This definition theoretically excludes patients with glycogenosis, or those taking contraceptives (e217), although some authors feel that this may be an unduly restrictive definition (22).

Histopathology

HCAs can be solitary or multiple. They represent a heterogeneous group of tumors in which histopathological features may vary according to the etiological background (e31). Microscopically, the tumor is composed of sheets of neoplastic cells in trabeculae that are one to three cells thick, separated by compressed sinusoidal spaces lined by endothelial cells and some Kupffer cells (Figure 15-47C). The tumor cells are the same size as or slightly larger than the normal hepatocytes and may be either normal, clear (glycogen-rich), or fatty. Some lesions may be almost entirely steatotic, prompting a differential diagnosis including angiomyolipoma. The tumor parenchyma is supplied by thin-walled arteries without other portal tract elements such as significant amounts of connective tissue, bile ducts, or ductular reaction. Bile may be present in intracellular canaliculi. Foci of dilated sinusoids may impart a "pelioid" appearance. Large vessels are often present near the periphery of the lesion, displaying arterial intimal thickening and elastic lamina reduplication. Smooth muscle proliferation may narrow or obliterate the lumen of veins, particularly in cases associated with contraceptive steroid use. Infarcts and hemorrhage are frequent, especially in larger lesions. Hemorrhage may be internal to the lesion, usually admixed with necrotic changes (this type is mostly observed in adenomas larger than 4 cm) or may result in spontaneous rupture with resultant subcapsular hematoma and/or hemoperitoneum (e425). Internal hemorrhage may heal with fibrosis, and this may simulate a central scar of FNH, making it difficult to differentiate the two, particularly in core biopsy material. Hemosiderin-laden macrophages may also be seen. Foci of extramedullary hematopoiesis as seen in cases of hepatoblastoma may be present, sometimes posing difficulty in differentiating the two lesions (150). Foci of dysplastic hepatocytes may be present within the lesion, especially in patients with Fanconi anemia, but malignant transformation is rare (150) (e208). Nuclear atypia, mitoses, and acinar ("pseudoglandular") growth pattern are rarely seen; these cases may also be extremely difficult to distinguish from HCC. The term "atypical adenoma" is often used in these settings to indicate that the distinction between HCA and HCC remains problematic and resection and/or close clinical follow-up may be needed. Cytogenetic techniques such as FISH and CGH may help distinguish HCA from HCC, since the former usually does not show chromosomal aberrations (e766). Resnick et al. suggest that immunostains for proliferating cell nuclear antigen (PCNA) may be used to help differentiate HCA from hepatoblastoma and HCC; the PCNA labeling index was significantly lower in hepatic adenomas (0.3% to 5.1%) than in HCCs (9.6% to 23.8%) and hepatoblastomas (21.8% to 44.3%), in their study (150). The range of PCNA labeling is even lower in patients with adenoma who do not have Fanconi anemia (0.3% to 1.7% for adenoma alone versus 3.2% to 5.1% for those with Fanconi anemia) (e70). Care must also be taken to distinguish the usual solitary HCA from the multiple nodules of NRH of the liver, which is associated with many other disorders.

As outlined above, the heterogeneous histopathology of HCA raises many differential diagnoses, the greatest overlap being with FNH. Until recently, the presence of bile ductules (characterized immunohistochemically as CK7 positive and usually CK19 negative) in a lesion precluded the diagnosis of HCA. However, molecular studies have shown that HCA may contain bile ductules, especially when associated with sinusoidal dilatation; these lesions traditionally referred to as telangiectactic FNH are being reclassified as adenomas (e70), although there is a lack of consensus at this time. The problem of differentiating HCA and FNH is further compounded by the fact that the two lesions are associated and may occur concurrently. Laurent et al. have shown that the presence of FNH is significantly higher than expected in at least two circumstances: adenomatosis and multiple inflammatory HCA (e373). Immunohistochemical stains with antibodies to CD34 (e252), cytokeratin 7, or hepatic transporters (e737) have been suggested as adjunct techniques to help differentiate between FNH and HCA.

Molecular Pathology

The past decade has seen numerous advances in understanding the molecular basis of HCA. Based on two molecular criteria (hepatocyte nuclear factor 1α [HNF1α] mutations and β-catenin mutations), and an additional histological criterion (the presence/absence of inflammation), a molecular/histologic classification correlating the genotype and phenotype of HCAs has been proposed (23) (e69,e791).

Typical HCA

These have classic histology with regular liver cell plates up to three cells thick and little cytologic atypia; thin-walled arteries without other portal tract elements, bile ducts, or ductular reaction; may be monoclonal; and overlap with FNH. They are negative for HNF 1α and β-catenin mutations.

Variant 1

HNF1α biallelic somatic mutations are observed in 35% of the HCA cases. These patients are almost always women. There is marked steatosis/clear cells and a lack of expression of liver fatty acid binding protein (LFABP) on immunohistochemistry. An HNF1α germline (constitutional) mutation is observed in less than 5% of HCA cases and is associated with MODY 3 diabetes, familial adenomatosis, and a younger age at presentation.

Variant 2

An activating β-catenin mutation is found in 10% of HCA. These β-catenin activated HCAs are observed in both men and women and are associated with specific risk factors such as male hormone administration or glycogenosis. There is cytological atypia and an acinar pattern (the so-called "atypical HCA" or "HCA/HCC borderline lesion") and steatosis is not prominent. Immunohistochemical studies show that these HCAs overexpress β-catenin (nuclear and cytoplasmic) and glutamine synthetase. This group of tumors has a higher risk of malignant transformation. The association in the same coalescent nodule of HCC and adenoma (β-catenin and glutamine synthetase positive) can be explained by either malignant transformation of adenoma, or an HCC with both very well differentiated and less differentiated areas. At present, this issue remains unresolved.

Variant 3

Inflammatory HCAs are observed in 40% of the cases; they are most frequent in women but are also found in men. In this group, GGT is frequently elevated, with a biological inflammatory syndrome present. Also, there are more overweight patients in this group. These lesions may be multiple and associated with other vascular or neurological disorders (e754). The histology is of the so-called "telangiectatic FNH" and is characterized by inflammatory infiltrates, dystrophic arteries, sinusoidal dilatation, and ductular reaction (CK7 positive ductules). Although definitionally there is no mutation, 10% of inflammatory HCAs also express β-catenin, and behave as variant 2, with higher risk of malignant transformation.

Variant 4

This group includes the (<10%) HCAs that are currently unclassified by the above schema. They lack any specific trait in that there are no known mutations or specific association.

There is a higher risk of bleeding in the variant forms, although the degree of this risk in each of the different categories is unknown. If molecular techniques are not available to test for β-catenin mutation on frozen or formalin-fixed tissue, immunostains for β-catenin (e682,e708) on paraffin sections may help identify variant two tumors, since these may have a higher risk of malignant transformation, although more studies are needed to confirm this.

MESENCHYMAL HAMARTOMA

Hepatic mesenchymal hamartoma (HMH) is an uncommon benign tumor of childhood. Historically, mesenchymal hamartoma has been described in the literature by various names including pseudocystic mesenchymal tumor, giant cell lymphangioma, cystic hamartoma, bile cell fibroadenoma, hamartoma, and cavernous lymphangiomatoid tumor; the unifying term mesenchymal hamartoma was coined by Edmondson in 1956 (e190). The lesion makes up approximately 8% of all pediatric tumors and, after hemangioma, is the second most common benign hepatic tumor in childhood.

Pathogenesis

The pathogenesis of HMH is still debated. A handful of series have shown an association with placental abnormalities including mesenchymal stem villous hyperplasia of the placenta, thrombosis, or transient honeycombed multicystic placental enlargement (56) (e105,e221,e347,e366,e712), raising the possibility of synchronous abnormal mesodermal development rather than a true developmental abnormality. Alternatively, placental dysplasia may be secondary to compression of the umbilical vein by the HMH. Given the similarities between the bile duct abnormalities in MHL and those in von Meyenburg complexes, bile duct hamartomas, Caroli disease, and CHF, a primary bile duct plate malformative etiology has also been proposed for MHL. In fact, serial dissection studies have demonstrated a single portal tract as being the source of the lesion (e384,e498).

Clinical Features, Laboratory Studies, and Imaging

Mesenchymal hamartoma is a lesion of infants; 55% of cases present in the 1st year of life and nearly 85% by 2 years of age (Figure 15-48A). Rare cases have been reported in children older than 5 years of age, with anecdotal reports in adults. Intrauterine HMHs have been well documented in several reports. Cornette et al. (43) reviewed 17 reported cases in the literature, with the earliest case having been incidentally detected on ultrasonography at 15 weeks' gestation (e398). However, only 4 of 17 had been correctly diagnosed antenatally, while in other cases, preoperative diagnoses entertained included ovarian masses, lymphangiomas, pseudocysts, enteric duplication cysts, and choledochal cysts. Mesenchymal hamartomas have also been noted as an incidental finding at autopsy.

Infants usually present with a history of a nontender enlarging abdomen over a period of days to months. Other symptoms that rarely present are vomiting, decreased appetite, and

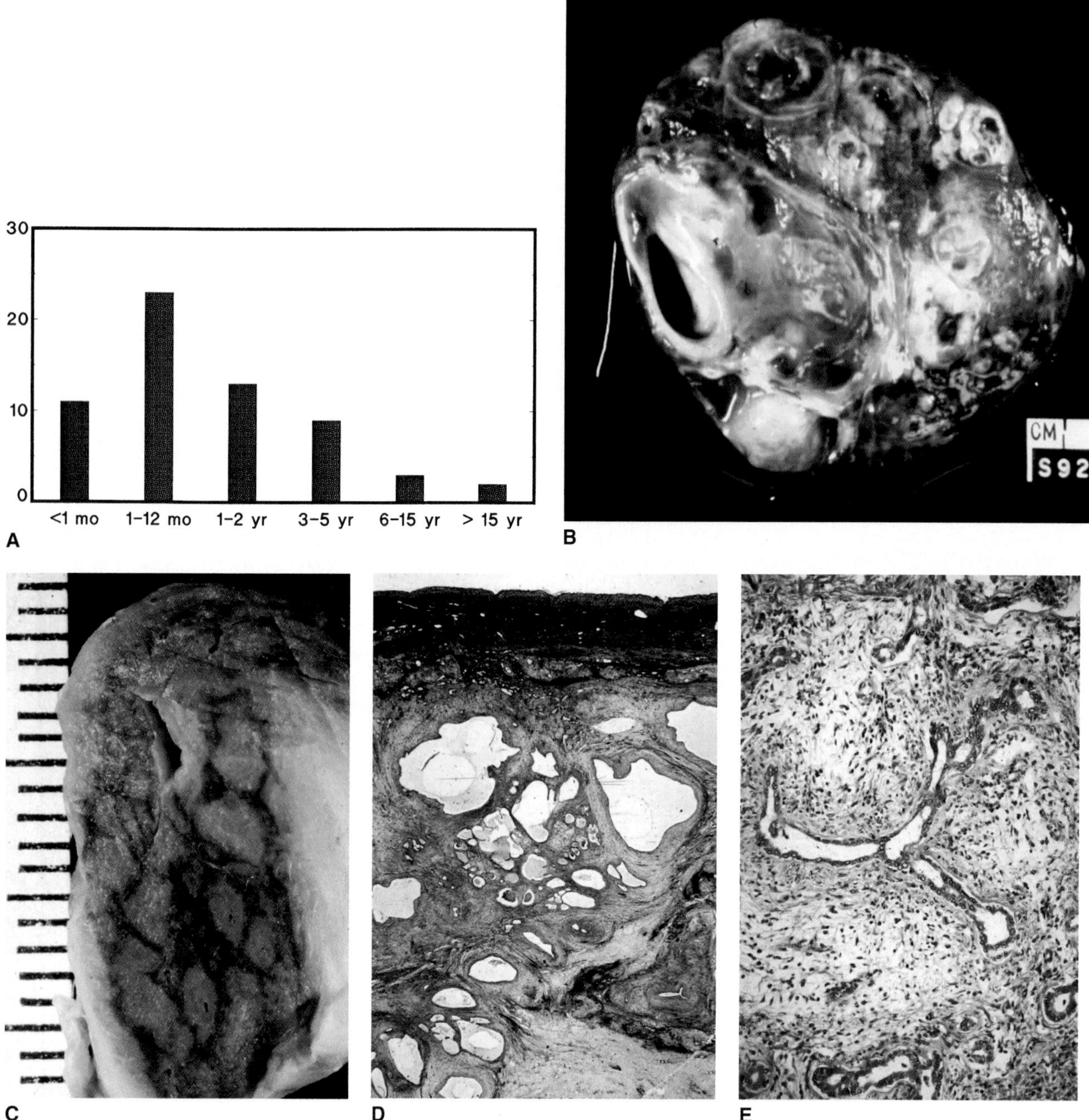

FIGURE 15-48 ■ Mesenchymal hamartoma. **A:** Age distribution in 71 cases. **B:** Multiple cysts of varying sizes (previously filled with clear yellow fluid) are surrounded by variegated, solid components. **C:** Near the edge of the cystic portion (on the left side of the image), the lesion displays a diffuse infiltration and widening of the portal areas (light tan areas), compressing the intervening hepatocytes lobules into thin brown strips. **D:** The cysts, with no discernible cellular lining, are surrounded by loose to compressed connective tissue, which contains scattered residual bile ducts. Note the compressed liver at top (Masson trichrome stain, original magnification 10×). **E:** Residual bile ducts within the lesion are surrounded by loose mesenchymal tissue containing scattered neutrophils, lymphocytes, and small foci of extramedullary hematopoiesis (H&E stain, original magnification 75×).

respiratory distress. There is a slight male predominance but no apparent racial predilection. Physical findings are those associated with the abdominal mass, including a protuberant abdomen and dilated superficial veins. Large masses may eventually produce a mass effect such as vena cava compression, feeding difficulties, and respiratory distress secondary to upward pressure on the diaphragm and may be complicated by ascites, jaundice, and even congestive heart failure (e305). Occasionally, the mass will expand rapidly, most likely because of rapid accumulation of fluid within cystic spaces (e316). Stocker and Ishak (172) reported other anomalies or diseases in 5 of 30 patients, including adrenal cytomegaly, neonatal hyperbilirubinemia, endocardial fibroelastosis of the left ventricle, idiopathic thrombocytopenic purpura, and diffuse endocrinopathy.

Laboratory findings are noncontributory; tumor markers including AFP, β-human chorionic gonadotropin (hCG), and vanillylmandelic acid are usually negative (e781), although rare cases may show elevated AFP levels (e99,e726). Ultrasonography, except in the youngest infants, displays an echogenic mass that may be pedunculated and which displays internal septation and cysts (e462,e781). MRI and CT also highlight the multicystic nature of the lesion and can suggest the fluid nature of the cyst contents (e295). The typical CT scan features are that of a well-circumscribed, multilocular, multicystic mass that contains low-density cysts separated by solid septae and stroma. The stroma and septae may be vascular and occasionally show contrast enhancement on CT scan similar to that seen in infantile hemangioma. When the cysts are small, the lesion may appear solid on imaging. Selective arteriography most frequently displays an avascular mass (172).

Treatment and Outcomes

Surgical resection of the lesion or partial hepatectomy is the treatment of choice. Partial resection with drainage of the cysts and marsupialization has been successful in managing large lesions believed to be impossible to resect completely, but may be associated with recurrence (e462). Less invasive techniques, such as laparoscopic fenestration, have also been used successfully (e293). Spontaneous regression of the lesion has been described, prompting some authors to suggest a policy of watchful waiting (e44,e324,e398). Others, on the other hand, have used liver transplantation for lesions in those children who are highly symptomatic or are considered to have an unresectable lesion (e693).

Prognosis is favorable in patients who undergo complete resection. Of 104 patients who underwent follow-up examination, six had died from intraoperative and postoperative complications; the remaining 98 were alive and well up to 15 years after surgery, except a 4-year-old boy who died of leukemia 2 years after surgery (e659). In neonates with large antenatal tumors, vascular compression of great vessels may lead to ischemia complicated by congestive cardiac failure, intraventricular hemorrhage, cystic encephalomalacia, and renal failure (e717). Fluid loss to the cysts and reduced fetal albumin production by the liver can further increase the risk of hydrops (e62,e324). Polyhydramnios is associated with upper intestinal tract obstruction, and elevation of the diaphragm poses the fetus at risk for pulmonary hypoplasia. In their literature review, Cornette et al. observed intrauterine demise or early neonatal mortality in 5 of 17 (29%) antenatally detected cases (43). In antenatally detected cases, fetal intervention in the form of ultrasound-guided percutaneous cyst aspiration has been reported to dramatically improve outcome (e717). Isaacs reports on 45 patients with mesenchymal hamartoma in the fetal and neonatal period, of which 29 (64%) had surgical resections and 23 (79%) survived (75).

Gross Appearance

The lesions vary in size from a few centimeters, an incidental finding at autopsy, to as large as 30 cm in older patients. The average weight is 1,300 to 1,900 g, but weights of 5,400 g have been reported (172). Cooper et al. (e141) noted a 3,500 g lesion in a 1-month-old boy whose birth weight had been 8,300 g. The right lobe is involved in 75% of cases, the left lobe in 22%, and both lobes in 3%. The tumor may bulge from the surface or even be pedunculated in about 20% of cases, attached to the liver by a thin to broad pedicle (e659).

On cut surface, multiple cysts are present, ranging in size from a few millimeters to 15 cm in over 85% of cases (Figure 15-48B, C). Clear amber to yellow fluid or gelatinous material fills the cyst and is similar to serum, except for lower concentrations of total protein, albumin, immunoglobulin, cholesterol, and glucose (e182). The cysts have gray-tan to yellow linings that may be smooth, long, or ragged. The surrounding tissue is yellow-tan to brown and loose to moderately dense. Only in the youngest patients are the lesions without cysts.

Histopathology

Microscopically, the lesion consists of an admixture of mesenchyme, bile ducts, hepatocyte cords, and variable-sized cysts (Figure 15-48D). The cysts may be no more than a loose, fluid-filled area of mesenchyme or dilated lymphatics or bile ducts. More often, the cysts that are discernible grossly consist of an "unlined" wall of loose to dense mesenchyme. In older patients, however (e.g., those older than 1 to 2 years of age), the cysts may be lined by cuboidal epithelium. The mesenchyme consists of scattered stellate cells in a rich matrix. Collagen in the form of fibrils or small bundles is often associated with vessels and bile ducts within the mesenchyme. Extramedullary hematopoiesis is a consistent finding (more than 85% of cases) (Figure 15-48E), and scattered plasma cells and lymphocytes, although rarely prominent, are seen throughout the lesion. In older patients, more mature collagen bundles may be present. Nodules of mesenchyme may be separated by dense, highly vascular connective tissue. Hepatocytes appear to be a passive component of the lesion, often seen near the periphery of the lesion or as thin compressed strips between collections of mesenchymal tissues within the lesion. Bile ducts, however, appear to be an active or proliferative component, with single ducts or intricately branching ducts primarily near the periphery of the lesion. Bile is rarely present within the ducts. Atypical mitoses and invasion of adjacent liver are absent. Cytologic sampling may result in misdiagnosis due to the heterogeneous nature of the lesion. Although clusters of normal bile duct epithelium and hepatocytes admixed with bland mesenchymal cells in a myxoid background are highly suggestive of HMH on fine needle aspiration, rare cases with elevated AFP levels have been misdiagnosed as hepatoblastoma due to limited sampling of the hepatocellular component (e99,e726). In a series of 17 cases of HMH, Chang et al. found 7 (41%) to be solid. The solid "variant" was associated with higher serum AFP levels, smaller bile ducts, and more frequent vascular proliferation. Serum AFP level correlated with the proportion of hepatocytes. Two of seven solid cases harbored a larger amount of evenly distributed hepatocytes and proliferation of small ducts with focal hepatocyte–bile duct transition, suggesting that hepatocytes within HMH may be a truly neoplastic rather than an entrapped component (37).

Immunohistochemistry may be used to rule out other entities. In HMH, bile ducts and hepatocytes are cytokeratin positive, whereas the mesenchyme and pseudocysts are vimentin positive. Myxomatous infantile hemangioendotheliomas can resemble HMH on fine-needle aspiration (FNA) biopsy, but the plump endothelium of the former is positive for factor VIII-related antigen, CD31, and CD34 immunohistochemical stains; however, a localized vascular proliferation within an HMH will stain similarly. Immunostains may not be helpful in differentiating HMH from biphasic hepatoblastomas.

Molecular Pathology

Various authors have noted a balanced translocation involving chromosome 11 (band q11, q13 or q15) and chromosome 19 (band 19q13.4) (e78,e430,e493,e555,e651). Talmon et al. (e684) reported a case with a deletion involving chromosome 19q13.4. Sharif et al. (e622) reported tumor recurrence associated with chromosome 19q translocation and suggested that these cases may require more radical surgical resection. In a case of an undifferentiated (embryonal) sarcoma putatively arising from an HMH, Lauwers et al. demonstrated that the transformed component had the 19q13.4 breakpoint in addition to several other numerical and structural chromosomal abnormalities. Taken together, these findings suggest that a subset of HMH may be truly neoplastic rather than hamartomatous (e374).

Relationship to Undifferentiated Embryonal Sarcoma

Ramanujam (e557) reported the "malignant transformation" of a mesenchymal hamartoma of the liver into a "malignant mesenchymoma," and de Chadarevian et al. (e164) noted an "undifferentiated (embryonal) sarcoma arising in conjunction with mesenchymal hamartoma." Lauwers et al. (e374) also described an undifferentiated (embryonal) sarcoma (UES) "arising in" a mesenchymal hamartoma. In their case, the mesenchymal hamartoma component was diploid by flow cytometry, while the UES showed a prominent aneuploid peak. Karyotypic analysis of the UES showed structural alterations of chromosome 19, which have been implicated as a potential genetic marker of mesenchymal hamartoma. We have also seen a case of UES surrounded with large areas of more bland mesenchymal tissue but without the characteristic bile ducts and cysts of a mesenchymal hamartoma. The question yet to be resolved in all these cases is whether the UES truly arises in a preexisting "benign" mesenchymal hamartoma or if the entire lesion is primarily an UES with areas of bland-appearing stroma. Begueret et al. reported a case of a large, cystic hepatic mass in a 17-year-old girl that had areas characteristic of both embryonal sarcoma and HMH, with the intervening "transition zone" showing the architectural features of a HMH but with the atypical mesenchymal cells of an embryonal sarcoma (19). Flow cytometric analysis of DNA aneuploidy showed that all three areas had similar DNA indices, suggesting a common lineage. O'Sullivan et al. have also described a case of UES arising within a mesenchymal hamartoma. The mesenchymal hamartoma in their case had unusual features including large mesothelial-lined cysts and adrenal cortical heterotopy (e493). While the association of UES and mesenchymal hamartoma is still tenuous, it would be prudent, in practice, to extensively sample all mesenchymal hamartomas for histologic evaluation, so as not to miss a focus of UES.

CAVERNOUS HEMANGIOMA

Although 1% of the population may harbor cavernous hemangiomas of the liver, the lesion is rare in children and is usually asymptomatic when it does occur (e659). The lesions are often small (<2 cm), single, red-purple, and spongy. Microscopically, the lesions are well-circumscribed collections of large channels with a thin layer of endothelial cells. Fibrosis, thrombosis, and calcification may be present. Infantile hemangioendotheliomas frequently contain foci of large vascular channels, resembling cavernous hemangioma.

INFANTILE HEMANGIOENDOTHELIOMA (IHE)

Infantile hemangioendothelioma is the most common benign hepatic neoplasm in the pediatric age group, accounting for 17.7% of all liver tumors/pseudotumors, and 40% of all benign tumors/pseudotumors in children (e305). It is a vascular tumor that is almost always seen in the 1st year of life.

Pathogenesis

The pathogenesis of infantile hemangioendothelioma is unclear.

Clinical Features, Laboratory Studies, and Imaging

Infantile hemangioendothelioma is seen most frequently in the first 6 months of life (86%) (Figure 15-49A) with 33% presenting in the neonatal period (e305). Patients are rarely older than 3 years of age (see Table 15-14); only one such patient (a 15-year-old female) was noted among 91 patients seen at the Armed Forces Institute of Pathology (163). There is a slight female predominance (1.7:1) but no racial predilection.

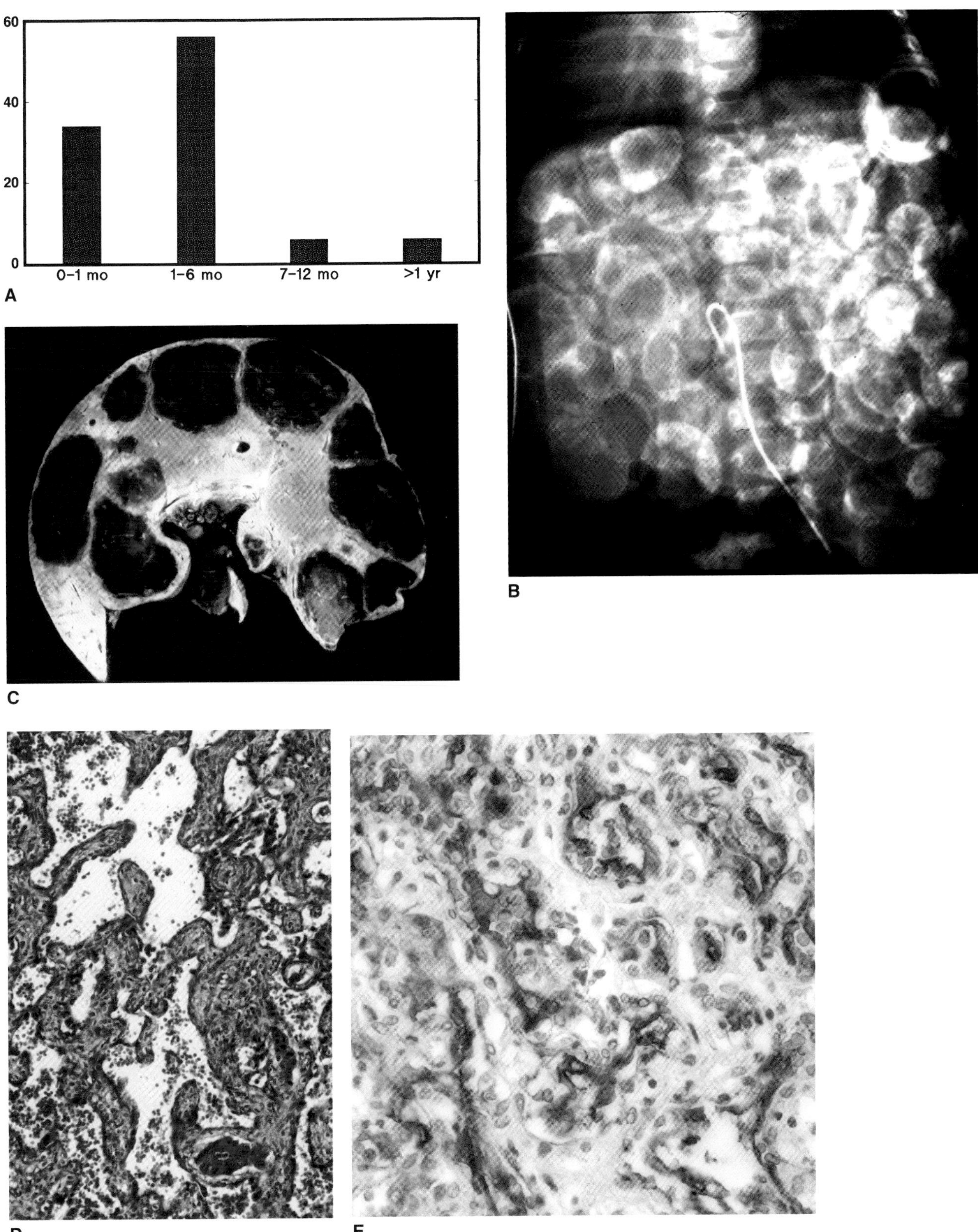

FIGURE 15-49 ■ Infantile hemangioendothelioma. **A:** Age distribution in 102 cases. **B:** Following injection of a radio-opaque dye, the liver displays numerous nodules throughout both lobes. **C:** On cut section of the liver, multiple blood-filled nodules are visible. **D:** The lesions of C are composed of trabeculae of loose fibrous connective tissue covered by a single layer of uniform endothelial cells (Masson trichrome stain, original magnification 75×). **E:** The epithelial cells lining the sinusoid of the lesion stain positively with the GLUT1 stain, a feature seen most prominently in patients with asymptomatic hepatomegaly and multiple small hepatic lesions (GLUT1 Immunoperoxidase stain, original magnification 100×).

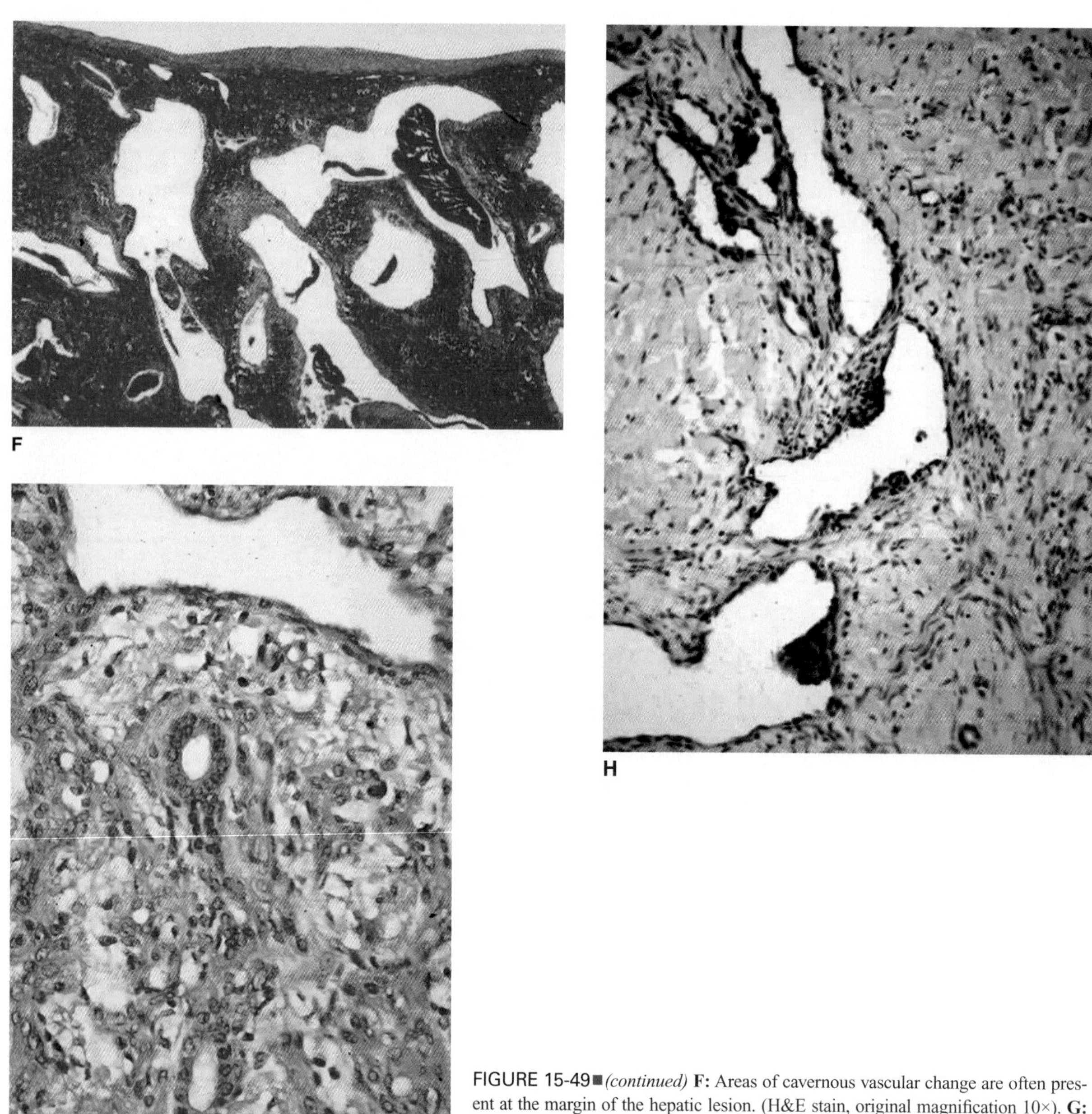

FIGURE 15-49 *(continued)* **F:** Areas of cavernous vascular change are often present at the margin of the hepatic lesion. (H&E stain, original magnification 10×). **G:** Entrapped bile ducts (**center**) can often be found within the fibrous septa. Note the thin covering of endothelial cells at top (H&E stain, original magnification 75×). **H:** Some lesions display dense clusters or "tufts" of endothelial cells felt by many to represent involutional changes within the lesion (H&E stain, original magnification 40×).

The classic presentation is a triad of hepatomegaly, congestive heart failure, and anemia (163). Most patients present with an abdominal mass or distension. Congestive heart failure may be present in 10% to 15% of cases, with increased cardiac output, elevated right and left end-diastolic pressure, small systolic pressure gradient across the pulmonary outflow tract, and mild elevation of pulmonary artery pressure (e156). Other presenting symptoms include failure to thrive, fever, jaundice (up to 20%), and (rarely) liver failure or tumor rupture with death (163) (e156,e278). Skopec and Lakatua (e640) reported on a premature infant who presented with nonimmune fetal hydrops, thrombocytopenia, and hypofibrinogenemia in association with an infantile hemangioendothelioma. This association, the Kasabach-Merritt syndrome, is attributed to trapping and increased destruction of platelets within the vascular tumor, often resulting in progression to disseminated intravascular coagulation with activation of both clotting and fibrinolytic pathways (e773). Fetal hydrops is attributable to large arteriovenous shunts created by the neoplastic vascular channels. In these cases, prenatal US can depict a liver mass together with polyhydramnios, cardiomegaly, anasarca, and ascites. In general, the prognosis is determined mainly by the amount of the shunt volume. Among 117 diagnosed antenatally (n = 33) and at birth (n = 84), the most common initial finding in the fetus was a hepatic mass detected by antenatal sonography followed in rank by anemia, hydrops, hydramnios, congestive heart failure, thrombocytopenia, and disseminated intravascular coagulation, which contributed to its demise. In the neonate, hepatomegaly was the leading finding, followed by congestive heart failure, cutaneous hemangiomas, a murmur (bruit), respiratory distress, cardiomegaly, and thrombocytopenia (75).

Hemangiomas of the skin have been reported in up to 70% of cases, but in an experience with 91 cases, they were noted in only 11% (163). Isaacs noted cutaneous hemangiomas in 4 (5%) of 76 patients with focal liver tumors, compared to 20 (49%) of 41 patients with multifocal liver lesions (75). Associated extrahepatic hemangiomas may also be present in the brain, placenta, lungs, eyes, lymph nodes, pancreas, retroperitoneum, adrenal, or bone as single or multiple lesions (75,163) (e429). Pereyra et al. (e523) described the death of a child from airway obstruction by a laryngotracheal hemangioma 4 months after resolution of a hepatic hemangioma treated with steroids and radiotherapy.

Significant laboratory findings in infantile hemangioendothelioma include anemia in about 50% of cases, hyperbilirubinemia in 20% of cases, and elevated aspartate transaminase (over 100 U/dL) in 32% of cases (163) (e52). Although in Isaacs' review (75) AFP levels were elevated in 5 fetuses and in 11 neonates (16/117 or 14%) with hemangiomas, the importance of this finding is unclear since even otherwise normal neonates may have elevated AFP levels (e331). Even in the absence of a liver lesion, "adult" levels of AFP (<25 ng/mL) are not reached until 6 months of age, and infants under 1 month of age may normally have levels as high as 2,500 ng/mL (e487). When adjusted for the age of the infant, AFP levels are not elevated with infantile hemangioendothelioma. Hemangioendotheliomas have been reported to express type 3 iodothyronine deiodinase and cause severe hypothyroidism (64). The hypothyroidism may be resistant to medical treatment, but resolves following OLT (e378).

Diagnostic imaging is helpful in the evaluation of infantile hemangioendotheliomas. Hepatomegaly with a soft tissue mass is usually visible on plain film of the abdomen, and speckled calcification of the lesion is present in 15% to 37% of cases (86). Chest radiography may demonstrate cardiomegaly with or without prominent pulmonary vascular markings. Ultrasound examination may show single or multiple hyperechoic, complex, or hypoechoic lesions. If significant arteriovenous shunting is present, a prominent Doppler signal flow is seen. On CT imaging, hepatic hemangioendtheliomas manifest as a well-defined, hypoattenuating mass. Contrast enhancement demonstrates peripheral pooling and central enhancement with variable delay. MRI is the most useful single modality because it shows not only the extent of the hemangioendothelioma but also the flow characteristics and the surrounding vascular structures (e572). Technetium-99m scans display a characteristic early "blush". Imaging studies demonstrate the hepatic origin of the lesion, multifocality, and extrahepatic lesions (e55,e286,e295,e515,e545). Selective arteriography displays a diffuse angiomatous lesions with rapid filing of the hepatic vein (e52) and can be used to determine the extent of the lesion and possible surgical approaches to the large feeder vessels.

Treatment and Outcomes

Infantile hepatic hemangioendotheliomas are vascular lesions that show a clinical course intermediate between a hemangioma and an angiosarcoma. Treatment is determined by the severity of the presenting symptom and whether the lesion is single or multifocal. Patients with congestive heart failure and a multifocal lesion are treated with digitalis and diuretics. Although spontaneous regression may occur, steroid therapy is thought by some to hasten the regression of the lesion and improve the platelet count but is considered by others not to be helpful (e546,e591). Alpha-interferon therapy has also been used as a component of medical management. Radiation therapy has been used in the past but is infrequently employed now, because of the potential long-term side effects. Interventional therapies include hepatic artery ligation or embolization, resectional surgery, or OLT (e5). Surgical excision of single lesions, even in the face of congestive heart failure, is frequently successful. Becker and Heitler noted the survival of 46 of 50 infants (92%) who had localized lesions treated with hepatic lobectomy or localized resection (52). For large single lesions or multifocal tumors, success has been achieved through OLT, hepatic artery ligation, or transarterial embolization, often in association with the use of digitalis, diuretics, and steroids (e5,e100,e435,e574).

Both success and complete failure have been reported variously with many agents including epsilon-aminocaproic acid (e755), tranexamic acid (e455), low-molecular-weight heparin (e692), vincristine (e524), cyclophosphamide (e418), and interferon-alpha (e692,e772). A treatment algorithm has been published by the vascular tumors study group at Boston Children's Hospital (40).

Patients with infantile hepatic hemangioendothelioma usually have an excellent prognosis, especially with spontaneous regression after the 1st year of life. Survival in 26 cases reviewed by Becker and Heitler was 65% (e52). Of 71 patients studied at the AFIP who had been followed for at least 6 months, 50 (70%) were alive and well approximately 24 years after diagnosis (mean 7.7 years). Of the 21 deaths, 19 occurred in the 1st month after diagnosis, and two deaths occurred at 3 and 7 months after diagnosis. Presence of congestive heart failure, jaundice, multiple tumor nodules, and absence of cavernous differentiation were significant predictors of death at 6 months (163). Because of the uncertainty about the behavior of "type 2", resection if possible, is advisable.

Gross Appearance

The tumors are single in about 55% of cases and multiple in 45%. Single tumors measure from smaller than 0.5 cm to as large as 13 cm and are located equally in the right and left lobes, with an occasional single lesion involving both lobes (163). When more than one lesion is present, they may be limited to one lobe but frequently involve large portions of the liver (Figure 15-49B). Lesions near the hepatic surface often show central umbilication. In his review of fetal and neonatal cases, Isaacs found 76 solitary and 41 multifocal lesions, the latter also including diffuse or disseminated hemangiomatosis. Most focal hemangiomas, 33 (43%) of 76, were found in the right lobe of the liver and 18 (24%) of 76 in the left. Among the 41 multifocal lesions, 11 were limited to the liver, 20 also had cutaneous hemangiomas, and 10 cases showed noncutaneous extrahepatic involvement (75). On cut section, they are well demarcated, reddish brown to light tan, and soft and spongy (Figure 15-49C). In large lesions, central areas of infarction, hemorrhage, fibrosis, and yellowish gritty specks of calcification may be present. In cases preoperatively treated with hepatic artery ligation or embolization, the entire lesion(s) may be infarcted.

Histopathology

Histologically, hemangioendotheliomas have traditionally been classified as type 1 or type 2 lesions (e169). Hemangioendotheliomas are composed of vascular channels lined by a single continuous layer of plump endothelial cells in a supporting fibrous stroma (Figure 15-49D to H), reflecting the "type 1" lesion defined by Dehner and Ishak (e169). Also, in about 20% of cases, larger pleomorphic and hyperchromatic cells are present along poorly formed vascular spaces, often displaying tufting or branching, the "type 2" lesion (Figure 15-49H). However, the so-called "type 2" lesions are now grouped together with angiosarcomas. Well-preserved bile ducts may be present in the supporting stroma, most frequently near the periphery of the lesion. Foci of extramedullary hematopoiesis are noted within the vascular spaces in over 60% of patients. Mitoses are infrequent but rarely may number 5 to 10 per high-power field. Larger vascular channels resembling cavernous hemangioma may be found in 50% to 65% of patients (Figure 15-49F). Areas of hemorrhage, infarction, fibrosis, and calcification may occupy small to large areas of the lesion, occasionally obliterating all but the margin of the lesion. When hemorrhage or fibrovascular reaction dominates the biopsy, it is difficult to differentiate the stroma of an infantile hemangioendothelioma from that of a mesenchymal hamartoma, and a discussion with the pediatric radiologist may help sort this differential diagnosis (46). One should also remember that hemorrhagic necrosis can be seen in IHE but is uncommon in mesenchymal hamartoma. The presence of hemorrhagic necrosis in a biopsy should also raise the possibility of a hepatoblastoma. Another vascular lesion with a myxoid stroma is hepatic epithelioid hemangioendothelioma, albeit rare in children. This is a multifocal tumor, comprised of strands, clusters, and nests of CD31-positive epithelioid cells with intracellular lumina and sinusoidal infiltraton (117).

Immunohistochemically, the endothelial cells of the lesion are positive for CD31, CD34, factor VIII–related antigen, von Willebrand factor, vimentin, and Ulex europaeus I lecten (e108,e780). Cerar et al. (e108) noted that the cells beneath the endothelial cells contained cytoplasm that was positive for alpha–smooth muscle actin and antimuscle actin, negative for desmin, and were enveloped with basement membrane (BM) that they believed were characteristic of pericytes. Electron microscopy displays vascular channels lined by endothelial cells with irregular fine cytoplasmic processes along the luminal surface (e205). Fibroblasts and collagen fibers are present in the stroma. The "type 2 lesion" with multilayered, hyperchromatic endothelial cells in a tufted or branching pattern is now thought to represent a form of angiosarcoma (see later), but could represent degenerative change.

Mo et al. (125) use the presence or absence of GLUT1 immunoreactivity of the endothelial lining in separating the "true infantile hemangioma" (hemangioendothelioma) from a "hepatic vascular malformation with capillary proliferation." They note that with the GLUT1-positive infantile hemangioma patients have asymptomatic hepatomegaly and an incidental finding of the lesion in the first few weeks or months of age. The lesion is present in the liver as multiple small nodules of closely packed capillary vessels with involutional features. These tumors undergo spontaneous involution over months or years and are usually unresponsive to corticosteroids or interferon treatment. The GLUT1-negative hepatic vascular malformation with capillary proliferation is usually symptomatic at birth or in the first few weeks of life with severe edema and congestive heart failure. The lesion is usually a single mass with malformed irregular vessels commonly associated with infarction, hemorrhage, calcification, and peripheral reactive capillary proliferation. Surgical resection is often required.

Molecular Pathology

Flow cytometry performed by Selby et al. on 21 cases showed 16 to be diploid, 3 to be aneuploid, and 2 with a wide coefficient of variation (163). Ito et al. described an interstitial deletion of chromosome 6q in a 6-month old boy with hepatic infantile hemangioendothelioma, microcephaly, hypertelorism, low-set ears, prominent nasal bridge, cubitus valgus, overlapping fingers, cryptorchidism, and micropenis (e310). Other anomalies reported in association with infantile hemangioendothelioma include trisomy 21, extranumerary digit, hydrocele, and congenital heart disease (163). Shah et al. noted a newborn girl with a large left-sided diaphragmatic hernia who had a heterotopic liver with an infantile hemangioendothelioma in the left hemithorax attached by a pedicle through the diaphragm to the left lobe of the liver (e619).

TERATOMA

Teratoma is a rarely occurring benign neoplasm composed of a mixture of tissue of mesodermal, ectodermal, and endodermal origin. Most pediatric cases occur in the 1st year of life, presenting as an abdominal mass, which on plain film frequently

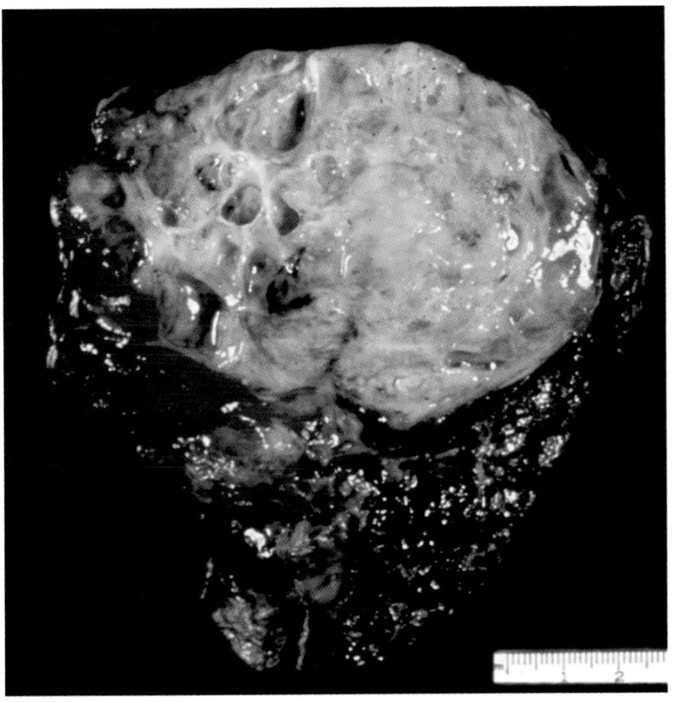

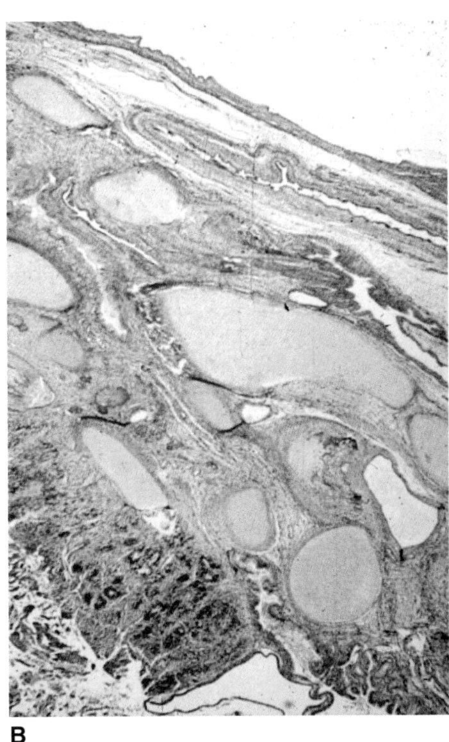

FIGURE 15-50 ▪ Teratoma. **A:** A large irregular mass contains both solid and cystic components of varying color. **B:** Random sampling of the lesion displays tissues of various somatic lines including, in this image, cartilage, epithelial-lined ducts, and "immature" tissue (**lower left**). (H&E stain, original magnification 15×).

displays areas of calcification (e559,e705,e757,e769). AFP may be elevated. Associated conditions include anencephaly and trisomy 13. Resection may be curative. Care should be taken not to confuse teratoma with a mixed hepatoblastoma with teratoid features (e139,e170). Intrahepatic fetus-in-fetu has been reported (e409).

The lesions are large, with a variegated cut surface reflecting the various tissues of the tumor (Figure 15-50). Microscopically, benign tissues of all three germ cell layers may be found, including well-differentiated squamous epithelium, bone, cartilage, gastrointestinal mucosa and muscularis propria, renal glomeruli and tubules, respiratory epithelium, and neural tissue. The presence of embryonal or fetal hepatoblastoma cells precludes the diagnosis of teratoma and instead favors mixed hepatoblastoma with teratoid features or teratoid hepatoblastoma.

HEPATOBLASTOMA

The incidence rate of primary hepatic malignancies in children 0 to 14 years of age is approximately 0.2 per 100,000 children in the United States, with hepatoblastomas accounting for 47% of the malignancies and nearly 27% of all pediatric hepatic tumors (42). By age group, hepatoblastoma accounts for 1% of all pediatric malignancies in children under 15 years age, 1.5% of all malignancies in children younger than 5 years of age, and 3.3% of all malignancies in white and black children under 1 year of age (e420,e575). The reported incidence is 11.2 cases per million during the 1st year of life; nearly 90% of hepatoblastomas are seen in the first 5 years of life, with 68% discovered in the first 2 years and 4% present at the time of birth (Figure 15-51). Of 271 primary hepatic malignancies reported in the United States to Surveillance, Epidemiology and End Results (SEER) data between 1973 and 1997 in patients below 20 years of age, 67% and 31% were HB and HCC, respectively. In the group less than 5 years of age, HB accounted for 91%, whereas among those 15 to 19 years of age, HCC represented 87% of the cases (45). The relative frequency of hepatoblastomas in younger children is most apparent when noting that hepatoblastomas account for over 40% of all hepatic tumors (benign and malignant) in children younger than 2 years of age, but only 7.5% of liver tumors in children 5 to 20 years old. Although

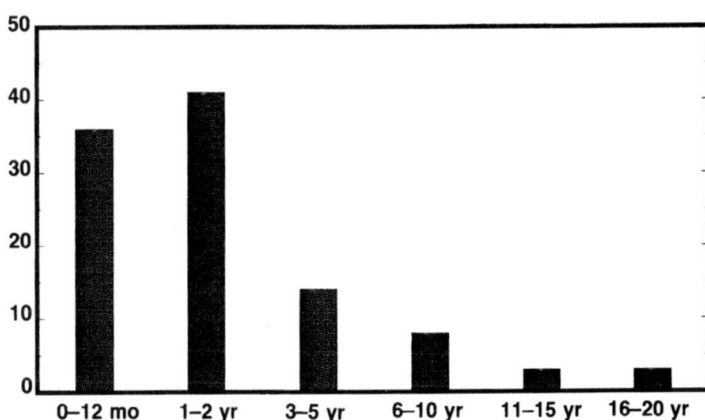

FIGURE 15-51 ▪ Hepatoblastoma. Age distribution in 105 cases.

there is no racial predilection for hepatoblastoma, there is a distinct male predominance from 1.2:1 to 3.6:1 (e93).

Pathogenesis

There appears to be a genetic predisposition to hepatoblastomas, with an increased incidence in a setting of Beckwith-Wiedemann syndrome (macrosomia, macroglossia, visceromegaly, abdominal wall defects, hemihypertrophy), hemihypertrophy, and familial adenomatous polyposis (FAP). The relative risk for the development of hepatoblastoma in Beckwith-Wiedemann syndrome is 22.80 (e166,e654), while that for FAP is 12.20 (e236), suggesting a role for genetic aberrations of chromosomes 11 and 5, respectively, in the pathogenesis of hepatoblastoma. Inactivation of the APC tumor-suppressor gene (found on chromosome 5) is found in 67% to 89% of sporadic hepatoblastoma (e34,e291,e317,e761). This gene is known to regulate beta-catenin and modulate the *wnt* signaling pathway, suggesting a role for this signaling pathway in the development of hepatoblastoma (e725). Additional biologic markers may include trisomies 2, 8, and 20 and translocation of the NOTCH2 gene on chromosome 1. There is also an association of prematurity/low birth weight and hepatoblastoma, with a relative risk of up to 15.64 in patients weighing less than 1,000 g, compared with patients weighing 2,500 g (e505). In Japan, Ikeda et al. (e300) have noted an increasing incidence of hepatoblastoma in very low birth weight infants from 0.7% of patients with birth weights less than 1,500 g with tumors in 1985 to 1989 to 8.6% of patients with similar low birth weights in 1990 to 1993. In the United States, Ross and Gurney (e576) have observed a similar increasing trend of 5.2% in hepatoblastoma incidence in children 4 years and younger during the most recent two decades, a period corresponding with improved survival for low birth weight children. Hepatoblastoma has been described in association with trisomy 18, including some cases with abdominal wall defects. Hepatoblastoma has been noted in a number of sibling pairs including identical male twins and two siblings with GSD type 1a (e309,e475,e563,e677). There are no known environmental risk factors (e605). Zimmermann has recently reviewed putative pathways from ontogenesis to oncogenesis as a possible basis for a molecular classification of hepatoblastomas (199).

Table 15-19 ■ CLINICAL SYNDROMES, CONGENITAL MALFORMATIONS AND OTHER CONDITIONS ASSOCIATED WITH HEPATOBLASTOMA

Absence of left adrenal gland
Aicardi syndrome
Alcohol embryopathy
Beckwith-Wiedemann syndrome
Beckwith-Wiedemann syndrome with opsoclonus, myoclonus
Bilateral talipes
Budd-Chiari syndrome
Cleft palate, macroglossia, dysplasia of ear lobes
Cystathioninuria
Down syndrome, malrotation of colon, Meckel diverticulum, pectum excavatum, intrathoracic kidney, single coronary artery
Duplicated ureters
Fetal hydrops
Gardner syndrome
Goldenhar syndrome oculoauriculovertebral dysplasia, absence of portal vein
Hemihypertrophy
Heterotopic lung tissue
Heterozygous A1AT deficiency
HIV or HBV infection
Horseshoe kidney
Hypoglycemia
Inguinal hernia
Isosexual precocity
Maternal clomiphene citrate and Pergonal
Meckel diverticulum
Oral contraceptive, mother
Oral contraceptive, patient
Osteoporosis
Persistent ductus arteriosus
Polyposis coli families
Prader-Willi syndrome
Renal dysplasia
Right-sided diaphragmatic hernia
Schinzel-Geidion syndrome
Synchronous Wilms tumor
Trisomy 18
Type 1a glycogen storage disease
Umbilical hernia
Very low birth weight

From Ishak KG, Goodman Z, Stocker JT. Tumors of the liver and intrahepatic bile ducts. In: Rosai J, Sobin L, eds. *Atlas of tumor pathology*, 3rd series, Washington, DC: Fascicle; Armed Forces Institute of Pathology, 2000.

Clinical Features, Laboratory Studies, and Imaging

Most patients present with an enlarged abdomen noted by a parent or discovered on routine physical examination. Other symptoms such as anorexia, weight loss (less frequently), nausea, vomiting, and abdominal pain may indicate advanced disease (e525). Jaundice is noted in about 5% of cases. Physical examination reveals a firm, often irregular mass in the right upper abdomen that may cross the midline and extend down to the pelvic rim. A variety of malformations and clinical presentations have been described in patients with hepatoblastoma (Table 15-19). A striking presentation of hepatoblastoma is seen in children (particularly young boys) whose tumors produce hCG, leading to precocious puberty with genital enlargement, the appearance of pubic hair, and a deepening voice. The increased levels of hCG correlate with immunohistochemical staining and are accompanied by increases in serum luteinizing hormone and plasma testosterone (e284,e285,e457,e469,e478,e758).

Anemia is common (70%) in patients with hepatoblastoma as is thrombocytosis (50% of cases). Platelet counts of greater than 500 × 10^6/L were noted in 35% of 99 cases by Shafford and Pritchard (e618), with 29% having counts over

800 × 10^6. Along with AFP, thrombocytosis has been used as a measure of disease activity (e220,e777). Approximately 90% of patients demonstrate elevated serum AFP levels, and there is a correlation between AFP levels and extent of disease (e736), with a return to normal levels after complete resection of the tumor and a re-elevation with recurrence (e658). However, the least well-differentiated hepatoblastomas, that is, the small cell undifferentiated type, may in some cases show little or no elevation in AFP (e720). Van Tornout et al. (e736) have noted that for unresectable or metastatic hepatoblastoma, AFP levels can reliably predict outcome and identify poor responders to treatment. In studying patients who had undergone an initial surgery and chemotherapy, those patients whose AFP failed to decrease by at least two logs had a much poorer prognosis. In contrast, a large early decrease in AFP levels was a strong independent predictor of favorable outcome. It is important to remember, however, that AFP is present at levels of 25,000 to 50,000 ng/mL at birth and does not fall to "adult" levels of less than 25 ng/mL until 5 to 6 months of age (e487). AFP levels in infants with tumors resected in the first 6 months of life may therefore be "appropriately" elevated even though the tumor has been completely resected.

Isaacs reviewed 32 cases of hepatoblastomas reported in fetuses and neonates (75). Nine cases were diagnosed antenatally and 23 at birth, with a female predominance (female to male ratio 1.6). Although the most common presenting finding was an elevated AFP, this finding was present only in 50% of the patients, suggesting that AFP levels may not be a reliable indicator of the tumor in the fetus and neonate as compared with older children. Abdominal distension was the second common presenting finding followed in rank by a palpable abdominal mass, hepatic or abdominal mass detected on antenatal sonography, and hepatomegaly. Anemia, fetal hydrops, and respiratory distress were other initial findings. The most common site of origin was the right lobe of the liver (47%) compared with the left (16%), or both lobes (6%). Four patients had more than one hepatic tumor at the time of diagnosis. Most patients were classified as stage 1 (12 of 32, 37.5%), none as stage 2, 4 (12.5%) as stage 3, and 6 (18.8%) as stage 4. In 10 patients (31.2%) the stage of disease was not mentioned in the report. Survival rates for stages 1, 3, and 4 were 50%, 50%, and 0%, respectively. Sixty-three percent of the patients were treated by the following modalities: surgical resection alone, surgical resection plus chemotherapy, and surgical resection with hepatic artery embolization and chemotherapy; survival rates were 3 of 9 (33%), 3 of 5 (60%), and 1 of 1 (100%), respectively. Only one of four infants who received chemotherapy alone after a biopsy survived. Fetal survival was slightly less than the neonatal diagnosed cases, 22% and 26%, respectively. All 12 untreated patients died. Of the 20 treated infants, 8 (40%) lived. The overall survival for hepatoblastoma group was poor, 8 of 32 (25%) survived. The main cause of death from hepatoblastoma was mass effect by the tumor, producing abdominal distension, compression of portal vein and inferior vena cava, fetal hydrops leading to stillbirth, and severe respiratory distress. Metastases to the placenta with occlusion of umbilical vessels and to the lungs were other terminal events. Anemia resulting from bleeding into the tumor and rupture of the tumor during delivery occurred in seven and four patients, respectively. There were a few perioperative deaths related to immaturity and clinical condition of the patients. Female/male ratio was 1.6:1. Of 32 cases, 9 (28%) were diagnosed antenatally and 23 (72%) in the neonatal period. Tumors were more common in the right (15/32, 47%) than in the left (5/32, 16%) lobe, with two patients (6%) having tumors in both lobes. Tumors ranged in size from 3 to 16 cm (mean 8 cm) and weighed from 21 to 429 cm (mean 160 cm). The relation of histology and survival was as follows: fetal 3/10 (30%); embryonal 1/6 (17%); fetal and embryonal 1/2 (50%); and fetal, embryonal, and mesenchymal 3/8 (37.5%).

Imaging studies are helpful in diagnosing hepatoblastoma and differentiating it from other liver disorders seen in young children (e286). CT demonstrates a solitary or occasionally multifocal mass(es) with attenuation values between those of water and normal liver parenchyma. Speckled or amorphous calcification may be seen on CT in more than 50% of cases (e446). Ultrasonography displays a mass with increased, inhomogeneous echogenicity, punctate or amorphous calcification, and occasional cystic areas (e162). On antenatal ultrasonography, hepatoblastomas are described as well-defined, solid, echogenic lesions, with a "spoked-wheel" appearance (e631). Calcifications may be present, and a pseudocapsule gives the lesion(s) a characteristic well-demarcated appearance (75). Using pulsed Doppler ultrasonography, Bates et al. (e47) found peak systolic Doppler frequency shifts equal to or greater than 4 kHz and were also able to demonstrate antegrade diastolic flow. Differentiation of hepatoblastoma from other childhood hepatic solid, cystic, or vascular lesions such as mesenchymal hamartoma, infantile hemangioendothelioma and HCC can be aided by MRI with standard spin-echo T1- and T2-weighted imaging enhanced by the application of advanced sequences such as gradient-echo, fast spin–echo, and fat suppression techniques (e545). The histologic features of hepatoblastomas can be differentiated by MRI as well, with the homogenous character of an "epithelial" lesion contrasting with the heterogeneous character of a "mixed" hepatoblastoma with its fibrotic bands. Decreased signal intensity compared with normal liver is noted on T1-weighted images, whereas increased signal intensity is seen on T2-weighted images. Hypointense bands on MRI identify fibrotic bands, and the presence of vascular invasion may be detected by gradient-echo MRI (e545).

Staging

Most patients in the United States are staged postoperatively according to the Children's Cancer Study Group

Table 15-20 ■ STAGING OF HEPATOBLASTOMAS

Stage I	Complete resection
Stage II	Microscopic residual tumor
	Intrahepatic
	Extrahepatic
Stage III	Gross residual tumor
	Primary completely resected, nodes positive and/or tumor spill
	Primary not completely resected, and/or nodes positive and/or tumor spill
Stage IV	Metastatic disease
	Primary completely resected
	Primary not completely resected

From King D, Ortega J, Campbell J. The surgical management or children with incompletely resected hepatic cancer is facilitated by intensive chemotherapy. *J Pediatr Surg* 1991;26:1074–1081, with permission.

(CCSG) classification (see Table 15-20) (e268,e501). Other classifications include the TNM or variations of the CCSG staging classification (173) (e279,e645). Based on these classifications, approximately 38% of hepatoblastomas are stage I at the time of initial diagnosis and before any chemotherapy is administered. At this same point, about 9% are stage II, 24% stage III, and 29% stage IV (42) (e211,e268). However, this traditional staging system has been criticized for being rather subjective, depending to a large extent on the surgeon rather than the tumor (e36,e439). In 1990, the International Society of Pediatric Oncology Liver Study Group (SIOPEL-1) adopted a new preoperative staging system, Pretreatment Extent of Disease (PRETEXT), based exclusively on images obtained *prior to surgery*, based on the branching pattern of the portal vein, which divides the liver into eight segments. The system divides the liver into four sectors: (a) lateral sector (Couinaud segments 2 and 3); (b) medial sector (segment 4); (c) anterior sector (segments 5 and 8) and; (d) posterior sector (segment 6 and 7). Tumors are classified as one of four categories (PRETEXT-I to PRETEXT IV) by determining the number of affected liver sector(s) on imaging. Extrahepatic growth of the tumor is indicated by adding a letter (V involvement of hepatic vein, P involvement of portal vein, E for extrahepatic extension, M for the presence of distant metastasis). The PRETEXT system has prognostic value for overall and disease-free survival and is useful in defining treatment (27) (e606). Although the PRETEXT system was developed mainly to assess the efficacy of neoadjuvant chemotherapy and to predict surgical resectability, it also had highly prognostic value for both overall survival and event-free survival (27). Conceptually, however, both preoperative and postoperative staging systems use the same parameters for staging, namely, size, vascular invasion, extension and complexity of the primary tumor, and the absence or presence of metastases. Metastatic spread of hepatoblastoma is seen most frequently to the lung but may also spread to bone, brain, eye, and ovaries (e79,e197,e255,e448,e567). Local extension into hepatic vessels and the inferior vena cava may also occur (e681).

Treatment and Outcomes

Although complete resection of hepatoblastoma is the mainstay of treatment and is the only chance of cure, improvements in survival that have occurred over the last three decades have been a function of standardized chemotherapy regimens that reduce tumor size and enable complete tumor excision, even permitting cure in the presence of initially unresectable or metastatic disease. Treatment strategies currently combine surgery, transplantation, and chemotherapy (adjuvant and neoadjuvant), as defined by the PRETEXT stage of the tumor. Surgery remains the mainstay in the treatment of hepatoblastoma, with prognosis directly related to tumor stage. Small, solitary lesions localized to a single lobe can be adequately treated by lobectomy. Larger lesions, including those requiring preoperative chemotherapy to allow resection, may require more extensive surgery or transplantation (e5,e193,e212,e234). Surgical complications, particularly hemorrhage, are noted in 14% of primary resections and 29% of second resections (e744). If resection is possible and safe, an attempt to obtain clear resection margins is essential; positive margins on pathology warrant a re-resection if possible. Although elevated AFP immediately after resection is common, persistently elevated or rising AFP levels indicate the need to evaluate further for disease recurrence or search for distant metastasis. Contraindications to immediate resection include extensive bilateral liver involvement, presence of vascular invasion of major hepatic veins or inferior vena cava, diffuse multifocal disease, and distant metastasis (e289).

At the time of diagnosis, 40% to 60% of hepatoblastomas are considered to be unresectable and 10% to 20% of patients are found to have pulmonary metastases. Preoperative chemotherapy converts nearly 85% of these "unresectable" lesions to ones that can be entirely grossly removed, that is, to stage I or II lesions (see Table 15-20) with subsequent long-term survival (e193,e533,e658). Even if unresectable at diagnosis, most hepatoblastomas are unifocal and chemosensitive, with cisplatin and adriamycin being the most commonly used agents. Chemotherapy has been proven effective in both an adjuvant and neoadjuvant treatment and can shrink tumors. It makes them less prone to bleed and delineates the tumor from the surrounding normal parenchyma and vascular structures facilitating resection. In rare cases, patients may survive with chemotherapy alone (e782). On the other hand, some tumors may become resistant to prolonged courses of chemotherapy (e747), and the highest survival rates have historically been observed in patients with initially resected tumors—although these tumors also tend to be the smaller more favorable tumors. Further, prolonged (>4 cycles) courses of neoadjuvant chemotherapy are discouraged, since this may lead to cumulative chemotherapy toxicity and cause tumor cells to become resistant to chemotherapy (122).

The 5-year survival rate for hepatoblastomas has improved to over 75% compared with a 5-year survival rate of 35% almost 30 years ago (122) (e201,e547). Preoperative chemotherapy has increased resectability of hepatoblastoma from 40% to 60%, to 90%, with the more extensive tumors requiring transplantation to remove the involved portions of liver (e196,e669). In fact, primary liver transplantation with neoadjuvant chemotherapy may result in an 80% 5- to10-year disease-free survival rate, whereas the 10-year survival falls to 40% in those undergoing transplantation as "rescue therapy" (135). The SIOPEL-1 study showed that, in patients undergoing transplantation, only macroscopic venous invasion had a significant prognostic effect on survival (e504). A worldwide electronic registry for liver transplant in childhood liver tumors (hepatoblastoma, HCC, and hemangioendothelioma) has been established; this "pediatric liver unresectable tumor observatory (PLUTO)" registry can be reached at http://transplant.test.cineca.it/.

Traditionally, tumor stage at the time of initial resection has been the key prognostic factor in determining the survival of children and adults with hepatoblastoma (42) (e193,e268,e669,e745). Data from the recent COG study, 9,645, show 3-year event-free survival of 90% for stage I to II, 50% for stage III, and only 20% for stage IV (122). However, as noted earlier, preoperative and postoperative chemotherapy and aggressive treatment of pulmonary and central nervous system metastases have significantly changed the survival rate in patients with stage IV tumors (e209,e518,e567). Survival is independent of histologic subtype when adjusted for age, sex, and stage (42) (e745). Only small cell undifferentiated hepatoblastoma may have a worse prognosis than others, but the small number of cases of this unusual type makes analysis uncertain. More recently, two broad categories of risk stratification have been advocated, namely standard risk and high risk. Standard risk tumors are PRETEXT I, II, or III. SIOPEL high-risk tumors are defined as tumors involving all four hepatic sectors (PREVEXT IV), or any tumor with metastasis (m), ingrowth of the vena cava (v), ingrowth of the portal vein (p) or contiguous extrahepatic disease (e), and tumors that fail to express AFP with AFP less than 100 at diagnosis (155).

Gross Appearance

Hepatoblastomas are single masses in approximately 80% of cases. They occur in the right lobe in 58% of cases, in the left in 15%, and in both lobes in the remaining 27%, either as a large single lesion extending across the midline or as multiple lesions (e659). Distant metastasis are present in 20% of patients at the time of diagnosis, with the lung as the most common site of metastasis; other common sites are the brain and bone and metastasis occurs more commonly with disease relapse (e209).

Tumors may measure 15 cm or more in diameter and weigh in excess of 1,000 g. Grossly, they are coarsely lobulated and frequently bulge from the surface of the liver (Figure 15-52A). On cut section, the lesions are tan to light brown to green and display frequent areas of hemorrhage and necrosis. Various types of mesenchymal tissues (e.g., osteoid, cartilaginous, fibrous) in the mixed type of hepatoblastoma may alter the color and consistency of the gross appearance.

Table 15-21 ■ HISTOLOGIC CLASSIFICATION OF HEPATOBLASTOMA

I. Epithelial type
   A. Fetal pattern
   B. Embryonal and fetal pattern
   C. Macrotrabecular pattern
   D. Small-cell undifferentiated pattern
II. Mixed epithelial and mesenchymal type
   A. Without teratoid features
   B. With teratoid features

Histopathology

Histologically, the tumor is traditionally classified into six patterns (Table 15-21) (Figures 15-52 to 15-54). The epithelial types account for approximately 56% of cases, including pure fetal (31%), embryonal (19%), macrotrabecular (3%), and small cell undifferentiated (3%). The mixed pattern of epithelial and mesenchymal components accounts for 44% of the cases, including 34% without teratoid features and 10% with such components as squamous epithelium and striated muscle (see later).

The fetal pattern refers to cases in which 100% of the tumor is composed of small, round, uniform cells with abundant cytoplasm and distinct cytoplasmic membranes (Figure 15-52B). The cells are arranged into thin trabeculae, usually two to three cells thick, with alternating light and dark areas.

The embryonal pattern refers to cases of epithelial hepatoblastoma in which, in addition to fetal cells, part of the tumor has cells arranged into sheets of irregular, angulated cells with a high nucleocytoplasmic ratio, increased nuclear chromatin, and indistinct cytoplasmic membranes (Figure 15-52C). Pseudorosette and acinar formation are common features. Foci of extramedullary hematopoiesis (EMH) are seen in both the fetal and embryonal areas.

The macrotrabecular pattern refers to cases in which trabeculae more than 10 cells in thickness are present as a repetitive pattern within the tumor (Figure 15-52D). The large trabeculae contain either fetal- or embryonal-type cells; a third, larger cell type with cytoplasm that is more abundant than in normal hepatocytes or fetal-type cells; or a combination of all three cell types. Thus, the term "macrotrabecular" refers more to a growth pattern rather than a distinct subtype and these lesions form a heterogeneous group. Cases that have embryonal or mesenchymal cells with an isolated macrotrabecular focus are classified based on the embryonal or mesenchymal cell present and not as macrotrabecular. Tumors where the third (hepatocyte-like) cell type predominates may be very difficult to distinguish from HCC. The presence of EMH is useful in a diagnosis of hepatoblastoma.

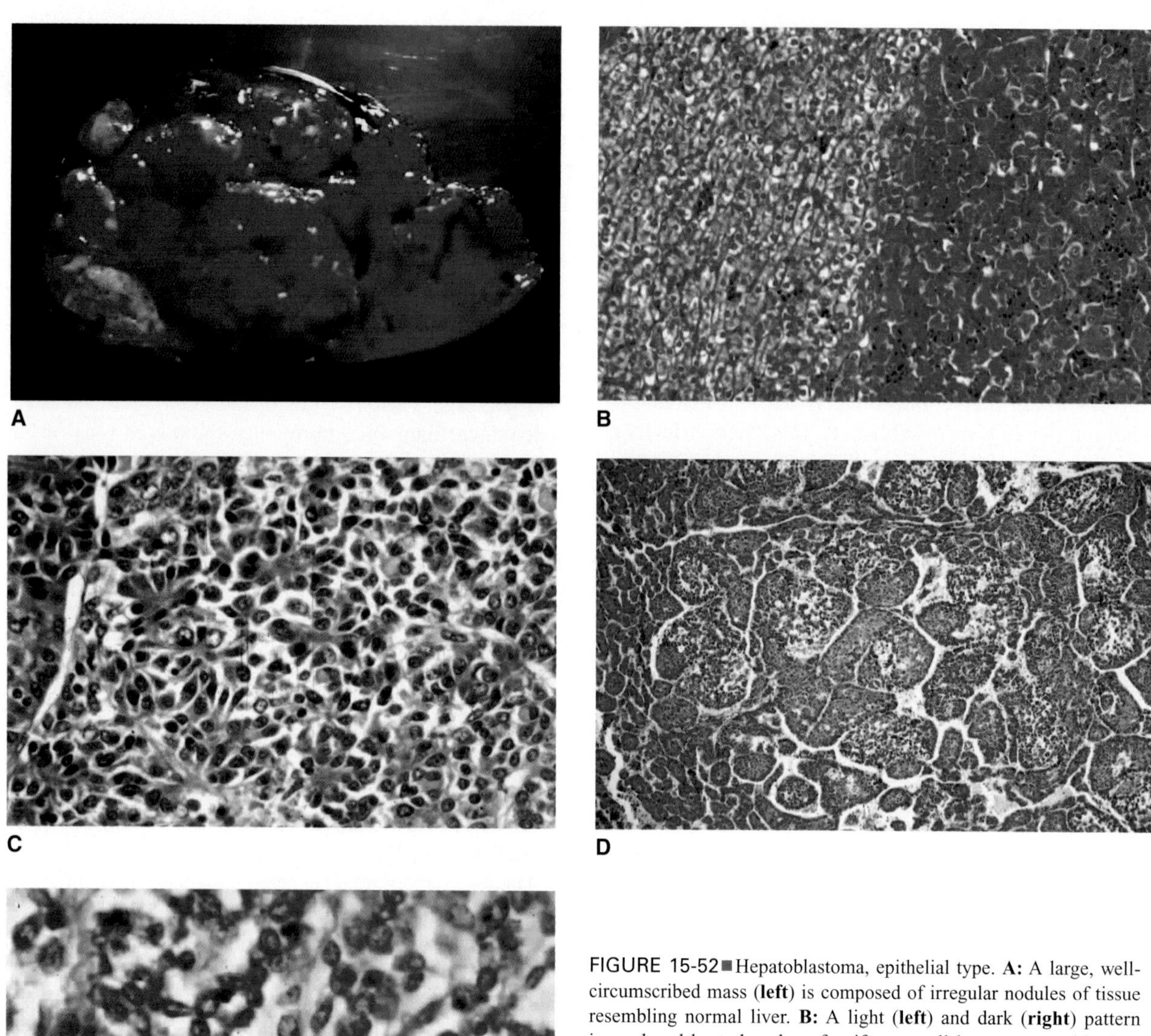

FIGURE 15-52 Hepatoblastoma, epithelial type. **A:** A large, well-circumscribed mass (**left**) is composed of irregular nodules of tissue resembling normal liver. **B:** A light (**left**) and dark (**right**) pattern is produced by trabeculae of uniform small hepatocytes with clear (*light*) or granular (*dark*) cytoplasm. Note the foci of extramedullary hematopoiesis in this well-differentiated fetal epithelial lesion (H&E stain, original magnification 100×). **C:** The embryonal component of the epithelial lesion is composed of single or small clusters of oval or tapered cells with mild anisonucleosis and nuclear hyperchromasia. (H&E stain, original magnification 150×). **D:** A "macrotrabecular" pattern is formed by solid sheets of hepatocytes, some with central areas of necrosis (H&E stain, original magnification 40×). **E:** With "anaplastic" hepatoblastoma, sheet of small, round blue cells resemble neuroblastoma cells (H&E stain, original magnification 200×).

The small cell undifferentiated or anaplastic pattern is composed of cells reminescent of neuroblastoma or other small round blue cell tumors, with scanty cytoplasm and hyperchromatic nuclei (Figure 15-52E). Round or ovoid cells predominate, with the occasional presence of spindle or stellate cells within a mucoid matrix. These cells grow in sheets but lack cohesiveness. Mitoses are occasionally present, but the cells do not produce glycogen, fat droplets, or bile pigment. Abortive or incompletely formed bile ductules may be present, but electron microscopy or immunohistochemical studies, or both, may be needed to confirm the diagnosis of hepatoblastoma. Particularly helpful in establishing the diagnosis is the presence of cytoplasmic staining with polyclonal anticytokeratin antibodies. Gonzalez-Crussi believes that the small cell form represents the subtype with the least differentiation within the highly variable morphologic spectrum of hepatoblastomas (e245). Medium- and large-sized cells have been reported in undifferentiated hepatoblastomas; some undifferentiated tumors have shown intermediate or large cells, leading to a proposal to subclassify undifferentiated hepatoblastomas as small cell, intermediate cell, and large cell subtypes (94,199). Immunostains are required to

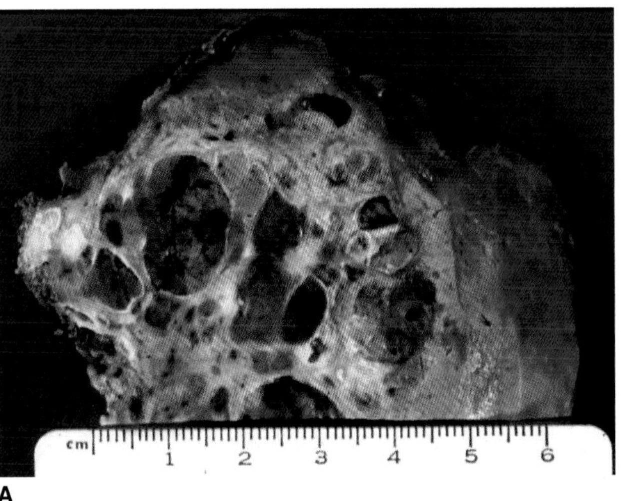

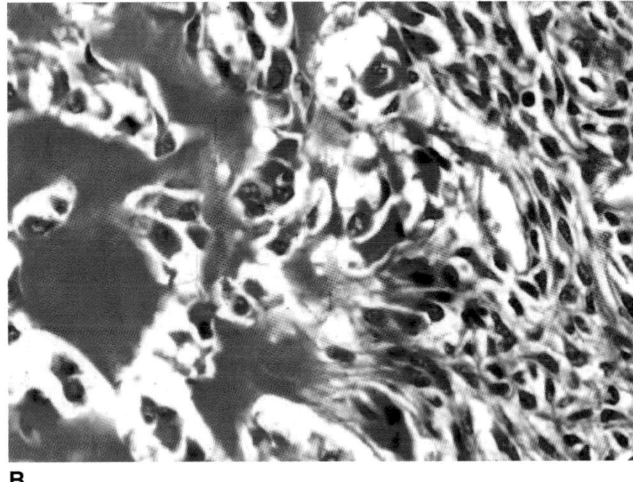

A B

FIGURE 15-53 ■ Mixed epithelial and mesenchymal hepatoblastoma. **A:** The tumor within the liver displays a highly variegated appearance reflecting the presence of mesenchymal tissue and epithelial cells. **B:** Osteoid-like material (**left**) contains cells similar to the fetal and embryonal epithelial cells (**right**). The cells associated with the "osteoid" are cytokeratin positive (H&E stain, original magnification 125×).

differentiate these from other large cell tumors such as lymphoma, large cell medulloblastoma (e235), large cell neuroblastoma (e709), and Ewing sarcoma family tumors, although some hepatoblastomas may be positive for CD99 (199). The histogenesis of these undifferentiated tumors is not known. Although hepatic stem cells have been invoked in their pathogenesis (e583), this has been refuted by other authors (13). An alternative pathway might involve regression to a primitive cell lineage of the hepatogenic foregut endoderm (199). These tumors may show loss of INI1.

The mixed epithelial and mesenchymal type of tumor contains cells admixed with primitive mesenchyme and various mesenchymally derived tissues (Figure 15-53). The highly cellular primitive mesenchyme consists of elongated, spindle-shaped cells with a scanty cytoplasm, and elongated pump nuclei with rounded ends, resembling fibroblastoid/ myofibroblastoid tissue. Some areas may display parallel orientation of cells with definite collagen fibers and young fibroblasts; other areas may have more loosely arranged cells leading to a myxomatous appearance. Mature fibrous septa are also seen, along with areas of osteoid and cartilaginous tissue. Cells within the osteoid foci have an irregular, angular outline and short processes that make them indistinguishable from osteoblasts. Immunohistochemical studies, however, have identified this osteoid-like material as being produced though a process of epithelial differentiation (e3). Osteoid stromal component is reportedly more prominent following chemotherapy (e283,e598). The prognostic significance of these stromal elements is unclear with studies reporting both improved survival or no effect on survival (e268). Approximately 20% of the mixed types of hepatoblastomas contain a variety of tissues, including stratified squamous epithelium, melanin pigment, mucinous epithelium, cartilage, bone, and striated muscle in addition to the epithelial cells, fibrous tissue, and osteoid-like material (Figure 15-54). These tumors have been termed teratoid hepatoblastomas by Manivel et al. (e419).

In view of the histologic heterogeneity of hepatoblastomas, rare tumors with unique morphologies may be seen that are difficult to classify into one of the above categories. This has led to anecdotal descriptions of "new" variants of hepatoblastomas including mucoid anaplastic hepatoblastoma (e322), hepatoblastomas with endocrine/neuroendocrine differentiation (e578,e579), cholangiocytic/cholangioblastic hepatoblastoma (e789), and hamartoma-like hepatoblastoma/ hepatoblastoma with organoid configuration or to the allocation of problematic cases into a neutral category, such as hepatoblastoma, not otherwise specified (199). The biologic significance, if any, of these morphologic variants is not known. Tumors that show mainly mesenchymal/stromal tissue with apparent lack of an epithelial component have been termed "pediatric hepatic stromal tumors" and have been proposed to resemble similar lesions described in childhood kidney cancer, that is, metanephric stromal tumor/MST (199). It is likely that these may be related to the so-called nested epithelial and stromal tumors (see later).

Notwithstanding the morphological differences in mixed HBs between epithelial components of any kind and the stromal components, there is evidence that both have a common lineage. This is suggested by the observation that β-catenin mutations visualized by nuclear reactivity occur in epithelial and mesenchymal components. The pathogenic pathways causing the development of both epithelial and mesenchymal/stromal lineages within the same tumor are not yet known. However, epithelial-mesenchymal transition or mesenchymal-to-epithelial transition has been hypothesized to play a role in pathogenesis.

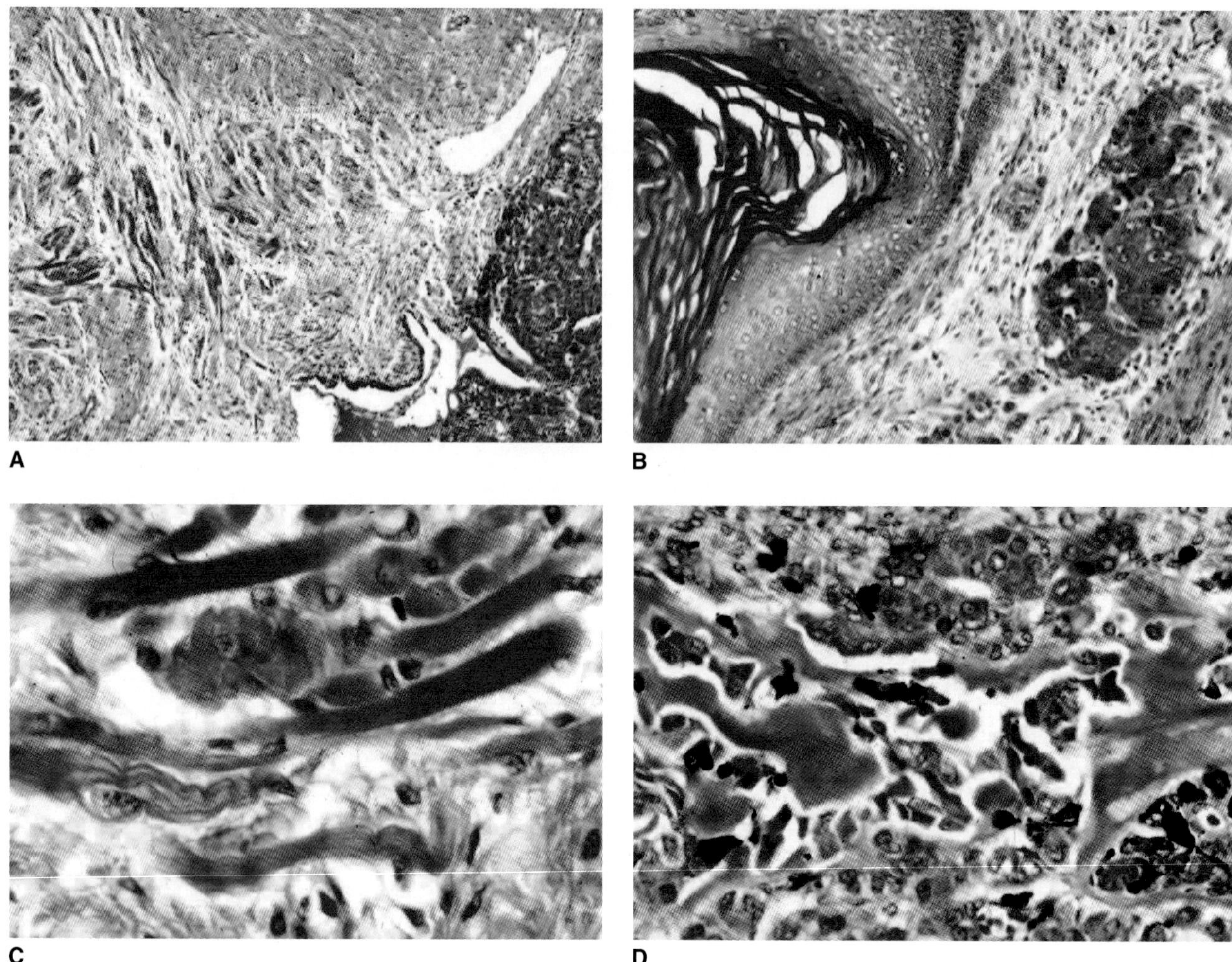

FIGURE 15-54 ■ Mixed hepatoblastoma with teratoid features. **A, B:** Together with the typical epithelial component (**right**), the tumor is composed of mesenchymal tissue showing differentiation into fibrous tissue (**left**) and stratified squamous epithelium (**right**). **C, D:** Striated muscle cells, and osteoid-like material containing melanin pigment. (H&E stains, original magnification 30× [**A**], 100× [**B**], 300× [**C**], and 200× [**D**]).

Although open biopsy and needle biopsy often are adequate in establishing the diagnosis, the use of FNA may prove difficult, particularly in cases of small cell undifferentiated or embryonal epithelial lesions. FNA has been reported to be accurate in diagnosing hepatoblastoma in approximately 65% (19 of 29) of cases, primarily fetal epithelial and mixed hepatoblastomas (e66,e172,e263,e647,e728,e749). The diagnosis was most frequently confused with metastatic tumor including Wilms tumor, neuroblastoma, and rhabdomyosarcoma (e647,e749). Weir et al. have reported the cytologic features of hepatoblastoma in serous cavity fluids. All six specimens examined showed hypercellular smears in a relatively clean background. Mixed embryonal and fetal subtypes of HBL disclosed three-dimensional clusters of neoplastic cells that formed straight or branched cords and acinus-like structures. The cells were moderately pleomorphic, had high nuclear-to-cytoplasmic ratios, rare intranuclear inclusions, and numerous mitoses. The small cell subtype showed tight clusters of small, round, primitive cells with hyperchromatic nuclei, high N/C ratios, and prominent nuclear molding. In addition, there were numerous single cells with naked nuclei, often in an Indian-file configuration. Bile pigment, osteoid, and other mesenchymal components were absent in all their specimens (191).

The prognostic impact of histology has been analyzed in a few studies (27,42) (e226,e267,e268,e415,e440,e746). Of the five histologic subtypes (pure fetal, embryonal, mixed epithelial-mesenchymal, macrotrabecular, and small cell undifferentiated), the fetal subtype carries the most favorable prognosis, and small cell undifferentiated the worst. In general, pure fetal histology is associated with an improved prognosis, while undifferentiated histology is associated with a poor prognosis, with macrotrabecular histology probably having an intermediate prognosis. In a study of 168 patients the estimated 24-month survival probability was 50% with the macrotrabecular type in comparison with 92%, 63%, and 0% for the purely foetal, embryonal, and SCUD histologies, respectively (e268). Small cell undifferentiated histology predicts an increased risk of relapse (184) (e502). Even a focal (partial or predominant) expression of small cell histology in completely resected HBL may have an unfavourable effect on outcome (e267), drawing a corollary with focal versus diffuse anaplasia in nephroblastoma. Small cell undifferentiated tumors appear to be biologically different from tumors with non–small cell histology and have been reported to be similar to rhabdoid tumors at the immunohistochemical (INI1 negative), cytogenetic and molecular level and in terms of their adverse adverse outcomes (184). Among the mixed epithelial/mesenchymal type tumors, the presence of mesenchymal elements may be associated with improved prognosis (e268).

Immunohistochemistry

The various patterns of hepatoblastoma display differing immunoreactivity, probably based on their degree of differentiation, with the fetal cell areas of an epithelial hepatoblastoma staining positively for a broad range of epithelial markers and small cell undifferentiated hepatoblastomas showing positivity for only a few markers (Table 15-22) (e3,e101,e490,e538,e580–e583,e643,e660,e734). Ruck et al. (e582) noticed a correlation between the cytokeratin staining of normal biliary epithelium and liver parenchymal cells and the types of epithelial cells in hepatoblastoma, with CK19 more prominent in small cell and embryonal epithelial cell areas (and in biliary epithelium) and CK18 more prominent in fetal epithelial areas (and in normal hepatocytes). Osteoid areas were positive for both CK18 and CK19, whereas spindle cells areas were not immunoreactive for any of the cytokeratins. These characteristics have suggested to some authors that the primitive small cells give rise to embryonal hepatoblastoma cells and, after further maturation, fetal hepatoblastomas (e3,e582). In a study of 12-needle core biopsies in proven hepatoblastomas, Ramsay et al. reported variable antigen expression with positivity for cytokeratins (10/12 cases), alpha-1-antitrypsin (5/12 cases) and AFP (7/12 cases), MIC-2 (CD99) (8/12 cases), NCAM (CD56) (4/12 cases), neuroblastoma marker NB84 (3/12), desmin (2/12 cases), BCL2 (2/12 cases), and one case each for vimentin, NSE, and PGP 9.5. However, all tumors were negative for CD45, WT1, and S-100. The authors concluded that hepatoblastoma shows no distinct immunohistochemical profile, and the diagnosis requires a combination of the clinical, imaging, and pathologic findings, since they can express antigens normally seen in other childhood malignancies (143). Insulin-like growth factor 2 and insulin-like growth factor–binding protein expression have been noted in 11 hepatoblastomas, with their expression inversely correlated with the degree of tumor cell differentiation. Akmal et al. (e11) suggest that these markers may be used as an assessment of the degree of differentiation of the tumor. Interestingly, hypoglycemia has been noted as a rare presenting symptom of hepatoblastoma with the hypoglycemia disappearing after removal of the tumor (e266). Glypican 3, a heparin sulfate proteoglycan bound to the cell surface, is overexpressed both at the genomic (by microarray studies) and at the protein (by IHC) levels in hepatoblastoma. In their series, Zynger et al. found that 65 of 65 hepatoblastomas had cytoplasmic immunoreactivity for GPC3 with greater than 90% of cases showing strong, diffuse positivity. There was no reactivity in benign

Table 15-22 ■ IMMUNOHISTOCHEMICAL FINDINGS IN HEPATOBLASTOMA

	Fetal Cell Areas	Embryonal Cell Areas	Small-cell Areas	Mesenchymal Areas	"Osteoid" Areas
Keratin	++	++	++	±	+
α fetoprotein	++	++	–		+
α_1-antitrypsin	++	++	±	+	++
α_1-antichymotrypsin	++	++	+	+	+
Ferritin	++	+	+		+
Carcinoembryonic antigen	++	++	–	–	±
Epithelial membrane antigen		+	–		++
Transferrin	+	++			
Human chorionic gonadotropin	+	+			
Vimenten	–	–	–	++	++
Serotonin	±	±	–	–	–
Somatostatin	±	±	–	–	–
NSE	–	±	–	+	++
S-100	±	+	±	+	++
Desmin	–	–		–	–
Chromogranin A	±	±	–	–	+

Symbols: ++, Majority of cases strongly positive; +, moderately or weakly positive in some cases; ±, positive in some reports and negative in others; –, negative in all reports.

From Ishak K, Goodman Z, Stocker J. Tumors of the liver and intrahepatic bile ducts. In: Rosai J, Sobin L, eds. *Atlas of tumor pathology*, 3rd series ed. Washington, DC: Armed Forces Institute of Pathology, 2001.

liver tissue. Fetal, embryonal, and small cell undifferentiated patterns were diffusely positive in almost all cases, whereas mesenchymal and teratoid patterns were nearly all negative (200). Immunohistochemical studies have identified putative stem cells in hepatoblastomas. Cells in atypical ducts were found to express simultaneously stem cell markers and hepatocytic or biliary lineage markers, suggesting a direct role for stem cells in the histogenesis of hepatoblastoma (e210). The presence of stem cells in these tumors is also supported by the occurrence of teratoid variant of hepatoblastoma.

Molecular Pathology

Deregulation of the APC/beta-catenin pathway occurs in a consistent fraction of hepatoblastomas, with mutations in the APC and beta-catenin genes implicated in FAP-associated and sporadic hepatoblastomas, respectively. Mutations of the beta-catenin gene are present in over 90% of hepatoblastomas, leading to activating transcription of a number of target genes. β-Catenin is central to the convergence of the Wnt, β-catenin, and cadherin signaling pathways, where it forms a signaling complex with axins, APC tumor suppressor protein, glycogen synthase kinase 3β, and other proteins (e479). The Wnt signalling pathway prevents proteosomal degradation of β-catenin and allows β-catenin to translocate to the nucleus and initiate gene transcription. In fact, β-catenin can be immunohistochemically detected in the nucleus, following its translocation. Nuclear staining for β-catenin in hepatoblastomas has been reported to correlate with poor histologic phenotype, higher stage disease, and poor survival (e517,e683). Other components of the Wnt signaling pathway including Axin gene mutation (e442) and loss of APC function (e700) have also been have been implicated in hepatoblastoma tumorigenesis. Giardiello et al. (e237) identified an APC gene mutation in all eight hepatoblastoma patients of seven FAP kindreds. Oda et al. (e495) have also noted genetic alterations in the APC (loss of heterozygosity [LOH] or somatic mutations) in 9 of 13 cases of hepatoblastoma in non-FAP patients. Interestingly, a distinct male predominance (nearly 75%) is seen in APC gene-related hepatoblastomas.

A host of other genetic alterations have been described in hepatoblastomas involving cell cycle–related genes (e14,e776), apoptosis pathways (e621), p53 mutations (e151), mismatch repair defects (e151), FOXG1 overexpression (e7), and signal transduction pathways (e466), to name a few. It is possible that many of these molecular aberrations may be late events in the clonal evolution of these tumors that indicate progressive genomic instability rather than primary events (199). López-Terrada et al. have hypothesized that histologic microheterogeneity in hepatoblastoma may correlate with molecular heterogeneity, reflecting different stages of developmental arrest. They found Wnt activation to be most prevalent in embryonal and mixed types, whereas Notch activation, needed for cholangiocytic differentiation at a more differentiated state, was predominant in pure fetal hepatoblastomas (105). p53 protein expression is seen less frequently in hepatoblastoma than in other childhood tumors. In 10 cases of hepatoblastoma, Chen et al. noted only one case of overexpression of p53 protein in a macrotrabecular type at stage IV (e122). Ruck et al. (e580) noted p53 protein immunoreactivity in two small cell hepatoblastomas and in the embryonal areas of two fetal and embryonal epithelial hepatoblastomas, but not in the fetal areas of eight fetal or fetal and embryonal epithelial tumors or the mesenchymal areas of four mixed tumors. Somatic mutations, however, were detected in 9 of 10 cases of hepatoblastoma in the five to eight exons of the p53 gene by Oda et al. (e494), who suggest that environmental mutagens may be involved in some cases of hepatoblastoma.

Many aberrations have also been reported at the chromosomal level in hepatoblastomas. Genome-wide allelotyping of hepatoblastomas have shown frequent allelic losses at many microsatellite loci implicating chromosome instability as an important factor in development and progression of hepatoblastoma (178). Trisomy 2, trisomy 20, and 4q structural rearrangement are the most common chromosomal abnormalities in hepatoblastoma (e13,e41,e43,e98, e218,e269,e272,e361,e397,e431,e511,e569,e608,e649, e658,e680,e689,e707) (see Table 15-23). A derivative chromosome 4 from an unbalanced translocation between the long arms of chromosomes 1 and 4 has been noted as a recurring abnormality in hepatoblastoma, while it is rarely seen in other types of neoplasms (e608). In 32 cases, Kraus et al. have shown LOH on chromosome 1p in seven cases, LOH on 1q in seven cases, and LOH on both 1p and 1q in three more, suggesting that tumor suppressor genes at the telomeric region of chromosome arm 1p and different regions of chromosome arm 1q may be involved in the pathogenesis of hepatoblastoma (e361). Albrecht et al. (e13) noted LOH in 6 of 18 hepatoblastomas in 11p restricted to the telomeric region 11p15.5 and determined that the parental origin was exclusively maternal. DNA analysis by flow cytometry has been reported in more than 70 cases, with a diploid pattern noted in the well-differentiated (fetal) portions of the tumors and an aneuploid pattern present in embryonal portions or in small cell (anaplastic) tumors (e140,e280,e363,e604). Krober et al. (e363) noted an aneuploid peak in tumors with embryonal and fetal components when the areas were analyzed together and encouraged analysis of all differing areas of a tumor if ploidy is to be used in drawing conclusions about the prognosis in individual cases. Hata et al. (e280) noted an increased incidence of vascular invasion and a poorer prognosis in patients with an aneuploid tumor. Terracciano et al. studied 35 hepatoblastoma specimens by CGH and found significant gains of genetic material. The most frequent alterations were gains of Xp (15 cases, 43%) and Xq (21 cases, 60%), while other common alterations were 1p−, 2q+, 2q−, 4q−, and 4q+. There was no difference between different histologic subtypes, suggesting a common clonal origin for the different components (179).

Table 15-23 ■ CYTOGENETIC FINDINGS IN HEPATOBLASTOMAS

Case No.	Karyotype	Histologic Type
1.	46,XY,-2,der(19)t(4,19),+mar	Epithelial; embryonal
2.	47,XY,+20,dmin	Mixed mesenchymal-epithelial; fetal
3.	47,XY,+20,dmin	Epithelial; primary embryonal, foci of fetal areas
4.	93,XXXX,+I(8q)/93,XXXX,del(1)(p22),+I(8q)	Mixed mesenchymal-epithelial; fetal
5.	50,XY,+2,+8,+20,+dic(1)(p12)	Mixed mesenchymal-epithelial; fetal and embryonal
6.	47,XX,+20,del(1)(q32.2)dup(2)(q21q35),dmin/50, XX,+5,+7,+ 20,+22,del(1),dup(2),I(8q),dmin	Mixed mesenchymal-epithelial; fetal and embryonal
7.	47,XX,+20,dup(2)(q23q35)/47,XX,+20,dup(2),dup(6)(p11p24)	Mixed mesenchymal-epithelial; fetal
8.	54,Y,der(X)t(X;1)(p22;q21),+2,+6,+8,+8,+12,+15,+17, +20,inv(9)(p11q21)[a]	Mixed mesenchymal-epithelial; fetal and embryonal
9.	46,XYder(4)t(2;4)(q21;q35),t(9;?)(p24;?)/47,XY,+20, der(4),t(9?)	Mixed mesenchymal-epithelial; fetal
10.	51,XY,+2,+12,+20,+der(5)t(1;5)(q25;q35),+del(6)(q15)	Epithelial; fetal
11.	48,XX,+2,+r/48,XX,+20,+der(2)t(1;2)(q23;p21),inv(5) (q22q35)/ 49,XX,+20,+der(2),inv(5),+r47,XX,+2	Epithelial; fetal
12.	47,XX,+2	Epithelial; primary fetal, foci of embryonal areas
13.	47,XX,2q+,t(3;5)(p25;q31),dup(4)(q12q26),+20	Mixed mesenchymal-epithelial
14.	46,XY,t(10;22)(q26;q11)	Small cell undifferentiated
15.	47,XY,+2	Fetal and embryonal, possible macrotrabecular
16.	47,XX,+20	Mixed mesenchymal-epithelial fetal and embryonal
17.	46,XX,del(17)(p12)/46,XX	Mixed with teratoid features

[a]inv(9)(p11q21) was constitutional.
Modified from Stocker J, Conran R, Selby D. Tumor and pseudotumors of the liver. In: Stocker J, Askin F, eds. *Pathology of solid tumors in children.* London: Chapman & Hall, 1998:83–110, with permission.

HEPATOCELLULAR CARCINOMA

HCC is the third most frequently seen pediatric liver tumor and represents up to 20% of all pediatric liver neoplasms (44,95). It occurs primarily in the older pediatric patient, with over 65% of cases seen in children older than 10 years of age (Figure 15-55A) (see Tables 15-14 and 15-16). Rare cases, however, have been reported even in infants (e268,e332,e368). However, the fibrolamellar variant has not been reported in infants (84) (e148). There is a slight male predominance, but no specific racial predilection, although there is an increased incidence in populations with a high number of HBV carriers.

Pathogenesis

Underlying liver dysfunctions, especially viral hepatitis (HBV and HCV) and cirrhosis, are known predisposing conditions, although children are less likely to have associated chronic liver disease than adults (44). In areas hyperendemic for HBV, almost all children with HCC are HBV seropositive (e121,e775). In a study of 20 Taiwanese patients aged 8 months to 16 years (all but one older than 8 years of age) with HCC, Wu et al. (e775) noted HBsAg positivity in all the patients, 70% of their mothers, and 52.9% of their siblings. In these children, HBV is commonly acquired from their mothers, with malignancy developing in 7 to 8 years (e119). However, exposure time may be less in immunocompromised hosts; an exposure time of only 3 years has been described in a 10-year-old boy with HCC who contracted HBV in the course of chemotherapy for acute lymphoblastic leukemia at age 7 (e120). The incidence of HBsAg seropositivity is higher in children with the usual histologic type of HCC than in patients with the fibrolamellar variant (see later) in whom the incidence of HBsAg positivity is only 5%. Unlike in adults, integration of HBV-DNA into the host genome may be a late event in children with chronic HBV infection. Huang et al. found that HBV-DNA integration increased in parallel with the progress of liver histology toward the neoplastic transformation, with 0% in the liver of chronic hepatitis, 22.2% in nontumor livers of HCC patients, and 66.7% in tumor liver tissues of HCC patients. Fortunately, the introduction of the hepatitis B vaccine has markedly reduced the incidence of HCC, especially in males. HCV, while becoming more frequently associated with adult HCC, is only occasionally associated with that tumor in children (e277).

HCC is also associated with inborn metabolic errors such as alpha-1-antitrypsin deficiency, hereditary tyrosinemia, Gaucher disease, urea cycle defects, CESD, glycogen storage disease, Alagille syndrome, and congenital biliary atresia (e175,e343,e368,e564,e629). Recently, a familial cholestasis syndrome caused by a bile salt export pump deficiency has been described as a previously unrecognized risk for HCC in children (e354).

Clinical Features, Laboratory Studies, and Imaging

Most patients (nearly 80%) present with abdominal pain, an abdominal mass, or both. Other symptoms include anorexia, malaise, fever, nausea, vomiting, and jaundice. Symptomatic patients (with abdominal discomfort or mass) often have

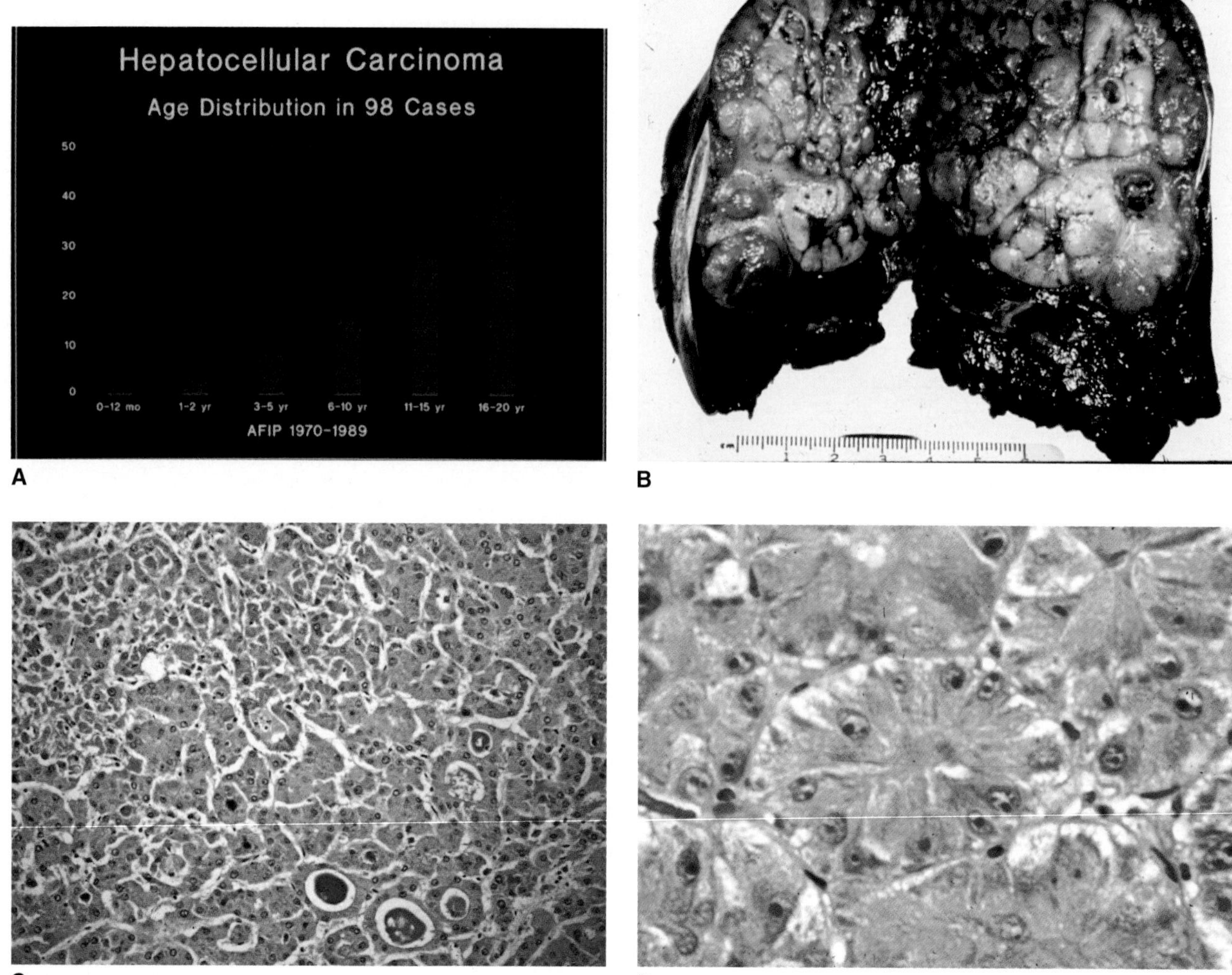

FIGURE 15-55 ■ Hepatocellular carcinoma. **A:** Age distribution on 98 cases. **B:** A single, large mass displays foci of hemorrhage and necrosis. **C:** The tumor is composed of broad trabeculae of poorly to moderately well-differentiated hepatocytes. Note the pseudogland appearance of some trabeculae with central necrosis of cells (H&E stain, original magnification 40×). **D:** The individual hepatocellular carcinoma cells may be moderately differentiated and cluster around a canaliculus (**center**), but note the nuclear anisocytosis and multiple nucleoli (H&E stain, original magnification 300×).

advanced stage disease at presentation (189). Tumor rupture with hemoperitoneum may be seen rarely. A wide variety of associated conditions are seen in 20% to 25% of cases (e659) (Table 15-24), including a recent association between Gardner syndrome and the fibrolamellar form of HCC (e258). One of the closest associations is with hereditary tyrosinemia, with a 37% incidence of HCC in tyrosinemia patients surviving beyond 2 years of age, and liver transplantation before 2 years of age has been suggested for these patients (e171,e421).

Laboratory findings in patients with HCC include mild anemia or erythrocytosis, and thrombocytosis. Serum transaminases (ALT and AST), lactate dehydrogenase (LDH), ALP, and lipid levels may be elevated (e659). Serum bilirubin levels may be increased in 15% to 20% of cases. Unlike in adults with HCC, where biochemical liver function tests are often abnormal, abnormal results of ALT, bilirubin, and albumin are infrequent in pediatric patients as well as in patients with advanced stage (189) (e121). Further, unlike in adults, elevated ALP in the presence of a liver mass did not correlate with metastatic disease (189). Serum AFP is elevated in 50% to 100% of children with HCC (189) (e482,e607), although AFP may be normal or only mildly elevated in patients with the fibrolamellar variant (e56,e436,e659). Elevated AFP levels are especially common in Taiwanese children and this has been attributed to the almost universal association with HBV in this cohort. HBV is both carcinogenic and also independently reactivates the gene encoding AFP within hepatocytes (e454,e653). Alternatively, extremely high levels of AFP may also be due to the advanced tumor stage in these HCC patients (e219).

Table 15-24 ■ CONDITIONS ASSOCIATED WITH HEPATOCELLULAR CARCINOMA IN CHILDREN
Acute lymphoblastic leukemia
A1AT deficiency
Ataxia-telangiectasia
Anomalies of abdominal venous drainage
Arteriohepatic dysplasia
Atypical retinitis pigmentosa
Biliary atresia
CHF
Cystinosis
Familial cholestatic cirrhosis (Byler disease)
Familial hepatocellular carcinoma
Familial polyposis
Fanconi anemia
Focal nodular hyperplasia of liver
Galactosemia
Gardner syndrome
Hepatic adenoma
Hepatitis B infection
Hepatitis C infection
Hereditary tyrosinemia
Hyperalimentation
Methotrexate therapy
Neurofibromatosis
Oral contraceptives
Osteogenesis imperfecta
Polycythemia
Soto syndrome
Types I and III glycogenoses
Wilms tumor
Wilson disease

Modified from Stocker JT: Hepatic tumors. In: Balistreri WF, Stocker JT, ed. *Pediatric hepatology*. New York, NY: Hemisphere Publishing Company, 1990:399–488, with permission.

Imaging studies can delineate the mass and often help in determining whether resection is possible (Figure 15-55B) (e545). Soyer et al. (e650) used CT scans to study patients with the fibrolamellar variant and noted a hypodense single, bilobed, or multilobulated mass that was hypervascular and variable enhancement after injection. Calcification was present in 40% of cases. McLarney et al. (e436) noted the appearance of the fibrolamellar variant as a lobulated heterogeneous mass with a central scar in an otherwise normal liver and cautioned that it not be confused with an FNH of the liver. Recently, PET/CT scan has been reported to be helpful for preoperative staging, selection of appropriate site for biopsy, identification of occult metastatic disease, follow-up for residual or recurrent disease, and assessment of response to chemotherapy in HCC and other pediatric abdominal neoplasms (e461). Sevmis et al. recommend mandatory serial AFP screening and combined imaging studies in the follow-up of children with chronic liver disease (e617). Imaging studies may also be helpful in differentiating metastatic tumors from primary malignant liver tumors, in that the former are more likely to show hypoechogenicity on abdominal ultrasound examination, while the latter are more likely to show vascular invasion and contrast enhancement on CT scan (189).

Staging

Multiple staging systems have been proposed for HCC. Lu et al. found the TNM staging system to be superior to the Okuda, Cancer of the Liver Italian Program (CLIP), and the Chinese University Prognostic Index (CUPI) staging systems for prognostication in HCC patients undergoing curative resection (106). On the other hand, Seo et al. found the CLIP system to have better predictive power than the TNM and Barcelona Clinic Liver Cancer (BCLC) staging systems (164). In yet another study comparing seven prognostic staging systems (including CLIP score, BCLC staging, the Groupe d'Etude et de Traitment du Carcinome Hépatocellulaire [GETCH] classification, CUPI grade, the Japan Integrated Staging [JIS] score, modified JIS [mJIS] score, and Tokyo score), Kondo et al. found the JIS score to be the best system in patients undergoing hepatectomy for HCC (92). More recently, in pediatric cases, the PRETEXT system devised for hepatoblastomas (44) has gained popularity.

Treatment and Outcome

The usual strategy for pediatric HCC is the combination of surgery and neoadjuvant chemotherapy. However, the relative chemoresistance of HCC makes surgery essential (44) (e332). Unfortunately, resectability at the time of diagnosis is possible in only 10% to 30% of cases (e121). Neoadjuvant chemotherapy may improve tumor resectability (e785). The most frequent chemotherapy regimen used in children is doxorubicin and cisplatin (44) (e485), although its effects are potent especially in resectable disease. For tumors still not resectable after chemotherapy, locoregional ablative therapies such as transarterial chemoembolization have been used (e332,e414). Tumor size and serum AFP level, alone or in combination, are reportedly useful in predicting the presence or absence of vascular invasion before hepatectomy for HCC (159). Liver transplantation may be helpful when resection is impossible and transplantation should be considered as soon as possible in these patients (e81,e183,e332). The presence of extrahepatic disease, nodal involvement, macroscopic vascular invasion, and/or distant metastases are obvious contraindications to transplantation. The experience with liver transplantation for HCC is still scarce in children. Although Sevmis et al. claim excellent results with both cadaveric and living-donor transplants (e617), Otte et al. have observed relatively poor results, similar to those in adults with HCC, except in a few highly selective series (135). In a recent study, patients with larger (3 to 5 cm) tumors, high serum AFP levels (>455 ng/mL), or a high MELD score (of 20 or more) had poor posttransplantation survival (74).

The prognosis of HCC is poor with an overall survival rate at 3 years below 25% (44) (e121,e330), notoriously worse than that of hepatoblastoma despite similar multidisciplinary approaches. Major prognostic factors are the presence of metastatic disease and the extent of disease, especially surgical resectability. In the SIOPEL-1 study that included 40 children with HCC, 33% were associated with cirrhosis, multifocal tumors were common (56%), as were metastases (31%), and extrahepatic tumor extension, vascular invasion, or both in 39%. Preoperative chemotherapy achieved a partial response in 49% of patients, complete tumor resection was achieved in 36% of patients, whereas 51% never became operable. Overall survival at 5 years was 28%, and event-free survival was 17%. Most deaths resulted from tumor progression. Resectability, presence of metastases, and high PRETEXT score predicted poor outcomes (44). In a Korean study of 16 pediatric HCC, estimated 5-year survival rate of all patients was 27.3%, but 62.5% for patients who underwent complete tumor resection versus 0% for those who underwent palliative resection or no operation (e785). The statistically significant prognostic factors were tumor stage, presence of metastasis, and complete tumor resection.

Childhood hepatoblastoma and HCC differ with respect to age (18 months versus 10.2 years), sex (females versus males), HBsAg status (none versus 64%), tumor stage (low versus high), tendency to rupture (36% versus 9%), chemosensitivity (more for hepatoblastoma), and tumor respectability (91% versus 45%), with considerably worse survival for HCC than hepatoblastoma (36). Postovsky et al. have reported a case of combined hepatoblastoma and HCC, where the HCC component recurred more than 5 years after initial diagnosis, suggesting that prolonged follow-up may be required for these tumors (e543).

Traditionally, patients with the fibrolamellar variant of HCC (FL-HCC) have been considered to have a somewhat better prognosis (e659). However, this is probably true in adults due to lack of association of this histologic form with cirrhosis. In children, FL-HCC may be biologically similar in behavior to classic HCC. Controversy exists whether FL-HCC has a better prognosis than classic HCC. Although some series have shown a better survival for FL-HCC than usual HCC (51) (e57,e84,e148,e368), this is due to a larger number of FL-HCC patients with localized and resectable tumors in these studies. Others, including recent studies of children and young adults with FL-HCC, have not shown favorable outcomes, with no difference in the rate or surgical respectability (44,84) (e268,e332,e456). In a study of 46 children with HCC, Katzenstein et al. found 10 cases (22%) of FL-HCC. Although the median survival was longer in patients with FL-HCC than for patients with typical HCC, the 5-year survival rate was similar for both groups. There was also no difference in the number of patients with advanced-stage disease, the incidence of surgical resectability at diagnosis, or the response to treatment between patients with FL-HCC and patients with typical HCC. Children with initially resectable HCC had a good prognosis irrespective of histologic subtype, whereas outcomes were uniformly poor for children with advanced-stage disease (84).

Gross Appearance

Grossly, HCC may be single or multicentric masses, with involvement of both the right and left lobes in over 70% of cases. The tumors weigh 800 to 1,500 g and vary in size from 2 to 25 cm. The lesions on cut section are tan to red and soft to firm with areas of hemorrhage and necrosis (Figure 15-55B). The surrounding lever may exhibit a micronodular or macronodular cirrhosis in up to 60% of cases, which is somewhat less than the 48% to 92% incidence seen in adults with HCC (e121). The cirrhosis may be related to biliary atresia or hereditary tyrosinemia, among other causes. The fibrolamellar variant is more often a single mass that is firm and gray. Cirrhosis is less frequent (4%) in patients with the fibrolamellar variant (120) FNH may be present in or adjacent to the HCC in about 4% of patients with the fibrolamellar variant (e56).

Histopathology

Microscopically, the "usual" HCC and the fibrolamellar variant present distinctly different features. The usual HCC is composed of trabeculae 2 to 10 or more cell layers in thickness (Figure 15-55C, D). The larger trabeculae may display central necrosis, imparting an acinar or pseudoglandular appearance. Individual cells are larger than normal hepatocytes, with nuclear hyperchromasia, anisocytosis, multiple nucleoli, and frequent and bizarre mitoses (e659). Large, multinucleated osteoclast-like giant cells or "tumor giant" cells (the so-called epithelial syncytial giant cells) may also be seen (10). Bile pigment may be present within the cytoplasm of tumor cells or within the canaliculi between cells. Vascular invasion may be prominent, and metastases to lung and lymph nodes may occur. Children with malignant liver tumors, especially with HCC, may have extensive angiogenesis that induces a rapid tumor growth and leads to a poor prognosis (175). Pathologic factors including tumor size greater than 2 cm, multifocality, and vascular invasion have been reported to be independent predictors of poor survival after resection (132).

The fibrolamellar variant was originally described in 1956 by Edmondson (e190). FL-HCC accounts for 1% of all HCC but 13% to 22% of HCC in younger patients, as it preferentially develops in children and young adults (51,84). It has not been linked with viral infection, or other risk factors for HCC, and patients usually have normal serum AFP (44,84). Histologically, FL-HCC is characterized by large, deeply eosinophilic (oncocytic) hepatocytes embedded within lamellar fibrosis (Figure 15-56) (e56). Individual cells vary from polygonal to spindle shaped and often contain discrete, pale eosinophilic bodies. Clusters of these cells are separated by narrow to broad bands of laminated collagen. Although rare, the most common variant of FL-HCC shows areas of glandular type differentiation with mucin production (182). Immunohistochemically, they may stain positive for fibrinogen, hepar, ferritin, and alpha-1-antitrypsin, but are negative

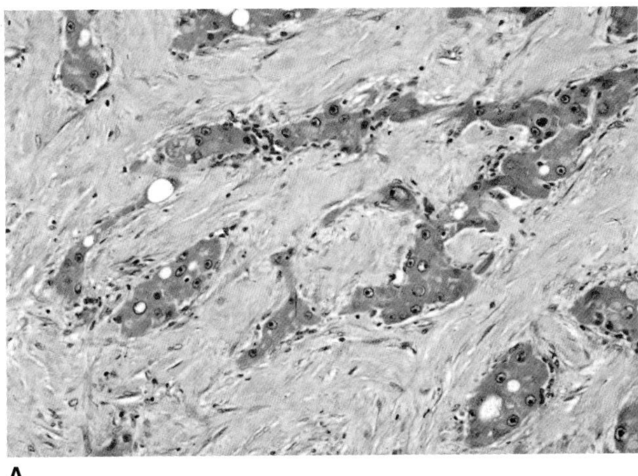
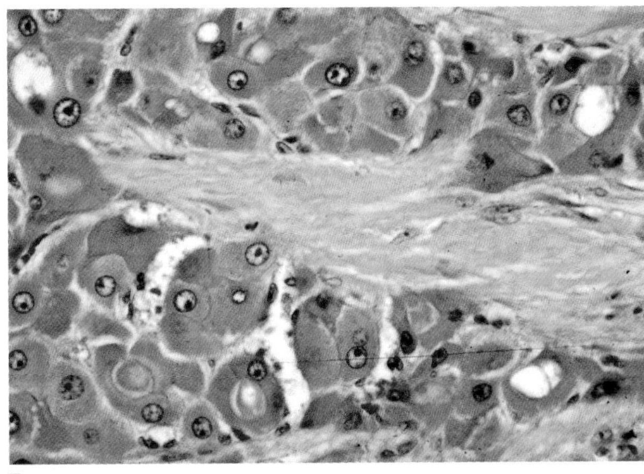

A B

FIGURE 15-56 ■ Fibrolamellar hepatocellular carcinoma. **A:** Broad bands of "plump" collagen separate clusters of large hepatocytes with prominent eosinophilic cytoplasm and large nucleoli (H&E stain, original magnification 60×). **B:** The hepatocytes contain abundant smooth to finely granular cytoplasm. Note the bile within the canaliculi between hepatocytes (H&E stain, original magnification 200×).

for HBsAg (e659). AFP staining has been noted in 21% of fibrolamellar cases and 40% of the usual HCC cases (e56); the latter 27% cases are also positive for HBsAg.

It may, on occasion, be difficult to differentiate the macrotrabecular variant of hepatoblastoma from HCC (199). Computerized image analysis has been claimed to help distinguish hepatoblastoma from HCC (185). Also, hepatoblastoma is rarely multiple and vascular invasion is uncommon even in advanced stage tumors (189). Prokurat et al. have even described a novel group of hepatocellular neoplasias in older children and adolescents, with an intermediate histology between HCC and HB, and a distinctive β-catenin pattern, that they term "transitional liver cell tumors" (142).

Recently, glypican-3 has been claimed to be a specific immunomarker for HCC and has been used to distinguish HCC from benign hepatocellular mass lesions, particularly HCA. However, the diagnosis of HCC should not rely entirely on positive glypican-3 immunostaining because focal immunoreactivity can be detected in a small subset of cirrhotic nodules. Also, glypican-3 expression in HCC can also be focal and thus, the lack of glypican-3 staining does not exclude the diagnosis of HCC (189). Further, glypican-3 may also be positive in hepatoblastomas (200). However, in a tissue microarray study of 4,387 tissue samples from 139 tumor categories and 36 nonneoplastic and preneoplastic tissue types, glypican-3 expression (using a 10% cut-off score) was detected in 9.2% of nonneoplastic liver samples (11/119), 16% of preneoplastic nodular liver lesions (6/38), 63.6% of HCCs (140/220), and in several nonhepatic tumors including squamous cell carcinoma of the lung (27/50 [54%]), testicular nonseminomatous germ cell tumors (32/62 [52%]), and liposarcoma (15/29 [52%]) (17). HCCs of higher histologic grade have been reported to have loss of E-cadherin, nonnuclear overexpression of β-catenin, and overexpression of osteopontin, with overexpression of osteopontin independently correlating with vascular invasion (93). Yamaoka et al. (196) found 17/17 pediatric HCCs to be positive for nuclear/cytoplasmic β-catenin in all childhood HCCs and suggest that β-catenin immunohistochemistry may be helpful in identifying malignancy in an otherwise borderline lesion. They also observed E-cadherin expression in all malignant pediatric liver tumors, while cyclin D1 expression was significantly detected in tumors of advanced stage, suggesting that cyclin D1, a gene downstream of beta-catenin, might play a role in tumor progression (196). EGFR overexpression is also reported in a majority of HCCs, suggesting a role for EGFR antagonists in therapy. However, the increased expression does not correlate with an increase in the EGFR gene copy number (30). Klein et al. report that although HCCs in children are morphologically similar to those in adults, the former are more likely to be CK7-positive (89).

Molecular Pathology

In contradistinction to many other childhood tumors (e.g., neuroblastomas, rhabdomyosarcomas, and ganglioneuroblastomas), amplification or overexpression of the oncogenes N-MYC, ERB A, ERB B, N-RAS, or Shb is not seen with HCC or hepatoblastoma (e423). Fibrolamellar carcinomas show fewer chromosomal abnormalities compared with those reported in literature for conventional HCC. The most common abnormalities in FL-HCC occur in chromosomes 7 and 8, and tumors with chromosomal changes appear to behave more aggressively compared with cases with no cytogenetic abnormalities. However, chromosomal changes do not correlate with age, gender, and tumor size (81). Terracciano et al. have reported the occurrence of FL-HCC in a young girl with a prior resection of a HCA; although there was no genetic alteration in the adenoma, several chromosomal aberrations were detected in the FL-HCC (e698).

The β-catenin pathway has been implicated in HCC (e778). MicroRNA profiling may help identify patients with HCC who are likely to develop metastases/recurrence (31). The uniqueness of FL-HCC extends to their molecular findings, as they show no evidence for involvement of many of the major pathways and genes that are dysregulated in typical HCC, including AFP, TP53 mutations, and β-catenin mutations. However, much of their molecular biology remains poorly described and awaits future investigation (182). The molecular pathology of HCCs in children is probably similar to that in adults. The topic has been the subject of excellent recent reviews (53,54,73,124,137,158,187,194) and is beyond the scope of detailed discussion in this text.

UNDIFFERENTIATED EMBRYONAL SARCOMA

UES is the fourth or fifth most common pediatric liver tumor (102) (e661). The term "undifferentiated (embryonal) sarcoma" was given to this lesion by Stocker and Ishak in 1978, prior to which the tumor was known as embryonal sarcoma, mesenchymoma, primary sarcoma, fibromyxosarcoma, or malignant mesenchymoma.

Pathogenesis

The histogenesis of undifferentiated sarcoma of the liver remains unresolved. Suggestions that UES is a sarcomatoid variant of hepatoblastoma (e445) have not found acceptance. The observation of UES occurring in association with mesenchymal hamartoma has suggested that the former may arise in a setting of the latter (see discussion above, in the section on mesenchymal hamartoma). This concept of malignant transformation occurring in a dysgenetic or hamartomatous lesion is similar to what has been described for other malignancies such as adenocarcinomas arising in bronchogenic and choledochal cysts, Wilms tumor from perilobar nephrogenicrests, and pleuropulmonary blastoma from presumed congenital lung cysts (not the case).

UES has been associated with the Li-Fraumeni syndrome (e369). An embryonal or congenital origin has been considered unlikely by some authors, because UES has also been reported in adults. The histogenesis of UES is probably from a mesenchymal lineage. There is no clear differentiation into rhabdomyosarcoma or fibrosarcoma, although myogenic differentiation has been suggested in a few cases based on immunohistochemical findings. The overlap of immunohistochemical staining patterns and ultrastructural features shown by UES and hepatic rhabdomyosarcoma has led Parham et al. to suggest a common histogenesis, perhaps from a multipotential mesenchymal stem cell (e513).

Clinical Features, Laboratory Studies, and Imaging

UES occurs primarily in children aged 6 to 10 years (Figure 15-57A), with 88% of cases occurring in those under 15 years of age (e149). Others have reported a median age of 9.5 to 12 years, with 63% occurring in children 6 to 10 years of age (32,138). In most reported series, there is an almost equal incidence in both sexes (96,102). In a large reviewed series of 113 cases in literature, 46 were males and 31 were females. There is no racial predilection.

Abdominal pain or an abdominal mass is seen at presentation in 87% of cases. Unusual presentations include dyspnea/cardiac murmur (due to extension of the tumor through the inferior vena cava into the right atrium and ventricle), jaundice, chest pain, and fever (96) (e131,e661). The abdominal mass and pain are often accompanied by anorexia, vomiting, lethargy, and malaise. Tumor rupture may lead to an acute abdomen (96) (e297,e661). Sakellaridis et al. report a presentation mimicking acute appendicitis (e587). Laboratory findings display a variety of abnormalities of SGOT, LDH, and alkaline phophatase, but serum AFP is uniformly negative and serum bilirubin is rarely elevated (96) (e661).

UES appears predominantly as a solid lesion on sonographic studies. The tumor is isoechoic or hyperechoic relative to the surrounding liver parenchyma. Cystic areas comprise an average of 19% of tumor volume. Sonographic findings are usually in agreement with gross pathologic findings in terms of proportion of solid and cystic components (32). Computed tomographic scans reveal predominantly

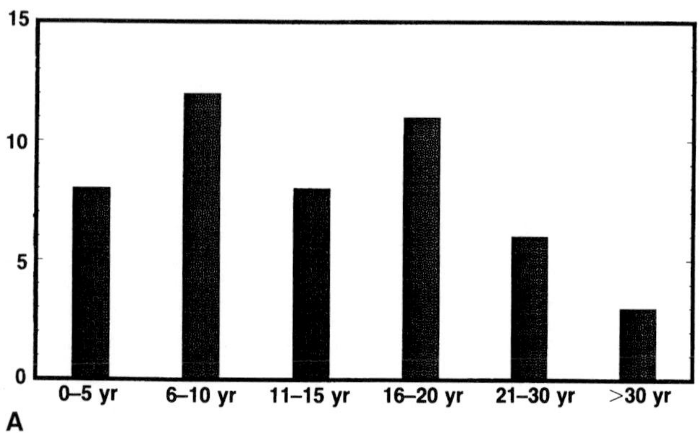

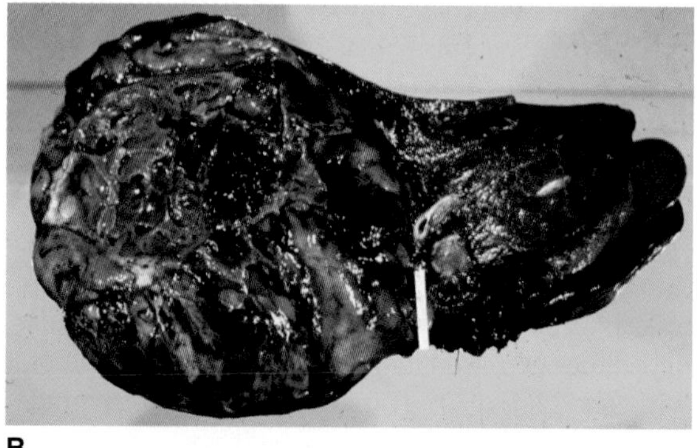

FIGURE 15-57 ■ Undifferentiated embryonal sarcoma. **A:** Age distribution in 48 cases. **B:** The tumor mass contains multiple cystic areas filled with gelatinous or hemorrhagic material.

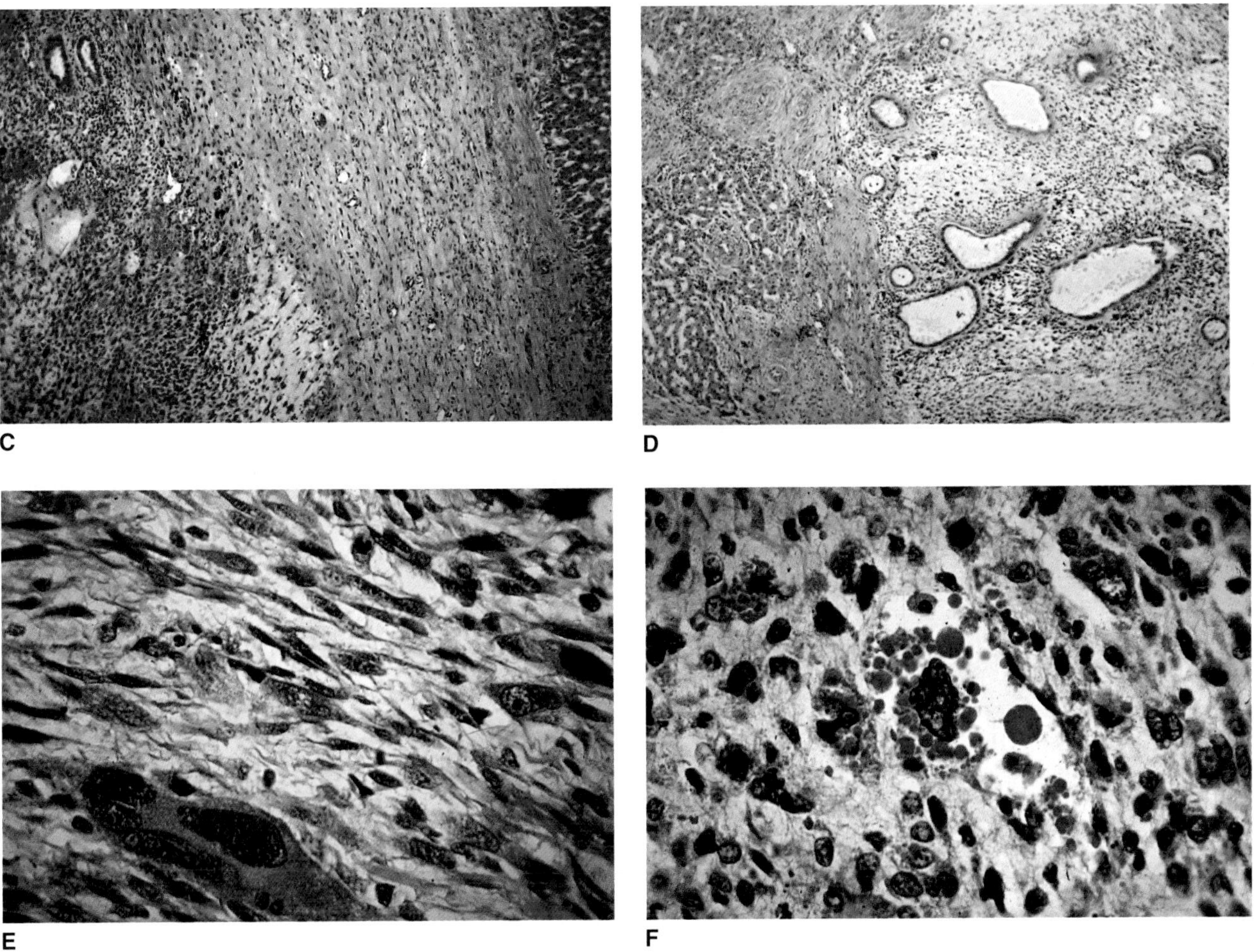

FIGURE 15-57 *(continued)* **C:** Loose and usually incomplete fibrous tissue separates the normal liver (**right**) from the malignant tumor (**left**) (H&E stain, original magnification 30×). **D:** Entrapped and degenerating bile ducts surrounded by anaplastic cells in a loose mesenchymal matrix lie next to the pseudocapsule separating the tumor from the normal liver (**left**) (H&E stain, original magnification 40×). **E:** Bizarre tumor giant cells with large and multiple nuclei are scattered throughout the lesion (H&E stain, original magnification 200×). **F:** Smooth eosinophilic globules are present in the cytoplasm of small and large tumor cells (H&E stain, original magnification 200×).

water attenuation. As determined by unenhanced scans and bolus contrast-enhanced scans, an average of 88% of the tumor volume shows water attenuation. Areas of intermediate or soft attenuation are also noted around the periphery of all lesions. On MRI, the tumor appears predominantly hypointense relative to the liver on T1-weighted images, with areas of high signal intensity present centrally, corresponding to areas of recent hemorrhage. T2-weighted images show predominantly high signal intensity, cystic foci, internal debris, and septations (32). A fibrous pseudocapsule of low signal intensity on T1-weighted and T2-weighted images is sometimes seen (e545). MRI and CT may show a misleading cystlike appearance of an UES compared with ultrasonography and pathologic findings in which the tumors are predominantly solid (>85% of tissue mass) (32) (e286). This discrepancy with gross appearances following tumor resection probably results from the abundant myxoid stroma in these tumors. A cystic appearance on imaging may lead to a misdiagnosis of hydatid disease, especially in areas endemic for this parasitic infestation (e10,e117,e321,e620). On angiography, UES commonly appears as an avascular or hypovascular hepatic mass (e573). Angiograms have shown that the tumor derives its vascular supply from the hepatic arterial system. Angiography has been helpful in delineating hepatic vein invasion and in vascular mapping for surgery (e341).

Pachera et al. have reviewed the clinicopathologic features of UES in adults based on 51 cases in literature. The mean age of affected adults is 31 years (range 15 to 86 years), with a female preponderance (28 F, 19 M). The right lobe is more commonly affected than the left lobe (59% versus 22%), with both lobes involved in 20% of cases. Tumors often exceeded 10 cm in size, with an average weight of 1,400 g. Spontaneous rupture was reported in only two cases. Results of liver function tests are usually normal, whereas high AFP levels have been reported only in five adults, and raised CA-12 in one. In adults, the appearance of a cystic lesion on imaging has led to a mistaken diagnosis of a benign lesion with a delay in diagnosis in 24% of cases (138).

Treatment and Outcomes

Although UES was uniformly considered to have a very poor prognosis in the past, complete resection and aggressive chemotherapy have changed the outcome favorably in recent years. In their original series, Stocker and Ishak documented an average survival time of only 11 months. Patients who undergo an incomplete tumor resection have a tendency toward poorer outcomes (96) (e385) and radical excision of the tumor provides the only chance of cure. However, a complete resection was possible to achieve in only 65% (33 patients) of the cases reported in the literature (138). Moon et al. observed a 50% to 90% reduction in tumor volume with preoperative chemotherapy, rendering the tumors respectable (e452). Polychemotherapy has been practiced with agents such as doxorubicin, cis-diaminodichloroplatinum, cyclophosphamide, dacarbazine, 5-FU, and vincristine (e526). The Soft Tissue Sarcoma Italian and German Cooperative Groups treated 17 children with UES using the same multimodal approach as for patients with other sarcomas including conservative surgery at diagnosis, multiagent chemotherapy, and second-look operation in cases of residual disease, with additional radiotherapy in 2 of 17 patients. Twelve patients were alive with follow-up ranging from 2.4 to 20 years (e71).

The tumor usually spreads by direct extension into adjacent organs and sometimes extends into the right atrium via the inferior vena cava. Rupture of the tumor can occur and massive intraperitoneal spread has sometimes been found (96). Metastases are rare, but have been reported in the lung, bone, pleura, and peritoneum (102) (e4,e78).

Gross Appearance

UES is a large tumor with an average weight of more than 1,200 g (range 90 to over 4,000 g) (96) (e661). The tumor ranges from 10 to 35 cm in diameter (32,96). The mass is in the right lobe of the liver in 69% of cases, in the left lobe in 14%, and involves both lobes in 17%. Pedunculated or exophytic tumors have been documented. The tumor is well demarcated from the adjacent liver by a compressed incomplete fibrous pseudocapsule. The cut section is variegated and soft. Myxoid gelatinous areas alternate with confluent areas of necrosis and hemorrhage (Figure 15-57B). Foci of hemorrhage or necrosis are present in over 50% of the cases and may constitute up to 80% of the tumor. The tumor is predominantly solid; the mean percentage of the solid component is 83%. An average 17% of cross-sectional areas of the tumors are composed of empty cavities (32). These cysts are up to 4 cm in diameter and contain gelatinous brown contents (96). Calcification is rare to absent (32) (e573). The uninvolved liver is normal in appearance. Pathological features are similar in adults and children (138).

Histopathology

Microscopically, the tumor is separated from the normal liver by an incomplete fibrous pseudocapsule of varying thickness (Figure 15-57C). This tumor pseudocapsule and the tumor immediately adjacent to it may contain remnants of normal-appearing hepatocytes and bile ducts (Figure 15-57D). The bile ducts may extend 0.5 to 1.0 cm into the lesion and show hyperplastic or reactive epithelial changes that may even appear anaplastic. These bile ducts are not present deeper in the tumor, nor within metastases, and are considered to represent entrapped or residual bile ducts rather than neoplastic elements of the tumor. The major component of the tumor consists of loose to dense foci of stellate or spindle-shaped cells with ill-defined outlines in a myxoid stroma (Figure 15-57D). Multinucleated cells with hyperchromatic nuclei are frequently scattered throughout the lesion (Figure 15-57E) or may only be a minor component. These cells may contain eosinophilic globules that are PAS-positive and diastase-resistant (Figure 15-57F); the globules may also be seen extracellularly. Histology may appear varied due to differing proportions of myxoid stroma, cellularity, hemorrhage, and necrosis. There is marked disparity in individual cell size and anisonuclsosis. Mitoses are abundant, with both atypical and bizarre mitotic forms. Proliferation index ranges from 30% to 95% (87). Some densely cellular areas have small round cells with hyperchromatic nuclei without nucleoli. Anaplastic malignant cells occur closer to the duct epithelium elements, as mentioned above. Numerous reticular fibers surround small groups of cells, and focal collagenization and hyalinization are present. Extramedullary hematopoiesis may be present. In a few tumors there are foci of direct invasion into hepatic sinusoids. Eosinophilic hyaline globules are present both intracellularly and extracellularly. These globules are PAS-positive and diastase-resistant. Patterns mimicking a sarcoma as a minor component of the tumor have been recorded, including osteoidlike matrix (96,102), "leiomyoblastic" (e244), and lipoblastic differentiation (e147,e231). The neoplastic cells may resemble fibroblastic, histiocytoid, fibrohistiocytoid, and myofibroblastic cells, occasionally suggesting a malignant fibrous histiocytoma, a tumor reported only in the liver of adults. Following chemotherapy, resected pathologic specimens show central necrosis, fibrosis, and dystrophic calcification (e452). Histologic dedifferentiation has been described following multiple recurrences (e127). In a comparative study of 14 primary and two recurrent UES, recurrent tumors showed greater cellularity, anaplasia, and pluripotential differentiation compared with primary tumors (197).

FNA cytology commonly yields a combination of polygonal and spindle cells. Polygonal cells are large with round or lobulated nuclei and occasionally are multinucleated with one or several nucleoli and variable cytoplasm with poorly defined borders. A few intracytoplasmic and extracytoplasmic eosinophilic globules are also observed (e232,e362,e539). Similar cytologic findings have also been described in peritoneal washings (e19). Findings on FNAC have been considered distinctive from other childhood liver tumors, allowing a confident preoperative diagnosis (e362,e646).

Immunohistochemistry shows evidence of widely divergent differentiation into mesenchymal and epithelial phenotypes, suggesting that immunostains have no specific or diagnostic relevance, but, by using a panel of antibodies, may help exclude other tumors. Variable positivity has been described for vimentin, BCL-2, pancytokeratin, CD10, calponin, desmin, smooth-muscle actin, muscle-specific actin, p53, alpha-1-antitrypsin, alpha-1-antichymotrypsin, desmin, CD56, and CD68 (96,138,139,197). The tumors are usually negative for myoglobin, myogenin, muscle-specific actin, h-caldesmon, S-100, ALK-1, nonspecific enolase (NSE), carcinoembryonic antigen (CEA), F-VIII, and AFP (87,102), although these could be anecdotally positive. Aberrant cytokeratin expression has been explained on the basis of genetic deregulation rather than differentiation (96).

Ultrastructurally, Agaram et al. have described the hallmark features to include dilated RERs and secondary lysosomes with dense precipitates, which correlate with the eosinophilic globules seen on light microscopy. Dilated mitochondria and mitochondrial-RER complexes are often seen. Other features include intracytoplasmic fat droplets, scant actin microfilaments, and focal glycogen pools (4). Primitive fibroblasts, small mesenchymal cells, and membrane-bound bodies that are alpha-1-antitrypsin or alpha-1-antichymotrypsin positive have been described by others (e4).

Molecular Pathology

Leuschner et al. undertook DNA ploidy studies in five cases and found that four tumors were diploid and one was hypodiploid (102). Chou et al. reported an aneuploid DNA stemline with high proliferative S phase in two patients studied with flow cytometry (e130).

In the first description of the chromosomal changes in UES, Iliszko et al. reported near-triploid and near-hexaploid clones with several chromosomal rearrangements (e302). Sowery et al. analyzed six cases of UES by both conventional cytogenetics and CGH. Although CGH demonstrated several chromosomal gains and deletions in each case, there was no specific abnormality seen in every case and no critical event important in tumorigenesis could be identified. Patterns of chromosomal changes included gains of chromosome 1q (four cases), 5p (four cases), 6q (four cases), 8p (three cases), and 12q (three cases), and losses of chromosome 9p (two cases), 11p (two cases), and chromosome 14 (three cases) (170). Other cytogenetic abnormalities have also been reported in UES, including near-triploid and near-hexaploid clones with several chromosomal rearrangements (e302). A clonal telomeric association (a cytogenetic phenomenon in which chromosome ends fuse to form dicentric, multicentric, and ring chromosomes) has been observed in UES (e597).

Mutation of TP53 gene but not the Wnt or telomerase pathways have been suggested to be involved in pathogenesis (e389). In fact, Lack et al. (96) described a 9-year-old boy, who was a member of a kindred with the family cancer syndrome (Li-Fraumeni syndrome), including a sister with soft tissue sarcoma of the wrist, a father with osteogenic sarcoma of the jaw, a mother with soft tissue sarcoma of the pectoralis muscle, and a half-brother with osteogenic sarcoma of the femur. Tawa et al. (e691) analyzed the expression of a multidrug-resistance (mdrl) gene in a UES of the liver in a 4-year-old boy, and noted a 7- and 11-fold increase in the gene expression level at the time of a first and second intracranial relapse. They suggested that acquired drug resistance as seen in their patient may correlate with overexpression of the mdrl gene.

NESTED STROMAL EPITHELIAL TUMOR OF THE LIVER

Nested stromal epithelial tumor is a recently described primary pediatric hepatic neoplasm that has been variably called "ossifying stromal-epithelial tumor," "calcifying nested stromal-epithelial tumor," "desmoplastic nested spindle cell tumor," and "nested stromal-epithelial tumor" (26,67,68,115,121) (e306). Less than 30 cases have been described in literature at the time of writing this section.

Pathogenesis

The tumors are of uncertain histogenesis; a possible origin in a hepatic mesenchymal precursor cell with primitive differentiation along the bile duct lineage has been suggested (67).

Clinical Features

Patients have ranged from 2 to 33 years of age; however, most tumors have been described in the first decade of life. Makhlouf et al. noted that four of their nine cases had a history of calcified hepatic nodules since early childhood (115). Ectopic ACTH production can lead to Cushing syndrome that abates following tumor excision. Most patients, however, are asymptomatic and are discovered to have the tumor incidentally. Meir et al. report a case that was associated with hydronephrosis. The hydronephrosis was discovered on antenatal ultrasound, whereas the hepatic neoplasm was incidentally discovered on routine follow-up abdominal imaging at 2 years of age (121). In Heerema-McKenney series, one 2-year-old patient subsequently developed nephroblastomatosis and Wilms tumor of the kidney, while another patient had a history of omphalocele, bowel obstruction due to postoperative adhesions, hypoplastic left kidney, and developmental delay (67).

Treatment and Outcomes

Partial hepatectomy is probably curative, although local recurrences have been reported in a few patients. Local recurrences are successfully treated with either surgery or radiofrequency ablation (115). Makhlouf et al. have suggested that this tumor is best considered a low-grade malignancy. Long-term prognosis appears to be good; six of eight patients in one series were alive and well up to 22 years after surgery (115). However, Brodsky et al. have reported a case in a 17-year-old girl with aggressive clinical behavior with multiple hepatic recurrences and an extrahepatic lymph node metastasis, suggesting that close follow-up is essential in these patients (26).

Gross Appearance

Based on the reported cases, the tumors are well circumscribed but not encapsulated and range in size from 4 to 30 cm. The tumors are intrahepatic; a pedunculated mass has also been described. On cut surface they appear multinodular, with a homogeneous, tan, granular-appearing cut surface. Variably sized foci of softening, cyst formation, calcification, or gritty ossification may be observed.

Histopathology

Nested stromal-epithelial tumors have been described as nonhepatocytic, nonbiliary tumors with nests of epithelial and spindle cells, an associated myofibroblastic stroma, as well as variable calcifications and ossifications (67,68). Architecturally, the tumor-liver interface is well-defined and the tumors consistently display an organoid arrangement of cellular nests comprised of spindled and/or epithelioid cells surrounded by a variably prominent collar of delicate myofibroblasts (Figure 15-58A). The stroma between the nests is usually desmoplastic. The periphery of the tumor shows a (probably entrapped) bile duct component. Psammomatous calcification may be sparse to prominent; when present, they are usually within or adjacent to cellular nests. Focal osteoid formation or ossification is common. The cellular nests have rounded edges and are relatively uniform in size in a given case; older children may show larger nests, suggesting that the tumor may grow slowly with age. Focal

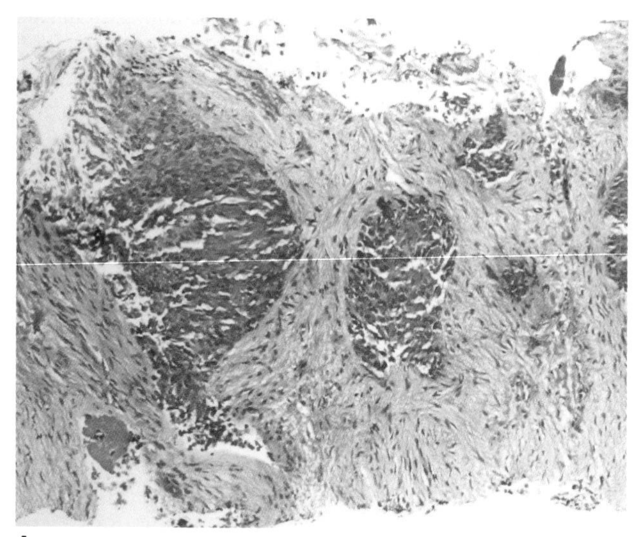

A

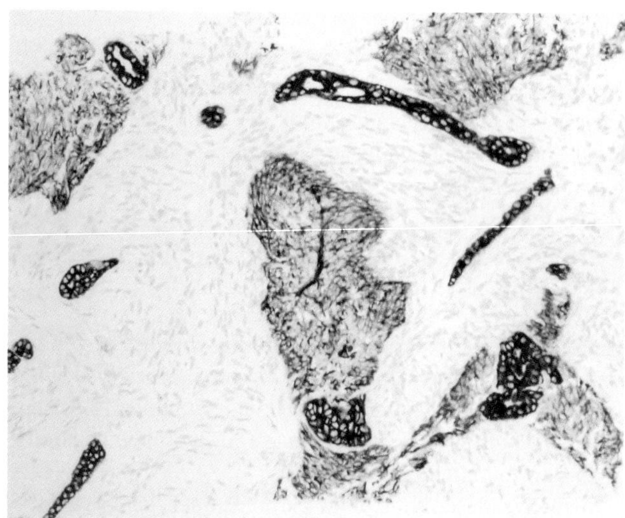

B

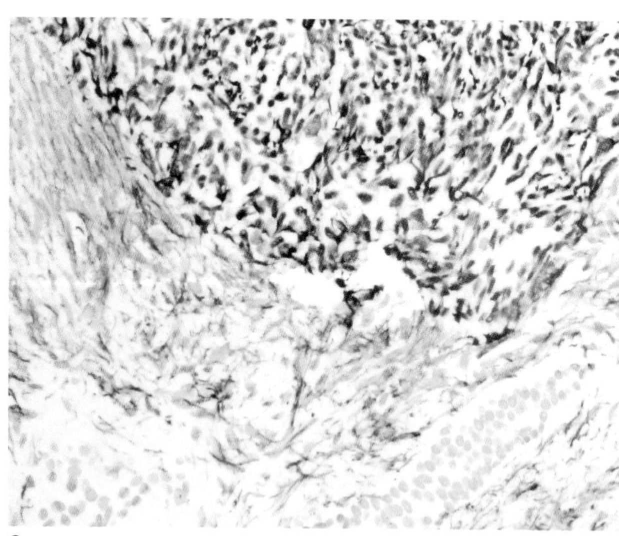

C

FIGURE 15-58 ■ Nested stromal epithelial tumor. **A:** The tumor is comprised of variably sized distinct nests of epithelioid cells embedded in variably myofibroblastic to desmoplastic stroma (H&E, 100×). **B, C:** The tumor cells in the nests are positive for cytokeratin (**B:** 100×) and WT-1 (**C:** 200×) immunostains.

neuroendocrine-appearing architecture has been described in cases with Cushing syndrome. The nests are composed predominantly of plump to fusiform spindled cells with centrally placed or scattered epithelioid cells. Epithelioid cells may predominate in cases with extensive calcification. Both spindle and epithelioid cells have bland oval nuclei with well-defined nuclear membrane, stippled chromatin, and variably conspicuous nucleoli. The cytoplasm is predominantly eosinophilic, with focal cells containing clear cytoplasm; epithelioid cells have distinct cellular borders. Mitoses are rare to scattered. Delicate osteoid formation may be present between the epithelioid nests. The desmoplastic stroma, a prominent feature in all four tumors, variably cellular, and composed of cells with morphologic features of myofibroblasts is not seen. Hill et al. specifically mentioned the lack of evidence of a ductal plate abnormality and lack of vascular invasion (68).

Immunohistochemically (Figures 15-58B, C), the tumor cells coexpress vimentin and cytokeratins, at least focally. They also exhibit moderate to strong diffuse nuclear staining for WT-1, using either the C-terminal or N-terminal antibodies (67,68,115,121). There is variable staining for EMA, CD56, CD57, S-100, and other mesenchymal markers. Synaptophysin and chromogranin stains are reportedly negative in all cases (67,68). ACTH immunohistochemistry may be positive in tumors associated with Cushing syndrome (154). The desmoplastic stroma has been reported to prominently display collagen type IV and smooth muscle actin (68).

Hill et al. performed ultrastructural studies in three cases and observed bland spindled and polygonal cells with focal basal lamina and focally well-developed cell junctions. Few mitochondria and sparse profiles of rough endoplasmic reticulum were seen in the cytoplasm. The polygonal cells contained focal collections of intermediate filaments and had interdigitating cell membranes. No neurosecretory granules were identified (68). On the other hand, Brodsky et al. report an abundance of rough endoplasmic reticulum and mitochondria in a tumor that behaved aggressively with intrahepatic recurrence and lymph node metastasis (26).

Molecular Pathology

Molecular studies for Ewing sarcoma family transcripts and SYT-SSX fusion transcripts have been negative in the cases studied (68,115). Hill et al. found a normal karyotype in the single case that they evaluated (68). Brodsky et al. report a cytogenetically complex tumor that later recurred and metastasized (26).

EMBRYONAL RHABDOMYOSARCOMA OF THE BILIARY TRACT

Although it is the most common sarcoma in the pediatric patient, rhabdomyosarcoma of the liver accounts for only 0.8% of all rhabdomyosarcomas and 1.0% of all liver tumors. At the same time, rhabdomyosarcoma is the most common malignant tumor of the biliary tree in childhood. It is difficult to diagnose and delayed diagnosis influences the prognosis. The occurrence of rhabdomyosarcoma of the liver and biliary tree was first reported in 1875 (e767). Almost 85 cases of biliary rhabdomyosarcoma have been reported in the literature; 75% of patients are under 5 years of age (85). The lesion is seen primarily (75% of cases) in children younger than 5 years of age and rarely in those older than 15 years (Figure 15-59A) (e396,e540,e593).

Jaundice is seen as the presenting symptom in 60% to 80% of cases and may be accompanied by cholemia, pale stools, and hepatomegaly, often confused with infectious hepatitis. Other symptoms include fever, abdominal distension, nausea, and vomiting (e367). The jaundice is reflected in moderate elevations of conjugated and unconjugated bilirubin, with total bilirubin of 1.5 to 9.0 mg/dL. ALP may also be elevated, along with a mild rise in SGOT. Imaging studies, including CT, MRI, ultrasonography (Figure 15-59B), and cholangiography may clearly demonstrate the site of obstruction within the intrahepatic ductal structures. Due to its rarity, it may be misdiagnosed as a choledochal cyst (7) (e480,e702).

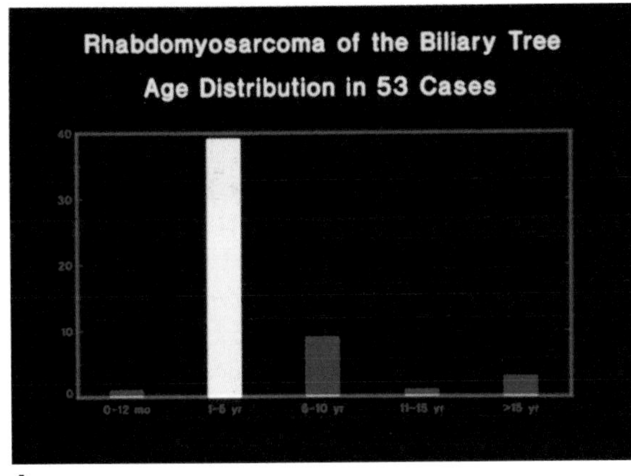

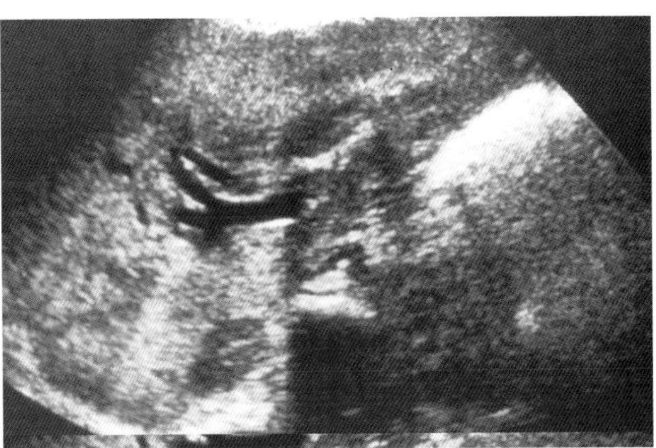

A B

FIGURE 15-59▪Embryonal rhabdomyosarcoma of the biliary tract. **A:** Age distribution. **B:** Ultrasonography displays the dilated ducts proximal to the tumor mass.

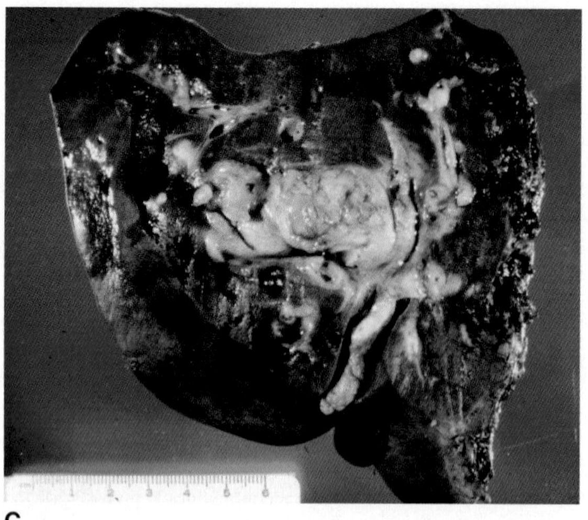

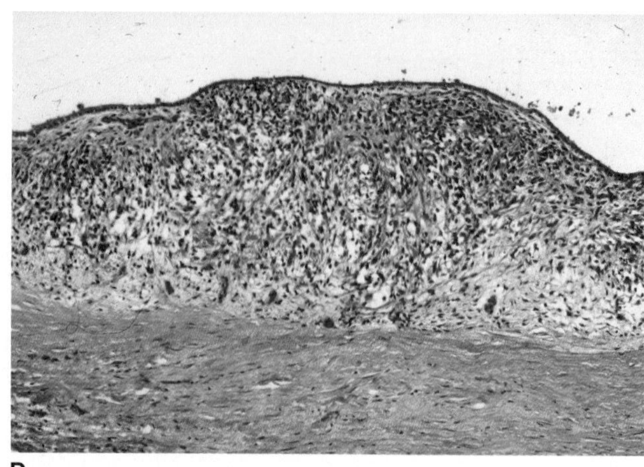

C D

FIGURE 15-59 *(continued)* **C:** The tumor occupies the major ducts within the porta hepatis (**center**) and extends proximally along the intrahepatic ducts. **D:** The tumor cells form a "cambium" layer of rhabdomyoblasts between the bile duct epithelium (**top**) and wall (**bottom**) (H&E stain, original magnification 75×).

Treatment is aimed at surgical resection, although complete resection is possible in only 20% to 40% of patients because of extension of the tumor into the liver, regional metastasis, and local extension to the duodenum, stomach, and pancreas. Recent preoperative therapy using standard protocols for embryonal rhabdomyosarcoma has proved effective, with Pollono et al. (e540) reporting complete remission using a multidrug protocol as the initial treatment of a 3-year-old girl after obtaining adequate transparietohepatic biliary drainage. Long-term survival of approximately 20% in previous years has risen for patients treated with preoperative chemotherapy and surgical "second-look" (e540,e570,e593).

Grossly, the tumor often presents as a botryoid, gelatinous mass occluding the lumen of the right and left or common bile duct (Figure 15-59C). The ducts proximal to the lesion are frequently dilated, and the walls of the duct containing the lesion are thickened. The tumor may extend into the liver as a soft lobulated mass. Occasional cases arise in the intrahepatic bile ducts (85).

Microscopically, the botryoid masses within the bile ducts are covered by a layer of cuboidal epithelium (bile duct epithelium) that may be inflamed or ulcerated. Beneath the epithelium lies a dense layer of tumor cells, the upper portion of the cambium layer (Figure 15-59D). Cells within this area are small and hyperchromatic, with scant cytoplasm. Deeper to the bile duct epithelium, the cells lie in a loose myxoid stroma and exhibit the typical features of embryonal rhabdomyosarcoma with round, spindle, or straplike shapes; elongate nuclei: scant acidophile cytoplasm; and frequent mitoses. As with other rhabdomyosarcomas, cross-striations may occasionally be found, but immunohistochemistry studies are consistently positive for desmin, with myoglobin and myosin identified in more differentiated cells (e659). The tumor is usually highly vascular, and areas of recent and remote hemorrhage and acute and chronic inflammation may be found throughout the lesion. The adjacent hepatic parenchyma is often compressed, and bile may be present within canaliculi and hepatocytes.

Nicol et al. have compared the clinicopathologic features of UES and hepatobiliary rhabdomyosarcoma (134). Although similarities do exist between the two lesions, UES has a male:female ratio of 1:1, a median age of occurrence of 10.5 years, and histology showing hyaline globules and diffuse anaplasia. Rhabdomyosarcoma, on the other hand, has a male:female ratio of 1.8:1 with a median age of 3.4 years and routinely lacks diffuse anaplasia and hyaline globules. Polyclonal desmin and muscle-specific actin are variably immunoreactive in both tumors; however, myogenin and myogenic regulatory protein D1 (MyoD1) is mostly negative in UES, but positive in rhabdomyosarcoma. With a median follow-up of 8 months, 11 of 18 patients with UES were still alive, whereas the estimated 5-year survival for biliary tract rhabdomyosarcoma was 66%. Establishing the correct diagnosis of these distinct clinical and pathologic entities is important, as surgery alone may be curative in UES, whereas initial chemotherapy is often recommended for the treatment of biliary tract rhabdomyosarcoma (see Chapter 24).

ANGIOSARCOMA

Angiosarcoma of the liver accounts for less than 2.5% of liver tumors in children (see Table 15-14). Selby et al. (162) studied 10 patients (six girls and four boys) ranging in age from 18 months to 7 years, and noted the presence of three older cases at 13, 17, and 18 years (Figure 15-60A). There is a reported predominance in females (female:male ratio of 2:1) and a mean age at presentation of near 4 years (162) (e486). This is in contrast to infantile hemangioendothelioma, which almost always occurs in the 1st year of life. However, hepatic angiosarcoma has also been reported in neonates (133). The most frequent presenting symptom is a rapidly enlarging abdominal mass, which may be accompanied by jaundice, diarrhea, abdominal pain, or vomiting. Congestive heart failure commonly seen with hepatic hemangioendotheliomas is absent with hepatic angiosarcomas (e196). An association with environmental exposure to Thorotrast, vinyl chloride, androgenic and anabolic steroids, oral contraceptives, and diethylstilbestrol, as reported in adults, has not been observed in children (e467). There is also no established syndromic or genetic association. Angiosarcoma arising in a child previously treated for infantile hemangioendothelioma has been described but is unusual (11) (e346). Treatment, including resection, radiation, transplantation, and a variety of chemotherapeutic agents, has been unsuccessful, and patients have rarely survived for more than 2 years (11). Gunawardena

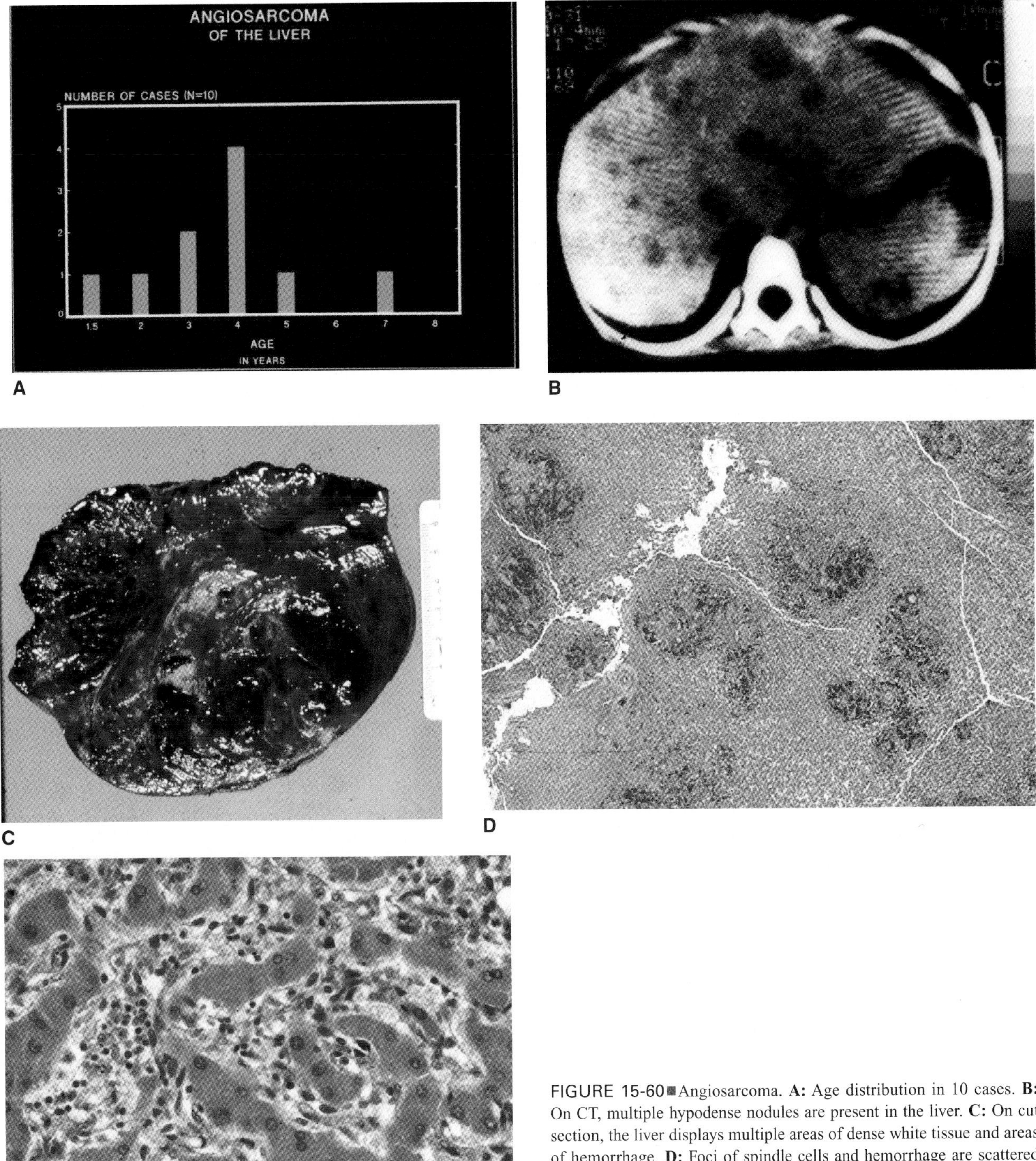

FIGURE 15-60 ■ Angiosarcoma. **A:** Age distribution in 10 cases. **B:** On CT, multiple hypodense nodules are present in the liver. **C:** On cut section, the liver displays multiple areas of dense white tissue and areas of hemorrhage. **D:** Foci of spindle cells and hemorrhage are scattered throughout the liver parenchyma (H&E stain, original magnification 40×). **E:** Bizarre endothelial cells fill and greatly distend the sinusoids of the liver, compressing and destroying hepatic trabeculae (H&E stain, original magnification 200×).

et al. (e260), however, report the 44-month survival without recurrence of a 4-year-old girl following surgical resection and postoperative chemotherapy with alternating cycles of ifosfamide and etoposide, cisplatinum and adriamycin, and vincristine and actinomycin D and cyclophosphamide for 18 months.

Hepatic angiosarcomas are often large multicentric lesions composed of well-demarcated, fleshy, tan nodules approximately 7 cm in diameter displaying areas of hemorrhage and necrosis (Figure 15-60B, C). Microscopically, the tumor is characterized by nodules of spindled cells in a whorled pattern (Figure 15-60D). Larger nodules composed of malignant vascular channels may also be present. Tumor cells are large, with hyperchromatic nuclei and frequent mitoses (Figure 15-60E). Intracytoplasmic and extracellular eosinophilic globules that are PAS-positive are present in most cases. Dimashkieh et al. have observed that the histology of pediatric hepatic angiosarcoma is distinct from adult angiosarcoma, with the former displaying hypercellular whorls of sarcomatous cells, or "kaposiform" spindle cells, in addition to the general features of angiosarcoma (50). Immunohistochemical stains are positive with vascular markers, alpha-1-antichymotrypsin, and Ulex europaeus but negative for keratin and AFP (162). Metastases to lungs, pleura, bone, adrenals, mesentery, and kidney have been described (11,162).

OTHER NEOPLASMS SEEN IN THE LIVER

Metastatic lesions such as neuroblastoma, Wilms tumor, and lymphoma are the most common neoplasms seen in the liver, but a variety of other primary neoplasms have been described. EBV-associated leiomyosarcoma has been described following liver transplantation in two children—the first, a 9-year-old boy who developed a tumor in his allografted liver 2 years after transplantation, and the second, in a 12-year-old girl, who, after transplantation, developed the leiomyosarcoma in the retroperitoneum involving the superior mesenteric vein (180). Malignant neoplasms that are rarely seen include malignant rhabdoid tumor, endodermal sinus (yolk sac) tumor, and lymphoma (e659).

GALL BLADDER

Congenital anomalies of the gallbladder include agenesis, duplication, bilobation, multiseptation, diverticula, ectopia, and congenital fistula (173). Agenesis occurs as an isolated anomaly in the majority of cases and is an incidental finding at autopsy in childhood. The gallbladder may be reduced to a fibrous cord or be diminutive in EHBA. In the neonate, a small or hypoplastic extrahepatic biliary tree may reflect a low-flow state in severe cholestatic liver disease. Alagille syndrome, A1AT, INH, and familial cholestatic syndromes are some of the conditions in which gallbladder hypoplasia may be seen. In CF, the gallbladder may be small and contain viscid mucus. Rarely, the bile ducts may be obstructed by biliary sludge.

The most common acquired disease of the gallbladder is cholelithiasis (Figure 15-61) (e659). This condition may be a complication of hemolytic disease, including congenital spherocytosis, sickle cell disease, and thalassemia. In most cases, the condition has been idiopathic. As in adults, there is a female preponderance in childhood cases, and cholecystitis is often associated. Some other conditions predisposing to cholelithiasis include TPN, biliary stasis, ileal disease, sepsis, prolonged fasting, inflammatory bowel disease, short gut syndrome, ileal resection, PSC, prematurity, dehydration, immaturity of the hepatic glucuronyl transferase, ceftriaxone therapy, CF, cirrhosis, Wilson disease, porphyria, biliary

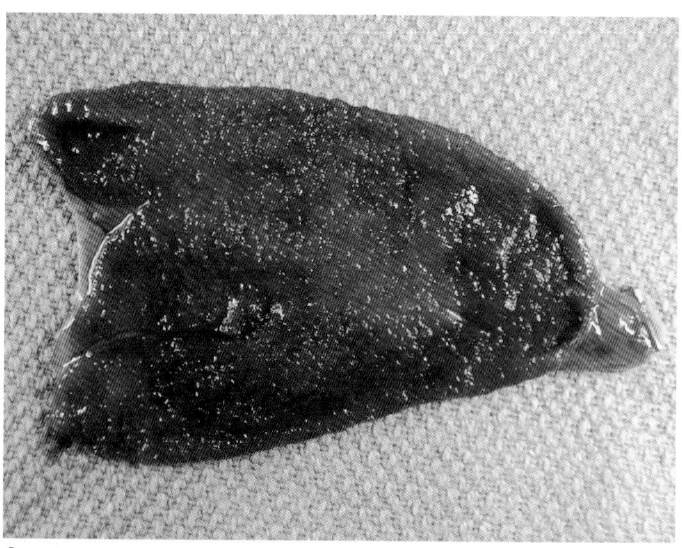
A

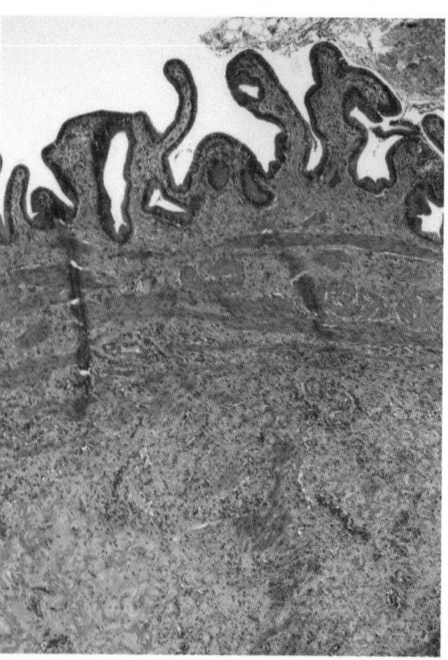
B

FIGURE 15-61 ■ Cholecystitis and cholelithiases. **A:** Gallbladder with red finely granular mucosa. **B:** Chronic cholecystitis with markedly thickened gallbladder wall and scattered chronic inflammatory cells (H&E, 40×).

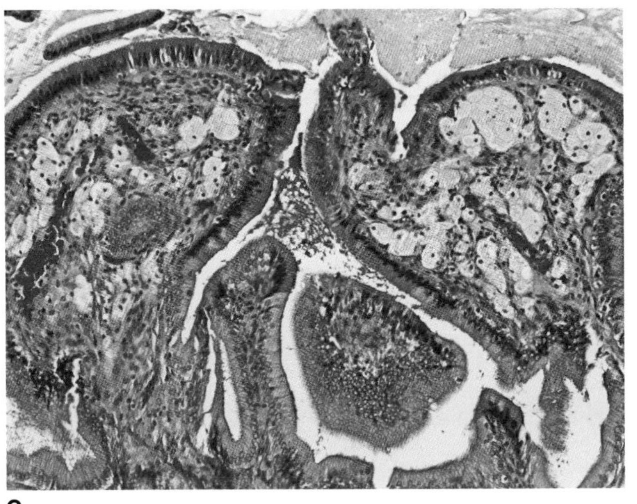
C

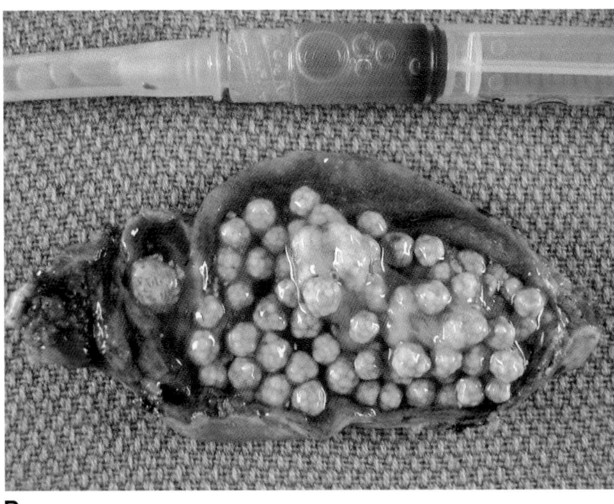
D

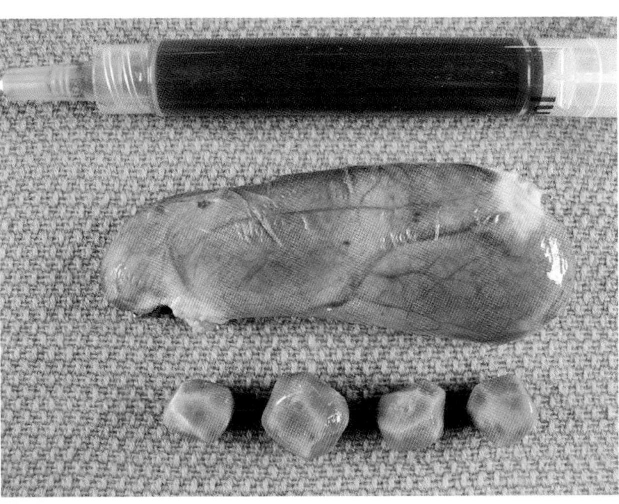
E

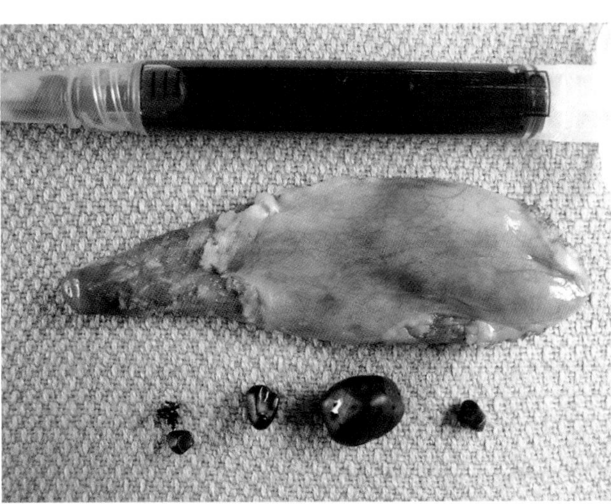
F

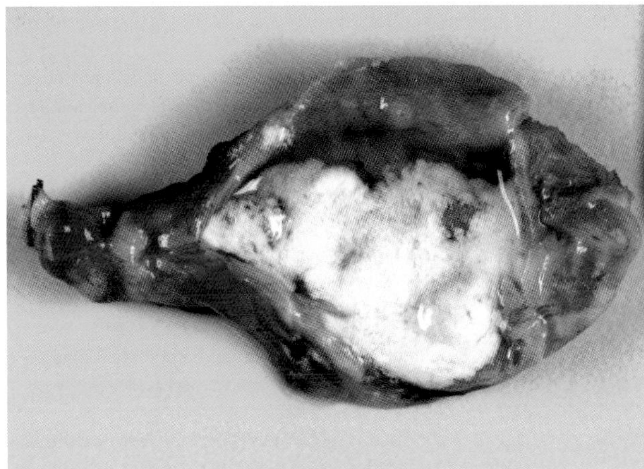
G

FIGURE 15-61 ■ *(continued)* **C:** Cholesterolosis characterized by foamy macrophages in lamina propria (H&E, 400×). **D–G:** Cholelithiases vary from cholesterol choleliths (**D**, **E**), ebonized choleliths (**F**), and calcium choleliths with milk-like bile (**G**).

dyskinesia, medications, and biliary tract anomalies, such as choledochal cyst. Cholelithiasis with cholesterol stones is seen in obese adolescents, both male and female. Tumors of the gallbladder are extremely rare in children; biliary rhabdomyosarcomas have been discussed above.

REFERENCES

1. Terminology of nodular hepatocellular lesions. International Working Party. *Hepatology* 1995;22(3):983–993.
2. Terminology of chronic hepatitis. International Working Party. *Am J Gastroenterol* 1995;90(2):181–189.

3. Acharya SK, Panda SK. Hepatitis E virus: epidemiology, diagnosis, pathology and prevention. *Trop Gastroenterol* 2006;27(2):63–68.
4. Agaram NP, Baren A, Antonescu CR. Pediatric and adult hepatic embryonal sarcoma: a comparative ultrastructural study with morphologic correlations. *Ultrastruct Pathol* 2006;30(6):403–408.
5. Albores-Saavedra J, Galliani C, Chable-Montero F, et al. Mucin-containing Rokitansky-Aschoff sinuses with extracellular mucin deposits simulating mucinous carcinoma of the gallbladder. *Am J Surg Pathol* 2009;33(11):1633–1638.
6. Alexander J, Kowdley KV. Hereditary hemochromatosis: genetics, pathogenesis, and clinical management. *Ann Hepatol* 2005;4(4):240–247.
7. Ali S, Russo MA, Margraf L. Biliary rhabdomyoscarcoma mimicking choledochal cyst. *J Gastrointestin Liver Dis* 2009;18(1):95–97.
8. Anthony PP, Vogel CL, Barker LF. Liver cell dysplasia: a premalignant condition. *J Clin Pathol* 1973;26(3):217–223.
9. Anthony PP, Ishak KG, Nayak NC, et al. The morphology of cirrhosis. Recommendations on definition, nomenclature, and classification by a working group sponsored by the World Health Organization. *J Clin Pathol* 1978;31(5):395–414.
10. Atra A, Al-Asiri R, Wali S, et al. Hepatocellular carcinoma, syncytial giant cell: a novel variant in children: a case report. *Ann Diagn Pathol* 2007;11(1):61–63.
11. Awan S, Davenport M, Portmann B, et al. Angiosarcoma of the liver in children. *J Pediatr Surg* 1996;31(12):1729–1732.
12. Bach N, Thung SN, Schaffner F. The histological features of chronic hepatitis C and autoimmune chronic hepatitis: a comparative analysis. *Hepatology* 1992;15(4):572–577.
13. Badve S, Logdberg L, Lal A, et al. Small cells in hepatoblastoma lack "oval" cell phenotype. *Mod Pathol* 2003;16(9):930–936.
14. Balistreri WF, Bezerra JA. Whatever happened to "neonatal hepatitis"? *Clin Liver Dis* 2006;10(1):27–53, v.
15. Balistreri WF, Grand R, Hoofnagle JH, et al. Biliary atresia: current concepts and research directions. Summary of a symposium. *Hepatology* 1996;23(6):1682–1692.
16. Batts KP. Iron overload syndromes and the liver. *Mod Pathol* 2007;20(Suppl 1):S31–S39.
17. Baumhoer D, Tornillo L, Stadlmann S, et al. Glypican 3 expression in human nonneoplastic, preneoplastic, and neoplastic tissues: a tissue microarray analysis of 4,387 tissue samples. *Am J Clin Pathol* 2008;129(6):899–906.
18. Bayraktar UD, Seren S, Bayraktar Y. Hepatic venous outflow obstruction: three similar syndromes. *World J Gastroenterol* 2007;13(13):1912–1927.
19. Begueret H, Trouette H, Vielh P, et al. Hepatic undifferentiated embryonal sarcoma: malignant evolution of mesenchymal hamartoma? Study of one case with immunohistochemical and flow cytometric emphasis. *J Hepatol* 2001;34(1):178–179.
20. Belghiti SD, Paradis V, Vilgrain V, et al. Specific management for multiple liver cell adenoma: is it justified? *Hepatology* 2005;42(Suppl.):297A.
21. Bioulac-Sage P, Balabaud C, Wanless IR. Diagnosis of focal nodular hyperplasia: not so easy. *Am J Surg Pathol* 2001;25(10): 1322–1335.
22. Bioulac-Sage P, Balabaud C, Bedossa P, et al. Pathological diagnosis of liver cell adenoma and focal nodular hyperplasia: Bordeaux update. *J Hepatol* 2007;46(3):521–527.
23. Bioulac-Sage P, Rebouissou S, Thomas C, et al. Hepatocellular adenoma subtype classification using molecular markers and immunohistochemistry. *Hepatology* 2007;46(3):740–748.
24. Bosma PJ. Inherited disorders of bilirubin metabolism. *J Hepatol* 2003;38(1):107–117.
25. Bove KE, Heubi JE, Balistreri WF, et al. Bile acid synthetic defects and liver disease: a comprehensive review. *Pediatr Dev Pathol* 2004;7(4):315–334.
26. Brodsky SV, Sandoval C, Sharma N, et al. Recurrent nested stromal epithelial tumor of the liver with extrahepatic metastasis: case report and review of literature. *Pediatr Dev Pathol* 2008;11(6):469–473.
27. Brown J, Perilongo G, Shafford E, et al. Pretreatment prognostic factors for children with hepatoblastoma—results from the International Society of Paediatric Oncology (SIOP) study SIOPEL 1. *Eur J Cancer* 2000;36(11):1418–1425.
28. Brunetti-Pierri N, Scaglia F. GM1 gangliosidosis: review of clinical, molecular, and therapeutic aspects. *Mol Genet Metab* 2008;94(4):391–396.
29. Brunt EM. Nonalcoholic steatohepatitis. *Semin Liver Dis* 2004;24(1):3–20.
30. Buckley AF, Burgart LJ, Sahai V, et al. Epidermal growth factor receptor expression and gene copy number in conventional hepatocellular carcinoma. *Am J Clin Pathol* 2008;129(2):245–251.
31. Budhu A, Jia HL, Forgues M, et al. Identification of metastasis-related microRNAs in hepatocellular carcinoma. *Hepatology* 2008;47(3):897–907.
32. Buetow PC, Buck JL, Pantongrag-Brown L, et al. Undifferentiated (embryonal) sarcoma of the liver: pathologic basis of imaging findings in 28 cases. *Radiology* 1997;203(3):779–783.
33. Bull LN, Carlton VE, Stricker NL, et al. Genetic and morphological findings in progressive familial intrahepatic cholestasis (Byler disease [PFIC-1] and Byler syndrome): evidence for heterogeneity. *Hepatology* 1997;26(1):155–164.
34. Burt AD, Mutton A, Day CP. Diagnosis and interpretation of steatosis and steatohepatitis. *Semin Diagn Pathol* 1998;15(4):246–258.
35. Casteels-Van Daele M, Van Geet C, Wouters C, et al. Reye syndrome revisited: a descriptive term covering a group of heterogeneous disorders. *Eur J Pediatr* 2000;159(9):641–648.
36. Chan KL, Fan ST, Tam PK, et al. Paediatric hepatoblastoma and hepatocellular carcinoma: retrospective study. *Hong Kong Med J* 2002;8(1):13–17.
37. Chang HJ, Jin SY, Park C, et al. Mesenchymal hamartomas of the liver: comparison of clinicopathologic features between cystic and solid forms. *J Korean Med Sci* 2006;21(1):63–68.
38. Chatelain D, Chailley-Heu B, Terris B, et al. The ciliated hepatic foregut cyst, an unusual bronchiolar foregut malformation: a histological, histochemical, and immunohistochemical study of 7 cases. *Hum Pathol* 2000;31(2):241–246.
39. Chen M, Wang J. Gaucher disease: review of the literature. *Arch Pathol Lab Med* 2008;132(5):851–853.
40. Christison-Lagay ER, Burrows PE, Alomari A, et al. Hepatic hemangiomas: subtype classification and development of a clinical practice algorithm and registry. *J Pediatr Surg* 2007;42(1):62–67; discussion 7–8.
41. Colombo C, Battezzati PM. Liver involvement in cystic fibrosis: primary organ damage or innocent bystander? *J Hepatol* 2004;41(6):1041–1044.
42. Conran RM, Hitchcock CL, Waclawiw MA, et al. Hepatoblastoma: the prognostic significance of histologic type. *Pediatr Pathol* 1992;12(2):167–183.
43. Cornette J, Festen S, van den Hoonaard TL, et al. Mesenchymal hamartoma of the liver: a benign tumor with deceptive prognosis in the perinatal period. Case report and review of the literature. *Fetal Diagn Ther* 2009;25(2):196–202.
44. Czauderna P, Mackinlay G, Perilongo G, et al. Hepatocellular carcinoma in children: results of the first prospective study of the International Society of Pediatric Oncology group. *J Clin Oncol* 2002;20(12):2798–2804.
45. Darbari A, Sabin KM, Shapiro CN, et al. Epidemiology of primary hepatic malignancies in U.S. children. *Hepatology* 2003;38(3): 560–566.
46. Dehner LP. The challenges of vasoformative tumors of the liver in children. *Pediatr Dev Pathol* 2004;7(5):A5–A7.
47. Desmet VJ. What is congenital hepatic fibrosis? *Histopathology* 1992;20(6):465–477.
48. Desmet VJ, Gerber M, Hoofnagle JH, et al. Classification of chronic hepatitis: diagnosis, grading and staging. *Hepatology* 1994;19(6):1513–1520.

49. Desmet VJ. Ludwig symposium on biliary disorders—part I. Pathogenesis of ductal plate abnormalities. *Mayo Clin Proc* 1998;73(1):80–89.
50. Dimashkieh HH, Mo JQ, Wyatt-Ashmead J, et al. Pediatric hepatic angiosarcoma: case report and review of the literature. *Pediatr Dev Pathol* 2004;7(5):527–532.
51. El-Serag HB, Davila JA. Is fibrolamellar carcinoma different from hepatocellular carcinoma? A US population-based study. *Hepatology* 2004;39(3):798–803.
52. Fabre A, Audet P, Vilgrain V, et al. Histologic scoring of liver biopsy in focal nodular hyperplasia with atypical presentation. *Hepatology* 2002;35(2):414–420.
53. Fabregat I. Dysregulation of apoptosis in hepatocellular carcinoma cells. *World J Gastroenterol* 2009;15(5):513–520.
54. Feo F, Frau M, Tomasi ML, et al. Genetic and epigenetic control of molecular alterations in hepatocellular carcinoma. *Exp Biol Med (Maywood)* 2009;234(7):726–736.
55. Feranchak AP. Hepatobiliary complications of cystic fibrosis. *Curr Gastroenterol Rep* 2004;6(3):231–239.
56. Francis B, Hallam L, Kecskes Z, et al. Placental mesenchymal dysplasia associated with hepatic mesenchymal hamartoma in the newborn. *Pediatr Dev Pathol* 2007;10(1):50–54.
57. Fridovich-Keil JL. Galactosemia: the good, the bad, and the unknown. *J Cell Physiol* 2006;209(3):701–705.
58. Gautier M, Jehan P, Odievre M. Histologic study of biliary fibrous remnants in 48 cases of extrahepatic biliary atresia: correlation with postoperative bile flow restoration. *J Pediatr* 1976;89(5):704–709.
59. Gilbert-Barness E, Barness L. *Metabolic diseases: Foundations of clinical management, genetics and pathology*. Natick, MA: Eaton Publishing, 2000.
60. Gopaul KP, Crook MA. The inborn errors of sialic acid metabolism and their laboratory investigation. *Clin Lab* 2006;52(3–4):155–169.
61. Grisaru-Granovsky S, Rabinowitz R, Ioscovich A, et al. Congenital diaphragmatic hernia: review of the literature in reflection of unresolved dilemmas. *Acta Paediatr* 2009;98(12):1874–1881.
62. Guglielmi FW, Regano N, Mazzuoli S, et al. Cholestasis induced by total parenteral nutrition. *Clin Liver Dis* 2008;12(1):97–110, viii.
63. Gunay-Aygun M. Liver and kidney disease in ciliopathies. *Am J Med Genet C Semin Med Genet* 2009;151C(4):296–306.
64. Guven A, Aygun C, Ince H, et al. Severe hypothyroidism caused by hepatic hemangioendothelioma in an infant of a diabetic mother. *Horm Res* 2005;63(2):86–89.
65. Hardwick D, Dimmick JE. Metabolic cirrhosis of infancy and childhood. *Perspect Pediatr Pathol* 1976;3:103–144.
66. Hartley JL, Davenport M, Kelly DA. Biliary atresia. *Lancet* 2009;374(9702):1704–1713.
67. Heerema-McKenney A, Leuschner I, Smith N, et al. Nested stromal epithelial tumor of the liver: six cases of a distinctive pediatric neoplasm with frequent calcifications and association with Cushing syndrome. *Am J Surg Pathol* 2005;29(1):10–20.
68. Hill DA, Swanson PE, Anderson K, et al. Desmoplastic nested spindle cell tumor of liver: report of four cases of a proposed new entity. *Am J Surg Pathol* 2005;29(1):1–9.
69. Hochman J, Balistreri WF. Neonatal cholestasis: differential diagnosis, evaluation and management. In: Balistreri W, Ohi R, Todani T, et al., eds. *Hepatobiliary, pancreatic and splenic disease in children: medica and surgical management*. Amsterdam: Elsevier Science, 1997:157–191.
70. Hoffmann B. Fabry disease: recent advances in pathology, diagnosis, treatment and monitoring. *Orphanet J Rare Dis* 2009;4:21.
71. Hussain SM, Terkivatan T, Zondervan PE, et al. Focal nodular hyperplasia: findings at state-of-the-art MR imaging, US, CT, and pathologic analysis. *Radiographics* 2004;24(1):3–17; discussion 8–9.
72. Hussain N, Feld JJ, Kleiner DE, et al. Hepatic abnormalities in patients with chronic granulomatous disease. *Hepatology* 2007;45(3):675–683.
73. Iizuka N, Hamamoto Y, Tsunedomi R, et al. Translational microarray systems for outcome prediction of hepatocellular carcinoma. *Cancer Sci* 2008;99(4):659–665.
74. Ioannou GN, Perkins JD, Carithers RL, Jr. Liver transplantation for hepatocellular carcinoma: impact of the MELD allocation system and predictors of survival. *Gastroenterology* 2008;134(5): 1342–1351.
75. Isaacs H, Jr. Fetal and neonatal hepatic tumors. *J Pediatr Surg* 2007;42(11):1797–1803.
76. Israeli R, Jule JE, Hom J. Pediatric pyogenic liver abscess. *Pediatr Emerg Care* 2009;25(2):107–108.
77. Jevon GP, Dimmick JE. Histopathologic approach to metabolic liver disease: Part 1. *Pediatr Dev Pathol* 1998;1(3):179–199.
78. Jevon GP, Dimmick JE. Histopathologic approach to metabolic liver disease: Part 2. *Pediatr Dev Pathol* 1998;1(4):261–269.
79. Kahn E, Daum F, Markowitz J, et al. Nonsyndromatic paucity of interlobular bile ducts: light and electron microscopic evaluation of sequential liver biopsies in early childhood. *Hepatology* 1986;6(5):890–901.
80. Kahn E. Biliary atresia revisited. *Pediatr Dev Pathol* 2004;7(2): 109–124.
81. Kakar S, Chen X, Ho C, et al. Chromosomal changes in fibrolamellar hepatocellular carcinoma detected by array comparative genomic hybridization. *Mod Pathol* 2009;22(1):134–141.
82. Kamath BM, Piccoli DA. Heritable disorders of the bile ducts. *Gastroenterol Clin North Am* 2003;32(3):857–875, vi.
83. Karrer FM, Bensard DD. Neonatal cholestasis. *Semin Pediatr Surg* 2000;9(4):166–169.
84. Katzenstein HM, Krailo MD, Malogolowkin MH, et al. Fibrolamellar hepatocellular carcinoma in children and adolescents. *Cancer* 2003;97(8):2006–2012.
85. Kebudi R, Gorgun O, Ayan I, et al. Rhabdomyosarcoma of the biliary tree. *Pediatr Int* 2003;45(4):469–471.
86. Keslar PJ, Buck JL, Selby DM. From the archives of the AFIP. Infantile hemangioendothelioma of the liver revisited. *Radiographics* 1993;13(3):657–670.
87. Kiani B, Ferrell LD, Qualman S, et al. Immunohistochemical analysis of embryonal sarcoma of the liver. *Appl Immunohistochem Mol Morphol* 2006;14(2):193–197.
88. Kirsch R, Yap J, Roberts EA, et al. Clinicopathologic spectrum of massive and submassive hepatic necrosis in infants and children. *Hum Pathol* 2009;40(4):516–526.
89. Klein WM, Molmenti EP, Colombani PM, et al. Primary liver carcinoma arising in people younger than 30 years. *Am J Clin Pathol* 2005;124(4):512–518.
90. Knisely AS. Progressive familial intrahepatic cholestasis: a personal perspective. *Pediatr Dev Pathol* 2000;3(2):113–125.
91. Kobayashi S, Murayama S, Takanashi S, et al. Clinical features and prognoses of 23 patients with chronic granulomatous disease followed for 21 years by a single hospital in Japan. *Eur J Pediatr* 2008;167(12):1389–1394.
92. Kondo K, Chijiiwa K, Nagano M, et al. Comparison of seven prognostic staging systems in patients who undergo hepatectomy for hepatocellular carcinoma. *Hepatogastroenterology* 2007;54(77): 1534–1538.
93. Korita PV, Wakai T, Shirai Y, et al. Overexpression of osteopontin independently correlates with vascular invasion and poor prognosis in patients with hepatocellular carcinoma. *Hum Pathol* 2008;39(12):1777–1783.
94. Lack EE, Neave C, Vawter GF. Hepatoblastoma. A clinical and pathologic study of 54 cases. *Am J Surg Pathol* 1982;6(8):693–705.
95. Lack EE, Neave C, Vawter GF. Hepatocellular carcinoma. Review of 32 cases in childhood and adolescence. *Cancer* 1983;52(8): 1510–1515.
96. Lack EE, Schloo BL, Azumi N, et al. Undifferentiated (embryonal) sarcoma of the liver. Clinical and pathologic study of 16 cases

with emphasis on immunohistochemical features. *Am J Surg Pathol* 1991;15(1):1–16.
97. Lamps LW. Hepatic granulomas, with an emphasis on infectious causes. *Adv Anat Pathol* 2008;15(6):309–318.
98. LaRusso NF, Shneider BL, Black D, et al. Primary sclerosing cholangitis: summary of a workshop. *Hepatology* 2006;44(3):746–764.
99. Lee WM, Squires RH Jr, Nyberg SL, et al. Acute liver failure: summary of a workshop. *Hepatology* 2008;47(4):1401–1415.
100. Lefton HB, Rosa A, Cohen M. Diagnosis and epidemiology of cirrhosis. *Med Clin North Am* 2009;93(4):787–799, vii.
101. Leone N, Saettone S, De Paolis P, et al. Ectopic livers and related pathology: report of three cases of benign lesions. *Dig Dis Sci* 2005;50(10):1818–1822.
102. Leuschner I, Schmidt D, Harms D. Undifferentiated sarcoma of the liver in childhood: morphology, flow cytometry, and literature review. *Hum Pathol* 1990;21(1):68–76.
103. Lewis MJ, Lewis EH III, Amos JA, et al. Cystic fibrosis. *Am J Clin Pathol* 2003;120(Suppl):S3–S13.
104. Loomba R, Sirlin CB, Schwimmer JB, et al. Advances in pediatric nonalcoholic fatty liver disease. *Hepatology* 2009;50(4): 1282–1293.
105. Lopez-Terrada D, Gunaratne PH, Adesina AM, et al. Histologic subtypes of hepatoblastoma are characterized by differential canonical Wnt and Notch pathway activation in DLK+ precursors. *Hum Pathol* 2009;40(6):783–794.
106. Lu W, Dong J, Huang Z, et al. Comparison of four current staging systems for Chinese patients with hepatocellular carcinoma undergoing curative resection: Okuda, CLIP, TNM and CUPI. *J Gastroenterol Hepatol* 2008;23(12):1874–1878.
107. Lu BR, Mack CL. Inflammation and biliary tract injury. *Curr Opin Gastroenterol* 2009;25(3):260–264.
108. Luketic VA, Shiffman ML. Benign recurrent intrahepatic cholestasis. *Clin Liver Dis* 2004;8(1):133–149, vii.
109. Madjov R, Chervenkov P, Madjova V, et al. Caroli's disease. Report of 5 cases and review of literature. *Hepatogastroenterology* 2005;52(62):606–609.
110. Maegawa GH, Stockley T, Tropak M, et al. The natural history of juvenile or subacute GM2 gangliosidosis: 21 new cases and literature review of 134 previously reported. *Pediatrics* 2006;118(5):e1550–e1562.
111. Maggiore G, Riva S, Sciveres M. Autoimmune diseases of the liver and biliary tract and overlap syndromes in childhood. *Minerva Gastroenterol Dietol* 2009;55(1):53–70.
112. Mahamid J, Miselevich I, Attias D, et al. Nodular regenerative hyperplasia associated with idiopathic thrombocytopenic purpura in a young girl: a case report and review of the literature. *J Pediatr Gastroenterol Nutr* 2005;41(2):251–255.
113. Mak CM, Lam CW. Diagnosis of Wilson's disease: a comprehensive review. *Crit Rev Clin Lab Sci* 2008;45(3):263–290.
114. Makhlouf HR, Abdul-Al HM, Goodman ZD. Diagnosis of focal nodular hyperplasia of the liver by needle biopsy. *Hum Pathol* 2005;36(11):1210–1216.
115. Makhlouf HR, Abdul-Al HM, Wang G, et al. Calcifying nested stromal-epithelial tumors of the liver: a clinicopathologic, immunohistochemical, and molecular genetic study of 9 cases with a long-term follow-up. *Am J Surg Pathol* 2009;33(7):976–983.
116. Mancini GM, Havelaar AC, Verheijen FW. Lysosomal transport disorders. *J Inherit Metab Dis* 2000;23(3):278–292.
117. Mani H, Van Thiel DH. Mesenchymal tumors of the liver. *Clin Liver Dis* 2001;5(1):219–257, viii.
118. Mani H, Kleiner DE. Liver biopsy findings in chronic hepatitis B. *Hepatology* 2009;49(5 Suppl):S61–S71.
119. McAdams AJ, Hug G, Bove KE. Glycogen storage disease, types I to X: criteria for morphologic diagnosis. *Hum Pathol* 1974;5(4):463–487.
120. McLarney JK, Rucker PT, Bender GN, et al. Fibrolamellar carcinoma of the liver: radiologic-pathologic correlation. *Radiographics* 1999;19(2):453–471.
121. Meir K, Maly A, Doviner V, et al. Nested (ossifying) stromal epithelial tumor of the liver: case report. *Pediatr Dev Pathol* 2009;12(3): 233–236.
122. Meyers RL. Tumors of the liver in children. *Surg Oncol* 2007;16(3):195–203.
123. Mieli-Vergani G, Vergani D. Autoimmune hepatitis in children: what is different from adult AIH? *Semin Liver Dis* 2009;29(3):297–306.
124. Minguez B, Tovar V, Chiang D, et al. Pathogenesis of hepatocellular carcinoma and molecular therapies. *Curr Opin Gastroenterol* 2009;25(3):186–194.
125. Mo JQ, Dimashkieh HH, Bove KE. GLUT1 endothelial reactivity distinguishes hepatic infantile hemangioma from congenital hepatic vascular malformation with associated capillary proliferation. *Hum Pathol* 2004;35(2):200–209.
126. Mohan N, Gonzalez-Peralta RP, Fujisawa T, et al. Chronic hepatitis C virus infection in children. *J Pediatr Gastroenterol Nutr* 2010;50(2):123–131.
127. Moran CA, Mullick FG, Ishak KG. Nodular regenerative hyperplasia of the liver in children. *Am J Surg Pathol* 1991;15(5):449–454.
128. Moyer K, Balistreri W. Hepatobiliary disease in patients with cystic fibrosis. *Curr Opin Gastroenterol* 2009;25(3):272–278.
129. Muenzer J. The mucopolysaccharidoses: a heterogeneous group of disorders with variable pediatric presentations. *J Pediatr* 2004;144(5 Suppl):S27–S34.
130. Nakanuma Y, Terada T, Ueda K, et al. Adenomatous hyperplasia of the liver as a precancerous lesion. *Liver* 1993;13(1):1–9.
131. Nakanuma Y, Hoso M, Sasaki M, et al. Histopathology of the liver in non-cirrhotic portal hypertension of unknown aetiology. *Histopathology* 1996;28(3):195–204.
132. Nathan H, Schulick RD, Choti MA, et al. Predictors of survival after resection of early hepatocellular carcinoma. *Ann Surg* 2009;249(5):799–805.
133. Nazir Z, Pervez S. Malignant vascular tumors of liver in neonates. *J Pediatr Surg* 2006;41(1):e49–e51.
134. Nicol K, Savell V, Moore J, et al. Distinguishing undifferentiated embryonal sarcoma of the liver from biliary tract rhabdomyosarcoma: a Children's Oncology Group study. *Pediatr Dev Pathol* 2007;10(2):89–97.
135. Otte JB, de Ville de Goyet J. The contribution of transplantation to the treatment of liver tumors in children. *Semin Pediatr Surg* 2005;14(4):233–238.
136. Ozen H. Glycogen storage diseases: new perspectives. *World J Gastroenterol* 2007;13(18):2541–2553.
137. Ozturk M, Arslan-Ergul A, Bagislar S, et al. Senescence and immortality in hepatocellular carcinoma. *Cancer Lett* 2009;286(1):103–113.
138. Pachera S, Nishio H, Takahashi Y, et al. Undifferentiated embryonal sarcoma of the liver: case report and literature survey. *J Hepatobiliary Pancreat Surg* 2008;15(5):536–544.
139. Perez-Gomez RM, Soria-Cespedes D, de Leon-Bojorge B, et al. Diffuse membranous immunoreactivity of CD56 and paranuclear dot-like staining pattern of cytokeratins AE1/3, CAM5.2, and OSCAR in undifferentiated (embryonal) sarcoma of the liver. *Appl Immunohistochem Mol Morphol* 2010;18(2):195–198.
140. Perlmutter DH. Alpha-1-antitrypsin deficiency: diagnosis and treatment. *Clin Liver Dis* 2004;8(4):839–859, viii–ix.
141. Phillips M, Pucell S, Patterson Jea. Metabolic liver disease. In: Phillips MJ, Poucell S, Patterson J, et al., eds. *The liver: An atlas and text of ultrastructural pathology*. New York: Raven Press, 1987:239.
142. Prokurat A, Kluge P, Kosciesza A, et al. Transitional liver cell tumors (TLCT) in older children and adolescents: a novel group of aggressive hepatic tumors expressing beta-catenin. *Med Pediatr Oncol* 2002;39(5):510–518.
143. Ramsay AD, Bates AW, Williams S, et al. Variable antigen expression in hepatoblastomas. *Appl Immunohistochem Mol Morphol* 2008;16(2):140–147.
144. Rana SS, Bhasin DK, Nanda M, et al. Parasitic infestations of the biliary tract. *Curr Gastroenterol Rep* 2007;9(2):156–164.

145. Rastogi A, Krishnani N, Pandey R. Dubin-Johnson syndrome—a clinicopathologic study of twenty cases. *Indian J Pathol Microbiol* 2006;49(4):500–504.
146. Rebouissou S, Bioulac-Sage P, Zucman-Rossi J. Molecular pathogenesis of focal nodular hyperplasia and hepatocellular adenoma. *J Hepatol* 2008;48(1):163–170.
147. Reiser DJ. Neonatal jaundice: physiologic variation or pathologic process. *Crit Care Nurs Clin North Am* 2004;16(2):257–269.
148. Reshamwala PA, Kleiner DE, Heller T. Nodular regenerative hyperplasia: not all nodules are created equal. *Hepatology* 2006;44(1):7–14.
149. Reshetnyak VI, Karlovich TI, Ilchenko LU. Hepatitis G virus. *World J Gastroenterol* 2008;14(30):4725–4734.
150. Resnick MB, Kozakewich HP, Perez-Atayde AR. Hepatic adenoma in the pediatric age group. Clinicopathological observations and assessment of cell proliferative activity. *Am J Surg Pathol* 1995;19(10):1181–1190.
151. Rizzetto M. Hepatitis D: thirty years after. *J Hepatol* 2009;50(5):1043–1050.
152. Roberts EA. Primary sclerosing cholangitis in children. *J Gastroenterol Hepatol* 1999;14(6):588–593.
153. Roberts EA. Neonatal hepatitis syndrome. *Semin Neonatol* 2003;8(5):357–374.
154. Rod A, Voicu M, Chiche L, et al. Cushing's syndrome associated with a nested stromal epithelial tumor of the liver: hormonal, immunohistochemical, and molecular studies. *Eur J Endocrinol* 2009;161(5):805–810.
155. Roebuck DJ, Aronson D, Clapuyt P, et al. 2005 PRETEXT: a revised staging system for primary malignant liver tumours of childhood developed by the SIOPEL group. *Pediatr Radiol* 2007;37(2):123–132; quiz 249–250.
156. Roels F, Espeel M, De Craemer D. Liver pathology and immunocytochemistry in congenital peroxisomal diseases: a review. *J Inherit Metab Dis* 1991;14(6):853–875.
157. Russo PA, Mitchell GA, Tanguay RM. Tyrosinemia: a review. *Pediatr Dev Pathol* 2001;4(3):212–221.
158. Sakamoto M, Mori T, Masugi Y, et al. Candidate molecular markers for histological diagnosis of early hepatocellular carcinoma. *Intervirology* 2008;51(Suppl 1):42–45.
159. Sakata J, Shirai Y, Wakai T, et al. Preoperative predictors of vascular invasion in hepatocellular carcinoma. *Eur J Surg Oncol* 2008;34(8):900–905.
160. Schwimmer JB, Behling C, Newbury R, et al. Histopathology of pediatric nonalcoholic fatty liver disease. *Hepatology* 2005;42(3):641–649.
161. Scott CR. The genetic tyrosinemias. *Am J Med Genet C Semin Med Genet* 2006;142C(2):121–126.
162. Selby DM, Stocker JT, Ishak KG. Angiosarcoma of the liver in childhood: a clinicopathologic and follow-up study of 10 cases. *Pediatr Pathol* 1992;12(4):485–498.
163. Selby DM, Stocker JT, Waclawiw MA, et al. Infantile hemangioendothelioma of the liver. *Hepatology* 1994;20(1 Pt 1):39–45.
164. Seo YS, Kim YJ, Um SH, et al. Evaluation of the prognostic powers of various tumor status grading scales in patients with hepatocellular carcinoma. *J Gastroenterol Hepatol* 2008;23(8 Pt 1):1267–1275.
165. Sharma S, Dean AG, Corn A, et al. Ciliated hepatic foregut cyst: an increasingly diagnosed condition. *Hepatobiliary Pancreat Dis Int* 2008;7(6):581–589.
166. Silverman EK, Sandhaus RA. Clinical practice. Alpha1-antitrypsin deficiency. *N Engl J Med* 2009;360(26):2749–2757.
167. Singham J, Yoshida EM, Scudamore CH. Choledochal cysts: part 2 of 3: Diagnosis. *Can J Surg* 2009;52(6):506–511.
168. Singham J, Yoshida EM, Scudamore CH. Choledochal cysts: part 1 of 3: classification and pathogenesis. *Can J Surg* 2009;52(5):434–440.
169. Singham J, Yoshida EM, Scudamore CH. Choledochal cysts. Part 3 of 3: management. *Can J Surg* 2010;53(1):51–56.
170. Sowery RD, Jensen C, Morrison KB, et al. Comparative genomic hybridization detects multiple chromosomal amplifications and deletions in undifferentiated embryonal sarcoma of the liver. *Cancer Genet Cytogenet* 2001;126(2):128–133.
171. Stocker JT, Ishak KG. Focal nodular hyperplasia of the liver: a study of 21 pediatric cases. *Cancer* 1981;48(2):336–345.
172. Stocker JT, Ishak KG. Mesenchymal hamartoma of the liver: report of 30 cases and review of the literature. *Pediatr Pathol* 1983;1(3):245–267.
173. Stocker JT. An approach to handling pediatric liver tumors. *Am J Clin Pathol* 1998;109(4 Suppl 1):S67–S72.
174. Stocker JT. Hepatic tumors in children. *Clin Liver Dis* 2001;5(1):259–281, viii–ix.
175. Sun XY, Wu ZD, Liao XF, et al. Tumor angiogenesis and its clinical significance in pediatric malignant liver tumor. *World J Gastroenterol* 2005;11(5):741–743.
176. Taddei T, Mistry P, Schilsky ML. Inherited metabolic disease of the liver. *Curr Opin Gastroenterol* 2008;24(3):278–286.
177. Tazawa Y, Abukawa D, Maisawa S, et al. Idiopathic neonatal hepatitis presenting as neonatal hepatic siderosis and steatosis. *Dig Dis Sci* 1998;43(2):392–396.
178. Terada Y, Matsumoto S, Bando K, et al. Comprehensive allelotyping of hepatoblastoma. *Hepatogastroenterology* 2009;56(89):199–204.
179. Terracciano LM, Bernasconi B, Ruck P, et al. Comparative genomic hybridization analysis of hepatoblastoma reveals high frequency of X-chromosome gains and similarities between epithelial and stromal components. *Hum Pathol* 2003;34(9):864–871.
180. Timmons CF, Dawson DB, Richards CS, et al. Epstein-Barr virus-associated leiomyosarcomas in liver transplantation recipients. Origin from either donor or recipient tissue. *Cancer* 1995;76(8):1481–1489.
181. Tomer G, Shneider BL. Disorders of bile formation and biliary transport. *Gastroenterol Clin North Am* 2003;32(3):839–55, vi.
182. Torbenson M. Review of the clinicopathologic features of fibrolamellar carcinoma. *Adv Anat Pathol* 2007;14(3):217–223.
183. Tovo PA, Lazier L, Versace A. Hepatitis B virus and hepatitis C virus infections in children. *Curr Opin Infect Dis* 2005;18(3):261–266.
184. Trobaugh-Lotrario AD, Tomlinson GE, Finegold MJ, et al. Small cell undifferentiated variant of hepatoblastoma: adverse clinical and molecular features similar to rhabdoid tumors. *Pediatr Blood Cancer* 2009;52(3):328–334.
185. Tsai HW, Tsai HH, Kuo FY, et al. Computerized analyses of morphology and proliferative activity differentiate hepatoblastoma from paediatric hepatocellular carcinoma. *Histopathology* 2009;54(3):328–336.
186. Tsokos M, Erbersdobler A. Pathology of peliosis. *Forensic Sci Int* 2005;149(1):25–33.
187. Varnholt H. The role of microRNAs in primary liver cancer. *Ann Hepatol* 2008;7(2):104–113.
188. Wanders RJ. Metabolic and molecular basis of peroxisomal disorders: a review. *Am J Med Genet A* 2004;126A(4):355–375.
189. Wang JD, Chang TK, Chen HC, et al. Pediatric liver tumors: initial presentation, image finding and outcome. *Pediatr Int* 2007;49(4):491–496.
190. Wanless IR. Micronodular transformation (nodular regenerative hyperplasia) of the liver: a report of 64 cases among 2,500 autopsies and a new classification of benign hepatocellular nodules. *Hepatology* 1990;11(5):787–797.
191. Weir EG, Ali SZ. Hepatoblastoma: cytomorphologic characteristics in serious cavity fluids. *Cancer* 2002;96(5):267–274.
192. Whitington PF. Neonatal hemochromatosis: a congenital alloimmune hepatitis. *Semin Liver Dis* 2007;27(3):243–250.
193. Wong D. Hereditary fructose intolerance. *Mol Genet Metab* 2005;85(3):165–167.
194. Wong CM, Ng IO. Molecular pathogenesis of hepatocellular carcinoma. *Liver Int* 2008;28(2):160–174.
195. Wraith JE. Lysosomal disorders. *Semin Neonatol* 2002;7(1):75–83.

196. Yamaoka H, Ohtsu K, Sueda T, et al. Diagnostic and prognostic impact of beta-catenin alterations in pediatric liver tumors. *Oncol Rep* 2006;15(3):551–556.
197. Zheng JM, Tao X, Xu AM, et al. Primary and recurrent embryonal sarcoma of the liver: clinicopathological and immunohistochemical analysis. *Histopathology* 2007;51(2):195–203.
198. Zimmerman MA, Cameron AM, Ghobrial RM. Budd-Chiari syndrome. *Clin Liver Dis* 2006;10(2):259–273, viii.
199. Zimmermann A. The emerging family of hepatoblastoma tumours: from ontogenesis to oncogenesis. *Eur J Cancer* 2005;41(11): 1503–1514.
200. Zynger DL, Gupta A, Luan C, et al. Expression of glypican 3 in hepatoblastoma: an immunohistochemical study of 65 cases. *Hum Pathol* 2008;39(2):224–230.

CHAPTER 16

The Pancreas

MARIKO SUCHI

ORGANOGENESIS AND EXOCRINE HISTOGENESIS

During week 4 of gestation, the ventral foregut gives rise to two pancreatic buds at the junction of the hepatic duct. The dorsal primordium develops in the mesentery. The ventral pancreatic bud rotates with the gut and fuses with the larger dorsal anlage and with the duodenum, and the fused primordia take up their normal position against the posterior abdominal wall in the concavity of the duodenum. The ventral bud gives rise to the uncinate process and the inferior portion of the head of the pancreas, and the dorsal primordium gives rise to the body, tail, and superior portion of the head (Figure 16-1). The duct of the dorsal pancreas opens more proximally into the duodenum and the ventral duct more distally, together with the common bile duct. Fusion of the primordia during the middle of week 6 of gestation leads to fusion of the duct systems. The duct of the ventral pancreas becomes the main pancreatic duct of Wirsung. The duct of the dorsal pancreas usually remains patent as the minor duct of Santorini.

During week 7 of gestation, simple, undifferentiated epithelial tubules grow into a loose mesenchyme. The epithelium rapidly forms a ramifying duct system, from which buds of cuboidal cells form the first recognizable acinar units by week 10; endocrine elements are also present by this time. The pancreas, from week 10 to term, continues to ramify and gives rise to exocrine and endocrine elements. Ductal elements, especially the centroacinar cells, can be hard to identify definitively from acinar and endocrine cells at this stage, but they express keratins 7 and 19 in addition to the keratins 8 and 18, which are found on acinar and endocrine cells after week 16 (17). Mucin glycoprotein gene messenger RNA (mRNA) studies reveal MUC6 in the pancreatic ducts from 13 weeks of gestation, and MUC3 is detected transiently at 13 weeks only (e201). Pancreatic exocrine development, like pulmonary alveolar maturation, is largely a postnatal event. The appearance of the pancreas at birth is one of underdeveloped acinar elements in a mesenchymal stroma (Figure 16-2). Acinar tissue increases rapidly after birth. Imrie et al. (74) showed that the ratio of acinar to connective tissue volume increases in a linear manner from 0.5 at week

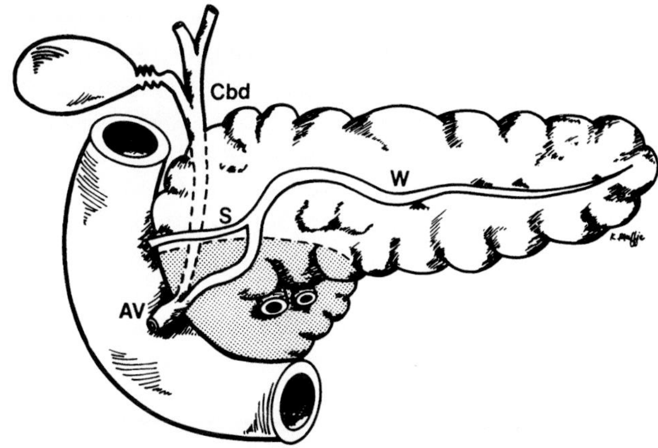

FIGURE 16-1 ■ Pancreas, ducts, and derivation. The pancreatic duct of Wirsung (*W*) drains most of the pancreas, joining the common bile duct (*Cbd*) proximal to the ampulla of Vater (*AV*). The accessory duct of Santorini (*S*) may drain part of the gland through a separate opening. A portion of the head and the uncinate lobe (stippled area) are derived from the ventral bud of the pancreas.

32 to 2.0 at week 52 after conception. In an assessment of the morphologic maturation of an infant pancreas, the length of postnatal survival is more important than the gestational age. The embryology of the pancreas is reviewed in detail by Cubilla and Fitzgerald (e46).

CONGENITAL ANOMALIES AND MALFORMATIONS

Agenesis and Hypoplasia

Agenesis of the pancreas refers to a complete absence of the gland, rather than a lack of the endocrine or exocrine portions alone. Insulin promoter factor-1 (IPF1), a homeodomain protein, is important for pancreatic development in the mouse, and its targeted disruption results in agenesis (e109). A homozygous point deletion in the *IPF1* at 13q12.1 has been identified in a patient with pancreatic agenesis (165), and heterozygosity has been associated with neonatal diabetes mellitus (164). The clinical presentation of pancreatic

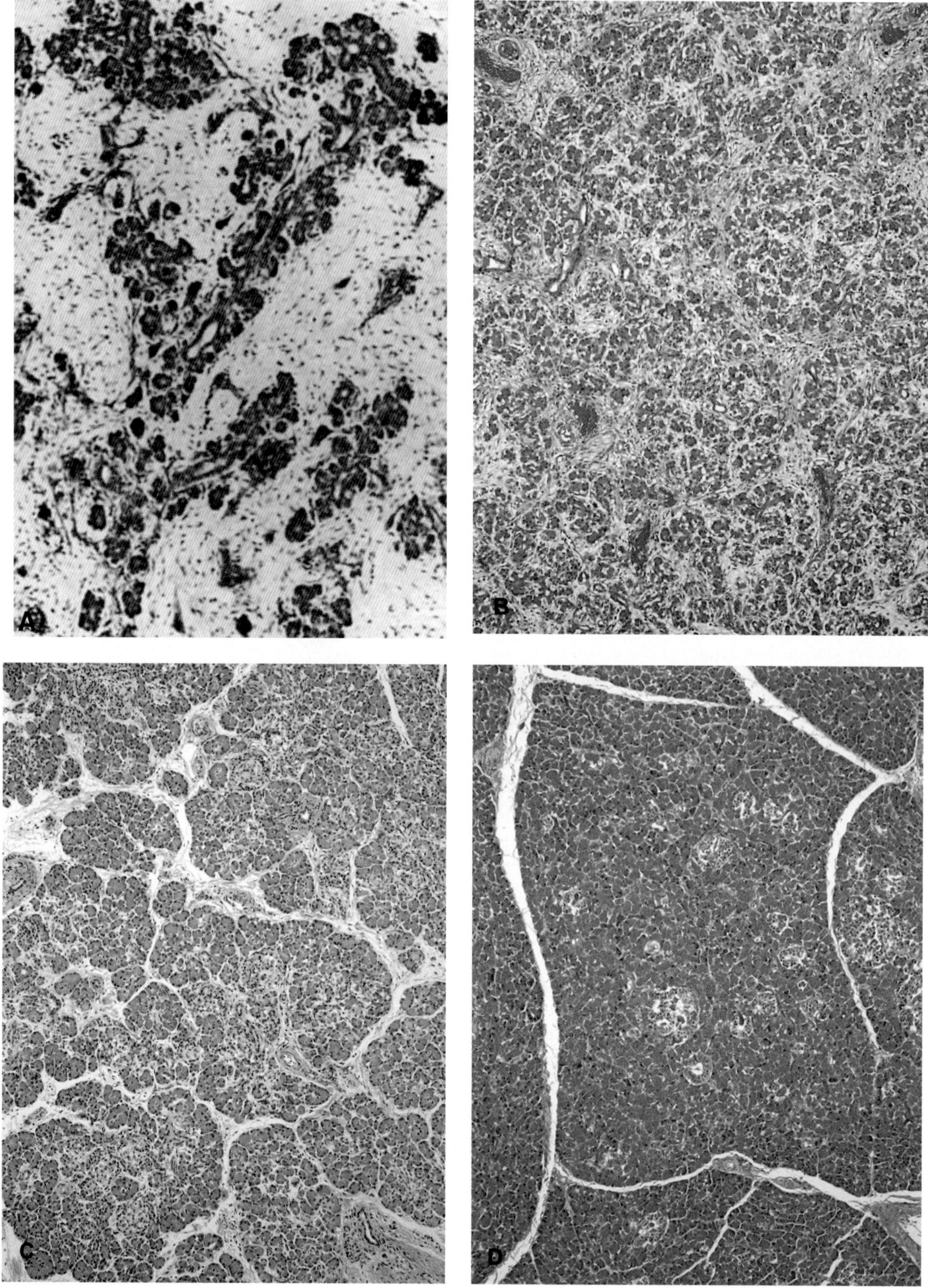

FIGURE 16-2 ■ Pancreatic development during gestation. **A:** At week 10 of gestation, the pancreas consists of rudimentary buds projecting from a central tube set in a loose mesenchymal stroma. Endocrine cells are already demonstrable. (Hematoxylin and eosin stain, original magnification ×155.) **B:** At week 17 of gestation, small lobules of acini and islets are visible. **C:** By week 40 of gestation (in a child who lived 1 day after birth), the endocrine elements lie centrally within the stalk of the lobule, and undeveloped acinar tissue is located peripherally. **D:** At the age of 22 months, the remarkable development of acinar tissue is obvious. (**B–D:** Hematoxylin and eosin stain, original magnification ×100.)

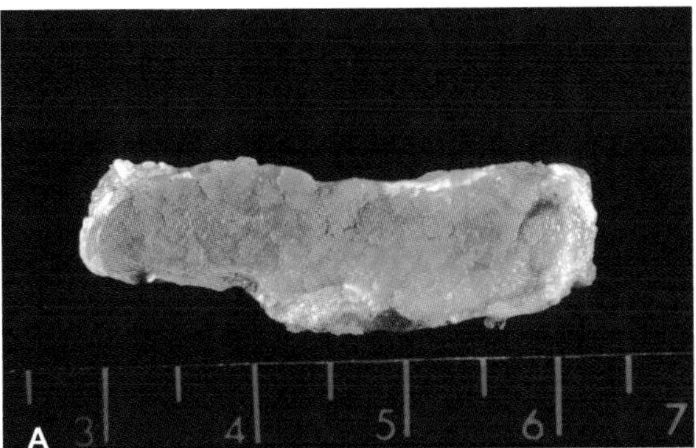

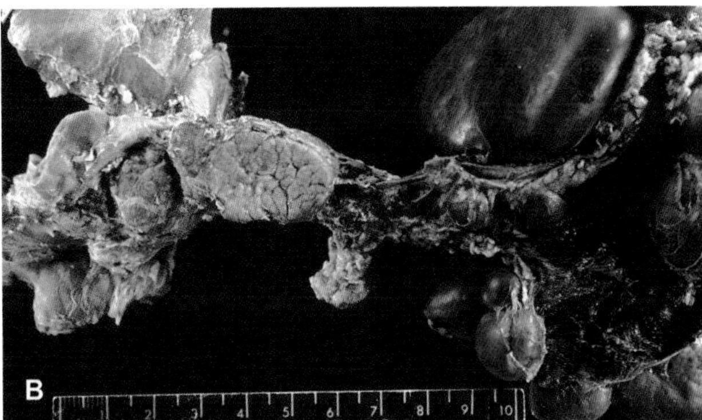

FIGURE 16-3▪Small pancreas. **A:** Hypoplastic pancreas (2.7 g, 3-cm long) from a 5-month-old child with probable tyrosinemia. **B:** Short pancreas (3-cm long) from a 2.5-year-old child with multiple spleens, intestinal malrotation, left bronchopulmonary isomerism, and extrahepatic biliary atresia.

agenesis is that of diabetes mellitus and malabsorption (185,e49,e155). Congenitally absent pancreas may be associated with diaphragmatic hernia (e138). Some infants have also lacked a gallbladder or intrahepatic bile ducts (e58,e242).

Functional pancreatic agenesis refers to organ failure without anatomic evidence of gland absence (e94). A functionally hypoplastic pancreas may be familial and can also lead to exocrine and endocrine insufficiency (e260). Severe pancreatic hypoplasia has been described in the Wolcott-Rallison syndrome (176).

Partial agenesis has been ascribed to failure of development of the dorsal or ventral primordium and may be familial (196,e94). More commonly, the pancreas is misshapen and described as short, stubby, or globular. These variants are not associated with hypofunction. Short pancreas may be an isolated finding, but it is seen with complex congenital heart disease and as part of a wider malformation complex that includes congenital heart disease, multiple spleens, and intestinal malrotation (e87). Figure 16-3 illustrates a short pancreas in association with syndromic extrahepatic biliary atresia. It has also been observed in the complete trisomy 22 syndrome (e50). Pancreatic anomalies, including agenesis, have been seen in some fetuses and infants with triploidy (e57).

Pancreatic Enlargement

Pancreatic weights are given in Appendix, Organ Weights. The noncystic pancreas is sometimes larger than usual or hyperplastic. Some infants with an enlarged pancreas have the Beckwith-Wiedemann syndrome (e224). Marked fatty replacement of the exocrine portion with preservation of the islets is found in the lipomatous pseudohypertrophy of the Shwachman-Diamond syndrome (66,81). Immune and nonimmune hydrops fetalis can lead to pancreatic enlargement through extramedullary hematopoiesis, and infiltration with leukemia can cause massive pancreatic enlargement (Figure 16-4). Down syndrome with congenital megakaryoblastic leukemia and pancreatic fibrosis has been

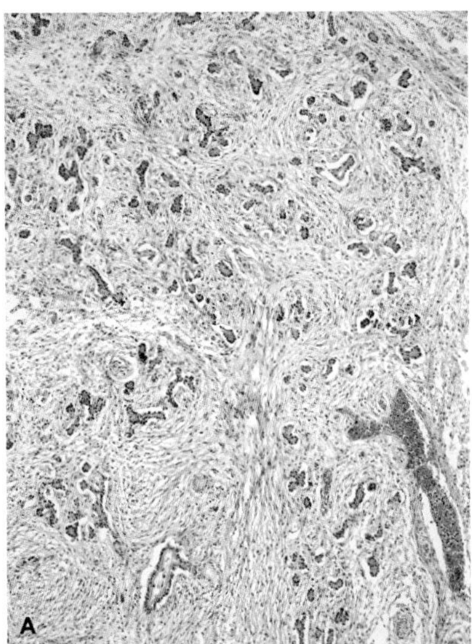

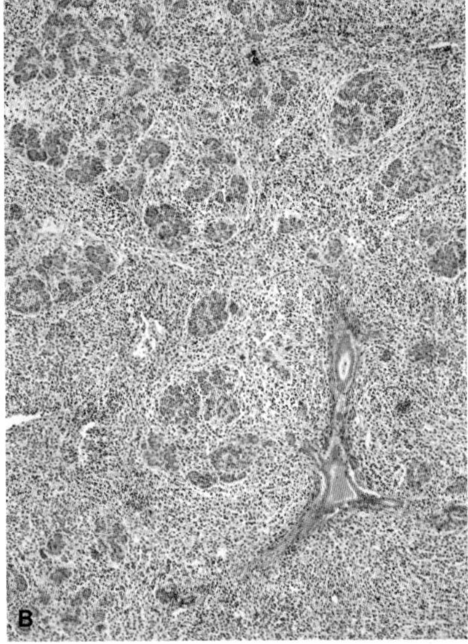

FIGURE 16-4▪Large pancreas. **A:** Congenital syphilis. An extensive, fine fibrosis distorts the pancreas. **B:** Congenital leukemia. Acinar elements are widely separated by the leukemic infiltrate, which is granulocytic in this instance. (**A,B:** Hematoxylin and eosin stain, original magnification ×100.)

reported (e19). In congenital syphilis, pancreatomegaly is a consequence of extensive interstitial fibrosis and inflammation (e178) (Figure 16-4).

Abnormalities of Position

The pancreas and the duodenum are retroperitoneal and separated from the posterior abdominal wall by an avascular plane. Abnormalities of fixation or position are often associated with left-sided diaphragmatic hernias. A "floating" pancreas on a mesentery, in the absence of a diaphragmatic hernia, has been reported (e117). Partial situs inversus with normal cardiac situs but inversion of the abdominal viscera, including the pancreas, has been seen with annular pancreas (e3).

Annular Pancreas

A ring of pancreatic tissue can encircle the second portion of the duodenum completely or partially (Figure 16-5). Johnston described two forms, extramural and intramural (e107). In the extramural form, a flattened band of normal pancreatic tissue can be separated from the duodenum. A duct originating anteriorly runs around the duodenum to join the main pancreatic duct. In the intramural form, ectopic pancreatic tissue is located within the duodenal wall, and small ducts drain directly into the duodenum. Duodenal obstruction is an associated malformation in this form of annular pancreas, not simply a mechanical constriction (e60). Several mechanisms have been proposed to explain the pathogenesis of the extramural form of annular pancreas. Two main hypotheses share the basis that the annular pancreas forms from the ventral anlage. The presence of large amounts of pancreatic polypeptide in islets of extramural annular pancreas supports this view (169,e215). Lecco postulated fixation of the tip of the single central ventral bud before rotation with subsequent persistence of the ventral lobe around the duodenum (e135), and this hypothesis is generally accepted. A recent report (e175), on the other hand, supports persistence and hypertrophy of the left portion of the paired ventral bud, suggested by Baldwin (e13).

As many as 20% of infants with annular pancreas are said to have trisomy 21 (104), and annular pancreas may be associated with cardiac defects or other intestinal malformations, such as tracheoesophageal fistula, Meckel diverticulum, absence of the gallbladder, and imperforate anus (e89,e116,e159,e200). Annular pancreas in a mother and three of her four children has been reported (e103), and the documentation of other familial instances (139,e41,e90,e146,e163) suggests an autosomal dominant inheritance or an involvement of an autosomal recessive sex-influenced gene (98).

Annular pancreas may present in the fetus with polyhydramnios or in the neonate with bile-stained vomiting if the constriction is below the ampulla. In older children and adults, annular pancreas may become symptomatic if duodenal ulceration or pancreatitis develops.

Ectopic Pancreas

Ectopic (heterotopic) pancreas is widely distributed, largely within the gastrointestinal tract. This condition has been discovered in 2% to 15% of all autopsies (97,147). Pancreatic tissue is most frequently found in the wall of the duodenum, jejunum, or stomach (e182). It is not unusual to find a nodule in the stomach consisting of a centrally ulcerated pit with localized thickening of the gastric wall (Figure 16-6).

Seifert (147) describes three types of ectopic pancreatic tissue. The first is similar to normal pancreas, with a full complement of acinar, ductal, and islet constituents. The second is characterized by incomplete lobular arrangement, few acini, many ducts, and an absence of endocrine elements. In the third type of ectopic pancreas, only proliferating ducts are present, without acinar or endocrine elements. This form is usually interpreted as an "adenomyoma" or "myoepithelial hamartoma" of the bowel wall (144). Immunohistochemistry of islet tissue in heterotopic pancreas has demonstrated a normal distribution of all cell types (e85).

Pancreatic tissue can be seen in the hilum of the liver or within the liver substance (e160). Although on occasion

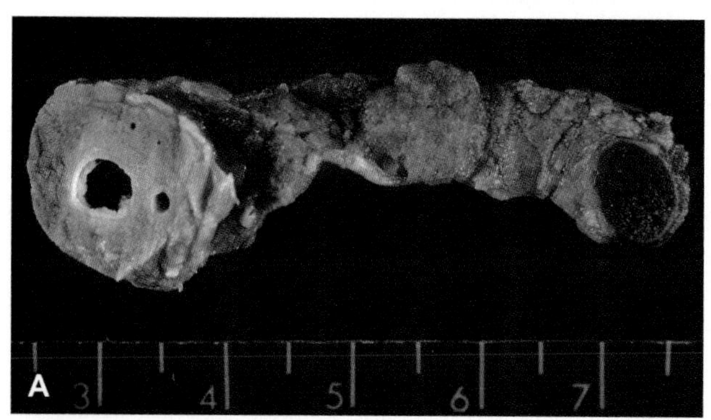

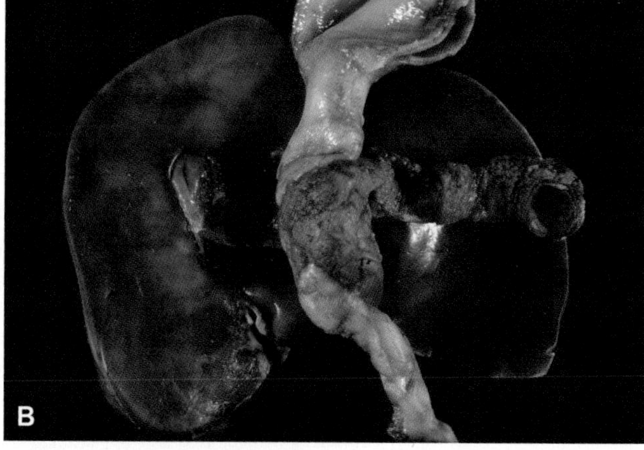

FIGURE 16-5 ■ Annular pancreas. **A,B:** An annular pancreas completely surrounds the second portion of the duodenum. An accessory spleen is present within the tail of the pancreas (trisomy 6).

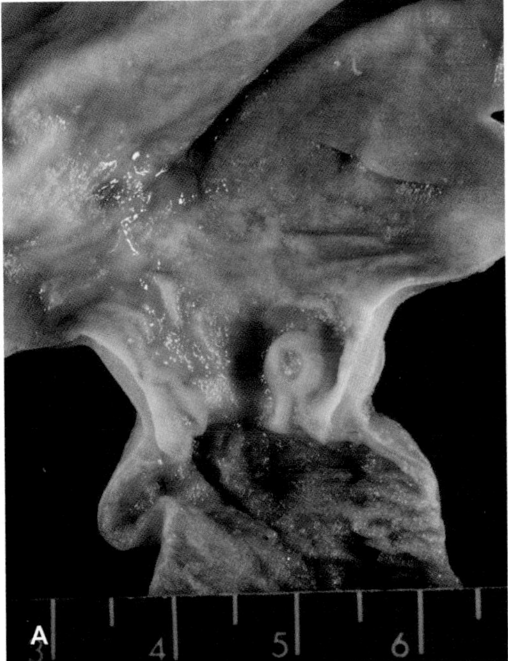

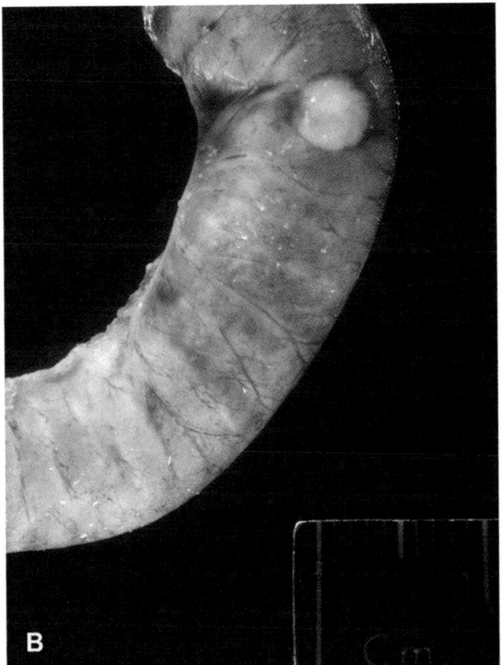

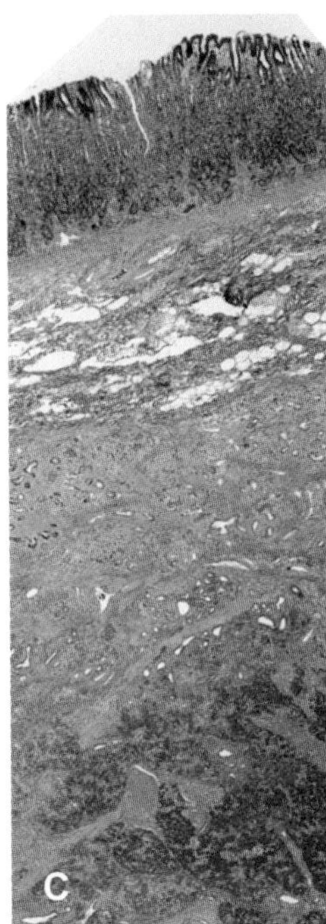

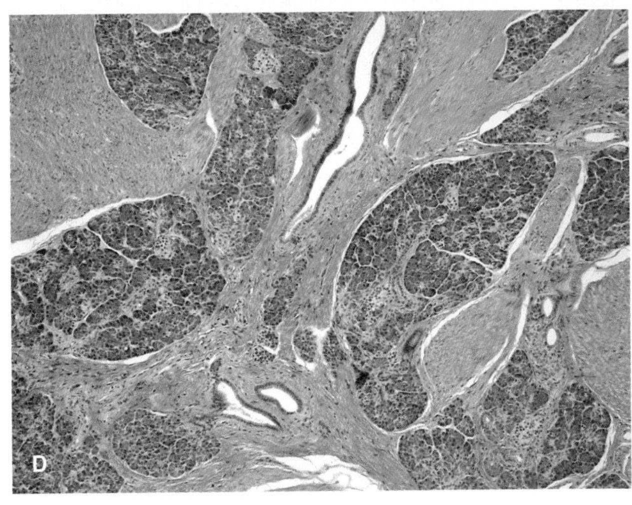

FIGURE 16-6 ■ Ectopic pancreas. **A:** Umbilicated mucosal nodule of the pyloric area. **B:** A jejunal subserosal nodule. **C:** An ectopic intramural (gastric) pancreas has ducts, exocrine acini, and endocrine component. **D:** Higher magnification of **C.** Islands of pancreatic tissue are separated by smooth muscle bundles. (**C,D:** Hematoxylin and eosin stain, original magnification, ×25 and ×100, respectively.)

a metaplastic process has been suggested for microscopic focus of exocrine pancreatic tissue in a posthepatitic cirrhotic liver (e264), it is unlikely to be metaplastic when endocrine cells are seen. Pancreas has also been described in the omentum, mesentery, Meckel diverticulum, vitelline duct, and umbilicus (e258). Ectopic pancreas has been associated with duplication cysts of the gut and has been reported in fallopian tubes, abdominal lymph nodes, and adjacent to the thyroid (99,e36,e167,e225). Intrasplenic islands of pancreas are found in trisomy 13–15 syndrome (59). Although heterotopic pancreas is often an incidental finding, it may present clinically as peptic ulceration, massive hemorrhage, biliary obstruction, cholecystitis, pyloric obstruction, intestinal obstruction, intussusception, or cystic degeneration (12). Hyperinsulinism (HI) associated with islet cell adenomatous hyperplasia in the ectopic pancreas has been described (129,195,e193). Rarely, it may present with neoplastic transformation (57). Solid-pseudopapillary neoplasms have been identified in ectopic pancreas (75,e61).

Jaffe et al. (e104) indicated that mediastinal pancreatic pseudocysts often arise from below the diaphragm, but isolated mediastinal pancreatic pseudocysts do exist (e258). Examination of intrapulmonary enteric cysts has revealed pancreatic elements (e44).

Pancreatic Cysts and Cystic Pancreatic Dysplasia

Congenital cysts of the pancreas are usually incidental findings and are rarely symptomatic (32). Simple epithelium-lined cysts may be solitary and unassociated with cystic diseases of other organs or complex malformation syndromes, but a review of older cases reveals that underlying disorders were probably present, such as a trisomy or

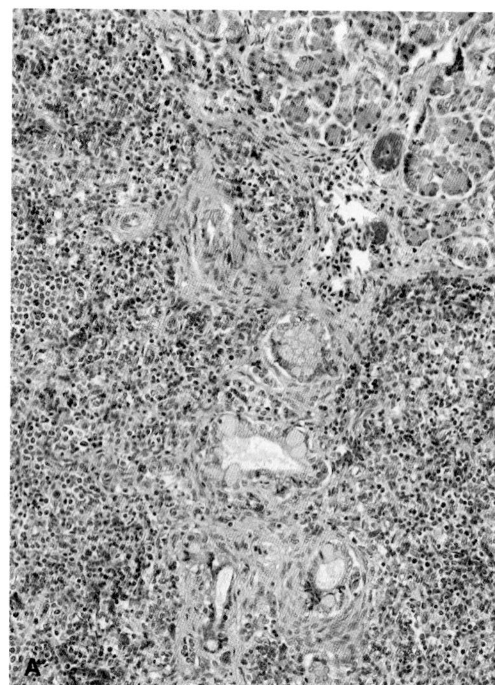

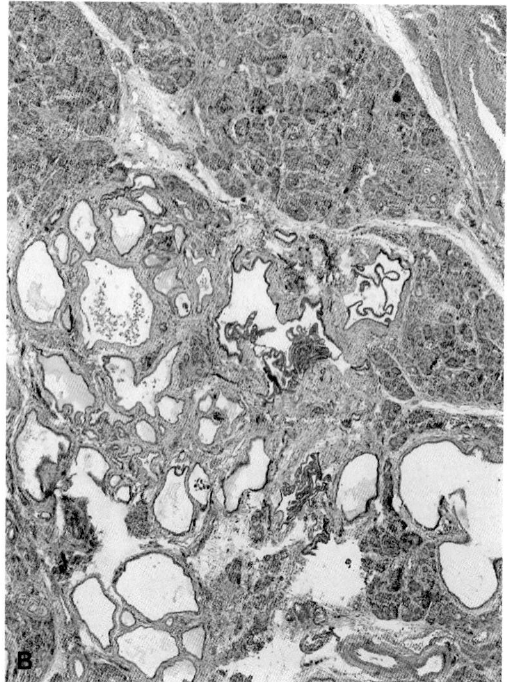

FIGURE 16-7 ■ Trisomies. **A:** Trisomy 13. Poorly circumscribed areas of splenic stroma extend into the pancreas, entrapping pancreatic ducts with mucoid lining cells. (Hematoxylin and eosin stain, original magnification ×200.) **B:** Trisomy 18. Numerous pancreatic cysts lined by duct-type epithelium are scattered. (Hematoxylin and eosin stain with immunohistochemistry for neuron-specific enolase, original magnification ×50.)

tuberous sclerosis (59,88,e149,e177,e190) (Figures 16-7 and 16-8; eFigure 16-1). Dermoid cysts have been described in children (e11). The abnormal pancreas of Beckwith-Wiedemann syndrome may contain cysts (162,e68) (Figure 16-8). Lymphatic malformation (184) (Figure 16-9) and intestinal duplications that communicate with the ductal system of the pancreas may present as "pancreatic cysts" (e7,e26,e225).

Polycystic kidney disease, of the autosomal dominant or recessive type, may involve the pancreatic ductal system, but pancreatic involvement appears to be uncommon. Potter and Craig (e188) noted pancreatic cysts in only 2 of 370 cases. Pancreatic cysts are seen in the Meckel-Gruber syndrome (e199,e212) (eFigure 16-1).

Ivemark et al. (e100) and others (178,e45) have described a familial form of renal, hepatic, and pancreatic cystic dysplasia, which is now generally included under the rubric of polycystic kidney and hepatic disease-1 (PKHD-1). Of all the reported cases, only 50% are familial, and the condition is associated with anomalies in other organ systems (100). Bernstein et al. (e23) emphasized that the triad is not unique but also occurs in trisomy 9, Meckel-Gruber syndrome, Jeune syndrome, Saldino-Noonan syndrome, Elejalde syndrome, and glutaric aciduria type II, all of which must be excluded first (e232,e270). Severe cystic involvement of the pancreas may occur in von Hippel-Lindau disease, and polycystic pancreas can be the main or only manifestation of von Hippel-Lindau disease in young patients who have no prior history of pancreatic disease (51,e99). Minor cystic dysplastic changes are sometimes present in tuberous sclerosis.

Two reports have been published of microcystic cystadenomas of the head of the pancreas in children with disseminated cytomegalovirus infection (e9,e37). The cystic dilation appears to be secondary to obstruction.

Cystic fibrosis in the older child can be associated with large, single or multilocular cysts (20,e39,e244). The pancreatic pseudocyst, caused by rupture of a duct into the lesser sac or abdominal cavity, consists of a fibrous inflammatory wall around an autodigested cavity. The entity is usually caused by trauma, surgery, or inflammation (pancreatitis). The fibrous wall of the cyst has no epithelial lining.

Variations in the Pancreatic Ducts

After the dorsal and the ventral pancreatic anlage fuse, the dorsal duct becomes the accessory duct of Santorini, and the ventral duct becomes the main draining duct of the pancreas, the duct of Wirsung. The fusion can occur at a single point proximally or at two points, both proximally and more distally (170). The normal architecture varies widely. The dorsal duct may regress completely, or the dorsal and ventral ducts may not communicate at all (pancreas divisum) (e21).

In pancreas divisum, the pancreas is separated into two portions. The pancreatic ducts fail to fuse, and the dorsal duct of Santorini drains most of the gland through

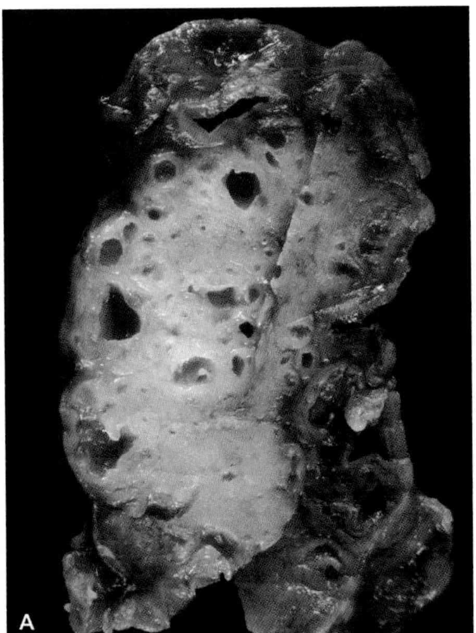

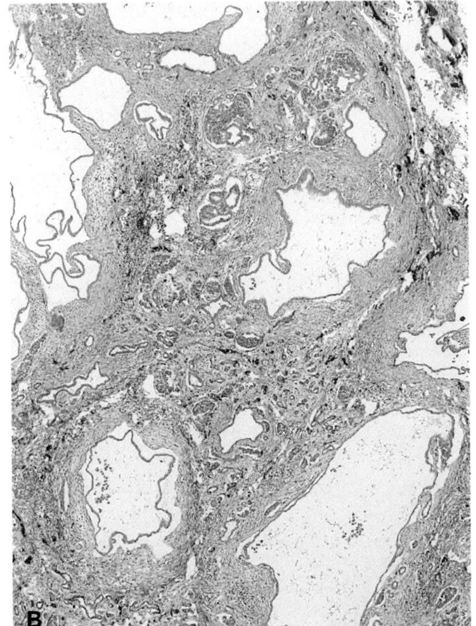

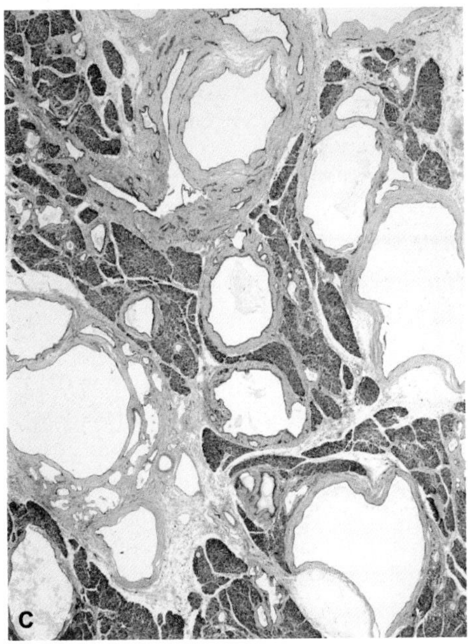

FIGURE 16-8 ■ Pancreatic cysts. **A:** A large pancreas (120 g) presented as an abdominal mass in a newborn baby with Beckwith-Wiedemann syndrome. Multiple cystic spaces are seen on cut surfaces. (Color version of Copyright 1990 from Beckwith-Wiedemann syndrome with unusual hepatic and pancreatic features: A case expanding the phenotype by Steigman CK, Uri AK, Chatten J, et al. *Pediatr Pathol* 1990;10:593. Reproduced with permission of Taylor & Francis Group, LLC., http://www.taylorandfrancis.com) **B:** Microphotograph of **A.** No normal pancreatic tissue is identified. Numerous ectatic ducts, clusters of endocrine cells, and few acini are in loose fibrous connective tissue. (Hematoxylin and eosin stain, original magnification ×50.) **C:** 15-year-old child with oral-facial-digital syndrome type I. Cystically dilated pancreatic ducts with periductal fibrosis (Hematoxylin and eosin, original magnification ×25.)

the minor papilla. The ventral duct of Wirsung drains only the smaller pancreatic remnant. Because of the recent advances in endoscopy, particularly endoscopic retrograde cholangiopancreatography, pancreas divisum is diagnosed with greater frequency (163,e236). Some investigators believe that pancreas divisum is clinically significant (e81), whereas others are more skeptical (40,e6,e236). The combination of acute pancreatitis and pancreas divisum is treated by endoscopic retrograde cholangiopancreatographic sphincteroplasty (133,e137).

The anatomy of the pancreaticobiliary junction varies noticeably (e234). The pancreatic duct can join the common bile duct within the duodenal wall, or it can enter the duodenum separately. The common channel can be short or long. If it is longer than 2 cm, the ducts join outside the duodenal wall, and this construction has been implicated in the pathogenesis of choledochal cyst (e265).

Stenosis of the ampulla may present with pancreatitis, but in the newborn it more commonly manifests as bile duct perforation (e52).

Pancreatic Pathology in Trisomies

Lesions of the pancreas characteristic of trisomy 13 were illustrated long before the chromosomal defect was identified (e212). Hashida et al. (59) demonstrated the multiple, poorly demarcated aggregates of splenic tissue in the tail and the body of the pancreas (Figure 16-7). These splenic islands

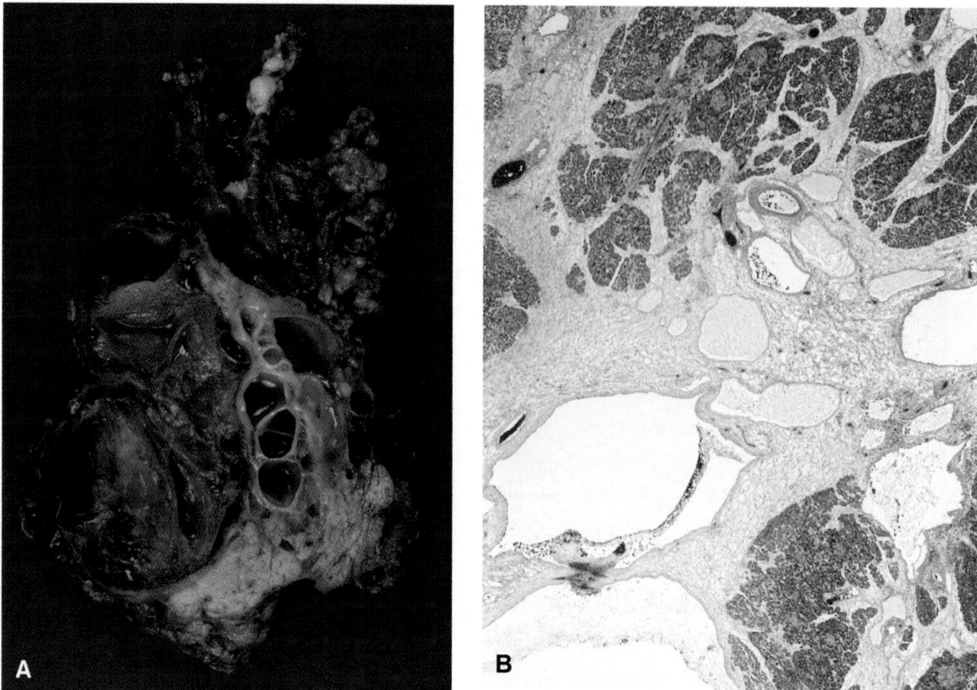

FIGURE 16-9 ■ Lymphatic malformation. **A:** Lymphatic malformation presented as a cystic pancreatic mass in a 12-year-old child. (Courtesy of Pierre Russo, M.D., Philadelphia, Pennsylvania.) **B:** Lymphatic channels of variable sizes are embedded within the pancreatic lobular septa and parenchyma. A small number of mononuclear cell infiltrates are present in the walls. (Hematoxylin and eosin stain, original magnification ×25.)

contain pancreatic acini, islets, and knots of ducts lined by tall columnar epithelium rich in goblet cells. Microcystic changes may be focal or quite widespread with inspissation, features that suggest a duct obstruction as the pathogenesis (e150). Ectopic splenic tissue in the gastric fundus and upper pole of the kidney has contained pancreatic elements (e166).

The pancreas in trisomy 18 often exhibits lobular fibrosis (59) and focal fibrotic nodules in which clusters of ducts and atrophic acini are found (e204). An area of cystadenomatous changes with back-to-back cysts is seen less frequently (Figure 16-7). These cysts along with inflammatory aggregates suggest an obstructive etiology (59).

Annular pancreas may occur in as many as 8% of infants with trisomy 21 (e159). A short pancreas has been described in trisomy 22, and pancreatic anomalies, including agenesis, are described in infants with triploidy (e57). Marked enlargement of the somatostatin-producing D cells has been reported in the pancreas of triploid fetuses (141).

EXOCRINE PANCREAS

Functional Development

Proteolytic activity is demonstrable in pancreatic homogenates from 500-g fetuses, and the levels of trypsin, chymotrypsin, and lipases increase during intrauterine life, accelerating before term (e141). Fetal mRNA levels of trypsinogen and lipase are much lower than adult levels (118). The presence of these enzymes suggests that the fetus can use swallowed amniotic fluid for nutritional purposes (e247). Secretory trypsin inhibitors are demonstrable in the fetal pancreas and in the gastrointestinal, urinary, and respiratory tracts by week 10 of gestation (e70).

Amylase is absent in the fetal pancreas, and salivary amylase predominates in amniotic fluid (e176,e247). Although trypsin and chymotrypsin levels are near normal adult levels by birth, lipase and, in particular, amylase levels in the intestinal tract remain low and increase slowly during the first year of life (103).

Zymogen granules are first evident in the developing pancreas by week 12 as elliptic and round structures (e132). By week 20 of gestation, basal round granules predominate, and the complex basolateral cell interdigitations are established (103) (eFigure 16-2). Developing ductal cells are filled with glycogen during the first 20 weeks of gestation, after which the glycogen disappears, first from the larger ducts and then from progressively smaller ones. Pancreatic secretion is influenced largely by neural cholinergic stimulation, cholecystokinin, pancreozymin, and secretin. In the adult, pancreozymin is responsible for pancreatic enzyme release, and secretin promotes fluid and electrolyte release. Lebenthal et al. (102,103) demonstrated that the pancreas of a neonate is unresponsive to exogenous cholecystokinin or secretin earlier before 1 month of age and not fully responsive before 2 years of age. The functional aspects of the developing pancreas, with particular reference to the perinatal period, have been summarized by Lee and Lebenthal (103).

Abnormalities of the Exocrine Pancreas Without Fibrosis

Isolated Enzyme Deficiencies

Trypsinogen deficiency is rare. It is characterized by malabsorption, growth failure, anemia, and hypoproteinemia, beginning in the neonatal period (e245,e246). An association with imperforate anus suggests that these cases are actually instances of Johanson-Blizzard or Shwachman-Diamond syndrome (50). Congenital enterokinase deficiency may mimic cystic fibrosis in that the infants fail to thrive and have diarrhea, hypoproteinemia, and edema (102). Isolated congenital lipase deficiency presents with severe steatorrhea soon after birth without failure to thrive or anemia; nonpancreatic lipases, such as lingual lipase, may be effective in preventing fatty acid deficiency (e64). Because the maturation of amylase production is normally delayed, alleged cases of isolated amylase deficiency are controversial (111). Lerner et al. (e139) established criteria that must be satisfied to document amylase deficiency. The pancreatic morphology is not described in the cases of isolated enzyme deficiency, although Townes (e245) described the pancreas of the sibling of a child with trypsinogen deficiency as having "immature acini," and zymogen granules were not observed.

Exocrine Atrophy Without Fibrosis

Exocrine atrophy is also called *lipomatous atrophy* or *lipomatous pseudohypertrophy* because the shape of the gland is preserved but the acinar component is replaced by fat (66,e213). This appearance may be common to a number of pathologic processes.

Shwachman-Diamond Syndrome

With an incidence estimated at 1 in 200,000 births, the Shwachman-Diamond syndrome is the most common cause of pancreatic insufficiency after cystic fibrosis. The clinical condition is described in a number of reports (14,e56,e145,e173,e213). Pancreatic exocrine insufficiency is accompanied by growth retardation, short stature, bone marrow depression with neutropenia, and skeletal changes, predominantly metaphyseal dysostosis.

Cases with anal atresia, Hirschsprung disease, and possibly asphyxiating thoracic dystrophy have been described (e34,e111,e145,e246). The marrow dysfunction, neutropenia in most instances, may be fixed or cyclical and is associated with the development of myelodysplasia and later leukemias, usually acute myelogenous leukemia (156,e5,e173,e267). The pancreatic insufficiency is invariable, may be profound, and appears shortly after birth; less often, it is mild and improves and normalizes with age in about half the patients (14,e91,e145).

Bodian et al. (14) and Shwachman et al. (153) reviewed the cases for which histologic evidence of pancreatic disease was obtained. Biopsies were occasionally performed. Postmortem reports on older children indicated that replacement of the bulk of the pancreas by fatty tissue gives the

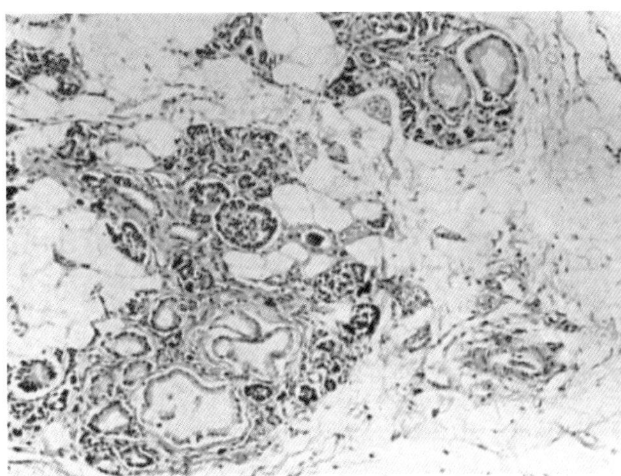

FIGURE 16-10■Exocrine atrophy in Shwachman-Diamond syndrome. The acinar elements are almost completely replaced by fat (lipomatous pseudohypertrophy), with only small aggregates of endocrine tissue left around ducts. (Hematoxylin and eosin stain, original magnification ×120.)

appearance of a lipomatous pseudohypertrophy (66). Acinar tissue is absent, without scarring or fibrosis, and the pancreatic ducts and endocrine elements are preserved (Figure 16-10). The characteristic lipomatous pancreas can be demonstrated by magnetic resonance imaging (e129).

Shwachman-Diamond syndrome is an autosomal recessive disorder, and the genetic basis has recently been reported (15). The gene involved (*SBDS*) is an uncharacterized gene, and resides at 7q11. Its 1.6-kb transcript encodes a predicted protein of 250 amino acids. A pseudogene copy (*SBDSP*) with 97% nucleotide sequence identity is in a locally duplicated genomic segment. Recurring mutations resulting from gene conversion (substitution of genetic material from another gene) were found in 89% of unrelated individuals of Shwachman-Diamond syndrome. The converted segments include pseudogene-like sequence changes that result in protein truncation. In a study including 23 unrelated patients, molecular genetic and hematologic evaluations demonstrated a poor genotype/phenotype correlation (e128).

Johanson-Blizzard Syndrome

First reported in 1971 (79), the Johanson-Blizzard syndrome comprises congenital aplasia of the ala nasi, deafness, hypothyroidism, dwarfism, absence of permanent teeth, and malabsorption resulting from pancreatic insufficiency. Subsequent reports described urogenital abnormalities (e180) and imperforate anus (50) associated with this syndrome. Postmortem examination reveals a total absence of acini with complete replacement of the pancreas by adipose tissue and a few remaining islets with connective tissue around the ducts (31,e79,e161). Mutations in the gene *UBR1* have been recently detected in affected individuals from 12 of 13 families (197). *UBR1* encodes one of E3 ubiquitin ligases of the N-end rule pathway, a conserved proteolytic system. The UBR1 protein substrate, presumably impaired degradation of which causes Johanson-Blizzard syndrome, is not yet known.

Immunofluorescence pattern for trypsinogen indicated that there was no primary defect of zymogen synthesis. Hypoplasia of the exocrine pancreas in association with facial anomalies, micrognathia, posterior cleft palate, and dental hypoplasia has been referred to as the *Donlan syndrome* (e53), but overlap with the Johanson-Blizzard syndrome seems likely (e84).

Other Abnormalities

Pancreatic acinar replacement by fat was observed in a 13-month-old girl with clinical features of leprechaunism, developmental delay, and abnormalities of gonadotropin regulation (e238). The pancreas contained multiple islets and ductules embedded in a matrix of adipose tissue but without acinar tissue. The morphology resembled that of children with the Shwachman-Diamond or Johanson-Blizzard syndrome, but no other features of these syndromes were present.

Abnormalities of the Exocrine Pancreas with Fibrosis

Sideroblastic Anemia and Exocrine Pancreatic Insufficiency: Pearson Syndrome

Pearson et al. (128) described a syndrome characterized by pancreatic insufficiency, refractory sideroblastic anemia, and variable neutropenia in which the marrow is normocellular but the cells are vacuolated.

Rötig et al. (e207) documented changes in the mitochondrial DNA, and a number of mitochondrial deletions have since been reported. Morikawa et al. (117) described a neonate with Pearson syndrome and diabetes mellitus and postulated a connection with Kearns-Sayre syndrome. The features of Kearns-Sayre syndrome, a mitochondrial myopathy, may develop later in life in patients who survive the early manifestations of Pearson syndrome (e134,e154). The most common deletion involves 4,977 base pairs of mitochondrial DNA, and Pearson syndrome can be diagnosed by blood tests from Guthrie cards (179).

The pancreatic pathologic features differ from those of the Shwachman-Diamond or Johanson-Blizzard syndrome in that acinar atrophy with fibrosis, not lipomatosis, is present (117,128).

Neonatal Hemochromatosis

Acinar deposition of iron in adult primary hemochromatosis is associated with interlobular and intralobular fibrosis (168). In neonatal hemochromatosis, hemosiderin deposition in the pancreatic acini is massive, although fibrosis is mild, and the islets are generally spared, at least in the early stages (e27,e77,e122,e221) (Figure 16-11). Acinar iron deposition in the absence of reticuloendothelial iron deposition is not pathognomonic of primary hemochromatosis; it was also seen in some control cases (154). Two sibs with a neonatal hemochromatosis phenotype that included pancreatic iron deposition also had hypertelorism and trichomalacia, a trichohepatoenteric syndrome (183).

Cystic Fibrosis

Fanconi et al. (45) and then Anderson (e10), while investigating causes of malabsorption, discovered in some of their patients a condition they termed *cystic fibrosis of the pancreas*. Recognition of the pancreatic lesion preceded the clinical delineation of the disease. Farber (e63) proposed mucous plugging of all secretory glands (mucoviscidosis) to be the pathogenetic key.

Cystic fibrosis is caused by defects in the cystic fibrosis conductance regulator gene (*CFTR*), localized to 7q31.2 (138,e114,e205). Pancreatic insufficiency is not obligatory, and 15% of patients are clinically pancreas "sufficient." The degree of pancreatic disease varies widely at any age, although the disease is progressive and leads to increasingly more severe changes with time. The final stage of cystic fibrosis is characterized by an obstruction of the pancreatic ducts by viscous secretion leading to complete acinar atrophy accompanied by fibrosis and lipomatosis (125,e56,e233).

The tissue alteration can be recognized even before 40 weeks of gestation (74,e233,e237). The ratio of acinar to connective tissue volume is 0.5 at 32 weeks after conception,

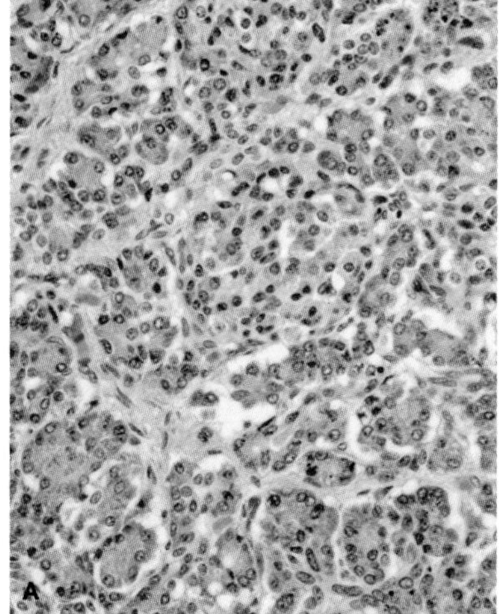

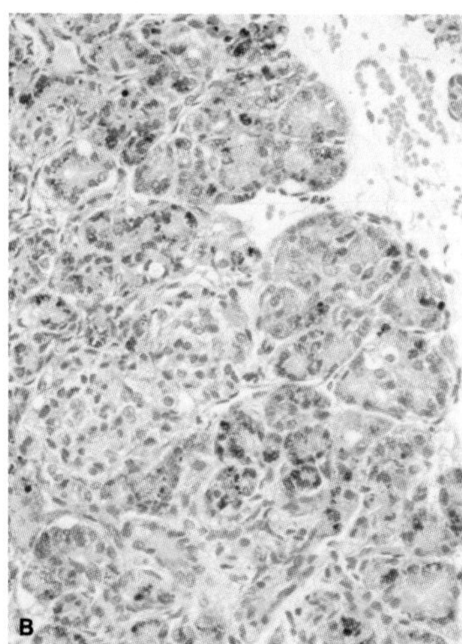

FIGURE 16-11 ■ Neonatal hemochromatosis. **A:** Exocrine acinar cells contain brown refractile pigment. (Hematoxylin and eosin stain, original magnification ×400.) **B:** The islets are devoid of iron, but acinar lobules have a marked intracytoplasmic iron deposition. (Prussian blue stain, original magnification ×400.)

increasing to 2.0 at 52 weeks in normal controls (74). In the cystic fibrosis pancreas, the ratio of acinar to connective tissue, low to begin with, decreases from 0.5 at 35 weeks to 0.3 at 52 weeks after conception. Further degeneration of exocrine tissue supervenes postnatally.

The earliest visible lesions are eosinophilic concretions in acini and ductules, which may lead to acinar or ductular dilation and flattening of the lining epithelium (125). These concretions generally stain with periodic acid–Schiff (PAS) and contain calcium. The changes may be focal in preterm infants and in mildly affected cases. Postnatal acceleration of the pathogenetic train of inspissation, obstruction, dilation, epithelial damage, atrophy, cell destruction, and fibrosis with minimal inflammation leads to progressive acinar loss with replacement by fibrous tissue (Figure 16-12; eFigure 16-3) and adipose tissue.

Even though acinar tissue may disappear, islet tissue is preserved until very late. The endocrine changes in cystic fibrosis are considered later in this chapter, and the appearance of large cysts in cystic fibrosis has already been discussed (e39).

Inspissation and Other Changes of Pancreatic Ducts

Baggenstoss (e12) described the widespread inspissation of secretions in centroacinar cell-lined ductules in patients with uremia. The finding is not restricted to uremia but is also seen in children dying with acidosis, dehydration, cardiac failure, or sepsis (e212). Inspissation may also be seen in the pancreas of children who have experienced prolonged hyperalimentation, but they usually have many of the other conditions listed.

Striking oncocytic changes of the ducts and centroacinar cells have been observed in an infant with mitochondrial myopathy, lactic acidosis, and "ragged red" muscle fibers (MELAR syndrome). Centroacinar hyperplasia of an impressive degree was observed in a young adult with HIV infection (eFigure 16-4).

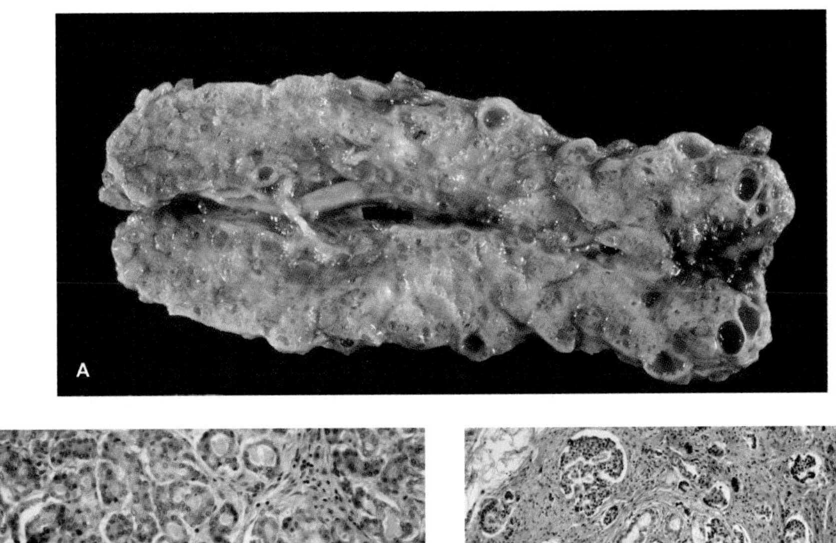

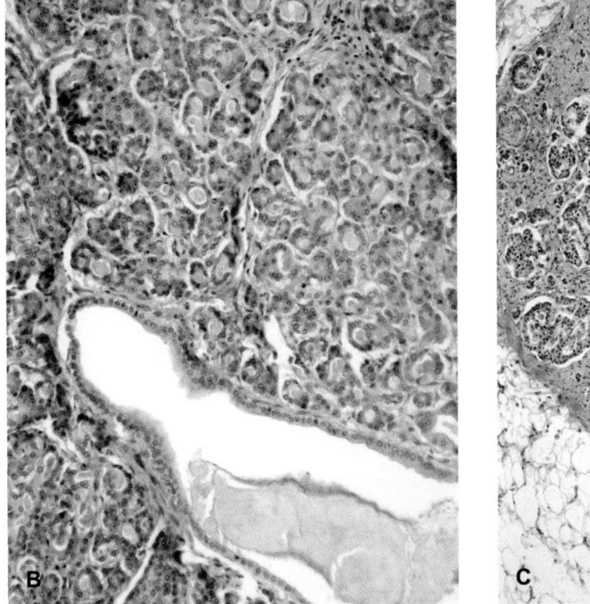

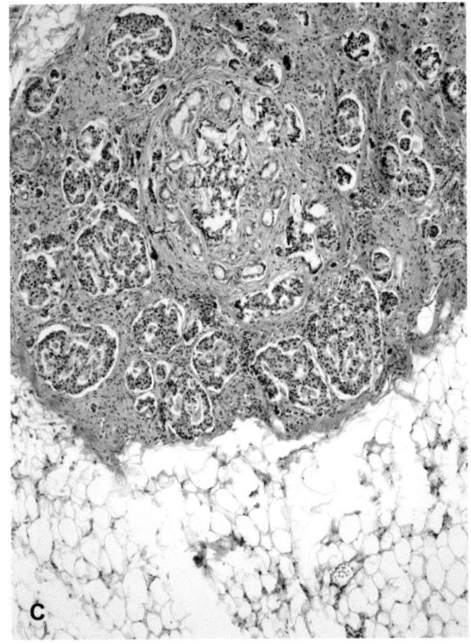

FIGURE 16-12■Cystic fibrosis. **A:** The pancreas of this 12-year-old child is lipomatous with scattered cysts. **B:** An 8-year-old child with a strong family history of cystic fibrosis was asymptomatic and, at autopsy, had only cystic dilation with inspissation of ducts, and acini with minimal fibrosis. (Hematoxylin and eosin stain, original magnification ×200.) **C:** A 10-year-old child with advanced acinar atrophy and fatty replacement has periductal endocrine overgrowth. (Hematoxylin and eosin stain, original magnification ×100.)

Pancreatitis in Childhood

In contrast to pancreatitis in adulthood frequently related to alcohol intake, the common causes of pancreatitis in children are trauma, multisystemic diseases, drug induced, infections, and biliary tract diseases while what are included in the "multisystem" category vary among the studies (36,188,e144,e254). Pancreatitis can also be seen in children with branched-chain organic acidemias, methylmalonic acidemia, isovaleric acidemia, maple syrup urine disease (83), and the Pearson syndrome. When all causes are excluded and the etiology remains undetermined, the pancreatitis has been traditionally labeled *idiopathic*. This group accounts for 8% to 34%, and leads the "cause" of childhood pancreatitis in some series (36,e254). Except for patients with cystic fibrosis, hereditary pancreatitis, and pancreatitis secondary to congenital structural or metabolic abnormalities, most children have a single, self-limited episode of pancreatitis, and few cases progress to chronicity (188). On the other hand, children with recurrent or so-called idiopathic chronic pancreatitis may possess mutations and sequence variations in modifier genes (8) as discussed below.

Acute pancreatitis of any cause varies from interstitial edema to necrotizing hemorrhagic inflammation depending on the severity and time point of the process. Fat necrosis is the characteristic finding, and results from sequential reactions including release of fatty acids from triglyceride esters by lipase and combination of the fatty acids with calcium (saponification). The formed insoluble salts produce grossly visible chalky white to yellow areas. Microscopically, outlines of degenerated fat cells with basophilic calcium deposits are seen along with acute inflammatory infiltrate (Figure 16-13).

Recurrent pancreatitis and chronic pancreatitis produce fibroinflammatory changes of the parenchyma (94). The pancreas shows extensive fibrosis, acinar atrophy characterized by reduced number and size of acini, and variable dilatation of the ducts with calcification (Figure 16-14). The endocrine islets are generally relatively spared and embedded in the fibrotic tissue. They may appear fused and enlarged, but in end-stage diseases, they eventually disappear.

Traumatic Pancreatitis

Blunt trauma is recognized as a cause of immediate or delayed pancreatitis in children (Figure 16-13) and an important cause of pancreatic pseudocyst. A pancreatic pseudocyst may occur as the result of child abuse, but bicycle injuries are the most common cause in children (e18,e28).

Infectious Pancreatitis

The pancreas may be the seat of any disseminated infection, such as herpes simplex, cytomegalovirus infection (Figure 16-13), or bacterial sepsis, but it is unusual to encounter clinically relevant pancreatitis (78). In some instances, the late consequences of a previous infectious pancreatitis are serious.

Rubella may cause an interstitial pancreatitis as part of the expanded rubella syndrome, and pancreatic insufficiency or even diabetes mellitus can ensue (e33,e55,e105). Mumps is a classic cause of pancreatitis in late childhood (e220). Coxsackievirus may selectively involve the exocrine or

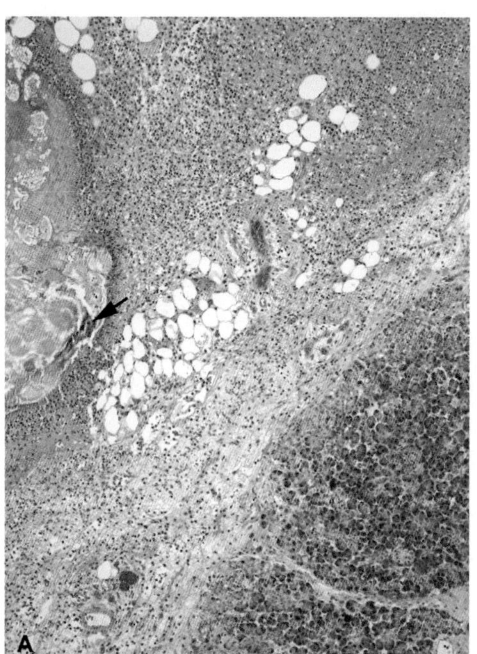

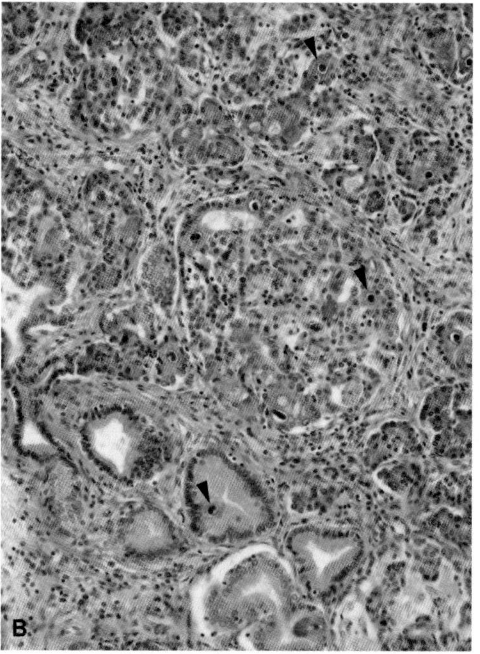

FIGURE 16-13■Acute pancreatitis. **A:** Traumatic pancreatitis in a 7-year-old child showing fat necrosis with saponification (*arrow*) and acute inflammatory infiltrate. (Hematoxylin and eosin stain, original magnification ×100.) **B:** Cytomegalovirus pancreatitis with inclusions in acinar, ductal, and endocrine cells (*arrow heads*). (Hematoxylin and eosin stain, original magnification ×200; courtesy of James E. Dimmick, M.D., Vancouver, British Columbia.)

endocrine components of the pancreas (78). Parainfluenza 3 pancreatitis, confirmed by immunohistochemical labeling, produced multinucleated giant cells in the pancreas of a child with severe combined immunodeficiency (186). Chronic coxsackievirus B interstitial pancreatitis in the absence of a meningoencephalomyocarditis and acute pancreatitis in a child with α_1-antitrypsin deficiency have been reported (e113). In most cases of pancreatitis in children with acquired immunodeficiency syndrome (AIDS), the disease is mild and opportunistic infections are absent, although nonspecific inflammatory changes such as focal lymphoplasmacytic aggregates are common (85); in one child with AIDS and clinical malabsorption, chronic pancreatitis was noted at autopsy without an identified opportunistic organism (e243). *Escherichia coli* pancreatitis usually accompanies septicemia, and congenital syphilis usually causes a pancreatitis in which ductular obliteration, acinar loss, and exuberant interstitial fibrosis with concentric perivascular accentuation are noted (e27,e69,e178) (Figure 16-4). Gummas are rare (e194).

Inflammatory Pancreatitis

Pancreatitis can accompany childhood collagen vascular diseases, such as lupus, but it may be hard to distinguish between the effects of disease and those of treatment, particularly drugs (155). Pancreatitis has been described in Henoch-Schönlein purpura, Reye syndrome, hemolytic-uremic syndrome, and Crohn disease (e30,e74,e127,e211).

Immunodysregulation, polyendocrinopathy, enteropathy, X-linked syndrome (IPEX) is a rare X-linked recessive disorder of immune regulation manifesting with neonatal onset diabetes mellitus, severe enteropathy, eczema, anemia, thrombocytopenia, and hypothyroidism. The disorder had been known by alternative names including X-linked polyendocrinopathy, immune dysfunction, and diarrhea and X-linked autoimmunity and allergic dysregulation. A mutant mouse strain, scurfy (*sf*) resembles IPEX (e76), and the disease-causing gene *Foxp3* encoding scurfin was identified (e32). Subsequently, the human IPEX locus was mapped to Xp11.23-q13.3 (10), and mutations have been identified in the human orthologue (*JM2, FOXP3*) (22,e20,e257). Patients with protein-truncating mutations have been reported to demonstrate an absence of FOXP3-nuclear positive lymphocytes in their small and large intestines (61). Postmortem pancreatic histology is almost always abnormal. Findings include mild-to-dense lymphocytic infiltrate, acinar loss with fibrosis (chronic sclerosing pancreatitis), dilated ducts, and cystic changes (132,191,e168,e203) (Figure 16-14). Islets of endocrine cells are decreased or absent in most cases with severe diabetes mellitus (105,e108,e203).

Obstructive Pancreatitis

Some of the causes of obstructive pancreatitis in children have already been mentioned in the section on congenital malformations, such as annular pancreas, pancreas divisum, gastric duplications that connect to the pancreatic duct system, and anomalies of the pancreaticobiliary junction (e7). Gallstone pancreatitis in children occurs only in the presence of a predisposing condition, such as myelomeningocele or hyperalimentation (e8). Cystic fibrosis is the prototype of a chronic obstructive pancreatitis.

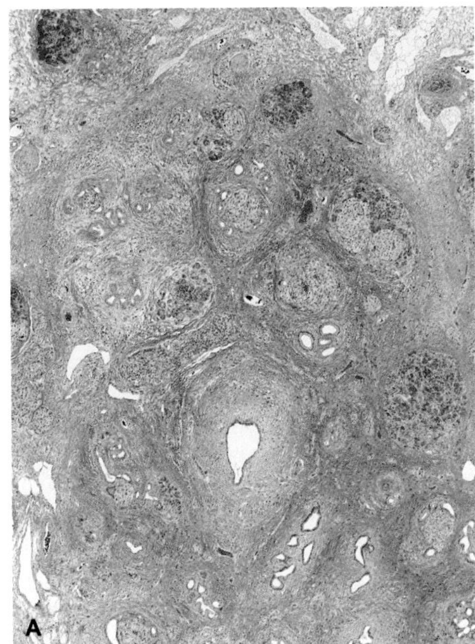

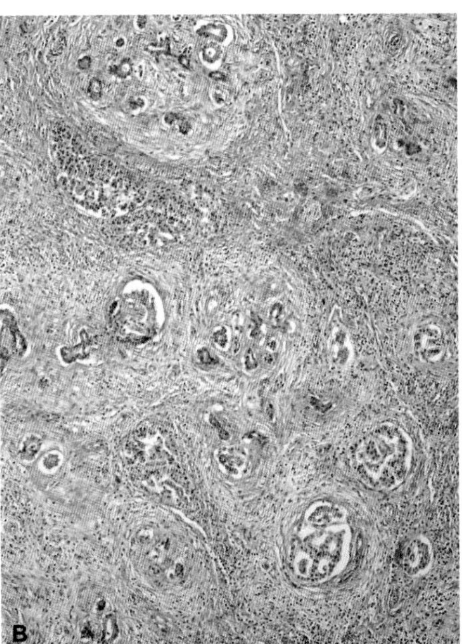

FIGURE 16-14 ■ Chronic pancreatitis. **A:** Obstructive pancreatitis with fibrosis, duct ectasia, acinar atrophy, and relative abundance of endocrine islets. Several pancreatic stones were also recovered. (Hematoxylin and eosin stain, original magnification ×50) **B:** Pancreas of a 79-day-old infant (born at 30 weeks of gestation) with immunodysregulation, polyendocrinopathy, and enteropathy, X-linked inheritance syndrome (IPEX) shows diffuse mononuclear cell infiltrate, fibrosis, and acinar loss. Residual endocrine islets are present.

Drug-induced Pancreatitis

Unlike drug-induced hepatitis detected by elevated transaminases that are part of the routine metabolic profile, pancreatitis may be often ignored among adverse drug reactions. This is also because of the difficulty in pointing to a drug as the cause of pancreatitis. A recent review categorizes the effects of drugs on pancreas (180) (Table 16-1) and incorporates voluminous data published by Biour et al. (13). Class I is reserved for medications implicated in greater than 20 reported cases of acute pancreatitis with at least one documented re-exposure. Eleven drugs listed in this class have been linked to pancreatitis in individuals less than 15 years of age. Class II comprises medications implicated in more than 10 cases of acute pancreatitis with or without positive rechallenge. Class III includes all medications reported to be associated with pancreatitis, too numerous to be listed in this chapter. In a study among hospitalized children, valproic acid was the most common drug associated with acute pancreatitis, followed by asparaginase (188).

Hereditary Pancreatitis

Classic hereditary pancreatitis follows an autosomal dominant inheritance pattern with incomplete penetrance and a highly variable disease expression (65,e43). Attacks of acute pancreatitis usually begin in childhood, but age of onset ranges from infancy to the fifth or sixth decade of life (101,e112,e206). The disorder is relatively rare, but is most commonly caused by one of the two mutations (R122H and N29I) of the cationic trypsinogen gene (*PRSS1*) located at 7q35 (56,190,e256). In the early literature, the mutation nomenclature was based on the chymotrypsin numbering system (87,189). The genetic numbering system, which designates the initiator methionine as position 1, has been subsequently adopted (171). Cationic trypsinogen is one of the three isoforms of the digestive proenzyme trypsinogen, and represents approximately two-third of total trypsinogen in the pancreatic juice. Activation of trypsinogen to trypsin normally occurs in the duodenum by the brush-border localized enterokinase and also by autoactivation by trypsin. The mutations either increase stability or increase autoactivation of trypsin (145,189). Pseudocysts of the pancreas develop in about 10% of patients with hereditary pancreatitis, and pancreatic insufficiency and diabetes mellitus are late occurrences (e206).

Table 16-1 ■ MEDICATIONS ASSOCIATED WITH PANCREATITIS

Class I	Class II
Didanosine	Rifampin
Asparaginase	Lamivudine
Azathioprine	Octreotide
Valproic acid	Carbamazepine
Pentavalent antimonials	Acetaminophen
Pentamidine	Phenformin[a]
Mercaptopurine	Interferon Alpha-2b
Mesalamine	Enalapril
Various estrogens	Hydrochlorothiazide
Opiates	Cisplatin
Tetracycline	Erythromycin
Cytarabine	Cyclopenthiazide[a]
Steroids	
Sulfamethoxazole/trimethoprim	
Sulfasalazine	
Furosemide	
Sulindac	

Listed from top by the order of number of reported cases.
[a]Drugs not currently FDA approved in the United States.
Table modified from Trivedi CD, Pitchumoni, CS. Drug-induced pancreatitis: an update. *J Clin Gastroenterol* 2005;39:709.

Genetic Risk Factors in so-called Idiopathic Chronic Pancreatitis

Identification of genetic alteration in hereditary pancreatitis has provided a significant tool to investigate other pathogenic factors of acute and chronic pancreatitis. Subsequent studies revealed a different *PRSS1* mutation detected almost exclusively in patients without a family history of chronic pancreatitis (e38,e261). In addition, Witt et al. (192) reported a close linkage of sequence alterations in *SPINK1* to idiopathic chronic pancreatitis. *SPINK1* encodes a natural antagonist of trypsinogens, serine protease inhibitor, Kazal type I, also known as *pancreatic secretory trypsin inhibitor*, which binds reversibly to trypsin and inhibits its activity. Sequence variations of *CFTR*, the gene responsible for cystic fibrosis, are also associated with idiopathic chronic pancreatitis (e42,e216). A recent review provides the role of *CFTR* compound heterozygosity and mild-to-variable mutations in idiopathic chronic pancreatitis (28). Transheterozygous status with sequence variations in different genes in certain individuals demonstrates additive effects of these modifier genes on pancreatitis risk (8,172). Idiopathic chronic pancreatitis has been a traditional clinical diagnosis describing the lack of an identifiable cause. As more genes and/or more mutations are identified that cause or predispose to chronic pancreatitis, the number of patients with "idiopathic" disease is reduced. At the same time, criteria of hereditary pancreatitis have been changing over the years (173), and the spectrum of disease associated with the *CTFR* mutant genes keeps expanding (8). The differentiation between hereditary and idiopathic chronic pancreatitis becomes difficult.

Exocrine Tumors

Primary pancreatic tumors are rare in children. The scarcity of cases and evolving nomenclature hinder us from studying these tumors and comparing current cases and remote published cases. Three epithelial pancreatic tumors, pancreatoblastoma, acinar cell carcinoma, and solid-pseudopapillary neoplasm, appear in a recent review of malignant pancreatic neoplasms in childhood and adolescence (152), and are discussed here. Ductal adenocarcinoma, the common tumor type in adults, has been reported in children mostly in the older literature (e130,e239). As the pediatric pancreatic neoplasms have been better characterized, this category has become exceedingly rare (23,152). Tumors and masses that may occur, but not specifically, in pancreas, include vascular lesions (184), lymphomas, and other childhood sarcomas (e.g., rhabdomyosarcoma). Tumors of endocrine cell origin will be discussed later.

Pancreatoblastoma

Pancreatoblastoma (e93), also called *pancreaticoblastoma*, is an epithelial neoplasm that exhibits multiple lines of differentiation including acinar differentiation, often with a lesser degree of endocrine and ductal differentiation, and is associated with squamoid corpuscles (68,90). A distinct mesenchymal component can also be seen. Some view this as the infantile or "blastomatous" form of acinar cell carcinoma. In support of this interpretation, a considerable overlap exists among pancreatoblastoma and acinar cell carcinoma (24). Pancreatoblastomas are usually large, solitary masses (Figure 16-15), ranging from 1.5 to 20 cm with a mean of 10.6 cm (92) and partially encapsulated. Microscopically, they are highly cellular, and the epithelial tumor cells are arranged in solid sheets and as small acini. The acinar differentiation is demonstrated by immunohistochemical positivity for pancreatic enzymes such as trypsin and chymotrypsin (119) and the presence of zymogen granules by electron microscopy (e110). The tumor usually has a lobular pattern, separated by stromal bands that may be hypercellular. The squamoid corpuscle is the characteristic feature of pancreatoblastoma (Figure 16-15). The structures may

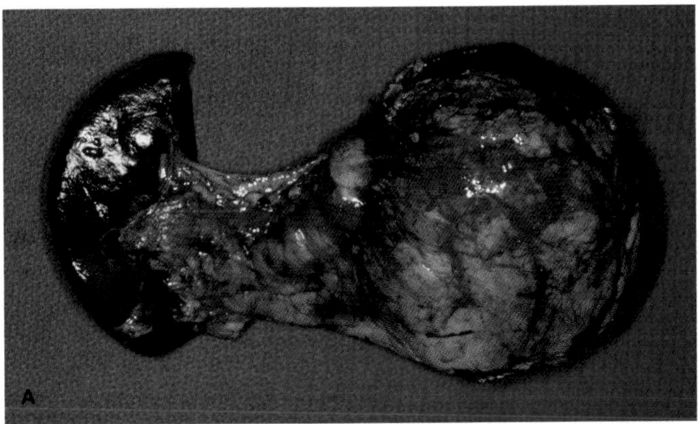

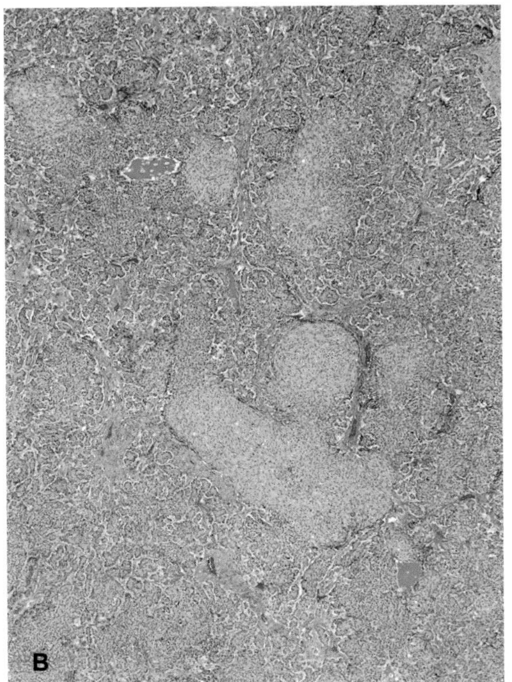

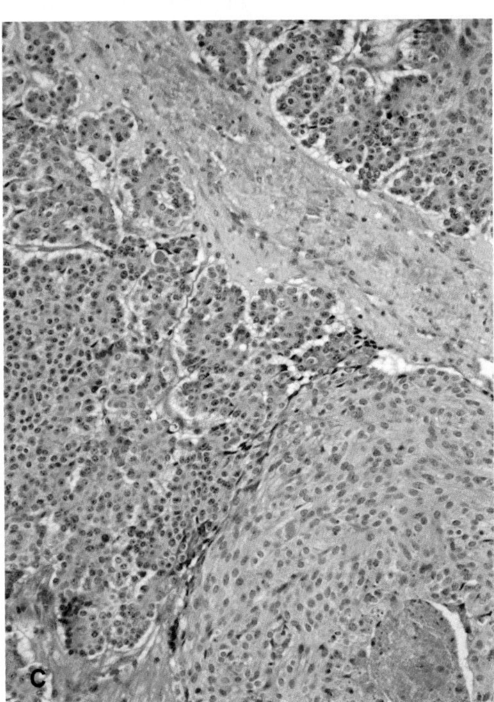

FIGURE 16-15 ■ Pancreatoblastoma. **A:** A 9.3-cm tumor removed with the tail of pancreas and the spleen from a 4-year-old girl. (Courtesy of James F. Southern, M.D., Milwaukee, Wisconsin.) **B:** Tumor consists of a mixture of areas with acinar arrangement and squamoid corpuscles. **C:** A squamoid corpuscle with central necrosis is on the lower right corner. A stromal band separates the areas of acinar differentiation with pinpoint lumina and cells showing darker cytoplasm and basally located nuclei. (**B,C:** hematoxylin and eosin stain, original magnifications, ×50 and ×200, respectively.)

be loose aggregates of larger spindle cells, or more frankly squamous, with keratinization. The cells forming squamoid corpuscles are not immunoreactive to antibody against cytokeratin 7, while acinar and solid areas are positively labeled (123) (eFigure 16-5). Alpha-fetoprotein production has been reported (24,e164), a character shared with cases of acinar cell carcinoma in childhood. It is common to detect endocrine and ductal differentiation by immunohistochemistry as a minor component of the tumor (92). The data on genetic alterations in pancreatoblastoma are limited, but allelic loss of chromosome 11p has been described (3,e115). Abnormalities involving adenomatous polyposis coli (APC)/β-catenin pathway are demonstrated (3) (eFigure 16-5). Pancreatoblastomas in children are usually detected before developing metastatic diseases and are curable by surgery (152). Marked responses to preoperative chemotherapy have been described (e250). This is in contrast to pancreatoblastomas in adults that are, in most instances, fatal.

Pancreatoblastoma has been described in association with the Beckwith-Wiedemann syndrome (41,120,e123). It is probably important to distinguish the adenomatous endocrine nodules of some infants with Beckwith-Wiedemann syndrome from pancreatoblastoma.

Acinar Cell Carcinoma

Acinar cell carcinoma is a malignant epithelial neoplasm that shows features of exocrine enzyme production by the neoplastic cells. By definition, endocrine and ductal components are minimal and do not exceed 25% of the neoplastic cells (67). The histology and the clinical behavior in the pediatric population of acinar cell carcinoma are very similar to pancreatoblastoma, and in some cases the pathologic distinction between the two can be difficult (24,152). Acinar cell carcinomas are usually large, solid, circumscribed tumors that sometimes show necrosis and cystic degeneration (91). They are microscopically highly cellular lesions that characteristically lack the desmoplastic stroma commonly seen with the ductal carcinomas (Figure 16-16, eFigure 16-6). The tumor cells show solid, trabecular, or glandular growth patterns as well as acinar formation. The cytoplasm tends to be abundant and granular. Immunoreactivity for trypsin, lipase, and chymotrypsin and ultrastructural demonstration of zymogen granules confirm acinar differentiation (67). As both acinar cell carcinoma and pancreatoblastoma share a densely cellular morphology, can exhibit a minor endocrine component, and demonstrate acinar differentiation, it is sometimes impossible to decide whether a tumor is a "squamoid corpuscle-free" pancreatoblastoma or an acinar cell carcinoma (24). It is therefore advised and practical to define pancreatoblastoma as a tumor with the characteristic squamoid corpuscles and is distinguished from acinar cell carcinoma (90). Genetic alterations in acinar cell carcinomas also points toward the similarity between the two tumors (2).

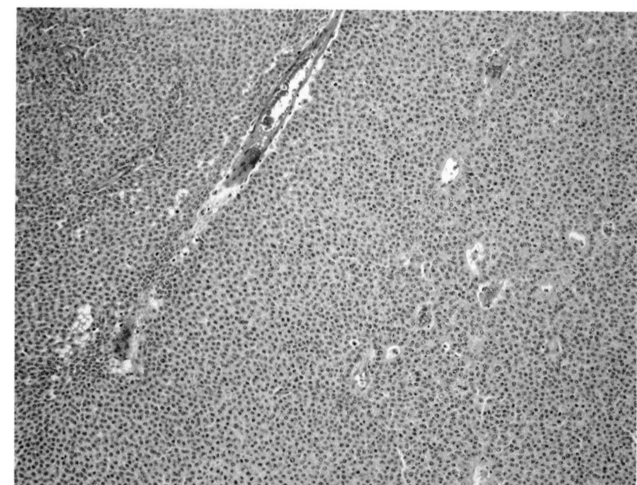

FIGURE 16-16■Acinar cell carcinoma. The tumor is highly cellular with virtually no stroma. The tumor cells are arranged in solid sheets and nests with small luminal spaces. (Hematoxylin and eosin, original magnification ×100.)

Solid-Pseudopapillary Neoplasm

This tumor is also known as *solid-pseudopapillary tumor, papillary cystic tumor of the pancreas, solid and papillary epithelial neoplasm, and papillary-cystic neoplasm*, but *solid-pseudopapillary neoplasm* is currently the preferred term (69). Most cases are found in females in the second and the third decades of life (137), but a few male patients have been reported (21,e148).

The tumors are generally large, both solid and cystic (Figure 16-17), and located anywhere in the pancreas. Solid sheets of epithelial cells may have an endocrine appearance, with uniform cells that have sharply defined cell borders. Perivascular pseudopapillae are interspersed with cystic degenerated areas. PAS-positive globules may be present in the cytoplasm (Figure 16-17). Despite recent studies, the line of differentiation of solid-pseudopapillary neoplasm is still unknown (93,96,119,e48). Consistently positive markers by immunohistochemistry are CD56, vimentin, α_1-antitrypsin, nuclear β-catenin, and CD10 (1,124) (eFigure 16-7). Some tumors show positive labeling by synaptophysin, but chromogranin is negative. The presence of progesterone receptors is frequently reported (e136,e268), while there are conflicting results on estrogen receptors (e71). The prognosis for patients with this neoplasm is excellent (93); most are cured by excision, but 10% to 15% have recurred locally (137) or metastasized (e48).

ENDOCRINE PANCREAS

Histogenesis, Maturation, and Morphology

During weeks 6 and 7 of intrauterine life, the dorsal and ventral pancreatic buds fuse. A simple epithelial tube of endodermal origin grows into the mesenchyme and gives rise to the endocrine and exocrine pancreas. It has been demonstrated in the rat that disaggregated and presumably single islet cells can regenerate new islets in culture that differentiate

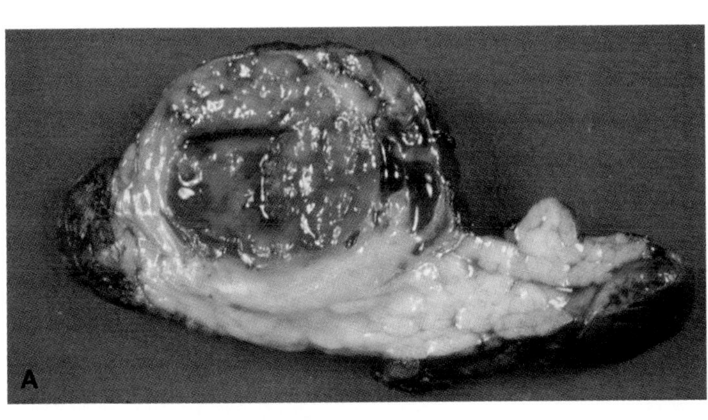

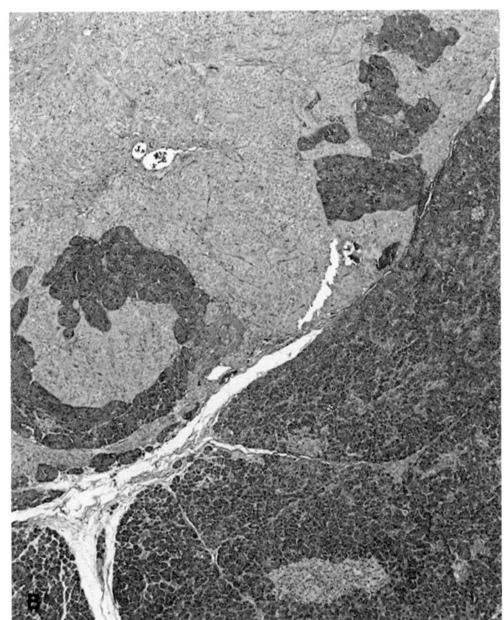

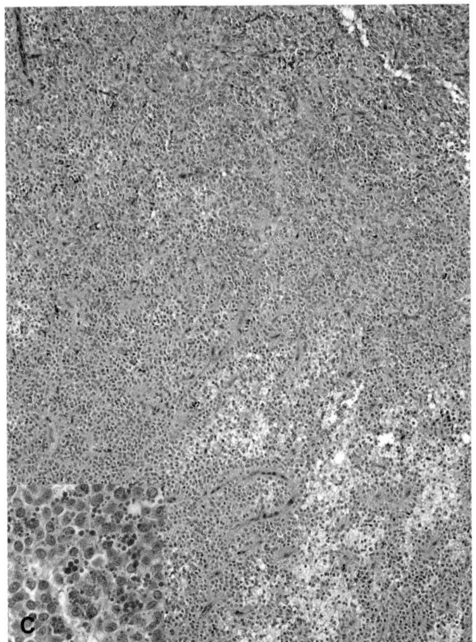

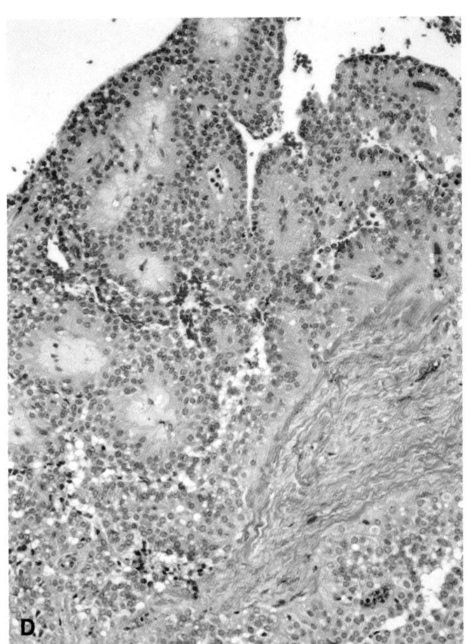

FIGURE 16-17 ■ Solid-pseudopapillary neoplasm. **A:** A 2.5-cm tumor removed from the tail of the pancreas in a 14-year-old girl (Courtesy of Marta E. Guttenburg, M.D., Philadelphia, Pennsylvania.) **B:** Despite the grossly circumscribed appearance, microscopic infiltrative growth is common, especially into the adjacent non-neoplastic pancreas. (Hematoxylin and eosin stain, original magnification ×50.) **C:** The basic architecture is solid cellular nests with small vessels. Some cells show cytoplasmic vacuolization. (Hematoxylin and eosin stain, original magnification ×100.) **Inset:** Eosinophilic "hyaline globules" are periodic acid-Schiff positive and diastase resistant, and typically found in the cytoplasm. (Periodic acid-Schiff with diastase stain, original magnification ×400.) **D:** The tumor cells situated away from the vessels degenerate, resulting in pseudopapillae. (Hematoxylin and eosin stain, original magnification ×200.)

into insulin- and glucagon-producing cells (e187). *Pax4* and *Pax6* are required for normal islet cell development in mice (e208,e231).

Microdissection studies in the mouse have shown that both the exocrine and endocrine cells of the pancreas develop from foregut endoderm; expression of both acinar enzyme and islet hormone genes is detected. Without mesenchyme, the primordial cells develop into endocrine cells only, but in the presence of mesenchyme, ducts and acini also form (e231).

Robb (e202) described the budding of islet cells from the pancreatic duct into the adjacent mesenchyme, visible after 10.5 weeks of gestation. The endocrine cells then lose their connection with the duct and become vascularized by a central capillary. In the study of Stefan and colleagues (e229), glicentin-containing cells were the first to appear, becoming detectable at week 8 of gestation in the wall of the developing duct. This pattern virtually disappeared by week 12 or 13 and was replaced by one in which the cells were reactive for adult glucagon and glicentin. By week 9, primitive islets were found to contain insulin (B) cells, somatostatin (D) cells, and glucagon (A) cells; pancreatic peptide (PP) cells were found only in the region of the duct of Wirsung, presumably in the ventral lobe (e40).

Between weeks 16 and 20 of gestation, the bipolar islets of Robb have insulin at one pole and somatostatin or glucagon at the other, except in the ventral lobe, in which PP predominates (e229). A central core of insulin cells develops in the mantle islet, surrounded by somatostatin and glucagon cells in the body and the tail and PP cells in the ventral head. The mature islets exhibit a trabecular arrangement, in which inner cells contain insulin and more peripheral cells contain glucagon or somatostatin; this arrangement is thought to be important in paracrine cell-to-cell control (e179). Gap junctions mediate cell-to-cell communication for the biosynthesis, storage, and release of insulin and other hormones, and connexin CX43 is expressed in islets (110).

Fetoscopy between weeks 19 and 21 of gestation has shown that levels of insulin, glucagon, and PP are similar in fetal and maternal blood (e4).

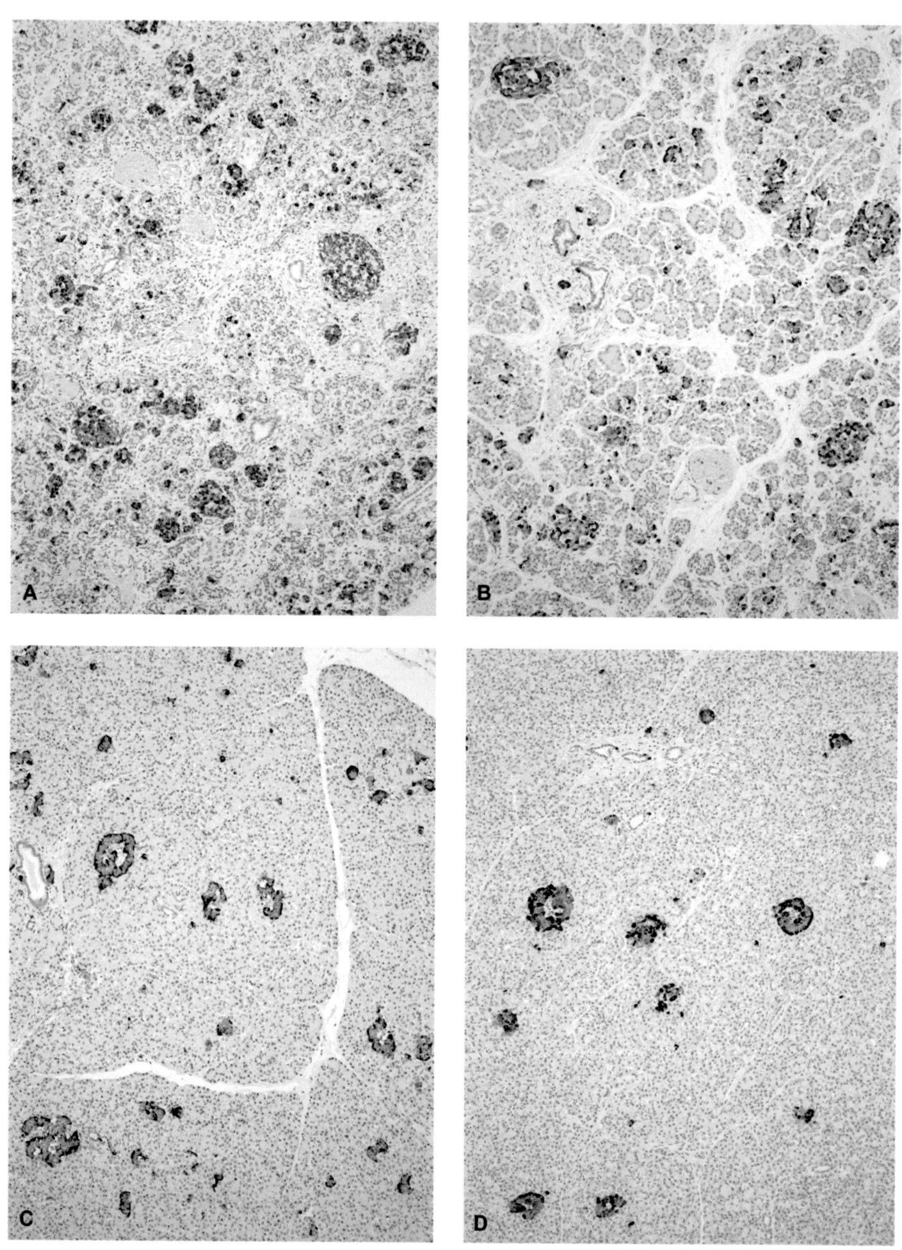

FIGURE 16-18 ■ Distribution of endocrine cells, which are revealed by immunohistochemistry for chromogranin A. Respective survival dates are as follows: **A:** Stillbirth at 25 weeks. **B:** Forty weeks of gestation, 8 days of postnatal survival. **C:** Twenty-two months. **D:** Eight years. (**A–D:** original magnifications ×100.)

The distribution of the various cell types is not homogeneous within the pancreas, nor are they stable from fetal to adult life. A portion of the head of the pancreas, ostensibly derived from the ventral primordium, is rich in islets containing PP (136,e147). The number of somatostatin-containing D-cells is greater in the fetal and neonatal period than later in life, reaching a peak between week 17 of gestation and 5 months of age (e198,e229). The distribution of endocrine cells in the fetus and neonate is characterized by a greater number of single cells and small clusters of cells outside the islets (76) (Figure 16-18).

The endocrine tissue in the developing pancreas lies centrally within the lobule, close to the ductal system from which it buds. The larger and better-formed islets of Langerhans form the stalk of the lobule, and smaller aggregates and single cells bud off within the more peripheral centroacinar tissues, resulting in the characteristic distribution of the endocrine tissue in late fetal life. At term, the smaller peripheral clusters of endocrine cells may be numerous, and the extrainsular endocrine cells may constitute much of the endocrine component of the newborn pancreas. This is often confused with the diffuse form of congenital HI, formerly *diffuse nesidioblastosis*, by the uninitiated.

A large body of literature has been published on the quantification of the endocrine content of the pancreas at various ages. The endocrine content of the pancreas can be expressed as a ratio of endocrine to acinar tissue. This is easy to quantify in a mature pancreas, in which confluent acinar tissue is present around islets. It is much more problematic in the pancreas of an infant, which consists mostly of mesenchyme and in which many of the largest islets are "septal" (Figure 16-18).

The amount of endocrine tissue present at birth, in a rough compilation of available estimates, is 10%; this decreases during acinar development to 5% by 6 months of age, and then gradually to the adult volumes of 1% to 2% (76,77,116,e82,e262). Figure 16-19 illustrates histologic features of normal pancreas in children often confused to be abnormal, including abundant endocrine tissue, endocrine cell clusters budding off ducts, and large septal islets.

The amount of endocrine tissue is not fixed. Ductal obstruction, with chronic pancreatitis and fibrosis, may be associated with a resurgence of endocrine development. This situation can mimic endocrine neoplasia (e17). Because volumetric determinations of endocrine mass are usually expressed relative to the acinar mass and because a decrease in exocrine tissue produces a relative increase in the mass of islet cells, the observer should determine whether an apparent excess of endocrine cells is absolute or secondary to acinar loss.

Abnormalities of the Endocrine Pancreas

Islet Hypertrophy

Islet size varies with age. Jaffe et al. (76) found that before the age of 2 months, only 3.5% of all islets are larger than 200 μm in diameter. Single septal islets at any age can be much larger, measuring as much as 700 μm in diameter (Figure 16-19). The term *islet hypertrophy* should be used to describe a generalized phenomenon in which the percentage of islets larger than 200 μm is excessive for a particular age.

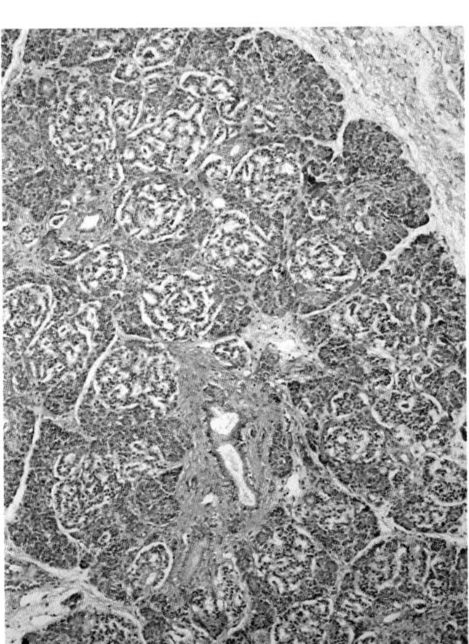

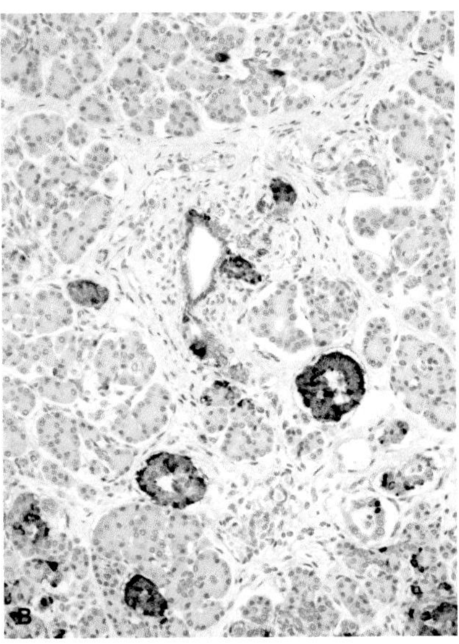

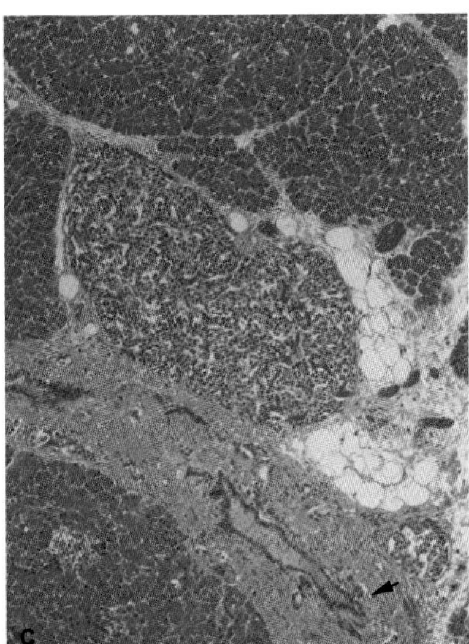

FIGURE 16-19 ▪ Histologic features of pancreas from individuals less than 2 years of age. **A:** Abundant islets/endocrine tissue is seen in the pancreas of a 5-month-old normoglycemic infant, especially in the head. (Hematoxylin and eosin stain, original magnification ×100.) **B:** Endocrine cells budding off a duct (nesidioblastosis) in an 8-day-old infant born at 40 weeks of gestation (Immunohistochemistry for chromogranin A, original magnification ×200.) **C:** Very large septal islets, such as this one in a 22-month-old child, are not uncommon. A small cluster of endocrine cells is budding off a duct (nesidioblastosis) in the lower right corner (*arrow*). (Hematoxylin and eosin stain, original magnification ×100.)

Borchard and Müntefering (16) provide values for islet size at different stages of gestation. True islet hypertrophy is seen in infants of diabetic mothers and, less commonly, in infants with erythroblastosis fetalis (16,71,e255).

Endocrine Aplasia and Hypoplasia

Combined exocrine and endocrine hypoplasia was mentioned previously (e58,e94,e138,e155,e242). A child with metabolic acidosis and diabetes shortly after birth had a pancreas in which exocrine elements appeared normal but no islets were seen on conventional histologic examination; a sibling had a similar clinical story (e51). A congenital absence of glucagon cells has been reported (but not illustrated), and an infant with normoinsulinemic hypoglycemia had few glucagon-containing cells (e16,e78). A generalized paucity of somatostatin cells has been implicated in some cases of neonatal hypoglycemia (e25). Some growth-retarded fetuses have been previously reported to show endocrine paucity (e249), but a more recent study demonstrated no differences between intrauterine growth retardation and control fetuses in insulin-positive areas or islet organization (11).

Infant of the Diabetic Mother

Maternal insulin and glucagon do not cross the placenta, although maternally derived or animal-derived antigen-antibody complexes of insulin do (113). The changes in the endocrine pancreas of a child born to a diabetic mother are a response to maternal hyperglycemia (e2,e106) and anti-insulin antibodies (113). The various changes in the pancreas of the diabetic offspring are ascribed to variations in the severity of maternal disease, the stringency of the therapeutic control, and the presence or absence of diabetic vascular complications (113,182,e88). Most infants of diabetic mothers have islet hypertrophy (>10% of islets larger than 200 μm), an increased total islet cell volume, pleomorphism of B-cell nuclei, eosinophilic insulitis (Figure 16-20), and periinsular or intrainsular fibrosis (71). Similar features may be present in the pancreata of infants born to prediabetic mothers.

Hultquist and Olding (71) stated that the pancreas of the infant whose mother is diabetic weighs less than that of a normal infant when corrected for total body weight. This is particularly true of the infants of mothers with the most severe diabetic complications. After week 34 of gestation, infants with a birth weight of 2.25 kg or more have an excess islet cell volume. This correlation was stronger for the offspring of mothers with uncomplicated diabetes because they had the largest babies. No difference was detected between islet cell volume in normal infants and the volume in the offspring of mothers with severely complicated diabetes. Borchard and Müntefering (16) claimed that an increased mean islet diameter is more characteristic of the diabetic infant than an increased number of islets.

The islet cell increase is largely the consequence of expansion of the B-cell mass from 40% of endocrine cells to 63.8% (182). This expansion is observed in the dorsal lobe-derived pancreatic polypeptide poor portion of the pancreas

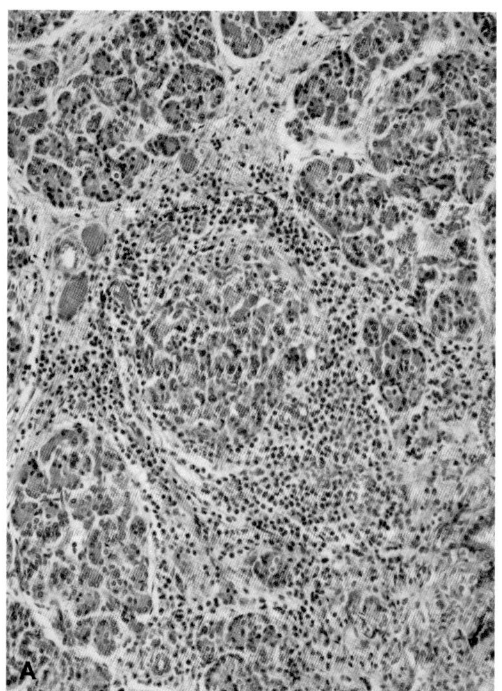

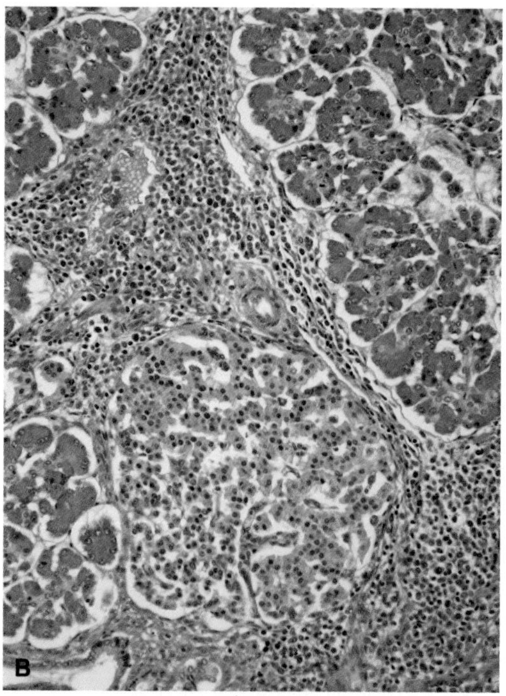

FIGURE 16-20 ■ Infant of diabetic mother and nonimmune hydrops fetalis. **A:** Eosinophilic insulitis in an infant of a diabetic mother. (Hematoxylin and eosin stain, original magnification ×200.) **B:** In this pancreas from an infant with nonimmune hydrops, an islet is associated with extramedullary hematopoiesis. (Hematoxylin and eosin stain, original magnification ×200.)

(e.g., tail) (182) as well as in the pancreatic polypeptide rich (ventral lobe-derived) region of the pancreas. Milner et al. (116) demonstrated that A-cell and PP-cell increases accompany B-cell hyperplasia in a diabetic pregnancy, with the A-cell increase occurring only in the pancreatic polypeptide poor and the PP-cell increase in the pancreatic polypeptide-rich regions. Pleomorphism of the B-cell nuclei is seen with the increase in endocrine volume and is also marked in the pancreata of the infants of mothers with complicated diabetes.

Wellman and Volk (e255) reviewed the issue of mesenchymal inflammatory infiltrate. Eosinophilic periinsulitis, the most characteristic finding, occurs in about 50% of infants of diabetic mothers, whether or not the mother is receiving insulin. The infiltrate is rich in eosinophilic myelocytes, may contain Charcot-Leyden crystals, and is said to disappear within days of birth. Charcot-Leyden crystals can be seen in the macerated pancreas. Klöppel (e119) suggested that the infiltrate is a local reaction to insulin-containing immune complex. Fibrosis within and around islets is seen in association with hypertrophy and eosinophilia, but it is also described as an early *in utero* finding independent of eosinophilic accumulation (71,e170).

Other, less constant findings in the islets of infants of diabetic mothers include an increase in the mitotic rate, degranulation of B-cells, islet edema, hydropic swelling of islet cells, ribbon-like transformation of islet cells, necrosis, and thickened extrainsular and intrainsular capillaries. Lymphocytic infiltration is not specific to these children.

A suggestion by Van Assche and Gepts (182) was that an intact hypothalamic-hypophyseal axis is required for the development of pathologic pancreatic changes because they are not seen in the anencephalic offspring of diabetic mothers.

It has been predicted that the prenatally affected islets of infants of diabetic mothers become insufficient through the stress of postnatal life and that infants of diabetic mothers are more likely to develop diabetes mellitus. Several epidemiological data show that consequences extend to adult life and even to the next generation through the maternal line (63). Family histories secured from consecutive pregnant diabetic women (e151) indicated that patients with gestational diabetes are more likely to have a mother with diabetes than gravidas with normal carbohydrate metabolism. The studies on Pima Indians (e47,e185) have shown that, besides a genetic transmission of diabetes, the diabetic intrauterine milieu can also induce a diabetogenic tendency in the offspring.

Hydrops Fetalis

The accumulation of fluid in the fetus results from various congenital and acquired/maternal conditions. Immune hydrops is caused by blood-group incompatibility, mostly of ABO and certain Rh types, between mother and child. The endocrine pancreas of Rh-positive infants born to Rh-negative mother with anti-Rh antibody has been described to partly resemble that of infants of diabetic mother but with some differences. The amount of endocrine tissue is increased in the tail of the pancreas (181), and it is parallel to the increased number of endocrine cells per islet. In contrast to infants of diabetic mothers, the proportion of B-cells and the contribution of the different cell types are unchanged. Milner et al. (115) report that the increased volume fraction of B, A, PP, and D cells is seen only in the pancreatic polypeptide-rich (ventral lobe) part of the pancreas.

Prevention of Rh immunization in at-risk mothers has reduced the incidence of this disorder, and nonimmune hydrops has become more prevalent. The causes of nonimmune hydrops are manifold. Excess endocrine tissue and islet cell hyperplasia (without morphometric confirmation) have been described in nonimmune hydrops fetalis (e165). An islet associated with extramedullary hematopoiesis is depicted in Figure 16-20.

Diabetes Mellitus

Diabetes mellitus is a group of metabolic diseases characterized by hyperglycemia resulting from defects in insulin secretion, insulin action, or both. Deficient insulin action is due to diminished tissue responses to insulin at one or more points in the complex pathways of hormone action. The recently revised classification reflects our understanding of the pathogenesis of diabetes mellitus (48). Four main forms are in the classification: type 1 diabetes mellitus, type 2 diabetes mellitus, other specific types, and gestational diabetes mellitus. Patients with any form of diabetes may require insulin treatment at some stage of their disease. Such use of insulin does not, of itself, classify the patient. The third category, other specific types, accounts for less than 10% of all diabetic patients, and includes diabetes mellitus caused by monogenetic defects of B-cell function and insulin action, diseases of the exocrine pancreas, endocrinopathies, drugs, infections, uncommon immune-mediated forms, and other genetic syndromes. Some in this category are described elsewhere in this chapter. Provided below are descriptions of type 1 and type 2 diabetes, which are the two principal types of diabetes, followed by neonatal diabetes and maturity-onset diabetes of the young (MODY) of which new insights have been delineated recently.

Type 1 Diabetes Mellitus

Type 1 diabetes mellitus is associated with an absolute insulin deficiency caused by destruction of insulin-producing B cells of the pancreas. This form used to be designated as insulin-dependent diabetes mellitus or juvenile onset diabetes mellitus, and, until recently, was considered the most prevalent type in children. It results from a cellular-mediated autoimmune process (7). Antibodies detected in 70% to 80% of patients are autoantibodies to islet cells, insulin, glutamic acid decarboxylase, and tyrosine phosphatase IA-2 and IA-2 β (130). The rate of B-cell destruction is variable, but when it is rapid as seen in infants and children, severe hyperglycemia and/or ketoacidosis may be the first manifestation. Type 1 diabetes mellitus has a complex pattern of genetic associations, and putative susceptibility genes have been mapped.

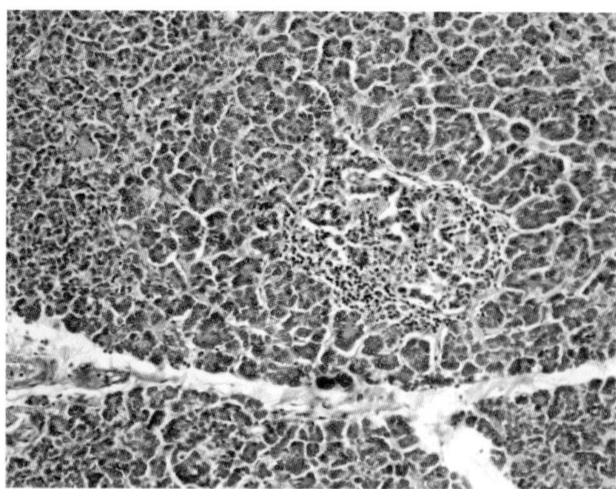

FIGURE 16-21 ■ Type 1 diabetes mellitus of recent onset. An active insulitis is present within and around an islet. Residual endocrine cells were demonstrable in this islet. (Hematoxylin and eosin stain, original magnification ×200.)

The most important is the class II MHC (HLA) locus at 6p21 (109). It is influenced by the DRB genes (e95), with linkage to the DQA and B genes. These *HLA-DR/DQ* alleles can be either predisposing or protective (e192).

Morphologic changes in the pancreas of diabetic individuals are not consistent, and they rarely contribute to diagnosis. The pancreas of classic type 1 diabetes may show a reduction in the number and the size of islets and insulitis (49,95) (Figure 16-21). Insulitis is characterized by islets infiltrated primarily by T-lymphocytes (112) and is confined to those islets in the recent-onset diabetic that still contain B cells (e67). Other early features include cellular vacuolation and nuclear pleomorphism (e72). Later in the course of the disease, insulitis is no longer seen and B-cells become sparse (49). Interlobular fibrosis is a feature in some diabetics. Trophic changes of the exocrine cells can be marked, with diffuse or, in the early stages, patchy, focal acinar atrophy (142,e120) (eFigure 16-8).

Type 2 Diabetes Mellitus

Patients with type 2 diabetes have insulin resistance and usually relative (rather than absolute) insulin deficiency. Relative insulin deficiency implies an inadequate secretory response by the pancreatic B-cells to compensate for insulin resistance. The specific etiologies are not known, but autoimmune destruction of B-cells does not occur. Patients should not have any of the other causes of diabetes listed under other specific types (48). Nevertheless, environmental factors, such as a sedentary life style and dietary habits, play a role in the pathogenesis. Most patients with this form of diabetes are obese, and the link between obesity and diabetes is mediated by insulin resistance (84). The incidence of type 2 diabetes mellitus, previously considered to be a disease of adult, has recently risen remarkably in children in different geographic areas of the world (5,e62,e118,e186,e248). Although type 2 diabetes is often associated with a strong genetic predisposition, more so than type 1 diabetes (e15, e172), its genetics are complex and not clearly defined.

The pancreas generally shows no change other than islet amyloid deposition (148), which becomes more frequent with age in both diabetics and nondiabetics (e120). Islet amyloid is formed from islet amyloid polypeptide, which is secreted with insulin, and is seen in longstanding adult cases of type 2 diabetes (26). Animal studies have shown some evidence of a direct role for amyloid in the pathogenesis of type 2 diabetes (70,e253). Figure 16-22 shows amyloid replacement of islets in a 4.5-year-old boy with diabetes, but also with dwarfism and genital hypertrophy. B-cell mass is

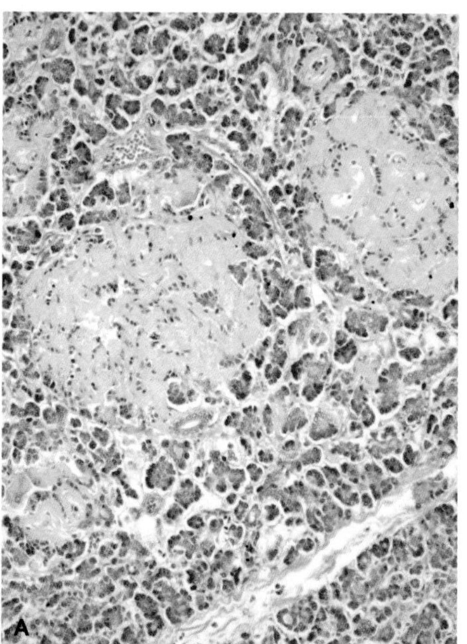

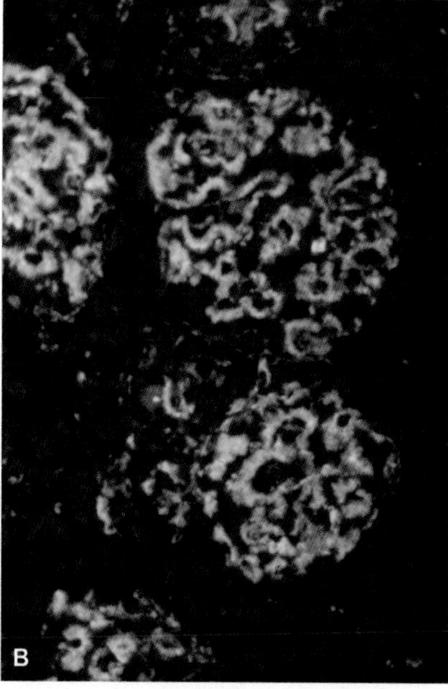

FIGURE 16-22 ■ Islet amyloid deposition. **A,B:** A 4.5-year-old boy with dwarfism, genital hypertrophy, and diabetes mellitus had amyloid in the islets. (**A:** Hematoxylin and eosin stain, original magnification ×200, **B:** Thioflavine T stain, original magnification ×200.)

suggested to be decreased in type 2 diabetes mellitus, but this remains controversial (19,26,148,e83,e197,e230).

Neonatal Diabetes Mellitus

Neonatal diabetes is rare, with a reported incidence of 1 in 400,000 live births (151), and may be defined as insulin-requiring hyperglycemia that is diagnosed within the first three months of life (54,131). It is a heterogeneous group of disorders, therefore, not part of the etiology-based classification recently proposed (48), but is a useful category when faced with infants with diabetes mellitus of neonatal onset.

The disease may be transient, remitting by 18 months of age but relapsing during adolescence in a significant proportion of patients (151,e252). Most patients are full-term, but growth-retarded, infants. Three inter-related genetic mechanisms have been ascribed to more than 50% of transient neonatal diabetes mellitus (174): paternal uniparental isodisomy of chromosome 6, paternal duplication of 6p24, and a methylation defect at a CpG island overlapping exon 1 of *ZAC* (zinc finger protein associated with apoptosis and cell cycle arrest)/*HYMAI* (imprinted in hydatidiform mole). These observations suggest that transient neonatal diabetes may result from overexpression of an imprinted gene on 6p24 and displaying paternal expression. Pancreatic morphology has not been described specifically for this form.

Permanent neonatal diabetes requires lifelong therapy, and a variety of causes and associations have been identified. They include pancreatic hypoplasia or aplasia (e49,e58,e138,e155,e242), Wolcott-Rallison syndrome (18,e263), homozygous inactivating mutations of insulin promoter factor 1 (IPF1) affecting proteins involved in pancreas formation (165), homozygous or compound heterozygous glucokinase mutations with complete enzymatic loss (e174), and immunodysregulation, polyendocrinopathy, enteropathy, X-linked (IPEX) syndrome (191,e20,e257). Pancreatic findings at autopsy from patients with Wolcott-Rallison syndrome and IPEX syndrome are described elsewhere in the chapter. The most common genetic cause, accounting for 34% to 64% of permanent neonatal diabetes mellitus, is activating mutations in the *KCNJ11*, which encodes Kir6.2, a subunit of the adenosine triphosphate (ATP)-sensitive potassium channel of the B cell (54,e66,e152,e251). This finding has a significant impact on management because many patients can be switched from insulin to oral sulfonylureas (e181). Most recently, activating mutations in *ABCC8* encoding the other component of the potassium channel have been reported to cause neonatal diabetes (9). The channel abnormality is also responsible for congenital HI discussed later.

Maturity-Onset Diabetes of the Young (MODY)

MODY is characterized by autosomal dominant inheritance and early-onset diabetes mellitus (60). Early onset is defined as at least one to two members of the family being diagnosed before age 25. These patients have monogenetic defects resulting in B-cell dysfunction, are not known to be insulin resistant, and do not need to be obese to develop diabetes. Although an earlier definition of MODY included early-onset *type 2* diabetes and autosomal dominant inheritance (60), MODY is under other specific types in the recent classification (48), and not part of type 2 diabetes mellitus. Nevertheless, childhood type 2 diabetes can be confused with MODY as both have insulin secretion, and are not usually insulin dependent or prone to ketoacidosis. Of 112 non–type 1 children reported in a survey performed in the United Kingdom, 25 had type 2 diabetes and 20 had MODY (e59). The rest was secondary and unclassifiable due to incomplete data. In contrast to type 2 diabetes, MODY patients were younger (10.8 vs. 12.8 years), less likely to be overweight, and none were from ethnic minority groups. Fifty-six percent of type 2 patients were of ethnic minority groups.

To date, six genetic defects that cause MODY have been uncovered, five of which correspond to transcription factors expressed in pancreatic B-cells: hepatic nuclear factor (HNF)-4α (193), HNF-1α (194), IPF1 (164), HNF-1β (64), and neurogenic differentiation 1/B-cell E-box transactivation 2 (108) for MODY 1, 3, 4, 5, and 6, respectively. Loss-of-function mutations of glucokinase that catalyzes the first step in glucose metabolism cause MODY 2 (46). In addition to their effects on B-cell function, deficiency of some of these transcription factors affects function of other organ systems (e101). Patients with HNF-1α mutations have decreased renal reabsorption of glucose and glycosuria (e158). The deficiency of HNF-4α affects triglyceride and apolipoprotein biosynthesis (e218). Families with HNF-1β mutations presenting with renal cysts and diabetes have been described (e24,e124).

Hyperinsulinism

HI is the most common cause of hypoglycemia in infants and children (158). Clinically transient forms of HI are seen in neonates born to diabetic mothers, infants with birth asphyxia and/or small for gestational age (158), and Beckwith-Wiedemann infants (43). The histologic features of pancreas in some of these conditions are mentioned elsewhere in this chapter.

Persistent HI in children, unlike adults, is rarely due to islet cell adenoma (insulinoma) (Table 16-2), but most often

Table 16-2 ■ FINDINGS IN PANCREAS RESECTED FROM CHILDREN WITH HI

Histology of Pancreas	Percentage of Children Affected (%)
Diffuse endocrine abnormality (large nuclei in islets)	45
Adenomatosis/ adenomatous hyperplasia (focal, multifocal, or generalized)	45
Adenoma	1
Normal	5
Equivocal/difficult to classify	4

Note: All known and unknown underlying genetic abnormality inclusive.
The Children's Hospital of Philadelphia (1983–2005, n = 159).

represents a congenital genetic disorder. The incidence of congenital HI in the general population ranges from one in 27,000 to 50,000 live births (53). In communities with high rates of consanguinity, the incidence may be as high as one in 2,500 live births (e153). As described below, the disorder is quite heterogeneous. Insulin levels are not usually dramatically elevated, but rather there is inadequate suppression of insulin secretion at low plasma concentrations of glucose (i.e., HI rather than hyperinsulinemia) (159). The diagnosis is based on evidence of the effects of excess insulin, which includes inappropriate suppression of lipolysis and ketogenesis and an inappropriately positive glycemic response to glucagon at times of hypoglycemia (e65,e227). Uncontrolled hypoglycemia may lead to seizures or permanent brain damage, and immediate medical intervention is required.

Infants with congenital HI were once believed to have abnormal pancreatic development associated with persistence of packets of islet cells (B-cells) budding off ducts, termed *nesidioblastosis* (e131,e269). Observations based on immunohistochemical investigations have shown that nesidioblastosis, as defined above, is a common feature of the pancreas in normoglycemic neonates and infants (76,e196,e262), and nesidioblastosis by itself is no longer considered the underlying histologic basis of congenital HI (114,134,159,e195). A supplemental discussion on nesidioblastosis and HI is provided at the end.

Congenital HI is caused by a number of genetic abnormalities in the pathways regulating insulin secretion by pancreatic islets (Table 16-3). A standardized nomenclature system has been proposed to facilitate communication among investigators/clinicians and identification of the precise clinical, biochemical, genetic, and physiological characteristics of each specific disease (53). The use of *HI* is recommended as a general term (instead of *hyperinsulinemic hypoglycemia*). If the genetic etiology is known, the mutated gene is added to the name, such as KATP-HI for HI due to mutations in the ATP-sensitive potassium channel genes and HI-GCK for HI due to mutations of glucokinase gene. When other clinical or histological characteristics are known, these should be stated, such as hyperinsulinism-hyperammonemia syndrome (HI/HA) for HI/HA and focal HI for focal disease (see below). This proposal has been conceptually accepted, but many variations of the term are still seen in publications.

Hyperinsulinism with B-cell ATP-Sensitive Potassium Channel Abnormalities (KATP-HI)

As a group, the ATP-sensitive potassium channel abnormalities are by far the most common cause of congenital HI. Three genetic mechanisms, recessive mutation, paternally inherited mutation with somatic loss of maternal 11p15, and dominant mutation, are known to cause insulin dysregulation. Children often present with severe hypoglycemia in the newborn period, with the exception of the rare dominantly inherited form. Because the channel is impaired, that is, channelopathy, they often do not respond to medical therapy with a channel agonist diazoxide, requiring further treatment including, but not limited to, pancreatectomy. Each one of the three is discussed separately along with its histology.

HI caused by recessive ATP-sensitive potassium channel mutations and associated diffuse histologic abnormality (diffuse HI): One of the most common forms of HI is associated with recessive mutations in one of the two adjacent genes on chromosome 11p that comprise the B-cell ATP-sensitive potassium channel: the high-affinity sulfonylurea receptor 1 (*ABCC8*, formerly *SUR1*) (175,e171) and its regulated ion pore, potassium inward rectifier 6.2 (*KCNJ11*, formerly *Kir6.2*) (121,e240). Loss-of-function mutations cause closure of the channel, leading to depolarization of the membrane and activation of a voltage-gated calcium channel that results in exocytosis of insulin granules.

The pancreatic histology of this form is characterized by the presence of abnormally large islet cell nuclei that are distributed throughout the pancreas. Frequency and easiness of finding enlarged endocrine cell nuclei vary from case to case. Large nuclei are empirically determined to be nuclei four times that of the nearby acinar cell nuclei (135) or nuclei occupying an area more than three times larger than the surrounding endocrine nuclei (e235) (Figure 16-23). A morphometric analysis revealed that the mean nuclear radius of the 50 largest nuclei of this type is significantly larger than the mean nuclear radius measured in islets that are present outside or away from the adenomatous (focal) lesions in the focal form described next (149). The cytologic changes also include "bizarre" crescent-shaped or ovoid nuclei with occasional nuclear pseudoinclusions (intranuclear cytoplasmic invagination). It is important to note that not all islets contain these abnormal nuclei, and the number of islets with characteristic nuclei may be small. Ductuloinsular complex composed of endocrine cells in the epithelium of the ducts and in connection with the endocrine cell clusters may be present (Figure 16-23). The B-cell proliferation rate is not higher when the fraction of Ki-67 positive B-cells was compared to a control group (149). Moreover, the mean total endocrine area and the volume density of B-cells are not increased in this form (76,134,e196,e262). The major source of confusion is the lack of familiarity with the histologic features of the normal newborn and infant pancreas, in which endocrine tissue is abundant, and smaller peripheral clusters of endocrine cells may constitute much of the endocrine component (Figures 16-18 and 16-19). These are the features that were previously interpreted as excessive "nesidioblastosis."

HI caused by paternally inherited ATP-sensitive potassium channel mutations together with somatic loss of maternal 11p15 and associated focal histologic abnormality (focal HI): An equally common and histologically distinct form of HI results from a paternally inherited mutation in the channel genes (*ABCC8* and *KCNJ11*) together with a sporadic somatic loss of the maternal 11p15 that contains

Table 16-3 ■ GENETICS AND PATHOLOGY OF CONGENITAL HI

Gene	Protein	Genetic Abnormality Clinical Information	Pathologic Findings	Examples of Suggested Nomenclature	
ABCC8	SUR1	Recessive mutation	Diffuse changes with large islet cell nuclei	HI-SUR1 Diffuse HI	
KCNJ11	Kir6.2	Recessive mutation	Diffuse changes with large islet cell nuclei	HI-Kir6.2 Diffuse HI	
ABCC8	SUR1	Paternally inherited mutation and loss of maternal 11p	Focal changes with adenomatous hyperplasia/ adenomatosis	HI-SUR1 Focal HI	KATP-HI
KCNJ11	Kir6.2	Paternally inherited mutation and loss of maternal 11p	Focal changes with adenomatous hyperplasia/ adenomatosis	HI-Kir6.2 Focal HI	
ABCC8	SUR1	Dominant mutation	Anecdotal Large islet cell nuclei	dominant SUR1-HI	
KCNJ11	Kir6.2	Dominant mutation	No pancreatectomy	dominant Kir6.2-HI	
GCK	glucokinase	Dominant mutation	Anecdotal Normal or large islet size and infrequent large islet cell nuclei	HI-GCK	
GLUD1	glutamate dehydrogenase	Dominant mutation Hyperammonemia	Anecdotal	HI/HA	HI-GLUD1
HADH (SCHADH)	SCHADH	Recessive mutation	No pancreatectomy	HI-SCHADH	
Not known		Dominantly inherited Physical exercise induced	No pancreatectomy	EIHI	

SUR1, sulfonylurea receptor 1; Kir6.2, inward rectifier 6.2; SCHADH, short-chain L-3-hydroxylacyl coenzyme A dehydrogenase.

imprinted genes involved in cell proliferation. The unbalanced expression of the imprinted growth factor (*IGF2*) and tumor-suppressor genes (*H19* and *CDKN1C*) leads to adenomatous hyperplasia; the expression of the mutated paternal gene causes unregulated insulin secretion from the hyperplastic lesion (33). $p57^{kip2}$ is the product of one of the imprinted genes (*CDKN1C*) that are normally expressed from the maternal allele and is lost in endocrine cells within the adenomatous lesions. The loss of $p57^{kip2}$ expression can be visualized by immunohistochemical labeling (86,166) (eFigure 16-9). Identification of this form of disease has major clinical implications because this form, if detected, can be surgically excised and cured without near-total pancreatectomy (4,35).

The pancreatic histology is characterized by a lesion formed by the confluence of hyperplastic but apparently normally structured islets occupying greater than 40% of the cross-sectional area of pancreatic lobules (76) (Figure 16-24). The lesion pushes the exocrine elements aside or haphazardly incorporates them. There is recapitulation of islet structure, with peripherally located A- and D-cells and B-cells aggregating more centrally. Other histologic terms frequently used and accepted are *adenomatosis* and *adenomatous hyperplasia*. In contrast to insulinomas, the lesions are difficult to identify grossly (Figure 16-24) because they do not distort the normal lobular architecture. The boundary between the uninvolved portion of the pancreas and the lesion may be sharp (Figure 16-24), but may also be vague and ill defined (eFigure 16-10). The lesions are generally small, thus their designation as *focal HI*. In one series, 24 of 35 lesions were less than 1 cm in the greatest dimension (161). However, the lesion may be multifocal and/or occupy a large portion of the pancreas to even the entire pancreas (76,167). The genetic pathogenesis of the latter is the same as smaller typical lesions, as demonstrated by the loss of expression of $p57^{kip2}$ (166). In these rare cases, the designation *focal lesion* or *focal HI* causes confusion, yet using the word *diffuse* is equally troublesome. A better terminology is being sought and *generalized adenomatosis* may be an option (76). Cases with ectopic pancreatic tissue harboring this type of lesions

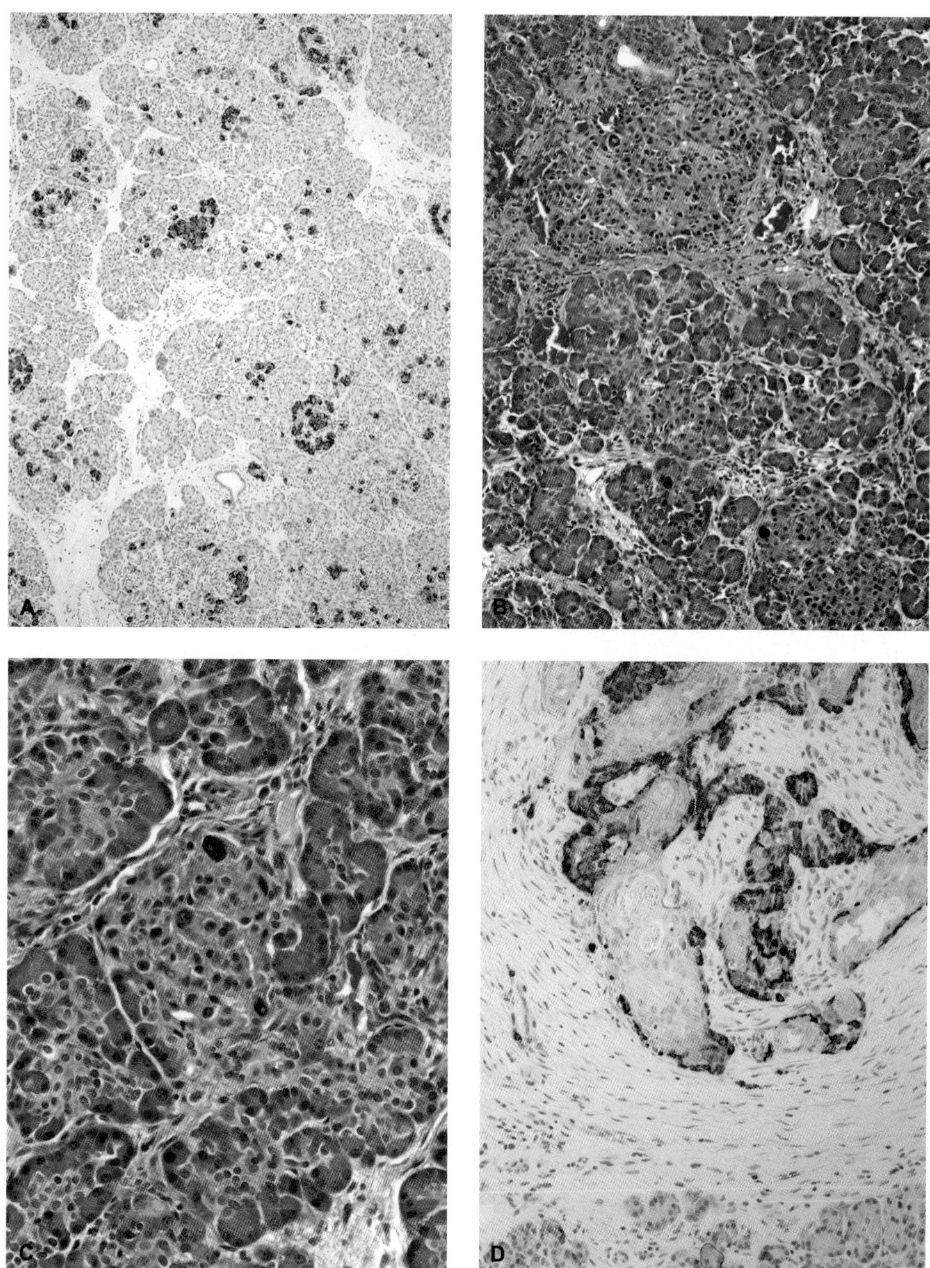

FIGURE 16-23 ■ ATP-sensitive potassium channel HI, diffuse form. **A:** Quantity of endocrine component is not significantly different from pancreas of normoglycemic individuals of similar age (2 months). (Immunohistochemistry for insulin. Original magnification ×50.) **B:** On a low-to-medium power field, a few large and hyperchromatic endocrine cell nuclei can be spotted. (Hematoxylin and eosin stain, original magnification ×200.). **C:** Enlarged islet cell nuclei are defined as those occupying an area at least three times larger than the neighboring endocrine nuclei, for diagnostic purposes. (Hematoxylin and eosin stain, original magnification ×400.) **D:** Ductuloinsular aggregates may be present in some cases, but they are seen too seldom to use as a diagnostic criterion. (Immunohistochemistry for chromogranin A, original magnification ×200.)

have also been described (129,e193). Although there are large nuclei in the confluent islet tissue of the adenomatous focal lesions, the islets in uninvolved portions of pancreas are reported to have a "resting" appearance with B-cells showing little cytoplasm and nucleus (135). B-cell nuclear crowding expressed as the number of B-cell nuclei/1,000 μm^2 of B-cell cytoplasm is higher in islets outside the lesion of this focal form as compared to islets of the diffuse form described above (150). This difference may be subtle and is not appreciated by other retrospective studies without morphometric measurements (e102,e222,e235).

In a limited number of institutions, intraoperative frozen sections are performed to identify patients with the focal form and further guide the extent of pancreatic resection (135,167). The presence of islet cell nuclear abnormalities (e.g., enlarged more than three times, "bizarre" shaped)

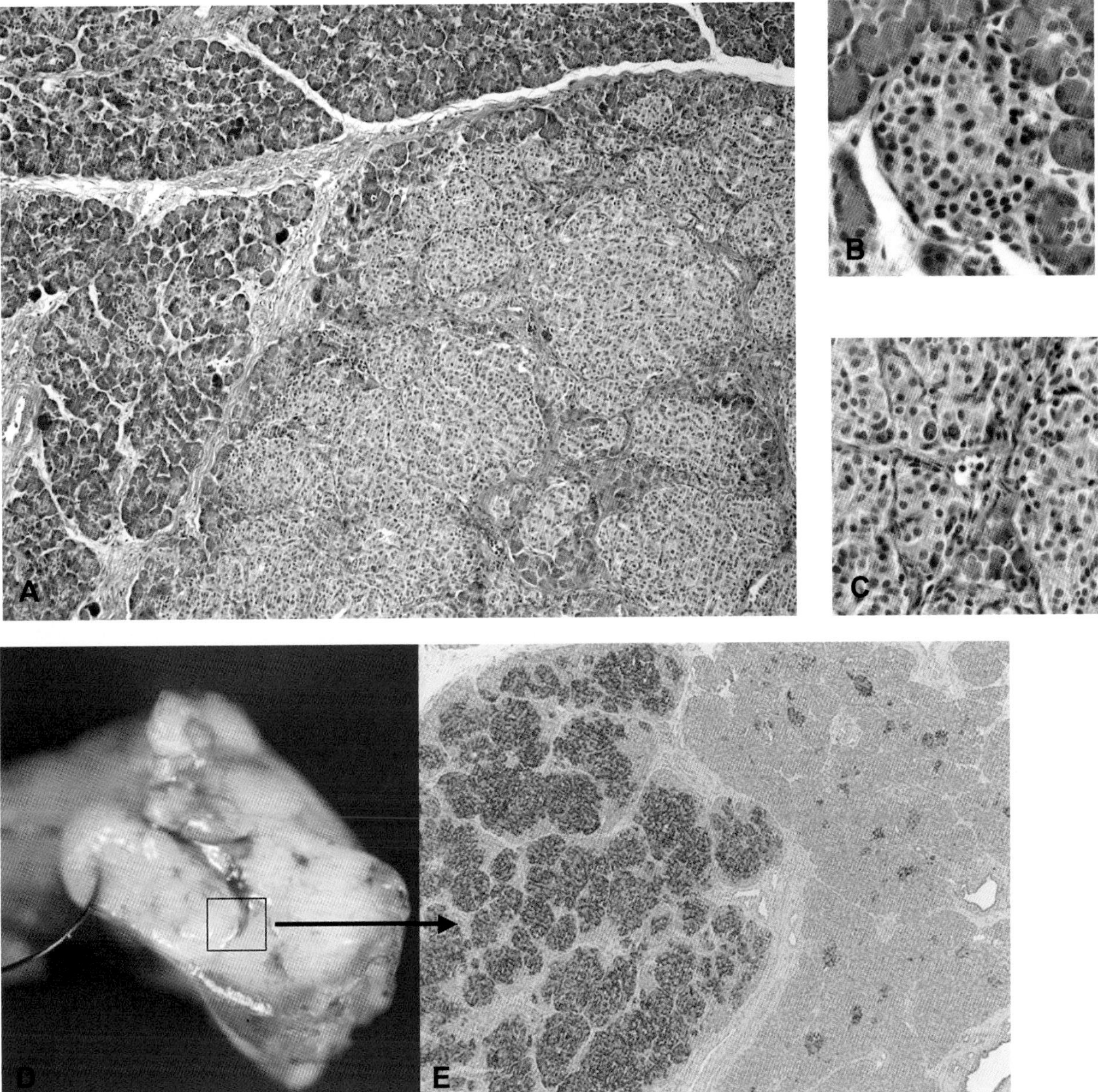

FIGURE 16-24 ■ ATP-sensitive potassium channel HI with loss of maternal 11p15 (focal form). **A:** Much of the lobule in the right lower half is occupied by endocrine tissue (adenomatosis). (Hematoxylin and eosin stain, original magnification ×200.) **B:** Islets outside the adenomatous lesion contain nuclei of normal size. **C:** There may be large endocrine cell nuclei within the adenomatosis. (**B,C:** Hematoxylin and eosin stain, original magnification ×400.) **D:** The adenomatous lesion is difficult to distinguish from the neighboring pancreas grossly. **E:** Immunohistochemistry confirms the abundance (>40%) of endocrine elements within the lobules. (Immunohistochemistry for chromogranin A, original magnification ×200.) (**D,E:** Copyright 2004 from A multidisciplinary approach to the focal form of congenital HI by partial pancreatectomy by Adzick NS, Thornton PS, Stanley CA, et al. *J Pediatr Surg* 2004;39:270–275. Reproduced with permission of Elsevier.)

suggests the recessively inherited diffuse form, and a near-total pancreatectomy follows. The absence of nuclear changes *in islets* is indicative of the focal form, and a search for a focal lesion continues until the lesion is identified. Examples of difficult cases are those with an ill-defined border of the focal form, with generalized adenomatosis, and with infrequently encountered and/or localized islet cell nuclear abnormality (167). Most recently, preoperative diagnosis of patients with the focal form is aided by fluorine-18 L-3,4-dihydroxyphenylalanine ([18F]-DOPA) positron emission tomography (58,127). This technique localizes the lesion within the pancreas and can detect even an extrapancreatic ectopic lesion (129,e97).

Hyperinsuminism caused by dominant ATP-sensitive potassium channel mutations: Rare dominantly expressed *ABCC8* and *KCNJ11* mutations have been described (72,e142,e241) with a milder clinical presentation. Pancreatic pathology is anecdotally reported to be similar to the recessively inherited form (72,e241).

Hyperinsulinism Caused by Defects of Other Genes

Abnormalities in three other genes are associated with generally milder forms of HI that usually respond to medical therapy with diazoxide. Patients with these disorders tend not to have their pancreas resected, and therefore, histologic descriptions are scarce.

Glucokinase, a hexokinase with a low affinity for glucose, controls the rate-limiting step of B-cell glucose metabolism and is responsible for glucose-mediated regulation of insulin secretion. The gene, *GCK*, is at 7p13–15. The enzyme with a gain-of-function mutation has a higher affinity for glucose, so that glycolysis and inappropriate insulin secretion take place at relatively low blood concentration of glucose (52). Several dominantly inherited mutations of the glucokinase gene have been described with variable clinical presentations (34). Some are mild and can be controlled by diazoxide while others may present with extremely severe HI that cannot be managed by diazoxide. Pathologic descriptions remain anecdotal. The pancreas of one case was reported to be normal (e75) while a systematic study of another case demonstrated moderately enlarged islet cell nuclei and increased average size of islet profiles compared to the control and cases caused by recessive ATP-sensitive potassium channel mutations (30). Of note, mutations in glucokinase that decrease enzymatic activity result in MODY 2 (46) as mentioned earlier in the chapter.

Another autosomal dominant form of HI is caused by gain-of-function mutations of the glutamate dehydrogenase gene, *GLUD1* (160), located at 10q23.3. Glutamate dehydrogenase is a mitochondrial enzyme, and catalyzes the reaction converting glutamate to α-ketoglutarate, a substrate for the TCA cycle. This form of HI is known as the *HI/HA* and is distinguished by persistently elevated plasma ammonia concentrations to three to five times normal, as a result of the enzymatic abnormality being expressed in the liver as well as in the pancreas (e226). A pancreatectomy specimen has been described (not illustrated) as showing "unusual islet cells arranged in ribbon pattern (islet cell dysplasia)" (187).

The most recently described metabolic abnormality resulting in HI is short-chain L-3-hydroxylacyl coenzyme A dehydrogenase (SCHADH) deficiency (27,e162). Each proband had a homozygous mutation, and the patients were medically managed.

There is an additional form of dominant HI that is physical exercise induced (126,e156,e157). Two families, Finnish and German, have been reported. The patients have abnormal insulin response to infusion of pyruvate, but the specific defect has not been elucidated. Sequence analysis of genes encoding monocarboxylate transporters did not identify sequence variants that cosegregate with the phenotype in the families.

Adenoma

Adenomas are rare in the pediatric population (Table 16-2). When HI manifests as a noncongenital manner after 6 to 12 months of age, an insulinoma needs to be considered. Adenomas are generally well demarcated (Figure 16-25), and differ from the lesions of adenomatosis in that they do not have intermixed acinar elements and do not recapitulate mini-islets. An adenoma does not contain all the cell types in normal proportions, although more than one cell type may be represented. Most lesions previously described as adenomas in the pediatric literature represent adenomatosis (adenomatous hyperplasia) when the illustrations are critically reviewed (e29).

Hyperinsulinism and Nesidioblastosis

To explain the origin of islet cell tumors of the pancreas, Laidlaw referred to the continuity of duct epithelium and islet cells observed in normal pancreas, speculating islet tumor formation to be an exaggeration of normal processes involving totipotent "nesidioblasts" (e131). He proposed a condition, termed *nesidioblastosis*, wherein islet cell proliferation from ducts becomes disseminated, as the putative cause for hypoglycemia. Yakovac investigated the histopathology of then *idiopathic hypoglycemia of infancy* and reported that a defining feature was B-cell nesidioblastosis (e269). Nesidioblastosis was thereafter used to support the hypothesis that neonatal hypoglycemia-HI is a developmental problem. The word *nesidioblastosis* subsequently acquired a clinical connotation essentially equating it to the disorder presenting with persistent hypoglycemia, particularly in neonates (114). The term has also been used frequently to describe the diverse histopathology found among pancreata obtained from patients with HI. Microscopic anatomy included in nesidioblastosis has been the presence of endocrine cells closely associated with ducts, small clusters of endocrine cells scattered throughout the exocrine pancreas, large islets with or without hypertrophic islet cell nuclei, and a proposed but not proven increase in endocrine cell mass. As a result, it has become increasingly difficult to ascribe specific meaning when authors provide statements such as "the pancreas showed nesidioblastosis." Other terms, for example, islet cell dysplasia and nesidiodysplasia, were subsequently put forward to compromise over objections raised in the use of nesidioblastosis, which is seen in normal developing pancreas. Pathologists who recognized the frequent association of endocrine cells and ducts in fetal and pediatric material were among the first to challenge conventional wisdom regarding the pathologic basis of congenital HI (76,e195,e262). Then followed endocrinologists, biochemists, and geneticists, who further delineated an understanding that HI is a functional defect in insulin regulation, one not simply due to islet development. Several genetic abnormalities are now described underlying congenital HI, and the pancreatic histology varies according to these alterations and subtypes of HI. The use of nesidioblastosis as a histologic finding in HI is therefore confusing, and it does not provide or characterize distinct anatomic or

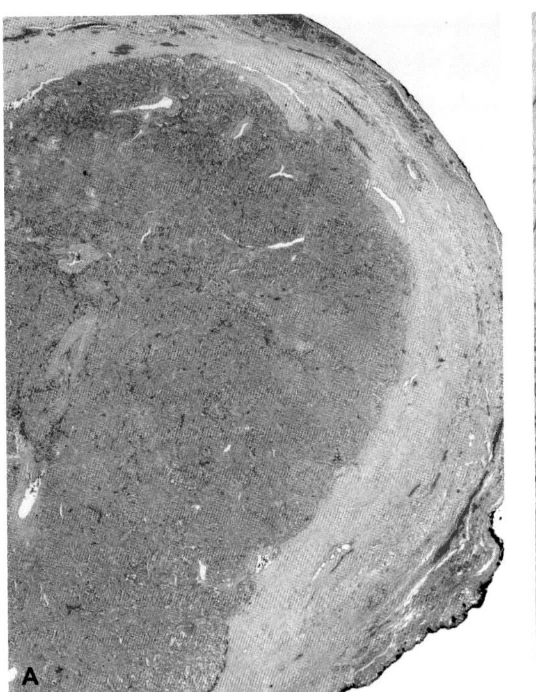

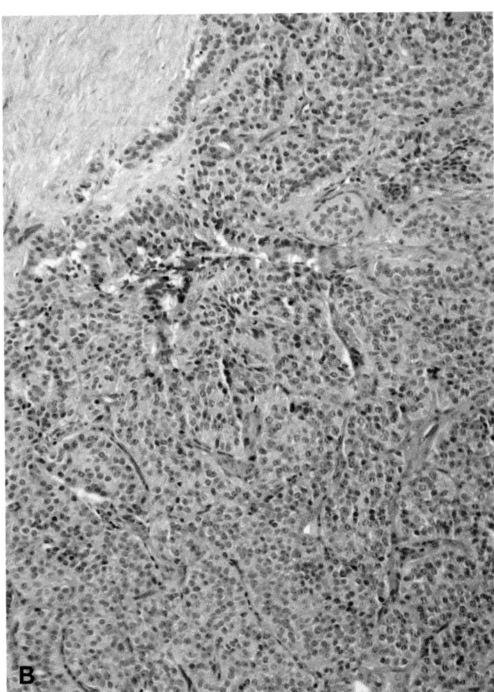

FIGURE 16-25 ▪ Islet cell adenoma from a 10-year-old boy. The tumor is composed of a monotonous population of endocrine cells arranged in trabeculae and cords, and has a relatively sharp border. (**A,B:** Hematoxylin and eosin stain, original magnification ×25 and ×200, respectively.)

clinical information. Moreover, lumping various histologic changes to a single term hinders objective description of pathology, which is the key in recognizing different pathological processes.

Pancreatic Islets in Shock

Bernstein (e22) described three newborns dying shortly after birth in whom renal tubular and selective pancreatic islet necrosis was found. Asphyxia was implicated. Seemayer et al. (146) found the same pattern in only 10% of infants with other severe manifestations of shock.

Viral Infections

Nonselective involvement of the pancreas is seen in disseminated herpesvirus, cytomegalovirus, varicella-zoster virus, and rubella virus infections (78). Selective damage to islet cells has been seen in coxsackievirus B infection (78,e73), although caution should be exercised in distinguishing viral effects from the changes of shock, described earlier. The onset of diabetes after coxsackievirus B infection has been documented, although direct evidence for virally induced diabetes is lacking (e271).

Malformation Syndromes

Beckwith-Wiedemann Syndrome

Beckwith-Wiedemann syndrome is a congenital overgrowth syndrome that is clinically and genetically heterogeneous. A number of complex genetic and epigenetic abnormalities resulting in dysregulation of imprinted growth regulatory genes clustered at 11p15 have been demonstrated (38,e140). Phenotypical features include macrosomia, macroglossia, omphalocele, visceromegaly (80), and, in about one-third to half of cases, hypoglycemia that is attributed to HI (37,43). The hypoglycemia is transient in the majority of infants and resolves within the first few days of life. In about 5% of children, the HI persists and extends beyond the neonatal period, requiring either continuous feeding, medical therapy, or partial pancreatectomy in rare cases.

The available pancreatic histology is, therefore, usually limited to the severe cases in which the patient has died or had partial pancreatectomy. The pancreatic parenchyma is composed of small endocrine cell clusters, well-formed islets, and large, confluent, and complex islet-like aggregates of endocrine cells in a background of a relatively narrow rim of exocrine acini (77) (Figure 16-26). The endocrine cells often show large cytoplasm and large nuclei. Focal areas of necrosis may be found in the larger endocrine nodules. When immunohistochemical reaction is applied, the islet-like aggregates recapitulate islet topography with the insulin-positive B-cells residing in the center and the non-B-cell being at the periphery of the "macroislets" (e228) (eFigure 16-11). A lack of segregation of pancreatic polypeptide-rich islets to the head of pancreas (ventral pancreas origin) has been described. In a Beckwith-Wiedemann patient with a Meckel diverticulum, the heterotopic pancreas within the diverticulum showed numerous enlarged islets or islet-like aggregates, some with a diameter of up to 1,600 μm,

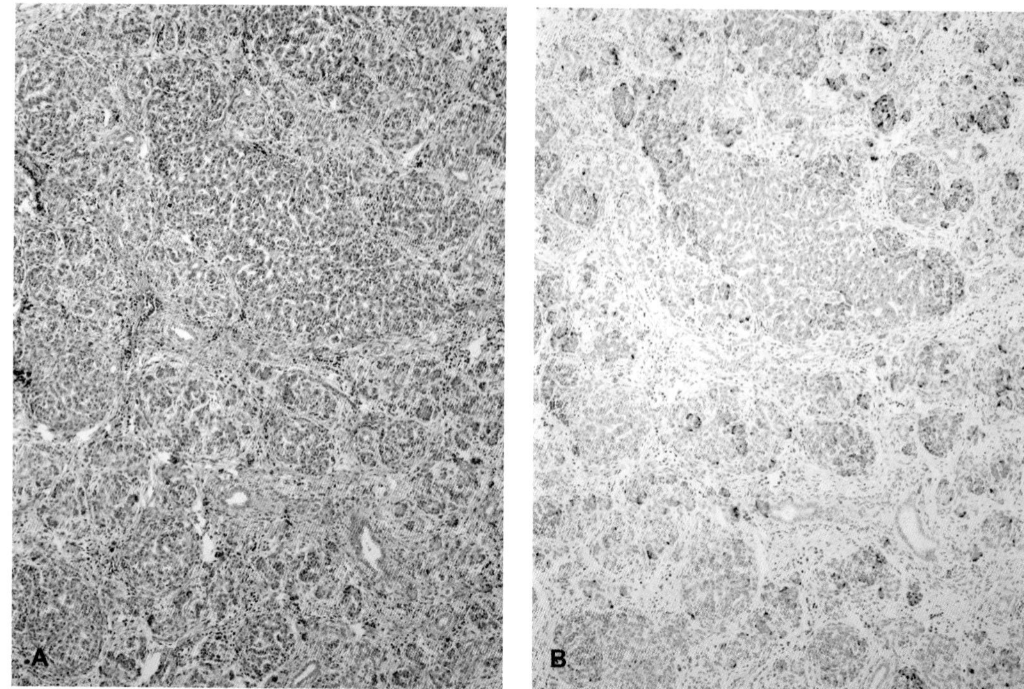

FIGURE 16-26 ■ Beckwith-Wiedemann syndrome. **A,B:** Much of the pancreatic lobule is formed of complex islet-like aggregates of endocrine cells. Exocrine acini are poorly developed. (**A:** Hematoxylin and eosin stain, **B:** Immunohistochemistry for chromogranin A, original magnification ×100.)

comprising approximately 15% of the pancreatic tissue (e209). The abundance of endocrine tissue forming irregular nodules and aggregates is reminiscent of the appearances seen in adenomatous hyperplasia (adenomatosis, focal HI) associated with paternally inherited ATP-sensitive potassium channel mutations together with loss of maternal 11p. The difference is, however, that the abnormality is present throughout the pancreas in Beckwith-Wiedemann syndrome (Figure 16-26). In one case with mosaic paternal uniparental disomy for 11p15, $p57^{kip2}$ protein was readily identified within the large islets, which is in contrast to the loss of $p57^{kip2}$ expression in the B-cells within the adenomatous lesions of focal HI (73).

A pancreas examined at 11 months of age at the time of death of a patient with Beckwith-Wiedemann syndrome shows significantly more acinar differentiation and proliferation as compared to the partial pancreatectomy specimen at one month of age (47). Another report by Sotelo-Avila and Gooch (e223) describes islet cell hyperplasia in five children who died of their disease-associated tumors, even though the earlier hypoglycemia had been transient.

Steigman et al. (162) reported a 2-day-old autopsy case with an enlarged and solely cystic pancreas containing numerous irregularly shaped ectatic ducts with sparse islands of endocrine tissue and exocrine acini (Figure 16-8). The pancreatic histology seen in Beckwith-Wiedemann syndrome may not be uniform as the underlying genetic and epigenetic abnormalities are highly variable.

Beckwith-Wiedemann syndrome with hemihypertrophy is associated with a striking tendency toward the development of embryonal tumors in a number of organs, and pancreatoblastoma is one of them (41,e123,e189).

Perlman Syndrome

Beckwith-Wiedemann syndrome and the syndrome of renal hamartomas, nephroblastomatosis, and fetal gigantism overlap to some degree. One-half of the cases are said to have islet cell hyperplasia (62,e183), hypoglycemia occurs (e80), and HI may be responsible. We have seen a large pancreas associated with Perlman syndrome (Figure 16-27).

Wilcott-Rallison Syndrome

Wilcott-Rallison syndrome is an autosomal recessive disorder that is characterized by permanent neonatal insulin requiring diabetes mellitus and multiple epiphyseal dysplasia (e263). Other features include osteopenia, mental and growth retardation, hepatic and kidney dysfunction, cardiac abnormalities, exocrine pancreatic dysfunction, and neutropenia (42,e214). The syndrome results from mutations in the gene encoding the eukaryotic initiation factor 2-α kinase 3 (*EIF2AK3*, also called *PERK*) (18,39). The transmembrane kinase EIF2AK3 is localized in the endoplasmic reticulum and phosphorylates EIF2A (e217), preventing B-cell death and relieve endoplasmic reticulum stress by reducing the number of unfolded proteins in the endoplasmic reticulum (198,e126). Autopsy of one case revealed a markedly hypoplastic pancreas with only a narrow cord of tissue (176). Histology showed a reduction of acinar tissue and increased

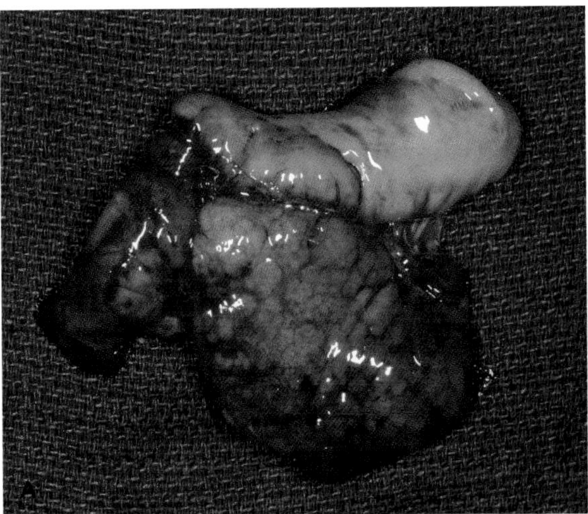

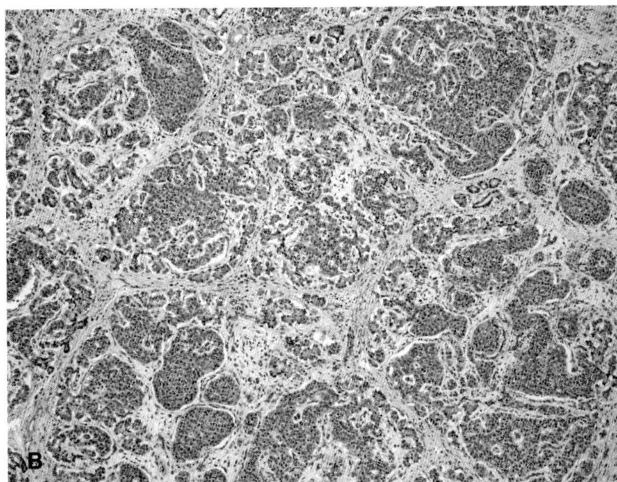

FIGURE 16-27 ■ Perlman syndrome. **A:** An 11-day-old infant delivered at 30 weeks of gestation presented with hypoglycemia and constellations of malformations consistent with Perlman syndrome. The pancreas was large and weighed 20 g. (Courtesy of Ralph A. Franciosi, M.D., Milwaukee, Wisconsin.) **B:** The pancreatic lobules appear disorganized, and are composed of irregularly shaped cords and islands of endocrine cells and poorly developed acini.

interstitial fibrosis. The islets appeared prominent with more glucagon staining cells than insulin staining cells.

Leprechaunism

Donohue (e54) described infants with a characteristic facies, hirsutism, enlarged genitalia, decreased muscle and subcutaneous tissues, and "dysendocrinism." An autosomal recessive defect in the insulin receptor gene (*INSR*) has been documented in some patients (44), and leprechaunism is listed in the recent diabetes classification under genetic defects in insulin action (48). On the other hand, intermittent hypoglycemia with HI has been described, and in a selective review of the literature, Rosenberg et al. (140) found that islet hyperplasia was reported in 67% of the cases at autopsy. An unusual case described by Szilagyi et al. (e238) had the features of lipomatous pseudoatrophy with preserved islets and is mentioned earlier in the chapter.

Other Disorders Affecting Endocrine Pancreas

Cystic Fibrosis

In the pancreas, cystic fibrosis primarily affects the exocrine component causing pancreatic insufficiency. However, diabetes mellitus has been recognized as a complication that commonly develops around 20 years of age. The prevalence increases with age, and, with improved survival and prospective screening by glucose tolerance test, approaches to 30% (107,e133,e272).

Several studies have been published focusing on islet changes in cystic fibrosis (106,157,e1,e98,e125). Although qualitative and quantitative methods differed among the studies and the pathology was always accompanied by exocrine and interstitial alterations, a decrease in the fraction of insulin-positive B-cells in islets was generally demonstrated in advanced cystic fibrosis. A "qualitative" islet number (e98) and the volume density of endocrine tissue to pancreatic tissue (106) were decreased in cystic fibrosis patients as compared to the control groups. Endocrine cell composition was not significantly different between pancreas showing predominantly fibrotic pattern and lipoatrophic pattern (106).

In diabetic young adults, islets were described as having a disorganized and lobulated appearance with thin fibrous septa enclosing the capillaries and subdividing the islets (157). Large amount of amyloid deposition was also demonstrated (29).

In contrast, an early endocrine increase has been also mentioned (e125). Multiple foci of neoformation of islets illustrated by islet cells arising from and around the ductal lumen were reported in all 11cystic fibrosis patients (age: 3 months to 7 years) as compared to less frequent encounters in the control subjects (e31). Neoislet formation from a small duct was present in nondiabetic children, but not in nondiabetic and diabetic young adults in a different series (e98).

The morphologic alterations may provide the basis for the glucose intolerance and overt diabetes mellitus eventually developing in some with cystic fibrosis. However, not all patients with advanced cystic fibrosis become diabetic. Other late complications of cystic fibrosis such as liver damage and peripheral insulin resistance might contribute to the changes in glucose metabolism seen in cystic fibrosis patients (106,177).

Hereditary Tyrosinemia Type I

Tyrosinemia may be associated with glycosuria and refractory hypoglycemia. The pancreas in some infants has been shown to contain many large islets (e184,e219), but this is not a constant feature in this disease (143). The variability likely comes from the difficulty in accurately assessing islet hypertrophy in infant (true increase in the percentage of islets larger than 200 μm for a given age). Mitotic activity within islets and hyalinization of islets have been seen in some cases (e86).

Ataxia-Telangiectasia

The familial disease with cerebellar ataxia, oculocutaneous telangiectasia, and immune disorder with IgA deficiency is associated with insulin-resistant diabetes mellitus (25). Islet cell hyperplasia may be impressive; however, the marked nuclear cytomegaly is not confined to islets but is a systemic manifestation of the disease (e14).

Sudden Infant Death Syndrome (SIDS)

In a retrospective review of infants with SIDS, examination of the pancreas did not divulge endocrine pathology (e143,e169). Hisaoka et al. (e92) claimed to have found "endocrine cell dysplasia" in 2 of 15 infants with SIDS, but no glucose or insulin determinations were available to support an etiologic connection. In a review of 112 pancreata from victims of sudden infant death, Klensang et al. (89) found no morphologic or morphometric differences between them and 19 controls. It is not unreasonable to assume that some infants or even older children with HI may present as instances of sudden death (6), but the diagnosis must rely on laboratory documentation of the HI. The morphologic features of normal infant pancreas may appear abnormal or similar to a form of HI if qualitative and quantitative differences from the adult pancreas are not taken into consideration (55,77).

Endocrine Tumors in Childhood

Most of the descriptions of endocrine adenomas in childhood appear to represent adenomatosis (76,e29,e121). True adenomas (Figure 16-25) have traditionally been classified according to the hormone produced. Adenomas may be part of the multiple endocrine neoplasia type I syndrome; even in this syndrome, functioning adenomas of the pancreas are unusual in childhood. Adenomas that produce gastrin and the Zollinger-Ellison syndrome are described in the adolescent pancreas (e259). Carney et al. (e35) described the occurrence of pheochromocytoma(s) or pancreatic islet cell tumor(s) or both, in two or more members of three unrelated families with a pattern consistent with autosomal dominant inheritance, and suggested a syndrome different from multiple endocrine neoplasia. Another 18-year-old with pheochromocytoma and a nonfunctioning islet cell adenoma of the pancreas has also been described (e273). Some of these patients may have had von Hippel-Lindau disease, which is associated with islet cell tumors, adenomatosis, pancreatic cysts and, in some instances, pheochromocytoma (122,e96,e191).

Malignant islet cell tumors are diagnosed on the basis of distant metastasis to distinguish them from multiple adenomas. Rare examples in childhood have been noted: a metastasizing insulinoma in a 14-year-old (e266) and a corticotropin-producing tumor of the head of the pancreas (e210). Judson et al. (82) reported a well-differentiated pancreatic endocrine neoplasm of an 18-year-old that metastasized to the breast with intraductal spread. Overall, malignant, metastasizing tumors of the pediatric endocrine pancreas are extremely uncommon (e266).

ACKNOWLEDGMENT

The author wishes to acknowledge the significant contribution to this chapter as portions were adapted from the previous edition, authored by Dr. Ronald Jaffe, Professor, University of Pittsburgh School of Medicine, and former Pathologist-in-Chief, Children's Hospital of Pittsburgh, Pittsburgh, Pennsylvania. His generosity in providing additional illustrative materials for figures, constructive advice, and encouragement is deeply appreciated.

REFERENCES

1. Abraham SC, Klimstra DS, Wilentz RE, et al. Solid-pseudopapillary tumors of the pancreas are genetically distinct from pancreatic ductal adenocarcinomas and almost always harbor β-catenin mutations. *Am J Pathol* 2002;160:1361–1369.
2. Abraham SC, Wu TT, Hruban RH, et al. Genetic and immunohistochemical analysis of pancreatic acinar cell carcinoma: frequent allelic loss on chromosome 11p and alterations in the APC/ β-catenin pathway. *Am J Pathol* 2002;160:953–962.
3. Abraham SC, Wu TT, Klimstra DS, et al. Distinctive molecular genetic alterations in sporadic and familial adenomatous polyposis-associated pancreatoblastomas: frequent alterations in the APC/ β-catenin pathway and chromosome 11p. *Am J Pathol* 2001;159:1619–1627.
4. Adzick NS, Thornton PS, Stanley CA, et al. A multidisciplinary approach to the focal form of congenital hyperinsulinism leads to successful treatment by partial pancreatectomy. *J Pediatr Surg* 2004;39:270–275.
5. American Diabetes Association. Type 2 diabetes in children and adolescents. *Diabetes Care* 2000;23:381–389.
6. Asmundo A, Aragona M, Gualniera P, et al. Sudden death from hypoglycemia [Italian]. *Pathologica* 1995;87:603–616.
7. Atkinson MA, Maclaren NK. The pathogenesis of insulin-dependent diabetes mellitus. *N Engl J Med* 1994;331:1428–1436.
8. Audrézet M-P, Chen JM, Le Maréchal C, et al. Determination of the relative contribution of three genes-the cystic fibrosis transmembrane conductance regulator gene, the cationic trypsinogen gene, and the pancreatic secretory trypsin inhibitor gene-to the etiology of idiopathic chronic pancreatitis. *Eur J Hum Genet* 2002;10:100–106.
9. Babenko AP, Polak M, Cave H, et al. Activating mutations in the ABCC8 gene in neonatal diabetes mellitus. *N Engl J Med* 2006;355:456–466.
10. Bennett CL, Yoshioka R, Kiyosawa H, et al. X-linked syndrome of polyendocrinopathy, immune dysfunction, and diarrhea maps to Xp11.23-Xq13.3. *Am J Hum Genet* 2000;66:461–468.
11. Beringue F, Blondeau B, Castellotti MC, et al. Endocrine pancreas development in growth-retarded human fetuses. *Diabetes* 2002;51:385–391.
12. Bethel CA, Luquette MH, Besner GE. Cystic degeneration of heterotopic pancreas. *Pediatr Surg Int* 1998;13:428–430.
13. Biour M, Delcenserie R, Grangé J-D, et al. Pancréatotoxicité des médicaments. Première mise à jour publiée du fichier bibliographique des atteintes pancréatiques aiguës et des médicaments responsables. *Gastroenterol Clin Biol* 2001;25:1S22–1S27.

14. Bodian M, Sheldon W, Lightwood R. Congenital hypoplasia of the exocrine pancreas. *Acta Paediatr* 1964;53:282–293.
15. Boocock GR, Morrison JA, Popovic M, et al. Mutations in SBDS are associated with Shwachman-Diamond syndrome. *Nat Genet* 2003;33:97–101.
16. Borchard F, Müntefering H. Beitrag zur quantitativen Morphologie der Langerhansschen Inseln bei Früh- und Neugeborenen. *Virchows Arch [A]* 1969;346:178–198.
17. Bouwens L. Cytokeratins and cell differentiation in the pancreas. *J Pathol* 1998;184:234–239.
18. Brickwood S, Bonthron DT, Al-Gazali LI, et al. Wolcott-Rallison syndrome: pathogenic insights into neonatal diabetes from new mutation and expression studies of EIF2AK3. *J Med Genet* 2003;40:685–689.
19. Butler AE, Janson J, Bonner-Weir S, et al. β-cell deficit and increased β-cell apoptosis in humans with type 2 diabetes. *Diabetes* 2003;52: 102–110.
20. Cahill ME, Parmentier JM, Van Ruyssevelt C, et al. Pancreatic cystosis in cystic fibrosis. *Abdom Imaging* 1997;22:313–314.
21. Casanova M, Collini P, Ferrari A, et al. Solid-pseudopapillary tumor of the pancreas (Frantz tumor) in children. *Med Pediatr Oncol* 2003;41:74–76.
22. Chatila TA, Blaeser F, Ho N, et al. JM2, encoding a fork head-related protein, is mutated in X-linked autoimmunity-allergic dysregulation syndrome. *J Clin Invest* 2000;106:R75–R81.
23. Chung EM, Travis MD, Conran RM. Pancreatic tumors in children: radiologic-pathologic correlation. *Radiographics* 2006;26:1211–1238.
24. Cingolani N, Shaco-Levy R, Farruggio A, et al. Alpha-fetoprotein production by pancreatic tumors exhibiting acinar cell differentiation: study of five cases, one arising in a mediastinal teratoma. *Hum Pathol* 2000;31:938–944.
25. Claret Teruel G, Giner Muñoz MT, Plaza Martín AM, et al. Variability of immunodeficiency associated with ataxia telangiectasia and clinical evolution in 12 affected patients. *Pediatr Allergy Immunol* 2005;16: 615–618.
26. Clark A, de Koning EJ, Hattersley AT, et al. Pancreatic pathology in non-insulin dependent diabetes (NIDDM). *Diabetes Res Clin Pract* 1995;28(Suppl):S39–S47.
27. Clayton PT, Eaton S, Aynsley-Green A, et al. Hyperinsulinism in short-chain L-3-hydroxyacyl-CoA dehydrogenase deficiency reveals the importance of β-oxidation in insulin secretion. *J Clin Invest* 2001;108:457–465.
28. Cohn JA, Noone PG, Jowell PS. Idiopathic pancreatitis related to CFTR: complex inheritance and identification of a modifier gene. *J Investig Med* 2002;50:247S–255S.
29. Couce M, O'Brien TD, Moran A, et al. Diabetes mellitus in cystic fibrosis is characterized by islet amyloidosis. *J Clin Endocrinol Metab* 1996;81:1267–1272.
30. Cuesta-Muñoz AL, Huopio H, Otonkoski T, et al. Severe persistent hyperinsulinemic hypoglycemia due to a de novo glucokinase mutation. *Diabetes* 2004;53:2164–2168.
31. Daentl DL, Frias JL, Gilbert EF, et al. The Johanson-Blizzard syndrome: case report and autopsy findings. *Am J Med Genet* 1979;3:129–135.
32. Daher P, Diab N, Melki I, et al. Congenital cyst of the pancreas. Antenatal diagnosis. *Eur J Pediatr Surg* 1996;6:180–182.
33. de Lonlay P, Fournet JC, Rahier J, et al. Somatic deletion of the imprinted 11p15 region in sporadic persistent hyperinsulinemic hypoglycemia of infancy is specific of focal adenomatous hyperplasia and endorses partial pancreatectomy. *J Clin Invest* 1997;100:802–807.
34. de Lonlay P, Giurgea I, Sempoux C, et al. Dominantly inherited hyperinsulinaemic hypoglycaemia. *J Inherit Metab Dis* 2005;28:267–276.
35. de Lonlay-Debeney P, Poggi-Travert F, Fournet JC, et al. Clinical features of 52 neonates with hyperinsulinism. *N Engl J Med* 1999;340: 1169–1175.
36. DeBanto JR, Goday PS, Pedroso MR, et al. Acute pancreatitis in children. *Am J Gastroenterol* 2002;97:1726–1731.
37. DeBaun MR, King AA, White N. Hypoglycemia in Beckwith-Wiedemann syndrome. *Semin Perinatol* 2000;24:164–171.
38. DeBaun MR, Niemitz EL, McNeil DE, et al. Epigenetic alterations of H19 and LIT1 distinguish patients with Beckwith-Wiedemann syndrome with cancer and birth defects. *Am J Hum Genet* 2002;70: 604–611.
39. Delépine M, Nicolino M, Barrett T, et al. EIF2AK3, encoding translation initiation factor 2-α kinase 3, is mutated in patients with Wolcott-Rallison syndrome. *Nat Genet* 2000;25:406–409.
40. Delhaye M, Cremer M. Clinical significance of pancreas divisum. *Acta Gastroenterol Belg* 1992;55:306–313.
41. Drut R, Jones MC. Congenital pancreatoblastoma in Beckwith-Wiedemann syndrome: an emerging association. *Pediatr Pathol* 1988;8:331–339.
42. Durocher F, Faure R, Labrie Y, et al. A novel mutation in the EIF2AK3 gene with variable expressivity in two patients with Wolcott-Rallison syndrome. *Clin Genet* 2006;70:34–38.
43. Elliott M, Bayly R, Cole T, et al. Clinical features and natural history of Beckwith-Wiedemann syndrome: presentation of 74 new cases. *Clin Genet* 1994;46:168–174.
44. Elsas LJ, Endo F, Strumlauf E, et al. Leprechaunism: an inherited defect in a high-affinity insulin receptor. *Am J Hum Genet* 1985;37: 73–88.
45. Fanconi G, Uelinger E, Knauer C. Das Coeliakiesyndrom bei angeborener zystischer Pankreas fibromatose und bronchiektasien. *Wien Med Wochenschr* 1936;86:753–756.
46. Froguel P, Zouali H, Vionnet N, et al. Familial hyperglycemia due to mutations in glucokinase. Definition of a subtype of diabetes mellitus. *N Engl J Med* 1993;328:697–702.
47. Fukuzawa R, Umezawa A, Morikawa Y, et al. Nesidioblastosis and mixed hamartoma of the liver in Beckwith-Wiedemann syndrome: case study including analysis of H19 methylation and insulin-like growth factor 2 genotyping and imprinting. *Pediatr Dev Pathol* 2001;4:381–390.
48. Gavin JRI, Alberti KGMM, Davidson MB, et al. Report of the expert committee on the diagnosis and classification of diabetes mellitus. *Diabetes Care* 2003;26(Suppl 1):S5–S20.
49. Gepts W, De Mey J. Islet cell survival determined by morphology. An immunocytochemical study of the islets of Langerhans in juvenile diabetes mellitus. *Diabetes* 1978;27(Suppl 1):251–261.
50. Gershoni-Baruch R, Lerner A, Braun J, et al. Johanson-Blizzard syndrome: clinical spectrum and further delineation of the syndrome. *Am J Med Genet* 1990;35:546–551.
51. Girelli R, Bassi C, Falconi M, et al. Pancreatic cystic manifestations in von Hippel-Lindau disease. *Int J Pancreatol* 1997;22:101–109.
52. Glaser B, Kesavan P, Heyman M, et al. Familial hyperinsulinism caused by an activating glucokinase mutation. *N Engl J Med* 1998;338: 226–230.
53. Glaser B, Thornton P, Otonkoski T, et al. Genetics of neonatal hyperinsulinism. *Arch Dis Child Fetal Neonatal Ed* 2000;82:F79–F86.
54. Gloyn AL, Pearson ER, Antcliff JF, et al. Activating mutations in the gene encoding the ATP-sensitive potassium-channel subunit Kir6.2 and permanent neonatal diabetes. *N Engl J Med* 2004;350:1838–1849.
55. Goossens A, Gepts W, Saudubray JM, et al. Diffuse and focal nesidioblastosis. A clinicopathological study of 24 patients with persistent neonatal hyperinsulinemic hypoglycemia. *Am J Surg Pathol* 1989;13: 766–775.
56. Gorry MC, Gabbaizedeh D, Furey W, et al. Mutations in the cationic trypsinogen gene are associated with recurrent acute and chronic pancreatitis. *Gastroenterology* 1997;113:1063–1068.
57. Guillou L, Nordback P, Gerber C, et al. Ductal adenocarcinoma arising in a heterotopic pancreas situated in a hiatal hernia. *Arch Pathol Lab Med* 1994;118:568–571.
58. Hardy OT, Hernandez-Pampaloni M, Saffer JR, et al. Diagnosis and localization of focal congenital hyperinsulinism by 18F-fluorodopa PET scan. *J Pediatr* 2007;150:140–145.
59. Hashida Y, Jaffe R, Yunis EJ. Pancreatic pathology in trisomy 13: specificity of the morphologic lesion. *Pediatr Pathol* 1983;1:169–178.
60. Hattersley AT. Maturity-onset diabetes of the young: clinical heterogeneity explained by genetic heterogeneity. *Diabet Med* 1998;15:15–24.

61. Heltzer ML, Choi JK, Ochs HD, et al. A potential screening tool for IPEX syndrome. *Pediatr Dev Pathol* 2007;10:98–105.
62. Henneveld HT, van Lingen RA, Hamel BC, et al. Perlman syndrome: four additional cases and review. *Am J Med Genet* 1999;86:439–446.
63. Holemans K, Aerts L, Van Assche FA. Lifetime consequences of abnormal fetal pancreatic development. *J Physiol* 2003;547:11–20.
64. Horikawa Y, Iwasaki N, Hara M, et al. Mutation in hepatocyte nuclear factor-1 β gene (TCF2) associated with MODY. *Nat Genet* 1997;17:384–385.
65. Howes N, Lerch MM, Greenhalf W, et al. Clinical and genetic characteristics of hereditary pancreatitis in Europe. *Clin Gastroenterol Hepatol* 2004;2:252–261.
66. Høyer A. Lipomatous pseudohypertrophy of the pancreas with complete absence of exocrine tissue. *J Pathol Bacteriol* 1949;61:93–100.
67. Hruban RH, Pitman MB, Klimstra DS. Acinar neoplasms. In: *Tumors of the pancreas, Fascicle 6*. Washington, DC: American Registry of Pathology, 2007;191–218.
68. Hruban RH, Pitman MB, Klimstra DS. Pancreatoblastoma. In: *Tumors of the pancreas, Fascicle 6*. Washington, DC: American Registry of Pathology, 2007;219–229.
69. Hruban RH, Pitman MB, Klimstra DS. Solid-pseudopapillary neoplasms. In: *Tumor of the pancreas, Fascicle 6*. Washington, DC: American Registry of Pathology, 2007;231–250.
70. Hull RL, Westermark GT, Westermark P, et al. Islet amyloid: a critical entity in the pathogenesis of type 2 diabetes. *J Clin Endocrinol Metab* 2004;89:3629–3643.
71. Hultquist GT, Olding LB. Endocrine pathology of infants of diabetic mothers. A quantitative morphological analysis including a comparison with infants of iso-immunized and of non-diabetic mothers. *Acta Endocrinol Suppl (Copenh)* 1981;241:1–202.
72. Huopio H, Reimann F, Ashfield R, et al. Dominantly inherited hyperinsulinism caused by a mutation in the sulfonylurea receptor type 1. *J Clin Invest* 2000;106:897–906.
73. Hussain K, Cosgrove KE, Shepherd RM, et al. Hyperinsulinemic hypoglycemia in Beckwith-Wiedemann syndrome due to defects in the function of pancreatic β-cell adenosine triphosphate-sensitive potassium channels. *J Clin Endocrinol Metab* 2005;90:4376–4382.
74. Imrie JR, Fagan DG, Sturgess JM. Quantitative evaluation of the development of the exocrine pancreas in cystic fibrosis and control infants. *Am J Pathol* 1979;95:697–707.
75. Ishikawa O, Ishiguro S, Ohhigashi H, et al. Solid and papillary neoplasm arising from an ectopic pancreas in the mesocolon. *Am J Gastroenterol* 1990;85:597–601.
76. Jaffe R, Hashida Y, Yunis EJ. Pancreatic pathology in hyperinsulinemic hypoglycemia of infancy. *Lab Invest* 1980;42:356–365.
77. Jaffe R, Hashida Y, Yunis EJ. The endocrine pancreas of the neonate and infant. *Perspect Pediatr Pathol* 1982;7:137–165.
78. Jenson AB, Rosenberg HS, Notkins AL. Pancreatic islet-cell damage in children with fatal viral infections. *Lancet* 1980;2(8190):354–358.
79. Johanson A, Blizzard R. A syndrome of congenital aplasia of the alae nasi, deafness, hypothyroidism, dwarfism, absent permanent teeth, and malabsorption. *J Pediatr* 1971;79:982–987.
80. Jones KL. Beckwith-Wiedemann syndrome (exomphalos-macroglossia-gigantism syndrome). In: *Smith's recognizable patterns of human malformation*. Philadelphila, PA: Elsevier Saunders, 2006;174–175.
81. Jones KL. Schwachman-Diamond syndrome. In: *Smith's recognizable patterns of human malformation*. Philadelphia, PA: Elsevier Saunders, 2006;436.
82. Judson K, Argani P. Intraductal spread by metastatic islet cell tumor (well-differentiated pancreatic endocrine neoplasm) involving the breast of a child, mimicking a primary mammary carcinoma. *Am J Surg Pathol* 2006;30:912–918.
83. Kahler SG, Sherwood WG, Woolf D, et al. Pancreatitis in patients with organic acidemias. *J Pediatr* 1994;124:239–243.
84. Kahn BB, Flier JS. Obesity and insulin resistance. *J Clin Invest* 2000;106:473–481.
85. Kahn E, Anderson VM, Greco MA, et al. Pancreatic disorders in pediatric acquired immune deficiency syndrome. *Hum Pathol* 1995;26:765–770.
86. Kassem SA, Ariel I, Thornton PS, et al. p57^{KIP2} expression in normal islet cells and in hyperinsulinism of infancy. *Diabetes* 2001;50:2763–2769.
87. Keim V, Teich N, Mossner J. Trypsinogen mutations in hereditary pancreatitis: which nomenclature is convenient? *Gut* 2000;46:873.
88. Kennedy SM, Hashida Y, Malatack JJ. Polycystic kidneys, pancreatic cysts, and cystadenomatous bile ducts in the oral-facial-digital syndrome type I. *Arch Pathol Lab Med* 1991;115:519–523.
89. Klensang U, Hagemann S, Saeger W, et al. Morphology, immunohistochemistry and morphometry of pancreatic islets in cases of sudden infant death syndrome (SIDS). *Int J Legal Med* 1997;110:199–203.
90. Klimstra DS, Adsay NV. Benign and malignant tumors of the pancreas. In: Odze RD, Goldblum JR, Crawford JM, eds. *Surgical pathology of the GI tract, liver, biliary tract, and pancreas* Philadelphia, PA: Saunders, 2004;699–736.
91. Klimstra DS, Heffess CS, Oertel JE, et al. Acinar cell carcinoma of the pancreas. A clinicopathologic study of 28 cases. *Am J Surg Pathol* 1992;16:815–837.
92. Klimstra DS, Wenig BM, Adair CF, et al. Pancreatoblastoma. A clinicopathologic study and review of the literature. *Am J Surg Pathol* 1995;19:1371–1389.
93. Klimstra DS, Wenig BM, Heffess CS. Solid-pseudopapillary tumor of the pancreas: a typically cystic carcinoma of low malignant potential. *Semin Diagn Pathol* 2000;17:66–80.
94. Klöppel G. Progression from acute to chronic pancreatitis. A pathologist's view. *Surg Clin North Am* 1999;79:801–814.
95. Klöppel G, Löhr M, Habich K, et al. Islet pathology and the pathogenesis of type 1 and type 2 diabetes mellitus revisited. *Surv Synth Pathol Res* 1985;4:110–125.
96. Kosmahl M, Seada LS, Jänig U, et al. Solid-pseudopapillary tumor of the pancreas: its origin revisited. *Virchows Arch* 2000;436:473–480.
97. Lai EC, Tompkins RK. Heterotopic pancreas. Review of a 26 year experience. *Am J Surg* 1986;151:697–700.
98. Lainakis N, Antypas S, Panagidis A, et al. Annular pancreas in two consecutive siblings: an extremely rare case. *Eur J Pediatr Surg* 2005;15:364–368.
99. Langlois NE, Krukowski ZH, Miller ID. Pancreatic tissue in a lateral cervical cyst attached to the thyroid gland–a presumed foregut remnant. *Histopathology* 1997;31:378–380.
100. Larson RS, Rudloff MA, Liapis H, et al. The Ivemark syndrome: prenatal diagnosis of an uncommon cystic renal lesion with heterogeneous associations. *Pediatr Nephrol* 1995;9:594–598.
101. Le Bodic L, Schnee M, Georgelin T, et al. An exceptional genealogy for hereditary chronic pancreatitis. *Dig Dis Sci* 1996;41:1504–1510.
102. Lebenthal E, Antonowicz I, Shwachman H. Enterokinase and trypsin activities in pancreatic insufficiency and diseases of the small intestine. *Gastroenterology* 1976;70:508–512.
103. Lee PC, Lebenthal E. Prenatal and postnatal development of the human exocrine pancreas. In: Go VLW, DiMagno EP, Gardner JD, et al., eds. *The exocrine pancreas: biology, pathobiology and diseases*. New York: Raven Press, 1993;57–73.
104. Levy J. The gastrointestinal tract in Down syndrome. *Prog Clin Biol Res* 1991;373:245–256.
105. Levy-Lahad E, Wildin RS. Neonatal diabetes mellitus, enteropathy, thrombocytopenia, and endocrinopathy: Further evidence for an X-linked lethal syndrome. *J Pediatr* 2001;138:577–580.
106. Löhr M, Goertchen P, Nizze H, et al. Cystic fibrosis associated islet changes may provide a basis for diabetes. An immunocytochemical and morphometrical study. *Virchows Arch A Pathol Anat Histopathol* 1989;414:179–185.
107. Mackie AD, Thornton SJ, Edenborough FP. Cystic fibrosis-related diabetes. *Diabet Med* 2003;20:425–436.
108. Malecki MT, Jhala US, Antonellis A, et al. Mutations in NEUROD1 are associated with the development of type 2 diabetes mellitus. *Nat Genet* 1999;23:323–328.

109. McDevitt H. The role of MHC class II molecules in the pathogenesis and prevention of type I diabetes. *Adv Exp Med Biol* 2001;490:59–66.
110. Meda P. Gap junction involvement in secretion: the pancreas experience. *Clin Exp Pharmacol Physiol* 1996;23:1053–1057.
111. Mehta DI, Wang HH, Akins RE, et al. Isolated pancreatic amylase deficiency: probable error in maturation. *J Pediatr* 2000;136: 844–846.
112. Meier JJ, Bhushan A, Butler AE, et al. Sustained beta cell apoptosis in patients with long-standing type 1 diabetes: indirect evidence for islet regeneration? *Diabetologia* 2005;48:2221–2228.
113. Menon RK, Cohen RM, Sperling MA, et al. Transplacental passage of insulin in pregnant women with insulin-dependent diabetes mellitus. Its role in fetal macrosomia. *N Engl J Med* 1990;323:309–315.
114. Milner RD. Nesidioblastosis unravelled. *Arch Dis Child* 1996;74:369–372.
115. Milner RD, Dinsdale F, Wirdnam PK, et al. Pancreatic endocrine cell fractions in erythroblastosis fetalis. *Diabetes* 1983;32:313–315.
116. Milner RD, Wirdnam PK, Tsanakas J. Quantitative morphology of B, A, D, and PP cells in infants of diabetic mothers. *Diabetes* 1981;30:271–274.
117. Morikawa Y, Matsuura N, Kakudo K, et al. Pearson's marrow/pancreas syndrome: a histological and genetic study. *Virchows Arch A Pathol Anat Histopathol* 1993;423:227–231.
118. Moriscot C, Renaud W, Carrere J, et al. Developmental gene expression of trypsinogen and lipase in human fetal pancreas. *J Pediatr Gastroenterol Nutr* 1997;24:63–67.
119. Morohoshi T, Kanda M, Horie A, et al. Immunocytochemical markers of uncommon pancreatic tumors. Acinar cell carcinoma, pancreatoblastoma, and solid cystic (papillary-cystic) tumor. *Cancer* 1987;59:739–747.
120. Muguerza R, Rodriguez A, Formigo E, et al. Pancreatoblastoma associated with incomplete Beckwith-Wiedemann syndrome: case report and review of the literature. *J Pediatr Surg* 2005;40:1341–1344.
121. Nestorowicz A, Inagaki N, Gonoi T, et al. A nonsense mutation in the inward rectifier potassium channel gene, Kir6.2, is associated with familial hyperinsulinism. *Diabetes* 1997;46:1743–1748.
122. Neumann HP, Dinkel E, Brambs H, et al. Pancreatic lesions in the von Hippel-Lindau syndrome. *Gastroenterology* 1991;101:465–471.
123. Nishimata S, Kato K, Tanaka M, et al. Expression pattern of keratin subclasses in pancreatoblastoma with special emphasis on squamoid corpuscles. *Pathol Int* 2005;55:297–302.
124. Notohara K, Hamazaki S, Tsukayama C, et al. Solid-pseudopapillary tumor of the pancreas: immunohistochemical localization of neuroendocrine markers and CD10. *Am J Surg Pathol* 2000;24: 1361–1371.
125. Oppenheimer EH, Esterly JR. Pathology of cystic fibrosis review of the literature and comparison with 146 autopsied cases. *Perspect Pediatr Pathol* 1975;2:241–278.
126. Otonkoski T, Kaminen N, Ustinov J, et al. Physical exercise-induced hyperinsulinemic hypoglycemia is an autosomal-dominant trait characterized by abnormal pyruvate-induced insulin release. *Diabetes* 2003;52:199–204.
127. Otonkoski T, Nanto-Salonen K, Seppanen M, et al. Noninvasive diagnosis of focal hyperinsulinism of infancy with [18F]-DOPA positron emission tomography. *Diabetes* 2006;55:13–18.
128. Pearson HA, Lobel JS, Kocoshis SA, et al. A new syndrome of refractory sideroblastic anemia with vacuolization of marrow precursors and exocrine pancreatic dysfunction. *J Pediatr* 1979;95:976–984.
129. Peranteau WH, Bathaii SM, Pawel B, et al. Multiple ectopic lesions of focal islet adenomatosis identified by positron emission tomography scan in an infant with congenital hyperinsulinism. *J Pediatr Surg* 2007;42:188–192.
130. Pietropaolo M, Eisenbarth GS. Autoantibodies in human diabetes. *Curr Dir Autoimmun* 2001;4:252–282.
131. Polak M, Shield J. Neonatal and very-early-onset diabetes mellitus. *Semin Neonatol* 2004;9:59–65.
132. Powell BR, Buist NR, Stenzel P. An X-linked syndrome of diarrhea, polyendocrinopathy, and fatal infection in infancy. *J Pediatr* 1982;100:731–737.
133. Quest L, Lombard M. Pancreas divisum: opinio divisa. *Gut* 2000;47:317–319.
134. Rahier J, Guiot Y, Sempoux C. Persistent hyperinsulinaemic hypoglycaemia of infancy: a heterogeneous syndrome unrelated to nesidioblastosis. *Arch Dis Child Fetal Neonatal Ed* 2000;82:F108–F112.
135. Rahier J, Sempoux C, Fournet JC, et al. Partial or near-total pancreatectomy for persistent neonatal hyperinsulinaemic hypoglycaemia: the pathologist's role. *Histopathology* 1998;32:15–19.
136. Rahier J, Wallon J, Gepts W, et al. Localization of pancreatic polypeptide cells in a limited lobe of the human neonate pancreas: remnant of the ventral primordium? *Cell Tissue Res* 1979;200:359–366.
137. Rebhandl W, Felberbauer FX, Puig S, et al. Solid-pseudopapillary tumor of the pancreas (Frantz tumor) in children: report of four cases and review of the literature. *J Surg Oncol* 2001;76:289–296.
138. Riordan JR, Rommens JM, Kerem B, et al. Identification of the cystic fibrosis gene: cloning and characterization of complementary DNA. *Science* 1989;245:1066–1073.
139. Rogers JC, Harris DJ, Holder T. Annular pancreas in a mother and daughter. *Am J Med Genet* 1993;45:116.
140. Rosenberg AM, Haworth JC, Degroot GW, et al. A case of leprechaunism with severe hyperinsulinemia. *Am J Dis Child* 1980;134: 170–175.
141. Rowlands CG, Hwang WS. Cytomegaly of pancreatic D cells in triploidy. *Pediatr Pathol Lab Med* 1998;18:49–55.
142. Rozin L, Perper JA, Jaffe R, et al. Sudden unexpected death in childhood due to unsuspected diabetes mellitus. *Am J Forensic Med Pathol* 1994;15:251–256.
143. Russo P, O'Regan S. Visceral pathology of hereditary tyrosinemia type I. *Am J Hum Genet* 1990;47:317–324.
144. Ryan A, Lafnitzegger JR, Lin DH, et al. Myoepithelial hamartoma of the duodenal wall. *Virchows Arch* 1998;432:191–194.
145. Sahin-Tóth M, Tóth M. Gain-of-function mutations associated with hereditary pancreatitis enhance autoactivation of human cationic trypsinogen. *Biochem Biophys Res Commun* 2000;278:286–289.
146. Seemayer TA, Osborne C, de Chadarevian JP. Shock-related injury of pancreatic islets of Langerhans in newborn and young infants. *Hum Pathol* 1985;16:1231–1234.
147. Seifert G. Congenital anomalies. In: Klöppel G, Heitz PU, eds. *Pancreatic pathology*. New York: Churchill Livingstone, 1984; 22–26.
148. Sempoux C, Guiot Y, Dubois D, et al. Human type 2 diabetes: morphological evidence for abnormal beta-cell function. *Diabetes* 2001;50(Suppl 1):S172–S177.
149. Sempoux C, Guiot Y, Dubois D, et al. Pancreatic B-cell proliferation in persistent hyperinsulinemic hypoglycemia of infancy: an immunohistochemical study of 18 cases. *Mod Pathol* 1998;11:444–449.
150. Sempoux C, Guiot Y, Jaubert F, et al. Focal and diffuse forms of congenital hyperinsulinism: the keys for differential diagnosis. *Endocr Pathol* 2004;15:241–246.
151. Shield JP, Gardner RJ, Wadsworth EJ, et al. Aetiopathology and genetic basis of neonatal diabetes. *Arch Dis Child Fetal Neonatal Ed* 1997;76:F39–F42.
152. Shorter NA, Glick RD, Klimstra DS, et al. Malignant pancreatic tumors in childhood and adolescence: The Memorial Sloan-Kettering experience, 1967 to present. *J Pediatr Surg* 2002;37:887–892.
153. Shwachman H, Diamond LK, Oski FA, et al. The syndrome of pancreatic insufficiency and bone marrow dysfunction. *J Pediatr* 1964;65:645–663.
154. Silver MM, Valberg LS, Cutz E, et al. Hepatic morphology and iron quantitation in perinatal hemochromatosis. Comparison with a large perinatal control population, including cases with chronic liver disease. *Am J Pathol* 1993;143:1312–1325.
155. Simons-Ling N, Schachner L, Penneys N, et al. Childhood systemic lupus erythematosus. Association with pancreatitis, subcutaneous fat necrosis, and calcinosis cutis. *Arch Dermatol* 1983;119:491–494.

156. Smith OP, Hann IM, Chessells JM, et al. Haematological abnormalities in Shwachman-Diamond syndrome. *Br J Haematol* 1996;94: 279–284.
157. Soejima K, Landing BH. Pancreatic islets in older patients with cystic fibrosis with and without diabetes mellitus: morphometric and immunocytologic studies. *Pediatr Pathol* 1986;6:25–46.
158. Stanley CA. Hyperinsulinism in infants and children. *Pediatr Clin North Am* 1997;44:363–374.
159. Stanley CA. Advances in diagnosis and treatment of hyperinsulinism in infants and children. *J Clin Endocrinol Metab* 2002;87:4857–4859.
160. Stanley CA, Lieu YK, Hsu BY, et al. Hyperinsulinism and hyperammonemia in infants with regulatory mutations of the glutamate dehydrogenase gene. *N Engl J Med* 1998;338:1352–1357.
161. Stanley CA, Thornton PS, Ganguly A, et al. Preoperative evaluation of infants with focal or diffuse congenital hyperinsulinism by intraoperative acute insulin response tests and selective pancreatic arterial calcium stimulation. *J Clin Endocrinol Metab* 2004;89:288–296.
162. Steigman CK, Uri AK, Chatten J, et al. Beckwith-Wiedemann syndrome with unusual hepatic and pancreatic features: a case expanding the phenotype. *Pediatr Pathol* 1990;10:593–600.
163. Stimec B, Bulajic M, Korneti V, et al. Ductal morphometry of ventral pancreas in pancreas divisum. Comparison between clinical and anatomical results. *Ital J Gastroenterol* 1996;28:76–80.
164. Stoffers DA, Stanojevic V, Habener JF. Insulin promoter factor-1 gene mutation linked to early-onset type 2 diabetes mellitus directs expression of a dominant negative isoprotein. *J Clin Invest* 1998;102: 232–241.
165. Stoffers DA, Zinkin NT, Stanojevic V, et al. Pancreatic agenesis attributable to a single nucleotide deletion in the human IPF1 gene coding sequence. *Nat Genet* 1997;15:106–110.
166. Suchi M, MacMullen CM, Thornton PS, et al. Molecular and immunohistochemical analyses of the focal form of congenital hyperinsulinism. *Mod Pathol* 2006;19:122–129.
167. Suchi M, Thornton PS, Adzick NS, et al. Congenital hyperinsulinism: intraoperative biopsy interpretation can direct the extent of pancreatectomy. *Am J Surg Pathol* 2004;28:1326–1335.
168. Suda K. Hemosiderin deposition in the pancreas. *Arch Pathol Lab Med* 1985;109:996–999.
169. Suda K. Immunohistochemical and gross dissection studies of annular pancreas. *Acta Pathol Jpn* 1990;40:505–508.
170. Tadokoro H, Kozu T, Toki F, et al. Embryological fusion between the ducts of the ventral and dorsal primordia of the pancreas occurs in two manners. *Pancreas* 1997;14:407–414.
171. Teich N, Hoffmeister A, Keim V. Nomenclature of trypsinogen mutations in hereditary pancreatitis. *Hum Mutat* 2000;15:197–198.
172. Teich N, Ockenga J, Keim V, et al. Genetic risk factors in chronic pancreatitis. *J Gastroenterol* 2002;37:1–9.
173. Teich N, Rosendahl J, Tóth M, et al. Mutations of human cationic trypsinogen (PRSS1) and chronic pancreatitis. *Hum Mutat* 2006;27:721–730.
174. Temple IK, Shield JP. Transient neonatal diabetes, a disorder of imprinting. *J Med Genet* 2002;39:872–875.
175. Thomas PM, Cote GJ, Wohllk N, et al. Mutations in the sulfonylurea receptor gene in familial persistent hyperinsulinemic hypoglycemia of infancy. *Science* 1995;268:426–429.
176. Thornton CM, Carson DJ, Stewart FJ. Autopsy findings in the Wolcott-Rallison syndrome. *Pediatr Pathol Lab Med* 1997;17:487–496.
177. Tofé S, Moreno JC, Maiz L, et al. Insulin-secretion abnormalities and clinical deterioration related to impaired glucose tolerance in cystic fibrosis. *Eur J Endocrinol* 2005;152:241–247.
178. Torra R, Alos L, Ramos J, et al. Renal-hepatic-pancreatic dysplasia: an autosomal recessive malformation. *J Med Genet* 1996;33:409–412.
179. Toth T, Bokay J, Szonyi L, et al. Detection of mtDNA deletion in Pearson syndrome by two independent PCR assays from Guthrie card. *Clin Genet* 1998;53:210–213.
180. Trivedi CD, Pitchumoni CS. Drug-induced pancreatitis: an update. *J Clin Gastroenterol* 2005;39:709–716.
181. Van Assche FA, Aerts L, Holemans K, et al. The endocrine pancreas in nonimmune hydrops fetalis. *Am J Obstet Gynecol* 1994;171:236–238.
182. Van Assche FA, Gepts W. The cytological composition of the foetal endocrine pancreas in normal and pathological conditions. *Diabetologia* 1971;7:434–444.
183. Verloes A, Lombet J, Lambert Y, et al. Tricho-hepato-enteric syndrome: further delineation of a distinct syndrome with neonatal hemochromatosis phenotype, intractable diarrhea, and hair anomalies. *Am J Med Genet* 1997;68:391–395.
184. Vogel AM, Alesbury JM, Fox VL, et al. Complex pancreatic vascular anomalies in children. *J Pediatr Surg* 2006;41:473–478.
185. Voldsgaard P, Kryger-Baggesen N, Lisse I. Agenesis of pancreas. *Acta Paediatr* 1994;83:791–793.
186. Washington K, Gossage DL, Gottfried MR. Pathology of the pancreas in severe combined immunodeficiency and DiGeorge syndrome: acute graft-versus-host disease and unusual viral infections. *Hum Pathol* 1994;25:908–914.
187. Weinzimer SA, Stanley CA, Berry GT, et al. A syndrome of congenital hyperinsulinism and hyperammonemia. *J Pediatr* 1997;130: 661–664.
188. Werlin SL, Kugathasan S, Frautschy BC. Pancreatitis in children. *J Pediatr Gastroenterol Nutr* 2003;37:591–595.
189. Whitcomb DC. Hereditary pancreatitis: new insights into acute and chronic pancreatitis. *Gut* 1999;45:317–322.
190. Whitcomb DC, Preston RA, Aston CE, et al. A gene for hereditary pancreatitis maps to chromosome 7q35. *Gastroenterology* 1996;110:1975–1980.
191. Wildin RS, Smyk-Pearson S, Filipovich AH. Clinical and molecular features of the immunodysregulation, polyendocrinopathy, enteropathy, X linked (IPEX) syndrome. *J Med Genet* 2002;39:537–545.
192. Witt H, Luck W, Hennies HC, et al. Mutations in the gene encoding the serine protease inhibitor, Kazal type 1 are associated with chronic pancreatitis. *Nat Genet* 2000;25:213–216.
193. Yamagata K, Furuta H, Oda N, et al. Mutations in the hepatocyte nuclear factor-4α gene in maturity-onset diabetes of the young (MODY1). *Nature* 1996;384:458–460.
194. Yamagata K, Oda N, Kaisaki PJ, et al. Mutations in the hepatocyte nuclear factor-1α gene in maturity-onset diabetes of the young (MODY3). *Nature* 1996;384:455–458.
195. Yasoshima H, Nakata Y, Ohkubo E, et al. An autopsy case of pancreatic and ectopic nesidioblastosis. *Pathol Int* 2001;51:376–379.
196. Yorifuji T, Matsumura M, Okuno T, et al. Hereditary pancreatic hypoplasia, diabetes mellitus, and congenital heart disease: a new syndrome? *J Med Genet* 1994;31:331–333.
197. Zenker M, Mayerle J, Lerch MM, et al. Deficiency of UBR1, a ubiquitin ligase of the N-end rule pathway, causes pancreatic dysfunction, malformations and mental retardation (Johanson-Blizzard syndrome). *Nat Genet* 2005;37:1345–1350.
198. Zhang P, McGrath B, Li S, et al. The PERK eukaryotic initiation factor 2α kinase is required for the development of the skeletal system, postnatal growth, and the function and viability of the pancreas. *Mol Cell Biol* 2002;22:3864–3874.

CHAPTER 17

The Kidney and Lower Urinary Tract

ALIYA N. HUSAIN
THEODORE J. PYSHER

Rapid advances in the field of genetics and molecular biology are leading to a better understanding of normal embryology, congenital malformations, glomerular and tubulointerstitial diseases, and neoplasia of the kidney and lower urinary tract. Approximately one-third of all congenital malformations are found in the urogenital system, many of which are part of complex multisystem anomalies with cumulative effects that are lethal in the neonatal period (e33,e35,e37,e88). Almost 80% of congenital uropathies seen in second-trimester fetuses are associated with other anomalies—both chromosomal and nonchromosomal, either syndromic or in casual combination (e53). Malformations of the bladder are often accompanied by major anomalies of the male and female genital tract because of the inter-related embryologic development of these organ systems. Glomerular diseases, reflux nephropathy, and infections are important causes of morbidity in childhood. Although cancer of the kidney is relatively uncommon in the pediatric age group, 5-year survival from Wilms tumor has increased from 73% in patients diagnosed in 1975 to 1977 to 92% in the period 1996 to 2002 (81), thus establishing a successful model for national multicenter study groups.

EMBRYOLOGY

Functionally, the urinary and the genital systems can be divided into two entirely separate systems; however, embryologically and anatomically they are intimately interwoven. Both develop from a common mesodermal ridge (intermediate mesoderm) along the posterior wall of the abdominal cavity, and initially the excretory ducts of both systems enter a common cavity, the cloaca. In humans, three separate but overlapping renal systems form. The pronephros, which is the most caudal and nonfunctional, regresses completely by the end of the 4th week of gestation, during which time the first excretory tubules of the mesonephros appear that may function for a short period. While the caudal tubules are still differentiating, the cranial tubules and glomeruli show degenerative changes, and by the end of the second month, most have disappeared. In the male, a few of the caudal tubules and the mesonephric duct persist and participate in the formation of the genital system, but they disappear in the female, leaving a few vestigial structures only (156).

The metanephros, or permanent kidney, appears in the fifth week at the level of the upper sacral segment, with its blood supply coming from the lateral sacral branches of the aorta. By the eighth week, it "ascends" to the lumbar region, mainly secondary to differential growth of the embryo, and derives its blood supply from progressively higher levels of the aorta. In the pelvic ectopic kidney, the renal arteries arise from a lower level of the aorta or from the iliac arteries. The nephrons develop from the caudal end of the nephrogenic cord (now termed the *metanephric blastema*), while the renal excretory system (collecting duct, calyces, pelvis, and ureter) develops from the ureteric bud, which is an outgrowth of the mesonephric duct close to its entrance into the cloaca. The proximal tip or the ampulla of the ureteric bud grows dorsally and cranially, pushes the metanephric blastema, and undergoes a series of dichotomous branching, the ampulla of each of which ultimately induces nephron formation. Each division proceeds more rapidly at the poles, so that the kidney acquires its characteristic shape. The first few generations of branches coalesce to form the renal pelvis and calyces (e240).

Nephrons form from condensation of the metanephric blastema, which develops a cyst-like cavity, elongates, and folds back to become S-shaped. One end fuses with the ampulla that induced it, while at the other end a mesh of capillaries develops and invaginates the nephrogenic vesicle to form a glomerulus. The upper and middle limbs of the nephrogenic vesicle elongate and differentiate into the proximal and distal convoluted tubules and the loop of Henle.

The process of nephrogenesis can be divided into four periods (e240,e241). From 7 to 14 weeks of gestation, the ureteric bud branches dichotomously for six to eight generations, with each branch inducing the formation of a new nephron. From 14 to 22 weeks, nephron arcades are formed, with the innermost nephron formed first (juxtamedullary nephron) (eFigure 17-1). From 22 to 36 weeks, no branching of the ureteric bud occurs. The ampulla extends to the subcapsular cortex to induce four to seven nephrons (eFigure 17-2). Thus, the nephrons formed last are subcapsular (the nephrogenic zone seen in sections of fetal kidneys)

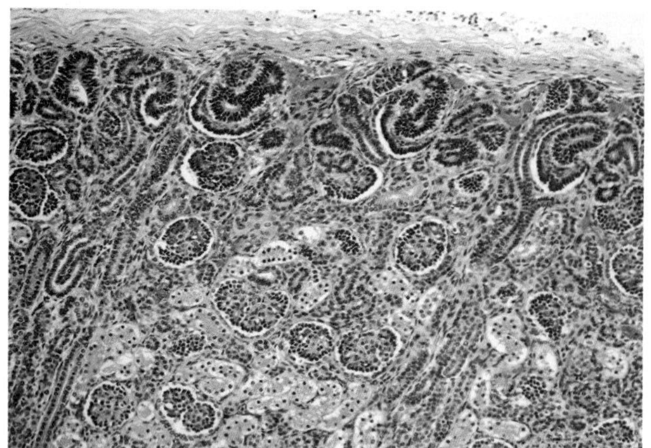

FIGURE 17-1 ■ Early third-trimester kidney with subcapsular nephrogenic zone. (Hematoxylin and eosin stain, original magnification ×100.)

(Figure 17-1). From 36 weeks of gestation through birth and up to maturity, the nephrons grow, but no new nephrons are formed. In extremely premature infants, nephrogenesis continues after birth until the kidney reaches maturity.

Evidence from studies by Potter (e251) indicates that nephrons in the developing metanephros may begin functioning as early as the eleventh or 12th week after conception. In fact, it has been suggested that the formation of a tubule fluid is essential to ensure the normal development of the renal pelvis and calyces.

Molecular Regulation of Kidney Development

As with most organs, differentiation of the kidney involves epithelial-mesenchymal interactions. Epithelium of the ureteric bud from the mesonephros interacts with mesenchyme of the metanephric blastema. The mesenchyme expresses *WT-1*, a transcription factor that makes this tissue competent to respond to induction by the ureteric bud. *WT-1* also regulates production of glial-derived neurotrophic factor (GDNF) and hepatocyte growth factor (HGF or scatter factor) by the mesenchyme, and these proteins stimulate branching and growth of the ureteric buds. The tyrosine kinase receptors RET, for GDNF, and MET, for HGF, are synthesized by the epithelium of the ureteric buds, establishing signaling pathways between the two tissues. In turn, the buds induce the mesenchyme via fibroblast growth factor 2 and bone morphogenetic protein 7. Both these growth factors block apoptosis and stimulate proliferation in the metanephric mesenchyme while maintaining production of WT1. Conversion of the mesenchyme to an epithelium for the nephron formation is also mediated by the ureteric buds, in part through modification of the extracellular matrix. Thus, fibronectin, collagen I, and collagen III are replaced with laminin and type IV collagen, characteristic of an epithelial basal lamina. In addition, the cell adhesion molecules, syndecan and E-cadherin, which are essential for condensation of the mesenchyme into an epithelium, are synthesized. Regulatory genes for conversion of the mesenchyme into an epithelium appear to involve *PAX2* and *WNT4* (156).

CONGENITAL MALFORMATIONS OF THE KIDNEY

If all malformations are considered, ranging from incidental findings with no clinical significance to major lethal anomalies, it is estimated that congenital abnormalities of the kidney and urinary tract are present in 10% of all newborns (93,98). Worldwide, a substantial percentage of children develop chronic kidney disease early in life, with congenital renal disorders such as obstructive uropathy and aplasia/hypoplasia/dysplasia being responsible for almost one-half of all cases (188). Table 17-1 lists the relative frequency of

Table 17-1 ■ RENAL MALFORMATIONS SEEN IN PEDIATRIC AUTOPSIES

Anomaly	No. of Cases		
	Series 1*	Series 2+	Total (%)
Renal agenesis, bilateral	16	13	29 (12)
Renal agenesis, unilateral	10	6	16 (6.6)
Renal dysplasia, bilateral	45	33	78 (32)
Renal dysplasia, unilateral	4	5	9 (2.1)
Renal dysplasia, unilateral, with contralateral renal agenesis	9	3	12 (5)
Autosomal recessive polycystic kidney disease	5	10	15 (6.2)
Autosomal dominant polycystic kidney disease	1	1	2 (0.8)
Renal fusion	20	12	32 (13.2)
Renal ectopia	4	1	5 (2.1)
Congenital hydronephrosis, bilateral	6	5	11 (4.5)
Congenital hydronephrosis, unilateral	4	8	12 (5)
Ureteral duplication	10	5	15 (6.2)
Renal hypoplasia	1	3	4 (1.7)
Other	0	6	6 (2.5)
Total	135	111	246 (~100)

Series 1* compiled from 1,442 consecutive autopsies performed at Minneapolis Children's Medical Center from 1977 to 1987, including stillborn infants and children younger than 1 year of age.

Series 2+ compiled from 1,242 pediatric autopsies performed at Loyola University Medical Center from 1978 to 1998, including stillbirths and children up to 18 years (Unpublished data from Aliya N. Husain, M.D.).

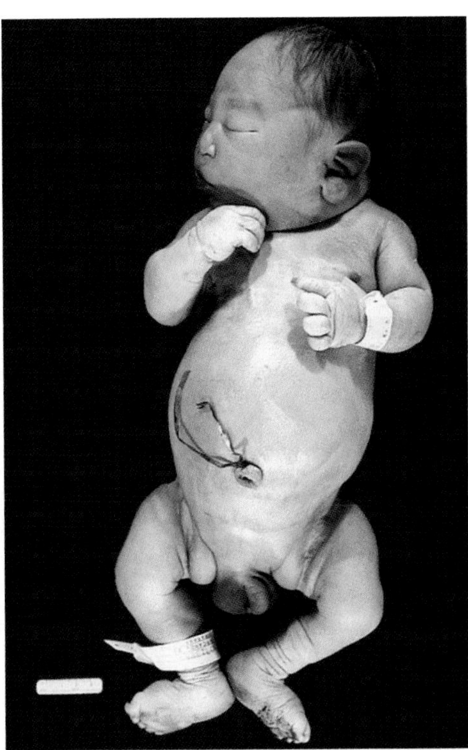

FIGURE 17-2 ■ Oligohydramnios (Potter sequence) is associated with low-set and deformed ears, beaked nose, receding chin, and lower limb positional deformity.

malformations seen in two series of pediatric autopsies—one from a children's hospital and the other from a tertiary care university medical center. Forty-one (38%) of the 107 renal malformations in series No. 2 were associated with major malformations of at least one other organ system.

A wide variety of renal malformations result in the oligohydramnios (Potter) sequence (i.e., characteristic facies, including low-set ears, beaked nose, prominent epicanthic folds, receding chin, limb deformities, growth retardation, and pulmonary hypoplasia) (Figure 17-2). These abnormalities are the result of decreased amniotic fluid rather than renal malformations per se. When these findings are associated with renal agenesis, the term *Potter syndrome* (as initially described by Potter in 1946) is used. Renal findings in children with oligohydramnios sequence are listed in Table 17-2. It has become clear that this sequence can result from even a relatively short duration of oligohydramnios, including persistent leakage of amniotic fluid (e147).

Most urogenital abnormalities are now diagnosed antenatally on high-resolution ultrasound scans. This has enabled recognition of those that are not compatible with survival and these can be managed with termination of pregnancy (82). Congenital anomalies of the kidney and urinary tract are responsible for approximately 40% of cases of childhood end-stage renal failure in the United States (150). The classification of congenital and developmental anomalies of the kidney given in Table 17-3 includes cystic diseases because many of these are inheritable disorders or are secondary to malformations of the kidney parenchyma and lower urinary tract (20).

Renal Ectopia

Permanent malposition of one or both kidneys is seen in 2% of pediatric autopsies (Table 17-1). The incidence is even higher in perinatal autopsies because renal ectopia is commonly associated with multiple other malformations. The ectopic kidney(s) may be located in the pelvis (most common), on the other side (crossed renal ectopia) with or without fusion, or even in the thorax (rare) (e223,177). Prenatal ultrasonographic diagnosis of pelvic kidney is possible, usually after 24 weeks of gestation (e210). Although renal function is normal in the neonatal period in patients with renal ectopia without other associated malformations, hydronephrosis eventually develops in 56% secondary to obstruction, reflux, or malrotation (28). Pseudocrossed renal ectopia occurs when an enlarging retroperitoneal mass displaces the kidney to the contralateral side of the abdomen.

Renal Fusion

Renal fusion, often with ectopia, was seen in 32 (1.2%) of 2,684 pediatric autopsies (Table 17-1). The most common fusion anomaly is horseshoe kidney, in which both kidneys are normally lateralized but have fused lower poles (Figure 17-3) and are located in a lower than normal position. The incidence of horseshoe kidney is reported to be 1 in 600 in the general population (156). One-third of persons with this

Table 17-2 ■ RENAL FINDINGS IN CHILDREN WITH OLIGOHYDRAMNIOS SEQUENCE

	No. of Cases		
Renal Abnormality	**Series 1**	**Series 2**	**Total (%)**
Bilateral renal agenesis	16	32	48 (30)
Bilateral cystic dysplasia	17	30	47 (29)
Unilateral agenesis with contralateral dysplasia	9	8	17 (10)
Obstructive uropathy	13	—	13 (8)
Autosomal recessive polycystic kidney disease	4	2	6 (4)
Renal ectopia and fusion	1	1	2 (1)
Autosomal dominant polycystic kidney disease	1	1	2 (1)
Other	13	13	26 (16)
Total	74	87	161 (~100)

Table 17-3 ■ CLASSIFICATION OF MALFORMATIONS OF THE KIDNEY, INCLUDING CYSTIC DISEASES

I. Renal position and form
  A. Ectopia
  B. Fusion
II. Renal quantity
  A. Agenesis (bilateral, unilateral)
  B. Hypoplasia
  C. Renal tubular dysgenesis
  D. Renomegaly
  E. Duplication
  F. Supernumerary
III. Hydronephrosis
IV. Renal dysplasia/cystic diseases (gross and/or microscopic)
  A. Renal dysplasia
    1. Sporadic (bilateral, unilateral)
    2. Hereditary
    3. With malformation syndromes
  B. Polycystic kidney disease
    1. Autosomal recessive (infantile type)
    2. Autosomal dominant (adult type)
  C. Medullary cysts
    1. Medullary sponge kidney
    2. Medullary cystic diseases
  D. Cortical cysts
    1. Glomerulocystic disease (s)
    2. Simple cysts
    3. Microcysts associated with syndromes
  E. Renal cysts with hereditary syndromes

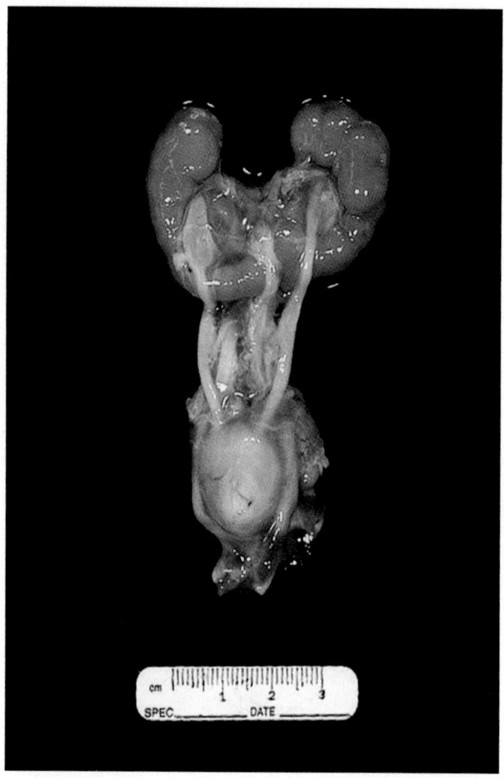

FIGURE 17-3 ■ Horseshoe kidney with fused lower poles.

condition have associated congenital malformations of other organs, including Turner syndrome (18,33,68); two-third have a major urologic complication, most of which require surgery, although newer techniques such as laparoscopic robotic-assisted management allow for minimally invasive procedures (31). Individuals with horseshoe kidney are at higher risk for the development of stones (56,61) and tumors (50,121,161), including carcinoids (151). The association of extrarenal Wilms tumor (WT) with horseshoe kidney has led to the theory that there is a nexus between the fusion of the metanephric blastema during weeks 6 and 7 of intrauterine life and that "ectopic" metanephric blastema cells may give rise to extrarenal Wilms tumor (e163). Rare cases of renal-adrenal fusion have been described, which may present as a renal mass in the upper pole (49).

Renal Agenesis/Hypoplasia

Inadequate renal tissue can be considered as a continuum, ranging from renal agenesis to subtle congenital nephron deficits. Renal agenesis (i.e., the complete absence of one or both kidneys) is commonly accompanied by other malformations of the genitourinary tract and various lower body defects, which has led to the theory that it is part of a field defect (e250). Although the exact cause of human renal agenesis/hypoplasia remains unknown, recent literature supports that one or more genetic mutations result in molecular dysregulation of nephrogenesis. Homozygous null mice for *c-Ret* (e276), *Gdnf* (e215,e248,e270), and *Gfrα-1* (e49) all exhibit bilateral renal agenesis due to the inhibition of ureteric bud growth and branching morphogenesis. Pax2 plays an integral role in the initiation and maintenance of the Ret/Gdnf pathway by not only activating the ligand of the pathway, but by also enhancing the expression of the pathway receptor Ret (36). Since an exhaustive review is beyond the scope of this chapter, one can focus on Pax2, one of the earliest genes expressed widely during fetal kidney development in the nephric duct, the metanephric mesenchyme, the ureteric bud, and in the S-shaped body. Early failure in the first two developmental stages (e.g., homozygous inactivation of Pax2) precludes formation of metanephric kidneys and causes bilateral renal agenesis, incompatible with life. Interference with the later stages affects the extent of branching morphogenesis (e.g., heterozygous Pax2 mutations). Although the resulting nephron deficits are compatible with life, they may be moderately severe and account for up to 40% of the children in dialysis and transplant units around the world. Finally, the effect of Pax2 on apoptosis in the branching ureteric bud seems to imply a quantitative process that is finely tuned. Modest changes in this program could account for subtle nephron deficits in "normal" humans and increased risk of hypertension or susceptibility to acquired renal disease later in life (44,139).

Bilateral Renal Agenesis

Uniformly fatal, bilateral renal agenesis, although less common than unilateral renal agenesis (URA), is seen more frequently in pediatric autopsies (1.1% of total autopsies in Table 17-1). The incidence of bilateral renal agenesis varies from 0.1/1,000 to 0.3/1,000 births (e310). It accounts for one-third of births with the oligohydramnios sequence (Table 17-2). The male-to-female ratio is 2.5:1. It is usually associated with severe oligohydramnios (Potter syndrome), intrauterine growth restriction, extrarenal anomalies, and malpresentation. The ureters and renal arteries are also absent, and the urinary bladder is hypoplastic or absent. The adrenals are disc-shaped secondary to lack of molding from the kidneys (eFigure 17-3). Forty percent of affected infants are stillborn, and the remainder die in the immediate postnatal period, generally of pulmonary hypoplasia (e249).

Bilateral renal agenesis is usually sporadic, although familial cases have been described (e228,e263,e274). Hereditary renal adysplasia (agenesis/dysplasia syndrome) is manifested as various combinations of unilateral or bilateral agenesis, unilateral or bilateral renal dysplasia, or dysplasia of one kidney and agenesis of the other, for which autosomal dominant inheritance with varying expression has been suggested (e44,e213). An increased prevalence of congenital renal anomalies was identified in the relatives of index patients with bilateral renal agenesis/adysplasia (14.7%) compared to controls (2.2%), with a recurrence risk of 6.2 for first-degree relatives (163).

Other reported malformations associated with bilateral renal agenesis include congenital pulmonary airway malformation type 2 (cystic adenomatoid malformation), left-heart hypoplasia (e50), sirenomelia (3), and urorectal septum malformation sequence (e325). A case of sirenomelia, limb reduction defects, cardiovascular malformations, and renal agenesis has been reported in a fetus born to an insulin-dependent diabetic mother (e197).

Bilateral renal agenesis has been described in mice homozygous for a trap mutation in the gene encoding heparan sulfate 2-sulfotransferase (Hs2st) (e45). Analysis of kidney development in Hs2st mutants reveals that the gene is not required for two early events—ureteric bud outgrowth from the Wolffian duct and initial induction of Pax2 expression in the metanephric mesenchyme. It is required, however, for mesenchymal condensation around the ureteric bud and initiation of branching morphogenesis. It is possible that the Hs2st mutant phenotype is a consequence of compromised interactions between growth factors and their signal transducing receptors.

Unilateral Renal Agenesis

URA is a common developmental defect in humans, occurring at a frequency of approximately 1 in 500 to 1,000 births (168). Although compatible with normal life, URA is still seen twice as often in pediatric autopsies (0.6%) than in the general population (0.3%) owing to its frequent association with other complex malformations (e266). The male-to-female ratio is about 1:1. Long-term follow-up of patients with URA has shown that these patients are at higher risk for the development of proteinuria, hypertension, and renal insufficiency (e8).

Malformations of the genitalia are commonly associated with URA. These include ipsilateral absence of fallopian tube, unicornuate and bicornuate uterus (e134), cysts of the epididymis and seminal vesicle (e206), agenesis of vas deferens, cystic dysplasia of testis (e330) and rete testis (e326), ectopia of vas deferens (e75), and urorectal septum malformation sequence (ambiguous genitalia with absence of perineal and anal openings) (e325). Single cases of various chromosomal anomalies have been reported in patients with URA associated with complex anomalies (e79, e 84,e175,e327,e328).

Cystic dysplasia of the testis appears to be associated consistently with renal malformations, most frequently ipsilateral renal agenesis; both conditions could be explained by failure of development of the ureteric bud (e40). Blind-ending ureteric bud remnant has been described in association with URA and renal dysplasia (e198).

Renal Hypoplasia

Renal hypoplasia, defined as histologically normal kidneys with a weight that is less than two standard deviations below the norm, is extremely rare. In the older literature, any small kidney was labeled *hypoplastic*, irrespective of the cause. Currently, small kidneys that are also dysplastic are considered with the dysplastic group, and those with scarring, inflammation, and hypertensive changes are end-stage kidneys assigned to the "underlying disease" category. Segmental renal hypoplasia (so-called Ask-Upmark kidney), which may be unilateral or bilateral and is characterized by localized atrophic scarring, is now thought to be secondary to vesicoureteral reflux and a form of reflux nephropathy.

In true renal hypoplasia, the absolute number of nephrons is reduced, possibly as a consequence of inadequate branching of the ureteric ducts that results in a decreased number (<5) of reniculi (e28,e34); however, the renal shape is normal. Unilateral hypoplasia is a sporadic condition, only rarely associated with lower urinary tract anomalies; patients present with hypertension and are predisposed to reflux nephropathy (e28). Bilateral hypoplasia results in renal insufficiency and early death in severe cases; less severe cases manifest growth retardation, chronic renal insufficiency, and mental retardation (e28).

Bilateral oligomeganephronic renal hypoplasia is a nonfamilial form of congenitally small kidneys characterized by slowly progressive renal insufficiency. The absolute number of nephrons is reduced. The glomeruli and tubules that are present are larger than normal. Infection, dysplasia, and obstructive uropathy are absent. Although several causes, including toxic factors, renal infection, vascular insufficiency, and disseminated intravascular coagulation, have been mentioned, it is not known what factors arrest the development of the metanephric renal blastema, presumably between weeks 14 and 20 of fetal life (e43). Abnormalities of chromosome 4 (e5) and mutations in hepatocyte nuclear factor-1beta (HNF-1beta) (157) and PAX2 (158) have been reported in patients with oligomeganephronia.

Significantly decreased glomerular number without decreased renal weight, thought to be due to impaired renal development in utero, has been reported in adult patients with primary hypertension (86). Considering how common primary hypertension is worldwide, this form of renal "hypoplasia" may be the most frequent renal "malformation."

Renal Tubular Dysgenesis

Familial renal tubular dysgenesis (RTD) is a rare autosomal recessive congenital disorder of renal tubular development associated with late-onset oligohydramnios, Potter sequence, skull ossification defects, and neonatal respiratory and renal failure with normal kidneys on ultrasonography (e1,e2,e255) that makes prenatal diagnosis difficult (142). In some cases, only hypoplasia of the proximal convoluted tubules is reported (167), while in others, microdissection has demonstrated marked shortening of all the nephron segments, from the glomeruli to the collecting tubules, rather than an isolated abnormality of the proximal convoluted tubules (e10). Despite the lack of normal proximal tubules, the major site of water resorption in the kidney, the principal clinical manifestations are caused by fetal and neonatal oliguria. Increased accumulation of renin has been demonstrated in the affected kidneys of three patients, which may reflect local vasoconstriction leading to reduced glomerular perfusion (e31).

The clinical, pathologic, and radiologic features of familial RTD and skull ossification defect are similar to the phenotype associated with fetal exposure to angiotensin-converting enzyme inhibitors, which suggests an abnormality of the renin-angiotensin-aldosterone system (e178,94). Mutations in the genes for the renin-angiotensin system have been reported with RTD (60,182). Tubular lesions similar to those of RTD have been described in twin-twin transfusion syndromes, acardia, unilateral lesion in renal artery stenosis, end-stage renal disease of various causes (e182), in utero exposure to nonsteroidal antiinflammatory drugs (NSAIDs) (e161) and piroxicam (e314), fetal renal vein thrombosis (e239), and severe congenital liver disease resembling neonatal hemochromatosis (e14). A similar staining pattern with various lectins suggests that at least some of the conditions studied are the result of renal ischemia, which could be acquired in utero or in early or later postnatal life (e182).

Renomegaly

The most common form of renal enlargement is compensatory hypertrophy, in which a single functioning kidney may reach twice the normal size and can be detected in utero. Bilateral renomegaly secondary to an increased number or size of normally developed nephrons is seen in growth-related disorders (172) such as Beckwith-Wiedemann syndrome (e252,e265,e291), hemihypertrophy, Perlman syndrome (e244), and congenital nephrosis of the Finnish type (e148).

Renal Duplication (Duplex Kidney)

Duplex kidneys are the most common anomalies of the upper urinary tract in childhood with an estimated incidence of 0.8% (39). The term *renal duplication* denotes the presence of two separate pelves in the same kidney accompanied by complete or partial duplication of the ureter (e227) (Figure 17-4). These kidneys usually have greater than normal number of reniculi. The anatomical and functional divisions between upper and lower moieties of duplex kidney are extremely variable. The underlying pathological condition associated with a lower moiety is usually massive vesicoureteral reflux to the lower collecting system and only rare obstruction. The nonfunctioning upper moiety is usually associated with obstructive ectopic ureter (with or without ureterocele) (39). Bilateral duplex kidneys have recently been reported in a boy with a mutation in the X-chromosomal gene (L1CAM) for cell adhesion molecule L1 (100).

Supernumerary Kidney

Supernumerary kidney is one of the rarest of renal malformations with some 80 cases reported so far (39). In addition to the normal two kidneys, an additional, usually small kidney is present within the renal fascia caudal to and completely

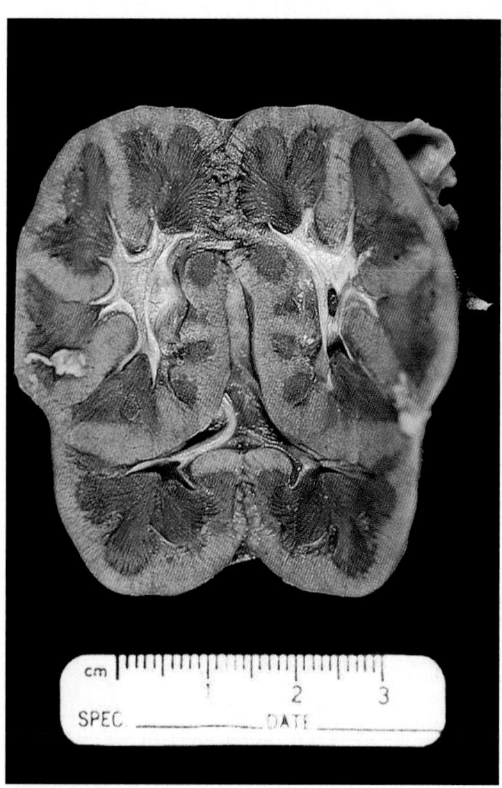

FIGURE 17-4 ■ Renal duplication (duplex kidney) with two separate pelves in the same kidney and more than the normal number of reniculi.

separate from the ipsilateral kidney (92). An ectopic ureterocele or common distal ureter may be associated with this condition (e51).

Hydronephrosis

Hydronephrosis may be congenital or acquired, unilateral or bilateral, and mild to severe. Renal dysplasia may or may not be present. Hydronephrosis is readily seen on antenatal ultrasonography but does not necessarily imply obstruction. Although most cases will resolve spontaneously (17), the probability of a significant pathology is related to the degree of pyelectasis, as seen on the third trimester ultrasound study. Criteria of obstruction are difficult to define with precision, but two that are well-accepted are size of the renal pelvis (>15 mm) and relative renal function (77,183).

Hydronephrosis is the most common cause of an abdominal mass of genitourinary tract origin in neonates (e167,e211,e318). It is most frequently caused by obstruction of the ureteral-pelvic junction, which leads to dilation of the renal pelvis and calyceal system. Depending on the severity and timing of the obstruction, the appearance of the renal parenchyma varies from relatively normal to markedly atrophic, with fibrosis and a scant chronic inflammatory infiltrate.

The specimen most commonly seen in surgical pathology is a portion of the ureteral-pelvic junction that shows remarkably little pathology on microscopic examination. When end-stage nonfunctioning hydronephrotic kidneys are removed, marked dilation of the pelvis and calyces with only microscopic foci of residual renal parenchyma can be seen (Figures 17-5 and 17-6). Neonatal hydronephrotic kidneys seen at autopsies usually have a histologically normal, although grossly compressed, cortex and medulla.

Hydronephrosis is often associated with renal dysplasia, so that the definition of these two entities often overlaps. Also, because urinary tract obstruction is a common underlying condition, it is best to consider them as the opposite ends of a spectrum. When severe obstruction occurs early in fetal development, it results in renal dysplasia; when it occurs late, one sees hydronephrosis; when it develops in between, both hydronephrosis and dysplasia are apparent to varying degrees. Hydronephrosis associated with reflux disease is discussed later in this chapter in the section on tubulointerstitial diseases.

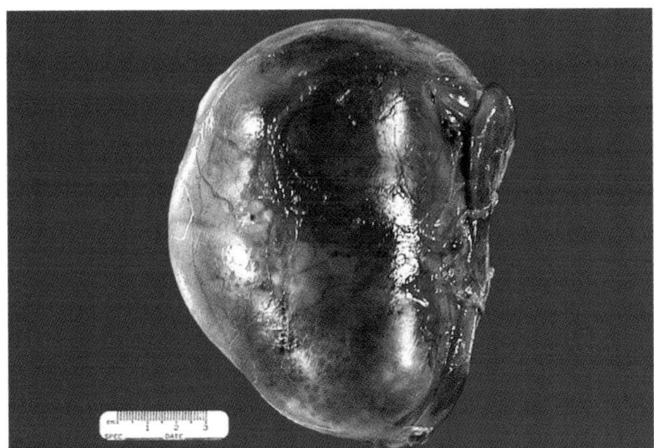

FIGURE 17-5▪Nephrectomy specimen from a 5-year-old who presented with a unilateral renal mass. The kidney appears to be one large cystic structure.

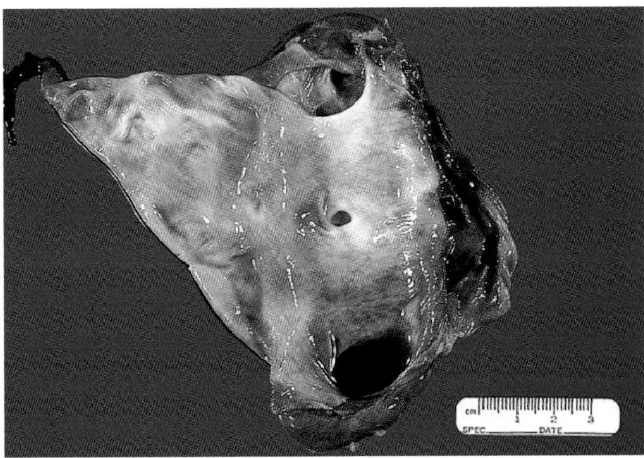

FIGURE 17-6▪Cut section of the kidney in Figure 17-5 shows a markedly dilated pelvis and calyces and very little residual renal parenchyma.

Although the vast majority of cases of hydronephrosis are sporadic, some syndromic associations have been reported (47,e247,e304,187). Hydronephrosis should also be distinguished from the rare disorder of megacalycosis (Puigvert disease), which is characterized by calyceal dilation, an increased number of calyces, hypoplasia of the pyramids of Malpighi, a normal renal pelvis, and, most importantly, normal renal function (e111).

RENAL DYSPLASIA/CYSTIC DISEASES

Cystic diseases of the kidney are a heterogeneous group of congenital (sporadic and genetic) and acquired disorders characterized by multiple cysts. In view of our better understanding of the genetic basis for some of the cystic renal diseases, the original "Potter classification" into types I to IV is no longer widely used (e242). There is no universally accepted classification for cystic diseases. Also, some authors classify renal dysplasia under abnormal renal differentiation or developmental defects (e106,93,97), whereas others place it with cystic diseases (e257,e283).

The term *multicystic* is reserved for a category of renal dysplasia characterized by multiple unilateral or bilateral cysts, while *polycystic* is conventionally used for hereditary autosomal recessive and autosomal dominant kidney diseases.

Renal Dysplasia

Multicystic dysplastic kidneys (probably more accurately called *dysgenetic* kidneys) are the most common type of malformed kidneys seen in pediatric autopsies (Table 17-1),

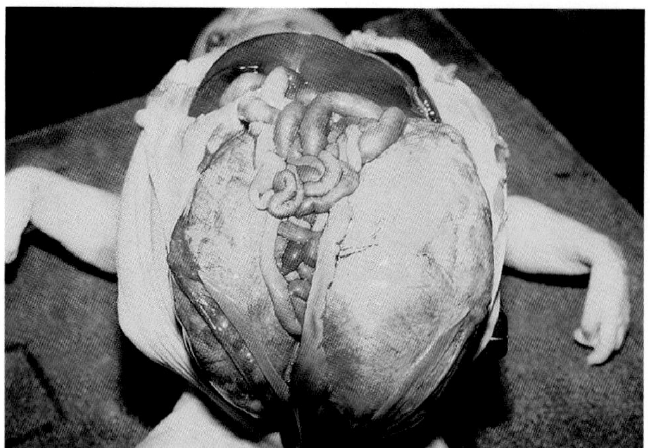

FIGURE 17-7 ■ Massively enlarged cystic dysplastic kidneys.

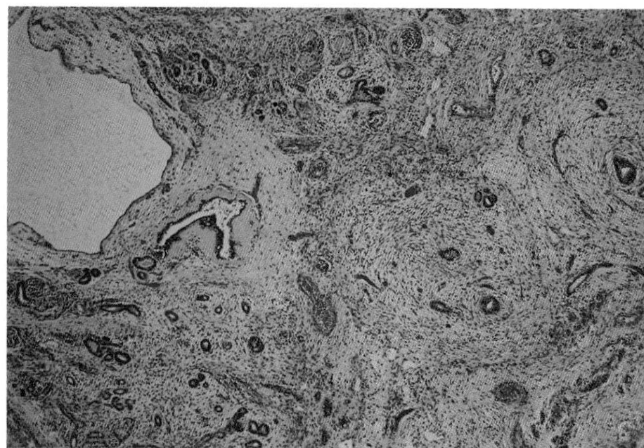

FIGURE 17-9 ■ Cystic dysplastic kidney with disorganized renal parenchyma in which immature tubules are surrounded by collarettes of condensed mesenchyme. (Hematoxylin and eosin stain, original magnification ×40.)

with bilateral dysplasia accounting for 32% and unilateral dysplasia (with or without contralateral agenesis) for 7.1% of patients with renal malformations. It may involve one or both kidneys or part of one kidney, with or without enlargement of the affected kidney and with or without grossly visible cysts. Renal dysplasia is one of the most common causes of an abdominal mass in children younger than 1 year (e129), although it may present in older children and adulthood (84).

The most common form of dysplasia is sporadic; however, a genetic contribution to its cause is being increasingly recognized (159). It is associated with obstruction of the ureteropelvic junction and bilaterally enlarged distorted kidneys (Potter type IIA) that are no longer reniform (Figure 17-7). Cysts of varying sizes can be appreciated through the capsule, and on sectioning are seen to be irregularly distributed throughout the parenchyma, with no identifiable cortex or medulla left (Figure 17-8).

The microscopic hallmark is the presence of immature dysplastic-appearing tubules surrounded by collarettes of condensed mesenchyme (Figure 17-9) that stains with periodic acid–Schiff. The tubules are lined by a single layer of cuboidal epithelium that often appears to be excessive, so that it is folded and may fill the lumen (Figure 17-10). The cells are not differentiated and tend to have a relatively high nuclear-to-cytoplasmic ratio (thus the term *dysplasia*). The basement membrane may be thick and eosinophilic. A myxoid, moderately cellular condensation of spindle cells is seen around the tubules. The remaining connective tissue is loose and contains many blood vessels, lymphatics, and peripheral nerves. Islands of immature-appearing cartilage can be identified in a majority of cases (depending on the number of sections examined), but their presence is not required for the diagnosis of dysplasia (Figure 17-11). Cysts of varying sizes with a markedly flattened lining epithelium or no identifiable lining are formed by the dilated, dysplastic tubules (positive for keratin and negative for CD31). Cysts can occur in any part of the nephron. Varying numbers of normal glomeruli and tubules can be identified between the dysplastic areas.

The terms *renal adysplasia* and *hypoplastic dysplasia* are used to describe small kidneys with extensive dysplasia

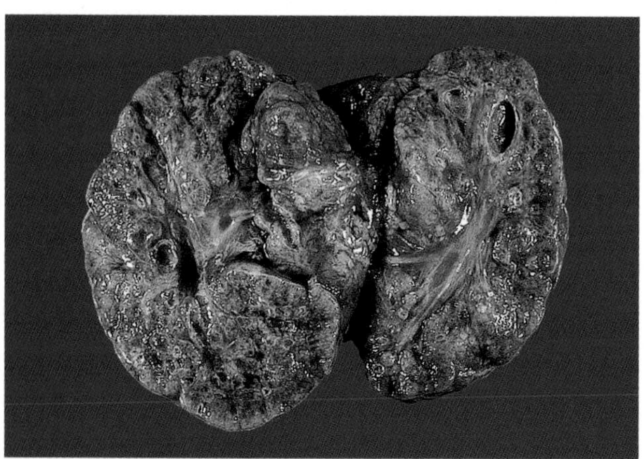

FIGURE 17-8 ■ Cut surface of cystic dysplastic kidney with multiple small, variably sized cysts involving both cortex and medulla.

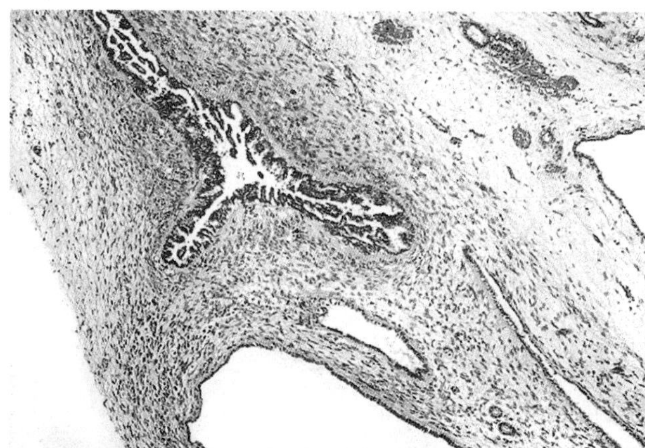

FIGURE 17-10 ■ Dysplastic tubules with an excessive amount of lining epithelium, which is thrown into papillary folds. (Hematoxylin and eosin stain, original magnification ×40.)

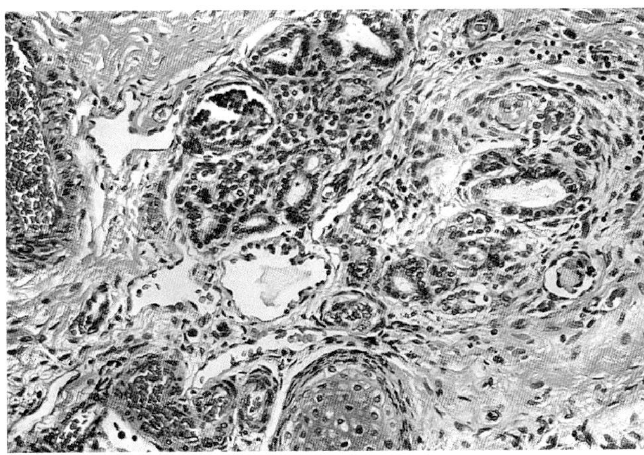

FIGURE 17-11 ■ Disorganized renal parenchyma and island of immature cartilage in cystic dysplastic kidney disease. (Hematoxylin and eosin stain, original magnification ×100.)

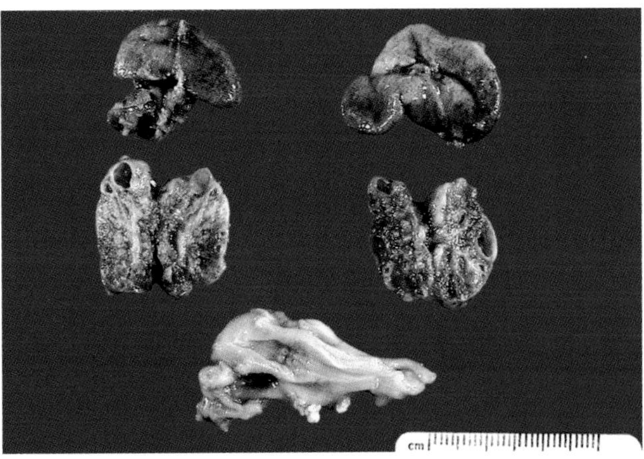

FIGURE 17-12 ■ Cystic dysplastic kidneys, shown bisected in the middle of the picture, are smaller than the adrenals above (Potter type IIB).

(Figure 17-12) that are totally nonfunctioning or minimally functioning, respectively. The essential histologic features are the same regardless of the size of the kidney or the extent of involvement.

The vast majority of sporadic multicystic dysplastic kidneys are associated with congenital urinary tract obstruction, which is often at the ureteropelvic junction but may occur at any level. Several animal models for renal dysplasia after gestational ureteral obstruction have been described (97). An ultrasonographically guided fetal kidney biopsy may rarely be used to detect the histologic features distinctive of dysplasia (e46,e114). Occasionally, open renal biopsies are performed in patients with renal insufficiency and lower urinary tract anomalies, which most often show renal dysplasia (e41). Grading of dysplasia has been described based on renal glomerular count and degree of dysplasia and correlated with lung development in patients with Potter sequence (e282).

In patients who survive the immediate postnatal period, clinical complications include hypertension, febrile urinary tract infection, vesicoureteral reflux, progressive scarring, and renal failure (8,128). In 3% to 5% of cases of dysplastic kidney, nodular renal blastema is also present (e68), and although Wilms tumor developing in dysplastic kidney has been reported (e219), a systematic review of 26 published studies with follow-up showed no increased risk of development of WT (119).

A multitude of genetic diseases, malformation syndromes, and chromosomal disorders have been described in which renal dysplasia is a major or a minor component. An excellent tabulation of these can be found at the end of Chapter 22 in Potter Pathology of the Fetus, Infant and Child (93). A brief summary is provided in Table 17-4.

Numerous genetic defects involving various transcription factors (WT-1, PAX-2, EYA-1, HNR-1β) growth factors (increased expression of TGFβ1 and increased β-catenin/SMAD1 signaling), survival factors (BCL2 and PAX-2 are upregulated in cystic epithelia in dysplastic kidneys), and adhesion molecules (KAL-1, glypican-3, FRAS1 and FREM-2) are being described in syndromic and nonsyndromic cases of renal dysplasia (97).

Winyard et al. (191) have shown that apoptosis is prominent in undifferentiated cells around dysplastic tubules, which perhaps explains the tendency of these organs to regress. In contrast, apoptosis was rare in dysplastic epithelia thought to be ureteric bud malformations. A high rate of proliferation has been demonstrated postnatally in dysplastic tubules, and PAX2, a potentially oncogenic transcription factor, is expressed in these epithelia (192). In contrast, both cell proliferation and PAX2 are downregulated during normal maturation of human collecting ducts. Ectopic expression of BCL2, which encodes a protein that prevents apoptosis during renal mesenchymal to epithelial conversion, has been observed in dysplastic kidney epithelia. Thus, dysplastic cyst formation may be understood in terms of aberrant temporal and spatial expression of master genes that are tightly regulated in normal human nephrogenesis.

Failure of normal insulinlike growth factor (IGF) and IGF-binding protein gene expression in the development of multicystic renal dysplasia suggests a role for the IGF system in the progressive histopathologic changes of this disorder (e204). Tubular epithelial production of platelet-derived growth factor A (PDGF-A) may induce collagenous matrix production by adjacent fibroblasts, and marked upregulation of PDGF-A by interstitial cells may be responsible for sustainable fibrogenic effects in the fetal kidney that contribute to renal maldevelopment (e194).

Polycystic Kidney Disease

According to current concepts, the term *polycystic kidneys* should be used to describe only two forms of inherited disease, autosomal recessive (ARPKD) and autosomal dominant (ADPKD) polycystic kidney disease, and not for any other disease in which multiple renal cysts are present. Despite different patterns of inheritance, clinical presentation and

Table 17-4 ■ SYNDROMES AND DISEASES ASSOCIATED WITH RENAL DYSPLASIA

Name	Heredity	Chromosomal Defect/Locus	Major Features	Congenital Hepatic Fibrosis
Meckel-Gruber syndrome (e392)	AR	17q22-q24	Posterior encephalocele, polydactyly, microcephaly	Yes
Zellweger syndrome (e402)	AR	UK	Peroxisomal deficiency, cerebrohepatorenal syndrome	Yes
Ivemark (II) syndrome[a] (e246,e292,e363, e409,e505)	AR	UK	Renal, pancreatic, hepatic dysplasia	Yes
Jeune syndrome (e65,e83,e316)	AR	UK	Asphyxiating thoracic dystrophy	Yes
Carnitine palmitoyltransferase deficiency (e369)	AR	UK	Myopathy	No
Short-rib polydactyly syndrome (e355)	AR	UK	Lethal skeletal dysplasias, multiple anomalies	Yes
Hereditary renal adysplasia (e169)	AD, XL	UK	URA with contralateral dysplasia	No
Nail-patella syndrome (e134)	AD	LMX1b mutation	Hypoplastic nails, absent patellae, glomerular changes	No
Tuberous sclerosis complex (e254,e514,e553)	AD	TSC1:9q34 TSC2:16p13.3	Tumors of skin, brain, heart, and kidney	No
von Hippel-Lindau syndrome (e364) carcinoma, pheochromocytoma, pancreatic islet cell tumors	AD mutations	VHL gene	Retinal and CNS hemangioblastomas, renal cysts-clear cell carcinoma	No
Beckwith-Wiedemann syndrome (e307,e394)	Usually sporadic	11p15.5 alterations	Organomegaly, nephroblastomatosis, WT	No
DiGeorge syndrome (e453)	Sporadic	DGS1 del(22q11) DGS2 del(10p)	Hypoplasia of thymus and aortic arch defects	No
Prune-belly sequence	Sporadic	UK	Deficient abdominal wall musculature, urinary tract dilation, cryptorchism	No
Trisomy 13, 18, 21 (e368)	Risk factor: advanced maternal age	13,18,21		No
Fetal alcohol syndrome (e534)	In utero exposure	UK	CNS dysfunction, growth deficits	No
Diabetic embryopathy (e81)	In utero exposure	UK	Macrosomia, congenital malformations, stillbirth	No

[a]Not to be confused with asplenia and cardiac malformations, also known as *Ivemark (I) syndrome.*
AR, autosomal recessive; AD, autosomal dominant; XL, X-linked; UK, unknown; CNS, central nervous system.

typical appearance of the kidneys, these two diseases have some similarities. Both diseases are caused by mutations in proteins located in primary cilia resulting in renal concentrating defect and both are characterized by increased rates of tubular epithelial proliferation and apoptosis (181). Elucidation of the pathogenic mechanisms of PKDs has been aided by the availability of several animal models. Rodent models have arisen by spontaneous mutation, random mutagenesis, transgenic technologies, or gene-specific targeting. Many of the proteins encoded by these mutated genes are expressed in the primary cilium or the centrosome—indicating the importance of the ciliary–centrosomal axis to normal tubular epithelial cell differentiation—or at sites of cell–cell or cell–matrix adhesion. Cytogenesis results from loss-of-function mutations in these genes or from loss-of function or gain-of-function mutations in genes that encode downstream signaling molecules and transcription factors in the cystogenic pathway (180).

Autosomal Recessive Polycystic Kidney Disease

ARPKD is rare, with an incidence of 1 in 20,000 live births and extreme variability in its severity. The gene abnormality has been mapped to the short arm of chromosome 6 named *polycystic kidney and hepatic disease* (PKHD1) *gene* because of the consistent hepatic involvement. The PKHD1 gene (6p12.2) and related protein named *polyductin* or *fibrocystin* are highly expressed in the epithelial cells of the collecting ducts and to a lesser extent in the biliary ducts and pancreas. Analogous to autosomal dominant PKD, polyductin (fibrocystin) localizes in the primary cilia of renal epithelial cells (20). Almost every vertebrate cell has a specialized cell surface projection called a primary cilium. Although these structures were first described more than a century ago, the full scope of their functions remains poorly understood. There is emerging evidence that in addition to their well-established roles in sight, smell, and mechanosensation, primary cilia are key participants in intercellular signaling. This new appreciation of primary cilia as cellular antennae that sense a wide variety of signals could help explain why ciliary defects underlie such a wide range of human disorders, including retinal degeneration, polycystic kidney disease, Bardet-Biedl syndrome, and neural tube defects (170).

In ARPKD, nephrogenesis proceeds normally, and the earliest abnormality involves the medullary ducts. Oligohydramnios occurs subsequently (usually before 20 to 21 weeks of gestation). These observations suggest that in severe fetal ARPKD, medullary collecting duct dilation occurs first and is successively followed by cortical collecting duct dilation, increased renal echogenicity, and diminution of urine production (e119).

Thirty to 50% of patients present with oligohydramnios (Potter sequence): massively enlarged, symmetric, reniform kidneys (Figure 17-13); and pulmonary hypoplasia. Death occurs in the perinatal period. The gross and microscopic hallmark is the presence of tubular cysts with a diameter of 1 to 2 mm arranged radially. The cysts are uniformly distributed and can be appreciated through the capsule of the markedly enlarged kidneys, which retain their shape (Figure 17-14). On cut section, the cortex and the medulla are often unrecognizable. The cysts represent tubular dilation of presumably normally formed collecting ducts; normal glomeruli and tubules are seen between the cysts (Figure 17-15). In the medulla, the cysts are more rounded. Significant fibrosis, inflammation, and obstruction are absent.

In cases with a later presentation, the degree of renal enlargement is less and the cystic change is less diffuse. However, all forms of ARPKD are associated with congenital hepatic fibrosis, more recently termed *ductal plate malformation* (see Chapter 15). Dilation of the interlobular bile ducts is associated with a variable degree of portal fibrosis (e78).

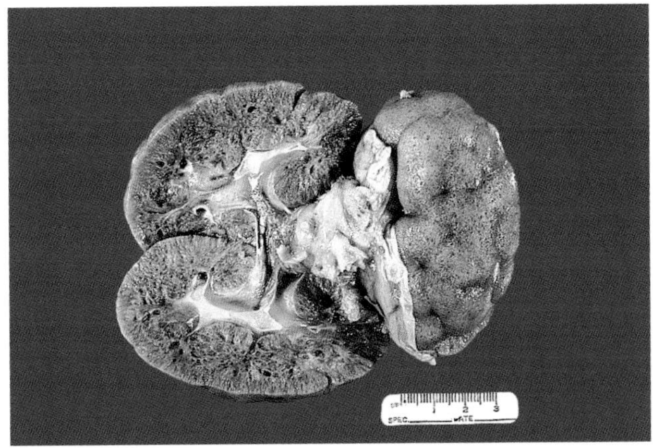

FIGURE 17-14 ■ Cysts of autosomal recessive polycystic kidney disease can be appreciated on the cortical surface. The cut section shows radially oriented cysts in the cortex and more rounded cysts in the medulla.

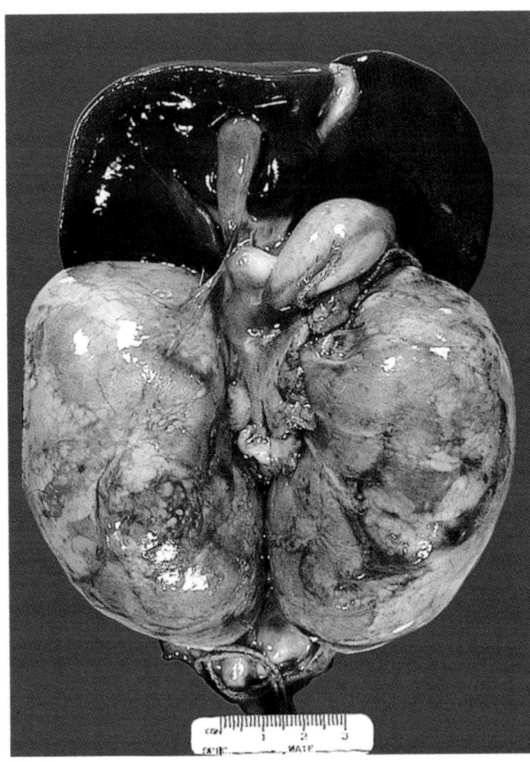

FIGURE 17-13 ■ Autosomal recessive polycystic kidney disease with massively enlarged symmetric reniform kidneys.

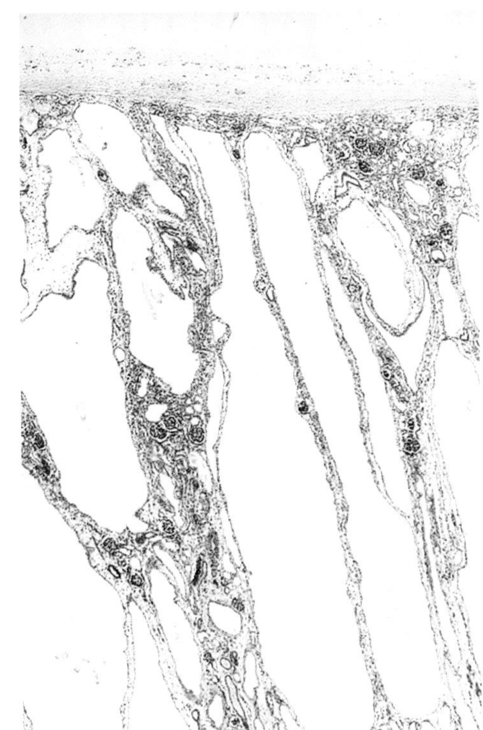

FIGURE 17-15 ■ Radially arranged cysts of autosomal recessive polycystic kidney disease. Normal glomeruli and tubules are seen between the cysts. (Hematoxylin and eosin stain, original magnification ×40.)

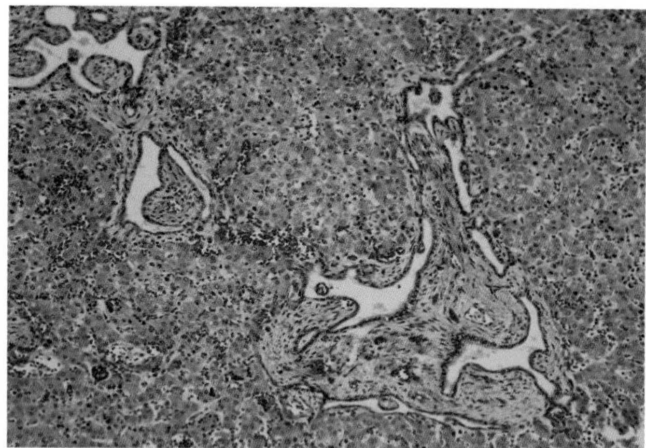

FIGURE 17-16 ▪ Ductal plate malformation of the liver with expanded portal area, peripheral tortuous dilated bile ducts, and blood vessels in the middle. (Hematoxylin and eosin stain, original magnification ×40.)

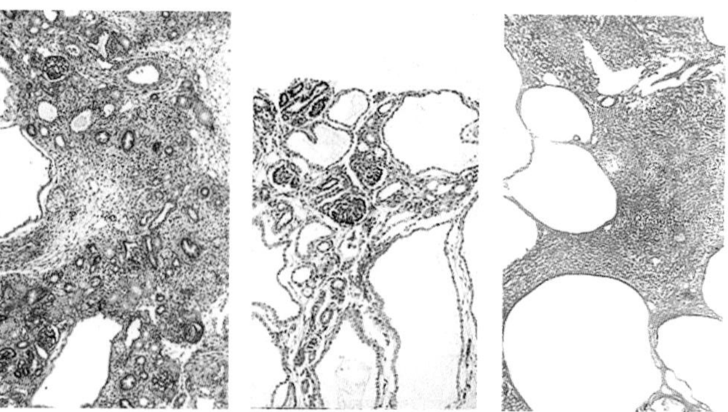

FIGURE 17-17 ▪ Low-power photomicrographs illustrate the differences between cystic dysplastic kidney (**left**), autosomal recessive polycystic kidney disease (**middle**), and autosomal dominant polycystic kidney disease (**right**). (Hematoxylin and eosin stain, original magnification ×40.)

The lobular architecture of the liver is preserved, but all portal areas are expanded and contain tortuous, slightly dilated ducts at the periphery with blood vessels in the middle (Figure 17-16). Stereologic studies have indicated that what appear as ducts on histologic section are in fact cisterns communicating with each other (e158). Similar hepatic changes are seen in Meckel, Zellweger, and Jeune syndromes, medullary cystic disease complex, and tuberous sclerosis (e183).

Mutational analysis of ARPKD presenting as infants and congenital hepatic fibrosis presenting in later childhood or adulthood with minimal or no renal disease has defined a broader spectrum of ARPKD. Congenital hepatic fibrosis with minimal kidney involvement can result from missense mutations in PKHD1 (2).

The clinical course of children with ARPKD who survive the neonatal period is variable and appears to be age dependent; however, the long-term prognosis in the majority of cases is better throughout childhood and youth than is often stated with a mean life expectancy of 27 years (64). Early detection and appropriate management of renal failure and systemic portal hypertension are important.

Autosomal Dominant Polycystic Kidney Disease

Commonly referred to as *adult PKD* because the vast majority of cases become symptomatic in the fourth and into the fifth decade of life, ADPKD is more common than ARPKD, with an incidence between 1/200 and 1/1,000 of the general population. ADPKD accounts for about 10% of adult kidney transplant recipients but is rare in children.

ADPKD has two disease loci, PKD1 and PKD2 that encode the membrane glycoproteins, polycystin-1 and -2, which have been localized to the primary cilia of renal epithelial cells (181). The primary cilia are finger-like projections on the surface of all kidney cells, except acid-base transporting intercalated cells in the collecting duct. Cilia have been proposed to serve as mechano- or chemosensors, responding to and interacting with the microenvironment. Abnormal cilia structure or function or both may lead to abnormalities in cell proliferation and tubular differentiation, ultimately leading to cyst formation (101).

Approximately 85% of affected families have mutations in PKD1 gene (e245), which has been mapped to chromosome 16p13.3 (e258) and the remaining 15% have mutations in PKD2, which has been localized to chromosome 4q13–23 (e170,e212,e246). Affected persons in these families appear to have a phenotype similar to that in PKD1 families, but the onset of cystic disease, hypertension, and renal insufficiency is delayed. A third gene, PKD3, is suspected in a few families but has been identified on chromosome 2p (20).

Autosomal dominant polycystic kidney disease diagnosed in utero or in the first year of life is reportedly associated with more severe renal cystic disease (e119). Although the majority of ADPKD infants survive, they tend to have more significant hypertension and a more rapid decline in renal function than do their affected adult relatives (e55). The kidneys vary in size from normal to enlarged, and rounded cysts range in size from microscopic (in asymptomatic children with disease detected on screening performed because of a positive family history) to about 3 cm in diameter. Some infants present with unilateral renal cysts. In contrast to the cysts seen in ARPKD, these cysts occur in any part of the nephron and are present in both the cortex and the medulla (Figure 17-17, eFigure 17-4).

Medullary Cysts

Cysts in the medulla can occur as part of several cystic kidney diseases (e.g., multicystic dysplasia, ARPKD, and ADPKD). The term *medullary cystic disease* encompasses two clinically and pathologically distinct entities.

Medullary Sponge Kidney

Also referred to as *precalyceal canalicular ectasia*, medullary sponge kidney is a generally sporadic disease with an equal sex distribution. It most commonly presents in adults, although some cases have been described in children and even infants. Medullary sponge kidney is a developmental disorder characterized by ectatic and cystic malformation of the papillary collecting ducts in the renal medulla; the condition is most often bilateral, but it may involve only one kidney or only one or several reniculi. Medullary sponge kidney remains symptomless unless complicated by urinary tract infection, renal stones, or hematuria—hence its presentation in later life. It is best diagnosed by intravenous pyelography, which shows dilated medullary tubules and the so-called papillary blush or bouquet of flowers.

Juvenile Nephronophthisis-Medullary Cystic Kidney Disease Complex

Originally described as two separate diseases, juvenile nephronophthisis (JNPH) and medullary cystic kidney disease (MCKD) are now considered to be part of the same complex, with similar clinicopathologic features. They are both inherited progressive tubulointerstitial diseases characterized by medullary cyst formation and secondary glomerular sclerosis. The main differences are that JNPH has a younger onset (average age, 11.5 years) with recessive inheritance and MCKD has an adult onset (average age, 28.5 years) with dominant inheritance (e139). JNPH, linked to mutations in more than one gene, occurring at different ages, has been mapped to chromosome 2q (juvenile form, NHPH1, with nephrocystin as a gene product), chromosome 9q (infantile form, NHPH2), chromosome 3q (adolescent form, NHPH3), and chromosome 1p36 (juvenile form, NHPH4), accounting for 70% of all cases of the JNPH-MCKD group (20).

MCKD usually occurs in the third to fourth decades of life, sharing the same clinical renal presentation with JNPH, except for the growth retardation and extrarenal malformations, which are absent in MCKD, and for the later age of occurrence of uremia. Two forms are recognized: MCKD1 and MCKD2, which have been mapped to chromosomes 1q and 16p, respectively. In approximately 15% of the cases of JNPH-MCKD complex, no family history is found, possibly representing a new mutation (20).

Polyuria, polydipsia, salt wasting, anemia, and growth retardation precede end-stage renal disease. Cysts 1 to 15 mm in diameter, located primarily at the corticomedullary junction, are seen in only 70% of the patients (e139). The remaining patients have no cysts. All cases have in common a chronic sclerosing tubulointerstitial disease, which is usually more severe than the cystic component (e135,e181). JNPH-MCKD complex is a major cause of end-stage renal disease in children, accounting for 10% to 25% of these patients. Associations with retinitis pigmentosa, hepatic fibrosis, skeletal defects, and central nervous system abnormalities have been described with familial JNPH but are typically absent in medullary cystic disease (e139).

Cortical Cysts

Glomerulocystic kidney disease (GCKD) and glomerulocystic kidney (GCK) are associated with cortical cysts.

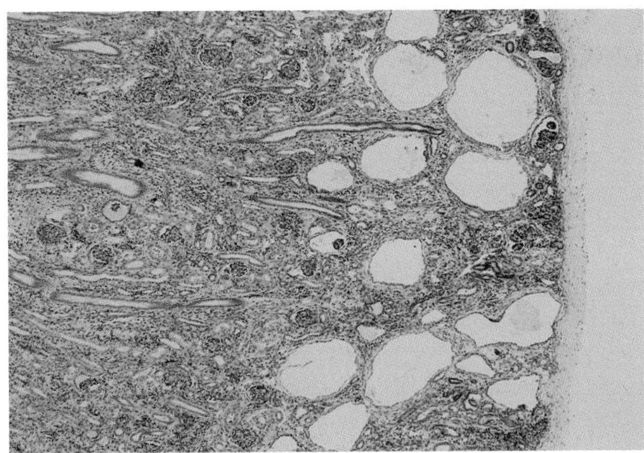

FIGURE 17-18 ■ GCKD with cystic dilation of Bowman spaces; the medulla is uninvolved. (Hematoxylin and eosin stain, original magnification ×40.)

GCKD, first described by Taxy and Filmer in 1976 (e302), is characterized histologically by cystic dilation of Bowman spaces and atrophy of the glomerular tufts (Figure 17-18). The term *disease* is suitable only for the familial autosomal dominant or sporadic GCK. It is now recognized that GCK is not a single disease entity but can be divided into five categories: (i) familial, (ii) associated with heritable diseases, (iii) syndromic, nonhereditary, (iv) sporadic, and (v) acquired GCK (98).

Most GCKD cases are transmitted according to an autosomal-dominant mode of inheritance, but the responsible gene has not been mapped yet to a specific locus, which, however, is not linked to the PKD1 and PKD2 loci, although a higher incidence has been noted among members with ADPKD. This disease is usually discovered in infants more often within the context of a familial history of ADPKD and less often as sporadic GCKD of young infants, although presentations occurring in older children and adults have also been observed of both familial and sporadic type with the latter reflecting the occurrence of new mutations (20).

Ultrasonographically, minute cysts, smaller than those occurring in autosomal-dominant polycystic kidney disease, are seen in the echogenic renal cortex. No cysts are observed in the renal medulla. Kidneys in GCKD of ADPKD phenotype are bilaterally enlarged and diffusely cystic, in which the main microscopic finding is represented by glomerular cysts, but asymmetric onset of this disease has also been seen. Kidneys in sporadic GCKD of non-ADPKD phenotype may be seen with either clustered or diffuse cysts. Kidneys in familial-dominant GCKD of older patients are normal in size, although occasionally they have been observed of enlarged size.

Finally, familial hypoplastic GCKD is probably a different type of GCKD, in which kidneys are smaller than normal and often associated with medullocalyceal abnormalities. Familial hypoplastic GCKD is associated with mutations in the hepatocyte nuclear factor-1-*b* gene (HNF1B or TCF2); its gene locus is at 17cen-q21.3 and is also found in some families with maturity-onset diabetes of the young, type V, which is the result of heterozygous mutations of the same HNF1B gene (193).

Glomerular cysts in all types of GCKD are less than 1 cm in size and located in the cortex from the subcapsular zone to the inner cortex (eFigure 17-5), histologically similar to glomerular cysts seen in other disease conditions. Familial and sporadic GCKD of young infants may also show renal medullary dysplasia and biliary dysgenesis ("ductal plate malformation") in the liver (20).

GCK may be a major component of heritable syndromes such as tuberous sclerosis, orofaciodigital syndrome, brachymesomelia-renal syndrome, trisomy 13, and short-rib polydactyly syndrome. This category also includes glomerular cysts in several syndromes, namely Jeune syndrome and familial JNPH, better known for chronic progressive tubulointerstitial disease. Glomerular cysts occur as a minor component (i.e., scattered cortical cysts) in several other syndromes, among them Zellweger syndrome, in which cysts are typically present but usually inconsequential, only occasionally serious enough to affect renal function. In all the syndromes, the cysts are inconsistently expressed (e29).

Acquired GCK disease has been described, following hemolytic-uremic syndrome (e3,e306) and in progressive systemic sclerosis (e281).

Simple Cysts

Simple cortical cysts, or retention cysts, which are very common in adults, are rarely seen in children. They are important because they may present as an abdominal mass, or their appearance ultrasonographic or radiologic images may raise the diagnostic consideration of cystic WT. Simple cysts arise from the cortex, are unilocular, contain yellow clear fluid, and are lined by a single layer of cuboidal epithelium.

Cysts Associated with Syndromes

Cysts of the cortex (sometimes referred to as *pluricystic kidney*), usually asymptomatic, have been described as a minor component of multiple malformation syndromes, both inheritable and noninheritable, including tuberous sclerosis, von Hippel-Lindau disease, Meckel-Gruber syndrome, orofaciodigital syndrome-type I, trisomies 9, 13, 18, 21, short-rib-polydactyly syndrome, Jeune asphyxiating thoracic dystrophy syndrome, Zellweger cerebrohepatorenal syndrome, VATER association, lissencephaly, renal-hepatic-pancreatic dysplasia, glutaric aciduria type II, Ellis-van Creveld syndrome, Elejalde syndrome, Peutz-Jeghers syndrome, Robert syndrome, phocomelia syndrome or pseudothalidomide syndrome), and Bardet-Biedl syndrome (20). In the following diseases, the renal cysts are histologically distinct from dysplasia.

Tuberous Sclerosis

Tuberous sclerosis complex is an autosomal dominant systemic malformation syndrome, linked to TSC1- and TSC2-suppressor genes, mapped on chromosome 9q and chromosome 16p, respectively, with the former encoding hamartin and the latter, which accounts for two-third of the mutations, encoding tuberin (20). It is characterized by hamartomatous proliferations of skin, brain, kidney, eye, bone, liver, and lung. In addition to the well-recognized association with renal angiomyolipomas, which occur in 40% to 80% of patients with tuberous sclerosis (e23), characteristic cortical cysts are present in about 50% of patients. The extent of involvement varies; small cysts may be diagnosed on imaging, or "polycystic kidneys" may lead to renal failure. The cysts vary in size and are lined by hyperplastic epithelium, which is often multilayered and papillary, with abundant eosinophilic granular cytoplasm (Figure 17-19). Solid nodules of these cells may also form. Mitotic activity evident in these cells may be related to the increased risk for neoplasia (e32). The histologic findings are so characteristic as to be virtually diagnostic of tuberous sclerosis when seen in an early biopsy performed before the onset of other stigmata of the disease (e30).

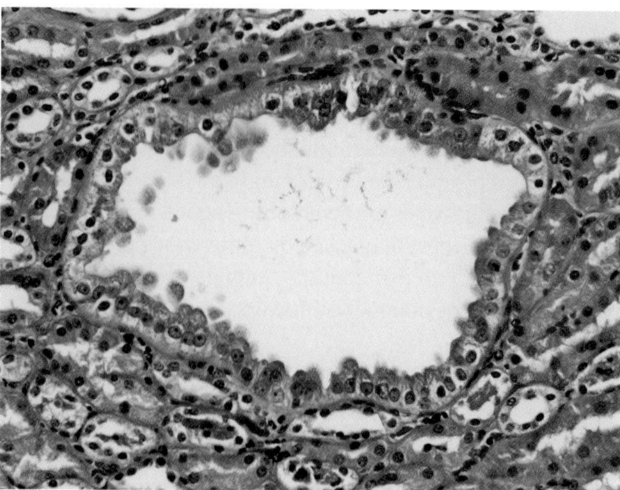

FIGURE 17-19 ■ Renal cysts of tuberous sclerosis lined by characteristic hyperplastic epithelium with abundant eosinophilic granular cytoplasm. (Hematoxylin and eosin stain, original magnification ×200.) (Courtesy of Dr. John Hicks, Houston, TX).

Von Hippel-Lindau Disease

Von Hippel-Lindau disease is an autosomal dominant multisystem (pre)neoplastic disorder genetically linked to a germline mutation of a tumor-suppressor gene (VHL gene) located on chromosome 3p. It is characterized by retinal angiomas, cerebellar hemangioblastomas, and cysts and tumors of the pancreas (microcystic adenoma), kidneys, and, less frequently, other abdominal organs. Renal cysts lined by hyperplastic epithelium with clear cytoplasm and a "hobnail" appearance are associated with a markedly increased risk for the development of renal cell carcinoma (RCC); multifocal cystic adenocarcinomas develop in 45% to 50% of patients beyond the third decade of life (e104,e145,e259). Less frequently, the cysts are numerous enough to simulate ADPKD.

Meckel-Gruber Syndrome

Meckel-Gruber syndrome has an autosomal recessive inheritance; is mapped to the long arms of chromosomes 17, 11, and 8; and occurs in 1/10,000 births (20,e268). It is characterized by posterior encephalocele, cystic kidneys, congenital hepatic fibrosis (ductal plate malformation), and polydactyly; additional features constituting several variants have been described. The kidneys are always bilaterally involved, although they may occasionally be variably involved. Round cysts arise from any part of the nephron, with microcysts seen in the subcapsular area and larger cysts in the medulla. The cysts are lined by a single layer of low-to-high cuboidal epithelium and are separated by loose, immature mesenchyme that may bulge into the cysts. Metaplastic cartilage is not usually present.

The pathogenesis of renal cysts in Meckel syndrome remains unknown. Study of midterm fetuses has shown that the kidneys are already enlarged by 11 to 20 weeks of gestation (110). Nephrogenesis is more or less normal at the periphery of the kidney. It appears that the nephrons are formed normally and the tubules and ducts are secondarily converted to cysts.

GLOMERULAR DISEASES

Metanephric blastema condenses around the end of the ureteric bud at about day 32 of development, and elongation, branching, and subsequent fusion of proximal generations of the bud give rise to the pelvicalyceal system and collecting ducts. The first glomerulotubular structures appear during week 8 as a result of the interaction of subcortical blastema with the ampullary ends of the collecting ducts, and glomerulogenesis continues until gestational week 36 when the neogenic (nephrogenic) zone disappears and nine to eleven generations of glomeruli are present (e19). The number of glomeruli in human kidneys varies from 250,000 to 1.8 million. This marked interindividual difference may be genetically programmed or due to perinatal factors such as low birthweight (estimated relation: 250,000 glomeruli per kilogram at birth), and may predispose persons with lesser numbers of glomeruli to renal failure in adulthood (104). Immature (fetal) glomeruli are characterized by their small size and prominent corona of visceral epithelial cells, and normally this corona disappears during the first year (e19). Mean glomerular diameter increases from 112 μm at birth to 167 μm at 15 years (e214), and enlarged (hypertrophied) glomeruli suggest a compensatory response to reduced nephron mass (e277). The thicknesses of the glomerular capillary wall and the lamina densa increase from 169 ± 30 nm and 98 ± 23 nm, respectively, at birth to 285 ± 39 nm and 219 ± 42 nm, respectively, at 11 years (e312). The molecular structure of the glomerular basement membrane also changes with age. Collagen α1 or α1 and α2 (IV) synthesized by podocytes, endothelial cells, and mesangial cells of immature glomeruli is replaced by collagen and α3 and α4 and α5 (IV) produced exclusively by podocytes (1).

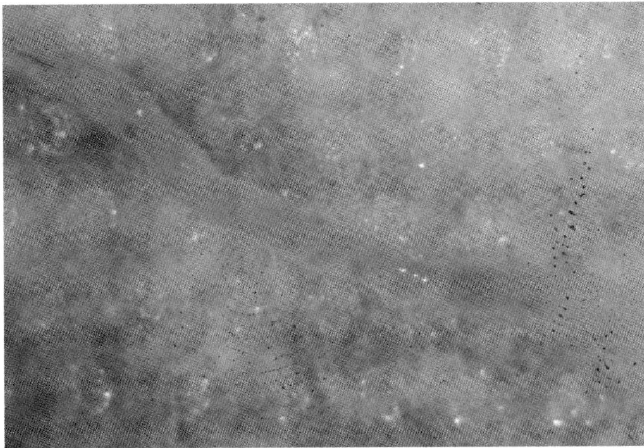

FIGURE 17-20 ■ Needle biopsy specimen of kidney viewed through a dissecting microscope. Glomeruli appear as red dots in the central region, and vasa recta in the outer medulla as linear striations at either end. (Original magnification, 5×.)

The pathologist most often encounters glomerular diseases in renal biopsy specimens collected with biopsy guns having needles of 18 gauge or less, and may be asked to examine the gross specimen for the presence of glomeruli with a magnifying lens or dissecting microscope (Figure 17-20). The presence of renal cortex may be inferred if one sees capsule and fat at one end of the biopsy specimen and architecture consistent with medulla at the other, but the macroscopic recognition of glomeruli requires sufficient blood flow within glomerular capillaries, and this may be reduced by disease. Definitive identification of glomeruli may rarely require rapid frozen section, or the pathologist may be asked to perform a rapid frozen section to determine if crescents are present. In either case, the tissue submitted for frozen section can also be utilized for immunofluorescent (IF) studies. Whenever possible, tissue should be sampled for light, IF, and electron microscopy (EM), even if all those studies are not initially requested, and with the smaller-gauge biopsy needles now used by pediatric nephrologists, two or three cores are usually required. The specimen submitted for light microscopy (LM) should contain as much cortex as possible along with the corticomedullary junction, whereas only cortical tissue is ordinarily required in the specimens submitted for IF and EM.

Our understanding of pediatric renal pathology has been greatly facilitated by contributions from two multi-institutional collaborative studies, the International Study of Kidney Disease in Children (ISKDC) and the Southwest Pediatric Nephrology Study Group (SPNSG), which have resulted in several seminal publications that are cited at the end of the chapter. The terms most commonly used to describe the lesions encountered in renal biopsy specimens are listed in Table 17-5. Children with renal disease usually present with proteinuria or hematuria, alone or in combination, with or without associated systemic disease.

Table 17-5 TERMS USED IN DESCRIBING GLOMERULAR LESIONS

Term	Description
Focal	Involvement of <50% of all glomeruli
Diffuse	Involvement of ≥80% of all glomeruli
Segmental	Involvement of <50% of a glomerulus
Global	Involvement of <50% of a glomerulus
Hyalinosis	Accumulation of eosinophilic, PAS-positive, silver-negative, structureless material that stains red with trichrome stains (glycoproteins and lipids)
Sclerosis	Accumulation of eosinophilic, PAS-positive, silver-positive structureless material that stains blue or green with trichrome stains (collagen IV)
Fibrosis	Accumulation of eosinophilic, PAS-negative, silver-negative fibrillar material that stains blue or green with trichrome stains (collagen I, III)
Mesangial proliferation	More than three mesangial cells per peripheral mesangial area
Mesangiocapillary (membranoproliferative) glomerulonephritis	A combination of mesangial proliferation and capillary wall thickening
Adhesion (senechia)	Attachment of part or all of the circumference of a glomerular tuft to Bowman capsule. Adhesions may be fibrous or fibrinous.
Crescent	A proliferation of glomerular epithelial cells and inflammatory cells that fills part (segmental) or all (circumferential) of Bowman space. Crescents may be cellular, fibrocellular, or fibrous.

PAS, periodic acid-Schiff stain.

Less commonly, patients present with a nephritic syndrome that includes proteinuria, hematuria, red blood cell and white blood cell casts, and decreased plasma levels of complement components, or with acute renal failure, renal concentration defects or chronic renal failure without known antecedent disease. Isolated proteinuria and hematuria do not usually warrant biopsy study, and most children with nephrotic syndrome responsive to steroid therapy or acute glomerulonephritis attributable to streptococcal disease do not undergo biopsy unless the course is atypical or the response to therapy is suboptimal. Typically, the glomeruli in patients with isolated proteinuria or hematuria are optically normal or show focal and segmental glomerulosclerosis (Figure 17-21A) or mesangial hypercellularity (Figure 17-21B). Diffuse and global mesangial hypercellularity with thickening of capillary walls and obliteration of capillary loops resulting in accentuation of the lobular architecture of the glomerulus (Figure 17-21C) or the presence of crescents, proliferations of parietal epithelial cells and inflammatory cells in Bowman space (Figure 17-21D) are usually associated with a nephritic syndrome or acute renal failure. IF and electron microscopic studies are usually necessary to arrive at a more precise diagnosis. A granular pattern of immunofluorescence—along capillary loops (Figure 17-22A), within mesangia (Figure 17-22B), or both (Figure 17-22C)—indicates immune complex deposition; and the site and the composition of the immunoreactant(s) depend on the disease. Crescents stain brightly for fibrinogen (Figure 17-22D). Linear staining along the capillary wall may indicate antiglomerular basement membrane disease (usually only IgG) or dense deposit disease (usually only C3) (Figure 17-22D). The histologic, IF, and ultrastructural lesions for specific diseases are described later, but a careful inventory of the lesions in all renal compartments—glomeruli, tubules, interstitium, and vessels—and correlation of the morphologic findings with the clinical history and the results of renal function tests and serologic studies are necessary for the proper clinicopathologic interpretation of renal biopsy specimens from patients of any age.

Glomerulopathies that Usually Present with Proteinuria or Nephrotic Syndrome

The incidence of idiopathic nephrotic syndrome is two to seven per 100,000 children, 95% of whom respond to steroid therapy, although 60% to 80% of these will experience one or more relapses (45). The distribution of lesions in untreated children with nephrotic syndrome in the ISKDC, conducted from January 1967 through June 1974, was minimal change disease (MCD), 76.4%; membranoproliferative glomerulonephritis (MPGN), 7.5%; focal segmental glomerulosclerosis (FSGS), 6.9%; mesangial proliferative glomerulonephritis, 4.6%; focal global glomerulosclerosis, 1.7%; membranous glomerulonephritis (MGN), 1.5%; and chronic or unclassified glomerulonephritis, 1.4%. Patients with MCD were younger than those with FSGS or MPGN (80% versus 50% versus 3% under 6 years old at diagnosis), showed a different sex ratio (male-to-female ratios of 60:40, 70:30, and 36:64), and presented less frequently with hypertension (21%, 49%, and 51%) or hematuria (23%, 48%, and 59%) in addition to nephrotic syndrome (e232). A response to prednisone at 8 weeks was seen in 93% of patients with MCD, 75% with focal global glomerulosclerosis, 30% with FSGS, 56% with diffuse mesangial hypercellularity, 7% with MPGN, and none with MGN (e254). MCD is under-represented in current biopsy practice because most patients with this lesion respond to steroid therapy and do not undergo biopsy; however, even allowing for the changes in biopsy practice, the

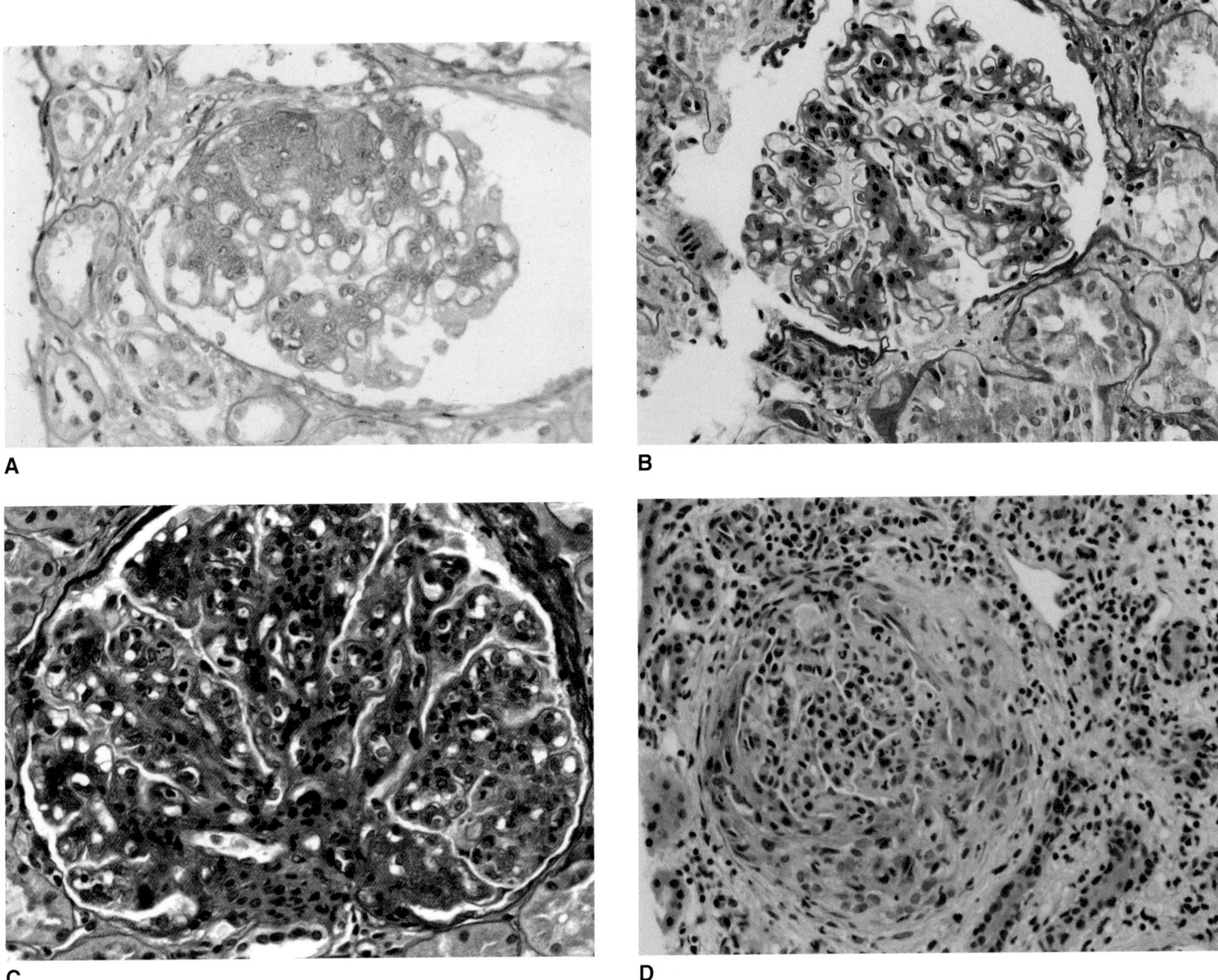

FIGURE 17-21 ▪ Glomerular lesions observed in pediatric renal biopsy specimens. **A:** FSGS with the sclerotic tuft in the 11 o'clock position adherent to Bowman's capsule, and segmental proliferation of visceral epithelial cells at the 2 o'clock to 4 o'clock position. **B:** Mesangial proliferation is defined as more than three mesangial cell nuclei per peripheral mesangial focus. **C:** Mesangiocapillary or membroproliferative glomerulonephritis shows both mesangial proliferation and thickening of capillary loops. **D:** In crescentic glomerulonephritis, a segmental, or in this case, circumferential proliferation of epithelial and inflammatory cells in Bowman space compresses the underlying glomerular tuft. (**A** and **D:** Hematoxylin and eosin, **B** and **C:** Periodic acid-Schiff stain, original magnifications ×400.)

incidence of FSGS in children appears to be increasing in all ethnic groups (e39,52), becomes more apparent in patients over 6 years of age at presentation (e296), and appears to be more common and more aggressive in African-American (e151,e290) and possibly Japanese (e329) children. Familial FSGS has been attributed to mutations that alter the membrane (podocin), cytoskeleton (α–actinin-4, CD2-AP), extracellular matrix adhesion molecules (β4 integrin), sialylated surface proteins, or nuclear proteins (WT1, LMX1B, SMARCAL1) of the visceral epithelial cell (38,45,145), though many of these patients do not present until adulthood and there is considerable variability in the clinical severity and response to therapy, especially among heterozygotes, implying that other genes or nongenetic triggers may be involved (27). Altered expression or distribution of these and other podocyte proteins have been found in studies of nonfamilial FSGS (e.g., dystroglycans reduced in MCD but not FSGS (27), and reduced podocin (63) and synaptopodin (174) in FSGS), suggesting that reorganization of podocyte proteins in response to injury is a key step in the pathogenesis of proteinuria (e16,146) Microarray analysis of RNA from renal biopsy specimens of 10 children with FSGS compared with five controls found a "gene expression fingerprint" of 429 genes, many of which had not been previously implicated in the pathogenesis of FSGS (162). FSGS, often with lesser (non-nephrotic) levels of proteinuria, is also the lesion seen in cyanotic congenital heart disease, sickle cell anemia, massive obesity, HIV, and other viral infections (parvovirus,

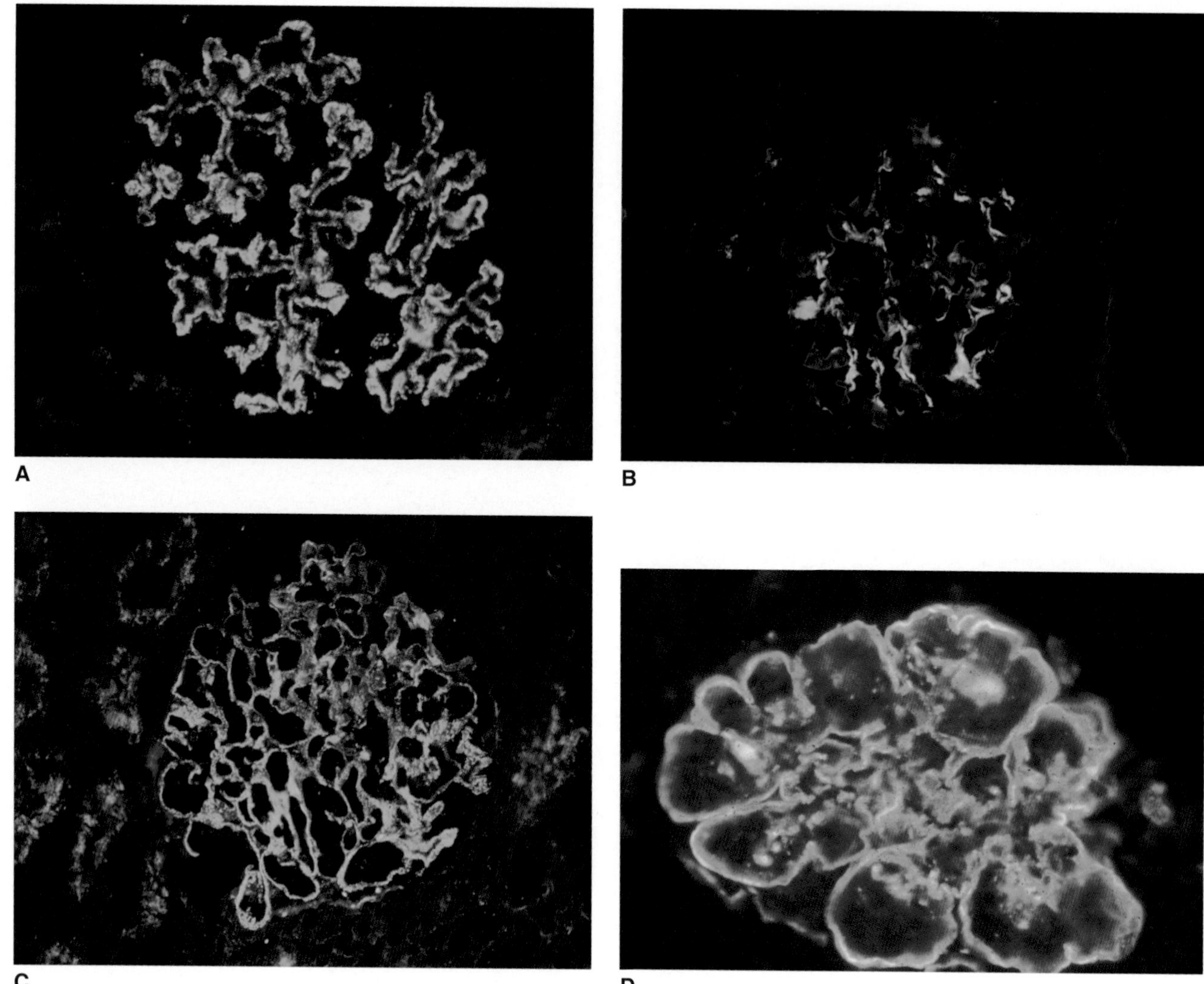

FIGURE 17-22 ■ Immunofluorescence patterns observed in pediatric renal biopsy specimens. **A:** Granular staining along capillary loops. **B:** Confluent granular staining in mesangia. **C:** Combination of capillary and mesangial granular staining. **D:** Linear staining for C3 along the capillary wall and bright rings with mesangia in dense deposit disease (type II membranoproliferative glomerulonephritis). [Fluorescein isothiocyanate-conjugated anti-IgG (**A–C**) or anti-C3 (**D**), original magnifications 400×].

SV40, and some cases of hepatitis C). Nephrotic syndrome in the first year of life may be associated with lesions that occur in older children but is more often caused by one of two lesions unique to this age group—congenital nephrotic syndrome of the finnish type (CNF) and diffuse mesangial sclerosis (DMS) that are discussed later. Medical complications of nephrotic syndrome include acute infections and thromboembolic disease related to the nephrotic state, and long-term effects on bones, growth, and the cardiovascular system related to the disease and its treatment (45).

Minimal Change Disease, Focal Segmental Glomerulosclerosis, and Diffuse Mesangial Hypercellularity

By definition, MCD should show no significant abnormalities by LM; FSGS should show segmental tuft sclerosis with adhesion to Bowman's capsule in a minority of glomeruli (Figure 17-21A), and diffuse mesangial hypercellularity should show three or more mesangial cells in most tufts of most glomeruli (Figure 17-21B). Slight segmental increases in mesangial matrix and cellularity and focal interstitial fibrosis are within the spectrum of "minimal change," but segmental proliferation of visceral epithelial cells (Figure 17-21A, 2 o'clock to 4 o'clock position) may be the earliest lesion of FSGS. D'Agati et al. (38) have subdivided FSGS into five categories: FSGS, NOS, and cellular, perihilar, tip and collapsing variants. NOS is the most common form seen in children and adults, and the collapsing variant confers a more guarded prognosis in children as well as adults (169). The classic ultrastructural findings in patients with the nephrotic syndrome include diffuse retraction of foot processes of visceral epithelial cells, microvillous transformation along the cell membrane, and vacuolization and lipid droplets within visceral epithelial cell cytoplasm, the prognostic significance of which is not certain (e269). Most authors consider any segmental glomerulosclerosis significant, but rare globally sclerotic or hyalinized glomeruli are occasionally seen in otherwise normal infant kidneys. It has been speculated that these may represent the residua of a population of large glomeruli that develop early in gestation, serve some unknown function during fetal life, and involute shortly after birth (e19). Emery and MacDonald found hyalinized glomeruli in the kidneys of 75 of 200 (38%) infants and children up to 15 years of age (0.5% to 30% of glomeruli in affected kidneys, but in most cases the range was 1% to 2%) and noted that rare sclerotic glomeruli were present in many of the kidneys that had no such glomeruli in the selected field (e95). Kohaut et al. found focal segmental hyalinosis in 9 of 29 autopsy specimens from children without apparent renal dysfunction and focal global sclerosis in 22, but the percentages of involved glomeruli were 0.7% for the segmental lesion and 1.9% for the global lesion (e177). Thus, a rare globally sclerotic glomerulus might be within normal limits but should initiate a search of serial sections through the block for a segmentally sclerotic glomerulus. Examination of serial sections is also recommended if focal tubular atrophy, interstitial fibrosis, enlarged glomeruli, segmental hyalinosis, segmentally positive immunofluorescence, collagen in glomeruli by EM, or an incomplete therapeutic response is found (e225).

Arguing that FSGS is a lesion with prognostic significance, but not a single disease, McAdams et al. classified biopsy material from 134 children with nephrotic syndrome as MCD (normal light and fluorescent microscopy, diffuse foot process retraction by EM), mesangial proliferation (at least two to three cells in most mesangia by LM and diffuse foot process retraction and thinning of the glomerular basement membrane by EM), or "primary" FSGS (segmental tuft sclerosis by LM and preservation of foot processes by EM). FSGS with foot process retraction ("fusion") was considered a "secondary" lesion in MCD or diffuse mesangial hypercellularity. Thus defined, the mean age at onset of MCD was 8.6 years; the racial distribution was similar to that of the region in which the hospital was located, and "secondary" FSGS developed in 41% of cases. Progression to end-stage renal disease occurred in 14% of all patients with MCD but in 30% of those with "secondary" FSGS, and FSGS recurred in two of eight transplants. The mean age at onset of mesangial proliferation was 7.0 years; African-American patients were under-represented, and "secondary" FSGS developed in 55% of cases. Progression to end-stage renal disease occurred in 13% of all patients with mesangial proliferation but 23% of those with "secondary", and FSGS recurred in 5 of 12 transplants. The mean age at onset of "primary" FSGS was 13 years; the proportion of African-American patients was more than twice that in the region in which the hospital was located, and FSGS was by definition present in all cases. Progression to end-stage renal disease occurred in 34% of these patients, but this lesion did not recur in any of nine transplants (e207).

IF microscopy in this group of diseases is usually negative or reveals only segmentally variable, non-pattern staining for IgM with or without C3 or C1q, bright staining for C1q, or, rarely, a pattern suggestive of IgA nephropathy. The reader is referred to the exhaustive reviews by Nadasdy et al. (e225) and Olson and Schwartz (e238) for a discussion of the significance of IgM nephropathy. In the above- report of pathologic findings of 134 children with nephrotic syndrome described earlier, McAdams et al. concluded that there was insufficient evidence to consider IgM nephropathy or C1q nephropathy, discussed below, valid categories of childhood nephrotic syndrome (e207). However, in a review of biopsies of 121 children with steroid-resistant or dependent nephrotic syndrome and 331 with nonnephrotic proteinuria and/or hematuria, Zeis et al. (198) found mesangial IgM in 20 of the 85 nephrotic syndrome biopsies and 44 of the 331 nonnephrotic proteinuria biopsies, and noted evolution to FSGS in six of the former (30%) and seven of the latter (16%), compared to 4.6% and 0% for the IgM-negative biopsies in those groups.

Jennette et al. described a proliferative glomerulonephritis with mesangial granular C1q as the dominant or codominant immunoreactant in 15 adolescents and young adults who presented with proteinuria or nephrotic syndrome (e155). In a report of 20 children (<18 years old at presentation) with C1q nephropathy, Lau et al. noted that 40% presented with nephrotic syndrome and another 30% with nephrotic range proteinuria, that 55% were boys and 60% were African-Americans, that the most common histologic finding was FSGS (40%) or MCD (30%), and that renal survival was best predicted by nephrotic syndrome at presentation (49% at 5 years for those with and 78% for those without nephrotic syndrome) (96) Markowitz et al. described 19 cases of C1q nephropathy in a series of 8,909 native kidney biopsies and noted that it was a disease of children and young adults (age range: 3 to 42 years, mean: 24.2 years) with a female and African-American preponderance. Renal biopsies showed FSGS in 17 and MCD in two patients, always with codeposits of IgG and many with codeposits of IgM (84%), C3 (53%), or IgA (32%), and these authors concluded that C1q nephropathy fell within the spectrum of MCD/FSGS (106). Rarely in children with nephrotic syndrome and MCD by LM, one finds a fluorescent antibody pattern characteristic of IgA nephropathy. These patients may have coexistent MCD and mild IgA nephropathy, and they usually respond to steroid therapy for MCD. In contrast, most patients with IgA nephropathy who present with nephrotic syndrome show segmentally proliferative, necrotizing, or sclerotic lesions by LM; do not respond to steroid therapy; and have a guarded prognosis (e6).

Membranous Glomerulonephritis

MGN is seen in 1.5% of children (e232) and 18.5% of adolescents with nephrotic syndrome. In children, the age at onset is usually 8 to 16 years and the sex ratio is equal. Most patients

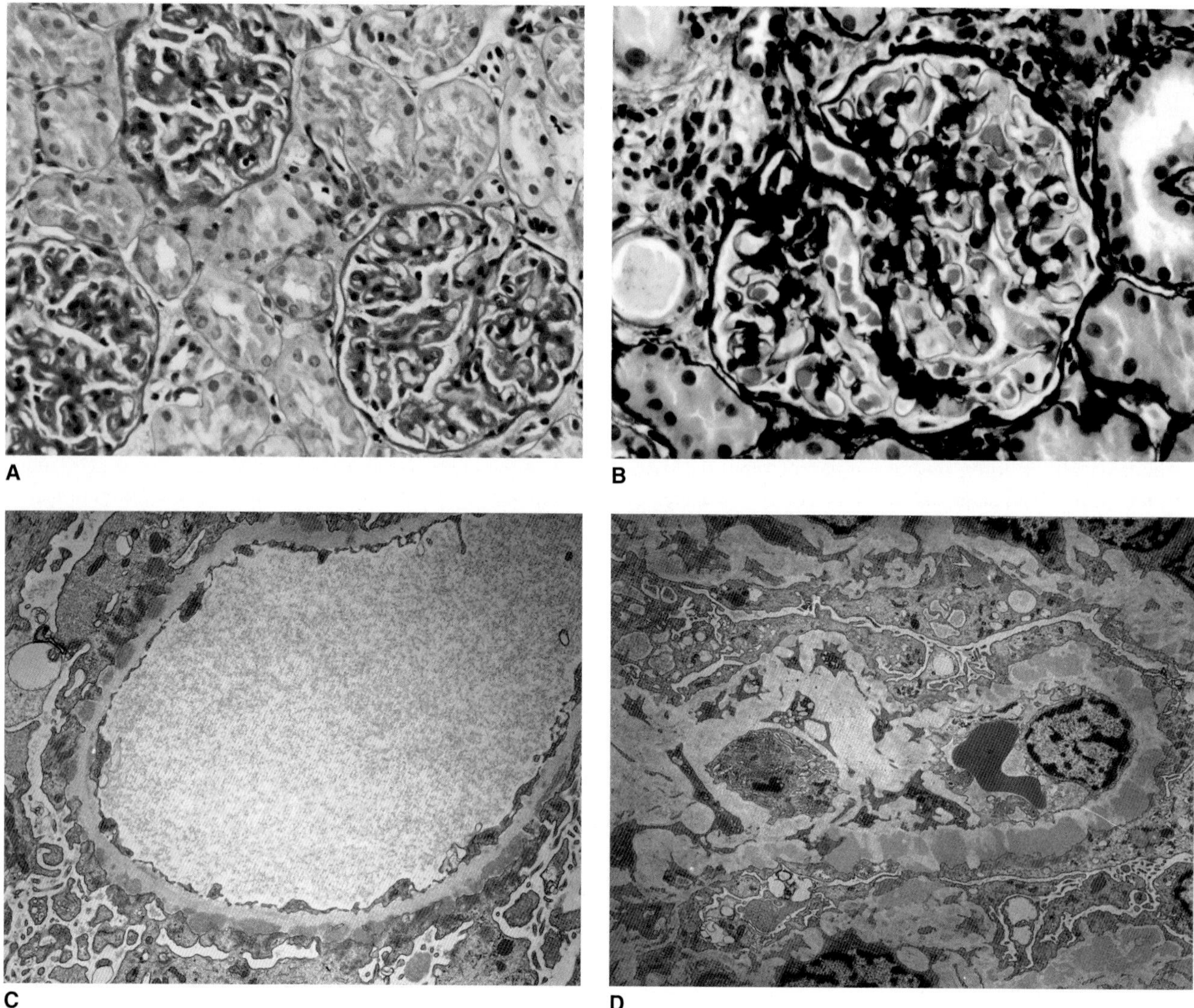

FIGURE 17-23■**AB:** MGN with diffuse thickening of capillary walls that in some stages exhibit short "spikes" extending from the outer surface of the capillary. **CD:** On Ehrenreich and Churg stage I small electron-dense deposits are present along the outer aspect of the basement membrane, but in stage III, larger deposits are incorporated into the basement membrane. (Periodic acid-Schiff stain, original magnification ×400. **B:** Jones methenamine silver stain, original magnification ×600. **C,D:** lead citrate and uranyl acetate.)

have microscopic hematuria in addition to proteinuria, but macroscopic hematuria is uncommon. Thirty-five percent of cases of MGN in children are secondary to systemic diseases, whereas the incidence of secondary MGN in adults is 23% (e107). Kleinknecht et al. found that more than 50% of children with secondary MGN had an underlying infectious disease, such as hepatitis B or congenital syphilis, and that another 27% of cases were secondary to lupus or another autoimmune disorder. However, the proportion of both "secondary" MGN and of MGN due to hepatitis B is decreasing as a result of the availability of hepatitis B vaccine. Drugs and neoplasia were very uncommon causes of secondary MGN in that series (e174). Following the description in 2002 of a remarkable case of antenatal MGN due to maternal antibodies directed against neutral endopeptidase, a podocyte and tubular brush border protein, which was present in the fetus but not the mother (40), Ronco and coworkers have reported other cases of MGN in early life attributable to alloimmunization (153). Primary MGN in children and adults appears to be an autoimmune disease against a podocyte or a basement membrane antigen (14).

Histologically, glomeruli in MGN appear large and have uniformly thickened capillary walls but patent capillary lumens (Figure 17-23A). The diagnostic "spikes" seen on silver stains (Figure 17-23B) represent notches along the outer aspect of the normally argyrophilic basement membrane due to immune complexes that do not take up the silver. Spikes cannot be detected when the deposits are small or sparse (Figure 17-23C) or when they have been fully incorporated into the basement membrane (Figure 17-23D). Mesangial hypercellularity, glomerular lobulation, and segmental inflammation, necrosis, or sclerosis are more common in secondary MGN (164). Glomerulosclerosis indicates advanced disease and interstitial fibrosis and tubular atrophy correlate with the degree of proteinuria and stage of disease (e199). However, FSGS (43) or interstitial fibrosis in the absence of glomerulosclerosis or tubular atrophy (e321) may portend an unfavorable course.

IF microscopy reveals granular staining along capillary walls (Figure 17-22A) and occasionally also within mesangia (Figure 17-22C). IgG and C3 are very commonly present, but a "full house" of immunoreactants suggests lupus or another systemic disease. Mesangial deposits also suggest systemic disease but are seen in 31% of children with idiopathic MGN (e66). Ehrenreich and Churg described four stages in MGN: stage I, small subepithelial deposits (Figure 17-23C); stage II, larger and more numerous deposits bordered by projections of the lamina densa; stage III, incorporation of deposits into the lamina densa (Figure 17-23D); and stage IV, a thickened and irregular basement membrane without recognizable deposits (e89). Patients may present at any stage and may have deposits characteristic of more than one stage. Foot process retraction is typically extensive in all stages. The SPNSG found that younger children tend to have more advanced disease (stage III or IV) and that lower stages were associated with a shorter clinical duration of disease before biopsy (e66).

Diabetic Nephropathy

Diabetic nephropathy develops in 40% to 50% of patients with insulin-dependent diabetes mellitus. Long-standing disease, poor metabolic control, smoking, male sex, non-Caucasian race, and other genetic factors predispose patients to the development of nephropathy (127). It is unusual for clinical nephropathy to develop in less than 10 years, but mesangial expansion and basement membrane thickening begin to appear within 2 to 5 years, even before the onset of microalbuminuria (e98). Ellis and Pysher found diffuse intercapillary glomerulosclerosis in 11 children and nodular intercapillary glomerulosclerosis (Kimmelstiel-Wilson lesion) in one child, all of whom had had insulin-dependent diabetes mellitus for only 4 to 10 years (e94). This and the other glomerular lesions of diabetic nephropathy, hyalinosis fibrin caps and capsular drops, and hyaline arteriolosclerosis, may also be seen in kidney biopsy specimens from massively obese adolescents (Figure 17-24). IF microscopy shows a characteristic linear staining along the glomerular capillary walls and tubular basement membranes for IgG and albumin, and hyalinotic lesions often stain with IgM and C3. The earliest and most characteristic ultrastructural lesion is thickening of the lamina densa of the glomerular basement membrane, but with time the width of the membrane varies as thinner areas develop as a result of microaneurysms and the deposition of neomembrane (e313). Other ultrastructural findings include increased mesangial matrix, variable effacement of foot processes, and subendothelial accumulations of electron-dense material that correspond to fibrin caps and should not be confused with the deposits seen in immune complex diseases.

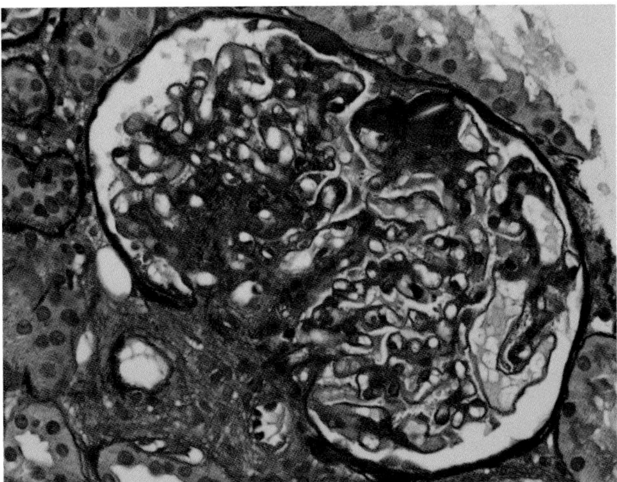

FIGURE 17-24 ■ Obesity-related glomerulonephritis. Nodular mesangial sclerosis, hyaline caps, capsular drops, and arteriosclerosis, all features of diabetic nephropathy, are also present in this adolescent with obesity-related nephropathy. (Periodic acid-Schiff stain, original magnification ×400.)

Nephrotic Syndrome in the First Year of Life

The term *congenital nephrotic syndrome* is used to describe either the clinical occurrence of nephrotic syndrome in the first 3 months of life, regardless of etiology, or a specific disease that was first recognized and is most common in Finland, commonly referred to as *Congenital Nephrotic Syndrome of the Finnish type* (CNF) (e121). In 1998, this autosomal recessive disorder was mapped to the *NPHS1* gene at 19q13.1 that encodes nephrin, a 185-kDA transmembrane protein in the slit diaphragm of podocytes (e168). In 2000, autosomal recessive steroid-resistant nephrotic syndrome (SRNS), a disorder of older children and adults, was mapped to the *NPHS2* gene that encodes podocin, another component of the slit diaphragm (24). In a review of patients with onset of proteinuria before 3 months of age and histologic and ultrastructural findings consistent with CNF, Koziell et al. (91) found that this phenotype could result from either *NPHS1* or *NPHS2* mutations but that triallelic mutations involving both genes resulted in congenital nephrosis with an FSGS phenotype. It is of interest that decreased expression of podocin (63), but not nephrin (74) has been described in children with nonfamilial nephrotic syndrome. A second disorder, DMS, is also unique to this age group, but approximately 5% of children with MCD, 5% with focal glomerulosclerosis, and 5% with MGN present in the first year of life (e123). Nephrosis or proteinuria in infants has been reported in conjunction with several genetic disorders (Denys-Drash, Frasier, Galloway-Mowat syndrome, Lowe and nail-patella syndromes (129), other disorders of neuronal migration (e144), and type I carbohydrate-deficient glycoprotein syndrome (e308), infections (cytomegalovirus, hepatitis B and C,

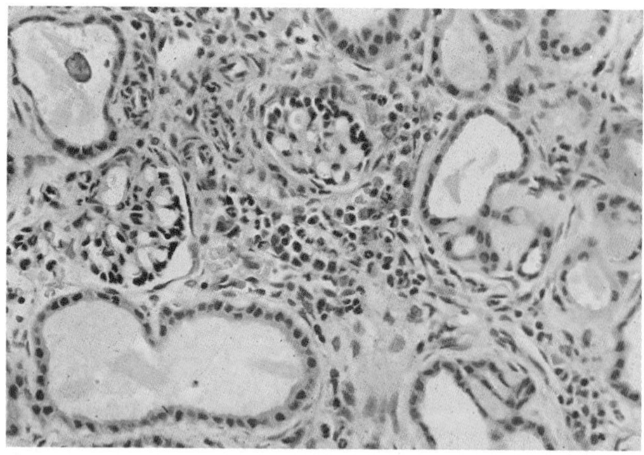
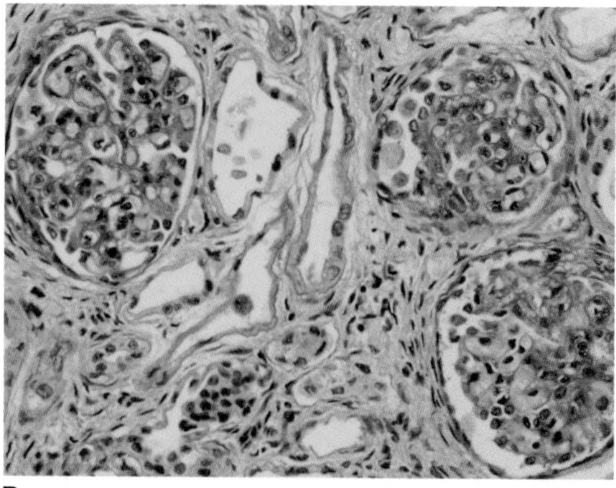

FIGURE 17-25 ■ Congenital nephropathies. **A:** Tubular ectasia, interstitial inflammation, and variable mesangial hypercellularity are nonspecific features seen in CNF. **B:** Increased mesangial matrix and segmental tuft sclerosis are seen in the early stages of DMS in this newborn infant with Denys-Drash syndrome. (**A:** Hematoxylin and eosin, original magnification 200×, **B:** Periodic acid-Schiff stain, original magnification 400×.)

HIV, malaria, rubella, syphilis, and toxoplasmosis), infantile systemic lupus erythematosus (SLE), mercury toxicity, hemolytic-uremic syndrome (HUS), WT, drug reactions, and, as described above, alloimmunization to podocyte proteins. However, it is likely that some patients in the reports of "secondary" congenital nephrosis may have had unrecognized *NPHS1* or *NPHS2* mutations (129). Sibley and colleagues, first in a study of 48 infants from their own institution (e285) and then in a literature review that included 502 infants (e286), showed that except for patients with DMS, which progressed to end-stage renal disease regardless of the patient's age at onset, patients in whom a lesion presented after 3 months of age had a much better outcome than those in whom the same lesion presented before 3 months of age, regardless of the type of lesion.

CNF is most common in Finland, where it occurs in 1/8,000 births, but many non-Finnish familial and sporadic cases have been reported (e231). Affected infants are typically small for gestational age and are born at 35 to 38 weeks of gestation with deformations of the skull, hips, knees, and elbows, which are ascribed to the markedly enlarged placenta that weighs more than 25% of the infant's birth weight. Other abnormalities (small nose with low bridge, widely separated cranial sutures, large fontanelles, delayed ossification) may be secondary to hypothyroidism as a consequence of urinary loss of thyroid-binding globulin (e286). Proteinuria in utero also leads to increased levels of a-fetoprotein in the amniotic fluid and maternal serum. Although proteinuria is present at birth in CNF, renal function is usually normal during the first 6 months, and no extrarenal disorders are present. In contrast, congenital nephrotic syndrome due to other causes typically presents later in the first year of life with less massive proteinuria, extrarenal manifestations are evident in congenital infections and syndromes with urogenital or neurologic components, and the rate of renal deterioration is much faster with DMS or interstitial nephritis (e144). The histologic hallmark of CNF is patchy dilation of the proximal tubules (Figure 17-25A), but this may not be present in biopsy specimens, especially those obtained before 6 months of age (e144), and is neither sensitive nor specific for CNF (e121). Glomeruli may show mesangial hypercellularity or crescents, and larger than normal glomeruli appear to be too closely spaced, but no glomerular lesion is diagnostic by light, IF, or EM (e121,e286). An interstitial lymphoid or myeloid infiltrate may be present. Proteinuria recurs in 25% of patients after transplantation, all of whom in one report had the same Fin-major *NPHS1* mutation, and may be due to the development of antinephrin antibodies (131).

DMS usually presents between 3 and 11 months, somewhat later than CNF, but the characteristic lesion has been reported in an 18-week fetus (e293). Mesangial sclerosis begins as an increase in fibrillar matrix but not cellularity (Figure 17-25B), and it progresses to transform the entire tuft into a shrunken hyalinized ball surrounded by a rim of visceral epithelium within a prominent Bowman space that may contain crescents (e286). A zonal distribution of small simplified glomeruli and undifferentiated tubules beneath the capsule, and relatively normal glomeruli but dilated tubules near the medulla may be present (e121). Immunofluorescence studies may be negative or show mesangial staining for IgM, C3, and C1q in intact glomeruli, and IgM and C3 outline the sclerotic glomeruli. By EM, endothelial and especially mesangial cells appear hypertrophic, and there is a marked increase in mesangial matrix (e121).

Habib et al. reported DMS as the usual renal lesion in patients with the Denys-Drash syndrome (e126). Initially, only genetic males with pseudohermaphroditism, nephropathy, and WT were included in this syndrome; however, since the recognition of patients who do not express the full syndrome, females with the full syndrome and patients with the characteristic nephropathy who also have either genital abnormalities or WT have been included (e67). The genital abnormality in Denys-Drash syndrome is either ambiguous genitalia or normal female genitalia with an XY karyotype, and children in whom WTs develop generally manifest bilateral tumors at a mean age of 18 months (e77). Several mutations in the WT-suppressor gene, WT1, have been reported in patients with Denys-Drash syndrome (e67). Moorthy et al. suggested that some patients previously reported to have Denys-Drash syndrome had, in fact, the Frasier syndrome of streak gonads and male pseudohermaphroditism associated with XY gonadal dysgenesis and nephrotic syndrome progressing to end-stage renal disease (e216). Patients with Frasier syndrome are at risk for gonadoblastoma but not WT (e216), and the glomerular lesion in Frasier syndrome is FSGS. Frasier syndrome is due to a mutation in intron 9 of the WT1 gene, but the tumor risk is much less than in Denys-Drash syndrome because Frasier patients have one normal copy of WT1 (e15). WT1 mutations were found in four of ten patients with DMS who did not have evidence of a urogenital abnormality or WT ("isolated diffuse mesangial sclerosis"), but in two of these patients, the mutations were different from those described in Denys-Drash syndrome (e153). WT1 mutations characteristic of Frasier or Denys-Drash syndrome were found in three of 32 girls with SRNS, but in none of 54 males with SRNS or 114 males and females with steroid-dependent nephrotic syndrome (9).

Nail-Patella Syndrome, Collagen Type III Glomerulopathy, Pierson Syndrome

Nail-patella syndrome may be a cause of proteinuria in infancy, childhood, or adulthood. The cardinal features of this condition are dysplasia of the nails and absent or hypoplastic patellas, but most patients also have iliac horns and dysplasia of the elbows. A nephropathy develops in some kindreds. LM may show patchy tubular atrophy and interstitial fibrosis, but the glomeruli are normal or show only irregular thickening of the capillary wall or mesangial expansion or segmental or global sclerosis. Immunofluorescence studies are usually negative. EM reveals prominent thickening of the glomerular basement membrane, which has a mottled appearance caused by irregular but sharply defined electron-lucent areas containing fibers that have the periodicity of collagen, especially if the grids have been stained with phosphotungstic acid. Progression to renal failure occurs in about 30% of patients with renal disease, but the course in an individual patient is unpredictable (65). Nail-patella syndrome is due to mutations in the LIM-homeodomain protein LMX1B at 9q34 that regulates transcription of collagen IV subtypes $\alpha3$ and $\alpha4$ (e85), and mutation analysis has shown correlation of mutations in this domain with proteinuria but not to the extra-renal manifestations of the disease (22). Collagen type III glomerulopathy presents with progressive proteinuria in late infancy to adulthood and most affected children go on to renal failure. Glomeruli are markedly enlarged and show expanded mesangia and thick capillary walls, and by EM the mesangia and the subendothelial space are electron lucent or mottled. Collagen fibers can be demonstrated with phosphotungstic acid staining, but patients do not have the extra-renal manifestations of nail-patella syndrome (65). Pierson syndrome, congenital nephrotic syndrome and microcoria, is due to mutations of LAMB2 on chromosome 3p that encodes laminin $\beta2$ that anchors the podocyte foot process to the basement membrane. Pathologically, it may show DMS or glomerular hypercellularity with variable thickening, thinning, rarefaction and lamination of the glomerular basement membrane on EM (65).

Glomerulopathies that Usually Present with Hematuria with or without Proteinuria

The most important diseases in this category in children include the primary IgA nephropathies—Berger disease and Henoch-Schönlein purpura (HSP) nephritis, and the basement membrane nephropathies—Alport syndrome and thin glomerular basement membrane disease. Hematuria is a well-known complication of hypercalciuria, but no specific pathologic lesion is associated with this condition (e298), and the histopathologic abnormalities in loin-pain hematuria syndrome are nonspecific. In all these conditions, the finding of red cell casts or hemosiderin in tubular epithelial cells lends support to a diagnosis of hematuria originating in the kidney rather than in the lower urinary tract. The primary IgA nephropathies are defined by the presence of IgA as the dominant or codominant immunoreactant in the absence of clinical or laboratory features of systemic lupus erythematosis. Characteristic but not always pathognomonic ultrastructural lesions are observed in many cases of Alport syndrome, and an ultrastructural lesion defines thin glomerular basement membrane disease.

IgA Nephropathy (Berger Disease)

IgA nephropathy was described by Berger and Hinglais in 1968 (e27), but the association of recurrent hematuria and focal glomerulonephritis, often in patients with a recent history of upper respiratory infection, had been recognized many years earlier. Today, IgA nephropathy is the most common glomerulopathy worldwide, accounting for 5% to 10% of cases of glomerular disease in North America, 15% to 30% in Europe, and up to 50% in Japan (69). These wide regional variations in incidence may be due, in part, to differences in ascertainment. For example, children of school age in Japan undergo an annual screening urinalysis, and three quarter of cases of IgA nephropathy in Japan are detected when only microscopic hematuria is present. In Europe and North America, 75% of children with IgA nephropathy present with gross hematuria (e146). In the SPNSG compilation of 83 children from the United States with IgA nephropathy who were 18 years of age or younger at first presentation, 59 were boys (71%) and the mean age at clinical presentation was 9.9 years (range, 3 to 17.3 years) (e142). In the 91 patients less than 15 years of age reported by Levy and coworkers in France, 63 were boys (69%), and the age range was 3.3 to 14 years (e191). Many cases of IgA nephropathy occur within a few days after an upper respiratory or a gastrointestinal infection; in contrast, several weeks usually separate the antecedent infection from the onset of postinfectious glomerulonephritis. Serum levels of IgA are significantly elevated in up to 50% of adults but in only 8% to 16% of children with IgA nephropathy (e146), but serum levels of IgA or of IgA-fibronectin cannot be used in lieu of renal biopsy for the diagnosis of these conditions (69). Recent studies have implicated aberrant glycosylation of the hinge region of the IgA1 molecule in the pathogenesis of IgA nephropathy. The abnormal molecule is not cleared by the reticuloendothelial system, elicits the formation of complement fixing IgG-IgA complexes, and can bind to mesangial cells and activate complement via lectin pathways. The IgG-IgA complexes show promise as biomarkers (124).

Classically, IgA nephropathy is characterized by focal segmental to global mesangial hypercellularity by LM (Figure 17-21B), confluent granular mesangial deposits that stain more brightly for IgA than for other immunoglobulins by IF microscopy (Figure 17-22B), and electron-dense deposits within and especially along the periphery of mesangia and adjacent to mesangial cells. However, the histologic picture is quite variable. In the SPNSG study, the initial biopsy specimens from 28 of the 83 (34%) patients showed mesangial hypercellularity (focal and segmental in 24 and mild to moderate in 23), but the specimens from 25 patients (30%) were histologically normal (50% of the biopsies from girls and 22% of those from boys), and those from 30 patients (36%) showed segmental necrosis, collapse, sclerosis (focal segmental sclerosis with or without proliferation in 18 patients), synechiae, or crescents (>50% of glomeruli involved in two patients) (e142). In an earlier report of 62 of these patients, this group found global sclerosis of 10% or more glomeruli in 10% of the biopsy specimens, more often but not exclusively in specimens that also had segmental lesions. Tubulointerstitial lesions were seen in 38% of specimens with normal glomeruli, 60% of those with segmental mesangial hypercellularity, and 70% of those with the more severe segmental lesions (e220). Levy et al. found histologically normal glomeruli in 26 of 91 specimens (29%), diffuse mesangial hypercellularity in 3 (3%), segmental mesangial hypercellularity in 41 (45%), and more severe segmental lesions in 21 (23%) (e191).

Mesangial deposits with IgA as the predominant immunoreactant define this disease, but 23% of biopsy specimens in the SPNSG series (e220) and 16% to 22% in the report of Levy et al. (e191) also showed capillary wall deposits by immunofluorescence. In addition, IgG was present in 52% (e142) to 60% (e191) of specimens, C3 in 76% (e142) to 87% (e191) IgM in 19%, C4 in 15% and C1q in 13% (e142). In addition to IgA nephropathy and HSP nephritis, the differential diagnosis of dominant or codominant mesangial IgA deposits includes lupus nephritis (LN), C1q nephropathy, HIV-associated glomerulonephritis, post-staphylococcal glomerulonephritis, and combinations of IgA nephropathy with MCD, MGN, and ANCA-associated glomerulonephritis (69). Mesangial electron-dense deposits were detected in 56 of 58 specimens in the SPNSG series, and 16% also showed small, usually juxtamesangial subendothelial deposits, 10% showed subepithelial deposits, and 9% showed intramembranous deposits (e220). Variations in the contour, caliber, or consistency of the glomerular basement membrane were noted in 40% of biopsy specimens in the SPNSG series, almost exclusively in those with relatively severe mesangial hypercellularity or segmental necrotic or sclerotic lesions by LM (e220). In an ultrastructural study of 34 patients with IgA nephropathy, Vogler et al. noted focal and segmental attenuation, splitting, duplication, paramesangial microaneurysms, and subepithelial protrusions of the glomerular basement membrane—features that were more marked in specimens with relatively severe lesions by LM and capillary wall deposits by IF microscopy (e311).

The SPNSG found a correlation of proteinuria and episodic gross hematuria with the more severe histologic and ultrastructural lesions (e142). Levy et al. found that patients with normal glomeruli by LM presented with macroscopic hematuria that might recur with upper respiratory infections but that proteinuria or elevation of blood urea nitrogen or creatinine levels was transient or absent in these patients, and renal failure, nephrotic syndrome, or hypertension did not develop. Patients with mesangial hypercellularity had a similar presentation and course, but more significant proteinuria was noted at presentation or developed later. In contrast, end-stage disease developed in 6 of 21 patients with more significant segmental lesions, including five of ten in whom more than 50% of glomeruli displayed such lesions; moderate renal failure and hypertension developed in two patients, severe hypertension in two, and significant proteinuria in three (e191). In a review of biopsy specimens from 65 children in whom IgA nephropathy was diagnosed during a 15-year period, Welch et al. noted that renal failure developed in only five, all of whom were severely hypertensive and three of whom were nephrotic at presentation; and the biopsy specimens from these five patients showed crescents in 50% to 90% of glomeruli (e322). A recent study of 250 adults and children with IgA nephropathy followed for a median of 5 years found that mesangial and intracapillary hypercellularity, segmental glomerulosclerosis, and tubular atrophy and interstitial fibrosis independently predicted renal outcome, but crescents did not, possibly because patients with more severe disease were excluded. (30)

Henoch-Schönlein Purpura Nephritis

HSP is a clinical syndrome involving the skin, joints, gastrointestinal tract, and, in 20% to 50% of cases, the kidneys. The heart, lungs, central nervous system, and muscles may also be affected. Although the incidence peaks at 4 to 5 years, older children and adolescents seem to be at higher risk for the development of renal disease. There are no specific laboratory tests for HSP, but titers for galactose-deficient IgA are elevated if renal disease is present, and, serologic studies are useful in excluding the other leading causes of rash and renal disease in children—lupus and microscopic polyarteritis nodosa (polyangiitis) (e6). Renal involvement in HSP is heralded by asymptomatic gross or microscopic hematuria, but proteinuria may also be present, and in some series from referral centers, a nephrotic syndrome is present in 50% of patients with renal disease. Renal failure develops in up to 20% of patients in these series, but the course appears to be less ominous in unselected patients (e127). After a mean follow-up of 23 years, Goldstein and coworkers found no evidence of renal disease in 82% of children with HSP who had presented with hematuria with or without proteinuria, but hypertension and impairment of renal function developed in 44% of those who had presented with an acute nephritic or nephrotic syndrome (e109).

The renal lesions in HSP are similar to those in IgA nephropathy by light, IF and EM, but the glomerular disease tends to be more severe and to more often include crescents, and the proportion of glomeruli with crescents is the basis for the ISKDC classification of HSP nephritis (69). In a summary of three series, children with minimal (ISKDC grade I) or purely mesangial proliferative (ISKDC grade II) lesions had a 3% chance of developing chronic renal insufficiency or dying within 6 years, while for children with crescents in 50% or more of glomeruli or membranoproliferative-like lesions (ISKDC grades IV, V, or VI) the risk was 35% (69). The skin lesion in HSP is a leukocytoclastic vasculitis, and deposits of IgA are seen in the walls of blood vessels in biopsies of fresh purpuric lesions, but they are not seen in skin specimens from patients with IgA nephropathy and may disappear in later stages of HSP (e191). As in IgA nephropathy, the outcome is worse in patients with severe segmental lesions and crescents (e127).

Alport Syndrome

Alport syndrome includes various combinations of lesions of the kidney, inner ear, eye, skin, smooth muscle, platelets, and granulocytes that are caused by mutations in genes coding for type IV collagen (e116). Proceeding from the observation that the antiglomerular basement membrane antibodies from patients with Goodpasture syndrome did not stain glomeruli from patients with Alport syndrome, it was learned that type IV collagen in all basement membranes is made up of a triple helix of two alpha-1 chains and one alpha-2 chain, but that with maturation in certain basement membranes this structure is replaced by a triple helix composed of various combinations of four other chains, alpha-3 through alpha-6, and that the genes for these chains are arranged in head-to-head pairs on chromosome 13 (*COL4A1* and *COL4A2*), chromosome 2 (*COL4A3* and *COL4A4*), and the X chromosome (*COL4A5* and *COL4A6*) (508). Approximately 80% of cases of Alport syndrome are X-linked secondary to mutations in the gene at Xq22 that encodes the alpha-5 chain of type IV collagen; and other patients have autosomal recessive or, less frequently, autosomal dominant disease secondary to mutations in the alpha-3 and alpha-4 genes on chromosome 2 (e189). The distribution of the alpha-3 through alpha-6 isomers in the body accounts for the organs involved in Alport syndrome.

Most authorities recommend that several criteria be met before a diagnosis of Alport syndrome is assigned to an individual or a family. Persistent unexplained hematuria; a history of nephritis, unexplained hematuria, or gradual progression to end-stage renal disease in a first-degree relative; bilateral sensorineural hearing loss in the 2,000- to 8,000-Hz range; anterior lenticonus or other characteristic ocular lesions; macrothrombocytopenia or granulocyte inclusions; widespread ultrastructural alterations in the glomerular basement membrane or immunohistochemical evidence of complete or partial loss of the Alport epitope in glomerular or epidermal basement membranes (Figure 17-26 A,B); or demonstration of a mutation in one of the type IV collagen genes listed above are examples of such criteria, but none alone is considered necessary or sufficient for a diagnosis of Alport syndrome (e116). Hematuria is demonstrable by 5 years of age in affected boys with X-linked Alport syndrome and in homozygotes and many heterozygotes of either sex with autosomal recessive disease, but renal disease may not be evident until adulthood in autosomal dominant disease (e102). The progression to end-stage renal disease is rapid in persons with autosomal recessive disease, often occurring between 5 and 15 years of age, and these patients typically are deaf but have no ocular abnormalities (e102). The progression to end-stage renal disease in X-linked Alport syndrome is more variable but roughly similar within kindreds, which show a bimodal distribution of the mean age at which end-stage renal disease develops in affected members. Hearing loss is universal, and ocular lesions are confined to "juvenile" kindreds, which have a mean age at onset of end-stage renal disease of less than 31 years. In contrast, only half of affected patients in "adult" kindreds (in whom end-stage renal disease occurs later) have hearing loss (e116). In a study of 195 families with X-linked Alport syndrome, a genotype-phenotype correlation could be demonstrated with males (90% chance of developing end-stage renal disease before age 30 with large rearrangements compared to a 50% chance with missense mutations) (80), but not females (79).

Histologic findings in children under 10 may be minimal, and at any age they are nonspecific. The number of fetal glomeruli may be increased, and there may be variable degrees of segmental or global mesangial hypercellularity, thickening of capillary walls, tuft sclerosis, patchy tubular atrophy, red cell casts or hemosiderin in tubular epithelial cells, and aggregates of foam cells in the interstitium (e116). Results of the standard immunofluorescence studies are negative, an important finding in ruling out IgA nephropathy or an immune complex glomerulonephritis, and in many (but not all) kindreds, the glomerular or epidermal basement membrane fails to stain with fluorescein-tagged antiglomerular basement membrane antibodies obtained from patients with Goodpasture syndrome or monoclonal antibodies to collagen IV chains (Figure 17-26C,D).

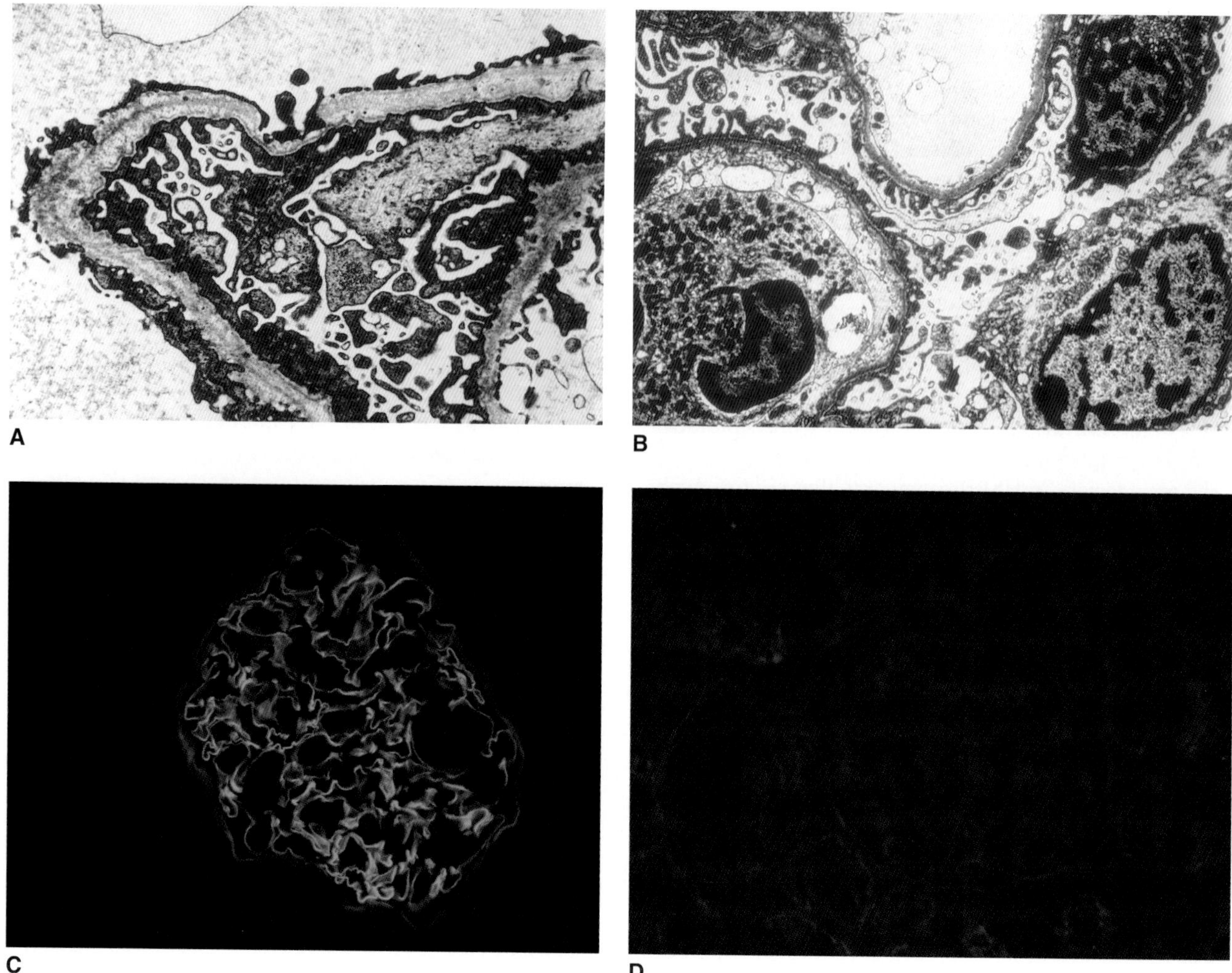

FIGURE 17-26 ■ Basement membrane nephropathies. **A:** Marked thinning, fraying, intersecting lamination, and granularity of the glomerular capillary basement membrane are characteristic of hereditary nephritis (Alport syndrome), but are not seen in all cases. **B:** Diffuse thinning of the capillary basement membrane is seen in familial hematuria, and may be the only ultrastructural lesion in Alport syndrome. **C,D:** Staining for collagen IVα5 is seen along the glomerular capillary basement membrane and, to a lesser extent, Bowman capsule in control **(C)** but not patient **(D)** glomeruli. (**A,B:** Lead citrate and uranyl acetate, **C,D:** Fluorescein isothiocyanate-conjugated anti-collagen IVα5, original magnification 400×.)

The characteristic ultrastructural abnormalities of Alport syndrome include irregular thinning, thickening, splitting, and a wavy intersecting lamellation known as the *basket weave* pattern (Figure 17-26A), often with 50-nm-diameter electron-dense granules between lamellae. However, renal specimens obtained early in life may show no abnormalities, and the most common observation in children is thinning of the basement membrane to less than 150 nm (Figure 17-26B) (65). The immunofluorescence studies and variable ultrastructural findings are consistent with the hypothesis that affected basement membranes contain an abnormal type IV collagen in which the chain that normally contains the product of the mutated gene is defective or absent, and the structural and functional consequences of this abnormal collagen are progressive (e165).

Thin Glomerular Basement Membrane Disease

The only significant abnormality in the renal biopsy specimens of 20% to 25% of children or adults evaluated for isolated hematuria is thinning of the glomerular basement membrane on ultrastructural study (Figure 17-26B) (e166) The term *benign familial hematuria* is applied when this lesion is the only abnormality, the family has a history of isolated hematuria that follows an autosomal dominant pattern, and affected persons do not manifest the progressive renal disease or extrarenal manifestations of Alport syndrome (e116). The term *thin glomerular basement membrane disease* describes a pathologic finding that may be familial or sporadic and may be associated with a benign or progressive course (e166). Heterozygous mutations in the *COL4A3* and *COL4A4* genes have been found in some, but not all, children from kindreds with benign familial hematuria (143). Furthermore, thinning of the glomerular basement membrane may be the only abnormality in a renal specimen from a child with Alport syndrome, even after a careful search for proteinuria and extra-renal lesions in the patient and abnormal collagen distribution in the biopsy, underscoring the need for close clinical follow-up and consideration of type IV collagen mutation analysis (65). Diffuse thinning of the glomerular basement membrane has also been described in the mesangial proliferative form of childhood nephrotic syndrome (e207) and other glomerulopathies associated with mesangial proliferation (e69).

Almost by definition, renal specimens with thin glomerular basement membrane disease are normal by light and IF microscopy. Focal immature or globally sclerotic glomeruli, areas of tubular atrophy, and variable staining for immunoglobulin or complement components along the glomerular capillary loop have been reported (e166); however, global sclerosis of 25% or more glomeruli was a feature in 9 of 16 patients with thin basement membrane disease who were subsequently reclassified as Alport syndrome variants on the basis of collagen IVα3, α4, and α5 expression and ultrastructural study (97). The cardinal finding in this group of diseases is diffuse thinning of the glomerular basement membrane by EM (Figure 17-26B). The widths of the lamina densa and capillary wall increase throughout childhood, but reported measurements of these structures have shown considerable interlaboratory variation, emphasizing the need for each facility to establish its own reference range (65). The mean thicknesses of the glomerular basement membranes in published reports of thin basement membrane disease have ranged from 150 to 300 nm, but most pediatric series have used a cut-off of 250 nm (65). Dische has suggested that a threshold of glomerular basement membrane thickness may exist below which hematuria occurs with increased frequency, and that physiologic variation in basement membrane thickness may account for some cases of asymptomatic microscopic hematuria in children of school age (e82).

Loin Pain–Hematuria Syndrome

Gross hematuria is accompanied by loin pain in many adults with IgA nephropathy, but such pain is encountered less often in children with IgA nephropathy (e150). *Loin pain–hematuria syndrome* refers to gross or microscopic hematuria accompanied by unilateral or bilateral loin pain, often severe enough that opiates are required. Most patients are women between 20 and 40 years of age, but adolescent boys and girls and an occasional younger child are included in reported series. Subtle biochemical or renovascular lesions have been described in some reports, and several reports have included patients with psychiatric disorders or an altered perception of pain (e47). By LM, a renal biopsy specimen may show a slight segmental proliferation of mesangial cells, mild interstitial fibrosis, especially near the corticomedullary junction, and minimal thickening of the walls of intracortical arteries and arterioles. Immunofluorescence often reveals linear or flecklike staining for C3 in the walls of arterioles, but not in the glomeruli. However, such staining in arterioles is not uncommon in specimens from patients with hematuria of many causes. EM shows no electron-dense deposits or diagnostic abnormality of the glomerular capillary basement membrane. Since none of these findings have any diagnostic specificity, the pathologist's role in the evaluation of these patients is to confirm, if possible, the renal origin of hematuria and exclude other conditions that might present with hematuria.

Glomerulopathies that Usually Present with a Nephritic Syndrome of Hypertension, Impaired Renal Function, Hypocomplementemia, and Cellular Casts, Protein, and Blood in the Urine

The most important causes of the "nephritic syndrome" in children include postinfectious glomerulonephritis, MPGN, and LN. These three conditions constitute the differential diagnosis of mesangiocapillary or endocapillary proliferative glomerulonephritis because they can produce a similar histologic lesion characterized by marked glomerular hypercellularity with accentuation of the lobular architecture and thickened capillary walls (Figure 17-21C). However, variations related to the stage or age of the lesion do exist. A similar clinical picture can be seen in crescentic glomerulonephritides (Figure 17-21D). Although crescents can occasionally be seen in almost any glomerulopathy, the major differential diagnosis of crescentic glomerulonephritis in children and adolescents includes immune complex diseases, such as postinfectious glomerulonephritis and LN, dense deposit disease, and antiglomerular basement membrane disease, which are discussed in this section; the small-vessel vasculitides, which are discussed in the section on renovascular diseases; and IgA nephropathy and HSP nephritis, discussed previously (e76).

Postinfectious Glomerulonephritis

The incidence of acute glomerulonephritis following throat or skin infections with group A streptococci in the United States and Europe has been declining for nearly 50 years, but poststreptococcal glomerulonephritis is still a relatively common disease worldwide, especially in tropical countries (116). Renal biopsies are usually obtained only if gross hematuria persists beyond 1 month; hypocomplementemia persists beyond 6 weeks; hypertension persists beyond 2 months; progressive deterioration of renal function or evidence of extrarenal disease is present; nephritis occurred within 48 hours of pharyngitis; age is less than 2 years, or there is a family history of renal disease (e141). Infections with organisms other than group A streptococci can produce morphologic features similar to that seen in poststreptococcal acute glomerulonephritis (hence the more generic term *postinfectious glomerulonephritis*), but many of these organisms can also elicit other forms of glomerular disease (116).

Histologically, poststreptococcal glomerulonephritis evolves over several weeks from an endocapillary proliferative (mesangiocapillary) (Figure 17-21C) and exudative (increased neutrophils within tufts) glomerulonephritis to a mesangial proliferative glomerulonephritis (Figure 17-21B) with patent capillary loops and normally thin capillary walls (e192). The immunofluorescence pattern also evolves from a coarse capillary granular (Figure 17-22A) staining for IgG and C3, with lesser amounts of other immunoreactants, to a mesangial granular (Figure 17-22B) staining for C3, typically without staining for other immunoreactants. Sorger et al. observed the capillary granular pattern, which they termed *starry sky*, in 13 of 42 patients, typically in specimens obtained within 2 weeks of the onset of symptoms, and noted the mesangial pattern in 19 patients who underwent biopsy later (e289). These authors also noted a third immunofluorescence pattern—confluent lumpy staining along capillary loops and lesser staining within and around mesangia—that they termed *garland* that was observed in both early and later biopsy specimens and tended to occur in older patients (median age, 21 years) and those who presented with significant proteinuria or the nephrotic syndrome (e288). Ultrastructurally, patients with the capillary wall (starry sky) pattern by immunofluorescence showed domed electron-dense deposits on the epithelial side of the basement membrane over which the foot processes of visceral epithelial cells characteristically arch (Figure 17-27). These subepithelial "humps" can be sparse to numerous and were flattened and focally confluent in specimens that showed the garland pattern by immunofluorescence (e288). An association between atypical humps and unfavorable outcome had also been noted in other reports (e140,e192). Basement membrane deposits may persist for years in some patients

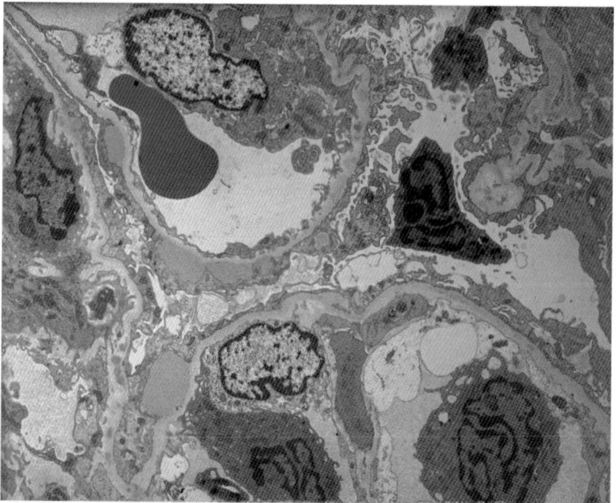

FIGURE 17-27 ■ Postinfectious glomerulonephritis. The foot processes of an epithelial cell arch over large subepithelial "humps." (Lead citrate and uranyl acetate).

(e13), but few if any humps are typically seen in later biopsy specimens from children (e192). Thus, the absence of humps in a later specimen does not exclude the diagnosis of postinfectious glomerulonephritis, and because structures consistent with humps, have been described in other conditions, the finding of a rare hump, typically above the junction of the capillary loop and mesangium, suggests (70), but does not necessarily establish this diagnosis.

Nearly all children with well-documented acute poststreptococcal glomerulonephritis recover completely (e253). However, Lewy et al. reported persistent clinical abnormalities in 5 of 46 children, and follow-up renal biopsies after 735 to 2,753 days demonstrated persistent mesangial hypercellularity in three of five patients, glomerulosclerosis in three of five, and tubular injury in four of five. The patients who died in the acute phase of disease or who developed persistent clinical abnormalities initially manifested markedly reduced renal function and prominent cellular proliferation, exudation of leukocytes, and crescent formation. However, other patients with equally marked reduction in renal function and equally severe glomerular lesions recovered completely. Patients with milder clinical disease had uniformly good outcomes, and this led these authors to conclude that it is unlikely that chronic glomerulonephritis such as MPGN evolves from mild or unrecognized acute poststreptococcal glomerulonephritis (10, e192).

Not unexpectedly, nonstreptococcal postinfectious glomerulonephritides manifest a more varied morphology. Staphylococcal infections often show a predominance of mesangial deposits with IgA as the dominant immunoreactant. The glomerulonephritis associated with subacute bacterial endocarditis may be diffuse and proliferative, but the classic lesion is a focal and segmental fibrinoid necrosis or thrombosis that evolves to similarly distributed sclerotic lesions in glomeruli by LM, but diffuse global, predominantly mesangial and subendothelial deposits by immunofluorescence and EM. Acute bacterial endocarditis can produce a variety of renal lesions ranging from a proliferative glomerulonephritis, often with crescents, to interstitial inflammation to infarction, and glomeruli show mesangial and intramembranous deposits as well as subepithelial humps that seem to persist longer than those in poststreptococcal glomerulonephritis. The glomerulonephritis associated with infected ventriculoatrial shunts is similar to that seen in acute poststreptococcal glomerulonephritis, including the presence of increased numbers of neutrophils, but typically shows mesangial and subendothelial rather than subepithelial deposits (116).

Membranoproliferative Glomerulonephritis

Type I MPGN was initially described in children by West et al. (e324) and Gotoff et al. (e113) in 1965, but it also occurs in adults, and the median age at onset is 21 years. Type II MPGN, or dense deposit disease, was first described by Berger and Galle in 1963 (e26) and is more common in children than adults, with a median age at onset of 11.5 years. The designation type III MPGN has been applied to several lesions over the years (e48,e173,e301) but is now generally reserved for the disorder with disruption of the glomerular basement membrane described by Strife et al. (e301) This lesion is probably lumped with type I disease in most reports, but the frequencies of types I, II, and III MPGN in children in range from 44% to 54%, 20% to 32%, and 14% to 36%, respectively (e323). In addition to these idiopathic forms of MPGN, a glomerular lesion essentially identical to MPGN type I is seen in the nephritis associated with infected ventriculoperitoneal shunts, hepatitis C, sickle cell disease, and α_1-antitrypsin deficiency (201).

Up to 70% of children with idiopathic MPGN present with nephrotic syndrome (e124), but a persistent nephrotic syndrome is a poor prognostic sign (e323). Most patients have hematuria that is often gross, but asymptomatic proteinuria or hematuria was the only sign at presentation in 65% of patients with type III and 22% of those with type I MPGN (e152). Extrarenal abnormalities, especially partial lipodystrophy and densities in the retinal epithelium, are seen in patients with type II MPGN (e6). Decreased levels of the third component of complement (C3) are seen in all forms of MPGN, and recent studies suggest that MPGN II and, possibly, MPGN I are due to dysregulation of the complement cascade due to mutations in the genes for factor H or another regulatory protein, or stabilization of C3 convertase against these regulatory proteins by C3 nephritic factor. (99) Evidence for a genetic basis for MPGN types I and III includes an increased incidence of the HLA haplotypes B8, DR3, SC01, and GL02; and partial defects of the complement system, rare familial cases, and the low frequency of the disease in African-Americans (e323).

Histologically, type I MPGN shows uniformly enlarged and hypercellular glomeruli with expanded and hypercellular mesangia (Figure 17-21C), compressed capillary lumens, and thickened capillary walls with segmental double contours ("tram tracks") on silver stains. Increased numbers of neutrophils are seen in glomeruli in 25% of cases (e157) and crescents in 10% (e169). Hyaline "thrombi," large eosinophilic globules in glomerular capillaries, raise the question of cryoglobulinemia and hepatitis C (e72). The interstitium shows edema, lymphocytic infiltrates, and patchy fibrosis. Type II disease shows more variable cellularity but more uniformly thickened capillary walls, and type III MPGN generally has a less pronounced and more variable cellularity. Immunofluorescence microscopy in type I disease shows coarse granular staining along capillary loops and the periphery of expanded mesangia, the "peripheral pattern" for C3 and, less often, IgM, IgG, C1q, and IgA. Type II MPGN shows a linear or a ribbonlike staining of capillary walls and hollow rings in mesangia for C3 (Figure 17-22D), and, less intensely and less often, for other immunoreactants (e284). Type III MPGN shows finely granular to confluent capillary wall and central mesangial staining for C3 (e301).

The three types of idiopathic MPGN are defined by their ultrastructure. In type I, the lamina densa of the glomerular capillary wall is normal, but numerous electron-dense deposits and cytoplasmic processes (interposition) are seen in the subendothelial space (Figure 17-28A). The two lines of the histologic "tram track" are the original lamina densa and the new membrane deposited between the interposed material and the endothelial cell (e323). Mesangial deposits are infrequent, but subepithelial deposits are seen in 30% to 50% of cases (200). Type II MPGN is characterized by extensive ribbonlike densities in the glomerular basement membrane (Figure 17-28B), mesangia, and, in some cases, tubular basement membranes, and similar deposits have been observed in extrarenal locations (202). Type III MPGN shows a thickened basement membrane with subendothelial and subepithelial deposits that are less electron-dense than those in MPGN I, and silver impregnation reveals a frayed and laminated basement membrane (e301).

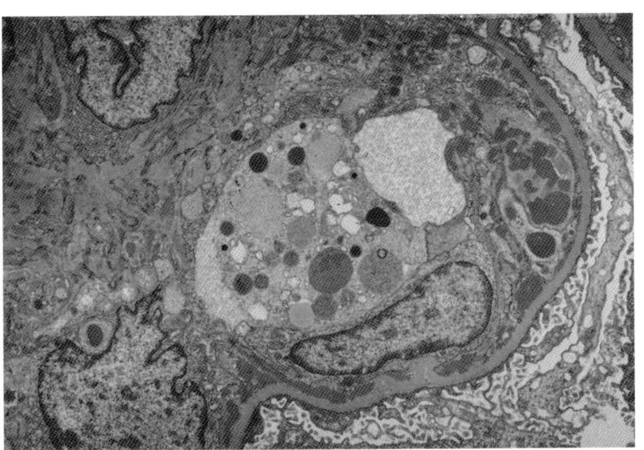

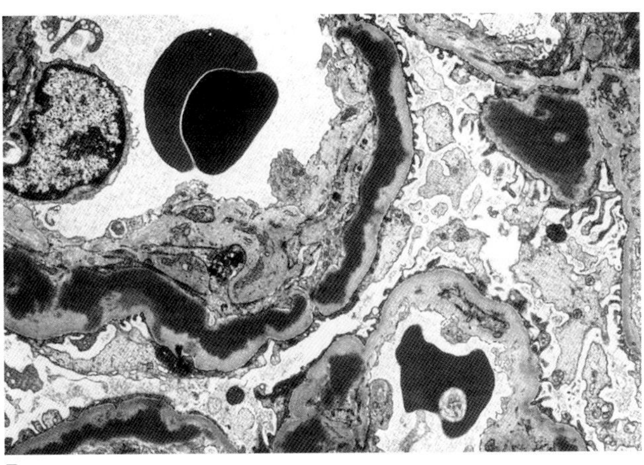

FIGURE 17-28 ▪ **A:** Type I MPGN with subendothelial electron-dense deposits and interposed mesangial cell cytoplasm. **B:** Type II MPGN (dense deposit disease) is defined by irregular ribbons of electron-dense material along the glomerular capillary basement membrane (**A,B**, lead citrate and uranyl acetate stain, original magnifications ×3,000.)

If MPGN is untreated, renal failure develops within 10 years in 50% of children, and within 20 years in 80% to 90% (e6). Crescents, sclerotic glomeruli, extensive double contours, and tubulointerstitial disease have been associated with a poor outcome in type I MPGN (199). In the study of Habib et al., 18 of 44 children with type II MPGN progressed to end-stage renal disease within 10 years, and end-stage renal disease developed in ten of these children within 2 years. Factors that seemed to predict a poor outcome included nephrotic syndrome, macroscopic hematuria, and decreased renal function at the time of presentation (e122). In contrast, only 2 of the 16 children with type II MPGN studied by the SPNSG had a rapidly progressive course, and only six evidenced progressive disease after a mean follow-up of 10 years. Pathologic rather than clinical features best predicted progressive disease in that report, and these included a mesangiocapillary pattern, mesangial sclerosis, and electron-dense deposits in mesangia (e63).

Lupus Nephritis

Dubois estimated that 20% to 25% of all cases of SLE present in childhood or adolescence (e86). The most common presenting complaints in children with SLE are arthritis, arthralgia, rash and fever, but renal, cardiac, and central nervous system involvement becomes evident as the disease progresses (e101,e108,e171,e208), and urinary or renal function abnormalities develop in 60% to 80% of children with SLE, usually within 2 years from the onset of disease (133). Most patients are girls, but the female predominance may be less striking in children under 12 than in adolescents (e171). The frequency of SLE is increased in Hispanic, Asian, and African-American children (e188), and the course of LN is more severe in Hispanics and African-Americans, possibly because of socioeconomic as well as biological factors (13,32,90). Renal involvement in SLE is heralded by hematuria, proteinuria, and hypertension, and these findings may prompt a renal biopsy before the diagnosis of SLE has been made. In children with an established diagnosis, renal biopsy may be performed to characterize the extent of renal disease or response to therapy.

LN is generally categorized by some variation on the World Health Organization (WHO) classification originally formulated in 1974 coupled with an indication of the activity and the chronicity of disease. The 2004 International Society of Nephrology/Renal Pathology Society (ISN/RPS) Classification maintains the emphasis on the appearance of glomeruli but incorporates information from IF and EM and includes subdesignations for activity and chronicity. In Class I, minimal mesangial LN, glomeruli are normal by LM but have mesangial immune deposits by IF (such findings qualified for Class IIa in the original WHO classification, in which Class I glomeruli were normal by LM, IF, and EM, or Class Ib in the 1982 modification). In Class II in the ISN/RPS scheme, mesangial proliferative LN, glomeruli show mesangial hypercellularity or matrix expansion without histologic alterations of capillary 1974 WHO Class IIb, 1982 WHO Class IIa or IIb), and the ISN/RPS classification allows very rare small subendothelial or subepithelial deposits by IF or EM in Class II. Class III, focal LN, and Class IV, diffuse LN, show focal (<50% of glomeruli) or diffuse glomerulonephritis, respectively, typically with subendothelial immune deposits by IF and EM, and the lesions may be active (A) or chronic (C) (or both—A/C), and, in Class IV, segmental (IV-S) or global (IV-G) to indicate whether the majority (>50%) of affected glomeruli show segmental or global involvement. Class V, membranous LN, is diagnosed, alone or in combination with class III or IV, when there are subepithelial immune deposits or their sequelae over greater than 50% of the capillary wall; and Class VI indicates global sclerosis of 90% or more of glomeruli without evidence of activity (189). Lesions indicative of active disease include endocapillary hypercellularity, leukocyte infiltration, subendothelial hyaline material, fibrinoid necrosis, karyorrhexis, cellular crescents and interstitial inflammation. Lesions indicative of chronic disease include glomerulosclerosis, fibrous crescents, tubular atrophy and interstitial fibrosis (e11).

The incidence of the various categories in published reports depends on the population studied, the indications for biopsy, and the specific criteria used for classification, but after pooling data from several large pediatric series and using the modified WHO classification, Lehman and Mouradian found mild or no glomerulitis in 26%, focal proliferative LN in 25%, diffuse proliferative LN in 42%, and membranous LN in 6% (e188). Applying the INS/RPS criteria to a group of 39 children, Marks et al. found class I in 2%, class II in 13%, class III in 15%, class IV in 51%, and class V in 20% with 12% of cases overlapping between classes III or IV and class V (107). In a series of 25 children with LN, Zappitelli et al. noted good correlation with clinical and laboratory parameters for biopsies obtained at the time of diagnosis, but not for follow-up biopsies (197). Electron-dense deposits with curvilinear patterning, so-called fingerprint deposits, and tubuloreticular aggregates in the cytoplasm of glomerular endothelial cells (Figure 17-29) are characteristic of LN and easiest to find in class IV disease.

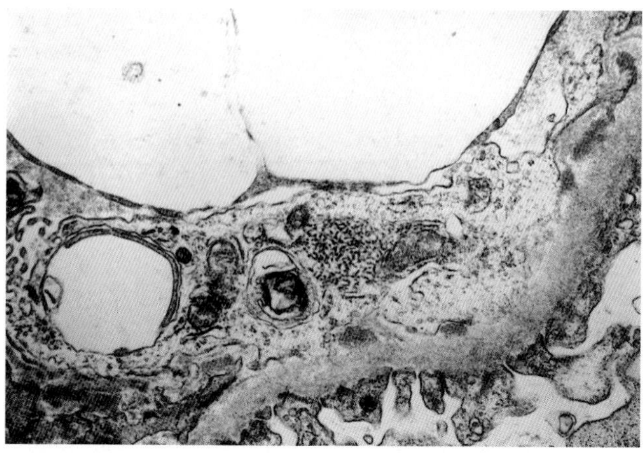

FIGURE 17-29 ■ LN may show tubuloreticular aggregates within endothelial cells (Lead citrate and uranyl acetate stain, original magnification ×5,000.)

Immunofluorescence microscopy reveals IgG in nearly all cases of LN, regardless of WHO class, and IgM and IgA in most (coexpression of these three immunoreactants is referred to as a "full house"). C3 is detected in most and C1q or C4 in many cases. Unlike IgA staining in IgA nephropathy, that in LN is generally less intense than IgG staining. In patients without an established diagnosis, a "full house" of immunoreactants, numerous mesangial deposits in an otherwise typical MGN, immune deposits along tubular basement membranes or in tubular nuclei, "fingerprint deposits," or tubuloreticular aggregates raise the possibility of SLE.

Crescentic Glomerulonephritis

During the influenza pandemic of 1919, Goodpasture described the development of hemoptysis and renal failure in an 18-year-old young man (e112), and the eponym Goodpasture syndrome was applied to the combination of pulmonary hemorrhage and glomerulonephritis by Stanton and Tange in 1958 (e297). Linear staining for immunoglobulin along the glomerular basement membrane was described in 1964 (e272), the role of antiglomerular basement membrane antibody in the pathogenesis of this form of glomerulonephritis was elucidated in 1967 (e190), and the recommendation to limit the term *Goodpasture syndrome* to a pulmonary-renal syndrome caused by antiglomerular basement membrane antibodies was made in 1971 (e203). Antiglomerular basement membrane disease accounts for only 6% (e154) to 15% (e63) of crescentic glomerulonephritis in children; immune complex diseases account for 50% (e154) to 70% (e63) of cases; and the small-vessel vasculitides associated with antineutrophil cytoplasmic antibodies (ANCA) account for 20% (e63) to 35% (e154) (see discussion of systemic vasculitides in the section on renovascular diseases). In patients of all ages, 95% of biopsy specimens from patients with antiglomerular basement membrane disease contain some crescents, and an average of 70% of glomeruli are involved. Comparable figures for other glomerulopathies are 90% of specimens and 48% of glomeruli for antineutrophil cytoplasmic antibody-associated vasculitides, 40% of specimens and 31% of glomeruli for classes III and IV LN, 53% of specimens and 24% of glomeruli for HSP nephritis, 27% of specimens and 24% of glomeruli for IgA nephropathy, 25% of specimens and 17% of glomeruli in poststreptococcal glomerulonephritis, 20% of specimens and 21% of glomeruli in type I MPGN, 12% of specimens and 17% of glomeruli in membranous LN, and 5% of specimens and 17% of glomeruli in MGN (e154). The presence of crescents portends a worse prognosis regardless of underlying disease, with the possible exception of poststreptococcal glomerulonephritis in children, in which some studies show no worsening of outcome (e63); but others find that most patients with this lesion progress to chronic renal insufficiency or end-stage renal disease (e295).

Crescents are initially cellular (Figure 17-21D) and resolve or organize into fibrocellular or fibrous forms. The constituent cells are predominantly macrophages or epithelial cells, and the proportion of each appears to be a function of the age of the lesion and the cause of the glomerulonephritis. Epithelial cells predominate in older lesions and in those caused by immune complex diseases (e154). Glomerular tufts beneath crescents may be compressed, necrotic, or sclerotic, but the better-preserved tufts in antiglomerular basement membrane disease and the pauciimmune glomerulonephritis secondary to small vessel vasculitis are generally normal, whereas in immune complex glomerulonephritis, they may show mesangial hypercellularity and thickening of the capillary wall. Extensive disruptions of the capillary wall and Bowman capsule may be seen in the vicinity of crescents, and the interstitium can show a mixed cellular infiltrate of varying intensity and distribution or patchy tubular atrophy and interstitial fibrosis in cases of longer duration. Crescents stain brightly with labeled antibody to fibrin in all forms of crescentic glomerulonephritis, but the staining pattern observed in the underlying glomerulus depends on the primary disease. In antiglomerular basement disease, there is linear staining along glomerular capillary walls for IgG and usually C3, but only rarely for IgA or IgM. In immune complex-mediated diseases, there is granular staining characteristic of the underlying disease and in vasculitis-related crescentic glomerulonephritis there is absent or very weak staining. By EM, all forms of crescentic glomerulonephritis can show endothelial cell swelling, expansion of the subendothelial space, disruptions of the glomerular basement membrane and Bowman capsule, and effacement of the foot processes of visceral epithelial cells, and in immune complex-mediated disease, there are dense deposits. The SPNSG found a correlation between large gaps in the glomerular basement membrane and fibrocellular or fibrous as opposed to cellular crescents, and between these findings and a poor clinical outcome (e63).

TUBULOINTERSTITIAL DISEASES

The renal tubule, consisting of the proximal convoluted tubule, loop of Henle, and distal convoluted tubule, is derived from the metanephric blastema through a process of elongation between the developing glomerulus and the collecting duct. The renal interstitium is composed of extracellular matrix and two or three types of interstitial cells whose function is poorly understood. Ordinarily, the interstitium is inapparent in the cortex, comprising less than 10% of the volume, but it occupies progressively more volume as one proceeds through the medulla to the papillary tip (e162). In addition to the diseases that primarily affect the tubules and interstitium, tubular injury and atrophy and interstitial inflammation and fibrosis are components of many glomerular and vascular diseases, and an increasing interstitial volume, which reflects tubular loss and interstitial fibrosis, is the best morphologic correlate of deteriorating renal function and progressive renal failure (e36).

Acute Tubular Necrosis

Isolated acute tubular necrosis (ATN) is seen infrequently in biopsy specimens because a biopsy is not performed if the diagnosis can be established clinically. However, it is not unusual to see ATN in conjunction with other lesions, especially in allograft biopsies performed because of a sudden decline in renal function. The two classic categories of ATN are ischemic and toxic (e61). The former, also known as *acute vasomotor nephropathy*, follows renal hypoperfusion of any cause, and in children, it most often occurs in conditions associated with massive fluid shifts, such as shock, sepsis, and trauma. Toxic ATN is defined as dose-dependent toxic renal injury, and in children, it is most often caused by an antibiotic, such as an aminoglycoside or amphotericin-B, or an antineoplastic agent, such as cisplatin or ifosfamide. However, clinically many patients have risk factors for both types, and though the two types of ATN differ in the extent and the location of injury along the tubule, it can be difficult to make this distinction on a biopsy specimen. In renal biopsy specimens, one initially sees swelling of tubular epithelial cells and loss of the brush border in proximal tubules (best appreciated in sections stained with periodic acid–Schiff). Cell death is indicated by nuclear dropout, hypereosinophilia, and apoptosis; and the cells exfoliate into the lumen along with proteinaceous material (Figure 17-30). Two key histopathologic clues to ATN are mitotic figures in tubular epithelial cells, rarely seen if there is not tubular injury, and ectasia of tubular lumens. One may also see casts and refractile crystals in distal tubules, mild interstitial edema, mononuclear cell infiltration, and accumulation of nucleated cells in the vasa recta (e236).

Interstitial Nephritis

Inflammation of the renal interstitium is known as *interstitial nephritis* or *tubulointerstitial nephritis* because extension of inflammatory cells into the epithelium of tubules (tubulitis) and associated tubular injury are frequently present. Such inflammation is most often caused by infection or a drug, but it is also the renal lesion in obstructive and reflux uropathies and in several immunologically mediated metabolic and familial diseases, as well a cellular rejection of a renal allograft. Acute interstitial nephritis is characterized by interstitial edema and an infiltrate of activated lymphocytes, predominantly T cells, variably admixed with neutrophils and eosinophils. This condition is rare in childhood, but a compilation of the data on 55 patients in reports from Pittsburgh (13 patients) (e92), Tokyo (21 patients) (89), and Serbia (21 patients) (123) reveals that 45% of cases could be ascribed to infections (predominantly streptococci in the report from Pittsburgh, *Yersinia pseudotuberculosis* in the report from Tokyo, and hantavirus in the report from Serbia), 13% to drugs, 20% to the tubulointerstitial nephritis and uveitis syndrome, and 22% were unclassified. Presenting symptoms included fatigue, fever, gastrointestinal disturbances and weight loss, laboratory studies documented acute renal failure with low urinary specific gravity or glucosuria suggesting tubular dysfunction, and in many of the cases the diagnosis was initially made on the renal biopsy. Pyelonephritis is a subset of interstitial nephritis, caused by hematogenous or ascending bacterial infection, in which the collecting system is involved in addition to the interstitium. Chronic interstitial nephritis is characterized by interstitial fibrosis, tubular atrophy, and an infiltrate of small lymphocytes. Plasma cells, macrophages, and granulomas may be seen in acute or chronic interstitial nephritis (e65). Renal biopsy is necessary to establish the diagnosis of interstitial nephritis, but because the histologic response is not specific, clinical and laboratory findings must be correlated to determine a cause.

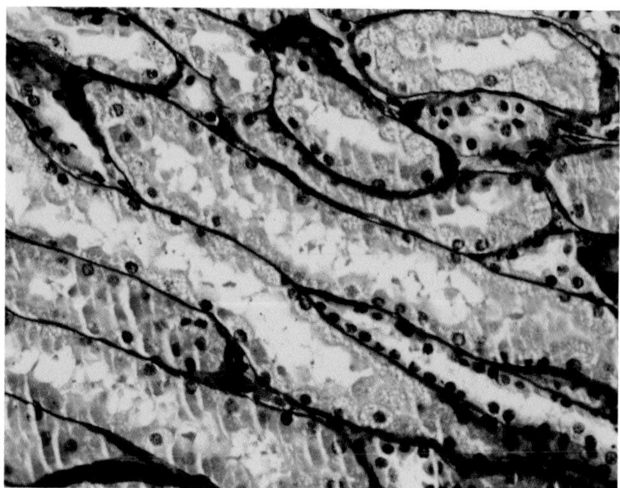

FIGURE 17-30 ▪ ATN is characterized by variable ectasia of lumina and necrosis and desquamation of epithelial cells. (Jones methenamine silver, original magnification 40×.)

Interstitial Nephritis Caused by Infectious Agents

It seems that almost any organism can cause acute interstitial nephritis. Historically, β-hemolytic streptococci were the most important bacteria and measles virus was the most important virus associated with this condition (e160). However, these are examples of reactive interstitial nephritis in which organisms do not directly infect the kidney, and other organisms with a similar pathogenesis include *Brucella, Legionella, Yersinia*, Epstein-Barr virus, HIV, *Leishmania donovani*, and *Toxoplasma gondii*. In contrast, *Escherichia coli, Staphylococcus aureus*, invasive streptococci, *Leptospira*, fungi, mycobacteria, rickettsiae, cytomegalovirus, herpes simplex virus, Asian and European hantaviruses, BK polyomavirus, and adenovirus do infect the kidney. *E. coli* may cause acute pyelonephritis (see later) or, in rare circumstances, malakoplakia of the kidney. Bacteria and fungi can be demonstrated with histologic stains; cytomegalovirus, herpes simplex virus, BK polyomavirus, and adenovirus produce characteristic inclusions and can be identified with specific immunohistochemical stains or molecular probes.

Rickettsiae require specific IF staining and hantavirus infection must be diagnosed serologically (e54,e65).

Acute pyelonephritis is a clinical diagnosis made in an infant with fever and evidence of a urinary tract infection or in an older child with significant bacteriuria, systemic symptoms, or renal tenderness. Hematogenous infection may occur in the first 2 months of life, but thereafter acute pyelonephritis results from ascending infection. The usual pathogen is *E. coli*, but *Klebsiella, Proteus, Pseudomonas, Enterobacter*, and *Enterococcus* species, group B or group A streptococci, and coagulase-negative staphylococci can also cause urinary tract infections (UTIs) in infants and children (e136). The pathologic features of acute pyelonephritis include patchy interstitial infiltrates of neutrophils that may form abscesses and eventually involve tubules with the formation of white blood cell casts in the urine. However, because prompt clinical diagnosis and treatment typically lead to resolution, these lesions are only rarely encountered in pathology specimens.

Chronic pyelonephritis is characterized by inflammation and fibrosis that involves the pelvicalyceal system in addition to the interstitium, features shared with the analgesic and sickle cell nephropathies but not other forms of interstitial nephritis. Failure to make that distinction in autopsy series in the past led to an overestimate of the likelihood that urinary tract infection would progress to chronic renal disease (e260). The relationship between vesicoureteral reflux and renal scarring has also been called into question by cortical imaging studies. Scans performed with technetium 99mTc dimercaptosuccinic acid (DMSA) have a sensitivity of 89% and a specificity of 100% for histologically confirmed pyelonephritis in studies in piglets (which have a collecting system similar to that of humans), and results are positive in 50% to 85% of children with a clinical diagnosis of acute pyelonephritis. Fifty percent of these lesions resolve on imaging studies in 4 to 6 months, and the remainder appear to develop into segmental parenchymal scars. Vesicoureteral reflux was present in 25% to 40% of children with acute pyelonephritis and positive DMSA scan findings, but renal scarring occurred as often in patients without as in patients with vesicoureteral reflux (e136). The fact that sites of renal scarring conformed to the distribution of composite papillae, which have a more patulous pore than simple papillae, supports the notion that scarring is caused by intrarenal reflux (e256). However, many children have parenchymal scarring at the time of their first imaging study, which suggests that they had an earlier unrecognized infection or that damage might have occurred in utero (e262). In kidneys that are small and scarred as a consequence of obstruction, the severity of inflammation and scarring often varies markedly between renal lobules, and when dysplastic features are also present, such as islands of cartilage and primitive collecting ducts, early intrauterine reflux seems certain. Congenital or acquired intrarenal reflux, rather than segmental hypoplasia, is the explanation for the segmental scarring in Ask-Upmark kidney (e7). Recognition of intrauterine vesicoureteral reflux and dysplasia is important because children with such lesions are more likely to develop hypertension and end-stage renal disease than are the renal scars acquired as a result of postnatal obstructive pyelonephritis (e136). Sclerotic glomeruli are seen in scarred areas, and FSGS can develop in the remaining glomeruli as a result of hyperperfusional injury.

Complications of acute pyelonephritis that are unusual in children include pyonephrosis and perinephric abscess. In pyonephrosis, an acute inflammatory exudate fills the renal calyces and pelvis because of a high-grade obstruction, and perinephric abscesses develop when the inflammation penetrates the renal capsule. Complications of chronic urinary tract infection that are also uncommon in children are xanthogranulomatous pyelonephritis and malakoplakia. Xanthogranulomatous pyelonephritis, which occurs in the setting of urinary obstruction or stone disease, presents clinically in affected children with abdominal pain, fever, weight loss, and anorexia, often with a palpable flank mass, and is characterized by orange-yellow foci or distinct masses that are composed of foamy macrophages, neutrophils, lymphocytes, plasma cells, and multinucleated giant cells with frequent calcification (19,e62,e128). Malakoplakia, in which yellow-brown nodules composed of foamy macrophages contain round laminated Michaelis-Gutmann bodies, has been described in the urinary bladder (165), kidney (72), colon (87), soft tissues and bone (35), and skin (e96) in children.

Drug-Induced Interstitial Nephritis

Many commonly used therapeutic agents can cause an acute interstitial nephritis. This allergic reaction is generally unpredictable and may be associated with other systemic symptoms. Antibiotics, especially β-lactams and NSAIDs, are most often implicated, but other antibacterial and antiviral agents, anticonvulsants, and diuretics have produced interstitial nephritis (e65). Other drugs, including some of the above-listed agents, can produce glomerular, tubular, or renovascular lesions. Only a minority of patients with drug-induced interstitial nephritis have eosinophilia of blood or urine, and eosinophils, if present, usually constitute 10% or fewer of the infiltrating cells in biopsy specimens (e224). They are most often seen in reactions to antibiotics, especially methicillin, and least often in reactions to NSAIDs and cimetidine. The majority of cells are T lymphocytes. Neutrophils and basophils are rare. Epithelioid granulomas were initially observed in reactions associated with sulfonamides but have subsequently been reported in association with numerous drugs (e65) and have been described in children (179).

Immune-Mediated Tubulointerstitial Nephritis

Antitubular basement membrane antibodies are usually identified in the context of glomerular or interstitial disease. However, Helczynski and Landing found antitubular basement membrane antibodies in 3 of 13 cases originally classified as nephronophthisis/medullary cystic disease and suggested that they were the cause of the renal injury (e135). Similarly, tubulointerstitial nephritis with granular deposits of immunoglobulin and complement components along tubular basement membranes or in the interstitium is usually seen in conjunction with an immune complex disease that also affects glomeruli, most commonly SLE; however, rare cases of apparent primary immune complex-mediated tubulointerstitial nephritis have been reported in children and adults (e91,e172). The predominant cell in most interstitial nephritides is the T-lymphocyte, but a primary abnormality of T-cells is suspected in tubulointerstitial nephritis with uveitis (66). Because uveitis and interstitial nephritis are found in Sjögren syndrome, Behçet syndrome, sarcoidosis, and several infections, these conditions must be excluded before a diagnosis of tubulointerstitial nephritis with uveitis is made (e65).

Tubulointerstitial Nephritis in Hereditary Diseases

Tubulointerstitial nephritis is an important component of Alport syndrome (e116), Alagille syndrome (arteriohepatic dysplasia) (e149), and Bardet-Biedl syndrome (mental retardation, pigmentary retinopathy, polydactyly, obesity, and hypogenitalism), formerly known as *Laurence-Moon-Biedl syndrome* (e271). The nephronophthisis-medullary cystic disease complex is likely a combination of several diseases, including two autosomal recessive conditions—familial infantile nephronophthisis, which maps to 9q22 to 31 (e229), and familial JNPH, which maps to 2q13 (e230)—and an adult-onset autosomal dominant medullary cystic disease that maps to 1q21 (e209). All forms are characterized by shrunken kidneys with cysts up to 2.0 cm at the corticomedullary junction or in the medulla and extensive tubular atrophy and interstitial fibrosis with a variable infiltrate of lymphocytes and plasma cells (e54). Colvin and Fang have summarized the reports of five families with an HLA-linked familial interstitial nephritis and 10 infants with a progressive tubulointerstitial nephropathy that may or may not have a genetic basis (e65).

RENOVASCULAR DISEASES

Hemolytic Uremic Syndrome

HUS is the most common cause of acute renal failure in childhood (e287). In 1925, Moschcowitz described a 16-year-old girl with clinical and pathologic features of what we would now recognize as *thrombotic thrombocytopenic purpura* (e217). In 1955, Gasser et al. introduced the term *HUS* to describe the disease they reported in five children with hemolytic anemia, thrombocytopenia, and acute renal failure (e105). Subsequently, Riley et al. reported the association of two outbreaks of hemorrhagic colitis with the rare *E. coli* O157:H7 serotype (e261), and Karmali et al. recognized the association between toxins produced by *E. coli* and sporadic cases of HUS (e164). Microangiopathic hemolytic anemia, thrombocytopenia, and acute renal failure constitute the diagnostic criteria for HUS, and approximately 90% of pediatric cases are preceded by a diarrheal prodrome. Enteropathogenic *E. coli* have been linked to 75% of cases of postdiarrheal HUS. These organisms asymptomatically inhabit the intestines of cattle, and contaminated beef products are implicated in most epidemics. However, most cases of HUS occur sporadically and may be acquired by drinking water or consuming products contaminated by cattle feces and by person-to-person spread (e287). Damage to colonic tissue is enhanced by an influx of neutrophils attracted by the release of cytokines from colonic epithelial cells when the toxin binds to these cells. The toxin is transported in the plasma or on the surface of monocytes or platelets and binds to receptors on susceptible cells, and is then internalized and causes the death of these cells. Toxin binds to glomerular endothelial and mesangial cells and glomerular and tubular epithelial cells, which release cytokines that upregulate the expression of receptors on endothelial cells. Cell death occurs as a result of inhibition of protein synthesis or apoptosis, the endothelium becomes procoagulant, and a thrombotic microangiopathy (TMA) ensues (111). Involvement of brain, liver, pancreas, heart, lung, skeletal muscle, skin, parotid gland, and retina has been reported in HUS, but central nervous system dysfunction occurs in one-third of cases, and central nervous system hemorrhage is the most common cause of death. Interindividual variations in the presence or density of receptors, especially in the brain, may account for the seemingly unpredictable extrarenal complications of HUS (e287).

Three major categories of pathologic lesions have been described in the kidney in HUS—cortical necrosis, glomerular TMA, and arterial TMA (e125). Tubular and interstitial injury are most likely secondary, possibly through endothelial injury in peritubular capillaries (141), and striking degrees of apoptosis have been described in tubular epithelial cells (178). Cortical necrosis is discussed in a subsequent section of this chapter, but the histologic lesion noted in the noninfarcted portions of the renal cortex in patients with cortical necrosis associated with HUS is usually glomerular TMA (e9). In glomerular TMA obliteration of the capillary loops by a combination of fibrin and platelet thrombi result in the fragmentation of red blood cells (Figure 17-31), and swelling, necrosis, and detachment of endothelial cells and expansion of the subendothelial space by electron-lucent "fluff." Neomembrane beneath the endothelial cell and the normal lamina densa on the other side of the fluffy material may impart a double contour to the capillary wall in histologic sections stained with silver methenamine. IF microscopy shows granular deposits of fibrin-reactive antigen, apparently within capillary loops. Mesangia often show a decreased amount of matrix (mesangiolysis) but are usually normocellular. Early arterial TMA is characterized by narrowing of the lumens of interlobular (intracortical) arteries and arterioles by endothelial cell swelling and fibrinoid

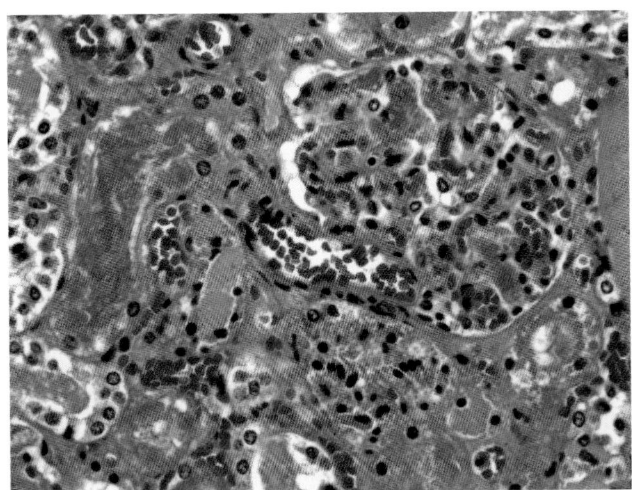

FIGURE 17-31 Hemolytic uremic syndrome. Fibrin thrombi and fragmented red blood cells occlude glomerular capillaries, and fibrin is seen in an areriole. (Hematoxylin and eosin, original magnification 400×.)

mural necrosis, and later lesions show intimal fibrosis or laminar proliferation ("onion skinning"). Red blood cells and fibrin thrombi may accumulate in the lumina and walls of affected vessels at any stage. Glomerular and arterial TMA can be present in the same biopsy specimen, but usually one or the other predominates, and the most common glomerular lesions seen with arterial TMA are collapse or retraction of the glomerular tuft and "paralysis" (exaggerated congestion) of capillary loops, presumably reflecting obstructive lesions in afferent and efferent arterioles, respectively. Habib et al. noted that in cases in which arterial TMA predominated, the superficial glomeruli were collapsed, but glomerular TMA could be seen at deeper levels (e125).

The prevalence of one or another pathologic lesion may be a function of the age of the patient or the evolution of the disease. In the series of 70 consecutive patients reported by Habib et al., 55 were less than 28 months old and 15 ranged in age from 3 to 16 years. Of the 55 infants, 45 had a preceding diarrheal illness, 42 had oliguria (21 for longer than 7 days), and 18 had central nervous system symptoms. Nine of the ten patients with cortical necrosis were infants (the tenth patient was 3 years old), and 26 of the 29 patients with predominantly glomerular TMA were infants. Of the 15 older children, five had a preceding diarrheal illness, seven had oliguria (all episodes lasted for 6 days or longer), none had central nervous system symptoms, and 10 of the 13 patients with predominantly arterial TMA were older children. Two of the nine infants and all ten of the older children who did not have a diarrheal prodrome had arterial TMA and progressed to renal failure, and four of the five older children with a diarrheal prodrome had glomerular TMA or cortical necrosis and recovered. Oliguria and hypertension occurred whether glomerular or arterial TMA predominated; anuria was observed only if glomerular TMA was present (and patients with a greater proportion of glomeruli so involved had anuria of longer duration and a worse outcome). Hypertension was more severe with arterial TMA regardless of the patient's age (e125). Arterial TMA is the predominant lesion in adults with HUS (95). In a series of biopsy or autopsy specimens from 24 children, 6 months to 12 years of age at presentation, glomerular TMA was the predominant lesion in 8 of 15 specimens obtained within 16 days of hospitalization, and arterial TMA was seen in all nine obtained 17 days to 3 months after presentation, but not in any of the specimens obtained earlier (e9). In follow-up biopsy specimens obtained after 1 year, patients who had had predominantly glomerular TMA showed varying degrees of glomerulosclerosis but generally normal vessels, whereas those who had had predominantly arterial TMA showed mainly vascular lesions (e125).

Atypical HUS may follow nonenteric infections, such as streptococcal pneumonia, and has been described as a complication of other glomerulopathies, several drugs, pregnancy, bone marrow transplantation, neoplasms, collagen vascular disorders, and HIV infection (e287). Many of these patients have mutations in the complement regulatory proteins—membrane cofactor protein (MCP), complement factor H (CFH), and factor I (IF), and patients with MCP mutations have a better prognosis and more favorable outcome following transplantation than do those with CFH or IF mutations (85). Factor H deficiency is also found in some cases of familial HUS (e316) and deficiency or inhibition of Factor 11 is implicated in dense deposit disease (99). HUS has been reported to recur in transplants in up to 41% of patients (e133), but was not observed in any of 62 children whose primary disease was Shiga-toxin associated HUS (51), suggesting that recurrences develop in patients with a genetic predisposition to HUS.

Renal Involvement in Systemic Vasculitides

Renal involvement in vasculitis in children is seen most often in HSP, microscopic polyarteritis (polyangiitis), Wegener granulomatosis, Churg-Strauss syndrome, and (macroscopic) polyarteritis nodosa, but kidney disease can also occur in Kawasaki disease and Takayasu arteritis (e264). Jennette noted that no classification of the systemic vasculitides has been universally accepted but outlined a functional approach to the diagnosis of those that involve the kidney. Giant cell arteritis and Takayasu arteritis cause granulomatous inflammation in larger arteries and may involve the aorta and main renal artery, with subsequent luminal narrowing and development of hypertension. Macroscopic polyarteritis nodosa and Kawasaki disease cause segmental necrosis in medium-sized vessels, including the interlobar and the arcuate arteries in the kidney, which can result in renal hemorrhage, ischemia, or infarction. Small-vessel vasculitis is characterized by a focal and segmental glomerulonephritis, often with segmental necrosis of the glomerular tuft and segmental cellular crescents. Such glomerular lesions are further categorized by IF microscopy. If immunoglobulin and complement components are deposited in glomeruli, the likely diagnosis is lupus or another immune complex-mediated vasculitis, Henoch-Shönlein purpura nephritis, or cryoglobulinemic vasculitis. If immunoglobulin or complement components are not present, the so-called pauci-immune glomerulonephritides include microscopic polyangiitis (microscopic polyarteritis nodosa), Wegener granulomatosis, and Churg-Strauss syndrome (e54).

Macroscopic polyarteritis nodosa can occur in children, and Kawasaki disease is a childhood illness with a peak incidence in the first year of life (e81,e264). Kawasaki disease preferentially involves the coronary arteries, but medium-sized renal arteries are the next most frequently affected site (e226), and it can also cause renal artery stenosis (48,53). The early histologic lesion in renal arteries in both these diseases involves the media, but in polyarteritis nodosa it is characterized by fibrinoid necrosis, whereas in Kawasaki disease, medial edema with myocyte degeneration, subintimal edema, and leukocytic infiltration are seen (e154). Microscopic polyangiitis, Wegener granulomatosis, and Churg-Strauss syndrome share many clinical features, and most affected patients have ANCA antibodies. Recent studies suggest that these diseases develop as a result of molecular mimicry when antibodies directed toward an epitope on an infectious agent, such as FimH on fimbriated bacteria, cross react with lysosomal membrane protein-2 and cause pauci-immune focal necrotizing glomerulonephritis (83), and there has been a single case report of pulmonary hemorrhage and renal disease in a newborn infant due to transplacental passage of ANCA antibodies (11).

Ear, nose, and throat involvement is more common in Wegener granulomatosis, and Churg-Strauss syndrome is characterized by allergic rhinitis or asthma and peripheral blood eosinophilia (e193). Histopathologically, all three conditions produce segmental fibrinoid necrosis that can involve glomerular and alveolar capillaries, arterioles in many organs, and venules in the skin and sinuses (e154). As noted above, the most common lesion in renal biopsy specimens is segmental necrosis of the glomerular tuft with crescent formation, and fluorescent antibody and ultrastructural studies show no immune complexes, a key negative that excludes the immune complex vasculitides that may have similar histologic features. A minority of specimens show fibrinoid necrosis of interlobular arteries, and the predominant tubulointerstitial lesion is periglomerular inflammation. Interstitial eosinophils suggest, but are not diagnostic of, Churg-Strauss syndrome (e154).

Renal Vein Thrombosis

Renal vein thrombosis occurs in the fetus or the neonate under conditions of dehydration, sepsis, maternal diabetes, birth asphyxia, or polycythemia (e138), and less frequently in the infant or the older child with nephrotic syndrome (e60) or leukemic hyperleukocytosis (e222). It may present as a flank mass or with hematuria, hypertension, or renal failure, and it can be readily diagnosed by renal ultrasonography (e138). Entrapment of the left renal vein between the aorta and the superior mesenteric artery (nutcracker phenomenon) may be a cause of renal congestion and postural proteinuria (e187). Grossly, the involved kidney is enlarged, hemorrhagic, and friable. Histology reveals intense congestion of veins and capillaries in the interstitium, interstitial edema or hemorrhage, variable degrees of necrosis of tubular epithelial cells, and margination of leukocytes in glomerular capillaries.

Renal Artery Stenosis

Renal artery stenosis in children is most often caused by fibromuscular dysplasia (175). It has also been reported in neurofibromatosis, Takayasu arteritis, Williams syndrome (e70), Kawasaki disease (48,53), and Alagille syndrome (e24). In addition, renal artery thrombosis has been reported in a dehydrated infant (e93). Fibromuscular dysplasia, or renal artery dysplasia, typically affects girls and women in the second or the third decade but can be seen in younger children. It is classified according to the layer of the vessel wall that is affected, but nearly 90% of cases show medial fibroplasia with aneurysms in which a longitudinal section of the artery shows thickened fibrotic ridges alternating with almost full-thickness defects resulting from a loss of smooth muscle and elastic laminae, or perimedial fibroplasia in which much of the outer portion of the media is fibrotic (e196). Renal artery stenosis in neurofibromatosis may be caused by compression by an encircling neurofibroma, adventitial or intimal compression in larger vessels by a proliferation of Schwann cells, or mesodermal dysplasia by nodular proliferations of smooth muscle cells in the intima or media of smaller vessels, and hypertension in neurofibromatosis may also be due to proliferative lesions in the aorta causing coarctation, or to an associated pheochromocytoma (e237).

Renal Cortical Necrosis and Papillary Necrosis

Renal cortical necrosis occurs in response to a sudden and sustained loss of renal perfusion caused by arterial thrombosis, as in the HUS, or shock, as in acute blood loss, overwhelming sepsis, or severe perinatal asphyxia. It is characterized by coagulative necrosis. Thrombi in glomeruli suggest that a TMA, such as disseminated intravascular coagulation or HUS, may be present, but correlation with clinical information is usually necessary to determine a cause.

Papillary necrosis in adults is usually a complication of analgesic abuse or diabetes, but it has been reported, often in conjunction with renal cortical necrosis, in neonates following asphyxia or shock (e4), infants following gastroenteritis (e59), and children with sickle cell disease (e202), disseminated candidiasis (e307), Wegener granulomatosis (e317), and meningococcal sepsis (59). The affected papillary tips are grossly yellow and show coagulative necrosis with a neutrophilic infiltrate at the junction with viable tissue, and necrotic papillae may slough into the collecting system and cause acute obstruction.

Radiation Nephritis

Radiation therapy can cause acute or chronic renal injury. Fibrinoid necrosis in arteries and arterioles progresses to subintimal fibrosis, which may be the only clue that the associated glomerulosclerosis, tubular atrophy, and interstitial fibrosis were caused by radiation (e447).

Bartter Syndrome

Bartter syndrome is an unusual secondary hyperaldosteronism in which patients have hypokalemic alkalosis with hypercalciuria and hyperreninemia but normal or low blood pressure. The characteristic renal lesion is hyperplasia of the juxtaglomerular apparatus in the hilum of the glomerulus, which is markedly enlarged and shows more than the allowable eight cells (e237). Both sporadic and familial forms have been described. The latter have an autosomal recessive pattern of inheritance and have been mapped to the region of the Na-K-2Cl cotransporter gene at 15q15 to 21 (e17).

Table 17-6 ■ PRIMARY RENAL TUMORS OF CHILDHOOD

Tumors	Relative Percentage
WT, favorable histology[a]	80
Anaplastic WT	5
Mesoblastic nephroma	5
Clear-cell sarcoma	4
Rhabdoid tumor	2
Miscellaneous	4
Neuroblastoma	
Peripheral neuroectodermal tumor	
Synovial sarcoma	
RCC	
Angiomyolipoma	
Lymphoma[b]	<1

[a]Includes cystic, partially differentiated nephroblastoma, and cystic nephroma, which together comprise fewer than 5% of cases of favorable WT cases.
[b]Includes only cases presenting as renal tumors. In many patients with leukemia/lymphoma, renal lesions develop later.

RENAL NEOPLASMS

During the past 40 years, cooperative groups have been remarkably successful at targeting pediatric renal tumors that comprise only 7% of all childhood cancers. They have enabled the development of accurate diagnostic criteria, stage and histology-based therapeutic stratifications, and appropriate surgical techniques. In addition, they have demonstrated that irradiation in conjunction with several active chemotherapeutic agents are effective. The overall result has been a dramatic improvement in the prognosis for most patients with WT (the most common pediatric renal tumor), from approximately 8% at the beginning of the century to approximately 50% in 1960 to greater than 90% in 2000. Most children in European countries are registered as patients in the International Society of Pediatric Oncology cooperative group protocols, which rely on the use of preoperative neoadjuvant chemotherapy and the provision of postoperative chemotherapy based on pathologic response. In contrast, the pediatric cooperative groups centered in North America have favored primary nephrectomy, with postoperative chemotherapy based on pathologic analysis of untreated tumors. Although these two approaches are difficult to compare, both have met with similar success in treating children with WT. During the 40 years of its existence, the National Wilms Tumor Study (NWTS), currently enrolling 85% of all new cases diagnosed in North America, has contributed greatly to the increase in long-term survivorship. The results of the NWTS clinical trials are widely published, and many complete detailed reviews are available. The pathologist seeking guidelines for managing pediatric renal tumor specimens is referred to any of the current recommendations by Perlman (134,135).

The classification of pediatric renal tumors and their relative percentages are given in Table 17-6. As more is being discovered about the underlying genetic defects in these tumors, classifiers based on gene expression provide diagnostic confidence and accuracy greater than that of pathologic analysis alone; however, these have to be used in the appropriate histopathologic context (76). This chapter only summarizes the salient features of these rare neoplasms, the study of which has answered many questions also relevant to other neoplasms.

Nephroblastoma (Wilms Tumor)

Nephroblastoma is one of the most common malignant, solid, extracranial tumor of childhood, with an incidence of 1/10,000 white children (the incidence is higher among blacks and lower in Orientals) (e300). The estimated yearly occurrence of WT is 400 to 500 cases in the United States with only 15 cases a year in the Chicago area for instance (134,135). It is slightly more common in girls (e56), in whom it tends to present at an older age (mean age, 36 months in boys versus 42 months in girls) (e221). It is uncommon in neonates and infants and is only occasionally reported in adults. Most cases of "adult WT" are primitive neuroectodermal tumors, synovial sarcomas, or metanephric adenomas. Approximately 10% of nephroblastomas develop in association with one of several well-characterized dysmorphic syndromes (e.g., WT, aniridia, genitourinary malformation, mental retardation, the WAGR syndrome; Denys-Drash syndrome, a syndrome characterized by mesangial sclerosis, pseudohermaphroditism; Beckwith-Wiedemann syndrome, characterized by hemihypertrophy, macroglossia, omphalocele, and visceromegaly). Five percent of cases are bilateral, with the bilateral tumors more likely to be associated with one of these syndromes as well as with nephrogenic rests. A positive family history is found in 2% of patients with WT (e42).

Molecular and Cellular Biology

Advances in the genetics of renal tumors are driving diagnosis and therapy stratification (29). The genetics of WT are very complex with multiple genetic events (some mutually exclusive) leading to tumor formation.

1. WT1: The first genetic locus was identified in patients with the WAGR syndrome, which carries a 30% risk of developing WT (135). Abnormalities involving WT1 are consistently found in the tumors of WAGR patients as well as in patients with Denys-Drash syndrome, which carries a 90% risk of nephroblastoma. Different WT1 abnormalities are associated with these different syndromes. WT1 is an important regulatory molecule involved in cell growth and development. It is expressed in a tissue-specific manner. In the developing embryo, WT1 expression is found primarily in the urogenital system. In adult tissues, WT1 expression is found in the urogenital system, central nervous system, and in tissues involved in hematopoiesis, including the bone marrow and the lymph nodes. The WT1 gene is located in the p13 region of chromosome 11. WT1 encodes a zinc finger DNA-binding transcription factor that is essential for normal genitourinary development, and mutations or deletions are found in 15% of sporadic cases of WT. An additional one-third of all nephroblastomas show loss of heterozygosity (LOH) at this locus. β-catenin is a cellular adhesion molecule that promotes overexpression of the c-myc and cyclin D1. Activating mutations in the β-catenin gene (CTNNB1 on chromosome 3p22) have been detected in 15% of patients with WT. There is a strong correlation between reduced expression of the WT1 gene and the β-catenin mutation (185). However, the majority of WT express wild-type WT1, sometimes to high levels. Furthermore, in WT that express wild-type WT1, it is not known whether the persistent expression of WT1 contributes to the development of the disease or is just a reflection of tumor ontogeny (148). Identical WT1 mutations and LOH patterns have been reported in both nephroblastomas and their associated nephrogenic rests. This suggests that WT1 inactivation may result in the formation of a nephrogenic rest and that at least some nephroblastomas are the result of subsequent genetic events occurring in a nephrogenic rest (135).

   The uncontrolled growth of cancer cells can be due to the loss of function of tumor suppressors and/or the activation of oncogenes. Although these are opposite functions that would be intuitively mutually exclusive for a single protein, evidence is emerging that one protein can exhibit both properties under different cellular conditions. An example of this is the oncogene Myc.1. The WT1 protein has a similar dual behavior depending upon the cell type in which it is expressed. There is evidence that WT1 can behave either as a tumor suppressor or an oncogene in the development of the malignancies (195). The presence or absence of regulatory protein partners (e.g., Par-4, p53, EGFR, FGFR1) may account for the variable behavior of WT1 in different malignancies. In addition to protein–protein interactions, other mechanisms that can affect the function of WT1 include alternate splicing, usage of alternate promoters, and posttranslational modification of WT1 (113,195). Adding to the complexity of WT1 is the fact that it has multiple layers of regulatory activity that are both DNA- and RNA mediated (46).
2. WT2: The second locus, 11p15 (WT2), is associated with Beckwith-Wiedemann syndrome, which carries a 5% risk of developing WT (173). The WT2 locus, comprising the two independent imprinted domains IGF2/H19 and KIP2/LIT1, can undergo maternal deletion or alterations associated with imprinting (160). Some functions of this gene are related to IGF-2, which encodes embryonal growth factor (185).
3. FWT1 and FWT2: Approximately 2% of WT patients have a family history of WT. Familial WT cases generally have an earlier age of onset and an increased frequency of bilateral disease, although there is variability among WT families, with some families displaying later than average ages at diagnosis. Only a minority of tumors carries detectable mutations in WT1, and it can be excluded as the predisposition gene in most WT families. Two familial WT genes have been localized, FWT1 at 17q12–q21 and FWT2 at 19q13.4; lack of linkage in some WT families to either of these loci implies the existence of at least one additional familial WT gene (154).
4. WTX: Recently, a gene located at Xq11.1, and named WTX, was shown to be inactivated in WTs (149). WTX inactivation appears to follow a "one hit hypothesis" since males only have one copy, and females only need to lose the copy on the active X chromosome. One-hit inactivation of a tumor-suppressor gene on the X chromosome is a departure from the traditional biallelic Knudson model and has been postulated but never documented until this study. WTX appears to participate in the WNT signaling pathway and to promote the ubiquitination and degradation of β-catenin (105,126). Previously WTX mutations, both small deletions and point mutations, were observed in 15/51 (29.4%) of WTs, and the mutation frequency was approximately equal in males and females (149). This study also noted that WTX alterations were never seen in tumors carrying mutations in either WT1 or CTNNB1. The implication of these data was that the etiology of approximately 50% of WTs involved mutations in either WT1 or WTX. A more recent study assessed 125 tumors and showed that WTX alterations were approximately equally frequent in WTs with mutations in WT1 and/or CTNNB1 and in tumors with no mutation in either WT1 or CTNNB1, and that WTX mutations occurred with about the same frequency as WT1 mutations. Thus, about one-third of tumors carry mutations at WT1, CTNNB1, and/or WTX (155).

5. p53: The tumor-suppressor gene p53 on chromosome 17p is thought to play a role in a subset of patients with WT. The high correlation of p53 mutations and anaplastic WT suggests that p53 alterations are required for progression to the anaplastic phenotype (88,132). They have also been shown to correlate with recurrence/metastasis in tumors that are not anaplastic (73,e180).
6. LOH 1p, 11p, and 16q: Grundy and Coppes (e117) studied the relationship of tumor-specific LOH and phenotype in a total of 286 cases enrolled in the NWTS. LOH has been thought to represent a "second hit" affecting a tumor-suppressor gene (loss of the remaining, normal allele following mutation or deletion of the first allele). Preliminary analysis of their data suggests an association between LOH at 11p, age at diagnosis, and histopathologic grade. A young age of the patient at diagnosis was observed for tumors with LOH at 11p13, and these tumors were less likely to have anaplastic histology (e117,e118). Despite a favorable outcome for most patients with favorable histology WT, the LOH for chromosomes 1p and 16q is an adverse prognostic factor (62). High telomerase expression is also an adverse prognostic factor in favorable histology WT (42). The presence of LOH for chromosomes 1p and 16q will direct therapy stratification among favorable histology Wilms tumor patients in the current COG renal study (AREN0532, AREN0533) (134).
7. Other loci, including 1q, 2q, 7p, 9q, 14q, and 22, have also been implicated in the etiology of Wilms tumor through studies of LOH, loss of imprinting, and constitutional chromosomal defects (155).

WT is believed to originate from the metanephric blastema and is histopathologically characterized by a triphasic pattern of blastemal, epithelial, and stromal elements that can show a wide variety of patterns and differentiation. LOH and clonality studies have shown that the different histologic components are of tumor origin (e331,67).

Gross Features

Nephroblastoma commonly presents as a solitary, more or less rounded mass arising from any part of the kidney. The tumor origin is multicentric in 7% of cases (Figure 17-32), and 5% of cases are bilateral (135). The tumor kidney specimen weight ranges from 60 to 6,350 g, with a median of 550 g (e221). The bulging cut surface is pale gray, soft, friable, and lobulated, and areas of hemorrhage, necrosis, and cyst formation are often apparent (Figure 17-33). The tumor is sharply demarcated from the adjacent renal tissue by a pseudocapsule (eFigure 17-6). The tumor may protrude into the calyces and sometimes the ureter, forming polypoid excrescences resembling botryoid rhabdomyosarcoma. It often invades the renal vein, from which it may extend up through the vena cava to the right atrium.

Adequate sampling is critical. One tissue block for each centimeter in the maximal dimension is recommended.

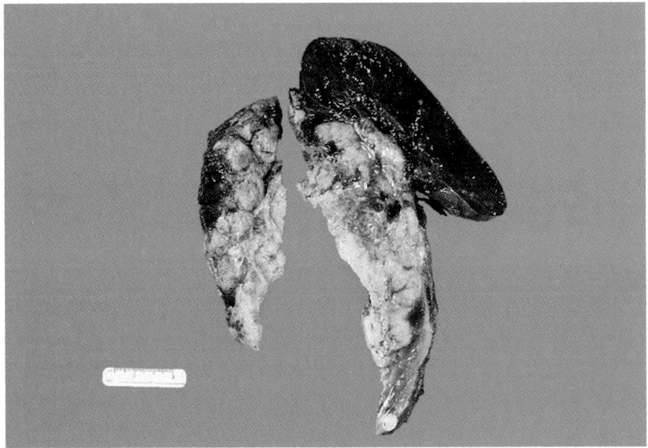

FIGURE 17-32 ■ Multicentric WT, cut surface. The larger, dominant mass invaded the spleen, and a second small round tumor is seen in the lower pole.

Evaluation of the renal pelvis and sinus, vein, capsule, and all lymph nodes is needed for staging. Beckwith and Perlman's suggestions for handling pediatric renal tumors include the following: receiving the specimen intact, avoiding frozen sections, not stripping the capsule, inking the surface, bivalving to demonstrate the relationship of tumor to kidney and renal sinus, taking initial sections for diagnosis and special studies (cytogenetic, molecular, and ultrastructural), fixing overnight in refrigerator, taking most of the sections from the periphery, including any areas that appear different (eFigure 17-7), documenting the exact source of each section, and generously sampling uninvolved

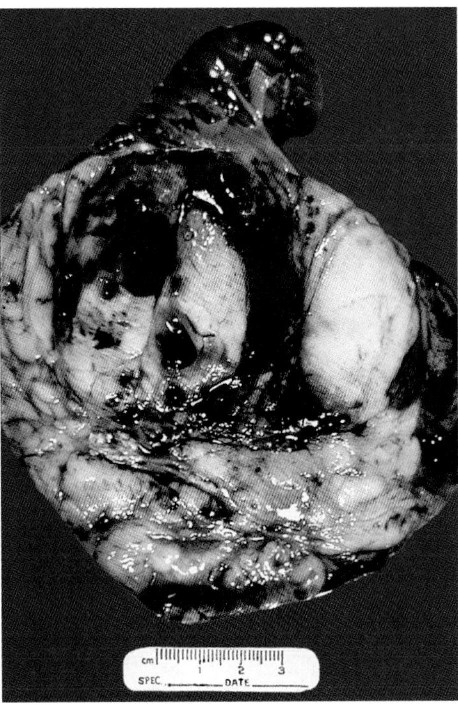

FIGURE 17-33 ■ Cut surface of WT is bulging, soft, and friable and has a nodular variegated appearance with areas of hemorrhage and necrosis. Normal kidney can be identified at the one pole.

kidney (e20). In addition submit sections that include the triangular interface between the intrarenal tumor pseudocapsule, the extrarenal tumor pseudocapsule, and the renal capsule. Careful consideration must be given to the renal sinus, which extends into the kidney following its medial contour and carries blood vessels and nerves within its fat and connective tissue (134).

Microscopic Features

The type of histologic pattern seen in WTs was of prognostic significance before the era of modern chemotherapy. Within the same specimen, the pattern tends to be uniform; however, it varies greatly from tumor to tumor. Classical triphasic WT is composed of blastemal, epithelial, and stromal components (Figure 17-34, eFigure 17-8), but biphasic and monophasic tumors are not uncommon. When one component comprises more than two-third of the tumor, the tumor is designated accordingly. The mixed type, in which no component predominates, is most common (41%), followed by blastema-predominant (39%) and epithelium-predominant (18%). Stroma-predominant WT is rare (1.4%) (e273). With adequate sampling, microscopic foci of all three components can be recognized in most cases.

Metanephric blastema is the most primitive cell type in WT and is characterized by densely packed primitive cells lacking identifiable features of differentiation by LM (Figure 17-35). Tumors with a diffuse blastemal pattern and noncohesive, infiltrative margins are highly aggressive but usually respond to current therapy (e22). The organoid blastemal patterns (serpentine, nodular, and basaloid) are characterized by regularly defined aggregates of blastemal cells set in a myxoid mesenchymal background, without aggressive infiltration and with a clearly demarcated edge, as is usual in all WT patterns.

The epithelial component of WT is most often of nephrogenic type, in which various stages of tubular and glomeruloid differentiation are seen (Figures 17-36 and 17-37). Heterologous epithelial patterns include mucinous, squamous, and neuroepithelial and neuroendocrine cells. Similarly, stromal patterns may be nephrogenic (myxoid, fibrous, smooth muscle, and adipose cells) or heterologous (skeletal muscle, which is most common, cartilage, and bone) (Figure 17-38).

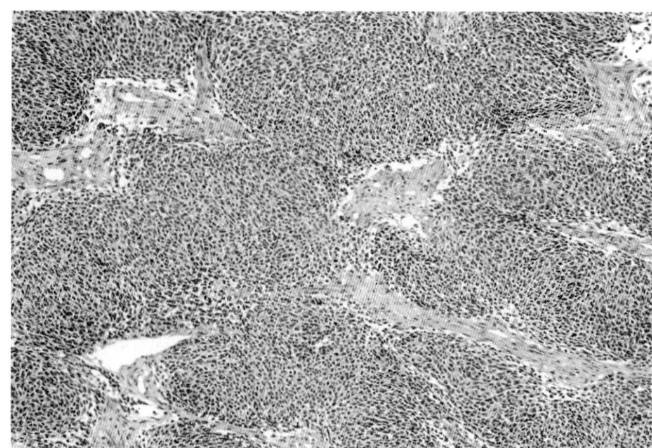

FIGURE 17-35 ■ Classic WT showing a predominantly blastemic appearance. (Hematoxylin and eosin stain, original magnification ×100.)

Anaplastic nuclear change is the only marker of "unfavorable histology" in WT. Other pediatric renal tumors with an unfavorable histology or in the high-risk category of the International Society of Pediatric Oncology (e273), such as clear-cell sarcoma and rhabdoid tumor, are separate neoplastic entities and not variants of WT. Anaplastic nuclear changes refer to extreme cytologic atypia, not minor variations in nuclear shape or size. Anaplasia is defined as a threefold increase in nuclear diameter, hyperchromasia of the enlarged nuclei, and multipolar mitotic figures (Figure 17-39A,B). These changes are severe enough to be detected when scanned with a ten times objective.

Anaplastic nuclear changes are a marker of resistance to therapy and do not imply aggressiveness. All patients are

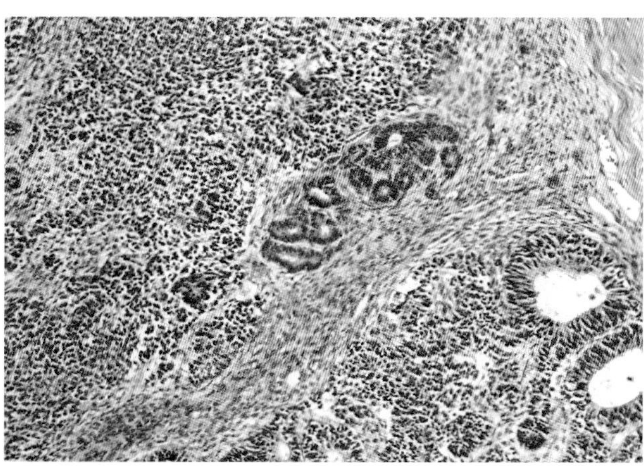

FIGURE 17-34 ■ Classic WT showing a triphasic pattern of blastema, tubules, and a glomerulus. (Hematoxylin and eosin stain, original magnification ×200.)

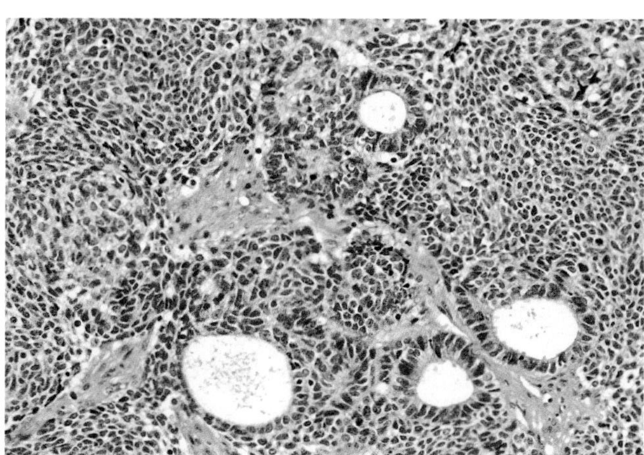

FIGURE 17-36 ■ Classic WT showing neoplastic tubules in a blastemal background. (Hematoxylin and eosin stain, original magnification ×200.)

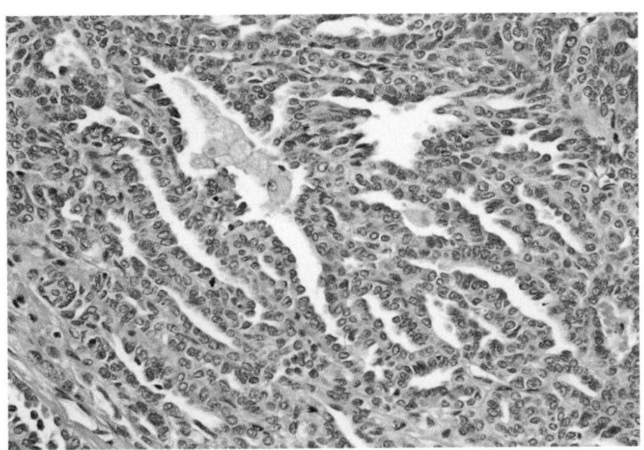

FIGURE 17-37 ■ WT showing a predominantly tubular or epithelial pattern. (Hematoxylin and eosin stain, original magnification ×200.)

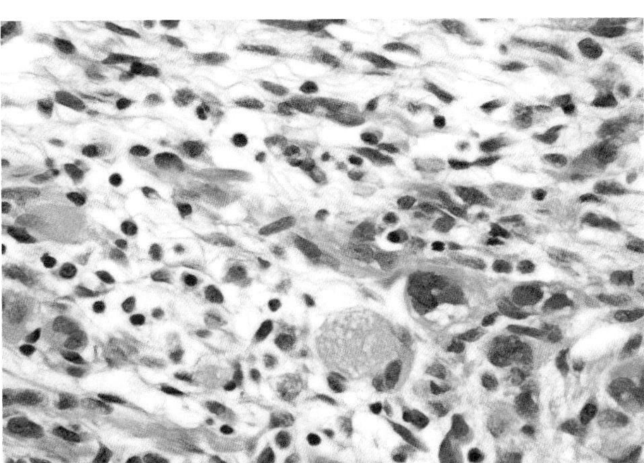

FIGURE 17-38 ■ WT with area of skeletal muscle differentiation in the stromal component. (Hematoxylin and eosin stain, original magnification ×400.)

staged irrespective of presence or absence of anaplasia. Patients with anaplastic stage I WT generally do well with conventional therapy (Table 17-7). Anaplasia is currently designated as focal when it is limited to one or a few discretely demarcated foci within the primary tumor and limited to the kidney. An adverse prognosis for anaplastic nuclear changes is associated only with stages II through IV tumors with diffuse anaplasia (e97).

It appears that therapy neither obscures nor produces anaplasia (e332). WT can be accurately staged in nephrectomy specimens obtained following chemotherapy. Staging based on the extent of viable tumor cells is directly related to outcome (e273). Post-therapy specimens may have extensive residual mature skeletal muscle (eFigure 17-9).

Regional lymph node metastasis is the most common site of noncontiguous spread of a WT. Benign inclusions in regional lymph nodes should not be misinterpreted as metastatic WT. Peritoneum, liver, and lung are the other common metastatic sites. Peritoneal metastases with desmoplasia can simulate a desmoplastic small round cell tumor. Bone marrow and skeletal metastases are rare; fewer than 2% of classic WTs metastasize to bone.

Bilateral Wilms tumors occur in 5% of patients and are designated as *stage V disease*, but the prognosis depends on the substage, that is, the stage of the largest tumor and presence or absence of anaplasia. The largest clinical experience is that of the NWTS (166). Several clinical and pathologic features characterize this group of tumors; genitourinary tract anomalies (16%), younger age at diagnosis, presence of nephroblastomatosis (67%), multicentricity (61%), and favorable histology (90%) are findings that tend to differentiate the stage V cases from all others. The overall 3-year survival was 76% in the NWTS.

Immunohistochemistry, EM, and molecular cytogenetics are useful in those cases in which the diagnostic material is limited, predominantly in differentiating Wilms tumor from other childhood small blue cell tumors (e.g., PNET, rhabdomyosarcoma, and neuroblastoma).

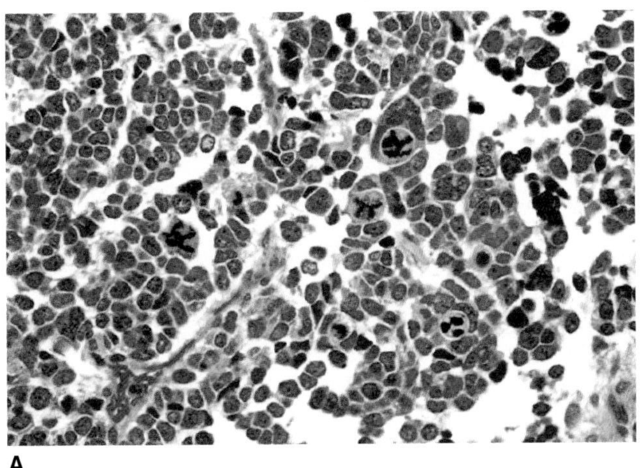

A

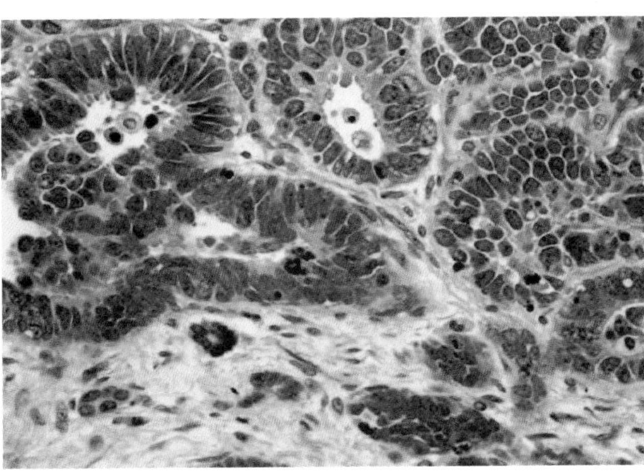

B

FIGURE 17-39 ■ WT showing anaplasia in the form of atypical multipolar mitotic figures; **A:** Within the blastomatous component and **B:** within the epithelial component (Hematoxylin and eosin stain, original magnification ×400.) (Courtesy of Dr. John Hicks.)

Table 17-7 ■ NATIONAL WILMS TUMOR STUDY STAGING DEFINITIONS

Stage	Definition
I	Tumor confined to kidney parenchyma and completely resected. Renal capsule intact, not penetrated by tumor. No involvement of vessels of renal sinus. No biopsy before nephrectomy (fine-needle aspiration biopsy is acceptable).
II	Tumor extends beyond kidney parenchyma but is completely resected. Tumor penetration of renal capsule into vessels of the renal sinus, including the renal vein, or localized spillage confined to the flank. Specimen margins uninvolved by tumor.
III	Residual nonhematogenous tumor confined to abdomen. Tumor in abdominal nodes, tumor spillage involving peritoneum, peritoneal implants, tumor involvement of resection margin.
IV	Hematogenous metastases or nodal deposits outside abdomen.
V	Bilateral renal tumors. In such cases, whenever possible, the lesions on each side should be staged individually, with a substage designation according to the highest individual tumor stage (e.g., stage V, substage 1).

From Beckwith JB. Renal tumors. In: Stocker JT, Askin FB, eds. *Pathology of solid tumors in children.* London: Chapman and Hall, 1998, with permission.

Cystic Variants of Nephroblastic Tumors

Cystic nephroma and cystic partially differentiated nephroblastoma are benign neoplasms currently considered to be a part of the spectrum of nephroblastoma (103,135). Both are well-circumscribed tumors composed entirely of cystic spaces separated by delicate septa (Figure 17-40A). The solid component conforms to the contours of the cystic spaces. In cystic nephroma (formerly known as *unilateral multilocular cyst*), it is composed of mature cell types (Figure 17-40B), whereas in cystic partially differentiated nephroblastoma, the cystic septa contain embryonal cell types without anaplasia (Figure 17-41A,B). If larger, solid, expansile regions are present, the tumor should be considered a conventional WT.

Nephrogenic Rests and Nephroblastomatosis

Nephrogenic rests are abnormally persistent foci of embryonal cells with the potential of developing into WT. They are encountered in 25% to 40% of WT and in 1% of routine postmortem examinations in infants (16,135). When these are multifocal or diffuse, the term *nephroblastomatosis* is used (Figure 17-42). They are classified into perilobar (Figure 17-43) and intralobar types (eFigure 17-10), which exhibit different biologic behaviors and have been shown to be genetically different, which may explain the ethnic differences in the epidemiology of WT (25,54). They consist of variable amounts of blastemal, epithelial, and stromal components but do not show the same potential to evolve into WT. The rests may be dormant, sclerosing, or hyperplastic (eFigure 17-11) (e18). The majority regresses and becomes fibrotic, and some give rise to WT, with the remnants of nephrogenic rest visible at the periphery of the neoplasm.

Perilobar rests occur in hemihypertrophy (Figure 17-44) and Beckwith-Wiedemann syndrome and also in association with some sporadic tumors. Perilobar rests are occasionally seen in cystic renal dysplasia and are rarely associated with mesoblastic nephroma. Intralobar rests are seen with the WAGR and Denys-Drash syndromes (Figure 17-45). Hyperplastic rests and Wilms tumors comprise a morphologic

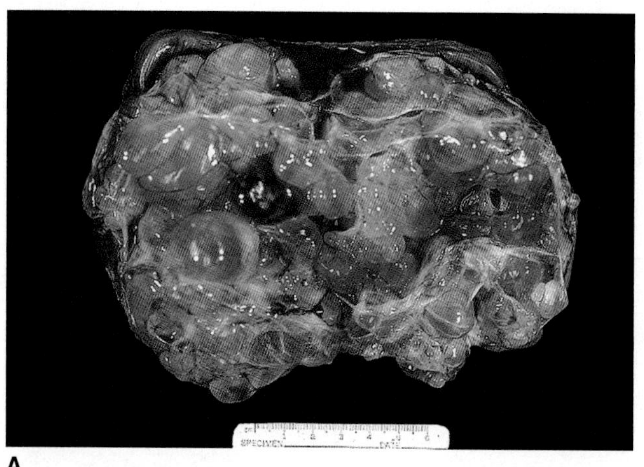

A

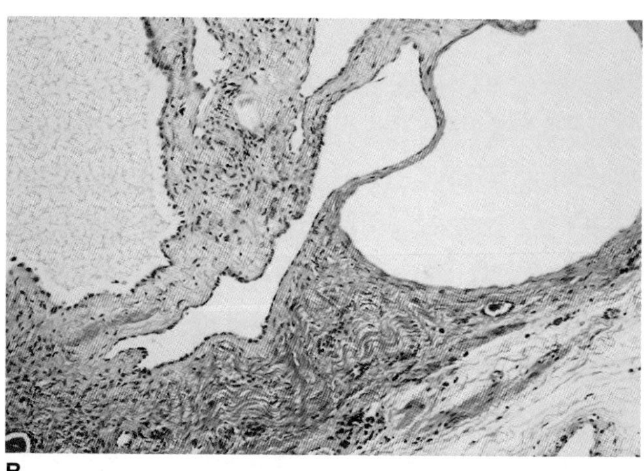

B

FIGURE 17-40 ■ Cystic nephroma (unilateral multilocular cyst) of the kidney. **A:** Gross picture of the cut surface shows multiple thin-walled cysts. Only a small amount of residual kidney present at the top. **B:** Typical cysts are lined by cuboidal or flat cells and a nondescript spindle cell stroma. (Hematoxylin and eosin stain, original magnification ×200.)

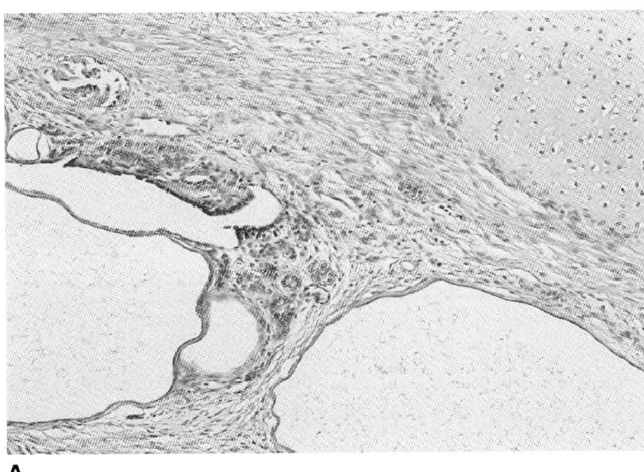

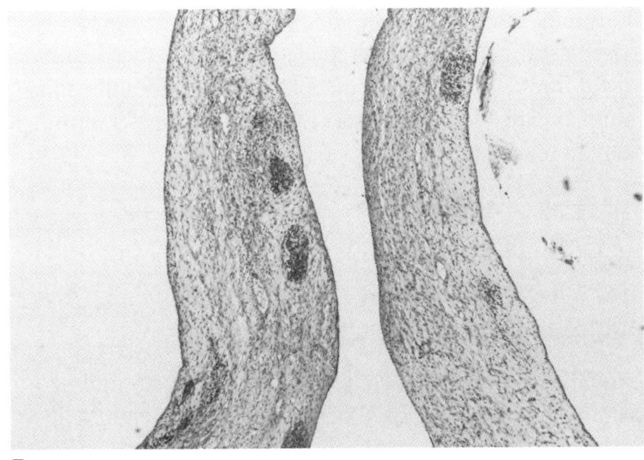

A B

FIGURE 17-41 ■ Cystic partially differentiated WT. Cysts have features very similar to those of cystic nephroma, but the surrounding stroma has immature tubules and cartilage in **(A)**, and islands of blastoma in **(B)**. (Hematoxylin and eosin stain, original magnification ×200.) (**B**: Courtesy of John Hicks. M.D. Houston, TX).

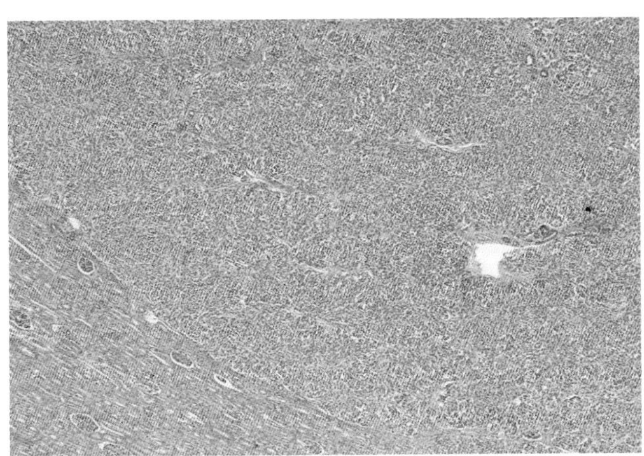

FIGURE 17-42 ■ Perilobar nephroblastomatosis in an infant with massive enlargement of the kidneys. The compact, uniform blastema with a nodular configuration and the discrete interface with the adjacent parenchyma are characteristic features. (Hematoxylin and eosin stain, original magnification ×40.)

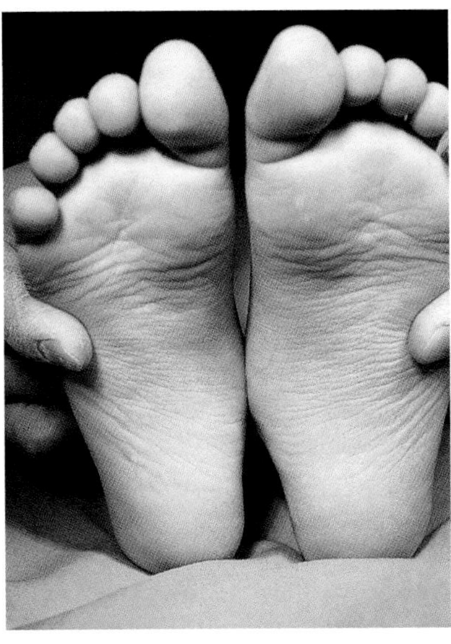

FIGURE 17-44 ■ Seven-year-old boy with hemihypertrophy that was diagnosed only after he was found to have a large WT (Figure 17-36). (Courtesy of David Hatch, M.D., Loyola University Medical Center, Maywood, Illinois.)

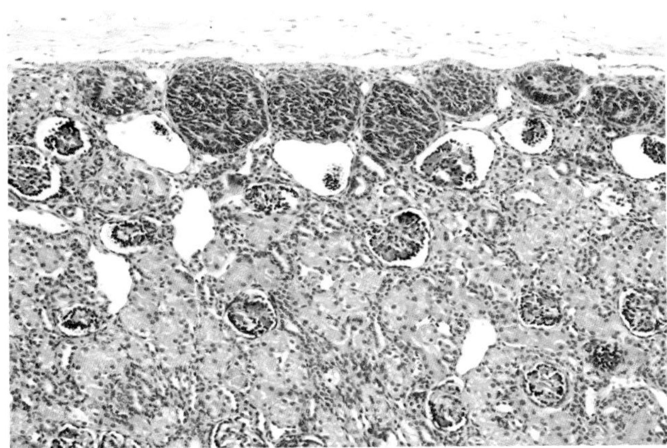

FIGURE 17-43 ■ Typical appearance of perilobar nephrogenic rests. (Hematoxylin and eosin stain, original magnification ×100.)

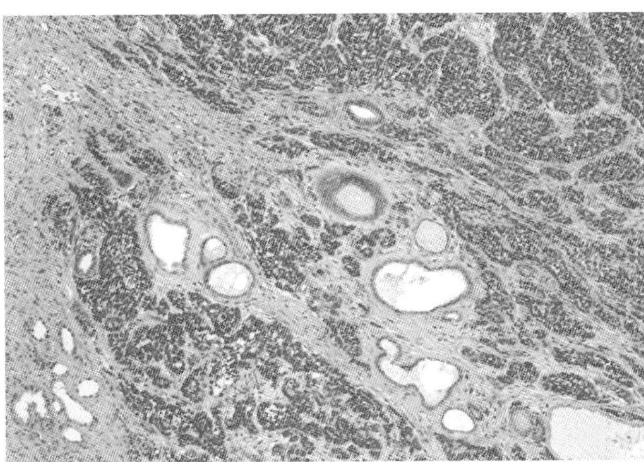

FIGURE 17-45 ■ Intralobar nephroblastomatosis with blastema and immature tubules blending into the surrounding kidney. (Hematoxylin and eosin stain, original magnification ×100.)

continuum that cannot be distinguished cytologically. Hyperplastic perilobar rests tend to preserve the original shape of the rest and have a distinct interface with the adjacent renal parenchyma, whereas the intralobar rest intermingles with the adjacent kidney.

OTHER CHILDHOOD NEOPLASMS

Congenital Mesoblastic Nephroma

Congenital mesoblastic nephroma (CMN) is a stromal neoplasm of infancy, composed of myofibroblasts, and is most commonly diagnosed in the first 3 months of life. First described by Bolande et al. (e38), it was thought to be a variant of WT but, based on the cytogenetic data available currently, is now considered to be distinct from WT. The classic variant of CMN shows no consistent genetic abnormality and probably represents infantile fibromatosis of the kidney. In contrast, the cellular variant is identical to infantile fibrosarcoma with the same t(12;15)(p13;q25) chromosomal translocation resulting in ETV6-NTRK3 gene fusion (e176). CMN is the most common renal tumor of infancy, with no sex predilection and only an occasional association with Beckwith-Weidemann syndrome. Most cases are detected because of an abdominal mass (eFigure 17-12), although polyhydramnios, premature delivery, and nonimmunologic hydrops have been reported. Hypertension secondary to renin production by entrapped renal elements, which may be immature and dysplastic, is not uncommon (135).

Grossly, the tumor is solitary, unilateral, characteristically whorled or trabeculated, and gray-white to yellow, with a rather indistinct tumor-kidney interface and a softly bulging cut surface (Figure 17-46). Cysts, hemorrhage, and necrosis are common and have no prognostic significance. The tumor tends to arise centrally within the kidney and extensively involves the renal sinus; thus, the medial margin needs to be carefully sampled.

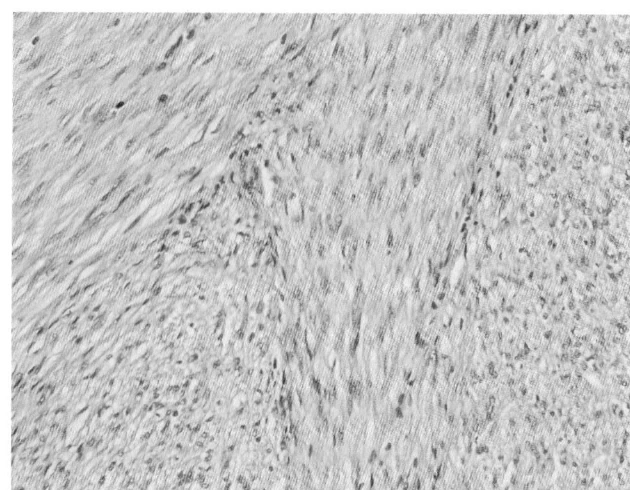

FIGURE 17-47 ▪ Classic pattern of CMN with intersecting bundles of uniform, bland spindle cells with minimal atypia. (Hematoxylin and eosin stain, original magnification ×200.)

Microscopically, classic, cellular, and mixed patterns are recognized with frequencies of 24%, 66%, and 10%, respectively, and a mean age at presentation of 7 days, 4 months, and 2 months, respectively. The classic pattern, originally described by Bolande, is characterized by intersecting bundles of spindle cells with minimal atypia and infrequent mitoses (Figure 17-47). At the periphery, the tumor infiltrates extensively into the renal parenchyma, so that wide margins of excision are necessary (Figure 17-48). Dysplastic entrapped tubules and islands of cartilage are often seen. The cellular mesoblastic nephroma has a distinct pushing border and is characterized by dense cells, mitoses, and a "sarcomatous" appearance (Figure 17-49A,B). Areas of cellular mesoblastic nephroma may be seen in an otherwise classic tumor, with eventual overgrowth of the former evidenced by the finding of compressed remnants of the classic pattern at the periphery of a cellular mesoblastic nephroma (e21).

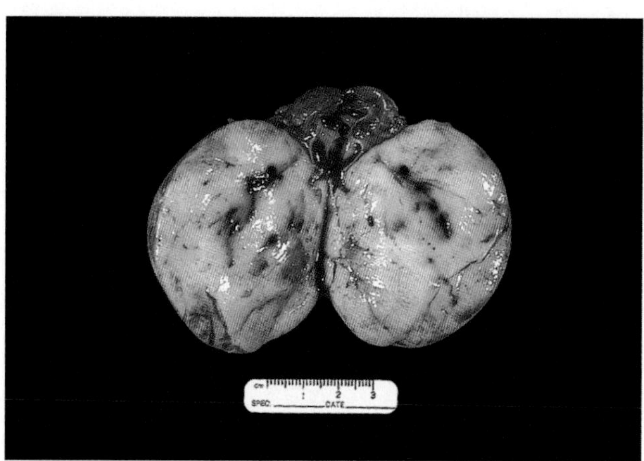

FIGURE 17-46 ▪ Cut surface of CMN shows yellow-white bulging cut surface with focal hemorrhage.

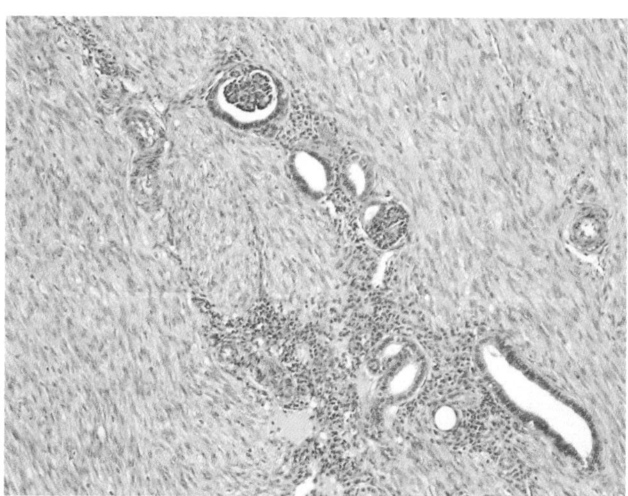

FIGURE 17-48 ▪ CMN infiltrates and overgrows renal elements. (Hematoxylin and eosin stain, original magnification ×200.)

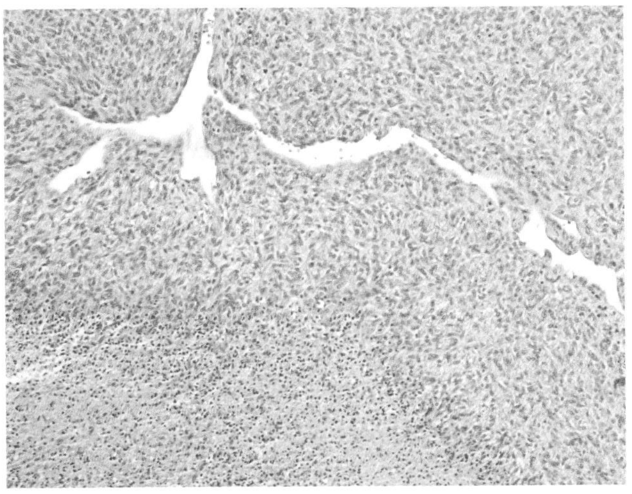
A

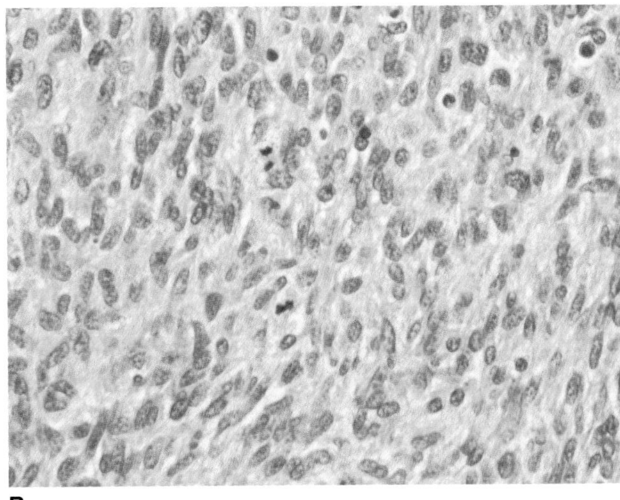
B

FIGURE 17-49 ■ Cellular mesoblastic nephroma. **A:** Low power shows high cellularity with hemangiopericytoma-like vessel and area of necrosis. **B:** High power shows mitoses and some pyknotic cells. (Hematoxylin and eosin stain, original magnification: **A**, ×200; **B**, ×400.)

However, all mixed tumors studied so far have shown no ETV6-NTRK3 gene fusion (5). By immunohistochemistry, both types of tumors react with antibodies directed toward myofibroblasts. Recurrences and metastases occur in about 5% to 10% of patients, risk factors for which are cellular histology, stage III or higher, and involvement of intrarenal or sinus vessels (55,135).

Clear-Cell Sarcoma of the Kidney

Although a rare tumor (~20 cases occur in the United States every year), the diagnosis of clear-cell sarcoma of the kidney (CCSK) is clinically important because it is a tumor with "unfavorable histology" that responds to chemotherapeutic regimens containing doxorubicin, actinomycin, and vincristine. In addition, it has been called the *great masquerader* because it can mimic, or be mimicked by every other pediatric renal neoplasm. The age distribution is similar to that of Wilms tumor, with a peak incidence during the second year of life; however, the age ranges from 2 months to 54 years (7). There is no association with any anomaly or syndrome.

CCSK is always unilateral, unicentric, and generally irregularly shaped with a distinct tumor-kidney junction (e21). It has a variable color and a glistening gelatinous surface (Figure 17-50). Cysts are often present. It seems to arise deep within the renal parenchyma.

Microscopically, various patterns can be seen; however, most tumors are quite monomorphous with a characteristic tumor-kidney interface. At low magnification, this appears scalloped and irregular but usually sharp. Under high magnification, the interface is less sharp because the tumor infiltrates between and around renal structures (eFigure 17-13), which may show metaplastic changes. In the classic pattern, an evenly distributed network of vascular septa with parallel capillary-sized vessels subdivides the tumor into cords and nests that are six to 10 cells wide (Figure 17-51A). The tumor cells are polygonal, with indistinct cell-cell borders, finely granular nuclear chromatin (hence the pale nuclei), and small or absent nucleoli (Figure 17-51B). Mitoses are variable but less than in other renal malignancies. The cytoplasm usually consists of delicate tendrils surrounding intercellular space (hence the "clear-cell" appearance), although it is important to recognize that not all CCSKs are clear. Histologic variations include epithelioid (eFigure 17-14), spindle cell (eFigure 17-15),

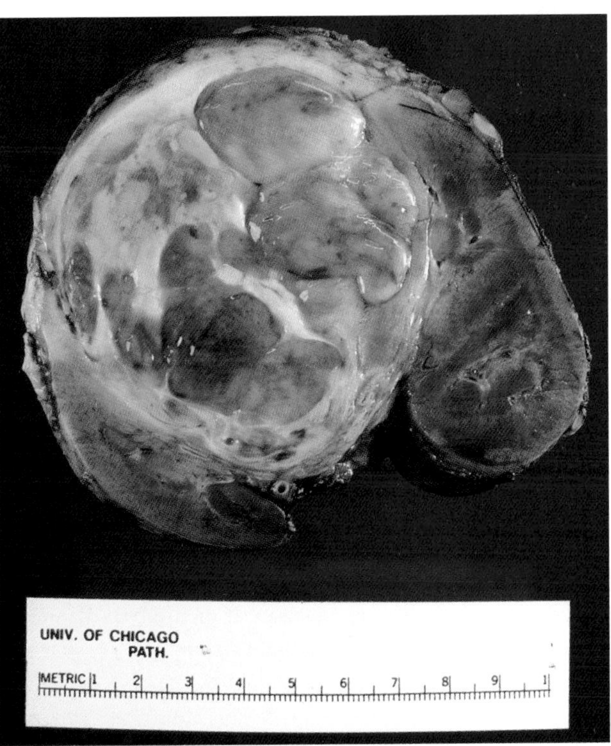

FIGURE 17-50 ■ CCSK showing distinct tumor-kidney junction, gelatinous nodular cut surface, and yellow areas of necrosis. (Courtesy of Christopher Weber, M.D., Ph.D., University of Chicago, Chicago, IL).

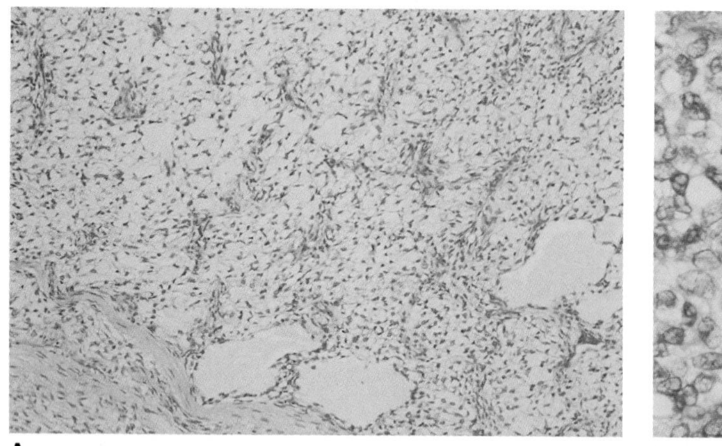

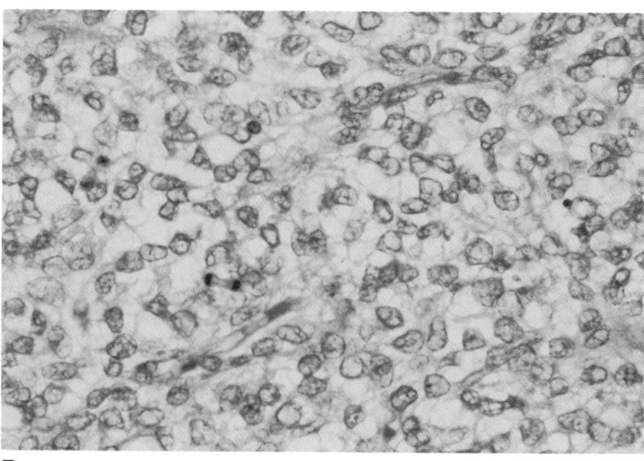

FIGURE 17-51 ■ **A:** CCSK showing a characteristic vascular or plexogenic pattern in which ill-defined groups of uniform tumor cells are separated by a capillary network of vessels. (Hematoxylin and eosin stain, original magnification ×100.) **B:** The nuclei often have an optically clear appearance, as in papillary carcinoma of the thyroid. (Hematoxylin and eosin stain, original magnification ×300.)

sclerosing, myxoid, cystic, pericytomatous, palisading, and monstrocellular patterns. However, most CCSKs exhibit the classic pattern, and even in those with a variant pattern, some areas with the classic pattern can be found.

One study of 14 CCSKs showed the genetic expression profile of CCSK to be highly distinctive as compared to WT. The finding that many of the genes upregulated in CCSK are involved with neural differentiation, development, or function may be an important reflection of the cell of origin of CCSK. Additionally, two pathways activated in CCSK (Sonic hedgehog and phosphoinositide-3-kinase/Akt) have also been implicated in other pediatric neural tumors. Lastly, potential therapeutic targets (nerve growth factor receptor, CD117 and epidermal growth factor receptor) were identified that may prove to be useful in the treatment of CCSK (37). So far, three cases of CCSK have been reported to have translocations at t(10;17) (26).

CCSKs are strongly positive for vimentin (eFigure 17-16) and vascular markers highlight the typical distribution of small vessels. Positivity for CD99 (Mic-2) (eFigure 17-17) and CD56 (eFigure 17-18) may also be seen. The differential diagnosis includes WT, rhabdoid tumor, and cellular variant of mesoblastic nephroma.

Almost 40% of cases metastasize to bone, hence the original term *bone-metastasizing renal tumor of childhood* (e201). It can also metastasize to other unusual sites, including skeletal muscle, orbit, brain, meninges, and spinal cord. Late recurrences have been described as many as 5 to 8 years after diagnosis (e115,e179). In contrast to WTs, even stage I CCSKs have relatively high recurrence rates, presumably because of occult micrometastases at the time of diagnosis. Prognosis varies with stage at presentation: 97% 6-year survival for stage I to 50% for stage IV (7).

Rhabdoid Tumor of the Kidney

The histogenesis of this rare (2.5% of NWTS cases) and highly malignant (80% mortality) tumor of the infantile kidney remains unknown despite extensive study. What is known is that it is not related to WT or to any syndrome except the familial rhabdoid tumor predisposition syndrome. The only known associations are with hypercalcemia in a few cases and, in 15% of cases, primitive neuroectodermal tumor of the brain (e221). It is seen in infants and children, with a 1.5:1 male-to-female ratio (e21). Metastases are generally widespread at the time of diagnosis (e315,e319). Primary extrarenal rhabdoid tumors can be seen in both children and adults, particularly in the central nervous system. The unifying feature at all sites is the presence of a mutation or deletion of the *INI1* gene located at chromosome 22q11.

Grossly, rhabdoid tumor is usually round, pale, soft, and unencapsulated. Satellite tumors may be present. Microscopically, the pattern is monomorphous; sheets of large, loosely cohesive tumor cells are characterized by intracytoplasmic hyaline inclusion and vesicular nuclei containing prominent central nucleoli (Figure 17-52). These features may be focal and should be looked for carefully

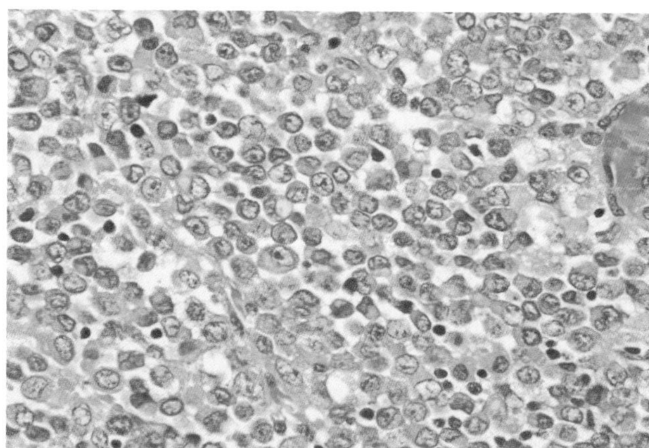

FIGURE 17-52 ■ Rhabdoid tumor of the kidney showing sheets of large, atypical mononuclear cells with a prominent nucleolus in each nucleus. There are characteristic intracytoplasmic hyaline inclusions indenting some of the nuclei. (Hematoxylin and eosin stain, original magnification ×300.)

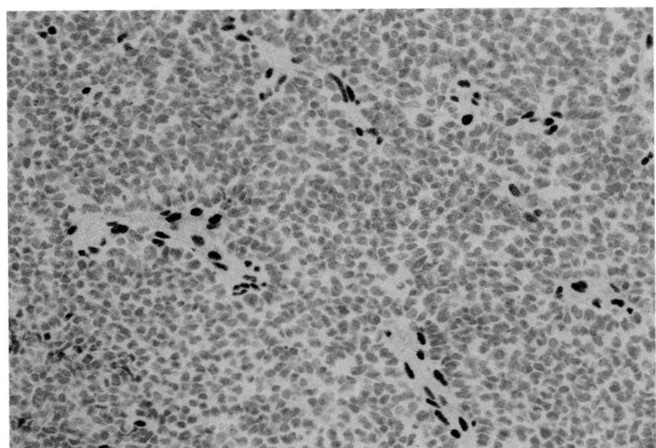

FIGURE 17-53 ■ Rhabdoid tumor of the kidney showing lack of immunoreactivity for BAF47. Note normally positive endothelial cells and scattered lymphocytes. (Peroxidase-antiperoxidase stain, original magnification ×200.)

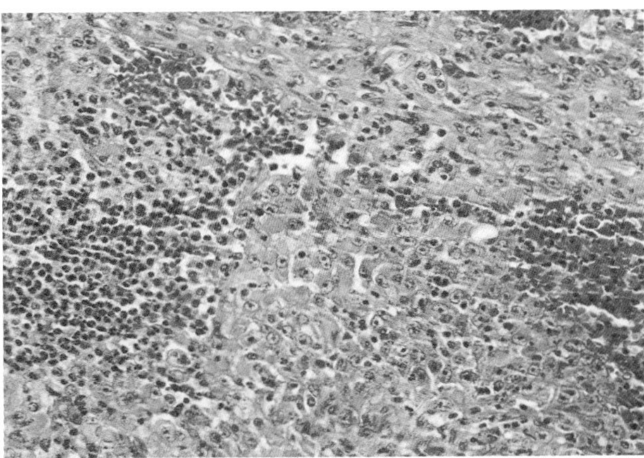

FIGURE 17-54 ■ Renal medullary carcinoma. Tumor cells have dark cytoplasm, clear nuclei, and very prominent nucleoli. Note acute inflammation and sickled red blood cells. (Hematoxylin and eosin stain, original magnification ×200.)

in any undifferentiated tumor of the kidney. The finding of rhabdoid features in other tumors, such as Wilms tumor and mesoblastic nephroma, does not imply the same poor prognosis (e320).

Immunohistochemically, the tumor cells are consistently positive for vimentin with frequent coexpression of cytokeratin (eFigures 17-19 and 17-20), epithelial membrane antigen, desmin, and neurofilament. The staining pattern is characteristically patchy and strong, with small clusters of positive cells in a background of nonreactive tumor cells, seen in over 90% of cases. Other markers, including CD99 and CD56 (eFigure 17-21), have been reported but are not found consistently (e56). They may represent nonspecific antibody entrapment by the filamentous arrays seen ultrastructurally to correspond to the cytoplasmic inclusion (e21).

All rhabdoid tumors appear to contain mutations or deletions that inactivate the *hSNF5/INI1* gene, whose role is to alter the conformation of the DNA-histone complex so that transcription factors have access to target genes (e309). Immunohistochemical staining using antibody to hSNF5/INI1, BAF47 has been shown to be very sensitive and highly specific for the detection of hSNF5/INI1 loss-of-function, which correlates well with the biallelic inactivation of this tumor suppressor gene (23). (Figure 17-53)

Renal Cell Carcinoma

Malignant epithelial tumors are rare in children and in part appear to be intrinsically different than those in adults. Clear-cell RCC is quite rare in the absence of a predisposing genetic condition such as von Hippel-Lindau syndrome. Papillary RCC is the most common histologic subtype of RCC with the same pathologic appearance and genetic changes as seen in adults. Foamy macrophages are present in over 80% of tumors. There is strong positivity for cytokeratin 7 and epithelial membrane antigen (EMA). Typically, the stage at presentation is low, surgery is the treatment of choice and any residual tumor is unresponsive to chemotherapy.

Renal medullary carcinoma is a rare highly malignant tumor associated with sickle cell trait that occurs in adolescents and young adults (e74). It appears to have a distinct molecular signature that clusters closely with urothelial (transitional cell) carcinoma of the renal pelvis, rather than RCC (196). Presenting symptoms are flank pain, hematuria, and a palpable abdominal mass. It is usually a lobulated neoplasm arising in the renal medulla. Histologically, it often shows cribriform and reticular growth patterns, reminiscent of yolk sac tumor (eFigure 17-22). The cells have dark cytoplasm, clear nuclei, and prominent nucleoli (Figure 17-54). Focally, rhabdoid features (eFigure 17-23) and intracytoplasmic lumens may be present. The stroma is often prominently desmoplastic and marked acute and chronic inflammation is characteristic (eFigure 17-24). It is widely metastatic at diagnosis, is unresponsive to chemotherapy and radiotherapy, and has a mean survival of only four months. There is overlap with rhabdoid tumor.

Translocation-associated renal tumors are defined by their genetic features (majority have translocations involving the TFE3 gene located at Xp11.2 and a number of variant partner genes). These tumors have a nested or a tubulopapillary pattern composed of cells with voluminous clear-to-acidophilic cytoplasm and distinct cell borders separated by thin fibrovascular septa (Figure 17-55). The tumor cells, in contrast to other RCCs, are negative or only focally positive for EMA, cytokeratin CAM5.2 and vimentin, but show nuclear reactivity for TFE3 or TFEB proteins (eFigure 17-25) (57).

Other Rare Renal Tumors

Ossifying renal tumor of kidney is a rare neoplasm, characteristically seen in infant boys, that presents with hematuria. A calcified mass in the renal pelvis grossly resembles calculi and is microscopically composed of proliferating

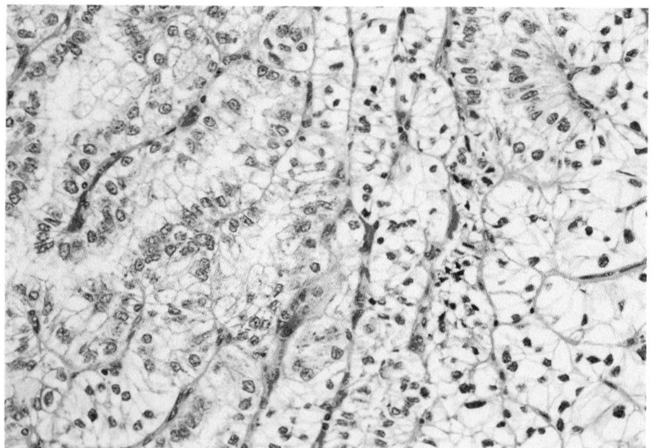

FIGURE 17-55 ■ RCC with translocation at Xp11.2. There are distinct cell borders and abundant clear cytoplasm. (Hematoxylin and eosin stain, original magnification ×200.)

spindle cells admixed with partially calcified osteoid matrix. The prognosis is excellent, with no known recurrences or metastases (e57,e156).

Metanephric tumors are rare benign tumors that have a pathologic spectrum from adenoma (most common of the group, occurring mainly in females with a mean age of 41 years) to adenofibroma (containing both epithelial and stromal components, occurring at a mean age of 82 months with 2:1 male-to-female ratio) to stromal tumor (mean age of 2 years) (135). All are unencapsulated and show distinctive morphology (eFigures 17-26 and 17-27).

Primitive neuroectodermal tumor occasionally occurs in the kidney in older children and adults. It is a small blue cell tumor, the diagnosis of which rests on the findings of pseudorosettes (Figure 17-56), CD99 and FLI-1 positivity, and t(11;22).

Angiomyolipomas and oncocytomas may occur in children, almost always in association with tuberous sclerosis. Primary neuroblastoma and lymphoma of the kidney also occur rarely.

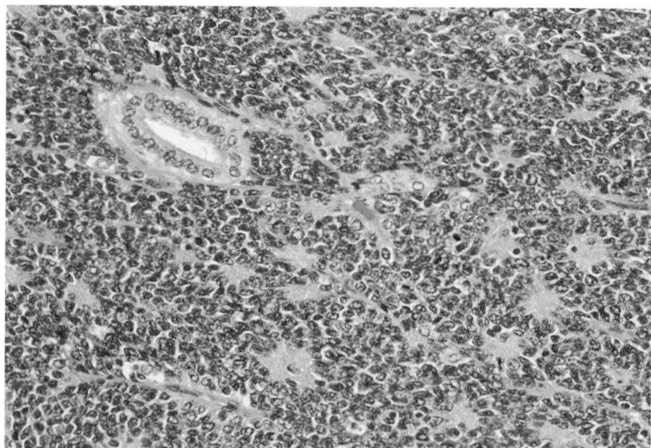

FIGURE 17-56 ■ Primitive neuroendocrine tumor of kidney showing pseudorosettes and an entrapped tubule. (Hematoxylin and eosin stain, original magnification ×200.)

DISEASES OF THE URETERS, BLADDER, AND URETHRA

Congenital Malformations of the Ureter

Malformations of the ureter are common and often occur in combination (e.g., duplication and ectopia, or ectopia and ureterocele with or without obstruction).

Ureteral Agenesis

Unilateral or bilateral ureteral agenesis is almost always seen with renal agenesis. Whenever a ureter is present, some renal tissue can usually be identified.

Ureteral Duplication

The vast majority of cases of ureteral duplication are sporadic, although a few cases have been reported with syndromic associations (e120,e275). All types of ureteral duplication are much more common in girls (male-to-female ratio of 6:1) (171). Duplication of the upper part of the ureter and renal pelvis occurs in association with premature branching of the ureteric bud; complete duplication occurs when two ureteric buds form. Partial unilateral duplication is the most common form and is associated with duplication of the renal pelvis and a duplex kidney. Often, the upper pole is smaller and dysplastic, with the associated ureter tortuous and dilated. In cases with complete duplication, the upper pole ureter inserts ectopically.

Ureteral Ectopia

Ureteral ectopia is more common in girls, often associated with ureteral duplication, and frequently presents with symptoms of urinary tract infection (e100). In boys, the ectopic orifice is located more often in the urinary tract than in the seminal tract (e303). That part of the kidney drained by the ectopic ureter is often dysplastic. The severity of the dysplasia is apparently determined by the position of the ectopic ureteric orifice; the more lateral the ectopia, the more severe the degree of dysplasia and hypoplasia of the kidney (e278–e280). Nonfunctioning renal segments are treated by laparoscopic nephroureterectomy of the upper pole (137), and functioning renal segments are conservatively treated, usually with ureterovesical reimplantation (117).

Ureterocele

Ureterocele is a congenital cystic dilation of the intravesical portion of the distal ureter. It is commonly detected by prenatal ultrasound (41). In childhood it usually presents with symptoms of vesicoureteral reflux and chronic infection. The ureteral orifice may be normally positioned or ectopic at the neck of the bladder or ureter, in which case it is most often associated with the upper pole of a duplex kidney (171).

Ureteral Obstruction

Intrinsic ureteral obstruction, bilateral in 20% of cases, is most often seen at the ureteropelvic junction, causing hydronephrosis (Figure 17-57), or associated with multicystic dysplasia, in which case the ureter(s) may be atretic. The obstruction of the ureteropelvic junction may be caused by stenosis, valves, or functional constriction (138). Extrinsic obstruction is seen in retrocaval ureters, and less often in retroiliac ureters. In obstruction of the vesicoureteral junction, the presence of an additional smooth muscle collar surrounding the terminal ureter has been demonstrated (e83). A number of experimental studies have shown that the younger the age of the patient at the time of unilateral ureteral obstruction, the more severe the growth impairment of the ipsilateral kidney and the greater the compensatory growth of the opposite kidney. Renal growth and development are impaired through complex interactions between regulators of cell proliferation, cell destruction, and extracellular matrix (e58).

Vesicoureteric Reflux

Vesicoureteric reflux is a congenital defect of the urinary tract that causes urine to flow retrogradely from the bladder to the kidneys due to short intravesical ureter(s), poorly developed trigone, and ectopic abnormally large ureteral orifice(s). It is associated with recurrent urinary tract infections, hypertension, and renal failure (third most common cause in children). Prevention of recurrent UTIs is believed to significantly reduce the risk of reflux nephropathy. However, despite medical and surgical therapy, the incidence of renal failure in these patients has not decreased. Thus, it is proposed that the renal damage associated with reflux is congenital and arises from a defect that affects both renal and urinary tract development (115).

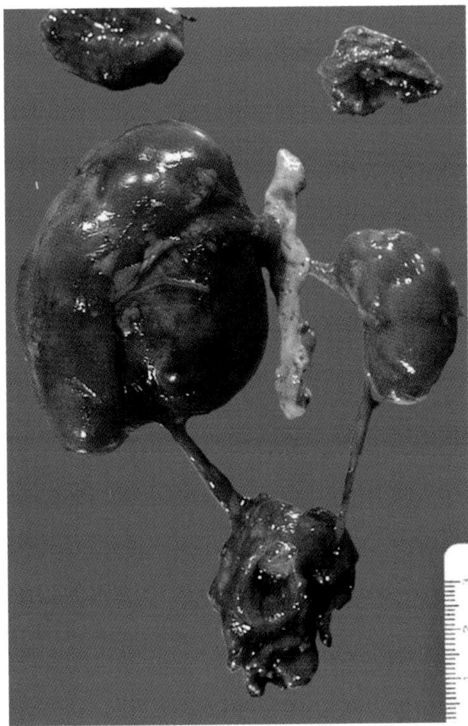

FIGURE 17-57▪Left hydronephrosis secondary to unilateral ureteropelvic junction obstruction.

Acquired Lesions of the Ureter

Inflammation and neoplasia primarily involving the ureter are rarely, if ever, seen by the pediatric pathologist. Chronic inflammation and fibrosis may be seen in association with pyelonephritis and vesicoureteral reflux. The ureter may be secondarily involved by rhabdomyosarcoma arising in the urinary bladder and other retroperitoneal tumors. Transitional cell carcinoma of the ureter is seen only in adults.

Congenital Lesions of the Bladder and Urethra

Most patients with bilateral agenesis of the kidneys also have agenesis of the bladder, although a small, contracted bladder may be identified in some. Agenesis is also seen as part of severe malformations (e.g., sirenomelia, caudal regression syndrome, and limb-body wall defects). Hypoplasia of the bladder is commonly seen with bilateral multicystic dysplastic kidneys. Duplication of the bladder is uncommon and rarely occurs as an isolated anomaly; rather, it is generally part of a complex malformation, as in the VACTERL (vertebrae, anal, tracheoesophageal, renal, and limb) association (Chapter 4).

Bladder Exstrophy

Bladder exstrophy is an uncommon anomaly with an even sex ratio (120). Epispadias, exstrophy of the bladder, and cloacal exstrophy are a spectrum of related malformations that result from a failure of the primitive streak mesoderm to invade the anterior part of the cloacal membrane (156). The size of the exstrophic bladder varies from patient to patient, ranging from a small hole in the anterior abdominal wall through which the bladder trigone protrudes on straining at micturition to a large defect through which the entire posterior wall of the bladder is exposed (Figure 17-58). The pubic symphysis remains open. Epispadias, in which the opening of the urethra is on the upper surface of the penis, is present in males, and bifid clitoris in females. In cloacal exstrophy, the bladder is separated into two halves by the central exstrophic bowel; other urogenital anomalies are also present.

Even after surgical repair, bladder function is often not normal. Complications include vesicoureteral reflux, cystitis cystica, squamous metaplasia, and an increased risk for the development of squamous cell carcinoma or adenocarcinoma.

Obstructive Lesions

Obstruction of the urinary tract results in a series of changes referred to as *obstructive uropathy* is a leading cause of renal

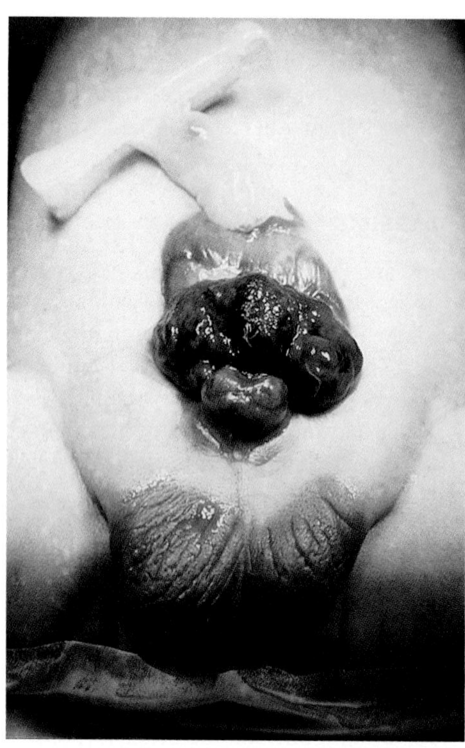

FIGURE 17-58 ■ Newborn boy with bladder exstrophy. (Courtesy of David Hatch, M.D., Loyola University Medical Center, Maywood, Illinois.)

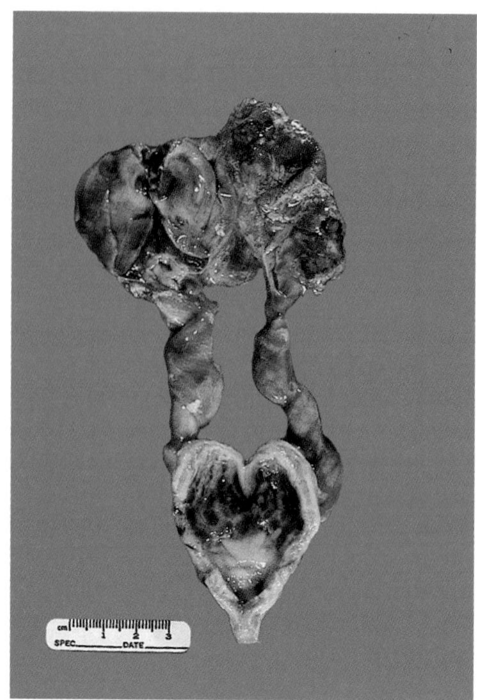

FIGURE 17-59 ■ Severe obstruction secondary to posterior urethral valve was diagnosed in utero and a vesicoamniotic shunt placed. A thick-walled, dilated bladder, bilateral hydroureters, and hydronephrosis were found at autopsy in this newborn boy, who died of pulmonary hypoplasia.

failure in childhood and adolescence. It accounts for 16.3% of pediatric renal transplantations (15). The obstruction can occur at multiple levels of the urinary tract, including the urethra, bladder outlet, and ureters. Renal lesions in obstructive uropathy vary from bilateral hydronephrosis to severe and diffuse hypodysplasia in which variably sized cysts mimic polycystic disease. A less severe renal change, characterized by the conservation of normal renal structure and the presence of subcapsular cysts (Potter type IV), is seen less frequently (e73).

The causes of bladder outlet obstruction include posterior urethral valves in males, urethral stenosis or atresia, and functional neck obstruction. Posterior urethral valves are the most common cause of lower urinary tract obstruction in male infants with an incidence of 1 in 5,000 to 8,000 live births (15). Severe obstruction can be detected in utero and treated by vesicoamniotic shunt placement, the efficacy of which decreases in the latter part of gestation (Figure 17-59).

Prune Belly Syndrome

Also called triad *syndrome* or *Eagle-Barett syndrome*, prune belly syndrome is rare, with an incidence of 1/40,000 live births (21), and often fatal. It predominantly affects boys and consists of absence or hypoplasia of the abdominal wall musculature, cryptorchism, and urinary tract anomalies. Findings include hypoplasia of the prostate, urethral obstruction in many but not all cases, markedly distended bladder, megaureters, bilateral hydronephrosis with atrophy, and often renal dysplasia and cyst formation. The condition is named for the characteristically lax and wrinkled appearance of the abdominal wall (Figure 17-60). The earliest manifestations are fetal ascites and Potter syndrome.

The pathogenesis of prune belly syndrome is not known; it may simply arise from the effects of early urethral obstruction (176) or else from a basic defect of the mesoderm from which the triad of abnormalities develop. In a study of the urethra and genital tracts of 21 patients with prune belly syndrome and 23 patients with posterior urethral valve, the seminal ducts and vesicles and prostatic glands were abnormal

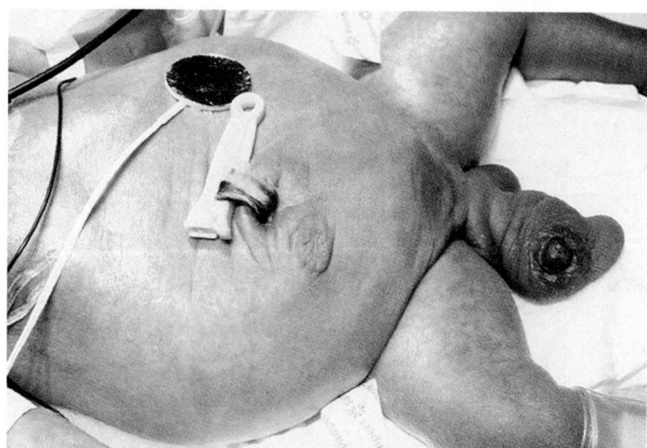

FIGURE 17-60 ■ Newborn boy with prune-belly syndrome; note the lax anterior abdominal wall and redundant scrotal skin. (Courtesy of David Hatch, M.D., Loyola University Medical Center, Maywood, IL.)

in the former group and normally developed in the latter (e299). According to the authors of the study, this major difference stems from a primary defect of the intermediate and lateral plate mesoderm in prune belly syndrome, affecting the embryogenesis not only of the mesonephric and paramesonephric ducts but also of the musculature of the abdominal wall and urinary organs, and prune belly valves, when present, are intrinsic components of the mesodermal defect of the urethra in prune belly syndrome.

Megacystic Microcolon Intestinal Hypoperistalsis Syndrome

Megacystic microcolon intestinal hypoperistalsis syndrome (MMIHS) is a rare congenital disorder characterized by a massively enlarged urinary bladder without mechanical outlet obstruction, microcolon, and a hypoperistaltic bowel with normal ganglion cells in a majority of cases (140). Absence of interstitial cells of Cajal, vacuolar degeneration of smooth muscle, neuronal dysplastic changes associated with increased laminin and fibronectin, and excessive smooth muscle cell glycogen storage with severely reduced contractile fibers displaced to the extreme periphery of cells have been reported (140). A lack of functional α3 subunit of nicotinic acetylcholine receptor has been demonstrated in most MMIHS tissues, which may prove to be the underlying pathogenesis of this rare syndrome (147).

Urachal Remnants

The patent urachus, which connects the developing urinary bladder with the allantoic duct, normally becomes a solid cord by month 4 of gestation. Patency may persist either completely, so that a fistula forms between the umbilicus and the bladder, or partially, in which case a sinus forms that usually opens into the umbilicus (Figure 17-61). A cyst develops if the urachus remains partially patent anywhere along its length. Persistence of the distal urachus where it joins the bladder produces a variably sized diverticulum.

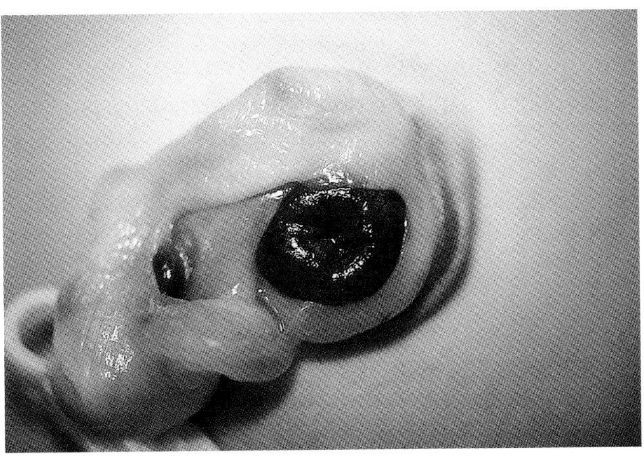

FIGURE 17-61 ▪ Patent urachus with sinus opening into the umbilicus. (Courtesy of Preston Black, M.D., Loyola University Medical Center, Maywood, IL.)

These remnants can be lined by transitional, intestinal, or squamous epithelium. There is a membrane to an ostomy site. Symptoms and complications include persistent umbilical discharge, infections, and development of carcinoma in adulthood.

ACQUIRED LESIONS OF THE BLADDER AND URETHRA

Cystitis

Cystitis in children can be broadly classified into two main categories: specific, in which the cause is known (e.g., bacteria, fungi, viruses, drugs, or radiation), and nonspecific, in which the cause is unknown (e.g., proliferative, interstitial, and eosinophilic cystitis and malakoplakia).

The etiology of UTIs is affected by underlying host factors such as age, diabetes, spinal cord injury, or catheterization. Consequently, complicated UTI has a more diverse etiology than uncomplicated UTI, and organisms that rarely cause disease in healthy patients can cause significant disease in hosts with anatomic, metabolic, or immunologic underlying disease. Most uncomplicated UTIs in children are caused by enterobacteria, mainly *E coli* 90% of which possess P fimbriae that allow the bacteria to adhere to the uroepithelial cell lining. *S. aureus* is more commonly seen among children with indwelling catheters. Coagulase-negative staphylococci and *Candida* app. are commonly associated with infections after instrumentation of the urinary tract. In nosocomial UTI, half of whom have had prior instrumentation, the organisms are *E coli* (28%), *Candida* spp. (18%), *Enterococcus* (13%), Gram-negative fermenters (13%), *Enterobacter* (10%), and *Pseudomonas* (10%). Although there have been minimal changes in the predominant uropathogens over the past decades, there have been significant changes in resistance patterns to antimicrobials that need to be considered when determining the most appropriate empiric therapy (152).

Granulomatous Cystitis

Granulomatous cystitis may be idiopathic or associated with a specific infection (e.g., tuberculosis, schistosomiasis, fungal infections in the immunocompromised). It may also be seen as part of chronic granulomatous disease of childhood, which is a rare congenital abnormality of the phagocyte NADPH (reduced nicotinamide adenine dinucleotide phosphate) oxidase system (e87,e294).

Cystitis Cystica and Glandularis

Cystitis cystica and cystitis glandularis are two forms of chronic proliferative cystitis, cystitis cystica being more common, that are often seen together in patients with chronic inflammation of the bladder. Proliferative cystitis eventually develops in patients with bladder exstrophy and may be a preneoplastic change, which would explain the increased risk for adenocarcinoma in these patients (125).

Cystoscopically, small rounded projections of the bladder mucosa are seen. Microscopically, cystic structures are apparent in the submucosa, composed of transitional and glandular epithelium (eFigure 17-28). When the lining resembles intestinal epithelium and the cysts become dilated with mucin, the condition is called *cystitis glandularis*. Chronic inflammatory infiltrate is usually minimal. A case with a 15-cm botryoid-like polyp has been described (4).

Interstitial Cystitis

Interstitial cystitis (IC) is a chronic noninfectious, probably inflammatory disorder of the bladder that primarily affects female adults. Occasionally, it can be seen in adolescent girls (122). Classic IC is characterized by frequency, nocturia, and suprapubic pain with ulceration (Hunner ulcer); in the nonclassic form, ulceration does not occur. The etiology and the pathogenesis are still undetermined, and the pathologic diagnosis is essentially one of exclusion. IC appears to be a syndrome with neural, immune, and endocrine components in which activated mast cells play a central role (e90,e305). The bladder transitional cell epithelium is normally covered by a mucin layer composed of glycosaminoglycans. This layer is thought to be almost impermeable, thereby preventing urine solutes from diffusing into the subepithelial components of the bladder. IC might affect this layer by increasing solute permeability, possibly leading to irritation, inflammation, and sensory-nerve sensitization of the bladder. Potassium could be the main offending substance and its diffusion across the permeable transitional epithelium the primary irritant; hence the development of the potassium sensitivity test for the diagnosis of IC (136).

Eosinophilic Cystitis

Eosinophilic cystitis is a rare disorder. In children, it may be associated with parasites, food allergens, or drugs. Associated risk factors include bronchial asthma, atopic diseases, and environmental allergens (184). It has also been reported in association with chronic granulomatous disease (12). The bladder mucosa may be markedly polypoid, so that embryonal rhabdomyosarcoma must be included in the differential diagnosis (144). Histologically, extensive eosinophilic inflammation of the bladder wall is present.

Malakoplakia

Malakoplakia is a chronic inflammatory disease that was originally described in the urinary bladder but can involve many other organs and soft tissues. It is rarely seen in children (109,165). Histologically, it is characterized by chronic inflammation, histiocytes, and poorly formed granulomas. A diagnostic feature is the Michaelis-Guttmann body, which is a laminated calcospherite present in the cytoplasm or extracellularly (Figure 17-62). It stains with period acid–Schiff, iron, and von Kossa stains and may represent bacterial degradation products (190).

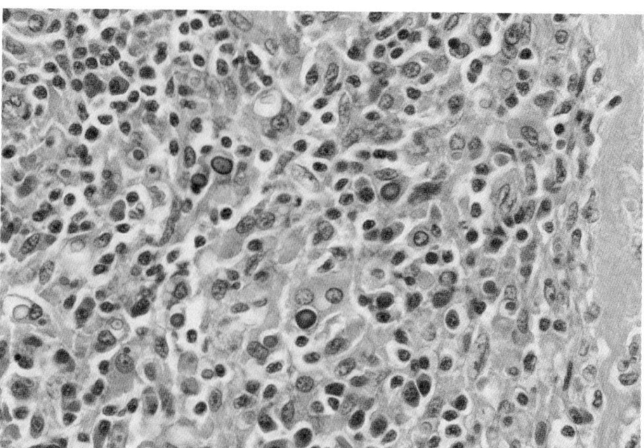

FIGURE 17-62 ■ Malakoplakia of the bladder in a child with a surgically repaired exstrophy. The inflammatory infiltrate is composed of lymphocytes, plasma cells, and macrophages, some with purple stained Michaelis-Guttmann bodies. (Hematoxylin and eosin stain, original magnification ×200.)

Hemorrhagic Cystitis

Acute hemorrhagic cystitis may be infectious or sterile. BK virus has been shown to be the main cause of viral hemorrhagic cystitis in bone marrow transplant patients (58). BK virus cystitis has also been reported in nonimmunocompromised hosts (e267). In patients receiving hematopoietic stem cell transplantation older age at transplant, allogeneic transplant, cyclophosphamide-containing conditioning, moderate-to-severe acute graft-versus-host disease (GVHD) and hepatic GVHD were associated with higher risks of HC (34). Adenovirus type 11 is responsible for acute, self-limiting cystitis with the sudden onset of gross hematuria, dysuria, and urinary frequency (e218). *E. coli* and occasionally Candida albicans may also cause hemorrhagic cystitis.

Cyclophosphamide therapy is complicated by ulceration of the bladder mucosa and massive hemorrhage into the submucosa in 7% of patients receiving the drug (e185). During high-dose therapy, up to 35% of patients have severe hemorrhagic cystitis (e52). Ifosfamide produces hemorrhagic cystitis even more commonly, which is its main dose-limiting toxicity (e195). The cytokines, tumor necrosis factor-a and interleukin-1, nitric oxide, nitric oxide synthetase, and platelet-activating factor have been shown to be involved in the pathogenesis of hemorrhagic cystitis (e110,e292). The blood loss may be so severe that blood transfusions and even surgical intervention are warranted. Marked cytologic atypia can be seen in the regenerating epithelium. The incidence of urothelial neoplasms is increased in patients receiving long-term cyclophosphamide therapy. Mesna is a drug that protects urothelium and prevents hemorrhagic cystitis and may even decrease the risk for urothelial carcinoma (e25,e200).

Tumors of the Bladder and Urethra

All tumors of the bladder and urethra are rare in children; benign tumors are even more infrequent. Benign tumors in children described in case reports include polyps, papilloma, hemangioma (4,78,e186), neurofibroma (e159), leiomyoma (114), paraganglioma (118), granular cell tumor (e243), nephrogenic adenoma (eFigure 17-29) (186), and inverted papilloma (194).

Rare cases of transitional cell carcinoma, leiomyosarcoma and secondary involvement by leukemia, lymphoma, and WT have been reported.

Inflammatory Myofibroblastic Tumor (Pseudosarcomatous tumor)

Inflammatory myofibroblastic tumor (IMT) is occasionally seen in the bladder. Myxoid, leiomyomatous, and sclerosing matrix patterns are seen, with the myxoid type being most common (eFigures 17-30,17-31) (e143). The proliferating cells stain with vimentin, muscle-specific actin, smooth muscle actin, desmin, and occasionally keratin and, rarely, Epstein-Barr virus (e80,e103,108). Although this tumor was long considered a benign proliferative response to inflammation, the frequent anaplastic lymphoma kinase gene alterations indicate that it is a neoplastic process (112). Some of the pathologic aspects occurring in a few of these tumors that support this view include local recurrence, development of multifocal noncontiguous tumors, infiltrative local growth, vascular invasion, and, rarely, malignant transformation (e64,71). However, a recent review of 35 pediatric cases showed no recurrence or metastasis (75). IMT should be regarded as a soft tissue-mesenchymal tumor with an indeterminate or low potential for malignancy (see Chapter 24).

Rhabdomyosarcoma

Although the term *rhabdomyosarcoma* indicates a mesenchymal tumor derived from striated muscle, rhabdomyosarcoma typically arises in sites lacking striated muscle. Approximately 250 new cases of rhabdomyosarcoma are diagnosed in the United States each year (e184), 15% to 30% of which are found in the genitourinary tract (e99,e205,e235). Thus, although rhabdomyosarcoma is the most common tumor of the lower genitourinary tract in the first two decades of life (e12), only a handful of cases occurring in the bladder are seen in the United States each year. The majority of cases are sporadic; however, rhabdomyosarcoma has an association with the familial cancer syndromes, including Li-Fraumeni, Beckwith-Wiedemann, neurofibromatosis type 1, and Gorlin syndrome (130). The mean age at diagnosis is 5 years, with a male-to-female ratio of 3:2 (e130,e131). Symptoms include hematuria, signs of bladder outlet obstruction (abdominal pain and distension, dysuria) and, occasionally, abdominal mass (102).

The vast majority of cases of rhabdomyosarcoma of the bladder are of the botryoid subtype of embryonal rhabdomyosarcoma. The gross configuration in most cases is grapelike. The tumor cells form a distinct layer with a thickness of several cells, at least focally, near the epithelium. The superficial stroma next to the epithelium is loose. The condensed tumor cells or cambian layer of Nicholson (e234) varies in thickness and extent (Figure 17-63). Some grossly grapelike lesions do not show the cambian layer under the epithelium. By this definition, these would not be called *botryoid rhabdomyosarcoma*, but rather *embryonal rhabdomyosarcoma* (e233). Cytogenetic and molecular features are discussed in the soft tissue chapter (Chapter 24).

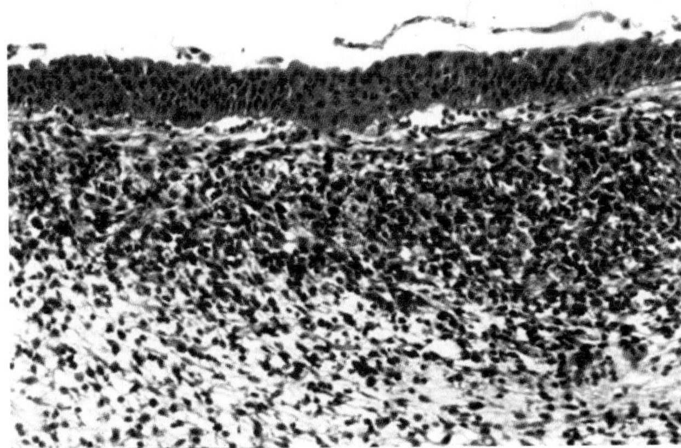

FIGURE 17-63 ■ Embryonal rhabdomyosarcoma as a polypoid urethral mass from an 8-week-old girl. The concentration of small, primitive tumor cells beneath the mucosal surface is typical of sarcoma botryoides. (Hematoxylin and eosin stain, original magnification ×200.)

In the vast majority of cases, the stroma of the botryoid lesion consists of a very loosely cellular tissue with a myxoid appearance. In the remainder, the stroma is more cellular. The appearance of the tumor cells also varies. In about 50% of the cases, the tumor cells are small and primitive, show very little myogenesis, and often demonstrate stellate cytoplasmic processes. In the remainder, the tumor cells are somewhat larger and more definitive myogenesis is present, consistent with rhabdomyoblasts. The cytoplasm of the rhabdomyoblasts varies from slight to abundant with cross-striations.

The importance of recognizing the botryoid subtype lies in the fact that these patients have a very good prognosis (95% survival at 5 years); in contrast, patients with embryonal rhabdomyosarcoma have a 5-year survival of 67%, and those with alveolar and undifferentiated sarcoma have 5-year survival rates of 54% and 47%, respectively (e233).

The goal of multimodality therapy is to improve outcome while preserving organ and function; therapy is intensified according to a risk-based study design (e71,e132). Bladder rhabdomyosarcoma is responsive to chemotherapy and radiotherapy. A complete loss of tumor cells was observed in 12 of 26 patients after induction therapy. Cystectomy specimens showed diminished tumor cells with varying degrees of cellular maturation (e137). There is lack of agreement concerning the significance of mature-appearing cells in post-treatment biopsies.

REFERENCES

1. Abrahamson DR, Hudson BG, Stroganova L, et al. Cellular origins of type IV collagen networks in developing glomeruli. *J Am Soc Nephrol* 2009;20(7):1471–1479.
2. Adeva M, El-Youssef M, Rossetti S, et al. Clinical and molecular characterization defines a broadened spectrum of autosomal recessive polycystic kidney disease (ARPKD). *Medicine (Baltimore)* 2006;85(1):1–21.
3. Akl MN, Saleh AA. Sirenomelia in a monoamniotic twin: a case report. *J Reprod Med* 2006;51(2):138–140.
4. Al-Ahmadie H, Gomez AM, Trane N, et al. Giant botryoid fibroepithelial polyp of bladder with myofibroblastic stroma and cystitis cystica et glandularis. *Pediatr Dev Pathol* 2003;6(2): 179–181.
5. Anderson J, Gibson S, Sebire NJ. Expression of ETV6-NTRK in classical, cellular and mixed subtypes of congenital mesoblastic nephroma. *Histopathology* 2006;48(6):748–753.
6. Argani P and Beckwith JB. Metanephric stromal tumor: report of 31 cases of a distinctive pediatric renal neoplasm. *Am J Surg Pathol* 2000;24(7):917–926.
7. Argani P, Perlman EJ, Breslow NE, et al. Clear cell sarcoma of the kidney: a review of 351 cases from the National Wilms Tumor Study Group Pathology Center. *Am J Surg Pathol* 2000;24(1):4–18.
8. Aslam M, Watson AR. Unilateral multicystic dysplastic kidney: long term outcomes. *Arch Dis Child* 2006;91(10):820–823.
9. Aucella F, Bisceglia L, De Bonis P, et al. WT1 mutations in nephrotic syndrome revisited. High prevalence in young girls, associations and renal phenotypes. *Pediatr Nephrol* 2006;21(10):1393–1398.
10. Baldwin DS, Gluck MC, Schacht RG, et al., The long-term course of poststreptococcal glomerulonephritis. *Ann Intern Med* 1974;80(3):342–358.
11. Bansal PJ, Tobin MC. Neonatal microscopic polyangiitis secondary to transfer of maternal myeloperoxidase-antineutrophil cytoplasmic antibody resulting in neonatal pulmonary hemorrhage and renal involvement. *Ann Allergy Asthma Immunol* 2004;93(4):398–401.
12. Barese CN, Podesta M, Litvak E, et al. Recurrent eosinophilic cystitis in a child with chronic granulomatous disease. *J Pediatr Hematol Oncol* 2004;26(3):209–212.
13. Barr RG, Seliger S, Appel GB, et al. Prognosis in proliferative lupus nephritis: the role of socio-economic status and race/ethnicity. *Nephrol Dial Transplant* 2003;18(10):2039–2046.
14. Beck LH Jr, Bonegio RG, Lambeau G, et al. M-type phospholipase A2 receptor as target antigen in idiopathic membranous nephropathy. *N Engl J Med* 2009;361(1):11–21.
15. Becker A, Baum M. Obstructive uropathy. *Early Hum Dev* 2006;82(1):15–22.
16. Beckwith JB, Management of incidentally encountered nephrogenic rests. *J Pediatr Hematol Oncol* 2007;29(6):353–354.
17. Belarmino JM, Kogan BA. Management of neonatal hydronephrosis. *Early Hum Dev* 2006;82(1):9–14.
18. Bilge I, Kayserili H, Emre S, et al. Frequency of renal malformations in Turner syndrome: analysis of 82 Turkish children. *Pediatr Nephrol* 2000;14(12):1111–1114.
19. Bingol-Kologlu M, Ciftci AO, Senocak ME, et al. Xanthogranulomatous pyelonephritis in children: diagnostic and therapeutic aspects. *Eur J Pediatr Surg* 2002;12(1):42–48.
20. Bisceglia M, Galliani CA, Senger C, et al. Renal cystic diseases: a review. *Adv Anat Pathol* 2006;13(1):26–56.
21. Bogart MM, Arnold HE, Greer KE. Prune-belly syndrome in two children and review of the literature. *Pediatr Dermatol* 2006;23(4):342–345.
22. Bongers EM, Huysmans FT, Levtchenko E, et al. Genotype-phenotype studies in nail-patella syndrome show that LMX1B mutation location is involved in the risk of developing nephropathy. *Eur J Hum Genet* 2005;13(8):935–946.
23. Bourdeaut F, Freneaux P. Thuille B, et al. hSNF5/INI1-deficient tumours and rhabdoid tumours are convergent but not fully overlapping entities. *J Pathol* 2007;211(3):323–330.
24. Boute N, Gribouval O, Roselli S, et al. NPHS2, encoding the glomerular protein podocin, is mutated in autosomal recessive steroid-resistant nephrotic syndrome. *Nat Genet* 2000;24(4):349–354.
25. Breslow NE, Beckwith JB, Perlman EJ, et al. Age distributions, birth weights, nephrogenic rests, and heterogeneity in the pathogenesis of Wilms tumor. *Pediatr Blood Cancer* 2006;47(3):260–267.
26. Brownlee NA, Perkins LA, Stewart W, et al. Recurring translocation (10;17) and deletion (14q) in clear cell sarcoma of the kidney. *Arch Pathol Lab Med* 2007;131(3):446–451.
27. Caridi G, Bertelli R, Di Duca M, et al. Broadening the spectrum of diseases related to podocin mutations. *J Am Soc Nephrol* 2003;14(5):1278–1286.
28. Cascio S, Sweeney B, Granata C, et al. Vesicoureteral reflux and ureteropelvic junction obstruction in children with horseshoe kidney: treatment and outcome. *J Urol* 2002;167(6):2566–2568.
29. Castellino SM, McLean TW, Pediatric genitourinary tumors. *Curr Opin Oncol* 2007;19(3):248–253.
30. Cattran DC, Coppo R, Cook HT, et al. The Oxford classification of IgA nephropathy: rationale, clinicopathological correlations, and classification. *Kidney Int* 2009;76(5):534–545.
31. Chammas M Jr, Feuillu B, Coissard A, et al. Laparoscopic robotic-assisted management of pelvic-ureteric junction obstruction in patients with horseshoe kidneys: technique and 1-year follow-up. *BJU Int* 2006;97(3):579–583.
32. Chan TM. Determinants of patient survival in systemic lupus erythematosus—focusing on lupus nephritis. *Ethn Dis* 2006;16(2 suppl 2):S2-66-69.
33. Chang P, Tsau YK, Tsai WY, et al. Renal malformations in children with Turner's syndrome. *J Formos Med Assoc* 2000;99(10):796–798.
34. Cheuk DK, Lee TL, Chiang AK, et al. Risk factors and treatment of hemorrhagic cystitis in children who underwent hematopoietic stem cell transplantation. *Transpl Int* 2007;20(1):73–81.
35. Choudhury M, Bajaj P, Jain R, et al. Malakoplakia of bone. A case report. *Acta Cytol* 2001;45(3):404–406.
36. Clarke JC, Patel SR, Raymond RM Jr, et al. Regulation of c-Ret in the developing kidney is responsive to Pax2 gene dosage. *Hum Mol Genet* 2006;15(23):3420–3428.
37. Cutcliffe C, Kersey D, Huang CC, et al. Clear cell sarcoma of the kidney: up-regulation of neural markers with activation of the sonic hedgehog and Akt pathways. *Clin Cancer Res* 2005;11(22):7986–7994.
38. D'Agati V. Pathologic classification of focal segmental glomerulosclerosis. *Semin Nephrol* 2003;23(2):117–134.
39. De Caluwe D, Chertin B, Puri P. Long-term outcome of the retained ureteral stump after lower pole heminephrectomy in duplex kidneys. *Eur Urol* 2002;42(1):63–66.
40. Debiec H, Guigonis V, Mougenot B, et al. Antenatal membranous glomerulonephritis due to anti-neutral endopeptidase antibodies. *N Engl J Med* 2002;346(26):2053–2060.
41. Direnna T, Leonard MP. Watchful waiting for prenatally detected ureteroceles. *J Urol* 2006;175(4):1493–1495; discussion 1495.
42. Dome JS, Bockhold CA, Li SM, et al. High telomerase RNA expression level is an adverse prognostic factor for favorable-histology Wilms' tumor. *J Clin Oncol* 2005;23(36):9138–9145.
43. Dumoulin A, Hill GS, Montseny JJ, et al. Clinical and morphological prognostic factors in membranous nephropathy: significance of focal segmental glomerulosclerosis. *Am J Kidney Dis* 2003;41(1):38–48.
44. Dziarmaga A, Quinlan J, Goodyer P. Renal hypoplasia: lessons from Pax2. *Pediatr Nephrol* 2006;21(1):26–31.
45. Eddy AA, Symons JM. Nephrotic syndrome in childhood. *Lancet* 2003;362(9384):629–639.
46. Ehrlich PF. Wilms tumor: progress and considerations for the surgeon. *Surg Oncol* 2007;16(3):157–171.
47. Ekinci S, Ciftci AO, Senocak ME, et al. Waardenburg syndrome associated with bilateral renal anomaly. *J Pediatr Surg* 2005;40(5):879–881.
48. Falcini F, Calabri GB, Simonini G, et al. Bilateral renal artery stenosis in Kawasaki disease: a report of two cases. *Clin Exp Rheumatol* 2006;24(6):719–721.

49. Fan F, Pietrow P, Wilson LA, et al. Adrenal pseudocyst: a unique case with adrenal renal fusion, mimicking a cystic renal mass. *Ann Diagn Pathol* 2004;8(2):87–90.
50. Fazio L, Razvi H, Chin JL. Malignancy in horseshoe kidneys: review and discussion of surgical implications. *Can J Urol* 2003;10(3):1899–1904.
51. Ferraris JR, Ramirez JA, Ruiz S, et al. Shiga toxin-associated hemolytic uremic syndrome: absence of recurrence after renal transplantation. *Pediatr Nephrol* 2002;17(10):809–814.
52. Filler G, Young E, Geier P, et al. Is there really an increase in non-minimal change nephrotic syndrome in children? *Am J Kidney Dis* 2003;42(6):1107–1113.
53. Foster BJ, Bernard C, Drummond KN. Kawasaki disease complicated by renal artery stenosis. *Arch Dis Child* 2000;83(3):253–255.
54. Fukuzawa R, Reeve AE. Molecular pathology and epidemiology of nephrogenic rests and Wilms tumors. *J Pediatr Hematol Oncol* 2007;29(9):589–594.
55. Furtwaengler R, Reinhard H, Leuschner I, et al. Mesoblastic nephroma–a report from the Gesellschaft fur Padiatrische Onkologie und Hamatologie (GPOH). *Cancer* 2006;106(10):2275–2283.
56. Gambaro G, Fabris A, Puliatta D, et al. Lithiasis in cystic kidney disease and malformations of the urinary tract. *Urol Res* 2006;34(2):102–107.
57. Geller JI, Argani P, Adeniran A, et al. Translocation renal cell carcinoma: lack of negative impact due to lymph node spread. *Cancer* 2008;112(7):1607–1616.
58. Gorczynska E, Turkiewicz D, Rybka K, et al. Incidence, clinical outcome, and management of virus-induced hemorrhagic cystitis in children and adolescents after allogeneic hematopoietic cell transplantation. *Biol Blood Marrow Transplant* 2005;11(10):797–804.
59. Gordon M, Cervellione RM, Postlethwaite R, et al. Acute renal papillary necrosis with complete bilateral ureteral obstruction in a child. *Urology* 2007;69(3):575 e511–e572.
60. Gribouval O, Gonzales M, Neuhaus T, et al. Mutations in genes in the renin-angiotensin system are associated with autosomal recessive renal tubular dysgenesis. *Nat Genet* 2005;37(9):964–968.
61. Gross AJ, Fisher M. Management of stones in patients with anomalously sited kidneys. *Curr Opin Urol* 2006;16(2):100–105.
62. Grundy PE, Breslow NE, Li S, et al. Loss of heterozygosity for chromosomes 1p and 16q is an adverse prognostic factor in favorable-histology Wilms tumor: a report from the National Wilms Tumor Study Group. *J Clin Oncol* 2005;23(29):7312–7321.
63. Guan N, Ding J, Zhang J, et al. Expression of nephrin, podocin, alpha-actinin, and WT1 in children with nephrotic syndrome. *Pediatr Nephrol* 2003;18(11):1122–1127.
64. Guay-Woodford LM, Desmond RA. Autosomal recessive polycystic kidney disease: the clinical experience in North America. *Pediatrics* 2003;111(5 Pt 1):1072–1080.
65. Gubler MC, Heidet L, Antignac C. Alport's syndrome, thin basement membrane nephropathy, nail-patella syndrome, and type III collagen glomerulopathy. In: Jennette JC, Olson JL, Schwartz MM, et al. eds. *Heptinstall's pathology of the kidney*. Philadelphia, PA: Lippincott Williams & Wilkins, 2007:506–508.
66. Guerriero S, Vischi A, Giancipoli G, et al. Tubulointerstitial nephritis and uveitis syndrome. *J Pediatr Ophthalmol Strabismus* 2006;43(4):241–243.
67. Guertl B, Leuschner I, Harms D, et al. Genetic clonality is a feature unifying nephroblastomas regardless of the variety of morphological subtypes. *Virchows Arch* 2006;449(2):171–174.
68. Gunther DF, Eugster E, Zagar AJ, et al. Ascertainment bias in Turner syndrome: new insights from girls who were diagnosed incidentally in prenatal life. *Pediatrics* 2004;114(3):640–644.
69. Haas M. IgA nephropathy and Henoch-Schonlein purpura nephritis. In: Jennette JC, Olson JL, Schwartz MM et al. eds. *Heptinstall's pathology of the kidney*. Philadelphia, PA: Lippincott Williams & Wilkins, 2007:424–431.
70. Haas M. Incidental healed postinfectious glomerulonephritis: a study of 1012 renal biopsy specimens examined by electron microscopy. *Hum Pathol* 2003;34(1):3–10.
71. Harik LR, Merino C, Coindre JM, et al. Pseudosarcomatous myofibroblastic proliferations of the bladder: a clinicopathologic study of 42 cases. *Am J Surg Pathol* 2006;30(7):787–794.
72. Hegde S, Coulthard MG. End stage renal disease due to bilateral renal malakoplakia. *Arch Dis Child* 2004;89(1):78–79.
73. Hill DA, Shear TD, Liu T, et al. Clinical and biologic significance of nuclear unrest in Wilms tumor. *Cancer* 2003;97(9):2318–2326.
74. Hingorani SR, Finn LS, Kowalewska J, et al. Expression of nephrin in acquired forms of nephrotic syndrome in childhood. *Pediatr Nephrol* 2004;19(3):300–305.
75. Houben CH. Pseudosarcomatous myofibroblastic proliferations of the bladder: a clinicopathologic study of 42 cases. *Am J Surg Pathol* 2007;31(4):642; author reply 642.
76. Huang CC, Cutcliffe C, Coffin C, et al. Classification of malignant pediatric renal tumors by gene expression. *Pediatr Blood Cancer* 2006;46(7):728–738.
77. Hubert KC, Palmer JS. Current diagnosis and management of fetal genitourinary abnormalities. *Urol Clin North Am* 2007;34(1):89–101.
78. Isaac J, Lowichik A, Cartwright P, et al. Inverted papilloma of the urinary bladder in children: case report and review of prognostic significance and biological potential behavior. *J Pediatr Surg* 2000;35(10):1514–1516.
79. Jais JP, Knebelmann B, Giatras I, et al. X-linked Alport syndrome: natural history and genotype-phenotype correlations in girls and women belonging to 195 families: a "European Community Alport Syndrome Concerted Action" study. *J Am Soc Nephrol* 2003;14(10):2603–2610.
80. Jais JP, Knebelmann B, Giatras I, et al. X-linked Alport syndrome: natural history in 195 families and genotype- phenotype correlations in males. *J Am Soc Nephrol* 2000;11(4):649–657.
81. Jemal A, Siegel R, Ward E, et al. Cancer statistics, 2007. *CA Cancer J Clin* 2007;57(1):43–66.
82. Joseph VT. The management of renal conditions in the perinatal period. *Early Hum Dev* 2006;82(5):313–324.
83. Kain R, Exner M, Brandes R, et al. Molecular mimicry in pauci-immune focal necrotizing glomerulonephritis. *Nat Med* 2008;14(10):1088–1096.
84. Kalyoussef E, Hwang J, Prasad V, et al. Segmental multicystic dysplastic kidney in children. *Urology* 2006;68(5):1121. e9–11.
85. Kavanagh D, Goodship TH, Richards A. Atypical haemolytic uraemic syndrome. *Br Med Bull* 2006;77–78:5–22.
86. Keller G, Zimmer G, Mall G, et al. Nephron number in patients with primary hypertension. *N Engl J Med* 2003;348(2):101–108.
87. Kianifar H, Sharifi N, Talebi S, et al. Malakoplakia of colon in a child with celiac disease and chronic granulomatous disease. *Indian J Gastroenterol* 2006;25(3):163–164.
88. Knudson A. Summary, conclusions, and commentary on the molecular genetics of childhood renal tumors. *Med Pediatr Oncol* 1996;27:498.
89. Kobayashi Y, Honda M, Yoshikawa N, et al. Acute tubulointerstitial nephritis in 21 Japanese children. *Clin Nephrol* 2000;54(3):191–197.
90. Korbet SM, Schwartz MM, Evans J, et al. Severe lupus nephritis: racial differences in presentation and outcome. *J Am Soc Nephrol* 2007;18(1):244–254.
91. Koziell A, Grech V, Hussain S, et al. Genotype/phenotype correlations of NPHS1 and NPHS2 mutations in nephrotic syndrome advocate a functional inter-relationship in glomerular filtration. *Hum Mol Genet* 2002;11(4):379–388.
92. Kusuma V, Hemalata M, Suguna BV, Ectopic supernumerary kidney presenting as inguinal hernia. *J Clin Pathol* 2005;58(4):446.
93. Lacson A, Bernstein J, Risdon RA, et al. Renal system: Part 1 kidneys and urinary tract. In: Gilbert-Barness E. ed. *Potter's pathology of the fetus infant and child*. Philadelphia, PA: Mosby/Elsevier, 2007:1281–1344.

94. Lambot MA, Vermeylen D, Noel JC. Angiotensin-II-receptor inhibitors in pregnancy. *Lancet* 2001;357(9268):1619–1620.
95. Laszik ZG, Silva FG. Hemolytic uremic syndrome, thrombotic thrombocytopenic purpura, and other thrombotic microangiopathies. In: Jennette JC, Olson JL, Schwartz MM, et al. eds. *Heptinstall's pathology of the kidney.* Philadephia, PA: Lippincott Williams & Wilkins, Philadelphia, 2007:704–721.
96. Lau KK, Gaber LW, Delos Santos NM, et al. C1q nephropathy: features at presentation and outcome. *Pediatr Nephrol* 2005;20(6): 744–749.
97. Liapis H, Gokden N, Hmiel P, et al. Histopathology, ultrastructure, and clinical phenotypes in thin glomerular basement membrane disease variants. *Hum Pathol* 2002;33(8):836–845.
98. Liapis H, Winyard PJ. Cystic diseases and developmental kidney defects (chapter 26). In: Jennette JC, Olson JL, Schwartz MM, et al., eds. *Heptinstall's pathology of the kidney*. Philadelphia, PA: Lippincott Williams & Wilkins, 2007:1258–1306.
99. Licht C, Fremeaux-Bacchi V. Hereditary and acquired complement dysregulation in membranoproliferative glomerulonephritis. *Thromb Haemost* 2009;101(2):271–278.
100. Liebau MC, Gal A, Superti-Furga A, et al. L1CAM mutation in a boy with hydrocephalus and duplex kidneys. *Pediatr Nephrol* 2007;22(7):1058–1061.
101. Lin F, Satlin LM. Polycystic kidney disease: the cilium as a common pathway in cystogenesis. *Curr Opin Pediatr* 2004;16:171–176.
102. Lott S, Lopez-Beltran A, Montironi R, et al. Soft tissue tumors of the urinary bladder Part II: malignant neoplasms. *Hum Pathol* 2007;38(7):963–977.
103. Luithle T, Szavay P, Furtwangler R, et al. Treatment of cystic nephroma and cystic partially differentiated nephroblastoma—a report from the SIOP/GPOH study group. *J Urol* 2007;177(1):294–296.
104. Luyckx VA, Brenner BM. Low birth weight, nephron number, and kidney disease. *Kidney Int Suppl* 2005;97:S68–S77.
105. Major MB, Camp ND, Berndt JD, et al. Wilms tumor suppressor WTX negatively regulates WNT/beta-catenin signaling. *Science* 2007;316(5827):1043–1046.
106. Markowitz GS, Schwimmer JA, Stokes MB, et al. C1q nephropathy: a variant of focal segmental glomerulosclerosis. *Kidney Int* 2003; 64(4):1232–1240.
107. Marks SD, Sebire NJ, Pilkington C, et al. Clinicopathological correlations of paediatric lupus nephritis. *Pediatr Nephrol* 2007;22(1):77–83.
108. Mergan F, Jaubert F, Sauvat F, et al. Inflammatory myofibroblastic tumor in children: clinical review with anaplastic lymphoma kinase, Epstein-Barr virus, and human herpesvirus 8 detection analysis. *J Pediatr Surg* 2005;40(10):1581–1586.
109. Minor L, Lindgren BW. Malacoplakia of the bladder in a 16-year-old girl. *J Urol* 2003;170(2 Pt 1):568–569.
110. Mittermayer C, Lee A, Brugger PC. Prenatal diagnosis of the Meckel-Gruber syndrome from 11th to 20th gestational week. *Ultraschall Med* 2004;25(4):275–279.
111. Moake JL. Thrombotic microangiopathies. *N Engl J Med* 2002;347(8):589–600.
112. Montgomery EA, Shuster DD, Burkart AL, et al. Inflammatory myofibroblastic tumors of the urinary tract: a clinicopathologic study of 46 cases, including a malignant example inflammatory fibrosarcoma and a subset associated with high-grade urothelial carcinoma. *Am J Surg Pathol* 2006;30(12):1502–1512.
113. Morrison AA, Viney RL, Ladomery MR. The post-transcriptional roles of WT1, a multifunctional zinc-finger protein. *Biochim Biophys Acta* 2008;1785(1):55–62.
114. Moyano Calvo JL, Maqueda Marin Mde L, Davalos Casanova G, et al. Bladder leiomyoma in a 17-year-old male patient. *Arch Esp Urol* 2005;58(9):954–956.
115. Murawski IJ, Gupta IR. Vesicoureteric reflux and renal malformations: a developmental problem. *Clin Genet* 2006;69(2):105–117.
116. Nadasdy T, Silva FG. Acute postinfectious glomerulonephritis and glomerulonephritis caused by persistent bacterial infection. In: Jennette JC, Olson JL, Schwartz MM et al. eds. *Heptinstall's pathology of the kidney*. Philadelphia, PA: Lippincott Williams & Wilkins, 2007: 322–349.
117. Nakai H, Asanuma H, Shishido S, et al. Changing concepts in urological management of the congenital anomalies of kidney and urinary tract, CAKUT. *Pediatr Int* 2003;45(5):634–641.
118. Naqiyah I, Rohaizak M, Meah FA, et al. Phaeochromocytoma of the urinary bladder. *Singapore Med J* 2005;46(7):344–346.
119. Narchi H. Risk of Wilms' tumour with multicystic kidney disease: a systematic review. *Arch Dis Child* 2005;90(2):147–149.
120. Nelson CP, Dunn RL, Wei JT, et al. Surgical repair of bladder exstrophy in the modern era: contemporary practice patterns and the role of hospital case volume. *J Urol* 2005;174(3):1099–1102.
121. Neville H, Ritchey ML, Shamberger RC, et al. The occurrence of Wilms tumor in horseshoe kidneys: a report from the National Wilms Tumor Study Group (NWTSG). *J Pediatr Surg* 2002;37(8):1134–1137.
122. Newsome G, Interstitial cystitis. *J Am Acad Nurse Pract* 2003; 15(2):64–71.
123. Nikolic V, Bogdanovic R, Ognjanovic M, et al. Acute tubulointerstitial nephritis in children. *Srp Arh Celok Lek* 2001;129(suppl 1): 23–27.
124. Novak J, Julian BA, Tomana M, et al. IgA glycosylation and IgA immune complexes in the pathogenesis of IgA nephropathy. *Semin Nephrol* 2008;28(1):78–87.
125. Novak TE, Lakshmanan Y, Frimberger D, et al. Polyps in the exstrophic bladder. A cause for concern? *J Urol* 2005;174(4 pt 2):1522–1526; discussion 1526.
126. Nusse R. Cancer. Converging on beta-catenin in Wilms tumor. *Science* 2007;316(5827):988–989.
127. Olson JL, Laszik ZG, Diabetic nephropathy. In: Jennette JC, Olson JL, Schwartz MM, et al. eds. *Heptinstall's pathology of the kidney*. Philadelphia: Lippincott Williams & Wilkins, 2007:803–806.
128. Onal B, Kogan BA. Natural history of patients with multicystic dysplastic kidney-what followup is needed? *J Urol* 2006;176(4 pt 1): 1607–1611.
129. Papez KE, Smoyer WE. Recent advances in congenital nephrotic syndrome. *Curr Opin Pediatr* 2004;16(2):165–170.
130. Parham DM, Ellison DA. Rhabdomyosarcomas in adults and children: an update. *Arch Pathol Lab Med* 2006;130(10):1454–1465.
131. Patrakka J, Ruotsalainen V, Reponen P, et al. Recurrence of nephrotic syndrome in kidney grafts of patients with congenital nephrotic syndrome of the Finnish type: role of nephrin. *Transplantation* 2002;73(3):394–403.
132. Peres EM, Savasan S, Cushing B, et al. Chromosome analyses of 16 cases of Wilms tumor: different pattern in unfavorable histology. *Cancer Genet Cytogenet* 2004;148(1):66–70.
133. Perfumo F, Martini A. Lupus nephritis in children. *Lupus* 2005;14(1):83–88.
134. Perlman EJ. Pediatric renal tumors: practical updates for the pathologist. *Pediatr Dev Pathol* 2005;8(3):320–338.
135. Perlman EJ. Tumors of the kidney, bladder, and related urinary structures. In: Murphy WM, Grignon DJ, Perlman EJ, eds. *AFIP atlas of tumor pathology*. Washington, DC: American Registry of Pathology, 2004:10–90.
136. Phatak S, Foster HE Jr. The management of interstitial cystitis: an update. *Nat Clin Pract Urol* 2006;3(1):45–53.
137. Piaggio L, Franc-Guimond J, Figueroa TE, et al. Comparison of laparoscopic and open partial nephrectomy for duplication anomalies in children. *J Urol* 2006;175(6):2269–2273.
138. Pontincasa P, Bartoli F, Di Ciaula A, et al. Defective in vitro contractility of ureteropelvic junction in children with functional and obstructive urine flow impairment. *J Pediatr Surg* 2006;41(9): 1594–1597.

139. Porteous S, Torban E, Cho NP, et al. Primary renal hypoplasia in humans and mice with PAX2 mutations: evidence of increased apoptosis in fetal kidneys of Pax2(1Neu) +/- mutant mice. *Hum Mol Genet* 2000;9(1):1–11.
140. Puri P, Shinkai M. Megacystis microcolon intestinal hypoperistalsis syndrome. *Semin Pediatr Surg* 2005;14(1):58–63.
141. Pysher TJ, Siegler RL, Tesh VL, et al. von Willebrand Factor expression in a Shiga toxin-mediated primate model of hemolytic uremic syndrome. *Pediatr Dev Pathol* 2002;5(5):472–479.
142. Ramalho C, Matias A, Brandao O, et al. Renal tubular dysgenesis: report of two cases in a non-consanguineous couple and review of the literature. *Fetal Diagn Ther* 2007;22(1):10–13.
143. Rana K, Wang YY, Powell H, et al. Persistent familial hematuria in children and the locus for thin basement membrane nephropathy. *Pediatr Nephrol* 2005;20(12):1729–1737.
144. Redman JF, Parham DM. Extensive inflammatory eosinophilic bladder tumors in children: experience with three cases. *South Med J* 2002;95(9):1050–1052.
145. Regele HM, Fillipovic E, Langer B, et al. Glomerular expression of dystroglycans is reduced in minimal change nephrosis but not in focal segmental glomerulosclerosis. *J Am Soc Nephrol* 2000;11(3):403–412.
146. Reiser J, Mundel P. Danger signaling by glomerular podocytes defines a novel function of inducible B7–1 in the pathogenesis of nephrotic syndrome. *J Am Soc Nephrol* 2004;15(9):2246–2248.
147. Richardson CE, Morgan JM, Jasani B, et al. Megacystis-microcolon-intestinal hypoperistalsis syndrome and the absence of the alpha3 nicotinic acetylcholine receptor subunit. *Gastroenterology* 2001;121(2):350–357.
148. Rivera MN, Haber DA. Wilms' tumour: connecting tumorigenesis and organ development in the kidney. *Nat Rev Cancer* 2005;5(9):699–712.
149. Rivera MN, Kim WJ, Wells J, et al. An X chromosome gene, WTX, is commonly inactivated in Wilms tumor. *Science* 2007;315(5812): 642–645.
150. Rodriguez MM. Developmental renal pathology: its past, present, and future. *Fetal Pediatr Pathol* 2004;23(4):211–229.
151. Romero FR, Rais-Bahrami S, Permpongkosol S, et al. Primary carcinoid tumors of the kidney. *J Urol* 2006;176(6 pt 1):2359–2366.
152. Ronald A. The etiology of urinary tract infection: traditional and emerging pathogens. *Am J Med* 2002;113(Suppl 1A):14S–19S.
153. Ronco P, Debiec H. New insights into the pathogenesis of membranous glomerulonephritis. *Curr Opin Nephrol Hypertens* 2006;15(3):258–263.
154. Ruteshouser EC, Huff V. Familial Wilms tumor. *Am J Med Genet C Semin Med Genet* 2004;129C(1):29–34.
155. Ruteshouser EC, Robinson SM, Huff V. Wilms tumor genetics: mutations in WT1, WTX, and CTNNB1 account for only about one-third of tumors. *Genes Chromosomes Cancer* 2008;47(6):461–470.
156. Sadler TW. Urogenital system. In: *Langman's medical embryology*, 10th ed. Philadelphia, PA: Lippincott Williams & Wilkins, 2006: 229–239.
157. Sagen JV, Bostad L, Njolstad PR, et al. Enlarged nephrons and severe nondiabetic nephropathy in hepatocyte nuclear factor-1beta (HNF-1beta) mutation carriers. *Kidney Int* 2003;64(3):793–800.
158. Salomon R, Tellier AL, Attie-Bitach T, et al. PAX2 mutations in oligomeganephronia. *Kidney Int* 2001;59(2):457–462.
159. Sanna-Cherchi S, Caridi G, Weng PL, et al. Genetic approaches to human renal agenesis/hypoplasia and dysplasia. *Pediatr Nephrol* 2007;22(10):1675–1684.
160. Satoh Y, Nakadate H, Nakagawachi T, et al. Genetic and epigenetic alterations on the short arm of chromosome 11 are involved in a majority of sporadic Wilms' tumours. *Br J Cancer* 2006;95(4):541–547.
161. Sawicz-Birkowska K, Apoznanski W, Kantorowicz-Szymik S, et al. Malignant tumours in a horseshoe kidney in children: a diagnostic dilemma. *Eur J Pediatr Surg* 2005;15(1):48–52.
162. Schwab K, Witte DP, Aronow BJ, et al. Microarray analysis of focal segmental glomerulosclerosis. *Am J Nephrol* 2004;24(4):438–447.
163. Schwaderer AL, Bates CM, McHugh KM, et al. Renal anomalies in family members of infants with bilateral renal agenesis/adysplasia. *Pediatr Nephrol* 2007;22(1):52–56.
164. Schwartz MM. Membranous glomerulonephritis. In: Jennette JC, Olson JL, Schwartz MM et al., eds. *Heptinstall's pathology of the kidney*. Philadelphia, PA: Lippincott Williams & Wilkins, 2007: 208–211.
165. Shah A, Chandran H, Malakoplakia of bladder in childhood. *Pediatr Surg Int* 2005;21(2):113–115.
166. Shamberger RC, Haase GM, Argani P, et al. Bilateral Wilms' tumors with progressive or nonresponsive disease. *J Pediatr Surg* 2006;41(4):652–657; discussion 652–657.
167. Shirakawa T, Kondoh T, Takahashi R, et al. Renal tubular dysgenesis complicated with severe cranium hypoplasia. *Pediatr Int* 2004;46(1):88–90.
168. Shull JD, Lachel CM, Strecker TE, et al. Genetic bases of renal agenesis in the ACI rat: mapping of Renag1 to chromosome 14. *Mamm Genome* 2006;17(7):751–759.
169. Silverstein DM, Craver R. Presenting features and short-term outcome according to pathologic variant in childhood primary focal segmental glomerulosclerosis. *Clin J Am Soc Nephrol* 2007;2(4):700–707.
170. Singla V, Reiter JF. The primary cilium as the cell's antenna: signaling at a sensory organelle. *Science* 2006;313(5787):629–633.
171. Siomou E, Papadopoulou F, Kollios KD, et al. Duplex collecting system diagnosed during the first 6 years of life after a first urinary tract infection: a study of 63 children. *J Urol* 2006;175(2):678–681; discussion 681–672.
172. Smith AC, Choufani S, Ferreira JC, et al. Growth regulation, imprinted genes, and chromosome 11p15.5. *Pediatr Res* 2007;61 (5 pt 2):43R–47R.
173. Sparago A, Russo S, Cerrato F, et al. Mechanisms causing imprinting defects in familial Beckwith-Wiedemann syndrome with Wilms' tumour. *Hum Mol Genet* 2007;16(3):254–264.
174. Srivastava T, Garola RE, Whiting JM, et al. Synaptopodin expression in idiopathic nephrotic syndrome of childhood. *Kidney Int* 2001;59(1):118–125.
175. Stanley JC, Criado E, Upchurch GR Jr, et al. Pediatric renovascular hypertension: 132 primary and 30 secondary operations in 97 children. *J Vasc Surg* 2006;44(6):1219–1228; discussion 1228–1219.
176. Strand WR. Initial management of complex pediatric disorders: prunebelly syndrome, posterior urethral valves. *Urol Clin North Am* 2004;31(3):399–415, vii.
177. Sundaram V, Vidhyashree SA, Pratap B, et al. A male patient with right-sided thoracic kidney, diabetes mellitus, hearing loss and renal dysfunction. *Int Urol Nephrol* 2007;39(3):959–962.
178. Te Loo DM, Monnens LA, van den Heuvel LP, et al. Detection of apoptosis in kidney biopsies of patients with D+ hemolytic uremic syndrome. *Pediatr Res* 2001;49(3):413–416.
179. Tong JE, Howell DN, Foreman JW. Drug-induced granulomatous interstitial nephritis in a pediatric patient. *Pediatr Nephrol* 2007;22(2):306–309.
180. Torres VE, Harris PC. Mechanisms of Disease: autosomal dominant and recessive polycystic kidney diseases. *Nat Clin Pract Nephrol* 2006;2(1):40–55; quiz 55.
181. Torres VE, Harris PC. Polycystic kidney disease: genes, proteins, animal models, disease mechanisms and therapeutic opportunities. *J Intern Med* 2007;261(1):17–31.
182. Uematsu M, Sakamoto O, Nishio T, et al. A case surviving for over a year of renal tubular dysgenesis with compound heterozygous angiotensinogen gene mutations. *Am J Med Genet A* 2006;140(21): 2355–2360.
183. Van Cangh PJ. Is it always necessary to treat a ureteropelvic junction syndrome? *Curr Urol Rep* 2007;8(2):118–121.

184. van den Ouden D. Diagnosis and management of eosinophilic cystitis: a pooled analysis of 135 cases. *Eur Urol* 2000;37(4):386–394.
185. Varan A. Wilms' tumor in children: an overview. *Nephron Clin Pract* 2008;108(2):c83–c90.
186. Vemulakonda VM, Kopp RP, Sorensen MD, et al. Recurrent nephrogenic adenoma in a 10-year-old boy with prune belly syndrome: a case presentation. *Pediatr Surg Int* 2008;24(5):605–607.
187. Wallerstein R, Shih LY, Fong MH, et al. A new case of Okamoto syndrome. *Clin Dysmorphol* 2005;14(2):85–87.
188. Warady BA, Chadha V. Chronic kidney disease in children: the global perspective. *Pediatr Nephrol* 2007;22(12):1999–2009.
189. Weening JJ, D'Agati VD, Schwartz MM, et al. The classification of glomerulonephritis in systemic lupus erythematosus revisited. *Kidney Int* 2004;65(2):521–530.
190. Weiss M, Liapis H, Tomaszewski JE, et al. Pyelonephritis and other infections, reflux nephropathy, hydronephrosis, and nephrolithiasis (chapter 22). In: Jennette JC, Olson JL, Schwartz MM, et al., eds. *Heptinstall's pathology of the kidney*. Philadelphia, PA: Lippincott Williams & Wilkins, 2007:991–1081.
191. Winyard PJ, Nauta J, Lirenman DS, et al. Deregulation of cell survival in cystic and dysplastic renal development. *Kidney Int* 1996:49(1):135–146.
192. Winyard PJ, Risdon RA, Sams VR, et al. The PAX2 transcription factor is expressed in cystic and hyperproliferative dysplastic epithelia in human kidney malformations. *J Clin Invest* 1996;98(2):451–459.
193. Woolf AS. Diabetes, genes, and kidney development. *Kidney Int* 2000;57(3):1202–1203.
194. Xambre L, Prisco R, Carreira F, et al. Inverted papillomas—cases at our service and review of the literature. *Actas Urol Esp* 2003;27(8):605–610.
195. Yang L, Han Y, Suarez Saiz F, et al. A tumor suppressor and oncogene: the WT1 story. *Leukemia* 2007;21(5):868–876.
196. Yang XJ, Sugimura J, Tretiakova MS, et al. Gene expression profiling of renal medullary carcinoma: potential clinical relevance. *Cancer* 2004;100(5):976–985.
197. Zappitelli M, Duffy C, Bernard C, et al. Clinicopathological study of the WHO classification in childhood lupus nephritis. *Pediatr Nephrol* 2004;19(5):503–510.
198. Zeis PM, Kavazarakis E, Nakopoulou L, et al. Glomerulopathy with mesangial IgM deposits: long-term follow up of 64 children. *Pediatr Int* 2001;43(3):287–292.
199. Zhou XJ, Silva FG. Membranoproliferative glomerulonephritis. In: Jennette JC, Olson JL, Schwartz MM, et al., eds. *Heptinstall's pathology of the kidney*. Philadelphia, PA: Lippincott Williams & Wilkins, 2007c:287–290.
200. Zhou XJ, Silva FG. Membranoproliferative glomerulonephritis. In: Jennette JC, Olson JL, Schwartz MM, et al., eds. *Heptinstall's pathology of the kidney*. Phildelphiam, PA: Lippincott Williams & Wilkins, 2007a:255–267.
201. Zhou XJ, Silva FG. Membranoproliferative glomerulonephritis. In: Jennette JC, Olson JL, Schwartz MM, et al., eds. *Heptinstall's pathology of the kidney*. Philadelphia, PA: Lippincott Williams & Wilkins, 2007d:300–306.
202. Zhou XJ, Silva FG. Membranoproliferative glomerulonephritis. In: Jennette JC, Olson JL, Schwartz MM et al., eds. *Heptinstall's pathology of the kidney*. Philadelphia, PA: Lippincott Williams & Wilkins, 2007b:272–282.

CHAPTER 18

The Female Reproductive System

ELIZABETH J. PERLMAN
MICHAEL K. FRITSCH

Abnormalities confined to the genital tract are quite unusual in prepubertal girls and such disorders seldom come to the attention of pediatricians or pediatric pathologists. Major developmental abnormalities affecting the reproductive system are often eclipsed by concomitant urinary tract abnormalities, which are more immediately clinically significant. Abnormal gonadal development is an important group of diseases that may also result in abnormal development of secondary sexual characteristics. The most frequently acquired diseases of the female genital tract include infections and neoplasms. Infections confined to the female reproductive tract are seldom life threatening in childhood, yet they may result in reproductive sequelae during adulthood. Neoplasms are dominated by those arising in primordial germ cells.

ANATOMY AND EMBRYOLOGY

The female reproductive tract consists of the gonads, a ductal system (Fallopian tubes, uterus, cervix, vagina) and the external genitalia (clitoris, labia majora, labia minora, vestibule, mons pubis). The process of sexual differentiation can be divided into various phases. Chromosomal (genetic) sex is determined by the XY or XX genotype, with the potential for abnormal deletion or addition of sex chromosomal material such as in Turner and Klinefelter syndromes. Gonadal sex refers to gonadal differentiation into testis or ovary and is predominantly dependent on the expression of the sex-determining region on Y gene (SRY). SRY begins a cascade of molecular signals, resulting in male gonadal differentiation; the absence of these male-specific signals and the presence of several female-specific signals result in normal female differentiation. Phenotypic sex refers to the differentiation of the ductal system and of the external genitalia, a process that is regulated by production of the Müllerian inhibitory substance/antiMüllerian hormone (MIS/AMH) by the Sertoli cells of the testis and steroid hormone production by the testis (testosterone/dihydrotestosterone) and the ovary (estrogen/progesterone). Lastly, the assigned or adopted sex is usually determined by the chromosomal, gonadal, and phenotypic sex at birth but may be altered postnatally in a variety of the intersex disorders [also referred to as *disorders of sex development* (DSD)]. These processes occur predominantly *in utero*, with the final phenotypic changes being initiated by the onset of puberty.

Primordial Germ Cells

The primordial germ cells first appear in the wall of the yolk sac at about 3 to 4 weeks after fertilization and migrate through the hindgut and mesonephric ridge to the genital ridge beginning about week 4 to 5, a process mediated by a number of molecular factors (140,154,163). Germ cells that do not reach the genital ridge are thought to disappear, but they have also been proposed as the cell of origin of extragonadal germ cell tumors. The initial events in testicular and ovarian differentiation are independent of the presence or genotype of primordial germ cells in the gonad (19). However, completion of appropriate ovarian development depends upon the presence of meiotic germ cells. In the absence of meiotic germ cells, the ovarian structure degenerates leaving streak ovaries (15,166).

Early Gonadal Development

The gonadal ridge develops at the ventromedial aspect of the mesonephros by a proliferation of mesodermal cells and thickening of the overlying coelomic epithelium at 4 to 5 weeks' gestation. Between 4.5 and 6 weeks, the indifferent gonad is indistinguishable as male or female (Figure 18-1). Within the developing gonads, the somatic cells express a number of genes that maintain the indifferent gonad and dictate sex-specific gonad development. In mice, these include the homeobox gene Emx2, the polycomb group gene Cbx2, and the LIM homeodomain gene Lhx9 (152). In both humans and mice, the Wilms tumor gene isoform WT1-KTS and the steroidogenic factor 1 (previously referred to as SF-1 and now designated NR5A1) genes are important in maintaining the indifferent gonad. Mutations in NR5A1 can lead to adrenal-gonadal failure, mostly affecting male gonad development, as maintenance of NR5A1 expression is also critical

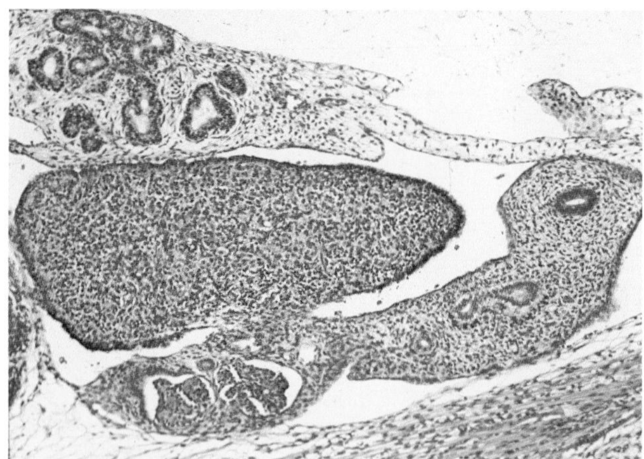

FIGURE 18-1 ■ The undifferentiated gonad lies adjacent to the mesonephros and the Wolffian and Müllerian ducts. The mesonephros has a profound effect on normal gonadal differentiation.

in testis development. The WT-KTS isoform is required for cell survival and proliferation within the bipotential gonad in both males and females (15,105,152,166,169). Mutations are associated with three syndromes characterized by gonadal dysgenesis [Wilms tumor/aniridia/gonadal dysgenesis/retardation—WAGR (OMIM 194072), Denys-Drash (OMIM 194080), and Frasier (OMIM 136680)] [reviewed in (81,129) and at OMIM, http://www.ncbi.nlm.nih.gov/entrez/query.fcgi?db=omim]. The phenotype of affected individuals includes genital and kidney defects as well as an increased risk for the development of Wilms tumors. At about 7 weeks' gestation, in XY embryos, a Y-linked genetic switch, SRY, is expressed by pre-Sertoli cells (15,19). The expression of SRY is necessary and sufficient to trigger male testis development; however, both the timing and the level of SRY expression are critical for normal development. In an XY embryo, the lack of SRY results in ovarian development. The SRY protein contains a highly conserved DNA-binding domain that allows specific genes to be turned on or off (19). One such gene is SOX-9, which is thought to be a Sertoli cell differentiation factor. Mutation in SOX-9 leads to the human dwarfism syndrome camptomelic dysplasia (OMIM 114290), which is often associated with XY sex reversal (69). Duplication of SOX-9 causes XX female-to-male sex reversal. NR5A1 expression in the developing testis regulates expression of several male-specific genes, including MIS/AMH (106) (see Chapter 27).

Ovarian Differentiation

The ovary can be identified at 7 to 8 weeks' gestation by the absence of testicular cords. After their arrival in the gonad, germ cells in the female continue to undergo active mitotic cell division, a process that continues until birth. It is estimated that approximately 3 to 4 million germ cells are present in each ovary by 20 weeks' gestation, and then the number decreases to about 0.5 to 1 million at term (102). The mechanism leading to the loss of oocytes remains poorly understood. At approximately 12 weeks' gestation, the first germ cells begin to enter into meiosis, a process first seen close to the medullary region (Figure 18-2). On entering meiosis, the primary oocyte will arrest at the diplotene stage of the first meiotic prophase and become enclosed by follicular cells to form primordial follicles. Follicular, or granulosa cells are in direct contact with the germ cells and are thought to play a role in regulating the continued meiotic arrest in the germ cells. Oogenesis is a gradual process that is generally complete by the third trimester, and there is no further increase in the number of primary oocytes thereafter (Figure 18-3). However, this has recently been questioned, at least in the mouse, where germ or stem cell replication may continue into adulthood (140). In addition to the germ cells, the ovary is populated by stromal cells that continue to remodel during the early first trimester, resulting in the formation of the ovarian cortex and the medulla. During the second trimester, a subepithelial collagenous connective tissue layer develops within the ovarian cortex beneath the basement membrane. The interstitial (thecal) cells can be detected during the first half of the second trimester, although estrogen production begins as early as 8 to 10 weeks' gestation. The importance of the production of estrogen by the developing fetus remains somewhat controversial with some evidence that significant estrogen production does not occur until following birth (166). The histology of the developing ovary has been previously described in detail (107,128).

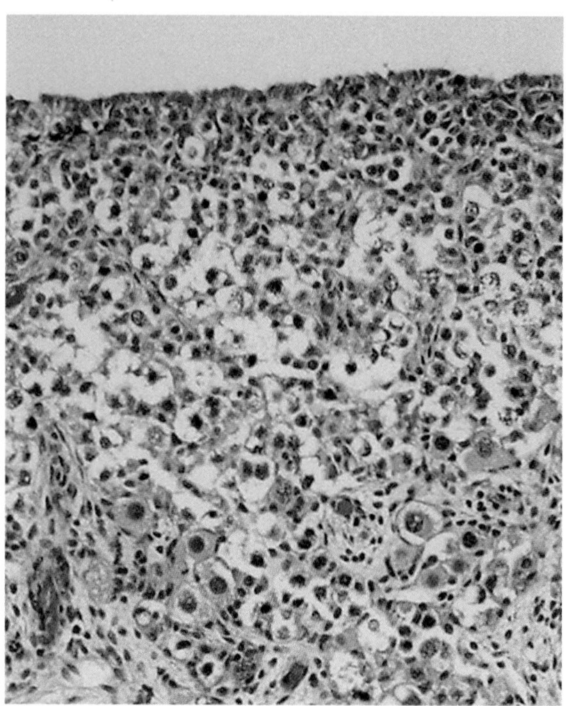

FIGURE 18-2 ■ Developing ovary at approximately 22 weeks' gestation showing formation of primordial follicles containing oocytes arrested in meiosis I in the deep ovarian cortex and premeiotic oogonia in the superficial cortex. Germ cell proliferation continues within the premeiotic oogonia until term.

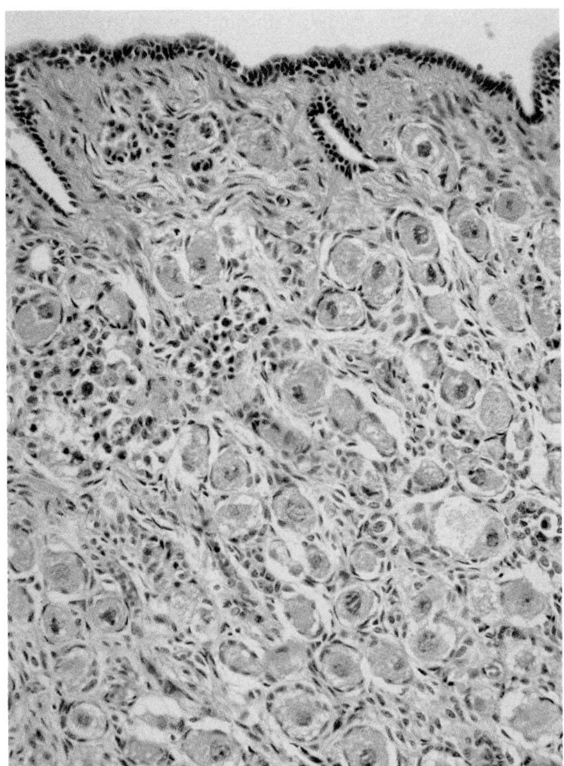

FIGURE 18-3 ■ Developing ovary at term showing numerous primordial follicles, and early development of the subepithelial stromal layer that will become more prominent with age. The number of germ cells will decrease progressively with age.

While many of the molecular details of testis development have been clearly established, the details regulating molecular ovarian development are still being explored. The NR0B1 gene, previously designated DAX-1, is a dosage-sensitive gene locus on the X chromosome that encodes an orphan nuclear receptor protein. This gene was initially thought to be a specific ovary-determining gene but has since been shown to be more essential for normal testicular development and is not required for normal ovarian development. NR0B1 is expressed in the normally developing ovary but turned off in the developing testis (15,140,152,166). Mutations of NR0B1 lead to hypogonadotropic hypogonadism with primary testicular defects and are associated with adrenal insufficiency. Loss of function of NR0B1 in XX females does not alter normal ovarian development. Overexpression of NR0B1, however, leads to ovarian development even if SRY is expressed. NR0B1 therefore appears to be more important in normal testis development. Recent evidence suggests that intact WNT4 signaling is necessary for normal development of the Müllerian duct, suppression of the interstitial cell lineage in the developing ovary, as well as oocyte maintenance (151,152,166). WNT4 is expressed in the bipotential gonad of both sexes, but it remains highly expressed only in the ovary. Without WNT4 expression in XX individuals, male-specific changes occur that include the presence of steroid producing cells within the ovary, persistence of the Wolffian ducts, loss of the Müllerian ducts, and the development of a male-specific coelomic blood vessel to the ovary. In the absence of WNT4, germ cells can still enter meiosis, but there is massive apoptosis of the germ cells prior to birth. WNT4 expression seems to provide a protective niche in the ovarian cortex for female germ cell survival. Other genes proposed to be involved in ovary-specific development include FOXL2, Pisrt1, and follistatin (Fst), although only FOXL2 has been shown to be important in human ovarian development thus far (152,166). Mutations in the forkhead transcription factor 2 (FOXL2) gene in humans are associated with eyelid defects and premature ovarian failure [blepharophimosis, ptosis and epicanthus inversus syndrome—BPES (OMIM 110100)]. FOXL2 is expressed by pregranulosa cells.

The ovary differs from the testis in that the presence of germ cells is essential for normal ovarian development. In the developing testis, the male germ cells do not play a significant role in the structural development of the organ. Female germ cells appear to follow an intrinsic clock to enter the first meiosis and arrest prior to completion. Once female germ cells have entered meiosis, they have committed to the oocyte fate. During fetal development, the oocyte becomes surrounded by a single layer of granulosa cells to form the primordial follicle. Figla (factor in germ line a) is an oocyte-specific basic helix-loop-helix transcription factor that is critical for recruiting granulosa cells to form the primordial follicles. In the absence of Figla expression, primordial follicles do not form and oocytes are rapidly depleted after birth. Figla is not expressed in male germ cells and does not appear to directly regulate meiosis (reviewed in ref. 166).

At birth, the ovary is tan, flat, and elongated and measures about 1.3 × 0.5 × 0.3 cm. and weighs less than 0.3 g (113). Before birth, some primordial follicles can develop further. The ovum enlarges and the surrounding follicular cells become more cuboidal to columnar and thereby form a primary follicle. This may be followed by stratification of the granulosa cells and increased granulosa cell proliferation, resulting in a preantral follicle (Figure 18-4). The Graafian follicle demonstrates a cavity within the granulosa cell layer.

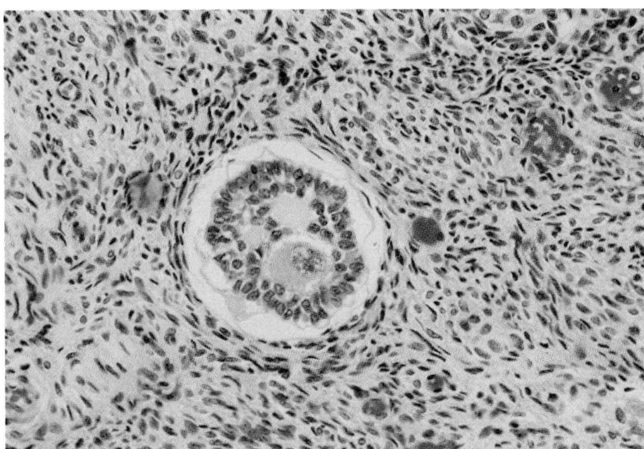

FIGURE 18-4 ■ Primary follicle, preantral stage, showing a thick layer of granulosa cells surrounding the oocyte. Several Call-Exner bodies containing acellular hyaline material are present.

The granulosa cells in these follicles have scant cytoplasm and often surround cavities filled with deeply eosinophilic material, known as *Call-Exner bodies* that may result in microscopic structures resembling gonadoblastoma or annular tubule-like profiles (83). These likely represent abnormal folliculogenesis. Thecal cells, which differentiate from the stromal cells at the periphery of developing follicles, may be seen. Throughout childhood, the ovaries enlarge to reach the size and the shape of an adult ovary (4 × 2 × 1 cm, 5 to 8 g). During the prepubertal period, the number of oocytes and primordial follicles continues to decrease and the amount of ovarian stroma increases. Like the testicular Leydig cells, ovarian hilus cells disappear during childhood and reappear during puberty.

The Ductal System

The development of the urinary and reproductive systems is highly interdependent, which explains the high incidence of coexisting genital and urinary tract anomalies in several syndromes. Early in development (~week 4) paired mesonephric (Wolffian) ducts arise from the intermediate mesoderm and nephrogenic cord (Figure 18-5). In the female embryo, the mesonephric duct is needed for induction of paramesonephric (Müllerian) duct development from invaginations of the coelomic epithelium. The mesonephric and the paramesonephric ducts are enclosed in a peritoneal fold that gives rise to the broad ligament of the uterus. In the male embryo AMH/MIS produced by fetal Sertoli cells leads to regression of the ipsilateral paramesonephric duct between weeks 8 and 10. AMH/MIS is proposed to have multiple functions in women (115,140). After the sensitivity of the paramesonephric ducts to AMH/MIS has disappeared, the ovarian granulosa cells begin to produce AMH/MIS with increasing levels that peak at about 10 years of age. AMH/MIS is thought to maintain meiotic arrest in the oocyte of the developing follicle in prepubertal females (9).

In the female embryo, the paramesonephric ducts fuse caudally before reaching the urogenital sinus, a process that is completed by week 10 (Figure 18-5). The unfused paramesonephric ducts become Fallopian tubes and the fused portions the uterus and the upper vagina. The distal tip of the Müllerian duct abuts the posterior wall of the urogenital sinus within a patch of mesoderm. This point is the future site of the hymenal membrane. The patch of mesodermal urogenital sinus epithelium begins to proliferate, forming a column of squamous cells called the *vaginal plate* that eventually gives rise to the vaginal epithelium. The vaginal plate and the Müllerian duct become patent by canalization early in the second trimester (by week 18). Mesonephric ducts in the female embryo begin to regress if not stimulated by testosterone by about week 10; however, mesonephric remnants in the broad ligament and lateral wall of the uterus and vagina can persist as Gartner ducts. By 13 weeks' gestation, the body (corpus) of the uterus and the cervix begin to be distinguished. In the fetus and the newborn, the cervix is twice as long as the corpus, whereas in the adult, the corpus is about two times longer than the cervix. At birth, the cervix and uterus together measure about 4 cm in length. The effects of maternal hormones (estrogens and progestins) result in a proliferative-to-weakly secretory endometrium at birth and cervical squamous cell maturation. These changes rapidly disappear after birth. During childhood, the endometrium is usually thin, with inactive glands in a spindled inactive stroma. The uterus reaches a plateau of growth in the second year of life, until the premenarchal uterine growth increase. The final adult (nulliparous) uterus measures 7 to 8 cm in longest dimension and weighs between 40 and 80 g.

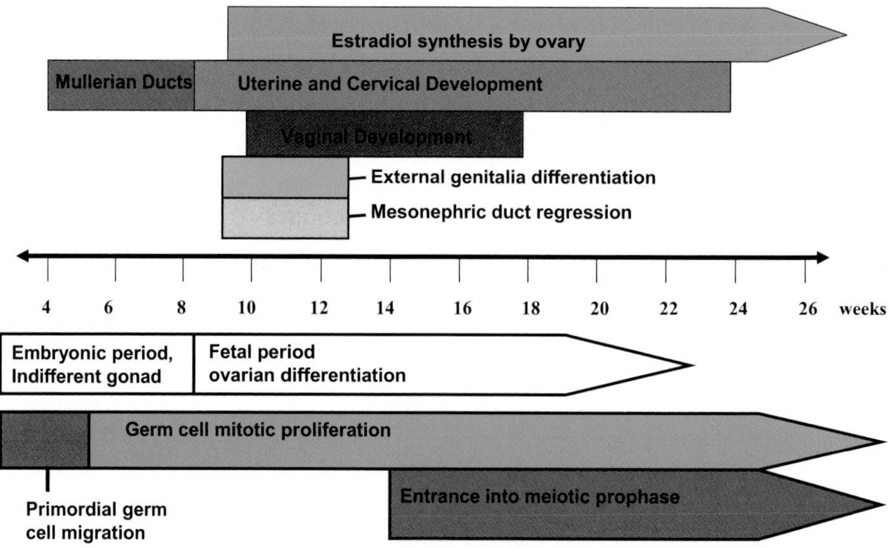

FIGURE 18-5 ■ Diagram indicating the gestational period of development of the ovary, ducts, and external genitalia.

The final maturation of the female reproductive tract is at the beginning of uterine bleeding (menarche), which occurs between 11 and 15 years of age. Menarche appears to be occurring earlier in US females, which has been proposed to be associated with the increased incidence of childhood obesity. The early menstrual cycles are often anovulatory and can result in disordered proliferative endometrium. By midadolescence, regular menstrual cycles should be occurring, along with the monthly histologic changes that are well described for the adult female reproductive tract.

A number of genes have been reported as important in regulating normal internal female genital development. WNT4 expression is essential for normal Müllerian development. A few patients have recently been described with mutations in WNT4 that present with phenotypes similar to that seen in Mayer-Rokitansky-Kuster-Hauser syndrome (Müllerian agenesis). In addition, spatial and temporal expression patterns of members of the HOXA gene locus are essential for normal development of the Fallopian tubes (HOXA9), uterus (HOXA10), cervix (HOXA11), and upper vagina (HOXA13). In mice, other transcription factors that have also been implicated in normal Müllerian duct formation include Lim1, Pax2, Emx2, Wnt5a, Wnt7a, and p63 (a p53 homolog) (169). Recently, it has been shown that expression of the Msx2 gene in mice is essential for normal vaginal development and that alterations in Msx2 levels may account for some of the female reproductive tract phenotypes seen with diethylstilbestrol exposure *in utero* (168). In the mouse, normal uterine gland development (uterine adenogenesis) and branching involve several important genes including Lif, calcitonin, several Wnt-signaling genes, matrix metalloproteinases, and their inhibitors, insulin-like growth factors, estrogen receptor α, and prolactin (reviewed in ref. 169).

Female External Genitalia

The external female genitalia begin to form during the fourth week of embryonic development. The genital tubercle forms ventral to the cloacal plate as two stromal elevations of the ectoderm. Lateral to the cloacal plate on each side, two parallel folds develop, the labia majora and the minora. As the labioscrotal folds extend cranially around the genital tubercle, they fuse and become the mons pubis (164). The role of estrogen in the development of any and all of the female reproductive tract is unknown. Levels of maternal estrogens are high throughout pregnancy, and local production by the fetal ovaries begins early, but is currently thought to be of little consequence. While estrogen secretion *in utero* does not appear to be important for sex determination, estrogen signaling does appear to be critical in the maintenance of the maturing ovary later during puberty. Blocking estrogen signaling in puberty results in transdifferentiation of the ovary and expression of Sertoli cell markers (27). Estrogen signaling appears to be critical in maintaining the mature ovarian structure by suppressing testicular development during early adult development. If a female fetus is exposed to elevated androgens before 10 to 12 weeks of gestation, the external genitalia may become ambiguous or resemble a phenotypic male. The vagina will often open into the membranous portion of the urethra. If androgens become elevated after week 20, the only effect will be an enlarged clitoris.

The entire vulva, with the exception of the vestibule, is lined by keratinized, stratified squamous epithelium. The vestibule and the vagina are lined by nonkeratinizing squamous epithelium, which becomes glycogenated in women of reproductive years, which should not be confused with koilocytotic change. The vaginal vestibule contains the orifices of the paraurethral (Skene) glands, the major (Bartholin) and minor vestibular glands, and the urethral meatus. The paired paraurethral glands are located on either side of the urethral meatus, are composed of pseudostratified mucous-secreting columnar epithelium, and are drained by ducts lined by transitional epithelium. The vestibular glands contain acini composed of simple columnar, mucous-secreting epithelium. The major vestibular (Bartholin) glands are drained by ducts lined proximally by mucous-secreting epithelium, and more distally by transitional epithelium with terminal lining by squamous epithelium on their exit just external to the hymenal ring. The minor vestibular glands are located close to the surface and ring the vestibule.

PREMATURE OVARIAN FAILURE

Premature ovarian failure can occur before or after the onset of menarche. Premature ovarian failure is defined by a deficiency of sex steroid production, high gonadotropin levels, and amenorrhea in any woman less than 40 years old. Chromosomal and genetic abnormalities including gonadotropin ligand or receptor defects, cholesterol desmolase deficiency, galactosemia, Turner syndrome, Fragile-X syndrome, Swyer syndrome, and blepharophimosis syndrome (FOXL2 gene mutation) are all associated with premature ovarian failure (91). In addition, infections, autoimmune disorders, and iatrogenic causes can lead to premature ovarian failure (91). In particular, treatment of childhood malignancies can result in a variety of disorders of abnormal puberty including premature puberty or hypogonadotrophic hypogonadism with premature ovarian failure (95).

STRUCTURAL ABNORMALITIES OF THE FEMALE REPRODUCTIVE ORGANS

The phenotypic abnormalities that can occur in the development of the female reproductive tract are numerous. These may represent isolated poorly understood variations in normal development, or they may be associated with major malformation syndromes; either may be related to chromosomal abnormalities or defects in known and unknown genes. Additionally, teratogens have been associated with abnormalities of the reproductive tract. DSD are discussed separately.

The Ductal System

Müllerian duct anomalies are frequently associated with intersexual disorders, discussed below. In patients with normal ovaries, Müllerian duct malformation occurs in about 0.5% of women and is frequently accompanied by anomalies of the urinary tract (122). These Müllerian duct anomalies include lateral and vertical fusion defects, hypoplasia, or absence of Fallopian tubes, uterus, or the upper vagina. Uterine abnormalities can be structurally and morphologically divided into three categories. These include (a) complete failure of formation of the Müllerian duct unilaterally (resulting in unicornuate uterus) or bilaterally (absent uterus), (b) arrested Müllerian duct development (hypoplastic uterus), or (c) abnormal lateral fusion of the Müllerian ducts to varying extents, resulting in paired uteri and cervices, accompanied by a vaginal septum (uterus didelphys), paired uteri and one cervix (bicornuate uterus), or a uterine septum (septate uterus) (45). Affected patients may be asymptomatic or may present with infertility, repeated abortions, breech delivery, preterm delivery, dyspareunia, or dysmenorrhea. Because the Wolffian ducts are essential for inducing the Müllerian ducts, defects in Wolffian duct development may likewise lead to uterine abnormalities. Isolated abnormalities of the Fallopian tubes (duplication or absence) are rare. Abnormalities of the cervix are also very rare and include atresia or hypoplasia, which is due to failure of canalization of the Müllerian ducts. The molecular events regulating the later events of Müllerian development including lateral fusion remain largely unknown.

Absence of the vagina occurs in 1 in 4,000 to 5,000 women and is often associated with Müllerian anomalies. In the Mayer-Rokitansky-Kuster-Hauser sequence, there is an absent vagina and often poorly formed uterus and Fallopian tubes (37,45,48). These patients are genotypic (46,XX) and phenotypic (normal external genitalia) females with normal endocrine status and they often present with amenorrhea. Some cases are associated with upper urinary tract abnormalities and/or spine and skeletal abnormalities. MURCS (MUllerian, Renal, Cervical, Somite) association appears to be an extreme presentation of these clustered anomalies (OMIM 601076) (48). It has been suggested that this sequence may be due to abnormal development of the Wolffian duct, with resulting abnormal Müllerian duct development. It has also been proposed that the etiology is related to abnormal HOXA gene expression during Müllerian development; however, despite numerous studies looking for mutations in the HOXA gene cluster none have been found to date in patients with Mayer-Rokitansky-Kuster-Hauser sequence. The Mayer-Rokitansky-Kuster-Hauser sequence usually occurs in a sporadic manner, and therefore aberrant HOXA gene expression may be related to temporally altered gene expression levels by exogenous factors. Other anomalies of the vagina result from developmental defects involving the cloaca or urogenital sinus. As previously discussed, the lower third of the vagina and the hymen are thought to be derived from ectoderm. If the urogenital sinus develops normally, the vagina can be present as a blind pouch even in the absence of normal Müllerian duct development. A variety of miscommunications between the urethra, rectum, and vagina have been described (42). Vaginal obstruction can result from absence of communication between the introitus and the vaginal canal, related to defects in vertical fusion. Etiologies include imperforate hymen, atresia of the lower vagina, or a transverse vaginal septum (failure of vertical canalization of the vaginal plate at the site of fusion between the urogenital sinus and the Müllerian ducts). Imperforate hymen, formed where the urogenital sinus and canalized, fused sinuvaginal bulbs meet, is the most common cause, and if there is complete obstruction this leads to a marked dilatation of the vagina and the uterus (hydrometrocolpos—retention of secreted mucous). If the person is asymptomatic until the onset of menses, the obstruction can result in hematocolpos.

The External Genitalia

Abnormalities in the development of the perineum, labia, and clitoris are not uncommon. The normal variations and structural abnormalities of the vulva have been extensively reviewed (141). Complete absence of the external genitalia is rare and occurs as part of malformation syndromes such as sirenomelia, limb-body wall defects, Robinow syndrome, multiple pterygia syndrome, Fryns syndrome, or CHARGE association. Vulvar duplication is rare and is associated with multiple congenital anomalies. Abnormalities of the clitoris and labia may cause problems in assigning the correct sex at birth. Clitoral hypertrophy may resemble male hypospadias. Exposure of the female fetus to excess male hormones, such as in congenital adrenal hyperplasia (reviewed in ref. 90), a maternal or fetal virilizing tumor, or maternal medication, can result in clitoral hypertrophy and may result in partial fusion of the posterior portion of the labia. Complete absence of the clitoris is rare. Many of the molecular events involved in early genital tubercle (anlage for the penis and clitoris) development, especially related to penile development, have recently been reviewed (165).

DISORDERS OF SEX DEVELOPMENT (INTERSEX DISORDERS)

Intersex disorders are characterized by congenital conditions associated with abnormal development of the gonads or secondary sex organs, or both, either with normal or abnormal sex chromosomes (Table 18-1) (44,63,78). In patients with normal sex chromosomes, these disorders are primarily associated with excess androgens in women and abnormal androgen or MIS action in males. Patients with abnormal sex chromosomes are divided into those with and without sexual ambiguity. These disorders are often associated with reproductive failure, and certain groups are at increased risk for the development of gonadal neoplasms. Classification schemes have been delineated based primarily on phenotype and genotype, including pseudohermaphroditism, mixed gonadal dysgenesis, true hermaphroditism, and pure gonadal dysgenesis. However, it is important to note that many of these conditions reflect a spectrum of phenotypic changes within a single genotype, or a spectrum of genotypic changes within a single phenotype. Therefore, disorders of sexual development are discussed by underlying etiology, when known. A new consensus statement regarding intersex disorders, now referred to as DSD, was recently published (78). This includes numerous changes in nomenclature provided in Table 18-1.

Female Pseudohermaphroditism (46,XX DSD)

Female pseudohermaphroditism results from excessive androgen exposure in 46,XX females with two ovaries and normal Müllerian duct development. The process is characterized by a spectrum of virilization of the external genitalia varying from clitoral enlargement, if androgen exposure begins after the 12th week of fetal life, to complete masculinization of the external genitalia if the process begins very early in fetal life. The source of androgen excess is most commonly related to enzymatic defects in the biosynthetic pathways of steroid hormone production from cholesterol. Glucocorticoids, mineralocorticoids, and sex hormones are synthesized through common intermediates; therefore, a defect in one enzyme can lead to overproduction of other products (90,93).

Table 18-1 ■ CLASSIFICATION OF DSD

I. Normal sex chromosomes
- A. Female pseudohermaphroditism (excess androgens in females)—**(46,XX DSD)**
  1. Adrenogenital syndrome (21-hydroxylase deficiency, 11-β-hydroxylase deficiency)
  2. Maternal ingestion of androgenic hormones
  3. Maternal virilization
- B. Male pseudohermaphroditism (deficient androgens in males)—**(46,XY DSD)**
  1. Testicular regression syndrome
  2. Gonadotropin-Leydig cell defects
  3. Steroid enzyme deficiencies (testosterone/dihydrotestosterone)
  4. Androgen insensitivity syndromes
  5. Persistent Müllerian duct syndrome

II. Abnormal sex chromosomes
- A. Sexual ambiguity frequently present
  1. Mixed gonadal dysgenesis—**(45,X/46,XY MGD)**
  2. True hermaphroditism—**(ovotesticular DSD)**
- B. Sexual ambiguity infrequently present
  1. Pure gonadal dysgenesis—**(46,XY complete gonadal dysgenesis)**
  2. Klinefelter syndrome—**(47,XXY)**
  3. Turner syndrome—**(45,X)**
  4. XX male syndrome—**(46,XX testicular DSD)**

Shown in **bold** is the new nomenclature.
From Lee PA, Houk CP, Ahmed SF, et al. Consensus statement on management of intersex disorders. International Consensus Conference on Intersex. *Pediatrics* 2006;118:e488–e500.

Adrenogenital syndrome (congenital adrenal hyperplasia) is the most common cause of female pseudohermaphroditism and is most commonly an autosomal recessive disorder. 21-Hydroxylase deficiency (OMIM 201910) accounts for more than 90% of cases of congenital adrenal hyperplasia and occurs in about 1:50,000 births. Lack of 21-hydroxylase prevents conversion of progesterone to 11-deoxycorticosterone and 17-hydroxyprogesterone to 11-deoxycortisol, thereby resulting in deficiencies of cortisol and aldosterone, which can be life threatening in the neonatal period. As a result, adrenocorticotropic hormone levels are high and the biosynthetic intermediates shift the equilibrium reaction toward overproduction of androgenic sex steroids, in particular testosterone. Estrogen levels do not increase because conversion of testosterone to estrogen is dependent on the presence of aromatase that is only found in specific target organs. The degree of virilization varies depending on the severity of the enzymatic defect and the timing of the onset of the endocrine effects. Another enzyme deficiency in this pathway leading to a similar phenotype involves 11-β-hydroxylase (OMIM 202010). Some girls with congenital adrenal hyperplasia can present late with delayed menarche, oligomenorrhea, hirsutism, and polycystic ovaries (90).

Other causes for female pseudohermaphroditism include maternal ingestion of synthetic androgens or progestins during pregnancy or the presence of a maternal virilizing tumor such as a primary or metastatic ovarian tumor and the luteoma of pregnancy, a hyperplastic lesion of the theca-lutein or stroma-lutein cells. The degree of masculinization in the latter is usually mild, suggesting that the luteoma does not become functional until the second half of gestation. The fetal gonads and Müllerian duct structures are unaffected, and normal secondary female sex characteristics, ovulation, and menstruation develop at puberty.

Disorders of Sex Development Associated with Abnormal Sex Chromosomes

Abnormalities in the sex chromosomes include deletions, additions, and mosaicisms, all of which can result in a wide variety of effects on gonadal development and thereby phenotypic expression. The gonads in these patients can range from a streak gonad to a relatively normal ovary or testis (11). As a result, sexual ambiguity may or may not be present. Interestingly, within a single genotypic abnormality and genetic background, the phenotype may vary widely, likely due to small differences in genetic expression within the very restricted time periods characterized by many of the steps of gonadal differentiation (11).

Mixed gonadal dysgenesis (45,X/46,XY MGD; OMIM 233420) refers to patients with at least one testis, persistent Müllerian duct structures, and incomplete development of Wolffian duct structures. The external genitalia are usually ambiguous with abnormalities of the labioscrotal swellings. The disorder is heterogeneous, with the most frequent karyotypes being 45,X/46,XY or 46,XY. Many 45,X/46,XY

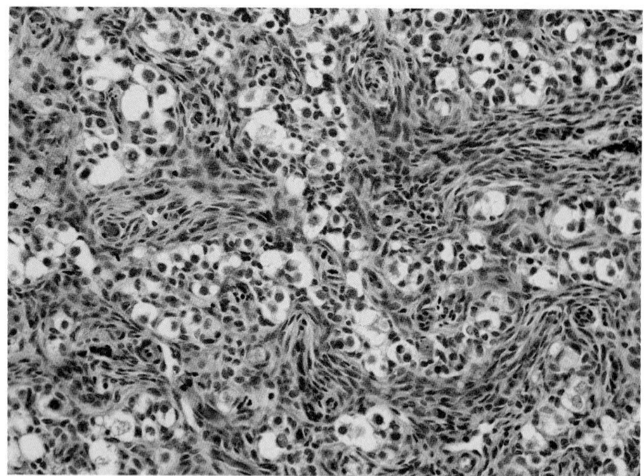

FIGURE 18-6 ■ Dysgenetic gonad removed from a 3-year-old child with ambiguous genitalia. Ovarian-like stroma is intermixed with abnormally developed sex-cord like structures containing primitive germ cells.

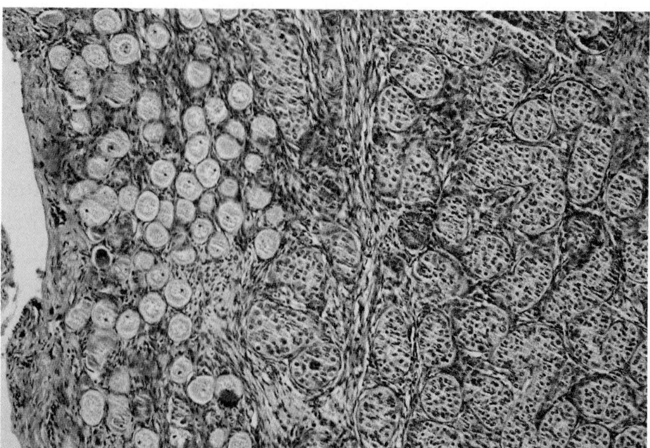

FIGURE 18-7 ■ Ovotestis removed from a 6-year-old child with ambiguous genitalia and an undescended left testicle. Peripheral lymphocyte karyotype 46,XY. The gonad demonstrates two distinct regions: the area on the right composed of ovarian stroma and numerous primordial follicles, and the area on the left lower corner shows normally developed seminiferous tubules with reduced numbers of germ cells.

individuals are phenotypically normal males, and only a small percentage present with mixed gonadal dysgenesis (121). About two-third of patients with mixed gonadal dysgenesis are raised as females. The gonads may have a wide variety of appearances depending upon the chromosomal complement present. They often demonstrate a disorganized arrangement of testicular and ovarian elements that do not resemble either gonadal type (Figure 18-6).

True hermaphrodites (ovotesticular DSD; OMIM 235600) are quite rare and contain both fully developed ovarian and testicular tissues either separately or combined as an ovotestis. The external phenotype can be either male or female, but usually the genitalia are ambiguous. Phenotypic men usually have incomplete virilization, gynecomastia, and monthly hematuria secondary to menstruation into a persistent urogenital sinus. The most common karyotypes include 46,XX (50% to 70%), 46,XY or mosaic 46,XX/46,XY, 46,XY/47,XXY, 45,X/46,XY (78,93). The testis is usually in the scrotum or labia, and the ovary is always abdominal. The ovotestis can be anywhere along the descent pathway but is most commonly abdominal. The ovotestis is frequently arranged with the ovarian and testicular tissues immediately adjacent to each other, usually with a sharp demarcation (155) (Figure 18-7). By reproductive age, the ovarian portion of an ovotestis usually appears to be normal, complete with follicles, corpora lutea, and corpora albicans. The testicular portion, however, is usually abnormal, with loss of germ cells and tubular sclerosis. The type of ductal organ that develops adjacent to a gonad often depends on the type of gonad present at that site. In true hermaphrodites, an epididymis or a vas deferens is next to a testes and a Fallopian tube is adjacent to an ovary. A Müllerian or a Wolffian structure develops adjacent to an ovotestis but not both. A variety of uterine anomalies can be present, although most true hermaphrodites with a uterus menstruate. The underlying defect leading to true hermaphroditism is not yet completely established.

Pure or complete gonadal dysgenesis or XY sex reversal (46,XY complete gonadal dysgenesis) includes a number of conditions and is characterized by phenotypic females with Müllerian ductal structures (uterus and Fallopian tubes) and streak gonads. The most common karyotype is 46,XY (Swyer syndrome; OMIM 306100), and the defect is due to an X-linked recessive mutation or deletion of the SRY gene on the short arm of the Y chromosome (35,97,104). Patients with Swyer syndrome have a female phenotype with a uterus and Fallopian tubes, but the karyotype is 46,XY and two dysgenetic gonads in the abdomen. In the rare patients with 46,XX gonadal dysgenesis or XX sex reversal (46,XX testicular DSD; OMIM 278850), the disorder is usually an autosomal recessive one, with or without an abnormality of the X chromosome (72,132). An autosomal dominant form also exists (OMIM 154230). The gonad is that of a streak, with ovarian-like stroma and no oocytes. Other genetic defects leading to 46,XX testicular DSD include a translocation of the SRY gene (OMIM 480000) or a duplication of SOX9 gene (OMIM 608160) that can both result in a male phenotype (78).

Turner syndrome occurs in about 1 in 3,000 live female births and is most commonly due to mosaic or nonmosaic 45,X karyotype. It is estimated that the vast majority of fetuses with nonmosaic 45,X karyotype spontaneously abort. Common features of this syndrome include phenotypic females with short stature, webbing of the neck (cystic hygroma *in utero*), congenital lymphedema of the hands and feet, preductal coarctation of the aorta, ventricular septal defects, micrognathia, renal anomalies (horseshoe kidney, hydronephrosis secondary to ureteropelvic obstruction), congenital nevi, short fourth metacarpal, and streak gonads (by adulthood) (47). Not all of these features appear in every patient, and other occasional anomalies have also been described. Most recently, haploinsufficiency for the short stature homeobox gene (SHOX), located on the X and Y chromosomes, has been proposed to account for some of the phenotypic findings in Turner syndrome patients (reviewed in ref. 47). The fetal ovary in a patient with Turner syndrome is normal histologically until about 16 to 18 weeks' gestation. Following entry into meiosis, however, without the second X chromosome the germ cells disappear, resulting in a streak ovary by adulthood. These patients have primary amenorrhea by adolescence. The internal genitalia are normal female. Germ cell tumors in pure Turner syndrome are very rare due to the absence of germ cells and the absence of the Y chromosome. Epithelial ovarian tumors can arise in these ovaries but at a rate no greater than that in normal females.

Tumors Associated with Gonadal Dysgenesis

Patients with dysgenetic gonads are at risk for the development of ovarian neoplasms. More than 50% of these neoplasms are gonadoblastomas, which are benign tumors, found only in patients with Y chromosomal material and dysgenetic gonads (Figure 18-8) (131). The frequency of occurrence of gonadoblastoma in the abovementioned clinical populations correlates with the frequency of the Y chromosome; gonadoblastoma is seen in approximately 30% of patients with mixed gonadal dysgenesis, less than 3% of individuals with true hermaphroditism, and over 50% of patients with 46,XY pure gonadal dysgenesis (23). Patients with 46,XX pure gonadal dysgenesis and patients with Turner syndrome only very rarely develop gonadal tumors; however, hilus cell hyperplasia and hilus cell tumors have been reported (132). The significance of the development of gonadoblastoma is that it is associated with a very high frequency of concurrent or future development of a malignant germ cell tumor, most commonly dysgerminoma (146). The risk of developing a germ cell malignancy with various forms of DSD has recently been summarized (23,39) and the groups with the highest risks include patients with gonadal dysgenesis (+Y), partial androgen insensitivity syndrome (nonscrotal gonad), Frasier syndrome or Denys-Drash syndrome (those with +Y). Dysgerminoma has been discovered as early as 6 months of age (146), and patients as old as 60 years of age have been seen by the authors. Because of the high incidence of gonadoblastoma in women with XY gonadal dysgenesis, a susceptibility locus on the Y chromosome has been proposed, located on the proximal long arm (23,126,147). The pathology of gonadoblastoma is described later.

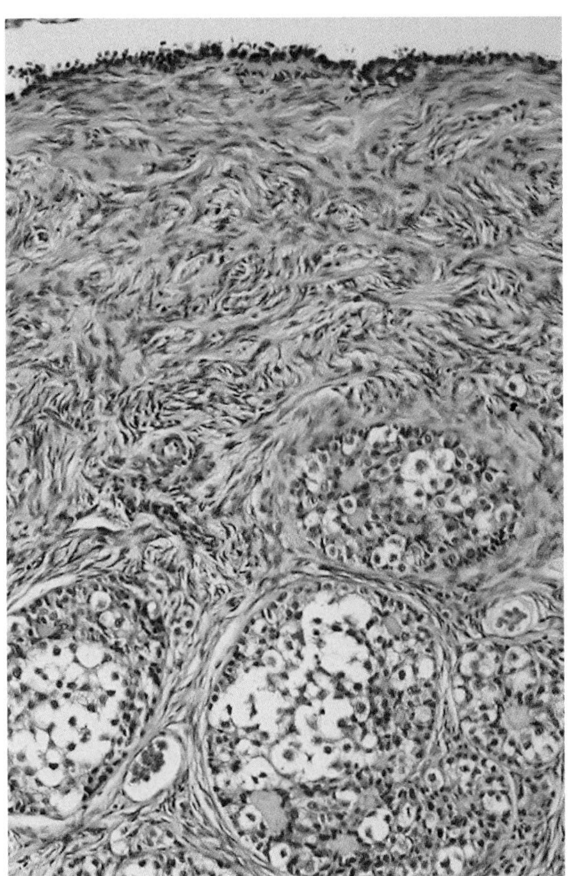

FIGURE 18-8 ▪ Small, streak gonad from a 46,XY phenotypic female that is composed of wavy ovarian-type stroma and no primordial follicles. Deep within the cortex, well-defined nests composed of a mixture of germ cells and granulose-like cells, consistent with gonadoblastoma.

ACQUIRED ABNORMALITIES AND OTHER LESIONS

Infections

Infections of the lower genitourinary tract account for the majority of genital lesions in premenarchal girls. These infections are most commonly due to a variety of bacterial organisms that do not penetrate the mucosa and are not related to a specific disease. Infections common in the sexually active, such as Gardnerella vaginalis and molluscum contagiosum, are quite rare in young children and should raise the suspicion of sexual abuse (Chapter 7). Specific infections of the vulvovagina include human papillomavirus (HPV), herpes simplex virus, syphilis, and molluscum contagiosum.

***Human Papillomaviruses*:** Condyloma acuminata are sexually transmitted lesions caused by papilloma viridae, most commonly the HPV types 6 or 11, although HPV 2 may also be seen (49). These lesions may involve the vulva, vagina, cervix, urethra, and perianal skin. Vulvar and vaginal lesions are commonly papillary and are almost always multiple; cervical lesions are often flat, white lesions surrounded by hyperemic mucosa. Uncommonly, the involved epithelium may extend into the endocervical glands and, therefore, have an endophytic appearance. Most lesions are asymptomatic unless secondarily infected. Histologically, parakeratosis, acanthosis, hyperkeratosis, and dyskeratosis are evident (Figure 18-9). The typical koilocytic cells with perinuclear cytoplasmic halos surrounding irregularly contoured ("raisinoid") nuclei may be seen in the more superficial or intermediate layers. Although intranuclear and cytoplasmic inclusions are not found by light microscopy, electron microscopy has

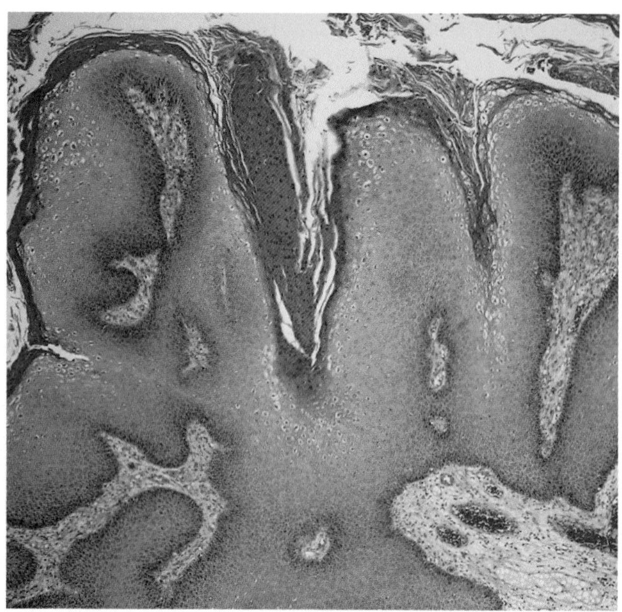

FIGURE 18-9 Condyloma acuminatum showing parakeratosis, ancanthosis, and numerous koilocytic cells with nuclear irregularity and prominent perinuclear vacuolization. No dysplasia is present.

shown intranuclear viral particles. Condyloma acuminata are commonly associated with pregnancy, and may result in laryngeal papillomas of infants exposed during delivery. Regression may occur after pregnancy; however, the clinical course may be quite protracted without treatment. In rare cases, progression to carcinoma *in situ*, verrucous carcinoma, and squamous carcinoma of the vulva may occur. Condyloma acuminata may at times be difficult to distinguish from vulvar intraepithelial neoplasia. The presence of a flat, macular growth pattern, abnormal mitoses, atypical nuclei, marked variation in nuclear size and shape, and hyperchromasia are all characteristics of vulvar intraepithelial neoplasia. The modes of transmission of HPV include perinatal, autoinoculation, heteroinoculation, and sexual abuse (49,94). Cervical infections with HPV types 16, 18, 31, 33, 35, and 45 are associated with the development of intraepithelial neoplasia (7). Only a small number of sexually active teenagers have dysplastic cells on cervicovaginal cytologies requiring colposcopically directed cervical biopsies. Invasive cervical carcinoma has rarely been reported in teenagers (65). The FDA approved an HPV vaccine in June 2006 for women aged 9 to 26 years that is effective against several high-risk subtypes of HPV (123). Despite clear evidence of effectiveness in reducing infection by high-risk HPV, the proposed mandatory use of this vaccine in young girls (prior to the beginning of sexual activity) has raised an ethical debate.

***Herpes*:** Patients with genital infection with herpes simplex virus types I or II present with dysuria and vulvar pain, often accompanied by generalized malaise and fever. The clinical picture is dominated by the appearance of vesicles and shallow ulcers that are often secondarily infected. Only two thirds of culture-positive women show diagnostic genital lesions. Histologically, the ulcers typically demonstrate extension deep into the epidermis, with the characteristic intranuclear inclusions present at the periphery of the lesion. Late in the evolution of the ulcer, the infected cells undergo karyorrhexis and lysis, and therefore, infected cells may not be identifiable in biopsy material. Cytologic evaluation of scrapings from a fresh ulcer or freshly opened vesicle will usually show the characteristic viral cytopathic effects. Recurrent episodes of herpetic vulvitis are common; however, these episodes decrease in frequency over time whether or not acyclovir is given. Anogenital herpes in children raises the concern of sexual abuse, but is not definitive evidence (61). Varicella infection of the lower genital tract is rare and most commonly detected in postmenopausal women.

***Syphilis*:** The primary lesion of syphilis is the chancre, a painless, shallow ulcer with raised edges that usually presents within 10 to 90 days of initial contact. These lesions often occur on inconspicuous surfaces, such as the cervix, and in about 50% of patients, the primary lesion is never seen (60). Histologically, the chancre is characterized by ulceration of the epidermis with acute and chronic inflammation within the dermis. There is a marked perivascular inflammatory response with a large number of plasma cells. The lack of specificity of these findings raises the importance of considering syphilis in the differential diagnosis of inflammatory lesions. Lymphadenopathy may develop 3 to 4 days after the chancre appears. If the primary stage is left untreated, the secondary stage of the disease will become evident within 6 weeks to 6 months when the patient will show elevated plaques measuring up to 3 cm, especially on the vulva. These plaques are known as *condylomata lata* and demonstrate marked acanthosis, epithelial hyperplasia, and hyperkeratosis. The inflammatory response within the dermis is similar to that seen in the chancre. Both the chancre and the condyloma lata are rich in spirochetes, which may be detected by the Dieterle or Warthin-Starry silver stains. However, these stains may be negative even with active infection. Serologic studies should be performed if syphilis is considered clinically or pathologically; even these studies may be negative for weeks after the presentation of the primary chancre. Other methods used for detecting spirochetes include dark field examination of serum expressed from the base of the ulcer or by a fluorescent-conjugated antibody technique. These methods are more sensitive and specific than the silver stain on paraffin-embedded tissue (60).

***Molluscum Contagiosum*:** Molluscum contagiosum is usually an asymptomatic infection caused by a moderately contagious virus often passed through sexual contact. The lesions are generally multiple, small, smooth 3- to 6-mm papules with a central umbilication. Diagnosis rarely requires biopsy. Cytologic identification of the typical intracytoplasmic inclusion bodies (molluscum bodies) within scrapings or in biopsy material is adequate to confirm the diagnosis (Figure 18-10).

***Chlamydia Trachomatis*:** The most common sexually transmitted disease in adolescent girls is Chlamydia trachomatis (119). Approximately 22% of urban adolescent girls

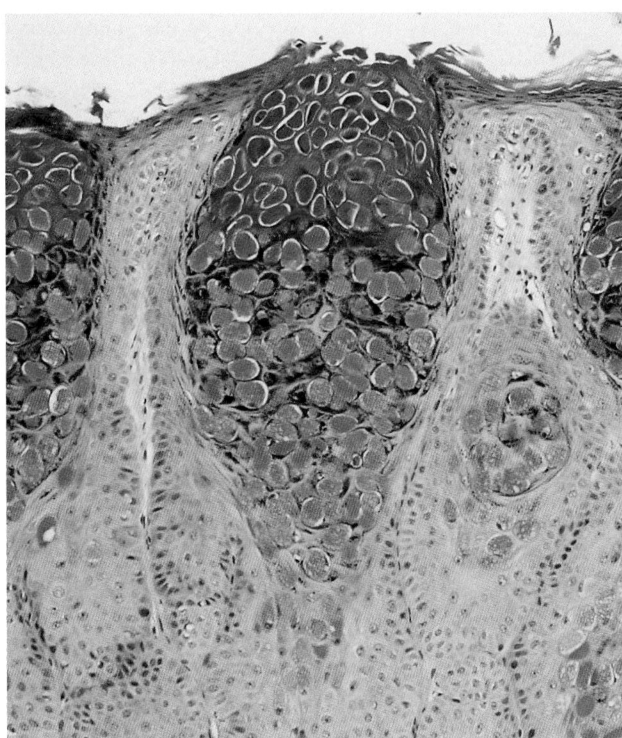

FIGURE 18-10 ■ Molluscum contagiosum with numerous epidermal cells containing large intracytoplasmic inclusion bodies, the so-called molluscum bodies, which are typically found in the lower cells of the stratum malpighii. The molluscum body compresses the nucleus, which appears as a thin crescent at the periphery of the cell.

have endocervical cultures positive for this organism, and the majority are asymptomatic (10). The organism most commonly infects the columnar and immature squamous cells of the endocervix; however, salpingitis and endometritis may be seen, which often leads to infertility (10). Cell culture is the optimum diagnostic test and has an accuracy rate of about 90%. Infected patients show lymphocytic inflammation and reactive epithelial changes by cytology. Some observers have reported cytoplasmic inclusion bodies in infected cells; however, others interpret these bodies as nonspecific cytoplasmic vacuoles. Therefore, the finding of lymphocytes, reactive epithelial cells, often dyskeratotic cells, and vacuolization of metaplastic cells should be considered suggestive but not diagnostic for chlamydial infection. Chlamydial infection of the vulva or vagina may result in lymphogranuloma venereum, a skin lesion characterized first by painless skin erosion, followed by lymphadenitis involving superficial groin lymph nodes, which may ulcerate and rupture. Over time, the chronic inflammatory process and chronic lymphatic obstruction may result in stricture, fibrosis, and nonpitting edema of the vagina and rectum.

Miscellaneous Infectious Diseases

Cytomegalovirus, Epstein-Barr virus, Candida, and other fungal and bacterial infections may cause acute or chronic inflammatory lesions of the lower genital tract, most commonly without ulceration. Chancroid is a rare genital ulcer caused by *Haemophilus ducreyi*, which is identified by culture alone. Histologically, chancroid shows a granulomatous inflammation with Gram-negative organisms. Tuberculosis of the vulva is rare and is usually associated with the disease at other sites. Sexual transmission is most uncommon in the absence of immunosuppression. Enterobius vermicularis (pinworm) may cause a severe vulvovaginal pruritus in infected children. Granuloma inguinale is caused by *Calymmatobacterium granulomatous*, a Gram-negative encapsulated rod. Primary lesions may present anywhere in the lower genitourinary tract as painless papules or necrotizing ulcers. The diagnosis depends on the identification of large, vacuolated histiocytes containing the characteristic cytoplasmic encapsulated bacilli called *Donovan bodies*, demonstrated by Warthin-Starry or Giemsa stains.

Noninfectious Inflammatory Diseases

***Behçet Syndrome*:** Behçet syndrome is characterized by the triad of recurrent oral ulcers, vulvar ulcers, and various ophthalmologic inflammations (OMIM 109650). Acne, cutaneous nodules, thrombophlebitis, encephalopathy, and colitis may also be present. The vulvar ulcers, seen in postmenarchal females, may be deep and characteristically relapse. Histologic examination reveals chronic inflammation and necrotizing vasculitis, which is considered a cardinal finding. Vascular endothelial cell swelling may result in arteriolar occlusions and venous thrombosis. Behçet disease is presumed to be autoimmune in etiology (125). Healing of the ulcers may result in severe scarring. Childhood Behçet may run a less severe course (71).

***Crohn Disease*:** Vulvar involvement by Crohn disease is rare and characterized by ulcerations that are often multiple, deep, and secondarily infected. The diagnosis may be difficult, particularly if this is the presenting site of the disease (130). Histology demonstrates noncaseating granulomatous inflammation with extensive granulation tissue within the dermis (Chapter 14).

***Lichen Sclerosus*:** Lichen sclerosus is a dermatosis of unknown etiology characterized pathologically by thinning of the epithelial layer, blunting or loss of the rete ridges, and a homogeneously collagenized or edematous subepithelial layer in the dermis with a band of chronic inflammatory cells beneath (Chapter 25). There is an absence of melanosomes and disappearance of the melanocytes, resulting in a hypopigmented patch that may be pruritic. The microscopic findings may vary considerably, depending on the age of the lesions, excoriation, and treatment. Lichen sclerosus is not limited to the elderly population and may be seen in the reproductive years, and has been reported in children as young as 18 months of age (OMIM 151590) (111). In children, symptoms include dysuria, painful defecation, and rectal bleeding (12). This may lead to anal fissures and genital and perianal ulcers, which may be confused with sexual abuse. Although lichen sclerosus is sometimes associated with vulvar squamous carcinoma, it is not considered to be a premalignant condition.

***Bullous Diseases (See Chapter 25)*:** The vulva may be involved with virtually any dermatologic disease; however, some of the bullous diseases may have their first manifestations in the vulva and in childhood. Darier-White disease (keratosis follicularis) is an autosomal dominant skin disorder that frequently involves the vulva (OMIM 124200). Patients present anytime after late childhood with crusted, hyperkeratotic papules that often appear darker than the surrounding skin. Histologically, these papules show acantholysis of the suprabasal epithelial cells resulting in clefts that extend from the basal layer through the granular layer. Corps ronds, nuclear grains, and dyskeratotic cells can be found in the granular layer. Hyperkeratosis, acanthosis, and papillomatosis are seen, along with keratotic plugs. Inflammation is minimal unless the lesions are secondarily infected. The affected gene is ATP2A2, which encodes a sarco/endoplasmic reticulum Ca^{2+}-ATPase. Hailey-Hailey disease (familial benign pemphigus or benign chronic pemphigus) is an autosomal dominant disease that may also be sporadic (OMIM 169600). Onset often occurs during adolescence, and several cases confined exclusively to the vulva have been reported. The lesions are characterized by clusters of acantholytic vesicles resulting in suprabasalar lacunae. Unlike Darier disease, vesicles and bullae are found. Acantholysis is more prominent than in Darier disease, and the basal cells maintain their orientation to the basement membrane. Minimal dyskeratosis is seen. Mutations in the ATP2C1 gene have been identified in several kindreds. ATP2C1 encodes a human homolog of an ATP pump in yeast that accumulates calcium into the Golgi. Benign chronic bullous disease of childhood (linear IgA bullous dermatosis) commonly involves the genital region of children. It presents as clusters of annular pruritic lesions that evolve into tense bullae, which may then ulcerate. Patients may have fever and anorexia, and a preceding infection is identified in 50% the cases. These lesions may be mistaken for evidence of child abuse. Biopsy reveals subepithelial vesicles that may contain granulocytes and eosinophils, and epidermal microabscesses may occur. The diagnosis depends on the identification of linear deposition of IgA in the basement membrane, which may react against the bullous pemphigoid antigens 180 or 230, members of the dermoepidermal adhesion complex (158). The differential diagnosis includes dermatitis herpetiformis (which shows granular IgA deposition) and bullous pemphigoid (which shows linear IgG basement membrane deposits to the above BP180, BP230 antigens) (40,158).

Vulvar involvement may be seen in Stevens-Johnson syndrome, the severe form of erythema multiforme. This disease may be associated with herpes virus or mycoplasma infection, drug therapy, malignancy, or radiotherapy and is characterized by involvement of the mouth, eyes, and skin with associated fever and other systemic symptoms. The histologic features include necrotic keratinocytes, cellular edema, and intraepithelial vesicles. The dermis shows a prominent chronic inflammatory infiltrate with extravasated red blood cells. Recent reports suggest that activation of Fas on keratinocytes by FasL secreted by peripheral blood mononuclear cells represents the initial step leading to diffuse apoptotic cell death of epidermal cells (1).

TUMORS OF THE FEMALE GENITAL TRACT

Benign Cystic Lesions

***Bartholin Cyst*:** Bartholin glands produce a clear mucoid secretion that continually lubricates the vestibular surface. The ducts of Bartholin glands are prone to obstruction, resulting in cystic dilatation of the duct and secondary infection. The epithelium lining the cyst may be squamous, transitional, or low cuboidal mucinous, and is immunoreactive for carcinoembryonic antigen.

***Mucous Cysts*:** Vulvar mucous cysts are lined by tall-to-cuboidal Alcian blue positive mucous-secreting epithelium. Squamous metaplasia may be present. Mucous cysts likely arise from the urogenital sinus epithelium, and they lack both myoepithelial cells and muscle fibers.

***Gartner Duct Cysts*:** Commonly seen are remnants of the mesonephric duct within the lateral wall of the vagina known as *Gartner duct cysts*. They are thin-walled cysts lined by low cuboidal epithelium that may or may not be ciliated. Smooth muscle may be present in the submucosal region.

***Cysts of the Canal of Nuck (Peritoneal Lined Cysts)*:** These cysts are found in the superior aspect of the labia majora or inguinal canal and are believed to arise from inclusions of the peritoneum at the inferior insertion of the round ligament into the labia majora, analogous to the hydrocele of the spermatic cord. They may get quite large and must be distinguished from an inguinal hernia.

***Müllerian Cyst*:** Of uncertain genesis, Müllerian cysts can be located anywhere within the vagina and are lined by any of the epithelia of the Müllerian duct, including mucinous, endocervical, endometrial, and ciliated tubal types. Squamous metaplasia may also be observed. The majority of vaginal cysts represent Müllerian remnant cysts or epidermal inclusion cysts (37).

Benign Solid Tumors

***Hidradenoma Papilliferum*:** Papillary hidradenoma is a benign tumor of apocrine sweat gland origin that presents as an asymptomatic small mass in the labia majora or the lateral labia minora. This tumor has not been described before puberty and almost all cases have occurred in white women (8,157). Histologically, the papillary hidradenoma is composed of tubules and acini lined by cuboidal epithelial cells with an outer layer of myoepithelial cells. These cells may simulate a well-differentiated adenocarcinoma, and entrapped epithelial cells may create a pseudoinfiltrative appearance. Mitotic figures are rare, and only mild nuclear pleomorphism is present (153). Therapy requires only local excision.

***Müllerian or Mesonephric Papilloma*:** Several tumors that are composed of complex, arborizing papillae with a fibrovascular core supporting bland-appearing epithelial cells (92) have been reported within the vagina of young girls. In some areas, the tumor may appear as either a solid mass or may contain glandular lumina and eosinophilic hyaline globules. Their embryologic origin remains uncertain (139).

Fibroepithelial Polyp (Mesodermal Stromal Polyp): Fibroepithelial polyps are uncommon hamartomatous polypoid masses of the vagina that are of interest to pathologists because of their inclination to show bizarre stromal cells that may be confused with embryonal rhabdomyosarcoma (100,114). The age at presentation ranges from 16 to 75 years and while the majority of the lesions arise in the vagina, they may be found in the cervix and the vulva (100). The lesions are usually asymptomatic and discovered incidentally. They resemble an acrochordon and microscopically show a stratified squamous epithelium covering an edematous stroma with variable numbers of fibroblasts. The lesions often demonstrate marked hypercellularity, pleomorphism, mitotic counts of more than ten mitoses per ten high-power fields, and atypical mitoses. The immunolocalization of steroid receptors in these bizarre cells and the frequent relationship to pregnancy raise the possibility that these may be hormonally induced.

Miscellaneous Lesions: As with virtually all other soft tissue neoplasms, capillary and cavernous hemangiomas and lymphangiomas may occur in the lower female genitourinary tract and are similar to those in other anatomic sites. These lesions should be distinguished from entities such as Kaposi sarcoma (which may have a hemangioma-like appearance) and bacillary angiomatosis. Angiokeratomas are variants of hemangiomas that occur almost exclusively in the scrotum and the vulva. Histologically, the dilated vascular channels are separated by strands of squamous epithelial cells growing down from the overlying epithelium. This may be accompanied by various degrees of acanthosis and papillomatosis. Neurofibromas, leiomyomas, granular cell tumors, hemangiopericytomas, inflammatory pseudotumors, Langerhan cell histiocytosis, and alveolar soft part sarcoma have likewise been described.

MALIGNANCIES OF THE LOWER GENITAL TRACT

Malignancies of the lower female genital tract are rare, with an incidence of about 0.5 cases per million female children per year (74). The majority of these malignancies (more than 80%) are sarcomas, most commonly rhabdomyosarcoma; approximately 10% are carcinomas and 5% extragonadal germ cell tumors. These malignancies are discussed below in greater detail.

Rhabdomyosarcoma

Embryonal rhabdomyosarcoma is the most common malignancy of the lower genital tract in girls. Although these lesions may arise in the vulva and the uterus, by far the most common genital site is the vagina. Most patients present before the age of 5 years, with a peak incidence between 1 and 2 years (24,54,79). Patients often present with vaginal bleeding or discharge, a palpable abdominal mass, or gross protrusion of a polypoid mass at the introitus. The site of origin is often the anterior vaginal wall, with extension into the bladder and the rectum. The initial size of the tumor has little prognostic significance (see Chapters 17 and 24).

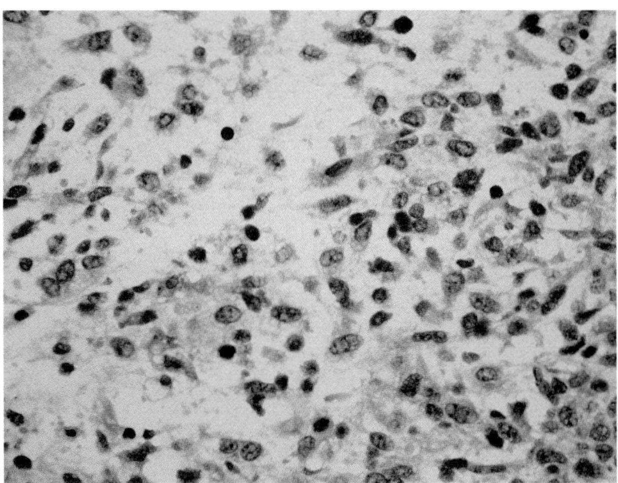

FIGURE 18-11 ▪ Embryonal rhabdomyosarcoma of the genitourinary tract may be deceptively hypocellular, with inapparent cytoplasm.

The most common histologic appearance of female genital rhabdomyosarcomas is that of the botryoid embryonal subtype, with round-to-spindled cells of varying size in a loose, myxoid stroma (Figure 18-11). Eosinophilic cytoplasm may or may not be apparent, and cytoplasmic cross-striations may occasionally be seen. The tumor cells often crowd around blood vessels, and a cambium layer may be present with condensation of tumor cells beneath the vaginal epithelium. The myxoid stroma may in some cases be rather hypocellular, resulting in a tumor mass that may resemble a benign polyp. Rhabdomyosarcomas of the cervix provide a greater diagnostic challenge histologically owing to the presence of islands of mature metaplastic cartilage in more than 40% of the cases (29). This histologic manifestation appears to be unique to cervical rhabdomyosarcomas for unknown reasons. An uncommon histologic pattern in the childhood genital tract is the diffuse form of embryonal rhabdomyosarcoma. The differential diagnosis of rhabdomyosarcoma in the female genital tract includes fibroepithelial polyps, Müllerian papillomas, and rhabdomyomas.

The clinical presentation and prognosis varies with the site of involvement. The majority of patients with vaginal rhabdomyosarcomas present before the age of 5, and the lesions are localized. These tumors are treated by chemotherapy, most commonly vincristine, dactinomycin, cyclophosphamide, and often adriamycin, followed by resection (88). Given this therapy, among 26 patients with localized vaginal tumors treated according to the Intergroup Rhabdomyosarcoma Study (IRS) protocols, six relapsed, five of whom were successfully salvaged; the remaining patients were cured (53). There is now a broad consensus that primary chemotherapy after an initial biopsy is the recommended therapeutic plan, followed

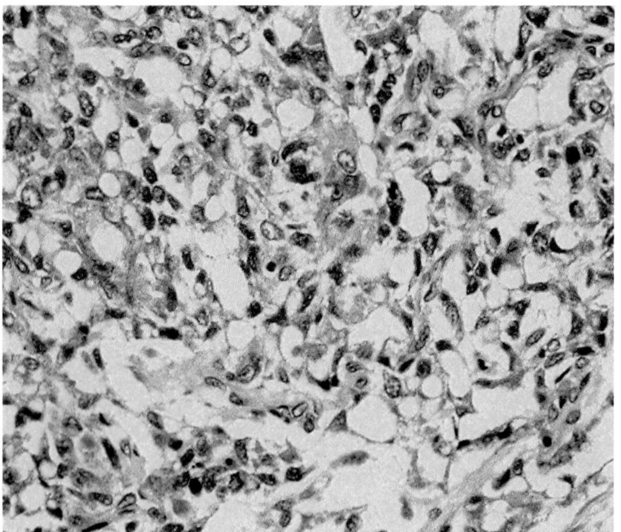

FIGURE 18-12 ■ EST of the vagina may demonstrate the entire histologic spectrum, similar to that seen in the ovary and testis. Many lack the characteristic Schiller-Duval bodies and other architectural features, such as the tumor illustrated. The histologic clues are the reticular pattern, the course chromatin, and the occasional cytoplasmic pink globules.

by local excision (2,86). Rhabdomyosarcomas of the uterus and cervix are rare and have been considered to be distinct from those of the vagina, with a mean age of presentation of greater than 14 years and a seemingly better prognosis (54). However, recent studies relying on more conservative management using preoperative chemotherapy and radiotherapy has resulted in increased survival (26,179).

Endodermal Sinus Tumor

The lower female genital tract is one of the more common sites for extragonadal, nonsacral endodermal sinus (yolk sac) tumor. This is presumably due to abnormal migration of primordial germ cells early in gestation; however, this does not explain the predilection for the vagina. These tumors present in children younger than 3 years of age, with the peak incidence between 8 and 11 months of age (25,172). Presenting symptoms usually include bloody vaginal discharge and a polypoid tumor filling the vagina. Microscopically, these tumors show the same histologic patterns as those seen in the sacral region, infantile testis, and ovary (Figure 18-12). Although reports before 1970 indicate an aggressive tumor with poor outcome, current chemotherapeutic regimens containing cyclophosphamide, vincristine, and actinomycin have resulted in a 95% disease-free survival (25). Several reports of children treated only with chemotherapy with complete response suggest that surgery may not always be required (76).

TUMORS OF THE OVARY

Benign Cystic Lesions of the Ovary

The most common ovarian lesions detected radiographically are cysts derived from follicles at different stages of maturation in prepubertal girls (32). Congenital ovarian cysts may be diagnosed *in utero* by ultrasound and are associated with resolution; however, their evolution is variable and may require intervention (120,176). Complications such as torsion and rupture usually occur in cysts larger than 5 cm in diameter. Cysts that develop *in utero* are most often lined by luteinized cells, whereas those in older children are more often lined by granulosa cells. Premature infants born before the 30th week of gestation may have multiple follicular cysts associated with estradiol production. These cysts are secondary to elevated follicle-stimulating hormone (FSH) and luteinizing hormone (LH) secretion, and they may be associated with relative insensitivity of the hypothalamus and anterior pituitary to negative feedback by estradiol (133).

Follicular cysts are commonly found in the ovaries of prepubertal females as an incidental finding. Rarely, multiple follicular cysts may be the cause of pseudoprecocious puberty (138), although more often they are the result of central causes of pseudoprecocity (110). As many as 75% of girls with juvenile hypothyroidism have multicystic ovaries, and, rarely, the ovarian enlargement may be the presenting sign leading to a diagnosis of hypothyroidism. Clinically, affected patients may show varying degrees of sexual precocity and galactorrhea due to increased secretion of pituitary gonadotropins and prolactin. Treatment with thyroxin results in regression of the ovarian cysts as well as the other symptoms (135).

Multiple follicular cysts should be distinguished from polycystic ovary syndrome (PCOS), which involves 3% to 8% of the female population. PCOS is responsible for 25% of cases of primary amenorrhea and is the most common cause of delayed puberty and heavy anovulatory bleeding in adolescent females (16). It is characterized by inappropriate gonadotropin secretion, hyperandrogenemia, increased peripheral conversion of androgens to estrogens, chronic anovulation, and sclerocystic ovaries. The diagnostic criteria for PCOS were established in 2004 by the Rotterdam criteria (145), although this has been heavily debated subsequently. Affected patients often have a history of premenarcheal obesity, secondary amenorrhea or oligomenorrhea, infertility, and hirsutism. These features may occur alone or in any combination and the clinical spectrum is broad (6). The unopposed estrogenic stimulation may cause menometrorrhagia and endometrial hyperplasia. Currently, the underlying etiology of PCOS is widely debated; however, the resulting clinical manifestations are known to be heavily impacted by environmental factors such as diet. While several genes have been linked with PCOS, the evidence supporting this linkage is weak (34). Grossly, the ovaries of PCOS are enlarged two- to fivefold and have smooth or nodular white surfaces, with multiple cysts located beneath the thickened cortex. Histologically, multiple follicle cysts, atretic follicles, a prominent theca interna with luteinization, and medullary stromal overgrowth are the principal histologic features. The superficial cortex is fibrotic and hypocellular (62). Maturing follicles up to midantral stage and atretic follicles showing prominent luteinization of the theca interna may be twice as numerous as in normal ovaries. Primordial follicles are often decreased in number (160). It is important to remember that these findings are not specific and may accompany adrenal lesions such as Cushing syndrome, congenital adrenal hyperplasia, virilizing adrenal tumors, primary hypothalamic disorders, ovarian lesions that produce excessive quantities of estrogens or androgens and hypothyroidism. Long-term sequelae of PCOS include infertility, endometrial carcinoma, an increased risk for cardiovascular disease due to type II diabetes mellitus, dyslipidemia, and systolic hypertension.

NON-NEOPLASTIC OVARIAN TUMORS

Endometriosis, or endometrioma, of the ovary may cause an adnexal mass in reproductive age females. Pigmented foci on an otherwise normal ovary or a large solitary hemorrhagic cyst are the gross findings. Histologic findings include columnar-to-plump cuboidal epithelium with condensed subepithelial stroma, hemosiderin-laden macrophages, fibrosis, and inflammation. Rare cases may also contain smooth muscle. Patients with uterine anomalies may develop severe endometriosis (127). Acute torsion of the adnexal structures is an uncommon event but is a surgical emergency. The severity of the symptoms varies widely and includes fever, nausea or vomiting, and abdominal pain (159). The correct diagnosis is rarely made preoperatively. The preoperative radiograph commonly shows a pelvic mass with a cystic or solid texture, often with thin internal septae, and may simulate an ovarian mass. Because the sigmoid colon cushions and secures the left adnexa, the right adnexa is more often affected than the left. The Fallopian tube and ovary have usually undergone hemorrhagic necrosis by the time of the surgery, often with secondary calcification. As a result, the cause of the torsion is not clear in most cases. Massive ovarian edema is an unusual clinical entity most often occurring in adolescence. It is characterized by marked enlargement of one or both ovaries due to marked accumulation of edema fluid in the ovarian stroma. Massive ovarian edema may result from partial or intermittent torsion of the mesovarium, interfering with venous and lymphatic drainage, but not with arterial blood flow (18,167).

OVARIAN NEOPLASMS

Ovarian neoplasms account for approximately 1% of all childhood cancers. Although the most common ovarian cancers in adults are epithelial, the distribution of histologic tumor types differs in children, with the majority being derived from primordial germ cells (Table 18-2). Ovarian tumors are most frequently found from 10 to 14 years of age, suggesting that hormonal factors may play a role in many. The most common symptoms at presentation include abdominal pain that often simulates acute appendicitis, resulting in emergency laparotomy. Recent advances in the management of these tumors have resulted in increased cure rates as well as preservation of future fertility. Examples include new disease-specific chemotherapeutic regimens as well as the advent of surgical staging (Table 18-3) (177).

Table 18-2 ▪ RELATIVE FREQUENCY OF OVARIAN NEOPLASMS IN CHILDREN AND ADOLESCENTS

Histogenetic Category	No. (%)
Germ cell	205 (58)
Coelomic epithelium	67 (19)
Sex cord–stromal	62 (18)
Supportive stroma and miscellaneous	19 (5)
Total	353 (100)

Ovarian Germ Cell Tumors

The ovary is the site of approximately 30% of all germ cell tumors. Ovarian germ cell tumors in children show a higher frequency of malignancy than those in adults (98). The vast majority are diagnosed in postpubertal adolescents; malignant germ cell tumors in the ovaries of very young children are exceedingly rare. Ovarian germ cell tumors show a biologic and clinical heterogeneity not seen in their testicular or extragonadal counterparts, with at least four distinct subgroups. These include mature teratomas, immature teratomas, malignant germ cell tumors, and germ cell tumors arising in dysgenetic gonads.

Mature Teratoma: Teratomas are defined as neoplasms containing a haphazard growth of one or more types of

Table 18-3 ▪ FEDERATION OF INTERNATIONAL GYNECOLOGISTS AND OBSTETRICIANS (FIGO) STAGING OF OVARIAN CARCINOMA

I. Tumor limited to ovaries
- A. Tumor limited to one ovary; no ascites
  1. Capsule intact
  2. Capsule ruptured or tumor present on the external surface
- B. Tumor limited to both ovaries; no ascites
  1. Capsule intact
  2. Capsule ruptured or tumor present on the external surface
- C. Tumor limited to ovaries; ascites present or positive peritoneal washings

II. Tumor involving ovaries with pelvic extension
- A. Extension and/or metastases to uterus and/or tubes; no ascites
- B. Extension to other pelvic tissues; no ascites
- C. Tumor either IIA or IIB with ascites or positive peritoneal washings

III. Tumor involving ovaries with intraperitoneal metastases outside the pelvis and/or positive retroperitoneal lymph nodes

IV. Distant metastasis, including parenchymal liver metastasis

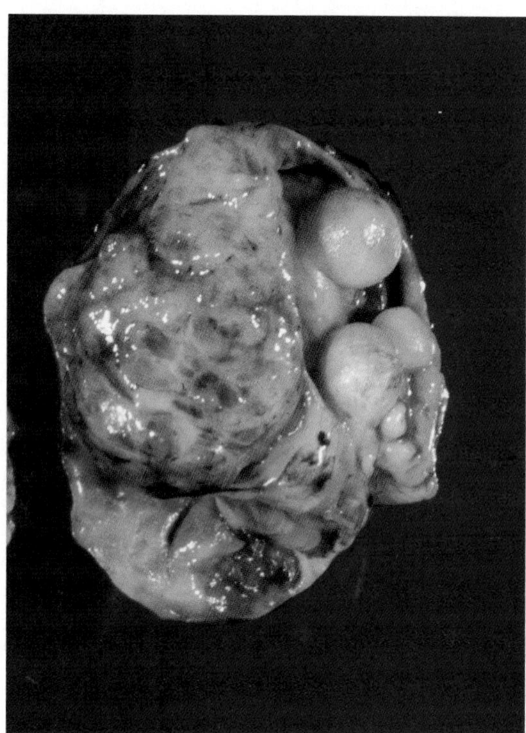

FIGURE 18-13 ■ Mature teratoma demonstrating multiple large and small cysts separated by heterogeneous solid nodules.

tissue derived from the three embryonic layers (ectoderm, mesoderm, and endoderm). Mature ovarian teratomas represent 40% to 60% of all childhood ovarian neoplasms, and patients with these tumors most commonly present at 13 to 15 years of age (30,161). There is a 10% incidence of bilaterality. Mature teratomas can be subdivided into those that are predominately cystic and those that are predominately solid. Cystic teratomas characteristically contain the copious hair and sebaceous material characteristic of those in adults; however, this type is less common in children (Figure 18-13). Immature elements are rarely found in predominately cystic teratomas, and the malignant potential of cystic teratomas in children is minimal unless the child has a constitutional genetic abnormality resulting in increased risk of development of neoplasms (such as Li-Fraumeni syndrome). The solid mature teratoma, which is more common in children, may show a closer biologic relationship to immature teratomas than to cystic mature teratomas, and it should be carefully sectioned to exclude immature elements. Neuroglial tissue is the predominant component in these lesions.

The development of a somatic malignancy within a teratoma is a rare event in childhood. This malignant transformation is thought to occur within differentiated teratomatous elements rather than from totipotent embryonal cells. Within childhood ovarian teratomas, 7/246 tumors developed somatic malignancies (13). The types of nongerm cell malignancies most commonly encountered were epithelial, glial, and embryonal. Such nongerm cell malignancies are associated with a worse prognosis owing to poor response to therapy. In the past, these events were referred to as *teratocarcinoma* or *malignant teratoma*, terms that are confusing and best avoided.

Ovarian mature teratomas have been the most thoroughly studied biologically owing to their abundant numbers. More than 325 cases have been cytogenetically analyzed, demonstrating 95% to be karyotypically normal and the remainder to show nonrecurrent numeric abnormalities (80,143). Studies of molecular loci show that the majority of mature ovarian teratomas have entered, but have not completed, meiosis (64,143). These studies suggest that mature ovarian teratomas arise from germ cells arrested in meiosis I.

Immature Teratoma: Immature teratomas are the third most common germ cell tumor seen in the adolescent female ovary. These are considered to be of intermediate malignancy, a concept that is controversial. Although immature teratomas have rarely been reported to metastasize, those that do so almost invariably contain endodermal sinus tumor (EST) components in the original tumor. This raises the possibility that the metastasizing component is the EST, which subsequently undergoes differentiation. Immature teratomas are predominately unilateral solid tumors that may be quite large and are most often confined to the ovary. Immature teratomas can be graded histologically according to the quantity of immature elements, most commonly the quantity of immature neuroectoderm (Figure 18-14) (99). Many variants of this grading system have been proposed; however, the differences between these systems are not substantive. Grade 1 lesions are those with immature tissue limited to rare low magnification fields, with not more than one field in any one slide. Grade 2 lesions contain immature neuroectoderm not exceeding three low power fields (10X objective, with a 4X to 10X ocular for a total magnification of 40X to 100X per slide). Grade 3 tumors show extensive immature neural epithelium in more than three low power fields per slide. This grading system is based on the presence of immature neuroectoderm; the significance of immaturity of non-neural elements (fetal muscle, cartilage, or kidney) is somewhat controversial. In practice, this seldom presents

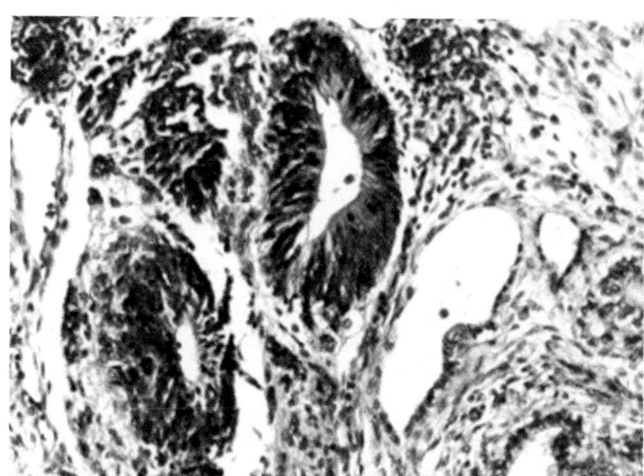

FIGURE 18-14 ■ Immature teratoma of the ovary with several immature neuroepithelial tubules composed of proliferating, primitive cells.

difficulties because the immature elements are almost invariably accompanied by immature neural elements. A common approach is to consider immature non-neural elements of any quantity as grade I. This grading system has been most successfully applied to ovarian immature teratomas, in which the grade correlates with metastatic potential as well as with behavior (101). The treatment of choice is unilateral oophorectomy. The reported prognosis of immature ovarian teratomas in adults depends on the histologic grade of the tumor, the size of the tumor, the age of the patient, and the stage at presentation. Analysis of the outcome of 41 pediatric ovarian immature teratomas treated by surgery alone (19 grade 1, 13 grade 2, and 9 grade 3), 10 of which also showed small foci of EST, suggests that pediatric tumors have a much better prognosis than adults. This study documents only one recurrence of a grade 1 lesion that contained EST in the initial tumor (85). Other recent reports also suggest that low-stage immature ovarian teratomas do not require chemotherapy (28,82).

In the pediatric age group, the most significant pathologic event that occurs within an immature teratoma is the development of a malignant component, most commonly EST. Such occurrences may be multifocal and may be very difficult to confidently identify (Figure 18-15). A valuable indicator of this event is an elevated serum α-fetoprotein (AFP) level. Most observers consider elevated AFP in "pure" immature teratomas to represent unrecognized, small foci of EST. However, some reports of carefully examined tumors have suggested that immature neural tissue or intestinal tissue may be a source of elevated levels of AFP. This is supported by the immunoreactivity of these tissue types with AFP (108). The judgment of most experienced observers has been that although these tissue elements may, in a minority of cases, explain a small, stable increase in serum AFP, a large or rapidly increasing elevation in a patient without liver failure must be assumed to represent the presence of EST (52).

Cytogenetic studies show a higher frequency of chromosomal abnormalities in immature teratomas (60%) when compared with mature teratomas; however, no consistent abnormalities have been identified (103,118,143). Most immature ovarian teratomas are diploid; however, occasional tumors are aneuploid in the triploid to tetraploid range. Most of these high-level aneuploid tumors harbor foci of EST (4).

Gliomatosis Peritonei: Gliomatosis peritonei is a rare condition that occurs almost exclusively in the setting of solid ovarian mature or immature teratoma. It is characterized by small gray-white nodules of mature glial tissues on peritoneal surfaces. The pathogenesis of these nodules has been debated. They may arise from small capsular ruptures of the ovarian mass, resulting in implantation on the peritoneal surfaces. Alternatively, they may represent independent lesions arising within the subcoelomic mesenchyme. Studies comparing the DNA of the glial implants with DNA of the associated ovarian teratomas and normal tissues demonstrate that gliomatosis peritonei is genetically unrelated to the associated teratoma, supporting the second hypothesis (41) (Figure 18-16). Mature nodules, whether peritoneal or in lymph nodes, may require additional surgery but have no adverse prognostic significance and do not impact the staging of the ovarian lesion (50,109). It is important that these peritoneal nodules be adequately examined to exclude foci of immaturity.

Ovarian Dysgerminoma: Dysgerminoma is the most common malignant germ cell tumor in the ovary, comprising 48% of such lesions. It is the most common ovarian malignancy in children and adolescents, and it is the pathologic and biologic equivalent of the testicular seminoma. There is a 10% to 15% incidence of bilaterality. Most dysgerminomas are pure and are composed of aggregates or nests of uniform neoplastic cells with distinct, nonoverlapping cellular borders (Figure 18-17). Germinomas often show a lymphocytic infiltrate and occasionally multinucleated giant cells.

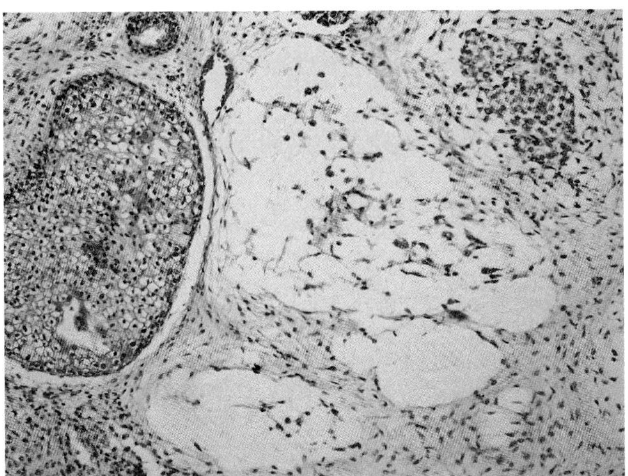

FIGURE 18-15 ■ Teratoma of the ovary with a microscopic focus of EST. The reticular pattern and the enlarged nuclei with course chromatin provide histologic clues. The serum AFP was moderately elevated before surgery.

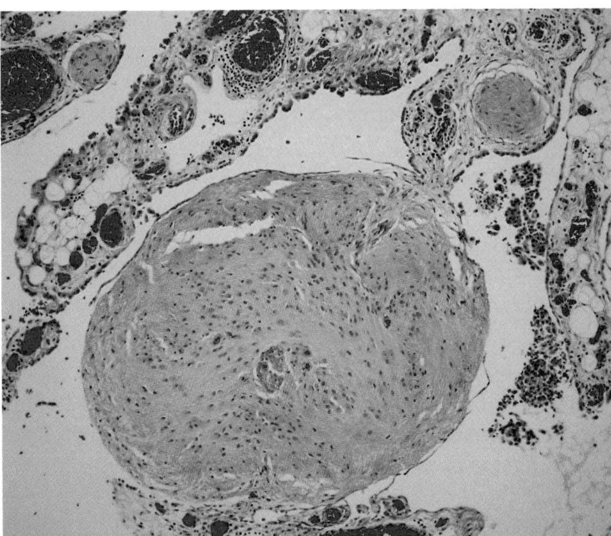

FIGURE 18-16 ■ Gliomatosis peritonei characterized by nodules of mature glial tissue in the omentum.

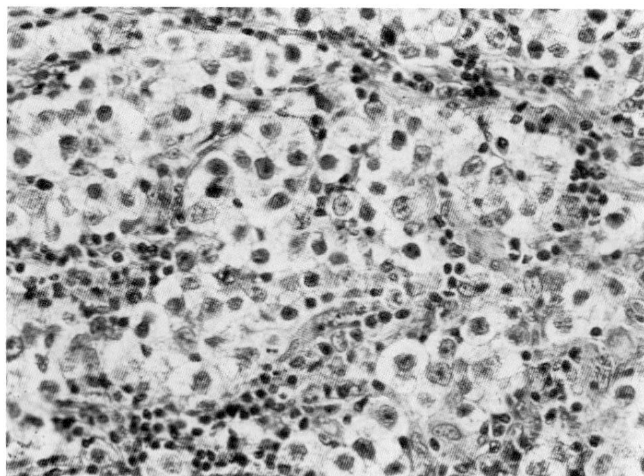

FIGURE 18-17 ■ Dysgerminomas are often arranged in nests of cells with well-defined cytoplasmic membranes and rounded nuclei with prominent nucleoli. Lymphocytes and occasional multinucleate cells may be seen in the stroma.

Although anaplastic variants of germinomas (seminomas and dysgerminomas) have been rarely reported, these foci may represent areas of solid embryonal carcinoma. Synciotrophoblastic cells may be scattered individually throughout germinomas and may be responsible for human chorionic gonadotropin (hCG) production, but unless they are accompanied by cytotrophoblastic cells, these cells do not represent choriocarcinoma and have no effect on prognosis (148). Immunohistochemically, the majority of germinomas are positive for placental-like alkaline phosphatase (PLAP), a cell surface glycoprotein. While PLAP is a valuable marker for germinomas, it may also be present focally in embryonal carcinomas and ESTs as well as in a wide variety of somatic tumors (17,84). A more specific antibody has been reported recently that strongly and specifically recognizes germinomas, embryonal carcinomas, and intratubular germ cell neoplasia, namely OCT4. This protein is highly expressed in pluripotent stem cells and has been demonstrated to be useful in the distinction of metastatic GCT from other tumor types (22). It is negative in ESTs.

The majority of patients with dysgerminomas (70% to 80%) present as stage I (162). Dysgerminomas are exquisitely radiosensitive, and the 5-year survival rate with radiotherapy ranges from 90% in stage I disease to 60% to 90% in patients with more advanced disease. Properly evaluated patients with stage Ia ovarian pure dysgerminoma who desire fertility can be safely treated without radiotherapy by unilateral oophorectomy after careful lymph node sampling alone (82). The tumor subsequently recurs in 17% of patients, but more than 90% of these patients may be successfully treated with chemotherapy. Bilateral dysgerminoma may be treated with bilateral oophorectomy and chemotherapy, with the uterus left *in situ* for future embryo transfer.

Endodermal Sinus Tumor: The second most common histologic subtype (22%) of malignant ovarian germ cell tumor in children is EST, also called *yolk sac tumor*. Grossly, these

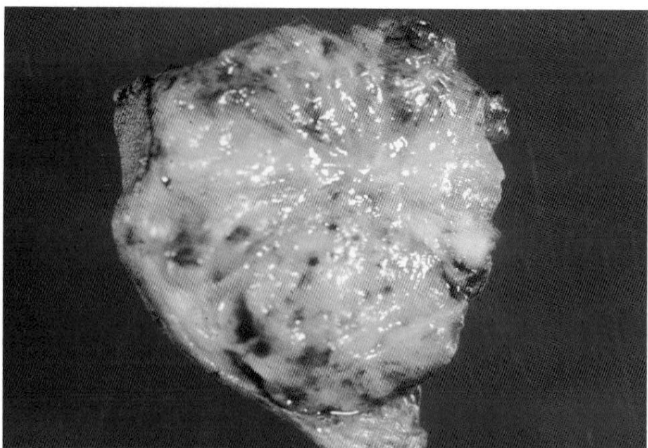

FIGURE 18-18 ■ Ovarian ESTs are often white, mucoid appearing, with microcysts.

lesions are most often tan to white and mucoid in appearance, often with small cystic regions (Figure 18-18). EST has only been reliably distinguished from other patterns of malignant germ cell tumor for the last two decades. Therefore, caution is advised when evaluating earlier studies of malignant ovarian germ cell tumors; these studies often equated EST with embryonal carcinoma and underappreciated the presence of EST within immature teratomas. The histology and cytology of ESTs vary widely, often causing difficulty in diagnosis. For detailed description of the protean manifestations of EST, many excellent reviews are available (144,150). Several histologic subtypes of EST have been described; most tumors contain several subtypes, and none of these subtypes have prognostic implication (Figures 18-19 to 18-21). The prototypic Schiller-Duvall bodies of EST (Figure 18-21) are present in 50% to 75% of tumors. ESTs are commonly associated with highly elevated serum AFP levels, which may be monitored clinically for recurrence and/or metastasis (136). Aggressive monitoring of serum AFP levels constitutes one of the important improvements in the

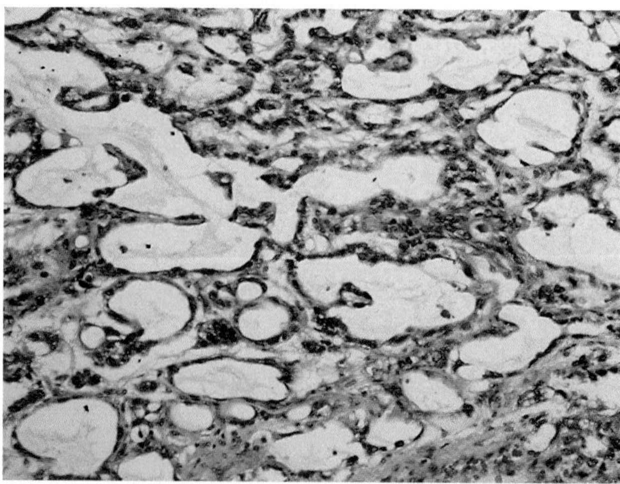

FIGURE 18-19 ■ ESTs often show a mixture of histologic types. The reticular pattern shows a network of communicating spaces.

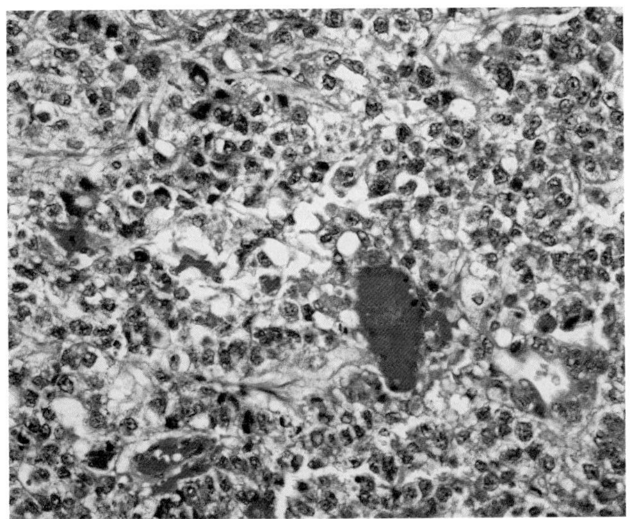

FIGURE 18-20 ■ Solid regions may be seen within ESTs; however, they are usually a minority component. The cells may contain large intracellular vacuoles. Hyaline bodies are occasionally seen.

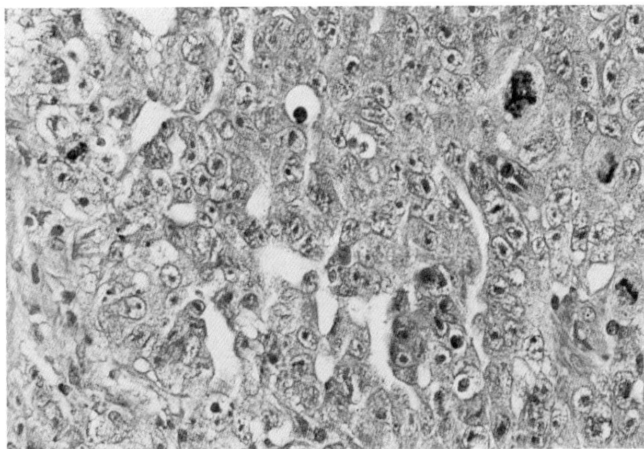

FIGURE 18-22 ■ Embryonal carcinoma is composed of large, overlapping nuclei with very large, prominent nucleoli and prominent individual cell necrosis. The cytoplasm is characteristically amphophilic.

management of patients with germ cell tumor, particularly those with EST. The AFP should fall into the normal range 5 to 7 weeks following surgery if resection of the tumor is complete. Rarely bilateral, ESTs are rapidly growing, yet most present as stage Ia tumors.

Other Histologic Types of Nongerminomatous Tumors: Pure embryonal carcinomas are rare ovarian neoplasms (4%) that should be differentiated from the more common EST. These are more commonly seen as a minor component of a mixed germ cell tumor. Like ESTs, embryonal carcinomas may show papillary, glandular, and solid areas. The cells are large, epithelioid, and often anaplastic with large nucleoli, abundant mitotic activity, hemorrhage and necrosis (Figure 18-22). Embryonal carcinomas show immunoreactivity for cytokeratin, but not for epithelial membrane antigen, a feature that may help to distinguish embryonal carcinoma from other epithelial neoplasms (149). A minority of embryonal carcinomas show focal, weak immunoreactivity for PLAP, as well as for AFP (73,84). It has been noted that embryonal carcinomas, but not other germ cell tumor histologic types, show immunopositivity for CD30, a marker more conventionally utilized for Hodgkin lymphoma (77). CD30 is a member of the tumor necrosis factor receptor superfamily whose expression protects against apoptosis (56). Embryonal carcinomas are reliably positive for OCT4 (5).

Ovarian choriocarcinoma is rarely seen as the sole histologic type, but may constitute a minor component within a mixed germ cell tumor. Choriocarcinomas are composed of both medium-sized cytotrophoblastic and multinucleate syncytiotrophoblastic cells with frequent evidence of hemorrhage (Figure 18-23). Immunohistochemical stains for hCG identify syncytiotrophoblastic cells, with unreliable staining of cytotrophoblasts. The prognosis of nongerminomatous germ cell tumors prior to the chemotherapy era was dismal. With the advent of bleomycin, etoposide, and cisplatin protocols, survival rates of 70% to 90% have been reported (46,67).

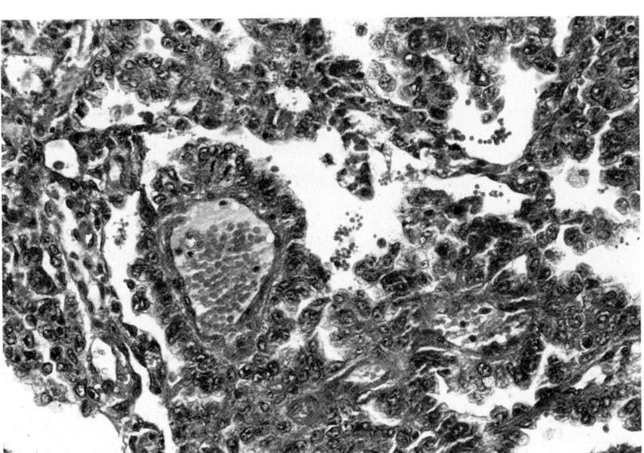

FIGURE 18-21 ■ Schiller-Duval bodies are present in many ESTs. These bodies are composed of a central vascular core lined by tumor cells, a space, and then an outer rim of tumor cells.

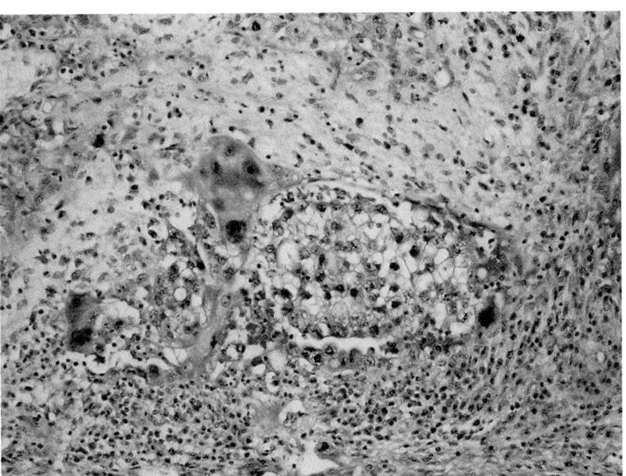

FIGURE 18-23 ■ Choriocarcinoma is composed of both multinucleate syncytiotrophoblastic cells and cytotrophoblastic cells. This histologic subtype can often be found associated with areas of hemorrhage.

Genetic studies of malignant ovarian germ cell tumors involving normal gonads show no difference from their testicular counterparts. Most malignant ovarian germ cell tumors are aneuploid or near-tetraploid. Most contain the i(12p) by classic cytogenetics and amplification of 12p by comparative genomic hybridization (3,58,118). As previously mentioned, ESTs frequently develop in the context of immature teratomas. The biologic changes associated with this histologic transformation have not been adequately studied; however, ploidy analyses have suggested a genetic change is associated with the histologic transformation (4). The absence of the i(12p) in immature teratomas and the presence of the i(12p) in ESTs associated with immature teratomas suggest that one genetic change may be the acquisition of the i(12p) (59,118). Recent studies have demonstrated c-kit mutation in a substantial minority of ovarian dysgerminomas, similar to findings seen in testicular germinomas (57).

Gonadoblastoma: Gonadoblastoma is a rare tumor that arises in the dysgenetic gonads of phenotypic females having Y chromosomal determinants, as discussed earlier (14,131). Gonadoblastomas are usually quite small and recognizable only on microscopic examination. Histologically, gonadoblastomas are characterized by nests containing both germ cells and stromal cells of granulosa-Sertoli cell type (Figures 18-24 and 18-25). These nests may be separated by stroma that often contains Leydig cells. Gonadoblastomas often show extensive hyalinization. A common feature is the presence of laminated calcific concretions. Numerous calcifications identified within a dysgerminoma should suggest the possibility that the patient may have gonadal dysgenesis and may be at a high risk for developing a contralateral dysgerminoma. While dysgerminoma is the most common histologic subtype of malignancy following gonadoblastoma, EST and embryonal carcinoma are also reported. Recently, TSPY has been reported as a candidate gene involved in the development of gonadoblastoma. The TSPY protein is expressed, along with PLAP and OCT4, in germ cells within gonadoblastoma (68).

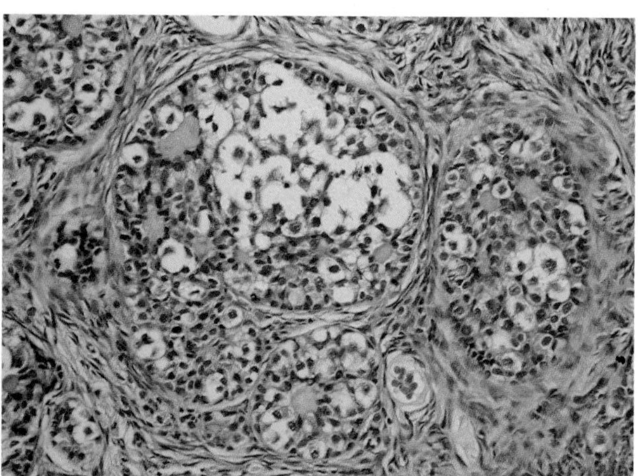

FIGURE 18-24 ■ Gonadoblastomas are seen as small nodules within streak gonads that contain eosinophilic hyaline bodies composed of basement membrane material. Calcifications are frequent.

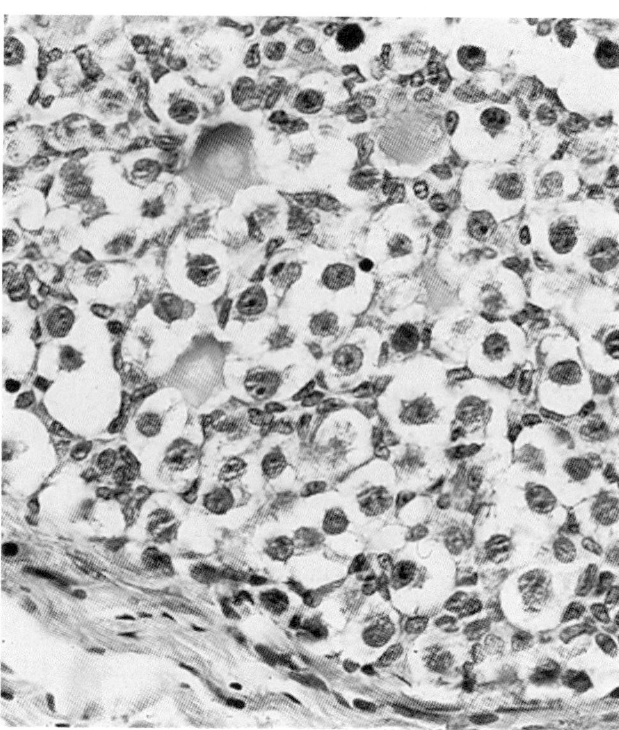

FIGURE 18-25 ■ Nodules of gonadoblastoma contain both germ cells and stromal cells, in varying proportions.

Serologic Markers: Serum and CSF concentrations of AFP and hCG are useful as markers of certain types of germ cell tumors. AFP is expressed at high levels by over 85% of ESTs (66) and at lower levels in other histologic types. The predominant utility is for monitoring for recurrence or metastasis in AFP-secreting tumors. The half-life of AFP is 5 to 7 days. Other neoplastic and non-neoplastic disorders may result in elevation of AFP, for example, hepatitis, cirrhosis, and other malignancies. The beta subunit of hCG is secreted by the syncytiotrophoblastic cells of the placenta and thus is characteristically markedly elevated in choriocarcinomas. However, virtually all histologic subtypes of malignant germ cell tumors may show rare or scattered syncytiotrophoblastic cells that may result in mildly elevated hCG but do not indicate a worse prognosis. Elevations above 100 ng/mL are unusual and suggest the true presence of choriocarcinoma. The half-life of hCG is approximately 20 to 30 hours.

Hematologic Malignancies Associated with Germ Cell Tumors: The association between germ cell tumors and hematologic malignancy is well established but uncommon. The vast majority of germ cell tumors that subsequently develop hematologic malignancies are malignant mediastinal germ cell tumors in men (21,33,70,87,96). The associated hematologic abnormalities have included erythroleukemia, histiocytic sarcoma, acute nonlymphocytic leukemia, myelodysplasia, and systemic mast cell disease. Three ovarian germ cell tumors have been reported in association with hematologic abnormalities, two of these were in 46,XY phenotypic females. The median interval between the diagnosis of the germ cell tumor and that of the hematologic malignancy is 6 months, much shorter than the 25- to 60-month interval commonly seen in chemotherapy-related hematologic malignancies. It has been proposed that the germ cells tumor may provide the stem line of the hematologic malignancy. This is supported by the presence of the i(12p) in both the germ cell tumor and the hematopoietic malignancy in several cases (20). Primary resections of germ cell tumors that show proliferating hematopoietic cells should raise the suspicion of an associated hematologic abnormality; however, more often this process is not detected at the initial resection.

Ovarian Sex Cord–Stromal Tumors

In addition to germ cells, the ovary is populated by granulosa cells, theca cells, interstitial (hilus) cells, and stromal fibroblasts. Each of these components may give rise to a neoplasm, and such lesions are grouped together as sex cord–stromal tumors. They account for 10% of all ovarian neoplasms in children and adolescents. Most are composed of ovarian cell types, but some contain only elements of testicular type (such as Sertoli cell tumors). Precocious puberty and virilization are the major clinical manifestations. Before 9 years of age, most sex cord–stromal tumors are feminizing, and after 9 years of age, there is a predominance of virilizing neoplasms. On occasion, it may be difficult or impossible to identify accurately a lesion as a stromal tumor or to determine to which of the stromal tumor categories a tumor belongs. Younger age and early-stage disease are important predictors for improved survival in patients with ovarian sex cord stromal tumors (180). Immunohistochemistry has been used to verify the diagnosis of sex cord–stromal tumors. Inhibin, calretinin, and CD99 are useful markers that positively mark the majority of sex cord-stromal tumors, while most are negative for epithelial membrane antigen (51,116).

Juvenile granulosa cell tumors constitute the most common type of functioning ovarian neoplasm. Although these are commonly composed almost entirely of granulosa cells, they may also contain theca cells or fibroblasts singly or in any combination. Fewer than 10% of all granulosa cell tumors are diagnosed in the first two decades of life (142). The majority (80% to 85%) of granulosa cell tumors in children are histologically distinct from the adult-type granulosa cell tumors described later. These juvenile granulosa cell tumors typically present with precocious pseudopuberty or virilization in a child younger than 10 years old, although infants and elderly patients have been reported (156,170). A few cases have been associated with Ollier disease, Potter syndrome, and other forms of dysmorphisms (170). Grossly, juvenile granulosa cell tumors are solid with fibrous bands separating yellow nodules and are usually confined to the ovary (Figure 18-26). Microscopically, juvenile granulosa cell tumors have a rather complex growth pattern with nodules of incompletely luteinized cells. Follicles may be

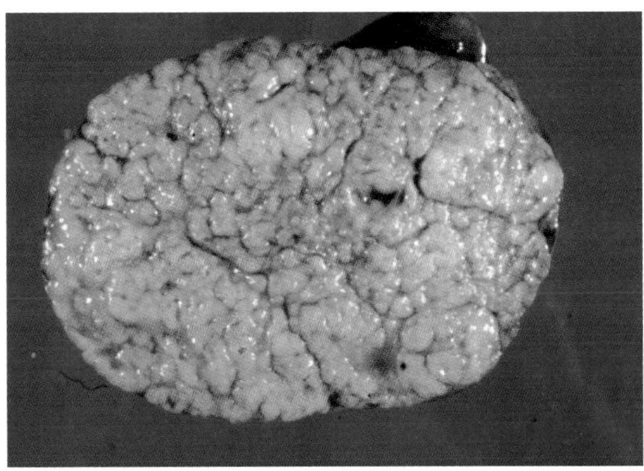

FIGURE 18-26 ▪ Juvenile granulosa cell tumor in a 7-year-old girl who presented with precocious puberty and a pelvic mass.

present that are irregular and resemble large Graafian follicles (Figure 18-27). The luminal contents contain mucicarmine-positive secretions. The stromal cells resemble fibroblasts or have polygonal outlines and pale cytoplasm containing abundant lipid (Figure 18-28). Luteinization is commonly greater and the nuclei are more hyperchromatic and immature than those in the adult-type granulosa cell tumors. Call-Exner bodies are not a feature of these tumors and the nuclear grooves typical of adult granulosa cell tumors are infrequent. Some mitotic activity and nuclear atypia is often present and is more pronounced than that seen in adult-type granulosa cell tumors, resulting in their frequent misdiagnosis as malignant germ cell tumors (Figure 18-28). Although juvenile granulosa cell tumors commonly present as stage 1, it is not uncommon for these tumors to rupture (170). Low-stage tumors have an excellent prognosis; however, the outcome for patients with nonconfined tumors may be poor (156). Although the adult granulosa cell tumor has a local recurrence of 20%, 92% of patients with juvenile granulosa cell tumors were free of disease following surgical removal

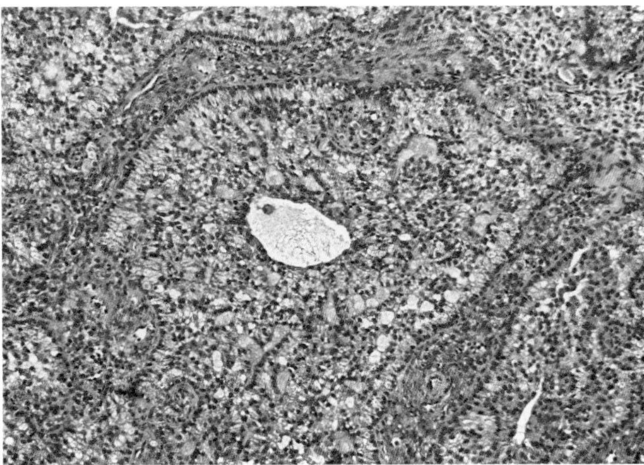

FIGURE 18-27 ▪ Juvenile granulosa cell tumor of the ovary showing a smaller cyst lined by clear cells and resembling a large, irregular Graafian follicle.

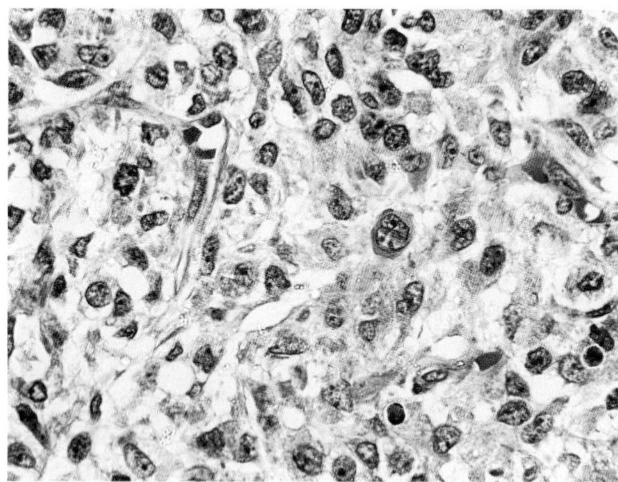

FIGURE 18-28 ■ Juvenile granulosa cell tumor of the ovary with ovoid-to-elliptical cells with pale eosinophilic cytoplasm and polygonal cells with clear cytoplasm are found in the nodules. Nuclear atypia and mitoses are often present.

(156). However, those that recur tend to do so within 3 years and have a rapid course (170). There is no known benefit from adjuvant chemotherapy or radiotherapy.

Adult-type granulosa cell tumors may also occur in the first two decades of life. These tumors are characterized by rounded follicles of varying sizes, minimal luteinization, and rare mitoses. The most differentiated forms show Call-Exner bodies, which consist of granulosa cells in a radial arrangement around a small cystic cavity containing a central rounded mass of eosinophilic material (142). Adult granulosa cell tumors may demonstrate a wide range of histologic appearances, which are commonly mixed within a single specimen, often making their diagnosis a challenge. Different patterns include microfollicular, macrofollicular, trabecular, insular solid-tubular, diffuse (sarcomatous), and luteinized. Some show branching columns of cells, whereas others are more diffuse; all show characteristic nuclear grooves (Figure 18-29).

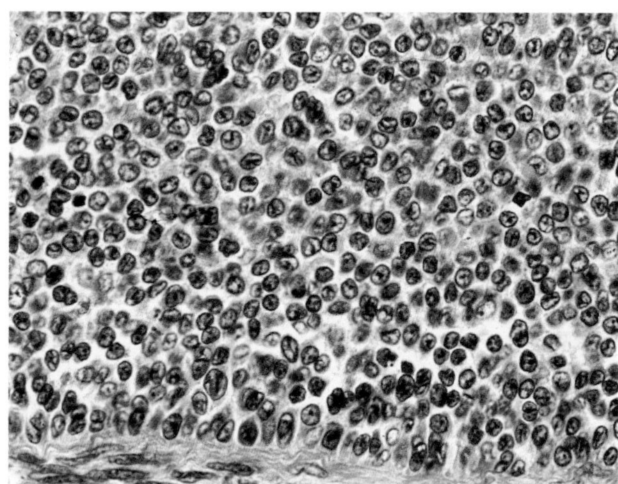

FIGURE 18-29 ■ Adult-type granulosa cell tumors at times show a predominately solid pattern, which may cause diagnostic difficulty. However, the prominent nuclear groves are seen in all tumors.

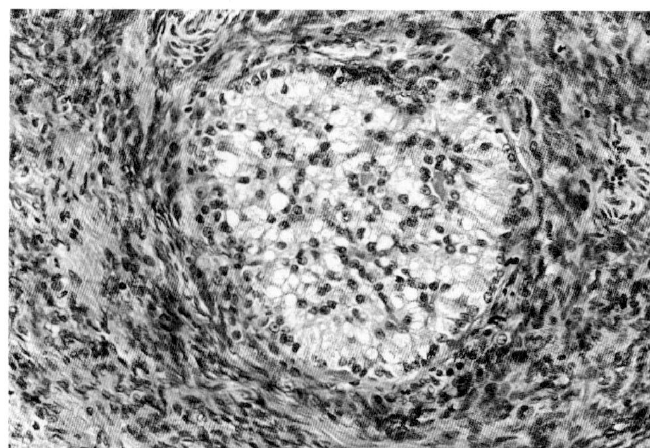

FIGURE 18-30 ■ Sex cord tumor with annular tubules is composed of rounded epithelial units containing cells with abundant eosinophilic cytoplasm that surrounds multiple hyaline bodies.

These tumors are commonly estrogenic and may cause endometrial hyperplasia and carcinoma in 5% to 25% of women of reproductive age.

Sex cord tumors with annular tubules (SCTAT) is a distinctive ovarian neoplasm with morphologic features intermediate between granulosa cell tumor and Sertoli cell tumor. SCTATs demonstrate multifocal cortical stromal tumors that contain epithelial nests with single or multiple hyaline bodies, representing annular tubules (Figure 18-30). These bodies may resemble the hyaline bodies seen in gonadoblastomas; however, the cells of the annular tubules have more abundant, pale, and vacuolated cytoplasm and lack germ cells. Hyperestrinism is common. Approximately one third of patients with SCTAT have Peutz-Jeghers syndrome (43,175).

Sclerosing stromal tumors are rare neoplasms that most commonly present in younger women (14 to 19 years of age) with irregular menses and abdominal pain (124). Grossly, the tumors are unilateral, firm, and gray to white; areas of edema, necrosis, and cystic degeneration are common (Figure 18-31). Microscopic features include spindled cells arranged in lobules separated by edematous stroma. Polygonal cells are scattered among the spindle cells and may have

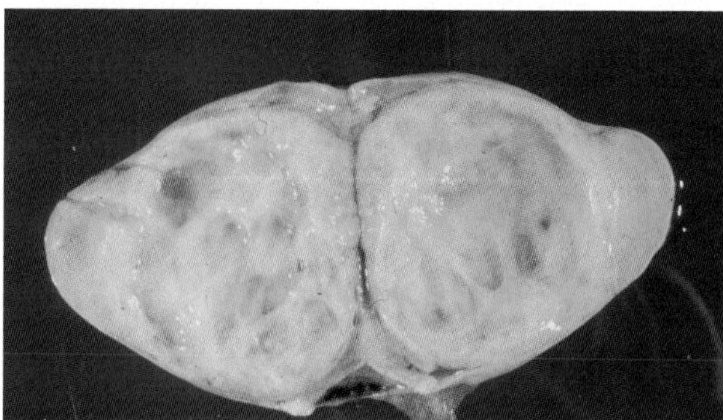

FIGURE 18-31 ■ Sclerosing stromal tumors show pseudolobulation at low power due to areas with differing cellularity, collagen, and edema.

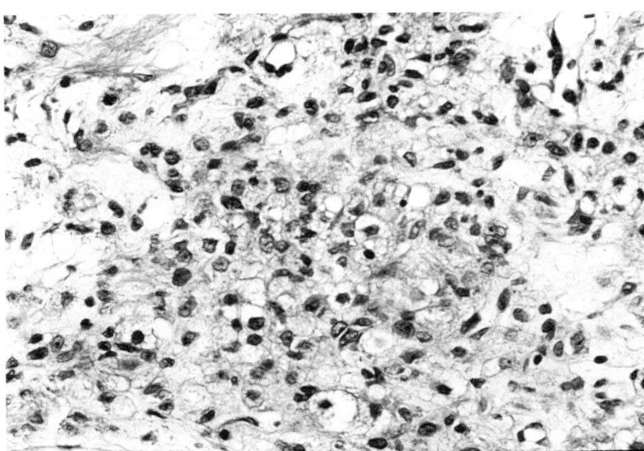

FIGURE 18-32 ■ Sclerosing stromal tumors are composed of an admixture of spindle cells forming collagen and lipid-laden theca-like cells with shrunken nuclei.

signet ring–like features; however, these cells contain oil red O–positive lipid and not mucin (Figure 18-32). None of these tumors has behaved in a malignant fashion.

Sertoli cell tumors of the ovary are exceedingly rare. The predominant pattern is tubular, with a minority of tumors demonstrating retiform or diffuse patterns. The tumors are most often virilizing, but may produce estrogen.

Sertoli-Leydig cell tumors contain various proportions of Sertoli, Leydig, and indifferent stromal cells, often similar to that seen in various phases of testicular development. These represent only 0.5% of ovarian neoplasms and are the most commonly virilizing of all ovarian tumors (173,174). Half have symptoms of androgen excess or virilization, but a few have estrogenic manifestations. Survival is excellent, with tumor-related deaths in only 5%, likely due to the fact that they are stage I at presentation in over 97% of patients (174,178). Sertoli-Leydig cell tumors have been classified on the basis of degree of differentiation and the presence or absence of heterologous elements. The well-differentiated or pure Sertoli cell tumors are the least common. These are composed of well-developed tubules or solid cords of cells with or without Leydig cells. Intermediate tumors comprise poorly formed tubules in a cellular stroma with a nodular or a diffuse configuration (Figure 18-33). Poorly differentiated or sarcomatoid tumors are composed of undifferentiated mesenchyme, poorly formed cords of Sertoli cells, and a paucity of Leydig cells. Sertoli-Leydig cell tumors with heterologous elements comprise 25% of all Sertoli-Leydig cell tumors and may contain cysts or glands with intestinal-type mucosa, carcinoid tumor, rhabdomyoblasts, cartilage, or neuroblastoma (112). These seem to be more common in Sertoli-Leydig cell tumors of younger patients and may be difficult to distinguish from immature teratomas. In recent years, the retiform pattern has received increased attention due to their younger age at presentation (median age of 15 years) and their often lack of androgenic manifestations, increasing the risk of misdiagnosis. Occasional retiform Sertoli Leydig cell tumors may be associated with elevated serum levels of AFP.

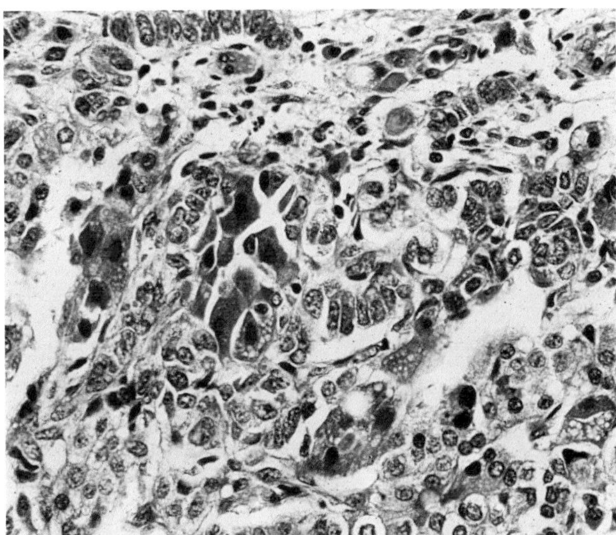

FIGURE 18-33 ■ Sertoli-Leydig cell tumor composed of irregular poorly formed tubules and cords lined by cells containing moderate amounts of cytoplasm; occasional clusters of Leydig cells demonstrating atypia and eosinophilic cytoplasm are seen.

Rare Tumors: A few examples of mixed germ cell–sex cord–stromal tumors have been described, but are quite rare (75). Other abdominal soft tissue tumors have presented in the ovary, including desmoplastic small round cell tumor, peripheral neuroectodermal tumors, and alveolar soft part sarcoma, to name a few.

Epithelial Neoplasms

Ovarian epithelial neoplasms arise from the surface epithelium of the ovary and, therefore, may express the multipotential nature of the embryonic coelomic epithelium, including mucous, serous, endometrioid, and mesenchymal appearances. These tumors comprise about 15% of ovarian neoplasms of patients younger than 20 years of age, and in this population, they occur after menarche and are virtually exclusively mucinous or serous, with mucinous tumors comprising the majority (77%) (57). The majority are unilateral and benign; approximately 15% are malignant. The pathologic categorization of these epithelial lesions is based on an evaluation of epithelial proliferative changes. These subgroups are benign, atypically proliferating ("borderline" tumors), and malignant. The intermediate group is defined as showing greater proliferation (including epithelial budding and nuclear stratification, mitotic activity, and nuclear atypia) but showing no destructive invasion of the stromal component. The criteria for inclusion into the intermediate group, and the nomenclature used, remain controversial.

Serous neoplasms are usually composed of multiple cysts with watery and clear contents. Characteristic is the presence of nodular papillary excrescences scattered over the lining of the cysts. These may be few and barely visible or numerous. Microscopically, the cysts are lined by papillary processes covered by a single layer of columnar-to-cuboidal cells

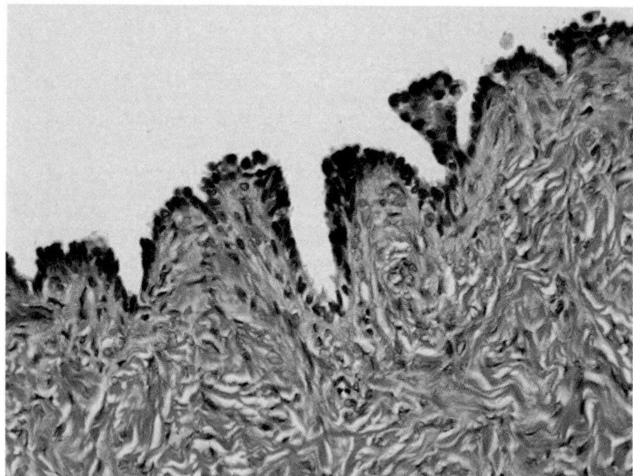

FIGURE 18-34 ■ Serous cystadenomas are lined by an epithelium resembling that of either the Fallopian tube or the surface epithelium of the ovary, and therefore may be ciliated or nonciliated.

(Figure 18-34). Intermediate neoplasms show more extensive and complex papillary patterns with stratification of the epithelial lining. The neoplastic cells show loss of polarity, nuclear pleomorphism, and increased mitotic activity. Most important, and required for the diagnosis of carcinoma, is the presence of stromal invasion. Ovarian borderline serous tumors show an increased risk of recurrence, and histologic features have been proposed and disputed that may define a subset of tumors with a greater risk of aggressive behavior (micropapillary serous carcinoma) (38,134,137).

Mucinous neoplasms are also usually multicystic tumors containing thick mucinous material. The lining of the cysts is smooth and glistening, with infrequent papillary excrescences. Microscopically, the cysts are lined by columnar nonciliated cells with faintly basophilic cytoplasm and the small, basally oriented nuclei (Figure 18-35A). Some tumors show scattered goblet cells. The supportive stroma is cellular and commonly has a thecal and even luteal appearance. Intermediate neoplasms are characterized by stratification of epithelial cells, loss of nuclear polarity, nuclear pleomorphism, and frequent mitoses (Figure 18-35B). The assessment of the clinical behavior of ovarian mucinous tumors demonstrates the importance of stromal invasion in predicting a poor prognosis and defining the category of ovarian mucinous carcinoma (31,55,117).

Small cell carcinomas of the ovary are often confused histologically with granulosa cell tumors and/or germ cell tumors. These are highly aggressive tumors and should not be treated conservatively. They are often associated with paraendocrine hypercalcemia. The patients range from 9 to 43 (average: 23.9) years of age, and the tumors often present at a high stage (51,171). The tumor is composed of poorly differentiated small cells with scant cytoplasm and nuclei with clumped chromatin. Therefore, it must be distinguished from other primary and metastatic small cell tumors that may involve the ovary, particularly in young patients. The cells may be diffuse or arranged in nests or cords. Rounded follicles containing eosinophilic fluid and lined by neoplastic cells have been demonstrated in over 75% of tumors. Mitotic figures are abundant. In one series of 15 cases, the tumors were reliably positive for p53, WT1, and EMA. Of concern, the majority were positive for calretinin and 4/15 were positive for CD56. All cases were negative with CK5/6, chromogranin, CD99, NB84, desmin, α-inhibin, and TTF-1. Therefore, the combination of EMA and WT-1 nuclear positivity, the latter usually intense and diffuse, may be of positive diagnostic value (89). Long-term survival is rare once the tumor has spread beyond the ovary, and even stage 1A tumors have a survival rate of only 30%. Recent studies suggest that newer aggressive, multiagent therapeutic regimens may improve survival somewhat (36). The cell lineage remains unknown. The age

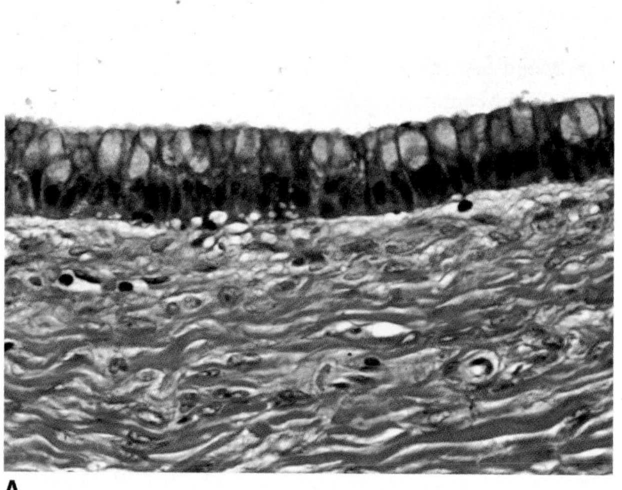

A

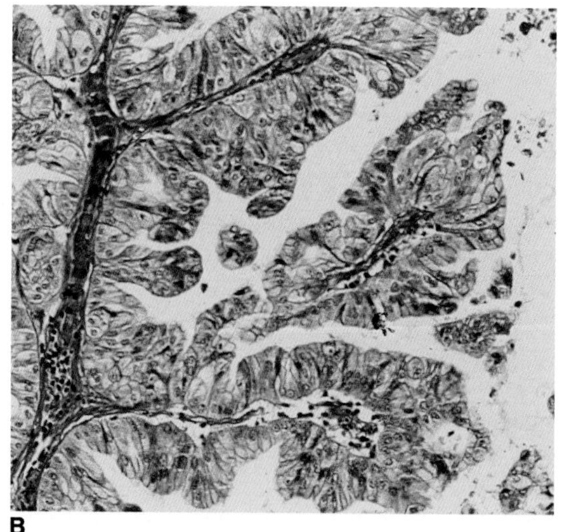

B

FIGURE 18-35 ■ Well-differentiated mucinous tumors most commonly show epithelium similar to that seen in the endocervix, consisting of a single row of mucin-filled column cells with basal nuclei (**A**). Borderline mucinous lesions show multiple fine papillary processes with stratification of cells and loss of polarity (**B**).

distribution, the presence of follicle formation, and calretinin positivity suggest the possibility of a sex cord origin (89).

REFERENCES

1. Abe R, Shimizu T, Shibaki A, et al. Toxic epidermal necrolysis and Stevens-Johnson syndrome are induced by soluble Fas ligand. *Am J Pathol* 2003;162:1515–1520.
2. Andrassy RJ, Wiener ES, Raney RB, et al. Progress in the surgical management of vaginal rhabdomyosarcoma: a 25-year review from the Intergroup Rhabdomyosarcoma Study Group. *J Pediatr Surg* 1999;34:731–734.
3. Atkin NB, Baker MC. Abnormal chromosomes including small metacentrics in 14 ovarian cancers. *Cancer Genet Cytogenet* 1987;26:355–361.
4. Baker BA, Frickey L, Yu IT, et al. DNA content of ovarian immature teratomas and malignant germ cell tumors. *Gynecol Oncol* 1998;71:14–18.
5. Baker PM, Oliva E. Immunohistochemistry as a tool in the differential diagnosis of ovarian tumors: an update. *Int J Gynecol Pathol* 2005;24:39–55.
6. Baldwin CY, Witchel SF. Polycystic ovary syndrome. *Pediatr Ann* 2006;35:888–896.
7. Barrasso R, De Brux J, Croissant O, et al. High prevalence of papillomavirus-associated penile intraepithelial neoplasia in sexual partners of women with cervical intraepithelial neoplasia. *N Engl J Med* 1987;317:916–923.
8. Basta A, Madej JG, Jr. Hydradenoma of the vulva: incidence and clinical observations. *Eur J Gynaecol Oncol* 1990;11:185–189.
9. Behringer RR. The in vivo roles of mullerian inhibiting substance. *Curr Top Develop Biol* 1994;29:171–187.
10. Bell TA. Chlamydia trachomatis infections in adolescents. *Med Clin North Am* 1990;74:1225–1233.
11. Berkovitz GD, Fechner PY, Zacur HW, et al. Clinical and pathologic spectrum of 46,XY gonadal dysgenesis: its relevance to the understanding of sex differentiation. *Medicine (Baltimore)* 1991;70:375–383.
12. Berth-Jones J, Graham-Brown RA, Burns DA. Lichen sclerosus et atrophicus: a review of 15 cases in young girls. *Clin Exp Dermatol* 1991;16:14–17.
13. Biskup W, Calaminus G, Schneider DT, et al. Teratoma with malignant transformation: experiences of the cooperative GPOH protocols MAKEI 83/86/89/96. *Klin Padiatr* 2006;218:303–308.
14. Brant WO, Rajimwale A, Lovell MA, et al. Gonadoblastoma and Turner syndrome. *J Urol* 2006;175:1858–1860.
15. Brennan J, Capel B. One tissue, two fates: molecular genetic events that underlie testis versus ovary development. *Nat Rev Genet* 2004;5:509–521.
16. Buggs C, Rosenfield RL. Polycystic ovary syndrome in adolescence. *Endocrinol Metab Clin North Am* 2005;34:677–705, x.
17. Burke AP, Mostofi FK. Placental alkaline phosphatase immunohistochemistry of intratubular malignant germ cells and associated testicular germ cell tumors. *Hum Pathol* 1988;19:663–670.
18. Bychkov V, Kijek M. Massive ovarian edema: four cases and some pathogenetic considerations. *Acta Obstet Gynecol Scand* 1987;66:397–399.
19. Capel B. Sex in the 90s: SRY and the switch to the male pathway. *Annu Rev Physiol* 1998;60:497–523.
20. Chaganti RSK, Ladanyi M, Samaniego F, et al. Leukemic differentiation of a mediastinal germ cell tumor. *Genes Chromosomes Cancer* 1989;1:83–87.
21. Chariot P, Monnet I, LeLong F, et al. Systemic mast cell disease associated with primary mediastinal germ cell tumor. *Am J Surg Pathol* 1991;90:381–385.
22. Cheng L. Establishing a germ cell origin for metastatic tumors using OCT4 immunohistochemistry. *Cancer* 2004;101:2006–2010.
23. Cools M, Drop SL, Wolffenbuttel KP, et al. Germ cell tumors in the intersex gonad: old paths, new directions, moving frontiers. *Endocr Rev* 2006;27:468–484.
24. Copeland LJ, Gershenson DM, Saul PB, et al. Sarcoma botryoides of the female genital tract. *Obstet Gynecol* 1985;66:262–266.
25. Copeland LJ, Sneige N, Ordonez NG, et al. Endodermal sinus tumor of the vagina and cervix. *Cancer* 1985;55:2558–2565.
26. Corpron CA, Andrassy RJ, Hays DM, et al. Conservative management of uterine pediatric rhabdomyosarcoma: a report from the Intergroup Rhabdomyosarcoma Study III and IV pilot. *J Pediatr Surg* 1995;30:942–944.
27. Couse JF, Hewitt SC, Bunch DO, et al. Postnatal sex reversal of the ovaries in mice lacking estrogen receptors alpha and beta. *Science* 1999;286:2328–2331.
28. Cushing B, Giller R, Ablin A, et al. Surgical resection alone is effective treatment for ovarian immature teratoma in children and adolescents: a report of the Pediatric Oncology Group and the Children's Cancer Group. *Am J Obstet Gynecol* 1999;181:353–358.
29. Daya DA, Scully RE. Sarcoma botryoides of the uterine cervix in young women: a clinicopathological study of 13 cases. *Gynecol Oncol* 1988;29:290–304.
30. De Backer A, Madern GC, Oosterhuis JW, et al. Ovarian germ cell tumors in children: a clinical study of 66 patients. *Pediatr Blood Cancer* 2006;46:459–464.
31. de Nictolis M, Montironi R, Tommasoni S, et al. Benign, borderline, and well-differentiated malignant intestinal mucinous tumors of the ovary: a clinicopathologic, histochemical, immunohistochemical, and nuclear quantitative study of 57 cases. *Int J Gynecol Pathol* 1994;13:10–21.
32. de Silva KS, Kanumakala S, Grover SR, et al. Ovarian lesions in children and adolescents: an 11-year review. *J Pediatr Endocrinol Metab* 2004;17:951–957.
33. DeMent SH. Association between mediastinal germ cell tumors and hematologic malignancies: an update. *Hum Pathol* 1990;21:699–703.
34. Diamanti-Kandarakis E, Kandarakis H, Legro RS. The role of genes and environment in the etiology of PCOS. *Endocrine* 2006;30:19–26.
35. Disteche CM, Casanova M, Saal H, et al. Small deletions of the short arm of the Y chromosome in 46,XY females. *Proc Natl Acad Sci U S A* 1986;83:7841–7844.
36. Distelmaier F, Calaminus G, Harms D, et al. Ovarian small cell carcinoma of the hypercalcemic type in children and adolescents: a prognostically unfavorable but curable disease. *Cancer* 2006;107:2298–2306.
37. Edmonds DK. Congenital malformations of the genital tract and their management. *Best Pract Res Clin Obstet Gynaecol* 2003;17:19–40.
38. Eichhorn JH, Bell DA, Young RH, et al. Ovarian serous borderline tumors with micropapillary and cribriform patterns: a study of 40 cases and comparison with 44 cases without these patterns. *Am J Surg Pathol* 1999;23:397–409.
39. Fallat ME, Donahoe PK. Intersex genetic anomalies with malignant potential. *Curr Opin Pediatr* 2006;18:305–311.
40. Farrell AM, Kirtschig G, Dalziel KL, et al. Childhood vulval pemphigoid: a clinical and immunopathological study of five patients. *Br J Dermatol* 1999;140:308–312.
41. Ferguson AW, Katabuchi H, Ronnett BM, et al. Glial implants in gliomatosis peritonei arise from normal tissue, not from the associated teratoma. *Am J Pathol* 2001;159:51–55.
42. Fleming SE, Hall R, Gysler M, et al. Imperforate anus in females: frequency of genital tract involvement, incidence of associated anomalies, and functional outcome. *J Pediatr Surg* 1986;21:146–150.
43. Foley TR, McGarrity TJ, Abt AB. Peutz-Jeghers syndrome: a clinicopathologic survey of the "Harrisburg family" with a 49-year follow-up. *Gastroenterology* 1988;95:1535–1540.
44. Frimberger D, Gearhart JP. Ambiguous genitalia and intersex. *Urol Int* 2005;75:291–297.
45. Gell JS. Mullerian anomalies. *Semin Reprod Med* 2003;21:375–388.

46. Gershenson DM, Morris M, Cangir A, et al. Treatment of malignant germ cell tumors of the ovary with bleomycin, etoposide, and cisplatin. *J Clin Oncol* 1990;8:715–720.
47. Gravholt CH. Clinical practice in Turner syndrome. *Nat Clin Pract Endocrinol Metab* 2005;1:41–52.
48. Guerrier D, Mouchel T, Pasquier L, et al. The Mayer-Rokitansky-Kuster-Hauser syndrome (congenital absence of uterus and vagina): phenotypic manifestations and genetic approaches. *J Negat Results Biomed* 2006;5:1.
49. Handley J, Hanks E, Armstrong K, et al. Common association of HPV 2 with anogenital warts in prepubertal children. *Pediatr Dermatol* 1997;14:339–343.
50. Harms D, Janig U, Gobel U. Gliomatosis peritonei in childhood and adolescence: clinicopathological study of 13 cases including immunohistochemical findings. *Pathol Res Pract* 1989;184:422–430.
51. Harrison ML, Hoskins P, du BA, et al. Small cell of the ovary, hypercalcemic type: analysis of combined experience and recommendation for management. A GCIG study. *Gynecol Oncol* 2006;100:233–238.
52. Hawkins E, Isaacs H, Cushing B, et al. Occult malignancy in neonatal sacroccygeal teratomas: a combined POG and CCG study. *J Pediatr Hematol* 1993;15:406–409.
53. Hays DM, Shimada H, Raney RBJ, et al. Clinical staging and treatment results in rhabdomyosarcoma of the female genital tract among children and adolescents. *Cancer* 1988;61:1893–1903.
54. Hays DM, Shimada H, Raney RBJ, et al. Sarcomas of the vagina and uterus: the Intergroup Rhabdomyosarcoma Study. *J Pediatr Surg* 1985;20:718–724.
55. Hendrickson MR, Kempson RL. Well-differentiated mucinous neoplasms of the ovary. *Pathol State Art Rev* 1993;1:307–334.
56. Herszfeld D, Wolvetang E, Langton-Bunker E, et al. CD30 is a survival factor and a biomarker for transformed human pluripotent stem cells. *Nat Biotechnol* 2006;24:351–357.
57. Hoei-Hansen CE, Kraggerud SM, Abeler VM, et al. Ovarian dysgerminomas are characterised by frequent KIT mutations and abundant expression of pluripotency markers. *Mol Cancer* 2007;6:12.
58. Hoffner L, Deka R, Chakravarti A. Cytogenetics and origins of pediatric germ cell tumors. *Cancer Genet Cytogenet* 1994;74:54–58.
59. Hoffner L, Shen-Schwarz S, Deka R, et al. Genetics and biology of human ovarian teratomas. III. Cytogenetics and origins of malignant ovarian germ cell tumors. *Cancer Genet Cytogenet* 1992;62:58–65.
60. Hollier LM, Cox SM. Syphilis. *Semin Perinatol* 1998;22:323–331.
61. Hornor G. Ano-genital herpes in children. *J Pediatr Health Care* 2006;20:106–114.
62. Hughesdon PE. Morphology and morphogenesis of the Stein-Leventhal ovary and of so- called "hyperthecosis". *Obstet Gynecol Surv* 1982;37:59–77.
63. Hyun G, Kolon TF. A practical approach to intersex in the newborn period. *Urol Clin North Am* 2004;31:435–443, viii.
64. Inoue M, Fujita M, Azuma C, et al. Histogenetic analysis of ovarian germ cell tumors by DNA fingerprinting. *Cancer Res* 1992;52: 6823–6826.
65. Jones DE, Russo JF, Dombroski RA, et al. Cervical intraepithelial neoplasia in adolescents. *J Adolesc Health Care* 1984;5:243–247.
66. Kaplan GW, Cromie WC, Kelalis PP, et al. Prepubertal yolk sac testicular tumors—report of the testicular tumor registry. *J Urol* 1988;140:1109–1112.
67. Kapoor G, Advani SH, Nair CN, et al. Pediatric germ cell tumor. *J Pediatr Hematol Oncol* 1995;17(4):318–324.
68. Kersemaekers AM, Honecker F, Stoop H, et al. Identification of germ cells at risk for neoplastic transformation in gonadoblastoma: an immunohistochemical study for OCT3/4 and TSPY. *Hum Pathol* 2005;36:512–521.
69. Kobayashi A, Chang H, Chaboissier MC, et al. Sox9 in testis determination. *Ann N Y Acad Sci* 2005;1061:9–17.
70. Koo CH, Reifel J, Kogut N, et al. True histiocytic malignancy associated with a malignant teratoma in a patient with 46XY gonadal dysgenesis. *Am J Surg Pathol* 1992;16:175–183.
71. Krause I, Uziel Y, Guedj D, et al. Childhood Behcet's disease: clinical features and comparison with adult-onset disease. *Rheumatology (Oxford)* 1999;38:457–462.
72. Krauss CM, Turksoy RN, Atkins L, et al. Familial premature ovarian failure due to an interstitial deletion of the long arm of the X chromosome. *N Engl J Med* 1987;317:125–131.
73. Kurman RJ, Ganjei P, Nadji M. Contributions of immunocytochemistry to the diagnosis and study of ovarian neoplasms. *Int J Gynecol Pathol* 1984;3:3–26.
74. La Vecchia C, Draper GJ, Franceschi S. Childhood nonovarian female genital tract cancers in Britain, 1962–1978. Descriptive epidemiology and long-term survival. *Cancer* 1984;54:188–192.
75. Lacson AG, Gillis DA, Shawwa A. Malignant mixed germ-cell-sex cord-stromal tumors of the ovary associated with isosexual precocious puberty. *Cancer* 1988;61:2122–2133.
76. Lacy J, Capra M, Allen L. Endodermal sinus tumor of the infant vagina treated exclusively with chemotherapy. *J Pediatr Hematol Oncol* 2006;28:768–771.
77. Latza U, Fossa SD, Durkop H, et al. CD30 antigen in embryonal carcinoma and embryogenesis and release of the soluble molecule. *Am J Pathol* 1995;146:463–471.
78. Lee PA, Houk CP, Ahmed SF, et al. Consensus statement on management of intersex disorders. International Consensus Conference on Intersex. *Pediatrics* 2006;118:e488–e500.
79. Leuschner I, Harms D, Mattke A, et al. Rhabdomyosarcoma of the urinary bladder and vagina: a clinicopathologic study with emphasis on recurrent disease—a report from the Kiel Pediatric Tumor Registry and the German CWS Study. *Am J Surg Pathol* 2001;25: 856–864.
80. Linder D, McCaw BK, Hecht F. Parthenogenic origin of benign ovarian teratomas. *N Engl J Med* 1975;292:63–66.
81. Little M, Wells C. A clinical overview of WT1 gene mutations. *Hum Mutat* 1997;9:209–225.
82. Lu KH, Gershenson DM. Update on the management of ovarian germ cell tumors. *J Reprod Med* 2005;50:417–425.
83. Manivel JC, Dehner LP, Burke B. Ovarian tumorlike structures, biovular follicles, and binucleated oocytes in children: their frequency and possible pathologic significance. *Pediatr Pathol* 1988;8:283–292.
84. Manivel JC, Jessurun J, Wick MR, et al. Placental alkaline phosphatase immunoreactivity in testicular germ-cell neoplasms. *Am J Surg Pathol* 1987;11:21–29.
85. Marina NM, Cushing B, Giller R, et al. Complete surgical excision is effective treatment for children with immature teratomas with or without malignant elements: A Pediatric Oncology Group/Children's Cancer Group Intergroup Study. *J Clin Oncol* 1999;17:2137–2143.
86. Martelli H, Oberlin O, Rey A, et al. Conservative treatment for girls with nonmetastatic rhabdomyosarcoma of the genital tract: a report from the Study Committee of the International Society of Pediatric Oncology. *J Clin Oncol* 1999;17:2117–2722.
87. Mascarello JT, Cajulis TR, Billman GF, et al. Ovarian germ cell tumor evolving to myelodysplasia. *Genes Chromosomes Cancer* 1993;7:227–230.
88. Maurer HM, Beltangady M, Gehan EA, et al. The Intergroup Rhabdomyosarcoma Study-I. A final report. *Cancer* 1988;61:209–220.
89. McCluggage WG, Oliva E, Connolly LE, et al. An immunohistochemical analysis of ovarian small cell carcinoma of hypercalcemic type. *Int J Gynecol Pathol* 2004;23:330–336.
90. Merke DP, Bornstein SR. Congenital adrenal hyperplasia. *Lancet* 2005;365:2125–2136.
91. Meskhi A, Seif MW. Premature ovarian failure. *Curr Opin Obstet Gynecol* 2006;18:418–426.
92. Mierau GW, Lovell MA, Wyatt-Ashmead J, et al. Benign mullerian papilloma of childhood. *Ultrastruct Pathol* 2005;29:209–216.
93. Migeon CJ, Wisniewski AB. Human sex differentiation and its abnormalities. *Best Pract Res Clin Obstet Gynaecol* 2003;17:1–18.
94. Moscicki AB. Genital HPV infections in children and adolescents. *Obstet Gynecol Clin North Am* 1996;23:675–697.

95. Muller J. Disturbance of pubertal development after cancer treatment. *Best Pract Res Clin Endocrinol Metab* 2002;16:91–103.
96. Nichols CR, Roth BJ, Heerema N, et al. Hematologic neoplasia associated with primary mediastinal germ-cell tumors. *N Engl J Med* 1990;322:1425–1429.
97. Nikolova G, Vilain E. Mechanisms of disease: transcription factors in sex determination—relevance to human disorders of sex development. *Nat Clin Pract Endocrinol Metab* 2006;2:231–238.
98. Norris HJ, Jensen RD. Relative frequency of ovarian neoplams in children and adolescents. *Cancer* 1972;30:713–719.
99. Norris HJ, Zirkin HJ, Benson WL. Immature (malignant) teratoma of the ovary: a clinical and pathologic study of 58 cases. *Cancer* 1976;37:2359–2372.
100. Nucci MR, Young RH, Fletcher CD. Cellular pseudosarcomatous fibroepithelial stromal polyps of the lower female genital tract: an underrecognized lesion often misdiagnosed as sarcoma. *Am J Surg Pathol* 2000;24:231–240.
101. O'Connor DM, Norris HJ. The influence of grade on the outcome of stage I ovarian immature (malignant) teratomas and the reproducibility of grading. *Int J Gynecol Pathol* 1994;13:283–289.
102. O'Rahilly R, Muller F. *Human embroyology and teratology*, 3rd ed. New York: Wiley-Liss, 2001.
103. Ohama K, Nomura K, Okamoto E, et al. Origin of immature teratoma of the ovary. *Am J Obstet Gynecol* 1985;152:896–900.
104. Page DC, Mosher R, Simpson EM, et al. The sex-determining region of the human Y chromosome encodes a finger protein. *Cell* 1987;51:1091–1104.
105. Park SY, Jameson JL. Minireview: transcriptional regulation of gonadal development and differentiation. *Endocrinology* 2005;146:1035–1042.
106. Parker KL. The roles of steroidogenic factor 1 in endocrine development and function. *Mol Cell Endocrinol* 1998;140:59–63.
107. Pelliniemi LJ, Frojdman K, Sundstrom J, et al. Cellular and molecular changes during sex differentiation of embryonic mammalian gonads. *J Exp Zool* 1998;281:482–493.
108. Perrone T, Steeper TA, Dehner LP. Alpha-fetoprotein localization in pure ovarian teratoma: an immunohistochemical study of 12 cases. *Am J Clin Pathol* 1987;88:713–717.
109. Perrone T, Steiner M, Dehner LP. Nodal gliomatosis and alpha-fetoprotein production: two unusual facets of grade I ovarian teratoma. *Arch Pathol Lab Med* 1986;110:975–977.
110. Pescovitz OH, Comite F, Hench K, et al. The NIH experience with precocious puberty: diagnostic subgroups and response to short-term luteinizing hormone releasing hormone analogue therapy. *J Pediatr* 1986;108:47–54.
111. Powell JJ, Wojnarowska F. Lichen sclerosus. *Lancet* 1999;353: 1777–1783.
112. Prat J, Young RH, Scully RE. Ovarian Sertoli-Leydig cell tumors with heterologous elements. II. Cartilage and skeletal muscle: a clinicopathologic analysis of twelve cases. *Cancer* 1982;50: 2465–2475.
113. Pryse-Davies J. The development, structure and function of the female pelvic organs in childhood. *Clin Obstet Gynaecol* 1974;1:483–508.
114. Pul M, Yilmaz N, Gurses N, et al. Vaginal polyp in a newborn: a case report and review of the literature. *Clin Pediatr (Phila)* 1990;29:346.
115. Rey R. Anti-Mullerian hormone in disorders of sex determination and differentiation. *Arq Bras Endocrinol Metabol* 2005; 49:26–36.
116. Riopel M, Perlman EJ, Seidman JD, et al. Inhibin and epithelial membrane antigen immunohistochemistry assist in the diagnosis of sex cord-stromal tumors and provide clues to the histogenesis of hypercalcemic small cell carcinomas. *Int J Gynecol Pathol* 1998;17:46–53.
117. Riopel MA, Ronnett BM, Kurman RJ. Evaluation of diagnostic criteria and behavior of ovarian intestinal-type mucinous tumors: atypical proliferative (borderline) tumors and intraepithelial, microinvasive, invasive, and metastatic carcinomas [In Process Citation]. *Am J Surg Pathol* 1999;23:617–635.
118. Riopel MA, Spellerberg A, Griffin CA, et al. Genetic analysis of ovarian germ cell tumors by comparative genomic hybridization. *Cancer Res* 1998;58:3105–3110.
119. Risser WL, Bortot AT, Benjamins LJ, et al. The epidemiology of sexually transmitted infections in adolescents. *Semin Pediatr Infect Dis* 2005;16:160–167.
120. Rizzo N, Gabrielli S, Perolo A, et al. Prenatal diagnosis and management of fetal ovarian cysts. *Prenat Diagn* 1989;9:97–103.
121. Robboy SJ, Miller T, Donahoe PK, et al. Dysgenesis of testicular and streak gonads in the syndrome of mixed gonadal dysgenesis: perspective derived from a clinicopathologic analysis of twenty-one cases. *Hum Pathol* 1982;13:700–716.
122. Rock JA, Azziz R. Genital anomalies in childhood. *Clin Obstet Gynecol* 1987;30:682–696.
123. Roden R, Wu TC. How will HPV vaccines affect cervical cancer? *Nat Rev Cancer* 2006;6:753–763.
124. Saitoh A, Tsutsumi Y, Osamura RY, et al. Sclerosing stromal tumor of the ovary: immunohistochemical and electron-microscopic demonstration of smooth-muscle differentiation. *Arch Pathol Lab Med* 1989;113:372–376.
125. Sakane T, Takeno M, Suzuki N, et al. Behcet's disease. *N Engl J Med* 1999;341:1284–1291.
126. Salo P, Kaariainen H, Petrovic V, et al. Molecular mapping of the putative gonadoblastoma locus on the Y chromosome. *Genes Chromosomes Cancer* 1995;14:210–214.
127. Sanfilippo JS, Wakim NG, Schikler KN, et al. Endometriosis in association with uterine anomaly. *Am J Obstet Gynecol* 1986;154:39–43.
128. Satoh M. Histogenesis and organogenesis of the gonad in human embryos. *J Anat* 1991;177:85–107.
129. Schedl A, Hastie N. Multiple roles for the Wilms' tumour suppressor gene, WT1 in genitourinary development. *Mol Cell Endocrinol* 1998;140:65–69.
130. Schrodt BJ, Callen JP. Metastatic Crohn's disease presenting as chronic perivulvar and perirectal ulcerations in an adolescent patient. *Pediatrics* 1999;103:500–502.
131. Scully RE. Gonadoblastoma: a review of 74 cases. *Cancer* 1970;25:1340–1356.
132. Scully RE. Gonadal pathology of genetically determined diseases. In: Kraus FT, and Damjanov I, eds. *The pathology of reproductive failure*. International Academy of Pathology Monograph #33. Baltimore: Williams and Wilkins, 1991.
133. Sedin G, Bergquist C, Lindgren PG. Ovarian hyperstimulation syndrome in preterm infants. *Pediatr Res* 1985;19:548–552.
134. Seidman JD, Kurman RJ. Ovarian serous borderline tumors: a critical review of the literature with emphasis on prognostic indicators. *Hum Pathol* 2000 May;31(5):539–557.
135. Sharma Y, Bajpai A, Mittal S, et al. Ovarian cysts in young girls with hypothyroidism: follow-up and effect of treatment. *J Pediatr Endocrinol Metab* 2006;19:895–900.
136. Shebib S, Sabbah RS, Sackey K, et al. Endodermal sinus (yolk sac) tumor in infants and children. *Am J Pediatr Hematol Oncol* 1989;11:36–39.
137. Silva EG, Tornos C, Zhuang Z, et al. Tumor recurrence in Stage I ovarian serous neoplasms of low malignant potential. *Int J Gynecol Pathol* 1998;17:1–6.
138. Sinnecker G, Willig RP, Stahnke N, et al. Precocious pseudopuberty associated with multiple ovarian follicular cysts and low plasma oestradiol concentrations. *Eur J Pediatr* 1989;148:600–602.
139. Smith YR, Quint EH, Hinton EL. Recurrent benign mullerian papilloma of the cervix. *J Pediatr Adolesc Gynecol* 1998;11:29–31.
140. Sobel V, Zhu YS, Imperato-McGinley J. Fetal hormones and sexual differentiation. *Obstet Gynecol Clin North Am* 2004;31:837-xi.
141. Spence JEH, Dewhurst SJ. The vulva and its anomalies in the newborn. *Pediatr Adolesc Gynecol* 1984;2:83.

142. Stenwig JT, Hazekamp JT, Beecham JB. Granulosa cell tumors of the ovary: a clinicopathological study of 118 cases with long-term follow-up. *Gynecol Oncol* 1979;7:136–152.
143. Surti U, Hoffner L, Chakravarti A, et al. Genetics and biology of human ovarian teratomas. I. Cytogenetic analysis and mechanism of origin. *Am J Hum Genet* 1990;47:635–643.
144. Talerman A. Germ cell tumors. In: Talerman A, Roth LM, eds. *Pathology of the testis and its adnexa*. New York: Churchill Livingstone, 29–65, 1986.
145. The Rotterdam ESHRE/ASRM-Sponsored PCOS consensus workshop group. Revised 2003 consensus on diagnostic criteria and long-term health risks related to polycystic ovary syndrome (PCOS). *Hum Reprod* 2004;19:41–47.
146. Troche V, Hernandez E. Neoplasia arising in dysgenetic gonads. *Obstet Gynecol Surv* 1986;41:74–79.
147. Tsuchiya K, Reijo R, Page DC, et al. Gonadoblastoma: molecular definition of the susceptibility region on the Y chromosome. *Am J Hum Genet* 1995;57:1400–1407.
148. Ulbright T, Roth L. Recent developments in the pathology of germ cell tumors. *Semin Diagn Pathol* 1987;4:304–319.
149. Ulbright TM. Germ cell neoplasms of the testis. *Am J Surg Pathol* 1993;17:1075–1091.
150. Ulbright TM, Roth LM, Brodhecker CA. Yolk sac differentiation in germ cell tumors. *Am J Surg Pathol* 1986;10:151–164.
151. Vainio S, Heikkila M, Kispert A, et al. Female development in mammals is regulated by Wnt-4 signalling. *Nature* 1999;397:405–409.
152. Val P, Swain A. Mechanisms of disease: normal and abnormal gonadal development and sex determination in mammals. *Nat Clin Pract Urol* 2005;2:616–627.
153. van der Putte SC. Mammary-like glands of the vulva and their disorders. *Int J Gynecol Pathol* 1994;13:150–160.
154. Van Doren M, Broihier HT, Moore LA, et al. HMG-CoA reductase guides migrating primordial germ cells [see comments]. *Nature* 1998;396:466–469.
155. van Niekerk WA, Retief AE. The gonads of human true hermaphrodites. *Hum Genet* 1981;58:117–122.
156. Vassal G, Flamant F, Caillaud JM, et al. Juvenile granulosa cell tumor of the ovary in children: a clinical study of 15 cases. *J Clin Oncol* 1988;6:990–995.
157. Virgili A, Marzola A, Corazza M. Vulvar hidradenoma papilliferum: a review of 10.5 years' experience. *J Reprod Med* 2000;45:616–618.
158. Walsh SR, Hogg D, Mydlarski PR. Bullous pemphigoid: from bench to bedside. *Drugs* 2005;65:905–926.
159. Warner MA, Fleischer AC, Edell SL, et al. Uterine adnexal torsion: sonographic findings. *Radiology* 1985;154:773–775.
160. Webber LJ, Stubbs S, Stark J, et al. Formation and early development of follicles in the polycystic ovary. *Lancet* 2003;362:1017–1021.
161. Westhoff C, Pike M, Vessey M. Benign ovarian teratomas: a population-based case-control study. *Br J Cancer* 1988;58:93–98.
162. Williams SD. Current management of ovarian germ cell tumors. *Oncology* 1994;8:53–60.
163. Wylie C. Germ cells. *Cell* 1999;96:165–174.
164. Yamada G, Satoh Y, Baskin LS, et al. Cellular and molecular mechanisms of development of the external genitalia. *Differentiation* 2003;71:445–460.
165. Yamada G, Suzuki K, Haraguchi R, et al. Molecular genetic cascades for external genitalia formation: an emerging organogenesis program. *Dev Dyn* 2006;235:1738–1752.
166. Yao HH. The pathway to femaleness: current knowledge on embryonic development of the ovary. *Mol Cell Endocrinol* 2005;230:87–93.
167. Yilmaz Y, Turkyilmaz Z, Sonmez K, et al. Massive ovarian oedema in adolescents. *Acta Chir Belg* 2005;105:106–109.
168. Yin Y, Lin C, Ma L. MSX2 promotes vaginal epithelial differentiation and Wolffian duct regression and dampens the vaginal response to diethylstilbestrol. *Mol Endocrinol* 2006;20:1535–1546.
169. Yin Y, Ma L. Development of the mammalian female reproductive tract. *J Biochem (Tokyo)* 2005;137:677–683.
170. Young RH, Dickersin GR, Scully RE. Juvenile granulosa cell tumor of the ovary: a clinicopathological analysis of 125 cases. *Am J Surg Pathol* 1984;8:575–596.
171. Young RH, Oliva E, Scully RE. Small cell carcinoma of the ovary, hypercalcemic type: a clinicopathological analysis of 150 cases. *Am J Surg Pathol* 1994;18:1102–1116.
172. Young RH, Scully RE. Endodermal sinus tumor of the vagina: a report of nine cases and review of the literature. *Gynecol Oncol* 1984;18:380–392.
173. Young RH, Scully RE. Well-differentiated ovarian Sertoli-Leydig cell tumors: a clinicopathological analysis of 23 cases. *Int J Gynecol Pathol* 1984;3:277–290.
174. Young RH, Scully RE. Ovarian Sertoli-Leydig cell tumors: a clinicopathological analysis of 207 cases. *Am J Surg Pathol* 1985;9: 543–569.
175. Young RH, Scully RE. Ovarian sex cord-stromal and steroid cell tumors. In: Roth LM, Czernobilsky B, eds. *Tumors and tumorlike conditions of the ovary*. New York: Churchill-Livingstone, 1985.
176. Zachariou Z, Roth H, Boos R, et al. Three years' experience with large ovarian cysts diagnosed in utero. *J Pediatr Surg* 1989;24:478–482.
177. Zaloudek C, Kurman RJ. Recent advances in the pathology of ovarian cancer. *Clin Obstet Gynaecol* 1983;10:155–185.
178. Zaloudek C, Norris HJ. Sertoli-Leydig tumors of the ovary: a clinicopathologic study of 64 intermediate and poorly differentiated neoplasms. *Am J Surg Pathol* 1984;8:405–418.
179. Zeisler H, Mayerhofer K, Joura EA, et al. Embryonal rhabdomyosarcoma of the uterine cervix: case report and review of the literature. *Gynecol Oncol* 1998;69:78–83.
180. Zhang M, Cheung MK, Shin JY, et al. Prognostic factors responsible for survival in sex cord stromal tumors of the ovary: an analysis of 376 women. *Gynecol Oncol* 2007;104:396–400.

CHAPTER 19

The Male Reproductive System, Including Intersex Disorders

HIKMAT A. AL-AHMADIE

THE TESTIS

Testicular Development and Disorders

Normal sexual development and differentiation is the result of a complex process of genetic, molecular, and endocrine mechanisms that are necessary for the development of the genitourinary system including the kidneys as well as the adrenals. Chromosomal sex (genotype) is established at fertilization, and from the bipotential gonads the male genotype (46,XY) leads to the development of the testis through a series of sex chromosome–linked and autosomal genes. The testis in turn secretes essential hormones for the development of the external male genitalia (phenotype) (36). A normal 46,XX female has ovarian and müllerian duct development because the Y chromosome is instrumental in the suppression of the female reproductive tract. Of the genes involved in the formation of the bipotential gonads, *WT1* (Wilms tumor gene), *NR5A1* (nuclear receptor subfamily 5, which encodes the steroidogenic factor-1, *SF-1*), and *LIM1* are perhaps the most important (36,52) These events are triggered by *SRY* (sex-determining region of the Y) located on the distal tip of the short arm of the Y chromosome (e77,25,31,52,e323,60).

The *SRY* gene encodes a protein that acts on the HMG (high mobility group) DNA-binding domain in somatic cells in the urogenital ridge to differentiate into Sertoli cells, the first differentiated cell type of the testis (36,e317,e541). Although *SRY* is the essential determinant of testicular development, various autosomal genes, downstream from *SYR*, are involved in this process including *WT1*, *SF-1*, *DAX-1* (dosage-sensitive sex reversal, adrenal hypoplasia critical region, on chromosome X, gene 1), and *SOX9* (SRY-box 9) (e208,e223,e270,e354,e418,70,e419).

Embryologically, the urogenital ridges appear at around the 4th week of gestation and are initially devoid of germ cells. By the 5th week, primordial germ cells migrate to the genital ridge and are arranged into the seminiferous cords. Up to the 6th week, both male and female gonads appear relatively similar. By the 7th week of gestation, the testes are formed with recognizable short, straight cellular tubules and are functioning with the synthesis of antimüllerian hormone (AMH, müllerian-inhibiting substance, müllerian-inhibiting factor) by the Sertoli cells, which develop from the somatic sex cord cells; and subsequently testosterone by the Leydig cells, which develop from the intercordal gonadal mesenchyme in the 8th week (6,9,e78,e355). The intercordal mesenchyme is composed of cells that migrate from the mesonephric stroma that eventually differentiate into testicular stromal cells and blood vessels in addition to Leydig cells. The produced hormones are essential as AMH plays a major role in the process of regression of the müllerian ducts and upper vagina, whereas testosterone is crucial for the differentiation of the wolffian ducts, epididymis, vas deferens, and seminal vesicles. The rete testis develops from the mesonephric remnants in proximity to the seminiferous cords. Development of a dense fibrous tunica albuginea in the 8th week of gestation is definitive for testis formation. Testosterone synthesis peaks at 12 to 16 weeks of gestation, allowing for male secondary sexual development concurrent with the appearance of AMH (75,e593). The remaining structures of the male genital system are derived from the urogenital sinus through the differentiation of the endoderm-derived epithelium into prostate, urethra, bulbourethral, and periurethral glands. In contrast, the wolffian duct derivatives are of mesodermal origin (20). The differentiation of the wolffian duct occurs under the influence of testosterone secreted by the ipsilateral testis. The differentiation of the urogenital sinus into male external genitalia occurs under the influence of dihydrotestosterone (DHT), which derives from testosterone by enzymatic conversion by 5α-reductase. Two additional hormones FSH (follicle-stimulating hormone) and LH (luteinizing hormone) play important roles in the development of the male genital system mainly in the last months of gestation, regulating androgen production and Sertoli cell activity (e138,e144).

The actions and the timing of these hormones are closely and precisely coordinated during development (20,e228,e588). After birth, the testis continues to develop until puberty with changes affecting all testicular components until puberty.

Congenital and Developmental Anomalies

A congenital or a developmental anomaly in the testis may be an insolated finding or it may be associated with a sexual maldevelopment syndrome that may or may not have an underlying cytogenetic defect. The most common presentation of these conditions is an "undescended" testis or an ambiguous external genitalia. Monorchidism, or the presence of a single testicle, may be due to a testicular regression syndrome (TRS) (discussed later), vascular injury, cryptorchidism, or another congenital anomaly.

Polyorchidism, or duplication of the testis, is a rare condition, with about 100 cases reported in the literature. This condition usually manifests as triorchidism but bilateral duplication has been also reported (42,e291). Clinically, two masses within the hemiscrotum, inguinal swelling and an undescended testis, or pain, are the usual presentations. Associated conditions include those related to anomalies in the processus vaginalis (hernia, hydrocele), testicular maldescent, intermittent torsion, epididymitis and varicocele, as well as malignant neoplasms (e72,e620). The duplicate testis develops due to a division or duplication in the genital ridge and is suggested to result from an abnormal division of the urogenital ridge before the 8th week of gestation (e85). The most common variant is that of a supernumerary testis sharing an epididymis with the primary testis, but other variants include a vascular pedicle with no epididymis, an independent blind epididymis, or a shared vas deferens (e85,e537). The duplicate testis is smaller than a normal testis and its torsion is more frequent. The microscopic appearance ranges from normal testicular tissue with intact spermatogenesis to disorganized seminiferous tubules with diminished spermatogenesis. Rare associated chromosomal anomalies have been reported (e72).

Cystic dysplasia of the testis is a rare congenital malformation first reported by Leissring and Oppenheimer in 1973 (e304), presenting as testicular enlargement due to cystic dilation of the rete testis. It is thought to result from an embryologic defect around the 5th week of gestation preventing the connection of the rete testis (afferent seminiferous tubule derived) with the efferent tubules (mesonephric or wolffian derived). The failure of such connection leads to degeneration of the mediastinum testis into small cysts with progressive dilation compressing and replacing the adjacent testicular parenchyma. Ipsilateral renal agenesis and multicystic dysplasia of the kidney are the most common associated anomaly (e141,e322). Histopathologic features include multiple, anastomosing, irregular cystic spaces of varying sizes and shapes predominantly located in the region of the mediastinum testis but also displacing the testicular parenchyma, which becomes subsequently compressed under the tunica albuginea. The cystic lining is flat epithelial resembling that of the rete testis (e184). Spontaneous regression of this lesion has been recently reported after conservative management in one case (e555).

Prepubertal macroorchidism is an idiopathic condition in most cases but may be associated with McCune-Albright syndrome, juvenile hypothyroidism, and fragile X syndrome (e524,e586). Histopathologic findings include some enlargement of the seminiferous tubules and thickening of tubular basement membrane. The tubules contain Sertoli cells and scattered Leydig cells are usually present in the interstitium. Focal mild interstitial fibrosis, occasional tubules containing only Sertoli cells, and focal paucity of Leydig cells are some of the pathological findings. Some have attributed the testicular enlargement in the absence of other findings to interstitial edema and obstruction. In one report, continuous splenogonadal fusion was reported in association with macroorchidism (e528).

Vascular anomalies of the testis are rare and include angiomatous malformations and congenital lymphangiectasis. Angiomatous malformation is a rare cause of testicular enlargement and consists of numerous thin-walled vascular channels (e505). Congenital lymphangiectasis has been reported with bilateral cryptorchidism and with Noonan syndrome, manifested by numerous ectatic and irregular lymphatic channels with frequent anastomoses and seminiferous tubules with decreased diameter, immature Sertoli cells, reduced spermatogenesis, and peritubular fibrosis (e397). Similar finding, however, have also been reported in the testes of infants without other abnormalities at autopsy (e393).

Cryptorchidism or undescended testis, where either one or both testes fail to migrate to the base of the scrotum, is one of the most common genitourinary disorders in male children, affecting 4% to 5% of full-term and 9% to 30% of premature males at birth (28,e231,86). Based on many recently published series, there has been an increase in the incidence of cryptorchidism over recent decades in North America and Europe (87). The cryptorchid testis can be found in any position along its usual line of descent including intra-abdominally; however, approximately 80% will be located in the inguinal region, just outside the inguinal canal and 20% to 27% of cryptorchid testes are impalpable (e86,e273,e564). Rarely, ectopic locations outside the normal line of descent have been reported that included the perineum, base of penis, abdominal wall, pubic region, and upper thigh (e230). The majority of undescended testes will achieve full spontaneous descent by 1 year of age, predominantly within the first 3 months, and only 0.8% of infants would have incomplete descent 12 months after birth. Spontaneous testicular descent after the first year is very unlikely (19,e342,86,91). A number of studies have reported an increased rate of undescended testis with low birth weight, maternal pre-eclampsia, mild gestational diabetes, and breech presentation (e249,e591). Bilateral testicular maldescent was reported in as high as 39% of babies with cryptorchidism, which was also more likely to occur in babies with low birth weights.

In addition to the presence of a patent processus vaginalis in most cryptorchid patients, other abnormalities can occur especially those pertaining to the genitourinary tract, which includes dysgenetic testis, duplication of the ureter, hypospadias, renal dysplasia, and inguinal hernia (e111,e163,93). Of the most common associations with cryptorchidism are malformations in the paratesticular structures such as the epididymis and its attachment to the vas deferens and gubernaculum (e1,3,e151). In a study by Favorito et al. (e150), the reported incidence of epididymal abnormalities in normal male fetuses was only 4% compared with 35% in patients with cryptorchidism. The most common of these anomalies is detachment between the epididymis and the testis followed by separation of the epididymis from the vas deferens and the long looping epididymis (e206).

Outside the genitourinary tract, abnormalities may include gastroschisis, omphalocele, imperforate anus, cardiac anomalies, lower limb anomalies, and caudal spinal malformations (e109,e277,e300). It has been reported that the etiologies of cryptorchidism and hypospadias are partly shared and the presence of both conditions simultaneously is associated with increased risk for ambiguous external genitalia and intersex disorders (e8,e255,93).

Multiple causes for testicular maldescent have been suggested including an abnormal differentiation of the male sexual organs, midline abnormalities, anatomical anomalies of the gubernaculum testis, hormonal dysfunction affecting the hypothalamo-pituitary-testicular axis (hypogonadotropic hypogonadism), mechanical impairment (insufficient intra-abdominal pressure, short spermatic cord, underdeveloped processus vaginalis), and heredity (e109,e232).

The prepubertal undescended testis is usually smaller than the contralateral one and the difference becomes even more significant with progressive lesions (e86). Generally, there is correlation between the age at the time of orchiopexy or orchiectomy and the severity of the histologic alterations in the testis. The isolated cryptorchid testis in the prepubertal child has only subtle quantitative abnormalities such as decreased percentage of tubules containing germ cells (low tubular fertility index), decreased mean tubular diameter, apparent tubular loss, and early interstitial fibrosis (e83,e361,67) (Figure 19-1). The postpubertal and adult cryptorchid testis usually exhibits abnormalities in all testicular structures characterized by tubular sclerosis, maturational arrest in spermatogenesis, and interstitial fibrosis (e432). Tubules with immature Sertoli cells only (Sertoli cell nodules) may also be found (Figure 19-2), and areas of Leydig cell hyperplasia are frequent (e396,e416). Granular transformation and degeneration of Sertoli cells have been

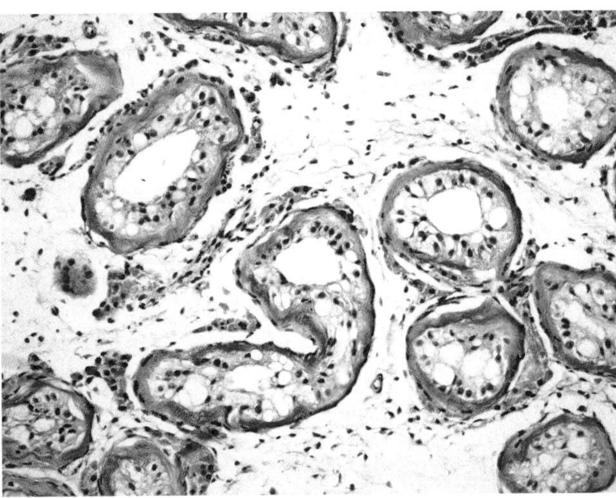

FIGURE 19-1 ■ Cryptorchid testis. Atrophic seminiferous tubules characterized by irregular contour, thickened basement membrane, and lack of spermatogenesis with Sertoli-only pattern. Loose fibrous interstitial stroma is evident.

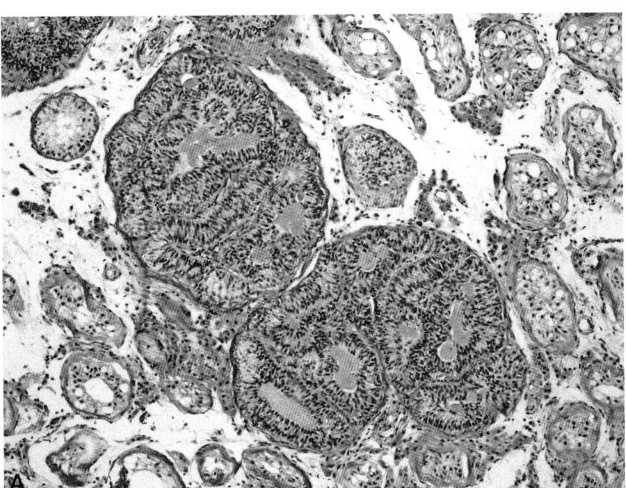

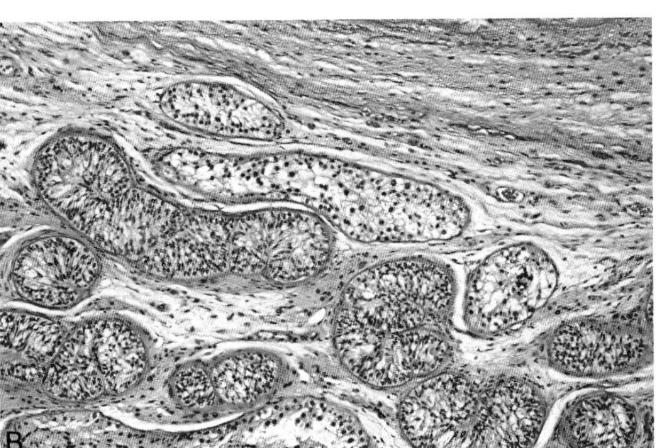

FIGURE 19-2 ■ **A:** Sertoli cell nodule in a cryptorchid testis. A well-circumscribed, nodular proliferation of immature Sertoli cells filling the seminiferous tubules with central hyaline foci. The surrounding testicular tissue is atrophic. Note the presence of Leydig cells in the interstitial area. **B:** We have encountered similar proliferation adjacent to a MGCT in an adolescent.

reported in the cryptorchid testis, as well as in other testicular disorders (e392,78). Similar histopathologic features were also identified in retractile testis, indicating that these conditions may share some causal relationships and that they may require similar management approach (e100,e207). Some changes in the rete testis have been reported particularly in postpubertal cryptorchid testis including adenomatous features or dysgenesis with hypoplastic changes (e106,e395).

The relationship between cryptorchidism and male infertility has been extensively studied, and links between the two conditions have been made in a number of series. Cryptorchidism was reported as the cause of infertility in up to 9% of cases (e80). Biopsies from cryptorchid testes may reveal lack of germ cells as early as 18 months of age, the incidence of which increases with advanced age and with bilaterality (15). Similar trends were observed even in patients who underwent orchiopexy, implying that the actual development of germ cells in cryptorchidism might also be impaired (15,37,59). Some authors, however, cast some doubt on the level of certainty of this causative relationship between cryptorchidism and infertility and advocate that while it is certain that untreated men with bilateral abdominal testes will be infertile, the levels of fertility are unpredictable in other less severe scenarios (unilateral cryptorchidism, inguinal testes, orchiopexy) (e563).

Another important association with cryptorchidism is the increased risk of developing testicular germ cell tumors (GCT), especially seminoma, compared with normally descended testes. It is estimated that the risk of testicular cancer in cryptorchid males is four times higher than that of the general population and approximately 10% of testicular cancer patients had cryptorchidism. The unrepaired cryptorchid testis has a 7% to 35% likelihood of developing a malignant germ cell tumor, especially seminoma (4,5,e50,e163,e183,e438,e542). It has been shown that the risk of developing a malignancy increases with an abdominal testis compared with an inguinal testis and also with those treated with orchiopexy postpubertal (15,e434,e598). In the latter case, the tubules are arrested in maturation.

Disorders of Sex Development (Intersex Disorders)

The term *intersex disorders* has been largely used to refer primarily to a clinical scenario of an infant born with external genitalia sufficiently ambiguous that sex assignment is not possible. However, the mechanisms underlying such a clinical scenario are variable and some disorders in sex development do not necessarily present with genital ambiguity. It has been recently recommended to use the term disorders of sex development (DSD) to replace such terms as *intersex*, *hermaphrodite*, and *pseudohermaphrodite* (38,76). DSD represents a congenital condition characterized by discordance between phenotypic sex and chromosomal sex and in which development of chromosomal, gonadal, or anatomic sex is atypical. Recent advances in molecular biology have enabled us to further our understanding of the processes involving normal sexual differentiation and the inborn errors that result in sexual ambiguity, which has led to improvement in diagnosing and managing patients with DSD (49,e324,76). It is estimated that two-third of sexually ambiguous neonates are female pseudohermaphrodites with congenital adrenal hyperplasia (e607). The remaining DSD are associated with some abnormality in male gonadal development or persistence of the müllerian tract with or without an abnormal constitutional karyotype.

Currently, the classification of DSD can be organized by broader categories in which the intersexual disorders are divided into "abnormalities of genital differentiation," due largely to the abnormal production or sensitivity of a single hormone, or "abnormalities in sex determination," due to abnormal gonadal differentiation, usually testicular, with or without chromosomal aberration (see Table 19-1) (e369,76) (see Chapter 18).

Disorders of Genital Differentiation

These disorders are generally associated with a normal chromosomal composition and normal gonads. This includes female and male pseudohermaphroditism.

Female pseudohermaphroditism occurs as a result of relative androgen excess *in utero* in an individual with two ovaries and a 46,XX genotype. The elevated levels of androgen present during embryogenesis usually result in genital ambiguity and may result in a male phenotype. The most common cause is the **adrenogenital syndrome** (AGS, congenital adrenal hyperplasia). The manifestations of AGS in genotypically female patients are related to defects in the biosynthetic pathways of mineralocorticoid, glucocorticoid, and sex steroids (e81). In males with AGS, usually there is no evidence of genital ambiguity, but they may have an enlarged phallus. They may also develop clinically detectable bilateral testicular nodules during childhood or young adulthood that may be confused with true Leydig cell tumors (LCTs) and are designated as testicular *tumors* of the AGS (e468,80) (see Chapters 18 and 21).

A rare condition, **placental aromatase deficiency**, causes maternal virilization during pregnancy and pseudohermaphroditism of the female fetus. Due to mutations in the aromatase gene *CYP19* and the resulting lack of aromatase activity, fetal androstenedione cannot be converted to estrogen by the placenta and instead is converted to testosterone peripherally, resulting in virilization of both fetus and mother (e248,e512).

Other conditions that might be associated with female pseudohermaphroditism are related to maternal factors such as **maternal ingestion of synthetic progestins or androgens** or the presence of **maternal virilizing lesions** during pregnancy including a luteoma of pregnancy (e166,e343,76,e585).

Male pseudohermaphroditism represents a heterogeneous group of intersex conditions that occur in individuals with normal 46,XY karyotype and either identifiable testes or evidence that testes were present during fetal development

Table 19-1 ■ DISORDERS OF SEXUAL DEVELOPMENT

Disorders of genital differentiation	Female pseudohermaphroditism (female intersex)	Adrenogenital syndrome —21 α-hydroxylase deficiency —11 β-hydroxylase deficiency Placental aromatase defect Maternal ingestion of progestins or androgens Maternal virilizing lesions
	Male pseudohermaphroditism (male intersex)	Testicular regression syndrome Leydig cell deficiency (Defective hCG–LH receptor) Defects in testosterone synthesis: a. Testosterone and adrenocorticoid insufficiency —Defect in cholesterol synthesis (Smith–Lemli–Opitz syndrome) —Congenital lipoid adrenal hyperplasia (defect StAR gene) —Congenital adrenal hyperplasia (3 β-hydroxylase dehydrogenase deficiency, 17 α-hydroxylase deficiency) b. Testosterone insufficiency only —17, 20-desmolase deficiency —17 β-hydroxysteroid (17-ketosteroid reductase) dehydrogenase deficiency Defect in mullerian inhibiting system End-organ defects: a. Androgen receptor disorders (androgen insensitivity syndromes) —Complete testicular feminisation (androgen receptor insufficiency) —Partial androgen receptor insufficiency b. Disorder of peripheral testosterone metabolism —5-α-reductase type 2 deficiency
Disorders of sex determination		Klinefelter syndrome (47 XXY) Turner syndrome and Turner-like (45 XO and X mosaicism) XX male and XY female syndrome (sex reversal) Pure gonadal dysgenesis (bilateral) Defect in the Wilms tumour suppressor (WT1) gene —Denys–Drash syndrome —Frasier syndrome Mixed gonadal dysgenesis (Turner-like, dysgenetic male pseudohermaphroditism, gonadoblastoma) True hermaphroditism

Adapted with modification from Robboy SJ, Jaubert F. Neoplasms and pathology of sexual developmental disorders (intersex). *Pathology* 2007;39(1):147–163.

but the external genitalia are usually female or ambiguous (7,e386). The responsible defect may be: (a) at the gonad level, leading to disorders of testosterone biosynthesis and metabolism or testosterone receptor abnormalities; or deficiency in MIS gene, or (b) at the end organ level, where the developing tissues are unresponsive to androgen stimulation leading to an abnormal phenotype. Other less well-defined causes may also be responsible.

Gonadal defects responsible for male pseudohermaphroditism include TRS, agenesis or deficiency of the Leydig cells, defects in specific enzymes in the pathway of testosterone or DHT biosynthesis or receptors to these hormones, or a defect in elaboration or action of MIS.

Testicular regression syndrome (TRS, congenital anorchia, vanishing testis) is a condition in which a testis is thought to have once existed but has atrophied and disappeared during early development (34,47). The testis is clinically impalpable and no normal testicular tissue can be identified following exploration. Generally, congenital absence of the testis, or testicular agenesis, is an uncommon anomaly as it was detected in less than 1% of testis both in fetuses and cryptorchid patients (e151). This condition results from the irreversible destruction of one or both testes during fetal life in an XY individual, resulting in variable hormonal deficiencies and developmental anomalies based on the stage at which testicular damage occurred (e333,62). Unilateral testicular destruction does not result in TRS. By histopathologic examination, the testis may be completely absent or represented by only a microscopic remnant. In addition to having no gonadal tissue, pathologic findings include a collection of vascularized fibroconnective tissue (85%), hemorrhage or hemosiderin deposition (70%), calcification (60%) or giant cells near the residual vas deferens or epididymis, the expected site of the gonad (e87,34,47,62,e526). The vas deferens ends blindly and a small and circumscribed nodule of tissue may be located in the retroperitoneum, the iliac fossa, or in the scrotum. By definition, no evidence of preserved remnants of seminiferous tubules should be present.

The clinical presentation of individuals with TRS is variable and is reflective of the specific stage of fetal development during which the testes were damaged. Generally, at one end of the spectrum, when gonadal regression occurs early in embryonic life before the testes release androgenic or antimullerian hormones, the testes are absent and the phenotype is female. At the other end, regression occurring later and through fetal life would allow for a male phenotype with infantile to nearly normal male genitalia and differentiated wollfian-derived structures. Affected individuals commonly have ambiguous genitalia. A number of etiologies have been proposed for TRS including inherited genetic defect, intrauterine infection, and infarction (e227,76).

It is presumed that testicular regression develops late in the fetal period after the mullerian structures regressed under the influence of the mullerian inhibitory substance and the male gonads and genitalia developed under the influence of the androgens. Despite the familial occurrences of TRS suggesting a genetic etiology, no specific genes have been identified to be associated with it and in particular those related to the opening reading frame sequence of SRY (e417). Unlike cryptorchidism, there is no increased risk of gonadal neoplasia, because there is little, if any, residual gonadal tissue.

Leydig cell deficiency (agenesis or hypoplasia) is a rare condition of male pseudohermaphroditism thought to be due to a defect in the human chorionic gonadotropin-LH receptor, primary agenesis or hypoplasia of the Leydig cells, or an abnormal LH receptor molecule (e26,e478,e497,e514). Affected individuals are genotypically males (46,XY) with female phenotype and unremarkable or ambiguous external genitalia. Bilateral, slightly small to normal-size cryptorchid testes are present with fully or partially developed epididymides and vasa deferentia, indicating that testosterone production by Leydig cells was intact early in embryonic development. The testes exhibit interstitial fibrosis, but no mature Leydig cells are present and no testosterone production is noted. LH levels are elevated in affected individuals. Tubules with Sertoli cells are found and mullerian structures are typically absent, indicating appropriate testicular production of MIS by Sertoli cells during fetal life (76,e487).

Familial occurrence of this condition has been reported and a number of mutations in the transmembrane domain of LH receptor gene, resulting in Leydig cell deficiency, have been identified (44,e307,e469,e618).

Defects in testosterone synthesis may be due to inborn errors of the enzymes involved in testosterone biosynthesis in the testis or the adrenal gland that may result in subnormal levels of testosterone and DHT during embryogenesis (relative estrogen excess) resulting in female or ambiguous external genitalia (e324,e388). These defects may involve cholesterol synthesis (mutations in 7-dehydrocholesterol reductase gene) as in Smith-Lemli-Opitz syndrome (e401,e615) or mutations in the steroidogenic enzymes responsible for the conversion of cholesterol to testosterone and DHT, which include: (a) steroidogenic acute regulatory protein (*StAR*) gene responsible for congenital lipoid adrenal hyperplasia (e34,e59,e97,e534), (b) 17α-hydroxylase (e65,e133) and 3β-hydroxylase dehydrogenase (e371,e517) responsible for congenital adrenal hyperplasia, and (c) 17-ketosteroid reductase (e426).

The degree to which the external genitalia develop depends upon the type and the severity of the defect. The microscopic features of testes in patients with these conditions vary and may show large clusters of Leydig cells surrounding seminiferous tubules. Germ cells (spermatogonia) are often normal in children but disappear by puberty resulting in Sertoli-only syndrome. Some germ cells, however, can persist and rarely develop into intratubular germ cell neoplasia (e280). Mullerian-derived structures are absent but wolffian duct structures may be present (76).

Defect in mullerian inhibiting system or the **persistent müllerian duct syndrome (PMDS)**, also referred to as *hernia uteri inguinale*, is a rare form of male pseudohermaphroditism characterized by the presence of mullerian duct structures in 46,XY phenotypic males. The age at diagnosis ranges from a neonate to the fourth decade. Most patients have unilateral or bilateral cryptorchid testes, normal or almost normal male external genitalia, and an inguinal hernia containing a prolapsed infantile uterus and fallopian tubes (8,e253,e334,e472). The testes may be histologically normal and the wolffian duct structures are developed with the vas deferens embedded in the wall of the upper vaginal structure in most cases. Inguinal hernias occur in almost 40% of cases (e583). Malignant testicular tumors such as intratubular germ cell neoplasia and seminoma have been rarely reported in cases of adult PMDS patients with uncorrected cryptorchid testis (e29,e258,e338,e611). More recently, rare examples of clear-cell adenocarcinoma of the müllerian duct and uterine adenosarcoma in a boy with PMDS have been reported (e511,e554). PMDS has been reported with a familial occurrence and rarely in identical male twins (e44,e149,e234,e359,e605).

PMDS is currently considered a heterogeneous group of disorders caused by at least two different defects in the mullerian inhibiting system. The most common is a defect in the *MIS* (mullerian inhibiting substance) gene, also known as *AMH* (anti-mullerian hormone) gene preventing it from producing any biologically functional MIS. The second defect involves an abnormal AMH type II receptor resulting in end-organ insensitivity to MIS despite the presence of biologically active MIS. In other patients, an abnormality in the timing of MIS secretion may exist (e45,e234,e252).

End-Organ Defects

As mentioned earlier, responsiveness to androgen is required to the normal development of the external genitalia and

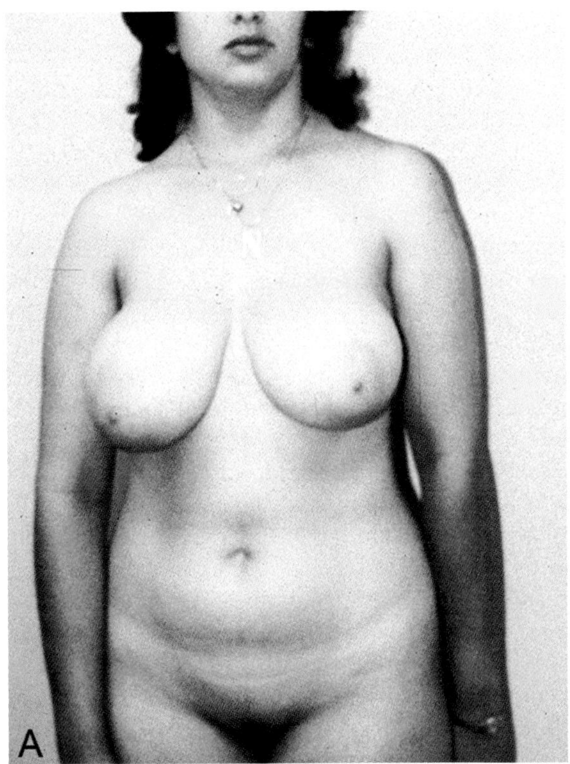

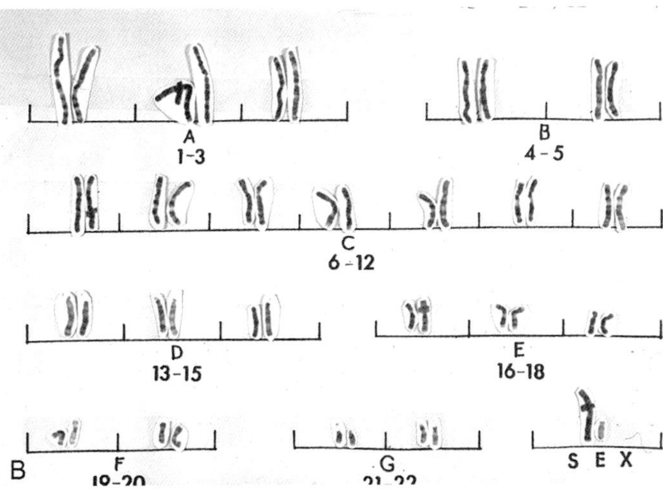

FIGURE 19-3■Testicular feminization. **A:** In this example of complete testicular feminization, a fully developed female phenotype is evident. **B:** The karyotype is that of a male (Contributed by Dr. Jerome Taxy, Chicago, Illinois).

wolffian duct–derived structures. The presence of the enzyme 5α-reductase in the anlage of the prostate and external genitalia is also required for the conversion of testosterone to DHT. An absent or unstable androgen receptor in 46,XY individuals leads to impaired development of both wolffian duct–derived structures as well as external genitalia. If only 5α-reductase is absent or defective, abnormalities confined to the external genitalia and prostate will be observed.

Androgen receptor disorders (androgen insensitivity syndromes) result in variable phenotypes ranging from a female phenotype with intra-abdominal testes to ambiguous genitalia to a male phenotype with minimal clinical abnormalities.

Complete testicular feminization due to **complete androgen insensitivity** (e.g., testicular feminization, Goldberg-Maxwell-Morris syndrome, hairless women, androgen receptor insufficiency) is the most common form of male pseudohermaphroditism occurring in 1 of 20,000 newborns (e6,e386,e422,e486,e601). It is caused by failure of androgen receptor binding despite its production and secretion by the fetal testis. The underlying mechanisms have been identified as mutations in the androgen receptor gene including point mutations resulting in amino acid substitutions or premature stopcodons, frame shift mutations by nucleotide insertions or deletions, complete or partial gene deletion, or intronic mutations affecting the splicing of the androgen receptor RNA (e63).

Due to the presence of phenotypically female external genitalia (Figure 19-3), the condition is rarely diagnosed before puberty unless an inguinal hernia or labial mass is encountered or unless the disorder is known to be familial (e14,e589). Primary amenorrhea is the most common complaint leading to evaluation and subsequent diagnosis. The wolffian tract involutes resulting in cystic epididymides that are usually not connected to the testes. The vasa differentia, seminal vesicles, and prostate are absent. As a rule, both the cervix and the uterine corpus are absent. A fragment of fallopian tube may be found in up to one-third of cases (76,e486).

The testes are cryptorchid and may be intra-abdominal or inguinal, or in the labia majora and 50% are found in inguinal hernias. Overall, the testes in androgen insensitivity syndrome are histologically similar to the cryptorchid testis except that the tubules are less mature with possible spermatogonia but no spermatogenesis. Leydig cells are absent or replaced by collagenized interstitial tissue in portions of the gonad, whereas sheets of Leydig cells may be found near the hilus and nerves. Ovarian-like stroma replaces the testicular interstitium. Hamartomas and Sertoli cell adenomas were reported in the majority of cases in the postpubertal testis (e381,e463,e486,e514). These hamartomatous nodules are multiple, bilateral, tan, yellow, or white in appearance with bulging cut surface and may be composed of immature Sertoli cells, germ cells, Leydig cells, ovarian-type stroma, nonspecific fibrous stroma, and smooth muscle. The typical size varies from 1 to 10 mm, but may occasionally be up to 40 mm (e486). Sertoli cell adenomas consist of nodules of predominantly or exclusively packed seminiferous tubules with immature Sertoli cells that are 3 cm in average size but range up to 25 cm (e486). A rare example of a testicular tumor resembling the sex cord with annular tubules has been reported (e457). GCT, particularly seminoma and less commonly intratubular germ cell neoplasia, can sometimes be encountered in patients with this syndrome and, rarely, sex cord–stromal tumors have been reported (e158,76,e404,e619). The development of malignant gonadal tumors in patients with testicular feminization usually occurs later in adulthood (e332).

Partial androgen insensitivity syndrome due to partial androgen receptor insufficiency accounts for 10% of all cases of androgen insensitivity (e487) and encompasses several different phenotypes, ranging from individuals with a predominantly female appearance to persons with ambiguous genitalia, or individuals with a predominantly male phenotype (e63). Affected patients typically present at birth with genital ambiguity but severe hypospadias, micropenis, bifid scrotum, and bilateral cryptorchidism are also common. Alternatively, the external genital phenotype may be predominantly female with partial labial fusion and clitoromegaly (e610). The underlying mechanism involves a qualitative defect in the androgen receptor (e195,e440,e498). Additionally, a number of syndromes and conditions are characterized by partial androgen insensitivity including Reifenstein, Lubs, Gilbert-Dreyfus, Rosewater and the infertile male syndromes, and Kennedy disease (e196,e295,e430,e614).

A disorder of peripheral testosterone metabolism is caused by mutation in the enzyme 5α-reductase type 2, which is responsible for converting testosterone to DHT to exert its effect on differentiating the urogenital sinus into external male genitalia and prostate (e19,e235,e613). Affected males usually have female to ambiguous external genitalia at birth (e153,e519,e522). The penis is small (clitoris-like) and lacks a urethral orifice. A blind vaginal pouch and inguinal or labial testes may be observed. Wolffian-derived structures are normal but no mullerian-derived structures are present. Due to activation of type 1 isoenzyme, some virilization occurs at puberty demonstrated by penile enlargement, scrotal rugation and hyperpigmentation, and testicular enlargement and descent. Microscopic findings of testicular tissue may include spermatogenesis, tubular atrophy, no spermatogenesis, or Leydig cell hyperplasia. The prostate remains rudimentary and the seminal vesicles remain underdeveloped (76).

Disorders of Sexual Determination

These disorders are generally associated with sex chromosome abnormalities resulting in abnormal gonad formation. Affected individuals characteristically have additions, deletions, or mosaicism of the sex chromosomes and the appearance of the gonads is variable, ranging from a streak gonad to a nearly normal female or male both grossly and microscopically.

Mixed gonadal dysgenesis (MGD) is one of the most frequent causes of male sexual ambiguity in individuals usually with a 45,X/46,XY or 46,XY karyotype. In one series, MGD was the diagnosis in approximately 8% of children with intersex conditions (e53). It represents a heterogeneous group of abnormalities characterized by persistent mullerian duct structures, a dysgenetic testis and a contralateral streak gonad (e15,7,e353,e369). The phenotypical heterogeneity of MGD is attributed to the presence of a variety of different genetic abnormalities causing the syndrome mostly related to deletions of both the short and the long arms of chromosome Y (e92,e224,e551).

The loss of testicular functions leads to incomplete inhibition of mullerian development, incomplete differentiation of wolffian duct structures, and incomplete male development of the external genitalia. Testicular maldescent may also occur (e369,e474) and some patients have phenotypical features of a Turner-like syndrome (e275,e551). An infantile or rudimentary uterus and at least one fallopian tube are found on the side with the uncommitted streak gonad. An intra-abdominal or inguinal cryptorchid testis or fibrous streak dysgenetic testis without an accompanying fallopian tube is present on the contralateral side. Organs of wolffian duct derivation may be present with variable frequency. An epididymis is identified in two-third of cases and is usually present on the side where there is a testis. The vas deferens is encountered less frequently and the seminal vesicle is identified only rarely.

The gonad may be a testis or a streak gonad (Figure 19-4). Streak gonads may show partial differentiation into testicular phenotype, or may exhibit features toward ovarian differentiation with the characteristic ovarian type stroma and rare primordial follicles. However, no true ovary is present, which requires the presence of differentiation with follicles in at least the antral stage (76). A unilateral macroscopic testis is found in 60% of cases, whereas bilateral testes may be seen in about 15% of cases usually with an asynchronous degree of maturity.

The testicular architecture is consistently abnormal in these individuals as the region of the tunica albuginea or cortex contains widely spaced seminiferous tubules with ovarian-like stroma or immature primary sex cords indeterminate between female and male structures. The medullary region may contain normal seminiferous tubules and interstitium, but in some cases it is difficult to distinguish between female and male structures. Occasional narrow closed seminiferous tubules are lined by Sertoli cells and in other examples the germ cells may be seen directly lining the basement membrane of the seminiferous tubule without the Sertoli cell layer that usually normally surrounds them. Leydig cells may be present in small clusters of varying size. Occasionally, broad zones of the cortex may exhibit a degree of differentiation toward streak-like ovary, even displaying rare primordial follicles. By puberty, the germ cells present in

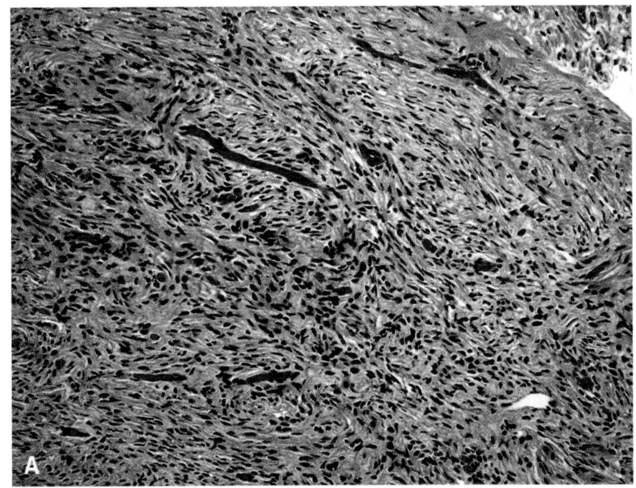

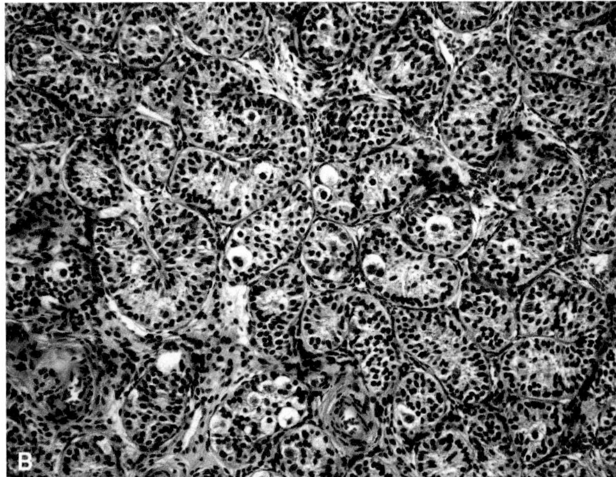

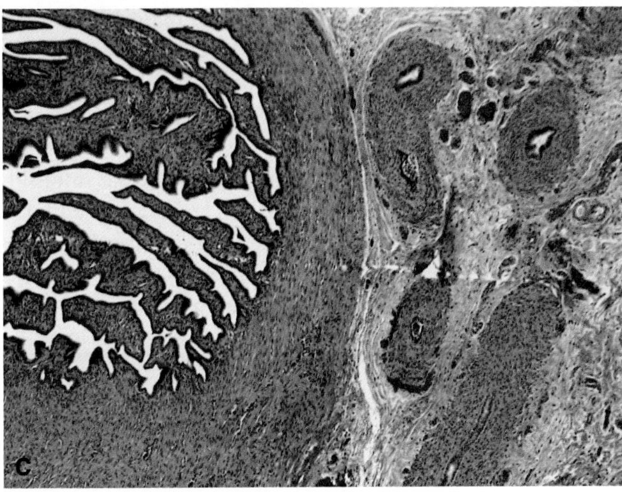

FIGURE 19-4 ■ Mixed gonadal dysgenesis in a 3-year-old patient with a female phenotype. **A:** On one side, an intra-abdominal streak gonad was present consisting of vascularized fibrous stroma. **B:** The contralateral side contained an immature cryptorchid testis with predominant Sertoli cells and only occasional spermatogonia. **C:** Bilaterally, structures of both wolffian (vas deferens) and mullerian (fallopian tube) origins were present.

a streak gonad may degenerate and disappear, resulting in a gonad composed exclusively of fibrous tissue and a few rete tubules. The hilar region of the streak gonad or streak testis is populated by hilus cells and rete or mesonephric tubules. Hyperplasia of the hilus cells in response to pituitary gonadotropins may result in clinical virilization. Tumors develop in about 10% of those with MGD and the dysgenetic gonads of which 25% to 30% are malignant, the most common of which is gonadoblastoma accounting for 75% to 80% of all germ cell neoplasms in this disorder. However, other GCT have been also reported including germinoma, yolk sac tumor (YST), teratoma, embryonal carcinoma (EC), and choriocarcinoma (e102,e165,e427,e474). These tumors may be unilateral or bilateral. Occasionally, Sertoli cell tumor and SCT-like proliferations of sex-cord elements have been also reported (e102,e399). Early gonadal resection is recommended in order to avoid the development of an invasive germ cell tumor and to avoid the consequences of onset of virilization in a patient who has been raised as a female.

Pure gonadal dysgenesis (PGD) refers to phenotypically female individuals with streak gonads and internal genitalia that include mullerian structures (uterus and fallopian tubes). It occurs with both 46,XX and 46,XY karyotypes and has both familial and sporadic patterns of inheritance (e199,e336). The stroma of the gonads has an ovarian-like appearance (e451) and primary amenorrhea is the usual clinical presentation. PGD patients with 46,XX karyotype only rarely develop gonadal tumors, examples of which include GCT and mucinous epithelial tumors (e298,e370,e383). Some have hilus cell hyperplasia and hilus cell tumors with the usual associated virilizing effects.

PGD patients with 46,XY karyotype are at higher risk for gonadoblastoma and other GCTs that may develop in 10% to 25% of cases and can be unilateral or bilateral (e139,285, e486,e487,82,e451,88).

True hermaphroditism (TH) is a disorder of gonadal differentiation defined by the concurrence of both ovarian and testicular tissue, with coexistent ovarian follicles (not just connective tissue stroma) and seminiferous tubules (not just Leydig cells). The gonads may be ovary and testis separately or combined in an ovotestis (76,95). Affected individuals may have either a female or a male phenotype with variable degrees of sexual ambiguity. The clinical manifestations are variable and depend on the gonadal tissue present and the age at the time of diagnosis. TH is a rare condition both in North American and Europe but is more commonly encountered in Africa, especially in South Africa (e198,30,45,e581).

The architecture and the distribution of gonadal tissues in TH take several forms with asymmetry of the gonads in the majority of cases. An ovotestis represents the most frequently encountered type of gonad in this condition (1,45,e581,95). Patterns of gonadal development include an ovary on one side and a testis on the other (30% of cases), or an ovary on one side and a contralateral ovotestis (30%). Bilateral ovotestes are found in 20% or more of true hermaphrodites and a testis-ovotestis combination is found in 10% of cases. In the majority of cases (80%), the ovarian and the testicular tissues are arranged in an end-to-end fashion with a distinct line demarcating the two tissues. The ovary, which is the second most common gonad in TH, preferentially develops on the left side whereas the testis, which is the least common gonad encountered in TH, develops preferentially on the right (76). The location of the gonad is influenced by the type and the quantity of gonadal tissue present. Increasing amounts of ovarian tissue increase the probability that the gonad will be in an ovarian position, and as a result it is very unlikely for female gonadal tissue (either ovary or ovotestis) to be situated in the inguinal canal or in the labioscrotal fold. The position of the testis is less constant as most reside in the scrotum but can be encountered in the inguinal region or in the normal ovarian position. The nature of the genital structure adjacent to a gonad in TH follows that of the ipsilateral gonad, which is characterized by having a fallopian tube adjacent to an ovary and an epididymis or vas deferens adjacent to a testis. Either a mullerian (more commonly) or wolffian structure, but not both, is adjacent to an ovotestis.

In young patients, the microscopic appearance of the gonadal tissue is often normal with the ovarian tissue containing numerous follicles, whereas the testicular parenchyma has normal appearing seminiferous tubules with spermatogonia. In older patients, ovarian tissue with structures indicative of ovulation (follicles, corpora lutea, and corpora albicantia) may be seen, but the testicular tissue (in testis or ovotestis) is usually abnormal with incomplete development, lack of spermatogenesis, loss of germ cells, and tubular sclerosis. Scrotal testes in these patients show less severe changes, sometimes showing faulty spermatogenesis (76).

The prevalence of gonadal neoplasms, mainly gonadoblastoma and other types of malignant germ cell neoplasms, is estimated at 2% to 3% of cases (e272,50,e487,e545). A rare case of juvenile granulosa cell tumor (JGCT) in this setting has been reported (e547).

The causes of TH are probably as varied as the karyotypic expressions and genetic aberrations appear to play a key role in its development. Patients with a "Y" chromosome have a 2- to 3-fold increased frequency of having a testis as opposed to an ovotestis, and nearly 75% of true hermaphrodites with an ovary and an ovotestis have a 46,XX karyotype. A 46,XX/46,XY karyotype represents true genetic chimerism, whereas the 46,XX karyotype is very likely to represent a crossing over of the X and Y chromosome during first meiotic division in the primary spermatocyte, or the presence of hidden mosaicism for *SRY* (30,e121,e413,e449,e488,e558). There are examples where the patients were 46,XX and lacked the *SRY* gene in usual cells examined (leukocytes) but cells from the gonad itself demonstrated *SRY* (e243). Autosomal dominant mutations that mimic *SRY* have been suggested as one possibility where *SRY* was absent (e459,e523). The 46,XY karyotype probably contains a hidden 46,XX cell line or that *SRY*, if present, may act at a time too late to stimulate the development of a testis, hence permitting ovarian tissue to develop.

Klinefelter syndrome (KS) is one of the most common causes of prepubertal delay and primary hypogonadism in males, occurring in about 1 of every 500 to 1 of every 1,000 live newborn males and accounting for about 3% of infertile males (e55,46,69,76,e608). In the majority of cases, the karyotype is 47,XXY, which usually results from nondisjunction occurring during meiosis of either paternal or maternal gametes. The clinical picture varies depending on the age when the diagnosis is first suspected. Men with KS present with sequels of androgen deficiency like infertility, low testosterone, erectile dysfunction, and low bone mineral density. They typically are tall men with narrow shoulders, broad hips, sparse body hair, gynecomastia, small testicles, and azoospermia. Infants with KS may have normal external male genitalia at birth, which may cause a delay in its discovery. However, in some individuals, other findings may be indicative of this syndrome such as hypospadia, micropenis, and small, soft testes or cryptorchidism. In adults with KS, the testes are small and rarely exceed 2 cm in greatest dimension. Histologically, the seminiferous tubules may show some degenerative changes during fetal life, which increases with age to the point that by late childhood the primary spermatogonia are greatly decreased in number. This degenerative process may dramatically accelerate shortly before the expected time of puberty (e9). In adults, the testes are largely atrophic with hyalinized seminiferous tubules and prominence of Leydig cells. Some tubules may be preserved, but lined only by Sertoli cells. Functionally, the Leydig cells are abnormal, as evidenced by low levels of serum testosterone with elevated levels of serum LH and FSH.

A variety of neoplasms have been associated with KS including both gonadal and extragonadal GCTs. Most extragonadal tumors occur in the mediastinum as teratoma and EC (e5,e48,e118,e296,e350), but rare examples of primary intrapelvic seminoma have been reported (e293). In the testis, seminoma, teratoma, and EC have been encountered (e340,e462,e532). LCTs are rare (e408,e525). Men with KS are at a higher risk of developing breast carcinoma than men without KS. (e179,84). Additionally, various hematological malignancies have been reported in individuals with KS, including acute leukemia, chronic myeloid leukemia, and malignant lymphoma (e43,e159,e365,e405,e506).

Turner syndrome is a disorder of sexual differentiation that is discussed in detail elsewhere in the book, whereas

Turner-like mosaicism (45,X/46,XY) is part of the mixed gonadal dysgenesis discussed earlier (see Chapter 18).

XX Male and XY Female Syndrome (Sex Reversal)

The XX male syndrome is one of the rarest of all sex chromosome anomalies, occurring in about 1 of 24,000 newborn males and is characterized by a nearly normal but infertile phenotypical male with a 46,XX karyotype (e473,e549). Genotypically, XX males share many characteristics of men with KS as both groups have a generally masculine appearance, normal or near-normal external genitalia and azoospermia with associated small testes, prominent Leydig cells, and tubules lined only by Sertoli cells. XX males, however, are generally shorter in height, and the frequency of hypospadias and gynecomastia is higher. Prenatal diagnosis of this syndrome is currently possible due to the increasing application of prenatal ultrasonography and genetic analyses (e178). In some cases, the mechanism underlying this disorder has been identified as translocation of the *SRY* gene from the Y chromosome to the X chromosome during meiosis (e178,e578).

Rare cases of male-to-female sex reversal have been identified in which phenotypically female individuals with 46,XY karyotype are identified, with some of these cases involving duplication and translocations of the short arm of the "Y" chromosome (e41,e435,e584).

Defects in the Wilms Tumor (WT1) Suppressor Gene

Syndromic male pseudohermaphroditism with gonadal dysgenesis and other genitourinary tract anomalies is intertwined with several genes that are active in male sexual differentiation, and one of these is *WT1* on chromosome 11p13 (e580). The product of *WT1* is a zinc finger transcriptional factor for many growth factor genes and is expressed in the developing kidney, especially in the condensing mesenchyme, and elsewhere in the genital ridge, in particular the Sertoli cells of the fetal gonad and mesothelium (e219,e424,73). Constitutional mutations in *WT1* are found in the following syndromes: Denys-Drash syndrome (90% or more of cases), Frasier syndrome, and WAGR syndrome (e23,e38,13,e313).

Patients with **Denys-Drash syndrome** have the clinical triad of early renal failure secondary to diffuse mesangial sclerosis, Wilms tumor in most cases (20% bilateral), and male pseudohermaphroditism in children with a 46,XY karyotype (i.e., dysgenetic testes, cryptorchidism, and severe hypospadias with micropenis) (e240,e378). Multiple gonadal abnormalities are reported in association with this syndrome and include normal ovaries with signs of early ovarian failures, normal mullerian and wolffian ducts, and normal to dysgenetic testes (e241,e242). Gonadoblastoma(s) are known to develop in the dysgenetic gonads of a child with a 46,XY karyotype. Constitutional heterozygosity in *WT1* represents missense point mutations within exons 8 and 9 in this gene (e58,e108).

Frasier syndrome is rare and results from a mutated *WT1* gene, specifically mutation of intron 9 resulting from abnormal splicing that leads to an unbalanced ratio of the WT1 isoforms needed for normal development of the glomeruli and gonads (e38,e431). It is phenotypically similar to Denys-Drash syndrome with male pseudohermaphroditism (normal female external genitalia, streak gonads, and XY karyotype) and progressive nephropathy (e282,e543). The nephropathy is usually focal segmental glomerulosclerosis, which differs from the diffuse mesangial sclerosis seen in Denys-Dash syndrome. As a rule, Wilms tumors do not develop in the Frasier syndrome patients because the loss of KTS-positive isoform of the WT1 protein retains its tumor suppressor function (e389), but gonadoblastoma develops in the dysgenetic testis in the child with a 46,XY karyotype (e494,e600). Mutations in the donor splice site in intron 9 of *WT1* distinguish Frasier syndrome from Denys-Drash syndrome (e38).

WAGR syndrome, which includes Wilms tumor, aniridia, genitourinary anomalies, and mental retardation, is the phenotypic expression of the constitutional chromosomal deletion within the short arm of one copy of chromosome 11p13 that includes both *WT1* and *PAX6* (e173,e219,e475).

Acquired Abnormalities and Other Lesions

Torsion of the testis or its appendage occurs with a yearly incidence of approximately one in 4,000 males younger than 25 years and accounts for 60% to 90% of cases of acute scrotal pain and swelling in men up to 18 years of age (e76,e254,e437,e471). Torsion of the testicular appendages may be more common than actual torsion of the testis, especially in prepubertal males, whereas torsion of the testis is seen more often in adolescence, at the time when acute epididymoorchitis also becomes an important consideration in the differential diagnosis (e254,e471). Torsion of the testis in infancy is rare but is well documented, including its detection in the prenatal period (e32,e262,e441). Testicular torsion should be suspected in every boy with testicular pain and must be diagnosed quickly and accurately in order not to risk testicular viability. Imaging studies, including color Doppler ultrasonography and scintigraphy, can be very helpful especially in clinically equivocal cases (e382,e402,e471,603). Torsion usually occurs in the absence of any precipitating event (e400). However, in 4% to 8% of cases, it may be associated with trauma (e499) or other possible predisposing factors including an increase in testicular volume (often associated with puberty), testicular tumor, testicles with horizontal lie, a history of cryptorchidism, and a spermatic cord with a long intrascrotal portion (e22).

The pathology of testicular torsion is testicular ischemia whose degree depends on the duration of torsion and the degree of rotation of the spermatic cord. Ischemia can occur as soon as 4 hours after torsion and is almost certain after 24 hours. It has been reported that testicular salvage can be

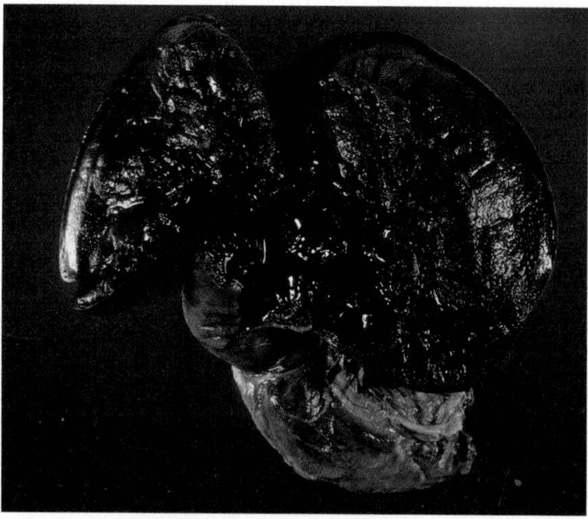

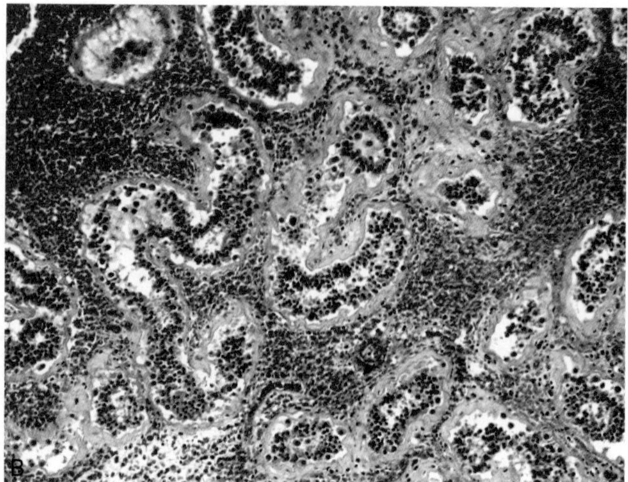

FIGURE 19-5 ■ Testicular torsion. **A:** The testis is congested with hemorrhagic cut section (Courtesy: Dr. Jerome Taxy, Chicago, Illinois). **B:** Microscopically, ischemic changes and features of hemorrhagic infarction are evident with sloughing of the seminiferous tubules and interstitial edema and hemorrhage.

achieved in approximately 90% of cases if treated within 6 hours from the onset of symptoms, but this rate falls to 50% after 12 hours and to less than 10% after 24 hours (e123). Greater degrees of rotation lead to a more rapid onset of ischemia (e471). Intermittent torsion with spontaneous resolution within 2 hours or less is a known clinical event (e114,e533).

Grossly, the testis is enlarged with a tense, bluish tunica albuginea and a dark, hemorrhagic appearance on cross sections (Figure 19-5). The epididymis has a similar appearance, and a spiral twist may or may not be seen in the spermatic cord. Little if any testicular parenchyma is appreciated through the hemorrhage. There is a sequence of microscopic changes in the testis that precede the final acute stage of near-total hemorrhagic infarction, starting with interstitial edema and hemorrhage and premature sloughing of germinal cells into the tubular lumina followed by diffuse interstitial hemorrhage and necrosis of germinal cells except for some viable seminiferous tubules beneath the tunica albuginea (e191,e192,e193,e360). Total necrosis of the testis is present in almost all cases of continuous torsion after 24 hours. Torsion of the testicular appendage results in a hemorrhagic cystic structure measuring up to 5 mm in diameter.

Two types of testicular torsion are recognized, with different ages at clinical presentation and anatomic location of the torsion. Extravaginal torsion (neonatal torsion, torsion of the spermatic cord) involves the testis, epididymis, and peritoneal coverings and results from spiraling on a vertical axis in the area of the external inguinal ring. This type accounts for approximately 6% of all torsion cases in childhood and occurs predominantly in neonates because the testis and the gubernaculum are free to rotate (e122). Most cases are unilateral, but some may occur bilaterally and may present as neonatal testicular enlargement if it occurred *in utero* (e261).

Intravaginal torsion (adolescent torsion) occurs when the testis, usually accompanied by the epididymis, is abnormally suspended and twists within the tunica vaginalis. This is caused by an abnormality of the processus vaginalis in which the tunica vaginalis covers not only the testis and the epididymis but also the spermatic cord. This creates a bell-clapper deformity, present in approximately 10% of all men (e74), which allows the testis to rotate freely within the tunica vaginalis (e471). The peak age of incidence of this type of torsion is between 12 and 18 years of age, and it accounts for up to 90% of torsions in later childhood and adolescence (e471,e616).

Epididymoorchitis produces symptoms very similar to those of torsion and generally manifests in adolescence (e471,e559). Acute scrotal pain on the basis of acute epididymoorchitis is found in 15% to 35% of cases in various pediatric series with this clinical presentation. Epididymoorchitis is uncommon in prepubertal boys, but has been reported in association with urinary tract infections with reflux or with an accompanying anorectal or related anomaly (e406,e483). A Gram-negative organism, such as *Salmonella* or *Escherichia coli*, may be identified as the causative pathogen (e123,e205). Tuberculous epididymoorchitis is reported in children in the less developed regions of the world (e344). Viral orchitis, especially mumps orchitis, has diminished with vaccination (e314,e331,e407). Testicular pain related to a vasculitis-associated orchitis has been reported in up to 22% of boys with Henoch-Schönlein purpura (e46,e124,e201).

Testicular microliths and calcified nodules are being more frequently identified recently due to the increased use of ultrasound as they produce hyperechogenic signals (e433) in up to 5% of healthy individuals. Histologically, they are concentric calcifications and their presence has been linked to cryptorchidism, testicular regression, silent torsion, and testicular GCT (e130,e168,e467).

Toxic injury to the testis in childhood can result in loss of germ cells, atrophy, and possible subfertility. Systemic chemotherapy and radiation of the testes or central nervous system are significant causes of testicular damage in survivors of childhood malignancy and in children who receive cyclophosphamide for renal diseases (e148,e290,e305,e502,e516). The prepubertal state of the testis does not protect the gonad from the late effects of treatment (e453). Decreased or absent spermatogenesis with Sertoli-only tubules, interstitial fibrosis, and testicular atrophy are the principal histologic findings. The effects of these medications are related to their cumulative doses (e132,e414,e576). Decreased testicular size correlates with decreased sperm production and inhibin B levels and increased levels of LH, FSH (e57,e516,e574). It has been suggested that despite these histologic effects, there is some recovery of spermatogenesis following aggressive chemotherapy when pharmacologic protection has been instituted (e287). Additionally, testicular tissue cryopreservation in prepubertal boys before chemotherapy and radiotherapy is now possible (e33,e560). Children with renal failure may experience a significant loss of spermatogonia per seminiferous tubule, which tends to increase with age but is not seen in all children with renal failure (e70).

Neoplasms of the Testis

Prepubertal testicular tumors are rare with an incidence of only between 0.5 and 2 per 100,000 children, accounting for approximately 1% to 2% of all pediatric solid neoplasms (40,e260,e303). They represent a diverse heterogeneous group of tumors of germ cell and non–germ cell origins (Table 19-2). Some of these tumors are associated with sexual maldevelopment syndromes with dysgenetic gonads, or cryptorchidism. As a result of the rarity of such tumors, the Section of Urology of the American Academy of Pediatrics established the Prepubertal Testicular Tumor Registry (PTTR) in order to compile clinical and pathological data from multiple institutions. Data from this registry have been published in a number of excellent studies and review papers (e211,51,e482). It was reported that approximately 30% of these tumors occur in the first year of life and about 7% occur in the neonatal period (51,e482). In earlier studies, the age of distribution was reported to be bimodal, with a peak in the first 5 years of life and a gradually increasing frequency in late adolescence (e2,e3,e194,e315).

The majority of pediatric testicular tumors are of germ cell origin followed in frequency by gonadal stromal tumors (e303,63,72,e482), whereas rhabdomyosarcoma (RMS) represents the most common tumor of the spermatic cord and paratesticular soft tissues (e372). In the newborn, however, the most frequent testicular tumor is JGCT (e89,33,48). A painless nontender scrotal mass is the presentation of the majority of prepubertal testicular neoplasms although, less commonly, the presentation may be that of testicular pain or trauma (e99,e303,e572,e573). Incidental testicular tumors during work-up for gynecomastia or precocious puberty have been reported in up to 10% of patients in one institution (e572). Adequate work-up of a testicular mass is important to determine its nature, first to select the appropriate management approach, and second to avoid misdiagnosis as a non-neoplastic condition that can potentially mimic testicular and paratesticular tumors. It has been reported that 5% to 23% of pediatric testicular tumors were misdiagnosed as torsion or hydrocele (e99,e103,e260,63,e572). Other conditions to be included in the differential diagnosis of a scrotal mass include hernia, hydrocele, hematoma/trauma, torsion, epididymitis, mumps orchitis, Henoch-Schönlein purpura, and paratesticular tumors.

A staging scheme by the Pediatric Oncology Group applies to pediatric GCT and is distinct from the adult counterpart (Table 19-3). The protocol for the examination of specimens from patients with malignant germ cell and sex cord–stromal tumors of the testis, exclusive of paratesticular malignancies, is useful in selected pediatric cases (89).

Table 19-2 ■ TESTICULAR TUMORS IN CHILDREN

Germ cell tumors	Yolk sac tumor	856
	Teratoma	439
	Epidermoid cyst	48
	Mixed germ cell tumor[a]	51
	Embryonal carcinoma	20
	Seminoma	7
	Dermoid cyst	5
	Choriocarcinoma	1
Gonadal-stromal tumors	Leydig cell tumor	27
	Sertoli cell tumor	29
	Juvenile granulosa cell tumor (JGCT)	12
	Stromal tumors, unspecified	37
Gonadoblastoma		5
Paratesticular tumors	Rhabdomyosarcoma	115
	Other sarcomas	5
	Other tumors, unspecified	26
Miscellaneous tumors		34
Total		1717

Compiled data from 12 series (e3, 10, e99, e152, e194, e260, e303, e306, 63, 72, e482, e538).
[a]Some of these tumors were designated *teratocarcinoma* in their original reports.

Table 19-3 ■ STAGING OF PEDIATRIC GCT BY THE PEDIATRIC ONCOLOGY GROUP

Stage I	Tumor limited to the testis. No clinical, radiographic, or histologic evidence of disease beyond the testis. Appropriate decline in serum AFP (AFP half-life = 5 days).
Stage II	Microscopic disease located in scrotum or high in spermatic cord (≤0.5 cm from proximal end). Retroperitoneal lymph node involvement (≤2 cm). Serum AFP persistently elevated.
Stage III	Retroperitoneal lymph node involvement (>2 cm). No visceral or extra-abdominal involvement.
Stage IV	Distant metastases.

Germ Cell Tumors

GCT are the most common primary tumors of the testis in the first two decades of life, 50% to 60% of which occur in the first 2 years (e152,e327). Significant differences exist between prepubertal testicular GCT and their adult (postpubertal) counterparts. While adult tumors usually comprise a mixed histology of seminomatous and nonseminomatous components, are most often malignant, and are almost always associated with intratubular germ cell neoplasia, prepubertal tumors typically contain only one histologic type (either teratoma or YST), can be benign or malignant, do not usually occur in undescended testes, and lack the intratubular germ cell neoplasia component (e260,54,74). These differences are also reflected in their respective genetic abnormalities. Prepubertal GCT are diploid (teratoma) or aneuploid (YST). Postpubertal GCT are hypertriploid (seminoma) or hypotriploid (nonseminoma) and consistently have one or more copies of the short arm of chromosome 12 [i(12p)]or other forms of 12p amplification (e260,53,74). Staging of pediatric GCT is distinct from that of the adult counterparts (Table 19-3) (22,39).

The most current World Health Organization (WHO) classification of testicular GCT divides them into tumors of one histological type, which includes seminoma, EC, YST, trophoblastic tumors and teratoma; and tumors with more than one histological type, which can contain any combination of any proportions of the pure forms (22). Consensus has now been reached concerning the prognostic factors that determine the outlook for patients with metastatic disease (39,71).

Despite the weak correlation of most etiologic factors with testicular GCT, it is generally believed that these tumors are associated with abnormal conditions in fetal life. A number of contributing factors are recognized including cryptorchidism, prior testicular GCT, family history of testicular GCT, and certain somatosexual ambiguity syndromes. Most of these factors, however, are important only in postpubertal boys and adults (e161,e577).

In GCT of the testis, generally three clinicopathologic entities are recognized: the teratomas—YSTs of the infantile testis, the seminomas and nonseminomas of adolescents and adults, and the spermatocytic seminomas. This chapter will focus on the former with highlights on the other entities as they relate to the pediatric population.

Yolk Sac Tumor

Formerly known as *endodermal sinus tumor*, YST is characterized by numerous patterns that recapitulate the yolk sac, allantois, and extraembryonic mesenchyme. The nosology has evolved from the concept of infantile adenocarcinoma, orchioblastoma, EC, and infantile EC to the current concept of a neoplasm with morphologic features recapitulating the extraembryonic yolk sac or endodermal sinus.

YST is the most common testicular GCT in childhood, accounting for as much as 75% of prepubertal testicular GCT (e152,40,e599). Despite its occurrence in all races, it is much more common in Whites than in Blacks, Native Americans, and Indians (e107,e311) and may be more common in Orientals when compared to Caucasians (e257). The median age at presentation is 16 to 19 months (40,e482,e552). YST is more commonly present in the right testis and the most common presenting symptom is a painless scrotal mass (40). Other possible complaints include a history of trauma, acute onset of pain, and hydrocele. At least one case has been reported in an intra-abdominal testis (e113). Serum α-fetoprotein (AFP) levels are elevated in more than 90% of tumors in a number of studies including those that are based on data from the PTTR (40,e482,e552). It is important to remember that normal AFP ranges in young infants are higher than those in older patients. Usually, YST is not hormonally active rendering precocious puberty an unlikely presentation. Most tumors are not associated with cryptorchidism or a dysgenetic gonad. Intratubular germ cell neoplasia is not observed in the adjacent testis in children with pure YST in contrast to its ubiquitous presence in testicular GCT in adolescents and young adults (57). By ultrasonography, YST is typically solid hypoechoic and devoid of cystic structures, which when present within the mass, argue against the diagnosis of YST (e210). Approximately 10% to 20% of children with YST will present with metastases (29,40,e482), which can occur hematogenously or via lymphatic drainage, unlike adult YST, which metastasizes predominantly through lymphatics. Hematogenous spread alone can occur in up to 40% of cases (29). YST metastases to the lung occur in 20% of cases compared with 4% to 6% to the retroperitoneal lymph nodes (e66,29,e617). The lungs represent the most common site of metastasis followed by retroperitoneal lymph nodes, liver, and bones (83). When metastases develop, they usually appear within 14 months of initial presentation (29,e221,40).

Grossly, pure YST is solid and soft with a pale gray to pale yellow cut surface, which can sometimes be gelatinous or mucoid (32,40). Hemorrhage and necrosis may be observed in large tumors; however, their presence (and/or that of cysts) should raise the possibility of a mixed GCT, especially in the adolescent (e544).

Microscopically, the histopathological appearance of YST is similar in both the pre- and postpubertal age groups. Several patterns are recognized that are usually admixed in variable proportions (Figure 19-6). It is not unusual for one pattern to predominate; however, it is rare that an entire tumor comprises a pure single histologic pattern (32,40,e544). The most common histologic pattern is the *microcystic or reticular pattern*, which consists of meshwork of vacuolated cells producing a honeycomb appearance, often with hyaline globules. Tumor cells are usually small and may contain pale eosinophilic secretions (32,e550). The *endodermal sinus pattern* consists of papillary structures known as *Schiller-Duval bodies*, which are considered the hallmark of YST, even though they are not required for the diagnosis. These structures consist of a stalk of connective tissue with thin-walled blood vessels lined on the surface by a layer of cuboidal cells with clear cytoplasm and prominent nucleoli. Other recognized microscopic patterns include: *solid, macrocystic, glandular-alveolar, papillary,*

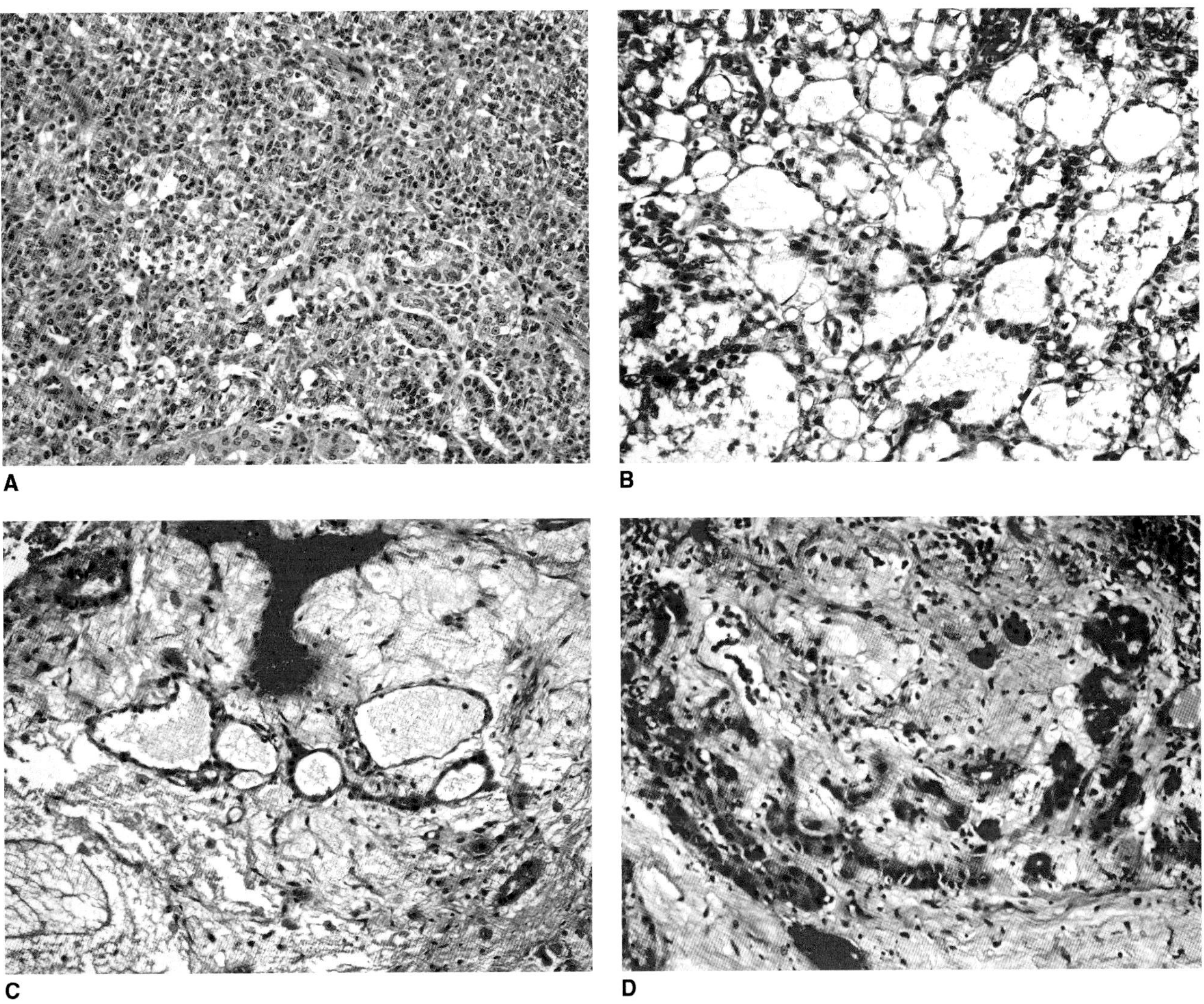

FIGURE 19-6 ■ Yolk sac tumor. **A-D:** Predominantly solid and focal glandular pattern (**A**), microcystic pattern (**B**), tubular/macrocystic pattern (**C**), and hepatoid pattern (**D**). Note the myxoid and hypocellular background (**C**,**D**).

myxomatous, polyvesicular vitelline, hepatoid and enteric patterns (Figure 19-6). Mitotic activity can be brisk in any of these patterns. Hyaline globules may be seen especially in the hepatoid and enteric patterns (e239,e570). By immunohistochemistry, expression of AFP is helpful but can be variable and sometimes weak. Its absence, however, does not exclude the diagnosis of YST. Low molecular weight cytokeratin is usually strongly expressed. A number of proteins, usually present in the fetal liver, may also be expressed in YST such as α-1-antitrypsin, albumin, and ferritin (e237,e239). Genetic analysis of infantile YST did not identify a specific gene or genes involved in its development. However, a number of recurrent genetic anomalies are known to occur including losses of the short arm of chromosome 1 (particularly the 1p36 region), the long arm of chromosomes 6 (6q21–26) and 16 and gains in the long arms of chromosomes 1 and 20 (20q13), the short arm of chromosome 3 (3p21-pter), and the complete chromosome 22 (e225,64,71,e579,90).

The treatment of choice for prepubertal YST is surgical excision (i.e., radical orchiectomy). Metastatic work-up is required for adequate staging of tumor and serum AFP is important in establishing the preoperative diagnosis and also as a follow-up postoperatively for possible tumor recurrence (e103,e210,e482).

Teratoma

Teratoma is a tumor composed of several types of tissue representing different germinal layers (endoderm, mesoderm, and ectoderm), forming somatic-type tissue in various stages of maturation and differentiation (11) for which the term *mature* or *immature* (fetal-like) apply. However, based on findings of genetic studies, it is now recommended to consider teratoma as a single entity regardless of the degree of maturation and differentiation of the tissue comprising it (22). Tumors consisting of ectoderm, mesoderm, or endoderm only are classified as monodermal teratomas. In its pure form, teratoma comprises approximately 3% of testicular GCT in adults and up to 38% of the prepubertal GCT (11,e597) with a reported incidence that ranges from 0.5 to 2.0

cases per 100,000 boys (e66). Teratoma is the second most common testicular tumor in children and adolescents following YST with a relative frequency ranging from 13% to 60% (e66,e67,10,29,e315,e482). About 65% of prepubertal teratomas occur in the first 2 years of life with a mean age of 20 months and represent 50% of GCT seen in the first decade of life (e373).

Most patients present with a firm, irregular, nodular, and nontender scrotal mass that usually does not transilluminate. Approximately 2% to 3% of prepubertal teratomas may be associated with or misdiagnosed as hydroceles, especially if the tumor has a cystic component. Teratomas usually present as a unilateral scrotal mass (e66), but rare examples of bilaterality in infancy and childhood have been reported (e3,e216,e320,e548,85). Teratomas in undescended, intra-abdominal testes may present with abdominal pain due to torsion, as calcification or ossification on imaging studies, or as an abdominal mass (e12,e142). Prenatal sonographic diagnosis might be possible in cases of fetal abdominal mass, especially when the testis cannot be detected in the scrotum by the 8th month (e345,e508). It is speculated that the undescended testis did not cause the neoplasia, but was induced by it (e379). Teratomas are hormonally inactive; hence, precocious puberty is not a common presentation and serum AFP levels are helpful in distinguishing them from YST (29,e485).

By imaging studies, teratomas are generally well-circumscribed and heterogeneous masses and a cystic component is commonly demonstrated (26). On gross examination, teratomas are usually nodular and firm with a variably cystic and solid cut surface (Figure 19-7A). The cysts may be filled with keratinous material or clear serous or mucoid fluid. The solid areas may contain translucent, gray-white nodules representing cartilage. Rarely, hair or melanin-containing tissue may also be seen. Areas of immature tissue are mostly solid and may have an encephaloid, hemorrhagic, or necrotic appearance.

Microscopically, mature elements resemble normal postnatal tissue and typically include structures derived from the three germ layers (Figure 19-7B). Structures of ectodermal origin are usually manifested by nests of squamous epithelium

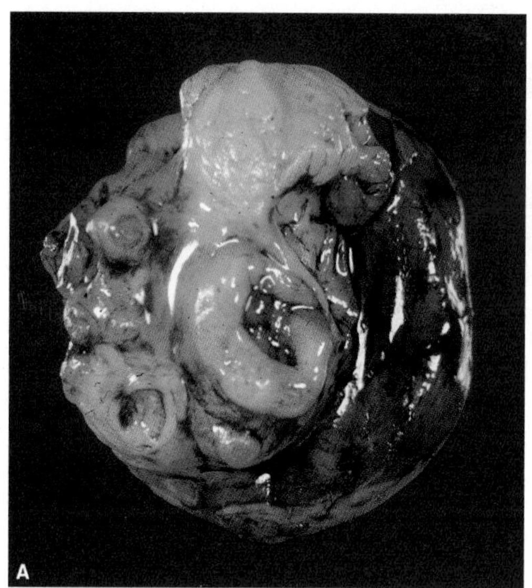

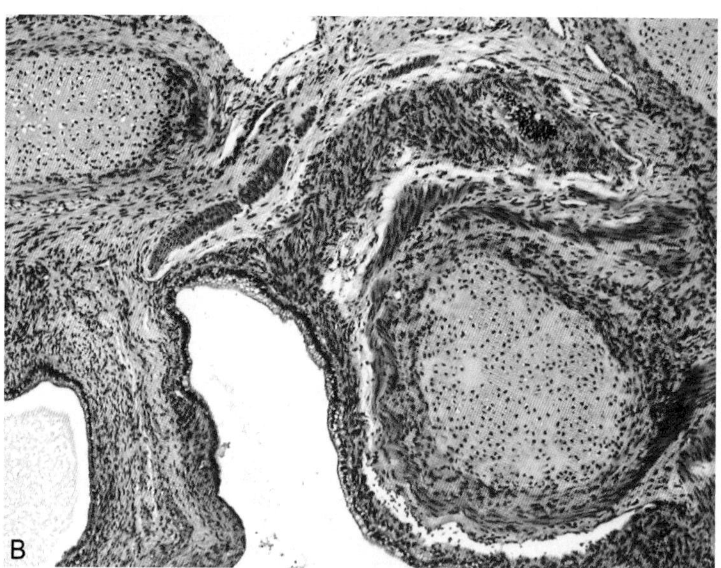

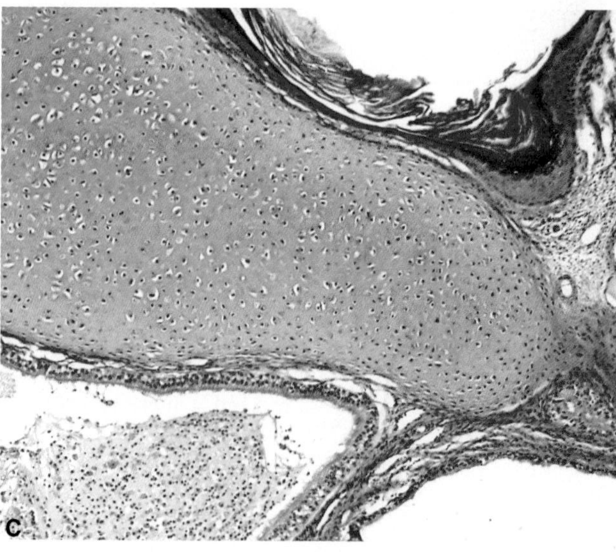

FIGURE 19-7 ■ Teratoma in a prepubertal testis. **A:** Grossly, the tumor has a heterogeneous multinodular appearance with cystic and solid areas. (Courtesy: Dr. Jerome Taxy, Chicago, Illinois). **B, C:** Microscopically, a mixture of mature structures derived from ectoderm, mesoderm, and endoderm is noted, characterized by keratinizing squamous epithelium, ciliated respiratory type epithelium, and mature cartilage.

with or without cyst formation and keratinization. Neural tissue may be encountered as foci of neuroglia. Structures of endodermal origin are represented by glandular epithelium of enteric or respiratory type. Other glandular tissue such as pancreatic, mucus producing epithelium, prostate, and thyroid may be found. Mesodermal elements are represented by cartilage, bone, adipose tissue, fibrous tissue, and, most commonly, muscle. Attempts at organ formation are frequently identified with smooth muscle encircling glands of respiratory or enteric morphology. Immature, fetal-type tissue may also consist of ectodermal, endodermal, and/or mesodermal elements. It usually occurs as islands of immature neuroepithelium resembling that of the developing embryonic neural tube. Immature tissue may also have an organoid arrangement with blastomatous and primitive tubular structures resembling that of the developing kidney or lung. Embryonic skeletal muscle, cartilage, and nonspecific cellular stroma may also be encountered (32,11,e337,e373). The so-called *fetus in fetu* is an expression of extreme maturation and organization of a teratoma or a form of pathologic monozygotic twinning (e12). A number of somatic type malignancies have developed in pediatric testicular teratomas some of which developed following irradiation for a testicular teratoma with metastases. These included Wilms tumor, leiomyosarcoma, angiosarcoma, and RMS (e568,e569).

Infantile teratomas are diploid. Genetic studies (karyotyping and comparative genomic hybridization) have failed to demonstrate chromosomal changes in these tumors. In contrast, teratomas in adult testes are hypotriploid and have genetic changes similar to those seen in other components of adult GCT (e367,64,71,90).

The prognosis is excellent in children since teratomas are universally benign tumors, unlike their adult counterpart (11,e211,e450). Pure teratoma of the prepubertal testis has not been reported to metastasize and does not develop, at least in the overwhelming majority of cases, from the lesion recognized as intratubular germ cell neoplasia, unclassified (89). Although orchiectomy has been considered the treatment of choice for prepubertal testicular teratomas, recent studies with long-term follow-up have demonstrated the safety and efficacy of testis-sparing surgery (77,e485).

Epidermoid Cyst

Epidermoid cyst is a benign tumor of ectodermal origin, characterized by its keratin-producing epithelium and lack of other germinal layer components, differentiating it from teratoma (e501). It accounts for less than 1% of all testicular tumors and 3% to 14% of pediatric testicular tumors with 25% occurring in the first two decades of life (e134,e303,63,e482,e513). The nosology and the pathogenesis are uncertain. A germ cell origin is most likely; however, intratubular germ cell neoplasia is not an accompanying feature (e134,e328). This lesion usually presents as a firm, well-defined intratesticular nodule, with or without symptoms. On ultrasonography, it appears as a central hypoechoic mass with an echogenic rim (e214,e503). Grossly, the cyst is confined to the testicular parenchyma and is filled with flaky yellow-white keratinous material (Figure 19-8A). Orderly, stratified squamous epithelium, a dense fibrous tissue wall, focal calcifications, and acellular keratinous debris are the histologic findings (Figure 19-8B). The cyst and the surrounding tissue should be examined carefully for teratomatous or dermal adnexal elements, a testicular scar or intratubular germ cell neoplasia, the presence of which should lead to reclassification of the lesion as a mature teratoma. A conservative surgical approach with simple enucleation has been advocated for this benign lesion (e49,e134,26,56,e481).

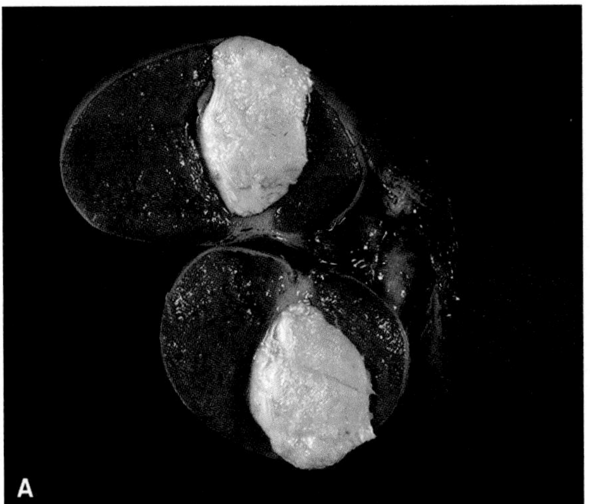

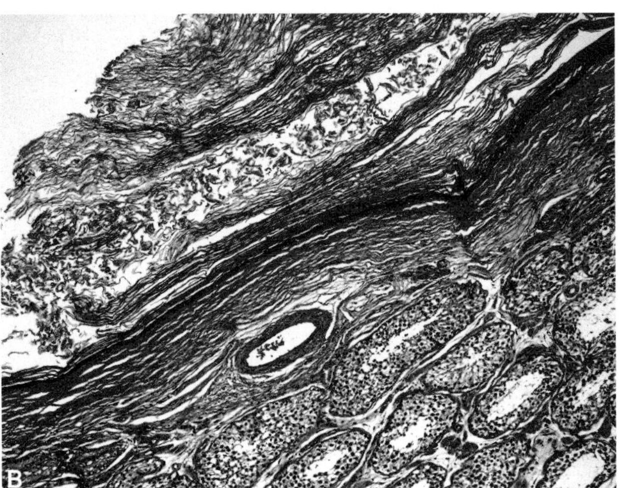

FIGURE 19-8 ■ Epidermoid cyst. **A:** The cyst is well circumscribed and completely intratesticular. It contains flaky yellow-white keratinous material (Courtesy: Dr. Jerome Taxy, Chicago, Illinois). **B:** Microscopically, abundant lamellated keratinous material is filling the cyst with a fibrous wall separating it from the adjacent testicular parenchyma. No intratubular germ cell neoplasia is noted in the adjacent seminiferous tubules.

Intratubular Germ Cell Neoplasia, Unclassified Type

Intratubular germ cell neoplasia, unclassified type (IGCNU) is a microscopic precursor lesion composed of germ cells within the seminiferous tubules with abundant clear cytoplasm, large irregular nuclei, and prominent nucleoli (22). This term refers to the lesion initially described by Skakkebaek as "carcinoma *in situ*" as well as to other "differentiated" forms of intratubular germ cell neoplasia (e135,e187,e368,e520). IGCNU is present in up to 4% of cryptorchid testes, in up to 5% of contralateral gonads in patients with unilateral GCT, and in up to 1% of biopsies from oligospermic infertile men (e51,e69,e160,e182,e222, e391,e423,e452,e477,e627). Additionally, it can be found in virtually all cases adjacent to invasive GCT in adult testes when residual testicular parenchyma is present (e135,e238). Contrastingly, the association with GCT arising in prepubertal testes is still a source of controversy and its true incidence is difficult to assess (e226,54,57). It is generally believed, however, that IGCNU is not associated with teratomas and pure YST in early childhood, in keeping with a different pathogenesis for this subset of testicular GCT. Rarely, IGCNU has been described in association with maldescended testes, intersex states and rare infantile YST and teratoma (e226,e283,e420,e466,e529,e530). In one series, IGCNU was reported in four patients with gonadal dysgenesis (65). In 12 patients with androgen insensitivity (testicular feminization), three were found to have unexpected IGCNU when no tumor was clinically apparent (e380). In another study of 102 cases of various intersex states, the authors reported IGCNU in 0 of 23 patients with androgen insensitivity syndrome (testicular feminization), 3 of 38 with gonadal dysgenesis, 1 of 12 with TH, 1 of 22 with male pseudohermaphroditism, and 1 of 7 with multiple congenital anomalies and ambiguous genitalia (e456).

IGCNU is not reliably detected in the prepubertal at-risk patients (e110,e409,e420). Conversely, the identification of atypical germ cells in prepubertal biopsies does not correlate with tumor risk. Although abnormal germ cell morphology has been described in prepubertal patients with cryptorchidism (e16,67), the findings are different from IGCNU, and their significance is not established, unlike the known significance of IGCNU. One large study found no intratubular germ cells adjacent to GCT in prepubertal children to be positive for PLAP or c-kit; five of seven were positive for PCNA and p53 was present in the two examined cases. These results indicate that germ cells adjacent to infantile GCT are proliferative but not neoplastic and offer additional evidence that intratubular germ cells and GCT in prepubertal boys are different from those of adolescents and adults (e212). Similar studies have reported morphologic and immunohistochemical features of normal prepubertal germ cells that resemble those of IGCNU that can persist up to 1 year of life (e25). Therefore, little or no benefit is derived from the routine biopsy of cryptorchid testes at the time of orchidopexy in prepubertal boys, and, if biopsy is to be performed, it should be delayed until after puberty. The assessment of risk by testicular biopsy in most prepubertal patients is not currently possible. An important exception to this general rule applies to prepubertal patients with intersex syndromes in whom the reliable identification of IGCNU or gonadoblastoma can be accomplished in early childhood (e325,e381,65,e456).

Microscopically, the seminiferous tubules are partially or completely filled by large cells with round nuclei, coarse chromatin, mitoses, and abundant clear cytoplasm (Figure 19-9A). A PAS stain demonstrates abundant glycogen. Immunohistochemical markers that are reliably positive include PLAP, CD117, and OCT4 (Figure 19-9B,C) (e69,e93,e236,e250,e266,e330,e390,e536). In contrast to invasive GCT in adult testis, the presence of i(12p) in IGCNU has not been universally confirmed with most investigators suggesting it is not present (e410,74).

Embryonal Carcinoma

EC is a rare tumor in the first decade of life and has a peak incidence in the 15- to 34-year old age group (e152,e594). Although very common in mixed GCT, occurring in greater than 80% of them, pure EC is rare with a rate of approximately 2.5% (e374). An adolescent or young adult presents with an enlarging painful scrotal mass or metastases in the regional lymph nodes, abdomen, or mediastinum. The testis contains a gray, focally necrotic, and hemorrhagic mass. The tumor is often poorly demarcated and the cut surface bulges markedly. Microscopically, sheets of large, pleomorphic undifferentiated cells with enlarged irregular and vesicular nuclei, distinct nuclear membranes, prominent nucleoli, and frequent mitoses are seen (Figure 19-10). Tumor necrosis is evident. Primitive gland formation and papillary structures with or without fibrovascular cores may be encountered. The characteristic immunohistochemical profile is: cytokeratin-positive, CD30-positive, OCT4-positive, PLAP-positive (focal), and epithelial membrane antigen (EMA) negative (24,e250,e566). EC shares similar genetic abnormalities with other adult GCT. Tumor stage is the single most important prognostic indicator and pure or predominant EC in a testicular tumor is associated with increased risk of advanced disease (e64,e147,e376).

Seminoma

Seminoma is a malignant GCT composed of relatively uniform cells, typically with clear or dense collagen containing cytoplasm, well-defined cell borders, and large regular nuclei with one or more prominent nucleoli; the cells resemble primitive germ cells. There is almost always an associated lymphoid infiltrate and frequently a granulomatous inflammatory response (89). While seminoma is the most common primary testicular tumor in adults, it is rare in prepubertal boys but is found more frequently in late adolescence (e2,e147,e590). In pediatric cases, the average age of presentation is 9.7 years (e590). It remains crucial to

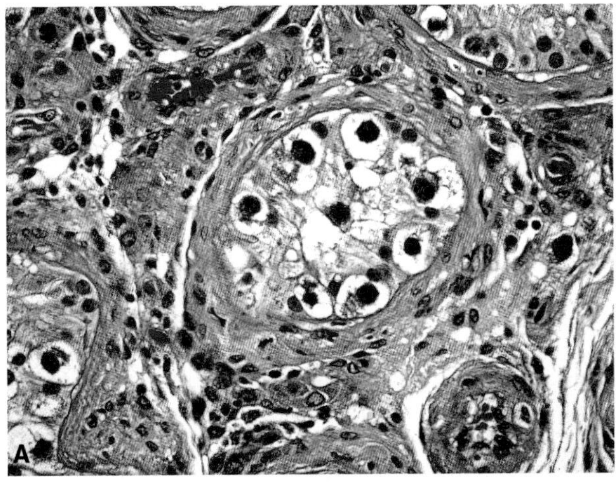

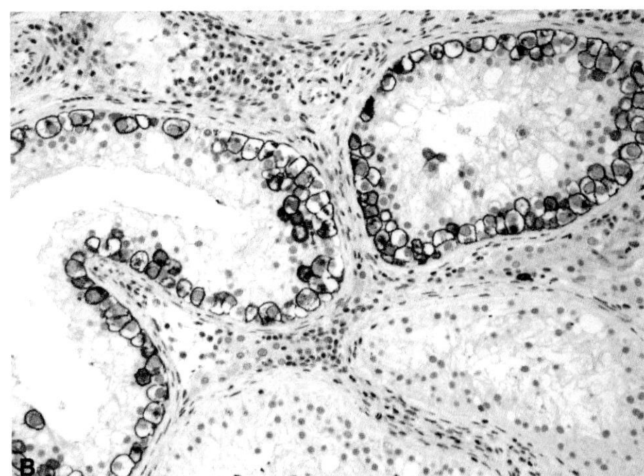

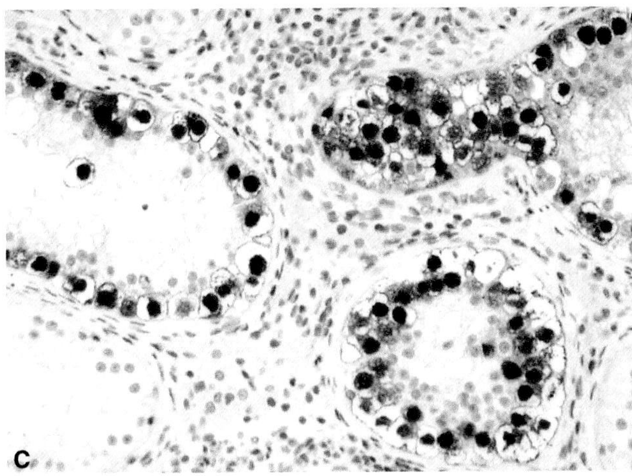

FIGURE 19-9 ▪ Intratubular germ cell neoplasia, unclassified type. **A:** The lesion consists of large cells with round-to-irregular nuclei, coarse chromatin, and occasional nucleoli. A mitotic figure is present. The cytoplasm is abundant and clear. **B,C:** The presence of lesional cells can be further facilitated by membranous expression of CD117 and nuclear labeling by OCT4.

distinguish seminoma from other forms (nonseminomatous) of GCT because of different treatments.

Grossly, a seminoma characteristically forms a gray, cream to pale pink, soft, homogeneous, lobulated, and well-defined mass that may have irregular yellow foci of necrosis. The tumor may occasionally present as multiple macroscopically distinct nodules. Microscopically, the uniform cells of seminoma are arranged in sheets, clusters, or columns and associated with lymphocytic infiltrate of variable density. Pseudoglandular, tubular, and cribriform morphologies have been reported, but the basic cell morphology of seminoma remains the same. The immunoprofile of seminoma is typically reactivity with vimentin, PLAP, CD117, and OCT4 (24,e250).

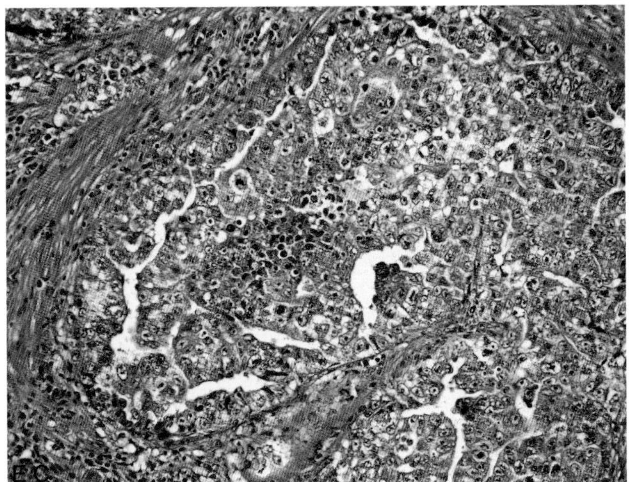

FIGURE 19-10 ▪ Embryonal carcinoma. Tumor cells are large and pleomorphic with enlarged irregular and vesicular nuclei, distinct nuclear membranes, prominent nucleoli, and frequent mitoses. Numerous apoptotic cells are present. Necrosis is a common finding.

Choriocarcinoma almost never occurs in childhood (e147) in its pure form but maybe found as a component of mixed GCT, especially in adolescents (e152). The pathologic features and treatment are similar to those of the same tumor in adults. Metastatic choriocarcinoma rarely occurs in infants from a primary tumor in the mother.

Mixed Germ Cell Tumor

Mixed germ cell tumor (MGCT) includes tumors containing two or more GCT components (22,89). The individual components are microscopically identical to those seen in pure GCT. While accounting for up to 54% of tumors in the adult testis (e375), MGCT is rarely seen in prepubertal children and becomes increasingly common in the second and third decades of life (e2,e147,e337). In one study, it accounted for 3% of prepubertal testicular tumors (e303). A common pattern is EC with one or more components of teratoma, seminoma, and YST, but virtually any combination can be seen. For diagnosis, similar to tumors of the adult testis, these tumors should be termed "mixed germ cell tumor, composed of…" followed by a tabulation of their percentage. The adjacent testis usually exhibits intratubular germ cell neoplasia. The combination of EC and teratoma has been previously termed *teratocarcinoma*, but it is currently preferable to include these under the MGCT category and list the components separately.

Sex Cord–Stromal Tumors

Sex cord–stromal tumors resemble the specialized supportive structures of the male or the female gonad and include LCTs, SCTs, granulosa cell tumors, and tumors of the theca/fibroma group (22). They account for 4% to 6% of tumors of the adult testis and up to 12% of prepubertal testicular tumors (41,e303,63,e482,e513). Sex cord–stromal tumors are generally benign with only rare cases of SCTs reportedly behaving in a malignant fashion (e279,e504). Additionally, a number of stromal tumors have been reported without evidence of differentiation toward any of the specific entities mentioned here and are referred to as *undifferentiated sex cord–stromal tumors*. Some of these tumors have occurred in pediatric age patients; some also developed metastasis (e556).

Leydig Cell Tumor

LCT, also known as *interstitial cell tumor*, is rare in children, accounting for up to 8% of pediatric testicular tumors and 14% of stromal tumors (e442,22). Generally, approximately 20% of LCT occur in the first decade of life. In this patient population, the tumor is most common between 3 and 9 years with a mean age at presentation of 7 years (e185,e269). Although it typically presents with a painless testicular mass, patients usually display signs of precocious puberty and elevated levels of serum testosterone and androstenedione and dehydroepiandrosterone (e61,e99,e612). Gynecomastia may be seen in 10% to 15% of patients (e95,14,e202,e352). LCT may be seen in patients with KS and 5% to 10% may have a history of cryptorchid testis (e269). Ultrasonography typically shows a well-defined hypoechoic small solid mass. Grossly, the tumor is well circumscribed and may be encapsulated. The cut surface is homogeneous yellow-brown, with possible areas of hyalinization and calcification. Microscopically, the tumor is composed of large polygonal or round cells with abundant granular, eosinophilic cytoplasm, forming sheets, trabeculae, and cords that displace seminiferous tubules (Figure 19-11). Nuclei may vary in size and shape but atypia and mitoses are not reliable for predicting aggressive behavior. Two other cell types seen occasionally are small round cells with scanty cytoplasm and an eccentric, hyperchromatic nucleus and clear cells resembling the adrenal zona fasciculata. Occasional spindling of tumor cells may be present. Lipofuscin pigment may be seen in up to 15% of cases. Crystals of Reinke are present only in 30% to 40% of cases (e269). Abundant smooth endoplasmic reticulum and lipid are identified ultrastructurally. By immunohistochemistry, LCT stains strongly and diffusely with antibodies to vimentin, inhibin, calretinin, and melan-A (A103) and shows variable staining with cytokeratins, EMA, desmin, S-100 protein, chromogranin, and synaptophysin (e71,e233,e346,e622). Immunostains for carcinoembryonic antigen and PLAP are consistently negative. LCT in prepubertal patients is benign and can be adequately treated by either radical orchiectomy or testis-sparing surgery (e210).

In contrast to LCT, Leydig cell hyperplasia occurs in neonates, is bilateral, and shows a transition between nodular and diffuse Leydig cell proliferation (68). Seminiferous

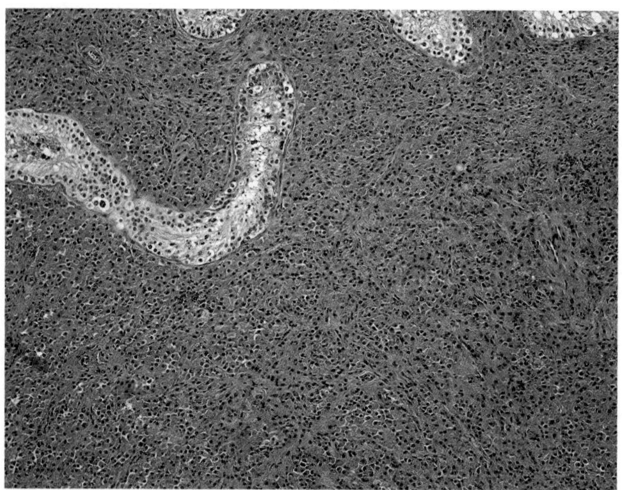

A

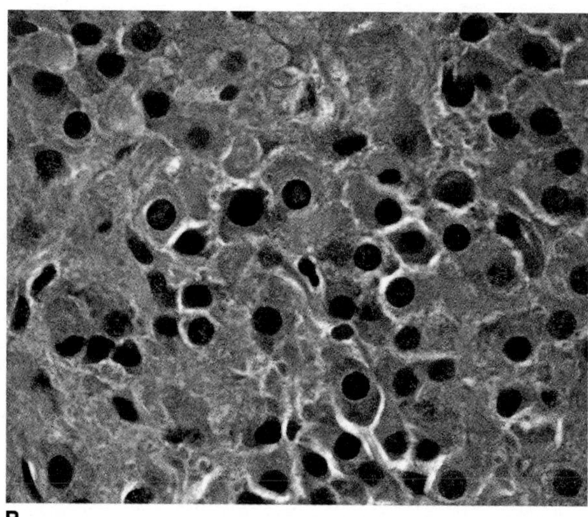

B

FIGURE 19-11 ■ Leydig cell tumor. **A:** Sheets of polygonal or round cells with abundant granular, eosinophilic cytoplasm are evident, displacing seminiferous tubules. **B:** The cytoplasm is typically finely granular and eosinophilic with mild variation in nuclear size and shape (inset).

tubules intermingle with Leydig cells throughout, and spermatogenesis is evident in tubules adjacent to nodules. An important differential diagnosis to consider is the testicular "tumor" of the AGS. These lesions are usually discovered in early adult life in patients with congenital adrenal hyperplasia but in up to one-third of cases are found in children as small nodules. Similar lesions are typically seen in Nelson syndrome (e244). This condition consists of bilateral, dark brown nodules with pleomorphic pigmented cells and hyalinized fibrotic stroma. Although small lesions may involve the testicular hilum only, larger nodules almost always involve the testicular parenchyma (e362,80). Awareness of this entity is important since these lesions usually decrease in size following corticosteroid therapy and may be managed conservatively but surgical removal, either by tumor enucleation or orchiectomy, may become necessary in refractory cases (e27,e468).

Sertoli Cell Tumor

SCT is a sex cord–stromal tumor of the testis composed of cells with features of Sertoli cells at variable degrees of development. This is a rare neoplasm accounting for less than 1% of all testicular tumors and typically occurring in adults and only exceptionally reported in males younger than 20 (96). Some variant forms, however, are more common in infants and children, especially those with syndromic and/or genetic associations such as androgen insensitivity syndrome (79), Carney syndrome (e602), and Peutz-Jeghers syndrome (94,96,e625).

Painless and slow testicular enlargement is a common presentation (e164,96). Elevated estradiol levels, sexual precocity, and gynecomastia may occur in patients with SCT of the Peutz-Jeghers syndrome (e11,e625). Although this tumor is usually unilateral, those associated with syndromic conditions may be multiple and bilateral (e286,e625). By ultrasonography, SCT is generally hypoechoic but can demonstrate variable echogenicity with possible cystic areas. In general, no imaging characteristics would allow distinction from a GCT. An exception is the large cell calcifying variant (see below), which is characterized by large areas of calcifications that can be readily suspected by ultrasound, especially when this tumor presents as multiple and bilateral masses (e91,e174).

The gross appearance of the enlarged testis is variable, ranging from a firm, circumscribed, lobulated, gritty, tan or yellow nodule to a multicystic mass. Foci of hemorrhage may be seen but necrosis is uncommon. Microscopically, SCT may vary in appearance ranging from tubular arrangement to retiform or solid growth pattern to cords of tumor cells (Figure 19-12). The intervening stroma is fibrotic and moderately to sparsely cellular or hyalinized. Tumor cells have round, oval, or elongate nuclei. The chromatin pattern is vesicular; nucleoli are not prominent and nuclear grooves or inclusions may be seen. The cytoplasm can be pale-to-eosinophilic, clear, or vacuolated due to lipids. Mild nuclear pleomorphism and atypia may be seen in the minority of cases. By immunohistochemistry, SCT is consistently reactive with antibodies against vimentin and cytokeratins with variable expression reported with antibodies against inhibin and S-100 (e233,e346,e546,96). It is typically negative for placental alkaline phosphatase, α-fetoprotein, and EMA (e94). Electron microscopy reveals the characteristic features of Sertoli cells: tubular structures with well-defined basement membrane, complex cytoplasmic interdigitations, numerous intercellular junctions, prominent Golgi apparatus, large lipid droplets, abundant smooth endoplasmic reticulum, and Charcot-Böttcher crystals in some examples.

In children, SCTs typically follow a benign course. However, metastatic potential does exist especially in older children (e279,e504,e556). Radical orchiectomy is the preferred treatment (e210). In older boys when the tumor is suspected of behaving in a malignant fashion, patients should undergo evaluation for metastatic disease. The latter condition should be treated aggressively with a combination of chemotherapy,

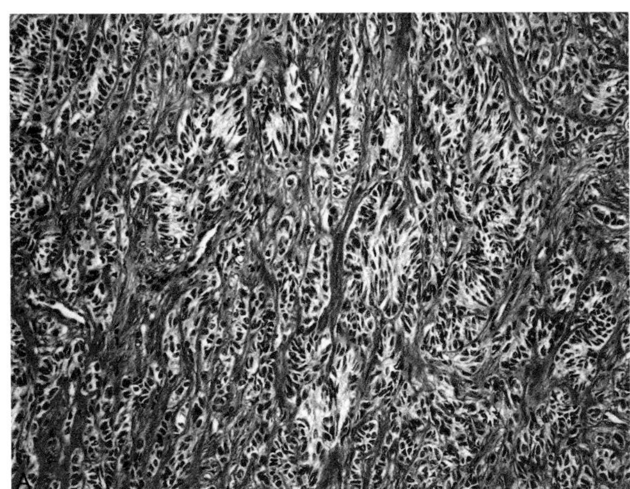

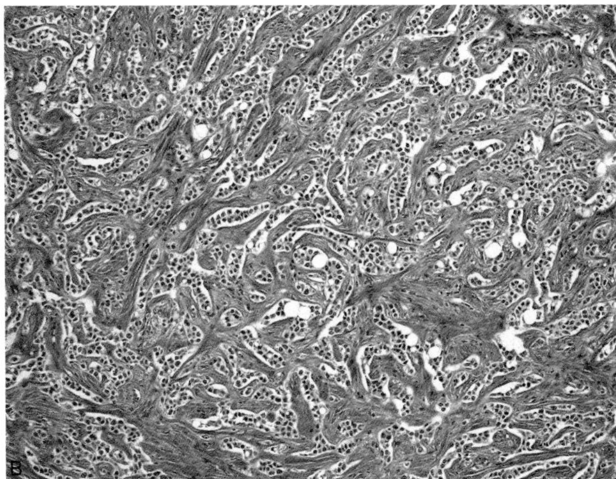

FIGURE 19-12 ▪ Sertoli cell tumor. **A,B:** This tumor exhibits variable morphology characterized by solid nests in a dense fibrotic background, compressed tubular arrangement (trabecular) with a resemblance to a carcinoid.

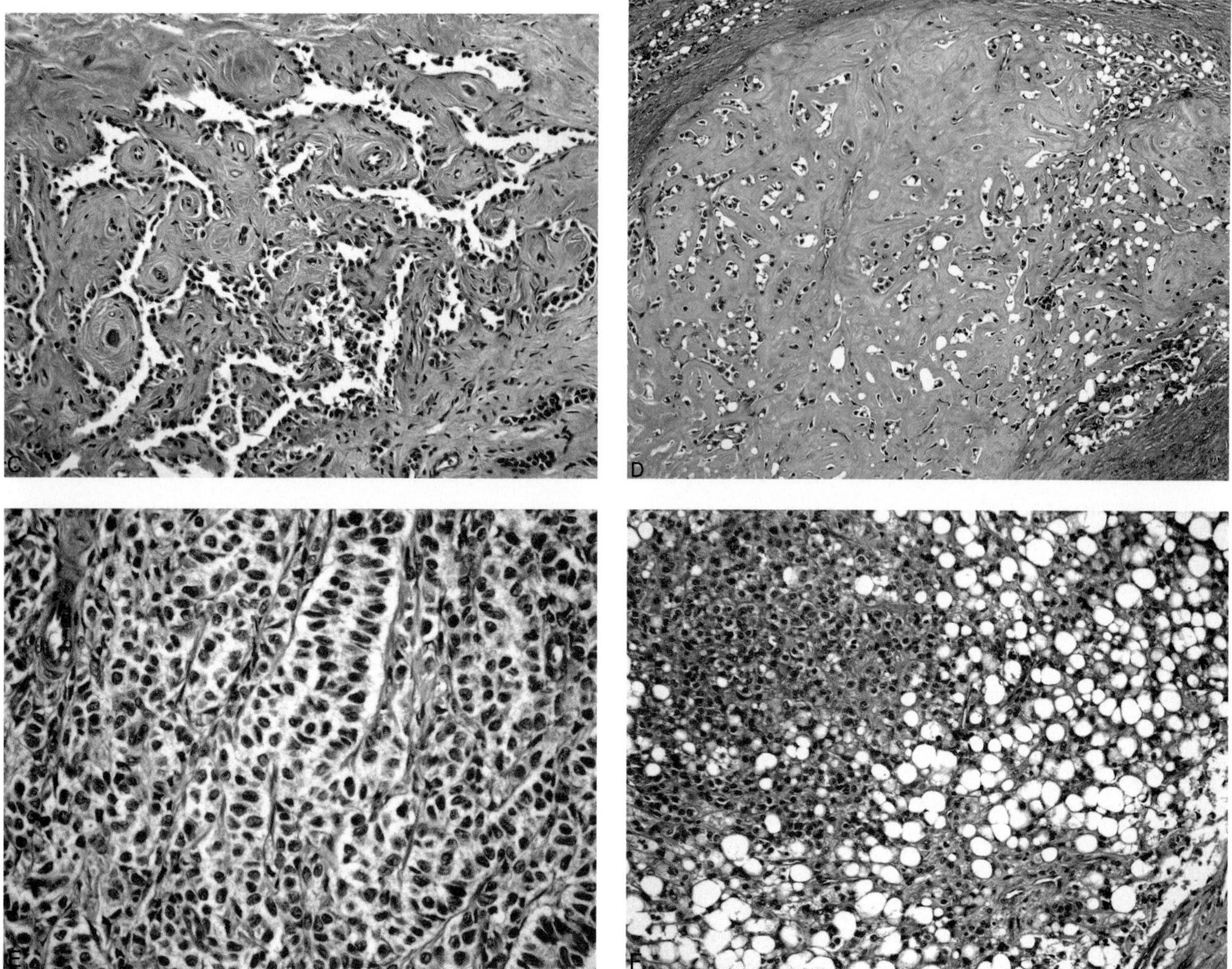

FIGURE 19-12 ■ *(continued)* **C:** Complex and anastomosing tubular structures "retiform", or cord-like structures in a sclerotic to hyalinized stroma. **D,E:** Tumor cells with round, oval, or elongate nuclei, vesicular chromatin pattern, occasional grooves, and inconspicuous nucleoli. **F:** The cytoplasm is pale-to-eosinophilic but can also exhibit prominent clearing or vacuolization.

radiation therapy, and retroperitoneal lymph node dissection (e211,77).

Large cell calcifying SCT (LCCSCT), as mentioned above, is a unique variant of SCT that can be sporadic (60%), but can also be part of Peutz-Jehgers and Carney syndromes (40%) (e286). This variant tends to occur in young individuals with an average age of 16 years and can be bilateral in 40% of cases. Associated features include multiple endocrine disorders manifested by precocious puberty, gynecomastia, acromegaly, bilateral primary adrenocortical hyperplasia, and pituitary adenomas. Cardiac myxomas and mucocutaneous pigmentations are reported features in Carney syndrome (e82,e623). Microscopically, this tumor consists of nests, trabeculae, small clusters, and cords of large polygonal cells with abundant eosinophilic finely granular cytoplasm embedded in a myxohyaline stroma, which typically contains large areas of calcifications (Figure 19-13). The nuclei are round to oval with vesicular chromatin pattern and inconspicuous nucleoli (e623). Intratubular spread of tumor cells is usually present.

Interestingly, multifocal intratubular proliferations of Sertoli cells distinct from those observed in LCCSCT have been recently reported in patients with Peutz-Jeghers syndrome in two separate studies. Eleven of the 14 patients from both studies did not have an associated SCT (e567,e587).

Juvenile Granulosa Cell Tumor

JGCT is a rare tumor consisting of structures resembling Graafian follicles. Despite its rarity, this tumor is the most frequent congenital testicular neoplasm and most common tumor in the first 6 months of life (33,48,e538). The reported incidence ranges from 3% (e482) to 6.6% of all prepubertal testicular tumors (41), with 50% of tumors occurring in the neonatal period and 90% within the first year of life (e90,18,48,66,e455,e565), making it exceptional to observe this tumor after the first year of life. Most of these tumors present as painless testicular mass and typically are not hormonally active (26,e513). JGCT can be associated with

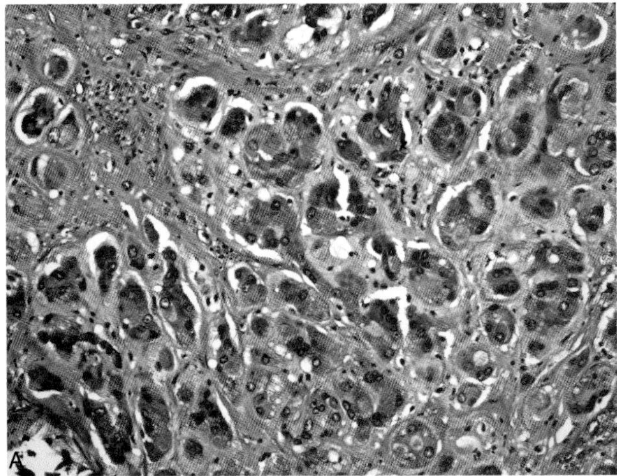

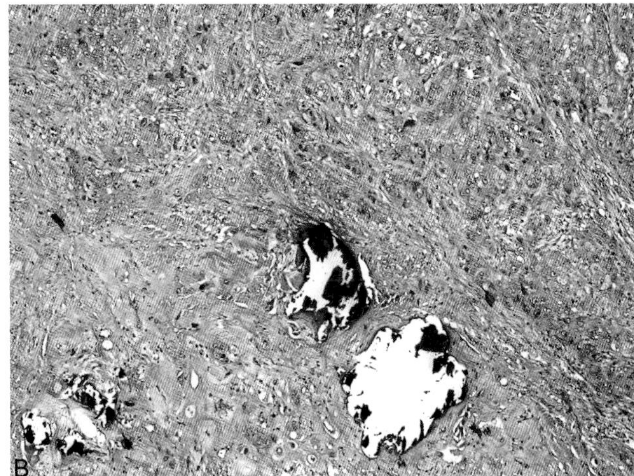

FIGURE 19-13▪Large cell calcifying SCT. **A:** Sheets and cords of large polygonal cells with abundant eosinophilic cytoplasm in a background of loose fibrous to myxohyaline stroma. **B:** Adjacent large areas of calcifications are present.

abnormal karyotypic mosaicism and structural abnormalities in chromosome Y, especially in patients with ambiguous external genitalia (16). Other associated abnormalities include MGD and hypospadias. JGCT can occasionally occur in the undescended testes of infants with intersex disorders (e455,e624). All the reported cases have had a benign course.

By ultrasonography, JGCT is a cystic and septate hypoechoic mass (e565). Grossly, solid and cystic patterns are present and hemorrhage may be observed (Figure 19-14). The cysts are usually thin walled and filled with viscous or gelatinous fluid. Microscopically, it is identical to its ovarian counterpart. The tumor consists of variably prominent solid and follicular or cystic patterns. The lining of the cysts consists of several layers of cells that resemble the granulosa (inner) or the theca cells (outer). The follicles contain basophilic or eosinophilic fluid that stains with mucicarmine. In nonfollicular areas, tumor growth can be in the form of sheets, nodules, or irregular clusters. Hyalinization may be prominent. The tumor cells have round-to-oval hyperchromatic nuclei with occasional nucleoli, and the cytoplasm is moderate to large with pale-to-eosinophilic appearance (Figure 19-14). Mitoses, which are often readily seen, and atypia do not adversely influence the favorable prognosis (68). By immunohistochemistry, the granulosa-like cells stain positive for cytokeratins, vimentin, and S-100. The theca-like cells are positive for vimentin, smooth muscle actin, and focally for desmin (e197,e428,e547). The main differential diagnosis is with YST, which can be solved by applying the appropriate immunostains (26,e341,e565).

Gonadoblastoma

Gonadoblastoma belongs to the category of testicular tumors containing both germ cells and sex cord elements.

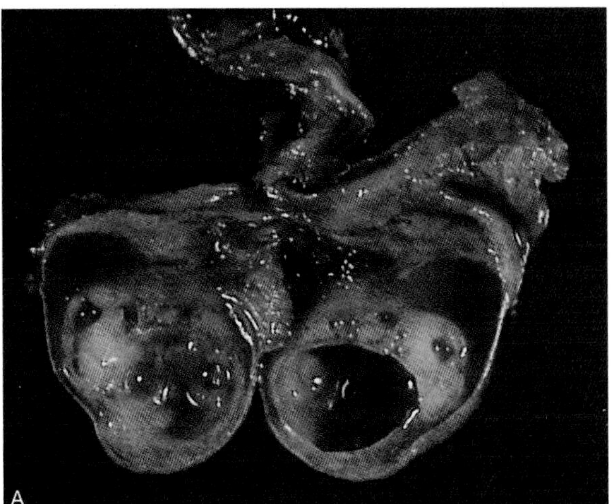

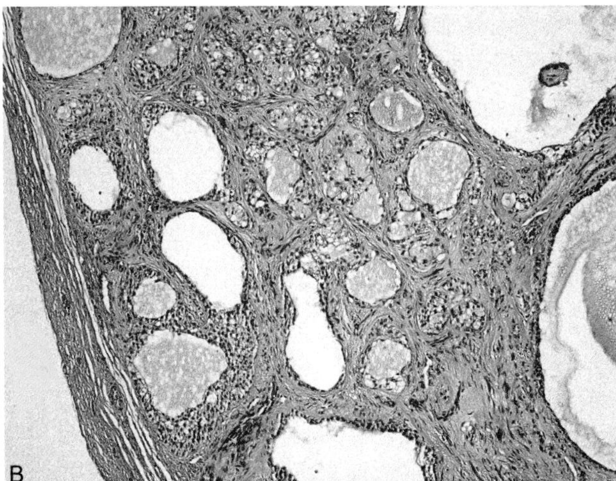

FIGURE 19-14▪Juvenile granulosa cell tumor. **A:** The tumor is relatively well circumscribed and has both solid and cystic areas. The solid areas are tan-white to yellow and the cysts can be prominent. **B:** Solid and follicular to cystic patterns are evident.

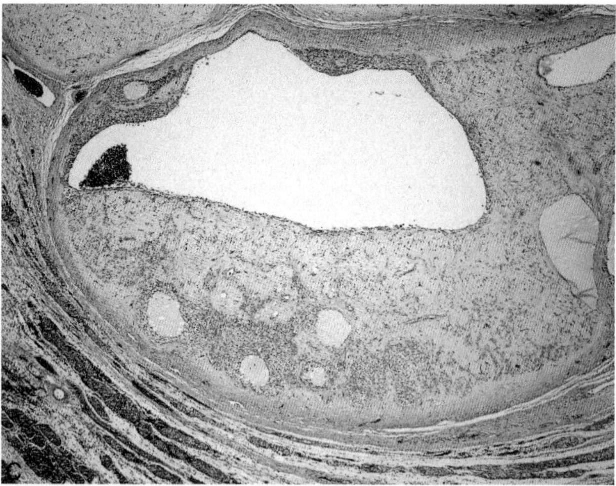

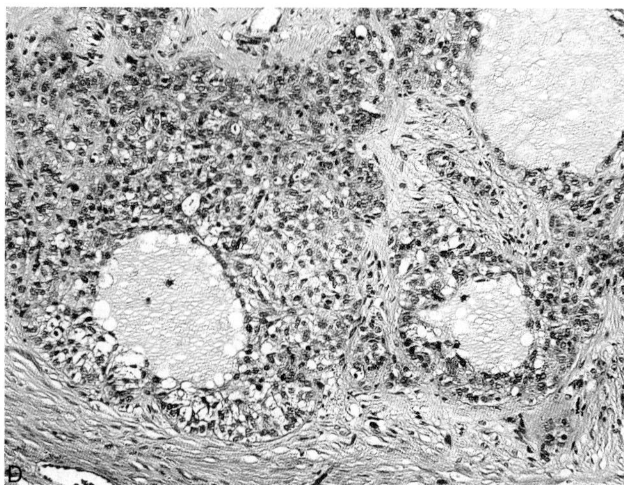

FIGURE 19-14 (*continued*) **C:** Areas with stromal hyalinization may predominate. **D:** Tumor cells have round-to-oval hyperchromatic nuclei and moderate-to-large amount of pale-to-eosinophilic cytoplasm (Courtesy of Dr. Jerome Taxy, Chicago, Illinois).

It is composed of a mixture of seminoma-like, large germ cells and sex cord cells having features of immature Sertoli cells and granulosa cells. Gonadoblastoma is most commonly seen in MGD associated with ambiguous genitalia (e284,43,79,81). The risk of developing gonadoblastoma in this setting is estimated to be 15% to 25% (e421). Surgical exploration of the cryptorchid testis often demonstrates persistence of female-type internal genital structures stemming from failure of involution of the müllerian ductal system (79). Bilateral involvement by gonadoblastoma occurs in about one-third of cases (81). Karyotypic analysis of the patients, regardless of sexual phenotype, almost always reveals a Y chromosome, with 46XY and 45X/46XY occurring most commonly (79).

Grossly, gonadoblastoma usually forms solid, yellow-tan nodules with gritty calcifications. The tumor size ranges from microscopic foci to large masses up to 8 cm (81). Microscopically, the nodules usually consist of well-defined, rounded nests of large, pale seminoma-like cells admixed with small, dark, angular, sex cord cells that may form a peripheral palisade around the cellular nests (Figure 19-15). Nodular foci of hyalinized basement membrane can be seen in the center of these nests and at the periphery. The stromal cells may become polygonal, resembling Leydig cells, mostly in postpubertal patients. Calcifications appear initially on this basement membrane and may become quite prominent. By immunohistochemistry, the germ cells stain similar to those in ITGNU including reactivity with PLAP, CD117, and OCT4 (e93,e104,e251), while the stromal cells express inhibin and WT-1 (e229).

Gonadoblastoma is a premalignant lesion from which invasive GCT can develop, most commonly as seminoma, but any nonseminomatous GCT may occur (81). Excision of a gonad with gonadoblastoma prior to development of an invasive lesion is curative.

A number of cases have been reported in which the tumors consisted of a combination of neoplastic germ cells and neoplastic sex cord–stromal elements arranged in a diffuse pattern rather than the nested pattern of gonadoblastoma (e56,e339,e458). These tumors have been designated germ cell–sex cord/gonadal stromal tumors, unclassified. In some of these tumors, at least according to a recent report, the neoplastic nature of the germ cells has been disputed (e571), suggesting that some of these tumors might in fact represent sex cord–stromal tumors with entrapped germ cells rather than unclassified mixed germ cell sex cord–stromal tumors.

Miscellaneous Tumors of the Testis

Congenital neuroblastoma may present as a testicular mass without evidence of disseminated disease until months later (e75,e264). A subset of patients with neuroblastoma originating below the diaphragm or with advanced stage disease may be more prone to testicular metastases and in some cases tumor relapse can occur in a scrotal location (e294,e518). It has been also recently suggested that neuroblastoma can arise *de novo* from the paratesticular tissue, presumably from sympathetic tissue remnants, as part of a multicentric disease rather than metastasis (e575).

Nephroblastoma (Wilms tumor) can metastasize to the testis from a renal primary (e30,e492,e562) but can also occur as a paratesticular, scrotal, or inguinal tumor (e7,e24,e412).

Carcinoid tumor has been rarely reported in the testis, especially those of children (e47,e156). Its microscopic features are identical to those reported in other sites with predominance of the trabecular and the insular patterns.

Tumors of hematopoietic origin may involve the testis. Overall, leukemia and lymphoma account for 2% to 5% of all pediatric testicular tumors. They are the most common metastatic malignancies to the testicle in children and

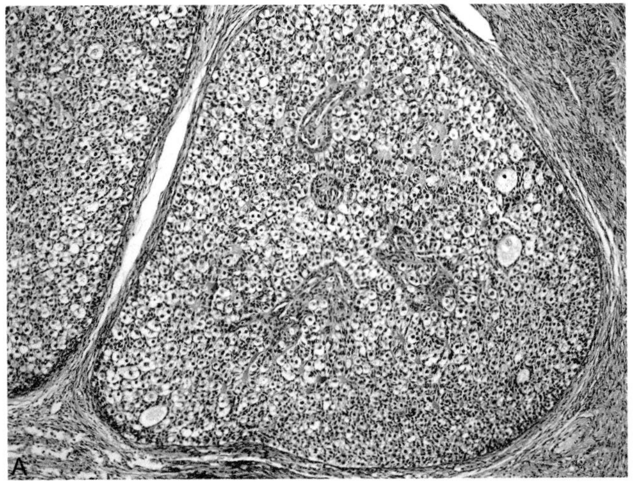

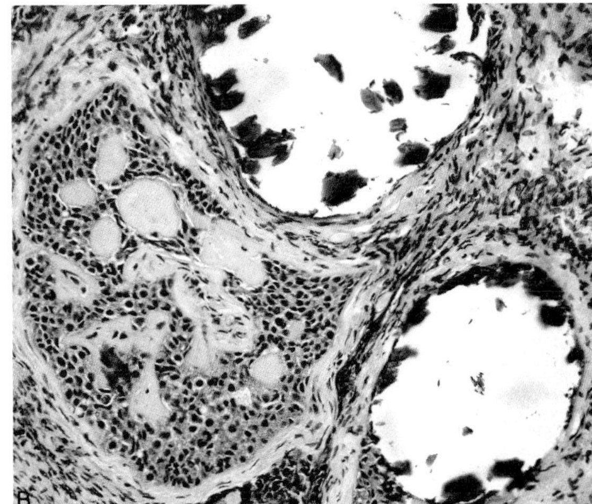

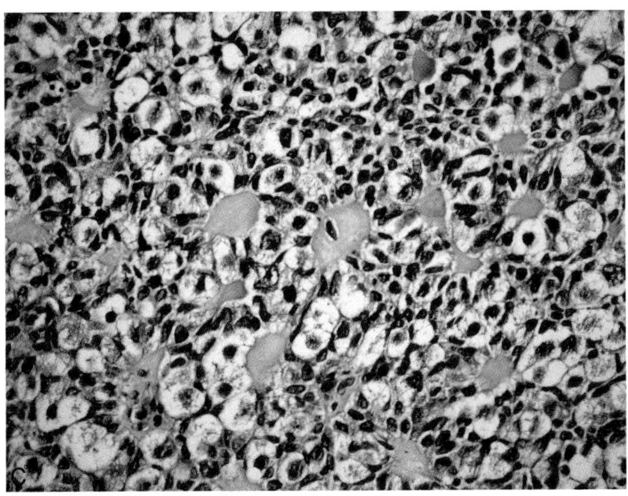

FIGURE 19-15 ■ Gonadoblastoma. **A:** Nodules of tumor consisting of a mixture of nests of large and pale seminoma-like cells admixed with sex cord cells with small, dark, angular nuclei. **B:** A focus with prominent calcifications. **C:** Hyalinized nodules of basement membrane material are surrounded by tumor cells.

account for the majority of the tumors that present bilaterally (e210,e306). Primary testicular lymphoma in children is rare and typically occurs prepubertally at 3 to 10 years of age (e 157,e203,e215,e319,e366,e415,e436). Secondary testicular involvement in children may also occur in approximately 5% of systemic lymphomas (e120,e263). Leukemic involvement of the testis is more commonly seen in acute lymphocytic leukemia (ALL) but can also develop in myelogenous leukemias (e181,e595). In a postmortem survey of children with leukemia and lymphoma, the overall incidence of testicular involvement was found in 25 of 39 cases (65%). In the majority of those cases, ALL was also identified in other organs, supporting the view that testicular infiltration is indicative of widespread disease (e465). Although testicular involvement by ALL may be clinically evident in about 8% of cases (e535), microscopic involvement may be as high as 21% (e271). The testis may also be the site of relapse after bone marrow remission is established and may signal a systemic relapse (e278,e292,e387).

In clinically evident cases, the testis has a bulging, pale tan surface with diffuse and nodular pattern of infiltration. Microscopically, there is diffuse interstitial infiltrate of small cells with scanty cytoplasm, surrounding and infiltrating the seminiferous tubules (e28,e292). The diagnosis can be established by needle or open wedge testicular biopsy (e210). Juvenile xanthogranuloma rarely occurs in the testis of infants.

EPIDIDYMIS, SPERMATIC CORD, AND PARATESTICULAR TISSUES

Congenital and Developmental Anomalies

A number of congenital anomalies of the mesonephric duct system can occur. These anatomic defects are usually identified either at the time of orchidopexy for an undescended testis or during an investigation for infertility. The spectrum of morphologic manifestations ranges from total absence of the epididymis, vas deferens, seminal vesicles, and ejaculatory ducts to selective atresia, cysts, diverticula, and ectopias (17,e326,e351). Complete absence of the vas deferens is the most common congenital obstructive abnormality of the male mesonephric duct system and is found in 3.5% to 8% of males evaluated for infertility (17); cystic fibrosis should be considered in the diagnosis. Absence of the seminal vesicles and ejaculatory ducts often accompanies absence of the vas deferens. Epididymal abnormalities are present in 36% to 43% of patients with maldescent of the testis. These include agenesis; atresia of the head, body, or tail; and a loop or an elongated epididymis (e176,e276,e288). This association is especially common in the presence of an undescended testis and a complete hernia sac (23,e213). Seminal vesicle cysts may simulate prostatitis clinically and are associated with ipsilateral upper urinary tract abnormalities (e476). Spermatic cord cysts may be of mesothelial or mesonephric origin (e394). Those of mesothelial origin are typically unilocular and lined by flat poorly cohesive epithelium with chronic inflammation and hyalinization in the wall, while mesonephric cysts are multilocular and lined by cohesive attenuated or columnar epithelium and may contain spermatozoa if in continuity with the sperm-excretory ducts. In approximately 10% of cases, the origin of spermatic cord cysts maybe indeterminate due to the lack of recognizable epithelium.

Small glandular or tubular inclusions, which probably represent embryonal remnants of müllerian ducts, are found in 0.53% to 6% of hernia sacs from males in the first two decades (12,e175,e443,e531,e596). The ciliated low columnar epithelial cells have eosinophilic cytoplasm and basal nuclei and are surrounded by a mantle of fibrous tissue without smooth muscle. Due to their morphologic overlap, it is important to distinguish these embryonal remnants in hernia sacs from the true vas deferens or epididymis because of the implications for fertility and potential medicolegal ramifications (e175,e557). These embryonal tubular structures have a smaller diameter than the vas deferens, often lack smooth muscle, and do not increase in diameter with advancing age (e443). Tortuous blood vessels and tangentially oriented, mesothelial-lined spaces are other pseudoglandular structures observed in hernia sacs.

Abnormalities of the epididymis and spermatic cord structures can also occur as a result of prenatal conditions. Exposure to diethylstilbestrol *in utero* is associated with epididymal cysts and varicoceles in addition to hypotrophic testes and capsular induration (e177,e606). Congenital rubella, in addition to causing cryptorchidism, may be associated with absence or obstruction of the vas deferens or epididymis (e447). Cystic fibrosis is a condition that, in addition to other complications in other organs, contributes to infertility in adult males. The disease may additionally be associated with aplasia or hypoplasia of the vas deferens or epididymis (e220,e312,e357). Moreover, congenital bilateral absence of the vas deferens has been linked to defects in the cystic fibrosis transmembrane conductance regulator (*CFTR*) gene (e96,e358,e510).

A number of heterotopic tissues may be encountered in the paratesticular region such as in splenogonadal fusion, ectopic immature renal tissue, ectopic adrenal rests, and rarely ectopic prostatic tissue. These lesions should be considered in the differential diagnosis of a scrotal mass. Splenogonadal fusion consists of a spectrum of malformations of unknown etiology involving abnormal fusion between the spleen and the gonad or mesonephric derivatives such as the epididymis and vas deferens (e35,e189,e256,e268,e289,e363). This entity was first mentioned by German pathologist, E. Bostroem in 1883 and later described in detail by G. Pommer in 1889 (e268).

There are two main morphologic types of this malformation: the continuous and the discontinuous type, depending on the presence or the absence of a structural connection between the regular spleen and the ectopic splenic tissue that is fused to the gonad (e448). Splenogonadal fusion occurs much more frequently in males than females and is almost always left sided (e42,e411). Patients, typically younger than 20 years, usually present with left scrotal swelling, left inguinal hernia, or cryptorchidism (e84). In about one-third of reported cases, other congenital defects are additionally present, predominantly in the continuous type. The most common of these anomalies is cryptorchidism; other associated anomalies include bilateral absent legs, imperforate anus, spina bifida, diaphragmatic hernia, and hypospadias (e112,e140). Microscopically, normal splenic tissue and testicular tissue are identified, but atrophy or immaturity may be seen. The cordlike structure present in the continuous type is composed of an admixture of splenic and fibrous tissues.

Nodules of ectopic immature renal tissue (e186,e347,e621), ectopic adrenocortical tissue (adrenal rests) (e267,e335,e539), and rarely ectopic prostatic tissue (e582) may be found incidentally along the spermatic cord and adjacent to the epididymis (Figure 19-16).

Acquired Abnormalities and Other Lesions

A variety of acquired disorders of the epididymis and spermatic cord may present as an "acute scrotum" and may simulate testicular torsion or neoplasia. Acute nonspecific epididymitis in prepubertal and early adolescent boys presents with slow onset of scrotal pain, erythema, and edema (e180). Although coexistent anatomic anomalies with this condition are rare in the pediatric age group, further work-up may be warranted if this condition recurs (e79,e204). Infants have a higher rate of associated acute epididymitis and genitourinary malformations than older children (e356,e515). Tuberculous epididymitis, probably due to hematogenous spread of infection, mimics malignancy because of the combination of painless testicular swelling and an abnormal chest radiograph (e73,e344). This condition should be included in the differential diagnosis of testicular swelling in endemic regions. Epididymal sarcoidosis causes granulomatous epididymitis and scrotal swelling mimicking a neoplasm (e146,e604). Spermatic vein thrombosis may simulate intermittent testicular torsion, with acute pain and swelling of the scrotum, spermatic cord, and epididymis (e105).

Henoch-Schönlein purpura may cause acute scrotum and scrotal swelling in up to 38% of patients and usually resolves spontaneously and does not require surgery (e101,e116,e209). If the scrotum is explored, edema, petechiae, and purpura of the scrotum, epididymis, and testis are the morphologic manifestations. Scrotal abscess formation has been reported following appendectomy performed both by laparoscopic and open approach (e167,e553).

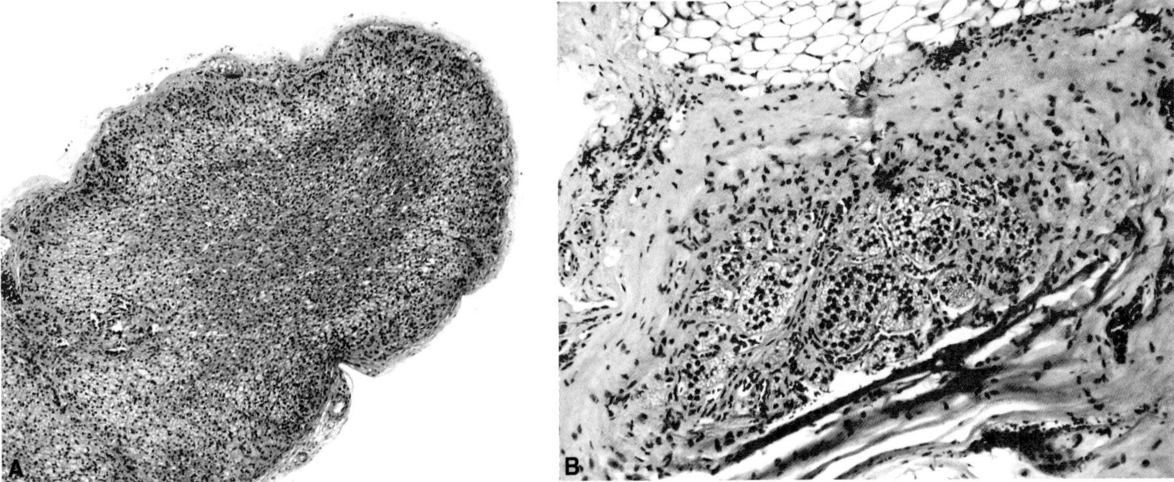

FIGURE 19-16 ▪ Ectopic adrenal tissue. **A:** One example of adrenocortical tissue presented as a palpable paratesticular nodule. The lesion is well circumscribed and encapsulated and exhibits zonation similar to the normal adrenal cortex. **B:** Another example of ectopic adrenal tissue incidentally discovered in an inguinal hernia sac.

Varicocele results from dilatation of veins in the pampiniform plexus of the spermatic cord and is found in 16% of boys between the age of 10 to 15 years, being uncommon in boys younger than 10 years (e218). In order to prevent the progressive and irreversible damage to the testis, surgical correction of varicocele should be performed soon after diagnosis regardless of the degree of severity and the presence or absence of symptoms (e68,e321). The pathogenesis is venous stasis and reflux with vascular insufficiency and consequent progressive tubular damage. Hydrocele is a lower abdominal and scrotal cystic mass resulting from accumulation of fluid in the processus vaginalis or tunica vaginalis (e461,e527).

Meconium periorchitis presents as a large solitary paratesticular mass or several small nodules along the spermatic cord and is frequently associated with a hydrocele (e60,e127). It may be the rare initial manifestation of cystic fibrosis or result from volvulus, intestinal atresia, or ischemia (e470). A rare case of scrotoschisis associated with meconium periorchitis has been also reported (e98). For this condition to occur, it requires an *in utero* perforation of the gastrointestinal tract, allowing meconium to leak into the peritoneal cavity and then into the tunica vaginalis via the processus vaginalis. The perforation may resolve antenatally with the scrotal lesion as the only clue and manifestation of the process. Scrotal and abdominal calcifications on plain films and hyperechogenic areas on scrotal ultrasound are the imaging abnormalities (e470,e491). The gross appearance is a yellowish green, gritty mass with focal dystrophic calcifications. Microscopically, the lesion consists of loose myxoid to irregular fibrous connective tissue. Aggregates of macrophages with multinucleated giant cells containing brown bile pigment or cholesterol clefts and scattered calcifications may be seen. The mass may spontaneously resolve without surgery (e127). A case of barium peritonitis secondarily causing an acute scrotal lesion in an infant has been reported (e190).

Tumors of the Paratesticular Structures

Mesothelial proliferations have been reported in the paratesticular region in the pediatric age group ranging from mesothelial hyperplasia to malignant mesothelioma.

Nodular mesothelial hyperplasia is a benign reactive process that may mimic a malignant process. It is typically incidentally encountered in hernia sacs, the majority of which occur in the pediatric age group (e480). It could also be associated with hydrocele or hematocele. The persistent irritation may easily result in histology that mimics malignant mesothelioma such as papillae and small tubules, solid nests and cords extending into the underlying reactive connective tissue simulating invasion (e17). However, the overall morphology is devoid of overtly malignant features.

Malignant mesothelioma of the paratesticular region is rare and even rarer in young patients with only 10% occurring in patients younger than 25 years (e17,e247,e429). Grossly, the tumor typically presents as thickening of the tunica vaginalis with multiple friable nodular lesions. The histopathologic features are variable with the majority of tumors showing pure epithelial phenotype. The biphasic tumors contain a variable proportion of sarcomatoid morphology, basically resembling their pleural and intra-abdominal peritoneal counterparts. The entire spectrum of differentiation may be seen ranging from well-differentiated tumors characterized by tubulopapillary architecture and variably invasive tubules to poorly differentiated tumors with solid sheets, cords, and nests of highly infiltrative epithelioid cells with necrosis.

Rarely, tumors of the ovarian epithelial types have been reported in the paratesticular region of adolescent patients. Their histopathologic features and classification are identical to their ovarian counterparts (e247,e624).

Desmoplastic small round cell tumor (DSRCT) consists of proliferation of small round cells with an epithelial growth pattern and a desmoplastic stroma. Although typically affecting the pelvic and abdominal cavities of adolescent males, involvement of the paratesticular region is not uncommon (e117,e171). It may present in the paratesticular soft tissue, serosal surfaces, and the epididymis near the junction with the rete testis. Grossly, the tumor is firm and has a white-to-tan appearance. Microscopically, it consists of nests and anastomosing cords of uniformly small blue cells with scant cytoplasm embedded in a densely fibrotic stroma. Focal tubular formation may be seen. Mitoses are readily seen and tumor necrosis is commonly present. By immunohistochemistry, the tumor typically exhibits dual reactivity with keratin and desmin. Additionally, neuron-specific enolase (NSE), EMA, and vimentin are expressed. DSRCT is typically nonreactive for muscle common actin, myogenin, and chromogranin and is variably reactive for MIC2 (CD99) and p53 (27,e297). DSRCT is characterized by a specific chromosomal abnormality, t(11;22)(p13;q12), resulting in the fusion of the Ewing sarcoma gene *EWS* on 22q12 and the Wilms tumor gene *WT1* on 11p13 (e172). The detection of this gene fusion EWS-WT1 is both a sensitive and a specific marker of DSRCT (27,e10) and its EWS-WT1 chimeric protein product is expressed in over 90% of tumors. Most patients with DSRCT develop metastasis to regional lymph nodes or to distant sites (e117).

Mesenchymal paratesticular tumors in infants and children are rare and include a variety of neoplasms such as hemangioma, juvenile xanthogranuloma, and RMS.

Paratesticular RMS is one of the relatively common tumors that involve the scrotal contents that are not of germ cell origin and is the most common paratesticular sarcoma in children (e308,55,e460). The mean age of occurrence in one large study was 6.6 years. Most paratesticular RMS are of embryonal subtype including the spindle cell variant (e308), although alveolar subtype has been also reported. Their histopathologic features are identical to their soft tissue counterpart. Metastases have been reported from these tumors to retroperitoneal lymph nodes and distant sites (e460).

Of the vascular tumors, cavernous hemangioma predominates and usually follows a benign course (e318,e425). A case involving the testis of a stillborn has been reported (e540). Bilateral testicular **hemangiomas** in neonates have been associated with cystic hygromas and may regress spontaneously (e505). **Juvenile xanthogranuloma** presents as a hard, irregularly enlarged testis with a circumscribed yellow nodule on cut surface (e484,e561).

Other tumors of the connective tissue surrounding the testicle include benign (leiomyoma, fibroma, lipoma, calcifying fibrous tumor/pseudotumor) and malignant entities (leiomyosarcoma, fibrosarcoma, liposarcoma, rhabdoid tumor, and malignant peripheral nerve sheath tumor). These tumors are extremely rare, being mostly the subject of case reports, and their morphologic features are similar to their soft tissue counterparts (2,e37,e155,e259,e385,e445).

Melanotic neuroectodermal tumor (*retinal anlage tumor*) is a rare melanin-containing tumor typically affecting the facial and skull bones. This tumor, however, has been reported in the epididymis and is seen mainly in infants (35). Grossly, these are circumscribed firm epididymal tumors with a white-to-gray cut surface that may show darker areas of pigmentation. Microscopically, the tumor consists of two components: the melanin-containing epithelioid cells arranged in cords, nests, or glandular structures, and the small neuroblast-like cells in a variably cellular stroma. These two components are usually intermixed. This tumor generally follows a benign clinical course but may recur locally. No distant metastases have been reported but regional lymph nodes (inguinal, retroperitoneal) have been rarely involved (e126,e245).

Adenomatoid tumor, the second most common tumor of the epididymis and cord in adults, can rarely be found in children as a scrotal nodule (e52,e398,e496). The mass is gray, dense, and homogeneous, with a mucoid cut surface. Microscopically, tubules and cords of flattened or cuboidal eosinophilic mesothelial cells in a fibrous stroma are characteristic of this tumor (e129,e377).

Papillary cystadenoma of the epididymis is a rare benign epithelial tumor of the epididymal ducts and, rarely, the spermatic cord. This tumor can be associated with von Hippel-Lindau disease especially when it is bilateral, which can happen in about 30% to 40% of cases. The tumor is solid and cystic with occasional papillary formation and is composed of cuboidal-to-columnar cells with clear or vacuolated cytoplasm (e246,e446).

THE PENIS

Most congenital abnormalities of the penis are related to defects in urethral closure, such as hypospadia and epispadia, and meatal stenosis. Hypospadia, with an incidence of 1:300 male newborns, is an anomaly involving the ventral aspect of the penis in the form of an abnormal ventral opening of the urethral meatus, an abnormal ventral curvature of the penis (chordee), and/or an abnormal distribution of the foreskin. The extent of the malformation is variable as the ectopic urethral opening (meatus) can be located anywhere from the tip of the glans penis, along the penile shaft and scrotum, to the perineum. The form and the extent of the malformed urethral opening can be variable but is rarely stenotic (e40,e136). Epispadia refers to the congenital absence of the dorsal aspect of the urethra, resulting in a urethral opening on the dorsum of the penis. The most frequent location of the opening is penopubic but can be penile or glanular. The incidence of male epispadia is 1 in 117,000 live male births. Associated urinary incontinence is frequently observed with penopubic epispadias and occasionally with penile type, but is not associated with glanular epispadias. Congenital anomalies that have been associated with epispadias include diastasis of the pubic symphysis, bladder exstrophy, renal agenesis, and ectopic pelvic kidney (e170).

Other rare malformations of the penis include penile agenesis, or aphallia, diphallia, accessory scrotum, and transposition of the penis and scrotum (penoscrotal transposition) (e88,e145, e200,e281,e299,e403,e464,e521). Some of these conditions may have familial predisposition and may be associated with other anomalies mostly in organs of the genitourinary tract (e31,e439).

Cutaneous viral infections and balanitis xerotica obliterans (BXO) are the principal acquired penile lesions in children and adolescents. The presentation of human papillomavirus (HPV) infection is variable ranging from asymptomatic infection to condyloma acuminata to bowenoid papulosis. Although DNA from certain known pathogenic HPV strains was detected in foreskins from newborns undergoing routine circumcision, there was no correlation with their respective mothers who had abnormal cervicovaginal cytologic smears (e479). In young children with clinically evident condyloma acuminata, a sexual etiology was determined in more than half of them, and occasionally these patients were found to have a mother with extensive condylomata observed at the time of childbirth (e507). It has been also noted that condylomata acuminata in young people are associated with the same HPV types found in anogenital lesions in adults (e626). Bowenoid papulosis, histologically identical to preinvasive squamous carcinoma, is usually a condition of young adults but may affect young children and is associated with HPV-16 (e62).

BXO is a chronic dermatitis of unknown etiology most often involving the glans and prepuce but sometimes extending into the urethra. BXO is relatively common in children and occurs in approximately 9% of all circumcised foreskins and in 19% to 40% of circumcisions performed for phimosis (e36,e169,e274). It may be seen in boys as young as 2 years of age and appears clinically as a thick, white plaque on the prepuce, with occasional involvement of the glans and meatus. The gross pathologic findings are subtle ranging from loss of skin wrinkling to change in skin color and texture (thick and white or thin and pink) compared with the adjacent skin. The microscopic features are identical to those of lichen sclerosus et atrophicus, which are characterized by a thick subepidermal zone of acellular eosinophilic hyaline material underlying the keratotic and atrophic epidermis. Slight basal liquefaction is characteristic, with occasional formation of bullae or ulcers. A dense bandlike or patchy lymphoid infiltrate is present toward the deep border of the hyalinized zone, and clusters of plasma cells are sometimes seen.

Fournier disease is a form of necrotizing fascitis affecting the penis and has been reported in children only rarely (e4). Staphylococcal and streptococcal infections are responsible for the condition.

Overall, neoplasms of the penis are exceptionally rare in the first two decades of life. Squamous cell carcinoma is rare in children in the United States but has been reported in several adolescents who were not circumcised during childhood (e39,e188,e364,e384). Rare examples of endodermal sinus tumor of the penis have been reported, with histopathologic features identical to their testicular counterpart (e13,e265). Benign and malignant mesenchymal tumors such as cavernous hemangioma, neurofibroma, dermatofibroma, glomus tumor, malignant lymphoma, malignant peripheral nerve sheath tumor, embryonal RMS, and clear-cell sarcoma have been also rarely reported in the penis (e21,e119,e128,e489,e493,e500). The histopathologic features of these tumors are identical to their soft tissue counterparts. Malignant peripheral nerve sheath tumor in this site has been usually reported in the clinical setting of von Recklinghausen neurofibromatosis.

THE PROSTATE

Congenital and Developmental Anomalies

Congenital abnormalities of the prostate are rare. Hypoplasia and dilation of the prostate are consistent findings in the prune-belly syndrome (e329,e444,e592). The epithelium of the prostatic glands and ducts, prostatic utricle, and prostatic urethra can undergo squamous metaplasia, in response to maternal estrogenic stimulation, during prenatal life. This histologic feature gradually disappears in the early postnatal months (e20). Focal hyperplasia of glandular epithelium, cystic dilatation of tubules, and intraluminal secretions are other histologic changes that are observed in the fetal and neonatal prostate. Congenital abnormalities of the prostate are rare. Hypoplasia and dilation of the prostate are consistent findings in the prune-belly syndrome (57,e444,e592). Cysts of the prostatic utricle (mullerian duct cyst) are an unusual cause of lower urinary tract obstruction and inflammation in boys (e137,e309).

Fibroepithelial polyps of the urethra have been reported typically in males younger than 10 years but can also occur in older men. These are benign growths that can cause a variety of symptoms in young boys including obstructive uropathy, infection, and/or hematuria. They typically occur in the posterior urethra near the verumontanum and consist of a fibrovascular core with loose stroma covered by urothelial lining (e18,e125,e131,e162). Surface ulceration, reactive atypia, and squamous metaplasia may develop in these polyps, which are considered developmental anomalies and are treated by simple transurethral resection.

Acquired Abnormalities and Other Lesions

Overall, lesions and tumors of the prostate are rare in infants and children. A few reports of periprostatic abscesses or hematomas appeared in the literature in which a midline pelvic mass was present accompanied by scrotal abscess and fever and caused lower urinary tract obstruction in infants (e217,e609). *Staphylococcus aureus* and *E. coli* were implicated as causative organisms in these cases.

RMS is by far the most common neoplasm of the prostate in children and adolescents (e316). Approximately 5% of all pediatric RMS primarily involve the prostate (e115). RMS can occur anytime from infancy to early adulthood

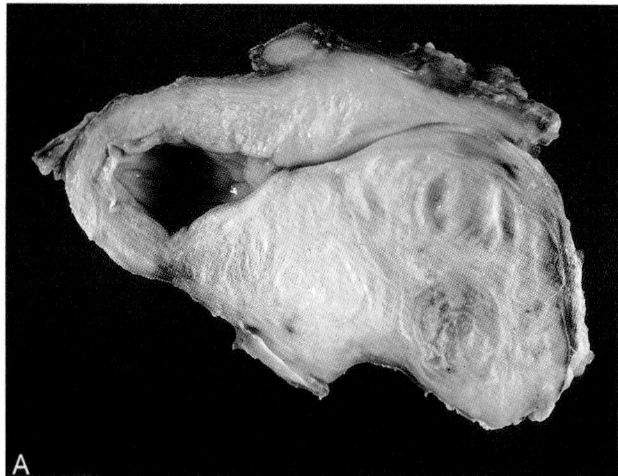

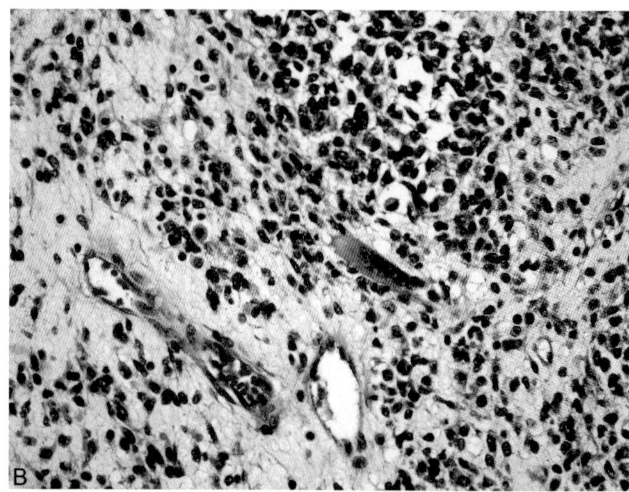

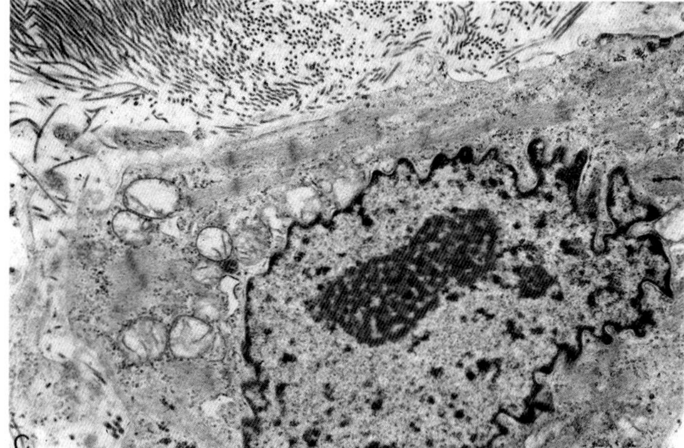

FIGURE 19-17 ■ Embryonal RMS. **A:** The tumor involves the prostatic and the bladder region. **B:** The tumor has variable cellularity with small hyperchromatic cells and scant cytoplasm in a loose stroma. **C:** An occasional giant cell with abundant eosinophilic cytoplasm is depicted. By ultrastructural examination, the cytoplasm contains thin and thick filaments with densities representing the z-bands (Courtesy of Dr. Jerome Taxy, Chicago, Illinois).

but has a peak incidence during the first 4 years of life (10) and a mean age of presentation of 5.3 years (e316). Overall, genitourinary involvement by RMS was found to more commonly affect infants younger than 1 year compared to older children (e454). Like soft tissue RMS, another peak of incidence may be observed during adolescence at 15 to 19 years. The presenting symptoms include bladder outlet obstruction, hematuria, incontinence, infection, and a pelvic or an abdominal mass (e143,348,e349). Large tumors can be difficult to assign a prostatic or a bladder origin, especially since both structures are frequently involved. An association between RMS in genitourinary sites and neurofibromatosis (NF-1) has been reported in one study (e154).

In the pretreatment clinical staging for pediatric RMS, prostatic or bladder involvement, unlike the favorable overall genitourinary location, is regarded as unfavorable site of involvement and assigned a higher clinical stage (58,61). Regional lymph nodal metastasis (usually iliac and para-aortic) can occur in up to 20% of prostate and bladder RMS, necessitating adequate nodal sampling for proper staging of the tumor (e301).

Microscopically, the majority of prostatic RMS is of the embryonal type and is considered of favorable histology (Figure 19-17). It remains important, however, to identify the rare cases of alveolar RMS in this location due to its unfavorable histologic subtype and the additional need for more aggressive chemotherapy. For further review, please refer to the soft tissue section for detailed histopathologic, immunohistochemical and molecular and genetic evaluation of RMS. Multimodality treatment combining surgery, chemotherapy, and radiation therapy is currently applied to pediatric RMS and has greatly improved the prognosis (61,e301,e316) (see Chapter 24).

Rare examples of other tumors occurring in the prostate or prostatic region have been the subject of case reports only. These include a malignant rhabdoid tumor (21), an undifferentiated carcinoma with disseminated metastasis (e509), non-Hodgkin lymphomas (e54,e310), a pheochromocytoma (92), a teratoma with angiosarcoma component (e302), and a case of fibromatosis (e495). Conventional prostatic adenocarcinoma was not detected before the fourth decade in a study of 152 young male patients (e490).

REFERENCES

1. Aaronson IA. True hermaphroditism: a review of 41 cases with observations on testicular histology and function. *Br J Urol* 1985;57(6): 775–779.
2. Agarwal PK, Palmer JS. Testicular and paratesticular neoplasms in prepubertal males. *J Urol* 2006;176(3):875–881.

3. Barteczko KJ, Jacob MI. The testicular descent in human; origin, development and fate of the gubernaculum Hunteri, processus vaginalis peritonei, and gonadal ligaments. *Adv Anat Embryol Cell Biol* 2000;156:III-X, 1–98.
4. Batata MA, Chu FC, Hilaris BS, et al. Testicular cancer in cryptorchids. *Cancer* 1982;49(5):1023–1030.
5. Benson RC, Jr, Beard CM, Kelalis PP, et al. Malignant potential of the cryptorchid testis. *Mayo Clin Proc* 1991;66(4):372–378.
6. Blyth B, Duckett JW, Jr. Gonadal differentiation: a review of the physiological process and influencing factors based on recent experimental evidence. *J Urol* 1991;145(4):689–694.
7. Borer JG, Nitti VW, Glassberg KI. Mixed gonadal dysgenesis and dysgenetic male pseudohermaphroditism. *J Urol* 1995;153(4):1267–1273.
8. Buchholz NP, Biyabani R, Herzig MJ, et al. Persistent Mullerian duct syndrome. *Eur Urol* 1998;34(3):230–232.
9. Byskov AG. Differentiation of mammalian embryonic gonad. *Physiol Rev* 1986;66(1):71–117.
10. Cangir A. Malignant genital tract tumors in children. *Curr Probl Cancer* 1986;10(6):301–341.
11. Carver BS, Al-Ahmadie H, Sheinfeld J. Adult and pediatric testicular teratoma. *Urol Clin North Am* 2007;34(2):245–251.
12. Cerilli LA, Sotelo-Avila C, Mills SE. Glandular inclusions in inguinal hernia sacs: morphologic and immunohistochemical distinction from epididymis and vas deferens. *Am J Surg Pathol* 2003;27(4):469–476.
13. Clericuzio CL. Clinical phenotypes and Wilms tumor. *Med Pediatr Oncol* 1993;21(3):182–187.
14. Coppes MJ, Rackley R, Kay R. Primary testicular and paratesticular tumors of childhood. *Med Pediatr Oncol* 1994;22(5):329–340.
15. Cortes D, Thorup JM, Visfeldt J. Cryptorchidism: aspects of fertility and neoplasms. A study including data of 1,335 consecutive boys who underwent testicular biopsy simultaneously with surgery for cryptorchidism. *Horm Res* 2001;55(1):21–27.
16. Cortez JC, Kaplan GW. Gonadal stromal tumors, gonadoblastomas, epidermoid cysts, and secondary tumors of the testis in children. *Urol Clin North Am* 1993;20(1):15–26.
17. Cromie WJ. Congenital anomalies of the testis, vas epididymis, and inguinal canal. *Urol Clin North Am* 1978;5(1):237–252.
18. Crump WD. Juvenile granulosa cell (sex cord-stromal) tumor of fetal testis. *J Urol* 1983;129(5):1057–1058.
19. John Radcliffe Hospital Cryptorchidism Study Group. Cryptorchidism: a prospective study of 7500 consecutive male births, 1984–8. *Arch Dis Child* 1992;67(7):892–899.
20. Cunha GR, Alarid ET, Turner T, et al. Normal and abnormal development of the male urogenital tract: role of androgens, mesenchymal-epithelial interactions, and growth factors. *J Androl* 1992;13(6):465–475.
21. Ekfors TO, Aho HJ, Kekomaki M. Malignant rhabdoid tumor of the prostatic region: immunohistological and ultrastructural evidence for epithelial origin. *Virchows Arch A Pathol Anat Histopathol* 1985;406(3):381–388.
22. Elbe JL. Tumors of the testis and paratesticular tissue, Chapter 4. In: Eble JN, Sauter G, Epstein JI, Sesterhenn I, eds. *World Health Organization classification of tumours, pathology and genetics; tumours of the urinary system and male genital organs*. IARC Press: Lyon, 2004.
23. Elder JS. Epididymal anomalies associated with hydrocele/hernia and cryptorchidism: implications regarding testicular descent. *J Urol* 1992;148(2 Pt 2):624–626.
24. Emerson RE, Ulbright TM. The use of immunohistochemistry in the differential diagnosis of tumors of the testis and paratestis. *Semin Diagn Pathol* 2005;22(1):33–50.
25. Fechner PY. The role of SRY in mammalian sex determination. *Acta Paediatr Jpn* 1996;38(4):380–389.
26. Garrett JE, Cartwright PC, Snow BW, et al. Cystic testicular lesions in the pediatric population. *J Urol* 2000;163(3):928–936.
27. Gerald WL, Ladanyi M, de Alava E, et al. Clinical, pathologic, and molecular spectrum of tumors associated with t(11;22)(p13;q12): desmoplastic small round-cell tumor and its variants. *J Clin Oncol* 1998;16(9):3028–3036.
28. Gill B, Kogan S. Cryptorchidism: current concepts. *Pediatr Clin North Am* 1997;44(5):1211–1227.
29. Grady RW, Ross JH, Kay R. Patterns of metastatic spread in prepubertal yolk sac tumor of the testis. *J Urol* 1995;153(4):1259–1261.
30. Hadjiathanasiou CG, Brauner R, Lortat-Jacob S, et al. True hermaphroditism: genetic variants and clinical management. *J Pediatr* 1994;125(5 Pt 1):738–744.
31. Harley VR, Clarkson MJ, Argentaro A. The molecular action and regulation of the testis-determining factors, SRY (sex-determining region on the Y chromosome) and SOX9 [SRY-related high-mobility group (HMG) box 9]. *Endocr Rev* 2003;24(4):466–487.
32. Harms D, Janig U. Germ cell tumours of childhood:report of 170 cases including 59 pure and partial yolk-sac tumours. *Virchows Arch A Pathol Anat Histopathol* 1986;409(2):223–239.
33. Harms D, Kock LR. Testicular juvenile granulosa cell and Sertoli cell tumours: a clinicopathological study of 29 cases from the Kiel Paediatric Tumour Registry. *Virchows Arch* 1997;430(4):301–309.
34. Hegarty PK, Mushtaq I, Sebire NJ, Natural history of testicular regression syndrome and consequences for clinical management. *J Pediatr Urol* 2007;3(3):206–208.
35. Henley JD, Ferry J, Ulbright TM. Miscellaneous rare paratesticular tumors. *Semin Diagn Pathol* 2000;17(4):319–339.
36. Hiort O, Holterhus PM. The molecular basis of male sexual differentiation. *Eur J Endocrinol* 2000;142(2):101–110.
37. Huff DS, Fenig DM, Canning DA, et al. Abnormal germ cell development in cryptorchidism. *Horm Res* 2001;55(1):11–17.
38. Hughes IA, Acerini CL. Factors controlling testis descent. *Eur J Endocrinol* 2008;159 (Suppl 1):S75–S82.
39. International Germ Cell Cancer Collaborative Group. International Germ Cell Consensus Classification: a prognostic factor-based staging system for metastatic germ cell cancers. *J Clin Oncol* 1997;15(2):594–603.
40. Kaplan GW, Cromie WC, Kelalis PP, et al. Prepubertal yolk sac testicular tumors–report of the testicular tumor registry. *J Urol* 1988;140(5 Pt 2):1109–1112.
41. Kaplan GW, Cromie WJ, Kelalis PP, et al. Gonadal stromal tumors: a report of the Prepubertal Testicular Tumor Registry. *J Urol* 1986;136(1 Pt 2):300–302.
42. Khedis M, Nohra J, Dierickx L, et al. Polyorchidism: presentation of 2 cases, review of the literature and a new management strategy. *Urol Int* 2008;80(1):98–101.
43. Krasna IH, Lee ML, Smilow P, et al. Risk of malignancy in bilateral streak gonads: the role of the Y chromosome. *J Pediatr Surg* 1992;27(11):1376–1380.
44. Kremer H, Kraaij R, Toledo SP, et al. Male pseudohermaphroditism due to a homozygous missense mutation of the luteinizing hormone receptor gene. *Nat Genet* 1995;9(2):160–164.
45. Krob G, Braun A, Kuhnle U. True hermaphroditism: geographical distribution, clinical findings, chromosomes and gonadal histology. *Eur J Pediatr* 1994;153(1):2–10.
46. Lanfranco F, Kamischke A, Zitzmann M, et al. Klinefelter's syndrome. *Lancet* 2004;364(9430):273–283.
47. Law H, Mushtaq I, Wingrove K, et al. Histopathological features of testicular regression syndrome: relation to patient age and implications for management. *Fetal Pediatr Pathol* 2006;25(2):119–129.
48. Lawrence WD, Young RH, Scully RE. Juvenile granulosa cell tumor of the infantile testis: a report of 14 cases. *Am J Surg Pathol* 1985;9(2):87–94.
49. Lee PA, Houk CP, Ahmed SF, et al. Consensus statement on management of intersex disorders. International Consensus Conference on Intersex. *Pediatrics* 2006;118(2):e488–e500.
50. Levin HS. Tumors of the testis in intersex syndromes. *Urol Clin North Am* 2000;27(3):543–551, x.

51. Levy DA, Kay R, Elder JS. Neonatal testis tumors: a review of the Prepubertal Testis Tumor Registry. *J Urol* 1994;151(3):715–717.
52. Lim HN, Hawkins JR. Genetic control of gonadal differentiation. *Baillieres Clin Endocrinol Metab* 1998;12(1):1–16.
53. Looijenga LH, de Munnik H, Oosterhuis JW. A molecular model for the development of germ cell cancer. *Int J Cancer* 1999;83(6):809–814.
54. Looijenga LH, Oosterhuis JW. Pathogenesis of testicular germ cell tumours. *Rev Reprod* 1999;4(2):90–100.
55. Loughlin KR, Retik AB, Weinstein HJ, et al. Genitourinary rhabdomyosarcoma in children. *Cancer* 1989;63(8):1600–1606.
56. Malek RS, Rosen JS, Farrow GM. Epidermoid cyst of the testis: a critical analysis. *Br J Urol* 1986;58(1):55–59.
57. Manivel JC, Simonton S, Wold LE, et al. Absence of intratubular germ cell neoplasia in testicular yolk sac tumors in children: a histochemical and immunohistochemical study. *Arch Pathol Lab Med* 1988;112(6):641–645.
58. Maurer HM, Gehan EA, Beltangady M, et al. The Intergroup Rhabdomyosarcoma Study-II. *Cancer* 1993;71(5):1904–1922.
59. McAleer IM, Packer MG, Kaplan GW, et al. Fertility index analysis in cryptorchidism. *J Urol* 1995;153(4):1255–1258.
60. McElreavey K, Fellous M. Sex determination and the Y chromosome. *Am J Med Genet* 1999;89(4):176–185.
61. McLean TW, Castellino SM. Pediatric genitourinary tumors. *Curr Opin Oncol* 2008;20(3):315–320.
62. Merry C, Sweeney B, Puri P. The vanishing testis: anatomical and histological findings. *Eur Urol* 1997;31(1):65–67.
63. Metcalfe PD, Farivar-Mohseni H, Farhat W, et al. Pediatric testicular tumors: contemporary incidence and efficacy of testicular preserving surgery. *J Urol* 2003;170(6 Pt 1):2412–2415; discussion 2415–2416.
64. Mostert M, Rosenberg C, Stoop H, et al. Comparative genomic and in situ hybridization of germ cell tumors of the infantile testis. *Lab Invest* 2000;80(7):1055–1064.
65. Muller J, Skakkebaek NE, Ritzen M, et al. Carcinoma in situ of the testis in children with 45,X/46,XY gonadal dysgenesis. *J Pediatr* 1985;106(3):431–436.
66. Nistal M, Gonzalez-Peramato P, Paniagua R. Congenital Leydig cell hyperplasia. *Histopathology* 1988;12(3):307–317.
67. Nistal M, Paniagua R, Diez-Pardo JA. Histologic classification of undescended testes. *Hum Pathol* 1980;11(6):666–674.
68. Nistal M, Redondo E, Paniagua R. Juvenile granulosa cell tumor of the testis. *Arch Pathol Lab Med* 1988;112(11):1129–1132.
69. Paduch DA, Fine RG, Bolyakov A, et al. New concepts in Klinefelter syndrome. *Curr Opin Urol* 2008;18(6):621–627.
70. Parker KL, Schedl A, Schimmer BP. Gene interactions in gonadal development. *Annu Rev Physiol* 1999;61:417–433.
71. Perlman EJ, Hu J, Ho D, et al. Genetic analysis of childhood endodermal sinus tumors by comparative genomic hybridization. *J Pediatr Hematol Oncol* 2000;22(2):100–105.
72. Pohl HG, Shukla AR, Metcalf PD, et al. Prepubertal testis tumors: actual prevalence rate of histological types. *J Urol* 2004;172(6 Pt 1): 2370–2372.
73. Pritchard-Jones K, Fleming S, Davidson D, et al. The candidate Wilms' tumour gene is involved in genitourinary development. *Nature* 1990;346(6280):194–197.
74. Reuter VE. Origins and molecular biology of testicular germ cell tumors. *Mod Pathol* 2005;18 (Suppl 2):S51–S60.
75. Rey R, Picard JY. Embryology and endocrinology of genital development. *Baillieres Clin Endocrinol Metab* 1998;12(1):17–33.
76. Robboy SJ, Jaubert F. Neoplasms and pathology of sexual developmental disorders (intersex). *Pathology* 2007;39(1):147–163.
77. Ross JH, Kay R. Prepubertal testis tumors. *Rev Urol* 2004;6(1): 11–18.
78. Rune GM, Mayr J, Neugebauer H, et al. Pattern of Sertoli cell degeneration in cryptorchid prepubertal testes. *Int J Androl* 1992;15(1):19–31.
79. Rutgers JL. Advances in the pathology of intersex conditions. *Hum Pathol* 1991;22(9):884–891.
80. Rutgers JL, Young RH, Scully RE. The testicular "tumor" of the adrenogenital syndrome: a report of six cases and review of the literature on testicular masses in patients with adrenocortical disorders. *Am J Surg Pathol* 1988;12(7):503–513.
81. Scully RE. Gonadoblastoma: a review of 74 cases. *Cancer* 1970;25(6):1340–1356.
82. Seraj IM, Chase DR, Chase RL, et al. Malignant teratoma arising in a dysgenetic gonad. *Gynecol Oncol* 1993;50(2):254–258.
83. Skoog SJ. Benign and malignant pediatric scrotal masses. *Pediatr Clin North Am* 1997;44(5):1229–1250.
84. Swerdlow AJ, Schoemaker MJ, Higgins CD, et al. Cancer incidence and mortality in men with Klinefelter syndrome: a cohort study. *J Natl Cancer Inst* 2005;97(16):1204–1210.
85. Taskinen S, Fagerholm R, Aronniemi J, et al. Testicular tumors in children and adolescents. *J Pediatr Urol* 2008;4(2):134–137.
86. Thong M, Lim C, Fatimah H. Undescended testes: incidence in 1,002 consecutive male infants and outcome at 1 year of age. *Pediatr Surg Int* 1998;13(1):37–41.
87. Thonneau PF, Gandia P, Mieusset R. Cryptorchidism: incidence, risk factors, and potential role of environment; an update. *J Androl* 2003;24(2):155–162.
88. Uehara S, Funato T, Yaegashi N, et al. SRY mutation and tumor formation on the gonads of XP pure gonadal dysgenesis patients. *Cancer Genet Cytogenet* 1999;113(1):78–84.
89. Ulbright TM. Protocol for the examination of specimens from patients with malignant germ cell and sex cord-stromal tumors of the testis, exclusive of paratesticular malignancies: a basis for checklists. Cancer Committee, College of American Pathologists. *Arch Pathol Lab Med* 1999;123(1):14–19.
90. Veltman I, Veltman J, Janssen I, et al. Identification of recurrent chromosomal aberrations in germ cell tumors of neonates and infants using genomewide array-based comparative genomic hybridization. *Genes Chromosomes Cancer* 2005;43(4):367–376.
91. Virtanen HE, Tapanainen AE, Kaleva MM, et al. Mild gestational diabetes as a risk factor for congenital cryptorchidism. *J Clin Endocrinol Metab* 2006;91(12):4862–4865.
92. Voges GE, Wippermann F, Duber C, et al. Pheochromocytoma in the pediatric age group: the prostate–an unusual location. *J Urol* 1990;144(5):1219–1221.
93. Weidner IS, Moller H, Jensen TK, et al. Risk factors for cryptorchidism and hypospadias. *J Urol* 1999;161(5):1606–1609.
94. Wilson DM, Pitts WC, Hintz RL, et al. Testicular tumors with Peutz-Jeghers syndrome. *Cancer* 1986;57(11):2238–2240.
95. Yordam N, Alikasifoglu A, Kandemir N, et al. True hermaphroditism: clinical features, genetic variants and gonadal histology. *J Pediatr Endocrinol Metab* 2001;14(4):421–427.
96. Young RH, Koelliker DD, Scully RE. Sertoli cell tumors of the testis, not otherwise specified: a clinicopathologic analysis of 60 cases. *Am J Surg Pathol* 1998;22(6):709–721.

CHAPTER 20

The Breast

JEFFREY MUELLER
REBECCA WILCOX
JEROME B. TAXY

The breast is often regarded as a modified sweat gland. Dichotomous branching of ductal structures ending as lobules and acini characterizes its embryology. Mammary gland development begins during the fourth week of embryonic life as mammary crests, thickened symmetric ridges of ectoderm on the ventral wall extending from the axillary to inguinal regions all of which involute except in the region of eventual breast development. Mammary buds, the solid downgrowths of cuboidal ectoderm in the mammary crest, penetrate into the underlying mesenchyme during the sixth week. The subsequent mammary buds develop into the lactiferous sinuses, which are then canalized when induced by placental sex hormones. By term, approximately 15 to 20 lactiferous ducts are formed. Progressive branching of this system eventually forms the ductal-lobular architecture.

Late in gestation, the nipples arise from the primitive epidermis in the form of shallow pits. These are depressed in the newborn but soon elevate due to the proliferation of the surrounding fibrovascular connective tissue of the areola. The mammary glands of the newborn, irrespective of gender, are rudimentary but responsive to maternal gestational hormones. They are clinically palpable and histologically characterized by secretory ducts and edematous stroma. Secretions known as "witch's milk" may be produced secondary to maternal hormones in the fetal circulation or production of prolactin in the infant pituitary.

From birth until puberty, the mammary glands remain undeveloped. In pubertal females, elevated levels of estrogens, progestogens, and growth hormone result in breast enlargement (thelarche) due to the accumulation of fat and the development of the ductal lobular units. Thelarche is classified by imaging modalities, principally ultrasound, into Tanner stages 1 to 5, with 1 being the least and 5 being the most developed. In males, breast tissue remains hormonally unstimulated, histologically characterized by ducts without lobular development throughout life (91,92,100).

Palpable breast lesions are infrequent. In addition, the pectoral soft tissues are not typically sampled during the course of a pediatric autopsy. Histology and cytology samples are therefore rare. This may result in a lack of familiarity with the morphology of the breast in children. Among those lesions surgically excised, there is a predominance of benign lesions, with fibroadenoma and gynecomastia together constituting 50% to 70% of all cases (14,15,35,36,47,58,65, 115,134,135,138) (Table 20-1). Most lesions of the breast in the first two decades of life are clustered in the adolescent age group (25). Neinstein and associates (104) reported the presence of newly detected masses in 3.25% of female adolescents. Most masses were unilateral, well circumscribed, and solitary at clinical presentation. Pettinato and colleagues (115) reviewed the experiences of three institutions, focusing on breast lesions in children and adolescents other than gynecomastia and fibroadenomas and many were, by their infrequent nature, diagnostic and therapeutic dilemmas. West and associates (160) reported unilateral thelarche in 26 (35%) of 74 children and adolescents with a symptomatic breast mass, so that the clinical approach should be a cautious one.

ANOMALIES

Congenital Absence of the Breast

The presence of a nipple may be accompanied by absent or hypoplastic breast tissue due to the failure of the pectoral portion of the mammary ridge to develop (150). This rare lesion has been subdivided into several clinical categories based on distribution, associated defects, and inheritance as an autosomal dominant, sex-linked recessive, or incompletely defined familial trait (18,105,144,150). Alopecia, saddle nose deformity, underdeveloped or missing teeth, absence of pectoral muscles, and anhidrotic ectodermal dysplasia are some of the accompanying defects (18). Some of these children have the clinical manifestations of Poland syndrome (aplasia of the pectoral muscle). Agenesis of breast lobules has been reported in cystic fibrosis (53).

Table 20-1 ■ BREAST LESIONS IN CHILDREN AND ADOLESCENTS: REVIEW OF EIGHT SERIES AND TWO CHILDREN'S HOSPITALS

	Eight Series from Literature (30,79,93, 108,121,194,239,247)	Primary Children's Hospital 1970–1989	St. Louis Children's Hospital 1989–1998	Total %
Fibroadenoma	524	13	166	703 (55)
Gynecomastia	38	34	81	153 (12)
Cysts/fibrocystic changes	77	4	27	108 (8)
Macromastia	26	9	52	87 (7)
Other	19	3[a]	26[b]	48 (4)
Inflammation[c]	39	2	1	42 (3)
Papilloma/papillomatosis[d]	24	—	3	27 (2)
Hyperplasia, NOS	18	—	4	22 (2)
Hemangioma	12	—	1	13 (1)
Fat necrosis	10	—	1	11 (1)
Cystosarcoma phyllodes	7	—	4	11 (1)
Rhabdomyosarcoma	7	1	1	9 (< 1)
Accessory breast tissue	8	1	—	9 (< 1)
Lipoma	5	—	2	7 (< 1)
Supernumerary nipple	2	4	—	6 (< 1)
Fibrosis	2	4	—	6 (< 1)
Granular cell tumor	1	—	3	4 (< 1)
Carcinoma	3	—	1	4 (< 1)
Fibromatosis	1	—	1	2 (< 1)
Total	825	75	374	1,274 (~100)

[a]Includes tubular adenoma (1), plexiform neurofibroma (1), lymphangioma (1).
[b]Includes tubular adenoma (10), lactating adenoma (5), keloid (2), neurofibroma (2), angiosarcoma (2), nipple duct adenoma (1), lymphangioma (1), hamartoma (1), stromal sarcoma (1), giant cell fibroblastoma (1).
[c]Includes mastitis and abscess.
[d]Includes juvenile papillomatosis and intraductal papilloma. NOS, not otherwise specified.

Supernumerary Nipple and Accessory Breast Tissue

Supernumerary Nipple

Supernumerary nipple (polythelia, accessory nipple) occurs in 2.5% of systematically examined neonates with a slight male predominance (98,155). Fewer than 10% are bilateral, and fewer than 5% arise at sites other than along the embryonic mammary line, such as the back, shoulder, posterior thigh, face, and neck. Familial supernumerary nipples have been reported (20,151). The clinical features are those of a small pigmented macule with a tiny umbilication (95) that histologically exhibits components of a normal nipple with occasional hyperplastic duct epithelium, capillary proliferation, pilosebaceous units with intraluminal keratinous material, and bundles of smooth muscle. Lactiferous ducts and terminal duct-lobular units may be inconspicuous (62,73,75,94,153).

Accessory Breast Tissue

Accessory breast tissue is unusual (1% to 2% of the white population), occasionally familial (159), presenting as a mass in the axilla or vulva. In the vulva, this may be inseparable from hidradenoma papilliferum (27). Both supernumerary nipples and accessory breast tissue have been noted more commonly in the Native American population (56). The mass is ill defined and composed of histologically unremarkable predominately breast ducts and subareolar structures. A variety of histologic and pathologic findings have been described in accessory breast tissue, including fibroadenomas and ductal carcinoma (31,64,78,115).

Breast Asymmetry

Breast asymmetry is common between Tanner stages 2 and 4, and it may persist to a mild degree in as many as 25% of young adults (60,145). Unilateral breast enlargement with its attendant asymmetry is seen in neonates as a response to maternal and placental hormones. This condition often spontaneously corrects; if no underlying endocrine abnormalities are present, the asymmetry is correctable by augmentation mammoplasty.

BREAST LESIONS

Fibroproliferative (Fibrocystic) Disease

Fibrocystic Changes

The term *fibrocystic change* has been historically used to refer to the spectrum of cysts, fibrosis, and epithelial proliferation reflective, in part, of hormonal-induced changes related to the menstrual cycle (59). Although more common in adults, it is occasionally seen in middle-to-late adolescence. Similar to adults, these are characterized by diffuse cysts and masses with size fluctuations correlating with the menstrual cycle and often manifesting perimenstrual tenderness. Biopsy may not be warranted, as the clinical presentation and physical exam without imaging is probably diagnostic. In children, solitary cysts are more common than multiple cysts (23). The histopathologic changes include dense hypocellular to moderately cellular stromal fibrosis, cystic dilation, apocrine metaplasia, adenosis, and usual ductal hyperplasia. Atypical ductal hyperplasia is rare in young women and is associated with an increase in risk of subsequent ductal carcinoma (42,45,63). Treatments include improved breast support, steroids, oral contraceptives, vitamin E, and avoidance of caffeine (33).

Dense fibrosis, occasionally termed *fibrous mastopathy*, is a localized and ill-defined fibrous proliferation of the breast stroma and may represent the fibrous end of the fibrocystic spectrum. It compromises and eventually obliterates the lobular breast parenchyma. Although a hormonal etiology is suspected, grossly the lesions are described as "stony-hard" and lack cysts, distinguishing them from typical fibrocystic changes as noted above. Microscopically, the lesions are divided into three groups based on the relationship of acinar tissue to stroma. Type I shows prominent acinar tissue with scant concentric collagen bundles encircling the epithelial units. Type II shows partial replacement of acini with dense bundles of collagen in an uneven manner. Type III reveals almost complete replacement of the acinar tissue. Type I is most commonly seen in the younger age group. Excisional biopsy is the treatment of choice (99,121,122).

Papillary Duct Hyperplasia

Among epithelial proliferations, papillary duct hyperplasia is uncommon, occurring almost exclusively in females, with a median age of 17 years, although these are occasionally reported in neonates and young children. The most common presenting symptom is a mass, less commonly accompanied by clear or bloody nipple discharge. Intraductal papilloma may be clinically considered. The size of the lesion varies but up to 5 cm has been reported. The cut surface grossly shows numerous cysts with papillary excrescences. Histologic examination shows three different patterns including true papilloma, sclerosing papilloma, and papillomatosis. All show fronds of epithelial cells in single or multiple layers with a fibrovascular stroma. Myoepithelial hyperplasia may be present. The sclerosing papilloma pattern may show a radial scar lesion with small clusters of epithelial cells trapped within the sclerotic stroma, probably representing lesional regression but histologically mimicking carcinoma (124,161).

Diabetic Mastopathy

Diabetic mastopathy is a complication of uncertain etiology associated with longstanding type 1 diabetes. The patients typically present in late adolescence with a firm mass in one or both breasts. The histologic findings are typified by lymphocytic lobulitis and ductitis, perivasculitis, and dense keloidal fibrosis (43). Recurrences are common (77,147).

Juvenile Papillomatosis

Juvenile papillomatosis is a benign proliferative lesion that despite the name also occurs in adults. The patients are typically postpubertal, with a firm, solitary mass at the periphery of the breast. Bilaterality or multifocality in the same breast is rare. When performed, mammography shows an area of increased density with poorly defined borders. A risk for breast carcinoma has been reported in maternal female family members of young patients with juvenile papillomatosis. Grossly, the tumor is a firm, discrete mass, which ranges from 1 to 8 cm, with slightly irregular borders (Figure 20-1). The cut surface shows numerous cysts, 1 mm to 2 cm giving rise to the term *Swiss-Cheese breast*. The intercystic tissue shows yellow-white flecks, similar in appearance to that of comedo-type necrosis. Although histologic examination shows a variety of benign proliferative changes typically associated with conventional fibrocystic disease, e.g., apocrine metaplasia, usual ductal hyperplasia, papillomas with involutional features, and cysts, there is nothing to suggest a common etiology or clinical association. Within the dilated ducts and cysts are numerous lipid-laden macrophages, consistent with stasis (Figures 20-2 to 20-4). Microcalcifications are sometimes present. The ductal proliferation is typically usual or florid hyperplasia, occasionally associated with sclerosis producing a radial scar pattern. Atypical ductal hyperplasia has been reported within juvenile papillomatosis in up to 40% of cases. In situ carcinoma is rare in young adults. Since fibroadenoma is the common preoperative diagnosis, the excisional biopsy margins may be inadequate and recurrences may ensue (55,67,129,139,140).

Infection and Fat Necrosis

Infections

Infections of the breast occur at any age during childhood, including the neonatal period. Adolescents may develop

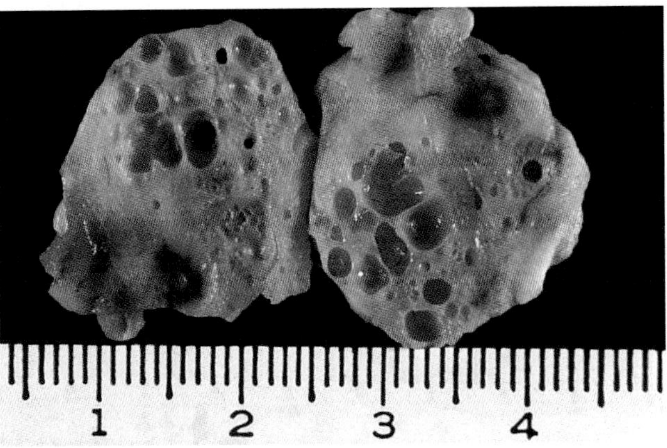

FIGURE 20-1 ▪ Juvenile papillomatosis. Gross appearance (the so-called Swiss cheese disease) with multiple small cysts in a densely fibrotic background.

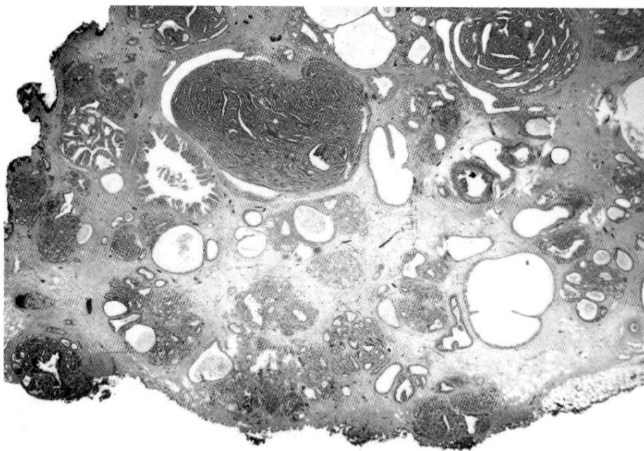

FIGURE 20-2 ■ Juvenile papillomatosis. Low-power section showing fibrosis, multiple cysts, and prominent papillary duct hyperplasia. Note that the lesion extends to the inked margin, a frequent feature in this lesion often clinically mistaken for fibroadenoma.

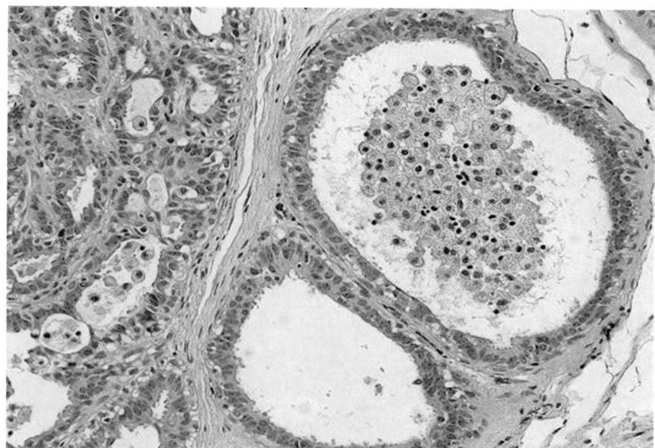

FIGURE 20-4 ■ Juvenile papillomatosis. Dilated cysts containing foamy macrophages.

mastitis or breast abscess due to foreign bodies, trauma, nipple piercing, and infection of an epidermal cyst. Localized tenderness, induration, and erythema may be followed by a fluctuant mass indicating abscess formation. *Staphylococcus aureus* is the most common organism involved, but the spectrum of organisms is wide, including Mycobacteria (34). Fine-needle aspiration may be diagnostic, precluding surgical biopsy. The histologic picture is variable, ranging from acute and chronic inflammation to abscess formation, granulomatous inflammation, and squamous metaplasia. Larger abscesses may need formal incision and drainage.

Fat Necrosis

Fat necrosis, possibly related to previous surgery or trauma, is a localized mass with or without tenderness. Grossly the nodules have a gritty yellow surface. The histology shows chronic inflammation with lipophages, fibrosis, and dystrophic calcifications (34,45).

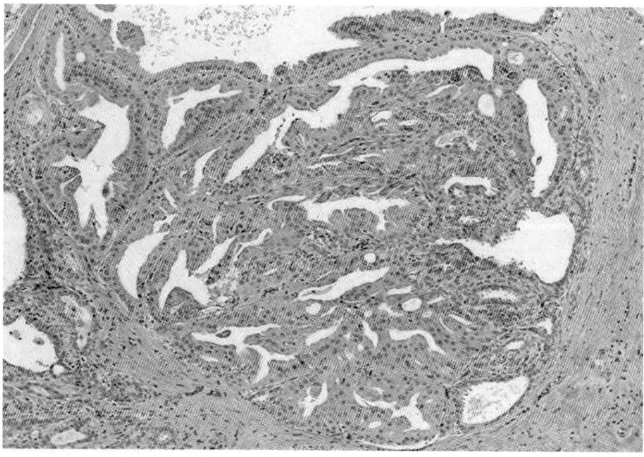

FIGURE 20-3 ■ Juvenile papillomatosis. Histologic features include apocrine metaplasia and papillary duct hyperplasia.

Gynecomastia and Juvenile Hypertrophy

Gynecomastia

Gynecomastia, idiopathic excessive development of the breast in males, is the most common breast abnormality in adolescent boys and a frequent source of surgical specimens (Table 20-1). The etiology may be an imbalance between estrogen and androgen, along with end-organ response factors, although many conditions are associated with gynecomastia (Table 20-2), including hyperthyroidism, hypogonadism, and drugs such as exogenous hormones that may be used by athletes for performance enhancement. When an underlying clinical endocrine abnormality is present, the gynecomastia is typically bilateral with a female pattern of enlargement and areolar hyperpigmentation. Pseudogynecomastia is breast enlargement that is caused by increases in other tissues such as muscle enlargement, obesity, or diffuse neurofibromatosis in the pectoral region. In addition, pseudoangiomatous stromal hyperplasia

Table 20-2 ■ SPECIFIC CONDITIONS ASSOCIATED WITH GYNECOMASTIA IN CHILDREN AND ADOLESCENTS
Adrenocortical adenoma and carcinoma
Choriocarcinoma and other gonadotropin-producing germ cell neoplasms
Congenital adrenal hyperplasia
Familial gynecomastia with aromatase excess
Fibrolamellar hepatocellular carcinoma with aromatase excess
Growth hormone therapy
Hepatoblastoma
Hypergonadotropic hypogonadism
Large-cell calcifying Sertoli cell tumor with and without Peutz-Jegher syndrome
Prolactinoma
Pseudohermaphroditism (5-α-reductase deficiency)
Spinal cord disorders
von Recklinghausen neurofibromatosis
X-linked mental retardation
Drugs

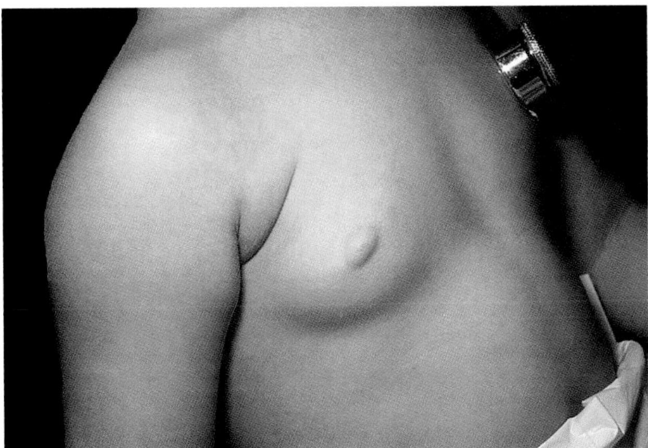

FIGURE 20-5 ■ Gynecomastia in a prepubertal boy.

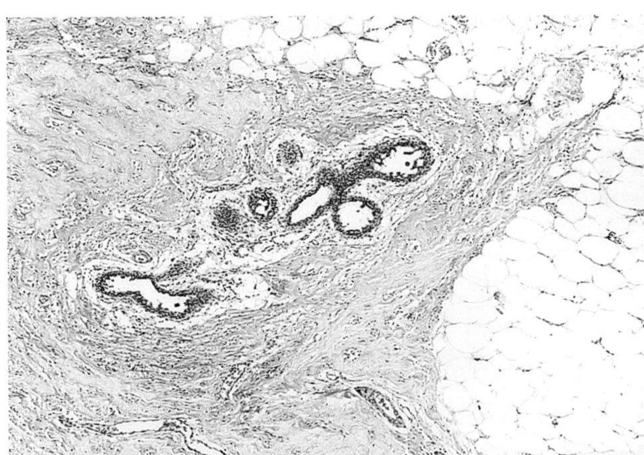

FIGURE 20-7 ■ Gynecomastia. Ducts cuffed by an edematous stromal "halo" and surrounding hyalinized stroma. No lobules are present.

(PASH) has also been described as a mimic of gynecomastia. The central subareolar region is typically affected but it may be eccentric, unilateral or bilateral, ranging from 2 to 10 cm. Nipple retraction is rare (Figure 20-5). The swelling is often painful and may interfere with participation in sports activities, but resolves over time. Grossly the tissue is rubbery, white, and ill-defined (Figure 20-6), mixed with mature yellow adipose tissue. Histologically, gynecomastia and juvenile hypertrophy are similar. The changes center on ductal epithelial hyperplasia and a cellular, myxoid stroma. In early phases, there is a ductal epithelial proliferation with papillary and/or cribriform patterns and accompanying myoepithelial hyperplasia. The periductal stroma is cellular and edematous (Figures 20-7 and 20-8). With time, there may be less epithelial proliferation and more collagenous stroma (59,81,108,126). Some lobular formation may be seen in Klinefelter syndrome.

Juvenile Hypertrophy and Macromastia

Juvenile hypertrophy is restricted to the female breast as a spontaneous, rapid, massive growth, unilateral or bilateral (Figure 20-9), probably secondary to increased sensitivity to gonadal hormones. Macromastia, deforming, painful overgrowth of the female breast, may be synonymous with juvenile hypertrophy. The usual age of onset is menarche. An association with Hashimoto thyroiditis, rheumatoid arthritis, and myasthenia gravis has been noted and therefore an autoimmune etiology has been alleged. The treatment primarily involves antiestrogen therapy and/or surgical reduction. Grossly, the tissue shows a homogeneous tan-yellow cut surface without a discrete mass. Histologic sections reveal an irregular proliferation of ducts with hyperplasia in a hypocellular edematous stroma. Pseudoangiomatous stromal hyperplasia may be present (29,34,45,87,137).

Epithelial-Stromal Lesions

Fibroadenoma, juvenile fibroadenoma, and cystosarcoma phyllodes (phyllodes tumor) are biphasic, fibroepithelial tumors that may be regarded as a clinicopathologic spectrum. While fibroadenoma in children and adolescents may be morphologically similar to its counterpart in adults, juvenile fibroadenoma is a term not employed in the adult population. Juvenile fibroadenoma has effectively subsumed the benign phyllodes tumor in this age group, since the morphologic characteristics and clinical behavior are similar (23). The term *cystosarcoma phyllodes*, or *phyllodes tumor*, in children is used in reference to at least a low-grade malignancy.

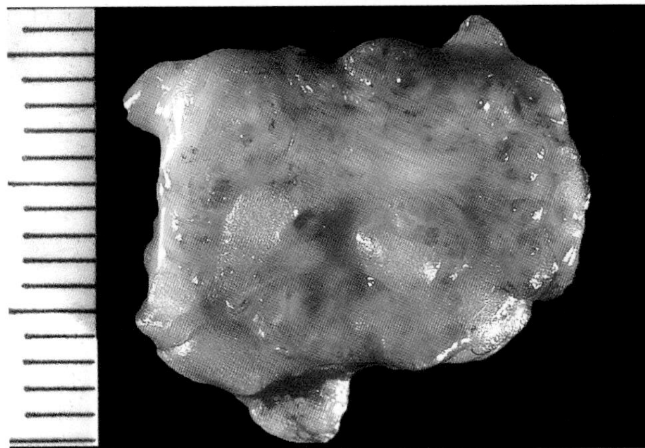

FIGURE 20-6 ■ Gynecomastia. Cut surface of gross specimen shows ill-defined dense white tissue and fat.

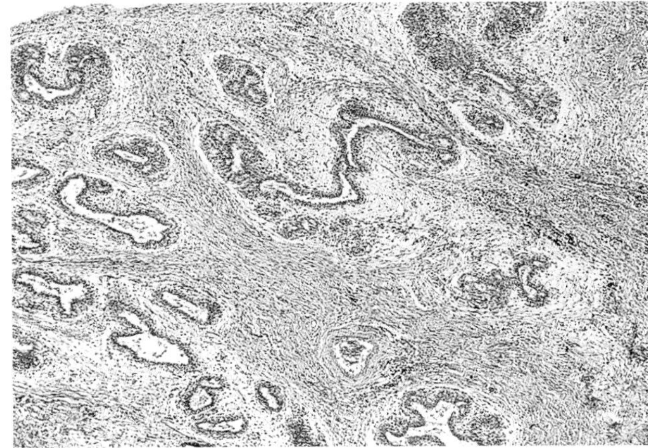

FIGURE 20-8 ■ Neonatal breast tissue. Ducts and edematous stroma. Note the histologic similarity to gynecomastia.

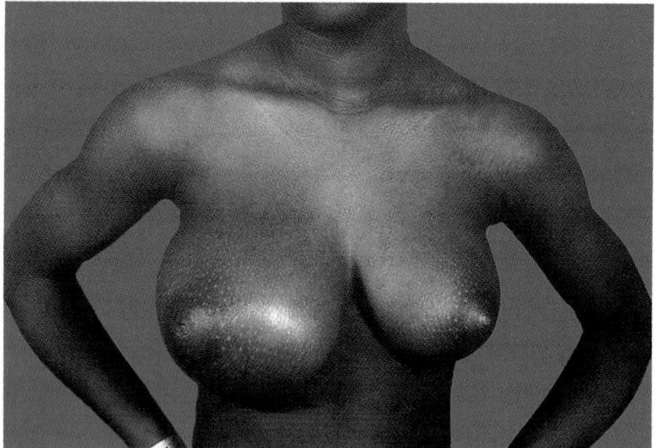

FIGURE 20-9 ■ Juvenile hypertrophy. Asymmetric enlargement of right breast. Histologically, the features are similar to gynecomastia.

Fibroadenoma and Tubular Adenoma

Fibroadenoma is the most common breast mass in adolescent females and as such accounts for most of the excisional breast biopsies in this age group (Table 20-1). The tumors come to attention in late adolescence (23) with a slowly enlarging, painless mass (59). Fibroadenomas are more common in African-American patients (33) and range from 2 to 5 cm. Physical exam reveals a firm, freely mobile, well-circumscribed mass. As these tumors are estrogen sensitive, growth may accelerate during pregnancy. Grossly, tumors are well circumscribed and have a rubbery, bulging and lobulated cut surface with a myxoid or a gelatinous appearance. Occasionally, cystic areas may be apparent. Histologically, fibroadenomas exhibit a proliferation of epithelial, myoepithelial, and stromal elements. Two acknowledged histologic patterns of fibroadenoma are recognized based on variations of the stromal and epithelial components but are not mutually exclusive. In the intracanalicular pattern, the stroma surrounds and compresses epithelial-lined ducts into anastomosing strands with slit-like lumens (Figure 20-10). Open acinar and ductal structures simulating normal breast tissue characterize the pericanalicular pattern (Figure 20-11). The different architectural patterns are frequently admixed and have no known prognostic or clinical significance. The epithelial component of fibroadenoma typically exhibits ductal hyperplasia of the usual or florid types. The stroma may be more cellular than is seen in adults; however, mitotic figures are rare. Stromal differentiation may rarely take the form of muscle, adipose tissue as well as osteochondroid metaplasia (148).

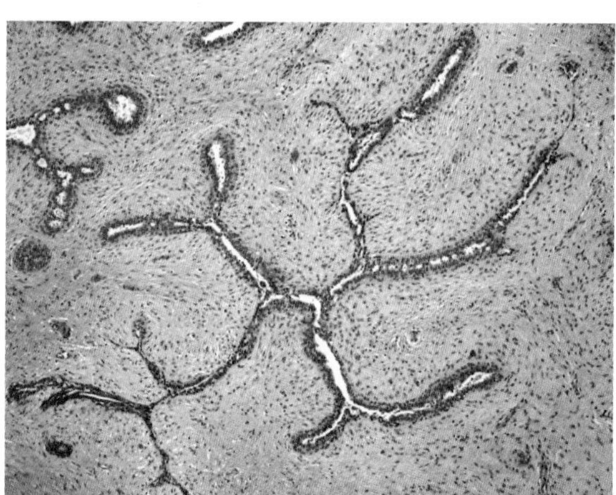

FIGURE 20-10 ■ Fibroadenoma. This tumor shows an intracanalicular pattern with ductal structures compressed by a bland stroma. The stromal cells have a spindle-to-stellate appearance.

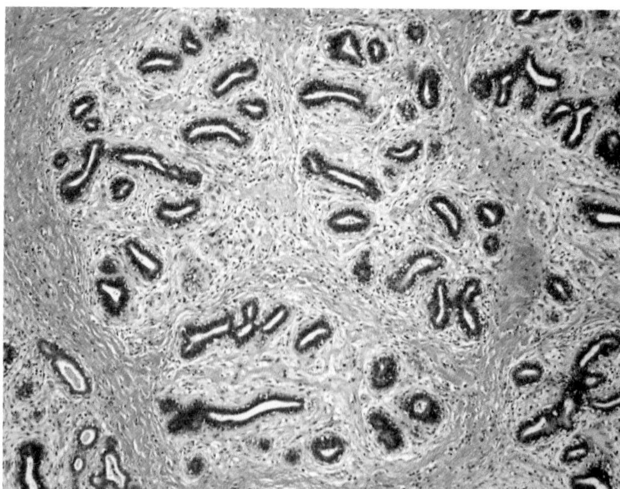

FIGURE 20-11 ■ Fibroadenoma. Pericanalicular pattern. Individual tubules have a clear zone of myoepithelial cells adjacent to the basement membrane. Stromal cells are uniformly distributed and exhibit a myxoid background adjacent to the ducts.

Tubular adenoma is a variant of fibroadenoma clinically and macroscopically. In one series, there was one tubular adenoma for 16 fibroadenomas (36). The solitary, well-circumscribed tumor has a firm, tan, and homogeneous surface (Figure 20-12). As in fibroadenoma, the interface with the adjacent parenchyma is discrete (Figure 20-13). This may be regarded as a fibroadenoma with a minimal stromal component. Small tubules are lined by an inner

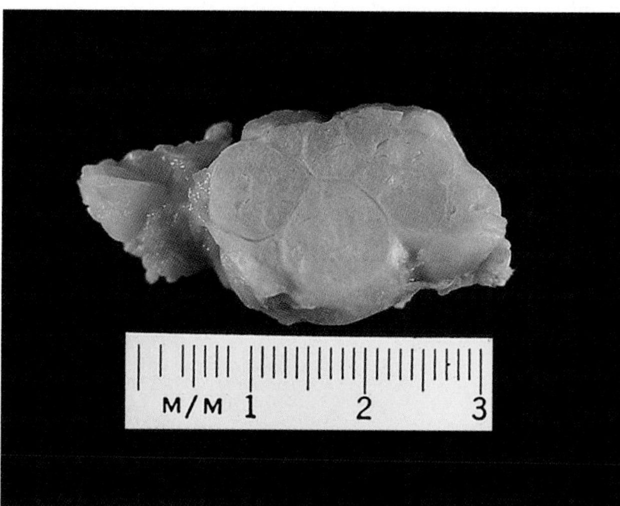

FIGURE 20-12 ■ Tubular adenoma. Circumscribed and lobulated light tan lesion. Grossly, fibroadenoma is similar.

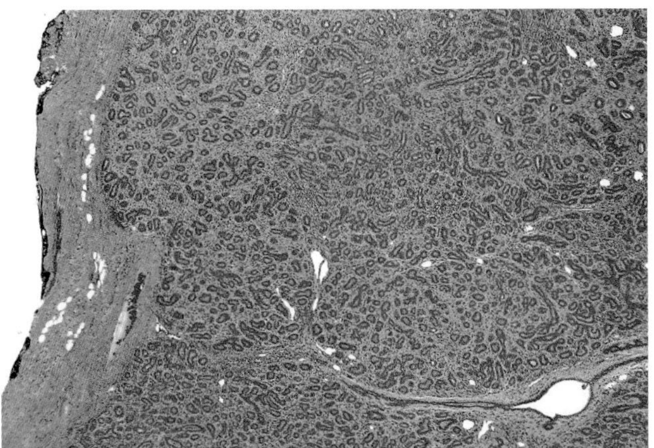

FIGURE 20-13 ■ Tubular adenoma. Uniform proliferation of closely packed small tubules and elongated ducts. This pattern is similar to the pericanalicular pattern of fibroadenoma. Patterns mixed with fibroadenoma are common.

layer of columnar epithelial cells and an outer layer of myoepithelial cells which are indistinguishable from small ductules (66,85). There may be occasional large ducts, mild fibrosis, sparse mononuclear inflammation, and even lactational changes. Emphasizing the connection to fibroadenoma is the occasional histologic admixture of tubular adenoma and fibroadenoma. Multiple bilateral tubular adenomas and fibroadenomas have been reported in adolescent identical twins (101). Lactating adenoma may represent a third variant of fibroadenoma. These adenomas, consisting entirely of lactational change, are unusual and are related to pregnancy. An excessively myxoid fibroadenoma should raise the possibility of Carney Syndrome.

Juvenile Fibroadenoma

Juvenile or cellular fibroadenoma is a rapidly enlarging tumor, sometime referred to as *giant fibroadenoma* due to the large size (>5 cm) it achieves. This variant is more common in African-Americans (59). Grossly, the larger tumors have a multilobulated, bosselated cut surface (Figure 20-14). Histologic features differ from the typical fibroadenoma by exhibiting a hypercellular stroma and more epithelial hyperplasia (Figure 20-15A,B). Nevertheless, the degree of stromal cellularity separating one from the other has never been defined or quantitated. In addition to pericanalicular and intracanalicular patterns similar to those encountered in routine fibroadenoma, there is a "leaf-like" pattern, i.e., clefts lined by hyperplastic epithelium similar to that seen in benign phyllodes tumor, suggesting that juvenile or cellular fibroadenomas may in fact represent a benign phyllodes tumor (23). Distinguishing between juvenile fibroadenoma and benign phyllodes tumor is difficult if not arbitrary relying in part on a more cellular and heterogeneously distributed stroma adjacent to the ducts in a benign phyllodes tumor and a more uniform stromal distribution in juvenile fibroadenoma. The clinicopathologic difference between the two is not certain. The stromal cells in juvenile fibroadenoma lack atypia and mitoses are sparse (<1 to 3 per 10 high-power fields). There

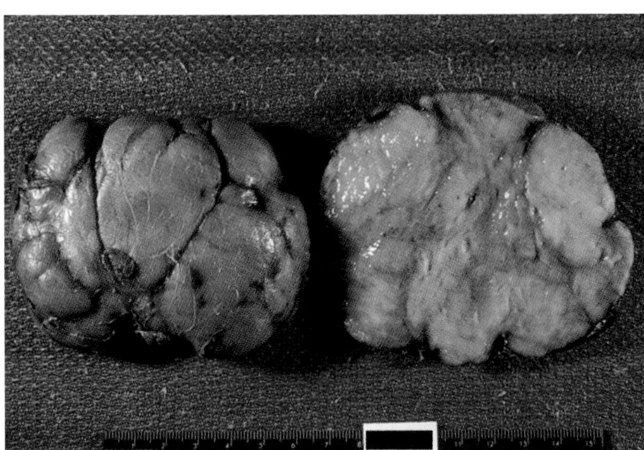

FIGURE 20-14 ■ Juvenile fibroadenoma. Adolescent girl with a solitary 6cm mass. The cut surface demonstrates depressed clefted spaces defining a lobulated pattern. The lesion has been incompletely removed. (Courtesy of Wendy Recant, M.D.)

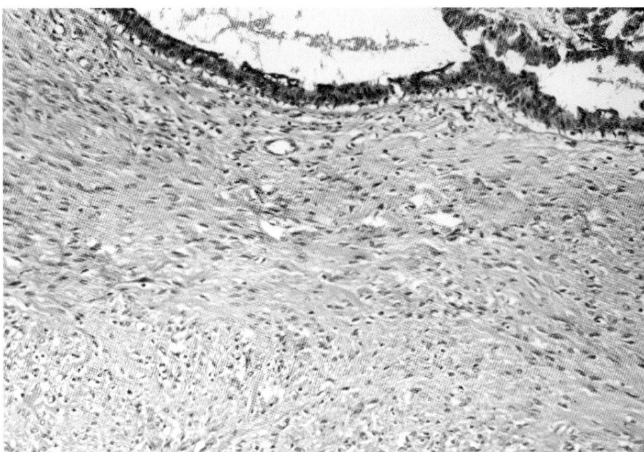

A

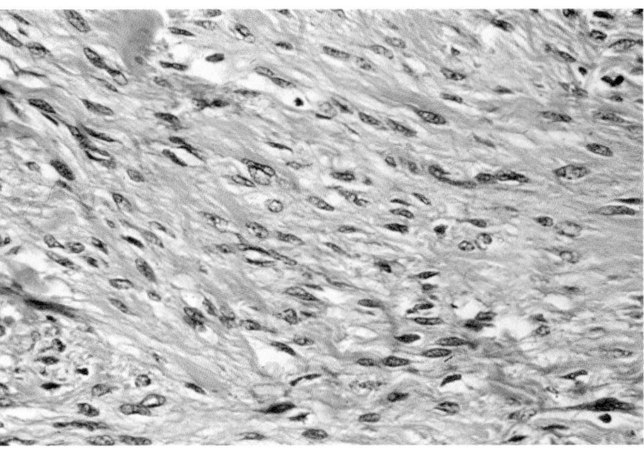

B

FIGURE 20-15 ■ Juvenile fibroadenoma in a 16-year-old girl. **A:** This field shows a portion of a leaf-like duct with mild hyperplasia (**right side**). **B:** The surrounding stroma has a cellular appearance with an occasional mitotic figure, but no cytologic atypia. (Courtesy of Wendy Recant, M.D.)

may also be proliferation of the myoepithelial cells. These lesions are benign with recurrent potential.

Phyllodes Tumor (Cystosarcoma Phyllodes)

In adults, cystosarcoma phyllodes is regarded as a tumor with three subtypes based on the histopathologic features of the spindle cell stroma that are presumed to correspond to biologic potential, that is, benign, intermediate (low malignant potential), and malignant. The fibroepithelial pathology has a morphologic relationship to fibroadenoma; the distinction is based on stromal cellularity and an irregular stromal distribution. In children, phyllodes tumor is an even less common fibroepithelial neoplasm for which the benign variant in its clinical, radiographic, and pathologic features has been absorbed into the entity and concept of juvenile fibroadenoma. Recent evidence from cytogenetic and molecular studies supports the hypothesis that fibroadenoma and phyllodes tumor are related neoplasms and that progression of the former to the latter may result from a biologic course of multiple recurrences (38,106).

If the benign variant is excluded, phyllodes tumor or cystosarcoma phyllodes in children may be best regarded as at least a low-grade malignancy that accounts for only 1% of breast lesions in children and adolescents (23) (Table 20-1). The clinical presentation is that of a discrete and palpable mass, often circumscribed on mammography. Commonly, there is a history of rapid enlargement and some patients may report rapid growth of a pre-existing lesion (112). Ulceration, fixation, nipple retraction, discharge, and skin discoloration are not typical (7).

Grossly the mass has a tan to gray, bulging, and clefted firm cut surface (Figure 20-16). The sizes have been reported in the range of 1 cm to more than 15 cm and while a tumor less than 4 cm is often cited as a favorable feature, the size of the lesion does not reliably correlate with clinical behavior (90). The margin of the tumor may be locally infiltrative histologically even though it grossly appears circumscribed; those with invasive rather than pushing borders have an increased risk of local recurrence. Inking practices for fibroadenomas vary, so that the unsuspected phyllodes tumor may not be appropriately managed initially (16,109,119). Histologically, the appreciation of a sarcomatous stroma may be a sampling issue, given the potential for distributional irregularities (Figure 20-17A,B). The typical low-grade spindle cell stroma seldom overgrows the epithelial component. Stromal density and mitoses are particularly noticeable adjacent to the branching ducts (110).

As a low-grade neoplasm with recurrent potential, most phyllodes tumors have a favorable outcome with 10-year survival close to 90% (61). No single criterion is reliable for predicting clinical behavior although the mitotic rate may be a significant factor in the evolution of metastatic disease (23), especially if there are more than 3 mitoses per 10 high-power fields. Intracytoplasmic inclusion bodies composed of actin may be seen in stromal cells, similar to those seen in infantile digital fibromatosis (13,68). In this regard, the spindle cells have the immunophenotype of myofibroblasts (8).

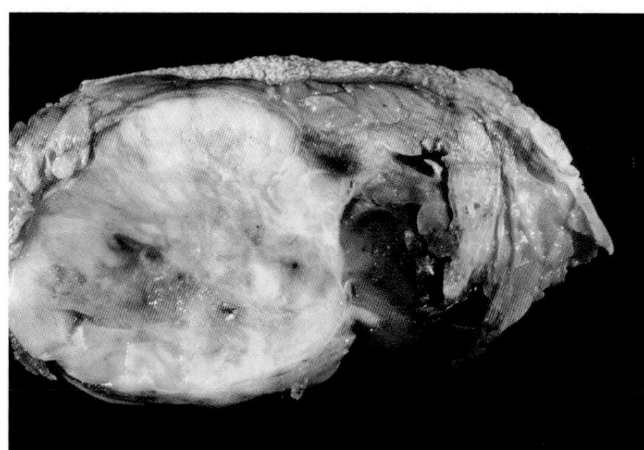

FIGURE 20-16 ■ Phyllodes tumor. Mastectomy specimen with a large firm white mass with areas of hemorrhage and clefts on cut surface.

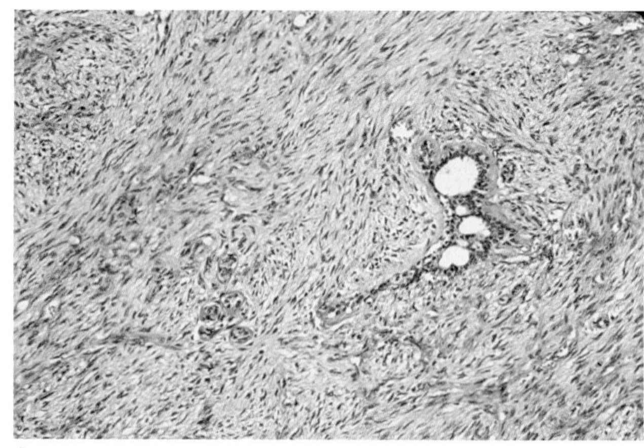

A

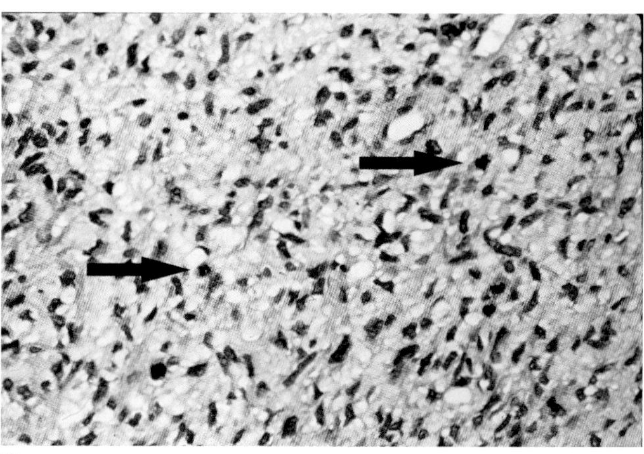

B

FIGURE 20-17 ■ Phyllodes tumor. **A:** Low power of a phyllodes tumor shows cellular stroma crowding the epithelial component. **B:** Higher-power view of densely cellular and myxoid stroma in which the stellate-shaped cells show occasional mitotic figures (*arrows*).

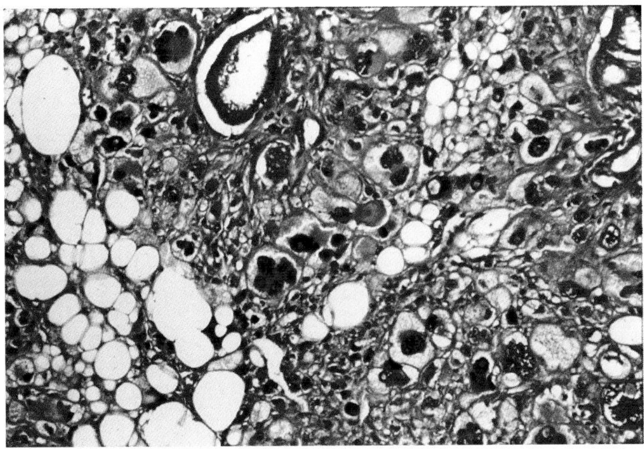

FIGURE 20-18 ■ Malignant stroma of a phyllodes tumor with lipoblasts indicating liposarcomatous differentiation.

If the sarcomatous component has features of an undifferentiated sarcoma or alveolar rhabdomyosarcoma, it should be anticipated that the tumor would behave accordingly regardless of the epithelial component. Liposarcoma or chondrosarcoma may be more favorable (Figure 20-18) (72,115,116,118). The overall recurrence rate of cystosarcoma phyllodes is 7% to 15%; metastases are exceptionally rare (3,7,16,79,119,152). One example of metastasis was in a 14-year-old girl who had a very aggressive spindle cell sarcoma that metastasized to the skin, soft tissue, and lungs (69). Another child, a 12-year-old girl, died with metastatic embryonal rhabdomyosarcoma (115).

Nipple Duct Adenoma and Hamartoma

Nipple Duct Adenoma

Nipple duct adenoma (florid papillomatosis, erosive adenomatosis) is a lesion of adults only rarely reported in children (114,115,127). A rapidly enlarging unilateral subareolar mass with erosion of the overlying skin and a nipple discharge are the clinical features. Three histologic patterns are seen: sclerosing papillomatosis, papillomatosis, and adenosis. Syringocystadenoma papilliferum resembles the nipple duct adenoma except for the fact that the former lesion exhibits an epithelial transition to the skin surface and a conspicuous plasma cell infiltration.

Hamartoma

Hamartomas include two entities: hamartoma of the breast and myoid hamartoma. These lesions are uncommon at any age. In a review of 5,834 breast biopsy specimens, hamartomas accounted for 1.2% of benign breast lesions (21). Most hamartomas present in adults, but they are also seen in middle-to-late adolescence as a sharply demarcated mass thought clinically to represent a fibroadenoma. Dense fibrous stroma or adipose tissue is the dominant component, the lobular-ductular units in the fibrous stroma do not have any appreciable abnormalities, and the histologic interpretation may be fibrous mastopathy or normal breast tissue (30,32). Hamartomas have been characterized as a breast within the breast (83). Fibroadenomas with heterologous cartilage or bone have been interpreted appropriately in the past as hamartomas (74).

Myoid (muscular) hamartoma is even less common, also reported more often in adults, and is paradoxical for a true maldevelopment (22,84). These lesions are smaller than 1 cm and are composed of plump stromal cells with a myogenic phenotype in association with small ducts.

Carcinoma

Carcinoma of the breast is exceedingly rare in children (111,112). Invasive carcinoma was found in 32 patients with 6 DCIS and 3 LCIS in a recent study using SEER data between 1973 and 2004 (61). No cases of carcinoma were found in 113 breast tumors in children in one study, and there was only one carcinoma of the breast in 234 cases of carcinomas in children in another series (93,115). Most pediatric carcinomas occur after age 15; the adult cases begin rising after age 25 (5,28,49,61,130). Secretory carcinoma, one of the rarest types of breast carcinoma, was initially termed *juvenile breast carcinoma* as initial studies found the average onset to be in childhood. Recently, there has been an association with a balanced translocation, t(12;15), as seen in several pediatric mesenchymal tumors (76). Grossly, the tumor is 1 to 2.5 cm in diameter, separate from the nipple, circumscribed, gray white, and firm. Nodules or lobules of tumor are separated by prominent bands of connective tissue (Figure 20-19). The presence of extracellular secretions imparts a micromulticystic appearance to the individual tumor nodules. Intracytoplasmic vacuoles are noted in most cells that otherwise have only mild-to-moderate cytologic atypia. Secretory carcinoma (juvenile carcinoma) is often cited as the principal type of breast carcinoma in the first two decades. However, in the SEER study, secretory carcinoma

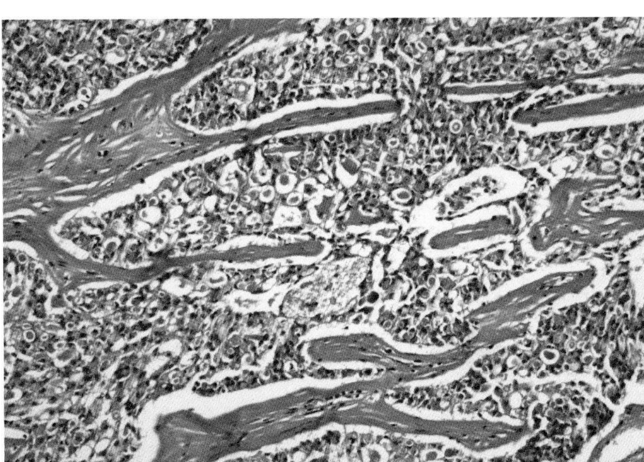

FIGURE 20-19 ■ Secretory carcinoma. Thick fibrous bands separate the lobules of tumor cells showing abundant eosinophilic cytoplasm and secretions with intracytoplasmic vacuoles. (Courtesy Thomas Kravszim, D.)

accounted for less than 10% of carcinomas (61). This variant also occurs in boys and adults (89,128,132,143). Secretory carcinoma in children and adolescents has been reported in association with juvenile papillomatosis (50,107,149). In the few cases available for follow-up, only one of the original seven cases recurred, and only a few have metastasized to regional lymph nodes (89). This indolent clinical behavior has been confirmed in other reports (47,111,142,143). Other types of infiltrating ductal carcinomas in young women generally are associated with a poor outcome with overall 10-year survival of 54% (24,61,162).

A spectrum of histologic variants of breast carcinoma have been reported (1,2,57,89,120,123,142,157). Carcinoma of the breast is a recognized type of second malignant neoplasm, certainly not the most common, that occurs later in life but earlier than expected in long-term survivors of other childhood malignancies (12). In the past decade, remarkable advances have been made in understanding the genetic basis of breast cancer, and breast cancer family syndromes have been identified with inherited mutations of the p53 gene or BRCA genes (26,41,86,133,146). Some breast carcinomas in young patients are related to these conditions, and other early childhood neoplasms may be manifestations of an inherited proclivity to breast and other cancers (19,52,80,113).

MESENCHYMAL LESIONS

Lipoma

Lipomas are uncommon and may be associated with lipoblastomatous foci in young children (115).

Fibromatosis

Desmoid-type fibromatosis of the breast, as in other soft tissues, is a firm, deceptively discrete mass that may produce skin fixation and dimpling. About 20% of all cases are encountered in the second decade; the condition is rare in infancy (115). The gross appearance is a gray-white, fibrous mass measuring 1 to 10 cm with ill-defined edges. Irregular bundles of mitotically inactive spindle cells are arranged in broad sheets or bands with open, thin-walled vessels and variable collagenization surrounding normal breast parenchyma. Myxoid foci, calcification, and lymphoid aggregates may be seen. Local invasion of soft tissue beyond the grossly apparent margin of the mass may account for the frequent recurrence rate of up to 20% and emphasizes the importance of careful evaluation of the tissue margins (158). The differential diagnosis in children includes nodular fasciitis (6) and pseudoangiomatous stromal hyperplasia (PASH), also a presumed myofibroblastic proliferation (71,117). Immunohistochemical staining for vimentin and focally for smooth muscle actin is consistent with a myofibroblastic lesion; the delicate spindle cells are also reactive for CD34 (163). Fibromatosis has been observed in gynecomastia, most frequently in children (97). β-catenin is a useful marker for desmoid tumors.

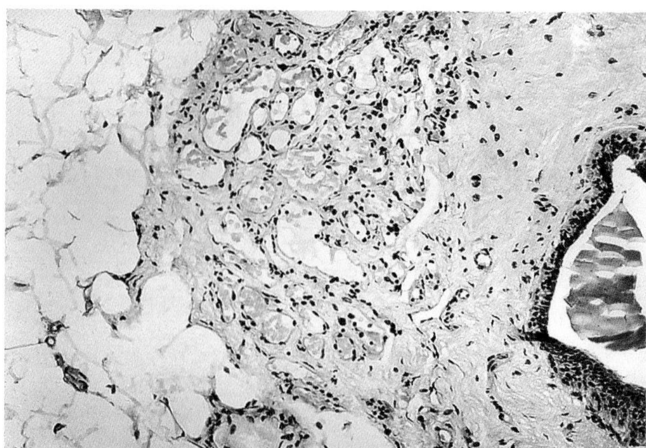

FIGURE 20-20 ■ Perilobular hemangioma. Collection of thin vascular channels adjacent to duct.

Vascular Tumors

Vascular tumors are soft tissue tumors that may originate in or near the breast or skin (23). Infantile or capillary *hemangiomas* are typically multilobular infiltrating masses exhibiting lobular architecture defined by fibrous septation and composed of small capillaries with little-to-absent thrombosis and canalization. Over time, the vascular spaces eventually regress or involute as evident by an increase in fibrotic stroma (23) (Figure 20-20). *Angiomatosis*, rare in children, is a diffuse, benign vascular lesion that may be associated with platelet trapping syndromes. Histologically, vascular channels are distributed throughout the breast parenchyma (102,125). The vascular spaces are lined by flat endothelium without atypia. Both hemangiomatous and lymphangiomatous channels may be seen. Although angiosarcoma may be considered morphologically, primary mammary or soft tissue angiosarcoma in children is even more rare than angiomatosis. Angiomatosis is not a precursor lesion and if possible should be excised with negative margins. *Angiosarcoma* is exceedingly rare in the pediatric age group mostly appearing as case reports. A recent review includes two cases in the breast (37). Both epithelioid and spindle cell morphology in a vasoformative pattern are apparent (see Chapter 24).

Granular Cell Tumor

Granular cell tumor of the breast is a benign lesion that presents a diagnostic challenge because of its clinical, mammographic, and macroscopic resemblance to infiltrating duct carcinoma (51,88,103,156). These uncommon tumors represent less than 1% of breast lesions in young persons. Both boys and girls are affected. The lesion arises in the deep dermis and subcutaneous tissue, infiltrating and surrounding adnexal and breast parenchymal structures. Grossly, it is a yellow, gritty, infiltrative lesion measuring 1 to 2 cm (Figure 20-21). Microscopically, large polygonal cells with abundant pale granular cytoplasm and central vesicular

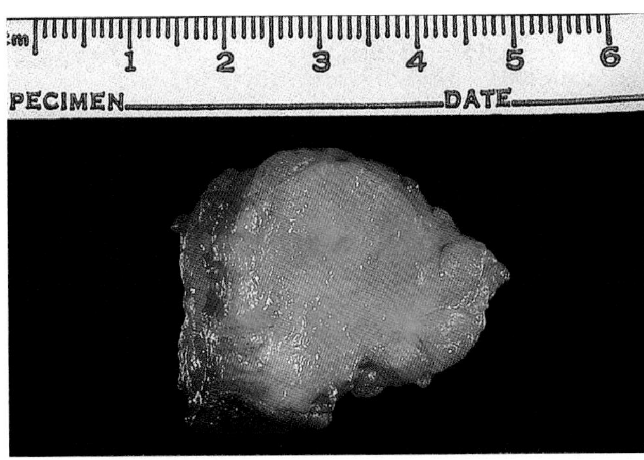

FIGURE 20-21 ■ Granular cell tumor. Pale yellow cut surface with infiltrative borders. The excision is incomplete.

nuclei with prominent nucleoli are arranged in sheets or cords (Figure 20-22). The granularity is PAS positive, diastase resistant, and S100 positive. Electron microscopy demonstrates the cytoplasm filled with lysosome-like structures (Figure 20-23).

Sarcoma

Sarcomas in or near the breast are rare and mostly related to phyllodes tumors (61). Other sarcomas are primary lesions of the chest wall and are discussed in the soft tissue chapter. The tumors mostly behave in a low-grade fashion, amendable to surgical excision with a 10-year survival close to 90% (61). Sarcomas, especially alveolar rhabdomyosarcoma, are known to metastasize to the breast.

Hematopoietic Lesions

The entire range of Hodgkin and non-Hodgkin lymphomas and leukemias rarely present as primary in the breast or even as a site of extramedullary relapse, perhaps more frequent in leukemias (39,46,82,96,136). Lymphomatous involvement of the breast in children is seen mainly in the setting of small noncleaved cell lymphoma or Burkitt's lymphoma with bilateral involvement. The latter seems to occur in young pregnant or lactating women (9,44,70,154). Neither diffuse large cell nor mucosa-associated lymphoid tissue (MALT) lymphoma is seen in children (17). The breast is an uncommon but well-documented site for granulocytic sarcoma as an initial manifestation or relapse of acute myeloid leukemia (4,10,11,40,54). An association has been noted with the t(8;21) (q22;q22) translocation in cases of primary acute myeloid leukemia with M2 morphology in children (48,131,141). Histologically, complete immunohistochemical studies, including myeloperoxidase, are required to demonstrate the discohesive infiltrate of malignant small round cells and establish the diagnosis.

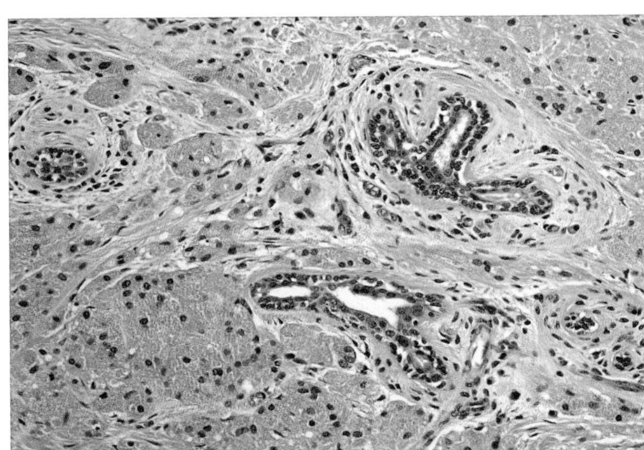

FIGURE 20-22 ■ Granular cell tumor. Small breast ducts surrounded by cords of polygonal cells with poorly defined cell borders, small round nuclei, and uniform finely granular cytoplasm.

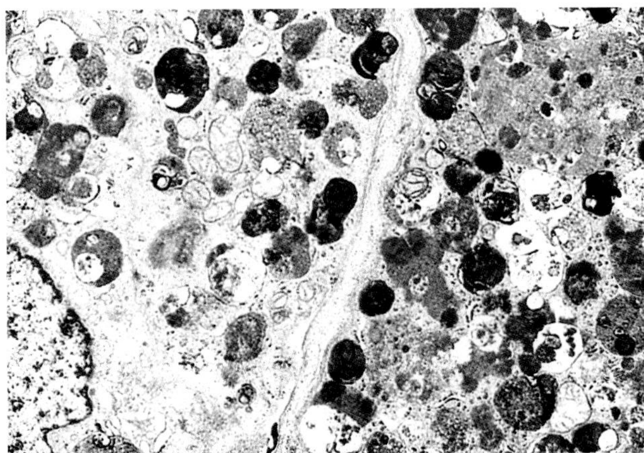

FIGURE 20-23 ■ Granular cell tumor. Electron microscopy reveals cytoplasm packed with numerous lysosome-like structures, corresponding to the histologic cytoplasmic granularity.

REFERENCES

1. Ackerman BL, Otis C, Stueber K. Lobular carcinoma in situ in a 15-year-old girl: a case report and review of the literature. *Plast Reconstr Surg* 1994;94(5):714–718.
2. Ackerman J, Gilbert-Barness E. Malignancy metastatic to the products of conception: a case report with literature review. *Pediatr Pathol Lab Med* 1997;17(4):577–586.
3. Adami HO, Hakelius L, Rimsten A, et al. Malignant, locally recurring cystosarcoma phyllodes in an adolescent female. A case report. *Acta Chir Scand* 1984;150(1):93–100.
4. Ahrar K, McLeary MS, Young LW, et al. Granulocytic sarcoma (chloroma) of the breast in an adolescent patient: ultrasonographic findings. *J Ultrasound Med* 1998;17(6):383–384.
5. Akhtar M, Robinson C, Ali MA, et al. Secretory carcinoma of the breast in adults. Light and electron microscopic study of three cases with review of the literature. *Cancer* 1983;51(12):2245–2254.
6. Al-Nafussi A. Spindle cell tumours of the breast: practical approach to diagnosis. *Histopathology* 1999;35(1):1–13.
7. Amerson JR. Cystosarcoma phyllodes in adolescent females. A report of seven patients. *Ann Surg* 1970;171(6):849–856.
8. Aranda FI, Laforga JB, Lopez JI. Phyllodes tumor of the breast. An immunohistochemical study of 28 cases with special attention to the role of myofibroblasts. *Pathol Res Pract* 1994;190(5):474–481.
9. Arber DA, Simpson JF, Weiss LM, et al. Non-Hodgkin's lymphoma involving the breast. *Am J Surg Pathol* 1994;18(3):288–295.

10. Au WY, Ma SK, Kwong YL, et al. Acute myeloid leukemia relapsing as gynecomastia. *Leuk Lymphoma* 1999;36(1–2):191–194.
11. Barker TH. Granulocytic sarcoma of the breast diagnosed by fine needle aspiration (FNA) cytology. *Cytopathology* 1998;9(2): 135–137.
12. Bhatia S, Robison LL, Oberlin O, et al. Breast cancer and other second neoplasms after childhood Hodgkin's disease. *N Engl J Med* 1996;334(12):745–751.
13. Bittesini L, Dei Tos AP, Doglioni C, et al. Fibroepithelial tumor of the breast with digital fibroma-like inclusions in the stromal component. Case report with immunocytochemical and ultrastructural analysis. *Am J Surg Pathol* 1994;18(3):296–301.
14. Boothroyd A, Carty H. Breast masses in childhood and adolescence. A presentation of 17 cases and a review of the literature. *Pediatr Radiol* 1994;24(2):81–84.
15. Bower R, Bell MJ, Ternberg JL. Management of breast lesions in children and adolescents. *J Pediatr Surg* 1976;11(3):337–346.
16. Briggs RM, Walters M, Rosenthal D. Cystosarcoma phylloides in adolescent female patients. *Am J Surg* 1983;146(6):712–714.
17. Brogi E, Harris NL. Lymphomas of the breast: pathology and clinical behavior. *Semin Oncol* 1999;26(3):357–364.
18. Burck U, Held KR. Athelia in a female infant—heterozygous for anhidrotic ectodermal dysplasia. *Clin Genet* 1981;19(2):117–121.
19. Burke E, Li FP, Janov AJ, et al. Cancer in relatives of survivors of childhood sarcoma. *Cancer* 1991;67(5):1467–1469.
20. Casey HD, Chasan PE, Chick LR. Familial polythelia without associated anomalies. *Ann Plast Surg* 1996;36(1):101–104.
21. Charpin C, Mathoulin MP, Andrac L, et al. Reappraisal of breast hamartomas. A morphological study of 41 cases. *Pathol Res Pract* 1994;190(4):362–371.
22. Chiacchio R, Panico L, D'Antonio A, et al. Mammary hamartomas: an immunohistochemical study of ten cases. *Pathol Res Pract* 1999;195(4):231–236.
23. Chung EM, Cube R, Hall GJ, et al. From the archives of the AFIP: breast masses in children and adolescents: radiologic-pathologic correlation. *Radiographics* 2009;29(3):907–931.
24. Chung M, Chang HR, Bland KI, et al. Younger women with breast carcinoma have a poorer prognosis than older women. *Cancer* 1996;77(1):97–103.
25. Ciftci AO, Tanyel FC, Buyukpamukcu N, et al. Female breast masses during childhood: a 25-year review. *Eur J Pediatr Surg* 1998;8(2):67–70.
26. Claus EB, Risch N, Thompson WD. Autosomal dominant inheritance of early-onset breast cancer. Implications for risk prediction. *Cancer* 1994;73(3):643–651.
27. Cogswell HD, Czerny EW. Carcinoma of aberrant breast of the axilla. *Am Surg* 1961;27:388–390.
28. JL C, RE F, Kempson RL. Recommendations for the reporting of breast carcinoma. Association of Directors of Anatomic and Surgical Pathology. *Am J Clin Pathol* 1995;104(6):614–619.
29. Corriveau S, Jacobs JS. Macromastia in adolescence. *Clin Plast Surg* 1990;17(1):151–160.
30. Daroca PJJ, Reed RJ, Love GL, et al. Myoid hamartomas of the breast. *Hum Pathol* 1985;16(3):212–219.
31. Das DK, Gupta SK, Mathew SV, et al. Fine needle aspiration cytologic diagnosis of axillary accessory breast tissue, including its physiologic changes and pathologic lesions. *Acta Cytol* 1994;38(2): 130–135.
32. Daya D, Trus T, D'Souza TJ, et al. Hamartoma of the breast, an underrecognized breast lesion. A clinicopathologic and radiographic study of 25 cases. *Am J Clin Pathol* 1995;103(6):685–689.
33. De Silva NK, Brandt ML. Disorders of the breast in children and adolescents, Part 2: breast masses. *J Pediatr Adolesc Gynecol* 2006;19(6):415–418.
34. De Silva NK, Brandt ML. Disorders of the breast in children and adolescents, Part 1: Disorders of growth and infections of the breast. *J Pediatr Adolesc Gynecol* 2006;19(5):345–349.
35. Dehner LP. *Pediatric surgical pathology,* 2nd ed. Baltimore, MD: Williams & Wilkins, 1987.
36. Dehner LP, Hill DA, Deschryver K. Pathology of the breast in children, adolescents, and young adults. *Semin Diagn Pathol* 1999;16(3):235–247.
37. Deyrup AT, Miettinen M, North PE, et al. Angiosarcomas arising in the viscera and soft tissue of children and young adults: a clinicopathologic study of 15 cases. *Am J Surg Pathol* 2009;33(2): 264–269.
38. Dietrich CU, Pandis N, Rizou H, et al. Cytogenetic findings in phyllodes tumors of the breast: karyotypic complexity differentiates between malignant and benign tumors. *Hum Pathol* 1997;28(12):1379–1382.
39. Domanic N, Akman N, Muftuoglu AU. Massive breast involvement in acute leukemia. Case report. *Helv Paediatr Acta* 1972;27(6): 601–605.
40. Dufour C, Garaventa A, Brisigotti M, et al. Massively diffuse multifocal granulocytic sarcoma in a child with acute myeloid leukemia. *Tumori* 1995;81(3):222–224.
41. Elger BS, Harding TW. Testing adolescents for a hereditary breast cancer gene (BRCA1): respecting their autonomy is in their best interest. *Arch Pediatr Adolesc Med* 2000;154(2):113–119.
42. Eliasen CA, Cranor ML, Rosen PP. Atypical duct hyperplasia of the breast in young females. *Am J Surg Pathol* 1992;16(3):246–251.
43. Ely KA, Tse G, Simpson JF, et al. Diabetic mastopathy. A clinicopathologic review. *Am J Clin Pathol* 2000;113(4):541–545.
44. Fahmy JL, Wood BP, Miller JH. Bilateral breast involvement in a teenage girl with Burkitt lymphoma. *Pediatr Radiol* 1995;25(1): 56–57.
45. Fallat ME, Ignacio RCJ. Breast disorders in children and adolescents. *J Pediatr Adolesc Gynecol* 2008;21(6):311–316.
46. Farah RA, Timmons CF, Aquino VM. Relapsed childhood acute lymphoblastic leukemia presenting as an isolated breast mass. *Clin Pediatr (Phila)* 1999;38(9):545–546.
47. Farrow JH, Ashikari H. Breast lesions in young girls. *Surg Clin North Am* 1969;49(2):261–269.
48. Felice MS, Zubizarreta PA, Alfaro EM, et al. Good outcome of children with acute myeloid leukemia and t(8;21)(q22;q22), even when associated with granulocytic sarcoma: a report from a single institution in Argentina. *Cancer* 2000;88(8):1939–1944.
49. Ferguson CM, Powell RW. Breast masses in young women. *Arch Surg* 1989;124(11):1338–1341.
50. Ferguson TBJ, McCarty KSJ, Filston HC. Juvenile secretory carcinoma and juvenile papillomatosis: diagnosis and treatment. *J Pediatr Surg* 1987;22(7):637–639.
51. Friedman RM, Hurwitt ES. Granular cell myoblastoma of the breast. *Am J Surg* 1966;112(1):76–79.
52. Garber JE, Burke EM, Lavally BL, et al. Choroid plexus tumors in the breast cancer-sarcoma syndrome. *Cancer* 1990;66(12):2658–2660.
53. Garcia FU, Galindo LM, Holsclaw DSJ. Breast abnormalities in patients with cystic fibrosis: previously unrecognized changes. *Ann Diagn Pathol* 1998;2(5):281–285.
54. Gartenhaus WS, Mir R, Pliskin A, et al. Granulocytic sarcoma of breast: aleukemic bilateral metachronous presentation and literature review. *Med Pediatr Oncol* 1985;13(1):22–29.
55. Gill J, Greenall M. Juvenile papillomatosis and breast cancer. *J Surg Educ* 2007;64(4):234–236.
56. Gilmore HT, Milroy M, Mello BJ. Supernumerary nipples and accessory breast tissue. *S D J Med* 1996;49(5):149–151.
57. Gogas J, Sechas M, Skalkeas G. Surgical management of diseases of the adolescent female breast: a clinicopathologic study. *Am J Surg* 1979;137(5):634–637.
58. Goldstein DP, Miler V. Breast masses in adolescent females. *Clin Pediatr (Phila)* 1982;21(1):17–19.
59. Greydanus DE, Matytsina L, Gains M. Breast disorders in children and adolescents. *Prim Care* 2006;33(2):455–502.

60. Greydanus DE, Parks DS, Farrell EG. Breast disorders in children and adolescents. *Pediatr Clin North Am* 1989;36(3):601–638.
61. Gutierrez JC, Housri N, Koniaris LG, et al. Malignant breast cancer in children: a review of 75 patients. *J Surg Res* 2008;147(2): 182–188.
62. Halper S, Rubenstein D. Aplasia cutis congenita associated with syndactyly and supernumerary nipples: report of a second family with similar clinical findings. *Pediatr Dermatol* 1991;8(1):32–34.
63. Harrison GM, Taylor FM. Diagnosis and management of fibrocystic disease in infants and children. *Tex State J Med* 1958;54(5): 296–298.
64. Hassim AM. Bilateral fibroadenoma in supernumerary breasts of the vulva. *J Obstet Gynaecol Br Commonw* 1969;76(3):275–277.
65. Hein K, Dell R, Cohen MI. Self-detection of a breast mass in adolescent females. *J Adolesc Health Care* 1982;3(1):15–17.
66. Hertel BF, Zaloudek C, Kempson RL. Breast adenomas. *Cancer* 1976;37(6):2891–2905.
67. Hidalgo F, Llano JM, Marhuenda A. Juvenile papillomatosis of the breast (Swiss cheese disease). *AJR* 1997;169(3):912.
68. Hiraoka N, Mukai M, Hosoda Y, et al. Phyllodes tumor of the breast containing the intracytoplasmic inclusion bodies identical with infantile digital fibromatosis. *Am J Surg Pathol* 1994;18(5): 506–511.
69. Hoover HC, Trestioreanu A, Ketcham AS. Metastatic cystosarcoma phylloides in an adolescent girl: an unusually malignant tumor. *Ann Surg* 1975;181(3):279–282.
70. Hubner KF, Littlefield LG. Burkitt lymphoma in three American children. Clinical and cytogenetic observations. *Am J Dis Child* 1975;129(10):1219–1223.
71. Ibrahim RE, Sciotto CG, Weidner N. Pseudoangiomatous hyperplasia of mammary stroma. Some observations regarding its clinicopathologic spectrum. *Cancer* 1989;63(6):1154–1160.
72. Jimenez JF, Gloster ES, Perrot LJ, et al. Liposarcoma arising within a cystosarcoma phyllodes. *J Surg Oncol* 1986;31(4):294–298.
73. Jojart G, Seres E. Supernumerary nipples and renal anomalies. *Int Urol Nephrol* 1994;26(2):141–144.
74. Jones MW, Norris HJ, Wargotz ES. Hamartomas of the breast. *Surg Gynecol Obstet* 1991;173(1):54–56.
75. Kenney RD, Flippo JL, Black EB. Supernumerary nipples and renal anomalies in neonates. *Am J Dis Child* 1987;141(9):987–988.
76. Lae M, Freneaux P, Sastre-Garau X, et al. Secretory breast carcinomas with ETV6-NTRK3 fusion gene belong to the basal-like carcinoma spectrum. *Mod Pathol* 2009;22(2):291–298.
77. Lakshmanan R, Clarke MJ, Putti TC. Diabetic fibrous mastopathy. *Singapore Med J* 2007;48(6):579–581.
78. Lesavoy MA, Gomez-Garcia A, Nejdl R, et al. Axillary breast tissue: clinical presentation and surgical treatment. *Ann Plast Surg* 1995;35(4):356–360.
79. Leveque J, Meunier B, Wattier E, et al. Malignant cystosarcomas phyllodes of the breast in adolescent females. *Eur J Obstet Gynecol Reprod Biol* 1994;54(3):197–203.
80. Li FP, Corkery J, Vawter G, et al. Breast carcinoma after cancer therapy in childhood. *Cancer* 1983;51(3):521–523.
81. Li RZ, Xia Z, Lin HH, et al. Childhood gynecomastia: a clinical analysis of 240 cases. *Zhongguo Dang Dai Er Ke Za Zhi* 2007;9(5): 404–406.
82. Lin Y, Govindan R, Hess JL. Malignant hematopoietic breast tumors. *Am J Clin Pathol* 1997;107(2):177–186.
83. Linell F, Ostberg G, Soderstrom J, et al. Breast hamartomas. An important entity in mammary pathology. *Virchows Arch A Pathol Anat Histol* 1979;383(3):253–264.
84. Magro G, Bisceglia M. Muscular hamartoma of the breast. Case report and review of the literature. *Pathol Res Pract* 1998;194(5): 349–355.
85. Maiorano E, Albrizio M. Tubular adenoma of the breast: an immunohistochemical study of ten cases. *Pathol Res Pract* 1995;191(12):1222–1230.
86. Malone KE, Daling JR, Thompson JD, et al. BRCA1 mutations and breast cancer in the general population: analyses in women before age 35 years and in women before age 45 years with first-degree family history. *JAMA* 1998;279(12):922–929.
87. Marconi F, Gallucci A, Marra M, et al. Macromastia in adolescents: notes on clinical aspects and therapy. *Chir Ital* 1993;45(1–6):85–92.
88. McCracken M, Hamal PB, Benson EA. Granular cell myoblastoma of the breast: a report of 2 cases. *Br J Surg* 1979;66(11):819–821.
89. McDivitt RW, Stewart FW. Breast carcinoma in children. *JAMA* 1966;195(5):388–390.
90. McDivitt RW, Urban JA, Farrow JH. Cystosarcoma phyllodes. *Johns Hopkins Med J* 1967;120:33–45.
91. McKiernan J, Coyne J, Cahalane S. Histology of breast development in early life. *Arch Dis Child* 1988;63(2):136–139.
92. McKiernan JF, Hull D. Breast development in the newborn. *Arch Dis Child* 1981;56(7):525–529.
93. McWhirter WR, Stiller CA, Lennox EL. Carcinomas in childhood. A registry-based study of incidence and survival. *Cancer* 1989;63(11):2242–2246.
94. Mehes K, Pinter A. Minor morphological aberrations in children with isolated urinary tract malformations. *Eur J Pediatr* 1990;149(6):399–402.
95. Mehregan AH. Supernumerary nipple. A histologic study. *J Cutan Pathol* 1981;8(2):96–104.
96. Meis JM, Butler JJ, Osborne BM. Hodgkin's disease involving the breast and chest wall. *Cancer* 1986;57(9):1859–1865.
97. Milanezi MF, Saggioro FP, Zanati SG, et al. Pseudoangiomatous hyperplasia of mammary stroma associated with gynaecomastia. *J Clin Pathol* 1998;51(3):204–206.
98. Mimouni F, Merlob P, Reisner SH. Occurrence of supernumerary nipples in newborns. *Am J Dis Child* 1983;137(10):952–953.
99. Minkowitz S, Hedayati H, Hiller S, et al. Fibrous mastopathy. A clinical histopathologic study. *Cancer* 1973;32(4):913–916.
100. Moore KL, Persaud TVN. *The developing human: Clinically oriented embryology*, 7th ed ed. Philadelphia: Saunders, 2003.
101. Morris JA, Kelly JF. Multiple bilateral breast adenomata in identical adolescent Negro twins. *Histopathology* 1982;6(5):539–547.
102. Morrow M, Berger D, Thelmo W. Diffuse cystic angiomatosis of the breast. *Cancer* 1988;62(11):2392–2396.
103. Mulcare R. Granular cell myoblastoma of the breast. *Ann Surg* 1968;168(2):262–268.
104. Neinstein LS, Atkinson J, Diament M. Prevalence and longitudinal study of breast masses in adolescents. *J Adolesc Health* 1993;14(4):277–281.
105. Nelson MM, Cooper CK. Congenital defects of the breast - an autosomal dominant trait. *S Afr Med J* 1982;61(12):434–436.
106. Noguchi S, Yokouchi H, Aihara T, et al. Progression of fibroadenoma to phyllodes tumor demonstrated by clonal analysis. *Cancer* 1995;76(10):1779–1785.
107. Nonomura A, Kimura A, Mizukami Y, et al. Secretory carcinoma of the breast associated with juvenile papillomatosis in a 12-year-old girl. A case report. *Acta Cytol* 1995;39(3):569–576.
108. Nordt CA, DiVasta AD. Gynecomastia in adolescents. *Curr Opin Pediatr* 2008;20(4):375–382.
109. Norris HJ, Taylor HB. Relationship of histologic features to behavior of cystosarcoma phyllodes. Analysis of ninety-four cases. *Cancer* 1967;20(12):2090–2099.
110. Oberman HA. Breast lesions in the adolescent female. *Pathol Annu* 1979;14(Pt 1):175–201.
111. Oberman HA, Stephens PJ. Carcinoma of the breast in childhood. *Cancer* 1972;30(2):470–474.
112. Ozumba BC, Nzegwu MA, Anyikam A, et al. Breast disease in children and adolescents in eastern Nigeria–a five-year study. *J Pediatr Adolesc Gynecol* 2009;22(3):169–172.
113. Paulino AC, Wen BC, Brown CK, et al. Late effects in children treated with radiation therapy for Wilms' tumor. *Int J Radiat Oncol Biol Phys* 2000;46(5):1239–1246.

114. Perzin KH, Lattes R. Papillary adenoma of the nipple (florid papillomatosis, adenoma, adenomatosis). A clinicopathologic study. *Cancer* 1972;29(4):996–1009.
115. Pettinato G, Manivel JC, Kelly DR, et al. Lesions of the breast in children exclusive of typical fibroadenoma and gynecomastia. A clinicopathologic study of 113 cases. *Pathol Annu.* 1989;24 (Pt 2):296–328.
116. Pietruszka M, Barnes L. Cystosarcoma phyllodes: a clinicopathologic analysis of 42 cases. *Cancer* 1978;41(5):1974–1983.
117. Powell CM, Cranor ML, Rosen PP. Pseudoangiomatous stromal hyperplasia (PASH). A mammary stromal tumor with myofibroblastic differentiation. *Am J Surg Pathol* 1995;19(3):270–277.
118. Powell CM, Rosen PP. Adipose differentiation in cystosarcoma phyllodes. A study of 14 cases. *Am J Surg Pathol* 1994;18(7):720–727.
119. Rajan PB, Cranor ML, Rosen PP. Cystosarcoma phyllodes in adolescent girls and young women: a study of 45 patients. *Am J Surg Pathol* 1998;22(1):64–69.
120. Ramirez G, Ansfield FJ. Carcinoma of the breast in children. *Arch Surg* 1968;96(2):222–225.
121. Ratner I, Liubina NI, Kuz'min VI, et al. Pathogenesis, diagnosis and therapy of fibrous mastopathy. *Sov Med* 1969;32(8):82–87.
122. Rivera-Pomar JM, Vilanova JR, Burgos-Bretones JJ, et al. Focal fibrous disease of breast. A common entity in young women. *Virchows Arch A Pathol Anat Histol* 1980;386(1):59–64.
123. Robinson JH, Dudley AG, Thompson FH. Infiltrating ductal carcinoma of the breast in the postpubertal adolescent: a case report. *Am Surg* 1976;42(3):219–222.
124. Rosen PP. Papillary duct hyperplasia of the breast in children and young adults. *Cancer* 1985;56(7):1611–1617.
125. Rosen PP. Vascular tumors of the breast. III. Angiomatosis. *Am J Surg Pathol* 1985;9(9):652–658.
126. Rosen PP. *Rosen's breast pathology*. Philadelphia, PA: Lippincott Williams & Wilkins, 2001.
127. Rosen PP, Caicco JA. Florid papillomatosis of the nipple. A study of 51 patients, including nine with mammary carcinoma. *Am J Surg Pathol* 1986;10(2):87–101.
128. Rosen PP, Cranor ML. Secretory carcinoma of the breast. *Arch Pathol Lab Med* 1991;115(2):141–144.
129. Rosen PP, Kimmel M. Juvenile papillomatosis of the breast. A follow-up study of 41 patients having biopsies before 1979. *Am J Clin Pathol* 1990;93(5):599–603.
130. Schnitt SJ, Connolly JL. Processing and evaluation of breast excision specimens. A clinically oriented approach. *Am J Clin Pathol* 1992;98(1):125–137.
131. Schwyzer R, Sherman GG, Cohn RJ, et al. Granulocytic sarcoma in children with acute myeloblastic leukemia and t(8;21). *Med Pediatr Oncol* 1998;31(3):144–149.
132. Serour F, Gilad A, Kopolovic J, et al. Secretory breast cancer in childhood and adolescence: report of a case and review of the literature. *Med Pediatr Oncol* 1992;20(4):341–344.
133. Sidransky D, Tokino T, Helzlsouer K, et al. Inherited p53 gene mutations in breast cancer. *Cancer Res* 1992;52(10):2984–2986.
134. Siegal A, Kaufman Z, Siegal G. Breast masses in adolescent females. *J Surg Oncol* 1992;51(3):169–173.
135. Simpson JS, Barson AJ. Breast tumours in infants and children: a 40-year review of cases at a children's hospital. *Can Med Assoc J* 1969;101(2):100–102.
136. Soyupak SK, Sire D, Inal M, et al. Secondary involvement of breast with non-Hodgkin's lymphoma in a paediatric patient presenting as bilateral breast masses. *Eur Radiol* 2000;10(3):519–520.
137. Sridhar GR, Sinha MJ. Macromastia in adolescent girls. *Indian Pediatr* 1995;32(4):496–499.
138. Stone AM, Shenker IR, McCarthy K. Adolescent breast masses. *Am J Surg* 1977;134(2):275–277.
139. Taffurelli M, Santini D, Martinelli G, et al. Juvenile papillomatosis of the breast. A multidisciplinary study. *Pathol Annu. 26 Pt* 1991; 1:25–35.
140. Talisman R, Nissim F, Rothstein H, et al. Juvenile papillomatosis of the breast. *Eur J Surg* 1993;159(5):317–319.
141. Tallman MS, Hakimian D, Shaw JM, et al. Granulocytic sarcoma is associated with the 8;21 translocation in acute myeloid leukemia. *J Clin Oncol* 1993;11(4):690–697.
142. Tanimura A, Konaka K. Carcinoma of the breast in a 5 years old girl. *Acta Pathol Jpn* 1980;30(1):157–160.
143. Tavassoli FA, Norris HJ. Secretory carcinoma of the breast. *Cancer* 1980;45(9):2404–2413.
144. Tawil HM, Najjar SS. Congenital absence of the breasts. *J Pediatr* 1968;73(5):751–753.
145. Templeman C, Hertweck SP. Breast disorders in the pediatric and adolescent patient. *Obstet Gynecol Clin North Am* 2000;27(1):19–34.
146. Thompson WD. Genetic epidemiology of breast cancer. *Cancer* 1994;74(1 Suppl):279–287.
147. Thorncroft K, Forsyth L, Desmond S, et al. The diagnosis and management of diabetic mastopathy. *Breast J* 2007;13(6):607–613.
148. Tiryaki T, Senel E, Hucumenoglu S, et al. Breast fibroadenoma in female adolescents. *Saudi Med J* 2007;28(1):137–138.
149. Tokunaga M, Wakimoto J, Muramoto Y, et al. Juvenile secretory carcinoma and juvenile papillomatosis. *Jpn J Clin Oncol* 1985;15(2):457–465.
150. Trier WC. Complete breast absence. Case report and review of the literature. *Plast Reconstr Surg* 1965;36(4):431–439.
151. Tsukahara M, Uchida M, Uchino S, et al. Male to male transmission of supernumerary nipples. *Am J Med Genet* 1997;69(2):194–195.
152. Turalba CI, el-Mahdi AM, Ladaga L. Fatal metastatic cystosarcoma phyllodes in an adolescent female: case report and review of treatment approaches. *J Surg Oncol* 1986;33(3):176–181.
153. Urbani CE, Betti R. Accessory mammary tissue associated with congenital and hereditary nephrourinary malformations. *Int J Dermatol* 1996;35(5):349–352.
154. van Hoeven KH, Hibbard CA, Flax H, et al. Metastatic malignant neoplasms and secondary lymphomatous involvement of the breast: a study of 43 cases. *Pathol Annu* 1993;2(Pt 28):221–241.
155. Velanovich V. Ectopic breast tissue, supernumerary breasts, and supernumerary nipples. *South Med J* 1995;88(9):903–906.
156. Ventura L, Guadagni S, Ventura T, et al. Benign granular cell tumor of the breast: a misleading disease. *Tumori* 1999;85(3):194–198.
157. Wallgren A, Silfversward C, Hultborn A. Carcinoma of the breast in women under 30 years of age: a clinical and histopathological study of all cases reported as carcinoma to the Swedish Cancer Registry, 1958–1968. *Cancer* 1977;40(2):916–923.
158. Wargotz ES, Norris HJ, Austin RM, et al. Fibromatosis of the breast. A clinical and pathological study of 28 cases. *Am J Surg Pathol* 1987;11(1):38–45.
159. Weinberg SK, Motulsky AG. Aberrant axillary breast tissue: A report of a family with six affected women in two generations. *Clin Genet* 1976;10(6):325–328.
160. West KW, Rescorla FJ, Scherer LR Jr, et al. Diagnosis and treatment of symptomatic breast masses in the pediatric population. *J Pediatr Surg* 1995;30(2):182–186; discussion 186–187.
161. Wilson M, Cranor ML, Rosen PP. Papillary duct hyperplasia of the breast in children and young women. *Mod Pathol* 1993;6(5):570–574.
162. Winchester DP. Breast cancer in young women. *Surg Clin North Am* 1996;76(2):279–287.
163. Zanella M, Falconieri G, Lamovec J, et al. Pseudoangiomatous hyperplasia of the mammary stroma: true entity or phenotype? *Pathol Res Pract* 1998;194(8):535–540.

CHAPTER 21

The Pineal, Pituitary, Parathyroid, Thyroid, and Adrenal Glands

RICHARD M. CONRAN
ELLEN CHUNG
LOUIS P. DEHNER
HIROYUKI SHIMADA

The endocrine system represents a diverse group of organs and cell types involved in the maintenance of a homeostatic environment. It is composed of the pineal gland, the pituitary gland, the thyroid gland, the parathyroid glands, the adrenal glands, the islets of Langerhan, and a diffuse network of neuroendocrine cells distributed throughout the respiratory and gastrointestinal tracts (eFigure 21-1). Endocrine function mediated through endocrine, autocrine, and paracrine signaling mechanisms is also seen in other organs including the hypothalamus, heart, thymus, kidneys, adipose tissue, skin, gonads, and the placenta.

Disorders related to pituitary (growth abnormalities), thyroid, or adrenal dysfunction or sexual maldevelopment and obesity are many of the diagnoses made in large pediatric endocrine clinics. Many endocrine disorders recognized in childhood often require life-long treatment and are also a substantial component of adult endocrine practice (e834,e405, e643,e1122,e528,e529). The study of endocrine disorders has been facilitated through molecular techniques with the identification of genetic aberrations in the afferent and efferent limbs of hormonal actions, with loss of a critical enzyme in the biosynthetic or biodegradative scheme, or with the absence of a hormonal receptor. Recent advances in imaging techniques combined with molecular diagnostics have also led to recognition of new disorders and new diagnostic and prognostic criteria, and the identification of new familial inherited syndromes (Table 21-1) (e643,e333,e723,e1174). This chapter incorporates these newer modalities while continuing to focus on the developmental, acquired, and neoplastic disorders involving the pineal, pituitary, parathyroid, thyroid, and adrenal glands in the pediatric age population. Disorders of the pancreas, ovary, and testis are discussed in Chapters 16, 18, and 19, respectively.

The opinions and assertions contained herein are the private views of the authors and are not to be construed as official or as representing the views of the Uniformed Services University or the Department of Defense.

PINEAL GLAND

Anatomy and Physiology

The pineal gland is a small, cone-shaped, 50- to 150-mg tan-brown structure attached to the superior aspect of the posterior border of the third ventricle. It develops at approximately 7 weeks' gestation from an evagination of the ependymal lining covering the caudal portion of the roof of the third ventricle (142,e980,e1108). Based on magnetic resonance (MR) imaging studies, the pineal gland increases in size from birth through 2 years of age, at which time it remains constant in size through adolescence (e1158). No size difference has been noted between male and female children. In children older than 2 years of age, the average pineal gland measures 6.5 × 4.8 × 4 mm (e1158).

At approximately 5 years of age, calcifications, in the form of corpora arenacea, develop. These calcifications increase with age giving the pineal gland a hyperdense appearance on computed tomography (CT) imaging at puberty (e1307). Pineal calcifications are observed in 8% of children by age 10, 20% at puberty, and 40% by age 20 (e313,e1307).

Histologically, the pineal gland is composed of nests of cells in lobular profiles, with a resemblance to the "zellballens" of paraganglia, surrounded by connective tissue septa containing blood vessels and nerve fibers (21,78,171). The pinealocytes, or chief cells, have basophilic cytoplasm with large irregular nuclei and prominent nucleoli and are arranged in cords or follicles within the lobules. Randomly distributed throughout the pineal gland in perivascular areas and between pinealocytes is a second cell population of astrocytes. In the late third-trimester fetus and neonate, two populations of pineal parenchymal cells are identified with the small cell population disappearing with advancing age (e980). The pinealocytes are immunoreactive for synaptophysin (SYN), chromogranin (CHR), and neurofilament protein (NFP), and the interstitial astrocytes are immunoreactive for S-100 and glial fibrillary acidic protein (GFAP) (142,e1051).

Table 21-1 ■ ENDOCRINE ORGANS INVOLVED IN SELECTED FAMILIAL TUMOR SYNDROMES

Syndrome	Inheritance	Gene	Pituitary	Parathyroid	Thyroid	Adrenal	Other Manifestations
Beckwith-Wiedemann		*CDKN1C/NSD1*				ACN	
Carney complex	AD	*PRKAR1A*	Adenoma		PTC	ACN	
Cowden		*PTEN*			FTC/PTC		
Familial adenomatosis polyposis coli		*APC*			PTC		
Familial medullary thyroid carcinoma		*RET*			MTC		
Familial paraganglioma-pheochromocytoma		*SDHD, SDHC, SDHB*				PHEO	Paraganglioma
Hyperparathyroidism-jaw tumor	AD	*HRPT2*		Adenoma/ carcinoma			
Li-Fraumeni		*TP53*				ACN	
McCune-Albright		*GNAS*	Adenoma		Hyperplasia	Hyperplasia/ adenoma	
MEN 1	AD	*MEN1*	Adenoma	Adenoma/ hyperplasia		ACN	Islet cell neoplasia
MEN 2	AD	*RET*		Adenoma/ hyperplasia	MTC	PHEO	Paraganglioma
Neurofibromatosis type 1	AD	*NF1*				PHEO	Paraganglioma
Von Hippel-Lindau	AD	*VHL*				PHEO	Islet cell neoplasia Paraganglioma

ACN, adrenocortical neoplasm; AD, autosomal dominant; FTC, follicular thyroid carcinoma; MTC, medullary thyroid carcinoma; PHEO, pheochromocytoma; PTC, papillary thyroid carcinoma.
Modified from Table 5.01. Eng C. Inherited tumor syndromes. Introduction. In: DeLellis RA, Lloyd RV, Heiz PU, eds. *World Health Organization classification of tumors: pathology and genetics. Tumors of endocrine organs.* Lyons: IARC, 2004;210.

The major hormone produced by the pineal gland is the indoleamine, melatonin, which plays a role in circadian rhythm regulation and gonadal steroidogenesis. Destruction of the pineal gland by a benign cyst or tumor has led to precocious puberty. Interference with the inhibitory effect of melatonin on gonadal steroidogenesis represents one mechanism (e307). Other physiologic functions attributed to the pineal gland include a role in modulating the hypothalamic-pituitary-gonadal axis, hormonal rhythms, the sleep cycle, and body temperature (e298,e923,e1242). Melatonin levels have been reported elevated in some children with primary pineal tumors (106,e755,e1237). Melatonin levels may be useful in determining the adequacy of pineal tumor resection when the level was increased before surgery (e1237). Other aspects of the anatomy and function of the pineal gland are discussed in more detail by Reiter (142).

Imaging

The normal pineal gland is less than 1 cm in size and isoattenuating to brain. Pineal lesions may be detected on CT, if large, but the pineal gland is best evaluated on MR imaging, particularly in the sagittal plane. Imaging helps to distinguish pineal region neoplasms from common pineal cysts. Pineal cysts are isodense to cerebrospinal fluid (CSF) on CT and are not associated with hydrocephalus (e426). The normal adult pineal gland is often centrally calcified on CT, but this process usually does not begin until age 10 to 12 (e1307), so the finding of calcification in the pineal gland of a child less than 10 years of age should be viewed with concern. Calcification may be seen at the periphery of the pineal gland in the older child or adult (eFigure 21-2). On MR, pineal cysts are optimally visualized in the sagittal plane, are homogeneous, and parallel the signal of CSF. Cysts greater than 1 cm in diameter that are heterogeneous may indicate the presence of hemorrhage (e371). Following intravenous administration of gadolinium chelate, a rim of compressed normal pineal tissue typically enhances, but the cyst itself does not enhance (e82).

Pineal germ cell neoplasms appear on CT as solid masses often with dense calcifications (eFigure 21-3A to C). On MR, the solid portion is isodense to brain on T1-weighted images and hyperintense to brain on T2-weighted images, while calcifications are hypointense on both pulse sequences. Pineocytomas on CT appear solid and may contain calcifications, but calcifications are less common in pineocytomas than in germ cell neoplasms (e347). Pineal tumors may compress the tectum and aqueduct of Sylvius causing findings of hydrocephalus (eFigure 21-3). Pineocytomas are hypo- to isointense to brain on T1-weighted images and hyperintense to brain on T2-weighted images (eFigure 21-4). Pineoblastomas are variable in their MR appearance since these tumors are aggressive, may be large and lobulated, and have areas of necrosis (Figure 21-1A) causing a heterogeneous appearance. Pineal parenchymal tumors generally enhance markedly after intravenous gadolinium contrast administration (e82).

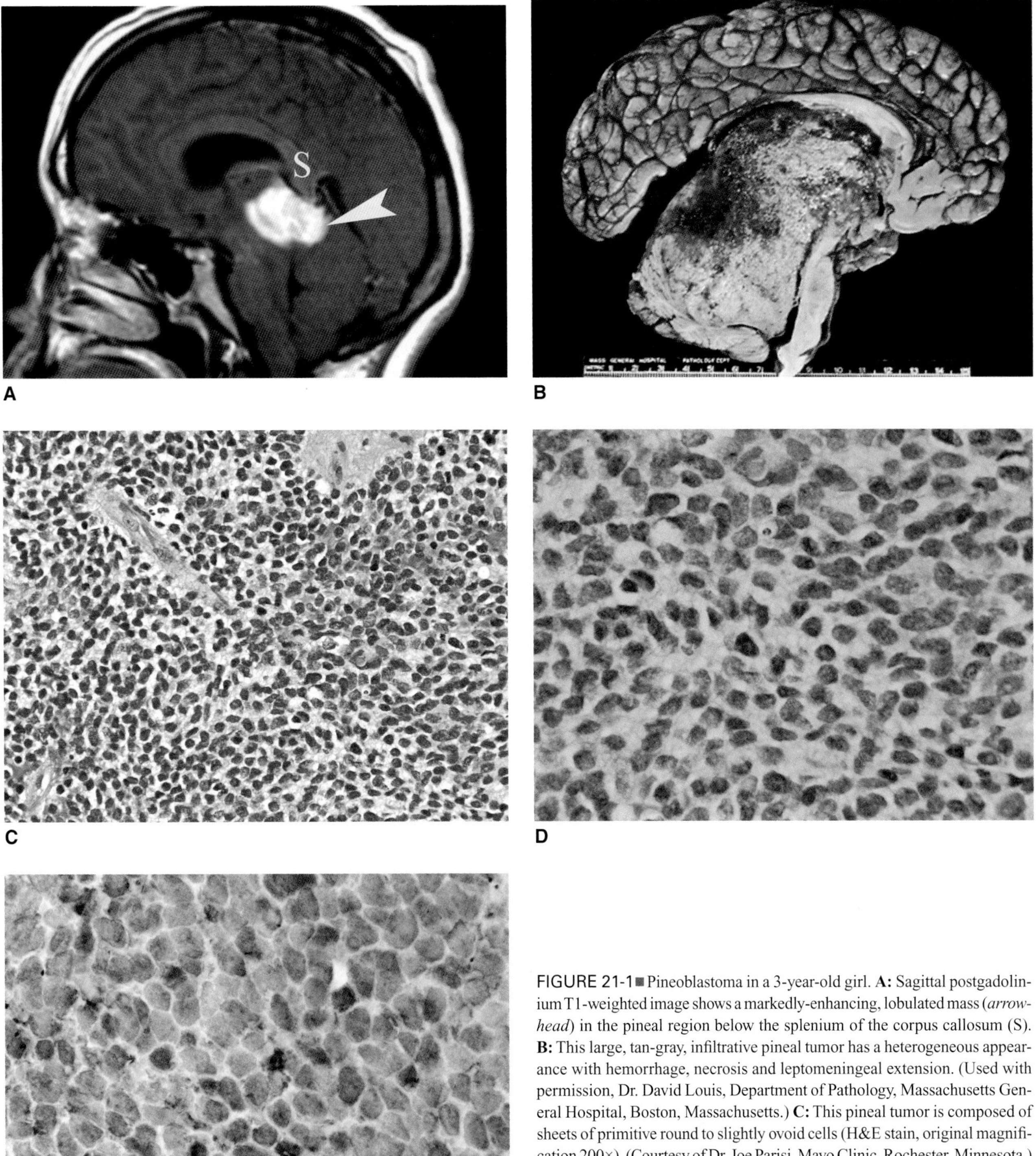

FIGURE 21-1 ■ Pineoblastoma in a 3-year-old girl. **A:** Sagittal postgadolinium T1-weighted image shows a markedly-enhancing, lobulated mass (*arrowhead*) in the pineal region below the splenium of the corpus callosum (S). **B:** This large, tan-gray, infiltrative pineal tumor has a heterogeneous appearance with hemorrhage, necrosis and leptomeningeal extension. (Used with permission, Dr. David Louis, Department of Pathology, Massachusetts General Hospital, Boston, Massachusetts.) **C:** This pineal tumor is composed of sheets of primitive round to slightly ovoid cells (H&E stain, original magnification 200×). (Courtesy of Dr. Joe Parisi, Mayo Clinic, Rochester, Minnesota.) **D:** The tumor cells have irregular, hyperchromatic nuclei and scant cytoplasm. Mitotic figures were also present (H&E stain, original magnification 400×). (Courtesy of Dr. Joe Parisi, Mayo Clinic, Rochester, Minnesota.) **E:** The tumor cells demonstrate immunoreactivity with synaptophysin (immunostain for synaptophysin, original magnification 400×). (Courtesy of Dr. Joe Parisi, Mayo Clinic, Rochester, Minnesota.)

Developmental Disorders

Pineal agenesis has been reported as a component of other midline central nervous system developmental syndromes with absence of the corpus callosum, such as in Aicardi syndrome (151,e398,e918). The contrasting abnormality, pineal gland hyperplasia, has been reported in children with genital enlargement (151,e1166).

Pineal cysts (glial cyst) are a relatively common radiological finding on MR and as an incidental finding in 25% to 40% of autopsies. There is a female predilection (eFigure 21-5) (21,106,171,e348,e371,e475,e754,e787, e824,e852,e1108). A pineal cyst larger than 1 cm in diameter may cause symptoms (headache, vertigo, and visual disturbances) in an adolescent or young adult (142,e348,e307). Symptomatic cysts have been treated by surgical excision (113,192,e892,e1132). Possible mechanisms for pineal cyst development include persistence of the ependymal-lined pineal diverticulum, secondary cavitation within the pineal gland, or as sequelae to hemorrhage in the gland (142,e787,e978,e1108). An ependymal lining often accompanied by reactive-appearing astrocytes are the microscopic features. (eFigure 21-6) Approximately 5% of children with hereditary retinoblastomas have pineal cyst as a benign variant of trilateral retinoblastoma (141,e94). Cyst formation is also seen in pineal neoplasms (50,106,e585).

Acquired Disorders

Neoplasms of the pineal gland region account for 2% or less of all primary CNS tumors in children and are discussed in more detail by Burger and Scheithauer (21) and in Chapter 10. Classically, there are three histogenetic categories: tumors of pineal parenchyma (true pinealomas) (eFigure 21-7), glial-derived tumors, and germ cell neoplasms, which account for 50% to 60% of cases. The germ cell tumors have a variety of patterns ranging from germinomas and teratomas to malignant mixed germ cell neoplasms (eFigures 21-8 to 21-10) (48,111,e1,e33,e264,e321,e346,e484,e582,e907). Imaging studies have not been found diagnostic in differentiating among these tumors and do not distinguish between a pineal neoplasm and a glial cyst (e977).

Pineal parenchymal tumors (PPT) are represented by the pineocytoma, pineoblastoma, and pineal parenchymal tumor (PPT) of intermediate differentiation (19,21,79,105, e135,e625,e798,e1064). Pineoblastomas, like germ cell tumors, preferentially occur in the first decade of life in contrast to pineocytomas, which are seen in the second decade and into adulthood. Almost 60% of PPTs are pineoblastomas (mean age, 2 to 3 years) and another 10% are pineocytomas (mean age 10 to 12 years) in the pediatric population (48,52). The M:F sex incidence for pineoblastomas varies among series from 5:1 to 1:2 for children 16 or younger (48,79,e264).

Pineoblastoma, like the other central primitive neuroectodermal tumors (PNET), is a tan-gray, soft, infiltrative tumor with or without hemorrhage and necrosis and often extends into the leptomeninges (21) (Figure 21-1B). Sheets of primitive round to slightly ovoid cells with irregular, hyperchromatic nuclei and scant cytoplasm are observed on histological examination. Mitotic figures and apoptotic bodies are readily identified (Figure 21-1C, D, eFigures 21-11 and 21-12). Focal necrosis and Homer-Wright rosettes are present in some cases. Infrequently, photoreceptor differentiation is indicated by the presence of Flexner-Wintersteiner–like rosettes. Tumor cells are immunoreactive for SYN (Figure 21-1E, eFigure 21-13), CHR and NFP to a lesser degree and to retinal S-antigen in about 50% of cases (21,34).

Trilateral retinoblastoma syndrome is defined by the development of a midline intracranial malignancy, usually a pineoblastoma, in the setting of hereditary retinoblastoma (21,141,e94,e72,e124,e502,e759,e955). The rhabdoid tumor predisposition syndrome with a germline mutation in the *INI1* gene is also associated with primary pineal neoplasms (19,e133). Astrocytomas, discussed in chapter 10, involving the pineal gland also occur throughout the first and second decades. Pineal astrocytomas have been reported in association with tuberous sclerosis and neurofibromatosis type 1 (e277,e893,e264). Papillary tumors presumably arising from the ependymal lining, usually seen in adults, have also been reported in children (19,e176,e364,e478).

Pineocytoma, unlike the pineoblastoma, has a lobular appearance like other examples of endocrine or neuroendocrine neoplasms, is well circumscribed and displaces surrounding structures. The tumor cells are uniform with small central nuclei and conspicuous eosinophilic cytoplasm with an absence of pleomorphism, necrosis and mitotic figures in most cases. Homer-Wright and Flexner-Wintersteiner rosettes and large GFAP-positive fibrillary areas, referred to as pineocytomatous rosettes, are observed in these tumors (eFigures 21-14A, B and 21-15). Like the pineoblastoma, tumor cells are immunoreactive for SYN, CHR, NFP and neuron specific enolase (NSE), in addition to retinal S-antigen in approximately 30% of cases (eFigure 21-16) (34,e798,e1292). Neurosecretory granules are identified ultrastructurally in contrast to their usual absence in pineoblastomas (e820).

The PPT of intermediate differentiation shows histological features of both pineoblastoma and pineocytoma with variable mitotic activity, necrosis and NFP immunoreactivity. Comparative genomic hybridization suggests that this tumor more closely resembles the pineoblastoma, but generally has the favorable prognosis of a pineocytoma (e363,e987,e1292).

Prognosis of PPTs is dependent on stage, tumor volume, histological type, and NFP immunostaining (52,79,e171,e499,e1293). These tumors are assigned to the following grades: pineocytoma (WHO grade 1), pineoblastoma (WHO grade 4) and the PPT of intermediate differentiation (WHO grade 2 or 3) (19,52,79,105). Pineocytoma has a favorable survival (85% to 90%, 5 years), whereas the pineoblastoma is below 25% (19,52,79,e1052,e1053). Among the pineoblastomas, those tumors with mutated *Rb1* gene are more aggressive with decreased survival rate, if possible, when compared to the sporadic pineoblastoma (e947).

Other neoplastic lesions involving the pineal gland include Langerhans cell histiocytosis (LCH) (e440), cavernous angioma (e631), lipoma (e1118), craniopharyngioma (e1215), and meningioma (e775). Pineal involvement with acute lymphocytic leukemia is reported (e657). Infections, vascular malformations, epidermoid cyst, hemorrhage, and apoplexy are nonneoplastic lesions of the pineal gland in children (e216,e660,e743,e752).

PITUITARY GLAND

Anatomy and Physiology

Posterior to the optic chiasma, the pituitary gland extends by a narrow stalk from the hypothalamus into the sella turcica, a small concavity in the sphenoid bone (9,101,134,e317). The pituitary gland is a small ovoid structure which is divided into a red-brown anterior lobe (adenohypophysis), a gray-white posterior lobe (neurohypophysis), and an indistinct intermediate lobe. The adenohypophysis is subdivided into the pars distalis, pars intermedia, and pars tuberalis, with the pars distalis accounting for the bulk of the anterior lobe. More prominent in the fetal pituitary gland, the pars intermedia is inconspicuous in adolescents and adults. The neurohypophysis is subdivided into the pars nervosa, the infundibulum, and the median eminence. The infundibulum and pars tuberalis comprise the pituitary stalk (eFigure 21-17).

The pituitary gland weighs approximately 100 mg at birth and increases in weight during adolescence to its adult weight of 500 to 600 mg (e37,e206), with the adenohypophysis accounting for 80% of the gland (9,101). Some populations, however, demonstrate a weight less than 500 mg (e1022). The pituitary gland of the neonate is especially prominent owing to its stimulation by maternal hormones, but it undergoes some involution in the postnatal period, followed by increased growth through the age of 3 years (e638). A notable increase in the size of the gland occurs with menarche and pregnancy (e366,e1022). Generally, the pituitary gland in women after puberty weighs more than the gland in men (e227,e330,e1022). Suprasellar extension of the pituitary gland during puberty has been reported as a normal variant (e587).

The pituitary gland receives its vascular supply from two hypophysial arteries that branch from the internal carotid arteries and give rise to two anastomosing networks of capillaries that surround the stalk and adenohypophysis. The hypophyseal-portal circulation, which arises from the second capillary plexus, supplies the adenohypophysis (9,101,e317). A thin diaphragm, arising from the dura, covers the opening to the sella turcica, but in the center of the diaphragm the pituitary stalk passes through an aperture. The pituitary gland is not covered by meninges. The periosteal dura lines the sella turcica.

The adenohypophysis is composed of three cell types on histological examination: the chromophobes, acidophils, and basophils, accounting for 50%, 40%, and 10% of adenohypophyseal cells, respectively (eFigure 21-18) (e518). Based on immunohistochemistry and ultrastructural observations, six distinct hormonally active cell types are identifiable in the adult gland. The cell types and their respective hormones are the somatotrophs (growth hormone), lactotrophs (prolactin), corticotrophs (ACTH), gonadotrophs (FSH/LH), and thyrotrophs (TSH), accounting for 40% to 50%, 10% to 30%, 10% to 20%, 5% to 10%, and 5% of the adenohypophyseal cells, respectively (101,134). Stimulating and inhibitory hypothalamic factors released into the hypophyseal-portal circulation regulate the release of ACTH, TSH, FSH, LH, growth hormone, and prolactin from the adenohypophysis (eFigure 21-19). Mammosommatotrophs (prolactin/growth hormone) are uncommon. Immunostaining reveals CK 7 and 8 positivity in these cells in addition to their respective hormones (10,33).

The folliculostellate cells are agranular, immunostain for S-100, GFAP and vimentin (VIM) and extend between the other adenohypophyseal cells. They are thought to have a paracrine regulatory function on the hormone-producing cells (101). Calcified concretions are an incidental finding in the anterior pituitary of ostensibly normal fetuses and neonates (e441,e442).

The posterior pituitary (neurohypophysis) contains the axonal processes of neurosecretory neurons that originate in the supraoptic and paraventricular nuclei of the hypothalamus and are GFAP positive (eFigure 21-19). Vasopressin and oxytocin, produced in the neurohypophysis are stored in secretory granules (Herring bodies) in the nerve endings (101).

The pituitary gland arises developmentally from two anlages (e634). Ectoderm from the roof of the oral stomatodeum gives rise to the adenohypophysis, whereas neuroectoderm from the floor of the diencephalon is the progenitor of the neurohypophysis. During the 4th week of gestation, an outpouching of ectoderm from the roof of the stomatodeum (primitive mouth cavity) grows dorsally toward the diencephalon as Rathke pouch. Along this route of migration, progenitor cells of the future adenohypophysis may lag behind as potential sources of ectopic anterior pituitary (e518). Constriction and disappearance of Rathke pouch during the 5th to 6th gestational week separate the adenohypophysis from the stomatodeum. Concurrently, the elongating Rathke pouch passes between the developing presphenoid and basisphenoid bones of the skull and joins with the infundibulum, a diverticulum arising from the diencephalon as the future neurohypophysis. The first vestiges of the hypothalamic-hypophyseal portal circulation are seen at 7 weeks' gestation, and the process is completed at 18 to 20 weeks' gestation.

Somatotrophs and corticotrophs are identified immunohistochemically in the adenohypophysis between the 5th and 12th gestational week; by 12 to 13 weeks' gestation, thyrotrophs and gonadotrophs are seen, and at 13 to 16 weeks' gestation, lactotrophs first appear. During the sixth gestational month, innervation of the neurohypophysis with axonal processes from the supraoptic and paraventricular nuclei takes place.

The differentiation of the oral ectoderm into the terminal anterior pituitary cell types, their hormones and receptors is under the control of a large complement of genes and transcription factors (eFigure 21-20). Several excellent reviews discuss the role of these factors in pituitary organogenesis in more detail (10,33,44,110,e83,e646,e900,e1068,e1288). The physiology of the different cell types, their hormones and the mechanisms of action of their respective hormones is beyond the scope of this chapter, but is detailed by others (9,33,101, 110,143,e1049,e1050,e1298).

Imaging

Due to its small size and location within the bony sella, the pituitary is best evaluated with dedicated MR imaging. The adenohypophysis is isointense to gray matter and has a flat superior margin until puberty when the margin becomes slightly convex, especially in girls. Due to the fat content of the hormones elaborated there, the neurohypophysis is hyperintense compared to brain on T1-weighted images, producing the posterior pituitary "bright spot." The pituitary stalk (infundibulum) is normally midline and no larger than the basilar artery on axial images (e82). Developmental lesions may be detected on imaging. Ectopia of the posterior pituitary is seen as an abnormal location of the posterior pituitary bright spot along the infundibulum or near the infundibular recess of the third ventricle (eFigure 21-21). Rathke cleft cysts are well-circumscribed, round or lobulated, and isodense to CSF on CT. The signal intensity of the cyst on MR is variable depending on the protein content of the fluid. They are generally iso- to slightly hyperintense to CSF on T1-weighted images and iso to slightly hypointense to CSF on T2-weighted images (eFigure 21-22) (e82).

Inflammatory or infiltrative disorders are optimally demonstrated on MR images. Lymphocytic and granulomatous hypophysitis and LCH appear similar on imaging studies. The hypothalamus and infundibulum appear enlarged. Generally, uniform enhancement is seen following intravenous administration of gadolinium (eFigures 21-23 to 21-26) (e504,e746,e1187,e1188). Primary pituitary tumors are best evaluated with dedicated MR imaging with and without contrast material. Microadenomas do not distort the gland but are hypointense to the normal gland on T1-weighted images and enhance less than the gland on early dynamic postgadolinium imaging (eFigure 21-27). Macroadenomas distort the gland and the infundibulum and enhance uniformly and intensely (e866).

Developmental Disorders

Anomalies in pituitary gland development are uncommon and outlined in Table 21-2 (133,e150,e227,e229,e590,e1055, e1111,e1119). Agenesis, complete absence of the pituitary gland is rare as an isolated finding. Isolated agenesis of the pituitary has been noted in infants of diabetic mothers as a presumed form of diabetic embryopathy. Pituitary dysfunction in neural tube defects is well documented (e329). Agenesis is usually associated with other midline and craniofacial abnormalities (101,e53,e1067,e1157). In the presence of pituitary agenesis, the thyroid gland, the adrenal glands, and gonads are expectedly diminutive. The posterior pituitary or neurohypophysis may be present.

Table 21-2 ■ CONGENITAL AND DEVELOPMENTAL ANOMALIES OF THE PITUITARY GLAND

Agenesis
Hypoplasia
Ectopic pituitary
Duplication
Rathke cleft cysts
Pars intermedia cyst
Dermoid cyst
Empty sella syndrome
Hamartoma
Teratoma
Isolated growth hormone deficiency
Combined pituitary hormone deficiency
Cranial vault abnormalities involving sella turcica
Transphenoidal encephalocele
Persistent craniopharyngeal canal

Modified from Parks JS, Felner EI. Hypopituitarism. In: Kliegman RM, Behrman RE, Jenson HB, Stanton BF, eds. *Nelson textbook of pediatrics*, 18th ed. Philadelphia, PA: Elsevier, 2007; Chapter 558.

Adenohypophyseal hypoplasia with congenital hypopituitarism is reported in the presence of mutations in the genes controlling early development such as in POUF1 (pit-1) (e150, e168,e172,e373,e386,e608,e800,e916,e917,e965,e1107, e1130,e1179,e1251). The adenohypophysis is absent or markedly hypoplastic, with an intact neurohypophysis (e53,e641). Vascular malformations leading to pituitary hypoplasia represent another etiologic consideration (e544,e1095).

Hypopituitarism, defined as diminution or absence of one or more anterior pituitary hormones, is estimated to occur in 1:4,000 to 10,000 live births. A number of genetic syndromes, conditions with widespread structural abnormalities, and midline CNS anomalies involving the hypothalamus are associated conditions. Mutations in various genes in pituitary development are present in approximately 13% of isolated pituitary hormone deficiency (IPHD) and 20% of combined pituitary hormone deficiency (CPHD) cases and other structural malformations (Table 21-3) (95,133,e916,e965,e1179). Hypopituitarism may be a complication of traumatic brain injury (TBI) (e78,e324,e868).

Various CNS anomalies are associated with pituitary malformations: holoprosencephaly (associated with rudimentary neurohypophysis and central diabetes insipidus), septo-optic dysplasia, and hypothalamic-hypophyseal dysgenesis in bilateral anophthalmia (e161,e162,e481,e492,e1165). Many of these anomalies with pituitary dysfunction are linked to genetic mutations including deletions of a portion of chromosome 14 that codes for several genes including *BMP4* and *OTX2* that are associated with ocular and pituitary development. Bilateral anopthalmia is seen in association with *BMP4* mutations (e703,e884). Mutations in the *OTX2* gene may be associated with CPHD, a hypoplastic pituitary gland, ectopic neurohypophysis, and Chiari malformation. Other syndromes in which hypopituitarism is a feature include

Table 21-3 ■ MANIFESTATIONS ASSOCIATED WITH MUTATIONS IN SELECTED GENES INVOLVED IN PITUITARY DEVELOPMENT

Gene	Function	Manifestations
LHX3, LHX4	Development and maintenance of adenohypophysis	CPHD, IPHD, pituitary hypoplasia, ectopia of neurohypohysis, Arnold-Chiari I malformation
HESX1	Early development of pituitary gland	CPHD, IPHD, pituitary hypoplasia, ectopia of neurohypohysis, septo-optic dysplasia
POUF1 (pit 1)	Differentiation of the somatotrophs, lactotrophs and thyrotrophs	Growth hormone, prolactin and TSH deficiency
PROP 1	Differentiation of the sommatotrophs, lactotrophs, thyrotrophs and gonadotrophs	30%–50% of cases of familial CPHD
Tpit	Differentiation of corticotrophs	ACTH deficiency
Gli 2, Gli3		Holoprosencephaly and panhypopituitarism, Hall-Pallister syndrome
PTX2		Reiger syndrome

CPHD, combined pituitary hormone deficiency; IPHD, isolated pituitary hormone deficiency; ACTH, adrenocorticotropic hormone; TSH, thyroid-stimulating hormone.
Based on data from Lap-Yin Pang A, Martin MM, Martin ALA, et al. Molecular basis of diseases of the endocrine system. In: Coleman WB, Tsongalis GJ, eds. *Molecular pathology: the molecular basis of human disease.* Amsterdam: Elsevier, 2009:435–463.

MELAS syndrome, Kallmann syndrome, Rieger syndrome, trisomy 18, trisomy 13, Pallister-Hall syndrome, neurofibromatosis, Fanconi anemia, and ataxia-telangiectasia (e458, e538,e542,e618,e620,e994,e1020,e1087).

Anencephaly is characterized by the presence of an anterior pituitary tissue within the mass of cerebrovasculosa tissue (eFigure 21-28A, B). The presence of somatotrophs, lactotrophs, and gonadotrophs is demonstrated by immunohistochemistry. Corticotrophs and thyrotrophs, present in the pituitary in the second trimester, disappear owing to lack of hypothalamic stimulation during the third trimester (e317,e618). A distinct neurohypophysis is absent. The adrenal glands are hypoplastic at birth (e945) (eFigure 21-28C, D).

Ectopia of anterior pituitary type tissue is common and invariably an incidental finding, generally, in the roof of the nasopharynx or as a pharyngeal pituitary (e147,e250,e515,e749,e782). Persistence of Rathke pouch in the roof of the oronasopharynx is the source of the pharyngeal pituitary gland which has been reported in a number of conditions including the anencephalic fetus, spina bifida, trisomy 18, and Meckel syndrome (e619,e621–e623,e1257). Ectopia of the posterior pituitary has been associated with mutations in the genes responsible for pituitary organogenesis (eFigure 21-21) (95,e822,e851,e1165). Ectopic pituitary adenomas (PAs) are documented in the suprasellar region, clivus, nasopharynx, and paranasal sinuses mainly in adults, but also in children (e31,e247,e276,e428,e451,e463,e520 e616,e996,e1248).

Rathke cleft cyst, with the formation of microcysts in the pars intermedia, is usually well circumscribed and is seen in normal pituitary glands in 2% to 26% of autopsies (e1235). Usually asymptomatic, fluid accumulation in these epithelial-lined cysts may be symptomatic on the basis of compression of intrasellar or suprasellar structures with growth retardation in children (the so-called pituitary dwarfism) (eFigure 21-22) (e230,e1235). Central precocious puberty has also been observed (e7). The cyst is filled with thickened mucoid secretions or dark fluid (eFigure 21-29). Ciliated columnar or low cuboidal epithelium lines the cyst (e152). Other cystic lesions in the region of the pituitary include the craniopharyngioma and intrasellar arachnoid cyst (e1091). A distinguishing feature of the craniopharyngioma is mixed cystic and solid areas with the presence of palisading and squamoid-type epithelium (Figure 21-2A, B). Because the craniopharyngioma and Rathke cleft cyst have a shared histogenesis, ciliated columnar epithelium may be seen on occasion in a craniopharyngioma. Abscess formation and hypophysitis are rare complications in Rathke cleft cysts.

Pituitary duplication is a rare disorder that is ascribed to a duplication of the prechordal plate and anterior aspect of the notochord. Two distinct pituitaries, each with a stalk, are the typical presentation (e634). This anomaly has been seen with partial twinning; the median cleft facial syndrome, precocious puberty, and fetal exposure to meclizine (teratogenic effect) (e283,e462,e998,e1016,e1231). A midline hypothalamic mass of disorganized neurons is accompanied by other midline developmental anomalies including a duplicated sella, cleft palate, hypertelorism, agenesis of corpus callosum, and vertebral anomalies (e634). Nasopharyngeal teratomas have been reported in association with pituitary duplication in infancy (e462,e530,e853,e1075,e1106).

Empty sella syndrome (ESS) is usually an incidental finding in young children in contrast to adults (e110,e183,e191,e325,e1272). The primary form of ESS results from a defect in the diaphragm covering the opening to the sella turcica, and arachnoid tissue extends through the diaphragmatic defect. Increased CSF pressure leads to enlargement of the sella turcica and compression of the pituitary gland along the floor of the sella turcica, giving the appearance of an empty sella turcica (eFigures 21-30 and 21-31) (e114). Pituitary infarction, pituitary atrophy from

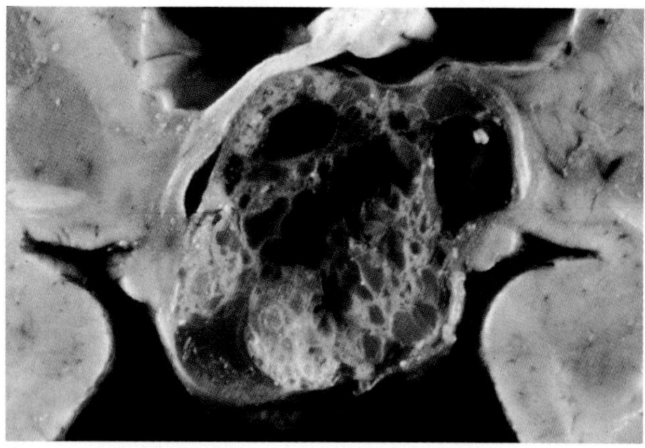
A

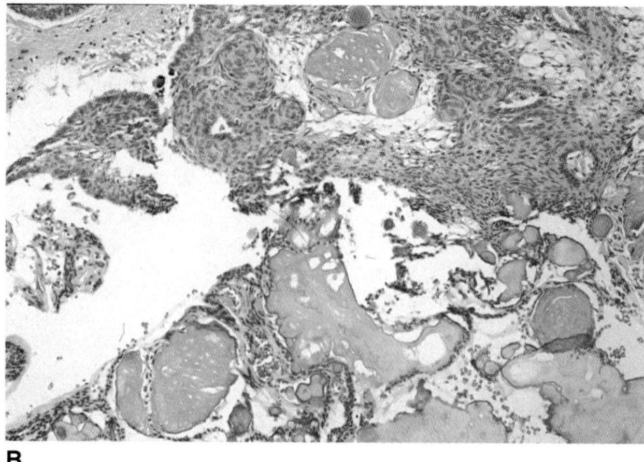
B

FIGURE 21-2■Craniopharyngioma. **A:** This gross brain image shows a suprasellar cystic lesion filled with a dark brown fluid containing cholesterol debris. **B:** This adamantinomatous variant consists of ribbons of epithelial cells with pseudopalisaded nuclei at the periphery of the lobules surrounding cystic spaces. The inner cells in the more solid areas have a loose, stellate appearance. The so-called wet keratin is seen as intermixed stacks of necrobiotic squames. This image is from a 7-year-old girl, who presented with headaches and decreased visual acuity and was found to have a suprasellar mass (H&E stain).

a tumor or other mass lesion, or prior hypophysectomy account for secondary ESS (e477).

Acquired Disorders

Inflammatory and infiltrative disorders are known to involve the pituitary gland including infections, noninfectious inflammatory conditions, and infiltrative processes. Examples of these diseases are congenital syphilis, mycobacteriosis, lymphocytic-granulomatous hypophysitis, LCH, sarcoidosis, Wegener granulomatosis, iron overload, storage disorder, Rosai-Dorfman disease (RDD), and Hurler syndrome (e105,e109,e127,e208,e228,e267,e424,e731, e1043,e1061,e1083,e1282). In addition to the PA and craniopharyngioma, the most common neoplasms of the sellar, parasellar, and suprasellar regions in children, germ cell neoplasms of the types seen more often in the pineal gland (60% to 70% of all primary intracranial germ cell tumors) also present in the suprasellar-sellar region (30% to 40% of cases). Visual field defects, diabetes insipidus, and panhypopituitarism are the principal clinical manifestations of suprasellar germ cell tumors.

Lymphocytic hypophysitis, typically observed in young women in the postpartum period with hypopituitarism, is seen in children as young as 9 years old; however, the condition is generally uncommon in children (e208,e406,e504,e747,e780). It is regarded as an autoimmune condition because of its association with Hashimoto or lymphocytic thyroiditis (e960,e1113). The adenohypophysis (lymphocytic adenohypophysitis) and neurohypophysis (lymphocytic infundibulo-neurohypophysitis) may be involved, and generically, the designation of lymphocytic hypophysitis is used to describe both conditions (e1043,e1227,e1260). The pituitary is enlarged with a firm consistency and contains an inflammatory infiltrate of small lymphocytes commingled with plasma cells (eFigure 21-32A to C). Eosinophils and some macrophages are also seen. Fibrosis is common, but may be inapparent in a small biopsy. Hypopituitarism, diabetes insipidus, and symptoms of a mass are the usual clinical manifestations in both children and adults (e1260). Because the pituitary and sella are enlarged, a PA is often the clinical impression.

Granulomatous hypophysitis with epithelioid or caseous granulomas has the differential diagnosis of infection (tuberculosis), sarcoidosis, rupture of a Rathke cleft cyst, LCH and idiopathic granulomatous hypophysitis (e535,e541,e650,e1002,e1151). Granulomas are not a feature of lymphocytic hypophysitis, although a nosologic and etiologic relationship may exist between these idiopathic inflammatory disorders (e504).

Xanthogranulomatous inflammation (cholesterol granuloma) of the sellar region is an inflammatory reaction characterized by cholesterol clefts, lymphoplasmacytic infiltrates, hemosiderin deposits, fibrosis, foreign body giant cells, histiocytes, and eosinophilic necrotic debris. Although this pattern of xanthogranulomatous inflammation may be seen in association with an adamantinomatous craniopharyngioma, Paulus et al. (e377,e922) have observed this pattern in idiopathic cases, mainly in adolescents and young adults, which is not on the basis of a craniopharyngioma (e922).

Vascular lesions with hypopituitarism are uncommon in children, but hemorrhagic infarction of a pituitary macroadenoma, referred to as pituitary apoplexy or pituitary tumor apoplexy is one such example (Figure 21-3A, B) (109,e280, e369,e370,e700,e856,e953). Sheehan syndrome is associated with severe maternal intrapartum hypotension with pituitary infarction in the postpartum period (e1191,e1192). Presumed ischemia of the pituitary in sickle cell crisis is associated with decreased growth hormone secretion and impaired growth in affected children (e1115). Some cases of septo-optic

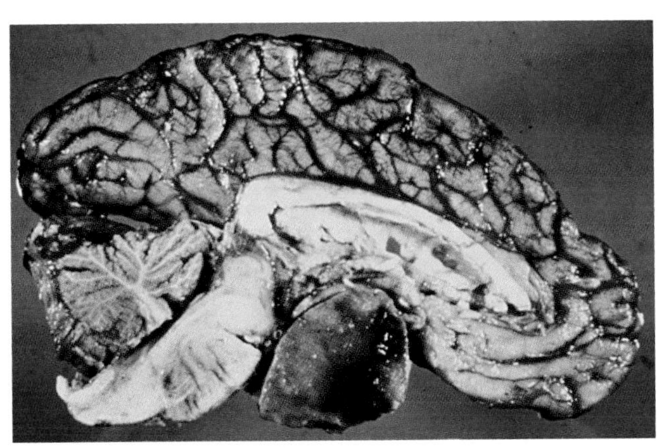
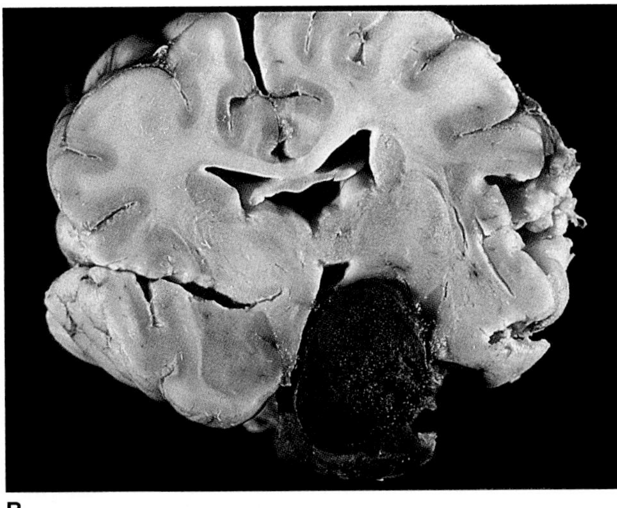

A B

FIGURE 21-3▪Pituitary apoplexy. **A:** Saggital section of brain showing hemorrhage within a pituitary macroadenoma. **B:** Coronal section showing hemorrhagic infarction of a 2-cm diameter well-circumscribed pituitary macroadenoma.

dysplasia, classified as a developmental anomaly, are thought to represent a vascular disruption of the anterior cerebral artery (e162,e736,e838,e999). Vascular lesions due to stalk transection may occur secondary to trauma (e640,e816,e1291).

Nonneoplastic cysts identified in children on radiological studies, are not clinically evident unless the sella turcica is expanded, leading to hypopituitarism and diabetes insipidus (e473,e829). Cystic dilatation of Rathke pouch remnants is common; however, these cysts are usually smaller than 5 mm in diameter (eFigures 21-22 and 21-29) (e858). Rathke cleft cysts arise from the squamous epithelium of the Rathke cleft, and infrequently become enlarged with symptoms resembling a craniopharyngloma (e230,e550). Arachnoid and dermoid cysts are also regarded by some as congenital defects (e218). An intrasellar arachnoid cyst must also be distinguished from a craniopharyngioma (e226,e829,e1091,e1109).

Pituitary hyperplasia is a nonneoplastic proliferation of one of the functional adenohypophyseal cell types (e55,e516,e1048). It is a polyclonal proliferation leading to pituitary enlargement and may produce a suprasellar mass (e988). In children, somatotroph hyperplasia is reported in the McCune-Albright syndrome (MAS) and gigantism (e644,e664,e696,e836,e915,e1303). Pituitary hyperplasia has also been reported in primary hypothyroidism (e372,e514). During pregnancy the pituitary gland doubles in size due to the proliferation of the lactotrophs (responsible for prolactin secretion) and decreases in size postpartum (101).

Pituitary adenoma (PA) is a monoclonal neoplasm of the adenohypophysis. As many as 10% of all PAs present in the first two decades of life (e242,e899). Tumors arising in the sellar region account for approximately 11% of all CNS tumors with PAs comprising 7.5% and craniopharyngiomas (CRPs) 3.2% (25). Most PAs are diagnosed in the second decade (90% or so of cases) and less than 10% before 10 years of age. Between the ages of 15 and 19 years, PAs are the most common CNS tumor and were twice as common in girls as boys (9,109,115,187, e1175). Reports of adenomas occurring in children less than 4 years are uncommon. One of the youngest examples of a PA occurred in a 7-month-old infant with Cushing disease and an ACTH-secreting PA (e720). Most PAs are sporadic, but they are one of the tumors observed in multiple endocrine neoplasia, type 1 (MEN 1), MAS, familial acromegaly syndrome, and Carney complex (61,129,e394,e450,e487,e488, e788,e796,e966,e1090,e1144,e1256,e1268). The three mutated genes associated with these familial tumors are *MEN 1* in MEN 1 syndrome, *PRKAR1A* in Carney complex and the gene for aryl hydrocarbon receptor-interacting protein in familial acromegaly syndrome (10,e407,e722,e1131,e1148).

In terms of function, the majority of PAs in children are prolactinomas (53%), and the remaining tumors are ACTH-secreting tumors (31%), growth hormone secreting tumors (9%), and endocrine-inactive (null cell tumors) (3%) (115,e245,54,188). ACTH-secreting adenomas are more common before puberty in contrast to prolactinomas and growth-hormone secreting tumors which are more common after puberty.

The clinical manifestations of PAs in children are variable and have been thoroughly documented (e173,e581,e661,e678). Headaches and visual field defects are the most common findings due to mass effect. In functional hormonally active tumors, girls with prolactinomas present with amenorrhea and galactorrhea, whereas, gynecomastia and hypogonadism are seen in boys. Children with ACTH-secreting adenomas present with Cushing disease and children with somatotropin or growth hormone–secreting adenomas present with gigantism.

Most prolactinomas, growth hormone-secreting tumors, and endocrine-inactive PAs are macroadenomas (tumor larger than 10 mm in diameter) (Figure 21-4A, B) in contrast

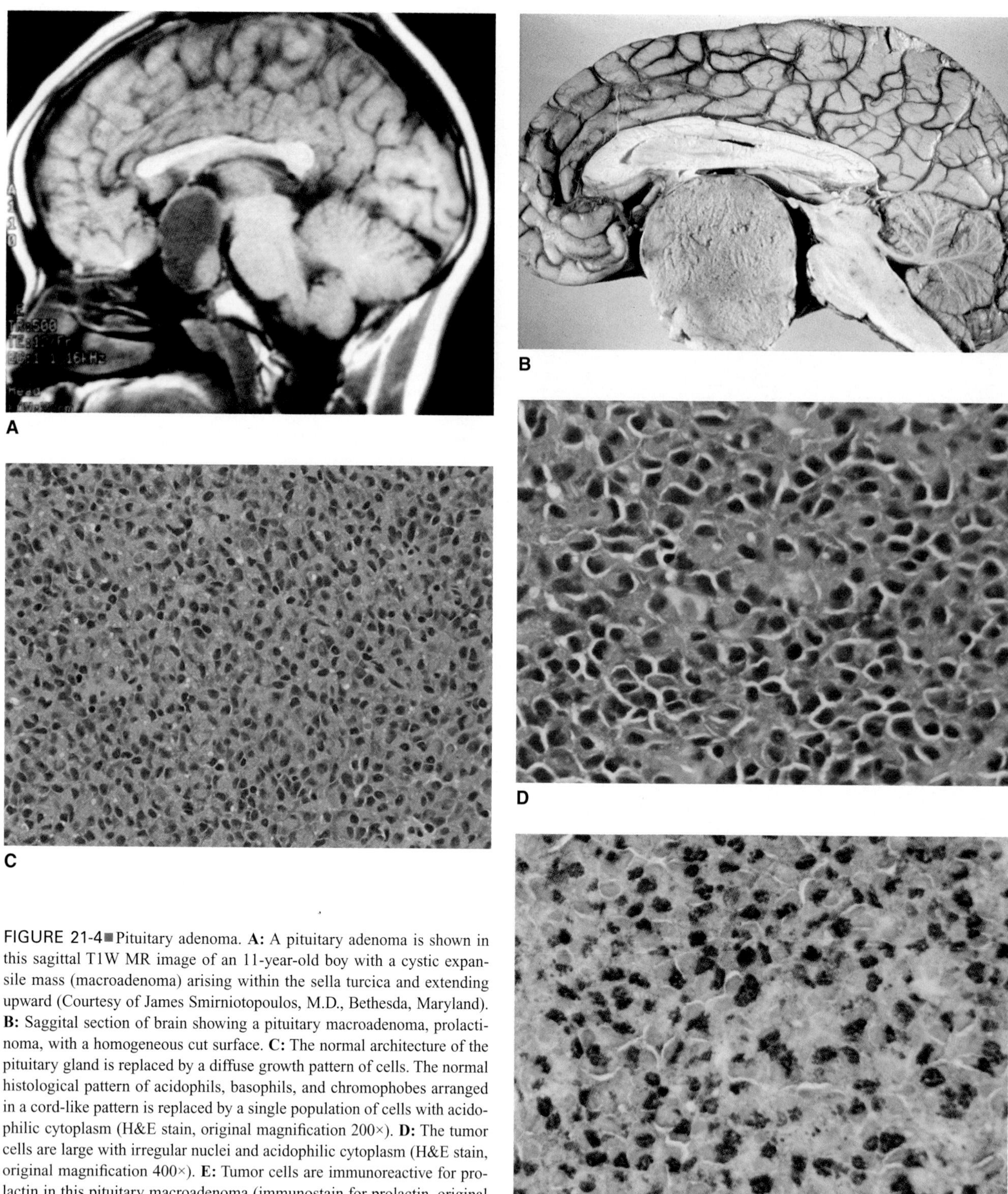

FIGURE 21-4 ■ Pituitary adenoma. **A:** A pituitary adenoma is shown in this sagittal T1W MR image of an 11-year-old boy with a cystic expansile mass (macroadenoma) arising within the sella turcica and extending upward (Courtesy of James Smirniotopoulos, M.D., Bethesda, Maryland). **B:** Saggital section of brain showing a pituitary macroadenoma, prolactinoma, with a homogeneous cut surface. **C:** The normal architecture of the pituitary gland is replaced by a diffuse growth pattern of cells. The normal histological pattern of acidophils, basophils, and chromophobes arranged in a cord-like pattern is replaced by a single population of cells with acidophilic cytoplasm (H&E stain, original magnification 200×). **D:** The tumor cells are large with irregular nuclei and acidophilic cytoplasm (H&E stain, original magnification 400×). **E:** Tumor cells are immunoreactive for prolactin in this pituitary macroadenoma (immunostain for prolactin, original magnification 400×). (Images **C–E**, courtesy of Dr. Joe Parisi, Mayo Clinic, Rochester, Minnesota.)

to the ACTH-secreting adenomas, which are more often microadenomas (tumor smaller than 10 mm in diameter) (eFigures 21-33 and 21-34) (9, e (272). Macroadenomas are more common than microadenomas in children, consistent with the finding that prolactinomas are more common than ACTH-secreting tumors. Pathologically, PAs are classified on the basis of five-tiered features: endocrine activity, imaging studies and operative findings, histology, immunohistochemistry, and ultrastructure (42,e645). PAs are soft and grayish-red, measuring 2 cm or less in diameter. On the basis of imaging criteria, four grades of tumors are recognized: grade I (smaller than 1 cm in diameter); grade II (intrasellar lesion larger than 1 cm in diameter or with suprasellar expansion without invasion); grade III (small or large locally invasive tumor with bony invasion of the sella turcica), and grade IV (large invasive tumor involving bone, the hypothalamus or cavernous sinus) (9). Larger aggressive tumors are more likely to be cystic, hemorrhagic, and necrotic (Figure 21-3A, B). One or more concurrent histological patterns, diffuse, trabecular, or papillary, may be evident. The degree of cellularity is variable from highly cellular to more scantily cellular tumors with a hyaline or amyloid-like stroma. The tinctorial quality of the cytoplasm has given rise to the characterization of PAs as basophilic, acidophilic or chromophobe with some limitations. The tumor cells are generally rounded with some spindling on occasion; the rounded nucleus is central or eccentric, and the tumor cells may have plasmacytoid qualities in the presence of an eccentric nucleus and prominent basophilic, acidophilic, or amphophilic cytoplasm. Prolactinomas are typically composed of chromophobes or slightly acidophilic cells, have a solid or papillary pattern, and have a hyalinized stroma with or without microcalcifications (Figure 21-4C, D, eFigure 21-35). PAs, in general, do not have a capsule (eFigure 21-33). Electron microscopy and immunohistochemistry are adjuncts to the characterization of these tumors (Figure 21-4E, eFigure 21-36) (e517,e518,e1034). In addition to specific hormonal immunostaining, PAs are positive for SYN, CHR, and NSE (33).

In terms of clinical behavior, macroadenomas are more likely to be invasive rather than the smaller expansile microadenomas. It is debatable whether PAs in children are more aggressive than their adult counterparts (e272,e340,e751). Invasive adenomas are characterized by extension into the dura, bone, and cavernous sinus; these features are generally not documented in the pathological examination. There is some correlation between the proliferative activity as determined by MIB-2 nuclear immunostaining and the observed invasiveness of the tumor (e188,e353,e770).

CRPs, thought to be derived from remnants of the Rathke pouch, account for 3% to 4% of primary CNS tumors in children (25). Generally, the tumor is found between the pharynx and floor of the sella turcica and is suprasellar in most cases (e5,e10,e400,e1261) (Figure 21-2A, eFigures 21-37 to 21-39). They may be parasellar or ectopic in the region of the pineal gland (e4,e327,e385,e606,e1033,e1215). The differential diagnosis includes PA, infection, inflammatory processes, vascular malformations, and Rathke cleft cyst (e400). Imaging has been found helpful in distinguishing among CRPs, PAs and Rathke cleft cysts (e226,e483).

Craniopharyngiomas (CRPs) in children are diagnosed between the ages of 5 and 14 years and have an equal male to female ratio (25). Tumors occurring during infancy are uncommon (e67,e74,e549,e573,e732). Compressive symptoms including pituitary dysfunction with retarded growth are the principal clinical manifestations (75,e456,e457,e1105). Diabetes insipidus due to posterior pituitary involvement is infrequent.

A calcified cystic suprasellar mass is the characteristic appearance on CT and MR scans (eFigure 21-39). Surgical resection may be followed by a recurrence (21,e26,e288, e368,e704,e1104,e1233). These tumors are typically characterized as a calcified suprasellar mass or cyst that measure 1 to 10 cm in diameter by imaging studies. The gross specimen consists of fragments of the cyst, and has a yellowish to dark brown appearance. Fluid contents have a dark oily appearance with cholesterol crystals and fragments of keratinous debris (e1109). In children, the histological features are adamantinomatous or ameloblastic in appearance (e385,e1033); the papillary squamous pattern is seen more often in adults (9,10,e400,e815). Beta-catenin mutations are seen in the adamantinomatous pattern (9,10). Epithelial lobules are arranged in a cloverleaf-like pattern (e71,e112). Palisading of the cells adjacent to the randomly distributed fluid-filled cyst-like spaces is another characteristic feature. Aggregates of necrotic, keratinized cells, or "wet" keratin accompanied by dystrophic calcification are other features (Figure 21-2B, eFigure 21-40). Fibrosis, chronic inflammation, and cholesterol clefts are observed in the solid areas (e589). A xanthogranulomatous reaction is prominent in some cases, especially in the presence of a ruptured cyst. Although CRPs are regarded as clinically benign, adherence to the hypothalamus and extension into the surrounding brain parenchyma are found in some cases. Cytokeratin expression has been used to distinguish CRP from Rathke cleft cyst (e1290). An uncommon variant of CRP is one with adamantinomatous features together with elements of a PA in a so-called collision tumor (e1296). In many of these "collision tumors," the adenoma is nonfunctional; however, immunohistochemistry displays gonadotropin, prolactin, ACTH, and TSH staining (e423,e586,e844,e1296).

Other tumefactive lesions of the pituitary and sellar region include the ganglion cell tumor (the so-called gangliocytoma), LCH, granular cell tumor, RDD, and salivary gland hamartoma. Gangliocytomas are regarded as neoplasm by most observers, but hamartoma, by others; they may be found in association with PAs, pituitary hyperplasia, or as a distinct mass (e404,e1204). Towfighi et al. have classified these lesions as either a mixed adenoma-gangliocytoma or pure gangliocytoma (e1204).

LCH is well documented in the CNS with involvement of the brain parenchyma or the hypothalamic-pituitary axis, in which case there is central diabetes insipidus. The pituitary stalk is thickened on imaging studies (e155,e701,e714,e746) (eFigures 21-24 to 21-26). Almost 15% of those with multisystem LCH have hypothalamic-pituitary involvement (e522). There is limited documentation of the pathology in such cases because the diagnosis is usually established on the basis of a biopsy from a more accessible site. A mixture

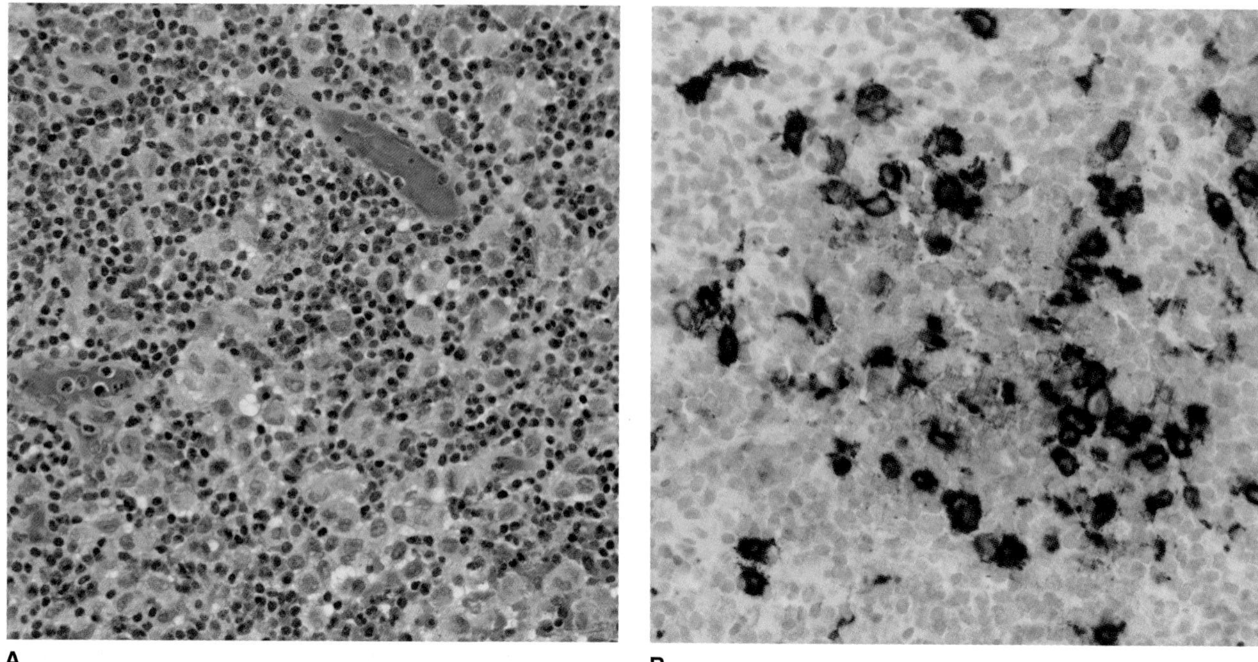

FIGURE 21-5■Langerhans cell histiocytosis. **A:** Biopsy from the pituitary stalk in an adolescent with diabetes insipidus. The infiltrate is composed of foamy histiocytes that were immunoreactive with CD1a, in a background of lymphocytes, eosinophils, and plasma cells (H&E stain, original magnification, 400×). (Courtesy of Dr. Joe Parisi, Mayo Clinic, Rochester, Minnesota.) **B:** CD1a positivity in histiocytic cells in a patient with LCH (immunostain for CD1a, original magnification 400×). (Courtesy of Dr. Joe Parisi, Mayo Clinic, Rochester, Minnesota.)

of Langerhans cells, characterized by large, convoluted and indented nuclei, that are CD1a positive, mixed with an infiltrate of lymphocytes, plasma cells and eosinophils is the characteristic appearance of LCH (Figure 21-5A, B, eFigure 21-41A to C).

RDD has craniospinal manifestations in a minority of cases, including the sellar-suprasellar region (e1284). In 50% of such cases, the RDD is limited to this site with obvious problems in diagnosis. **Salivary gland rest or heterotopia** is an incidental microscopic finding on the surface of the posterior pituitary (e464). Other neoplasms of presumed salivary gland type, granular cell tumor of the pituitary and pituitary stalk (e438,e1046), leukemia, lymphoma, and metastatic involvement of the pituitary are restricted to adults in most cases (e444,e470,e1056,e1296). Both primary and metastatic germ cell neoplasms also occur in the pituitary.

PARATHYROID GLANDS

Anatomy/Physiology

The parathyroid glands, usually four in number, are pinkish, oval 4- to 6-mm in diameter glands located in proximity to the thyroid gland or even embedded within the thyroid. The inferior and superior parathyroid glands arise as endodermal outpouchings from the dorsal bulbar portion of the third and fourth pharyngeal pouches, respectively, during the fifth gestational week (e6). Concurrently, the thymus arises from the ventral aspect of the third pharyngeal pouches. Both the thymus and inferior parathyroid glands initially migrate together caudally with the heart. During the descent, the thymus and inferior parathyroid glands separate and the inferior parathyroid glands localize to the inferior aspect of the thyroid gland (e1065).

In children, the combined parathyroid gland weight for all four glands increases with age from a mean weight of 5 to 10 mg each in the neonatal period to an adult combined weight of 120 mg for adult males and 140 mg for adult females by age 30 (e34,e938,e1065). In children younger than 10 years old, the mean weight of all four glands is less than 60 mg (e416). In individuals between the ages of 11 and 20 years, the mean weight of all four glands has been recorded as less than 100 mg, but more recently a study of parathyroid gland weight in children between the ages of 9 and 19 years indicated individual gland weights can range between 10 and 80 mg (e410).

The parathyroid glands in children tend to be solid and cellular with minimal fat. A connective tissue capsule encloses the gland. Chief cells arranged in sheets are the predominant cell type. Blood vessels are intermixed among the parenchymal cells, and small delicate capillaries are present between the cells. The polyhedral chief cells have a small central nucleus and clear cytoplasm. Oxyphil cells are not observed generally until puberty, if at all. Adipocytes within the gland initially appear around puberty with fatty infiltration gradually accounting for 25% to 30% of total gland weight after age 18 (41,e18,e416).

Calcium homeostasis is regulated by the interaction of parathormone (PTH), calcitonin, and vitamin D (eFigure 21-42) (24,46,e1003). In response to hypocalcemia, PTH is released from the chief cells, which is accompanied by an increase in PTH mRNA within hours of the onset of hypocalcemia. Hyperplasia of chief cells occurs within weeks. In contrast, hypercalcemia inhibits the release of PTH by activation of the chief cell calcium receptor. Serum phosphate levels, independent of vitamin D_3, also affect PTH release (24,46,e1003). The anatomy and physiology of the parathyroid glands is discussed in more detail by Lloyd et al. (102).

Imaging

The parathyroid glands are small and difficult to appreciate on imaging studies when not enlarged. Patients with hyperparathyroidism (HPT) are best evaluated with ultrasonography (US) and/or radionuclide scintigraphy. In children, high resolution US should be the first line imaging modality (e339). Enlarged parathyroid glands in the neck are typically identified posterior to the thyroid gland. As parathyroid glands are best identified based on proximity to the thyroid gland, ectopic glands pose a diagnostic challenge. Radionuclide scintigraphy is more accurate than US (87% versus 80%), particularly for ectopic glands (e574). The combination of nuclear scintigraphic studies and US provides the highest accuracy for preoperative localization of hyperfunctioning glands.

Nuclear medicine studies utilize ^{99m}Tc sestamibi, which localizes to hyperfunctioning parathyroid glands as well as the thyroid gland and salivary glands. Sestamibi scans can be performed in several ways. In dual isotope, single phase imaging, the patient is administered labeled sestamibi and ^{123}I or ^{99m}Tc pertechnetate, which are taken up by the thyroid gland. The images are subtracted to show the activity only in the hyperfunctioning parathyroid glands (eFigure 21-43). Alternatively, a single isotope, dual phase technique may be employed. Sestamibi washes out of the thyroid and salivary glands faster than the parathyroid glands, so delayed images show relatively greater uptake in the hyperfunctioning parathyroid gland (e339). SPECT imaging in addition to planar imaging helps to localize the abnormality in the anterior-posterior plane. Further, the fusion of SPECT imaging to x-ray based CT adds additional anatomic information that aids in precise localization of the parathyroid gland, which may be particularly useful in recurrences after surgery (e20).

Parathyroid adenomas may also be demonstrated on CT and MR, but the accuracy of these studies for preoperative localization is no greater than for US. On CT, adenomas are usually well-defined and they enhance intensely following intravenous contrast administration (eFigure 21-44). On MR, adenomas are generally of intermediate signal on T1-weighted images and high signal intensity on T2-weighted images and enhance intensely following intravenous administration of gadolinium chelate (Figure 21-6A) (e574). Prior to the advent of laboratory screening, patients with undiagnosed, prolonged HPT developed characteristic findings on bone radiographs as well as nephrocalcinosis and nephrolithiasis, but these findings are now rarely encountered (eFigures 21-45 and 21-46).

Developmental Disorders

Supernumerary parathyroid glands are found in up to 16% of the population, with an additional single gland the most common presentation (e17,e414,e415,e954). Supernumerary glands, with as many as 12 glands, may be of normal size or rudimentary. Parathyroid adenomas and carcinoma have been reported in ectopic parathyroid glands in children (eFigure 21-44) (2,e989,e1059).

Ectopic parathyroid tissue or a normally formed gland is relatively common within the thyroid or thymus (e100,e468,e956). Ectopic parathyroid tissue has also been observed as scattered small nests in the soft tissues of the neck and mediastinum owing to aberrant migration or premature separation of parathyroid primordial during fetal development (e1247). Not surprisingly, nests of parathyroid tissue may be accompanied by equally diminutive nests of thymic tissue. Aberrant parathyroid and thymus are known to present as a recurrent lateral neck mass in children (e275). Heterotopic parathyroid tissue has also been observed at remote sites, including the vagina (e663).

Agenesis-hypoplasia of the parathyroids, due to a defect in pharyngeal pouch development or defective neural crest migration, is uncommon as an isolated finding with associated congenital hypoparathyroidism (e596). Agenesis-aplasia is more frequently associated with other syndromes, having been reported in the 22q11.2 deletion syndrome (DiGeorge anomaly, DiGeorge syndrome), Smith-Lemli-Opitz syndrome type II, X-linked recessive hypoparathyroidism, Kenny syndrome, Kearns-Sayre syndrome, and trisomy 18 (e266,e349,e439,e1201,e1275). The parathyroid glands may be absent in as many as 50% of patients with 22q11.2 deletion syndrome (e995). Anomalies of the aortic arch, thymus, thyroid, and C-cells in addition to abnormal facial development are also observed (e505,e506,e507,e524,e1017,e1180). Parathyroid hemorrhage is reported in osteogenesis imperfecta and refractory hypocalcemia (e628) (see Chapter 3).

Cyst(s) of the parathyroid are rare in children and usually asymptomatic; these cysts may represent cystic degeneration of an adenoma, or due to a presumed aberration in development (e186,e336,e1246,e779). Other cysts in the neck may contain both parathyroid and thymic tissue as developmental cysts of the third pharyngeal pouch (e198).

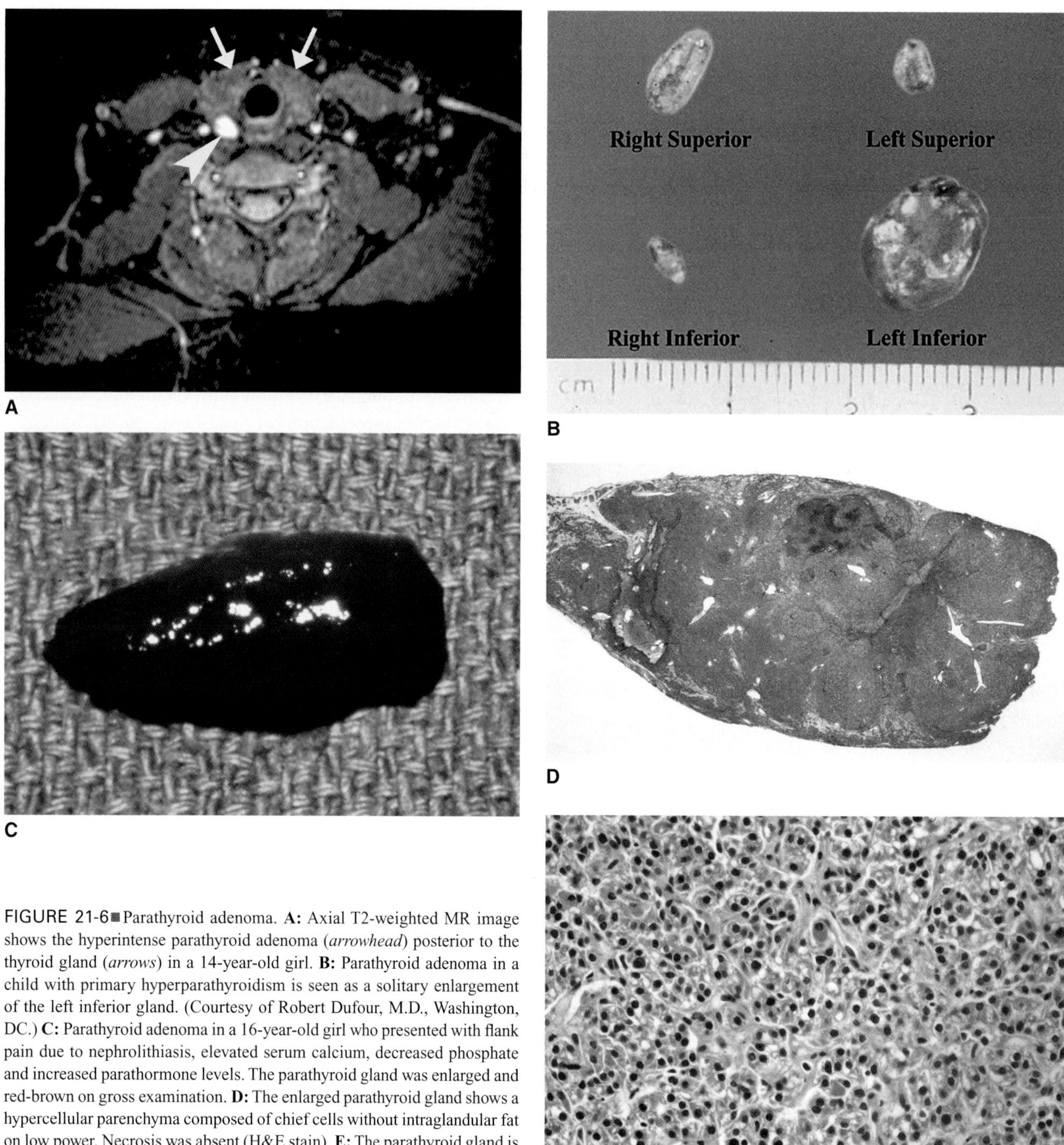

FIGURE 21-6■Parathyroid adenoma. **A:** Axial T2-weighted MR image shows the hyperintense parathyroid adenoma (*arrowhead*) posterior to the thyroid gland (*arrows*) in a 14-year-old girl. **B:** Parathyroid adenoma in a child with primary hyperparathyroidism is seen as a solitary enlargement of the left inferior gland. (Courtesy of Robert Dufour, M.D., Washington, DC.) **C:** Parathyroid adenoma in a 16-year-old girl who presented with flank pain due to nephrolithiasis, elevated serum calcium, decreased phosphate and increased parathormone levels. The parathyroid gland was enlarged and red-brown on gross examination. **D:** The enlarged parathyroid gland shows a hypercellular parenchyma composed of chief cells without intraglandular fat on low power. Necrosis was absent (H&E stain). **E:** The parathyroid gland is composed of a monotonous population of chief cells with no intraglandular fat. Mitotic figures were absent (H&E stain).

Acquired Disorders

Hypercalcemia in childhood may be a manifestation of increased PTH secretion by an adenoma or hyperplasia (primary HPT) or PTH-related peptide-induced hypercalcemia of malignancy, mutations involving the calcium-sensing receptor gene (*CASR*) [familial hypocalciuric hypercalcemia (FHH), neonatal HPT] or PTH receptor, conditions associated with vitamin D excess (sarcoidosis, tuberculosis, granulomatous disorders), medications, immobilization, and other endocrine disorders (46,47,145,e166,e682). Anorexia, fatigue, constipation, weight loss, weakness, and mental status changes are some of the clinical manifestations. Metastatic calcifications in various organs may result

Table 21-4 ■ PRIMARY HYPERPARATHYROIDISM ETIOLOGY IN CHILDHOOD

Parathyroid adenoma
Sporadic (nonsyndromic)
Hyperparathyroidism-jaw tumor syndrome
Parathyroid hyperplasia
Sporadic (nonsyndromic)
Neonatal hyperparathyroidism
Familial isolated hyperparathyroidism
MEN 1
MEN 2a
Parathyroid carcinoma

MEN, multiple endocrine neoplasia.
Based on data from DeLellis RA, Mazzaglia P, Mangray S. Primary hyperparathyroidism: a current perspective. *Arch Pathol Lab Med.* 2008;132:1251–1262.

in organ damage if the hypercalcemia is not recognized (145).

Primary HPT is uncommon in children with an incidence of two to five cases: 100,000 (Table 21-4) (83). Most children are older than 10 years at diagnosis and there is a male predilection in contrast to the female predilection in adults (Figure 21-6B) (69,83,e123,e136,e262,e417,e500,e692,e729, e756,e886,e970). A solitary adenoma is the etiology in 80% to 90% of cases. The serum calcium level is usually elevated to greater than 12 mg/dL (e1214).

In neonatal HPT and MEN syndromes, four gland hyperplasia is the common finding (eFigure 21-47). Other heredofamilial settings of HPT are HPT with or without fibro-osseous tumor of the jaws, MEN 1 and MEN, type 2a (MEN 2a) (e34, e202,e299,e471,e486,e523,e525,e647–e649) (Chapter 27).

Multiple endocrine neoplasia 1, an autosomal dominant disorder, is characterized by parathyroid gland hyperplasia, PA, pancreatic endocrine tumors, extrapancreatic neuroendocrine tumors, adrenocortical neoplasms, angiofibromas and lipomas (43). The *MEN 1* gene, a tumor suppressor gene, has been mapped to chromosome 11q13 where it encodes the protein, menin, that is involved in transcriptional regulation, genome stability, and cell division (95,e345,e498,e608, e637,e766,e767,e912,e1078,e1079). In addition to parathyroid gland hyperplasia, medullary thyroid carcinoma (MTC) and pheochromocytoma (PHEO) are the other associated tumors of MEN 2a, an autosomal dominant disorder with mutations in the *RET* gene (10q11.2) that encodes for a tyrosine kinase receptor. HPT-jaw tumor (HPT-JT) syndrome, an autosomal dominant disorder, is associated with inactivating mutations in the tumor suppressor gene *HRPT2* (1q25–32) that encodes for the protein, parafibromin (e85,e547,e1170,e1253). Solitary or multiple enlarged parathyroid glands are accompanied by fibro-osseous lesions of the mandible or maxilla (95). Parathyroid carcinoma is reportedly more common in this syndrome. Renal cysts, hamartomas, renal cell carcinoma, and Wilms tumor are other accompanying lesions and tumors (e243,e413,e1181). Isolated familial HPT, distinct from HPT-JT syndrome, is a rare disorder without other associated endocrinopathies with germline mutations involving the *CASR*, *MEN 1*, and *HRPT2* genes. All four glands show chief cell hyperplasia (e599,e913).

Osteopenia, subperiosteal phalangeal bone resorption, bone cyst formation, and genu valgum are some of the skeletal anomalies in long-standing unrecognized HPT (e58,e102,e802) (eFigures 21-46 and 21-48). Hypercalciuria and nephrolithiasis are frequent manifestations of primary HPT in childhood (69,e698). Pulmonary calcinosis has also been observed (e1200). Measurement of intact serum PTH distinguishes primary HPT from other causes of hypercalcemia in most cases; however, cases of HPT with apparent normal PTH levels have been reported (e92). Preoperative US and radionuclide scan may be helpful in the localization of an enlarged gland but is more limited in a case of a small adenoma or multigland hyperplasia (e939,e954). Intraoperative PTH testing has an important role in the differentiation of a solitary adenoma from multiglandular hyperplasia in primary HPT (83,e580,e939,e954).

Neonatal primary HPT is an uncommon disorder associated with FHH (e73,e390). Hypotonia, failure to thrive, and respiratory distress are the clinical manifestations (e185,e500). Severe hypercalcemia and elevated PTH levels are present (e393). Osteopenia, subperiosteal bone resorption, and multiple pathological fractures of long bones are some of the overlapping skeletal findings with osteogenesis imperfecta. FHH, an autosomal dominant condition, has an estimated prevalence of 1:15,000 to 30,000 individuals. It is usually asymptomatic with hypercalcemia, normal PTH levels, and decreased urine calcium excretion (69). Mutations in the *CASR* gene, which encodes for the calcium sensing receptor in the parathyroid gland and renal tubular epithelium, are found in FHH and neonatal primary HPT (e282,e393,e485,e944,e1249,e1250).

Secondary HPT is a multiglandular hyperplasia of the parathyroid to hypocalcemia (102,e1007,e1027). Chronic renal failure is the major cause, with malabsorption, vitamin D deficiency, and X-linked hypophosphatemic rickets as other less common causes (e629,e705,e773,e1030,e1138). Secondary HPT is also a feature of mucolipidoses type II and maternal hypoparathyroidism (e32,e1042). Multiglandular hyperplasia is additionally seen in tertiary HPT, an uncommon entity in children, which is characterized by hypercalcemia after renal function is restored after renal transplantation in children who had secondary HPT (e765,e828).

Parathyroid adenomas account for 80% of parathyroid tumors in primary HPT in children which is somewhat lower than the adult experience once familial HPT and other inherited endocrinopathies are included. Several different genetic alterations involving parathyroid hormone, *RET*, *MEN I*, *PRAD 1*, *p53*, *HRPT2*, and G protein genes have been identified as different pathogenetic mechanisms (24,41,43). Clonal analysis of sporadic parathyroid adenomas reveals a monoclonal cell population in contrast to the polyclonal population seen in diffuse hyperplasia, except for some cases of hyperplasia in secondary HPT due to chronic renal failure (24,e1079,e1193). It is usually not possible to distinguish the single gland adenoma from hyperplasia morphologically without the benefit of a second parathyroid gland to examine by frozen section. This differentiation can be accomplished with an intraoperative determination of PTH level which normalizes within a few minutes in the case of a single gland adenoma whereas it will initially fall and return to elevated levels in the presence of hyperplasia (83,e512,e938,e983,e1159). An enlarged gland may be hidden in the thymus, thyroid, or around the esophagus (e239,e417).

Parathyroid adenomas and hyperplasia have similar gross features with a reddish-brown appearance, weight in excess of 60 mg and dimension of 1 to 2 cm in greatest diameter (Figure 21-6B, C). Any parathyroid gland weighing more than 40 mg in a child should be considered abnormal (41). In one study, the mean weight of an adenoma in a child was 597 mg with a range between 170 and 1550 mg (69). A nodular or diffuse pattern of chief cells with minimal interstitial fat interspersed is the usual microscopic finding (e970) (Figure 21-6D, E, eFigure 21-49). Cellular pleomorphism, necrosis, and increased mitotic activity are usually not present, but some mitotic activity should not be viewed with any undue concern. A well-formed capsule is usually not present, but the adenomatous portion of the gland is distinguishable from remnants of compressed and suppressed parathyroid gland at the periphery if present. The chief cells often contain glycogen which is demonstrable by a periodic acid-Schiff stain with diastase digestion and for PTH and CHR by immunohistochemistry. Normal glands demonstrate greater immunoreactivity to PTH compared to hyperplastic glands and adenomas (35). Adenomas involving two glands are uncommon and have been reported in children with an increased frequency in the HPT-JT syndrome (43,69,e262,e1160,e1211).

Parathyroid carcinoma is a rare cause of primary HPT in adults and even more so in children (e460,e784,e795). Screening for germline *HRPT2* mutations should be undertaken in any child with either a personal or family history of parathyroid carcinoma (e599). Unlike the smaller adenoma, the carcinoma is a neoplasm that infiltrates into the soft tissues of the neck and has vascular and capsular invasion (e1289,e795).

Hypocalcemia in children is multifactorial. It is due to decreased PTH production (hypoparathyroidism), PTH receptor defects, pseudohypoparathyroidism as in Albright hereditary osteodystrophy, mitochondrial DNA mutations as in the Kearns-Sayre syndrome, dietary imbalances in vitamin D, calcium and magnesium, or increased inorganic phosphate consumption (47,102,e35,e1276). Hypocalcemia is also observed with pancreatitis, sepsis, increased serum phosphate levels, renal failure, and antineoplastic therapy. Impaired renal and bone response to PTH accounts for the hypocalcemia seen in premature infants (e655).

Hypoparathyroidism is due to a developmental anomaly of the parathyroid glands as in 22q11.2 microdeletion syndrome and 10p13 deletion as well as autoimmune disorders, infiltrative disorders, prior thyroidectomy, or parathyroidectomy (102,e25,e153,e1210). Clinically, children are either asymptomatic or present with paresthesias, tetany, muscle cramps, or seizures. Polyglandular autoimmune syndrome, type I, is an autosomal recessive multisystem autoimmune disorder due to a mutation in the autoimmune regulatory gene (*AIRE*) on chromosome 21q22.3. It presents during infancy, childhood, or adolescence with hypoparathyroidism in 80% to 85% of patients, hypoadrenalism (Addison disease), and chronic mucocutaneous candidiasis (80,e15). Parathyroid autotransplantation is effective in preventing the hypoparathyroidism associated with total thyroidectomy (e1102).

THYROID GLAND

The thyroid gland, a bilobed structure connected by an isthmus of thyroid tissue at the level of the trachea, is located in the mid-anterior neckline and is adherent to the larynx and trachea (103,e383). The weight of the thyroid varies with sex and age through the fetal, infantile, and childhood periods of life. There are also differences in thyroid weight on the basis of geography in the United States and elsewhere. As an approximation, the thyroid gland at birth weighs 1 to 2 g; by 2 years of age, it approaches 3 g; at 4 years of age, 4 to 5 g; and by 15 years of age or so, 15 to 20 g, which is near the adult weight of the gland.

As some measure of its importance, the thyroid gland is the first endocrine organ to develop as a proliferation of endodermal cells on the floor of the pharynx at approximately 3 weeks' gestation. Two small lateral and a larger median anlagen from the foramen cecum at the base are formed. Through a process of elongated cephalad embryonic growth rather than active descent, the thyroid diverticulum resides between the first pharyngeal pouches. A thyroglossal duct as an attenuated canal is maintained until 6 to 7 weeks' gestation, at which time it normally disappears as an intact structure, but its remnants are retained to become one of the most common anomalies of the neck, the thyroglossal duct cyst (TDC). The endodermal cells differentiate into follicular cells in the eighth gestational week. Diminutive follicles without colloid are identifiable by 8 to 9 weeks' gestation. Well-defined follicles containing colloid are observed by the end of the first trimester.

With the incorporation of the ultimobranchial body into the thyroid, the follicles acquire C-cells and solid cell nests in the interstitium (e189,e443,e763). A remnant of the thyroglossal duct is the pyramidal lobe, a narrow ribbon of thyroid tissue, which is attached to the isthmus and is present in 40% to 65% of individuals (e128,e1004). More detailed discussions of the embryology of the thyroid gland are found elsewhere (136,179,e292,e1199). In addition to *POU1F1*, several distinct genes, *TITF1*, *TTIF2*, *PAX8*, *TSH*, and *TSHR* are involved in its development and migration (17,94,136,179,184).

Thyroid follicles are the basic morphologic and functional unit of the thyroid gland, and comprise the majority of the thyroid parenchyma. The follicular cells are responsible for the synthesis of thyroid hormone. Both the growth and synthetic function of the thyroid gland are under the control of thyroid-stimulating hormone (TSH) synthesized by the thyrotrophs of the anterior pituitary gland; this hormone mediates its action by cyclic AMP following attachment to receptor sites on the follicular cell membrane. Through a classic feedback mechanism, peripheral levels of thyroxine (T4) have a positive or negative effect on hypothalamic thyrotropin-releasing hormone with the release or not of TSH from the pituitary thyrotrophs (103,e1163) (eFigure 21-50). Excess TSH as a response to low T4 in congenital hypothyroidism is the mechanism by which hyperplasia of the thyroid gland is mediated.

Stimulation or activation of the follicular cells by TSH results in the production of thyroid hormone from thyroglobulin. Several enzymes, localized to the follicular cell, are required for thyroid hormone synthesis and loss of one of these enzymes on the basis of an autosomal recessive defect leads to dyshormonogenic goiter (Figure 21-7). The physiology and biochemistry of the thyroid gland in the context of the various inherited disorders with clinical manifestations of congenital hypothyroidism or hereditary hyperthyroidism have been reviewed by others (17,103,136,e292,e1223).

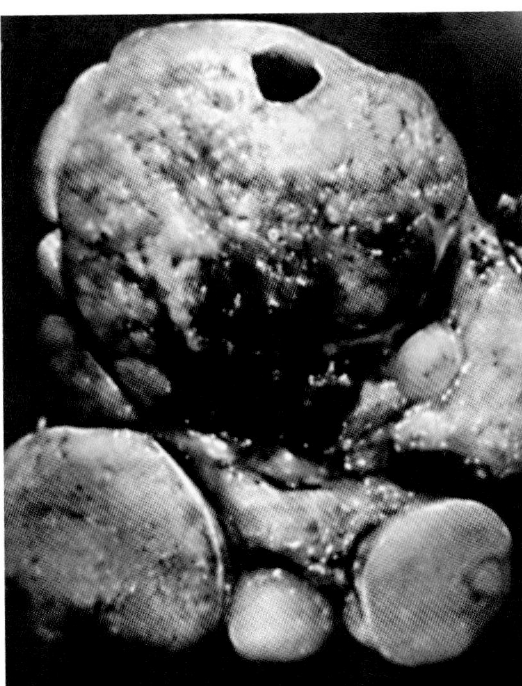

FIGURE 21-7 ■ Dyshormonogenic goiter. This image is a section through the thyroid gland of an individual who presented with a dyshormonogenic goiter. The thyroid parenchyma has a nodular pattern with retrogressive and hyperplastic changes including hemorrhage and fibrosis. (From Lloyd RV, Douglas BR, Young WF. Endocrine diseases. *Atlas of nontumor pathology*. Washington, DC: American Registry of Pathology. Originally published in *Atlas of tumor pathology, tumors of the thyroid gland*, Fascicle 5, Third Series. Washington, DC: Armed Forces Institute of Pathology).

The C-cell (parafollicular cell) is the other hormonally active cell of the thyroid, representing less than 0.5% of the total epithelial population. These neuroendocrine cells are identifiable immunohistochemically by their reactivity for CHR, SYN, and calcitonin (103). Like the dominant follicular cell, the C-cell is enclosed within the basement membrane of the follicle, but at the periphery of the follicle without any contact with the colloid. Unlike the endodermally-derived follicular cell, the C-cell progenitor migrates from the vagal or cephalic region of the neural crest to the fourth and fifth pharyngeal pouches, one of whose derivatives is the ultimobranchial body (103,e1278). The greatest number of C-cells is found in the upper two-thirds of the lateral lobes of the thyroid, along the central axis (103). The neonatal gland contains a tenfold number of C-cells as compared to the adult thyroid as the number of C-cells diminishes with age (e1283). A paucity of C-cells in the thyroid is reported in DiGeorge anomaly (syndrome) on the presumed basis of a developmental field defect in the formation of pharyngeal pouch derivatives (e179). Hyperplasia of C-cells in children is divided into physiologic hyperplasia, seen in neonates, after a hemithyroidectomy, in the presence of autoimmune (Hashimoto) thyroiditis and in association with MEN 2a or 2b and neoplastic hyperplasia (103). Hyperplasia is defined as the presence of 50 or more C-cells in one 10× magnification field. Medullary thyroid carcinoma (MTC) MTC in MEN 2a, MEN, type 2b (MEN 2b) and familial (non-MEN) MTC (FMTC) are the consequences of *RET* gene germline mutations and are characterized by the presence of multifocal C-cell hyperplasia and often with multifocal MTCs (59,81,103,e1267).

Solid cell nests, a remnant of the ultimobranchial body, are the third cell type identified in the thyroid gland. They are localized to the upper and middle third of the thyroid gland and have a parafollicular or intrafollicular location. These solid, squamoid appearing cells are immunoreactive with low molecular weight keratin and carcinoembryonic antigen. Cells with follicular or C-cell differentiation are present within these nests and may account for the rare mixed follicular-medullary carcinoma.

More detailed comprehensive reviews of the functional and morphologic aspects of the thyroid gland have been detailed by others (39,93,96,103184,e36,e39,e850).

Imaging

Imaging studies are an integral component of the diagnostic evaluation of a child with an enlarged thyroid or other mass-producing process in the neck. US is a basic modality and provides for a confident diagnosis of a TDC, which appears as midline or paramedian cyst with or without debris when complicated by infection or hemorrhage (e574) (Figure 21-8A, B). TDCs are commonly near the hyoid bone. Branchial cleft cysts have a similar imaging appearance, but are positioned away from the midline (eFigure 21-51).

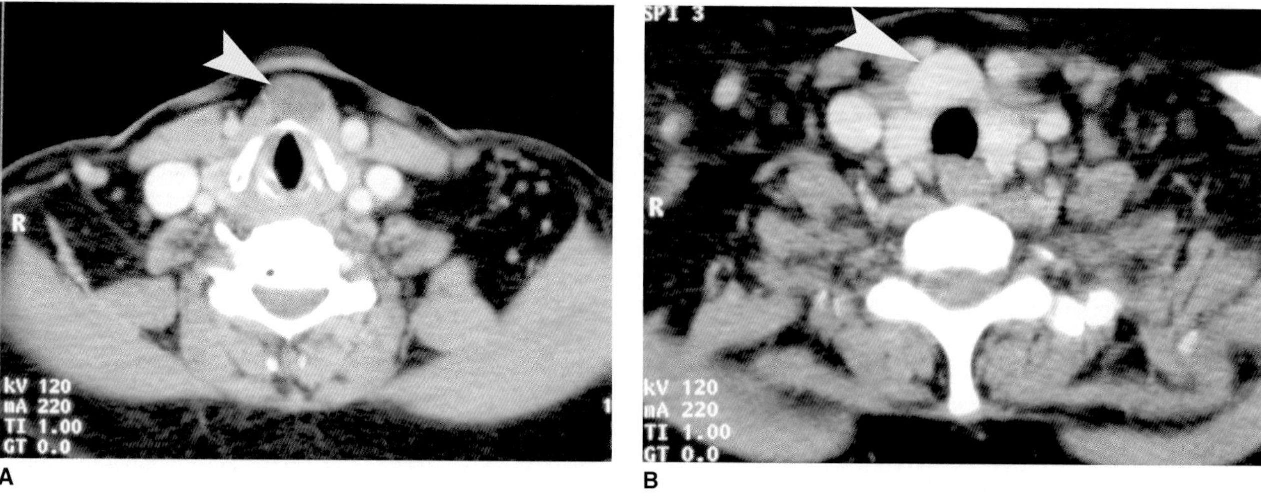

FIGURE 21-8 ■ Thyroglossal duct cyst in an adult complicated by papillary thyroid carcinoma. **A:** Axial contrast-enhanced CT image shows a midline cyst (*arrowhead*). **B:** Axial CT image caudal to (a) shows markedly-enhancing, midline mass (*arrowhead*).

Ultrasound is also useful in depicting thyroid nodules in patients with thyroid dysfunction or goiter. Complex cases may require MR (e574). CT is less desirable for the evaluation of thyroid lesions because the use of iodinated contrast will preclude later radioactive thyroid ablation therapy if necessary for several weeks (e574). Thyroid carcinomas appear well-defined and heterogeneous on US, CT, or MR. Papillary thyroid carcinoma (PTC) is more likely to contain cystic-appearing, necrotic areas compared to follicular thyroid carcinoma (FTC) (e574) (Figure 21-9A). Most MTCs are solid and may contain coarse calcifications (Figure 21-9B).

Radionuclide scintigraphy with ^{99m}Tc pertechnetate or ^{123}I is very useful in the evaluation of thyroid dysfunction and nodules or in localization of ectopic thyroid tissue (eFigure 21-52A to C). Nodules with decreased radiotracer uptake ("cold" nodules) are more likely to be malignant than nodules that are inapparent or take up more of a radiopharmaceutical agent than normal thyroid ("hot" or hyperfunctioning nodule). When ectopic thyroid tissue is identified, it is important to evaluate the neck base for an orthotopic thyroid gland (Figure 21-10A, B, eFigure 21-52A to C).

Developmental Disorders

Dysmorphism of the thyroid gland is a structural phenomenon with several morphologic expressions from absence or incomplete formation of a normal gland, failure in the normal anatomic localization of the gland, or persistence of embryologic remnants with a branching lobular pattern of immature follicles rather than the dense formation of individual follicles.

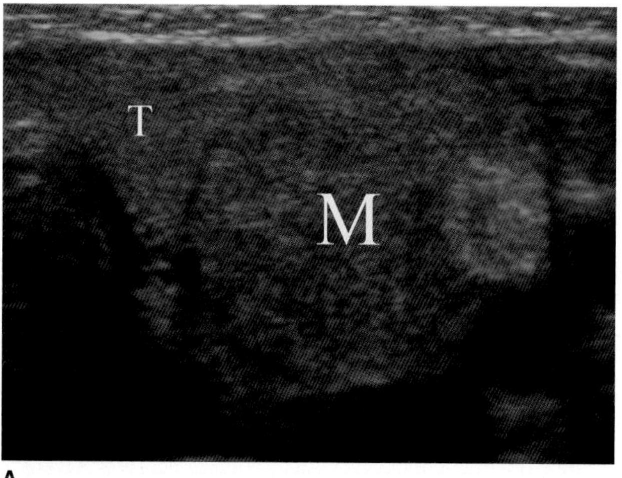

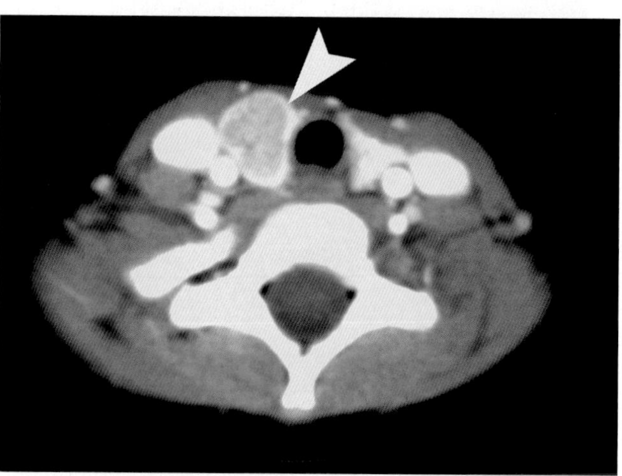

FIGURE 21-9 ■ Papillary thyroid carcinoma in 15-year-old girl. **A:** Transverse sonographic image showing a heterogeneous mass (M) within the homogeneous thyroid gland (T). **B:** Medullary thyroid carcinoma in an 8-year-old girl with family history of MEN 2a. Axial contrast-enhanced CT shows a mass within the left thyroid lobe which enhances less than the surrounding thyroid gland (*arrowhead*).

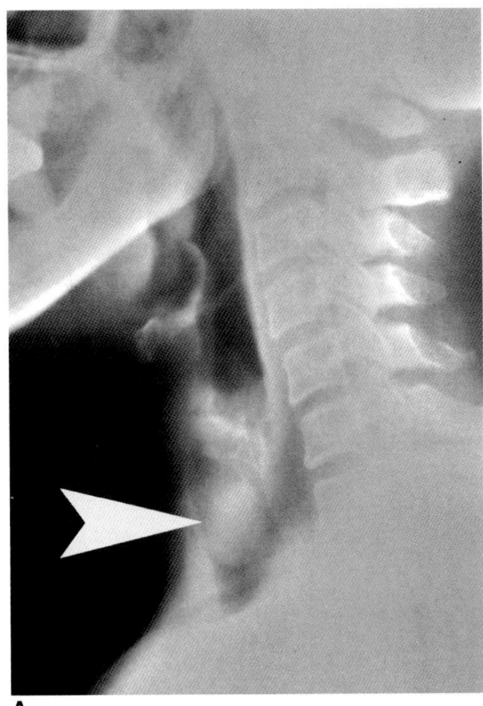

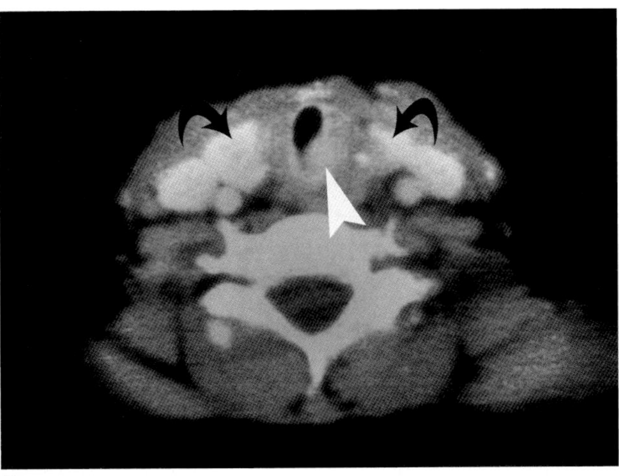

FIGURE 21-10 ■ Ectopic thyroid gland in the trachea of an adult. **A:** Lateral tomogram shows an ovoid mass within the tracheal air column (*arrowhead*). **B:** Axial CT image shows markedly enhancing eccentric mass in the trachea (*arrowhead*) and normal thyroid lobes in the orthotopic location (*curved arrows*).

The recessively inherited defects in the enzymes responsible for thyroid hormone synthesis are another developmental disorder but are not characterized by a primary structural anomaly of the thyroid gland (eFigure 21-53); however, the elevated TSH levels lead to multinodular hyperplasia with the formation of the so-called dyshormonogenic goiter (Figure 21-7) (e36,e39,e119). Clinically, these various developmental disorders present with congenital hypothyroidism, a mass at the base of the tongue or in the neck, or congenital hypothyroidism with development of a goiter (e403). Many of these developmental anomalies also affect first-degree relatives indicating a familial component (e12,e203,e204,e702).

Dysgenesis of the thyroid is a generic designation for various anatomic developmental anomalies that include complete failure in gland formation (agenesis), decreased amount of thyroid tissue (hypoplasia), absence of a lobe (hemiagenesis), or ectopic location. Dysgenesis is an important etiology of congenital hypothyroidism whose incidence in the United States is 1:3,000 to 5,000 live births (e446,e117,e449,e534, e626,e652,e679,e1202,e1243). Most causes of congenital hypothyroidism are due to dysgenesis or one of the inherited defects in thyroid hormone synthesis (e104,e122,e192,e193, e338,e343,e388,e445,e545,e801,e837,e940,e941,e992,e993, e1128,e1212,e1219,e1243) (Table 21-5). Congenital hypothyroidism has been also been observed in Williams and Down syndromes (e122,e445,e1128).

Congenital hypothyroidism in 80% to 85% of cases is associated with one of several types of dysgenesis. The prevalence of hypothyroidism in the neonatal period is 1:4,000 live births for thyroid dysgenesis in contrast to dyshormonogenesis in 1:30,000 live births, transient hypothyroidism 1:40,000 live births and central hypothyroidism, hypothalamic/pituitary

Table 21-5 ■ ETIOLOGIC CLASSIFICATION OF CONGENITAL HYPOTHYROIDISM

- I. Primary Hypothyroidism
  - A. Dysgenesis (85%) (1:4,000)
    - Idiopathic or genetic (*TITF-1, TITF-2, FOXE1, PAX-8,* and *TSHR* defects)
      - Agenesis
      - Hemiagenesis
      - Hypoplasia
      - Ectopia
        - Lingual thyroid (90% of thyroid ectopia) (1:10,000)
  - B. Dyshormonogenesis (10–15%) (1:30,000)
    - Iodide transport (sodium-iodide symporter defect (*NIS* gene)
    - Iodide organification and coupling defect
      - Thyroid peroxidase defect (*TPO* gene) (Pendred defect)
      - Thyroid oxidase 2 defect (*DUOX1/THOX1 DUOX/THOX2* genes)
    - Defect in thyroglobulin synthesis or transport (*Tg* gene)
    - Iodotyrosine deiodinase defect (*DEHAL1* gene)
  - C. Other (5%)
- II. Secondary/Tertiary Hypothyroidism (Hypothalamic-Pituitary-Thyroid Axis Dysfunction) (1:100,000)
  - Genetic defects involving *LHX3, LHX4, PROP 1, POUF1, HESX1, TRHR, TSHB*
- III. Peripheral Thyroid Hormone Resistance
  - Genetic defects involving *MCT8, THRB*
- IV. Transient Hypothyroidism (1:40,000)
  - Maternal antithyroid antibodies, goitrogenic drugs, iodine deficiency

Based on data from Peter, F, Muzsnai A. Congenital disorders of the thyroid: hypo/hyper. *Endocrinol Metab Clin North Am.* 2009;38:491–507; LaFranchi S. Section 2: Disorders of the thyroid gland. In: Kliegman RM, Behrman RE, Jenson HB, Stanton BF, eds., *Nelson textbook of pediatrics*, 18th ed. Philadelphia, PA: Elsevier, 2007; Bettendorf M. Thyroid disorders in children from birth to adolescence. *Eur J Nucl Med Mol Imaging.* 2002;29(Suppl 2):S439–S446.

defect in 1:100,000 live births (17,93). In one study of 230 children with congenital hypothyroidism, scintigraphy revealed the following findings: ectopia in 61%, goiter in 18%, agenesis in 16%, normal in 4% and hemiagenesis in less than 1% (e303). In another series of 800,000 neonates with increased TSH and normally positioned thyroid glands, an enlarged gland or goiter was observed in 55% of cases, a normal gland in 29% of cases, and hypoplasia in 16% of cases (e403). If the thyroid gland is anatomically orthotopic in the presence of congenital hypothyroidism, a defect exists in thyroid hormone biosynthesis with the development of a dyshormonogenic nodular goiter or an inability of the gland to respond to TSH (e287,e403,e1217,e1223). Dysgenesis is more common in females than in males (3:1) and is sporadic in most cases (85% of all cases) (136). Affected infants with agenesis/hypoplasia have permanently elevated levels of TSH and low levels of circulating thyroid hormone. A number of mutations have been identified in the genes responsible for thyroid development, including *PAX8*, *TITF-1* (thyroid transcription factor 1), *TITF-2* (thyroid transcription factor 2), and *TSHR* (TSH receptor) and are pathogenetically involved in thyroid dysgenesis (17,94,136,140,179,184,e107,e117,e205,e253,e305,e341,e495, e496,e566,e635,e651,e658,e739,e741,e740,e757,e794,e883, e1173,e1196,e1198,e1232). These genetic defects and their association with other diseases are reviewed elsewhere (136).

Hemiagenesis is another form of dysgenesis with failure in the formation of the left lobe in most cases. This anomaly occurs in less than 0.5% of the population and is more common in females (e1072). Thyroid function is within normal limits (e750,785).

Ectopia of the thyroid gland, which also has a female predominance, is more thoroughly documented on a morphologic basis than the other types of dysgenesis, as judged by the descriptions in the literature (eFigure 21-54). The lingual thyroid occurs at the base of the tongue in approximately 1:10,000 individuals and is detected in most cases during a diagnostic evaluation for congenital hypothyroidism or as an incidentally discovered mass (Figure 21-11A, eFigure 21-52) (e21,e89). The lingual thyroid accounts for approximately 90% of all thyroid ectopias (e742,e887). Most lingual thyroids are accompanied by an orthotopic thyroid (e532); however, a minority of lingual thyroids constitute the only site of thyroid tissue (e532). Some cases classified as agenesis have a lingual remnant. Ectopic thyroid tissue including dual ectopia (location at different sites) and the exclusion of its occurrence in a teratoma, has been documented in the submandibular region, trachea, heart, mediastinum, and various intra-abdominal sites (e22, e43, e273,e304,e461,e663,e742). The presence of thyroid follicles in lymph nodes as so-called lateral aberrant thyroid represents metastatic thyroid carcinoma in many cases (103). Thyroid neoplasia arising in ectopic thyroid, usually in a TDC, is recognized in children (e490,e1006,e1176).

Ectopic thyroid may be represented by individual microfollicles or small foci of multiple microfollicles or solid nests of follicular cells without apparent colloid formation. The follicles are interspersed between bundles of skeletal muscle in the tongue or within the tissues of the other ectopic sites (Figure 21-11B, eFigure 21-55). In some instances, the epithelial structures are not readily identifiable as thyroid

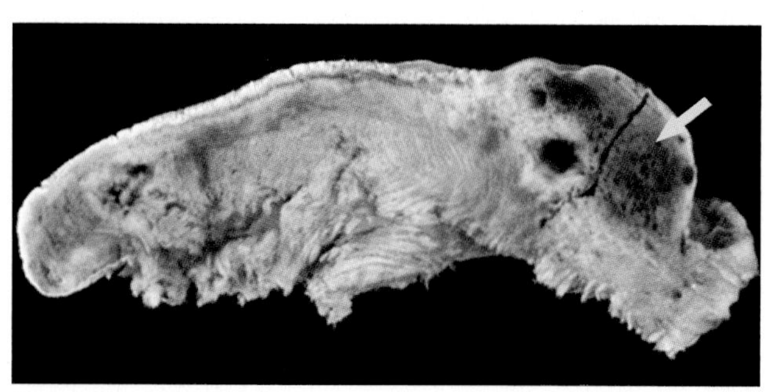

A

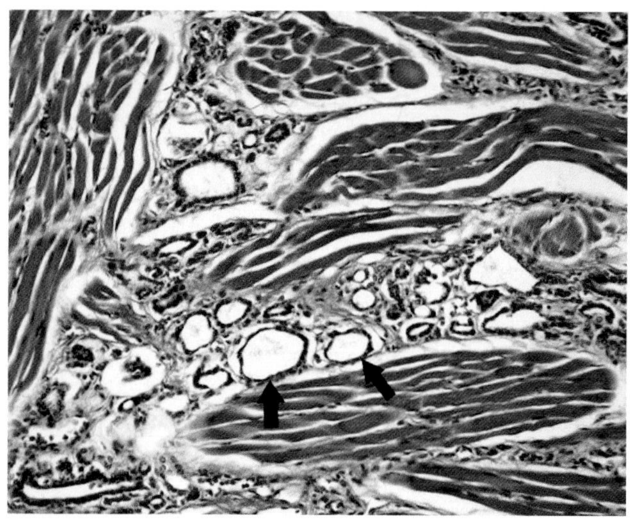

B

FIGURE 21-11 ■ Lingual thyroid. **A:** Sagittal section through the tongue, which shows a smooth, ovoid, 2 cm diameter mass in the posterior third of the tongue (*arrow*). Small and large cysts with adjacent red-brown thyroid tissue are present in the mass. Incidental finding at autopsy in a 69-year-old man who died from cerebral hemorrhage. (From Turk JL, Fletcher CDM, eds. *Endocrine system*. Royal College of Surgeons of England Slide Atlas of Pathology, 1985. Originally published by Gower Medical Publishing, Ltd. Reprinted with permission of Elsevier Inc. and C.D.M. Fletcher, M.D.). **B:** This section of tongue shows the presence of thyroid follicles between the muscle fibers (*arrows*). This was an incidental finding at autopsy in a stillborn infant (H&E stain, original magnification 100×).

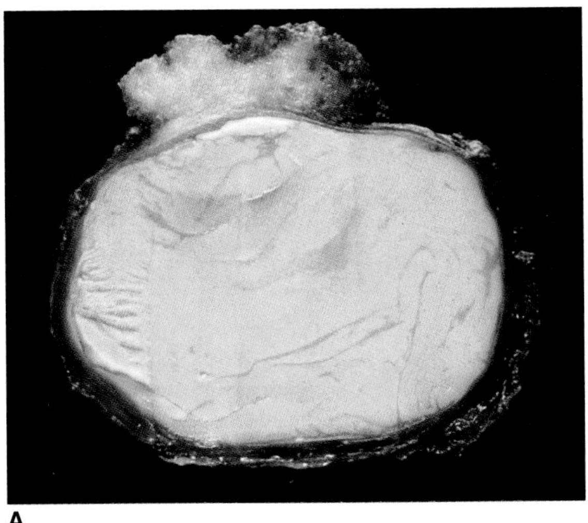
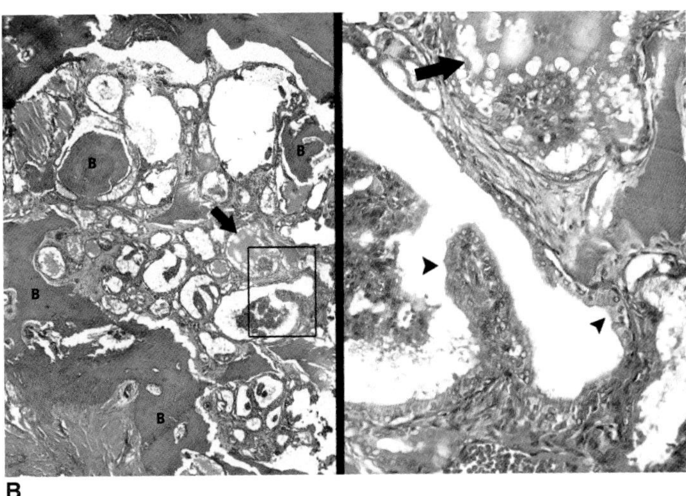

FIGURE 21-12■Thyroglosssal duct cyst. **A:** This midline cyst was filled with tan-white mucoid fluid on gross examination. Fibrosis of soft tissue adjacent to the cyst was present. **B:** This composite image shows the resected hyoid bone on the left with entrapped thyroid follicles (*arrow*). The area within the rectangle is magnified on the right side and shows a cuboidal epithelium (*arrowheads*) lining the cystic spaces. A thyroid follicle is also present in this image (*arrow*). Lymphoid aggregates not shown were also present (H&E stain).

tissue and may require immunohistochemical staining for thyroglobulin or thyroid transcription factor 1. In addition to the immature or nonfunctioning appearance of the ectopic follicles, the ectopia is also hypoplastic because the total tissue volume of thyroid is less than normal for the age and sex of the patient.

Another form of thyroid dysgenesis is an enlarged lobe composed of immature lobules of fetal-appearing follicles separated by an immature mesenchyme. Nodules of immature cartilage or other heterologous tissues present within the lobule may suggest the interpretation of a teratoma.

Thyroglossal duct cyst (TDC) is the consequence in the failure of the thyroglossal duct to undergo complete obliteration and regression during fetal life (54,e898). Approximately 15% of all neck masses in children are TDCs with the clinical presentation of a midline anterior neck mass overlying the hyoid bone (54,100,e167,e295,e716). Rather than a midline location, 10% to 25% of TDCs are found laterally, usually on the left side, and a minority occur at the base of the tongue, floor of the mouth, or within the thyroid itself. The TDC differential includes branchial cleft cyst, lymphoepithelial cyst, lymphadenopathy including lymphoma, epidermal inclusion cyst, and other thyroid malformations (100,e716,e387,e930,e1077, e1155,e1169). Most cysts are diagnosed at or before 5 years of age but are recognized throughout life (54,100,e24,e716). A familial association has been reported (e627). A rare presentation of TDC is sudden death due to asphyxiation (54,e337,e467,e578,e659). Infected cysts may lead to fistula formation to the skin surface or pharynx (54).

The pathologic findings of TDC vary from case to case with a dominant cyst or several smaller cysts in the soft tissues superior, inferior, or anterior to the hyoid bone (e318,e1185) (Figure 21-8A, eFigure 21-56). The dominant cyst usually measures 1 to 2 cm; however it may be in excess of 4 to 5 cm in diameter. The contents may have a mucoid or purulent appearance. TDCs are known to become infected. In some cases, it may be difficult to identify any cysts, but rather a firm, ill-defined fibrotic area that represents prior episodes of chronic inflammation is present in the soft tissues (Figure 21-12A). Thyroid tissue is generally not appreciated in the gross examination and can be difficult to identify even microscopically. Individual follicles or larger islands of well-formed follicles are found in less than 50% of cases. Cuboidal to stratified columnar epithelium with cilia lines the cysts in 50% or more of cases (Figure 21-12B). Nonkeratinizing squamous epithelium is present in 25% of cases. The type of epithelium may vary from one cystic structure to another in any one specimen. The background stroma varies from a mucoid to a dense fibrotic appearance. Lymphoid aggregates adjacent to the cyst or cysts and the ciliated respiratory-type epithelium have a resemblance to a branchial cleft cyst; however, the branchial cleft cyst typically occurs in the lateral portion of the neck. Psammomatous calcification may be found in TDCs without accompanying PTC (e65). Fine-needle aspiration biopsy (FNAB) had a positive predictive value of almost 70% in cases of TDC (e1077). Follicular adenomas and PTCs are reported in 1% to 4% of TDCs (Figure 21-8B) (54,e30,e134,e490,e904,e921, e929,e1006,e1176).

Branchial apparatus–associated anomalies are represented principally by the branchial cleft cyst (eFigures 21-51 and 21-57) (e198,e713,e1019,e1089,e1241). A similar lesion, the lymphoepithelial cyst, is recognized in the thyroid (e46). The cyst is accompanied by chronic lymphocytic thyroiditis (CLT) in most cases. A bronchogenic cyst has also been reported in the thyroid. Another type of branchial anomaly is the cyst or sinus from the oropharynx and/or hypopharynx with extension into the thyroid with the complication of recurrent acute thyroiditis.

Heterotopias in the thyroid gland include parathyroid, salivary gland, and thymic tissue (e13,e748) (eFigures 21-58 and 21-59).

Acquired Disorders

Persistent diffuse or nodular enlargement of the thyroid gland, regardless of its underlying nature, is referred to clinically as a goiter without any specific pathologic implications. Through a variety of noninvasive and invasive techniques, including FNAB, an attempt is generally made to ascertain whether the pathological process is inflammatory, hyperplastic, or neoplastic in nature before a decision is made about the need for surgical intervention (e737,e1271,e1297,e1244). US is helpful in the characterization of a nodule or nodules as predominantly cystic, cystic and solid, or solid (e302,e1297).

Thyroid nodules are detected in 1% to 1.5% of children with the entire range of pathology from developmental to neoplastic processes [congenital hypothyroidism due to dyshormonogenesis or ectopia, hemiagenesis, TDC, simple goiter, cystic lesions, nodular hyperplasia, follicular adenoma, Graves disease, and chronic lymphocytic (Hashimoto) thyroiditis] (45,59,71,77,123,e556,e1279). Nodular hyperplasia (adenomatous hyperplasia) with a dominant nodule, followed by follicular adenoma, is the most common cause of a thyroid nodule(s) in children (185). Studies have suggested that approximately 20% to 25% of solitary thyroid nodules are malignant with the overwhelming majority representing PTCs (123,145). Management of the solitary thyroid nodule is reviewed elsewhere (45,123,185,190). Several studies have addressed the efficacy of ultrasound-guided FNAB of the thyroid in the pediatric age group with comparable results to those in adults with a diagnostic accuracy in excess of 85% in most cases (e27,e40,e519,e556). Others have reported a lower diagnostic accuracy rate (e1277).

One of the most common referrals to a pediatric endocrinologist is an enlarged thyroid gland (goiter) (e281). Most cases of a diffusely enlarged thyroid gland (nontoxic goiter) on physical examination in children are due to autoimmune-associated inflammatory conditions of the thyroid: CLT, juvenile lymphocytic thyroiditis, juvenile variant of Hashimoto thyroiditis, autoimmune thyroiditis, and diffuse toxic hyperplasia (Graves disease) (e281,e289,e301,e355,e560,e967).

Chronic lymphocytic thyroiditis (CLT), which accounts for 40% of goiters in adolescents, affects females more commonly than males with a male: female ratio of 1:2 to 1:4, compared to a 1:10 male:female ratio in adults (17,93,e281,e289). The mean age at diagnosis is 11 to 12 years (range: 1 to 19 years) (e289,e1010).

Rather than a smooth, enlarged gland, in most cases, nodularity may be present in 25% to 30% of cases. Most children (50% to 70%) are euthyroid, or asymptomatic with laboratory values in the hypothyroid range, whereas 20% to 40% are clinically hypothyroid. Thyrotoxicosis is present in less than 5% of cases (e355,e964). Thyroid peroxidase (TPO) antibodies are present in 80% to 90% of cases, and antithyroglobulin antibodies in 50% to 60% of cases (e309). Several mechanisms including T-cell mediated cytotoxicity, cytokine-mediated, and antibody–dependent cell-mediated cytotoxicity directed against follicular epithelial cells are implicated in the pathogenesis of CLT (eFigure 21-60) (e309,e559,e656,e745,e786).

Most cases of CLT in children are sporadic, but there is an increased association of CLT with HLA haplotypes, DR3, DR4, and DR5 (17,93). HLA-DR2 and HLA-DQ1 apparently have a protective effect against autoimmune thyroid disease (103). Polyglandular autoimmune syndrome type I, due to a defect in the autoimmune regulatory gene on chromosome 21q22.3, is defined in part by the presence of CLT; polyglandular autoimmune syndrome type II and type III are uncommon in the pediatric population (80). Systemic lupus erythematosus, chronic juvenile arthritis, Sjögren syndrome, celiac disease, vitilgo, alopecia, mixed connective tissue disease, Bannayan-Riley-Ruvalcaba syndrome and type I diabetes mellitus may be accompanied by CLT as part of an autoimmune diathesis (e42,e66,e120,e169,e217,e384,e445, e501,e537,e576,e609,e639,e665,e666,e687,e797,e891,e962, e963,e433,e630,e814,e821). Approximately 4% of children with type I diabetes mellitus have CLT (e963). Trisomy 21 syndrome, Klinefelter syndrome, and Turner syndrome are three chromosomal disorders associated with CLT (e217,e445,e962). Approximately 25% of young individuals with Turner syndrome have antithyroid antibodies and 10% have enlarged thyroids (e962,e217).

The pathological diagnosis of CLT is more often established by FNAB than by histological examination. Surgical resection is reserved for specific clinical circumstances, such as a possible thyroid neoplasm (e867,e895,e1063). The thyroid is symmetrically enlarged and weighs more than 25 to 30 g. A pale, vaguely nodular, tannish-gray appearance with a resemblance to lymph nodal tissue is noted on cross section after fixation (Figure 21-13A). On occasion, one or the other lateral lobe or the pyramidal lobe is larger with the loss of symmetry. Any areas of discrete firmness, sclerosis, or nodularity may indicate the presence of PTC or scarring as in the fibrosing stage of CLT. Microscopically, lymphoid follicles with reactive germinal centers are interspersed throughout the gland with destructive replacement of parenchyma (Figure 21-13B, eFigure 21-61B, C). An intermixture of mature plasma cells is also apparent in a predominant population of B- and T-lymphocytes. The follicles are typically small and uniform, although some larger follicles with papillary infoldings may be seen. Some of the intact thyroid follicles may contain intrafollicular histiocytes and giant cells as evidence of so-called palpation thyroiditis or the presence of giant cells and lymphoid aggregates where follicles once resided. The diminutive follicles are lined by cuboidal or flattened epithelial cells or by epithelial cells with optically clear nuclei and grooves as seen in PTC. The diagnosis of PTC is made in the presence of a discrete lesion(s). Classic Hürthle

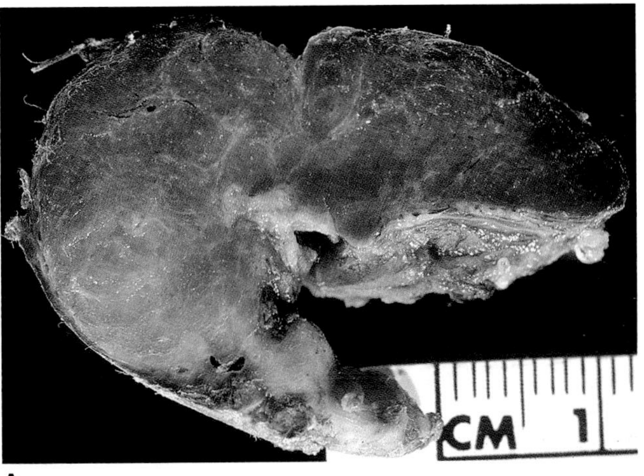

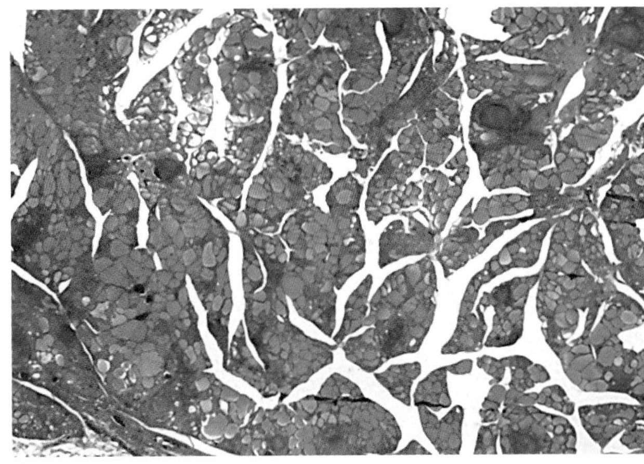

FIGURE 21-13 ■ Chronic lymphocytic thyroiditis. **A:** This specimen shows the characteristic diffuse thyroid gland enlargement seen in chronic lymphocytic thyroiditis on gross examination. A vaguely nodular pattern corresponding to the presence of lymphoid follicles is seen in this cut section. **B:** Chronic lymphocytic thyroiditis in this low power magnification image shows prominent lymphoid aggregates interspersed between the thyroid follicles. Plasma cells and lymphocytes were present in the interstitium (H&E stain).

or oncocytic follicular cells as a diffuse finding are uncommon in CLT in children and, in this respect, do not fulfill the classic morphologic definition of Hashimoto thyroiditis (eFigure 21-62). However, CLT and Hashimoto thyroiditis are pathogenetically identical forms of autoimmune thyroiditis in all other respects. Mizukami et al. found no morphologic difference in the types of chronic thyroiditis between adults and children younger than 10 years old (e827).

The fibrosing or end-stage of CLT with marked loss and atrophy of follicles, fibrosis with a finely nodular pattern and a diminution of the lymphocytic infiltrate is infrequently encountered in children. As noted earlier, the morphologic diagnosis of CLT is usually based on FNAB (e256,e951). A mixture of individual and small nonpapillary groups of benign-appearing follicular epithelial cells in a background of many dispersed small lymphocytes, some plasma cells, and histiocytes is the cytological finding. Hürthle cells are infrequent, and even less common are papillary profiles of cells, whose presence should raise the possibility of PTC. Approximately 30% of cases of CLT in children had distinct nodules and 3% had a PTC (e44,e256,e688).

Other types of thyroiditis, infections and noninfections types occur in children infrequently (e75,e494,e735,e971,e1076). Abscess of the thyroid has been reported in children, and opportunistic infections are seen in the immunocompromised setting (e432). Recurrent acute suppurative thyroiditis with or without abscess formation should suggest the presence of a branchial pouch anomaly such as a pyriform sinus cyst or TDC remnant (54,e224,e452,e825,e826,e848,e1024). Most cultures demonstrate a mixed flora containing a *Streptococcus* species (e164). Common features of acute suppurative thyroiditis include a painful/tender neck mass associated with fever. Involvement of the left lobe is more common. A left hemithyroidectomy may need to be performed for recurrent infections (e224). An infectious etiology should be excluded in granulomatous thyroiditis in a child because subacute giant cell or deQuervain thyroiditis is extremely rare in childhood.

Hyperplasia of the thyroid gland is either diffuse or multinodular in appearance. Diffuse hyperplasia is often associated with hyperthyroidism or thyrotoxicosis. The so-called simple goiter is defined clinically as diffuse or nodular enlargement of the thyroid gland without obvious evidence of hyperthyroidism (e376,e380). Children with a simple goiter are predominantly young adolescent females and do not experience any further gland enlargement. A small percentage, however, may develop CLT (e562).

The simple or colloid goiter is a more or less symmetrically enlarged thyroid gland with a diffuse or multinodular appearance (eFigure 21-63). The follicles vary in size with one or more colloid-filled macrofollicles lined by a flattened layer of epithelial cells (eFigure 21-64). Formation of colloid cysts occurs in some cases. Multiple variably sized follicular nodules with or without dense fibrous bands, cystic degeneration, hemorrhage, and nonspecific chronic inflammation are some of the contrasting gross and microscopic features of nodular or adenomatous hyperplasia (e52). The follicles of the adenomatous nodules may be quite uniform to the extent that on the basis of a small nodule, it may be difficult to differentiate a follicular adenoma from a dominant nodule in isolation from the other pathological findings. Alternatively, an individual nodule may have cystic changes with hemorrhage, histiocytes, hyaline-type fibrosis, and calcifications. Papillary profiles are a source of concern in areas of degeneration, but the follicular cells do not have the requisite nuclear features of PTC. On the other hand, PTC does arise infrequently in children and adolescents within one or more of the adenomatous nodules. A peripheral hyperplastic nodule may be found in the surrounding soft tissues and even embedded in skeletal muscle as an example of a sequestered nodule.

Multinodular hyperplasia is the pathological finding associated with the dyshormonogenic goiter (Figure 21-7). One example is Pendred syndrome with a goiter and hearing loss in adolescence due to a defect in the *PDS* gene (*SLC26A4* gene) on chromosome 7 that encodes for the protein, pendrin, which is involved in iodide transport across the cell membranes whose absence results in decreased organification of iodide with disruption in thyroid hormone synthesis (e973,e1013). The follicular nodules of a dyshormonogenic goiter tend to be cellular with the formation of microfollicles, trabecular profiles, and papillary formations with (eFigure 21-65) cellular pleomorphism, nuclear hyperchromatism, and mitotic figures. Some of these features in a dyshormonogenic goiter can be worrisome with the addition of apparent angioinvasion at the periphery of the nodules. The thyroid has especially atypical histological features in the presence of deiodinase deficiency. Well-differentiated thyroid carcinoma has been reported in dyshormonogenic goiters, but it is difficult to judge whether the risk of malignancy is increased in these glands (e29,e36,e316,e791).

Diffuse hyperplasia with clinical hyperthyroidism (Graves disease) is an autoimmune disorder of the thyroid, with some overlapping immunological and pathological findings with CLT. Hyperthyroidism also occurs infrequently on the basis of "toxic" nodular hyperplasia, functioning follicular adenoma, autosomal dominant nonimmune hyperthyroidism, and congenital hyperthyroidism (e1194,e1195,e1197). The latter two disorders have been reported with activating germline mutations in the TSH-receptor gene (e284,e389,e448). Sporadic congenital hyperthyroidism occurs in the presence of maternal autoimmune thyroid disease with the transplacental passage of maternal thyroid-stimulating immunoglobulins. Only 1% of neonates whose mothers have active Graves disease during pregnancy have evidence of hyperthyroidism at birth (e948,e1306). Most cases of hyperthyroidisim in children are on the basis of Graves disease (17,e533,e932,e933). Other etiologies of hyperthyroidism in children have been tabulated by LaFranchi (93,94).

A screening study of school-age population children between 11 and 18 years of age revealed that almost 4% had clinical or laboratory evidence of "thyroid abnormalities" and approximately 5% of those with abnormalities had hyperthyroidism (e968). This figure compares with other studies in which 10% to 15% of all pediatric thyroid disease is diagnosed as hyperthyroidism (e690). Juvenile hyperthyroidism typically presents in girls (6:1, female-to-male ratio) who are usually 11 years of age and older (11 to 18 years) and have diffuse enlargement of the thyroid (95% of cases) or less often have a dominant "toxic" or autonomous nodule (17). Hyperthyroidism occurs in families and is associated with MAS with activating mutations in the stimulatory G protein (e1305,e1306). Germline mutations in the TSH receptor account for cases of toxic multinodular goiter and toxic thyroid adenoma.

Graves disease is characterized by hyperthyroidism, ophthalmopathy (exopthalmos), and dermopathy (pretibial myxedema) in the pediatric population. It has its peak incidence in adolescence (11 to 15 years of age) and is three to five times more common in girls (17). The pathogenesis of Graves disease involves T- and B-cell dysregulation leading to the production of several anti-TSH receptor antibodies, thyroid-stimulating immunoglobulin, thyroid growth-stimulating immunoglobulin and TSH-binding inhibitor immunoglobulin (eFigure 21-60) (e140–e142). Thyroid-stimulating immunoglobulin mimics TSH and binds to the follicular cell TSH receptor leading to hypersecretion of thyroid hormones. The thyroid growth-stimulating immunoglobulin also binds to the TSH receptor and stimulates follicular cell hyperplasia with the development of increased serum levels of thyroxine or triiodothyronine and decreased TSH. The presence of anti-TSH receptor antibodies confirms the diagnosis of Graves disease versus other causes of hyperthyroidism. Total or subtotal thyroidectomy is performed in those cases of medical failure or intolerance. The clinical management of Graves disease in children is the subject of continued study and controversy (e447,e972,e991,e1305,e1125,e1153,e1116,e1240,e1280).

Pathologically, the thyroid gland is symmetrically enlarged without apparent nodules in most cases (Figure 21-14A, eFigure 21-66A) (e194). A red-brown color without an appreciation of translucent colloid is noted on cut surface. The weight of the gland is generally more than 25 to 30 g, but this varies somewhat with the age of the patient. In the unsuppressed gland, the follicular cells have a tall columnar appearance. Crowding of these cells leads to intrafollicular papillary infoldings on histological examination (Figure 21-14B, eFigure 21-66B). The colloid has a pale watery appearance and is absent in some follicles. Those follicles with colloid often show peripheral scalloping of the colloid. These latter findings are usually attenuated with preoperative suppression to diminish the function and vascularity of the gland (eFigure 21-67). Epithelial hyperplasia, through the action of TSH, leading to more prominent intrafollicular papillary infoldings is seen in the gland treated by thiouracil. Iodine administration before surgery results in the accumulation of colloid and the formation of macrofollicles. Rather than cuboidal to columnar epithelium lining the intrafollicular papillae, flattened epithelial cells cover the slender papillae. Marked follicular cell pleomorphism can be seen in pretreated glands.

Lymphocytic infiltrates in the interstitium and lymphoid nodules with reactive germinal centers are prominent in some glands. Without the clinical history of Graves disease, a diagnosis of CLT may be the preferred interpretation based on histological examination. The intrafollicular papillae may cause concern about PTC; however, the follicular cells lack the typical cytomorphology of a PTC. At least in the pediatric age population, PTC is rarely found in the midst of diffuse toxic hyperplasia.

Neoplasms

The 2004 World Health Organization classification of thyroid tumors contains a number of histological types but the

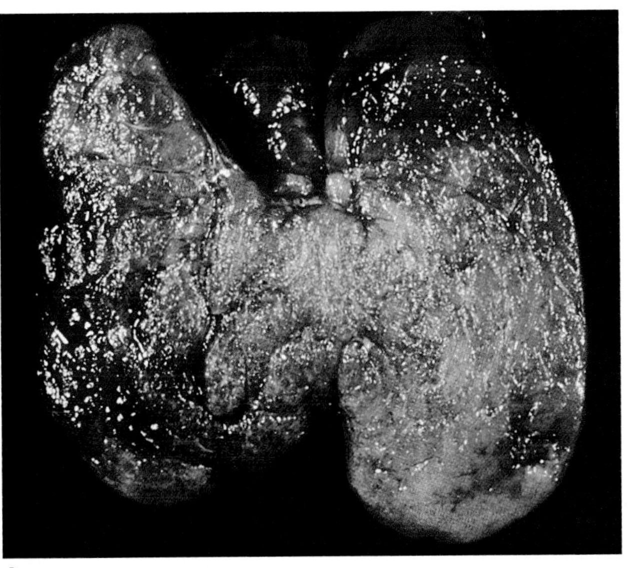
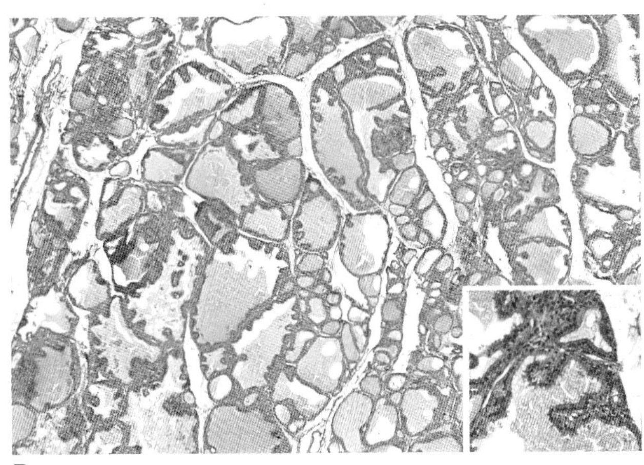

A B

FIGURE 21-14■ Graves disease. **A:** This image shows diffuse symmetrical enlargement of the thyroid gland from a patient with Graves disease. The parenchyma has a deep red color due to increased vascularity within the gland. (Reprinted with permission from Lloyd RV, Douglas BR, Young WF. Endocrine diseases. *Atlas of nontumor pathology*. Washington, DC: American Registry of Pathology.) **B:** This section of thyroid gland from a patient with untreated Graves disease shows follicles with hyperplastic epithelium and papillary infoldings. Pale watery colloid and an interstitial lymphocytic infiltrate (not pictured) were observed. The papillary infoldings (inset) lack the optically clear nuclei seen in papillary thyroid carcinoma (H&E stain).

overwhelming majority of differentiated carcinomas of the thyroid in children are PTC. Institutional referral patterns may affect the proportion of MTC in children with *RET* mutations in affected kindreds with MEN 2a or MEN 2b. Almost 30% of children with differentiated carcinomas at St. Louis Children's Hospital are MTCs because of MEN 2 referrals to the institution. FTC and MTC comprise less than 10% of thyroid carcinomas in the experience of most other institutions. Undifferentiated (anaplastic) carcinomas are rare in children in contrast to adults (e248,e1004).

Differentiated carcinomas of the thyroid gland account for only 1% to 3% of all malignant neoplasms in the pediatric age group in North America (e314,e790,e1012). It has an annual incidence of 2.4:100,000 children, less than 19 years of age (66). The most common histological type is PTC representing approximately 85% to 90% of all thyroid malignancies in children. The follicular variant of PTC accounts for approximately 25% of PTCs (42,e57,e185,e138,e207, e274,e351,e354,e418,e421,e469,e497,e548,e564,e671,e686, e769,e830,e1028,e1080,e1097,e1097,e1137,e1208,e1254, e1304). Other than PTC, FTC, and MTC, follicular adenomas, hemangiomas, lymphangiomas, teratomas, and plexiform neurofibromas are the other types of tumors involving the thyroid in children. FTC and follicular adenoma have been observed in patients with congenital goitrous hypothyroidism (e29,e36). Follicular adenoma is a relatively frequent cause of a solitary thyroid nodule in children (71). RDD, LCH, and hematolymphoid malignancies are examples of infiltrative processes involving the thyroid in children (e306,e434,e684,e926,e1023,e1152,e1182,e1209). There is also the spindle-epithelial tumor with thymus-like differentiation that presents in the thyroid.

Most carcinomas of the thyroid in children are diagnosed between 13 and 16 years of age, but individual cases have been reported throughout childhood, even in the newborn (e175,e342,e791,e819). The female:male incidence is approximately 1:1 in carcinomas diagnosed prior to adolescence, but with a 3–6:1 female predominance during adolescence.

Many recent studies have looked at the molecular events underlying the development of thyroid cancer (59,e258, e300,e1071,e1114). A number of somatic mutations involving the *RET* gene have been identified in sporadic PTC (42,59,e328,e721,e874,e1071); *RET/PTC1* and the *RET/PTC3* gene arrangements are found in a variable proportion of PTCs in children (e258,e360). In children not exposed to radiation, the *RET/PTC1* rearrangement is more frequent than the *RET/PTC3* rearrangement, which is more common in radiation-induced thyroid cancer (42,185,e360,e721). The "classic" papillary pattern is associated with *RET/PTC1* rearrangement whereas the *RET/PTC3* is found more often in the follicular variant of PTC. In terms of behavior, PTCs with the *RET/PTC3* gene rearrangement appear to have a somewhat more aggressive course than PTCs with the *RET/PTC1* rearrangement (e694). Mutations involving *BRAF* are uncommon in PTCs in children less than 15 years of age at diagnosis (59,e924). FTC and follicular adenoma are associated with *RAS* and *PAX8-PPAR*γ (peroxisome proliferator-activated receptor gamma) mutations but these mutations do not distinguish between the two neoplasms (59,185,e367,e1114).

MTCs, in contrast, demonstrate distinct mutations in the *RET* gene. Mutations in the RET proto-oncogene in the pericentromeric region of chromosome 10q11.2 have been identified in three autosomal dominant syndromes, MEN 2a, MEN 2b, and FMTC (42,59,81,e772,e225,e299,e331,e332,e431,e942). The *RET* gene codes for a transmembrane receptor tyrosine kinase that is involved in development of the kidney and nervous system. The gene spans 21 exons. Each of these syndromes involves mutations with different codons (eFigure 21-68). MEN 2a and FMTC more frequently involve missense mutations in exons 10 and 11 involving codons 609,611,618,620, and 634. MEN 2b has a characteristic mutation in exon 16 (codon 918) in 95% of cases and in codon 883 in exon 15 (42,e772).

PTC presents with a painless or a tender mass in the thyroid gland. Palpable cervical adenopathy at diagnosis is common since regional lymph node metastasis is present in 30% to 80% of children at diagnosis (45,132,185, e1080). Most cases of PTC are sporadic, but a family history should be sought since there are several familial-associated tumor predisposition syndromes (e286). There is an increased incidence of PTC in children who have received radiation therapy for a prior neoplasm in the head and neck (e125,e132,e358,e806,e1074,e1234). In one study, the average interval between the delivery of radiation and the diagnosis of carcinoma was 8.5 years, with approximately 75% of patients exposed between 3.5 and 14 years before the development of the carcinoma (e99). An increased incidence of thyroid cancer with the signature *RET/PTC* gene rearrangement was detected in children as early as 4 years after exposure to fallout from the Chernobyl nuclear reactor explosion in 1986 (e45,e391,e553,e554,e557,e870–e873,e875, e876,e905,e909,e1037,e1208,e1252). Ten to thirty percent of children with PTC and no history of radiation exposure demonstrate *RET/PTC* gene rearrangement in contrast to 50% to 70% in children with a history of radiation exposure (59). Nonneoplastic abnormalities such as multinodularity, fibrosis, and lymphocytic infiltrates have also been reported in the thyroid gland after prior neck irradiation (e873).

PTC, as well as the follicular adenoma and carcinoma, is found in association with MAS (e249) and MEN 1 (parathyroid hyperplasia, islet cell hyperplasia, and PA) but not in MEN 2a or MEN 2b, in which MTC is the rule (e636). Other familial settings of non-MTC are Carney complex, familial adenomatous polyposis, and Cowden syndrome (42,e189, e210,e211,e212,e213,e710,e721,e727,e931,e1140).

The gross features of PTC are variable from one or more solid, grayish-tan nodules; dense, poorly circumscribed foci of fibrous effacement of the normal gland; a cyst(s) with a mural nodule or solid, reddish glistening nodule with a fibrous capsule (e254) (Figure 21-15A, B). Calcifications may be present. The classic papillary and follicular variants of PTC usually present as a well-circumscribed, encapsulated tumor, whereas (e1004,e1186) the diffuse sclerosing variant is a poorly circumscribed focus of dense fibrosis replacing the thyroid parenchyma and often extending into the surrounding soft tissues including the skeletal muscle. The sclerosing variant, though uncommon, is seen more often in children than in adults. Among PTCs in children, the classic papillary type, follicular variant, solid type, mixed papillary and follicular pattern, and sclerosing variant were present in 11%, 35%, 30%, 17%, and 8% of cases, respectively and among adolescents, 26%, 28%, 24%, 20%, and 2% of cases, respectively (e1208).

The classic PTC is composed of branching fronds or papillae with fibrovascular stalks (Figure 21-15C, eFigure 21-69). Regardless of the particular histological pattern, the pathologic diagnosis of PTC is based largely upon nuclear features including crowded and overlapping nuclei with an elongated cleaved appearance, often with prominent nuclear grooves or folds, margination of chromatin with clearing of the nucleoplasm ("optically clear" or "Orphan Annie" nuclei) (e215) and cytoplasmic invaginations or nuclear pseudoinclusions (Figure 21-15D, eFigure 21-70). Small concentric whorls of calcification (i.e., psammoma bodies) are present more commonly in the classic and sclerosing variants of PTCs than in the other variants, especially the follicular variant (Figure 21-15E). Multifocal gross lesions, but more commonly multiple microscopic foci of PTC, are identified in the ipsilateral and the contralateral lobe in 20% to 25% of cases. The latter finding is the rationale for subtotal-total thyroidectomy (e151,e472,e592,e1070, e1127,e1265).

Squamous metaplasia is a feature of PTC in the pediatric age group, which may cause some concern about the possibility of a higher grade thyroid carcinoma (42,e721). In other cases, varying degrees of a desmoplastic stromal reaction may be encountered, which is so prominent as to superficially resemble the "amyloid stroma" of MTC; in other instances, the fibrosis is associated with the infiltrative growth pattern of the sclerosing variant, which is associated with angiolymphatic invasion and numerous psammoma bodies. The architecture of the follicular variant of PTC is exclusively follicular but diminutive intrafollicular micropapillae are seen with some frequency. Focal areas of classic PTC may be present in some cases in other areas of the thyroid. The follicular variant of PTC is distinguished from the well-differentiated FTC by the presence of the characteristic nuclear morphology of PTC. Capsular and vascular invasion are present in both PTC and FTC.

Lymphocytic infiltration of the surrounding thyroid is a common feature in PTC regardless of age, and its presence has been associated with an improved prognosis (185,e730,e895). Regional lymph node metastasis is present in 30% to 80% or more of cases overall. Pulmonary metastasis is found in 6% to 8% of pediatric cases at diagnosis (45,185,e672,e1029,e1224) although some series report a higher incidence (45).

The diagnosis of pediatric thyroid cancer is made for the most part on specific histopathological criteria.

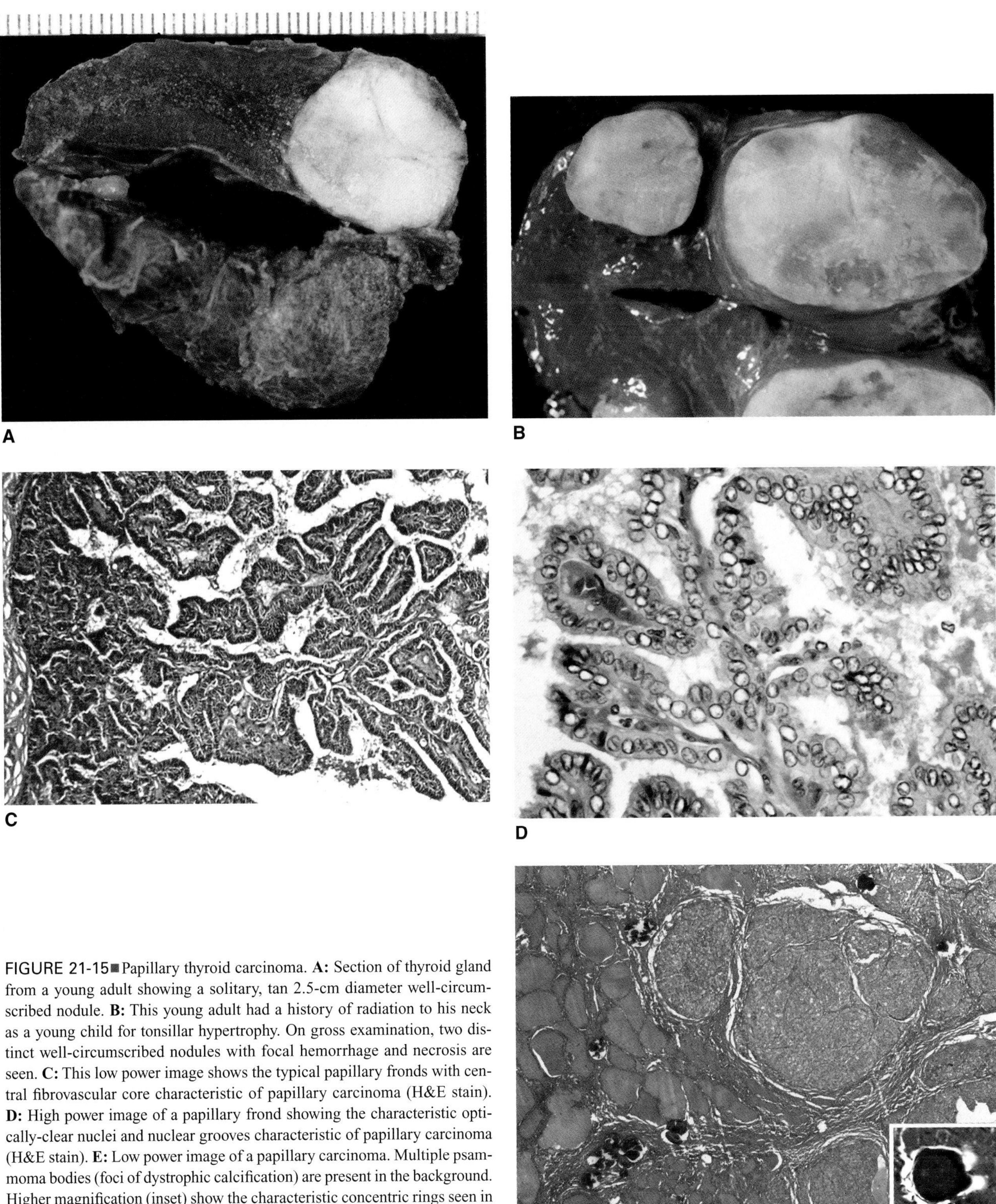

FIGURE 21-15 ■ Papillary thyroid carcinoma. **A:** Section of thyroid gland from a young adult showing a solitary, tan 2.5-cm diameter well-circumscribed nodule. **B:** This young adult had a history of radiation to his neck as a young child for tonsillar hypertrophy. On gross examination, two distinct well-circumscribed nodules with focal hemorrhage and necrosis are seen. **C:** This low power image shows the typical papillary fronds with central fibrovascular core characteristic of papillary carcinoma (H&E stain). **D:** High power image of a papillary frond showing the characteristic optically-clear nuclei and nuclear grooves characteristic of papillary carcinoma (H&E stain). **E:** Low power image of a papillary carcinoma. Multiple psammoma bodies (foci of dystrophic calcification) are present in the background. Higher magnification (inset) show the characteristic concentric rings seen in a psammoma body. Their presence strongly suggests a diagnosis of papillary carcinoma (H&E stain).

Immunohistochemistry is not usually necessary in most cases of non-MTC although the occasional solid PTC or FTC may require differentiation from MTC (e367). The tumor cells in PTC are immunoreactive for cytokeratins, thyroglobulin, and TITF-1 (thyroid transcription factor-1) (42,e367,e721). Cytokeratin 19 is strongly expressed in PTCs. Staining for RET/PTC rearrangements has also been utilized, but availability of sensitive antibodies is a limiting factor (42,e367,e721).

The prognosis in children with PTC is excellent despite the presence of local extrathyroidal spread (40% to 50% of cases) and lymph node metastasis (e175,e459,e563,e670, e865,e1056,e1302). The presence of invasion in the soft tissues of the neck from the primary or extranodal site contributes substantially to the local morbidity of the disease.

The extent of disease and age at diagnosis are important prognostic features. Management is surgical resection in most cases with additional modalities in some cases (45). Prognostically unfavorable histological variants of PTC are uncommon in children such as the tall cell, dedifferentiated, and poorly differentiated variants. Postoperative staging is based on a combination of factors. The MACIS (metastasis-age-completeness of resection-invasion-size) system has been found useful in children (45). In children less than 10 years of age, PTC is more locally aggressive and more likely to have pulmonary metastasis. Overall, the long-term survival rate for PTC is excellent in children with a 98% 10-year survival, regardless of the pathologic stage.

Follicular neoplasms of the thyroid present several problems in pathological diagnosis without regard for age. One of the less consequential ones is the differentiation of a follicular adenoma from a dominant nodule of multinodular or adenomatous hyperplasia. In some cases, it is a distinction without a difference in terms of prognosis. Follicular lesions diagnosed pathologically as an adenoma have a delicate continuous or interrupted fibrous capsule separating the relatively monotonous follicular architecture to larger, more variably sized follicles (eFigure 21-71). Follicular adenoma is a sporadically occurring tumor in most cases in children, but is reported in young individuals with Cowden syndrome and pleuropulmonary blastoma familial tumor predisposition syndrome (e470,e1000).

FTC is diagnosed pathologically, not on the basis of nuclear features which are often quite bland, but on the presence of a well-defined thickened, circumscribed fibrous capsule with preferably more than one focus of transcapsular invasion as a "mushroom" of neoplastic follicles protruding through the capsule. Microvascular invasion in the capsule is another diagnostic feature, but there should be adherence of tumor cells to the endothelium of the vessel or vessels and not free-floating tumor cells or pressing into a vascular space with an interposed intact endothelium (Figure 21-16A to C, eFigure 21-72). It is common to identify groups of follicles pressing on capsular vascular spaces in a follicular adenoma or dominant adenomatous nodule, which should not be interpreted as vascular invasion. An accurate diagnosis of an encapsulated, well-differentiated FTC often requires extensive sampling of the fibrous capsule with well-oriented sections and the use of vascular endothelial markers or an elastic stain to confirm "bona fide" vascular invasion. The distinctive nuclear features of PTC distinguish the follicular variant of PTC from FTC.

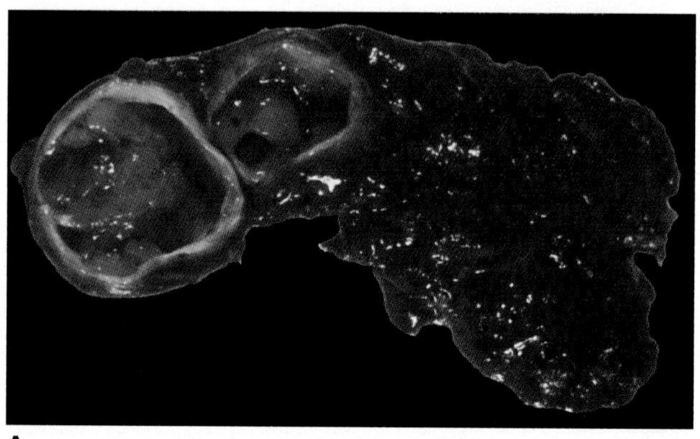

A

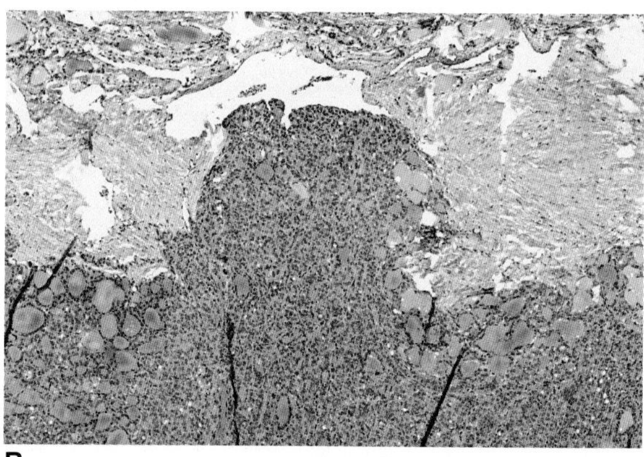

B

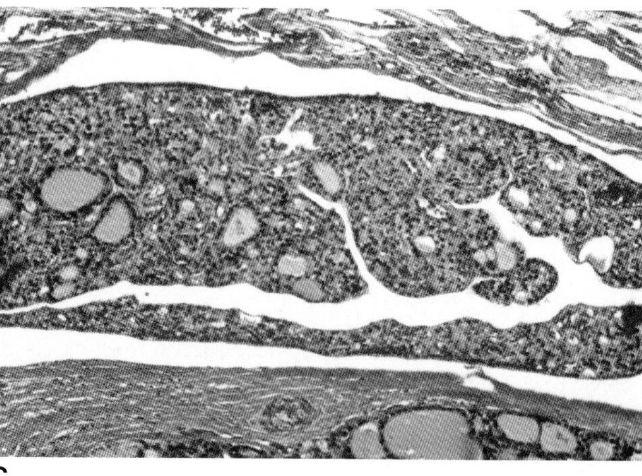

C

FIGURE 21-16■ Follicular thyroid carcinoma. **A:** This section of thyroid gland shows a well-circumscribed nodule with a thick irregular capsule within the thyroid parenchyma. The neoplasm was composed of small well-defined follicles on histological examination. No well formed papillae or psammoma bodies were present. The nuclei did not have the optically-clear appearance or nuclear grooves characteristic of the follicular variant of papillary carcinoma. **B,C:** Invasion of the adjacent capsule and blood vessels was present (H&E stain).

FTC is immunoreactive for thyroglobulin, TITF-1, and low molecular weight cytokeratins (e367).

Moderate to poorly differentiated carcinomas of the follicular and papillary types are distinct yet uncommon neoplasms in children (e190,e479,e611,e642,e725,e997, e1026,e1096,e1301). Some of these solid nested tumors are examples of insular-like carcinomas. These tumors present as well-defined neoplasms grossly with invasion often appreciated during gross examination.

In general, intraoperative frozen section examination is often a frustrating exercise to resolve the differential diagnosis among the follicular variant of PTC, follicular adenoma, dominant adenomatous nodule, and well-differentiated FTC. The characteristic optically clear nuclei of PTC are not seen in frozen sections or touch preparations, and although nuclear grooves are helpful, they are insufficient alone for a specific diagnosis of PTC. Furthermore, the separation of the encapsulated, well-differentiated FTC from follicular adenoma may require processing multiple blocks of tumor with capsule, and then multiple levels through individual blocks which is unsuitable for frozen section analysis.

MTC in children occurs almost exclusively in the familial setting with or without the other features of MEN 2a (MTC, diffuse parathyroid hyperplasia, and PHEO) or MEN 2b (MTC, PHEO, intestinal ganglioneuromatosis, and mucosal neuromas) (e197,e345,e498,e543,e833,e890,e919,e1145).

Only 1% to 3% of differentiated thyroid carcinomas in children are MTCs except in some specialized medical centers (59,145,e1266). Sporadic MTCs, which are palpable, unifocal neoplasms without C-cell hyperplasia, account for 80% to 90% of all MTCs in adults and children, however, are uncommon in children. The aggressive nature of MTC is evident in adults who have regional lymph node metastasis in 50% or more of cases and distant metastasis (lung, liver) in 15% of cases at diagnosis (42,e772,e969,e1172). It is noteworthy that approximately 20% of adults with apparent sporadic MTCs have germline *RET* mutations with its obvious familial implications (45).

Syndromic-associated MTCs in children are typically small, often microscopic, multifocal tumors in association with diffuse C-cell hyperplasia in the upper two-thirds of the lateral lobes (e493). The small size of the tumor or tumors in syndromic MTC is in part a reflection of genetic screening of children in affected kindreds using molecular diagnostic techniques (e680,e683,e719,e1101,e1218). Virtually all resected thyroids in the setting of MEN 2a, MEN 2b, and FMTC have microscopic multifocal C-cell hyperplasia, if not microscopic or infrequently grossly visible tumors (e653).

On gross examination, MTCs present as a well-circumscribed or infiltrative mass that is gray-white to tan in appearance. The individual tumors range from 1 mm or less to 4 to 5 cm in diameter (Figure 21-17A, B). The several histological patterns include the common, compact solid-rounded nests to lobular, insular, or trabecular profiles. Whether the tumor cells are rounded or spindled, the polygonal nuclei have finely dispersed chromatin and a prominent nucleolus. There are also small cell and even pigmented variants of MTC. Mitotic activity and anaplasia are inapparent in most cases. Intersecting bands of fibrosis and/or an amyloid stroma are generally found in those tumors in excess of 2 cm in diameter (Figure 21-17C, eFigure 21-73).

One of the challenges in the pathological examination in syndromic cases is the differentiation between C-cell hyperplasia and microscopic MTC. The degree and extent of C-cell hyperplasia can vary markedly from one prophylactic thyroidectomy to another. Foci of C-cell hyperplasia can be relatively inconspicuous without the assistance of immunohistochemistry. In other cases, the C-cell hyperplasia is not only apparent, but extensive to the degree that there is concern about microscopic MTC. The hyperplasia is recognized by a collection of C-cells partially filling the colloid space of the follicle and/or bulging into the perifollicular, interstitial space without breaching of the basement membrane of the follicle (not always readily apparent). A microscopic MTC has a similar bulging growth from the follicle as C-cell hyperplasia, but more importantly, there is interstitial infiltration and the displacement, if not the overgrowth, of contiguous follicles or coalescence of aggregates of enlarged, atypical cells. The tumor cells are larger than those of the surrounding smaller hyperplastic C-cells, and the nucleoli are prominent in comparison to the inapparent or micronucleoli of the hyperplastic C-cells.

Immunohistochemical staining for calcitonin is helpful in the identification of inconspicuous foci of C-cell hyperplasia, or in the confirmation of the thyroid carcinoma as MTC (Figure 21-17D, eFigure 21-74). C-cells and MTC are also immunoreactive for SYN, CHR, and CEA, and nonreactive for thyroglobulin and TITF-1 as in PTC and FTC (103). In keeping with the distribution of C-cells in the thyroid, hyperplasia and MTC have a predilection for the upper two-thirds of the lateral lobes. It is helpful to submit multiple sections from the superior to the inferior pole of the resected gland.

Early prophylactic thyroidectomy with lymph node dissection and serum calcitonin levels in children with germline *RET* mutations is the recommended management (81,e1103). Based on the specific *RET* codon involved, specific risk groups have been established with recommended surgical intervention dependent on the risk group (45,81,e1103,e1162). In young children, most cases of MTC are associated with MEN 2b, and for this reason, thyroidectomy is recommended as soon as possible in MEN 2b *RET*-positive infants, whereas in MEN 2a, surgery is recommended between 3 and 5 years of age (81). Prognosis is dependent on stage and postoperative calcitonin levels. Syndromic MTC with total thyroidectomy and negative postoperative serum calcitonin levels at 6 and 12 months postsurgery have a recurrence rate of 5% and a 10-year survival rate of 98% (45).

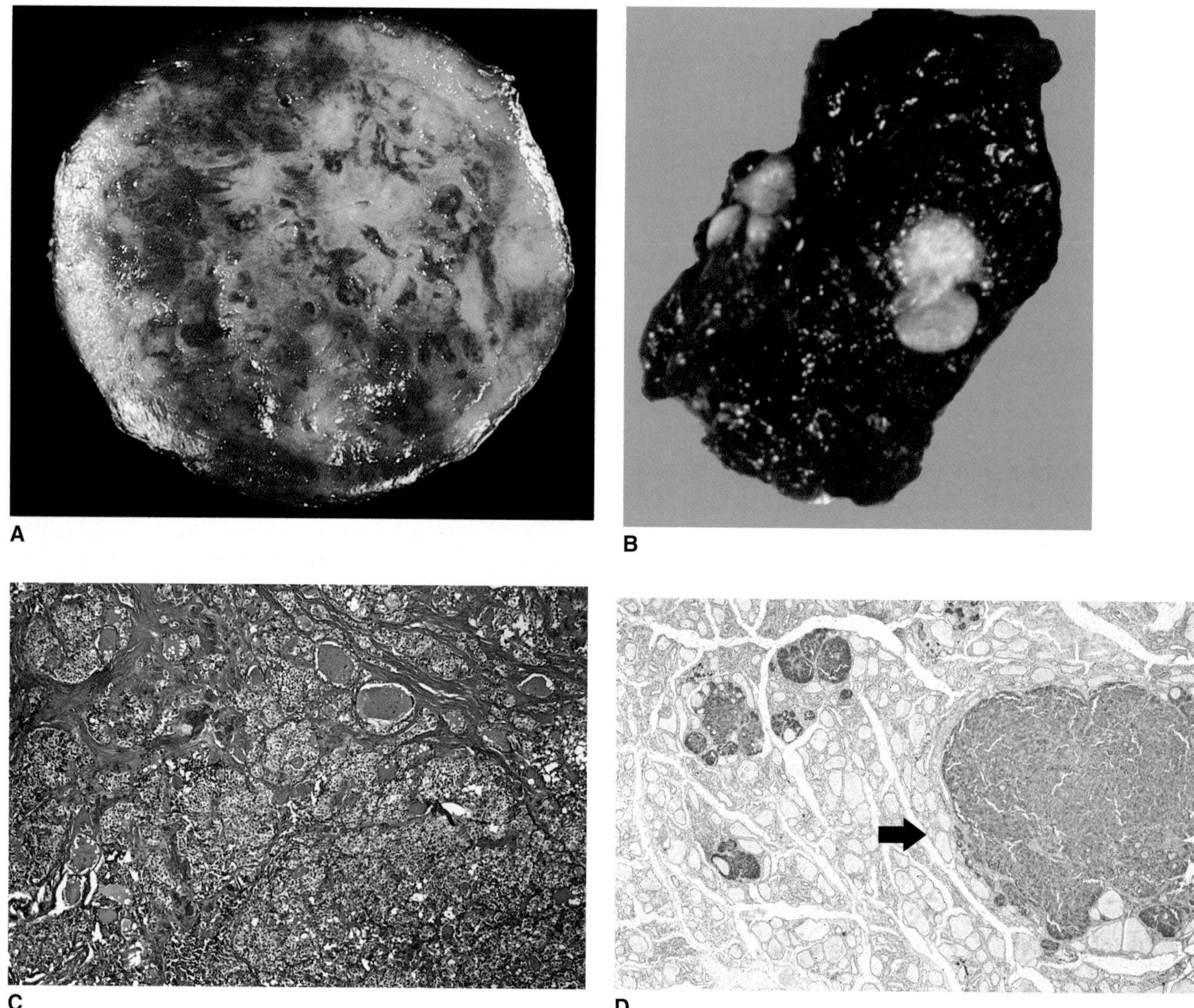

FIGURE 21-17 ■ Medullary thyroid carcinoma. **A:** This image from a sporadic (nonsyndromic) medullary carcinoma shows a large tan-yellow, non-encapsulated mass that had a firm gritty consistency on sectioning. **B:** Syndromic medullary carcinoma tends to be small and multifocal. This 0.4 cm in diameter tumor nodule (**right**) in a patient with MEN 2 is demarcated from the red-brown thyroid parenchyma. A smaller nodule of medullary carcinoma (**left**) is also seen. **C:** This tumor on low power demonstrates the characteristic lobular pattern. Nests of tumor cells with round nuclei were surrounded by bands of connective tissue. The round to polygonal tumor cells has an abundant eosinophillic or clear cytoplasm. The nuclei are predominantly round to oval with coarse chromatin. The cells were immunoreactive for calcitonin (H&E stain). **D:** This section of thyroid gland from a child with MEN 2 shows a small focus of medullary carcinoma (*arrow*) and several foci of C-cell hyperplasia that were immunoreactive for calcitonin (immunostain for calcitonin).

Cervical-thyroidal teratoma (CTT) accounts for 3% or less of thyroid resections in children especially in the infancy period. Approximately 2% to 5% of germ cell neoplasms in children present in the head and neck region, and the anterior portion of the neck including the thyroid gland is one of several specific sites in this anatomic region (e200,e396,e604,e1255). There is an equal male to female ratio (68,182,1183). These tumors are typically congenital and are not subtle clinically given their size. Byard et al. reported that 6 of 14 (43%) of cases were detected in stillborn infants or neonates who died within 2 days of birth (e182). Compression of the upper airway is the major complication requiring early surgical intervention. A minority of cases are known to present beyond the infancy period. The mass fills the soft tissues of the anterior and lateral portions of the neck. An attachment to the thyroid and its infiltration is not always demonstrable due to the size and extensive replacement of normal tissues. Grossly, these tumors are soft and often cystic, measuring several centimeters in greatest dimension and microscopically are composed of a range of immature and some mature somatic elements. Immature neuroepithelium with primitive neural tubules and sheets of neuroblasts are often the dominant microscopic pattern and should not be mistaken for neuroblastoma (NB) which can present in the cervical region but more lateral and with an exclusive neuroblastic appearance, usually poorly differentiated NB (e1238). One confounding aspect is the presence of immature or mature teratoma in regional lymph nodes in some cases, which we have preferred to designate as "nodal gliomatosis" and others have referred to nodal "deposits" rather than metastasis (e91,e293,e597,e1203). The excellent clinical outcome of CTT is usually not affected by the presence of nodal deposits. As in sacrococcygeal teratomas, microscopic foci of endodermal sinus may be detected (e293,e669). If these foci of endodermal sinus tumor represent only a minor component and are not in regional lymph nodes, the excellent prognosis may be affected in only a marginal fashion, but the decision about further management is complicated.

ADRENAL GLANDS

The adrenal glands are composed of an outer cortex and an inner medulla. Functionally, they are two separate endocrine organs, with the cortex responsible for steroid hormone synthesis and the medulla for catecholamine production. In children and adolescents, the pyramidal-shaped right and crescent-shaped left adrenal glands have an average combined weight of 4 to 6 g, similar to adults with combined adrenal weights ranging between 2 and 8 g (87,104). There is no difference in the weight of the adrenals between male and female children. A coarse connective tissue capsule with attached periadrenal fat surrounds the gland. The fat in the vicinity of the adrenals has immature features of finely vacuolated adipocytes in infants resembling those of a lipoblastoma. On sectioning, the adrenal cortex consists of a yellow subcapsular layer that corresponds to the zona glomerulosa and zona fasciculata. A thin brown layer, the zona reticularis, separates the zona fasciculata from the gray-white central medulla. The adrenals receive their blood supply from the inferior phrenic artery, aorta, and renal artery.

In the fetus, a prominent provisional (fetal) cortex is present. Adrenal weight ranges upward with the gestational age. There is rapid growth of the provisional cortex during the third trimester. The average combined weight of the adrenals is about 2 g at 30 weeks' gestation compared to 6 g at birth in a term infant. Following birth, the provisional cortex involutes and rapidly disappears, leaving the permanent cortex and central medulla (87) (see Appendices: *Weights of Organs of 1- to 12- Month-old Girls*. and *Weights of Organs of 1- to 12-Month-old Boys*). The involuted remnant of the fetal cortex can be observed throughout the first 6 months of life. In the newborn, the adrenal gland on sectioning has a dark red-brown appearance beneath a thin yellow cortical rim due to degeneration of the provisional cortex. The adrenal medulla, which makes up less than 1% of the fetal adrenal compared with 10% of the adult adrenal, is generally not recognized on gross examination.

The definitive adrenal cortex is divided into three distinct zones. The zona glomerulosa, which accounts for approximately 10% of the adult adrenal gland, consists of islands of haphazardly distributed cells beneath the connective tissue capsule. Individual cells contain small amounts of eosinophilic cytoplasm and have rounded nuclei. The zona fasciculata located beneath the zona glomerulosa accounts for 70% to 80% of the adult adrenal cortex and consists of large polyhedral, lipid-laden cells arranged in columns 1- to 2-cells thick separated by thin sinusoidal capillaries in the nonstressed adrenal gland. The nuclei are round, pale staining, and occasionally binucleated. The zona reticularis, which accounts for less than 10% of the cortex, consists of anastomosing cords of small eosinophilic cells with deeply staining closely apposed nuclei. The adrenal medulla, which occupies the center of the gland, consists of large, pale staining, polyhedral cells, known as chromaffin cells, which are arranged in cords and small islands. These cells, innervated by preganglionic sympathetic nerve fibers, are modified postganglionic neurons.

In the fetus, the provisional (fetal) zone accounts for 70% to 80% of the total weight of the gland (eFigure 21-75) (e129,e130,e437). The fetal zone, composed of cords of large eosinophilic cells surrounded by sinusoidal capillaries, is located beneath the permanent cortex. A distinct adrenal medulla is not identifiable in the fetal gland. Chromaffin cells, however, are haphazardly scattered throughout the fetal cortex. In fact, neuroblastic cells from the neural crest migrate through the cortex as individual and small nests of primitive appearing cells. These cells should not be interpreted as evidence of congenital NB.

Adrenal gland development is dependent on a number of factors. Steroidogenic factor (SF-1) encoded on chromosome 9q33, and DAX1, encoded on chromosome Xp21, are two critical transcription factors required for adrenal gland development and steroidogenesis (95,188,e115,e715). Growth and maturation of the gland is also dependent on ACTH stimulation.

The adrenal cortex is responsible for the synthesis of three classes of steroids, glucocorticoids, mineralocorticoids, and androgens. A series of cytochrome P450 enzymes are involved in adrenal steroid synthesis (eFigure 21-76). The rate-limiting step is the transfer of cholesterol from the cytosol across the mitochondrial membrane. Several proteins, including the steroidogenic acute regulatory protein (StaR) induced by ACTH, are involved in this rate-limiting step. In response to ACTH stimulation, cholesterol is metabolized through a series of enzymatic steps in the zona fasciculata and reticularis into cortisol, the major glucocorticoid (eFigure 21-77). Once secreted, cortisol provides negative feedback on the pituitary gland to inhibit further ACTH secretion. Aldosterone, synthesized in the zona glomerulosa, is a mineralocorticoid. Dihydroepiandrosteindione sulfate is the major androgen and is primarily synthesized in the zona reticularis. During early fetal development, androgens of adrenal origin are responsible for differentiation of the male external genitalia.

The cathecholamines, epinephrine, and norepinephrine, are formed from tyrosine and secreted in response to sympathetic neural stimulation by the chromaffin cells. Extensive reviews of adrenal steroidogenesis and catecholamine production are beyond the scope of this chapter but are widely available (12,87,96,e312,e1189).

Imaging

The visualization of the adrenal in infants is accomplished optimally by US. In older children, US is useful as a screening method for an adrenal mass. If an adrenal mass is discovered, further imaging with MR or CT is indicated.

The normal adrenal glands of an infant on US are Y- or V-shaped on longitudinal images. The medulla is seen as an echogenic (bright) central line surrounded by the thin hypoechoic (dark) cortex. A long straight adrenal gland may be seen in cases of renal agenesis or ectopia. In the presence of congenital adrenal hyperplasia, the adrenal glands are enlarged with an abnormal undulating surface and/or replacement of the central echogenic line by a stippled pattern throughout the gland (e23). An adrenal mass in the neonate is a cyst, hemorrhage, or congenital NB. In the case of adrenal hemorrhage, US provides the most useful modality in the follow-up period without the need for CT or MR (e823). The echogenicity of the hemorrhage varies with the age of the hemorrhage and is usually heterogeneous. No flow is demonstrated to the mass on Doppler evaluation. On follow-up the mass becomes smaller and more hypoechoic (dark) over time. The adrenal gland may become calcified, appearing as a dense focus with posterior acoustic shadowing (e823). NB should be suspected if the mass fails to diminish in size on short interval follow-up. It should be noted that NB in neonates are more likely to be cystic than in an older child and these cystic NBs may become smaller over time, but do not entirely resolve as a cystic hemorrhage. Calcifications may be identified in both lesions. The neonate may present with the particular pattern of metastases of stage 4S disease with diffuse involvement of the liver, nodules of the skin, and infiltration of the bone marrow. Adrenal cysts have a varied appearance on imaging depending on the presence or absence of complicating hemorrhage or infection. Simple cysts are anechoic (black) on US and of fluid attenuation on CT or MR. Hemorrhage or infection causes a heterogeneous appearance to the internal structure of the cyst and the wall of the cyst may be calcified (Figure 21-18A to C).

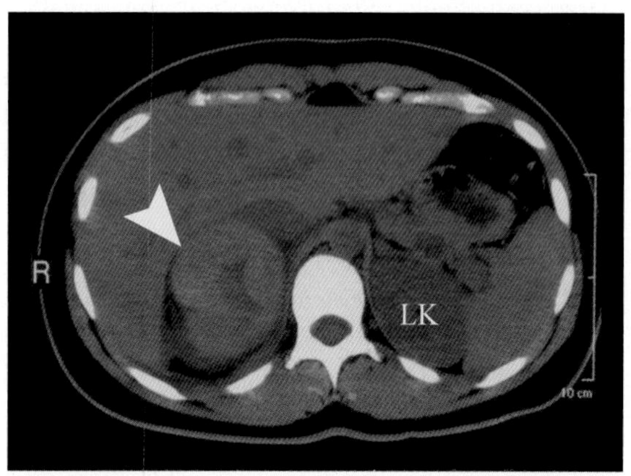

A

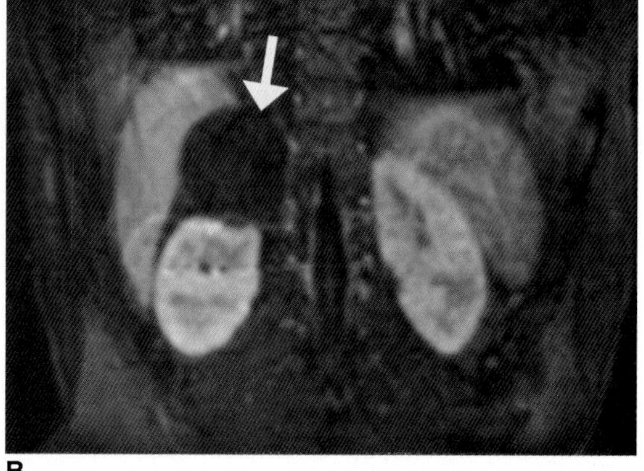
B

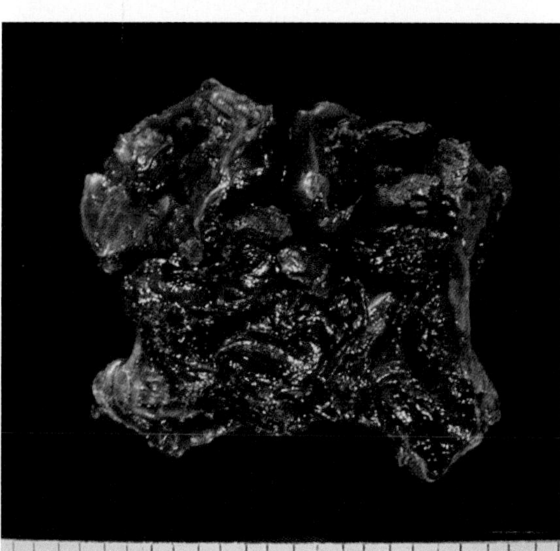
C

FIGURE 21-18 ■ **A:** Hemorrhagic adrenal cyst in an 18-year-old girl. Axial unenhanced CT image shows a mass in the right suprarenal region (*arrowhead*) which is denser than the left kidney (LK) indicating acute hemorrhage. **B:** Coronal postgadolinium T1-weighted image showing no enhancement of the cyst (*arrow*) above the enhancing right kidney. **C:** Image of the sectioned resected specimen showing hemorrhage.

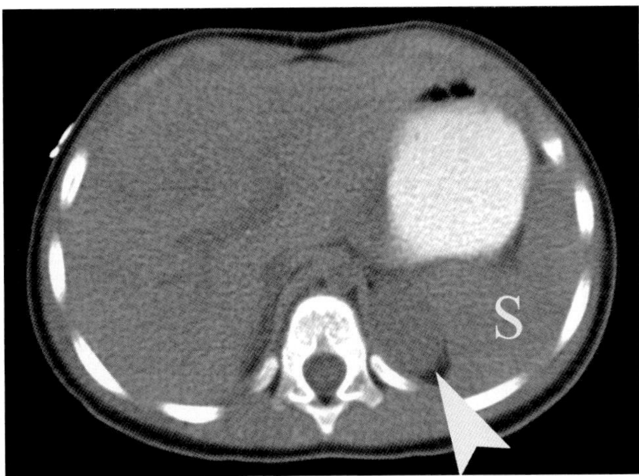

FIGURE 21-19 ▪ Adrenal cortical tumor in 18-month-old girl with virilization. CT image without intravenous contrast material shows a mass in the region of the left adrenal fossa (*arrowhead*) adjacent to the spleen (S).

If an adrenal mass is initially discovered by US, further imaging with CT or MR is necessary to characterize the nature of the mass. The imaging appearance of adrenal cortical tumors on US, CT, and MR depends on their size (e920). Small tumors tend to appear homogeneous, whereas in larger tumors, central necrosis, calcification, or scar causes a heterogeneous appearance (Figure 21-19, eFigure 21-78). Local spread or metastatic disease may be evident indicating an aggressive tumor. Extension into the vena cava should be sought.

NB typically appears as a mass in excess of 2 cm in most cases (Figure 21-20). Calcifications are relatively frequent, which is particularly evident on CT but may also be seen on US as echogenic foci possibly with posterior acoustic shadowing. Cystic areas from old hemorrhage or cystic or necrotic changes are anechoic (black) on US and of fluid attenuation on CT and MR. After injection of contrast material, the tumor generally enhances heterogeneously. CT and MR are useful in evaluating the extent of disease. The primary tumor frequently crosses the midline and surrounds the aorta and other vessels (Figure 21-21). Adjacent organ involvement may be seen and enlarged lymph nodes and liver metastases may be identified (Figure 21-22). MR is particularly useful in demonstrating neural foraminal and spinal canal invasion (eFigure 21-79). PHEO appears as a soft-tissue mass on CT with homogeneous, heterogeneous or rim-like enhancement postcontrast (e920). On MR, PHEOs are hypointense (dark) on T1-weighted images and hyperintense on T2-weighted images. Postgadolinium images typically show intense enhancement with slow washout (Figure 21-23) (e1073). As lesions are frequently multiple, the radionuclide scan using ^{131}I-MIBG may be helpful in the preoperative localization of lesions.

Developmental Disorders

Agenesis, congenital adrenal hypoplasia (CAHP), congenital adrenal hyperplasia, and adrenal gland heterotopia are the major structural and biochemical disorders of a congenital or developmental nature (Table 21-6). Except in the setting of anencephaly or other syndromes in which there is adenohypophyseal dysfunction or absence, bilateral adrenal agenesis is rare (e319). **Unilateral adrenal agenesis** may be seen in combination with other malformational syndromes and in the setting of unilateral renal agenesis. **Adrenal fusion**, characterized by the midline union of the adrenal glands giving the fused glands a horseshoe or butterfly shape (horseshoe adrenal gland), is rare and is associated with other congenital anomalies (e624,e1150,e1294) (Figure 21-24A). Renal-adrenal fusion (accreta) and hepatic-adrenal and renal-adrenal union, characterized by

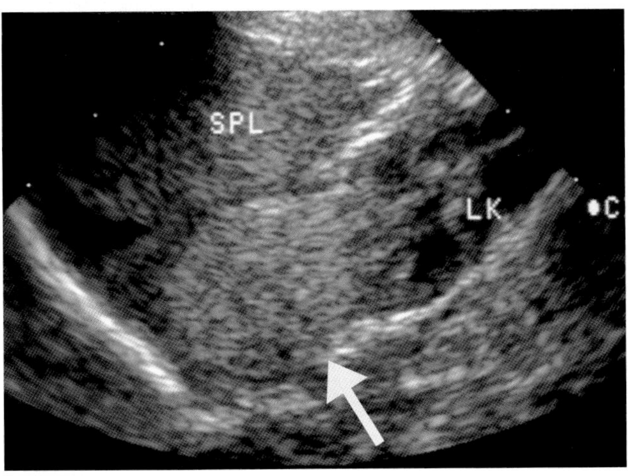

A

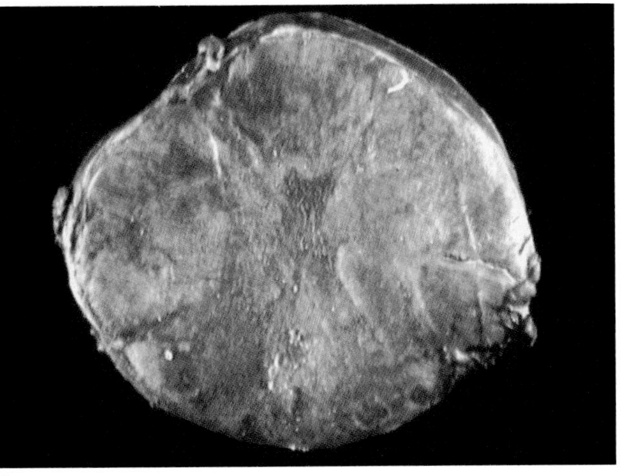

B

FIGURE 21-20 ▪ Neuroblastoma in 2-month-old boy. **A:** Longitudinal ultrasound image demonstrating a homogeneous mass (*arrow*) between the upper pole of the left kidney (LK) and the spleen (SPL). **B:** The sectioned gross specimen shows a homogeneous yellowish-tan tumor and calcifications.

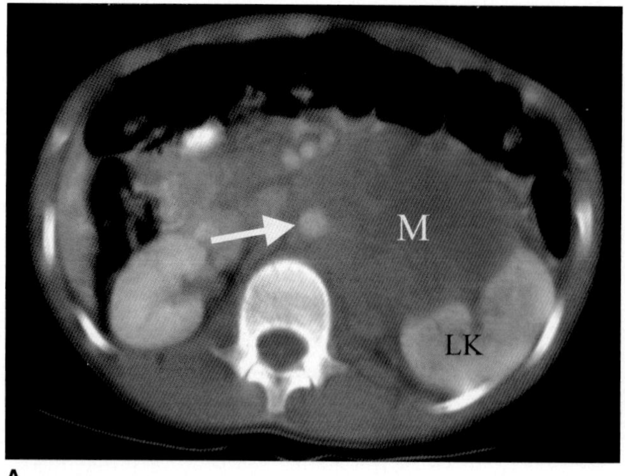

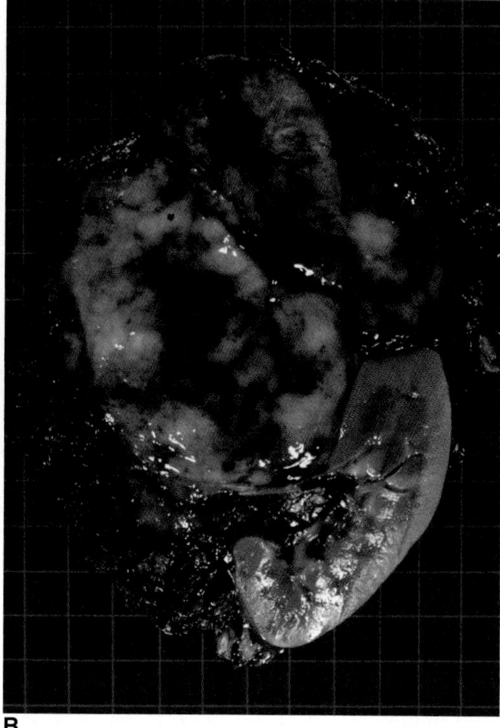

FIGURE 21-21 ■ Neuroblastoma in 9-month-old boy. **A:** Contrast-enhanced CT image of the abdomen demonstrates a mass (M) pushing the left kidney (LK) laterally and surrounding the aorta (*arrow*). **B:** The sectioned gross specimen shows a multinodular, whitish-tan tumor with hemorrhage.

intermingling of parenchymal cells of both organs, are uncommon in childhood (Figure 21-24B, eFigure 21-80) (e508). Alteration of adrenal shape occurs in the presence of renal agenesis where the adrenal gland acquires a flat disk-shape in contrast to its normal triangular appearance (eFigure 21-81).

Ectopic adrenal tissue is usually observed in the abdominal cavity along the celiac axis or along the pathway of

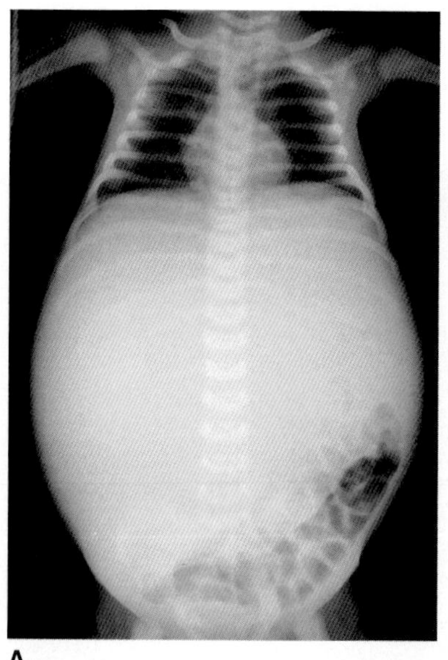

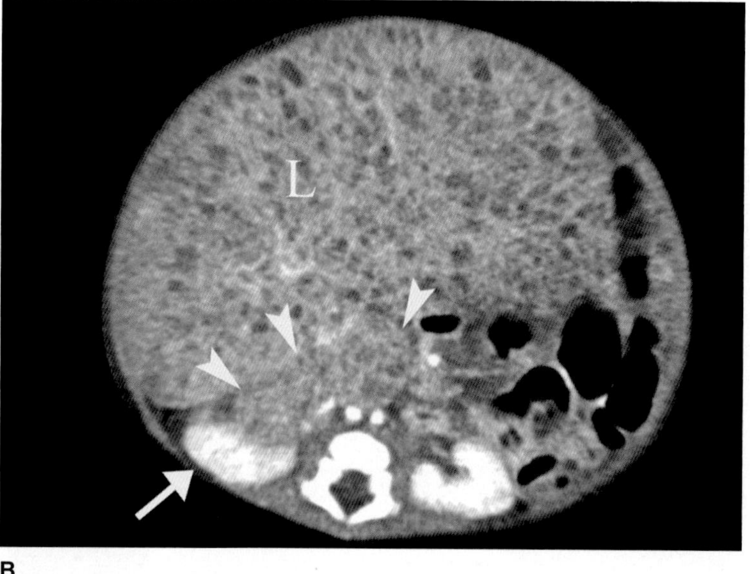

FIGURE 21-22 ■ Congenital stage 4 neuroblastoma with Pepper syndrome. **A:** KUB shows marked enlargement of the liver pushing up on the hemidiaphragms and pushing the air-filled bowel to the left lower quadrant. **B:** Contrast-enhanced CT scan of the abdomen shows a markedly enlarged liver diffusely infiltrated with small hypoattenuating masses (L). Anterior to the right kidney (*arrow*) is an adrenal mass (*arrowheads*).

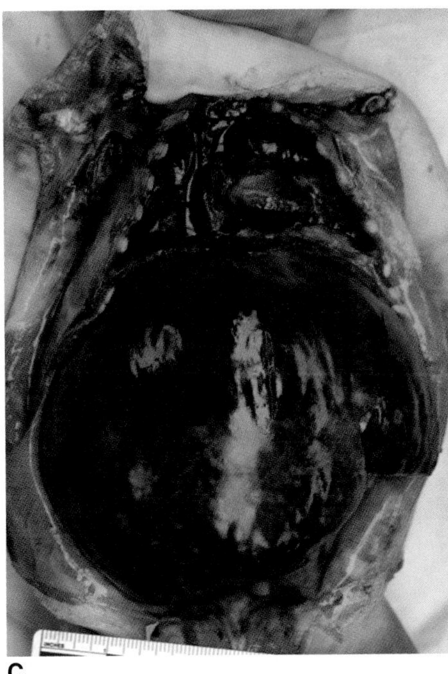

FIGURE 21-22 ■ *(continued)* **C:** Massive hepatomegaly reflects the diffuse infiltration by neuroblastoma.

gonadal descent (e436). Intrarenal ectopia can simulate renal cell carcinoma or an invasive adrenal neoplasm (e1294). Adrenal ectopia is found in as many as 10% of orchiopexies and in approximately 4% of inguinal herniorrhaphies (e605,e760,e799,e894) (see Chapter 19). Ectopic adrenal has also been observed in the lung, liver, brain, ovary, and placenta as a rare isolated event (eFigure 21-82) (e11,e149,e510,e673, e1230,e1262,e1287). Most ectopic adrenal tissue, especially at distant sites, includes only adrenocortical tissue with distinct cortical zonation in some instances. Small islands or nodules of adrenal cortical tissue can be found with some frequency in the fat surrounding the orthotopic adrenal gland. True adrenal gland heterotopia, in which the adrenal gland is absent from its normal location and an adrenal gland with both cortex and medulla is identified, is usually present in the vicinity of the celiac axis but has also been found at distant sites including the brain.

Wolman disease together with the related cholesterol ester storage disease is a heritable disorder characterized by an inborn error of acid lipase A deficiency (10q23.2–q23.3). Vomiting, steatorrhea, failure to thrive, hepatosplenomegaly, and adrenomegaly with bilateral adrenal calcifications visible radiographically are seen in the neonatal period (Figure 21-25A) (e56,e412,e777). Cholesterol and triglycerides accumulate in the lysosomes of the liver, spleen, adrenal glands, gastrointestinal tract, hematopoietic organs, and brain. The adrenal glands are symmetrically enlarged, yellow, and firm. There is a prominent yellow cortical rim and gray-white center (Figure 21-25B). The zona glomerulosa and outer zona fasciculata are histologically unremarkable, but the fetal zone, zona reticularis and inner zona fasciculata have been replaced by haphazardly arranged foamy cells,

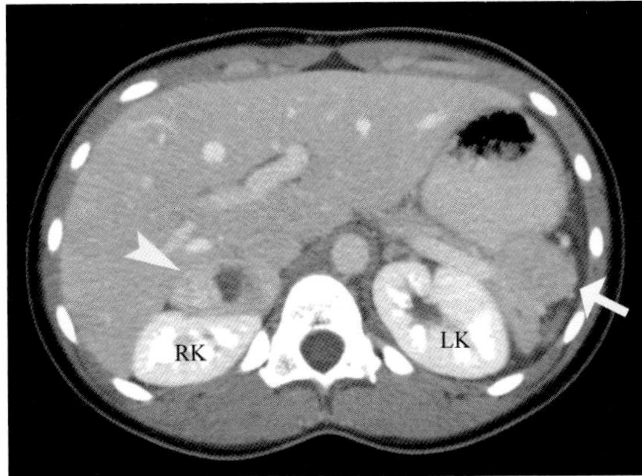

A

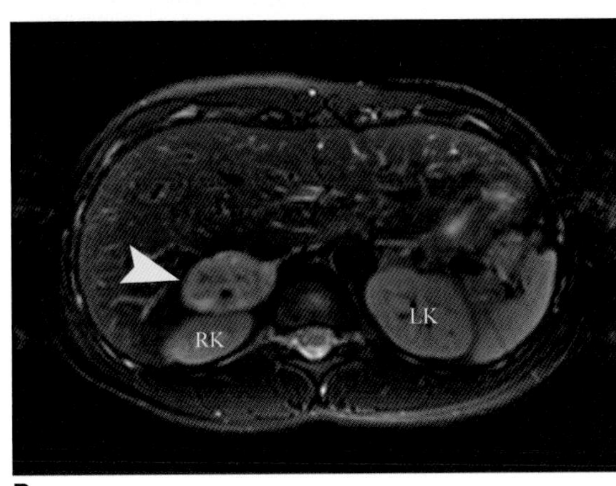

B

FIGURE 21-23 ■ Pheochromocytoma in a 12-year-old girl with hypertension. **A:** Axial contrast-enhanced CT image shows a heterogeneous mass (*arrowhead*) anterior to the right kidney (RK). Also noted is a mass of the pancreatic tail which was a neuroendocrine tumor (*arrow*). **B:** Axial T2-weighted MR image demonstrates a heterogeneous, predominantly-hyperintense mass in the right suprarenal fossa (*arrowhead*).

Table 21-6 ■ CONGENITAL DISORDERS OF THE ADRENAL GLAND

- Agenesis
- Adrenal cytomegaly
- Adrenal fusion
- Congenital adrenal hypoplasia
  - Anencephalic form
  - Cytomegalic form (*NROB1* gene defect, DAX1 mutation)
  - Miniature form
- Congenital adrenal hyperplasia
  - 21-hydroxylase deficiency (*CYP21A2* gene defect)
  - 11 β-hydroylase deficiency (*CYP11B1* gene defect)
  - 17 α-hydroxylase deficiency (*CYP17A1* gene defect)
  - 3β-hydroxysteroid dehydrogenase deficiency (*HSD3β2* gene defect)
  - Cholesterol desmolase deficiency (StAR protein defect) (congenital lipoid adrenal hyperplasia)
- Ectopia
- Metabolic disorders
  - Adrenoleukodystrophy
  - Wolman disease

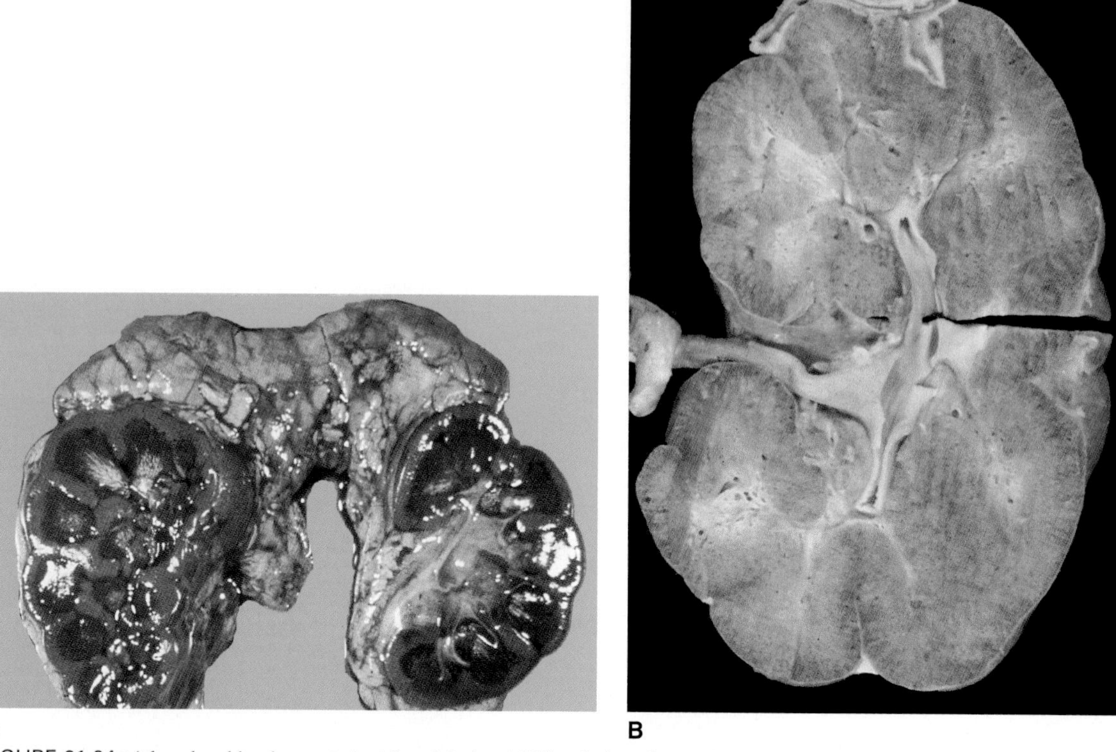

FIGURE 21-24 ■ Adrenal maldevelopment. **A:** Adrenal fusion. Midline fusion of two otherwise normal adrenal glands was found at autopsy in a newborn infant with multiple malformations. **B:** Adrenal accreta. The adrenal gland (*arrow*) was firmly adherent to the adjacent kidney at autopsy. Both organs were separated by a joint band of connective tissue on histological examination.

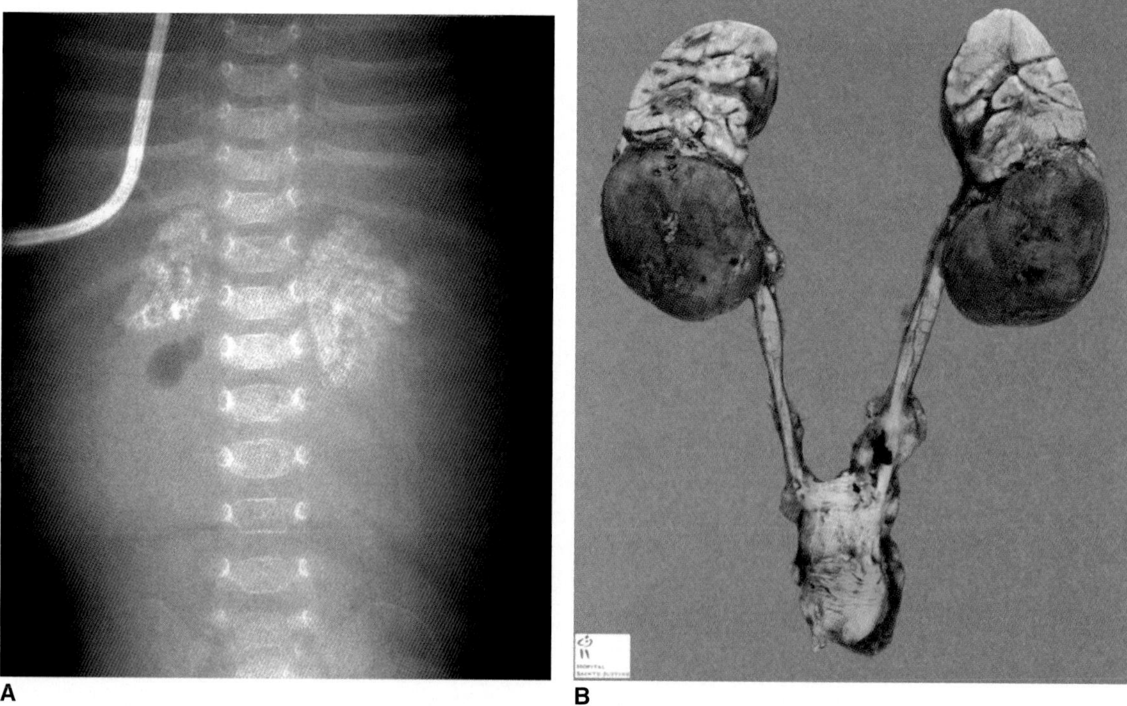

FIGURE 21-25 ■ Wolman disease. **A:** Plain radiograph of the abdomen reveals triangular-shaped collections of mottled calcifications in the expected location of the adrenal glands. **B:** Both adrenals are enlarged and deep yellow in color due to accumulation of cholesterol esters within the adrenal cortex in this autosomal-recessive inherited disease. Image from www.humpath.com. (Reprinted with permission, Dr. Jean-Christophe Fournet, CHU Sainte-Justine, Montreal, Canada.)

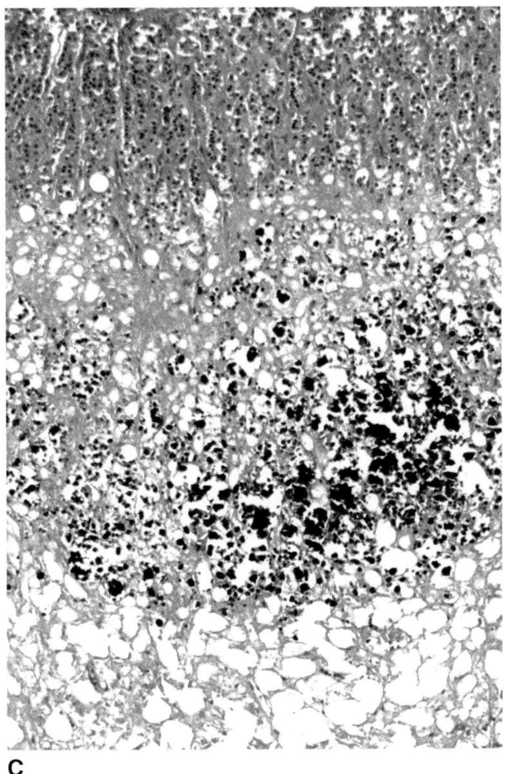

FIGURE 21-25■*(continued)* **C:** Wolman disease was diagnosed in this 3-month-old boy with bilateral adrenal calcifications. The cortical cells of the zona reticularis and inner zona fasciculata are swollen with vacuolated cytoplasm due to cholesterol ester accumulation. Dystrophic calcification is present in the foci of necrosis. (Reprinted with permission from Lack EE, Tumors of the adrenal glands and extraadrenal paraganglia. *AFIP atlas of tumor pathology*, Fourth Series. Washington, DC: American Registry of Pathology).

which are accompanied by focal areas of necrosis and calcifications (Figure 21-25C). Cholesterol clefts may be identified as well (eFigure 21-83) (see Chapter 5).

Adrenoleukodystrophy (ALD), a peroxisomal disorder with defective fatty acid β-oxidation leading to accumulation of very long chain-saturated fatty acids, is associated with inflammatory demyelination of axons and loss of oligodendrocytes and atrophy of the adrenal glands (16,e108, e116,e220,e320,e401,e402,e567,e600,e610,e783,e843, e1092–e1094). A neonatal autosomal recessive form that presents with hypotonia and seizures, and a childhood X-linked recessive form are recognized (e220,e610,e843) The adrenals are atrophic and normal cortical zonation is absent (Figure 21-26A, B, eFigure 21-84). The adrenal medulla appears unremarkable (e108). Cortical nodules of ballooned cells with waxy cytoplasm are observed and between the nodules are macrophages with phagocytized lipid and mild fibrosis. Membrane-bound lipid vacuoles with cholesterol clefts are seen on ultrastructural examination (eFigure 21-85) (e108) (see Chapter 5).

In the X-linked form of ALD [mutations in ABCD1 gene on Xp28 that codes for transporter protein (ALDP) in the peroxisome membrane], estimated to occur in 1:17,000 male infants (hemizygotes and heterozygotes), the adrenals usually weigh 2 g or less (e108,e116). Quantitative (absent) and qualitative defects in ALDP lead to the accumulation of very long chain saturated fatty acids (e108). There are more than 400 recognized mutations leading to variations in the clinical presentation. The morphologic appearance of the adrenal is variable. The zona glomerulosa is recognized but decreased in thickness. The zona fasciculata and reticularis are markedly reduced in thickness so that the zona glomerulosa occupies about half of the adrenal cortex thickness. The medulla is otherwise normal.

Adrenal cytomegaly is usually an incidental finding observed in the fetal cortex, focally or diffusely, in approximately 6% of normal adrenal glands (e61). It is more frequently seen in stillborn, premature and newborn infants; however, it is also observed in older children. The cytomegalic cells contain large (two to three times the normal size),

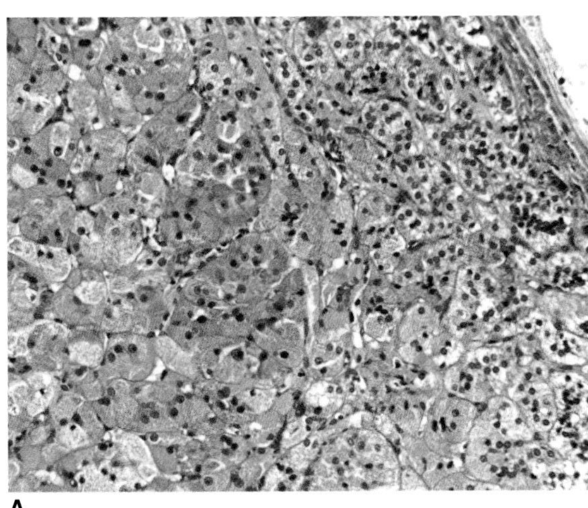

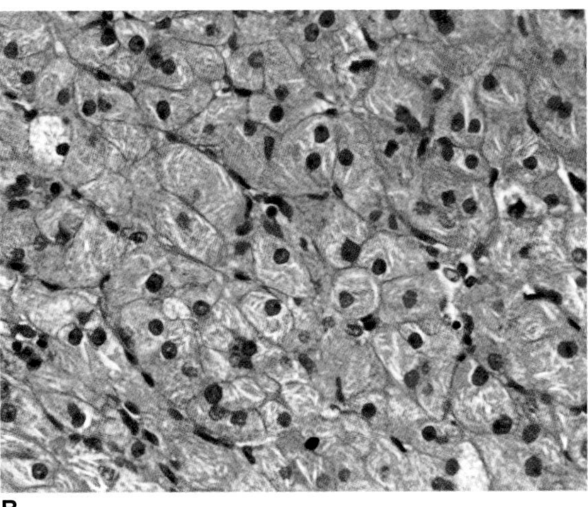

FIGURE 21-26■X-linked adrenoleukodystrophy in a young male child. **A:** There was prominent atrophy of the adrenal cortex at autopsy. The inner cortical cells are enlarged with abundant pale cytoplasm (H&E stain, original magnification 100×). **B:** Cortical nodules of ballooned cells with a waxy cytoplasm and faint striations are observed in this peroxisomal disorder with defective fatty acid β-oxidation leading to accumulation of very long chain-saturated fatty acids within cells (H&E stain, original magnification 200×).

hyperchromatic, pleomorphic nuclei, often with prominent nucleoli and "pseudoinclusions" of cytoplasm and abundant vacuolated eosinophilic cytoplasm (Figure 21-27A, B). Mitoses are absent. These cells have been reported in association with a number of malformational syndromes including trisomies 13 and 18 and in various perinatal-maternal conditions including hemolytic disease of the newborn, nonimmune hydrops, eclampsia, intrauterine infection, sepsis, multifetal gestations, congenital lupus erythematosus, and polyhydramnios (e59,e855). It has also been associated with Rh incompatibility and in utero fetal distress and as an incidental finding in approximately 1% of pediatric autopsies (e357). Adrenal cytomegaly is one of the characteristic features of the Beckwith-Wiedemann syndrome (BWS), which (e365,e896) is a congenital disorder characterized by exomphalos, macroglossia, and giantism. The estimated frequency is 1:13,000 live births. Dysregulation of several genes encoded on chromosome 11p15.5 is thought to be the pathogenetic mechanism (104). Most cases are sporadic (85%); however, an autosomal dominant inheritance with variable expressivity is reported in familial cases (e869,e888,e889). Wilms tumor, hepatoblastoma, adrenocortical neoplasms, NB, pancreaticoblastoma, and PHEO are some of the childhood neoplasms associated with BWS (104). The adrenal glands in BWS are enlarged and may have a combined weight of 16 g or more. Grossly, the glands have cerebriform contours due to cortical hyperplasia (Figure 21-27C, eFigure 21-86). Large cells with bizarre nuclei (adrenal cytomegaly) are a prominent feature and are observed bilaterally. Diffuse sheets of such cells cause marked expansion of the fetal zone (Figure 21-27D, eFigure 21-87). Hemorrhagic cysts may also occur with the formation of an abdominal mass in the neonate (e41,e778).

Congenital adrenal hypoplasia (CAHP) is an uncommon condition with an estimated incidence of 1:12,500 births (e69,e356,e603,e691). Three distinct histological patterns, so-called cytomegalic, anencephalic, and miniature, are recognized (e180). A combined adrenal weight of less than 2 g in a term infant qualifies as hypoplasia. Use of a combined adrenal weight–body weight ratio of less than 1:1000 improves diagnostic accuracy. Utilizing these criteria, CAHP is present in 2% or so of fetopsies and perinatal autopsies. Prenatally, maternal plasma levels of dehydroepiandrosterone sulfate and estriol are useful in detecting CAHP in families at risk (e19,e935). Decreased maternal estriol levels are an important diagnostic clue. X-linked, autosomal recessive, variable, or sporadic inheritances are reported (e121). Most infants with CAHP present with signs of adrenocortical insufficiency and may present as sudden infant death syndrome (e88,e1014).

The cytomegalic type, which is the most common pattern, with X-linked inheritance is due to a deletion or inactivating mutation of *NROB1* (Xp21.3-p21.2) that encodes for DAX-1 which is critical for adrenal gland development. Over 100 mutations involving the *NROB1* gene have been reported accounting for the phenotypic variability (95,139,e3, e8,e80,e503,e934,e936,e1164,e1270). In one series, DAX-1 mutations were found in almost 60% of 46,XY phenotypic boys referred with adrenal hypoplasia and in all boys with hypogonadotropic hypogonadism and a family history of adrenal failure (99,e144). The cytomegalic pattern has also been reported in association with other inheritance patterns (e654). As part of a contiguous gene syndrome, a number of affected males also have glycerol kinase deficiency and Duchenne muscular dystrophy without any CNS anomalies (e246). Grossly, the adrenals are small and lack a definitive cortex (Figure 21-28A). The fetal cortex has a disorganized architectural pattern consisting of clusters of large adenocortical cells with variable nuclear hyperchromasia. The eosinophilic cytoplasm is vacuolated and intranuclear cytoplasmic inclusions may be seen in these cells (Figure 21-28B).

The anencephalic type with autosomal recessive inheritance in many cases resembles the adrenal glands of anencephalic infants but in the absence of anencephaly (eFigure 21-28C, D) (e437). The pituitary and CNS are either normal or may have developmental anomalies. Adrenal insufficiency is noted at birth and hypogonadism may develop at puberty with survival beyond infancy. The small adrenal glands have a definitive, but attenuated cortex and the fetal zone is markedly diminished. An autosomal recessive pattern of inheritance is often present.

The miniature type with a sporadic occurrence or autosomal recessive inheritance is seen in infants without any karyotypic abnormalities or developmental anomalies, although this pattern has been reported in association with triploidy, and trisomies 13 and 18 (e577). Clinical manifestations are dependent upon the degree of hypoplasia. The miniature pattern is associated with the onset of pregnancy-induced hypertension (e170). Grossly, the adrenals are small with a definitive cortex but a diminutive or absent fetal cortex. Otherwise there is normal zonation and an absence of any cellular abnormalities (eFigure 21-88). Hereditary unresponsiveness to ACTH due to mutations involving the ACTH receptor gene may mimic CAHP (95,188).

Congenital adrenal hyperplasia (CAH), also known as adrenogenital syndrome, is a group of autosomal recessive disorders of adrenal steroid biosynthesis with similar morphologic features (29,30,86,95,188,e412,e526,e708, e803–e805,e817,e864,e990,e1122,e1123,e1258,e1259,e1274). The incidence of CAH is 1:500 to 1:16,000 live births, dependent on the population sampled, and is the most frequent cause of ambiguous genitalia in the neonate and/or of primary adrenal insufficiency in the pediatric population (29,30,86,95,188, e579,e934,e1178). Approximately 90% to 95% of CAH cases are due to 21-hydroxylase deficiency and 5% to 8% due to 11 β-hydroxylase deficiency (29,30,86,95,188,e803,e864,e214, e269,e427,e527,e536,e571,e598,e607,e662,e681,e697,e699, e937,e1120,e1121,e1178,e1273). Decreased cortisol production interrupts the normal feedback inhibition on the pituitary gland, leading to persistent ACTH secretion and continued synthesis of cortisol precursors up to the level of the enzymatic

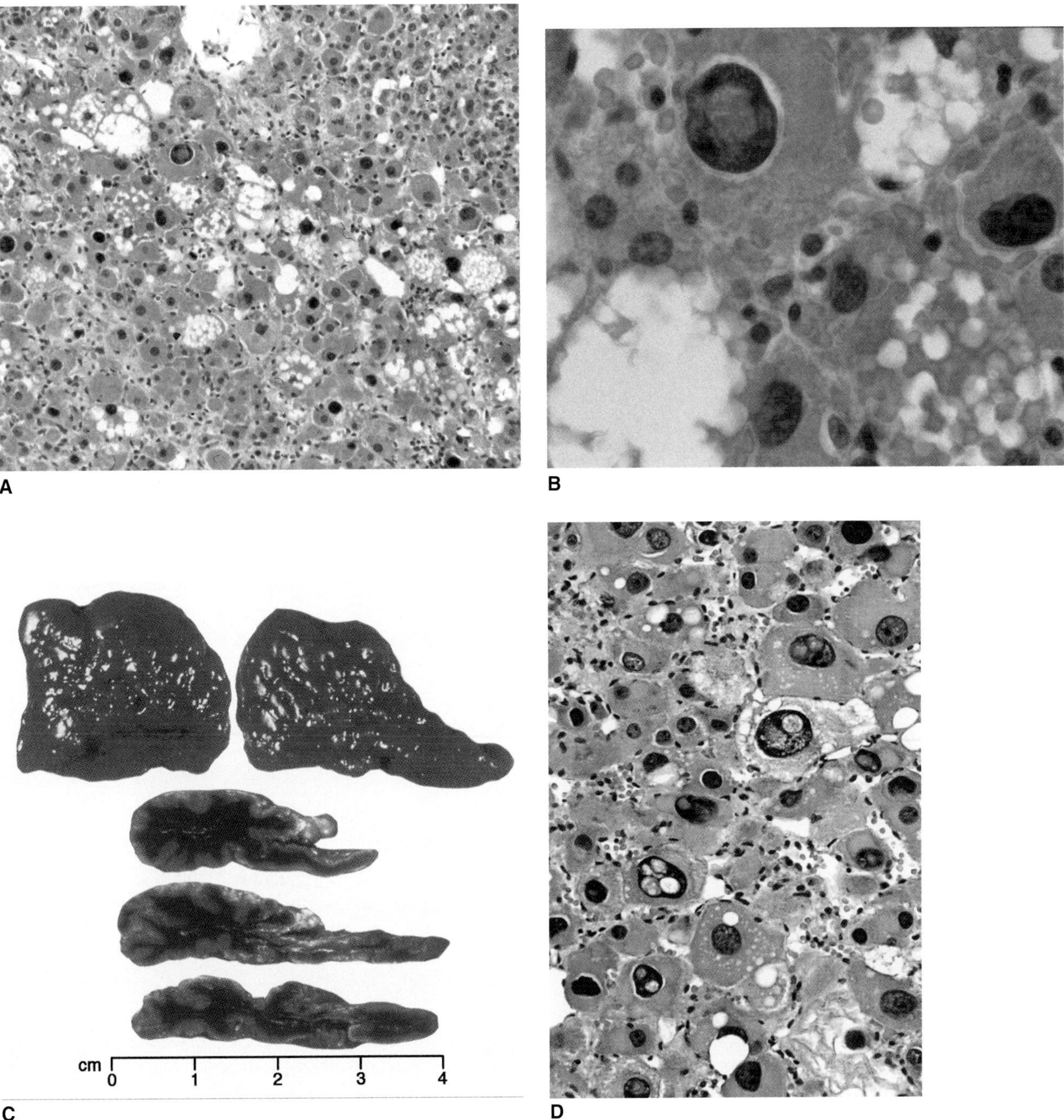

FIGURE 21-27 ■ Adrenal cytomegaly. **A:** Cytomegaly of the fetal adrenal cortex characterized by large cells with hyperchromatic nuclei is seen in this term infant with in utero fetal demise due to a cord accident (H&E stain). **B:** Nuclear pseudoinclusion (cytoplasmic invagination into the nucleus) are seen in this image of adrenal cytomealy from a term infant with in utero fetal demise (H&E stain). **C:** The adrenal glands from a 3-week-old infant with Beckwith-Wiedemann syndrome are hyperplastic with increased cortical nodularity and redundant folds. (Reprinted with permission from Lack EE, Tumors of the adrenal glands and extraadrenal paraganglia. *AFIP atlas of tumor pathology*, 4th Series. Washington, DC: American Registry of Pathology). **D:** There is marked cytomegaly with nuclear enlargement, hyperchromasia and nuclear "pseudoinclusions" in this section of fetal cortex from an infant with Beckwith-Wiedemann syndrome on histological examination (H&E stain). (Reprinted with permission from Lack EE. Tumors of the adrenal glands and extraadrenal paraganglia. *AFIP atlas of tumor pathology*, Fourth Series. Washington, DC: American Registry of Pathology).

defect. Symptoms and laboratory findings are dependent on which enzyme is absent. The diagnosis of CAH can be made prenatally by chorionic villus sampling during the first trimester (29,30,86,e143,e209,e511,e846,e861–e863,e877–e879, e881,e885,e1124). Many states have neonatal screening programs for 17-hydroxyprogesterone to detect 21-hydroxylase deficiency. The administration of dexamethasone which crosses the placenta before 8 weeks gestation, has been

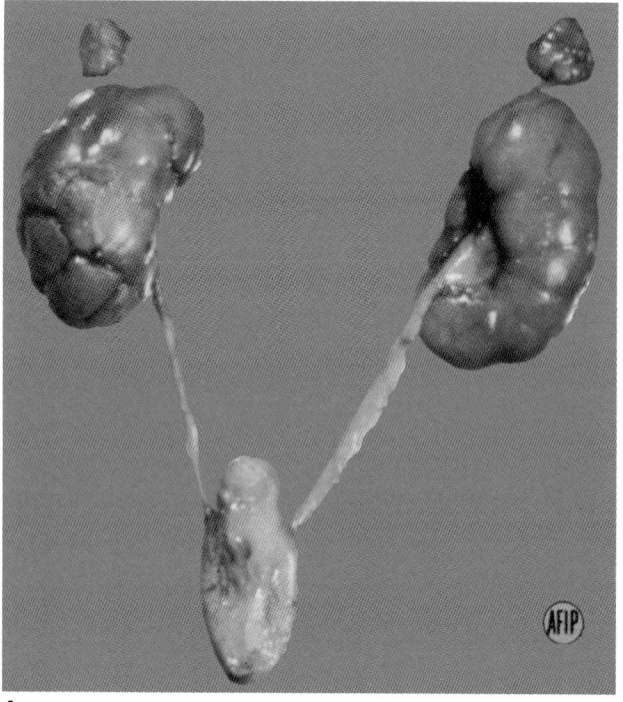

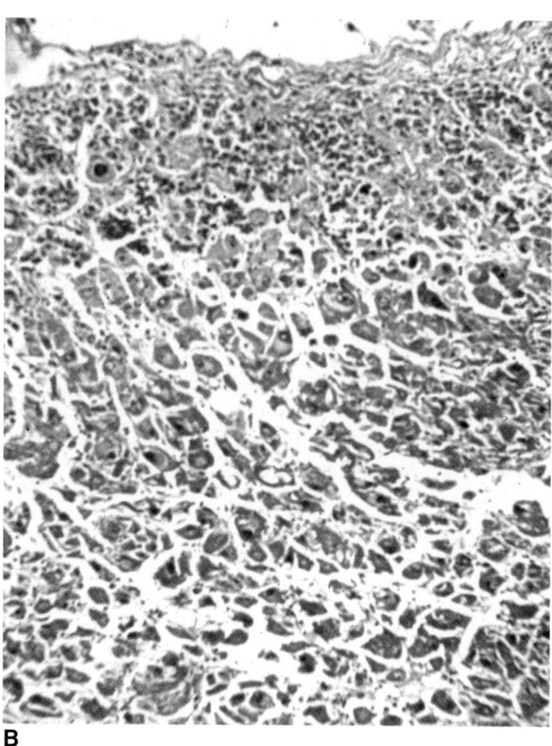

A B

FIGURE 21-28 ▪ Congenital adrenal hypoplasia. **A:** Section of bladder, kidneys, and adrenals from a 470 g preterm male infant. The combined adrenal weight was 0.147 g (versus expected of 2.5 g). The brain and pituitary were normal on gross examination. A normal component of acidophilic cells was present in the pituitary. **B:** The adrenal glands consisted of large cells with abundant eosinophillic cytoplasm. The nuclei were large and bizarre with eosinophillic inclusions similar to adrenal cytomegaly. (From James Arey, M.D., Luther Youngs, M.D. Pediatric pathology: congenital malformations [Slide collection, 1966]. Washington, DC: The Armed Forces Institute of Pathology.)

helpful in preventing virilization of the external genitalia in utero (29,30,86). The clinical, laboratory and genetic features are beyond the scope of this chapter but are reviewed at length by others (29,30,86,188,e412,e526,e708,e803–e805,e817, e864,e990,e1122,e1123,e1259,e1274).

The 21-hydroxylase deficiency (21-OHD) is the most common form of CAH (29,30,86,95,188,e880e269,e427, e527,e536,e579,e598,e1121,e1178,e1258,e1273). Clinical manifestations vary with the severity of the enzymatic deficiency (e1120). The affected gene, *CYP21A2*, is located in the region of the major histocompatibility complex III on chromosome 6p21.3 (29,30,86,95,e311,e427,e813,e990). Intergenic recombinations occur between *CYP21A2* and the pseudogene *CYP21A1P*; these events account for most of the mutations (80% of cases), and the remainder are deletions in *CYP21* (29,30,86,e352,e709,e839,e1136,e1273). Three distinct clinical patterns of 21-OHD are recognized, classic salt-wasting, simple virilizing (70% and 30% of classic subtypes, respectively), and nonclassic milder subtypes (29,30,86,95,188,e880,e70,e817). It is thought that these three types represent a continuum from mild to severe rather than three distinct phenotypes. Greater than 50 *CYP21A2* mutations have been described and these determine the particular phenotypic expression (86). The incidence for the classic salt-wasting form is 1:10,000 to 1:16,000 live births, and the milder form may be as frequent as 1:500 to 1:1,000 individuals which makes this condition one of the most common autosomal recessive disorders (29,30,86,188, e70,e860,e1273). In the classic form, failure to convert progesterone to the mineralocorticoids, deoxycorticosterone and aldosterone, leads to decreased sodium reabsorption by the kidney, resulting in hyponatremia, hyperkalemia, acidosis, shock, and death. Decreased glucocorticoid production due to the failure to convert 17-hydroxyprogesterone to 11-deoxycortisol leads to lack of negative feedback on the pituitary gland and subsequent unimpeded ACTH secretion. The increased production of adrenal androgens causes virilization of the external genitalia, with fusion of the labioscrotal fold in the most severe form in which case the female infant has a male-appearing external genitalia at birth. Hydrops of fetal stem villi has been reported in CAH (e392). Signs of androgen excess, characterize the nonclassic form at puberty, with premature adrenarche, menstrual irregularities, acne, hirsutism, and sclerocystic ovaries (29,30). Mineralocorticoid activity is adequate. An attenuated pattern with biochemical abnormalities only is also recognized.

The 11-β-hydroxylase deficiency is the second most frequent pattern and accounts for 5% to 8% of cases

(29,30,86,95,188,e214,e571,e662,e846,e937). The incidence is approximately 1:100,000 to 1:200,000 live births. Greater than 50 different inactivating mutations involving the 11 β-hydroxylase gene (*CYP11B1*) on chromosome 8q21 are identified (29,30,86,95,188). Failure to convert 11-deoxycortisol to cortisol and 11-deoxycorticosterone to corticosterone results in increased mineralocorticoid activity, leading to hypernatremia, hypokalemia, and hypertension. Lack of negative feedback inhibition by cortisol leads to increased androgen production. Female pseudohermaphroditism and virilization of male and female infants postnatally are the other major manifestations (see Chapter 18).

The 17-α-hydroxylase deficiency (*CYP17A1*) accounts for approximately 1% of cases. Deficiency leads to failure to hydroxylate pregnenolone and progesterone, resulting in decreased synthesis of androgens and cortisol (29,30,86,95,188,e118,e397,e1041). Increased synthesis of corticosterone may cause hypertension. Affected females may present at puberty with primary amenorrhea and males are incompletely masculinized (29,30,86,95,188, e118,e397,e1041).

The 3β-hydroxysteroid dehydrogenase deficiency and steroidogenic acute regulatory protein (StAR; cholesterol desmolase deficiency) are rare causes of CAH (29,30,86, 95,188,e9,e76,e139,e430,e570,e818,e911,e914,e1021, e1098). The 3β-hydroxysteroid dehydrogenase (*HSD3β2*) deficiency leads to salt wasting and female pseudohermaphroditism and precocious masculinization in male infants. The so-called congenital lipoid adrenal hyperplasia is the only one of this group of disorders that is not caused by a defective steroidogenic enzyme but is rather a defect in the StAR protein which is required for the transport of cholesterol to the inner mitochondrial membrane for conversion to pregnenolone. Greater than 34 different mutations are present in the gene encoding for the StAR protein. Korean and Japanese populations are notably affected with these mutations. These infants have adrenal insufficiency and a female phenotype (29,30,86,188,e1295).

Bilateral hyperplasia of the adrenal glands, with weights two to four times normal size, is the typical finding; however, normal-size glands are reported (104,e1041) (Figure 21-29A, B). The external surfaces have a cerebriform appearance. Depletion of the lipid-rich cells of the zona fasciculata to compact eosinophilic cells, identical to those observed normally in the zona reticularis, gives the glands a dark, tan-brown color on sectioning (Figure 21-29C, D, eFigure 21-89). The exception occurs in the adrenals of those individuals who have been partially treated with steroids. The zone fasciculata under ACTH stimulation shows the greatest degree of hyperplasia among the three zones of the cortex. In contrast to the other forms of CAH, cholesterol accumulated in the cytoplasm of the cortical cells imparts a bright yellow, nodular appearance to the cortex in congenital lipoid adrenal hyperplasia (104,e422,e1167). Lipid-rich cells, cholesterol clefts, foreign body giant cells, and calcifications are the principal histological features. There is some resemblance in the latter respect to the adrenals in Wolman disease. The presence of bilateral adrenal incidentaloma (unsuspected, nonhyperfunctional adrenal nodule), adrenal adenomas and the development of adrenocortical carcinoma has been reported in association with CAH (88,89,e28,e111,e667, e1001,e1220).

Bilateral nodular hyperplasia of testicular adrenal rests [testicular adrenal rest tumors (TART)] is reported with some frequency in CAH in as many as 90% or more of adult males (27,88,e62–e64,e103,e106,e236–e238,e240,e265, e411,e588,e706,e764,e849,e984,e985,e1126,e1133,e1134, e1133). Male infertility secondary to primary gonadal failure is associated with TART. The testis has a firm multilobular, tan-brown appearance on cross-section and is commonly localized in the rete testis (eFigure 21-90). Confluent sheets of polygonal cells with eosinophilic cytoplasm resembling adrenocortical tissue are present on microscopic examination (eFigure 21-91). These cells have the biochemical attributes of adrenocortical cells. Morphological differentiation of TART from the Leydig cell tumor is difficult but TART tends to be bilateral in contrast to Leydig cell tumor. Reinke crystals are absent in TART but present in up to 35% of Leydig cells tumors. These nodules can be locally resected in an attempt to preserve testicular parenchyma (e1126) (see Chapter 19). Bilateral ovarian steroid cell tumors and malignant Leydig cell tumors have also been reported in the setting of CAH (see Chapters 18 and 19) (e86,e279,e1015).

Primary pigmented (micronodular) adrenocortical disease (PPAD) is associated with Cushing syndrome and 25% to 35% of cases have the manifestations of Carney complex with myxomas, spotty skin pigmentation, and endocrine hyperactivity (89,104,e195,e196,e231,e362,e540, e1086,e1138,e1139,e1141,e1142,e1147). In addition to PPAD in 45% of cases, growth hormone secreting PAs are present in about 10% of cases (e906). Two affected genetic loci in this autosomal recessive disorder have been mapped to chromosomes 2p16 and 17q22,24 (PRKAR1A) (89,104, e444,e614,e615,e753,e1147,e776,e1031). Pathologically, the adrenals are decreased, normal, or slightly increased in size. Multiple pigmented nodules less than 4 mm in diameter occupy an otherwise atrophic appearing cortex with loss of normal zonation (eFigure 21-92). Nodules may be present in the periadrenal fat (e613,e633). The enlarged cortical cells have an eosinophilic cytoplasm with abundant lipofuscin pigment (eFigure 21-93). These cells are immunoreactive for SYN but fail to stain for CHR (e1143). In this respect, the cortical nodules of PPAD react in a similar manner to adrenocortical neoplasms.

Adrenocortical hyperplasia is also seen in BWS, MAS, and MEN 1. Cushing syndrome in the setting of MAS is associated with autonomously functioning multinodular hyperplasia of the adrenals (e612). Cushing syndrome is present in 30% to 40% of cases of MEN 1 (e345).

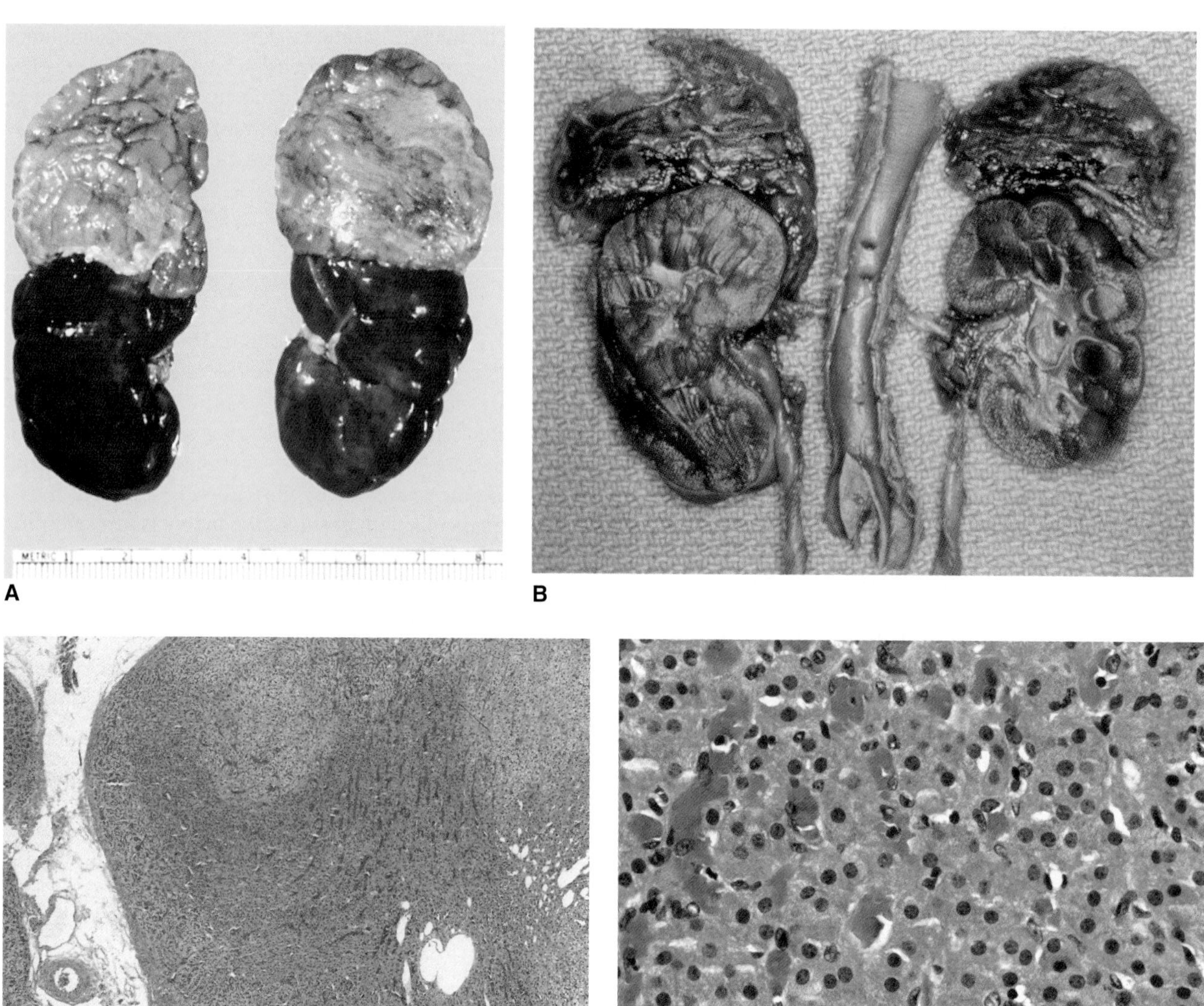

FIGURE 21-29 Congenital adrenal hyperplasia in a 7-week-old boy who had signs of intestinal obstruction. **A:** The kidneys and adrenal glands are shown, and the enlarged adrenals (combined weight 16.8 g) have a convoluted cerebriform appearance due to the hyperplastic cortex. (From James Arey, M.D., Luther Youngs, M.D. Pediatric pathology: congenital malformations Slide collection, 1966. Washington, DC: The Armed Forces Institute of Pathology.) **B:** This image of kidneys, adrenals and aorta is from another child with congenital adrenal hyperoplasia showing enlarged cerebriform adrenals. **C:** The adrenal cortex is enlarged due to marked expansion of the zona fasciculata in congenital adrenal hyperplasia. The cortex is predominantly characterized by a pattern of compact cells with focal collections of clear cells with lipid-rich cytoplasm interspersed (H&E stain). (Reprinted with permission from Lloyd RV, Douglas BR, Young WF. Endocrine diseases. *Atlas of nontumor pathology*. Washington, DC: American Registry of Pathology.) **D:** High power image showing lipid depletion of zona fasciculata cells with compact eosinophillic cytoplasm in congenital adrenal hyperplasia (H&E stain). (Reprinted with permission from Lloyd RV, Douglas BR, Young WF. Endocrine diseases. *Atlas of nontumor pathology*. Washington, DC: American Registry of Pathology.)

Adrenocortical insufficiency can be congenital or acquired (188,e902,e934). ALD, CAHP, and CAH are the primary adrenal disorders with accompanying adrenal insufficiency. Other inherited syndromes with adrenal insufficiency include Smith-Lemli-Opitz syndrome, Kearns-Sayre syndrome, and ACTH insensitivity syndrome. Infections, autoimmune disorders, adrenal hemorrhage, and drugs represent acquired etiologies. In children autoimmune involvement can be isolated or part of an autoimmune syndrome. Autoimmune polyglandular syndrome, type 1, a multisystem autoimmune disease, is associated with adrenal insufficiency and hypoparathyroidism. Pituitary and other CNS diseases, as discussed previously, are secondary causes. In one review, CAH was the most common etiology of adrenal insufficiency which accounted for about 70% of cases with autoimmune adrenalitis as the second most common etiology (e944). These findings are similar to the study by Osuwannaratana et al. who observed that greater than 85% of cases were examples of CAH with panhypopituitarism as the most common cause of secondary adrenal insufficiency (e902,e934).

Acquired Disorders

Adrenal cysts are relatively uncommon in children (104,e84,e174). There are four histopathogenetic types: epithelial, endothelial, pseudocystic, and parasitic (e98,e379). Adrenal neoplasms can undergo cystic necrosis and simulate a large benign cyst, especially the cystic NB in the infant (e61,e261). Cystic cortical degeneration with microcysts may be seen in stillborn infants exposed to substantial stress in utero. Adrenal cysts are also present in a number of syndromes including BWS, autosomal recessive polycystic kidney disease, prune-belly syndrome, and Gorlin-Goltz syndrome (e16,e87,e234,e509,e551,e778,e842). Idiopathic adrenal cysts are reported from the neonatal period into adolescence (e156).

Bacterial, fungal, parasitic, and viral infections can involve the adrenal glands. Adrenal infections with or without necrosis are found in congenital intrauterine infections (*Herpes simplex* with necrosis, cytomegalovirus with adrenalitis or necrosis), *Varicella-zoster* and congenital or acquired immunodeficiency disorders (eFigures 21-94 and 21-95) (e1011). Histoplasmosis and tuberculosis are also recognized causes of Addison disease (e432,e454,e593,e1039). Paracoccidioidomycosis has been observed in children in South America (e927) (see Chapter 6).

Adrenal hemorrhage occurs in a wide spectrum of lesions in children and adults (e1228). The hemorrhage may range from massive involvement of the gland to focal segmental necrosis. Unilateral or bilateral involvement is dependent in some cases on the etiology. Fetal adrenal hemorrhage occurs with some frequency and has been observed as early as the second trimester (e350,359). Although many lesions in the perinatal period are ascribed to birth trauma and in utero asphyxia, the etiology for most adrenal hemorrhages is uncertain in many cases (e595). Trauma, sepsis, shock, underlying coagulopathy, arterial thrombosis secondary to umbilical artery catheterization, extracorporeal membrane oxygenation (ECMO), neonatal stress, and renal vein thrombosis have been reported in association with neonatal adrenal hemorrhage (eFigure 21-96) (e48,e178,e552,e809,e897, e943,e1066,e1100,e1117,e1177). Massive adrenal hemorrhage is one of several sources of an abdominal mass in an infant. Imaging studies are helpful in the diagnosis (e219,e810). Resolution of a hemorrhage with progressive calcifications is well documented (eFigure 21-97). One should keep in mind the possibility of a NB (e310). Spontaneous resolution after birth is a feature of the adrenal hemorrhage in contrast to an adrenal tumor (e1236). Transient adrenocortical insufficiency has been observed. Rarely, adrenal abscess formation complicates adrenal hemorrhage (e60).

Trauma, adrenal tumors, stress, and infection are important considerations in the differential diagnosis of adrenal hemorrhage in older children and adolescents. The trauma-associated adrenal hemorrhage is unilateral with a preference for the right adrenal gland (eFigure 21-98) (e1099). Child abuse must be considered in the differential diagnosis of traumatic adrenal hemorrhage. Unilateral involvement of the right adrenal gland with adrenal medullary hemorrhage on histological examination has been found in child abuse cases (e882). Bilateral adrenal hemorrhagic necrosis in the setting of sepsis with rapid onset of circulatory collapse, petechial rash (noninflammatory microangiopathy), and coagulopathy is known as the Waterhouse-Friderichsen syndrome (WFS), and is most commonly associated with meningococcemia (e558,e695,e1222). Other common infectious agents in children associated with WFS include group A β-*hemolytic streptococci* and *Haemophilus influenza* (e409,e419,e558). Congenital asplenia or splenic atrophy in the setting of sickle cell anemia is a risk association for bacterial septicemia and development of WFS in children (e583,e726). Acute adrenal insufficiency is common (e480). Adrenal hemorrhage in WFS begins in the adrenal reticular plexus and extends toward the capsule (Figure 21-30A). There is a loss of the adrenal cortical parenchyma with hemorrhage as well as partial or complete cortical necrosis (Figure 21-30B). Subcapsular hematomas may form and extend into the periadrenal fat and surrounding tissues in severe cases. Histological examination reveals compression of the sinusoidal capillaries with occasional rupture. Small fibrin thrombi may be seen in the sinusoidal capillaries as features of a microangiopathy (e131).

Calcifications of the adrenal glands are found in several defined settings but most notably Wolman disease and resolving adrenal hemorrhage (eFigure 21-97) (104, e56,e310,e412). There are also individual reports of adrenal calcifications in association with congenital nephrotic syndrome, as a sequela to congenital infections, congenital heart disease and BWS (eFigure 21-94B) (104,e539,e546,e841, e903,e952,e1018,e1221).

Adrenal cortical neoplasms (ACNs) include the adrenocortical adenoma (AA) and carcinoma (ACC), and are rare in the pediatric age group (90,189,e137,e315,e474,e807, e1032,e1146,e1171). The clinicopathological features of ACN in children, their behavior and epidemiology contrast nominally with the same neoplasms in adults. However, one of the consistent observations is that these neoplasms in children, though having several morphologic features associated with ACC in adults, do not have the same unfavorable prognostic implications, especially in children under 6 years of age (40,90). Because these atypical histological features are commonly found

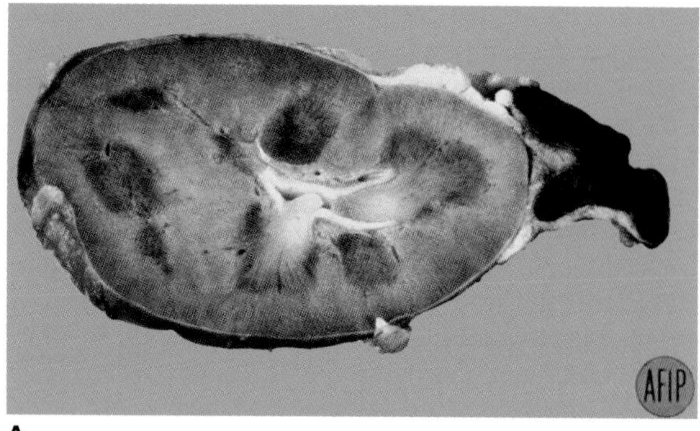

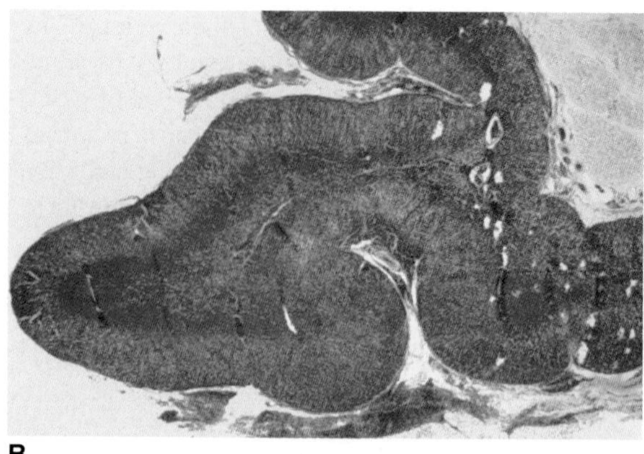

A B

FIGURE 21-30■**A,B:** Waterhouse-Frederichsen syndrome in a young child who died of meningococcal sepsis is manifested by adrenal hemorrhage on gross examination and diffuse hemorrhage throughout the cortex and medulla on histological examination (H&E stain).

in ACNs in children, they are disproportionately interpreted as ACCs. The incidence of cases classified as ACCs in children in the United States was 0.2 cases: 1,000,000 individuals less than 19 years of age (67). ACC accounts for less than 0.5% of all pediatric malignancies but is the third most common carcinoma in children exceeded by PTC and salivary gland carcinoma (40,90,e575).

There is a bimodal age distribution of ACNs and they are more common in females in the pediatric population. In a report of 256 cases from the International Pediatric Adrenocortical Tumor Registry (IPATR), the male to female ratio was 1:1.6 (112). Two age distributions were noted by the IPATR, an infantile group with a peak incidence in the first year of life and an adolescent group with a peak incidence between 9 and 16 years. A female predilection with a mean age at diagnosis of 4.6 years and nearly 50% of cases diagnosed in the first 4 years of life has been documented by others (40,e181,e237,e450,e681,e723,e857). The experience of Dehner and Hill is similar (40). In a review of 39 cases, ACN presented in children between 7 days and 12 years of age with a mean age of 3 years and median of 2 years (40). Seventy-six percent of children were less than 4 years. The male:female ratio was 1:2.5. Others have reported similar findings (e177,e233,e444,e676,e718). There are congenital examples of ACNs (90,e181,e555,e1040). One of the highest incidences of purported ACCs in children (4.7 cases:1,000,000) has been identified in southern Brazil where a distinct germline *p53* mutation has been found in the population, but whose other features are not those of classic Li-Fraumeni syndrome (e177,e444,e781,e981,e982).

There are several syndromic associations with ACNs including BWS (hemihypertrophy, splanchnomegaly, macroglossia, and intraabdominal neoplasms), the Li-Fraumeni syndrome, and Carney complex (40,90,e335,e365,e513, e555,e693,e712,e869,e888,e889,e976,e1129,e1147,e1269). Adrenal hyperplasia and ACN have been reported in MEN 1 syndrome, MAS, and neurofibromatosis 1 (e187,e1239,e1263). Examples of ACN have been seen in the setting of CAH (e667,e1001). Bilateral ACNs, often seen in syndromic-associated cases, and ectopic ACNs are uncommon (40, e601,e555).

Adrenocortical neoplasms in children account for 50% to 70% of cases of Cushing syndrome, in contrast to only 20% of cases in adults (e137,e315,e1161). Less often does an ACN present with feminizing and masculinizing manifestations in children. Conn syndrome, due to an aldosterone-producing ACN, is rare in childhood. Most tumors in Conn syndrome are benign and characterized by their lipid-rich clear cells (e81,e291,e711).

The most important initial step in the pathologic examination of an ACN in childhood is weighing the tumor, since all other gross and histopathologic attributes of the tumor itself are in a sense secondary, if the tumor is confined to the gland and does not have evidence of metastatic spread to regional lymph nodes or to more distant sites such as the liver and lungs. In some cases, it may be difficult to judge whether a circumscribed mass in the adrenal is part of multinodular hyperplasia of the cortex or even a PHEO (eFigure 21-99) (e49,e758).

Cortical neoplasms, not only in children but in adults, vary in size, weight, coloration, consistency (solid and/or cystic), presence or absence of hemorrhage, and presence or absence of necrosis (Figures 21-31 to 21-33, eFigure 21-100). A complete or incomplete fibrous capsule may be apparent at the periphery of the tumor, or the tumor appears to compress the adjacent parenchyma without a capsule. As noted earlier, the size and weight, especially the latter, are closely correlated with the clinical outcome of an ACN in a child. The cut surface in the absence of hemorrhage and necrosis often has a pale to bright yellow to yellow-brown appearance which may or may not be uniform throughout because of cystic changes (Figure 21-31A, eFigure 21-100). Uncommonly, the tumor may have a brownish-black appearance due to lipofuscin accumulation in the cytoplasm of tumor cells as in the case of the PPAD. A hemorrhagic mass may be difficult to differentiate from a NB.

A number of pathologic studies in the literature have examined every conceivable microscopic feature of ACN for their

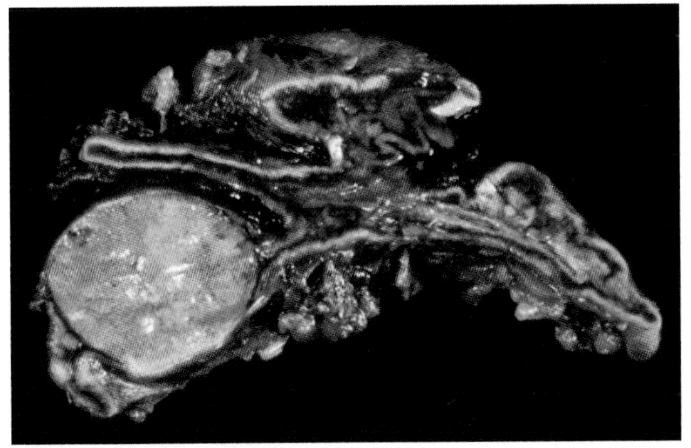

A

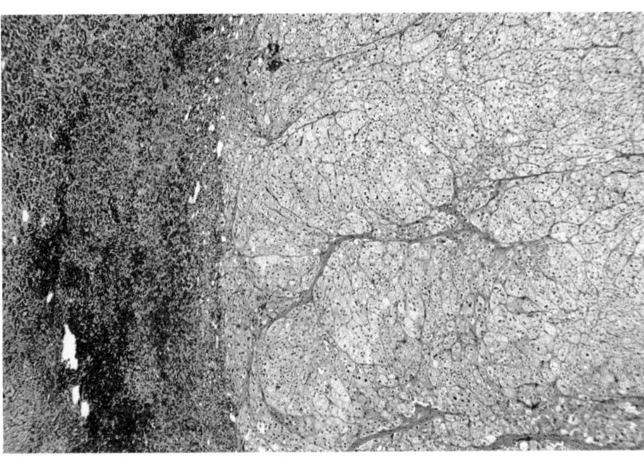

B

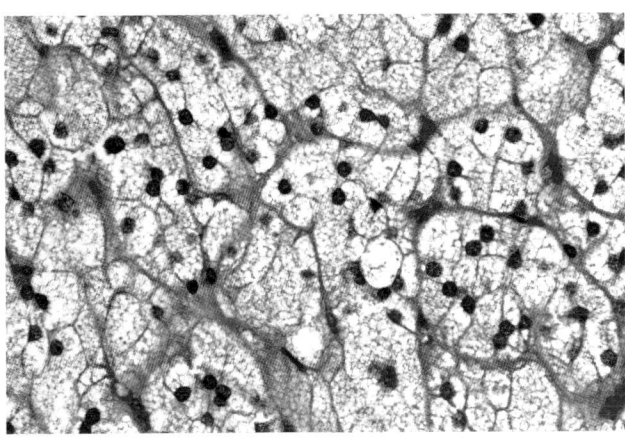

C

FIGURE 21-31 ■ Adrenal adenoma. **A:** This adrenalectomy specimen that weighed 35 g was from a 17-year-old male who presented with hypertension. A 2-cm diameter yellow cortical nodule surrounded by a thin rim of stretched uninvolved adrenocortical tissue is present. The remainder of the adrenal gland shows the typical zonation and was unremarkable. **B:** Low power magnification demonstrating an adrenal adenoma with lipid-laden cells (balloon cells) arranged in small clusters that are surrounded by a thin delicate vascular network. A rim of uninvolved (nonneoplastic) adrenocortical tissue compressed by the mass with focal hemorrhage is on the left (H&E stain). **C:** High power magnification shows the typical clear lipid-laden cells arranged in small clusters. Cellular and nuclear pleomorphism was not present. Mitotic figures were absent (H&E stain). This tumor would be classified as an adrenocortical neoplasm, low risk in Dehner and Hill's proposed classification (see Table 21-7 reproduced from Dehner LP, Hill A. Adrenal cortical neoplasms in children: Why so many carcinomas and yet so many survivors? *Pediatr Dev Pathol* 2009;12:284–291).

predictive prognostic value, but most of the studies have consisted principally of tumors in adults where cytologic atypia, mitotic activity, zonal necrosis and transecting fibrous bands have predictive value in terms of outcome when several of these features are present in the ACN. Some of these same histological features are found with some frequency in ACNs in children yet lack any significant correlation with prognosis. The classic pattern of an ACN is a neoplasm which is composed of clear or pale polygonal cells with abundant lipid-rich cytoplasm or cells with more homogeneous eosinophilic cytoplasm, all arranged in short cords or trabecular profiles (Figure 21-31B, C, eFigure 21-101). The nuclei are uniform and centrally positioned in the cell. The adjacent cortex is often compressed and atrophic (eFigure 21-102). Other histological patterns include diffuse, formless sheets of relatively monotonous polygonal cells, alveolar pattern of loosely cohesive cells, glandular profiles, a yolk sac tumor-like pattern and delicate ribbons of cells in a hyaline myxoid stroma, either as an exclusive pattern or component of the ACN (40,189,e184,e294,e344,e521,e792,e1264).

If polymorphism is the theme for the various patterns in ACNs in children, then pleomorphism applies to the individual cellular features (Figures 21-32 and 21-33, eFigure 21-103). In some ACNs, monomorphism is an appropriate characterization in the presence of uniform tumor cells. Especially prominent in cases of ACNs in children who are usually 4 years old or less is pleomorphism in terms of individual cell size as bordering on tumor giant cells with bizarre nuclear configurations and intense hyperchromatism; these latter cell types when present can constitute a minor or major component of a particular tumor (Figure 21-33).

By contrast, some tumors can have substantial mitotic activity yet are small (less 100 g) and confined to the gland. Other features of ACNs in children can include necrosis, either as individual cells, or microfoci or macrofoci of necrosis which may have been appreciated in the gross examination. Intratumoral microinvasion of blood vessels and apparent microscopic breaching of the capsule are additional histological findings (Figure 21-33).

It would appear from the preceding paragraph that an ACN with some of these features has attained the threshold for the pathologic diagnosis of ACC and for that reason many studies of ACNs in children are represented by a majority of cases with a diagnosis of ACC (40). However, the paradox is that the prognosis for ACCs in children, especially those under 5 years of age, are remarkably favorable with a 5-year event-free survival (EFS) of 70% to 80% (40).

Adrenocortical carcinoma indisputably occurs in children and these tumors usually weigh in excess of 400 g and in

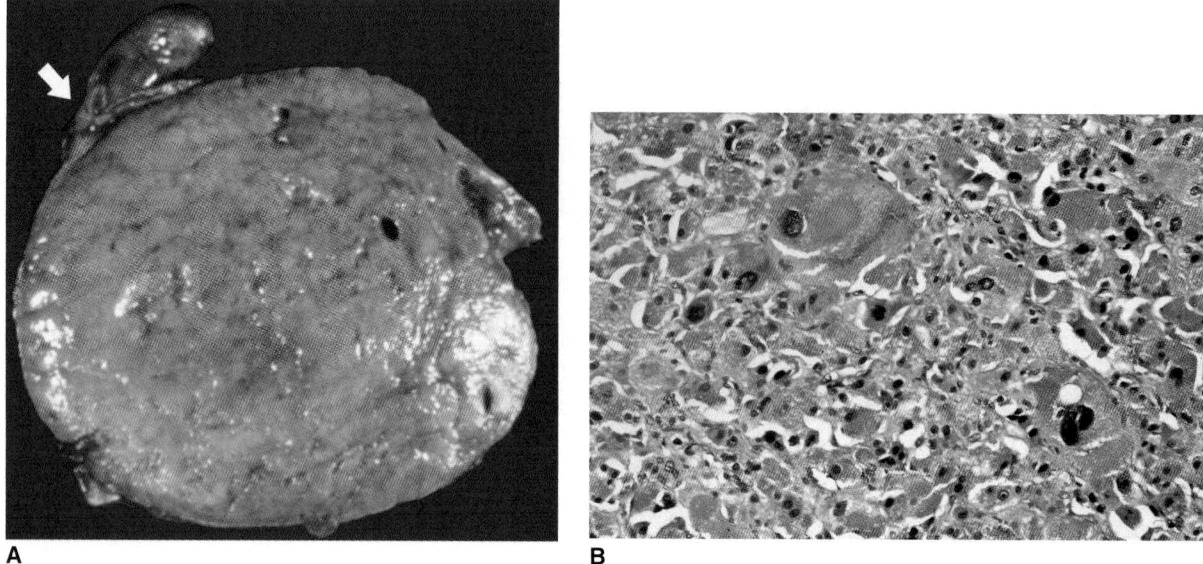

FIGURE 21-32 ■ Adrenocortical neoplasm. **A:** This 250-g adrenal gland from an adolescent who presented with hypertension and signs of virilization had a homogenous tan appearance on gross examination. A small portion of normal adrenal gland (*arrow*) is present. **B:** On histological examination there was prominent cellular pleomorphism with enlarged atypical nuclei. Occasional mitotic figures were present. There was no capsular or vascular invasion. There were no signs of metastatic disease at the time of surgery. This lesion was diagnosed as an atypical adenoma. This tumor would be classified as an adrenocortical neoplasm, intermediate risk in Dehner and Hill's proposed classification (see Table 21-7 reproduced from Dehner LP, Hill A. Adrenal cortical neoplasms in children: Why so many carcinomas and yet so many survivors? *Pediatr Dev Pathol* 2009;12:284–291).

some cases may exceed 1 kg. These tumors have irregular contours, extensive areas of hemorrhage and/or necrosis and invasion beyond the capsule, into the surrounding soft tissues and organs. The various histopathologic features associated with ACCs in adults are present throughout these tumors (40,189,e184,e294,e344,e521,e792,e1264). These obviously malignant neoplasms are found in children beyond 10 years of age whose 5-year EFS ranges from 20% to 35%. These tumors metastasize to the liver (>90% of cases), lungs (80%), retroperitoneal soft tissues and regional lymph

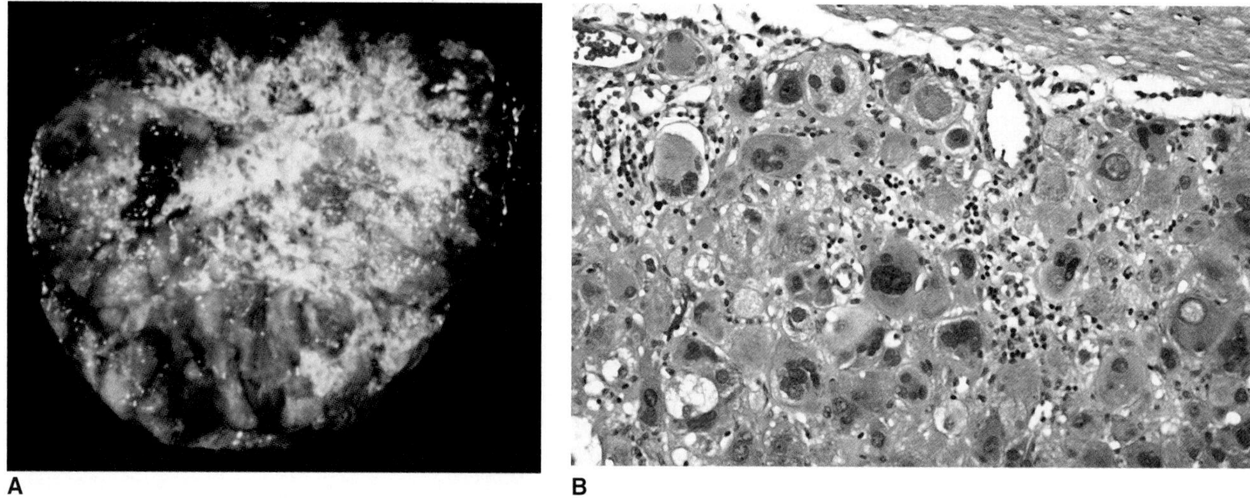

FIGURE 21-33 ■ Adrenocortical neoplasm. **A:** A 2-year-old-male child with precocious puberty and accelerated bone age was found to have a 9.6 × 8 × 6.2 cm mass arising from the right adrenal gland. There was no sign of metastatic disease at the time of surgery. The 215-g adrenal gland had extensive necrosis and calcification on gross examination. **B:** On histological examination the tumor was composed of large, pleomorphic, eosinophillic cells. Nuclear enlargement with hyperchromasia, intranuclear inclusions and increased mitotic rate were present. Capsular invasion (not shown) was also observed. This tumor was classified as an adrenocortical carcinoma. This tumor would be classified as an adrenocortical neoplasm, intermediate risk in Dehner and Hill's proposed classification (see Table 21-7 reproduced from Dehner LP, Hill A. Adrenal cortical neoplasms in children: Why so many carcinomas and yet so many survivors? *Pediatr Dev Pathol* 2009;12:284–291).

Table 21-7 ▪ PROPOSED RISK GROUPS FOR ADRENOCORTICAL NEOPLASMS IN CHILDREN

Risk Group	Criteria
Low	Any cortical neoplasm confined to the adrenal gland and weighing less than 200 g.
Intermediate	Any cortical neoplasm confined to the adrenal gland and weighing between 200 and 400 g.
	Any cortical neoplasm weighing <400 g with microscopic invasion into surrounding soft tissues, completely resected, and no evidence of metastatic spread.
High	Any cortical neoplasm weighing in excess of 400 g or with direct gross invasion into adjacent organs like the liver, spleen, or kidney or with metastatic spread.

Reproduced with permission from Dehner LP, Hill DA. Adrenal cortical neoplasms in children: Why so many carcinomas and yet so many survivors? *Pediatr Dev Pathol.* 2009;12:289.

nodes with less common spread to the bone and brain (189, e676,e946,e1239). Most children with "bona fide" ACCs are usually dead from tumor within 2 years of the diagnosis. As another measure that putative ACCs in young children behave in a different fashion compared to adults are the observations that BWS-associated ACCs are not aggressive neoplasms and that a congenital ACC is reported to have undergone spontaneous regression (e1038,e1060,e1226).

Three risk groups based on tumor localization and weight have been proposed as an alternative means of predicting the clinical behavior of a particular ACN in a child (40) (Table 21-7). Because of the unreliable correlation of histological features to prognosis of ACNs in children, some have gone so far as to eliminate histological features altogether in the prognostic assessment. The three risk groups include those ACNs weighing less than 200 g and confined to the gland as "low risk" for malignant behavior and these tumors are interpreted as adenomas (Figure 21-31, eFigures 21-101 and 21-102), to be contrasted with ACNs weighing in excess of 400 g with a high risk of malignant behavior and are commonly associated with the various histopathologic features of ACCs in adults. The most problematic group consists of those ACNs that are confined to the gland but weigh between 200 and 400 g; these neoplasms are designated "atypical" adenomas with uncertain malignant potential (Figures 21-32 and 21-33, eFigure 21-103). Some of these tumors have invaded beyond the adrenal gland into adjacent tissues and/or have major vascular invasion, not simply microinvasion of vessels within the tumor itself; these tumors are clearly behaving in a malignant fashion. Most of the "atypical" adenomas have a favorable outcome in our experience (40).

The immunophenotype of an ACN in a child is identical to its counterpart in the adult as the tumor cells are reactive with VIM, melan-A, inhibin, and calretinin. There are no immunophenotypic differences between an adenoma and carcinoma (36,e50,e51,e374,e375,e395). ACNs, typically adenomas, may demonstrate immunoreactivity for cytokeratin; carcinomas are usually nonreactive (36,e395). Ploidy analysis has limited value in the discrimination of an adenoma from a carcinoma. In one study of 50 ACNs in children, 21 of 29 patients (73%) with aneuploid tumors remained disease-free (e835,e1229).

The distinction between a cortical neoplasm and PHEO is not clear in every case, especially in a tumor with large, bizarre-appearing cells, granular basophilic cytoplasm, and a nested growth pattern. The challenge is further heightened by the fact that the results of pertinent biochemical studies are usually not available to correlate with the pathological findings. The tumor is more likely to be cystic and hemorrhagic, and the tumor cells are devoid of some of the tinctorial attributes that are useful in the differentiation of a cortical from a medullary neoplasm. In these cases, immunohistochemistry is helpful with the differential diagnosis.

SYN and NSE are commonly immunoreactive in both PHEOs and adrenal cortical tumors, whereas CHR is nonreactive in adrenocortical tumors, but is consistently expressed in PHEOs and paragangliomas (36,e90,e455,e811,e1058). Cytokeratin is typically not found in either PHEOs or paragangliomas with rare exceptions, but they are often immunoreactive for VIM (36,e222,e221,e675). S-100 protein and HMB-45 staining is useful in the labeling of the sustentacular cells of PHEOs. It is necessary to acknowledge that the results of bcl-2, cytokeratin, and VIM expression have not proven to discriminate between a cortical and medullary neoplasm in every case.

Peripheral NB Group Tumors. Classic or peripheral neuroblastic tumors are represented by the NB, ganglioneuroblastoma (GNB), and ganglioneuroma (GN) as a group of histogenetically-related neoplasms of neural crest origin (eFigure 21-104). These tumors are histogenetically distinct from the central primitive neuroectodermal tumor (cPNET) and Ewing sarcoma-primitive neuroectodermal tumor (EWS-PNET) despite the presence of overlapping morphologic and immunophenotypic features (see Chapters 10 and 24).

Epidemiology: NB is the most common extracranial solid neoplasm of childhood and is surpassed in incidence only by the acute leukemias and primary brain tumors, principally astrocytoma and medulloblastoma; SEER Program for 1975 to 2000 reported that NB accounted for 7.2% of all cancers among children younger than 15 years of age in the United States, and the total incidence was 10.2 to 10.3:1,000,000 for males and 10.1 for females (155). The incidence rates by age are the following: 19.6:1,000,000 for ages 1 to 4 years, 2.9 for ages 5 to 9 years, and 0.7 for 10 to 14 years. The rates by race and ethnicity are the following: 10.8:1,000,000 for whites, 8.4 for blacks, and 7.5 for children in other racial/ethnic groups. In the United States, approximately 650 children are newly diagnosed each year (57). Based on the SEER data, the 5-year relative survival rate is 65%, a figure which has remained more or less static for the past several decades.

In the past, NB was referred to as "enigmatic" because of its unpredictable behavior since these tumors manifest a wide range of clinical courses from an excellent prognosis due to complete resectability, tumor involution, spontaneous regression and/or maturation or a fatal outcome due to tumor progression despite intensive treatment. Now NB is believed to be biologically heterogeneous, and is composed of at least two subgroups, clinically favorable and unfavorable; these two subgroups have distinct molecular/genetic attributes closely correlated with their clinical behaviors. Several epidemiological studies in the past have not identified any causal factors for NB; however, it may be necessary to analyze neuroblastic tumors in each biological subgroup separately to elucidate any possible extrinsic factors.

Familial or hereditary NB, first recognized in 1945, is a rare entity (e (308) and has offered an opportunity to identify any hereditary NB predisposition genes: Maris et al. have reported a hereditary NB predisposition gene (*HNB1*) on the distal short arm of chromosome 16p (16p12-13), (108) and Perri et al. have identified another gene on the distal short arm of chromosome 4p (4p16) (135). Recently, activating mutations in the anaplastic lymphoma kinase (*ALK*) oncogene (2p23) have been found in hereditary NB cases as well as a smaller subset of sporadic tumors (26,118,125,128, e561). The same gene has an important oncogenic role in anaplastic large cell lymphoma and inflammatory myofibroblastic tumor. DICER1 has even been questioned as having a role.

Beckwith and Perrin used the term of NB *in situ* to describe an exclusively microscopic finding in neonatal and infant autopsies, histologically identical to NB, as an incidental finding in or around the adrenal medulla. The incidence of these lesions has been calculated as 40 to 100 times that of clinically overt NBs (e95). Most NBs *in situ* during life are asymptomatic (e453,e476). Since similar neuroblastic nodules are seen during the fetal development of the adrenal medulla, some have questioned the neoplastic potential if any of NB *in situ*. It has not yet been demonstrated whether these lesions are clonal proliferations of genetically abnormal cells. Therefore, the premalignant or neoplastic nature of these lesions remains unproven to date.

The anatomic sites of predilection for NB are related to the distribution of neural crest cells. They include the paravertebral region from the neck to the pelvis (3% to 5% of cases), the adrenal medulla (35% of cases), the extra-adrenal retroperitoneum (30% to 35% of cases), and the posterior mediastinum (20% of cases) (20,e278,e840,e1025). Less common primary sites include the cephalic, paratesticular, or para-ovarian tissues, and the inguinal region; one concern about these various sites is whether they represent a primary tumor or metastasis (1,23,70,182). Rarely, NB presents as apparent multifocal tumors (64,e1084). A primitive appearing neuronal tumor may occur as the only or predominant element of a sacrococcygeal or ovarian teratoma, in which case, the neuroblastic cells usually have the characteristics of the central nervous system rather than the peripheral nervous system or neural crest.

Occasionally, some difficulty is encountered in distinguishing an adrenal or perirenal NB from Wilms tumor (WT). Most WTs are well-demarcated intra-renal masses. Biologically favorable perirenal NB usually grows outside of the kidney, while biologically unfavorable perirenal NB often shows a direct invasion into the renal parenchyma. The blastema-predominant WT may frequently require immunohistochemical differentiation from NB: the blastemal cells of WT are positive for VIM and WT-1 and are negative for CHR and SYN. In the case of EWS-PNET, the tumor may be positive for neuroendocrine markers as well as MIC2 (CD99) and FLI-1, but is negative for WT-1 and TH [tyrosine hydroxylase (TH)] (131,e569).

Clinical Features: Signs and symptoms at presentation are related to the location of the primary tumor and the extent of disease. The most common presentation of NB is an abdominal mass in which radiological imaging studies demonstrate a suprarenal or retroperitoneal mass with or without calcification (e145). Orbital metastasis also causes periorbital ecchymosis and edema with the so-called raccoon or panda eyes. Invasion or circumscription of the kidney by a NB in the adrenal, retroperitoneum or the perihilar region can mimic a WT. NB may cause renal artery stenosis due to compression leading to systemic hypertension.

Patients with localized disease are often asymptomatic. A localized NB may be discovered incidentally in a routine well-baby examination or by a caregiver. Metastatic spread is seen in patients with "progressive" stage 4 disease and "regressive" stage 4S (S stands for "special") disease (Table 21-8). Major metastatic sites in stage 4 disease include bone marrow and bone. To find a metastatic nodule in the brain parenchyma is rare: CNS metastasis, when present, often show a form of diffuse meningeal spread. Lung metastasis at initial diagnosis is also extremely rare (49). In stage 4S disease, liver, skin, and/or bone marrow (without bone destruction) are the sites of metastasis (e268). Congenital NB can be diagnosed perinatally by US and placental examination. Most congenital NBs are stage 1 or 4S with an excellent clinical outcome (73,148,e268). It is interesting to note that neuroblastic cells may be found in the fetal capillaries of the chorionic villi in the presence of a congenital NB, suggesting that the placenta as a source of dissemination (eFigure 21-105) (126,e565,e1110,e1149). Another presentation is nonimmune fetal hydrops. Placental metastasis is often present in these cases (125,e572,e855). Spinal cord compression is caused by a paravertebral tumor growing into the spinal canal through neural foramina ("dumbbell lesion") or osteolytic metastasis with vertebral collapse (38,e958). Neurological abnormalities include motor deficit, radicular or back pain, sphincter abnormalities, and sensory deficit.

Table 21-8 ■ INTERNATIONAL NEUROBLASTOMA STAGING SYSTEMA

Stage 1	Localized tumor with complete gross excision, with or without microscopic residual disease; representative ipsilateral lymph nodes negative for tumor microscopically (nodes attached to and removed with the primary tumor may be positive).
Stage 2A	Localized tumor with incomplete gross excision; representative ipsilateral nonadherent lymph nodes negative for tumor microscopically.
Stage 2B	Localized tumor with or without complete gross excision, with ipsilateral nonadherent lymph nodes positive for tumor. Enlarged contralateral lymph nodes must be negative microscopically.
Stage 3	Unresectable unilateral tumor infiltrating across the midline,[a] with or without regional lymph node involvement; or localized unilateral tumor with contralateral regional lymph node involvement; or midline tumor with bilateral extension by infiltration (unresectable) or by lymph node involvement.
Stage 4	Any primary tumor with dissemination to distant lymph nodes, bone, bone marrow, liver, skin, and/or other organs (except as defined for stage 4S).
Stage 4S	Localized primary tumor (as defined for stage 1, 2A, or 2B), with dissemination limited to skin, liver and/or bone marrow[b] (limited to infants <1 year of age).

Multifocal primary tumors (e.g., bilateral adrenal primary tumors) should be staged according to the greatest extent of disease, as defined previously, followed by a subscript "M" (e.g., 3_M).
[a]The midline is defined as the vertebral column. Tumors originating on one side and "crossing the midline" must infiltrate to or beyond the opposite side of the vertebral column.
[b]Marrow involvement in stage 4S should be minimal, that is, < 10% of total nucleated cells identified as malignant on bone marrow biopsy or on marrow aspirate. More extensive marrow involvement would be considered to be stage 4. The MIBG scan (if done) should be negative in the marrow.
International Neuroblastoma Staging System. Reproduced with permission from Brodeur GM, Maris, JM. Neuroblastoma. In: Pizzo PA, Poplack DG, editors. *Principles and practice of pediatric oncology*, 5th ed. Philadelphia, PA: Lippincott-Williams & Wilkins Publishers, 2006;1997:761–797.

Other uncommon clinical manifestations of NB are listed in Table 21-9. A small proportion of cases may have a so-called paraneoplastic syndrome including the opsoclonus-myoclonus-ataxia syndrome (Kinsbourne syndrome) with "dancing eyes" (rapid and irregular movement of the eyes) and/or myoclonus and ataxia of the limbs, trunk, and eyelids (32,55,144). An immune-mediated pathogenesis is suggested by the presence of a prominent lymphocytic infiltrate and lymphoid follicle formation in the primary site along with antineuronal antibodies. The prognosis in terms of tumor behavior itself is generally excellent, but cognitive and motor developmental delay and language deficit often persist even after complete resection of the NB. Horner syndrome (ptosis, miosis, enophthalmos) and heterochromia (difference in color) of the iris may occur in the presence of a NB involving the cervical sympathetic ganglia. Intractable diarrhea with hypokalemia and dehydration are the manifestations of vasoactive intestinal peptide-producing neuroblastic tumor with differentiating neuroblasts or a GN (e255,e326,e584,e1047). Differentiating neuroblasts may also produce somatostatin and other neuropeptides (e959). Cushing syndrome and systemic hypertension are other clinical presentations (51). Extremely rare cases of vilirizing adrenal GN with Leydig cells have been reported (e14,e420). The so-called neuroblastic "leukemia" in the peripheral blood with extensive bone marrow involvement is an uncommon hematological event (e148,e925). Another hematopathological finding is myelofibrosis in the absence of demonstrable metastatic NB in the bone marrow (e668,e674).

Table 21-9 ■ UNCOMMON AND UNUSUAL CLINICAL MANIFESTATIONS OF NEUROBLASTOMA

Opsoclonus-myoclonus ataxia syndrome
Horner syndrome and heterochromia of iris
Intractable watery diarrhea with hypokalemia and dehydration (VIP secretion)
Cushing syndrome
Systemic hypertension
Virilizing, masculinization (ganglioneuroma)
Neuroblastoma "leukemia"
Myelofibrosis
Fetal hydrops with placental involvement

VIP, vasoactive intestinal peptide.

There are several distinct associations of NB with other disorders including neurofibromatosis, BWS, Hirschsprung disease, musculoskeletal and cardiovascular malformations, and Turner syndrome (Table 21-10) (e96,e97,e126,e241, e244,e408,e808,e1009,e1281). Molecular studies of cases of familial NB have failed to provide any linkage with the genes responsible for neurofibromatosis 1 and 2 (108,e761). The relationship of congenital NB to the syndrome of central failure of ventilation (incorrectly referred to as Ondine curse—the curse actually involved the loss of all autonomic and perceptive function) often accompanied by Hirschsprung disease has been explained on the basis of a widespread abnormality of neural crest cell development and migration (152,178,e252,e1005,e1135). An excess of thyroid carcinomas (histological type not stated) is reported in individuals who received radiation therapy for NB; this excess persisted when the study was analyzed for radiation dose to the thyroid in other childhood neoplasms (e285). An unusual type of renal cell carcinoma with oncocytoid features is reported as a second primary neoplasm in survivors of NB

Table 21-10 ■ ASSOCIATION OF NEUROBLASTOMA WITH OTHER DISORDERS

von Recklinghausen neurofibromatosis
Beckwith-Wiedemann syndrome
Hirschsprung disease
Musculoskeletal and cardiovascular malformations
Turner syndrome
Central failure of ventilation ("Ondine curse")
Increased incidence of thyroid carcinoma in irradiated neuroblastoma patients (in comparison with patients irradiated for other childhood neoplasms)
Renal cell carcinoma (oncocytoid variant)

(13,53,e793). *Biochemical Markers:* NB is characterized biochemically by catecholamine synthesis with metabolites that are detected in the serum and urine; this property is utilized in the initial diagnosis and clinical follow-up as a measure of therapeutic response (e435). The precursor amino acids for catecholamine synthesis are phenylalanine and tyrosine. A series of enzymes, such as TH, DOPA decarboxylase, dopamine β-hydroxylase, and phenylethanolamine N-methyltransferase, are involved in the pathway of catecholamine catabolism and production of norepinephrine and epinephrine. NB cells usually lack the last enzyme, phenylethanolamine N-methyltransferase, which is present in adrenal chromaffin cells and PHEOs. Degradation of L-DOPA and dopamine by catechol-O-methyltransferase and norepinephrine by monoamine oxidase, are primarily responsible for production of the metabolites, homovanillic acid (HVA) and vanillylmandelic acid (VMA). These two metabolites, VMA and HVA, are the most widely measured serum and urinary products for the diagnosis of NB and GNB, because GN is not a biochemically active neoplasm in most cases. When the VMA/HVA ratio is less than 1, these tumors seem to have a less favorable clinical outcome than those with a ratio of 1 or greater (e689). Elevated tissue levels of the neuropeptides, VIP and somatostatin, have been correlated with cellular differentiation and low stage disease (e959). An elevated serum level of neuron-specific enolase is reported not only in NB, but also in other tumors such as EWS-PNET, small cell neuroendocrine carcinoma, PHEO, acute lymphoblastic leukemia, and non-Hodgkin lymphoma (60). Although detecting NSE in serum is less specific for the diagnosis of NB, high levels at diagnosis have been correlated with a poor clinical outcome in several studies; this marker has some value for monitoring of recurrent tumor (165,e1299,e1300). Elevated serum ferritin levels are also observed in NB, Hodgkin lymphoma, leukemia, and carcinoma of the breast (60). Higher serum ferritin levels at diagnosis are associated with metastatic NB and its poor prognosis (e113,e465,e466). Ferritin is not suitable for monitoring disease activity, since it becomes elevated from frequent blood transfusions during the clinical course. High serum lactate dehydrogenase (LDH) has some prognostic value, although LDH is not tumor specific but elevated levels reflect tumor load and rapid cell turnover (98,164,e113). Other tumor markers reported to correlate with disease stage and/or prognosis include serum CHR A levels (68) and serum neuropeptide Y levels (e632). Recently detection of circulating *MYCN* DNA in serum has shown some promise in unmasking *MYCN* amplified NBs (31).

Morphologic features: The bone marrow (BM) biopsy is one of the essential procedures in the staging of a newly diagnosed NB, but it is also important in the monitoring of disease activity (163,e154,e845,e975). It is generally recognized that both BM needle and aspiration biopsies have their complimentary value (7). An adequate aspirate may be difficult to obtain when the marrow is densely replaced by tumor or with fibrosis after therapy. Paratrabecular nests of metastatic NB are the characteristic findings in the involved biopsy, but micrometastatic disease may require immunohistochemistry, flow cytometry, and even RT-PCR in an attempt to establish the presence of tumor cells in a posttreatment specimen (14,84,154,e223,e334). TH, PGP9.5, and MAP2 immunostaining are useful with limitations on the basis of specificities and sensitivities for detecting the rare malignant cell. Metastatic NB in BM from a newly diagnosed case typically demonstrates collections of poorly differentiated neuroblasts with only a hint of neuropil in the background. On the other hand, differentiating neuroblasts, individually distributed or forming small clusters, with abundant neuropil are often seen in the BM after chemotherapy. Schwannian stroma is rarely encountered in BM biopsies.

The International Neuroblastoma Pathology Committee (INPC) made recommendations in 1999 for terminology and morphologic criteria of neuroblastic tumors by adopting and modifying the original Shimada classification (156,157,159). The recommendations were based on the hypothesis that these tumors provided one of the better models for analyzing the biological relationship between molecular/genomic alterations and morphology. As outlined below, peripheral neuroblastic tumors are classified into four categories: (Table 21-11) NB, GNB-intermixed, GNB-nodular, and ganglioneuroma (GN).

NBs are further subclassified into undifferentiated, poorly differentiated, and differentiating subtypes. Grossly (Figure 21-34A, B, eFigure 21-106), NB usually presents as a solid circumscribed or multinodular mass, measuring 10 cm or less in greatest dimension, with considerable variation in appearance depending on the anatomic location, histological subtype, and secondary changes. A deep reddish hemorrhagic appearance with or without scattered foci of glistening gray-white tissue is a common gross presentation for NB of the undifferentiated or poorly differentiated subtype. Punctate or coarse calcifications or yellowish areas of coagulative necrosis are other relatively common macroscopic features in these latter two subtypes. Cystic degeneration with or without hemorrhage is another feature; the cystic NB, commonly arising in the adrenal gland, may require extensive sampling to identify microscopic foci of tumor. On the other hand, NB of the differentiating subtype is usually tan-yellow and less hemorrhagic with only limited areas of necrosis, if any.

Table 21-11 ▪ CATEGORY AND SUBTYPES RECOMMENDED BY THE INTERNATIONAL NEUROBLASTOMA PATHOLOGY COMMITTEE

Category	Subtype
Neuroblastoma (Schwannian stroma-poor)[a]	Undifferentiated Poorly differentiated Differentiating
Ganglioneuroblastoma, intermixed (Schwannian stroma-rich)	
Ganglioneuroma (Schwannian stroma-dominant)	Maturing Mature
Ganglioneuroblastoma, nodular[b] (Schwannian stroma-dominant/stroma-rich and stroma-poor)	

[a]MKI (mitosis-karyorrhexis index; Low, Intermediate, or High) is assigned along with subtype of each neuroblastic tumor.
[b]Subtype (undifferentiated, poorly differentiated, or differentiating) and MKI are assigned to the neuroblastomatous nodule of each ganglioneuroblastoma, nodular tumor.
From Peuchmaur M, d'Amore ESG, Joshi VV, et al. Revision of the international neuroblastoma pathology classification: confirmation of favorable and unfavorable prognostic subsets in ganglioneuroblastoma, nodular. *Cancer.* 2003;98:2274–2281; Shimada H, Ambros IM, Dehner LP, et al. Terminology and morphologic criteria of neuroblastic tumors: Recommendation by the International Neuroblastoma Pathology Committee. *Cancer.* 1999;86:349–363.

NBs are further defined as Schwannian stroma-poor, and composed of neuroblasts forming lobules which are completely or incompletely separated by delicate fibrovascular septa. Putative Schwannian blasts may be detected as slender S-100 positive cells in the septal area (158). The typical neuroblast is round or slightly ovoid with a round to oval nucleus with salt-and-pepper chromatin and scanty cytoplasm. With the formation of neurites, an eosinophilic fibrillary network or neuropil becomes apparent, but is not regarded as "stroma." Homer-Wright rosettes are arranged around a central tangle of neurofibrillary processes without a central lumen or canal. Differentiating neuroblasts, a transitional form of neuroblastic differentiation toward ganglion cells, are characterized by synchronous changes in both the nucleus (enlarged, eccentrically located with vesicular chromatin pattern, and a single prominent nucleolus) and cytoplasm (eosinophilic/amphophilic with a diameter usually two or more times larger than the nucleus). Neuritic processes or neuropil becomes less prominent with ganglionic differentiation.

The undifferentiated subtype of NB is composed of undifferentiated neuroblasts without clearly identifiable neuropil or rosettes (Figure 21-35). In fact, there is very little to differentiate these tumor cells from the nonneuroblastic round cell neoplasms of childhood without the assistance of immunohistochemistry and molecular/cytogenetic studies. Preliminary data suggest that undifferentiated neuroblasts lack the potential for differentiation. S-100 protein staining demonstrates no or very few putative Schwannian blasts in the septal areas of the tumor when septation is present. Some tumors in this subtype show a diffuse growth pattern without a lobular architecture.

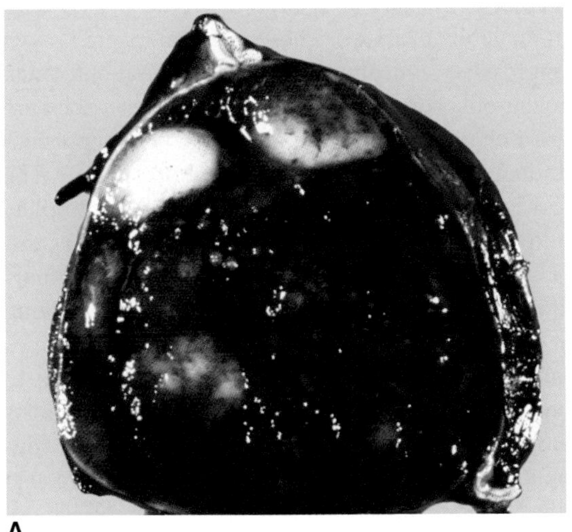
A

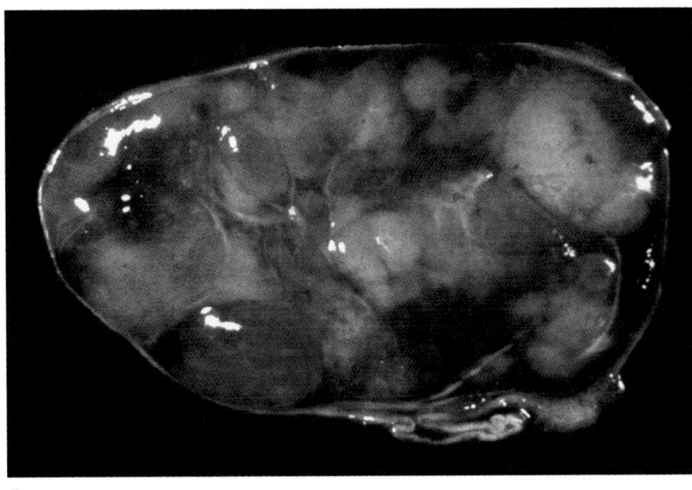
B

FIGURE 21-34 ▪ Neuroblastoma. **A:** Adrenal neuroblastoma (Schwannian stroma-poor), poorly differentiated subtype, measuring 5 cm × 4.5 cm in the greatest dimension, shows a friable and hemorrhagic appearance. **B:** Adrenal neuroblastoma (Schwannian stroma-poor), differentiating subtype, measuring 6 cm × 4 cm in the greatest dimension, shows a soft and less hemorrhagic appearance.

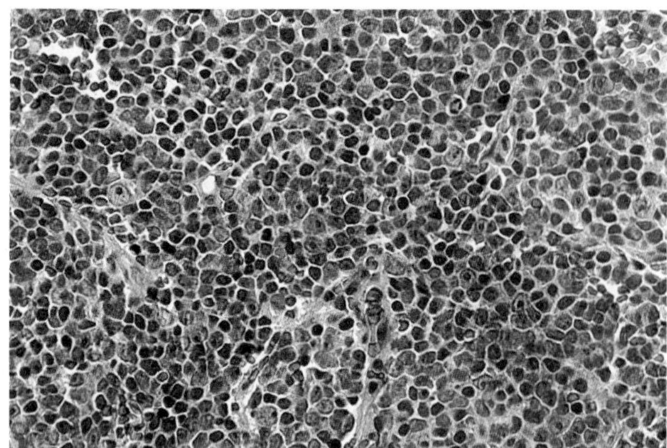

FIGURE 21-35 ■ Neuroblastoma (Schwannian stroma-poor), undifferentiated subtype is composed of primitive cells without clearly recognizable neurite formation. Tumor cells in this case often have one or few prominent nucleoli. Note that tumor cells are irregularly demarcated by thin fibrovascular septal tissue.

The poorly differentiated subtype is the most common pattern of NB in this group, and is diagnosed in most cases without difficulty since neuropil and/or Homer-Wright rosettes are commonly present (Figure 21-36) (eFigure 21-107). Most tumor cells are typical neuroblasts, and less than 5% of the population is pursuing ganglionic differentiation. Lobular formations of neuroblasts with thin fibrovascular septa are evident in many of these tumors. S-100 protein positive slender Schwann cells or putative Schwannian blasts are detectable especially in the biologically favorable tumors of this subtype. It has been postulated that those Schwann cells/Schwannian blasts are recruited into the tumor by the biologically favorable neuroblasts, rather than as end-stage product differentiation from the neural crest cells (e38).

NB, differentiating subtype contains 5% or more of tumor cells with the features of differentiating neuroblasts (Figure 21-37). These tumors also have a prominent neuropil. It is

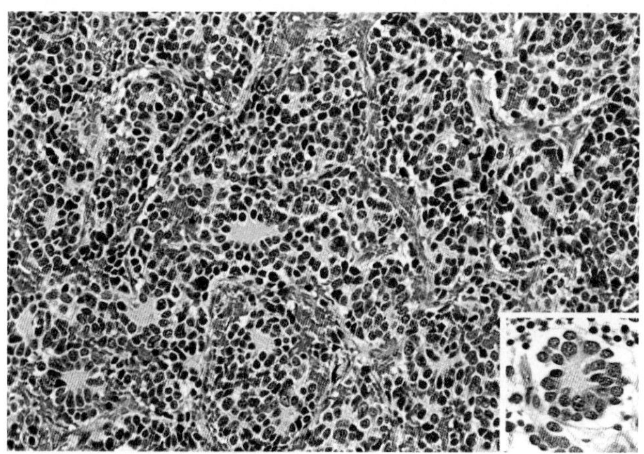

FIGURE 21-36 ■ Neuroblastoma (Schwannian stroma-poor), poorly differentiated subtype is the most common form of tumor in the neuroblastoma group. Neuroblastoma cells produce neurites and can show rosette formations. Inset: Typical Homer-Wright rosette.

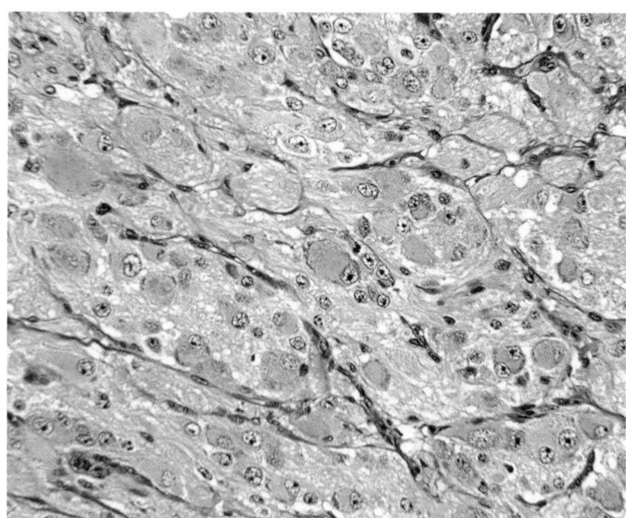

FIGURE 21-37 ■ Neuroblastoma (Schwannian stroma-poor), differentiating subtype (containing more than 5% of the tumor cells showing an appearance of differentiating neuroblast by definition) is often characterized by abundant neuropil formation. Tumor cells are irregularly separated by thin fibrovascular septa, but significant Schwannian stromal development is not observed.

thought that biologically favorable NBs of the poorly differentiated subtype can either regress or mature in the direction of the differentiating subtype. To date, among the biologically favorable NBs, there is no clear distinction in molecular characteristics between tumors with a potential for regression and those with presumed potential for maturation. In fact, during the process of tumor maturation from a poorly differentiated subtype to a differentiating subtype, the vast majority of neuroblasts undergo programmed cell death or apoptosis before or after attaining a certain degree of neuroblastic differentiation.

Some NBs have unique morphologic features including anaplastic appearing tumor cells which are characterized by the presence of enlarged, bizarre cells and atypical mitotic figures (120,e259). There is a large cell type of NB with prominent nucleoli (175,176). These rare tumors are known for their aggressive clinical course and often fatal outcome.

Ganglioneuroblastoma-intermixed is defined as a Schwannian stroma-rich tumor whose Schwannian component occupies more than 50% of the tumor area (Figure 21-38). The histological features seem to imply that there is incomplete transition to a fully mature GN, but the process is not complete, as evidenced by the presence of scattered “residual” microscopic foci or collections in neuroblasts in varying stages of differentiation with a background of neuropil. These neuroblasts, many with differentiating features to immature ganglion cells, are in a process of either apoptosis or continuous maturation to mature ganglion cells. Individually distributed mature and maturing ganglion cells are also found in the Schwannian stroma with the pattern of GN.

Ganglioneuroma is a Schwannian stroma-dominant neoplasm without any aggregates of neuroblasts in a neuropil background. The exclusive cellular elements are Schwann cells with accompanying individually distributed or small

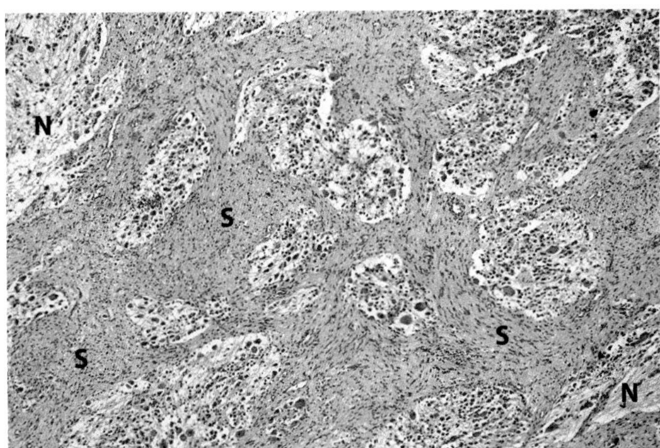

FIGURE 21-38 ■ Ganglioneuroblastoma, intermixed (Schwannian stroma-rich) is characterized by an extensive Schwannian stromal development (S) occupying more than 50% of tumor tissue. Pockets of naked neuropil (N) area containing tumor cells of various stages of neuronal differentiation are found. Tumor cells in those pockets are composed of a mixture of differentiating neuroblasts and maturing ganglion cells with or without poorly differentiated neuroblasts.

groups of maturing/mature ganglion cells. Two subtypes, GN-maturing (Figure 21-39A) and GN-mature (Figure 21-39B), are included in this category. The GN-maturing, previously designated as "GNB, well differentiated" in the original Shimada classification (159), contains scattered individual immature ganglion cells and/or neuroblasts in addition to mature ganglion cells. The mature GN (GN-mature) is the fully mature peripheral neuroblastic tumor, and is composed of Schwannian stroma and mature ganglion cells which are surrounded by satellite cells. Fully developed Schwannian stroma is seen in GNs and focally in the GNB-intermixed. Mature unmyelinated type of Schwann cells characteristically forming multiple fascicles which are covered with perineurial cells are present. These areas of a mature GN without ganglion cells resemble a schwannoma. A well-formed capsule is more characteristic of the schwannoma, whereas, the GN tends to blend into the adjacent soft tissues with some circumscription of the peripheral margins.

Both the GNB-intermixed and GN have similar gross features with a firm consistency, and a cut surface with a tan-yellow, homogenous appearance with or without fibrous bands (Figure 21-40).

Ganglioneuroblastoma-nodular is a composite tumor characterized by the presence of one or more grossly visible, often hemorrhagic/necrotic neuroblastic nodule(s) coexisting with GNB-intermixed or GN (Figure 21-41A, B). There is typically an abrupt demarcation (pushing border or pseudo-capsular formation) between the neuroblastic nodule(s) and the ganglioneuromatous component (GNB-intermixed or GN). Some neuroblastic nodules may not be clearly demarcated, but rather there is neuroblastic infiltration into the Schwannian stromal component of GNB-intermixed or GN component. It is possible that some neuroblastic nodules are intratumoral metastasis into the ganglioneuromatous areas. Infrequently, a neuroblastic nodule grows so large that the ganglioneuromatous component (GNB-intermixed or GN) can only be recognized microscopically, often at the periphery of the tumor, as a narrow ribbon of GN. Neuroblastic nodules are usually evident in the gross examination of the primary tumor; however, they may be overlooked. For that reason, those primary tumors with the features of GNB-intermixed or GN, but with metastatic NB

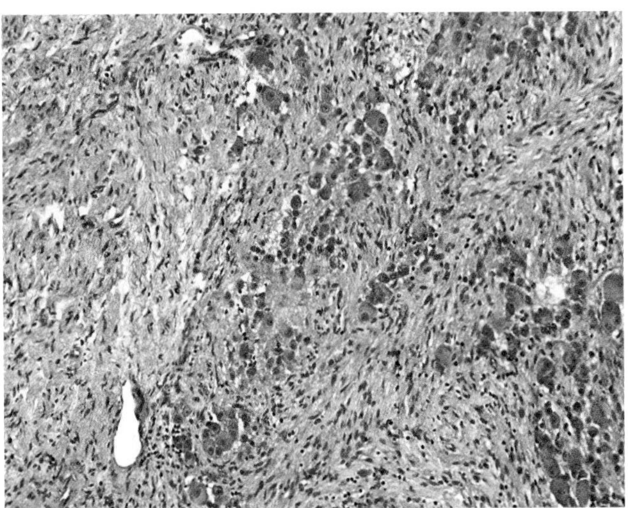

A

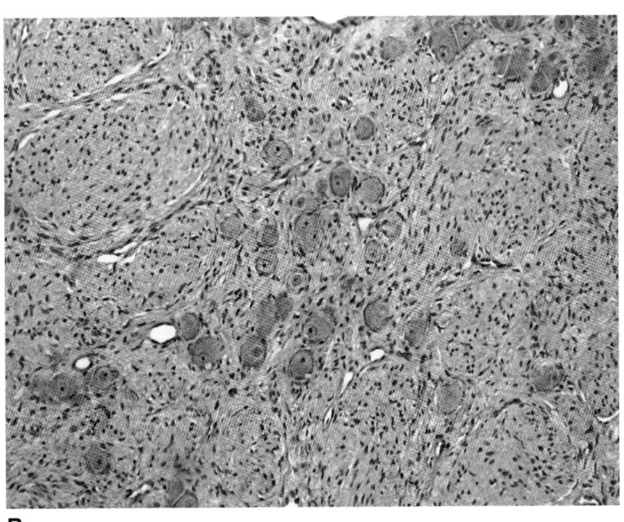

B

FIGURE 21-39 ■ **A:** Ganglioneuroma (Schwannian stroma-dominant), maturing is a tumor predominantly composed of Schwannian stromal tissue. Differentiating neuroblasts and maturing/mature ganglion cells are distributed without clearly recognizable pockets of neuropil. **B:** Ganglioneuroma (Schwannian stroma-dominant), mature, is a completely mature form in the neuroblastoma group. Fully mature ganglion cells are covered with satellite cells. Stroma component is well organized and shows multiple fascicular formations composed of Schwann cells of unmyelinated type surrounded by perineurial cells.

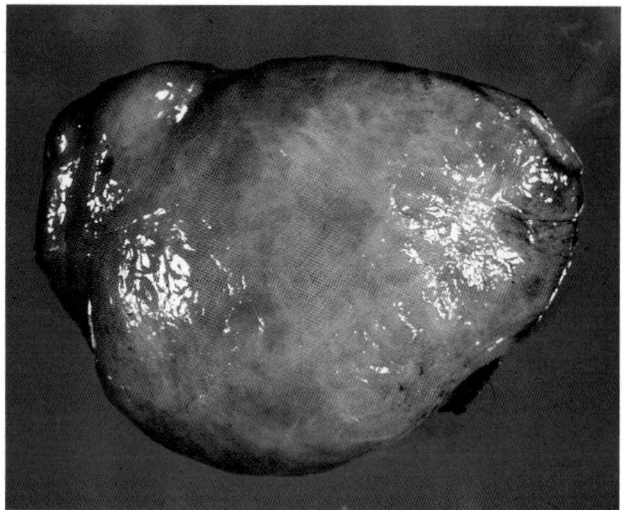

FIGURE 21-40 ■ Ganglioneuroblastoma, intermixed (Schwannian stroma-rich), in the mediastinum measuring 9 cm × 7 cm in the greatest dimension, is rubbery in consistency and has no grossly visible nodule of neuroblastomatous growth. Tumors in both ganglioneuroblastoma, intermixed (Schwannian stroma-rich) and ganglioneuroma (Schwannian stroma-dominant) category present a gross appearance similar to a Schwannoma.

to lymph node, bone or other sites are also included in the category of GNB-nodular (137).

As a component of the pathologic evaluation of a NB, the INPC has recommended a determination of the mitotic and karyorrhectic activities by the mitosis-karyorrhexis index (MKI) which has been defined by three semiquantitative levels: low (<2% or <100 mitotic and karyorrhectic cells per 5,000 neuroblasts), intermediate (2% to 4%) or 100 to 200 mitotic and karyorrhectic cells per 5,000 neuroblasts), and high (>4% or >200 mitotic and karyorrhectic cells per 5,000 neuroblasts). The MKI is determined by counting the number of tumor cells in mitosis and in the process of karyorrhexis, and should reflect an average for all tumor sections available. Cells in karyorrhexis, one of the apoptotic processes and individual cell death due to severe genomic instability, are characterized by condensed and fragmented nuclear chromatin without nuclear membrane, usually accompanied by condensed eosinophilic cytoplasm. Hyperchromatic nuclei without chromatin fragmentation are not included in the MKI count. It has been reported that increased mitotic and karyorrhectic activity is correlated with *MYCN* amplification and excess production of *MYCN* protein (58,161).

Ultrastructure, Immunohistochemistry, Molecular Diagnostics: Ultrastructural features characteristic of neuroblastic cells include the presence of membrane-bound neurosecretory granules in the cytoplasm and neuritic processes with typically arranged microtubules which are parallel to each other (e491,e1205,e1206). Rudimentary attachment structures are found between adjacent neuroblasts. These features, however, are also detectable in EWS-PNETs. Nissl bodies composed of rough endoplasmic reticulum and free ribosomes are found in the periphery of the cytoplasm of differentiating neuroblasts and ganglion cells. Neuromelanin can be detected in some of the differentiating neuroblasts (e429). Mature Schwannian cells found in the GNB-intermixed and GN are the unmyelinated cells and contain multiple neurites in the individual cell bodies.

Immunohistochemically, neuroblastic cells are positive for NSE, NB84, PGP9.5, SYN, CHR, Leu 7 (CD57), a variety of NFPs, NCAMs, and other neural antigens (191, e163,e201,e399,e812,e832,e901). TH is a useful marker for identifying neural crest cells, and is positive in both NB and PHEO/paraganglioma (74). In most cases, application of

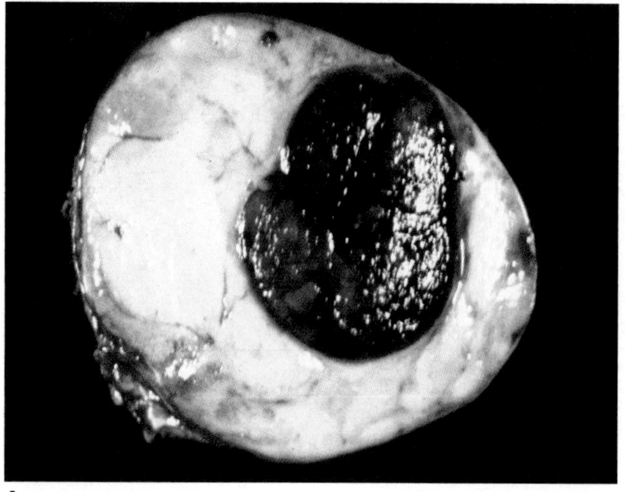

A

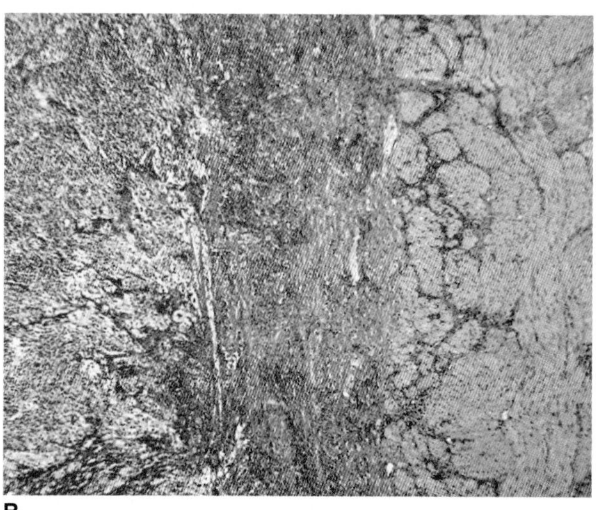

B

FIGURE 21-41 ■ Ganglioneuroblastoma, nodular (composite, Schwannian stroma-dominant/stroma-rich and stroma-poor) arising the retroperitoneum. **A:** The tumor measuring 8 cm × 7 cm in the greatest dimension, is tan-yellow and rubbery in consistency, and contains a grossly visible hemorrhagic nodule. There are two (or multiple) distinct tumor types/clones coexisting in the same tumor tissue of this category. **B:** As shown in this example, one tumor type (**left side**) has an appearance of neuroblastoma (Schwannian stroma-poor) forming a grossly visible and often hemorrhagic nodule, and other (**right side**) has a feature of ganglioneuroma (Schwannian stroma-dominant).

immunohistochemistry is more adjunctive to the histological examination, since the accumulative data of clinical and laboratory findings generally support a straightforward diagnosis of NB. In our own practice (HS), PGP9.5, TH, MIC2 (CD99), desmin, MyoD1, myogenin, and lymphoid markers are applied as the immunohistochemical panel for distinguishing an undifferentiated NB from the other malignant round cell neoplasms of childhood. Undifferentiated NBs are diffusely positive for PGP9.5, often sporadically positive for TH, and negative for the other markers. While EWS-PNET is positive for PGP9.5 and MIC2 (CD99) but negative for TH, rhabdomyosarcoma is positive for desmin, MyoD1, and myogenin. Hematolymphoid malignancies can be screened with CD43 and CD45 to be followed by additional specific lineage markers. When only VIM is immunoreactive, one should think in terms of an undifferentiated NB or a hematolymphoid malignancy. Putative Schwannian blasts are positive for S-100 (use of monoclonal antibody against β-chain recommended) and located in the thin fibrovascular septa demarcating groups/clusters of NB cells of especially the biologically favorable NB tumors (158). Ganglioneuroblastoma and GN are characterized by the S-100 positive Schwannian stromal development. Satellite cells around the fully mature ganglion cells are also positive for S-100.

Frequently used molecular markers in a setting of differential diagnosis include EWS-ETS translocation (EWS-FLI1, EWS-ERG) and PAX-FKHR translocation. NBs are negative for those translocations. Demonstrating EWS-ETS translocation by FISH and detecting its chimeric protein are diagnostic of EWS-PNET (8,76). The presence of PAX-FKHR translocation, detectable in around 80% alveolar rhabdomyosarcomas (130), is reported to indicate an aggressive clinical behavior of the disease (37).

International NB Pathology Classification: A morphological classification designed to be prognostically significant and biologically relevant, was established by the INPC in 1999 (156,157) and revised in 2003 (137). This classification distinguishes two pathologic -prognostic groups: favorable histology (FH) and unfavorable histology (UH) group (Table 21-12) (3,5,22,56,72,97,119,121,146,162). This classification is age-linked and utilizes three morphologic indicators: status of Schwannian stromal development (stroma-poor,

Table 21-12 ■ PROGNOSTIC DISTINCTION ACCORDING TO THE INTERNATIONAL NEUROBLASTOMA PATHOLOGY CLASSIFICATION

Age	Favorable Histology Group	Unfavorable Histology Group
Any	Ganglioneuroma (Schwannian stroma-dominant) • Maturing • Mature Ganglioneuroblastoma, intermixed (Schwannian stroma-rich)	Neuroblastoma (Schwannian stroma-poor) • Undifferentiated and any MKI
Less than 1.5 years	Neuroblastoma (Schwannian stroma-poor) • Poorly differentiated and low or intermediate MKI • Differentiating and low or intermediate MKI	Neuroblastoma (Schwannian stroma-poor) Poorly differentiated and high MKI Differentiating and high MKI
1.5 years up to less than 5 years	Neuroblastoma (Schwannian stroma-poor) • Differentiating and low MKI	Neuroblastoma (Schwannian stroma-poor) • Poorly differentiated and any MKI • Differentiating and intermediate or high MKI
Equal to or greater than 5 years		Neuroblastoma (Schwannian stroma-poor) • Any subtype and any MKI
	Ganglioneuroblastoma, nodular (composite, Schwannian stroma-rich/stroma-dominant and stroma-poor), favorable subset[a]	Ganglioneuroblastoma, nodular (composite, Schwannian stroma-rich/stroma-dominant and stroma-poor), unfavorable subset[a]

[a]All tumors in the category of ganglioneuroblastoma, nodular were once classified into an unfavorable histology group according to the original Shimada classification (159) and the original International Neuroblastoma Pathology Classification (INPC) (156). However, the revised INPC distinguishes two prognostic subsets, favorable, and unfavorable, by applying the same age-linked histopathology evaluation to the nodular (neuroblastoma) components of the tumors in this category (137).

MKI, Mitosis-karyorrhexis index.

From Peuchmaur M, d'Amore ESG, Joshi VV, et al. Revision of the International Neuroblastoma Pathology Classification: confirmation of favorable and unfavorable prognostic subsets in ganglioneuroblastoma, nodular. *Cancer.* 2003;98:2274–2281; Shimada H, Ambros IM, Dehner LP, et al. Terminology and morphologic criteria of neuroblastic tumors: Recommendation by the International Neuroblastoma Pathology Committee. *Cancer.* 1999;86:349–363.

stroma-rich and stroma-dominant), grade of neuroblastic differentiation (undifferentiated, poorly differentiated, and differentiating), and MKI (low, intermediate, high). The histological features should be evaluated on a resected specimen or biopsy before the initiation of chemotherapy/irradiation therapy. Metastatic sites except for bone marrow are eligible for evaluation of all these histological features since a BM biopsy is not informative for MKI determination. FH NBs fall within the conceptual framework of an age-appropriate maturational sequence starting with NB (Schwannian stroma-poor), poorly differentiated subtype (up to 1.5 years of age at diagnosis) to NB-differentiating subtype (up to 5 years of age at diagnosis) to GNB-intermixed (Schwannian stroma-rich) to GN (Schwannian stroma-dominant). All GNs, the final end of tumor maturation, are thought to have had a neuroblastic component in their early developmental stage. In this regard, most GNs are diagnosed in later childhood and into adulthood. FH neuroblastic tumors should have a low (when diagnosed <5 years old at diagnosis) or an intermediate (when diagnosed <1.5 years old at diagnosis) MKI. In contrast, the histological features of UH neoplasms are immature or inappropriate for the age at diagnosis, and include NB, undifferentiated subtype (at any age), poorly differentiated NB (≥1.5 years of age), and all NB subtypes (≥5 years of age). Among tumors in the NB category, those with high MKI (at any age), or an intermediate MKI (≥1.5 years of age) are also assigned to the UH group. Ganglioneuroblastoma-intermixed and GN, usually diagnosed in older children, are examples of FH tumors with an excellent prognosis (127). Tumors in the GNB-nodular (composite, Schwannian stroma-rich/stroma-dominant and stroma-poor) category are further subclassified into two subsets, favorable and unfavorable, by application of the same criteria of age-linked evaluation of histological features (grade of neuroblastic differentiation and MKI) to the nodular (NB-, Schwannian stroma-poor) component (137,181).

Ganglioneuroblastoma-intermixed or GN are usually resected surgically. These tumors may encase the great vessels and/or organs, so that complete surgical excision with tumor-free margins is often difficult and unnecessary in most cases since local recurrences are uncommon. When only a biopsy is available and shows features of GNB-intermixed or GN, the pathologic diagnosis should be qualified by the comment, "the diagnosis is made based on review of limited material." In this circumstance, careful reassessment of the primary tumor site as well as a metastatic workup are recommended since there is the possibility of GNB-nodular in which case an unsampled neuroblastic nodule may exist. An unsampled neuroblastic nodule, if present, is often hemorrhagic and necrotic or may show invasive growth into the surrounding tissues which may be apparent by imaging studies. Metastatic foci may be demonstrable as well. Catecholamine determination is also advisable.

Histological changes after chemotherapy/irradiation therapy especially in the UH tumors do not provide any reliable information in predicting clinical outcome. These changes include extensive necrosis, hemorrhage, hemosiderin deposition, fibrosis, and calcification along with varying degrees of tumor maturation, often presenting different histological features from area to area, while, in the FH tumors, chemotherapy often seems to facilitate/expedite uniform tumor maturation without extensive necrosis, hemorrhage, and marked hemosiderin deposition. According to the Children's Oncology Group (COG) Neuroblastoma Study, the INPC evaluation of either FH or UH, once determined based on the review of prechemotherapy specimen, will not be altered during the clinical course of individual cases.

Molecular/Genetic Alterations: One of the more remarkable aspects of NB is the biological heterogeneity which is reflected in its tumorigenesis and diverse clinical behaviors. Structural genetic alterations often detected in NB include genomic amplification of *MYCN* oncogene on chromosome 2p24 (e157,e158,e1069), allelic deletion of the short arm of chromosome 1p36 (del 1p) (11,170,e158), allelic deletion of the long arm of chromosome 11q23 (del 11q) (11,167,169), and unbalanced gain of genetic material of the long arm of chromosome 17q21 (17q-gain) (e146). Besides these alterations, allelic losses of genetic material on 3p, 4p, 9p, 14q, 16p, and 19q, as well as segmental gains of 1q, 5q, and 18q have been detected in varying numbers of NBs (153). Most of these alterations are associated with unfavorable clinical behavior. Among these changes, 17q-gain is the most frequent alteration in some two-thirds of NBs, and may be related to the tumorigenesis. Spitz et al. could not confirm the prognostic impact of 17q-gain in children with NB (168). PHOX2B transcription factor (a homeobox gene functioning as an important regulator in development of normal autonomic nervous system) is mutated in a small proportion of NBs (117,177,183).

MYCN amplification, one of the strongest indicators for aggressive tumor progression, is observed in 15% to 20% of all NBs; the result is excess *MYCN* protein production. *MYCN-MAX* heterodimer formation in the tumor nuclei seems to prevent cellular differentiation, to promote cellular proliferation, and to effect genomic instability (e738,e1225). There is a reproducible correlation between the molecular event of *MYCN* amplification and the morphologic features of a NB. Those tumors with amplified *MYCN* typically have undifferentiated or poorly differentiated features with a high MKI reflecting increased cellular proliferation and apoptosis due to genomic instability (Figure 21-42) (58,161). The presence of prominent nucleoli in neuroblastic cells of undifferentiated or poorly differentiated tumor cells is reported to be an additional hallmark of *MYCN* amplification with a high sensitivity and a relatively lower specificity (82,172,176).

MYCN status of the individual tumors is now tested by fluorescent *in situ* hybridization (FISH) analysis in many institutions. The International Neuroblastoma Risk Group (INRG) Biology Committee has defined *MYCN* amplification by FISH analysis as "More than fourfold increase in the *MYCN* signal number compared with the reference probe located on the chromosome 2q." Furthermore, *MYCN*

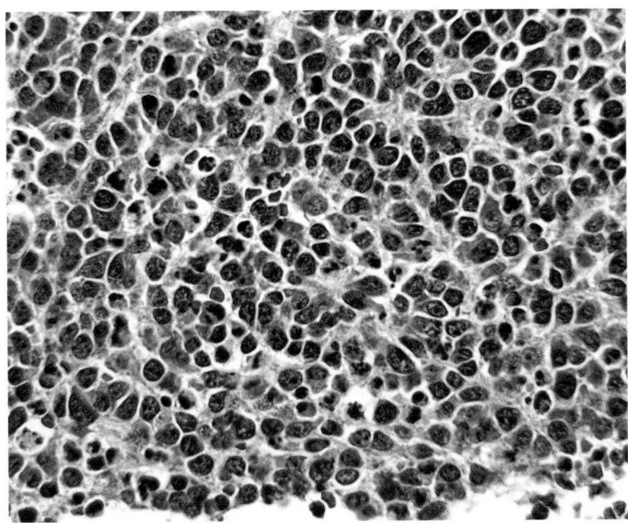

FIGURE 21-42 ▪ Neuroblastoma. Typical histological features of the MYCN amplified neuroblastoma include no Schwannian stroma development, no or limited neuroblastic differentiation, and markedly increased mitotic and karyorrhectic activities (high MKI—mitosis-karyorrhexis index).

gain has been defined as a signal increase but not up to the amplified status, whose clinical significance is yet to be determined (6). It is also noted that *MYCN* amplified status usually remains unchanged after chemotherapy.

Activating mutations in the ALK oncogene appear to be responsible for many of the hereditary NBs and could also be relevant for some fraction of sporadic cases. Interestingly, 20% to 25% of primary NBs present copy number increases at the *ALK* locus on 2p23, and elevated ALK gene-expression levels are reported in aggressive neuroblastic tumors (26,118,125,128,186,e561). Genetic variation at chromosome 6p22 has been identified for NB susceptibility. Additionally, patients who are homozygous for the risk alleles at 6p22 are likely to have metastatic disease, *MYCN* amplification, and decrease relapse (107).

Gene expression-based analyses show that elevated levels of TrkA, CD44, and CAMTA1 correlate with favorable clinical outcome (62,160,e251,e854), while elevated levels of expression of survivin, repp86, and PRAME are reported to correlate with adverse outcome (85,114,124). However, anyone of those candidates alone cannot sufficiently explain the diverse clinical behaviors of NBs, and is not considered as an independent prognostic factor in clinical trials.

DNA ploidy patterns, diploid ("near-diploid") or hyperdiploid ("near-triploid"), are reported to distinguish prognostic categories (92,166,e733,e734). A near-triploid DNA content due to whole chromosomal gain (lack of structural chromosomal aberration) has been reported as a favorable prognostic indicator. In contrast, a near-diploid DNA content predicts a poor clinical outcome for patients especially when they are infants.

Risk Grouping (INRG): Because of the biological complexity of tumors in the NB group, it is essential to establish a risk-group system for patient stratification and protocol assignment in the clinical management. Those risk factors or so-called prognostic factors include age at diagnosis, clinical stage, histopathologic classification according to the INPC, and molecular/genetic alterations.

Historically, 1 year of age at diagnosis has been utilized as a cutoff for predicting the prognosis. Recent analysis, however, demonstrates that the prognostic contribution of age to clinical outcome is continuous in nature. There is a gradual worsening of prognosis with increasing age, and there is statistical support for any choice of age cutoff between 15 and 19 months for use of risk stratification (e689). Based on these results, the COG NB study is currently using two age cutoffs, 12 months (365 days) and 18 months (547 days), at diagnosis in their risk-grouping scheme.

The International Neuroblastoma Staging System (INSS), a postsurgical staging system, has been used for prognostic purposes (Table 21-8) (e159,e160). Recently the INRG proposed a pretreatment staging system, based on clinical criteria and image-defined risk factors (116). In order to facilitate the comparison of risk-based clinical trials conducted in different regions and countries, the INRG defined four risk groups based on the combination of INRG stage (L1, L2, M, MS) (28,116) age at diagnosis (cutoffs at 12 and 18 months), histopathology (tumor category and grade of neuroblastic differentiation according to the recommendation by the INPC, *MYCN* status, 11q aberration, and ploidy: very low (>85% 5-year EFS); low (>75% to ≤85% 5-year EFS); intermediate (≥50% to ≤75% 5-year EFS), and high (<50% 5-year EFS) (186). In contrast, the COG NB studies distinguish three risk groups for the purpose of patient stratification and protocol assignment based on the combination of INSS stage [1, 2, 3, 4, 4S] (e158,e160), age at diagnosis (cutoffs at 12 and 18 months), histopathology (INPC; FH versus UH), *MYCN* status, ploidy, 1pLOH, and unb11qLOH. Their projected 5-year EFS rates are greater than 95% for the low-risk patients with surgery alone, greater than 90% for the intermediate-risk patients with surgery/biopsy and chemotherapy, and approximately 40% for the high-risk patients with intensive treatment including bone marrow transplantation (e1088).

Mass Screening: A mass screening program for preclinical detection of NB by measuring catecholamine metabolites was initiated in Japan 35 years ago (e1044) and then introduced to other countries including England, Germany, France, Austria, and Canada (149,e260,e602,e771). This program was based on the assumption that NB begins as a nonaggressive disease and would eventually progress to a more aggressive disease, and secondly that one-time screening in early life could detect all or many of the NBs in their nonaggressive state. In Japan, nationwide screening began in 1984 based on the significantly increased survival that could have been artificially raised due to increased incidence of newly (and unnecessarily) diagnosed cases through the screening (147,e1045,e1154). Whereas controlled studies from Quebec (screened at the age of 3 weeks and 6 months) (193,e594,e1168,e1285,e1286) and Germany (screened at the age of 1 year) (150,e1054) both reported similar and widely accepted results: (a) Screening almost doubled the incidence of NB and (b) cumulative mortality in the screened population was not reduced compared with an appropriate control population. NB is composed of at least two distinct clinical-biologic favorable and unfavorable behavior; tumors in the former group, once established, typically favorable clinical course and do not progress into the latter group. It had also been known that certain NBs in the biologically favorable group have the potential to spontaneously regress. However, the magnitude of such regression was not anticipated by the screening program. Screening failed to detect substantial numbers of biologically unfavorable tumors before their progression. Beside these biological and clinical issues, mass screening for NB yielded many clinical, psychological, and economic problems (the law of unanticipated consequences). In Japan, screening was finally terminated in 2004 because of the many pitfalls (180). Recently they reported a Japanese experience of a screening program at 6 months of age, and introduced an on-going screening at 18 months of age (63,65). Unfortunately their retrospective study contains major methodological issues (e762), such as changes in diagnostic standards and treatment modalities over the study period.

PHEO is a relatively rare neoplasm whose annual incidence ranges from two to eight cases:1,000,000 population. The term pheochromocytoma is derived from the brown color observed when the tumor is immersed in a dichromate solution (Figure 21-43A, B) (e789). Approximately 5% to 10% of incidentally-discovered adrenal masses, mainly in adults, are PHEOs (e728). Although 10% to 15% of cases present in the first two decades of life, some of the special clinical settings of PHEOs in children include the greater likelihood of a syndromic association, estimated at 15% to 25% of tumors (to include BWS, von Hippel-Lindau syndrome, MEN 2a (50% of cases), MEN 2b, Carney complex, familial PHEO and neurofibromatosis (1), bilaterality (commonly an association with one of the predisposing inherited disorders), and extraadrenal paraganglioma (25% to 40% of children) (Table 21-1) (4,15,18,91,122,138,173,174,e2,e79,e93,e101,e235, e263,e290,e323,e361,e425,e482,e489,e707,e744,e859,e986, e1008,e1035,e1207,e1245).

Genetic testing in 314 PHEOs in 56 patients with a family history and 258 patients with "sporadic" tumors, 27% had a hereditary tumor; among the 56 patients with a positive family history, NF1 and germline mutations in *VHL*, *RET*, and *SDHB* (succinate dehydrogenase subunit B) and *SDHD* (succinate dehydrogenase subunit D) were identified (4). In patients with apparent sporadic PHEOs, 11% had germline mutations in *VHL*, *RET SDHB* and *SDHD*. In a similar study of 271 patients with "sporadic" PHEOs, 24% had germline mutations in *VHL*, *RET*, *SDHB*, and *SDHD*; younger age, multifocality, and extra-adrenal sites (paragangliomas) (122). Havekes et al. have recently reported that 40% of PHEOs (adrenal and extra adrenal) had a hereditary basis (e482).

The WHO defines PHEO as a tumor of chromaffin cells of the adrenal medulla, and paraganglioma as a tumor arising from the extra-adrenal paraganglia; both tumors are neural crest in origin (eFigure 21-104) (42,e724,e789). A number of studies, however, combine both adrenal medullary tumors and extra-adrenal tumors under the diagnosis "pheochromocytoma." When combined, 80% of these tumors arise in the adrenal medulla and the remainder in the extra-adrenal paraganglia (20%) (15,e482). In a review of 520 PHEOs, 50 PHEOs (9.6%) occurred in children less than 16 years of age (15). Among these 50 childhood cases, the male:female ratio was 2:1, bilaterality was present in 32% of cases and extra-adrenal location in 18% of cases. A hereditary syndrome was identified in 7% of cases. Local recurrence or metastasis after initial excision occurred in 12% of children.

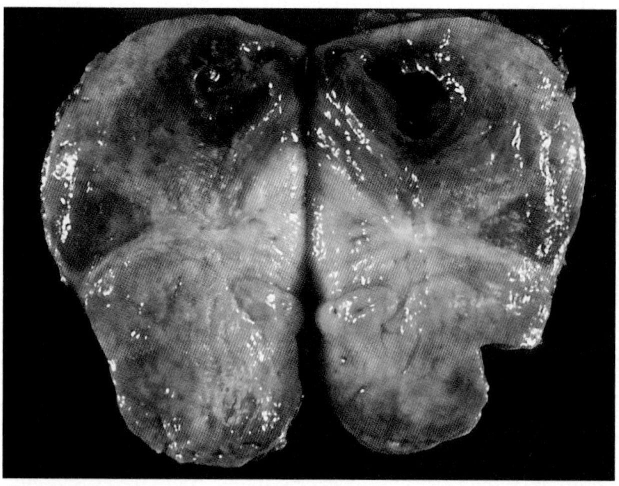
A

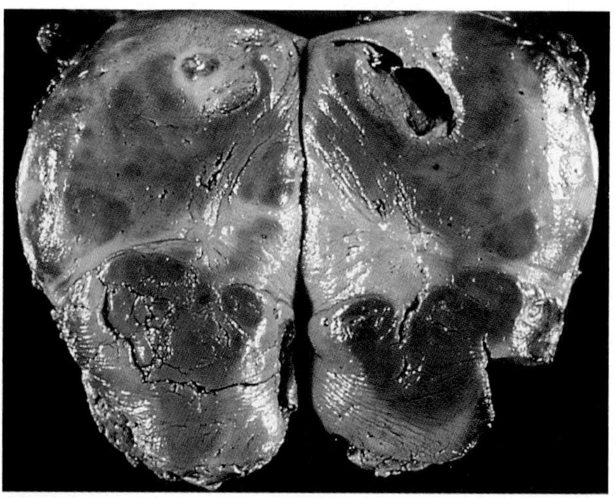
B

FIGURE 21-43 ■ Pheochromocytoma. **A:** This adrenal gland from a patient with episodic hypertension is replaced with a tan-white tumor with focal area of hemorrhage and necrosis and fibrosis. The tumor cells were immunoreactive for chromogranin. **B:** Immersion of this tumor in a dichromate-containing fixative yielded a dark-brown color. This positive chromaffin reaction is due to oxidation of the catecholamines, epinephrine and norepinephrine.

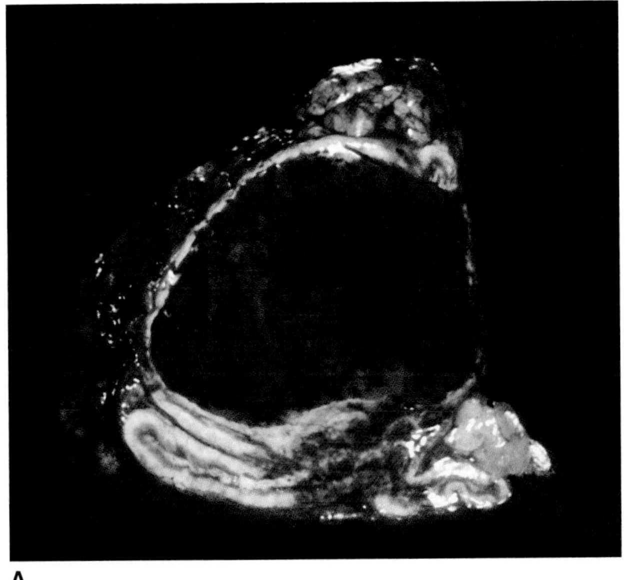

A

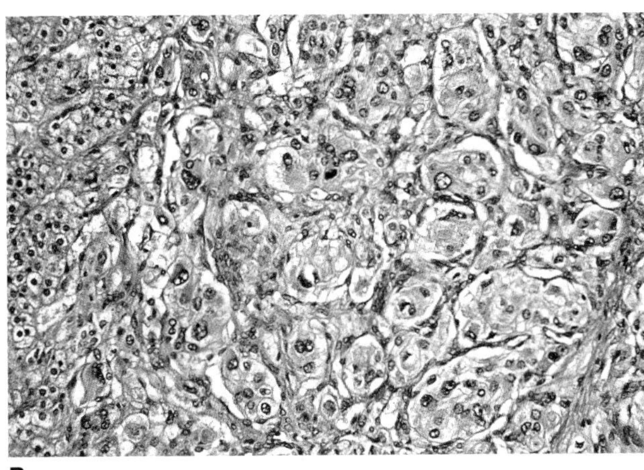

B

FIGURE 21-44 ▪ Pheochromocytoma. **A:** This adrenal gland demonstrates a central brown 3 cm diameter tumor replacing the adrenal medulla. The adrenal cortex (*yellow*) is seen at the periphery of this tumor. This tumor was resected from a patient with a chief complaint of paroxysmal attacks of headache, blurred vision, tachycardia and diaphoresis. **B:** The tumor cells are arranged in a characteristic alveolar "zellballen" or nesting pattern. They are surrounded by thin fibrovascular septate. The polyhedral tumor cells vary in shape and size. Most cells have an eosinophillic granular cytoplasm. The ovoid nuclei have a dispersed stippled chromatin pattern with inconspicuous nucleolus. Mitotic figures were infrequent in this tumor (H&E stain).

The major clinical signs and symptoms are related to the release of epinephrine with hypertension, paroxysms (headaches, palpitations and sweating) and either tachycardia (epinephrine) or reflex bradycardia (norepinephrine) (18,e79,e232,e1156). Cerebral infarction, cardiomyopathy, and catecholamine crisis have been observed in children (e270,e617). A female predilection is seen in some studies and others report a male preference (e322,e974). The average age at diagnosis in childhood is 12 to 15 years (e290,e378,e928,e979).

Sporadic PHEO is typically a solitary, well-circumscribed mass with either a true capsule or a pseudocapsule related to the tumor expansion and compression of adjacent connective tissue. Most tumors range in size from 3 to 5 cm, and the average weight is about 100 g (Figure 21-43A). Periadrenal brown fat is often seen. Because medullary tissue is concentrated in the head and body of the adrenal, the smaller PHEO arises in the latter locations (Figure 21-44A). On cut section, the tumor is firm and gray or dark red or is extensively hemorrhagic with cystic degeneration and friability. The chromaffin reaction is a manifestation of the catecholamines in the tissue and is produced by exposure of the unfixed specimen to a dichromate solution, which leads to a deep brown coloration (Figure 21-43B).

Three principal histological patterns are found in PHEO: a trabecular pattern with anastomosing cords of cells, an alveolar or nesting pattern with "zellballen" formation, and a diffuse or solid growth pattern (Figure 21-44B, eFigure 21-108). Spindle cells, angiomatoid foci, prominent interstitial and perivascular sclerosis, pseudopapillary formations and small spaces filled with eosinophilic proteinaceous debris are focal or generalized features in any one tumor (e685). Nuclear pseudoinclusions and eosinophilic hyaline intracytoplasmic globules are common. The individual tumor cells range from eosinophilic and granular to intense basophilia.

Immunohistochemistry has superseded many of the classic silver stains. These tumors are typically immunoreactive for VIM, CHR, VIP, and, infrequently HMB-45 (36, e381,e768,e1213). Antibodies to S-100 protein stain the sustentacular cells. Electron microscopy reveals cells with interdigitating borders and poorly formed cells junctions. Membrane-bound dense-core neurosecretory granules are prominent; these granules appear to be norepinephrine with a prominent eccentric electron-lucent space surrounding the dense core.

The incidence of malignancy in childhood PHEOs is difficult to ascertain due to the inclusion of paragangliomas in many studies; however, it is estimated that 2% to 12% of these tumors behave in a malignant fashion (91,e531). With inclusion of paragangliomas, the incidence is even higher, since paragangliomas especially in sites other than in the head and neck region are more prone to malignant behavior. When paragangliomas are included in the assessment of prognosis, the incidence of malignancy approaches 50% in some series inclusive of pediatric series (138,e257). Except for the presence of metastasis, no single histological feature of the tumor itself including local invasion is predictive of malignant behavior (eFigure 21-109,173,174, e974,e1057,e1184). Risk factors for malignancy include the diagnosis of paraganglioma and tumor size greater than 6 cm.

However, tumor size is not always predictive of malignancy (e1085). The 5- and 10-year survival rates for malignant tumors is 78% and 31%, respectively (138). In aggregate, extra-adrenal location, coarse nodularity, confluent necrosis, and absence of hyaline globules are features associated with malignancy (e717). An increased MIB-1 index (nuclear immunopositivity) correlated with malignant behavior in some but not all studies (173,174,e165,e910,e1062,e1216).

Adrenal medullary hyperplasia is found in the setting of the MEN 2 syndromes as the presumed precursor of PHEOs. It has also been reported as an isolated finding in the nonfamilial setting of hypertension and biochemical studies suggesting PHEO; however, no discrete adrenal medullary tumor is found at surgery (104,e961). Criteria for the pathological diagnosis of adrenal medullary hyperplasia include an increase in adrenal weight which is accompanied by diffuse or nodular extension of the medulla into the alae (e677,e908). Morphometric criteria include a decrease in the overall ratio of cortex to medulla (normal is 10:1) and an increase in the calculated medullary weight and volume (eFigures 21-110 and 21-111).

Composite adrenal medullary neoplasms are rare entities that are composed in part of a PHEO, one of the three patterns of the neuroblastic tumors or a peripheral nerve sheath neoplasm (e77,e382,e1189,e1190). Most of these tumors have been reported in adults, but have been infrequently observed in children.

Other tumor and tumor-like lesions of the adrenal gland include a variety of cysts of a presumed vascular nature. Extramedullary hematopoiesis in the setting of β-thalassemia may present as an adrenal incidentaloma in childhood (e (949). Myelolipoma, one of the more common "incidentalomas" of the adrenal gland in adults, is extremely unusual in children and slightly more frequent than the lipoma and leiomyoma (e47,e271,e296,e568,e847,e950,e1081,e1082). Hemangioma or hemangioendothelioma of the adrenal has been observed in infancy (e297,e1112). One other unusual tumor of the adrenal gland that we have had an opportunity to study was an extrarenal Wilms tumor presenting in a 4-year-old boy (e1036). Molberg et al. reported the occurrence of a primitive epithelial and mesenchymal neoplasm of the adrenal in an infant with virilizing signs, which was interpreted as an adrenal blastoma (90,e831). Primitive neuroectodermal tumor family tumor has been reported in the adrenal gland of children (e591,e774). Though not an adrenal lesion per se, subdiaphragmatic extralobar sequestration may simulate an adrenal tumor when it presents as a suprarenal mass (see Chapter 12) (e199,e957).

REFERENCES

1. Akramipour R, Zargooshi J, Rahimi Z. Infant with congenital presence of hernia/hydrocele and primary paratesticular neuroblastoma: a diagnostic and therapeutic challenge. *J Pediatr Hematol Oncol* 2009;31:349.
2. Alizzi AM, Hemil JM, Diger A, et al. Primary solitary mediastinal mass lesions: a review of 37 cases. *Heart Lung Circ* 2006;15: 310–313.
3. Altungoz O, Aygun N, Tumer S, et al. Correlation of modified Shimada classification with MYCN and 1p36 status detected by fluorescence in situ hybridization in neuroblastoma. *Cancer Genet Cytogenet* 2007;172;113–119.
4. Amar L, Bertherat J, Baudin E, et al. Genetic testing in pheochromocytoma or functional paraganglioma. *J Clin Oncol* 2005;23: 8812–8818.
5. Ambros IM, Hata J, Joshi VV, et al. Morphologic features of neuroblastoma (Schwannian stroma-poor tumors) in clinically favorable and unfavorable groups. *Cancer* 2002;94:1574–1583.
6. Ambros PF, Ambros IM, Brodeur GM, et al. International consensus for neuroblastoma molecular diagnostics: report from the International Neuroblastoma Risk Group (INRG) Biology Committee. *Br J Cancer* 2009;100:1471–1482.
7. Aronica PA, Pirrotta VT, Yunis EJ, et al. Detection of neuroblastoma in the bone marrow: biopsy versus aspiration. *J Pediatr Hematol Oncol* 1998;20:330–334.
8. Arvand A, Danny CT. Biology of EWS/ETS fusions in Ewing's family tumors. *Oncogene* 2001;20:5747–5754.
9. Asa SL. Tumors of the pituitary gland. *Atlas of tumor pathology*, 3rd series. Washington: Armed Forces Institute of Pathology, 1998: 47–150.
10. Asa SL, Ezzat S. The pathogenesis of pituitary tumors. *Annu Rev Pathol Mech Dis* 2009;4:97–126.
11. Attiyeh EF, London WB, Mosse YP, et al. Chromosome 1p and 11q deletions and outcome in neuroblastoma. *N Engl J Med* 2005;353:2243–2253.
12. Auchus RJ, Miller WL. The principles, pathways, and enzymes of human steroidogenesis. In: DeGroot LJ, Jameson JL, eds. *Endocrinology*, 5th ed. Philadelphia, PA: Elsevier, 2006.
13. Bassal M, Mertens AC, Taylor L, et al. Risk of selected subsequent carcinomas in survivors of childhood cancer: a report from the Childhood Cancer Survivor Study. *J Clin Oncol* 2006;24:476–483.
14. Beiske K, Burchill SA, Cheung IY, et al. Consensus criteria for sensitive detection of minimal neuroblastoma cells in bone marrow, blood and stem cell preparations by immunocytology and QRT-PCR: recommendations by the International Neuroblastoma Risk Group Task Force. *Br J Cancer* 2009;100:1627–1637.
15. Beltsevich DG, Kuznetsov NS, Kazaryan AM, et al. Pheochromocytoma surgery: epidemiologic peculiarities in children. *World J Surg* 2004;28:592–596.
16. Berger J, Gartner J. X-linked adrenoleukodystrophy: clinical, biochemical and pathogenetic aspects. *Biochim Biophys Acta* 2006;1763:1721–1732.
17. Bettendorf M. Thyroid disorders in children from birth to adolescence. *Eur J Nucl Med Mol Imaging* 2002;29(suppl 2):S439–S446.
18. Bhansali A, Rajput R, Behra A, Rao KL, et al. Childhood sporadic pheochromocytoma: clinical profile and outcome in 19 patients. *J Pediatr Endocrinol Metab* 2006;19:749–756.
19. Brat DJ, Parisi JE, Kleinschmidt-DeMasters BK, et al. Surgical neuropathology update: a review of changes introduced by the WHO Classification of Tumours of the Central Nervous System, 4th edition. *Arch Pathol Lab Med* 2008;132:993–1007.
20. Brodeur GM, Maris JM. Neuroblastoma. In: Pizzo PA, Poplack DG, eds. *Principles and practice of pediatric oncology*, 4th ed. Philadelphia, PA: Lippincott-Williams & Wilkins, 2002;895–937.
21. Burger PC, Scheithauer BW. *AFIP atlas of tumor pathology, series 4, Tumors of the central nervous system*. Washington: American Registry of Pathology, 2007;295–308.
22. Burgues O, Navarro S, Noguera R, et al. Prognsotic value of the International Neuroblastoma Pathology Classification in Neuroblastoma (Schwannian stroma-poor) and comparison with other prognostic factors: a study of 182 cases from the Spanish Neuroblastoma Registry. *Virchows Arch* 2006;449:410–420.
23. Calonge WM, Heitor F, Castro LP, et al. Neonatal paratesticular neuroblastoma misdiagnosed as in utero torsion of testis. *J Pediatr Hematol Oncol* 2004;26:693–695.

24. Carling T. Molecular pathology of parathyroid tumors. *Trends Endocrinol Metab* 2001;12:53–58.
25. CBTRUS (2009). *CBTRUS statistical report: primary brain and central nervous system tumors diagnosed in the United States in 2004–2005*. Source: Central Brain Tumor Registry of the United States, Hinsdale, IL. Website: www.cbtrus.org.
26. Chen Y, Takita J, Choi YL, et al. Oncogenic mutations of ALK kinase in neuroblastoma. *Nature* 2008:455;971–974.
27. Claahsen-van der Grinten HL, Otten BJ, Stikkelbroeck MM, et al. Testicular adrenal rest tumours in congenital adrenal hyperplasia. *Best Pract Res Clin Endocrinol Metab* 2009;23:209–220.
28. Cohn SL, Pearson ADJ, London WB, et al. The International Neuroblastoma Risk Group (INRG) Classification System: An INRG Task Force Report. *J Clin Oncol* 2009;27:289–297.
29. Collett-Solberg PF. Congenital adrenal hyperplasia: from genetics and biochemistry to clinical practice, part 1. *Clin Pediatr (Phila)* 2001;40:1–16.
30. Collett-Solberg PF. Congenital adrenal hyperplasia: from genetics and biochemistry to clinical practice, part 2. *Clin Pediatr (Phila)* 2001;40:125–132.
31. Combaret V, Bergeron C, Noguera R, et al. Circulating MYCN DNA predicts MYCN-amplification in neuroblastoma. *J Clin Oncol* 2005;23:8919–8920.
32. Cooper R, Khakoo Y, Matthay KK, et al. Opsoclonus-myoclonus-ataxia syndrome in neuroblastoma: histopathologic features—a report from the Children's Cancer Group. *Med Pediatr Oncol* 2001;36:623–629.
33. Dabbs D. *Diagnostic immunohistochemistry*, 2nd ed. Philadelphia, PA: Elsevier, 2006;265–267.
34. Dabbs D. *Diagnostic immunohistochemistry*, 2nd ed. Philadelphia, PA: Elsevier, 2006;267, 782–783.
35. Dabbs D. *Diagnostic immunohistochemistry*, 2nd ed. Philadelphia, PA: Elsevier, 2006;276–278.
36. Dabbs D. *Diagnostic immunohistochemistry*, 2nd ed. Philadelphia, PA: Elsevier, 2006;278–283.
37. Davicioni E, Anderson MJ, Finckenstein FG, et al. Molecular classification of rhabdomyosarcoma—genotypic and phenotypic determinants of diagnosis: a report from the Children's Oncology Group. *Am J Pathol* 2009;174:550–564.
38. DeBernardi B, Pianca C, Pistamiglio P, et al. Neuroblastoma with symptomatic spinal cord compression at diagnosis: treatment and results with 76 cases *J Clin Oncol*. 2001;19:183–190.
39. DeGroot LJ, Jameson JL, eds. *Endocrinology*, 5th ed. Philadelphia, PA: Elsevier, 2006.
40. Dehner LP, Hill A. Adrenal cortical neoplasms in children: Why so many carcinomas and yet so many survivors? *Pediatr Develop Pathol* 2009;12:284–291.
41. DeLellis RA. *Tumors of the parathyroid gland*, Third series. Washington: Armed Forces Institute of Pathology, 1993:2.
42. DeLellis RA, Lloyd RV, Heitz PU, et al. eds. World Health Organization classification of tumors. *Pathology and genetics: tumors of endocrine organs*. Lyon: IARC Press, 2004.
43. DeLellis RA, Mazzaglia P, Mangray S. Primary hyperparathyroidism: a current perspective. *Arch Pathol Lab Med* 2008;132: 1251–1262.
44. Diamond FB Jr. Pituitary adenomas in childhood: development and diagnosis. *Fetal Pediatr Pathol* 2006;25:339–356.
45. Dinauer C, Francis GL Thyroid cancer in children. *Endocrinol Metab Clin North Am*. 2007;36: 779–806.
46. Doyle DA, DiGeorge AM. Hormones and peptides of calcium homeostasis and bone metabolism. In: Kliegman RM, Behrman RE, Jenson HB, Stanton BF, eds., *Nelson textbook of pediatrics*, 18th ed., Chapter 571. Philadelphia, PA: Elsevier, 2007.
47. Doyle DA, DiGeorge AM. Hyperparathyroidism. In: Kliegman RM, Behrman RE, Jenson HB, Stanton BF, eds. *Nelson textbook of pediatrics*, 18th ed., Chapter 574. Philadelphia, PA: Elsevier, 2007.
48. Drummond KJ, Rosenfeld JV. Pineal region tumors in childhood: a 30-year experience. *Childs Nerv Syst* 1999;15:119–127.
49. DuBois S. London W, Zhang Y, et al. Lung metastases in neuroblastoma at initial diagnosis: a report from the International Neuroblastoma Risk Group (INRG) Project. *Pediatr Blood Cancer* 2008;51:589–592.
50. Engel U, Gottschalk S, Niehaus L, et al. Cystic lesions of the pineal region—MRI and pathology. *Neuroradiology* 2000;42: 399–402.
51. Espinasse-Holder M, Defachelles AS, Weill J, et al. Paraneoplastic Cushing syndrome due to adrenal neuroblastoma. *Med Pediatr Oncol* 2000;34:231–233.
52. Fauchon F, Jouvet A, Paquis P, et al. Parenchymal pineal tumors: A clinicopathological study of 76 cases. *Int J Radiat Oncol Biol Phys* 2000;46:959–968.
53. Fleitz JM, Wootton-Gorges SL, Wyatt-Ashmead J, et al. Renal cell carcinoma in long-term survivors of advanced neuroblastoma in early childhood. *Pediatr Radiol* 2003;33:540–545.
54. Foley DS, Fallat ME. Thyroglossal duct and other congenital midline cervical aanomalies. *Semin Pediatr Surg* 2006;15:70–75.
55. Gambini C, Conte M, Bernini G, et al. Neuroblastic tumors associated with opsoclonus-myoclonus syndrome: histological, immunohistochemical and molecular features of 15 Italian cases. *Virchow Arch* 2003;442:555–562.
56. George RE, Variend S, Cullinane C, et al., United Kingdom Children Cancer Study Group. United Kingdom Children Cancer Study Group: Relationship between histopathological features, MYCN amplification, and prognosis: a UKCCSG study. *Med Pediatr Oncol* 2001;36:169–176.
57. Goodman MT, Gurney JG, Smith MA, et al. Sympathetic nervous system tumors, chap IV. In: Ries LAG, Smith MA, Gurney JG, Linet M, Tamra T, Young JL, Bunin GR, eds. *Cancer incidence and survival among children and adolescents: United States SEER program 1975–1995, National Cancer Institute, SEER Program*. NIH Publ # 00–4649, Bethesda, MD, 1999.
58. Goto S, Umehara S, Gerbing RB, et al. Histopathology and MYCN Status in peripheral neuroblastic tumors: a report from the Children's Cancer Group. *Cancer* 2001;92:2699–2708.
59. Halac I, Zimmerman D. Thyroid nodules and cancers in children. *Endocrinol Metab Clin North Am*. 2005;34:725–744.
60. Hann HW, Bombardieri E. Serum markers and prognosis in neuroblastoma: Ferritin, LDH, NSE. In Brodeur G, Sawada T, TSuchida Y, Voute PA, eds. *Neuroblastoma*. Amsterdam: Elsevier, 2000; 371–381.
61. Hemminki K, Forsti A., Ji J. Incidence and familial risks in pituitary adenoma and associated tumors. *Endocr Relat Cancer* 2007;14: 103–109.
62. Henrich KO, Fischer M, Mertens D, et al. Reduced expression of CAMTA1 correlates with adverse outcome in neuroblastoma patients. *Clin Cancer Res* 2006;12:131–138.
63 Hiyama E, Iehara T, Sugimoto T, et al. Effectiveness of screening for neuroblastoma at 6 months of age: a retrospective population-based cohort study. *Lancet* 2008;371:1173–1180.
64. Hiyama E, Yokoyama T, Hiyama K, et al. Multifocal neuroblastoma: biologic behavior and surgical aspects. *Cancer* 2000;88: 1955–1963.
65. Hiyama E. Neuroblastoma screening in Japan: population-based cohort study and future aspects of screening. *Ann Acad Med (Singapore)* 2008;37(12 suppl):88–94.
66. Horner MJ, Ries LAG, Krapcho M, et al., eds. *Table 26.6: Cancer of the thyroid (invasive), SEER incidence and US Death Rates, age-adjusted and age-specific rates, by race and sex*. SEER Cancer Statistics Review, 1975–2006, National Cancer Institute, Bethesda, MD, http://seer.cancer.gov/csr/1975_2006/, based on November 2008 SEER data submission, posted to the SEER web site, 2009.

67. Horner MJ, Ries LAG, Krapcho M, et al., eds. *Table 29.1: Age-adjusted and age-specific SEER cancer incidence rates, 2002–2006*. National Cancer Institute, Bethesda, MD, http://seer.cancer.gov/csr/1975_2006/, based on November 2008 SEER data submission, posted to the SEER web site, 2009.
68. Hsiao RJ, Seeger RC, Yu AL, et al. Chromogranin A in children with neuroblastoma. Serum concentration parallels disease stage and predicts survival. *J Clin Invest* 85:1555–1559.
69. Hsu SC, Levine MA. Primary hyperparathyroidism in children and adolescents: the Johns Hopkins Children's Center experience 1984–2001. *J Bone Miner Res* 2002;17(suppl 2):N44–N50.
70. Hua X, Mao-Sheng X, Hong-Quan G, et al. Primary paratesticular neuroblastoma: a case report and review of literature. *J Pediatr Surg* 2008;43:E5–E7.
71. Hung W. Solitary thyroid nodules in 93 children and adolescents: a 35-years experience. *Horm Res* 1999;52:15–18.
72. Ikeda H, Iehara T, Tsuchida Y, et al. Experience with international neuroblastoma staging system and pathology classification. *Br J Cancer* 2002;86;1110–1116.
73. Isaacs H. Fetal and Neonatal neuroblastoma: retrospective review of 271 cases. *Fetal Pediatr Pathol* 2007;26:177–184.
74. Iwase K, Nagasaka A, Nagatsu I, et al. Tyrosine hydroxylase indicates cell differentiation of catecholamine biosynthesis in neuroendocrine tumors. *J Endocrinol Invest* 1994;17:235–239.
75. Jane JA Jr, Laws ER. Craniopharyngioma. *Pituitary* 2006;9:323–326.
76. Janknecht R. EWS-ETS oncoproteins: the linchpins of Ewing's tumors. *Gene* 2005;363:1–14.
77. Josefson J, Zimmerman D. Thyroid nodules and cancers in children. *Pediatr Endocrinol Rev* 2008;6:14–23.
78. Jouvet A, Fevre-Montange M, Besancon R, et al. Structural and ultrastructural characteristics of human pineal gland, and pineal parenchymal tumors. *Acta Neuropathol* 1994;88:334–348.
79. Jouvet A, Saint-Pierre G, Fauchon F, et al. Pineal parenchymal tumors: a correlation of histological features with prognosis in 66 cases. *Brain Pathol* 2000;10:49–60.
80. Kahaly GJ. Polyglandular autoimmune syndromes. *Eur J Endocrinol* 2009;161:11–20.
81. Kloos RT, Eng C, Evans DB, et al. Medullary thyroid cancer: management guidelines of the American Thyroid Association. *Thyroid* 2009;19:565–612.
82. Kobayashi C, Monforte-Munoz HL, Gerbing RB, et al. Enlarged and prominent nucleoli may be indicative of MYCN amplification: a study of neuroblastoma (Schwannian stroma-poor), undifferentiated /poorly differentiated subtype with high mitosis-karyorrhexis index. *Cancer* 2005;103:174–180.
83. Kollars J, Zarroug AE, van Heerden J, et al. Primary hyperparathyroidism in pediatric patients. *Pediatrics* 2005;115:974–980.
84. Komada Y, Zhang XL, Zhou YW, et al. Flow cytometric analysis of peripheral blood and bone marrow for tumor cells in patients with neuroblastoma. *Cancer* 1998;82:591–599.
85. Krams M, Heidebrecht HJ, Hero B, et al. Repp86 expression and outcome in patients with neuroblastoma. *J Clin Oncol* 2003;21:1810–1818.
86. Krone N, Arlt W. Genetics of congenital adrenal hyperplasia. *Best Pract Res Clin Endocrinol Metab* 2009;23:181–192.
87. Lack EE. Tumors of the adrenal gland and extra-adrenal paraganglia. *AFIP atlas of tumor pathology*, Ser. 4. Washington: American Registry of Pathology, 2007:1–37.
88. Lack EE. Tumors of the adrenal gland and extra-adrenal paraganglia. *AFIP atlas of tumor pathology*, Ser. 4. Washington: American Registry of Pathology, 2007:39–55.
89. Lack EE. Tumors of the adrenal gland and extra-adrenal paraganglia. *AFIP atlas of tumor pathology*, Ser. 4. Washington: American Registry of Pathology, 2007:57–97.
90. Lack EE. Tumors of the adrenal gland and extra-adrenal paraganglia. AFIP atlas of tumor pathology, Ser. 4. Washington: American Registry of Pathology, 2007:161–179.
91. Lack EE. Tumors of the adrenal gland and extra-adrenal paraganglia. *AFIP atlas of tumor pathology*, Ser. 4. Washington: American Registry of Pathology, 2007:241–282.
92. Ladenstein R, Ambros IM, Potschger U, et al. Prognostic significance of di-tetraploidy in neuroblastoma. *Med Pediatr Oncol* 2001;36:83–92.
93. LaFranchi S. Section 2: disorders of the thyroid gland. In: Kliegman RM, Behrman RE, Jenson HB, Stanton BF, eds. *Nelson textbook of pediatrics*, 18th ed. Philadelphia, PA: Elsevier, 2007.
94. LaFranchi S. Thyroid hormone in hypopituitarism, Graves' disease, congenital hypothyroidism, and maternal thyroid disease during pregnancy. *Growth Horm IGF Res* 2006;16(suppl A): S20–S24.
95. Lap-Yin Pang A, Martin MM, Martin ALA, et al. Molecular basis of diseases of the endocrine system. In: Coleman WB, Tsongalis GJ, eds. *Molecular pathology: the molecular basis of human disease*. Amsterdam: Elsevier, 2009;435–463.
96. Larsen PR, Kronenberg HM, Melmed S, et al. eds. *Williams textbook of endocrinology*, 10th ed. Philadelphia, PA: Saunders, 2003.
97. Lastowska M, Cullinane C, Variend S, et al. United Kingdom Children Cancer Study Group and United Kingdom Cancer Cytogenetics Group. Comprehensive genetic and histopathologic study reveals three types of neuroblastoma tumors. *J Clin Oncol* 2001;19: 3080–3090.
98. Lau L. Neuroblastoma: a single institution's experience with 128 children and an evaluation of clinical and biological prognostic factors. *Pediatr Hematol Oncol* 2002;19:79–89.
99. Lin L, Gu WX, Ozisik G, et al. Analysis of DAX1 (NR0B1) and steroidogenic factor-1 (NR5A1) in children and adults with primary adrenal failure: ten years' experience. *J Clin Endocrinol Metab* 2006;91:3048–3054.
100. Lin S, Tseng F, Hsu C, et al. Thyroglossal duct cyst: a comparison between children and adults. *Am J Otolaryngol* 2008;29:83–87.
101 Lloyd RV, Douglas BR, Young WF. *Endocrine diseases: atlas of nontumor pathology*, Fascicle 1. Washington, DC: American Registry of Pathology, 2001:1–44.
102. Lloyd RV, Douglas BR, Young WF. *Endocrine Diseases: Atlas of Nontumor Pathology*, Fascicle 1. Washington, DC: American Registry of Pathology, 2001:45–90.
103. Lloyd RV, Douglas BR, Young WF. *Endocrine diseases: atlas of nontumor pathology*, Fascicle 1. Washington, DC: American Registry of Pathology, 2001:91–170.
104. Lloyd RV, Douglas BR, Young WF. *Endocrine diseases: atlas of nontumor pathology*, Fascicle 1. Washington, DC: American Registry of Pathology, 2001:171–258.
105. Louis DN, Ohgaki H, Wiestler OD, et al. The 2007 WHO classification of tumors of the central nervous system. *Acta Neuropathol (Berl)* 2007;114:97–109.
106. Mandera M, Marcol W, Bierzynska-Macyszyn G, et al. Pineal cysts in childhood. *Childs Nerv Syst* 2003;19:750–755.
107. Maris JM, Mosse YP, Bradfield JP, et al. Chromosome 6p22 locus associated with clinically aggressive neuroblastoma. *N Engl J Med* 2008;358:2585–2593.
108. Maris JM, Weiss MJ, Mosse Y, et al. Evidence for hereditary neuroblastoma predisposition locus at chromosome 16p12–13. *Cancer Res* 2002;62:6651–6658.
109. Mehrazin, M. Pituitary tumors in children: clinical analysis of 21 cases. *Childs Nerv Syst* 2007;23:391–398.
110. Melmed S, Kleinberg DL. Anterior pituitary. In: Larsen PR, Kronenberg HM, Melmed S, Polonsky KS. eds. *Williams Textbook of Endocrinology*, 10th ed. Philadelphia, PA: Saunders, 2003;177–280.
111. Mena H, Nakazato Y, Jouvet A, Scheithauer B. Pineal parenchymal tumours. In: Kleihues P, Cavenee WK, eds. *Pathology and genetics of tumours of the nervous system*. Lyon: IARC Press 2000; 115–121.
112. Michalkiewicz E, Sandrini R, Figueiredo B, et al. Clinical and outcome characteristics of children with adrenocortical tumors: a report

from the International Pediatric Adrenocortical Tumor Registry. *J Clin Oncol* 2004;22:838–845.
113. Michielsen G, Benoit Y, Baert E, et al. Symptomatic pineal cysts: clinical manifestations and management. *Acta Neurochir (Wien)* 2002;144:233–242.
114. Miller MA, Ohashi K, Zhu X, et al. Survivin mRNA levels are associated with biology of disease and patient survival in neuroblastoma: a report from the Children's Oncology Group. *J Pediatr Hematol Oncol* 2006;28:412–417.
115. Mindermann T, Wilson CB. Pediatric pituitary adenomas. *Neurosurgery* 1995;36:259–268; discussion 269.
116. Monclair T, Brodeur GM, Ambros PF, et al. The International Neuroblastoma Risk Group (INRG) Staging System: an INRG Task Force Report. *J Clin Oncol* 2009;27:298–303.
117. Mosse YP, Laudenslager M, Khazi D, et al. Germline PHOX2B mutations in hereditary neuroblastoma. *Am J Hum Genet*. 2004;75: 727–730.
118. Mosse YP, Laudenslager M, Longo L et al. Identification of ALK as a major familial neuroblastoma predisposition gene. *Nature* 2008;455:930–935.
119. Munchar MJ, Sharifah NA, Jamal R, et al. CD44s expression correlates with the International Neuroblastoma Pathology Classification (Shimada system) for neuroblastic tumours. *Pathology* 2003;35: 125–129.
120. Navarro S, Noguera R, Pellin A, et al. Pleomorphic anaplastic neuroblastoma. *Med Pediatr Oncol* 2000;35:498–502.
121. Navarro S, Amann G, Beiske K, et al. European Study Group 94.01 Trial and Protocol. Prognostic value of International Neuroblastoma Pathology Classification in localized resectable peripheral neuroblastic tumors: a histopathologic study of localized neuroblastoma European Study Group 94.01 Trial and Protocol. *J Clin Oncol* 2006;24:695–696.
122. Neumann HP, Bausch B, McWhinney SR, et al. Germ-line mutations in nonsyndromic pheochromocytoma. *N Engl J Med* 2002;346: 1459–1466.
123. Niedziela, M. Pathogenesis, diagnosis and management of thyroid nodules in children. *Endocr Relat Cancer* 2006;13:427–453.
124. Oberthuer A, Hero B, Spitz R, et al. The tumor-associated antigen PRAME is universally expressed in high-stage neuroblastoma and associated with poor outcome. *Clin Cancer Res* 2004;10(13) 4307–4313.
125. Oberthuer A, Kaderali L, Kahlert Y, et al. Subclassification and individual survival time prediction from gene expression data of neuroblastoma patients by using CASPAR. *Clin Cancer Res* 2008;14:6590–6601.
126. Ohyama M, Kobayashi S, Aida N, et al. Congenital neuroblastoma diagnosed by placental examination. *Med Pediatr Oncol* 1999;33:430–431.
127. Okamatsu C, London WB, Naranjo A, et al. Clinicopathological characteristics of ganglioneuroma and ganglioneuroblastoma: a report from the CCG and COG. *Pediatr Blood Cancer* 2009;53: 563–569.
128. Osajima-Hakomori Y, Miyake I, Ohira M, et al. Biological role of anaplastic lymphoma kinase in neuroblastoma. *Am J Pathol* 2005;167:213–222.
129. Pandey P, Ojha BK, Mahapatra AK. Pediatric pituitary adenoma: a series of 42 patients. *J Clin Neurosci* 2005;12:124–127.
130. Parham DM, Qualman SJ, Teot L, et al. Soft Tissue Sarcoma Committee of the Children's Oncology Group: correlation between histology and PAX/FKHR fusion status in alveolar rhabdomyosarcoma: a report from the Children's Oncology Group. *Am J Surg Pathol* 2007;31:895–901.
131. Parham DM, Roloson GJ, Feely M, et al. Primary malignant neuroepithelial tumors of the kidney: a clinicopathological analysis of 146 adult and pediatric cases from the National Wilms' Tumor Study Group Pathology Center. *Am J Surg Pathol* 2001;25: 133–146.
132. Parisi MT, Mankoff D. Differentiated pediatric thyroid cancer: correlates with adult disease, controversies in treatment. *Semin Nucl Med* 2007;37:340–356.
133. Parks JS, Felner EI, Hypopituitarism. In: Kliegman RM, Behrman RE, Jenson HB, Stanton BF, eds. *Nelson textbook of pediatrics*, 18th ed., Chapter 558. Philadelphia, PA: Saunders, 2007.
134. Pernicone P, Scheithauer BW, Horvath E, et al. Pituitary and sellar region. In: Sternberg S, ed. *Histology for pathologists*, 2ed. New York: Raven Press, 1997:1053–1074.
135. Perri P, Longo L, Cusano R, et al. Weak linkage at 4p16 to predisposition for human neuroblastoma. *Oncogene* 2002;21:8356–8360.
136. Peter, F, Muzsnai A. Congenital disorders of the thyroid: hypo/ hyper. *Endocrinol Metab Clin North Am* 2009;38:491–507.
137. Peuchmaur M, d'Amore ESG, Joshi VV, et al. Revision of the International Neuroblastoma Pathology Classification: confirmation of favorable and unfavorable prognostic subsets in ganglioneuroblastoma, nodular. *Cancer* 2003;98:2274–81.
138. Pham TH, Moir C, Thompson GB, et al. Pheochromocytoma and paraganglioma in children: a review of medical and surgical management at a tertiary care center. *Pediatrics* 2006;118: 1109–1117.
139. Phelan JK, McCabe ER. Mutations in NR0B1 (DAX1) and NR5A1 (SF1) responsible for adrenal hypoplasia congenita. *Hum Mutat* 2001;18:472–487.
140. Polak M, Sura-Trueba S, Chauty A, et al. Molecular mechanisms of thyroid dysgenesis. *Horm Res* 2004;62(suppl 3):14–21.
141. Popovic MB, Diezi M, Kuchler H, et al. Trilateral retinoblastoma with suprasellar tumor and associated pineal cyst. *J Pediatr Hematol Oncol* 2007;29:53–56.
142. Reiter RJ. The pineal gland. In: Lechago J, Gould VE, eds. *Bloodworth's endocrine pathology*, 3rd ed. Baltimore, MD: Williams & Wilkins, 1997:153–170.
143. Robinson AG Verbalis JG. Posterior pituitary gland. In: Larsen PR, Kronenberg HM, Melmed S, Polonsky KS. eds. *Williams textbook of endocrinology*, 10th ed. Philadelphia, PA: Saunders, 2003: 177–280.
144. Rudnick E, Khakoo Y, Antunes N, et al. Opsoclonus-myoclonus-ataxia syndrome in neuroblastoma: clinical outcome and antineuronal antibodies—a report from the Children's Cancer Group Study. *Med Pediatr Oncol* 2001;36:612–622.
145. Safford SD, Skinner MA. Thyroid and parathyroid disease in children. *Semin Pediatr Surg*. 2006;15:85–91.
146. Sano H, Bonadio J, Gerbing RB, et al. International Neuroblastoma Pathology Classification adds independent prognostic information beyond the prognostic contribution of age. *Eur J Cancer* 2006;42:1113–1119.
147. Sawada T, Takeda T. Screening for neuroblastoma in infancy in Japan. In: Brodeur GM, Sawada T, Tsuchida Y, Voute PA, eds. *Neuroblastoma*. Amsterdam: Elsevier, 2000:245–264.
148. Schiavetti A, Foco M, Ingrosso A, et al. Congenital stage 1 neuroblastoma evolved into stage 4s. *J Pediatr Hematol Oncol* 2009;31:59–60.
149. Schilling F, Oberrauch W, Schanz F, et al. Evaluation of a rapid and reliable method for mass screening for neuroblastoma in infants. *Prog Clin Biol Res* 1991;366:579–583.
150. Schilling F, Spix C, Berthold F, et al. Neuroblastoma screening at one year of age. *N Engl J Med* 2002;346:1047–1053.
151. Schimke RN. The endocrine glands. In: Stevenson RE, Hall JG, Goodman RM, eds. *Human malformations and related anomalies*. New York: Oxford University Press, 1993:1017–1029.
152. Schor NF. Neuroblastoma as a neurobiological disease. *J Neurooncol* 1999;41:159–166.
153. Schwab M, Westermann F, Hero B, et al. Neuroblastoma: biology and molecular and chromosomal pathology. *Lancet Oncol* 2003;4:472–80.
154. Seeger RC, Reynolds CP, Gallego R, et al. Quantitative tumor cell content of bone marrow and blood as a predictor of outcome in

Stage IV neuroblastoma: a Children's Cancer Group study. *J Clin Oncol* 2000;18:4067–4076.

155. SEER. *Surveillance, Epidemiology, and End Results Program, SEER*Stat Data-base: Incidence – SEER 9 Regs, Nov 2002 Sub (1973–2000)*. National Cancer Institute, DCCPS, Surveillance Research Program, Cancer Statistics Branch, released April 2003, based on the November 2002 submission, www.seer.cancer.gov.
156. Shimada H, Ambros IA, Dehner LP, et al. Establishment of the International Neuroblastoma Pathology Classification (Shimada System). *Cancer* 1999;86:364–372.
157. Shimada H, Ambros IM, Dehner LP, et al. Terminology and morphologic criteria of neuroblastic tumors: Recommendation by the International Neuroblastoma Pathology Committee. *Cancer* 1999;86:349–363.
158. Shimada H, Aoyama C, Chiba T, et al. Prognostic subgroups for undifferentiated neuroblastoma: immunohistochemical study with anti-S-100 protein antibody. *Hum Pathol* 1985;16: 471–476.
159. Shimada H, Chatten J, Newton WA Jr, et al: Histopathologic prognostic factors in neuroblastic tumors: definition of subtypes of ganglioneuroblastoma and an age-linked classification of neuroblastoma. *J Natl Cancer Inst* 1984;73:405–416.
160. Shimada H, Nakagawa A, Peters J, et al. TrkA expression in peripheral neuroblastic tumors: prognostic significance and biological relevance. *Cancer* 2004;101:1873–1881.
161. Shimada H, Stram D, Chatten J, et al. Identification of subsets of neuroblastomas combined histopathologic and N-myc analysis. *J Natl Cancer Inst* 1995;87:1470–1476.
162. Shimada H, Umehara S, Monobe Y, et al. International Neuroblastoma Pathology Classification for prognostic evaluation of patients with peripheral neuroblastic tumors: a report from the Children's Cancer group. *Cancer* 2001;92:2451–2461.
163. Shono K, Tajiri T, Fujii Y, et al. Clinical implications of minimal disease in the bone marrow and peripheral blood in neuroblastoma. *J Pediatr Surg* 2000;35:1415–1420.
164. Shuster JJ, McWilliams NB, Castleberry R, et al. A Pediatric Oncology Group recursive partitioning study. Serum lactate dehydrogenase in childhood neuroblastoma. *Am J Clin Oncol* 1992;15:295–303.
165. Simon T. Tumour markers are poor predictors for relapse or progression in neuroblastoma. *Eur J Cancer* 2003;39:1899–1903.
166. Spitz R, Betts DR, Simon T, et al. Favorable outcome of triploid neuroblastomas: a contribution to the special oncogenesis of neuroblastoma cells. *Cancer Genet Cytogenet* 2006;167:51–56.
167. Spitz R, Hero B, Ernestus K, et al. Deletions in chromosome arms 3p and 11q are new prognostic markers in localized and 4s neuroblastoma. *Clin Cancer Res* 2003;9:52–58.
168. Spitz R, Hero B, Ernestus K, et al. Gain of distal chromosome arm 17q is not associated with poor prognosis in neuroblastoma. *Clin Cancer Res* 2003;9:4835–4840.
169. Spitz R, Hero B, Simon T, et al. Loss in chromosome 11q identifies tumors with increased risk for metastatic relapses in localized and 4s neuroblastoma. *Clin Cancer Res* 2006;12:3368–3373.
170. Spitz R, Hero B, Westermann F, et al. Fluorescence in situ hybridization analysis of chromosome band 1p36 in neuroblastoma detect two classes of alterations. *Genes Chromosomes Cancer* 2002;34:299–305.
171. Tapp E. Huxley M. The histological appearance of the human pineal gland from puberty to old age. *J Pathol* 1972;108:137–144.
172. Thorner PS, Ho M, Chilton-MacNeill S, et al. Use of chromogenic in situ hybridization to identify MYCN gene copy number in neuroblastoma using routine tissue sections. *Am J Surg Pathol* 2006;30:635–642.
173. Tischler AS, Kimura N, McNicol AM. Pathology of pheochromocytoma and extra-adrenal paraganglioma. *Ann N Y Acad Sci* 2006;1073:557–570.
174. Tischler AS. Pheochromocytoma and extra-adrenal paraganglioma updates. *Arch Pathol Lab Med* 2008;132:1272–1284.
175. Tornoczky T, Kalman E, Kajtar PG, et al. Large cell neuroblastoma: A distinct phenotype with aggressive clinical behavior. New entity? *Cancer* 2004;100:390–397.
176. Tornoczky T, Semjen D, Shimada H, et al. Pathology of peripheral neuroblastic tumors: significance of prominent nuclei in undifferentiated/poorly differentiated neuroblastoma. *Pathol Oncol Res* 2007;13:269–275.
177. Trochet D, Bourdeaut F, Janoueix-Lerosey I, et al. Germline mutations of the paired-like homeobox 2B (PHOX2B) gene in neuroblastoma. *Am J Hum Genet* 2004;74:761–764.
178. Trochet D, O'Brien LM, Gozal D, et al. PHOX2B genotype allows for prediction of tumor risk in congenital central hypoventilation syndrome. *Am J Hum Genet* 2005;76:421–426.
179. Trueba SS, Auge J, Mattei G, et al. PAX8, TITF1, and FOXE1 gene expression patterns during human development: new insights into human thyroid development and thyroid dysgenesis-associated malformations. *J Clin Endocrinol Metab* 2005;90:455–462.
180. Tsubono Y, Hisamichi S. A halt to neuroblastoma screening in Japan. *N Engl J Med* 2004;350:2010.
181. Umehara S, Nakagawa A, Matthay KK, et al. Histopathology defines prognostic subsets of ganglioneuroblastoma, nodular: a report from the Children's Cancer Group. *Cancer* 2000;89:1150–1161.
182. van den Berg H, Caron HN. Paratesticular neuroblastoma: a case against metastatic disease? *J Pediatr Hematol Oncol* 2007;29: 187–189.
183. van Limpt V, Schramm A, van Lakemen A, et al. The Phox2B homeobox gene is mutated in sporadic neuroblastomas *Oncogene* 2004;23:9280–9288.
184. van Vliet G, Polak M, eds. Thyroid gland development and function. *Endocr Dev* 2007;10.
185. Vasko V, Bauer AJ, Tuttle RM, et al. Papillary and follicular thyroid cancers in children. In: Van Vliet G, Polak M, eds. *Thyroid gland development and function*. Basel: Karger. *Endocr Dev* 2007;10: 140–172.
186. Wang Q, Diskin S, Rappaport E, et al. Integrative genomics identifies distinct molecular classes of neuroblastoma and shows that multiple genes are targeted by regional alterations in DNA copy number. *Cancer Res* 2006;66:6050–6062.
187. Webb C, Prayson RA. Pediatric pituitary adenomas. *Arch Pathol Lab Med* 2008;132:77–80.
188. White PC. Section 4: Disorders of the adrenal gland. In: Kliegman RM, Behrman RE, Jenson HB, Stanton BF, eds., *Nelson textbook of pediatrics*, 18th ed. Philadelphia, PA: Elsevier, 2007.
189. Wieneke JA, Thompson LD, Heffess CS. Adrenal cortical neoplasms in the pediatric population: a clinicopathologic and immunophenotypic analysis of 83 patients. *Am J Surg Pathol* 2003;27:867–881.
190. Wiersinga WM. Thyroid cancer in children and adolescents—consequences in later life. *J Pediatr Endocrinol Metab* 2001;14(suppl 5): 1289–1296.
191. Wirnsberger GH, Becker H, Ziervogel K, et al. Diagnostic immunohistochemistry for neuroblastic tumors. *Am J Surg Pathol* 1992;16:49–57.
192. Wisoff JH, Epstein F. Surgical management of symptomatic pineal cysts. *J Neurosurg* 1992;77:896–900.
193. Woods WG, Gao R, Shuster J, et al. Screening of infants and mortality due to neuroblastoma. *N Engl J Med* 2002;346:1041–1046.

CHAPTER 22

The Lymph Nodes, Spleen, and Thymus

THOMAS L. McCURLEY
MARY M. ZUTTER
ANDREA M. SHEEHAN

LYMPH NODES

The lymph node is a remarkable structure that serves as (a) a meeting place for antigen, antigen-presenting cells, and naïve B- and T-cells to initiate the adaptive immune response, and (b) the site of clonal expansion and differentiation of effector B- and T-lymphocytes (58). These processes so essential to normal immune function also require a number of genetic events (DNA replication, class switching, somatic mutation, receptor editing, etc.) that underlie most lymphomas (both Hodgkin and non-Hodgkin) (73).

Lymph Nodes (Normal Structure and Function)

The normal lymph node is a round or an ovoid encapsulated structure. It is usually small (2 to 3 mm) to modest (~1 cm) in size, but it may attain dramatic dimensions if the lymph draining into it is particularly rich in immunogenic material. Macroscopically, normal lymph nodes are tan or creamy white in color, and the cut surface may be homogeneous or vaguely nodular. In reactive lymph nodes, the hilum is visible on gross examination. Microscopically, four anatomic compartments are present (Figure 22-1) (e314). The most readily identified are the primary and secondary follicles, which are spherical collections of small and large B-lymphocytes in the periphery of the lymph node. Although rich in B-cells, the follicles also contain T helper cells and follicular dendritic cells (e205). Morphologically, the follicular center has a dark zone where proliferation (clonal expansion) and somatic mutation occur, and an adjacent light zone that is the site of selection of high-affinity B-cells and differentiation to plasma cells and memory B-cells (Figure 22-2). Surrounding the follicle is a rim of uniformly sized small lymphocytes, the mantle, which is polarized toward the subcapsular sinus and blends imperceptibly into the cortex. Like the follicles, the mantle is composed largely of B-cells. Beyond the mantle and between the follicles is a T-cell–rich zone, the paracortex, which contains a heterogeneous population of cells, including macrophages, interdigitating reticulum cells, scattered B-cells, and abundant T-cells in various stages of activation (e313). High endothelial venules in this area serve as the site of entry for naïve T-cells and B-cells (Figure 22-3). The medullary cords, not always evident in tissue sections as a discrete zone, are located in the central portion of the lymph node and consist of elongated arrays of lymphoplasmacytoid cells that surround the sinuses.

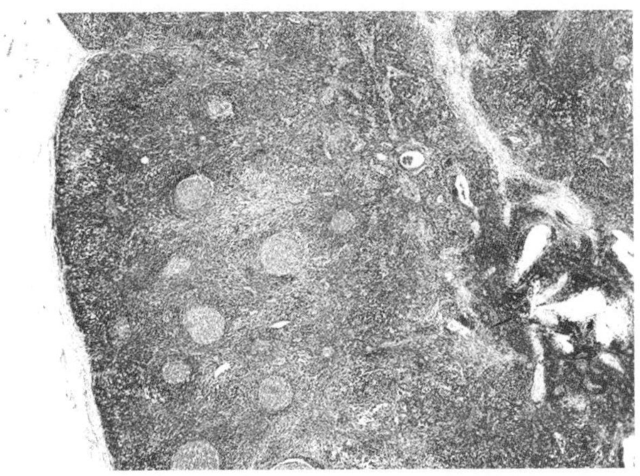

FIGURE 22-1 ■ In this reactive lymph node with follicular hyperplasia, the germinal centers are widely spread, vary in size, and are demarcated by a rim of small lymphocytes, the mantle zone. (Hematoxylin and eosin stain 4×.)

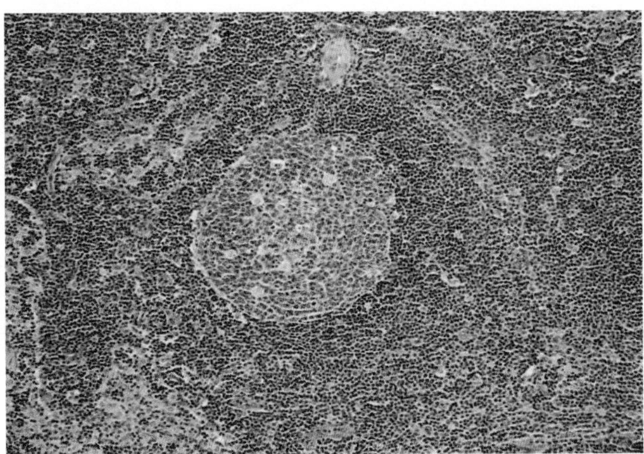

FIGURE 22-2 ■ Polarization of the benign germinal center reflects the segregation of centrocytes to the light zone and mitotically active centroblasts to the dark zone. (Hematoxylin and eosin stain 10×.)

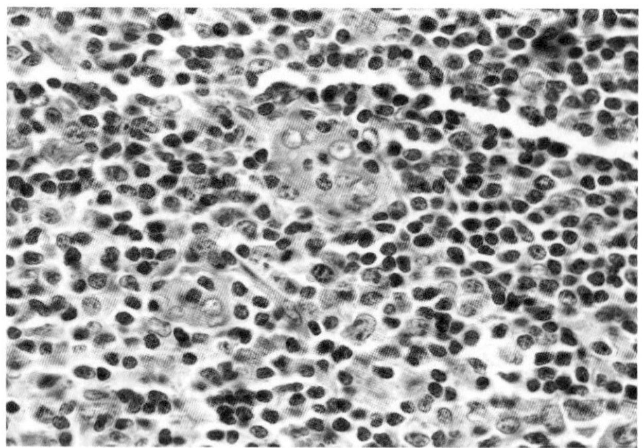

FIGURE 22-3 ■ Interfollicular T-cell zone demonstrating high endothelial venules and dendritic cells. (Hematoxylin and eosin stain 40×.)

The sinuses, endothelium-bounded spaces containing macrophages and antigen-presenting cells, form the fourth anatomic compartment and converge on the hilum from multiple points along the subcapsular sinus.

Clinical Significance of Lymphadenopathy in Children

Palpable lymphadenopathy is more common in children and adolescents than in adults. The most common cause of adenopathy in children is a benign lymphoid proliferation, and in many patients, some evidence of a self-limiting infectious or inflammatory process can be found to explain the enlarged nodes (e234). The presence of certain clinical factors suggests that biopsy may disclose a condition requiring specific treatment, including fevers unresponsive to antibiotics, generalized adenopathy or massive localized adenopathy, mediastinal disease, weight loss, peripheral blood cytopenias, and elevated serum levels of lactate dehydrogenase (e227). Slap et al. (e288) defined three simple variables that identified lymph nodes which should be biopsied: (a) size greater than 2 cm in diameter, (b) abnormalities on chest x-ray, and (c) absence of symptoms of recent otolaryngologic disease in patients with cervical adenopathy.

Approach to Diagnosis in Patients with Lymphadenopathy

The availability of a broad array of new diagnostic techniques in hematopathology offers the opportunity for making faster diagnoses with more precision on smaller samples using less invasive procedures such as fine-needle aspiration (FNA) cytology and needle biopsy. The success of such efforts (if they are to be cost effective) depends in part on the quality of communication between hematologists and hematopathologists so that the most appropriate studies are ordered in a timely fashion.

The basic approach that we use in our practice is that we examine touch preps or smears on biopsies or aspirates of lymph nodes immediately after staining (Table 22-1). Since the most common pediatric non-Hodgkin hematopoietic lymphoid neoplasms are recognizable as malignant on touch preps/smears (anaplastic large cell lymphoma, diffuse large B-cell lymphoma, Burkitt lymphoma, lymphoblastic lymphoma), these entities can be quickly triaged to flow cytometric and cytogenetic analysis. Similarly, most reactive proliferations, metastatic tumors, and those lymphomas with only a few dysplastic cells (as in Hodgkin lymphoma) would not benefit flow cytometry but may require cultures, cytogenetics, and other studies can be triaged as well. This approach often allows the definitive diagnosis of many malignancies within hours and prevents substantial waste in resources.

Immunophenotypic Studies of Lymph Node Biopsy Specimens

Flow cytometry is an essential part of the diagnosis and classification of non-Hodgkin lymphoma involving lymph nodes. The rapid availability of results (1 to 3 hours) allows triage to appropriate ancillary genetic studies while viable material is still available (32). In Hodgkin lymphoma and in non-Hodgkin lymphoma in which flow cytometry is not

Table 22-1 ■ APPROACH TO DIAGNOSIS AT THE TIME OF BIOPSY

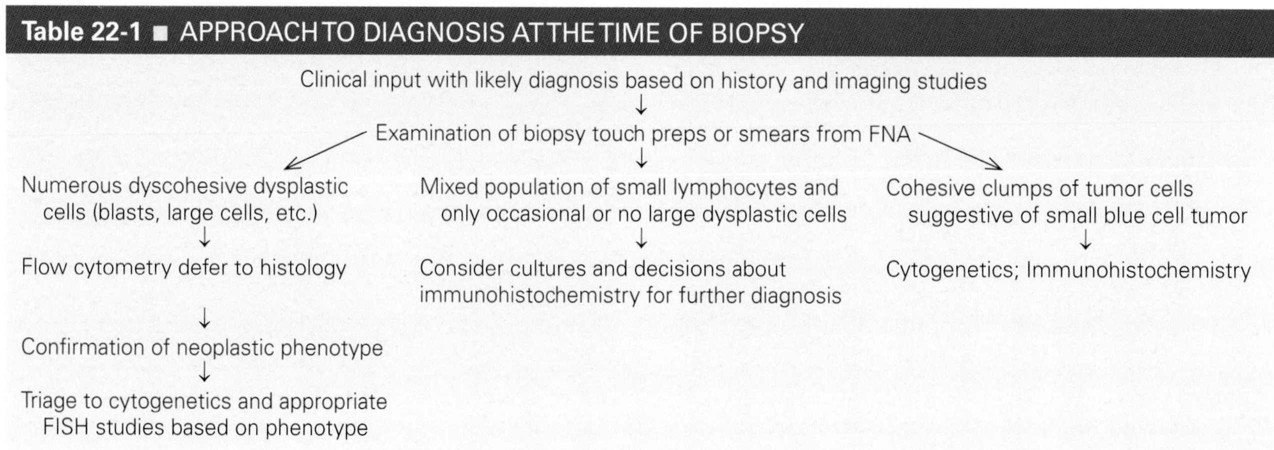

Clinical input with likely diagnosis based on history and imaging studies
↓
Examination of biopsy touch preps or smears from FNA

Numerous dyscohesive dysplastic cells (blasts, large cells, etc.)	Mixed population of small lymphocytes and only occasional or no large dysplastic cells	Cohesive clumps of tumor cells suggestive of small blue cell tumor
↓	↓	↓
Flow cytometry defer to histology	Consider cultures and decisions about immunohistochemistry for further diagnosis	Cytogenetics; Immunohistochemistry
↓		
Confirmation of neoplastic phenotype		
↓		
Triage to cytogenetics and appropriate FISH studies based on phenotype		

Table 22-2 ■ IMMUNOPHENOTYPIC MARKERS USED IN LYMPHOMA DIAGNOSIS

Cluster Designation	Antibody	Antigen
General markers		
CD45	LCA	Leukocyte common antigen (+ almost all NHL negative/DIM in most acute leukemias, – in CHL, and many ALCL)
CC	TdT	Terminal deoxynucleotidyl transferase (+ >95% LBL 20% ANLL, – in all NHL)
CD34	HPCA	Human progenitor cell antibody (50% of blasts in ALL/ANLL) endothelial cells
B-cell lineage markers		
CD10	J5	CALLA; positive in follicle center cell NHL (+ >95% B-ALL, 100% BL, 25% of DLBL)
CD19	B4	Pan B-cell marker (present on all B-cell NHL including B-LBL)
CD20	L26	Mature B-cell marker (not present on most B-LBL)
	CD23	Activated B-cells; follicular dendritic cells, low-affinity FcR for IgE
T-cell lineage markers		
CD1a	O10	Thymic T-cells, Langerhans cells
CD2	Leu5	T-cells; E-rosette receptor
CD3	Leu4	T-cells; TcR complex component NK cells (cytoplasm only)
CD4	Leu3	Helper/suppressor T-cells; MHC class II receptor, monocyte/macrophages, 60% of ANLL
CD5	Leu1	Preferential T-cell marker, B-cell subset
CD7	Leu9	T-cells, some NK cells; FcR for IgM, 25% of ANLL
CD8	Leu2, T8	Cytotoxic T-cells; MHC class I receptor
CD16	Leu11	NK cells, granulocytes; IgG FcR III
CD43	MT1	Pan T-cell marker, blasts in ANLL, T and B-LBL
CD45ro	UCHL-1	T-cells, some macrophages
CD56	Leu7	NK and T-cells; N-CAM isoform, neuroendocrine tumors
CD57		T and NK cells
Monocyte/macrophage/accessory cell markers		
CD1a	O10	Some T-cells, Langerhans cells
CD15	LeuM1	Granulocytes, also positive in RS cell in classic Hodgkin lymphoma
CD21	1F8, B2	Dendritic cells, some B-cells; C3d/EBV receptor
CD68	KP1	Macrophages, monocytes, blasts in ANLL
	S100	Langerhans cells, melanoma, other cell types

ALCL, anaplastic large cell lymphoma; ANLL, acute nonlymphocytic leukemia; BL, Burkitt lymphoma; B-LBL, precursor B-cell lymphoblastic leukemia; CALLA, common acute lymphocytic leukemia antigen; CHL, classic Hodgkin lymphoma; EBV, Epstein-Barr virus; Fcr, Fc receptor; MHC, major histocompatibility complex; NHL, non-Hodgkin lymphoma; NK, natural killer; Tcr, T-cell receptor; T-LBL, T-lymphoblastic lymphoma.

performed, the wide variety of CD markers, which mark well in fixed tissue, allow immunohistochemical characterization of most hematopoietic lymphoid neoplasms (Table 22-2).

Cytogenetic Studies of Lymph Node Biopsy Specimens

For routine cytogenetic analysis, which is helpful in securing an accurate diagnosis in some cases, viable, fresh tissue must be taken by sterile technique at the time of biopsy and placed into culture so that metaphase spreads can be generated. In the appropriate clinical setting, some karyotypic abnormalities may be pathognomic for certain types of malignancies (Table 22-3) and can therefore be used for diagnostic purposes (24,65,e178). In other settings, especially precursor B-cell lymphoblastic lymphoma/acute lymphoblastic leukemia, the results of cytogenetic studies can also be used for prognostic purposes (45,e248). The most common karyotypic changes related to lymphoproliferative disorders in children include translocations of immunoglobulin and T-cell receptor loci, which are frequently paired with loci involved in normal development and hematopoiesis (6,e153,68). A major advance in diagnostic cytogenetics is the widespread availability of FISH studies for these translocations. Two major advantages of FISH techniques over routine cytogenetics are (a) rapid turnaround (<24 hours) and (b) they can be done on fixed tissues including touch preps or cytospin preps and in paraffin-embedded tissues (Table 22-3) (12,19).

Reactive Lymphadenopathy

The two major patterns of reactive lymphadenopathy are usually dominated either by follicular hyperplasia or interfollicular expansion (immunoblastic, granulomatous, or histiocytic). Occasional reactive processes produce an apparent diffuse alteration of architecture (Table 22-4) (e32). In practice, a single lymph node is constantly exposed to a diversity of immunogens and therefore exhibits more than one pattern of response, but when the degree of adenopathy is sufficient to warrant a biopsy, a single pattern usually dominates. Additional factors that assist in the differential diagnosis include the age-specific nature of some disorders; certain reactive processes affecting lymph nodes are rare in children (e.g., luetic lymphadenitis, Kimura disease), whereas others affect them primarily (e.g., acute infectious mononucleosis, autoimmune lymphoproliferative disorder) (e280).

Table 22-3 ■ KARYOTYPIC AND GENETIC CHANGES ASSOCIATED WITH NON-HODGKIN LYMPHOMA

Disease	Abnormality	Implicated Loci
Precursor B-cell LBL/B-cell ALL	t(1;19)(q23;p13)	pbx1-e2a
	t(4;11)(p21;q23)	AF4-MLL
	Hyperdiploidy (>50 chr)	
	Hyperdiploidy (47;50 chr)	
	Hypodiploidy	
B-cell large-cell lymphoma	t(3q27;var)	BCL-6
Burkitt lymphoma	t(2;8) (p11;q24)	IgL-lambda-myc
	t(8;14) (q24; q32)	c-myc-IgH
	t(8;22) (q24;q11)	c-myc-IgL-kappa
Precursor T-cell LBL/T-cell ALL	t(1;14-15)(p12;q11)	TAL1;TcR gamma
	t(1;14)(p32;p14–15)	TAL1;TcR delta
	t(1;7)(p32;q34)	TAL1;TcR beta
T-cell anaplastic large-cell lymphoma	t(2;5)(p23;q35)	NPM-ALK

ALL, acute lymphoblastic leukemia; IgH, immunoglobulin heavy chain; IgL, immunoglobulin light chain; LBL, lymphoblastic leukemia; TcR, T-cell receptor.

Table 22-4 ■ REACTIVE LYMPHADENITIS IN CHILDREN

Follicular hyperplasia
Nonspecific
HIV
Progressive transformation of follicular centers
Toxoplasmosis
Castleman disease/angiofollicular hyperplasia

Interfollicular reactions
Paracortical immunoblastic reactions
EBV
Hypersensitivity reactions (phenytoin)
Juvenile rheumatoid arthritis 1
Systemic lupus erythematosus 1,3
Kikuchi histiocytic necrotizing lymphadenitis 1,3
Autoimmune lymphoproliferative syndrome (ALPS) 1
Kawasaki disease

Granulomatous
Mycobacterial infection (MTB and atypical mycobacterial) 1,2
Cat-scratch disease 1,2,4
Fungal infection

Histiocytic
Sinus histocytosis
Lysosomal storage disorders
Hemophagocytic syndromes (Hemophagocytic lymphohistiocytosis)
Rosai-Dorfman
Dermatopathia
Langerhans cell histocytosis

Diffuse alteration of architecture
Sarcoidosis
Post-transplant lymphoproliferative disease
Other features
1. Follicular hyperplasia
2. Necrosis with neutrophils
3. Necrosis with apoptosis
4. Capsulitis

FOLLICULAR HYPERPLASIAS

Nonspecific Germinal Center Hyperplasia

Nonspecific germinal center hyperplasia is the most common of all benign histologic findings. The bulk of the lymph node is composed of round or irregularly shaped germinal centers that vary in size. These contain small, intermediate, and large mitotically active lymphocytes, tingible body macrophages, and apoptotic cells. The hyperplastic follicles tend to remain in the cortical regions of the affected node, but in particularly robust cases, the paracortex and the medulla may be compressed by the process (e60,e159). Immunophenotypic studies show that the follicles contain a predominance of $CD20^+$, $CD10^+$, 6^+ B-cells that do not stain for bcl2 (e205,e310). Differential diagnostic considerations in children are few but include Castleman disease, HIV-related adenopathy, and progressive transformation of germinal centers.

HIV-related Adenopathy

Most series treating the subject of HIV-related persistent generalized lymphadenopathy are based on a patient population of homosexual young adult men at risk for HIV (e17,e37,e143). Reports of this condition in children at risk for HIV because of maternal-fetal transmission or hemophilia present similar data (e41,e280,e336). A spectrum of histologic findings may be seen in this context, with two clearly recognizable extremes. Florid follicular hyperplasia, the earliest change of HIV-related persistent generalized lymphadenopathy, has many features in common with nonspecific follicular hyperplasia, although the germinal centers are larger, often serpiginous, and tend to fuse with focal follicular lysis (Figure 22-4) (e106,e228). Regressively

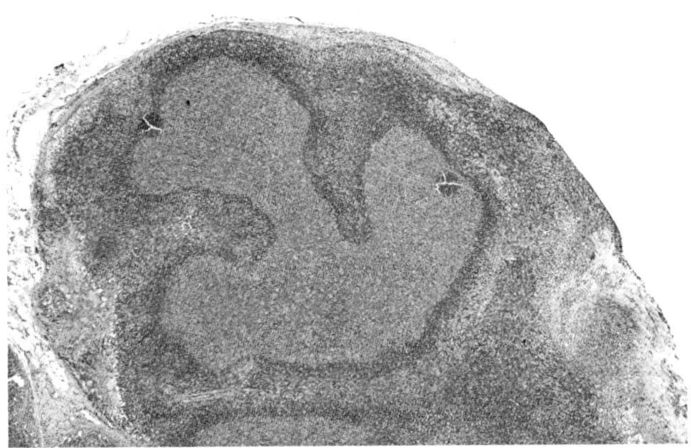

FIGURE 22-4 ■ Serpentine follicular center in a patient with HIV infection and a generalized adenopathy. (Hematoxylin and eosin stain 4×.)

transformed germinal centers typify late persistent generalized lymphadenopathy and are characterized by small size, lymphoid depletion, and numerous dendritic cells, vessels, and amorphous eosinophilic deposits (e143,e144,e159). The mantle is absent or very poorly formed, and the paracortex is proportionally rich in histiocytes, plasma cells, and high endothelial venules because of the paucity of lymphocytes. The morphologic features associated with persistent generalized lymphadenopathy (i.e., large and irregularly shaped follicles, follicular lysis, follicular involution) are distinctive but not specific for HIV infection, and they have been seen in 5% to 10% of otherwise entirely unremarkable lymph nodes obtained as part of carcinoma staging before the beginning of the AIDS era (e215,e287,e294).

Progressively Transformed Germinal Centers

For unknown reasons, when clinically significant lymphadenopathy develops in some patients, the biopsy specimen shows progressively transformed germinal centers (PTFC). Most patients are asymptomatic male adolescents or young adults with isolated inguinal or cervical adenopathy (99,e225). The bulk of the lymph node, which can be up to 5 cm in size, exhibits florid follicular hyperplasia; however, what makes this disorder distinctive is the presence of scattered, very large (three to five times the size of surrounding germinal centers) follicles that are dramatically expanded by an influx of small lymphocytes (Figure 22-5) with mantle cell-like morphology and IgM+, IgD+ phenotype (e94,e224,e280). The borders of these "transformed" germinal centers with the surrounding paracortex are blurred, and they may be encircled by wreaths of histiocytes (e94). Relative to normal follicles, the transformed follicles exhibit a disrupted and dispersed dendritic cell network on CD21 or CD23 staining (99). An important feature is the absence of variant Reed-Sternberg cells since the major concern in differential diagnosis is lymphocyte predominant Hodgkin lymphoma that rarely may precede, follow, or be concurrent with PTFC (e37,e129).

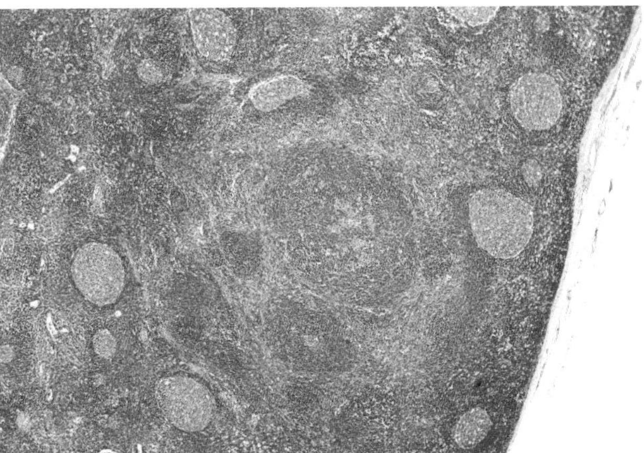

FIGURE 22-5 ■ Progressively transformed follicular center (with disrupted follicle infiltrated by small mantle zone lymphocytes) in a background of follicular hyperplasia. (Hematoxylin and eosin stain 4×.)

Toxoplasmosis

Acute toxoplasmosis, an infectious disease, is often accompanied by lymphadenopathy. This is usually limited to the cervical lymph nodes, although occasionally patients with typical histology and serologic confirmation have isolated inguinal or axillary lymph node enlargement (e103). Florid follicular hyperplasia dominates the histology at low power and is invariably accompanied by patches of epithelioid histiocytes and parasinusoidal accumulations of monocytoid B-cells. The histiocytic aggregates, randomly distributed throughout, abut and even infiltrate the germinal centers (e70,e192,e283). Immunophenotypic studies play no role in confirming the diagnosis but may be helpful in excluding conditions such as nodular lymphocyte-predominant Hodgkin lymphoma, which may superficially resemble Toxoplasma-related lymphadenitis. The triad of florid follicular hyperplasia, hyperplasia of parasinusoidal B-cells, and histocytic aggregates (variably encroaching on follicular centers) has a high degree of sensitivity and specificity for diagnosis of toxoplasmosis (Figure 22-6) (34,82).

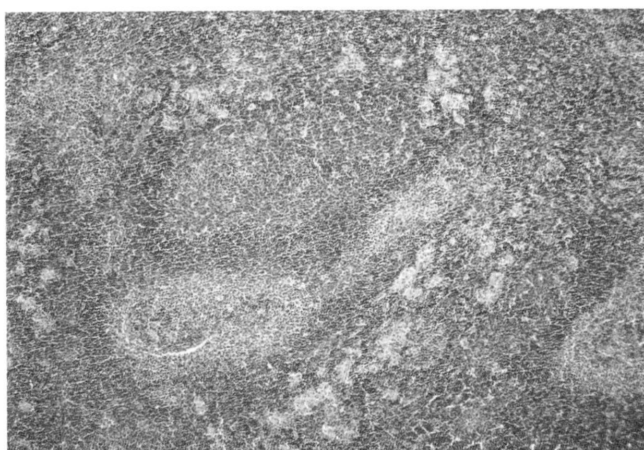

FIGURE 22-6 ■ Low power of toxoplasmosis demonstrating the triad of hyperplastic follicles, monocytoid B-cell proliferation, and histiocytic aggregates encroaching of follicles. (Hematoxylin and eosin stain 4×.)

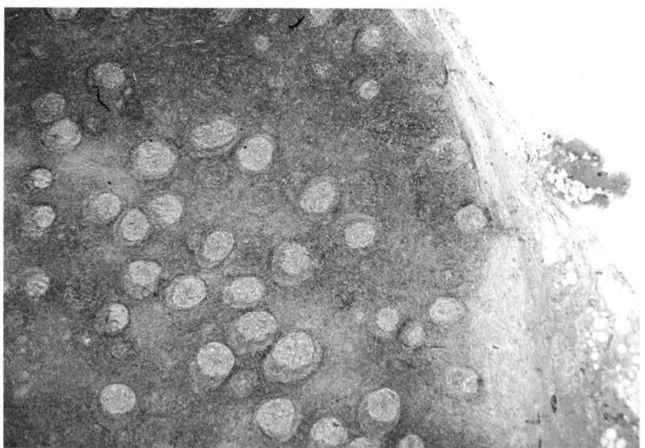

FIGURE 22-7 ■ Low power of hyaline vascular angiofollicular hyperplasia with "bag of marbles" small uniform follicles evenly dispersed throughout the cortex and the medulla. (Hematoxylin and eosin stain 4×.)

Castleman Disease/Angiofollicular Hyperplasia

Most patients with hyaline vascular Castleman disease (HV-CD) present with cervical or mediastinal involvement, or both (e142,e281). At low power, the architecture of HV-CD is nodular (Figure 22-7) with small and involuted germinal centers throughout the node (bag of marbles). The mantles are expansive and composed of small lymphocytes often in a laminated (orbiting) or "onion skin" pattern (e67,e101,e191). Multiple germinal centers may be found within the boundaries of a single mantle zone, and in some sections, radially penetrating hyalinized high endothelial venules are seen passing from the germinal centers into the adjacent paracortex (lollypops) (Figure 22-8). The germinal centers are depleted of lymphocytes and contain both extracellular matrix and abundant follicle dendritic cells (e159,e209). The cellular components of the interfollicular zone include plasmacytoid monocytes, myoid cells, histiocytes, dendritic cells, and lymphocytes, which vary in proportion from case to case (e209). Cuffing of sinuses by collagen may be prominent. Immunophenotypic studies lend little to the diagnosis, although CD21 and CD23 highlight the dense aggregates of dendritic cells, which are in contrast to the circumscribed but loose meshwork seen in normal germinal centers. Both HV-CD and PC-CD may show monotypic plasma cells (usually lambda light chain) by immunohistochemistry (e218). Although differential diagnostic considerations in adults include mantle cell lymphoma and follicle center cell lymphoma, these malignancies are very rare in children. Partial nodal involvement by Hodgkin lymphoma may be overlooked if a significant concomitant Castleman disease-like proliferation is present (e179) and small biopsy specimens of mediastinal HV-CD may be mistaken for thymoma if involuted germinal centers are misinterpreted as Hassall corpuscles.

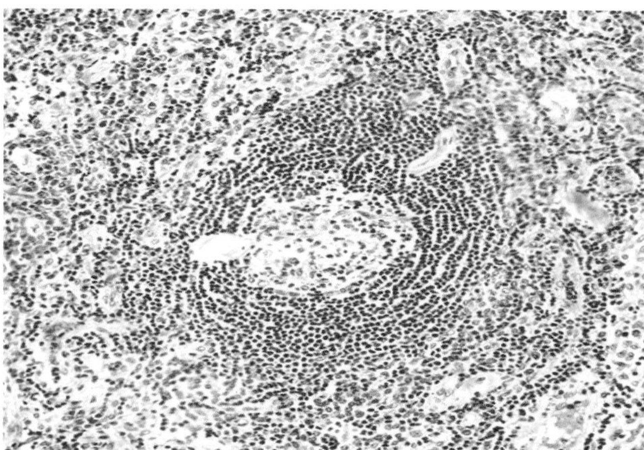

FIGURE 22-8 ■ The mantle zone has a laminated or "onion skin" appearance in the hyaline vascular type of Castleman disease. Note the radially penetrating vessel. (Hematoxylin and eosin stain 10×.)

The plasma cell variant of Castleman disease (PV-CD) is usually a systemic disorder that has also been reported in children (e142,e186). Patients present with fever and weight loss, and laboratory studies may show immune-mediated cytopenia, an elevated erythrocyte sedimentation rate, and hypergammaglobulinemia (e40). When localized, the adenopathy of PV-CD is typically axial (mediastinum or abdomen) like HV-CD. When the adenopathy is multicentric, patients often have hepatosplenomegaly and symptoms fitting the POEMS (polyneuropathy, organomegaly, endocrinopathy, M protein, skin changes) syndrome may be present (8,e110,e182,e203). The low-power appearance of PV-CD is that of follicular hyperplasia with a marked interfollicular plasmacytosis (e101,e152,e159,e209). The germinal centers are large and hypercellular, contain dense eosinophilic material, and have a discrete, if thinned, mantle zone (e191,e323). As in the hyaline vascular variant of Castleman disease (HV-CD), the secondary follicles may contain more than one germinal center within the same mantle. The subcapsular and medullary sinuses remain patent, and extracapsular extension is distinctly unusual. Rheumatic lymphadenitis, luetic lymphadenitis, immunocytoma, autoimmune lymphoproliferative syndrome (ALPS), and HIV-related lymphadenopathy all are plausible diagnostic considerations, and correlation with clinical and immunophenotypic studies is a successful means of excluding these possibilities. PC-MCD in HIV-positive patients is usually associated with infection with human herpes virus 8 (e109). A subset of these patients may evolve into frank plasmablastic lymphoma (33).

INTERFOLLICULAR/PARACORTICAL REACTIONS—IMMUNOBLASTIC

Epstein-Barr Virus Infection (Infectious Mononucleosis)

Acute illness secondary to Epstein-Barr virus (EBV) infection (acute infectious mononucleosis) is common in young children and is usually self-limited. In those few cases that culminate in biopsy, the clinical features are often atypical—advanced

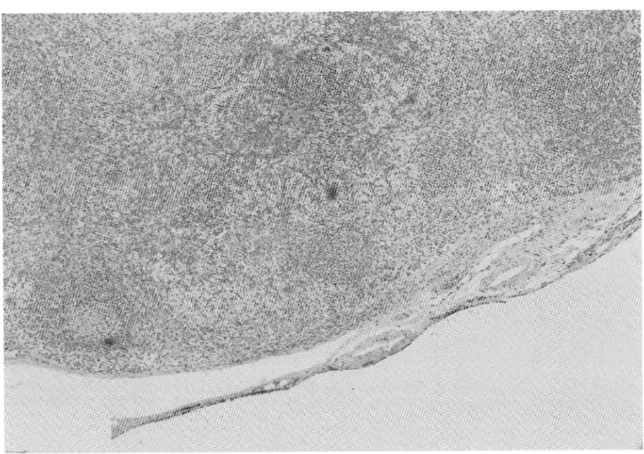

FIGURE 22-9■The immunoblastic proliferation in acute infectious mononucleosis localizes to the paracortex and may compress or distort residual germinal centers. (Hematoxylin and eosin stain 4×.)

age, the presence of "B" symptoms, a negative monospot test [uncommon except in very young children (<4 years) or early in infection], localized adenopathy, or persistent adenopathy, hepatosplenomegaly, or splenic rupture (e174). Patients with X-linked lymphoproliferative disorder (Duncan syndrome) present with rapidly progressive and usually fatal disease because of an inability to mount a successful immune response against EBV-infected cells (e52).

At low power, architecture is obscured but generally preserved with moth-eaten follicles and prominent paracortical expansion (Figure 22-9) by immunoblasts, plasma cells, and plasmacytoid lymphocytes (Figure 22-10). Similar large cells pack the sinuses. Occasionally, large cells with a bilobed or multilobed nuclei and prominent nucleoli are present, reminiscent of Reed-Sternberg cells (e5,e296,e306). Histiocytes may be scattered singly or in small clusters, and increased numbers of capillaries and high endothelial venules also contribute to the polymorphic appearance of the paracortex. Normal landmarks—germinal centers, subcapsular and paratrabecular sinuses—are generally present

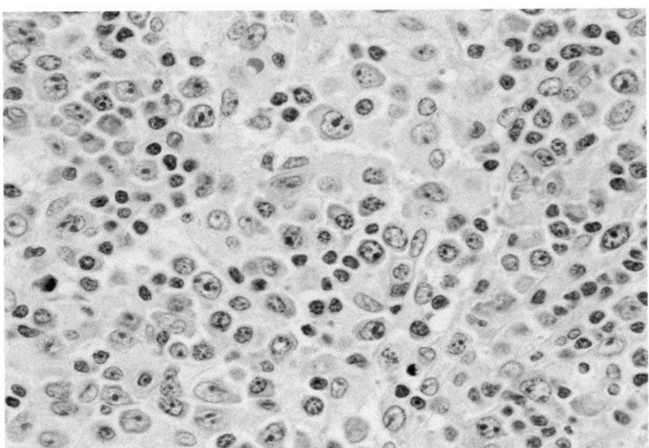

FIGURE 22-10■Small, intermediate and large cells fill the paracortex in acute infectious mononucleosis, often with a predominance of immunoblasts. (Hematoxylin and eosin stain 40×.)

but may be compressed or distorted by the immunoblastic proliferation (e40,e286). In very early cases of EBV infection, monocytoid B-cell proliferations may be prominent (5). Staining with CD20 and CD3 highlights the presence of a mixture of interfollicular B- and T-immunoblasts, and a polytypic pattern of light-chain expression is always seen. The Reed-Sternberg–like cells are characteristically $CD20^+$, $CD15^-$, and show variable reactivity for the activation antigen CD30 (e279) as well as markers of EBV infection such as latent membrane protein (LMP) or EBV, RNA transcripts (EBER) (e93,e210,e252). Difficult cases may exhibit sheet-like arrays of immunoblasts, a brisk mitotic rate, or extensive necrosis and may closely mimic large cell lymphoma (e40,e226). In such cases, examination of the peripheral blood smear for atypical lymphocytes, viral serology, and immunohistochemistry to better define architectural preservation and establish the presence of EBV is helpful.

Non-EBV Viral Adenopathy

Lymphadenopathy may occur as a result of herpes simplex (e79) and cytomegalovirus infection (e311). Children with some form of immune deficiency are the most frequently affected (e104,e112). Paracortical hyperplasia with discrete foci of necrosis is the typical histologic finding in these cases (e194). In comparison with acute EBV-related lymphadenopathy, the proportion of immunoblasts is less, and interfollicular areas are expanded by a mixture of mature lymphocytes, plasma cells, histiocytes, plasmacytoid monocytes, and lesser numbers of immunoblasts (e141). Viral inclusions that appear as smudged or hyperchromatic alterations of the nucleus (herpes simplex virus) or very large eosinophilic structures within the nucleus (cytomegalovirus) can be identified and may be most numerous adjacent to zones of necrosis (e303). Immunohistochemistry is helpful in excluding neoplasia and can also document the presence of infected cells (e338). The viral inclusions in enlarged cells of cytomegalovirus lymphadenitis are $CD15^+$, a potential pitfall in the safe exclusion of Hodgkin lymphoma (e266). Attention to clinical parameters will assist in discriminating viral lymphadenitis from other causes of necrotizing lymphadenitis, which include Kikuchi-Fujimoto disease and lupus erythematosus.

Hypersensitivity Reactions Emphasizing Phenytoin (Dilantin) Reactions

Hypersensitivity-related lymphadenopathy is quite rare and has been associated most commonly with phenytoin (Dilantin) therapy (e2,e271) and vaccines (small pox, measles, tetanus) (e9,e12,e71). In phenytoin hypersensitivity, the architecture of the lymph node is distorted by a paracortical proliferation of immunoblasts, lymphocytes, plasma cells, and eosinophils. Germinal centers persist, and in some cases, a florid follicular hyperplasia may accompany the immunoblastic reaction. Purely diffuse architectural effacement (e2) is rare. The immunoblasts represent a mixture of $CD20^+$ B-cells and $CD3^+$ T-cells. Progression to lymphoma is well described (e2,e271). The pattern of paracortical expansion may be seen in T-cell lymphomas such as angioimmunoblastic T-cell lymphoma (112), which is a major problem in differential diagnosis. A detailed history as well as immunophenotypic studies is usually helpful.

Juvenile-onset Rheumatoid Arthritis Emphasizing Still Disease

Several different histologies have been described in juvenile rheumatoid arthritis including the classic findings associated with adult RA of follicular hyperplasia, interfollicular plasma cells, and intrasinusoidal neutrophils (e213). In Still disease, a pattern of paracortical immunoblastic proliferation mimicking lymphoma is occasionally described as well as interfollicular necrosis similar to that seen in Kikuchi disease (64,67,e217,e312).

Systemic Lupus Erythematosus

Systemic lupus erythematosus is an autoimmune disease that affects both adolescents and young adults. When lymphadenopathy occurs, it is typically peripheral and multifocal or generalized. Classically follicular hyperplasia with patchy paracortical necrosis dominates the low-power appearance of the lymph node (e26,e189). The germinal centers are well formed with a discrete mantle zone, and they are separated by an expanded paracortex in which pockets of necrosis are randomly distributed (e77). The necrotic foci are composed of amorphous eosinophilic material and apoptotic debris. Neutrophils and plasma cells are scarce. In addition, "hematoxylin bodies" (round or oblong blue structures, 5 to 15 μm long, which stain with periodic acid–Schiff and the Feulgen method) and vascular encrustations (Azzopardi effect) may be present (e98). Less commonly, necrosis dominates the morphology, and follicles may be few and more widely spaced; in these circumstances, the lymph node findings may resemble those of Kikuchi-Fujimoto disease (e68). Other patterns described in systemic lupus erythematosus include follicular hyperplasia without necrosis resembling Castleman disease.

Histiocytic Necrotizing Lymphadenitis/ Kikuchi-Fujimoto Disease

Kikuchi-Fujimoto disease (histiocytic necrotizing lymphadenitis) is uncommon in children. The median age is in the third decade in most large series, although the age range is great (e15). Rare fatal cases in children have been reported often associated hemophagocytic syndrome (e44). These nodes exhibit follicular hyperplasia, but the histologic hallmark of this disease is zonal karyorrhexis with scant neutrophil response (e67,e68,e161). At low power, the paracortex is distorted by pale-staining patchy zones of necrotic debris with a cellular rim composed of apoptotic cells, histiocytes, small lymphocytes, plasmacytoid dendritic cells, and immunoblasts (e81,e82,e254). The areas of necrosis may coalesce, but a serpiginous contour rarely develops. Beyond the necrotic zone is a mottled paracortex, rich in small lymphocytes, immunoblasts, apoptotic debris and plasmacytoid monocytes and high endothelial venules (Figure 22-11) (e307,e309). In children, the differential diagnostic considerations for the early proliferative lesions of histiocytic necrotizing lymphadenitis include non-Hodgkin lymphoma (e42). and mixed-cellularity Hodgkin lymphoma. Fully developed lesions may mimic Kawasaki disease or herpetic lymphadenitis, and lupus-related lymphadenitis may be difficult or even impossible to exclude. A third pattern is characterized by dominance of foamy histiocytes (e218). Immunophenotypic characterization of the large cells at the periphery of karyorrhexis areas shows that they represent CD8 T-cells and plasmacytoid dendritic cells (81). One report suggests that the sparsity of CD8 T-cells in SLE may be helpful in differential diagnosis (54).

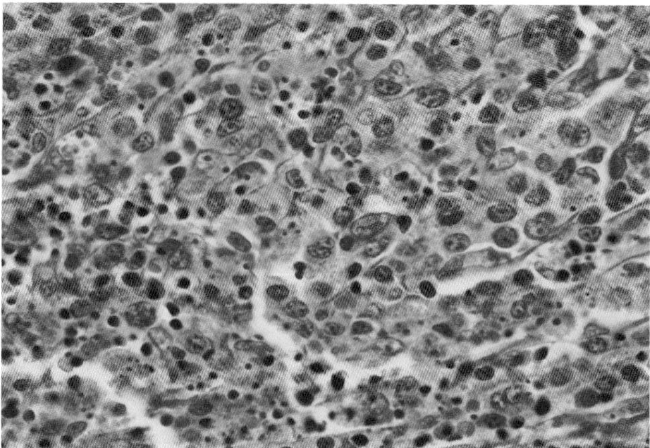

FIGURE 22-11 ■ The border of necrosis shows apoptotic debris admixed with histiocytes small lymphocytes, plasmacytoid dendritic cells, and immunoblasts in Kikuchi disease. (Hematoxylin and eosin stain 40×.)

Autoimmune Lymphoproliferative Syndrome

Lymphadenopathy secondary to loss of Fas or Fas ligand mediated apoptosis is a rare cause of non-neoplastic lymphadenopathy, known as *autoimmune lymphoproliferative disorder* (ALPS). Patients with ALPS present within the first 2 years of life with bulky generalized adenopathy and hepatosplenomegaly (e38,e73,e291,e292). Enlarged lymph nodes show generally intact architecture with follicles ranging from floridly hyperplastic to small involuting follicles with compressed mantle zones like those seen in hyalinized vascular Castleman disease. The proliferation that occurs in the interfollicular areas consists of immunoblasts and transformed large cells with scant-to-moderate cytoplasm (80,e291). Small lymphocytes, plasma cells, and histiocytes may be present. On flow cytometry, $CD2^+$, $CD3^+$, $CD4^-$, $CD8^-$ T-cells with an α-β T-cell receptor predominate. B-cells are phenotypically normal (e63,e292). On tissue section, the immunoblasts in the interfollicular zones are virtually all $CD3^+$, double negative T-cells, with only a few showing reactivity for CD4, CD8, or CD20 (71,e247,e291). T-zone lymphoma may mimic ALPS, but the former typically contains more small-to-intermediate cells and rarely has a CD4−, CD8− phenotype. Gene sequencing is necessary to confirm the diagnosis of ALPS, which may be caused by mutations in Fas, Fas ligand, or the caspase 10 gene (e73,138).

Kawasaki Disease

Kawasaki disease is endemic in Japan but rare in Western countries (e19). A slight male predominance has been noted, and the peak incidence is in children 3 to 4 years old. Histologic descriptions are quite variable, and it is clear that lymph node biopsy seldom yields findings on which a firm diagnosis of Kawasaki disease can be made independent of clinical parameters. The main findings are patchy paracortical necrosis with phlebitis and fibrin microthrombi (e111). Germinal centers are inconstantly present, as is an immunoblast-rich paracortical expansion. If perinodal tissues are represented, an acute necrotizing arteritis similar to infantile polyarteritis nodosa may be identified even in early phases; in established cases, a measure of luminal dilation is also present in larger-caliber vessels, with medial destruction (see Chapter 13).

INTERFOLLICULAR GRANULOMATOUS PROCESSES

Cat-Scratch Disease

Cat-scratch disease frequently affects children and adolescents, although in recent, large, population-based studies, nearly half of all patients have been over the age of 20 (e39). The adenopathic phase of the disease is dominated by follicular hyperplasia, capsulitis, paracortical monocytoid B-cell hyperplasia, and small, neutrophil-rich microabscesses (e195). As the lesions develop, the microabscesses coalesce, forming serpiginous and stellate zones of eosinophilic necrosis (Figure 22-12) (e165). In the late stage, the microabscesses take on a granulomatous appearance, with a well-formed rim of palisading histiocytes and scattered multinucleated giant cells (Figure 22-13). Warthin-Starry staining may highlight pleomorphic and bow-shaped rods and cocci, both in the center of abscesses and around blood vessels in the early phases of disease (e195). However, Warthin-Starry staining is technically difficult and problematic in interpretation. PCR techniques that detect the organism in a majority of patients with a high degree of specificity are preferred for confirmation of diagnosis (e278).

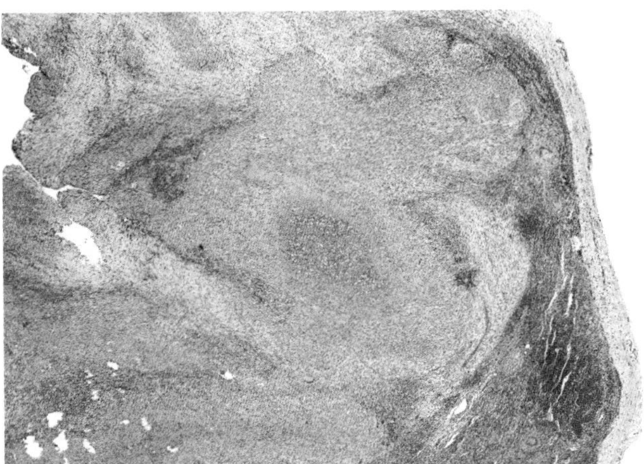

FIGURE 22-12 ■ The abscesses in cat-scratch disease have a serpiginous or stellate contour. (Hematoxylin and eosin stain 4×.)

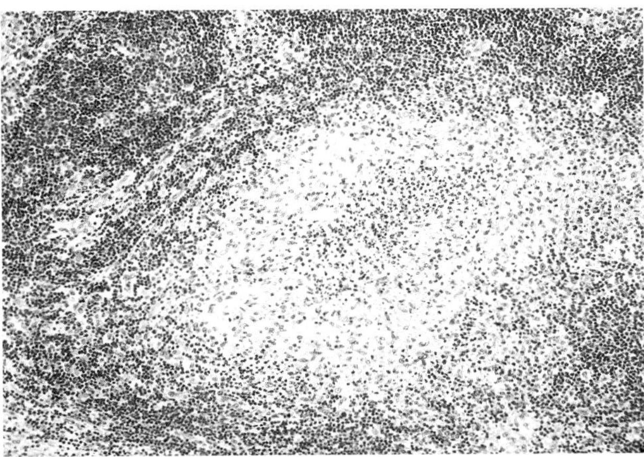

FIGURE 22-13 ■ In well-developed cases, the abscesses of cat-scratch disease have a broad, histiocyte-rich rim with abundant neutrophils forming a so-called pyogranuloma. (Hematoxylin and eosin stain 10×.)

Histologically similar lesions may also be seen in yersinia infection, lymphogranuloma venereum, tularemia, and infection with MAI in young children (see the following section) (66,75,105).

Mycobacterial Infections

The most common cause of granulomatous lymphadenitis in small children (1 to 5 years old) is infection by nontuberculous "atypical" mycobacteria (NTM), most commonly *Mycobacterium avium-intracellulare* (MAI) or *Mycobacterium scrofulaceum* (2,e21,e240,60). Diagnosis may be made by FNA or excisional lymph node biopsy. Cytologically, smears show epithelioid histiocytes and granulomata with reactive lymphocytes and plasma cells in the background as well as amorphous necrosis or necrosis associated with abundant neutrophils (140). Histologically, the nodal architecture is partially distorted or entirely effaced by follicular hyperplasia with well-formed granulomas composed of epithelioid histiocytes and multinucleated giant cells, which rim central areas of caseous necrosis (eFigures 22-1 and 22-2) or necrosis containing abundant neutrophils similar to lesions in cat-scratch disease (eFigures 22-3 and 22-4) (e88,132,e313). According to one study, well-defined granulomas with caseous necrosis and numerous giant cells are more characteristic of Mycobacterium tuberculosis while microabscesses are more predictive of NTM, although there is significant overlap of features (70). Small lymphocytes are evenly distributed throughout lesional areas, and immunoblasts are rare or lacking. Immunocompromised patients may lack the classical granulomas and instead show looser aggregates of histiocytes with a foamy appearance and more abundant organisms on special stains (eFigures 22-5 and 22-6) (60). Rare cases in immunocompetent patients may show mycobacterial organisms on acid-fast stain, although greater sensitivity may be obtained using fluorescence microscopy using auramine orange (15) or immunohistochemistry against the MPT64 mycobacterial antigen (more specific for the *Mycobacterium tuberculosis complex*) (97,109). The remainder of cases may be diagnosed via one of several polymerase chain reaction–based techniques (7,11,106,108,135) or microbiologic culture. Most of these techniques, except for culture, have the advantage of being applicable to fresh as well as paraffin-embedded tissue and may be performed using cytology specimens as well as core needle biopsies or whole lymph node biopsies. Other causes of caseating and noncaseating granulomatous lymphadenitis include infection by agents other than mycobacteria (e147,e304,e335) and neoplastic disease, including peripheral T-cell lymphoma, nodular lymphocyte-predominant Hodgkin lymphoma, and classical Hodgkin lymphoma (e126,e140,e246).

Chronic Granulomatous Disease

Chronic granulomatous disease of childhood, a congenital disorder caused by defective components of the NADPH (reduced nicotinamide adenine dinucleotide phosphate) oxidase pathway (e57,e255,121), is an extremely rare form of granulomatous lymphadenitis in which lymph nodes and other tissues are extensively infiltrated by granulomas and neutrophil-rich abscess-like foci. Catalase-positive bacteria, specifically *Staphylococcus aureus* and Gram negative bacilli, and *Aspergillus* are the most common agents to be recovered in culture (e57,121) and a test for nitroblue tetrazolium reduction or other assessment of the respiratory burst by peripheral blood leukocytes by either chemiluminescence or flow cytometry should be performed in suspected cases (e56,128,e318). Molecular diagnostic testing may be performed to confirm the gene involved (128) (see Chapter 5).

In 11% to 25% of cases, a careful review of clinical, radiologic, histologic, and laboratory data fails to identify a cause of the granuloma formation (e21,e30,95), and a diagnosis of idiopathic granulomatous lymphadenitis is rendered. In such circumstances, with all secondary causes excluded, sarcoidosis can be considered a possibility (e180,e229,123) (Chapter 12). This disease is most common in young adults, although it is seen occasionally in adolescents and rarely in children. Lymph node architecture is often totally effaced with no or few residual follicles. Necrosis is rare, but when present, it is more commonly fibrinoid than caseating. Recent studies have demonstrated an increased CD4+ FoxP3+ regulatory T-cell (Treg) population both in the peripheral blood and the lymph nodes of patients with sarcoidosis (94,131). Noncaseating granulomatous lymphadenitis may also be seen in benign lymph nodes draining organs involved by tumor, and histiocytic proliferations mimicking granulomas may be present in lymph nodes involved by lymphoma (20,e140,e239).

Interfollicular Processes with Histiocytic Proliferation

Sinus histiocytosis is a nonspecific reactive pattern that may be seen in lymph nodes draining inflammatory or malignant processes of the skin, bowel, or lungs. In particularly striking cases, only compressed primary follicles are seen, and germinal centers are either diminutive or absent. The subcapsular and paratrabecular sinuses are expanded by a cellular infiltrate composed of large polygonal cells with bland nuclei and abundant pale eosinophilic cytoplasm, some with phagocytosed debris (26). These histiocytes can be distinguished from Langerhans cells and Rosai-Dorfman cells by their $CD68^+$, lysozyme-positive, $S100^-$, $CD1a^-$, $CD207^-$ phenotype.

Sinus Histiocytosis with Massive Lymphadenopathy

Sinus histiocytosis with massive lymphadenopathy (SHML), also known as *Rosai-Dorfman disease*, affects young patients (e257). Germinal centers are atrophic or lacking in most cases, and the paracortex is similarly diminished secondary to the compressive effects of the expanded sinusoids (e258) (Figure 22-14). A polymorphous array of lymphocytes, plasma cells, histiocytes, xanthoma cells, and "SHML" cells distend the sinusoids, with the proportions varying from case to case. The SHML cells, which are the hallmark of this disorder, have oval nuclei with condensed chromatin and abundant cytoplasm, which ranges from eosinophilic to xanthomatous (e97) (Figure 22-15 and eFigure 22-7). Invariably, engulfed lymphocytes ("emperipolesis") can be found in the SHML cells, although this feature may be focal in some cases. Several groups have demonstrated the utility of FNA in the diagnosis of SHML. Smears generally

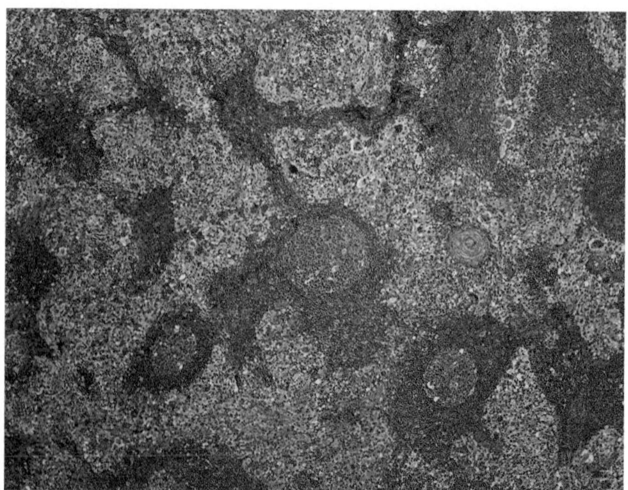

FIGURE 22-14■As a result of massive sinusoidal expansion by histiocytes, germinal centers are compressed in Rosai-Dorfman disease (SHML). (Hematoxylin and eosin stain 40× magnification.)

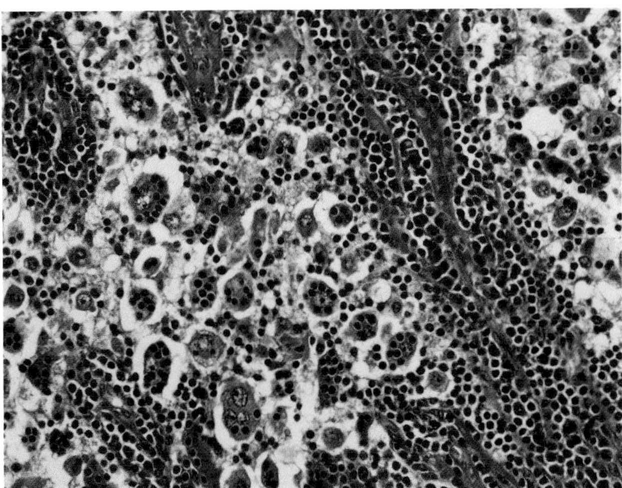

FIGURE 22-15 ■ The lesional cell in Rosai-Dorfman disease (SHML) has a small, cytologically bland nucleus and abundant eosinophilic cytoplasm containing one or more lymphocytes (emperipoplesis). Although obvious in this case, emperipolesis may be difficult to detect on routine sections. (Hematoxylin and eosin stain 200× magnification.)

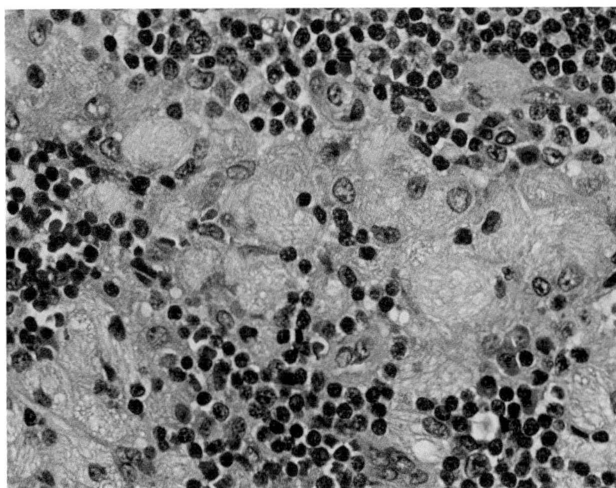

FIGURE 22-16 ■ Histiocytic proliferations caused by congenital storage disorders have a sinusoidal, often paracortical distribution in lymph nodes. The histiocytes seen in storage disorders often have coarsely vacuolated, ("bubbly") or fibrillar ("crumpled tissue paper") cytoplasm, as seen in this case of Gaucher disease. (Hematoxylin and eosin stain 400× magnification.)

demonstrate the presence of small lymphocytes, plasma cells, few neutrophils, and SHML cells (25,30,72,118). The phenotype of the SHML cell is $S100^+$, $CD68^+$, but the cells lack markers for Langerhans cells (CD1a and CD207) or dendritic cells (DRC, CD23, CNA42) (9,e75). SHML has been seen in association with neoplasms, including mixed cellularity and lymphocyte-predominant Hodgkin lymphoma as well as non-Hodgkin lymphoma, and in patients with immune dysregulation such as post–bone marrow transplant or in the setting of the ALPS that should be taken into account in the evaluation of unusual cases (3,85,e97,86,119).

Foreign Body Sinusoidal Histiocytic Reactions

Histiocytic lymphadenopathy secondary to foreign (nonnodal) material accumulations occurs in the setting of primary metabolic disease, in lymph nodes draining ulcerated or tumoral areas (e102,e119,e124), or adjacent to joint prostheses (e11,e18,e137,e162,134), or after lymphangiography, although current radiographic techniques have largely replaced lymphangiography. There is no specific manner, and the adenopathy in these patients is rarely worrisome. In the case of accumulated contrast media, the sinusoids are dilated by foamy macrophages, histiocytes, and multinucleated giant cells containing large lipid vacuoles (eFigure 22-8). A similar pattern may be seen in cases of lymphadenopathy due to silicone from leaking or ruptured implants (eFigures 22-9–22-11). In the case of joint replacement, sinuses contain pale-staining vacuolated macrophages with refractile or birefrigent material that may be oil red O positive, depending on whether metallic particles or polyethylene particles are present. Associated granulomas, giant cells, and fibrosis may be seen in some cases (134). Similar findings may be noted in patients with Gaucher disease or other metabolic storage diseases (Figure 22-16). In such cases, histiocytes resemble those seen in the bone marrow in storage diseases with either fibrillar "crumpled tissue paper" or bubbly foamy macrophages (see Chapter 23). Little of the material is found outside the sinusoids, and the remainder of the lymph node, although compressed or atrophic, is normal. Morbidity and mortality may be associated with the primary process causing the accumulation of foreign material, but not with the adenopathy itself.

Dermatopathia

Because of the distribution of the predisposing dermatologic conditions (mycosis fungoides, psoriasis, eczema) (e34,e326,139) dermatopathic lymphadenopathy is more frequently seen in adults. Children with dermatopathic lymphadenopathy commonly have eczema or another chronic exanthematous disorder, and they present with enlarged axillary or inguinal lymph nodes. At low power, involved lymph nodes show a mixed pattern of follicular hyperplasia and sinusoidal expansion caused by an influx of histiocytes, Langerhans cells (40,e282), and variable numbers of eosinophils (e36,e134) (Figure 22-17 and eFigure 22-12). The paracortex is expanded and may have a pink mottled appearance because of infiltrating histiocytes and Langerhans cells ($S100^+$, $CD1a^+$), some of which may contain coarsely granular brown-black melanin pigment that is positive on Fontana staining. Occasional hemosiderin pigment is also seen. FNA of lymph nodes with dermatopathia show large clusters of histiocytes, histiocytes with melanin pigment, few tingible body macrophages, and histiocytes with elongated or grooved nuclei (56).

Hemophagocytic Lymphohistiocytosis

The disease profile of hemophagocytic lymphohistiocytosis may be idiopathic, familial, infection related (e50,55,83), rheumatologic, malignancy related (e14,e91,38), related to

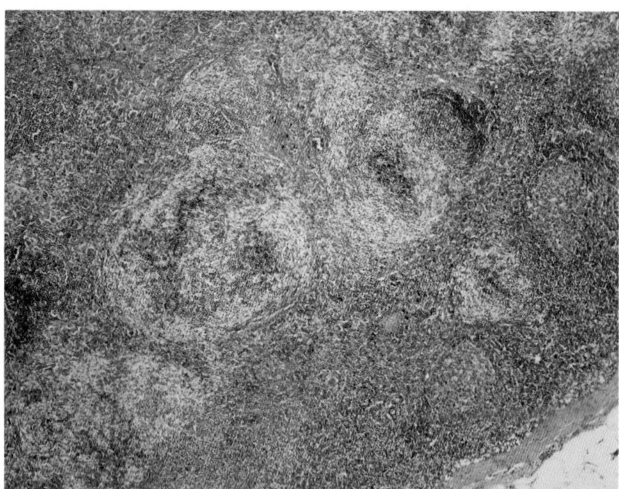

FIGURE 22-17 ■ The paracortical regions in dermatopathic lymphadenitis are expanded and show a pale pink swirled appearance due to the collections of abundant histocytes and Langerhans cells admixed with small lymphocytes. Some histiocytes contain brown melanin pigment. (Hematoxylin and eosin stain 40× magnification.)

antineoplastic therapy (74), or rarely preceded by Kikuchi disease (41,79). It results from uncontrolled activation of $CD8^+$ T cells, macrophages, and histiocytes associated with decreased NK cell function and increased levels of circulating proinflammatory cytokines (38,59). Clinically significant lymphadenopathy is uncommon in patients with hemophagocytic lymphohistiocytosis, which is diagnosed on clinical grounds when specific clinical, laboratory, and histopathologic criteria are met, according to HLH-2004 guidelines established by the Histiocyte Society (49). A lymph node biopsy, if performed, is generally done to exclude lymphoma. In most cases, the follicles are small, and the germinal centers are few in number. The paracortex is depleted and has a mottled appearance because of the presence of increased numbers of pale-staining histiocytes. The sinusoids are distended by histiocytes, many phagocytic. The nuclear features are bland, and the cells have abundant eosinophilic cytoplasm containing variable numbers of red blood cells and red blood cell fragments (eFigure 22-13). Leukophagocytosis is uncommon relative to erythrophagocytosis in this condition, and, in further contrast to SHML cells, the histiocytes in hemophagocytic lymphohistiocytosis exhibit a $CD68^+$, $S100^-$, $CD1a^-$, $CD207^-$ phenotype. Erythrophagocytosis and hemophagocytosis can be seen as a secondary phenomenon outside the context of primary hemophagocytic lymphohistiocytosis, and all these conditions must be considered as part of the differential diagnostic assessment. For instance, it has been reported in patients with a robust autoimmune hemolytic anemia (e160), active systemic lupus erythematosus (e200,110,e334), X-linked lymphoproliferative disease, ehrlichiosis (e3,31), typhoid fever (e87,126), the accelerated phase of Chediak-Higashi disease (e134,59,e265), SHML, acute myelogenous leukemia (e267), acute lymphoblastic leukemia (101), juvenile myelomonocytic leukemia (41,125), and peripheral T-cell lymphoma (e51,e114,e222,122,124,e334). In some cases, there may be a spectrum of histiocytic disorders with macrophage activation syndrome or secondary hemophagocytic syndrome seen in patients with Langerhans cell histiocytosis (37), and patients with T-lymphoblastic leukemia have rarely shown subsequent involvement by Langerhans cell histiocytosis or hemophagocytic lymphohistiocytosis (116,133).

Langerhans Cell Histiocytosis

The majority of children with Langerhans cell histiocytosis present with systemic multiorgan disease, and most have palpable adenopathy. Common sites of involvement include bone, skin, lung, liver, spleen, bone marrow, and pituitary (98,120). In most cases, the disease is accurately diagnosed after biopsy of a painful bone lesion or skin biopsy (e20,e330,120). When biopsied, lymph nodes may show a spectrum from subtle focal sinus or paracortical involvement to total effacement of the nodal architecture involving the sinuses and/or the paracortex (35) (eFigure 22-14). The sinuses, when involved, are expanded by an array of Langerhans cells, non-Langerhans histiocytes, dendritic cells, lymphocytes, eosinophils, and actively phagocytic macrophages (e92) (eFigures 22-15 and 22-16). Older lesions may have a proportional increase in non–Langerhans-type histiocytes and xanthoma cells, and eosinophils may be scarce (e92). By immunohistochemical analysis, Langerhans cells are reactive for CD1a (e78) and S100 (e337) but less so for CD68 (e125). A relatively new marker, CD207, or Langerin, is a lectin associated with the Birbeck granule and is more specific for Langerhans cells than CD1a (16,77). Ultrastructural studies demonstrate Birbeck granules, a pathognomonic finding (e90).

MALIGNANT LYMPHADENOPATHY

The most common nodal malignancies in children are of lymphoid lineage, although mesenchymal (e201), histiocyte/macrophage (e145,e190), and metastatic tumors (e132) may also present initially as node-based disease. Immunophenotypic analysis is always required for an accurate diagnosis, and cytogenetic studies in non-Hodgkin lymphomas are frequently helpful.

Like its benign counterparts, malignant adenopathy can be categorized morphologically by the architectural changes seen in affected lymph nodes (Table 22-5). The most widely accepted current classification from the World Health Organization (WHO) adopts a diagnostic and biologically meaningful approach based on the lineage of the malignant cell. Within each lineage of the WHO classification, distinct diseases are defined based on a combination of clinical, morphologic, immunophenotypic, and molecular genetic features (Table 22-6) (48).

The vast majority of pediatric cases of non-Hodgkin lymphoma fall into one of the four categories: diffuse large B-cell lymphoma, Burkitt lymphoma, lymphoblastic lymphoma (T-cell or B-cell), and anaplastic large cell lymphoma.

Table 22-5 ▪ MALIGNANT CAUSES OF LYMPH NODE ENLARGEMENT CLASSIFIED ACCORDING TO HISTOLOGIC PATTERNS

Nodular proliferations
Hodgkin lymphoma, nodular sclerosis type
Hodgkin lymphoma, lymphocyte-predominant type
Follicle center cell lymphoma
Mantle cell lymphoma (mantle zone pattern)
Diffuse and paracortical proliferations
Chloroma (granulocytic sarcoma)
Lymphoblastic lymphoma
Burkitt lymphoma
Diffuse large B-cell lymphoma
Peripheral T-cell lymphoma
Small lymphocytic lymphoma
Mantle cell lymphoma
Marginal zone lymphoma
Hodgkin lymphoma, mixed-cellularity type
Partial nodal involvement by lymphoma (any type)
Solid tumor metastasis
Posttransplant lymphoproliferative disorders
Necrotizing proliferations
Nodal infarction secondary to lymphoma or leukemia
Granulomatous or histiocyte-rich proliferations
Hodgkin lymphoma, mixed-cellularity type (some cases)
Sinusoidal proliferations
T γ/δ hepatosplenic lymphoma
T-cell anaplastic large-cell lymphoma
Solid tumor metastasis

Table 22-6 ▪ ABBREVIATED WHO CLASSIFICATION AS APPLIED TO PEDIATRICS

Precursor B- and T-cell neoplasms
Precursor B-lymphoblastic leukemia/lymphoma
Precursor T-lymphoblastic leukemia/lymphoma
Mature B-cell neoplasms
Marginal zone B-cell lymphoma
Follicular lymphoma
Diffuse large B-cell lymphoma
Mediastinal (thymic) large B-cell lymphoma
Burkitt lymphoma
Mature T-cell and NK-cell neoplasms
Hepatosplenic T-cell lymphoma[a]
Primary cutaneous CD30+ T-cell lymphoproliferative disorders[a]
Primary cutaneous anaplastic large cell lymphoma (C-ALCL)
Lymphomatoid papulosis
Angioimmunoblastic T-cell lymphoma
Peripheral T-cell lymphoma, unspecified
Anaplastic large cell lymphoma
Hodgkin lymphoma
Classical Hodgkin lymphoma
Nodular sclerosing Hodgkin lymphoma
Mixed-cellularity Hodgkin lymphoma
Lymphocyte-depleted Hodgkin lymphoma
Lymphocyte-rich classical Hodgkin lymphoma
Nodular lymphocyte-predominant Hodgkin lymphoma

[a]Not discussed in this chapter.

Indolent lymphomas composed of small lymphocytes (e.g., small lymphocytic lymphoma, marginal zone lymphoma, mantle cell lymphoma, follicle center cell lymphoma) are extremely rare in children, and they should be diagnosed with caution.

Precursor B Lymphoblastic Lymphoma

B-cell lymphoblastic lymphoma, which represents approximately 15% of all cases of lymphoblastic lymphoma, is most common in older children and young adults. Patients with this type of lymphoma present with rapidly enlarging lymph nodes or soft tissue masses. In contrast to T-cell lymphoblastic lymphoma, the B-lymphoblastic lymphoma rarely involves the mediastinum. The distinction between B-cell lymphoblastic lymphoma and precursor B-cell acute lymphoblastic leukemia is made through examination of the bone marrow biopsy specimen; in cases in which fewer than 25% of the marrow cells are blasts, a diagnosis of B-cell lymphoblastic lymphoma should be made (e132). One feature typical of lymphoblastic lymphoma (B or T) is infiltration through perinodal fat and linear infiltrates in the capsular collagen (Figure 22-18). The nodal architecture is effaced by a diffuse proliferation of small and intermediate cells (12 to 14 mm) with fine or speckled chromatin, small or indistinct nucleoli, and scant cytoplasm (e23,e123,e203) (Figure 22-19). The mitotic rate is frequently elevated, and necrosis may be present. A CD45 (dim to negative), terminal deoxynucleotidyl transferase (TdT) positive, $CD19^+$, $CD20^-$, sIg^- phenotype sets these tumors apart from lymphomas composed of mature (nonblastoid) B-cells, including Burkitt lymphoma (e 284) (Figure 22-19). Almost all cases are positive for CD10 (common acute lymphocytic leukemia antigen or CALLA) (111). Important in the differential diagnosis in children are other small blue cell tumors including

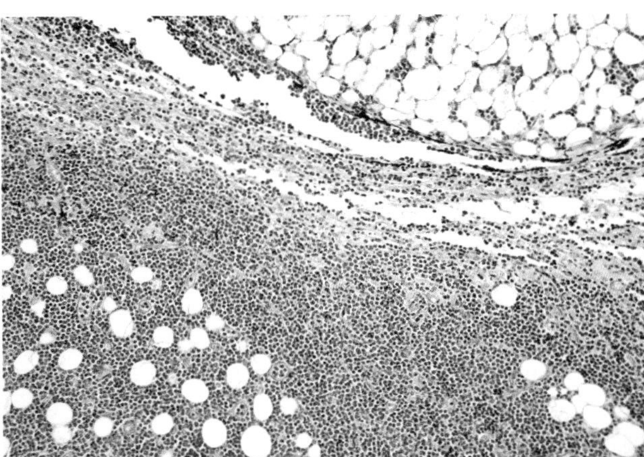

FIGURE 22-18 ▪ Precursor B lymphoblastic lymphoma demonstrating diffuse architectural effacement of the node in infiltration into adjacent perinodal fat and linear infiltrates of the capsular collagen. (Hematoxylin and eosin stain 10×.)

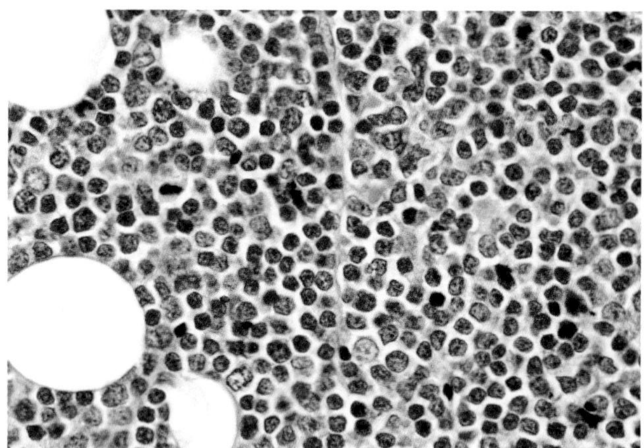

FIGURE 22-19 The chromatin is fine and nucleoli are indistinct in lymphoblastic lymphoma. (Hematoxylin and eosin stain 40×.)

granulocytic sarcoma/chloroma, Ewing sarcoma/primitive neuroectodermal tumor (104), embryonal rhabdomyosarcoma that can be distinguished by phenotype, although care should be taken not to overvalue results from any single stain (e187). For example, like Ewing sarcoma, lymphoblastic lymphomas are often $CD45^-$ and $CD99^+$.

Diffuse Large B-Cell Lymphoma

Diffuse large B-cell lymphoma (DLBCL) is disproportionately common relative to other types of lymphoma in patients with congenital, iatrogenic, or acquired immune deficiency states (e235). Patients with B-cell diffuse large cell lymphoma may present with steadily enlarging peripheral lymphadenopathy or extranodal disease (soft tissue, bone, oropharynx). Although rare, a primary mediastinal B-cell diffuse large cell lymphoma has also been described in children (e238). DLBCL has a diffuse growth pattern and may have intermixed fibrosis (particularly in the mediastinum). Cytoplasm is abundant and may be either amphophilic or densely eosinophilic (e320). The cytology of the tumor cells ranges from that of reactive immunoblasts (round nucleus, thick nuclear membrane, single large eosinophilic nucleolus, abundant cytoplasm), to polylobate and even frankly anaplastic multilobate cells. Immunophenotypically, tumor cells mark with pan B-cell markers (CD19, CD20, CD79A, CD22) and are surface Ig+ (except in mediastinal large B-cell lymphoma). CD10 is positive in a minority.

Burkitt Lymphoma

Burkitt lymphoma takes three epidemiologic forms (140). Endemic Burkitt lymphoma most commonly affects children and exhibits a male predominance. It is common in equatorial Africa and New Guinea and is strongly associated with EBV infection. Sporadic Burkitt lymphoma is less commonly related to EBV infection and affects both children and adults, with a bimodal age distribution. Immunodeficiency-related Burkitt lymphoma is seen in the setting of congenital immunodeficiency, HIV infection, and posttransplant. Burkitt lymphoma is one of the most rapidly replicating of all human tumors, and patients frequently present with the sudden development of large tumor masses (57). In endemic Burkitt lymphoma, the tumor shows an unexplained predilection for areas of growth, including the sockets around deciduous teeth of young (2- to 4-year-old) children, and hormonally responsive locations, such as the breasts of pubertal and pregnant women, ovaries, testes, and thyroid. In sporadic and immunodeficiency-associated Burkitt lymphoma, visceral involvement, particularly of the small bowel, is common, with initial symptoms related to obstruction or perforation.

Burkitt lymphoma diffusely effaces the nodal architecture. A monomorphic proliferation of intermediate-sized cells is seen (nuclear size similar to that of histiocytes or endothelial cells); the round or oval nuclei have a thick nuclear membrane and two to four nucleoli, and the cytoplasm is moderately amphophilic (65,e230). Many Burkitt lymphomas have a somewhat cohesive appearance, and the cell borders maintain a molded contour, particularly at the periphery. The mitotic rate is high (MIB-1/KI-67 is positive in >95% of cells), and necrosis is often present, particularly at the periphery. Evenly distributed macrophages containing cellular debris give a mottled ("starry sky") appearance to Burkitt lymphoma at low power. Some classification systems make a distinction between "Burkitt" and "non-Burkitt" morphology of small noncleaved cell lymphomas; however, the criteria are subjective, and because of the lack of reproducibility, this histologic point is of limited clinical relevance (e331). The immunophenotype is that of a mature surface Ig+ B-cell, and both CD19 and CD20 are expressed. CD10 is positive. BCL-2 expression is not present. TdT expression is lacking (e8). Differential diagnostic considerations include lymphoblastic lymphoma and rapidly replicating large cell lymphomas. Cytogenetic analyses play a key role in confirming the diagnosis. FISH studies are very helpful in demonstrating translocations that deregulate expression of the protooncogene c-myc (chromosome 8) paired with either the heavy-chain loci (chromosome 14) or light-chain locus (chromosome 2 and 22) (e25,e231) (Table 22-3).

Other Rare B-Cell Lymphoma in Children

Two small B-cell lymphomas are worthy of note but only rarely seen in children—follicular lymphoma and nodal marginal zone lymphoma. Follicular lymphoma in children affects males more than females and, unlike their adult counterparts, often presents with limited stage disease. Even though most are grade 2 or 3, many are curable. Morphologically, they range from the typical low-power pattern of crowded monomorphic small-to-medium size follicles to large expansive follicles and even "floral variant." Phenotypically like adults, most cases are $CD10^+$ and $BCL\text{-}6^+$, but unlike adults, are often $BCL\text{-}2^-$ and most do not have underlying BCL-2/IgH (14;18) translocation. The small minority with BCL-2 translocations appear to have a worse prognosis (84,e243).

Pediatric nodal marginal zone lymphoma, like its adult counterpart, can be particularly difficult to diagnose in that these lymphomas often only partially efface architecture with an interfollicular distribution. The neoplastic cells are frequently a mix of classic monocytoid B-cells with small somewhat folded nuclei and abundant cytoplasm, small lymphocytes with little cytoplasm, large lymphocytes, and variable numbers of plasma cells and plasmacytoid lymphocytes. Follicular colonization may be present as well as follicles resembling those of progressive transformation of follicular centers. Most cases have CD5–CD10-phenotype with monotypic surface Ig. Many have monotypic cytoplasmic immunoglobulin in plasma cells on paraffin immunoperoxidase stains. Like pediatric follicular lymphoma, these patients are predominantly males with limited stage disease (usually cervical nodes) and have an apparently good prognosis (130).

T-Lymphoblastic Leukemia

T-cell lymphoblastic lymphoma is commonly seen in adolescents and young adults. Although a rare type of lymphoma in the adult population, it represents approximately 30% of all pediatric non-Hodgkin lymphomas, and, like B-cell lymphoblastic lymphoma, T-cell lymphoblastic lymphoma is distinguished from T-cell acute lymphoblastic leukemia by the demonstration of limited bone marrow disease (<25% involvement). Because it is frequently located in the mediastinum (e132), a rapidly growing T-cell lymphoblastic lymphoma may compress the heart and great vessels or cause a pleural or pericardial effusion. The morphology of T-cell lymphoblastic lymphoma is identical in every respect to B-cell lymphoblastic lymphoma, and the immunophenotype is that of an immature T-cell with CD45 (dim-to-negative), TdT^+, cytoplasmic $CD3^+$, usually surface $CD3^-$, $CD2^+$, $CD7^+$ with variable expression of CD1a, CD4, CD5, and CD8 (e283,e324). HLA-DR is negative. CD10 is expressed in 25% of cases. Other entities in the differential diagnosis, including B-cell lymphoblastic lymphoma, Ewing sarcoma/primitive neuroectodermal tumor, and embryonal rhabdomyosarcoma, can be excluded with immunophenotype studies. Tumor karyotype is less helpful in the prognosis of T-cell lymphoblastic lymphoma than of B-cell lymphoblastic lymphoma (43). Many (although not all) translocations involve either the α and the δ T-cell receptor locus at 14q11.2, the β locus at 7q35, or the γ locus at 7p14–15 (e221).

Peripheral T-Cell Lymphoma

Peripheral T-cell lymphomas including angioimmunoblastic T-cell lymphoma represent only a small fraction of lymphomas in children (e7,e133,e235), and heterogeneity is their histologic hallmark (Table 22-7). At low power, the lymph node architecture is either diffusely effaced or shows interfollicular expansion. Thick-walled vessels are more prominent in peripheral T-cell lymphomas than in B-cell non-Hodgkin lymphomas, and the even mixture of atypical small, intermediate, and large lymphoid elements is another clue to the lineage of this type of lymphoma (e118,e168). Scattered eosinophils and plasma cells may also be seen. Irregularity of the nuclear contour may be particularly prominent, and, in further contrast to lymphomas of B-cell lineage, these tumors in many cases have cells with a clear cytoplasm. Detailed phenotypic studies have shown that peripheral T-cell lymphomas are uniformly TdT^-, $CD45^+$ with most having a $CD3^+$, $CD45Ro^+$, $CD4^+$, $CD8^-$ helper T-cell phenotype (e241). Other T-cell antigens (e.g., CD2, CD5, CD7) are variably expressed, and the loss of these markers is characteristic of peripheral T-cell lymphoma (e241). Virally mediated or drug hypersensitivity immunoblastic reactions may mimic peripheral T-cell lymphoma, as can Hodgkin lymphoma, B-cell lymphomas rich in T-cells ("T-cell-rich B-cell lymphomas"), and Fas mutation-related (ALPS).

Table 22-7 ▪ CATEGORIES OF PERIPHERAL T-CELL LYMPHOMA

Phenotype-specific
CD56 + (NK-like) PTCL
CD30 + PTCL (ALCL)
Organ-specific subtypes
Enteropathy-associated PTCL
Angiocentric PTCL
T γ/δ hepatosplenic PTCL
Subcutaneous panniculitic PTCL
Peripheral T-cell lymphoma, NOS
Predominantly small-cell
Mixed small- and large-cell
Predominantly large-cell
Histology-specific
Lennert PTCL
AILD type PTCL
Virally mediated
HTLV-1–related
EBV-related

NK, natural killer; PTCL, peripheral T-cell lymphoma; AILD, angioimmunoblastic lymphadenopathy with dysproteinemia; HTLV, human T-cell leukemia/lymphoma/lymphotrophic virus; EBV, Epstein-Barr virus; NOS, not otherwise specified.

Anaplastic Large Cell Lymphoma

T-cell anaplastic large cell lymphoma, a special type of peripheral T-cell lymphoma, affects patients of all ages, from children to the elderly (e121,e219,e275). Cervical lymphadenopathy is particularly common in some series, and the skin, bone, and soft tissue may be secondarily involved. Involved lymph nodes may exhibit either a diffuse or a sinusoidal pattern (Figure 22-20) of tumor cell infiltration, and the latter may be mistaken for metastases of a solid tumor. The tumor cells of T-cell anaplastic large cell lymphoma are often very large (>20 mm) and have bizarre, lobulated, or wreath-like nuclei (hallmark cells) with small-to-large nucleoli and abundant eosinophilic cytoplasm (e6) (Figure 22-21). Pleomorphic (e49), sarcomatoid (e43), histiocyte-rich (e239), neutrophil-rich (90,127), and even monomorphic/small

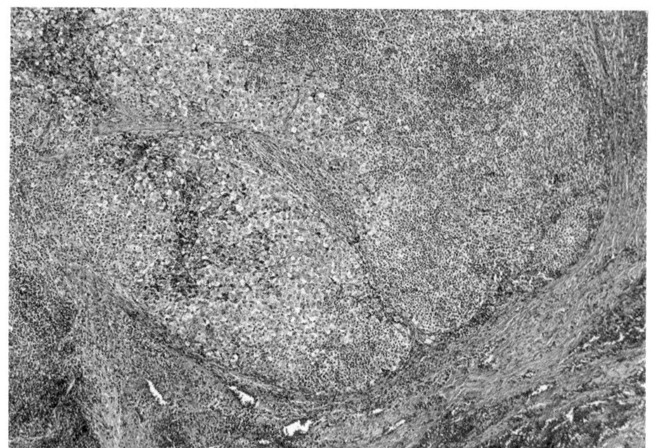

FIGURE 22-20 ■ Anaplastic large cell lymphoma may resemble metastatic carcinoma when it remains localized to the sinusoids. (Hematoxylin and eosin stain 4×.)

cell variants (51,e156) have been described. The common denominator in most pediatric cases being the t(2;5) karyotype abnormality with ALK positivity (e167). Membranous staining (usually associated with Golgi positivity) for CD30 is required for the diagnosis. Anaplastic large cell lymphoma exhibits a variable expression of pan T-cell markers CD3, CD7, and CD5. Epithelial membrane antigen (EMA) and CD45 are usually but not always positive (e83,65). CD4, CD2, CD43, and CD45 RO are often helpful. Most cases are positive for cytotoxic molecules like TIA-1, granzyme B, and perforin. Only a minority are CD8$^+$. Stains for EBV-like LMP and EBER are consistently negative (28,e158,129). Staining for EBV, ALK, PAX-5, and a battery of T-cell and cytotoxic granule markers is helpful in evaluating CD45$^-$, CD30$^+$ cases of ALCL in which the major consideration is Hodgkin lymphoma with a syncytial growth phase.

Hodgkin Lymphoma

Hodgkin lymphoma is a primary nodal tumor of B-cell lineage (22). Recent studies in which microdissected tissue and single-cell polymerase chain reaction methods were used have shown that the Reed-Sternberg cells in most cases of Hodgkin lymphoma have clonal rearrangements of the immunoglobulin heavy-chain locus and exhibit intraclonal point mutations, indicative of ongoing somatic hypermutation (e183,e216). These findings have allowed assignment to a B-cell lineage and germinal center status to the cell of origin of Reed-Sternberg cells (22).

Hodgkin lymphoma manifests a bimodal age distribution, with peaks in young adults and older adults, and is more common overall in males than in females (e13). The key pathological characteristic of Hodgkin lymphoma is that the bulk of the tumor is composed of reactive leukocytes and histiocytes, with very few neoplastic cells (46,e175). The diagnosis of Hodgkin lymphoma requires (a) the presence of neoplastic Reed-Sternberg cells of appropriate phenotype and (b) a cytologically bland population of background inflammatory cells (e131). The WHO classification of Hodgkin lymphoma divides these lymphomas into lymphocyte-predominant Hodgkin lymphoma and classic Hodgkin lymphoma, which includes nodular sclerosing, mixed cellularity, lymphocyte-rich, and lymphocyte-depleted subtypes (Fig 22-22).

In classic Hodgkin lymphoma, typical Reed-Sternberg cells are large (20 to 40 μm), with a range of appearances. The classic type has a bilobed or a multilobed nucleus, with a thick nuclear membrane and one or several very large nucleoli, and abundant eosinophilic cytoplasm (47) (Figure 22-23). In the mononuclear type, the nucleus has a single lobe and often a single central nucleolus, which may be so large that it mimics a cytomegalovirus inclusion. The lacunar type of Reed-Sternberg cell characteristic of nodular sclerosing Hodgkin has a single-lobed or a multilobed nucleus, usually with small nucleoli and a water clear cytoplasm that is fragmented and retracted from the surrounding cells (Table 22-8). Phenotypically, the Reed-Sternberg cells of the different subtypes of classic Hodgkin lymphoma share a CD45$^-$, CD30$^+$, CD15$^\pm$, CD20$^\pm$ and PAX5$^+$ (weak) phenotype. In up to one-half of cases, Reed-Sternberg

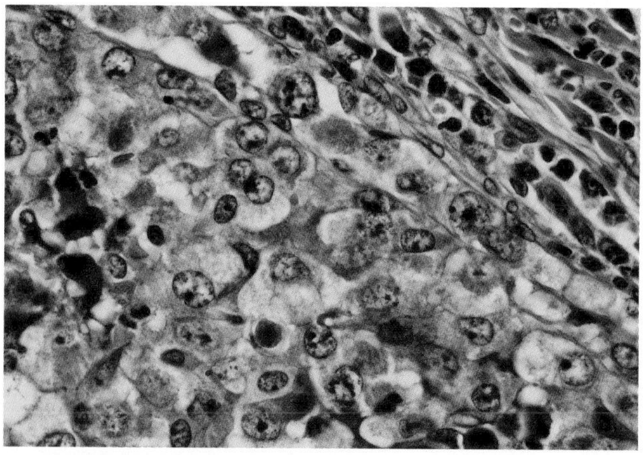

FIGURE 22-21 ■ Anaplastic large cell lymphoma with large bizarre tumor cells with multilobated nuclei with small-to-large nucleoli and abundant cytoplasm. (Hematoxylin and eosin stain 40×.)

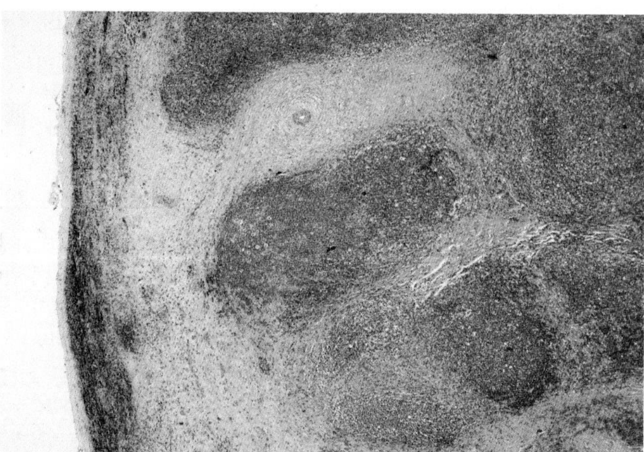

FIGURE 22-22 ■ Broad bands of frequently paucicellular collagen dissect the lymph node into cellular nodules in nodular sclerosis Hodgkin lymphoma. (Hematoxylin and eosin stain 4×.)

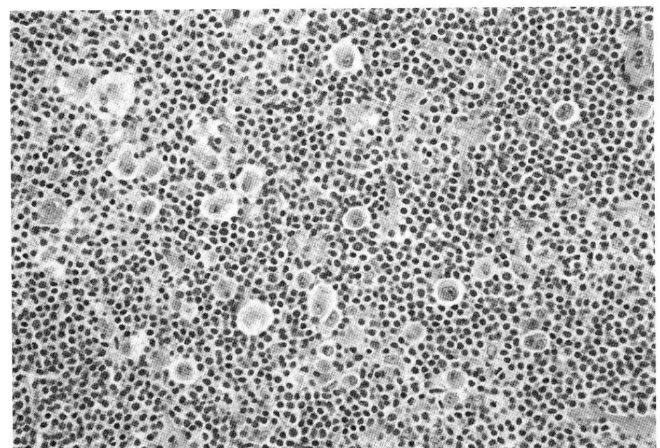

FIGURE 22-23 Lacunar Reed-Sternberg cells have vesicular chromatin, small nucleoli, multilobed nuclei, and abundant cytoplasm. (Hematoxylin and eosin stain 10×.)

cells-stain for Epstein Barr virus products LMP or EBER, particularly in cases associated with immunodeficiency (17,42) (Table 22-9).

Nodular Sclerosing Hodgkin Lymphoma

Nodular sclerosing Hodgkin lymphoma is the most common type of Hodgkin lymphoma in children and is slightly more common in girls than in boys. Common sites of primary disease are the cervical, mediastinal, and supraclavicular lymph nodes. The presentation may be secondary to a mass effect (e.g., superior vena cava syndrome, palpable adenopathy) or not directly referable to the tumor bulk ("B" symptoms). In most cases of nodular sclerosis Hodgkin lymphoma, the low-power view is diagnostic. Broad bands of birefringent fibrosis dissect the node into cellular nodules containing both lacunar Reed-Sternberg cells and a mixed inflammatory infiltrate (Figures 22-22 and 22-23). The background cellularity in this subtype of Hodgkin lymphoma is quite variable and may include a mixture of granulocytes, eosinophils, lymphocytes, and histiocytes, in which one of these cell types may predominate (Table 22-10). Mononuclear Reed-Sternberg cell variants may be numerous, but "classic" or "diagnostic" forms are in the minority (Table 22-8). With rare exceptions, all exhibit the typical CD15$^+$, CD30$^+$, PAX5$^+$ (weak), CD45$^-$, and CD20$^\pm$ profile (e131,e242). Other entities in the differential diagnosis, include ALCL, inflammatory myofibroblastic tumor, cat-scratch disease, and large cell lymphoma with or without sclerosis (e48,e238), can be distinguished from nodular sclerosis Hodgkin lymphoma by light microscopic features and immunohistochemistry.

Table 22-8 ■ CORRELATION OF REED-STERNBERG CELL TYPE AND SPECIFIC SUBTYPE OF HODGKIN LYMPHOMA

	NSHL	MCHL	LPHL	LDHL
Classic	+	++	−/+	++
Mononuclear	++	++	+	++
Lacunar	++	0	0	0
L&H	0	0	++	0

L&H, lymphocyte and histiocyte; NSHL, nodular Sclerosis Hodgkin lymphoma; MCHL, mixed cellularity Hodgkin lymphoma; LPHL, lymphocyte predominance Hodgkin lymphoma; LDHL, lymphocyte depletion Hodgkin lymphoma; +, present; ++, numerous; 0, absent; −/+, rare to absent.

Table 22-9 ■ IMMUNOPHENOTYPE IN HODGKIN LYMPHOMA

	NSHL	MCHL	LPHL	LDHL
Classic[a]	+	+	0	+
B-cell[b]	0	0	+	0

[a]CD15+, CD30+, CD20−, CD45−.
[b]CD15−, CD30−, CD20+, CD45+.
NSHL, nodular sclersis Hodgkin lymphoma; MCHL, mixed cellularity Hodgkin lymphoma; LPHL, lymphocyte predominance Hodgkin lymphoma; LDHL, lymphocyte depletion Hodgkin lymphoma.

Mixed Cellularity Hodgkin Lymphoma

The other common type of classic Hodgkin lymphoma is the mixed-cellularity Hodgkin lymphoma. This is seen in all age groups, although it is more common than nodular sclerosis Hodgkin lymphoma in older patients, and shows a male predominance. Patients present with either isolated disease or multiple contiguous sites of involvement centered in the neck and mediastinum. The architecture of the lymph node in mixed-cellularity Hodgkin lymphoma is usually diffuse or interfollicular, although the cellular composition of the background population varies from an even mixture of lymphocytes, plasma cells, eosinophils, neutrophils, and histiocytes to a monotony of one of these elements (Table 22-10). Only rarely do the Reed-Sternberg cells in mixed-cellularity Hodgkin lymphoma deviate from the classic phenotypic profile. Because of a close morphologic overlap with T-cell–rich B-cell large cell lymphoma (e48,e225) and peripheral T-cell lymphoma, all cases of mixed-cellularity Hodgkin lymphoma should be evaluated by immunohistochemistry.

Lymphocyte-Depleted Hodgkin Lymphoma

Lymphocyte-depleted Hodgkin lymphoma is exceedingly rare, if it occurs at all, in children and most often seen in adults over 50 years of age. Involved lymph nodes are diffusely overrun by small, intermediate, and numerous large cells, the latter representing classic and variant forms of Reed-Sternberg cells (e175,e208). The proliferation is embedded within a fibrillary and fibrotic matrix (diffuse fibrosis type), or a collagenous background and increased numbers of fibroblasts may be present (reticular type) (e122,e150). The Reed-Sternberg cells have a classic immunophenotype profile, and the background infiltrate is composed largely of T-cells (e150) (Table 22-9).

Table 22-10 ■ CORRELATION OF BACKGROUND CELLULAR AND METRIC COMPOSITION WITH SPECIFIC TYPE OF HODGKIN LYMPHOMA

	NSHL	MCHL	LPHL	LDHL
Lymphocytes	+	++	++	+
Neutrophils	++	++	0	+
Eosinophils	++	++	0	0
Histiocytes	+	++	+	–/+
Bands of fibrosis	++	0	0	0
Architecture	Nodular	Diffuse	Nodular[a]	Diffuse

[a]The exixtence of a diffuse form of LPHL is controversial.
L&H, lymphocyte and histiocyte; NSHL, nodular sclerosis Hodgkin lymphoma; MCHL, mixed cellularity Hodgkin lymphoma; LPHL, lymphocyte predominance Hodgkin lymphoma; LDHL, lymphocyte depletion Hodgkin lymphoma; +, present; ++, numerous; 0, absent; –/+, rare to absent.

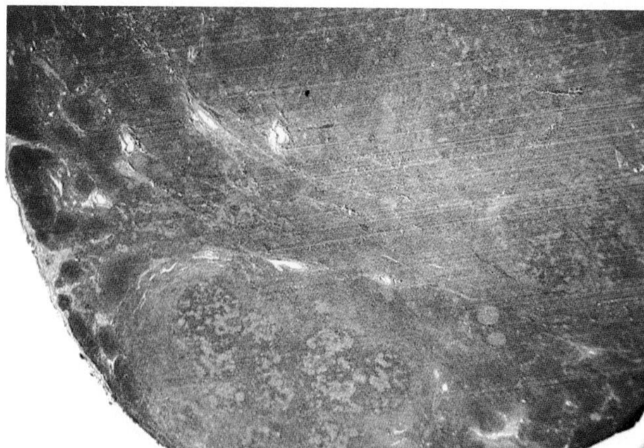

FIGURE 22-24■In lymphocyte-predominant Hodgkin lymphoma, the nodularity is created by contrasting populations of basophilic small mature lymphocytes centrally and eosinophilic histiocytes and compressed high endothelial venules peripherally. (Hematoxylin and eosin stain 4×.)

Lymphocyte-Rich Classic Hodgkin Lymphoma

This is a rare and recently recognized subtype of Hodgkin lymphoma, which at low power has a nodular growth pattern like nodular LPHL. Also like LPHL, the background lymphocyte population is predominantly small B-cells (usually IgD+), unlike other subtypes of classic Hodgkin lymphoma in which CD4 small T-cells predominate. However, the neoplastic Reed-Sternberg cells maintain a CD45$^-$, CD30$^+$, CD20$^-$, CD15$^\pm$ phenotype unlike the CD45$^+$, CD20$^+$, CD30$^-$ phenotype of LPHL (4).

Lymphocyte-Predominant Hodgkin Lymphoma

Lymphocyte-predominant Hodgkin lymphoma has a unimodal age distribution, a predilection for males, with a peak incidence in the fourth decade. Most patients present with isolated and asymptomatic adenopathy and very few are at an advanced stage at presentation (100,117). The architecture is distorted by nodules of small B-lymphocytes that are bounded by a compressed, reticulin-rich rim of blood vessels and histiocytes (117) (Figure 22-24). Scattered within the nodules are lymphocytic and histiocytic (L&H), Reed-Sternberg cell variants, many of which are ringed by T-cells (e47). L&H cells are multinucleated (popcorn-like) with a thin nuclear membrane, delicate chromatin, and inconspicuous nucleoli, and the cell has a variable quantity of cytoplasm (Figure 22-25).

Diagnostic Reed-Sternberg cells are rare (if present at all), and mononuclear variants are few in number. Typically, the L&H cells are evenly spaced throughout the nodules, although on occasion they are present in tighter clusters or form small aggregates. In the diffuse form of lymphocyte-predominant Hodgkin lymphoma, a controversial entity (e244), nodule formation is minimal, and the morphologic and immunophenotypic overlap with B-cell large cell lymphomas rich in T-cells is considerable (e130). The L&H variants exhibit a B-cell phenotype (CD20$^+$, CD45$^+$) (Figure 22-25) and do not express the usual Hodgkin markers, CD15 and CD30 (e185). The majority of the background lymphocytes are CD20$^+$ B-cells; CD57$^+$ T cells commonly form a collarette pattern around the L&H cells. Transformation to DLBCL is occasionally seen. Differential diagnostic considerations are numerous and include T-cell–rich B-cell large cell lymphoma (e46,e149,e276), lymphocyte-rich classic Hodgkin lymphoma (e188), progressive transformation of germinal centers (e37,e48,99,e308), and florid toxoplasmosis-related lymphadenopathy (e67).

Tumors of Monocyte/Macrophage Lineage

Chloroma/granulocytic sarcoma occurs more frequently in patients with simultaneous or subsequent acute myelogenous leukemia (27), and it may also be the first sign of relapse in patients with a previous diagnosis of acute myelogenous leukemia (e322). Lymphadenopathy or bulk disease

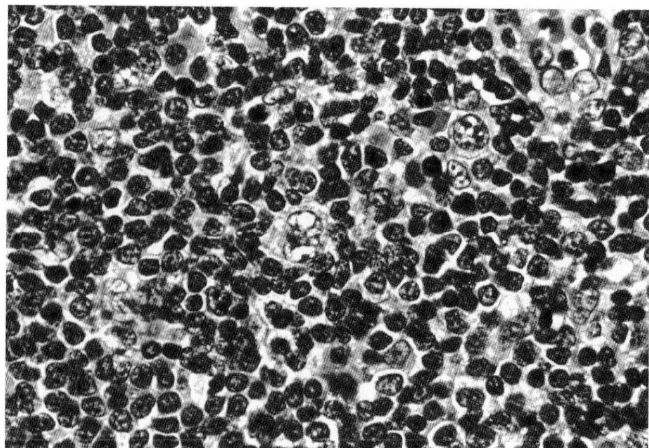

FIGURE 22-25■The "lymphocytic and histiocytic" cell of lymphocyte-predominant Hodgkin lymphoma has a thin nuclear membrane, distinct nucleoli, and scant-to-moderate quantities of cytoplasm. (Hematoxylin and eosin stain 40×.)

in nodal groups is less common than visceral or soft tissue involvement, but when it is present, a biopsy is often performed (e31,21,e96,e171,89,e301). The architecture of the lymph node is diffusely effaced by a proliferation of cells of uniformly intermediate size with oval or folded nuclei, fine chromatin, and scant-to-moderate quantities of pale or amphophilic cytoplasm. Cytoplasmic granules may be faint or absent, although a Leder stain accentuates their presence in some cases (e207). Most cells are positive for myeloperoxidase and CD45, and some aberrantly express macrophage markers such as CD68 or lysozyme. Rare cases may be of apparently mixed lineage and show reactivity for polyclonal CD3 (e250,e253), CD30 (e95), or CD99 (e66), some cases may be positive for TdT (53,e223,e250). Examinations of touch preparations of involved nodes should disclose a blast morphology, which effectively excludes a mature B- or T-cell lymphoma. Immunohistochemistry and correlation with clinical and laboratory parameters (92) are important in excluding nodal metastasis of Ewing sarcoma/primitive neuroectodermal tumor or involvement by lymphoma (e328) or Langerhans cell histiocytosis.

SPLEEN

Embryology

The spleen develops from mesenchyme located between the two layers of the dorsal mesentery of the stomach (the dorsal mesogastrium). As the stomach rotates during development, the dorsal mesogastrium becomes fused to the peritoneum of the left kidney to form the lienorenal ligament, which envelops the splenic artery and vein and the tail of the pancreas.

Normal Structure and Function

In contrast to lymph nodes, which filter lymphatic fluid, the spleen is the major site of blood filtration. In the microenvironment of the spleen, antibody-antigen binding takes place and immune complexes, such as opsonized bacteria, are removed. The spleen is also a major site of removal of red cells with decreased flexibility or increased osmotic fragility. The filtering function of the spleen is a dual-edged sword. Although the spleen protects against life-threatening infections caused by encapsuled bacteria, the destruction of antibody-coated platelets or red blood cells makes it necessary to remove the spleen in certain diseases.

The spleen is subdivided into the areas of red and white pulp (Figure 22-26). This division is useful for surgical pathologists because most diseases primarily affect one compartment or the other. The red pulp comprises most of the splenic volume and is the major site of removal of senescent and antibody-coated red cells and platelets and of red cell inclusions, such as Howell-Jolly bodies (nuclear fragments) and Pappenheimer bodies (siderotic granules). Blood enters the spleen via splenic arteries. The splenic arteries branch into progressively smaller arteries and arterioles that ultimately empty into a network of thin-walled, endothelium-lined capillaries. These terminate in sheathed capillaries that are lined not by endothelium but by specialized phagocytic mononuclear cells. Blood cells traverse the sheathed capillaries and basement membrane to enter the splenic sinuses and ultimately drain into the splenic veins. While crossing the sheathed capillaries, red blood cells with decreased flexibility become trapped in the splenic cords and are destroyed by the phagocytic lining cells.

The white pulp of the spleen, which grossly appears as numerous gray-white spots within the red pulp, is composed of masses of T- and B-lymphocytes. The T-lymphocytes

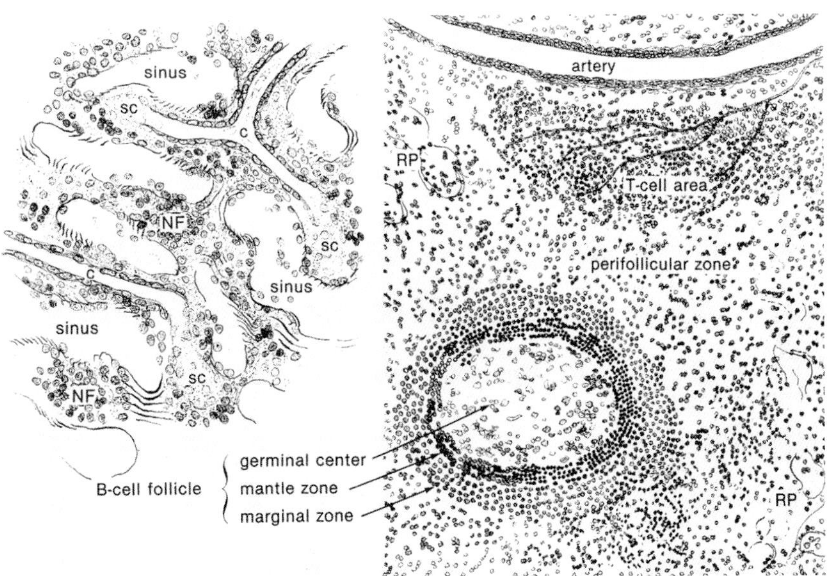

FIGURE 22-26 ■ Schematic representation of the splenic red pulp (**left**) and white pulp (**right**) showing the main compartments and structures of the human spleen. (From Van Krieken JH, Orazi A. Spleen. In Mills SE, ed. *Histology for Pathologists*, 3rd ed. Philadelphia: Lippincott Williams & Wilkins, 2007:783–798).

surround the arterioles and become less plentiful around the more distant arteriolar branches. Within these areas are the B-cell areas, which may contain germinal centers, particularly in the spleens of children and persons with autoimmune disorders. Germinal centers in the spleen, as in other sites, are surrounded by a mantle zone. This in turn is surrounded by a marginal zone of cells with relatively abundant pale cytoplasm that is usually appreciable only in the spleen. In a retrospective review of splenic histopathology from 205 children dying unexpectedly, there was a significant increase in reactive germinal centers in the spleen of children dying unexpectedly in comparison to other children of the same age (e10). Germinal centers in the spleen develop in response to immunological stimulation. The existence of a high number of germinal centers in the spleen is evidence that an immune reaction has occurred. The histology of the normal spleen is described in greater detail by van Krieken and te Velde (e315).

Examination of the Spleen

Many pathological processes affect the spleen of children, including congenital anomalies, benign cysts, trauma, infection, malignancies, and other hematological disorders (50). Splenectomies in children are performed for many reasons. The most common reasons from splenectomy include hereditary spherocytosis, hemolytic anemias, trauma, idiopathic thrombocytopenic purpura, hypersplenism, and trauma (e45,e58,e80,136,e319). Splenectomies to stage Hodgkin lymphoma, once the most common indication, have become rare as chemotherapy has become the primary modality of therapy. Common causes of splenomegaly are listed in Table 22-11.

Regardless of the indication for splenectomy, all surgically removed spleens should be measured and weighed (e204). After the capsule has been examined for color, irregularities, and tears, the spleen is sliced transversely into thin sections. For the pathologic staging of Hodgkin lymphoma, the sections should be cut as thinly as possible, typically about 3 mm (e154). Sections of abnormal-appearing areas should be taken (typically six to eight sections) in addition to a section of normal-appearing spleen. We routinely order periodic acid–Schiff staining of the section of normal spleen, as this highlights the splenic cords and makes it easier to recognize other hematopoietic elements. If hilar lymph nodes are present, these should be dissected off and processed as a regular fresh lymph node biopsy.

Table 22-11 ■ CAUSES OF SPLENOMEGALY IN CHILDHOOD

Nonspecific infections	
Acute splenitis	Hodgkin lymphoma
Autoimmune disorders	Malaria
Autoimmune hemolytic anemia	Myeloproliferative disorders (CML, JMML, chronic myelofibrosis)
Acute leukemias (AML, ALL)	Niemann-Pick disease
Brucellosis	Non-Hodgkin lymphoma
Cardiac failure	Portal or splenic vein thrombosis
Congestion	Rheumatoid arthritis
Cytomegalovirus infection	Schistosomiasis
Echinococcosis	Sickle cell anemia
Gaucher disease	Storage diseases
Hematologic malignancies	Systemic lupus erythematosus
Hemolytic anemias	Thalassemias
Hepatic cirrhosis	Toxoplasmosis
Hereditary elliptocytosis	Trypanosomiasis
Hereditary spherocytosis	Tuberculosis
Histoplasmosis	Typhoid fever
Other causes	
Vascular tumors (hemangioma, lymphangioma, angiosarcoma)	
Myofibroblastic tumor (inflammatory pseudotumor)	
Metastatic tumors	
Hamartomas	
Cysts	

AML, acute myelogenous leukemia; ALL, acute lymphocytic leukemia; CML, chronic myelogenous leukemia; JMML, juvenile myelomonocytic leukemia.

CONGENITAL ANOMALIES

Asplenia

Asplenia, congenital absence of the spleen, occurs in about 1/40,000 live births (e4). It is more common in boys and is often associated with cardiac anomalies, such as dextrocardia, transposition of the great vessels, and bilateral superior venae cavae, and development defects in other organs, including the liver, lungs, and intestines (e99,e100). Primarily because of these associated defects, the prognosis of patients with congenital asplenia is poor. In one series, nearly 80% of the patients died in infancy of cardiac failure or complications of surgery (e259). Asplenia of any cause is associated with characteristic peripheral blood findings, including Howell-Jolly bodies, Pappenheimer bodies, and dysmorphic and nucleated red blood cells.

Polysplenia

In contrast to asplenia, polysplenia is more common in girls (e259). The multiple small splenic masses are located in the right upper quadrant and are often associated with dextrocardia, a right-sided aortic arch, and pulmonary and hepatic defects (e232). The histology of the splenic tissue is normal. Although less likely to die of cardiopulmonary defects in infancy, patients with polysplenia nonetheless have a high mortality rate. In one series, only 25% of patients were alive at 5 years (e232).

Accessory Spleen

Accessory spleen is the most common congenital anomaly, encountered in about 16% of pediatric splenectomies (e80). Accessory spleens are usually solitary and are most commonly located in the splenic hilum, although they may be found in the omentum, gastrosplenic and splenocolic ligaments, or retroperitoneum (e80,e128,e197,e214). The primary importance of accessory spleens is that they must be removed along with the spleen in therapeutic splenectomies for diseases such as idiopathic thrombocytopenic purpura to prevent recurrence.

Fusion

Most cases of splenic fusion occur in white males, and most often, the spleen is fused with the left testis (e249). Very rare cases of splenorenal or splenohepatic fusion have also been reported (e55,e113).

Hamartoma

Hamartomas of the spleen are uncommon benign tumors located primarily within the red pulp (1). They are usually discovered incidentally after a splenectomy or at autopsy. Most are reported in the adult population, but recent reviews suggest that 20% of reported hamartomas occur in children (1,e85). The lesions are associated with congenital abnormalities such as tuberosis sclerosis. Often patients present with hematologic conditions including refractory microcytic anemia, sickle cell anemia, hereditary spherocytosis, and dyserythropoietic hemolytic anemia.

A recent report of four pediatric patients with splenic hamartomas described children ranging in age from 4 to 11 years, who presented with splenomegaly and hematological abnormalities. In each case, the spleen was enlarged (315 to 724 g). On cut surface, single or multiple discrete bulging nodules ranging from 1.3 to 7 cm were identified. In other studies, the nodules have been reported as large as 15 cm in diameter (e85). Microscopically, the lesions are composed of vascular channels that resemble splenic sinusoids and lack malpighian corpuscles. They are usually associated with histiocytic proliferations, extramedullary hematopoiesis, lymphoplasmacytosis, fibrosis, and siderotic-calcific deposits.

Cysts

Congenital splenic cysts are rare. Hydatid or echinococcal cysts are the most common splenic cysts worldwide but are very rare in the United States. True or primary cysts are lined by epithelium, whereas false cysts or pseudocysts lack a cellular lining and are thought to arise after trauma (e76,e107). Splenic cysts can become quite large (>20 cm) and are typically filled with serous fluid. Although most congenital cysts are asymptomatic, cases of rupture associated with granulomatous peritonitis have been reported (e172).

Diseases of the Red Pulp

Diseases primarily involving the red pulp include congestion, hereditary hemolytic anemias, hemoglobinopathies, infections, histiocytic proliferations, acute and chronic leukemias, and nonhematopoietic (particularly vascular) tumors.

Congestion

Chronic passive congestion of the spleen is commonly the result of portal hypertension or right-sided cardiac failure. The spleen is grossly enlarged, and microscopically the findings are nondescript. The splenic sinuses are distended with red cells, and the capsule and splenic cords may be thickened and fibrotic. Splenic congestion is also common in hereditary hemolytic anemias and hemoglobinopathies, which are discussed in the following sections.

Thrombocytopenia

The spleen is the major site of both antiplatelet antibody production and platelet removal from the bloodstream. Splenectomy is performed in patients with refractory thrombocytopenia when the disorder is refractory to steroid or other immunosuppressive therapy (107). Refractory thrombocytopenia is defined as persistent and severe thrombocytopenia (platelet count $<20 \times 10^9$/L) and the inability of therapies to increase and sustain the platelet count increase. Multiple factors have been identified to lead to refractoriness. These include some cases of drug-induced thrombocytopenia. In addition, infection with HIV, hepatitis C virus, Epstein Barr virus, cytomegalovirus, parvovirus, herpes virus 6 and 8, and Helicobacter are all chronic infections that are associated with refractory thrombocytopenia. In China, acute thrombocytopenia in childhood is often associated with CMV infection (107). Secondary thrombocytopenia can arise from systemic lupus as well as a number of congenital syndromes and abnormalities seen in childhood including common variable immune deficiency, Evans syndrome, autoimmune lymphoproliferative disorder, and paroxysmal nocturnal hemoglobinuria. Splenectomy offers a 60% to 70% chance of cure in patients with chronic ITP.

Surgically removed spleens of patients with thrombocytopenia are usually of normal size or mildly enlarged. Microscopically, the white pulp of spleens from patients with idiopathic thrombocytopenic purpura is usually prominent; numerous reactive follicles are present unless the patient has recently been treated with steroids. The red pulp shows myeloid hyperplasia and increased numbers of foamy histiocytes containing platelets and phospholipid debris (e333).

Hereditary Hemolytic Anemias

Common inherited causes of hemolytic anemia include hereditary spherocytosis and elliptocytosis, and hemoglobinopathies such as the thalassemias and sickle cell anemia. Many of the clinical problems of hereditary hemolytic disorders can be controlled by splenectomy. However the use of splenectomy in a young child exposes the patient to lifelong risk of overwhelming infections and other complication. Vasilescu et al. (136) have proposed and demonstrated that subtotal splenectomy controls the hemolysis and maintains the splenic function. This new model preserves the lower pole of the spleen.

Most patients with hereditary spherocytosis and elliptocytosis have splenomegaly (e163,e177). The erythrocytes in these conditions are inflexible and become trapped as they attempt to pass through the splenic cords. Spleens removed for these diseases typically weigh from 250 to 500 g and are firm and dark red as a result of congestion (e329). Microscopically, the venous sinuses are distended with red cells and are surrounded by hemosiderin-laden macrophages and endothelial cells. Often, the splenic white pulp is hyperplastic, with increased numbers of germinal centers. Patients usually respond well to splenectomy. Refractory cases are most commonly the result of an unrecognized accessory spleen (e268).

Splenomegaly is also present in the majority of young children with sickle cell anemia. In patients more than 10 years old, however, the spleen is usually decreased in size as a result of infarction and scarring (e321). Acute rapid enlargement of the spleen may be the result of a sequestration crisis. Ultimately, the organ undergoes "autosplenectomy," and only a fibrotic remnant is left. Microscopically, early in the course of the disease, the sinusoids are distended with sickled red blood cells, and the splenic cords are thickened and fibrotic; later, the splenic parenchyma is replaced by fibrous scars containing multicolored deposits of minerals and hemosiderin (Gamna-Gandy bodies).

Occasionally, progressive splenomegaly develops in patients with β-thalassemia who have undergone splenectomy, and the spleen may weigh as much as 750 to 1,000 g by adolescence. The histologic findings resemble those of the other hereditary hemolytic anemias, with extramedullary hematopoiesis a particularly common finding.

Infection

Acute splenitis can arise as a result of many blood-borne infections. The spleen typically becomes congested, with infiltration of the red and white pulp by neutrophils and plasma cells. Sometimes, necrotic foci develop. Abscess formation is uncommon. Granulomatous inflammation may be seen in the spleen in disseminated fungal or mycobacterial infections. As previously mentioned, echinococcal infections, although rare in the United States, are the most common cause of splenic cysts worldwide.

Bartonella henselae infection usually results in self-limited lymphadenitis, cat-scratch disease, primarily a disease of children (10,e157,e173,114). Bartonella species are small, intracellular Gram-negative rods. Bacillary infection can also result in an unusual vascular lesion called *bacillary angiomatosis*. Bacillary angiomatosis usually occurs in the skin, bone, and the brain, but a related proliferative lesion called *vascular peliosis* occurs in the liver and the spleen. Bacillary angiomatosis-peliosis was first identified in HIV-infected patients with AIDS. In most children and adolescents with intact immune systems, cat-scratch disease is confined to the lymph nodes. But numerous examples of the systemic manifestation have been reported (10,e157,e173,114).

Splenomegaly is seen in about half of patients with infectious mononucleosis and is occasionally complicated by fatal splenic rupture (e120,e176). Microscopically, the red pulp cords and sinuses are infiltrated by a polymorphic population of T- and B-immunoblasts that may include large multinucleated forms resembling Reed-Sternberg cells (e306). The clinical setting is most helpful in avoiding a misdiagnosis of Hodgkin lymphoma. Immunohistochemically, the immunoblasts in acute EBV infection may be $CD30^+$ but are usually $CD15^-$) and negative for leukocyte common antigen (e1).

DISEASES OF THE WHITE PULP

Histiocytic Proliferations

Splenomegaly is a common feature of a variety of inborn errors of metabolism, including diseases ranging from sphingolipidosis to glucocerebrosidosis. The accumulation of storage histiocytes engorged with storage products within the spleen causes progressive enlargement (e164,e316).

Gaucher disease, which encompasses a spectrum of autosomal recessive disorders that result from glucocerebrosidase deficiency, is the most common metabolic cause of splenomegaly in childhood and the most prevalent lysosomal storage disorder (14). Of the three clinical types, type I (chronic non-neuropathic) is the most common, particularly in individuals of European Jewish descent. Although traditionally referred to as the "adult type," 66% of individuals with type I Gaucher disease presents in childhood as hypersplenism develops (e115,e124,65). In this form of Gaucher disease, macrophages containing glucosylceramide-laden lysosomes accumulate primarily in the bone marrow and spleen without involving the central nervous system. Hepatosplenomegaly is also seen in type II disease (acute neuropathic), but involvement of the central nervous system leads to death in early childhood. The spleen is also involved in type III disease (subacute neuropathic), where neurologic manifestations begin in early adult life.

The basic pathology of classic, type I Gaucher disease, includes hepatosplenomegaly, bone marrow infiltration, hematocytopenia, and bone disease. The disease is progressive and may ultimately lead to bleeding complications, liver and lung fibrosis, pulmonary hypertension, and bone disease (44,76,93). Macrophage-targeted enzyme replacement therapy has been shown to reverse or prevent many of the manifestations of Gaucher disease type I including hepatosplenomegaly, marrow infiltration, and cytopenia.

Microscopic evaluation of the spleen shows that the sinuses are diffusely expanded by clusters and sheet large macrophages. The storage macrophages or Gaucher cells are two to six times the size of a normal macrophage but maintain the cytologically bland, round, oval, vesicular nuclei. There is abundant cytoplasm with a wrinkled or a striated appearance. The cytoplasm stains with both periodic acid-Schiff and iron.

The disease is diagnosed by identifying the enzyme deficiency. The characteristic lysosomal β-glucocerebrosidase activity is decreased or absent in leukocytes. A targeted mutational analysis has identified four mutations (N370S, L44P, 84GG, and IVS2+1) that account for almost 90% of all disease (36). Pseudo-Gaucher cells can be seen in a number of disorders associated with hematopoietic destruction such as chronic myelogenous leukemia. In these cases, the macrophage cytoplasm contains insoluble lipid pigment that stains intensely blue (see Chapter 5).

Niemann-Pick disease is an autosomal recessive deficiency of sphingomyelinase that leads to the accumulation of sphingomyelin within cells and tissues. Niemann-Pick disease is subclassified into two subtypes, A and B, based on phenotypic manifestations (39,91). Type C Niemann-Pick disease shares the eponym but is now recognized to be a genetically distinct disorder resulting from defective intracellular trafficking of cholesterol (e327). Type A (infantile) Niemann-Pick disease accounts for about 80% of cases, and predominantly affects children of Jewish descent. Niemann-Pick disease type A presents as a severe neurodegenerative disease in infancy. Splenomegaly develops as macrophages containing sphingomyelin accumulate in the spleen and other organs. Niemann-Pick disease type B is panethnic and is characterized by hepatosplenomegaly, thrombocytopenia, *interstitial* lung disease, and dyslipidemia. Splenomegaly is the most common presenting manifestation. The spleen becomes significantly enlarged. Splenic volume directly correlates with liver volume and the patient's triglyceride level and inversely correlates with the patients HDL level, their height, hemoglobin concentration, and white cell count. Niemann-Pick cells have finely vacuolated cytoplasm that is yellow-green in hematoxylin and eosin-stained sections and blue-green in Wright-Giemsa-stained smears. The cells are usually positive for period acid–Schiff and lipid stains, such as Sudan black B (performed on air-dried smears or frozen tissue), but negative for iron stains (see Chapter 5).

The GM1 and GM2 gangliosidoses are associated with splenomegaly (e65), although the most marked effects are seen in the central nervous system (e193,e220). The GM2 gangliosidoses represent deficiencies in one of the three enzymes needed to catabolize GM2 gangliosides. The most common of these is Tay-Sachs disease, which is caused by deficiency of hexosaminidase A. The disease is seen relatively frequently in European Jews and begins in infancy; death by age 3 results from progressive dementia and motor deterioration. Microscopically, splenic macrophages are finely vacuolated and stain positively for lipids with oil red O and Sudan black B stains.

Hepatosplenomegaly is a common feature of the mucopolysaccharidoses, particularly Hurler syndrome (MPS I H) and Hunter syndrome (MPS II). The cells most affected in these disorders are macrophages and endothelial and intimal smooth muscle cells, which are distended by transparent vacuoles filled with mucopolysaccharide. These vacuoles stain positively with periodic acid–Schiff and are negative for lipids.

Chediak-Higashi Syndrome

Chediak-Higashi syndrome results in massive hepatosplenomegaly. Chediak-Higashi syndrome is an autosomal recessive disease characterized by oculocutaneous albinisms, bleeding abnormalities, bacterial infections, and neurologic systems. The disease results from the formation of abnormal cells containing giant, abnormal granules due to mutation in the LYST gene. As the disease accelerates, these abnormal lymphohistiocytes are deposited in the liver, spleen, lymph nodes, and bone marrow. The disease is treatable by bone marrow transplant (96).

Langerhans Cell Histiocytosis

Splenic involvement is common in multifocal-multisystemic Langerhans cell histiocytosis. Typically, the spleen is mildly enlarged, and the red pulp is infiltrated by histiocytes with bland cytologic features. The white pulp is spared. Although they are common in other involved organs, multinucleated histiocytes and eosinophils are infrequently seen in the spleen.

Virus-Associated Hemophagocytic Syndrome

Virus (infection)-associated hemophagocytic syndrome (VAHS) is often associated with splenomegaly, and occasionally splenectomy is warranted to relieve the pancytopenia or reduce the risk for rupture. Microscopically, spleens involved by VAHS show numerous erythrophagocytic histiocytes in the red pulp, so that sometimes the possibility of malignant histiocytosis, which is extraordinarily rare, is raised. The histiocytes, however, are cytologically bland and do not form grossly visible tumors.

Leukemia and Myeloproliferative Disorders

The spleen is frequently involved in many reactive and malignant hematopoietic disorders. The spleen is a common site of extramedullary hematopoiesis (102). Extramedullary hematopoiesis is seen in benign reactive conditions and hematologic and nonhematologic malignancies. It is important to distinguish the neoplastic disorders involving the spleen from those reactive conditions discussed above. Acute lymphocytic leukemia and acute myelogenous leukemia may result in splenomegaly. However, splenomegaly is most marked in the myeloproliferative disorders, including chronic myelogenous leukemia and juvenile myelomonocytic leukemia (e135,e196). O'Malley et al. (102) recently evaluated 80 splenectomy specimens to define the involvement of benign and neoplastic disorders. The patients ranged from 2 to 84 years of age. Of the 80 splenectomy samples, 43 were involved with a neoplastic myeloid disorder and 37 with reactive extramedullary hematopoiesis. The age of the patients in the neoplastic group was 4 to 81 years and the age of the reactive group ranged from 2 to 84 years. Only seven patients were within the pediatric age. Of the neoplastic myeloid disorders identified, 67% were chronic myeloproliferative disorders including CML, chronic idiopathic myelofibrosis, and essential thrombocythemia. Another 7% of patients had involvement by myelodysplasia or other myeloproliferative disorder including one patient with juvenile myelomonocytic leukemia and two patients with chronic

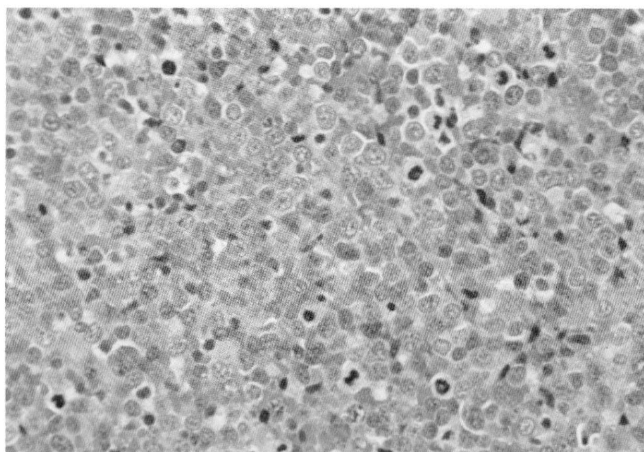

FIGURE 22-27 ■ Immature myeloid and megaloblastic erythroid progenitors effacing red pulp in spleen from a 2-year-old boy with juvenile myelomonocytic leukemia. Rapid splenic enlargement prompted splenectomy. (Hematoxylin and eosin stain, original magnification 20×.)

myelomonocytic leukemia. In addition, there were two other patients with myelodysplasia, nine patients with AML, and two patients with mastocytosis.

Although chronic myeloproliferative disorders such as idiopathic myelofibrosis are rare in children, there are several reports in the literature. One report describes three children, two of whom were siblings that presented at the ages of 9, 10, and 16 months of age with symptoms similar to those of idiopathic myelofibrosis (e181). All three patients progressed rapidly with a fatal course. The occurrence in siblings suggested that this may have a genetic cause.

Splenectomy is performed occasionally to reduce disease burden and pain, particularly in patients with chronic myelogenous leukemia. Microscopically, spleens involved with chronic myelogenous leukemia or juvenile myelomonocytic leukemia appear similar, with sheets of immature and maturing myeloid cells particularly concentrated around the central arteries (Figure 22-27). Erythroid elements may also be present, but megakaryocytes tend to be rare in chronic myelogenous leukemia (e135,e290).

Vascular Tumors

Vascular neoplasms are the most common nonhematopoietic proliferations to involve the spleen. Vascular neoplasms are usually easily distinguished from histocytic proliferations, inflammatory myofibroblastic tumors, and hematomas. Vascular tumors that involve the spleen include hemangiomas, lymphangiomas, littoral cell angiomas, hemangioendotheliomas, angiosarcomas, and myoid angioendotheliomas.

Lymphangiomas and hemangiomas are closely related benign vascular tumors that may involve the spleen, either as a solitary mass or as part of a disseminated disease (e16,e45). Splenic hemangiomas are usually solitary and less than 2 cm in diameter. Although most are asymptomatic, larger hemangiomas are prone to rupture or may result in a consumptive coagulopathy or thrombocytopenia (e285). Microscopically, splenic hemangiomas are composed of masses of dilated, endothelium-lined spaces filled with erythrocytes. By convention, tumors consisting of vessels filled with hypocellular proteinaceous fluid are considered lymphangiomas. In some cases, it is not possible to distinguish a hemangioma from a lymphangioma definitively. Peliosis of the spleen is usually associated with peliosis of the liver (e22,e163). In contrast to the dilated spaces of hemangiomas, the dilated blood-filled spaces in peliosis lack an endothelial lining and are diffusely dispersed throughout the spleen.

Littoral cell angiomas are benign vascular tumors composed of specialized tall endothelial cells that express both endothelial and histiocytic markers. The sinusoidal spaces of littoral cell angiomas are lined by tufts and papillary arrays of littoral cells that project into the lumen. The youngest reported patient was a 3-year-old boy. Other vascular tumors that involve the spleen include epithelioid hemangioendothelioma (e33,e151) and epithelioid and spindle cell hemangioendothelioma (e297).

Myoid angioendothelioma is a distinct vascular entity with features that differ from the other vascular neoplasms (61). This is a benign tumor as originally described as a composite tumor with areas of vascular stasis intermixed with stromal cells with myoid features. In the original description of three patients by Kraus and Dehner, two of the patients were children, 3 and 7 years of age (70). The one remaining patient was a 43-year-old patient. A recent publication describes a 51-year-old man with similar morphology. The reported lesions vary in size but were otherwise histologically quite similar and all were well circumscribed. There were scattered rounded or tubular spaces lined by cytologically bland cells throughout that documented the vascular nature of these lesions. The predominant cell was a large, polygonal-shaped epithelioid cell with abundant eosinophilic cytoplasm and indistinct cell borders. Nuclear configuration ranged from rounded to elongated or twisted and hyperchromatic, and eosinophilic nucleoli were present and occasionally prominent. In many cases, the fibroblastic-rich stroma was interspersed with chronic inflammatory cells.

Angiosarcomas of the spleen are extraordinarily rare in children and do not show the association with exposure to vinyl chloride, arsenic, or Thorotrast established for angiosarcomas involving the liver (e84,e245). Distinction from benign vascular tumors rests primarily on the presence of cytologic atypia and mitoses among the endothelial cells, in addition to an infiltrative pattern of growth. The prognosis is poor (29).

Other Nonhematopoietic Tumors

A variety of mesenchymal tumors or proliferations, including Kaposi sarcoma (e211,e273), mycobacterial spindle cell tumors (e298), and smooth muscle tumors (e74), tend to develop in patients infected with HIV.

Inflammatory myofibroblastic tumor, also known as *inflammatory pseudotumor*, is most common in the lungs or mesentery but also occasionally involves the spleen (e199,e305).

Inflammatory pseudotumors are well-circumscribed gray masses composed microscopically of spindle cells that on immunophenotyping are of myofibroblastic origin (positive for smooth muscle and muscle-specific actin, positive for cytokeratin) (e53). Although inflammatory pseudotumors are usually clinically benign, in rare cases, they may undergo malignant transformation (18). Metastatic tumors to the spleen in children are uncommon. We have seen splenic involvement by neuroblastoma or embryonal carcinoma. Direct invasion of the spleen is occasionally seen in neuroblastoma, hepatoblastoma, or Wilms tumor.

Follicular Hyperplasia

Splenic follicular hyperplasia is common in children and especially prominent in autoimmune diseases, including rheumatoid arthritis (e35), systemic lupus erythematosus (e333), autoimmune hemolytic anemia or idiopathic thrombocytopenic purpura (e28,e302), and HIV infection.

Localized Lymphoid Hyperplasia

In localized lymphoid hyperplasia, proliferations of lymphocytes form solitary nodules that are suspicious for lymphoma (e33). Two forms were originally described by Burke and Osborne (e35). In the first, the nodules are composed of aggregates of reactive germinal centers. In the other form, the aggregates are composed of small lymphocytes, immunoblasts, and plasma cells. The principal features distinguishing lymphoid hyperplasia from non-Hodgkin lymphoma are the polymorphic nature of the infiltrate and the absence of cytologic atypia. In addition, the nodules of localized lymphoid hyperplasia are usually less than 1 cm in diameter and rarely are multiple (e33).

Non-Hodgkin Lymphoma

Splenic involvement by non-Hodgkin lymphoma, although common in adults, is rare in children. Follicular lymphoma is so rare in childhood that the diagnosis should not be made without incontrovertible evidence of clonality. Small noncleaved cell lymphoma involves the spleen early by colonizing germinal centers, and later by diffusely effacing both red and white pulp. Lymphoblastic lymphoma rarely involves the spleen, usually as a diffuse infiltrate. Large cell lymphomas, usually of B-cell origin, involve the spleen as multiple macroscopic nodules (e86). Rare examples of hepatosplenic γ/δ T-cell lymphoma have been reported (e105,69).

Hodgkin Lymphoma

Splenectomies are seldom performed to stage Hodgkin lymphoma, in part because of the widespread use of chemotherapy and the risk for postsplenectomy septicemia (e251,e263,e274). When the spleen is processed (see section on "Examination of the Spleen"), foci of involvement should be sought carefully. These appear as fibrotic, usually well-circumscribed, gray-tan masses (Figure 22-28). The number of foci should be noted because the presence of five or more can denote a worse prognosis (e69,e89). Each nodule should be examined microscopically (a total of six to eight sections) to confirm that it represents Hodgkin lymphoma. The diagnostic criteria for involvement in patients with known Hodgkin lymphoma are the same as in other sites: the presence of diagnostic Reed-Sternberg cells or mononuclear variants in the appropriate cellular background. Early splenic involvement by Hodgkin lymphoma can be subtle, with small numbers of mononuclear variants confined to the periarteriolar lymphatic sheath or germinal center marginal zones. In more advanced involvement, the areas of white pulp become focally confluent and eventually extend into the red pulp, often with associated fibrosis or necrosis. Epithelioid granulomas are seen in about 9% of spleens from patients with Hodgkin lymphoma and do not by themselves signify splenic involvement or a worse prognosis (e148,e269).

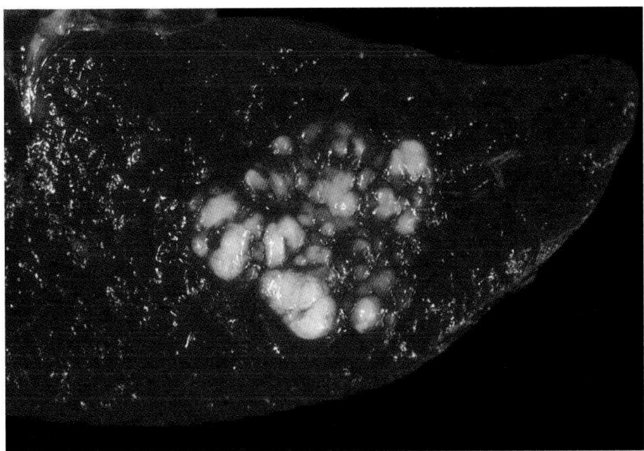

FIGURE 22-28 ■ Focal splenic involvement by Hodgkin lymphoma. The patient was a 9-year-old boy who underwent splenectomy for immune thrombocytopenic purpura. The spleen contains a circumscribed, whitish nodule, 2.1 cm in greatest dimension.

Primary Immunodeficiencies

The etiology and classification of the primary immunodeficiencies are discussed in detail in the section on the "Lymph Nodes." In severe combined immunodeficiency, the spleen is small, with a marked decrease in the number of lymphocytes in both the T- and the B-cell zones of the white pulp (e136,e198). In infantile-linked agammaglobulinemia, the B-cell zones containing B-lymphocytes and plasma cells are nearly absent, and the T-cell zones appear normal (e54,e169). In the spleens of patients with Wiskott-Aldrich syndrome, the white pulp is depleted, with decreased numbers of both T and B lymphocytes, and the thickness of the marginal zone is markedly reduced. These features have been proposed to be the cause of the defective response to T-cell–independent antigens in such patients (137).

THYMUS

The thymus is a lymphoepithelial organ located in the anterior mediastinum. The important role of the thymus in immune regulation was not appreciated until the 1960s, when thymus-dependent cell-mediated immunity was first described (19,e115,e116,e117). In 1965, DiGeorge (e64) described a syndrome in which congenital absence of the thymus is associated with severely impaired cell-mediated immunity. The very important role that the thymus plays in normal T-cell development and immunologic responses has been extensively explored in the subsequent decades.

Embryology

The thymus originates as paired epithelial anlage derived from coordinated outpouchings of the lateral pharyngeal pouches at invaginations of the external pharyngeal clefts (e317). The superior aspect of the third pharyngeal pouch forms the inferior lobes of the parathyroid glands. The inferior aspects of the third pharyngeal pouch and sometimes part of the fourth pharyngeal pouch develop into the thymus. Because the parathyroid glands and the thymus are derived from the same pharyngeal pouch, it is not unusual for the lower lobes of the parathyroid gland to be enmeshed within the thymus. Although they originate in the cervical region, the tubules of the thymic primordium elongate and descend into the superior mediastinum. The thymus passes behind the thyroid gland and the sternocleidomastoid muscle. Not uncommonly, remnants of the thymus remain in the neck and can develop into cysts or thymic tumors (e112,e212). In humans, circulating lymphoid stem cells arising from either the yolk sac or the liver subsequently populate the thymus by the ninth week of gestation. After this point, thymocyte differentiation begins. The organization of the thymus into the cortex and medulla begins around the twelfth gestational week.

Anatomy and Histology

Histologically, the thymus consists of two lobes that form a V-shaped structure extending from the thyroid gland into the anterosuperior mediastinum. The thymic lobes are joined in the midline by connective tissue at a site over the pericardium. The thymus weighs 10 to 35 g at birth and continues to grow to a maximum weight of 20 to 50 g at puberty (e295,e299). Normal thymic involution progresses from puberty through old age. In older adults and the elderly, a thymic weight of 5 to 15 g is finally achieved. Thymic growth and involution vary tremendously between persons, so that the thymic weight at any given age is variable.

Fibrous extensions of the thymic capsule divide the thymus lobes into numerous lobules; however, the lobules are not completely separated because the medullary lymphoid region is continuous throughout the thymus (e299). Each thymic lobule is separated into cortical and medullary regions, and both cortex and medulla are composed of lymphocytes and epithelial cells. In addition to the subspecialized thymic epithelial cells and T-lymphocytes, mononuclear phagocytes, myoid cells, mast cells, eosinophils, plasma cells, and a small population of mature B-cells are present within the normal thymus.

The border between the thymic cortex and medulla is not clearly delineated (e299). The lymphocytes in the cortex are much more closely packed than those in the medulla, so that a darker appearance of the cortex and a lighter, spacious appearance of the medulla are characteristic. As thymic maturation proceeds, the lymphocytes move from the outer cortex toward the medulla, where the thymocytes then enter the peripheral circulation (e202). The cortical thymocytes express markers of immature T-cell differentiation, whereas the medullary thymocytes express antigens representing mature, peripheral T-cells (e112,e202). Epithelial cells are located throughout the cortex and the medulla. The epithelial cells provide much of the stroma and framework for lymphocyte maturation. A number of distinct subtypes of thymic epithelial cells have been described. Some investigators have separated epithelial cells by morphology, with some cells characterized by electron-dense nucleoli and round or elongated spindle-shaped cytoplasmic processes. Others categorize the epithelial cells according to whether or not they express MHC determinants. Although many discrepancies are found in the literature, the epithelial cell component is essential for normal thymic development (e202). Hassall corpuscles are concentric whorls of keratinizing epithelial cells that have undergone cystic degeneration. Their location in the thymic medulla in addition to their function and significance are still unexplained.

Thymic Atrophy

Thymic atrophy occurs as part of normal aging and also in association with severe stress, malnutrition, and drug use (e72) (Table 22-12). Complete thymic agenesis is associated with primary immunodeficiency in a number of congenital defects. Similar defects in the thymus that result in immunodeficiency are seen in patients with AIDS. Accelerated thymic involution was reported in newborns born to mothers who smoked during the prenatal period. The thymic index and the thymic index to weight ratio of newborns from mothers who smoked greater than 1 cigarette per day were significantly lower (142).

Table 22-12 ■ THYMIC LESIONS

Lesion	Etiologic Factor
Atrophy (common finding)	Stress
Cortical lymphocyte	Endogenous or exogenous
Necrosis	Corticosteroids
Depletion→atrophy	Cyclophosphamide
Lymphoid proliferation (rare)	Antigenic stimulation, phytohemagglutinin, thyroxine, hormonal agents
Germinal center induction	As in myasthenia gravis, immunostimulants, antigenic response, hormonal
Epithelial proliferation	Diethylstilbestrol (mice)
Epithelial cysts	Estrogens (rats)

Adapted from Gopinath C. Pathology of toxic effects on the immune system. *Inflamm Res* 1996;45(Suppl 2):74–78, with permission.

Table 22-13 ■ IMMUNODEFICIENCY DISEASES ASSOCIATED WITH THYMIC ABNORMALITIES

	T-cell Areas (Lymphocytes in Paracortex or Germinal Plasma Periarteriolar Sheath)	Germinal Centers	Plasma Cells
DiGeorge syndrome	A	NL	NL
Severe combined immunodeficiency	↓	↓	↓
Autosomal recessive	A	A	A
X-linked	↓-A	↓-A	↓-A
Thymic hypoplasia	↓	↓	↓
Ataxia telangiectasia	↓-A	NL-↓	NL-↓

During normal aging, although the overall size of the thymus does not change dramatically, the cellular composition is markedly altered. The major change in the human thymus during aging is a replacement of the lymphoid cellular elements with adipocytes (e295,e299). Complete lymphoid atrophy is the most evident age-related change and represents the final state of involution. In the newborn infant, little adipose tissue surrounds the capsule or the septa. However, during aging, the perivascular spaces and the area surrounding the capsule and fibrous septa are gradually replaced by adipose tissue. At the same time, the number of lymphocytes progressively decreases, as described by Steinman (e295). The number of lymphocytes gradually diminishes until in the older person few remain. At this point, the cortical-medullary junction is poorly discriminated. A few TdT+ lymphocytes can be identified in elderly persons.

Acquired hypoplasia results from rapid involution in young patients during severe stress, malnutrition, or irradiation, or following the administration of cytotoxic agents (e277). The morphologic changes seen in the thymus are similar following a number of stressors. Experimental studies in animals have demonstrated that corticosteroid injection or the administration of radiation results in acute thymic involution immediately following the insult (e277). The lymphocytes undergo rapid karyorrhexis, and the cortex is infiltrated with macrophages and presents a "starry sky" appearance. The cellular destruction observed in experimental conditions also occurs in children after a number of acute insults that cause thymic atrophy, including malnutrition and the administration of corticotropin or radiation. Surprisingly, the Hassall corpuscles usually remain and become multicystic large structures within the medulla.

Thymic hypoplasia is associated with primary or secondary immunodeficiency. Primary immune deficiency disorders are a group of complex diseases characterized by abnormalities in the development and maturation of the immune system. Significant advances in understanding the defects underlying many subtypes of primary immunodeficiency have identified specific blocks in the normal schema of lymphoid maturation have been identified (e260). Each block in lymphoid maturation results in a distinct immunodeficiency state. The advances in the field have recently been reviewed by Rosen et al. (e260,e261) and Perez-Atayde and Rosen (e233). The Rosen classification provides the diagnostic pathologist with a readily usable system for evaluating the spleen, lymph nodes, and thymus of a child with a suspected or confirmed immunodeficiency state (e166,e233,e260,e261). The outline encompasses immunologic defects resulting from combined immunodeficiencies (i.e., deficiencies of both B-cells and T-cells), primary antibody (B-cell) deficiency, or primary T-cell deficiency. Disorders resulting in a primary T-cell deficiency are caused either by a defect in primary thymic maturation or by secondary thymic abnormalities associated with altered T-cell development. The primary immunodeficiencies that affect thymocyte maturation include DiGeorge syndrome, reticular dysgenesis, combined immunodeficiency disease, and ataxia-telangiectasia (Table 22-13).

DiGeorge anomaly was first identified as thymic agenesis associated with abnormalities of T-cell maturation (e64). DiGeorge syndrome results from a failure of the normal development of the third and fourth branchial arches, which results in abnormalities in multiple organs during the fourth to sixth weeks of embryogenesis. The major defects include aplasia or hypoplasia of the thymus and parathyroid glands, type I truncus arteriosis, and dysmorphic facies with micrognathia. Other associated conditions include esophageal atresia, thyroid aplasia/hypoplasia, absence of calcitonin-containing cells of the thyroid, and endocardial cushion defects. Although a few familial cases have been reported, the defect appears not to be hereditary but to result from an unknown defect occurring *in utero* during the first trimester of pregnancy.

In cases of "complete" DiGeorge syndrome, both the thymus and the parathyroid glands are completely absent. Most patients manifest a "partial" or "incomplete" DiGeorge syndrome, in which the thymus is hypoplastic and otherwise histologically normal. The degree of thymocyte hypoplasia is variable, but in most instances, thymic lobation is normal, corticomedullary differentiation is detected, and Hassall corpuscles are present. Although not all the genetic defects are defined, many patients have either partial monosomy or a deletion of chromosome 10q11 (e59,e62,e261,e276,e332). Recent progress has been made in treating the athymia by thymus transplantation (87). Markert et al. (87,88) report that transplantation of cultured postnatal thymus successfully restored many of the immune abnormalities in patients with complete DiGeorge syndrome.

Severe combined immunodeficiency diseases are represented by several distinctive disorders with similar clinical manifestations and distinct genetic bases. These include the lymphoid stem cell type (Swiss type) with autosomal recessive or X-linked modes of inheritance. Infants with severe combined immunodeficiency disease usually present by 3 months of age with thrush, monilial rashes, intractable diarrhea, and *Pneumocystis jiroveci* pneumonia. In some neonates, the symptoms are similar to those of graft-versus-host disease. Death results from overwhelming infection with herpesvirus, adenovirus, and cytomegalovirus. Hecht giant cell pneumonia, resulting from measles infection or live measles or smallpox vaccination, is lethal to the immunocompromised host. Laboratory evaluation of infants with severe combined immunodeficiency disease reveals a marked lymphopenia (<1,000 lymphocytes per cubic millimeter). In the X-linked form, the number of B-cells is normal, but the B-cells fail to mature properly. T-cells are rare and of maternal origin. One genetic defect responsible for X-linked severe combined immunodeficiency disease is a mutation of the gene coding for the γ chain of interleukin (IL) receptor, mapped to Xq13. The γ chain is a component of several IL receptors, including IL-4, IL-7, IL-11, and IL-16. Normal lymphocyte progenitors fail to differentiate because of a lack of appropriate growth factor stimulation. Other types of severe combined deficiency are recessive in inheritance. The most common enzyme defects that result in immunodeficiency are of enzymes in the purine degradation pathway. The accumulation of toxic metabolites in adenosine deaminase deficiency and purine nucleoside phosphorylase deficiency results in lymphocyte defects (e108,e136,e138,e139,e184,e198). The symptomatology is essentially identical to that in children with AIDS.

The difference in the lymphoid tissue among the various types of severe combined immunodeficiency disease is minimal. The lymphocytes are generally depleted in all lymphoid tissues, including the thymus, spleen, lymph nodes, tonsils, adenoids, and mucosa-associated lymphoid tissue. The thymus is small and dysplastic. A variable number of T-cells at the corticomedullary junction and scattered Hassall corpuscles are found early in most cases. Because of progressive lymphoid depletion, the thymic epithelium becomes prominent and may appear disorganized or acquire an organoid and pseudoglandular architecture (e233). The morphology of the thymus in other well-characterized immunodeficiencies, including ataxia-telangiectasia, Wiscott-Aldrich syndrome, and chronic mucocutaneous candidiasis, is variable. The thymus histology can be normal or show slight lymphocytic depletion or complete atrophy.

The Thymus in AIDS

Changes in the thymus in patients with AIDS have been controversial. In a report of 11 infants with AIDS, Joshi (e146) described histologic changes similar to those in patients subjected to severe stress. The thymus was located in the correct anatomic site and the lobation and blood vessels were normal, but the size, weight, and number of lymphocytes were reduced. In some cases, more severe abnormalities were noted, including complete involution or inflammatory changes. Animal studies suggest that transmission of the virus early in fetal development results in more severe immune destruction. A recent study demonstrated that HIV infection results in a high rate of spontaneous abortions, and that the thymus in spontaneously aborted fetuses demonstrates severe abnormalities of lymphocytic differentiation and corticomedullary demarcation and an absence of Hassall corpuscles (e146). The more severe thymic abnormalities develop earlier in gestation.

Thymic Tumors

The majority of tumors that occur in the mediastinum of children are lymphomas (41%) or tumors of neurogenic origin. True thymic lesions including cysts, thymolipomas, thymic hyperplasia, and thymic tumors represent approximately 2.5% of all mediastinal masses in children (13). Hyperplasia of the thymus is the most common anterior mediastinal mass found in infants. Histologically, two types of thymic hyperplasia are recognized. True thymic hyperplasia is characterized by increases in both the size and the depth of the gland with retention of the normal microscopic appearance. In the second type, lymphoid hyperplasia, reactive lymphoid follicles appear within the thymus (e293). The reactive germinal centers are identical to those seen in normal lymph nodes. Follicular hyperplasia of the thymus can occur *de novo* or in association with autoimmune diseases and chronic inflammatory states, most commonly myasthenia gravis. Approximately 70% to 80% of patients with myasthenia gravis have follicular hyperplasia of the thymus. Although myasthenia is usually a disease of older persons, Somnier (e293) identified a bimodal male and female age distribution. The incidence of early-onset myasthenia gravis peaked at 21 to 30 years, but persons as young as 5 to 10 years of age were affected. The peak for early-onset disease was approximately 10 years later in males than in females. Other autoimmune diseases, including Graves disease, Addison disease, systemic lupus erythematosus, scleroderma, and rheumatoid arthritis, are associated with thymic hyperplasia.

True thymic hypertrophy, enlargement of the thymus, has been reported in neonates and children up to 14 years of age. In most cases, an enlarged thymus is an incidental finding. In other cases, the mediastinal enlargement causes respiratory or gastrointestinal symptoms (e293). In some cases, the hypertrophy represents regeneration following stress. The thymus in cases of hypertrophy is normal, with a normal cortical-medullary junction and Hassall corpuscles. The diagnosis is based on the weight of the thymus at resection. Because the thymic weight varies widely, the thymus must weigh more than approximately 100 g to be considered hypertrophic.

Neoplastic Proliferation of the Thymus

Thymic tumors account for only 1.5% of all mediastinal masses in children and include thymomas, thymic carcinomas, and thymic carcinoids (13). Lymphomas are neoplastic proliferations of the lymphoid cells within the thymus and will be discussed separately. Thymomas are neoplastic proliferations of the thymic epithelium. Although thymomas are the most common primary neoplasms of the anterior mediastinum, they are the least frequent mediastinal tumors in children. Fewer than 2% of all thymomas are diagnosed in the first two decades of life. Small series of childhood cases occurring between 9 months and 15 years of life have been reported in the literature (13,63,103,113,115). Myasthenia gravis and other autoimmune disorders occur in 30% of adults with thymoma but are less frequent in children.

Morphologically, although thymomas are composed of neoplastic epithelial cells and lymphocytes, there is great morphologic heterogeneity. The role of histology in prognosis has been hotly debated. The WHO in 1999 defined the histologic criteria for distinct subtypes of thymic epithelial tumors (13,63,103,113,115). Thymic neoplasms are now subdivided into five entities: Type A, AB, B1, B2, and B3 thymomas. The classification is still based on the extent of lymphocytic infiltration. It is important to recognize the possibility of a thymoma because the lymphocytes express the antigens of immature thymocytes. These normal thymocytes can easily be confused with the malignant lymphoblasts of lymphoblastic lymphoma. A variety of distinct cellular features may be seen within the typical thymoma, including thymic cysts that may form papillary structures, germinal centers, squamous differentiation, and keratin pearls (52). As would be expected, the typical epithelial component of a thymoma expresses epithelium-associated antigens, including cytokeratin and EMA. The lymphocytes in a typical thymoma express the markers of normal cortical thymocytes, medullary thymocytes, or mixtures. Immature thymocytes express CD1, CD2, CD5, and CD7, coexpress CD4 and CD8, and express TdT.

Type C thymoma is considered thymic carcinoma. Thymic carcinomas represent 5% to 15% of all thymic neoplasms. In contrast to benign thymoma, thymic carcinoma shows cytologically malignant epithelial cells with nuclear prominence, increased mitotic activity, and areas of necrosis. Thymic carcinomas can present with squamous cell, basaloid, adenosquamous, small cell, clear cell, sarcomatoid, and anaplastic large cell features. Significant numbers of immature intraepithelial thymocytes are lacking. Type C thymoma is usually indistinguishable from a carcinoma observed elsewhere. These malignant lesions are more likely to invade and metastasize.

Malignant thymoma is very rare in children. In a current literature review by Yaris et al. only 14 cases of thymic carcinoma in patients younger than 18 years old were reported. In this series of children, the median age was 13 years and there was a male predominance. Although myasthenia gravis is frequently associated with benign thymoma, myasthenia gravis and other paraneoplastic disorders are rarely associated with thymic carcinomas (62,141). Dehner et al. reported that the mortality for children with thymoma is much higher than that for adults (e62). In this series, only 3 of 11 children survived for 6 months after diagnosis.

A number of the diseases associated with thymomas are similar to those associated with thymic hyperplasia, and they resolve following removal of the mass. Both thymic hyperplasia and thymomas are associated with numerous autoimmune diseases: myasthenia gravis, hypogammaglobulinemia, polymyositis, systemic lupus erythematosus, Hashimoto thyroiditis, and a variety of cytopenias, including pure red cell aplasia (e155,e293). A recent study reports the case of a 7-year-old child with a thymoma. The child presented with facial muscle weakness without ophthalmoplegia or ptosis. The patient had a benign thymoma. Following thymic resection, the patient became asymptomatic (23). Of the patients reported by Dehner et al. three presented with signs of superior vena cava syndrome (e62). Thymomas outside the thorax are seen in children when metastasis to the lungs, bone, liver, and lymph nodes has occurred.

Malignant Lymphomas

Hodgkin and non-Hodgkin lymphomas account for approximately one third of all childhood cancers, and lymphomas are the third most common group of cancers in children. Non-Hodgkin lymphomas represent 60% of the lymphomas of childhood, and Hodgkin lymphoma represents 40%. The classification of non-Hodgkin lymphomas and Hodgkin lymphoma has been discussed earlier in the section. Of all the tumors that occur in the mediastinum, malignant lymphoma, both Hodgkin and non-Hodgkin lymphoma, represent the second most common malignancy.

The classification system of non-Hodgkin lymphomas was developed primarily for adults. Only a relative few subtypes of non-Hodgkin lymphomas occur in childhood. In contrast to adult cases non-Hodgkin lymphoma, approximately 50% of childhood cases of non-Hodgkin lymphoma are of T-cell origin (e170). Low-grade and intermediate-grade lymphomas are rare in children. The high-grade lymphomas, small noncleaved cell lymphoma (Burkitt), and lymphoblastic lymphoma account for 70% to 80% of all non-Hodgkin lymphoma in children. Extranodal presentation of non-Hodgkin lymphoma in sites such as the mediastinum, gastrointestinal tract, and head and neck is much more common in children than in adults. Small noncleaved cell lymphoma in North America commonly presents in the abdomen. Lymphoblastic lymphoma most commonly arises within thymic remnants and presents with mediastinal involvement. Patients with mediastinal lymphomas usually present with signs of mediastinal compression—cough, chest pain, dysphagia, dyspnea, and superior vena cava syndrome.

Hodgkin Lymphoma

Hodgkin lymphoma involves the mediastinum in approximately 50% to 70% of patients younger than 40 years. Patients typically present with peripheral lymphadenopathy, mainly in the cervical region, and enlargement of the mediastinal lymph nodes. The lymphadenopathy is associated

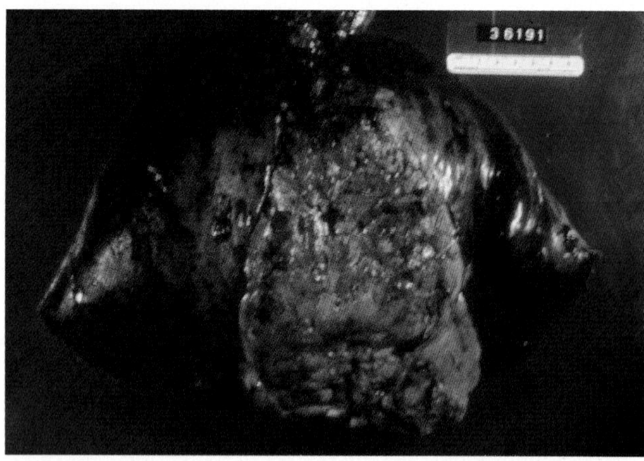

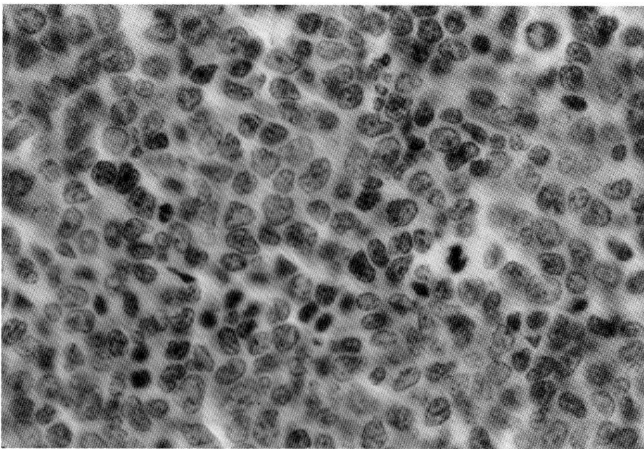

A B

FIGURE 22-29■ Lymphoblastic lymphoma results in massive enlargement of the thymus. **A, B:** Lymphoblastic lymphoma effaces the normal thymic architecture with sheets of uniform malignant lymphoid small-to-medium sized lymphocytes with very scant cytoplasm, irregular, convoluted, and inconspicuous nuclei. (Hematoxylin and eosin stain, original magnification 40×.)

with systemic symptoms, including fever, night sweats, and weight loss, in 25% to 30% of patients. Extreme mediastinal involvement, which is defined as enlargement of the mediastinum to more than one third of the diameter of the chest, is an adverse prognostic factor.

The classification scheme and the pathology of Hodgkin lymphoma have been discussed in detail in the section on "Lymph Nodes." In the United States, most cases of Hodgkin lymphoma in children are of the nodular sclerosis or mixed-cellularity types. The morphology of the mediastinum is that typical of nodular sclerosis Hodgkin lymphoma, in which the lymph nodes and the thymus are replaced by dense collagen bands that divide the tumor into discrete nodules. The typical cellular milieu of lymphocytes, plasma cells, eosinophils, classic or diagnostic Hodgkin cells, and Reed-Sternberg cells are identified. In many patients with Hodgkin lymphoma, it is unnecessary to obtain a biopsy specimen from the mediastinum because the disease spreads to contiguous lymph nodes. Often, a node can be identified in the cervical or the supraclavicular area that is easier to sample.

If mediastinal specimens are obtained, the diagnosis may be difficult. In many cases, dense fibrous and collagenous bands are infiltrated by lymphocytes. The identification of the cellular component of Hodgkin lymphoma may be difficult, and Reed-Sternberg cells must be identified for a diagnosis to be made. In some cases, immunohistochemistry may aid in the identification of the diagnostic Reed-Sternberg cells. In nodular sclerosis Hodgkin lymphoma, the Hodgkin cells typically react with antibodies against CD15 and CD30, and they fail to express CD45, the leukocyte common antigen, or CD20 or CD3, markers of B cells and T cells, respectively.

Lymphoblastic Lymphoma

The other primary malignant lymphoma involving the mediastinum is lymphoblastic lymphoma. Lymphoblastic lymphoma presents as a distinct clinicopathologic disorder and accounts for approximately 30% of non-Hodgkin lymphomas in childhood (e272). Among all the non-Hodgkin lymphomas of childhood, the mediastinum is involved in 26% of cases (Figure 22-29). The vast majority of these are lymphoblastic lymphomas. The classification schemes for non-Hodgkin lymphoma have undergone multiple revisions during the last several decades. The Revised European-American Classification of Lymphoma has generated a significant controversy in addition to identifying a number of new subtypes of lymphomas (e61,e131,e262). Although the revision has dramatically affected the subclassifications of non-Hodgkin lymphomas in adults, its effect on the diagnosis of lymphoblastic lymphoma in children and adults has been minimal. What was formerly known as lymphoblastic lymphoma is now categorized in the Revised European-American Classification as precursor T-lymphoblastic lymphoma/leukemia (e131). Lymphoblastic lymphoma presents with a typical clinical picture, including a large mediastinal mass (50% to 70% of cases) that causes symptoms associated with chest compression and cervical or axillary lymphadenopathy. Although the largest percentage of cases of lymphoblastic lymphoma occur in children, a bimodal age distribution has been identified, with the first peak at 16 years of age and the second at more than 40 years of age. A marked male predisposition has been noted, with a male-to-female ratio of 2.5:1.

Histologically, lymphoblastic lymphoma demonstrates diffuse effacement of the lymph nodes or thymus. The cells of lymphoblastic lymphoma are uniform in size and range from about 10 to 14 μm (about the size of a histiocyte nucleus). The cells have very scant cytoplasm, so that they often give the impression of having "bare" nuclei. The nuclei are small and inconspicuous. Mitoses are frequent. Folds or indentations in the nucleus produce convolutions that, despite the designation of "small convoluted cell lymphoma," are seen in only 50% of cases in the larger series. A particular tumor may be composed predominantly of convoluted cells, a mixture of convoluted and nonconvoluted cells, or exclusively of nonconvoluted cells. Nuclear convolutions are best appreciated in the smaller lymphocytes. Because studies comparing the convoluted and nonconvoluted subtypes show no clinically significant differences (e206), we do not attempt to distinguish between these subtypes.

As noted, about 80% to 90% of cases of lymphoblastic lymphoma are of T-cell lineage and commonly express the pan T-cell markers CD1a, CD2, CD3 (cytoplasmic), CD7, and CD43 (e246). T-cell lymphoblastic lymphomas most commonly express CD1a and both CD4 and CD8 or neither CD4 nor CD8, corresponding to stage II of thymocyte maturation. Less commonly, they lack CD1 expression and express either CD4 or CD8, corresponding to stage III of thymocyte maturation (e24,e256). In contrast, most cases of T-cell acute lymphoblastic leukemia correspond to stage I of thymocyte maturation (negative for CD4, CD8, and CD1) (e24,e256). Importantly, almost all cases of lymphoblastic lymphoma express TdT (e29), which can be detected immunohistochemically on air-dried imprints, frozen tissue, or paraffin-embedded tissue (e270). TdT can also be detected on permeabilized cells by flow cytometry (e127,e289,e300). Thus, expression of T-cell markers and TdT lends very strong support to a diagnosis of T-cell lymphoblastic lymphoma in association with blastic histology. One important caveat is that thymomas, which are rare in children and young adults, often contain lymphocytes that are indistinguishable on the basis of immunophenotype from those of lymphoblastic lymphoma (e264). The less common B-lineage lymphoblastic lymphomas typically express TdT, CD19, and CD10 without expression of surface immunoglobulin and with or without expression of CD20, an immunophenotype similar to that of precursor B-cell acute lymphoblastic leukemia (e237,e325).

With improved chemotherapy and aggressive management, the long-term survival of patients with lymphoblastic lymphoma overall is reported to be from 65% to 75% (e308). The biology of lymphoblastic lymphoma overlaps with that of acute lymphoblastic leukemia of T-cell origin. T-cell acute lymphoblastic leukemia and T-cell lymphoblastic lymphoma often express the same antigens and present with the same clinical features. Based on arbitrary criteria, lymphoblastic lymphoma and acute lymphoblastic leukemia are distinguished according to the percentage of lymphoblasts in the bone marrow (e27,e132). Cases of lymphoblastic lymphoma in which lymphoblasts comprise more than 25% of the bone marrow are subclassified as acute lymphoblastic leukemia. Not surprisingly, acute lymphoblastic lymphoma and acute lymphoblastic leukemia demonstrate the same molecular genetic abnormalities.

Large Cell Lymphoma

Mediastinal large cell lymphoma occurs relatively infrequently in children. Large cell lymphomas of the mediastinum also display a typical immunophenotype and clinical-morphologic spectrum. The majority of the patients are young women; the age range is 10 to 63 years, but the median is approximately 30 to 40 years (e236,e238). Mediastinal large cell lymphomas, which are almost always of B-cell origin, appear to arise within the thymus (e236,e238). The symptomatology at presentation is similar to that of a lymphoblastic lymphoma, with evidence of a mass in the anterior mediastinum.

The histopathology of mediastinal large cell lymphoma is the same as that of diffuse large cell lymphoma. Large cells have moderate-to-abundant amounts of pale to clear cytoplasm and vesicular nuclei with distinct to prominent nucleoli. Occasionally, immunoblastic or anaplastic morphology is seen. In addition, mediastinal large cell lymphoma frequently demonstrates compartmentalization, in which nodules of large cells are surrounded by fibrous septa. Mediastinal large cell lymphomas must be distinguished from seminomas (positive for placental alkaline phosphatase, negative for leukocyte common antigen), thymic carcinoma (positive for keratin, negative for leukocyte common antigen), anaplastic large cell lymphoma, and Hodgkin lymphoma, in particular the syncytial variant of nodular sclerosis Hodgkin lymphoma (positive for Reed-Sternberg cells, Ki-1, and Leu-M1; negative for leukocyte common antigen; usually negative for other B-cell markers).

Surprisingly, although T-cells are predominantly identified in the thymus, mediastinal large cell lymphoma typically involves mature B-cells. Large cell lymphomas within the mediastinum are classically positive for the CD19 and CD20 antigens. Mediastinal large cell lymphoma of T-cell origin is extremely rare.

Anaplastic large cell lymphoma represents another subtype of large cell lymphoma that occurs in children. ALCL accounts for 10% to 15% of childhood non-Hodgkin lymphomas. The diagnosis is based on proliferation of large pleomorphic cells of a T-cell phenotype that invade into the lymph node sinuses. As elsewhere, ALCLs usually exhibit t(2;5) translocation. Primary ALCL involves lymph nodes and extranodal sites including the skin, bone, soft tissue, lung, and liver. Mediastinal involvement is not very common. In a recent review of 225 children treated for anaplastic large cell lymphoma mediastinal involvement, as well as B symptoms, skin lesions, visceral involvement, St. Jude stage 3 to 4, and Ann Arbor stage 3 to 4, elevated lactate dehydrogenase correlated with the risk of progression and relapse (78). The overall 5-year progression-free survival rate of 81 patients with no risk factors was 89%. Progression for survival of patients with a risk factor was 61%. Therefore, the identification of mediastinal involvement in anaplastic large cell lymphoma is important for long-term prognosis.

REFERENCES

1. Abramowsky C, Alvarado C, Wyly JB, et al. "Hamartoma" of the spleen (splenoma) in children. *Pediatr Dev Pathol* 2004;7(3): 231–236.
2. Albright JT, Pransky SM. Nontuberculous mycobacterial infections of the head and neck. *Pediatr Clin North Am* 2003;50(2):503–514.
3. Ambati S, Chamyan G, Restrepo R, et al. Rosai-Dorfman disease following bone marrow transplantation for pre-B cell acute lymphoblastic leukemia. *Pediatr Blood Cancer* 2008;51(3):433–435.

4. Anagnostopoulos I, Hansmann ML, Franssila K, et al. European Task Force on Lymphoma project on lymphocyte predominance Hodgkin disease: histologic and immunohistologic analysis of submitted cases reveals 2 types of Hodgkin disease with a nodular growth pattern and abundant lymphocytes. *Blood* 2000;96(5): 1889–1899.
5. Anagnostopoulos I, Hummel M, Falini B, et al. Epstein-Barr virus infection of monocytoid B-cell proliferates: an early feature of primary viral infection? *Am J Surg Pathol* 2005;29(5):595–601.
6. Antillon F, Behm FG, Raimondi SC, et al. Pediatric primary diffuse large cell lymphoma of bone with t(3;22)(q27;q11). *J Pediatr Hematol Oncol* 1998;20(6):552–555.
7. Baek CH, Kim SI, Ko YH, et al. Polymerase chain reaction detection of Mycobacterium tuberculosis from fine-needle aspirate for the diagnosis of cervical tuberculous lymphadenitis. *Laryngoscope* 2000;110(1):30–34.
8. Belec L, Mohamed AS, Authier FJ, et al. Human herpesvirus 8 infection in patients with POEMS syndrome-associated multicentric Castleman's disease. *Blood* 1999;93(11):3643–3653.
9. Bernacer-Borja M, Blanco-Rodriguez M, Sanchez-Granados JM, et al. Sinus histiocytosis with massive lymphadenopathy (Rosai-Dorfman disease): clinico-pathological study of three cases. *Eur J Pediatr* 2006;165(8):536–539.
10. Bonatti H, Mendez J, Guerrero I, et al. Disseminated Bartonella infection following liver transplantation. *Transpl Int* 2006;19(8):683–687.
11. Bruijnesteijn Van Coppenraet ES, Lindeboom JA, Prins JM, et al. Real-time PCR assay using fine-needle aspirates and tissue biopsy specimens for rapid diagnosis of mycobacterial lymphadenitis in children. *J Clin Microbiol* 2004;42(6):2644–2650.
12. Buno I, Nava P, Alvarez-Doval A, et al. Lymphoma associated chromosomal abnormalities can easily be detected by FISH on tissue imprints: an underused diagnostic alternative. *J Clin Pathol* 2005;58(6):629–633.
13. Chen G, Marx A, Wen-Hu C, et al. New WHO histologic classification predicts prognosis of thymic epithelial tumors: a clinicopathologic study of 200 thymoma cases from China. *Cancer* 2002;95(2):420–429.
14. Chen M, Wang J. Gaucher disease: review of the literature. *Arch Pathol Lab Med* 2008;132(5):851–853.
15. Cheng AG, Chang A, Farwell DG, et al. Auramine orange stain with fluorescence microscopy is a rapid and sensitive technique for the detection of cervical lymphadenitis due to mycobacterial infection using fine needle aspiration cytology: a case series. *Otolaryngol Head Neck Surg* 2005;133(3):381–385.
16. Chikwava K, Jaffe R. Langerin (CD207) staining in normal pediatric tissues, reactive lymph nodes, and childhood histiocytic disorders. *Pediatr Dev Pathol* 2004;7(6):607–614.
17. Claviez A, Tiemann M, Luders H, et al. Impact of latent Epstein-Barr virus infection on outcome in children and adolescents with Hodgkin's lymphoma. *J Clin Oncol* 2005;23(18):4048–4056.
18. Coffin CM, Humphrey PA, Dehner LP. Extrapulmonary inflammatory myofibroblastic tumor: a clinical and pathological survey. *Semin Diagn Pathol* 1998;15(2):85–101.
19. Cook JR. Paraffin section interphase fluorescence in situ hybridization in the diagnosis and classification of non-hodgkin lymphomas. *Diagn Mol Pathol* 2004;13(4):197–206.
20. Corapcioglu F, Basar EZ, Demirel A, et al. Granulomatous reaction in mediastinal B-cell non-Hodgkin lymphoma and intracardiac thrombosis. *Pediatr Hematol Oncol* 2008;25(3):217–226.
21. Corpechot C, Lemann M, Brocheriou I, et al. Granulocytic sarcoma of the jejunum: a rare cause of small bowel obstruction. *Am J Gastroenterol* 1998;93(12):2586–2588.
22. Cossman J, Annunziata CM, Barash S, et al. Reed-Sternberg cell genome expression supports a B-cell lineage. *Blood* 1999;94(2): 411–416.
23. Coulter D, Gold S. Thymoma in the offspring of a patient with Isaacs syndrome. *J Pediatr Hematol Oncol* 2007;29(11):797–798.
24. Coventry S, Punnett HH, Tomczak EZ, et al. Consistency of isochromosome 7q and trisomy 8 in hepatosplenic gammadelta T-cell lymphoma: detection by fluorescence In situ hybridization of a splenic touch-preparation from a pediatric patient. *Pediatr Dev Pathol* 1999;2(5):478–483.
25. Das DK, Gulati A, Bhatt NC, et al. Sinus histiocytosis with massive lymphadenopathy (Rosai-Dorfman disease): report of two cases with fine-needle aspiration cytology. *Diagn Cytopathol* 2001;24(1):42–45.
26. De Petris G, Lev R, Siew S. Peritumoral and nodal muciphages. *Am J Surg Pathol* 1998;22(5):545–549.
27. Dehner LP, Hill DA, Deschryver K. Pathology of the breast in children, adolescents, and young adults. *Semin Diagn Pathol* 1999;16(3):235–247.
28. Delsol G, Ralfkiaer E, Stein H, et al. Anaplastic large cell lymphoma. In: Jaffe ES, Harris NL, Stein H, Vardiman JWE, eds. *World Health Organization classification of tumours pathology and genetics*. IRAC Press: Lyon, 2001:230–236.
29. den Hoed ID, Granzen B, Granzen B, et al. Metastasized angiosarcoma of the spleen in a 2-year-old girl. *Pediatr Hematol Oncol* 2005;22(5):387–390.
30. Deshpande AH, Nayak S, Munshi MM. Cytology of sinus histiocytosis with massive lymphadenopathy (Rosai-Dorfman disease). *Diagn Cytopathol* 2000;22(3):181–185.
31. Dierberg KL, Dumler JS. Lymph node hemophagocytosis in rickettsial diseases: a pathogenetic role for CD8 T lymphocytes in human monocytic ehrlichiosis (HME)? *BMC Infect Dis* 2006;6:121.
32. Dunphy CH, Applications of flow cytometry and immunohistochemistry to diagnostic hematopathology. *Arch Pathol Lab Med* 2004;128(9):1004–1022.
33. Dupin N, Diss TL, Kellam P, et al. HHV-8 is associated with a plasmablastic variant of Castleman disease that is linked to HHV-8-positive plasmablastic lymphoma. *Blood* 2000;95(4): 1406–1412.
34. Eapen M, Mathew CF, Aravindan KP. Evidence based criteria for the histopathological diagnosis of toxoplasmic lymphadenopathy. *J Clin Pathol* 2005;58(11):1143–1146.
35. Edelweiss M, Medeiros LJ, Suster S, et al. Lymph node involvement by Langerhans cell histiocytosis: a clinicopathologic and immunohistochemical study of 20 cases. *Hum Pathol* 2007;38(10): 1463–1469.
36. Elstein D, Abrahamov A, Dweck A, et al. Gaucher disease: pediatric concerns. *Paediatr Drugs* 2002;4(7):417–426.
37. Favara BE, Jaffe R, Egeler RM. Macrophage activation and hemophagocytic syndrome in langerhans cell histiocytosis: report of 30 cases. *Pediatr Dev Pathol* 2002;5(2):130–140.
38. Filipovich AH. Hemophagocytic lymphohistiocytosis and related disorders. *Curr Opin Allergy Clin Immunol* 2006;6(6):410–415.
39. Garver WS, Francis GA, Jelinek D, et al. The National Niemann-Pick C1 disease database: report of clinical features and health problems. *Am J Med Genet A* 2007;143A(11):1204–1211.
40. Geissmann F, Dieu-Nosjean MC, Dezutter C, et al. Accumulation of immature Langerhans cells in human lymph nodes draining chronically inflamed skin. *J Exp Med* 2002;196(4):417–430.
41. Gerritsen A, Lam K, Marion Schneider E, et al. An exclusive case of juvenile myelomonocytic leukemia in association with Kikuchi's disease and hemophagocytic lymphohistiocytosis and a review of the literature. *Leuk Res* 2006;30(10):1299–1303.
42. Gheorghe G, Albano EA, Porter CC, et al. Posttransplant Hodgkin lymphoma preceded by polymorphic posttransplant lymphoproliferative disorder: report of a pediatric case and review of the literature. *J Pediatr Hematol Oncol* 2007;29(2):112–116.
43. Goldsby RE, Carroll WL. The molecular biology of pediatric lymphomas. *J Pediatr Hematol Oncol* 1998;20(4):282–296.
44. Grabowski GA, Andria G, Baldellou A, et al. Pediatric non-neuronopathic Gaucher disease: presentation, diagnosis and assessment. Consensus statements. *Eur J Pediatr* 2004;163(2):58–66.

45. Green E, McConville CM, Powell JE, et al. Clonal diversity of Ig and T-cell-receptor gene rearrangements identifies a subset of childhood B-precursor acute lymphoblastic leukemia with increased risk of relapse. *Blood* 1998;92(3):952–958.
46. Harris NL. Hodgkin lymphoma: classification and differential diagnosis. *Mod Pathol* 1999;12(2):159–175.
47. Harris NL. Hodgkin's lymphomas: classification, diagnosis, and grading. *Semin Hematol* 1999;36(3):220–232.
48. Harris NL, Jaffe ES, Stein H, et al. Tumours of haematopoietic and lymphoid tissues: introduction. In Jaffe ES, Harris NL, Stein H, Vardiman JW, eds. *World Health Organization classification of tumours pathology & genetics*. IARC Press: Lyon, 2001:12–13.
49. Henter JI, Horne A, Arico M, et al. HLH-2004: diagnostic and therapeutic guidelines for hemophagocytic lymphohistiocytosis. *Pediatr Blood Cancer* 2007;48(2):124–131.
50. Hilmes MA, Strouse PJ. The pediatric spleen. *Semin Ultrasound CT MR* 2007;28(1):3–11.
51. Hodges KB, Collins RD, Greer JP, et al. Transformation of the small cell variant Ki-1+ lymphoma to anaplastic large cell lymphoma: pathologic and clinical features. *Am J Surg Pathol* 1999;23(1):49–58.
52. Honda S, Morikawa T, Sasaki F, et al. Cystic thymoma in a child: a rare case and review of the literature. *Pediatr Surg Int* 2007;23(10):1015–1017.
53. Hossain D, Weisberger J, Sreekantaiah C, et al. Biphenotypic (mixed myeloid/T-cell) extramedullary myeloid cell tumor. *Leuk Lymphoma* 1999;33(3–4):399–402.
54. Hu S, Kuo T-t, Hong H-S. Lupus lymphadenitis simulating Kikuchi's lymphadenitis in patients with systemic lupus erythematosus: a clinicopathological analysis of six cases and review of the literature. *Pathol Int* 2003;54(4):221.
55. Imashuku S, Ueda I, Teramura T, et al. Occurrence of haemophagocytic lymphohistiocytosis at less than 1 year of age: analysis of 96 patients. *Eur J Pediatr* 2005;164(5):315–319.
56. Iyer VK, Kapila K, Verma K. Fine needle aspiration cytology of dermatopathic lymphadenitis. *Acta Cytol* 1998;42(6):1347–1351.
57. Jaffe ES, Diebold J, Harris NL, et al. Burkitt's lymphoma: a single disease with multiple variants. The World Health Organization classification of neoplastic diseases of the hematopoietic and lymphoid tissues. *Blood* 1999;93(3):1124.
58. Janeway CA, Travers P, Walport M, et al. The generation of lymphocyte antigen receptors. In: *Immunobiology*. London: Taylor & Francis, 2004:136–164.
59. Janka GE. Familial and acquired hemophagocytic lymphohistiocytosis. *Eur J Pediatr* 2007;166(2):95–109.
60. Jarzembowski JA, Young MB. Nontuberculous mycobacterial infections. *Arch Pathol Lab Med* 2008;132(8):1333–1341.
61. Karim RZ, Ma-Wyatt J, Cox M, et al. Myoid angioendothelioma of the spleen. *Int J Surg Pathol* 2004;12(1):51–56.
62. Kertesz GP, Hauser P, Varga P, et al. Advanced pediatric inoperable thymus carcinoma (type C thymoma): case report on a novel therapeutic approach. *J Pediatr Hematol Oncol* 2007;29(11):774–775.
63. Kim DJ, Yang WI, Choi SS, et al. Prognostic and clinical relevance of the World Health Organization schema for the classification of thymic epithelial tumors: a clinicopathologic study of 108 patients and literature review. *Chest* 2005;127(3):755–761.
64. Kim YM, Lee YJ, Nam SO, et al. Hemophagocytic syndrome associated with Kikuchi's disease. *J Korean Med Sci* 2003;18(4):592–594.
65. Kinney MC, Kadin ME. The pathologic and clinical spectrum of anaplastic large cell lymphoma and correlation with ALK gene dysregulation. *Am J Clin Pathol* 1999;111(1 Suppl 1):S56–S67.
66. Kojima M, Morita Y, Shimizu K, et al. Immunohistological findings of suppurative granulomas of Yersinia enterocolitia appendicitis: a report of two cases. *Pathol Res Pract* 2007;203(2):115–119. Epub 2006 Dec 26.
67. Kojima M, Nakamura S, Morishita Y, et al. Reactive follicular hyperplasia in the lymph node lesions from systemic lupus erythematosus patients: a clinicopathological and immunohistological study of 21 cases. *Pathol Int* 2000;50(4):304–312.
68. Kramer MH, Hermans J, Wijburg E, et al. Clinical relevance of BCL2, BCL6, and MYC rearrangements in diffuse large B-cell lymphoma. *Blood* 1998;92(9):3152–3162.
69. Kraus MD, Crawford DF, Kaleem Z, et al. T gamma/delta hepatosplenic lymphoma in a heart transplant patient after an Epstein-Barr virus positive lymphoproliferative disorder: a case report. *Cancer* 1998;82(5):983–992.
70. Kraus MD, Dehner LP. Benign vascular neoplasms of the spleen with myoid and angioendotheliomatous features. *Histopathology* 1999;35(4):328–336.
71. Kraus MD, Shenoy S, Chatila T, et al. Light microscopic, immunophenotypic, and molecular genetic study of autoimmune lymphoproliferative syndrome caused by fas mutation. *Pediatr Dev Pathol* 2000;3(1):101–109.
72. Kumar B, Karki S, Paudyal P. Diagnosis of sinus histiocytosis with massive lymphadenopathy (Rosai-Dorfman disease) by fine needle aspiration cytology. *Diagn Cytopathol* 2008;36(10):691–695.
73. Kuppers R, Klein U, Hansmann ML, et al. Cellular origin of human B-cell lymphomas. *N Engl J Med* 1999;341(20):1520–1529.
74. Lackner H, Urban C, Sovinz P, et al. Hemophagocytic lymphohistiocytosis as severe adverse event of antineoplastic treatment in children. *Haematologica* 2008;93(2):291–294.
75; Lamps LW, Havens JM, Sjostedt A, et al. Histologic and molecular diagnosis of tularemia: a potential bioterrorism agent endemic to North America. *Mod Pathol* 2004;17(5):489–495.
76. Larsen EC, Connolly SA, Rosenberg AE. Case records of the Massachusetts General Hospital. Weekly clinicopathological exercises. Case 20–2003. A nine-year-old girl with hepatosplenomegaly and pain in the thigh. *N Engl J Med* 2003;348(26):2669–2677.
77. Lau SK, Chu PG, Weiss LM. Immunohistochemical expression of Langerin in Langerhans cell histiocytosis and non-Langerhans cell histiocytic disorders. *Am J Surg Pathol* 2008;32(4):615–619.
78. Le Deley MC, Reiter A, Williams D, et al. Prognostic factors in childhood anaplastic large cell lymphoma: results of a large European intergroup study. *Blood* 2008;111(3):1560–1566.
79. Lim GY, Cho B, Chung NG. Hemophagocytic lymphohistiocytosis preceded by Kikuchi disease in children. *Pediatr Radiol* 2008;38(7):756–761.
80. Lim MS, Straus SE, Dale JK, et al. Pathological findings in human autoimmune lymphoproliferative syndrome. *Am J Pathol* 1998;153(5):1541–1550.
81. Lin C-W, Liu T-Y, Lin C-J, et al. Oligoclonal T cells in histiocytic necrotizing lymphadenopathy are associated with TLR_9^+ plasmacytoid dendritic cells. *Lab Invest* 2004;85:267–275.
82. Lin MH, Kuo TT. Specificity of the histopathological triad for the diagnosis of toxoplasmic lymphadenitis: polymerase chain reaction study. *Pathol Int* 2001;51(8):619–623.
83. Lin MT, Chang HM, Huang CJ, et al. Massive expansion of EBV+ monoclonal T cells with CD5 down regulation in EBV-associated haemophagocytic lymphohistiocytosis. *J Clin Pathol* 2007;60(1):101–103.
84. Lorsbach RB, Shay-Seymore D, Moore J, et al. Clinicopathologic analysis of follicular lymphoma occurring in children. *Blood* 2002;99(6):1959–1964.
85. Lu D, Estalilla OC, Manning JT, Jr, et al. Sinus histiocytosis with massive lymphadenopathy and malignant lymphoma involving the same lymph node: a report of four cases and review of the literature. *Mod Pathol* 2000;13(4):414–419.
86. Maric I, Pittaluga S, Dale JK, et al. Histologic features of sinus histiocytosis with massive lymphadenopathy in patients with autoimmune lymphoproliferative syndrome. *Am J Surg Pathol* 2005;29(7):903–911.
87. Markert ML, Devlin BH, Chinn IK, et al. Factors affecting success of thymus transplantation for complete DiGeorge anomaly. *Am J Transplant* 2008;8(8):1729–1736.

88. Markert ML, Sarzotti M, Ozaki DA, et al. Thymus transplantation in complete DiGeorge syndrome: immunologic and safety evaluations in 12 patients. *Blood* 2003;102(3):1121–1130.
89. McCluggage WG, Boyd HK, Jones FG, et al. Mediastinal granulocytic sarcoma: a report of two cases. *Arch Pathol Lab Med* 1998;122(6):545–547.
90. McCluggage WG, Walsh MY, Bharucha H. Anaplastic large cell malignant lymphoma with extensive eosinophilic or neutrophilic infiltration. *Histopathology* 1998;32(2):110–115.
91. McGovern MM, Wasserstein MP, Giugliani R, et al. A prospective, cross-sectional survey study of the natural history of Niemann-Pick disease type B. *Pediatrics* 2008;122(2):e341–e349.
92. Menasce LP, Banerjee SS, Beckett E, et al. Extra-medullary myeloid tumour (granulocytic sarcoma) is often misdiagnosed: a study of 26 cases. *Histopathology* 1999;34(5):391–398.
93. Mistry PK, Sadan S, Yang R, et al. Consequences of diagnostic delays in type 1 Gaucher disease: the need for greater awareness among hematologists-oncologists and an opportunity for early diagnosis and intervention. *Am J Hematol* 2007;82(8):697–701.
94. Miyara M, Amoura Z, Parizot C, et al. The immune paradox of sarcoidosis and regulatory T cells. *J Exp Med* 2006;203(2):359–370.
95. Moore SW, Schneider JW, Schaaf HS. Diagnostic aspects of cervical lymphadenopathy in children in the developing world: a study of 1,877 surgical specimens. *Pediatr Surg Int* 2003;19(4):240–244.
96. Mottonen M, Lanning M, Baumann P, et al. Chediak-Higashi syndrome: four cases from Northern Finland. *Acta Paediatr* 2003;92(9):1047–1051.
97. Mustafa T, Wiker HG, Mfinanga SG, et al. Immunohistochemistry using a Mycobacterium tuberculosis complex specific antibody for improved diagnosis of tuberculous lymphadenitis. *Mod Pathol* 2006;19(12):1606–1614.
98. Narula G, Bhagwat R, Arora B, et al. Clinico-biologic profile of Langerhans cell histiocytosis: a single institutional study. *Indian J Cancer* 2007;44(3):93–98.
99. Nguyen PL, Ferry JA, Harris NL. Progressive transformation of germinal centers and nodular lymphocyte predominance Hodgkin lymphoma: a comparative immunohistochemical study. *Am J Surg Pathol* 1999;23(1):27–33.
100. Nogova L, Rudiger T, Engert A. Biology, clinical course and management of nodular lymphocyte-predominant Hodgkin lymphoma. *Hematol Am Soc Hematol Educ Program* 2006:266–272.
101. O'Brien MM, Lee-Kim Y, George TI, et al. Precursor B-cell acute lymphoblastic leukemia presenting with hemophagocytic lymphohistiocytosis. *Pediatr Blood Cancer* 2008;50(2):381–383.
102. O'Malley DP, Kim YS, Perkins SL, et al. Morphologic and immunohistochemical evaluation of splenic hematopoietic proliferations in neoplastic and benign disorders. *Mod Pathol* 2005;18(12):1550–1561.
103. Okumura M, Miyoshi S, Fujii Y, et al. Clinical and functional significance of WHO classification on human thymic epithelial neoplasms: a study of 146 consecutive tumors. *Am J Surg Pathol* 2001;25(1):103–110.
104. Ozdemirli M, Fanburg-Smith JC, Hartmann DP, et al. Precursor B-Lymphoblastic lymphoma presenting as a solitary bone tumor and mimicking Ewing's sarcoma: a report of four cases and review of the literature. *Am J Surg Pathol* 1998;22(7):795–804.
105. Pahwa R, Hedau S, Jain S, et al. Assessment of possible tuberculous lymphadenopathy by PCR compared to non-molecular methods. *J Med Microbiol* 2005;54:873–878.
106. Patzina RA, de Andrade HF, Jr, de Brito T, et al. Molecular and standard approaches to the diagnosis of mycobacterial granulomatous lymphadenitis in paraffin-embedded tissue. *Lab Invest* 2002;82(8):1095–1097.
107. Psaila B, Bussel JB. Refractory immune thrombocytopenic purpura: current strategies for investigation and management. *Br J Haematol* 2008;143(1):16–26.
108. Purohit MR, Mustafa T, Sviland L. Detection of Mycobacterium tuberculosis by polymerase chain reaction with DNA eluted from aspirate smears of tuberculous lymphadenitis. *Diagn Mol Pathol* 2008;17(3):174–178.
109. Purohit MR, Mustafa T, Wiker HG, et al. Immunohistochemical diagnosis of abdominal and lymph node tuberculosis by detecting Mycobacterium tuberculosis complex specific antigen MPT64. *Diagn Pathol* 2007;2:36.
110. Qian J, Yang CD. Hemophagocytic syndrome as one of main manifestations in untreated systemic lupus erythematosus: two case reports and literature review. *Clin Rheumatol* 2007;26(5):807–810.
111. Reaman GH, Sposto R, Sensel MG, et al. Treatment outcome and prognostic factors for infants with acute lymphoblastic leukemia treated on two consecutive trials of the Children's Cancer Group. *J Clin Oncol* 1999;17(2):445–455.
112. Ree HJ, Kadin ME, Kikuchi M, et al. Angioimmunoblastic lymphoma (AILD-type T-cell lymphoma) with hyperplastic germinal centers. *Am J Surg Pathol* 1998;22(6):643–655.
113. Rena O, Papalia E, Maggi G, et al. World Health Organization histologic classification: an independent prognostic factor in resected thymomas. *Lung Cancer* 2005;50(1):59–66.
114. Ridder-Schroter R, Marx A, Beer M, et al. Abscess-forming lymphadenopathy and osteomyelitis in children with Bartonella henselae infection. *J Med Microbiol* 2008;57(Pt 4):519–524.
115. Rios A, Torres J, Galindo PJ, et al. Prognostic factors in thymic epithelial neoplasms. *Eur J Cardiothorac Surg* 2002;21(2):307–313.
116. Rodig SJ, Payne EG, Degar BA, et al. Aggressive Langerhans cell histiocytosis following T-ALL: clonally related neoplasms with persistent expression of constitutively active NOTCH1. *Am J Hematol* 2008;83(2):116–121.
117. Rudiger T, Ott G, Ott MM, et al. Differential diagnosis between classic Hodgkin's lymphoma, T-cell-rich B-cell lymphoma, and paragranuloma by paraffin immunohistochemistry. *Am J Surg Pathol* 1998;22(10):1184–1191.
118. Ruggiero A, Attina G, Maurizi P, et al. Rosai-Dorfman disease: two case reports and diagnostic role of fine-needle aspiration cytology. *J Pediatr Hematol Oncol* 2006;28(2):103–106.
119. Sachdev R, Shyama J. Co-existent Langerhans cell histiocytosis and Rosai-Dorfman disease: a diagnostic rarity. *Cytopathology* 2008;19(1):55–58.
120. Satter EK, High WA. Langerhans cell histiocytosis: a review of the current recommendations of the Histiocyte Society. *Pediatr Dermatol* 2008;25(3):291–295.
121. Seger RA. Modern management of chronic granulomatous disease. *Br J Haematol* 2008;140(3):255–266.
122. Sevilla DW, Choi JK, Gong JZ. Mediastinal adenopathy, lung infiltrates, and hemophagocytosis: unusual manifestation of pediatric anaplastic large cell lymphoma: report of two cases. *Am J Clin Pathol*. 2007;127(3):458–464.
123. Shetty AK, Gedalia A. Childhood sarcoidosis: a rare but fascinating disorder. *Pediatr Rheumatol Online J* 2008;6:16.
124. Shimada A, Kato M, Tamura K, et al. Hemophagocytic lymphohistiocytosis associated with uncontrolled inflammatory cytokinemia and chemokinemia was caused by systemic anaplastic large cell lymphoma: a case report and review of the literature. *J Pediatr Hematol Oncol* 2008;30(10):785–787.
125. Shin HT, Harris MB, Orlow SJ. Juvenile myelomonocytic leukemia presenting with features of hemophagocytic lymphohistiocytosis in association with neurofibromatosis and juvenile xanthogranulomas. *J Pediatr Hematol Oncol* 2004;26(9):591–595.
126. Silva-Herzog E, Detweiler CS. Intracellular microbes and haemophagocytosis. *Cell Microbiol* 2008;10(11):2151–2158.
127. Simonart T, Kentos A, Renoirte C, et al. Cutaneous involvement by neutrophil-rich, CD30-positive anaplastic large cell lymphoma mimicking deep pustules. *Am J Surg Pathol* 1999;23(2):244–246.
128. Stasia MJ, Li XJ. Genetics and immunopathology of chronic granulomatous disease. *Semin Immunopathol* 2008;30(3):209–235.

129. Stein H, Foss HD, Durkop H, et al. CD30(+) anaplastic large cell lymphoma: a review of its histopathologic, genetic, and clinical features. *Blood* 2000;96(12):3681–3695.
130. Taddesse-Heath L, Pittaluga S, Sorbara L, et al. Marginal zone B-cell lymphoma in children and young adults. *Am J Surg Pathol* 2003;27(4):522–531.
131. Taflin C, Miyara M, Nochy D, et al. FoxP3+ regulatory T cells suppress early stages of granuloma formation but have little impact on sarcoidosis lesions. *Am J Pathol* 2009;174(2):497–508.
132. Tang YW, Procop GW, Zheng X, et al. Histologic parameters predictive of mycobacterial infection. *Am J Clin Pathol* 1998;109(3):331–334.
133. Trebo MM, Attarbaschi A, Mann G, et al. Histiocytosis following T-acute lymphoblastic leukemia: a BFM study. *Leuk Lymphoma* 2005;46(12):1735–1741.
134. Urban RM, Jacobs JJ, Tomlinson MJ, et al. Dissemination of wear particles to the liver, spleen, and abdominal lymph nodes of patients with hip or knee replacement. *J Bone Joint Surg Am* 2000;82(4):457–476.
135. Vago L, Barberis M, Gori A, et al. Nested polymerase chain reaction for Mycobacterium tuberculosis IS6110 sequence on formalin-fixed paraffin-embedded tissues with granulomatous diseases for rapid diagnosis of tuberculosis. *Am J Clin Pathol* 1998;109(4):411–415.
136. Vasilescu C, Stanciulea O, Tudor S, et al. Laparoscopic subtotal splenectomy in hereditary spherocytosis: to preserve the upper or the lower pole of the spleen? *Surg Endosc* 2006;20(5):748–752.
137. Vermi W, Blanzuoli L, Kraus MD, et al. The spleen in the Wiskott-Aldrich syndrome: histopathologic abnormalities of the white pulp correlate with the clinical phenotype of the disease. *Am J Surg Pathol* 1999;23(2):182–191.
138. Wang J, Zheng L, Lobito A, et al. Inherited human Caspase 10 mutations underlie defective lymphocyte and dendritic cell apoptosis in autoimmune lymphoproliferative syndrome type II. *Cell* 1999;98(1):47–58.
139. Winter LK, Spiegel JH, King T. Dermatopathic lymphadenitis of the head and neck. *J Cutan Pathol* 2007;34(2):195–197.
140. Wright DH. What is Burkitt's lymphoma and when is it endemic? *Blood* 1999;93(2):758.
141. Yaris N, Nas Y, Cobanoglu U, et al. Thymic carcinoma in children. *Pediatr Blood Cancer* 2006;47(2):224–227.
142. Zeyrek D, Ozturk E, Ozturk A, et al. Decreased thymus size in full-term newborn infants of smoking mothers. *Med Sci Monit* 2008;14(8):CR423–CR426.

CHAPTER 23

The Bone Marrow

JOCHEN K.M. LENNERZ
ANJUM HASSAN

Acute lymphocytic leukemia is the most common malignancy in children and classically presents with pancytopenia, bleeding, and signs of anemia or infection. Characterized by an almost complete loss of hematopoietic elements, this disease tragically illustrates the fragility of the otherwise harmonically orchestrated "fluid-organ," the bone marrow. Ultimately forming approximately 3% to 6% of the total body weight and reconstructing the peripheral blood throughout life, this organ undergoes a fascinating embryologic development. From midfetal development on and extending throughout life, the bone marrow is the site of origin of peripheral blood, the macrophages/dendritic cell system, mast cells, lymphocytes, NK cells, and osteoclasts (52). At this point, we know that the potency of some of the stem cells even extends this spectrum and that the bone marrow also contributes to solid/epithelial tissues.

DEVELOPMENT

Mesenchymal-derived primitive erythroblasts in the yolk sac are the earliest signs of hematopoiesis in the embryo at a crown rump length of 95 mm (30). While the presence of lymphoid elements in the yolk sac is controversial, it has been shown that the aorta [aorto-gonad-mesonephros (AGM)] (185) as well as the placenta contribute in this earliest phase to the lymphomyeloid stem cell pool (128,137,186). The proposed candidates for hematopoietic stem cells (HSCs) in the AGM express the following markers: CD34$^+$/CD45$^+$ and stem cell receptor c-kit (CD117) and the transcription factor GATA-2 (117). The cells arising in the yolk sac show myeloid restriction (184). At weeks 10 to 24, the liver is the primary hematopoietic organ with production of red cells, granulocytes, and megakaryocytes in the primitive sinusoids. At this time, the spleen also contributes with approximately 20% to hematopoiesis. Slowly, the production within the bone marrow takes over, and at 4 to 5 months it will be the primary site of hematopoiesis. Typically by birth, liver and spleen show minimal myelopoiesis. This switch is often referred to as *embryo-to-fetal-to-adult-type hematopoieses* (33). The development of the bone marrow continues in a topographically organized fashion. Hematopoiesis changes from the axial and radial skeleton (newborns) to the flat bones of the central skeleton by 12 to 16 years. Microscopically, the bone marrow is an inhomogeneous organ, which is often illustrated by higher cellularity within deeper areas of the medullary cavity than in subcortical zones. Due to the relatively short lifespan of peripheral blood elements, the production rates within the bone marrow are astronomic (111). The turnaround time of neutrophils (~2 hours) requires the production of approximately 700,000 cells per second to maintain the normal value of 5,000/μL; exponentially higher values are needed in neutrophilia or sepsis, illustrating the dynamics of this system.

With aging, hematopoietic tissue is replaced by fat and key figures for the hematopoietic elements are: approximately 80% until 9 years, approximately 50% until 70 years, and <30% beyond. Hematopoiesis (Table 23-1), its development and maintenance, is an exquisitely regulated, dynamic, and highly complicated system of cell production that

Table 23-1 ■ GENERAL FEATURES OF THE BONE MARROW AND HEMATOPOIESIS

- Microenvironment with regulatory factors for stem/progenitor cells and structural support via stromal framework and surrounding liquid matrix.
- Stem/progenitor cells localize to specific niches based on complementary adhesion molecule expression between hematopoietic cells, microenvironment and stromal cells.
- Stem/progenitor cell proliferation and maturation under exquisite regulatory control; regulated "cross talk" between stromal cells and hematopoietic cells maintains steady state.
- Stimulatory and suppressive factors within microenvironmental matrix; regulatory factors consist of CSFs, ILs, and inhibitory cytokines.
- Stem cells[a] are capable of self-renewal and multilineage differentiation.
- Committed progenitor cells[a] are destined to a specific lineage.

[a]Not morphologically distinct.

involves molecular control of cell division, differentiation commitment, and maturation carried out via the close interaction of bone marrow microenvironmental elements with precursor cells (26,29,200).

BONE MARROW STRUCTURE

Encased and protected by cortical bone, traversed and supported by trabecular bone, the bone marrow consists of a highly organized thin-walled capillary network, venous sinuses, and surrounding extracellular matrix. The capillary-venous sinus, which results from bifurcations of the nutrient or medullary arteries, is the basic structural unit of the bone marrow (202). Within this histologic compartment, HSC and progenitor cells are exposed to the extracellular matrix that comprises the bone marrow microenvironment (Figure 23-1). The outer adventitial reticular cells (ARCs) add connective tissue elements and form the outer sinusoidal wall, synthesize collagen, laminin, fibronectin, and proteoglycans. All regulatory factors, adhesion molecules, and other proteins necessary for the regulation of hematopoiesis are contained within this matrix (52,134). Furthermore, the ARCs are phagocytic and can become lipocytes. As outlined before, the fat/hematopoietic ratio ("marrow cellularity") is variable and a rough estimate can be calculated as: cellularity = 100% − age (see below). Mitotically active cells are normally found around the supporting bone, typically paratrabecular and perivascular from where cells mature progressively. All newly formed mature hematopoietic cells are released into the bone marrow capillary-venous sinuses. Most cells pass through the sinus wall, but megakaryocytes reside adjacent to sinuses and extend pseudopodia directly into the vascular space (146,177). The capillary-venous sinuses coalesce into venules and ultimately into veins that carry newly formed hematopoietic cells to the systemic circulation (202).

STEM CELLS AND PROGENITOR CELLS

HSC can be defined by their ability to regenerate long-term multilineage hematopoiesis in myeloablated recipients. Although not morphologically recognizable, stem cells can be detected by either functional features (the simultaneous capability of sustained self-renewal and multilineage differentiation potential) or immunophenotype ($CD34^+$, Thyr-1^+, c-kit^+, $CD38^-$, cytokine receptor and adhesion molecule expression) (52,123) (Figure 23-2). HSC are estimated to constitute 1 in 10^4 nucleated marrow cells. In contrast, progenitor cells are progressed stem cells with lineage commitment. The process of lineage commitment is incompletely understood; however, the resulting committed stem/progenitor cells are also morphologically unrecognizable but immunophenotypically defined by CD34, c-kit, and CD38 expression (123,127). Further, maturation is characterized by the acquisition of cytologic and immunophenotypic properties of the different morphologically recognizable hematopoietic lineages. Both proliferation and lineage maturation are regulated by the synergistic stimulatory activities of colony-stimulating factors (CSFs) and interleukins (ILs), whereas antagonistic effects are driven by inhibitory factors that include tumor necrosis factor (91,112). It is known that mature hematopoietic elements play a role in the regulation of lineage production and to maintain steady-state hematopoiesis. Even though molecular pathways for this homeostasis are fragmentary and complicated, endocrine, paracrine, mesenchymal, and autonomic nervous system contributions have been implicated (91,112). The molecular regulation of bone marrow contribution and feedback regulation during the regeneration in peripheral tissues is at this time uncharted.

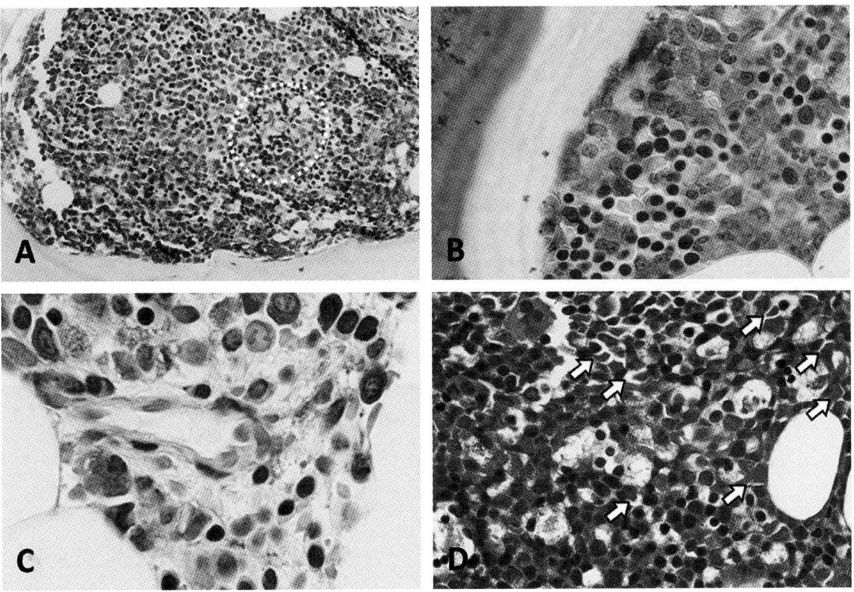

FIGURE 23-1 ■ Bone marrow microarchitecture. **A**: Bone marrow biopsy from a 1-day-old boy showing hematopoietic tissue that occupies approximately 90% of the marrow space. Only few regions of bone marrow fat are seen. The myeloid lineage is highlighted in red (Leder stain) and the *perivascular region* (*circle*) shows lack of myeloid cells. **B**: The *paratrabecular region* shows myeloid and erythroid precursors. **C**: Perivascular distribution of precursors in a bone marrow biopsy from an 18-year-old girl; note the delicate reticulum and extracellular matrix derived from *ARCs*. **D**: Highly cellular (>90%) bone marrow biopsy in a preterm girl shows numerous capillaries (*arrows*) interspersed between the hematopoietic cells and extracellular matrix.

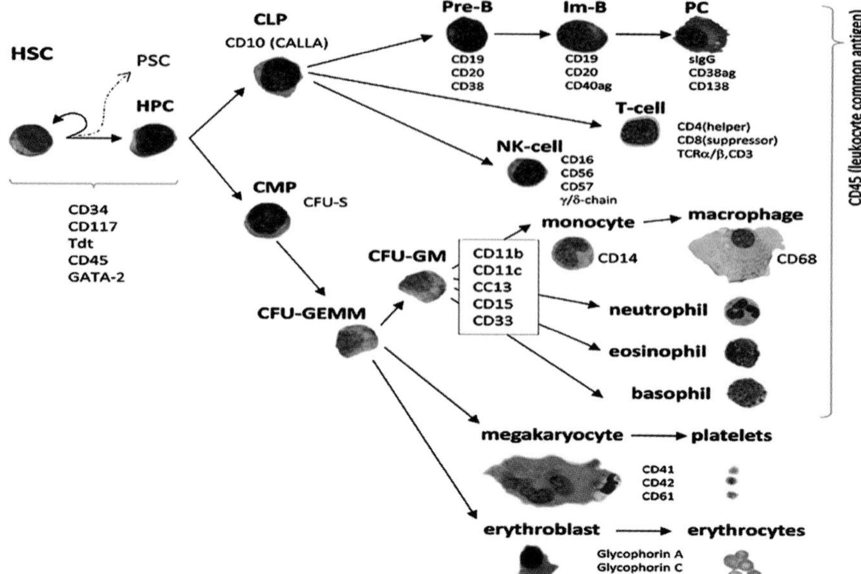

FIGURE 23-2 ■ Selected aspects of hematopoiesis. See text for details. CLP, committed lymphoid progenitor; CMP, committed myeloid progenitor (e.g., CFU-S: colony-forming unit—spleen); GEMM, granulo-erythro-megakaryo-monocytic; GM, granulo-monocytic (= myelomonocytic); HPC, hematopoietic progenitor committed; HSC, hematopoietic stem cell; Im-B, immature B-lymphocyte; PC, plasma cell; PSC, peripheral stem cell.

HEMATOPOIETIC LINEAGES

Granulopoiesis

The process of granulocytic maturation is characterized by a progressive nuclear segmentation, simultaneous decrease in the nucleus to cytoplasmic (*N*/*C*) ratio, as well as acquisition and increase of primary and later secondary cytoplasmic granules. The earliest morphologically recognizable cell in the granulocytic lineage is the myeloblast (20 μm; *N*/*C* ratio > 85%); the subsequent arbitrary stages of this continuous maturation process include promyelocytes, myelocytes, metamyelocytes, band neutrophils, and segmented neutrophils (Figure 23-3). The key regulatory factors involved in granulopoiesis are granulocyte-macrophage colony-stimulating factor (GM-CSF), granulocyte colony-stimulating factor (G-CSF), and interleukin-3 (IL-3) (167). G-CSF is an 813 amino acid membrane protein that functions by binding to its specific cell surface receptor (G-CSFr) and activates cytoplasmic tyrosine kinases (28). Granulopoiesis is also under the control of retinoic acid receptors (RAR), which bind to all-trans-retinoic acid and 9-cis-retinoic acid (28). The combination of four otherwise nonmyeloid restricted transcription factors is unique to the granulocyte lineage: C/EBPa (restricted to $CD34^+$/$CD33^+$ myeloid cells), PU.1 (Ets family member), CBF (AML1), and c-Myb (50,95,103,197). Other transcription factors (e.g., WT-1, Rb, and Hox) have also been implicated in granulopoiesis (197). Granulopoiesis occurs predominantly in paratrabecular and perivascular regions within the bone marrow (134). Thus, in normal bone marrow biopsy sections, immature granulocytic precursors selectively localize to the paratrabecular and, less conspicuously, the perivascular regions. This distribution may be altered after cytokine treatment, chemotherapy, as well as after bone marrow transplantation (see below). Normal localization can be highlighted by immunoperoxidase staining for myeloperoxidase.

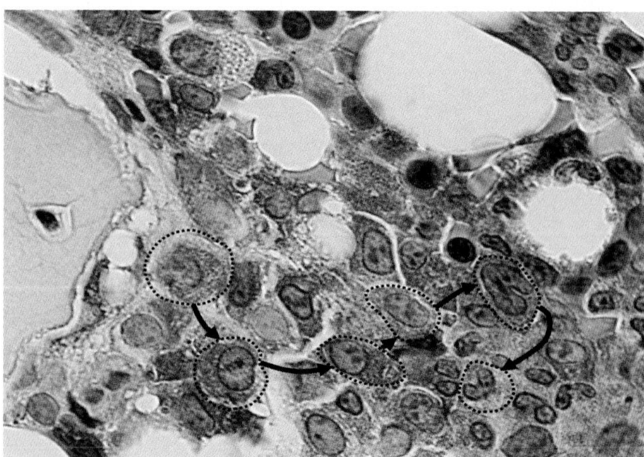

FIGURE 23-3 ■ Granulopoiesis. Immature granulocytic precursors (Leder positive) localize to the paratrabecular regions. Subsequent arbitrary stages are indicated (*circles*) and maturation progresses to, for example, band neutrophils.

Erythropoiesis

The earliest morphologically recognizable cell in the erythroid lineage is the erythroblast (normoblast). The subsequent maturation has been arbitrarily divided into the basophilic normoblast, polychromatophilic normoblast, orthochromic normoblast, reticulocyte, and mature erythrocyte stages (Figure 23-4). The maturational process is characterized by progressive nuclear condensation with ultimate extrusion of the pyknotic nucleus at the end of the orthochromic normoblastic stage, which results in the young erythrocyte (reticulocyte). Simultaneously, the cytoplasm gradually changes from a deeply basophilic, organelle-rich substance to one that consists almost entirely of hemoglobin. In addition to the general growth factors (GM-CSF, IL-3, and

IL-11), the primary growth factor responsible for red blood cell production is erythropoietin (EPO), a 30.4-kDa glycoprotein that induces proliferation and maturation of committed erythroid progenitor cells by binding to its specific cell receptor (R-EPO), which inhibits apoptosis and thereby regulates the rate of red cell production (65,138). EPO does not cross the placenta and therefore the fetus primarily controls erythropoiesis (138). Although erythroid and megakaryocytic lineages share several transcription factors such as GATA-1 and NF-E2 (6,118), specific growth factors act selective and allow committed cells to differentiate and proliferate. Erythropoiesis occurs in small colonies (erythroblast islands), and even though related to vascular structures, they appear randomly dispersed throughout the hematopoietic cavity. They are neither paratrabecular nor perivascular in distribution (16). Erythroid architecture can be highlighted by immunohistochemistry (Figure 23-4).

Megakaryocytopoiesis

Megakaryocytes are the largest (50 to 150 μm) nucleated cell in the bone marrow. Unlike the maturation of the other lineages, megakaryocyte maturation from the blast to the mature cell stage is not associated with mitotic divisions. Megakaryocyte differentiation occurs via endomitosis, resulting in increasing nuclear lobulations without cell division (194), controlled via thrombopoietin (TPO) (92,140,143). The earliest megakaryocyte precursor identified in cell culture studies is the promegakaryoblast. Subsequent maturational stages have been arbitrarily designated as megakaryoblast, basophilic megakaryocyte, granular megakaryocyte, and platelet-producing megakaryocyte (47). The maturational sequence is characterized by a progressive increase in the overall size, an increase in nuclear lobulations ($n = 8$, 16 or 32, without nucleoli, and the development of demarcation membranes and multiple types of (purple-red or pink) cytoplasmic granules. Megakaryocyte production is regulated by a variety of factors, including multilineage growth factors such as GM-CSF, stem cell factor, IL-3, IL-6, and lineage-selective factors such as IL-11 and TPO (92,140,143,196). TPO binds to c-Mpl and acts in synergy with other cytokines (see above, EPO, IFN-α, IFN-β) (129). Even though megakaryocytes appear randomly distributed in biopsy sections, they are localized selectively to the parasinusoidal regions within the bone marrow microanatomy. Megakaryocytes project pseudopodia into the vascular space, and proplatelets are directly released into the blood stream by this mechanism (189).

Monopoiesis and Dendritic Cell Development

Monocytes, at 12 to 20 μm the largest leukocyte, are derived from the same precursor cells that give rise to neutrophils, and M-CSF is instrumental in influencing the progenitor cells to differentiate into monocyte-macrophages (78). Gradual nuclear folding and the acquisition of cytoplasmic granules characterize the stages of maturation, designated as monoblast, promonocyte, and mature monocyte. Although characteristically monocytes have fewer and smaller granules than neutrophils, neither monoblasts nor promonocytes are generally recognizable in normal bone marrow. Monocytes circulate in the blood and subsequently migrate to solid tissues to become macrophages or various types of immune accessory cells. This accessory role and evidence that these cells play an integrated, multifaceted role in humoral and cellular immunity beyond simple phagocytosis, the former designation *mononuclear phagocyte system* (100) has been replaced. Foucar and Foucar (63) proposed the alternative name *mononuclear phagocyte and immunoregulatory effector* (M-PIRE) system as a more accurate descriptor. The M-PIRE system includes monocytes, macrophages, multiple dendritic cells (e.g., Langerhans and dendritic reticulum cells), and their bone marrow precursors. Some evidence suggests a common cell of origin (73). Because the constituent cells show unique immunophenotypic and functional properties and are therefore viewed as distinct cell lineages,

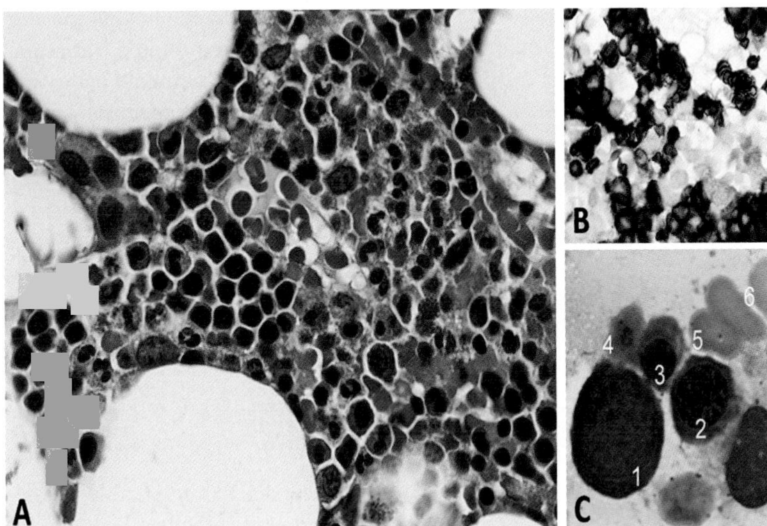

FIGURE 23-4 ■ **A**: Erythropoiesis occurs in small colonies (erythroblast islands) related to vascular structures. **B**: Glycophorin A; marker of erythrocytoid differentiation. **C**: Subsequent stages of erythroid differentiation.

the M-PIRE designation remains controversial. Regardless of the name, both macrophages (histiocytes) and dendritic cells are inconspicuous normal constituents of virtually all organ systems, and mature cells of monocyte-macrophage lineage also remain as a major constituent of the bone marrow microenvironment.

Lymphopoiesis

T- and B-lymphocytes are derived from the same stem cells that give rise to all hematopoietic elements. Factors that are known to influence B-cell proliferation, differentiation, and functional activities include IL-1, IL-2, IL-4, IL-10, adhesion molecules, and IFN-γ; analogous T-cell factors include IL-1 through IL-9 (163). The bone marrow microenvironment serves as the "bursal equivalent" in humans and is the primary site of postnatal B-cell development, whereas T-cell precursors migrate from the marrow to the thymus for maturation and differentiation. Antigenetically mature T- and B-cells can proliferate in response to a variety of cytokines.

The stages of maturation of both B- and T-lymphocytes are generally defined by the surface antigen profile rather than by morphologic features (Figure 23-2). The earliest immunologically recognizable B-cells express nuclear terminal deoxynucleotidyl transferase (TdT), surface CD34 (progenitor cell antigen), CD79a, and HLA-DR; CD10 expression is variable but common (59,108). Further maturation is characterized by the acquisition of cytoplasmic mu heavy chain, and later, surface immunoglobulin. B-cell precursors are generally infrequent in normal bone marrow, although these immature cells are much more prominent in specimens from infants and young children. When they are abundant, the term *hematogones* has been applied to immature lymphocytes (see below).

T-cell maturation is characterized by the presence of cytoplasmic and, later, surface CD3 together with the expression of many other antigens associated with T-cells (132). Terminal maturation is defined by the development of either a helper ($CD4^+$) or a suppressor surface antigen profile ($CD8^+$).

Although the terms *lymphoblast* and *prolymphocyte* have been applied to developing lymphoid cells and are utilized in leukemia classification, the distinction is not easy in normal bone marrow specimens. Lymphocytes migrate from blood to specific tissue sites throughout the body, selectively homing to B- or T-cell regions of lymph node, spleen, and thymus, and to widespread extranodal regions. T-lymphocytes are characteristically long lived and periodically recirculate.

Development of Natural Killer Cells

Natural killer (NK) cells are unique among mature cells in that they were initially defined by a functional activity, nonmajor histocompatibility complex-restricted cytotoxicity, before either morphologic or immunophenotypic characteristics were delineated (107). These cells were subsequently found to perform many other functions (132,171,192). Evidence suggests a common T/NK progenitor cell, and the thymus may be an additional site of NK-cell maturation.

On immunophenotype analysis, NK cells are defined by the expression of such adhesion molecules as CD56, CD57, and CD16. However, the expression of these adhesion molecules is not restricted to NK cells. The fact that true NK cells lack CD3 and CD8 expression facilitates their distinction from cytotoxic/suppressor T-cells, which share other features with true NK cells, including large granular lymphocyte morphology and adhesion molecule expression (CD57, CD16).

Cells with NK activity (both cytotoxic/suppressor T-cells and true NK cells) are concentrated within the large granular lymphocyte population of peripheral blood mononuclear cells. The mature cells have round nuclei, condensed chromatin, inconspicuous nucleoli, and moderate amount of pale blue cytoplasm that contains a small number of prominent, coarse, azurophilic granules. The granules contain cytolytic perforin and associated granule proteases (e.g., granzyme) essential for their cytolytic activity.

NORMAL HEMATOPOIETIC PARAMETERS

The peripheral blood and bone marrow profile are characterized by prominent age-related physiologic variations (Tables 23-2 and 23-3). As previously outlined, bone marrow cellularity decreases with age (115) and is classically best evaluated on biopsy sections or imprints. Particle sections are next best choice and aspirate smears may be difficult to evaluate; however, section imprints and aspiration smears are all reported as equally reliable (130). While earlier references specified 100% cellularity at birth, more recent studies show that bone marrow cellularity is somewhat lower than previously estimated (66); therefore, the percentage should be taken as a representative figure. The distribution of erythroid and lymphoid elements also varies by age, whereas the proportion of bone marrow devoted to granulopoiesis is generally stable. A dramatic decline in erythroid elements parallels the drop in EPO levels that occurs after birth in normal-term infants (139). Erythropoiesis returns to normal steady-state levels following resolution of this so-called physiologic anemia of infancy. Likewise, dramatic age-related variations occur in the proportion of bone marrow lymphoid cells, with up to 40% lymphocytes in bone marrow specimens from very young children and infants (18). The proportion of lymphocytes decreases in bone marrow specimens and B-cell production in general declines with age (2).

Age-related variations in peripheral blood values are well delineated (Table 23-2) and the most dramatic changes are found in erythrocyte, neutrophil, and lymphocyte parameters (17).

HEMATOLOGIC PROFILE OF THE NEONATE

The first month of life is characterized by remarkable physiologic changes in erythrocyte and white blood cell parameters

Table 23-2 ■ NORMAL VALUES FOR BONE MARROW AND DIFFERENTIAL CELL COUNTS

Parameter (Unit)	Cord Blood	Week 1	Week 4	1 year	Child	Adult
Hemoglobin (g/dL)	16.5	17	14	12	13.5	M-16 F-14
Hematocrit (%)	53	54	43	37	40	M-47 F-41
RBC (×106/μL)	5.3	5	4	4.6	4.6	M-5.2 F-4.6
MCV (μm^3)	115	100	98	80	84	90
MCHC (g/dL)	32	33	33	34	34	34
Reticulocytes (% of RBC)	3–7	0–1	0	0–1	0–1	0–1
Nucleated RBC (per 100 WBC)	500	0	0	0	0	0
WBC (×109/L)	20	12	10	10	7	6
Absolute neutrophil count (×109/L)	13	5	4	4	3	3
Absolute lymphocyte count (×109/L)	5	5	6	6–8	4	3
Platelet count (×109/L)	290	250	250	250	250	250

Cell Type	Normal Range (%)	Cell Type	Normal Range (%)
Myeloblasts	0–3	Basophils and precursors	0–1
Promyelocytes	2–8	Monocytes	0–1
Myelocytes	10–13	Erythroblasts	0–2
Metamyelocytes	10–15	Other erythroid elements	10–25
Band/neutrophils	25–40	Lymphocytes	10–35
Eosinophils and precursors	1–3	Plasma cells	0–1

(Table 23-3), and these parameters vary between term and preterm neonates (17). In the normal-term neonate, the hematocrit, mean corpuscular volume, red cell count, and white cell count are higher than normal at any age. The neonatal period is also the only time when circulating erythroid precursors are physiologic. The nucleated red blood cells are cleared rapidly from the blood and do not normally persist beyond the first 3 to 4 days of life (62). In healthy neonates, the relative hypoxia in utero is reversed at birth, so that a marked, transient, abrupt decline in erythropoiesis (so-called physiologic anemia of infancy) occurs. These physiologic changes are exaggerated in preterm infants (139).

The neonate assessment for a hematologic disorder is uniquely challenging because of the complex interplay between possible maternal, familial, and obstetric factors in conjunction with the pronounced physiologic variations (62), all of which must be included in the workup of any hematologic aberration.

Table 23-3 ■ HEMATOLOGIC PROFILE DURING THE FIRST MONTH OF LIFE AND IN YOUNG INFANTS

I. Term infants to 1 month
- Hgb and Hct drop from 16.5 g/dL and 53% at birth to an average of 14 g/dL and 43% at 1 month of age
- MCV declines from 115 μm^3 at birth to about 98 μm^3 at 1 month
- Reticulocyte count drops from 5% to 7% at birth to ~0% at 1 month
- Nucleated red blood cells are present at birth but disappear in first week of life
- Marked leukocytosis with neutrophilia is normal at birth and lymphocytes predominate by 1 month

II. Preterm infants
- Lower Hgb and Hct levels at birth than term neonates
- Higher MCV, more nucleated red blood cells and higher reticulocyte counts compared with term neonates
- More rapid and pronounced physiologic nadir
- Lower leukocyte counts than term neonates

III. Young infants
- Neonatal assessment complex because of dramatic physiologic variations in conjunction with potential maternal, familial, obstetric, and other fetal and neonatal factors
- Maternal factors: infections, medications, obstetrical complications, and underlying illnesses
- For example, maternal and paternal incompatibility for red blood cell antigens can result in hemolysis (hemolytic disease of the newborn)
- Numerous constitutional hereditary disorders of hematopoietic cell production and survival including:
  - Diamond Blackfan anemia (red cell aplasia)
  - Thalassemias (hemoglobinopathy)
  - Congenital neutropenia (granulocyte aplasia) ± thrombocytopenia with absent radii (megakaryocyte aplasia)
- Constitutional disorders can manifest at birth or in early infancy
- Fetomaternal hemorrhage or internal hemorrhage can produce neonatal anemia
- Other causes include various congenital malformations and congenital neoplasms

Hct, hematocrit; Hgb, hemoglobin; MCV, mean corpuscular volume.

Table 23-4 ■ INDICATIONS FOR BONE MARROW EXAMINATION IN CHILDREN

- Peripheral blood abnormality (undetermined after regular workup)
- Evaluation of possible constitutional hematopoietic disorder
- Evaluation for leukemia, myelodysplasia, myeloproliferative/myelodysplastic disorders, and chronic myeloproliferative disorders
- Evaluation for fever of unknown origin, storage diseases, and unexplained splenomegaly
- Staging and management of patients with certain types of neoplasms (e.g., Hodgkin and non-Hodgkin lymphoma, various other solid tumors)
- Evaluation of patient with atypical but nondiagnostic lymphoreticular process in other sites
- Evaluation of patient who does not follow predicted course of initial diagnosis (e.g., patient with presumed idiopathic thrombocytopenic purpura who does not respond to therapy)
- Ongoing monitoring of response to therapy in patients with a variety of hematologic and lymphoreticular disorders
- Bone marrow assessment prior to autologous bone marrow transplantation

EXAMINATION OF THE BONE MARROW IN CHILDREN

Indications for bone marrow examination in children are listed in Table 23-4. The decision to examine the bone marrow is made on an individual basis by correlating laboratory and hematologic findings with the clinical history. While the posterior iliac crest is the preferred site for the evaluation in older children, aspirates and even biopsy specimens can be obtained from the tibia in young infants (178). Before performing a bone marrow examination, careful consideration must be given to what types of specimens are necessary for optimal evaluation of the most likely differential diagnosis (Table 23-5). Except for cultures, as a general rule, all specialized studies should be delayed until the bone marrow aspirate smears have been reviewed. When verified as adequate, the appropriate specialized tests can be ordered. Flow cytometry is one of the routine techniques for immunophenotyping and aids in determining the lineage and stage of "maturation" of neoplastic bone marrow infiltrates. Cytogenetic evaluation provides essential diagnostic and prognostic information, not only in acute lymphoid and myeloid leukemias but also in other myeloid disorders. Other, special techniques are also useful to assess for minimal residual disease in patients with leukemias/lymphomas, and to evaluate metastatic processes (Table 23-5).

Constitutional Hematopoietic Disorders

Bone marrow biopsies for constitutional hematologic disorders are only rarely encountered in clinical practice. The different entities represent a heterogeneous group of diseases and involve individual lineage defects of, for example, erythroid, megakaryocytic, and histiocytic elements (Table 23-6). Many of these constitutional disorders (e.g., thrombocytopenia with absent radii, see below) are evident at birth or shortly thereafter, whereas the multilineage abnormalities that characterize the constitutional aplastic anemias usually develop more gradually, sometimes not until adulthood (40,41,125). Another interesting pattern is that constitutional hematologic disorders are frequently associated with a variety of abnormalities in other organ systems (Table 23-6), while the bone marrow

Table 23-5 ■ SPECIALIZED TECHNIQUES IN BONE MARROW EXAMINATIONS

Technique	Specimen Required	Indications
Culture	Aspirate, sterile	Workup for infection
Cytochemical stains	Air-dried aspirate smears	Lineage identification for immature cells
Immunohistochemical stains	Paraffin-embedded tissues	Numerous antibodies available to assess for lymphoid, myeloid, erythroid, and megakaryocytic antigens as well as to determine lineage of metastatic processes Selected antibodies to assess immaturity (e.g., CD34) also available
Immunophenotyping (by flow cytometry)	Aspirate, sterile	Useful in determining immunophenotypic profile of wide variety of neoplastic disorders (e.g., leukemias and lymphomas) as well as benign infiltrates (e.g., hematogones)
Cytogenetics	Aspirate, sterile	Yield prognostic and diagnostic information in acute leukemias, myeloid neoplasms, and lymphoma Essential in the evaluation of acute leukemias
Fluorescence in situ hybridization	Air-dried smears, cell culture smears	Assess for specific cytogenetic abnormality if probe available Useful in minimal residual disease assessment
Molecular analysis	Paraffin-imbedded tissues (PCR)	Useful in determining B- and T-cell clonality, as well as gene rearrangements and other genetic aberrations
	Aspirate, sterile (other methods)	Useful in detecting gene amplifications in metastatic neuroblastoma.

Table 23-6 ■ CONSTITUTIONAL HEMATOLOGIC DISORDERS

Fanconi anemia		
DNA repair defect (autosomal/X-linked recessive) with increased incidence of AML		
Aplastic anemia in >90%, prominent neonatal cytopenia; pancytopenia by midchildhood		
Gradual development of single and multilineage aplasia		
Associated congenital anomalies of bone, skin, kidney; mental retardation		
13 genes (A-N) identified—most common:	*FANCA* (16q24.3; exon 43) ~60% *FANCC* (9q22.3; exon 14) ~10% *FANCG* (9p13; exon 14) ~10%	
Dyskeratosis congenita		
DNA repair defect (uncharacterized genetic subtype in 50%)		
Gradual development of pancytopenia and aplastic anemia ~80%)		
Initial hypercellularity common		
Associated with congenital anomalies of skin, nails, mucosa; frequent mental retardation		
Four genes identified:	X-linked recessive (~30%)	dyskerin (Xq28; exon 15)
	Autosomal dominant (10%)	*TERC* (3q26; exon1) *TERT* (5p15; exon16)
	Autosomal recessive (~1%)	*NOP10* (15q14; exon 2) *TERT* (5p15; exon 16)
Diamond-Blackfan anemia[a]		
70% uncharacterized genetic subtypes (autosomal dominant and recessive described)		
Likely intrinsic progenitor cell defect		
Constitutional red cell aplasia (rare erythroblasts present)		
Some patients develop marrow failure		
Associated with congenital anomalies, especially skeletal (30%–40%)		
Three genes identified:	Autosomal dominant (~30%)	*RPS19* (19q13.2; exon 6) *RPS24* (10q22–23; exon 7) *RPS17* (15q25.2; exon 5)
Congenital dyserythropoietic/idiopathic aplastic anemia[a]		
Erythroid hyperplasia/aplasia		
Associated with distinctive bone marrow abnormalities including multinucleation, nuclear bridging, and megaloblastic changes/ bone marrow failure		
Chromosomal instability and increased incidence of malignancy (repair defect)		
Heterozygous mutations in *TERC* and *TERT* are risk factors for some cases		
Schwachman-Diamond syndrome[b]		
Constitutional neutropenia with frequent development of aplasia (~20%)		
Associated with congenital anomalies including exocrine pancreas insufficiency		
One gene identified:	Autosomal recessive (~90%)	*SBDS* (7q11; exon 5)
Thrombocytopenia with absent radii[c] **(TAR)**		
Constitutional thrombocytopenic disorder with reduced megakaryocytes and bone anomalies		
Probable autosomal recessive disorder	MPL (1q34; exon12)	
Congenital amegakaryocytic thrombocytopenia[c]		
Decreased megakaryocytes		
Different inheritance pattern than TAR, some cases X-linked		
High incidence of dysplasia		
Lysosomal enzyme defects/storage disorders (multiple types):		
Over 40 genetic disorders (~1 in 7,000 live births) with mostly secondary hematologic manifestations		
Accumulation of substrate protein within histiocytes/macrophages		
Increased bone marrow histiocytes with distinctive morphology		
Classification into six groups:	*Lipid storage disorders* (Gaucher, Niemann-Pick) *Gangliosidosis* (Tay-Sachs disease) *Leukodystrophies* (ADL, MLD, Krabbe, Refsum, Pelizaeus-Merzbacher) *Mucopolysaccharidosis* (Hunter syndrome, Hurler disease) *Glycoprotein* storage disorders (mucolipidosis, pseudo-Hurler) *Mucolipidoses* (ML type I–IV; sialidosis)	

[a]Considered a *constitutional erythrocyte disorder;* this group also includes hemoglobinopathies, membrane defects and enzyme defects; For example, thalassemias, sickle cell disorders, hereditary spherocytosis, and pyruvate kinase deficiency (not discussed here).
[b]Considered a *constitutional granulocyte disorder,* this group also includes Kostmann agranulocytosis syndrome, cyclic neutropenia, and Chédiak-Higashi syndrome (see Table 23-7).
[c]Considered a constitutional megakaryocytic disorder.
ALD, adrenal leukodystrophy; MLD, metachromatic leukodystrophy.

picture is largely one of individual aplasia or multilineage failure without distinctive morphologic aberrations (41). Exceptions include marked dyserythropoiesis in congenital dyserythropoietic anemia, and erythroid hyperplasia in various constitutional erythrocyte survival disorders (81,180).

The related group of storage diseases typically occurs as a consequence of lysosomal enzyme defects, affecting mainly histiocytes. Tissues throughout the body are affected and cells exhibit distinctive morphologic abnormalities caused by the accumulation of substrate proteins. Although not a primary hematologic disorder, the accumulation of abnormal histiocytes in the bone marrow produces secondary hematologic effects (41) (see Chapter 5).

Aplastic Anemia in Children

Aplastic anemia in children can be separated into constitutional/inherited versus acquired (173). This heterogeneous group of disorders, characterized by bone marrow failure with/without somatic abnormalities, typically presents with bone marrow failure in childhood. Eventually, severe trilineage hypoplasia develops; however, despite the name (aplastic), initial presentation is often trilineage hyperplasia, megaloblastic changes, or single lineage aplasia. It is noteworthy that some cases may not present until adulthood, highlighting the importance not only for pediatric pathologists. Since cloning of the first aplastic-anemia-related gene in 1992 [*Fanconi anemia* (*FA*)-gene], considerable advances in the syndromic entities have been made (41). It is clear that approximately 20% of bone marrow failure syndromes in children are inherited and approximately 10% represent secondary causes. The latter includes radiation, drugs (typically busulfan, chloramphenicol, nonsteroids), viruses (e.g., hepatitis), and immunological causes (e.g., systemic lupus erythematosus). The classic diepoxy-butane/mitomycin C-induced chromosome fragility testing in cytogenetics has been complemented by targeted molecular approaches (183). The former test assayed the underlying constitutional DNA repair defect in FA, which represents the most common genetic aplastic anemia (Table 23-6). Our current understanding of the molecular pathology underlying this group of diseases is convergence in the DNA repair-FBRCA pathway (41). The diseases affect telomere maintenance in dyskeratosis congenita–related genes (e.g., dyskerin, TERC, TERT, NOP10), ribosome biogenesis in Shwachman-Diamond syndrome and Diamond-Blackfan anemia genes (SBDS and RPS19/24/17, respectively) (67), or congenital amegakaryocytic thrombocytopenia-associated genes (e.g., MPL encoding for TPO) (38,69,174,183,188). Despite the availability of mutational information and mode of inheritance (Table 23-6), the majority (~70%) of "classical" bone marrow failures is "idiopathic" or uncharacterized and therefore the main/primary pathogenesis remains unknown (41,93). The peak incidence for secondary and idiopathic aplastic anemia in children is 3 to 5 years of age, and the morphologic features in the bone marrow are generally absent or severely reduced hematopoiesis.

Benign Erythroid Disorders in Children

Non-neoplastic erythroid disorders (also known as *pure red-cell aplasia*) consist primarily of congenital and acquired anemias (Table 23-6) (145). The congenital form is induced by intrauterine damage to early erythroid precursors (180). Although the uncommon familial or tumor-associated polycythemia/erythrocytosis can be seen in the neonatal period, the most common neonatal polycythemia is the physiological subtype, resulting from intrauterine hypoxia. The prevalence of specific types of anemia varies by patient age and ethnicity. In neonates, anemias secondary to blood loss predominate, followed by immune and nonimmune hemolytic processes. Anemias secondary to either maturation or proliferation defects are uncommon in infants and include constitutional red cell aplasia and congenital dyserythropoietic anemias (180).

Depending on the ethnic features in a given practice area, constitutional erythrocyte survival disorders, including hemoglobinopathies and erythrocyte membrane disorders (36), are relatively common causes of anemia in infants. However, bone marrow examination is generally not required for diagnosis.

A relatively common diagnostic challenge in bone marrow biopsies in children is the classification of red cell aplasia. The three primary causes of red cell aplasia in young children are Diamond-Blackfan anemia, transient erythroblastopenia of childhood, and red cell aplasia secondary to parvovirus infection (71). The latter (also-called acquired pure red-cell aplasia) is typically transient and self-limited. If a variety of clinical, laboratory, hematologic, and bone marrow morphologic findings are integrated, the types of red cell aplasia in young children can generally be distinguished. In all types of constitutional and acquired red cell aplasia, the bone marrow is characterized by a profound decrease in maturing erythroid elements, although usually a variable number of erythroblasts are apparent. In addition, distinctive intranuclear inclusions within the residual enlarged erythroblasts are the hallmark of parvovirus infection, but these may not be readily apparent in all cases and immunohistochemistry can be helpful (Figure 23-5). Consequently, acute parvovirus infection should always be excluded by serologic or molecular studies in cases of red cell aplasia, even when the morphologic features of parvovirus infection are lacking. Another distinctive bone marrow finding, increased hematogones (88,96), may accompany any type of red cell aplasia in children, especially in very young patients.

In older infants and children, the most common cause of anemia is iron deficiency; other causes of anemia in this age group include chronic disease, such as HIV-1 infection, and red cell aplasia. The frequency of constitutional hemolytic anemias varies by ethnicity. Other nutritional anemias, including vitamin B12 and folate deficiency, occur in both constitutional and acquired forms in children, but the incidence is low. For many of these types of anemia, the diagnosis can be established by integrating clinical and laboratory parameters, and bone marrow examination may not be required; however,

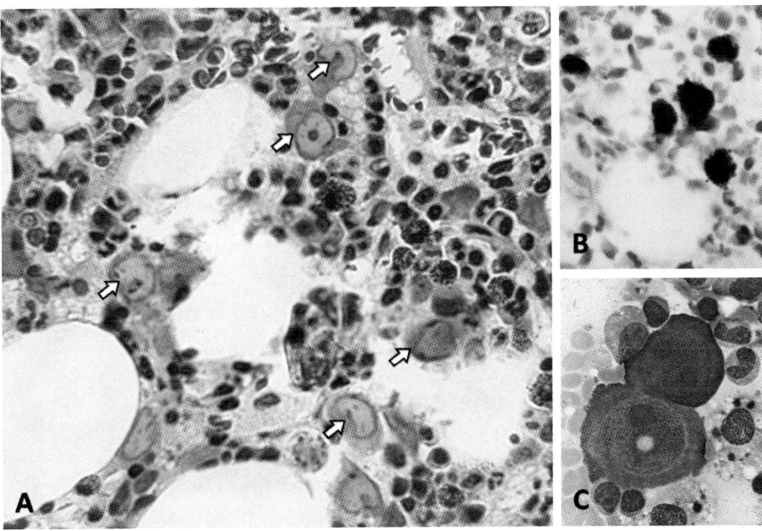

FIGURE 23-5 ■ Parvovirus. **A,B:** Intranuclear viral inclusions in a patient with Parvo B19 induced red cell aplasia (*arrows*) and corresponding Parvovirus immunohistochemistry. **C:** Morphology of intranuclear inclusion on smear (Wright-Giemsa stain).

bone marrow evaluation is necessary for diagnosis in most patients with red cell aplasia, pancytopenia, and suspected congenital dyserythropoietic anemia (55,203).

Finally, drugs and chemicals are associated with the development of pure red-cell aplasia (166). Common examples include ampicillin, azathioprine, carbamazepine, cephalothin, chlormadinone, cotrimoxazole, D-penicillamine, erythromycin, estrogens, furosemide, gold, indomethacin, rifampicin, and valproic acid (49).

Inherited and Congenital Hematopoietic Syndromes Affecting Granulocytes

Disorders affecting granulocytes result from known genetic patterns of inheritance, from known mutations and/or from mechanisms that are still poorly understood. Conventionally, if present at birth, these are designated as *congenital* and if diagnosed later in infancy, these are termed *inherited*. An important note of caution in the diagnosis of these disorders is the exclusion of much more common, reactive causes such as inflammatory conditions, infections, nutritional deficiencies, and/or therapy effect. These are much more common causes of marked changes in the peripheral blood counts, such as leukocytosis, monocytosis, and neutropenia.

In general, the congenital disorders of granulocytes are typically associated with isolated neutropenia and further subclassified into three categories: (a) severe congenital neutropenia, (b) cyclic neutropenia, and (c) chronic benign neutropenia. The inherited disorders, on the other hand, cause morphologic and/or functional changes in the leukocytes with or without cytopenias. Among the numerous disorders in this group, the more common ones are Pelger-Huet anomaly, May-Hegglin anomaly, and Chediak- Higashi syndrome (Table 23-7).

Table 23-7 ■ SELECTED CONSTITUTIONAL HEMATOLOGIC DISORDERS INVOLVING GRANULOCYTES

Immunodeficiency Disorder	Mode of Inheritance and Predominant Morphologic Findings	Clinical Observations
Phagocytic/motility/adhesion defects in granulocytes		
Chronic granulomatous disease (e23)	X-linked or autosomal recessive. Abscess and granulomas common; normal leukocyte morphology	Defective microbial killing by phagocytic cells; any site can be involved, most documented are GI lesions and lungs; incomplete response to infections
Leukocyte adhesion defect (e1,e13)	Autosomal recessive (mutations in chromosome 18). Distinct lack of neutrophils at sites of infection despite peripheral neutrophilia and myeloid hyperplasia in bone marrow; normal morphology	Delayed wound healing, delayed attachment of umbilical cord, recurrent infections
Chediak-Higashi syndrome (e2,e3)	Autosomal recessive; functionally defective neutrophils with giant cytoplasmic granules	Recurrent pyogenic infections, partial oculocutaneous albinism, progressive neuropathy
Cyclic neutropenia (e10,e19)	Autosomal dominant or sporadic; absence of granulocytic precursors in neutropenic phase; normal morphology	Cyclic hematopoiesis with periods of neutropenia lasting from 9 to 21 days followed by neutrophila. Increased infections correspond to neutropenic cycle
Kostman syndrome (e4,e5,e25)	Autosomal recessive or sporadic; severe neutropenia with sustained myeloid aplasia in bone marrow	Recurrent bacterial infections; myelodysplasia and acute myeloid leukemia may be seen in those treated with G-CSF therapy.

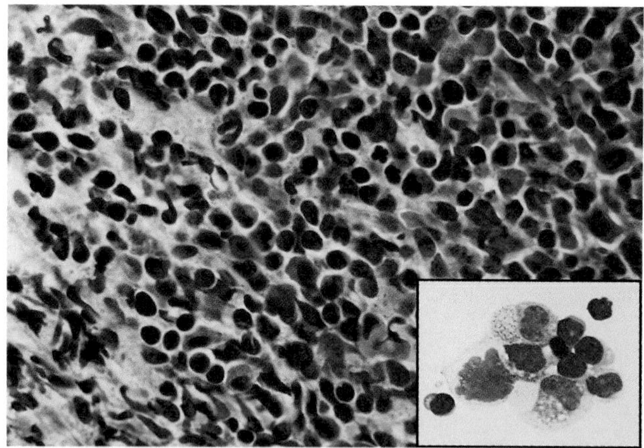

FIGURE 23-6 ■ Hematogones, in a bone marrow core biopsy; cells exhibit condensed nuclear chromatin (inset).

INHERITED IMMUNODEFICIENCY DISORDERS

General Considerations

In the peripheral blood and bone marrow of children, lymphocytes are a prominent component, constituting up to 40% of nucleated elements. Typically, these are evenly dispersed without formation of aggregates. If aggregation is encountered, autoimmune or inflammatory disorders should be considered.

Hematogones are a type of benign lymphocyte that can be found in very large numbers in the bone marrow of young children (106,195). These cells characteristically have round-to-irregular nuclei with homogeneously condensed chromatin, inconspicuous nucleoli, and a very high nuclear-to-cytoplasmic ratio (Figure 23-6). Bone marrow hematogones can be substantially increased in a variety of constitutional and acquired hematologic disorders, in children undergoing nonhematologic tumor staging, and in children recovering from bone marrow suppression (106,114). Immunophenotypically, hematogones are B-lymphocytes that express an antigenic spectrum ranging from immature B- to mature (polyclonal) B-cells (157) (Figure 23-7). This maturational spectrum is best evaluated by flow cytometry and useful in distinguishing hematogone-rich lymphocytosis from the chief differential diagnostic consideration, acute lymphoblastic leukemia (ALL) (157). In addition, although $CD34^+$, TdT^+ lymphocytes are evident on clot/biopsy sections, hematogones are generally dispersed rather than clustered, another feature useful in the distinction from ALL (157,158).

Specific Inherited Immunodeficiency Disorders

This group of disorders can be classified into deficiencies of B-cells, T- cells, or combined deficiencies. Some authors also include defects of the phagocytic and complement systems in this category (199). While several of the disorders in this group have been defined genetically (e.g., severe combined immunodeficiency, X-linked agammaglobulinemia adenosine deaminase deficiency), the classification and genetic basis of many other disorders remains to be determined (Table 23-8).

Platelet and Megakaryocytic Disorders

Transient thrombocytopenia of newborns affects up to 4% of new births and is most commonly seen in distressed neonates (43,135). In most cases, no cause is identified and remission is spontaneous. Known causes of neonatal thrombocytopenia include maternal illnesses, maternal drug therapy, maternal alloimmunization against fetal platelets, fetal or neonatal infections, and chromosomal abnormalities. If a bone marrow biopsy is deemed necessary, megakaryocytes are usually slightly increased in number and morphologically normal. Decreased number of bone marrow megakaryocytes is usually

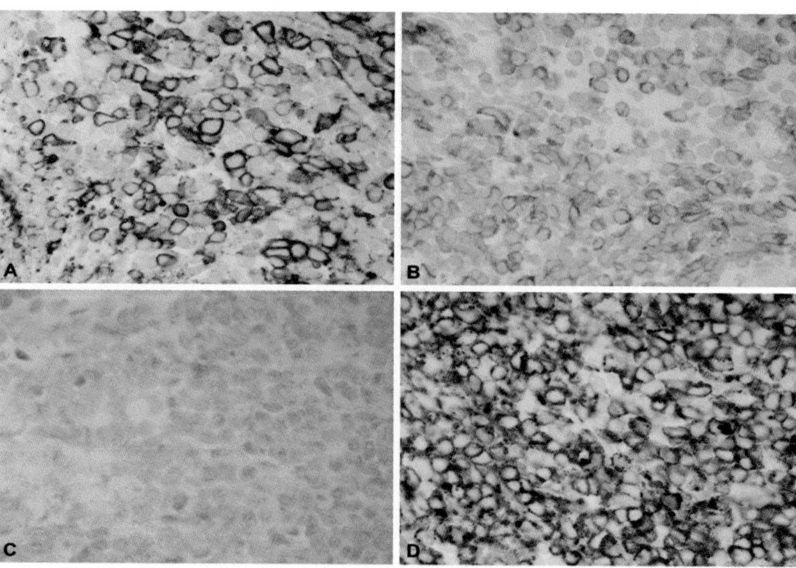

FIGURE 23-7 ■ **A-D:** Immunohistochemistry of hematogones (same case as Figure 24-6), showing variable CD20 (**A**) and CD79a (**B**) expression with no Tdt (**C**) and strong CD10 (**D**) expression.

Table 23-8 ■ SELECTED CONSTITUTIONAL HEMATOLOGIC DISORDERS INVOLVING B-CELLS AND T-CELLS

Antibody deficiency disorders		
Combined variable immunodeficiency (e7,e9,e12)	Heterogeneous group of disorders with intrinsic B-lymphocyte defect; T-lymphocyte defects described in some; lymphadenopathy with hyperplastic germinal centers, no plasma cells.	Recurrent sinupulmonary infections, malabsorption; complications like chronic lung disease, chronic gastroenteritis, or liver failure.
X-linked (Bruton)Agammaglobulinemia (e12,e16,e27)	Mutations in B-lymphocyte–specific tyrosine kinase gene; hypoplastic lymphoid organs with atritic germinal centers; decreased B-lymphocytes, absent plasma cells	Sinopulmonary, GI, skin and joint infections caused by pyogenic bacteria and enteroviruses
Selective IgA deficiency (e8,e24)	Most common and mildest; varying modes of inheritance; nonspecific findings of villous blunting and follicular hyperplasia in GI biopsies	Heterogeneous clinical presentation; mostly no significant illness; recurrent sinopulmonary infections; food allergy; celiac disease.
Hyper IgM syndromes (e21)	Mostly X-linked; inapparent germinal centers; B- lymphocytes are present with abundant plasma cells	Similar clinical findings to other antibody deficiency disorders
Predominantly T-cell deficiency disorders		
Severe combined immunodeficiency (e8,e9)	X-linked; defects in all stages of T-cell development; B-lymphocytes affected in some types; involuted thymus; decreased lymphocytes	Several subtypes with varied presentations; severe and recurrent systemic infections
Ataxia telangiectasia (e6,e17)	A single genetic defect localized to chromosome 11q22–23; loss of cerebellar Purkinje cells and granular layer; pneumonia; chronic hepatitis; hypoplastic lymph nodes	Sinopulmonary infections, telangiectasia; progressive ataxia, and hypersensitivity to ionizing radiation
Wiscott-Aldrich syndrome (e18,e26)	Deletions on Xp11.22–23; varying degrees of lymphoid depletion in lymphoid organs; poorly formed or absent germinal centers	Thrombocytopenia with petechiae or bleeding; recurrent infections, eczema; immunodeficiency

seen in constitutional disorders such as thrombocytopenia with absent radii or X-linked amegakaryocytic thrombocytopenia (Table 23-6). Down syndrome (DS) is associated with multiple platelet and megakaryocytic abnormalities including giant platelets, circulating megakaryocytes, and thrombocytopenia in some cases (4,10,22).

NEOPLASTIC DISORDERS IN BONE MARROW

Myeloproliferative Disorders in Down Syndrome (DS)

Transient myeloproliferative disorder (TMD) and acute mekaryoblastic leukemia (AMKL) are the two most common myeloid malignancies encountered in DS. Mutations in GATA-1 have been classically detected in DS-TMD and DS-AMKL; however, more recently the same mutations were found in blasts of non-DS TMD and AMKL, suggesting an etiologic and a clonal link between the two disorders (83,85,204).

Transient Myeloproliferative Disorder

TMD is the most frequently encountered myeloproliferative disorder in neonates. TMD generally occurs in the neonatal period but has been documented in utero (64). In newborns with DS or trisomy 21 mosaicism, it affects up to 10% of newborns (70,206). Although it resembles congenital acute leukemia (99) and can show up to 50% blasts and a clonal chromosome X inactivation in all lineages, it resolves spontaneously in 1 to 2 months (99,159). The white blood cell count is characteristically markedly elevated, exceeding 50,000/mm^3 and shows normal appearing neutrophils with an otherwise variable hemogram. The hallmark of TMD is the striking number of circulating heterogeneous blasts. Morphological, cytochemical, and immunophenotypic studies show a predominance of erythroblasts and megakaryoblasts (9,105) (Figure 23-8). Despite spontaneous resolution, a substantial portion of patients have been reported to develop acute myeloid leukemia, usually, acute megakaryoblastic leukemia (9,42,105,121).

Acute Leukemia

The incidence of overt acute leukemia is markedly increased in children with DS irrespective of an antecedent TMD (9,32,187,205). The affected children are generally older and present with evidence of severe bone marrow failure and hepatosplenomegaly. The type of acute leukemia seen in children with DS is age dependent. In children less than 3 years of age, acute megakaryoblastic leukemia generally develops with an admixed erythrocytic component, whereas ALL predominates in older children (32,85). In an overt acute leukemia, the bone marrow is replaced by blasts,

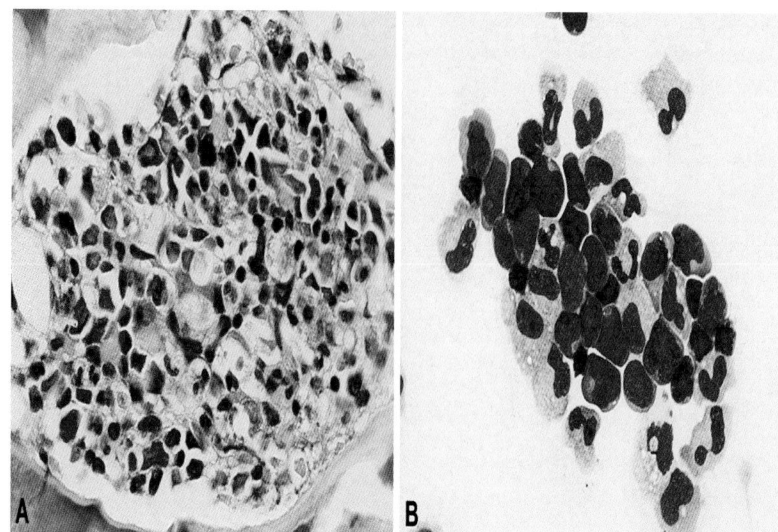

FIGURE 23-8 ■ **AB:** Bone marrow in a newborn with TMD associated with DS, showing myeloid left shift **(A)** and prominence of immature cells including blasts **(B)**.

which are generally cytochemically, morphologically, and phenotypically homogeneous. Additional clonal chromosomal abnormalities along with trisomy 21 are more common in acute leukemias than in TMD (32).

Congenital Acute Leukemias

Congenital leukemias are by definition acute leukemias presenting at birth until 1 month of age. Likely to have originated in utero, these are extremely rare and described with rates of one in 5 million births (151). Congenital leukemias are predominantly myeloid; however, lymphoid types have been described in biologic subsets associated with translocations involving 11q23 (MLL gene) (31,74,122,153,164). The myeloid leukemias typically demonstrate a prominent monoblastic component, marked leukocytosis, and extramedullary disease; hepatosplenomegaly and skin lesions are especially prominent (153,164). Distinctive features of 11q23-associated congenital ALL include central nervous system disease and a $CD10^-$, $CD15^+$ B-cell precursor phenotype with frequent myeloid antigen coexpression (31,153). The second biologic subset of congenital acute leukemias are associated with t(1;22)(p13;q13). This subtype is an acute megakaryoblastic leukemia that occurs in infants less than 1 year of age (198), and the clinical picture resembles a solid tumor. Both bone marrow and extramedullary infiltrates are extremely fibrotic and tumor cells often appear as isolated nests (25,104). On the hemogram t(1;22) associated leukemia presents typically with severe pancytopenia, while in contrast the 11q23 leukemia is characterized by marked leukocytosis. Although the prognosis is poor in all subtypes of congenital leukemia, those cases that present within the first month have the worst prognosis. Lineage switch in congenital acute leukemias is characterized by MLL gene rearrangements with t(4;11), t(9;11), and other translocation partners (98,175).

Acute Lymphoblastic Leukemia

ALL is a clonal B- or T-cell neoplasm characterized by a loss of normal hematopoietic elements and the predominance of immature B- or T-cells capable of minimal, if any, maturation. ALL represents the most prevalent of pediatric leukemias with an incidence of approximately 3/100,000 children annually. ALL predominates in children between 2 and 9 years of age and 75% of all ALL patients are younger than 15 years (1,97). Boys are affected more often, and a substantially increased incidence of ALL has been documented in patients with genetic disorders such as DS and 11q23 abnormalities (85).

Patients typically present with fever, bleeding, splenomegaly, or hepatosplenomegaly. In infants, remarkable organomegaly, high white cell count, and central nervous system involvement predominate. In older children, the typical presentation is a mediastinal mass with or without leukocytosis. Infection and bleeding are the consequence of cytopenias, and organomegaly is secondary to the infiltration of solid tissues by leukemic blasts (1). The white blood cell count is highly variable and ranges from less than $4,000/mm^3$ to more than $1,000,000/mm^3$. In cases with a low white blood cell count, careful blood smear and bone marrow examinations are necessary for diagnosis.

The most widely accepted classification system for ALL was initially proposed by the French-American-British (FAB) Working Group in 1976 and revised in 1981 to improve concordance (11,12) (Table 23-9). Although the

Table 23-9 ■ CLASSIFICATION OF ALL

French-American British	
L1a	High nuclear/cytoplasmic ratio
	Nuclei have inconspicuous nucleoli
	Blasts variable in size but often small
L2a	Moderate-to-abundant amounts of cytoplasm
	Nuclear have one or more distinct, prominent nucleoli
	Blasts, medium to large
L3b	Scant-to-abundant amounts of deeply basophilic cytoplasm
	Abundant cytoplasmic (distinct) vacuoles
	Nuclear chromatin homogeneous
	One or more, generally indistinct nucleoli
	Blasts, medium to large

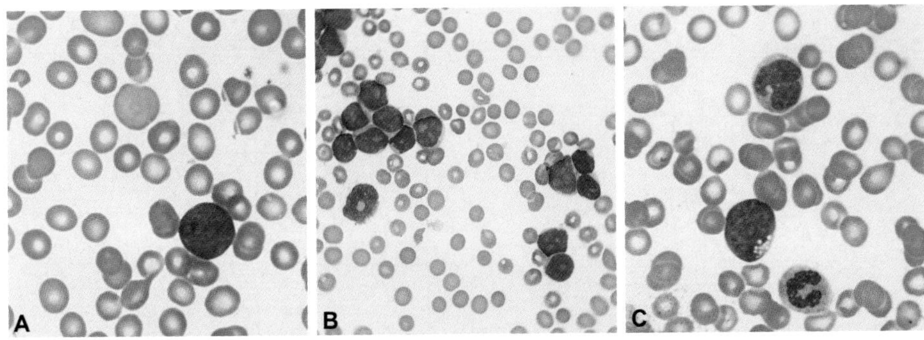

FIGURE 23-9■A-C: The three types of lymphoblasts (FAB classification) include FAB-L1 blasts with high nuclear cytoplasm ratio (**A**), FAB-L2 blasts with moderate-to-abundant cytoplasm (**B**) and FAB-L3 blasts with deeply basophilic and highly vacuolated cytoplasm (**C**).

FAB criteria are valid for identification and distinction of most myeloid from lymphoid processes, the lineage-based classification does not allow distinguishing biologic subsets of acute leukemia. In 2003, the World Health Organization (WHO) sponsored the development of a new classification system that focused on defining distinct clinicopathologic entities based on morphologic, immunophenotypic, genetic, and clinical features (77).

Morphologic Basis of ALL Classification

In ALL, the bone marrow blasts characteristically account for more than 90% of all nucleated cells. Whether B- or T-precursor derived, cases of prototypic ALL are morphologically indistinguishable (94). Lymphoblasts, termed L1 and L2 (FAB-criteria), consist of intermediate-to-large cells with variable amounts of cytoplasm and nuclei exhibiting finely dispersed chromatin and variably prominent nucleoli (11,12) (Figure 23-9A,B). The nuclei of prototypic lymphoblasts usually exhibit subtle irregularities and convolutions that are best appreciated on high power.

Although very rare (<1%), the abnormal ALL population can be indistinguishable from tissue infiltrates of Burkitt lymphoma. Burkitt cells are defined by both nuclear and cytoplasmic features, including deeply basophilic cytoplasm with distinct lipid vacuoles and moderately sized round nuclei with several indistinct nucleoli (19,35) (Figure 23-9C). Although Burkitt leukemia is, by convention, included in the FAB-classification of ALL, the morphologic and immunophenotypic profile is consistent with a mature B-cell lymphoma rather than the prototypic ALL. On bone marrow biopsy sections, cells of Burkitt leukemia/lymphoma are more homogeneous and have round nuclear contours with one to three small basophilic nucleoli (35). Mitotic activity is very brisk, and the abundance of tingible body macrophages may sometimes impart a "starry sky" appearance to bone marrow sections, similar to that seen in other solid tissue sites of disease (Figure 23-10). Cytoplasmic vacuolation is best appreciated in aspirate smears.

Granular ALL, comprising up to 7% of pediatric ALL cases, is characterized by coarse cytoplasmic granulation in at least 5% of the blasts. It can be mistaken for myeloid leukemia; however, the granules are myeloperoxidase negative. This morphologic subtype confers a poor prognosis (27).

Phenotypic Basis of ALL Classification

Most cases of ALL are B-lineage leukemias while T-lineage ALL accounts for only 10% to 25% of cases. In comparison with normal B- and T-cell maturation profiles, most cases of ALL display aberrant or asynchronous antigen expression, including adhesion molecule expression (68,75). The optimal flow cytometric panel for ALL should contain a variety of B-, T-, and myeloid monoclonal antibodies along with Tdt and CD34, which are assessed on the weak CD45+ blast population (15,34) (Figure 23-11).

Biologic Basis of ALL Classification

Combining cytogenetic and molecular techniques, chromosomal abnormalities are detected in 80% to 90% of ALL cases (53,119,161). The most frequent numeric chromosomal abnormality in ALL is hyperdiploidy (~50% of B-cell precursor ALL), with 15% having 47 to 50 chromosomes (119). Hyperdiploidy can be determined with

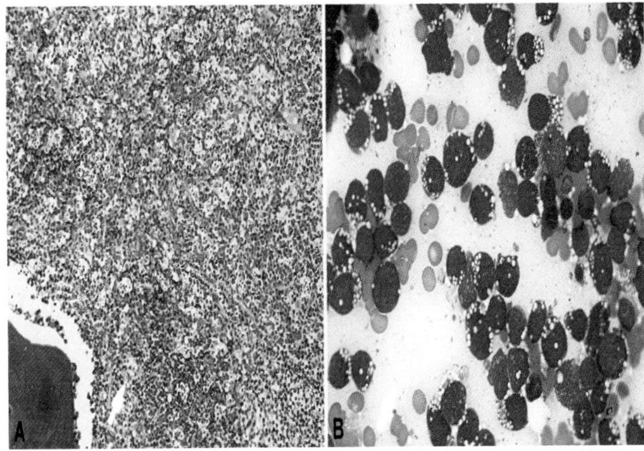

FIGURE 23-10■ **A, B:** A "starry sky" pattern is evident in this bone marrow showing extensive involvement by Burkitt lymphoma; bone marrow aspirate shows cytoplasmic vacuoles in malignant cells.

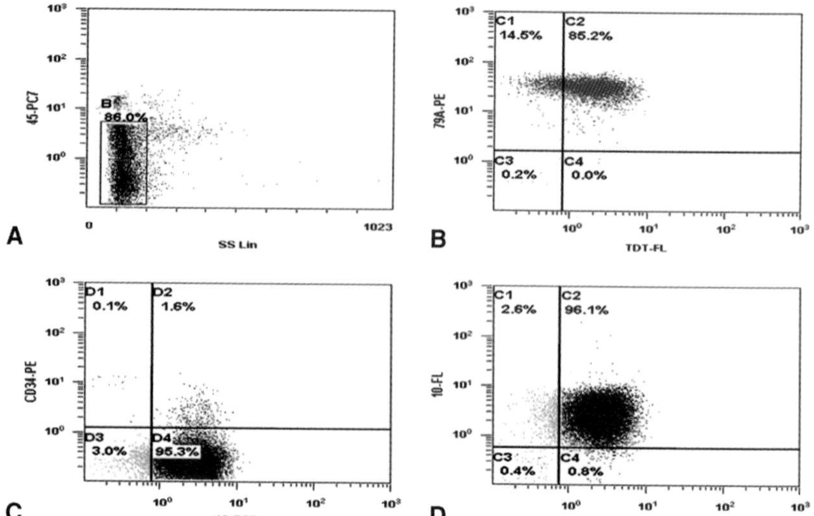

FIGURE 23-11 ■ **A-D:** Composite flow-cytometry histograms showing immunophenotypic profile of a precursor B-acute lymphoblastic leukemia. Note that the cells are dim CD45+ (**A**), TdT+ (**B**), CD34+ (**C**) and coexpressing CD10 and CD19 (**D**).

standard cytogenetic techniques or by flow cytometric measurement of DNA content. Hyperdiploidy, with a chromosome number of 50 or greater, or a DNA content index (ratio of patient DNA content to normal control DNA content) of 1.16 or greater is an established good prognostic indicator in ALL. This prognostic advantage has been attributed to higher response rates to antimetabolite-based therapy. However, cases with extreme hyperdiploidy (i.e., near triploidy, tetraploidy, or >65 chromosomes) exhibit a poor outcome (149,152).

Approximately 40% of pediatric ALL cases demonstrate chromosomal translocations by standard cytogenetic analysis (161). The most common translocation, t(12;21), can be detected by molecular methods in 20% to 25% but remains cryptic on routine cytogenetics (<0.5% detection). The prognosis of t(12;21) is similarly favorable to those of hyperdiploid ALL. In contrast, t(1;19) presents with high-risk disease and carries a worse prognosis. Blasts show a pre-B phenotype with negative CD34, cytoplasmic immunoglobulin positivity, and partial CD20 expression. ALL with t(5;14) and eosinophilia tends to occur in older children and is characterized by striking tissue eosinophilia with consequent organomegaly and usually an aggressive clinical course. The eosinophils exhibit striking dysplasia. (124,161). As illustrated above, a significant proportion of cases may be missed by classic cytogenetics, and PCR- or fluorescence in situ hybridization (FISH)-based analysis is strongly indicated for therapeutic stratification. Philadelphia chromosome (Ph)-positive ALL is another biologic subtype of ALL that results from the classic t(9;22)(q34;q11) translocation (Figure 23-12A,B). In most pediatric ALL cases, the chimeric bcr/abl transcript encodes for the p190 protein. Although Ph-positive ALL cases show no difference in terms of clinical presentation, these patients usually have poor responses to chemotherapy, necessitating alternative therapies including bone marrow transplant (156,168). With few exceptions, the prognosis in ALL can be determined by integrating age, white blood cell count, sex, genotype, and other parameters (Table 23-10). The clinical,

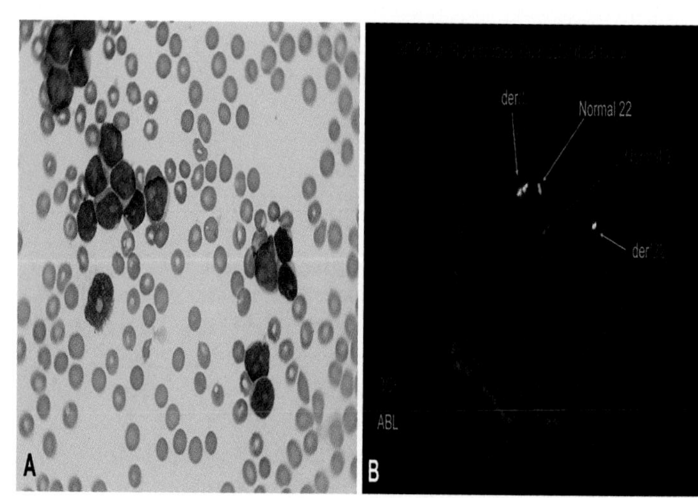

FIGURE 23-12 ■ **A, B:** Precursor B-acute lymphoblastic leukemia with translocation t (9;22) as demonstrated by dual color fusion FISH probes.

Table 23-10 ▪ CLINICAL AND LABORATORY FEATURES IN PEDIATRIC ALL ASSOCIATED WITH POOR PROGNOSIS

Clinical features
Age <1 year old or >10 years
Mediastinal mass[a]
Marked hepatosplenomegaly[a]
Non-Caucasian race[a]
CNS disease at the time of presentation
Suboptimal response to induction chemotherapy
Laboratory features
High white blood cell count (>50 × 10^9/L
Blast immunophenotype (T-cell, CD10−, L3 morphology)
Biologic factors (see Table 23-12)

[a]No longer considered statistically significant prognostic variables (e22).

immunophenotypic, and prognostic significance of a variety of these chromosomal translocations is summarized in Table 23-11.

Acute Myelogenous Leukemia

Acute myelogenous leukemia (AML) is a clonal hematopoietic disorder characterized by a predominance of immature cells capable of minimal, if any, maturation. AML can be derived from progenitors of any lineage and hence multilineage differentiation can be noted. AML occurs in patients of all ages but is more prevalent in adults. Nevertheless, most congenital leukemias are myeloid in origin. The incidence of AML is low throughout childhood and early adulthood, but the proportion of cases of acute leukemia that are myeloid steadily increases during these years. Factors linked to an increased incidence of AML include constitutional genetic disorders, acquired bone marrow diseases, smoking, occupational/environmental exposures, and therapeutic agents (13,85,141,179). Numerous studies have documented an increased incidence of AML in patients receiving chemotherapy, especially alkylating agents or topoisomerase II inactivators (13,144,151). Other environmental exposures associated with AML include radiation, benzene, and other chemicals (13,141,179).

Similar to ALL, the most widely accepted classification system for AML is the FAB-system (Table 23-12) (12). Subsequently, new classification strategies have been devised to include differing clinical features of de novo AML and therapy or myelodysplasia-related AML (79,87,151). The most significant change is the blast percentage (20%) required for diagnosis of AML (FAB: 30%). Several other features, however, both clinical and genetic, play a role in establishing the final diagnosis (51).

Table 23-11 ▪ INCIDENCE AND CLINICAL FEATURES ASSOCIATED WITH GENOTYPIC ABNORMALITIES IN PEDIATRIC ALL

Numerical Abnormalities	Incidence	Comments/Prognosis
Hypodiploid (1)	2%–8%;	Older than 10, poor risk by NCI criteria, Poor prognosis
Hyperdiploid	25%–40%	Most frequently seen genetic abnormality; low risk by NCI criteria, favorable response to antimetabolite therapy; trisomies 4 and 10 likely linked to improved outcome; outcome worse in cases of additional, worse outcome translocations (see below)
Structural abnormalities		
Cryptic t(12;21)(p13;q22)	20%–40%	TEL/AML 1; most commonly seen genetic translocation; good prognosis
t(9;22)(q34;q11)	3%–5%	BCR/ABL; may be cryptic; may be associated with additional abnormalities; poor response to therapy
t(1;19)(q23;p13)	≤5% by routine cytogenetics; 20%–25% if molecular techniques are employed	E2A/PBX 1; mostly in neonates and infants; high-risk disease at presentation; usually pre-B with cy immunoglobulin; poor outcome
t(v;11)(v;q23)(2,3)	2%–11%	High-risk presentation; inferior treatment outcome; predominates in therapy-related and congenital leukemias
t(8;14)(q24;q32) also t(2;8) and t(8;22)	<5%	MYC dysregulation; B-ALL with L3 (Burkitt) morphology; mature B-cell phenotype
t(11;14)(p15;q11), t(1;14)(p32;q11), and t(1;7)(p32;q35)	30% of T-ALL by molecular techniques	TAL1 dysregulation on chromosome 1p32 or TCR gene dysregulation; usually older patients; prominent extramedullary disease
t(5;14)(q31;q32)	Rare	Older patients; aggressive disease course; neural and cardiovascular complication due to striking eosinophilia secondary to IL-3 related stimulation

Modified from Foucar KM. The bone marrow. In: *Pediatric Pathology*, 2nd ed. Stocker JT, Dehner LP, eds. Philadelphia: Lippincott Williams & Wilkins. 2001;1135–1162.
v = variable.

Table 23-12 ■ ORIGINAL FAB CLASSIFICATION OF AML[a]

AML-M0	≥30% blasts <3% Sudan black B/myeloperoxidase positivity Myeloid antigen expression by immunophenotyping or myeloperoxidase expression by electron microscopy
AML-M1	≥30% blasts ≥3% Sudan black B/myeloperoxidase positivity in blasts <10% cells exhibiting maturation beyond blast stage
AML-M2	≥30% blasts ≥3% Sudan black B/myeloperoxidase positivity in blasts >10% granulocytic cells exhibiting maturation beyond blast stage <20% monocytic cells
AML-M3	≥30% blasts + hypergranular promyelocytes[b] Intense myeloperoxidase/Sudan black B reaction in virtually all cells
AML-M3m	Same criteria, except that granules within most promyelocytes very inconspicuous and nuclei highly grooved and reniform
AML-M4	Monocytosis (≥5 × 10^9/L); increased lysozyme ≥30% myeloblasts + monoblasts + promonocytes >20% Sudan black B/myeloperoxidase-positive cells >20% NSE positive cells
AML-M4 eos	Same criteria as AML-M4 + abnormal eosinophils in bone marrow
AML-M5 a,b	≥30% myeloblasts + monoblasts + promonocytes <20% Sudan black B/myeloperoxidase-positive cells >80% NSE positive cells Monoblasts predominate in M5a Promonocytes predominate in M5b
AML-M6 a,b	≥30% of nonerythroid cells are myeloblasts >50% erythroid elements Erythroblasts predominate (suggested AML-M6b category)
AML-M7	≥30% blasts (myeloblasts + megakaryoblasts) >30% megakaryocytic elements defined by immunophenotyping or ultrastructural electron microscopy

[a]Currently the required blast percentage for morphologic AML diagnosis is 20% or more.

Morphologic and Immunophenotypic Basis of AML Classification

The morphologic diagnosis of AML depends on the identification of a variety of types of blasts and other immature cells that define the subtype of AML. Accordingly, cytochemical stains are valuable in delineating specific types of immature myeloid cells and greatly enhance accuracy in the diagnosis of AML (Table 23-13). Flow cytometry is useful in determining the lineage and stage of maturation in many cases of AML; immunophenotyping is also critical in the successful identification of both undifferentiated myeloid leukemias and acute megakaryoblastic leukemias (198). Although marker selection is limited, paraffin immunoperoxidase techniques can be used to assess for immaturity (CD34, TdT), myeloid/monocytic maturation (myeloperoxidase, CD43, lysozyme, CD68, CD15), erythroid maturation (hemoglobin A), and megakaryocyte maturation (CD61, factor VIII) (126,160,191) (Figure 23-13A,B).

Table 23-13 ■ MORPHOLOGIC FEATURES OF BLASTS AND OTHER IMMATURE CELLS

Type of Cell	Key Morphologic Features	Cytochemistry	Immunophenotypic Features
Myeloblast	Large nucleus with finely dispersed chromatin and variably prominent nucleoli. Relatively high nuclear/cytoplasmic ratio Variable number of cytoplasmic granules, may be concentrated in limited portion of cytoplasm	SBB+, MPO+	HLA-DR, CD33, CD13, anti-MPO, CD34
Promyelocyte	Nuclear chromatin slightly condensed; nucleoli variably prominent; nucleus often eccentric and Golgi zone may be apparent Numerous cytoplasmic granules that may be more dispersed throughout cytoplasm In APL intense cytoplasmic granularity usually present, and nuclear configuration variable, but nuclear folding and lobulation characteristic of microgranular variant of APL	SBB+, MPO+	CD33, CD13, anti-MPO

(Continued)

Table 23-13 ■ MORPHOLOGIC FEATURES OF BLASTS AND OTHER IMMATURE CELLS *(Continued)*

Type of Cell	Key Morphologic Features	Cytochemistry	Immunophenotypic Features
Monoblast	Moderate-to-low nuclear to cytoplasmic ratio, nuclear chromatin finely dispersed with variably prominent nucleoli; nuclei round to folded Abundant, slightly basophilic cytoplasm containing fine granulation and occasional vacuoles	NSE+	HLA-DR, CD33, CD13, vCD14, CD4
Promonocyte	Slightly condensed nuclear chromatin; variably prominent nucleoli Abundant finely granular blue/gray cytoplasm that may be vacuolated Very monocytic appearance with nuclear immaturity	NSE+	HLA-DR, CD33, CD13, CD14, CD4
Erythroblast	Relatively high nuclear/cytoplasmic ratio Nucleus round with slightly condensed chromatin; nucleoli variably prominent Moderate amounts of deeply basophilic cytoplasm that may be vacuolated	PAS+	Glycophorin A, Hgb A
Megakaryoblast	Highly variable morphologic features Often not recognizable without special studies May be lymphoid-appearing with high nuclear to cytoplasmic ratio Nuclear chromatin fine to variably condensed Cytoplasm may be scant to moderate, is usually agranular or contains a few granules; blebbing or budding of cytoplasm may be evident Blasts may form cohesive clumps	PAS+	CD41, CD61, HLA-DR, v Factor VIII

SBB, Sudan black B; MPO, myeloperoxidase; APL, acute promyelocytic leukemia; NSE, neuron specific esterase; PAS, periodic acid-Schiff; Hgb, hemoglobin.

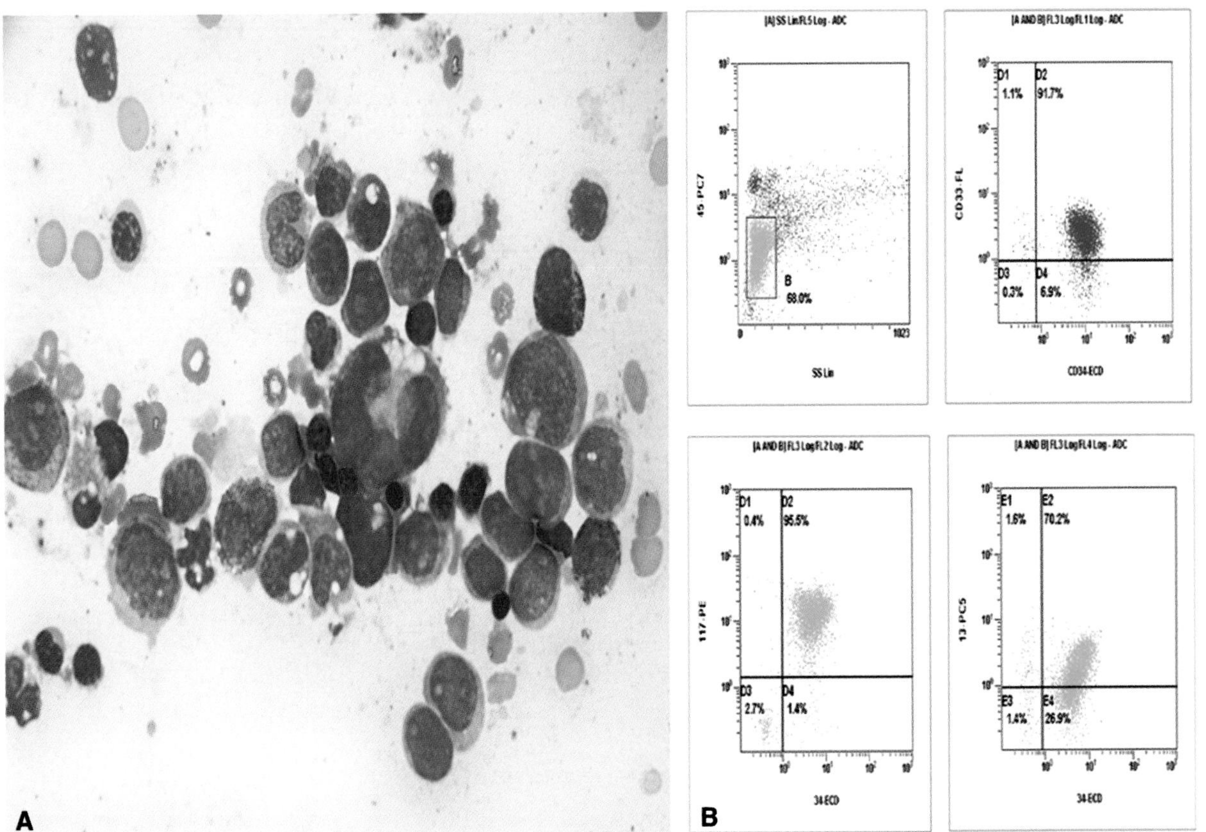

FIGURE 23-13 ■ **A**: Acute myeloid leukemia with maturation. **B**: Flow cytometry histograms show a dim CD45 population, coexpressing CD34, CD33, CD13, and CD117.

Table 23-14 ■ COMMON GENOTYPIC ABNORMALITIES IN AML

Numerical Abnormalities	Comments
−5,−7,−X,−Y,+8,del(5q), del(7q),+21	Found in 30%–40% of AML in children Linked to adverse outcome
Structural Abnormalities	
t(8;21)(q22;q22)	AML 1/ETO; 10%–15% of pediatric AML
t(15;17)(q22;q11–21)	PML/RARα; 8%–15% of pediatric AML
Inv16(p13q22)	CBFβ/MYH11; 5%–12% of pediatric AML
11q23	MLL (multiple partner genes); 5%–20% of pediatric AML

Biologic Basis of AML Classification

Because of the implications for treatment and prognosis, cytogenetic analysis is now a standard of care for patients with AML. Clonal cytogenetic abnormalities are identified less frequently than in ALL, approximating 50% to 80% of cases (161) (Table 23-14). Cytogenetic abnormalities, specific for a FAB subtype of AML, are rarely encountered. The strongest association between FAB-classification and karyotype is in AML-M3 with most cases demonstrating t(15;17). Less clear associations include t(8;21) with AML-M2, and inv(16) with AML-M4 and eosinophilia. Abnormalities of 11q23 have been correlated with AML of monocytic differentiation. In the WHO classification of AML, the traditional lineage-based classification is retained and distinct biologic subtypes based on genotype are integrated (Table 23-15). Cases of AML characterized by reciprocal translocations occur more commonly in children than in adults (119,161). The four most frequent types of translocation-induced AML represent distinct clinicopathologic entities with characteristic morphologic and clinical parameters.

AML with t(8;21)

The fusion gene AML1-ETO produced by t(8;21)(q22;q22) accounts for 10% to 15% of childhood AML cases and usually shows myeloid maturation (119,161). Patients may present with extramedullary myeloid tumors. The bone marrow is characteristically effaced by myeloblasts and maturing myeloid elements, which may exhibit an odd, salmon-colored cytoplasm with a peripheral basophilic rim. Dysplastic findings may lead to a mistaken diagnosis of myelodysplasia, especially if the blast count is less than 20%. Auer rods with tapered ends are typically readily apparent (136). Coexpression of CD19 and CD56 has been noted in cases of t(8;21) AML (86,148).

Table 23-15 ■ SUMMARY OF THE WHO CLASSIFICATION OF ACUTE MYELOID LEUKEMIAS

A. Acute myeloid leukemia with recurrent genetic abnormalities

Disease	Clinical	Morphology	Immunophenotype	Prognosis
Acute myeloid leukemia with t(8;21)(q22;q22); (*AML1/ETO*)	Often presents with extramedullary disease	Blasts with long slender Auer rods, abnormal granulation	CD13+, CD33+, MPO+, CD19+, CD34+, CD56+	Favorable
Acute myeloid leukemia with abnormal bone marrow eosinophils inv(16)(p13q22) or t(16;16)(p13;q22) (*CBFb/MYH11*)	Occasionally presents with extramedullary disease	Abnormal eosinophils with large basophilic granules, decreased lobation	CD13+, CD33+, MPO+; frequently CD4+, CD14+, CD11b+, CD11c+, CD64+, CD36+, lysozyme+	Favorable
Acute promyelocytic leukemia (AML with t(15;17)(q22;q12); (*PML/RARα* and variants)	Coagulopathy, normal/low WBC (hypergranular variant); high WBC (hypogranular variant)	Abnormal promyelocytes with multiple Auer rods predominate	CD13+ (heterogeneous), CD33+ (bright), HLA-DR−, CD34−	Favorable
Acute myeloid leukemia with 11q23 (*MLL*) abnormalities	Frequently occurs in children	Monocytic blasts predominate	Variable CD13 and CD33+, CD4+, CD14+, CD11b+, CD11c+, CD64+, CD36+, lysozyme+	Intermediate survival

B. Acute myeloid leukemia with multilineage dysplasia

- Following a myelodysplastic syndrome or myelodysplastic syndrome/myeloproliferative disorder
- Without antecedent myelodysplastic syndrome

C. Acute myeloid leukemia and myelodysplastic syndromes, therapy related

- Alkylating agent related
- Topoisomerase type II inhibitor-related (some may be lymphoid)
- Other types

(Continued)

Table 23-15 ■ SUMMARY OF THE WHO CLASSIFICATION OF ACUTE MYELOID LEUKEMIAS *(Continued)*

D. Acute myeloid leukemia not otherwise categorized

Disease	Clinical	Morphology/ Cytochemistry	Immunophenotype	Prognosis
Acute myeloid leukemia minimally differentiated	Usually presents in adulthood, cytopenias	<3% of blasts MPO+, <3% of blasts NBE+	Often CD13+, CD33+, CD117+, CD34+, CD38+, HLA-DR+	Unfavorable
Acute myeloid leukemia without maturation	Usually presents in adulthood, cytopenias, occasionally with markedly increased WBC	Blasts comprise ≥90% of nonerythroid cells; ≥3% of blasts MPO+, ≥3% of blasts NBE+	Often CD13+, CD33+, CD34+, CD117+, MPO+	Unfavorable
Acute myeloid leukemia with maturation	Variable age range and symptomatology	≥3% of blasts MPO+, ≤3% of blasts NBE+	Usually CD13+, CD33+, CD15+; variable CD117+, CD34+, HLA-DR+	Variable
Acute myelomonocytic leukemia	Anemia, fever, fatigue; WBC usually elevated	>20% blasts; ≥ monocytes and precursors; ≥neutrophils and precursors; ≥3% of blasts MPO+, ≥3% of blasts usually NBE+*	Usually CD13+, CD33+; Often CD4+, CD14+, CD11b+, CD11c+, CD64+, CD36+, lysozyme+	Variable
Acute monoblastic leukemia	Most common in children, often presents with extramedullary disease, bleeding disorders	≥80% monocytic cells, of which ≥80% are monoblasts; <20% neutrophils and precursors; <3% of blasts MPO+, ≥3% of blasts NBE+	Variable CD13+, CD33+, CD117+; Often CD14+, CD4+, CD11b+, CD11c+, CD64+, CD68+, CD36+, lysozyme+	Unfavorable
Acute monocytic leukemia	Most common in adults, often presents with extramedullary disease, bleeding disorders	≥80% monocytic cells, of which the majority are promonocytes; <20% neutrophils and precursors; <3% of blasts MPO+, ≥3% of blasts NBE+	Variable CD13+, CD33+, CD117+; Often CD14+, CD4+, CD11b+, CD11c+, CD64+, CD68+, CD36+, lysozyme+	Unfavorable
Acute erythroid leukemia (erythroid/myeloid)	Adults; anemia	≥50% of entire nucleated population is erythroid and ≥20% myeloblasts in nonerythroid population; >3% of blasts may be MPO+	Erythroblasts are glycophorin A+ and hemoglobin A+; myeloblasts are CD13+, CD33+, CD117+, and MPO+	Unfavorable
Pure erythroid leukemia	Extremely rare	>80% of cells are immature erythroid cells; no significant myeloblast component; <3% of blasts MPO+, ≥3% of blasts NBE+	Blasts are sometimes glycophorin A+ and hemoglobin A+	Unfavorable
Acute megakaryoblastic leukemia	Cytopenias	Dysplastic megakaryocytes, Blasts often have cytoplasmic pseudopods. Abnormal platelets and megakaryocyte fragments in peripheral blood; usually <3% of blasts MPO+ and <3% of blasts NBE+	Usually CD41+, CD61+; occasionally CD13+, CD33+; CD34−, CD45−, HLA-DR-	Poor

(Continued)

Table 23-15 ■ SUMMARY OF THE WHO CLASSIFICATION OF ACUTE MYELOID LEUKEMIAS *(Continued)*

Acute basophilic leukemia	Very rare	Blasts are toluidine blue+; usually <3% of blasts MPO$^+$, <3% of blasts NBE$^+$	Usually CD13$^+$, CD33$^+$, CD34$^+$, HLA-DR+, CD9$^+$	Difficult to predict due to low number of reported cases, probably poor
Acute panmyelosis with myelofibrosis	Very rare, adults, pancytopenia with no/minimal splenomegaly	Pan-hyperplasia, dysplastic megakaryocytes; increased reticulin fibrosis	CD13$^+$, CD33$^+$, CD117$^+$, MPO$^+$; some cases express erythroid or megakaryocytic antigens	Poor

MPO, myeloperoxidase; NBE, naphthyl butyrate esterase; WBC, white blood count (e14).

AML t(8;21) has a favorable prognosis in adults, however, additional KIT activating mutations confer poorer prognosis.

AML with t(15;17)

Acute promyelocytic leukemia (APL) is a distinct clinicopathologic entity with t(15;17)(q22;q11-12) resulting in a PML-RARa fusion gene (119, 161) (Figure 23-14). Older children and young adults are most commonly affected and present with pancytopenia, profound thrombocytopenia, and marked coagulopathy (12). In the common, hypergranular subtype, promyelocytes are inconspicuous in blood, whereas the bone marrow is effaced by intensely granulated promyelocytes (Figure 23-15). Auer rods are numerous and often stacked in bundles (Figure 23-15, inset). A microgranular variant accounts for about one-fourth of cases and is characterized by leukocytosis and hypogranular promyelocytes exhibiting marked nuclear folding. Intense staining with Sudan black B and myeloperoxidase characterizes both the common and the microgranular subtypes. Immunophenotypic studies show a CD34 and HLA-DR negative phenotype that indicates maturity, but is not diagnostic of APL. The clinical outcome is good if coagulopathy is arrested by all-trans retinoic acid therapy; conventional chemotherapy is also required (56,182).

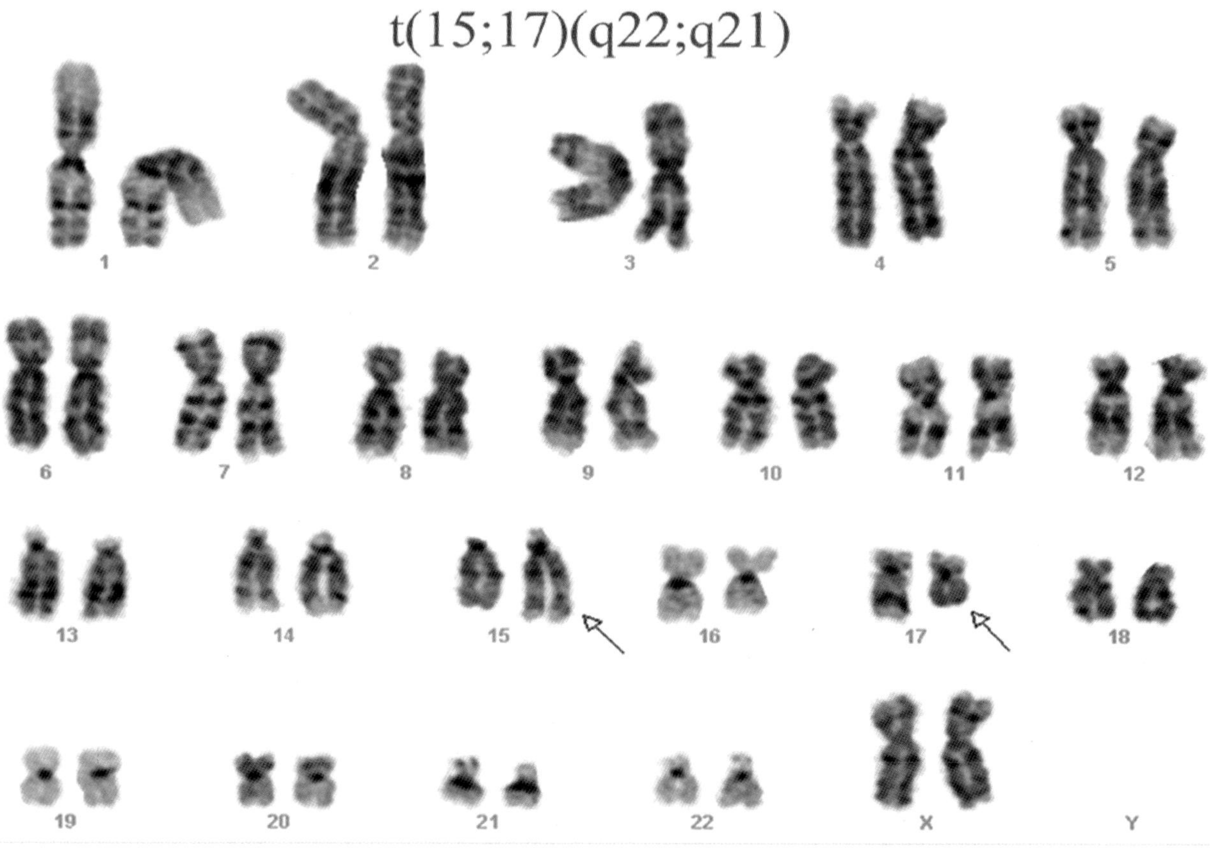

FIGURE 23-14 ■ The translocation (15;17) is exclusively observed in APL; *arrows* indicate breakpoints.

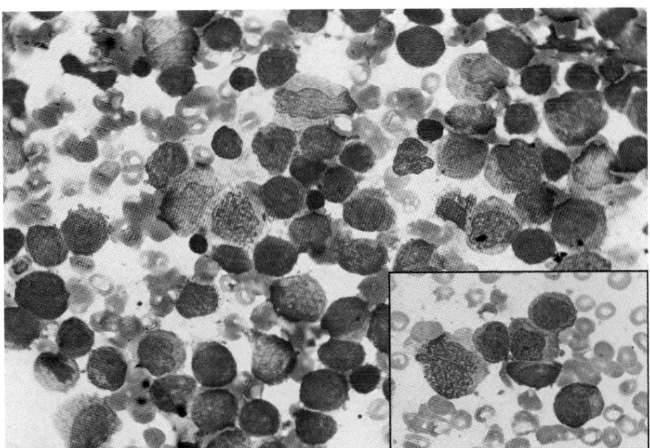

FIGURE 23-15 ■ Several intensely granular promyelocytes are evident in the aspirate smear showing APL; Auer rods can be seen (inset).

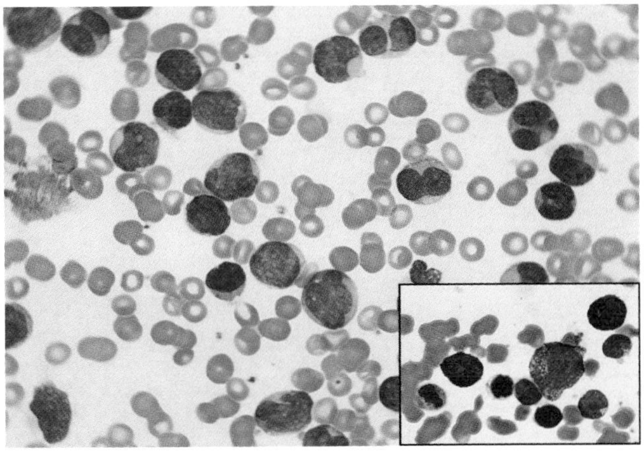

FIGURE 23-17 ■ AMML demonstrates myeloid blasts and immature monocytic cells; scattered cells with eo-baso- granules were evident **(inset)**.

Acute Myeloid Leukemia with inv (16)

Acute myelomonocytic leukemia (AMML) with bone marrow eosinophilia is often associated with inv16(p13q22) and CBFb-MYH11 fusion gene formation (Figure 23-16). Another translocation that is less commonly identified is t(16;16). Together, these are seen in approximately 10% of pediatric patients. This subtype may be associated with extramedullary myeloid cell tumors (myeloid sarcoma). The bone marrow eosinophils often exhibit mixed eosinophil-basophil granules (8) (Figure 23-17). However, not all cases with this cytogenetic abnormality exhibit eosinophilia or AMML morphology. Prognosis is good with high likelihood of cure by chemotherapy and prolonged disease free course (102,116).

AML with 11q23 Abnormalities

11q23 is the defining translocation in this AML with multiple partner genes. In children, the MLL gene rearrangement is most frequently noted in congenital myeloid leukemias, often monoblastic, especially in t(4;11) (31,74,164). The MLL gene rearrangement also typifies the therapy-related monocytic/monoblastic leukemias that occur following topoisomerase II inhibitor therapy (Figure 23-18). These occur 1 to 3 years after epipodophyllotoxin or related therapies and are characterized by the abrupt onset of cytopenias and bone marrow effacement by promonocytes/monoblasts. Although initial remissions are generally achieved, the overall outcome is poor in therapy-related AML with 11q23 translocations (150,153).

AML with Monosomy 7

This abnormality is much more commonly seen in pediatric myelodysplasias; however, approximately 5% to 7% of pediatric de novo AML cases are associated with monosomy 7. The vast majority occurs in patients with a preceding history of myelodysplasia, monosomy 7, or chronic myelomonocytic leukemia. (89,110,142). The prognosis is uniformly poor.

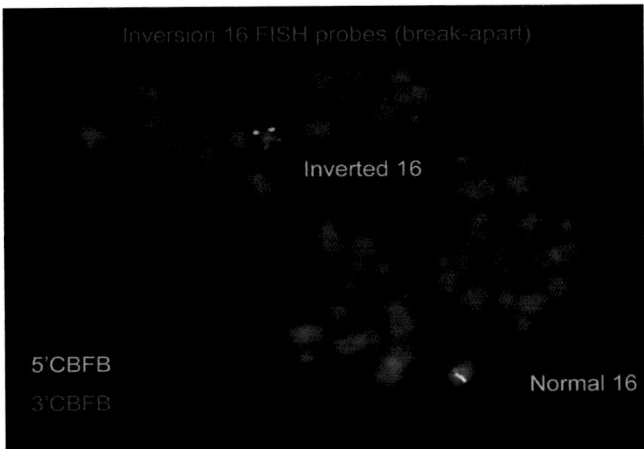

FIGURE 23-16 ■ Florescent *in situ* hybridization (FISH) analysis of the AMML cells demonstrates inversion of chromosome 16 utilizing break-apart FISH probes (*two green, two red signals*).

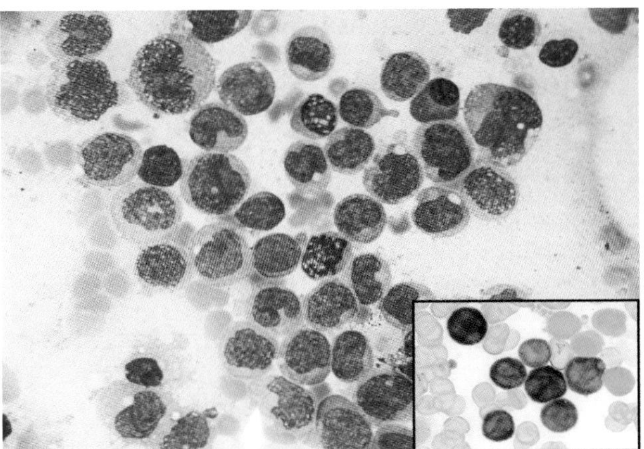

FIGURE 23-18 ■ 11q23-associated acute monocytic leukemia evolving in post-therapy setting; the monocytic nature is confirmed by NSE staining **(inset)**.

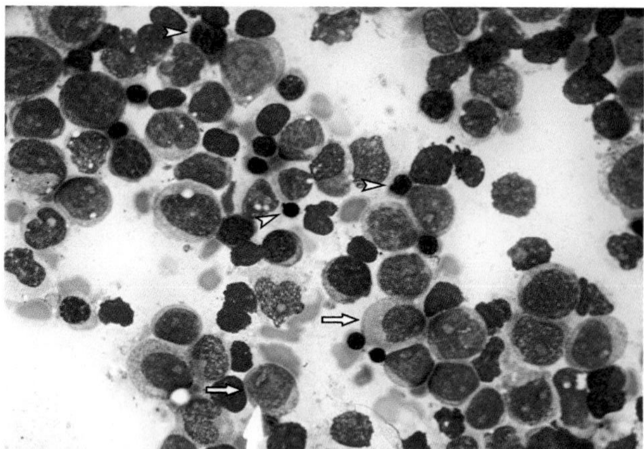

FIGURE 23-19 ■ Acute myeloid leukemia evolved from myelodysplastic syndrome. Note dyserythropoiesis (*arrowheads*) and abnormally granular myelocytes with nuclear cytoplasmic asynchrony (*arrows*).

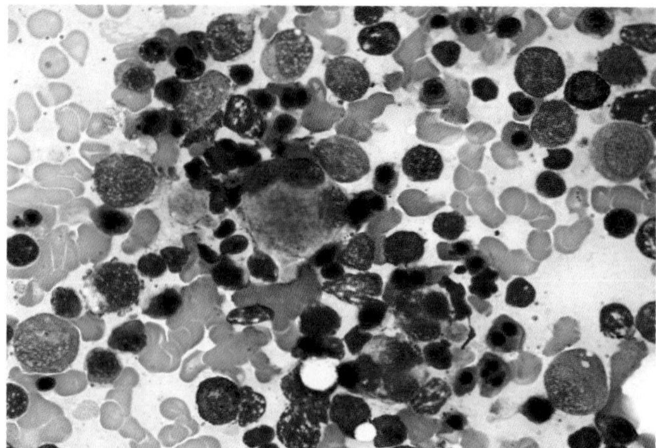

FIGURE 23-20 ■ Severe dyserythropoiesis and myeloid left shift in a young patient with leukocytosis, anemia, and thrombocytopenia. Note megakaryocyte with separate lobes (center field). Cytogenetic studies showed complex cytogenetics including del(7).

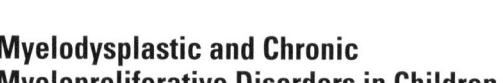

Myelodysplastic and Chronic Myeloproliferative Disorders in Children

In young children, a chronic myelodysplastic/myeloproliferative disorder is characterized by leukocytosis with both neutrophilia and monocytosis, a left shift to blasts, multilineage dyspoiesis, anemia, and thrombocytopenia (Figure 23-19; Table 23-16). Typically, hepatosplenomegaly and skin lesions also develop (48,109,120). In some children, a constitutional monosomy 7 has been identified, and the term *infantile monosomy 7 syndrome* has been utilized to describe such cases. In other infants, a very similar blood, bone marrow, and clinical picture develops in conjunction with increased levels of hemoglobin F and various RAS or NF1 gene mutations (48,57,176). The latter disease, originally termed *juvenile chronic myelogenous leukemia* (*CML*) and later called *juvenile myelomonocytic leukemia*, is differentiated from CML by the Philadelphia chromosome-breakpoint cluster region-abl gene rearrangement (58,60,61). Despite the disparate terminology, so-called infantile monosomy 7 syndrome and juvenile myelomonocytic leukemias are currently thought to comprise a spectrum of infantile myelodysplastic/myeloproliferative processes that are frequently associated with monosomy 7/del(7q) (109,120). The WHO Working Group placed these disorders into a hybrid "myelodysplastic/myeloproliferative disease" category to distinguish them from both conventional chronic myeloproliferative disorders and "adult-type" myelodysplasia (77).

Conventional chronic myeloproliferative disorders, including CML (Ph+), also occur in children. CML accounts for approximately 5% of childhood leukemias and usually affects adolescents; cases in earlier childhood have been reported (58,165). Clinical manifestations and course of Ph+ CML are similar to adult cases. In addition, rare reports describe familial/constitutional myeloproliferative disorders, including essential thrombocythemia and chronic idiopathic myelofibrosis (44,90,170). "Adult-type" myelodysplastic syndromes, characterized by cytopenias and multilineage dysplasia, also affect children (Figure 23-20). The children are typically older and, in some cases, the condition is therapy related.

Table 23-16 ■ MYELODYSPLASTIC DISORDERS IN CHILDHOOD

I. Patients ≤5 years
• Hybrid myelodysplastic/myeloproliferative picture
• Leukocytosis with monocytosis, left shift, dysplasia
• Frequent extramedullary disease with organomegaly, lymphadenopathy
• Association with constitutional genetic/immune disorders
• Striking incidence of monosomy 7
• Male predominance
• Terms infantile monosomy 7 syndrome, juvenile CML (JCML), CMML, and JMML used
• Variable disease course, overall poor prognosis
II. Patients ≥5 years
• Typical features of "adult" type MDS
• Includes therapy-related cases
• More high-grade forms of MDS predominate
• Monosomy 7 common finding but often have other cytogenetic

NEOPLASTIC HISTIOCYTIC DISORDERS IN BONE MARROW

Neoplastic Histiocytoses

Clonal disorders characterized by increased numbers of bone marrow monocytes/histiocytes include acute and chronic monocytic/myelomonocytic leukemias (described earlier), Langerhans cell histiocytosis, and malignant histiocytosis/histiocytic sarcoma. Minimal-to-extensive bone marrow involvement is evident in at least 20% of patients with multisystem Langerhans cell histiocytosis (7), and

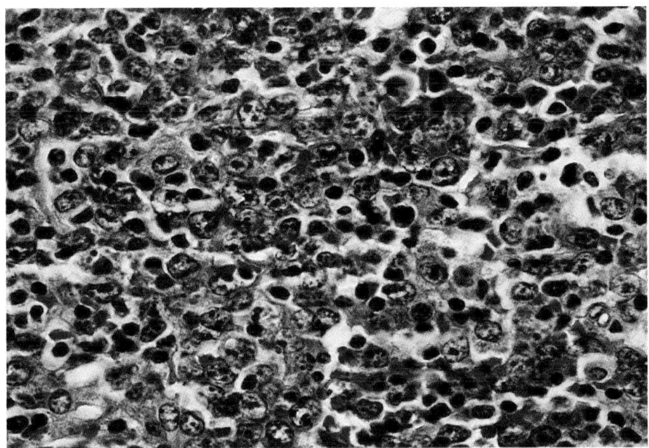

FIGURE 23-21 ■ Histiocytic sarcoma extensively involves spleen in a patient with disseminated malignant histiocytosis. Anaplastic large cell lymphoma must be ruled out.

patients with extensive bone marrow replacement often exhibit pancytopenia and extensive extramedullary disease, associated with a poor prognosis. On smear preparations, the nuclear chromatin of Langerhans cells is delicately clumped, and the cytoplasm is abundant and pale and may contain vacuoles or granules. More characteristic Langerhans cell morphology is appreciated on clot or biopsy sections in the form of small, inconspicuous clusters (169) or discrete collections of cells with admixed neutrophils, eosinophils, and multinucleated giant cells. Other nonspecific abnormalities, such as eosinophilia and mild reticulin fibrosis, may be present. S100 and CD1a are useful immunophenotypic markers for Langerhans cell histiocytosis, and both stains can be performed on paraffin sections (169).

The bone marrow infiltrates in cases of so-called malignant histiocytosis (proposed WHO designation of disseminated histiocytic sarcoma), unlike those in acute and chronic leukemias, are often inconspicuous, accounting for only a minority of the total nucleated cells (72). Malignant histiocytosis/histiocytic sarcoma is characterized by a diffuse admixture of hematopoietic elements, very large cells, and marked nuclear atypia (Figure 23-21). If present, phagocytosis is minimal. On biopsy sections, the cells are either individually dispersed or in small clusters and easily overlooked. The immunophenotypic features of malignant histiocytosis are somewhat variable, but most cells express myeloid and monocytic antigens, whereas others appear more akin to immune accessory cells, demonstrating S100, CD21, and/or CD35 reactivity (181). Although often weak, nonspecific esterase (NSE) activity is a useful marker for these cells.

The morphologic and clinical features of several disorders substantially overlap with those of malignant histiocytosis, including hemophagocytic lymphohistiocytosis, anaplastic large cell lymphoma expressing Ki-1 antigen, acute monoblastic leukemias, and rare NK-cell and B-cell lymphomas (46,131,133). The distinction between malignant histiocytosis and anaplastic large cell lymphoma is based on immunophenotypic, cytogenetic, and molecular studies. Unlike malignant histiocytosis/histiocytic sarcoma, anaplastic large cell lymphomas are usually T-cell neoplasms with a unique chromosomal abnormality, t(2;5)(p23;q35), if ALK positive (14). Because T-cell neoplasms, and more rarely NK-cell or B-cell neoplasms, can closely mimic histiocytic sarcoma, immunophenotyping and molecular techniques should be used to exclude more common T-, NK-, or B-cell neoplasm in cases of possible histiocytic sarcoma (20,46,133).

The distinction between malignant histiocytosis/histiocytic sarcoma and acute monoblastic leukemia is occasionally problematic and somewhat semantic, as both neoplasms are derived from the same hematopoietic lineage. Correct diagnosis of malignant histiocytosis reportedly occurs with a frequency of 0.5 to 1/1,000 compared to other malignant lymphomas (101). Some authors recommend using the percentage of neoplastic cells in bone marrow to distinguish between monocytic leukemia (≥25% blasts) and malignant histiocytosis/histiocytic sarcoma (<25% malignant cells in bone marrow) (20). Presence of a mass lesion, cytologic dysplasia, and immunophenotypic studies in addition to the clinical presentation are helpful in establishing the correct diagnosis. Historically, an incorrect diagnosis of malignant histiocytoses has been rendered in the setting of a histiocyte-rich lymphoma with a relatively small lymphoid component, or in the setting of anaplastic large cell lymphoma (histiocytic variant) or in the setting of hemophagocytic syndrome which causes life-threatening illness and raises concern of a hematopoietic malignancy (21,113).

Histiocytoses of Varied Biologic Behavior

This group of disorders is characterized by an unpredictable biologic behavior and includes dendritic cell–related disorders for example xanthogranuloma disseminatum (within the family of juvenile xanthogranuloma "JXG"; systemic JXG) and macrophage-related disorders ranging from benign hemophagocytic histiocytoses to solitary histiocytomas to name a few (24,54).

Metastatic Disorders in Bone Marrow

The incidence of metastasis of childhood solid tumors to bone marrow is quite variable. A significant contributing factor is the adequacy of the bone marrow biopsy sample for optimal staging. Marrow metastases are frequently seen in neuroblastomas, peripheral neuroectodermal tumor, rhabdomyosarcoma, synovial sarcoma, and lymphomas. The metastatic rates are extremely low for Wilms tumor, hepatoblastomas, and retinoblastomas (37,154,155). In children, metastatic small blue cell tumors, such as Ewing sarcoma, rhabdomyosarcoma, retinoblastoma, and neuroblastoma, may exhibit blast-like nuclear features and can be seen individually dispersed on aspirate smears, closely mimicking acute leukemia in bone marrow (3,37,45,76,80,147) (Figure 23-22). In fact, neuroblastoma ranks as the second most frequent cause of bone marrow infiltration in children;

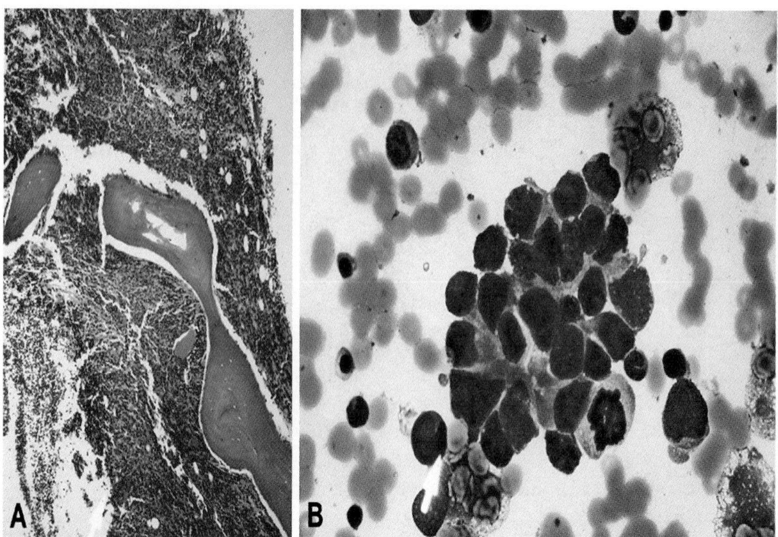

FIGURE 23-22 ■ **A, B:** Bone marrow biopsy shows extensive effacement by metastatic neuroblastoma. The malignant cells tend to form cohesive clusters in the smear; a mimic of leukemia.

the first being ALL. Confusion with acute leukemia is especially likely when the primary lesion is occult and when the bone marrow is extensively replaced by metastatic tumor. Although some evidence of tumor cell cohesion is usually apparent on aspirate smears or biopsy sections, a variety of immunologic techniques can be used to distinguish these metastatic lesions conclusively from a primary hematologic neoplasm. Immunoperoxidase staining for various solid tumor-associated antigens can be employed and bone marrow biopsies are considered more effective in diagnosis of metastatic disease as the aspirates are often "aspicular" due to fibrosis (201).

Bone Marrow Transplantation

Bone marrow transplantation is currently available as a therapeutic option for a variety of neoplastic and non-neoplastic disorders (5,82). It is particularly considered as an option in refractory acute leukemias and lymphomas and untreatable solid tumors (84). Two kinds of bone marrow transplants are usually available: autologous and allogeneic (HLA-matched donor). The concept behind bone marrow transplantation is reconstitution of normal bone marrow elements after cure of the pathologic marrow. In diseases involving clonal stem cell abnormalities, an allogeneic transplant is the best chance for curing the disease. This follows intense chemotherapy with or without total body irradiation to eradicate the bone marrow and immune cells as well as the neoplastic cells. In other instances, collections of bone marrow or peripheral blood stem cells from the patient may be used for an autologous bone marrow transplantation (172). This does not require marrow ablation and can be performed if the bone marrow is free of neoplastic process. Autologous transplantation does not carry the risk of serious complications associated with allogeneic transplants such as graft versus host disease, post-transplant lymphoproliferative disorders, myelodysplasia, secondary hematologic malignancies, solid tumors, and graft rejection (190).

Morphologic Expectations in Post-Transplant Bone Marrow Samples

In the immediate post-transplant period (1 to 7 days), findings resemble chemoablation, *that is*, bone marrow fibrosis, serous atrophy, and nonspecific edema with a predominance of stromal cells (162). Bone marrow engraftment starts as early as 7 days and is characterized by small colonies of red blood cells (which usually appear first), followed by white blood cells and megakaryocytes (39). Peripheral blood counts recover in the same general order (193). Failure of bone marrow cellularity to normalize (50% of normal cellularity by day 21) and persistent peripheral cytopenia is a significant cause for concern of graft failure (failure of transplanted cells to engraft by day 28). Significant increase in peripheral blood counts may, on the other hand, herald recurrence of primary disease or cytokine effect (23). Once graft failure has been excluded as a potential cause, engraftment status and recurrence of disease is monitored.

REFERENCES

1. Alexander FE, Chan LC, Lam TH, et al. Clustering of childhood leukaemia in Hong Kong: association with the childhood peak and common acute lymphoblastic leukaemia and with population mixing. *Br J Cancer* 1997;75(3):457–463.
2. Allman D, Miller JP. B cell development and receptor diversity during aging. *Curr Opin Immunol* 2005;17(5):463–467.
3. Almanaseer IY, Trujillo YP, Taxy JB, et al. Systemic rhabdomyosarcoma with diffuse bone marrow involvement. Case report of an unusual presentation. *Am J Clin Pathol* 1984;82(3):349–353.
4. Alter BP, Young, NS. The bone marrow failure syndromes. In: *Hematology of infancy and childhood.* Philadelphia, PA: WB Saunders, 1993:216.
5. Amylon MD, Co JP, Snyder DS, et al. Allogeneic bone marrow transplant in pediatric patients with high-risk hematopoietic malignancies early in the course of their disease. *J Pediatr Hematol Oncol* 1997;19(1):54–61.
6. Andrews NC, Erdjument-Bromage H, Davidson MB, et al. Erythroid transcription factor NF-E2 is a haematopoietic-specific basic-leucine zipper protein. *Nature* 1993;362(6422):722–728.

7. Arico M, Egeler RM. Clinical aspects of Langerhans cell histiocytosis. *Hematol Oncol Clin North Am* 1998;12(2):247–258.
8. Arthur DC, Bloomfield CD. Partial deletion of the long arm of chromosome 16 and bone marrow eosinophilia in acute nonlymphocytic leukemia: a new association. *Blood* 1983;61(5):994–998.
9. Avet-Loiseau H, Mechinaud F, Harousseau JL. Clonal hematologic disorders in Down syndrome. A review. *J Pediatr Hematol Oncol* 1995;17(1):19–24.
10. Beardsley D. Platelet abnormalities in infancy and childhood. In: *Hematology of infancy and childhood*. Philadelphia, PA: WB Saunders, 1993:216.
11. Bennett JM, Catovsky D, Daniel MT, et al. The morphological classification of acute lymphoblastic leukaemia: concordance among observers and clinical correlations. *Br J Haematol* 1981;47(4): 553–561.
12. Bennett JM, Catovsky D, Daniel MT, et al. Proposals for the classification of the acute leukaemias. French-American-British (FAB) co-operative group. *Br J Haematol* 1976;33(4):451–458.
13. Bhatia S, Neglia JP. Epidemiology of childhood acute myelogenous leukemia. *J Pediatr Hematol Oncol* 1995;17(2):94–100.
14. Bitter MA, Franklin WA, Larson RA, et al. Morphology in Ki-1(CD30)-positive non-Hodgkin's lymphoma is correlated with clinical features and the presence of a unique chromosomal abnormality, t(2;5)(p23;q35). *Am J Surg Pathol* 1990;14(4):305–316.
15. Borowitz MJ, Guenther KL, Shults KE, et al. Immunophenotyping of acute leukemia by flow cytometric analysis. Use of CD45 and right-angle light scatter to gate on leukemic blasts in three-color analysis. *Am J Clin Pathol* 1993;100(5):534–540.
16. Brown DC, Gatter KC. The bone marrow trephine biopsy: a review of normal histology. *Histopathology* 1993;22(5):411–422.
17. Brugnara C. Reference values in infancy and childhood. In: *Hematology of infancy and childhood*. Philadelphia, PA: WB Saunders, 1998.
18. Brunning R. Normal bone marrow. In: *Tumors of the bone marrow. Atlas of tumor pathology*. Washington, DC: Armed Forces Institute of Pathology, 1994:2–18.
19. Brunning R, McKenna RW. Acute leukemias. In: *Tumors of the bone marrow. Atlas of tumor pathology*. Washington, DC: Armed Forces Institute of Pathology, 1994:19–142.
20. Bucsky P, Egeler RM. Malignant histiocytic disorders in children. Clinical and therapeutic approaches with a nosologic discussion. *Hematol Oncol Clin North Am* 1998;2(2):465–471.
21. Bucsky P, Favara B, Feller AC, et al. Malignant histiocytosis and large cell anaplastic (Ki-1) lymphoma in childhood: guidelines for differential diagnosis–report of the Histiocyte Society. *Med Pediatr Oncol* 1994;22(3):200–203.
22. Bussel J, Corrigan JJ. Platelet and vascular disorders. In: *Blood disease of infancy and childhood*. Mosby: St. Louis, 1995:866.
23. Byrne JL, Haynes AP, Russell NH. Use of haemopoietic growth factors: commentary on the ASCO/ECOG guidelines. American Society of Clinical Oncology/Eastern Co-operative Oncology Group. *Blood Rev* 1997;11(1):16–27.
24. Calverly DC, Wismer J, Rosenthal D, et al. Xanthoma disseminatum in an infant with skeletal and marrow involvement. *J Pediatr Hematol Oncol* 1995;17(1):61–65.
25. Carroll A, Civin C, Schneider N, et al. The t(1;22) (p13;q13) is nonrandom and restricted to infants with acute megakaryoblastic leukemia: a Pediatric Oncology Group Study. *Blood* 1991;78(3): 748–752.
26. Case J, Horvath TL, Howell JC, et al. Clonal multilineage differentiation of murine common pluripotent stem cells isolated from skeletal muscle and adipose stromal cells. *Ann N Y Acad Sci* 2005;1044:183–200.
27. Cerezo L, Shuster JJ, Pullen DJ, et al. Laboratory correlates and prognostic significance of granular acute lymphoblastic leukemia in children. A Pediatric Oncology Group study. *Am J Clin Pathol* 1991;95(4):526–531.
28. Chambon P. A decade of molecular biology of retinoic acid receptors. *Faseb J* 1996;10(9):940–954.
29. Charbord P, Moore K. Gene expression in stem cell-supporting stromal cell lines. *Ann N Y Acad Sci* 2005;1044:159–167.
30. Chen LT, Weiss L. The development of vertebral bone marrow of human fetuses. *Blood* 1975;46(3):389–408.
31. Cimino G, Rapanotti MC, Rivolta A, et al. Prognostic relevance of ALL-1 gene rearrangement in infant acute leukemias. *Leukemia* 1995;9(3):391–395.
32. Creutzig U, Ritter J, Vormoor J, et al. Myelodysplasia and acute myelogenous leukemia in Down's syndrome. A report of 40 children of the AML-BFM Study Group. *Leukemia* 1996;10(11):1677–1686.
33. Dame C, Juul SE. The switch from fetal to adult erythropoiesis. *Clin Perinatol* 2000;27(3):507–526.
34. Davis BH, Foucar K, Szczarkowski W, et al. U.S.-Canadian Consensus recommendations on the immunophenotypic analysis of hematologic neoplasia by flow cytometry: medical indications. *Cytometry* 1997;30(5):249–263.
35. Dayton VD, Arthur DC, Gajl-Peczalska KJ, et al. L3 acute lymphoblastic leukemia. Comparison with small noncleaved cell lymphoma involving the bone marrow. *Am J Clin Pathol* 1994;101(2): 130–139.
36. Delaunay J. Red cell membrane and erythropoiesis genetic defects. *Hematol J* 2003;4(4):225–232.
37. Delta BG, Pinkel D. Bone marrow aspiration in children with malignant tumors. *J Pediatr* 1964;64:542–546.
38. Desai SR, Ranade SR. Congenital amegakaryocytic thrombocytopenia (CAMT): a case report with review of literature. *Indian J Pathol Microbiol* 2007;50(3):659–660.
39. Dick F, Gingrich RD. Biopsy analysis in bone marrow transplantation. In: *Transplant pathology*. Chicago: ASCP, Press, 1994: 281–292.
40. Dokal I. Fanconi's anaemia and related bone marrow failure syndromes. *Br Med Bull* 2006;77–78:37–53.
41. Dokal I, Vulliamy T. Inherited aplastic anaemias/bone marrow failure syndromes. *Blood Rev* 2008;22(3):141–153.
42. Doyle JJ, Thorner P, Poon A, et al. Transient leukemia followed by megakaryoblastic leukemia in a child with mosaic Down syndrome. *Leuk Lymphoma* 1995;17(3–4):345–350.
43. Dreyfus M, Kaplan C, Verdy E, et al. Frequency of immune thrombocytopenia in newborns: a prospective study. Immune Thrombocytopenia Working Group. *Blood* 1997;89(12):4402–4406.
44. Dror Y, Zipursky A, Blanchette VS. Essential thrombocythemia in children. *J Pediatr Hematol Oncol* 1999;21(5):356–363.
45. DuBois SG, Kalika Y, Lukens JN, et al. Metastatic sites in stage IV and IVS neuroblastoma correlate with age, tumor biology, and survival. *J Pediatr Hematol Oncol* 1999;21(3):181–189.
46. Egeler RM, Schmitz L, Sonneveld P, et al. Malignant histiocytosis: a reassessment of cases formerly classified as histiocytic neoplasms and review of the literature. *Med Pediatr Oncol* 1995;25(1):1–7.
47. Ellis MH, Avraham H, Groopman JE. The regulation of megakaryocytopoiesis. *Blood Rev* 1995;9(1):1–6.
48. Emanuel PD. Myelodysplasia and myeloproliferative disorders in childhood: an update. *Br J Haematol* 1999;105(4):852–863.
49. Erslev AJ, Soltan A. Pure red-cell aplasia: a review. *Blood Rev* 1996;10(1):20–28.
50. Ess KC, Witte DP, Bascomb CP, et al. Diverse developing mouse lineages exhibit high-level c-Myb expression in immature cells and loss of expression upon differentiation. *Oncogene* 1999;18(4): 1103–1111.
51. Estey E, Thall P, Beran M, et al. Effect of diagnosis (refractory anemia with excess blasts, refractory anemia with excess blasts in transformation, or acute myeloid leukemia [AML]) on outcome of AML-type chemotherapy. *Blood* 1997;90(8):2969–2977.
52. Evans T. Developmental biology of hematopoiesis. *Hematol Oncol Clin North Am* 1997;11(6):1115–1147.
53. Faderl S, Kantarjian HM, Talpaz M, et al. Clinical significance of cytogenetic abnormalities in adult acute lymphoblastic leukemia. *Blood* 1998;91(11):3995–4019.

54. Favara BE, Feller AC, Pauli M, et al. Contemporary classification of histiocytic disorders. The WHO Committee On Histiocytic/Reticulum Cell Proliferations. Reclassification Working Group of the Histiocyte Society. *Med Pediatr Oncol* 1997;29(3):157–166.
55. Federman N, Sakamoto KM. The genetic basis of bone marrow failure syndromes in children. *Mol Genet Metab* 2005;86(1–2):100–109.
56. Fenaux P, Chomienne C, Degos L. Acute promyelocytic leukemia: biology and treatment. *Semin Oncol* 1997;24(1):92–102.
57. Flotho C, Valcamonica S, Mach-Pascual S, et al. RAS mutations and clonality analysis in children with juvenile myelomonocytic leukemia (JMML). *Leukemia* 1999;13(1):32–37.
58. Foucar K. Chronic leukemias in childhood. In: *Pediatric hematopathology*. New York: Churchill Livingstone, 2001.
59. Foucar K. Hematopoiesis. In: *Bone marrow pathology*. Chicago, IL: ASCP Press, 2001:1–29.
60. Foucar K. Myelodysplastic syndrome. In: *Bone marrow pathology*. Chicago: ASCP Press, 2001:224–261.
61. Foucar K. Neonatal hematopathology: special considerations. In: *Pediatric hematopathology*. New York: Churchill Livingstone, 2001.
62. Foucar K. Special considerations for bone marrow evaluation in children. In: *Bone marrow pathology*. Chicago, IL: ASCP Press, 2001: 586–607.
63. Foucar K, Foucar E. The mononuclear phagocyte and immunoregulatory effector (M-PIRE) system: evolving concepts. *Semin Diagn Pathol* 1990;7(1):4–18.
64. Foucar K, Friedman K, Llewellyn A, et al. Prenatal diagnosis of transient myeloproliferative disorder via percutaneous umbilical blood sampling. Report of two cases in fetuses affected by Down's syndrome. *Am J Clin Pathol* 1992;97(4):584–590.
65. Freyssinier JM, Lecoq-Lafon C, Amsellem S, et al. Purification, amplification and characterization of a population of human erythroid progenitors. *Br J Haematol* 1999;106(4):912–922.
66. Friebert SE, Shepardson LB, Shurin SB, et al. Pediatric bone marrow cellularity: are we expecting too much? *J Pediatr Hematol Oncol* 1998;20(5):439–443.
67. Ganapathi KA, Shimamura A. Ribosomal dysfunction and inherited marrow failure. *Br J Haematol* 2008;141(3):376–387.
68. Geijtenbeek TB, van Kooyk Y, van Vliet SJ, et al. High frequency of adhesion defects in B-lineage acute lymphoblastic leukemia. *Blood* 1999;94(2):754–764.
69. Germeshausen M, Schulze H, Gaudig A, et al. Congenital amegakaryocytic thrombocytopenia (CAMT) - a defect of the thrombopoietin receptor c-Mpl. *Klin Padiatr* 2001;213(4):155–161.
70. Ghosh K. Transient abnormal myelopoiesis in Down's syndrome–are some of them truly leukaemic? *Leuk Res* 1992;16(5):545–546.
71. Giri N, Kang E, Tisdale JF, et al. Clinical and laboratory evidence for a trilineage haematopoietic defect in patients with refractory Diamond-Blackfan anaemia. *Br J Haematol* 2000;108(1):167–175.
72. Gogusev J, Nezelof C. Malignant histiocytosis. Histologic, cytochemical, chromosomal, and molecular data with a nosologic discussion. *Hematol Oncol Clin North Am* 1998;12(2):445–463.
73. Goordyal P, Isaacson PG. Immunocytochemical characterization of monocyte colonies of human bone marrow: a clue to the origin of Langerhans cells and interdigitating reticulum cells. *J Pathol* 1985;146(3):189–195.
74. Greaves MF. Infant leukaemia biology, aetiology and treatment. *Leukemia* 1996;10(2):372–377.
75. Griesinger F, Piro-Noack M, Kaib N, et al. Leukaemia-associated immunophenotypes (LAIP) are observed in 90% of adult and childhood acute lymphoblastic leukaemia: detection in remission marrow predicts outcome. *Br J Haematol* 1999;105(1):241–255.
76. Hachitanda Y, Hata J. Stage IVS neuroblastoma: a clinical, histological, and biological analysis of 45 cases. *Hum Pathol* 1996;27(11):1135–1138.
77. Harris NL, Jaffe ES, Diebold J, et al. World Health Organization classification of neoplastic diseases of the hematopoietic and lymphoid tissues: report of the Clinical Advisory Committee meeting-Airlie House, Virginia, November 1997. *J Clin Oncol* 1999;17(12):3835–3849.
78. Hashimoto S, Suzuki T, Dong HY, et al. Serial analysis of gene expression in human monocytes and macrophages. *Blood* 1999;94(3):837–844.
79. Head DR. Revised classification of acute myeloid leukemia. *Leukemia* 1996;10(11):1826–1831.
80. Head DR, Kennedy PS, Goyette RE. Metastatic neuroblastoma in bone marrow aspirate smears. *Am J Clin Pathol* 1979;72(6):1008–1011.
81. Heimpel H, Wilts H, Hirschmann WD, et al. Aplastic crisis as a complication of congenital dyserythropoietic anemia type II. *Acta Haematol* 2007;117(2):115–118.
82. Heslop HE. Haemopoietic stem cell transplantation from unrelated donors. *Br J Haematol* 1999;105(1):2–6.
83. Hitzler JK, Cheung J, Li Y, et al. GATA1 mutations in transient leukemia and acute megakaryoblastic leukemia of Down syndrome. *Blood* 2003;101(11):4301–4304.
84. Hongeng S, Krance RA, Bowman LC, et al. Outcomes of transplantation with matched-sibling and unrelated-donor bone marrow in children with leukaemia. *Lancet* 1997;350(9080):767–771.
85. Horwitz M. The genetics of familial leukemia. *Leukemia* 1997;11(8):1347–1359.
86. Hurwitz CA, Raimondi SC, Head D, et al. Distinctive immunophenotypic features of t(8;21)(q22;q22) acute myeloblastic leukemia in children. *Blood* 1992;80(12):3182–3188.
87. Jaffe ES. Acute myeloid leukemia and myelodysplastic syndrome, therapy related. In: Jaffe E, Harris NL, Stein H, et al., eds. *Pathology and genetics of tumours of haematopoietic and lymphoid tissues*. Lyon. IARC Press; 2001:75–104.
88. Jelic TM, Raj AB, Jin B, et al. Expression of CD5 on hematogones in a 7-year-old girl with Shwachman-Diamond syndrome. *Pediatr Dev Pathol* 2001;4(5):505–511.
89. Johnson E, Cotter FE. Monosomy 7 and 7q–associated with myeloid malignancy. *Blood Rev* 1997;11(1):46–55.
90. Kapoor G, Correa H, Yu LC. Essential thrombocythemia in an infant. *J Pediatr Hematol Oncol* 1996;18(4):381–383.
91. Katayama Y, Battista M, Kao WM, et al. Signals from the sympathetic nervous system regulate hematopoietic stem cell egress from bone marrow. *Cell* 2006;124(2):407–421.
92. Kaushansky K. The molecular mechanisms that control thrombopoiesis. *J Clin Invest* 2005;115(12):3339–3347.
93. Keohane EM. Acquired aplastic anemia. *Clin Lab Sci* 2004;17(3):165–171.
94. Khalidi HS, Chang KL, Medeiros LJ, et al. Acute lymphoblastic leukemia. Survey of immunophenotype, French-American-British classification, frequency of myeloid antigen expression, and karyotypic abnormalities in 210 pediatric and adult cases. *Am J Clin Pathol* 1999;111(4):467–476.
95. Klemsz MJ, McKercher SR, Celada A, et al. The macrophage and B cell-specific transcription factor PU.1 is related to the ets oncogene. *Cell* 1990;61(1):113–124.
96. Klupp N, Simonitsch I, Mannhalter C, et al. Emergence of an unusual bone marrow precursor B-cell population in fatal Shwachman-Diamond syndrome. *Arch Pathol Lab Med* 2000;124(9):1379–1381.
97. Krajinovic M, Labuda D, Richer C, et al. Susceptibility to childhood acute lymphoblastic leukemia: influence of CYP1A1, CYP2D6, GSTM1, and GSTT1 genetic polymorphisms. *Blood* 1999;93(5):1496–1501.
98. Krawczuk-Rybak M, Zak J, Jaworowska B. A lineage switch from AML to ALL with persistent translocation t(4;11) in congenital leukemia. *Med Pediatr Oncol* 2003;41(1):95–96.
99. Kurahashi H, Hara J, Yumura-Yagi K, et al. Monoclonal nature of transient abnormal myelopoiesis in Down's syndrome. *Blood* 1991;77(6):1161–1163.

100. Lasser A. The mononuclear phagocytic system: a review. *Hum Pathol* 1983;14(2):108–126.
101. Lauritzen AF, Ralfkiaer E. Histiocytic sarcomas. *Leuk Lymphoma* 1995;18(1–2):73–80.
102. Le Beau MM, Larson RA, Bitter MA, et al. Association of an inversion of chromosome 16 with abnormal marrow eosinophils in acute myelomonocytic leukemia. A unique cytogenetic-clinicopathological association. *N Engl J Med* 1983;309(11):630–636.
103. Levanon D, Negreanu V, Bernstein Y, et al. AML1, AML2, and AML3, the human members of the runt domain gene-family: cDNA structure, expression, and chromosomal localization. *Genomics* 1994;23(2):425–432.
104. Lion T, Haas OA, Harbott J, et al. The translocation t(1;22)(p13;q13) is a nonrandom marker specifically associated with acute megakaryocytic leukemia in young children. *Blood* 1992;79(12):3325–3330.
105. Litz CE, Davies S, Brunning RD, et al. Acute leukemia and the transient myeloproliferative disorder associated with Down syndrome: morphologic, immunophenotypic and cytogenetic manifestations. *Leukemia* 1995;9(9):1432–1439.
106. Longacre TA, Foucar K, Crago S, et al. Hematogones: a multiparameter analysis of bone marrow precursor cells. *Blood* 1989;73(2): 543–552.
107. Lotzova E. Definition and functions of natural killer cells. *Nat Immun* 1993;12(4–5):169–176.
108. Lucio P, Parreira A, van den Beemd MW, et al. Flow cytometric analysis of normal B cell differentiation: a frame of reference for the detection of minimal residual disease in precursor-B-ALL. *Leukemia* 1999;13(3):419–427.
109. Luna-Fineman S, Shannon KM, Atwater SK, et al. Myelodysplastic and myeloproliferative disorders of childhood: a study of 167 patients. *Blood* 1999;93(2):459–466.
110. Luna-Fineman S, Shannon KM, Lange BJ. Childhood monosomy 7: epidemiology, biology, and mechanistic implications. *Blood* 1995;85(8):1985–1999.
111. Lyman SD, Jacobsen SE. c-kit ligand and Flt3 ligand: stem/progenitor cell factors with overlapping yet distinct activities. *Blood* 1998;91(4):1101–1134.
112. Maestroni GJ. Sympathetic nervous system influence on the innate immune response. *Ann N Y Acad Sci* 2006;1069:195–207.
113. Malone M. The histiocytoses of childhood. *Histopathology* 1991;19(2):105–119.
114. Mandel M, Rechavi G, Neumann Y, et al. Bone marrow cell populations mimicking common acute lymphoblastic leukemia in infants with stage IV-S neuroblastoma. *Acta Haematol* 1991;86(2):86–89.
115. Marley SB, Lewis JL, Davidson RJ, et al. Evidence for a continuous decline in haemopoietic cell function from birth: application to evaluating bone marrow failure in children. *Br J Haematol* 1999;106(1):162–166.
116. Marlton P, Keating M, Kantarjian H, et al. Cytogenetic and clinical correlates in AML patients with abnormalities of chromosome 16. *Leukemia* 1995;9(6):965–971.
117. Marshall CJ, Thrasher AJ. The embryonic origins of human haematopoiesis. *Br J Haematol* 2001;112(4):838–850.
118. Martin DI, Zon LI, Mutter G, et al. Expression of an erythroid transcription factor in megakaryocytic and mast cell lineages. *Nature* 1990;344(6265):444–447.
119. Martinez-Climent JA. Molecular cytogenetics of childhood hematological malignancies. *Leukemia* 1997;11(12):1999–2021.
120. Martinez-Climent JA, Garcia-Conde J. Chromosomal rearrangements in childhood acute myeloid leukemia and myelodysplastic syndromes. *J Pediatr Hematol Oncol* 1999;21(2):91–102.
121. Massey GV, Zipursky A, Chang MN, et al. A prospective study of the natural history of transient leukemia (TL) in neonates with Down syndrome (DS): Children's Oncology Group (COG) study POG-9481. *Blood* 2006;107(12):4606–4613.
122. McCoy JP, Jr., Overton WR, Immunophenotyping of congenital leukemia. *Cytometry* 1995;22(2):85–88.
123. McKinstry WJ, Li CL, Rasko JE, et al. Cytokine receptor expression on hematopoietic stem and progenitor cells. *Blood* 1997;89(1):65–71.
124. Meeker TC, Hardy D, Willman C, et al. Activation of the interleukin-3 gene by chromosome translocation in acute lymphocytic leukemia with eosinophilia. *Blood* 1990;76(2):285–289.
125. Memon S, Shaikh S, Nizamani MA. Etiological spectrum of pancytopenia based on bone marrow examination in children. *J Coll Physicians Surg Pak* 2008;18(3):163–167.
126. Menasce LP, Banerjee SS, Beckett E, et al. Extra-medullary myeloid tumour (granulocytic sarcoma) is often misdiagnosed: a study of 26 cases. *Histopathology* 1999;34(5):391–398.
127. Metcalf D. Lineage commitment and maturation in hematopoietic cells: the case for extrinsic regulation. *Blood* 1998;92(2):345–347; discussion 352.
128. Mikkola HK, Gekas C, Orkin SH, et al. Placenta as a site for hematopoietic stem cell development. *Exp Hematol* 2005;33(9): 1048–1054.
129. Miyazaki R, Ogata H, Kobayashi Y. Requirement of thrombopoietin-induced activation of ERK for megakaryocyte differentiation and of p38 for erythroid differentiation. *Ann Hematol* 2001;80(5):284–291.
130. Moid F, DePalma L. Comparison of relative value of bone marrow aspirates and bone marrow trephine biopsies in the diagnosis of solid tumor metastasis and Hodgkin lymphoma: institutional experience and literature review. *Arch Pathol Lab Med* 2005;129(4):497–501.
131. Mongkonsritragoon W, Li CY, Phyliky RL. True malignant histiocytosis. *Mayo Clin Proc* 1998;73(6):520–528.
132. Moore TA, Zlotnik A. T-cell lineage commitment and cytokine responses of thymic progenitors. *Blood* 1995;86(5):1850–1860.
133. Murase T, Nakamura S, Tashiro K, et al. Malignant histiocytosis-like B-cell lymphoma, a distinct pathologic variant of intravascular lymphomatosis: a report of five cases and review of the literature. *Br J Haematol* 1997;99(3):656–664.
134. Naeim F. Topobiology in hematopoiesis. *Hematol Pathol* 1995;9(2):107–119.
135. Newland A, Evans T. ABC of clinical haematology. Haematological disorders at the extremes of life. *Br Med J* 1997;314:1262–1265.
136. Nucifora G, Dickstein JI, Torbenson V, et al. Correlation between cell morphology and expression of the AML1/ETO chimeric transcript in patients with acute myeloid leukemia without the t(8;21). *Leukemia* 1994;8(9):1533–1538.
137. Oberlin E, Tavian M, Blazsek I, et al. Blood-forming potential of vascular endothelium in the human embryo. *Development* 2002;129(17):4147–4157.
138. Orkin SH, Weiss MJ. Apoptosis. Cutting red-cell production. *Nature* 1999;401(6752):433, 435–436.
139. Palis J, Segel GB. Developmental biology of erythropoiesis. *Blood Rev* 1998;12(2):106–114.
140. Pang L, Weiss MJ, Poncz M. Megakaryocyte biology and related disorders. *J Clin Invest* 2005;115(12):3332–3338.
141. Pasqualetti P, Festuccia V, Acitelli P, et al. Tobacco smoking and risk of haematological malignancies in adults: a case-control study. *Br J Haematol* 1997;97(3):659–662.
142. Passmore SJ, Hann IM, Stiller CA, et al. Pediatric myelodysplasia: a study of 68 children and a new prognostic scoring system. *Blood* 1995;85(7):1742–1750.
143. Patel SR, Hartwig JH, Italiano JE, Jr. The biogenesis of platelets from megakaryocyte proplatelets. *J Clin Invest* 2005;115(12):3348–3354.
144. Pedersen-Bjergaard J, Pedersen M, Roulston D, et al. Different genetic pathways in leukemogenesis for patients presenting with therapy-related myelodysplasia and therapy-related acute myeloid leukemia. *Blood* 1995;86(9):3542–3552.
145. Perkins SL. Pediatric red cell disorders and pure red cell aplasia. *Am J Clin Pathol* 2004;122 (Suppl):S70–S86.
146. Peterson P, Ellis J. The development, morphology, and function of normal bone marrow: a review. In: *Polycythemia vera and the myeloproliferative disorders*. Philadelphia, PA: WB Saunders, 1995:1–13.

147. Pollak E, Miller H, Vye M. Medulloblastoma presenting as leukemia. *Am J Clin Pathol* 1981;76:98–103.
148. Porwit-MacDonald A, Janossy G, Ivory K, et al. Leukemia-associated changes identified by quantitative flow cytometry. IV. CD34 overexpression in acute myelogenous leukemia M2 with t(8;21). *Blood* 1996;87(3):1162–1169.
149. Pui CH, Crist WM. Biology and treatment of acute lymphoblastic leukemia. *J Pediatr* 1994;124(4):491–503.
150. Pui CH, Frankel LS, Carroll AJ, et al. Clinical characteristics and treatment outcome of childhood acute lymphoblastic leukemia with the t(4;11)(q21;q23): a collaborative study of 40 cases. *Blood* 1991;77(3):440–447.
151. Pui CH, Kane JR, Crist WM. Biology and treatment of infant leukemias. *Leukemia* 1995;9(5):762–769.
152. Pui CH, Raimondi SC, Dodge RK, et al. Prognostic importance of structural chromosomal abnormalities in children with hyperdiploid (greater than 50 chromosomes) acute lymphoblastic leukemia. *Blood* 1989;73(7):1963–1967.
153. Pui CH, Ribeiro RC, Campana D, et al. Prognostic factors in the acute lymphoid and myeloid leukemias of infants. *Leukemia* 1996;10(6):952–956.
154. Reid MM, Hamilton PJ. Histology of neuroblastoma involving bone marrow: the problem of detecting residual tumour after initiation of chemotherapy. *Br J Haematol* 1988;69(4):487–490.
155. Reid MM, Roald B. Adequacy of bone marrow trephine biopsy specimens in children. *J Clin Pathol* 1996:49(3):226–229.
156. Ribeiro RC, Abromowitch M, Raimondi SC, et al. Clinical and biologic hallmarks of the Philadelphia chromosome in childhood acute lymphoblastic leukemia. *Blood* 1987;70(4):948–953.
157. Rimsza LM, Larson RS, Winter SS, et al. Benign hematogone-rich lymphoid proliferations can be distinguished from B-lineage acute lymphoblastic leukemia by integration of morphology, immunophenotype, adhesion molecule expression, and architectural features. *Am J Clin Pathol* 2000;114(1):66–75.
158. Rimsza LM, Viswanatha DS, Winter SS, et al. The presence of CD34+ cell clusters predicts impending relapse in children with acute lymphoblastic leukemia receiving maintenance chemotherapy. *Am J Clin Pathol* 1998;110(3):313–320.
159. Robison LL, Nesbit ME, Jr., Sather HN, et al. Down syndrome and acute leukemia in children: a 10-year retrospective survey from Children's Cancer Study Group. *J Pediatr* 1984;105(2):235–242.
160. Roth MJ, Medeiros LJ, Elenitoba-Johnson K, et al. Extramedullary myeloid cell tumors. An immunohistochemical study of 29 cases using routinely fixed and processed paraffin-embedded tissue sections. *Arch Pathol Lab Med* 1995;119(9):790–798.
161. Rubnitz JE, Look AT. Molecular genetics of childhood leukemias. *J Pediatr Hematol Oncol* 1998;20(1):1–11.
162. Sale GE, Buckner CD. Pathology of bone marrow in transplant recipients. *Hematol Oncol Clin North Am* 1988;2(4):735–756.
163. Sanchez M, Alfani E, Visconti G, et al. Thymus-independent T-cell differentiation in vitro. *Br J Haematol* 1998;103(4):1198–1205.
164. Satake N, Maseki N, Nishiyama M, et al. Chromosome abnormalities and MLL rearrangements in acute myeloid leukemia of infants. *Leukemia* 1999;13(7):1013–1017.
165. Savage DG, Szydlo RM, Goldman JM. Clinical features at diagnosis in 430 patients with chronic myeloid leukaemia seen at a referral centre over a 16-year period. *Br J Haematol* 1997;96(1):111–116.
166. Sawada K, Fujishima N, Hirokawa M. Acquired pure red cell aplasia: updated review of treatment. *Br J Haematol* 2008;142(4):505–514.
167. Sawai N, Koike K, Mwamtemi HH, et al. Thrombopoietin augments stem cell factor-dependent growth of human mast cells from bone marrow multipotential hematopoietic progenitors. *Blood* 1999;93(11):3703–3712.
168. Schlieben S, Borkhardt A, Reinisch I, et al. Incidence and clinical outcome of children with BCR/ABL-positive acute lymphoblastic leukemia (ALL). A prospective RT-PCR study based on 673 patients enrolled in the German pediatric multicenter therapy trials ALL-BFM-90 and CoALL-05–92. *Leukemia* 1996;10(6):957–963.
169. Schmitz L, Favara BE. Nosology and pathology of Langerhans cell histiocytosis. *Hematol Oncol Clin North Am* 1998;12(2):221–246.
170. Sekhar M, Prentice HG, Popat U, et al. Idiopathic myelofibrosis in children. *Br J Haematol* 1996;93(2):394–397.
171. Shau H, Roth MD, Golub SH. Regulation of natural killer function by nonlymphoid cells. *Nat Immun* 1993;12(4–5):235–249.
172. Shen V, Woodbury C, Killen R, et al. Collection and use of peripheral blood stem cells in young children with refractory solid tumors. *Bone Marrow Transplant* 1997;19(3):197–204.
173. Shimamura A. Inherited bone marrow failure syndromes: molecular features. *Hematology Am Soc Hematol Educ Program* 2006:63–71.
174. Shimamura A. Shwachman-Diamond syndrome. *Semin Hematol* 2006;43(3):178–188.
175. Shimizu H, Culbert SJ, Cork A, et al. A lineage switch in acute monocytic leukemia. A case report. *Am J Pediatr Hematol Oncol* 1989;11(2):162–166.
176. Side LE, Emanuel PD, Taylor B, et al. Mutations of the NF1 gene in children with juvenile myelomonocytic leukemia without clinical evidence of neurofibromatosis, type 1. *Blood* 1998;92(1):267–272.
177. Sieff C, Nathan D, Clark S. The anatomy and physiology of hematopoiesis. In: *Hematology of infancy and childhood*. Philadelphia, PA: WB Saunders, 1998:161–236.
178. Sola MC, Rimsza LM, Christensen RD. A bone marrow biopsy technique suitable for use in neonates. *Br J Haematol* 1999;107(2):458–460.
179. Sorahan T, Prior P, Lancashire RJ, et al. Childhood cancer and parental use of tobacco: deaths from 1971 to 1976. *Br J Cancer* 1997;76(11):1525–1531.
180. Steiner LA, Gallagher PG. Erythrocyte disorders in the perinatal period. *Semin Perinatol* 2007;31(4):254–261.
181. Takeshita M, Kikuchi M, Ohshima K, et al. Bone marrow findings in malignant histiocytosis and/or malignant lymphoma with concurrent hemophagocytic syndrome. *Leuk Lymphoma* 1993.12(1–2):79–89.
182. Tallman MS. Differentiating therapy with all-trans retinoic acid in acute myeloid leukemia. *Leukemia* 1996;10(Suppl 1):S12–S15.
183. Tamary H, Alter BP. Current diagnosis of inherited bone marrow failure syndromes. *Pediatr Hematol Oncol* 2007;24(2):87–99.
184. Tavian M, Cortes F, Charbord P, et al. Emergence of the haematopoietic system in the human embryo and foetus. *Haematologica* 1999;84(Suppl EHA-4):1–3.
185. Tavian M, Peault B. Embryonic development of the human hematopoietic system. *Int J Dev Biol* 2005;49(2–3):243–250.
186. Tavian M, Zheng B, Oberlin E, et al. The vascular wall as a source of stem cells. *Ann N Y Acad Sci* 2005;1044:41–50.
187. Tchemia G. Eythroblastic and/or megakaryoblastic leukemia in Down's syndrome. *J Pediatr Hematol Oncol* 1996;18:59.
188. Tefferi A. JAK and MPL mutations in myeloid malignancies. *Leuk Lymphoma* 2008;49(3):388–397.
189. Thiele J, Kvasnicka HM, Fischer R, et al. Clinicopathological impact of the interaction between megakaryocytes and myeloid stroma in chronic myeloproliferative disorders: a concise update. *Leuk Lymphoma* 1997;24(5–6):463–481.
190. Thomas ED. A history of haemopoietic cell transplantation. *Br J Haematol* 1999;105(2):330–339.
191. Traweek ST, Arber DA, Rappaport H, et al. Extramedullary myeloid cell tumors. An immunohistochemical and morphologic study of 28 cases. *Am J Surg Pathol* 1993;17(10):1011–1019.
192. Uchida A, Fukata H. Role of NK cell cytotoxic factor against fresh human tumors. *Nat Immun* 1993;12(4–5):267–278.
193. Van den Berg H, Kluin PM, Vossen JM. Early reconstitution of haematopoiesis after allogeneic bone marrow transplantation: a prospective histopathological study of bone marrow biopsy specimens. *J Clin Pathol* 1990;43(5):365–369.
194. Vitrat N, Cohen-Solal K, Pique C, et al. Endomitosis of human megakaryocytes are due to abortive mitosis. *Blood* 1998;91(10):3711–3723.

195. Vogel PB, Frank AB. Sternal marrow of children in normal and in pathologic states. *Am J Dis Children* 1939;57:245–268.
196. Wang Z, Skokowa J, Pramono A, et al. Thrombopoietin regulates differentiation of rhesus monkey embryonic stem cells to hematopoietic cells. *Ann N Y Acad Sci* 2005;1044:29–40.
197. Ward AC, Loeb DM, Soede-Bobok AA, et al. Regulation of granulopoiesis by transcription factors and cytokine signals. *Leukemia* 2000;14(6):973–990.
198. Washio S, Ido M, Azuma E, et al. Acute megakaryoblastic leukemia with translocation t(1;22)(p13;q13) in a 10-week-old infant. *Am J Hematol* 1992;39(1):56–60.
199. Wedgewood RA, Primary immunodeficiency disease. *Clin Exp Immunol* 1995; 99 (suppl 1):1–24.
200. Weisel KC, Moore MA. Genetic and functional characterization of isolated stromal cell lines from the aorta-gonado-mesonephros region. *Ann N Y Acad Sci* 2005;1044:51–59.
201. Westerman MP. Bone marrow needle biopsy: an evaluation and critique. *Semin Hematol* 1981;18(4):293–300.
202. Wickramasinghe SN. Bone marrow. In: *Histology for pathologists*. New York: Raven Press, 1992:1–31.
203. Young NS, Scheinberg P, Calado RT. Aplastic anemia. *Curr Opin Hematol* 2008;15(3):162–168.
204. Zipursky A. Leukemia in Down syndrome. *Pediatr Hematol Oncol* 1992;9(2):139–149.
205. Zipursky A. Myelodysplasia and AMKL in Down's syndrome. *Leu Res* 1994;18:163.
206. Zipursky A, Brown EJ, Christensen H, et al. Transient myeloproliferative disorder (transient leukemia) and hematologic manifestations of Down syndrome. *Clin Lab Med* 1999;19(1):157–167, vii.

CHAPTER 24

Soft Tissue

LOUIS P. DEHNER

The pediatric surgical pathologist who is presented with a "soft-tissue tumor" in a child may be confronted with a wide spectrum of pathology ranging from an enlarged lymph node, fibroinflammatory process in the superficial soft tissues, maldevelopment of vessels or lymphatics, or a true neoplasm (Table 24-1). Some of the soft-tissue tumors (STTs) arise in the skin (infantile myofibroma) with involvement of the subcutis, subcutis (infantile fibromatosis or lipofibromatosis), or at the level of the fascia and the deep soft tissues. Soft-tissue sarcomas (STSs) in children may be organ based as in the case of embryonal rhabdomyosarcoma (ERMS), whereas others [such as Ewing sarcoma-primitive neuroectodermal tumor (EWS-PNET), alveolar rhabdomyosarcoma (ARMS), and synovial sarcoma (SS)] have the more familiar pattern of presenting in the peripheral soft tissues of the extremities. Immunohistochemistry (IHC) and molecular diagnostic studies have facilitated the diagnostic evaluation of STSs in children, but the entire exercise is initiated with a differential diagnosis.

One of the more common clinical diagnoses accompanying a pediatric surgical specimen is "rule out soft-tissue tumor." If this is the case, the neoplasm is benign in the majority of cases and more often than not is a vascular tumor of one type or another. Of course, there is the dilemma in some vascular tumors of a true neoplasm or malformation, which may or may not bear upon the surgical management. Vascular, neurogenic, fibrous-myofibroblastic, and myogenic tumors account for the majority (70% to 85%) of all soft-tissue neoplasms in children. Most of these tumors are benign (60% to 70% of cases) where there is a predilection for the trunk, extremities, and head and neck region in descending order of frequency; these tumors as a group generally come to clinical attention at or before 10 years of age. Some of the more aggressive STS are diagnosed in the second decade such as EWS-PNET, ARMS, and SS; however, like all generalizations, there are exceptions that each one of these neoplasms is recognized in the first 2 to 3 years of life (142). Arguably one of the most malignant and treatment-resistant soft-tissue neoplasms of childhood is the malignant rhabdoid tumor (MRT) with its many primary organ-based primary sites (kidney, liver, and central nervous system), which is also seen in a variety of nonorgans soft-tissue locations including the head and neck and mediastinum. Congenital STTs are mainly restricted to vasoformative proliferations, teratomas arising in the sacrococcygeal soft tissues, retroperitoneum, and head and neck without a specific localization to an organ. Other less common STTs presenting at birth or in the first month of life are congenital infantile fibrosarcoma (CIFS), myofibroma-myofibromatosis, granular cell tumor (GCT) (oral cavity), and embryonal or rarely ARMS. However, one should be prepared for the unanticipated when the clinical impression is a STT in a child.

Table 24-1 ■ SOME EXAMPLES OF "SOFT TISSUE TUMORS" IN CHILDREN

Developmental cyst (e.g., dermoid cyst)
Inflammatory process (e.g., granulomatous lymphadenitis, fibroinflammatory process in soft tissues, deep granuloma annulare)
Vascular malformation or neoplasm
Neoplasms (e.g., pilomatrixoma, myofibroma)

The classification of STTs in children is accommodated for the most part by the World Health Organization (WHO) classification (75). Traditionally, STTs are classified on the basis of tissue differentiation and phenotype as determined by IHC. Another ancillary technique, molecular genetics, has come to occupy an increasingly important role in the diagnosis of STSs in children (74,170,187) (Table 24-2). One of the first STS specific, nonrandom chromosomal abnormalities, t(11;22) (q24;q12) translocation, was identified in EWS-PNET, the second most common STS of childhood (92). Emerging from this initial observation is the appreciation that there is a family of STSs with a predilection for children, adolescents, and young adults in which the EWS gene on chromosome 22q is the fusion partner in a number of non–random translocations; these chromosomal perturbations can be detected utilizing fluorescent in situ hybridization (FISH) on nuclear preparations obtained from formalin-fixed, paraffin-embedded tissue.

Table 24-2 ■ SOFT TISSUE NEOPLASMS IN CHILDREN AND THEIR RECURRING CYTOGENETIC ABNORMALITIES

Tumor Type	Cytogenetic Abnormality	LOCI
EWS-PNET[a]	t(11;22)(q24;q12)	EWS-FLI1 (85%)
	t(21;22)(q22;q12)	EWS-ERG (10%)
	t(7;22)(p22;q12)	ETV1-EWS
	t(17;22)(q12;q12)	E1AF-EWS
	t(2;22)(q33;q12)	FEV-EWS
DSRCT[a]	t(11;22)(q13;q12)	EWS-WT1
CCS of soft tissue (melanoma of soft parts)[a]	t(12;22)(q13;q12)	EWS-ATF1
EMC[a]	t(9;22)(q22;q12)	EWS-CHN/TEC
	t(9;17)(q22;q11.2)	RBP56-CHN/TEC
	t(9;15)(q22;q21)	TCF12-CHN/TEC
AFH[a]	t(12;22)(q13;q12)	EWSR1-ATF1
	t(12;16)(q13;q11)	FUS-ATF1
Myxoid LPS[a]	t(12;16)(q13;p11)	FUS-CHOP
	t(12;22)(q13;p12)	EWSR1-CHOP
ERMS	LOH at 11p15, gains 2+, 7+, 8+, 11+, 12+, 20+, 21+, 13q 21+, 20+; Losses 1p35–36–, 3–, 7–, 6–, 9q22–, 14q 21–32–, 17–	
ARMS	t(2;13)(q35;q14)	PAX 3-FKHR
	t(1;13)(p36;q14)	PAX7-FKHR
CIFS	t(12;15)(p13;q25)	ETV6-NTRK3
SS	t(X;18)(p11;q11)	SYT-SSX1(biphasic)
		SYT-SSX2(monophasic)
		SYT-SSX4
ASPS	der(17)t(X;17)(p11.2;q25)	ASPL-TFE3
MRT	deletion and mutation in 22q11	SMAR CB1/INI1 (hSNF5/INI1)
Lipoblastoma	8q11–13	PLAG1
IMT	Translocations involving 2p23 (ALK) t(2;17)(p23;q23)	ALK-CLTC
		ALK-TPM3
		ALK-TPM4
		ALK-CAR5
		ALK-RANBP2
		ALK-TMP4
		ALK-SEC31L
LGFS	t(7;16)(q32–34;p11)	FUS-CREB3L2
	t(11;16)(p11;p11)	FUS-CREB3L1

[a]Extended EWS family of tumor.

The approach to the pathologic diagnosis of a STT from a child has the same starting point as one in an adult, a careful gross examination which is followed by the selection of tissue blocks from representative areas of the tumor based on the macroscopic features (if one has digital photographic capability, a gross illustration can often substitute for a long narrative description). The decision about the number of tissue blocks is guided by the size of the specimen and the variability of gross features from viable areas to those with a necrotic or hemorrhagic appearance. Many blocks may be required to identify any residual tumor in those cases with preoperative adjuvant therapy. If the specimen is submitted as a gross resection, the peripheral margins and any attached organs or bony structures should be identified and the margins tattooed with India ink or other dyes that will survive processing in order to evaluate the adequacy of the surgical margins. Margins of surgical resection are generally reported as "free of tumor" or not. Determining the distance between the tumor and the tumor-free margin by gross and microscopic examination is difficult in many cases. Some margins are limited by the constraints of the anatomy as it relates to neurovascular bundles or bony structures and can be even more challenging in an infant or small child.

If the specimen is a small biopsy and submitted for intraoperative frozen section consultation, very little tissue may remain for permanent sections; thus, another tissue sample should be obtained, if at all possible, as a contingency. Once the biopsy has been examined, it should be marked with an appropriate dye and placed in a small tea bag before routine tissue processing. If facilities are available and the tissue sample is judged to be more than adequate for histological examination, cytogenetics and tissue banking should be considered as well.

The world of STTs in children can be divided into three morphologic spheres: vascular structures of varying morphology, spindle cells, and small or not so small round cells (Table 24-3). Various spindle cell tumors are listed in this table, and many of them are familiar to the pediatric

Table 24-3 ■ MORPHOLOGIC THEMES IN SSTS IN CHILDREN SOME DIFFERENTIAL DIAGNOSTIC CONSIDERATIONS

Morphology	Tumor Types
Round and not so "rounded" small cells	RMS (both ERMS and ARMS)
	EWS-PNET
	Mononuclear histiocytic-like cells
	LCH and JXG
	Non-histiocytic hematolymphoid neoplasms (lymphoma, granulocytic sarcoma)
	MRT
	ASPS
	PEComa
	Epithelioid vascular tumor
	ES
Spindle cells	Fibrous tissue reaction
	NF
	Fibrous tumors—fibromatosis
	CIFS
	SS
	IMT
	DFSP
	Schwannoma
	KHE
	LGFS
	MPNST
	Spindle cell RMS
Blood vessels and lymphatics	Hemangiomas of diverse subtypes
	Vascular malformations
	Lymphangioma
	Cystic hygroma

pathologist. Some of the diagnoses are made with relative ease through one's own experience with the appreciation of certain histologic features, which separate that particular round cell or spindle cell proliferation from all of the other similar appearing tumors. As one peruses Table 24-3, it becomes apparent that some of these STTs occur almost exclusively in the first two decades of life whereas others are seen more often in adolescence or early adulthood (65).

Ancillary IHC studies have had a profound, determinant effect upon the practice of surgical pathology over the past 25 years, but especially so in the diagnosis of soft tissue and hematopoietic neoplasms; the same can be said about the role of cytogenetics and molecular genetics for these two phenotypic categories. In the case of malignancies in children, several of the more common neoplasms, soft tissue or otherwise, are morphologically similar from the perspective of their more or less uniform composition of small or large malignant round cells (Table 24-4). Of course, there are other accompanying features, which should be incorporated into the differential diagnosis without the need to utilize every commercially available antibody in one's IHC laboratory. However, it is acknowledged that there are those cases in which successive waves of newly ordered immunostains may be necessary in order to arrive at a final diagnosis or the realization for the need to send the case to an outside consultant. In the meantime, the titer of anxiety is on the rise for all concerned. A difficult case is a difficult case for no other reason than that it is a difficult case as an existential reality. Attention to the clinical aspects including clinical laboratory studies can be helpful in crafting the differential diagnosis and guiding the selection of stains. In the course of this chapter, there will be frequent references to Table 24-4, which should be familiar to most pathologists with some level of experience with the malignant round cell tumors of childhood, which are not necessarily all "small blue cells." Each of these tumor types, less the undifferentiated round cell sarcoma, has one or more molecular aberrations with diagnostic and prognostic implications in some cases.

There are other "round cell" neoplasms presenting in childhood, though also in adults, which are not included in Table 24-4 but are cited in Table 24-3. These are neoplasms with the added characterization as "epithelioid" whose cytomorphologic features are polygonal contours, a central nucleus, and abundant eosinophilic to clear cytoplasm. Alveolar soft part sarcoma (ASPS), perivascular epithelioid cell tumor (PEComa), epithelioid hemangioma and hemangioendothelioma (HE), and epithelioid sarcoma (ES) are among the principal tumor types in this category.

Table 24-4 ■ MALIGNANT ROUND CELL TUMORS AND THEIR IMMUNOPHENOTYPE

Tumor	VIM	CK	DES	MYOD1-MYOG	CD99	CD43	WT1	CHR	BAF47
RMS	+	–	+	+	–	–	–	–	–
NB	±	–	–	–	–	–	–	+	–
EWS/PNET	+	±	–	–	+	–	–	–	–
WT-BL	+	–	±	–	–	–	+	–	–
DSRCT	+	±	+	–	±	–	+	±	–
SS-PD	+	+	–	–	±	–	–	–	–
MRT	+	+	–	–	±	–	–	–	+
UDS	+	±	–	–	±	–	–	–	–
HPN	+	–	–	–	±	+	–	–	–

RMS, rhabdomyosarcoma; NB, neuroblastoma; EWS/PNET, Ewing sarcoma—primitive neuroectodermal tumor; WT-BL, Wilms tumor—blastemal predominant; DSRCT, desmoplastic small round cell tumors; SS—PD, synovial sarcoma—poorly differentiated; MRT, malignant rhabdoid tumor; UDS, undifferentiated sarcoma; HPN, hematopoietic neoplasm to include lymphoid and non-lymphoid tumors; VIM, vimentin; CK, cytokeratin; DES, desmin; MyoD1-Myog, MyoDl—myogenin; WT1, Wilms tumor; CHR, chromogranin.

STSs in adults are commonly graded pathologically on the basis of mitotic activity [mitoses per 10 or 50 high power fields (×400)], nuclear pleomorphism, and necrosis. Pleomorphic sarcoma (formerly many of these sarcomas were interpreted as "malignant fibrous histiocytoma") and leiomyosarcomas are the two most common STSs in adults, which lend themselves to this traditional grading scheme. Pathologic grading of nonrhabdomyosarcomas (RMSs) in the Children Oncology Group (COG) system relies on a combination of specific histologic types of sarcomas in the grade 1 and grade 3 categories together with an assessment of mitotic activity [<5 mitoses per 10 high-power fields (40× objective) and <15% of surface area necrosis, grade 2]. Those sarcomas not included in the grade 3 category but with an excess of 5 mitoses and/or greater than 15% surface area necrosis are grade 3 sarcomas. Needless to say, differences in pathologic grading may arise between observers in a particular soft-tissue sarcoma. CIFS has a low risk for metastasis and is a COG grade 1 sarcoma but can have considerable mitotic activity and extensive necrosis. Only a malignant peripheral nerve sheath tumor (MPNST) with rhabdomyoblastic elements is a grade 3 sarcoma, but other MPNSTs are presumably graded on mitotic activity and/or necrosis. The COG system of grading STS is less than satisfactory in our opinion. Pathologic staging of STSs in children differs in several respects from its adult counterpart and especially so in the case of RMSs in children where the primary site may have a significant impact upon the stage and prognosis. Whether metastatic disease is detected or not in the unfavorable histology STS in children, like ARMS and EWS-PNET, the assumption is made that micrometastases already exist and their presumed presence serves as the rationale for systemic chemotherapy whether the tumor is localized at the time of clinical presentation or not. A final point in these introductory comments about STSs in children is whether there is a difference in the clinical behavior of the pathologically identical neoplasms, based upon age at diagnosis (65,93,191). There are some data to support that argument in the case of SS.

VASCULAR TUMORS

Vascular tumors of one type or another are among the most common STTs in children and account for 20% to 30% of all cases (40). As many as one third of all vascular tumors in childhood are diagnosed in the first year of life and are one of the most frequently recognized tumors at or shortly after birth (39). Cutaneous and even deep organ vascular tumors may present with multifocal sites of involvement in infancy. One such example is the infant with a HE of the liver with multiple extrahepatic hemangiomas, often in the skin and less often in the spleen.

Traditionally, vascular lesions (or tumors) have been divided on the basis of their resemblance or appearance to blood vessels or lymphatics. In some cases, this distinction between the two types of vessels may require IHC. A pathologic distinction is also made between a vascular neoplasm and malformation, which has been incorporated into a classification of "vascular anomalies" (33,45) (Table 24-5). This classification is probably more widely utilized by clinicians whereas the WHO classification of vascular tumors is more familiar to most pathologists (75) (Table 24-5). The latter classification does not include vascular malformations or a separate category for lymphatic or lymphangiomatous lesions. The rationale for the latter is the stated difficulty in reliably differentiating vascular from lymphatic endothelium on the basis of histology alone; however, the monoclonal antibody D2-40 is directed against a specific epitope on lymphatic endothelium (Fig 24-1). In regard to vascular anomalies and malformations, a number of mutations have been identified in genes, which are important in vasculogenesis.

Benign tumors. Hemangioma or HE with any number of qualifying prefixes was found to be the most common pathologic diagnosis of a STT seen in the first two decades of life during a 20-year period with an excess of 1,500 cases (40). The most common site is the skin in 25% of all vascular tumors. There is a preference for the head and neck region in the case of the skin and soft tissue. Other sites include the deep soft tissues, bone, orbit, parotid gland, skeletal muscle, and upper air passages including the nasal cavity and larynx. The overwhelming majority (70% to 90%) of hemangiomas, and HEs for that matter, are initially recognized in the first 6 months (38).

Lobular capillary hemangioma (LCH) and hemangioma with the designation of "infantile," "juvenile," or "capillary" are the two most commonly diagnosed vascular lesions in the skin and subcutaneous and/or deeper soft tissues in children, respectively (153,154). Both types of vascular tumors are characterized by a lobular growth pattern, but hemangiomas in the subdermal soft tissues may have a more infiltrative pattern, often with extension into the overlying dermis. The LCH or so-called pyogenic granuloma of the skin is a raised, erythematous nodule with or without epidermal ulceration. Lobules of diminutive, hypercellular vascular spaces with mitotic figures to the formation of patent capillaries with a fibrous stroma reflect the proliferative and involutional stages in the evolution of LCH (Figure 24-1). Within the vascular lobules, this process can be appreciated with the formation of patent capillaries. Arcades of feeding vessels are found at the base of the LCH. The polypoid configuration of the LCH makes it prone to trauma with ulceration and inflammation to the point that the underlying pathology may be obscured.

Hemangiomas of the soft tissues are found in the subcutis with or without a dermal component and may extend into the fascia or less often into skeletal muscle. Though these tumors may appear well circumscribed clinically, microscopic examination frequently demonstrates a more diffuse pattern. One of the characteristic features is the superimposition of the vascular growth on existing structures such as lobules of subcutaneous fat or lymph nodes. In addition to the circumscribed lobular foci, a more diffuse pattern of small and even larger vessels is often present at the margins of excision. Like the LCH, the cellularity of these vascular

Table 24-5 ■ CLASSIFICATION OF VASCULAR ANOMALIES

	ISSVA	WHO
Tumors		
	Hemangioma	Hemangiomas (benign)
	Infantile	Subcutaneous—deep
	Tufted angioma	Capillary
	Epithelioid	Cavernous
	Spindle cell	Arteriovenous
	Capillary	Venous
	Lobular capillary (pyogenic granuloma)	Intramuscular
	HE	Synovial
	Kaposiform	Epithelioid
	Papillary intralymphatic (Dabska tumor)	Angiomatosis
	Retiform	Lymphangioma
	Spindle cell	HE (intermediate)
	Epithelioid	Kaposiform HEA
	Angiosarcoma	Retiform HEA
		Papillary intralymphatic angioendothelioma
		Composite HEA
		KS
		Malignant
		Epithelioid HEA
		Angiosarcoma
Malformations		
	Simple (slow flow)	
	Capillary (portwine, angiokeratoma)	
	Lymphatic (lymphangioma)	
	Venous (cavernous hemangiomas)	
	Simple (fast flow)	
	Arterial (arteriovenous hemangiomas)	
	Combined	
	AVM	
	Capillary—venous	
	Capillary—lymphatic venous	
	Lymphatic—venous	
	Capillary AVM	

lobules and the presence of patent vascular spaces are a manifestation of the proliferative phase of growth. It is in the involutional or regressive phase that there is the formation of thrombi in varying stages of organization and subsequent dystrophic calcifications and fibrosis. The latter process is well documented in the infantile HEs of the liver. Organization of the clot may be associated with papillary endothelial hyperplasia (PEH, vegetant hemangioma of Masson), which is also seen in hematomas. Though referred to as a hemangioma, most examples of PEH are simply an exuberant organization of a thrombohematoma and should not be mistaken for an angiosarcoma. Lack of nuclear pleomorphism and marked atypism in the PEH should give pause to the diagnosis of angiosarcoma.

Other morphologic variants of hemangioma include the epithelioid, arteriovenous, and tufted types. The cavernous and arteriovenous hemangiomas are considered examples of malformations in the International Society for the Study of Vascular Anomalies (ISSVA) classification (Figure 24-2) (Table 24-5). Epithelioid hemangioma is recognized in the skin (angiolymphoid hyperplasia with eosinophilia), in blood vessel in soft tissues (vasocentric) and bone. The histologic hallmark is a prominent polygonal endothelial cell resembling an epithelial cell. The endothelial cells may have cytoplasmic vacuoles that form small, capillary-sized vascular spaces, which may resemble small glands (Figure 24-3). Lymphocytes and/or eosinophils accompany the vascular proliferation and their presence is a useful clue to the diagnosis. However, epithelioid endothelial cells have some similarity to Langerhans cells as well so that one may wish to include CD1a for Langerhans cells in addition to CD31, CD34, and factor VIII–related antigen (endothelial markers) in the panel of IHC stains. Pericytes are present at least focally around these small vessels, which can be demonstrated by smooth muscle actin (SMA) positivity.

Hemangiomas in children are known to occur in specific sites in the soft tissues such as the synovium and skeletal muscle. A network of capillary-sized vascular spaces occupies the supporting stroma of the synovium and surrounding periarticular soft tissues, thus explaining hemarthrosis as the clinical presentation. Prominent hemosiderin deposition and synovial hyperplasia are also features

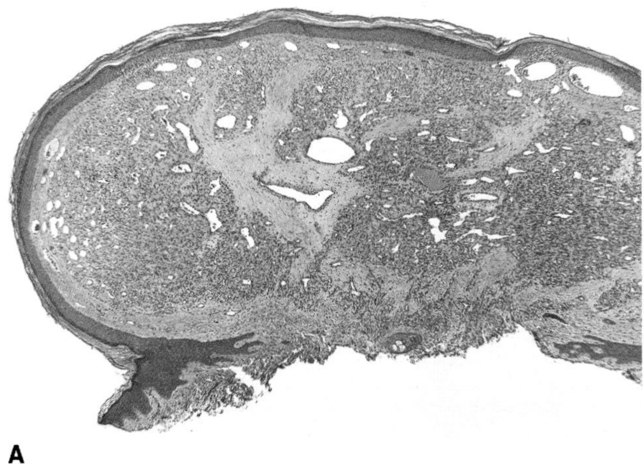

A

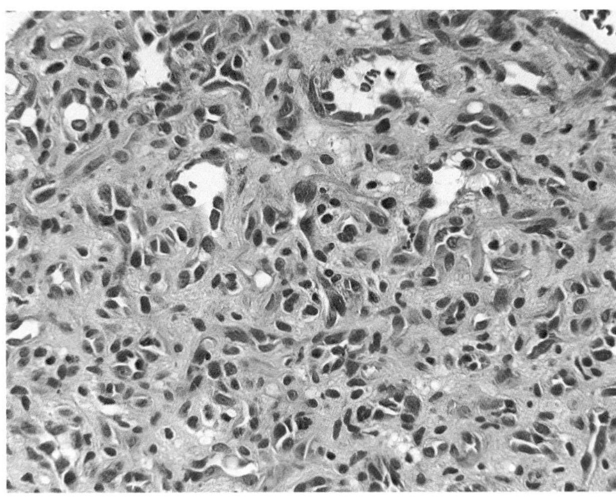

B

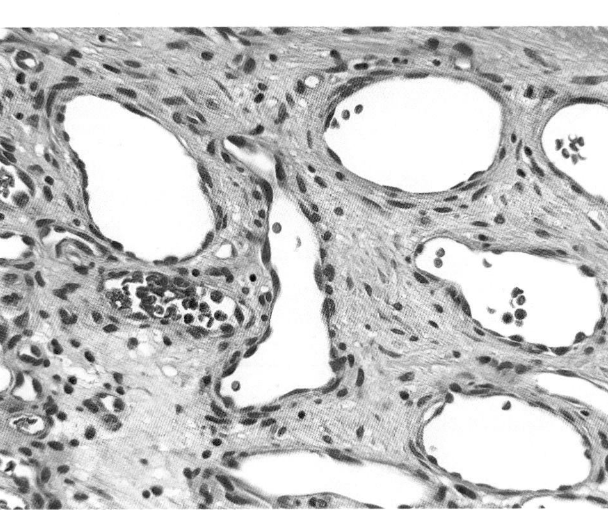

C

FIGURE 24-1 ■ LCH presented on the shoulder of this young female. **A:** A polypoid mass is composed of lobules of capillary-sized vascular spaces. **B:** In the more cellular or proliferating areas, vascular spaces are difficult to appreciate and mitotic figures are found with ease. **C:** The involuting areas are characterized by well formed, patent capillaries. Some congenital hemangiomas do not involute.

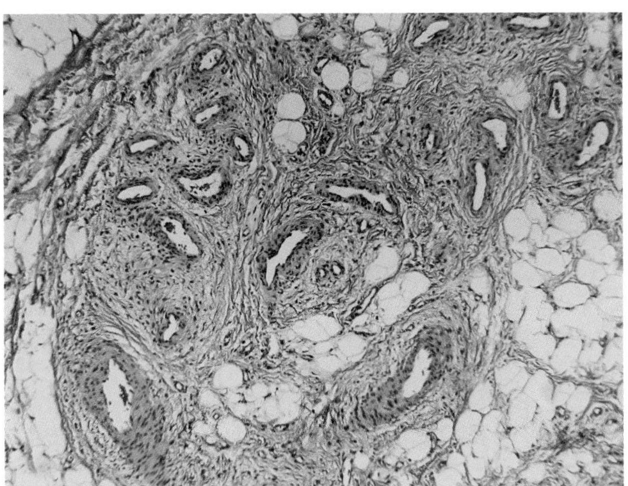

FIGURE 24-2 ■ Arteriovenous hemangioma presented in a 3-year-old female with an enlarging mass on the heel of the left foot. Vascular nodules are composed of venous and arteriole-like structures. This vascular lesion is probably a malformation.

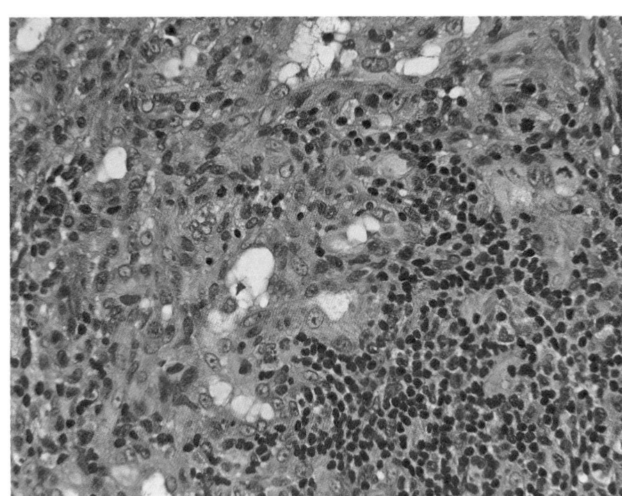

FIGURE 24-3 ■ Epithelioid hemangioma presented as a cutaneous mass on the arm of a 3-year-old male. Compact small vessels lined by epithelioid or histiocytoid endothelial cells, some with vacuolated cytoplasm and an accompanying lymphocytic infiltrate characterize this lesion.

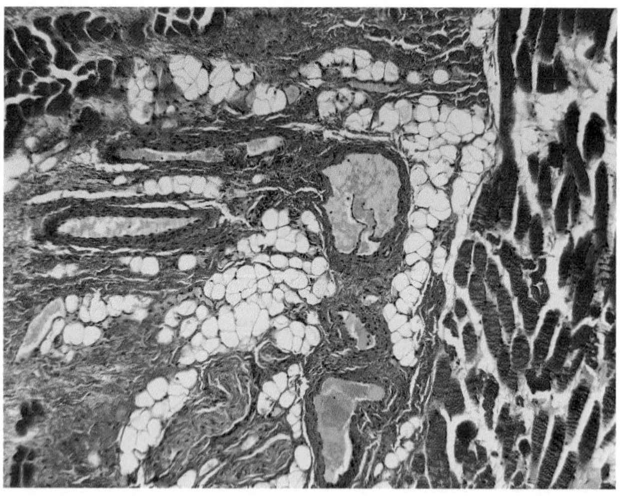

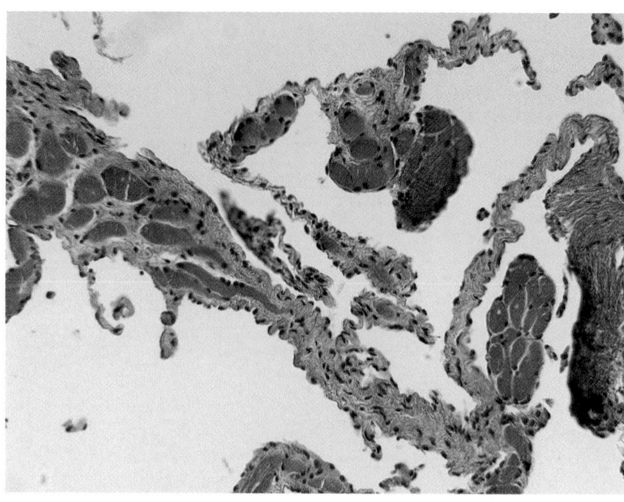

A B

FIGURE 24-4 ■ Skeletal muscle hemangioma presented as a soft tissue mass on the back of a 2-year-old female. **A:** Vascular spaces and adipose tissue are present in the skeletal muscle. **B:** Other areas consist of vascular spaces within the skeletal muscle.

of hemophiliac synoviopathy–arthropathy and pigmented villonodular synovitis, which should be considered in the differential diagnosis. Skeletal muscle hemangioma presents in the muscles of the head and neck region and extremities, usually in children older than 10 years of age. All or a portion of the skeletal muscle is occupied by an infiltrative process consisting of capillary-sized vascular spaces with or without a component of larger blood vessels and adipose tissue, which has resulted in the alternative designation of infiltrating angiolipoma (Figure 24-4). The vessels occupy the interstitial tissues and occur within the muscle itself as small vessels infiltrating between skeletal muscle fibers. An entire muscle can be involved by this diffusely infiltrative process. The distinction from an angiomatosis is not always clear; however, the latter tends to involve multiple tissue layers from the skin to bone. When an extremity is the site of involvement, as it is in cases of angiomatosis, the differentiation between the skeletal muscle hemangioma and the latter may be one of degree or diagnostic preference. The pathogenesis of both is more in the realm of a malformation than a neoplasm. Venous malformations of skeletal muscle also have a predilection for the head and extremities and most cases (70% to 80%) are noted at birth (95). Often some smooth muscle accompanies the vessels as appropriate for veins. In contrast to vascular neoplasms, glucose transporter-1 is not expressed by the endothelial cells of vascular malformations (147).

Intermediate tumors. This category of vascular neoplasms includes several entities, which are designated as HEs whose clinical behavior is characterized as *locally aggressive* or *rarely metastatic* in the WHO classification (75) (Table 24-5). Some HEs have complex mixed pattern features as in the case of the so-called composite HE (80).

Kaposiform hemangioendothelioma (KHE) occurs almost exclusively in children with a mean age at diagnosis between 2 and 4 years old, but as early as antenatally, with nonimmune hydrops or pericardial effusion (133). The extremities and head and neck are the anatomic sites of predilection. However, KHE has been reported in the retroperitoneum, mediastinum, intestinal tract, middle ear, or as diffuse multifocal sites. As many as 50% of cases are complicated by the Kasabach-Merritt syndrome and also have evidence of lymphangiomatosis. The tumor may be confined to the skin or present in the deeper soft tissues as multiple nodules with a diffusely infiltrating pattern. Though a mass may be palpable, KHE usually does not form a well-circumscribed, solitary mass, which is also generally true for most "vascular anomalies." Microscopically, the nodules have a distinctive spindle cell appearance (thus the designation of Kaposi sarcoma [KS]-like) (Figure 24-5). The tumor cells have uniformly bland features in the absence of nuclear hyperchromatism and mitotic figures. Erythrocytes may or may not be present among the spindle cells, but the small eosinophilic globules of KS are usually not seen. Nodules may also have the morphology of a more conventional capillary hemangioma. A lymphangiomatous component may be present as well. Glomeruloid nodules have a resemblance to the formations of a tufted angioma, which is usually confined to the dermis with the formation of so-called cannonball-like lesions. It has been reported that D2-40 expression may assist in the differentiation of KHE from tufted angioma (4). Unlike KS, KHE does not harbor HHV-8.

Spindle cell and retiform HEs occur throughout life without a particular predilection to children. Papillary intralymphatic angioendothelioma (PILA, Dabska tumor) presents in not only older children and adolescents, but also in young adults (60). A dermal nodule is a poorly circumscribed lesion whose size varies from a few centimeters to more than 30 cm. Papillary or glomeruloid structures with the phenotype of lymphatics are found in enlarged thin-walled vascular

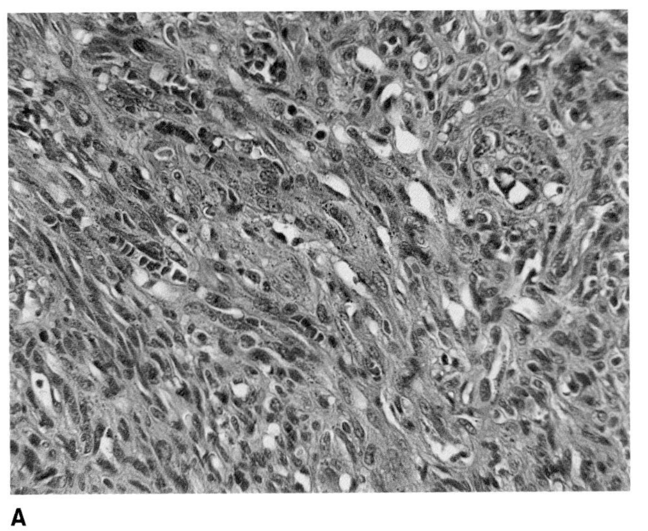

A

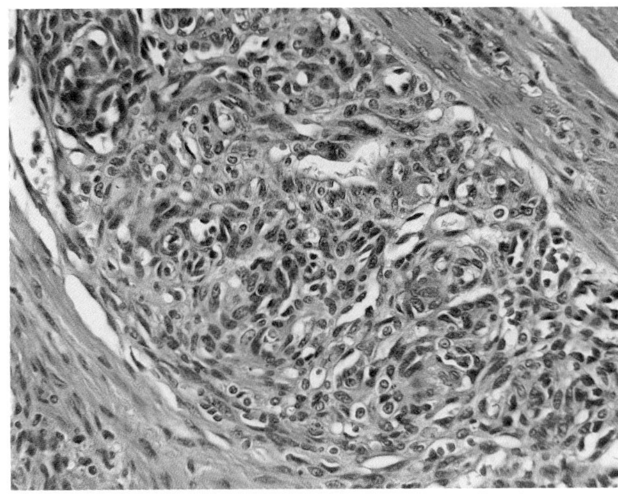

B

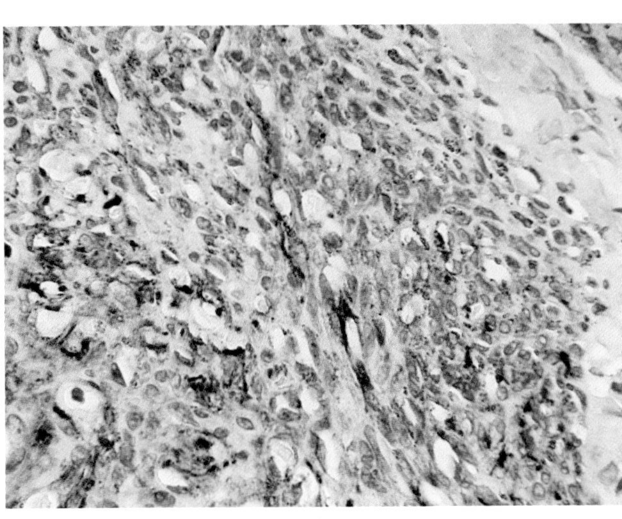

C

FIGURE 24-5 ■ KHE presented as multiple masses in the intestinal tract and retroperitoneum in a 7-year-old female. **A:** Many of the nodules are composed of compact spindle cells with interposed erythrocytes resembling KS. **B:** Other nodules had a more lobulated and tufted appearance. **C:** Factor VIII-related antigen immunostaining labeled the spindle cells.

structures. Though initially considered a malignant vascular tumor, PILA rarely metastasizes and infrequently recurs.

Malignant vascular tumors. Epithelioid hemangioendothelioma (EHE) is a low-grade vascular neoplasm with microscopic features, which are similar to the benign counterpart, but with more cytologic atypia and an aggressive infiltrating pattern. The one example of EHE, which we have seen most often in the first two decades of life has presented in the liver. Small groups and individual tumor cells with a cytoplasmic vacuole are surrounded by a pale hyaline to almost chondroid appearing stroma unlike the more compact pattern of vascular spaces in the epithelioid hemangioma. Overall, EHE has a metastatic rate of 15% to 20%. The lung is the favored site of metastasis of the hepatic EHE where the pulmonary lesions were once referred to as intravascular bronchoalveolar tumor of Leibow.

Conventional high-grade **angiosarcoma** is uncommon in adults and rarer yet in children. Though reported in the peripheral soft tissues, the few angiosarcomas in children that we have seen presented in the liver. These tumors, usually in children 10 years old or less, had the characteristic sinusoidal growth pattern by atypical endothelial cells with hyperchromatic nuclei and the occasional mitotic figure. We acknowledge that there are examples of "infantile hemangioendothelioma" of the liver with the so-called type II pattern whose microscopic features are borderline to a degree of uncertainty about the potential for malignant behavior. However, we have not encountered yet as infantile HE with an exclusive, small vessel type I pattern, which has pursued a malignant course. However, the type II endovascular papillary pattern is less reliably reassuring in terms of ultimate outcome.

Kaposi sarcoma (KS) is known to occur in childhood as either lymph node–based disease or in a variety of extranodal sites in an immunocompromised child with AIDS or an organ transplant recipient. There is the same association with HHV-8 as in adults. The lesions of KS occur in mucosal sites of the oral cavity, gastrointestinal tract, and lung. Cutaneous lesions or inguinal lymphadenopathy are other presentations. Hepatosplenic KS is also known to occur in children.

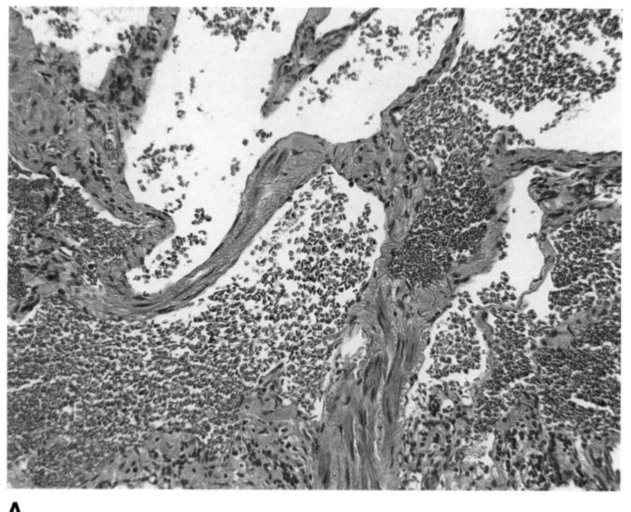

A

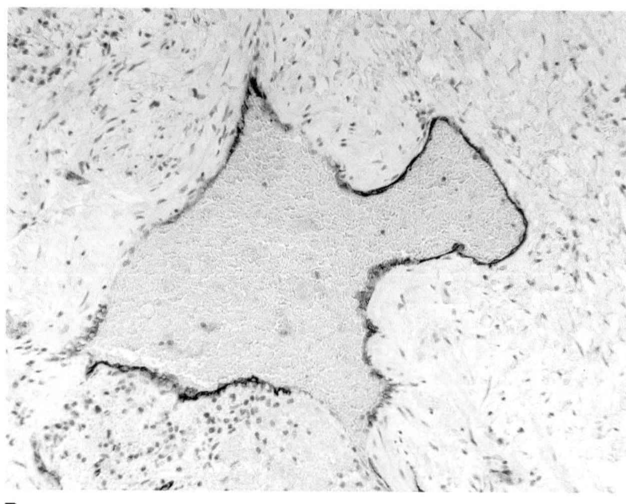

B

C

FIGURE 24-6 ■ Mixed venous and lymphatic malformation presented as a mass on the chest wall of a 17-year-old female. **A:** A mixture of muscle associated venous structures are intermixed with thin-walled lymphatic-like spaces. **B:** Some of these spaces stain positively for D2-40, a lymphatic marker. **C:** Many of the vascular channels are associated with SMA positivity.

The histopathologic features are those of a relatively low-grade spindle cell proliferation and entrapped erythrocytes. These spindle cells have membrane immunoreactivity for CD31 and CD34, and the nuclei are positive for HHV-8.

Lymphatic Tumors

Cystic lymphangioma (hygroma) and the other variants of lymphangioma are classified simple, low flow malformations in the ISSVA classification (Table 24-5). A compressible soft-tissue mass in the neck or more extensive involvement of surrounding anatomic structures such as the orbit, parotid gland, bone or into the mediastinum, and/or axilla in the clinical presentation. Solitary or more generalized cystic lesions may be present in the retroperitoneum and/or mesentery. Bone involvement may result in so-called disappearing bone disease (Gorham-Stout syndrome). Variably sized lymphatic spaces lined by inconspicuous endothelium and a watery eosinophilic coagulum in some lumina are the basic microscopic features. These spaces are irregularly distributed in the soft tissues with extension along septal planes and into the interstitium between lobules of salivary gland in the neck or the thymus when there is involvement of the mediastinum. Some of these malformations may include capillary or venous elements (Figure 24-6). In the latter case, smooth muscle may accompany some of the larger vascular spaces. Another complication in the pathology of a lymphangioma is in the recurrence whose vascular pattern has been altered by a reactive fibrous stroma with some resemblance to a fibromatosis.

The ISSVA classification reflects the fact that some vascular malformations are a collage of vessels of different types from capillaries to arteries (21,22,153) (Table 24-5). The classic arteriovenous malformation (AVM), usually encountered in the central nervous system or extremities, is a racemose of arteries and veins often accompanied by secondary features such as thrombi in various stages of organization, fibrosis, hemosiderin deposition, and dystrophic calcifications. There are several hereditary disorders whose predominant feature is the formation of AVMs, which have been reviewed by Tille and Pepper (201). Mutations in several genes, which are involved in angiogenesis have been

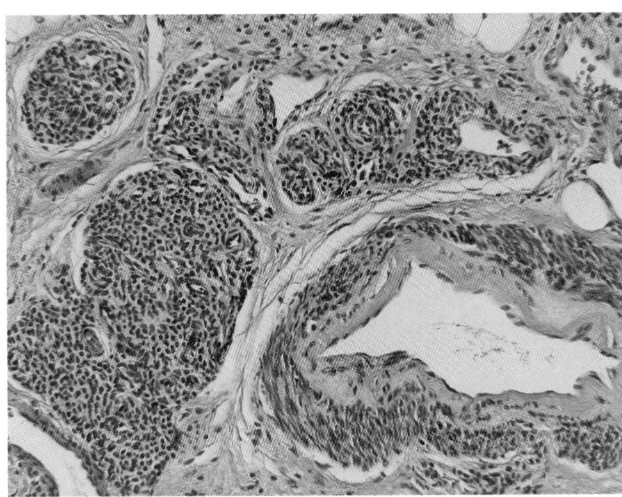

FIGURE 24-7 ■ Glomangioma (glomuvenular malformation) in a 20-year-old female presented as paraspinal and retroperitoneal masses. The vascular spaces are accompanied by a circumferential population of small, basophilic appearing cells beneath the endothelium.

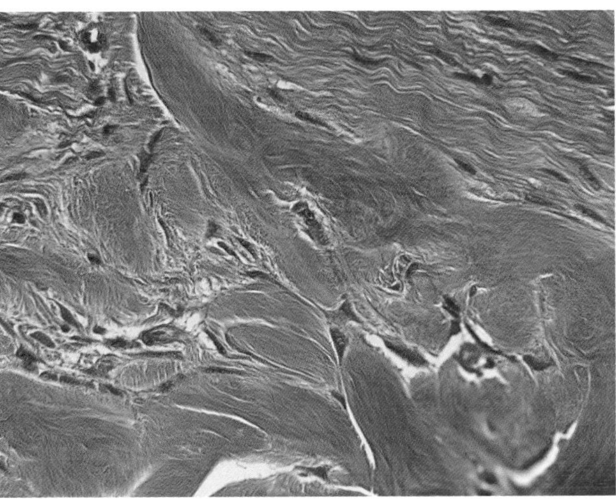

FIGURE 24-8 ■ Keloid presented as a mass in the posterior auricular region of a 5-year-old female. Dense acellular bundles of collagen are separated by fibroblasts.

detected in hereditary hemorrhagic telangiectasia (three subtypes, each with a different mutation), Klippel-Trenaunay syndrome (AGGF1 mutation) mutation, and other disorders with AVMs (37,45,103,209). Rarely, AVMs are complicated by the development of angiosarcoma.

Glomus tumor (glomuvenous malformation) is variably regarded as a neoplasm or malformation of the neuromyoarterial body. Solitary glomus tumors (90% of cases) have a predilection for subungual sites on the hand. Autosomal dominant multiple glomus tumors or glomangiomas (10% of cases) are characterized by a germ-line mutation in GLMN gene on 1p22. It is also of interest that there may be an increase in glomus tumors in the setting of neurofibromatosis type 1 (NF1). Approximately 10% to 15% of solitary glomus tumors present before the age of 20 years, usually in the second decade. The glomus cell is a modified smooth muscle cell. Cuffs of small uniform, basophilic cells are present beneath an intact, inconspicuous endothelium (Figure 24-7).

FIBROUS, MYOFIBROBLASTIC, AND PERICYTIC TUMORS

This section is concerned with a category of non–neoplastic and neoplastic entities which have in common a spindle cell with the morphologic and phenotypic features of a fibroblast, and/or a transitional type mesenchymal cell with the composite attributes of a fibroblast and smooth muscle cell, the myofibroblast, a cell with a smooth muscle phenotype and vascular perithelial localization (75). In the setting of one of the unique fibrous tumors of childhood, infantile myofibromatosis-myofibroma, the proliferating subintimal myofibroblasts have the capacity to differentiate into a cell with the morphology and immunophenotype of pericytes with contractile attributes of smooth muscle.

Scars, keloids, and fasciitis. The scar, a reactive fibrous and myofibroblastic proliferation, occurs in all tissue types and organs (brain excepted with its reactive gliosis) and is a programmed process of repair. Morphologically, the myofibroblasts and fibroblasts can acquire a degree of atypia, especially in a field of radiation, which can be a source of concern about its benign or malignant nature. A resected sarcoma after radiation therapy is one circumstance when a highly atypical fibroblastic reaction can be mistaken for persistent tumor.

Keloids and hypertrophic scars are similar in many respects with the formation of nodules of reactive fibroblasts in the dermis, whose presence has obliterated or replaced the normal microanatomy. Keloids are additionally characterized by groups of thickened intensely eosinophilic bundles of collagen (Figure 24-8). Similar bundles of collagen may be seen in desmoids fibromatosis in the mesentery or nodular fasciitis (NF). The formation of keloids and hypertrophic scars is regarded as an abnormality in the normal wound-healing process; the frequency of both processes is increased in some families and is more common in individuals of African descent (12,185). There has been considerable interest in attempting to understand the pathogenesis of these presumably related processes (118).

Nodular fasciitis (NF) and other pseudosarcomatous myofibroblastic lesions remain important because of their potential for misdiagnosis as a sarcoma despite the many admonitions in the literature over the last 50 to 60 years (180). It remains underappreciated for the most part that NF occurs in children including those in the first few years of life (47). One of the more dramatic examples of a fasciitis in infancy is cranial fasciitis presenting as a large mass with compression of the underlying brain in some cases (171). In our experience, approximately 40% of all cases of NF present in the first two decades, particularly in the first

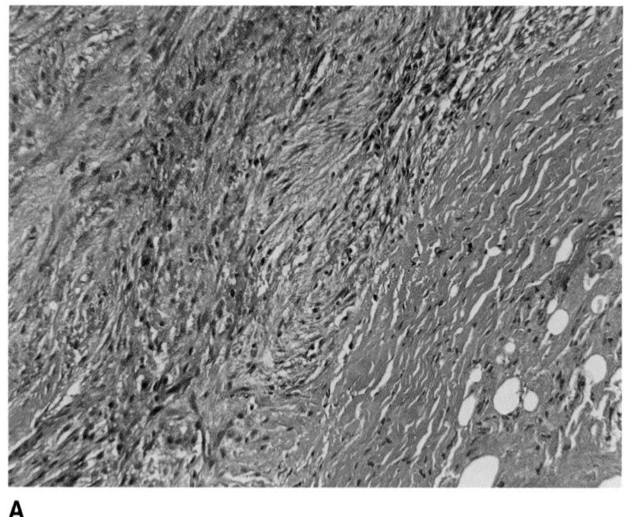

A

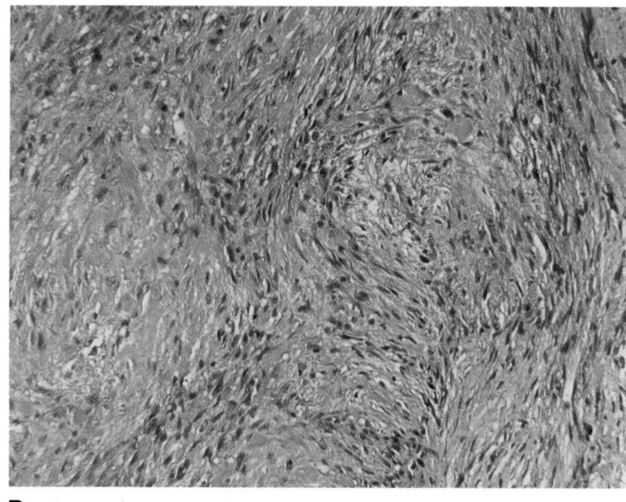

B

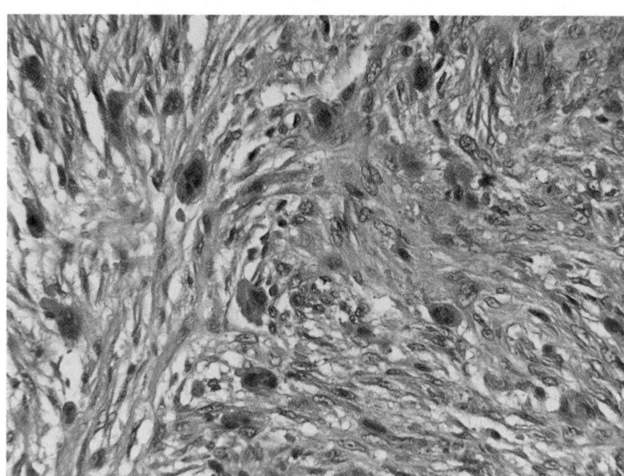

C

FIGURE 24-9 ■ NF in a 10-year-old female presented as a 2 cm mass in the posterior triangle of the neck. **A:** The abrupt interface exists between the spindle cells and the adjacent nonlesional collagen. Note the presence of interstitial hemorrhage. **B:** Intersecting fascicles and nodules of loosely arranged spindle cells and interstitial mucin are some of the characteristic features. The nuclei failed to immunostain for β-catenin. **C:** The presence of multinucleated cells may cause confusion with a fibrohistiocytic lesion.

decade of life, as a mass with a predilection for the head and neck region in 35% to 40% of our cases. Often NF arises as a rapidly developing mass, generally measuring less than 3 cm, in the orbital and periorbital, periparotid, premaxillary and intramaxillary, auditory canal, and intraoral soft tissues. There is often clinical concern about ERMS, which may not abate even after a biopsy due to its pseudosarcomatous features. The subcutis is the tissue level of origin for most NFs, followed by the fascia, lower dermis, muscle, and rarely the joint space. Grossly, a circumscribed, nonencapsulated nodule with a glistening mucoid appearance is reflected in the histologic features. Several histologic patterns coexist in the nodule with dense, spindle cell areas forming short fascicles adjacent to less cellular foci with separation of the spindle cells by mucoid-myxoid extracellular material (so-called tissue culture pattern) and transitional areas with both patterns (Figure 24-9). Mitotic figures are readily identified with some nuclear atypia (absent atypical mitotic figures and anaplasia). Microcysts with mucin, a variable number of histiocytes, foci of interstitial hemorrhage, and scattered inflammatory cells in the background are the constellation of diagnostic features. Scattered multinucleated cells and a storiform-like pattern may suggest a fibrohistiocytic proliferation; the compact spindle cell proliferation with mitotic figures serves to raise concern for fibrosarcoma (FS) or leiomyosarcoma; and immature fibroblasts in the tissue culture–like foci are the features to suggest the possibility of ERMS. The myofibroblasts of NF express vimentin and SMA but desmin, myoD1, and myogenin are all nonreactive by IHC. In general, NF is regarded as a nonrecurring process and if there is a recurrence, one should consider the likelihood of a misdiagnosis. The difficulty in the differentiation of cranial fasciitis from a fibromatosis is presented in a study where β-catenin was expressed in the nuclei of a putative recurring cranial fasciitis. Similarly, this may explain the local recurrence of 20% in a series of NF in children, which are in reality examples of desmoid type fibromatosis. However, β-catenin nuclear positivity may be seen infrequently in NF. Proliferative fasciitis and myositis are regarded as related entities to the more common NF.

Myositis ossificians (MO), either the solitary, sporadically occurring soft-tissue mass or the multifocal fibrodysplasia ossificans progressiva (FOP), has its own potential

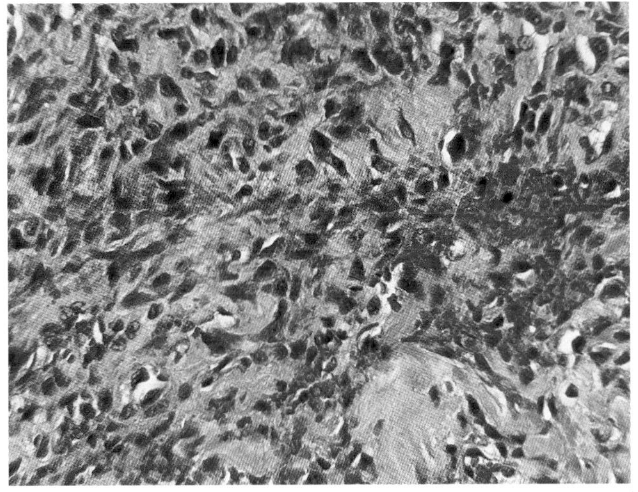

A

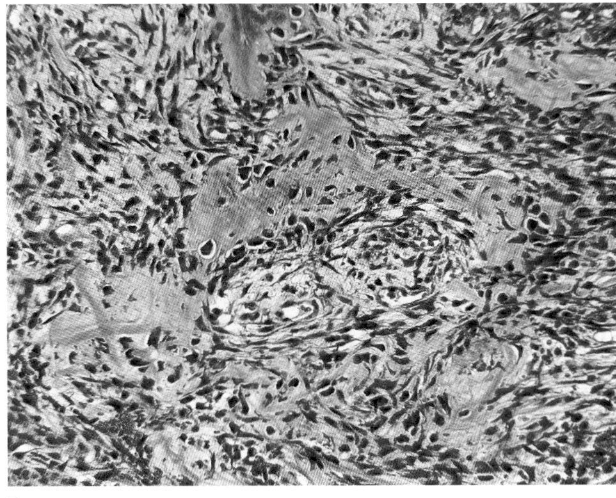

B

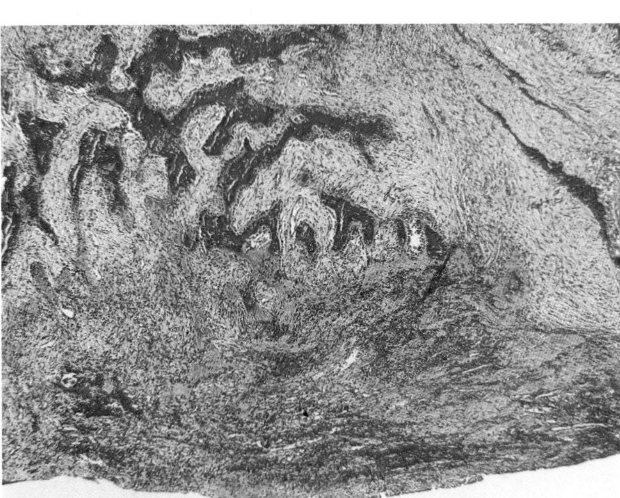

C

FIGURE 24-10 ▪ Myositis ossificans presenting as a soft tissue mass in the posterior neck of a 10-year-old male. **A:** The center of this mass is composed of compact spindle cells with some nuclear atypia but in the absence of atypical mitotic figures. **B:** The transition zone is between the central spindle cells and osteoid formation. **C:** The peripheral zone is represented by the active new bone formation.

for diagnostic miscues. Most cases of MO are sporadic, solitary, and may or may not be accompanied by a history of trauma to possibly explain the male predominance. It is seen uncommonly in the first decade of life and more often in later childhood or adolescence in which case there may be a history of incidental or organized (sports) blunt trauma. The classic presentation is a circumscribed intramuscular mass, or alternatively the formation of a parosteal, calcified mass, or a mass attached to the surface of the bone by a pedicle. The sites of predilection are the thigh, buttock, and abdominal wall (50). In terms of size, MO can measure in excess of 10 to 15 cm. The inner portion of the 3-zone mass is composed of plump spindle and polygonal myofibroblasts, blood vessels and histiocytes, which are surrounded by a zone of immature osteoid and an outer shell of mature bone (Figure 24-10). The diagnostic trap is set if a biopsy is obtained from the central, proliferating zone (180). Despite the initial impression of marked cellularity and some degree of atypia, the realization is that there are few mitotic figures and certainly no atypical mitoses. Nuclear anaplasia is absent.

Heterotopic ossification with fibro-osseous features has been reported in the auditory canal of young individuals. Cutaneous osteoma occurs sporadically or may be a manifestation of Albright hereditary osteodystrophy (AHO) or pseudohypoparathyroidism type Ia with or without the AHO phenotype. There are inactivating mutations of the GNAS gene (20q13).

FOP is an autosomal dominant disorder, which is characterized by the progressive transformation of soft tissues and skeletal muscle to heterotopic bone (112). The mutation has been mapped to chromosome 2q23-24, the site of activin A type I receptor/activin-like kinase 2 (ACVR1/ALK2), a bone morphogenetic protein type I receptor. In addition to the characteristic great toe malformations, there is the development of soft-tissue swelling or masses on the back, which are described as "spreading" through the subcutaneous tissues and deeper. Biopsy reveals a spindle cell and myxoid transformation of the subcutis with a resemblance to infantile subcutaneous fibromatosis or lipofibromatosis, more so than NF. A biopsy site may enlarge due to metaplastic ossification, which appears to accelerate in foci of trauma.

Other forms of so-called **pseudosarcomatous proliferations** of the soft tissues and periosteum are florid reactive periostitis, fibrous pseudotumor of the digit, a form of localized MO, and bizarre parosteal osteochondromatous proliferation (Nora lesion) (180). These various lesions are problematic if the specimen is a biopsy without adequate clinical information and characterization of the imaging features. Once again, the atypical histology is not accompanied by overtly malignant features, as discussed in the previous sections on NF and myositis ossificans, in particular as it relates to the absence of atypical mitoses and anaplasia.

Fibroblastic-myofibroblastic tumors in the WHO classification include both NF and myositis ossificans. However, this section focuses upon a group of neoplasms or presumed neoplasms, some of which occur predominantly in children, and others that are seen in adults as well (41,75,211).

Most of the unique fibroblastic-myofibroblastic tumors of childhood with some exceptions are recognized in the first 5 years of life and many at or before 2 years of age. These fibrous tumors of childhood include the following: fibromatosis colli, myofibroma-myofibromatosis, fibrous hamartoma of infancy (FHI), inclusion body fibromatosis (infantile digital fibroma), infantile fibromatosis (lipofibromatosis), Gardner-nuchal fibroma, juvenile aponeurotic fibroma, nasopharyngeal angiofibroma, congenital-infantile FS. Palmar and plantar fibromatoses (superficial fibromatosis) and desmoid-type fibromatosis are seen in all age groups. Desmoid-type fibromatosis, Gardner fibroma, and nasopharyngeal angiofibroma are known manifestations of familial adenomatous polyposis (FAP) including Gardner syndrome (43). Infantile myofibromatosis has an autosomal dominant pattern of inheritance in a minority of cases whereas juvenile hyaline fibromatosis (JHF) with its allelic syndrome, systemic hyalinosis, is an autosomal recessive disorder (2).

Infantile myofibromatosis (myofibroma), the most common of various fibrous tumors of childhood, accounts for 20% to 25% of all cases. A solitary cutaneous or subcutaneous nodule (90% of cases) measures less than 3 cm in most cases, presents in the first 5 years of life, and may be noted at birth and occurs in the head and neck region (40% to 60% of cases) followed by the trunk and extremities (192). However, the bone and various organs including the brain, dura, liver, intestinal tract, lung, and testicle are some of the other less common sites. Multifocal lesions, usually restricted to the skin-subcutis and/or bone, are seen in 5% to 8% of cases, and in 1% to 2% of cases, there are more widespread skin, soft tissue, and visceral lesions, which are recognized in an infant less than 6 months old. The clinical outcome is poor in these infants because of pulmonary venous occlusion by the formation of intravascular myofibromas. On the other hand, solitary lesions are known to undergo spontaneous regression.

A firm nodular non–encapsulated mass measuring 1 to 3 cm in greatest dimension may also be accompanied by calcifications, cysts, and central hemorrhage with a microscopic pattern of a hemangiopericytoma (HPC) with hemorrhage and coagulative type necrosis. The cellularity is most apparent toward the periphery where the compact spindle cells are arranged in short fascicles or within hyaline-myxoid, almost chondroid-appearing stroma, which separates or largely replaces the spindle cells (Figure 24-11). If the nodule is located in the dermis, there are often multiple discrete nodules with normal intervening cutaneous structures and dermal collagen and if in the subcutis, there is overgrowth and entrapment of fat. A more infiltrative pattern may be seen in the dermis, but the small, SMA positive nodules are best seen in the superficial dermis. However, the myofibroma does not have the infiltrative growth of a desmoid-type fibromatosis. At the periphery

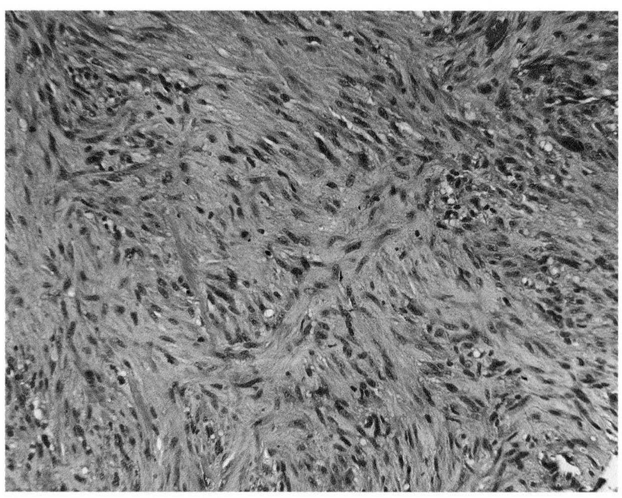

A

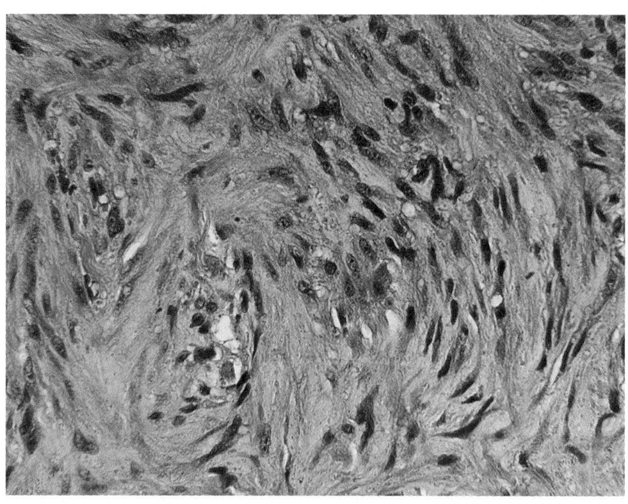

B

FIGURE 24-11 ■ Infantile myofibroma (myofibromatosis) presented as deep mass in the posterior neck of a 3-month-old female. **A:** The sharply demarcated mass measuring 3.0 cm is composed of uniform spindle cells in a pale eosinophilic stroma. **B:** Sweeping arrays of spindle cells are present in a fibrohyaline stroma with a small vascular space which has been compressed by spindle cells.

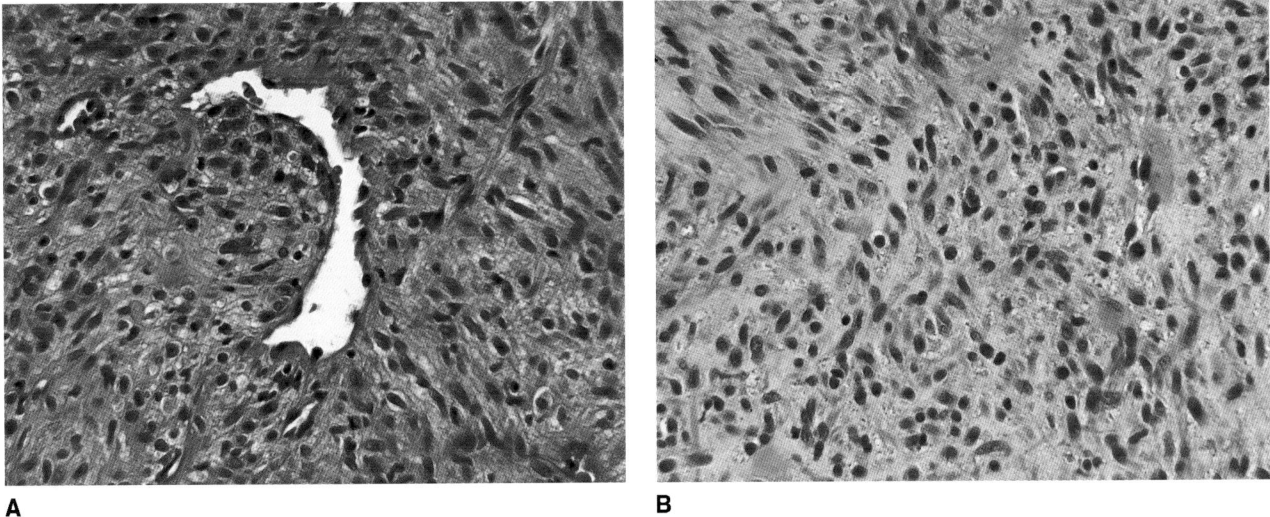

FIGURE 24-12 ■ Infantile myofibroma (myofibromatosis) presented as a soft tissue mass in the neck of a 3-month-old boy. **A:** The smaller nodules of spindle cells are associated with a compressed vessel at the periphery which is useful in the recognition of a myofibroma. **B:** Other fields are composed of fascicles and nodules with a fibromyxoid appearance.

of some nodules, a compressed vessel is a hallmark feature of the myofibroma and can be identified in many cases (Figure 24-12). The associated HPC-like pattern can be dominant in some tumors with only peripheral, nodular myofibromatous foci (Figure 24-13). Central degeneration without overt necrosis is yet another feature. The myofibromatous pattern is immunopositive for SMA whereas the HPC-like foci are positive for CD34. In addition to the HPC-like areas, dense spindle cell foci can simulate CIFS but without the potential implications nor cytogenetics of the latter tumor (Figure 24-14) (see Table 24-2). Local recurrence is seen in less than 10% of cases. It should be noted that the myofibroma is seen in older children and even adults.

The myofibroblast and pericyte also coexist in skin tumor and STT, the **myopericytoma (MPC)**, with its resemblance to infantile myofibromatosis (59). This tumor occurs in older children and adolescents though mainly in adults. The nodular pattern of MPC consists of small vessels surrounded by concentric collarettes of spindle cells with a resemblance to the metanephric stromal tumor of the kidney. On the theme of pericytes, there is the solitary fibrous tumor (SFT), initially described in the pleura, but now recognized in many extrapleural sites and the classic HPC (64). These two neoplasms are regarded as a single spectrum entity, and both tumors are distinct from the fibroblastic-myofibroblastic tumors (71).

Infantile fibromatosis includes three pathologic patterns based in part on the level of tissue involvement: subcutis with the alternative designation of lipofibromatosis; skeletal muscle with diffuse infiltration of the muscle by immature appearing spindle cells and desmoid-type fibromatosis without any specific microscopic features to differentiate it from any other desmoid tumor without respect to age (211). Infantile subcutaneous fibromatosis (lipofibromatosis) accounts for approximately 5% to 10% of fibrous tumors of childhood with a predilection for the distal extremities, though it may occur on the trunk and head and neck region (70). The growth pattern of variably dense spindle cells with a collagenous background extends along and around the interlobular septa of the subcutaneous fat and is not well circumscribed either clinically or pathologically (Figure 24-15). There is partial overgrowth of the fat by the spindle cells with a remote resemblance to dermatofibrosarcoma protuberans (DFSP). In fact, a fibrous-appearing DFSP should be considered in the differential diagnosis even in a young child. CD34 expression may be present focally in the infantile subcutaneous fibromatosis (usually diffuse in DFSP), but the spindle cells of infantile fibromatosis are variably positive for SMA. These tumors are known to recur which is not surprising, given their diffuse growth pattern. Infiltration into the deep soft tissues is uncommon. The diffuse pattern of infantile fibromatosis is recognized as an infiltrating tumor involving a skeletal muscle in the head and neck and often the tongue. Immature spindle cells sweep through the interstitum of the muscle with retention of some architectural landmarks of the separated bundles of muscle (Figure 24-16). Because of the relatively immature appearance of the tumor cells, a fetal rhabdomyoma (FRM) or RMS may be considered in the differential diagnosis. Appropriate immunohistochemical stains for myoD1 and/or myogenin should resolve the dilemma since these are only expressed in rhabdomyoblasts. Complete surgical resection is complicated by the morbidity of tumor location and its diffuse pattern. The desmoid-type fibromatosis rarely occurs in infants but its fibrous, spindle cell pattern with irregular infiltration and replacement of skeletal muscle along the invasive borders are identical to those of desmoid tumors in older children and adolescents. Any one of the infantile fibromatoses can involve the lower dermis, whereas

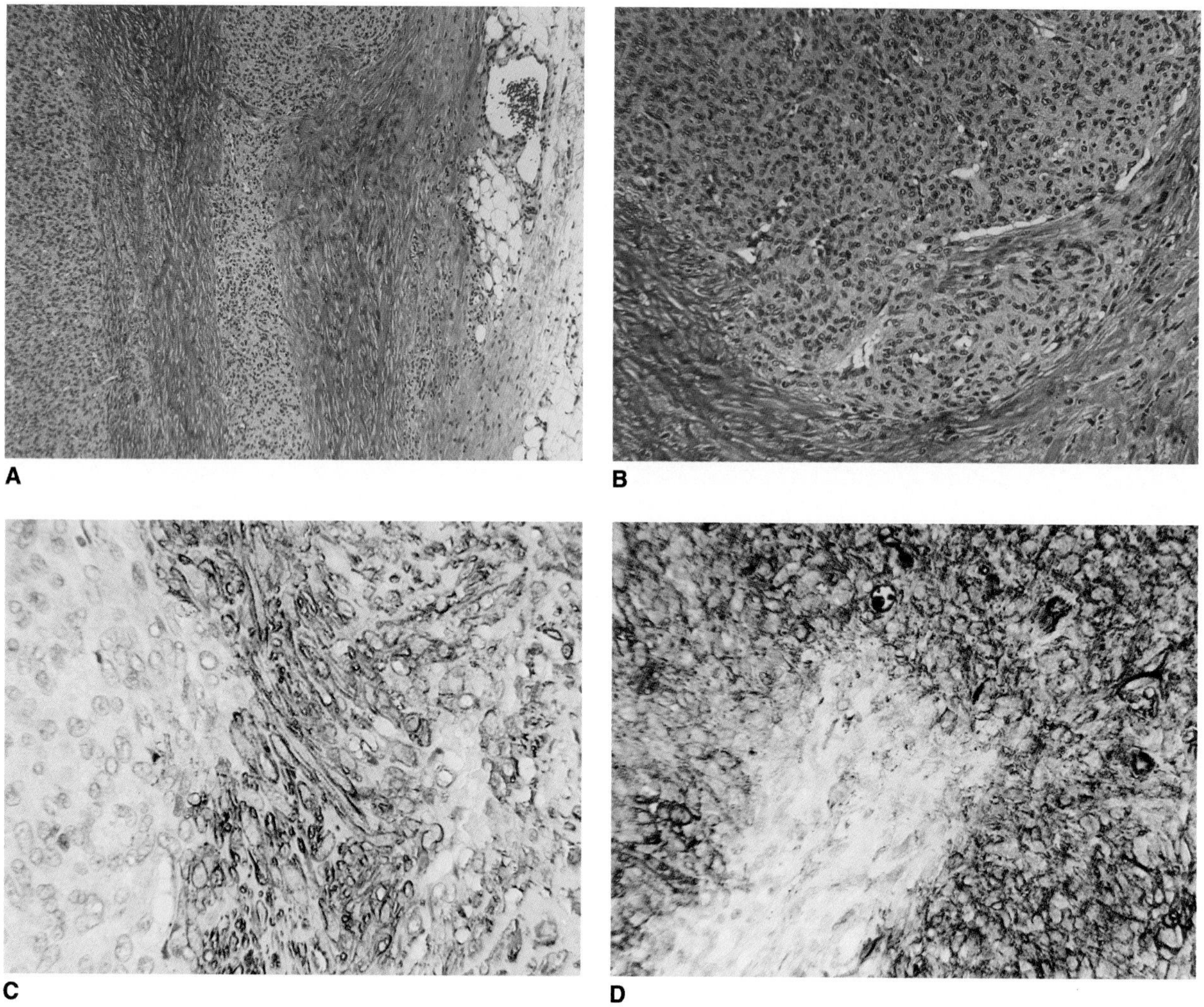

A

B

C

D

FIGURE 24-13 ■ Infantile myofibroma (myofibromatosis) presented as a mass in the groin of a 4-month-old male. **A:** This tumor has a mixed pattern of myofibroma and HPC which in this field has the former features. **B:** The HPC areas are usually present centrally with more ovoid cells surrounding small, clefted vascular spaces. **C:** Immunohistochemical staining for SMA highlights the myofibromatous pattern without reactivity in the contiguous HPC-like foci. **D:** A contrasting pattern of immunoreactivity for CD34 is seen in the CD34-positive HPC-like foci and absence of staining in myofibromatous focus.

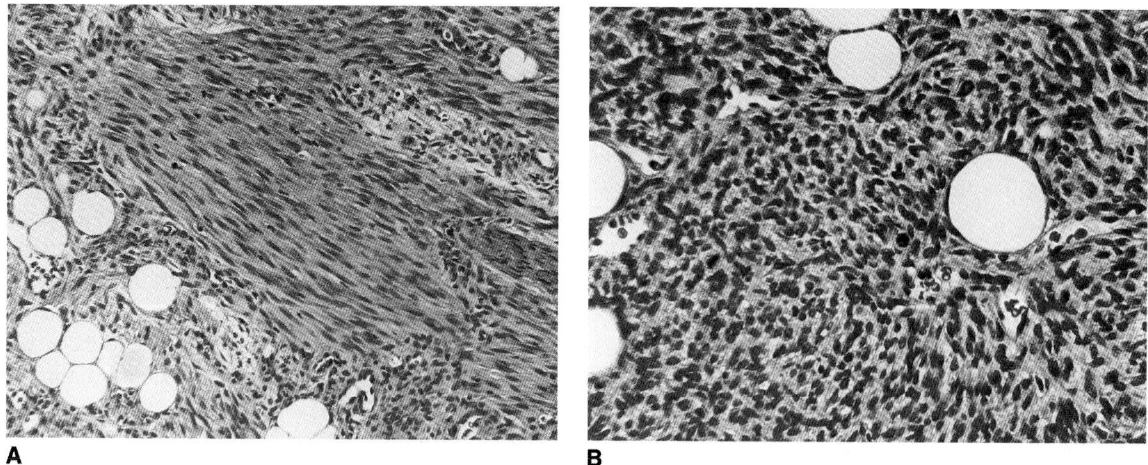

FIGURE 24-14 ■ Infantile myofibroma (myofibromatosis) presented in a 7-day-old female as a mass on the back. **A:** One of the two patterns in this tumor includes uniform spindle cells in a pale, eosinophilic background. **B:** Other foci are more hypercellular and mitotically active with a resemblance to CIFS. Despite the similarities, a t(12;15) is not found in these worrisome foci.

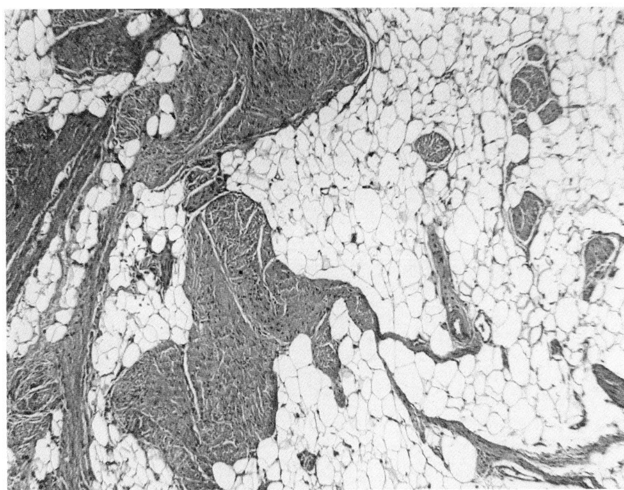

FIGURE 24-15 ■ Infantile subcutaneous fibromatosis (lipofibromatosis) in this 3-day-old boy in the head and neck region shows a proliferation of immature appearing spindle cells within the subcutaneous fat. The entrapment rather than overgrowth distinguishes this fibromatosis from DFSP-GCF which is also seen in infancy.

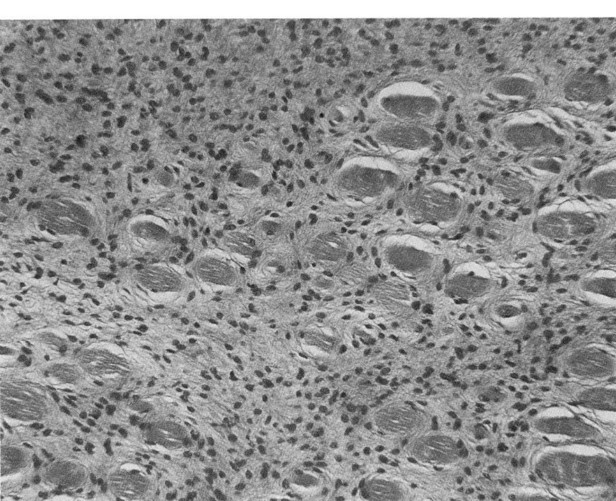

FIGURE 24-16 ■ Infantile fibromatosis of the diffuse type presented on the upper back of a 4-month-old boy. The loosely arrayed immature spindle cells are infiltrating through the skeletal muscle rather than its destructive overgrowth as in desmoid fibromatosis.

involvement of the deeper soft tissues including the skeletal muscle is confined to the diffuse and desmoid types.

Fibrous hamartoma of infancy (FHI), another unique fibrous tumor of childhood, accounts for no more than 5% of all such neoplasms (41). This tumor occurs almost exclusively in the 2 to 3 years of life, often in the first few months where the trunk, axilla, inguinal region, and extremities are the sites of predilection in descending order (28,55). The subcutaneous, poorly circumscribed fibrofatty tumor generally measures less than 5 cm. It shares many of the same gross and microscopic features with the infantile subcutaneous fibromatosis except for the small nodules of immature, spindled mesenchymal cells in a pale basophilic background (Figure 24-17). These may be found as isolated structures in the fat or along the periphery or within bundles of more mature appearing spindle cells. Focal extension may be found in the overlying dermis in which case the predominantly subcutis nature of the tumor is not readily apparent. The local recurrence rate is only 10% to 15%, which is low in light of the fact that FHI is incompletely resected in most cases.

Inclusion body fibromatosis (infantile digital fibroma) presents on the lateral and/or dorsal aspect of finger and/or toe with usual sparing of the thumb and great toe as a firm nodule(s) in an infant or child 5 years of age or less at diagnosis (124). More than one digit is involved in 25% to 30% of cases. This tumor measures 1 to 2 cm in most cases and has a uniform

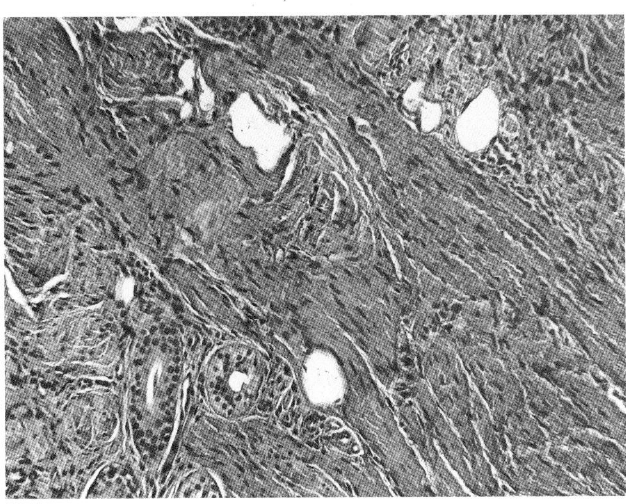

A

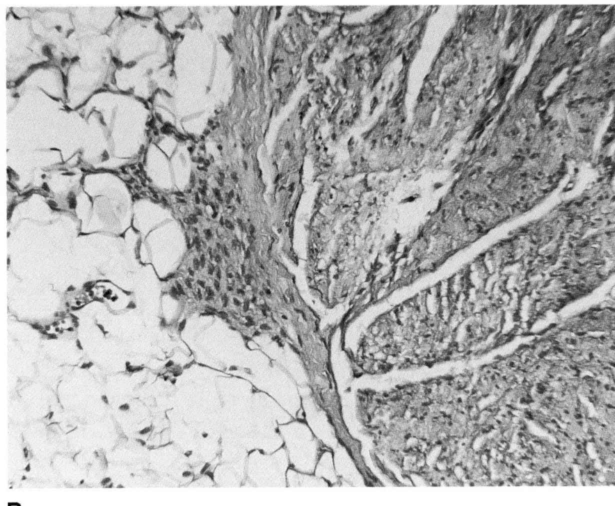

B

FIGURE 24-17 ■ FHI presented in the axillary region of a 4-month-old boy. **A:** The pattern of subcutaneous infiltration by bland appearing spindle cells resembles infantile subcutaneous fibromatosis. **B:** The presence of small bundles of immature spindle cells at the periphery or within the midst of the more mature fibroblasts is the diagnostic feature.

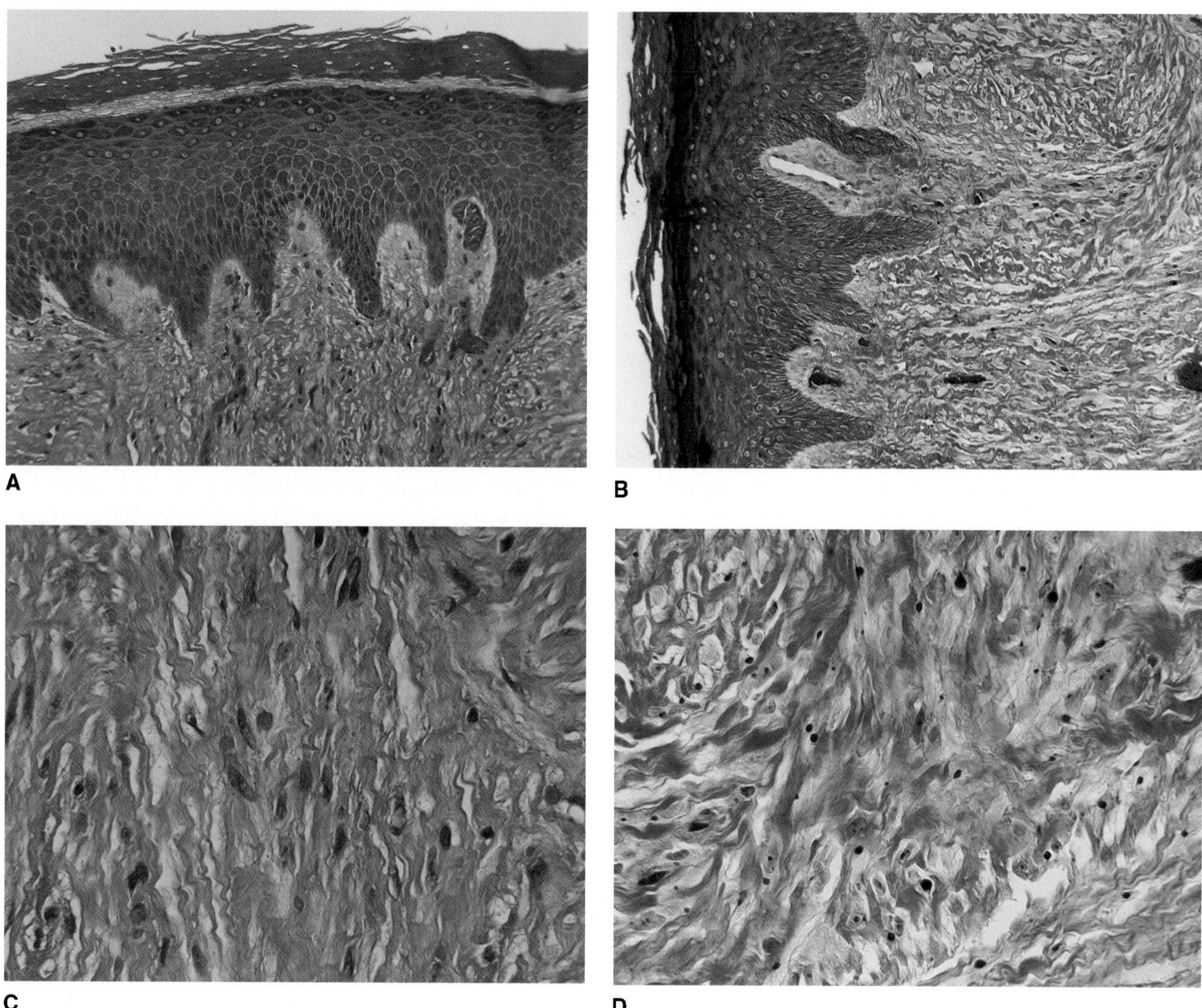

FIGURE 24-18 ■ Inclusion body fibromatosis (infantile digital fibroma) presented on the fifth toe of a 7-month-old female. **A:** The dense, relatively hypocellular spindle cell proliferation has effaced the dermis. **B:** Trichrome stain demonstrates uniform pattern of collagen deposition. **C:** Paranuclear eosinophilic bodies are best seen at higher magnification. **D:** These filamentous bodies of actin are demonstrated to better advantage in the trichrome stain.

white, fibrous appearance similar to a desmoid-type fibromatosis. The dermis is commonly effaced by a uniform spindle cell proliferation, forming short fascicles, and with a collagenous background with isolated hair follicles or sweat glands (Figure 24-18). Confluent, contiguous extension into the subcutis is associated with overgrowth of fat. There is a microscopic resemblance to the desmoid-type fibromatosis, except for the presence of eosinophilic, paranuclear inclusions in variable numbers; these inclusions are usually more readily identified in a trichrome stain (Figure 24-18) (15). The infiltrative growth around and through neurovascular structures in the digit limits complete resection in most cases, which accounts for a local recurrence rate in excess of 50%. It is important to take note of the fact that more than one digit may be involved.

A small subset of fibroblastic-myofibroblastic tumors, typically presenting in the first 2 years of life, are seemingly composed of more than one histologic pattern (composite fibrous tumor). The most common example is the infantile myofibromatosis—HPC with concurrent patterns of both. Other combinations are the infantile fibromatosis with CIFS-like foci and infantile myofibroma. These tumors demonstrate the morphologic plasticity of the fibroblast-myofibroblast and its capacity to simultaneously express itself with several microscopic patterns and in a sense reflect the relationship of these separate fibrous tumors of childhood to each other. We have seen examples of composite fibrous tumor behave in the fashion of multifocal or generalized infantile myofibromatoses.

Desmoid-type fibromatosis (desmoid tumor, musculoaponeurotic fibromatosis) is the most common fibrous neoplasm presenting in the first two decades of life (60% to 70% of all fibrous tumors) with cases presenting throughout

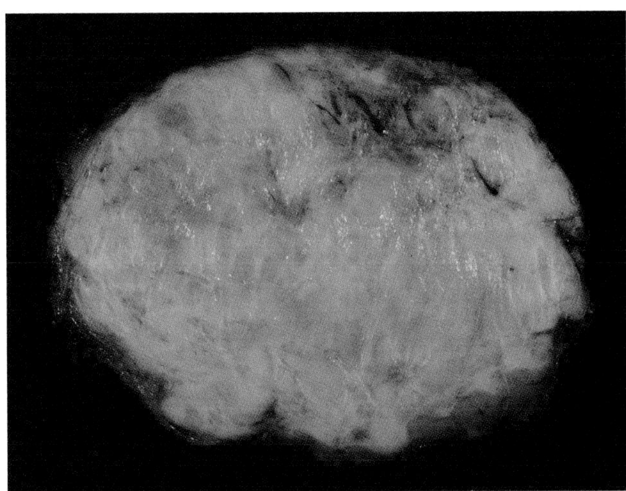

FIGURE 24-19 ■ Desmoid fibromatosis (desmoid tumor) presented as a deep soft tissue mass in the posterior thigh of a 15-year-old female. The cut surface of this 12 cm circumscribed mass has a tan-white trabecular appearance. Note the pushing growth into the skeletal muscle at the periphery.

childhood and adolescents with a bimodal age distribution in the first 2 years and later in older children (41). The extremities (including brachial plexus) and trunk are the sites of predilection in older children, but these tumors are also seen in the head and neck (orbit, paranasal sinus, mandible), intrathoracic, and abdominal (mesentery and pelvis) sites. Desmoid tumors arising in the shoulder-axilla or gluteal-thigh region have a local recurrence rate of 30% or greater (23). Most tumors occur sporadically (90% to 97% of cases), but there is a strong association with Gardner syndrome—FAP in less than 5% of cases.

A small incisional or needle biopsy can be challenging since other non–neoplastic and neoplastic fibrous proliferations arise in the differential diagnosis. An operative resection yields a gray-white mass with a uniform mucoid to trabeculated appearance whose dimensions range from a few centimeters to >10 cm (Figure 24-19). When skeletal muscle is present at the periphery of the resection, irregular infiltration by the usually bland spindle cell proliferation into the muscle can be appreciated; this same feature is seen to a more limited extent in some cases of NF arising in a muscle. The periphery of the mass should be tattooed with India ink (or other appropriate dye) since the status of surgical margins correlates with a local recurrence rate of 35% to 70%.

Fascicles of spindle cells or a loosely organized pattern of spindle cells are accompanied by a variably pale, myxoid to edematous or more collagenized background. The spindle cells may have the features of mature fibroblasts or display variation in the size and configuration of the stromal cells to reflect their less mature, more myofibroblastic attributes, which is manifested by immunopositivity for SMA (Figure 24-20). Mitotic figures can be identified among the myofibroblasts. A myxoid background, proliferating myofibroblasts, and some interstitial hemorrhage and edema portray a more NF-like appearance. The infiltrative margins rather than peripheral nodularity characterize the desmoid tumor in contrast to NF in most cases. Scattered lymphoid nodules at the interface with the surrounding normal soft tissues also usefully distinguish a desmoid tumor from other fibrous proliferations. There is little to differentiate a recurrent desmoid from the newly diagnosed tumor except for the findings of earlier surgery including scarring and foreign body giant cells and a more circumscribed margin in the primary tumor.

The relationship of the desmoid tumor to FAP has provided the opportunity to understand some of the molecular pathology of this neoplasm. Sporadic desmoid tumors have somatic mutations in the β-catenin gene (CTNNB1 on 3p21), which regulates the Wnt signaling pathway whereas the FAP-associated desmoids have an APC gene (5q22) mutation. Nuclear expression of a β-catenin is a useful marker to differentiate the sporadic and familial desmoid tumor from other fibrous tumors including NF in most cases (Figure 24-20) (13,26). However, some of the other fibrous tumors may have nuclear positivity for β-catenin so that it is not absolutely specific for desmoid tumors (200).

Gardner-nuchal fibroma is a distinctive paucicellular, densely collagenized mass presenting in the first decade of life with a predilection for the posterior truncal-paraspinal region (43). Other sites of involvement include the head and neck and extremities (144). Approximately 70% of affected individuals have a family history of FAP or represent a new mutation (43). The tumor is poorly circumscribed with a plaque-like growth in the subcutis or deeper soft tissues. It can be difficult to judge the peripheral margins of a fibroma from the normal fibrous connective tissues. A desmoid tumor may accompany a fibroma or evolve from a recurrent fibroma. Like the desmoid tumor, there is nuclear positivity for β-catenin in 60% to 70% of cases. Cyclin-D1 is expressed in the nuclei in virtually all cases. Nuchal and Gardner fibromas have virtually identical pathologic features.

Palmar-plantar fibromatosis is seen in children but more commonly in adults. These are poorly circumscribed fibrous tumors with a pattern of spindle cell foci separated by bland hypocellular collagenized stroma (69).

JHF is an autosomal recessive disorder, which is allelically related to **infantile systemic hyalinosis (ISH)** with a loss of function mutation in the capillary morphogenesis gene-2 (CMG2 on 4q21) (2,128). Large, painful nodules in the head and neck region (including marked gingival hypertrophy) and around joints evolve from small cutaneous papules, which are first noted in infancy and accelerate in growth throughout childhood. Osteolytic bone lesions develop, as do joint contractures. Firm, white nodules in the soft tissues and dense fibrous effacement of the dermis, resembling to some extent morphea-scleroderma, are some of the pathologic features (Figure 24-21). The nodules are circumscribed and consist of homogeneously dense hyaline collagen with focal paucicellular and more cellular foci, consisting of ovoid stromal cells residing in apparent lacunae with a chondrocyte-like appearance (Figure 24-22). Unlike JHF, ISH has

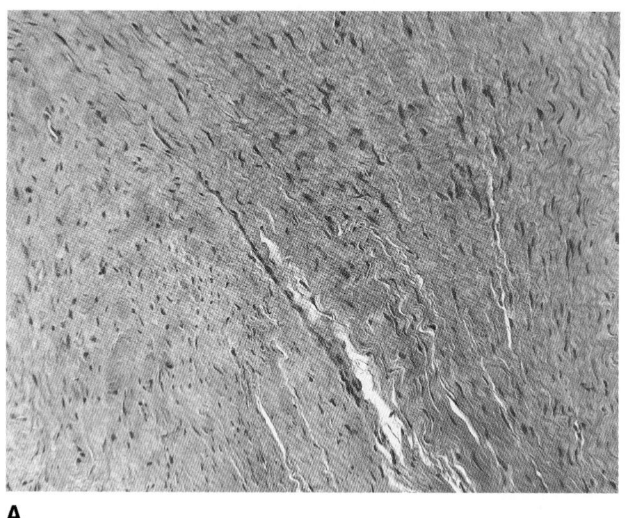

A

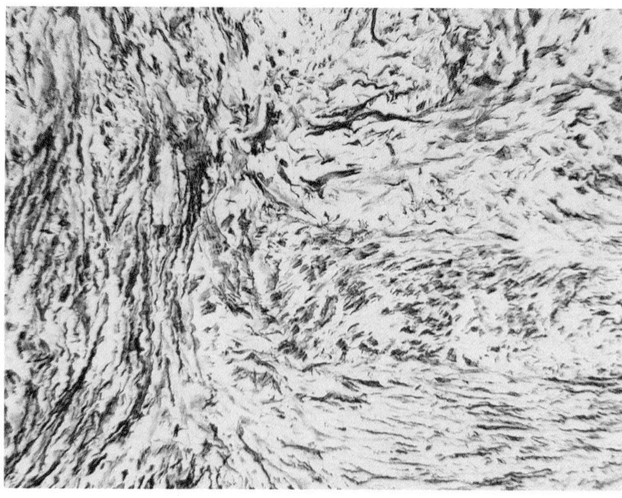

B

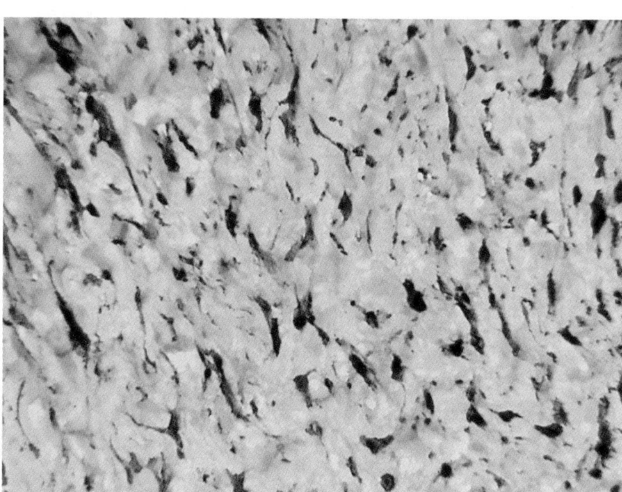

C

FIGURE 24-20 ■ Desmoid fibromatosis (desmoid tumor) presented in the posterior thigh of a 15-year-old female. **A:** A bland proliferation of fibroblasts is seen in a non-homogeneous collagenous background. **B:** The fibroblasts maintain their myofibroblastic phenotype with immunostaining for SMA. **C:** Most desmoids express nuclear β-catenin by IHC.

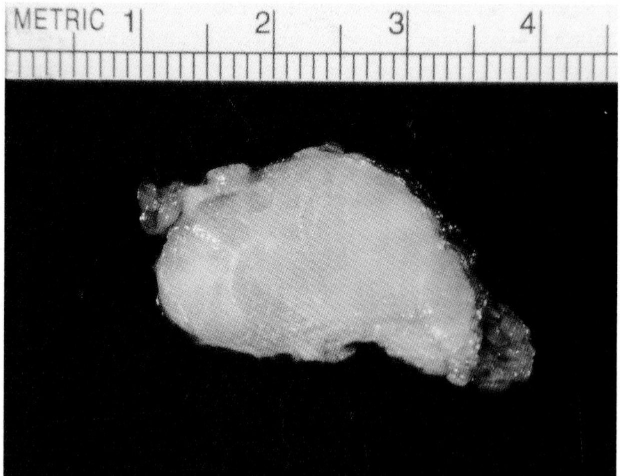

FIGURE 24-21 ■ JHF presented as a firm mass around the knee of a 17-year-old female who had several other similar masses excised previous to this one. This well-circumscribed mass had a glistening, slightly nodular appearance on cut surface. The consistency of the mass was described as firm with a chondroid-like quality.

visceral involvement in addition to papulonodular lesions of the skin and soft tissues. The heart, intestinal tract, spleen, and skeletal muscle are infiltrated by the fibrohyaline tissue with a resemblance to amyloid. Protein-losing enteropathy is a complication of small intestinal hyalinosis. Only infantile myofibromatosis among the other fibrous proliferations has visceral involvement by a more cellular, vasocentric nodular proliferation than the diffuse interstitial hyalinosis of ISH.

Calcifying aponeurotic fibromatosis (juvenile aponeurotic fibroma) is one of the least common of the fibrous tumors of childhood (1% to 2% of all cases) with a predilection for the distal extremities (75). Usually, older children and adolescents present with a mass in the ankle or wrist in the deep subcutis, fascia, or tendon. A poorly circumscribed mass measuring less than 5 cm has a firm, gritty, gray-white appearance of cut surface. An infiltrative process of spindle cells (fibroblasts) is accompanied by less cellular, hyalinized areas in which foci of granular calcifications are found. Without the calcifications, there is a resemblance to infantile subcutaneous

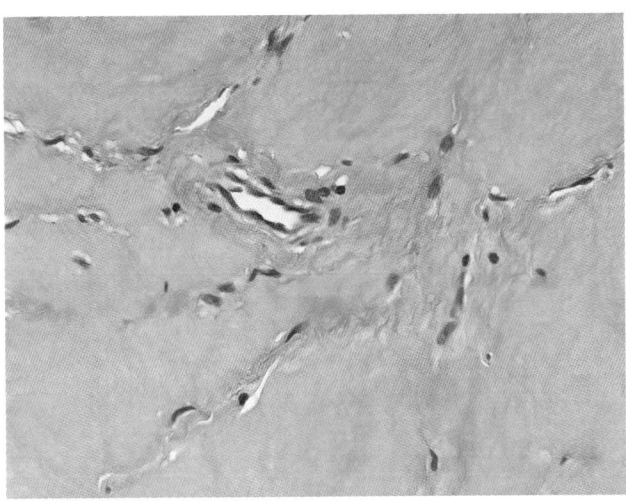

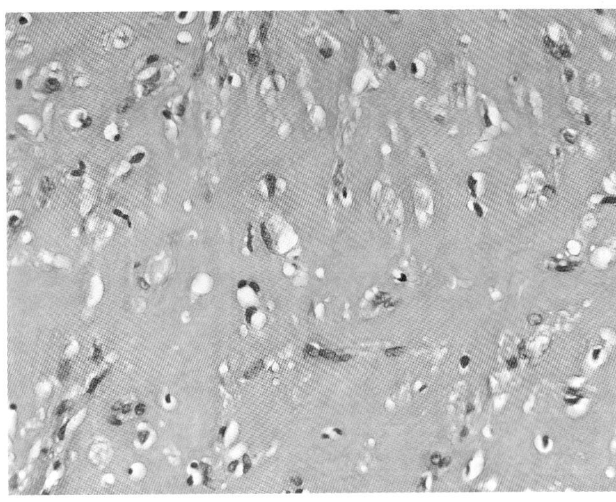

A B

FIGURE 24-22 ■ JHF presented as multiple masses in this 17-year-old female. **A:** The dense, hypocellular nodules of collagen are characteristic of this tumor. **B:** Rounded stromal cells within lacunar spaces resembling chondrocytes is another histologic feature. No other fibrous lesion in childhood approaches this degree of dense, uniform hyalinization with the possible exception of a Gardner fibroma which lacks nodularity.

fibromatosis. Recurrences are reported in 50% or more of cases. Because of the distal, periarticular localization, monophasic SS may be briefly considered in the differential diagnosis.

Juvenile nasopharyngeal angiofibroma (JNA) is a tumor whose ambiguous histogenesis has resulted in its uncertain classification in the past as a fibroma or vascular tumor. Most cases present in older male children or adolescents with epistaxis. These tumors are seen in the setting of FAP. Like desmoid-type fibromatosis, the nuclei of JNA express β-catenin. A firm lobulated or pedunculated mass measuring 5 to 10 cm is the gross appearance. A uniform population of spindled to stellate fibroblasts lacks a fasciculated pattern and is interrupted by evenly distributed thin-walled vascular spaces. Mast cells are commonly distributed within the background. These tumors have pushing rather than the infiltrating borders of a desmoid-type fibromatosis.

Fibromatosis colli is infrequently seen as a surgical specimen though it is one of the more common fibrous tumors of childhood since spontaneous regression occurs in more than 90% of cases (39). A firm, white lobulated fibrous mass measuring 1 to 3 cm typically arises in the lower one-third of the sternocleidomastoid muscle where it has infiltrative borders like the desmoid-type fibromatosis though fibromatosis colli is usually more cellular with a less collagenized stroma. There is some similarity to NF, which only rarely arises in skeletal muscle.

Inflammatory myofibroblastic tumor (IMT) is a distinctive clinicopathologic entity, which has emerged from a somewhat poorly defined group of idiopathic fibroinflammatory processes collectivity known as inflammatory pseudotumors (88). In the WHO Classification, the IMT is regarded as an "intermediate, rarely metastasizing" neoplasm, which principally occurs in the first three decades with cases seen as early as the first year of life into early adulthood with a mean age at diagnosis between 10 and 15 years without the inclusion of older adults (42,75). The lung, gastrointestinal tract, mesentery, liver, and bladder are the principal primary sites, which in aggregate account for 70% to 75% of all cases in children (Table 24-6). This tumor is also ubiquitous in terms of its other less common sites of presentation including the dura, orbit, kidney, uterus, and upper respiratory tract. Peripheral soft tissues and bones are rarely affected. In a small proportion of cases, multiple lesions may be detected at presentation or develop over a prolonged clinical course. It is not always clear whether multiple IMTs are metastatic lesions or independently developing multifocal tumors (149). Constitutional or B-symptoms with fever, failure to thrive, and weight loss together with microcytic hypochromic anemia and polyclonal gammopathy are present in 5% to 15% of cases; these children may be a diagnostic dilemma for weeks to months. There is IL-6 production in association with IMTs, which often falls to normal levels after surgical resection.

The tumors range in size from less than 1 to 15 cm in greatest dimension, with the larger IMTs arising in the abdomen. In the lung, IMT measures 4 to 6 cm, but in the mesentery or retroperitoneum, IMT is generally in excess of 10 cm. A well-circumscribed, non–encapsulated tumor has a glistening tan-white to gray-tan homogeneous and nodular appearance, with minimal hemorrhage and absence of necrosis in most cases. Calcifications are seen more often in the pulmonary IMTs (where it is the most common primary neoplasm of the lung in childhood) but occur in extrapulmonary sites as well. Microscopically, three basic patterns are recognized; they are not necessarily in equal proportions nor is each represented in every case. The first of these is characterized by a dense spindle cell proliferation with some fascicular formation in association with a variably prominent population of lymphocytes and mature plasma cells in the background.

Table 24-6 ■ SITE OF IMT IN THE FIRST TWO DECADES OF LIFE

Sites	No.	Mean Age and Range	Sex (M/F)	Total (%)
Abdomen				61 (50)
Small Intestine	36	9 years (3 months–17 years)	13/23	
Omentum-mesentery				
Liver	11	4 years (2 months–9 years)	6/5	
Stomach	5	9 years (6 years–14 years)	2/3	
Retroperitoneum	5	7 years (4 months–14 years)	3/2	
Pancreas	2	12 years, 7	1/1	
Spleen	2	16 years, 9 years	2/0	
Genitourinary Tract				16 (13)
Bladder	13	11 years (4 years–17 years)	6/7	
Scrotum	2	7 years, 15 years	2/0	
Prostate	1	17 years	1/0	
Thorax				32 (26)
Lung	17	10 years (2 years–20 years)	13/4	
Larynx-Trachea	6	7 years (12 days–12 years)	3/3	
Heart	9	2 ½ years (1 month–12 years)	6/3	
Superficial and Deep Soft Tissues				12 (10)
Extremities–trunk	5	6 years (1 month–13 years)	3/2	
Head and neck	3	2 years(1 year–3 years)	2/1	
Perirectal–pelvic	4	8 years (3 years–13 years)	1/3	
Brain				2 (2)
	2	1 year, 15 years	0/2	123 (~100)

From the files of the Lauren V. Ackerman Laboratory of Surgical Pathology, St. Louis Children's Hospital, Washington University Medical Center, St. Louis, MO.

Adjacent foci may be composed of loosely arranged spindled to plump stromal cells in a myxoedematous background resembling NF to yet a third pattern of paucicellular dense fibrosis with some inflammatory cells in the background (Figure 24-23A). Dystrophic calcifications, osseous metaplasia, and collections of histiocytes are other features. Mitotic figures are found in the spindle cell foci; however, atypical mitotic figures and anaplasia should suggest a high-grade pleomorphic sarcoma. Necrosis is present in those IMTs, which have undergone sarcomatous changes and may be accompanied by overt nuclear pleomorphism and hyperchromatism. Most IMTs are immunoreactive for vimentin, SMA (Figure 24-23B), and cytokeratin in a minority of cases in children. Approximately 50% to 60% of IMTs are ALK-1 positive with a membrane or cytoplasmic pattern to reflect a specific ALK-1 translocation (Figure 24-23C) (53,168,215) (Table 24-2). Coffin and associates found that ALK-1-positive IMTs pursue a less aggressive course than those which are ALK-1-negative (42). Surgical resection is the treatment of choice with a recurrence-free survival of 80% or greater.

The differential diagnosis includes low-grade myofibroblastic sarcoma, NF, inflammatory leiomyosarcoma, myxofibrosarcoma and calcifying fibrous pseudotumor, desmoid-type fibromatosis, and gastrointestinal stromal tumor (GIST). The latter two neoplasms, when arising in the mesentery or intestine, display β-catenin (nuclear) and CD117 immunopositivity, respectively. Calcifying fibrous tumor is thought to be a distinctively different entity from IMT; this tumor is recognized more commonly in adults than IMT but also occurs in the mesentery-omentum and intestinal tract like the latter. Irregular dystrophic and/or psammomatous calcifications are found in a uniform fibrous background. These tumors are CD34-positive, show sparse reactivity for SMA, and are uniformly ALK-1-negative.

Myxoinflammatory fibroblastic sarcoma and myxofibrosarcoma are tumors of the peripheral soft tissues typically seen in adults (71). Inflammatory leiomyosarcoma is likewise a sarcoma of adults, which is desmin- and SMA-positive. NF shares a histologic pattern with IMT but is small (2 cm or less), and superficial in most cases. SMA is positive in both, but ALK-1 is not expressed in NF. Low-grade myofibroblastic sarcoma is a rare sarcoma with many overlapping morphologic and immunohistochemical features in common with IMT except for the fact that it generally does not occur in children and adolescents and is seen in the head and neck region and extremities rather than the lung and abdomen as in the case of IMT. Finally, we acknowledge that it is not always clear in some cases when the diagnosis of inflammatory pseudotumor should be applied to a fibroinflammatory mass. However, there are other entities in addition to the IMT, which were designated as inflammatory pseudotumors in the past such as the dendritic cell (DC) tumor. Most deep circumscribed mass lesions in children composed of myofibroblasts and inflammatory cells, which are either ALK-1-positive or -negative are probably examples of IMT.

Fibrosarcoma (FS) includes several specific pathologic entities: congenital infantile FS, low-grade fibromyxoid sarcoma (LGFS), and sclerosing epithelioid FS, all of which are seen in children and one, congenital infantile FS, which occurs almost exclusively in the first few years of life and is

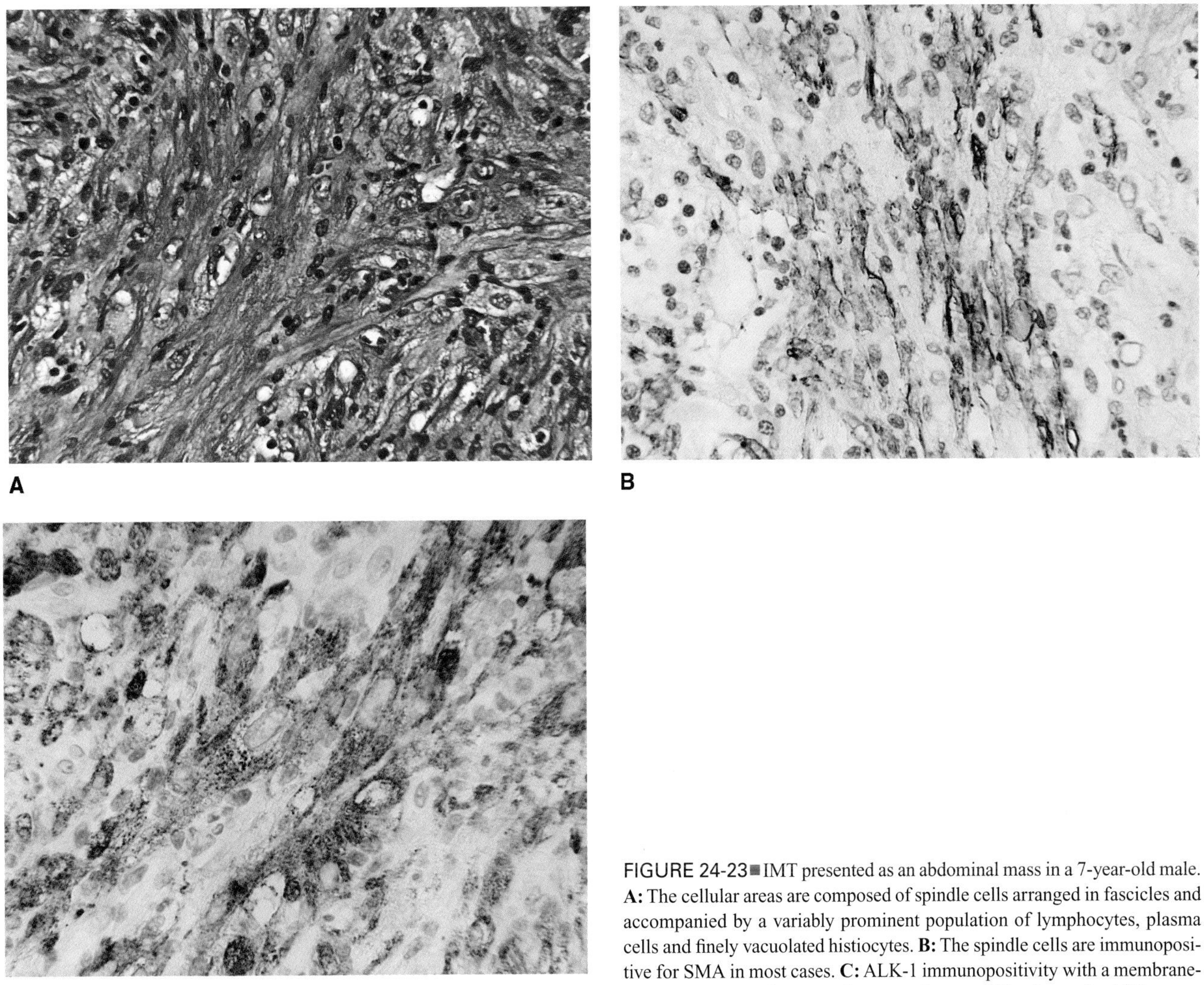

A

B

C

FIGURE 24-23 ■ IMT presented as an abdominal mass in a 7-year-old male. **A:** The cellular areas are composed of spindle cells arranged in fascicles and accompanied by a variably prominent population of lymphocytes, plasma cells and finely vacuolated histiocytes. **B:** The spindle cells are immunopositive for SMA in most cases. **C:** ALK-1 immunopositivity with a membraneous and cytoplasmic pattern is present in over 50% of cases in children.

distinguished pathologically from the adult-type FS (75). In other diagnostic settings, FS or spindle cell sarcoma is the differential diagnosis for monophasic SS, MPNST, leiomyosarcoma, spindle cell RMS, and the disputed infantile rhabdomyofibrosarcoma when the latter five neoplasms have been excluded after a through immunohistochemical and molecular-cytogenetic evaluation. In other words, adult-type FS is in a sense a pathologic diagnosis of exclusion. However, there is a CD34-positive variant of adult-type FS, which occurs in children and adults (68,72). Adult FSs in most cases in children are grade 2 neoplasms based upon a mitotic count of five mitoses or fewer per 10 high-power fields (Figure 24-24). These tumors tend to be less than 6 cm in diameter, are well circumscribed, and lack necrosis (Figure 24-25).

Congenital infantile fibrosarcoma (CIFS) generally presents in the first year or two of life as a large mass occupying a substantial portion of the involved site (hand, foot or entire extremity, trunk) or an obstructing mass in the small or

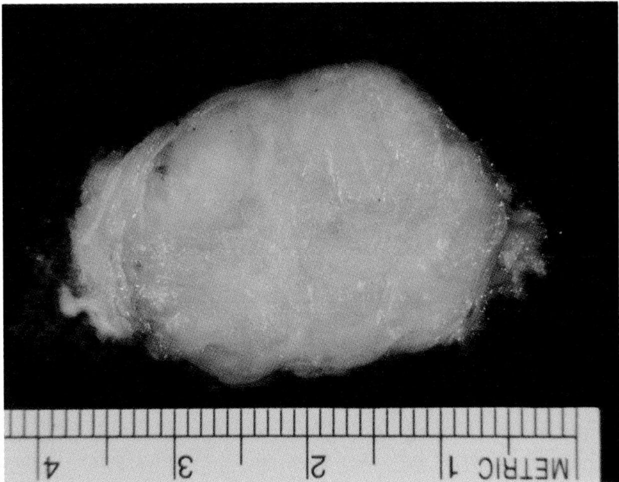

FIGURE 24-24 ■ FS (adult type) presented in the region of the right ankle in this 7-year-old male. The cut surface of this 4.5 cm mass has a faintly multinodular tan-white glistening appearance.

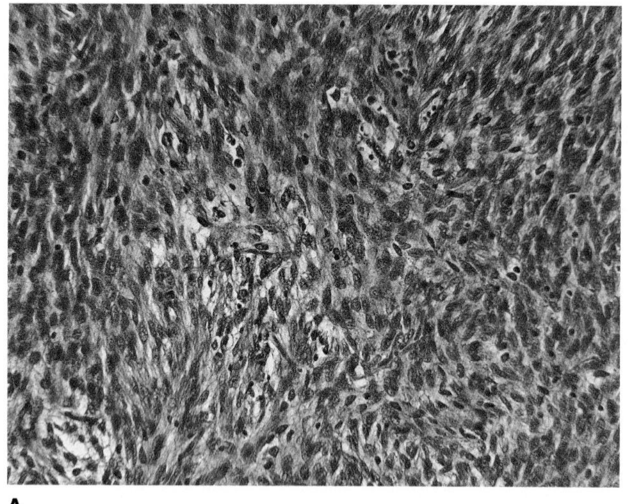

A

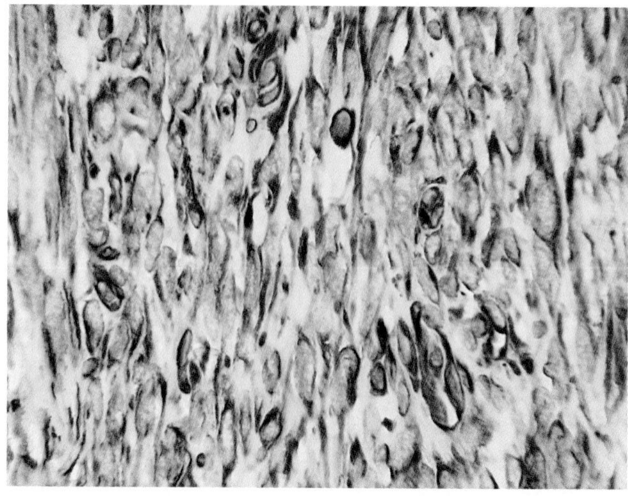

B

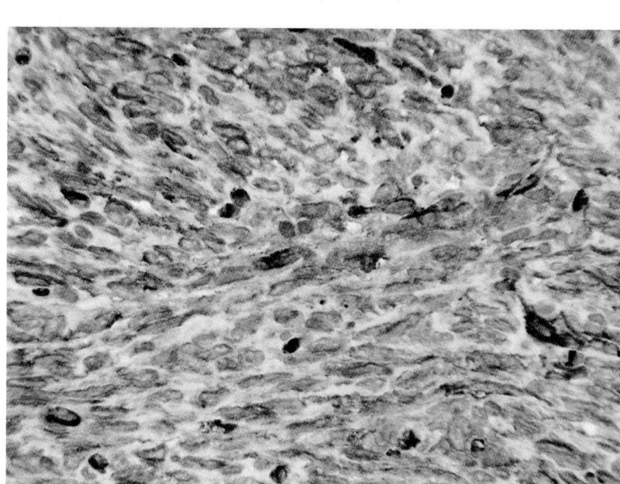

C

FIGURE 24-25 FS (adult type) presented in the ankle of a 7-year-old male. **A:** The pattern is that of densely apposed spindle cells with fusiform nuclei with prominent nucleoli. Mitotic activity is brisk. **B:** The tumor cells are uniformly positive for vimentin. **C:** There is diffuse membrane positivity for CD34 and negative for all other markers and did not have the t(x;18) translocation of SS.

large intestine of an infant. These tumors can be quite hemorrhagic and may be mistaken for a vascular tumor clinically. In the past, this tumor was managed by extensive surgery including amputation, but today CIFS is treated by low dosage adjuvant chemotherapy with often impressive reduction in its size. A circumscribed, but non–encapsulated mass measuring 6 to 15 cm in greatest dimension has either uniform, glistening tan-white cut surface or a cystic, hemorrhagic, and friable character whose features may suggest something other than CIFS. Fascicles of uniform spindle cells with or without the so-called herringbone pattern are the classical features, but we have been impressed by the histologic diversity of these tumors that have a poorly organized pattern of immature and even primitive mesenchymal cells; the more primitive appearing CIFSs can be more aggressive in behavior than their typical spindle cell counterpart (Figure 24-26). A primitive RMS or an undifferentiated sarcoma (US) may be considered in the differential diagnosis before IHC and/or molecular genetic studies are applied to sort out the diagnosis. Though the histologic pattern may be problematic, CIFS has the ETV6-NTRK3 fusion transcript, t(12;15)(p13;q25), in most cases (136) (Table 24-2). Other cytogenetic abnormalities include trisomy 11, t(12;13), gains in chromosomes 8, 11, 17, and 20; and deletion of 17q. Foci resembling CIFS may be found in other fibrous tumors of childhood including infantile myofibromatosis, but the characteristic translocation is not present in these cases. The other neoplasm with the t(12;15) translocation is the cellular mesoblastic nephroma or infantile FS of the kidney. After chemotherapy, the resected specimen may have minimal residual tumor with only fibrosis, histiocytes, and hemosiderin deposition. Metastasis occurs in less than 5% of cases. In the lung, the infantile peribronchial myofibroblastic tumor has a histologic resemblance to CIFS but lacks the signature translocation of the latter tumor.

Low-grade fibromyxoid sarcoma (LGFS) (Evans tumor) is a generally slow-growing soft-tissue neoplasm with a preference for the lower extremity and trunk (78,156). Approximately 20% of cases are discovered before the age of 20 years and have been seen as early as 4 years old (89). A well-circumscribed, nonencapsulated fibrous-appearing tumor has a distinctive microscopic appearance of bland spindle cells with an alternating pale myxoid background to a

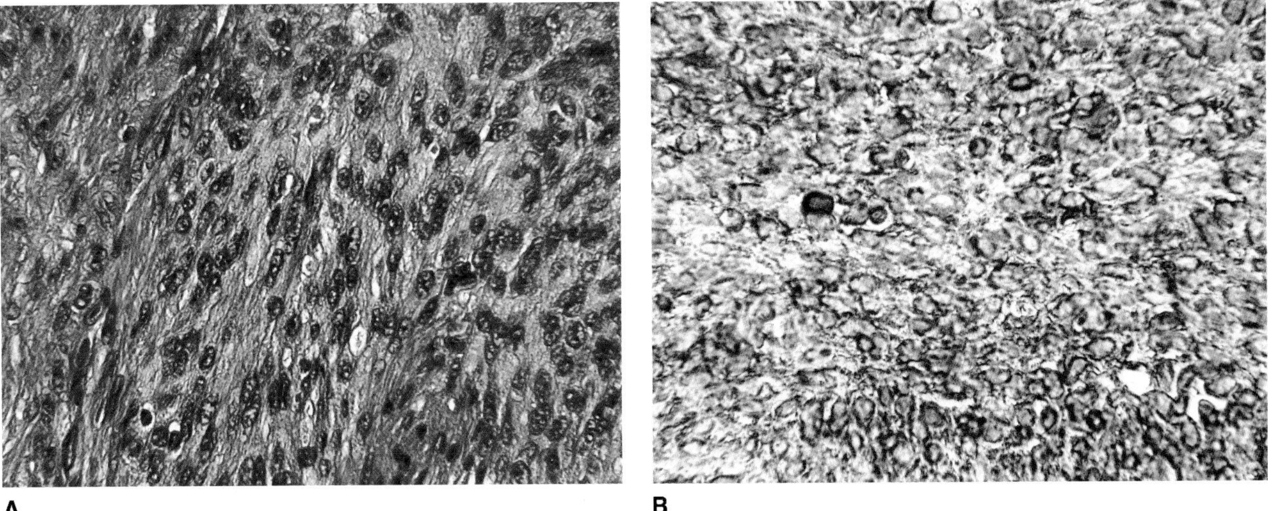

A B

FIGURE 24-26 ■ CIFS presented as a mass in the jejunum of a 3-month-old female. **A:** A uniform proliferation of spindle cells with and without a fascicular growth pattern is the characteristic appearance of this tumor. **B:** The spindle cells are consistently immunopositive for vimentin, but little else. This tumor was translocation positive.

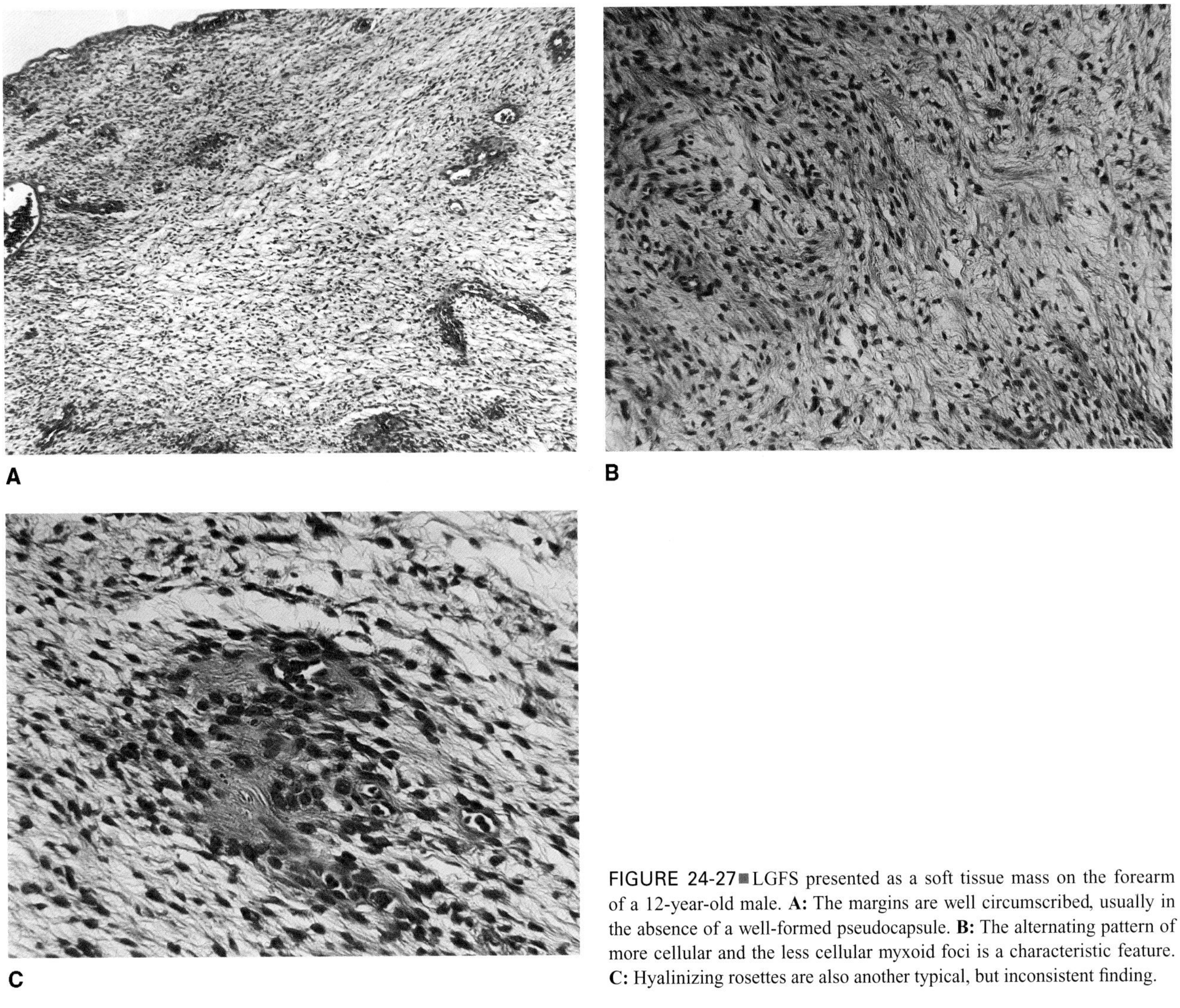

A B

C

FIGURE 24-27 ■ LGFS presented as a soft tissue mass on the forearm of a 12-year-old male. **A:** The margins are well circumscribed, usually in the absence of a well-formed pseudocapsule. **B:** The alternating pattern of more cellular and the less cellular myxoid foci is a characteristic feature. **C:** Hyalinizing rosettes are also another typical, but inconsistent finding.

more collagenous stroma (Figure 24-27). Foci of epithelioid cells are found in those tumors with a hyalinized stroma and in some of these cases, hyalinizing giant rosettes are present to establish the linkage between LGFS and the hyalinizing spindle cell tumor with giant rosettes (205) (Figure 24-27C). A shared translocation, t(7;16)(q34;p11), has been identified in 90% of cases as well as a second less common translocation, t(11;16) (p11;q11). Immunohistochemically, LGFS is diffusely positive for vimentin and focally for epithelial membrane antigen (EMA) in greater than 75% of cases.

Sclerosing epithelioid fibrosarcoma (SEFS), an uncommon subtype of FS, is seen on occasion in adolescents but more often in the latter decades of life (75,162). The lower extremity and pelvis are the preferred sites of presentation and reside in the deep soft tissue where bone involvement may be present. A hyalinized matrix like stroma contains the small aggregates and individual epithelioid cells, which are only immunoreactive for vimentin. The SEFS is an aggressive neoplasm, which metastasizes to the lungs in 50% to 70% of cases. A rearrangement of chromosome 10p11 is reported. Sclerotic areas in LGFS have a resemblance to SEFS.

Solitary fibrous tumor (SFT) and **hemangiopericytoma (HPC)** have been wedded as a pathologic continuum and classified with the fibroblastic-myofibroblastic tumors in the same WHO category of intermediate, rarely metastasizing neoplasms (75). The relationship of SFT and HPC to each other has been reviewed by Gengles and Guillou (85). Most cases of SFT arise from the pleura in adults, but any number of nonpleural sites of origin have been documented in both children and adolescents so that it is important to consider this diagnosis when presented with a bland appearing spindle cell neoplasm with a collagenous stroma (172). The cellular foci may alternate with less cellular fibrous areas. Some SFTs may be more uniformly cellular with a variety of patterns associated with FS (fascicular or herringbone), nerve sheath neoplasm especially in the presence of a myxoid background or LGFS (palisading) or storiform (fibrous histiocytoma and dermatofibrosarcoma). Both SFT and HPC are immunoreactive for vimentin and CD34; this immunophenotype is shared with DFSP, but in most cases, a distinction is made by the clinical presentation of a dermal-subcutaneous-based neoplasm in the case of DFSP rather than a deep soft tissue or serosal-based mass in the case of a SFT. In terms of HPC, a differentiation is made between infantile myofibromatosis–associated HPC and HPC presenting in the soft tissues in older children, adolescents, and adults. The HPC-like pattern may be encountered in other soft-tissue neoplasms including monophasic SS, congenital infantile FS, mesenchymal chondrosarcoma (MCS) and MPNST.

Dermatofibrosarcoma protuberans (DFSP) and the related **giant cell fibroblastoma (GCF)** have been regarded variously as fibrohistiocytic or fibroblastic neoplasms. Given the fibrosarcomatous progression in some DFSPs, the tumor may have declared itself in a histogenetic sense. Approximately 8% to 10% of DFSPs are diagnosed in the first two decades of life, but some tumors, which are finally diagnosed in adults have been present clinically since childhood (35,36). The early suggestion that GCF is the juvenile variant of DFSP has been validated by the demonstration of a shared translocation, t(17;22)(q22;q13) as well as concurrent histologic patterns of DFSP and GCF in the same tumor (107) (Table 24-2). The earliest clinical presentation is a tumor noted shortly after birth (10% of cases) (86). A nodule or hypertrophic or atrophic plaques on the trunk or proximal extremity are two of the more common presentations. Other less common sites include an acral or inguinal-perineal localization. Except for the more frequent pattern of GCF in children (75% or so of cases <20 years old), DFSP is a tumor that occupies the mid-to-lower dermis with contiguous extension into the subcutis with overgrowth of fat and extension along fibrous septa and into the deep fascia.

Three basic histologic patterns account for the microscopic variation and the diagnostic challenge offered by DFSP: uniform low-grade compact spindle cell proliferation with or without storiform profiles, spindle cells with fibroblastic features, and a collagenous stroma resembling a fibrous tumor and a pale myxoid background with separation of spindle cells (Figure 24-28). GCF has a similar pattern of infiltration as the classic DFSP. Pigmented cells are found in the so-called Bednar tumor or pigmented DFSP (176). The floret-like giant cells of GCF appear to reside in tissue clefts and spaces. The mesenchymal cells can display substantial cytologic variability and have a somewhat primitive appearance in a fibromyxoid background. A more fibrous appearance may suggest a fibromatosis. The diagnosis is eased if there are areas of classic storiform DFSP. Perivascular lymphocytes in GCF are useful in the diagnosis. Vimentin and CD34 are expressed by the tumor cells (Figure 24-28C) (197). It has been reported that DFSP and GCFs can be immunopositive for CD99 (in addition to SS, angiomatoid fibrous histiocytoma (AFH) and other EWS family of tumors, MRT, SFT, HPC, and MCS).

The differential diagnosis of DFSP includes fibrohistiocytic tumors of the skin, and in some cases, even after thorough immunohistochemical evaluation, there may remain some uncertainty about the final diagnosis. Factor XIIIa immunoreactivity is often useful to establish the identity of a fibrohistiocytic tumor whereas CD34 is negative in most cases. Juvenile xanthogranuloma (JXG) with a predominant spindle cell pattern can be mistaken for DFSP when Touton giant cells are not present. The medallion-like dermal dendrocyte hamartoma must be considered in any rounded, atrophic lesion on the upper trunk, which has a congenital clinical presentation. A spindle to oval cell proliferation replaces the dermis with concentric proliferation around small vessels and nerve. There is extension into the subcutis like the DFSP; these tumors are immunopositive for factor XIIIa and CD34 but lack the t(17;22) translocation of DFSP.

FIBROHISTIOCYTIC TUMORS

WHO classification of fibrohistiocytic tumors conveys a certain element of skepticism in referring to them as the

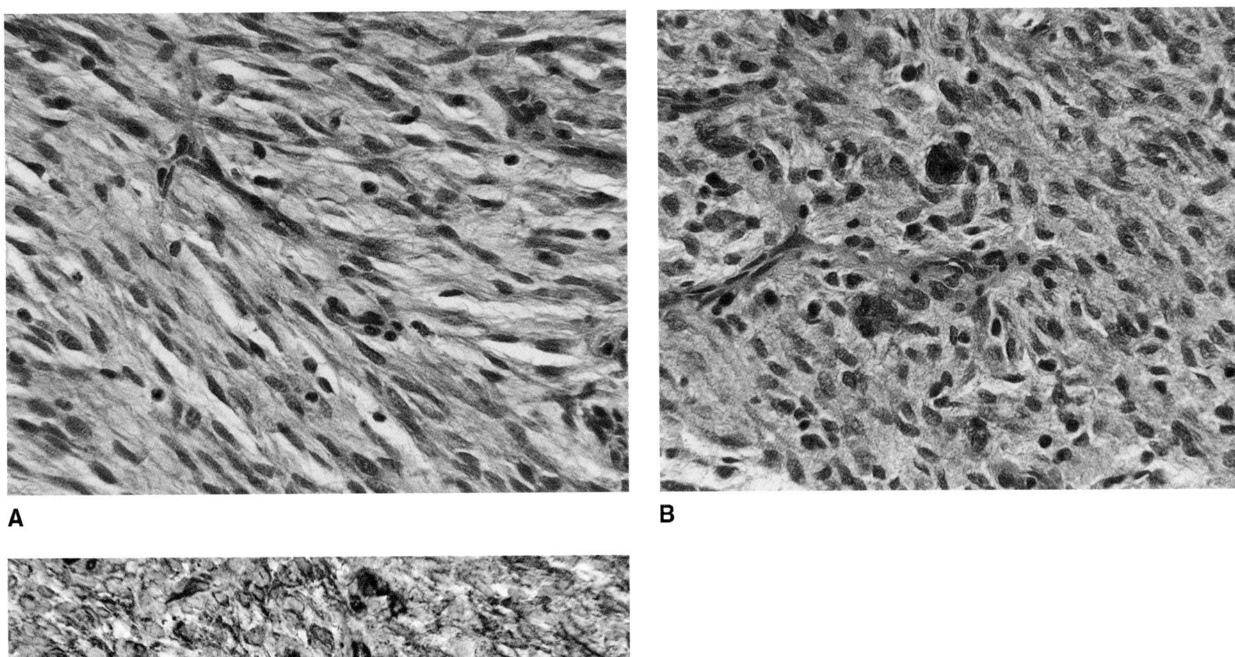

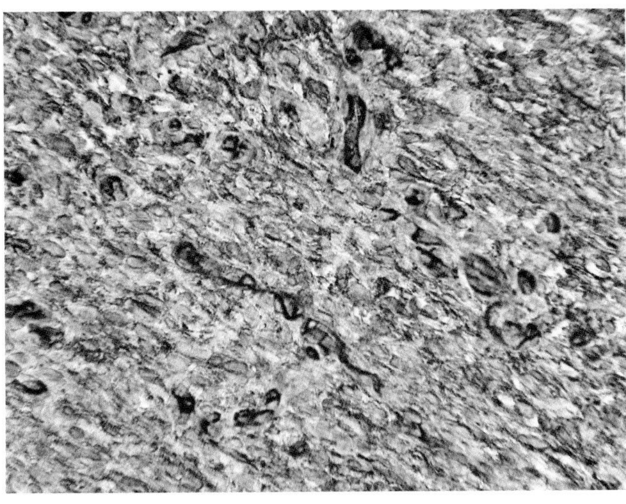

FIGURE 24-28 ■ DFSP presented as a soft tissue mass in the breast of a 2-year-old female. **A:** Uniform spindle cells with pale staining nuclei are arranged in broad fascicles. **B:** Among the spindle cells, there are scattered giant cells similar to those in the GCF. **C:** The tumor cells are diffusely immunoreactive for CD34.

"so-called fibrohistiocytic tumors (75)." The pathway to this state of affairs was the result of the decline and fall of the malignant fibrous histiocytoma (MFH) as it reemerged as the "undifferentiated pleomorphic sarcoma," which was premised on the argument that MFH was nothing more than the final common morphologic and biologic pathway for several specific types of STSs mainly in adults (54). Pleomorphic sarcomas are uncommonly encountered in children and some of these have been second malignant neoplasms in a survivor of a first childhood malignancy. In a review of STSs in children exclusive of RMS, Hayes-Jordan and associates reported that 11% of cases were diagnosed as MFHs in addition to the more common SS (24% of cases) and MPNST (15% of cases) (93).

Fibrous histiocytoma in some respects appears as often as a histogenetic concept as a specific diagnosis in a child or adult. Dermatofibroma (DF) of the skin (benign cutaneous fibrous histiocytoma) is the most common "conceptual" representative of fibrohistiocytic tumors in children and adults in our experience. Even the latter statement is the subject of disagreement by Zegler and associates who refer to DF as "fibrosing dermatitis" rather than a true neoplasm (218). Another viewpoint is that the DF is a neoplasm of dermal dendrocytes, which explains some of its overlapping microscopic and immunohistochemical features to those of JXG (52). In addition to a pure spindle cell proliferation in the dermis with its characteristic collagen trapping at its CD34-immunopositive lateral margins, DF may contain hemosiderin-laden macrophages (hemosiderotic DF) with focal hemorrhage, prominent erythrocyte-filled lakes (aneurysmal DF), multinucleated giant cells, or epithelioid histiocytes (Figure 24-29). The histiocytic component among the spindle cells may have finely xanthomatized or foamy cytoplasm. Touton-like giant cells may raise the possibility of JXG which cannot be resolved with IHC since the latter and DF both express factor XIIIa. However, JXG in the skin has a "pushing" rather than infiltrating margins into the dermis of a DF. DF can extend into the deep dermis and subcutis to cause concern about DFSP, but infiltration into the subcutaneous fat is not a feature of DF (14).

A problematic fibrohistiocytic lesion is the so-called **benign fibrous histiocytoma (BFH)** of the subcutis and

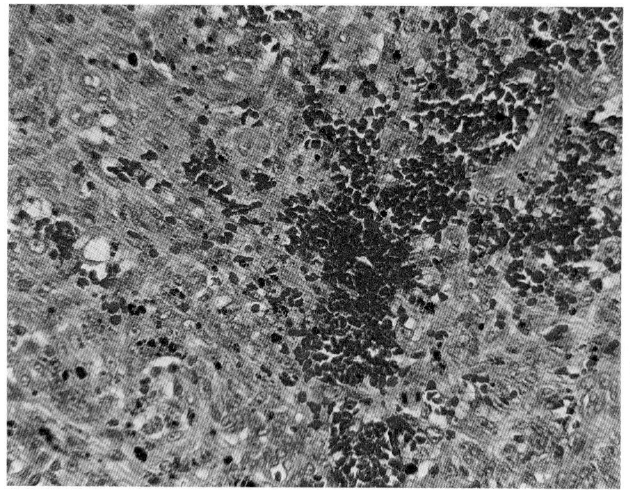
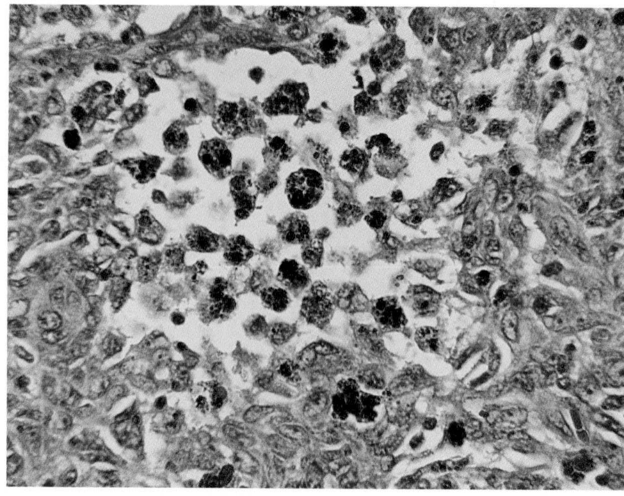

A B

FIGURE 24-29 ■ Hemosiderotic DF in the lower extremity of a 16 year old male. **A:** The tumor is composed of plump spindle cells with interstitial hemorrhage. **B:** In this field there are collections of hemosiderin laden macrophages.

deep soft tissues with a recurrence rate of 15% (compared to the DF with a local recurrence rate of 5% or less) and a rarely expressed potential for metastasis (87). Microscopically, BFH is a hypercellular spindle cell neoplasm, more so than a DF, whose cells tend to have more cytoplasm but can resemble the more common DF. Multinucleated giant cells and mitotic figures may be present in BFH. Atypical mitoses and anaplasia are present in the rare atypical fibroxanthoma of skin in a child. If metastasis develops, it is more often than not after multiple local recurrences of a BFH.

The differential diagnosis of a suspected fibrous histiocytoma is determined to some degree on the presenting site. In the skin, DFSP and JXG are the principal diagnostic considerations whereas in the subcutis or deeper soft tissues, NF with a storiform pattern with or without multinucleated giant cells has a resemblance to a fibrous histiocytoma. In the bone, fibrous histiocytoma and nonossifying fibroma are often a microscopic distinction without a difference. Fibrous histiocytoma in the airway or lung has some features in common with the IMT. JXG also rarely presents as a solitary mass in the upper airway.

Giant cell tumor (GCT) of tendon sheath has two patterns: the more common nodular (nodular tenosynovitis) and the less common diffuse (extra-articular pigmented villonodular tenosynovitis) types (51,183). The diffuse GCT may be composed almost exclusively of mononuclear cells despite its appellation and is located in the deep soft tissues, often in or around a large joint, but extra-articular in location (188). The localized nodular GCT presents in the finger or wrist as a firm nodule, measuring 2 cm or less and well circumscribed by a fibrous capsule. The nodule is composed of bland appearing mononuclear cells with a variable number of multinucleated cells. Spindle cells, xanthomatized histiocytes, and hemosiderin are other features.

Pigmented villonodular synovitis is reported in children, typically over the age of 10 years, presenting in the knee joint with a chronic joint effusion (129). Papillary-appearing hemorrhagic tissues are characterized by synovial cell hyperplasia with a hypercellular stroma and hemosiderin-laden mononuclear cells. Chronic hemarthropathy of hemophilia and synovial hemangiomatosis are other considerations in the differential diagnosis.

Two fibrohistiocytic tumors, AFH and plexiform fibrohistiocytic tumor (PFHT), occur predominantly in children and are both regarded as intermediate or low malignant potential neoplasms (75).

Angiomatoid fibrous histiocytoma (AFH) is a slowly enlarging tumor of the extremities or trunk in a child older than 10 years or in a young adult (61). The tumor may present in the vicinity of a lymph node so that an apparent lymphoid-based neoplasm may be the initial microscopic impression in the presence of nodular collections of lymphocytes around the periphery of the mass but in the absence of a fibrous capsule and subcapsular sinusoids. Constitutional manifestations like those of the IMT have been observed in a small minority of cases. A sharply demarcated, but nonencapsulated mass measures from 1 to 8 cm in diameter. Cystic areas of hemorrhage are commonly seen on cut surface but may be absent either grossly or microscopically with the seeming contradiction of a nonangiomatoid AFH (Figure 24-30). An incomplete fibrous pseudocapsule contains prominent collections of small lymphocytes and plasma cells. The tumor cells are ovoid to spindle shape and are arranged in densely cellular nodular cells with faint storiform configuration. There is minimal nuclear atypia and mitotic figures in most cases, but some tumors can display individual nuclear pleomorphism and considerable mitotic activity, even atypical mitotic figures. Occasionally, giant cells are present. Immunohistochemically, these tumors are reactive for

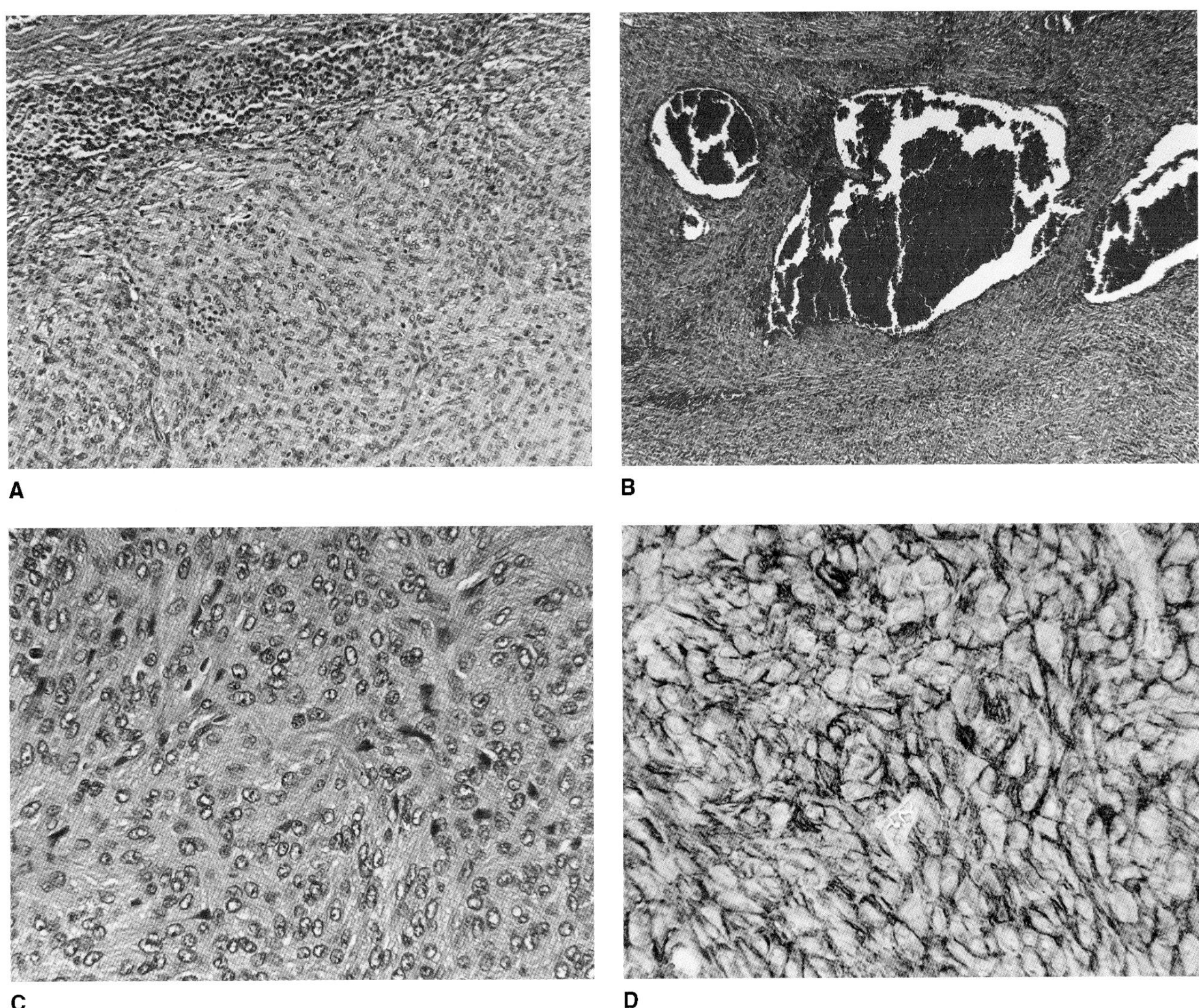

FIGURE 24-30 ■ AFH in a 14-year-old male presented in the upper arm. **A:** A lymphocytic infiltrate is present at the periphery of the mass in addition to lymphoid follicles can be mistaken for a lymph node-based neoplasm. **B:** The angiomatoid characterization of this tumor is based upon the presence of red cell filled spaces. These spaces are seen in most but not all cases which can lead to diagnostic difficulties. **C:** The tumor cells have ovoid to polygonal-shaped nuclei and eosinophilic cytoplasm. The cell borders are poorly defined. Scattered mitotic figures are present and in some cases, atypical mitotic figures may be seen. **D:** Immunohistochemical staining for CD99 shows diffuse membrane positivity. This tumor had an EWS breakapart by FISH.

vimentin (100% of cases), desmin (40% to 50% of cases), CD68, EMA (5% to 10% of cases), and CD99 (diffuse membrano-cytoplasmic staining similar to EWS-PNET in 50% or more of cases) (Figure 24-30D). The CD99 positivity is interesting in light of the molecular genetics of EWS gene fusion in the EWSR1-ATF1 translocation (186,199) (Table 24-2). There is a local recurrence rate of 10% to 15% and distant metastasis in 5% or less of cases. The rare case may have metastatic involvement of a regional lymph node upon initial clinical presentation.

Plexiform fibrohistiocytic tumor (PFHT) is a distinctive neoplasm of the dermis and/or subcutis whose morphologic variability contributes to some of its difficulties in pathologic diagnosis (148). A firm nodule on the forearm, lower extremity, or trunk in a child over 10 years of age and into early adulthood is the clinical presentation. The multinodular growth pattern at low magnification is characteristic; these nodules may be composed of fibroblast-like cells and/or mononuclear cells with osteoclast-like giant cells whose numbers can vary from inapparent to several in the midst of the mononuclear cells. In those PFHTs with a predominant fibroblastic pattern, an inflammatory component is often present (Figure 24-31). Infiltration of the subcutaneous fat has some similarities to infantile subcutaneous fibromatosis. Adding to the challenge is that the fibroblasts are often immunoreactive for SMA. Overall, PFHT has a locally nonaggressive appearance in contrast to a fibromatosis and has minimal mitotic activity in most cases. A background of hyalinized collagen can accentuate the nested character of the tumor and can have some resemblance to the clear cell sarcoma (CCS) of tendon sheath. The mononuclear cells of

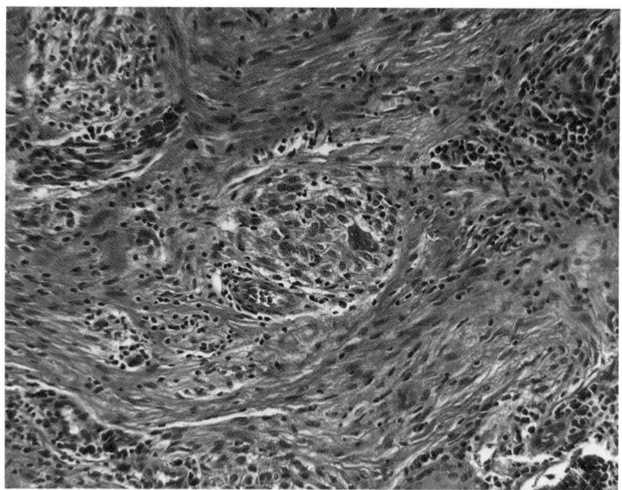
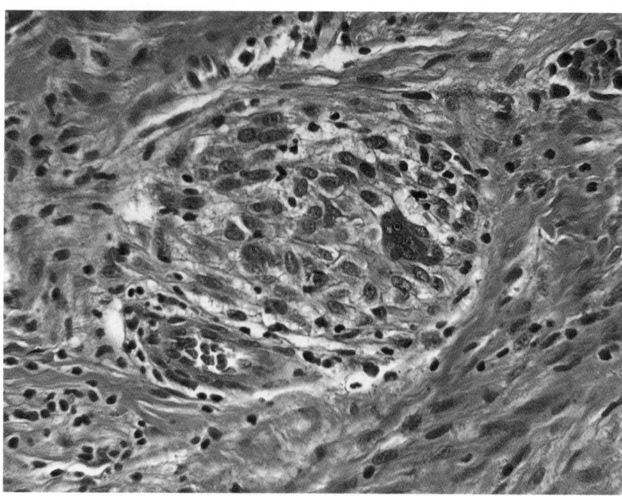

A B

FIGURE 24-31 ■ PFHT in a 5-year-old female presented on the lower extremity. **A:** A mass measuring 2 cm in greatest dimension involved the lower dermis and underlying subcutis and composed of nodules of pale staining histiocyte-like cells with lymphocytes. **B:** Some or many of the nodules have one or several multinucleated giant cells.

PFHT are immunoreactive for CD68 whereas the tumor cells in the CCS express S100 proteins and HMB-45 (196). Other considerations in the differential diagnosis when the dermis is involved by multiple nodules of histiocytic cells is a melanocytic proliferation (Spitz or cellular blue nevus) and neurothekeoma especially in those PFHTs with myxoid features. One histogenetic perspective is that PFHT and cellular neurothekeoma may be related neoplasms. Like other fibrohistiocytic neoplasms, PFHT has a reported local recurrence rate of 15% to 40%, but a metastatic rate of less than 2% of cases.

Dendritic cell (DC) neoplasms are composed of cells whose normal function is antigen presentation represented by four distinctive types: follicular DC, interdigitating DC (IDC), Langerhans cell, and histiocytic-fibroblastic cell. The latter cell may serve as the neoplastic progenitor for the DF and JXG. The Langerhans cell and Langerhans cell histiocytosis (LCH) are familiar topics in pediatric pathology. **JXG** is likewise well known as a cutaneous lesion in a young child, but approximately 5% of cases of JXG in children present as a mass in the subcutis or within the skeletal muscle (52,106). These children are less than 1-year-old at diagnosis and the mass may even be present at birth. The head and neck and trunk are the sites of predilection for a nodule measuring 3 cm or less. A well-circumscribed, nonencapsulated proliferation may be composed predominantly of mononuclear cells, a combination of mononuclear and spindle cells or infrequently only of bland appearing spindle cells (Figure 24-32). The presence of xanthomatized mononuclear cells should alert to the possibility of JXG since classic Touton giant cells are often not present in the extracutaneous lesions of JXG. Eosinophils can be prominent and their presence may lead to concern about LCH but the cells of JXG do not express CD1a; however, like most DC proliferations, there is often S100 protein reactivity. Pseudorheumatoid nodule or deep granuloma annulare, a nonneoplastic lesion of the soft tissues of the head and lower extremities in young children, can be mistaken for a histiocytic proliferation (Figure 24-33).

Follicular DCs are found in the germinal centers where they are characterized by CD21, CD35, CD138, and clusterin positivity and less often for S100 protein and nonreactive for CD1a. These spindle cell tumors with concentric whorls of cells can be mistaken for a fibrohistiocytic neoplasm of unspecified type or IMT. Though a rare neoplasm, follicular DC tumor is recognized in children.

IDC tumors are seemingly less common than the follicular DC tumors and have been documented in children. There is a report of a histiocytic sarcoma with IDC differentiation in a 3-month-old boy (121). These tumors may be composed of highly pleomorphic large polygonal cells whose features have some resemblance to the cells of the MRT as well as a spindle cell component, which is not a feature of MRT. Multinucleated giant cells have been observed as well. The tumor cells are reactive for vimentin, CD68, and S-100 protein but not for CD30 (positive in anaplastic large cell lymphoma), ALK-1, CD1a, or CD21.

ADIPOCYTIC (LIPOMATOUS) TUMORS

Just as there is a "gray zone" between what constitutes a vascular neoplasm versus a malformation, an analogous dilemma is encountered in some examples of adipocytic or lipomatous tumors. Since lipomatous lesions in children are resected for a number of reasons other than the presence of a mass, it may be the case that the pathologist is not always provided with a complete clinical profile on the patient. However, there are several important and well-characterized syndromes in which the specimen is not just another "lipoma" (Table 24-7). Each of these syndromes is associated with multiple lipomatous tumors with the less than

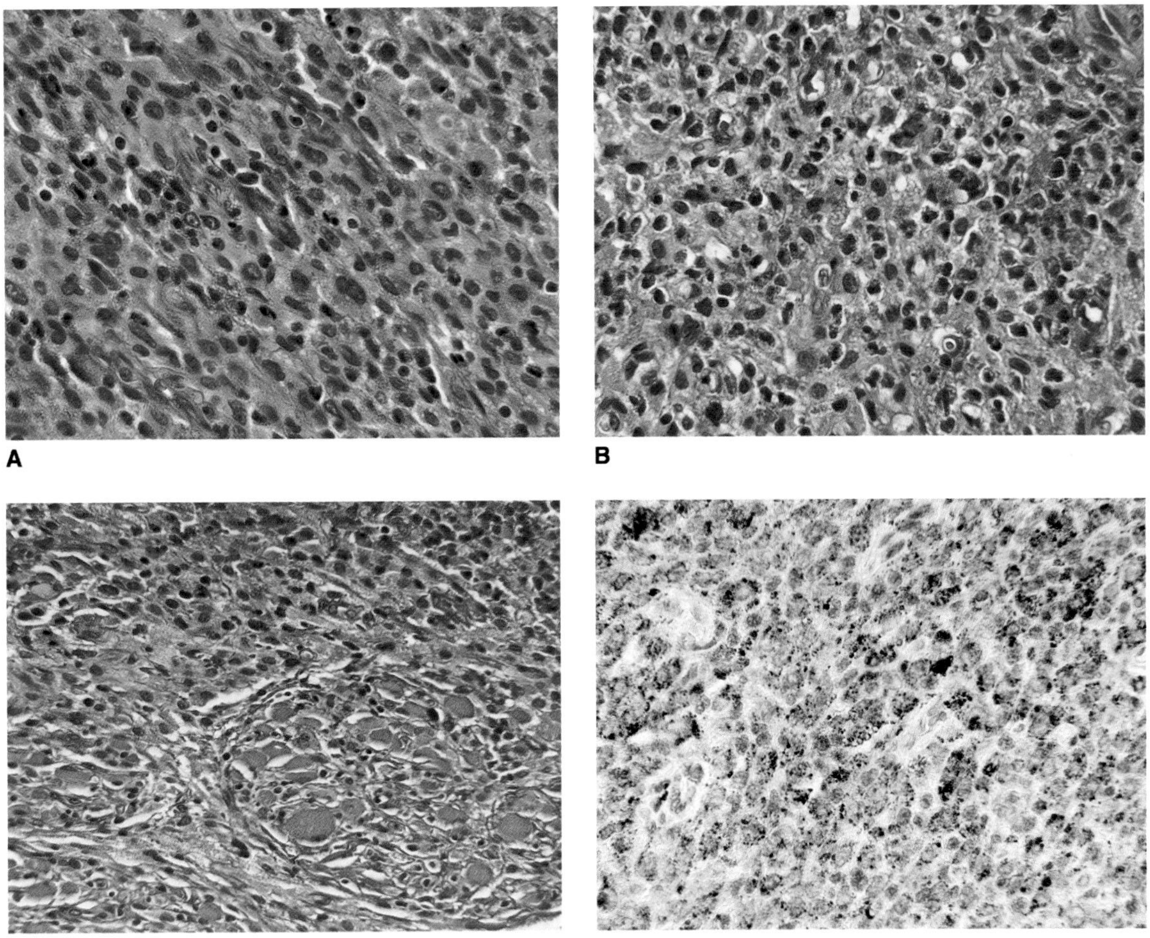

FIGURE 24-32 ■ JXG presented as a soft tissue mass in the posterior thigh of a 10-week-old male. **A:** Mononuclear, pale staining histiocyte-like cells and Touton giant cells are the classic microscopic features. **B:** Other foci are composed of xanthoma-like cells. **C:** A spindle cell component is infiltrating into the skeletal muscle. **D:** Factor XIIIa and CD68 (shown) are expressed by the tumor cells which are immunonegative for CD1a.

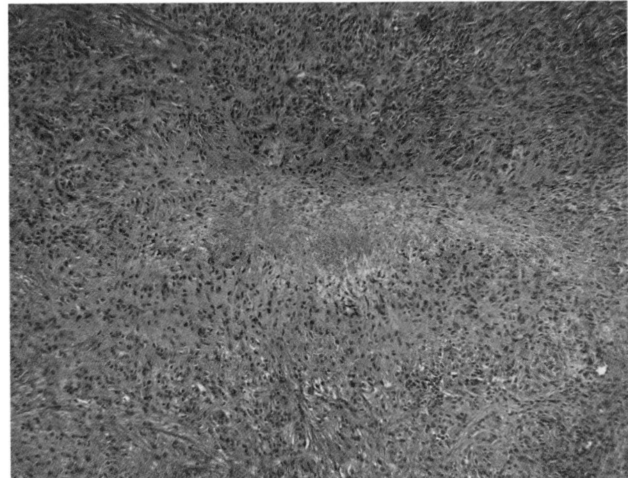

FIGURE 24-33 ■ Deep granuloma annulare presented in the ankle region of a 4-year-old male who also had a second similar mass over the tibia. A central focus of necrobiotic collagen is surrounded by a densely cellular mantle of histiocytes. Numerous such lesions comprise the mass effect. This diagnosis may be elusive when the central necrobiosis is relatively inconspicuous in which case a histiocytic proliferation or vascular lesion is often considered in an involuting lesion.

settled question whether these fatty masses are hamartomas or neoplasms. The lipomatosis in encephalocraniocutaneous lipomatosis (ECCL) is diffuse overgrowth of subcutaneous fat of the scalp and eyelids, and ipsilateral to unilateral porencephalic cysts (193). It has been questioned whether another syndrome, oculocerebral syndrome, may not represent a milder variant of ECCL. There is also the possible relationship of congenital infiltrating lipomatosis to multiple familial lipomatosis.

Phosphatase, tensin homologue, and deleted on chromosome TEN (PTEN) hamartoma tumor syndromes comprise four entities, all of which are characterized to a greater or less degree by a germ-line mutation in the tumor suppressor gene PTEN on 10q23.3; these syndromes, all phenotypically distinctive, are associated with hamartomatous overgrowths to include the development of lipomas. Lipomatous lesions develop in over 90% of those with **Proteus syndrome**. Some of these tumors have features of well-circumscribed mature lipomas whereas others are more diffuse with overgrowth of mature fat with accompanying fibrous septa resembling the microanatomy of the subcutis

Table 24-7 ■ SYNDROMIC-ASSOCIATED LIPOMA—LIPOMATOSIS

Congenital infiltrating lipomatosis (Slavin-Cols)
ECCL (Haberland)
Congenital lipomatous overgrowth, vascular malformations and epidermal nevi (Sapp)
PTEN (10q23.3) hamartoma tumor syndromes
Cowden syndrome
Bannayan-Kiley-Ruvaleaba syndrome
Proteus and proteus-like syndrome
Bannayan-Zonana syndrome
Multiple familial lipomatosis
Macrodystrophia lipomatosa

with associated nerves and blood vessels. Infiltration of skeletal muscle by mature adipose tissue is another feature. Vascular lesions with hemangioma and lymphangioma-like features occur as well.

Macrodystrophia lipomatosa and **macrodactyly** are characterized by an overgrowth of an entire extremity or a digit. A substantial component of the overgrowth phenomenon is mature adipose tissue in all tissue layers below the dermis. In addition to the fatty overgrowth, fibrous, vascular, and neural components either in excess or resembling other lesions such as fibromatosis, hemangioma, and neuromatous proliferations can lead to uncertainty about a neoplastic or hamartomatous process. We have elected to refer to these as "soft-tissue dysplasia-overgrowth." Lipofibromatous hamartoma of the median nerve or other nerves in the upper extremity is found in association with 25% to 30% of cases of macrodactyly.

Congenital intraspinal lipoma is seen with some frequency in those institutions with an active neural tube defect-spinal dysraphia program (158,214). One-third to one-half of all lipomas in children in our own experience are diagnosed in the latter setting. A mass in the subcutis is detected in the midline of the lower back. A circumscribed, multinodular mass of pale tan to yellow tissue is composed predominantly of lobules of mature adipose tissue with neural elements and a variety of other tissues indigenous to this site including bone and cartilage. Microscopic foci of immature nephrogenic tissue and enteric- and/or respiratory-lined cysts offer the possibility of a teratoma as an alternative interpretation, but the context of a spinal defect and the predominance of adipose tissue should be kept in mind before a diagnosis of a sacral teratoma is made. One potential problem in the differential diagnosis is the Currarino syndrome (point mutations in the HLXB9 homeobox gene, 7q36) with sacral anomalies, tethered spinal cord or lipoma, various anorectal malformations and presacral teratoma. The spinal lipoma is distinct from the mature teratoma. In some cases, the presacral cyst can have some limited features of an enteric duplication.

Lipomas are neoplasms and perhaps more hyperplasias or hamartomas in some cases which in either instance are circumscribed masses of lobules of mature adipocytes. In adults, lipomas comprise 50% or more of all STTs whereas in children lipomas constitute only 5% of all STTs compared to vascular tumors at 30% in this age group. Other than the sacral lipomas in association with spinal dysraphia, lipomas in children have a preference for the superficial soft tissues of the head and neck and trunk. Deep and intramuscular lipomas are uncommon in children. The differential diagnosis of the intramuscular lipoma includes the skeletal muscle hemangioma, which can have a substantial component of adipose tissue. Angiolipoma presents in the subcutis of the extremities (forearm predilection) or trunk, usually in adolescents and young adults. Multiple angiolipomas, often tender, may have an autosomal dominant or recessive pattern of inheritance. Deep angiolipomas, as an apparent hamartoma, is seen in Proteus syndrome. Angiolipoma, like the common lipoma, is composed of one or more lobules of mature adipose tissue but with small peripheral capillaries, which are congested or contain fibrin thrombi. Although rarely performed as an ancillary study, cytogenetic analysis of a true lipoma demonstrates supernumerary rings and giant rod chromosomes reflecting amplification of 12q14-15, the site of the MDM2 oncogene (91). Myxoid foci at the periphery of a fatty lobule(s) in an otherwise mature lipoma in a child may represent the residual immature fat in a lipoma-like lipoblastoma or alternatively myxoid degeneration (Figure 24-34). There are a number of morphologic subtypes of lipomas, which are largely seen in adults.

Lipoblastoma is the distinctive lipomatous neoplasm of childhood, presenting between early infancy to 10 years of age (one-third of cases at or before 1 year old) with a predilection for the extremities (60% to 65% of cases) (Table 24-8). Individual cases have been detected in utero by fetal ultrasonography. There are two growth patterns, localized, and diffuse (so-called lipoblastomatosis), but most lipoblastomas are a well-circumscribed mass in the subcutis rather than diffusely infiltrating into the deeper soft tissues (56,96). A well-circumscribed, lobulated yellow-tan to grayish mucoid mass measures from 1 to 10 cm in greatest dimension (Figure 24-35). The lobules are composed of immature lipocytes with or without central mature lipocytes in a background of delicate, branching capillaries whose vascular pattern has a resemblance to myxoid liposarcoma (LPS) (Figure 24-36). Pools of acellular, basophilic mucoid matrix are another feature, which is also seen in myxoid LPSs. IHC generally does not provide any assistance in the diagnosis, which may be vexed by a positive desmin stain in a population of immature mesenchymal cells. The local recurrence rate is reportedly as high as 50% but is closer to 20% to 25% in our experience. We have had to resort to molecular diagnostic studies in some cases to confirm that the immature-appearing lipomatous neoplasm, especially in the older child, is not a myxoid LPS. Lipoblastoma is characterized by a chromosomal rearrangement of 8q11-13 region (8q12), which harbors the developmentally regulated zinc finger gene, PLAG1 (11,18). Lipoblastoma-like hamartoma

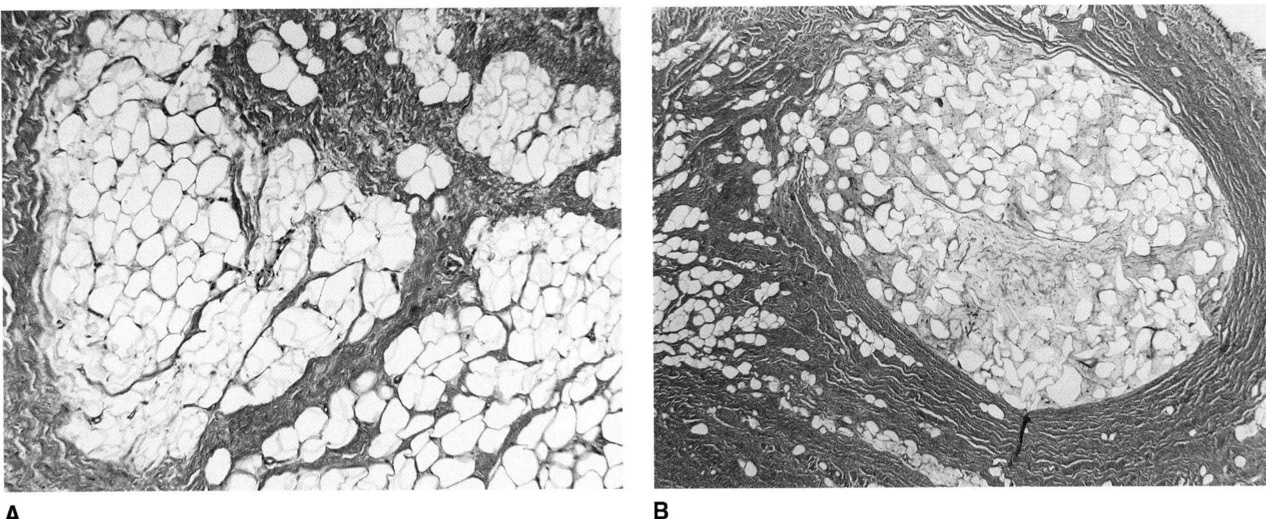

FIGURE 24-34 ■ Lipoma with myxofibrous features presented as a soft tissue mass on the foot of an 8-year-old male. **A:** Lobules of mature lipocytes are separated by prominent fibrous septa. **B:** Some of the lobules of fat have a myxomatous appearance. In the presence of immature lipocytes, it may support the interpretation of a lipoma-like lipoblastoma.

is seen in soft tissues of the extremity in young child in a focus of lipoatrophy. A final note is that children with a lipoblastoma may have neurodevelopmental problems as well as other systemic manifestations (Coffin, *personal communication*, 2009).

Liposarcoma (LPS) is a rare soft-tissue sarcoma of childhood, which accounts for approximately 3% of all STSs in children; less than 5% of all LPSs are diagnosed in the first two decades of life; LPS in children typically presents in the second decade (average age of 15 to 17 years), has a female predilection (2F:1M), and has a preference for the lower extremity (60% to 70% of cases) (1). Myxoid LPS accounts for 80% to 90% of cases and most of these tumors are conventional myxoid-round cell types (Figure 24-37). Variation in the morphology includes spindle cell foci and pleomorphic features. Lipoma-like or well-differentiated and pleomorphic LPSs that together account for 65% to 70% of LPSs in adults represent 10% or less of cases in children. The prognosis of LPS in children is similar to the experience in adults. Cytogenetics is helpful in those cases of myxoid LPS with the differential diagnosis of lipoblastoma with the demonstration of the t(12;16) (q13;p11) (FUS-CHOP fusion transcript) or EWSR1-CHOP rearrangement (141). The latter translocation would seem to qualify some myxoid LPSs as a distant cousin in the extended EWS family (Table 24-2). In the COG grading scheme of STSs in children, myxoid LPS is a grade I neoplasm.

Another distinctive lipomatous tumor is the **hibernoma,** which infrequently presents before 20 years of age (<10% of cases). The extremities and head and neck region are the sites of predilection. A lobulated, yellowish-brown mass is composed of lipocytes with eosinophilic, finely

Table 24-8 ■ SITES AND AGE AT PRESENTATION OF LIPOBLASTOMAS FROM THE FILES OF LAUREN V ACKERMAN LABORATORY OF SURGICAL PATHOLOGY (1989 TO 2009)

Site	No. (%)	Age (Range and Mean)	Sex (Male:Female)
Lower extremity[a]	16 (32)	1–10 years (3.5 years)	8M/8F
Trunk	10 (20)	3 months–9 years (2.7 years)	6M/4F
Neck[b]	6 (12)	1–5 years (3 years)	2M/4F
Axilla—upper extremity	6 (12)	6 months–4 years (2 years)	2M/4F
Retroperitoneum—omentum	3 (6)	1–2 years (1.6 years)	1M/2F
Scrotum	3 (6)	2 years–6 years (5 years)	1M/2F
Mediastinum	2 (4)	8 months, 6 years	1M/1F
Orbit	2 (4)	1 year, 1 year	2M
Scalp	1 (2)	1 year	1M
Vulva	1 (2)	1 year	1F
	50 (100)	Mean (2.8 years)	26M/24F

[a]Gluteal region, thigh, foot.
[b]Parotid (1 case).
From the files of the Lauren V. Ackerman Laboratory of Surgical Pathology, St. Louis Children's Hospital, Washington University Medical Center, St. Louis, MO.

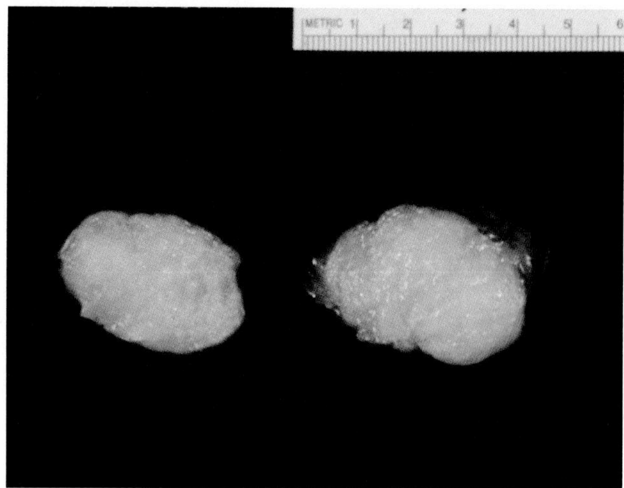

FIGURE 24-35 ■ Lipoblastoma in the neck of a 5-year-old female has a well circumscribed, yellowish-white, has a faintly lobulated appearance on cut surface and measures 8 × 4 × 1.5 cm. This tumor recurred several months after the initial excision.

vacuolated cytoplasm resembling immature adipocytes in the retroperitoneum of infants. Not surprisingly, lipoblastoma may have hibernoma-like foci.

A lipomatous lesion whose pathologic features are characterized by fatty infiltration and replacement of the right ventricle of the heart by mature adipose tissue is **arrythmogenic right ventricular cardiomyopathy** (dysplasia). There is progressive replacement of the entire thickness of the apical, inferior, and infundibular wall of the right ventricle by mature adipose tissue, which begins from the epicardium or from the midmyocardium as a seeming metaplasia rather than fatty infiltration (198).

PERIPHERAL NERVE SHEATH TUMORS

This category of tumor accounts for as many as 15% of all soft-tissue neoplasms in childhood with neurofibroma (NF) and schwannoma as the two most common types. There are several morphologic subtypes in the latter two categories reflecting variability in the histologic features from the growth pattern (localized, diffuse, and plexiform in the case of NF) to cellularlity and regressive atypia (in the case of the schwannoma). Both NF and schwannoma have pigmented variants; the psammomatous melanotic schwannoma arises in spinal nerve roots, bone, skin, and upper intestinal tract and may be a manifestation of the Carney complex. Also included among the peripheral nerve sheath tumors (PNSTs) are the perineurioma, GCT, and neurothekeoma or nerve sheath myxoma (75). Although Weiss and Goldblum have listed CCS of tendon and aponeuroses as a malignant PNST, it is discussed with the extended EWS family of neoplasms in this chapter (211). MPNST occurs as a sporadic tumor or in the setting of NF1 in children and adults alike (8,82). In children, MPNST is the second or third most common non-rhabdomyosarcomatous STS, accounting for 15% of all sarcomas compared to SS, representing 25% of cases in the pediatric age group (63,92,93). There is also a category of tumefactions of a reparative-reactive type, which includes the traumatic neuroma, postamputation nerve hypertrophy, and presumed hamartomatous lesions such as the neuromuscular hamartoma and the neural lipofibroma involving the median nerve (Figure 24-38).

Neurofibroma (NF) is the most common PNST in children, accounting for almost 70% of cases. Localized NFs are restricted to the dermis whereas the diffuse NF with involvement of the dermis and subcutis as well as the deeper

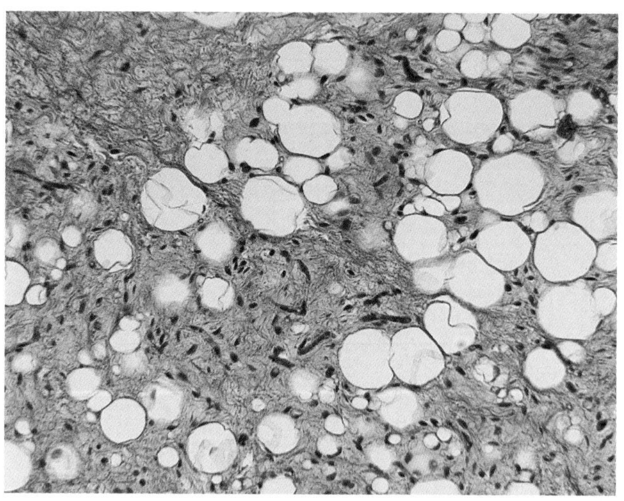

A

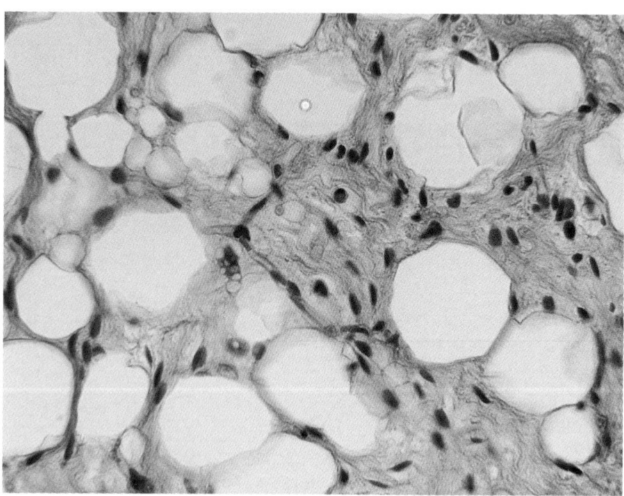

B

FIGURE 24-36 ■ Lipoblastoma in the neck of a 5-year-old female presented some difficulty in the differential diagnosis from myxoid LPS. **A:** The background is composed of immature mesenchymal cells with pale staining features. These cells may stain positively for desmin. The interspersed lipocytes show varying stages of maturation. **B:** A pale myxoid background with a delicate arborizing network of capillaries separate both immature and more mature lipocytes.

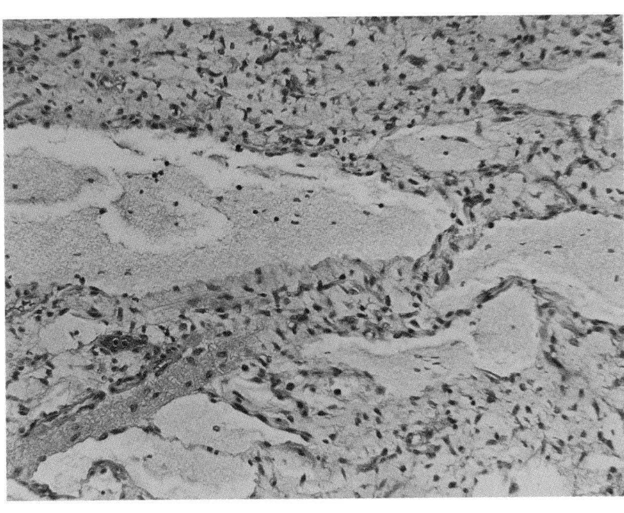

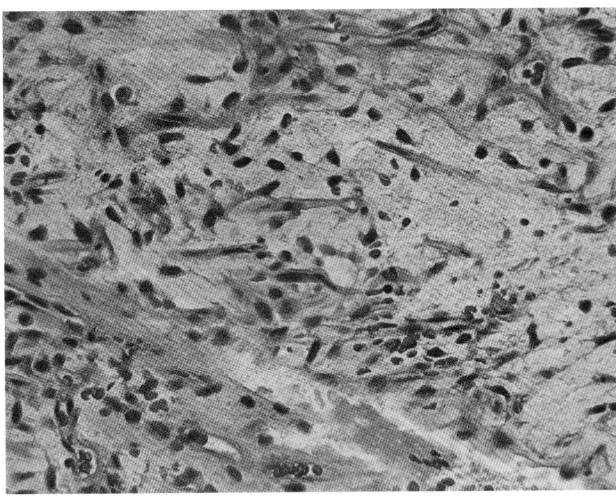

A B

FIGURE 24-37 ■ Myxoid LPS presented on the anterior abdominal wall of a 13-year-old male. **A:** Mucinous filled cysts are separated by moderately cellular foci with a myxoid and vascularized background. **B:** The individual tumor cells have enlarged nuclei which are moderately hyperchromatic. The delicate network of capillaries is present in the background.

plexiform NF are invariably a manifestation of NF1 with the development of multiple cutaneous, subcutaneous, and deep soft-tissue masses (62,181). Plexiform NFs in NF1 are detected in 40% to 50% of children by 5 years of age with a anatomic preference for the trunk and extremities, although the infiltrative plexiform NF may involve deep anatomic structures in the head and neck region (203,204,207) (Table 24-9). NFs are less common in NF2, where the characteristic tumor type is the schwannoma, which can have plexiform features to be differentiated from the plexiform NF. Diffuse NF is composed of uniform, bland appearing spindle cells in a pale staining eosinophilic background.

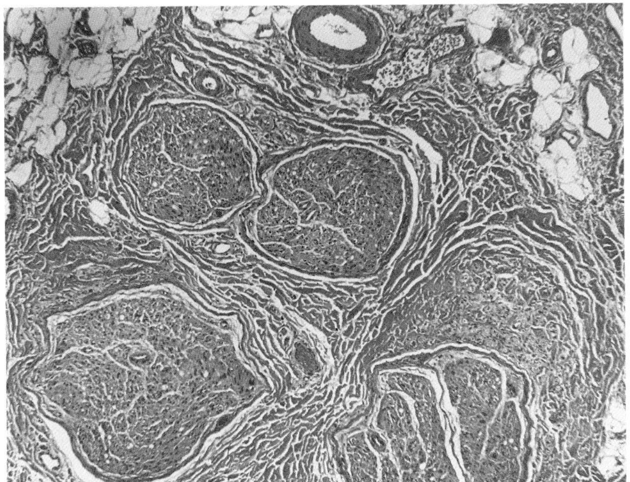

FIGURE 24-38 ■ Traumatic neuroma of the peroneal nerve occurred in a 17-year-old female who had sustained deep soft tissue injury to the lower extremity. Several nerve fascicles are present in the soft tissues as individual structures separated by collagen. Smaller nerve bundles are adjacent to one of the larger nerve bundles.

There is often overgrowth of the dermis with contiguous growth into the subcutis. Plexiform NF is composed of rounded to more serpentine nodules of spindle cells in a pale staining myxoid background. These nodules are found in the skin and/or subcutis with or without an accompanying pattern of diffuse NF (Figure 24-39). The nodules can be found in and around salivary glands in the head and neck region or grossly as thickened and tortuous peripheral nerves. The smaller plexiform NFs are less readily traceable to a peripheral nerve. The presence of enlarged, pleomorphic nuclei and even a few mitotic figures should be viewed with concern about sarcomatous transformation of a plexiform NF. These pleomorphic nuclei often display p53 staining whose presence should be correlated with any other features to suggest malignant transformation (127).

Schwannoma is a neoplasm with morphologic and immunophenotypic features of Schwann cells forming the nerve sheath (122). There is a predilection for the head and neck region and upper extremity in the case of sporadic schwannomas in children (114,115). It is unusual for a schwannoma to present before the age of 10 years (182). In children with NF2, nodular or plaque lesions in the skin or subcutis are well circumscribed, encapsulated spindle cell neoplasms with or without plexiform features; these tumors show strong diffuse S100 protein positivity unlike the less uniform pattern of S100 protein staining of the NF (182). Grossly, the schwannoma varies in size from 1 to 10 cm in greatest dimension, is encapsulated, and has a glistening, mucoid, and a pale tannish to yellowish-tan appearance (Figure 24-40). Hemorrhage, cystic degeneration, and fibrosis are uncommon secondary features in schwannomas in children in contrast to schwannomas in adults. The challenge in the pathologic diagnosis is the variability in the

Table 24-9 ■ GENETICS AND MANIFESTATIONS OF NFTOSES TYPE 1 AND 2 AND SCHWANNOMATOSIS

	NF Type 1	NF Type 2	Schwannomatosis
Incidence	1:3,000	1:30–40,000	1:1.7 million (Finnish)
Gene	NF1: 17q11.2	NF2: 22q12.2	Possible 22q 11 which harbors SMARCB1/INI1
	Neurofibromin, negative regulator of RAS-MAPK	Merlin, inhibits cell proliferation in response to cellular adhesion	
Phenotype	Café au lait macules (infancy) Diffuse and plexiform NFs Optic nerve glioma (pilocytic astrocytoma) MPNST (lifetime risk 8%–13%) Pseudarthrosis Vascular dysplasias	Schwannomas Bilateral VIII nerve schwannomas Ependymoma	Two or more schwannomas without VIII nerve schwannomas

Compiled from Yohay, K. *Neurologist* 2006;12:86–93; McClatchey AI. Neurofibromatosis. *Annu Rev Pathol* 2007;2:191–216; MacCollin M, Chiocca EA, Evans DG, et al. Diagnostic criteria for schwannomatosis. *Neurology* 2005;64(11):1838–1845; Hadfield KD, Newman WG, Bowers NL, et al. Molecular characterisation of SMARCB1 and NF2 in familial and sporadic schwannomatosis. *J Med Genet* 2008;45(6):332–339; Brems H, Beert E, de Ravel T, et al. Mechanisms in the pathogenesis of malignant tumours in neurofibromatosis type 1. *Lancet Oncol* 2009;10(5):508–515.

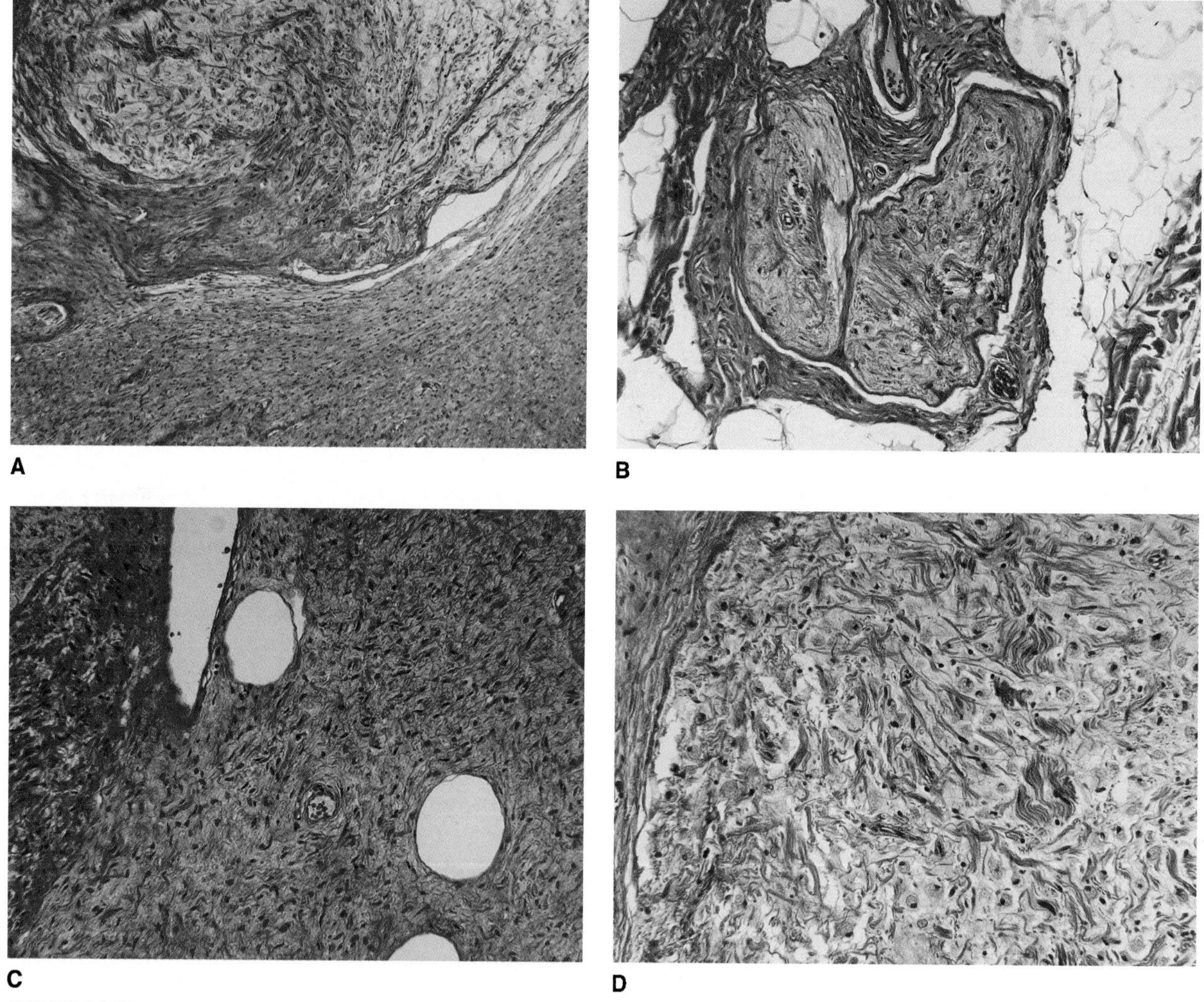

FIGURE 24-39 ■ Plexiform NF arose in soft tissues of the lower back in a 14-year-old female with a history of NF1. **A:** This field discloses both the plexiform and diffuse pattern of growth, both characteristic of NF1. **B:** Plexiform transformation occurs in peripheral nerves at all levels of the nerve. **C:** Diffuse pattern is often found in association with plexiform tumors. **D:** The plexiform nodules are usually hypocellular with or without coarse eosinophilic bundles. Increased cellularity and mitotic figures should be viewed with concern about malignant progression.

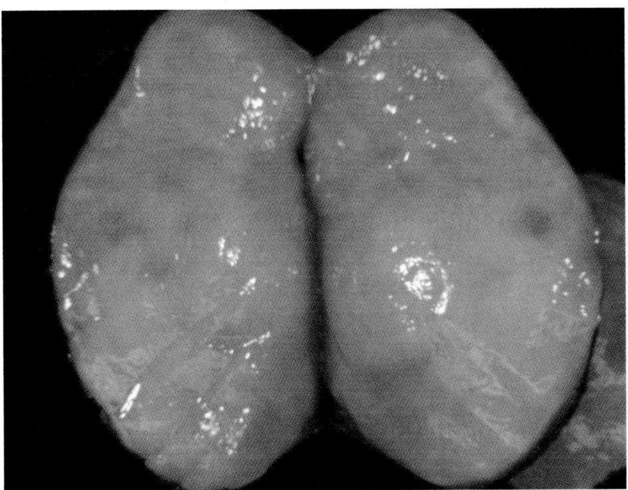

FIGURE 24-40 ■ Schwannoma presented as a paraspinal mass in a 17-year-old male. This encapsulated tumor measured 10 cm in greatest dimension and had a uniform, glistening yellowish-tan cut surface.

histologic patterns, but the two basic ones are the spindle cell pattern with or without Verocay body formation (Antoni A) and the alternating less cellular myxoid foci (Antoni B) (Figure 24-41). Foci resembling a NF may be seen in some cases, but keep in mind the presence of a capsule in the schwannoma. Lymphocytes and foamy histiocytes may be more or less apparent in a particular schwannoma. Mast cells are present in variable numbers. Nuclear enlargement and hyperchromatism are present in some cases and should not be viewed with concern about potential malignancy. Sporadically schwannomas can have a hypercellular spindle cell pattern, and mitotic figures can be seen in the cellular variant. In the setting of NF2, caution is advisable with a diagnosis of MPNST when the schwannoma is both cellular and mitotically active. Rather than a diffuse pattern, a multinodular pattern is also documented in children and these tumors are mistaken for a NF (213). Bilateral schwannoma of the VIII cranial nerve is a diagnostic manifestation of NF2 (138,166) (Table 24-9). Finally without the presence of ganglion cells, a ganglioneuroma with its predominant neuromatous-stromal component has a convincing resemblance to a schwannoma or NF (Figure 24-42).

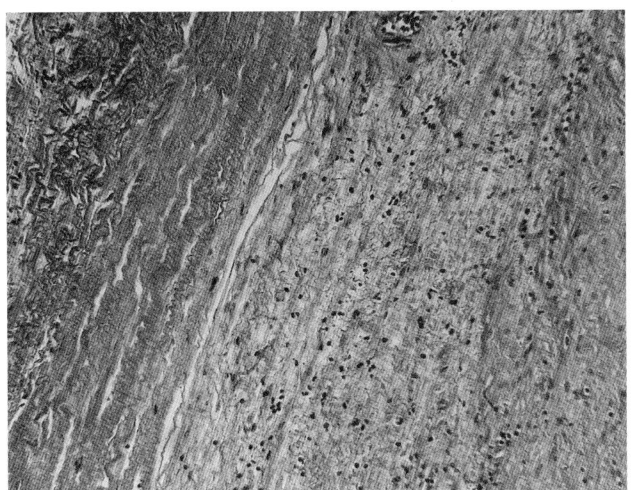

FIGURE 24-41 ■ Schwannoma presented in the paraspinal region of a 17-year-old male. The encapsulated tumor had a predominant Antoni B pattern of loosely arrayed spindle cells in an edematous to myxoid background.

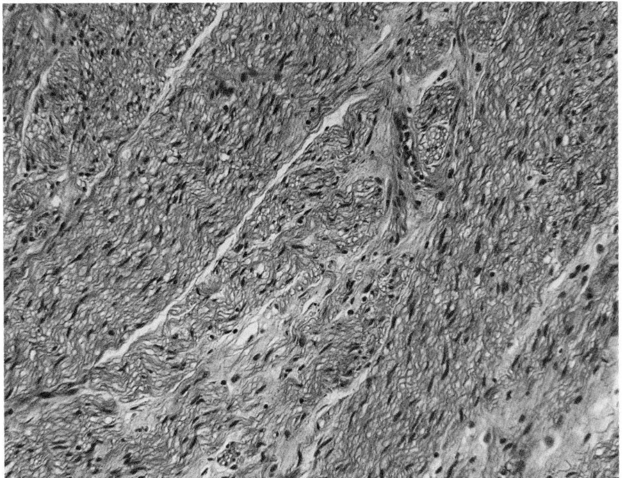

A

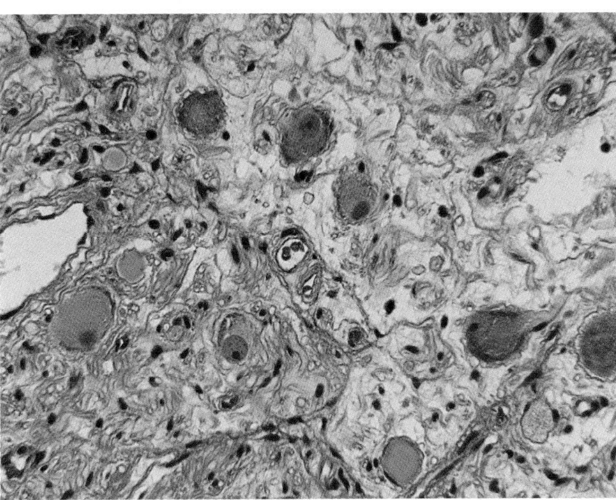

B

FIGURE 24-42 ■ Ganglioneuroma presented in the lumbosacral region of a 12-year-old female. **A:** The tumor is well circumscribed with a capsule or pseudocapsule and is composed of bundles of fusiform spindle cells with a resemblance to a schwannoma. **B:** Other microscopic fields contain individual or small groups of mature ganglion cells.

Schwannomatosis, like NF2, is characterized clinically by the presence of two or more schwannomas, but unlike NF2, vestibular nerve involvement is not a feature (135) (Table 24-9). Some 15% of affected individuals develop schwannomas in the first two decades of life. The suspected genetic mutation is near the NF2 gene locus at 22q11 where the INI1 gene resides as an important oncogenic site (90).

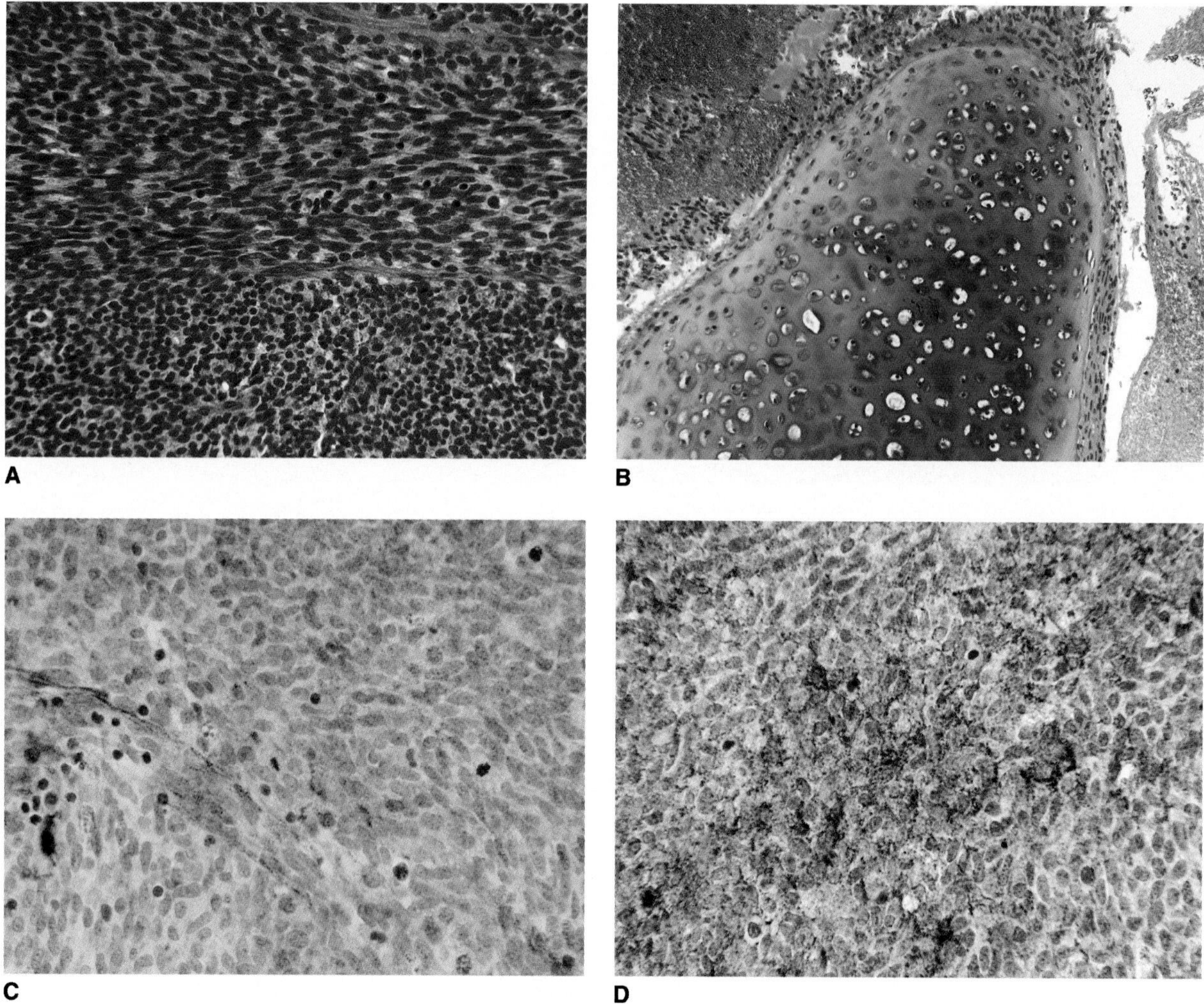

FIGURE 24-43 MPNST presented in a 5-year-old male with NF1 with an intracranial presentation of a large mass arising in the region of the frontal lobe. **A:** A high grade spindle cell sarcoma consists of uniform cells with enlarged, elongated hyperchromatic nuclei. **B:** Nodules of hypercellular cartilage are present focally. **C:** The tumor cells are uniformly reactive for vimentin, but only focally for S100 protein. **D:** The CD57 immunostaining is diffuse throughout all microscopic fields.

Malignant peripheral nerve sheath tumor (MPNST) presents as a sporadic neoplasm or as a complication of NF1. The other STS in the setting of NF1 is ERMS, which presents earlier in life than does the MPNST in most cases. It is rare for a MPNST in NF1 to develop before 5 years of age, but the incidence increases in subsequent decades with a lifetime risk of 10% to 15% (20,63). Most MPNSTs generally measure in excess of 5 cm and have a gelatinous grayish-tan to white surface with or without necrosis and hemorrhage. When the MPNST arises as a plexiform NF, as it often does in NF1, there is often widespread sarcomatous involvement of the nerve with the formation of one or more masses. The mass(es) is usually not sharply demarcated from the plexiform component. The basic histologic pattern of a MPNST is a spindle cell sarcoma with fascicular profiles of interweaving cells. At low magnification, the fascicles may have an alternating "light cell-dark cell" quality due to more cellular and less cellular foci with lucency between the cells, often with a pale mucoid to myxoid appearance. Fusiform to more ovoid nuclei display varying degrees of hyperchromatism and mitotic activity. Anaplasia is uncommon. Residual foci of plexiform NF are often present in NF1-associated MPNSTs; overgrowth or infiltration by the sarcoma is appreciated in these transitional zones with residual NF. It is for this reason that a biopsy may yield equivocal findings for MPNST other than scattered atypical spindle cells intermixed with a plexiform NF. Though the biopsy may not be satisfactory for an unequivocal diagnosis of MPNST, it should prompt a re-biopsy especially in the presence of an enlarging, previously stable deep soft-tissue mass. In addition to the features of a spindle cell sarcoma, other findings include individual and small collections of rhabdomyoblasts (Triton tumor), gland-like structures, a multinodular pattern with overgrowth of a plexiform NF, an epithelioid pattern with tumor cells resembling those of a MRT, nodules of cartilage or a small cell, rosette-like pattern with a resemblance to EWS-PNET, or neuroblastoma (Figure 24-43).

Formations resembling tactile bodies are found in both NFs and MPNSTs. Sporadically occurring MPNSTs are more difficult to diagnose with certainty when major nerve involvement is not obvious. IHC is not always helpful but is useful in the differentiation of MPNST from monophasic SS or adult-type FS. In addition to vimentin, MPNST is immunoreactive for S100, CD57, and collagen type IV in some but not all cases (Figure 24-43). Another issue in the prognostic assessment of MPNST is the histologic grade and outcome; however, there is the opinion that all MPNSTs should be viewed as high-grade sarcomas regardless of their individual pathologic features even in the presence of "low-grade" histology. More relevant is the adequacy of the surgical resection, which can be problematic when a major nerve is the primary site.

Other types of PNSTs of the soft tissues include the perineurioma, nerve sheath myxoma, and neurothekeoma. **Perineurioma** is an uncommon neoplasm, which is seen in children and adults alike (134). Extraneural and intraneural variants are recognized (17). A well-circumscribed subcutaneous mass measuring less than 7 cm is composed of spindle cells or more epithelioid appearing cells in a fibrous and emptier appearing background. Tight whorls of spindle cells and storiform profiles have some resemblance to DFSP. These tumors may be immunoreactive for CD34 like DFSP but are also positive for EMA and vimentin (both markers are positive in meningiomas) as well as collagen type IV. Unlike schwannomas, these tumors do not express S100 protein. Intraneural perineurioma is even less common than extraneural or soft-tissue variant. Over 50% of cases are diagnosed by 20 years of age as a soft-tissue mass arising in a major nerve or the brachial plexus. There is some resemblance to a plexiform NF in terms of gross involvement. The spindle cell areas like those in the extraneural perinerioma are EMA-positive and S100 protein–negative. **Nerve sheath myxoma** is a predominant myxoid neoplasm of the dermis and subcutis (68). It is composed of spindled and epithelioid cells arranged in cords and nests. These Schwann-like cells are immunoreactive for S100 protein, glial fibrillary acidic protein, and CD57 with some EMA-positive, presumed perineural cells. **Neurothekeoma** is a neoplasm of young individuals with 60% of cases presenting before the age of 20 years, and also a tumor whose features overlap with the nerve sheath myxoma (67). These tumors have been histologically subtyped as cellular, myxoid, and mixed (102). Multiple, small nodules of spindled to epithelioid cells with or without a prominent myxoid matrix are accompanied by osteoclast-like giant cells. The immunophenotype of these tumors includes expression of NK1-C3, neuron specific enolase, CD10, and CD68 whereas they are nonreactive for S100 protein. Quite frankly, some of these cases are difficult to distinguish from the plexiform fibrohisticytic tumor (104).

Granular cell tumor (GCT) is one of the ubiquitous neoplasms in terms of its anatomic distribution whose phenotype characterizes it as either neural (S100 protein positive) or nonneural (S100 negative) in type. Two examples of the latter are the so-called congenital epulis or GCT presenting on the anterior alveolar border of the maxilla or mandible of a neonate and the so-called primitive polypoid GCT of the dermis (Figure 24-44) (19,34). The skin, oral cavity, and upper respiratory tract are among the more frequent primary sites in children (Table 24-10). Multifocal GCTs occur in the presence of a positive family history or in the setting of Noonan syndrome. A firm, poorly demarcated yellowish-tan to white mass measuring less than 2 cm in most cases is the usual gross appearance. Nests of granular cells of varying sizes and shapes are composed of polygonal to more ovoid cells with prominent eosinophilic cytoplasm and a central nucleus (Figure 24-45). The cytoplasm contains eosinophilic or granular bodies representing lysosomes; these bodies account for the CD68-granular positivity (Figure 24-44). Nuclear pleomorphism is present in some cases without any implications about outcome, but mitotic figures should be viewed with concern. Perineural involvement with plexiform features is seen in a small minority of cases (Figure 24-45). With the noted exceptions, most GCTs are diffusely immunoreactive for S100 protein as well as inhibin-α (125). Malignancy in GCT is rare, especially in children. Mitotic activity, nuclear pleomorphism, spindle cell morphology, and deep invasion of soft tissues should alert to the possibility of malignancy. We have seen malignant GCT in the vulva of a 4-year-old female and in the thigh of a 17-year-old female.

Table 24-10 ■ GCTS IN CHILDREN AND ADOLESCENTS

Site	No. (%)	Age Range (Mean)	M:F
Solitary skin	21 (34)	2–16 years (10 years)	7/14
Soft tissue[a]	9 (15)	11–17 years (12.5 years)	4/5
Oral cavity (congenital)[b]	9 (15)	1 day–1 month (10 days)	0/9
Breast	5 (8)	14–18 years (17 years)	0/5
Orbit	4 (7)	15–17 years (16 years)	1/3
Lip	4 (7)	9–14 years (12 years)	2/2
Multiple skin	4 (7)	5–16 years (13 years)	2/2
Larynx	3 (5)	4–18 years (11 years)	1/2
Tongue	1 (2)	10 years	0/1
Esophagus	1 (2)	16 years	1/0
	61 (~100)		18:43

[a]One case in the thigh of 13M with regional lymph node metastasis.
[b]Anterior maxilla (5 cases), anterior mandible (2 cases), hard palate (1 case), frenulum of tongue (1 case).
From the files of the Lauren V. Ackerman Laboratory of Surgical Pathology, St. Louis Children's Hospital, Washington University Medical Center, St. Louis, MO.

Glioneuronal heterotopia, usually presenting in the head and neck region as a polypoid or mass, is usually seen in early childhood. One example is the so-called nasal glioma. Islands of heterotopic glial tissue are accompanied by a fibrous stroma in the nasal glioma. Neurons are identifiable in some cases. Glial heterotopias have been described on the trunk as a soft-tissue mass in children. Extramedullary soft tissue ependymomas and myxopapillary ependymomas are forms of a heterotopic neoplastic process.

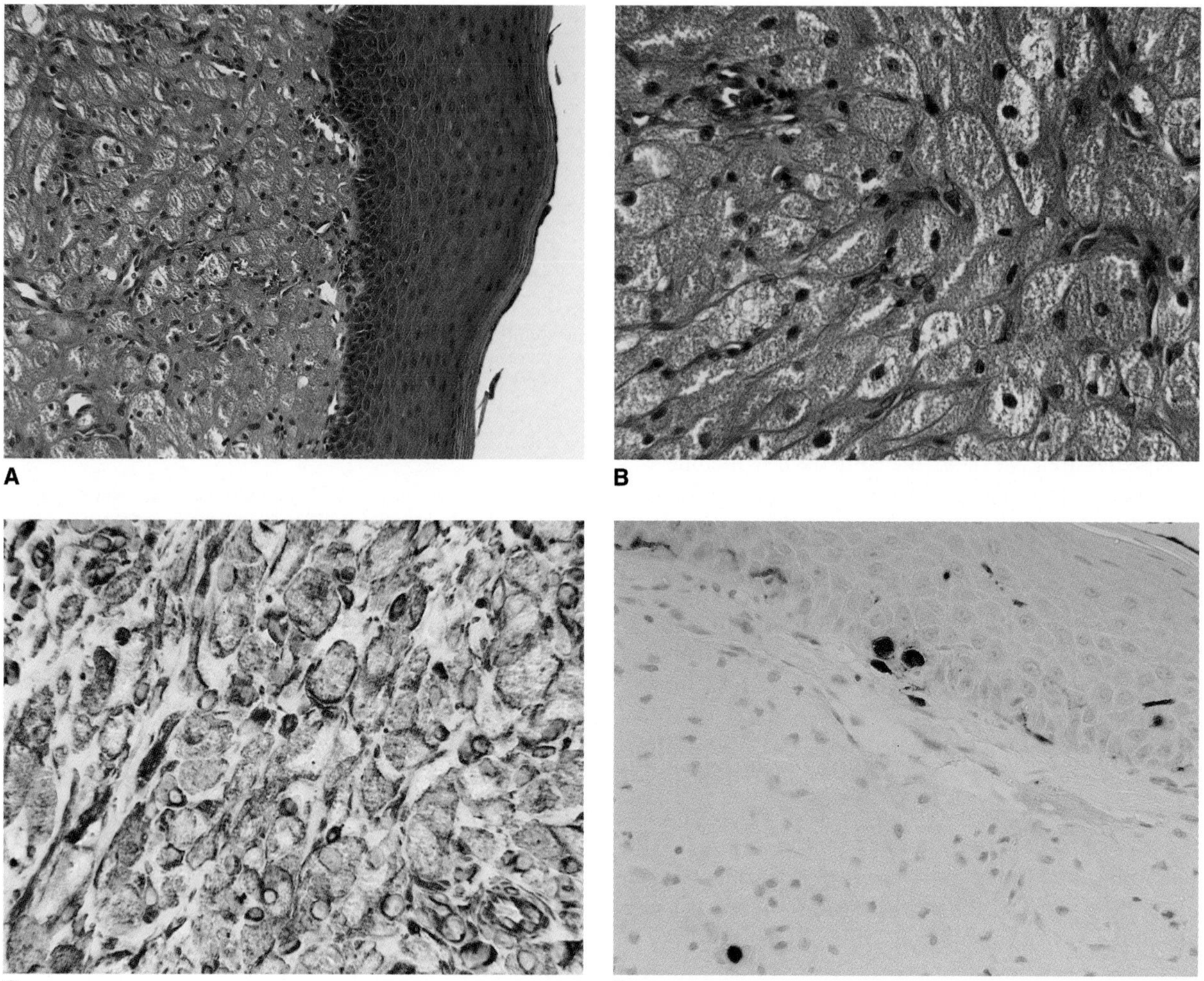

FIGURE 24-44 ■ Congenital GCT (congenital epulis) presented as an intraoral mass attached to maxillary gingival ridge in a neonatal female. **A:** The tumor cells are compactly arranged against the overlying squamous mucosa. **B:** The individual tumor cells are characterized by the pale eosinophilic granular cytoplasm. **C:** The tumor cells are immunoreactive for CD68 with a granular pattern of positivity. **D:** This tumor is regarded as a "non-neural" type of GCT since the S100 protein is nonreactive in the tumor cells. Note the positivity of the Langerhans and DCs in the mucosa.

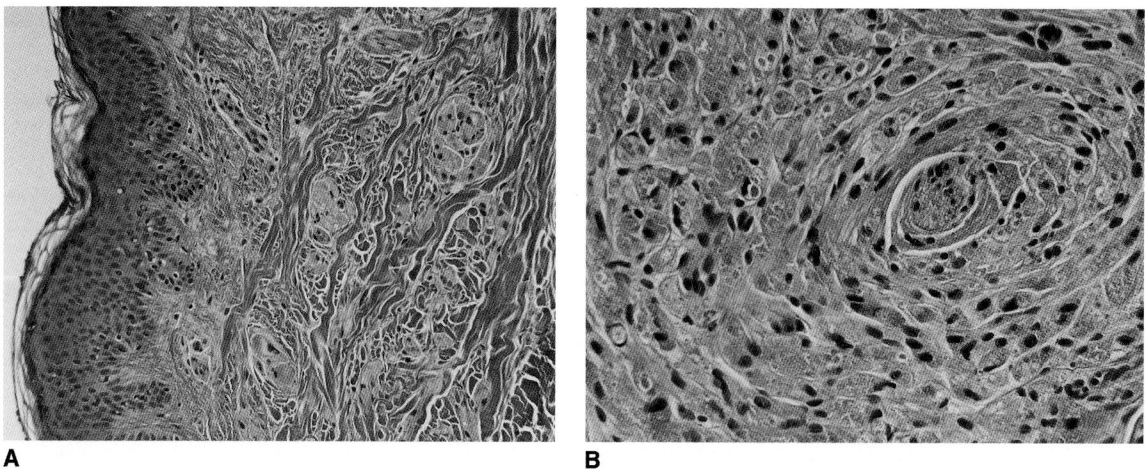

FIGURE 24-45 ■ GCT presented on the arm of a 7-year-old female. **A:** Small collections of granular cells are seen in the superficial dermis. **B:** This tumor also had a plexiform growth pattern with its intraneural and perineural involvement (see *J Cutan Pathol* 2009;36:1174–1176).

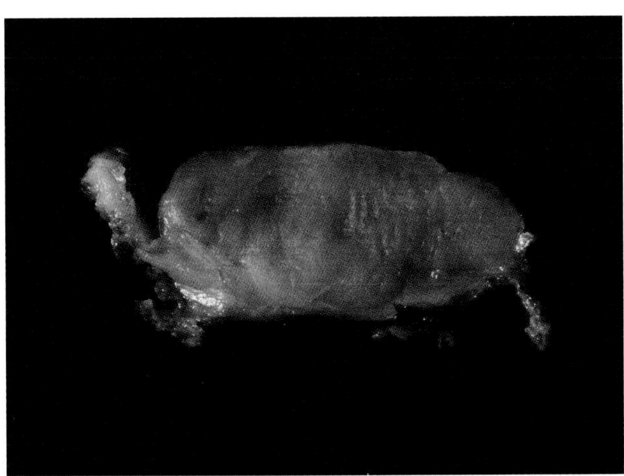

FIGURE 24-46■PEComa presented as a mass in the abdominal mid-line and was associated with the umbilical vein-ligamentum teres in a 4-year-old female. The tumor on cut surface has a well circumscribed appearance with a slightly nodular tannish-brown appearance. It measured 3.5 cm in greatest dimension.

PERIVASCULAR EPITHELIOID CELL NEOPLASM (PECOMA)

This category of neoplasms is a histogenetic concept in a sense since there is no known normal counterpart cell at the present (101). What has emerged from the concept is a group of neoplasms that includes the angiomyolipoma of the kidney and the so-called sugar tumor of the lung. Although these tumors lack morphologic homogeneity, they share a unique immunophenotype of smooth muscle (SMA, calponin) and melanocytes (HMB-45, melan-A, and microphthalmic transcription factor) (79). The S100 protein is often nonreactive.

The PEComa arises in soft tissues and various visceral structures and organs including the falciform ligament (so-called myomelanocytic tumor), uterus, vagina, and liver where the epithelioid angiomyolipoma can be mistaken for a hepatic adenoma (Figure 24-46) (159). The tumor cells of the PEComa can have a predominantly clear cell appearance or large epithelioid cells with abundant eosinophilic cytoplasm (Figure 24-47). The differential diagnosis includes malignant melanoma, ASPS, and CCS of tendon sheath and aponeuroses. There is the conundrum of the histogenetic relationship of the PEComa to the Xp11.2 translocation renal neoplasm with its TFE3 gene fusion, ASPS (der TFE3 fusion), and melanoma. The PEComa, though having some immunophenotypic overlap with the CCS of tendon sheath, is not one of the extended EWS family neoplasms.

GASTROINTESTINAL STROMAL TUMOR

The GIST is a well-established clinicopathologic entity with its signature activating pathway mutations of KIT (type III tyrosine receptor kinase) or PDGFRA (platelet-derived growth factor receptor α) on 4q12 with resulting immunohistochemical positivity for CD117 (c-kit) and CD34 (145,167). These tumors are uncommon in the first two decades of life accounting for only 1% of all cases. However, GISTs in younger individuals have some distinctive features in contrast to the adult counterpart. The general experience with sporadic GISTs in all age groups is that the stomach (50% to 60% of cases) and small intestine (20% to 30%) are the two most common primary sites. In individuals 21 years of age or less, the stomach is the preferred site of presentation (>80% of cases). A small subset of GISTs in children (usually over the age of 10 years at diagnosis) is associated with the Carney triad (pulmonary chondroma, paraganglioma, and GISTs in addition to adrenal adenomas in young females) and NF1 (58,137,212). Most GISTs have an activating mutation in KIT (85% to 90% of cases) or PDGFRA (10% or less of cases), but in children and those with NF1, the wild type KIT without mutations is the rule rather than the exception and the gastric tumors tend to be multifocal rather than solitary as in adults (105,146). Histopathologically, GISTs have a predominant spindle or epithelioid or mixed morphology. An epithelioid pattern has been observed with greater frequency in GISTs in the children. Spread into the peritoneal cavity and regional lymph node, metastases are reportedly more common in children, but paradoxically the clinical course is more indolent despite this aggressive behavior by the tumor. In some respects, the risk assessment based upon the size of the tumor and mitotic rate loses some of its predictive value in GISTs in children. Though not likely to be confused with a GIST, CCS of the kidney may be immunopositive for CD117.

SKELETAL AND SMOOTH MUSCLE NEOPLASMS

Not surprisingly, the subject of myogenic tumors in children is dominated by one neoplasm, RMS, which accounts for 40% to 60% of all STSs in the first two decades of life (92). Benign myogenic tumors represented by the adult, fetal and cardiac rhabdomyomas, and leiomyoma are uncommon by comparison with RMS in children.

Rhabdomyomas in children present either in the heart or as a mass in the subcutis of the head and neck region or chest wall in children in the first 2 years of life. Over 50% of cardiac tumors in children are rhabdomyomas and 50% to 80% of those cases are associated with the tuberous sclerosis complex (25). These tumors are diagnosed in utero in 0.1% to 0.2% of prenatal ultrasounds. Fetal hydrops and findings to suggest hypoplastic left heart syndrome are among some of the clinical presentations. Well-circumscribed solitary mass or multifocal pale tan masses in the left or right ventricle are the two most common sites of involvement but not restricted to the ventricle. Histologically, the enlarged myocytes have clear to vacuolated to eosinophilic cytoplasm with scattered cells having strands of cytoplasm from the nuclear to cell membrane producing the so-called spider cell (Figuer 24-48).

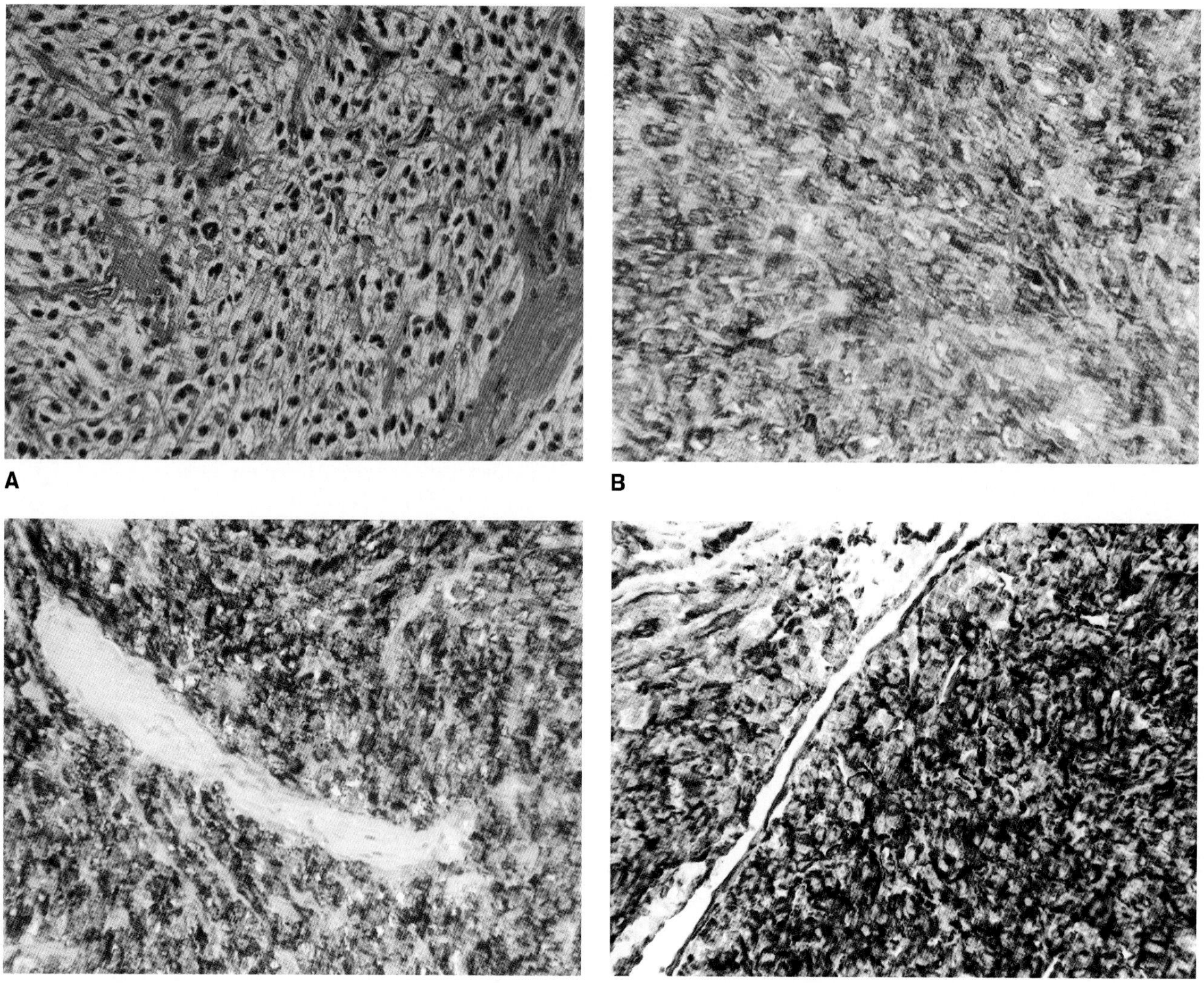

FIGURE 24-47 ■ PEComa has characteristic microscopic and immunophenotypic features. **A:** A uniformly nested neoplasm is composed of rounded to ovoid tumor cells with uniform clear cytoplasm. **B:** The immunohistochemical profile included positivity for vimentin. **C:** The tumor cells are immunoreactive for SMA. **D:** A similar diffuse pattern of positivity is seen for HMB-45.

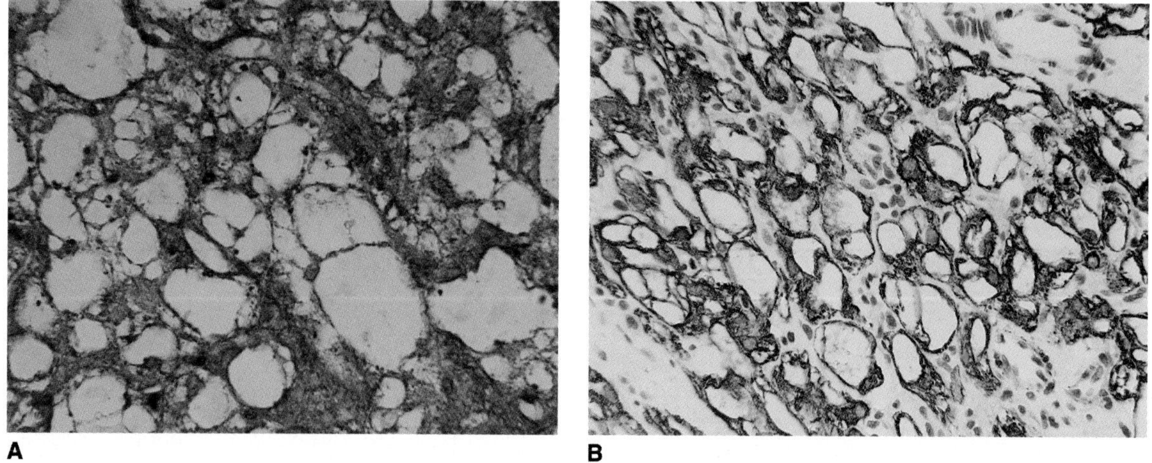

FIGURE 24-48 ■ Cardiac rhabdomyoma in a 3-week-old female presented as an obstructing mass in the left ventricle. **A:** Large tumor cells with abundant clear cytoplasm are accompanied by interspersed cells with strands of cytoplasm producing the features of the so-called spider cells. **B:** The tumor cells are strongly immunopositive for desmin.

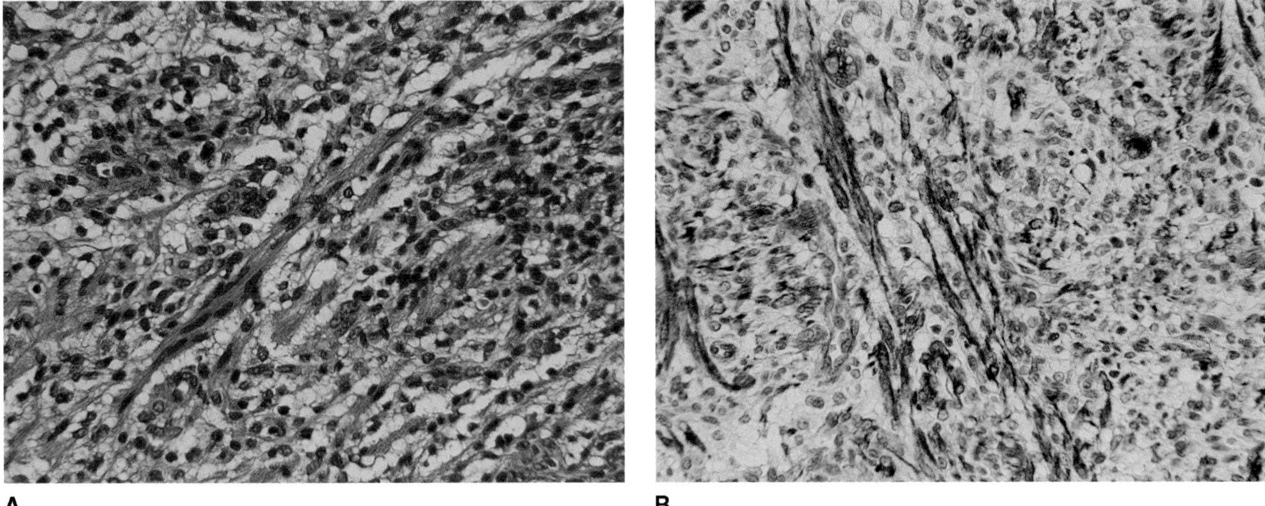

A B

FIGURE 24-49 ■ FRM presented in a 4-month-old female with a 2.7cm mass on the upper chest wall. **A:** The pattern consists of fetal appearing myotubes separated by uniform immature mesenchymal cells without appreciable atypia, rhabdomyoblastic differentiation nor mitotic figures. **B:** Desmin immunostaining enhances the pattern of positively staining myotubes and non reactive immature mesenchymal cells.

Fetal rhabdomyoma (FRM) is a rare, sporadic tumor (also known to occur in the basal cell carcinoma syndrome) with two histologic patterns: myxoid and cellular (111). Unlike RMS with its presentation in deep soft tissue or visceral-based tumors, FRM presents in the deep dermis and/or subcutis (208). A vague multinodular pattern is composed of an orderly, almost layered, arrangement of small immature cells with interposed immature myotubes (Figure 24-49). The nuclei of both cell types are uniform and are neither enlarged nor hyperchromatic. The presence of any mitotic figures warrants reconsideration of a diagnosis of FRM to a well-differentiated ERMS. **Adult rhabdomyoma** is a rare tumor overall, but even more so in children (119). Over 90% of all cases present in the head and neck region are known to form multifocal masses occurring almost exclusively in males. These tumors have some resemblance to the cardiac rhabdomyoma. The differential diagnosis includes a nonneoplastic disorder of skeletal muscle, **focal myositis**, presenting as a mass or masses in the deep soft tissues of the extremities (9,83). This inflammatory process forms a well-circumscribed mass in the skeletal muscle with a combination of inflammatory and myopathic changes (Figure 24-50). The adjuvant muscle often has accompanying injury with degenerative and regenerative features.

Smooth muscle tumors in children include the rare smooth muscle hamartoma arising on the lower trunk usually in infants. Leiomyoma of the soft tissues is a rare soft-tissue

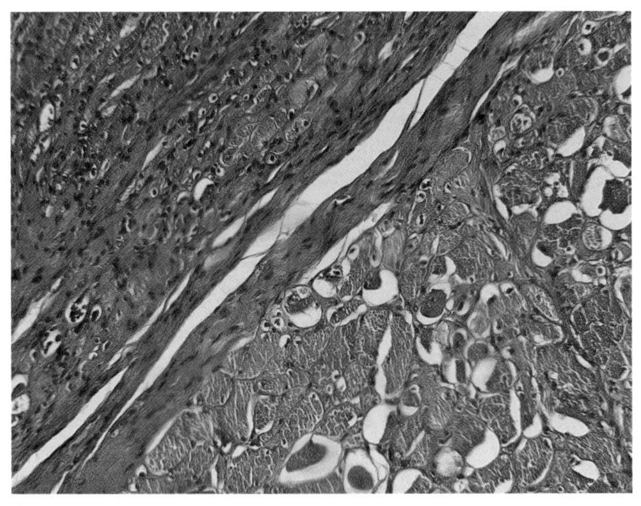

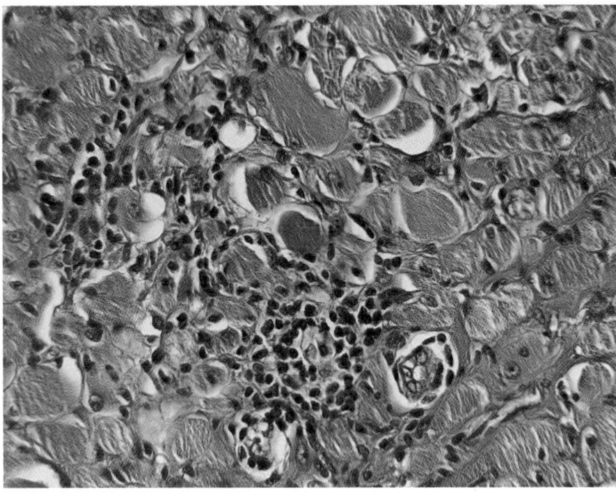

A B

FIGURE 24-50 ■ Focal myositis in an 11-year-old female presented with multiple soft tissue masses in the lower extremity. **A:** The biopsy shows a circumscribed multinodular pattern of skeletal muscle with atrophy and myopathic changes. **B:** Multifocal lymphocytic infiltrates are found among muscle fibers with degenerating features.

neoplasm regardless of age (210). Multifocal smooth muscle tumors of undetermined malignant potential and leiomyosarcoma have been reported in the immunosuppressed child and in some cases; these tumors are another example of Epstein-Barr virus–associated neoplasm. A variant of Alport syndrome is associated with diffuse smooth muscle masses in the esophagus and perineal region (84).

Rhabdomyosarcoma (RMS), together with neuroblastoma and Wilms tumor, is one of the most familiar and well-studied malignant neoplasms of childhood. Its two distinctive subtypes, ERMS (65% to 75% of cases) and ARMS (20% to 25%), constitute approximately 45% to 55% of all STSs in children and 6% to 8% of all malignancies in the first two decades of life (139,164). In the United States, approximately 900 newly diagnosed cases are seen per year compared to 60 cases per year in the United Kingdom. In common with several other solid malignancies of childhood, the majority of cases (65% to 79%) are diagnosed before the age of 10 years with an initial age peak between 1 and 4 years and a later smaller age peak between 15 and 19 years to reflect the more numerous ERMS in the younger children and ARMS in older children and adolescents (194). However, it should be kept in mind that ARMS can present in infancy and early childhood just as an ERMS occurs in adolescence as in a case of paratesticular embryonal RMS. The anatomic distribution of RMS is well established in the following sites and organ systems: genitourinary tract (25% to 30% of all cases) to include the bladder, prostate, vagina, cervix and pelvic soft tissues, head and neck (30% to 35% of all cases) to include oral cavity, oropharynx, nasal cavity and nasopharynx, pterygopalatine fossa, middle ear and orbit (Figure 24-51), extremities (15% to 20% of all cases), and miscellaneous other sites (15% to 30% of all cases). Some of the miscellaneous sites are ones in which there is minimal clinical suspicion about RMS such as in the skin, common bile duct, chest wall, retroperitoneum, and perianal-perineum. In a small minority of cases, there is widespread disease with involvement of bone and lymph node upon initial clinical presentation as in the case of ARMS but rarely in embryonal RMS. Both ERMS and ARMS spread to regional lymph nodes and beyond to the lungs and bone marrow. Approximately 15% to 20% of children who present with RMS have evidence of regional or distant metastatic disease. In the specific instance of ARMS, a higher proportion of children will have lymph node and/or bone marrow involvement at diagnosis (30% to 35% of cases). Regardless of the pathologic stage of RMS at presentation, the decision for chemotherapy is based on the premise that there is at least micrometastatic disease at the time without specific pathologic documentation.

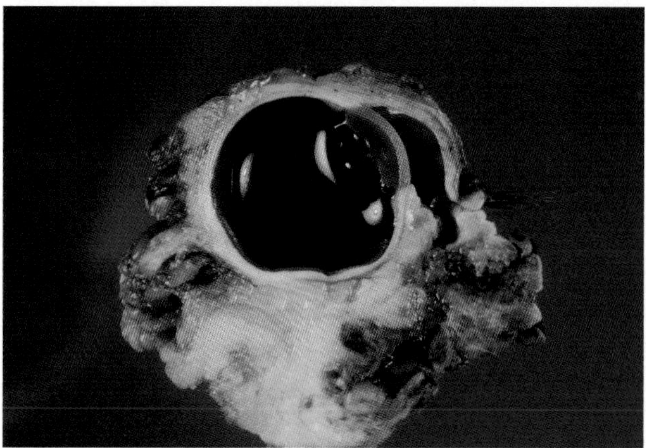

FIGURE 24-51 ■ ERMS arising in the soft tissues of the orbit. Though rarely necessary today, this specimen from an orbital exenteration shows a soft, glistening, whitish neoplasm infiltrating around the globe.

Most children with RMS do not have any predisposing genetic conditions or risk factors (95% to 98% of cases) except in the minority of children with Li-Fraumeni syndrome, NF1, Beckman-Wiedemann syndrome, Costello syndrome, Noonan syndrome, and the familial pleuropulmonary blastoma tumor predisposition syndrome (216).

Other neoplasms of childhood may have a malignant rhabdomyoblastic component, yet are not regarded as RMSs per se: triton tumor (MPNST with RMS component), malignant ectomesenchymoma (PNET with RMS component) or gangliorhabdomyosarcoma (Figure 24-52), pleuropulmonary blastoma in its three pathologic subtypes (Figure 24-53), RMS arising in a germ cell neoplasm, Sertoli-Leydig cell tumor of the ovary with heterologous elements in the form of RMS and congenital melanocytic nevus with RMS elements (76).

The staging of RMS, as with any other solid malignancy, is a combined clinical and pathologic endeavor, which incorporates the extent of disease beyond the primary site, but it also includes the specific primary site since the latter influences outcome in addition to the presence or absence of regional lymph node metastasis and distant metastasis to the bone marrow and/or lungs as well as to other sites. Those tumors arising in the head and neck region may be parameningeal (nasopharynx, middle ear, or pterygopalatine fossa) or not (orbit). Parameningeal RMS is more likely to spread to the meninges and brain (174).

Though the pathologic subtype of RMS is not formally incorporated into the staging of the disease, ARMS is known to have advanced stage disease at presentation more often than ERMS, as a manifestation of the more aggressive behavior of ARMS. RMS is divisible into three pathologic-prognostic categories: favorable, intermediate, and unfavorable (169) (Table 24-11). In addition to favorable, intermediate, and unfavorable pathologic subtypes of RMS, these tumors have also been subclassified on the basis of genotype, which correlates with the histologic subtype (48) (Table 24-2).

The overall 5-year disease-free survival for RMS in children is 70% to 75% today compared to 15% or less 30 years ago. As Dr. Jesse Ternberg, chief of pediatric surgery at St. Louis Children's Hospital from 1972 to 1990, summarized the outcome for these children in the early years, "If I could not cut it out entirely, the child was a goner."

Embryonal RMS constitutes slightly over 80% of all RMSs in our experience with the head and neck region and

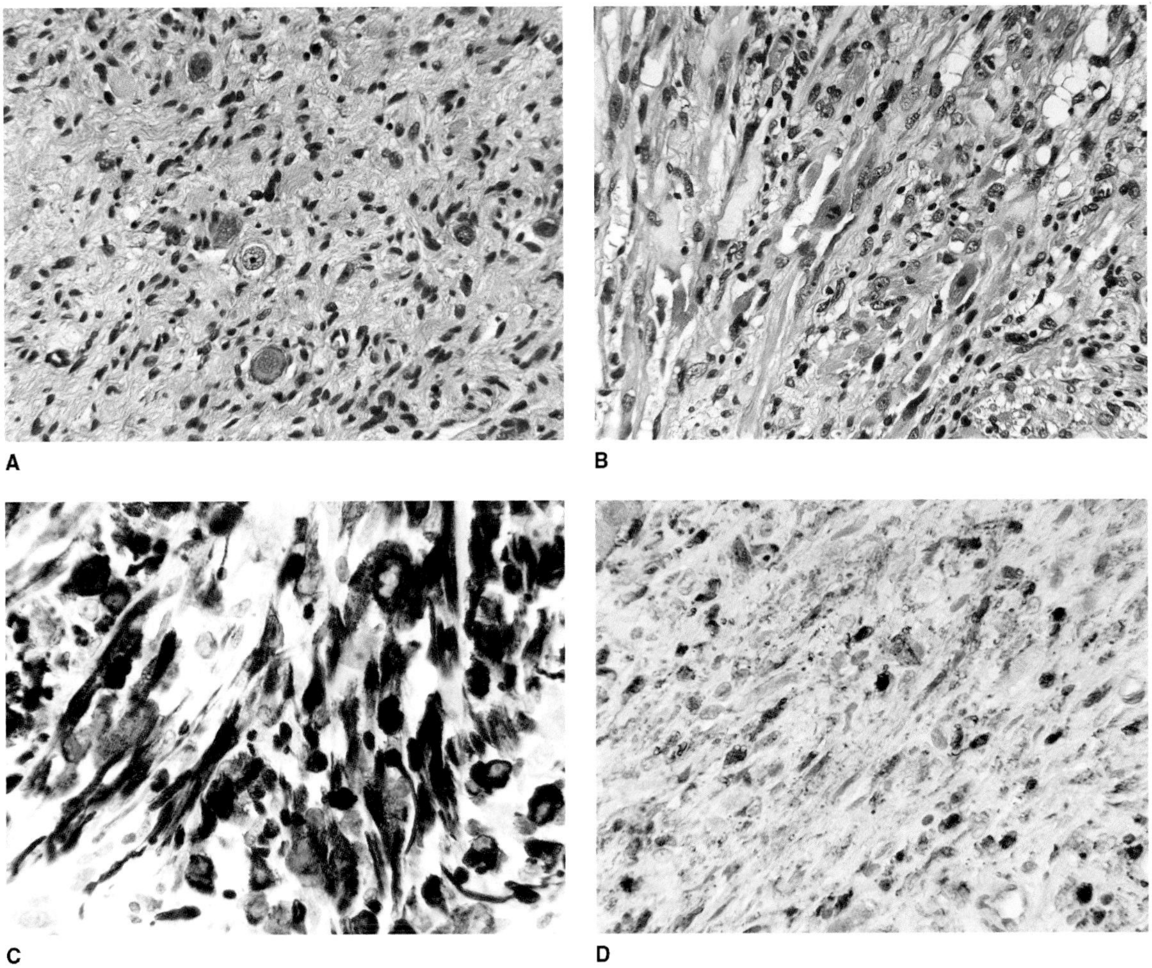

A B C D

FIGURE 24-52 ■ Gangliorhabdomyosarcoma (malignant ectomesenchymoma) presented as an extratesticular scrotal mass in a 2-year-old boy. **A:** Focal areas of the tumor are composed in part of mature ganglion cells in a background with a neuromatous appearance. **B:** Other foci show an ERMS with differentiated rhabdomyoblasts accompanied by less mature appearing malignant cells. **C:** Desmin immunostaining is shown in the rhabdomyosarcomatous areas. **D:** The neuromatous stroma is strongly positive for S100 protein.

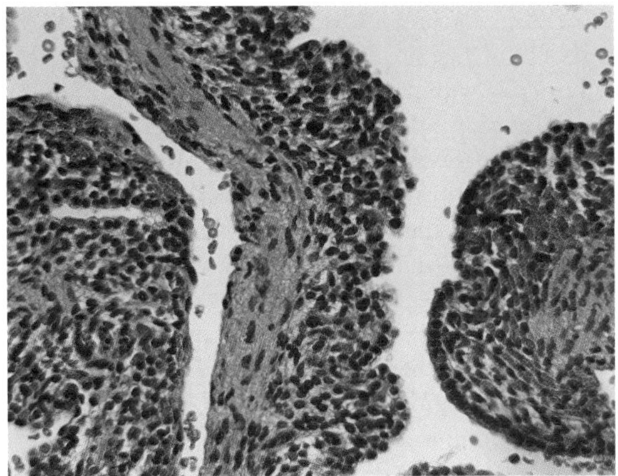

FIGURE 24-53 ■ Pleuropulmonary blastoma, cystic or type I presented as a cystic lung lesion in a 2-day-old male. Beneath the epithelial lining of the cysts, there is a cambium layer-like population of primitive round cells, some of which have the bright eosinophilic cytoplasm of rhabdomyoblasts. Previously these neoplasms were considered as an example of embryonal RMSs arising in a congenital lung cyst.

genitourinary tract together accounting for 80% of all cases (143). The nasal cavity and nasopharynx were the most common primary sites in the head and neck region (23 of 76 cases, 30%) and the paratesticular soft tissues (17 of 59 cases, 29%) and vagina (15 of 59 cases, 25%) together were the most common sites in the genitourinary tract (Table 24-12).

Grossly, the size of ERMS correlates with the primary site with the largest tumors presenting in the abdomen-pelvis and extremities where the mass commonly exceeds 6 to 8 cm in greatest dimension. The typical macroscopic appearance of an untreated ERMS is a soft gelatinous mass with a glistening, mucoid grayish-white cut surface with or without hemorrhage and necrosis. Most tumors are well circumscribed in the absence of a well-formed capsule. Since a primary resection is generally unusual today, most RMSs are unlikely to have the latter features but rather reflect the effects of preoperative chemotherapy which can reduce the tumor to no more than a small yellowish-white scar composed of histiocytes and fibrosis with or without any remnants of

Table 24-11 ■ PATHOLOGIC–PROGNOSTIC CATEGORIES OF CHILDHOOD RMS

	Incidence
Favorable	
Embryonal RMS, sarcoma botryoides	4%–6%
Embryonal RMS, spindle cell	2%–3%
Intermediate	
Embryonal RMS, patterns other than sarcoma botryoides and spindle cell types	45%–50%
Unfavorable	
Alveolar RMS	25%–30%
US	3%–5%
Pleomorphic RMS 1%–2%	

the tumor other than differentiated rhabdomyoblasts (7,44). When residual tumor is identified, a fibrous capsule may surround a cystic and/or solid focus with focal hemorrhage and fibrosis.

The usual initial encounter with a RMS by the pathologist is a needle or open biopsy, which can establish the terms of the diagnostic challenge. In some respects, ERMS is one of the most histologically diverse of the solid neoplasms of childhood, which reflects the broad range in the differentiation of the rhabdomyoblasts from small primitive cells displaying considerable heterogeneity in nuclear size and shape with minimal evidence as to the exact nature of the tumor (Figure 24-54). In fact, the cytologic diversity of individual tumor cells, which may be accompanied by a pale, mucoid to myxoid background is an important clue to the diagnosis. The nuclei are densely hyperchromatic, and mitotic figures are variably prominent. Scattered among the smaller tumor cells, larger individual cells with eosinophilic cytoplasm may be present; these latter cells are the ones most likely to demonstrate positivity for desmin, muscle specific actin, myoD1, and myogenin whereas the small primitive tumor cells may stain diffusely for vimentin, only focally for desmin if at all

Table 24-12 ■ EXPERIENCE WITH RMS IN CHILDREN AND ADOLESCENTS FROM 1989 TO 2009

Anatomic Sites	ERMS	ARMS	Total (%)
Head and neck	68	8	76 (34)
Genitourinary tract	58	1	59 (26)
Chest wall-trunk	11	4	15 (7)
Extremity	11	18	29 (13)
Abdomen-pelvis	19	6	25 (11)
Perianal region	5	5	10 (4)
Retroperitoneum	6	—	6 (3)
Skin	3	—	3 (1)
	181 (81)	**42 (19)**	**223**

From the files of the Lauren V. Ackerman Laboratory of Surgical Pathology, St. Louis Children's Hospital, Washington University Medical Center, St. Louis, MO.

and may have limited nuclear reactivity for myoD1 and/or myogenin (31,184). Other microscopic patterns include condensation of small primitive cells beneath an epithelial-lined surface in the sarcoma botryoides or solid sheets of tumor cells interspersed by nested collections of primitive tumor cells resembling the blastemal pattern of Wilms tumor; the blastema-like pattern is composed predominantly of polygonal-shaped tumor cells with scattered rhabdomyoblasts with clear to eosinophilic cytoplasm. A spindled population can be seen in association with the blastemal-like pattern, but one and possibly a second type of ERMS is composed almost exclusively of spindle cells with a differential diagnosis inclusive of CIFS and leiomyosarcoma. However, most spindled ERMS have scattered immature rhabdomyoblasts within the background or other minor foci of more primitive appearing small tumor cells. In the uterine cervix, ERMS is often seen in association with heterologous cartilage (Figure 24-55). When the primary site is the paratesticular region, ERMS of the spindle cell type is the tumor to be excluded on the basis of IHC. The other presumed type of RMS with an exclusive spindle cell pattern is the infantile rhabdomyofibrosarcoma with its usual bland microscopic features unlike the spindle cell embryonal RMS. These tumors can have a resemblance to CIFS, but unlike the latter tumor, there is immunopositivity for myoD1 and myogenin and they do not have the ETV6-NTRK3 translocation.

Anaplasia may be seen on occasion and if the suspected RMS is a tumor in or near the chest or lung, it is likely that the neoplasm is a pleuropulmonary blastoma especially in the presence of a collage of high-grade sarcomatous patterns including nodules of malignant-appearing cartilage. Nodules of immature cartilage or other teratoid elements are present with some frequency in sarcoma botryoides of the uterine cervix. Another uncommon feature of ERMS is the presence of a hyalinized or sclerotic stroma. Virtually all ERMSs are immunoreactive for vimentin, but the number of tumor cells, which express desmin and muscle specific actin is quite variable from one tumor to another as a manifestation of the spectrum of myogenic differentiation. Likewise, the number of tumor cells with nuclear positivity for myoD1 and myogenin varies from case to case. One ERMS demonstrates diffuse nuclear positivity, whereas another, especially the more immature or primitive ones, may have only a few labeled nuclei. Myogenin and myoD1 have a high degree of sensitivity exceeding 95% and a specificity of virtually 100%.

The molecular genetics of ERMS is different from those of alveolar RMS in that there is no signature or non–random translocations. Rather there is loss of heterozygosity on 11p15.5 in the region of IGF-2. Gains and losses of chromosomes or chromosomal regions have also been identified (Table 24-2).

ARMS is the less common of the two subtypes and in our series accounted for 19% of cases with the soft tissues of the extremities, lower greater than upper, as the preferred primary site of 43% of our cases (Table 24-12). In the perianal region, ARMS accounted for 50% of cases.

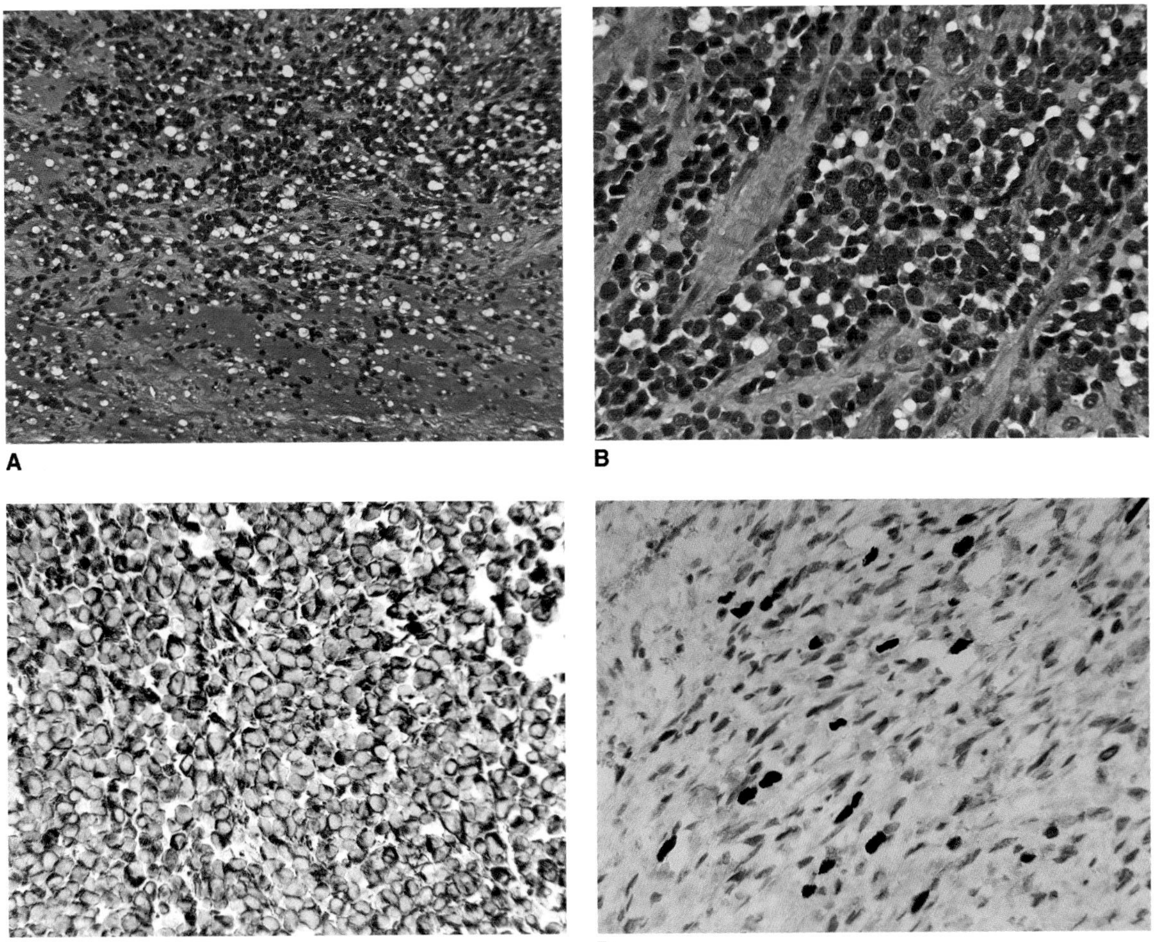

FIGURE 24-54 ■ ERMS presented in the paratesticular soft tissues of a 7-year-old male. **A:** One pattern consists of small, polymorphic appearing cells including spindle cells with embryonal features. **B:** Other foci are composed of more monotonous pleomorphic round cells arranged in loosely cohesive groups with an alveolar-like appearance. **C:** Rhabdomyoblasts are staining for desmin. **D:** The areas concerning for ARMS show only scattered nuclear positivity for myogenin unlike ARMS with its diffuse nuclear positivity. FISH studies failed to demonstrate a FKHR breakapart.

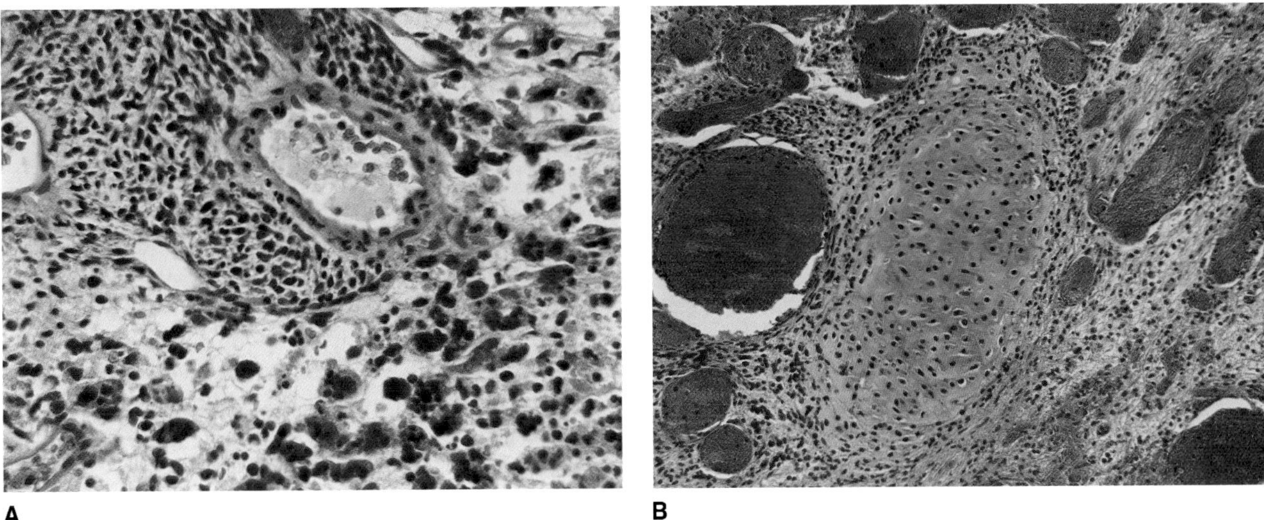

FIGURE 24-55 ■ ERMS presented as a polypoid mass arising from the uterine cervix of a 15-year-old female. **A:** Primitive appearing rhabdomyoblasts are present with population of enlarged, more pleomorphic malignant cells. **B:** Unique among ERMS is the presence of nodules of cartilage when this tumor presents in the cervix. There is the question of the relationship of this tumor to the adenosarcoma of the uterus. This tumor may be found in association with the pleuropulmonary blastoma complex with DICER1 mutation.

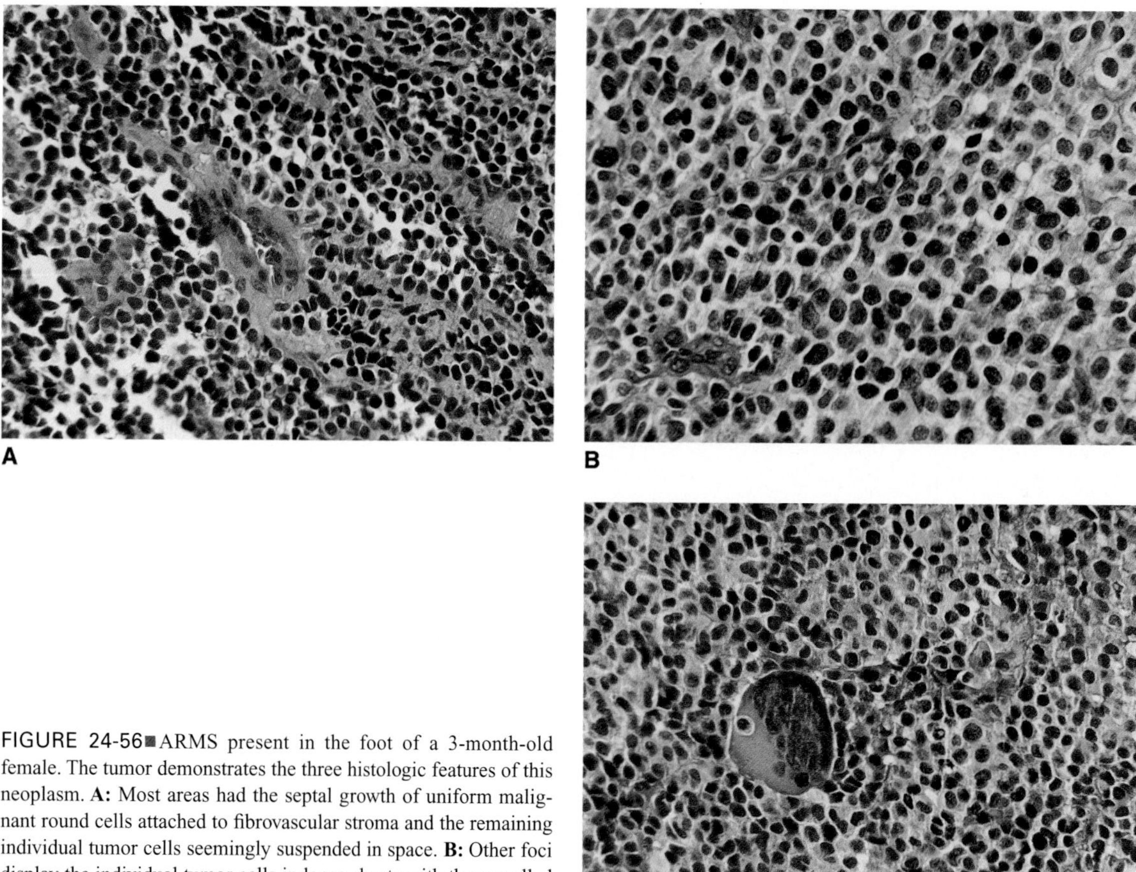

FIGURE 24-56■ARMS present in the foot of a 3-month-old female. The tumor demonstrates the three histologic features of this neoplasm. **A:** Most areas had the septal growth of uniform malignant round cells attached to fibrovascular stroma and the remaining individual tumor cells seemingly suspended in space. **B:** Other foci display the individual tumor cells in loose sheets with the so-called nascent alveolar pattern. **C:** Large, multinucleated tumor cells are seen in a background of monotonous round cells. FISH studies identified a FKHR breakapart.

This tumor more so than ERMS accommodates to the characterization of a malignant round cell neoplasm in that the cells are uniformly polygonal with high-grade rounded nuclei and variably prominent cytoplasm. Mitotic figures and nuclear debris are more prominent than in ERMS. The tumor cells may form solid sheets of nonoverlapping cells with foci in which the tumor cells tend to fall away from each other, producing the so-called nascent alveolar pattern (Figure 24-56). When the biopsy is a more generous one with stroma in the background, the tumor is more likely to have a nested-septal pattern in which the alveolar pattern of central disaggregated individual tumor cells is surrounded by individual tumor cells attached to the septal stroma. A similar alveolar pattern is seen in some cases of EWS-PNET (Figure 24-57). The presence of larger multinucleated tumor cells with prominent eosinophilic cytoplasm among the mononuclear tumor cells in these solid or more obvious septal-alveolar foci is virtually diagnosis of ARMS. In a minority of cases, one may encounter foci of ARMS with a pattern resembling ERMS; these cases are very uncommon in our experience and molecular genetic studies are very helpful in terms of diagnosis, but one complication is the emergence of the fusion-negative ARMS, now accounting for over 40% of currently diagnosed ARMS, unlike the historic figure of 20% of all ARMS as fusion-negative tumors.

Most ARMSs are consistently immunopositive for vimentin and desmin as well as myoD1 and myogenin (150,184). The latter three markers are diffusely positive in most cases of ARMS and less consistently so in ERMS. Diffuse nuclear staining for myogenin in ARMS has been described as a useful discriminating reaction from the more limited nuclear positivity in ERMS, and the diffuse nuclear staining is correlated with an unfavorable outcome (94).

There are two well-documented translocations in ARMS involving PAX3-FKHR (FOX01) and PAX7-FKHR (FOX01) gene fusions, t(2;13) (q35;q14) and t(1;13) (p36;q14) in 60% and 20% of fusion-positive cases, respectively (48,165). PAX3-FKHR-positive ARMS is associated with a poorer outcome than the PAX7-FKHR-positive and fusion-negative ARMS. Amplification of 12q13-q14 has an adverse effect upon prognosis. The t(1;13) ARMS is seen more often in younger children (190).

What is clear about ARMS is that it is prognostically unfavorable. Because ARMS can present with a lymph node metastasis or as disseminated disease in bones and bone marrow, the pathologic diagnosis can be challenging if ARMS is not considered in the differential diagnosis.

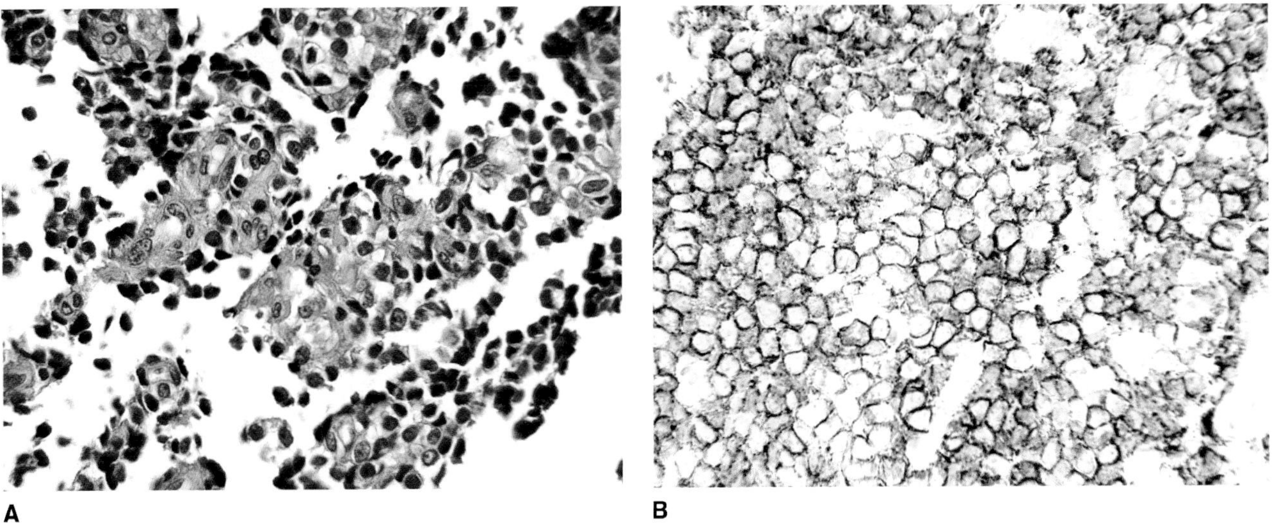

FIGURE 24-57 ■ EWS-PNET can have microscopic features with rosette formation to suggest a classic neuroblastoma. **A:** This tumor displays a septal pattern resembling ARMS. **B:** Diffuse CD99 membrane positivity and the EWS breakapart by FISH corroborated the diagnosis.

A nonlymphoid hematopoietic neoplasm, MRT, EWS-PNET, and neuroblastoma are other childhood malignancies, which are candidate neoplasms with some qualified clinical and pathologic overlap with ARMS. Pleomorphic RMS is recognized in childhood as a rarely occurring tumor (81). A sclerosing variant of RMS has been reported but is probably not a specific pathologic subtype with prognostic implications.

SARCOMAS OF UNCERTAIN HISTOGENESIS

Undifferentiated sarcoma (US) with various descriptors such as "round cell," "small blue cell," "anaplastic," or "spindle cell" existed for generations in the past and still does in a more limited sense for those malignant neoplasms in children whose morphological and immunohistochemical features as well as cytogenetic and molecular diagnostic studies are not diagnostic for a known tumor entity (175). At one time, as many as 25% of all STSs in children were assigned to the US or a similar category of "sarcoma of undetermined differentiation or histogenesis." This latter category was only exceeded by RMS, which accounted for 50% to 60% of STSs in children. Over the past 20 to 25 years, the diagnosis of US has steadily declined with the application of IHC and cytogenetics to establish the identity of such tumors as primitive embryonal RMS, myeloid-monocytic neoplasms, the various representative tumor types in the extended EWS family and MRT. The pathologic classification of RMS in children has a category of "unfavorable histology undifferentiated sarcoma." Somers and associates were among the first to report their experience with 13 cases of US in children between the ages of 1 month and 16 years at diagnosis; these tumors were described as "diffuse sheets of tumor cells with high cellularity" with round or spindle cell features (189). The diagnostic "full court press" on these tumors failed to establish a specific tumor type. In our own experience, the diagnosis of US is made in the presence of a malignant round cell neoplasm with high-grade nuclear features, often more atypical and pleomorphic than those of EWS-PNET and more like the MRT (Figure 24-58). Some of these tumors closely resemble EWS-PNET with periodic acid-Schiff (PAS)-positive granular cytoplasm, which is diastase sensitivity, but without the EWS breakapart by FISH. Possibly, some of these US are examples of a primitive round cell sarcoma with translocation t(4;19) (q35;q13.1). We are aware of another round cell "sarcoma" with the t(15;19) translocation of the undifferentiated carcinoma of the upper aerodigestive tract in children (Figure 24-59). Other examples of USs in children include the entities undifferentiated embryonal sarcoma of the liver and anaplastic sarcoma of the kidney (152,173,206). The specific tumor types with primitive round cell features are the primitive ERMS (with only rare cells positive for desmin and myoD1 or myogenin), MRT (usually <5 years old and few, if any, rhabdoid cells by microscopic examination but microscopically are more obvious in the vimentin and/or cytokeratin immunostain and lack BAF47 nuclear positivity to indicate an INI1 deletion) or a nonlymphoid hematopoietic neoplasm (vimentin and CD43 positivity). One would question whether some of the USs in the study of Orbach and associates were possibly MRTs (160).

Ewing sarcoma-primitive neuroectodermal tumor (EWS-PNET) and the extended EWS family of tumors have evolved as a result of the recognition that EWS and several other neoplasms are chacterized by an EWS breakapart to form a number of unique non–random translocations. Soon after the initial reports of an EWS-equivalent neoplasm in the soft tissues and a malignant small cell tumor of the chest wall and paraspinal region (Askin tumor), cytogenetic studies established that these two presumably separate entities

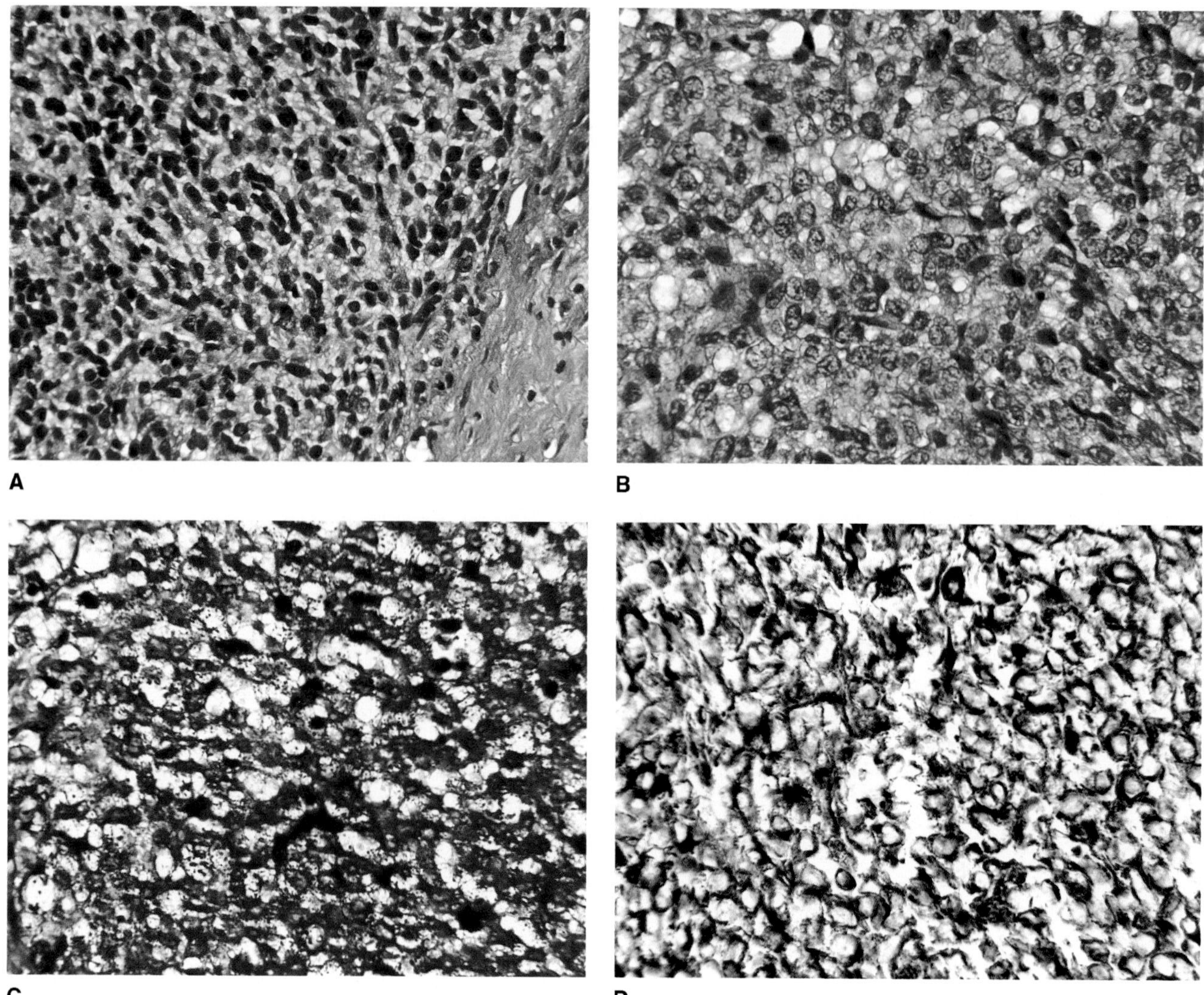

FIGURE 24-58 ■ Undifferentiated round cell sarcoma presented as a mass in the inguinal region of an 11-year-old male. **A:** These neoplasms are most commonly round cell neoplasms whose features resemble EWS-PNET though with somewhat more polymorphic and pleomorphic features. **B:** The nuclei tend to be more irregular than EWS-PNET but are accompanied by a clear to vacuolated cytoplasm. **C:** A PAS stain demonstrates the granular positivity of glycogen. **D:** Vimentin immunopositivity is a consistent finding, but CD99, if reactive, does not display the diffuse positivity of EWS-PNET. An EWS breakapart was not identified in this case by FISH studies.

had the same t(11;22) (q24;q12) translocation (24,131,177). Eventually, it became apparent that there was no longer any reason to maintain the dichotomy between EWS and the peripheral PNET from a pathologic, therapeutic, or prognostic perspective so that today these cases are diagnosed as "EWS-PNET." The past category of "sarcoma of uncertain histogenesis," the second most common STS of childhood, is now largely occupied by EWS-PNET (92).

EWS-PNET of soft tissues, the archetype of the extended EWS family of tumors, is a neoplasm whose origin is probably a mesenchymal stem cell whose oncogenesis is triggered with the formation of unique fusion genes consisting of the transactivation domain of EWS and the DNA finding domain of one of five ETS family transcription factors (178). EWS was originally described in the bone of young individuals in the 1920s and almost 50 years later was recognized in the soft tissues with a predilection for the chest wall, extremities, and paraspinal region (179) (Table 24-13). It is now recognized that the EWS-PNET can present in the kidney, lung, salivary gland, skin, and any number of other sites including the vulva, dura, and brain, which requires its inclusion in the differential diagnosis of any malignant round cell neoplasm in a young individual. Most cases of EWS-PNET present in the second decade with an average age at diagnosis of 12 years. However, almost 40% of tumors presented at or before 10 years of age with the two youngest cases, 1-year-old males with paraspinal and floor of the mouth tumors, respectively (Table 24-13). When EWS-PNET presents in the retroperitoneum and paravertebral locations, the tumor must be differentiated from undifferentiated and poorly differentiated neuroblastoma, especially in a child less than 6 years old.

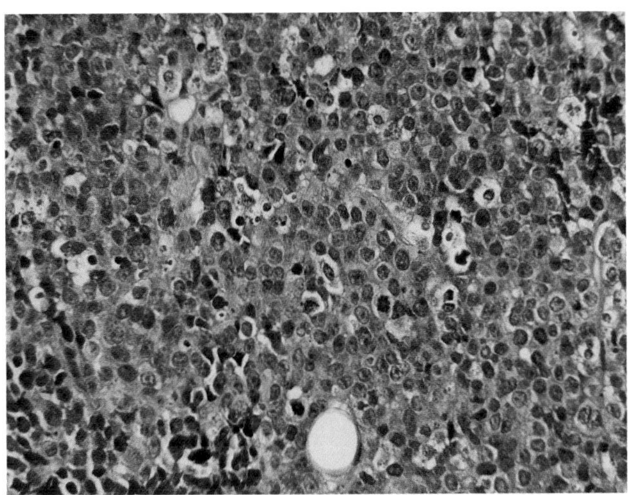

FIGURE 24-59 ■ Malignant round cell neoplasm presented in the abdomen of a 2-year-old male. A biopsy consists of crowded, uniform malignant round cells infiltrating through mesenteric fat. MRT, nonlymphoid hematopoietic neoplasm (granulocytic sarcoma) and undifferentiated neuroblastoma were considered in the differential diagnosis. The tumor cells only expressed vimentin and cytogenetic studies revealed a t(15;19) translocation (BRD4-NUT fusion) of the type associated with the childhood upper airway carcinoma. (Contributed by Bahig M. Shehata, M.D., Atlanta, Georgia).

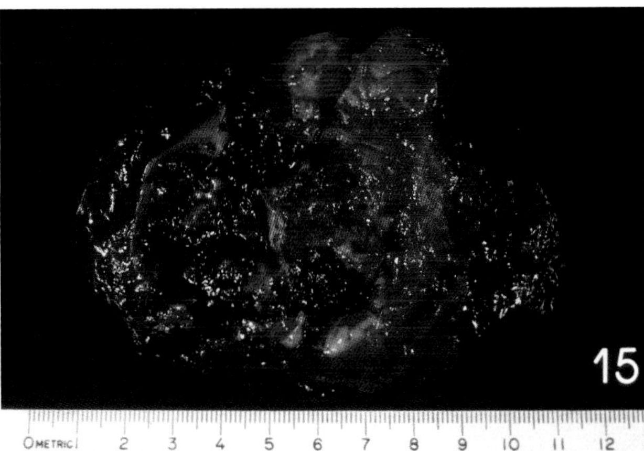

FIGURE 24-60 ■ EWS-PNET presented in the paraspinal region of a 15-year-old male. This 10 cm mass with cystic and hemorrhagic features has soft, gray-white viable tumor at the periphery. Hemorrhage and necrosis are common gross features.

The pathologic evaluation of a suspected EWS-PNET of soft tissue and bone has been thoroughly outlined by Carpentier and associates who have appropriately stated that the "first priority should always be given to formalin-fixed tissues for morphologic evaluation" (27). The biopsy specimen is more often than not "small" by most measures plus the fact that there may be as much hemorrhage and necrosis as

Table 24-13 ■ EWS-PNET OF SOFT TISSUE AND BONE IN CHILDREN AND ADOLESCENTS

Soft Tissue[a]		Bone[b]	
Site	**No. (%)**	**Site**	**No. (%)**
Chest wall	14 (39)	Pelvic bones	14 (40)
Extremity	7 (19)	Humerus	5 (14)
Paraspinal	4 (11)	Tibia	4 (11)
Scalp, face, floor of mouth, submandibular gland	4 (11)	Femur	4 (11)
Neck	3 (8)	Rib	3 (8)
Retroperitoneum	2 (5)	Radius	2 (6)
Nasopharynx	1 (3)	Fibula	2 (6)
Trachea	1 (3)	Mandible	1 (3)
	36 (100)		**35 (100)**

[a]Average age at diagnosis, 12 years, (age range 1 to 20 years), 14 (39%) children 10 years or less at diagnosis; 22 males and 14 females.
[b]Average age at diagnosis, 14 years (age range 2 to 20 years), 6 (17%) children 10 years old at diagnosis, 17 males and 18 females.
From the files of the Lauren V. Ackerman Laboratory of Surgical Pathology, St. Louis Children's Hospital, Washington University Medical Center, St Louis, MO.

viable, well-preserved neoplastic tissue (Figure 24-60). The other reality is that the biopsy may be the last opportunity to document the pathologic features since preoperative chemotherapy often results in total or near-total ablation of tumor.

A well-preserved and fixed biopsy demonstrates a diffuse and/or nested-lobular pattern of a monotonous, monolayer of rounded or polygonal tumor cells. Where there is an apparent nested or lobular pattern, there is an accompanying fibrous stroma. Other features can include focal necrosis, pools, or lakes of erythrocytes with a pelioid appearance and collections of tumor cells with apparent loss of cohesion with an alveolar-like quality reminiscent of ARMS. As a monolayer of nonoverlapping tumor cells, the central nuclei are similar with a uniformly dispersed or subtly clumped chromatin with one or more micronucleoli (Figure 24-61). The cytoplasm is clear to finely vacuolated and often contains abundant PAS-positive, diastase-digestible glycogen granules (Figure 24-62A,B). Any compression of the tissue results in the loss of the latter cytologic features with more hyperchromatic nuclei with fusiform contours and inapparent cytoplasm. Mitotic figures are usually modest in number, and anaplasia is absent. Some tumors may display the presence of pyknotic, shrunken tumor cells scattered in the background of better preserved tumor cells. On occasion, diminutive extracellular pools of a mucoid to an almost chondrohyaline stroma material are noted. The characteristic immunophenotype includes diffuse vimentin and CD99 positivity with a dot-like and/or perinuclear reactivity and a uniform cytoplasmic-membranous pattern, respectively (Figure 24-62C,D). A similar pattern of cytoplasmic positivity for cytokeratin is present in 20% to 25% of cases; many fewer cells are reactive compared to vimentin. It is well to keep in mind that these two markers alone will not differentiate EWS-PNET from lymphoblastic lymphoma, desmoplastic small round cell tumor (DSRCT), or MRT (Table 24-2). It is unusual for a EWS-PNET not to express CD99; however, we have seen several examples, which subsequently were shown

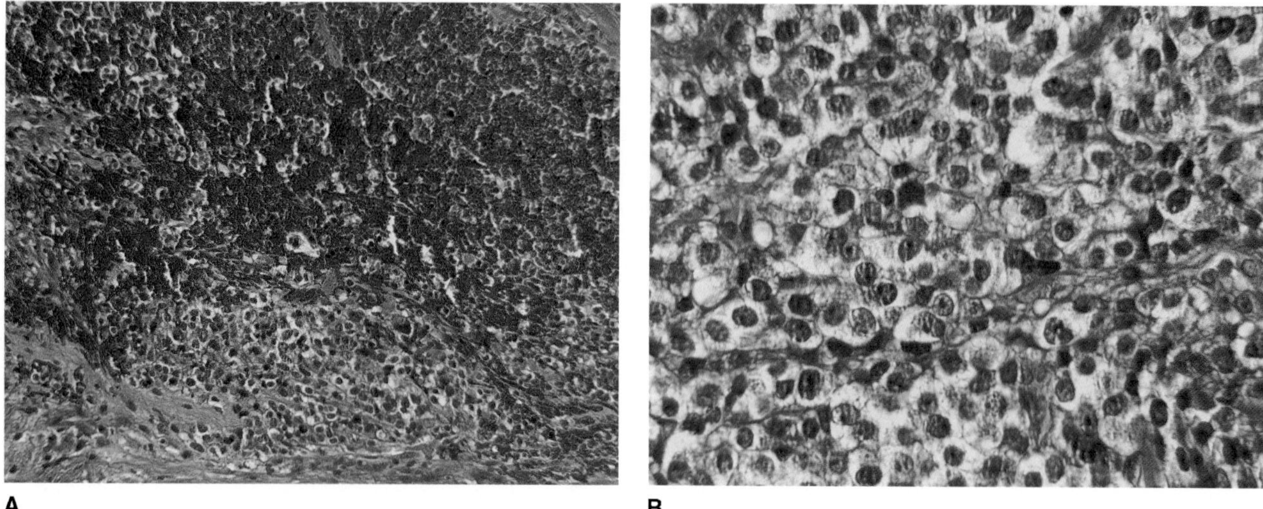

FIGURE 24-61 ■ EWS-PNET presented as a deep soft tissue mass in the paraspinal retroperitoneum. **A:** Substantial hemorrhage and necrosis can accompany these tumors in which some microscopic fields may contain few tumor cells. **B:** These tumors like ARMS and hematolymphoid neoplasms qualify as pure round cell neoplasms. Well-preserved areas of tumor show cells with uniform central nuclei surrounded by clear to vacuolated cytoplasm.

to have an EWS breakapart to emphasize that FISH has an important role in the evaluation of any suspected EWS fusion-associated neoplasm.

Desmoplastic small round cell tumor (DSRCT) is the second neoplasm to have been recognized as a member of the extended EWS family with an EWS fusion partner, but with WT1 rather than FLI1. Originally described as a multifocal, multinodular neoplasm arising from the peritoneum, DSRCT is known to occur in the posterior fossa, pleura, scrotum, ovary, and kidney (15). Because of its unique immunophenotype of vimentin, cytokeratin, desmin, and WT1 positivity, it was suggested initially that the DSRCT might be a primitive mesothelial neoplasm since this phenotype is shared with mesothelial cells (32,161). The most common presenting site is the abdomen, which coincides with our own experience in 19 cases, of which 16 (84%) occurred in the abdominal cavity as multiple peritoneal nodules. The remaining three cases presented on the pleura and in the pancreas and parotid gland. The patients ranged in age from 3 to 18 years (mean age 10 years) with 11 tumors presenting in the second decade, but this tumor is well documented into the third decade and beyond. The male-to-female ratio in our experience was 9 males and 10 females. Virtually all of our cases were seen as biopsies since the clinical presentation does not lend itself to primary surgical resection. The basic microscopic features are summarized in the name of the tumor with a dense

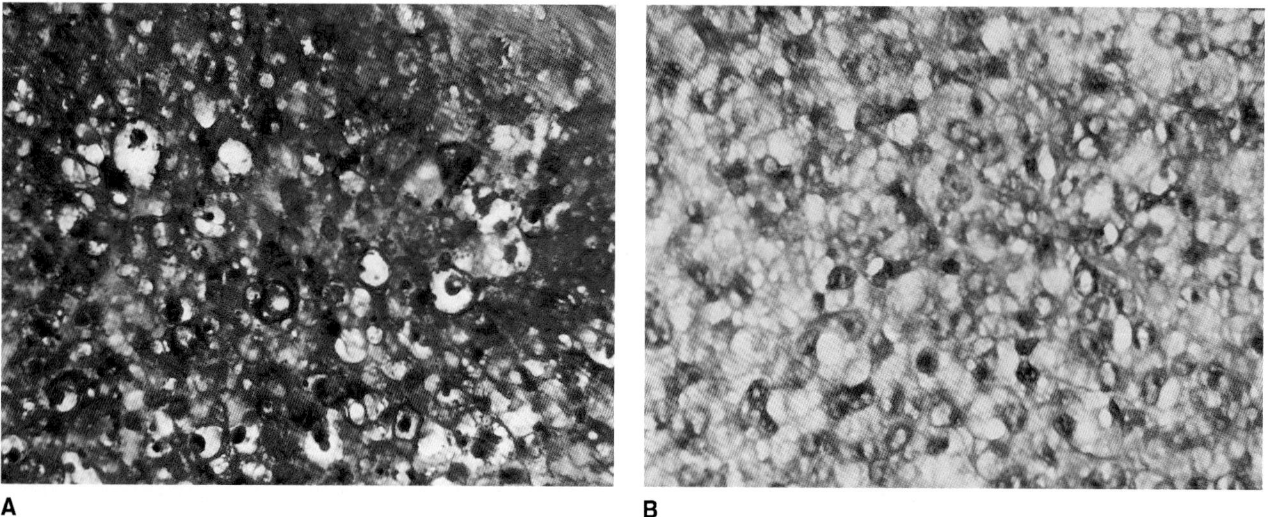

FIGURE 24-62 ■ EWS-PNET can be characterized histochemically and immunohistochemically. **A:** The clear cytoplasm of the tumor cells reflects the abundant glycogen as seen in this PAS stain. **B:** Following diastase digestion of the PAS stain, the tumor cells reacquire the clear cytoplasm.

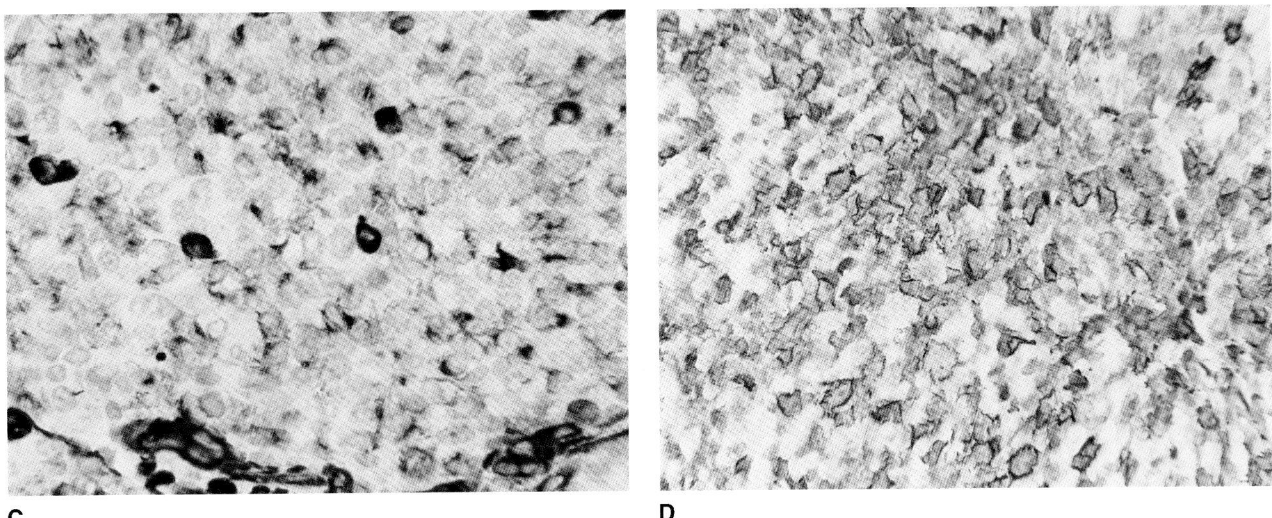

FIGURE 24-62■*(continued)* **C:** Virtually all tumors are immunopositive for vimentin with a perinuclear cytoplasmic or dot-like pattern of reactivity. **D:** These tumors are uniformly positive for CD99 with a diffuse pattern of reactivity.

fibrous background containing numerous, variably sized nests of undifferentiated small cells, which are not necessarily all rounded or polygonal (Figure 24-63). Gland-like structures, solid squamoid nests, and even rhabdoid cells can be seen. However, a desmoplastic fibrous stroma is also a feature of metastatic Wilms tumor and RMS, which can create a microscopic and immunohistochemical dilemma with DRSCT, which may be resolved by MyoD1 or myogenin staining in the case of RMS and the lack of an EWS breakapart in the case of Wilms tumor.

Clear cell sarcoma (CCS) of soft tissues (malignant melanoma of soft parts), another member of the extended EWS family, is characterized by an EWS translocation, t(12;22)(q13;q12), which is found in 75% or more of cases; this same translocation is found in AFH (98) (Table 24-2). Though the CCS is phenotypically a melanoma as defined by the presence of melanosomes and the expression of S100 protein, HMB-45, melan-A, and micropthalmic transcription factor, it does not have the activating mutations of BRAF kinase, which are the basic molecular events of cutaneous melanoma. A slowly enlarging soft-tissue mass in the distal extremities (lower more often than upper) and rarely in bone, small intestine, and kidney in adolescents or young adults is the clinical presentation (57,109). This tumor is infrequent in children 5 years old or less. A mass in the region of a tendon or aponeurosis, measuring 5 cm or less, is firm and well circumscribed with a grayish-tan surface. Like the cutaneous melanoma, the spindled or more epithelioid cells are arranged in cohesive

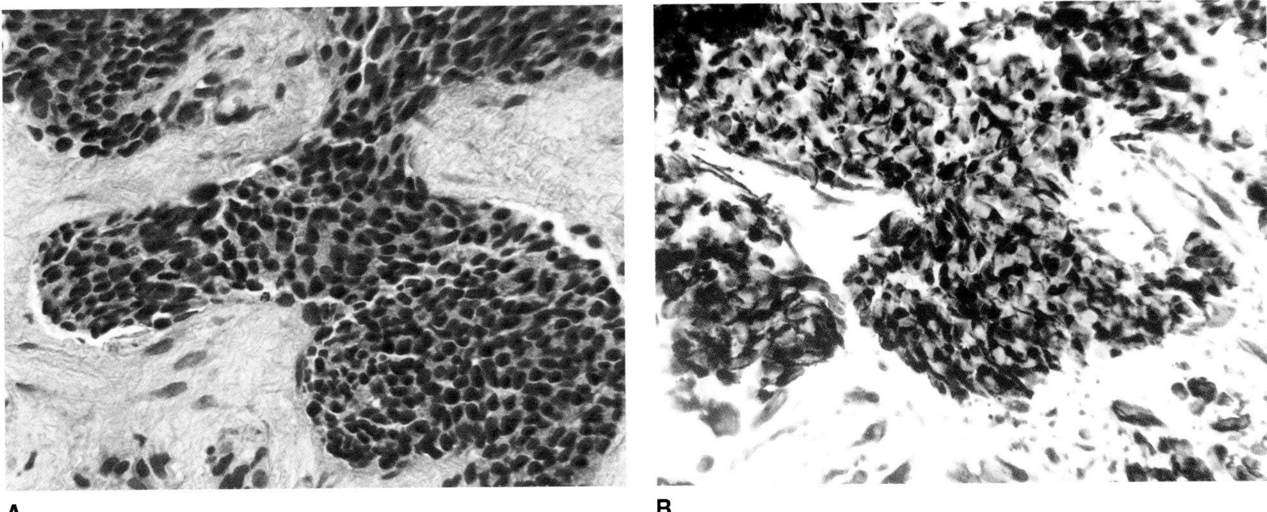

FIGURE 24-63■DSRCT in a 17-year-old male presented with abdominal pain. Multiple masses were identified by imaging studies. **A:** A biopsy shows the presence of discrete and interconnecting nests of crowded malignant small basophilic tumor cells surrounded by a fibrous stroma. **B:** The tumor shows strong diffuse positivity for vimentin.

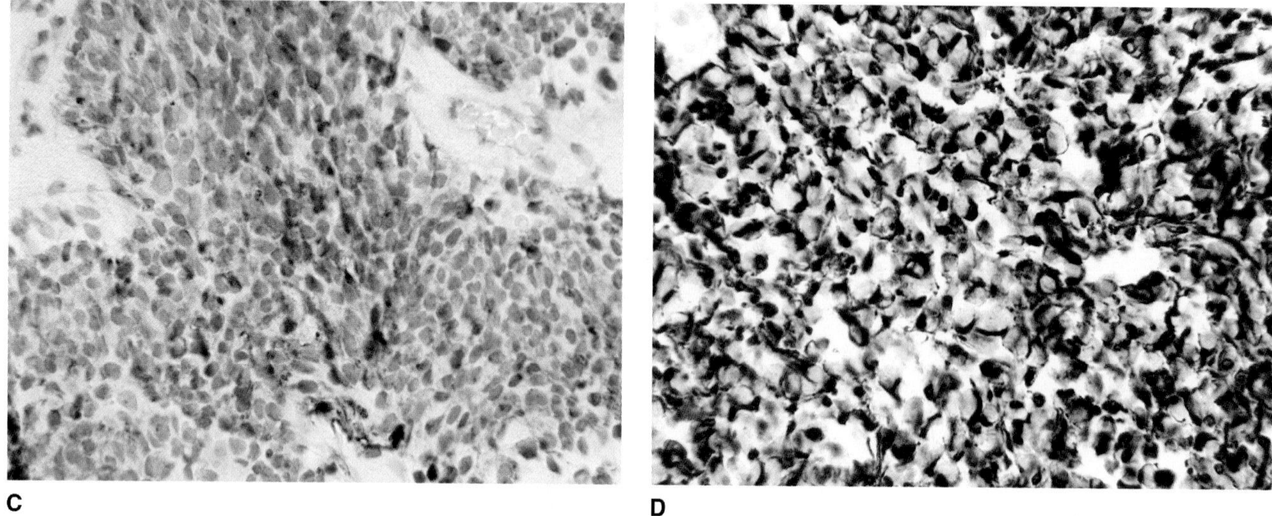

FIGURE 24-63 *(continued)* **C:** Scattered tumor cells show dot-like and perinuclear pattern of cytokeratin positivity. **D:** Desmin expression may be strong and diffuse as in this case or may be more limited. These tumors also show strong nuclear positivity for WT1 (not illustrated). The EWS breakapart was identified by FISH.

groups with a delicate fibrous stromal network in the background or with a more prominent hyalinized stroma and can be highly infiltrative (140). Other patterns have a resemblance to the disaggregated cells of an ARMS or EWS when the tumor cells are more polygonal in appearance. Multinucleated giant cells are seen with some frequency. Clear to eosinophilic cytoplasm can add to the EWS-like appearance. The rounded to ovoid nuclei are modestly hyperchromatic and vesicular with amphophilic nucleoli (Figure 24-64). Pseudoinclusions are more or less prominent. Mitotic figures are not especially numerous. Other immunophenotypic attributes include the expression of CD99 and neuron-specific enolase. Tumors larger than 5 cm and those with necrosis are regarded as having unfavorable prognosis. Regional lymph node metastasis is a common mode of spread. Overall survival is approximately 50%. The differential diagnosis includes SS (common sites of presentation), PEComa (similarities in immunophenotype, but without EWS breakapart), paraganglioma (similar immunophenotype, but absence of HMB-45 or melan-A expression) and cutaneous melanoma (similar immunophenotype, but absence of EWS breakapart).

Extraskeletal myxoid chondrosarcoma (EMC) is seemingly the least common representative of the extended EWS family tumors and the least frequently of these neoplasms in children and adolescents. A large combined institutional experience revealed no cases in the first decade and only 2

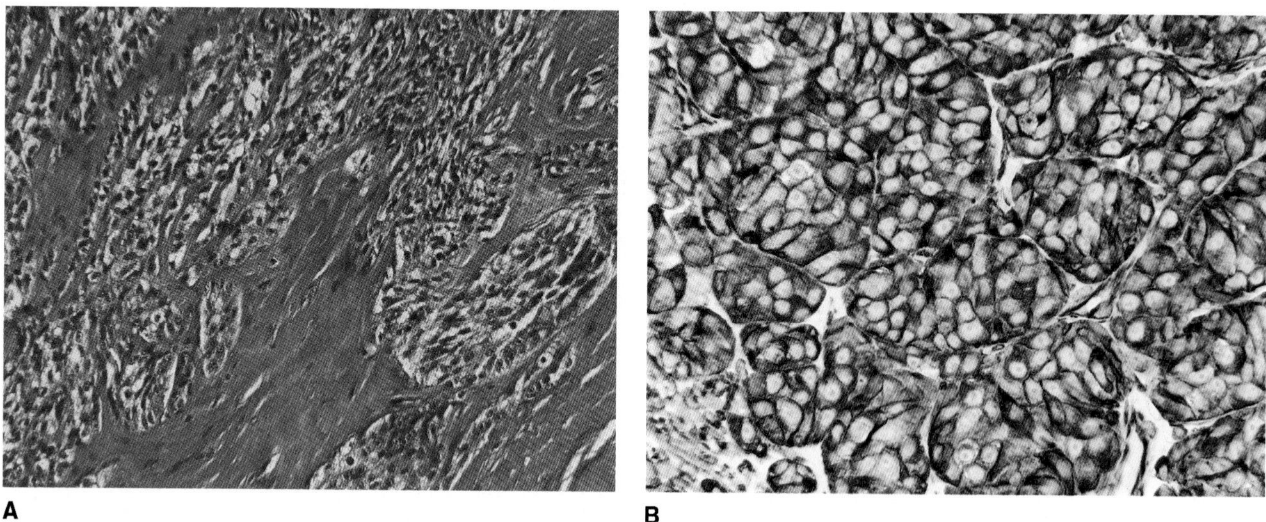

FIGURE 24-64 CCS of tendon sheath (melanoma of soft part) presented as a mass over the clavicle in a 10-year-old male. **A:** A nodular tan-white mass measuring 2.5 cm consisted of ill-defined nests of rounded to spindled-shaped tumor cells in a background of fibrous stroma. **B:** Immunohistochemical staining showed strong positivity for HMB-45.

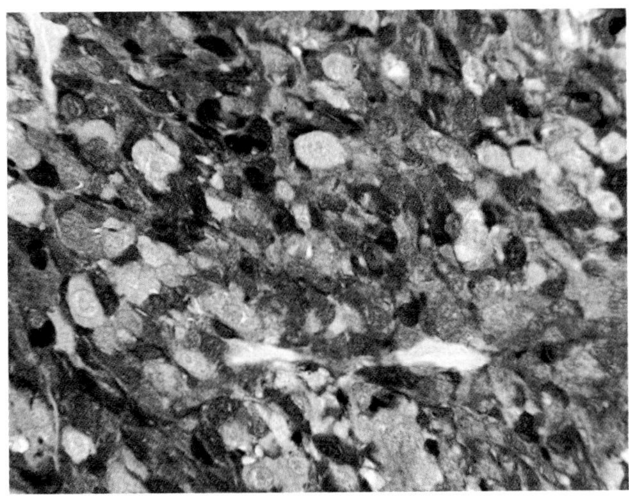

C

FIGURE 24-64■ *(continued)* **C:** The tumor cells are also positive for S100 protein. An EWS breakapart was demonstrated by FISH.

(2%) of 86 cases in individuals between 11 and 20 years old, though the individual case has been seen in younger children. Three translocations have been identified to date and one of these is an EWS fusion partner (Table 24-2). The proximal lower extremity is the most common site of presentation in all age groups (3). These tumors arise in the subcutis or deeper soft tissues as a well-circumscribed, multinodular mass with a complete or incomplete fibrous capsule, usually less than 10 cm in diameter and have a gelatinous whitish-tan to tannish appearance. Cartilage is generally not identified grossly or microscopically leading to question whether EMC should be regarded as chondrosarcoma since it is also inconsistently immunoreactive for S100 protein. Fibrous septa separate the tumor into lobules, which are composed of delicate lacelike strands, more solid appearing nests, spindle cells, and high-grade round cells. The background has a variable myxoid or mucoid appearance. In some cases, it is the multilobulated architecture at low magnification, which provides the subtle clue to the diagnosis while other SSTs are under consideration in the differentiated diagnosis like poorly differentiated or monophasic SS, MRT (rhabdoid cells in EMC), neurothekeoma, myoepithelial tumor of soft tissues, chordoma, parachordoma (if it exists as a distinct entity), and EWS-PNET (117). Immunohistochemically, EMC is reactive for vimentin (75% to 80% of cases), neuron-specific enolase (50% to 95%), EMA (10% to 15%), S100 protein (15% to 20%), synaptophysin (40% to 50%), and glial fibrillary acidic protein (2% to 5%) (97). These tumors are generally nonreactive for CD99, c-MET, and CAM 5.2 (the two latter markers are also positive in chordomas) and have normal expression of BAF47 (INI1).

Mesenchymal chondrosarcoma (MCS), like myxoid chondrosarcoma and EWS-PNET, has a primary soft tissue and skeletal presentation (30,46). Its relationship to the other extended EWS family of tumors is not entirely clear, though a t(11;22) translocation has been reported in addition to other karyotypic abnormalities (trisomy 8, 20−, 12+) (151). Most MCSs present in children beyond the age of 10 years and into the third decade (30). Very rarely, MCS is seen in the neonate (49). Approximately 60% to 70% of MCSs arise in the soft tissues or nonosseous sites like the dura, orbit, pelvis, sinonasal tract, peripheral soft tissues, and kidney. The tumor is characterized microscopically by nodules or islands of atypical hyaline cartilage and an accompanying population of primitive round cells resembling EWS or a more spindle cell stroma with clefted vascular spaces resembling HPC. We have seen cases of MCS in which the two patterns appeared to segregate from each other. These tumors are immunopositive for vimentin, CD99, and reportedly desmin and myogenin (155). The 5-year survival is 40% to 50%, and MCSs arising in the soft tissues and with the HPC-like pattern fared worse than tumors arising in the bone and with EWS-like features (30).

Myoepithelial tumor of soft tissue is a neoplasm presenting predominantly in the extremities but not to the exclusion of other regional sites. The largest series to date reported that approximately 20% of tumors are diagnosed before the age of 20 years (100). The multilobulated and reticulated growth pattern of epithelioid and spindle cells has some overlapping features with EMC, proximal type epithelioid sarcoma (ES), and parachordoma. These tumors are immunoreactive for cytokeratin (AE1/AE3) and/or EMA, S100 protein, calponin, p63, and glial fibrillary acidic protein. Pathologic grade and resectability are the two principal correlates of outcome.

Synovial sarcoma (SS) is one of the most common non-RMSs in the first two decades of life together with the MPNST. There is some variance from one series to another, but 15% to 30% of SSs are diagnosed at or before 20 years of age (66,74,191). Less than 15% of all SSs in children and adolescents are diagnosed before the age of 10 years. In our own experience with SSs, there were 57 cases, which were diagnosed between 4 and 20 years of age (mean age, 14 years) with 12 (20%) of the cases seen in children 10 years old or less. Approximately 60% of cases presented in the extremities, which is in accord with other larger series, which have reported up to 70% of tumors in the extremities (Table 24-14). Various sites in the head and neck region accounted for 10% of our cases. With molecular genetic testing for the t(X;18) translocation, SS has been documented in a number of previously unrecognized sites such as the lung-pleura, heart, and intestinal tract as some examples. Several cases of pleuropulmonary SS were originally submitted for review as possible examples of type I or cystic pleuropulmonary blastomas (PPB), but four of the patients were adolescents between 13 and 15 years of age whereas the median age for type I PPB is 9 months. A firm, well-circumscribed fibrous appearing mass may be accompanied by focal hemorrhagic cysts and dystrophic calcifications or metaplastic bone (Figure 24-65). In those tumors with minimal fibrous stroma, the consistency is soft and the cut surface has a glistening, mucoid appearance resembling an ERMS or CIFS. Attention to the dimensions of the tumor

Table 24-14 ■ SS IN CHILDREN AND ADOLESCENTS

Anatomic Site	No.	(%)
Lower extremity	22	(39)
Proximal	14	
Distal	8	
Upper extremity	11	(19)
Proximal	6	
Distal	5	
Chest wall	7	(12)
Lung-Pleura	5	(9)
Abdominal wall	3	(5)
Retroperitoneum	2	(3)
Neck	2	(3)
Paranasal sinus—pharynx	2	(3)
Scalp	1	(2)
Orbit	1	(2)
Posterior mediastinum	1	(2)
	57	(100)

37 males, 20 females (mean age, 14 years).
From the files of the Lauren V. Ackerman Laboratory of Surgical Pathology, St. Louis Children's Hospital, Washington University Medical Center, St. Louis, MO.

is important since there is a consistent correlation between size (> or <5 cm) and outcome; those tumors in excess of 5 cm have a significantly poorer prognosis (non-RMSs in children, regardless of pathologic type, have a poor outcome if >5 cm in greatest dimension) (126).

There are two basic histologic patterns of SS: monophasic spindle cell proliferation and biphasic spindle-glandular type (Figure 24-66). A third poorly differentiated pattern, constituting 5% or less of cases, has some similarities to EWS-PNET including a similar immunophenotype of vimentin, cytokeratin, and CD99 positivity but in the absence of a EWS breakapart but with a SYT-SSX breakapart. The fourth purely glandular pattern resembling well-differentiated adenocarcinoma is very rare. Necrosis and rhabdoid cells are

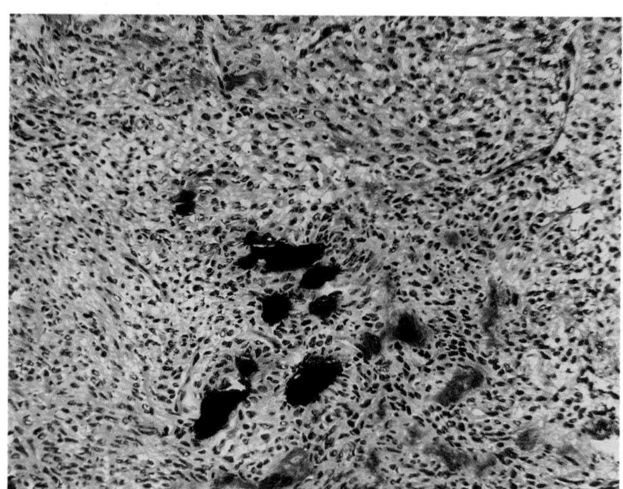

FIGURE 24-65 ■ This SS presented in the ankle of an 8-year-old male. Some tumors are associated with dystrophic calcifications.

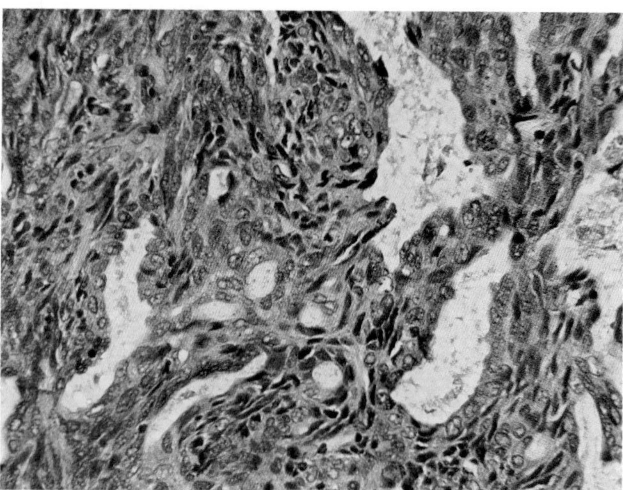

FIGURE 24-66 ■ SS presented in the left foot of this 18-year-old male. This neoplasm had a classic biphasic pattern of gland formation in a spindle cell background.

other features of poorly differentiated SS. Uniform spindle cells with either ovoid or fusiform contours are arranged in dense sheets or short fascicles (Figure 24-67). The nuclei have a pale, finely granular chromatin, and the cytoplasm is inconspicuous. Mitotic figures are not prominent. Like the MPNST, which the monophasic spindle cell SS resembles, there may be alternating "light cell-dark cell" areas reflecting variable cellular density. A HPC-like pattern is another useful clue to the diagnosis. In addition, myxoid foci convey an impression of MPNST or DFSP. Mast cells are nonspecific, but their presence should evoke concern about SS or MPNST in the appropriate setting. The glandular profiles are either subtle, residing as small tubular structures interspersed in a predominant spindle cell background or are overly obvious large glands or cysts. Immunohistochemically, SS is diffusely positive for vimentin in the spindle cell component whereas the epithelial component expresses cytokeratin AE1/AE3, cytokeratin 7, and EMA; the cytokeratins may be limited to individual tumor cells or entirely nonreactive (Figure 24-68). The EMA is more likely to stain small groups of tumors cells with a membranous pattern. Both CD99 and bcl2 are consistently expressed in SS. An antibody to TLE1 has shown some diagnostic value in cases of SS. SS is also known to be immunopositive for S100 protein. Though most SSs have the t(X;18) translocation, whether it is the fusion transcript, SYT-SSX1 (present more often in biphasic SS) or SYT-SSX2 (more often monophasic SS) does not seem to have prognostic significance though there is some evidence to suggest that the latter fusion transcript is correlated with a less favorable outcome. All SSs are at least grade 2 sarcomas but increased mitotic activity and necrosis are grade 3 features. However, COG regards all SSs as grade 3 based upon the tumor type. A spindle cell sarcoma with marked nuclear pleomorphism, anaplasia, and extensive necrosis is unlikely to represent a SS. The overall survival of children and adolescents is approximately 80%, whereas it is lower in adults (60%) (195).

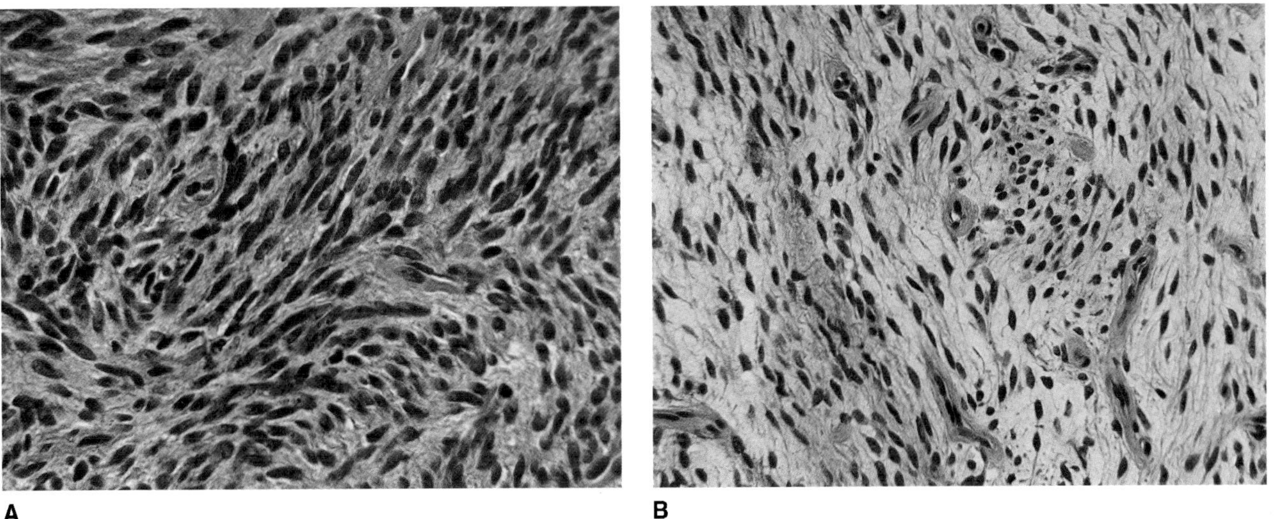

FIGURE 24-67 ■ SS presented in the wrist of an 11-year-old male. **A:** A monotonous population of uniform spindle cells characterizes this monophasic neoplasm. **B:** Some areas had a more myxoid appearance with the separation of tumor cells.

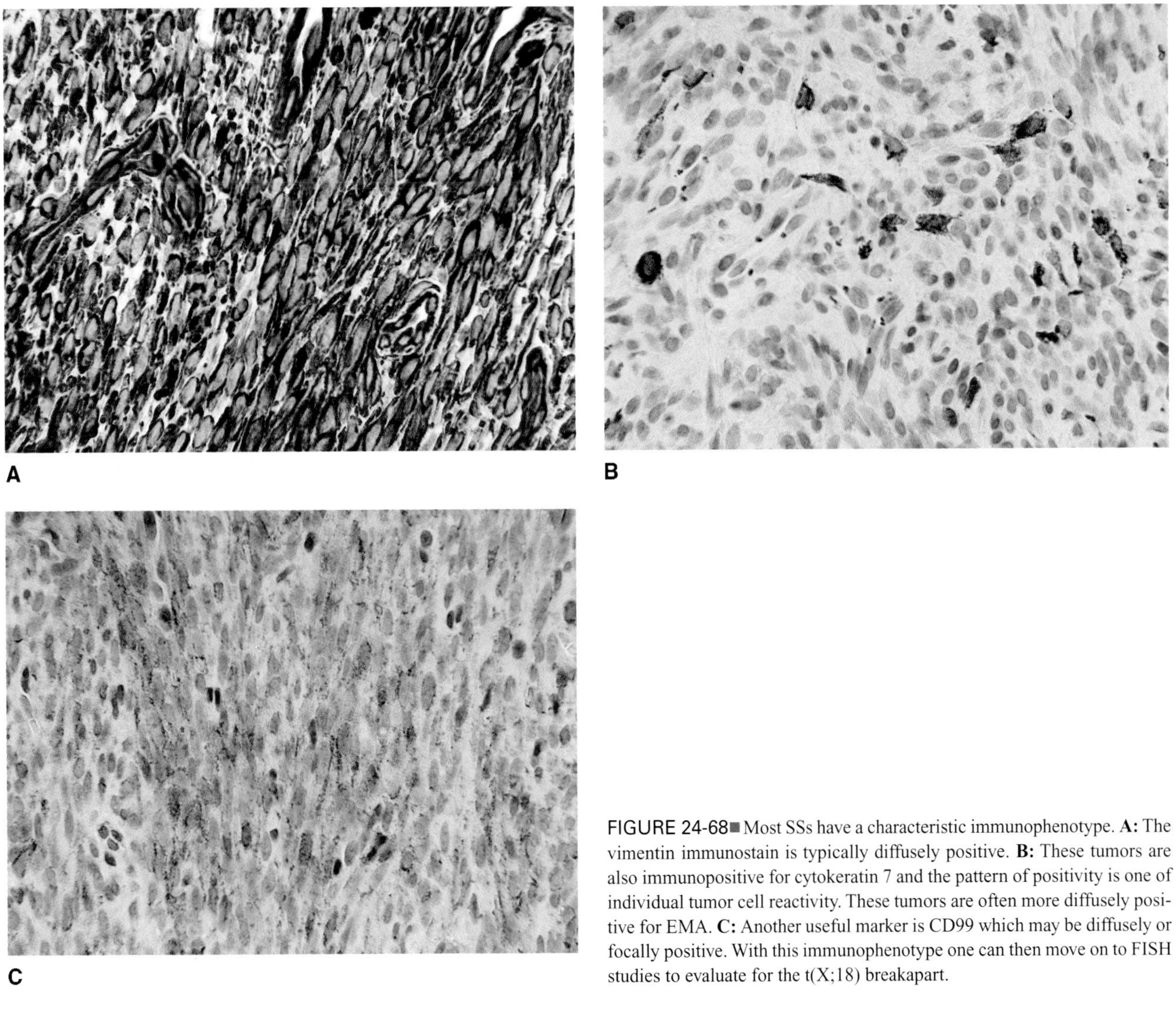

A

B

C

FIGURE 24-68 ■ Most SSs have a characteristic immunophenotype. **A:** The vimentin immunostain is typically diffusely positive. **B:** These tumors are also immunopositive for cytokeratin 7 and the pattern of positivity is one of individual tumor cell reactivity. These tumors are often more diffusely positive for EMA. **C:** Another useful marker is CD99 which may be diffusely or focally positive. With this immunophenotype one can then move on to FISH studies to evaluate for the t(X;18) breakapart.

Table 24-15 ■ EXTRARENAL AND RENAL MRTs IN CHILDREN (1989 TO 2009)

	No.	(%)
Soft tissue (1 week–16 years, mean 3.9 years)	47	(48)
Neck (16)		
Paraspinal region (11)		
Axilla (5)		
Abdominal wall (3)		
Arm (3)		
Back (2)		
Other (7)		
Central nervous system (1 year–18 years, mean 5 years)	15	(15)
Kidney (3 days–5 years, mean 1.3 years)	12	(12)
Liver (3 months–8 years, mean 1.6 years)	11	(11)
Abdomen (2 months–2 years, mean 1 year)	4	(4)
Mediastinum (7 months–3 years, mean 1.2 years)	4	(4)
Dessiminated (3 days–3 weeks, mean 1.5 weeks)	3	(3)
Bladder (5 years, 10 years)	2	(2)
	98	**(100)**

53 males and 45 females.
From the files of the Lauren V. Ackerman Laboratoryears of Surgical Pathology, St. Louis Children's Hospital, Washington University Medical Center, St. Louis, MO.

Malignant rhabdoid tumor (MRT) and its counterpart in the brain and spinal cord, atypical teratoid/rhabdoid tumor (ATRT), have evolved into a single pathologic and molecular genetic entity, which is characterized by biallelic inactivation of the hSNF5/INI1/SMARCB1 on 22q11.2 through deletion or mutation (EWS gene is located on 22q12) (110,157). Though the MRT was initially described in the kidney, our experience revealed that almost 50% of cases presented in a variety of extrarenal sites in the soft tissues with a preference for the neck and paraspinal region (Table 24-15). Three neonates had disseminated disease including the soft tissues of the head and neck and multiple organs. Like congenital neuroblastoma, the placenta may contain micrometastases in the chorionic villi. The ATRTs presented as a supratentorial (nine cases), posterior fossa (four cases), and spinal cord (two cases) mass. The MRT, regardless of the primary site, is a neoplasm of early childhood and 53 (54%) of our cases presented in children 1-year-old or less with the youngest, a 3-day-old female with a renal MRT and another 3-day-old infant with disseminated MRT with disfiguring facial masses and widespread metastases including the placenta. Approximately 80% of our cases were diagnosed at or before 5 years of age.

The gross features of a MRT are optimally demonstrated in a resected mass from the kidney or liver; these tumors are soft and have a bosselated, glistening tan-white surface. In the soft tissues, fibrous stroma can accompany these tumors so that there is a nesting pattern or a fibromyxoid alteration with remote resemblance to chondroid matrix. The number and prominence of rhabdoid cells with intensely eosinophilic filamentous inclusion in the cytoplasm can vary considerably from one MRT to another and from one microscopic field to another in the same tumor. Small biopsies can be especially problematic without appropriate immunohistochemical stains and/or molecular studies (Figure 24-69). Another important morphologic attribute is the large, eccentric vesicular nucleus with its prominent nucleolus. Rhabdoid cells may be inconspicuous in a background of more epithelioid appearing cells without inclusions to populations of smaller, lymphoid-like cells, which are seen with some frequency in ATRTs, which have led to a diagnosis of a central PNET or medulloblastoma in the past. It is advisable to consider MRT in the differential diagnosis of a malignant round cell neoplasm in a child before

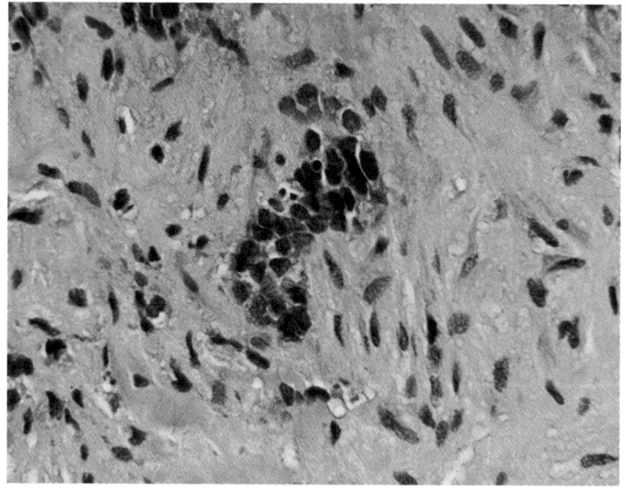
A

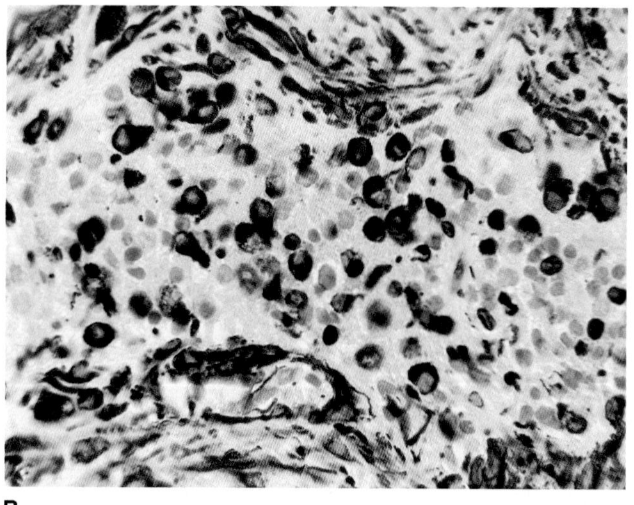
B

FIGURE 24-69 ■ MRT as in this case of a 2-year-old male proved to be an elusive diagnosis when it presented as a anterior and middle mediastinal mass which involved the thymus. **A:** Small nests of uniform polygonal malignant cells are separated by a dense fibromyxoid stroma. Though filamentous cytoplasmic inclusions were not identified histologically, prominent nucleoli are seen. **B:** Dense vimentin-positive inclusions are noted by IHC and they correspond to the rhabdoid inclusions by routine light microscopy.

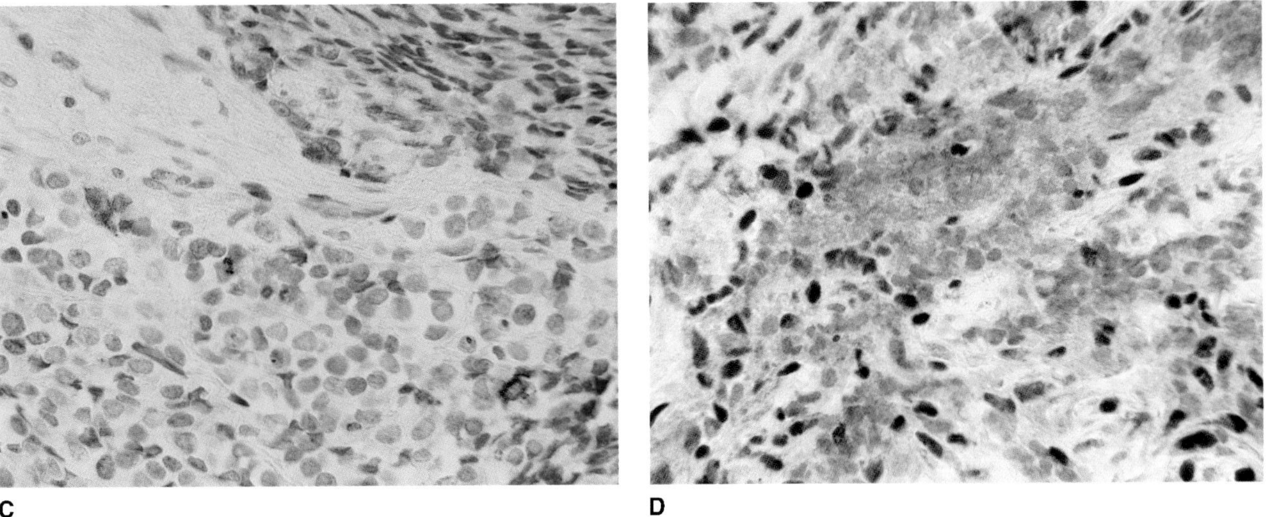

FIGURE 24-69 ■ *(continued)* **C:** Cytokeratin staining is sparing but the tumor cells are strongly immunopositive for EMA. **D:** BAF47 IHC demonstrates nuclear positivity in stromal and inflammatory cells in the background, but the nuclei of the tumor cells are nonreactive. INI1 deletion was confirmed by FISH.

settling on an interpretation of "undifferentiated round cell sarcoma." IHC for vimentin and cytokeratin demonstrates intense cytoplasmic positivity in the configuration of a spherical inclusion that totally occupies the cytoplasm (Figure 24-68). In general, vimentin staining produces the more diffuse pattern of positivity, but the cytokeratin staining of the rhabdoid inclusions often stands out in a background of nonreactive tumor cells. Membrane-cytoplasmic positivity for CD99 does not produce the diffuse pattern of a EWS-PNET. SMA positivity is consistently present in the ATRT in contrast to nonneural MRTs. The nuclei fail to stain for BAF47 to reflect the inactivated INI1 gene, but the interpretation can be complicated by the presence of numerous inflammatory cells or fibroblasts with their functioning INI1 gene with intense nuclear staining as the internal control, but these cells may also obscure small groups of nonreactive tumor cells in the background (99) (Figure 24-68). Originally reported as INI1-negative small cell hepatoblastoma, these tumors are now considered primary MRTs of the liver. Other round cell neoplasms of infancy and young children with INI1 loss but without the dire clinical outcome of MRT have been reported (16,120,202). It remains to be determined how these relate to MRT.

Epithelioid sarcoma (ES) is a rare STS regardless of age at diagnosis. It accounts for 1% to 2% of all STSs overall, but because it has a predilection for adolescents and young adults, it may represent as many as 5% to 8% of non-RMStous STSs in the first two decades of life. There are two types of ES: the classic or the distal type presenting as slow-growing nodule or nodules in the hand or forearm in almost 50% of cases and the proximal or axial presenting type (6,73). The latter type of ES is a neoplasm whose pathologic, immunophenotype, and molecular genetic features are very similar to the MRT with an abbreviated aggressive clinical course like the MRT and unlike the classic ES (116,130). The classic ES is a more superficial neoplasm in the dermis or subcutis in contrast to the proximal ES in the deep soft tissues. Classic ES has a multinodular or diffuse pattern of uniform epithelioid cells with abundant eosinophilic or clear, but vacuolated cytoplasm with or without a spindle cell component. The nodules are composed of a mantle of epithelioid cells with central necrosis or hyalinization. In the presence of nodules with central necrosis, necrobiotic granulomas of the granuloma annulare type may arise in the differential diagnosis, both clinically and pathologically. IHC can settle the diagnostic dilemma in that the histiocytes of granuloma annulare are CD68-positive whereas the cells of ES coexpress vimentin and pancytokeratin as well as EMA (123). In at least one series, 93% of all ESs (both classic and proximal types) had loss of INI1 staining blurring the distinction from MRT (219). Approximately 50% of ES are CD34-positive, which can be problematic if the differential diagnosis includes an epithelioid vascular tumor since there is a variant of the latter, which can mimic ES.

Alveolar soft part sarcoma (ASPS) is a neoplasm, which occurs in a similar age group as ES and also represents only 1% of all STSs in the first two decades of life. Unlike ES, ASPS may present in early childhood as a mass in the base of the tongue (113,217). The head and neck region are preferred sites for the presentation of ASPS in children. The deep soft tissue of the proximal lower extremity is the single most common primary site (29). There are a number of diverse sites in which ASPS has been documented including heart, lung, bone, and uterus as a sampling of some of the non-soft tissue primary sites (132). There is a female predilection in contrast to most other STSs in childhood. Although the histogenesis of ASPS remains uncertain, it has a non-random unbalanced translocation, der(17)t(x;17)(p11;q25),

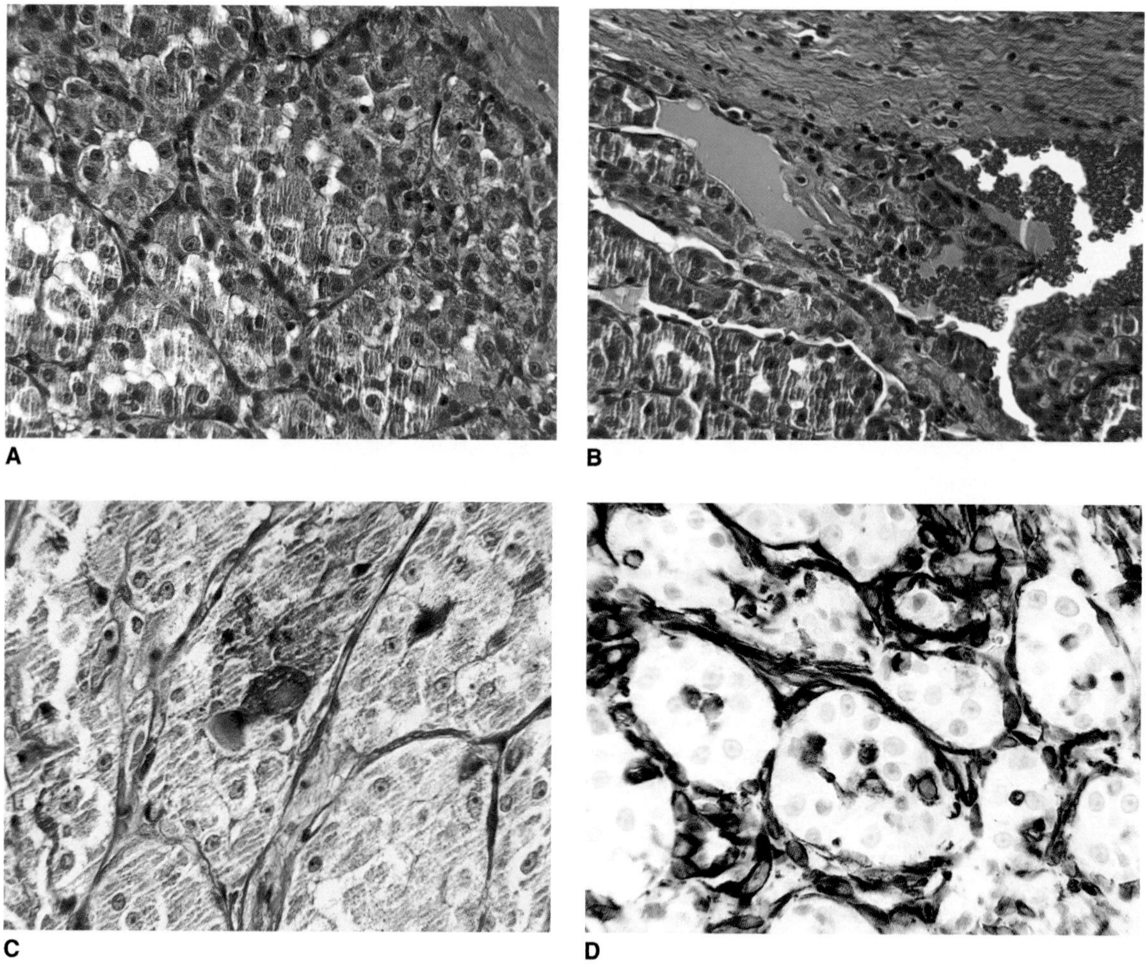

A

B

C

D

FIGURE 24-70 ■ ASPS presented as a soft tissue mass in the lower leg of a 9-year-old male. **A:** The circumscribed 7 cm tumor is composed of uniform polygonal cells with prominent nucleoli surrounded by delicate stromal envelopes. **B:** Microvascular invasion is found at the periphery of the tumor. **C:** Pale granular cytoplasmic staining was present in the PAS stain. **D:** Only isolated tumor cells are immunoreactive for vimentin. Note the prominent staining of the stromal envelopes.

which produces an ASPL-TFE3 fusion gene; the balanced fusion translocation involving the same fusion partners is present in the Xp11.2 renal cell carcinoma (nonmelanotic and melanotic types) of childhood (5,10,77,163).

Grossly, a circumscribed mass with a grayish to yellowish to hemorrhagic cut surface is the rather nonspecific appearance. The alveolar characterization refers to distinct collections of uniform polygonal cells with eosinophilic to granular cytoplasm surrounding a central nucleus with a variably sized nucleolus, which is surrounded by delicate vascular envelopes (Figure 24-70). Larger groups of tumor cells may be separated by dense, hyaline stroma or the overall pattern may be one of sheets of tumor cells without the alveolar architecture (Figure 24-71). The latter appearance has been seen with some frequency in ASPSs in children in our experience and can be the source of some diagnostic perplexity. Other variations include the presence of more gigantiform rounded or elongated tumor cells in a background of smaller but more typical appearing cells identifiable by routine histology or PAS staining after diastase digestion.

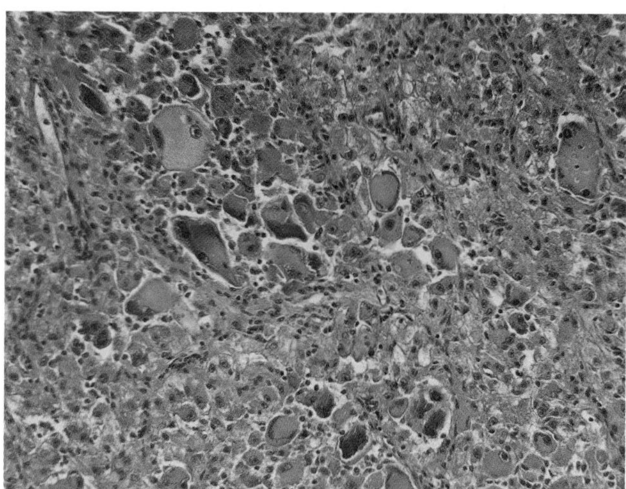

FIGURE 24-71 ■ ASPS presented as a mass in the right atrium of the heart of an 11-year-old female. The tumor has a diffuse pattern of tumor cells more like the nascent alveolar pattern of ARMS. This diffuse pattern can be confusing initially but is not uncommon in those tumors presenting in childhood.

Necrosis, hemorrhage, and an inflammatory infiltrate are other secondary findings. In the presence of a classic alveolar pattern, the diagnosis is reasonably straightforward together with corroborating IHC, which includes reactivity for vimentin, muscle specific actin, and desmin. On the other hand, the only immunoreactivity is for vimentin, which outlines the delicate vascular envelope around groups of tumor cells and tumor cells may or may not be positive. The most specific marker is TFE3 nuclear positivity. The differential diagnosis of ASPS includes ARMS, but in most cases, the distinction is made without difficulty given the absence of true organized alveolar pattern, the presence of marked nuclear hyperchromatism, and mitotic activity in the ARMS; these features contrast with those of ASPS. Desmin is diffusely positive in ARMS and only focally so, if at all, in ASPS. If the cells of ASPS have vacuolated cytoplasm and a less than obvious alveolar pattern, diffuse GCT of tendon sheath is worthy of consideration. The emergence of the PEComa is another neoplasm in the differential diagnosis of ASPS. The short-term survival is relatively favorable, but ASPS is known for its delayed metastatic behavior to the brain and/or lung as long as 5 to 10 years after the original diagnosis. This tumor is an example of a grade 3 sarcoma in the COG grading scheme based on its pathologic type rather than individual pathologic features, which are commonly low grade.

REFERENCES

1. Alaggio R, Coffin CM, Weiss SW, et al. Liposarcomas in young patients: a study of 82 cases occurring in patients younger than 22 years of age. *Am J Surg Pathol* 2009;33(5):645–658.
2. Antaya RJ, Cajaiba MM, Madri J, et al. Juvenile hyaline fibromatosis and infantile systemic hyalinosis overlap associated with a novel mutation in capillary morphogenesis protein-2 gene. *Am J Dermatopathol* 2007;29(1):99–103.
3. Antonescu CR, Argani P, Erlandson RA, et al. Skeletal and extraskeletal myxoid chondrosarcoma: a comparative clinicopathologic, ultrastructural, and molecular study. *Cancer* 1998;83(8):1504–1521.
4. Arai E, Kuramochi A, Tsuchida T, et al. Usefulness of D2–40 immunohistochemistry for differentiation between kaposiform hemangioendothelioma and tufted angioma. *J Cutan Pathol* 2006;33(7): 492–497.
5. Argani P, Aulmann S, Karanjawala Z, et al. Melanotic Xp11 translocation renal cancers: a distinctive neoplasm with overlapping features of PEComa, carcinoma, and melanoma. *Am J Surg Pathol* 2009;33(4):609–619.
6. Armah HB, Parwani AV. Epithelioid sarcoma. *Arch Pathol Lab Med* 2009;133(5):814–819.
7. Arndt CA, Hammond S, Rodeberg D, et al. Significance of persistent mature rhabdomyoblasts in bladder/prostate rhabdomyosarcoma: Results from IRS IV. *J Pediatr Hematol Oncol* 2006;28(9): 563–567.
8. Arun D, Gutmann DH. Recent advances in neurofibromatosis type 1. *Curr Opin Neurol* 2004;17(2):101–105.
9. Auerbach A, Fanburg-Smith JC, Wang G, et al. Focal myositis: A clinicopathologic study of 115 cases of an intramuscular mass-like reactive process. *Am J Surg Pathol* 2009;33(7):1016–1024.
10. Aulmann S, Longerich T, Schirmacher P, et al. Detection of the ASPSCR1-TFE3 gene fusion in paraffin-embedded alveolar soft part sarcomas. *Histopathology* 2007;50(7):881–886.
11. Bartuma H, Domanski HA, Von Steyern FV, et al. Cytogenetic and molecular cytogenetic findings in lipoblastoma. *Cancer Genet Cytogenet* 2008;183(1):60–63.
12. Bayat A, Bock O, Mrowietz U, et al. Genetic susceptibility to keloid disease and hypertrophic scarring: transforming growth factor beta1 common polymorphisms and plasma levels. *Plast Reconstr Surg* 2003;111(2):535–543.
13. Bhattacharya B, Dilworth HP, Iacobuzio-Donahue C, et al. Nuclear beta-catenin expression distinguishes deep fibromatosis from other benign and malignant fibroblastic and myofibroblastic lesions. *Am J Surg Pathol* 2005;29(5):653–659.
14. Billings SD, Folpe AL. Cutaneous and subcutaneous fibrohistiocytic tumors of intermediate malignancy: an update. *Am J Dermatopathol* 2004;26(2):141–155.
15. Bisogno G, Roganovich J, Sotti G, et al. Desmoplastic small round cell tumour in children and adolescents. *Med Pediatr Oncol* 2000;34(5):338–342.
16. Bourdeaut F, Freneaux P, Thuille B, et al. hSNF5/INI1-deficient tumours and rhabdoid tumours are convergent but not fully overlapping entities. *J Pathol* 2007;211(3):323–330.
17. Boyanton BL Jr, Jones JK, Shenaq SM, et al. Intraneural perineurioma. A systematic review with illustrative cases. *Arch Pathol Lab Med* 2007;131(9):1382–1392.
18. Brandal P, Bjerkehagen B, Heim S. Rearrangement of chromosomal region 8q11–13 in lipomatous tumours: correlation with lipoblastoma morphology. *J Pathol* 2006;208(3):388–394.
19. Brannon RB, Anand PM. Oral granular cell tumors: an analysis of 10 new pediatric and adolescent cases and a review of the literature. *J Clin Pediatr Dent* 2004;29(1):69–74.
20. Brems H, Beert E, de Ravel T, et al. Mechanisms in the pathogenesis of malignant tumours in neurofibromatosis type 1. *Lancet Oncol* 2009;10(5):508–515.
21. Brouillard P, Vikkula M. Genetic causes of vascular malformations. *Hum Mol Genet* 2007;16 Spec No. 2:R140–R149.
22. Bruder E, Perez-Atayde AR, Jundt G, et al. Vascular lesions of bone in children, adolescents, and young adults. A clinicopathologic reappraisal and application of the ISSVA classification. *Virchows Arch* 2009;454(2):161–179.
23. Buitendijk S, van de Ven CP, Dumans TG, et al. Pediatric aggressive fibromatosis: a retrospective analysis of 13 patients and review of literature. *Cancer* 2005;104(5):1090–1099.
24. Burchill SA. Ewing's sarcoma: diagnostic, prognostic, and therapeutic implications of molecular abnormalities. *J Clin Pathol* 2003;56(2):96–102.
25. Burke A, Virmani R. Pediatric heart tumors. *Cardiovasc Pathol* 2008;17(4):193–198.
26. Carlson JW, Fletcher CDM. Immunohistochemistry for beta-catenin in the differential diagnosis of spindle cell lesions: analysis of a series and review of the literature. *Histopathology* 2007;51(4): 509–514.
27. Carpentieri DF, Qualman SJ, Bowen J, et al. Protocol for the examination of specimens from pediatric and adult patients with osseous and extraosseous Ewing sarcoma family of tumors, including peripheral primitive neuroectodermal tumor and Ewing sarcoma. *Arch Pathol Lab Med* 2005;129(7):866–873.
28. Carretto E, Dall'Igna P, Alaggio R, et al. Fibrous hamartoma of infancy: an Italian multi-institutional experience. *J Am Acad Dermatol* 2006;54(5):800–803.
29. Casanova M, Ferrari A, Bisogno G, et al. Alveolar soft part sarcoma in children and adolescents: A report from the Soft-Tissue Sarcoma Italian Cooperative Group. *Ann Oncol* 2000;11(11):1445–1449.
30. Cesari M, Bertoni F, Bacchini P, et al. Mesenchymal chondrosarcoma. An analysis of patients treated at a single institution. *Tumori* 2007;93(5):423–427.
31. Cessna MH, Zhou H, Perkins SL, et al. Are myogenin and myoD1 expression specific for rhabdomyosarcoma? A study of 150

cases, with emphasis on spindle cell mimics. *Am J Surg Pathol* 2001;25(9):1150–1157.

32. Chang F. Desmoplastic small round cell tumors: cytologic, histologic, and immunohistochemical features. *Arch Pathol Lab Med* 2006;130(5):728–732.
33. Chang MW. Updated classification of hemangiomas and other vascular anomalies. *Lymphat Res Biol* 2003;1(4):259–265.
34. Chaudhry IH, Calonje E. Dermal non-neural granular cell tumour (so-called primitive polypoid granular cell tumour): a distinctive entity further delineated in a clinicopathological study of 11 cases. *Histopathology* 2005;47(2):179–185.
35. Checketts SR, Hamilton TK, Baughman RD. Congenital and childhood dermatofibrosarcoma protuberans: a case report and review of the literature. *J Am Acad Dermatol* 2000;42(5 pt 2):907–913.
36. Chien CR, Chang YL, Lin DT, et al. Excellent survival of pediatric dermatofibrosarcoma protuberans in Taiwanese. *Pediatr Surg Int* 2007;23(3):211–214.
37. Chiller KG, Frieden IJ, Arbiser JL. Molecular pathogenesis of vascular anomalies: classification into three categories based upon clinical and biochemical characteristics. *Lymphat Res Biol* 2003;1(4): 267–281.
38. Chiller KG, Passaro D, Frieden IJ. Hemangiomas of infancy: clinical characteristics, morphologic subtypes, and their relationship to race, ethnicity, and sex. *Arch Dermatol* 2002;138(12): 1567–1576.
39. Coffin CM, Dehner LP. Soft tissue tumors in first year of life: a report of 190 cases. *Pediatr Pathol* 1990;10(4):509–526.
40. Coffin CM, Dehner LP. Vascular tumors in children and adolescents: a clinicopathologic study of 228 tumors in 222 patients. *Pathol Annu* 1993;28(pt1):97–120.
41. Coffin CM, Dehner LP. Fibroblastic-myofibroblastic tumors in children and adolescents: a clinicopathologic study of 108 examples in 103 patients. *Pediatr Pathol* 1991;11(4):569–588.
42. Coffin CM, Hornick JL, Fletcher CDM. Inflammatory myofibroblastic tumor: comparison of clinicopathologic, histologic, and immunohistochemical features including ALK expression in atypical and aggressive cases. *Am J Surg Pathol* 2007;31(4):509–520.
43. Coffin CM, Hornick JL, Zhou H, et al. Gardner fibroma: a clinicopathologic and immunohistochemical analysis of 45 patients with 57 fibromas. *Am J Surg Pathol* 2007;31(3):410–416.
44. Coffin CM, Lowichik A, Zhou H. Treatment effects in pediatric soft tissue and bone tumors: practical considerations for the pathologist. *Am J Clin Pathol* 2005;123(1):75–90.
45. Cohen MM Jr. Vascular update: morphogenesis, tumors, malformations and molecular dimensions. *Am J Med Genet A* 2006;140(19):2013–2038.
46. Dantonello TM, Int-Veen C, Leuschner I, et al. Mesenchymal chondrosarcoma of soft tissues and bone in children, adolescents, and young adults: experiences of the CWS and COSS study groups. *Cancer* 2008;112(11):2424–2431.
47. Dauendorffer JN, Ortonne N, Bodemer C, et al. Nodular fasciitis of childhood: a clinicopathological analysis of 10 cases. *Ann Dermatol Venereol* 2008;135(8–9):553–558.
48. Davicioni E, Anderson MJ, Finckenstein FG, et al. Molecular classification of rhabdomyosarcoma–genotypic and phenotypic determinants of diagnosis. A report from the Children's Oncology Group. *Am J Pathol* 2009;174(2):550–564.
49. DeCecio R, Migliaccio I, Falleti J, et al. Congenital intracranial mesenchymal chondrosarcoma: case report and review of the literature. *Pediatr Dev Pathol* 2008;11 (4):309–313.
50. de Silva MV, Reid R. Myositis ossificans and fibroosseous pseudotumor of digits: a clinicopathological review of 64 cases with emphasis on diagnostic pitfalls. *Int J Surg Pathol* 2003;11(3): 187–195.
51. de Visser E, Veth RP, Pruszczynski M, et al. Diffuse and localized pigmented villonodular synovitis: evaluation of treatment of 38 patients. *Arch Orthop Trauma Surg* 1999;119(7–8):401–404.
52. Dehner LP. Juvenile xanthogranulomas in the first two decades of life: a clinicopathologic study of 174 cases with cutaneous and extracutaneous manifestations. *Am J Surg Pathol* 2003;27(5):579–593.
53. Dehner LP. Inflammatory myofibroblastic tumor: the continued definition of one type of so-called inflammatory pseudotumor. *Am J Surg Pathol* 2004;28(12):1652–1654.
54. Dei Tos AP. Classification of pleomorphic sarcomas: where are we now? *Histopathology* 2006;48(1):51–62.
55. Dickey GE, Sotelo-Avila C. Fibrous hamartoma of infancy: current review. *Pediatr Dev Pathol* 1999;2(3):236–243.
56. Dilley AV, Patel DL, Hicks MJ, et al. Lipoblastoma: pathophysiology and surgical management. *J Pediatr Surg* 2001;36(1): 229–231.
57. Dim DC, Cooley LD, Miranda RN. Clear cell sarcoma of tendons and aponeuroses: a review. *Arch Pathol Lab Med* 2007;131(1): 152–156.
58. Diment J, Tamborini E, Casali P, et al. Carney triad: case report and molecular analysis of gastric tumor. *Hum Pathol* 2005;36(1): 112–116.
59. Dray MS, McCarthy SW, Palmer AA, et al. Myopericytoma: a unifying term for a spectrum of tumours that show overlapping features with myofibroma. A review of 14 cases. *J Clin Pathol* 2006;59(1):67–73.
60. Fanburg-Smith JC, Michal M, Partanen TA, et al. Papillary intralymphatic angioendothelioma (PILA): a report of twelve cases of a distinctive vascular tumor with phenotypic features of lymphatic vessels. *Am J Surg Pathol* 1999;23(9):1004–1010.
61. Fanburg-Smith JC, Miettinen M. Angiomatoid "malignant" fibrous histiocytoma: a clinicopathologic study of 158 cases and further exploration of the myoid phenotype. *Hum Pathol* 1999;30(11): 1336–1343.
62. Ferner RE. Neurofibromatosis 1 and neurofibromatosis 2: a twenty first century perspective. *Lancet Neurol* 2007;6(4):340–351.
63. Ferrari A, Bisogno G, Macaluso A, et al. Soft-tissue sarcomas in children and adolescents with neurofibromatosis type 1. *Cancer* 2007;109(7):1406–1412.
64. Ferrari A, Casanova M, Bisogno G, et al. Hemangiopericytoma in pediatric ages. A report from the Italian and German Soft Tissue Sarcoma Cooperative Group. *Cancer* 2001;92(10):2692–1698.
65. Ferrari A, Casanova M, Collini P, et al. Adult-type soft tissue sarcomas in pediatric-age patients: experience at the Istituto Nazionale Tumori in Milan. *J Clin Oncol* 2005;23(18):4021–4030.
66. Ferrari A, Gronchi A, Casanova M, et al. Synovial sarcoma: a retrospective analysis of 271 patients of all ages treated at a single institution. *Cancer* 2004;101(3):627–634.
67. Fetsch JF, Laskin WB, Hallman JR, et al. Neurothekeoma: an analysis of 178 tumors with detailed immunohistochemical data and long-term patient follow-up information. *Am J Surg Pathol* 2007;31(7):1103–1114.
68. Fetsch JF, Laskin WB, Miettinen M. Nerve sheath myxoma: a clinicopathologic and immunohistochemical analysis of 57 morphologically distinctive, S-100 protein- and GFAP-positive, myxoid peripheral nerve sheath tumors with a predilection for the extremities and a high local recurrence rate. *Am J Surg Pathol* 2005;29(12):1615–1624.
69. Fetsch JF, Laskin WB, Miettinen M. Palmar-plantar fibromatosis in children and preadolescents. A clinicopathologic study of 56 cases with newly recognized demographics and extended follow-up information. *Am J Surg Pathol* 2005;29(8):1095–1105.
70. Fetsch JF, Miettinen M, Laskin WB, et al. A clinicopathologic study of 45 pediatric soft tissue tumors with an admixture of adipose tissue and fibroblastic elements, and a proposal for classification as lipofibromatosis. *Am J Surg Pathol* 2000;24(11):1491–1500.
71. Fisher C. Myofibroblastic malignancies. *Adv Anat Pathol* 2004;11(4):190–201.
72. Fisher C. Low-grade sarcomas with CD34-positive fibroblasts and low-grade myofibroblastic sarcomas. *Ultrastruct Pathol* 2004;28(5–6): 291–305.

73. Fisher C. Epithelioid sarcoma of Enzinger. *Adv Anat Pathol* 2006;13(3):114–121.
74. Fisher C. Soft tissue sarcomas with non-EWS translocations: molecular genetic features and pathologic and clinical correlations. *Virchows Arch* 2010;456(2):153–166.
75. Fletcher CDM, Unni KK, Mertens F. *World Health Organization Classification of Tumours. Pathology and Genetics of Tumours of Soft tissue and Bone*. Lyon, France: IARC Press; 2002.
76. Floris G, Debiec-Rychter M, Wozniak A, et al. Malignant ectomesenchymoma: genetic profile reflects rhabdomyosarcomatous differentiation. *Diagn Mol Pathol* 2007;16(4):243–248.
77. Folpe AL, Deyrup AT. Alveolar soft-part sarcoma: a review and update. *J Clin Pathol* 2006;59(11):1127–1132.
78. Folpe AL, Lane KL, Paull G, et al. Low-grade fibromyxoid sarcoma and hyalinizing spindle cell tumor with giant rosettes. A clinicopathologic study of 73 cases supporting their identity and assessing the impact of high-grade areas. *Am J Surg Pathol* 2000;24(10):1353–1360.
79. Folpe AL, Mentzel T, Lehr HA, et al. Perivascular epithelioid cell neoplasms of soft tissue and gynecologic origin: a clinicopathologic study of 26 cases and review of the literature. *Am J Surg Pathol* 2005;29(12):1558–1575.
80. Fukunaga M, Suzuki K, Saegusa N, et al. Composite hemangioendothelioma. Report of 5 cases including one with associated Maffucci syndrome. *Am J Surg Pathol* 2007;31(10):1567–1572.
81. Furlong MA, Fanburg-Smith JC. Pleomorphic rhabdomyosarcoma in children: four cases in the pediatric age group. *Ann Diagn Pathol* 2001;5(4):199–206.
82. Furniss D, Swan MC, Morritt DG, et al. A 10-year review of benign and malignant peripheral nerve sheath tumors in a single center: clinical and radiographic features can help to differentiate benign from malignant lesions. *Plast Reconstr Surg* 2008;121(2):529–533.
83. Gaeta M, Mazziotti S, Minutoli F, et al. MR imaging findings of focal myositis: a pseudotumour that may mimic muscle neoplasm. *Skeletal Radiol* 2009;38(6):571–578.
84. Garcia-Torres R, Cruz D, Orozco L, et al. Alport syndrome and diffuse leiomyomatosis. Clinical aspects, pathology, molecular biology and extracellular matrix studies. A synthesis. *Nephrologie* 2000;21(1):9–12.
85. Gengler C, Guillou L. Solitary fibrous tumour and haemangiopericytoma: evolution of a concept. *Histopathology* 2006;48(1):63–74.
86. Gerlini G, Mariotti G, Urso C, et al. Dermatofibrosarcoma protuberans in childhood: two case reports and review of the literature. *Pediatr Hematol Oncol* 2008;25(6):559–566.
87. Gleason BC, Fletcher CDM. Deep "benign" fibrous histiocytoma: clinicopathologic analysis of 69 cases of a rare tumor indicating occasional metastatic potential. *Am J Surg Pathol* 2008;32(3): 354–362.
88. Gleason BC, Hornick JL. Inflammatory myofibroblastic tumours: where are we now? *J Clin Pathol* 2008;61(4):428–437.
89. Guillou L, Benhattar J, Gengler C, et al. Translocation-positive low-grade fibromyxoid sarcoma: clinicopathologic and molecular analysis of a series expanding the morphologic spectrum and suggesting potential relationship to sclerosing epithelioid fibrosarcoma: a study from the French Sarcoma Group. *Am J Surg Pathol* 2007;31(9):1387–1402.
90. Hadfield KD, Newman WG, Bowers NL, et al. Molecular characterisation of SMARCB1 and NF2 in familial and sporadic schwannomatosis. *J Med Genet* 2008;45(6):332–339.
91. Hameed M. Pathology and genetics of adipocytic tumors. *Cytogenet Genome Res* 2007;118(2–4):138–147.
92. Harms D. Soft tissue malignancies in childhood and adolescence. Pathology and clinical relevance based on data from the Kiel Pediatric Tumor Registry. *Handchir Mikrochir Plast Chir* 2004;36(5):268–274.
93. Hayes-Jordan AA, Spunt SL, Poquette CA, et al. Nonrhabdomyosarcoma soft tissue sarcomas in children: is age at diagnosis an important variable? *J Pediatr Surg* 2000;35(6):948–953.
94. Heerema-McKenney A, Wijnaendts LC, Pulliam JF, et al. Diffuse myogenin expression by immunohistochemistry is an independent marker of poor survival in pediatric rhabdomyosarcoma: a tissue microarray study of 71 primary tumors including correlation with molecular phenotype. *Am J Surg Pathol* 2008;32(10):1513–1522.
95. Hein KD, Mulliken JB, Kozakewich HP, et al. Venous malformations of skeletal muscle. *Plast Reconstr Surg* 2002;110(7):1625–1635.
96. Hicks J, Dilley A, Patel D, et al. Lipoblastoma and lipoblastomatosis in infancy and childhood: histopathologic, ultrastructural, and cytogenetic features. *Ultrastruct Pathol* 2001;25(4):321–333.
97. Hisaoka M, Hashimoto H. Extraskeletal myxoid chondrosarcoma: updated clinicopathological and molecular genetic characteristics. *Pathol Int* 2005;55(8):453–463.
98. Hisaoka M, Ishida T, Kuo TT, et al. Clear cell sarcoma of soft tissue. A clinicopathologic, immunohistochemical, and molecular analysis of 33 cases. *Am J Surg Pathol* 2008;32(3):452–460.
99. Hoot AC, Russo P, Judkins AR, et al. Immunohistochemical analysis of hSNF5/INI1 distinguishes renal and extra-renal malignant rhabdoid tumors from other pediatric soft tissue tumors. *Am J Surg Pathol* 2004;28(11):1485–1491.
100. Hornick JL, Fletcher CDM. Myoepithelial tumors of soft tissue. A clinicopathologic and immunohistochemical study of 101 cases with evaluation of prognostic parameters. *Am J Surg Pathol* 2003;27(9):1183–1196.
101. Hornick JL, Fletcher CDM. PEComa: what do we know so far? *Histopathology* 2006;48(1):75–82.
102. Hornick JL, Fletcher CDM. Cellular neurothekeoma: detailed characterization in a series of 133 cases. *Am J Surg Pathol* 2007;31(3): 329–340.
103. Hu Y, Li L, Seidelmann SB, et al. Identification of association of common AGGF1 variants with susceptibility for Klippel-Trenaunay syndrome using the structure association program. *Ann Hum Genet* 2008;72(pt 5):636–643.
104. Jaffer S, Ambrosini-Spaltro A, Mancini AM, et al. Neurothekeoma and plexiform fibrohistiocytic tumor. Mere histologic resemblance or histogenetic relationship? *Am J Surg Pathol* 2009;33(6):905–913.
105. Janeway KA, Liegl B, Harlow A, et al. Pediatric KIT wild-type and platelet-derived growth factor receptor alpha-wild-type gastrointestinal stromal tumors share KIT activation but not mechanisms of genetic progression with adult gastrointestinal stromal tumors. *Cancer Res* 2007;67(19):9084–9088.
106. Janssen D, Harms D. Juvenile xanthogranuloma in childhood and adolescence: a clinicopathologic study of 129 patients from the kiel pediatric tumor registry. *Am J Surg Pathol* 2005;29(1):21–28.
107. Jha P, Moosavi C, Fanburg-Smith JC. Giant cell fibroblastoma: an update and addition of 86 new cases from the Armed Forces Institute of Pathology, in honor of Dr. Franz M. Enzinger. *Ann Diagn Pathol* 2007;11(2):81–88.
108. Jimenez RE, Folpe AL, Lapham RL, et al. Primary Ewing's sarcoma/primitive neuroectodermal tumor of the kidney: a clinicopathologic and immunohistochemical analysis of 11 cases. *Am J Surg Pathol* 2002;26(3):320–327.
109. Joo M, Chang SH, Kim H, et al. Primary gastrointestinal clear cell sarcoma: report of 2 cases, one case associated with IgG4-related sclerosing disease, and review of literature. *Ann Diagn Pathol* 2009;13(1):30–35.
110. Judkins AR. Immunohistochemistry of INI1 expression: a new tool for old challenges in CNS and soft tissue pathology. *Adv Anat Pathol* 2007;14(5):335–339.
111. Kapadia SB, Meis JM, Frisman DM, et al. Fetal rhabdomyoma of the head and neck: a clinicopathologic and immunophenotypic study of 24 cases. *Hum Pathol* 1993;24(7):754–765.
112. Kaplan FS, Xu M, Glaser DL, et al. Early diagnosis of fibrodysplasia ossificans progressiva. *Pediatrics* 2008;121(5):e1295–e1300.
113. Kayton ML, Meyers P, Wexler LH, et al. Clinical presentation, treatment and outcome of alveolar soft part sarcoma in children, adolescents, and young adults. *J Pediatr Surg* 2006;41(1):187–193.

114. Kim DH, Murovic JA, Tiel RL, et al. A series of 397 peripheral neural sheath tumors: 30-year experience at Louisiana State University Health Sciences Center. *J Neurosurg* 2005;102(2):246–255.
115. Knight DM, Birch R, Pringle J. Benign solitary schwannomas. A review of 234 cases. *J Bone Joint Surg Br* 2007;89(3):382–387.
116. Kohashi K, Izumi T, Oda Y, et al. Infrequent SMARCB1/INI1 gene alteration in epithelioid sarcoma: a useful tool in distinguishing epithelioid sarcoma from malignant rhabdoid tumor. *Hum Pathol* 2009;40(3):349–355.
117. Kohashi K, Oda Y, Yamamoto H, et al. SMARCB1/INI1 protein expression in round cell soft tissue sarcomas associated with chromosomal translocations involving EWS: a special reference to SMARCB1/INI1 negative variant extraskeletal myxoid chondrosarcoma. *Am J Surg Pathol* 2008;32(8):1168–1174.
118. Kose O, Waseem A. Keloids and hypertrophic scars: are they two different sides of the same coin? *Dermatol Surg* 2008;34(3):336–346.
119. Koutsimpelas D, Weber A, Lippert BM, et al. Multifocal adult rhabdomyoma of the head and neck: a case report and literature review. *Auris Nasus Larynx* 2008;35(2):313–317.
120. Kreiger PA, Judkins AR, Russo PA, et al. Loss of INI1 expression defines a unique subset of pediatric undifferentiated soft tissue sarcomas. *Mod Pathol* 2009;22(1):142–150.
121. Krokowski M, Merz H, Thorns C, et al. Sarcoma of follicular dendritic cells with features of sinus lining cells–a new subtype of reticulum cell sarcoma? *Virchows Arch* 2008;452(5):565–570.
122. Kurtkaya-Yapicier O, Scheithauer B, Woodruff JM. The pathobiologic spectrum of schwannomas. *Histol Histopathol* 2003;18(3): 925–934.
123. Laskin WB, Miettinen M. Epithelioid sarcoma. New insights based on an extended immunohistochemical analysis. *Arch Pathol Lab Med* 2003;127(9):1161–1168.
124. Laskin WB, Miettinen M, Fetsch JF. Infantile digital fibroma/fibromatosis. A clinicopathologic and immunohistochemical study of 69 tumors from 57 patients with long-term follow-up. *Am J Surg Pathol* 2009;33(1):1–13.
125. Le BH, Boyer PJ, Lewis JE, et al. Granular cell tumor. Immunohistochemical assessment of inhibin-alpha, protein gene product 9.5, S100 protein, CD68, and Ki-67 proliferative index with clinical correlation. *Arch Pathol Lab Med* 2004;128(7):771–775.
126. Lewis JJ, Antonescu CR, Leung DH, et al. Synovial sarcoma: a multivariate analysis of prognostic factors in 112 patients with primary localized tumors of the extremity. *J Clin Oncol* 2000;18(10):2087–2094.
127. Liapis H, Marley EF, Lin Y, et al. p53 and Ki-67 proliferating cell nuclear antigen in benign and malignant peripheral nerve sheath tumors in children. *Pediatr Dev Pathol* 1999;2(4):377–384.
128. Lindvall LE, Kormeili T, Chen E, et al. Infantile systemic hyalinosis: case report and review of the literature. *J Am Acad Dermatol* 2008;58(2):303–307.
129. Llauger J, Palmer J, Roson N, et al. Pigmented villonodular synovitis and giant cell tumors of the tendon sheath: radiologic and pathologic features. *Am J Roentgenol* 1999;172(4):1087–1091.
130. Lualdi E, Modena P, Debiec-Rychter M, et al. Molecular cytogenetic characterization of proximal-type epithelioid sarcoma. *Genes Chromosomes Cancer* 2004;41(3):283–290.
131. Ludwig JA. Ewing sarcoma: historical perspectives, current state-of-the-art, and opportunities for targeted therapy in the future. *Curr Opin Oncol* 2008;20(4):412–418.
132. Luo J, Melnick S, Rossi A, et al. Primary cardiac alveolar soft part sarcoma. A report of the first observed case with molecular diagnostics corroboration. *Pediatr Dev Pathol* 2008;11(2):142–147.
133. Lyons LL, North PE, Mac-Moune Lai F, et al. Kaposiform hemangioendothelioma: a study of 33 cases emphasizing its pathologic, immunophenotypic, and biologic uniqueness from juvenile hemangioma. *Am J Surg Pathol* 2004;28(5):559–568.
134. Macarenco RS, Ellinger F, Oliveira AM. Perineurioma. A distinctive and underrecognized peripheral nerve sheath neoplasm. *Arch Pathol Lab Med* 2007;131(4):625–636.
135. MacCollin M, Chiocca EA, Evans DG, et al. Diagnostic criteria for schwannomatosis. *Neurology* 2005;64(11):1838–1845.
136. Marino-Enriquez A, Li P, Samuelson J, et al. Congenital fibrosarcoma with a novel complex 3-way translocation t(12;15;19) and unusual histologic features. *Hum Pathol* 2008;39(12):1844–1848.
137. Matyakhina L, Bei TA, McWhinney SR, et al. Genetics of Carney triad: recurrent losses at chromosome 1 but lack of germline mutations in genes associated with paragangliomas and gastrointestinal stromal tumors. *J Clin Endocrinol Metab* 2007;92(8):2938–2943.
138. McClatchey AI. Neurofibromatosis. *Annu Rev Pathol* 2007;2: 191–216.
139. McDowell HP. Update on childhood rhabdomyosarcoma. *Arch Dis Child* 2003;88(4):354–357.
140. Meis-Kindblom JM. Clear cell sarcoma of tendons and aponeuroses: a historical perspective and tribute to the man behind the entity. *Adv Anat Pathol* 2006;13(6):286–292.
141. Meis-Kindblom JM, Sjogren H, Kindblom LG, et al. Cytogenetic and molecular genetic analyses of liposarcoma and its soft tissue simulators: recognition of new variants and differential diagnosis. *Virchows Arch* 2001;439(2):141–151.
142. Meyer WH, Spunt SL. Soft tissue sarcomas of childhood. *Cancer Treat Rev* 2004;30(3):269–280.
143. Meza JL, Anderson J, Pappo AS, et al. Analysis of prognostic factors in patients with nonmetastatic rhabdomyosarcoma treated on Intergroup Rhabdomyosarcoma Studies III and IV: the Children's Oncology Group. *J Clin Oncol* 2006;24(24):3844–3851.
144. Michal M, Fetsch JF, Hes O, et al. Nuchal-type fibroma: a clinicopathologic study of 52 cases. *Cancer* 1999;85(1):156–163.
145. Miettinen M, Lasota J. Gastrointestinal stromal tumors: review on morphology, molecular pathology, prognosis, and differential diagnosis. *Arch Pathol Lab Med* 2006;130(10):1466–1478.
146. Miettinen M, Lasota J, Sobin LH. Gastrointestinal stromal tumors of the stomach in children and young adults: a clinicopathologic, immunohistochemical, and molecular genetic study of 44 cases with long-term follow-up and review of the literature. *Am J Surg Pathol* 2005;29(10):1373–1381.
147. Mo JQ, Dimashkieh HH, Bove KE. GLUT1 endothelial reactivity distinguishes hepatic infantile hemangioma from congenital hepatic vascular malformation with associated capillary proliferation. *Hum Pathol* 2004;35(2):200–209.
148. Moosavi C, Jha P, Fanburg-Smith JC. An update on plexiform fibrohistiocytic tumor and addition of 66 new cases from the Armed Forces Institute of Pathology, in honor of Franz M. Enzinger, MD. *Ann Diagn Pathol* 2007;11(5):313–319.
149. Morotti RA, Legman MD, Kerkar N, et al. Pediatric inflammatory myofibroblastic tumor with late metastasis to the lung: case report and review of the literature. *Pediatr Dev Pathol* 2005;8(2): 224–229.
150. Morotti RA, Nicol KK, Parham DM, et al. An immunohistochemical algorithm to facilitate diagnosis and subtyping of rhabdomyosarcoma: the Children's Oncology Group experience. *Am J Surg Pathol* 2006;30(8):962–968.
151. Naumann S, Krallman PA, Unni KK, et al. Translocation der (13:21) (q10;q10) in skeletal and extraskeoletal mesenchymal chondrosarcoma. *Mod Pathol* 2002;15(5):572–576.
152. Nicol K, Savell V, Moore J, et al. Distinguishing undifferentiated embryonal sarcoma of the liver from biliary tract rhabdomyosarcoma: a Children's Oncology Group study. *Pediatr Dev Pathol* 2007;10(2):89–97.
153. North PE, Waner M, Buckmiller L, et al. Vascular tumors of infancy and childhood: beyond capillary hemangioma. *Cardiovasc Pathol* 2006;15(6):303–317.
154. North PE, Waner M, James CA, et al. Congenital nonprogressive hemangioma: a distinct clinicopathologic entity unlike infantile hemangioma. *Arch Dermatol* 2001;137(12):1607–1620.
155. Nussbeck W, Neureiter D, Söder S, et al. Mesenchymal chondrosarcoma: an immunohistochemical study of 10 cases examining

prognostic significance of proliferative activity and cellular differentiation. *Pathology* 2004:36(3);230–233.

156. Oda Y, Takahira T, Kawaguchi K, et al. Low-grade fibromyxoid sarcoma versus low-grade myxofibrosarcoma in the extremities and trunk. A comparison of clinicopathological and immunohistochemical features. *Histopathology* 2004;45(1):29–38.
157. Oda Y, Tsuneyoshi M. Extrarenal rhabdoid tumors of soft tissue: clinicopathological and molecular genetic review and distinction from other soft-tissue sarcomas with rhabdoid features. *Pathol Int* 2006;56(6):287–295.
158. Oi S, Nomura S, Nagasaka M, et al. Embryopathogenetic surgicoanatomical classification of dysraphism and surgical outcome of spinal lipoma: a nationwide multicenter cooperative study in Japan. *J Neurosurg Pediatr* 2009;3(5):412–419.
159. Ong LY, Hwang WS, Wong A, et al. Perivascular epithelioid cell tumour of the vagina in an 8 year old girl. *J Pediatr Surg* 2007;42(3):564–566.
160. Orbach D, Rey A, Oberlin O, et al. Soft tissue sarcoma or malignant mesenchymal tumors in the first year of life: experience of the International Society of Pediatric Oncology (SIOP) Malignant Mesenchymal Tumor Committee. *J Clin Oncol* 2005;23(19): 4363–4371.
161. Ordonez NG. Desmoplastic small round cell tumor: II: an ultrastructural and immunohistochemical study with emphasis on new immunohistochemical markers. *Am J Surg Pathol* 1998;22(11): 1314–1327.
162. Ossendorf C, Studer GM, Bode B, et al. Sclerosing epithelioid fibrosarcoma: case presentation and a systematic review. *Clin Orthop Relat Res* 2008;466(6):1485–1491.
163. Pang LJ, Chang B, Zou H, et al. Alveolar soft part sarcoma: a bimarker diagnostic strategy using TFE3 immunoassay and ASPL-TFE3 fusion transcripts in paraffin-embedded tumor tissues. *Diagn Mol Pathol* 2008;17(4):245–252.
164. Parham DM, Ellison DA. Rhabdomyosarcomas in adults and children: an update. *Arch Pathol Lab Med* 2006;130(10):1454–1465.
165. Parham DM, Qualman SJ, Teot L, et al. Correlation between histology and PAX/FKHR fusion status in alveolar rhabdomyosarcoma. A report from the Children's Oncology Group. *Am J Surg Pathol* 2007;31(6):895–901.
166. Pothula VB, Lesser T, Mallucci C, et al. Vestibular schwannomas in children. *Otol Neurotol* 2001;22(6):903–907.
167. Prakash S, Sarran L, Socci N, et al. Gastrointestinal stromal tumors in children and young adults: a clinicopathologic, molecular, and genomic study of 15 cases and review of the literature. *J Pediatr Hematol Oncol* 2005;27(4):179–187.
168. Qiu X, Montgomery E, Sun B. Inflammatory myofibroblastic tumor and low-grade myofibroblastic sarcoma: a comparative study of clinicopathologic features and further observations on the immunohistochemical profile of myofibroblasts. *Hum Pathol* 2008;39(6): 846–856.
169. Qualman SJ, Coffin CM, Newton WA, et al. Intergroup Rhabdomyosarcoma Study: update for pathologists. *Pediatr Dev Pathol* 1998;1(6):550–561.
170. Qualman SJ, Morotti RA. Risk assignment in pediatric soft-tissue sarcomas: an evolving molecular classification. *Curr Oncol Rep* 2002;4(2):123–130.
171. Rakheja D, Cunningham JC, Mitui M, et al. A subset of cranial fasciitis is associated with dysregulation of the Wnt/beta-catenin pathway. *Mod Pathol* 2008;21(11):1330–1336.
172. Rakheja D, Wilson KS, Meehan JJ, et al. Extrapleural benign solitary fibrous tumor in the shoulder of a 9-year-old girl: case report and review of the literature. *Pediatr Dev Pathol* 2004;7(6):653–660.
173. Raney B, Anderson J, Arndt C, et al. Primary renal sarcomas in the Intergroup Rhabdomyosarcoma Study Group (IRSG) experience, 1972–2005: A report from the Children's Oncology Group. *Pediatr Blood Cancer* 2008;51(3):339–343.
174. Raney B, Anderson J, Breneman J, et al. Results in patients with cranial parameningeal sarcoma and metastases (Stage 4) treated on Intergroup Rhabdomyosarcoma Study Group (IRSG) Protocols II-IV, 1978–1997: report from the Children's Oncology Group. *Pediatr Blood Cancer* 2008;51(1):17–22.
175. Raney RB, Anderson JR, Barr FG, et al. Rhabdomyosarcoma and undifferentiated sarcoma in the first two decades of life: a selective review of intergroup rhabdomyosarcoma study group experience and rationale for Intergroup Rhabdomyosarcoma Study V. *J Pediatr Hematol Oncol* 2001;23(4):215–220.
176. Reis-Filho JS, Milanezi F, Ferro J, et al. Pediatric pigmented dermatofibrosarcoma protuberans (Bednar tumor): case report and review of the literature with emphasis on the differential diagnosis. *Pathol Res Pract* 2002;198(9):621–626.
177. Riggi N, Stamenkovic I. The biology of Ewing sarcoma. *Cancer Lett* 2007;254(1):1–10.
178. Riggi N, Suva ML, Suva D, et al. EWS-FLI-1 expression triggers a Ewing's sarcoma initiation program in primary human mesenchymal stem cells. *Cancer Res* 2008;68(7):2176–2185.
179. Rodriguez-Galindo C, Liu T, Krasin MJ, et al. Analysis of prognostic factors in Ewing sarcoma family of tumors: review of St. Jude Children's Research Hospital studies. *Cancer* 2007;110(2):375–384.
180. Rosenberg AE. Pseudosarcomas of soft tissue. *Arch Pathol Lab Med* 2008;132(4):579–586.
181. Rosser T, Packer RJ. Neurofibromas in children with neurofibromatosis 1. *J Child Neurol* 2002;17(8):585–591.
182. Ruggieri M, Iannetti P, Polizzi A, et al. Earliest clinical manifestations and natural history of neurofibromatosis type 2 (NF2) in childhood: a study of 24 patients. *Neuropediatrics* 2005;36(1):21–34.
183. Sciot R, Rosai J, Dal Cin P, et al. Analysis of 35 cases of localized and diffuse tenosynovial giant cell tumor: a report from the Chromosomes and Morphology (CHAMP) study group. *Mod Pathol* 1999;12(6):576–579.
184. Sebire NJ, Malone M. Myogenin and MyoD1 expression in paediatric rhabdomyosarcomas. *J Clin Pathol* 2003;56(6):412–416.
185. Seifert O, Mrowietz U. Keloid scarring: bench and bedside. *Arch Dermatol Res* 2009;301(4):259–272.
186. Shao L, Singh V, Cooley L. Angiomatoid fibrous histiocytoma with t(2;22)(q33;q12.2) and EWSR1 gene rearrangement. *Pediatr Dev Pathol* 2009;12(2):143–146.
187. Slater O, Shipley J. Clinical relevance of molecular genetics to paediatric sarcomas. *J Clin Pathol* 2007;60(11):1187–1194.
188. Somerhausen NS, Fletcher CDM. Diffuse-type giant cell tumor: clinicopathologic and immunohistochemical analysis of 50 cases with extraarticular disease. *Am J Surg Pathol* 2000;24(4): 479–492.
189. Somers GR, Gupta AA, Doria AS, et al. Pediatric undifferentiated sarcoma of the soft tissues: a clinicopathologic study. *Pediatr Dev Pathol* 2006;9(2):132–142.
190. Sorensen PH, Lynch JC, Qualman SJ, et al. PAX3-FKHR and PAX7-FKHR gene fusions are prognostic indicators in alveolar rhabdomyosarcoma: a report from the Children's Oncology Group. *J Clin Oncol* 2002;20(11):2672–2679.
191. Spunt SL, Pappo AS. Childhood nonrhabdomyosarcoma soft tissue sarcomas are not adult-type tumors. *J Clin Oncol* 2006;24(12): 1958–1959.
192. Stanford D, Rogers M. Dermatological presentations of infantile myofibromatosis: a review of 27 cases. *Australas J Dermatol* 2000;41(3):156–161.
193. Sugarman JL. Epidermal nevus syndromes. *Semin Cutan Med Surg* 2007;26(4):221–230.
194. Sultan I, Qaddoumi I, Yaser S, et al. Comparing adult and pediatric rhabdomyosarcoma in the Surveillance, Epidemiology and End Results program, 1973 to 2005: an analysis of 2,600 patients. *J Clin Oncol* 2009;27(20):3391–3397.

195. Sultan I, Rodriguez-Galindo C, Saab R, et al. Comparing children and adults with synovial sarcoma in the Surveillance, Epidemiology, and End Results program, 1983 to 2005: an analysis of 1268 patients. *Cancer* 2009;115(15):3537–3547.
196. Taher A, Pushpanathan C. Plexiform fibrohistiocytic tumor: a brief review. *Arch Pathol Lab Med* 2007;131(7):1135–1138.
197. Tardio JC. CD34-reactive tumors of the skin. An updated review of an ever-growing list of lesions. *J Cutan Pathol* 2009;36(1): 89–102.
198. Thiene G, Corrado D, Basso C. Arrhythmogenic right ventricular cardiomyopathy/dysplasia. *Orphanet J Rare Dis* 2007;2:45–60.
199. Thway K. Angiomatoid fibrous histiocytoma: a review with recent genetic findings. *Arch Pathol Lab Med* 2008;132(2):273–277.
200. Thway K, Gibson S, Ramsay A, et al. Beta-catenin expression in pediatric fibroblastic and myofibroblastic lesions: a study of 100 cases. *Pediatr Dev Pathol* 2008:12(4):292–296.
201. Tille JC, Pepper MS. Hereditary vascular anomalies: new insights into their pathogenesis. *Arterioscler Thromb Vasc Biol* 2004:24(9);1578–1590.
202. Trobaugh-Lotrario AD, Tomlinson GE, Finegold MJ, et al. Small cell undifferentiated variant of hepatoblastoma: adverse clinical and molecular features similar to rhabdoid tumors. *Pediatr Blood Cancer* 2009;52(3):328–334.
203. Tucker T, Friedman JM, Friedrich RE, et al. Longitudinal study of neurofibromatosis 1 associated plexiform neurofibromas. *J Med Genet* 2009;46(2):81–85.
204. Tucker T, Wolkenstein P, Revuz J, et al. Association between benign and malignant peripheral nerve sheath tumors in NF1. *Neurology* 2005;65(2):205–211.
205. Vernon SE, Bejarano PA. Low-grade fibromyxoid sarcoma: a brief review. *Arch Pathol Lab Med* 2006;130(9):1358–1360.
206. Vujanic GM, Kelsey A, Perlman EJ, et al. Anaplastic sarcoma of the kidney: a clinicopathologic study of 20 cases of a new entity with polyphenotypic features. *Am J Surg Pathol* 2007;31(10):1459–1468.
207. Waggoner DJ, Towbin J, Gottesman G, et al. Clinic-based study of plexiform neurofibromas in neurofibromatosis 1. *Am J Med Genet* 2000;92(2):132–135.
208. Walsh SN, Hurt MA. Cutaneous fetal rhabdomyoma: a case report and historical review of the literature. *Am J Surg Pathol* 2008;32(3):485–491.
209. Wang QK. Update on the molecular genetics of vascular anomalies. *Lymphat Res Biol* 2005;3(4):226–233.
210. Weiss SW. Smooth muscle tumors of soft tissue. *Adv Anat Pathol* 2002;9(6):351–359.
211. Weiss SW, Goldblum JR. *Enzinger and Weiss's Soft Tissue Tumors*. 5th ed. Philadelphia, PA: Mosby Elsevier, 2008.
212. Wilkes D, McDermott DA, Basson CT. Clinical phenotypes and molecular genetic mechanisms of Carney complex. *Lancet Oncol* 2005;6(7):501–508.
213. Woodruff JM, Scheithauer BW, Kurtkaya-Yapicier O, et al. Congenital and childhood plexiform (multinodular) cellular schwannoma: a troublesome mimic of malignant peripheral nerve sheath tumor. *Am J Surg Pathol* 2003;27(10):1321–1329.
214. Xenos C, Sgouros S, Walsh R, et al. Spinal lipomas in children. *Pediatr Neurosurg* 2000;32(6):295–307.
215. Yamamoto H, Yamaguchi H, Aishima S, et al. Inflammatory myofibroblastic tumor versus IgG4-related sclerosing disease and inflammatory pseudotumor: A comparative clinicopathologic study. *Am J Surg Pathol* 2009;33(9):1330–1340.
216. Yang P, Grufferman S, Khoury MJ, et al. Association of childhood rhabdomyosarcoma with neurofibromatosis type I and birth defects. *Genet Epidemiol* 1995;12(5):467–474.
217. Zarrin-Khameh N, Kaye KS. Alveolar soft part sarcoma. *Arch Pathol Lab Med* 2007;131(3):488–491.
218. Zelger B, Zelger BG, Burgdorf WH. Dermatofibroma-a critical evaluation. *Int J Surg Pathol* 2004;12(4):333–344
219. Hornick JL, Dal Cin P, Fletcher CD. Loss of INI1 expression is characteristic of both conventional and proximal-type epithelioid sarcoma. *Am J Surg Pathol* 2009;33(4):542–550.

CHAPTER 25

The Skin

VIJAYA B. REDDY
ALIYA N. HUSAIN

Although any adult dermatologic disease can be seen in children, there are several conditions that are of clinical significance that occur with greater frequency, or at times exclusively, in children and neonates. Table 25-1 lists the pediatric dermatologic diseases seen by the general pathologist at two tertiary care medical centers over a period of 19 years. Although the vast majority of the specimens were those of benign pigmented lesions and plastic repair and debridement, a variety of benign and malignant neoplasms as well as life-threatening inflammatory dermatoses can occur in children and require accurate diagnosis and timely management. This chapter, while covering the spectrum of dermatologic diseases, focuses specifically on the clinicopathologic features of the diseases encountered in children. Although a majority of the congenital diseases involving the skin are diagnosed clinically and rarely need biopsy, a significant number of diseases can only be diagnosed with specificity on histopathologic grounds. A specific diagnosis can be rendered by using a simple algorithmic approach based on low-power pattern analysis (Table 25-2). As in other areas of pathology, clinicopathologic correlation is an integral part of the diagnostic process.

EMBRYOLOGY

The epithelial structures of the skin, namely epidermis, folliculo-sebaceous units, and apocrine and eccrine sweat glands, are derived from the ectoderm. The dermis and its mesenchymal constituents, namely vessels, smooth muscle, and nerve bundles, originate from the mesoderm.

There is a third component of skin that is composed of the migratory cells that originate at different sites and populate the skin. The melanocytes, Merkel cells, and Langerhans histiocytes form an integral part of the epidermis, while the mast cells and dendritic cells are present in the dermis. Melanocytes, Merkel cells, and perineural cells are neural-crest derivatives. Mast cells and Langerhans cells are derived from mesenchymal precursors of bone marrow.

Skin development starts as a single layer of cells or periderm, which can be recognized in a 3-week-old

Table 25-1 ■ DISEASES SEEN IN CONSECUTIVE PEDIATRIC SKIN SPECIMENS AT LOYOLA UNIVERSITY MEDICAL CENTER OVER 10 YEARS (1986–96) AND AT RUSH UNIVERSITY MEDICAL CENTER OVER 9 YEARS (1996–2004)

	Loyola (%)		Rush (%)		Total (%)	
Benign pigmented lesions	742	(51.5)	554	(43.1)	1296	(47)
Scars, keloids, debridement, plastic repair	421	(29.1)	431	(33.5)	852	(31)
Viral infections	82	(5.7)	51	(4)	131	(4.8)
Inflammatory conditions	68	(4.7)	96	(7.5)	164	(6)
Vascular lesions	47	(3.25)	26	(2)	73	(2.7)
Cysts	42	(2.9)	47	(3.7)	89	(3.3)
Benign neoplasms	38	(2.6)	58	(4.5)	96	(3.5)
Malignant melanoma	2		13	(1)	15	(0.5)
Urticaria pigmentosa	2		0		2	
Langerhans cell histiocytosis	1		1		2	
Dermatofibrosarcoma protruberans	1		3		4	
Infantile fibrosarcoma	–		2		2	
Metastases	–		2		2	
Basal cell carcinoma	–		1		1	
Total	1446		1285		2731	

Table 25-2A ■ ALGORITHMIC APPROACH TO SPECIFIC DIAGNOSIS: INFLAMMATORY DERMATOSES

1. Superficial perivascular dermatitis
   - Consider: Urticaria
     Telangiectasia macularis eruptiva perstans
     Vitiligo
     Spongiotic dermatoses:
       Contact dermatitis
       Nummular dermatitis
       Atopic dermatitis
       Drug-hypersensitivity reaction (especially with eosinophils)
     Viral exanthem
     Dermatophytosis
2. Superficial and deep perivascular dermatitis
   - Consider: Mucha-Habermann disease – pityriasis lichenoides et varioliformis acuta (interface dermatitis)
     Lymphomatoid papulosis
     Insect bite reactions (with eosinophils)
3. Vasculitis
   Small vessels vasculitis with neutrophils–leukocytoclastic vasculitis
   Medium vessel vasculitis with neutrophils–polyarteritis nodosa
   Large vessel vasculitis–nodular vasculitis (erythema induratum):
4. Granulomatous dermatitis
   Palisading granulomas
     Granuloma annulare
     Necrobiosis lipoidica
     Rheumatoid nodule
   Caseating and noncaseating granulomas
     Infectious
     Sarcoidosis
5. Vesiculobullous dermatoses
   Subcorneal:
     Subcorneal pustular dermatosis of childhood
     Impetigo
   Intraepidermal:
     Staphylococcal scalded skin syndrome
     Pemphigus vulgaris
     Herpes virus infection
     Darier disease
   Subepidermal:
     Dermatitis herpetiformis/Linear IgA dermatosis
     Bullous cutaneous lupus erythematosus
6. Folliculitis and perifolliculitis
   - Consider: Dermatophytosis
     Eosinophilic pustular dermatosis
     Acne vulgaris
     Alopecia areata
     Lupus erythematosus
     Trichotillomania
7. Fibrosing dermatitis
   Scar
   Dermatofibroma
   Scleroderma/morphea
8. Panniculitis
   Septal panniculitis
     Erythema nodosum
     Scleroderma
     Eosinophilic fasciitis
   Lobular panniculitis
     Sclerema neonatorum
     Subcutaneous fat necrosis of newborn
     α-1-antitrypsin deficiency
     Weber-Christian disease
     Cytophagic panniculitis

Table 25-2B ■ ALGORITHMIC APPROACH TO SPECIFIC DIAGNOSIS: NEOPLASTIC CONDITIONS

1. Epithelial
2. Melanocytic
3. Mesenchymal
4. Hematopoietic

Benign	Malignant
Small	Large
Well circumscribed	Poorly circumscribed
Symmetric	Asymmetric
Smooth margins	Infiltrating margins
	May be ulcerated

embryo. There is progressive stratification of the epidermis, and by the end of the first trimester, several layers of glycogen-rich cells can be seen in the epidermis. Cornification of the epidermis is completed during the 6th month of gestation (Figure 25-1). Defects in cornification (ichthyoses) can be diagnosed through fetal skin biopsies at this stage. At about 12 weeks, folliculo-sebaceous units and sweat glands begin as buds of basal cells that protrude into the mesenchyme of the dermis. Ectodermal dysplasias, which are characterized by absence of follicles and sweat glands, can be detected through fetal skin biopsies after the second trimester.

By the end of the first trimester, the dermoepidermal junction can be recognized, and at about 6 months, the dermal papillae become recognizable. The dermis, which begins as loosely arranged mesenchymal cells in a myxoid background, continues to be modified throughout the third trimester and beyond.

Because fetal skin biopsies are becoming increasingly useful in the diagnosis of genodermatoses, an understanding of the embryology of skin is critical in not only selecting the time of biopsy but also in interpretation of the biopsy findings.

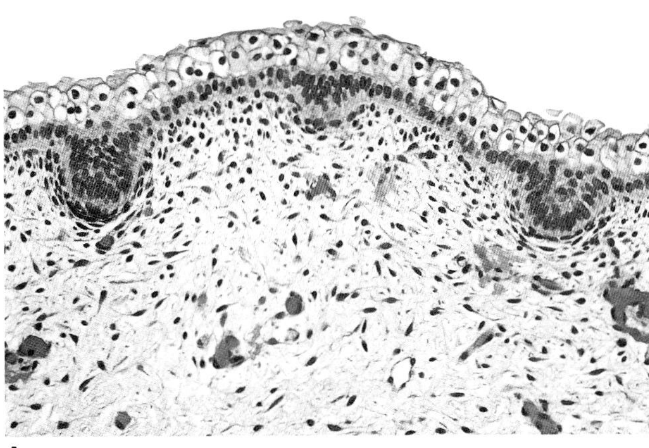

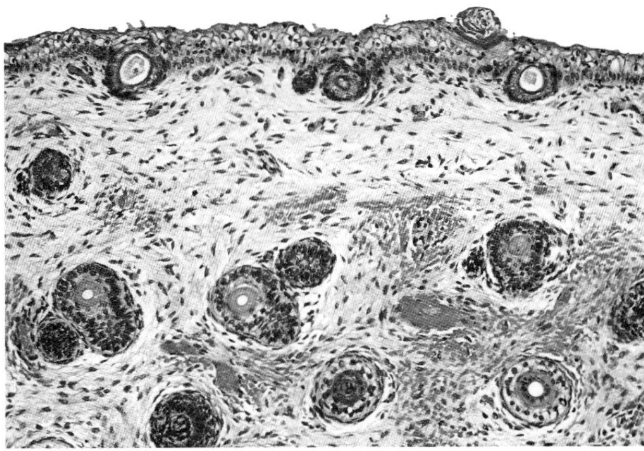

A B

FIGURE 25-1 ■ **A:** Skin of an early, second-trimester fetus showing stratification of epidermis, beginning of the follicular germs, and immature dermis. **B:** Skin from a 28-week fetus with stratum corneum and adnexal structures in a collagenized dermis. (Hematoxylin and eosin stain, original magnifications ×200.)

NORMAL HISTOLOGY

Fetal skin is characterized by a virtually absent stratum corneum and an epidermis that is only a few cell layers thick. Depending on the gestational age, the dermis is relatively hypocellular and myxoid. Rudiments of adnexa including hair follicles and sweat glands can be identified starting from 20 to 24 weeks of gestation. In a premature baby, subcutaneous fat is virtually absent.

The dermis is thin in children compared with that in adults, with proportionately larger amount of subcutaneous fat. With increasing age, the epidermis and the stratum corneum increase in thickness and the dermis becomes more compact and thick. Anatomic variations exist within the normal spectrum, and awareness of these features may prove helpful in localizing the site of biopsy when clinical information is lacking. These include numerous terminal hair follicles in the scalp, many vellus hair follicles and sebaceous lobules in facial skin, apocrine glands in the axilla and genitalia, and eccrine glands in acral skin. A prominent stratum granulosum and stratum corneum characteristic of chronic trauma are present in biopsies from the palm and sole.

BIOPSY TECHNIQUES

Skin samples can be obtained using various biopsy techniques, including punch, shave, excision, and curettage. Selection of the appropriate biopsy technique depends on the clinical impression and the kind of information anticipated by the clinician.

Punch biopsy is generally the choice of technique in evaluation of inflammatory dermatoses. This technique allows the histologic examination of the full thickness of the skin including the subcutaneous fat. A 4-mm punch biopsy provides an adequate sample. In small children and cosmetically important areas, a 3-mm punch may be substituted. The area selected for biopsy should be a well-developed lesion and representative of the pathologic process.

Shave biopsy is the technique used in the evaluation of lesions that appear to be confined to the epidermis and superficial dermis, and is best for the clinical diagnosis of keratoses and other benign neoplastic lesions. It may, on occasion, be used for diagnostic confirmation of basal cell or squamous cell carcinoma.

Excisional biopsy is the technique of choice for suspected malignancies or atypical pigmented lesions. Excisional biopsies generally allow for the evaluation of surgical margins, and as such, the lateral and deep margins should be inked before sectioning. Excisional biopsy or an incisional biopsy can also be used when panniculitis is clinically suspected.

Curettage is the technique some clinicians employ in examining clinically benign lesions. From a pathologist's point of view, this is not a preferred method because the fragments of tissue so obtained are often small and superficial, precluding accurate analysis. Furthermore, if a clinically benign lesion turns out to be malignant on histologic examination, vital information such as invasion or thickness cannot be obtained. Curette fragments are difficult to orient.

Scrape preparation is useful in evaluation of viral vesicles, when cells are scraped off a vesicular or pustular lesion and analyzed after a quick stain.

Fine-needle aspiration biopsy is a popular method of biopsy in the evaluation of subcutaneous bumps and lumps. However, it requires an experienced cytopathologist for proper handling and interpretation of the material obtained.

SPECIMEN HANDLING

Routine Processing

Biopsy specimens should be placed immediately in a fixative. The fixative of choice for the majority of the specimens is 10% buffered formalin. Punch and shave biopsies larger than 3 mm in diameter should be bisected for optimal fixation as well as for appropriate plane of sectioning through the lesion, which is usually located in the center of the specimen. Excisional biopsies should be inked and sectioned at 2- to 3-mm intervals. Sections cut at 3 to 5 μm are routinely stained with hemotoxin and eosin.

Special Processing

Specimens for direct immunofluorescence (IF) testing of bullous diseases are ideally obtained by biopsy of perilesional skin. A well-established lesion is best for suspected cases of lupus, whereas an early lesion is ideal for suspected case of vasculitis. Michel fixative is a good transport medium because IF testing can be performed for approximately 7 days. Alternatively, the specimen can be placed in normal saline and transported immediately to the laboratory. Frozen sections are incubated with fluorescein-labeled antibodies typically against IgG, IgA, IgM, C3, C1q, and fibrinogen and evaluated with IF microscope.

Electron microscopy may be of use in the diagnosis of undifferentiated neoplasms and can be invaluable in establishing the diagnosis of various types of epidermolysis bullosa and also in metabolic disorders like Fabry disease. Specimens for electron microscopy should be fixed immediately in 2% glutaraldehyde or paraformaldehyde.

Skin and subcutaneous tissue may be used for cytogenetic analysis. Sterile specimens should be placed in a transport medium such as RPMI.

ALGORITHMIC APPROACH TO SPECIFIC DIAGNOSES

A systematic approach in analysis of biopsy sections allows for a smooth and accurate diagnosis. The pattern analysis method, which was introduced by Wallace H. Clark Jr, popularized by A. Bernard Ackerman and followed widely by most dermatopathologists today, involves the evaluation of sections at a scanning magnification. Examination at scanning magnification can be highly informative and usually helps in classifying a disease process either as neoplastic or inflammatory. Table 25-2 is rather simplistic but representative of the more common dermatologic conditions that can be diagnosed with specificity in the pediatric patient. The following is a description of diseases grouped according to etiology and pathogenesis.

CONGENITAL DISEASES (GENODERMATOSES)

Genodermatoses are a large and diverse group of disorders presenting with cutaneous involvement and an underlying genetic defect. Only those genodermatoses that can be diagnosed in the fetus, neonate, or child will be discussed. It must be emphasized that some of these will be rarely seen by the pathologist, while others are not uncommon and are frequently included in the differential diagnosis.

Aplasia Cutis Congenita

Aplasia cutis congenita, or localized absence of skin, presents as a single or multiple skin defects typically involving the scalp. It presents at birth with a deep ulcer-like lesion, in which the subcutaneous fat is exposed. If the lesion occurs in utero, it manifests as a healed scar at birth. A sporadic lesion of aplasia cutis has no significant clinical consequences. More often, aplasia cutis may be a part of a variety of inheritable or noninheritable syndromes including trisomy 13, amniotic bands, and cardiac anomalies (29,159).

A histologic section of aplasia cutis shows a full-thickness skin defect with healing at the edges. A fully healed lesion shows scar with absence of adnexal structures. Formerly considered as synonymous, congenital absence of skin, characterized by absence of epidermis only, is now regarded as part of the epidermolysis bullosa group of disorders.

Ichthyosis

Ichthyoses are a heterogeneous group of disorders of epidermal cornification that are characterized by dryness and scaling of the skin. Ichthyoses are generally inherited, although acquired forms are described, especially in association with hematopoietic malignancies. The hereditary forms are divided into (a) the primary forms, which include ichthyosis vulgaris, recessive X-linked ichthyosis, epidermolytic hyperkeratosis (bullous congenital ichthyosiform erythroderma), classical lamellar ichthyosis, and nonbullous congenital ichthyosiform erythroderma; (b) ichthyosiform disorders such as Harlequin ichthyosis, erythrokeratoderma variabilis, and CHILD (congenital hemidysplasia with ichthyosiform erythrodermal and limb defects) syndrome; and (c) other related disorders of differentiation such as Darier disease, Hailey-Hailey disease, and porokeratosis (143).

Ichthyosis vulgaris is a common disorder, inherited in an autosomally dominant pattern that presents with fine white to larger scales involving large areas of the body but most prominent on the extensor surfaces of the extremities with relative sparing of the flexural areas. Histologically, there is moderate hyperkeratosis with a decreased or an absent granular layer and follicular plugging (Figure 25-2).

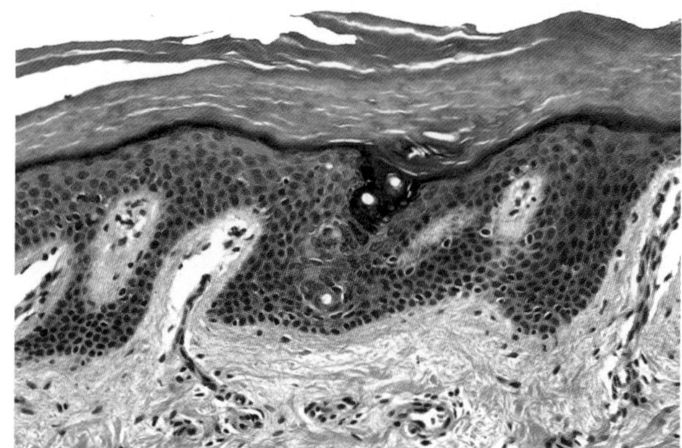

FIGURE 25-2 ■ Ichthyosis vulgaris showing hyperkeratosis and a prominent stratum corneum with a diminished granular cell layer. (Hematoxylin and eosin stain; original magnification ×200.)

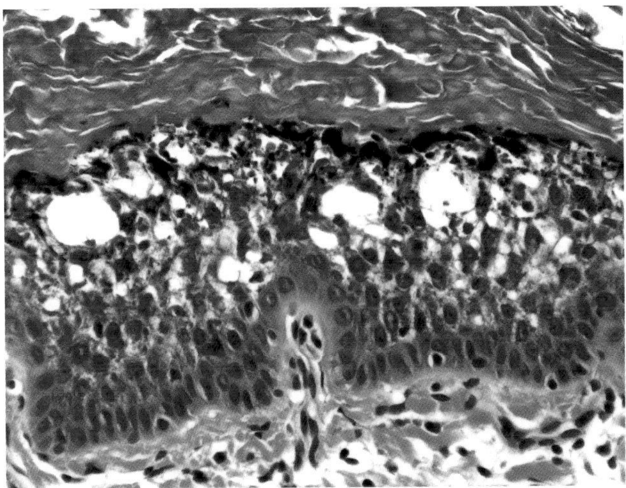

FIGURE 25-3 ■ Congenital bullous ichthyosiform erythroderma showing marked hyperkeratosis and epidermolytic hyperkeratosis with vacuolar degeneration of the stratum spinosum and granulosum, which is responsible for the formation of bullae. (Hematoxylin and eosin stain; original magnification ×200.)

X-linked ichthyosis inherited as a recessive disease presents early in infancy with large brown scales involving the entire body with accentuation on the neck and behind ears and relative sparing of the flexural areas. Histologically, there is hyperkeratosis with normal or thickened granular layer.

Bullous congenital ichthyosiform erythroderma or epidermolytic hyperkeratosis has an autosomal dominant pattern of inheritance and presents with generalized erythema and blistering at birth. Microscopic features include hyperkeratosis, a characteristic vacuolization of the cells in spinous and granular layers and prominent keratohyaline granules (Figure 25-3).

Lamellar ichthyosis is inherited as an autosomal recessive disorder and is characterized by large plate-like scales involving face, trunk, and extremities with a predilection for flexor areas. Microscopic changes are nonspecific and include hyperkeratosis with or without foci of parakeratosis and mild epidermal hyperplasia (Figure 25-4). Lamellar ichthyosis can present as a collodion baby, in which the infant is encased in a keratinous membrane and superficially resembles a harlequin fetus. However, the membrane is usually shed in 10 to 14 days, following which the clinical features of lamellar ichthyosis become apparent.

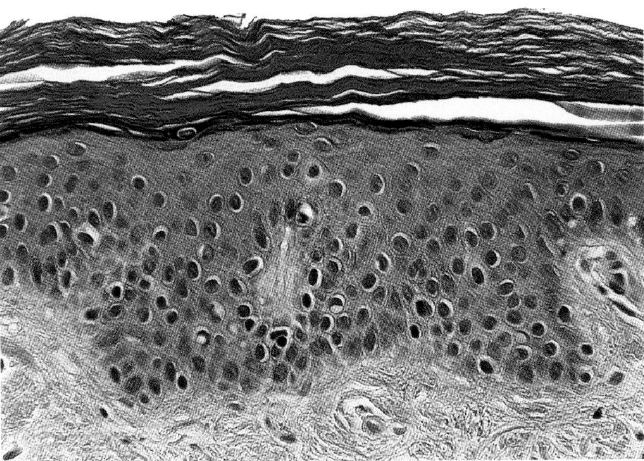

FIGURE 25-4 ■ Lamellar ichthyosis showing hyperkeratosis and mild psoriasiform changes. (Hematoxylin and eosin stain; original magnification ×200.)

Nonbullous congenital ichthyosiform erythroderma is inherited as autosomal recessive disorder, is milder than lamellar ichthyosis, and has a more prominent erythrodermic component.

Fetal harlequin ichthyosis is an autosomal recessive disorder that can be fatal. Fetal skin biopsy can be diagnostic and shows massive hyperkeratosis. In utero, the massive hyperkeratosis interferes with normal development. At birth, the child is encased in a thick, fissured, scaly cast, associated with ectropion.

Darier Disease

Darier disease, also known as *keratosis follicularis*, is a relatively uncommon disease that is inherited in an autosomal dominant pattern. Darier disease gene has been localized to chromosome 12 (201). It typically presents in children aged 5 to 15 years as keratotic papules distributed in the seborrheic areas such as face, neck, and upper trunk (28). Oral mucosa and nails can also be involved (78,208). The histopathologic findings are characterized by suprabasal acantholysis covered by dyskeratotic cells (corps ronds) and parakeratosis (corps grains), in addition to papillomatous epidermal hyperplasia and hyperkeratosis (Figure 25-5). Occasionally, these lesions are centered around the hair follicles.

Most cases of Darier disease have a benign but protracted course with exacerbations during summer.

Hailey-Hailey Disease

Hailey-Hailey disease is an autosomal dominant genodermatosis that initially manifests typically only after puberty (late

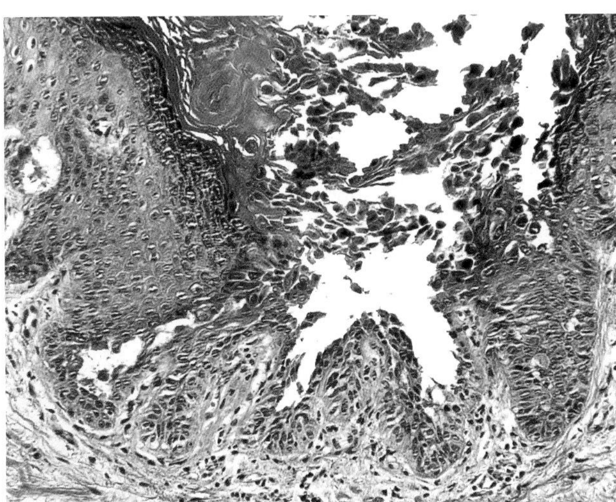

FIGURE 25-5 ■ Darier disease with focal intraepidermal acantholysis, dyskeratosis, and hyperkeratosis. (Hematoxylin and eosin stain, original magnification ×200.)

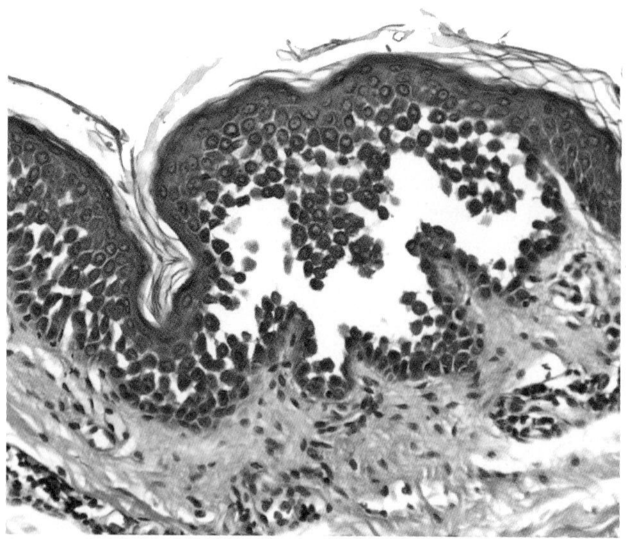

FIGURE 25-6 ■ Hailey-Hailey disease showing intraepidermal acantholysis with a dilapidated brick wall-like appearance. There is no significant dyskeratosis which helps in the differential diagnosis from Darier disease.

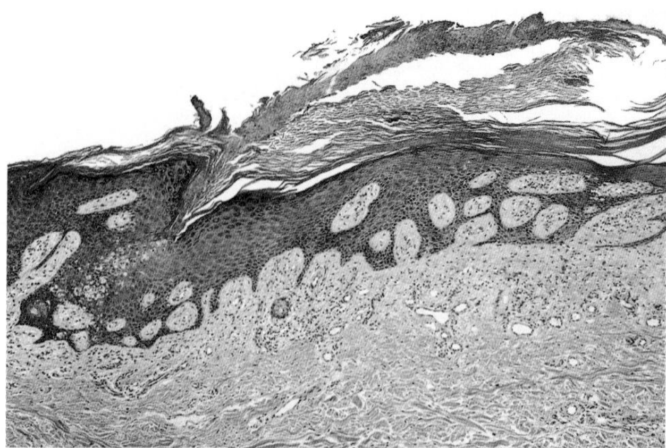

FIGURE 25-7 ■ Porokeratosis showing a column of parakeratosis that is inclined toward the center (cornoid lamella). Dyskeratotic keratinocytes may be seen at the base of the column. (Hematoxylin and eosin stain, original magnification ×100.)

teens or early 20s). It is characterized by recurrent vesicles and erosions on the neck, axillae, and groin. Mucosal involvement is uncommon. Histologic features include suprabasal acantholysis resulting in a dilapidated brick wall-like appearance (Figure 25-6). Most cases of Hailey-Hailey disease have a fairly stable course. The cutaneous lesions are exacerbated by heat, humidity, and bacterial and candidal infections.

Porokeratosis

Porokeratosis is inherited as an autosomal dominant disorder that manifests in childhood and infancy as asymptomatic keratotic papules that enlarge progressively to form plaques with peripheral keratotic ridges. Four variants of porokeratosis can be seen in the pediatric population and include the classic plaque type of Mibelli, linear porokeratosis, porokeratosis palmaris, plantaris et disseminata, and punctate porokeratosis that is limited to palms and soles. A fifth type, disseminated superficial actinic porokeratosis, is a disease of adulthood (36,91,141,168). Histopathologic features common to all types of porokeratoses include a cornoid lamella, which is a column of parakeratosis that corresponds to the peripheral keratotic ridges seen clinically (Figure 25-7). The cornoid lamella overlies an area of epidermal invagination where there is a diminished granular zone and vacuolated and dyskeratotic keratinocytes that correspond to an abnormal clone of keratinocytes. In porokeratosis of Mibelli, the epidermal invagination is more pronounced and deep compared with other types of porokeratosis.

In addition to the inherited form, porokeratosis has been described in various immunosuppressive states including Crohn disease, renal transplantation, and HIV infection. Squamous cell carcinoma and Bowen disease have been reported to develop in lesions of porokeratosis.

Restrictive Dermopathy

Restrictive dermopathy is an uncommon autosomal recessive disorder that presents with prematurity; rigid and tense skin with erosions, denudations, and multiple joint contractions; fixed facial expression; and perineal anomalies (Figure 25-8). Histologic features include a thickened epidermis with flattening of rete ridges and hyperkeratosis. The dermis is thin with absent elastic fibers, collagen bundles oriented parallel to the surface, and poorly developed adnexal structures (Figure 25-9). The disease is fatal, with most infants dying within weeks after birth. Abnormalities in collagen and abnormal synthesis of keratin have been proposed as the underlying defects.

Ectodermal Dysplasia

Ectodermal dysplasias form a large and heterogeneous group of congenital disorders that share the involvement of structures of ectodermal origin and may include trichodysplasia, odontodysplasia, onychodysplasia, and disorders of sweating. More than 100 syndromes encompassing all forms of Mendelian inheritance have been described clinically, two forms of ectodermal dysplasia are recognized: hidrotic and anhidrotic or hypohidrotic. The hidrotic form, with an autosomal dominant pattern of inheritance, is primarily a disorder of keratinization. It is characterized by hypotrichosis, dystrophic nails, and palmoplantar hyperkeratosis. The hypohidrotic form is an X-linked recessive disorder localized to the q11-q21.1 region of X-chromosome with full expression in men, who show the tetrad of anhidrosis or hypohidrosis, hypotrichosis, dental hypoplasia, characteristic facies, and frequently dystrophy of nails. In addition to aplasia and hypoplasia of sweat glands, the submucosal glands of the trachea and bronchus may be affected, leading to frequent respiratory infections. Histologically, both forms show hypoplasia of hair and sebaceous glands. In addition, the anhidrotic form shows aplasia or hypoplasia of eccrine glands and occasionally of apocrine glands.

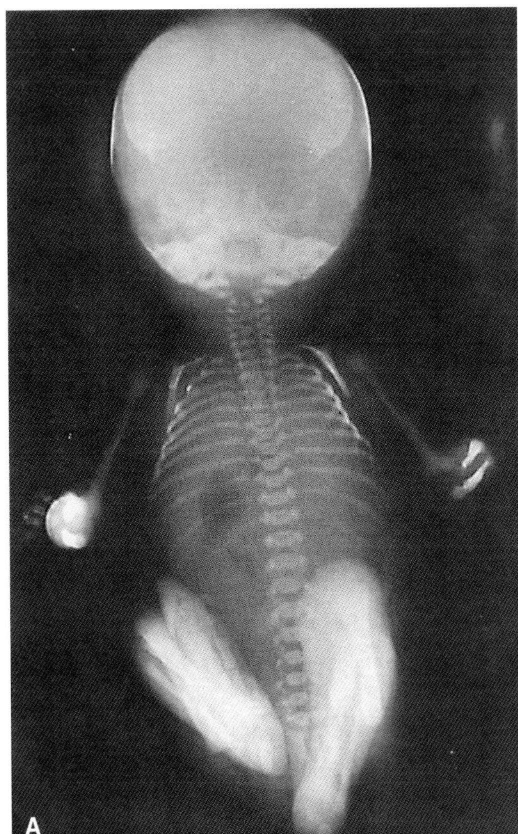

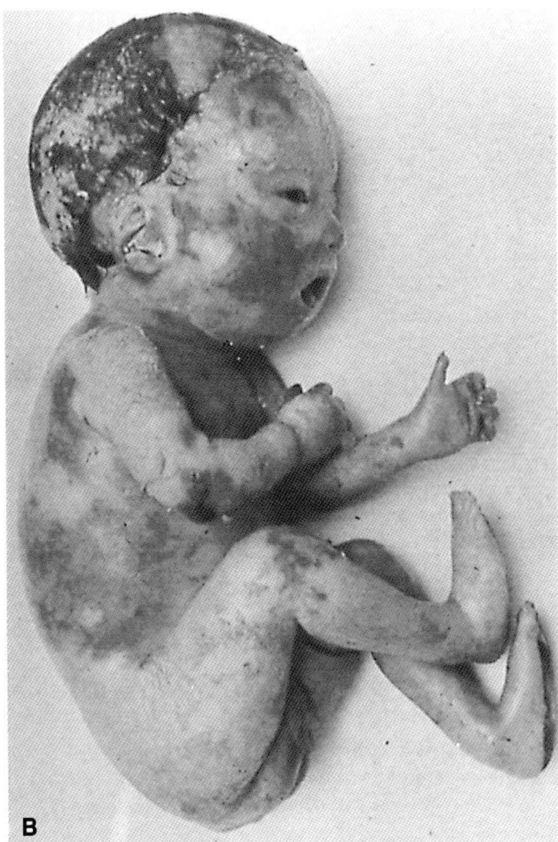

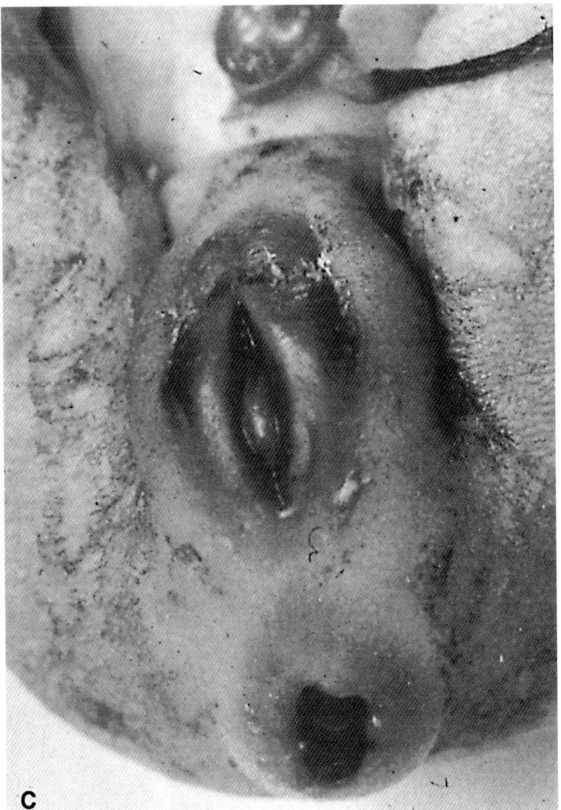

FIGURE 25-8■ **A:** Restrictive dermopathy showing severe contractures in the absence of overt bony abnormalities. **B,C:** The tight, shiny skin and characteristic fixation of the mouth and perineum.

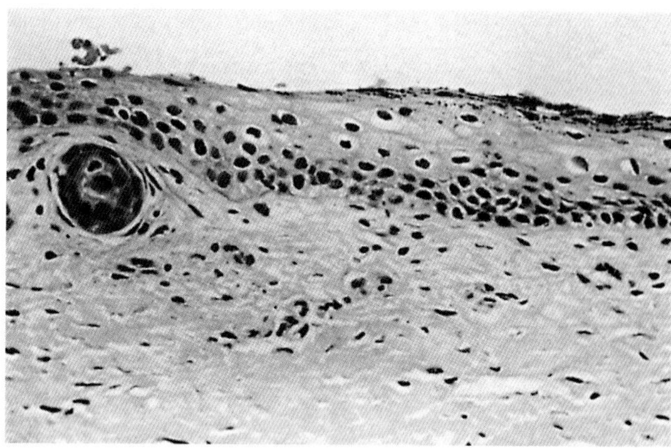

FIGURE 25-9 ■ Restrictive dermopathy without a stratum corneum, but the granular layer is prominent, indicating that the stratum corneum may have been lost in the postmortem interval. The rete ridges are flattened and most of the adnexal structures are atrophic. (Hematoxylin and eosin stain; original magnification ×250.)

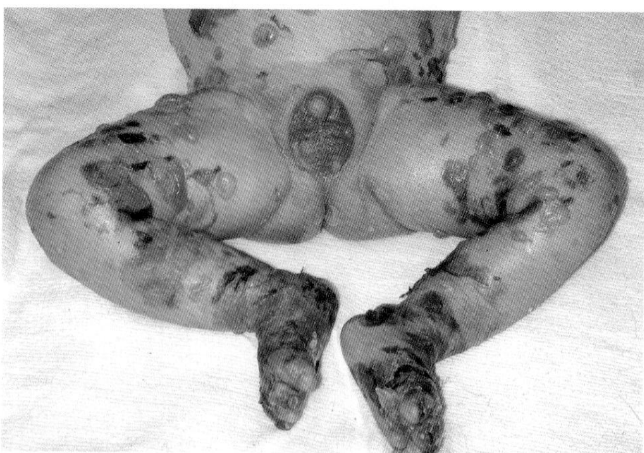

FIGURE 25-10 ■ Junctional epidermolysis bullosa in a 6-week old infant showing extensive blistering and sloughing of the skin. (Courtesy of Sarah Stein, M.D., Department of Medicine, University of Chicago Medical Center.)

Focal Dermal Hypoplasia

Focal dermal hypoplasia was originally described by Libermann (119) as part of ectodermal and mesodermal dysplasia in association with osseous defects. The cutaneous aspects were first detailed by Goltz et al. (76). Because a majority of the patients are women, it has been assumed to have X-linked dominant mode of inheritance. Focal dermal hypoplasia is a multisystem condition in which developmental defects of skin are associated with ocular, dental, and skeletal system abnormalities. The clinical course is dictated by the extent of systemic involvement. The skin findings, which are present from birth, consist of widely distributed asymmetric linear streaks of atrophy or hypoplasia of the skin, often with associated telangiectasia that follow Blaschko lines. Some lesions may present as soft yellow nodular outpouchings caused by herniation of fat through an atrophic dermis in linear array. Various mutations in X-linked PORCN, a putative regulator of Wnt signaling, have been identified in focal dermal hypoplasia (83,202).

Histological features of focal dermal hypoplasia include a marked decrease in the thickness of the dermis, with collagen distributed as thin fibrils rather than bundles, which may be interrupted by presence of adipocytes. The latter corresponds to the clinically apparent soft yellow nodules. The frequent presence of adipocytes high up in the dermis raises the possibility of nevus lipomatosus in the differential diagnosis. Nevus lipomatosus, however, lacks the collagen abnormalities and the frequent X-linked chromosomal abnormalities of focal dermal hypoplasia.

Epidermolysis Bullosa

Epidermolysis bullosa is a heterogeneous group of inherited disorders with variable modes of transmission, characterized by bullous lesions that develop spontaneously or secondary to minor trauma and includes approximately 20 subtypes (65). Based on the presence or absence of scarring, mode of inheritance, cleavage plane of the blister, and the presence or absence of structural elements of skin, epidermolysis bullosa is traditionally divided into three major forms: simplex, junctional, and dystrophic (19,196).

Epidermolysis bullosa simplex, including Cockayne, and Dowling-Meara forms, is typically transmitted in an autosomal dominant pattern and generally associated with good prognosis because the blisters heal without scar formation. Histologic sections show intraepidermal separation, generally within the basal cell layer. A periodic acid-Schiff (PAS) stain is helpful in localizing the level of cleavage above the basement membrane zone. Gene defects of keratins 5, 14 are implicated and may be identified with IF mapping.

Junctional epidermolysis bullosa is inherited as an autosomal recessive disorder and includes the fatal Herlitz type, in which blistering begins at birth and death occurs within the first 2 years (Figure 25-10), and the non-Herlitz type, which manifests similar to the Herlitz type but with a generally better overall prognosis. The cleavage plane occurs in the lamina lucida of the basement membrane at the dermoepidermal junction. Similar changes may involve the gastrointestinal, respiratory, and urinary tracts. Gene defects involving laminin 5 chain and collagen are identified.

Dystrophic epidermolysis bullosa includes the dominant form, which has a good prognosis, and the recessive form, which has a poor prognosis due to extensive erosions and ulcerations that heal with scarring. The level of cleavage is in the papillary dermis below the basement membrane (Figure 25-11). The principal gene defect involves collagen VII.

Immunomapping studies are useful in localizing the cleavage plane and determining the presence, increase, or absence of the structural protein for which the gene is mutated in epidermolysis bullosa. These studies are essential for accurate classification of the type of epidermolysis bullosa, which in conjunction with clinical presentation forms the basis of prognostic information and genetic counseling. Furthermore,

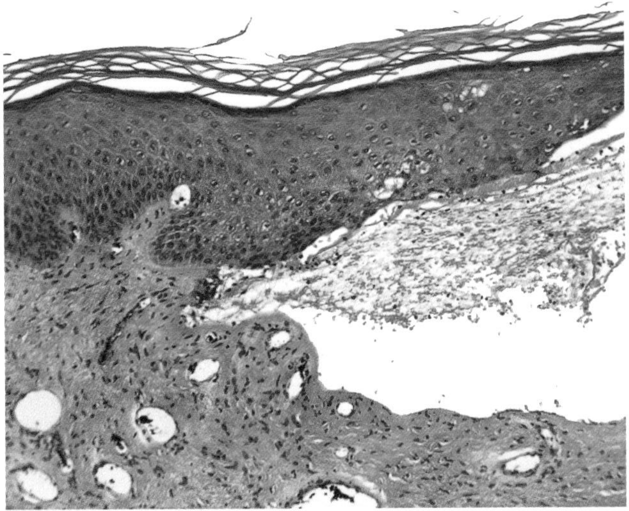

FIGURE 25-11 ■ Epidermolysis bullosa dystrophica has a subepidermal blister with mild dermal inflammation. (Hematoxylin and eosin stain, original magnification ×200.)

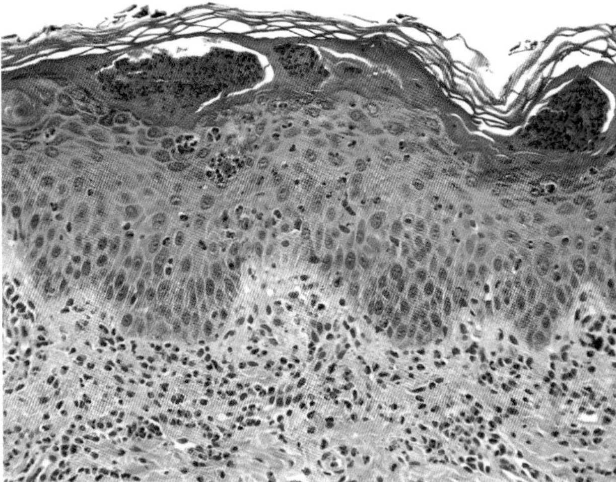

FIGURE 25-12 ■ Incontinentia pigmenti showing the initial skin changes with an intense eosinophilic infiltration within mildly spongiotic epidermis and the dermis. (Hematoxylin and eosin stain, original magnification ×200.)

fetal skin biopsies during the third trimester can be diagnostic in the most severe forms of epidermolysis bullosa.

Incontinentia Pigmenti

Incontinentia pigmenti (Bloch-Sulzberger syndrome) is an X-linked dominant dermatosis that affects mostly women (55,149). Affected hemizygous male fetuses are generally thought to die in utero although recent literature suggests that some male individuals may show cutaneous and extracutaneous features of incontinentia pigmenti in a limited distribution that allow survival (142). The characteristic cutaneous manifestations evolve from crops of vesicles and bullae on the extremities arranged in linear or whorled pattern at birth or shortly thereafter that heal with hyperkeratotic verrucous lesions. As the verrucous lesions subside, characteristic streaks and whorls of hyperpigmentation develop, being most pronounced on the trunk. Faint hypochromic or atrophic lesions in a linear pattern may be seen on the lower extremities in some women and rarely in children (20).

Histologically, the vesicular stage is characterized by eosinophilic spongiosis and intraepidermal vesicle formation and eosinophil-rich dermal inflammatory cell infiltrate (Figure 25-12). The verrucous stage is characterized by hyperkeratosis and papillomatous epidermal hyperplasia with focal dyskeratosis. The hyperpigmented stage corresponds to numerous melanophages in the dermis as in any other postinflammatory pigmentary change.

In approximately 80% of patients, systemic involvement, particularly of the central nervous system and the eye, and teeth abnormalities may be present. Although the skin manifestations are self-limiting, the clinical course is guided by the extent of systemic involvement.

Acrodermatitis Enteropathica

Acrodermatitis enteropathica is an autosomal recessive disorder characterized by defective intestinal absorption of zinc presenting with the triad of dermatitis, diarrhea, and alopecia in infancy at the time of weaning (128). Acquired acrodermatitis enteropathica–like syndromes can occur in exclusively breast-fed preterm infants, infants who are fed on breast milk low in zinc, infants with organic acid urea, and any other acquired zinc deficiency states including human immunodeficiency virus infection. Cutaneous manifestations are characterized by vesiculobullous lesions with acral and periorificial distribution. The histopathologic findings include intraepidermal bullae with epidermal necrosis or spongiosis and superficial perivascular mixed inflammatory cell infiltrate. A well-established lesion shows parakeratosis, marked pallor, ballooning of keratinocytes, and a markedly diminished granular zone. The histologic changes can be identical to those in glucagonoma syndrome and pellagra, conditions associated with nutritional deficiencies of factors essential for normal maturation and metabolism of epidermal keratinocytes.

NONINFFECTIOUS ACQUIRED VESICULOBULLOUS DISEASES

Linear IgA Bullous Dermatosis

Linear IgA bullous dermatosis, also known as *chronic bullous dermatosis of childhood*, presents with large tense bullae in prepubertal children often younger than 5 years of age. The lesions are widespread in distribution and vesicles and bullae, sometimes arranged like a string of pearls, occur at the periphery of a healing lesion. Areas of predilection include the lower part of the trunk, including the groin and genitalia and perioral areas. Rare cases have been described in neonates. Microscopic features are essentially indistinguishable from dermatitis herpetiformis and consist of neutrophilic microabscesses at the tips of dermal papillae in early lesions and subepidermal bulla filled with neutrophils or eosinophils in well-established lesions

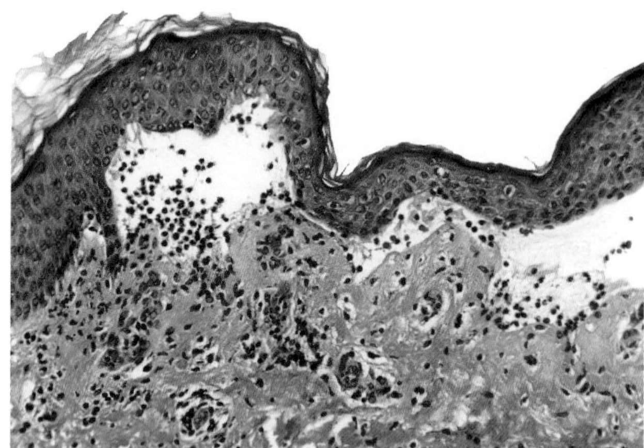

FIGURE 25-13■Linear IgA dermatosis with a subepidermal blister with neutrophils.

(Figure 25-13). Direct IF testing shows a distinct linear pattern of staining at the basement membrane zone with IgA, in sharp contrast to the granular IgA deposits seen in dermatitis herpetiformis. Direct IF testing is crucial in differentiating lupus erythematosus and chronic bullous dermatosis of childhood from other childhood bullous diseases like bullous pemphigoid and lichen planus. Chronic bullous disease of childhood has generally a benign course with a spontaneous remission before puberty. Rare cases heal with scarring when the disease process seems to overlap with childhood cicatricial pemphigoid, which some consider to be another morphologic expression of linear IgA dermatosis of childhood and adults. Linear IgA dermatosis of both children and adults is also similar, both IgA1-mediated diseases (204) with some cases of chronic bullous dermatosis of childhood relapsing into adulthood. Distinction of linear IgA bullous disease from dermatitis herpetiformis is important because linear IgA bullous disease is not typically associated with gluten-sensitive enteropathy.

Dermatitis Herpetiformis

Dermatitis herpetiformis presents as an intensely pruritic papulovesicular eruption that is typically distributed on the scalp, the extensor aspects of extremities, and the back. The lesions may be grouped in herpetiform fashion and symmetrical in distribution. They are characterized by small papules and tense vesicles that rupture easily (165). Although dermatitis herpetiformis generally manifests as a skin disease, approximately 75% to 90% of the children with this disorder have an associated gluten-sensitive enteropathy and a high frequency of HLA antigens, including HLA B8, DR3, and DqW2 (105,107). Histologic sections of a papular lesion show the characteristic neutrophilic microabscesses at the tips of the dermal papillae (Figure 25-14). Sections of a clinically apparent vesicle show a subepidermal bulla filled with neutrophils and a varying mixture of eosinophils and fibrin. Microabscesses are present at the edge of the blister. Direct IF testing is positive for granular deposits of IgA at the tips of dermal papillae in almost all patients (6). A gluten-free diet is effective in controlling the intestinal and cutaneous manifestations in most children.

Herpes Gestationis

Pemphigoid gestationis (herpes gestationis) is a rare acquired autoimmune bullous disease that affects pregnant women most commonly during the second trimester (32) and, in a small percentage of cases, can be transmitted to the neonates born to these women. The affected neonate may present with macules, or papulovesicular or bullous lesions at birth or shortly thereafter. In neonates, the condition is transient, with complete resolution of the lesions occurring within a month, and it is attributed to the transplacental transfer of maternal antibodies (9). Studies have failed to show significant association between pemphigoid gestationis and increased incidence

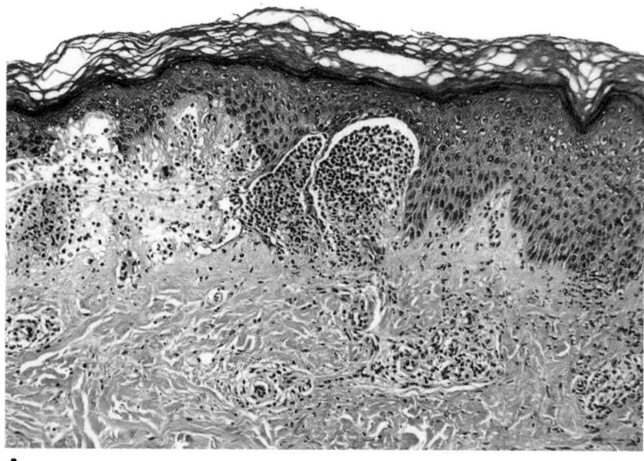

A

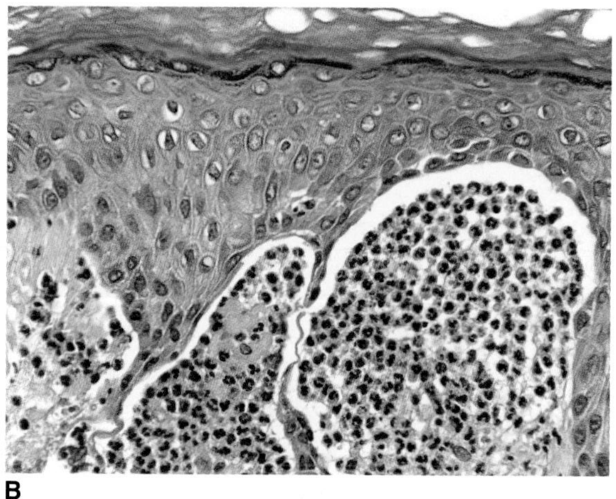

B

FIGURE 25-14■Dermatitis herpetiformis: **A,B:** subepidermal separation with neutrophilic microabscesses at the tips of dermal papillae. Differentiation from linear IgA dermatosis is possible only on IF studies. [Hematoxylin and eosin stains, original magnification ×200(**A**), ×400(**B**).]

and risk of fetal morbidity or mortality. Histopathologic and IF findings may be identical to those seen in bullous pemphigoid and consist of subepidermal bulla with eosinophils and linear deposits of C3 and IgG at the basement membrane zone. Additionally, sera from patients with pemphigoid gestationis like those with bullous pemphigoid are positive for antibodies against a 180-kD epidermal antigen (46).

Epidermolysis Bullosa Acquisita

Epidermolysis bullosa acquisita is an acquired form of epidermolysis bullosa that is seen more commonly in adults but can sometimes be seen in children (30,195). Clinically, it may resemble the autosomal dominant dystrophic type of epidermolysis bullosa acquisita and manifests with tense blisters on the extensor aspects that heal with scarring and milia formation. However, epidermolysis bullosa acquisita is an autoimmune disease characterized by IgG antibodies to type VII collagen of the basement membrane (129,205).

Light microscopic and IF findings are indistinguishable from bullous pemphigoid, which can also be seen in children (54). Both conditions are characterized by subepidermal bullae with linear deposits of IgG and C3 at the basement membrane zone. Indirect IF studies localize the IgG deposits to the roof of salt-split skin, in which the cleavage runs through the lamina lucida of the basement membrane in pemphigoid and the floor (beneath the lamina lucida) in epidermolysis bullosa acquisita.

Erythema Multiforme, Stevens-Johnson Syndrome, and Toxic Epidermal Necrolysis

Erythema multiforme, Stevens-Johnson (S-J) syndrome, and toxic epidermal necrolysis (TEN) (Lyell syndrome) form the clinical and histopathologic spectrum of a potentially life-threatening group of disorders characterized by epidermal necrosis with formation of bullae, which can involve a large part of the skin surface and mucosa. The high mortality rate in patients with TEN is directly related to the resultant fluid loss and sepsis. S-J syndrome is more common in childhood than erythema multiforme or TEN.

Erythema multiforme is distinguished clinically by the characteristic iris or targetoid lesions that can occur on any part of the body but most commonly on the palms and soles. Erythematous and purpuric macules that progress to flaccid bullae and detach from the underlying dermis are characteristic of S-J syndrome and TEN. The detachment is extensive in TEN while mucosal involvement is more prominent in S-J syndrome.

The majority of cases of erythema multiforme in children is etiologically related to herpes simplex virus infection; other viral infections including Epstein-Barr virus and orf and mycoplasma infections have also been implicated (115). Drugs such as sulfonamides and penicillins play an important role, especially in the more severe S-J syndrome and TEN (66,111). No cause can be identified in a significant number of cases.

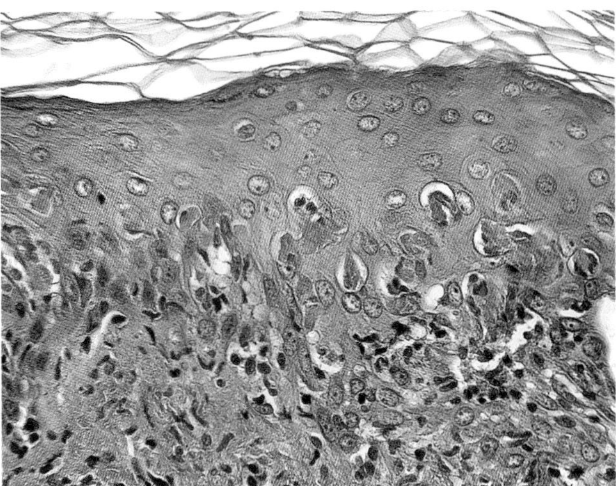

FIGURE 25-15 ▪ Erythema multiforme with basket-weave orthokeratosis, vacuolar alteration of the basal cell layer, necrotic keratinocytes, and mild superficial perivascular inflammation. (Hematoxylin and eosin stain, original magnification ×400.)

Histopathologic features include interface dermatitis with vacuolar alteration of the basal cell layer and mild perivascular infiltrate of lymphocytes, which are also present along the dermoepidermal junction. The histologic hallmark of this group of diseases is the necrotic keratinocyte, which may be few in milder forms and numerous with confluent areas of necrosis in more established lesions (Figure 25-15). In TEN, full-thickness epidermal necrosis leads to subepidermal separation and loss of epidermal surface with the eroded clinical appearance of skin originally described by Lyell (Figure 25-16). An unaltered stratum corneum in skin biopsies attests to the acute nature of the assault on the skin. Immune complex mediated reactions of type III and IV and helper T-cell–mediated immunoreactions are believed to play a role in the pathogenesis of erythema multiforme/TEN (198). Erythema multiforme/S-J syndrome/TEN are potentially life-threatening disorders that require hospitalization,

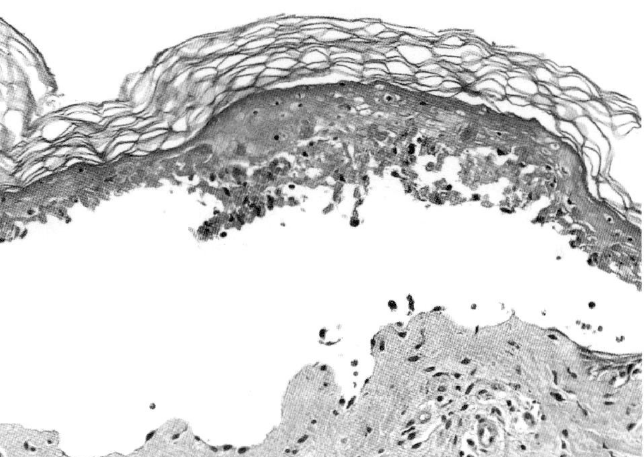

FIGURE 25-16 ▪ Toxic epidermal necrolysis with full-thickness epidermal necrosis with separation at the dermoepidermal junction and sparse inflammatory cell infiltrate. An unaltered cornified layer attests to the acuteness of the event. (Hematoxylin and eosin stain, original magnification ×400.)

withdrawal of recent drugs, and supportive care. Potential infectious causes should be sought and treated. The benefits of specific treatment including corticosteroids and intravenous administration of immunoglobulin are still under debate and further investigation (70,133,173,189).

MISCELLANEOUS NONINFECTIOUS VESICULOPUSTULAR DISEASES

A variety of benign vesiculopustular diseases are commonly seen in neonates and infants. It is important to differentiate these conditions from the more serious vesiculopustular diseases that can affect children (200).

Erythema Toxicum Neonatorum

Erythema toxicum neonatorum (toxic erythema of newborn) is an asymptomatic, transient, self-limiting, common eruption that occurs in the first 24 to 48 hours of life of full-term newborns. The lesions are characterized by macules, papules, and tiny pustules that can affect any part of the body but favor the trunk and proximal extremities. Classical clinical presentation rarely requires a skin biopsy that would reveal eosinophils in the pilosebaceous units and differentiate erythema toxicum neonatorum from other neonatal pustular dermatoses including incontinentia pigmenti (131,138).

TRANSIENT NEONATAL PUSTULAR MELANOSIS

Transient neonatal pustular melanosis is a benign, self-limiting condition that predominantly affects black infants. The skin eruption begins as superficial sterile pustules that rupture easily and typically heal with hyperpigmented macules with collarettes of fine scale. Similarities between transient neonatal pustular melanosis and erythema toxicum neonatorum are emphasized by some authors who proposed "sterile transient neonatal pustulosis" as a unifying term (63). However, the pustules in transient neonatal pustular melanosis show abundance of neutrophils.

Acropustulosis of Infancy

Acropustulosis of infancy presents as recurrent crops of pruritic vesicles and pustules on distal extremities with predilection for palms and soles, primarily in black infants during the 1st year of life. Most cases show spontaneous resolution by the age of 2 years (50).

Smears from the pustule or histologic sections of the subcorneal pustules will show abundant neutrophils.

ECZEMATOUS DERMATITIS

"Eczema" is the term often used to describe erythematous, scaling vesicular lesions with serum crust. Eczematous dermatitis is characterized histologically by epidermal spongiosis and, therefore, is often referred to interchangeably as spongiotic dermatitis. A specific diagnosis is based on clinical history, morphologic appearance, and distribution of lesions. This group of disorders includes nummular dermatitis, contact dermatitis, dyshidrotic dermatitis, and atopic dermatitis.

Nummular Dermatitis

Nummular dermatitis is characterized by coin-shaped, pruritic, erythematous, scaly crusted plaques on the extensor aspect of the extremities. It is believed to be a manifestation of xerosis and is more commonly seen in older patients.

Atopic Dermatitis

Atopic dermatitis is an inherited chronic pruritic skin disease and is the most common skin disease seen in children, with an estimated incidence of as high as 20% (147). About one-third of the cases are diagnosed before the age of 1 year and before 5 years of age in vast majority of patients (85). Sites of predilection are the face in young infants, extensor surfaces of extremities in children younger than 1 year of age, and the popliteal and antecubital fossae, face, and neck in older children and adolescents. The major abnormality in this disease appears to be the overproduction of allergen-specific IgE, and some authors suggest that demonstration of such antibodies be a requisite for the diagnosis of atopic dermatitis (184). Cytokines, T-cells, and antigen-presenting cells in addition to abnormalities of skin barrier appear to play a role in the pathogenesis (34).

Contact Dermatitis

Contact dermatitis includes primary irritant dermatitis and allergic contact dermatitis. Primary irritant dermatitis is frequently seen in children on the cheeks caused by saliva, extremities in response to harsh soaps or detergents, and the diaper area from toiletries (171). Allergic contact dermatitis presents with pruritic, edematous papules, plaques, and occasionally vesicles 12 to 24 hours after exposure to an allergen such as poison ivy, fragrances, nickel, and rubber compounds (16). Allergic contact dermatitis occurs more frequently in children with atopic tendencies (93).

Dyshidrotic Dermatitis

Dyshidrotic dermatitis (pompholyx) typically presents with numerous, pinpoint, recurrent, pruritic vesicles along the sides of the fingers and toes and on palms and soles that usually last a few weeks and frequently relapse.

Histopathology of Spongiotic Dermatitis

Irrespective of the specific type of disease, spongiotic dermatitis shows a similar spectrum of changes. In the acute phase, there is epidermal spongiosis, sometimes marked,

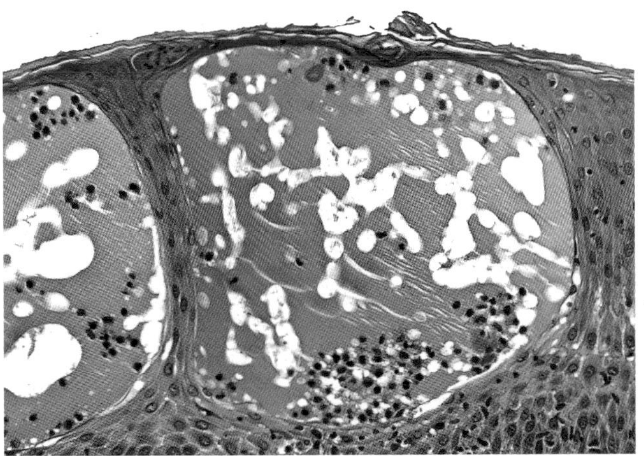

FIGURE 25-17 ■ Eczematous dermatitis showing marked epidermal spongiosis with formation of intraepidermal vesicles and moderate perivascular mixed inflammation. (Hematoxylin and eosin stain, original magnification ×400.)

with vesiculation (Figure 25-17). In the subacute phase, the spongiosis is milder, but associated parakeratosis with plasma cells, neutrophils, eosinophils and epidermal hyperplasia may be present. In the chronic phase, the spongiosis is mild to absent, but changes of chronicity are reflected in a hyperkeratotic cornified layer, marked epidermal hyperplasia, and fibrotic papillary dermis. Superficial perivascular lymphohistiocytic infiltrate is present to varying degrees in all the phases of spongiotic dermatitis.

NONINFECTIOUS PAPULOSQUAMOUS DERMATOSES

This includes a group of diverse disorders characterized by papular and scaling lesions and associated epidermal proliferation. Approximately 10% of the patients seen in a pediatric dermatology clinic present with papulosquamous skin disorders (170). The following is a brief discussion of the more common dermatoses traditionally regarded as the papulosquamous dermatoses.

Psoriasis Vulgaris

Psoriasis vulgaris accounts for 4% of all dermatoses encountered in children younger than the age of 16 years (176) and in about 30% of the patients, psoriasis manifests in the first or the second decade of life (18). Of the various forms of psoriasis, namely, plaque type, guttate, pustular and erythrodermic psoriasis, plaque type is the most common one seen in children followed by guttate psoriasis (61). Pustular psoriasis and psoriatic arthropathy are less common in children (161). The clinical presentation is characterized by asymptomatic scaly erythematous plaques in the plaque type and by slightly pruritic small red droplike scaly lesions in guttate psoriasis. Silvery scales that, on scraping, leave pinpoint areas of bleeding (Auspitz sign) are typical of psoriasis. Lesions are distributed in a bilaterally symmetrical pattern with predilection for scalp and extensor aspects of extremities. Involvement of

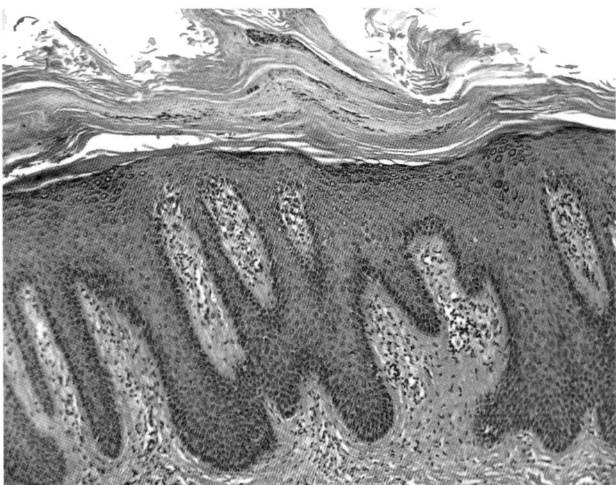

FIGURE 25-18 ■ Psoriasis showing confluent parakeratosis and a regular epidermal hyperplasia in which the rete ridges are of equal length. (Hematoxylin and eosin stain, original magnification ×200.)

face is more common in children than in adults and needs to be distinguished from atopic dermatitis. Similarly, psoriasis may involve the diaper area in up to 13% of patients where it must be differentiated from infantile seborrheic dermatitis and other causes of diaper dermatitis (24). Classic histologic features of psoriasis include confluent parakeratosis with neutrophils (Munro microabscesses), regular elongation of epidermal rete with thin suprapapillary plates, dilated vessels in dermal papillae, and mild superficial perivascular inflammation (Figure 25-18). Dermatophytes can produce a psoriasiform dermatitis.

Psoriasis, a multifactorial disorder with a genetic basis, typically runs a chronic course with remissions and flare-ups.

Seborrheic Dermatitis

A chronic dermatosis of unknown cause, seborrheic dermatitis is quite common in infants aged 2 to 10 weeks and in adolescents. In infants, seborrheic dermatitis begins as an erythematous scaly rash typically involving the scalp, face, and diaper area. In adolescents, it appears as a dry fine exfoliation of the scalp (dandruff) and expands to the face with the clinical features sometimes overlapping with those of psoriasis.

Histopathologic features overlap with psoriasis and spongiotic dermatitis and consist of epidermal hyperplasia and spongiosis with exocytosis and patchy parakeratosis, which is often present at the openings of the follicular infundibula. A mild superficial perivascular lymphohistiocytic inflammation is present in the dermis.

Infantile seborrheic dermatitis may clinically mimic Langerhans cell histiocytosis, which is a potentially serious disorder.

Lichen Planus

More commonly a disease of adulthood, lichen planus, generally a self-limiting pruritic eruption, is generally considered uncommon in children (120). However, children of

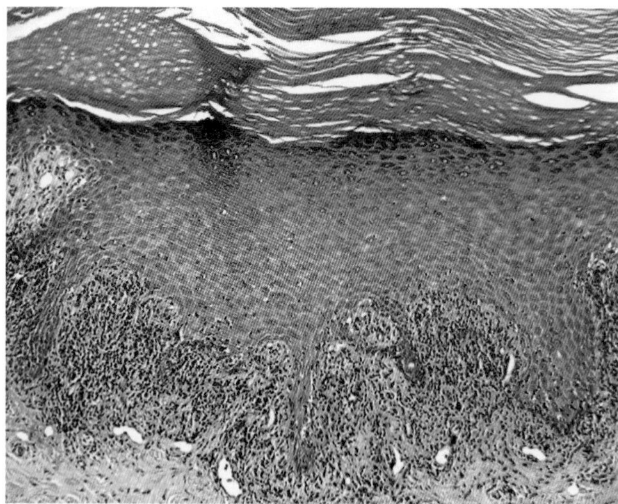

FIGURE 25-19 Lichen planus showing hyperkeratosis, hypergranulosis, irregular epidermal hyperplasia, and a bandlike lymphohistiocytic infiltrate that obscures the dermoepidermal junction. (Hematoxylin and eosin stain, original magnification ×400.)

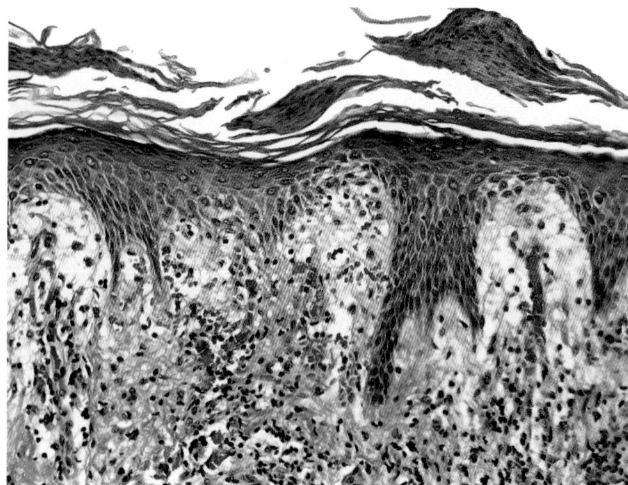

FIGURE 25-20 Pityriasis rosea showing patchy parakeratosis (mounding parakeratosis) and focal spongiosis and extravasated red cells and inflammatory cells in the superficial dermis. (Hematoxylin and eosin stain, original magnification ×200.)

South Asian subcontinent appear to be more susceptible to developing lichen planus (14). The clinical appearance of the eruption is distinctive and consists of flat-topped violaceous papules involving flexor aspects of the extremities and lower back. Lichen planus can also involve hair, nails, and mucous membranes in a significant number of cases. The histologic features are distinctive and consist of hyperkeratosis, hypergranulosis, irregular epidermal hyperplasia, and a bandlike lymphohistiocytic infiltrate that obscures the dermoepidermal junction (lichenoid dermatitis) where there are vacuolar alterations and colloid bodies (Figure 25-19). Melanophages are seen in the infiltrate in older lesions.

The etiology of lichen planus is unknown in most cases, whereas in others, various drugs have been implicated.

Pityriasis Rosea

Pityriasis rosea is an acute, self-limiting papulosquamous eruption appearing in children, especially adolescents, up to 45% of the time (40). It typically presents with a single large scaly plaque, the herald patch on the trunk that is followed within a week by more disseminated smaller oval scaly pink papules along the lines of skin cleavage. In addition to the trunk, the neck and proximal extremities may be involved. Histologic sections show focal parakeratosis, focal spongiosis, and a mild superficial perivascular lymphohistiocytic infiltrate. Extravasated red blood cells are often present in the papillary dermis and may extend into the epidermis (Figure 25-20). Biopsy of the herald patch also shows epidermal hyperplasia and denser infiltrate of inflammatory cells. A viral etiology has been suspected for a long time, and in recent years, viruses such as human herpes virus 7 and parvovirus have been implicated in the etiology (26). Most cases of pityriasis rosea resolve within 6 to 12 weeks with no specific treatment.

Pityriasis Rubra Pilaris

Pityriasis rubra pilaris is a chronic follicular-based erythematous papular eruption of unknown etiology that can manifest in children (5). Although most cases are acquired, a familial form is also recognized. Keratoderma of the palms and soles develops in a majority of the affected children and about 40% show cephalic involvement. Histologic findings include epidermal hyperplasia, alternating hyperkeratosis and parakeratosis oriented in both vertical and horizontal directions, and a mild superficial perivascular lymphocytic infiltrate. Follicular plugging is present in biopsies of the follicular papules (Figure 25-21).

Spontaneous resolution of the cutaneous rash is expected in a majority of the cases within 2 to 3 years, whereas recurrences and a protracted course may occur in others.

Pityriasis Lichenoides

Pityriasis lichenoides is a self-limiting cutaneous eruption of unknown cause that can occur in pediatric patients, commonly

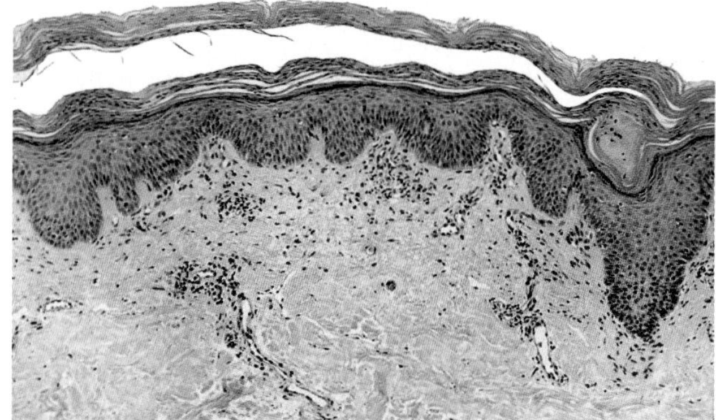

FIGURE 25-21 Pityriasis rubra pilaris showing mild epidermal hyperplasia with alternating layers of hyperketatosis and parakeratosis and follicular plugging. (Hematoxylin and eosin stain, original magnification ×200.)

during the first decade of life (59). The cutaneous eruption may be delineated along a spectrum including an acute, more severe form, pityriasis lichenoides et varioliformis acuta (PLEVA, Mucha-Habermann disease), and a chronic milder form, pityriasis lichenoides chronica. Transitional forms in between the two extremes are recognized in children. In addition, a more severe but rare variant, the acute febrile ulceronecrotic form, which is more common in children, has also been described (109). PLEVA is characterized by an extensive papular, papulonecrotic, and occasionally, vesiculopustular eruption on the trunk and proximal extremities that resolves within a few weeks. As the older lesions resolve, crops of newer lesions continue to appear, and the overall course may be protracted to several months. The ulceronecrotic form is characterized by large coalescing ulceronecrotic nodules and plaques associated with high fever.

The chronic form of pityriasis lichenoides chronica is characterized by recurrent crops of reddish-brown papules with an adherent scale that typically resolve within 3 to 6 weeks without scarring. Transient postinflammatory pigmentary changes may occur.

Histopathologic findings in pityriasis lichenoides include interface dermatitis with parakeratosis, epidermal spongiosis, necrotic keratinocytes, and a perivascular lymphocytic infiltrate. Papillary dermal edema and extravasated red cells may be present. In PLEVA, the inflammatory cell infiltrate is dense and deep, and spongiosis and epidermal necrosis are more marked with eventual erosion or ulceration of the epidermis with overlying parakeratotic scale crust containing neutrophils (Figure 25-22).

Clinical and histopathologic findings may show some overlap with lymphomatoid papulosis, a benign, recurrent self-healing dermatosis that falls within the spectrum of CD30-positive cutaneous lymphoproliferative disorders. Studies have shown T-cell clonality in pityriasis lichenoides, especially in the acute form (122,203), suggesting that host immune reaction prevents further progression to lymphoma. Although evolution to cutaneous T-cell lymphoma has been reported (144), in a long-term follow-up study of 89 children with pityriasis lichenoides, the clinical course was essentially benign, with no evolution into lymphomatoid papulosis or lymphoma (73).

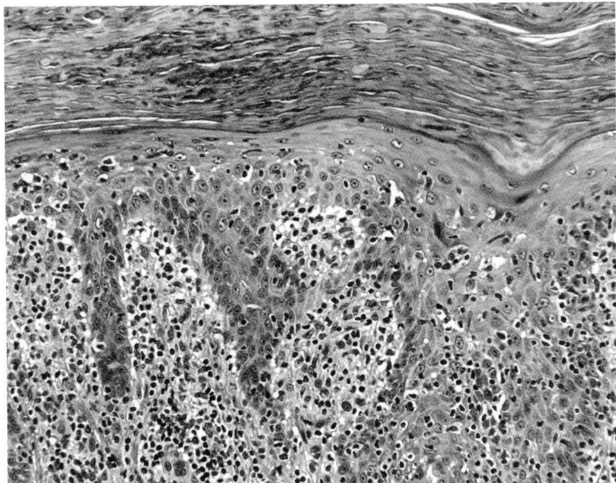

FIGURE 25-22 ■ Pityriasis lichenoides et varioliformis acuta with mounds of parakeratosis containing neutrophils and interface dermatitis with vacuolar alteration of the basal cell layer and necrotic keratinocytes. (Hematoxylin and eosin stain, original magnification ×200.)

Papular Acrodermatitis of Childhood

Papular acrodermatitis of childhood, or Gianotti-Crosti syndrome, is a self-limiting papular and papulovesicular eruption involving the face, extremities, and buttocks of children aged 2 to 6 years with an underlying viral infection. Since the original description of the cases in association with hepatitis B infection, a variety of other viruses including Coxsackie, Epstein-Barr, parainfluenza, pox, parvovirus B19, and HIV, and, certain bacteria as well as immunizations have been shown to be associated with similar cutaneous eruptions. In recent years, there has been a striking shift from HBV to EBV as the most common cause, although the exact mechanism of how the infectious agents cause the cutaneous eruption continues to reside in the realm of the unknown (25).

The histologic features are not specific and include focal parakeratosis, varying degrees of epidermal spongiosis with exocytosis, and a mild perivascular lymphohistiocytic infiltrate. Spongiotic vesicles, when present, contain lymphocytes and Langerhans cells.

The cutaneous eruption generally lasts for about 3 to 4 weeks, and relapses are not reported.

Lichen Sclerosus

Lichen sclerosus is generally a skin disease of adults of unknown etiology that can be seen in children (151). The majority of the affected children have involvement of the anogenital area by ivory-colored flattened papules and plaques. Human papillomavirus (HPV) has been shown to be present in some pediatric cases of lichen sclerosus (51), although the exact significance of this finding and the risk of squamous cell carcinoma in pediatric onset lichen sclerosus are undefined (150). The clinical and histopathologic findings are essentially similar to those seen in adults. The histologic features include hyperkeratosis, epidermal atrophy, and a zone of papillary dermal sclerosis, beneath which there may be a band of lymphocytes (Figure 25-23). Lichen sclerosus in childhood generally has a better prognosis, with spontaneous resolution occurring in up to 60% of the affected girls before puberty. There is some morphologic overlap with morphea.

INFECTIOUS DISEASES

Bacterial Infections

Bacterial infections of skin are a common cause for pediatric outpatient visits. Skin infection may be primary or a complication of an underlying skin disease. Occasionally, skin involvement may be a manifestation of a systemic infection.

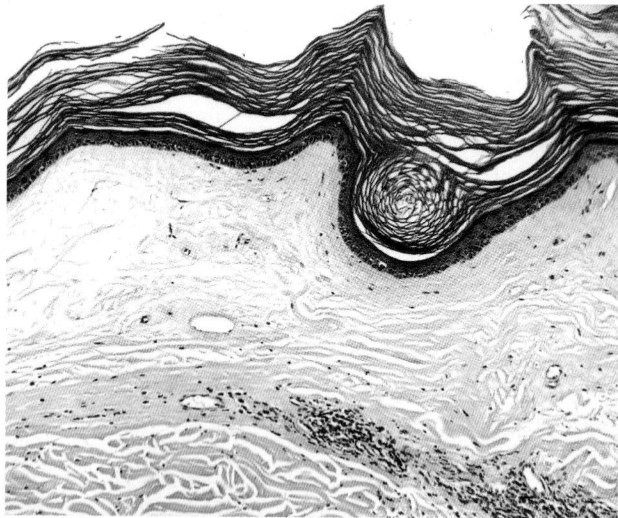

FIGURE 25-23 ■ Lichen sclerosus showing atrophy of the epidermis with zone of sclerosis underneath, which is a band of inflammatory cells. (Hematoxylin and eosin stain, original magnification ×200.)

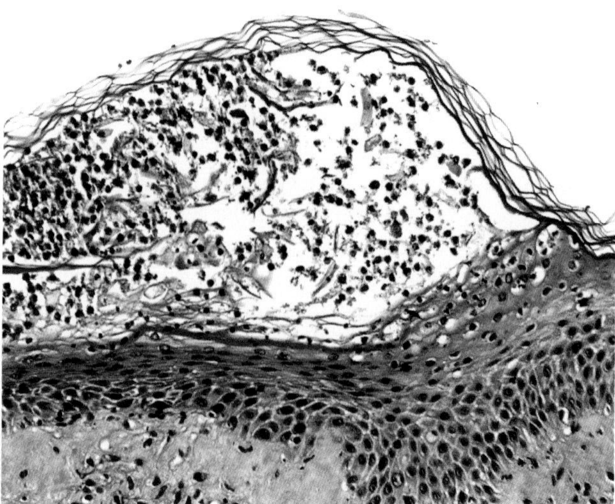

FIGURE 25-24 ■ Impetigo with its subcorneal pustule. Gram stain may show Gram-positive cocci. (Hematoxylin and eosin stain, original magnification ×200.)

Only the more common bacterial infections that often affect children are discussed.

Impetigo

Impetigo is the most common bacterial infection of the skin seen in children. Two clinical forms are recognized: nonbullous and bullous forms.

Nonbullous Impetigo (Impetigo Contagiosa)

Nonbullous impetigo or the crusted form of impetigo accounts for the majority of cases. It was historically often caused by group A β-hemolytic streptococci but now appears to be more commonly caused by *Staphylococcus aureus*. It is characterized by highly infectious 1 to 2 mm vesiculopustular lesions that quickly rupture to be covered by heavy yellow crusts. Lesions may involve any part of the body but occur most frequently on the exposed parts of the body such as face, neck, and extremities.

Histologic sections from a vesiculopustule show a subcorneal pustule, which may contain Gram-positive cocci (Figure 25-24). Sections of the crusted lesions show a neutrophilic scale crust covering the epidermis. Impetigo contagiosa may be superimposed on pre-existing skin diseases such as atopic dermatitis (4). Complete resolution of the lesions, either spontaneously or with treatment with antibiotics, occurs in most cases. Acute glomerulonephritis, a well-recognized sequela in a small percentage of patients, appears to be decreasing in incidence partly due to changing patterns in the infecting agents.

Bullous Impetigo

Bullous impetigo, caused almost always by *S. aureus*, generally affects newborn infants and children and can be thought of as a localized form of staphylococcal scalded skin syndrome (SSSS), caused by the same exfoliative toxins. It presents with small vesicles that may progress to flaccid bullae of more than 1 cm, with no associated erythema. The bullae are filled with clear fluid.

Histologic sections of the bullae show a cleavage plane in the uppermost part of the epidermis at or below the level of the granular layer, similar to the findings in SSSS. The underlying dermis shows a perivascular neutrophilic infiltrate that may also involve the epidermis. Unlike that in impetigo contagiosa, the bullous cavity contains few or no inflammatory cells.

When impetigo appears to be rapidly spreading, prompt treatment with systemic antibiotics avoids the risk of worsening infection or hospitalization (87). Although skin infections due to methicillin-resistant *S. aureus* (MRSA) are still relatively uncommon in children, given the evolving epidemiology, skin swabs should be cultured and sensitivity tests performed (21,114).

Staphylococcal Scalded Skin Syndrome

SSSS is a generalized blistering disease seen most often in neonates and children younger than 5 years of age. Like bullous impetigo, this disease is caused usually by epidermolytic toxin-producing *S. aureus*. The pathogen cannot be isolated from the lesions of SSSS; instead, a distant source of staphylococcal infection in the form of purulent pharyngitis, conjunctivitis, rhinitis, or umbilical infection may be present. Exfoliative toxins, ETA and ETB, produced by *S. aureus* target desmoglein 1, a cell-to cell-adhesion molecule found in the desmosomes of superficial epidermis and cause the cleavage in the superficial granular layer of the epidermis, typical of SSSS (7). The clinical manifestations appear to depend on serotypes of the exfoliative toxins with ETA associated with bullous impetigo and ETB with generalized SSSS (206).

SSSS is characterized by an abrupt onset of fever and diffuse erythema that evolves into large flaccid sterile bullae

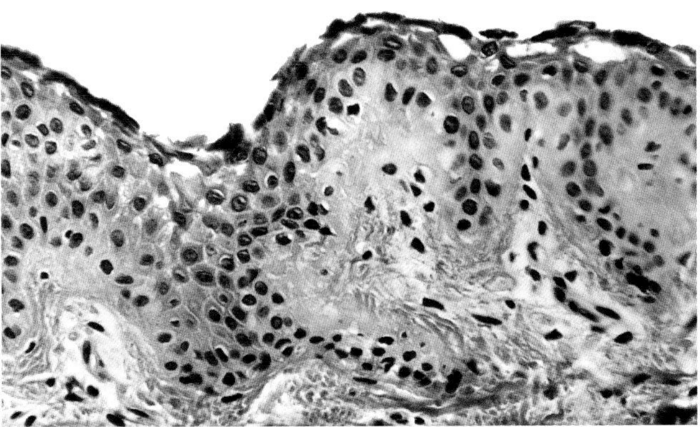

FIGURE 25-25▪Staphylococcus scalded skin syndrome showing intraepidermal clefting at the level of granular zone with minimal to absent inflammation is characteristic because the lesion is caused by toxin. [Hematoxylin and eosin stain, original magnification ×200(**A**), ×400(**B**).]

filled with clear fluid. Within a short time, the bullae rupture and large sheets of epidermis peel off, giving the typical scalded appearance. The scaly desquamation resolves within 3 to 5 days without scarring.

Histologic findings are identical to those seen in bullous impetigo, with the cleavage plane at or below the granular layer. However, in contrast to bullous impetigo, the superficial dermis in SSSS is usually free of inflammatory cells (Figure 25-25). Despite the clinical similarities, SSSS can be easily distinguished from TEN, a potentially fatal skin loss disorder, based on the histologic finding of full-thickness epidermal necrosis in the latter. In addition, mucosal involvement, often seen in TEN, is lacking in SSSS. Treatment is directed at eradicating the nidus of staphylococcus infection and management of fluids and electrolytes with complete recovery within 2 weeks expected in most pediatric patients. Fatalities are generally related to sepsis from the primary source.

Toxic Shock Syndrome

Toxic shock syndrome, although classically described in menstrual women, can occur in nonmenstrual form that is much more common now and occurs in a variety of clinical settings (98) It is an acute life-threatening multisystem disease characterized by fever, hypotension, a generalized rash, and involvement of three or more organ systems, caused by TSS toxin-1 and enterotoxins produced by a strain of *S. aureus*. In children, the most common sources of *S. aureus* infection are upper airway infections such as sinusitis and tracheitis, burns, and minor skin infections. Community-associated MRSA may be isolated from some patients (37). The cutaneous eruption is a diffuse macular erythroderma resembling scarlet fever or sunburn. The histologic findings are nonspecific and may include a spongiotic dermatitis with necrotic keratinocytes and exocytosis of neutrophils, papillary dermal edema, and perivascular and interstitial infiltrate of neutrophils and eosinophils (97). Toxic shock syndrome, similar to that caused by *S. aureus*, is occasionally caused by group A β-hemolytic streptococcus and may be associated with localized infection such as necrotizing fasciitis (127). TSS is managed with supportive therapy, identification, and aggressive treatment of source of infection.

Ecthyma

Ecthyma is an ulcerative pyoderma caused by group A β-hemolytic streptococci commonly affecting children. Like impetigo, it begins as a superficial vesicle that evolves into a vesiculopustule. This lesion enlarges and becomes crusted. Unlike impetigo, in ecthyma, the organism infects not only the epidermis but also the dermis, and consequently, the lesions heal with a scar. A history of antecedent trauma is present in most cases. Histologic features are those of ulcerative dermatitis with dense neutrophilic infiltrate. Gram-positive cocci may be identified.

Ecthyma Gangrenosum

Ecthyma gangrenosum is an ulcerative cutaneous lesion caused by *Pseudomonas aeruginosa* generally in association with pseudomonas sepsis (35). Underlying predisposing conditions such as immunodeficiency, cancer, chemotherapy, burns, and treatment with multiple antibiotics may be present. Rarely, ecthyma gangrenosum can occur in previously healthy children (212). The cutaneous lesions start as hemorrhagic bullae that rupture and form punched-out ulcers with a necrotic base. Nonulcerating nodules may be simultaneously present, which demonstrate cellulitis caused by the bacilli. Histologic sections of the ulcerated lesion demonstrate a necrotizing vasculitis at the base of the ulcer, with only a scant neutrophilic infiltrate. It is believed that the pseudomonas bacilli invade the walls of the deep subcutaneous vessels and spread along the periadventitial tissues to the dermal vessels, with resultant vascular necrosis and ulcer formation (49). The presence of Gram-negative bacilli can be demonstrated in and around the ulcer. Ecthyma gangrenosum in the absence of underlying bacteremia has a better prognosis. However, the presence of underlying pseudomonas sepsis can be rapidly fatal and requires early diagnosis, treatment with appropriate antibiotics, and surgical excision of progressive lesions to prevent mortality (110).

Erysipelas

Erysipelas is a form of superficial cellulitis of the skin caused most commonly by group A β-hemolytic streptococcus and rarely by non–group A streptococci, *S. pneumoniae* and other organisms (58). Factors that predispose pediatric patients to erysipelas included very young age, diabetes, immunocompromised states, and nephritic syndrome (33). The characteristic lesion is a well-demarcated, slightly indurated, dusky red area with an advancing border, typically on the face and recently more commonly seen on legs, especially in association with chronic lymphatic obstruction (82). Histologic sections show marked dermal edema with diffuse infiltrate of predominantly neutrophils. Dilated lymphatics and capillaries are present. Gram stain is positive for Gram-positive cocci. Septicemia, abscess formation, and rarely, necrotizing fasciitis may complicate some cases of erysipelas.

Viral Infections

Human Papillomavirus

HPV, a member of the Papovaviridae family, is a group of DNA viruses. With advances in molecular biology techniques, more than 67 types of HPV have been identified, some with specific cellular tropism. Transmission of HPV is by direct contact. Clinical patterns of HPV infection include verruca vulgaris or common wart, verruca plantaris or palmaris, verruca plana, and condyloma acuminatum. Certain HPV types manifest with characteristic type of lesions such as HPV types 2, 4, and 7 in verruca vulgaris; HPV type 3 in verruca plana; HPV types 1, 2, and 4 in palmoplantar warts; and HPV types 6 and 11 in condyloma acuminatum in children (140). However, more than one type can share the same cellular tropism.

The characteristic histologic changes of HPV infection, irrespective of the clinical pattern, are epithelial hyperplasia, which can be papillomatous, hyperkeratotic and parakeratotic, especially at the tips of the papillary projections. The cytopathic effect of HPV is manifested as an irregular and hyperchromatic nucleus surrounded by a halo of clear cytoplasm or koilocyte (Figure 25-26).

In children, verruca vulgaris is the most common pattern of HPV infection seen. In most immunocompetent hosts, spontaneous regression is the expected course. In immunocompromised patients, including patients with epidermodysplasia verruciformis (both autosomally inherited and acquired forms), widespread infection with HPV and progression to squamous cell carcinoma can occur. Oncogenetic types of HPV, such as HPV type 16, can be identified by DNA hybridization in these lesions. Sexual abuse can be a source of condyloma acuminatum in children and requires careful evaluation of the clinical findings and history (125,182). However, most cases of anogenital warts in children are likely to be the result of nonsexual transmission, that is prenatal mode and maternal history of warts may be obtained in a significant number (102).

Molluscum Contagiosum

Molluscum contagiosum is a common pediatric cutaneous infection caused by a DNA poxvirus that spreads through person-to-person contact or autoinoculation. It most commonly presents in children younger than 5 years of age with discrete, dome-shaped umbilicated waxy papules varying in size from 1 to 5 mm, involving the face, neck, axilla, abdomen, and thighs.

The histologic findings are classic and consist of epidermal hyperplasia with surface invaginations. Within the epidermal cells, there are large intracytoplasmic inclusion bodies—called *molluscum bodies*—that compress the nuclei to a thin crescent at the periphery of the cell (Figure 25-27). The molluscum bodies increase in size as the infected cells move toward the surface. Basophilic molluscum bodies are found along with the cornified layer within the invaginations. Occasionally, molluscum contagiosum can rupture into the dermis and induce an inflammatory response.

In most immunocompetent hosts, spontaneous regression of the lesions is seen without treatment. In the context of immunosuppressed states, especially HIV infection, hundreds of lesions of molluscum contagiosum may be seen with no tendency toward resolution. Hundreds of lesion in a child is cause for concern about immunodeficiency.

Herpes Virus Infection

Herpes viruses are a family of large DNA viruses that include herpes simplex virus, varicella zoster virus, cytomegalovirus, Epstein-Barr virus, and human herpesviruses 6–8.

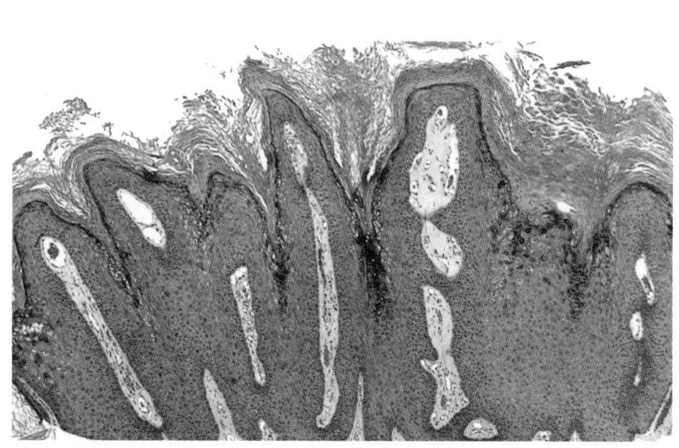

A

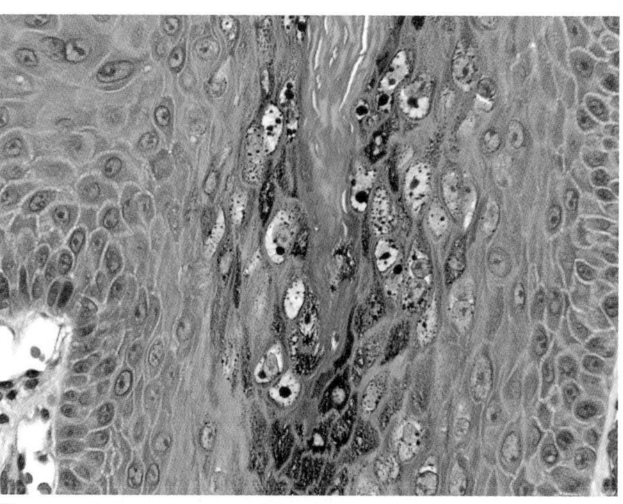

B

FIGURE 25-26 ■ Verruca vulgaris. **A:** Hyper- and parakeratosis and papillomatous epidermal hyperplasia. **B:** Hypergranulosis and koilocytosis typical of papilloma virus infection. As warts involute, koilocytes and papillomatosis become less apparent. (Hematoxylin and eosin stain, original magnification ×100.)

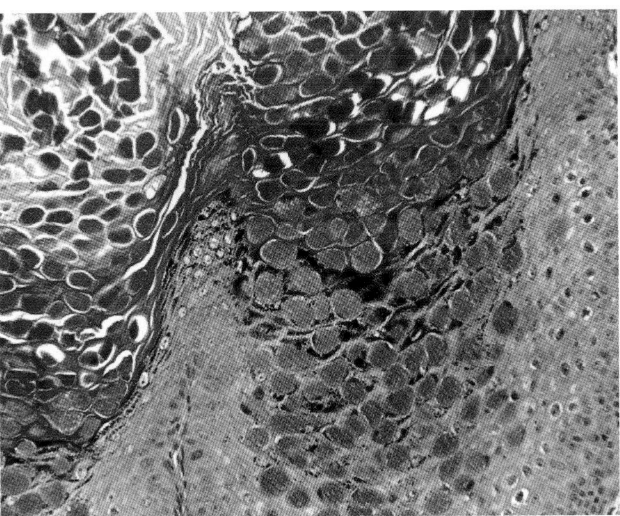

FIGURE 25-27 ▪ Molluscum contagiosum with characteristic eosinophilic round intranuclear and intracytoplasmic inclusions are seen within the hyperplastic epithelium of the follicular infundibula. (Hematoxylin and eosin stain, original magnification ×400.)

Herpes Simplex

Two forms of herpes simplex virus infections are recognized—orofacial type caused by herpes simplex virus type 1 and genital type caused by herpes simplex type 2—and both can present as primary or recurrent infections. Primary infection with HSV-I is largely a childhood disease that can manifest as gingivostomatitis and rarely as Kaposi varicelliform eruption and keratoconjunctivitis. HSV-2 is primarily acquired through sexual contact and can rarely be seen in infants owing to *in utero* infection or direct contact in the birth canal. Most primary HSV infections are asymptomatic. Recurrent HSV infection occurs in people with previous infections and is characterized by repeated episodes of lesions at the same site.

Varicella and Herpes Zoster

Herpes zoster virus commonly manifests in children as chicken pox due to primary infection with *varicella zoster* infection. Chicken pox is a highly contagious generalized vesiculopustular eruption that spreads centrifugally, with lesions in different stages of development. *Herpes zoster* is caused by reactivation of latent *varicella-zoster* virus that resides in a dorsal root ganglion and presents as grouped vesicles in a dermatomal distribution. *Herpes zoster* can develop any time after a primary infection and is often triggered by immunocompromised state. Because varicella vaccine is a live attenuated virus, *herpes zoster* can develop in a vaccine recipient. In young children, *herpes zoster* has a predilection for areas supplied by the cervical and sacral dermatomes (118).

The histologic findings are identical in herpes simplex and varicella-zoster infections. Intraepidermal vesicles with acantholysis are the characteristic feature. Balloon degeneration and multinucleated keratinocytes with eosinophilic intranuclear inclusions are seen. Epidermal necrosis with neutrophilic scale crust characterizes older lesions (Figure 25-28). Leukocytoclastic vasculitis may develop in some cases of herpes simplex.

Human Immunodeficiency Virus

In the acute stage, HIV can present with a transient viral exanthem not unlike other viral exanthems. More commonly, the cutaneous manifestations in HIV are related to immunocompromise and opportunistic infections. Mucocutaneous candidiasis, severe seborrheic dermatitis, eosinophilic pustular folliculitis, and lichenoid dermatitis of AIDS are some of the manifestations (152). In addition, a range of persistent infections including fungal infections, prolonged varicella, severe cases of herpes zoster, herpes gingivostomatitis, verrucae or condyloma acuminatum, and molluscum contagiosum can be seen in HIV-infected patients (79).

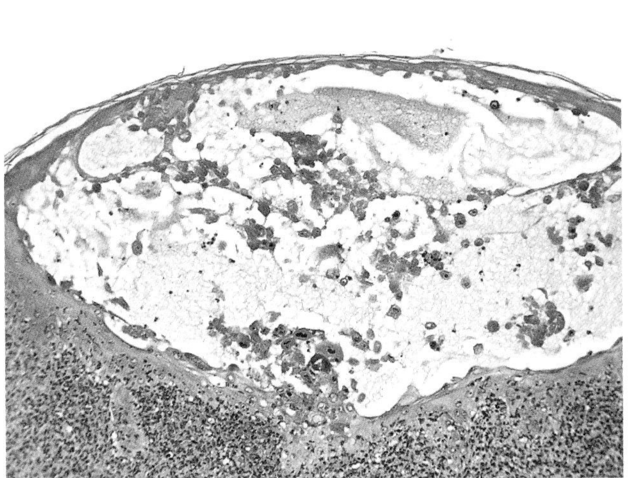

A

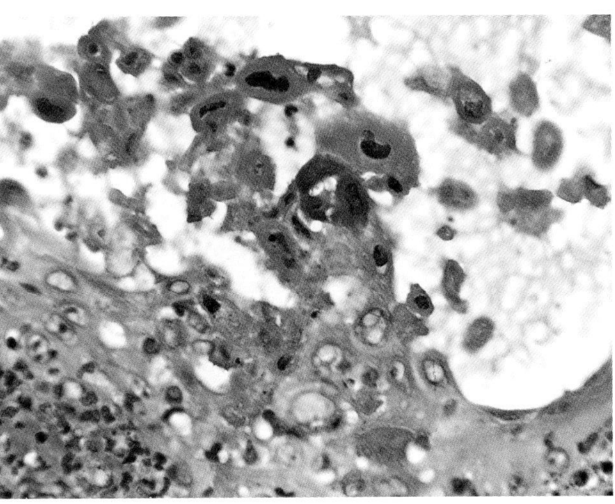

B

FIGURE 25-28 ▪ Herpetics lesions regardless of the specific virus have similar histologic features. **A:** An intraepidermal vesicle surrounded by multinucleated keratinocytes. **B:** Characteristic intranuclear inclusions are present at the margins of the vesicle. [Hematoxylin and eosin stain, original magnification ×200(**A**), ×400(**B**).]

Fungal Infections

Fungal infections of the skin can be classified as superficial and deep forms.

Superficial fungal infections of the skin include dermatophytosis (Tinea) typically caused by three genera, namely, *Trichophyton, Microsporum*, and *Epidermophyton*. In addition, *Pityrosporum* and *Candida* can also cause superficial fungal infections of the skin.

Tinea capitis is a fungal infection of the scalp and hair that is common in prepubertal children and is most often caused by *Tinea tonsurans* in the United States (57). Tinea capitis presents as one or more scaly patches of alopecia (167). With some species, such as *T. verrucosum* or *Microsporum canis*, large boggy swellings called *kerion* can develop in the infected areas. Tinea corporis is also common in children and characteristically presents with annular scaly lesions with an active inflammatory border (ringworm). The lesions can be seen anywhere on the body.

Tinea versicolor caused by *Pityrosporum ovale* involves upper trunk with areas of brownish discoloration that later appear hypopigmented.

Primary cutaneous infection with Candida is often seen in the diaper area of infants and characteristically presents as an eczematous dermatitis. Oral candidiasis (thrush) is not uncommon in infants, especially those born to HIV-positive mothers. The diagnosis of superficial fungal infections is best accomplished by demonstration of the organism by culture. KOH preparation offers a rapid method of diagnosis if the organism can be demonstrated. A biopsy of the lesion and demonstration of the organism is another reliable method of establishing diagnosis (1).

Histologically, dermatophytoses generally show mild nonspecific superficial perivascular inflammation and occasionally subcorneal neutrophilic pustules. Fungal hyphae, best seen with PAS stain, are present in the cornified layer in tinea corporis, and within the cornified layer as well as the follicle and hair shaft in tinea capitis (Figure 25-29). In kerion celsi, a marked, mixed inflammatory response with formation of dermal abscesses is seen. A granulomatous response to disrupted hair shafts may also be present.

Histologic sections from a biopsy of pityriasis versicolor show minimal inflammatory reaction. However, the short nonbranching hyphae and spores of Malassezia are easily identified within the cornified layer, even on hematoxylin and eosin–stained sections.

Deep mycosis can be primarily a cutaneous fungal infection with a propensity to involve deeper tissues or be part of systemic infections such as those involving the respiratory system or reticuloendothelial system. Primary subcutaneous mycoses often caused by saprophytic organisms include sporotrichosis, chromoblastomycosis, histoplasmosis, coccidioidomycosis, blastomycosis, and cryptococcosis. Most of these infections manifest with suppurative and granulomatous inflammation of the dermis and subcutis, with a frequent pseudoepitheliomatous epidermal hyperplasia. PAS and silver stains often reveal the characteristic morphology of the fungal organism (Figure 25-30). Deep mycosis may be part of a systemic infection, especially in immunocompromised children. Necrotizing skin lesions with vasculitis and granulomas can be seen with disseminated aspergillosis, mucormycosis, and fusarial infection. A deep necrotizing process in the subcutis should alert to a deep angioinvasive infection.

Infestations

Scabies is a highly contagious pruritic papular vesicular and pustular eruption caused by *Sarcoptes scabiei* (88). Children are often affected with rapid spread through person-to-person contact. The adult female mite lays eggs within burrows in the superficial epidermis, most commonly involving the soles, wrists, interdigital spaces, thenar eminences, and genitalia. Erythematous papules and pustules with intense pruritus and multiple excoriations characterize the clinical presentation.

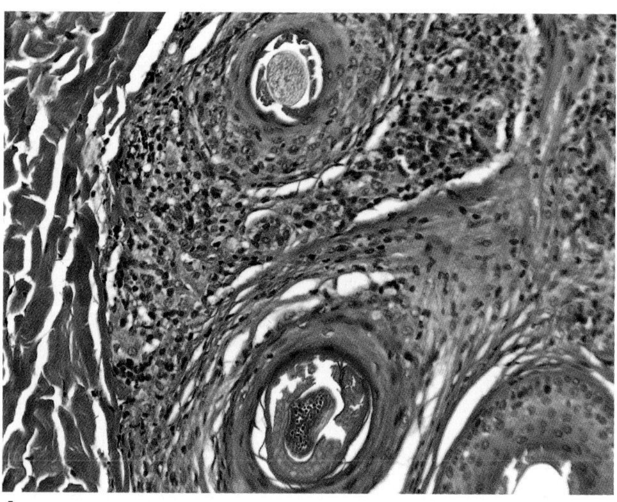
A

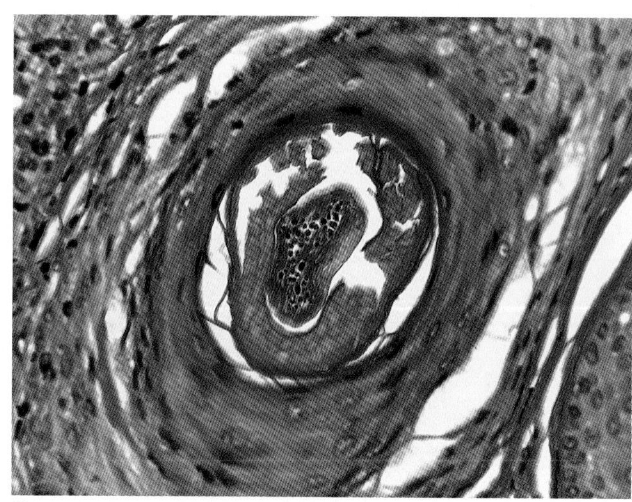
B

FIGURE 25-29 **A,B:** Tinea capitis showing involvement of a hair follicle and shaft by numerous spores. (Hematoxylin and eosin stain, original magnification ×200.)

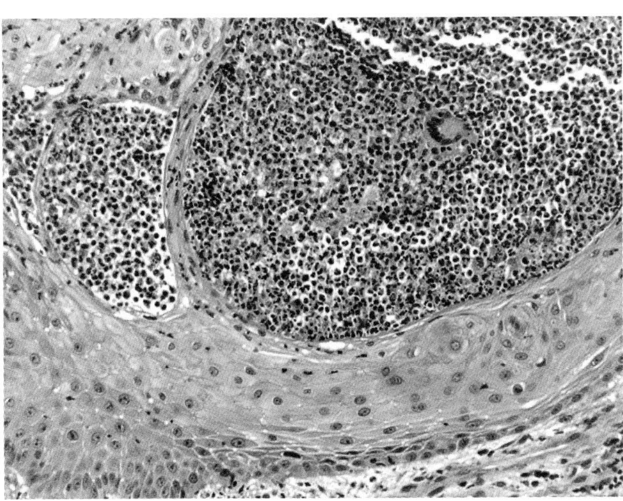
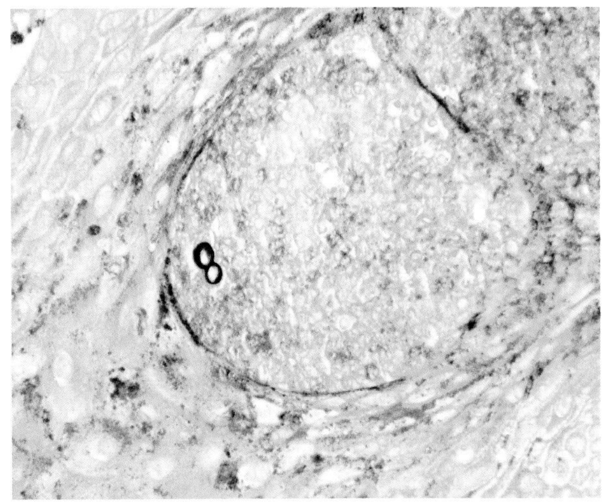

A B

FIGURE 25-30 ■ Blastomycosis. **A:** Pseudoepitheliomatous hyperplasia with suppurative and granulomatous inflammation. Broad-based budding yeast forms of blastomycosis can be seen within the cytoplasm of multinucleated giant cells or within the microabscesses, or both. (Hematoxylin and eosin stain, original magnification ×400.) **B:** GMS stain highlights the characteristic broad based budding yeast form.

A positive diagnosis can be made by scraping a burrow and examining the scrapings under a drop of mineral oil. A more aggressive approach is to biopsy a suspected lesion. Histologic sections show a superficial and deep perivascular mixed inflammatory cell infiltrate with frequent eosinophils suggestive of a hypersensitivity reaction. A definite diagnosis can be made only when the mite or eggs of *S. scabiei* are identified within the parakeratotic cornified layer.

NONINFECTIOUS INFLAMMATORY DERMATOSES

Acute Febrile Neutrophilic Dermatosis

Acute febrile neutrophilic dermatosis (Sweet syndrome) is generally a disease of adults characterized by fever, leukocytosis, violaceous plaquelike lesions on the face, trunk, and extremities, and a diffuse dermal neutrophilic infiltrate without vasculitis (42). Although the condition is rare, several reports of Sweet syndrome in children have been documented (89,96), and as in adults, many of these cases are associated with underlying malignancies or inflammatory diseases, which most often dictate the overall clinical prognosis.

Eosinophilic Cellulitis

Eosinophilic cellulitis, or Well syndrome, originally described in adults, is a rare, recurrent inflammatory dermatosis of uncertain pathogenesis. Cases of eosinophilic cellulitis have been reported in children (8) in association with various precipitating events such as viral infections and insect bites. A possible genetic factor is also suggested. Histologic features include a dense diffuse dermal infiltrate of eosinophils. Foci of collagen degeneration deposited with eosinophilic granules, referred to as *flame figures*, may be present.

Neutrophilic Eccrine Hidradenitis and Idiopathic Palmoplantar Hidradenitis

Neutrophilic eccrine hidradenitis is a generally self-limiting inflammatory dermatosis often seen in association with chemotherapy for various malignancies. Neutrophilic eccrine hidradenitis has been reported in children in association with chemotherapy for non-Hodgkin lymphoma and acute myelogenous leukemia (106). The condition is characterized by the appearance of numerous erythematous papules and plaques on the trunk and extremities within several weeks of beginning chemotherapy. Histologic sections show a dense neutrophilic infiltrate within and around the coils of eccrine glands and ducts.

Idiopathic palmoplantar hidradenitis was first described by Stahr et al. (186) primarily in otherwise healthy children and young people. It is characterized by the abrupt onset of tender erythematous papules, plaques, and nodules on the soles and, less often, palms of young patients. The ages of the patients range from 1.5 to 15 years, with increased prevalence in autumn and spring (163,179). Skin biopsy shows a dense neutrophilic infiltrate with abscess formation in and around the eccrine coil. However, special stains and microbiologic cultures are generally negative for organisms. The presence of neutrophilic abscesses and absence of squamous syringometaplasia in idiopathic palmoplantar hidradenitis aid in differentiation from neutrophilic eccrine hidradenitis. There is complete resolution of the lesions within 2 to 3 weeks with supportive therapy alone. Approximately 50% of the patients may experience a relapse that resolves spontaneously (181).

Pyoderma Gangrenosum

Pyoderma gangrenosum is an uncommon idiopathic ulceronecrotic skin disease that can present in children 4% to 5% of the time (22). A systemic illness, most often inflammatory bowel disease or hematologic disorder, is present in 50% to 74% of the patients (130). As in adults, the lower extremities are often involved. In addition, head and neck and anogenital areas appear to be more commonly involved in infants and children. A typical lesion of pyoderma gangrenosum consists of ulceration with a necrotic center, mucopurulent exudate, a violaceous undermined border, and an erythematous periphery. Histologic findings are nonspecific and vary depending on the area biopsied from a typical ulcer with necrosis and neutrophilic abscesses in the center of the lesion to endothelial swelling, fibrinoid necrosis, thrombosis, and extravasated red cells and a lymphocytic infiltrate at the erythematous periphery. Biopsy of the undermined edge shows mixed inflammatory cell infiltrate and early neutrophilic abscesses. A lymphocytic or a leukocytoclastic vasculitis was observed at the border of the lesion by some authors (199). Pyoderma gangrenosum is one in the family of neutrophilic dermatoses.

NONINFECTIOUS GRANULOMATOUS DERMATOSES

Granulomatous reaction may be seen in response to a variety of agents including infections, foreign body, and degenerative changes of collagen. In some cases, as in sarcoidosis, the inciting agent is not apparent. An infectious process should be appropriately excluded in all cases. Some granulomatous reactions such as those seen in response to ruptured cyst contents, degenerating collagen (necrobiotic granulomas), and sarcoidosis are so characteristic that a specific diagnosis can usually be rendered.

Granuloma Annulare

Granuloma annulare is a benign disorder of unknown etiology associated with degenerated collagen and is often seen in children. It is characterized by a single or multiple asymptomatic ringed papules most commonly on the dorsa of hands and feet and often mistaken for tinea.

Histologic findings are diagnostic of granuloma annulare. They consist of zones of degeneration of collagen within the upper half of the dermis, sometimes with mucinous deposits. These zones are surrounded by histiocytes arranged in a palisade (Figure 25-31). Perivascular lymphocytic infiltrates may also be present. A subcutaneous form of granuloma annulare, also known as *pseudorheumatoid nodule*, is more commonly seen in children than adults. This form presents commonly on the pretibial area or lower legs and head and neck as asymptomatic deep dermal or subcutaneous nodules. Histologic sections show large foci of myxoid degeneration of collagen surrounded by palisades of histiocytes within the deep dermis and subcutaneous tissue (187). Although mucinous degeneration rather than fibrinoid degeneration of the collagen and the absence of arthritis help differentiate subcutaneous granuloma annulare from rheumatoid nodule, this distinction is not always possible. However, the majority of patients with granuloma annulare show no serologic evidence of IgM rheumatoid factor. Deep granuloma annulare in a child may present as a soft tissue tumor.

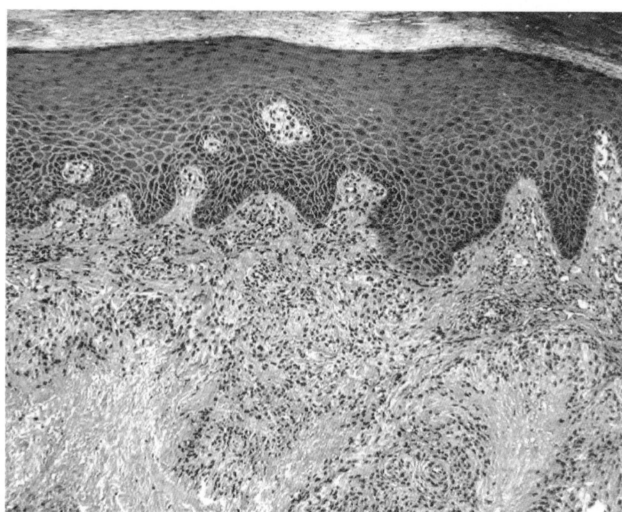

FIGURE 25-31 ■ Granuloma annulare as an upper dermal granuloma showing central myxoid degeneration of the collagen surrounded by a palisade of histiocytes. (Hematoxylin and eosin stain, original magnification ×200.)

Although an association of granuloma annulare with systemic diseases such as diabetes, lymphoma, and other malignancies and sarcoidosis has been suggested in adult patients, most of the children are otherwise healthy and progression to systemic disease of any kind is not common (62). Rare cases of underlying immune defects, such as IgA-IgG2 deficiency, have been reported in children (113). The clinical course of granuloma annulare is spontaneous regression with occasional recurrences.

Necrobiosis Lipoidica

Necrobiosis lipoidica is a degenerative disease of the dermal collagen often seen in association with diabetes. It is a disease of young adults and is rarely reported in children (148,197). Clinically, it is characterized by oval plaques, most commonly on the shins. The center of the plaque may later become atrophic with a distinctive yellow waxy hue. Histologic sections show a palisading granulomatous inflammation surrounding zones of degenerated collagen. The process may involve the entire dermis and extend up to the subcutaneous fat. Plasma cells are a frequent component of the inflammatory cell infiltrate. Late lesions show marked sclerosis and deposits of fat in the epidermis.

Rheumatoid Nodule

Juvenile rheumatoid arthritis is a chronic debilitating disease of childhood. Classic rheumatoid nodules are, however, uncommon in this form of rheumatoid arthritis. Rheumatoid nodules occur as subcutaneous nodules over the extensor surfaces. Histologically, the lesions are characterized by palisading granulomas surrounding large zones of fibrinoid degeneration of collagen. These lesions occur in patients with rheumatoid arthritis and elevated rheumatoid factors. Similar lesions occurring in the absence of rheumatoid arthritis and more commonly seen in children and referred to as *pseudorheumatoid nodule* most likely represent subcutaneous granuloma annulare (60).

Sarcoidosis

Sarcoidosis is a multisystem disorder characterized by noncaseating granulomas (Chapters 12 and 22). Although rare, sarcoidosis can be seen in children younger than the age of 15 years (132). Skin involvement is seen in approximately a 25% of the patients with sarcoidosis and up to 50% of patients have eye involvement. A subgroup of childhood sarcoidosis manifests in preschool children younger than 6 years of age with skin, joint, and eye involvement without any pulmonary lesions, which may be confused with juvenile rheumatoid arthritis (178). The cutaneous lesions of sarcoidosis are red to yellow or violaceous papules and plaques that, on histologic examination, show typical noncaseating epithelioid granulomas with little or no necrosis, similar to lesions seen in other organs. Sarcoidosis must be differentiated from infectious conditions particularly mycobacterial and deep fungal infections (124).

PANNICULITIS

Inflammation of the fat may predominantly involve either the lobules of the fat, that is, lobular panniculitis, or the fibrous septae, that is, septal panniculitis. It is important to recognize that, on histologic examination, considerable overlap may exist. Panniculitis may be a manifestation of underlying systemic disease, most notably connective tissue diseases such as lupus, dermatomyositis, polyarteritis nodosa, and juvenile rheumatoid arthritis. The histologic changes are typical and diagnostic in some entities, like erythema nodosum, whereas in others, they are nonspecific and require extensive clinical, microbiologic, and often serologic support.

Erythema Nodosum

Patients with erythema nodosum present with sudden onset of symmetric, tender, erythematous subcutaneous nodules on the extensor aspects of lower legs. A prodrome of sore throat and respiratory symptoms may be seen in some children. Histologic sections that contain subcutaneous fat show a predominantly septal pattern of inflammation with acute and chronic inflammation and thickening of the septae with some involvement of the periphery of lobules. In older lesions, granulomatous inflammation with multinucleated giant cells may be present (Figure 25-32). Necrosis within the granulomatous foci should prompt a search for microorganisms. Overt fat necrosis and vasculitis are uncommon findings.

Erythema nodosum–like reaction patterns can be seen in a variety of infections including tuberculosis, streptococcal infection, histoplasmosis, coccidioidomycosis, and occasionally mumps. Another well-recognized association is with inflammatory bowel disease.

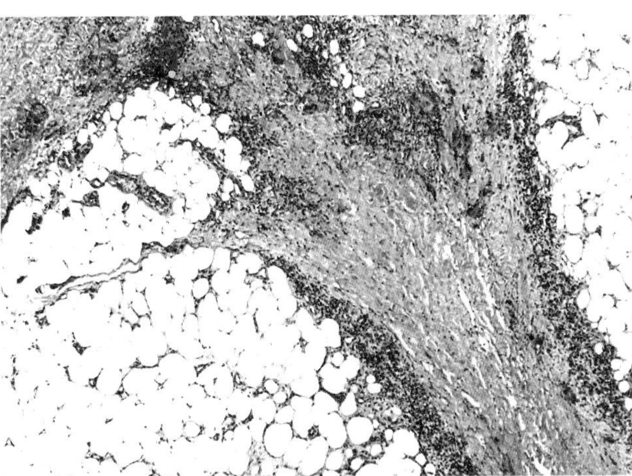

FIGURE 25-32 ▪ Erythema nodosum with a septal pattern of panniculitis and marked fibrous thickening of the septa and granulomatous inflammation. (Hematoxylin and eosin stain, original magnification ×200.)

In children, erythema nodosum is a self-limiting disease, with resolution of the lesions occurring within a few weeks. Elimination of the precipitating factor and treatment of infection, if identified, is generally sufficient (137).

Subcutaneous Fat Necrosis of the Newborn

Subcutaneous fat necrosis of the newborn is a relatively uncommon, painless, self-limiting disease that affects full-term and post-term infants (68). It manifests at 1 to 6 weeks of age as asymptomatic, firm nodules on cheeks, shoulder, back, buttocks, and thighs.

Histologic sections show a predominantly lobular involvement with foci of fat necrosis and infiltration by macrophages and multinucleated giant cells. Within the cytoplasm of the macrophages and giant cells, lipid is present as needle-shaped crystals arranged in a radial array (Figure 25-33). Deposits of calcium may be seen. The etiology of subcutaneous fat necrosis is largely unknown. Maternal factors and obstetric trauma are implicated in some cases. Spontaneous resolution of the lesions occurs within the first few months of life. Hypercalcemia is a rare complication, which if present, should be actively treated (123).

Sclerema Neonatorum

Sclerema neonatorum is a rare, rapidly spreading, diffuse hardening of the subcutaneous tissue of back, shoulders, and buttocks usually affecting premature, ill newborns. Histologic features include diffuse involvement of fat lobules by fat cells containing radially arranged crystals of lipid. Inflammation is minimal or absent, a feature that histologically distinguishes sclerema neonatorum from subcutaneous fat necrosis of newborn (209). The prognosis is generally poor, with a fatal outcome. In a case control study of neonates with sepsis and sclerema, exchange transfusion has been shown to improve survival (164).

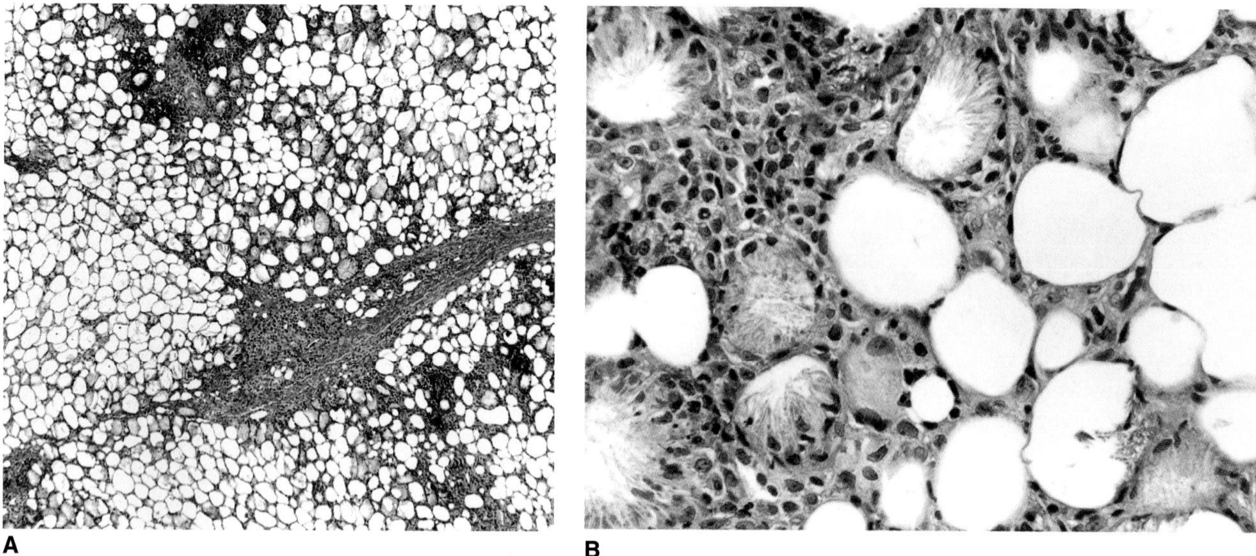

FIGURE 25-33 ■ Subcutaneous fat necrosis. **A:** Lobular pattern of panniculitis with lymphohistiocytic infiltrate. **B:** Multinucleated histiocytes contain characteristic needle-shaped crystals of lipid. Histologic differential diagnosis includes sclerema neonatorum. [Hematoxylin and eosin stain, original magnification ×200(**A**), ×400(**B**).]

VASCULITIS

Cutaneous vasculitis may be a primary disorder, but more commonly, it is a manifestation of an underlying systemic disease such as collagen vascular disease. A simple classification of vasculitis considers the type of blood vessel involved, namely, capillary, venule, or artery, and the type of inflammatory cell infiltrate involved, namely, lymphocytes and neutrophils. Although there is some debate regarding the actual classification schemes, it is generally agreed that the minimum criteria for the diagnosis of vasculitis include demonstration of actual damage to the vessel wall in the form of fibrinoid necrosis, a perivascular inflammatory cell infiltrate and red cell extravasation.

Leukocytoclastic Vasculitis

Henoch-Schönlein Purpura

Henoch-Schönlien purpura, a form of leukocytoclastic vasculitis, is the most common type of vasculitis seen in children (75,169) following streptococcal upper respiratory infection, with a peak incidence between 4 and 8 years of age. In addition to palpable purpura on buttocks and lower extremities, affected children often have arthralgias and arthritis, abdominal pain, and hematuria. A skin biopsy is of great value in the diagnostic workup of these patients. Histologic features typical of leukocytoclastic vasculitis are usually present and include superficial perivascular infiltrates of neutrophils, neutrophilic nuclear dust (leukocytoclasia), and extravasated red blood cells (Figure 25-34). The vessels show endothelial swelling and deposits of fibrin within the walls. IF studies are of help in differentiating other causes of leukocytoclastic vasculitis from Henoch-Schönlein purpura. Deposits of IgA in association with C3 and fibrinogen are present within the vessel walls (207).

Henoch-Schönlein purpura is a self-limiting immune complex disorder, with complete resolution occurring within 6 to 16 weeks (23).

Leukocytoclastic vasculitis may be seen secondary to infections due to either direct invasion of vessels or immune-mediated mechanisms. Meningococcal infection is a frequent cause of infectious leukocytoclastic vasculitis in children (53), in whom meningococci can be found within the endothelial cells and neutrophils. Leukocytoclastic vasculitis can also be seen in association with autoimmune diseases and secondary to use of certain drugs. An unusual variant of leukocytoclastic vasculitis, acute hemorrhagic edema of childhood (Finkelstein disease) generally affects children younger than of 3 years of age (77) and has many similarities to Henoch-Schönlein purpura (44). However, the lesions are larger and not associated with systemic symptoms. IgA may not be present by IF studies. Leukocytoclastic vasculitis in children has a relatively benign course, especially in those cases associated with infection and drugs.

Lymphocytic Vasculitis

A histologic diagnosis of lymphocytic vasculitis with authentic vascular damage and infiltration of the vessel walls with lymphocytes is only rarely documented. A lymphocytic vasculitis may be seen in insect bite reactions, PLEVA, lymphomatoid papulosis, and collagen vascular diseases. Lichen aureus and Schamberg-Majocchi purpura represent benign pigmented purpuras characterized by chronic petechiae in legs and elsewhere. Histologically, there is a superficial perivascular lymphocytic infiltrate and extravasated red cells. In older lesions, hemosiderin-laden macrophages may be seen that give the characteristic pigmented appearance. The lesions are asymptomatic and may last for months to years.

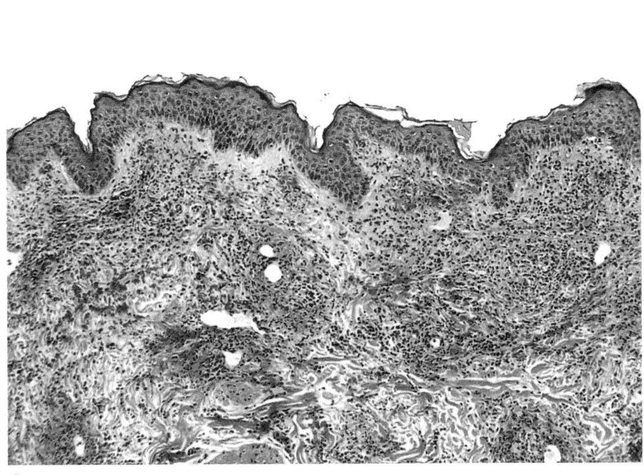

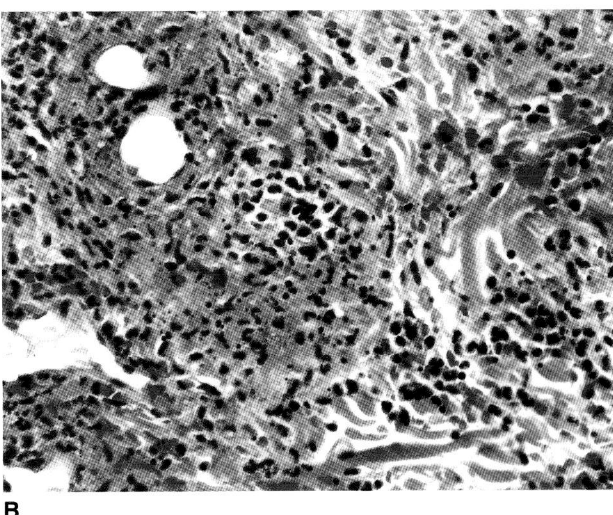

A B

FIGURE 25-34 ■ Henoch-Schönlein purpura. **A:** Superficial perivascular and interstitial infiltrate of neutrophils and extravasated red cells. **B:** Neutrophils, extravasated red blood cells, and neutrophilic dust are present. Fibrinoid necrosis of the vessel wall is seen only in later lesions. [Hematoxylin and eosin stain, original magnification ×200(**A**), ×400(**B**).]

Other rare causes of childhood vasculitis in children include polyarteritis nodosa, Wegener granulomatosis, and Churg-Strauss syndrome, which can rarely present with cutaneous symptoms (47,177). Some cases are a manifestation of a drug reaction.

FOLLICULITIS AND PERIFOLLICULITIS

Acne

Acne is a common cause of visits to the physician's office, especially among adolescents. Acne vulgaris is most common on the face and anterior and posterior trunk, where there are abundant sebaceous glands that produce more sebum in response to androgens. The primary lesion is intrafollicular hyperkeratosis, together with collection of desquamating cells and sebum with subsequent obstruction of the follicular infundibula leading to the formation of a comedone. Open comedones (blackheads) appear as large pores with central black-brown cores. Closed comedones (whiteheads) are often associated with inflammation and rupture to produce a pustule or nodule when the inflammation is deep. Nodulocystic acne and acne conglobata are severe expressions of acne vulgaris, whereas neonatal acne is a transient eruption in newborns secondary to maternal and infant androgen response (17). Persistent acne in an infant should raise suspicion of a possible androgen-producing neoplasm (100).

Eosinophilic Pustular Folliculitis

Eosinophilic pustular folliculitis, or Ofuji disease, originally described in healthy Japanese adults, can present in infancy with white-yellow pustules on the scalp and upper forehead (52). However, it is more likely that this is simply a histologic pattern that can be seen in association with a variety of diseases including scabies and insect bite reactions rather than a specific entity (211).

Histologic findings include eosinophilic spongiosis, subcorneal pustule with eosinophils, and a dense perifollicular inflammation with frequent eosinophils. Microbiologic cultures are generally negative for organisms. The eruption resolves without scarring. Eosinophilic pustular folliculitis may occur in association with HIV infection and other immunocompromised states.

SYSTEMIC DISEASES WITH CUTANEOUS MANIFESTATIONS

Collagen Vascular Diseases

Lupus erythematosus is the most common collagen vascular disease to present in childhood, followed by juvenile rheumatoid arthritis and dermatomyositis (175). Polyarteritis nodosa, scleroderma, and other collagen vascular diseases are less common.

Lupus Erythematosus

Although all forms of lupus can affect children, systemic lupus erythematosus is the most common form. Childhood systemic lupus erythematosus peaks in early adolescence, with about 60% of cases occurring between the ages of 11 and 15 years. Cutaneous manifestations are the second most frequent finding (77%) next to renal involvement (84%) in pediatric patients with systemic lupus erythematosus. Discoid lupus erythematosus without clinical serologic evidence of systemic disease can occur rarely in children (166). However, discoid lupus erythematosus may be a part of systemic lupus erythematosus syndrome. Cutaneous changes of lupus erythematosus include malar rash, oral ulcerations, photosensitivity, alopecia, and discoid lupus erythematosus (92).

Neonatal lupus erythematosus is seen in newborn infants born to anti-Ro (SS-A) antibody–positive mothers (117), with the development of skin lesions and or heart block at birth to 2 months of age (134). The skin lesions consist of erythematous, nonscaling, sharply demarcated lesions with a predilection for involvement around the eyes and sometimes annular polycyclic type of lesions commonly seen in subacute cutaneous lupus erythematosus.

Sections from early lesions of systemic lupus erythematosus corresponding to the erythematous malar rash show only nonspecific changes. The histologic changes seen in well-established systemic lupus erythematosus, subacute cutaneous lupus erythematosus, neonatal lupus erythematosus, and discoid lupus erythematosus are essentially similar, varying only in degree. The characteristic changes are those of interface dermatitis with marked vacuolar alteration of the basal cell layer, where there is also a lymphocytic infiltrate that obscures the dermoepidermal junction. Additional findings include hyperkeratosis with epidermal atrophy and follicular plugging, most prominent in discoid lesions, and perivascular and periadnexal lymphocytic infiltrate. A thickened basement membrane, best seen with PAS stain, and separation at the dermoepidermal junction are seen in older lesions (Figure 25-35). Interstitial dermal mucin is also seen. Direct IF reveals a continuous granular deposit of C3, IgG, and occasionally, IgM along the dermoepidermal junction in involved and uninvolved skin in systemic lupus erythematosus and only in involved skin in discoid lupus erythematosus.

Neonatal lupus erythematosus is a transient disorder, and prognosis is generally good in the absence of heart block (158). Some of these infants may develop systemic lupus erythematosus as young adults. The prognosis in childhood systemic lupus erythematosus, like that in adults, has improved with aggressive therapy. Renal complications generally dictate the survival (see Chapter 17).

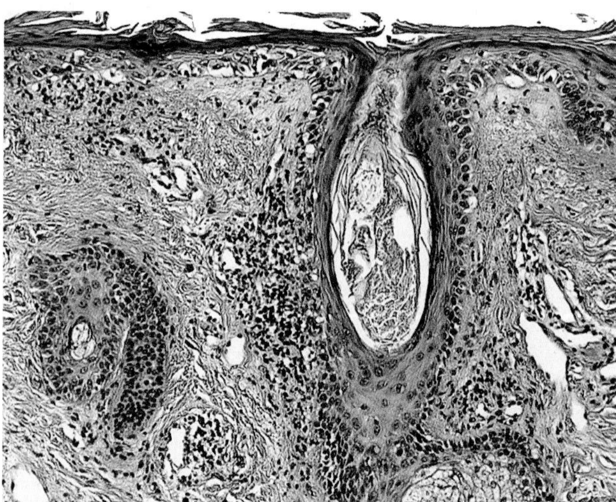

FIGURE 25-35■Lupus erythematosus: mild hyperkeratosis, atrophy of the epidermis with vacuolar alteration of the basal cell layer, smudging of the basement membrane and interface dermatitis extending around the hair follicle. (Hematoxylin and eosin stain, original magnification ×400.)

Scleroderma or Progressive Systemic Sclerosus

Scleroderma or progressive systemic sclerosus in children shows a significantly less frequent involvement of all organs, a higher prevalence of arthritis and myositis, and a better outcome than in adults (213). The localized form of scleroderma or morphea is a disease of children and young adults. It can present as plaque, linear, guttate, or generalized forms. Histologic findings vary according to the duration of the lesion. In active lesions, there is a superficial and deep perivascular and interstitial lymphocytic infiltrate that extends into the subcutaneous tissue associated with thickened collagen bundles. In older lesions, the inflammatory component is mild or absent, and hyalinized collagen bundles replace the entire dermis and extend into the septa of the subcutaneous fat (Figure 25-36). The prognosis of morphea is generally good, with the lesions healing with atrophy and eventual cessation of new lesions occurring. Sclerodermoid skin changes may occur in chronic graft-versus host disease.

GRAFT-VERSUS-HOST DISEASE

Graft-versus-host disease is a response seen in immunocompromised hosts to immunocompetent donor cells. In children, this is most often seen as a complication of hematopoietic stem cell transplantation in the treatment of acute leukemia or following a nonirradiated blood transfusion in an immunocompromised infant (99). The cutaneous findings of acute graft-versus-host disease include a pruritic maculopapular

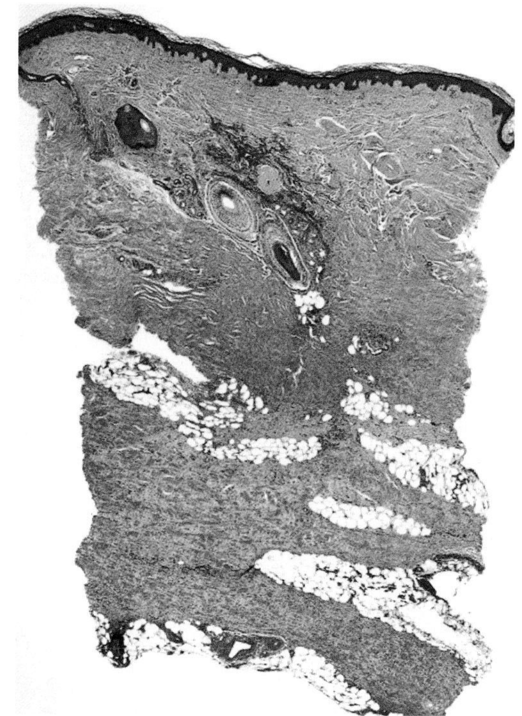

FIGURE 25-36■Scleroderma showing the characteristically rectangular biopsy with dense dermal sclerosis and thickening of the septae in the subcutaneous fat. (Hematoxylin and eosin stain, original magnification ×200.)

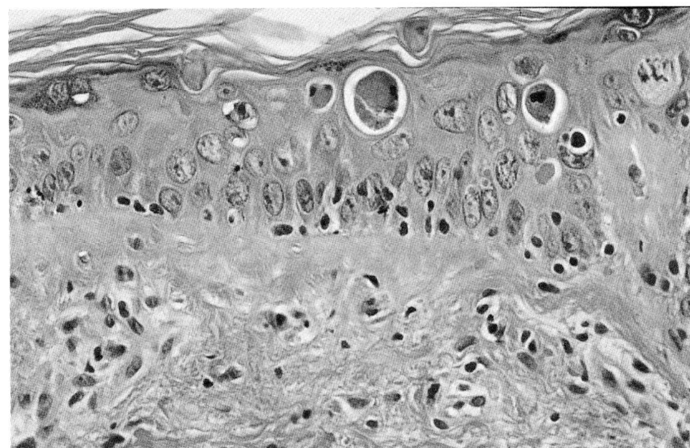

FIGURE 25-37 ■ Acute graft-versus-host disease showing vacuolar alteration of the basal cell layer with scattered "apoptotic" keratinocytes surrounded by few lymphocytes. The changes are those of an interface dermatitis. (Hematoxylin and eosin stain, original magnification ×400.)

eruption, which can become exfoliative. The histologic findings in acute graft-versus-host disease closely resemble those of erythema multiforme and TEN, and consist of vacuolar alteration of the basal cell layer with necrotic keratinocytes, some of which are surrounded by lymphocytes, the so-called satellite necrosis (Figure 25-37). In severe cases, there is marked epidermal necrosis with formation of subepidermal bullae. A subacute lesion of graft-versus-host disease resembles lichen planus, with a dense bandlike lymphocytic infiltrate that obscures the dermoepidermal junction. In the chronic form, the histologic changes closely resemble those of scleroderma, with hyalinization of collagen bundles. Vacuolar alteration at the basal cell layer and satellite necrosis, if present, may help in the differential diagnosis in all stages.

The prognosis for graft-versus-host disease is generally good when the disease is localized to skin alone. Early treatment may be of help in preventing joint contractures and disability associated with chronic graft-versus-host disease. In recent reports, a significantly higher mortality was observed in children with sclerodermatous graft versus host disease (194). The differential diagnosis includes host lymphocyte recovery and drug reaction in the first 30 days.

METABOLIC DISORDERS

Calcinosis Cutis

Cutaneous calcifications may be of the localized dystrophic type or systemic metastatic type. One type of localized calcinosis is subepidermal calcific nodules seen on the heels of infants following repeated heel sticks (Figure 25-38). Idiopathic subepidermal calcific nodules can be seen at birth (84). Calcinosis may be a manifestation of systemic disease such as dermatomyositis and, rarely, scleroderma and renal failure (193). Tumoral calcinosis seen around joint areas is mainly a disease of children which presents as a soft tissue tumor.

Other metabolic diseases like amyloidosis, porphyrias, and mucinoses can involve the skin but are not common in pediatric age groups.

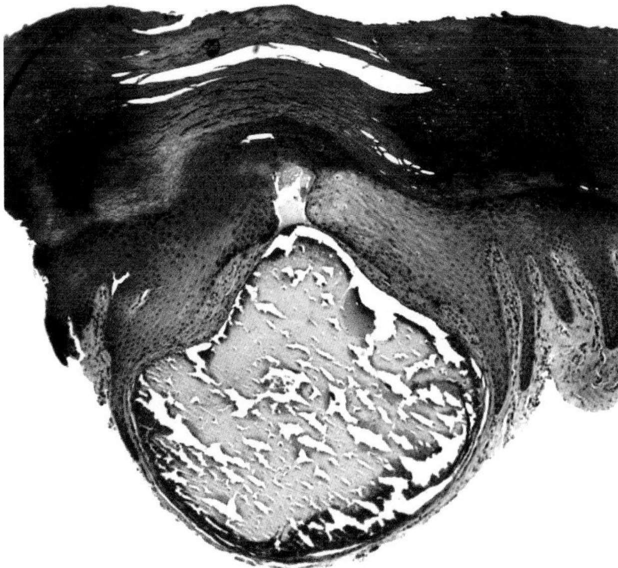

FIGURE 25-38 ■ Subepidermal calcified nodule at the site of a heel stick. (Hematoxylin and eosin stain, original magnification ×40.)

Mucopolysaccharidoses

Mucopolysaccharidoses are lysosomal enzyme deficiency disorders that manifest with abnormal accumulations of mucopolysaccharides in many organs including the skin. In all types of mucopolysaccharidoses, the skin may appear thickened and inelastic. Biopsy sections stained with Giemsa stain show metachromatic granules within fibroblasts. By electron microscopy, membrane-bound finely granular deposits can be seen in the cytoplasm of fibroblasts (Figure 25-39) (see Chapter 5).

CYSTS, NEOPLASMS, AND HAMARTOMAS

Epidermal Nevi

Epidermal nevi are proliferations of epidermal keratinocytes that present as rough-surfaced lesions at birth or shortly thereafter. Clinically, they may be localized to palms and soles, widespread or segmental in distribution. Clinical patterns of expression include linear, zosteriform, and whorled. Histologic sections usually show a single pattern throughout the lesion. Various histologic patterns that are seen in epidermal nevi include epidermolytic hyperkeratosis, focal acantholytic dyskeratosis, verrucous hyperkeratosis, inflammatory linear verrucous epidermal nevus, seborrheic keratosis-like (Figure 25-40), and veruciform xanthomatosis (190). Abnormally formed pilosebaceous units, often in excess numbers, are the features of nevus sebaceus of Jadassohn.

Epidermal nevi are generally stable benign lesions, and transformation to benign or malignant neoplasms is rare but well described in adults. Some epidermal nevi are associated with extracutaneous manifestations, notably of the central nervous, skeletal, and renal systems, and are called *epidermal nevus syndromes* that are likely due to specific genetic defects (162,191).

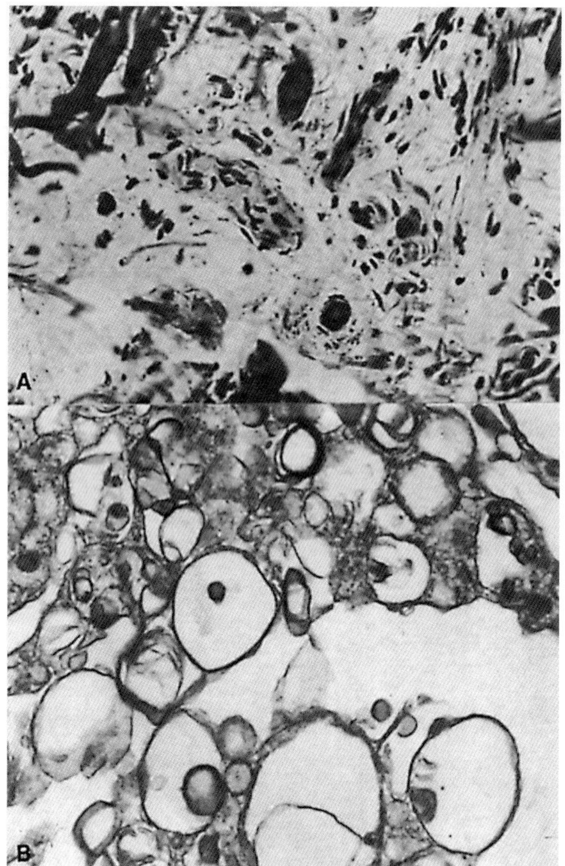

FIGURE 25-39 ■ **A:** Hurler syndrome showing a skin biopsy specimen with questionable increase in dermal metachromasia. (Toluidine blue stain, original magnification ×400.) **B:** Electron microscopy of fibroblasts, endothelial cells, and macrophages disclosed numerous membrane-bound vacuoles, some with granular and lamellar electron-dense contents. (Uranyl acetate and lead citrate stain, original magnification ×40,000.)

Non-neoplastic epithelial cysts are among the most common tumorous lesions seen in children.

Epidermal Inclusion Cyst

Epidermal inclusion cyst or keratinous cyst presents as a single firm dermal nodule that shows a keratinizing stratified squamous epithelial-lined cyst filled with laminated keratin or pilar keratin in the case of a tricholemmal cyst. Multiple epidermal inclusion cysts are seen in Gardner syndrome (71). Milia that can be seen occasionally on the face of a neonate are small epidermal inclusion cysts. Milial cysts are not associated with a formed hair follicle.

Dermoid Cyst

Dermoid cysts are developmental in origin and arise along lines of embryonic suture closures. Common sites of involvement are the periorbital region, midline of nose, scalp, and anterior neck (154). Dermoid cysts are lined by keratinizing squamous epithelium. In contrast to epidermal inclusion cysts, the lining also contains folliculosebaceous and apocrine

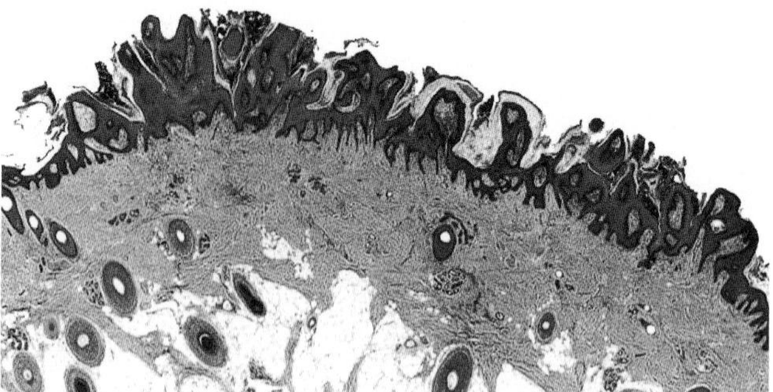

FIGURE 25-40 ■ Epidermal nevus showing hyperkeratosis and papillomatous epidermal hyperplasia. Note that the adnexal structures are normal. (Hematoxylin and eosin stain, original magnification ×200.)

units, and sebum and hair are seen in addition to laminated keratin in the cyst contents. There is a resemblance to a steatocystoma. Simple excision is the treatment of choice. Midline dermoid cysts may be accompanied by a sinus tract and should be evaluated radiologically before surgery.

Eruptive Vellus Hair Cyst

Eruptive vellus hair cysts occur as multiple soft asymptomatic follicular papules of sudden onset in children and young adults. The sites of predilection are anterior chest, extremities, face, neck, and posterior trunk. Histologic sections show a squamous epithelial-lined cyst filled with laminated keratin and numerous hairs cut transversely and obliquely. An autosomal dominant developmental abnormality of vellus hair follicles is believed to be the underlying etiology.

Steatocystoma Multiplex

Steatocystoma multiplex is an autosomal dominant disorder seen as multiple small cystic lesions most commonly in the axillae, sternal region, and on the arms. The cysts are lined by stratified squamous epithelium, with only two to three cell layers and covered with a thick homogeneous eosinophilic cuticle (Figure 25-41). Flattened sebaceous lobules can be

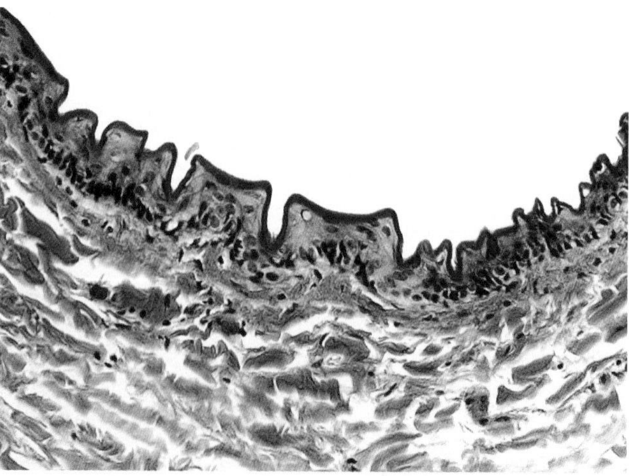

FIGURE 25-41 ■ Steatocystoma: cyst lined by stratified squamous epithelium with only two to three cell layers and a thick homogeneous eosinophilic cuticle. (Hematoxylin and eosin stain, original magnification ×200.)

seen in the vicinity. It is generally believed that eruptive vellus hair cysts and steatocystoma multiplex are variable expressions of the same disorder with overlapping clinical and histologic features (39,146).

ADNEXAL TUMORS

Adnexal tumors occur in children less commonly than in adults. Of the adnexal tumors, tumors with follicular differentiation account for the majority. Pilomatrixoma, also known as *calcifying epithelioma of Malherbe*, is perhaps the most common adnexal neoplasm seen in the pediatric age group (41). *Pilomatrixomas* present with increased frequency in the first and the sixth decades, with the head and neck area being the most common site. Clinically, they present as a hard dermal or a subcutaneous nodule (103). Familial occurrences and multiple lesions are documented (12,155).

Histologic changes follow a distinct chronologic sequence. Early lesions begin as cystic structures lined by matrical and supramatrical cells similar to those in the bulb of normal hair follicles. As the cells mature, the nuclei disappear and leave ghosts of completely cornified cells, or the "shadow cells." Fully developed lesions show irregularly shaped and sized lobules of matrical and supramatrical cells. Each lobule shows maturation toward the center in the form of masses of "shadow cells" (Figure 25-42). With time, the lesion shows signs of regression in the form of less apparent or even absent peripheral epithelial elements and consists mostly of the shadow cells, which may be surrounded by granulation tissue and granulomatous inflammation. Late lesions show no epithelial component and consist only of masses of cornified cells with extensive calcification and occasionally ossification (3).

At all times, the benign nature of the neoplasm is apparent from the sharp circumscription seen at the periphery. In early lesions, mitotic figures may be frequent in keeping with the proliferative phase of the neoplasm and do not imply malignancy.

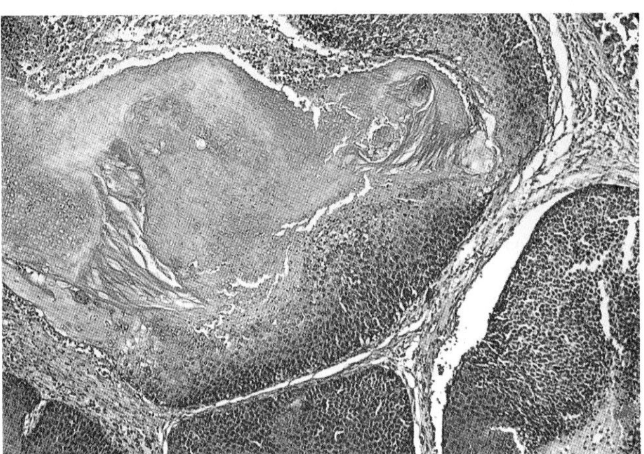

FIGURE 25-42 ■ Pilomatrixoma is a well-circumscribed cystlike lesion with proliferation of basaloid cells that cornify in a peculiar pattern resulting in formation of shadow or ghost cells. (Hematoxylin and eosin stain, original magnification ×40.)

Trichoepithelioma often presents as solitary, flesh-colored papules occurring on the face. Less commonly, it presents as multiple lesions, transmitted as an autosomal dominant disorder.

Histologically, the silhouette is that of a benign neoplasm composed of germinative cells embedded in a cellular fibrocytic stroma. The germinative cells can be arranged as nodules or cribriform and retiform patterns, and are usually encircled by mesenchymal cells like those of the embryonic perifollicular sheath. Infundibulocystic structures filled with cornified cells may be prominent trichoblastoma, a less differentiated follicular neoplasm composed of germinative cells, is another expression of trichoepithelioma.

Eccrine Neoplasms

Syringoma is a relatively common adnexal neoplasm that differentiates toward the acrosyringium of the eccrine duct. It is seen in children with greater frequency in association with trisomy 21 syndrome (172). It can present as a sudden onset eruption of small papules, usually on the face and sometimes on the vulva (72,183). Histologically, the lesions are characterized by multiple, small epithelial structures that may be solid or tubular. The tubular structures may contain granular material within the lumina. Some of the epithelial nests may have elongated or tadpole-like shapes. An important histologic feature is the confinement of the neoplasm to the upper half of the dermis, a feature helpful in distinguishing syringoma from microcystic adnexal carcinoma, especially in adults.

Other eccrine neoplasms such as eccrine poroma and eccrine acrospiroma occur infrequently in children.

Sebaceous and apocrine neoplasms: True sebaceous and apocrine neoplasms are uncommon in children. Nevus sebaceus of Jadassohn is a hamartoma that contains most elements of normal skin and subcutaneous fat and is best designated as an organoid nevus. Nevus sebaceus commonly occurs as a yellowish round-to-oval hairless plaque on the scalp, forehead, and lateral portions of the face. The clinical and histologic appearances vary considerably and follow a chronologic sequence. The yellowish pebbly appearance of these lesions at birth corresponds to prominent sebaceous lobules, a result of the effects of maternal hormones.

After infancy, the appearance and development of the sebaceous lobules in the lesions follow the growth of sebaceous units elsewhere. They are small and the epidermis is flat until puberty, when sebaceous lobules become greatly increased in number and arranged as clusters. The epidermis also becomes papillomatous. After puberty, the number of sebaceous lobules decreases but their size increases. The epidermis remains hyperplastic and verrucous (188). Rudimentary hair follicles and apocrine glands are common findings (Figure 25-43). In the postpubertal stage, nevus sebaceus can be the site of a variety of adnexal neoplasms, the most common

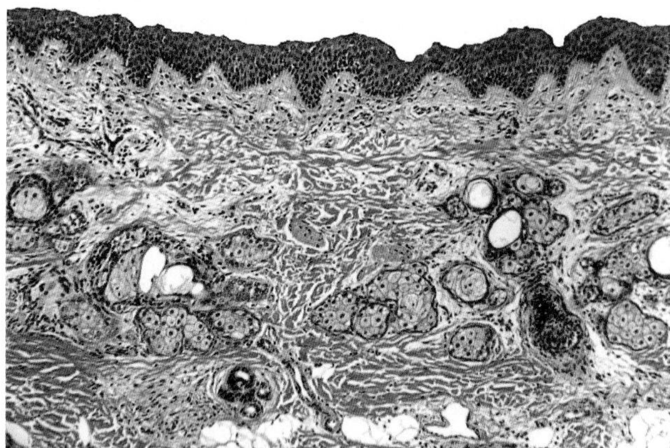

FIGURE 25-43 ■ Nevus sebaceus of Jadassohn is a broad lesion characterized by epidermal hyperplasia, numerous sebaceous lobules, poorly formed hair follicles and apocrine glands. (Hematoxylin and eosin stain, original magnification ×100.)

being trichoblastoma, followed by syringocystadenoma papilliferum and sebaceous tumors (43,108).

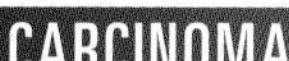

CARCINOMA

Carcinomas of the skin are extremely uncommon in childhood and usually are seen in association with hereditary syndromes. Based cell nevus syndrome, also known as *Gorlin and Gorlin-Goltz syndromes*, is an autosomal dominant disorder characterized by multiple jaw cysts, skeletal anomalies, intracranial calcifications, and multiple basal cell carcinomas that commonly appear after puberty (69). Medulloblastoma can occur in early childhood. Survivors face the problem of repeated cutaneous and internal malignancies. Many other patients affected with nevoid basal cell carcinoma can suffer from disfigurement secondary to multiple surgeries.

MELANOCYTIC NEOPLASMS

In normal skin, melanocytes are located within the basal cell layer, where they are separated by four to ten keratinocytes. A proliferation of these melanocytes may give rise to a variety of melanocytic lesions.

Melanocytic Nevi

Melanocytic nevi are of two main types, namely, congenital and acquired, and both types can be junctional, compound, or intradermal. Although melanocytic nevi may be present at birth in 1.5% to 2.0% of the population, the majority of the nevi are acquired during the first two decades of life.

Congenital Melanocytic Nevi

Congenital melanocytic nevi are first noticed at birth or shortly thereafter as variably sized pigmented lesions. Depending on the size, congenital melanocytic nevi have

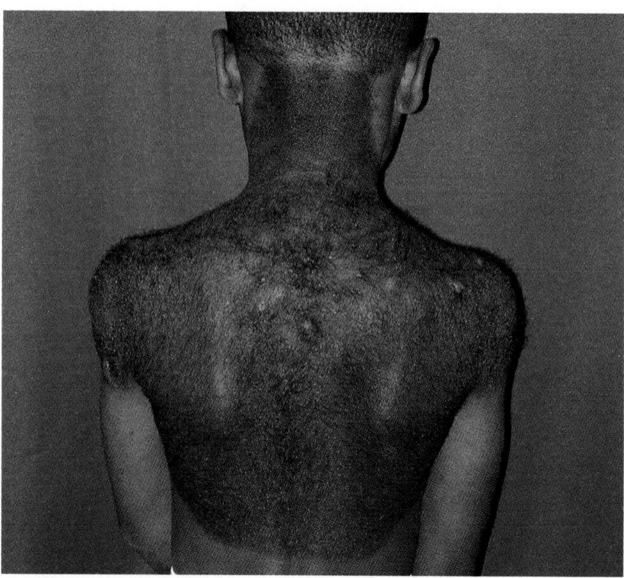

FIGURE 25-44 ■ Congenital melanocytic nevus showing a diffuse involvement of the upper trunk arms and neck. (Courtesy of Sarah Stein, M.D., Department of Medicine, University of Chicago Medical Center.)

been classified as giant (>20 cm), large (1.5 to 20 cm), and small (<1.5 cm). The bathing trunk–type giant congenital nevi are rare, and are characterized by an uneven verrucous surface, variations in shades of brown and blue, and moderate growth of hair throughout the lesions (Figure 25-44). Scattered similar but smaller satellite lesions are often present. Giant congenital nevi, when present on the head and neck region, may be associated with leptomeningeal melanocytosis and neurologic disorders (neurocutaneous melanosis). There is an increased risk of primary leptomeningeal melanoma in these cases. Large congenital nevi show mild-to-moderate variation in color and epidermal hyperplasia. Small congenital nevi are seen as solitary light tan to brown uniformly pigmented macules. Congenital nevi change with age with development of darker areas, nodules, and coarse hair.

Like acquired nevi, congenital nevi may be junctional, compound, or intradermal. It is believed that all nevi begin with increased numbers of melanocytes at the dermoepidermal junction with subsequent dropping down into the dermis. Eventually, the junctional component disappears and only the dermal component is left behind. Congenital nevi are histologically distinguished from acquired nevi by the presence of melanocytic nests and individual melanocytes around the adnexal and vascular structures as well as infiltration between the collagen bundles as individual cells. Deep infiltration into the reticular dermis, often with extension into the septa of subcutaneous fat, is a feature seen in giant congenital nevi (Figure 25-45). In smaller congenital nevi, the nests of melanocytes are located more superficially and have led some authors to classify congenital nevi on histologic grounds into superficial and deep types. Nests of larger melanocytes may be seen closer to the dermoepidermal junction with maturation to smaller monomorphous melanocytes toward the base.

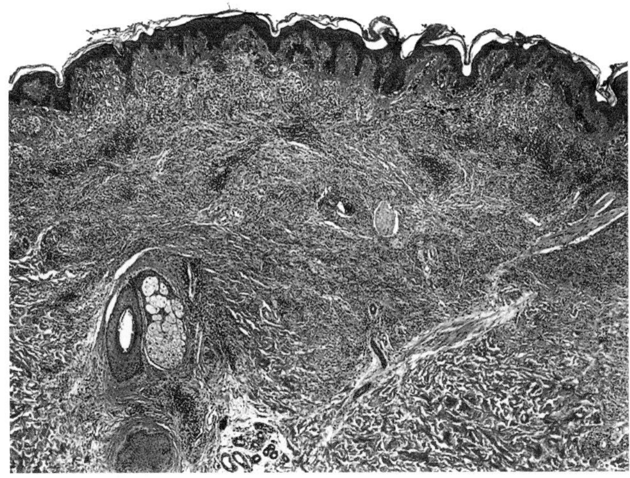

FIGURE 25-45 ▪ Compound congenital melanocytic nevus with nests of melanocytes at the dermoepidermal junction and deep in the dermis, where they infiltrate between the collagen bundles and surround the blood vessels and adnexal structures as individual cells. (Hematoxylin and eosin stain, original magnification ×100.)

Congenital Nevus and Malignant Melanoma

One of the complications of giant congenital nevus, especially when associated with leptomeningeal melanosis, is the development of malignant melanoma and other primitive malignancies such as rhabdomyosarcoma within the nevus. The estimated incidence of malignant transformation is between 4% and 12% in various reports (126), although a more recent study suggests a much lower overall risk of 0.7% (112). In one study, the relative risk of development of malignant melanoma in giant congenital nevi was 1,000 times greater than that in the general population, which supports a multistage excision approach in the treatment of giant congenital nevi. The incidence of melanoma in other congenital nevi correlates with the size of the lesion. When melanoma develops in a congenital nevus, it generally begins at the dermoepidermal junction. In some instances, especially in association with giant congenital nevus, it may begin deep in the dermis, where it consists of a nodule of undifferentiated cells which must be differentiated from "proliferative nodules", which are mistakenly diagnosed as melanomas. Heterologous differentiation and cytologic anaplasia do not necessarily imply poor prognosis.

Melanoma can appear at any time but occurs most often before puberty in giant congenital nevi and after puberty when associated with smaller congenital nevi.

Acquired Melanocytic Nevi

Most melanocytic nevi are acquired and appear within the first two decades of life and only rarely in midlife. Nevi generally begin as junctional nevi, characterized clinically by small tan to tan-brown macules and histologically by increased basal melanocytes that nest eventually at the dermoepidermal junction (56). This is followed by dermal migration of some melanocytes characteristic of a compound nevus that results in a papule formation. With progression, the junctional component eventually disappears, leaving only the dermal component of an intradermal nevus.

The number and distribution of acquired melanocytic nevi are influenced by genetics, sex, and hormonal and environmental factors. Clinically, acquired melanocytic nevi are characterized by small size, uniform color, and well-defined borders and histologically by a symmetric, well-circumscribed proliferation of monomorphous melanocytes that show well formed nests and maturation with progressive descent into the dermis. The following variations of acquired melanocytic nevi deserve special attention because some may have clinical or histologic features that make differentiation from malignant melanoma difficult.

Spitz Nevus

Spitz nevus, also known as *spindle and epithelioid cell nevus* (145), was originally described by Sophie Spitz in 1948 (185) as a juvenile form of malignant melanoma with a good prognosis. Although it is now apparent that Spitz nevus is a distinct type of nevus, distinguishing Spitz nevus from melanoma continues to be a challenge (136). Spitz nevus occurs more commonly in children before the age of 14 years as an acquired nevus and only rarely as a congenital nevus. Most Spitz nevi are solitary, small (<1 cm), and pink, and clinically mimic hemangioma or pyogenic granuloma. In rare instances, multiple lesions can occur (84). Histologically, Spitz nevus is symmetric and well circumscribed, and show maturation, features characteristic of a nevus. However, cytologically, the melanocytes are large, spindle-shaped, or epithelioid, with considerable cytologic and nuclear pleomorphism, that are features of an atypical Spitz nevus. Pagetoid spread of melanocytes into the epidermis and frequent mitotic figures further make distinction from melanoma difficult and sometimes impossible. Eosinophilic hyaline globules (Kamino bodies), often present in significant numbers, are more commonly seen in Spitz nevi. Pseudoepitheliomatous epidermal hyperplasia, hyperkeratosis and parakeratosis, patchy perivascular lymphohistiocytic inflammation, and papillary dermal vascular ectasia are other features commonly seen in Spitz nevus (Figure 25-46). Like other melanocytic nevi, Spitz nevus can be junctional, compound, or intradermal.

Halo Nevus

Halo nevus has a clinically distinct appearance characterized by the appearance of a zone of depigmentation surrounding a previously present nevus. A majority of them are seen on the back of children and young adults. Complete regression of the pigmented lesion may occur, leaving a depigmented macule. Histologically, halo nevi are characterized by the presence of dense lymphocytic inflammation with destruction of melanocytes. Destruction of the normal melanocytes at the periphery of the nevus results in the initial halo formation. Eventually, all melanocytes within the nevus may disappear and the inflammation subsides. In the earlier stage of inflammation,

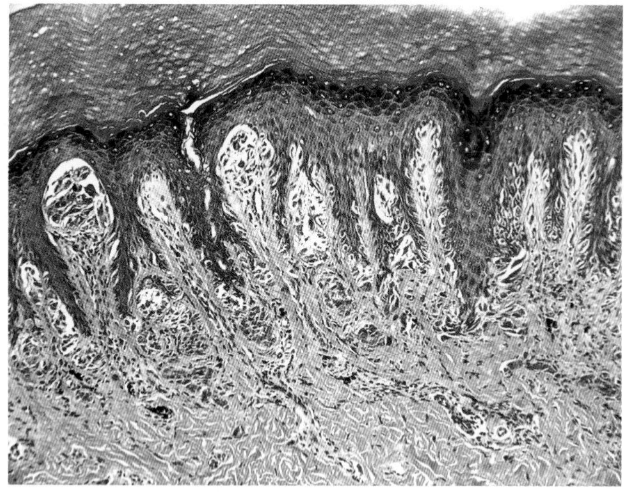

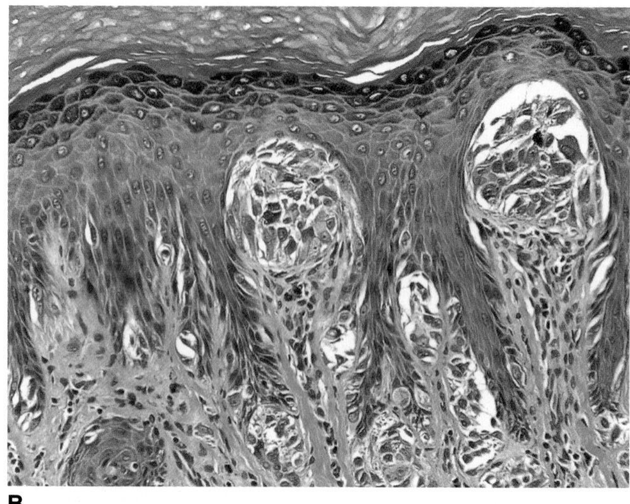

A B

FIGURE 25-46 **A:** Spindle-epithelioid (Spitz) nevus showing junctional and dermal nests of spindle- and epithelioid-shaped cells amelanocytes. The overlying epidermis is hyperkeratotic and somewhat hyperplastic. **B:** Clefts surround the vertically oriented nests of epithelioid melanocytes. (Hematoxylin and eosin stain, original magnification ×40.)

the melanocytes of the nevus may be enlarged and cytologically atypical and rare mitotic figures, when present, may cause some concern. However, the overall architecture is that of a nevus, and pagetoid spread of melanocytes is generally absent. Halo nevi are common in patients with vitiligo suggesting a common underlying immune-mediated mechanism. Occasionally, halo phenomenon may be observed around Spitz nevi and congenital nevi.

Blue Nevus

Blue nevi are rarely seen in children younger than 10 years of age. Clinically, blue nevi present as blue-gray papules. Histologically, dendritic melanocytes with melanin pigment are present as nests and fascicles extending into the deep reticular dermis. Cellular blue nevus is a variant of blue nevus, which often presents as a blue nodule on the scalp and lumbosacral region, and is histologically characterized by cellular islands of large oval cells with pale cytoplasm, in addition to the dendritic melanocytes (Figure 25-47). A variant of this nevus, the epithelioid blue nevus composed of deeply pigmented spindle-shaped cells and lightly pigmented oval to polygonal melanocytes were described in patients with Carney complex (31). Combined nevi, with features of both blue nevus and Spitz nevus, may fall within the spectrum of epithelioid blue nevus and more recently described *Pigmented epithelioid melanocytoma* (81,210). However, a combined nevus can have various patterns.

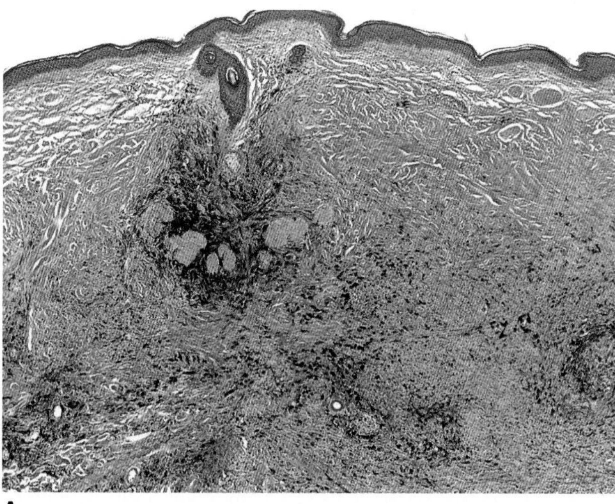

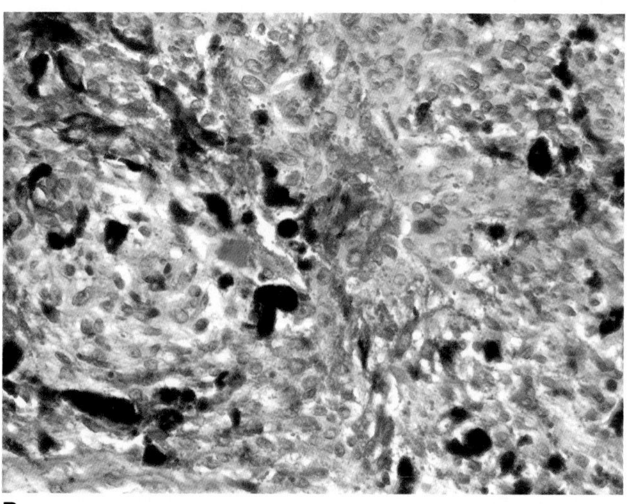

A B

FIGURE 25-47 Cellular blue nevus from the lumbosacral region of a 14-year-old girl. **A:** Interlacing spindle cells and nodular foci of cells with clear cytoplasm are shown. **B:** Pigmented spindle-shaped cells with dendritic processes are scattered throughout the lesion. (Hematoxylin and eosin stain, original magnification ×100.)

Clark Dysplastic Nevus

Originally described by Reimer et al. (156) dysplastic nevus has been the subject of considerable controversy over the last two decades. It is generally agreed now that a subgroup of population with a family history of melanoma and multiple clinically atypical-appearing nevi has a genetic predisposition to developing malignant melanoma. The histologic features of dysplastic nevi include a broad junctional or compound nevus, with nests of melanocytes bridging the adjacent rete ridges, concentric and lamellar fibroplasia and melanocytic atypia to include large size, enlarged nuclei, and abundant dusty melanin-laden cytoplasm. It must be emphasized that histologic diagnosis of dysplastic nevus is relevant in the context of appropriate clinical findings. Nevi when biopsied in very young children, particularly shortly after birth and those on genital skin, conjunctiva, palms, and soles, and recurrent nevi are notorious simulators of malignant melanoma and should be interpreted with caution in these circumstances (2). These nevi are also known as architecturally disordered nevi.

Malignant Melanoma

Less than 2% of malignant melanomas are diagnosed in children (13) and, in the absence of congenital nevus, are rare in the first decade of life. Congenital melanoma is a rare event (153,174) and can occur as a de novo process or as transplacental metastases. Malignant melanoma in children has similar clinical and histologic features as that in adults and is characterized clinically by large size, asymmetry, and irregular color and borders. Histologic features include asymmetry, poor circumscription, pagetoid melanocytes in pagetoid pattern, lack of maturation, and cytologic atypia with mitotic figures (Figure 25-48). Prognostic factors are likewise similar to those in adults and include maximum thickness of the lesion.

In addition, a distinct type of melanoma with capability for metastasis and features overlapping with Spitz nevus has been reported in prepubescent children (135). These lesions are characterized clinically by rapid growth and not conforming to the classic ABCD criteria of melanoma, and histologically by a vertical growth of large epithelioid melanocytes that fail to mature with progressive descent into the dermis. Presence of mitotic figures including atypical forms may be particularly helpful in making the correct diagnosis.

MESENCHYMAL NEOPLASMS

Neurothekeoma

Neurothekeoma are benign tumors of nerve sheath origin. In a recently published large series, 24% of the patients were 10 years old or less. The tumor presents as a solitary, superficial slow growing mass measuring 0.3 to 2 cm, most commonly involving the head and neck area and upper extremities (64). Histologically, the tumor is characterized by multinodular dermal mass composed of whorls of spindle-shaped and epithelioid cells with varying amounts of myxoid matrix in the background. The tumor cells are positive for vimentin, NKI/C3, and CD10 and negative for S-100 protein. Although the exact lineage of these tumors is uncertain, nerve sheath differentiation, as initially suggested, is not supported by the recent literature (94) (see Chapter 24).

Other neurogenic tumors in children include solitary neurofibroma and plexiform neurofibroma of von Recklinghausen disease (Figure 25-49). Rare complex neural tumors with heterologous elements have been described in neonates and infants. Metastatic neuroblastoma of the skin is seen in some children (see Chapter 24).

Vascular Tumors

True neoplasms with vascular differentiation as well as malformations of the vessels are common in children.

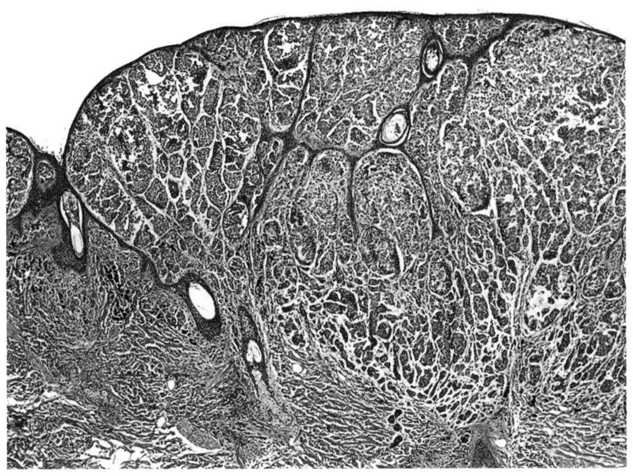

A

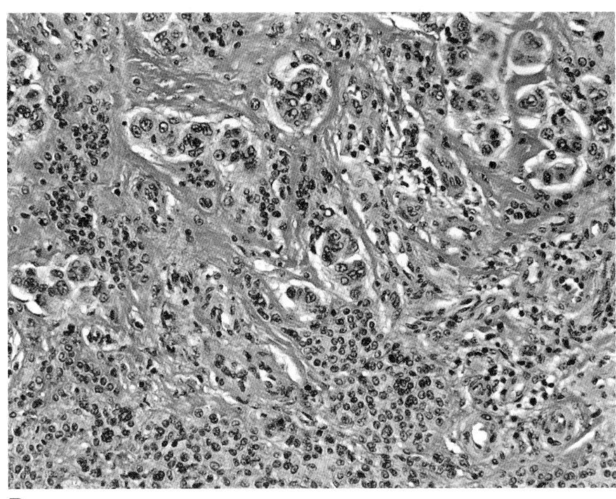

B

FIGURE 25-48 ▪ Malignant melanoma in association with congenital nevus. **A:** A nodular proliferation of large atypical melanocytes arranged in a sheet-like pattern. **B:** Atypical melanocytes of melanoma adjacent to smaller monomorphous nevus cells. Beware that this pattern may represent a non-malignant proliferation nodule.

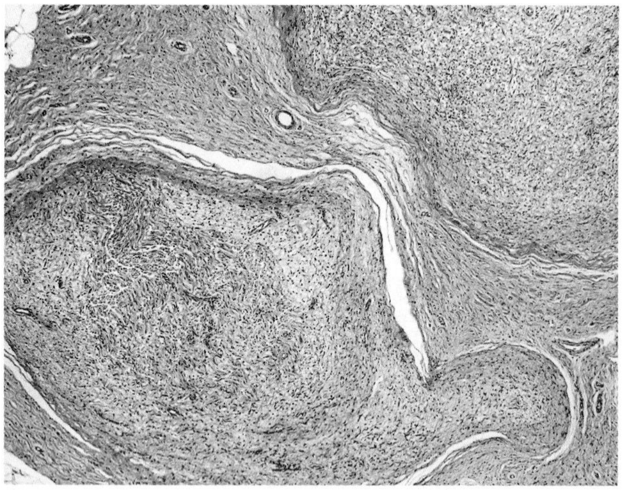

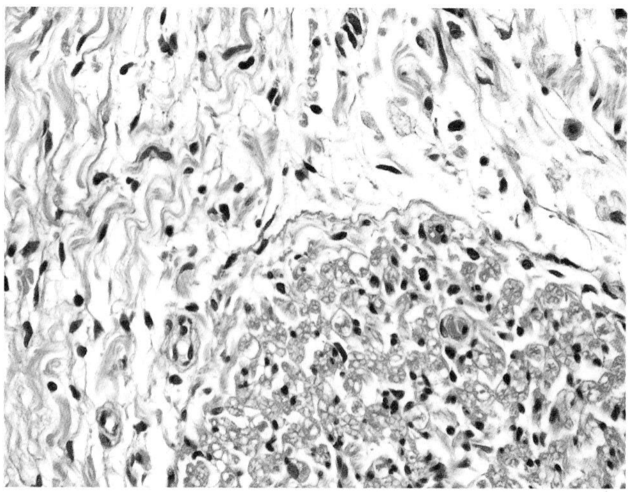

A B

FIGURE 25-49 ■ **A:** Plexiform neurofibroma from the forearm of an adolescent male showing multiple myxoid nodules in the dermis. (Hematoxylin and eosin stain; original magnification ×100.) **B:** Some cytologic atypia is present and should be furthered evaluated for possible sarcomatous transformation. (Hematoxylin and eosin stain; original magnification ×200.)

Hemangioma

Hemangioma is one of the most common benign tumors of childhood and can be superficial, deep, or mixed. It may present as a single or multiple lesions, which vary in size from 10 mm to several centimeters. The head and neck area is the most common site, with one-third being present at birth. Spontaneous regression occurs in most cases. Rarely, the large size of the lesion may cause distortion and dysfunction of neighboring structures (see Chapter 24).

Histology varies from dilated thin-walled vessels in the superficial dermis in superficial hemangioma (port-wine stain) to lobular clusters of spindle cells with barely recognizable vascular spaces in cellular hemangioma of infancy in which the endothelial cells are large and mitotically active, and may lead to a mistaken diagnosis of malignancy.

Pyogenic Granuloma

Pyogenic granuloma, also known as *lobular capillary hemangioma*, is common in children, and presents as a rapidly growing elevated bright red papule on the hand, finger, lip, or gum. Histologically, the lesion is a polypoid mass of vascular proliferation with myxoid and edematous stroma. Surface ulceration, acute and chronic inflammatory cell infiltrate, and a collarette of epidermis surrounding the lesion are other features. After an initial phase of rapid growth, the lesion persists as a stable mass unless it is surgically removed.

Tufted Hemangioma

Tufted hemangioma presents as angiomatous papules and plaques in children aged 1 to 5 years, most commonly on the upper trunk, neck, and extremities. In some patients, lesions may be present at birth (90). Histologically, the lesion is characterized by well-defined foci of closely set capillaries, discrete ovoid angiomatous lobules, or tufts within the dermis and occasionally the subcutis. Most of the lesions progress slowly over years, whereas some show spontaneous regression (27) (see Chapter 24).

Myogenic Tumors

Smooth muscle hamartoma and rhabdomyoma can be seen in children. Rhabdomyosarcomas infrequently metastasize to skin.

Congenital Infantile Myofibromatosis

Congenital infantile myofibromatosis presents generally as a solitary cutaneous or subcutaneous mass at birth or within the 1st year of life. A generalized or systemic variant with a poor prognosis is also recognized and in some cases a familial pattern of inheritance is reported (10). Histologically, both the solitary and the systemic variants show a nodular proliferation with biphasic pattern consisting of a central vascular area reminiscent of hemangiopericytoma surrounded by peripheral fascicles of spindle-shaped myofibroblasts and fibroblasts reconstructing smooth muscle tumors.

Cutaneous myofibroma has identical histologic features but presents as a well-circumscribed solitary mass in older children and adults (Figure 25-50) (see Chapter 24).

Infantile Digital Fibromatosis

Infantile digital fibromatosis is a distinctive benign tumor that occurs in the fingers and the toes of infants. It presents as a single or multiple dome-shaped lesions on the lateral or the dorsal aspect of the distal or middle phalangeal joint, most often in the fingers, sparing the thumb and the greater toes. The tumor consists of a uniform proliferation of fibroblasts surrounded by a dense collagenous stroma. Characteristic inclusion bodies, first described by Reye in 1965 (157), are present in the fibroblast cytoplasm, separated

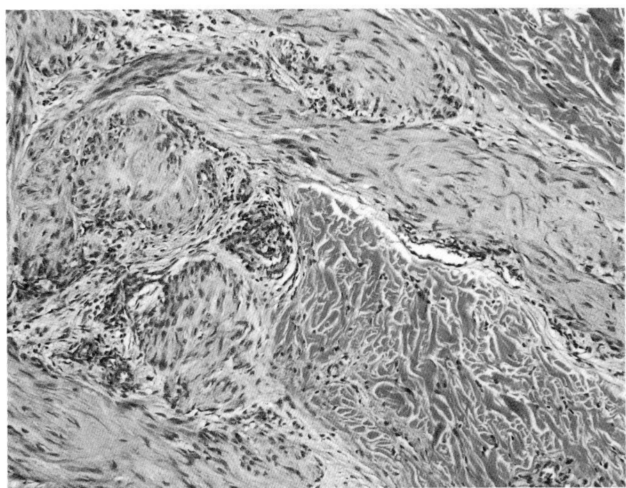

FIGURE 25-50 ■ Cutaneous myofibroma showing myofibroblastic nodules of loosely arrayed spindle cells within the dermis often noted in an infant. (Hematoxylin and eosin stain, original magnification ×100.)

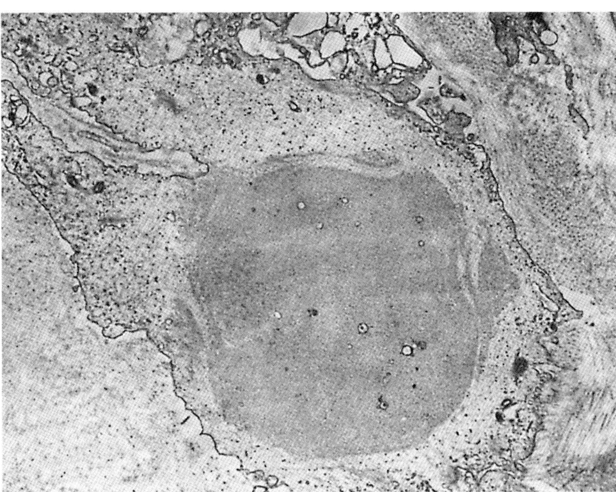

FIGURE 25-52 ■ Infantile digital fibromatosis showing an inclusion composed of a tangled network of filaments. (Uranyl acetate and lead citrate stain, original magnification ×14,400.)

from the nucleus by a narrow clear zone (Figure 25-51). The inclusions vary in number and range from 3 to 15 mm in diameter. They are round, eosinophilic, and resemble erythrocytes. They stain a deep red with Masson trichrome and are PAS negative. Ultrastructurally, the tumor cells are identified as fibroblasts and myofibroblasts. The inclusion bodies consist of fibrillary and granular material, which is often actin positive (Figure 25-52). Local recurrence is common; however, the vast majority of infantile digital fibromas regress over time (80) (see Chapter 24).

Giant Cell Fibroblastoma

Giant cell fibroblastoma, first described by Shmookler and Enzinger in abstract form in 1992, is now considered to be the juvenile form of dermatofibrosarcoma protuberans, as evidenced by the frequent presence of giant cell fibroblastoma–like areas in examples of conventional dermatofibrosarcoma protuberans. Furthermore, immunohistochemical studies have shown both areas to be reactive with CD34 (86,139,180) and CD99 (48). It presents at a median age of 3 years as a painless nodule or mass in the dermis or subcutis of the back of the thigh, inguinal region, or chest wall. Two-thirds of the patients are boys. The lesion is poorly circumscribed and measures from 1 to 8 cm. The tumor is composed of spindle cells, with moderate nuclear pleomorphism, infiltrating the deep dermis and subcutis. Cellularity varies with the formation of characteristic pseudovascular spaces lined by a discontinuous row of multinucleated cells that are the basic proliferating tumor cells (Figure 25-53). Both giant cell fibroblastoma and dermatofibrosarcoma protuberans share the same cytogenetic abnormality,

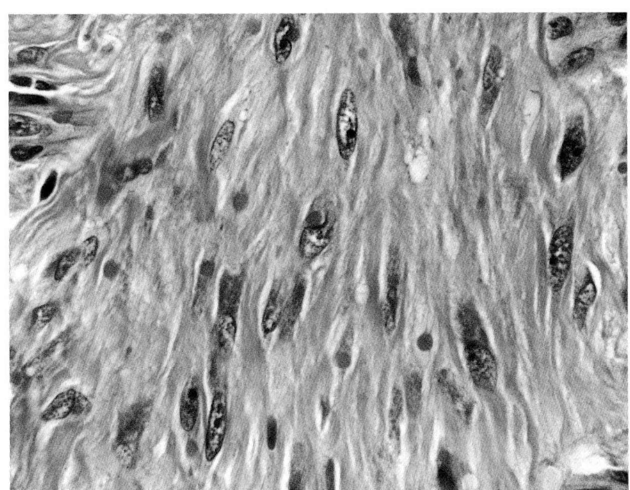

FIGURE 25-51 ■ Infantile digital fibromatosis showing paranuclear inclusions. (Hematoxylin and eosin stain, original magnification ×400.)

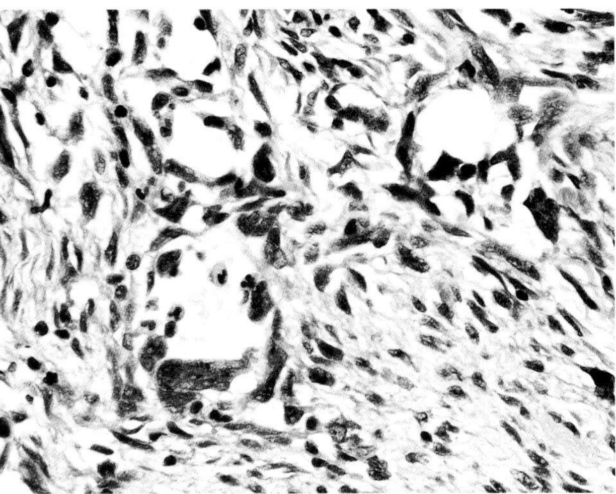

FIGURE 25-53 ■ Giant cell fibroblastoma is a spindle cell lesion with pseudovascular spaces, multinucleated giant cells, and occasional mitoses. (Hematoxylin and eosin stain, original magnification ×400.)

which include reciprocal translocation t or, more commonly, supernumerary ring chromosomes containing sequences from chromosomes 17 and 22. The tumor recurs locally in half the cases but has not been known to metastasize (101).

HEMATOPOIETIC

Mast Cell Diseases

Mastocytosis in children is generally a benign self-healing condition characterized by abnormal proliferation of mast cells, most often presenting as cutaneous lesions (95). Cutaneous mastocytosis can manifest as solitary mastocytoma usually present at birth, urticaria pigmentosa presenting as maculopapular eruption in children between the ages of 3 to 9 months, or as diffuse mastocytosis that presents with diffuse thickening of the skin in infants and is associated with a poor prognosis owing to systemic involvement. Of these lesions, urticaria pigmentosa is the most common manifestation and includes the telangiectatic form.

All variants of cutaneous mastocytosis are generally marked by wheal formation in response to rubbing, which is known as *Darier sign*. Occasional blister formation is also seen. A skin biopsy is diagnostic in all cases and demonstrates an infiltrate of monomorphous mononuclear cells (Figure 25-54) with oval bland nuclei and abundant amphophilic to pale cytoplasm. Eosinophils are present in varying numbers. The infiltrate may be of varying density and depends on the clinical appearance, with most cells being present in a nodule of solitary mastocytoma and least in telangiectasia macularis eruptiva perstans. Special stains such as Giemsa, toluidine blue, and Leder stain or immunohistochemical stain for mast cell tryptase can be helpful in confirming the diagnosis.

The prognosis is generally good for cutaneous mastocytosis, with solitary mastocytomas regressing spontaneously in a few years and urticaria pigmentosa resolving before puberty in the majority of patients. Diffuse mastocytosis has a guarded prognosis and may be complicated by tachycardia and shock.

Histiocytoses

Histiocytoses are a complex group of disorders best divided into Langerhans cell and non-Langerhans cell histiocytosis.

Langerhans Cell Histiocytosis (LCH)

Langerhans cell histiocytosis is characterized by a proliferation of Langerhans histiocytes that are immunoreactive with S100 protein, peanut agglutinin, and CD1a, and contain Birbeck granules by electron microscopy. Three clinical classes are recognized: an acute disseminated form with visceral involvement known as *Letterer-Siwe disease* presenting in the 1st year of life; a chronic multisystem disease with osseous involvement but less visceral involvement known as *Hand-Schüller-Christian syndrome* presenting in early childhood; and the chronic focal disease presenting with one or more bone lesions known as *eosinophilic granuloma* seen in late childhood and adults. Cutaneous involvement is encountered in all forms but is most common in the acute disseminated form, and a skin biopsy is often diagnostic. Cutaneous lesions may consist of petechiae, papules, and often diffuse eruption, particularly of the scalp and the anogenital areas, resembling seborrheic dermatitis. Occasionally, the lesions may be vesicular, ulcerated, or urticarial. Langerhans histiocytes are present in the papillary dermis, obscuring the dermoepidermal junction (Figure 25-55) and often extending into the overlying epidermis. The cells are characterized by abundant pale cytoplasm and characteristic reniform nucleus. Multinucleated histiocytes and eosinophils are present in varying numbers. Several dermatoses are associated with hyperplasia of Langerhans cells which should not be diagnosed as LCH.

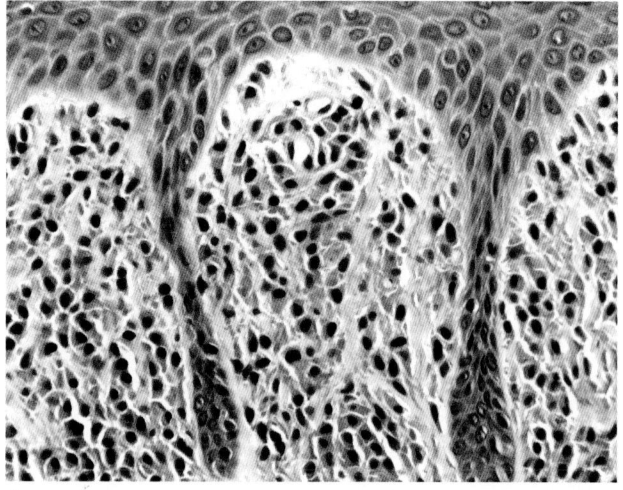
A

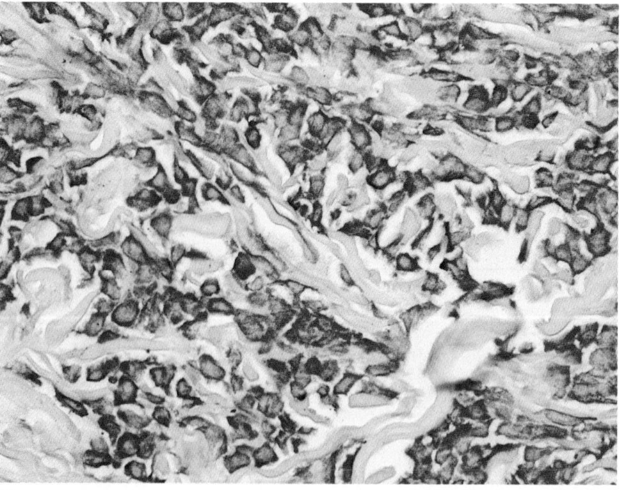
B

FIGURE 25-54 ■ Urticaria pigmentosa: **A:** Dense dermal infiltrate of monomorphic cells, which are mast cells. (Hematoxylin and eosin stain, original magnification ×400.) **B:** Giemsa stain shows the mast cells with purple, metachromatic granules. Most cells are also c-kit (CD117) positive.

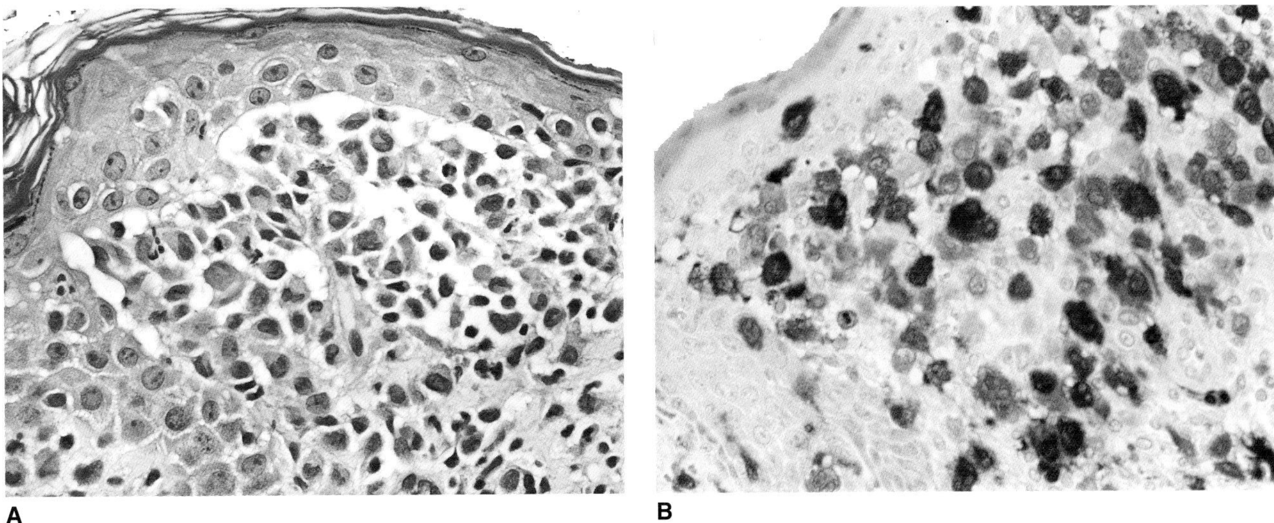

FIGURE 25-55 ■ Langerhans cell histiocytosis: **A:** Dense diffuse dermal infiltrate of atypical histiocytic cells with grooved nuclei and multinucleation, admixed with eosinophils. (Hematoxylin and eosin stain, original magnification ×400.) **B:** The histiocytic cells are positive for S100 protein and CD1a (not illustrated) by immunohistochemistry.

Congenital self-healing reticulohistiocytosis is considered to be on the benign end of the spectrum of Langerhans cell histiocytosis, presenting at birth or shortly after and resolving spontaneously (104). Microscopically, the histiocytes in this condition are distinguished by the presence of abundant eosinophilic cytoplasm with a ground-glass appearance.

Non-Langerhans Cell Histiocytoses

These histiocytoses are characterized by a proliferation of histiocytic cells that express a variety of macrophage markers but not CD1a or S100 protein.

Juvenile xanthogranuloma is the most common form of non-Langerhans cell histiocytosis seen in children. The clinical appearance is that of a solitary or multiple red-yellow papules or nodules appearing during the 1st year of life. Histologically, the lesions show a dense dermal infiltrate of histiocytes with varying degrees of lipidization, a variety of multinucleated cells including Touton giant cells, and an admixture of lymphocytes and eosinophils (Figure 25-56). Older lesions show proliferation of fibroblasts with fibrosis replacing the infiltrate. Deep forms with involvement of the subcutaneous tissue or muscle can occur.

Although juvenile xanthogranuloma is generally a benign disorder, several systemic complications, including ocular involvement, oral lesions, central nervous system and bone involvement, are seen in rare cases.

Benign cephalic histiocytosis is a clinically distinct self-healing disorder of children characterized by small papular eruptions on the face. Histologic features overlap with juvenile xanthogranuloma and eruptive histiocytoma of adults (74,160).

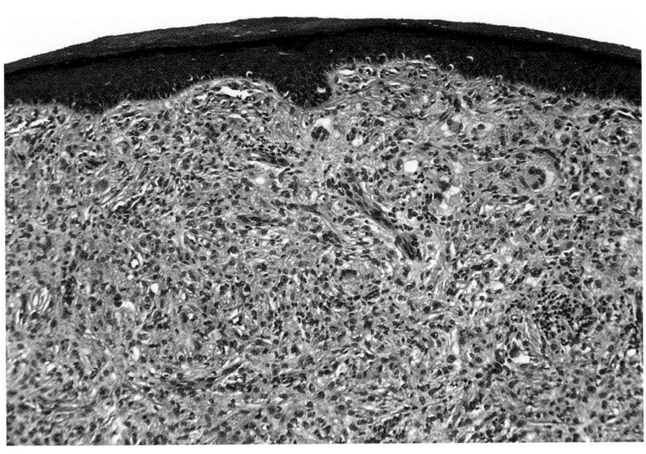

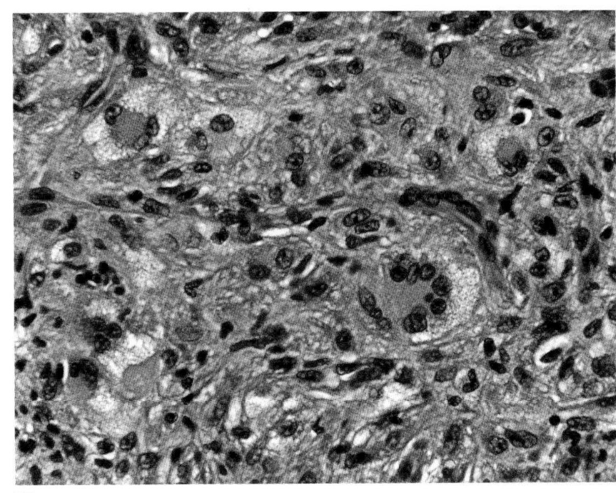

FIGURE 25-56 ■ Juvenile xanthogranuloma: **A:** A well-circumscribed dome-shaped papule. **B:** Diffuse infiltrate of histiocytic cells, many of which are multinucleated with nuclei arranged in a wreath-like pattern. Note also the lipidized features of the cytoplasm. [Hematoxylin and eosin stain, original magnification ×25(**A**), ×400(**B**).]

Sinus Histiocytosis with Massive Lymphadenopathy

Skin involvement may be seen in approximately 10% of cases and presents as papules or nodules that on biopsy show histiocytes with abundant cytoplasm and occasional multinucleation with emperipolesis of lymphocytes.

Leukemia and Lymphoma

Cutaneous involvement by leukemia and lymphoma is uncommon in childhood. Congenital monocytic leukemia has been reported in some patients (11,67). Anaplastic large cell lymphoma, now regarded as being of T-cell origin (45), may present with cutaneous involvement with or without lymph node involvement. Involvement of mediastinum, viscera, and skin is associated with increased risk of progression/relapse (116). The histologic features include a dense diffuse infiltrate of anaplastic mononuclear cells that are typically CD30 positive. The skin lesion may be ALK-negative. Lymphomatoid papulosis may show a population of cells identical to those seen in large cell anaplastic lymphoma but is generally regarded as a self-limiting benign disorder. Rare cases have shown progression to anaplastic large cell lymphoma and, therefore, require close follow-up.

A subset of lymphomatoid papulosis, which is likely to progress to malignant lymphoma and clinically resembles hydroa vacciniforme and histologically shows typical features of lymphomatoid papulosis, has also been described in children (192). A related entity is angiocentric cutaneous T-cell lymphoma of childhood that presents with a vesiculopapular eruption mimicking hydroa vacciniforme has been described. Most of the children are from Asia and Latin America (15,38,121). Patients present with vesicles, necrotic areas, and scars on the face and dorsa of the hands, forearms, and legs. Unlike hydroa vacciniforme, the lesions are not related to sun exposure and are larger and deeper. Histologically, atypical lymphoid infiltrates are present in the dermis and subcutaneous tissue with a tendency for angiocentricity and vascular destruction. Epstein-Barr virus has been detected in several cases, suggesting a possible etiologic role. These lymphomas are graded as any other angiocentric T-cell lymphoma. The prognosis correlates with grade and extent of disease. Higher grade and systemic involvement are associated with a high mortality rate.

REFERENCES

1. Abraham AG, Kulp-Shorten CL, Callen JP. Remember to consider dermatophyte infection when dealing with recalcitrant dermatoses. *South Med J* 1998;91(4):349–353.
2. Ackerman AB. Melanocytic proliferations that simulate malignant melanoma histopathologically. *Monogr Pathol* 1988;30:153–173.
3. Ackerman AB, Reddy VB, Soyer HP. Pilomatricoma and matricoma (Chapter 20), In: *Neoplasms with follicular differentiation*. New York: Ardor Scribendi, 2001:349–388.
4. Adachi J, Endo K, Fukuzumi T, et al. Increasing incidence of streptococcal impetigo in atopic dermatitis. *J Dermatol Sci* 1998;17(1):45–53.
5. Allison DS, El-Azhary RA, Calobrisi SD, et al. Pityriasis rubra pilaris in children. *J Am Acad Dermatol* 2002;47(3):386–389.
6. Alonso-Llamazares J, Gibson LE, Rogers RS III. Clinical, pathologic, and immunopathologic features of dermatitis herpetiformis: review of the Mayo Clinic experience. *Int J Dermatol* 2007;46(9): 910–919.
7. Amagai M. Desmoglein as a target in autoimmunity and infection. *J Am Acad Dermatol* 2003;48(2):244–252.
8. Anderson CR, Jenkins D, Tron V, et al. Wells' syndrome in childhood: case report and review of the literature. *J Am Acad Dermatol* 1995;33(5 Pt 2):857–864.
9. Aoyama Y, Asai K, Hioki K, et al. Herpes gestationis in a mother and newborn: immunoclinical perspectives based on a weekly follow-up of the enzyme-linked immunosorbent assay index of a bullous pemphigoid antigen noncollagenous domain. *Arch Dermatol* 2007;143(9):1168–1172.
10. Arcangeli F, Calista D. Congenital myofibromatosis in two siblings. *Eur J Dermatol* 2006;16(2):181–183.
11. Attal H, Kowal-Vern A, Husain AN, et al. Newborn infant with multiple purple skin nodules. *Arch Dermatol* 1996;132(3):343–346.
12. Avci G, Akan M, Akoz T. Simultaneous multiple pilomatrixomas. *Pediatr Dermatol* 2006;23(2):157–162.
13. Bader JL, Li FP, Olmstead PM, et al. Childhood malignant melanoma. Incidence and etiology. *Am J Pediatr Hematol Oncol* 1985;7(4):341–345.
14. Balasubramaniam P, Ogboli M, Moss C. Lichen planus in children: review of 26 cases. *Clin Exp Dermatol* 2008;33(4):457–459.
15. Barrionuevo C, Anderson VM, Zevallos-Giampietri E, et al. Hydroa-like cutaneous T-cell lymphoma: a clinicopathologic and molecular genetic study of 16 pediatric cases from Peru. *Appl Immunohistochem Mol Morphol* 2002;10(1):7–14.
16. Beattie PE, Green C, Lowe G, et al. Which children should we patch test? *Clin Exp Dermatol* 2007;32(1):6–11.
17. Bekaert C, Song M, Delvigne A. Acne neonatorum and familial hyperandrogenism. *Dermatology* 1998;196(4):453–454.
18. Benoit S, Hamm H. Childhood psoriasis. *Clin Dermatol* 2007;25(6):555–562.
19. Bergman R. Immunohistopathologic diagnosis of epidermolysis bullosa. *Am J Dermatopathol* 1999;21(2):185–192.
20. Berlin AL, Paller AS, Chan LS. Incontinentia pigmenti: a review and update on the molecular basis of pathophysiology. *J Am Acad Dermatol* 2002;47(2):169–187.
21. Bernard P. Management of common bacterial infections of the skin. *Curr Opin Infect Dis* 2008;21(2):122–128.
22. Bhat RM, Shetty SS, Kamath GH. Pyoderma gangrenosum in childhood. *Int J Dermatol* 2004;43(3):205–207.
23. Blanco R, Martinez-Taboada VM, Rodriguez-Valverde V, et al. Henoch-Schonlein purpura in adulthood and childhood: two different expressions of the same syndrome. *Arthritis Rheum* 1997;40(5):859–864.
24. Bowcock AM, Barker JN. Genetics of psoriasis: the potential impact on new therapies. *J Am Acad Dermatol* 2003;49(2 Suppl): S51–S56.
25. Brandt O, Abeck D, Gianotti R, et al. Gianotti-Crosti syndrome. *J Am Acad Dermatol* 2006;54(1):136–145.
26. Broccolo F, Drago F, Careddu AM, et al. Additional evidence that pityriasis rosea is associated with reactivation of human herpesvirus-6 and -7. *J Invest Dermatol* 2005;124(6):1234–1240.
27. Browning J, Frieden I, Baselga E, et al. Congenital, self-regressing tufted angioma. *Arch Dermatol* 2006;142(6):749–751.
28. Burge SM, Wilkinson JD. Darier-White disease: a review of the clinical features in 163 patients. *J Am Acad Dermatol* 1992;27(1):40–50.
29. Caksen H, Kurtoglu S. Our experience with aplasia cutis congenita. *J Dermatol* 2002;29(6):376–379.
30. Callot-Mellot C, Bodemer C, Caux F, et al. Epidermolysis bullosa acquisita in childhood. *Arch Dermatol* 1997;133(9):1122–1126.

31. Carney JA, Ferreiro JA. The epithelioid blue nevus. A multicentric familial tumor with important associations, including cardiac myxoma and psammomatous melanotic schwannoma. *Am J Surg Pathol* 1996;20(3):259–272.
32. Castro LA, Lundell RB, Krause PK, et al. Clinical experience in pemphigoid gestationis: report of 10 cases. *J Am Acad Dermatol* 2006;55(5):823–828.
33. Celestin R, Brown J, Kihiczak G, et al. Erysipelas: a common potentially dangerous infection. *Acta Dermatovenerol Alp Panonica Adriat* 2007;16(3):123–127.
34. Chan LS. Atopic dermatitis in 2008. *Curr Dir Autoimmun* 2008;10:76–118.
35. Chan YH, Chong CY, Puthucheary J, et al. Ecthyma gangrenosum: a manifestation of *Pseudomonas* sepsis in three paediatric patients. *Singapore Med J* 2006;47(12):1080–1083.
36. Chernosky ME. Porokeratosis. *Arch Dermatol* 1986;122(8): 869–870.
37. Chi CY, Wang SM, Lin HC, et al. A clinical and microbiological comparison of Staphylococcus aureus toxic shock and scalded skin syndromes in children. *Clin Infect Dis* 2006;42(2):181–185.
38. Cho KH, Kim CW, Lee DY, et al. An Epstein-Barr virus-associated lymphoproliferative lesion of the skin presenting as recurrent necrotic papulovesicles of the face. *Br J Dermatol* 1996;134(4): 791–796.
39. Cho S, Chang SE, Choi JH, et al. Clinical and histologic features of 64 cases of steatocystoma multiplex. *J Dermatol* 2002;29(3): 152–156.
40. Chuang TY, Ilstrup DM, Perry HO, et al. Pityriasis rosea in Rochester, Minnesota, 1969 to 1978. *J Am Acad Dermatol* 1982;7(1):80–89.
41. Cigliano B, Baltogiannis N, De Marco M, et al. Pilomatricoma in childhood: a retrospective study from three European paediatric centres. *Eur J Pediatr* 2005;164(11):673–677.
42. Cohen PR, Kurzrock R. Sweet's syndrome revisited: a review of disease concepts. *Int J Dermatol* 2003;42(10):761–778.
43. Cribier B, Scrivener Y, Grosshans E. Tumors arising in nevus sebaceus: a study of 596 cases. *J Am Acad Dermatol* 2000;42(2 Pt 1): 263–268.
44. Crowe MA, Jonas PP. Acute hemorrhagic edema of infancy. *Cutis* 1998;62(2):65–66.
45. d'Amore ES, Menin A, Bonoldi E, et al. Anaplastic large cell lymphomas: a study of 75 pediatric patients. *Pediatr Dev Pathol* 2007;10(3):181–191.
46. Di Zenzo G, Calabresi V, Grosso F, et al. The intracellular and extracellular domains of BP180 antigen comprise novel epitopes targeted by pemphigoid gestationis autoantibodies. *J Invest Dermatol* 2007;127(4):864–873.
47. Dillon MJ. Childhood vasculitis. *Lupus* 1998;7(4):259–265.
48. Diwan AH, Skelton HG III, Horenstein MG, et al. Dermatofibrosarcoma protuberans and giant cell fibroblastoma exhibit CD99 positivity. *J Cutan Pathol* 2008;35(7):647–650.
49. Dorff GJ, Geimer NF, Rosenthal DR, et al. Pseudomonas septicemia. Illustrated evolution of its skin lesion. *Arch Intern Med* 1971;128(4):591–595.
50. Dorton DW, Kaufmann M. Palmoplantar pustules in an infant. Acropustulosis of infancy. *Arch Dermatol* 1996;132(11):1365–1366, 1368–1369.
51. Drut RM, Gomez MA, Drut R, et al. Human papillomavirus is present in some cases of childhood penile lichen sclerosus: an in situ hybridization and SP-PCR study. *Pediatr Dermatol* 1998;15(2):85–90.
52. Duarte AM, Kramer J, Yusk JW, et al. Eosinophilic pustular folliculitis in infancy and childhood. *Am J Dis Child* 1993;147(2): 197–200.
53. Edwards MS, Baker CJ. Complications and sequelae of meningococcal infections in children. *J Pediatr* 1981;99(4):540–545.
54. Edwards S, Wakelin SH, Wojnarowska F, et al. Bullous pemphigoid and epidermolysis bullosa acquisita: presentation, prognosis, and immunopathology in 11 children. *Pediatr Dermatol* 1998;15(3):184–190.
55. Ehrenreich M, Tarlow MM, Godlewska-Janusz E, et al. Incontinentia pigmenti (Bloch-Sulzberger syndrome): a systemic disorder. *Cutis* 2007;79(5):355–362.
56. Elder DE, Clark WH Jr. Developmental biology of malignant melanoma. *Pigment Cell Res* 1987;8:1.
57. Elewski BE. Tinea capitis: a current perspective. *J Am Acad Dermatol* 2000;42(1 Pt 1):1–20; quiz 21–24.
58. Eriksson B, Jorup-Ronstrom C, Karkkonen K, et al. Erysipelas: clinical and bacteriologic spectrum and serological aspects. *Clin Infect Dis* 1996;23(5):1091–1098.
59. Ersoy-Evans S, Greco MF, Mancini AJ, et al. Pityriasis lichenoides in childhood: a retrospective review of 124 patients. *J Am Acad Dermatol* 2007;56(2):205–210.
60. Evans MJ, Blessing K, Gray ES. Pseudorheumatoid nodule (deep granuloma annulare) of childhood: clinicopathologic features of twenty patients. *Pediatr Dermatol* 1994;11(1):6–9.
61. Fan X, Xiao FL, Yang S, et al. Childhood psoriasis: a study of 277 patients from China. *J Eur Acad Dermatol Venereol* 2007;21(6): 762–765.
62. Felner EI, Steinberg JB, Weinberg AG. Subcutaneous granuloma annulare: a review of 47 cases. *Pediatrics* 1997;100(6):965–967.
63. Ferrandiz C, Coroleu W, Ribera M, et al. Sterile transient neonatal pustulosis is a precocious form of erythema toxicum neonatorum. *Dermatology* 1992;185(1):18–22.
64. Fetsch JF, Laskin WB, Hallman JR, et al. Neurothekeoma: an analysis of 178 tumors with detailed immunohistochemical data and long-term patient follow-up information. *Am J Surg Pathol* 2007;31(7):1103–1114.
65. Fine JD, Eady RA, Bauer EA, et al. The classification of inherited epidermolysis bullosa (EB): Report of the Third International Consensus Meeting on Diagnosis and Classification of EB. *J Am Acad Dermatol* 2008;58(6):931–950.
66. Forman R, Koren G, Shear NH. Erythema multiforme, Stevens-Johnson syndrome and toxic epidermal necrolysis in children: a review of 10 years' experience. *Drug Saf* 2002;25(13):965–972.
67. Francis JS, Sybert VP, Benjamin DR. Congenital monocytic leukemia: report of a case with cutaneous involvement, and review of the literature. *Pediatr Dermatol* 1989;6(4):306–311.
68. Fretzin DF, Arias AM. Sclerema neonatorum and subcutaneous fat necrosis of the newborn. *Pediatr Dermatol* 1987;4(2):112–122.
69. Friedrich RE. Diagnosis and treatment of patients with nevoid basal cell carcinoma syndrome [Gorlin-Goltz syndrome (GGS)]. *Anticancer Res* 2007;27(4A):1783–1787.
70. Fromowitz JS, Ramos-Caro FA, Flowers FP. Practical guidelines for the management of toxic epidermal necrolysis and Stevens-Johnson syndrome. *Int J Dermatol* 2007;46(10):1092–1094.
71. Gardner EJ, Richards RC. Multiple cutaneous and subcutaneous lesions occurring simultaneously with hereditary polyposis and osteomatosis. *Am J Hum Genet* 1953;5(2):139–147.
72. Garman M, Metry D. Vulvar syringomas in a 9-year-old child with review of the literature. *Pediatr Dermatol* 2006;23(4):369–372.
73. Gelmetti C, Rigoni C, Alessi E, et al. Pityriasis lichenoides in children: a long-term follow-up of eighty-nine cases. *J Am Acad Dermatol* 1990;23(3 Pt 1):473–478.
74. Gianotti R, Alessi E, Caputo R. Benign cephalic histiocytosis: a distinct entity or a part of a wide spectrum of histiocytic proliferative disorders of children? A histopathological study. *Am J Dermatopathol* 1993;15(4):315–319.
75. Golitz LE. The vasculitides and their significance in the pediatric age group. *Dermatol Clin* 1986;4(1):117–125.
76. Goltz RW, Peterson WC, Gorlin RJ, et al. Focal dermal hypoplasia. *Arch Dermatol* 1962;86:708–717.
77. Gonggryp LA, Todd G. Acute hemorrhagic edema of childhood (AHE). *Pediatr Dermatol* 1998;15(2):91–96.

78. Gorlin RJ, Chaudhry AP. The oral manifestation of keratosis follicularis. *Oral Surg Oral Med Oral Pathol* 1959;12:1468–1470.
79. Gottschalk GM. Pediatric HIV/AIDS and the skin: an update. *Dermatol Clin* 2006;24(4):531–536, vii.
80. Grenier N, Liang C, Capaldi L, et al. A range of histologic findings in infantile digital fibromatosis. *Pediatr Dermatol* 2008;25(1):72–75.
81. Groben PA, Harvell JD, White WL. Epithelioid blue nevus: neoplasm Sui generis or variation on a theme? *Am J Dermatopathol* 2000;22(6):473–488.
82. Grosshans EM. The red face: erysipelas. *Clin Dermatol* 1993;11(2):307–313.
83. Grzeschik KH, Bornholdt D, Oeffner F, et al. Deficiency of PORCN, a regulator of Wnt signaling, is associated with focal dermal hypoplasia. *Nat Genet* 2007;39(7):833–835.
84. Hamm H, Happle R, Brocker EB. Multiple agminate Spitz naevi: review of the literature and report of a case with distinctive immunohistological features. *Br J Dermatol* 1987;117(4):511–522.
85. Hanifin JM, Reed ML. A population-based survey of eczema prevalence in the United States. *Dermatitis* 2007;18(2):82–91.
86. Harvell JD, Kilpatrick SE, White WL. Histogenetic relations between giant cell fibroblastoma and dermatofibrosarcoma protuberans. CD34 staining showing the spectrum and a simulator. *Am J Dermatopathol* 1998;20(4):339–345.
87. Hedrick J. Acute bacterial skin infections in pediatric medicine: current issues in presentation and treatment. *Paediatr Drugs* 2003;5(Suppl 1):35–46.
88. Hengge UR, Currie BJ, Jager G, et al. Scabies: a ubiquitous neglected skin disease. *Lancet Infect Dis* 2006;6(12):769–779.
89. Herron MD, Coffin CM, Vanderhooft SL. Sweet syndrome in two children. *Pediatr Dermatol* 2005;22(6):525–529.
90. Herron MD, Coffin CM, Vanderhooft SL. Tufted angiomas: variability of the clinical morphology. *Pediatr Dermatol* 2002;19(5):394–401.
91. Himmelstein R, Lynfield YL. Punctate porokeratosis. *Arch Dermatol* 1984;120(2):263–264.
92. Hiraki LT, Benseler SM, Tyrrell PN, et al. Clinical and laboratory characteristics and long-term outcome of pediatric systemic lupus erythematosus: a longitudinal study. *J Pediatr* 2008;152(4):550–556.
93. Hogeling M, Pratt M. Allergic contact dermatitis in children: the Ottawa hospital patch-testing clinic experience, 1996 to 2006. *Dermatitis* 2008;19(2):86–89.
94. Hornick JL, Fletcher CD. Cellular neurothekeoma: detailed characterization in a series of 133 cases. *Am J Surg Pathol* 2007;31(3):329–340.
95. Horny HP, Sotlar K, Valent P. Mastocytosis: state of the art. *Pathobiology* 2007;74(2):121–132.
96. Howard R, Tsuchiya A. Adult skin disease in the pediatric patient. *Dermatol Clin* 1998;16(3):593–608.
97. Hurwitz RM, Ackerman AB. Cutaneous pathology of the toxic shock syndrome. *Am J Dermatopathol* 1985;7(6):563–578.
98. Iwatsuki K, Yamasaki O, Morizane S, et al. Staphylococcal cutaneous infections: invasion, evasion and aggression. *J Dermatol Sci* 2006;42(3):203–214.
99. Jacobsohn DA. Acute graft-versus-host disease in children. *Bone Marrow Transplant* 2008;41(2):215–221.
100. Jansen T, Burgdorf WH, Plewig G. Pathogenesis and treatment of acne in childhood. *Pediatr Dermatol* 1997;14(1):17–21.
101. Jha P, Moosavi C, Fanburg-Smith JC. Giant cell fibroblastoma: an update and addition of 86 new cases from the Armed Forces Institute of Pathology, in honor of Dr. Franz M. Enzinger. *Ann Diagn Pathol* 2007;11(2):81–88.
102. Jones V, Smith SJ, Omar HA. Nonsexual transmission of anogenital warts in children: a retrospective analysis. *Sci World J* 2007;7:1896–1899.
103. Julian CG, Bowers PW. A clinical review of 209 pilomatricomas. *J Am Acad Dermatol* 1998;39(2 Pt 1):191–195.
104. Kapur P, Erickson C, Rakheja D, et al. Congenital self-healing reticulohistiocytosis (Hashimoto-Pritzker disease): ten-year experience at Dallas Children's Medical Center. *J Am Acad Dermatol* 2007;56(2):290–294.
105. Karpati S, Kosnai I, Verkasalo M, et al. HLA antigens, jejunal morphology and associated diseases in children with dermatitis herpetiformis. *Acta Paediatr Scand* 1986;75(2):297–301.
106. Katsanis E, Luke KH, Hsu E, et al. Neutrophilic eccrine hidradenitis in acute myelomonocytic leukemia. *Am J Pediatr Hematol Oncol* 1987;9(3):204–208.
107. Katz SI, Hall RP III, Lawley TJ, et al. Dermatitis herpetiformis: the skin and the gut. *Ann Intern Med* 1980;93(6):857–874.
108. Kazakov DV, Calonje E, Zelger B, et al. Sebaceous carcinoma arising in nevus sebaceus of Jadassohn: a clinicopathological study of five cases. *Am J Dermatopathol* 2007;29(3):242–248.
109. Khachemoune A, Blyumin ML. Pityriasis lichenoides: pathophysiology, classification, and treatment. *Am J Clin Dermatol* 2007;8(1):29–36.
110. Khalil BA, Baillie CT, Kenny SE, et al. Surgical strategies in the management of ecthyma gangrenosum in paediatric oncology patients. *Pediatr Surg Int* 2008;24(7):793–797.
111. Khalili B, Bahna SL. Pathogenesis and recent therapeutic trends in Stevens-Johnson syndrome and toxic epidermal necrolysis. *Ann Allergy Asthma Immunol* 2006;97(3):272–280.
112. Krengel S, Hauschild A, Schafer T. Melanoma risk in congenital melanocytic naevi: a systematic review. *Br J Dermatol* 2006;155(1):1–8.
113. Kutukculer N, Tutuncuoglu S, Yilmaz D, et al. Subcutaneous granuloma annulare and IgA-IgG2 deficiency. *Turk J Pediatr* 1998;40(2):279–281.
114. Ladhani S, Garbash M. Staphylococcal skin infections in children: rational drug therapy recommendations. *Paediatr Drugs* 2005;7(2):77–102.
115. Lam NS, Yang YH, Wang LC, et al. Clinical characteristics of childhood erythema multiforme, Stevens-Johnson syndrome and toxic epidermal necrolysis in Taiwanese children. *J Microbiol Immunol Infect* 2004;37(6):366–370.
116. Le Deley MC, Reiter A, Williams D, et al. Prognostic factors in childhood anaplastic large cell lymphoma: results of a large European intergroup study. *Blood* 2008;111(3):1560–1566.
117. Lee LA, Weston WL. Neonatal lupus erythematosus. *Semin Dermatol* 1988;7(1):66–72.
118. Leung AK, Robson WL, Leong AG. Herpes zoster in childhood. *J Pediatr Health Care* 2006;20(5):300–303.
119. Libermann S. Atrophoderma linearis maculosa et papillomatosis congenita. *Acta Derm Venereol* 1935;16:476.
120. Luis-Montoya P, Dominguez-Soto L, Vega-Memije E. Lichen planus in 24 children with review of the literature. *Pediatr Dermatol* 2005;22(4):295–298.
121. Magana M, Sangueza P, Gil-Beristain J, et al. Angiocentric cutaneous T-cell lymphoma of childhood (hydroa-like lymphoma): a distinctive type of cutaneous T-cell lymphoma. *J Am Acad Dermatol* 1998;38(4):574–579.
122. Magro C, Crowson AN, Kovatich A, et al. Pityriasis lichenoides: a clonal T-cell lymphoproliferative disorder. *Hum Pathol* 2002;33(8):788–795.
123. Mahe E, Girszyn N, Hadj-Rabia S, et al. Subcutaneous fat necrosis of the newborn: a systematic evaluation of risk factors, clinical manifestations, complications and outcome of 16 children. *Br J Dermatol* 2007;156(4):709–715.
124. Mangas C, Fernandez-Figueras MT, Fite E, et al. Clinical spectrum and histological analysis of 32 cases of specific cutaneous sarcoidosis. *J Cutan Pathol* 2006;33(12):772–777.
125. Marcoux D, Nadeau K, McCuaig C, et al. Pediatric anogenital warts: a 7-year review of children referred to a tertiary-care hospital in Montreal, Canada. *Pediatr Dermatol* 2006;23(3):199–207.

126. Marghoob AA, Schoenbach SP, Kopf AW, et al. Large congenital melanocytic nevi and the risk for the development of malignant melanoma. A prospective study. *Arch Dermatol* 1996;132(2):170–175.
127. Martin JM, Green M. Group A streptococcus. *Semin Pediatr Infect Dis* 2006;17(3):140–148.
128. Maverakis E, Fung MA, Lynch PJ, et al. Acrodermatitis enteropathica and an overview of zinc metabolism. *J Am Acad Dermatol* 2007;56(1):116–124.
129. Mayuzumi M, Akiyama M, Nishie W, et al. Childhood epidermolysis bullosa acquisita with autoantibodies against the noncollagenous 1 and 2 domains of type VII collagen: case report and review of the literature. *Br J Dermatol* 2006;155(5):1048–1052.
130. Meissner PE, Jappe U, Niemeyer CM, et al. Pyoderma gangraenosum, a rare, but potentially fatal complication in paediatric oncology patients. *Klin Padiatr* 2007;219(5):296–299.
131. Mengesha YM, Bennett ML. Pustular skin disorders: diagnosis and treatment. *Am J Clin Dermatol* 2002;3(6):389–400.
132. Milman N, Hoffmann AL. Childhood sarcoidosis: long-term follow-up. *Eur Respir J* 2008;31(3):592–598.
133. Mittmann N, Chan BC, Knowles S, et al. IVIG for the treatment of toxic epidermal necrolysis. *Skin Therapy Lett* 2007;12(1):7–9.
134. Monari P, Gualdi G, Fantini F, et al. Cutaneous neonatal lupus erythematosus in four siblings. *Br J Dermatol* 2008;158(3):626–628.
135. Mones JM, Ackerman AB. Melanomas in prepubescent children: review comprehensively, critique historically, criteria diagnostically, and course biologically. *Am J Dermatopathol* 2003;25(3):223–238.
136. Mooi WJ, Krausz T. Spitz nevus versus spitzoid melanoma: diagnostic difficulties, conceptual controversies. *Adv Anat Pathol* 2006;13(4):147–156.
137. Moraes AJ, Soares PM, Zapata AL, et al. Panniculitis in childhood and adolescence. *Pediatr Int* 2006;48(1):48–53.
138. Nanda S, Reddy BS, Ramji S, et al. Analytical study of pustular eruptions in neonates. *Pediatr Dermatol* 2002;19(3):210–215.
139. O'Brien KP, Seroussi E, Dal Cin P, et al. Various regions within the alpha-helical domain of the COL1A1 gene are fused to the second exon of the PDGFB gene in dermatofibrosarcomas and giant-cell fibroblastomas. *Genes Chromosomes Cancer* 1998;23(2):187–193.
140. Obalek S, Misiewicz J, Jablonska S, et al. Childhood condyloma acuminatum: association with genital and cutaneous human papillomaviruses. *Pediatr Dermatol* 1993;10(2):101–106.
141. Otsuka F, Shima A, Ishibashi Y. Porokeratosis as a premalignant condition of the skin. Cytologic demonstration of abnormal DNA ploidy in cells of the epidermis. *Cancer* 1989;63(5):891–896.
142. Pacheco TR, Levy M, Collyer JC, et al. Incontinentia pigmenti in male patients. *J Am Acad Dermatol* 2006;55(2):251–255.
143. Paller AS, Mancini AJ. Hereditary disorders of cornification. In: *Hurwitz clinical pediatric dermatology*. Philadelphia, PA: Elsevier, 2006:107.
144. Panhans A, Bodemer C, Macinthyre E, et al. Pityriasis lichenoides of childhood with atypical CD30-positive cells and clonal T-cell receptor gene rearrangements. *J Am Acad Dermatol* 1996;35(3 Pt 1):489–490.
145. Paniago-Pereira C, Maize JC, Ackerman AB. Nevus of large spindle and/or epithelioid cells (Spitz's nevus). *Arch Dermatol* 1978;114(12):1811–1823.
146. Patrizi A, Neri I, Guerrini V, et al. Persistent milia, steatocystoma multiplex and eruptive vellus hair cysts: variable expression of multiple pilosebaceous cysts within an affected family. *Dermatology* 1998;196(4):392–396.
147. Peroni DG, Piacentini GL, Bodini A, et al. Prevalence and risk factors for atopic dermatitis in preschool children. *Br J Dermatol* 2008;158(3):539–543.
148. Pestoni C, Ferreiros MM, de la Torre C, et al. Two girls with necrobiosis lipoidica and type I diabetes mellitus with transfollicular elimination in one girl. *Pediatr Dermatol* 2003;20(3):211–214.
149. Phan TA, Wargon O, Turner AM. Incontinentia pigmenti case series: clinical spectrum of incontinentia pigmenti in 53 female patients and their relatives. *Clin Exp Dermatol* 2005;30(5):474–480.
150. Poindexter G, Morrell DS. Anogenital pruritus: lichen sclerosus in children. *Pediatr Ann* 2007;36(12):785–791.
151. Powell J, Wojnarowska F. Childhood vulvar lichen sclerosus: an increasingly common problem. *J Am Acad Dermatol* 2001;44(5):803–806.
152. Prose NS. Human immunodeficiency virus infection in childhood: the disease and its cutaneous manifestations. *Adv Dermatol* 1990;5:113–128; discussion 129.
153. Prose NS, Laude TA, Heilman ER, et al. Congenital malignant melanoma. *Pediatrics* 1987;79(6):967–970.
154. Pryor SG, Lewis JE, Weaver AL, et al. Pediatric dermoid cysts of the head and neck. *Otolaryngol Head Neck Surg* 2005;132(6):938–942.
155. Pujol RM, Casanova JM, Egido R, et al. Multiple familial pilomatricomas: a cutaneous marker for Gardner syndrome? *Pediatr Dermatol* 1995;12(4):331–335.
156. Reimer RR, Clark WH Jr, Greene MH, et al. Precursor lesions in familial melanoma. A new genetic preneoplastic syndrome. *JAMA* 1978;239(8):744–746.
157. Reye RD. Recurring digital fibrous tumors of childhood. *Arch Pathol* 1965;80:228–231.
158. Robles DT, Jaramillo L, Hornung RL. Neonatal lupus. *Dermatol Online J* 2006;12(7):25.
159. Rodrigues RG. Aplasia cutis congenita, congenital heart lesions, and frontonasal cysts in four successive generations. *Clin Genet* 2007;71(6):558–560.
160. Rodriguez-Jurado R, Duran-McKinster C, Ruiz-Maldonado R. Benign cephalic histiocytosis progressing into juvenile xanthogranuloma: a non-Langerhans cell histiocytosis transforming under the influence of a virus? *Am J Dermatopathol* 2000;22(1):70–74.
161. Rogers M. Childhood psoriasis. *Curr Opin Pediatr* 2002;14(4):404–409.
162. Rogers M, McCrossin I, Commens C. Epidermal nevi and the epidermal nevus syndrome. A review of 131 cases. *J Am Acad Dermatol* 1989;20(3):476–488.
163. Rubinson R, Larralde M, Santos-Munoz A, et al. Palmoplantar eccrine hidradenitis: seven new cases. *Pediatr Dermatol* 2004;21(4):466–468.
164. Sadana S, Mathur NB, Thakur A. Exchange transfusion in septic neonates with sclerema: effect on immunoglobulin and complement levels. *Indian Pediatr* 1997;34(1):20–25.
165. Safai B, Rappaport I, Matsuoka L, et al. Childhood dermatitis herpetiformis. Review of the new aspects and report of a case. *J Am Acad Dermatol* 1981;4(4):435–441.
166. Sampaio MC, de Oliveira ZN, Machado MC, et al. Discoid lupus erythematosus in children–a retrospective study of 34 patients. *Pediatr Dermatol* 2008;25(2):163–167.
167. Sarabi K, Khachemoune A. Tinea capitis: a review. *Dermatol Nurs* 2007;19(6):525–529; quiz 530.
168. Sasaki S, Urano Y, Nakagawa K, et al. Linear porokeratosis with multiple squamous cell carcinomas: study of p53 expression in porokeratosis and squamous cell carcinoma. *Br J Dermatol* 1996;134(6):1151–1153.
169. Saulsbury FT. Henoch-Schonlein purpura. *Curr Opin Rheumatol* 2001;13(1):35–40.
170. Schachner L, Ling NS, Press S. A statistical analysis of a pediatric dermatology clinic. *Pediatr Dermatol* 1983;1(2):157–164.
171. Scheinfeld N. Diaper dermatitis: a review and brief survey of eruptions of the diaper area. *Am J Clin Dermatol* 2005;6(5):273–281.
172. Schepis C, Siragusa M, Palazzo R, et al. Palpebral syringomas and Down's syndrome. *Dermatology* 1994;189(3):248–250.
173. Schneck J, Fagot JP, Sekula P, et al. Effects of treatments on the mortality of Stevens-Johnson syndrome and toxic epidermal necrolysis: a retrospective study on patients included in the prospective EuroSCAR Study. *J Am Acad Dermatol* 2008;58(1):33–40.
174. Schneiderman H, Wu AY, Campbell WA, et al. Congenital melanoma with multiple prenatal metastases. *Cancer* 1987;60(6):1371–1377.

175. See Y, Koh ET, Boey ML. One hundred and seventy cases of childhood-onset rheumatological disease in Singapore. *Ann Acad Med Singapore* 1998;27(4):496–502.
176. Seyhan M, Coskun BK, Saglam H, et al. Psoriasis in childhood and adolescence: evaluation of demographic and clinical features. *Pediatr Int* 2006;48(6):525–530.
177. Sheth AP, Olson JC, Esterly NB. Cutaneous polyarteritis nodosa of childhood. *J Am Acad Dermatol* 1994;31(4):561–566.
178. Shetty AK, Gedalia A. Pediatric sarcoidosis. *J Am Acad Dermatol* 2003;48(1):150–151.
179. Shih IH, Huang YH, Yang CH, et al. Childhood neutrophilic eccrine hidradenitis: a clinicopathologic and immunohistochemical study of 10 patients. *J Am Acad Dermatol* 2005;52(6):963–966.
180. Shmookler BM, Enzinger FM, Weiss SW. Giant cell fibroblastoma. A juvenile form of dermatofibrosarcoma protuberans. *Cancer* 1989;64(10):2154–2161.
181. Simon M Jr, Cremer H, von den Driesch P. Idiopathic recurrent palmoplantar hidradenitis in children. Report of 22 cases. *Arch Dermatol* 1998;134(1):76–79.
182. Sinclair KA, Woods CR, Kirse DJ, et al. Anogenital and respiratory tract human papillomavirus infections among children: age, gender, and potential transmission through sexual abuse. *Pediatrics* 2005;116(4):815–825.
183. Soler-Carrillo J, Estrach T, Mascaro JM. Eruptive syringoma: 27 new cases and review of the literature. *J Eur Acad Dermatol Venereol* 2001;15(3):242–246.
184. Somani VK. A study of allergen-specific IgE antibodies in Indian patients of atopic dermatitis. *Indian J Dermatol Venereol Leprol* 2008;74(2):100–104.
185. Spitz S. Melanomas of childhood. 1948. *CA Cancer J Clin* 1991;41(1):40–51.
186. Stahr BJ, Cooper PH, Caputo RV. Idiopathic plantar hidradenitis: a neutrophilic eccrine hidradenitis occurring primarily in children. *J Cutan Pathol* 1994;21(4):289–296.
187. Stefanaki K, Tsivitanidou-Kakourou T, Stefanaki C, et al. Histological and immunohistochemical study of granuloma annulare and subcutaneous granuloma annulare in children. *J Cutan Pathol* 2007;34(5):392–396.
188. Steffen C, Ackerman AB. Neoplasms with sebaceous differentiation. In: Steffen C, Ackerman AB, eds. *Nevus sebaceous*. Philadelphia: Lea & Febiger, 1994:89.
189. Stella M, Clemente A, Bollero D, et al. Toxic epidermal necrolysis (TEN) and Stevens-Johnson syndrome (SJS): experience with high-dose intravenous immunoglobulins and topical conservative approach. A retrospective analysis. *Burns* 2007;33(4):452–459.
190. Su WP. Histopathologic varieties of epidermal nevus. A study of 160 cases. *Am J Dermatopathol* 1982;4(2):161–170.
191. Sugarman JL. Epidermal nevus syndromes. *Semin Cutan Med Surg* 2007;26(4):221–230.
192. Tabata N, Aiba S, Ichinohazama R, et al. Hydroa vacciniforme-like lymphomatoid papulosis in a Japanese child: a new subset. *J Am Acad Dermatol* 1995;32(2 Pt 2):378–381.
193. Tan O, Atik B, Kizilkaya A, et al. Extensive skin calcifications in an infant with chronic renal failure: metastatic calcinosis cutis. *Pediatr Dermatol* 2006;23(3):235–238.
194. Tolland JP, Devereux C, Jones FC, et al. Sclerodermatous chronic graft-versus-host disease–a report of four pediatric cases. *Pediatr Dermatol* 2008;25(2):240–244.
195. Trigo-Guzman FX, Conti A, Aoki V, et al. Epidermolysis bullosa acquisita in childhood. *J Dermatol* 2003;30(3):226–229.
196. Uitto J, Richard G. Progress in epidermolysis bullosa: genetic classification and clinical implications. *Am J Med Genet C Semin Med Genet* 2004;131C(1):61–74.
197. Verrotti A, Chiarelli F, Amerio P, et al. Necrobiosis lipoidica diabeticorum in children and adolescents: a clue for underlying renal and retinal disease. *Pediatr Dermatol* 1995;12(3):220–223.
198. Villada G, Roujeau JC, Clerici T, et al. Immunopathology of toxic epidermal necrolysis. Keratinocytes, HLA-DR expression, Langerhans cells, and mononuclear cells: an immunopathologic study of five cases. *Arch Dermatol* 1992;128(1):50–53.
199. von den Driesch P. Pyoderma gangrenosum: a report of 44 cases with follow-up. *Br J Dermatol* 1997;137(6):1000–1005.
200. Wagner A. Distinguishing vesicular and pustular disorders in the neonate. *Curr Opin Pediatr* 1997;9(4):396–405.
201. Wakem P, Ikeda S, Haake A, et al. Localization of the Darier disease gene to a 2-cM portion of 12q23–24.1. *J Invest Dermatol* 1996;106(2):365–367.
202. Wang X, Reid Sutton V, Omar Peraza-Llanes J, et al. Mutations in X-linked PORCN, a putative regulator of Wnt signaling, cause focal dermal hypoplasia. *Nat Genet* 2007;39(7):836–838.
203. Weinberg JM, Kristal L, Chooback L, et al. The clonal nature of pityriasis lichenoides. *Arch Dermatol* 2002;138(8):1063–1067.
204. Wojnarowska F, Bhogal BS, Black MM. Chronic bullous disease of childhood and linear IgA disease of adults are IgA1-mediated diseases. *Br J Dermatol* 1994;131(2):201–204.
205. Woodley DT, Briggaman RA, Gammon WR. Acquired epidermolysis bullosa. A bullous disease associated with autoimmunity to type VII (anchoring fibril) collagen. *Dermatol Clin* 1990;8(4):717–726.
206. Yamasaki O, Yamaguchi T, Sugai M, et al. Clinical manifestations of staphylococcal scalded-skin syndrome depend on serotypes of exfoliative toxins. *J Clin Microbiol* 2005;43(4):1890–1893.
207. Yang YH, Chuang YH, Wang LC, et al. The immunobiology of Henoch-Schonlein purpura. *Autoimmun Rev* 2008;7(3):179–184.
208. Zaias N, Ackerman AB. The nail in Darier-White disease. *Arch Dermatol* 1973;107(2):193–199.
209. Zeb A, Darmstadt GL. Sclerema neonatorum: a review of nomenclature, clinical presentation, histological features, differential diagnoses and management. *J Perinatol* 2008;28(7):453–460.
210. Zembowicz A, Carney JA, Mihm MC. Pigmented epithelioid melanocytoma: a low-grade melanocytic tumor with metastatic potential indistinguishable from animal-type melanoma and epithelioid blue nevus. *Am J Surg Pathol* 2004;28(1):31–40.
211. Ziemer M, Boer A. Eosinophilic pustular folliculitis in infancy: not a distinctive inflammatory disease of the skin. *Am J Dermatopathol* 2005;27(5):443–455.
212. Zomorrodi A, Wald ER. Ecthyma gangrenosum: considerations in a previously healthy child. *Pediatr Infect Dis J* 2002;21(12):1161–1164.
213. Zulian F. Systemic sclerosis and localized scleroderma in childhood. *Rheum Dis Clin North Am* 2008;34(1):239–255; ix.

CHAPTER 26

Neuromuscular Diseases

KEVIN E. BOVE
LILI MILES

NORMAL MUSCLE DEVELOPMENT

Detailed reviews of skeletal muscle development provide a basis for understanding early events in myogenesis (114,222). In the first few weeks of embryonic life (Figure 26-1), primitive mesenchyme, under the influence of MyoD, Myf, and PAX genes, differentiates to muscle progenitor cells. Myofibrils form under the influence of myogenin. Myoblasts with disorganized sarcomeres fuse to form multinucleate myotubes in which oriented sarcomeres surround a central core that is rich in organelles but devoid of contractile filaments (Figure 26-2A). At this stage, muscle nuclei are centrally located, and there are no definable histochemical or structural subtypes. Prominent peripheral nuclei are those of satellite cells, located within the sarcolemmal basement membrane, or residual unfused myoblasts. Desmin and myogenin are strongly expressed in fetal myotubes: this immunohistochemical reactivity is markedly reduced by late gestation (210). Further growth and development of muscle is influenced by workload, growth factors such as myostatin, and steroid hormones.

The transition from myotubes, which average 8 to 10 μm in diameter, to larger muscle fibers with peripheral nuclei is completed between 22 and 26 weeks of gestation when most are typeable as IIc fetal fibers containing fetal myosin. During the third trimester (Figure 26-2B), type IIc fibers are replaced by type I fibers, type IIa fibers, and type IIb fibers (102). Type IIc fibers, defined as those with an intermediate level of myosin ATPase reactivity at low pH, evolve to mature subtypes and finally disappear during early infancy. Abnormal persistence of type IIc fibers occurs in both myopathic and neuropathic disorders of infancy and may indicate a maturation disturbance. Myofibers containing fetal myosin may transiently reappear during regeneration after muscle fiber injury at all ages.

A few widely scattered, relatively large type I fibers (the Wohlfart B fibers) with an uncertain role in development

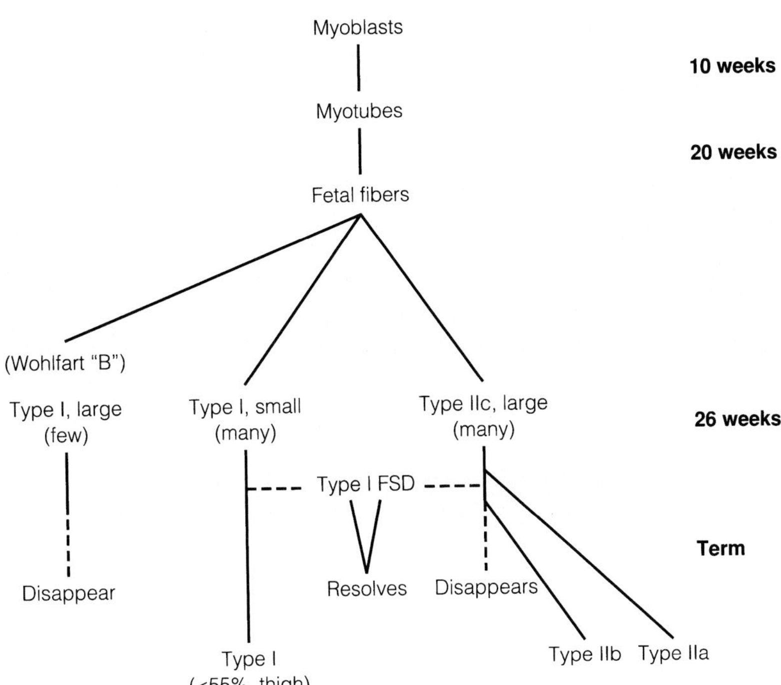

FIGURE 26-1 ■ Steps involved in prenatal and perinatal muscle fiber maturation. Fsd, fiber size disproportion.

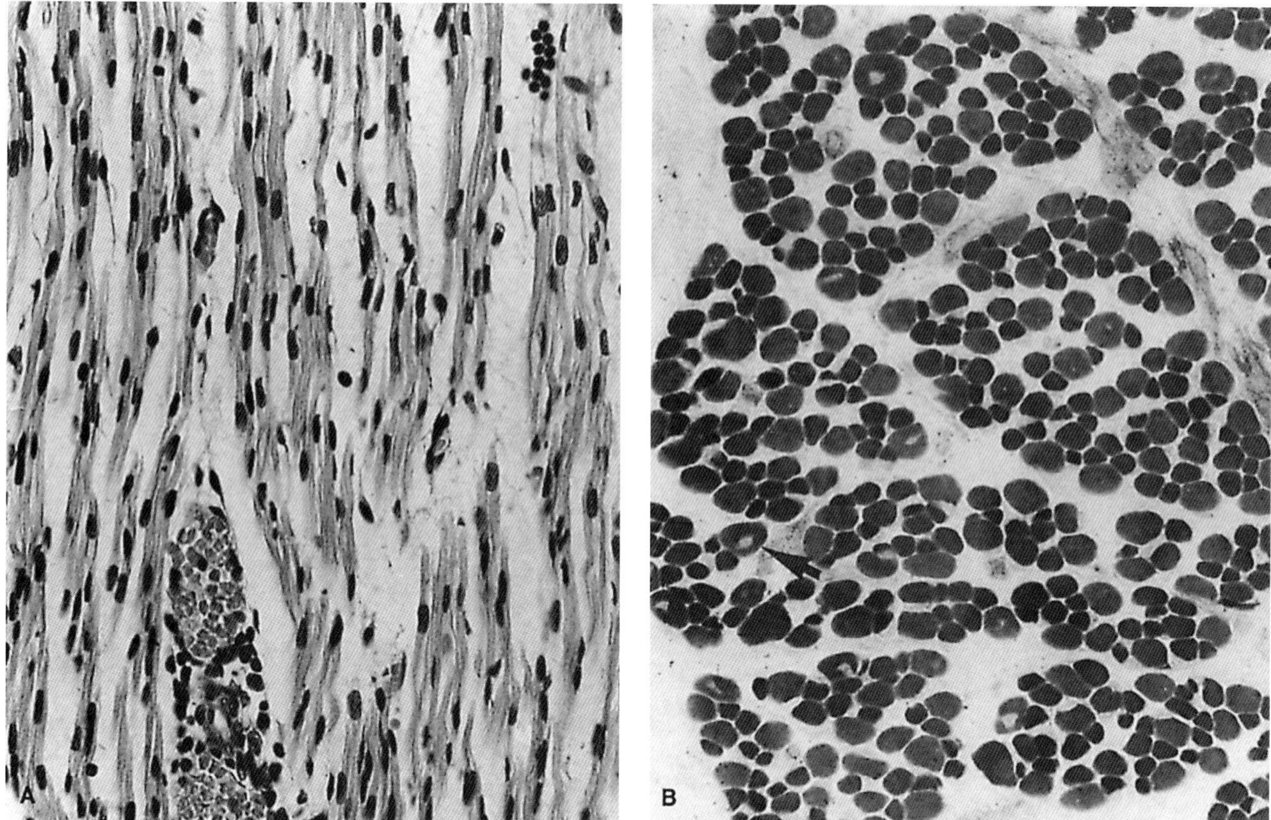

FIGURE 26-2■ **A:** Myotubular configuration of muscle fibers in a 19-week-old fetus. (Hematoxylin and eosin stain; original magnification ×400.) **B:** Normal deltoid muscle in a 29-week-old fetus contains small, dark, type I fibers and larger, intermediate-stained, type IIc fibers, many retaining central nuclei (*arrow*). (Myosin ATPase stain with preincubation at pH 4.3; original magnification ×250.)

make a brief appearance during late gestation and then rapidly regress. Most type I fibers are smaller than type IIc fibers until birth or slightly later in normal infants (259). Underlying the progressive disappearance of fetal fibers and appearance of mature fiber subtypes are poorly understood determinants of structural, enzymatic, and contractile proteins and of organelle populations including links between muscle and central nervous system maturation.

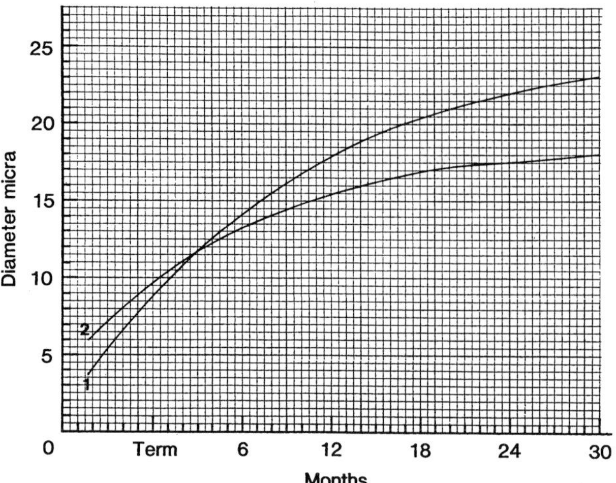

FIGURE 26-3■ Diameter of normal type I (1) and type II (2) fibers at various ages in young children.

Brooke and Engel published a useful review of muscle fiber subtype profiles for normal and abnormal muscle in children (31). They identified disproportionately small type I muscle fibers as a major finding in childhood neuromuscular disease, defining this state as a difference in diameter of type I and type II fibers of greater than 12%. Their nomogram relating normal muscle fiber diameter to age is valuable but falls short of the ideal because data for several muscles and for fiber subtypes were pooled and because of the paucity of data from young infants. A nomogram derived from frozen postmortem specimens of thigh muscles (Figure 26-3) is useful for assessment of fiber size in infants (259). Muscle fiber diameter in formalin-fixed paraffin sections is about 70% to 80% of that in sections of fresh-frozen muscle.

MUSCLE APLASIA AND HYPOPLASIA

Determination of whether muscles are small because of primary failure to develop or because of regression is always problematic for the pathologist. The best-documented examples of primary muscle aplasia or hypoplasia are secondary to spinal cord abnormalities. In the Poland anomaly, familial

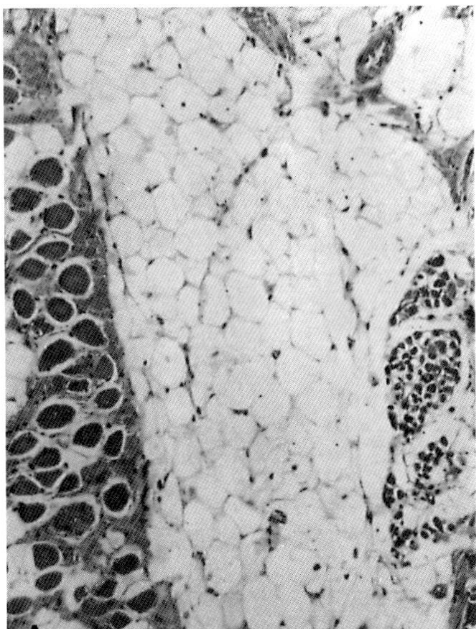

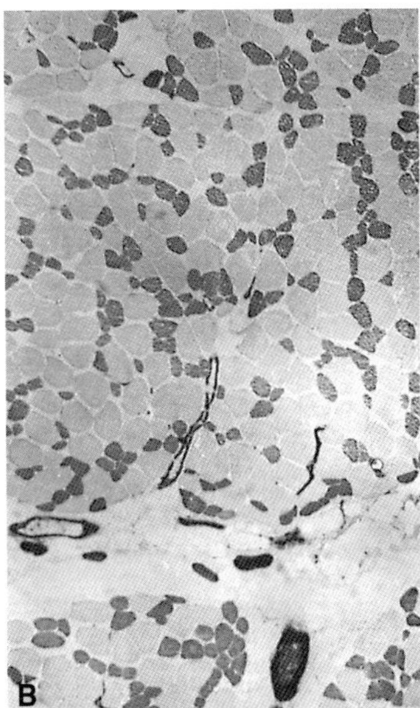

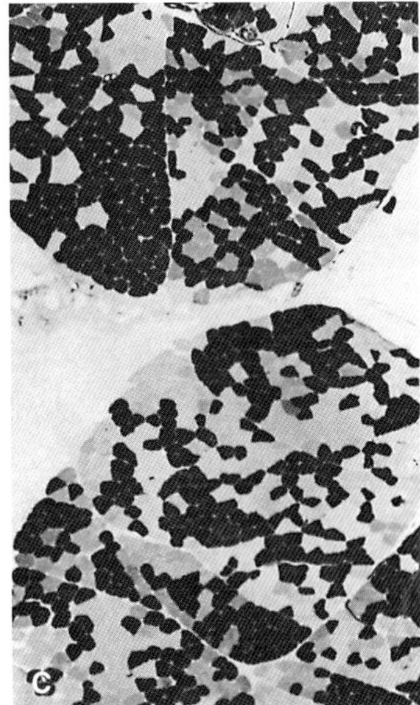

FIGURE 26-4■ **A:** Severely hypoplastic abdominal wall muscle in an infant with prune-belly syndrome typically contains few fibers and abundant fat. (Hematoxylin and eosin stain; original magnification ×70.) **B:** Thin rectus abdominis muscle in a 19-year-old patient with prune-belly syndrome exhibits type I FSD. (Myosin ATPase stain with preincubation at pH 4.3; original magnification ×80.) **C:** Thin rectus abdominis muscle in a 13-year-old child with prune-belly syndrome. Homogeneous-type groups suggest reinnervation. (Myosin ATPase stain with preincubation at pH 4.6; original magnification ×400.)

absence of pectoralis muscle is associated with local soft tissue and skeletal defects and syndactyly (57). Möbius syndrome may coexist with the Poland anomaly, suggesting that a primary lesion may exist in the central nervous system and interfere with development of specific muscles in some cases (177). Chromosome abnormalities influence muscle development in trisomy syndromes, but it is uncertain whether this is a defect in muscle specification from primitive mesenchyme or the result of abnormal organization at the level of the spinal cord (20,183,192). The alleged normality of the spinal cord in most patients with urinary tract dilatation and deficient abdominal wall musculature (so-called prune-belly syndrome) requires re-examination, but it tends to focus attention on alternate hypotheses for deficient numbers of fibers (Figure 26-4A), such as a mesodermal field defect, favored by the character of associated anomalies, and linkage to trisomy 18 (143). Compression secondary to abdominal distension may contribute to muscle atrophy by direct pressure, by limiting blood supply, or by interfering with innervation (Figure 26-4B, C).

Congenital diaphragmatic hernia is either an open defect or one covered only by a thin membrane lacking muscle fibers. Typically, it is located on the left side, and the phrenic nerve and the cervical spinal cord are normal. This form of hernia is thought to result from a primary defect in mesenchymal precursors involved in closure of the pleuroperitoneal canal. Eventration of the diaphragm is a unilateral or a bilateral thinning of the diaphragm that occurs as a consequence of neuromuscular disease, such as birth trauma to the spinal cord or brachial plexus, anterior horn cell disease, phrenic nerve agenesis, myotonic dystrophy, or congenital myopathy (CM) (87). Diaphragm muscle fibers usually display the lesion of the primary disorder (see Chapter 12) (27,44,146).

ARTHROGRYPOSIS

Congenital joint contractures (Figure 26-5A) typically do not progress and usually result from intrauterine disorders that restrict fetal movement, also known as fetal akinesia deformation sequence (91,155,267). The etiology is heterogeneous and includes chromosome abnormalities of various types (193), teratogens, restrictive skin diseases, neurogenic and myogenic disorders. Most cases are sporadic and of unknown etiology. A tentative pathogenic classification (Table 26-1) of arthrogryposis congenita includes subtypes due to external compression, primary muscle disease, primary or secondary disorders of the central nervous system, such as dysgenesis or disruption of the motor centers of the brain or spinal cord, or deficiencies in the number or organization of the lower motor neurons and their peripheral connections. Rare diseases of soft tissue, skin, or the skeleton may also restrict fetal movement (see Chapters 25 and 27) (133,266).

Specific neuromuscular diseases that cause contractures before birth usually are not associated with other major developmental defects. Notable exceptions are brain anomalies in patients with congenital muscular dystrophy (CMD) (158) and multiple anomalies in some patients with a type II glutaric acidemia (96). The consequences of poor muscle tone or diminished movement vary from minor to life threatening.

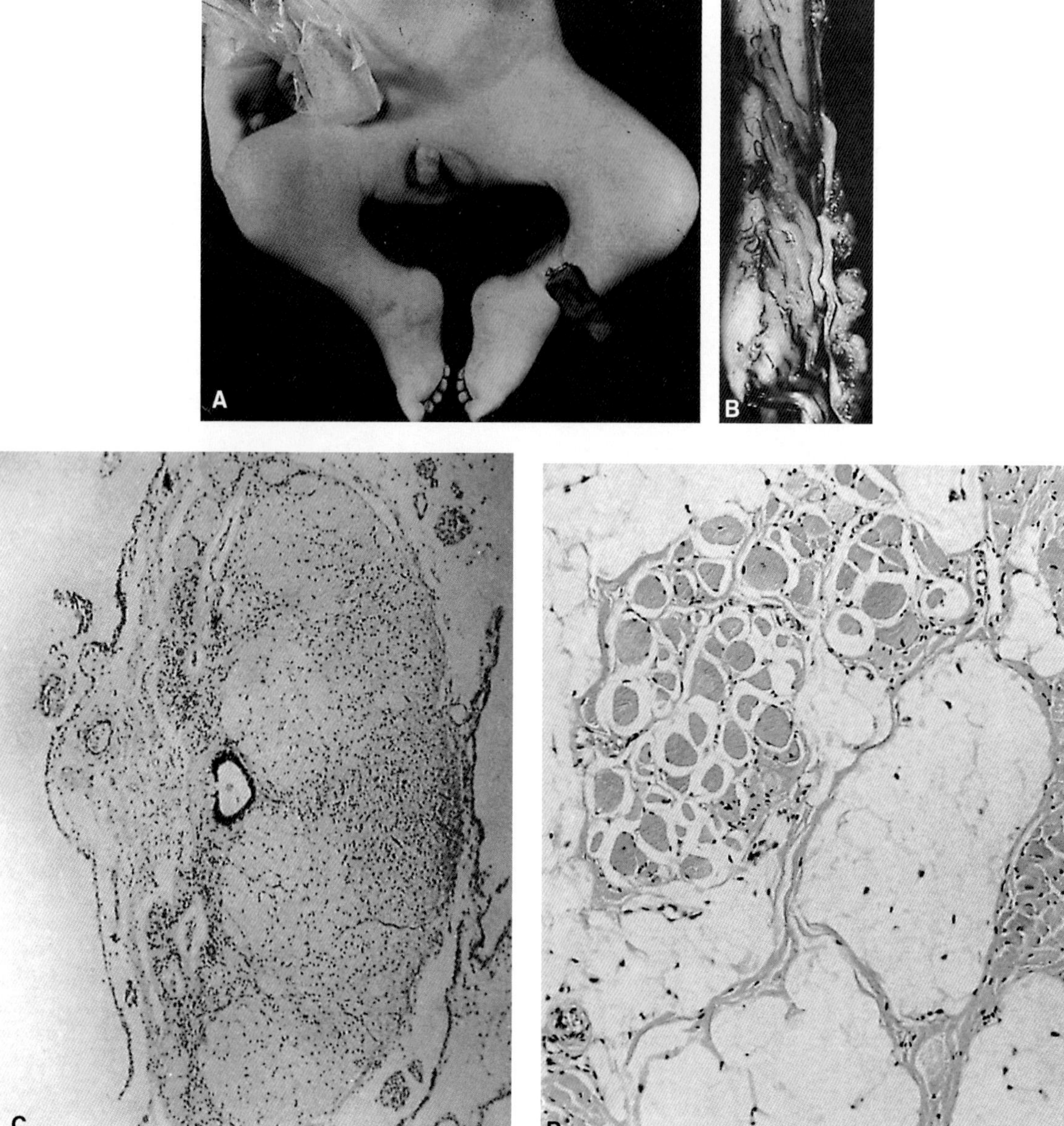

FIGURE 26-5 **A:** Congenital joint contractures due to distal spinal cord hypoplasia in caudal dysgenesis syndrome. **B:** The spinal cord in caudal dysgenesis is short and truncated, although it is histologically normal. **C:** Spinal cord in fetus with arthrogryposis multiplex is small, disorganized, and deficient in motor neurons. (Hematoxylin and eosin stain; original magnification ×64.) **D:** Thigh muscle in caudal dysgenesis is composed mainly of fat cells. A rare cluster of muscle fibers exhibits mixed hypertrophy and atrophy. (Hematoxylin and eosin stain; original magnification ×160.)

Diminished fetal movement is one of several causes of short umbilical cord (151):

- Short cord
- Contractures
- Gracile ribs
- Pectus excavatum
- High arched palate
- Laryngeal diaphragm
- Hydramnios
- Lung hypoplasia
- Eventration

Banker proposed that arthrogryposis congenita multiplex (ACM) is often the result of changes in muscle secondary to spinal cord disease (15). In a few arthrogrypotic fetuses, gross or microscopic malformation of the spinal cord is striking (Figure 26-5B and C), but the changes may be subtle (46). Autopsy studies after *in utero* diagnosis indicate a higher incidence of brain than spinal cord abnormalities (267). The histology of poorly developed muscle related to congenitally fixed limbs is highly variable, which has engendered considerable confusion. Whether congenital arthrogryposis is due to lesions of the nervous system, muscle, or other tissues, muscle histology may be

Table 26-1 ▪ PATHOGENETIC CLASSIFICATION OF ARTHROGRYOPSIS

Amyoplasia
Aplasia, isolated (talipes)
Aplasia/hypoplasia in trisomy syndromes
Aplasia/hypoplasia, neuropathic

Neuropathic
Meningomyelocele
Spinal cord dysgenesis
Motor neuron disease
Absence of peripheral myelin
Cerebral/spinal malformation (Pena-Shokeir syndrome)
Cerebral/spinal disruption

Myopathic
Congenital myopathies
Infantile myotonic dystrophy
CMD
Intrauterine myositis

Skeletal, connective tissue, or skin disease
Congenital arachnodactyly with contractures
Larsen syndrome
Restrictive dermopathy

External deformation (e.g., oligohydramnios)

determined as much by the degree and duration of intrauterine immobility as it is by other factors (see Chapter 10). Careful selection of cases for muscle biopsy may increase the yield of diagnostic information (116). Changes are most likely in muscles contiguous with the contracture; when several, fascial layers may enclose adipose tissue alone or with scattered muscle spindles or clusters of muscle fibers (Figure 26-5D). The hypoplastic muscle may collapse, producing condensation of stroma and an apparent increase in number of muscle spindles, often with extreme variation in muscle fiber size. Nonspecific myopathic changes seen focally may not be germane to pathogenesis. Recognizable denervation atrophy is uncommon. Theoretically, a marked deficit of muscle fibers could reflect primary deficiency of myoblasts, disturbed innervation at a critical early period, or loss of innervation due to circulatory disturbance or compression. Histological criteria for establishing these distinctions are unreliable. It is probably best to avoid arbitrary designation of histologic changes as myopathic or neuropathic when the major abnormality is too few muscle fibers and too much adipose tissue. When in doubt, the term *amyoplasia*, used by clinicians to designate common sporadic form of ACM, may suffice.

Contractures may be a component of complex phenotypes of genetic origin, particularly when mental retardation, developmental abnormalities and/or facial abnormalities coexist (193). Pena-Shokeir phenotype (3,138,173,154) consists of central nervous system lesions, facial anomalies, polyhydramnios, fetal growth restriction, pulmonary hypoplasia, and arthrogryposis. The brain lesions in some examples are acquired disruptions (43,65). The occasional concurrence of Pena-Shokeir phenotype in siblings confirms that genetic factors are sometimes involved. Muscle may be normal, atrophic, or denervated. Reduced numbers of anterior horn cells are reported (154). Exposure of fetal rats to curare produced a similar phenotype, suggesting that fetal akinesia can produce structural anomalies of the face, polyhydramnios due to decreased swallowing, pulmonary hypoplasia due to decreased fetal breathing movements, and multiple joint contractures (155). Hall analyzed the Pena-Shokeir phenotype and agreed (91).

Primary muscle diseases that produce congenital contractures include the congenital myopathies (CMs) and the congenital muscular dystrophies. In specific forms of CM, contractures usually are not severe, the muscles are not hypoplastic, and muscle fibrosis, if present, is usually minor. In contrast, CMD is a diverse group of diseases that may be associated with contractures at birth or progressive contractures later in life, and prominent connective tissue proliferation in muscle.

DIAGNOSTIC EVALUATION

Muscle Biopsy

Muscle biopsy is a deceptively simple procedure, the success of which requires the cooperation of a clinician who determines the need and selects the muscle to be biopsied, a surgeon who has learned the skills requisite to provide a nontraumatized specimen, a specially trained histotechnologist, and a pathologist who interprets the findings in conjunction with the responsible clinician. Skeletal muscle biopsy plays a central role in guiding the management of a child thought to have a neuromuscular disease. Muscle biopsy should not be performed until other, noninvasive diagnostic methods have been used to evaluate the patient. These include a complete history (including birth and family history), physical evaluation by a neurologist, electrodiagnostic tests of neuromuscular function, and measurement of serum levels of enzymes, such as creatine kinase and aldolase that are released by damaged skeletal muscle fibers.

Recommendations for muscle biopsy technique and processing are available from several sources (67,208). General anesthesia is necessary in small infants, but the risk of a malignant hypothermic reaction in patients with certain forms of muscle disease must be kept in mind. Local anesthesia may be used in older children, but the agent should not be directly injected into the muscle to be sampled.

Modified surgical biopsy using suction applied with a large-bore, reusable needle inserted through a small skin incision has been advocated as an alternative to open surgical biopsy (94). Applicable to patients of all ages except small infants, this technique produces a specimen of adequate size and quality for diagnostic studies for those neuromuscular diseases in which sampling error is not an issue. Major advantages are use at the bedside or in an outpatient setting, low cost, ease of scheduling, and a small scar, all of which focus the decision to perform or repeat a muscle biopsy on essential medical criteria.

Optimal specimens obtained by open surgical biopsy are strips of fresh skeletal muscle, 1 to 2 cm long and approximately 0.5 cm wide, which are excised by sharp dissection. This is ideal for snap freezing and for preparation of frozen sections for histochemical procedures. If only one specimen is obtained, as in some infants with poorly developed muscles, a small portion of it can be excised from an untraumatized area before freezing and placed in an appropriate fixative for resin embedding and ultrastructural study.

Muscle biopsy clamps are not recommended because clumsy application of clamps creates troublesome artifacts from twisting, tearing, and compression, and a portion of the specimen is destroyed by the clamps. Moreover, optimal fixation for ultrastructural studies is limited to the most superficial layers of muscle, which may be the most traumatized by the procedure. Available clamps are too large for convenient use in small infants.

A sample of every muscle biopsy performed should be prepared for ultrastructural studies, in case of need. If the status of the patient suggests a need for biochemical or molecular studies, an additional sample of fresh muscle should be obtained for immediate analysis or storage after snap freezing in liquid nitrogen. The specimen should be wrapped tightly to prevent desiccation.

Skeletal muscle cannot be slowly frozen in a cryostat chamber or a freezer without producing highly objectionable intracellular ice crystals. Skeletal muscle is particularly susceptible, because most of the sarcoplasm contains tough, dense, deformable fibrillar proteins, which, when stained, provide a stark contrast to the angular spaces remaining after ice crystals have formed and then melted. The standard procedure for freezing skeletal muscle uses liquid nitrogen or a halogenated hydrocarbon as the primary coolant and isopentane as a secondary coolant to facilitate heat transfer from the muscle specimen. We have effectively employed talc as a substitute for isopentane in our laboratory. A thick layer of talc around the muscle specimen is a good heat transfer agent, which consistently yields high-quality frozen sections. In our experience, freeze artifact is unavoidable in overly manipulated specimens, regardless of the method employed.

MUSCLE HISTOCHEMISTRY

Cross section is the preferred orientation of muscle fibers for diagnostic evaluation. In a minority of cases, useful supplementary information can be obtained by examining muscle fibers in longitudinal sections. Most laboratories no longer prepare paraffin sections of muscle because of limited tissue, the difficulty of preparing high-quality paraffin sections of skeletal muscle, and the necessity of frozen sections for the diagnostic methods described below.

Among the dozens of histochemical and immunohistochemical methods that may be applied to skeletal muscle, a few are essential while the others are best reserved for exploring specific questions raised by the clinical impression or based upon the initial microscopical findings, such as metabolic myopathy, inflammatory myopathy, or muscular dystrophy. The modified trichrome method provides an overview, highlights collagen, displays normal and pathological mitochondrial distribution, and reveals the myofibrillar network. Krebs cycle substrates, such as succinate, may be used to display mitochondrial activity and distribution, based on formazan deposition at sites of activity. DPNH reductase highlights areas of sarcoplasm lacking contractile elements. Alkaline phosphatase and reactions for fetal myosin assist in identification of injured or regenerating myofibers. Acid phosphatase helps to identify primary and secondary lysosomes.

The calcium-dependent myosin ATPase reactions, performed by varying the preincubation substrate pH, are the mainstay for delineation of at least four major fiber subtypes in diagnostic muscle specimens (Figure 26-6). All human muscles are composed of a mosaic of fiber subtypes; the composition depends on the particular muscle or muscle group and its functions, the position within the muscle, constitutional differences between individuals, physical training, and disease (99,206). Although to some extent a dynamic quality, fiber subtypes revealed by the myosin ATPase reaction can be relied upon in most situations to provide information useful for diagnosis.

Type I fibers are physiologic slow-twitch fibers that are richly endowed with mitochondria and contain relatively abundant, evenly dispersed lipid droplets, little glycogen, and lower concentrations of glycolytic enzymes, such as phosphorylase. Type II fibers are fast-twitch fibers that contain fewer mitochondria, relatively little lipid, abundant glycogen, and abundant phosphorylase activity. Fatigue-resistant muscles responsible for antigravity posture maintenance, such as the paraspinal and abdominal wall muscles, contain a high proportion of type I fibers. Muscles involved in rapid, repetitive movements, such as the intrinsic muscles of the larynx

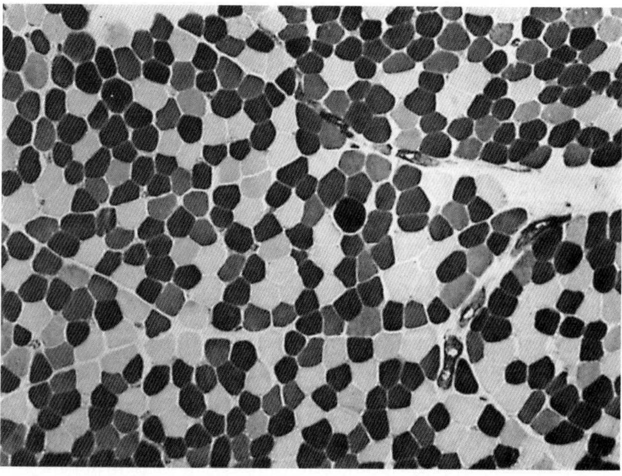

FIGURE 26-6 ■ Three major fiber subtypes are displayed by myosin ATPase reaction with preincubation at pH 4.6 in a normal thigh muscle from a 19-month-old boy. Type I fibers, dark; type IIa fibers, pale; type IIb fibers, intermediate density. (Persistent intermediate reaction after preincubation at pH 4.2 to 4.3 identifies type IIc fibers; original magnification ×200.)

and the superficial muscles of the face, are predominantly composed of type II fibers. Among common biopsy sites, the deltoid and the gastrocnemius muscles have a predominance of type I fibers, and the quadriceps muscle has a predominance of type II fibers. Information on composition of less commonly biopsied muscles is available (110,136).

HISTOPATHOLOGY IN MUSCLE DISEASE

Pathologic alterations in muscle fibers are conventionally classified as "myopathic" or "neuropathic" to signify respectively primary diseases of the muscle fiber alone and diseases of fibers as components of motor units. This approach is useful, but the narrow scope of muscle fiber reaction to injury limits diagnostic application. Many muscle specimens from infants or children show readily classifiable changes (Table 26-2), which correlate well with results of clinical investigations. However, troublesome discrepancies are common, requiring cooperation between the clinician and the pathologist, and considerable experience to resolve. The myopathy versus neuropathy paradigm seems to be particularly impotent in its application to congenital neuromuscular diseases, perhaps because of a failure to account for the dependence of maturation and architectural modeling of muscles on the normal development of the nervous system (209).

MUSCLE ATROPHY

Loss of muscle bulk is a common feature of chronic neuromuscular disease in all age groups. In congenital muscle disorders, overall bulk and size of individual muscle fibers may never have been normal. The term *hypotrophy* has been introduced to distinguish primary growth disturbance from secondary muscle fiber atrophy, but this distinction is difficult to make in practice. There is little information available on muscle fiber size in babies with intrauterine

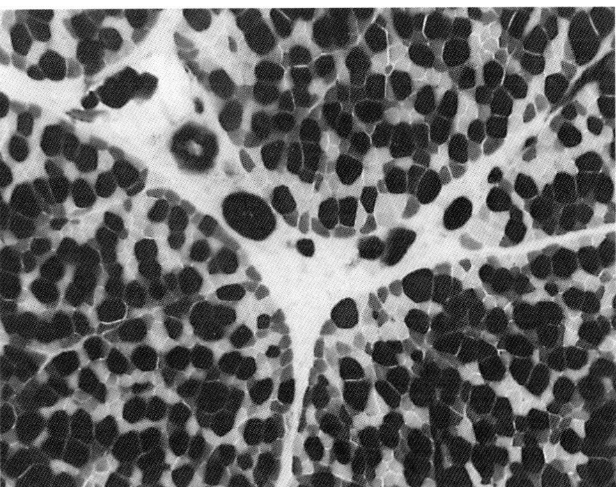

FIGURE 26-7■Selective atrophy of type IIa (pale) and type IIb (intermediate density) fibers in a child with idiopathic cardiomyopathy. (Myosin ATPase stain with preincubation at pH 4.6; original magnification ×400.)

growth restriction. Muscle fiber atrophy tends to be uniform in malnourished infants (56). Muscle atrophy associated with central nervous system disorders, myasthenic syndromes, neoplasia, cardiomyopathy, inflammatory myopathy, or steroid therapy often selectively affects type II fibers (Figure 26-7). It has been suggested that type II fibers are more dependent than type I fibers on the trophic stimulation provided by normal activity levels and more vulnerable to the catabolic effects of steroids when activity is reduced (198).

DISTURBANCES OF MUSCLE MATURATION

Features of muscle immaturity include persistent myotubes, central nuclei, prominent satellite cells, type I fiber size disproportion (FSD), large isolated type I Wohlfart fibers, a high percentage of fetal type IIc fibers, numeric predominance of type I fibers, and absence of type IIb fibers. Signs of muscle maturation disturbance are common in congenital

Table 26-2 ■ MUSCLE FIBER PATHOLOGY

Neuropathic Changes	Myopathic Changes	Changes of Indeterminate Cause
Motor unit distribution	Focal or general distribution	Muscle hypoplasia
No fiber subtype preference	May be influenced by fiber type	Delayed or arrested maturation
Loose or compact grouped atrophy		Poor fiber subtype display
	Fiber degeneration, many forms	Central nuclei
Grouped fibers of similar subtype		Type I atrophy
	Fiber necrosis, segmental	Type II atrophy
Angular atrophic fibers	Fiber regeneration	
Extreme fiber atrophy with nuclear aggregates	Replacement fibrosis	
	Inflammatory reaction	
Limited degeneration and regeneration	Organelle diseases	
Acute atrophy	Storage diseases	
Target fibers		
Condensation of structural collagen		

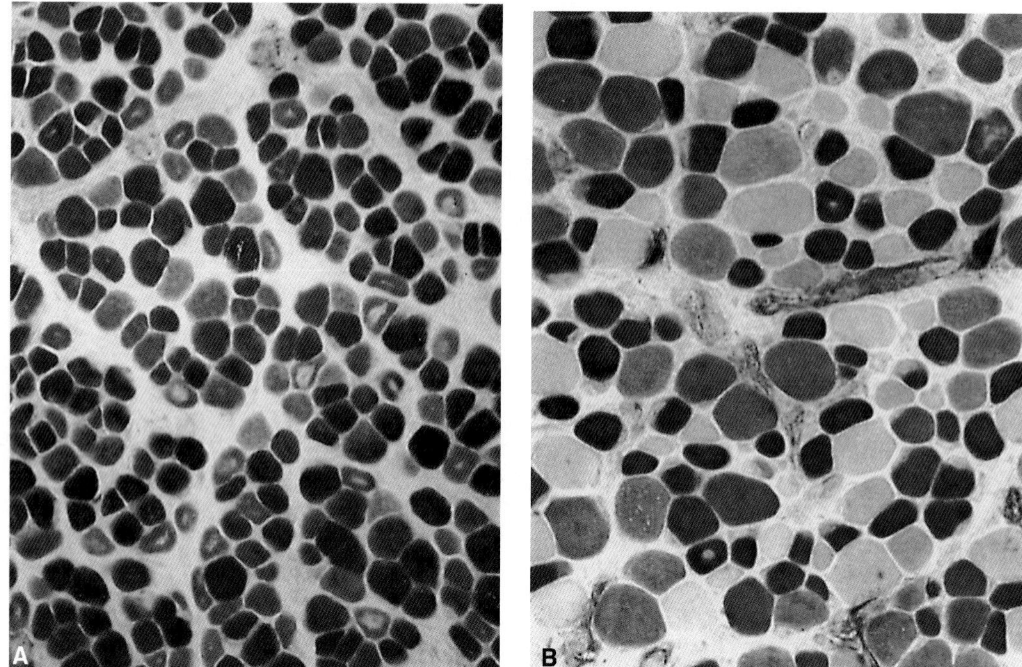

FIGURE 26-8 **A:** Severe immaturity in thigh muscle of a term baby with myotonic dystrophy. Type I fibers and type IIc fibers prevail. Nonstaining central zones are myotubes or central nuclei. (Myosin ATPase stain with preincubation at pH 4.3; original magnification ×740.) **B:** Thigh muscle of an improved 3-month-old infant with myotonic dystrophy syndrome exhibits near-normal composition with persistent small type I fibers. (Myosin ATPase stain with preincubation pH at 4.3; original magnification ×800.)

myopathies, infantile spinomuscular atrophy (ISMA), peripheral neuropathy manifested in infancy, and in central hypotonia (107). In the perinatal period, intramuscular myelopoiesis in perivascular connective tissue may accompany dysmaturation (28).

An important prototype for muscle maturation delay occurs in newborn infants of mothers with myotonic dystrophy, a dominantly inherited disease of variable severity (106,241,247). Even when severely affected, such infants usually improve clinically and in terms of muscle morphology (Figure 26-8). The causative mutation is an expansion of a trinucleotide repeat sequence in the myotonin gene, which is the basis for a reliable diagnostic test on blood DNA that has largely supplanted muscle biopsy. The degree of expansion correlates reasonably well with disease severity and tends to increase from one generation to the next, particularly in women.

CENTRAL HYPOTONIA

Central hypotonia designates a heterogeneous clinical group of infants and young children who display general poor muscle tone and various degrees of slowing of motor development accompanied by one or more signs of central nervous system dysfunction, such as motor delay, decreased alertness, delayed or dysarthric speech, seizures, learning disabilities, pyramidal tract signs, or ataxia. Some of these children have defined syndromes, but many do not. Central nervous system disorders associated with hypotonia and/or morphologic signs of muscle dysmaturity in infancy include

- Microcephaly, macrocephaly
- Ischemic encephalopathy
- Cerebral palsy
- Cerebellar hypoplasia
- CMD
- Cerebral dysgenesis

Imaging studies of the brain may be normal or show borderline abnormalities, including expansion of the subarachnoid space, atrophy of cortical gyri, polymicrogyria, ventricular dilatation, or cerebellar hypoplasia. Infants who are suspected of having central hypotonia are sometimes subjected to muscle biopsy for the purpose of ruling out specific causes of muscle hypotonia. Thigh muscle samples may be normal but often display signs of muscle dysmaturation with disturbances of fascicular composition, irregularities of fiber size, and distribution suggesting previous denervation and reinnervation or preferential atrophy or hypertrophy of type I or type II fibers (Figure 26-9) (9,61,240). A similar spectrum of changes has been described in specimens from spastic muscles in children with cerebral palsy (37). It is relevant that a history of perinatal asphyxia is obtained in some patients with central hypotonia, some of whom eventually develop spastic paresis (107).

Several authors have suggested that a suprasegmental determinant of normal skeletal muscle maturation may

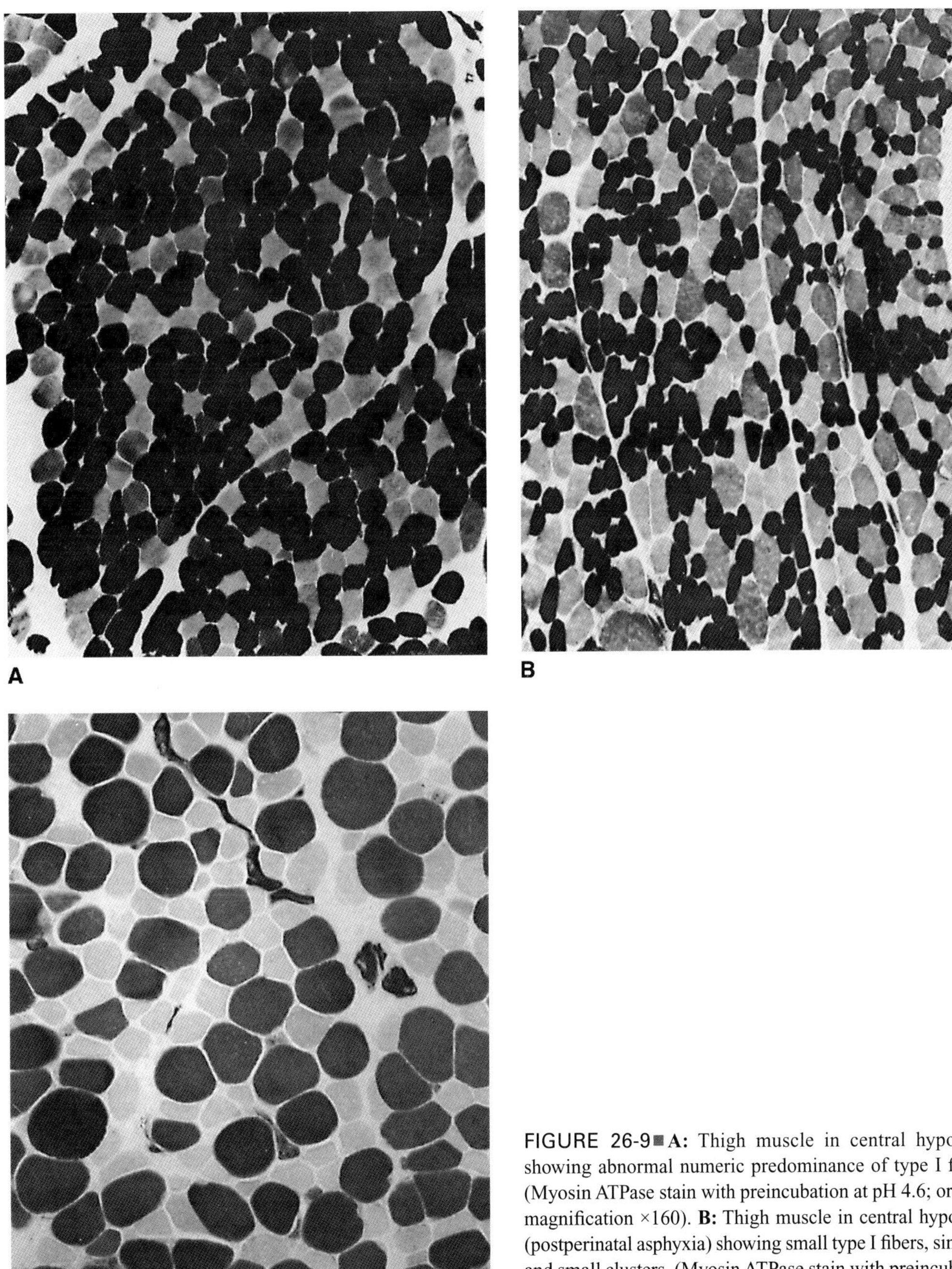

FIGURE 26-9▪**A:** Thigh muscle in central hypotonia showing abnormal numeric predominance of type I fibers. (Myosin ATPase stain with preincubation at pH 4.6; original magnification ×160). **B:** Thigh muscle in central hypotonia (postperinatal asphyxia) showing small type I fibers, singlets, and small clusters. (Myosin ATPase stain with preincubation at pH 4.6; original magnification ×160.) **C:** Thigh muscle in central hypotonia showing small type II fibers and hypertrophied type I fibers. (Myosin ATPase stain with preincubation at pH 4.6; original magnification ×400.)

be disturbed in some infants with central hypotonia or arthrogryposis multiplex congenita (77,209,267). However, skeletal muscle development is usually quite normal in infants with anencephaly, indicating that normal unmodified spinal cord function is sufficient for lower motor unit maturation. It is possible that sporadic central hypotonia results in some babies from simultaneous perinatal insult to the developing central nervous system and the peripheral motor units. Alternatively, a genetic defect may affect both brain and muscle development, as in some children with CMD.

NEUROMUSCULAR DISEASES

Detailed histochemical and ultrastructural investigation of muscle specimens from patients with neuromuscular dysfunction has increased dramatically the number of recognizable clinicopathologic entities. In recent years, the advent of more precise understanding of the cellular and genetic basis for many neuromuscular diseases has provided more sophisticated tools for the diagnosis of some disorders while at the same time narrowing the role for diagnostic histomorphology.

Table 26-3 ■ NEUROMUSCULAR DISEASES

Disorders of innervation
Spinal cord dysplasia
Motor neuron disease
Peripheral neuropathy
Combined central and peripheral neuropathy
Nutritional disorders
Disorders of neuromuscular transmission
Congenital myopathy
Central nuclear and myotubular myopathy
Nemaline myopathy
Central core disease
Minicore-multicore disease
CM with small type I fibers
CM with fingerprint bodies
CM, other
Metabolic myopathy
Lysosomal storage diseases
Glycogen storage diseases
Triglyceride storage diseases
Mitochondriopathies
Metabolic myopathy, other
Episodic myglobinuria
MH syndrome
Drug-induced myopathy
Muscular dystrophy
Dystrophinopathies, X-linked
DMD
BMD
Muscular dystrophies, autosomal recessive
Adhalin deficiency (dystrophin-associated complex)
Other limb-girdle types
Muscular dystrophies, dominant
Facioscapulohumeral type
Congenital muscular dystrophy
Merosin normal
Merosin absent
Fukuyama type
Walker-Warburg type
Inflammatory myopathy
Infectious myositis
Local myositis
Idiopathic inflammatory myopathy, childhood dermatomyositis
Skeletal myopathy and cardiomyopathy

Table 26-3 outlines the primary neuromuscular diseases presenting in infancy and childhood. Six generic categories are delineated:

1. Disorders of innervation
2. CM
3. Metabolic myopathy
4. Skeletal and cardiomyopathy
5. Muscular dystrophy
6. Inflammatory myopathy

DISORDERS OF INNERVATION

Denervation is expressed in all the muscle fibers of an affected motor unit, producing loss of tone and atrophy.

Table 26-4 ■ MAJOR CHILDHOOD DENERVATING DISORDERS

Spinal cord hypoplasia or dysplasia
Spinomuscular atrophy
Type I (infantile, Werdnig-Hoffmann)
Type II (late infantile)
Type III (juvenile, Kugelberg-Weylander)
ISMA, X-linked
Bulbar muscular atrophy (Fazio-Londe)
Scapuloperoneal spinal muscular atrophy
HSMNs, all types
Acquired myelopathy or neuropathy
Traumatic
Ischemic
Infectious (enterovirus)
Postinfectious (Guillian-BarrŽ)
Toxic/drug-induced
Nutritional

Denervated fibers often exhibit angulated contours as a result of molding by normotonic neighbors. The appearance of denervated muscle has no specificity for the underlying neurologic disorder (Table 26-4) and may depend on the chronologic relation of the biopsy to the onset of the disease (Figure 26-10A, B). Findings are further modified by expression *in utero* or during early infancy, a time when impairment of muscle maturation may be added to the effect of denervation (Figure 26-10C, D). Reinnervation occurs unpredictably as the distal nerve twigs of an intact motor unit expand to make new junctions with adjacent denervated fibers, resulting in abnormally large groups of fibers of one subtype (see Figure 26-9B). Recognition of clusters of reinnervated fibers in muscle that normally contains mostly one type of fiber may require a quantitative approach. Other features of chronic denervation are target and targetoid fibers, and central nuclei (213).

SPINAL CORD DISEASES

Deficiency of spinal neurons results from developmental deficiency (dysplasia or hypoplasia) or may result from degeneration or loss caused by genetic motor neuron diseases, trauma, ischemia, and viral infections (e.g., enterovirus) with affinity for spinal motor neurons. Microscopic dysplasia or malformation of the spinal cord is typically sporadic and may be generalized or limited to the distal cord, causing segmental deficiency of lower motor units, muscle hypoplasia, and contractures (15).

Spinal cord trauma occurs during difficult deliveries or as a result of accidents, and it does not selectively damage the anterior horn regions. Diaphragmatic paralysis in newborns is more often the result of unilateral brachial plexus injury than of spinal cord injury. Cervical spine instability or a narrow cervical canal, as in chondrodystrophy or other developmental disorders involving the spine, predisposes the individual to hyperextension injury of the spinal cord. Acute selective upper spinal motor neuron necrosis occasionally

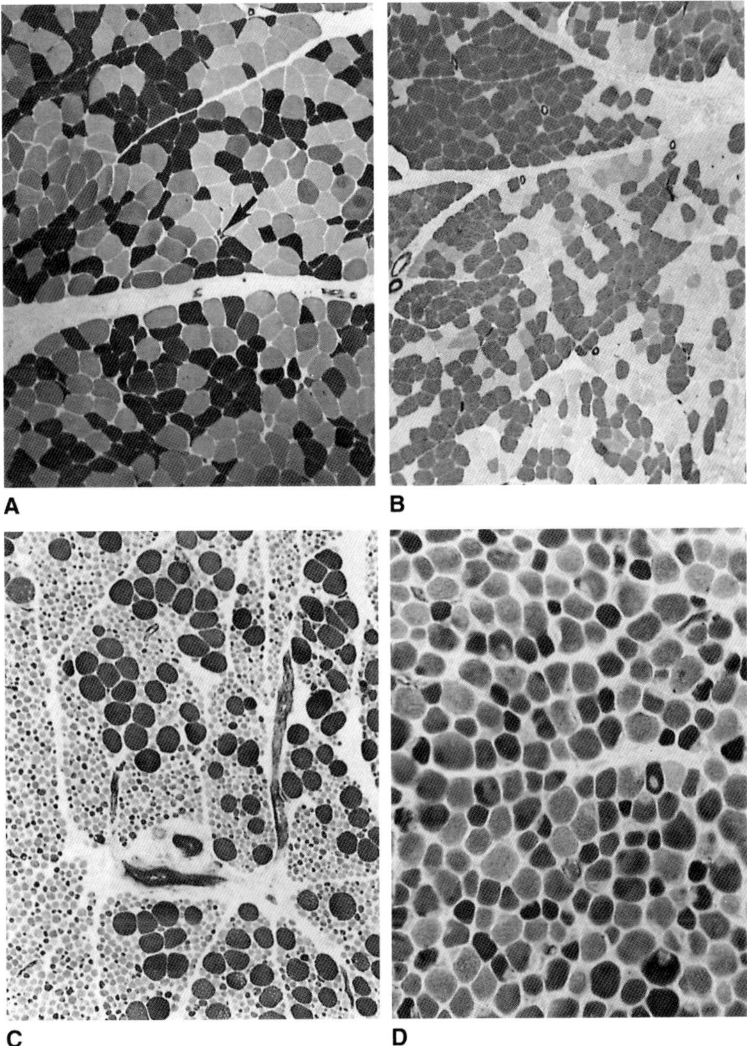

FIGURE 26-10 ■ **A:** Active denervation involves fibers of each subtype that causes atrophy, often with angulated profiles (*arrow*). (Myosin ATPase stain with preincubation at pH 4.6; original magnification ×64.) **B:** Reinnervation produces clusters of fibers of similar type in chronic peripheral neuropathy. (Myosin ATPase stain with preincubation at pH 4.6; original magnification ×80.) **C:** Infantile spinomuscular atrophy. Subtotal or panfascicular fiber atrophy with clusters of hypertrophied type I fibers. (Myosin ATPase stain with preincubation at pH 4.6; original magnification ×64.) **D:** Atrophic fibers in ISMA exhibit features of delayed maturation. (Myosin ATPase stain with preincubation at pH 4.3; original magnification ×640.)

accompanies widespread perinatal ischemic injury to brain stem nuclei (234). Spinal cord injury from compromise of the spinal arterial circulation is a recognized complication of surgical procedures on the aorta, such as coarctation repair.

MOTOR NEURON DISEASE

Hereditary motor neuron diseases of children and adults are characterized by progressive degeneration of the motor neurons of the spinal cord and brain stem nuclei. Typically, sensory neurons, upper motor neurons, and the cortical spinal tracts are not involved. Classification is based on factors such as age at presentation, rate of progression, milestones achieved, and distribution of neuronal lesions (274). Although imperfect, the following clinical classification currently enjoys wide usage:

Type 1: never able to sit
Type 2: able to sit but not to walk
Type 3: able to walk
  a. onset before 3 years
  b. onset 3 to 30 years
Type 4: onset after 30 years

Infantile Spinomuscular Atrophy (ISMA) may be recognized at birth, or the onset may be delayed. Early onset usually is followed by rapid progression (180). Weakness is generalized, but respiratory muscles are spared; diaphragmatic involvement is rarely observed at onset (27,146). Muscle biopsy discloses groups or entire fascicles composed of small rounded fibers displaying poor delineation of fiber subtypes, small immature type I fibers, variable persistence of type IIc fibers, and small clusters of hypertrophied type I fibers (see Figure 26-10C and D). Features of ISMA in muscle may be confused with the incomplete muscle maturation that prevails in late gestation. Spinomuscular atrophy (SMA) presenting in older children exhibits features similar to denervation in adults, including clusters of angulated atrophic fibers and groups of hypertrophied reinnervated type I and type II fibers.

ISMA has long been suspected to be an autosomal recessive trait. Linkage studies have now mapped the gene to a 5q deletion in more than 95% of cases of type 1 SMA, including many families with a pattern of later onset (274). Two important candidate genes have been identified: survival motor neuron (SMN) and neuronal apoptosis inhibitory protein gene. Specific deletions of SMN are found in more than 90% of children with types 1 and 2 SMA and about 80% with type 3 SMA, but they are absent in patients with type 4 SMA. Atypical variants of infantile SMA include a diaphragmatic form with early respiratory failure (27), and an X-linked arthrogrypotic form that lacks the 5q/SMN deletion (274). Inclusion of variant cases in previously reported series of infants with SMA may have suggested more heterogeneity than actually exists.

Genetic testing is a powerful tool for analysis of patients with SMA, eclipsing the role of muscle biopsy. However, because atypical SMA in infants may not be detected in currently employed genetic tests and because the SMN gene may be deleted in normal siblings, SMN deletion does not provide diagnostic certainty unless the patient has a typical clinical presentation.

Among patients with spinal muscular atrophy presenting in childhood is a subgroup (those with Kugelberg-Welander disease) in whom proximal muscle involvement may simulate muscular dystrophy. Muscle biopsy reveals changes of denervation, but focal myopathic changes may also be observed, as is true in other chronic denervating diseases. Single-fiber electromyography may help resolve the issue of pathogenesis in patients with mixed neuromyopathic biopsy findings by identifying enlarged motor units, a consequence of reinnervation (223).

PERIPHERAL NEUROPATHY

The diagnosis of the peripheral neuropathies affecting children is facilitated by electrophysiologic studies that distinguish myelinopathies from axonopathies, by evaluation of individual teased axons and ultrastructure of sural nerve specimens, and by genetic testing for mutations or duplications in genes related to myelin formation such as PMP22 and PO that are responsible for many familial and sporadic cases (242,186).

Hereditary sensory motor neuropathies (HSMNs) are much more common in children than acquired chronic neuropathies. Classic phenotypes include the usually autosomal dominant hypertrophic peroneal neuropathies of Charcot-Marie-Tooth [types I and II hereditary sensory motor neuropathy (HSMN)], the autosomal recessive hypertrophic hypomyelinating infantile neuropathy of Déjérine-Sottas (type III HSMN), and Refsum disease (type IV HSMN) (244).

Schwann cell proliferation that results in "onion bulb" formation (Figure 26-11A and B) is most prominent in type III,

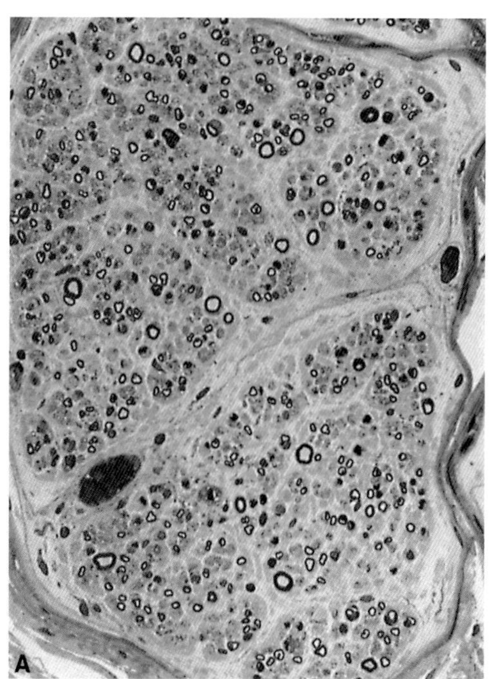

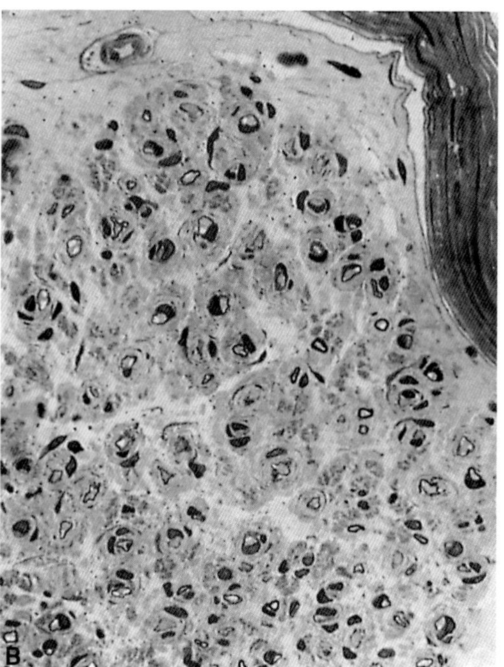

FIGURE 26-11 ■ **A:** Sural nerve in idiopathic childhood neuropathy, possibly type I HSMN, with scattered "onion bulbs" and variable myelin thickness. (Methylene blue and azure II stain; original magnification ×400.) **B:** Sural nerve in type III HSMN with prominent "onion bulbs" and uniform severe defect in myelin thickness. (Methylene blue and azure II stain; original magnification ×640.)

but it is not a specific feature for genetic disorders. Delayed nerve conduction velocity related to myelination disorder is a feature of all except type II. Denervation of muscle may occur with axonopathy. Genetic analyses have disclosed extreme heterogeneity with defects in different steps in myelin formation producing overlapping phenotypes. Neuropathy in infants with extreme hypomyelination and Schwann cell proliferation associates with multiple gene defects (127,255). Congenital absence of peripheral myelin is described in a lethal form of arthrogryposis congenita (41), and has also been observed in some infants with CMD (227).

Acquired demyelinating diseases of peripheral nerves include acute postinfectious polyneuritis (Guillain-Barré syndrome) and chronic idiopathic inflammatory polyneuropathy (118,233). Both cause hypotonia, weakness, hyporeflexia, and slow nerve conduction, more commonly in older children or adults and rarely in infancy. In both conditions, segmental demyelination and remyelination are accompanied by Schwann cell proliferation and mononuclear infiltrates of variable severity (Figure 26-12). Inflammation is often scanty, making distinction from genetic forms of peripheral neuropathy difficult. Perivascular infiltrates of macrophages may be helpful (238). In chronic cases, muscle wasting probably is due more to disuse than to denervation, which typically is lacking. Peripheral neuropathy caused by drugs, heavy metal intoxication (e.g., lead), or bacterial toxins (e.g., diphtheria) may be due to axonal degeneration alone or combination with demyelination.

COMBINED CENTRAL AND PERIPHERAL NEUROPATHY

Complex multisystem metabolic diseases and genetically determined diseases of central neurons or central white matter usually do not involve peripheral nerves, but exceptions are noteworthy. Rare patients with peripheral neuropathy and mitochondrial myopathy have complex crystalline inclusions in Schwann cell cytoplasm (Figure 26-13) (26). Lower motor neuron involvement in olivospinocerebellar atrophy, Friedreich ataxia, and ataxia-telangiectasia leads to axonal loss and muscle denervation and reinnervation (Figure 26-14), which usually is overshadowed clinically by the peripheral and central sensory deficits. Neuraxonal dystrophy involves central and peripheral axons in which focal expansile lesions accumulate complex tubulomembranous inclusions. Among the leukodystrophies, the metachromatic subtypes are most likely to involve peripheral nerves and may cause muscle denervation; peripheral neuropathy also occurs in Krabbe disease (see Chapter 5).

NUTRITIONAL DISORDERS

Neuropathies due to malnutrition are extremely rare in industrialized societies. However, deficient absorption of fat-soluble vitamins may produce neuropathy in infants with chronic cholestasis, in children with cystic fibrosis, or in patients with

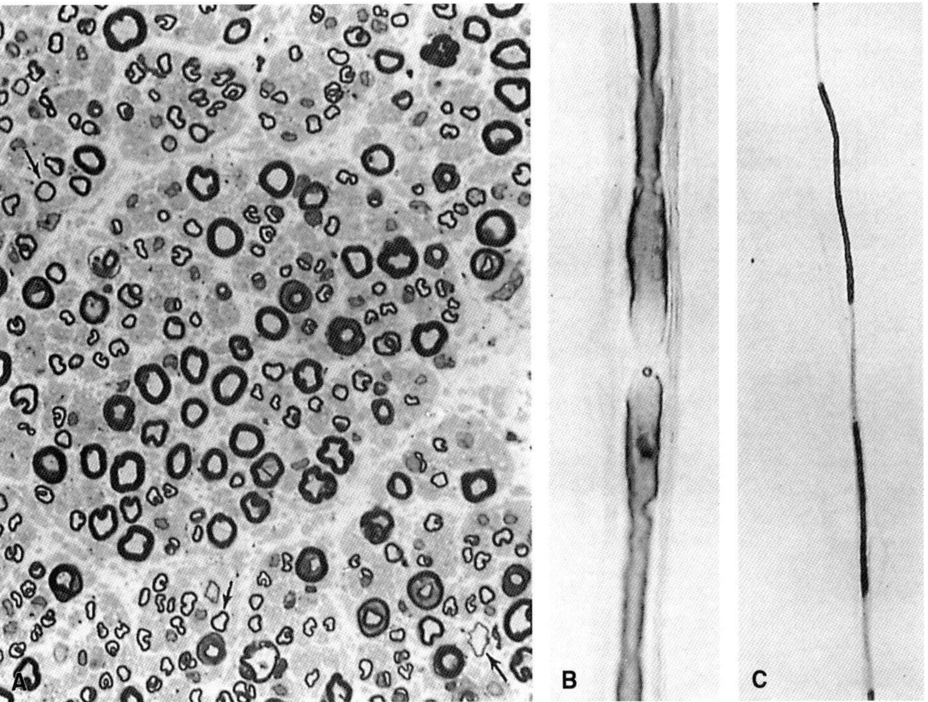

FIGURE 26-12 ■ **A:** Sural nerve in prolonged Guillain-Barre syndrome. Thin myelin sheaths are inconspicuous. There is no inflammation. (Methylene blue and azure II stain; original magnification ×640.) **B:** Teased isolated myelinated fiber. Demyelination begins at nodes of Ranvier. **C:** Teased isolated myelinated fibers with segmental demyelination, typical of postinfectious polyneuropathy.

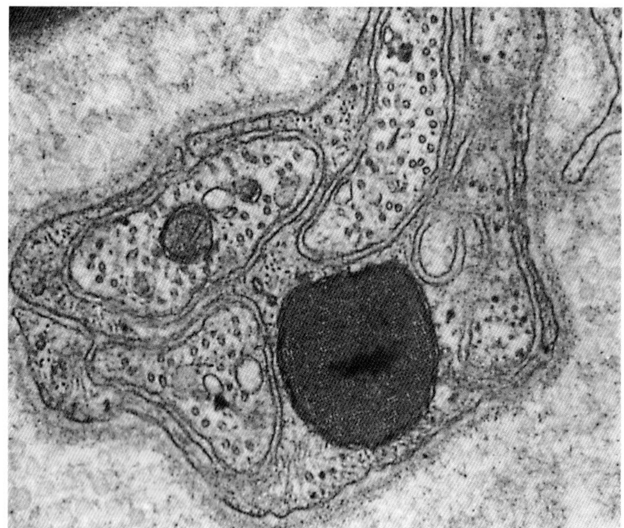

FIGURE 26-13■**A:** Schwann cell, enclosing several unmyelinated nerves, contains crystalline inclusion with double mitochondroid outer membrane. Patient had abnormal mitochondria in heart, skeletal muscle, and peripheral nerves. (Uranyl acetate and lead citrate stain; original magnification ×20,000.)

abetalipoproteinemia. Areflexia or progressive ataxia due to central dysfunction is likely to develop if prolonged, unrelenting cholestasis begins in early infancy, causing vitamin E deficiency (132). In these children, muscle fiber-type groups develop, residual bodies accumulate in muscle fibers (Figure 26-15) and in Schwann cells, and the serum creatine kinase may be elevated. This mixed neuromyopathy can be arrested with parenteral vitamin E therapy (236).

DISORDERS OF NEUROMUSCULAR TRANSMISSION

The neuromuscular junction is the target of many toxic, infectious, or autoimmune insults and the locus of several rare genetically transmitted defects. The specific site of impairment may be presynaptic or postsynaptic. The differential diagnosis of these conditions requires evaluation of response to acetylcholine esterase inhibition, detailed electromyography, measurement of circulating antibodies to acetylcholine receptors, and in selected cases, morphologic studies of motor end plates, which are best sampled in external intercostal muscle specimens. Muscle may be normal or show selective type II fiber atrophy or overt signs of denervation.

Neonatal myasthenia gravis is a transient condition expressed within the first few days after birth and continuing for several weeks thereafter in babies born to mothers with myasthenia gravis (49). Affected infants are otherwise normal, although the rare coexistence of congenital contractures suggests the possibility of an *in utero* injury. The mediator of the disease is thought to be transplacental maternal IgG antibody to acetylcholine receptors on the postsynaptic muscle membrane. High maternal levels of pathologic antibody increase the risk, but unknown factors, such as the rate of antibody degradation, may modify expression of the disease in neonates. Myasthenia gravis, similar to that in adults, also occurs in older children. Antibody to acetylcholine receptor is usually demonstrable, and acetylcholine esterase inhibitors relieve symptoms. Myasthenia-like syndromes include a number of very rare congenital disorders due to presynaptic, synaptic, or postsynaptic defects that result in abnormal neuromuscular transmission. The complex molecular basis for these disorders is rapidly being elucidated (75). Morphological studies usually are not helpful, an exception being congenital, paucity of postsynaptic clefts (235).

Acquired disorders of neuromuscular transmission in children are caused by neurotoxins associated with diphtheria or the infantile form of botulism, drugs such as magnesium sulfate or aminoglycoside antibiotics, and neoplasms or autoimmune disorders that cause motor conduction changes typical of the Eaton-Lambert syndrome. Infantile botulism is of particular interest because it results from endogenous production of a neurotoxin by gastrointestinal flora rather than ingestion of preformed toxin (10). Early signs may be constipation and various degrees of failure to thrive. In protracted cases, dysphagia, loss of head control, and progressive flaccid paralysis

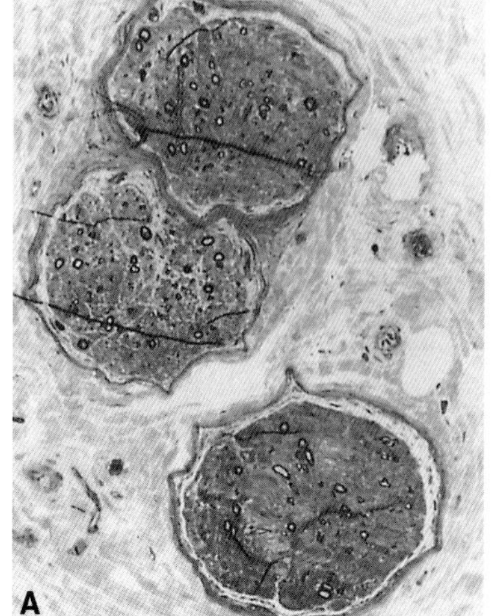

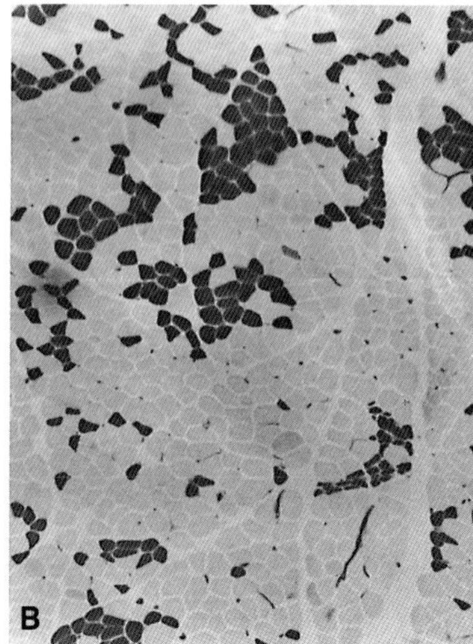

FIGURE 26-14■**A:** Marked reduction of fascicular area and number of myelinated axons in the sural nerve from an older child with Friedreich ataxia. (Original magnification ×00.) **B:** Denervation atrophy with type groups indicating reinnervation in Friedreich ataxia. (Myosin ATPase stain with preincubation at pH 4.3; original magnification ×64.)

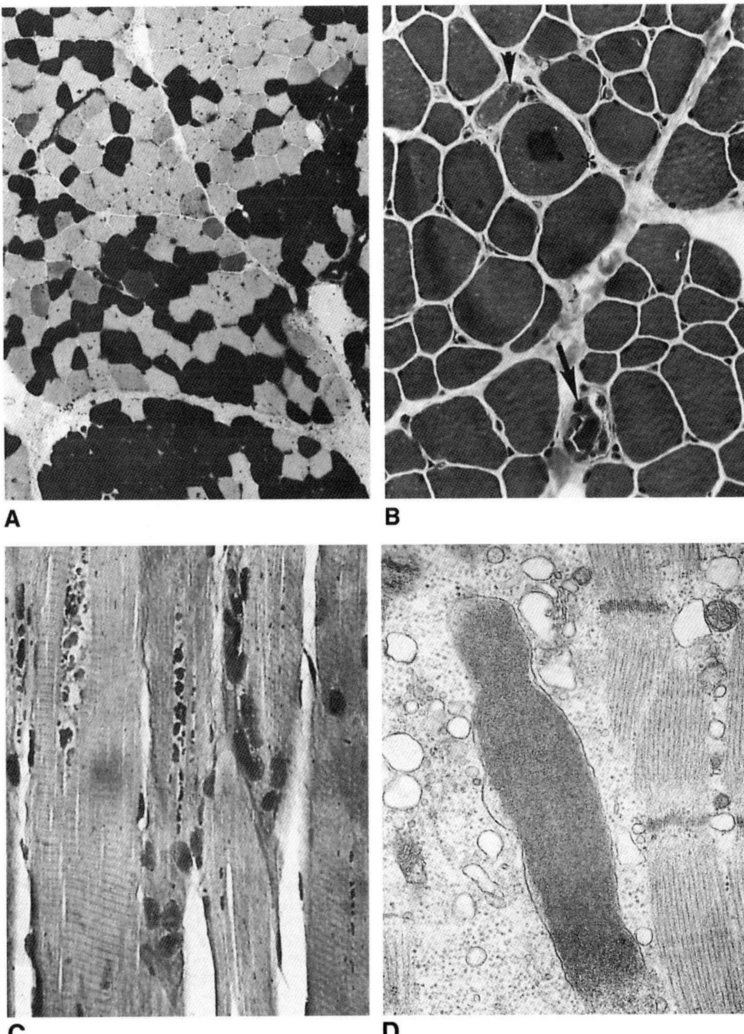

FIGURE 26-15 ▪ **A:** Reinnervation (type groups) in a child with chronic cholestasis from infancy causing central and peripheral neuropathy due to low levels of vitamin E. (Myosin ATPase stain with preincubation at pH 4.6; original magnification ×160.) **B:** Mixed neuromyopathic change in a child with prolonged vitamin E deficiency. Fiber necrosis (*arrow*), degeneration (*arrowhead*), and target fibers (*asterisk*) are shown. (Trichrome stain; original magnification ×500.) **C:** Massive deposition of residual bodies in a child with chronic cholestasis and low vitamin E levels. (Methylene blue and azure II stain; original magnification ×1,000.) **D:** Dense monomorphous residual body, typical of infantile vitamin E deficiency myopathy. (Uranyl acetate and lead citrate stain; original magnification ×10,500.)

develop. A few infants with sudden unexplained death have had clostridial endotoxin detected in the gut. The basis for transient susceptibility of infants to endogenous toxin production is unknown. Morphologic studies of terminal motor nerves in affected infants have not been reported.

Serious neuromuscular sequelae to intensive care may be due to excessive use of curare-like drugs, to concomitant exposure to aminoglycoside antibiotics or to corticosteroid drugs, or to severe underlying illness, such as sepsis. Among patients exposed for prolonged periods to curare-like drugs during mechanical ventilation, a few develop transient or permanent paralysis or contractures after withdrawal (171,232). In these patients, muscle biopsy may help exclude antecedent neuromuscular disease and identify the basis for prolonged weakness. We observed acute denervation of muscle, myopathic change, and a presynaptic abnormality of neuromuscular transmission in one child who eventually recovered (19). Clinically similar disorders, which may be differentiated on the basis of electrophysiologic and muscle biopsy findings, include critical illness polyneuropathy and critical illness myopathy (265). Autopsy evaluation of psoas muscle fiber diameter in infants who had been paralyzed for extended periods indicated smaller average muscle fiber diameter than expected, suggesting the possibility of muscle fiber growth retardation (205).

CONGENITAL MYOPATHY

The CMs are static or slowly progressive disorders of muscle of genetic origin that exhibit substantial clinical overlap. Definitions based on morphology are increasingly augmented by knowledge of gene mutations that, in some subtypes, cause defective contractile proteins to accumulate. However, a major limitation is poor correlation of disease severity with morphologic severity, character of abnormal inclusions, and specific gene defects. Typical characteristics are nonprogressive weakness often detected in infancy, normal serum levels of creatine kinase, absence of electrophysiologic or morphologic evidence for denervation, and no other definable primary muscle diseases, such as a dystrophy or myositis. The best established among the subtypes are myotubular-centronuclear myopathy, nemaline myopathy (NM), central core disease, minicore-multicore disease, and type I FSD myopathy. These conditions have distinctive morphologic features that are identifiable in a muscle biopsy examined by light or electron microscopy, or both.

Severity of CM is highly variable from patient to patient and within affected families. Some infants with CM are extremely hypotonic and weak at birth, and are weaned from mechanical ventilatory support with great difficulty owing to severe involvement of the diaphragm and accessory muscles of respiration. Muscles with cranial nerve innervation are sometimes involved, resulting in ptosis, ophthalmoplegia, facial weakness, and dysphagia. Muscle contractures may be congenital or may develop during infancy, but they are usually not severe. In less affected infants, modest motor progress may occur, but ambulation and acquisition of motor skills are delayed. Children who are older at the time of a recognized CM usually are thin, have reduced muscle bulk and strength, and tend to avoid strenuous activity, but they are able to perform ordinary tasks. Recurrent pneumonia or progressive scoliosis is frequent. Regardless of age at presentation, cerebral function is usually intact. Family studies have often identified minimally impaired or asymptomatic relatives with similar or related morphologic abnormalities in a muscle biopsy.

Prenatal morbidity is probably increased in infants with CM, although hypotonia may contribute to deceptively low Apgar scores. Maternal weakness or fetal hypotonia may prolong labor. Although myotonic dystrophy is not in the strict sense a CM, central nervous system injury is unusually prevalent in affected infants (Figure 26-16) and may overshadow the natural history of the primary myopathy, the principal early manifestations of which are delayed muscle maturation and weakness (see Figure 26-8). Myotonia in the mother is a helpful diagnostic sign.

Identification and classification of the patient with CM is often challenging. Serum levels of creatine kinase, though typically normal, may be mildly elevated. Autopsy studies suggest that variation among muscles is common. Muscle biopsy, including electron microscopy, is essential. In samples lacking specific structural markers, the various subtypes of CM exhibit overlapping features. Muscle fibrosis is exceptional in CM, but may be observed in central core disease and in severe infantile NM. To establish a genetic basis, it is helpful to examine close relatives of the patient and to perform other studies, such as electromyography and muscle biopsy. Specific gene defects have been identified for many types of CM.

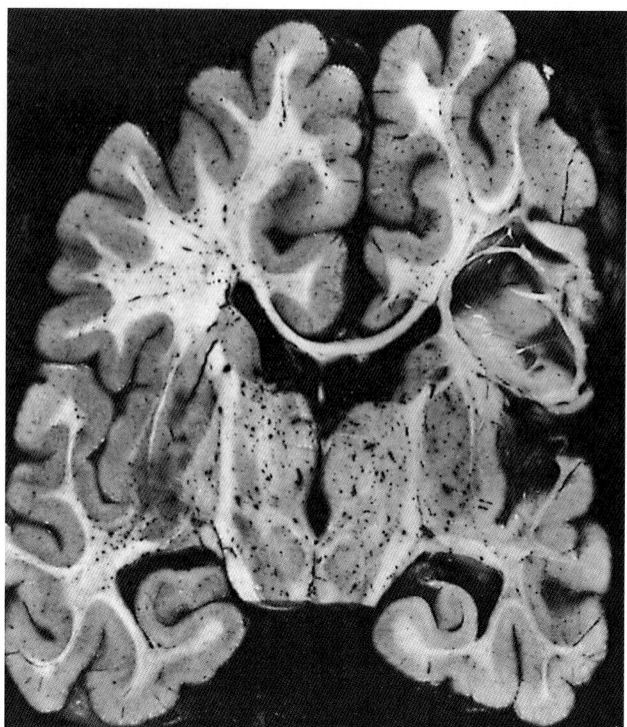

FIGURE 26-16 ■ Acquired porencephaly in a 2-year-old child who had symptomatic myotonic dystrophy with documented muscle maturation delay as an infant.

CENTRAL NUCLEAR AND MYOTUBULAR MYOPATHY

Central position of muscle nuclei occurs in muscle regeneration and is a nonspecific alteration in chronic neuromuscular diseases of all kinds. It is also the hallmark of a CM in which most fibers have central nuclei (Figure 26-17). Sex-linked recessive and dominant inheritance patterns of central nuclear myopathy are well documented (6,58,145,230). The autosomal recessive form is the most common. Severely affected infants are reported mainly in kindreds exhibiting an X-linked recessive inheritance pattern. Untypeable myotubes resembling the fetal myotube stage of development are usually prevalent in affected infants, but in contrast to the normal myotube, may extend for only a short distance on either side of the central nucleus. Overexpression of vimentin and desmin occurs only in the X-linked form (210). Mutations in the MTM1 gene that codes for myotubularin cause only the X-linked disease (185); genetic markers are not yet available for other subtypes. The major alternative histological diagnosis in infants is the neonatal form of myotonic dystrophy, a condition in which myotubes are also found. The juxtanuclear clear zone in both conditions contains glycogen, sarcoplasmic reticulum, mitochondria, and associated enzymes, but lacks myofibrils.

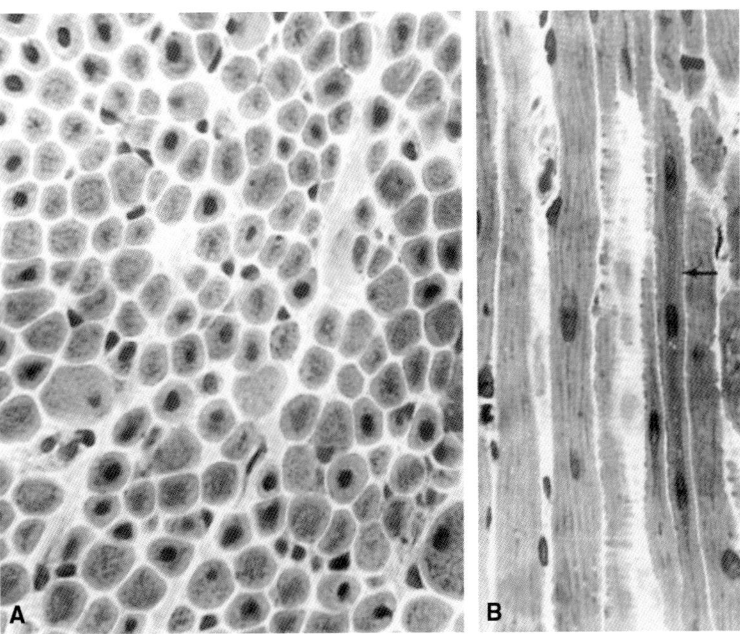

FIGURE 26-17▪**A:** Central nuclear and myotubular myopathy. Central nuclei and central concentration of organelles are prominent. (Hematoxylin and eosin stain; original magnification ×800.) **B:** Central nuclear and myotubular myopathy. Myotubular configuration (*arrow*) is demonstrable in a variable percentage of fibers. (Methylene blue and azure II stain; original magnification ×800.)

Nemaline Myopathy

NM is a distinctive and relatively common form of CM. Family data suggest two patterns of genetic expression: dominant with variable penetrance and autosomal recessive (134). Clinical subgroups include a rapidly fatal infantile form, a static or slowly progressive form with mild-to-moderate impairment, and a subclinical form in relatives. In most cases, the rods are readily observed by light microscopy (LM) using a modification of the trichrome stain (Figure 26-18) or the phosphotungstic acid–hematoxylin method, but rods are undetectable in sections stained with hematoxylin and eosin. Associated changes include type I fiber predominance and, in some instances, indistinct myosin ATPase reactions. Infants with NM usually have type I FSD.

Ultrastructural study of rods demonstrates discrete, electron-dense bodies with characteristic crystalline substructures (Figure 26-19). In some infants with severe CM, rods are difficult to detect by LM, but rodlike Z-band changes are prevalent in electron micrographs. Rods contain multiple proteins including a-actinin, a Z-band protein, and actin and are located in continuity with Z-bands, aggregated beneath the sarcolemma or in some patients, located within the nucleus (104). Molecular studies indicate that mutations in nebulin and skeletal muscle alpha-actin cause the majority of cases of autosomal recessive NM (4). Mutations in several other

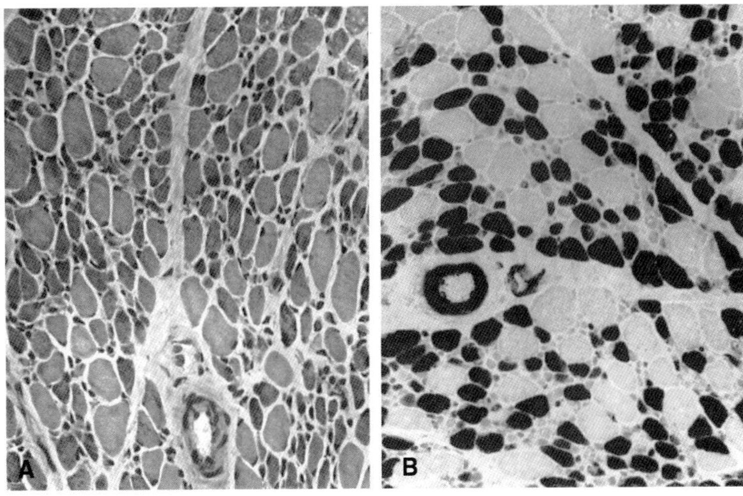

FIGURE 26-18▪**A:** NM, infantile form. Dark-stained, rodlike granules tend to be most prevalent in smaller muscle fibers in symptomatic infants. (Trichrome stain; original magnification ×400.) **B:** NM, infantile form. Type I fibers are smaller than type II fibers. Smallest fibers are untypeable. (Myosin ATPase stain with preincubation at pH 4.3; original magnification ×400.)

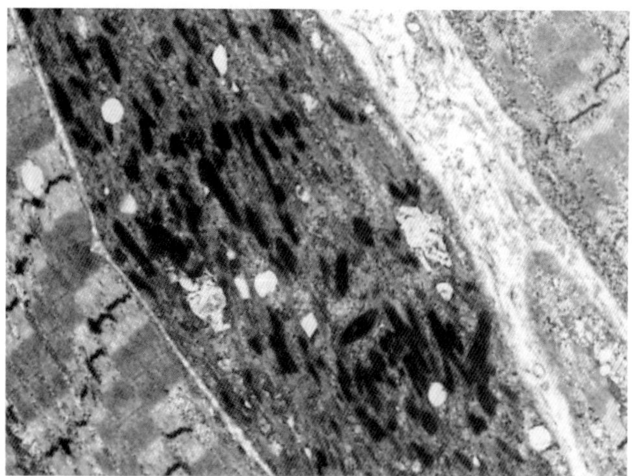

FIGURE 26-19 ■ Nemaline bodies are dense crystalline structures originating in the Z band. (Uranyl acetate and lead citrate stain; original magnification ×10,000.)

NM-associated genes such as tropomyosin and troponin are uncommon. Nebulin mutations associate only with autosomal recessive NM; in other respects, genotype-phenotype correlation is poor and not useful for prognosis.

Central Core Disease

Central core disease, the first defined form of CM, is usually detected in infancy or early childhood and may be mildly progressive. Dominant inheritance has been demonstrated, but many cases are sporadic. Severe involvement of the diaphragm is typical at autopsy. Cores have also been observed in the diaphragm in some patients with NM. Cores are well demarcated (Figure 26-20), more or less centrally located, long contiguous zones usually found within the interior of type I muscle fibers. In cores, oxidative enzyme activity, mitochondria, lipid, glycogen, and phosphorylase activity are deficient. Myofibrils in the core area are intact (structured core) or are in disarray (unstructured core). Unstructured cores resemble target fibers, an acquired lesion commonly seen in disorders of chronic innervation, particularly in type I fibers. Variation in the prominence of cores within a single sample and disturbed differentiation of myofiber subtypes is common. Morphologically, atypical cases with incompletely developed cores, or with both cores and nemaline bodies have been reported (212). Liability to malignant hyperthermia (MH) reaction associates with both central core disease and multi-minicore disease; most patients with these forms of CM have mutations in the RYR1 gene that codes for a calcium channel regulatory protein (140,199) located in the sarcoplasmic reticulum.

Multi-Minicore Disease

Minicore-multicore disease causes hypotonia that may be marked but most affected children ambulate. Axial weakness, scoliosis, and eventual respiratory insufficiency are the most common phenotype in older children (113). Tiny foci of myofibrillar and organellar depletion (Figure 26-21) resemble unstructured cores, except for their small dimensions and distribution less related than typical cores to the central region of muscle fibers. These lesions are demonstrable on frozen sections as random tiny foci of reduced myosin ATPase and oxidative enzyme activity, and in longitudinally oriented muscle fibers as foci of lost striations, a feature that is easily confirmed in plastic embedded tissue, and by electron microscopy.

Congenital Myopathy with Small Type I Fibers

Type I FSD is a common phenomenon in muscle specimens obtained during early infancy from hypotonic babies (107). Frequently associated with early-onset disorders of the nervous system and a component of many subtypes of CM, the clinical heterogeneity of patients with FSD has delayed acceptance of a CM characterized only by small size of type I fibers. In the absence of a structural marker, morphologic

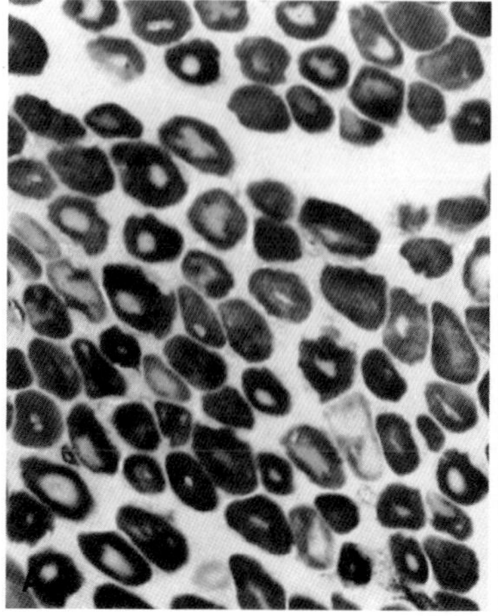

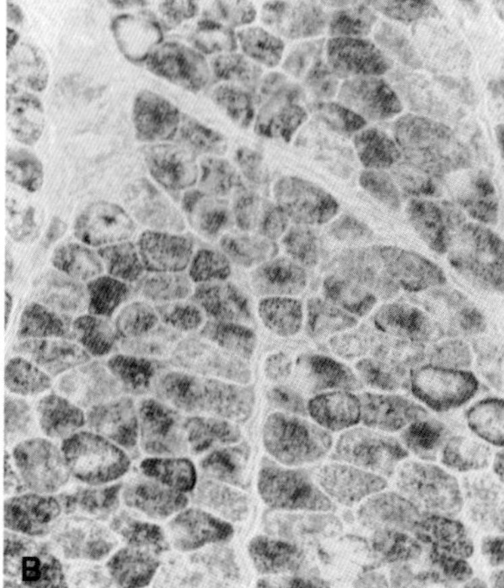

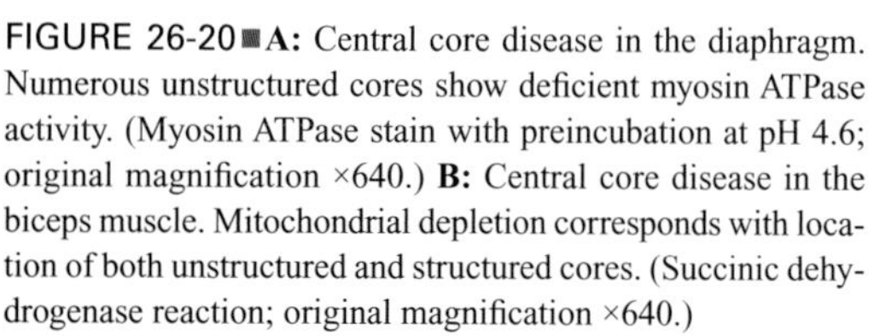

FIGURE 26-20 ■ **A:** Central core disease in the diaphragm. Numerous unstructured cores show deficient myosin ATPase activity. (Myosin ATPase stain with preincubation at pH 4.6; original magnification ×640.) **B:** Central core disease in the biceps muscle. Mitochondrial depletion corresponds with location of both unstructured and structured cores. (Succinic dehydrogenase reaction; original magnification ×640.)

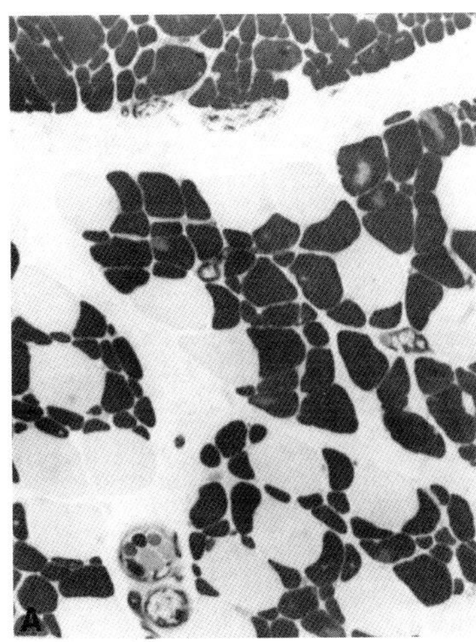

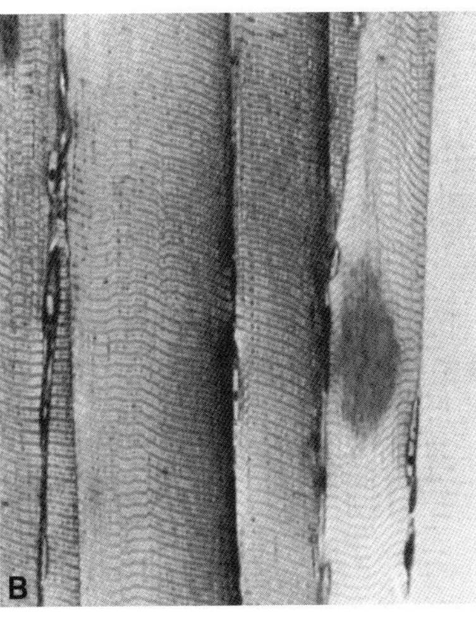

FIGURE 26-21■ **A:** Minicore-multicore disease. Limited cores in type I fibers display focally deficient myosin ATPase reaction. (Myosin ATPase stain with preincubation at pH 4.3; original magnification ×200.) **B:** Limited cores are focal zones of myofibrillar degeneration with loss of sarcomeres and deficient organelles. (Methylene blue and azure II stain; original magnification ×640.)

criteria less reliably distinguish primary myopathy with FSD from the more common secondary form. Nonetheless, CM with FSD typically has excessive numbers of type I fibers, defined as greater than 60% of the fibers in a thigh muscle sample. This feature alone is unreliable because numerical predominance may result from an acquired expansion of type I motor units caused by neuropathic injury. Despite these problems, after the age of 6 months, severe persistent FSD with uniformly small type 1 fibers, and numerical predominance, coupled with absence of clusters of type I fibers (Figure 26-22), may help identify cases of primary myopathy (Iannacone107). Based upon analysis of kindreds with dominant and recessive familial patterns of FSD, CM with FSD appears to be a distinct entity with a relatively homogeneous clinical phenotype that includes normal intelligence, contractures, ophthalmoplegia, facial weakness, and some cases with early respiratory failure (45). Unlike most other forms of CM, clinical and morphologic improvement has been observed in some familial cases. A relationship of pure FSD to NM is suggested by cases of FSD with rods limited to a few fibers and mutations in skeletal muscle actin (130).

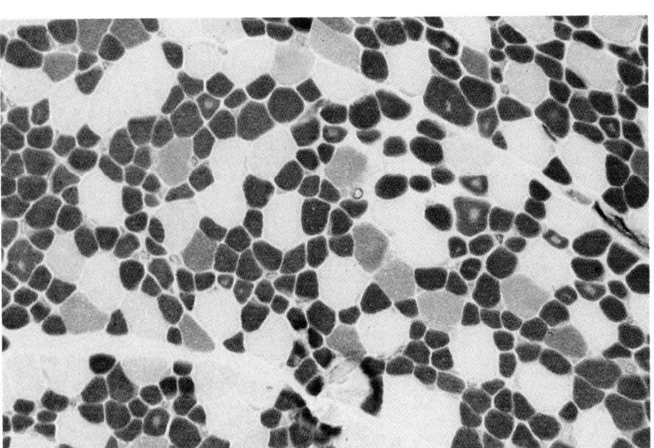

FIGURE 26-22■ CM with type I FSD. (Myosin ATPase stain with preincubation at pH 4.6; original magnification ×400.)

Other Congenital Myopathies

Additional putative subtypes of CM have been suggested, usually on the basis of clinical features, occasional familial occurrence and a prevalent unusual structural abnormality in muscle fibers, such as fingerprint bodies, zebra bodies, tubular aggregates, trilaminar fibers, and aggregates of intermediate filaments, as in cytoplasmic bodies or in myofibrillar myopathy with desmin accumulation (214). The ultimate nosologic status of these disorders depends upon additional observations and identification of a molecular basis that is specific to each structure and putative subtype. Knowledge of the myofibrillar myopathies in adults is expanding rapidly, but information about manifestations in children is meager. Excessive reliance on particular structural markers may lead to errors or misconceptions. Nemaline bodies may be acquired; target fibers, which resemble both cores and minicores, commonly develop in denervating disorders. Cytoplasmic bodies are found in a variety of acquired myopathic and denervating disorders of muscle, including ISMA (33) (Figure 26-23), but they also seem to be a marker for an extremely rare, dominantly inherited CM (178). Fingerprint bodies have been described in myotonic dystrophy, oculopharyngeal dystrophy, and dermatomyositis. In some cases of clinically typical CM, muscle biopsy may show minimal changes that suggest a CM, but not a specific subtype, possibly because of sampling error or incomplete expression.

METABOLIC MYOPATHY

Lysosomal Storage Diseases

Skeletal muscle involvement is mild in most lysosomal enzyme deficiency diseases, and clinical manifestations are slight or absent. With the exception of type II glycogenosis, which is associated with a vacuolar myopathy of variable severity (Figure 26-24), skeletal muscle biopsy has not been a major diagnostic method for defining storage disease. However, if hypotonia or weakness prompts a muscle biopsy

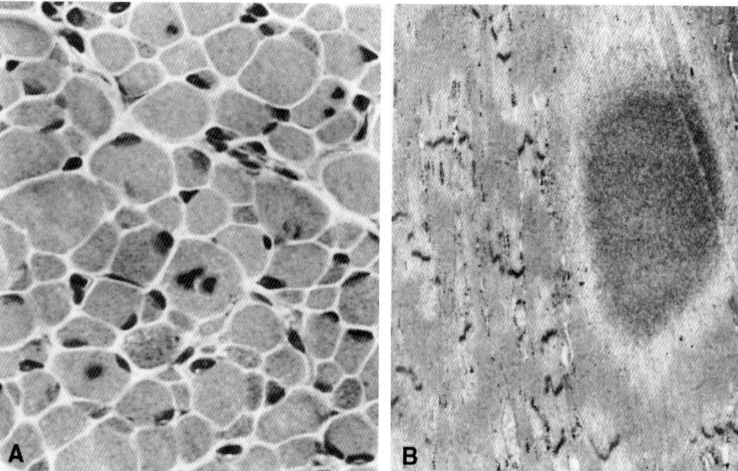

FIGURE 26-23 A: Cytoplasmic bodies, dense purple-staining inclusions with a discernible halo, occur in ISMA, as shown here, and in a rare CM. (Trichrome stain; original magnification ×800.) **B:** Ultrastructure of cytoplasmic body shows granular center surrounded by disorganized filaments. (Uranyl acetate and lead citrate stain; original magnification ×6,000.)

before a storage disease has been identified, morphologically specific types of lysosomal storage may be encountered (34). Usually, the storage vesicles are strongly positive for acid phosphatase, indicating the lysosomal nature of the disease. Infantile ceroid lipofuscinosis (Santavouri disease) is accompanied by dense homogeneously granular intramuscular inclusions, which are surprisingly similar to inclusions (see Figure 26-15D) that develop in the vitamin E deficiency–associated neuromyopathy complicating chronic cholestasis of infancy. Muscle fibers in the late infantile form (Jansky-Bielschowsky disease) contain inclusions with curvilinear profiles.

In the mucopolysaccharidoses, endomysial fibroblasts may show typical acid-phosphatase–positive vacuolar inclusions, but muscle fibers are usually normal. Characteristic inclusions of stored material occur in endothelium or smooth muscle cells in fucosidosis and Sandhoff disease. Storage inclusions occur in skeletal muscle fibers and vessel walls in Fabry disease and mannosidosis. Stored material accumulates in vascular endothelium and satellite cells but may not involve the muscle fibers of patients with I-cell disease and GM1 gangliosidosis (Figure 26-25A). In some of these rare conditions, too few patients have been studied to warrant conclusive statements. We have observed extensive intramuscular storage in one child with I-cell disease (Figure 26-25B; see Chapter 5).

Glycogen Storage Diseases

The glycogenoses are defined as metabolic disorders of glycogen metabolism in which tissue glycogen levels are excessive (100). Reduced availability of hepatic glycogen increases the risk of hypoglycemia in types I, III, and IX glycogenosis; impaired glycolysis results in cardiomyopathy in types III and IV and skeletal muscle hypotonia in types III, IV, V, VII, and X (Table 26-5).

Among the lysosomal storage diseases, only the infantile form (type IIa or Pompe disease) produces severe hypotonia. Type IIa glycogenosis is a systemic disorder primarily involving liver, brain, and skeletal, cardiac, and smooth muscle. Muscle fibers progressively enlarge owing to accumulation of glycogen in lysosomes and unidentified hematoxylinophilic acid mucins (in some cases) in secondary lysosomes (see Figure 26-23A). Until the storage vesicles become extremely distended, the acid phosphatase reaction is typically strong, indicating the lysosomal origin

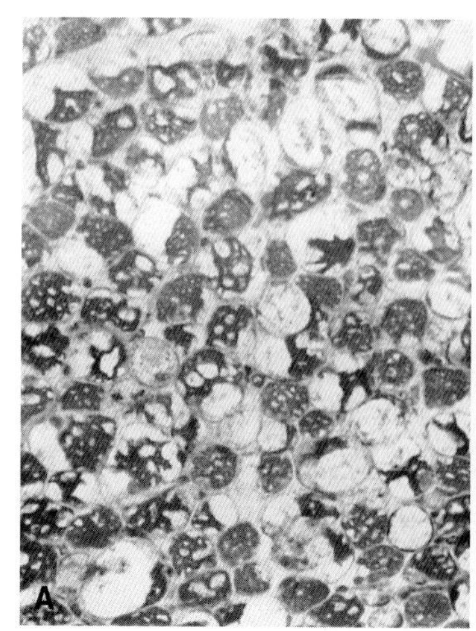

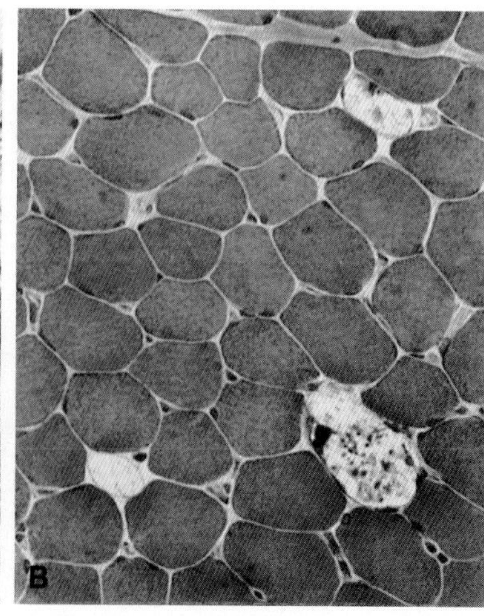

FIGURE 26-24 A: Type IIa lysosomal glycogenosis features severe confluent vacuolar degeneration affecting all muscle fibers. **B:** Type IIb lysosomal glycogenosis features confluent vacuolar degeneration of isolated fibers. Ultrastructural lysosomal changes are more prevalent. (Trichrome stain; original magnifications ×600.)

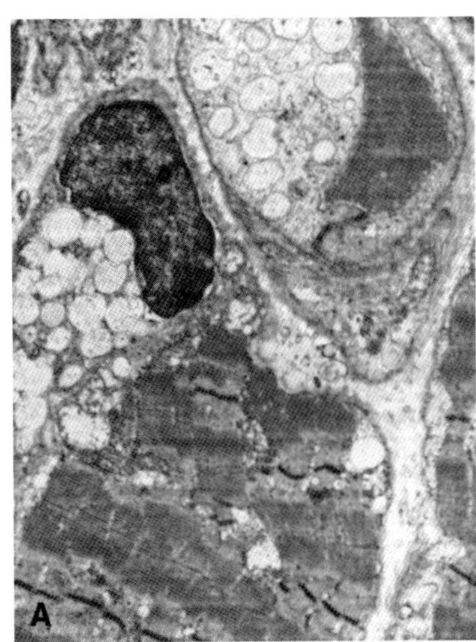

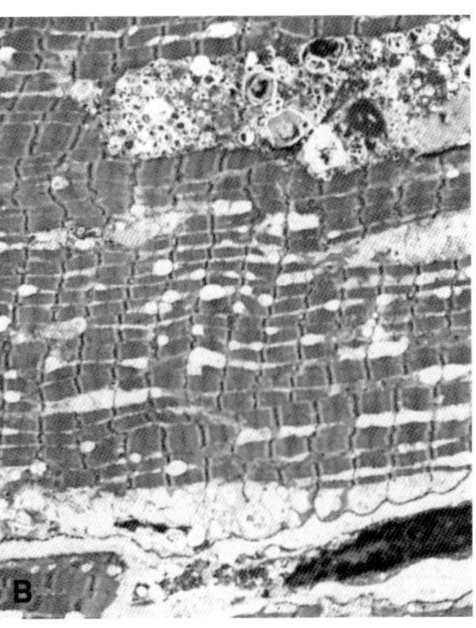

FIGURE 26-25 ■ **A:** Lysosomal inclusions containing amorphous material are located in endothelium and in muscle satellite cells of a patient with GM1 gangliosidosis. (Uranyl acetate and lead citrate stain; original magnification ×7,000.) **B:** Lysosomal inclusions containing polymorphous debris are present in skeletal muscle of this patient with I-cell disease. (Uranyl acetate and lead citrate stain; original magnification ×3,000.)

(see Chapters 5 and 15). The definitive morphologic diagnosis can be achieved by LM of muscle and liver, and by electron microscopy of dermal or amnionic fibroblasts (144). Acid a-glucosidase activity is low or absent in all tissues including circulating leukocytes. Antenatal diagnosis is possible using a biochemical or a morphologic approach (103). Because of multiple mutations, genetic analysis is only useful if an affected sibling has been previously analyzed. Early diagnosis of the infantile subtype is critically important now that both transgenic and recombinant enzyme replacement therapies have been shown to be effective if initiated in early infancy (190,245).

The precise mechanism responsible for hypotonia in type IIa glycogenosis is puzzling because nonlysosomal glycogen is abundant and the glycolytic pathway is intact. Possible mechanisms include absolute loss, rather than simple displacement of myofibrils, increased work due to the mass of accumulated glycogen, rupture of overdistended lysosomes with intramuscular proteolysis, and hypoinnervation secondary to glycogen storage in motor neurons.

Type II glycogenosis exists in less severe forms in older children or adults, who typically experience exercise intolerance associated with slowly progressive weakness (8). The deficiency of lysosomal glucosidase activity approximates that in the infantile form but residual activity may be somewhat greater. Skeletal muscle fibers show morphologic changes of variable severity and extent (see Figure 26-24B). Liver, heart, and leukocytes may contain only a few abnormal glycogen-laden lysosomes, despite low levels of acid a-glucosidase. Glycogen-filled lysosomes develop within a few weeks in cultured muscle or fibroblasts obtained from these patients and may also be seen in the resting fibroblasts (11). A biochemical test that identifies the infantile, childhood, and adult forms of type II glycogenosis is lacking.

Table 26-5 ■ GLYCOGENOSES AND ASSOCIATED MUSCLE ABNORMALITIES

Type	Enzyme Defect	Tissues Affected	Muscle Morphology
I	Glucose-6-phosphatase	Liver	Normal muscle; secondary increase of lipid in type I fibers (rare)
IIA	Acid a-glucosidase	Generalized	Severe progressive vacuolar degeneration secondary to lysosomal storage of undegraded glycogen; sarcoplasmic glycogen increased
IIB	Acid a-glucosidase	Muscle, liver, heart	Variable (less severe) vacuolar degeneration secondary to lysosomal storage of undegraded glycogen
III	Debrancher enzyme	Liver, heart, muscle	Increased intermyofibrillar and subsarcolemmal glycogen; rarely shows vacuolar degeneration
IV	Brancher enzyme	Liver, muscle, heart	Abnormal polysaccharide (amylopectin)
V	Myophosphorylase	Muscle	Excess intermyofibrillar and subsarcolemmal glycogen
VI	Liver phosphorylase	Liver	Normal muscle
VII	Phosphofructokinase	Muscle	Normal or similar to type V
VIII	Phosphorylase kinase activator	Liver, brain	Normal or similar to type V
IX	Phosphorylase kinase deficiency	Liver, muscle (rare)	Normal
X	Cyclic AMP-dependent phosphorylase kinase	Liver, muscle	Similar to type V

However, recent work suggests that this may be based upon immunoassay of both enzyme protein and specific activity, and lysosomal glycogen content of cultured fibroblasts (256). Approximately 100 mutations in the acid-a-glucosidase gene are known and have an unpredictable effect upon enzyme activity. Genotype-phenotype correlation is poor and does not explain the phenotype diversity in late-onset disease (175).

The pure myopathic phenotypes of type IV glycogenosis include fetal akinesia deformation sequence, CM, and juvenile myopathy. Another phenotype, progressive liver failure due to hepatic fibrosis in infancy or early childhood, often occurs without clinical cardiomyopathy or skeletal muscle disease. A morphologically abnormal form of unbranched glycogen (amylopectin) accumulates in liver and variably in heart and skeletal muscle owing to deficiency of the brancher enzyme, which regulates the formation of normally branched glycogen molecules. This amylopectin stains blue-brown with Lugol iodine in frozen sections and has a characteristic granulofibrillar ultrastructure. Expression of the defect in type IV glycogenosis is extremely heterogeneous (see Chapter 15) (32).

The other nonlysosomal glycogenoses feature accumulation of normal glycogen between myofibrils and in the subsarcolemmal region, areas where glycogen is normally found in small amounts (144). In these disorders (types III, V, VII, IX, X, XI), the periodic acid–Schiff (PAS) method applied to frozen or paraffin sections demonstrates mild glycogen excess between myofibrils or beneath the sarcolemma, particularly in type 2 fibers (Figure 26-26A). Assessment of glycogen content by ultrastructural means (Figure 26-26B) can be misleading because glycogen pools may be artifactually produced by hypercontraction or enhanced by tangential sectioning. Dense aggregates of morphologically abnormal glycogen may be seen in type VII. Direct measurement of glycogen and of glycolytic enzymes in muscle is a reliable approach and should be considered if the history is suggestive of metabolic myopathy, glycogen excess is suspected, and/or focal myopathic features are otherwise unexplained. Histochemical methods are available for detecting the enzyme defect in type V and type VII glycogenosis. In both disorders, low-grade myopathy is observed (see Figure 26-26B). Segmental necrosis or basophilic regeneration correlate with clinical myopathy or myoglobinuria precipitated by recent exercise.

Unusually early presentation of myophosphorylase deficiency (type V glycogenosis) is reported in one case of fatal infantile hypotonia, and delayed motor development and proximal weakness occurred in an older child, simulating CM (50,63). An exceptionally severe presentation of phosphofructokinase deficiency is recorded in a young child (216). Phosphorylase kinase deficiency (type VIb or IX glycogenosis) was described initially as a liver disease, but a variant with only skeletal muscle involvement has been implicated as the cause of muscle glycogen excess and hypotonia in an otherwise normal child (169). Exercise intolerance and glycogen excess have recently been described in several other defects in terminal glycolysis, such as phosphoglycerate kinase and mutase deficiencies, conditions not previously classified with the glycogenoses (64).

Nonglycogen polysaccharide storage diseases are poorly understood. First among these is Lafora disease, characterized by seizures, myoclonus, progressive dementia, and corpora amylacea–like deposits in neurons (Lafora bodies). Mutations in laforin, a unique phosphatase that contains a carbohydrate binding module necessary for the maintenance of normal cellular glycogen, appear to cause Lafora disease (268). A puzzling cardioskeletal myopathy resembles type IV glycogenosis except for normal levels of brancher enzyme (89). In both conditions, PAS-positive, diastase-resistant, variably metachromatic, granulofibrillar material called *polyglycosan*, accumulates in several tissues, including muscle. Ultrastructural study of muscle may help identify aggregates of material consistent with both conditions. However, typical well-formed Lafora bodies may be absent in skeletal muscle fibers in Lafora disease.

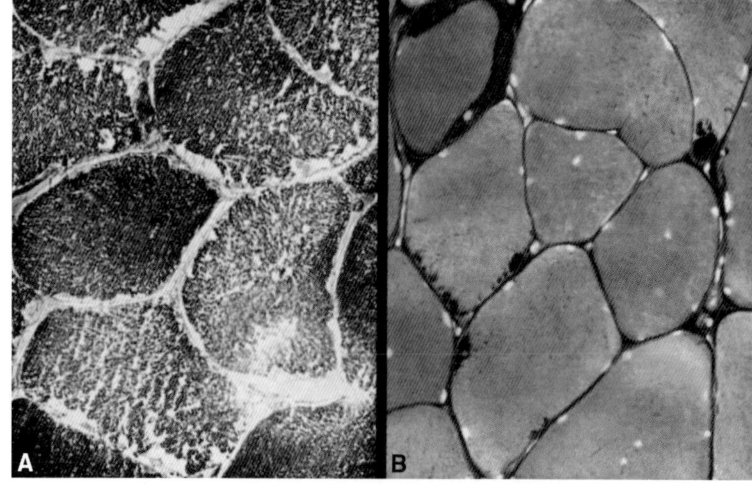

FIGURE 26-26 **A:** Type V glycogenosis in a young adult. Coarse clumps of glycogen beneath sarcolemma and within fibers are excessive. (PAS stain, alcohol-fixed frozen section; original magnification ×400.) **B:** Type V glycogenosis. Low-grade changes include central nuclei and subsarcolemmal clearing at sites of glycogen accumulation. (Hematoxylin and eosin stain; original magnification ×400.)

Triglyceride Storage Diseases

Beta-oxidation of free fatty acids derived from circulating triglycerides is the major energy source for skeletal muscle fibers, both at rest and during prolonged exercise. In normal muscle fibers, a storage pool of minute neutral lipid droplets are evenly dispersed between myofibrils, more prominently in type I muscle fibers, signifying primary reliance on fatty acids for energy supply in these mitochondria-rich fibers. Muscle lipid content is probably a relatively labile feature, dependent on plasma fatty acid concentration, which may be altered in fasting states, starvation, or disease (168).

After entry into muscle, free fatty acids, conjugated with coenzyme A, are transported across the mitochondrial membrane by a biochemical shuttle involving carnitine acyltransferases. Transient increase of muscle neutral lipid occurs in many primary metabolic diseases, Reye syndrome, and probably in other clinical crises as well. Therefore, diagnostic specificity seems doubtful.

Many inborn errors that disrupt neutral lipid catabolism have been identified in the last two decades (Table 26-6) (142,197,202). Symptoms related to episodes of nonketotic hypoglycemia may begin in the neonatal period, typically fluctuate, and may be precipitated in the form of a potentially lethal, metabolic crisis by a viral respiratory illness or low caloric intake (29,40,201,202). In older children, weakness and cramps may be precipitated by intense exercise, following which the serum level of creatine kinase rises, and myoglobinuria may appear (12).

Metabolic diseases cause multiorgan triglyceride storage especially in heart, liver, kidney, and skeletal muscle, and may be associated with recurrent episodes of acute encephalopathy resembling Reye syndrome, cardiac decompensation, or sudden death. A small subset of infants who die suddenly, and about 10% of cases of epidemic Reye syndrome, have been shown to have medium-chain acyl CoA dehydrogenase deficiency, a disorder that, during a crisis, promotes neutral lipid accumulation in liver, myocardium, and in some instances, skeletal muscle (5,201). This is caused by a common point mutation in 80% of cases. The mechanism of sudden death in affected infants has not been established (see Chapters 5 and 15).

Table 26-6 ■ DISORDERS WITH TRIGLYCERIDE EXCESS IN MUSCLE

Shock
Carnitine transporter deficiency
Carnitine-acylcarnitine translocase deficiency
Carnitine palmitoyltransferase deficiency
Acyl-CoA dehydrogenase deficiency
- Long-, medium-, and short-chain
- Multiple (glutaric aciduria II)

3-Hydroxy-3-methylglutaryl-CoA synthase deficiency
Krebs cycle defects
- Fumarase deficiency

Electron transport system defects
Complexes I, III, and IV

Specific metabolic defects that can lead to neutral lipid accumulation in muscle fibers (Figure 26-27A and B) include carnitine membrane transporter defect, carnitine palmitoyltransferase (CPT) II deficiency and defects in various components of the electron transport system, and (201,253). The pattern of acylcarnitine compounds excreted in urine has considerable diagnostic usefulness in disorders of lipid catabolism (39,253). Carnitine deficiency, based on the finding of low levels of carnitine in blood, usually is a secondary phenomenon caused by urinary loss of carnitine conjugated with organic acids resulting from defective lipid use. Carnitine transporter defect (142) is the basis for previously described cases of "primary" carnitine deficiency in which loss of carnitine in the urine is caused by failure of carnitine to transfer from blood to muscle after production in the liver. Among the listed disorders, muscle lipid accumulation is least likely to be seen in carnitine palmityl transferase II deficiency, the

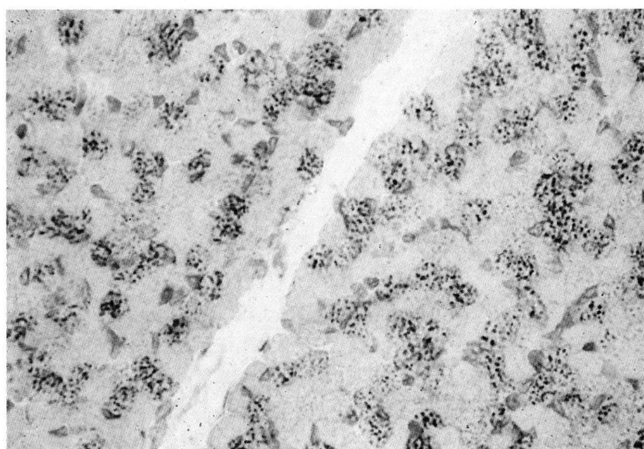

A

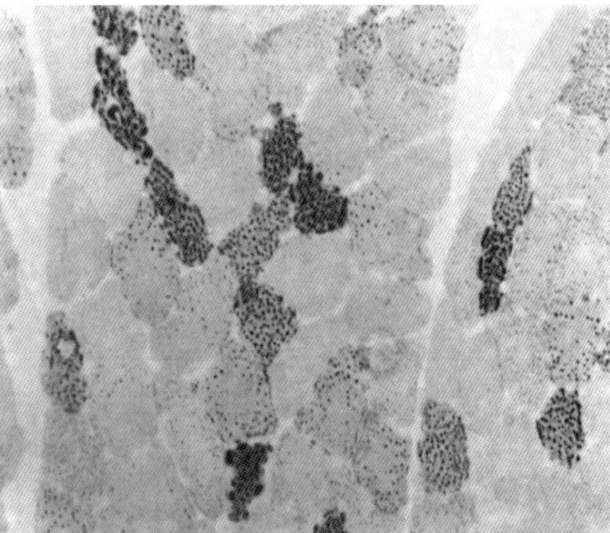

B

FIGURE 26-27■**A:** Neutral lipid accumulation, mainly in type I fibers of a young adult with defect in lipid oxidation. (Sudan black stain; original magnification ×200.) **B:** Neutral lipid accumulation, mainly in type I fibers of an infant with lethal CPT II deficiency. (Sudan black stain; original magnification ×200.)

most important cause of exercise-induced rhabdomyolysis in adults. In contrast, infants with this defect have prominent multiorgan lipid accumulation including intramuscular lipid droplets and lethal outcome (60,102). The phenotypic heterogeneity is explained by differing levels of residual enzyme activity and by extreme molecular genetic heterogeneity demonstrable in tissue and in fibroblast culture (172), consisting of several different point mutations in the infantile form and, in adults, relatively common polymorphisms that cause lesser reduction in enzyme activity.

Neutral lipid storage is inconstant in muscle fibers in mitochondrial myopathies. Ragged-red myofibers (RRF), a hallmark of many mitochondriopathies, often contain increased neutral lipid as well as clusters of pathological mitochondria. Muscle fibers in primary coenzyme Q_{10} deficiency, a rare encephalomyopathy, contain increased neutral lipid and aggregates of mitochondria that respond to replacement therapy (59). A few patients with type I glycogenosis have been described as having a neutral lipid storage myopathy associated with muscle weakness (270).

Recognition of focal or generalized neutral lipid storage in skeletal muscle fibers is only the first step in identification of these disorders. When a disorder of energy metabolism is suspected based on clinical history or muscle biopsy findings, useful laboratory studies include determination of blood lactate, pyruvate, and carnitine levels; evaluation of a fasting urine sample for ketone bodies or acylcarnitine compounds; determination of unusual organic acids; measurement of tissue levels of carnitine transporter, carnitine, carnitine palmityl transferase activity; and studies of fatty acid oxidation in fibroblast culture. Increasingly, molecular studies are used to delineate these conditions.

Mitochondrial Myopathy

Mitochondrial diseases are a heterogeneous group of multisystemic disorders, which are difficult to diagnose, especially in children. Mitochondrial myopathies are mainly disorders of oxidative phosphorylation (OXPHOS) caused by abnormalities in mtDNA, mtRNA, or nuclear determinants of OXPHOS proteins (62,156,203,226). Disorders of mtDNA may be maternally inherited duplications or point mutations. Sporadic cases of OXPHOS defects result from postzygotic somatic mutation of the mitochondrial genome or autosomal recessive nuclear gene defects. The diagnosis of mitochondriopathy is based on clinical history, laboratory, genetic and biochemistry testing, and muscle biopsy findings (18). Major clinical presentations are unexplained multisystemic involvement, signs of clinical progression, or exacerbation with intercurrent illnesses and positive family history. Organs or tissues that are highly dependent on energy metabolism such as skeletal muscle, brain, heart, and peripheral nerve are most likely to be affected. Other organs such as liver, kidney, eye, gastrointestinal tract, and pancreas may also be involved. Clinical and laboratory findings depend on the spectrum of organ involvement. In encephalomyopathy, a common combination, lactate and pyruvate levels may be elevated in both blood and spinal fluid. When skeletal muscle only is involved, unexplained weakness, lactic acidosis, episodic cramps, and rarely, myoglobinuria may occur. Measurement of activity of electron transport complexes in skeletal muscle samples plays a major role in the diagnosis of mitochondriopathy. Over 50 pathogenic point mutations and hundreds of large-scale deletions and duplications of mtDNA have been identified in a variety of mitochondriopathies (55,218). However, often in children who are suspected to have mitochondriopathy based upon currently accepted criteria, OXPHOS enzyme activity defects or pathogenic mutations are not identified (218).

Muscle biopsy is a primary investigative procedure in patients who are suspected to have a disorder of energy metabolism as a screening tool for morphological features, which support the clinical suspicion and as a source of tissue for biochemical and molecular genetic study. By LM, muscle from patients with mitochondriopathies may appear normal, show nonspecific focal myopathic changes, or a few scattered diagnostic features such as "ragged-red" myofibers. Histochemical methods for succinic dehydrogenase (SDH) and cytochrome *c* oxidase (COX) demonstrate mitochondrial distribution and are a crude but useful measure of activity. Impaired lipid utilization is assessed with stains for neutral lipid. SDH is a component of complex II of the respiratory chain. COX is a component of complex IV of the respiratory chain that is coded for by both nuclear and mDNA. Monoclonal antibodies to subunits of electron transport complexes can be used to differentiate deficiencies due to mDNA or nuclear DNA alone or in combination (92). This approach has not yet received wide use.

The most striking LM findings in mitochondriopathies are "ragged-red" myofibers; these are rare in infants but slightly more common in older children. RRF contain large aggregates of SDH reactive and COX reactive or negative mitochondria between myofibrils and beneath the sarcolemma. Best seen in cryostat sections stained with the modified trichrome method and SDH activity are "ragged-red" and "ragged-blue" fibers, respectively (Figure 26-28A and B). Small subsarcolemmal mitochondrial aggregates occur in up to 25% of myofibers in children and probably are of no consequence (Figure 26-29A). More than 2% of myofibers containing large subsarcolemmal mitochondrial aggregates based on the SDH reaction supports a diagnosis of mitochondriopathy (Figure 26-29B). Oil red O-stained slides may show focal accumulation of large coarse lipid droplets between myofibrils in mitochondrial myopathy. A general increase of lipid droplets in type 1 myofibers is more likely in disorders of lipid transport or oxidation.

Several different syndromes have been described in which activity of COX is reduced or absent in a few, most, or all muscle fibers (55). All skeletal muscle fibers lack COX activity in lethal cytochrome oxidase deficiency of infancy (Figure 26-30) (153). In our experience, the mitochondria display subtle abnormalities only. A benign reversible form

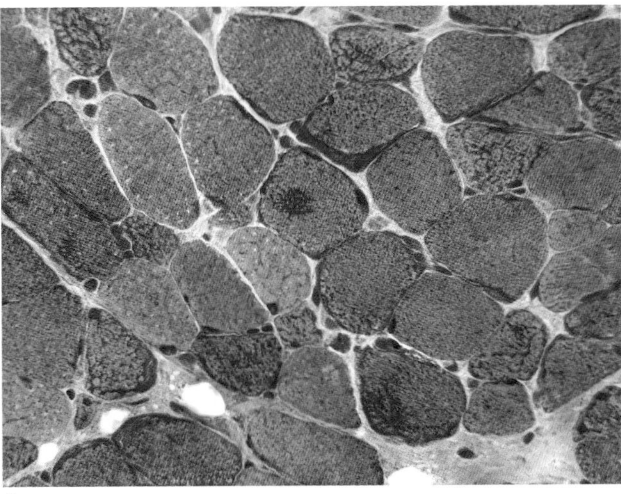

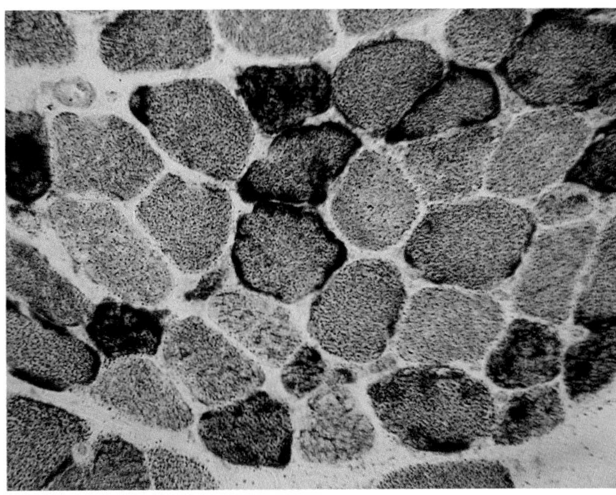

FIGURE 26-28 ■ **A:** RRF in KSS contain coarse aggregates of pathological mitochondria. (Modified trichrome stain; original magnification ×200.) **B:** Ragged-blue fibers in KSS contain coarse aggregates of pathological mitochondria. (SDH histochemistry; original magnification ×200.)

of this condition differs in histochemical characteristics (252). Isolated COX negative fibers, common in adults with mitochondrial disease, are rarely seen in young children.

The role of electron microscopic (EM) examination of myofibers for the diagnosis of mitochondriopathy is somewhat controversial. It is very helpful if unequivocally pathological mitochondria, as described in classical mitochondriopathies, are identified. These are mitochondria of normal or abnormal size or shape with paracrystalline inclusions, abnormal matrix density, and abnormal arrangements of cristae (Figure 26-31). Slight increase in apparent number, or variation in mitochondrial size, and mitochondrial budding and branching, or occurrence in small aggregates are not diagnostic features for pathological mitochondria and are too subjective to be assigned a major role in support of that diagnosis, especially when clinical suspicion is weak. Structurally abnormal mitochondria occur in both type I and type II fibers.

Mitochondrial disorders with muscle involvement in infants or children include Kearns-Sayre syndrome (KSS); myoclonic epilepsy with ragged-red fibers (MERRF); mitochondrial encephalomyopathy, lactic acidosis, and stroke-like episodes (MELAS); Leigh syndrome (LS); fatal infantile mitochondrial myopathy with lactic acidosis and de Toni-Fanconi-Debre syndrome; infantile cytochrome oxidase deficiency (fatal and benign subtypes); and myoclonic epilepsy with weakness, short stature, and ataxia (203) (see Chapter 5).

KSS is usually sporadic with onset before age 20. Most patients have mtDNA deletions. Common clinical presentations include progressive external ophthalmoplegia, pigmentary retinopathy, and cardiomyopathy. Muscle samples contain scattered RRF and variable numbers of COX-negative fibers. Pathological mitochondria are usually seen on EM. The disease is slowly progressive and most patients die before the fourth decade.

The onset of MERRF may be in childhood or in adult life with variable disease progression. Patients typically present with myoclonic seizures, cerebellar ataxia, and mitochondrial myopathy with RRF. COX negative fibers are also commonly seen. Biochemical studies may show defects in complex I, II, III, or IV. The discovery of a highly specific point mutation at nt 8344 (A8344G) in the $tRNA^{Lys}$ gene of mtDNA facilitates the diagnosis of MERRF.

The onset of MELAS is usually before the age of 15 years. Common clinical presentations include seizures, hemianopia, and cortical blindness. Serum and CSF lactate is significantly increased. Muscle biopsy may show RRF or COX negative fibers, but also may be normal. An interesting finding is mitochondrial accumulation in vascular smooth muscle detectable in the SDH reaction. Many patients have complex I deficiency. Demonstration of a point mutation at nt 3243 (A3243G) in the $tRNA^{LEU(UUR)}$ gene of mtDNA is very helpful in the diagnosis.

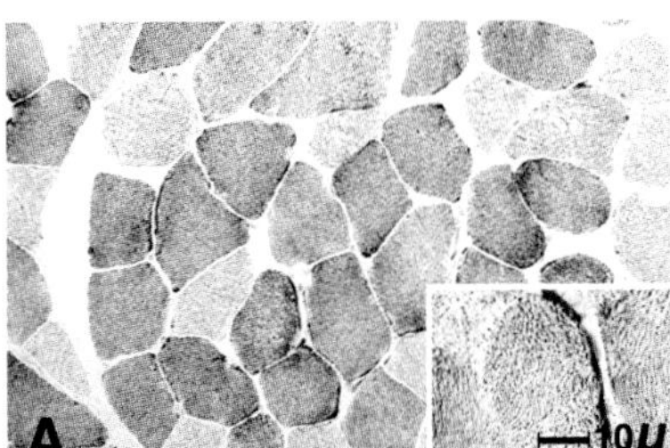

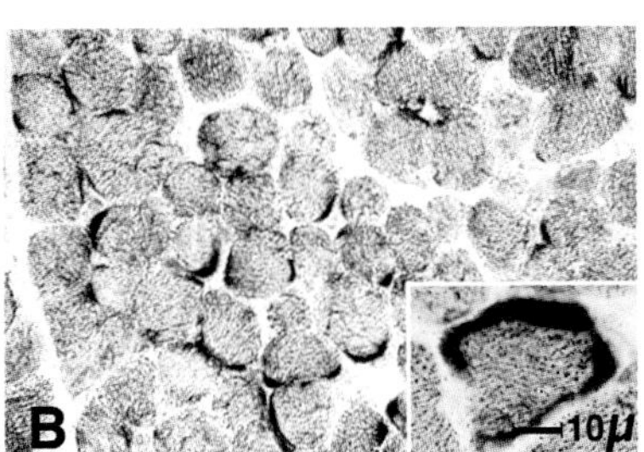

FIGURE 26-29 ■ **A:** Small subsarcolemmal mitochondrial aggregates but no intermyofibrillar aggregates are common in normal skeletal muscle fibers. (SDH histochemistry; original magnification ×200.) **B:** More than 2% Subsarcolemmal mitochondrial aggregates larger than 4 μm in depth support a diagnosis of mitochondriopathy. (SDH histochemistry; original magnification ×200.)

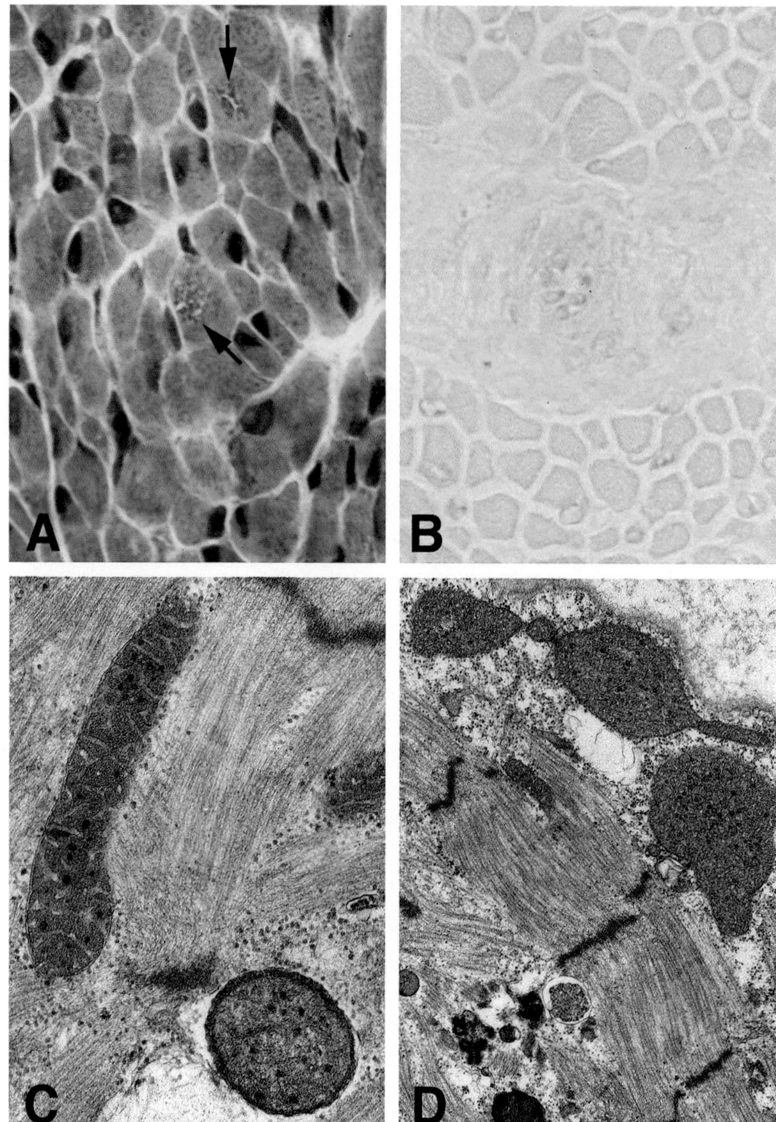

FIGURE 26-30 ■ **A:** Low-grade myopathic change with occasional near RRFs (*arrows*) in lethal infantile COX deficiency. (Hematoxylin and eosin stain; original magnification ×400.) **B:** Absent COX activity in muscle fibers and blood vessel. (Cytochrome oxidase histochemistry; original magnification ×400.) **C:** Pathological mitochondria with dense matrix, excess matrix dense granules, dilatation of cristae and fused outer membranes. (Uranyl acetate and lead citrate stain; original magnification ×15,000.) **D:** Pathological mitochondria with prominent proliferation by budding. (Uranyl acetate and lead citrate stain; original magnification ×15,000.)

Leigh syndome typically present with neuropathy, ataxia, and retinitis pigmentosa. Bilateral symmetric subacute necrotizing encephalomyelopathy is characteristic finding. Microscopy of muscle is normal in many cases, although myofibers that are COX negative or contain increased lipid are reported. RRF are consistently absent. Biochemical studies may show deficiencies in several of the electron transport complex complexes, the most common being complex IV. Although LS is usually inherited in autosomal recessive mode, sporadic, X-linked, and maternal modes of transmission also occur. Maternally inherited LS is associated with heteroplasmic point mutation of T8993G in the ATPase 6 gene of mtDNA. In these cases, genetic analysis of the muscle may be helpful.

The mtDNA depletion syndromes (MDSs) are autosomal recessive disorders with a decreased mitochondrial DNA copy number and a broad phenotypic spectrum. Mutations in thymidine kinase 2 (*TK2*), a nDNA gene, have been associated with a myopathic form of MDS with onset in childhood. Microscopy demonstrates myopathic features with RRF, COX deficient fibers, ultrastructural abnormalities in mitochondria and in a few cases, progressive loss of muscle fibers, mimicking muscular dystrophy (305).

In current practice, many infants with unexplained hypotonia, seizures, developmental delay, sporadic elevation of blood lactate and borderline abnormal brain imaging studies have a muscle biopsy to investigate for possible

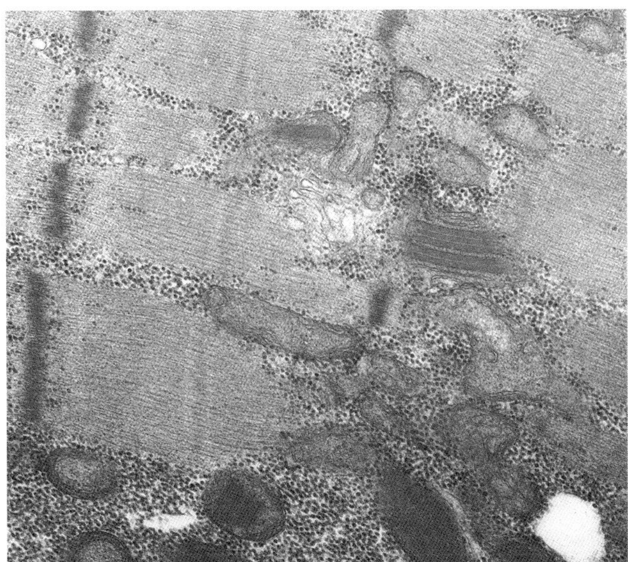

FIGURE 26-31 ■ Pathological mitochondria in KSS exhibit two patterns. Some have central matrix clearing with margination of cristae at the periphery near the outer membrane. Others contain paracrystalline inclusions located in the inner cristal space. Typically some mitochondria exhibit normal morphology. (Uranyl acetate and lead citrate stain; original magnification ×7,500.)

mitochondrial encephalomyopathy. The yield of diagnostic abnormality using a multimodal approach that includes light and electron microscopy, and measurement of electron transport activities is low (149). Better approaches for screening for disorders of energy metabolism are needed.

Other Metabolic Myopathies

Congenital lactic acidosis comprises a heterogeneous group of metabolic disorders characterized by generalized organ dysfunction, especially involving the brain, heart, skeletal muscle, and liver. The differential diagnosis includes defects in mitochondrial electron transport, especially in complex I, mDNA depletion, organic acidemia of various types, deficiency of enzymes involved in gluconeogenesis, defects in the pyruvate dehydrogenase complex, and type I glycogenosis. Hypotonia with lactic acidosis often prompts a muscle biopsy. Muscle fibers may exhibit increased neutral lipids, morphologically abnormal mitochondria, or both, but are often morphologically normal. Biochemical studies should be guided by clinical features.

Myoadenylate deaminase activity in skeletal muscle in the general population is variable due to prevalent gene polymorphisms that result in functional proteins with reduced activity (84,108). Partially reduced enzyme activity due to polymorphisms is typically asymptomatic, but is over-represented in patients with muscular weakness or cramping after strenuous exercise in adults, and rarely, in children (176). Diagnosis is based on histochemical and/or biochemical assays, and mutation analysis. Molecular genetic confirmation is desirable because the histochemical and biochemical methods (160) may not distinguish secondary deficiency due to common polymorphisms, from primary deficiency due to mutation. Myoadenylate deaminase deficiency has been reported in an infant with hypotonia and developmental delay, and in a child whose symptoms resembled those in adults (204,228). The concept of synergistic heterozygosity proposes that combinations of polymorphisms or susceptibility alleles may result in triggerable myopathies as a result of partial defects in two or more enzyme activities such as myoadenylate deaminase, CPT II, or myophosphorylase (170).

EPISODIC MYOGLOBINURIA

Myoglobinuria may be caused by sepsis, myositis, MH, severe transient electrolyte imbalance, drug reaction, or inherited metabolic disease (147). Repeated episodes precipitated by exercise or minor, usually febrile, viral illnesses signal the need for an investigation for an underlying metabolic disease or an unrecognized Becker dystrophinopathy (248,254). Major biochemical defects responsible for about half the cases of episodic myoglobinuria, in approximate order of frequency, involve CPT II; myophosphorylase; phosphorylase kinase; b-oxidation lipolytic enzymes of several types, of which medium-chain triglyceride acylCoA dehydrogenase is the most common; and phosphofructokinase. Other less frequent causes of recurrent myoglobinuria include phosphoglycerate kinase deficiency, myoadenylate deaminase deficiency, two types of muscle lactate dehydrogenase defect, lipoamide dehydrogenase deficiency, and most recently, as sophisticated molecular genetic tools are applied to this problem, defects in mitochondrial OXPHOS (72,117,120,211). Muscle biopsy is central to this formidable workup and requires that as much of the specimen as possible be frozen for biochemical and molecular studies. Several of the specific defects listed can be diagnosed on the basis of muscle morphology and histochemistry, and others, such as CPT II deficiency, can be determined in fibroblast culture. With application of genetic methods that identify potential for triggerable myopathies due to synergistic heterozygosity, the proportion of idiopathic cases may dwindle.

MALIGNANT HYPERTHERMIA

MH is an intraoperative catastrophe characterized by acute rigidity and rapid temperature elevation associated with necrosis of muscle, gross pigmenturia due to myoglobin, and renal failure. Susceptibility to MH when exposed to halothane anesthetics or membrane depolarizers, such as succinylcholine, may be observed in persons with no antecedent myopathy having elective surgery or after recent trauma. The definition of susceptibility and anesthetic risk in children with a previous episode or family history of malignant hyperthermic reaction has relied on *in vitro* testing of strips of fresh muscle for susceptibility to contracture when exposed directly to halothane, caffeine and/or ryanodine, a plant alkaloid. This method requires a special facility, and although the test is highly specific, it has a significant number of false-negative results (140). Noninvasive screening for common RYR1 mutations is a more practical method to detect susceptibility to MH (195), but sensitivity remains uncertain. Dantrolene, which inhibits calcium release from the sarcoplasmic reticulum, is effective in preventing or aborting malignant hyperthermic reactions, MH has been observed in patients with primary myopathies, especially central core disease and multi-mini core disease, but also in Duchenne muscular dystrophy (DMD), myotonic dystrophy, and CMD. Baseline alteration of creatine kinase levels, commonly found long after an attack, may be the only indication of underlying myopathy. The hazard of MH is magnified by the need for multiple orthopedic procedures engendered by the deformities that may develop in children with neuromuscular disease. The lesion of MH, segmental muscle fiber necrosis (Figure 26-32A), is not specific, and may be a final common pathway for any muscle injury (immune, drug, toxin, virus, extreme exercise) that triggers calcium-mediated proteolysis. This muscle lesion usually heals promptly with restoration of muscle fiber structure and no scarring.

SKELETAL MYOPATHY ASSOCIATED WITH CARDIOMYOPATHY

Patients with primary diseases of skeletal muscle sometimes exhibit cardiac dysfunction and have lesions in cardiac muscle similar to those in skeletal muscle (82). Predictable examples are type IIa glycogenosis and dystrophinopathies. Cardiac involvement has also been reported in Emery-Dreifuss muscular dystrophy, scapulohumeral, scapuloperoneal, and humeroperoneal syndromes myotonic dystrophy, and CMD (158,247). NM, centronuclear myopathy, central core disease, and FSD may be accompanied by cardiomyopathy (6,13,109). The genetic myofibrillinopathies, including desminopathies, are important cardioskeletal myopathies in adults (206) that are not well described in children. Metabolic diseases that may cause skeletal muscle and cardiac dysfunction include type III and IV glycogenosis, disorders of b-oxidation, carnitine transporter defect, the infantile form of CPT II deficiency, and several mitochondriopathies.

In early reports of cardioskeletal myopathy, no metabolic defect was defined, although mitochondriopathy was suspected on the basis of morphologic evidence such as expansion of the numbers of mitochondria in the perinuclear zone and ultrastructural evidence for pathological mitochondria (101). Since then, numerous examples are well documented. Mitochondrial encephalomyopathy and cardiomyopathy may be caused by complex 1 deficiency (163). Hypertrophic cardiomyopathy with unusually prominent left ventricular trabeculation occurs in the KSS, the prototype for mitochondrial cytopathy with ragged-red muscle fibers. Idiopathic cardiac hypertrophy, hypotonia, and RRF occur in a few patients with Leigh phenotype, a heterogeneous condition caused by at least six different biochemical defects. A maternally inherited myopathy and cardiomyopathy reported by Zeviani is due to an mDNA defect (275). X-linked cardioskeletal myopathy, originally identified in infants by Neustein (162), includes several genetically distinct disorders, Barth syndrome, and Danon disease. Barth syndrome mainly affects older children and young adults, and includes neutropenia and growth delay, morphologically abnormal mitochondria in heart and skeletal muscle, defects in OXPHOS and deficiency of cardiolipin, a constituent of the inner mitochondrial membrane. A gene, TAZ, is linked, but the encoded proteins are not known. The best diagnostic test is quantitation of cardiolipin in platelets or cultured fibroblasts (14). Danon disease is a vacuolar cardioskeletal myopathy caused by deficiency of a lysosomal-associated membrane protein, LAMP-2 (21). Autophagic vacuoles are a hallmark of the associated myopathy (164). Senger syndrome is characterized by congenital cataracts, hypertrophic cardiomyopathy, hypotonia, and abnormal mitochondria in heart and skeletal muscle. Results of investigations of mitochondrial energetics in these rare patients are inconsistent, suggesting that this phenotype may have multiple causes. Deficient activity of adenine nucleotide translocator is reported (157).

DRUG-INDUCED MYOPATHY

Examples of drug-induced muscle lesions include local acute or chronic myopathy at injection sites, acute or chronic proximal myopathy in myasthenic or polydermatomyositis-like disorders, myotonic syndromes, and MH reactions. In the setting of critical care units, a number of different drugs (curare-like paralytic agents, corticosteroids, and aminoglycoside antibiotics), possibly augmented by the effects of sepsis, are associated with the development of acute myopathy or polyneuropathy, as discussed previously. Some drugs, such as alcohol, may produce several different clinical syndromes; most important in the pediatric age group are characteristic embryo toxicity and fetal myopathy (see Chapter 3) (2,47). Habitual use of Emetine or syrup of ipecac, usually observed in girls with eating disorders, may cause a significant proximal myopathy, clinically simulating dermatomyositis (17). Ipecac-induced myopathy features a distinctive form of myofibrillar degeneration, with coarse clumps of degenerated contractile elements (Figure 26-32B). Both cimetidine and d-penicillamine have been associated with the emergence of polymyositis, possibly by modulating T-cell–mediated reactions (35,264). Myopathy associated with chronic HIV infection resembles polymyositis. The myopathy associated with zidovudine therapy is a mitochondriopathy possibly being related to mtDNA depletion (53).

The range of morphologic reaction to injury of muscle fibers is limited, and reactions in metabolic myopathy, inflammatory myopathy, and drug-induced injury often overlap. Necrosis of muscle fiber segments, the basic lesion in all myoglobinuric muscle diseases, may be precipitated by anesthetic agents and after exposure to ethanol or heroin (see Figure 26-32A). Low-grade, drug-induced myopathy often results in isolated basophilic muscle fibers, a manifestation of degeneration

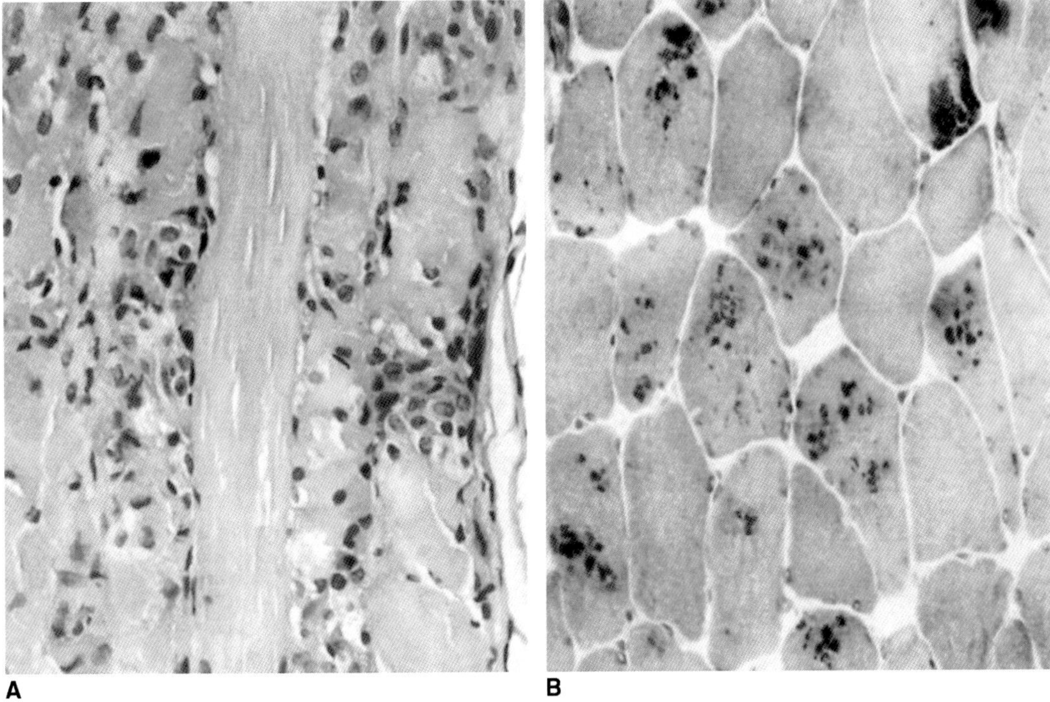

FIGURE 26-32■**A:** Segmental necrosis of muscle fibers following massive ethanol binge, leading to myoglobinuria. (Hematoxylin and eosin stain; original magnification ×400.) **B:** Clumps of degenerating myofibrils in this teenage girl with ipecac-induced myopathy resemble cytoplasmic bodies. (Trichrome stain; original magnification ×400.)

and regeneration cycles, without an inflammatory reaction. A common cause is electrolyte imbalance related to diuretic therapy. Overtly inflammatory drug-induced myopathies may be extremely difficult to distinguish from idiopathic inflammatory myopathy on the basis of histological features. Clinical improvement after withdrawal of the suspect drug may prevent unnecessary muscle biopsy.

MUSCULAR DYSTROPHIES

Duchenne and Becker Dystrophinopathies

The muscular dystrophies are genetically determined diseases of skeletal muscle characterized by cumulative muscle fiber injury, progressive fibrosis, and loss of function. By far, the most common form is DMD, an X-linked disorder with an incidence of approximately 1 per 3,500 to 5,000 live born males (73). As many as two-third of the new cases of DMD are thought to be the result of new mutations in the dystrophin gene either in the mother or in the affected boy (128).

Affected boys usually appear normal until about age 2 years, when clumsiness, proximal muscle weakness, and calf pseudohypertrophy prompt clinical investigation, which establishes the diagnosis. The serum creatine kinase level is usually very high at this stage, and electromyographic studies indicate widespread myopathy. Despite recent advances in experimental treatment of DMD in animal models (246), there is no cure for DMD. Most patients can no longer walk after the first decade, and few survive beyond the end of the second decade. Cardiac muscle involvement is a constant feature at autopsy and may cause clinical manifestations late in the course of the disease (see Chapter 13).

Becker muscular dystrophy (BMD) is a milder form of X-linked dystrophinopathy with a more protracted course and later onset of disease affecting 1 in 18,500 live born males. Despite milder skeletal muscle disease, patients with BMD are more likely to have clinical cardiomyopathy. An unusual presentation of the Becker form is recurrent myalgia with cramps (207). Both DMD and BMD are caused by deletions (in 60% to 65% of cases), duplications (in 5% to 10% of cases), or point mutations in the dystrophin gene. Until recently, it has been impractical to identify point mutations in families without deletions or duplications (42,159,189,239). Dystrophin, absent in DMD and present in an altered form or reduced amounts in BMD, is spatially related to muscle sarcolemma. Deletions and duplications, which are responsible for two-thirds of the cases, can be identified in leukocyte DNA, obviating the need for muscle biopsy. An important difference between DMD and BMD in deletion cases depends on whether the genetic reading frame has shifted, resulting in lack of dystrophin (DMD), or is maintained, resulting in coding for a truncated, partly functional protein that is reduced in amount (BMD).

Initial attempts at prenatal diagnosis of DMD by measuring creatine kinase levels in amniotic fluid or serum produced inconsistent results. Subsequently, polymorphic DNA sequences on the X chromosome, identified using restriction-enzyme digestion, were closely linked to expression of the DMD phenotype in families with one affected boy. This method remains useful for identifying carriers and affected

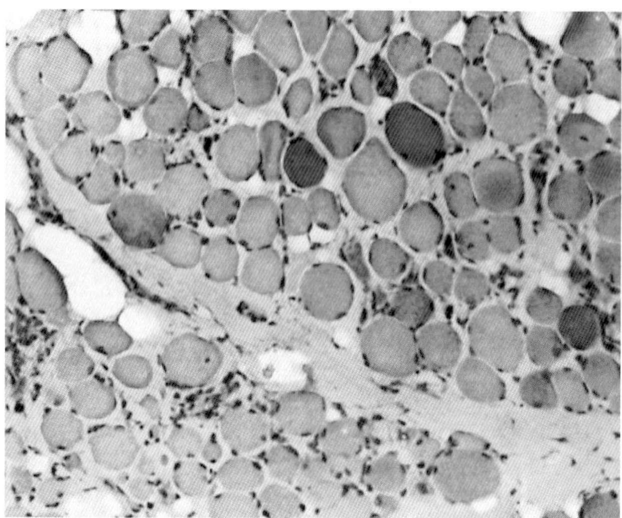

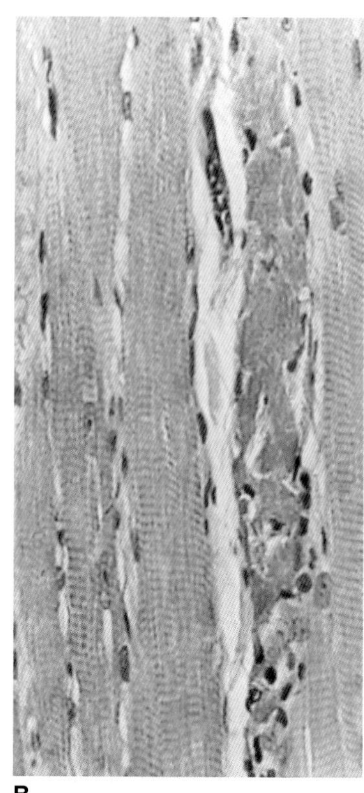

FIGURE 26-33 **A:** Duchenne muscular dystrophy. Replacement fibrosis, focal active myopathy, and scattered, dense, rounded, hypercontracted fibers are typical. (Hematoxylin and eosin stain; original magnification ×160.) **B:** Duchenne muscular dystrophy. Segmental necrosis of isolated fibers is a consistent feature. (Hematoxylin and eosin stain; original magnification ×400.)

fetuses when more specific methods are noninformative (1). Common deletions and duplications can be detected in chorionic villus samples and in amnion cells.

Muscle biopsy findings in DMD include random variation in muscle fiber size, with atrophic and isolated hypertrophic rounded, dense hypercontracted fibers with eosinophilic sarcoplasm; muscle fiber necrosis; fiber regeneration; and progressive increase in connective tissue and fat within and around muscle fascicles (Figure 26-33A, B). Inflammatory changes are typically minor, except during the early phase of the disease. All muscle fiber subtypes are affected. None of the changes are specific, but the constellation is typical and diagnostic in most cases. Muscle biopsy remains useful in nondeletion cases for histologic diagnosis of a dystrophic process. Using specific antibodies to three dystrophin domains, DMD muscle lacks sarcolemmal labeling in the vast majority of myofibers (Figure 26-34A). Muscle sections from BMD patients are characterized by subtle sarcolemmal labeling abnormalities (Figure 26-34B). BMD with an in-frame deletion may show strong sarcolemmal labeling of antibodies against the N- and C-termini but total absence of labeling using antibodies against the rod domain. These results may be further confirmed by western blots for quantitation and by more detailed characterization of mutations in the dystrophin gene.

Segmental necrosis of individual muscle fibers is the major feature in active DMD/BMD. A similar lesion in etiologically diverse skeletal muscle diseases is usually repaired without fibrosis, unlike DMD in which repeated breakdown of muscle fibers may exceed the capacity for repair. The prevalence of intact-appearing muscle fibers with highly stainable calcium content suggests that calcium-activated proteolysis may be exceptionally active in DMD (22).

Other Muscular Dystrophies

Other subtypes of muscular dystrophy that may be encountered in children are comparatively rare. Progressive muscle damage with fibrosis usually is less severe than in DMD. Classification, which is usually based on clinical information, is becoming more precise, as methods based on molecular genetics are developed. Myotonic dystrophy is notable because of myotonia, dominant inheritance, and its effect on infants, but it is not a dystrophic disease in the morphologic sense (106). Genetically heterogeneous autosomal recessive forms of muscular dystrophy, some of which are clinically similar to DMD, may be responsible for some instances of the Duchenne phenotype in girls with a normal karyotype (86). Limb-girdle muscular dystrophy (LGMD) is less severe and has a later onset. Both conditions are morphologically nonspecific. Mutations in sarcoglycan genes have been identified in a minority of patients in each of these clinical groups (69). The sarcoglycans are components of the dystrophin-associated complex of proteins that stabilize the

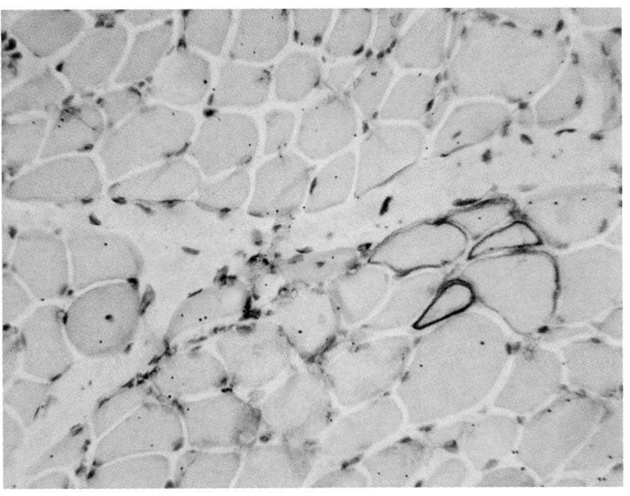
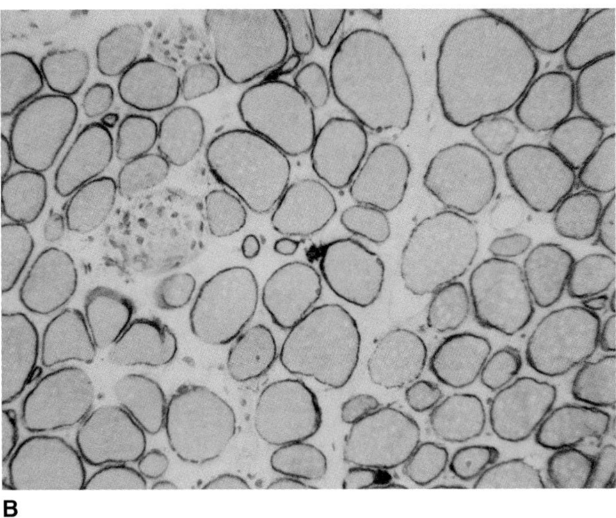

A B

FIGURE 26-34 **A:** In DMD, dystrophin is absent in the sarcolemma of 95% to 100% of myofibers. Rare positive myofibers may indicate partially successful transcription during muscle fiber regeneration. (Dystrophin immunostain; original magnification ×200.) **B:** In BMD, dystrophin is present in most muscle fibers but the sarcolemmal pattern is often weak or interrupted. Dystrophin is absent in the necrotic muscle fiber. (Dystrophin immunostain; original magnification ×200.)

sarcolemmal membrane. Both partial and complete deficiencies of sarcoglycans have been described. The diagnostic role of immunohistology using antibodies to the known sarcoglycans is not yet clear.

The fascioscapulohumeral form of muscular dystrophy often begins in childhood and a rare severe infantile phenotype is described (124). Affected children may have mental retardation and seizures. This dominantly inherited form of muscular dystrophy is recognized by careful attention to distribution of weakness and examination of relatives. Focal myositis is common, but the mechanism and the importance of inflammation are unclear. Deletion of tandem repeats at 4q35 is the basis for a reliable diagnostic test. The Emery-Dreifuss form of humeroperoneal muscular dystrophy is a rare disease recognizable in later childhood on the basis of an associated cardiac conduction disorder; both dominant and X-linked modes of inheritance are described. Defects in nuclear envelope proteins lamin A and emirin are demonstrable using immunostains (172).

CONGENITAL MUSCULAR DYSTROPHY

CMD is a heterogeneous group of disorders characterized by proximal muscle disease causing hypotonia, weakness, and a liability to contractures, which are often present at birth or develop soon thereafter (125). Affected infants are often floppy, and motor development is delayed. Involvement of the central nervous system is variable and helps define important subsets. This may take the form of gray matter migration defects or myelination disturbance. Elevations of the serum creatine kinase level vary. The clinical course of the disease ranges from severe, often with early demise, to mildly progressive with survival to adult life. Muscle fibrosis is often prominent and may be well developed at birth, but severe fibrosis in infants does not predict static versus progressive disease. Marked regional variations exist in incidence of different types of CMD, the highest being 0.46 per 10,000 live births in Japan making CMD one of the more common neuromuscular disorders. In recent years, great progress has been made in discerning the underlying molecular basis of congenital muscular dystrophies (148,158). The most recent classification of CMD is based on clinical presentation and immunohistologic, biochemical, and genetic defects (Table 26-7).

Muscle biopsy findings are generic in CMD and have no specificity for disease subtypes (see Figure 26-35, 26-36, and 26-37). The spectrum of pathological features includes myofiber atrophy, hypertrophy with eosinophilic sarcoplasm, and the presence of scattered split, degenerative, necrotic, and regenerative myofibers. Fibrofatty replacement of myofibers is variable in amount and may be absent in the early stages of disease. Inflammation is limited to foci of fiber degeneration and is typically minor. Many of these features overlap with other forms of muscular dystrophy. Electron microscopy has no proven value in the diagnosis of CMD.

CMD with α_2-laminin deficiency (merosin-deficient CMD) includes almost 50% of the cases of CMD and is the basis for convenient subclassification based upon merosin status. These patients have mutations in the α_2 chain of laminin that lead to complete or partial deficiency of α_2 laminin (merosin) (184,258). Merosin is an extracellular matrix protein linked to the dystrophin-associated glycoproteins in basement membranes of muscle, peripheral nerves, trophoblast, and intracerebral blood vessels and glia limitans that form the blood brain barrier (258). Most patients with merosin deficiency (MDC1) learn to sit unsupported but are unable to walk. Progressive scoliosis is common.

Table 26-7 ■ CONGENITAL MUSCULAR DYSTROPHY

Congenital Muscular Dystrophy	Gene Defects	Organ/Tissue Involvement	Defects in IHC Stain
1. Abnormal extracellular matrix protein			
a. Congenital muscular dystrophy type I (MDC1A)	*$LAMA_2$*	Skeletal muscle, brain, and peripheral nerve	Merosin
b. Ullrich congenital muscular dystrophy (UCMD)	*COL6A1, COL6A2, COL6A3*	Skeletal muscle	Collagen VI
2. Abnormal membrane receptors for the extracellular matrix			
a. Fukuyama congenital muscular dystrophy (FCMD)	*FUKUTIN*	Skeletal muscle, brain and heart	Glycosylated α-dystroglycan
b. Muscle-eye-brain disease	*POMGnT1*	Skeletal muscle, eye and brain	Glycosylated α-dystroglycan and merosin
c. Walker-Warburg syndrome	*POMT1, POMT2, FUKUTIN, FKRP*	Skeletal muscle, eye and brain	Glycosylated α-dystroglycan
d. Congenital muscular dystrophy type 1C (MDC1C)	*FKRP*	Skeletal muscle, heart and brain	Glycosylated α-dystroglycan
e. Congenital muscular dystrophy type 1D (MDC1D)	*LARGE*	Skeletal muscle and brain	Glycosylated α-dystroglycan
3. Abnormal endoplasmic reticulum protein			
a. Rigid spine with muscular dystrophy type 1 (RSMD1)	*SEPN1*	Skeletal muscle and heart	None

The majority have diffuse white matter abnormalities after 6 months of age. The internal capsule, corpus callosum, basal ganglia, thalami, and cerebellum are typically spared. Demyelinating motor neuropathy is common and sensory neuropathy may develop in older children. Merosin status can be determined using standard immunohistologic methods on frozen sections of skeletal muscle, skin, and trophoblast (Figures 26-36 and 26-37) (217). Most, but not all, patients with merosin deficiency have demonstrable mutations; in some patients, the merosin deficiency may be secondary (181).

Ullrich congenital muscular dystrophy (UCMD) is probably the second most common CMD, with a likely autosomal recessive pattern of inheritance. Patients present in the neonatal period with muscle hypotonia, kyphosis of the spine, proximal joint contractures, hyperelasticity of the distal joints, and hip dislocation. Mutation in the COL6A gene leads to collagen VI deficiency in these patients. Collagen VI is a ubiquitous extracellular matrix protein that forms a microfibrillar network associated with basement membranes.

Although typical dystrophic features are seen in the muscle biopsies from most UCMD patients, pathological findings may be limited to mild fiber size variation, myofibers

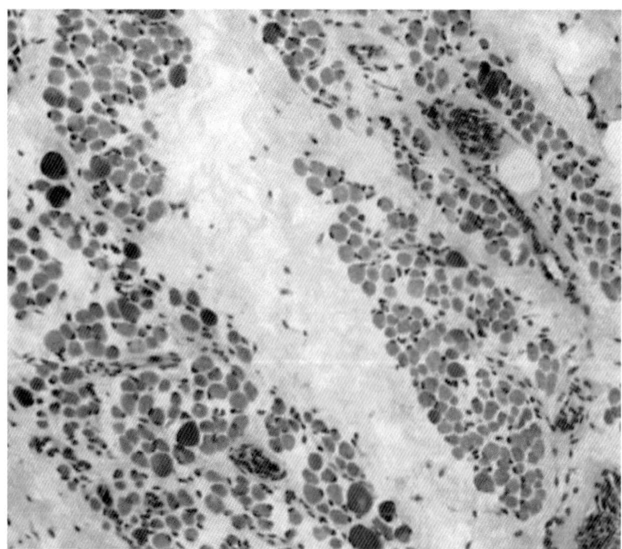

FIGURE 26-35 ■ **A:** CMD shows extensive fibrosis but little evidence of active myopathy. This case was clinically static. (Hematoxylin and eosin stain; original magnification ×160.)

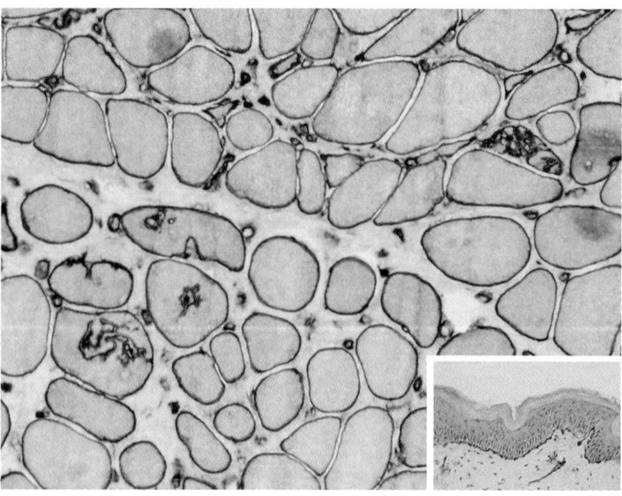

FIGURE 26-36 ■ CMD with normal merosin in basement membranes of skeletal muscle fibers and skin (inset). Internalization of basement membrane in skeletal muscle fibers is a striking feature in some cases. (Merosin immunostain; original magnification ×200.)

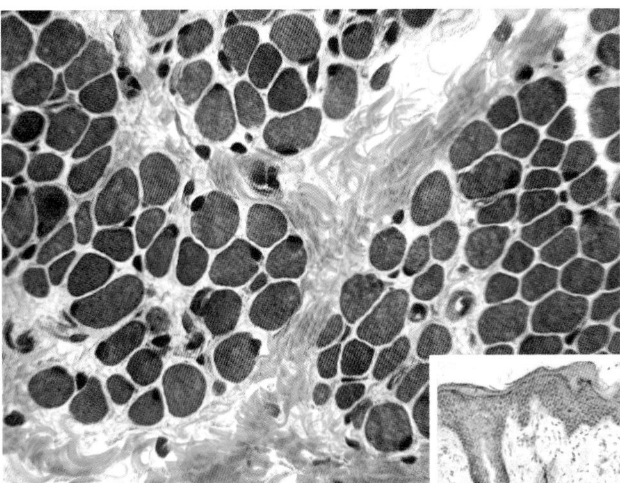

FIGURE 26-37 ■ CMD with absent merosin in basement membranes of skeletal muscle fibers and skin (**inset**). (Merosin immunostain; original magnification ×200.)

containing central nuclei, and minimal endomysial fibrosis. The immunostain for collagen VI is an important diagnostic tool that can be applied to skin, where the protein can be detected in the papillary dermis and around hair follicles. Collagen VI stain may be falsely positive in patients with partial collagen VI deficiency, or falsely negative in patients with secondary downregulation of collagen VI. In both cases, genetic testing for COL6A may provide the definitive diagnosis. Mutations in the gene encoding collagen VI (COL6A) may also cause Bethlem myopathy (BM), which has similar but milder clinical features. BM is likely inherited as an autosomal dominant trait.

CMD with abnormal glycosylation of α-dystroglycan includes three severe forms of CMD that are associated with brain and/or eye involvement: Walker-Warburg syndrome (WWS), muscle-eye-brain (MEB) disease, and Fukuyama congenital muscular dystrophy (FCMD). Also included are congenital muscular dystrophy 1C (MDC1C), a milder form of LGMD2I, congenital muscular dystrophy 1D (MDC1D), and the myodystrophy mouse. All are caused by mutations that affect glycosyltransferases and all share an abnormally glycosylated dystroglycan. Dystroglycan is an important component of the dystrophin-glycoprotein complex and the glycosylation of α-dystroglycan is crucial for basement membrane function.

Muscle biopsies typically show low-grade myopathy with dystrophic features. Immunostain for α-dystroglycan is helpful in recognition of deficiency, but subclassification of this group of diseases is based on the clinical presentation and genetic testing.

WWS is the most severe disease in this category. Patients present with severe early onset hypotonia, profound developmental delay, type II lissencephaly, pontocerebellar hypoplasia, defective central myelination, and ocular dysgenesis. Death usually occurs in infancy. Although there are reports of POMGnT1, fukutin, and FKRP gene mutations in a few patients (16), the primary gene defect in WWS is uncertain. Marked dystrophic features plus a tendency to type I fiber predominance and size disproportion and persistence of type IIc fibers are present in muscle biopsies. The diagnosis depends on clinical, radiological, and pathological findings.

FCMD is particularly frequent in Japan, but occurs in other ethnic groups and is characterized by dystrophic myopathy of early onset associated with central nervous system malformations, including cerebral and cerebellar microgyria, followed by the development of dilated cardiomyopathy (85). FCMD is caused by mutations of fukutin gene on chromosome 9q31 (126); evidence favors an autosomal recessive trait. Recognition depends on detection of appropriate central nervous system malformations, lack of sarcolemmal staining for α-dystroglycan and genetic testing. Merosin expression may be reduced, but linkage studies indicate a different genomic locus in Fukuyama dystrophy than the one assigned to α_2 laminin.

MEB disease is an autosomal recessive disorder with a heterogeneous clinical spectrum. Characteristic clinical findings include early onset hypotonia, congenital glaucoma, myopia, retinal hypoplasia, pachygyria, and cerebellar hypoplasia. The eye involvement is usually more severe than in FCMD. Mutation of POMGnT1, a gene encoding a glycotransferase, resulting in defective O-mannosyl glycan synthesis has been found in patients with MEB (272). Because POMGnT1 is a laminin-binding ligand of α-dystroglycan, muscle biopsies in these patients may lack sarcolemmal labeling with both α-dystroglycan and merosin antibodies.

MDC1C is caused by FKRP missense or null mutation. Broad variation in the clinical phenotype correlates with residual expression of α-dystroglycan. The severe form usually involves both muscle and brain, and LGMD2I represent the milder form with no brain involvement.

MDC1D is related to LARGE, an animal model of CMD with a loss of function mutation in the LARGE gene, encoding for a putative bifunctional glycosyltransferase. The human equivalent of the LARGE mutation was defined in a patient with muscular dystrophy, mental retardation, brain structural changes, and decreased muscle labeling for α-dystroglycan (141).

Included in the broad category of CMD are children with the rigid-spine syndrome (RSMD1) (70). These are usually boys, and they have a fibrosing myopathy manifested as weakness in infancy; biopsy may show type I fiber numeric predominance or size disproportion. Upper spinal stiffness, scoliosis, and in some cases, cardiomyopathy develop in later childhood. The disease is caused by selenoprotein N gene mutation. There is substantial overlap of clinical manifestations and muscle abnormalities with other forms of muscular dystrophy and with CM. SPEN1 gene mutation has been reported in patients with multi mini-core disease (80,81), which further complicates the diagnosis of RSMD1.

CMD may be considered when some other form of muscular dystrophy presents at an unusually early age.

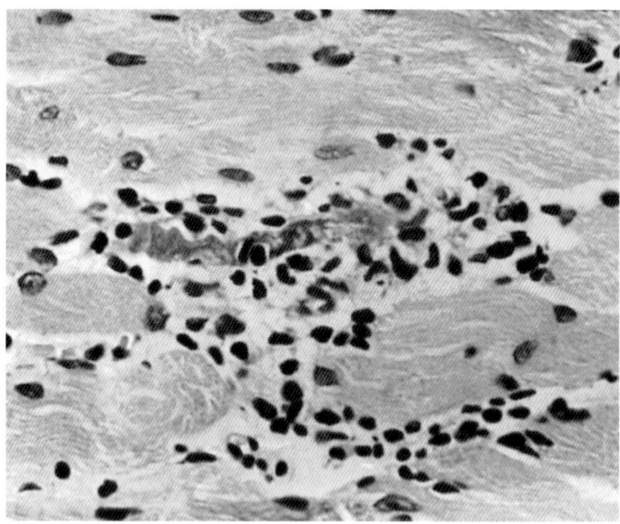

FIGURE 26-38 ■ Congenital polymyositis is indistinguishable from CMD except for occasional foci of necrotizing myositis. Contractures regressed and creatinine kinase normalized without therapy. (Hematoxylin and eosin stain; original magnification ×640.)

Another source of confusion may be the so-called congenital polymyositis (Figure 26-38), an incompletely defined condition that is distinguished from CMD mainly by foci of active "myositis" (221). This disorder has few clinical or morphologic features in common with childhood polydermatomyositis and is probably not an autoimmune disorder. Cerebral abnormalities in some of these infants suggest a nosologic relationship to CMD.

INFLAMMATORY MYOPATHY

Infectious Myositis

Acute, generalized myopathy may accompany acute bacterial or viral infections and may be severe enough to cause pigmenturia due to the release of myoglobin from damaged fibers. Local bacterial myositis may result by extension from cellulitis or acute necrotizing fasciitis, and it often follows trauma. A syndrome of "spontaneous" multifocal pyomyositis is prevalent in the tropics; most of these cases are due to Staphylococcus aureus sepsis (219).

Myalgia is a common component of the general malaise associated with flu-like respiratory illnesses and may be exceptionally severe (30). Viruses most often implicated in acute myopathy include influenza virus and enteroviruses, particularly coxsackievirus and echovirus. Muscle biopsy in these cases has shown focal muscle fiber necrosis without inflammation or overt myositis. Virus has been recovered directly from muscle only rarely, and putative morphologic evidence for acute viral infection of muscle fibers is unconvincing. A cautionary note: Muscle glycogen may be rearranged in a crystalline form, which resembles picornavirus particles in both antemortem and postmortem specimens (48,243). The serologic evidence that chronic inflammatory myopathy is associated with coxsackievirus type B is intriguing but inconclusive (249).

Focal Myositis

Primary, noninfectious fasciitis arises in a variety of circumstances more common in adults than in children. Significant fasciitis is most likely to be encountered in full-thickness biopsy specimens in linear scleroderma, morphea, rheumatic fever, systemic sclerosis, or rheumatoid arthritis or in the syndrome of fasciitis with eosinophilia (152,231). Focal interstitial lymphocytic myositis is limited to the connective tissue framework of muscle contiguous with the involved fascia. Muscle fibers tend to be spared. Overlying fasciitis is surprisingly uncommon in juvenile dermatomyositis (JDM).

Macrophagic myofasciitis is a recently described histologically distinctive focal lesion incidentally encountered in muscle biopsies from adults and children performed to investigate muscle pain, fatigue and, often to rule out an underlying metabolic disorder as a cause of developmental delay (129). The macrophages contain cytoplasmic deposits of slate gray material that contain aluminum salts. Controversy exists over possible relationship to systemic disease, but the lesion is probably an innocuous local reaction to insoluble components of injected vaccines (244).

Local myositis, unrelated to fasciitis, infection, or overt trauma, is a self-limited, histologically florid, true myositis of undetermined cause (95). Changes seen in biopsy specimens from these tender lesions may resemble those of polymyositis (see Chapter 24).

IDIOPATHIC INFLAMMATORY MYOPATHY

Idiopathic inflammatory myopathy is a generic category that includes the childhood and the adult forms of dermatomyositis, polymyositis as a component of systemic collagen-vascular disease, or in association with neoplasia (23). JDM and polymyositis are clinically and pathologically distinct diseases; the former is by far more common in children. Polymyositis also occurs in chronic HIV infection, certain drug reactions and in chronic graft-versus-host disease.

Juvenile dermatomyositis (JDM) is a clinically and morphologically distinct multisystem autoimmune disease, (24,51) that is more common in girls usually with onset after the age of 5 years. Links to HLA-B8, and more recently, to HLA-DQA1, are reported (194). In a typical case rash, insidious onset of fatigue, weight loss, and low-grade fever are accompanied by mucositis, arthralgia, myalgia, dysphonia, and dysphagia. Weakness, tenderness, and reduction in muscle mass most severely affect the proximal muscles. The skin lesion is a distinctive erythematous maculopapular rash involving the face and the extensor surfaces of the elbows, knees, and knuckles. The rash may be transient or subtle, but patients who never display it are rare. A few patients exhibit typical skin changes, but muscle involvement is delayed or never appears. Calcinosis cutis is common

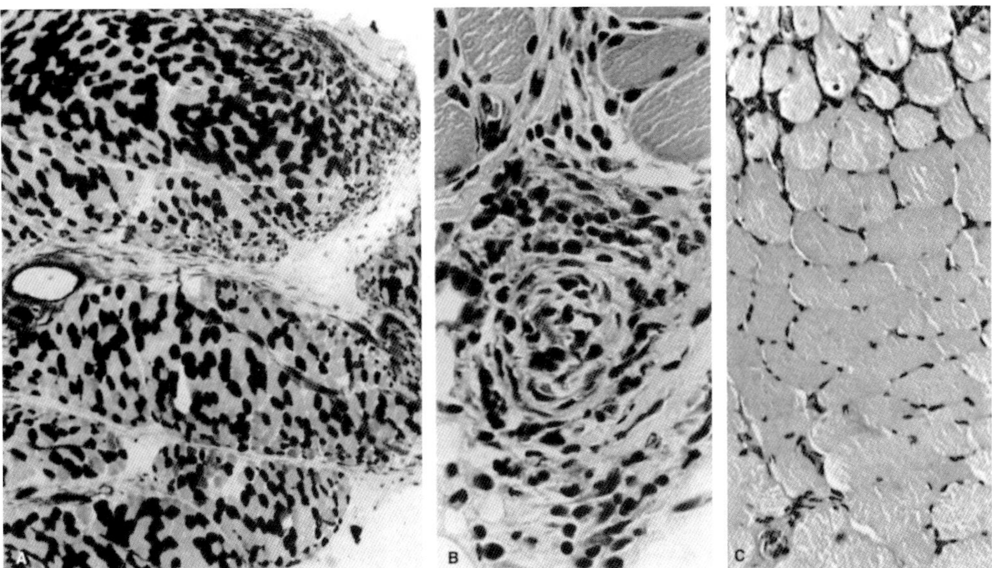

FIGURE 26-39■ **A:** Muscle in JDM exhibiting selective fiber atrophy at the periphery of fascicles. (Myosin ATPase stain with preincubation at pH 4.6; original magnification ×200) **B:** Mononuclear cell perivenulitis in JDM may coexist with true venulitis. CD68-positive macrophages, T-cells, and less commonly B-cells are demonstrable in this location. (Hematoxylin and eosin stain; original magnification ×800.) **C:** Endomysial mononuclear cell infiltrate in JDM is composed of T-cells or macrophages or both. (Hematoxylin and eosin stain; original magnification ×400.)

in chronic JDM, is usually not present initially, and has been linked to delay in diagnosis or therapy (174) (see Chapter 25).

Aids in establishing a diagnosis include elevated serum creatine kinase levels and electromyography, which usually reveals widespread signs of sarcolemmal membrane instability and nonuniform muscle fiber destruction. Noninvasive imaging methods help select a biopsy site and evaluate response to therapy (139), but lack the specificity required to justify a course of prolonged therapy. Tests for antinuclear antibodies, rheumatoid factor, and antimyoglobin are typically negative but may be transiently positive. A few patients eventually develop clinical and serologic features indicating another connective tissue disease, such as systemic lupus erythematosus or mixed connective tissue disease. Overlap occurs with some features of scleroderma (scleromyositis), but true systemic sclerosis is exceptionally rare in children.

Muscle biopsy is not routinely employed for diagnosis but is indicated in clinically uncertain cases, and would find greater use if findings had predictive value for chronic disease, as has been suggested (150,263) Nondiagnostic muscle biopsy in a patient with inflammatory myopathy can result from nonuniform distribution of myositis, but subtle changes are easily obscured by poor handling. Efficiency is maximized by careful technique, performing the muscle biopsy before starting therapy, sampling a muscle group that is clinically involved, and using electron microscopy and direct immunofluorescence, techniques that increase detection of diagnostic changes in small blood vessels. Selective expression on and beneath the sarcolemma of class II histocompatibility antigens (HLAs) in polymyositis (277) and class I HLAs in JDM (137) may be useful when muscle biopsy specimens do not display diagnostic features in patients suspected to have inflammatory myopathy.

Histology of muscle in new-onset JDM is highly variable and may be in part due to established chronicity; histological changes may be unexpectedly slight in patients who are profoundly weak. Muscle fiber atrophy, or degeneration, is usually more severe at the periphery of muscle fascicles (Figure 26-39A), possibly as a consequence of ischemia. Random fiber hypertrophy is never seen. Necrosis may be absent, or involve single fibers or small clusters of fibers with preservation of the sarcolemma, or it may be regional in the form of muscle infarction. Perifascicular collagen tends to be altered, often severely, owing to fibrinoid swelling of collagen bundles and accumulation of interstitial fluid. Inflammatory infiltrates are preferentially located around perimysial veins, with expansion into the surrounding muscle fascicles (Figure 26-39B, C). In most cases, the small muscular arteries appear normal; in a few patients, the small arteries in muscle and subcutaneous fat exhibit noninflammatory intimal cell swelling, degeneration, or lumen occlusion by cellular debris, often intermixed with fibrin (Figure 26-40A); rarely, fibrinoid degeneration of the media or arteritis is demonstrated. Intimal fibrosis with intact elastic lamina and luminal narrowing or occlusion, plus atrophy of the medial smooth muscle are features of chronic arteriopathy (Figure 26-40B). Severe vascular changes may contribute to treatment resistance in chronic JDM.

Small arteries and arterioles, whether histologically normal or not, often react (Figure 26-40C) with antisera to fibrin, IgM, Clq, C3, and C5 alone or as a component of C5-8 membrane attack complex (123). Similar immunoreactivity

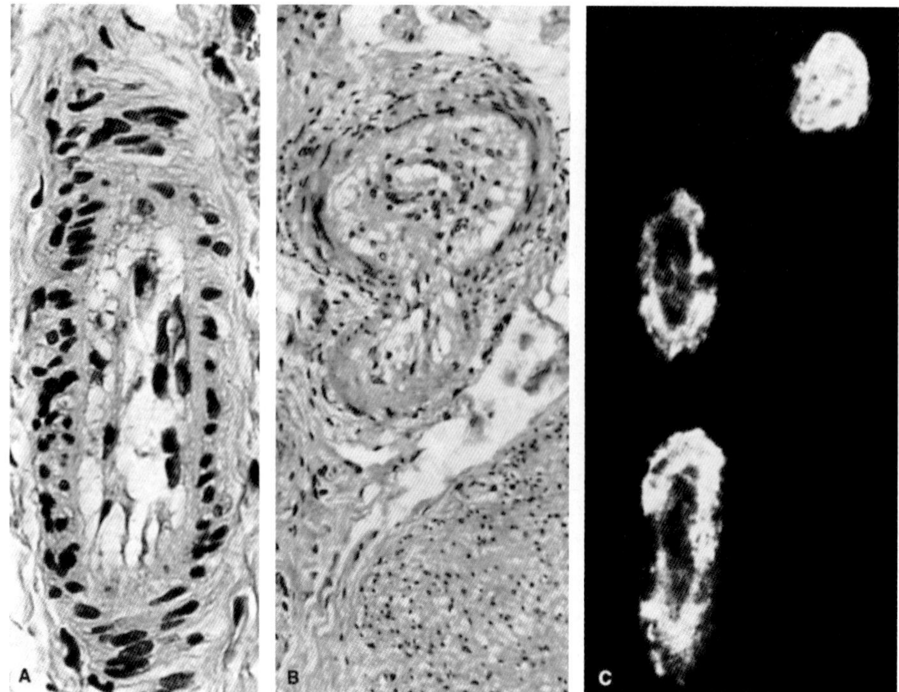

FIGURE 26-40 **A:** Acute intimal arteriopathy in JDM. Endothelial cells are reactive. Prominent vacuolar changes usually reflect neutral lipid deposition. (Hematoxylin and eosin stain; original magnification ×800.) **B:** Chronic arteriopathy in JDM. Occlusive changes resulting from subintimal proliferation cause ischemic damage to the gut, skin, and muscle. (Hematoxylin and eosin stain; original magnification ×400.) **C:** JDM involvement displays positive direct fluorescence reaction in intramuscular arteries. (Anti-C3 stain; original magnification ×400.)

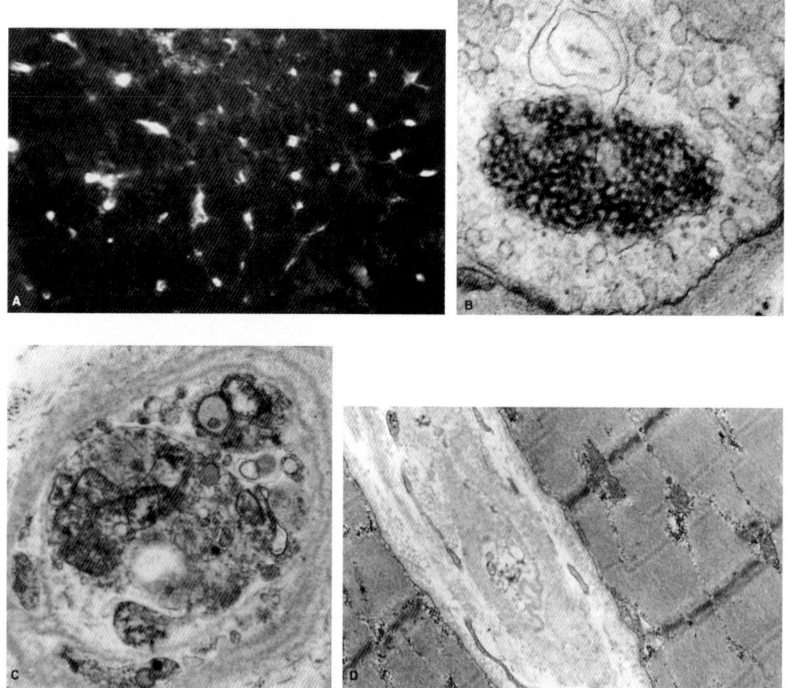

FIGURE 26-41 **A:** JDM is apparent with positive direct immunofluorescence reaction in the intrafascicular muscle capillary bed. (Antifibrin stain; original magnification ×400.) **B:** JDM tubuloreticular inclusions are present in the endothelial cytoplasm. (Uranyl acetate and lead citrate stain; original magnification ×20,000.) **C:** In JDM, a capillary is occluded by cell debris and marked basement membrane redundancy. (Uranyl acetate and lead citrate stain; original magnification ×950.) **D:** Capillary obsolescence is present in chronic JDM. (Uranyl acetate and lead citrate stain; original magnification ×4,500.)

may be demonstrable in the endomysial capillary bed (Figure 26-41A). Virtually all cases of acute JDM have ultrastructural evidence of endothelial cell alterations, including tubuloreticular inclusions, cytoplasmic swelling, and necrosis (Figure 26-41B, C). Similar inclusions also occur in lupus myositis and nephritis and occur in a variety of cell types, including circulating lymphocytes; it is possible that these inclusions result from immune-mediated cellular injury. The capillaropathy of JDM may resolve or permanent capillary obliteration may result (Figure 26-41D).

The distinctive vasculopathy of JDM features complement-mediated vascular immunoreactivity and a relatively high proportion of B-cells and helper T4 cells in the predominantly perimysial infiltrates. This suggests humoral factors are particularly important in the pathogenesis of the disease (76). In contrast, polymyositis (inflammatory myopathy without rash), which is seen much more commonly in adults than in children, displays less prominent perivascular infiltrates and a higher proportion of intrafascicular cytotoxic T8 cells and macrophages reactive to isolated necrotic muscle fibers (Figure 26-42) (74). That finding is compatible with a cell-mediated cytotoxicity model. The implied mechanisms of vascular or muscle fiber injury mediated by complement—B-cell–T-cell interaction, T-cells alone, or T-cell-macrophage interaction—are not mutually exclusive.

Favorable outcome of JDM correlates directly with early treatment, and is adversely influenced by the severity of the vasculopathy and prevalence of muscle fiber necrosis in pretreatment specimens (150,263). Cutaneous ulcers and gastrointestinal catastrophes, resulting from occlusive arteriopathy, are a common cause of morbidity and mortality. Many patients respond dramatically to therapy whereas others develop a chronic form of the disease. Management choices are unsettled. Dubowitz contends that prolonged high-dose steroid treatment may actually promote the development of debilitating or life-threatening complications (66).

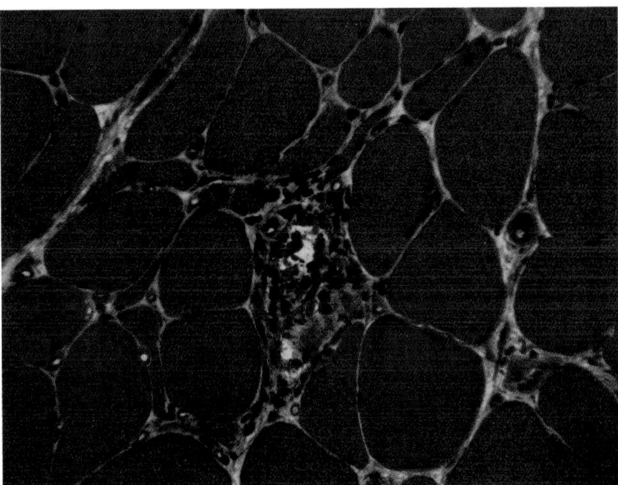

FIGURE 26-42 ■ Multifocal muscle fiber necrosis without histologic features of JDM in this child with arthritis/arthralgia, rheumatoid factor, anti-nuclear antibody and no rash suggests polymyositis associated with a connective tissue disease. (Hematoxylin and eosin stain; original magnification ×200.)

REFERENCES

1. Abbs S. Prenatal diagnosis of Duchenne and Becker muscular dystrophy. *Prenat Diagn* 1996;16:1187.
2. Adickes ED, Shuman RM. Fetal alcohol myopathy. *Pediatr Pathol* 1983;1:369.
3. Agapitos M, Georgiou-Theodoropoulu M, Koutselinis A, et al. Arthrogryposis multiplex congenita, Pena-Shokeir phenotype, with gastroschisis and agenesis of the leg. *Pediatr Pathol* 1988;8:409.
4. Agrawal PB, Greenleaf RS, Tomszak KK, et al. Nemaline myopathy with minicores caused by mutation of the CFL2 gene encoding the skeletal muscle actin-binding protein, cofilin2. *Am J Hum Genet* 2007;80:162.
5. Allison F, Bennett MJ, Variend S, et al. Acylcoenzyme A dehydrogenase deficiency in heart tissue from infants who die unexpectedly with fatty change in the liver. *Br Med J* 1988;296:11.
6. Al-Rawaishid A, Vaisar J, Tein I, et al. Centronuclear myopathy and cardiomyopathy requiring transplant. *Brain Dev* 2003;25:62.
7. Ambler MW, Neave C, et al. X-linked recessive myotubular myopathy: 1. Clinical and pathological findings in a family. *Hum Pathol* 1984;15:566.
8. Angelini C, Engel AG, Titus JL. Adult acid maltase deficiency. *N Engl J Med* 1972;287:948.
9. Argov Z, Gardner-Medwin D, Johnson MA, et al. Patterns of muscle fiber type disproportion in hypotonic infants. *Arch Neurol* 1984;41:53.
10. Arnon SS, Chin J. The clinical spectrum of infant botulism. *Rev Infect Dis* 1979;1:614.
11. Askanas V, Engel WK, DiMauro S, et al. Adult-onset acid maltase deficiency. Morphologic and biochemical abnormalities reproduced in cultured muscle. *N Engl J Med* 1976;284:573.
12. Bank WJ, DiMauro S, Bonilla E, et al. A disorder of muscle lipid metabolism and myoglobinuria: absence of carnitine palmityl transferase. *N Engl J Med* 1975;292:443.
13. Banwell BL, Becker LE, Jay V, et al. Cardiac manifestations of congenital fiber-type disproportion myopathy. *J Child Neurol* 1999;14:83.
14. Barth PG, Valianpour F, Bowen VM, et al. X-linked cardioskeletal myopathy and neutropenia (Barth Syndrome): an update. *Am J Med Genet* 2004;126:349.
15. Banker BQ. Arthrogryposis multiplex congenita: spectrum of pathologic changes. *Hum Pathol* 1986;17:656.
16. Beltran-Valero de Bernabe D, Currier S, Steinbrecher A, et al. Mutations in the O-mannosyltransferase gene POMT1 give rise to the severe neuronal migration disorder Walker-Warburg syndrome. *Am J Hum Genet* 2002;71:1033.
17. Bennett HS, Spiro AJ, Pollack MA, et al. Ipecac-induced myopathy simulating dermatomyositis. *Neurology* 1982;32:91.
18. Bernier FP, Boneh A, Dennett X, et al. Diagnostic criteria for respiratory chain disorders in adults and children. *Neurology* 2002;59:1406.
19. Benzing G III, Iannaccone ST, Bove KE, et al. Prolonged myasthenic syndrome after one week of muscle relaxants. *Pediatr Neurol* 1990;6:190.
20. Bersu ET. Anatomical analysis of the developmental effects of aneuploidy in man: the Down syndrome. *Ann J Med Genet* 1980;5:399.
21. Bertini E, Donati MA, Broda P, et al. Phenotypic heterogeneity in two unrelated Danon patients associated with LAMP-2 gene mutation. *Neuropediatrics* 2005;36:309–313.
22. Bodensteiner JB, Engel AG. Intracellular calcium accumulation in Duchenne dystrophy and other myopathies: a study of 567,000 muscle fibers in 114 biopsies. *Neurology* 1978;28:439.
23. Bohan A, Peter JB. Polymyositis and dermatomyositis (first of two parts). *N Engl J Med* 1975;292:344.

24. Bohan A, Peter JB. Polymyositis and dermatomyositis (second of two parts). *N Engl J Med* 1975;292:403.
25. Bookleman H, Trijbels JMF, Sengers RCA, et al. Measurements of cytochromes in human skeletal muscle mitochondria isolated from fresh and frozen stored muscle specimens. *Biochem Med* 1978;19:366.
26. Bouillot S, Martin-negrier ML, Vital A, et al. Peripheral neuropathy associated with mitochondrial disorders: 8 cases and review of the literature. *J Periph Nerv Syst* 2002;7:213.
27. Bove KE, Iannaccone ST. Atypical infantile spinomuscular atrophy presenting as acute diaphragmatic paralysis. *Pediatr Pathol* 1988;8:95.
28. Bove KE, Iannaccone ST, Vogler CA. Intramuscular hematopoiesis in hypotonic infants with type 1 muscle fiber dysmaturation. *Arch Pathol Lab Med* 1986;110:207.
29. Bove KE. The metabolic crisis: a diagnostic challenge. *J Pediatr* 1997;131:181
30. Bove KE, Partin JP, Farrell MK, et al. The morphology of myopathy associated with influenza B infection. *Pediatr Pathol* 1983;1:51.
31. Brooke MH, Engel WK. The histographic analysis of human muscle biopsies with regard to fiber type: IV. Children's biopsies. *Neurology.* 1969;19:591.
32. Bruno C, van Diggelen OP, Cassandrini D, et al. Clinical and genetic heterogeneity of branching enzyme deficiency (glycogenosis type IV). *Neurology.* 2004;63:1053.
33. Buchino JJ, Bove KE, Iannaccone ST. Transient cytoplasmic bodies in muscle of three infants with Werdnig-Hoffmann disease. *Pediatr Pathol* 1990;10:563.
34. Carpenter S, Karpati G. Lysosomal storage in human skeletal muscle. *Hum Pathol* 1986;17:683.
35. Carroll GJ, Will RK, Peter JB, et al. Penicillamine induced polymyositis and dermatomyositis. *J Rheumatol* 1987;14:995.
36. Carroll JE, Brooke MH. Infantile facioscapulohumeral dystrophy. In: Serratrice G, Roux H, eds. *Peroneal Atrophies and Related Disorders.* New York: Masson Publishing, 1979:305.
37. Castle ME, Reyman TA, Schneider M. Pathology of spastic muscle in cerebral palsy. *Clin Orthop Rel Res* 1979;142:223.
38. Cavanaugh NPC, Lake BD, McMeniman P. Congenital fiber type disproportion myopathy. *Arch Dis Child* 1979;54:735.
39. Chalmers RA, Roe CR, Stacey TE, et al. Urinary excretion of l-carnitine and acylcarnitines by patients with disorders of organic acid metabolism: evidence for secondary insufficiency of l-carnitine. *Pediatr Res* 1984;18:1325.
40. Chalmers RA, Stanley CA, English N, et al. Mitochondrial carnitine-acylcarnitine translocase deficiency presenting as sudden neonatal death. *J Pediatr* 1997;131:220.
41. Charnas L, Trapp B, Griffin J. Congenital absence of peripheral myelin: abnormal Schwann cell development causes lethal arthrogryposis multiplex congenita. *Neurology* 1988;38:966.
42. Chaturvedi LS, Mukherjee M, Srivastava S et al. Point mutation and polymorphism in Duchenne/Becker muscular dystrophy (D/BMD) patients. *Exp Mol Med* 2001;33:251.
43. Choi BH, Ruess WR, Kim RC. Disturbances in neuronal migration and laminar cortical organization associated with multicystic encephalopathy in Pena-Shokeir syndrome. *Acta Neuropathol* 1986;69:177.
44. Chudley AE, Barmada MA. Diaphragmatic elevation in neonatal myotonic dystrophy. *Am J Dis Child* 1979;133:1182.
45. Clarke NF, North KN. Congenital fiber type disproportion—30 years on. *J Neuropathol Exp Neurol* 2003;62:977.
46. Clarren SK, Hall JG. Neuropathologic findings in the spinal cords of 10 infants with arthrogryposis. *J Neurol Sci* 1983;58:89.
47. Clarren SK, Smith DW. The fetal alcohol syndrome. *N Engl J Med* 1978;198:1063.
48. Collins DN, Gilbert EF. Glycogen complexes in muscle in Reye's syndrome simulating virus-like particles. *Lab Invest* 1977;36:91.
49. Cornblath DR. Disorders of neuromuscular transmission in infants and children. *Muscle Nerve* 1986;9:606.
50. Cornelio F, Bresolin N, DiMauro S, et al. Congenital myopathy due to phosphorylase deficiency. *Neurology* 1983;33:1383.
51. Crowe WE, Bove KE, Levinson JE, et al. Clinical and pathogenetic implications of histopathology in childhood polydermatomyositis. *Arthritis Rheum* 1982;25:126.
52. Curless RG, Nelson MB, Crimmer F. Histologic patterns of muscle in infants with developmental brain abnormalities. *Dev Med Child Neurol* 1978;20:159.
53. Dalakas M, Illa I, Pezeshkpour GH, et al. Mitochondrial myopathy caused by long term zidovudine therapy. *N Engl J Med* 1990;332:1098.
54. Darin N, Oldfors A, Moslemi AR, et al. The incidence of mitochondrial encephalomyopathies in childhood: clinical features and morphological, biochemical, and DNA abnormalities. *Ann Neurol* 2001; 49:377.
55. Darin N, Moslemi AR, Lebon S, et al. Genotypes and clinical phenotypes in children with cytochrome-c oxidase deficiency. *Neuropediatrics* 2003;343:11.
56. Dastur DK, Daver SM, Manghani DK. Changes in muscle in human malnutrition with an emphasis on the fine structure in protein-calorie malnutrition. In: Zimmerman HM, ed. *Progress in Neuropathology*, vol 4. New York: Raven Press, 1979:29.
57. David TJ, Winter RM. Familial absence of the pectoralis major, serratus anterior and latissimus muscles. *J Med Genet* 1985;22:390.
58. DeAngelis MS, Palmucci L, Leone M, et al. Centronuclear myopathy: clinical, morphological and genetic characters. A review of 288 cases. *J Neurol Sci* 1991;103:2.
59. Di Giovanni S, Mirabella M, Spinazzola A, et al. Coenzyme Q_{10} reverses pathological phenotype and reduces apoptosis in familial Co Q_{10} deficiency. *Neurology* 2001;57:515.
60. Demaugre F, Bonnefont JP, et al. Infantile form of carnitine palmitoyl transferase II deficiency with hepatomuscular symptoms and sudden death. *J Clin Invest* 1991;87:859.
61. DeVito DC, DiMauro S. Mitochondrial defects of brain and muscle. *Biol Neonate* 1990;58(Suppl 1):54.
62. DiMauro S, Bonilla E, Zeviani M, et al. Mitochondrial myopathies. *Ann Neurol* 1985;17:521.
63. DiMauro S, Hartlage PL. Fatal infantile form of muscle phosphorylase deficiency. *Neurology* 1978;28:1124.
64. DiMauro S, Miranda AF, et al. Metabolic myopathies. *Am J Med Genet* 1986;25:635.
65. Dimmick JE, Berry K, MacLeod PM, et al. Syndrome of ankylosis, facial anomlies and pulmonary hypoplasia: a pathologic analysis of one infant. In: Bergsma D, ed. *Embryology and Pathogenesis and Prenatal Diagnosis*, vol 13. New York: Alan R. Liss, 1977:133.
66. Dubowitz V. Prognostic factors in dermatomyositis. *J Pediatr* 1984;105:336.
67. Dubowitz V, Brooke MH. *Muscle Biopsy: A Modern Approach.* London: WB Saunders, 1973:475.
68. Dubowitz V, Roy S. Central core disease of muscle: clinical, histochemical and electron microscopic studies of an affected mother and child. *Brain* 1970;93:133.
69. Duggan DJ, Gorospe JR, Fanin M, et al. Mutations in the sarcoglycan genes in patients with myopathy. *N Engl J Med* 1997;336:618.
70. Echenne B, Astruc J, et al. Congenital muscular dystrophy and rigid spine syndrome. *Neuropediatrics* 1983;14:97.
71. Egger J, Lake BD, Wilson J. Mitochondrial cytopathy. A multisystem disorder with ragged red fibers on muscle biopsy. *Arch Dis Child* 1981;56:741.
72. Elpeleg ON, Saada AB, Shaag A, et al. Lipoamide dehydrogenase deficiency: a new cause for recurrent myoglobinuria. *Muscle Nerve* 1997;20:238.
73. Emery AE. Population frequencies of inherited neuromuscular diseases-a world survey. *Neuromuscul Disord* 1991;1:19.
74. Emslie-Smith AM, Arahata K, Engel AG. Major histocompatability complex class I antigen expression, immunolocalization of interferon subtypes and T-cell mediated cytotoxicity in myopathies. *Hum Pathol* 1989;20:224.
75. Engel AG, Ohno K, Sine SM. Congenital myasthenic syndromes: recent advances. *Arch Neurol* 1999;56:163.

76. Engel AG, Arahata I. Mononuclear cells in myopathies: quantitation of functionally distinct subsets, recognition of antigen-specific cell-mediated cytotoxicity in some diseases and implications for the pathogenesis of the different inflammatory myopathies. *Hum Pathol* 1986;17:704.
77. Farkas-Bargeton E, Aicardi J, Arsenio-Nunes ML, et al. Delay in the maturation of muscle fibers in infants with congenital hypotonia. *J Neurol Sci* 1978;39:17.
78. Farrington ML, Haas JE, Nazar-Stewart V, et al. Eosinophillic fasciitis in children frequently progresses to scleroderma-like cutaneous fibrosis. *J Rheumatol* 1993;20:1.
79. Farrants GW, Hovmoller S, Stadhouders AM. Two types of mitochondrial crystals in diseased human skeletal muscle fibers. *Muscle Nerve* 1988;11:45.
80. Ferreiro A, Quijano-Roy S, Pichereau C, et al. Mutations of the selenoprotein N gene, which is implicated in rigid spine muscular dystrophy, cause the classical phenotype of multiminicore disease: reassessing the nosology of early-onset myopathies. *Am J Hum Genet* 2002; 71:739.
81. Ferreiro A, Ceuterick-de Groote C, Marks JJ, et al. Desmin-related myopathy with Mallory body-like inclusions is caused by mutation of the selenoprotein N gene. *Ann Neurol* 2004;55:676.
82. Finsterer J, Stollberger C. Cardiac involvement in primary myopathies. *Cardiology* 2000;94:1.
83. Fischer JC, Ruitenbeek W, et al. A mitochondrial encephalomyopathy: the first case with an established defect at the level of coenzyme Q. *Eur J Pediatr* 1986;144:441.
84. Fishbein WN, Armbrustmacher VW, Griffin JL. Myoadenylate deaminase deficiency: a new disease of muscle. *Science* 1978;200:545.
85. Fukuyama Y, Osawa M, Suzuki H. Congenital progressive muscular dystrophy of the Fukuyama type. Clinical, genetic and pathological considerations. *Brain Dev* 1981;3:1.
86. Gardner-Medwin D, Johnston HM. Severe muscular dystrophy in girls. *J Neurol Sci* 1984;64:79.
87. Goldstein JD, Reid LM. Pulmonary hypoplasia resulting from phrenic nerve agenesis and diaphragmatic amyoplasia. *J Pediatr* 1980; 97:282.
88. Greenberg F, Fenolio KR, et al. X-linked infantile spinal muscular atrophy. *Am J Dis Child* 1988;142:217.
89. Greene CM, Weldon DE, et al. Juvenile polysaccharidosis with cardioskeletal myopathy. *Arch Pathol Lab Med* 1987;111:977.
90. Greene HL, Brown BI, McClenathon DT, et al. A new variant of type IV glycogenosis: deficiency of branching enzyme activity without apparent progressive liver disease. *Hepatology* 1988;8:302.
91. Hall JG. Analysis of Pena Shokeir phenotype. *Am J Med Genet* 1986;25:99.
92. Hanson BJ, Capaldi RA, Marusich MF, et al. An immunohistochemical approach to detection of mitochondrial disorders. *J Histochem Cytochem* 2002;50:2181–1288.
93. Hart A, Chang C, Perrin E, et al. Familial poliodystrophy, mitochondrial myopathy and lactic acidemia. *Arch Neurol* 1977;34:180.
94. Heckmatt JZ, Moosa A, Hutson C, et al. Diagnostic needle muscle biopsy. A practical and reliable alternative to open biopsy. *Arch Dis Child* 1984;59:528.
95. Heffner RR, Armbrustmacher VW, Earle KM. Focal myositis. *Cancer* 1977;40:301.
96. Hoganson G, Berlow S, Gilbert E, et al. Glutaric acidemia type II and flavin-dependent enzymes in morphogenesis. *Pediatr Pathol* 1986;5:98.
97. Holliday PL, Climie ARW, Gilroy J, et al. Mitochondrial myopathy and encephalopathy: three cases—a deficiency of NADH-CoQ dehydrogenase? *Neurology* 1983,33:1619.
98. Holt IJ, Hardin AE, Morgan-Hughes JA. Deletions of mitochondrial DNA in patients with mitochondrial myopathies. *Nature* 1988; 331:717.
99. Howald H. Training induced morphological and functional changes in skeletal muscles. *Int J Sports Med* 1982;3:1.
100. Hug G. Glycogen storage disease. In: Kelly VC, ed. *Practice of Pediatrics*, vol 6. Philadelphia: Harper and Row, 1984:1.
101. Hug G, Schubert WK. Idiopathic cardiomyopathy. *Lab Invest* 1970;22:541.
102. Hug G, Bove K, Soukup S. Multiorgan deficiency of carnitine palmitoyl transferase II—a lethal neonatal disease. *N Engl J Med* 1991;325:1862
103. Hug G, Soukup S, Ryan M, et al. Rapid prenatal diagnosis of glycogen storage disease, type II, by electron microscopy of uncultured amniotic fluid cells. *N Engl J Med* 1984;310:1018.
104. Hutchinson DO, Charlton A, Laing NG, et al. Autosomal dominant nemaline myopathy with intranuclear rods due to mutation of skeletal muscle ACTA1 gene: clinical and pathological variability within a kindred. *Neuromuscul Disord* 2006;16:113.
105. Hoagland MH, Frank KA, Hutchins GM. Prune belly syndrome with prostatic hypolasia, bladder wall rupture and massive ascites in a fetus with trisomy 18. *Arch Pathol Lab Med* 1988;112:1126.
106. Iannaccone ST, Bove KE, Vogler CA, et al. Muscle maturation delay in infantile myotonic dystrophy. *Arch Pathol Lab Med* 1986;110:405.
107. Iannaccone ST, Bove KE, Vogler CA, et al. Type I fiber size disproportion. Morphometric data from 37 children with myopathic, neuropathic or idiopathic hypotonia. *Pediatr Pathol* 1987;7:395.
108. Isackson PJ, Bujnicki H, Harding, CO, et al. Myoadenylate deaminase deficiency caused by alternate splicing due to a novel intronic mutation in the AMPD1 gene. *Mol Genet Metab* 2005;86:250.
109. Ishibashi-Ueda H, Imakita M, Yutani C, et al. Congenital nemaline myopathy with dilated cardiomyopathy: an autopsy study. *Hum Pathol* 1990;21:77.
110. Johnson MA, Polgar J, Weightman D, et al. Data on the distribution of fiber types in thirty-six human muscles. *J Neurol Sci* 1973;18:111.
111. Johnson MA, Turnbull DM, Dick DJ, et al. A partial deficiency of cytochrome oxidase in chronic progressive external ophthalmoplegia. *J Neurol Sci* 1983;60:31.
112. Jongpiputvanich S, Walsh PJ, Kakulas BA. Minicores and congenital fibre type disproportion observed in a family. *J Paediatr Child Health* 1995;31:253.
113. Jungbluth H, Sewry C, Brown SC, et al. Minicore myopathy in children: a clinical and histopathological study of 19 cases. *Neuromuscul Disord* 2000;10:264.
114. Kablar B, Asakura A, Krastel K, et al. MyoD and Myf-5 define the specification of musculature of distinct embryonic origin. *Biochem Cell Biol* 1998;76:1079.
115. Kaimaktchiev V, Goebel H, Laing N, et al. Intranuclear nemaline rod myopathy. *Muscle Nerve* 2006;34:369.
116. Kang PB, Lidov HG, David WS, et al. Diagnostic value of electromyography and muscle biopsy in arthrogryposis multiplex congenita. *Ann Neurol* 2003;54:790.
117. Kanno T, Maekawa M. Lactate dehydrogenase M-subunit deficiencies: clinical features, metabolic background, and genetic heterogeneities. *Muscle Nerve* 1995;18:54.
118. Kararizou E, Karandreas N, Davaki P, et al. Polyneuropathies in teenagers: a clinicopathological study of 45 cases. *Neuromuscul Disord* 2006;16:304.
119. Keenaway NG, Buist NR, et al. Lactic acidosis and mitochondrial myopathy associated with deficiency of several components of complex III of the respiratory chain. *Pediatr Res* 1984;18:991.
120. Keightly JA, Hoffbuhr KC, Burton MD, et al. A microdeletion in cytochrome c oxidase (COX) subunit III associated with COX deficiency and recurrent myoglobinuria. *Nat Genet* 1996;12:410.
121. Kihira S, Nonaka I. Congenital muscular dystrophy: a histochemical study with morphometric analysis on biopsied muscles. *J Neurol Sci* 1985;70:139.
122. Kinoshita M, Satoyoshi E, Kumagai M. Familial type 1 atrophy. *J Neurol Sci* 1975;25:11.
123. Kissel JT, Mendell JR, Rammohan KW. Microvascular deposition of complement membrane attack complex in dermatomyositis. *N Engl J Med* 1986;314:329.

124. Klinge L, Eagle M, Haggerty ID, et al. Severe phenotype in infantile facioscapulohumeral muscular dystrophy. *Neuromuscul Disord* 2006;16:553.
125. Kobayashi O, Hayashi Y, Arahata K, et al. Congenital muscular dystrophy: clinical and pathological study of 50 patients with the classical (Occidental) form. *Neurology* 1996;46:815.
126. Kobayashi K, Nakahori Y, Miyake M, et al. An ancient retrotransposal insertion causes Fukuyama-type congenital muscular dystrophy. *Nature* 1998;23;394:388.
127. Kochanski A, Drac H, Kabzinska D, et al. A novel MPZ gene mutation in congenital neuropathy with hypomyelination. *Neurology* 2004;62:2122.
128. Kunkel LM. Analysis of deletions in DNA from patients with Becker and Duchenne myscular dystrophy. *Nature* 1986;322:72.
129. Lacson AG, D'Cruz CA, Gilbert-Barness E, et al. Aluminum phagocytosis in quadriceps muscle following vaccination in children: relationship to macrophagic myofasciitis. *Pediatr Dev Pathol* 2002 5:151.
130. Laing NG, Clarke NF, Dye DE, et al. Actin mutations are one cause of congenital fiber type disproportion. *Ann Neurol* 2004;56:689.
131. Lampe AK, Bushby KM. Collagen VI related muscle disorders. *J Med Genet* 2005;42:673.
132. Landrieu P, Selva J, Alvarez F, et al. Peripheral nerve involvement in children with chronic cholestasis and vitamin E deficiency. A clinical, electrophysiological and morphological study. *Neuropediatrics* 1985;16:194.
133. Latta RJ, Graham CB, Aase JM, et al. Larsen's syndrome: a skeletal dysplasia with multiple joint dislocations and unusual facies. *J Pediatr* 1971;78:291.
134. Lehtokari VL, Pelin K, Sandbacka M, et al. Identification of 45 novel mutations in the nebulin gene associated with recessive nemaline myopathy. *Hum Mutat* 2006;27:946.
135. Lenard HG, Goebel HH. Congenital fiber type disproportion. *Neuropediatrics* 1975;6:220.
136. Lexell J, Downham D, Sjostrom M. Distribution of different fibre types in human skeletal muscles. *J Neurol Sci* 1983;61:301.
137. Li CK, Varsani H, Holton JL, et al. MHC Class I overexpression on muscle in early juvenile dermatomyositis. *J Rheumatol* 2004;31:605.
138. Lindhout D, Hageman G, et al. The Pena-Shokeir syndrome: report of nine Dutch cases. *Am J Med Genet* 1985;21:655.
139. Lofberg M, Liewendahl K, Lamminen A, et al. Antimyosin scintography compared with magnetic resonence imaging in inflammatory myopathies. *Arch Neurol* 1998;55:987.
140. Loke J, MacLennon DH. Malignant hyperthermia and central core disease: disorders of Ca2+ release channels. *Am J Med* 1998;104:470.
141. Longman C, Brockington M, Torelli S, et al. Mutations in the human LARGE gene cause MDC1D, a novel form of congenital muscular dystrophy with severe mental retardation and abnormal glycosylation of alpha-dystroglycan. *Hum Mol Genet* 2003;12:2853.
142. Longo N, Amat di San Fillipo C, Pasquali M. Disorders of carnitine transport and the carnitine cycle. *Am J Med Genet C Semin Med Genet* 2006;142:77.
143. Manivel JC, Pettinato G, Reinberg Y, et al. Prune belly syndrome: clinicopathologic study of 29 cases. *Pediatr Pathol* 1989;9:691.
144. McAdams AJ, Hug G, Bove KE. Glycogen storage disease. Types I to X. *Hum Pathol* 1974;5:463.
145. Mcleod JG, Baker WC, Lethlean AK, et al. Centronuclear myopathy with autosomal dominant inheritance. *J Neurol Sci* 1972;15:375.
146. McWilliam RC, Gardner-Medwin D, Doyle D, et al. Diaphragmatic paralysis due to spinal muscular atrophy. *Arch Dis Child* 1985;60:145.
147. Melli G, Chaudry V, Cornblath DR. Rhabdomyolysis: an evaluation of 475 hospitalized patients. *Medicine* 2005;84:377.
148. Mendell JR, Boue DR, Martin PT. The congenital muscular dystrophies: recent advances and molecular insights. *Pediatr Dev Pathol* 2006;9:427.
149. Miles l, Bove KE, Wong B, et al. Investigation of children for mitochondriopathy confirms need for strict patient selection, improved morphological criteria, and better laboratory methods. *Human Pathol* 2006;37:173.
150. Miles L, Bove KE, Lovell D, et al. The clinical course of juvenile dermatomyositis is predictable based on initial muscle biopsy: a retrospective study of 72 patients. *Arthr Rheum: Care Res* 2007(In Press).
151. Miller ME, Higgenbottom MC, Smith DW. Short umbilical cord: its origin and relevance. *Pediatrics* 1981;67:618.
152. Miller JJ. The fasciitis-morphea complex in children. *Am J Dis Child* 1992;146:733.
153. Minchom PE, Dormer RL, et al. Fatal infantile mitochondrial myopathy due to cytochrome c oxidase deficiency. *J Neurol Sci* 1983;60:453.
154. Moerman PH, Godderis P, Lauwerijns JM. Multiple ankyloses, facial anomalies and pulmonary hypoplasia associated with antenatal spinal muscular atrophy. *J Pediatr* 1983;103:238.
155. Moessinger AC. Fetal akinesia deformation sequence. An animal model. *Pediatrics* 1983;72:857.
156. Morgan-Hughes JA, Hayes DJ, Clark JB. Mitochondrial myopathies. In: Serratrice G, Roux H, eds. *Neuromuscular Diseases*. New York: Raven Press, 1984:79.
157. Morava E, Sengers R, Ter Laak H, et al. Congenital hypertrophic myopathy, cataract, mitochondrial myopathy and defective oxidative phosphorylation in two siblings with Senger-like syndrome. *Eur J Pediatr* 2004;163:467.
158. Muntoni F, Voit T. The congenital muscular dystrophies in 2004: a century of exciting progress. *Neuromuscul Disord* 2004;14:635.
159. Muscarella LA, Piemontese MR, Barbano R, et al. Novel mutations of dystrophin gene in DMD patients detected by rapid scanning in biplex exons DHPLC analysis. *Biomol Eng* 2006 (elec pub).
160. Nagao H, Habara S, et al. AMD deaminase activity of skeletal muscle in neuromuscular disorders in childhood. Histochemical and biochemical studies. *Neuropediatrics* 1986;17:193.
161. Naomi D, Alessandro M, Sewry C, et al. The role of immunocytochemistry and linkage analysis in the prenatal diagnosis of merosin-deficient congenital muscular dystrophy. *Hum Genet* 1997;99:535.
162. Neustein HB, Lurie PR, Dahms B, et al. An X-linked recessive cardiomyopathy with abnormal mitochondria. *Pediatrics* 1979;64:24.
163. Nishizawa M, Tanaka K, et al. A mitochondrial encephalomyopathy with cardiomyopathy. A case revealing a defect of complex I in the respiratory chain. *J Neurol Sci* 1987;78:189.
164. Nishimo I. Autophagic vacuolar myopathy. *Semin Pediatr Neurol* 2006;13:90.
165. Nonaka I, Sugita H, Takada K, et al. Muscle histochemistry in congenital muscular dystrophy with central nervous system involvement. *Muscle Nerve* 1982;5:102.
166. North K. Congenital myopathies, Chapter 54 in Engel AG, Franzini-Armstrong C, eds. *Myology Basic and Clinical*, 3rd edn. New York: McGraw-Hill, 2004:1473.
167. Norman B, Mahnke-Zizleman DK, Vallis A, et al. Genetic and other determinants of AMP deaminase activity in healthy adult skeletal muscle. *J Appl Physiol* 1998;85:1273.
168. Odusote K, Karpati G, Carpenter S. An experimental morphometric study of neutral lipid accumulation in skeletal muscles. *Muscle Nerve* 1981;4:3.
169. Ohtani Y, Matsuda I, et al. Infantile glycogen storage myopathy in a girl with phosphorylase kinase deficiency. *Neurology* 1982; 32:833.
170. Olpin SE, Afifi A, Clarke S, et al. Mutation and biochemical analysis in carnitine palmitoyltransferase type II (CPT II) deficiency. *J Inherit Metab Dis* 2003;26:543.
171. Op de Coul AAW, Lambregts PCLA, et al. Neuromuscular complications in patients given Pavulon (pancuronium bromide) during artificial ventilation. *Clin Neurol Neurosurg* 1985;87:17.
172. Ostlund C, Worman HJ. Nuclear envelope proteins and neuromuscular disease. *Muscle Nerve* 2003;27:393.
173. Ouvrier RA, McLeod JG, Conchin TE. The hypertrophic forms of hereditary motor and sensory neuropathy. *Brain* 1987;110:121.

174. Pachman LM, Hayford JR, Chung A, et al. Juvenile dermatomyositis at diagnosis: clinical characteristics in 79 children. *J Rheumatol* 1998;25:1198.
175. Palmer RE, Amartino HM, Niizawa G, et al. Pompe disease (glycogen storage disease type II) in Argentineans: clinical Manifestations and identification of 9 novel mutations. *Neuromuscul Disord* 2006 (Epub ahead of print.)
176. Pantoja-Martinez J, Navarro Fernandez-Balbuena C, Gormaz-Moreno M, et al. Myooadenylate deaminase deficiency in a child with myalgias induced by physical exercise. *Rev Neurol* 2004;39:431.
177. Parker DL, Mitchell PR, Holmes GL. Poland-Mobius syndrome. *J Med Genet* 1981;18:317.
178. Patel H, Berry K, MacLeod P, et al. Cytoplasmic body myopathy: report on a family and review of the literature. *J Neurol Sci* 1983;60:281.
179. Pavlakis SG, Phillips PC, DiMauro S, et al. Mitochondrial myopathy, encephalopathy, lactic acidosis and stroke-like episodes (MELAS): a distinctive clinical syndrome. *Ann Neurol* 1984;16:481.
180. Pearn JH, Wilson J. Acute Werdnig-Hoffmann disease. Acute infantile spinomuscular atrophy. *Arch Dis Child* 1973;48:425.
181. Pegoraro E, Marks H, Garcia CA, et al. Laminin alpha2 muscular dystrophy: genotype/phenotype correlations of 22 patients. *Neurology* 1998;51:101
182. Pena SDJ, Shokeir MHK. Syndrome of camptodactyly, multiple ankylosis, facial anomalies and pulmonary hypoplasia: a lethal condition. *J Pediatr* 1974;85:373.
183. Petterson JC, Colacino SC, Koltis GG, et al. A muscle phenotype characteristic of trisomy 13 based upon 8 subjects. *Pediatr Pathol* 1986;5:109(abst).
184. Philpot J, Sewry C, Pennock J, et al. Clinical phenotype in congenital muscular dystrophy: correlation with expression of merosin in skeletal muscle. *Neuromusc Disord* 1995;5:301.
185. Pierson CR, Tomczak K, Agrawal P, et al. X-linked myotubular and centronuclear myopathies. *J Neuropathol Exp Neurol* 2005;64; 555.
186. Plante-Bordeneuve V, Parman Y, Guiochon-Mantel A, et al. The range of chronic demyelinating neuropathy of infancy: a clinico-pathological and genetic study of 15 unrelated cases. *J Neurol* 2001;248:795.
187. Popek EJ, Tyson RW, Miller GJ, et al. Prostate development in prune belly syndrome (PBS) and posterior urethral valves (PUV): etiology of PBS—lower urinary tract obstructiuon or primary mesenchymal defect? *Pediatr Pathol* 1991;11:1.
188. Poulton J, Sewrey C, Potter CG, et al. Variation in mitochondrial DNA levels in muscle from normal controls. Is depletion of mtDNA in patients with mitochondrial myopathy a distinct clinical syndrome? *J Inher Metab Dis* 1995;18:4.
189. Prior TW, Bartolo C, Pearl DK, et al. Spectrum of small mutations in the dystrophin coding region. *Am J Hum Genet* 1995;57:22.
190. Raben N, Fukuda T, Gilbert AL, et al. Replacing acid alpha-glucosidase in Pompe disease: recombinant and transgenic enzymes are equipotent, but neither completely clears glycogen from type II muscle fibers. *Mol Ther* 2005;11:48–56.
191. Radu H, Rosa-Serbis AM, Ionescu V, et al. Focal abnormalities in mitochondrial distribution in muscle. Two atypical cases of so-called "central core disease." *Acta Neuropathol (Berl)* 1977;39:25.
192. Ramirez-Castro JL, Bersu ET. Anatomical analysis of the developmental effects of aneuploidy in man—the trisomy 18 syndrome: II. Anomalies of the upper and lower limbs. *Am J Med Genet* 1978;2:285.
193. Reed SD, Hall JG, Riccardi VM, et al. Chromosomal abnormalities associated with congenital contractures (arthrogryposis). *Clin Genet* 1985;27:353.
194. Reed AM, Pachman LM, Hayford J, et al. Immunogenetic studies in families of children with juvenile dermatomyositis. *J Rheumatol* 1998;25:1000.
195. Reuffert H, Olthoff D, Deutrich C, et al. Determination of a positive malignant hyperthermia (MH) disposition without the in vitro contraction test in families carrying the RYR1 Arg614Cys mutation. *Clin Genet* 2001;60:117.
196. Reyes MG, Noronha P, Thomas W, Jr., et al. Myositis of chronic graft versus host disease. *Neurology* 1983;33:1222.
197. Rinaldo P, Matern D, Bennett MJ. Fatty acid oxidation disorders. *Annu Rev Physiol* 2002;64:477.
198. Robinson AJ, Clamann HP. Effects of glucocorticoids on motor units in cat hindlimb muscles. *Muscle Nerve* 1988;11:703.
199. Robinson R, Carpenter D, Shaw MA, et al. Mutations in RYR1 in malignant hyperthermia and central core disease. *Hum Mutat* 2006;27:977.
200. Robotham JL, Haddow JE. Rhabdomyolysis and myoglobinuria in childhood. *Pediatr Clin North Am* 1976;23:279.
201. Roe CR, Millington DS, Maltby DA, et al. Recognition of medium-chain acyl-CoA dehydrogenase deficiency in asymptomatic siblings of children dying of sudden infant death or Reye-like syndromes. *J Pediatr* 1986;108:13.
202. Roe CR, Coates PM. Mitochondrial fatty acid oxidation disorders. In: Scriver CR, Beaudet AL, Sly WS, et al., eds. *The Metabolic and Molecular Bases of Inherited Disease*, 7th edn, vol 1. New York: McGraw-Hill, 1995;1501.
203. Rosenberg RN, Prusiner SB, DiMauro S, et al., eds. Mitochondrial disorders, Part IV. *The Molecular and Genetic Basis of Neurological Disease*. Butterworth-Heinemann, Boston, 1997.
204. Rossi LN, Cornelio F, et al. Myoadenylate deaminase deficiency in a 5-year-old boy with intermittant muscle pain. *Helv Paediatr Acta* 1984;39:89.
205. Rutledge ML, Hawkins EP, Langston C. Skeletal muscle growth failure induced in premature newborn infants by prolonged pancuronium treatment. *J Pediatr* 1986;109:883.
206. Salmons S, Henriksson J. The adaptive response of skeletal muscle to increased use. *Muscle Nerve* 1981;4:94.
207. Samaha FJ, Quinlan JG. Dystrophinopathies: clarification and complication. *J Child Neurol* 1996;11:13.
208. Sarnat HB. *Muscle Pathology and Histochemistry*. Chicago: American Society of Clinical Pathologists Press, 1983.
209. Sarnat HB. Cerebral dysgeneses and their influence on fetal muscle development. *Brain Dev* 1986;8:495.
210. Sarnat HB. Vimentin and desmin in maturing skeletal muscle and developmental myopathies. *Neurology* 1992;42;1616.
211. Saunier P, Cretien D, Wood C, et al. Cytochrome c oxidase deficiency presenting as neonatal myoglobinuria. *Neuromuscul Disord* 1995;5:285.
212. Scacheri PC, Hoffman EP, Fratkin JD, et al. A novel ryanodine receptor gene mutation causing both cores and rods in congenital myopathy. *Neurology* 2000;12:1689.
213. Schmitt HP, Volk B. The relationship between target targetoid and targetoid/core fibers in severe neurogenic muscular atrophy. *J Neurol* 1975;210:167.
214. Selcen D, Ohno K, Engel AG. Myofibrillar myopathy: clinical morphologicaland genetic studies. *Brain* 2004;127:439.
215. Sengers RCA, Stadhouders AM, Trijbels JMF. Mitochondrial myopathies. Clinical morphological and biochemical aspects. *Eur J Pediatr* 1984;141:192.
216. Servidei S, Bonilla E, et al. Fatal infantile form of muscle phosphofructokinase deficiency. *Neurology* 1986;36:1465.
217. Sewry CA, Philpot J, Sorokin LM, et al. Diagnosis of merosin (laminin-2) deficient congenital muscular dystrophy by skin biopsy. *Lancet* 1996;347:582.
218. Shanske S, Wong LJ. Molecular analysis for mitochondrial DNA disorders. *Mitochondrion* 2004;4:403.
219. Shepherd JJ. Tropical myositis: is it an entity and what is its cause? *Lancet* 1983;2:1240.
220. Sherratt HSA, Watmough NJ, Johnson MA, et al. Methods for the study of normal and abnormal skeletal muscle mitochondria. *Meth Biochem Anal* 1988;33:243.
221. Shevell M, Rosenblatt B, Silver K, et al. Congenital inflammatory myopathy. *Neurology* 1990;40:111.
222. Shi X, Garry DJ. Muscle stem cells in development, regeneration and disease. *Genes Dev* 2006;20:1692.

223. Shields RW. Single fiber electromyography in the differential diagnosis of myopathic limb-girdle syndromes and chronic spinal muscular atrophy. *Muscle Nerve* 1984;7:265.
224. Siegrist CA. Vaccine adjunants and macrophagic myofasciitis. *Arch Pediatr* 2005;12:96.
225. Shoffner JM. Maternal inheritance and the evaluation of oxidative phosphorylation diseases. *Lancet* 1996;348:1283.
226. Shoffner JM, Wallace DC. Oxidative phosphorylation diseases. In: Scrivner CR, Beaudet AL, Sly WS, Valle D, eds. *The Metabolic And Molecular Bases Of Inherited Disease*, 7th edn. New York: McGraw-Hill, 1995:1566.
227. Shorer Z, Philpot J, Muntoni F, et al. Demyelinating peripheral neuropathy in merosin-deficient congenital muscular dystrophy. *J Child Neurol* 1995;10:472.
228. Shumate JB, Kaiser KK, Carroll JE, et al. Adenylate deaminase deficiency in a hypotonic infant. *J Pediatr* 1980;96:885.
229. Shy GM, Magee KR. A new congenital nonprogressive myopathy. *Brain* 1956;79:610.
230. Silver MM, Gilbert JJ, Stewart S, et al. Morphologic and morphometric analysis of muscle in X-linked myotubular myopathy. *Hum Pathol* 1986;7:1167.
231. Simon DB, Ringel SP, Sufit RL. Clinical spectrum of fascial inflammation. *Muscle Nerve* 1982;5:525.
232. Sinha SK, Levene ML. Pancuronium bromide induced joint contractures in the newborn. *Arch Dis Child* 1984;59:73.
233. Sladky JT, Brown MJ, Berman PH. Chronic inflammatory demyelinating polyneuropathy of infancy: a corticosteroid responsive disorder. *Ann Neurol* 1986;20:76.
234. Sladky JT, Rorke LB. Perinatal hypoxic/ischemic spinal cord injury. *Pediatr Pathol* 1986;6:87.
235. Smit LME, Hageman G, et al. A myasthenic syndrome with congenital paucity of secondary synaptic clefts: CPSC syndrome. *Muscle Nerve* 1988;11:337.
236. Sokol R, Guggenheim M, et al. Improved neurologic function after long-term treatment of vitamin E deficiency in children with chronic cholestasis. *N Engl J Med* 1985;313:1580.
237. Somer H, Voutilainen A, et al. Duchenne-like muscular dystrophy in two sisters with normal karyotypes: evidence for autosomal recessive inheritance. *Clin Genet* 1985;28:151.
238. Sommer C, Koch S, Lammens M, et al. Macrophage clustering as a diagnostic marker in sural nerve biopsies of patients with CIDP. *Neurology* 2005;65:1924.
239. Specht LA, Kunkel LM. Duchenne and Becker muscular dystrophies. In: Rosenberg RN, Prusiner SB, DiMauro S, et al., eds. *The Molecular And Genetic Basis Of Neurological Disease*. Boston: Butterworth-Heinnemann, 1993:613.
240. Stedman H, Sarkar S. Molecular genetics in basic myology: a rapidly evolving perspective. *Muscle Nerve* 1988;11:668.
241. Strong PN, Brewster BS. Myotonic dystrophy: molecular and cellular consequences of expanded DNA repeats are elusive. *J Metab Inher Dis* 1997;20:159.
242. Szigeti K, Garcia CA, Lupski JR. Charcot-Marie-Tooth disease and related hereditary neuropathies: molecular diagnostics determine aspects of medical management. *Genet Med* 2006;8:86.
243. Tang TT, Sedmak GV, Siegesmund KA, et al. Chronic myopathy associated with Coxsackie virus type A9. A combined electron microscopical and viral isolation study. *N Engl J Med* 1975;292:608.
244. Thomas PK. Inherited neuropathies. *Mayo Clin Proc* 1983;58:476.
245. Thurberg BL, Maloney CL, Vaccaro C, et al. Charactyerization of pre- and post-treatment pathology after enzyme replacement therapy for Pompe disease. *Lab Invest* 2006;86:1208.
246. Tidhall JG, Wehling-Henricks M. Evolving therapeutic strategies for Duchenne muscular dystrophy: targeting downstream events. *Ped Res* 2004;56:831.
247. Tokgozoglu LS, Ashizawa T, Pacifico A, et al. Cardiac involvement in a large kindred with myotonic dystrophy. Quantitative assessment and relation to size of CTG expansion. *JAMA* 1995;274:813.
248. Tonin P, Lewis P, Servidei S, et al. Metabolic causes of myoglobinuria. *Ann Neurol* 1990;27:181.
249. Travers RL, Hughs GRV, Cambridge G, et al. Coxsackie B neutralisation titres in polymyositis/dermatomyositis [Letter]. *Lancet* 1977;1:1268.
250. Treem WR, Stanley CA, Finegold DN, et al. Primary carnitine deficiency due to a failure of carnitine transport in kidney, muscle and fibroblasts. *N Engl J Med* 1988;319:1331.
251. Tritschler HJ, Andreeta F, Moraes CT, et al. Mitochondrial myopathy of childhood associated with depletion of mitochondrial DNA. *Neurology* 1992;42:209.
252. Trischler HJ, Bonilla E, Lombes A, et al. Differential diagnosis of fatal and benign cytochrome c oxidase myopathies of infancy. *Neurology* 1991;41:300.
253. Trumbull DM, Bartlett K, et al. Short chain acyl-CoA dehydrogenase deficiency associated with lipid storage myopathy and secondary carnitine deficiency. *N Engl J Med* 1984;311:1232.
254. Tsurui S, Sugie H, Ito M, et al. Clinical and biochemical analysis of 27 patients with myoglobinuria of unknown causes. *Clinical Neurol (Japan)* 1995;35:24.
255. Tyson J, Ellis D, Fairbrother U, et al. Hereditary demyelinating neuropathy of infancy. A genetically complex syndrome. *Brain* 1997;120:113.
256. Umapathysivam K, Hopwood JJ, Meikle PJ. Correlation of alpha-glucosidase and glycogen content in skin fibroblasts with age of onset in Pompe disease. *Clin Chim Acta* 2005;361:191.
257. VanBiervliet JPGM, Bruinvis L, et al. Hereditary mitochondrial myopathy with lactic acidemia, a DeToni-Fanconi-Debre syndrome and a defective respiratory chain in voluntary muscles. *Pediatr Res* 1977;11:1088.
258. Villanova M, Malandrini A, Sabatelli P, et al. Localization of laminin alpha 2 chain in normal human central nervous system: an immunofluorescence and ultrastructural study. *Acta Neuropathol (Berl)* 1997;94:567.
259. Vogler CA, Bove KE. Morphology of skeletal muscle in children. An assessment of normal growth and differentiation. *Arch Pathol Lab Med* 1985;109:238.
260. Voit T, Sewry CA, Meyer K, et al. Preserved merosin M-chain (or laminin alpha 2) expression in skeletal muscle distinguishes Walker-Warburg syndrome from Fukuyama muscular dystrophy and merosin-deficient muscular dystrophy. *Neuropediatrics* 1995;26:148.
261. Wallgren-Pettersson C. Genetics of the nemaline myopathies and myotubular myopathies. *Neuromuscul Disord* 1998;8:401.
262. Wallgren-Pettersson C, Pelin K, Nowak KJ, et al. Genotype-phenotype correlations in nemaline myopathy caused by genes for nebulin and skeletal muscle alpha-actin. *Neuromuscul Disord* 2004;14:461.
263. Wargula JC, Lovell DJ, Passo MH, et al. What more can we learn from muscle histopathology in children with dermatomyositis/polymyositis ?. *Clin Exp Rheumatol* 2006;24:333.
264. Watson AJS, Dalbow MH, et al. Immunologic studies in cimetidine induced nephropathy and polymyositis. *N Engl J Med* 1983;308:142.
265. Williams S, Horrocks IA, Ouvrier RA, et al. Critical illness polyneuropathy and myopathy in pediatric intensive care: a review. *Pediatr Crit Care Med* 2006 (Epub ahead of print).
266. Witt DR, Hayden MR, et al. Restrictive dermopathy: a newly recognized autosomal recessive skin dysplasia. *Am J Med Genet* 1986;24:631.
267. Witters I, Moerman P, Fryns JP. Fetal akinesia deformation sequence: a study of 30 consecutive in-utero diagnoses. *Am J Med Genet* 2002;15:23.
268. Worby CA, Gentry MS, Dixon JE. Laforin, a dual specificity phosphatase that dephosphorylates complex carbohydrates. *J Biol Chem* 2006;281:30412.
269. Xhou H, Yamaguchi N, Xu L, et al. Characterization of recessive RYR1 mutations in core myopathies. *Hum Mol Genet* 2006;15:2791.
270. Yamaguchi K, Santa T, Inoue K, et al. Lipid storage myopathy in von Gierke's disease. A case report. *J Neurol Sci* 1978;38:195.

271. Yang Z, McMahon CJ, Smith LR, et al. Danon disease as an unrecognized cause of hypertrophic cardiomyopathy in children. *Circulation* 2005;112:612.
272. Yoshida A, Kobayashi K, Manya H, et al. Muscular dystrophy and neuronal migration disorder caused by mutations in a glycosyltransferase, POMGnT1. *Dev Cell* 2001;1:717.
273. Zerres K, Rudnik-Schoneborn S. Natural history of proximal spinal muscular atrophy (SMA): clinical analysis of 445 patients and suggestions for a modification of existing classifications. *Arch Neurol* 1995;52:518.
274. Xerres K, Rudnik-Schoneborn S. 93rd ENMC international workshop: non-5q-spinal muscular atrophies (SMA). *Neuromuscul Disord* 2003;13:179.
275. Zeviani M, Gellera C, Antozzi C, et al. Maternally-inherited myopathy and cardiomyopathy: association with mutation in mitochondrial DNA tRNA. *Lancet* 1991;338:143.
276. Zinn AB, Kerr DS, Hoppel CL. Fumarase deficiency: a new cause of mitochondrial encephalomyopathy. *N Engl J Med* 1986;315:469.
277. Zuk JA, Fletcher A. Skeletal muscle expression of class II histocompatibility antigens (HLA-DR) in polymyositis and other muscle disorders with an inflammatory infiltrate. *J Clin Pathol* 1988;41:410.

CHAPTER 27

Skeletal System

LOUIS P. DEHNER

The complexity of the developing skeletal system was appreciated long before the advent of molecular biology. In the interval since the second edition, the molecular genetic understanding of skeletogenesis has expanded exponetially as evidenced by several excellent reviews (448,482,512,594,651,672). The morphologic events begin with the segregation of progenitor mesenchymal cells in the cranial portion of the neural crest (neuroectoderm) and mesoderm (craniofacial bone development, paraxial somite (axial skeleton) and lateral plate mesoderm (limb skeleton) (36). The blue print or patterning and migration are controlled by highly conserved transcriptional factors such as the HOX and PAX genes and their signaling pathways which are integral to cell-to-cell communication and intracellular signaling (283,327,328). The mesenchymal cells after migration to their specific sites undergo the process of condensation whose end result is the formation of the 206 or so bones of the human skeleton (109,258). Once condensation has taken place, the next event is osteoblastic and chondrogenic differentiation which is accompanied by a number of molecular events involved with lineage determination; SOX 9 (SRY-box 9), a transcriptional factor gene, is critical in the differentiation of an osteochondral progenitor to a chondrocyte (164,448). Goldring and associates have pointed out that chondrogenesis is the earliest phase of skeletogenesis (238). Not only is SOX 9 one of the earliest expressed genes in the condensation phase, but it is also necessary for the expression of COL2A1, which encodes the alpha-1 chain of type 2 collagen and other matrix proteins (56,240). The differentiation phase of chondrocytes occurs when two other members of the SOX family, SOX 5 (SRY-box 5) and SOX 6 (SRY-box 6), are expressed somewhat later than SOX 9. Extracellular matrix is synthesized with further chondrocyte differentiation to hypertrophic chondrocytes; these extracellular macromolecules include proteoglycans, aggrecan, decorin, biglycan, fibromodulin, and perelcan in addition to collagens type II, IX, and XI (404). The next stage is the process of cartilage undergoing metamorphosis to bone (400). Just as SOX 9 is critical in the development of chondroblasts, so the transcriptional factor, Runt-related 2 (Runx 2 or Cbfa-1) has a similar role in the differentiation of the osteoblast from the primordial osteochondral cell. The Runx 2 (Cbfa-1) is also involved in the development of the hypertrophic chondrocyte. In turn there are several regulators of Runx 2 function. The bones as the basic gross components of the skeleton develop by one of two processes, enchondral ossification in the formation of the appendicular and axial skeleton and membraneous ossification in the formation of the craniofacial bones and portions of the clavicle (116,133,325). Membranous ossification is characterized by the direct differentiation of the common progenitor mesenchymal cell to an osteoblast even before the condensation stage; there is osteoid deposition with the formation of ossification centers that fuse into the plate-like bone of the calvarium. The bone matrix proteins, osteocalcin, collagen type 1, bone sialoprotein and alkaline phosphatase, are induced by Runx 2 (Cbfa-1). However, Runx 2 does not induce osteoblastic differentiation alone, but interacts with TGF-β superfamily, bone morphogenic protein and specific SMADs (385,479). Other important signaling molecules include Wnt/β-catenin and Hedgehog pathways (156,259,390).

Enchondral ossification requires the coordination of chondrocytes, osteoblasts, and osteoclasts. The osteoclast is a bone marrow derived cell of the monocyte lineage which is critical in the process of bone remodeling. Following the stage of condensation (6 to 7 weeks of gestation), the formation of the cartilaginous anlage-template (18 to 19 weeks of gestation) occurs in a proximal to distal fashion and in anterior before posterior structures. The primary center of ossification is found in the mid-shaft of the bone anlage in the vicinity of the hypertrophied or terminally differentiated chondrocytes (95,133,485). There is also vascular invasion as the hypertrophied chondrocytes express vascular endothelial growth factor. A periosteal bone collar is formed by mesenchymal cells which undergo osteoblastic differentiation to initiate the process of cortical bone formation. With the vascular invasion, hematopoietic precursors including preosteoclasts have gained access to the bone. Secondary centers of ossification are formed at the proximal and distal ends of the bone and are separated from the primary center by the growth plate where the epiphyseal cartilage proliferates, hypertrophies, and undergoes apoptosis (95,102). This latter process is in part under the control of the gene, Indian hedgehog. The invading front of ossification from the primary and secondary centers of ossification and the proliferating cartilage together account for bone growth.

We have not mentioned the roles of parathyroid hormone (PTH)-related peptide and its receptor which is controlled by COL2A1 promoter and fibroblast growth factor receptor 3 (FGFR3) (359). The receptors are present on the cell membrane of the osteoblasts; the role of this receptor tyrosine kinase at the growth plate is an important one since activating mutations are involved in several types of skeletal dysplasia. The third basic cell type, the osteoclast, is a multinucleated cell of mononuclear phagocytic derivation whose function is bone matrix resorption through its resorptive organelle, the ruffled membrane (472). Defective function or differentiation of osteoclasts is the underlying pathogenesis of osteopetrosis (OP). Osteoblasts and osteoclasts interact through cytokines and growth factors which serve to choreograph the initial modeling and remodeling of bone through autocrine, paracrine, and endocrine (parathormone) mechanisms (26).

CONGENITAL AND DEVELOPMENTAL DISORDERS AND MALFORMATIONS

Skeletal anomalies consist of a broad range of anatomic defects, which may be an intrinsic abnormality in the development and growth of a single bone or a generalized process affecting the entire skeleton as the manifestation of a mutated constitutional genetic determinant or an extrinsic teratogen (469,537). Examples of the former include the various chromosomal syndromes, inheritable metabolic disorders, a multitude of congenital anomaly syndromes, and the numerous genetic skeletal disorders also know as skeletal dysplasias or osteochondrodysplasias. Several agents are well documented or highly suspected teratogens affecting normal skeletal development (42,370,438) (Table 27-1).

The estimated frequency of the various types of skeletal anomalies in children is derived from diverse sources including the experience of individual institutions, vital statistics, and registries (409,626). In one pediatric autopsy series that included children through 14 years of age, congenital anomalies and malformations were identified in 18% of cases; almost 20% of these were found in the skeletal system. Multiple organ anomalies were found in most of these children. Major musculoskeletal anomalies were documented at autopsy in 1.3% of previable fetuses and live born infants who died in the perinatal period with the exclusion of chromosomal syndromes (422). Major malformations of the limbs are found in approximately 2% of live born infants and minor limb abnormalities in another 5% to 7%. Overall, approximately 1:1,000 neonates have some defective development of the limbs, most commonly limb reduction defects (316,409).

Among the three most common trisomy syndromes, trisomy 18 is characterized by overlapping fingers, the less common rocker-bottom feet, and the equinovarus deformity, whereas trisomy 13 is associated with postaxial polydactyly. Clinodactyly of the fifth finger with a hypoplastic middle phalanx is found in 50% to 60% of infants with trisomy 21 (336,503,598). Additional malformations of the axial skeleton in these three trisomic syndromes have been documented by Kjaer and associates (345,346). Syndactyly and talipes equinovarus are the two most common limb anomalies in triploid fetuses (624).

Limb reduction defects (LRD) comprises one of the most common categories of congenital skeletal anomalies and is defined by the following anatomic categories: absence or hypoplasia of a phalanx, metacarpal, or metatarsal bone as a portion of any long bone with accompanying deformity; these anomalies are represented by the specific defects of amelia, aplasia to hypoplasia of individual long bones, oligodactyly, polydactyly, and syndactyly (Figure 27-1) (278,624,631). These developmental anomalies are seen as an isolated finding or as a component of a syndrome as one of several anomalies in other organ systems including the cardiovascular system, kidney, and intestinal tract. Approximately 70% to 75% of LRDs occur in the upper extremity, whereas 15% to 20% are present in the lower extremity alone and both upper and lower in 10% of cases (211,353,429,605). The incidence of these defects is approximately 1:1,000 to 2,000 live births (191,317,602). Limb reduction defects are estimated to be present in 2% of perinatal autopsies and in less than 1% of stillborns (241). The genetic and developmental aspects of LRDs are discussed at length elsewhere (250,273,602).

The morphology of LRDs include the following anatomic categories: terminal longitudinal defects (e.g., aplasia-hypoplasia of the radius with absence of the thumb); terminal transverse defects (loss of distal limb structure with preservation

Table 27-1 ■ TERATOGEN AND SKELETAL ANOMALIES

Agent	Phenotype
Thalidomide	Phocomelia
Valproic acid and other antiepileptics	Limb reduction defects Polydactyly
Retinoids	"Lower limb defects"
Cyclophosphamide	Craniosynostosis
Warfarin	"Short limbs," stippled calcification of epiphyses of long bones, brachydactyly
Aminopterin	Craniosynostosis, oligodactyly, syndactyly, mesomelic shortening of forearms, talipes, equinovarus

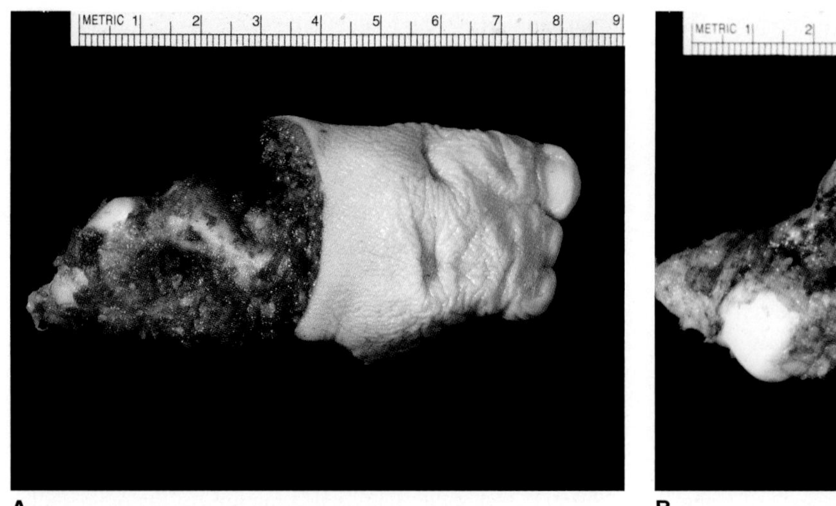

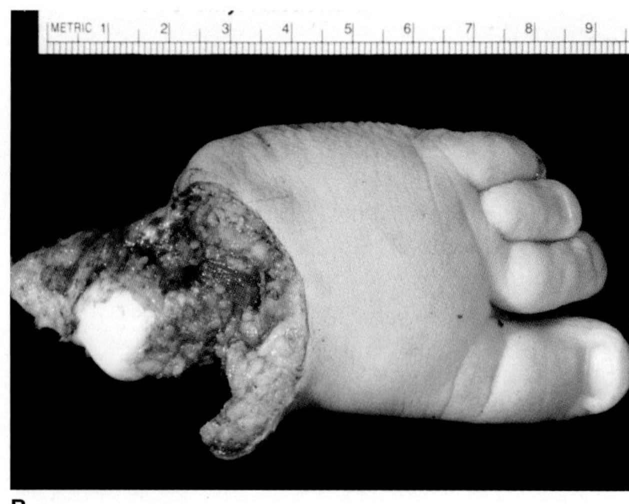

A B

FIGURE 27-1 ■ Limb reduction defects are shown in these two amputation specimens. **A**: Symes amputation of the foot demonstrates absence of the fourth and fifth toes as an example of postaxial ray deficiency together with proximal syndactyly in a 9-month-old male. **B:** This amputation specimen of the foot from a 10-month-old female shows only four toes with absence of the fifth digit. The fibula was absent as well.

of proximal structure); intercalary defects (aplasia or hypoplasia of proximal limb structure); split hand-foot defects (loss of radial ray or central ray of hand or foot); and complex defects with multiple types of LRDs. Lin and associates (387) reported the following distribution of 271 LRDs in live born infants from the Congenital Malformation Registry: terminal longitudinal (25%), terminal transverse (35%), intercalary (10%), split hand-foot (26%), and multiple (4%) defects.

The etiopathogeneses of LRDs are divisible into the following categories: dominant—recessive inheritance (15% to 20% of cases), chromosomal abnormalities (5% to 10%), known syndromes, some with a multiorgan pattern of anomalies (5% to 10%), and teratogens (3% to 5%). The latter four categories are collectively thought to account for 30% to 35% of all LRDs and another 30% to 35% of cases are ascribed to vascular disruption. A determination as to etiopathogenesis is inconclusive for almost one-third of cases. Among those LRDs associated with congenital anomalies (12% to 33% of cases), there are patterns or associations that repeat themselves (603). Seven specific anatomic categories of LRDs are defined in Table 27-2. The various LRDs have several associated major congenital anomalies, some of which are better known than others (602). Preaxial limb defects have the highest frequency according to Rosano et al. (542) and are recognized in the VATER-VACTERL association which acronymically refers to vertebra, anorectal atresia, congenital heart, tracheoesophageal fistula, renal and distal urinary tract and limb anomalies (85,114,335,572). These may be a consequence of perturbations in the sonic hedgehog homolog gene (7q36) and its signaling pathway since a murine knockout produces a similar pattern of anomalies as seen clinically (571). Vertebral anomalies including vertebral fusion and butterfly vertebra as examples are present in approximately 25% of VACTERL cases whereas limb defects are found in 10% of cases with the preaxial absence of the radius and/or thumb and first metacarpal. Tibial aplasia-hypoplasia, another preaxial defect, is less common than radial aplasia in the VACTERL association.

Transverse limb defects with the loss of fingers and toes are associated anorectal atresia, craniofacial anomalies,

Table 27-2 ■ ANATOMIC CATEGORIES OF LIMB DEFECTS

Type	Phenotype
Preaxial	Complete or partial absence of thumbs, first metacarpal and radius and/or absence of hallux, first metatarsal, and tibia
Transverse	Absence of distal metacarpal in phalanges with normal or deficient proximal structures
Postaxial	Complete or partial absence of fifth finger
Intercalary	Absence or hypoplasia of humerus or femur and remaining long bones as a single bone or multiple bones involvement, hands, and feet minimally involved
Split hand-foot	Defects in central ray including metacarpal-metatarsal with nearly normal lateral digits
Amelia	Complete or near complete limb absence
Mixed	Presence of multiple limb defects
Unspecified	Defects not included in previous definitions

syndactyly, and genital defects. Absence of fingers and toes, cleft palate, and constriction band acrosyndactyly are anomalies associated with the amniotic rupture sequence (ARS) or amniotic band syndrome whose prevalence varies from 1: 1,200 to 15,000 live births (88). Most cases of ARS are sporadic, but there is an apparent increased prevalence in type 4 Ehlers-Danlos syndrome and severe osteogenesis imperfecta (685). Similar distal limb defects are found in association with ventral body wall defects which are commonly accompanied by a short umbilical cord. A vascular disruption has been proposed as a possible pathogenetic factor in both ARS and ventral body wall defect (301,309,640,653). Whether the tethered threads of amnion after the rupture of the amniotic sac are the entire explanation remains an unresolved issue (38,205,210).

Another preaxial limb defect, radial hypoplasia-aplasia, occurs in a number of syndromic settings and it is estimated that as many as 50% to 80% of infants with absent radii have other anomalies as a component of a defined syndrome (145,236,242,311,419,580) (Table 27-3).

Lower limb deficiencies are considerably less common than those in the upper extremities accounting for 20% to 40% of cases which may or may not also have defects in the upper extremity. Isolated deficiencies or defects of the lower extremity are very uncommon, as illustrated by the fact that congenital deficiency of the tibia, or tibial hemimelia, is found in 1:1 million live births (197). In most cases, other anomalies are found in the same extremity, and often other extremities and visceral organ systems are the sites of additional development defects. One of the more common of these is congenital radial-tibial deficiency, which is defined by an absence or hypoplasia of the preaxial structures of the extremity including the thumb, first metacarpal, radius, hallux, first metatarsal, and tibia. This disorder is known to be familial and syndromic, as in the Poland sequence and Holt-Oram syndrome. Isolated femoral or fibular deficiency is equally uncommon. Somewhat more frequent is ulnar-fibular deficiency, which is typically manifested by postaxial ray deficiency in the hands and feet with defects of the ipsilateral ulna and fibula. In most cases, ulnar-fibular deficiency is an isolated defect without anomalies elsewhere.

Split hand-foot limb defect or malformation (SHFM) occurs as a sporadic or familial anomaly on the basis of a failure in the initiation and maintenance of the median apical ectodermal ridge (46,564). Four autosomal and one X-linked loci have been identified in various pedigrees with SHFM (SHFM1 on 7q21.2–22.1; SHFM 2 on Xq26; SHFM 3 on 10q24–25; SHFM 4 on 3q27,p63; SHFM 5 on 2q31) (182). The prevalence of SHFM is 1:18,000 live births. In addition to the split hand malformation, polydactyly, and syndactyly may be present. Congenital heart disease is found in almost 50% of those with a SHFM 5 mutation. Ectrodactyly, ectodermal dysplasia, and facial cleft syndrome are associated with a p63 (homologue of tumor suppressor gene, p53) mutation; p63 function is critical in the development of the limb bud and hair follicle.

Patellar aplasia (absence) and hypoplasia as a lower limb deficiency are found in a number of syndromes which are discussed at length by Bongers and associates (81,82). Some of these syndromes include neurofibromatosis type 1 (NF1), campomelic dysplasia (CD) with SOX9 (17q24.3) mutations and nail patella syndrome (NPS) with LMX1B (9q 34.1) mutation which has a downstream effect on collagen type 4 expression in the glomerular basement development. So-called iliac horns are triangular shaped outgrowths of the posterior ilium which are diagnostic of NPS (see Chapter 17).

Amelia denotes incomplete or absent limb. This rare anomaly is seen in 0.15:10,000 live births and occurs with equal frequency in the upper and lower extremities (212,416). Amelia is associated with encephalocele, gastroschisis, omphalocele, anorectal atresia, trisomy 8, VACTERL association, and splenogonadal fusion. Severe lower limb defects are found in association with an omphalocele and diaphragmatic defect. A seemingly related or similar phenotypic association is the omphalocele-exstrophy-imperforate anus-spinal defects complex with severe lower limb defects.

Caudal dysgenesis [(*CD*), *caudal regression syndrome*] *and sirenomelia* are pathogenetically related disorders of the caudal developmental field or axial mesodermal patterning (Figure 27-2) (2,96,601). Debate continues about the relationship between CD and sirenomelia (so-called mermaid syndrome) (176,635). Axial mesodermal dysplasia (oculo[facio]-auriculo-vertebral spectrum and CD), CD, and sirenomelia are seen more commonly in infants of diabetic mothers to support the hypothesis of a diabetic embryopathy (13,187,246,520). However, there is no consensus whether

Table 27-3 ▪ SYNDROMIC ASSOCIATIONS WITH ABSENCE OF RADII
Tubulocytopenia—absent radius syndrome (HOXA11-IGKV3D-20 mutation on 7p15-p14)
Holt-Oram syndrome (TBX5 mutations on 12q24.1)
Fanconi anemia (FANCD1/BIRCA2 on 13q12.3, FANCN/PALB2 on 16p12.3 and FANCJ/BRIP1, TORCA2 mutations on 17q 22–24)
Renal hypoplasia—bilateral/radial ray aplasia
Hypoteralanic hamartoblastoma syndrome
Multiple epiphyseal dysplasia (COL9A1 ON 6q12–q14, COL9A3 ON 20q13.3, COMP/TSP-5 on 5q31.2, MATS3 ON 1p33-p32)
Chromosome 22q11 deletion syndrome
Preaxial aerofacial dysostosis (Nager and de Reynier)
Trisomy 18
RAPADILINO syndrome (RECQ64 mutations on 8q24.3)
Baller-Gerold syndrome (craniosynostosis) (RECQ64 mutations on 8q24.3)

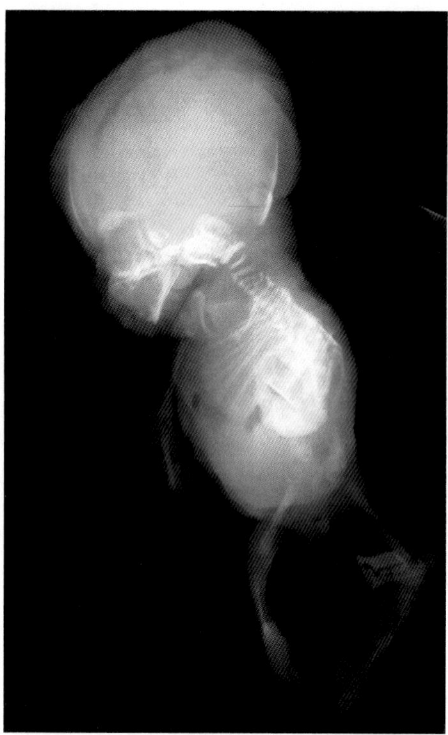

FIGURE 27-2■Caudal dysgenesis (caudal regression syndrome) shows a constellation of findings including absence of the lumbosacral spine, hypoplastic and flattened pelvis, and absence of the pubis. Bilateral radial agenesis, one of the more common terminal longitudinal defects, is also present and the ribs are hypoplastic and deficient. Bilateral equinovarus deformities are also noted.

the hyperglycemia itself is the teratogen. Limb deficiencies are another proposed manifestation of diabetic embryopathy. Dysgenesis or agenesis of the sacrum, renal agenesis, fused ectopic kidneys, ectopic ureters, müllerian duct agenesis or hypoplasia, agenesis of the bladder, cloacal exstrophy, cryptorchidism, anorectal atresia, penile-scrotal transposition, limb deficiencies, and fusion of a single dysmorphic lower limb are the range of anomalies in the genitourinary tract and lower extremities in sirenomelia. Other anomalies include holoprosencephaly and Alagille syndrome (417). The estimated frequency of CD-sirenomelia is 1:7,500 births. CD has been reported in i(18q), 18p-, and trisomy 18 syndromes, VACTERL association and heterotaxy. Retinoic acid and synthetic retinoids have been shown to cause CD experimentally. Currarino syndrome is considered by some to be a variant of caudal regression; hemisacrum, anorectal malformation, usually stenosis or atresia and presacral developmental cyst are the basic phenotypic features. The cyst has been interpretated as a cystic teratoma, but in some cases it is not always clear as to the exact nature of the cyst. Hirschsprung disease and spinal dysraphia are other findings. Mutations in the homeobox gene H9 (HLXB9, MNX1 on 7q 36) have been detected in Currarino syndrome with a pattern of autosomal dominant (AD) transmission, but not in CD (350,534).

Anomalies of the axial skeleton include various abnormalities in the ribs, vertebra, and sacrum. Some of these are important in their own right, whereas others are associated with more severe anomalies, such as CD including the Currarino syndrome, anorectal malformations, and the VATER-VACTERL association. It has been reported that approximately 60% of those with congenital vertebral anomalies also have major or minor abnormalities in other organ systems.

Polydactyly is defined by the presence of six or more digits on the hand(s) or foot (feet) or both and is the obvious antithesis to the previously discussed limb reduction defects (LRDs) (631). Anatomically, similar designations to limb reduction defects are applied to polydactyly: preaxial (lateral), postaxial (medial ray), and the rare central polydactyly. Polydactyly or duplication of the thumb (preaxial) is the most common example with an incidence of almost 1:100 live births (137). The development of the duplicate digit is either a partially formed or severely hypoplastic structure with minimal features to suggest a digit, but rather a small polyp (374). Histologically, the various fibrous, vascular, neural and adipose tissues are not well organized and have a similarity to the soft tissue dysplasia of macrodactyly. Isolated preaxial polydactyly is more common in those of European descent, and isolated postaxial polydactyly occurs more frequently in those of African than European descent with an incidences of 1:140 to 1,300 live birth, respectively (383). Postaxial polydactyly in a Caucasian infant has several syndromic associations (Table 27-4). Polydactyly can usually be observed by fetal ultrasonography at 14 to 16 weeks of gestation; one such study reported that 26 fetuses (0.15%) had polydactyly from a total of 17,760 examinations. It was an isolated finding in 16 infants and postaxial in 14 (88%) (687). There were two cases of in utero autoamputation.

Table 27-4 ■ SYNDROMIC ASSOCIATION WITH PREAXIAL AND POSTAXIAL POLYDACTYLY

Prexial	Postaxial
Carpenter	Ellis van Creveld
Orofaciodigital II	Orofaciodigital III
Short rib—polydactyly II	Short-rib polydactyly I
Townes Brock	McKusick-Kaufmann
NF1	Smith-Lemli-Opitz
Diabetic embryopathy[a]	Bardet-Biedl[b]
Femoral-facial syndrome	Meckel-Gruber
Greg[b]	Jeune
Apert	Pallister-Hall[c]
Partial trisomy 4q	NF1
WAGR syndrome	Orofaciodigital IV[d]
14q(22) deletion	Deletion 22q11 (DiGeorge)[c]
Partial trisomy 1q	
Distal trisomy 10q	
Laurin-Sandrow	
Triphalangeal thumb polysyndactyly	
Amniotic band, cleft lip plate	
Trisomy 21	
VACTERL	

[a]Preaxial hallucal polydactyly.
[b]Pre- and postaxial polydactyly.
[c]Central polydactyly.
[d]Postaxial upper and preaxial lower extremities.

Preaxial and postaxial polydactyly have differing genetic mechanisms by which these malformation develop. In the case of preaxial polydactyly, point mutations sonic hedgehog are expressed along the so-called zone of polarizing activity. Postaxial polydactyly has at least three different mutated genes: 7p13, 19p 13.2, and 13q21–32; there are also frameshift mutations in GL13. Two types of postaxial polydactyly have two genophenotypic expressions: type A with a well formed digit and a normal fifth digit and type B as a hypoplastic structure with a resemblance to a small papilloma or acrochordon. When these lesions autoamputate, a traumatic neuroma is a known sequel which is less common if the digit is surgically excised.

Syndactyly is defined by soft tissue fusion of fingers and toes with or without fusion of bones. Like the other anomalies in this section, syndactyly occurs as an isolated finding or as a manifestation of a syndrome including acrocephalosyndactyly with its several types (Apert, Waardenburg, Pfeiffer, Summitt and Sacthre-Chotzan syndromes), Poland, Fraser and F-syndrome (624). Syndactyly is also a well documented feature of the amniotic band syndrome without any specific pattern of digital or limb involvement. Polydactyly and syndactyly can also occur together with heterogeneous phenotypes (405).

Arthrogryposis or congenital contracture is represented by two phenotypes: isolated or limited with single area involvement and multifocal with two or more joint contractures (39). Multiple congenital contracture are further classified into amyoplasia, distal arthrogryposis and related syndromes (68). The latter category includes failure in forebrain development, chromosomal abnormalities and motor neuron disorders like spinal muscular atrophy, congenital myopathies and heritable peripheral neuropathies. It has been estimated that more than 300 disorders are accompanied by multiple joint contractures. The contractures are often symmetrical in both upper and lower extremities (Figure 27-3).

Fetal akinesia-hypokinesia deformation (FAD) sequence has an estimated prevalence of 1:12,000 to 19,000 live births and it can be recognized after the first trimester (256,257,440,669). These infants have the so-called Pena-Skokeir phenotype with limb contractures (arthrogryposis), intrauterine growth restriction, an attenuated umbilical cord because of diminished fetal activity, secondary pulmonary hypoplasia and craniofacial anomalies (515,648,649). The FAD sequence is itself a clinical phenotype with several specific genetic mutations including the Escobar syndrome (multiple pterygium syndrome) with multiple mutations involving the gamma subunit gene (CHRNG) of acetycholine receptor

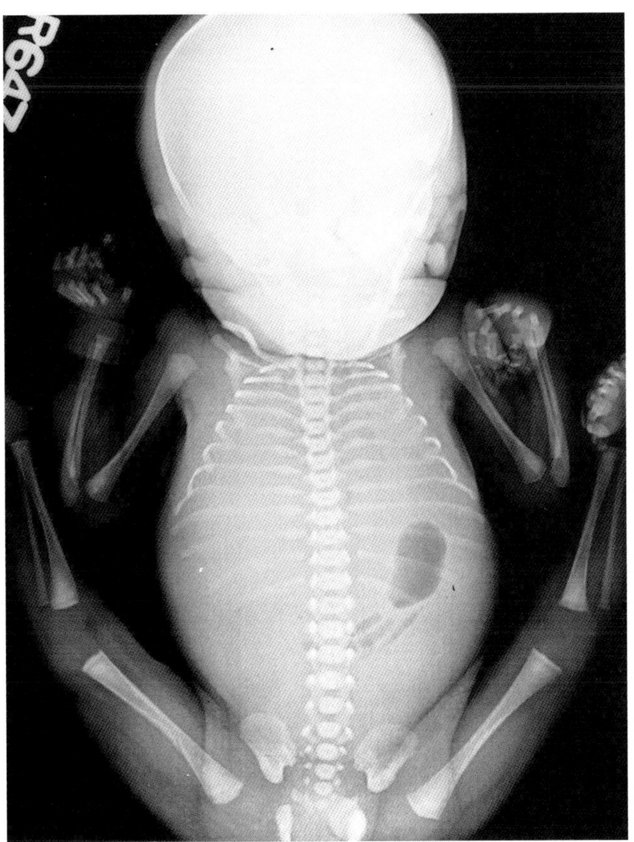

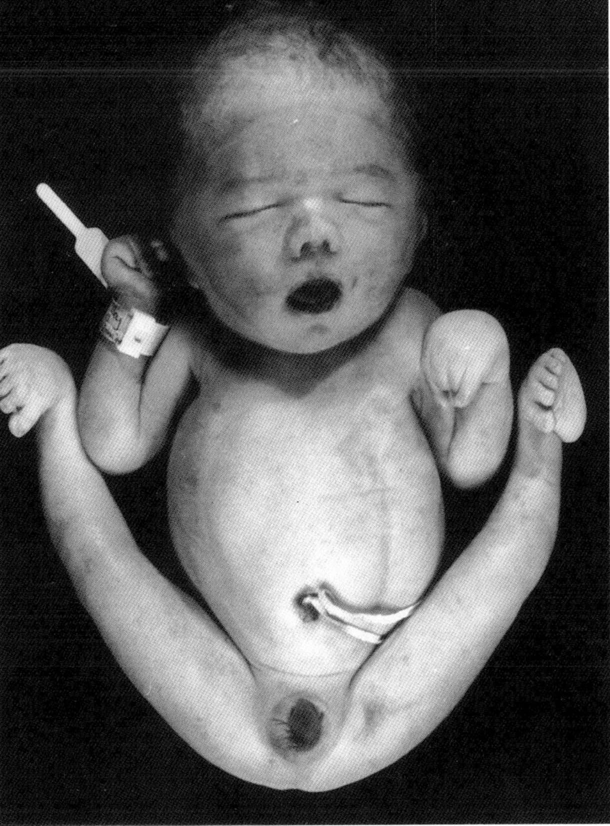

A B

FIGURE 27-3 **A,B:** Congenital arthrogryposis is characterized by deformities as in these postmortem images. Although associated with polyhydramnios, the severe pulmonary hypoplasia is secondary to a defective mechanical descent of the diaphragm, possibly the consequence of a neuromuscular disorder.

(437,451), the three types of lethal congenital contractures, and German syndrome.

Skeletal dysplasia or genetic skeletal disorders are an encompassing designation for the group of disorders which affect the normal development of bones and supporting tissues in terms of their shape and size, often with a reduction in normal stature (240,352,462,558). The number of recognized skeletal dysplasias now stands at more than 380 disorders with the frequent addition of newly described types or variants of existing types [see International Skeletal Dysplasia Registry (ISDR), www.csmc.edu]. Several modifications have been made in the classification of skeletal dysplasias over the past 20 years or so to reflect the addition of new types of disorders, often with their signature mutation (131). The latest revision of the International Classification refers to itself as "nosology and classification of genetic skeletal disorders: 2006 revision" and has a total of 37 groups or categories whose nosologic approach is one of common molecular and/or similar morphologic abnormalities (611) (Table 27-5). Three pathogenetic-morphologic distinctions still exist as a subtext to the International Classification: (a) defects of growth of tubular bones and spine referred to as the chondrodysplasias, (b) disorganized development of the fibrous and cartilagenous components of the skeleton, and (c) disorders in bone density or cortical-diaphyseal structure and metaphyseal modeling (536). The dysostoses, not previously considered in earlier classifications, are included and are defined as abnormalities in individual bones or groups of bones. Some of these disorders have been considered in the sections on limb reduction defects and polydactyly which are classified as dysostoses.

The prevalence rate of the skeletal dysplasias is approximated at 2 to 3:10,000 stillbirths and live births, but among infants who died in the perinatal period, the frequency is higher at 9 to 10:1,000 perinatal deaths (487,604,626,670). Several types of skeletal dysplasias are inconsistent with

Table 27-5 ▪ THE GROUPS OF GENETIC DISORDERS OF BONE WITH PHENOTYPIC EXAMPLES

1. FGFR 3 Group (Former Achondroplasia Group example, TD type 2)
2. Type 2 collagen group (e.g., achondrogenesis type 2)
3. Type 11 collagen group (e.g., Stickler syndrome type 2)
4. Sulphation disorders group (e.g, achondrogenesis type1 B)
5. Perlecan group (e.g., Schwartz-Jampel syndrome)
6. Filamin group (e.g., frontometaphyseal dysplasia)
7. Short-rib dysplasia (with or without polydactyly) group (e.g., EVC syndrome)
8. Multiple epiphyseal dysplasia and pseudochondroplasia (e.g., pseudochondroplasia)
9. Metaphyseal dysplasia (e.g., metaphyseal dysplasia Schmid type)
10. Spondylometaphyseal dysplasia (e.g., spondylometaphyseal dysplasia Kozlowski type)
11. Spondyloepi (-meta) physeal dysplasias (e.g., immune-osseous dysplasia, Schimke)
12. Severe spondylodysplastic dysplasias (e.g., achondrogenesis type 1A)
13. Moderate spondylodysplastic dysplasias (e.g., brachyolmia, Hoback/Toledo types)
14. Acromelic dysplasias (e.g., trichorhinophalengeal dysplasia types 1/3)
15. Acromesomelic dysplasias (e.g., acromesomelic dysplasia type Maroteaux)
16. Mesomelic and rhizo-mesomelic dysplasias (e.g., dyschondrosteosis, Leri-Weil)
17. Bent bone dysplasias (e.g., CD)
18. Slender bone dysplasias (e.g., Kenny-Caffey dysplasia type 1)
19. Dysplasias with multiple joint dislocations (e.g., Desbuquois dysplasia 259)
20. CDP group (e.g., Conradi-Hünermann type)
21. Neonatal osteosclerotic dysplasias (e.g., Blomstrand dysplasia)
22. Increased bone density group (without modification of bone shape) (e.g., OP)
23. Increased bone density group with metaphyseal and/or diaphyseal involvement (e.g., craniometaphyseal dysplasia, autosomal dominant)
24. Decreased bone density group (e.g., OI type 1)
25. Defective mineralization group (e.g., HP, perinatal lethal and infantile forms) (mucopolysacchoridosis type 1H/1S)
26. LSDs with skeletal involvement (dysostosis multiplex group)
27. Osteolysis group (e.g., infantile systemic hyalinosis)
28. Disorganized development of skeletal components group (e.g., cherubism)
29. Cleidocranial dysplasia group (e.g., cleidocranial dysplasia)
30. Craniosynostosis syndroms and other cranial ossification disorders [e.g., Pfeiffer xyndrome (FGFR1-related)]
31. Dysostoses with predominant craniofacial involvement (e.g., mandibulo-facial dysostosis of Treacher-Collins)
32. Dysostosis with predominant vertebral and costal involvement (e.g., Currarino syndrome)
33. Patellar dysostoses (e.g., nail-patella syndrome)
34. Brachydactylies (with or without extraskeletal manifestations) (e.g., AOH)
35. Limb hypoplasia-reduction defects group (e.g., Fanconi anemia)
36. Polydactyly-syndactyly-triphalangism group (e.g., Pallister-Hall syndrome)
37. Defects in joint formation and synotoses (e.g., radio-ulnar synostosis with amegakaryocytic thrombocytopenia)

Source: Adapted from Superti-Furga A, Unger S. Nosology and classification of genetic skeletal disorders: 2006 revision. *Am J Med Genet A* 2007;143A:1–18.

survival beyond the neonatal or early infancy period and are collectively referred to as lethal chondrodysplasias (126,368,487,570) (Table 27-6). The point prevalence at birth of the lethal chondrodysplasias was 15.4:100,000 births in one geographic region of Denmark (20,21,126). In a prospective study in a small middle eastern country, the birth prevalence rate of all skeletal dysplasias was 13.45:10,000 new borns (12). Fibrochondrogenesis and chondrodysplasia punctute were the most common recessive skeletal dysplasias. Whether the particular clinical observations are derived from prenatal diagnosis by ultrasonography or perinatal autopsies, thanatophoric dysplasia (TD), and osteogenesis imperfecta (OI) type 2 are the most common lethal skeletal dysplasias (169,239,254,351,655). Prenatal sonography has proven to be a highly reliable means of detecting skeletal dysplasias. In one of the larger studies by Schramm and associate, TD, and OI accounted for 35% and 31% of lethal dysplasias, respectively (562,592). This latter experience is similar to several other reports in the literature (Table 27-7). Short rib dysplasias (SRDs), achondrogenesis and CD comprise the next most common lethal disorders (126,132). A somewhat different experience in the context of ISDR which is based on referral cases with the following distribution: osteogenesis imperfect type 2 (20% of all cases), TD (11%), achondrogenesis type 2 (8%), CD (4%) and other specific disorders (36%) (356). Approximately 4.5% of cases were unclassified. In virtually all of the lethal skeletal dysplasias, there is a severe narrowing or reduction in the volume of the thoracic cavity with restricted lung growth and resulting secondary pulmonary hypoplasia (3,441).

Table 27-6 ■ VARIOUS LETHAL SKELETAL DISORDERS AND SITES OF GENE MUTATION (IF KNOWN)

Disorder	Mutated Gene
TD	FGFR3
Achondroplasia (homozygous)	FGFR3
Achondrogenesis type 2	COL2
Kneist-like dysplasia	COL2
Platyspondylic dysplasia (Torrance type)	COL2
Achondrogenesis type 1B (Fracco type)	DTDST
Diatrophic dysplasia	DTDST
Dyssegmental dysplasia, Silverman-Handmaker type	HSPG2 (1p36.1-p34)
AO2	FLNB
Boomerang dysplasia	FLNB
Short rib polydactyly	
Type 1 (Saldino-Noonan)	DYNC2H1 (11q21–q22.1)
Type 2 (Majewski)	—
Type 4 (Mohr-Majewski)	—
ATD	DYNC2H1 (11q21–q22.1)
Metaphyseal dysplasia, Jansen type	PTHRI
Metatrophic dysplasia, types 1 and 2	—
Achondrogenesis type 1A	TRIP11 (14q31–q32)
Spondylometaphyseal dysplasia, Sedaghatean type	—
Fibrochondrogenesis	—
Schneckenbecker dysplasia	—
CD	SOX9
Rhizomelic CDP	
Type 1	PEX7 (6q23.3)
Type 2	6NPAT (1q42)
Type 3	AGPS (2q31.2)
Astley-Kendall dysplasia	—
Blomstrand dysplasia	PTHR1 (3p22–p21.1)
Osteosclerotic bone dysplasia (Raine syndrome)	FAM20C (7p22.3)
OI, Type 2	CRTAP (3p22.3) LEPRE1 (1p34.1)
Spondylothoracic dysplasia (Jarcho-Levin syndrome)	—
HP, perinatal lethal	ALP (1p36.12)
Desbuquois dysplasia	CANT1 19q25.3

Postmortem examination in skeletal dysplasias. Although it may seem obvious, radiographs with anteroposterior and lateral views should be obtained as a prerequisite to the postmortem examination on any dysmorphic infant, including one with a suspected skeletal dysplasia (672). No conventional autopsy can hope to demonstrate the entire range of abnormalities in the skeletal system without a total body image (84). In fact, the skeletal dysplasias in the past have been classified primarily on the basis of their radiographic features, but the results of molecular genetic studies have served as the foundation for the current classification of these disorders (611).

Acquisition of tissues, mainly soft tissues rich in fibroblasts, is recommended for standard metaphase cytogenetics. Although a few hours may have lapsed since death, it is still possible to obtain cellular growth, provided that the body has been placed in a temperature-controlled environment. Samples of cartilage at the costochondral junction or joint space can be snap-frozen in liquid nitrogen. The utility of standardized sections from various specific sites for optimal pathologic examination has been discussed by Yang and associates (677). Certainly molecular genetic studies have introduced a level of diagnostic sophistication and specificity higher than was possible with traditional radiographs and pathologic examination, but the histopathologic features may become especially important in the atypical or unique skeletal dysplasias.

Before the internal examination is performed, a careful documentation of the various standard measurements in the perinatal autopsy and photographs from the anterior, posterior, and lateral profiles should be obtained (477). Various sites, with particular emphasis on the regions of the growth plate, have been recommended for the sampling of membranous bone, including the ribs, vertebral bodies, proximal and distal humerus and/or femur, and cranium (676,677). The costochondral junctions of the fourth through sixth ribs are regarded by some as the optimal sites for identifying disturbances in the growth plate (14,184,229). Decalcified and undecalcified sections have complementary value. It is helpful to have microscopic sections available from the osteochondral junction of an age-matched infant without any known skeletal abnormalities for purposes of reference and orientation.

Table 27-7 ■ TYPES OF SKELETAL DYSPLASIAS BY PRENATAL DETECTION AND PERINATAL AUTOPSY

	Schramm (562)[a]	Tretter (626)[a,d]	Witters (670)[a]	Wood and Dimmick (672)[e]	Lahmar-Bodfaroua (368)[f]	Konstantinidou (351)[f]
TD and other group 1	49[b]	58	13[e]	15	8	7[g]
OI and other group 24	35	50	9	11	9	5
Achondrogenesis and other group 2	14	20	—	2	3	2
SRD and other group 7	26[c]	16	—	3	3	5
CD and other group 17	8	20	—	1	—	4
CDP and other group 20	—	—	—	3	—	2
DD and other group 4	5	4	1	—	8	—
HP and other group 25	—	—	—	3	—	—
Metatrophic dysplasia and other group 11	—	—	—	1	—	—
Severe spondylodysplastic dysplasias and other group 25	—	—	—	—	4	—
Other	—	—	—	2	—	16
Total	137	168	23	41	35	41

[a]Prenatal diagnosis.
[b]Includes 40 TDs and 9 achondroplasia.
[c]Includes nine EVC and seven asphyxiating thoracic dystrophy.
[d]Tabulation includes Tretter and two other literature series.
[e]Includes seven TDs and six achondroplasia.
[f]Perinatal autopsy.
[g]Includes five TDs, one hypochondroplasia, one achondroplasia.

A particularly useful review of the morphologic aspects of the growth plate has been provided by Brighton (95). Many of the histologic abnormalities in a skeletal dysplasia are semiquantitative, in addition to individual cellular alterations. The cellularity of the various zones of cartilage (resting, proliferating, and hypertrophic) and their organization into columns in the hypertrophic zone and the actual chondro-osseous junction or zone of provisional ossification are the specific foci of histologic interest in this group of disorders. In some but not all disorders, the morphologic abnormalities are consistent from one case to another within a specific diagnostic entity. The discussion of chondrodysplasias by Gilbert-Barness with its high quality images which correlate the radiographic, gross, and microscopic features is recommended (228).

The following discussion of genetic skeletal disorders is based on the nosology "groups" as defined in the classification of the International Skeletal Dysplasia Society (ISDS) (611). Selected groups are considered based upon their frequency and models of morphologic and molecular pathology.

FGFR3 group, formerly the achondroplasia group (group 1 in the ISDS Classification) includes the platyspondylic lethal dysplasias, characterized by short limbs relative to a somewhat longer trunk (130,611). The individual entities are achondroplasia, hypochondroplasia, hypochondrodysplasia-like dysplasia and TD, type 1 and type 2 (15,80,380). Several mutations have been identified in the FGFR3 gene on chromosome 4p16.3 (472). FGFR3 mutations have been detected in some of the other nosologic groups (groups 2, 12, 30, and 36 in the ISDS Classification) (611).

Achondroplasia, the most common type of chondrodysplasia, is a nonlethal disorder in the heterozygote (AD inheritance), with a birth prevalence of 1:10,000 to 30,000 live births (49,111,577). Most cases are sporadic, with greater than 75% of cases representing a new mutation (116). The point mutation at nucleotide 1138 on FGFR3 (G38OR) amplifies its usual inhibitory effect on bone formation at the growth plate, so that rhizomelic shortening of the extremities is the result. Morphologically, the growth plate is regular with periosteal overgrowth.

Hypochondroplasia is also a nonlethal disorder of AD inheritance, with a prevalence of 1.5:100,000 live births. The point mutations on the FGFR3 gene (NS40K) in 50% to 60% of cases differ from those in achondroplasia, and other mutations in the FGFR3 gene have been identified in hypochondroplasia (511). Some families are not linked to FGFR3. Although the clinical and radiographic heterogeneity in hypochondroplasia is considerable, the condition can be diagnosed based on clinical and radiographic criteria. Compound carriers of the heterozygous mutations on the FGFR3 gene (G380R and N540K) appear to have a more morbid phenotype than those with either one or the other point mutations. Like achondroplasia, the growth plate is more or less normal microscopically.

TD occurs in 1:35,000 to 50,000 births and is the most common type of lethal chondrodysplasia in most series based upon prenatal ultrasonography and/or at autopsy (126,135,181). Nine point mutations on the FGFR3 gene have been detected and eight of these are present in the more common type 1 TD (angulated or curved humeri and femora and craniosynostosis in 28% and mild cloverleaf skull in 3%) and a single point mutation in type 2 (relatively straight femora, cloverleaf skull in 50%, and craniosynostosis in 90%) (Figure 27-4) (6,418,470). Angulated femora are also present in CD and OI type 2. Most infants die in the neonatal period because of respiratory failure on the basis of severe secondary

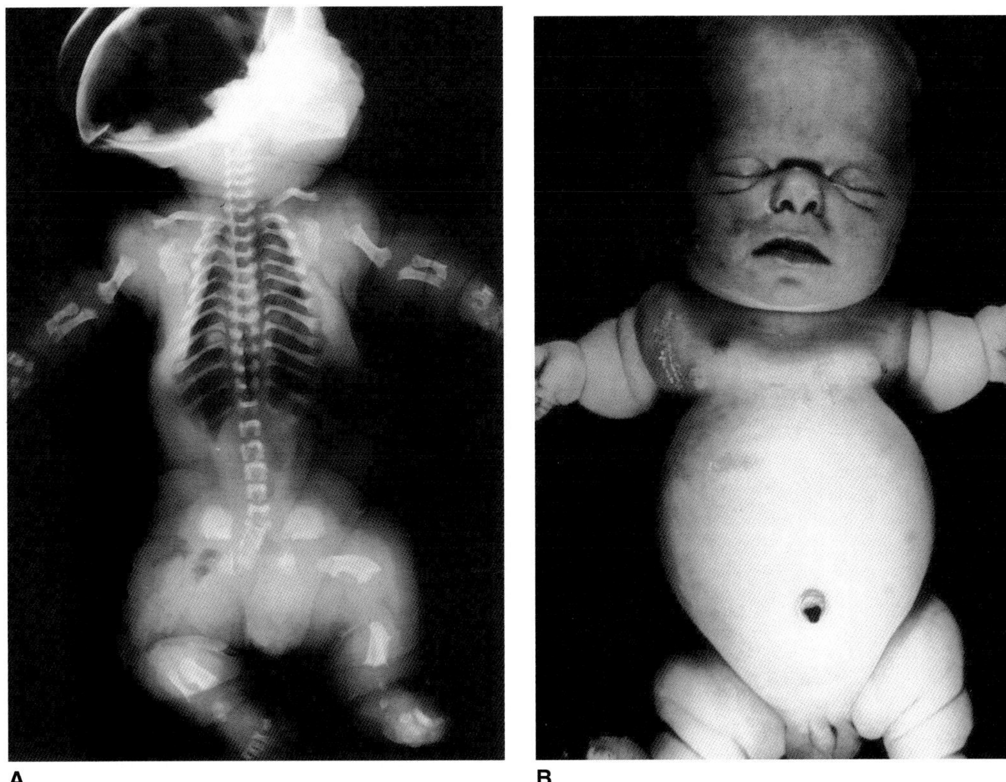

FIGURE 27-4 ■ Postmortem images of type 1 thanatophoric dysplasia. **A**: Radiographs show flattened, U-shaped vertebrae; short, squared iliac bones with small sacrosciatic notches; shortened long bones with metaphyseal flaring; a "French telephone receiver"-like left femur (right femur removed for special studies); and short ribs. **B**: The large head with frontal bossing, rhizomelic extremities, and narrow thorax are typical external findings.

pulmonary hypoplasia as a consequence of the reduced volume of the thoracic cavity which impedes normal lung growth. The chondro-osseous junction of the growth plate is substantially reduced in width with poor columnation and the presence of fibrous bands and fibrosis rather than regular chondroid ossification (284,657,666). Other findings include the flattening of ossification centers (platyspondyly). Polyhydraminios is present in 50% of cases. Severe achondroplasia—developmental delay-acanthosis nigricans is another in the FGFR3 group which has a mutation different fromTD type 2; this difference is manifested by survival into early childhood. In addition to the skeletal abnormalities, there is enlargement of the temporal lobes, deep sulci across the inferio-medial temporal surface and hippocampal dysplasia (271).

Homozygous achondroplasia is also a lethal disorder with a resemblance to TD. Severe pulmonary hypoplasia is similarly the cause of death. It is estimated that 90% of cases have a mutation in COL1A1 or COL1A2. In two of the autosomal recessive (AR) forms of OI type 3, there are mutations in the CRTAP or P3H1 genes.

Decreased bone density group (group 24 in the ISDS Classification) is largely represented by the seven types of OI with mutations in the COL1A1 (17q 21–22), COL1A2 (7q 22.1), CRTAP (3p22-p24.1), or LEPRE 1 (1p 34.1) genes (121,234). These genes are involved in collagen type 1 synthesis and assemblage which occurs in osteoblasts. OI type 2 accounts for 10% to 30% of lethal skeletal dysplasias and is second to TD in the category of lethal dysplasias. There is approximately one case of OI type 2 to three cases of TD. The overall incidence of OI, inclusive of all seven types, is 1:10,000 to 20,000 births. Five types have AD inheritance (types 1 to 5), and AR in types 7 and 8 (523). In the AR forms of OI, there are mutations in CRTAP or LEPRE 1 genes. Approximately 90% of cases of OI (types 1 to 4) have mutations in either of the genes which encode pro-α1 or pro-α2 chains of type I collagen. Most cases of perinatal lethal type 2 are AD with a new mutation since neither parent is a carrier in most cases.

OI type 2, known as the perinatal lethal type, is characterized by severe osteopenia, blue sclera, short and bowed or angulated extremities, a diminutive thorax, and crumpled or collapsed long bones, especially the femora (Figure 27-5) (134). The cranium is soft and intracranial hemorrhage is not uncommon. Shortened, deformed extremities are also features of achondrogenesis, TD, and hypophosphatasia (HP). A small thoracic cavity with its deformities results in severe secondary pulmonary hypoplasia with smaller than normal weight lungs for gestational age and structural abnormalities of the thoracic cage. The bones are shortened, with multiple fractures with minimal normal callus formation, and multinodular chondroid masses are present that resemble an endosteal cartilaginous neoplasm or enchondroma

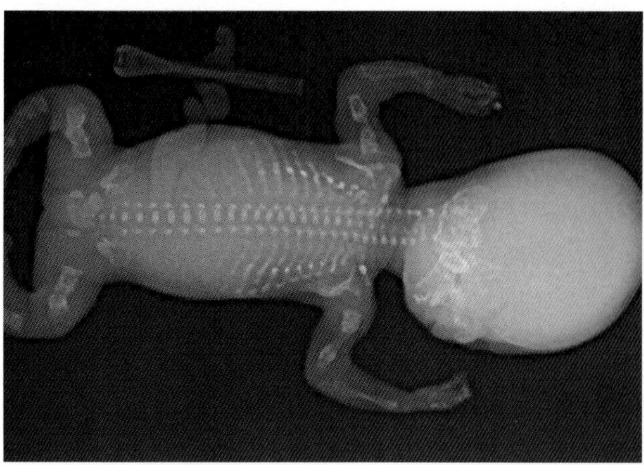
A

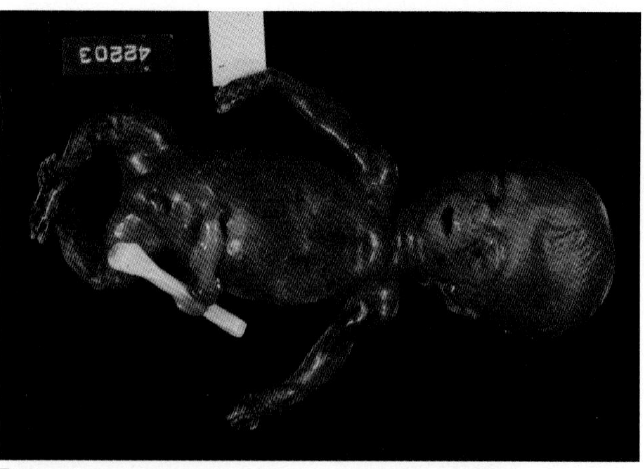

B

FIGURE 27-5 ■ Osteogenesis imperfecta, type 2 in a 21-week gestation male fetus was discovered in prenatal imaging. **A**: Postmortem roentgenogram demonstrates poor ossification of the cranium, multiple fractures of the ribs, long bones and pelvis and normal vertebra. **B**: Shortening of the femora secondary to fractures and marked curvature of the lower extremities are some of the more obvious external abnormalities. Note also the abnormal positioning of the upper extremities.

(101). The cortex is quite attenuated and the trabecular bone consists of delicate strands and is often disorganized, with an overall osteopenic appearance. The bone may appear hypercellular and the mosaic lines or osteoid seams are increased in number. The apparent hypercellularity is explained by a reduction in osteoid matrix secondary to defective type 1 collagen. The physis may be normal in many respects or may be disorganized (Figure 27-6) (113,556). Chondrocyte columnation often appears normal, but osteoid forms directly on the cartilage without orderly endochondral ossification (415,524,606). These infants also exhibit neuropathologic changes, including perivenous microcalcifications and impaired neuroblastic-neuromal migration (185).

OI type 3, unlike type 2, is usually not lethal in the perinatal period, but its severe phenotype is characterized by fractures and deformities of the lower extremities; these complications are present at birth and continue throughout life with the development of severe kyphoscoliosis (622). Lung infections occur throughout the first decade of life because of the thoracic cage abnormalities (424,585). Marrow fibrosis and disorganized trabecular bone in OI type 3 convey a fibrous dysplasia (FD)-like appearance to the bones. There are no specific histologic features to permit the differentiation of one type of OI from another (615). Immature woven bone is prominent, and lamellar bone is poorly formed.

Other pathologic features of OI include hyperplastic callus formation (in particular in OI type 5), especially in the femora, that may be mistaken for osteosarcoma (OS) (122,365,369). Pseudoarthrosis and aortic and mitral valvular insufficiency are other manifestations. Multiple fractures in the absence of a prior diagnosis of OI can be mistaken for child abuse (622). Rare examples of bone neoplasms and cysts have been reported in OI, including OS, ossifying fibroma (OF), and aneurysmal bone cyst (ABC) (53,599,616).

Bruck syndrome with OI-like skeletal changes and congenital joint contractures is grouped together with classic OI although this disorder has overlap features with arthrogryposis (41,262,381). This AR disorder has been mapped to chromosome 17q12 (type 1) and 3q 23-q24 (PLOD 2, type 2). Fibrous pterygia are present in addition to spontaneous fractures and wormian bones. Astley-Kendall syndrome is a lethal perinatal skeletal dysplasia with features of OI and chondrodysplasia punctata (CDP).

Defective mineralization group (group 25 in the ISDS Classification) includes HP, an inborn error of metabolism associated with a deficiency of tissue nonspecific alkaline phosphatase with mutations on 1p36.12 (611). The inheritance of the perinatal lethal and infantile forms of this disorder is AR with a prevalence of 1:100,000 births (445,578). There are six clinical forms of HP and these to some extent reflect the heterogeneity of the missense mutations on the ALPL gene (529). There are some overlapping radiographic features among HP, OI types 2 and 3 and achondrogenesis type IA, however, these conditions can be differentiated from each other by radiographic analysis of the entire skeleton. Approximately 2% to 4% of lethal osteochondrodysplasias are cases of perinatal HP. The histopathologic findings at the physis include a hypercellular, disordered osteochondral junction with cartilaginous overgrowth and minimal bone formation. Uncalcified osteoid with cores of cartilage are demonstrated in undecalcified sections; there is a similarity in this respect to the histology in OP. Some pathologic features of HP resemble those of rickets-osteomalacia.

Type 2 collagen group (group 2 in the ISDS Classification) comprise a phenotypically diverse category including lethal achondrogenesis type 2 (Langer-Saldino syndrome), hypochondrogenesis, nonlethal spondyloepiphyseal dysplasia congenita, Kniest dysplasia, and Stickler dysplasia (272,611). Czech dysplasia is a related disorder, since it like the others has mutations in the COL2A1 gene (12q13.1-q13.3) with faulty synthesis of type 2 collagen, a basic constituent of hyaline cartilage (632). Achondrogenesis type 2 (ACG 2) accounts

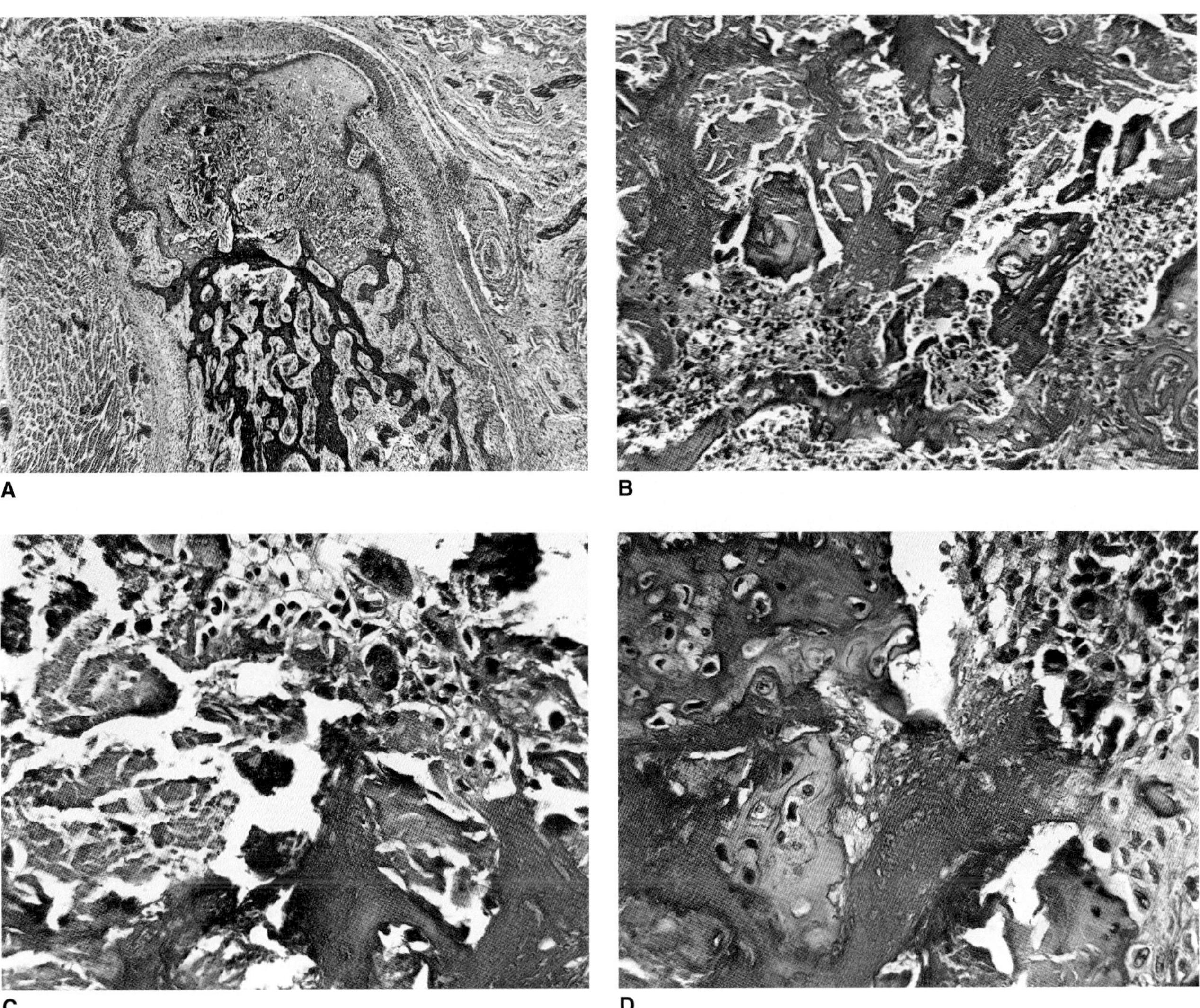

FIGURE 27-6 ■ Osteogenesis imperfecta, type 2 is a representative disorder of the "decreased bone density group." This type is associated with death in the perinatal-neonatal period. **A**: A long bone at low magnification shows the overall architecture and the physeal growth plate. **B**: Though there are few abnormalities in the physeal plate itself in terms of growth, a fracture is present at the lateral aspect of the growth plate. **C**: A higher magnification shows fragmentation and necrosis of the growth plate. **D**: Osteoclasts and macrophages are present in a focus of necrotic bone with very early callus formation.

for 5% to 7% of lethal skeletal dysplasias (Table 27-7). Hypochondrogenesis is a closely related entity with amino acid substitutions for glycine at different sites in type 2 procollagen. The inheritance in both disorders is autosomal dominant. In addition to absent or minimal vertebral body ossification, cystic hygroma and/or hydrops fetalis is often present. Severe pulmonary hypoplasia is the cause of death in the perinatal period. Complex congenital cardiovascular anomalies have been reported in hypochondrogenesis (509,654). A papillomatous epidermal proliferation of the scalp with central ulceration has been reported in an infant with ACG 2 whose features are those of an epidermal nevus with possible aplasia cutis congenita (653). Chondrocytes reside in enlarged lacunae, and the apparent hypercellularity is a consequence of diminished matrix in both ACG2 and hypochondrogenesis. Apparent "ballooning" of chondrocytes is described. Vascularity is increased in the reserve (resting) and proliferating zones of chondrocytes and the columns of chondrocytes in the hypertrophic zone are irregular. Persistent central cores of cartilage are found within the bony trabeculae, as in HP and OP.

SRDs with or without polydactyly (group 7 in the ISDS Classification) includes asphyxiating thoracic dysplasia (ATD, Jeune) and chondroectodermal dysplasia (Ellis-van Creveld syndrome, EVC) which have many clinical features in common; however, the latter condition is generally compatible with life through the perinatal-neonatal period (48,141,473,581,678). Saldino-Noonan (Verma-Naumoff types I and 3), Majewski (type 2), and Beemer (type 4) syndromes are the other entities in this morphologic group (Figure 27-7) (115). Postaxial hexadactyly is a common feature in EVC. Some minor histologic differences are noted in the physes in the various types of SRD, but in general,

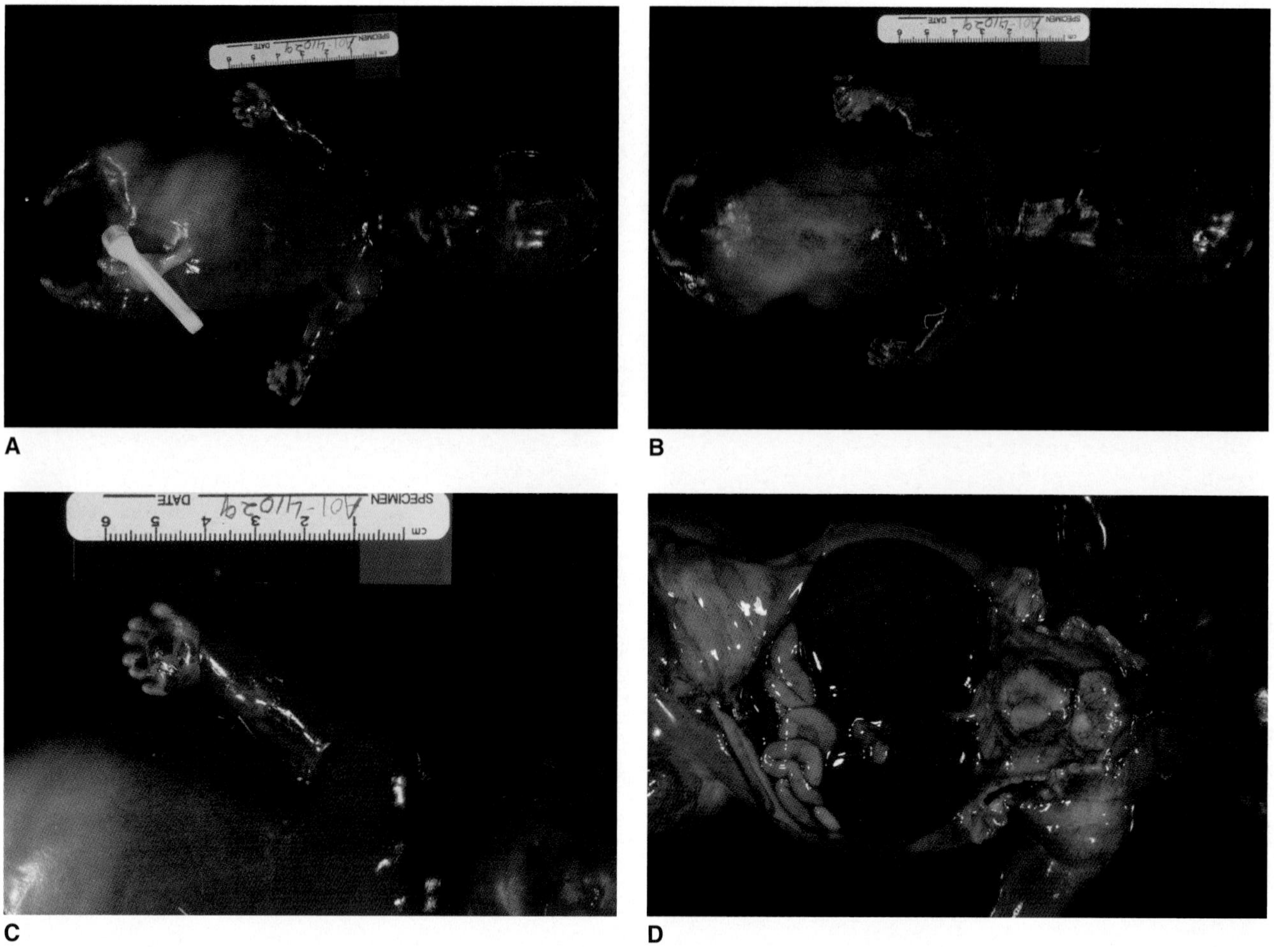

A B C D

FIGURE 27-7 ■ Short rib dysplasia with polydactyly is a group 7 skeletal disorder, which is shown in this case of Majewski syndrome. **A**: This stillborn fetus weighed 325 g. Various external anomalies are seen in this anterior view with a cleft lip, narrow thoracic cage, and severe shortening of the long bones of the upper and lower extremities. **B**: The posterior view demonstrates these same findings in addition to the bulging flanks. **C**: The upper extremity shows postaxial polydactyly and syndactyly. **D**: Exposure of the thoracic and abdominal organs reveals the extremely small thorax, which contributes to the severe secondary pulmonary hypoplasia, which is largely responsible for the lethal nature of this disorder.

chondrocytic proliferation is diminished, as evidenced by a reduction in thickness of the growth plate and disorganization of the columns of chondrocytes (Figure 27-8) (268,516,679). Overlapping pathologic features are seen in EVC, ATD, and renal-hepatic-pancreatic dysplasia of Ivemark (57,98). Both EVC and Weyers acrodental dysostosis share mutations on the EVC2 (EVC2, 4p16); ectodermal dysplasia with enamel hypoplasia, hypodontia and early eruption and exfoliation of teeth are seen on both disorders (546). Atrial septal or atrioventricular septal defects are present in 65% to 70% of EVC cases.

Severe spondylodysplasias (group 12 in the ISDS Classification) is a problematic category since these platyspondylic lethal skeletal dysplasias (PLSD) are differentiated from the other major category of platyspondylic dysplasias, the FGFR3 group (Group 1) (611). The San Diego type of PLSD has the same FGFR3 mutation as TD type 1. Likewise, Torrance and Luton types of PLSD have been considered in the past as variants of TD; however, the Torrance type has a mutation in the COL2A1 gene which places it into group

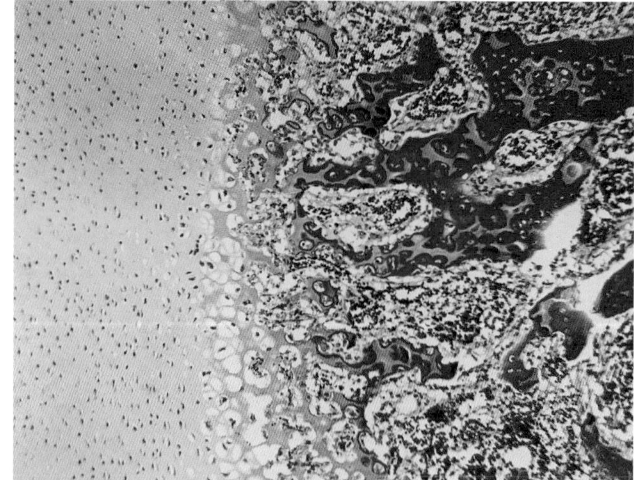

FIGURE 27-8 ■ Short rib dysplasia with polydactyly in a stillborn fetus is represented in this case of Majewski syndrome. The growth plate shows irregular columnation of chondrocytes and disordered maturation of bone with retention of central cartilage.

2 or type 2 collagenopathies (451). Achondrogenesis type 1A (ACG1A, Houston-Harris) is the other lethal dysplasia in group 12 (4,83). Occipital encephalocele has been reported in association with the latter disorder as well as in TD. These infants are often born prematurely with polyhydramnios and fetal hydrops. Microscopically, the growth plate in ACG1A is hypercellular, and the enlarged chondrocytes have a periodic acid–Schiff-positive, diastase-resistant inclusion within a cytoplasmic vacuole (4). Mutations in TRIP11 (14q31-q32) identified in ACG1A which results in apparent loss of function of the golgins GMAP-210 and there is reduced expression of COL10a1 (209,589). Schneckenbecken (snail pelvis) dysplasia, a PLSD with AR inheritance, is also characterized by a snail-like pelvis and short limbs. There is some resemblance to TD (467). Because of hypercellularity of the resting and proliferating zones of chondrocytes, the lacunar spaces are inapparent and the intercellular matrix is relatively inconspicuous. Reduced columnation of chondrocytes and hypervascularization are seen in the proliferating zones and the chondrocytes have uniformly centralized nuclei. Fibrochondrogenesis, a quite rare disorder, also has some phenotypic features resembling those of TD, but several radiographic differences are notable (11,190). The spindled chondrocytes in the poorly formed growth plate are surrounded by delicate envelopes of fibroblasts (664).

Spondylo-epi (-meta)physeal dysplasias (group 11 in ISDS Classification) accounts for 5% or fewer of skeletal dysplasias. The several types of metatrophic dysplasia, immune-osseous dysplasia (Schimke) and progressive pseudorheumatoid dysplasia (PPD) are included in group 11 (611). Metatropic dysplasia (MD) has at least four types: type 1 (perinatal lethal or lethal hyperplasic type), type 2 (perinatal lethal or lethal in early childhood MD), type 3 (severe, nonlethal) and type 4 (milder, nonlethal) (51,255,321). Types 1 and 2 have AR inheritance. Some of the basic features of MD are marked platyspondyly, halberd pelvis, short limbs and a narrow thorax with short ribs and expanded metaphyses with dumbbell shaped long bones (222). A caudal appendage or tail-like structure is another feature of MD, type I (Figure 27-9) (77,362,489). Pulmonary hypoplasia is a complication of a small, conical thorax. A disorganized primary spongiosa with irregular trabeculae, diminished ossification of epiphyseal cartilage in the tubular bones and vertebrae with poor chondroosseous columnation, hypercellular, and hyperplastic cartilage are some of the microscopic features of MD. PPD, an AR disorder, is caused by loss of function mutations of the WISP3 gene (6q22) (163,686). A progressive arthropathy with a clinical onset between 2 and 8 years of age resembles idiopathic juvenile arthropathy, but platyspondylia is the distinguishing feature of PPD. Swelling of both large and small

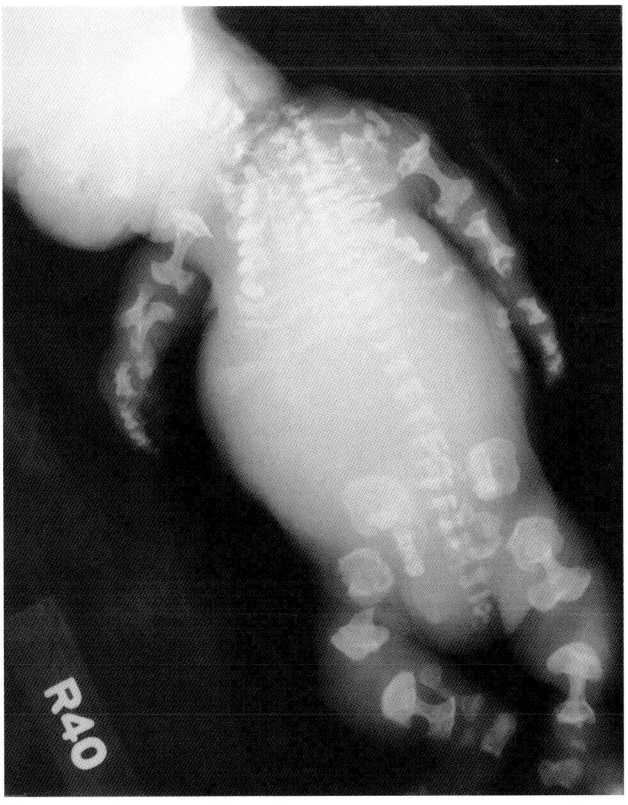

A

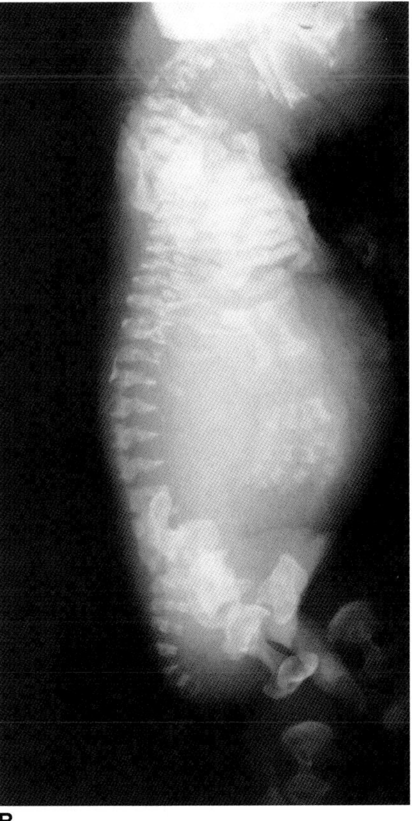

B

FIGURE 27-9 ■ Metatrophic dysplasia type I (lethal variant) is shown in (**A**) anteroposterior and (**B**) lateral radiographic views, which demonstrates shortened long bones with trumpet-like flaring of the metaphyses, accessory vertebrae with flattened vertebral bodies, a caudal appendage and a small, conical thorax with hyperossified ribs.

joints develops, but in the absence of apparent synovitis. The articular cartilage undergoes progressive degeneration, with early onset osteoarthropathy and the formation of osteocartilaginous loose bodies. Nesting of chondrocytes in the resting zone and an absence of chondrocyte columnation in the proliferating to provisional ossification zone are the principal histologic features. So-called Czech dysplasia has a similar clinical phenotype to PPD, but has AD inheritance and is caused by a missense mutation of the COL2A1 gene. Schimke immunoosseous dysplasia is an AR disorder with biallelic missense mutations in the SMARCA1 gene (2q34-q35); spondyloepiphyseal dysplasia is accompanied by a T-cell deficiency, focal segmental glomerulosclerosis and hyalinosis, dysmorphic facies, autoimmune enteropathy and cerebral ischemia (moya moya disease) (78,125). Intrauterine growth restriction and postnatal growth failure are other findings. The histologic findings in the physis are similar to those in PPD. The growth plate has a hypocellular appearance with an attenuated growth plate. There is little evidence of chondrocyte enlargement and poorly defined chondrocyte columnation.

Sulphation disorders group (group 4 in the ISDS Classification) includes achondrogenesis type 1B, atelosteogenesis type 2 (AO2) and diastrophic dysplasia (DD) (624). There is considerable phenotypic overlap between AO2 and DD (260,582). Five examples (2%) of these latter disorders were detected among 226 pathologically confirmed skeletal dysplasias and one case (4%) of AO2 was diagnosed among 28 infants with lethal dysplasias. Of note, AO1, the most severe form of AO, with death occurring in the neonatal period has been assigned to the filamin group (Group 6) together with AO3 and Larsen syndrome on the basis of molecular genetics (70,286). AO2, DD, AO1B, and AR multiple epiphyseal dysplasia have in common mutations in the SLC26A2 gene (5q32-q33.1) which encodes a protein in cartilage that transports inorganic sulfate whose absence results in undersulfation of proteoglycans (Figure 27-10) (168,461). McAlister dysplasia and another lethal dysplasia, de la Chapelle dysplasia, are probably related sulphation disorders (563). The pathologic features of DD and AO are similar: an attenuated growth plate, irregular clumping of chondrocytes in the resting zone, and foci of myxoid degeneration that are not necessarily confined to the resting zone. One of the hallmark features is a dense rim of matrix around each lacuna; the concentrically arranged collagen is demonstrable with a trichrome stain (399,401). Giant chondrocytes may be found as well. AO1B, in addition to severe micromelia with marked shortening of the femora and humeri, is characterized by minimal or absent ossification of the vertebral bodies and malformed tibiae and fibulae (Figure 27-11) (610).

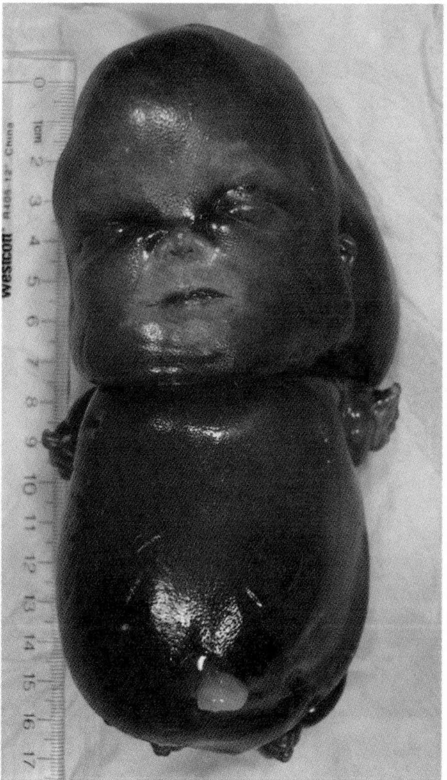

A

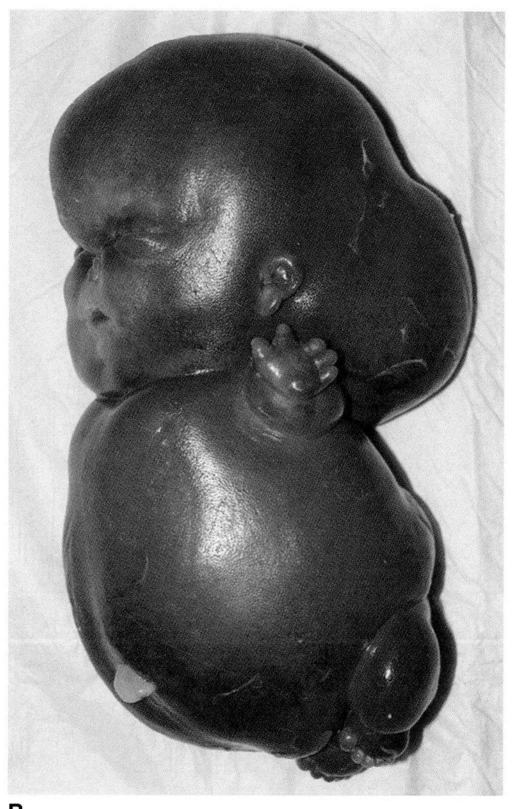

B

FIGURE 27-10■Achondrogenesis type 1B is a representative of group 4 or sulphation disorders. **A**: Severe micromelia and hydrops fetalis are noted in this anterior view. **B**: A profile view shows the severe micromelia and cystic hygroma. (Contributed by Bahig M. Shehata, MD, Atlanta, GA).

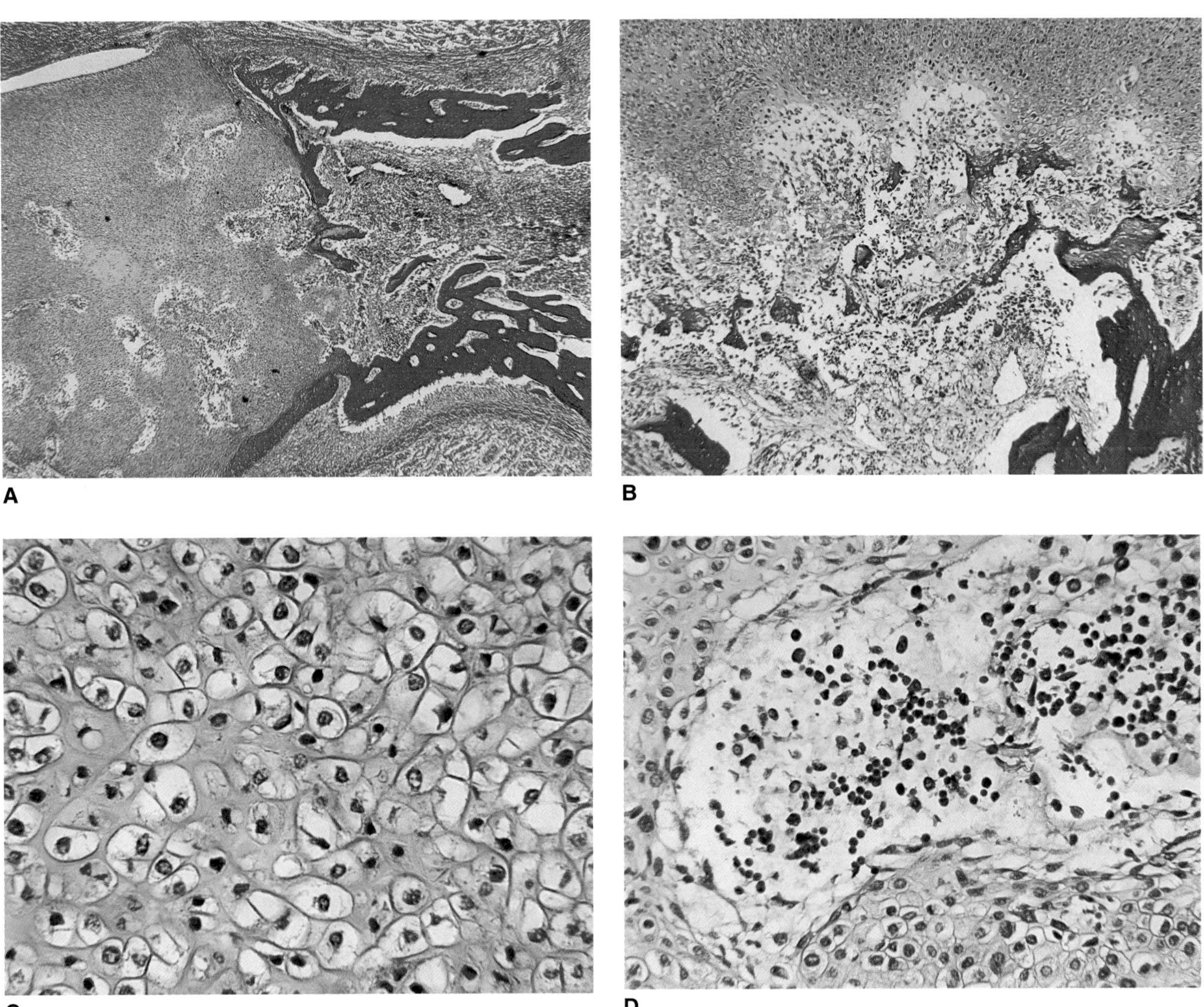

FIGURE 27-11 ▪ Achondrogenesis type 1B shows the several substantial abnormalities in the physis. **A**: This field shows the epiphyseal cartilage and growth plate with obvious absence of any resemblance to a normal growth plate. **B**: The growth plate in another micromelic long bone shows a complete absence of any physeal organization. **C**: The zone of proliferating chondrocytes demonstrates an eosinophilic stroma in the background, which is collagen surrounding each cell. **D**: The multifocal cystic degeneration present in panel A is seen in this higher magnification field with hemorrhage and degenerating chondrocytes in the background. (Contributed by Bahig M. Shehata, MD, Atlanta, Georgia.)

Filamin group (group 6 in the ISDS Classification) is defined by the presence of mutations in the FLNA gene (Xq28) that encodes filamin A and includes frontometaphyseal dysplasia, Melnick-Needles osteodysplasia and otopalatodigital syndromes types 1 and 2; these are all X-lined disorders (538,611). Mutations in FLNB gene (3p 14.3) are associated with AO1 and AO3, Larsen syndrome, spondylocarpotarsal syndrome and boomerang dysplasia (70,71,139,194,394). The filamins are cytoplasmic proteins that regulate the cytoskeletal network by cross-linking actin and link the cell membrane to the cytoskeleton. Otopalatodigital syndrome type 2 is a potentially lethal disorder with its thoracic and pulmonary hypoplasia. Other defects include hypomineralized calvarium, poorly formed small bones of the hands and feet, septal and right ventricular outflow tract defects, omphalocele, and genitourinary tract anomalies. Boomerang dysplasia and AO1 are lethal disorders due to the hypoplastic thorax and lungs (55,286). Multinucleated and giant chondrocytes may be seen in a focally hypocellular reserve or resting zone. Similar giant chondrocytes have been seen in Piepkorn dysplasia which may be allelic to boomerang dysplasia (108). There is near complete absence of ossification and mineralization in boomerang dysplasia. Overall there is marked disorganization in the columns of chondrocytes.

CDP group (group 20 in the ISDS Classification) comprises several rare skeletal dysplasias (611). There are other acquired disorders in children unrelated to the skeletal dysplasias with punctate stippled calcifications in the epiphyses and around the spine. For instance, prenatal exposures to warfarin or neonatal lupus erythematosus are two examples

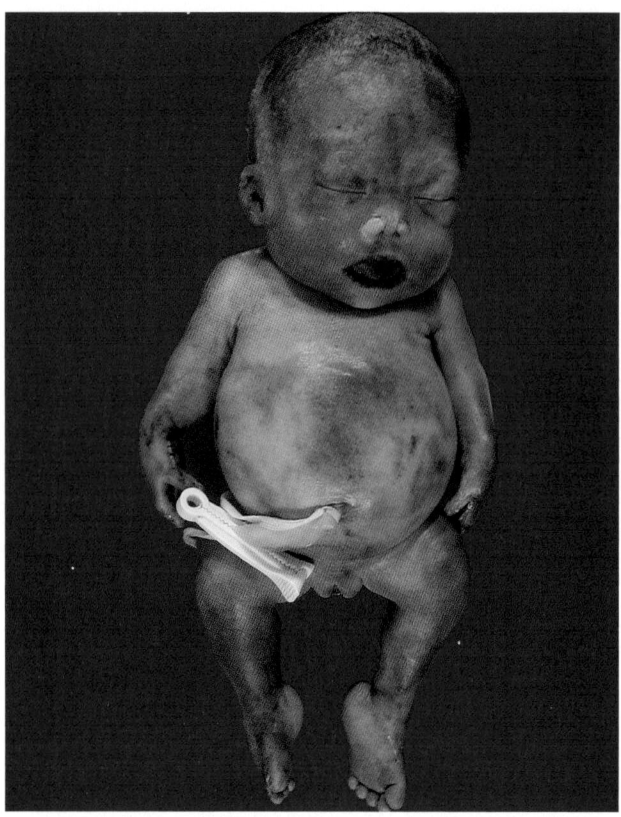

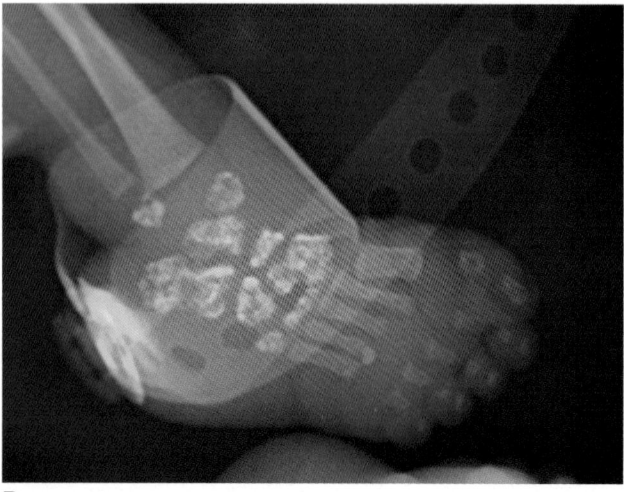

A B

FIGURE 27-12 ■ CDP, X-linked dominant (Conradi-Hunermann-Happle syndrome). **A**: The external examination reveals severe shortening of the upper and lower extremities with rhizomesoacromelic features. Note also the bilateral talipes equinovarus deformities. **B**: Multifocal stippled epiphyseal calcifications are the characteristic findings in CDP. This image of the foot shows the numerous calcifications in the epiphyses. (**Panel A** from *Pediatr Dev Pathol* 2007;10:142–148.)

with the presence of stippled epiphyses (568). In terms of pathogenesis, CDP can be classified into inborn errors of cholesterol biosynthesis, peroxisomal biogenesis disorders, disruption of vitamin K metabolism and chromosomal abnormalities (219,297,337). Among the skeletal dysplasias with stippled epiphyses, rhizomelic CDP type I, and Zellweger syndrome, both AR peroxisomal disorders, are lethal in most cases (50). Conradi-Hunermann-Happle (CHH) syndrome, with X-linked dominant inheritance (Xp11.23-p11.22), may be lethal in the affected neonate (Figure 27-12) (518). One of the characteristic and accessible pathologic findings in CHH syndrome is lamellar orthokeratosis and dystrophic calcifications in keratotic plugs in a skin biopsy (275). Rhizomelic CDP is represented by three AR disorders: peroxisomal CDP1 (PEX7 on 6q22-q24), CDP2 (DHAPAT on 1q 42) and CDP3 (AGPS on 2q 31) (663). The incidence is 1:100,000 live births. Severe shortening of proximal long bones (rhizomelia), cataracts, dysmorphic facies, and severe growth abnormalities are the various clinical features. Approximately 50% or more of children do not survive beyond the age of 6 years. The cause of death is usually respiratory in nature after multiple respiratory tract infections. Dystrophic calcifications in the region of an otherwise unremarkable growth plate and cystic myxoid degeneration in the subarticular cartilage are the principal histologic features in rhizomelic CDP (188). In other conditions association with stippled calcifications, dystrophic calcifications, and degenerative changes in the chondroid matrix are the microscopic findings (Figure 27-13).

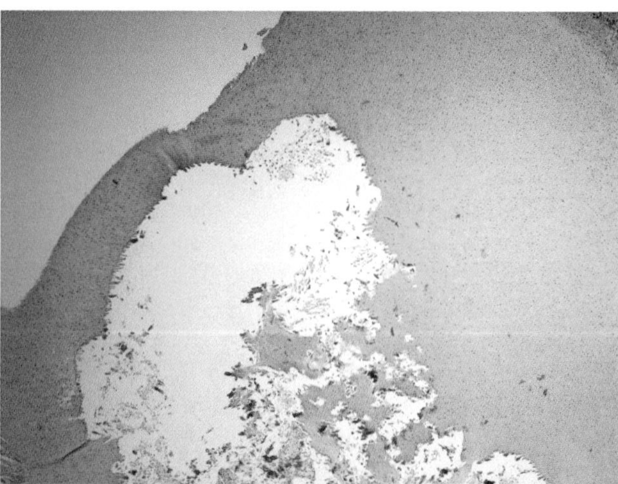

FIGURE 27-13 ■ Chondrodysplasia punctuate, X-linked dominant (Conradi-Hunermann-Happle syndrome) shows the presence of dystrophic calcifications and cystic degeneration of the epiphysis. (Contributed by Charles Timmons, MD, Dallas, Texas.)

Osteogenesis-like features are present in the lethal Astley-Kendall syndrome as one of the overlap syndromes which in this case is classified with the group 20 disorders (180).

Bent bone dysplasias (group 17 in the ISDS Classification) are characterized by short limb dysplasia and bowing of the long bones of the lower extremity (611). Four disorders, CD, kyphomelic dysplasia, Cumming syndrome, and Stuve-Wiedemann dysplasia, comprise this group of rare but radiographically distinctive conditions. CD has a reported incidence of 1:200,000 births and accounts for approximately 4% to 6% of all lethal skeletal dysplasias (230,410). Mutations in the SOX 9 gene (17q24-q25) is the molecular genetic defect in this AD disorder (650). Anterior bowing of the lower extremity long bones and a hypoplastic thorax with secondary pulmonary hypoplasia are the phenotypic abnormalities in addition to the characteristic sexual anomalies with so-called sex reversal, in which one-third of the phenotypic females have an XY karyotype (XY gonadal dysgenesis) (339,373,499). Abnormalities of both müllerian and wolffian duct structures and incomplete ovarian or testicular development are other findings. Gonadoblastoma may be seen in the dysgenetic testis (297). The physes of the long bones exhibit minimal histologic abnormalities; however, some alterations in the proliferative and hypertrophic zones of chondrocytes may be seen. In place of normal cortical bone, immature woven bone, osteoclastic activity, and vascularized intraosseous spaces are the microscopic features. Stuve-Wiedemann syndrome (SWS) is a severe AR disorder with mutations in the LIFR gene (5p13.1) (140,149). Cortical thickening is present in bowed long bones with flared metaphyses and progressive decalcification. Hyperthermia, respiratory complications on the basis of aspiration pneumonitis and cutaneous infections all contribute to death by 2 years of age (371). A variant of SWS is neonatal Schwartz-Jampel syndrome type 2 (see Chapters 5, 18 and 19).

Increased bone density is a feature of three categories of bone disorders: neonatal osteosclerotic dysplasias (group 21 in the ISDS Classification), increased bone density group without alteration in bone shape (group 22) and increased bone density group with metaphyseal and/or diaphyseal involvement (group 23) (160,611). Infantile cortical hyperostosis (ICH) is an example of a group 21 disorder, but is also an example of type 1 collagenopathy whose principal features are decreased bone density (see group 24) (451). Blomstrand dysplasia is an AR lethal neonatal disorder which is characterized by generalized osteosclerosis and advanced skeletal maturation (483). It shares group 21 with ICH, desmosclerosis and Raine dysplasia. Mutations in the PTH-related peptide type I receptor gene (3p22-21.1) are present in Blomstrand dysplasia (175,326). This same gene is mutated in Jansen chondrodysplasia. In addition to very short stature, the limbs are micromelic with accelerated ossification of virtually the entire skeleton. Like the other lethal skeletal dysplasias, the thorax is short and narrow. Early ossification of the epiphyseal center, a reduction in the epiphyseal cartilage, irregularity of the transformation zone, subperiosteal ossification, and cortical hyperostosis are some of the histologic findings.

OP (group 22 in the ISDS Classification) is a heritable osteosclerotic disorder in which one of several mutations is associated with defects in the differentiation and/or function of the osteoclast (244). The severe, neonatal forms with AR inheritance are seen in 1:250,000 births. Loss of functions mutations have been identified in five genes, TCIRG1 (11q13), CLCN7 (16p13), OSTM1(6q21), RANKL (TNFSF11, 13q14), and RANK (TNFRSF11A, 18q22.1) (162,597,652). The latter two mutations are associated with "osteoclast-poor" OP since there is a defect in osteoclastic differentiation, whereas the former three mutations are found in "osteoclast-rich" OP whose defect is a failure in osteoclastic function (645). Among these mutations in the AR-OP, the TCIRG1 mutation is detected in 50% to 60% of cases and CLCN7 mutation is 20% to 25% of cases (208). Leukopenia and hepatosplenomegaly are manifestations of bony overgrowth of the marrow space with phthisic anemia and organomegaly on the basis of extramedullary hematopoiesis. Early death may result from pathologic fractures, hydrocephalus, or anemia; the pathologic fractures are typically transverse breaks in the long bones. Those who survive beyond early infancy often succumb to pneumonia, intracerebral hemorrhage or phthisic anemia in the first decade. Other expressions of AR-OP are renal tubular acidosis (RTA) and cerebral calcification with mutations in the carbonic anhydrase 2 gene on chromosome 5 and the so-called intermediate form with the CLCN7 mutation (567). OP associated with RTA is usually detected in the first 2 years of life with growth failure, mental retardation, visual and auditory deficiencies, pathologic fractures, and metabolic acidosis. Cerebral calcifications are detectable after 18 months of age. Cortical bone thickening is present in all forms of OP, but in the most severe cases, the marrow cavity is obliterated and the corticomedullary demarcation is lost (Figure 27-14). Osteosclerosis may be uniform or alternating, as seen in the vertebrae, where transverse striations of alternating lucent and dense bone produce the so-called rugger jersey spine. Lucency of the central portions of bones may convey the appearance of "bone within bone." Coxa vara and lateral bowing of the long bones are common findings, and rachitic features may be observed in infants. The microscopic hallmark is the persistence of calcified cartilage, surrounded by dense woven or lamellar bone of endochondral origin (Figure 27-15) (265). The zone of proliferating cartilage is often extremely wide at sites of active endochondral ossification in infants which reflects the failure in remodeling of mineralized cartilage and bone. Woven bone persists in the absence of lamellar bone formation. The number of osteoclasts in a bone biopsy may depend on the sampling or the osteoclast-rich or poor nature of the particular type. Howship lacunae are often difficult to identify. Osteoblasts are generally present in normal numbers, but they often appear flattened and inactive. The marrow space is more or less obliterated by woven rather than lamellare bone, which is thought to account for the

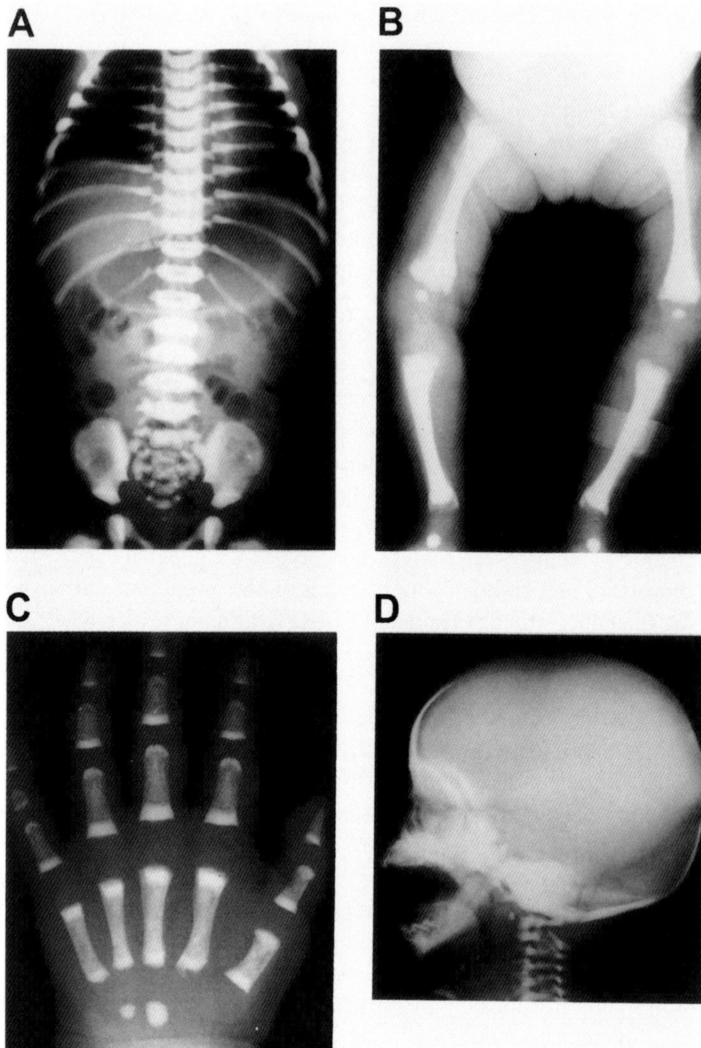

FIGURE 27-14 ■ Osteopetrosis, autosomal recessive lethal type, is manifested by diffuse skeletal osteosclerosis, as demonstrated in these radiographic views. **A**: The images of the chest, abdomen, and pelvis demonstrate the generalized increased bone density. **B**: Sclerosis of the long bones of the lower extremities shows metaphyseal fragmentation, mild metaphyseal expansion, periosteal new bone formation, and an absence of the medullary canal. **C**: Sclerosis of the bones in the hand shows the most marked changes at the proximal ends of the phalanges and distal ends of the metacarpals. **D**: Lateral view of the skull demonstrates diffuse sclerosis, especially marked at the base.

extreme fragility of the bone despite its increased density. Ultrastructurally, the osteoclasts adjacent to the bone surface may lack the ruffled membrane that is necessary for bony resorption which is impaired in all forms of OP. There are two AD expressions of OP, type I with mutations in low density lipoprotein receptor-related protein 5 gene (11q 13.4) and type 2 with CLCN7 gene mutations (267). However, there is some question whether type 1 AD-OP and Albers-Schonberg disease are separate entities from type 2 AD-OP.

Lysosomal storage diseases (*LSDs*) with skeletal involvement or dysostosis multiplex group (group 26 in the ISDS Classification) comprise a family of heritable metabolic diseases with a defect in a specific acid hydrolase or enzyme activator whose functional and morphologic consequences are an accumulation or storage of the catabolic product at the blocked biochemical step. Currently, 21 disorders with similar radiographic abnormalities are included in the ISDS Classification (611). The incidence of LSDs is approximately 1:1,500 to 7,000 live births (596). Hypoplastic iliac bones with pseudoenlargement of the acetabula, pointed proximal metacarpals, defective development of the anterosuperior portions of the vertebral bodies at the thoracolumbar junctions, and widened ribs that taper near the vertebral margins are among the various skeletal abnormalities of LSDs with some differences among the specific types (Figure 27-16) (9,497). The changes in the tubular bones, which are more pronounced in the upper extremities, include diaphyseal and metaphyseal expansion, delayed epiphyseal ossification, and osteopenia. Other changes include macrocrania, coxa valga, small carpal bones with V-shaped deformities of the distal radius and ulna, cardiomegaly and hepatosplenomegaly. A consistent histologic finding in a variety of parenchymal and mesenchymal cells, from hepatocytes to chondrocytes, is cellular enlargement which reflects the presence of numerous membrane-bound vacuoles representing distended lysosomes that are clear or contain finely granular material (Figure 27-17) (100,170,584) (see Chapter 5).

Mucopolysaccharidoses (*MPSs*) are the most familiar and common LSDs. Six eponymic types of MPS and a total of 14 subtypes are recognized. The overall incidence of the

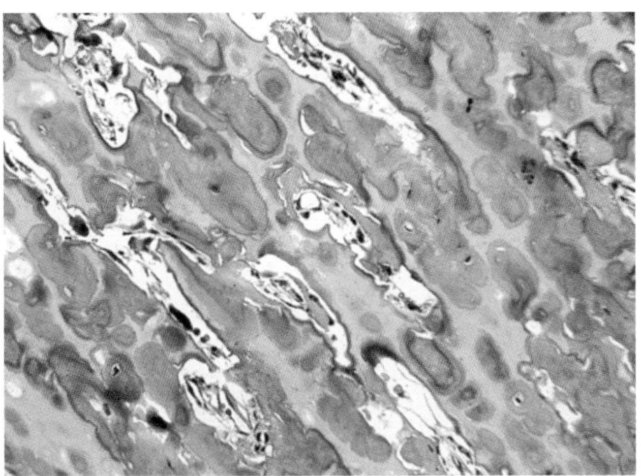
A

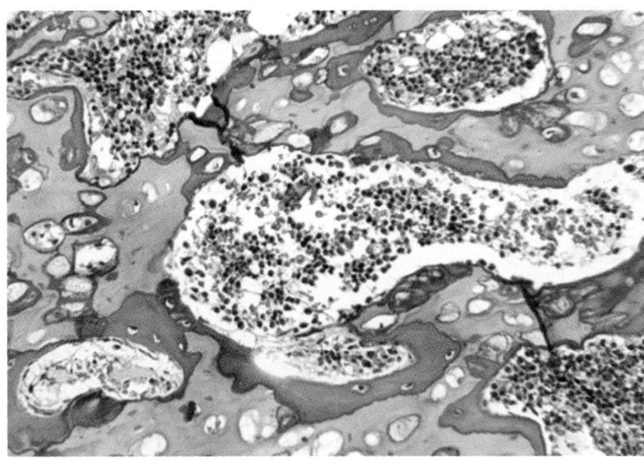
B

FIGURE 27-15 ■ Osteopetrosis, autosomal recessive type, is shown in these two photomicrographs from the same infant. **A**: The bone biopsy shows thickened trabeculae with retained central cores of cartilage. Note also the absence of bone marrow and hematopoiesis. **B**: A follow-up biopsy 2.5 years after a bone marrow transplant shows a reduction in the thickness of the trabeculae and the presence of hematopoiesis. A follow-up image at that time showed decreased bone density and an identifiable marrow. (From Tolar J, Teitelbaum SL, Orchard PJ. *N Engl J Med* 2004;351:2938–2949.)

AR MPSs ranges from 1:100,000 to 600,000 live births. A specific chromosomal defect has been identified in virtually all of the MPSs. Vieira and associates have studied the natural history in 113 individuals with MPSs (643). Shortened stature and progressive skeletal deformities are indicative of growth plate and bony abnormalities with subluxation of joints and progressive kyphoscoliosis, as in MPS type 7 (Sly syndrome). The cartilaginous growth plate is reduced or disorganized in appearance. The prominence of enlarged, vacuolated chondrocytes varies somewhat among the types of MPS. Abrupt calcification of the cartilage without the formation of primary trabeculae is another feature of the growth plate in several of these disorders, including MPS type 1H (Hurler syndrome), MPS type IH/1S (Hurler-Scheie syndrome), and MPS type 4A (Morquio syndrome) (426). In addition to abnormalities in the axial and appendicular skeleton, histologic changes in the temporal bone have been correlated with deafness in MPS type 1H, type 1 IS (Scheie syndrome), MPS type 1H/1S, and MPS type 2 (Hunter syndrome). Several LSDs distinct from MPS also are manifested by dyostosis multiplex, including mucolipidosis 2 (I-cell disease) and mucolipidosis 3 (pseudo-Hurler polydystrophy). Yet another category of metabolic disorders includes those in which glycoprotein degradation and structure are defective: fucosidosis, α-mannosidosis, β-mannosidosis, sialidosis, aspartylglycosaminuria, sialic acid storage disease, multiple sulfatase deficiency, and galactosialidosis (223,407). Carpal tunnel syndrome is a complication in both the MPSs and mucolipidoses secondary to the accumulation of material in swollen fibroblasts and the presence of foamy histiocytes (251).

Melorheostosis, osteopoikilosis, pyknodysostosis, and osteopathia striata are examples of group 22 in the ISDS Classification which are characterized by increased bone density or sclerosis (611). The estimated prevalence of melorheostosis is 1:1,000,000 individuals (245). The overwhelming majority of cases have been sporadic, but isolated examples have been reported in association with osteopoikilosis with mutations in the LEM domain containing 3 gene (12q14) (460). Mutations in this same gene are found in Buschke-Ollendorff syndrome. The diagnosis is rarely made in infancy, but 40% to 50% of cases are discovered before the age of 20 years (107). Any bone or bones may be affected; however, involvement is frequently unilateral, with one or more long bones, usually in the lower extremity, being hyperostotic (so-called flowing hyperostosis) (300). The fibrosing component in the contiguous soft tissues has fibromatosis-like or atypical decubital fibroplasia-like histologic appearance which results in contractures, a cause of substantial morbidity in this disorder (296). Fibrofatty and myositis ossificans-like lesions have also been observed (220). Unlike the marrow space in OP, the marrow space remains intact but the cortex is thickened and dense, with a paucity of haversian canals. Mosaic lines may be prominent. Osteoclastic activity is inapparent whereas osteoblasts are present, but not in appreciable numbers. Endochondral ossification extends well into the zone of articular cartilage. Osteopoikilosis is an AD disorder in which bone islands form at the ends of a bone and in the vicinity of the metaphysic. Histologically, the foci are identified as rounded expansions of hyperdense bone with some mosaic lines. Multiple dermal fibrous papules in association with osteopoikilosis are the features of Buschke-Ollendorff syndrome.

Metaphyseal dysplasias (MTD) (group 9 in the ISDS Classification) comprise a genetically heterogenous group of disorders which are characterized by a failure in enchondral

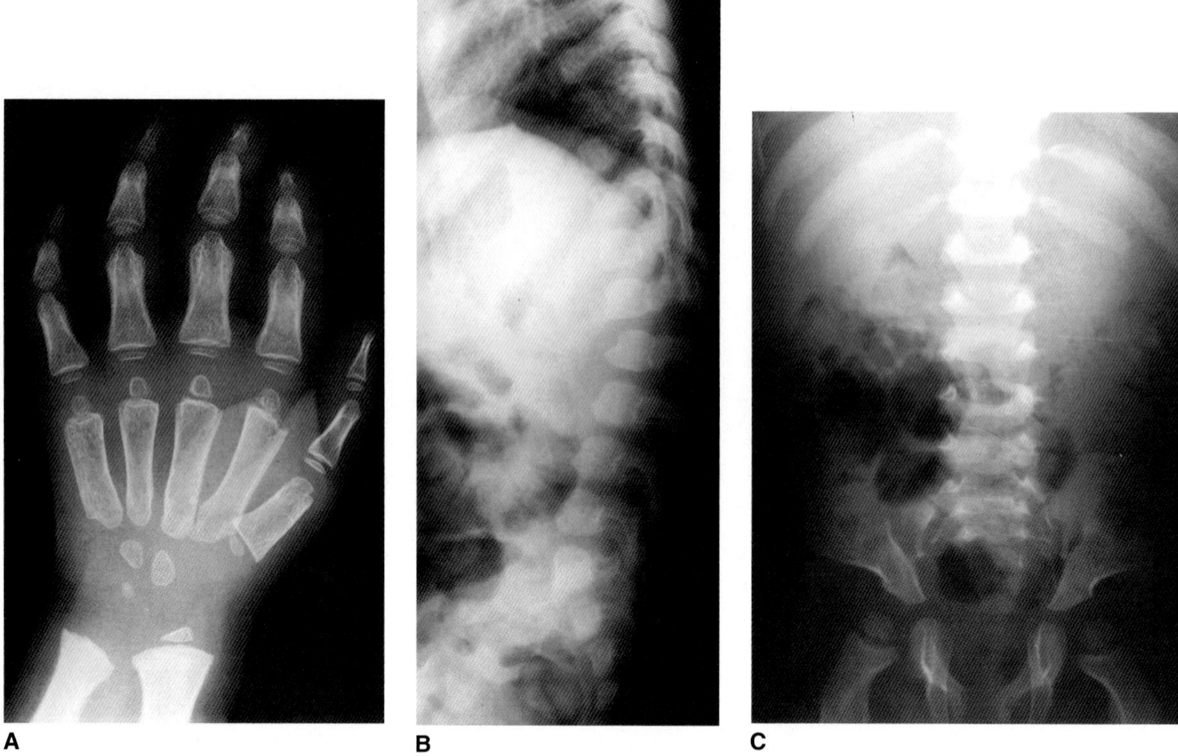

FIGURE 27-16 ■ Dyostosis multiplex congenita group (group 26) in radiographs of children with three of the specific disorders. **A**: A 7-year-old boy with Hunter syndrome demonstrates proximal pointing of the metacarpals, widening of the proximal phalanges, tapering of the distal phalanges, and poor carpal bone development. **B**: A 9-month-old boy with Hurler syndrome shows the gibbous deformity of the spine and anterior beaking of the L2 vertebra. **C**: This 2-year-old boy with mucolipidosis has underdevelopment of the superacetabular portions of the iliac bones, coxa valga, and widening and tapering of the lower ribs near the spine.

bone growth and remodeling of the end of the long bones with an Erlenmeyer flask-like deformity of the metaphysis with an increased diameter (193,642). The distal femur and proximal tibia are the most frequently affected sites. Other unrelated skeletal dysplasias may have similar deformaties.

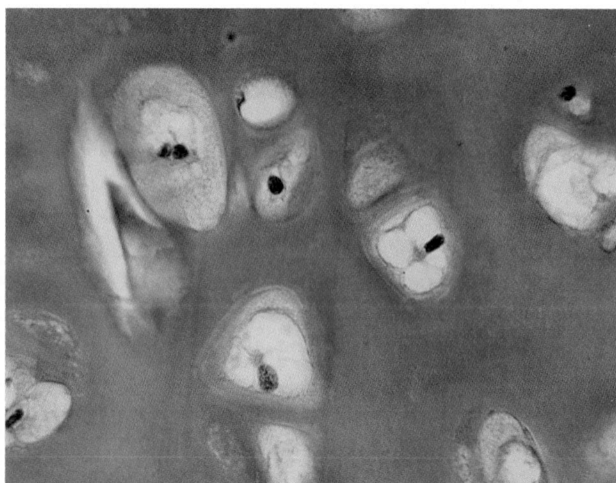

FIGURE 27-17 ■ Mucopolysaccharidosis, type 6 (Sly syndrome) is present in this 18-year-old male. This field shows several chondrocytes with distended, finely vacuolated cytoplasm.

Shwachman-Diamond syndrome, one of the four inherited bone marrow failure syndromes, is an AR disorder with an incidence of 1:75,000 births and 90% of cases have mutations in the SBDS gene (7q11) (174,431,468,544). Metaphyseal dysplasia of the femoral head is present in 50% of cases, but abnormalities in ribs (shortened with flared ends) can result in a hypoplastic thorax with lethal consequences in the neonatal period. There is an apparent failure in the formation of the zone of hypertrophic cartilage; however, a case has been reported with features of spondylometaphyseal dysplasia in a neonate with a SBDS gene mutation in which the hypertrophic zone was hypercellluar with minimal matrix extending into the metaphysis. Cartilage-hair hypoplasia (CHH, McKusick type) is one of four skeletal dysplasias with mutations in the RMRP gene (9p21-p13) (402,403). The incidence is 1:23,000 live births (471). Two other types of MTDs are the Jansen and Schmid types, the former has gene mutations in PTH/PTHrP receptor 1 (3p22-21.i) and the latter has mutations in the collagen 10 gene (COL10A1 on 6q21-22.3). Neonatal onset multisystem inflammatory disease (NOMID) is one of a family of inherited autoinflammatory syndromes which in the case of NOMID is the consequence of mutations in the CIAS1 gene (1q44) (5,171,274). This same gene whose pyrin-like protein regulates inflammation and the immune response is also mutated in Muckle-Wells syndrome with clinical similarities to NOMID. There are mass-like formations in distal femurs and/or proximal tibia, the common sites of MTDs. Progressive calcifications develop in these sites. The epiphyses are involved with bulging into the metaphyses. Poorly organized columns of chondrocytes are the rather nonspecific histologic features in the few reported biopsies.

Disorganized development of skeletal component group (group 28 in the ISDS Classification) constitute several tumefactive lesions of bone, some of which are familiar to pathologists including polyostotic FD, multiple osteochondromas (OCDs), or multiple hereditary exostoses (MHE), multiple giant cell reparative granulomas (GCRGs), and enchondromatosis with or without hemangiomas (611). These various tumor and tumor-like lesions are discussed in the subsequent section on neoplasms.

ACQUIRED DISORDERS

The major acquired disorders in children include infectious-inflammatory conditions involving bone or joint space, nutritional-metabolic conditions, and tumefactions of bone. Each of these three categories is related in the clinical differential diagnosis of a mass or swelling with or without pain and fever.

Metabolic and Nutritional Conditions

Vitamin deficiency disorders that have notable effects on the skeletal system include vitamin C or ascorbic acid deficiency, which causes scurvy, and vitamin D deficiency, which causes rickets-osteomalacia. At one time in the past, both vitamin deficiencies were found in infants.

Scurvy is characterized by a failure in the formation of the primary spongiosa, where the earliest recognizable bone formation at the growth plate takes place. The inability to form extracellular collagenous matrix is secondary to the loss of hydroxylation of lysine and proline, which depends on vitamin C as a cofactor. Rather than bone formation, fibroblastic proliferation with extravasation of red cells occurs, reminiscent of nodular fasciitis. Subperiosteal hemorrhage and microfractures through the metaphyses are other findings. The medullary trabecular bone is markedly osteopenic; these radiographic changes are found predominantly in infancy and early childhood. The radiographic findings in the long tubular bones include diffuse demineralization; some sclerosis and irregularity in the provisional zone of calcification, in part secondary to microfractures; metaphyseal spurs; transverse metaphyseal bands of diminished bone density ("scurvy line") with peripheral fractures ("corner sign"); epiphyses with marked central rarefaction and relatively sclerotic margins (Wimberger sign); and periosteal new bone. Swelling of the knees is a presenting sign, and metaphyseal microfractures and dislocation may be falsely interpreted as evidence of child abuse. However, the presence of severe demineralization together with lateral metaphyseal spurs and a dense irregular provisional zone of calcification makes differentiation relatively easy in most cases. Cupping of the epiphysis-metaphysis is a rare residual manifestation of infantile scurvy.

Rickets-osteomalacia is the consequence of deficient mineralization of bone matrix secondary to inadequate intake of calcium or a state of calciferol deficiency. Approximately 50 distinct disorders and conditions exhibit rachitic and osteomalacic features (221,397). In congenital rickets secondary to maternal vitamin D deficiency, elements of hyperparathyroidism are noted in the fetus in response to maternal hypocalcemia. A substantial proportion of the childhood cases of rickets-osteomalacia in the developed countries of the world are secondary to hereditary defects in vitamin D activation or phosphate reabsorption by the renal tubules (464). However, rickets has been seen in the United States and Canada in infants breast-fed for a prolonged period without vitamin D supplementation (69,413). In some parts of the underdeveloped world, calcium malnutrition in children is a cause of rickets. Malabsorption syndromes, chronic hepatic disease, and infantile OP in children are complicated by rickets-osteomalacia. Linear sebaceous nevus syndrome, hemangiomatosis of bone, nonossifying fibroma (NOF), osteoblastoma, and OS are some of the causes of oncogenic hypophosphatemic rickets-osteomalacia (110,201,531). The imaging and pathologic features of rickets-osteomalacia are discussed elsewhere. The radiographic appearance frequently differs according to the underlying disease. Infantile rickets is characterized by disruption of enchondral ossification and persistence of cartilage into the metaphysic (484). In undecalcified sections, the osteoid seams surrounding the bony trabeculae are widened and uncalcified (618). Myelofibrosis as a result of secondary hyperparathyroidism has been reported in an infant with vitamin D-deficient rickets.

Hyperparathyroidism in the pediatric age population is usually secondary to chronic renal failure (561,662). Primary hyperparathyroidism is seen in the neonatal period and is commonly associated with skeletal abnormalities and four gland hyperplasia (406,420). A classic but quite uncommon manifestation of hyperparathyroidism is the brown tumor, which has microscopic features overlapping with those of GCRG. Both osteoclastic and osteoblastic activity, often with medullary fibrosis, in a bone biopsy specimen should suggest the diagnosis of hyperparathyroidism. We have seen osteitis fibrosa cystica as an incidental finding in bone marrow specimens from children with chronic renal failure and anemia (see Chapter 21).

Pseudohypoparathyroidism (PHP) is an inherited disorder which is functionally characterized by peripheral characterized by resistance to PTH as a result of mutation in the imprinted gene, GNAS (20q13.3) (411). There are two subtypes of PHP: type 1a with maternal inheritance and the Albright hereditary osteodystrophy (AOH) phenotype (short stature, brachydactyly and extraskelatal osteomas in the dermis, subcutis and skeletal muscles and type 1b with paternal inheritance and AOH phenotype in the absence of the endocrinopathies. It has been noted that mutations in GNAS exons 1 to 13 are not present in all cases of PHP1a. Progressive osseous heteroplasia (POH) is another of the GNAS-inactivating mutation disorders with heterotopic ossification in the skin with extension into the underlying soft tissues whose onset may be seen in infancy or in later childhood (1,560,579). There is an absence of the AOH phenotype. In this respect, there is an overlap between PHP1b and POH. The formation of heterotopic bone resembles intramembrane bone with its direct development from mesenchymal-derived osteoblasts.

Primary hyperoxaluria 1 is an AR disorder with mutations in the alanine-glyoxlate aminotransferase (AGT) gene (2q36-q37) (144); AGT is responsible for the conversion of glyoxalate to glycine and in its absence glyoxalate is converted to oxalates which accumulate in the kidney and other organs including the skeletal system. Dense and lucent metaphyseal band develop in the tubular (long) bones are characteristic findings (179,486). There is depostion of oxalate crystals in the medullary space and osteoblastic and osteoclastic activity in the trabecular bone which reflects in part secondary hyperparathyroidism associated with chronic renal failure (see Chapter 5).

Tumor and Tumor-Like Conditions

Neoplasms and other tumefactions of the skeletal system comprise a largely unique clinicopathologic group of tumors which are generally restricted to the first two decades of life, but are seen in young adults and tend to diminish in frequency beyond the age of 40 years (646). OCD and OS account for 50% or more of all primary bone tumors in childhood whereas OS represents 8% to 10% of all cases (189,600,634,637). Over 50% of all benign bone lesions in children are OCDs. Almost 60% of all primary malignant neoplasms of bone in the same age group are OSs. The incidence of other primary skeletal lesions including bone cysts and FDs tend to increase in incidence throughout the first two decades of life. In a review of the experience of biopsy-proven bone tumors in children from the Dutch Pathology Registry, the incidence per million children between 10 and 18 years rose from 3.9 to 108 with a peak at 15 years of age (637). Primary bone tumors in the first 5 years of life are uncommon but some examples include Langerhans cell histiocytosis (LCH), melanotic neuroectodermal tumor of infancy (MNTI), myofibroma, chest wall hamartoma, ABC, hemangioma, and Ewing sarcoma-primitive neuroectodermal tumor (EWS-PNET) (354,423). The most common solid malignant neoplasm in the bone(s) of a child less than 5 years old is metastatic neuroblastoma (NB).

There are few areas in anatomic and surgical pathology in which the formulation of the differential diagnosis is so fundamentally important to the ultimate interpretation. For the pathologist, challenges and potential pitfalls encountered along the way to the correct diagnosis include the generally uncommon nature of these tumors and the often diminutive size of biopsy specimens, in some cases with associated artifacts, even to the point where the characteristic microscopic features of a specific entity are entirely absent. However, immunohistochemistry in a suspected malignant round cell neoplasm may rescue a diagnosis even in the presence of artifacts which have compromised the morphology. In many cases, especially in matrix-associated and "giant cell" lesions, a review of the skeletal images is imperative during the process of formulating a pathologic diagnosis that is reasonable and consistent with the imaging features.

In this section, our approach to pathologic diagnosis focuses on the principal histologic features(s) in a biopsy or resection specimen. Many lesions have mixed microscopic features, but in general, most skeletal tumors can be placed into one of three general morphologic categories: (a) osteoid and/or chondroid matrix-containing entities; (b) nonmatrix associated lesions with a spindle cell stroma, with or without giant cells and with or without cyst formation; and (c) round cell lesions with or without polymorphous features and an absence of matrix production in most cases.

MATRIX PRODUCING AND ASSOCIATED TUMORS

The overwhelming majority of benign and malignant neoplasms and tumor-like conditions of bone presenting clinically in the first two decades of life are matrix producing or associated tumors (159). Chondrogenic [OCD, chondroma, chondroblastoma (CHB), chondromyxoid fibroma (CMF)] and osteogenic (osteoma, osteoid osteoma, osteoblastoma) tumors account for 90% of all benign bone tumors in the first two decades and 80% of these lesions are diagnosed in the second decade of life; benign chondrogenic tumors alone comprise 60% to 70% of all benign tumors and the overwhelming of these are OCDs (189,650). The number of OCDs in our own files reflects the number of children who have had resections for MHE. Among primary malignant bone tumors in children, OS accounts for 60% to 70% of all cases; only 4% are chondrosarcomas (CSs). Approximately 20% to 30% of cases are EWS-PNET, but this figure can vary depending upon the relative proportion of Caucasian and African-American children in a particular population (152,192,439). According to United States Cancer Statistics for 2006 Childhood Cancers, primary malignant bone tumors represent 0.8 cases per 10^5 persons, compared to the incidence for leukemia and Hodgkin and non-Hodgkin lymphoma of 6.3 cases per 10^5 persons between the ages of 0 and 19 years (281).

In addition to the more common osteogenic and chondrogenic neoplasms, there are several other bone centered lesions which are familiar though uncommon in an epidemiologic sense, whose pathogenesis and nosology are somewhat ambiguous as in the case of the unicameral or simple bone cyst (UBC) and NOF (200). Some lesions are discovered incidentally and their imaging characteristics are virtually diagnostic to the extent that the pathologist may infrequently encounter them as a biopsy or resection unless some complication has occurred with surgical intervention like a pathologic fracture.

Osteosarcoma (OS) should be considered in the presence of any primary bone tumor in an individual between 10 and 25 years of age who has a radiologically poorly defined metaphyseal lesion with a mixed lytic and sclerotic pattern of permeative growth and cortical destruction in a long bone where the distal femur, proximal tibia, and proximal humerus account for 65% to 80% of all OSs (Figure 27-18); a contiguous mass in the soft tissues may or may not be present (Figure 27-19) (434,504). Less frequently, OS in children presents in the axial skeleton and head and neck region (155,216). So-called malignant osteoid, which has a fine, wispy, basophilic to eosinophilic appearance, may be inapparent or present as small extracellular eosinophilic deposits with or without obvious calcification or bone formation; it is often seen as deposits or strands around small groups or individual malignant round to spindle shaped cells (Figure 27-20). A biopsy may reveal only a high grade sarcoma composed of large rounded to epithelioid to spindle-shaped cells. Necrosis and hemorrhage without malignant osteoid can be suspected as representing OS since few other malignancies of bone or soft tissues in children have this constellation of high grade, pleomorphic features. Even in the presence of highly atypical, if not overtly malignant appearing cartilage, the tumor is more likely than not a chondrogenic or chondroblastic OS. The suspicion of OS can be corroborated in most cases by a review of the pertinent images with an experienced bone radiologist. Infrequently, an innocuous image may belie the obvious presence of an OS in a biopsy specimen. On the other hand, a highly destructive, osteolytic lesion may have imaging features more in keeping with EWS-PNET yet is an OS on biopsy.

OS of the "conventional" high grade type comprises 65% to 80% of cases in young individuals. These tumors typically arise in the medullary region with expansile and infiltrative growth through the cortex and directly into the soft tissues. A rare comparably high grade OS seemingly originates from the surface of the bone and has a circumferential growth in 50% to 60% of cases; these tumors often arise from the diaphysis of the femur or tibia (348,634). High grade OS displays other features including patterns of pleomorphic sarcoma, sheets of osteoclast-like giant cells resembling giant cell tumor (GCT) and/or nodules of malignant appearing cartilage (348). Malignant osteoblasts with epithelioid features

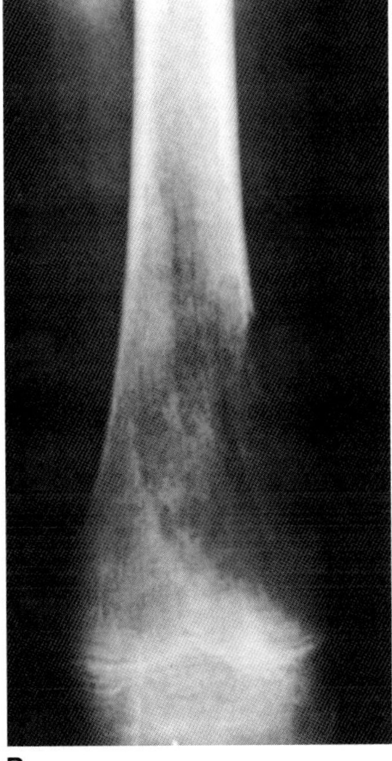

A B

FIGURE 27-18 ■ Radiographs of osteosarcomas in a 13-year-old girl and an 11-year-old girl show two patterns. **A**: Irregular poorly defined sclerotic lesion in the distal femur. **B**: Purely osteolytic lesion in the distal femur, which may be associated with hemorrhage and cystic changes in the telangiectatic variant of osteosarcoma.

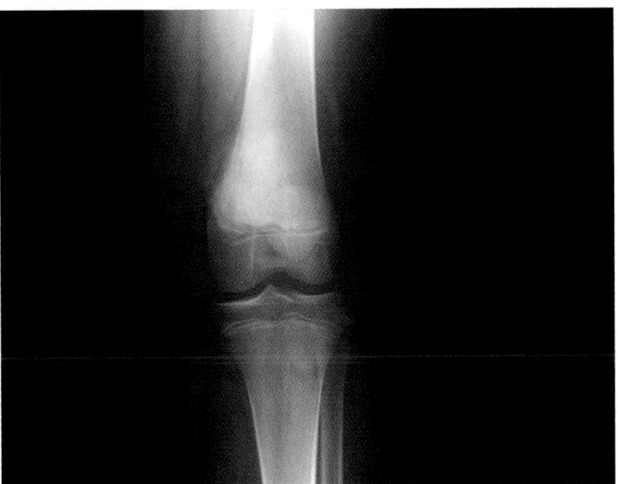

A

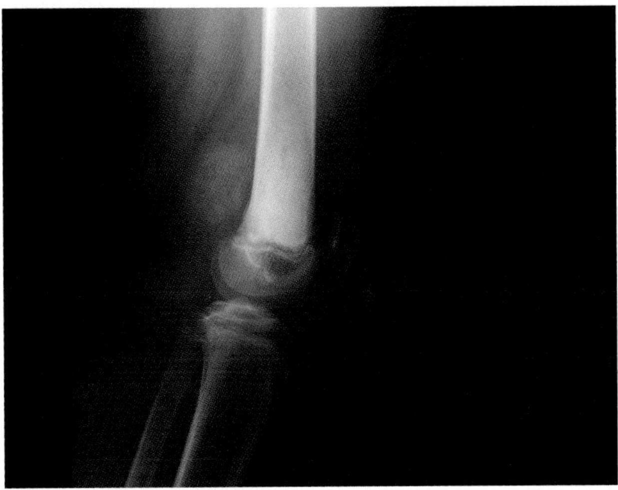

B

FIGURE 27-19 ■ Osteosarcoma presented in the distal femur of this 11-year-old female who presented with a history of pain in the area and a palpable mass. **A**: The anterior-posterior view of the distal femur shows the medullary sclerosis. **B**: The lateral view demonstrates the sclerosis and the suggestion of growth across the epiphyseal plate. There is a periosteal reaction with a prominent soft tissue mass.

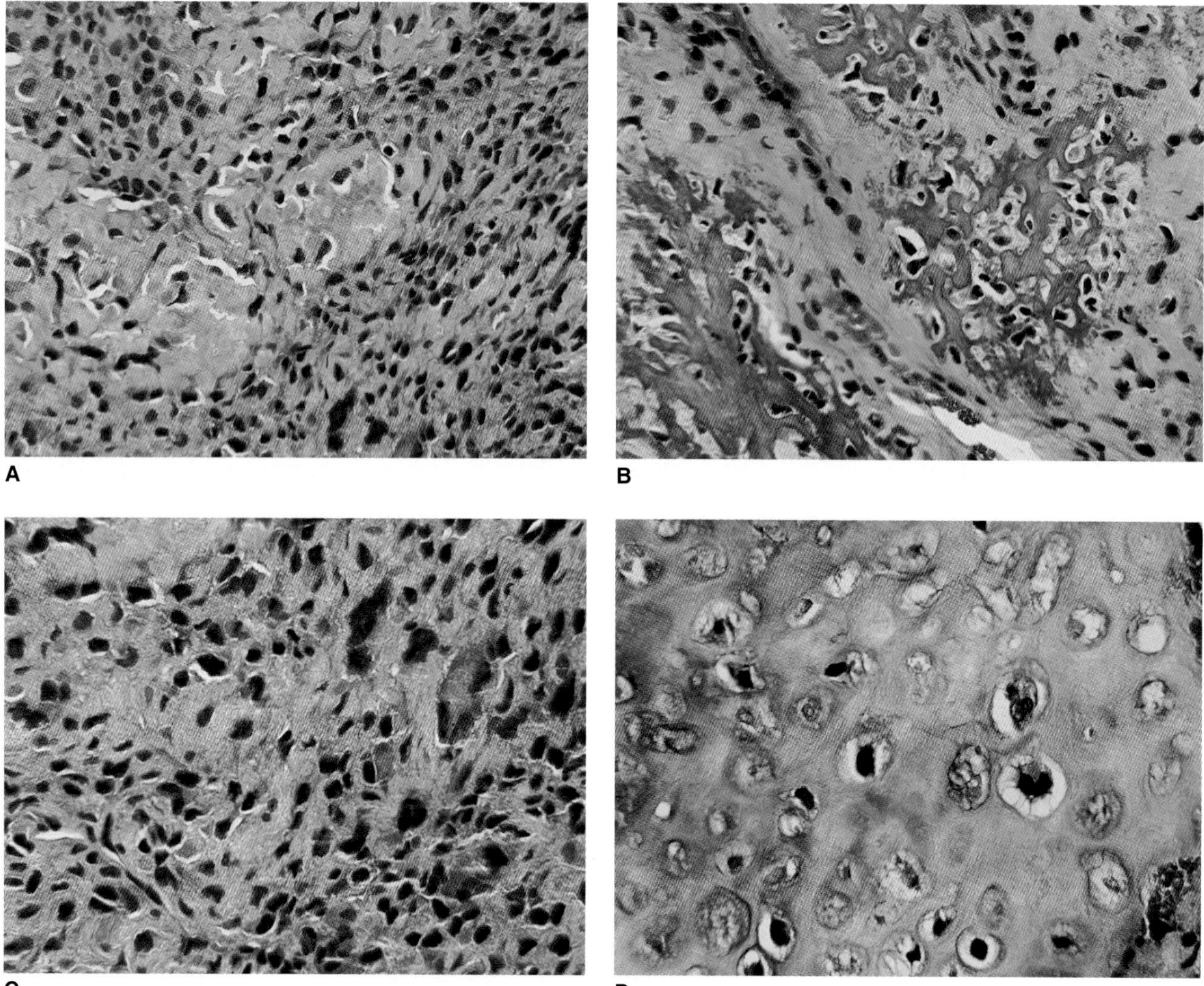

FIGURE 27-20 ■ Osteosarcoma of the distal femur in an 11-year-old female shows the several features, which is not unusual even in relatively small biopsies. **A**: This microscopic field shows the presence of high-grade malignant cells with nuclear hyperchromatism and a mixed population of ovoid and spindle-shaped cells. The appearance of the matrix may or may not qualify as osteoid. **B**: This microscopic field shows the presence of a lace-like pattern of formed osteoid with associated malignant osteoblasts. **C**: Another field contains high-grade malignant mesenchymal cells with pale staining matrix without clear osteoid formation. Tumor giant cells and atypical mitotic figures are also present. **D**: Another pattern of this tumor is the presence of malignant appearing cartilage with high-grade features. It should be kept in mind that classic chondrosarcomas are rare in children.

resembling rhabdoid cells are present as either isolated foci or a more diffuse pattern whose presence may be the source of a challenging differential diagnosis when "malignant" osteoid is inapparent. Additionally, unusual histologic patterns in conventional OS are those with osteoblastoma-like, CMF-like, clear cell, CHB-like, and pleomorphic (malignant fibrous histiocytoma-like) sarcoma-like features (33,200). Anaplasia and mitotic figures, often atypical, are present to a greater or lesser degree in most conventional OSs.

Dense osteoid formation rather than the more subtle intercellular eosinophilic matrix and appositional growth of "malignant bone" on the surface of nonneoplastic cancellous bone are common findings although less frequently observed in a biopsy, especially a small one.

The "nonconventional" OSs, representing 10% to 15% of cases, are represented by one of the following variants: telangiectatic, small cell, periosteal, parosteal, and low grade, central types (200,348,530,634). A predominantly lytic OS may have the telangiectatic features of an ABC, but anaplasia and pleomorphism of the mesenchyme within the septa are the diagnostic features and may be overlooked if the malignant cells are not uniformly distributed throughout the tumor or not sampled in a small biopsy. Pathologic fracture occurs in 40% to 50% of telangiectatic OSs at presentation and does not have the dire prognostic implications as once thought with improved management (658).

Small cell OS accounts for only 1% to 2% of all OSs and its differentiation from EWS-PNET of bone is the deposition of osteoid among the relatively monotonous rounded to subtly spindled cells; there is a degree of pleomorphism, mitotic activity, and cell size variation that helps to differentiate a small cell OS from a typical EWS-PNET (Figure 27-21) (454). The tumor cells in small cell OS are immunopositive for vimentin, but nonreactive for cytokeratin and only focal CD99 positivity if any reactivity at all. Small cell OS is a metaphyseal-based tumor with osteoid deposition in most cases.

Parosteal OS (3% to 4% of cases) is a markedly sclerotic tumor typically involving the distal posterior femur. A lobulated mass encircles the involved bone and may have a cartilaginous cap with OCD-like features. This variant is regarded as a low grade neoplasm but progression to telangiectatic OS is known to occur in small proportions of cases (32). The tibial diaphysis is the characteristic site of the periosteal OS (1% to 2% of all cases); this tumor, like the parosteal or juxtacortical OS, is associated with a more favorable prognosis than conventional type OS (Figure 27-22) (530). Low grade central OS (1% or less of all cases) is a neoplasm with imaging and microscopic features deceptively similar to those of FD (123,363). The spindle cell stroma, despite its bland appearance, shows a degree of mitotic activity that is not ordinarily encountered in FD. Intracortical or surface OS exists as individual reports of an otherwise conventional, high grade neoplasm (75,330,595).

In most cases, a segmental surgical resection is preceded by adjuvant chemotherapy, which affects the gross appearance of the surgical specimen (Figure 27-23) (34,127). An area of dense, intramedullary sclerosis and irregular trabecular islands of atypical appearing bone extend for some distance inferiorly and superiorly from the epicenter in the metaphysis is a common appearance of the treated OS which has had a positive response to chemotherapy. There is an "empty" quality to the focus of tumor with minimal cellularity (Figure 27-24). If the tumor is soft, friable, and hemorrhagic and has a viable-appearing periosteal and soft tissue component, it can be surmised that the tumor did not respond favorably to chemotherapy. After fixation and photography of the bisected specimen, grid-oriented sections should be obtained for semi-quantitative assessment of the effect of the chemotherapy on the tumor. Ablation of 90% or more of the tumor is considered a positive response. Another important parameter of

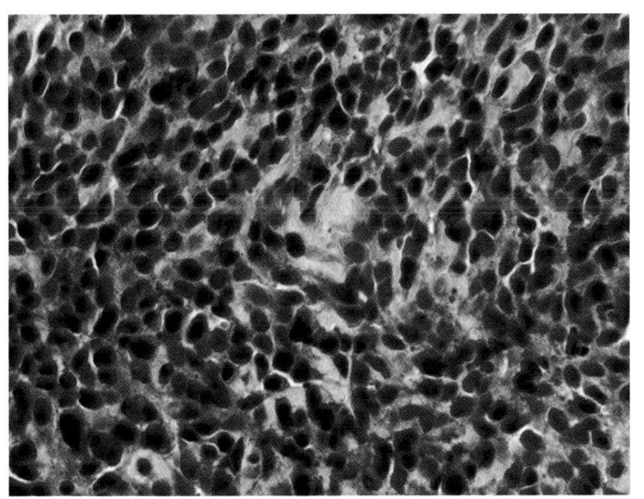

A

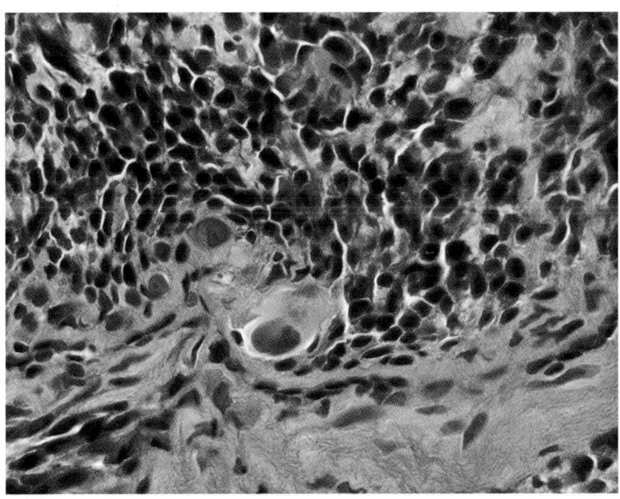

B

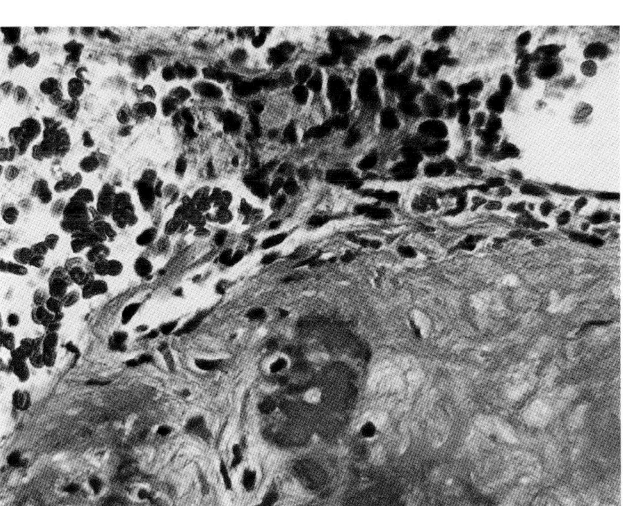

C

FIGURE 27-21 ■ Osteosarcoma presented in the distal femur of a 16-year-old male. **A**: Sheets of malignant round cells without apparent matrix were concerning for Ewing sarcoma-primitive neuroectodermal tumor. **B**: Large pleomorphic cells among the malignant round cells are unlikely findings in Ewing sarcoma—primitive neuroectodermal tumor whose presence should initiate concern about an osteosarcoma. **C**: Elsewhere the focal presence of osteoid confirmed the diagnosis of osteosarcoma with predominant small cell features or small cell osteosarcoma.

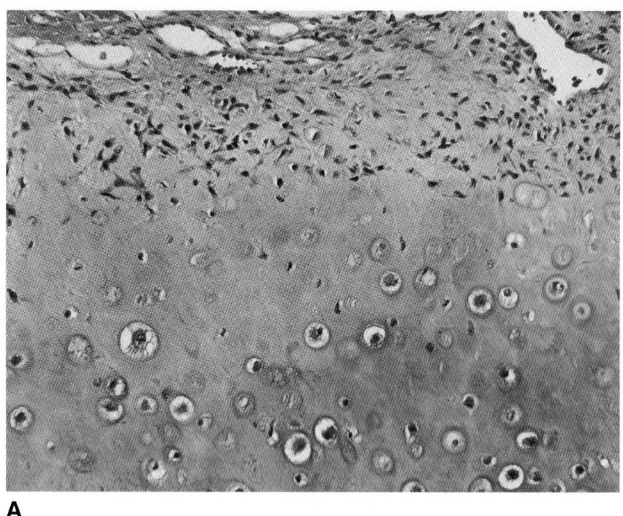

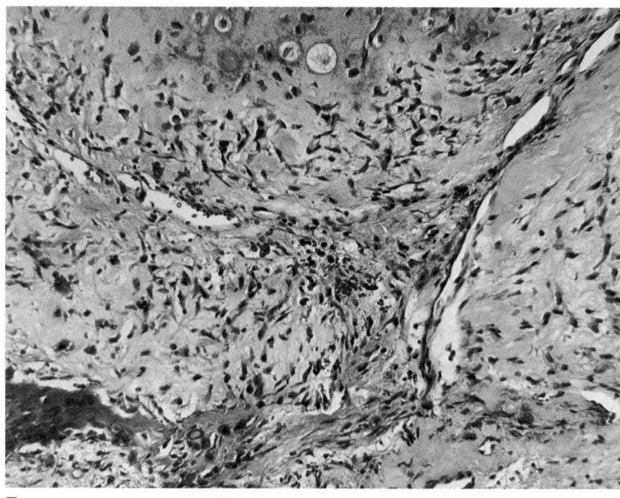

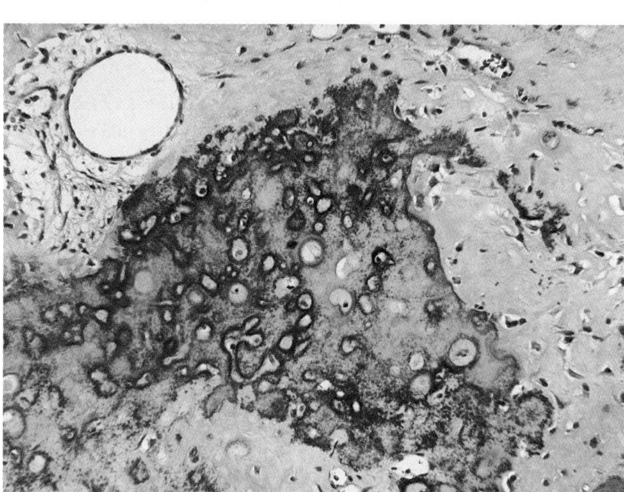

FIGURE 27-22 Osteosarcoma of the periosteal type presented in the diaphysis of the tibia in a 13-year-old female as a mass seemingly arising from the surface of the bone. This tumor type is still somewhat controversial because of its chondrogenic features. **A**: This microscopic field shows the surface of the tumor with a resemblance to an osteochondroma. **B**: Other areas of this tumor showed a multinodular growth pattern with spindle cell myxoid features. **C**: This focus shows the formation of malignant osteoid with the basophilic features resembling cartilage.

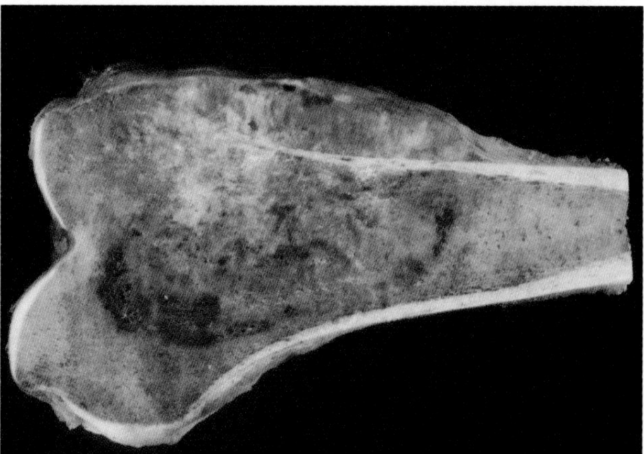

FIGURE 27-23 Osteosarcoma of the distal femur in a 17-year-old male is shown in this surgical resection specimen. The mass in the region of the metaphysis measures 9.5 cm in greatest dimension and has a firm, densely sclerotic almost marbleized quality. Most osteosarcomas, like the present one, have been resected after chemotherapy. The College of American Pathologists' protocol for the examination of bone tumor specimens should be consulted for details (see *Arch Pathol Lab Med* 2010;134(4):e1–e7).

prognosis which is optimally seen in the pretreatment images is tumor size or volume (72,375). Children with "larger" OSs have a poorer outcome than those with smaller neoplasms.

Approximately 45% to 50% OSs are diagnosed before 20 years of age and only 5% of cases are recognized in the first decade of life and only rarely in children under 5 years of age (396,547). By comparison, EWS-PNET is a more likely occurrence in the infant or young child. Most OSs are sporadic, but there are several hereditary diseases with a predisposition for OS including Li-Fraumeni syndrome (TP53 on 17p13.1), RECQL4gene (8q24.3) family syndrome (Rothmund-Thompson, Bloom, and Werner syndromes) and heritable retinoblastoma (RB1 on 13q14.2) (120,124,213,398). Approximately 3% of children with OS have the Li-Fraumeni syndrome. There may also be an increased risk for OS in association with Blackfan-Diamond anemia (388). RB and TP53 genes are inactive in OS cell lines whereas the RUNX 2 gene (6p21) is active (322,501).

Metastatic OS, most commonly to the lung(s) is present in 15% to 20% of cases at the time of initial clinical presentation;

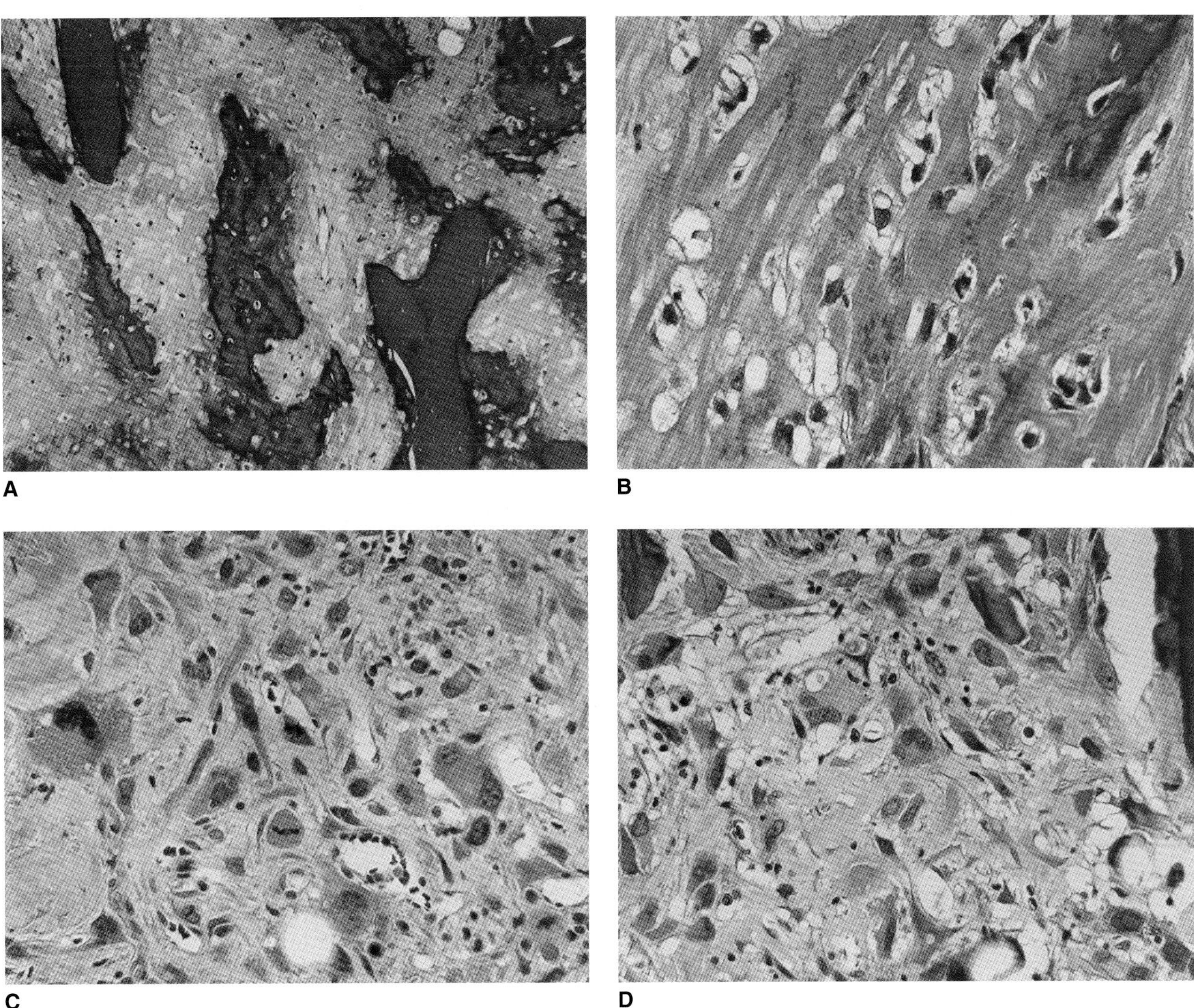

FIGURE 27-24▪Osteosarcoma in a postchemotherapy resection of the distal femur in a 17-year-old male has been examined thoroughly in order to judge the extent of viable tumor ablation. The sections require thorough decalcification especially in osteoblastic osteosarcomas and for that reason, the microscopic sections often have a pale eosinophilic quality. **A**: Acellular stroma and abnormal trabeculae identify this focus as largely ablated of any viable tumor. **B**: Another focus is composed of "malignant" appearing osteoid with atypical stromal cells. **C**: A focus of bizarre-appearing tumor cells and mitoses imply the presence of viable tumor. **D**: A comparison is made with the pretreatment biopsy demonstrates that there are apparent chemotherapy-related changes in the persistent tumor. There was less than 90% tumor ablation in this specimen and thus "a poor response."

there is an apparent association with osteoblastic histology which in turn accounts for the frequent presence of calcifications within metastatic lesions (331). Another pattern of presentation is multifocal skeletal lesions of OS without pulmonary metastasis in 1% to 2% of cases; the incompletely resolved issue is whether this phenomenon constitutes multifocal synchronous primary tumors or is a unique pattern of metastases (147,280). The presence of a dominant mass has argued for the metastatic theory. Yet another problematic lesion is the skip metastasis which is detected in 2% to 7% of cases of conventional OS. A skip metastasis is defined as a separate, small focus of OS in the same site as the primary tumor, in a second bone across a shared joint space, or in the distal portion of the involved bone (312,551). Regardless of the three scenarios of presumed metastatic OS, the clinical outcome is adversely affected. However, the overall prognosis of OS is now 70% from its earlier 5-year survival (393).

Osteoid osteoma and osteoblastoma are regarded as closely related benign osteogenic neoplasms which account for approximately 8% to 19% of all bone tumors in children (207). From the perspective of bone biopsies in children, osteoid osteoma and osteoblastoma accounted for 6% and 1.6% of all cases in one series (637). The microscopic similarities and examples of recurrent osteoid osteomas as larger, more locally aggressive osteoblatomas have served to support the hypothesis of a common histopathogenesis (67,446). Osteoid osteoma is the more common of the two tumors by a ratio of 4:1 overall, but in the first two decades, the ratio is 5:1 to 6:1, in favor of the osteoid osteoma (243). The male predilection is 2:1 to 4:1 for both tumors. These lesions are seen most commonly in the second decade; however, osteoid osteoma is more likely than osteoblastoma to present between the ages of 4 and 10 years although osteoblastoma is known to occur infrequently in quite young children (333,334,344). The blood supply and unique innervation of the osteoid osteoma may be responsible for the local pain (157,475).

The femur and tibia are sites of presentation of osteoid osteoma in 60% to 65% of cases, followed by the spine in 10% of cases (347,358). Beyond these preferred sites, osteoid osteoma is seen in the mandible, small bones of the hands and feet and even within a joint space (332). An intracortical ring of radiolucency surrounding the nidus, usually measuring 1 cm or less, is the typical imaging appearance of the osteoid osteoma, however, other imaging modalities, particularly computed tomography and may be required to identify the lesion since it is not apparent in plain radiographs in 25% to 30% of cases (Figure 27-25). In the long bones, there is a preference for the cortico-diaphyseal or metaphyseal location, but an osteoid osteoma may present in the medullary as well as in the periosteal site. In contrast to the osteoid osteoma, the osteoblastoma presents in the femur or tibia in only 15% to 20% of cases, but it has a predilection for the axial skeleton (60% to 65% of cases) and 5% to 8% of the tumors present in the head and neck region including the mandible, maxilla, skull, and orbit where the differential diagnosis includes juvenile ossifying fibroma (JOF) (309,458). The lumbo-sacral vertebra is the preferred site of presentation in the spine (31,60). A well-circumscribed, mixed sclerotic and lucent or predominantly sclerotic lesion with cortical expansion is the frequent plain view appearance of an osteoblastoma although sclerosis is not as common as it is in an osteoid osteoma (Figure 27-26) (360,395). Less often is the origin of an osteoblastoma from the medullary portion of bone. Cortical destruction and apparent expansion beyond the bone account for the aggressive appearance of an osteoblastoma. There may even be extension into a contiguous vertebra. On magnetic resonance imaging, increased signal intensity, interpreted as edema, is often noted both in the soft tissues surrounding the tumor and in

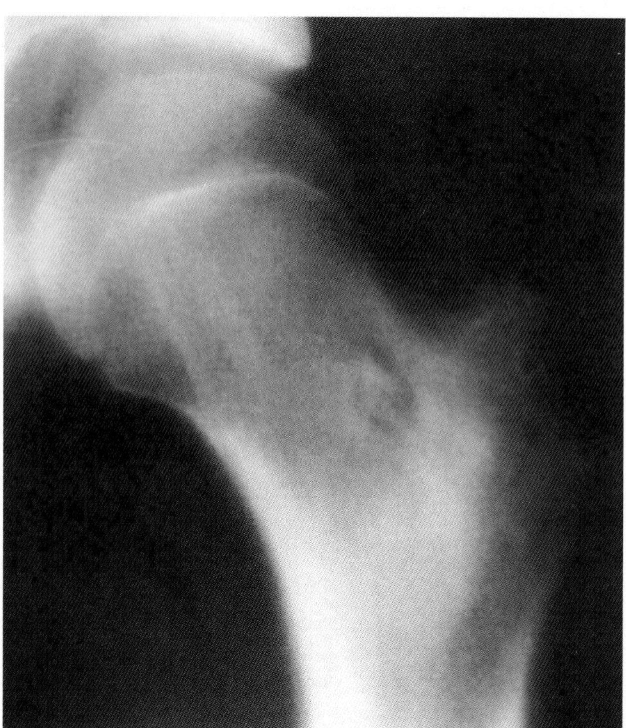

FIGURE 27-25 ■ Osteoid osteoma in the femoral neck of a 13-year-old shows a central, lucent nidus surrounded by sclerotic bone in this tomogram.

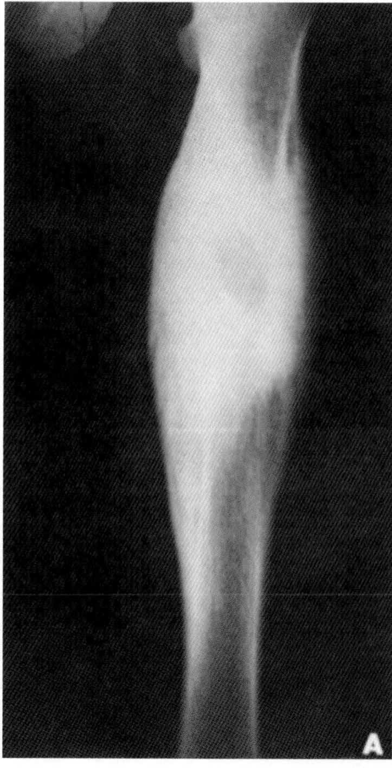

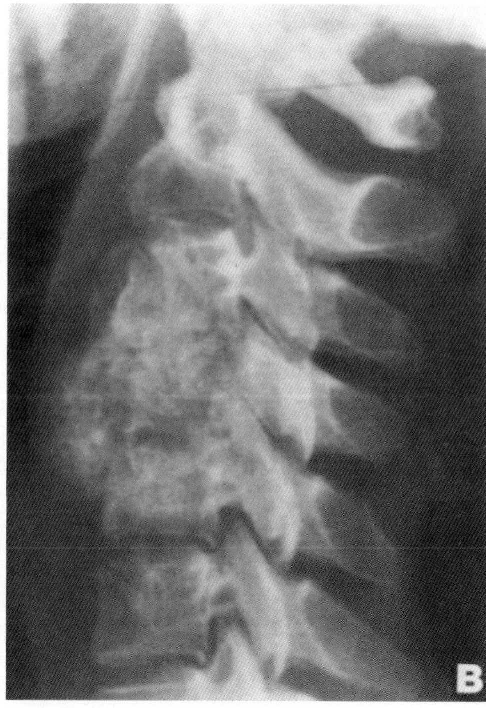

FIGURE 27-26 ■ Osteoblastomas generally have a benign radiographic appearance. Although most of the tumors are well circumscribed, approximately 25% appear poorly marginated so that a malignant process is suspected radiographically. **A**: A femoral lesion is shown with marked sclerosis. **B**: A lesion in the cervical vertebra is well circumscribed and composed of sclerotic and lucent areas.

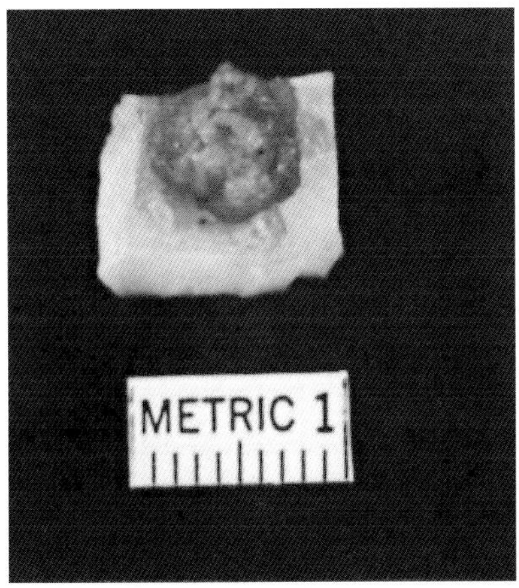

FIGURE 27-27 ■ Osteoid osteoma consists of an erythematous nidus surrounded by sclerotic bone. Very often, the specimen is fragmented, and the nidus is less apparent on gross examination. Current management of these lesions often yields minimal recognizable tumor.

the bone marrow proximal and distal to the lesion. The tissue reaction to an osteoblastoma may convey the impression of a larger tumor than is the actual case. Rarely is an osteoblastoma a multifocal tumor.

Pathologically, the nidus of the osteoid osteoma and the mass lesion of an osteoblastoma often have a hemorrhagic appearance, and both tumors are circumscribed and gritty with a surrounding zone of reactive-appearing sclerotic bone (Figure 27-27) (392). Although seemingly arbitrary, the principal distinction between the osteoid osteoma and osteoblastoma is the size of the nidus, which if smaller than 2 cm represents an osteoid osteoma and if larger than 2 cm is interpreted as an osteoblastoma (494). The nidus of both lesions is composed of a regularly irregular network of variably calcified osseous trabeculae which are accompanied by plump osteoblasts and some osteoclasts on the surfaces of the islands of osteoid (Figure 27-28). An inconspicuous or hypocellular fibrovascular stroma with multinucleated

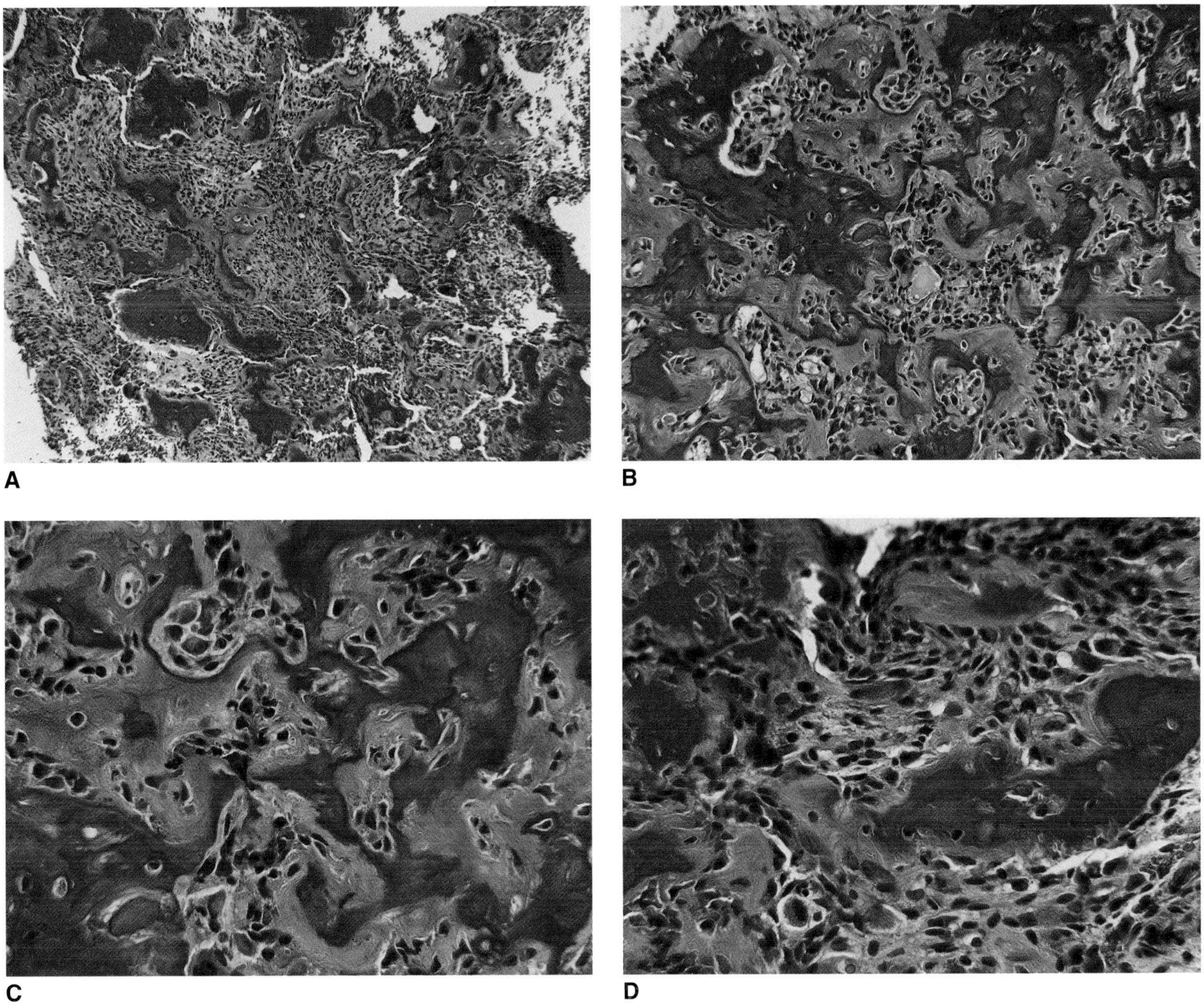

A B C D

FIGURE 27-28 ■ Osteoid osteoma in a 2-year-old male was identified in the right proximal tibia after he presented with pain in the area and fever. **A**: Bony trabeculae though varying in size and shape have an orderly appearance together and a uniformly cellular stroma in the background. **B**: The number of stromal cells is unevenly distributed in different fields. **C**: Some stromal cells are found in the background, and the bony trabeculae have a complex interconnecting pattern. **D**: In the more cellular foci, the osteoblasts and stromal cells show minimal cytologic atypia and mitoses are unapparent.

osteoclast-like cells is present in the intertrabecular spaces. The larger size and irregularly arranged osseous trabeculae of an osteoblastoma may lead to concern about an OS (481). However, the fine, lace-like osteoid and hypocellular, vascularized stroma importantly do not display the same degree of cellularity nor mitotic activity, or anaplasia of an OS. Plump epithelioid osteoblasts have been associated with the so-called aggressive osteoblastoma (Figure 27-29) (22). In most cases, the stroma is not especially cellular. Mitotic figures are present in limited numbers, but atypical mitotic figures and enlarged, pleomorphic and anaplastic cells should signal the likelihood of an OS. A chondroid matrix has been described in a minority of osteoblastomas (64). Osteoblastoma-like OS and malignant transformation of osteoblastoma exist as rarely reported entities (61).

Other osteoblastic proliferations with a resemblance to osteoid osteoma and osteoblastoma include reactive new bone, JOF, cemento-OF, and cementoblastoma. The latter three tumors are restricted to the mandible and maxilla. Juvenile (aggressive) ossifying fibroma and osteoblastoma have more similar than dissimilar microscopic features. Fewer osteoid osteomas are encountered in pathologic specimens given the minimally invasive procedures in vogue today which often yield small bony fragments with only a vague resemblance to an osteoid osteoma or any other diagnostic entity (225).

Osteoma is a benign osseous lesion whose histologic features are those of dense compact or cancellous bone with or without an accompanying osteoblastic or vascular component similar to an osteoid osteoma or osteoblastoma (243). There is almost exclusive involvement of craniofacial bones including the mandible and maxilla (323,372). The frontal sinus is the site of preference in some series where as in others it is the mandible (430). Only 5% or so of osteomas are diagnosed

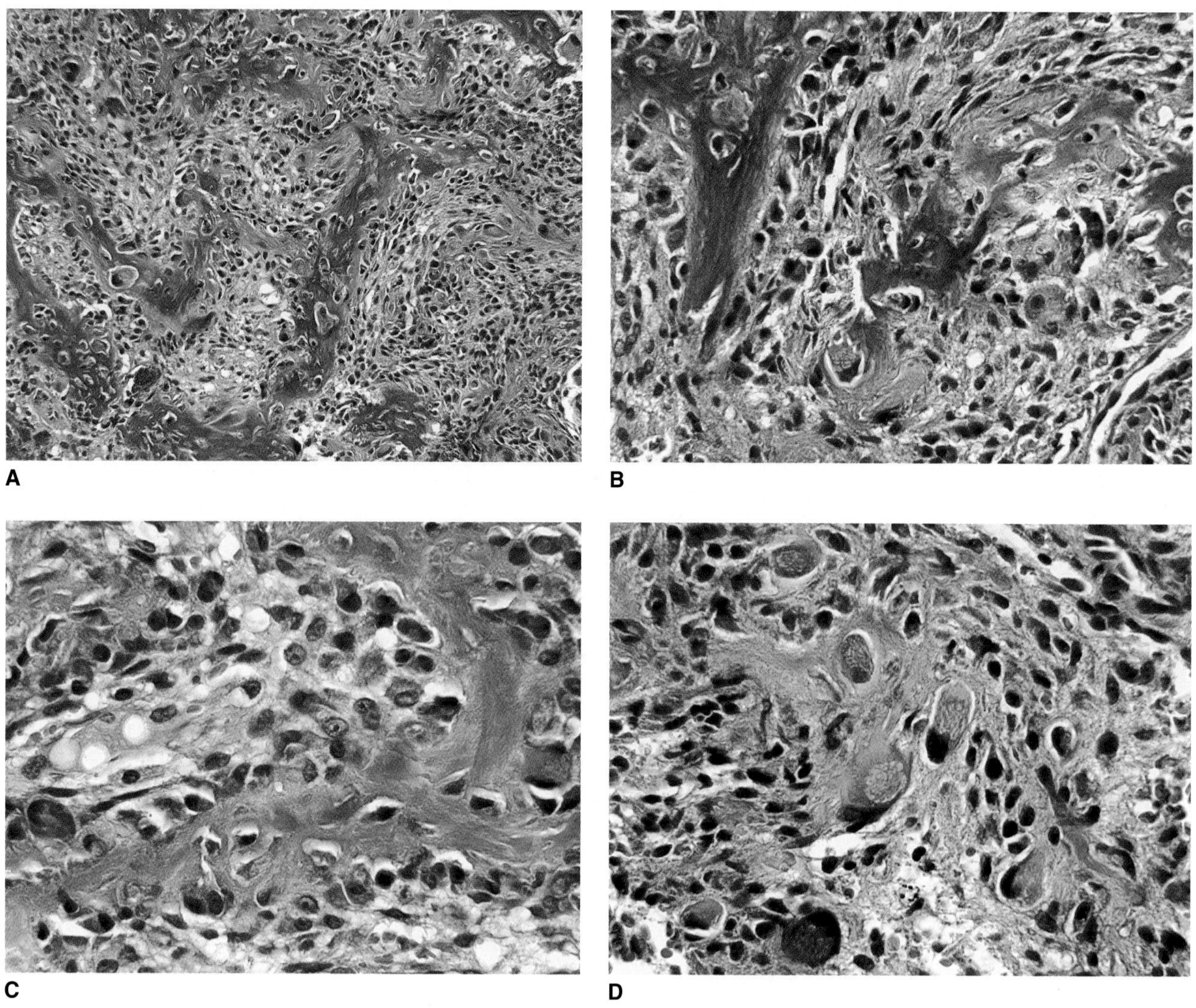

FIGURE 27-29 ■ Osteoblastoma presented in a 7-year-old male who developed pain in the hip. A 4-cm expansile medullary lesion was identified in the proximal femur. **A**: A mixed pattern of bony trabeculae with a regular pattern is accompanied by cellular stroma. **B**: Some bony trabeculae do not have osteoblasts. **C**: Other bony trabeculae are rimmed by polygonal osteoblasts. **D**: Epithelioid osteoblasts have abundant eosinophilic cytoplasm. Despite the cellularity of this tumor, anaplasia and mitotic figures are absent.

before 20 years of age. However, an osteoma may be the initial clinical presentation of Gardner syndrome in which case there are commonly multiple osteomas (10,617). Most osteomas are central with an origin from the cancellous bone and the remainder (peripheral osteoma) arise from the cortex.

Ossifying fibroma, osteofibrous dysplasia (OFD), and FD are the other osseous matrix associated lesions of children which have been collectively designated as "benign fibro-osseous lesions or tumors" (16,90,432,528,586). At least one of these, FD, is not regarded as a true neoplasm which may also be the case for OFD or OF of the tibia and fibula whose pathologic features overlap with those of congenital pseudarthrosis (CP) and adamantinoma (ADA). Because fibro-osseous lesions have a predilection for the facial and jaw bones, current classifications have tended to focus on maxillofacial fibro-osseous lesions which include the following three entities: (a) FD; (b) OF divisible into the three subtypes—conventional, juvenile trabecular, and juvenile psammomatoid; and (c) osseous dysplasia with four subtypes—periapical osseous dysplasia, focal osseous dysplasia, florid osseous dysplasia, and familial gigantiform cementoma (7,146,554). Osseous dysplasia is regarded as a hamartomatous lesion.

JOF includes the two distinct histopathologic patterns with psammamatoid or trabecular features (7,183). A rapidly enlarging mass whose radiographic features often depict a localized destructive process has come to be characterized as "aggressive" or "active" which is often incorporated into the diagnosis (308). It has been pointed out the trabecular JOF is seen more often in the mandible and maxilla whereas the psammomatoid JOF has a preference for the orbit and paranasal sinuses (Figure 27-30) (588). A fibroblastic stroma with islands of osteoid resembling cementicles or psammoma bodies (psammomatoid JOF) or a network of immature osteoid with prominent osteoblastic rimming merging with a spindle cell stroma are the two basic histopathologic patterns. The small well defined and smoothly contoured ossicles are distinct structures whose density can vary with the result that the compact spindle cell stroma is more or less prominent in the background of the psammomatoid JOF. The latter tumor is seen in a broader age group than the trabecular JOF which occurs in children less than 15 years old and even in those under 5 years of age (660). The maxilla is more commonly involved than the mandible. A large, locally destructive mass is composed of a vascularized, reactive appearing spindle cell stroma with some resemblance to nodular fasciitis and accompanying cellular osteoid forming trabecular profiles in the background (Figure 27-31). Both osteoblasts and osteoclasts are associated with trabecular osteoid. The presence of immature woven bone may raise the possibility of FD except for the osteoblastic rimming (Figure 27-32). Scattered typical mitoses in the stroma should not be viewed with concern. Incomplete resection can be followed by rapid re-growth or persistence for a period of time.

Hyperparathyroidism—jaw tumor syndrome is an AD syndrome with mutations in the HRPT2 gene (1q31.2), a tumor suppressor gene (261). In addition to hyperparathyroidism, JOFs develop in the mandible or maxilla in approximately 30% of affected individuals. There is also an increased risk for Wilms tumor and polycystic kidney disease. Another more generalized clinical setting in which psammomatoid JOF is reported in gnathodiaphyseal dysplasia (GDD); this AD syndrome is also characterized by bone fragility and sclerosis and bowing of tubular bones (629). The GDD gene has been mapped to 11p14.3-15.1

OFD presents as an expansile multilocated radiolucent lesion with sclerotic margins in the diaphysis of the tibia in a

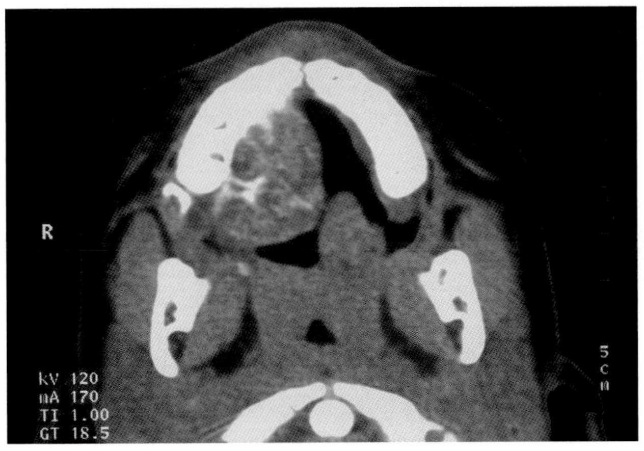

A

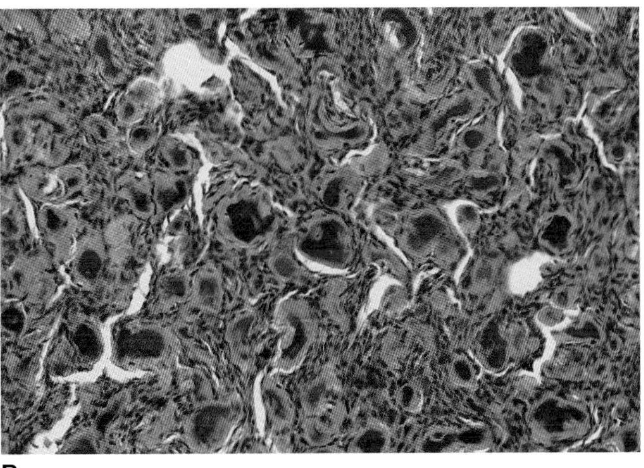

B

FIGURE 27-30 ■ Juvenile ossifying fibroma, psammomatoid type, is one of the two morphologic types. **A**: A well-circumscribed mass is present in the ethmoid sinus adjacent to the orbit in this computed tomographic image. These lesions have a mixed radiolucent and radiodense appearance. **B**: These tumors are composed of relatively uniform calcified ossicles, which have been interpreted in the past as cementicles giving rise to the designation of cementifying fibroma. The spindle cell stroma may be inconspicuous as in this microscopic field or as the predominant spindle cell pattern with fewer ossicles. (Contributed by Samir El-Mofty, DMD, PhD, St. Louis, Missouri.)

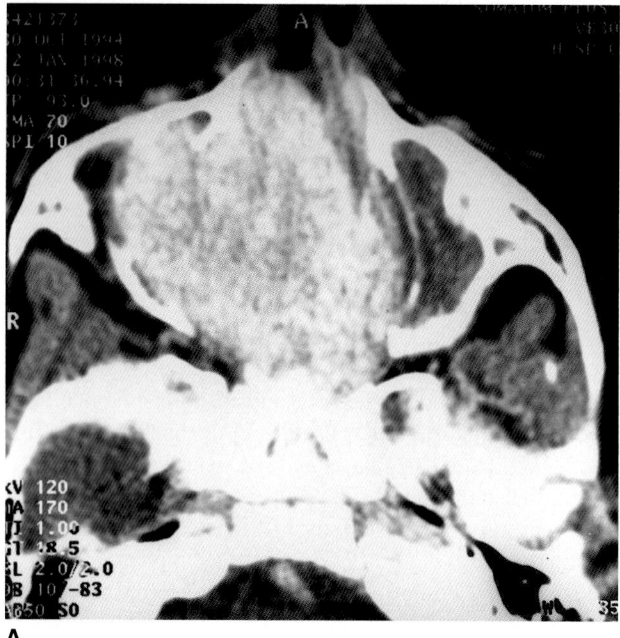

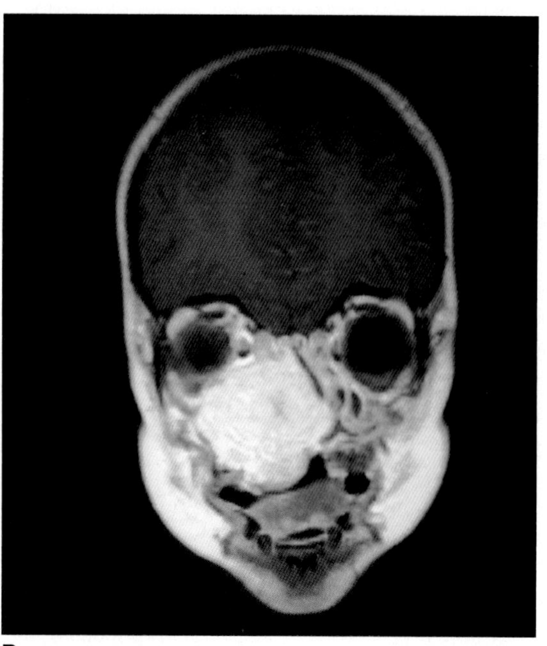

FIGURE 27-31 ■ Juvenile ossifying fibroma, trabecular type, presented in a 3-year-old boy as a rapidly enlarging mass filling the right maxillary sinus and depressing the palate inferiorly. **A**: Computed tomography shows the entire right maxilla and nasal cavity filled by a circumscribed, inhomogeneous mass. **B**: A frontal image shows the mass effect on the palate.

child less than 10 years old (Figure 27-33) (313,384,456,496). One still encounters the designation of cemento-OF or cementifying fibroma in the literature which has been largely superseded by the term OF. In addition to central OF arising within the bone, there is a peripheral OF that presents on the maxillary gingiva in the incisor-cuspid region, as a pedunculated lesion, typically measuring 2 cm or less and is diagnosed between 10 and 16 years of age. Calcified islands of bone are embedded in a variably compact spindle cell stroma.

FD is the most common of the fibro-osseous lesions of bone in children. In a biopsy series of bone tumors in children, approximately 6% of cases were FDs, whereas another series has shown as many as 10% of cases are FDs in children (637). Though discussed in terms of a bone tumor, FD is not considered a neoplasm but rather a localized defect in normal bone formation on the basis of somatic activating mutations effecting the stimulatory alpha subunit of G-protein on the GNAS gene (20q13.3) (119,508). The protein product of this

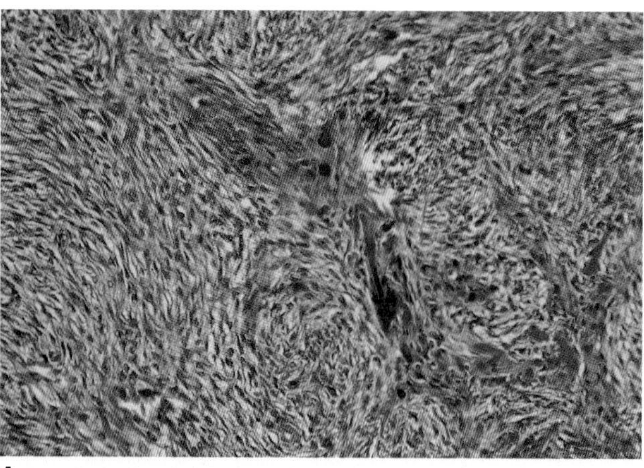

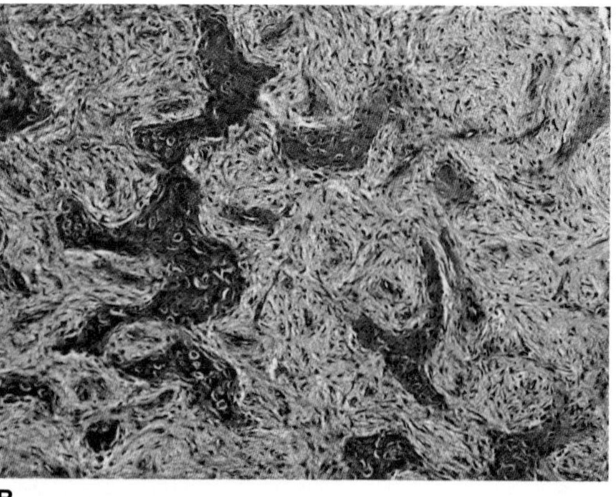

FIGURE 27-32 ■ Juvenile ossifying fibroma, trabecular type, occurs almost exclusively in children and is characterized by rapid and even locally aggressive expansile growth. **A**: The spindle cell stroma with the hint of osteoid formation in the background has a resemblance to the center of myositis ossificans and without the osteoid to nodular fasciitis. Mitotic figures may be identified without difficulty but are not atypical in form. **B**: Other foci are composed of immature woven bone, which is outlined in part by osteoblasts in a loose spindle cell stroma. Without the osteoblasts, there is a resemblance to fibrous dysplasia. (Contributed to Samir El-Mofty, DMD, PhD, St. Louis, Missouri.)

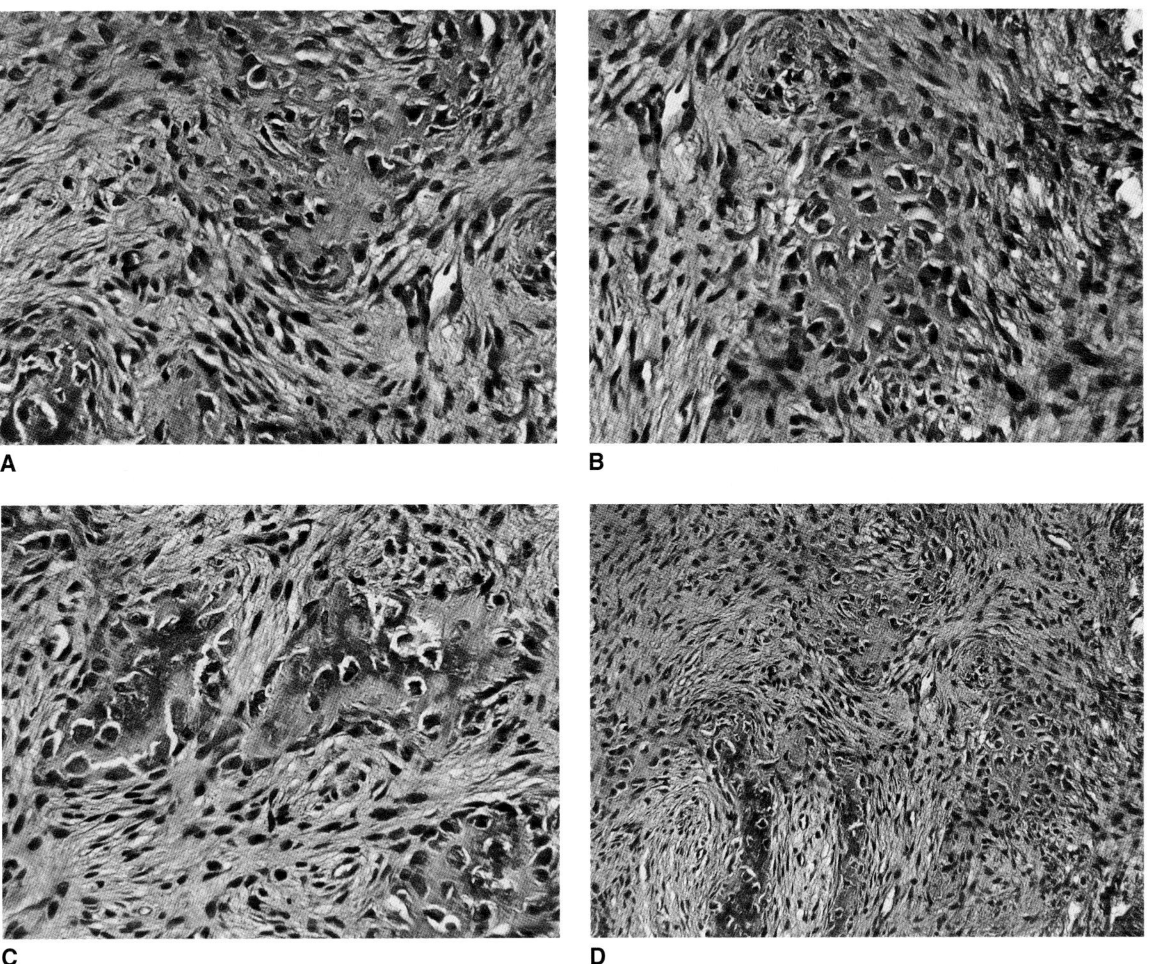

FIGURE 27-33▪Osteofibrous dysplasia of the tibia presented in the tibia of a 4-year-old male. The histologic features are somewhat variable in terms of the prominence of the spindle cell stroma and the focality of bone formation. **A**: The spindle stroma may only hint at the deposition of osteoid among the spindle cells. **B**: An adjacent focus demonstrates very early organization of bony trabeculae. **C**: This field shows bony trabeculae, which are outlined by osteoblasts. **D**: This lower magnification field shows an organizational pattern of spindle cells, osteoid formation, and bony trabeculae.

inprinted gene is an intermediate between receptor cuppling and cyclic adenosine monophosphate (cAMP) generation. Increased levels of cAMP result in defective osteoblastic differentiation. Somatic mosacism accounts for the highly variable expression in early development with differences in phenotype from solitary to multiple bone lesions and accompanying endocrinopathies including the McCune-Albright syndrome (MAS) (377). This accounts for the monostotic and polyostotic bone lesions with monostotic bone lesions in 70% to 80% of cases and the remainder as polyostatic lesions with more than one lesion in a bone or multiple bone involvement (142,166,495). Approximately 50% of cases of FD are diagnosed in the first two decades of life (294). The proximal femur, tibia, and ribs are the three most frequently involved sites, but craniofacial FD is the most common regional presentation in some series. FD of the proximal femur is one of the more common sites of pathologic fractures in children. The polyostotic presentation of FD may be recognized in the first decade of life with complications of severe bowing (so-called shepherd crook deformity in the proximal femur) and pathologic fractures. Various endocrine disorders with or without MAS and the Mazabraud syndrome have been reported in association with FD. The imaging features are those of a demarcated radiolucent or dense lesion within the medullary canal of the metaphysis or diaphysis. There is also the rare exophytic presentation (173). A so-called ground glass appearance is correlated with the density of woven bone spicules (307). These islands of immature woven bone of different sizes and shapes and devoid of osteoblasts are surrounded by a variably cellular fibrous stroma devoid of nuclear pleomorphism and mitotic figures (Figure 27-34) (535). There is an absence of osteoblasts in most cases and lack of differentiation to normal cancellous or trabecular bone. Polarization microscopy discloses the mosaic pattern of woven bone compared to normal bone. If an intramedullary FD-like tumor exhibits a sarcoma-like stroma and the radiographic features are not typical for FD, a well differentiated central OS is a possibility and likely accounts for

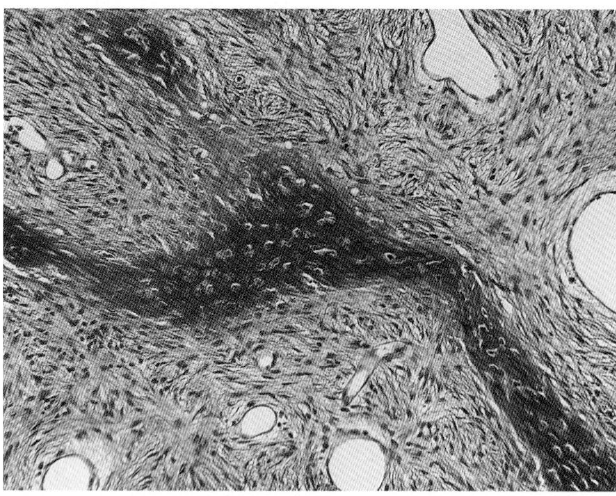

A

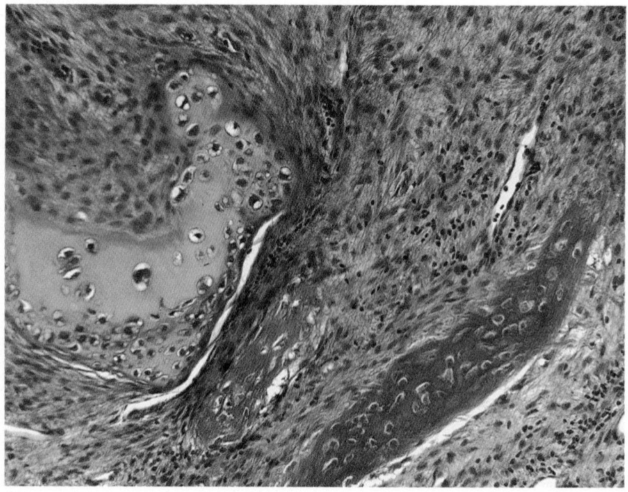

B

FIGURE 27-34■ Fibrous dysplasia presented in the femur of a 20-year-old male. **A**: Islands of woven bone with varied configurations are surrounded by a bland spindle cell stroma. **B**: Another feature is the presence of islands of metaplastic cartilage. (Contributed by Michael Kyriakos, MD, St. Louis, Missouri.)

those putative examples of sarcomatous transformation in a FD (545). However, stromal atypia in the absence of mitotic activity may be observed and is thought to be "degenerative" in nature much like the enlarged atpical cells seen in a schwannoma or leiomyoma (63). Hemorrhage and cystic changes with a resemblance to an ABC or a xanthomatous transformation of the stroma are other pathologic findings. Osteoblastic activity is inapparent in FD in long bones and ribs; however, in craniofacial lesions, osteoblastic activity is seen in some cases, to the extent that the distinction from other matrix-producing tumors, such as OF or osteoblastoma, may be problematic. Cartilaginous metaplasia in FD is a recognized feature most often seen in cases of polyostotic FD (367). The spindle cell stroma of FD expresses periostin as a reflection of c-FOS activation (329). When a fracture has occurred through FD, callus formation may cause concern for a more serious pathologic process, but the absence of pleomorphism and mitotic activity should dissipate some of the anxiety about a sarcoma. It is time to review the images with the radiologist.

Focal fibrocartilaginous dysplasia (FFCD), (fibrous periosteal inclusion) is not related to FD *per se*. The solitary FFCD lesion presents most frequently in the first 3 years of life as a varus deformity of the proximal medial tibia (310). A lytic lesion with sclerotic margins is the radiographic appearance. Dense fibrous tissue with or without associated cartilage and surrounding bone remodeling with osteoblastic and osteoclastic activity are the rather nonspecific microscopic findings.

Osteochondroma (OCD) of the solitary type is the most common benign cartilaginous tumor of childhood, comprising 70% to 75% of cases, followed by enchondroma (10% to 15% of all cases), CHB (10%), and CMF (2% to 5%) (540,559,634). Approximately 40% to 50% of all bone tumors in children are OCDs and it has been estimated that 0.5% to 1% of all individuals before the age of 20 may develop an OCD (542). The average age at diagnosis ranges between 10 and 15 years and there is a male predilection. Generally not included in a consideration of benign chondroid tumors are subungual exostosis, bizarre parosteal osteochondromatous proliferation of hands and feet (Nora lesion), and focal fibrocartilaginous dysplasia of long bones (see FD) (533). Brien et al. have comprehensively reviewed the entire range of cartilaginous tumors (93,94).

OCD in children present as a solitary tumor in 85% to 90% of cases and as MHE in the remaining 10% to 15%. A painless mass arising in the distal femoral or proximal tibial metaphysis in 55% to 60% of cases is the most common clinical presentation (343). The proximal humerus is the third most frequent site. One of the more common benign tumors of the rib in a child is OCD (Figure 27-35) (342). However, the OCD is ubiquitous in its distribution especially in the setting of MHE. The lesion, pedunculated or sessile, has a thin, translucent, bluish tinted cartilaginous cap. The stalk of cortical bone and its cartilaginous cap are in continuity with the underlying medullary bone (Figure 27-36). Microscopically, the cartilaginous cap and underlying region of enchondral ossification recapitulate the epiphyseal or growth plate (Figure 27-37). A periosteal OS also has a cartilaginous cap resembling that of an OCD, but the presence of an atypical appearing fibrous stroma in the intertrabecular spaces, rather than the fatty or hematopoietic marrow of an OCD, along with the imaging findings, are clues to the appropriate diagnosis. The differential diagnosis of OCD includes dysplasia epiphysealis hemimelica (Trevor disease) which presents as an asymmetrical enlargement of the epiphysis of long bones (solitary or multiple) in children between 3 and 15 years of age (35,232). Islands of cartilage with enchondral ossification are the microscopic features.

MHE is an AD disorder which is characterized by the presence of two or more OCDs. The incidence is 1:50,000 and is the most common inherited bone disorder (86). These

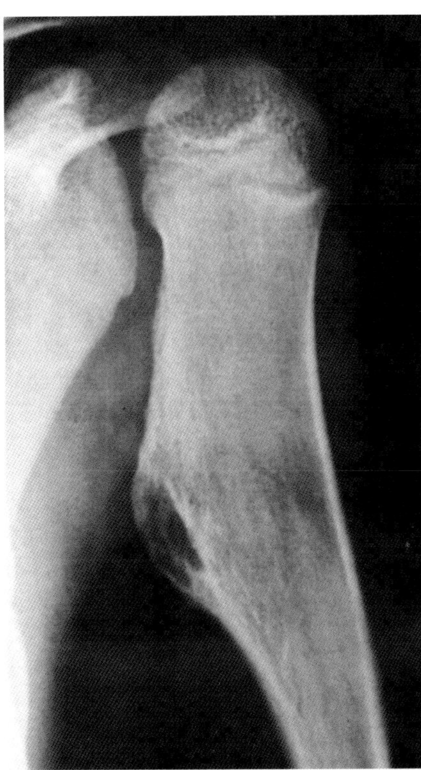

FIGURE 27-35 ■ Osteochondromas are either sessile, as in this radiograph, or pedunculated. The cortical bone and underlying medullary bone are in continuity.

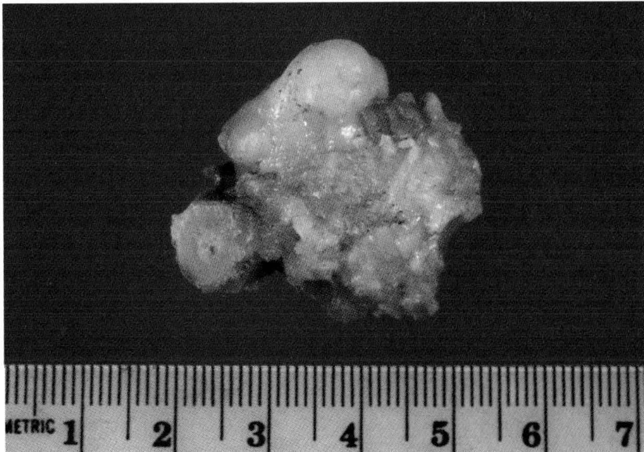

FIGURE 27-36 ■ Osteochondroma of the proximal humerus in a 13-year-old male shows a 3.5-cm mass with an irregular surface, which is particularly covered by a cartilaginous cap. Some concern was expressed about a chondrosarcomatous transformation but was not confirmed pathologically.

lesions develop earlier, 2 to 4 years of age on average, than the solitary OCD and are typically sessile rather than the pedunculated, sporadic OCD. Three genetic loci have been identified to date: EXT1 (8q24.1), EXT2 (11p11.2), and EXT3 (19p) (493,625). Malignant transformation, usually CS, is reported in 5% to 20% of those with MHE. Approximately 80% of all cases of hereditary multiple exostosis are linked to either EXT1 or EXT2. In the trichorhinophalangeal syndrome or Langer-Giedion syndrome, several dysmorphisms, including multiple exostoses, are associated with a hemizygous deletion in chromosome 8q23.3 to 24.11. One of the more serious complications of MEH is secondary malignant transformation of the cartilaginous cap; the incidence of CS ranges from 3% to 25% in MHE but 5% or less in the usual experience. A peripheral CS, in contrast to the more common central CS, should raise the possibility of MHE (507). Bilateral symmetric or unilateral sessile or pedunculated protuberances develop in the region of the tendinous insertions at the metaphyses of long bones (distal femur, proximal humerus, proximal tibia) (506). The small bones of the hands and feet may also be involved. The histologic features of an exostosis in MEH do not differ appreciably from those of a solitary lesion. Cystic changes in a

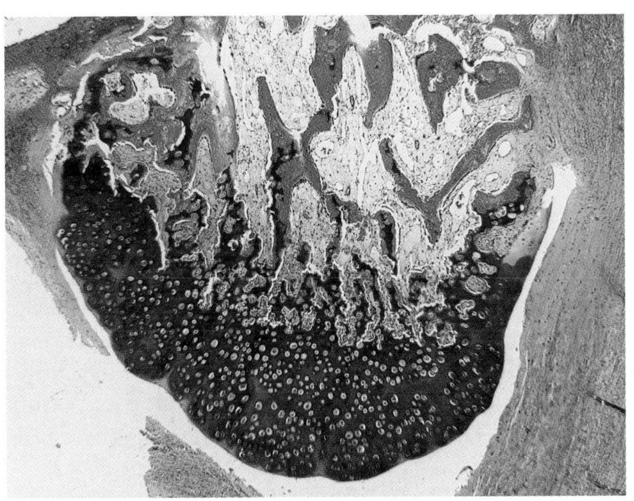

A

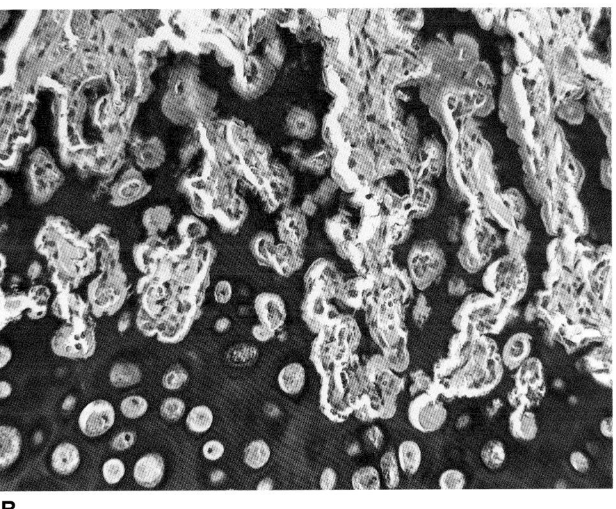

B

FIGURE 27-37 ■ Osteochondroma occurs as a sporadic or multifocal tumor. This tumor arose from the fifth metatarsal in a 17-year-old male with multiple hereditary exostosis. **A**: This tumor is one of several lesions and shows a sessile exostosis with the characteristic architecture of the growth plate associated with an osteochondroma. **B**: The irregular columnation of the chondrocytes and the retained cartilage are characteristic features.

cartilaginous cap with a thickness of more than 2 cm may indicate chondrosarcomatous transformation.

Chondroma presents as a solitary central intramedullary tumor in the case of an enchondroma, or less often as a periosteal or soft tissue based neoplasm (93,94,324). An enchondroma is infrequently diagnosed before the age of 8 to 10 years. The small bones of the hand, especially the phalanges, are the sites most frequently affected, and may present with a pathologic fracture. In the long bones or rib, the incidental finding of a radiographic abnormality—an expansile, sharply marginated radiolucency with punctuate and ring like calcifications—is the mode of detection of an enchondroma in 50% to 60% of cases (Figure 27-38). The small size (<4 cm) and well defined lobulated contours are the principal radiographic features differentiating a central enchondroma from the larger, low grade CS. The multifocal enchondromas of Maffucci syndrome and Ollier disease are defined in part by the presence of multifocal enchondromas (8,94,493,583). Other presentations of multifocal enchondromas include metachondromatosis or genochondromatosis (47,87,270,315). Some of these rare disorders are accompanied by exostoses (298).

Enchondroma is often submitted as multiple fragments of solid, blue-gray semitranslucent chondroid tissue intermixed with some cancellous bone from curettage. Nodules of hyaline cartilage show variable cellularlity without any accompanying fatty or marrow elements. In the long bones, the nodules of cartilage are often intermixed with marrow and cancellous bone. Secondary ossification is present when

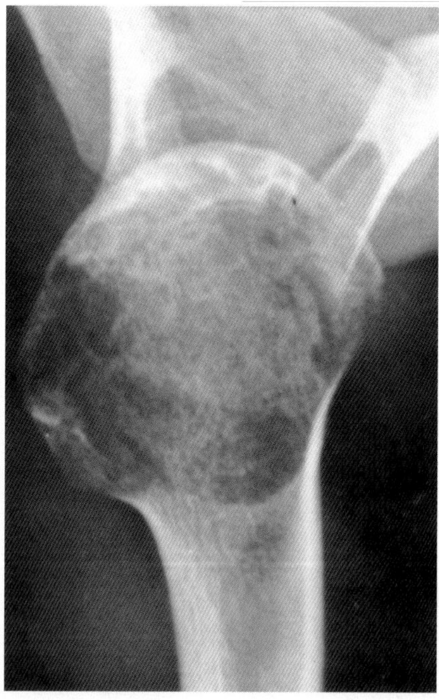

FIGURE 27-38■ Enchondroma is a central, expansile tumor with ring-like or punctate calcifications indicative of a cartilaginous matrix. Note the absence of cortical destruction and soft tissue extension and relatively small size and uniform distribution of the calcifications. These features are consistent with a benign, central cartilaginous tumor.

the tumor is located near the epiphysis (478,510). These tumors can be quite cellular but in the absence of cytologic atypia nor mitotic figures (Figure 27-39). It is acknowledged that the distinction between a low grade CS and enchondroma is based more on the radiographic than the histologic features. Periosteal chondroma occurs on the metaphysis of long bones, especially in the proximal humerus and less often the small bones of the hands and feet, in the second decade. A lobulated, cartilaginous mass measuring 1 to 4 cm in greatest dimension arising from the cortical surface and its growth may erode into the bone. Lobules of mature hyaline cartilage with calcification and ossification are the microscopic features. The fibrous periosteum is noted on the surface.

Chondroblastoma (CHB) is a neoplasm that could be considered equally well as a "round cell" neoplasm of bone because the chondroid matrix is not readily apparent in all cases. Only 1% to 2% of all primary tumors in children are CHBs, in contrast to chondromas which account for 10% of cases. In the first two decades of life, the average age at diagnosis is 12 to 15 years with 60% to 65% of all CHBs presenting before the age of 20 years (519,550). Males are more commonly affected than females. The epiphysis of the proximal tibia and humerus and distal femur are the preferred sites of presentation (Figure 27-40). Though representing only 5% to 7% of cases, CHB may arise in the tarsal bone, base of the skull, or temporal bone. Occasionally a CHB presents in the metaphysis. The tumor may be described by the surgeon as mucoid in texture and appearance. A fibrochondroid stroma with embedded polygonal mononuclear cells with or without calcifications, occasionally nodules of cartilage and osteoclast-like giant cells are the spectrum of histologic features; these features are not necessarily represented uniformly in any one tissue specimen or tumor (Figure 27-41) (630). The chondroblasts have features resembling those of Langerhans cells, including nuclear grooves. Mitotic activity may be prominent in the chondroblastic population but is of no particular prognostic importance. So-called chicken wire calcifications may occur in areas without an apparent chondroid stroma. Because of the substantial osteoclast-like giant cell component, CHB was originally designated as an epiphyseal GCT. Secondary ABC formation is another relatively common feature (Figure 27-42). The differential diagnosis of a CHB is LCH, GCT, and ABC. Like Langerhans cells, chondroblasts are immunoreactive for S100 protein but are CD1a negative. There is a CHB-like OS which should be suspected in the presence of substantial cytologic atypia and abnormal mitotic figures. Following curettage, the local recurrence rate ranges from 20% to 35%. There is a small risk for pulmonary metastasis to occur in the setting of one or more local recurrences.

Chondromyxoid Fibroma (CMF) is the other cartilaginous neoplasm with minimal matrix production. This uncommon neoplasm represents 1% or less of bone tumors in children (186). Fibromyxomatous lobules are typically interspersed by foci of multinucleated giant cells. Unlike

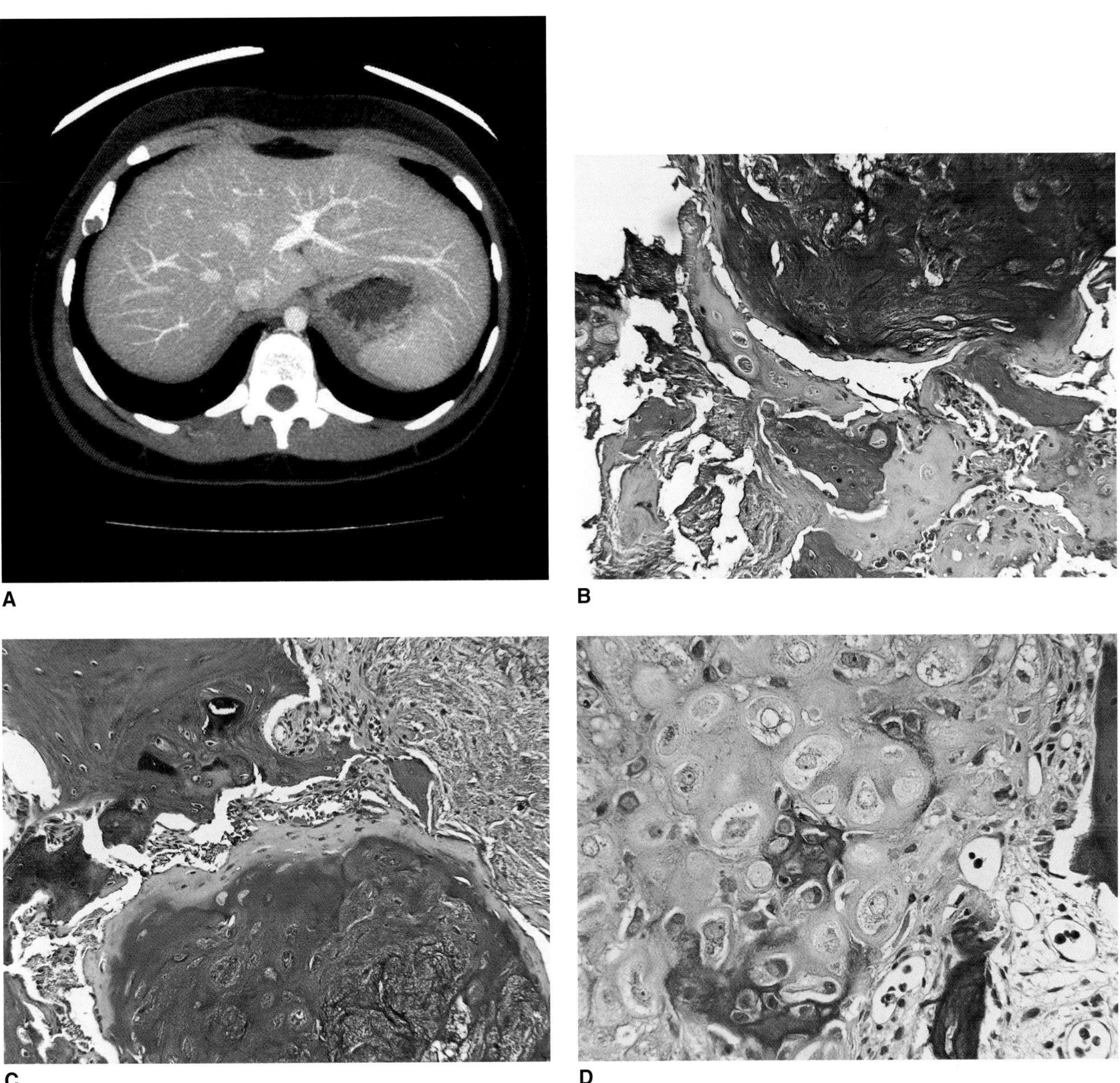

FIGURE 27-39■Enchondroma as its designation implies arises within the medullary portion of the bone and for that reason can be difficult in some cases to differentiate from well-differentiated chondrosarcoma but most cartilaginous tumors of bone in children arising centrally are examples of enchondroma. **A**: This central tumor arose in the 8th rib of a 10-year-old male. **B**: One of the essential features of an enchondroma is the growth through the intertrabecular spaces with expansion and infiltration. **C**: In this focus, the interaction between the neoplastic cartilage and bone is seen. **D**: Early enchondral ossification in a hypercellular focus of chondrocytes may cause concern about a malignant neoplasm; however, the chondrocytes in an enchondroma may show nuclear enlargement and atypia.

CHB, CMF exhibits a preference for the metaphysis (Figure 27-43). The tumor presents rarely as a juxtacortical or soft tissue lesion (414). Like CHB, it tends to affect the proximal tibia and other long bones, but CMF is also seen in the ilium and small bones of the hands and feet. Most tumors present in the second decade and it is rare to encounter a CMF in a child under 10 years of age (433). Most CMFs measure 4 to 5 cm, whereas the CHBs are generally larger. The margins are sharply defined from the adjacent sclerotic bone (667). Distinct lobulations are composed of fibromyxomatous stroma or have a fibrocartilaginous appearance (Figure 27-44) (673). The tumor cells are spindled to stellate rather than polygonal, as in CHB. The stromal cells of CMF are myofibroblasts to explain the fasciitis-like appearance. Giant cells are typically located at the interface between adjacent lobules and their numbers are variable from one tumor to another. Calcifications are uncommonly present in CMFs in children.

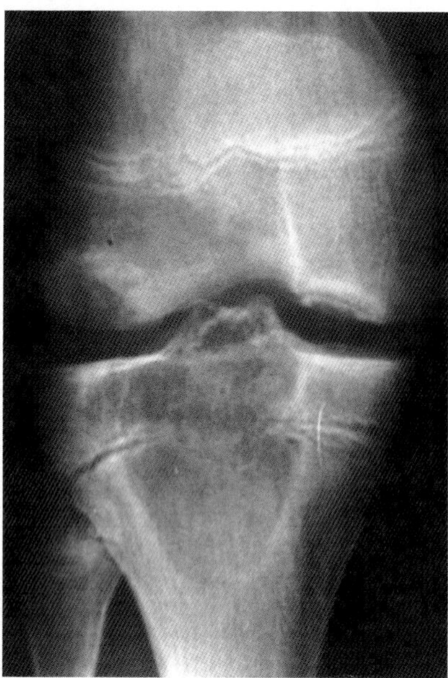

FIGURE 27-40 ■ Chondroblastoma in proximal tibia presents as a lytic, well-circumscribed defect in the epiphysis of a 17-year-old female.

Chest wall hamartoma (mesenchymal hamartoma or chondromatous hamartoma of chest wall) is a tumefaction of one or more ribs in young infants presenting as a mass with or without respiratory symptoms (Figure 27-45) (19,129). An expansile, intraosseous lesion measures 3 to 5 cm in greatest dimension and usually has a cystic and solid appearance (Figure 27-46) (247). Nodules of hypercellular hyaline cartilage and foci of enchondral ossification are separated by a spindle cell stroma with or without giant cells, with a resemblance to giant cell granuloma, and the blood-filled cysts have ABC-like features (Figure 27-47). The presence of woven bone imparts a similarity to FD. Local recurrence is uncommon, but is seen in those cases of incomplete resection. A seemingly comparable tumor is seen in the nasal-paranasal passages in infants or somewhat older children (427). There may be an association with pleuropulmonary blastoma of the lung.

Chondrosarcoma (CS) comprises 5% or less of all primary malignant skeletal tumors in the first two decades of life but approximately 25% of all such tumors when all age groups are

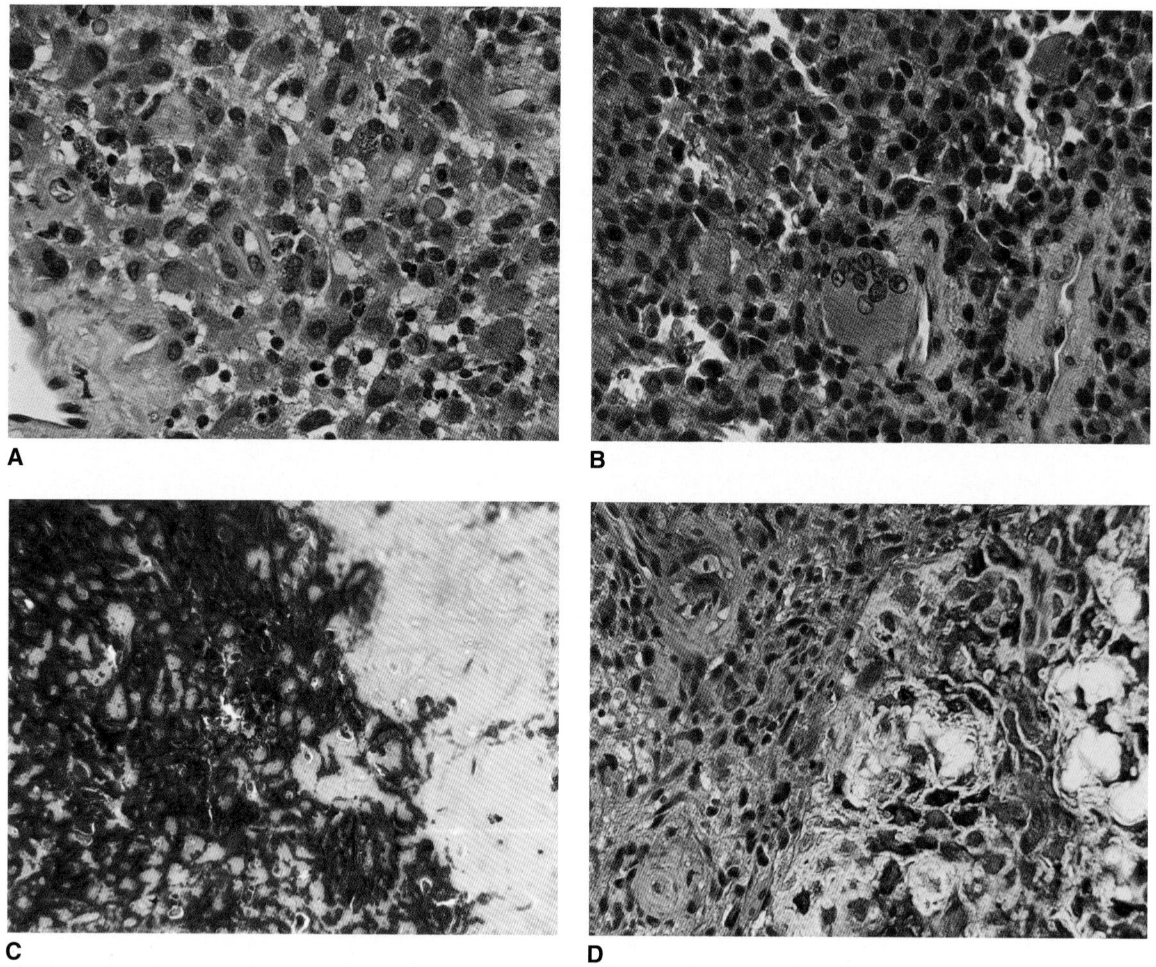

FIGURE 27-41 ■ Chondroblastoma can be a challenge in pathologic diagnosis because of its varied microscopic features. **A**: This field shows mononuclear cells with a resemblance to histiocytes or Langerhans cells. **B**: Multinucleated cells may be numerous to the extent that giant cell tumor is a consideration microscopically before the images are reviewed. **C**: This pattern of calcifications is helpful in the diagnosis. **D**: An island of tumor with a myxoid appearance is adjacent to a focus of more typical chondroblasts.

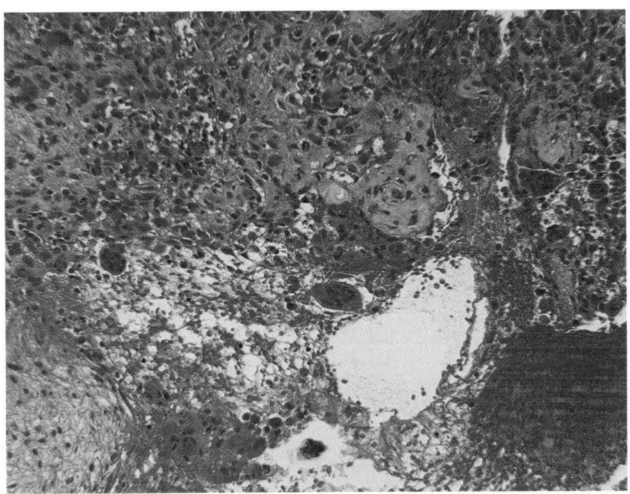

FIGURE 27-42■Chondroblastoma is commonly cystic and may be hemorrhagic. This field shows changes resembling those of aneurysmal bone cyst.

included. Most CSs of bone in children are sporadically occurring neoplasms except for those cases of peripheral CSs arising in OCDs in the setting of multiple hereditary exostosis in 0.5% to 5% of cases. Both enchondromas and CMFs can mimic CS microscopically. Malignant CHB is considered a type of CS; it represents less than 1% of cases. Conventional or central CS in the child, as in the adult, tends to develop in the proximal long and flat bones. The tumors are generally quite large and invade and destroy the cortex. The histologic features are those of a low to intermediate grade neoplasm in most cases, and if high grade or with dedifferentiated features, it may be necessary to consider whether the tumor is a chondroblastic or parosteal OS. Three subtypes of CS are recognized in children: clear cell, mesenchymal and myxoid; the latter two subtypes present as well in the soft tissues (288,684). Mesenchymal CS though accounting for only 4% to 5% of all CSs is the most common subtype in children with 25% to 30% of presenting before 20 years of age (455). The head and neck (skull, mandible, maxilla, and meninges), ribs and femur are the sites of predilection. The most important of the three variants of CS (mesenchymal, clear cell, and myxoid) in children in terms of frequency and a malignant small cell histology is mesenchymal CS. Approximately 25% to 30% of mesenchymal CSs are diagnosed before the age of 20 years in the skull, mandible, ribs, and femur (455). The pathologic features of mesenchymal CS are discussed in the soft tissue chapter (Chapter 24) as is myxoid CS. It is of interest that we have seen one example of myxoid CS in the metatarsal bone of an adolescent female whose tumor had a EWS breakapart (Figure 27-48). Clear cell CS constitutes only 1% to 2% of all CSs, but unlike most conventional CSs, this tumor occurs in the second and third decades of life with a predilection for the epiphysis of long bones, especially the proximal femur or humerus where it can be mistaken for CHB or GCT. Lobules of hyaline cartilage are occupied by sheets of chondrocytes with abundant clear cytoplasm. Small islands of woven bone may be interspersed among the clear cells. The presence of giant cells around lobules of cartilage can be mistaken for CHB or CMF.

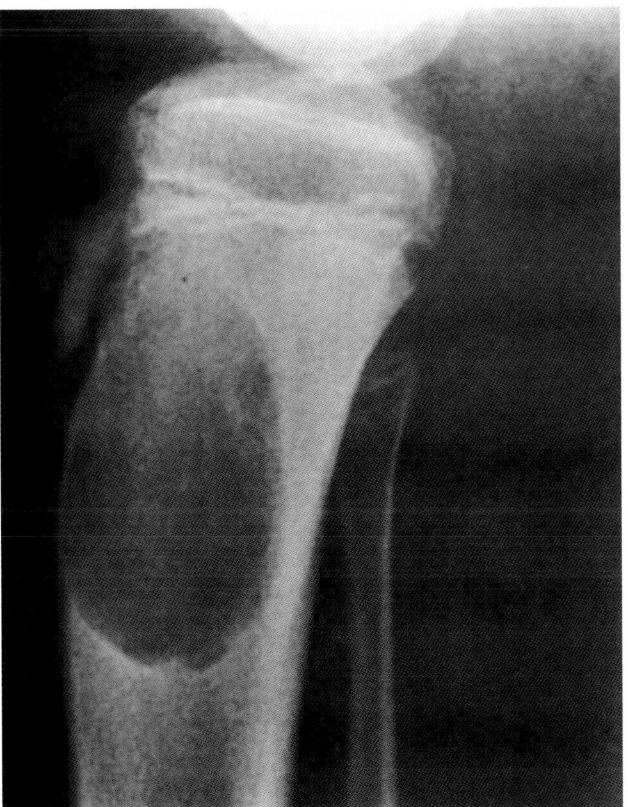

FIGURE 27-43■Chondromyxoid fibroma typically presents as an eccentric, purely lytic lesion in the metaphysis, as in this 9-year-old female with a tumor in the proximal tibia.

The pathologic diagnosis of CS in a child should be approached with caution and circumspection. When a biopsy of a bone neoplasm has features of high grade, malignant appearing cartilage, it is more likely than not that the tumor is a chondroblastic OS since even in children, the conventional CS has low to intermediate grade (grade 1 or 2) features. In the case of an enchondromatous neoplasm, the distinction from low grade CS is an acknowledged difficult and problematic differential diagnosis. Permeative growth through medullary bone is a reasonably reliable feature associated with CS in contrast to an enchondroma which is more circumscribed. A review of the images with a knowledgable radiologist is often rewarding.

NONMATRIX PRODUCING TUMORS AND CYSTS

Nonmatrix producing lesions, with or without giant cells with or without cyst formation, include a variety of benign tumors for the most part that in some cases may exhibit locally aggressive behavior (389). One pathologic subset comprises those lesions with giant cells and an accompanying stroma. The presence of giant cells in any osseous lesion may serve as a distraction in some cases with the consequence of overlooking the underlying pathology and diagnosis. In a wide

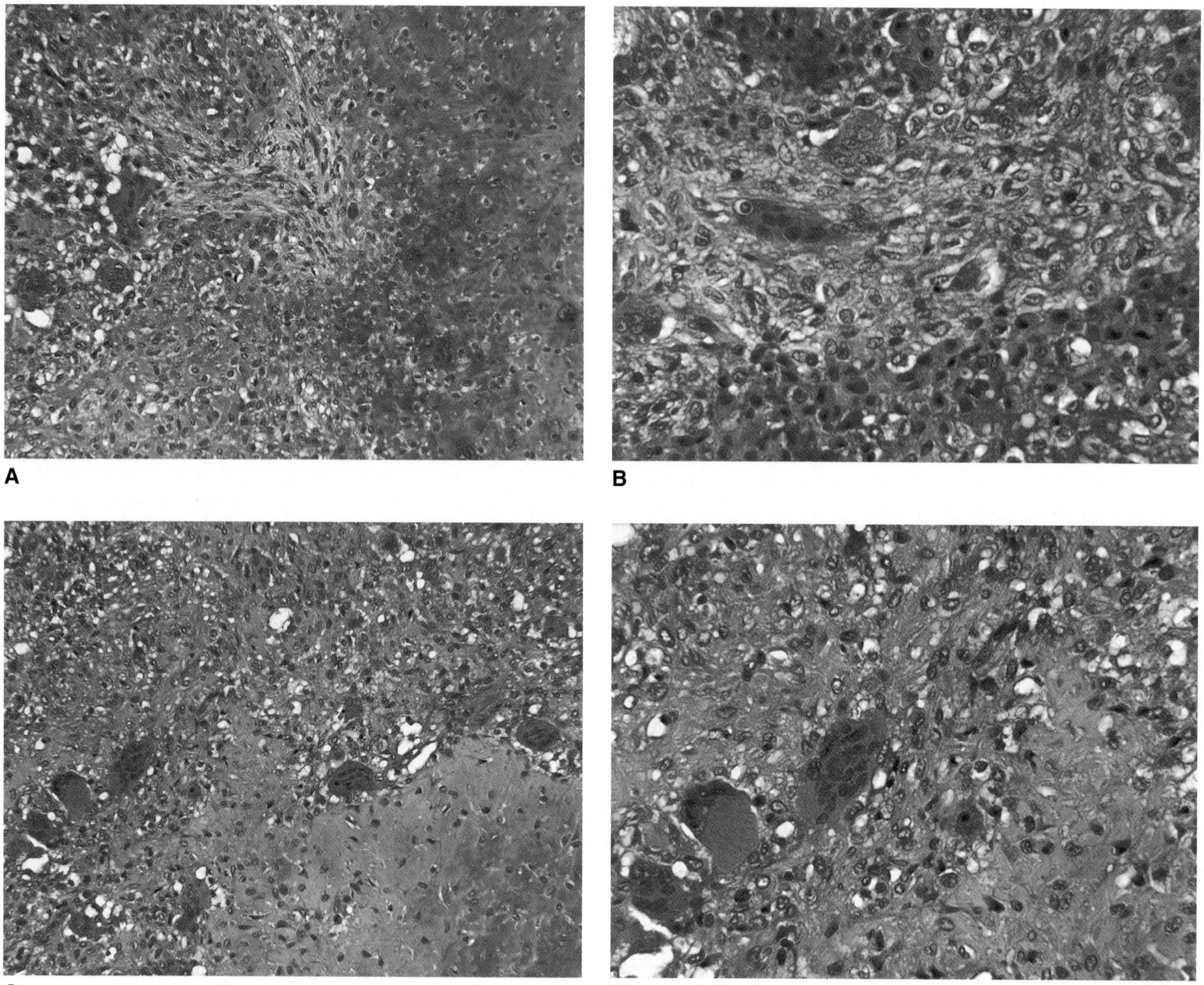

A B C D

FIGURE 27-44 ■ Chondromyxoid fibroma presented as a mass in the proximal tibia of a 14-year-old female. **A**: A chondroid focus is separated by a zone of cellular stroma and several osteoclast-like giant cells. **B**: A sheet of polygonal cells resembling chondroblasts is adjacent to stroma with osteoclast-like giant cells. **C**: Osteoclast-like giant cells are present at the periphery of a chondroid nodule. **D**: The three elements of this tumor are shown in this field: stroma, giant cells, and a portion of a chondroid nodule.

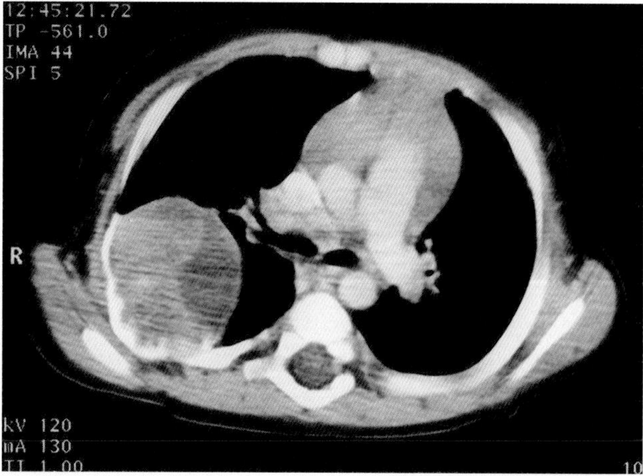

FIGURE 27-45 ■ Chest wall hamartoma in a 6-month-old male presents as a mass arising from the rib. More than a single rib may be involved as well as multifocal tumors.

variety of osseous lesions, osteoclast-like giant cells are a major or minor histologic component (Table 27-8). The giant cells may be the neoplastic elements or incidental to the pathologic process.

Giant Cell Tumor (GCT) comprises only 1% to 2% of primary osseous neoplasms in children and adolescents and because of their predilection for skeletally mature persons, they are quite uncommon in prepubertal children and for that reason are rare before the age of 12 years (428,505). An overall female preponderance of 1.5:1 is exaggerated in childhood, reflecting the earlier skeletal maturation of girls, who are more prone to the development of GCTs (276). The giant cells are formed through fusion of mononuclear cells of monocyte-macrophage derivation and exhibit osteoclastic differentiation. It should be kept in mind that most bone lesions in children are unlikely to be GCTs, especially in those 10 years old or less. The distal femur and proximal tibia

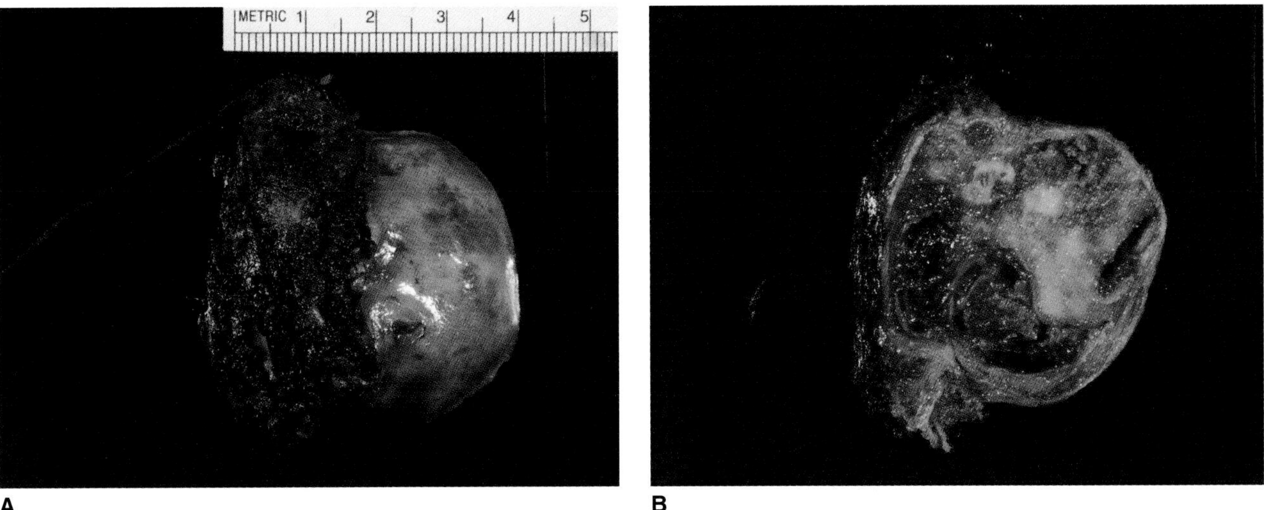

A B

FIGURE 27-46 ■ Chest wall hamartoma in a 3-day-old male presented with two masses arising from and involving several ribs. **A**: The external surface of the mass has the glistening appearance of cartilage. **B**: Cross section of this mass presents a varied appearance with cystic and solid foci with areas of apparent hemorrhage.

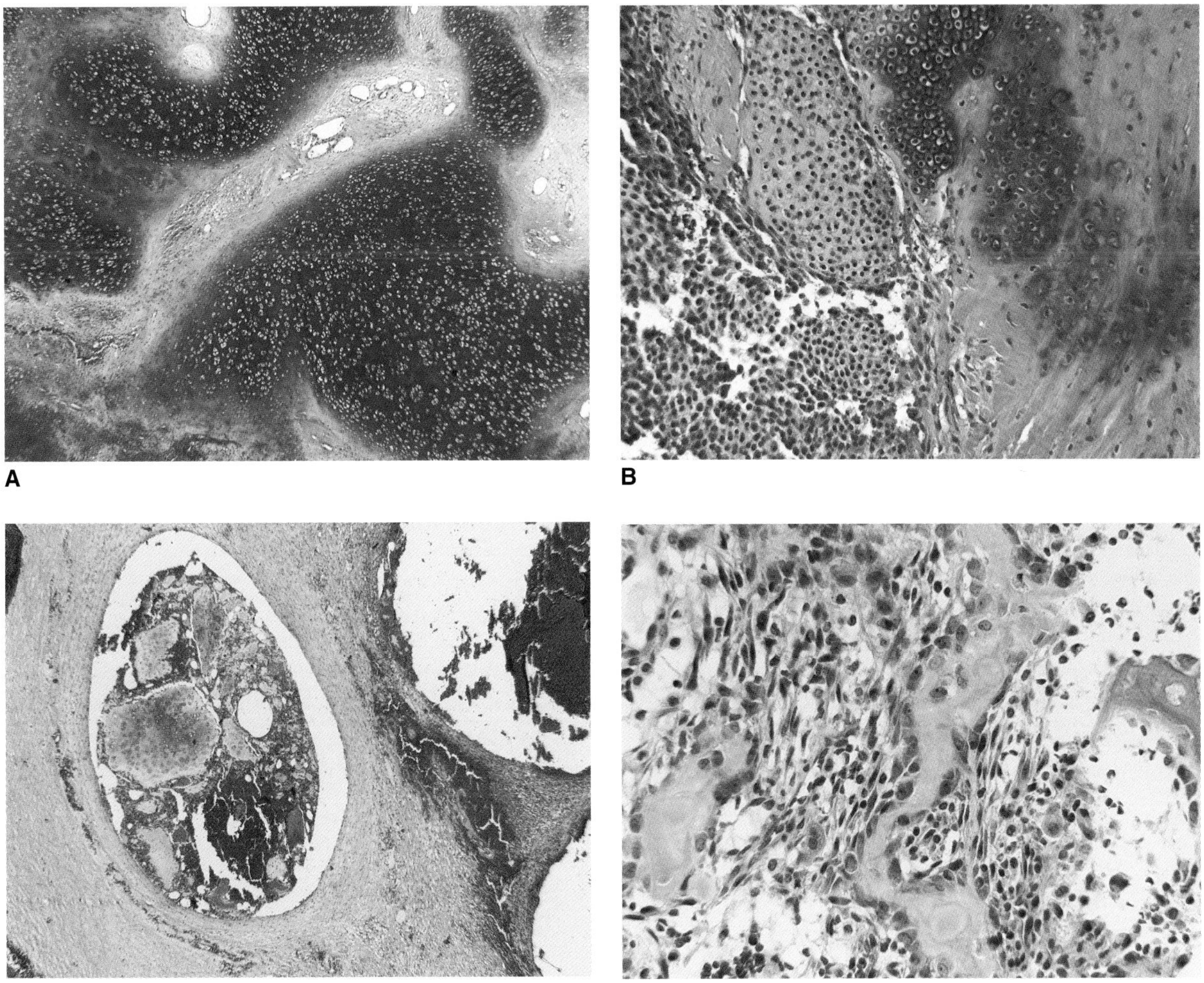

A B

C D

FIGURE 27-47 ■ Chest wall hamartoma has several patterns. **A**: Nodules of well-differentiated cartilage comprise a substantial portion of the solid foci. **B**: Other areas have a bimorphic pattern of cartilage and polygonal cells with a resemblance to chondroblasts. **C**: Cystic and hemorrhagic foci have features of aneurysmal bone cyst. **D**: Another pattern is represented by bony trabeculae with osteoblastic rimming.

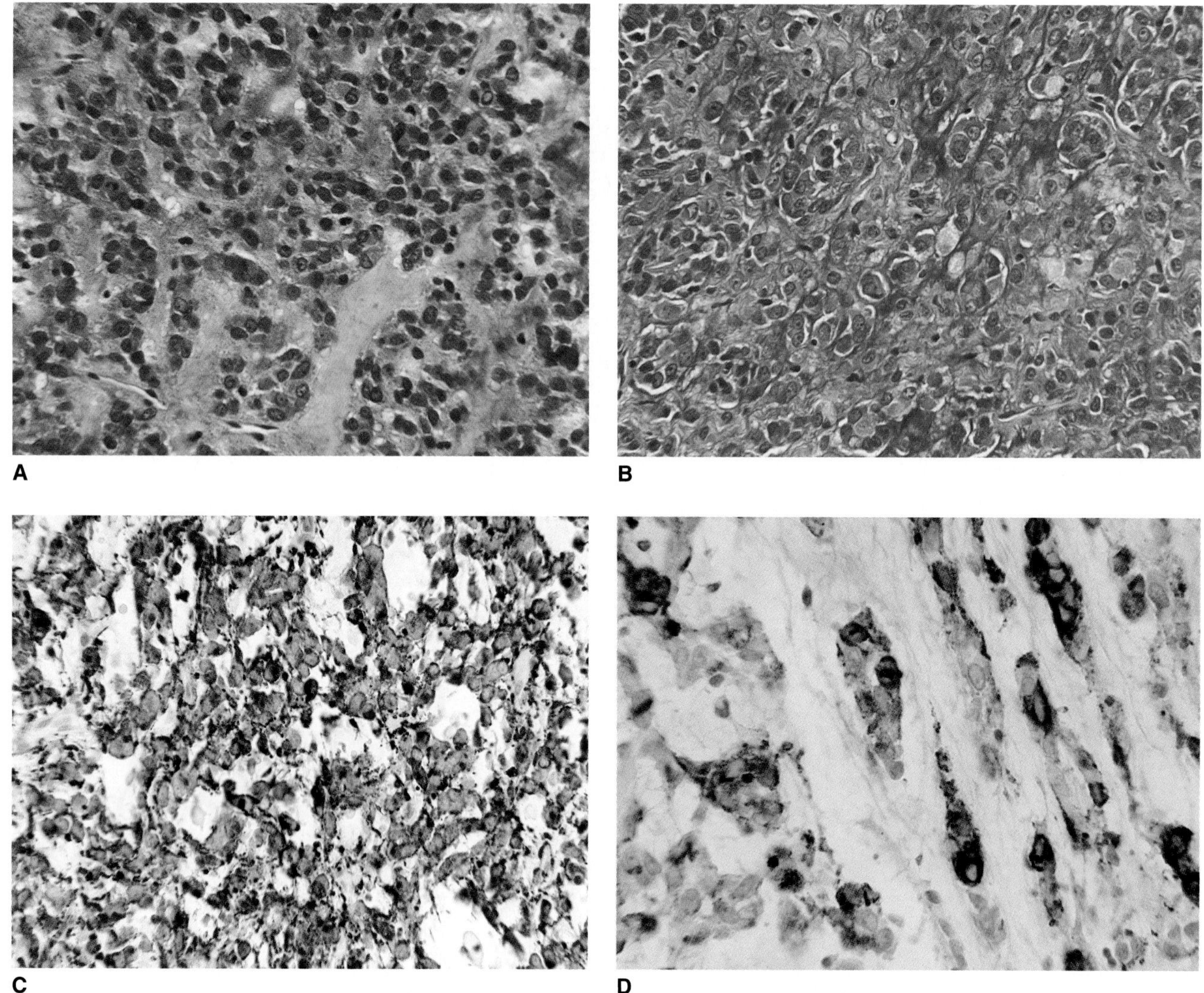

FIGURE 27-48 ■ Myxoid chondrosarcoma presented as an expansile osteolytic lesion in the middle phalanx of the right long finger in a 19-year-old female. **A**: The tumor has a multilobular or nodular pattern composed of cords and strands of tumor cells in a myxoid stroma. **B**: The other pattern is one of solid sheets of relatively uniform epithelioid cells with wisps of extracellular mucoid material among the tumor cells. **C**: The tumor cells are diffusely positive for synaptophysin. **D**: These cells are also immunoreactive for chromogranin. One other feature of this particular intraosseous tumor was the presence of an EWS breakapart by FISH studies, an unusual finding in a myxoid chondrosarcoma of bone.

Table 27-8 ■ CHARACTERIZATION OF GIANT CELLS IN VARIOUS BONE LESIONS

Bone Lesion	
GCT	Uniform appearance and distribution of large osteoclast-like cells
GCRG—brown tumor	Clusters of variably sized giant cells, focal hemorrhage and spindle cell stroma (features similar to brown tumor).
LCH	Variable in number and usually dispersed in a background of clustered Langerhan cells.
Aneursymal bone cyst	Scattered or grouped variably sized giant cells within loose spindle cell stroma or septa. More numerous in solid foci with a GCT appearance.
CHB	Osteoclast-like giant cells similar to GCT but with an irregular distribution in a background of chondroblasts.
Metaphyseal fibrous defect—NOF	Variably sized and distributed giant cells in a prominent spindle cell stroma with or without storiform pattern.
OS	Osteoclast-like giant cells usually focal and rarely numerous as well as pleomorphic multinucleated tumor giant cells.
CMF	Variably sized multinucleated giant cells at the margin of myxoid or chondroid lobules.

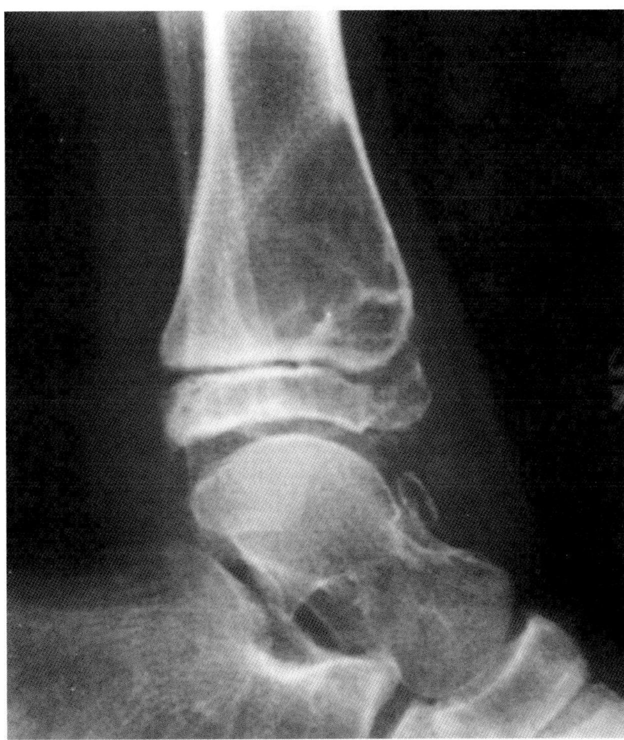

FIGURE 27-49■ Giant cell tumor of the distal tibia in an 8-year-old female is a lytic lesion that crosses the physis and lacks any bony sclerosis.

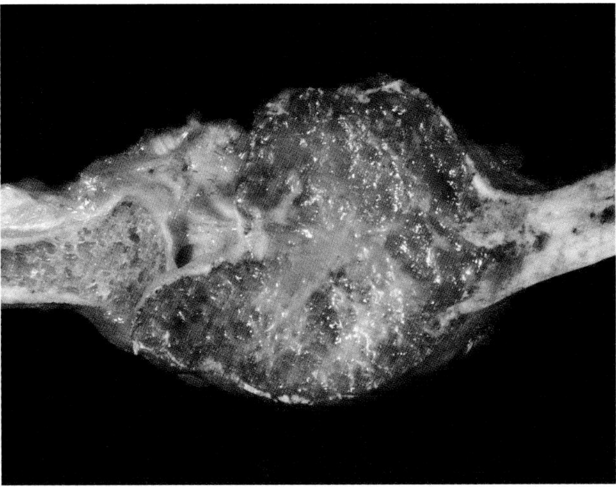

FIGURE 27-50■ Giant cell tumor of bone is an infrequent neoplasm in a prepubertal child. This tumor presented in the right index metacarpal bone of a 19-year-old male. An amputation was performed after an unsuccessful curettage. This mass measures 4.2 cm in greatest dimension and is situated beneath the articular cartilage. A brownish-tan, glistening tumor has destroyed the cortical bone.

together account for more than 50% of all cases, followed by the distal radius (Figure 27-49) (613). The short tubular bones and vertebral bodies are uncommonly affected overall, but both are more often involved in children than in adults (Figure 27-50) (355). Multicentric GCTs in 1% of cases have a particular predilection in the short tubular bones.

An eccentric osteolytic lesion extending to the subchondral bone and exhibiting expansion, cortical thinning is the characteristic radiographic appearance in tubular bones with metaphyseal extension in some cases. In the skeletally immature patient, the tumor may be based in the metaphysis like the NOF. Friable, reddish and hemorrhagic tissue is the gross appearance of the curetted fragments. A variably prominent and even inconspicuous spindle cell stroma accompanies the usually evenly distributed giant cells (Figure 27-51). The giant cells are relatively uniform in size and contain numerous overlapping nuclei (Table 27-8). These cells may be found in groups separated by stroma or as uninterrupted sheets. Mitotic activity may abound in the mononuclear cells but is lacking in atypical forms. The tumor has a vascularized background and although it produces no matrix, reactive bone may be observed at the

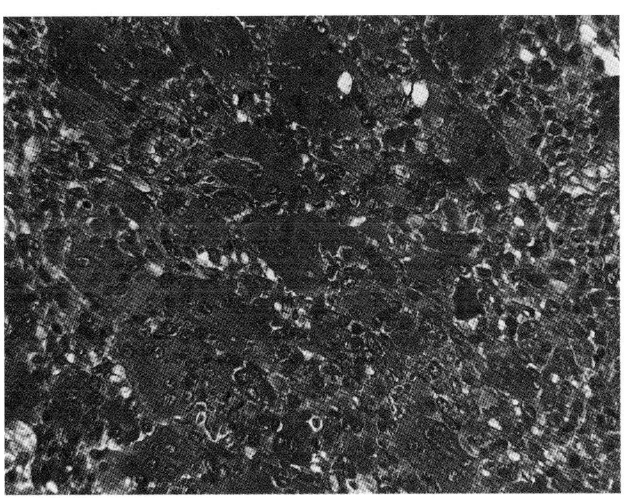

A

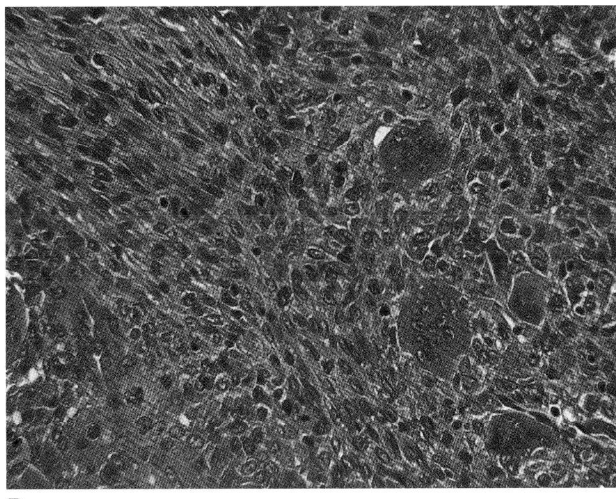

B

FIGURE 27-51■ Giant cell tumor of bone in a 17-year-old female presented in the right distal tibia. **A**: The focus as most foci in this tumor is composed of relatively uniform osteoclast-like giant cells. **B**: Other fields have a less concentrated population of giant cells in a fibrous stromal background.

advancing edge. Hemosiderin-laden macrophages reflect prior hemorrhage and ABC-like regions can be seen. A xanthomatous and fibrohistiocytic pattern may be seen focally in which case there is some microscopic overlap with NOF. In some cases, the microscopic distinction between a GCT and an ABC (cystic and solid variants) is not always readily apparent.

Giant Cell Reparative Granuloma (GCRG) is one of the several differential diagnoses of bone lesions containing giant cells (Table 27-8). Most cases are diagnosed between the ages of 10 and 25 years with 30% to 35% of cases in the first two decades of life. There is a female predilection. The most common sites of involvement are the jaw bones (mandible more common than maxilla), orbit, paranasal sinuses, and temporal bone (158,159,449). Lesions similar to GCRG are described in the short tubular bones (671). There is also the question about the relationship of GCRG to the solid variant of ABC. Most lesions in the head and neck region are solitary, but multiquadrant lesions in jaw bones should raise the distinct likelihood of familial cherubism (SH3BP2 gene mutation on 4p16) (112,289,591). Another syndromic association is the Cohen-Gorlin syndrome (Noonan-like phenotype with GCRG-like lesions) (177). Likewise, GCRG and other giant cell lesions of tendinous or synovial origin are found in NF1, Jaffe-Campanecci and Noonan-NF1 syndromes. A small apical lucency to a large, destructive multilocular, or unilocular lesion in the mandible or maxilla is the range of radiographic features. Friable, tan to red-brown tissue with accompanying hemorrhage and cystic changes is the gross appearance of the curetted tissue whose features resemble the GCT and ABC. A predominantly fibrous and variably cellular background with interspersed giant cells often forming small aggregates around lacunae is the typical histologic feature. The lack of a mononuclear background population and the irregular distribution and number of the giant cells throughout the various microscopic fields serve to differentiate GCRG from a GCT (27). It has been reported that p63 expression in GCTs is not found in GCRG (167). Secondary ABC-like changes are seen in GCRG. Brown tumor of hyperparathyroidism is indistinguishable from GCRG (59,627). Both LCH and juvenile xanthogranuloma (JXG) are considerations in the differential diagnosis. There remains some confusion in the literature but the lesions of cherubism are GCRGs and not FD (675).

Osteoglophonic dysplasia (OD) and *cherubism* are AD disorders in which abnormalities of the jaws have microscopic features resembling those of a GCRG and NOFs in long bones (30). Severe rhizomelic dysplasia and other craniofacial anomalies are present in OD as well as mutations in FGFR1 (8p11.2-p11.1) (54). Cherubism, or familial FD, is generally not recognized clinically until the 2nd or 3rd year of life; it presents as fullness of the lower face secondary to symmetrical cystic lesions of the mandible and maxilla and less often of the floor and lateral wall of the orbit (Figure 27-52). Point mutations in the SH3BP2 gene (4p16.3) have been detected in familial cherubism. Some cases of cherubism are sporadic while others are associated with Noonan syndrome and Ramon syndrome (gingival fibromatosis, juvenile rheumatoid arthritis, seizure disorders, and a retinal pigmentary disorder). Microscopically, osteoclast-like giant cells are present in a fibrous spindle cell stroma in the cherubic lesion and not the features of a fibroosseous lesion. The designation of cherubism as familial FD is a misnomer as it relates to the typical histologic findings, although some affected families may also have fibroosseous involvement of the jaws. The jaw lesions resolve through adolescence and early adulthood, with loss of dentition, and the development of severe bony abnormalities.

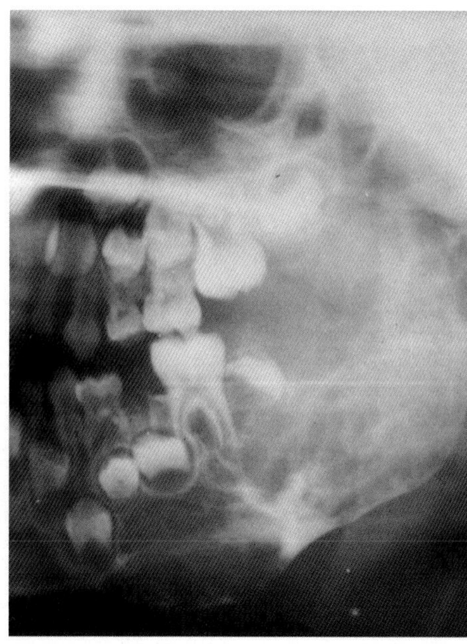

A

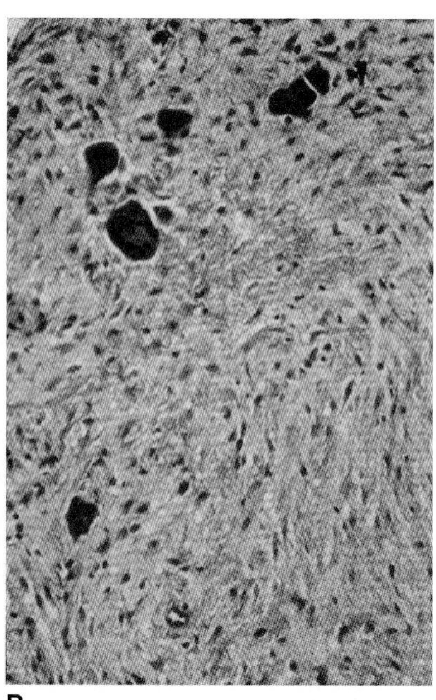

B

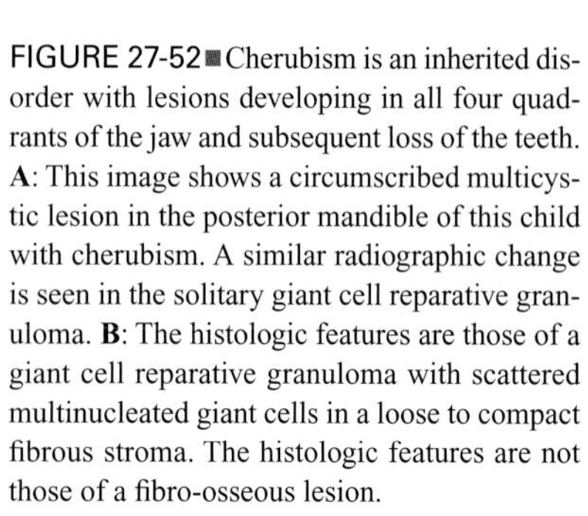

FIGURE 27-52 ■ Cherubism is an inherited disorder with lesions developing in all four quadrants of the jaw and subsequent loss of the teeth. **A**: This image shows a circumscribed multicystic lesion in the posterior mandible of this child with cherubism. A similar radiographic change is seen in the solitary giant cell reparative granuloma. **B**: The histologic features are those of a giant cell reparative granuloma with scattered multinucleated giant cells in a loose to compact fibrous stroma. The histologic features are not those of a fibro-osseous lesion.

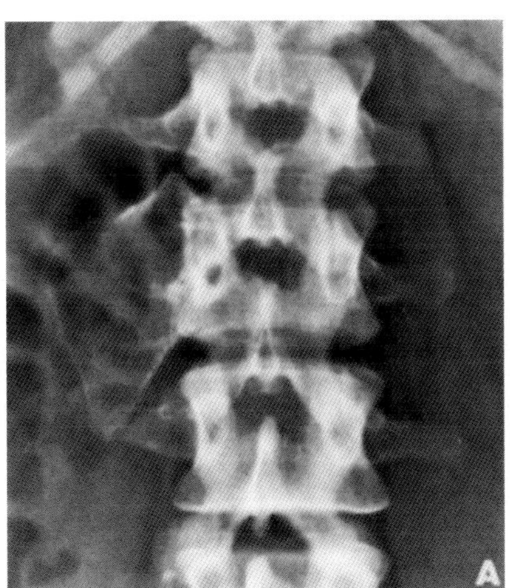

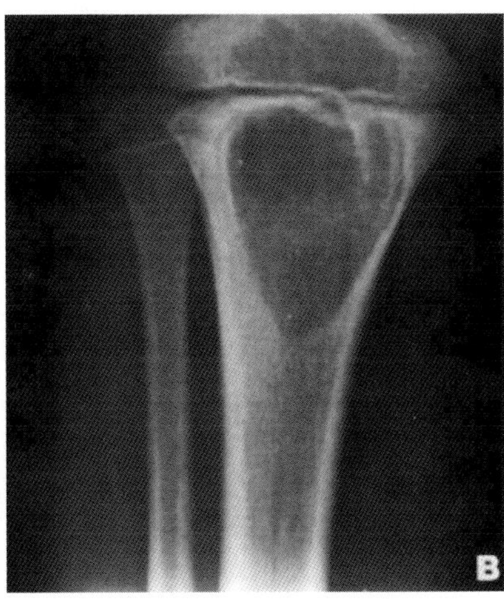

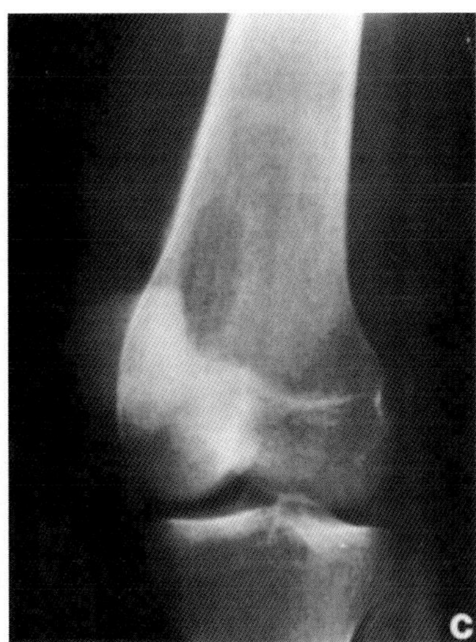

FIGURE 27-53 ▪ The radiographic features of ABC vary from well circumscribed and innocuous to a destructive process. **A**: The "blown-out" appearance of a vertebral lesion. **B**: A proximal tibial lesion crosses the open growth plate. **C**: A less well-defined distal femoral lesion with a periosteal reaction mimics an osteosarcoma.

Aneurysmal Bone Cyst (ABC) is predominantly a lesion of childhood, with a peak presentation in the second decade with a median age of 9 to 11 years and a male predilection (73,357,379). Approximately 10% to 15% of ABCs are diagnosed at or before 5 years of age. Overall, ABCs account for 5% to 8% of all bone "tumors" in children (637). The femur (20% to 25%), tibia (15% to 18%), spine (15% to 20%), humerus (8% to 10%), and fibula (5% to 6%) are the prefered sites with localization to the metaphysis of a long bone (641). However, ABCs are seen in the craniofacial bones and even the soft tissues (539). Rarely ABCs may present as multifocal lesions or in the soft tissues (465). The typical plain radiographic appearance is that of a lytic, "blow-out," eccentric lesion with a thin, expanded bony shell. Fluid levels often present within the loculated spaces are well shown on computed tomography (Figure 27-53). Friable hemorrhagic tissue fragments, often without intact cysts, are the non-specific features of the curetted tissues, but occasionally a multicystic hemorrhagic lesion is resected intact. Multiple cavernous blood-filled spaces are separated by fibrous septae containing multinucleated giant cells in a spindle background with or without osteoid or chondroid production (Figure 27-54). Although a vascular etiology is proposed for these lesions, the blood-filled cysts are not lined by endothelial cells. Aneurysmal cystic changes may occur secondarily in a wide variety of osseous lesions and the designation ABC should be reserved for cases lacking the diagnostic features of another primary bone lesion. The local recurrence rate is 20% to 25% after curettage. With the observation that the primary ABC has a translocation involving the fusion partners, USP6 oncogene (17p13) and the CDH11 promoter, this lesion is now regarded as neoplastic rather than reactive in nature (480). As a final note is the so-called solid variant of ABC which is considered by some as a GCRG presenting in a long bone (291).

Unicameral Bone Cyst (UBC) occurs almost exclusively in children; 80% of cases present in the first decade and a half of life and about two-thirds of all cases are found in adolescents with a male predilection. The proximal humerus and proximal femur are the most commonly affected bones; the talus, calcaneus and ilium comprise a second set of bones less commonly involved (Figure 27-55) (18). The cyst is intramedullary, generally in the metaphysis at or near the epiphysis; it frequently extends to the growth plate and may involve it which has raised the possibility of a growth disturbance in the pathogenesis of the UBC. Importantly, the cortex remains intact and soft tissue involvement does not occur unless there is a pathologic fracture which is seen with some frequency especially in large cysts of the proximal humerus (488). Although typically unilocular, the cyst may appear multiloculated radiographically because of the presence of trabeculations. An infrequent radiographic hallmark of the UBC is the "fallen fragment" sign, which appears when a small cortical bone fragment falls into the cyst (608). There are no specific diagnostic microscopic features so that one must rely on such non-specific findings as a variably thickened fibrovascular lining with or without a granulation tissue response, hemosiderin deposition and inflammatory infiltrates. Multinucleated giant cells may be inapparent or numerous, as may calcospherites, which are concentrically mineralized fibrin deposits with a resemblance to cementum (17,555). Recurrence rates after steroid injections, curettage, and packing range from 15% to 20%. EWS-PNET may present initially as a UBC.

Other bone cysts occur in specific sites such as the mandible and maxilla where a variety of odontogenic-related cysts are recognized. Epidermoid cysts present in the base of the skull or distal phalanx as a squamous lined cyst with keratin debris. So-called traumatic or hemorrhagic cysts are

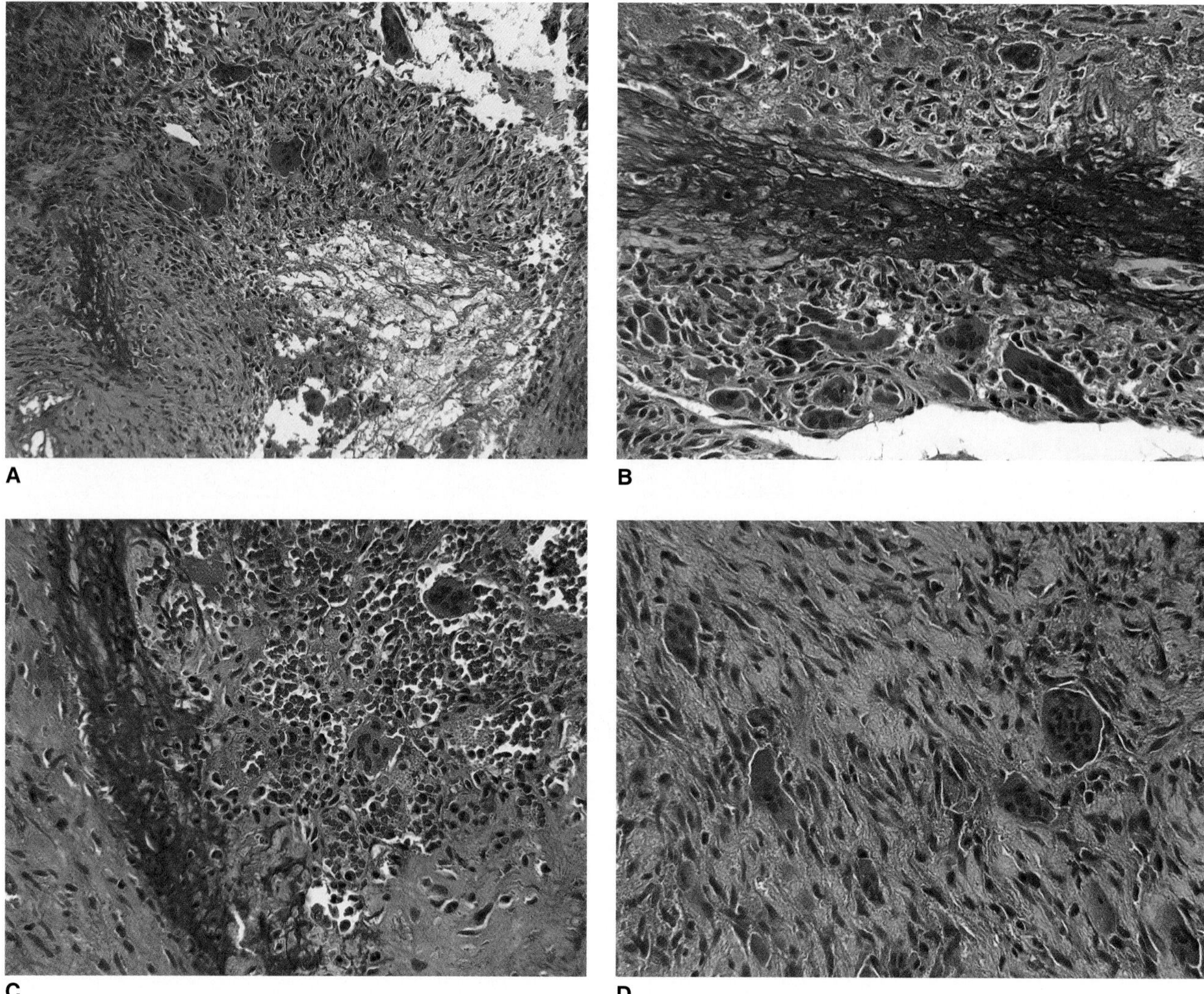

FIGURE 27-54■ABC has several characteristic microscopic features. **A**: Cystic spaces are filled with erythrocytes and fibrin and separated by variably thickened septae with multinucleated giant cells. **B**: Osteoid within the septa often undergoes lacey-like calcifications. Also, note the variability in the size and shapes of the multinucleated giant cells. **C**: This focus shows bone beneath the cyst lining with accompanying multinucleated giant cells. **D**: The thickened septa contain multinucleated giant cells and a reactive appearing spindle cell stroma without appreciable atypia, which is not the case in the telangiectatic osteosarcoma.

reported in the mandible or following a fracture especially in the region of the distal radius.

Primary vascular neoplasms and other vascular lesions of bone in children comprise a small pathologic category unlike their common occurrence in the skin and soft tissues. Several studies have examined vascular tumors in bone for the purpose of revising concepts about their pathogenesis as malformatious or neoplasms (97,659). One of the larger pediatric series on vascular lesion of bone has classified 44 (57%) of 77 cases as malformations of venous-lymphatic or arteriovenous types with an equal number of cases in these two histogenetic categories (97). Some of the issues on the terminology of vascular lesions have been discussed in the chapter on soft tissue tumors (Chapter 24). Overall it would appear that 5% to 10% of all "vascular tumors" of bone present in the first two decades. Craniofacial bones and vertebra are the most sites of cavernous hemangiomas or venous malformations (Figure 27-56). These lesions are uncommon in the long tubular bones. Most tumors are typically well-defined, radiolucent lesions. Uniform patent, thin-walled vascular spaces with minimal stroma are the basic microscopic features (Figure 27-57). Organizing thrombi may be present in some vessels with the presence of papillary endothelial hyperplasia (Masson lesion) in some cases. Bone resorption versus bone formation is found respectively in the vertebral and calvarial hemangiomas. These lesions are generally nonreactive for GLUT1 and D2-40. Less common than the hemangiomas are epithelioid hemangioma (EH) whose histologic features are identical to the soft tissue counterpart. Nielsen et al. reported that 10% of EHs occurred in individuals 20 years old or less and that these tumors are found in long bones (466). Epithelioid hemangioendothelioma, kaposiform

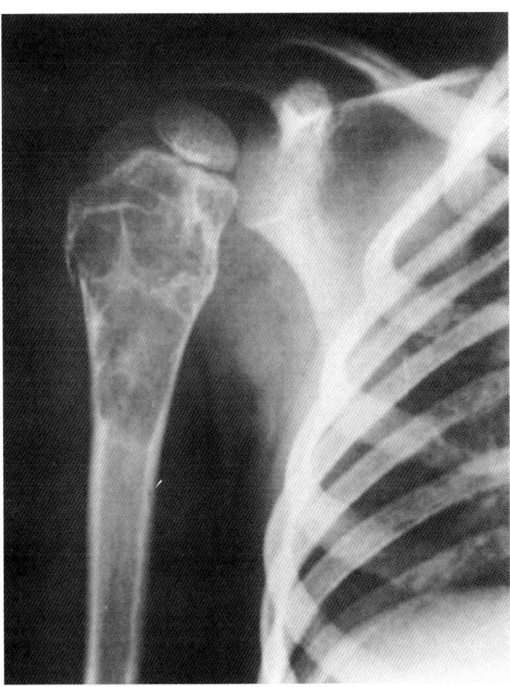

FIGURE 27-55■Unicameral or simple bone cyst is a well-circumscribed, expansile medullary lesion with a unilocular or septated appearance; in the latter case, ABC is included in the differential diagnosis.

hemangioendothelioma and angiosarcoma in aggregate are rare, but documented in the bones of older children and adolescents.

Gorham-Stout disease (disappearing bone disease) is characterized by a proliferation of lymphatic spaces in bone which results in substantial loss of bone or osteolysis in the axial and appendicular skeleton, but with a predilection for the humerus, scapula and pelvis (28,314,498). CD105 (endoglin) is expressed by the lymphatics in this disorder (206). Involvement of the pleura and/or thoracic duct may be accompanied by chylothorax. A more generalized form of the disease has been described with infiltration of soft tissues and splenic involvement. A defect in lymphatic formation, either acquired or maldeveloped, has been proposed in the pathogenesis (517). The relationship of cystic angiomatosis and Gorham-Stout disease remains somewhat ambiguous except that the latter tends to be more localized in distributions.

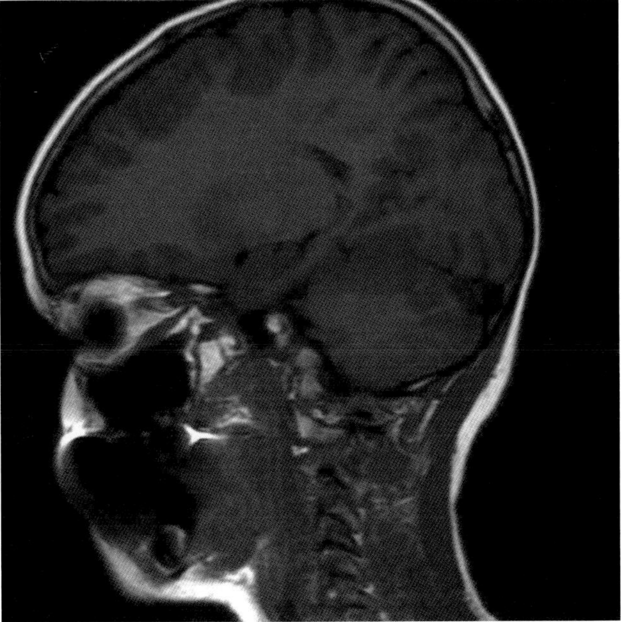

FIGURE 27-56■Hemangioma of the skull in a 9-year-old male was a concern about a possible metastasis from an "atypical adrenal adenoma" 2 years previously. A defect was identified in the parieto-occipital area.

Fibrous, spindle cell tumors of bone in children are represented by several clinicopathologic entities including NOF, myofibroma, and desmoplastic fibroma (DEF). Fibrosarcoma (FS) is an uncommon primary neoplasm in the bone overall and is rare in children. Only 5% to 10% of all FSs of bone are diagnosed in the first two decades.

Nonossifying Fibroma (NOF, metaphyseal fibrous defect, fibrous cortical defect) is a relatively common incidental finding in skeletally immature individuals and is seen more often by the radiologist than pathologist (66,103). In a pediatric bone tumor biopsy series, 3% of all cases were NOFs (637). Multifocal NOFs may be familial or associated with NF1, Jaffe-Campanacci syndrome, and osteoglophonic dysplasia with mutations in the FGFR1 gene (8p11.2-p11.1) (408). In the latter disorder there are cystic lesions in the proximal femurs with NOF-like microscopic features. Like the sporadic NOF these lesions are subject to pathologic fractures.

Although usually asymptomatic, these lesions may, when large, cause pain with or without a pathologic fracture. The distal femur and proximal tibia are the most common locations. This lesion is cortically based as an eccentric metaphyseal radiolucency in the long tubular bones with a densely sclerotic, scalloped border (Figure 27-58) (306). The lesion is generally well demarcated and tan-brown but aneurysmal cystic changes within may alter its gross appearance. The microscopic features are basically those of a bland, uniform spindle cell proliferation with a variable number of giant cells from single cells to small aggregates. Individual giant cells may be large and contain numerous nuclei and resemble those of a GCT. Others are smaller and more irregular in outline. Small collections of giant cells may be localized in areas of interstitial hemorrhage (Figure 27-59). Well organized fascicles of spindle cells are unusual, but storiform profiles may be prominent. Sheets or small aggregates of xanthoma cells tend to vary from one NOF to another. When xanthomatized histiocytes are prominent, some have chosen to designate the lesion as a fibroxanthoma (447). Hemorrhagic and cystic changes are present in some cases to the extent that the lesion resembles an ABC. Pathologic fracture through a NOF with early callus formation may replace too much of the underlying features of a NOF. At least microscopically, NOF is indistinguishable

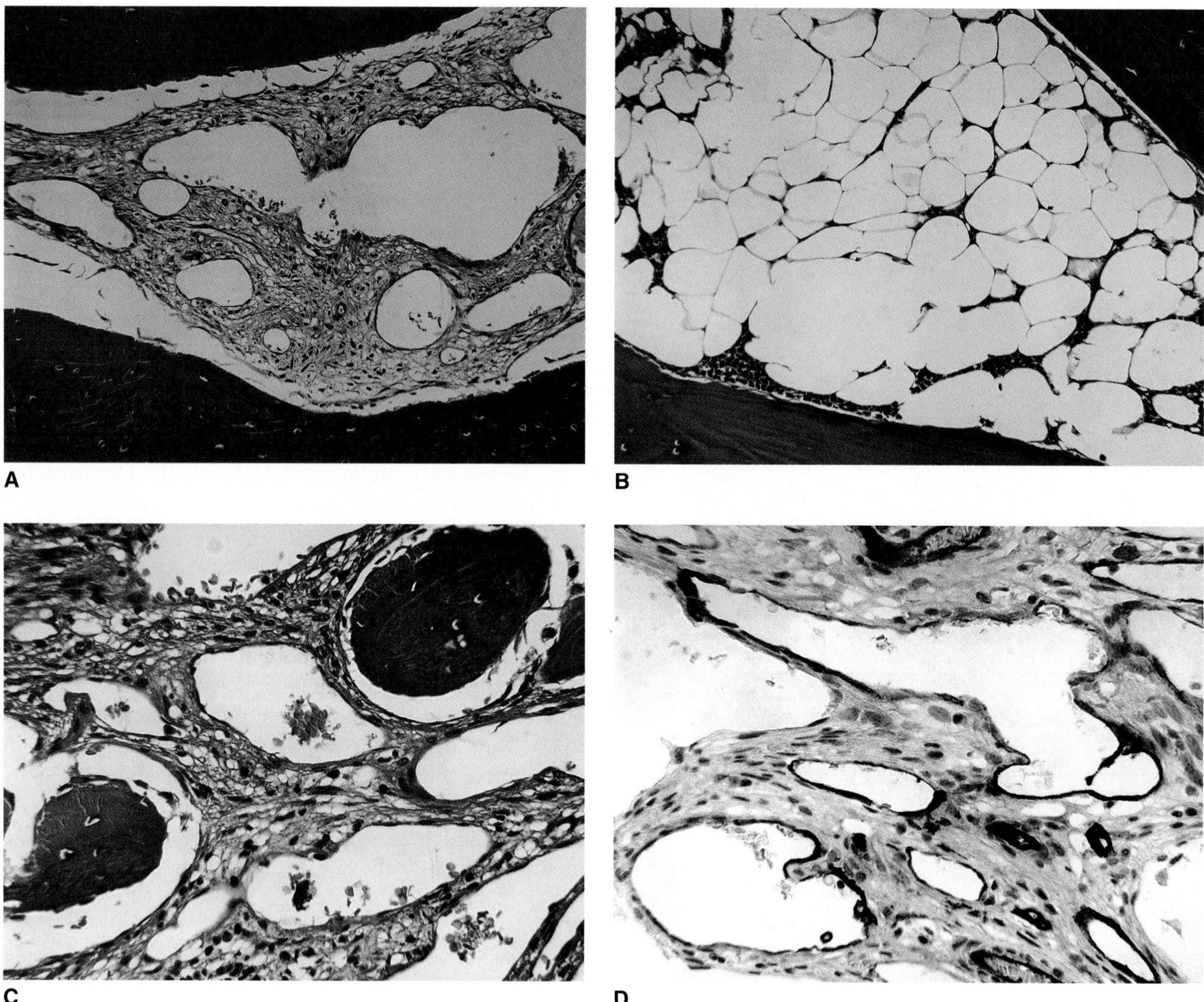

FIGURE 27-57 ■ Hemangioma of the skull from this 9-year-old male demonstrates the various diagnostic features. **A**: Widely dilated empty, vascular spaces are present within the intraosseous spaces. **B**: Elsewhere in the excision, fat and small foci of hematopoiesis are present away from the lesion. **C**: Thin-walled endothelial lined vascular spaces are accompanied by a bland appearing stroma. A vascular space has dissected around an island bone. **D**: Immunohistochemical staining for CD34 shows strong reactivity in the endothelial cells. (Contributed by Susan Simonton, MD, Minneapolis, Minnesota).

from benign fibrous histiocytoma of bone (62). There is at least one report of a translocation in NOF (457).

Desmoplastic Fibroma (DEF) and myofibroma have their respectively counterparts in the soft tissues in that the former tumor is regarded as an intraosseous desmoid type fibromatosis and the myofibroma of bone is either solitary or present in association with multifocal myofibromas in an infant. Less than 1% of all bone tumors in children are DEFs. In excess of 70% of all DEFs present in the first three decades of life with most cases diagnosed between 12 and 20 years of age, but are seen as early as the first years of life (79,587,680). The mandible is the most site of involvement (20% to 25% of cases), followed by the femur (12% to 15%), pelvic bones (10% to 13%), radius (10% to 12%), and tibia (8% to 10%) (549,557,639). In the mandible and maxilla, the tumor is located posteriorly in 20% to 80% of cases. A multiseptated (nucleated makes no sense) radiolucency or ill-defined mass are the imaging features in the jaw bones. An osteolytic focus in the metadiaphysis is the appearance of a DEF in the long bone. A juxtacortical mass with erosion into the bone is the other less common presentation (172). In 50% or more of cases, the tumor has extended into the adjacent soft tissues; this aggressive local growth accounts in part for the absence of a sclerotic border or an attenuated cortex. Pathologically, the DEF like the desmoid-type fibromatosis is composed of spindle cells which are separated by a pale eosinophilic or more densely collagenized stroma. The nuclei are relatively uniform nuclei are tapered or more plump appearing especially in foci with a fasciitis-like appearance. Nuclear pleomorphism and a more densely spindle cell appearance with readily identifiable

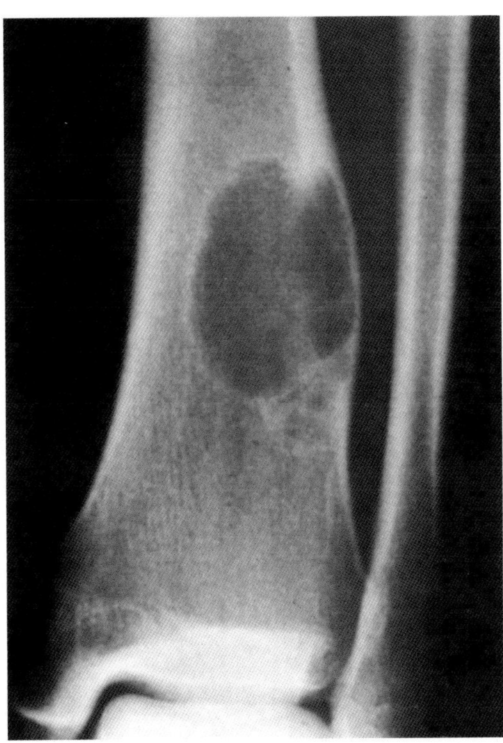

FIGURE 27-58 ■ Nonossifying fibroma or metaphyseal fibrous defect is eccentric and well circumscribed with sclerotic borders. Lesions occupying 50% or more of the diameter of the bone may be complicated by a pathologic fracture.

mitotic figures should be viewed with concern for FS or myofibrosarcoma. Typical mitotic figures in limited numbers may be found in a DEF just as they are in a desmoid fibromatosis. Multinucleated cells in the background are seen in DEF, but are a feature of GCRG. The local recurrence rate is 30% to 40% which is also similar to desmoid fibromatosis in the soft tissues. DEF may present in the periosteal or juxtacortical location. It can be difficult in some cases to determine whether a fibromatosis in the head and neck region has arisen in the bone as a DEF or invaded into the bone from the soft tissues. The management issues in either scenario remain the same.

The differential diagnosis of DEF in the mandible and maxilla is the **central odontogenic fibroma** (COF) which is not an insignificant distinction since the latter has a very low recurrence rate (159,299). The COF has a female predilection and is more likely to occur in individuals over 20 years of age (153). The mandible and maxilla are equally involved as a multilocular or unilocular lesion in the absence of local extension into the surrounding soft tissues. Histologically, the simple COF is a purely stromal, spindle cell proliferation with a myxoid stroma resembling a dental papilla.

Myofibroma of bone is one of the least common presentations of this fibrous tumor of childhood. Most examples are solitary lytic lesions with sclerosis of the skull, orbit or mandible in an infant or young child with the differential diagnosis of LCH, dermoid-epidermoid cyst or metastatic NB (151,203,226,293,628,681). Even less commonly is a presentation with myofibromas in the skin, soft tissues or multiple skeletal lesions in an infant with congential generalized myofibromatosis (118,128). Histologicaly, an infiltrative process expands and replaces the intraosseous space by nodules and bundles of bland appearing spindle cells (Figure 27-60). Some of the nodules have a juxtavascular orientation whereas the spindle cells form interrupted bundles or fascicles. Like myofibromas in the skin and soft tissues, the cells are immunpositive for smooth muscle actin. Recurrences are uncommon though the resection may be incomplete. Another fibroproliferative lesion presenting as a rapidly enlarging mass of the skull in an infant is cranial fasciitis. Its local growth may erode through the outer and inner table of the skull. Like the myofibroma, this lesion is composed of myofibroblasts, but its histologic features resemble nodular fasciitis (see Chapter 24).

Congenital Pseudoarthrosis (CP congenital tibial dysplasia) is rare disorder of the tibia, but also reported in the fibula and is rarer yet in the radius (318,378,384). The incidence is 1:190,000 live births. Approximately 1% of children with NF1 have CP, but 50% of those with CP have NF1 (58,264,382,638). Another association is with OFD of the tibia (620). There are varying degrees of severity from slight angulation to cystification to the most severe form of CP with tapered fragmented ends of bone merging into a fibrous mass-like area. The dense fibrous mass has a resemblance to an overly cellular desmoid fibromatosis. It has been claimed that schwannian elements are present among the fibroblasts, but the histologic features are not those of a neurofibroma. There are conflicting observations as to the nature of this stromal proliferation with the claim of a hamartomatous process in two cases of NF1-associated CP (412). Islands or spicules of woven bone with accompanying osteoblasts with maturation to lamellar bone and a fibroblastic stroma containing cytokeratin-positive cells are the features of an associated OFD (295).

Fibrosarcoma (FS) and *myofibrosarcoma* of bone in children are rare compared to the already rare DEF (40). The latter tumor has been reported in the bones of the jaw in children whereas most FSs occur in the metaphysis of long bones. If a biopsy from a tumor with a FS pattern is seen in a child, the possibility of a fibroblastic OS should be questioned whose answer may reside in the radiographic features. One other fibrous tumor which has been described in the bone is inflammatory myofibroblastic tumor which we have yet to see in our practice (565). In the differential diagnosis of an apparent primary spindle cell sarcoma of bone is malignant peripheral nerve sheath tumor (661).

Adamantinoma (ADA), like OFD and congenital pseudoarthrosis, occurs predominantly in the tibia (85% to 90% of cases) especially in the anterior diaphysis (106,299,384). Involvement of the fibula with or without a synchronous lesion in the tibia is present in 5% to 10% of cases. This tumor accounts for 0.5% or less of bone tumors in children (443). As many as 25% to 30% are diagnosed in the second decade of life with the infrequent example in a child under 10 years of age. A well-circumscribed, multiseptated lesion with peripheral sclerosis is typically located in the cortex in those

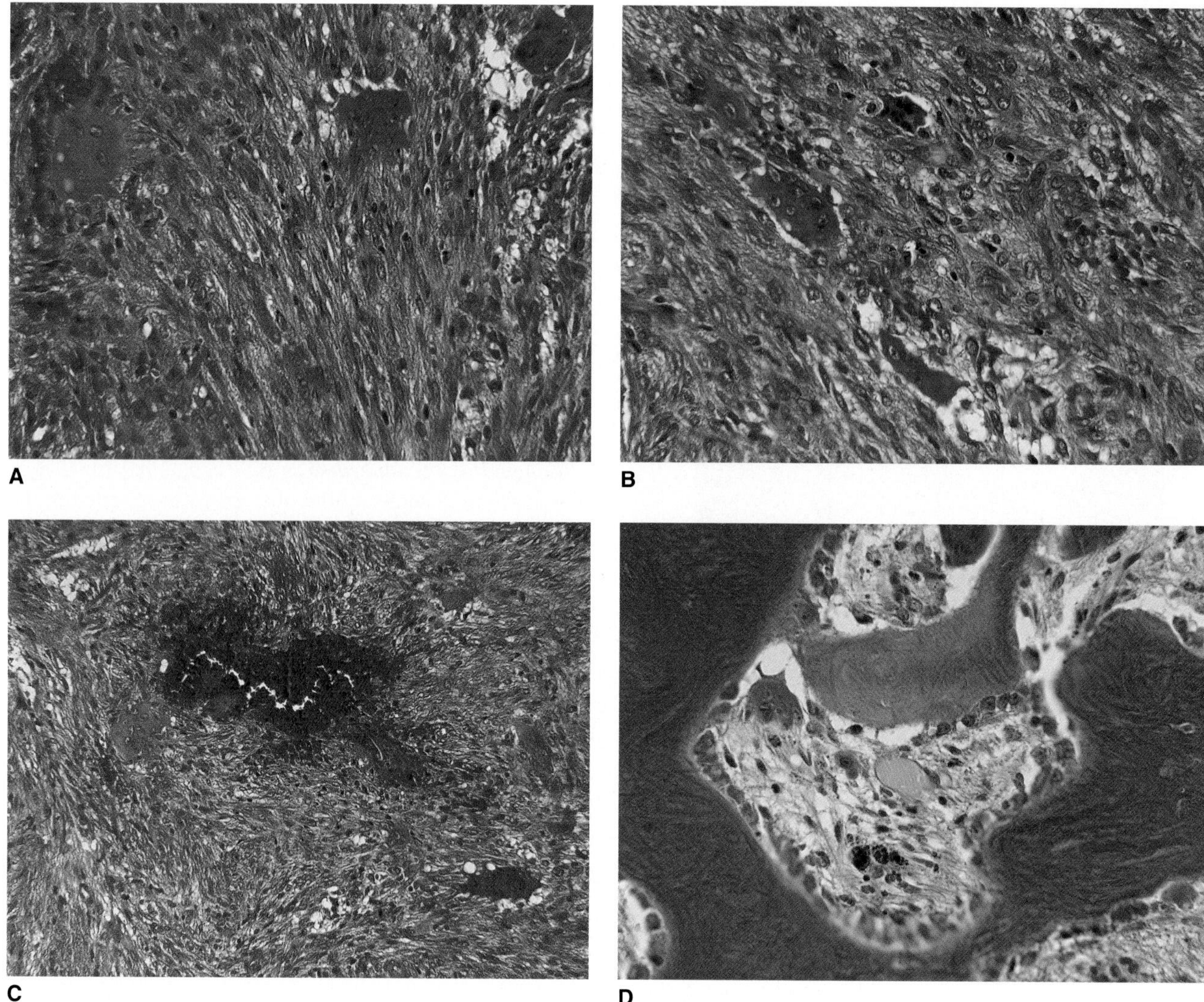

FIGURE 27-59 Nonossifying fibroma of the distal femur presented in an 18-year-old female. **A**: The basic microscopic features include multinucleated giant cells in a bland spindle cell stroma. **B**: The multinucleated cells vary in number from one focus to another as well as in size and shape. **C**: Secondary changes include hemorrhage with or without features resembling an aneurysmal bone cyst. **D**: As these tumors expand into the cortex, there is often the presence of osteoblastic and osteoclastic activity as the bone is remodeled.

tumors in children whereas the medullary based lesion are seen more commonly in adults (Figure 27-61) (165). The so-called differentiated ADA, the type seen in children, often is associated with OFD-like features which have been interpretated as secondary reparative changes (231,263,364,513,593). A bland spindle cell stroma contains a variable number of cytokeratin-positive cells. The other feature is the presence of trabeculae of woven bone to complete the OFD-like appearance. The other type is the so-called classic type which is seen on occasion in children, but more often in adults with its pattern of basaloid, squamoid, pseudoglandular and strand-like epithelial nests in a myxoid or modestly spindle cell stroma (Figure 27-62). ABC-like changes have been in ADAs with OFD-like features. Those OFD-like ADAs locally recur in 25% of cases, but have virtually no potential to metastasize unlike the classic ADA which may spread to regional lymph nodes and lung in 15% or more of cases (148). Trisomies 7, 8, and 12 have been identified in ADAs by Gleason and associates (237). When a biopsy of a tibial diaphyseal lesion in a young patient shows the presence of nests of small cells in the stromal background, the neoplasm may represent the ADA-like EWS with its signature t(11;22) translocation (92,214).

ROUND CELL NEOPLASMS OF VARIOUS TYPES

Ewing Sarcoma-Primitive Neuroectodermal Tumor (EWS-PNET) is the second most common primary sarcoma of bone in children and adolescents, but is third behind CS when all age groups are considered (152). It is estimated that there are approximately 250 newly diagnosed cases of EWS-PNET per year in the United States. The incidence has changed little

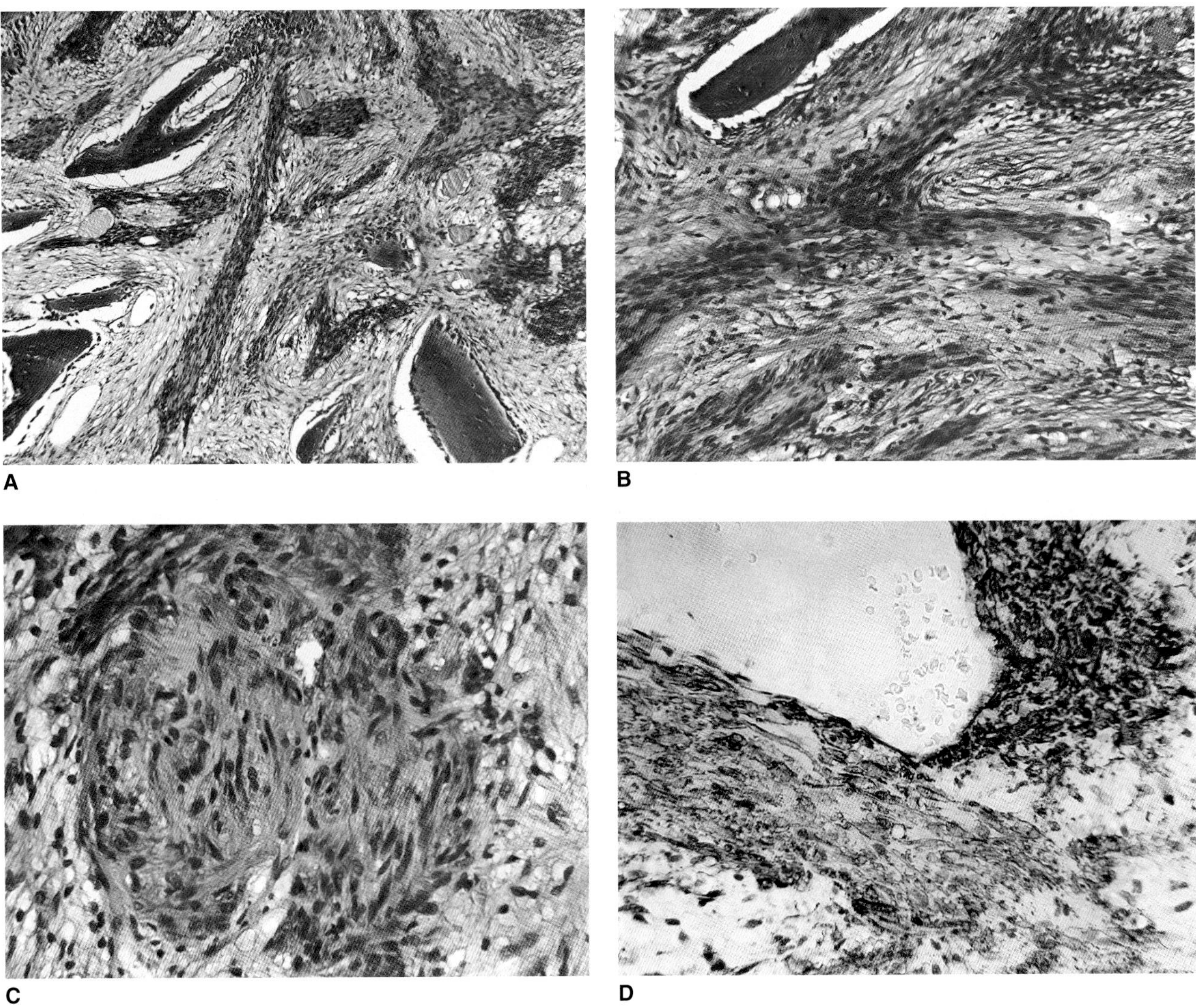

FIGURE 27-60 ■ Infantile myofibroma-myofibromatosis presented in the frontoparietal skull as an osteolytic focus in an 8-month-old male. **A**: A biopsy shows the presence of spindle cell proliferation filling the intramedullary spaces and separating islands of bone. **B**: Hypercellular bundles of spindle cells alternate with a less cellular background. **C**: Nodules of loosely arranged spindle cells surround a small central vessel. This vasocentric pattern is characteristic of myofibroma. **D**: Immunohistochemical staining for smooth muscle actin yields a strongly positive reaction. (Contributed by Christine Reyes, MD, Washington, DC.)

over the past 30 to 40 years with the most recent figure at 0.128 case per 100,000 populations (281). There is one case of EWS-PNET of bone for every two to three cases of OS. Approximately 80% of cases of EWS-PNET present in the bone and the remaining are seen in a variety of extraosseous sites. Among 1,474 newly diagnosed primary bone tumors in children and adolescents to the age of 18 years, van den Berg and associates reported that approximately 5% were EWS-PNET (637). Most cases are diagnosed between the ages of 10 and 25 years, but EWS-PNET in bone or soft tissue may be seen in infancy and early childhood (636). The femur and tibia are the primary sites in 30% to 35% of cases, pelvis in 20% to 25%, axial-spine and nonspine site in 25% to 30%, and the head and neck in 2% to 3% (Figure 27-63) (277). In the long bones, EWS-PNET has preference for the diaphysis where the tumor is a poorly marginated medullary lesion with permeative osseous destruction and cortical loss and a prominent periosteal, onion-skin-like reaction representing new bone formation (Figure 27-64). Rarely, the tumor may be located in the periosteum or as multifocal lesions (29,136,253). Histologic features of the reactive bone may be initially unsettling until it is realized that the osteoblasts have an orderly arrangement around the islands of osteoid and there is absence of anaplasia and mitotic figures, especially atypical mitotic figures (Figure 27-65). When EWS-PNET presents in the pelvis, the osteolytic focus in the pubis or ischium may be disproportionately small compared to a sizable soft tissue component.

The pathologic diagnosis of EWS-PNET is facilitated to a considerable degree with the availability of immunohistochemistry and molecular diagnostics since the basic

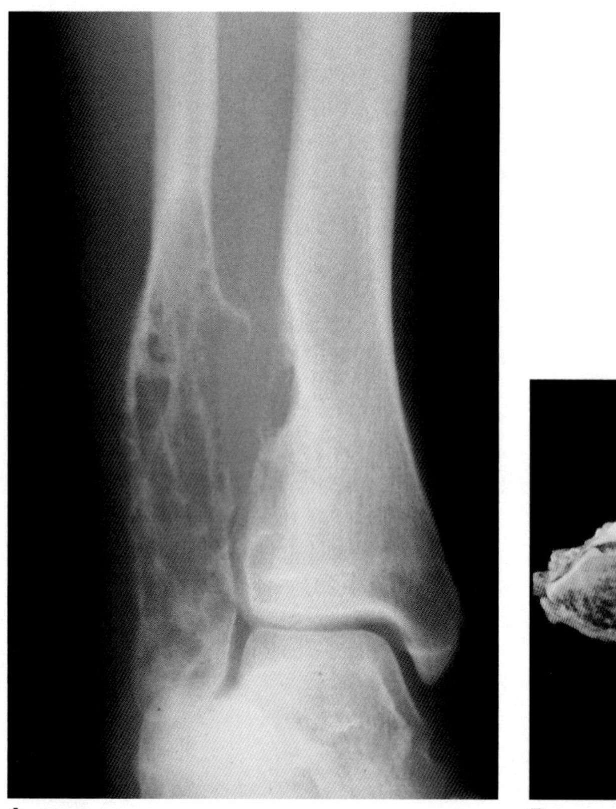

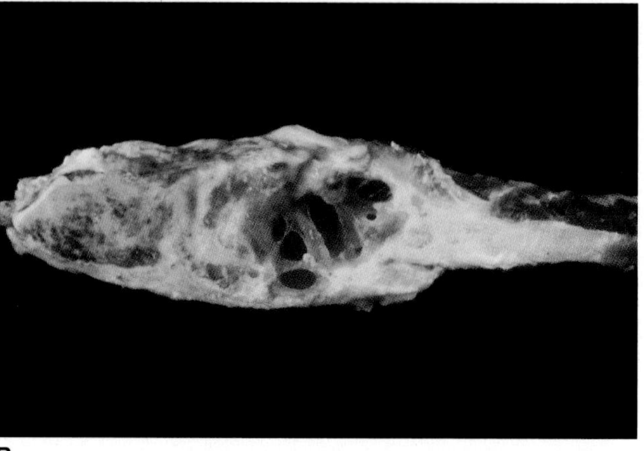

A B

FIGURE 27-61 ■ Adamantinoma of bone presented in the distal fibula of a 19-year-old male. **A**: The radiograph shows a multicystic and septated lesion. **B**: A resection of the distal fistula shows the same lesion and its corresponding gross appearance.

morphology may be distorted by artifacts created at the time of biopsy and subsequent processing for microscopic examination. Because these tumors may be extensively hemorrhagic and necrotic, the biopsy itself may be paucicellular. Otherwise, there are essentially no histopathologic differences between the osseous and extraosseous EWS-PNET. A monolayer of nonoverlapping polygonal cells have a distinct cell membrane, a uniform round to oval nucleus with finely dispersed chromatin and a small nucleolus, and clear to finely vacuolated cytoplasm in the well-preserved

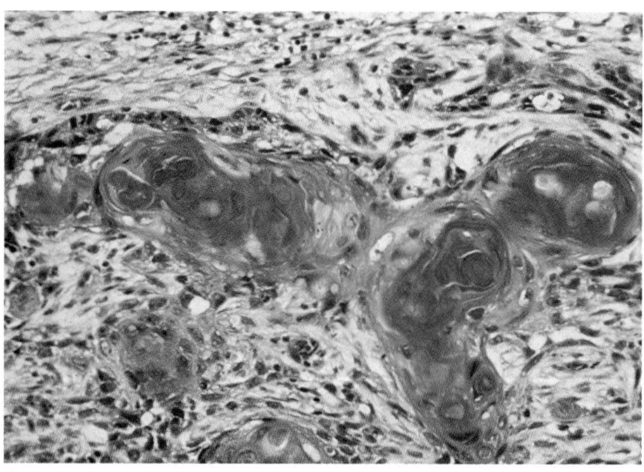

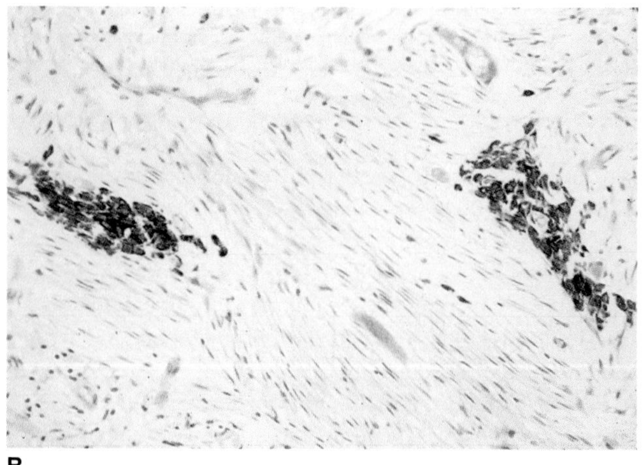

A B

FIGURE 27-62 ■ Adamantinoma of bone is associated with several patterns including the so-called tubular variant, basaloid variant, spindle cell variant and squamous variant. In children and adolescents, osteofibrous dysplasia and Ewing sarcoma-like variants are seen. **A**: The tumor is an example of the squamous variant with its resemblance to well-differentiated squamous cell carcinoma. **B**: The immunohistochemical stain for cytokeratin shows the presence of small positively staining nests in a spindle cell background, representing the pattern of the differentiated or osteofibrous dysplasia-like adamantinoma, which is the histologic type seen in children.

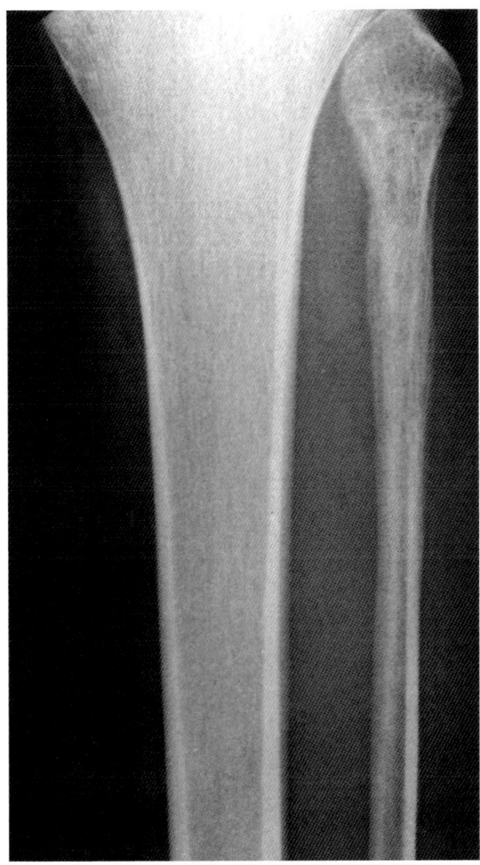

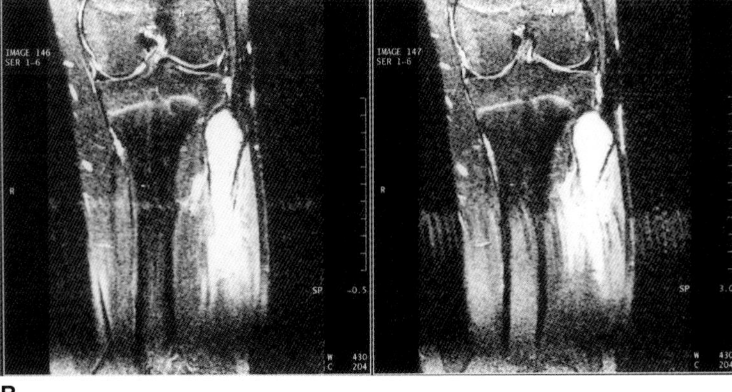

A B

FIGURE 27-63 ■ Ewing sarcoma-primitive neuroectodermal tumor presenting in the left proximal fibula of a 16-year-old boy. **A**: The anteroposterior radiographic view reveals a permeative, destructive medullary process with the so-called onionskin periosteal reaction and a soft-tissue mass in the space between the tibia and fibula. **B**: Magnetic resonance imaging shows an intense signal in the proximal fibula and adjacent soft tissues.

and prepared biopsy (Figure 27-66). Mitotic figures are generally inconspicuous, but not in all cases. Indistinct cell borders, overlapping cells, nuclear hyperchromatism, scattered mitotic figures and lobular-trabecular, or rosette-like profiles are other features. Any degree of anaplasia and substantial pleomorphism should be viewed with a question about the possibility of small cell OS, large cell lymphoma including anaplastic large cell lymphoma, or metastatic alveolar rhabdomyosarcoma (RMS). Foci of necrosis with or without a perithelial arrangement of tumor cells and hemorrhage with a pseudovascular or peliosis-like appearance are other common microscopic features. Small contracted pyknotic or secondary cells may be seen among the better preserved tumor cells. Whether an artifact or otherwise, the tumor cells may have more spindled features. If the biopsy has been obtained from the soft tissue component, fibrous stroma with reactive features is often present and some of these nonneoplastic changes can obscure some of the diagnostic findings. Infiltration of

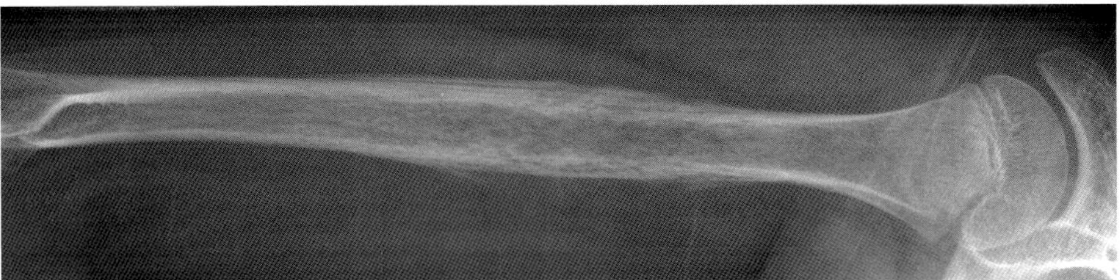

FIGURE 27-64 ■ Ewing sarcoma—primitive neuroectodermal tumor presented in the humerus of an 8-year-old female. The image shows the presence of a medullary-based process in the diaphysis with a prominent periosteal reaction with a classic onionskin-like appearance.

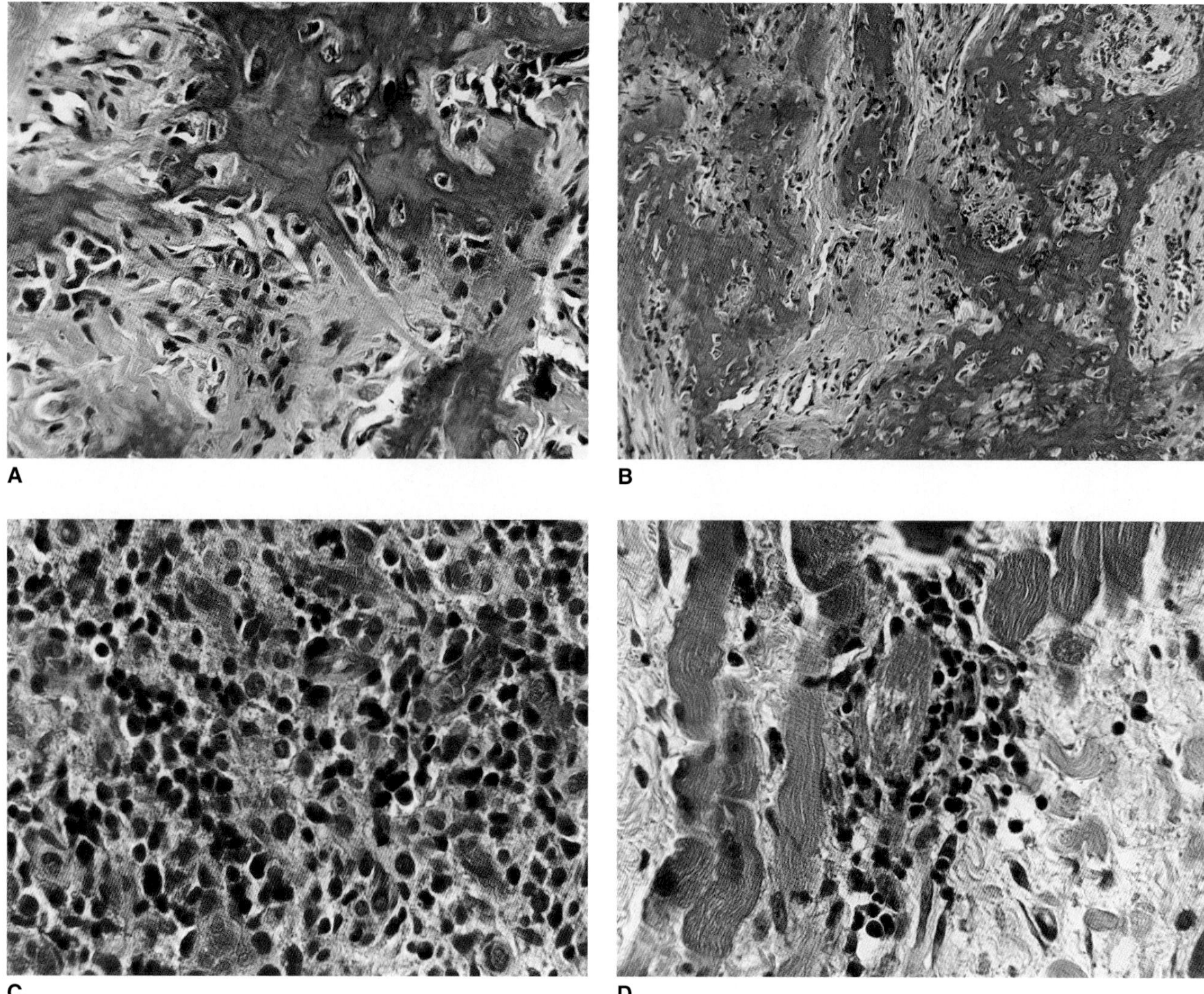

FIGURE 27-65 ■ Ewing sarcoma—primitive neuroectodermal tumor presented in the metaphyseodiaphyseal region of the proximal femur in a 3-year-old male. **A**: The biopsy shows extensive new bone formation with an accompanying population of osteoblasts and stromal cells with atypical features but in the absence of mitotic figures. **B**: Another field shows somewhat irregular sclerotic bone, which caused some concern about osteosarcoma yet in absence of anaplastic cells. **C**: A nodule in the adjacent soft tissues is composed of uniform hyperchromatic malignant round cells. **D**: Another focus consists of malignant round cells infiltrating skeletal muscle. The tumor cells were immunoreactive for vimentin, cytokeratin, and CD99. An EWS breakapart was demonstrated by FISH studies. (Contributed by D. Ashley Hill, MD, Washington, DC.)

surrounding skeletal muscle is present more commonly in the osseous-based tumor than one arising in the soft tissues. There is a rare histologic variant of EWS-PNET with features resembling those of an ADA so that possibility should be considered in the presence of the latter neoplasm (95). The immunohistochemical and molecular diagnostic studies and their anticipated results are the same as those in the soft tissues and other extraosseous examples of EWS-PNET (Figure 27-67) (43,202,514) (see Chapter 24).

The gross examination of the resected tumor occurs after preoperative chemotherapy in virtually all cases since primary resections are a treatment of the past. It is to be expected that the gross features are variable from a solid medullary focus of tumor to a hemorrhagic mass extending through the cortex into the subperiosteum of the diaphysis or beyond into the soft tissues (Figure 27-68). In some cases, the tumor may involve the medullary cavity along its length with associated cortical thickening (Figure 27-69). Though a substantial soft tissue component may have been present before chemotherapy, it is often reduced to a residual subcortical mass or no evidence at all of a mass. The presence of residual viable tumor should be assessed in a fashion similar to OS. Blocks are obtained from grossly visible tumor and surrounding bone so as to provide a semi-quantitative percentage of tumor death with an optimal index of necrotic tumor in the range of 90% or greater. Effectiveness of chemotherapy can be judged by imaging studies in particular the soft tissue component (386). Fibrosis, hemorrhage, and cyst

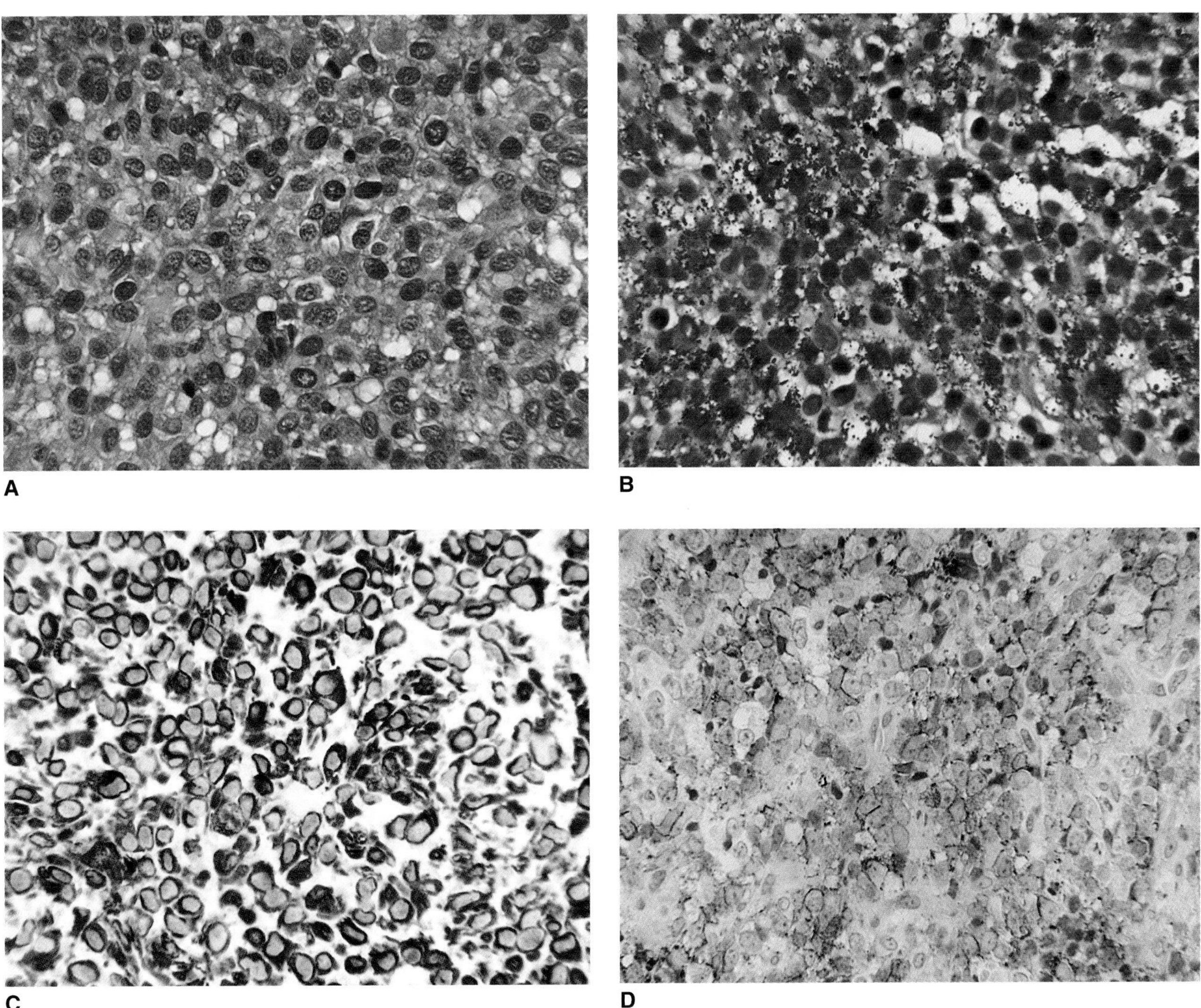

FIGURE 27-66 ■ Ewing sarcoma-primitive neuroectodermal tumor lends itself to several ancillary studies to confirm the suspected diagnosis in this case of a tumor arising in the humerus of an 8-year-old male. **A**: The tumor cells are uniform with clear to vacuolated cytoplasm on the basis of glycogen. **B**: The periodic acid-Schiff stain shows diffuse cytoplasmic positivity. **C**: The tumor cells demonstrate a diffuse cytoplasmic pattern of vimentin positivity by immunohistochemistry. The strongly positive cells are nonneoplastic stromal cells. **D**: CD99 or MIC2 immunopositivity shows a diffuse membrane-cytoplasmic pattern with mosaic-like features.

formation may be the only residual findings in the resected specimen. The prognostic determinants of outcome are location (axial, poor), size (8 cm or greater, poor), and complete surgical resection after chemotherapy, favorable) (198). Those tumors originating in the appendicular skeleton or in an extraosseous site have a more favorable outcome than tumor arising in the axial skeleton (277).

Melanotic Neuroectodermal Tumor of Infancy (MNTI), like some other neoplasms whose most common site of presentation is the bone (maxilla, mandible, or skull), is also seen in several nonosseous sites like the brain and epididymis (566). In fact, 90% or more of cases are diagnosed in children less than 1 year of age and present in the head and neck region (361). An expansile mass in the maxilla (60% to 70% of MNTIs) with slight discoloration and a nonulcerated mucosa is usually well circumscribed radiographically, but often has more infiltrative features as documented pathologically. Grossly, the tumor has a dense fibrous appearance and is variably pigmented from tan to an intense jet black. One of the notable microscopic features is the dense fibrous stroma with small cellular, angulated nests, some with an apparent large cell population with a central grouping of small hyperchromatic cells; the larger cells are the epithelioid appearing melanocyte-like cells and the small cells are neuroblasts. The composition of the nests can vary from those composed almost exclusively of neuroblasts to nests of variably pigmented epithelioid cells. The neuroblasts are immunoreactive for chromogranin and synaptophysin and the epithelioid cells express vimentin, cytokeratin AE1/AE3, HMB-45, and even desmin (Figure 27-70) (502). Most MNTIs do not recur after resection, but local recurrences develop in 10% to 15% of cases and 1% to 3% of tumors are known to metastasize with pathologic features usually indistinguishable from classic NB.

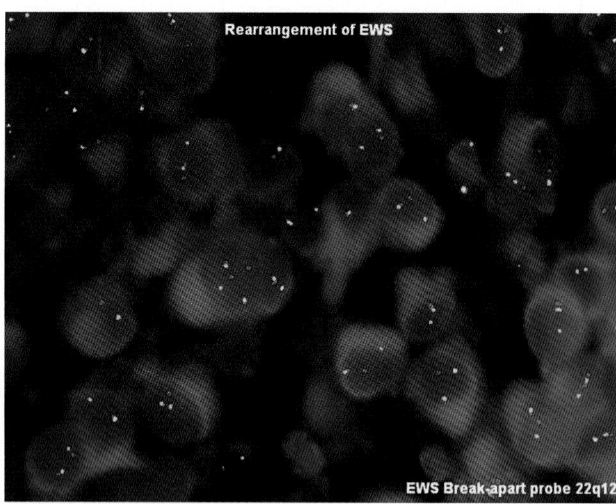

FIGURE 27-67 ■ Ewing sarcoma—primitive neuroectodermal tumor is characterized by its most common signature translocation, t(11;22)(q24;q12). This translocation of the EWS gene is demonstrated by fluorescent in situ hybridization by the presence of a split signal as shown in this study. Approximately 90% of tumors have an EWS breakapart and the remaining 10% of cases have variant translocations not involving the EWS gene as a fusion partner.

The differential diagnosis of MNTI is a limited given the age and clinical presentation in the head and neck region of an infant. Metastatic NB is the most immediate consideration especially in a biopsy with crush artifact of the small cells and without a readily recognizable population of melanin containing cells. If the immunohistochemical evaluation is restricted to "neural" markers, MNTI can not be discriminated from classic NB. Desmin and myogenin positivity in MNTI is another finding which is not entirely surprising given the neural crest-like character of this tumor. Desmoplastic small round cell tumor has been reported in the bone and its histologic and some of its immunophenotypic features overlap with EWS-PNET and MNTI (682).

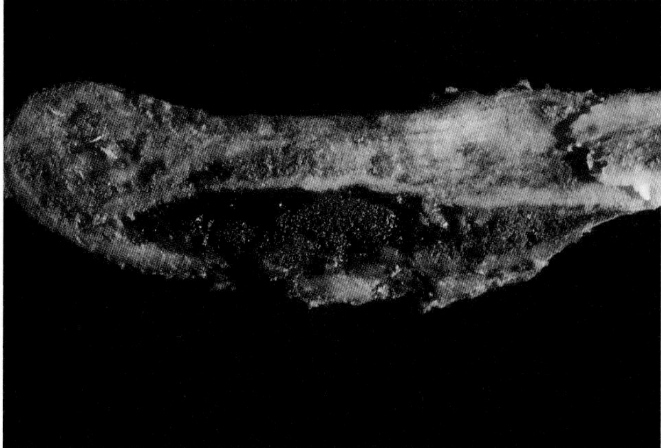

FIGURE 27-68 ■ Ewing sarcoma-primitive neuroectodermal tumor involving the clavicle as seen in this surgical specimen. The tumor has infiltrated through the cortex with the formation of a hemorrhagic mass elevating the periosteum.

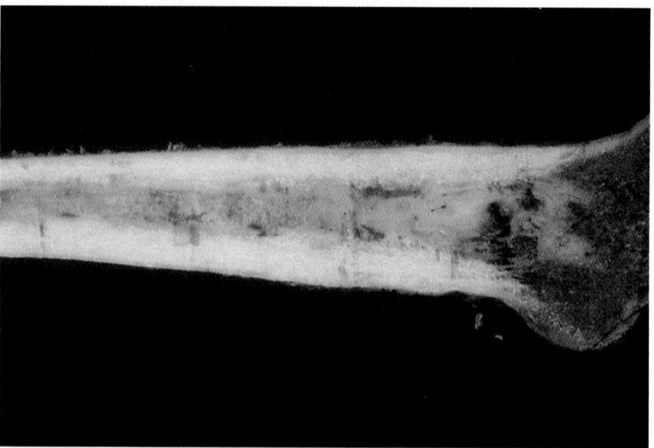

FIGURE 27-69 ■ Ewing sarcoma-primitive neuroectodermal tumor in this resection specimen demonstrates both the medullary growth pattern of tumor as well as the cortical permeation with thickening, which results in the periosteal "onion skin-like" reaction.

Primary lymphoma of bone constitutes only 1% or less of malignant skeletal neoplasms in the first two decades, but 5% to 10% of all lymphomas in children and adolescents present in the bone (37,215,235). An institutional review of 15 cases reported an average age at diagnosis of approximately 12 years. An axial distribution of lesions, either solitary or multifocal, present the differential diagnosis of LCH, EWS-PNET, and osteomyelitis (Figure 27-71). Diffuse large B-cell and lymphoblastic lymphomas are the most common types in that order (Figure 27-72). Approximately 10% of anaplastic large cell lymphomas (ALCL) are known to present in the bone with an axial skeletal and multifocal site distribution of lytic lesions (99,117,463). Children under 5-years of age may present with osseous lesions of ALCL in which case LCH or NB is often the favored clinical impression. Small biopsies can be problematic especially in the presence of necrosis. An ALCL with its nested pattern in some cases may suggest a nonhematopoietic malignancy of a probable metastatic nature. Lymphoblastic lymphoma is another potentially problematic diagnosis in the presence of CD99 positivity, but other ancillary studies should eliminate EWS-PNET from further consideration. Hodgkin lymphoma rarely involves the skeletal system as a primary or secondary manifestation. Acute lymphoblastic leukemia in children is associated with multifocal osteolytic lesions in 20% to 25% of cases which in most cases does not require a biopsy since the lesions have a characteristic appearance on imaging (526,575). Granulocytic sarcoma, as an extramedullary feature of acute myeloid leukemia, can present as a solitary osteolytic lesion in bone mimicking EWS-PNET or as multiple bone lesions in an infant to suggest metastatic NB (25). Hodgkin lymphoma is a rare presentation in the bone (501).

Multiple myeloma-plasma cell dyscrasia is the most common hematolymphoid malignancy to present in the bone(s), but almost exclusively in adults older than 40 years (74). Less than 2% of cases are diagnosed in individuals under 40 years

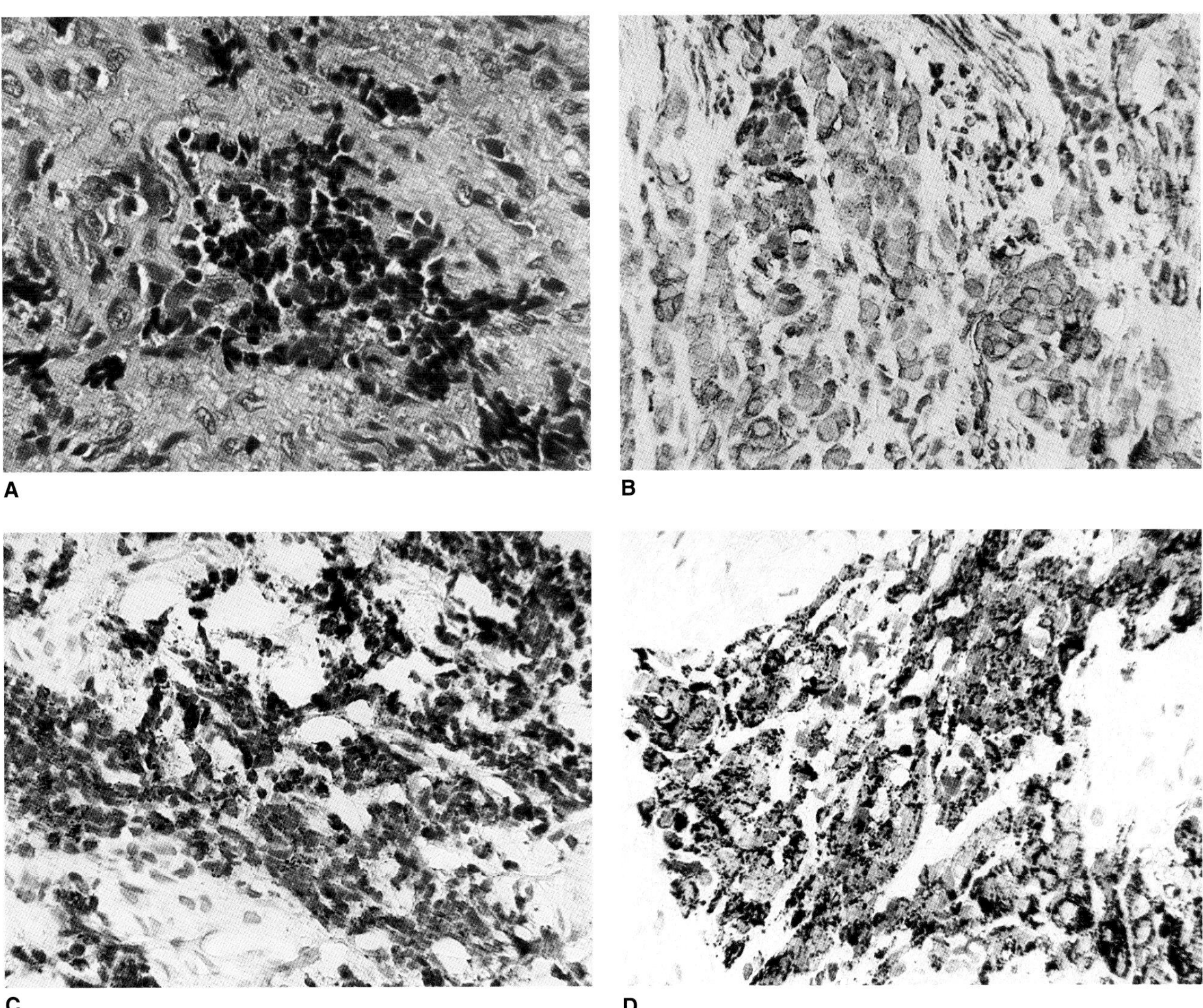

FIGURE 27-70 ■ Melanotic neuroectodermal tumor of infancy presented as a mass with a lytic defect in the skull of a 10-week-old male. **A**: The tumor is composed of multiple small nests of darkly staining cells within a dense fibrous background. Two populations of cells are shown, one population of larger, more epithelioid appearing cells with finely pigmented cytoplasm and a second population of smaller more darkly staining cells representing neuroblasts. **B**: The vimentin immunostain shows the presence of staining of the larger rounded cells as well as some of the smaller cells. Cytokeratin was positive in scattered cells (not shown). **C**: Chromogranin immunostaining shows diffuse granular cytoplasmic positivity in the small neuroblastic cells. This tumor is also positive for neuron-specific enolase and chromogranin (not shown). **D**: HMB45 immunostaining demonstrates diffuse cytoplasmic positivity in the larger epithelioid cells. This tumor also had a small population of cells staining for desmin (not shown). (Contributed by Deborah Perry, MD, Omaha, Nebraska.)

of age. It is estimated that 20 or so cases have been documented in children in the second decade of life (491).

Skeletal metastasis is well known and documented in the case of several childhood malignancies exclusive of hematolymphoid neoplasms, however, acute megakaryocytic leukemia in infancy can present with multiple osteolytic lesions to simulate metastatic NB (376). NB is the most common solid malignancy of childhood with skeletal metastasis either at the time of clinical presentation or during the clinical course, usually in setting of stage 3 disease. One or more osteolytic lesions are present in 75% to 80% of those who are found to have stage IV NB, mainly in children over 2 years of age at diagnosis. In an autopsy series of metastatic skeletal disease in children, 16 (41%) of 39 cases were NB. Clinically, it is important to differentiate between the metastasis to the bone marrow and a bone destructive lesion. The histologic features of metastatic NB are readily identifiable in most cases as nests or sheets of malignant small cells with a variably prominent fibrillary network of cytoplasmic processes. A ganglioneuromatous stroma may be seen in association with neuroblasts in some cases. Metastatic RB to bone is seen in 1% to 5% of those cases which have recurred usually with involvement of the central nervous system. Malignant small cells with minimal differentiation in the form of

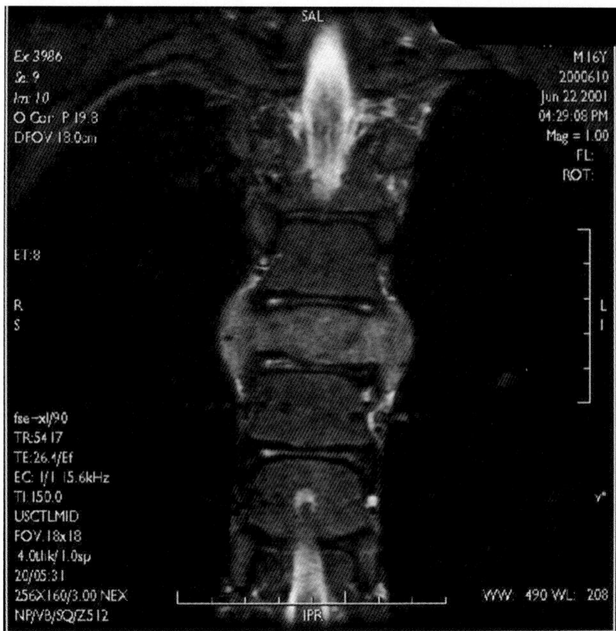

FIGURE 27-71 ■ Non-Hodgkin lymphoma with vertebral collapse presented with symptoms of spinal cord compression in a 17-year-old male. The collapsed vertebra or vertebra plana raised the possibility of Langerhans cell histiocytosis.

rosettes are the basic microscopic features. Unlike NB which can present with metastatic disease to the bone, this behavior is rare in RB. One point has been made that metastatic RB to bone has a predilection for the mandible (492).

RMS as the most common soft tissue sarcoma in childhood is also the one with the highest frequency of metastatic bone lesions (683). Approximately 15% of children with RMS have metastatic tumor at the time of presentation with the lung (47%), bone marrow (38%), bone (34%), and remote lymph node (26%) as the most common sites (474,569). Embryonal and alveolar RMS is equally likely to present with metastatic tumor (435). Alveolar RMS can completely replace the marrow spaces by a population of uniform, high grade malignant round cells which may initially raise the possibility of leukemia or another hematolymphoid neoplasm. This is less likely to be a problem in the case of embryonal RMS with its small elliptical and spindle-shaped cells. Other sarcomas known to metastasize to bone include OS (multifocal), EWS-PNET (both osseous and extraosseous types), malignant rhabdoid tumor, alveolar soft part sarcoma, and pleuropulmonary blastoma and clear cell sarcoma of the kidney unlike Wilms tumor which rarely metastasizes to bone. However, both RMS and desmoplastic small round cell tumor in the bone have been reported as primary osseous tumors (391,450).

Metastatic carcinoma to the bone is rare in children. Nasopharyngeal carcinoma is the epithelial malignancy seen with some frequency in older children with metastases beyond the head and neck to distant bony sites in 30% to 40% of cases (Figure 27-73) (104). The translocation carcinoma [t(15;17)] of the respiratory tract in children, like carcinoma of the lung in adults, metastasizes to bone. Sialoblastoma and poorly differentiated carcinoma of the salivary gland are other examples of epithelial malignancies with metastatic potential in children.

Histiocytic disorders with skeletal manifestations in children include LCH, JXG, and Rosai-Dorfman disease (RDD). These rare disorders are not only important in their own regard as entities, but the presentation of one or more predominantly osteolytic lesions is a concern from the perspective of the differential diagnosis inclusive of an infection or malignancy, especially metastatic disease.

Langerhans Cell Histiocytosis (LCH) is the most common of the histiocytic disorders with osseous involvement. Single systemic involvement is present in 75% to 80% of cases in children and the skeletal system is the most

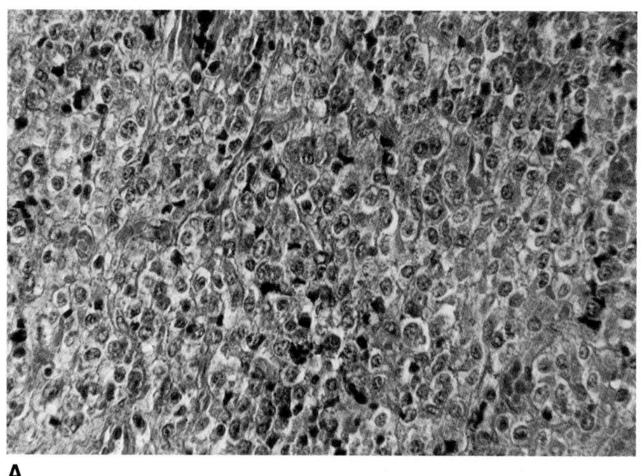

A

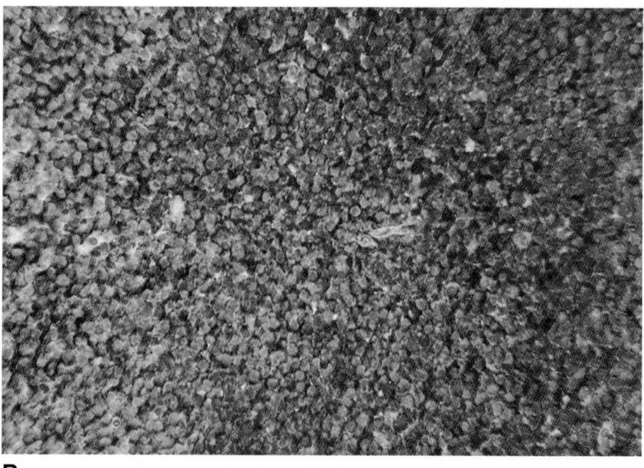

B

FIGURE 27-72 ■ Non-Hodgkin lymphoma presented in the vertebra of a 17-year-old male. **A**: A biopsy shows the presence of uniform round cells with sharply defined cell borders and clear cytoplasm. Ewing sarcoma-primitive neuroectodermal tumor and a nonlymphomatous hematopoietic neoplasm were the other considerations in the differential diagnosis. **B**: Immunohistochemical positivity for CD20 establishes the diagnosis of large B-cell lymphoma.

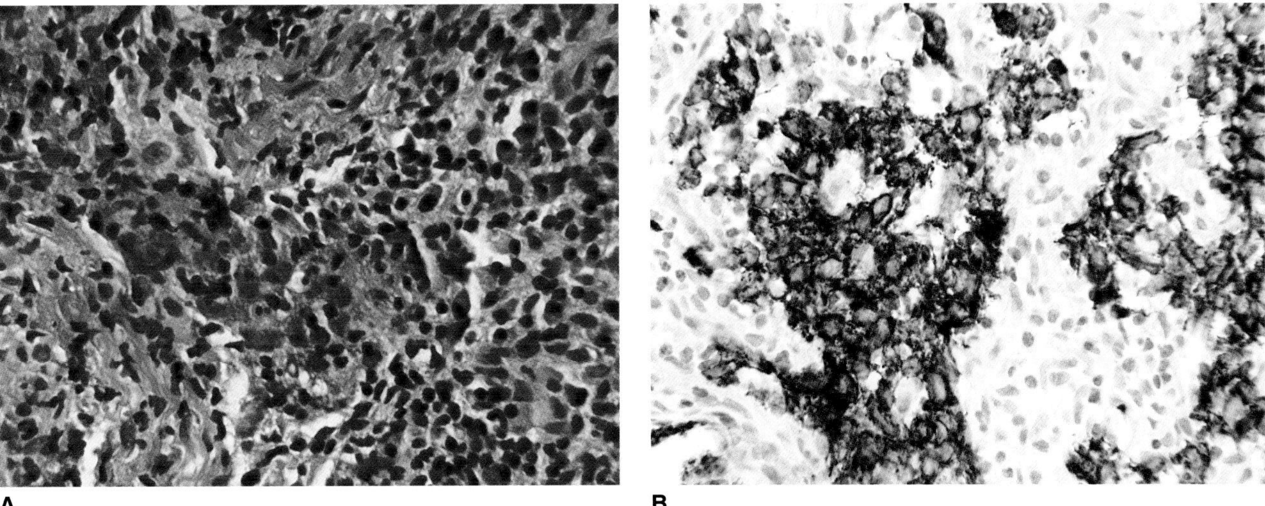

FIGURE 27-73 ▪ Nasopharyngeal carcinoma metastasized to the T12 vertebra in a 16-year-old male whose primary tumor was diagnosed earlier with the clinical presentation of cervical lymphadenopathy. **A**: A nest of malignant cells is accompanied by a dense lymphocytic infiltrate that is present in the primary and metastatic tumor in this disease, which is also known as lymphoepithelioma. **B**: Immunohistochemical stain for cytokeratin highlights the metastatic carcinoma in a dense background of lymphocytes.

commonly affected in 70% to 80% of single system LCH, followed by the skin, usually in a child with multisystemic disease (23,292,444,553,681). Approximately 60% of cases of osseous LCH have a single lesion and the remaining cases are found to have two or more involved bones (340). It is estimated that 10% to 15% of children with bone lesion(s) in fact have multisystem LCH. The average age at diagnosis with a solitary or multiple bone lesion is 7 to 8 years old, whereas those with multisystem LCH are 5 years old or less which also includes those cases in infancy with a more aggressive clinical course (674). There is validity to the statement that any bone may be involved, but there are preferred sites including the skull, axial skeleton (vertebra, pelvic bones), and facial bones (orbit, mandible and zygoma) (Table 27-9). Facial bone involvement is often present in children with multisystem LCH. A sharply demarcated osteolytic focus with a sclerotic bone margin in the diaphysis and metaphysis in a long bone or elsewhere is the appearance of a more chronic stage lesion whereas the presumed early stage lesion is poorly marginated and has a more aggressive, if not malignant appearance, to suggest EWS-PNET or acute osteomyelitis (AO) (Figure 27-74) (609). A sizeable soft tissue component may accompany the latter radiographic image.

A biopsy often accompanied by a request for frozen section consultation, consists of small fragments of otherwise nondescript tissue. When the clinical impression is LCH, touch imprints are useful to supplement the microscopic examination. Collections or aggregates of pale staining mononuclear cells with reniform nuclei and nuclear grooves are found in association with a background which is variable in terms other cell types and necrosis (Figure 27-75). In a site with an overlying mucous membrane which has undergone ulceration, neutrophils in association with a granulation tissue reaction can overwhelm and obscure the presence of Langerhans cells; these findings often accompany a biopsy from the middle ear or oral cavity with an underlying LCH in the mandible. Extensive necrosis and/or collection of eosinophils even with Charcot-Leyden crystals can also obscure the pathologic diagnosis, but should suggest the possibility of LCH as one attempts to correlate the histological and imaging features. Immunohistochemistry establishes the diagnosis with the demonstration of aggregates of CD1a-positive cells whose presence is often accentuated as variably sized groups of cells. In addition to the Langerhans cells, multinucleated giant cells including osteoclasts are often seen as well in the osseous lesions and these cells are strongly for

Table 27-9 ▪ LCH OF THE BONE (1989 TO 2009)

Site	No (%)	Age (Y) (Mean and Range)	Sex (M/F)
Skull	19 (19)	9 (1–19)	10/9
Temporal, mastoid, middle ear	16 (16)	6 (1–20)	9/7
Femur	15 (15)	8 (2–20)	11/4
Vertebra	12 (12)	6 (1–15)	8/4
Mandible (8) and maxilla (1)	9 (9)	5 (7 months-13)	3/6
Pelvis (Ilium 6; ischium 1)	7 (7)	7 (1–15)	6/1
Humerus	6 (6)	6 (1–12)	5/1
Orbit	6 (6)	7 (5–11)	4/2
Rib	4 (6)	8 (1–20)	3/1
Radius(2); Ulna (1)	3 (3)	2 (2–3)	0/3
Scapula	3 (3)	7 (4–8)	1/2
Clavicle	1 (≤1)	11	0/1
Total	101 (~100)		60/41

From the files of the Lauren V. Ackerman Laboratory of Surgical Pathology at Barnes-Jewish and St. Louis Children's Hospitals, Washington University Medical Center, St. Louis, MO.

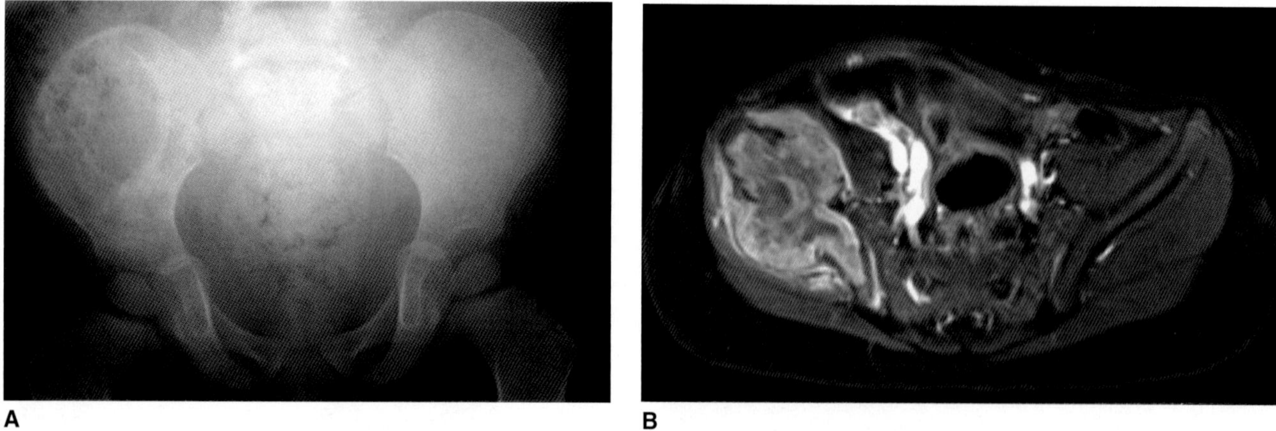

FIGURE 27-74 ■ Langerhans cell histiocytosis presented as a rapidly enlarging mass in the region of the hip of an 18-month-old male. **A**: The plane view image shows the presence of a large predominantly lytic lesion in the right iliac bone. **B**: Additional imaging demonstrates this mass with a mixed signal, which is largely occupying the right iliac bone. Because of its locally aggressive features, there was concern about the possibility of a malignant neoplasm. This case illustrates that Langerhans cell histiocytosis during its active growth phase can produce an unsettling appearance unlike the more established lesions in bone presenting as a sharply defined lytic defect with a sclerotic margin. (Contributed by William McAlister, MD, St. Louis, Missouri.)

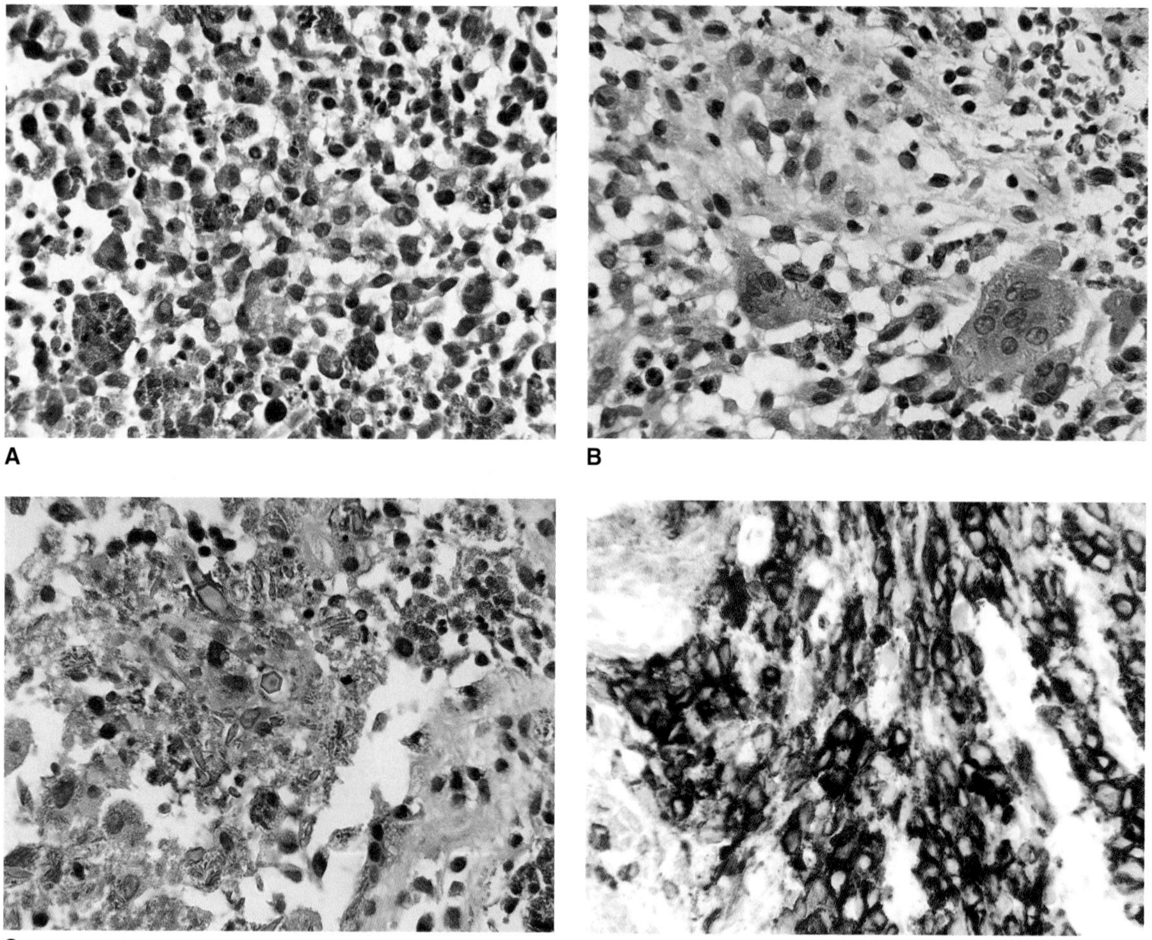

A B

C D

FIGURE 27-75 ■ Langerhans cell histiocytosis presented in the right iliac bone of an 18-month-old male. **A**: This focus shows the presence of Langerhans cells comprising the almost exclusive population of cells. **B**: Multinucleated giant cells can be found in Langerhans cell histiocytosis especially in the bone. In the background are Langerhans cells and scattered eosinophils. **C**: Numerous Charcot-Leyden crystals are present in this necrotic focus with degenerating eosinophils. **D**: CD1a immunostaining shows the diagnostic features of aggregates of positively staining Langerhans cells.

CD68. S100 protein stains the Langerhans cells, but the histiocytes in RDD and JXG are also immunopositive for this same marker.

Rosai-Dorfman Disease (RDD, sinus histiocytosis with lymphadenopathy) is characterized by prominent bilateral cervical lymphadenopathy, but as many as 35% to 40% of cases have extranodal sites of involvement in children and adolescents. In a minority of cases, these are the only extranodal manifestations. Approximately 2% have skeletal involvement with or without lymphadenopathy (204,249). A biopsy of a bone lesion has polymorphic features with a mixture of histiocytes, plasma cells and lymphocytes whose features are sufficiently nonspecific that chronic osteomyelitis may be the initial considedration especially in a child without obivous RDD elsewhere. Even in the presence of histiocytes, lymphocytes, and plasma cell are unusual in LCH and CD1a immunhistochemical staining fails to demonstrate aggregates of positive Langerhans cells (Figure 27-76). However, strong immunoreactivity in the histiocytes for S100 protein should suggest the possibility of RDD and emperiposesis may be enhanced with the demonstration of lymphocytes with a halo in the cytoplasm. The histiocytes in RDD have abundant pale staining cytoplasm and a central nucleus without the reniform contours of a Langerhans cell. Eosinophils are not usually present in RDD.

Juvenile Xanthogranuloma (JXG) is the least likely of the histiocytic disorders of childhood to have osseous manifestations. One of the difficulities in the diagnosis is the awareness that JXG may present as a solitary, noncutaneous lesion in the bone. Bone involvement has been observed in temporal bone and vertebra (196,303,521). In the related Erdheim-Chester disease (ECD) which occurs predominantly in adults, is characterized by bilateral sclerotic lesions in the metaphyses of long bones of the lower extremities, but has been reported in the jaw bones and elsewhere in children (452). Microscopically, a mononuclear infiltrate with or without xanthomatized histiocytes and few if any Touton giant cells are the histologic features in JXG. Xanthomatized mononuclear and multinucleated cells with or without features of Touton giant cells and a more prominent fibrous component imparts a fibrohistiocytic appearance in ECD and JXG (574).

Xanthoma of bone may or may not represent a distinct clinicopathologic entity. The presence of xanthomatized histiocytes may represent an involuted LCH without residual Langerhans cells or the primary features of JXG or ECD. If none of these primary histiocytic disorders or a chronic inflammatory process has been excluded, then the default interpretation is xanthoma. Xanthoma cells may be prominent in a NOF, FD, and a posttreatment EWS-PNET.

Chordoma is an uncommon axial-based osseous neoplasm whose histologic features and immunophenotype are similar to the embryonic notochord yet it is seen more often in adults than children (only 5% of all cases). In children, the chordoma is more likely to present in the region of the basicranial and cervical region in contrast to the lumbosacral region in adults. A soft, mucoid mass is typically composed of lobules of large, pale staining cells, and physaliferous cells with the classic pattern, but these tumors may be poorly differentiated consisting of high grade polygonal cells with a resemblance to rhabdoid cells. There is also a chondroid variant. Most chordomas co-express vimentin and cytokeratin as well as S100 protein and epithelial membrane antigen.

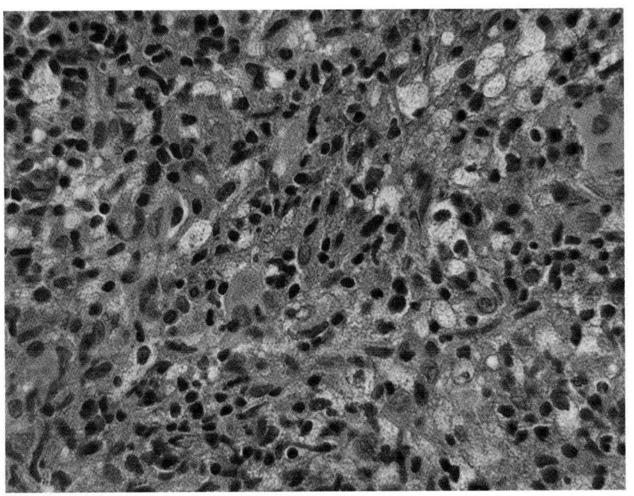

A

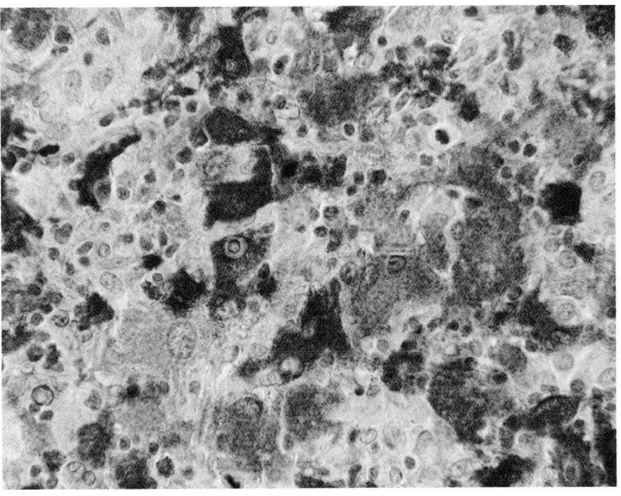

B

FIGURE 27-76■ Rosai-Dorfman disease infrequently presents in the bones but it may be the only manifestation of the disease as was the case in this 13-year-old male with a palpable scalp mass and a lytic defect in the left frontal bone. **A**: A biopsy shows the presence of a mixed inflammatory population consisting of histiocytes, plasma cells, and eosinophils. This histologic finding may easily be interpreted as Langerhans cell histiocytosis or chronic osteomyelitis until the finding of emperiopolesis. **B**: The histiocytes in Rosai-Dorfman disease are typically S100-positive but CD1a-negative. The S100 protein stain may highlight histiocytes with emperiopolesis, which may have been less apparent in the routine histology. Plasma cells and large foamy histiocytes are features to suggest the diagnosis of Rosai-Dorfman disease in the appropriate clinical setting.

INFECTION AND NONINFECTIOUS INFLAMMATORY CONDITIONS OF BONES AND JOINTS AND OSTEONECROSIS

The generic designation, osteomyelitis is defined pathologically by the character of the inflammatory infiltrate: predominantly neutrophils in the acute phase; a mixture of neutrophils, lymphocytes, and some plasma cells in the subacute phase; and lymphocytes, plasma cells, and histiocytes in the chronic phase (Figure 27-77). Histiocytes and plasma cells are features of RDD and a similar reaction may be seen in some cases of LCH. However, the composition of the inflammatory infiltrate does not necessarily correlate with the clinical course in all cases. Necrotic bone fragments (sequestra) are identified in cases of AO after a vigorous curettage, but less often in a specimen from a drainage procedure. New bone forms on the surface of sequestra (involucra) in the healing stage of osteomyelitis. The presence of inflammatory cells in a bone lesion does not imply that it is infectious in all cases. Often a bone specimen from a presumptive case of osteomyelitis may only demonstrate the presence of reactive new bone formation.

Acute Osteomyelitis (AO) in children is a bacterial infection in the overwhelming majority of cases, and *Staphylococcus aureus* (*S. aureus*) is the most common pathogen in both infants and older children with 60% or more of cases caused by *S. aureus*, with a variable proportion of methicillin-resistant *S. aureus* (MRSA) and methicillin sensitive strains (24,138,217). There has been a considerable increase in the number of MRSA infections. Other bacterial agents of note are Group-B streptococcus, *Streptococcus pneumoniae* and various Gram-negative organisms to include *Salmonella* in children with sickle cell disease (45,89,548). Many fewer cases of *Haemophilus influenza* are seen in this era of immunization. Approximately 40% to 50% of all cases of AO are diagnosed in the first two decades of life; children 5 years of age or less are most frequently affected, and boys more often than girls (476). Most children in whom AO develops do not have a predisposing condition like sickle cell disease and chronic granulomatous disease (CGD). A variety of organisms including *S. aureus*, *Serratia*, *Aspergillus*, *Candida*, and

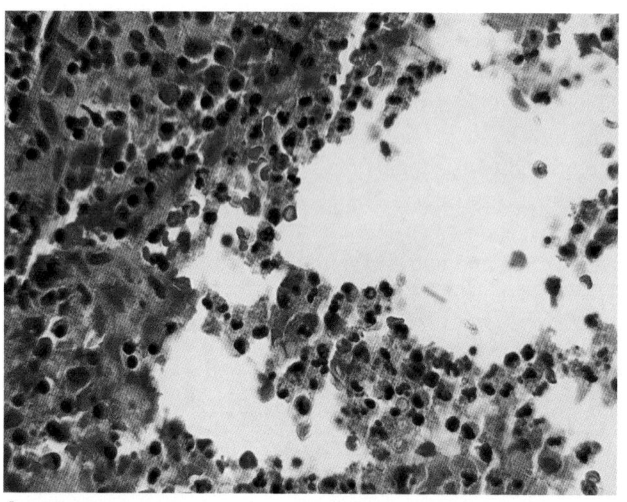
A

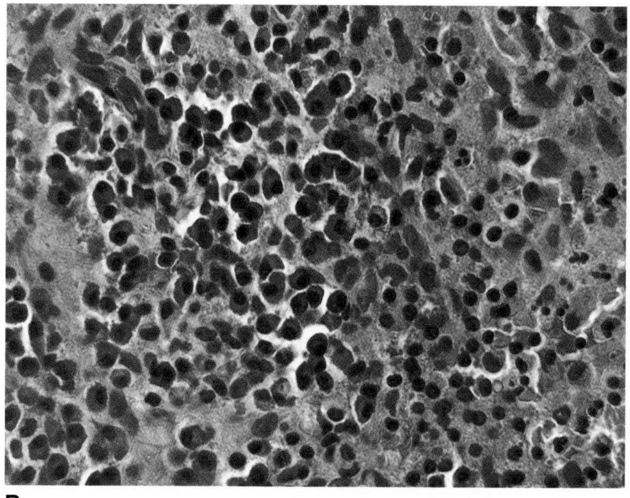
B

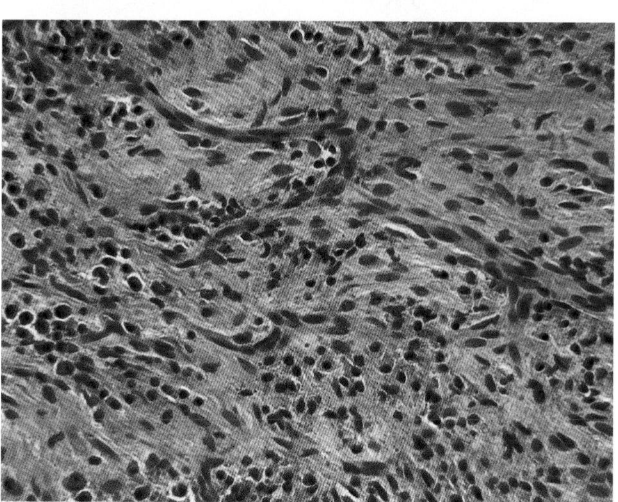
C

FIGURE 27-77 ■ Osteomyelitis presented in the mandible of a 13-year-old male. By the time of surgical intervention in a case of osteomyelitis, the process is often characterized by a mixed inflammatory population since it has often been present for some period of time. **A**: The center of this lesion contains neutrophils, necrosis, and some hemorrhage. **B**: Plasma cells are either intermixed with macrophages or as monomorphous collections of plasma cells. **C**: Sheets of histiocytes with accompanying plasma cells are features of subacute to chronic osteomyelitis, but Rosai-Dorfman and nonbacterial osteitis have similar features. There is essentially no difference in the histologic features of infection-associated osteomyelitis from nonbacterial osteitis.

Salmonella are responsible for osteomyelitis in CGD in addition to the other more common sites of infection (590,668). Many of these same pathogens are detected in children with primary or secondary immunodeficiency disorders. Tuberculous osteomyelitis has been on the increase in both developed and developing areas due to a host of epidemiologic factors. Skeletal involvement is present in 1% to 2% of all cases of tuberculosis, but seemingly higher in children (619). These infections are hematogenous in nature with a predilection for the anterior portion of the vertebral body. Joint space involvement may be present with metaphyseal lesions. Caseating granulomas are demonstrated on biopsy in 50% or more of cases. Nontuberculous mycobacterial osteomyelitis is either the consequence of puncture inoculation or in an immunosuppressed host including children with cystic fibrosis (76). Less than 1% of nontuberculous mycobacterial infections in children are associated with bone involvement alone. Though not an infection, *per se*, sarcoidosis with epithelioid granulomas are rarely seen in the small bones of the hands and feet also in children with cystic fibrosis (41). *Bartonella henselae*, the causative organism in cat-scratch disease, is a reported cause of localized or multifocal osteomyelitis (252). Fungal osteomyelitis caused by *Candida* species may be seen in premature infants. The femur and tibia are the most commonly involved bones in acute hematogenous osteomyelitis. Organisms typically are seeded at the junction of the epiphysis and metaphysis because of the unique pattern of vascular supply to this region. The infection and inflammatory reaction are more likely to breach the attenuated cortex of an infant, with the subsequent development of pyomyositis. Permeative bone destruction is centered in the metaphysis with periosteal new bone formation. Subacute osteomyelitis, with formation of a so-called Brodie abscess, develops in the metaphyseal cortex at a site contiguous with the epicenter of AO, but it can be found throughout the skeletal system. Plain radiographs usually show a lytic area surrounded by osteosclerosis which can resemble an osteoid osteoma or another neoplastic process (Figure 27-78) (143).

Nonbacterial osteitis (NBO) is a clinicopathologic entity which occurs in children and adults which is regarded as one in the family of so-called autoinflammatory disorders (227,237). Some of these cases have been classified in the recent past as examples of chronic recurrent multifocal osteomyelitis and SAPHO syndrome (synovitis, acne, pustulosis, hyperostosis, and osteitis) (623,665). An AR disorder with mutations of the IL1RN gene (2q14.2) has been described in several kindreds with the onset of multisystem inflammation as early as infancy (5,171,527). The multiple bone lesions may be symmetrical and widely distributed, but with a preference for the upper anterior chest wall (including the clavicle) and vertebrae. The bones of the feet are also involved. The differential diagnosis in children includes LCH, EWS, and bacterial osteomyelitis. HP, an inborn error of metabolism, with a low serum alkaline phosphatase, may mimick clinically NBO. The variable histologic changes include a predominantly neutrophilic or mixed type of inflammatory

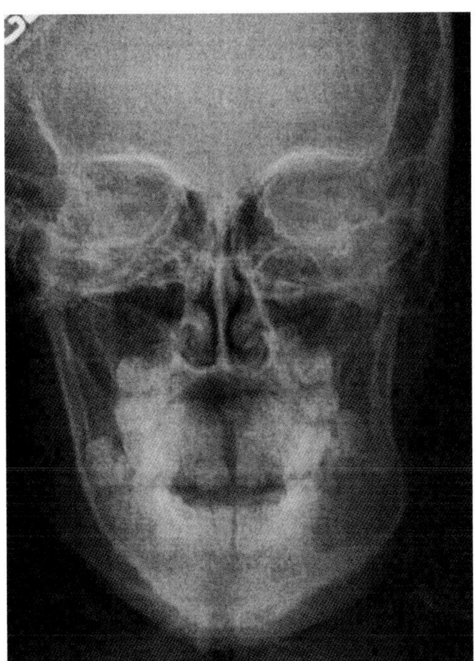
A

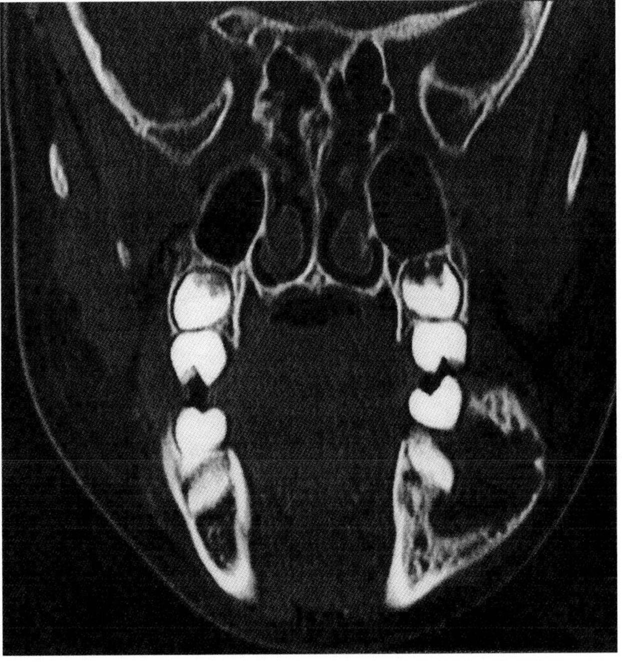
B

FIGURE 27-78■ Subacute to chronic osteomyelitis presents with a lytic lesion in the bone as it did in this 13-year-old male who presented with swelling in the left mandible. **A**: This frontal view shows a large lytic lesion in the left mandible, which was a concern for possible Langerhans cell histiocytosis versus a cyst of odontogenic origin including a cystic ameloblastoma. **B**: Another image shows the large lytic defect with some erosion of the bone.

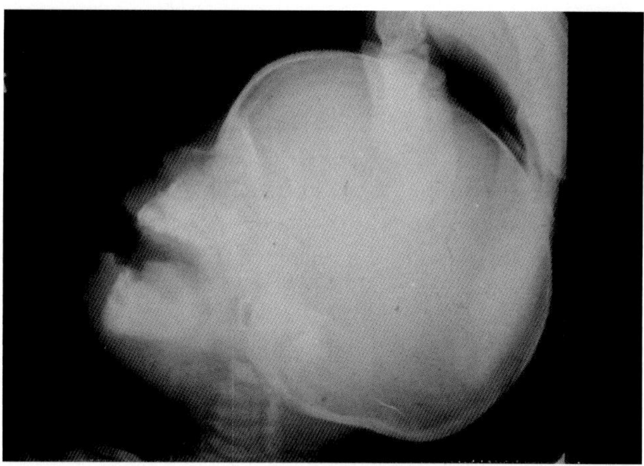

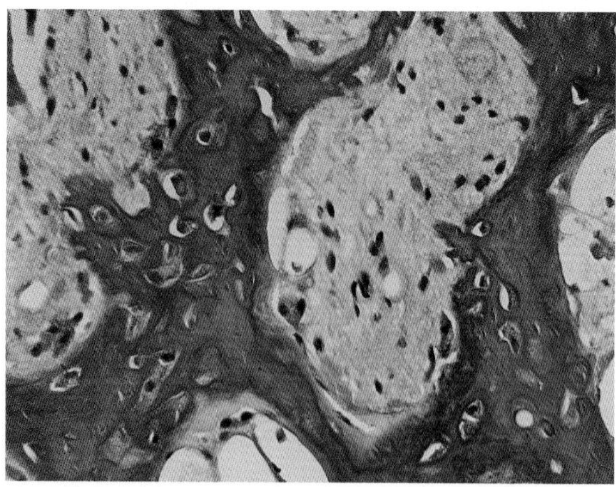

A B

FIGURE 27-79■Infantile cortical hyperostosis generally usually presents in the first year of life but may be seen in toddlers. This condition is either idiopathic or is an inherited collagenopathy, which is manifested by subperiosteal new bone formation with structural loss of the cortical bone. **A**: This image demonstrates the presence of a soft tissue mass in the region of the mandible whose cortical margins are indistinct. **B**: Irregular bony trabeculae with some osteoblastic activity and fibrosis are some of the nonspecific microscopic findings if a biopsy is performed. The fibrous reaction with some accompanying inflammation is present in the advancing front into the adjacent soft tissues, which accounts for the soft tissue swelling. (Contributed by Samir El-Mofty, DMD, PhD, St. Louis, Missouri).

reaction and irregular bony trabeculae with prominent mosaic lines. The presence of acute inflammation is microscopically indistinguishable from an acute infectious osteomyelitis. Fibrosis of the marrow space and a modest degree of chronic inflammation with histiocytes are alternative histologic findings. In the long tubular bones, a lytic area with larger areas of surrounding sclerosis is the usual radiographic finding. Expansion of the bone with sclerosis and small osteolytic areas is best seen in the clavicles and ribs. When the skin is involved, the histologic features are those of a neutrophilic dermatitis.

Infantile cortical hyperostosis (ICH, Caffey disease) has a familial or sporadic presentation, is manifested before 5 months of life and has an incidence of 3 cases per 1,000 infants less than 6 months of age. The familial form has AD inheritance and has been shown to have a missense mutation in COL1A1 gene on chromosome 17q and is a related collagenopathy with OI and Ehlers-Danlos syndrome (233). The clinical course may be a waxing and waning one through the first 3 years of life. Soft tissue swelling(s) with accompanying inflammatory signs and constitutional symptoms are the clinical manifestations. In sporadic ICH, the mandible is involved more often then in the familial form (319). Involvement of a single or multiple bones and bilateral symmetric involvement are the other patterns (612). Cortical thickening without bone destruction of the mandible, clavicles, and long tubular bones, often the ulna and ribs is the characteristic alteration of the bones (Figure 27-79). The ends of the bones are not involved. Reactive new bone formation with osteoblastic activity and a variably intense mixed inflammatory infiltrates with neutrophils are nonspecific in a sense, but whose features may suggest an acute to sub-AO (500). The inflammation with edema and accompanying fibroplasia extends into the surrounding soft tissues. A self-limited clinical course is the usual outcome, although premature infants seem to fare less well than term infants. The diagnosis of ICH with or without nonimmune hydrops has been made prenatally (269).

Osteonecrosis (aseptic or avascular necrosis) is a known complication of chronic corticosteroids and hemoglobinopathy particularly sickle cell disease. Children with acute lymphoblastic leukemia and non-Hodgkin lymphoma are especially at risk for osteonecrosis in which case, the steroid therapy is thought to have an important role in etiology (44,552). Other nontraumatic causes and associations with osteonecrosis in children include congenital hip dysplasia, slipped capital femoral epiphysis and Gaucher disease. Legg-Calve-Perthes (LCP) disease is defined by the presence of osteonecrosis of the capitol femoral epiphysis of the femoral head (305,532,607,647). The male to female ratio is 4–5:1 and median age at diagnosis is 7 to 8 years with a range of 3 to 12 years. Vascular occlusion to the subchondral cortical bone in LCP is possibly the complication of a primary thrombophilia as in the case of protein C deficiency, factor V Leiden and methylenetetrahydrofolate reductase C677T mutations (338,647). Gaucher disease is associated with bone involvement in 70% to 100% of individuals with type 1 or 3 (248,607). The osteonecrosis in the femoral head is identical to LCP disease. Infarcts also occur in the head of the humerus, femoral condyle, and tibial plateau. Necrosis is first identified in the tissues of the medullary cavity with fat necrosis and coagulative necrosis of the hematopoietic elements (644). The cancellous bone acquires a pale, homogeneous appearance and the osteocyte lacunae are empty. Often the architecture of the bone is irregular due to past episodes of remodeling.

Synovium

The joint space is at the junction of two contiguous bones and is lined by a synovial membrane which overlies the articular cartilage. Under normal circumstances, the synovinum is inconspicuous, but in the presence of inflammation, regardless of the etiology, the synovial membranes, and the underlying interstitial tissues are variably infiltrated by a range of inflammatory cells which reflect the nature of the etiology (infectious pathogens, metabolic abnormality, and autoimmunity) and the duration in some cases. Over a period of time as the integrity of the synovial membrane is functionally compromised, there are degenerative changes in the underlying articular cartilage. In most cases, the joint space pathology is a clinical concern which is unlikely to involve the pathology directly except in the clinical laboratory (224).

Acute synovitis is an infiltration of the interstitum by neutrophils and is seen most frequently in the presence of a pyogenic infection of the joint space in septic arteritis. The latter is a complication of acute hematogenous osteomyelitis and occurs most frequently in the hip or knee joint. Kang and associates noted that the incidence is considerably lower in children in developed versus developing countries (1:100,000 vs. 1:5,000 to 20,000) (320). Lyme arthritis is associated with an acute inflammatory reaction, but persistent lyme arthritis with the presence of lymphoid hyperplasia, histiocytes and mast cells resembles chronic idiopathic arthritis (266,621).

Chronic synovitis is characterized by an inflammatory reaction which is dominated by lymphocytes with a diffuse and/or nodular pattern and with or without plasma cells. There is hyperplasia of the synovial lining cells with or without a papillary architecture. Mast cells are conspicuous in the background whose presence can be demonstrated by an Leder stain. Fibrin deposition, lymphoid nodules and plasma cells in appreciable numbers in a synovial biopsy has been associated with rheumatoid arthritis (RA). The latter diagnostic category in reference to children as juvenile RA has been subsumed as a subset of juvenile idiopathic arthritis. The latter topic has been reviewed in two useful publications (154,525).

Hemophilic arthropathy is associated with chronic synovitis with proliferative features and a lymphocytic and histiocytic infiltrates, vascularized fibrosis and striking hemosiderin deposition within the synovial lining cells as wellas in the interstitium and withing histiocytes (541). Hemoarthrosis occurs when factor VIII or IX levels are below 1% of normal levels (302). The knee, ankle and elbow joints are most prone to a hemarthroses. There is progressive injury to the articular cartilage and bone especially in the knee and ankle joints in those with frequent episodes of hemarthroses (178). Since synovectomy is recommended in those children with progressive joint injury, these specimens are seen for pathologic examination. Another cause of nontraumatic hemarthrosis especially of the knee and joint is synovial hemangioma or hemangiomatosis.

Granulomatous synovitis is rarely observed in sarcoidosis in child and the inherited disease, Blau syndrome which is characterized clinically by granulomatous polyarthritis, uveitis and an exanthematous skin rash (52,199). There is a mutation in capase recruitment domain-15.

Histiocytic synovitis or histiocytic infiltration of the synovium is seen in the camptodactyly, arthropathy, coxa vera, pericarditis syndrome (573). The synovium contains CD68—positive multinucleated giant cells. Foamy histiocytes are found in the synovium in α-mannosidosis which is accompanied by destructive joint disease in young individuals. Nontuberculous mycobacterial synovitis may have a diffuse histiocytic reaction rather than well formed granulomas. A similar histiocytic reaction in the synovium with a destructive arthropathy is present in multicentric reticulohistiocytosis which is rare in childhood, but is documented in several cases (421,490). There is mixture of mononuclear and multinuclear histiocytes.

Tumefactive lesions within and around the joints in children constitute a heterogeneous group of uncommon conditions (459). Some of these are intraarticular and are seen frequently in adults such as synovial chondromatosis (349). The nodules of mature cartilage arise in the synovial membranes and/or free floating in the joint space of the knee, hip and elbow. Rounded to faceted nodules vary from 1 mm to over 1 cm in diameter. A fibrous membrane surrounds the individual cartilaginous nodules which are composed of haphazardly arranged chondrocytes with a chondroid matrix. Some degree of cytologic atypia may exist in the chondrocytes which does not appear to have any importance in terms of prognosis. Another tumefaction is synovial lipomatosis (lipoma arborescens) presenting as a suprapatellar mass (285). Involvement of the synovial sheath of the tendon has been reported. This rare process is seen in children in a variety of joint spaces and bursa. The interstitial tissues of the synovium are largely placed by lobules of mature adipose tissue which are nodular fasciitis; ganglion cyst and synovial sarcoma have also been documented with intraarticular presentation (436,450). Pigmented villonodular synovitis has been discussed in the chapter on soft tissues together with GCT of tendon sheath, another periarticular soft tissue tumor. Ganglion cysts occur in children and represent 5% to 10% of all cases in all age groups (105,656). Thye are seen as early as infancy and throughout childhood. Most cysts are located in the wrist on the volar or dorsal aspect. There are a number of other sites of presentation including the knee in the region of the anterior cruciate ligament, around the hip, spine and adjacent to the spine (341,453). Rarely ganglion cysts may be multifocal and referred to "cystic ganglionosis (576)." Though referred to as "synovial" cysts in some cases, most cysts arise in the tissues in and around tendons. One or more rounded to elongated cysts without lining cells and with or without pale mucoid material are located within a dense fibrous background. Nodular fasciitis has been reported in the joint space (282).

Osteoarthopathy (OAP) or degenerative joint disease is rarely encountered by the pathologist in a child who required a joint replacement. However, OAP is the consequence of any chronic inflammatory process, metabolic disorder with accompanying osteopenia, osteonecrosis and abnormal skeletal development with erosion and destruction of the articular cartilage. Some of these conditions include multiple epiphyseal dysplasia, pseudo HP, Marfan syndrome, Ehlers-Danlos syndrome, cystic fibrosis, hemophiliac-associated hemarthrosis, CDP, dysostosis multiplex, achondroplasia, and Gaucher disease (150,633).

REFERENCES

1. Adegbite NS, Xu M, Kaplan FS, et al. Diagnostic and mutational spectrum of progressive osseous heteroplasia (POH) and other forms of GNAS-based heterotopic ossification. *Am J Med Genet A* 2008;146A:1788–1796.
2. Adra A, Cordero D, Mejides A, et al. Caudal regression syndrome: etiopathogenesis, prenatal diagnosis, and perinatal management. *Obstet Gynecol Surv* 1994;49:508–516.
3. Aghabiklooei A, Goodarzi P, Kariminejad MH. Lung hypoplasia and its associated major congenital abnormalities in perinatal death: an autopsy study of 850 cases. *Indian J Pediatr* 2009;76:1137–1140.
4. Aigner T, Rau T, Niederhagen M, et al. Achondrogenesis Type IA (Houston-Harris): a still-unresolved molecular phenotype. *Pediatr Dev Pathol* 2007;10:328–334.
5. Aksentijevich I, Masters SL, Ferguson PJ, et al. An autoinflammatory disease with deficiency of the interleukin-1-receptor antagonist. *N Engl J Med* 2009;360:2426–2437.
6. Alanay Y, Krakow D, Rimoin DL, Lachman RS. Angulated femurs and the skeletal dysplasias: experience of the International Skeletal Dysplasia Registry (1988–2006). *Am J Med Genet A* 2007;143A:1159–1168.
7. Alawi F. Benign fibro-osseous diseases of the maxillofacial bones. A review and differential diagnosis. *Am J Clin Pathol* 2002;118(suppl):S50–S70.
8. Albregts AE, Rapini RP. Malignancy in Maffucci's syndrome. *Dermatol Clin* 1995;13:73–78.
9. Aldenhoven M, Sakkers RJ, Boelens J, et al. Musculoskeletal manifestations of lysosomal storage disorders. *Ann Rheum Dis* 2009;68:1659–1665.
10. Alexander AA, Patel AA, Odland R. Paranasal sinus osteomas and Gardner's syndrome. *Ann Otol Rhinol Laryngol* 2007;116:658–662.
11. Al-Gazali LI, Bakalinova D, Bakir M, et al. Fibrochondrogenesis: clinical and radiological features. *Clin Dysmorphol* 1997;6:157–163.
12. Al-Gazali LI, Bakir M, Hamid Z, et al. Birth prevalence and pattern of osteochondrodysplasias in an inbred high risk population. *Birth Defects Res A Clin Mol Teratol* 2003;67:125–132.
13. Allen VM, Armson BA, Wilson RD, et al. Teratogenicity associated with pre-existing and gestational diabetes. *J Obstet Gynaecol Can* 2007;29:927–944.
14. Alman BA. Skeletal dysplasias and the growth plate. *Clin Genet* 2008;73:24–30.
15. Almeida MR, Campos-Xavier AB, Medeira A, et al. Clinical and molecular diagnosis of the skeletal dysplasias associated with mutations in the gene encoding Fibroblast Growth Factor Receptor 3 (FGFR3) in Portugal. *Clin Genet* 2009;75:150–156.
16. Alsharif MJ, Sun ZJ, Chen XM, et al. Benign fibro-osseous lesions of the jaws: a study of 127 Chinese patients and review of the literature. *Int J Surg Pathol* 2009;17:122–134.
17. Amling M, Werner M, Posl M, et al. Calcifying solitary bone cyst: morphological aspects and differential diagnosis of sclerotic bone tumours. *Virchows Arch* 1995;426:235–242.
18. Amling M, Werner M, Posl M, et al. Solitary bone cysts. Morphologic variation, site, incidence and differential diagnosis. *Pathologe* 1996;17:63–67.
19. Amstalden EMI, Carvalho RB, Pacheco EM, et al. Chondromatous hamartoma of the chest wall: description of 3 new cases and literature review. *Int J Surg Pathol* 2006;14:119–126.
20. Andersen PE Jr. Prevalence of lethal osteochondrodysplasias in Denmark. *Am J Med Genet* 1989;32:484–489.
21. Andersen PE Jr, Hauge M. Congenital generalised bone dysplasias: a clinical, radiological, and epidemiological survey. *J Med Genet* 1989;26:37–44.
22. Angervall L, Persson S, Stenman G, et al. Large cell, epithelioid, telangiectatic osteoblastoma: a unique pseudosarcomatous variant of osteoblastoma. *Hum Pathol* 1999;30:1254–1259.
23. Arkader A, Glotzbecker M, Hosalkar HS, et al. Primary musculoskeletal Langerhans cell histiocytosis in children: an analysis for a 3-decade period. *J Pediatr Orthop* 2009;29:201–207.
24. Arnold SR, Elias D, Buckingham SC, et al. Changing patterns of acute hematogenous osteomyelitis and septic arthritis: emergence of community-associated methicillin-resistant Staphylococcus aureus. *J Pediatr Orthop* 2006;26:703–708.
25. Athale UH, Kaste SC, Razzouk BI, et al. Skeletal manifestations of pediatric acute megakaryoblastic leukemia. *J Pediatr Hematol Oncol* 2002;24:561–565.
26. Aubin JE, Heersche JNM. Bone cell biology osteoblasts, osteocytes, and osteoclasts. In: Glorieux FH, ed. *Pediatric Bone. Biology and Diseases.* San Francisco: Academic Press, 2002:43–76.
27. Auclair PL, Cuenin P, Kratochvil FJ, et al. A clinical and histomorphologic comparison of the central giant cell granuloma and the giant cell tumor. *Oral Surg Oral Med Oral Pathol* 1988;66:197–208.
28. Aviv RI, McHugh K, Hunt J. Angiomatosis of bone and soft tissue: a spectrum of disease from diffuse lymphangiomatosis to vanishing bone disease in young patients. *Clin Radiol* 2001;56:184–190.
29. Aymore IL Meohas W, Brito de Almeida AL, Proebstner D. Case report. Periosteal Ewing's sarcoma. Case report and literature review. *Clin Orthop Relat Res* 2005;434:265–272.
30. Azouz EM, Kozlowski K. Osteoglophonic dysplasia: appearance and progression of multiple nonossifying fibromata. *Pediatr Radiol* 1997;27:75–78.
31. Azouz EM, Kozlowski K, Marton D, et al. Osteoid osteoma and osteoblastoma of the spine in children. Report of 22 cases with brief literature review. *Pediatr Radiol* 1986;16:25–31.
32. Azura M, Vanel D, Alberghini M, et al. Parosteal osteosarcoma dedifferentiating into telangiectatic osteosarcoma: importance of lytic changes and fluid cavities at imaging. *Skeletal Radiol* 2009;38:685–690.
33. Bacchini P, Inwards C, Biscaglia R, et al. Chondroblastoma-like osteosarcoma. *Orthopedics* 1999;22:337–339.
34. Bacci G, Longhi A, Versari M, et al. Prognostic factors for osteosarcoma of the extremity treated with neoadjuvant chemotherapy: 15-year experience in 789 patients treated at a single institution. *Cancer* 2006;106:1154–1161.
35. Bahk WJ, Lee HY, Kang YK. Dysplasia epiphysealis hemimelica: radiographic and magnetic resonance imaging features and clinical outcome of complete and incomplete resection. *Skeletal Radiol* 2010;39:85–90.
36. Baker CV. The evolution and elaboration of vertebrate neural crest cells. *Curr Opin Genet Dev* 2008;18:536–543.
37. Bakhshi S, Singh P, Thulkar S. Bone involvement in pediatric non-Hodgkin's lymphomas. *Hematology* 2008;13:348–351.
38. Bamforth JS. Amniotic band sequence: Streeter hypothesis revisited. *Birth Defects Orig Artic Ser* 1993;29:279–289.

39. Bamshad M, Van Heest AE, Pleasure D. Arthrogryposis: a review and update. *J Bone Joint Surg Am* 2009;91 Suppl 4:40–46.
40. Bang G, Baardsen R, Gilhuus-Moe O. Infantile fibrosarcoma in the mandible: case report. *J Oral Pathol Med* 1989;18:339–343.
41. Bargagli E, Olivieri C, Penza F, et al. Rare localizations of bone sarcoidosis: two case reports and review of the literature. *Rheumatol Int* 2009, Dec 15; [Epub ahead of print].
42. Barnicoat AJ, Seller MJ, Bennett CP. Fetus with features of Crane-Heise syndrome and aminopterin syndrome sine aminopterin (ASSAS). *Clin Dysmorphol* 1994;3:353–357.
43. Barr FG, Womer RB. Molecular diagnosis of Ewng family tumors: too many fusions...? *J Mol Diagn* 2007;9:437–440.
44. Barr RD, Sala A. Osteonecrosis in children and adolescents with cancer. *Pediatr Blood Cancer* 2008;50:483–485; discussion 486.
45. Barton LL, Villar RG, Rice SA. Neonatal group B streptococcal vertebral osteomyelitis. *Pediatrics* 1996;98:459–461.
46. Basel D, Kilpatrick MW, Tsipouras P. The expanding panorama of split hand foot malformation. *Am J Med Genet A* 2006;140 A:1359–1365.
47. Bassett GS, Cowell HR. Metachondromatosis. Report of four cases. *J Bone Joint Surg Am* 1985;67:811–814.
48. Baujat G, Le Merrer M. Ellis-van Creveld syndrome. *Orphanet J Rare Dis* 2007;2:27.
49. Baujat G, Legeai-Mallet L, Finidori G, et al. Achondroplasia. *Best Pract Res Clin Rheumatol* 2008;22:3–18.
50. Baumgartner MR, Poll-The BT, Verhoeven NM, et al. Clinical approach to inherited peroxisomal disorders: a series of 27 patients. *Ann Neurol* 1998;44:720–730.
51. Beck M, Roubicek M, Rogers JG, et al. Heterogeneity of metatropic dysplasia. *Eur J Pediatr* 1983;140:231–237.
52. Becker ML, Rose CD. Blau syndrome and related genetic disorders causing childhood arthritis. *Curr Rheumatol Rep* 2005;7:427–433.
53. Bedi HS, Kaufman DV, Choong PF, Slavin JL. Osteosarcoma of the scapula arising in osteogenesis imperfecta. *Pathology* 1999;31:52–54.
54. Beighton P. Osteoglophonic dysplasia. *J Med Genet* 1989;26:572–576.
55. Bejjani BA, Oberg KC, Wilkins I, et al. Prenatal ultrasonographic description and postnatal pathological findings in atelosteogenesis type 1. *Am J Med Genet* 1998;79:392–395.
56. Bell DM, Leung KK, Wheatley SC, et al. SOX9 directly regulates the type-II collagen gene. *Nat Genet* 1997;16:174–178.
57. Bendon RW. Ivemark's renal-hepatic-pancreatic dysplasia: analytic approach to a perinatal autopsy. *Pediatr Dev Pathol* 1999;2:94–100.
58. Berber R, Berber O, Taguri N, Sekhar Maroju R, Abdulla S. Pseudarthrosis of the tibia: emergency department presentation of neurofibromatosis type 1 in a 4-month-old infant. *Emerg Med J* 2009;26:306–307.
59. Bereket A, Casur Y, Firat P, Yordam N. Brown tumour as a complication of secondary hyperparathyroidism in severe long-lasting vitamin D deficiency rickets. *Eur J Pediatr* 2000;159:70–73.
60. Berry M, Mankin H, Gebhardt M, Rosenberg A, Hornicek F. Osteoblastoma: a 30-year study of 99 cases. *J Surg Oncol* 2008;98:179–183.
61. Bertoni F, Bacchini P, Donati D, et al. Osteoblastoma-like osteosarcoma. The Rizzoli Institute experience. *Mod Pathol* 1993;6:707–716.
62. Bertoni F, Calderoni P, Bacchini P, et al. Benign fibrous histiocytoma of bone. *J Bone Joint Surg Am* 1986;68:1225–1230.
63. Bertoni F, Fernando Arias L, Alberghini M, et al. Fibrous dysplasia with degenerative atypia: a benign lesion potentially mistaken for sarcoma. *Arch Pathol Lab Med* 2004;128:794–796.
64. Bertoni F, Unni KK, Lucas DR, et al. Osteoblastoma with cartilaginous matrix. An unusual morphologic presentation in 18 cases. *Am J Surg Pathol* 1993;17:69–74.
65. Bertoni F, Unni KK, McLeod RA, Sim FH. Xanthoma of bone. *Am J Clin Pathol* 1988;90:377–384.
66. Betsy M, Kupersmith LM, Springfield DS. Metaphyseal fibrous defects. *J Am Acad Orthop Surg* 2004;12:89–95.
67. Bettelli G, Tigani D, Picci P. Recurring osteoblastoma initially presenting as a typical osteoid osteoma. Report of two cases. *Skeletal Radiol* 1991;20:1–4.
68. Bevan WP, Hall JG, Bamshad M, Staheli LT, Jaffe KM, Song K. Arthrogryposis multiplex congenita (amyoplasia). An orthopaedic perspective. *J Pediatr Orthop* 2007;27:594–600.
69. Bhowmick SK, Johnson KR, Rettig KR. Rickets caused by vitamin D deficiency in breast-fed infants in the southern United States. *Am J Dis Child* 1991;145:127–130.
70. Bicknell LS, Farrington-Rock C, Shafeghati Y, et al. A molecular and clinical study of Larsen syndrome caused by mutations in FLNB. *J Med Genet* 2007;44:89–98.
71. Bicknell LS, Morgan T, Bonafe L, et al. Mutations in FLNB cause boomerang dysplasia. *J Med Genet* 2005;42:e43.
72. Bieling P, Rehan N, Winkler P, et al. Tumor size and prognosis in aggressively treated osteosarcoma. *J Clin Oncol* 1996;14:848–858.
73. Biesecker JL, Marcove RC, Huvos AG, Mike V. Aneurysmal bone cysts. A clinicopathologic study of 66 cases. *Cancer* 1970;26:615–625.
74. Blade J, Kyle RA. Multiple myeloma in young patients: clinical presentation and treatment approach. *Leuk Lymphoma* 1998;30:493–501.
75. Blasius S, Link TM, Hillmann A, et al. Intracortical low grade osteosarcoma. A unique case and review of the literature on intracortical osteosarcoma. *Gen Diagn Pathol* 1996;141:273–278.
76. Blyth CC, Best EJ, Jones CA, et al. Nontuberculous mycobacterial infection in children. A prospective national study. *Pediatr Infect Dis J* 2009;28:801–805.
77. Boden SD, Kaplan FS, Fallon MD, et al. Metatropic dwarfism. Uncoupling of endochondral and perichondral growth. *J Bone Joint Surg Am* 1987;69:174–184.
78. Boerkoel CF, O'Neill S, Andre JL, et al. Manifestations and treatment of Schimke immuno-osseous dysplasia: 14 new cases and a review of the literature. *Eur J Pediatr* 2000;159:1–7.
79. Bohm P, Krober S, Greschniok A, et al. Desmoplastic fibroma of the bone. A report of two patients, review of the literature, and therapeutic implications. *Cancer* 1996;78:1011–1023.
80. Bonaventure J, Rousseau F, Legeai-Mallet L, et al. Common mutations in the fibroblast growth factor receptor 3 (FGFR 3) gene account for achondroplasia, hypochondroplasia, and thanatophoric dwarfism. *Am J Med Genet* 1996;63:148–154.
81. Bongers EMHF, Gubler MC, Knoers NV. Nail-patella syndrome. Overview on clinical and molecular findings. *Pediatr Nephrol* 2002;17:703–712.
82. Bongers EMHF, van Kampen A, van Bokhoven H, et al. Human syndromes with congenital patellar anomalies and the underlying gene defects. *Clin Genet* 2005;68:302–319.
83. Borochowitz Z, Lachman R, Adomian GE, et al. Achondrogenesis type I: delineation of further heterogeneity and identification of two distinct subgroups. *J Pediatr* 1988;112:23–31.
84. Borochowitz Z, Rimoin DL, The congenital chondroplasias. In: Reed GB, Claireaux AE, Cockburn F, eds. *Pathology, Imaging, Genetics and Management*, 2nd edn. London: Chapman and Hall, 1995:787–802.
85. Botto LD, Khoury MJ, Mastroiacovo P, et al. The spectrum of congenital anomalies of the VATER association: an international study. *Am J Med Genet* 1997;71:8–15.
86. Bovee JV. Multiple osteochondromas. *Orphanet J Rare Dis* 2008;3:3.
87. Bovee JV, Hameetman L, Kroon HM, et al. EXT-related pathways are not involved in the pathogenesis of dysplasia epiphysealis hemimelica and metachondromatosis. *J Pathol* 2006;209:411–419.
88. Bower C, Norwood F, Knowles S, et al. Amniotic band syndrome: a population-based study in two Australian states. *Paediatr Perinat Epidemiol* 1993;7:395–403.
89. Bradley JS, Kaplan SL, Tan TQ, et al. Pediatric pneumococcal bone and joint infections. The Pediatric Multicenter Pneumococcal Surveillance Study Group (PMPSSG). *Pediatrics* 1998;102:1376–1382.

90. Brannon RB, Fowler CB. Benign fibro-osseous lesions: a review of current concepts. *Adv Anat Pathol* 2001;8:126–143.
91. Breslau-Siderius EJ, Engelbert RH, Pals G, van der Sluijs JA. Bruck syndrome: a rare combination of bone fragility and multiple congenital joint contractures. *J Pediatr Orthop* B 1998;7:35–38.
92. Bridge JA, Fidler ME, Neff JR, et al. Adamantinoma-like Ewing's sarcoma: genomic confirmation, phenotypic drift. *Am J Surg Pathol* 1999;23:159–165.
93. Brien EW, Mirra JM, Kerr R. Benign and malignant cartilage tumors of bone and joint: their anatomic and theoretical basis with an emphasis on radiology, pathology and clinical biology. I. The intramedullary cartilage tumors. *Skeletal Radiol* 1997;26:325–353.
94. Brien EW, Mirra JM, Luck JV Jr. Benign and malignant cartilage tumors of bone and joint: their anatomic and theoretical basis with an emphasis on radiology, pathology and clinical biology. II. Juxtacortical cartilage tumors. *Skeletal Radiol* 1999;28:1–20.
95. Brighton CT. Morphology and biochemistry of the growth plate. *Rheum Dis Clin North Am* 1987;13:75–100.
96. Bruce JH, Romaguera RL, Rodriguez MM, et al. Caudal dysplasia syndrome and sirenomelia: are they part of a spectrum? *Fetal Pediatr Pathol* 2009;28:109–131.
97. Bruder E, Perez-Atayde AR, Jundt G, et al. Vascular lesions of bone in children, adolescents, and young adults. A clinicopathologic reappraisal and application of the ISSVA classification. *Virchows Arch* 2009;454:161–179.
98. Brueton LA, Dillon MJ, Winter RM. Ellis-Van Creveld syndrome, Jeune syndrome, and renal-hepatic-pancreatic dysplasia: separate entities or disease spectrum? *J Med Genet* 1990;27:252–255.
99. Brugieres L, Deley MC, Pacquement H, et al. CD30(+) anaplastic large-cell lymphoma in children: analysis of 82 patients enrolled in two consecutive studies of the French Society of Pediatric Oncology. *Blood* 1998;92:3591–3598.
100. Buchino JJ, Vogler C, Dimmick JE. Anatomical pathology and lysosomal storage diseases. In: Applegarth DA, Dimmick JE, Hall JG, eds. *Organelle Diseases*. London: Chapman and Hall, 2007:117–142.
101. Bullough PG, Davidson DD, Lorenzo JC. The morbid anatomy of the skeleton in osteogenesis imperfecta. *Clin Orthop Relat Res* 1981:42–57.
102. Burdan F, Szumilo J, Korobowicz A, et al. Morphology and physiology of the epiphyseal growth plate. *Folia Histochem Cytobiol* 2009;47:5–16.
103. Caffey J. On fibrous defects in cortical walls of growing tubular bones: their radiologic appearance, structure, prevalence, natural course, and diagnostic significance. *Adv Pediatr* 1955;7:13–51.
104. Caglar M, Ceylan E, Ozyar E. Frequency of skeletal metastases in nasopharyngeal carcinoma after initiation of therapy: should bone scans be used for follow-up? *Nucl Med Commun* 2003;24:1231–1236.
105. Calif E, Stahl S, Stahl S. Simple wrist ganglia in children: a follow-up study. *J Pediatr Orthop B* 2005;14:448–450.
106. Camp MD, Tompkins RK, Spanier SS, et al. Best cases from the AFIP: Adamantinoma of the tibia and fibula with cytogenetic analysis. *Radiographics* 2008;28:1215–1220.
107. Campbell CJ, Papademetriou T, Bonfiglio M. Melorheostosis. A report of the clinical, roentgenographic, and pathological findings in fourteen cases. *J Bone Joint Surg Am* 1968;50:1281–1304.
108. Canki-Klain N, Stanescu V, Stanescu R, et al. Lethal short limb dwarfism with dysmorphic face, omphalocele and severe ossification defect: Piepkorn syndrome or severe "boomerang dysplasia"? *Ann Genet* 1992;35:129–133.
109. Caplan AI. Bone development. *Ciba Found Symp* 1988;136:3–21.
110. Carey DE, Drezner MK, Hamdan JA, et al. Hypophosphatemic rickets/osteomalacia in linear sebaceous nevus syndrome: a variant of tumor-induced osteomalacia. *J Pediatr* 1986;109:994–1000.
111. Carter EM, Davis JG, Raggio CL. Advances in understanding etiology of achondroplasia and review of management. *Curr Opin Pediatr* 2007;19:32–37.
112. Carvalho VM, Perdigao PF, Amaral FR, et al. Novel mutations in the SH3BP2 gene associated with sporadic central giant cell lesions and cherubism. *Oral Dis* 2009;15:106–110.
113. Cassella JP, Stamp TC, Ali SY. A morphological and ultrastructural study of bone in osteogenesis imperfecta. *Calcif Tissue Int* 1996;58:155–165.
114. Castori M, Rinaldi R, Cappellacci S, et al. Tibial developmental field defect is the most common lower limb malformation pattern in VACTERL association. *Am J Med Genet A* 2008;146A:1259–1266.
115. Cavalcanti DP, Huber C, Le Quan Sang KH, et al. Mutation in IFT80 gene in a foetus with a phenotype of Verma-Naumoff provides molecular evidence for the Jeune-Verma-Naumoff dysplasia spectrum. *J Med Genet* 2009; Aug 11 [Epub ahead of press].
116. Chai Y, Maxson RE Jr. Recent advances in craniofacial morphogenesis. *Dev Dyn* 2006;235:2353–2375.
117. Chan JK, Ng CS, Hui PK, et al. Anaplastic large cell Ki-1 lymphoma of bone. *Cancer* 1991;68:2186–2191.
118. Chan YF, Lau JH, Tong CY. Congenital generalized fibromatosis with predominant osseous involvement in a Chinese newborn. *J Pediatr Orthop* 1989;9:64–68.
119. Chapurlat RD, Meunier PJ. Fibrous dysplasia of bone. *Baillieres Best Pract Res Clin* Rheumatol 2000;14:385–398.
120. Chauveinc L, Mosseri V, Quintana E, et al. Osteosarcoma following retinoblastoma: age at onset and latency period. *Ophthalmic Genet* 2001;22:77–88.
121. Cheung MS, Glorieux FH. Osteogenesis imperfecta: update on presentation and management. *Rev Endocr Metab Disord* 2008;9:153–160.
122. Cheung MS, Glorieux FH, Rauch F. Natural history of hyperplastic callus formation in osteogenesis imperfecta type V. *J Bone Miner Res* 2007;22:1181–1186.
123. Choong PF, Pritchard DJ, Rock MG, et al. Low grade central osteogenic sarcoma. A long-term followup of 20 patients. *Clin Orthop Relat Res* 1996:198–206.
124. Chowdhry M, Hughes C, Grimer RJ, et al. Bone sarcomas arising in patients with neurofibromatosis type 1. *J Bone Joint Surg Br* 2009;91:1223–1226.
125. Clewing JM, Antalfy BC, Lucke T, et al. Schimke immuno-osseous dysplasia: a clinicopathological correlation. *J Med Genet* 2007;44:122–130.
126. Cobben JM, Cornel MC, Dijkstra I, et al. Prevalence of lethal osteochondrodysplasias. *Am J Med Genet* 1990;36:377–378.
127. Coffin CM, Lowichik A, Zhou H. Treatment effects in pediatric soft tissue and bone tumors: practical considerations for the pathologist. *Am J Clin Pathol* 2005;123:75–90.
128. Coffin CM, Neilson KA, Ingels S, et al. Congenital generalized myofibromatosis: a disseminated angiocentric myofibromatosis. *Pediatr Pathol Lab Med* 1995;15:571–587.
129. Cohen MC, Drut R, Garcia C, et al. Mesenchymal hamartoma of the chest wall: a cooperative study with review of the literature. *Pediatr Pathol* 1992;12:525–534.
130. Cohen MM Jr. FGFs/FGFRs and associated disorders. Inborn errors of development. In: Epstein CJ, Erickson RP, Wynshaw-Boris A, eds. *The Molecular Basis of Clinical Disorders of Morphogenesis*. New York: Oxford University Press, 2004:380–400.
131. Cohen MM Jr. The new bone biology: pathologic, molecular, and clinical correlates. *Am J Med Genet A* 2006;140:2646–2706.
132. Cohen MM Jr. Some chondrodysplasias with short limbs: molecular perspectives. *Am J Med Genet* 2002;112:304–313.
133. Cole WG. Structure of growth plate and bone matrix. In: Glorieux FH, ed. *Pediatric Bone. Biology & Diseases*. San Francisco: Academic Press, 2003:1–41.
134. Cole WG, Dalgleish R. Perinatal lethal osteogenesis imperfecta. *J Med Genet* 1995;32:284–289.
135. Connor JM, Connor RA, Sweet EM, et al. Lethal neonatal chondrodysplasias in the West of Scotland 1970–1983 with a description of a thanatophoric dysplasialike, autosomal recessive disorder, Glasgow variant. *Am J Med Genet* 1985;22:243–53.
136. Coombs RJ, Zeiss J, McCann K, et al. Case report 360: multifocal Ewing tumor of the skeletal system. *Skeletal Radiol* 1986;15:254–257.

137. Cooney WP, Wolf J, Holtkamp K, et al. Congenital duplication of the thumb. *Handchir Mikrochir Plast Chir* 2004;36:126–136.
138. Copley LAB. Pediatric musculoskeletal infection: trends and antibiotic recommendations. *J Am Acad Orthop Surg* 2009;17:618–626.
139. Cordier AG, Mabille M, Delezoide AL, et al. Prenatal diagnosis of a rare skeletal dysplasia by ultrasound and scan tomography: atelosteogenesis III (AO III). Correlation with autopsy. *Prenat Diagn* 2008;28:975–977.
140. Cormier-Daire V, Superti-Furga A, Munnich A, et al. Clinical homogeneity of the Stuve-Wiedemann syndrome and overlap with the Schwartz-Jampel syndrome type 2. *Am J Med Genet* 1998;78:146–149.
141. Cortina H, Beltran J, Olague R, et al. The wide spectrum of the asphyxiating thoracic dysplasia. *Pediatr Radiol* 1979;8:93–99.
142. Cottalorda J, Haddad H, Bollini G, et al. [Fibrous dysplasia in children]. Pediatrie 1993;48:818–822.
143. Cottias P, Tomeno B, Anract P, et al. Subacute osteomyelitis presenting as a bone tumour. A review of 21 cases. *Int Orthop* 1997;21:243–248.
144. Coulter-Mackie MB, Lian Q, Applegarth DA, et al. Mutation-based diagnostic testing for primary hyperoxaluria type 1: survey of results. *Clin Biochem* 2008;41:598–602.
145. Cox H, Viljoen D, Versfeld G, Beighton P. Radial ray defects and associated anomalies. *Clin Genet* 1989;35:322–330.
146. Cuisia ZE, Brannon RB. Peripheral ossifying fibroma–a clinical evaluation of 134 pediatric cases. *Pediatr Dent* 2001;23:245–248.
147. Currall VA, Dixon JH. Synchronous multifocal osteosarcoma: case report and literature review. *Sarcoma* 2006;2006:53901.
148. Czerniak B, Rojas-Corona RR, Dorfman HD. Morphologic diversity of long bone adamantinoma. The concept of differentiated (regressing) adamantinoma and its relationship to osteofibrous dysplasia. *Cancer* 1989;64:2319–2334.
149. Dagoneau N, Scheffer D, Huber C, et al. Null leukemia inhibitory factor receptor (LIFR) mutations in Stuve-Wiedemann/Schwartz-Jampel type 2 syndrome. *Am J Hum Genet* 2004;74:298–305.
150. Dahlqvist J, Orlen H, Matsson H, et al. Multiple epiphyseal dysplasia. *Acta Orthop* 2009;80:711–715.
151. Damotte D, Peuchmaur M, Padovani JP, et al. Solitary infantile myofibromatosis of bone. *Ann Pathol* 1996;16:108–111.
152. Damron TA, Ward WG, Stewart A. Osteosarcoma, chondrosarcoma, and Ewing's sarcoma: National Cancer Data Base Report. *Clin Orthop Relat Res* 2007;459:40–47.
153. Daniels JSM. Central odontogenic fibroma of mandible: a case report and review of the literature. *Oral Surg Oral Med Oral Pathol Oral Radiol Endod* 2004;98:295–300.
154. Dannecker GE, Quartier P. Juvenile idiopathic arthritis: classification, clinical presentation and current treatments. *Horm Res* 2009;72(suppl 1):4–12.
155. Daw NC, Mahmoud HH, Meyer WH, et al. Bone sarcomas of the head and neck in children: the St Jude Children's Research Hospital experience. *Cancer* 2000;88:2172–2180.
156. Day TF, Yang Y. Wnt and hedgehog signaling pathways in bone development. *J Bone Joint Surg Am* 2008;90(suppl 1):19–24.
157. de Chadarevian JP, Katsetos CD, Pascasio JM, et al. Histological study of osteoid osteoma's blood supply. *Pediatr Dev Pathol* 2007;10:358–368.
158. de Lange J, van den Akker HP. Clinical and radiological features of central giant-cell lesions of the jaw. *Oral Surg Oral Med Oral Pathol Oral Radiol Endod* 2005;99:464–470.
159. de Lange J, van den Akker HP, van den Berg H. Central giant cell granuloma of the jaw: a review of the literature with emphasis on therapy options. *Oral Surg Oral Med Oral Pathol Oral Radiol Endod* 2007;104:603–615.
160. de Vernejoul MC. Sclerosing bone disorders. *Best Pract Res Clin Rheumatol* 2008;22:71–83.
161. Dehner LP. Juvenile xanthogranulomas in the first two decades of life: a clinicopathologic study of 174 cases with cutaneous and extracutaneous manifestations. *Am J Surg Pathol* 2003;27:579–593.
162. Del Fattore A, Peruzzi B, Rucci N, et al. Clinical, genetic, and cellular analysis of 49 osteopetrotic patients: implications for diagnosis and treatment. *J Med Genet* 2006;43:315–325.
163. Delague V, Chouery E, Corbani S, et al. Molecular study of WISP3 in nine families originating from the Middle-East and presenting with progressive pseudorheumatoid dysplasia: identification of two novel mutations, and description of a founder effect. *Am J Med Genet A* 2005;138A:118–126.
164. Deng ZL, Sharff KA, Tang N, et al. Regulation of osteogenic differentiation during skeletal development. *Front Biosci* 2008;13:2001–2021.
165. Desai SS, Jambhekar N, Agarwal M, Puri A, Merchant N. Adamantinoma of tibia: a study of 12 cases. *J Surg Oncol* 2006;93:429–433.
166. DiCaprio MR, Enneking WF. Fibrous dysplasia. Pathophysiology, evaluation, and treatment. *J Bone Joint Surg Am* 2005;87A:1848–1864.
167. Dickson BC, Li SQ, Wunder JS, et al. Giant cell tumor of bone express p63. *Mod Pathol* 2008;21:369–375.
168. Diez-Roux G, Ballabio A. Sulfatases and human disease. *Annu Rev Genomics Hum Genet* 2005;6:355–379.
169. Dighe M, Fligner C, Cheng E, et al. Fetal skeletal dysplasia: an approach to diagnosis with illustrative cases. *Radiographics* 2008;28:1061–1077.
170. Dimmick JE. Pathology of peroxisomal disorders. In: Applegarth DA, Dimmick JE, Hall JG, eds. *Organelle diseases*. London: Chapman and Hall, 1997:211–232.
171. Dinarello CA. Interleukin-1beta and the autoinflammatory diseases. *N Engl J Med* 2009;360:2467–2470.
172. Dong PR, Seeger LL, Eckardt JJ, et al. Case report 847. Juxtacortical aggressive fibromatosis (desmoplastic fibroma) of the forearm. *Skeletal Radiol* 1994;23:560–563.
173. Dorfman HD, Ishida T, Tsuneyoshi M. Exophytic variant of fibrous dysplasia (fibrous dysplasia protuberans). *Hum Pathol* 1994;25:1234–1237.
174. Dror Y. Shwachman-Diamond syndrome. *Pediatr Blood Cancer* 2005;45:892–901.
175. Duchatelet S, Ostergaard E, Cortes D, et al. Recessive mutations in PTHR1 cause contrasting skeletal dysplasias in Eiken and Blomstrand syndromes. *Hum Mol Genet* 2005;14:1–5.
176. Duesterhoeft SM, Ernst LM, Siebert JR, et al. Five cases of caudal regression with an aberrant abdominal umbilical artery: further support for a caudal regression-sirenomelia spectrum. *Am J Med Genet A* 2007;143A:3175–3184.
177. Dunlap C, Neville B, Vickers RA, et al. The Noonan syndrome/cherubism association. *Oral Surg Oral Med Oral Pathol* 1989;67:698–705.
178. Dunn AL, Busch MT, Wyly JB, et al. Arthroscopic synovectomy for hemophilic joint disease in a pediatric population. *J Pediatr Orthop* 2004;24:414–426.
179. El Hage S, Ghanem I, Baradhi A, et al. Skeletal features of primary hyperoxaluria type 1, revisited. *J Child Orthop* 2008;2:205–210.
180. Elcioglu N, Hall CM. A lethal skeletal dysplasia with features of chondrodysplasia punctata and osteogenesis imperfecta: an example of Astley-Kendall dysplasia. Further delineation of a rare genetic disorder. *J Med Genet* 1998;35:505–507.
181. Elejalde BR, de Elejalde MM. Thanatophoric dysplasia: fetal manifestations and prenatal diagnosis. *Am J Med Genet* 1985;22:669–683.
182. Elliott AM, Evans JA. Genotype-phenotype correlations in mapped split hand foot malformation (SHFM) patients. *Am J Med Genet A* 2006;140:1419–1427.
183. El-Mofty S. Psammomatoid and trabecular juvenile ossifying fibroma of the craniofacial skeleton: two distinct clinicopatho-

logic entities. *Oral Surg Oral Med Oral Pathol Oral Radiol Endod* 2002;93:296–304.

184. Emery JL, Kalpaktsoglou PK. The costochondral junction during later stages of intrauterine life, and abnormal growth patterns found in association with perinatal death. *Arch Dis Child* 1967;42:1–13.
185. Emery SC, Karpinski NC, Hansen L, et al. Abnormalities in central nervous system development in osteogenesis imperfecta type II. *Pediatr Dev Pathol* 1999;2:124–130.
186. Engels C, Priemel M, Moller G, et al. Chondromyxoid fibroma. Morphological variations, site, incidence, radiologic criteria and differential diagnosis. *Pathologe* 1999;20:224–229.
187. Eriksson UJ, Cederberg J, Wentzel P. Congenital malformations in offspring of diabetic mothers–animal and human studies. *Rev Endocr Metab Disord* 2003;4:79–93.
188. Erzen M, Stanescu R, Stanescu V, et al. Comparative histopathology of the growth cartilage in short-rib polydactyly syndromes type I and type III and in chondroectodermal dysplasia. *Ann Genet* 1988;31:144–150.
189. Estrada-Villasenor E, Delgado Cedillo EA, et al. Frequency of bone neoplasms in children. *Acta Ortop Mex* 2008;22:238–242.
190. Eteson DJ, Adomian GE, Ornoy A, et al. Fibrochondrogenesis: radiologic and histologic studies. *Am J Med Genet* 1984;19:277–290.
191. Evans JA, Vitez M, Czeizel A. Congenital abnormalities associated with limb deficiency defects: a population study based on cases from the Hungarian Congenital Malformation Registry (1975–1984). *Am J Med Genet* 1994;49:52–66.
192. Eyre R, Feltbower RG, Mubwandarikwa E, et al. Epidemiology of bone tumours in children and young adults. *Pediatr Blood Cancer* 2009;53:941–952.
193. Faden MA, Krakow D, Ezgu F, et al. The Erlenmeyer flask bone deformity in the skeletal dysplasias. *Am J Med Genet A* 2009;149A:1334–1345.
194. Farrington-Rock C, Firestein MH, Bicknell LS, et al. Mutations in two regions of FLNB result in atelosteogenesis I and III. *Hum Mutat* 2006;27:705–710.
195. Farrow EG, Davis SI, Mooney SD, et al. Extended mutational analyses of FGFR1 in osteoglophonic dysplasia. *Am J Med Genet A* 2006;140:537–539.
196. Farrugia EJ, Stephen AP, Raza SA. Juvenile xanthogranuloma of temporal bone—a case report. *J Laryngol Otol* 1997;111:63–65.
197. Fernandez-Palazzi F, Bendahan J, Rivas S. Congenital deficiency of the tibia: a report on 22 cases. *J Pediatr Orthop B* 1998;7:298–302.
198. Ferrari S, Bertoni F, Palmerini E, et al. Predictive factors of histologic response to primary chemotherapy in patients with Ewing sarcoma. *J Pediatr Hematol Oncol* 2007;29:364–368.
199. Fetil E, Ozkan S, Ilknur T, Kavukcu S, Kusku E, Lebe B. Sarcoidosis in a preschooler with only skin and joint involvement. *Pediatr Dermatol* 2003;20:416–418.
200. Fletcher CDM, Unni KK, Mertens F. *World Health Organization classification of tumours, pathology and genetics of tumours of soft tissue and bone*. Lyon: IARC Press, 2002.
201. Folpe AL, Fanburg-Smith JC, Billings SD, et al. Most osteomalacia-associated mesenchymal tumors are a single histopathologic entity: an analysis of 32 cases and a comprehensive review of the literature. *Am J Surg Pathol* 2004;28:1–30.
202. Folpe AL, Goldblum JR, Rubin BP, et al. Morphologic and immunophenotypic diversity in Ewing family tumors: a study of 66 genetically confirmed cases. *Am J Surg Pathol* 2005;29:1025–1033.
203. Foss RD, Ellis GL. Myofibromas and myofibromatosis of the oral region: A clinicopathologic analysis of 79 cases. *Oral Surg Oral Med Oral Pathol Oral Radiol Endod* 2000;89:57–65.
204. Foucar E, Rosai J, Dorfman R. Sinus histiocytosis with massive lymphadenopathy (Rosai-Dorfman disease): review of the entity. *Semin Diagn Pathol* 1990;7:19–73.
205. Foulkes GD, Reinker K. Congenital constriction band syndrome: a seventy-year experience. *J Pediatr Orthop* 1994;14:242–248.
206. Franchi A, Bertoni F, Bacchini P, et al. CD105/endoglin expression in Gorham disease of bone. *J Clin Pathol* 2009;62:163–167.
207. Frassica FJ, Waltrip RL, Sponseller PD, et al. Clinicopathologic features and treatment of osteoid osteoma and osteoblastoma in children and adolescents. *Orthop Clin North Am* 1996;27:559–574.
208. Frattini A, Pangrazio A, Susani L, et al. Chloride channel ClCN7 mutations are responsible for severe recessive, dominant, and intermediate osteopetrosis. *J Bone Miner Res* 2003;18:1740–1747.
209. Freeze HH. Achondrogenesis type 1A—from mouse to human. *N Engl J Med* 2010;362:266–267.
210. Froster UG, Baird PA. Amniotic band sequence and limb defects: data from a population-based study. *Am J Med Genet* 1993;46:497–500.
211. Froster UG, Baird PA. Upper limb deficiencies and associated malformations: a population-based study. *Am J Med Genet* 1992;44:767–781.
212. Froster-Iskenius UG, Baird PA. Amelia: incidence and associated defects in a large population. Teratology 1990;41:23–31.
213. Fuchs B, Pritchard DJ. Etiology of osteosarcoma. *Clin Orthop Relat Res* 2002:40–52.
214. Fujii H, Honoki K, Enomoto Y, et al. Adamantinoma-like Ewing's sarcoma with EWS-FLI1 fusion gene: a case report. *Virchows Arch* 2006;449:579–584.
215. Furman WL, Fitch S, Hustu HO, et al. Primary lymphoma of bone in children. *J Clin Oncol* 1989;7:1275–1280.
216. Gadwal SR, Gannon FH, Fanburg-Smith JC, et al. Primary osteosarcoma of the head and neck in pediatric patients: a clinicopathologic study of 22 cases with a review of the literature. *Cancer* 2001;91:598–605.
217. Gafur OA, Copley LA, Hollmig ST, et al. The impact of the current epidemiology of pediatric musculoskeletal infection on evaluation and treatment guidelines. *J Pediatr Orthop* 2008;28:777–785.
218. Galois L, Mainard D, Delagoutte JP. Polydactyly of the foot. Literature review and case presentations. *Acta Orthop Belg* 2002;68:376–380.
219. Gartner J. Disorders related to peroxisomal membranes. *J Inherit Metab Dis* 2000;23:264–272.
220. Garver P, Resnick D, Haghighi P, *Guerra J*. Melorheostosis of the axial skeleton with associated fibrolipomatous lesions. *Skeletal Radiol* 1982;9:41–44.
221. Gazit D, Tieder M, Liberman UA, et al. Osteomalacia in hereditary hypophosphatemic rickets with hypercalciuria: a correlative clinical-histomorphometric study. *J Clin Endocrinol Metab* 1991;72:229–235.
222. Genevieve D, Le Merrer M, Feingold J, et al. Revisiting metatropic dysplasia: presentation of a series of 19 novel patients and review of the literature. *Am J Med Genet A* 2008;146A:992–996.
223. Gerards AH, Winia WP, Westerga J, et al. Destructive joint disease in alpha-mannosidosis. A case report and review of the literature. *Clin Rheumatol* 2004;23:40–42.
224. Gerlag D, Tak PP. Synovial biopsy. *Best Pract Res Clin Rheumatol* 2005;19:387–400.
225. Ghanem I. The management of osteoid osteoma: updates and controversies. *Curr Opin Pediatr* 2006;18:36–41.
226. Gibson SE, Prayson RA. Primary skull lesions in the pediatric population: a 25-year experience. *Arch Pathol Lab Med* 2007;131:761–766.
227. Gikas PD, Islam L, Aston W, et al. Nonbacterial osteitis: a clinical, histopathological, and imaging study with a proposal for protocol-based management of patients with this diagnosis. *J Orthop Sci* 2009;14:505–516.
228. Gilbert-Barness E. Osteochondrodysplasia—constitutional diseases of bone. In: *Potter's Pathology of the Fetus, Infant and Child*, 2nd edn. Philadelphia: Mosby Elsevier, 2007:1836–1897.
229. Gilbert-Barness E, Opitz JM. Abnormal bone development: histopathology of skeletal dysplasias. *Birth Defects Orig Artic Ser* 1996;30:103–156.

230. Gimovsky M, Rosa E, Tolbert T, Guzman G, Nazir M, Koscica K. Campomelic dysplasia: case report and review. *J Perinatol* 2008;28:71–73.
231. Gleason BC, Liegl-Atzwanger B, Kozakewich HP, et al. Osteofibrous dysplasia and adamantinoma in children and adolescents: a clinicopathologic reappraisal. *Am J Surg Pathol* 2008;32:363–376.
232. Glick R, Khaldi L, Ptaszynski K, Steiner GC. Dysplasia epiphysealis hemimelica (Trevor disease): a rare developmental disorder of bone mimicking osteochondroma of long bones. *Hum Pathol* 2007;38:1265–1272.
233. Glorieux FH. Caffey disease: an unlikely collagenopathy. *J Clin Invest* 2005;115:1142–1144.
234. Glorieux FH. Osteogenesis imperfecta. *Best Pract Res Clin Rheumatol* 2008;22:85–100.
235. Glotzbecker MP, Kersun LS, Choi JK, et al. Primary non-Hodgkin's lymphoma of bone in children. *J Bone Joint Surg Am* 2006;88:583–594.
236. Goldfarb CA, Wall L, Manske PR. Radial longitudinal deficiency: the incidence of associated medical and musculoskeletal conditions. *J Hand Surg Am* 2006;31:1176–1182.
237. Goldfinger S. The inherited autoinflammatory syndrome: a decade of discovery. *Trans Am Clin Climatol Assoc* 2009;120:413–418.
238. Goldring MB, Tsuchimochi K, Ijiri K. The control of chondrogenesis. *J Cell Biochem* 2006;97:33–44.
239. Gordienko I, Grechanina E, Sopko NI, et al. Prenatal diagnosis of osteochondrodysplasias in high risk pregnancy. *Am J Med Genet* 1996;63:90–97.
240. Gordon CT, Tan TY, Benko S, et al. Long-range regulation at the SOX9 locus in development and disease. *J Med Genet* 2009;46:649–656.
241. Goutas N, Simopoulou S, Petraki V, Agapitos E. Limb reduction defects—autopsy study. *Pediatr Pathol* 1993;13:29–35.
242. Greenhalgh KL, Howell RT, Bottani A, et al. Thrombocytopenia-absent radius syndrome: a clinical genetic study. *J Med Genet* 2002;39:876–881.
243. Greenspan A. Benign bone-forming lesions: osteoma, osteoid osteoma, and osteoblastoma. Clinical, imaging, pathologic, and differential considerations. *Skeletal Radiol* 1993;22:485–500.
244. Greenspan A. Sclerosing bone dysplasias—a target-site approach. *Skeletal Radiol* 1991;20:561–583.
245. Greenspan A, Azouz EM. Bone dysplasia series. Melorheostosis: review and update. *Can Assoc Radiol J* 1999;50:324–330.
246. Grix A Jr., Curry C, Hall BD. Patterns of multiple malformations in infants of diabetic mothers. *Birth Defects Orig Artic Ser* 1982;18:55–77.
247. Groom KR, Murphey MD, Howard LM, et al. Mesenchymal hamartoma of the chest wall: radiologic manifestations with emphasis on cross-sectional imaging and histopathologic comparison. *Radiology* 2002;222:205–211.
248. Guggenbuhl P, Grosbois B, Chales G. Gaucher disease. *Joint Bone Spine* 2008;75:116–124.
249. Gupta P, Babyn P. Sinus histiocytosis with massive lymphadenopathy (Rosai-Dorfman disease): a clinicoradiological profile of three cases including two with skeletal disease. *Pediatr Radiol* 2008;38:721–728.
250. Gurrieri F, Kjaer KW, Sangiorgi E, et al. Limb anomalies: developmental and evolutionary aspects. *Am J Med Genet* 2002;115:231–244.
251. Haddad FS, Jones DH, Vellodi A, et al. Carpal tunnel syndrome in the mucopolysaccharidoses and mucolipidoses. *J Bone Joint Surg Br* 1997;79:576–582.
252. Hajjaji N, Hocqueloux L, Kerdraon R, Bret L. Bone infection in cat-scratch disease: a review of the literature. *J Infect* 2007;54:417–421.
253. Hakozaki M, Hojo H, Tajino T, et al. Periosteal Ewing sarcoma family of tumors of the femur confirmed by molecular detection of EWS-FLI1 fusion gene transcripts: a case report and review of the literature. *J Pediatr Hematol Oncol* 2007;29:561–565.
254. Hall BD. Lethality in Desbuquois dysplasia: three new cases. *Pediatr Radiol* 2001;31:43–47.
255. Hall CM, Elcioglu NH. Metatropic dysplasia lethal variants. *Pediatr Radiol* 2004;34:66–74.
256. Hall JG. Arthrogryposis multiplex congenita: etiology, genetics, classification, diagnostic approach, and general aspects. *J Pediatr Orthop B* 1997;6:159–166.
257. Hall JG. Pena-Shokeir phenotype (fetal akinesia deformation sequence) revisited. *Birth Defects Res A Clin Mol Teratol* 2009;85:677–694.
258. Hamilton WJ, Boyd JD, Mossman HW. *Human embryology*. Baltimore, MD: Williams & Wilkins, 1962.
259. Hartmann C. A Wnt canon orchestrating osteoblastogenesis. *Trends Cell Biol* 2006;16:151–158.
260. Hastbacka J, Superti-Furga A, Wilcox WR, et al. Atelosteogenesis type II is caused by mutations in the diastrophic dysplasia sulfate-transporter gene (DTDST): evidence for a phenotypic series involving three chondrodysplasias. *Am J Hum Genet* 1996;58:255–262.
261. Haven CJ, Wong FK, van Dam EW, et al. A genotypic and histopathological study of a large Dutch kindred with hyperparathyroidism-jaw tumor syndrome. *J Clin Endocrinol Metab* 2000;85:1449–1454.
262. Ha-Vinh R, Alanay Y, Bank RA, et al. Phenotypic and molecular characterization of Bruck syndrome (osteogenesis imperfecta with contractures of the large joints) caused by a recessive mutation in PLOD2. *Am J Med Genet A* 2004;131:115–120.
263. Hazelbag HM, Wessels JW, Mollevangers P, et al. Cytogenetic analysis of adamantinoma of long bones: further indications for a common histogenesis with osteofibrous dysplasia. *Cancer Genet Cytogenet* 1997;97:5–11.
264. Hefti F, Bollini G, Dungl P, et al. Congenital pseudarthrosis of the tibia: history, etiology, classification, and epidemiologic data. *J Pediatr Orthop* B 2000;9:11–15.
265. Helfrich MH, Aronson DC, Everts V, et al. Morphologic features of bone in human osteopetrosis. *Bone* 1991;12:411–419.
266. Hendrickx G, De Boeck H, Goossens A, Demanet C, Vandenplas Y. Persistent synovitis in children with Lyme arthritis: two unusual cases. An immunogenetic approach. *Eur J Pediatr* 2004;163:646–650.
267. Henriksen K, Gram J, Hoegh-Andersen P, et al. Osteoclasts from patients with autosomal dominant osteopetrosis type I caused by a T253I mutation in low-density lipoprotein receptor-related protein 5 are normal in vitro, but have decreased resorption capacity in vivo. *Am J Pathol* 2005;167:1341–1348.
268. Hentze S, Sergi C, Troeger J, et al. Short-rib-polydactyly syndrome type Verma-Naumoff-Le Marec in a fetus with histological hallmarks of type Saldino-Noonan but lacking internal organ abnormalities. *Am J Med Genet* 1998;80:281–285.
269. Herman TE. Antenatal-onset infantile cortical hyperostosis and non-immune hydrops. *J Perinatol* 1996;16:137–139.
270. Herman TE, Chines A, McAlister WH, et al. Metachondromatosis: report of a family with facial features mildly resembling trichorhinophalangeal syndrome. *Pediatr Radiol* 1997;27:436–441.
271. Hevner RF. The cerebral cortex malformation in thanatophoric dysplasia: neuropathology and pathogenesis. *Acta Neuropathol* 2005;110:208–221.
272. Hicks J, De Jong A, Barrish J, et al. Tracheomalacia in a neonate with Kniest dysplasia: histopathologic and ultrastructural features. *Ultrastruct Pathol* 2001;25:79–83.
273. Hill RE, Heaney SJ, Lettice LA. Sonic hedgehog: restricted expression and limb dysmorphologies. *J Anat* 2003;202:13–20.
274. Hill SC, Namde M, Dwyer A, et al. Arthropathy of neonatal onset multisystem inflammatory disease (NOMID/CINCA). *Pediatr Radiol* 2007;37:145–152.
275. Hoang MP, Carder KR, Pandya AG, Bennett MJ. Ichthyosis and keratotic follicular plugs containing dystrophic calcification in newborns: distinctive histopathologic features of x-linked dominant chondrodysplasia punctata (Conradi-Hunermann-Happle syndrome). *Am J Dermatopathol* 2004;26:53–58.

276. Hoeffel JC, Galloy MA, Grignon Y, et al. Giant cell tumor of bone in children and adolescents. *Rev Rhum Engl Ed* 1996;63:618–623.
277. Hoffmann C, Ahrens S, Dunst J, et al. Pelvic Ewing sarcoma: a retrospective analysis of 241 cases. *Cancer* 1999;85:869–877.
278. Holder-Espinasse M, Devisme L, Thomas D, et al. Pre- and postnatal diagnosis of limb anomalies: a series of 107 cases. *Am J Med Genet A* 2004;124A:417–422.
279. Hong JR, Barber M, Scott CI, et al. 3-Year-old phenotypic female with campomelic dysplasia and bilateral gonadoblastoma. *J Pediatr Surg* 1995;30:1735–1737.
280. Hopper KD, Moser RP Jr, Haseman DB, et al. Osteosarcomatosis. *Radiology* 1990;175:233–239.
281. Horner MJ, Ries, LAG, Krapcho, M, et al., eds. SEER Cancer Statistics Review, 1975–2006, National Cancer Institute, Bethesda, MD, http://seer.cancer.gov/csr/1975_2006, based on November 2008 SEER data submission, posted to the SEER web site, 2009.
282. Hornick JL, Fletcher CD. Intraarticular nodular fasciitis—a rare lesion: clinicopathologic analysis of a series. *Am J Surg Pathol* 2006;30:237–241.
283. Horton WA. Skeletal development: insights from targeting the mouse genome. Lancet 2003;362:560–569.
284. Horton WA, Hood OJ, Machado MA, et al. Abnormal ossification in thanatophoric dysplasia. *Bone* 1988;9:53–61.
285. Huang GS, Lee HS, Hsu YC, et al. Tenosynovial lipoma arborescens of the ankle in a child. *Skeletal Radiol* 2006;35:244–247.
286. Hunter AG, Carpenter BF. Atelosteogenesis I and boomerang dysplasia: a question of nosology. *Clin Genet* 1991;39:471–480.
287. Hurst JA, Firth HV, Smithson S. Skeletal dysplasias. *Semin Fetal Neonatal Med* 2005;10:233–241.
288. Huvos AG, Marcove RC. Chondrosarcoma in the young. A clinicopathologic analysis of 79 patients younger than 21 years of age. *Am J Surg Pathol* 1987;11:930–942.
289. Hyckel P, Berndt A, Schleier P, et al. Cherubism—new hypotheses on pathogenesis and therapeutic consequences. *J Craniomaxillofac Surg* 2005;33:61–68.
290. Ikeshima A, Utsunomiya T. Case report of intra-osseous fibroma: a study on odontogenic and desmoplastic fibromas with a review of the literature. *J Oral Sci* 2005;47:149–157.
291. Ilaslan H, Sundaram M, Unni KK. Solid variant of aneurismal bone cysts in long tubular bones: giant cell reparative granuloma. *AJR Am J Roentgenol* 2003;180:1681–1687.
292. Imashuku S, Kinugawa N, Matsuzaki A, et al. Langerhans cell histiocytosis with multifocal bone lesions: comparative clinical features between single and multi-systems. *Int J Hematol* 2009;90:506–512.
293. Inwards CY, Unni KK, Beabout JW, et al. Solitary congenital fibromatosis (infantile myofibromatosis) of bone. *Am J Surg Pathol* 1991;15:935–941.
294. Ippolito E, Bray EW, Corsi A, et al. Natural history and treatment of fibrous dysplasia of bone: a multicenter clinicopathologic study promoted by the European Pediatric Orthopaedic Society. *J Pediatr Orthop B* 2003;12:155–177.
295. Ippolito E, Corsi A, Grill F, et al. Pathology of bone lesions associated with congenital pseudarthrosis of the leg. *J Pediatr Orthop B* 2000;9:3–10.
296. Ippolito V, Mirra JM, Motta C, et al. Case report 771:melorheostosis in association with desmoid tumor. *Skeletal Radiol* 1993;22:284–288.
297. Irving MD, Chitty LS, Mansour S, et al. Chondrodysplasia punctata: a clinical diagnostic and radiological review. *Clin Dysmorphol* 2008;17:229–241.
298. Isidor B, Guillard S, Hamel A, et al. Genochondromatosis type II: report of a new patient and further delineation of the phenotype. *Am J Med Genet A* 2007;143A:1919–1921.
299. Jain D, Jain VK, Vasishta RK, Ranjan P, Kumar Y. Adamantinoma: a clinicopathological review and update. *Diagn Pathol* 2008;3:8.
300. Jain VK, Arya RK, Bharadwaj M, et al. Melorheostosis: clinicopathological features, diagnosis, and management. *Orthopedics* 2009;32:512.
301. Jamsheer A, Materna-Kiryluk A, Badura-Stronka M, et al. Comparative study of clinical characteristics of amniotic rupture sequence with and without body wall defect: further evidence for separation. *Birth Defects Res A Clin Mol Teratol* 2009;85:211–215.
302. Jansen NW, Roosendaal G, Lafeber FP. Understanding haemophilic arthropathy: an exploration of current open issues. *Br J Haematol* 2008;143:632–640.
303. Janssen D, Harms D. Juvenile xanthogranuloma in childhood and adolescence: a clinicopathologic study of 129 patients from the Kiel Pediatric Tumor Registry. *Am J Surg Pathol* 2005;29(1):21–28.
304. Jansson AF, Muller TH, Gliera L, et al. Clinical score for nonbacterial osteitis in children and adults. *Arthritis Rheum* 2009;60:1152–1159.
305. Jaramillo D. What is the optimal imaging of osteonecrosis, Perthes, and bone infarcts? *Pediatr Radiol* 2009;39(suppl 2):S216–S219.
306. Jee WH, Choe BY, Kang HS, et al. Nonossifying fibroma: characteristics at MR imaging with pathologic correlation. *Radiology* 1998;209:197–202.
307. Jee WH, Choi KH, Choe BY, et al. Fibrous dysplasia: MR imaging chacteristics with radiopathologic correlation. *AJR Am J Roentgenol* 1996;167:1523–1527.
308. Johnson LC, Yousefi M, Vinh TN, et al. Juvenile active ossifying fibroma. Its nature, dynamics and origin. *Acta Otolaryngol Suppl* 1991;488:1–40.
309. Jones AC, Prihoda TJ, Kacher JE, et al. Osteoblastoma of the maxilla and mandible: a report of 24 cases, review of the literature, and discussion of its relationship to osteoid osteoma of the jaws. *Oral Surg Oral Med Oral Pathol Oral Radiol Endod* 2006;102:639–650.
310. Jouve JL, Kohler R, Mubarak SJ, et al. Focal fibrocartilaginous dysplasia ("fibrous periosteal inclusion"). An additional series of eleven cases and literature review. *J Pediatr Orthop* 2007;27:75–84.
311. Kaariainen H, Ryoppy S, Norio R. RAPADILINO syndrome with radial and patellar aplasia/hypoplasia as main manifestations. *Am J Med Genet* 1989;33:346–351.
312. Kager L, Zoubek A, Kastner U, et al. Skip metastases in osteosarcoma: experience of the Cooperative Osteosarcoma Study Group. *J Clin Oncol* 2006;24:1535–1541.
313. Kahn LB. Adamantinoma, osteofibrous dysplasia and differentiated adamantinoma. *Skeletal Radiol* 2003;32:245–258.
314. Kai B, Ryan A, Munk PL, et al. Gorham disease of bone: three cases and review of radiological features. *Clin Radiol* 2006;61:1058–1064.
315. Kaissi AA, Roetzer K, Klaushofer K, et al. Acroform type of enchondromatosis associated with severe vertebral involvement and facial dysmorphism in a boy with a new variant of enchondromatosis type II of Spranger: case report and a review of the literature. *Cases J* 2008;1:324.
316. Kallen B. Population surveillance of multimalformed infants—experience with the Swedish Registry of Congenital Malformations. First Part. *J Genet Hum* 1987;35:205–215.
317. Kallen B. A prospective study of some aetiological factors in limb reduction defects in Sweden. *J Epidemiol Community Health* 1989;43:86–91.
318. Kameyama O, Ogawa R. Pseudarthrosis of the radius associated with neurofibromatosis: report of a case and review of the literature. *J Pediatr Orthop* 1990;10:128–131.
319. Kamoun-Goldrat A, le Merrer M. Infantile cortical hyperostosis (Caffey disease): a review. *J Oral Maxillofac Surg* 2008;66:2145–2150.
320. Kang SN, Sanghera T, Mangwani J, et al. The management of septic arthritis in children: systematic review of the English language literature. *J Bone Joint Surg Br* 2009;91B:1127–1133.
321. Kannu P, Aftimos S, Mayne V, et al. Metatropic dysplasia: clinical and radiographic findings in 11 patients demonstrating long-term natural history. *Am J Med Genet A* 2007;143A:2512–2522.
322. Kansara M, Thomas DM. Molecular pathogenesis of osteosarcoma. *DNA Cell Biol* 2007;26:1–18.

323. Kaplan I, Nicolaou Z, Hatuel D, et al. Solitary central osteoma of the jaws: a diagnostic dilemma. *Oral Surg Oral Med Oral Pathol Oral Radiol Endod* 2008;106:e22–e29.
324. Karabakhtsian R, Heller D, Hameed M, Bethel C. Periosteal chondroma of the rib—report of a case and literature review. *J Pediatr Surg* 2005;40:1505–1507.
325. Karaplis AC. Embryonic development of bone and the molecular regulation of intramembranous and endochondral bone formation. In: Bilezikian JP, John P, Raisz G, Rodan GA, eds. *Principles of Bone Biology*, Vol. 1, 2nd edn. San Francisco: Academic Press, 2002:33–58.
326. Karaplis AC, He B, Nguyen MT, et al. Inactivating mutation in the human parathyroid hormone receptor type 1 gene in Blomstrand chondrodysplasia. *Endocrinology* 1998;139:5255–5258.
327. Karsenty G. Transcriptional control of skeletogenesis. *Annu Rev Genomics Hum Genet* 2008;9:183–196.
328. Karsenty G, Wagner EF. Reaching a genetic and molecular understanding of skeletal development. *Dev Cell* 2002;2:389–406.
329. Kashima TG, Nishiyama T, Shimazu K, et al. Periostin, a novel marker of intramembranous ossification, is expressed in fibrous dysplasia and in c-Fos-overexpressing bone lesions. *Hum Pathol* 2009;40:226–237.
330. Kaste SC, Fuller CE, Saharia A, et al. Pediatric surface osteosarcoma: clinical, pathologic, and radiologic features. *Pediatr Blood Cancer* 2006;47:152–162.
331. Kaste SC, Pratt CB, Cain AM, et al. Metastases detected at the time of diagnosis of primary pediatric extremity osteosarcoma at diagnosis? Imaging features. *Cancer* 1999;86:1602–1608.
332. Kawaguchi Y, Sato C, Hasegawa T, et al. Intraarticular osteoid osteoma associated with synovitis: a possible role of cyclooxygenase-2 expression by osteoblasts in the nidus. *Mod Pathol* 2000;13:1086–1091.
333. Kaweblum M, Lehman WB, Bash J, et al. Diagnosis of osteoid osteoma in the child. *Orthop Rev* 1993;22:1305–1313.
334. Kaweblum M, Lehman WB, Bash J, et al. Osteoid osteoma under the age of five years. The difficulty of diagnosis. *Clin Orthop Relat Res* 1993:218–224.
335. Keckler SJ, St Peter SD, Valusek PA, et al. VACTERL anomalies in patients with esophageal atresia: an updated delineation of the spectrum and review of the literature. *Pediatr Surg Int* 2007;23:309–313.
336. Keeling JW, Hansen BF, Kjaer I. Pattern of malformations in the axial skeleton in human trisomy 21 fetuses. *Am J Med Genet* 1997;68:466–471.
337. Kelley RI. Inborn errors of cholesterol biosynthesis. *Adv Pediatr* 2000;47:1–53.
338. Kenet G, Ezra E, Wientroub S, et al. Perthes' disease and the search for genetic associations: collagen mutations, Gaucher's disease and thrombophilia. *J Bone Joint Surg Br* 2008;90:1507–1511.
339. Khoshhal K, Letts RM. Orthopaedic manifestations of campomelic dysplasia. *Clin Orthop Relat Res* 2002;401:65–74.
340. Kilpatrick SE, Wenger DE, Gilchrist GS, et al. Langerhans' cell histiocytosis (histiocytosis X) of bone. A clinicopathologic analysis of 263 pediatric and adult cases. *Cancer* 1995;76:2471–2484.
341. Kim MG, Kim BH, Choi JA, et al. Intra-articular ganglion cysts of the knee: clinical and MR imaging features. *Eur Radiol* 2001;11:834–840.
342. Kim S, Lee S, Arsenault DA, Strijbosch RA, Shamberger RC, Puder M. Pediatric rib lesions: a 13-year experience. *J Pediatr Surg* 2008;43:1781–1785.
343. Kitsoulis P, Galani V, Stefanaki K, et al. Osteochondromas: review of the clinical, radiological and pathological features. *In Vivo* 2008;22:633–646.
344. Kitsoulis P, Mantellos G, Vlychou M. Osteoid osteoma. *Acta Orthop Belg* 2006;72:119–125.
345. Kjaer I, Keeling JW, Fischer Hansen B. Pattern of malformations in the axial skeleton in human trisomy 13 fetuses. *Am J Med Genet* 1997;70:421–426.
346. Kjaer I, Keeling JW, Hansen BF. Pattern of malformations in the axial skeleton in human trisomy 18 fetuses. *Am J Med Genet* 1996;65:332–336.
347. Klein MH, Shankman S. Osteoid osteoma: radiologic and pathologic correlation. *Skeletal Radiol* 1992;21:23–31.
348. Klein MJ, Siegal GP. Osteosarcoma. Anatomic and histologic variants. *Am J Clin Pathol* 2006;125:555–581.
349. Ko E, Mortimer E, Fraire AE. Extraarticular synovial chondromatosis: review of epidemiology, imaging studies, microscopy and pathogenesis, with a report of an additional case in a child. *Int J Surg Pathol* 2004;12:273–280.
350. Kochling J, Karbasiyan M, Reis A. Spectrum of mutations and genotype-phenotype analysis in Currarino syndrome. *Eur J Hum Genet* 2001;9:599–605.
351. Konstantinidou AE, Agrogiannis G, Sifakis S, et al. Genetic skeletal disorders of the fetus and infant: pathologic and molecular findings in a series of 41 cases. *Birth Defects Res A Clin Mol Teratol* 2009;85:811–821.
352. Kornak U, Mundlos S. Genetic disorders of the skeleton: a developmental approach. *Am J Hum Genet* 2003;73:447–474.
353. Kozin SH. Upper-extremity congenital anomalies. *J Bone Joint Surg Am* 2003;85A:1564–1576.
354. Kozlowski K, Beluffi G, Cohen DH, et al. Primary bone tumours in infants. Short literature review and report of 10 cases. *Pediatr Radiol* 1985;15:359–367.
355. Krajca-Radcliffe JB, Thomas JR, Nicholas RW. Giant-cell tumor of bone: a rare entity in the hands of children. *J Pediatr Orthop* 1994;14:776–780.
356. Krakow D, Alanay Y, Rimoin LP, et al. Evaluation of prenatal-onset osteochondrodysplasias by ultrasonography: a retrospective and prospective analysis. *Am J Med Genet A* 2008;14A:1917–1924.
357. Kransdorf MJ, Stull MA, Gilkey FW, Moser Jr RP. Osteoid osteoma. *Radiographics* 1991;11:671–696.
358. Kransdorf MJ, Sweet De. Aneurysmal bone cyst: concept, controversy, clinical presentation, and imaging. *Am J Roentgenol* 1995; 164:573–580.
359. Kronenberg HM. PTHrP and skeletal development. *Ann N Y Acad Sci* 2006;1068:1–13.
360. Kroon HM, Schurmans J. Osteoblastoma: clinical and radiologic findings in 98 new cases. *Radiology* 1990;175:783–790.
361. Kruse-Losler B, Gaertner C, Burger H, et al. Melanotic neuroectodermal tumor of infancy: systematic review of the literature and presentation of a case. *Oral Surg Oral Med Oral Pathol Oral Radiol Endod* 2006;102:204–216.
362. Kumar B, Kannu P, Savarirayan R, et al. Lethal metatropic dysplasia: a case report. *Pathology* 2007;39:177–181.
363. Kurt AM, Unni KK, McLeod RA, et al. Low-grade intraosseous osteosarcoma. *Cancer* 1990;65:1418–1428.
364. Kuruvilla G, Steiner GC. Osteofibrous dysplasia-like adamantinoma of bone: a report of five cases with immunohistochemical and ultrastructural studies. *Hum Pathol* 1998;29:809–814.
365. Kutsumi K, Nojima T, Yamashiro K, et al. Hyperplastic callus formation in both femurs in osteogenesis imperfecta. *Skeletal Radiol* 1996;25:384–387.
366. Kuttesch JF Jr, Parham DM, Kaste SC, et al. Embryonal malignancies of unknown primary origin in children. *Cancer* 1995;75:115–121.
367. Kyriakos M, McDonald DJ, Sundaram M. Fibrous dysplasia with cartilaginous differentiation ("fibrocartilaginous dysplasia"): a review, with an illustrative case followed for 18 years. *Skeletal Radiol* 2004;33:51–62.
368. Lahmar-Boufaroua A, Yacoubi MT, Hmisssa S, et al. Lethal osteochondro-dysplasia: feto-pathological study of 32 cases. *Tunis Med* 2009;87:127–132.
369. Lamovec J, Mozina E, Baebler B. Hyperplastic callus formation in osteogenesis imperfecta. *Ann Diagn Pathol* 2003;7:231–235.

370. Langer B, Haddad J, Gasser B, et al. Isolated fetal bilateral radial ray reduction associated with valproic acid usage. *Fetal Diagn Ther* 1994;9:155–158.
371. Langer R, Al-Gazali L, Raupp P, et al. Radiological manifestations of the skeleton, lungs and brain in Stueve-Wiedemann syndrome. *Australas Radiol* 2007;51:203–210.
372. Larrea-Oyarbide N, Valmaseda-Castellon E, Berini-Aytes L, et al. Osteomas of the craniofacial region. Review of 106 cases. *J Oral Pathol Med* 2008;37:38–42.
373. Lazjuk GI, Shved IA, Cherstvoy ED, et al. Campomelic syndrome: concepts of the bowing and shortening in the lower limbs. *Teratology* 1987;35:1–8.
374. Leber GE, Gosain AK. Surgical excision of pedunculated supernumerary digits prevents traumatic amputation neuromas. *Pediatr Dermatol* 2003;20:108–112.
375. Lee JA, Kim MS, Kim DH, et al. Relative tumor burden predicts metastasis-free survival in pediatric osteosarcoma. *Pediatr Blood Cancer* 2008;50:195–200.
376. Leeson MC, Makley JT, Carter JR. Metastatic skeletal disease in the pediatric population. *J Pediatr Orthop* 1985;5:261–267.
377. Leet AI, Collins MT. Current approach to fibrous dysplasia of bone and McCune-Albright syndrome. *J Child Orthop* 2007;1:3–17.
378. Lehman WB, Abdelgawad AA, Sala DA. Congenital tibial dysplasia (congenital pseudoarthrosis of the tibia): an atypical variation. *J Pediatr Orthop B* 2009;18:211–213.
379. Leithner A, Windhager R, Lang S, et al. Aneurysmal bone cyst. A population based epidemiologic study and literature review. *Clin Orthop Relat Res* 1999:176–179.
380. Lemyre E, Azouz EM, Teebi AS, et al. Bone dysplasia series. Achondroplasia, hypochondroplasia and thanatophoric dysplasia: review and update. *Can Assoc Radiol J* 1999;50:185–197.
381. Leroy JG, Nuytinck L, De Paepe A, et al. Bruck syndrome: neonatal presentation and natural course in three patients. *Pediatr Radiol* 1998;28:781–789.
382. Leskela HV, Kuorilehto T, Risteli J, et al. Congenital pseudarthrosis of neurofibromatosis type 1: impaired osteoblast differentiation and function and altered NF1 gene expression. *Bone* 2009;44:243–250.
383. Lettice LA, Hill RE. Preaxial polydactyly: a model for defective long-range regulation in congenital abnormalities. *Curr Opin Genet Dev* 2005;15:294–300.
384. Levine SM, Lambiase RE, Petchprapa CN. Cortical lesions of the tibia: characteristic appearances at conventional radiography. *Radiographics* 2003;23:157–177.
385. Li X, Cao X. BMP signaling and skeletogenesis. *Ann N Y Acad Sci* 2006;1068:26–40.
386. Lin PP, Jaffe N, Herzog CE, et al. Chemotherapy response is an important predictor of local recurrence in Ewing sarcoma. *Cancer* 2007;109:603–611.
387. Lin S, Marshall EG, Davidson GK, Roth GB, Druschel CM. Evaluation of congenital limb reduction defects in upstate New York. *Teratology* 1993;47:127–135.
388. Lipton JM, Federman N, Khabbaze Y, et al. Osteogenic sarcoma associated with Diamond-Blackfan anemia: a report from the Diamond-Blackfan Anemia Registry. *J Pediatr Hematol Oncol* 2001;23:39–44.
389. Liu B, Yu SF, Li TJ. Multinucleated giant cells in various forms of giant cell containing lesions of the jaws express features of osteoclasts. *J Oral Pathol Med* 2003;32:367–375.
390. Liu F, Kohlmeier S, Wang CY. Wnt signaling and skeletal development. Cell Signal 2008;20:999–1009.
391. Locatelli F, Tonani P, Porta F, et al. Rhabdomyosarcoma with primary osteolytic lesions simulating non-Hodgkin's lymphoma. *Pediatr Hematol Oncol* 1991;8:159–164.
392. Loizaga JM, Calvo M, Lopez Barea F, et al. Osteoblastoma and osteoid osteoma. Clinical and morphological features of 162 cases. *Pathol Res Pract* 1993;189:33–41.
393. Longhi A, Errani C, De Paolis M, et al. Primary bone osteosarcoma in the pediatric age: state of the art. *Cancer Treat Rev* 2006;32:423–436.
394. Lu J, Lian G, Lenkinski R, et al. Filamin B mutations cause chondrocyte defects in skeletal development. *Hum Mol Genet* 2007;16:1661–1675.
395. Lucas DR, Unni KK, McLeod RA, O'Connor MI, Sim FH. Osteoblastoma: clinicopathologic study of 306 cases. *Hum Pathol* 1994;25:117–134.
396. Luiz CP, al Kharusi W, Sethu AU, et al. Osteosarcoma in a 26-month-old girl. *Cancer* 1992;70:894–896.
397. Ma NS, Malloy PJ, Pitukcheewanont P, et al.. Hereditary vitamin D resistant rickets: identification of a novel splice site mutation in the vitamin D receptor gene and successful treatment with oral calcium therapy. *Bone* 2009;45:743–746.
398. MacCarthy A, Bayne AM, Draper GJ, et al. Non-ocular tumours following retinoblastoma in Great Britain 1951 to 2004. *Br J Ophthalmol* 2009;93:1159–1162.
399. Macias-Gomez NM, Megarbane A, Leal-Ugarte E, et al. Diastrophic dysplasia and atelosteogenesis type II as expression of compound heterozygosis: first report of a Mexican patient and genotype-phenotype correlation. *Am J Med Genet A* 2004;129A:190–192.
400. Mackie EJ, Ahmed YA, Tatarczuch L, et al. Endochondral ossification: how cartilage is converted into bone in the developing skeleton. *Int J Biochem Cell Biol* 2008;40:46–62.
401. Maeda K, Miyamoto Y, Sawai H, et al. A compound heterozygote harboring novel and recurrent DTDST mutations with intermediate phenotype between atelosteogenesis type II and diastrophic dysplasia. *Am J Med Genet A* 2006;140:1143–1147.
402. Makitie O, Marttinen E, Kaitila I. Skeletal growth in cartilage-hair hypoplasia. A radiological study of 82 patients. *Pediatr Radiol* 1992;22:434–439.
403. Makitie O, Sulisalo T, de la Chapelle A, et al. Cartilage-hair hypoplasia. *J Med Genet* 1995;32:39–43.
404. Malemud CJ. Matrix metalloproteinases: role in skeletal development and growth plate disorders. *Front Biosci* 2006;11:1702–1715.
405. Malik S, Grzeschik KH. Synpolydactyly: clinical and molecular advances. *Clin Genet* 2008;73:113–120.
406. Mallet E. Primary hyperparathyroidism in neonates and childhood. The French experience (1984–2004). *Horm Res* 2008;69:180–188.
407. Malm D, Nilssen O. Alpha-mannosidosis. *Orphanet J Rare Dis* 2008;3:21.
408. Mankin HJ, Trahan CA, Fondren G, et al. Non-ossifying fibroma, fibrous cortical defect and Jaffe-Campanacci syndrome: a biologic and clinical review. *Chir Organi Mov* 2009;93:1–7.
409. Manouvrier-Hanu S, Holder-Espinasse M, Lyonnet S. Genetics of limb anomalies in humans. *Trends Genet* 1999;15:409–417.
410. Mansour S, Hall CM, Pembrey ME, et al. A clinical and genetic study of campomelic dysplasia. *J Med Genet* 1995;32:415–420.
411. Mantovani G, de Sanctis L, Barbieri AM, et al. Pseudohypoparathyroidism and GNAS epigenetic defects: clinical evaluation of Albright hereditary osteodystrophy and molecular analysis in 40 patients. *J Clin Endocrinol Metab* 2010;95(2):651–658.
412. Mariaud-Schmidt RP, Rosales-Quintana S, Bitar E, et al. Hamartoma involving the pseudarthrosis site in patients with neurofibromatosis type 1. *Pediatr Dev Pathol* 2005;8:190–196.
413. Marie PJ, Pettifor JM, Ross FP, et al. Histological osteomalacia due to dietary calcium deficiency in children. *N Engl J Med* 1982;307:584–588.
414. Marin C, Gallego C, Manjon P, et al. Juxtacortical chondromyxoid fibroma: imaging findings in three cases and a review of the literature. *Skeletal Radiol* 1997;26:642–649.
415. Marion MJ, Gannon FH, Fallon MD, et al. Skeletal dysplasia in perinatal lethal osteogenesis imperfecta. A complex disorder of endochondral and intramembranous ossification. *Clin Orthop Relat Res* 1993:327–337.

416. Martinez-Frias ML, Bermejo E, Aparicio P, et al. Amelia: analysis of its epidemiological and clinical characteristics. *Am J Med Genet* 1997;73:189–193.
417. Martinez-Frias ML, Bermejo E, Garcia A, et al. Holoprosencephaly associated with caudal dysgenesis: a clinical-epidemiological analysis. *Am J Med Genet* 1994;53:46–51.
418. Martinez-Frias ML, de Frutos CA, Bermejo E, et al. Review of the recently defined molecular mechanisms underlying thanatophoric dysplasia and their potential therapeutic implications for achondroplasia. *Am J Med Genet A* 2010;152A:245–255.
419. Maschke SD, Seitz W, Lawton J. Radial longitudinal deficiency. *J Am Acad Orthop Surg* 2007;15:41–52.
420. Masi G, Barzon L, Iacobone M, et al. Clinical, genetic, and histopathologic investigation of CDC73-related familial hyperparathyroidism. *Endocr Relat Cancer* 2008;15:1115–1126.
421. Matiz C, Ferguson PJ, Zaenglein A, et al. Papular xanthomas and erosive arthritis in a 3 year old girl, is this a new MRH variant? *Pediatr Rheumatol Online J* 2009;7:15.
422. Mattos TC, Giugliani R, Haase HB. Congenital malformations detected in 731 autopsies of children aged 0 to 14 years. *Teratology* 1987;35:305–307.
423. Maygarden SJ, Askin FB, Siegal GP, et al. Ewing sarcoma of bone in infants and toddlers. A clinicopathologic report from the Intergroup Ewing's Study. *Cancer* 1993;71:2109–2118.
424. McAllion SJ, Paterson CR. Causes of death in osteogenesis imperfecta. *J Clin Pathol* 1996;49:627–630.
425. McCaffrey M, Letts M, Carpenter B, et al. Osteofibrous dysplasia: a review of the literature and presentation of an additional 3 cases. *Am J Orthop* 2003;32:479–486.
426. McClure J, Smith PS, Sorby-Adams G, et al. The histological and ultrastructural features of the epiphyseal plate in Morquio type A syndrome (mucopolysaccharidosis type IVA). *Pathology* 1986;18:217–221.
427. McDermott MB, Ponder TB, Dehner LP. Nasal chondromesenchymal hamartoma: an upper respiratory tract analogue of the chest wall mesenchymal hamartoma. *Am J Surg Pathol* 1998;22:425–433.
428. McDonald DJ, Sim FH, McLeod RA, et al. Giant-cell tumor of bone. *J Bone Joint Surg Am* 1986;68:235–242.
429. McGuirk CK, Westgate MN, Holmes LB. Limb deficiencies in newborn infants. *Pediatrics* 2001;108:E64.
430. McHugh JB, Mukherji SK, Lucas DR. Sino-orbital osteoma: a clinicopathologic study of 45 surgically treated cases with emphasis on tumors with osteoblastoma-like features. *Arch Pathol Lab Med* 2009;133:1587–1593.
431. McLennan TW, Steinbach HL. Schwachman's syndrome: the broad spectrum of bony abnormalities. *Radiology* 1974;112:167–173.
432. Mehta D, Clifton N, McClelland L, et al. Paediatric fibro-osseous lesions of the nose and paranasal sinuses. *Int J Pediatr Otorhinolaryngol* 2006;70:193–199.
433. Meredith CC, Kepes JJ, Johnson P, et al. Chondromyxoid fibroma of the upper thoracic spine in a 7-year-old patient. A case report and review of the literature. *Pediatr Neurosurg* 2004;40:190–195.
434. Messerschmitt PJ, Garcia RM, Abdul-Karim FW, et al. Osteosarcoma. *J Am Acad Orthop Surg* 2009;17:515–527.
435. Micallef M, Devaney D, Donoghue V, et al. Alveolar rhabdomyosarcoma presenting with symmetrical bony and renal metastases in infancy. *Clin Radiol* 1999;54:693–695.
436. Michal M, Fanburg-Smith JC, Lasota J, et al. Minute synovial sarcomas of the hands and feet: a clinicopathologic study of 21 tumors less than 1 cm. *Am J Surg Pathol* 2006;30:721–726.
437. Michalk A, Stricker S, Becker J, et al. Acetylcholine receptor pathway mutations explain various fetal akinesia deformation sequence disorders. *Am J Hum Genet* 2008;82:464–476.
438. Milunsky A, Graef JW, Gaynor MF, Jr. Methotrexate-induced congenital malformations. *J Pediatr* 1968;72:790–795.
439. Mirabello L, Troisi RJ, Savage SA. International osteosarcoma incidence patterns in children and adolescents, middle ages and elderly persons. *Int J Cancer* 2009;125:229–234.
440. Moerman P, Fryns JP. The fetal akinesia deformation sequence. A fetopathological approach. *Genet Couns* 1990;1:25–33.
441. Mogayzel PJ, Marcus CL. Skeletal dysplasias and their effect on the respiratory system. *Paediatr Respir Rev* 2001;2:365–371.
442. Mohanty SK, Wazir S, Rajwanshi A, et al. Cytologic diagnosis of plasma myeloma in an 8-year-old child: case report. *Diagn Cytopathol* 2004;31:193–195.
443. Moon NF. Adamantinoma of the appendicular skeleton in children. *Int Orthop* 1994;18:379–388.
444. Morimoto A, Ishida Y, Suzuki N, et al. Nationwide survey of single-system single site Langerhans cell histiocytosis in Japan. *Pediatr Blood Cancer* 2009;54:98–102.
445. Mornet E. Hypophosphatasia. *Best Pract Res Clin Rheumatol* 2008;22:113–127.
446. Morton KS, Quenville NF, Beauchamp CP. Aggressive osteoblastoma. A case previously reported as a recurrent osteoid osteoma. *J Bone Joint Surg Br* 1989;71:428–431.
447. Moser RP Jr, Sweet DE, Haseman DB, et al. Multiple skeletal fibroxanthomas: radiologic-pathologic correlation of 72 cases. *Skeletal Radiol* 1987;16:353–359.
448. Murakami S, Akiyama H, De Crombrugghe B. The development of bone and cartilage. In: Epstein CJ, Erickson RP, Wynshaw-Boris A, eds. *Inborn Errors of Development: The Molecular Basis of Clinical Disorders of Morphogenesis*. New York: Oxford University Press, 2004:133–147.
449. Murphey MD, Nomikos GC, Flemming DJ, et al. From the archives of AFIP. Imaging of giant cell tumor and giant cell reparative granuloma of bone: radiologic-pathologic correlation. *Radiographics* 2001;21:1283–1309.
450. Murphy A, Stallings RL, Howard J, et al. Primary desmoplastic small round cell tumor of bone: report of a case with cytogenetic confirmation. *Cancer Genet Cytogenet* 2005;156:167–171.
451. Myllyharju J, Kivirikko KI. Collagens and collagen-related diseases. *Ann Med* 2001;33:7–21.
452. Nagatsuka H, Han PP, Taguchi K, et al. Erdheim-Chester disease in a child presenting with multiple jaw lesions. *J Oral Pathol Med* 2005;34:420–422.
453. Nahra ME, Bucchieri JS. Ganglion cysts and other tumor related conditions of the hand and wrist. *Hand Clin* 2004;20:249–260.
454. Nakajima H, Sim FH, Bond JR, Unni KK. Small cell osteosarcoma of bone. Review of 72 cases. *Cancer* 1997;79:2095–2106.
455. Nakashima Y, Unni KK, Shives TC, et al. Mesenchymal chondrosarcoma of bone and soft tissue. A review of 111 cases. *Cancer* 1986;57:2444–2453.
456. Nakashima Y, Yamamuro T, Fujiwara Y, et al. Osteofibrous dysplasia (ossifying fibroma of long bones). A study of 12 cases. *Cancer* 1983;52:909–914.
457. Nelson M, Perry D, Ginsburg G, et al. Translocation (1;4)(p31;q34) in nonossifying fibroma. *Cancer Genet Cytogenet* 2003;142:142–144.
458. Nemoto O, Moser RP Jr, Van Dam BE, et al. Osteoblastoma of the spine. A review of 75 cases. *Spine* (*Phila Pa 1976*) 1990;15:1272–1280.
459. Netscher DT, Baumholtz MA, Popek E, et al. Non-malignant fibrosing tumors in the pediatric hand: a clinicopathologic case review. *Hand* (*NY*) 2009;4:2–11.
460. Nevin NC, Thomas PS, Davis RI, et al. Melorheostosis in a family with autosomal dominant osteopoikilosis. *Am J Med Genet* 1999;82:409–414.
461. Newbury-Ecob R. Atelosteogenesis type 2. *J Med Genet* 1998;35:49–53.
462. Newman B, Wallis GA. Skeletal dysplasias caused by a disruption of skeletal patterning and endochondral ossification. *Clin Genet* 2003;63:241–251.
463. Ng A, Hobson R, Williams D, et al. Anaplastic large cell lymphoma of bone—is it a bad tumour? *Pediatr Blood Cancer* 2007;48:473–476.

464. Nicolaidou P, Tsitsika A, Papadimitriou A, et al. Hereditary vitamin D-resistant rickets in Greek children: genotype, phenotype, and long-term response to treatment. *J Pediatr Endocrinol Metab* 2007;20:425–430.
465. Nielsen GP, Fletcher CD, Smith MA, et al. Soft tissue aneurysmal bone cyst: a clinicopathologic study of five cases. *Am J Surg Pathol* 2002;26:64–69.
466. Nielsen GP, Srivastava A, Kattapuram S, et al. Epithelioid hemangioma of bone revisited. A study of 50 cases. *Am J Surg Pathol* 2009;33:270–277.
467. Nikkels PG, Stigter RH, Knol IE, et al. Schneckenbecken dysplasia, radiology, and histology. *Pediatr Radiol* 2001;31:27–30.
468. Nishimura G, Nakashima E, Hirose Y, et al. The Shwachman-Bodian-Diamond syndrome gene mutations cause a neonatal form of spondylometaphysial dysplasia (SMD) resembling SMD Sedaghatian type. *J Med Genet* 2007;44:e73.
469. Nissim S. Development of the limbs. In: Epstein, CJ, Erickson RP, Wynshaw-Boris A, eds. *Inborn Errors of Development: The Molecular Basis of Clinical Disocrders of Morphogenesis*. New York: Oxford University Press, 2004:148–167.
470. Norman AM, Rimmer S, Landy S, et al. Thanatophoric dysplasia of the straight-bone type (type 2). *Clin Dysmorphol* 1992;1:115–120.
471. Notarangelo LD, Roifman CM, Giliani S. Cartilage-hair hypoplasia: molecular basis and heterogeneity of the immunological phenotype. *Curr Opin Allergy Clin Immunol* 2008;8:534–539.
472. Novack DV, Teitelbaum SL. The osteoclast: friend or foe? *Annu Rev Pathol* 2008;3:457–484.
473. Oberklaid F, Danks DM, Mayne V, et al. Asphyxiating thoracic dysplasia. Clinical, radiological, and pathological information on 10 patients. *Arch Dis Child* 1977;52:758–765.
474. Oberlin O, Rey A, Lyden E, et al. Prognostic factors in metastatic rhabdomyosarcomas: results of a pooled analysis from United States and European cooperative groups. *J Clin Oncol* 2008;26:2384–2389.
475. O'Connell JX, Nanthakumar SS, Nielsen GP, et al. Osteoid osteoma: the uniquely innervated bone tumor. *Mod Pathol* 1998;11:175–180.
476. Offiah AC. Acute osteomyelitis, septic arthritis and discitis: differences between neonates and older children. *Eur J Radiol* 2006;60:221–232.
477. Offiah AC, Hall CM. Radiological diagnosis of the constitutional disorders of bone. As easy as A, B, C? *Pediatr Radiol* 2003;33:153–161.
478. Ojeda-Thies C, Bonsfills N, Albinana J. Solitary epiphyseal enchondroma of the proximal femur in a 23-month-old girl. *J Pediatr Orthop* 2008;28:565–568.
479. Okamoto M, Murai J, Yoshikawa H, et al. Bone morphogenetic proteins in bone stimulate osteoclasts and osteoblasts during bone development. *J Bone Miner Res* 2006;21:1022–1033.
480. Oliveira AM, Perez-Atayde AR, Inwards CY, et al. USP6 and CDH11 oncogenes identify the neoplastic cell in primary aneurysmal bone cysts and are absent in so-called secondary aneurysmal bone cysts. *Am J Pathol* 2004;165:1773–1780.
481. Oliveira CR, Mendonca BB, Camargo OP, et al. Classical osteoblastoma, atypical osteoblastoma, and osteosarcoma: a comparative study based on clinical, histological, and biological parameters. *Clinics (Sao Paulo)* 2007;62:167–174.
482. Olsen BR, Reginato AM, Wang W. Bone development. *Annu Rev Cell Dev Biol* 2000;16:191–220.
483. Oostra RJ, van der Harten JJ, Rijnders WP, et al. Blomstrand osteochondrodysplasia: three novel cases and histological evidence for heterogeneity. *Virchows Arch* 2000;436:28–35.
484. Oppenheimer SJ, Snodgrass GJ. Neonatal rickets. Histopathology and quantitative bone changes. *Arch Dis Child* 1980;55:945–949.
485. O'Rahilly R, Gardner E. The timing and sequence of events in the development of the limbs in the human embryo. *Anat Embryol (Berl)* 1975;148:1–23.
486. Orazi C, Picca S, Schingo PM, et al. Oxalosis in primary hyperoxaluria in infancy. Report of a case in a 3-month-old baby. Follow-up for 3 years and review of literature. *Skeletal Radiol* 2009;38:387–391.
487. Orioli IM, Castilla EE, Barbosa-Neto JG. The birth prevalence rates for the skeletal dysplasias. *J Med Genet* 1986;23:328–332.
488. Ortiz EJ, Isler MH, Navia JE, et al. Pathologic fractures in children. *Clin Orthop Relat Res* 2005;432:116–126.
489. O'Sullivan MJ, McAllister WH, Ball RH, et al. Morphologic observations in a case of lethal variant (type I) metatropic dysplasia with atypical features: morphology of lethal metatropic dysplasia. *Pediatr Dev Pathol* 1998;1:405–412.
490. Outland JD, Keiran SJ, Schikler KN, et al. Multicentric reticulohistiocytosis in a 14-year-old girl. *Pediatr Dermatol* 2002;19:527–531.
491. Ozdemirli M, Mankin HJ, Aisenberg AC, et al. Hodgkin's disease presenting as a solitary bone tumor. A report of four cases and review of the literature. *Cancer* 1996;77:79–88.
492. Pandya J, Valverde K, Heon E, et al. Predilection of retinoblastoma metastases for the mandible. *Med Pediatr Oncol* 2002;38:271–273.
493. Pannier S, Legeai-Mallet L. Hereditary multiple exostoses and enchondromatosis. *Best Pract Res Clin Rheumatol* 2008;22:45–54.
494. Papagelopoulos PJ, Galanis EC, Sim FH, et al. Clinicopathologic features, diagnosis, and treatment of osteoblastoma. *Orthopedics* 1999;22:244–247.
495. Parekh SG, Donthineni-Rao R, Ricchetti E, et al. Fibrous dysplasia. *J Am Acad Orthop Surg* 2004;12:305–313.
496. Park YK, Unni KK, McLeod RA, et al. Osteofibrous dysplasia: clinicopathologic study of 80 cases. *Hum Pathol* 1993;24:1339–1347.
497. Pastores GM. Musculoskeletal complications encountered in the lysosomal storage disorders. *Best Pract Res Clin Rheumatol* 2008;22:937–947.
498. Patel DV. Gorham's disease or massive osteolysis. *Clin Med Res* 2005;3:65–74.
499. Pazzaglia UE, Beluffi G. Radiology and histopathology of the bent limbs in campomelic dysplasia: implications in the aetiology of the disease and review of theories. *Pediatr Radiol* 1987;17:50–55.
500. Pazzaglia UE, Byers PD, Beluffi G, et al. Pathology of infantile cortical hyperostosis (Caffey's disease). Report of a case. *J Bone Joint Surg Am* 1985;67:1417–1426.
501. Pereira BP, Zhou Y, Gupta A, et al. Runx2, p53, and pRB status as diagnostic parameters for deregulation of osteoblast growth and differentiation in a new pre-chemotherapeutic osteosarcoma cell line (OS1). *J Cell Physiol* 2009;221:778–788.
502. Pettinato G, Manivel JC, d'Amore ES, et al. Melanotic neuroectodermal tumor of infancy. A reexamination of a histogenetic problem based on immunohistochemical, flow cytometric, and ultrastructural study of 10 cases. *Am J Surg Pathol* 1991;15:233–245.
503. Pfeiffer RA, Santelmann R. Limb anomalies in chromosomal aberrations. *Birth Defects Orig Artic Ser* 1977;13:319–337.
504. Picci P. Osteosarcoma (osteogenic sarcoma). *Orphanet J Rare Dis* 2007;2:6.
505. Picci P, Manfrini M, Zucchi V, et al. Giant-cell tumor of bone in skeletally immature patients. *J Bone Joint Surg Am* 1983;65:486–490.
506. Pierz KA, Stieber JR, Kusumi K, et al. Hereditary multiple exostoses: one center's experience and review of etiology. *Clin Orthop Relat Res* 2002:49–59.
507. Pierz KA, Womer RB, Dormans JP. Pediatric bone tumors: osteosarcoma, Ewing's sarcoma, and chondrosarcoma associated with multiple hereditary osteochondromatosis. *J Pediatr Orthop* 2001;21:412–418.
508. Pollandt K, Engels C, Kaiser E, et al. Gs α gene mutations in monostotic fibrous dysplasia of bone and fibrous dysplasia-like low-grade central osteosarcoma. *Virchows Arch* 2001;439:170–175.
509. Potocki L, Abuelo DN, Oyer CE. Cardiac malformation in two infants with hypochondrogenesis. *Am J Med Genet* 1995;59:295–299.
510. Potter BK, Freedman BA, Lehman RA Jr, et al. Solitary epiphyseal enchondromas. *J Bone Joint Surg Am* 2005;87A:1551–1560.
511. Prinster C, Carrera P, Del Maschio M, et al. Comparison of clinical-radiological and molecular findings in hypochondroplasia. *Am J Med Genet* 1998;75:109–112.
512. Provot S, Schipani E, Wu J, et al. Development of the skeleton. In: Marcus R, Feldman D, Nelson DA, Rosen CJ, eds. *Osteoporosis*, 3rd edn. San Francisco: Academic Press, 2008:241–269.

513. Putnam A, Yandow S, Coffin CM. Classic adamantinoma with osteofibrous dysplasia-like foci and secondary aneurysmal bone cyst. *Pediatr Dev Pathol* 2003;6:173–178.
514. Qian X, Jin L, Shearer BM, et al. Molecular diagnosis of Ewing's sarcoma/primitive neuroectodermal tumor in formalin-fixed paraffin-embedded tissues by RT-PCR and fluorescence in situ hybridization. *Diagn Mol Pathol* 2005;14:23–28.
515. Quinn CM, Wigglesworth JS, Heckmatt J. Lethal arthrogryposis multiplex congenita: a pathological study of 21 cases. *Histopathology* 1991;19:155–162.
516. Qureshi F, Jacques SM, Evans MI, et al. Skeletal histopathology in fetuses with chondroectodermal dysplasia (Ellis-van Creveld syndrome). *Am J Med Genet* 1993;45:471–476.
517. Radhakrishnan K, Rockson SG. Gorham's disease. An osseous disease of lymphangiogenesis? *Ann N Y Acad Sci* 2008;1131:203–205.
518. Rakheja D, Read CP, Hull D, et al. A severely affected female infant with x-linked dominant chondrodysplasia punctata: a case report and a brief review of the literature. *Pediatr Dev Pathol* 2007;10:142–148.
519. Ramappa AJ, Lee FY, Tang P, et al. Chondroblastoma of bone. *J Bone Joint Surg Am* 2000;82A:1140–1145.
520. Ramos-Arroyo MA, Rodriguez-Pinilla E, Cordero JF. Maternal diabetes: the risk for specific birth defects. *Eur J Epidemiol* 1992;8:503–508.
521. Rampini PM, Alimehmeti RH, Egidi MG, et al. Isolated cervical juvenile xanthogranuloma in childhood. *Spine (Phila Pa 1976)* 2001;26:1392–1395.
522. Rauch F. Watching bone cells at work: what we can see from bone biopsies. *Pediatr Nephrol* 2006;21:457–462.
523. Rauch F, Glorieux FH. Osteogenesis imperfecta. *Lancet* 2004;363:1377–1385.
524. Rauch F, Travers R, Parfitt AM, et al. Static and dynamic bone histomorphometry in children with osteogenesis imperfecta. *Bone* 2000;26:581–589.
525. Ravelli A, Martini A. Juvenile idiopathic arthritis. *Lancet* 2007;369:767–778.
526. Redaelli A, Laskin BL, Stephens JM, et al. A systematic literature review of the clinical and epidemiological burden of acute lymphoblastic leukaemia (ALL). *Eur J Cancer Care (Engl)* 2005;14:53–62.
527. Reddy S, Jia S, Geoffrey R, et al. An autoinflammatory disease due to homozygous deletion of the IL1RN locus. *N Engl J Med* 2009;360:2438–2444.
528. Regezi JA. Odontogenic cysts, odontogenic tumors, fibroosseous, and giant cell lesions of the jaws. *Mod Pathol* 2002;15:331–341.
529. Reibel A, Maniere MC, Clauss F, et al. Orodental phenotype and genotype findings in all subtypes of hypophosphatasia. *Orphanet J Rare Dis* 2009;4:6.
530. Revell MP, Deshmukh N, Grimer RJ, et al. Periosteal osteosarcoma: a review of 17 cases with mean follow-up of 52 months. *Sarcoma* 2002;6:123–130.
531. Reyes-Mugica M, Arnsmeier SL, Backeljauw PF, et al. Phosphaturic mesenchymal tumor-induced rickets. *Pediatr Dev Pathol* 2000;3:61–69.
532. Reynolds RAK. Diagnosis and treatment of slipped capital femoral epiphysis. *Curr Opin Pediatr* 1999;11:80–83.
533. Richardson RR. Variants of exostosis of the bone in children. *Semin Roentgenol* 2005;40:380–390.
534. Riebel T, Kochling J, Scheer I, et al. [Currarino syndrome: variability of imaging findings in 22 molecular-genetically identified (HLXB9 mutation) patients from five families]. *Rofo* 2004;176: 564–569.
535. Riminucci M, Liu B, Corsi A, et al. The histopathology of fibrous dysplasia of bone in patients with activating mutations of the Gs alpha gene: site-specific patterns and recurrent histological hallmarks. *J Pathol* 1999;187:249–258.
536. Rimoin DL. Chondrodysplasias. In: Rimoin DL, Connor JM, Pyeritz RE, Korf BR, eds. *Emery and Rimoin's Principles and Practice of Medical Genetics*, Vol. 3, 5th edn. Philadelphia: Elsevier, 2007:3709–3765.
537. Rizzo R, Lammer EJ, Parano E, et al. Limb reduction defects in humans associated with prenatal isotretinoin exposure. *Teratology* 1991;44:599–604.
538. Robertson SP. Molecular pathology of filamin A: diverse phenotypes, many functions. *Clin Dysmorphol* 2004;13:123–131.
539. Rodriguez-Peralto JL, Lopez-Barea F, Sanchez-Herrera S, et al. Primary aneurysmal cyst of soft tissues (extraosseous aneurysmal cyst). *Am J Surg Pathol* 1994;18:632–636.
540. Romeo S, Hogendoorn PCW, Dei Tos AP. Benign cartilaginous tumors of bone: from morphology to somatic and germ-line genetics. *Adv Anat Pathol* 2009;16:307–315.
541. Roosendaal G, van den Berg HM, Lafeber FP, et al. [Pathology of synovitis and hemophilic arthropathy]. *Orthopade* 1999;28:323–328.
542. Rosano A, Botto LD, Olney RS, et al. Limb defects associated with major congenital anomalies: clinical and epidemiological study from the International Clearinghouse for Birth Defects Monitoring systems. *Am J Med Genet*, 2000;93:110–116.
543. Rosenberg AE, Nielsen GP, Krishnasetty V, et al. Skeletal systems, Part 1. Disorders of the skeletal system including tumor. In: Gilbert-Barness E, ed. *Potter's Pathology of the Fetus, Infant and Child*, 2nd edn. Philadelphia: Mosby Elsevier, 2007:1797–1835.
544. Rossbach HC. Hereditary and familial syndromes of bone and blood. Genetic pathways, diagnostic pitfalls. *Fetal Pediatr Pathol* 2007;26:1–16.
545. Ruggieri P, Sim FH, Bond JR, et al. Malignancies in fibrous dysplasia. *Cancer* 1994;73:1411–1424.
546. Ruiz-Perez VL, Goodship JA. Ellis-van Creveld syndrome and Weyers acrodental dysostosis are caused by cilia-mediated diminished response to hedgehog ligands. *Am J Med Genet* C *Semin Med Genet* 2009;151C:341–351.
547. Rytting M, Pearson P, Raymond AK. Osteosarcoma in preadolescent patients. *Clin Orthop Relat Res* 2000;373:39–50.
548. Sadat-Ali M. The status of acute osteomyelitis in sickle cell disease. A 15-year review. *Int Surg* 1998;83:84–87.
549. Said-Al-Naief N, Fernandes R, Louis P, et al. Desmoplastic fibroma of the jaw: a case report and review of literature. *Oral Surg Oral Med Oral Pathol Oral Radiol Endod* 2006;101:82–94.
550. Sailhan F, Chotel F, Parot R. Chondroblastoma of bone in a pediatric population. *J Bone Joint Surg Am* 2009;91A:2159–2168.
551. Sajadi KR, Heck RK, Neel MD, et al. The incidence and prognosis of osteosarcoma skip metastases. *Clin Orthop Relat Res* 2004;426:92–96.
552. Sala A, Mattano LA Jr, Barr RD. Osteonecrosis in children and adolescents with cancer - an adverse effect of systemic therapy. *Eur J Cancer* 2007;43:683–689.
553. Salotti JA, Nanduri V, Pearce MS, et al. Incidence and clinical features of Langerhans cell histiocytosis in the UK and Ireland. *Arch Dis Child* 2009;94:376–380.
554. Salum FG, Yurgel LS, Cherubini K, et al. Pyogenic granuloma, peripheral giant cell granuloma and peripheral ossifying fibroma: retrospective analysis of 138 cases. *Minerva Stomatol* 2008;57:227–232.
555. Sanerkin NG. Old fibrin coagula and their ossification in simple bone cysts. *J Bone Joint Surg Br* 1979;61B:194–199.
556. Sanguinetti C, Greco F, De Palma L, et al. Morphological changes in growth-plate cartilage in osteogenesis imperfecta. *J Bone Joint Surg Br* 1990;72:475–479.
557. Sato K, Kawana M, Nonomura N, et al. Desmoid-type infantile fibromatosis in the mandible: a case report. *Am J Otolaryngol* 2000;21: 207–212.
558. Savarirayan R, Rimoin DL. The skeletal dysplasias. *Best Pract Res Clin Endocrinol Metab* 2002;16:547–560.
559. Scarborough MT, Moreau G. Benign cartilage tumors. *Orthop Clin North Am* 1996;27:583–589.

560. Schimmel RJ, Pasmans SG, Xu M, et al. GNAS-associated disorders of cutaneous ossification: Two different clinical presentations. *Bone* 2009; Nov 10. [Epub ahead of print].
561. Schlosser K, Schmitt CP, Bartholomaeus JE, et al. Parathyroidectomy for renal hyperparathyroidism in children and adolescents. *World J Surg* 2008;32:801–806.
562. Schramm T, Gloning KP, Minderer S, et al. Prenatal sonographic diagnosis of skeletal dysplasias. *Ultrasound Obstet Gynecol* 2009;34:160–170.
563. Schrander-Stumpel C, Havenith M, Linden EV, et al. De la Chapelle dysplasia (atelosteogenesis type II): case report and review of the literature [corrected]. *Clin Dysmorphol* 1994;3:318–327.
564. Schwabe GC, Mundlos S. Genetics of congenital hand anomalies. *Handchir Mikrochir Plast Chir* 2004;36:85–97.
565. Sciot R, Dal Cin P, Fletcher CD, et al. Inflammatory myofibroblastic tumor of bone: report of two cases with evidence of clonal chromosomal changes. *Am J Surg Pathol* 1997;21:1166–1172.
566. Selim H, Shaheen S, Barakat K, et al. Melanotic neuroectodermal tumor of infancy: review of literature and case report. *J Pediatr Surg* 2008;43:E25–E29.
567. Shah GN, Bonapace G, Hu PY, et al. Carbonic anhydrase II deficiency syndrome (osteopetrosis with renal tubular acidosis and brain calcification): novel mutations in CA2 identified by direct sequencing expand the opportunity for genotype-phenotype correlation. *Hum Mutat* 2004;24:272.
568. Shanske AL, Bernstein L, Herzog R. Chondrodysplasia punctata and maternal autoimmune disease: a new case and review of the literature. *Pediatrics* 2007;120:e436–e441.
569. Shapeero LG, Couanet D, Vanel D, et al. Bone metastases as the presenting manifestation of rhabdomyosarcoma in childhood. *Skeletal Radiol* 1993;22:433–438.
570. Sharony R, Browne C, Lachman RS, et al. Prenatal diagnosis of the skeletal dysplasias. *Am J Obstet Gynecol* 1993;169:668–675.
571. Shaw-Smith C. Genetic factors in esophageal atresia, tracheo-esophageal fistula and the VACTERL association: roles for FOXF1 and the 16q24.1 FOX transcription factor gene cluster, and review of the literature. *Eur J Med Genet* 2010;53:6–13.
572. Shaw-Smith C. Oesophageal atresia, tracheo-oesophageal fistula, and the VACTERL association: review of genetics and epidemiology. *J Med Genet* 2006;43:545–554.
573. Shayan K, Ho M, Edwards V, et al. Synovial pathology in camptodactyly-arthropathy-coxa vara-pericarditis syndrome. *Pediatr Dev Pathol* 2005;8:26–33.
574. Sheu SY, Wenzel RR, Kersting C, et al. Erdheim-Chester disease: case report with multisystemic manifestations including testes, thyroid, and lymph nodes, and a review of literature. *J Clin Pathol* 2004;57:1225–1228.
575. Shimonodan H, Nagayama J, Nagatoshi Y, et al. Acute lymphocytic leukemia in adolescence with multiple osteolytic lesions and hypercalcemia mediated by lymphoblast-producing parathyroid hormone-related peptide: a case report and review of the literature. *Pediatr Blood Cancer* 2005;45:333–339.
576. Shinawi M, Hicks J, Guillerman RP, et al. Multiple ganglion cysts ('cystic ganglionosis'): an unusual presentation in a child. *Scand J Rheumatol* 2007;36:145–148.
577. Shirley ED, Ain MC. Achondroplasia: manifestations and treatment. *J Am Acad Orthop Surg* 2009;17:231–241.
578. Shohat M, Rimoin DL, Gruber HE, et al. Perinatal lethal hypophosphatasia; clinical, radiologic and morphologic findings. *Pediatr Radiol* 1991;21:421–427.
579. Shore EM, Ahn J, Jan de Beur S, et al. Paternally inherited inactivating mutations of the GNAS1 gene in progressive osseous heteroplasia. *N Engl J Med* 2002;346:99–106.
580. Siitonen HA, Kopra O, Kaariainen H, et al. Molecular defect of RAPADILINO syndrome expands the phenotype spectrum of RECQL diseases. *Hum Mol Genet* 2003;12:2837–2844.
581. Sillence D, Kozlowski K, Bar-ziv J, et al. Perinatally lethal short rib-polydactyly syndromes. 1. Variability in known syndromes. *Pediatr Radiol* 1987;17:474–480.
582. Sillence D, Worthington S, Dixon J, et al. Atelosteogenesis syndromes: a review, with comments on their pathogenesis. *Pediatr Radiol* 1997;27:388–396.
583. Silve C, Juppner H. Ollier disease. *Orphanet J Rare Dis* 2006;1:37.
584. Silveri CP, Kaplan FS, Fallon MD, et al. Hurler syndrome with special reference to histologic abnormalities of the growth plate. *Clin Orthop Relat Res* 1991:305–311.
585. Singer RB, Ogston SA, Paterson CR. Mortality in various types of osteogenesis imperfecta. *J Insur Med* 2001;33:216–220.
586. Slootweg PJ. Lesions of the jaws. *Histopathology* 2009;54:401–418.
587. Smith SE, Kransdorf MJ. Primary musculoskeletal tumors of fibrous origin. *Semin Musculoskelet Radiol* 2000;4:73–88.
588. Smith SF, Newman L, Walker DM, et al. Juvenile aggressive psammomatoid ossifying fibroma: an interesting, challenging, and unusual case report and review of the literature. *J Oral Maxillofac Surg* 2009;67:200–206.
589. Smits P, Bolton AD, Funari V, et al. Lethal skeletal dysplasia in mice and humans lacking the golgin GMAP-210. *N Engl J Med* 2010;362:201–216.
590. Soler-Palacin P, Margareto C, Llobet P, et al. Chronic granulomatous disease in pediatric patients: 25 years of experience. *Allergol Immunopathol (Madr)* 2007;35:83–89.
591. Southgate J, Sarma U, Townend JV, et al. Study of the cell biology and biochemistry of cherubism. *J Clin Pathol* 1998;51:831–837.
592. Spranger J, Maroteaux P. The lethal osteochondrodysplasias. *Adv Hum Gent* 1990;19:1–103.
593. Springfield DS, Rosenberg AE, Mankin HJ, Mindell ER. Relationship between osteofibrous dysplasia and adamantinoma. *Clin Orthop Relat Res* 1994;309:234–244.
594. St.-Jacques B, Helms JA. Prenatal bone development otogeny and regulation. In: Glorieux FH, ed. *Pediatric Bone. Biology and Diseases*. San Francisco: Academic Press, 2003:77–117.
595. Staals EL, Bacchini P, Bertoni F. High-grade surface osteosarcoma: a review of 25 cases from the Rizzoli Institute. *Cancer* 2008;112:1592–1599.
596. Staretz-Chacham O, Lang TC, LaMarca ME, et al. Lysosomal storage disorders in the newborn. *Pediatrics* 2009;123:1191–1207.
597. Stark Z, Savarirayan R. Osteopetrosis. *Orphanet J Rare Dis* 2009;4:5.
598. Stempfle N, Huten Y, Fredouille C, et al. Skeletal abnormalities in fetuses with Down's syndrome: a radiographic post-mortem study. *Pediatr Radiol* 1999;29:682–688.
599. Stig Jacobsen F. Aneurysmal bone cyst in a patient with osteogenesis imperfecta. *J Pediatr Orthop B* 1997;6:225–227.
600. Stiller CA, Bielack SS, Jundt G, et al. Bone tumours in European children and adolescents, 1978-1997. Report from the Automated Childhood Cancer Information System project. *Eur J Cancer* 2006;42:2124–2135.
601. Stocker JT, Heifetz SA. Sirenomelia. A morphological study of 33 cases and review of the literature. *Perspect Pediatr Pathol* 1987;10:7–50.
602. Stoll C, Alembik Y, Dott B, et al. Risk factors in limb reduction defects. *Paediatr Perinat Epidemiol* 1992;6:323–338.
603. Stoll C, Clementi M. Prenatal diagnosis of dysmorphic syndromes by routine fetal ultrasound examination across Europe. *Ultrasound Obstet Gynecol* 2003;21:543–551.
604. Stoll C, Dott B, Roth MP, et al. Birth prevalence rates of skeletal dysplasias. *Clin Genet* 1989;35:88–92.
605. Stoll C, Wiesel A, Queisser-Luft A, et al. Evaluation of the prenatal diagnosis of limb reduction deficiencies. *Prenat Diagn* 2000;20:811–818.
606. Stoss H. Pathologic anatomy of osteogenesis imperfecta. Light and electron microscopic studies of supportive tissue and skin. *Veroff Pathol* 1990;134:1–88.

607. Stowens DW, Teitelbaum SL, Kahn AJ, et al. Skeletal complications of Gaucher disease. *Medicine (Baltimore)* 1985;64:310–322.
608. Struhl S, Edelson C, Pritzker H, et al. Solitary (unicameral) bone cyst. The fallen fragment sign revisited. *Skeletal Radiol* 1989;18:261–265.
609. Stull MA, Kransdorf MJ, Devaney KO. Langerhans cell histiocytosis of bone. *Radiographics* 1992;12:801–823.
610. Superti-Furga A. Achondrogenesis type 1B. *J Med Genet* 1996;33:957–961.
611. Superti-Furga A, Unger S. Nosology and classification of genetic skeletal disorders: 2006 revision. *Am J Med Genet A* 2007;143A:1–18.
612. Suphapeetiporn K, Tongkobpetch S, Mahayosnond A, et al. Expanding the phenotypic spectrum of Caffey disease. *Clin Genet* 2007;71:280–284.
613. Szendroi M. Giant-cell tumour of bone. *J Bone Joint Surg Br* 2004;86B:5–12.
614. Szendroi M, Antal I, Arato G. Adamantinoma of long bones: a long-term follow-up study of 11 cases. *Pathol Oncol Res* 2009;15:209–216.
615. Sztrolovics R, Glorieux FH, Travers R, et al. Osteogenesis imperfecta: comparison of molecular defects with bone histological changes. *Bone* 1994;15:321–328.
616. Takahashi S, Okada K, Nagasawa H, et al. Osteosarcoma occurring in osteogenesis imperfecta. *Virchows Arch* 2004;444:454–458.
617. Takeuchi T, Takenoshita Y, Kubo K, et al. Natural course of jaw lesions in patients with familial adenomatosis coli (Gardner's syndrome). *Int J Oral Maxillofac Surg* 1993;22:226–230.
618. Teitelbaum SL. Pathological manifestations of osteomalacia and rickets. *Clin Endocrinol Metab* 1980;9:43–62.
619. Teo HE, Peh WC. Skeletal tuberculosis in children. *Pediatr Radiol* 2004;34:853–860.
620. Teo HE, Peh WC, Akhilesh M, et al. Congenital osteofibrous dysplasia associated with pseudoarthrosis of the tibia and fibula. *Skeletal Radiol* 2007;36(suppl 1):S7–S14.
621. Thompson A, Mannix R, Bachur R. Acute pediatric monoarticular arthritis: distinguishing Lyme arthritis from other etiologies. *Pediatrics* 2009;123:959–965.
622. Tinkle BT, Wenstrup RJ. A genetic approach to fracture epidemiology in childhood. *Am J Med Genet* C *Semin Med Genet* 2005;139C:38–54.
623. Tlougan BE, Podjasek JO, O'Haver J, et al. Chronic recurrent multifocal osteomyelitis (CRMO) and synovitis, acne, pustulosis, hyperostosis, and osteitis (SAPHO) syndrome with associated neutrophilic dermatoses: a report of seven cases and review of the literature. *Pediatr Dermatol* 2009;26:497–505.
624. Tonkin MA. Failure of differentiation part I: Syndactyly. *Hand Clin* 2009;25:171–193.
625. Trebicz-Geffen M, Robinson D, Evron Z, et al. The molecular and cellular basis of exostosis formation in hereditary multiple exostoses. *Int J Exp Pathol* 2008;89:321–331.
626. Tretter AE, Saunders RC, Meyers CM, et al. Antenatal diagnosis of lethal skeletal dysplasias. *Am J Med Genet* 1998;75:518–522.
627. Triantafillidou K, Zouloumis L, Karakinaris G, et al. Brown tumors of the jaws associated with primary or secondary hyperparathyroidism. A clinical study and review of the literature. *Am J Otolaryngol* 2006;27:281–286.
628. Tsuji M, Inagaki T, Kasai H, et al. Solitary myofibromatosis of the skull: a case report and review of literature. *Childs Nerv Syst* 2004;20:366–369.
629. Tsutsumi S, Kamata N, Vokes TJ, et al. The novel gene encoding a putative transmembrane protein is mutated in gnathodiaphyseal dysplasia (GDD). *Am J Hum Genet* 2004;74:1255–1261.
630. Turcotte RE, Kurt AM, Sim FH, et al. Chondroblastoma. *Hum Pathol* 1993;24:944–949.
631. Turra S, Gigante C, Bisinella G. Polydactyly of the foot. *J Pediatr Orthop B* 2007;16:216–220.
632. Tzschach A, Tinschert S, Kaminsky E, et al. Czech dysplasia: report of a large family and further delineation of the phenotype. *Am J Med Genet A* 2008;146A:1859–1864.
633. Unger SL, Briggs MD, Holden P, et al. Multiple epiphyseal dysplasia: radiographic abnormalities correlated with genotype. *Pediatr Radiol* 2001;31:10–18.
634. Unni KK, Inwards CY, Bridge JA, et al. *Tumors of the Bones and Joints*. Washington, D.C.: American Registry of Pathology, 2005.
635. Valenzano M, Paoletti R, Rossi A, et al. Sirenomelia. Pathological features, antenatal ultrasonographic clues, and a review of current embryogenic theories. *Hum Reprod Update* 1999;5:82–86.
636. van den Berg H, Dirksen U, Ranft A, et al. Ewing tumors in infants. *Pediatr Blood Cancer* 2008;50:761–764.
637. van den Berg H, Kroon HM, Slaar A, et al. Incidence of biopsy-proven bone tumors in children: a report based on the Dutch pathology registration "PALGA". *J Pediatr Orthop* 2008;28:29–35.
638. Vander Have KL, Hensinger RN, Caird M, et al. Congenital pseudarthrosis of the tibia. *J Am Acad Orthop Surg* 2008;16:228–236.
639. Vanhoenacker FM, Hauben E, De Beuckeleer LH, et al. Desmoplastic fibroma of bone: MRI features. *Skeletal Radiol* 2000;29:171–175.
640. Vauthay L, Mazzitelli N, Rittler M. Patterns of severe abdominal wall defects: insights into pathogenesis, delineation, and nomenclature. *Birth Defects Res A Clin Mol Teratol* 2007;79:211–220.
641. Vergel De Dios AM, Bond JR, et al. Aneurysmal bone cyst. A clinicopathologic study of 238 cases. *Cancer* 1992;69:2921–2931.
642. Verloes A, Lesenfants S, Barr M, et al. Fronto-otopalatodigital osteodysplasia: clinical evidence for a single entity encompassing Melnick-Needles syndrome, otopalatodigital syndrome types 1 and 2, and frontometaphyseal dysplasia. *Am J Med Genet* 2000;90:407–422.
643. Vieira T, Schwartz I, Munoz V, et al. Mucopolysaccharidoses in Brazil: what happens from birth to biochemical diagnosis? *Am J Med Genet A* 2008;146A:1741–1747.
644. Vigorita VJ, Osteonecrosis. In: *Orthopaedic Pathology*, 2nd edn. Philadelphia: Lippincott Williams & Wilkins, 2008:546–573.
645. Villa A, Guerrini MM, Cassani B, et al. Infantile malignant, autosomal recessive osteopetrosis: the rich and the poor. *Calcif Tissue Int* 2009;84:1–12.
646. Vlychou M, Athanasou NA. Radiological and pathological diagnosis of paediatric bone tumours and tumour-like lesions. *Pathology* 2008;40:196–216.
647. Vosmaer A, Pereira RR, Koenderman JS, et al. Coagulation abnormalities in Legg-Calve-Perthes disease. *J Bone Joint Surg Am* 92:121–128.
648. Vuopala K, Herva R. Lethal congenital contracture syndrome: further delineation and genetic aspects. *J Med Genet* 1994;31:521–527.
649. Vuopala K, Leisti J, Herva R. Lethal arthrogryposis in Finland–a clinico-pathological study of 83 cases during thirteen years. *Neuropediatrics* 1994;25:308–315.
650. Wada Y, Nishimura G, Nagai T, et al. Mutation analysis of SOX9 and single copy number variant analysis of the upstream region in eight patients with campomelic dysplasia and acampomelic campomelic dysplasia. *Am J Med Genet A* 2009;149A:2882–2885.
651. Wagner EF, Karsenty G. Genetic control of skeletal development. *Curr Opin Genet Dev* 2001;11:527–532.
652. Waguespack SG, Hui SL, Dimeglio LA, et al. Autosomal dominant osteopetrosis: clinical severity and natural history of 94 subjects with a chloride channel 7 gene mutation. *J Clin Endocrinol Metab* 2007;92:771–778.
653. Wainwright H, Beighton P. Achondrogenesis type II with cutaneous hamartomata. *Clin Dysmorphol* 2008;17:207–209.
654. Wainwright H, Beighton P. Visceral manifestations of hypochondrogenesis. *Virchows Arch* 2008;453:203–207.
655. Waller DK, Correa A, Vo TM, et al. The population-based prevalence of achondroplasia and thanatophoric dysplasia in selected regions of the US. *Am J Med Genet A* 2008;146A:2385–2389.

656. Wang AA, Hutchinson DT. Longitudinal observation of pediatric hand and wrist ganglia. *J Hand Surg Am* 2001;26:599–602.
657. Weber M, Johannisson T, Thomsen M, et al. Thanatophoric dysplasia type I: new radiologic, morphologic, and histologic aspects toward the exact definition of the disorder. *J Pediatr Orthop B* 1998;7:1–9.
658. Weiss A, Khoury JD, Hoffer FA, et al. Telangiectatic osteosarcoma: the St. Jude Children's Research Hospital's experience. *Cancer* 2007;109:1627–1637.
659. Wenger DE, Wold LE. Benign vascular lesions of bone: radiologic and pathologic features. *Skeletal Radiol* 2000;29:63–74.
660. Wenig BM, Vinh TN, Smirniotopoulos JG, et al. Aggressive psammomatoid ossifying fibromas of the sinonasal region: a clinicopathologic study of a distinct group of fibro-osseous lesions. *Cancer* 1995;76:1155–1165.
661. Wesche WA, Khare V, Rao BN, et al. Malignant peripheral nerve sheath tumor of bone in children and adolescents. *Pediatr Dev Pathol* 1999;2:159–167.
662. Wesseling K, Bakkaloglu S, Salusky I. Chronic kidney disease mineral and bone disorder in children. *Pediatr Nephrol* 2008;23:195–207.
663. White AL, Modaff P, Holland-Morris F, et al. Natural history of rhizomelic chondrodysplasia punctata. *Am J Med Genet A* 2003;118A:332–342.
664. Whitley CB, Langer LO Jr, Ophoven J, et al. Fibrochondrogenesis: lethal, autosomal recessive chondrodysplasia with distinctive cartilage histopathology. *Am J Med Genet* 1984;19:265–275.
665. Whyte MP, Wenkert D, McAlister WH, et al. Chronic recurrent multifocal osteomyelitis mimicked in childhood hypophosphatasia. *J Bone Miner Res* 2009;24:1493–1505.
666. Wilcox WR, Tavormina PL, Krakow D, et al. Molecular, radiologic, and histopathologic correlations in thanatophoric dysplasia. *Am J Med Genet* 1998;78:274–281.
667. Wilson AJ, Kyriakos M, Ackerman LV. Chondromyxoid fibroma: radiographic appearance in 38 cases and in a review of the literature. *Radiology* 1991;179:513–518.
668. Winkelstein JA, Marino MC, Johnston RB Jr, et al. Chronic granulomatous disease. Report on a national registry of 368 patients. *Medicine (Baltimore)* 2000;79:155–169.
669. Witters I, Moerman P, Fryns JP. Fetal akinesia deformation sequence: a study of 30 consecutive in utero diagnoses. *Am J Med Genet* 2002;113:23–28.
670. Witters I, Moerman P, Fryns JP. Skeletal dysplasias: 38 prenatal cases. *Genet Couns* 2008;19:267–275.
671. Wold LE, Dobyns JH, Swee RG, et al. Giant cell reaction (giant cell reparative granuloma) of the small bones of the hands and feet. *Am J Surg Pathol* 1986;10:491–496.
672. Wood B, Dimmick JE. Skeletal system. In: Dimmick JE, Kalousek DK, eds. *Developmental Pathology of the Embryo and Fetus*. Philadelphia: JB Lippincott Co., 1992:662–706.
673. Wu CT, Inwards CY, O'Laughlin S, et al. Chondromyxoid fibroma of bone: a clinicopathologic review of 278 cases. *Hum Pathol* 1998;29:438–446.
674. Yagci B, Varan A, Caglar M, et al. Langerhans cell histiocytosis: retrospective analysis of 217 cases in a single center. *Pediatr Hematol Oncol* 2008;25:399–408.
675. Yamaguchi T, Dorfman HD, Eisig S. Cherubism: clinicopathologic features. *Skeletal Radiol* 1999;28:350–353.
676. Yang S. The skeletal system. In: Wigglesworth JS, Singer DB, eds. *Textbook of Fetal and Perinatal Pathology*, 2nd edn. Malden: Blackwell Science, 1998:1039–1082.
677. Yang SS, Kitchen E, Gilbert EF, et al. Histopathologic examination in osteochondrodysplasia. Time for standardization. *Arch Pathol Lab Med* 1986;110:10–12.
678. Yang SS, Langer LO Jr, Cacciarelli A, et al. Three conditions in neonatal asphyxiating thoracic dysplasia (Jeune) and short rib-polydactyly syndrome spectrum: a clinicopathologic study. *Am J Med Genet Suppl* 1987;3:191–207.
679. Yang SS, Lin CS, Al Saadi A, et al. Short rib-polydactyly syndrome, type 3 with chondrocytic inclusions: report of a case and review of the literature. *Am J Med Genet* 1980;7:205–213.
680. Yoon SH, Kim SH, Shin YS, et al. Desmoplastic fibroma of the skull in an infant. *Childs Nerv Syst* 2006;22:176–181.
681. Yoon SH, Park SH. A study of 77 cases of surgically excised scalp and skull masses in pediatric patients. *Childs Nerv Syst* 2008;24:459–465.
682. Yoshida A, Edgar MA, Garcia J, et al. Primary desmoplastic small round cell tumor of the femur. *Skeletal Radiol* 2008;37:857–862.
683. Yoshikawa H, Ueda T, Mori S, et al. Skeletal metastases from soft-tissue sarcomas. Incidence, patterns, and radiological features. *J Bone Joint Surg Br* 1997;79B:548–552.
684. Young CL, Sim FH, Unni KK, et al. Chondrosarcoma of bone in children. *Cancer* 1990;66:1641–1648.
685. Young ID, Lindenbaum RH, Thompson EM, et al. Amniotic bands in connective tissue disorders. *Arch Dis Child* 1985;60:1061–1063.
686. Yue H, Zhang ZL, He JW. Identification of novel mutations in WISP3 gene in two unrelated Chinese families with progressive pseudorheumatoid dysplasia. *Bone* 2009;44:547–554.
687. Zimmer EZ, Bronshtein M. Fetal polydactyly diagnosis during early pregnancy: clinical applications. *Am J Obstet Gynecol* 2000;183:755–758.

Index

Note: Page numbers followed by '*f*' indicate figures; those followed by '*t*' indicate tables.

A

Abetalipoproteinemia, 614, 615*f*
Abrasions
  brush-burn, child abuse, 268–269, 269*f*
  muzzle stamp, gunshot wounds, 283, 283*f*
Abruptio placentae
  chronic, 330
  marginal, 338
Abscess
  CNS, 393–394
  hepatic, 690–691
  perianal, 66
Acanthamoeba keratitis, 415–416, 415*f*
Achondroplasia, 1198
Aciduria, 282
Acinar cell carcinoma, 758, 758*f*
Acquired hypoplasia, 1001
Acquired melanocytic nevi, 1135
Acrocephalosyndactyly syndrome, 109–111, 110*t*
Acrodermatitis enteropathica, 1113
Acropustulosis of infancy, 1116
Actinomycotic infection, 238–239
Acute allograft rejection, 291–292
Acute antibody-mediated rejection (AMR), 309–310
Acute disease processes
  abruptio placenta, 344–345
  fetal hemorrhage, 347
  umbilical cord occlusion, 345–346
Acute interstitial pulmonary emphysema (AIPE), 477, 479*f*
Acute lymphoblastic leukemia (ALL)
  biologic basis, 1023–1025, 1024*f*
  classification, 1022–1023, 1022*t*
  clinical and laboratory features, 1025*t*
  incidence, 1022, 1025*t*
  morphologic basis, 1023, 1023*f*
  phenotypic basis, 1023, 1024*t*
Acute myelogenous leukemia (AML)
  biologic basis, 1028, 1030–1032
  classification, 1025, 1026*t*
  FAB classification, 1026*t*
  genotypic abnormalities, 1026, 1028*t*
  incidence, 1025
  inv (16), 1031, 1031*f*
  monosomy 7, 1031
  morphologic diagnosis, 1026, 1026*t*–1027*t*, 1027*f*
  11q23 abnormalities, 1031, 1031*f*
  t(8;21), 1028, 1030
  t(15;17), 1030, 1030*f*–1031*f*
  WHO classification, 1028*t*–1030*t*
Acute osteomyelitis (AO), 1252–1253, 1253*f*
Acute synovitis, 1255
Acute tubular necrosis, 810, 810*f*
Acyl-CoA dehydrogenase deficiency, 157–159, 159*f*
Acyl-CoA oxidase deficiency, 172
Adamantinoma (ADA), 1239–1240
Adenocarcinoma, 494
Adenoid cystic carcinoma, 493
Adenoma, 765*t*, 770, 771*f*
Adenomatoid tumor, 892
Adenovirus infection, 214
Adipocere, postmartem, 253
Adipocytic (lipomatous) tumors
  congenital intraspinal lipoma, 1070
  lipoblastoma, 1070–1071
  lipomas, 1070
  liposarcoma, 1071–1072
  macrodystrophia lipomatosa and macrodactyly, 1070
  phosphatase, tensin homologue, and deleted on chromosome TEN (PTEN), 1069–1070
Adnexal tumors, 1133–1134, 1133*f*
Adrenal cortical neoplasms (ACNs), 953–957, 955*f*, 956*f*
Adrenal cysts, 953
Adrenal cytomegaly, 947–948, 949*f*
Adrenal glands
  acquired disorders
    adrenal cortical neoplasms, 953–957
    adrenal cysts, 953
    adrenal hemorrhage, 953
    adrenal medullary hyperplasia, 970
    bacterial, fungal, parasitic, and viral infections, 953
    calcifications, 953
    composite adrenal medullary neoplasms, 970
    peripheral NB group tumors, 957–968
    pheochromocytoma, 968–970
  developmental disorders, 943–953
  imaging studies, 942–943
Adrenal medullary hyperplasia, 970
Adrenogenital syndrome, 843, 868
Adrenoleukodystrophy (ALD), 947, 947*f*
Adult-type granulosa cell tumors, 858, 858*f*
α-dystroglycan glycosylation, 1179
Aeromona, 606
Agenesis of the corpus callosum, 362, 362*f*
Agenesis-hypoplasia, 923
Alagille syndrome, 649–650, 651*f*
Alcohol embryopathy, 99, 100*t*
Algor mortis, definition of, 253
Allergic colitis, 627, 628*f*
Allograft
  acute rejection, 291–292
  hyperacute rejection, 291
  tolerance, 292–293
Alpers-Huttenlocher syndrome, 373
Alpha-1-antitrypsin deficiency, 669, 670*f*, 671
Alport syndrome, 419, 803–804, 804*f*
Alveolar soft part sarcoma, 1097–1099
Amelia, 1193
Amino acid disorders
  central nervous system, 373
  hepatic involvement in, 662–663, 663*f*
Aminoacidopathy, 150–152
  homocystinuria, 151
  maple syrup urine disease (MSUD), 152
  nonketotic hyperglycinemia, 152
  phenylketonuria, 150
  tyrosinemia type I (hepatorenal tyrosinemia, congenital tyrosinosis), 150–151, 151*f*
  tyrosinemia type II (oculocutaneous tyrosinemia, Richner-Hanhart syndrome), 151
Ammon horn sclerosis. *See* Mesial temporal sclerosis
Amnion, 58
Amnion rupture disruption sequence, 101–102, 102*f*, 103*t*
Amniotic fluid meconium, 341–343
  clinical correlation, 343
  in utero hypoxia, 341
  pathology, 343
AMR. *See* Acute antibody-mediated rejection
Anatomic landmarks, in forensic pathology, 255
Andersen disease, 156, 157*f*
Androgen receptor disorders, 871
Anembryonic pregnancy, 328
Anemia
  aplastic, 1018
  siderublastic, with exocrine pancreatic insufficiency, 752
Anencephaly
  neural tube defect, 359*f*
  in pituitary gland, 917
Aneuploidy. *See also* Sex chromosome aneuploidy
  definition, 73*t*
  early spontaneous abortion, 56
  incidence, 75*t*
  nondisjunction, 74–75, 75*t*
  partial. *See* Partial chromosomal aneuploidy
  PCS-MVA, 77
  somatic, 77
  spontaneous abortion, 75
  structural rearrangement, 75
Aneurysmal bone cyst (ABC), 1235, 1235*f*
Aneurysms
  aorta, 559–560, 559*t*–560*t*
  Galen, 402

Angiokeratoma corporis diffusum universale. *See* Fabry disease
Angiomatoid fibrous histiocytoma (AFH), 1041*t*, 1066–1067, 1067*t*
Angiomyolipomas, 826
Anisosplenia, bronchial isomerism syndrome, 452
Annular pancreas, 746
Anomalies
  breast
    accessory breast tissue, 898
    breast asymmetry, 898
    congenital absence, 897
    supernumerary nipple, 898
  in pituitary gland, 916
  spleen, congenital
    accessory of, 994
    asplenia, 994–995
    cysts, 995
    fusion, 995
    hamartoma, 995
    polysplenia, 994
Antenatal disruptive lesions, 366
Anthrax, 246
Antigens, 26–29
  alpha-1-antitrypsin (A1AT), 29
  cell cycle and apoptotic markers, 28–29
  cell surface, 26
  cytoskeleton, 26
  embryonal and cancer markers, 28
  hormones, 27–28
  limitations, 29
  pathogens, 27
  protooncogenes, 28
Antral web, 581
Anus
  condylomata acuminata, 66
  congenital abnormalities, 65–66, 65*f*
  imperforate, 65
  perianal abscess and anal fistula, 66
Aortic arch system malformation, 533–536
  branching anomalies
    left aortic arch with aberrant right subclavian artery, 535
    right-sided aortic arch, 535
    vascular rings, 535–536
  ductus arteriosus, 533
  obstructive anomalies, 534*t*
    coarctation of the aorta, 534–535, 535*t*
    interruption of the aortic arch, 535, 535*t*
    tubular hypoplasia, 535
  patent ductus arteriosus, 533–534
Aortopulmonary septal defect. *See* Aortopulmonary window
Aortopulmonary window, 525
Apendicitis, 62–63
Apert syndrome, 109
Aplasia, 1148–1149, 1149*f*
Aplasia cutis congenita, 1108
Aplastic anemia, 1018
Appendix
  carcinoid tumors, 65
  congenital and neuromuscular disorders, 62
  Crohn disease, 64–65
  cystic fibrosis, 64, 64*f*
  diverticula, 62
  infections, 63–64, 64*f*
  interval appendectomy, 63
  mucosal melanosis, 64
  neuroma, 62
  normal anatomy and histology, 634–635
  ulcerative colitis, 64–65
Argininosuccinic aciduria, 169
Arrhythmogenic right ventricular dysplasia (ARVD), 541–542, 541*f*
Arteriopathy, 558–559
Arterio-venous malformations (AVMs), 402
Arthrogryposis, 1149–1151
  contractures, 1149–1151, 1150*f*
  pathogenetic classification, 1151*t*
Askin tumor, 497
Aspartylglycosaminuria, 143
Asphyxia, 265–266
Aspiration, 479–482
  amniotic fluid, 479, 482*f*
  aspirated material, 481*t*
  foreign bodies, 481
  maternal blood, 481
  meconium, 480, 481*f*
Asplenia syndrome, 452
Assisted reproductive technologies (ARTs), 58
Asthma, 503–504, 503*f*
Astroblastoma, 383–384
Astrocytoma
  anaplastic, 382*f*
  diffusely infiltrating, 382, 382*f*
  pilocytic, 381–382, 381*f*
  subependymal giant cell, 384
Ataxia-telangiectasia, 774
Atherosclerosis, 560–561, 560*t*
Atopic dermatitis, 1116
Atresia
  bronchial, 450–451
  choanal, 444–445
  esophageal, 449–450, 450*f*–451*f*, 451*t*
  laryngeal, 446–447, 446*f*
Atrial appendages, juxtaposition, 538
Atrioventricular connection, univentricular, 529, 529*t*
Atrioventricular septal defect
  complete, 521, 521*f*
  partial, 520–521
Atrioventricular valves, straddling and overriding, 529
Atypical teratoid/rhabdoid tumor (ATRT), 386, 387*f*
Autism, 377
Autoimmune enteropathy, 615–616, 616*f*
Autoimmune hepatitis (AIH), 297*t*, 301, 301*f*, 302, 688–690, 690*f*
Autoimmune lymphoproliferative syndrome, 982–983
Autopsy, 180–181
  abdomen examination
    adrenals and kidneys, 13–14
    bowel, 14, 14*f*
    external, 5–6, 6*f*
    internal, 7–8, 7*f*–8*f*
    liver, 13, 13*f*
    spleen, 13
  blood culture, 8, 8*f*
  body cavity, 9–10, 10*f*
  brain, 15–16
  calvarium, 14–15
  cardiac-thoracic ratio, 9, 9*f*
  central nervous system, 14–17, 14*f*–16*f*
  chest examination
    external, 5, 5*f*
    internal, 7–8, 7*f*–8*f*
  crown-heel length measurement, 2, 3*f*
  cytogenetics, 8
  ears, 3, 5*f*
  external examination, 2, 3*f*
  eyes, 3, 4*f*, 436, 436*f*–437*f*
  face, 2–3, 4*f*
  forensic pathology
    collection of trace evidence and clothing, 253
    documentation of external evidence of injury, 253–255
    techniques and procedures, 256–257
  head measurement, 2, 3*f*
  heart/lung, 10–13, 11*f*–12*f*
  hydrops fetalis, 180*t*
  instruments, 1, 2*f*, 2*t*
  laboratory techniques, 6–7
  lower extremities, 6, 6*f*
  lung culture, 8
  mouth, 4
  neglected child, 262–263
  neonaticide, 259–261
  nose, 3, 4*f*
  organ removal, Rokitansky technique, 9
  palms of the hands, 4
  permit, 1
  photography, 6
  radiography, 6
  remains, disposition, 17
  respiratory system, 13
  scalp, 14
  specimen, 181*t*
  standard, 1–2, 2*f*–3*f*, 2*t*
  testes/ovaries, 9
  thymus, 8
  upper extremities, 4
  vertebral column/spinal cord, 10, 10*f*–11*f*
Autosomal dominant mutation, 108–109
  heterogenous dysplasia associated with, 115–116
Autosomal monosomy, 79
Autosomal recessive mutation, 111–115, 112*f*, 114*f*
  heterogenous dysplasia associated with, 115–116
Autosomal trisomy
  amplified developmental instability, 77
  critical region hypothesis, 77
  infants life expectancy, 77, 79
  malformations and postnatal disorders
    trisomy 13, 77, 80*t*, 82*f*
    trisomy 18, 77, 79*t*, 81*f*
    trisomy 21, 77, 78*t*, 81*f*
  nonmosaic, 77
  nonsex chromosomes, 77
  prenatal screening markers, 77, 82*t*
AV conduction disorders, 556
Avellino corneal dystrophy, 416
Axial mesodermal defects, 358–360, 360*f*
Axial skeleton anomalies, 1194
Axonal spheroids, 352, 353*f*, 373–374
Axons, disruption of in head injury, 272–276

B

Bacterial infection
  actinomycotic infection, 238–239
  Chlamydial infection, 237–238, 238*t*
  Citrobacter species, 224
  Clostridial infection, 231–232
  CNS
    abscess, 393–394
    acute meningitis, 392–393, 393*f*
    chronic infection, 394
  diphtheria, 224
  enterobacteriaceae, 222–223, 222*f*
  enterococci, 221
  hemophilus influenza, 223–224, 223*f*
  intestinal
    aeromona, 606
    Campylobacter jejuni, 605
    causes, 602–603
    Clostridium difficile, 605–606
    Escherichia coli, 604–605, 604*f*
    Salmonella, 603
    Shigella, 603
    Vibrio cholerae, 603–604
    Yersinia enterocolitica, 605
  leptospirosis, 229
  listeriosis, 225, 225*f*
  lyme disease, 229–231
  mycoplasma infection, 236–237, 237*f*
  Neisseria infections, 221, 221*f,* 222*f*
  neonatal sepsis, 216–218, 217*t*
  nonvenereal treponematoses, 231
  Pseudomonas aeruginosa, 224, 224*f*
  rickettsial infections, 235–236, 235*t,* 236*f*
  Salmonella infection (typhoid), 223
  Serratia marcescens, 224
  skin
    ecthyma, 1121
    erysipelas, 1121–1122
    impetigo, 1120
    staphylococcal scalded skin syndrome, 1120–1121
    toxic shock syndrome, 1121
  spontaneous abortion, 61, 62
  Staphylococcal infections, 218–219, 219*f*
  Streptococcal infections, 219–221, 220*f*
  syphilis, 225–229, 226*f,* 227*f*
  tuberculosis, 232–235, 234*f*
  zoonoses, 232
Balanitis xerotica obliterans (BXO), 893
Band keratopathy, 417, 418*f*
Barrett esophagus, 578–579, 578*f*
Barth syndrome, 168
Bartholin cyst, 848
Bartter syndrome, 815
Basal cell nevus syndrome, 409
Bat gio (skin), child abuse *vs.,* 281
Batten disease. *See* Neuronal ceroid lipofuscinoses
B-cell lymphoblastic lymphoma, 987
B-cell lymphomas, 988–989
Beckwith-Wiedemann syndrome, 104–105, 104*f,* 758
Behçet syndrome, 847
Benign fibrous histiocytoma, 1065–1066
Bent bone dysplasias, 1207
β-Amyloid precursor protein (β-APP), 275
Bile acid metabolism disorders, 667–669
Bile duct
  agenesis, 654
  congenital bronchobiliary fistula, 654
  congenital dilatation, 654–656, 654*f*–655*f*
  congenital hepatic fibrosis, 656–657, 657*f*
  development, 640–641
  extrahepatic biliary atresia, 645–649, 646*f*–649*f,* 646*t*
  hereditary hyperbilirubinemia, 643–644, 644*t*
  idiopathic neonatal hepatitis, 644–645, 645*f*
  persistent intrahepatic cholestasis, 649–653, 650*t,* 651*f*–653*f*
  physiologic jaundice, 643, 644*t*
  recurrent intrahepatic cholestasis, 653–654
  remnants, 649
Biopsy
  cornea, 414
  electron microscopic examination of specimens, 47–48, 48*f*
  fine-needle aspiration as, 18–20
  heart, 554–555, 554*t*–555*t*
  hepatic
    after liver transplantation, 689–690
    in chronic hepatitis, 685
    extrahepatic biliary atresia, 646, 646*f*
    fulminant failure, 686, 686*f*–688*f*
    triaging, 642–643, 643*f*
  intestinal
    celiac disease, 610–612
    Hirschsprung disease, 594–596, 594*f*–596*f*
    malabsorption, 608, 609*f*
  of lymph nodes
    cytogenetic studies, 977, 978*t*
    immunophenotypic studies, 976–977, 977*t*
  renal
    electron microscopic examination of, 47–48, 48*f*
Bioterrorism, systemic infectious agents
  anthrax, 246
  differential diagnosis, 245–246, 245*t*
  plague, 246–247
  smallpox, 245–246, 246*f*
Birbeck granules, 49, 50*f*
Birth trauma, 356, 356*f*
Bites, human, child abuse, 254
Bloch-Sulzberger syndrome, 1113
Blue nevus, 1136, 1136*f*
Bone marrow
  development, 1010–1011
  examination
    aplastic anemia, 1018
    benign erythroid disorders, 1018–1019, 1019*f*
    constitutional hematopoietic disorders, 1016, 1017*t,* 1018
    indications, 1016*t*
    inherited and congenital hematopoietic syndromes, granulocytes, 1019, 1019*t*
    specialized techniques, 1016*t*
  general features, 1010*t*
  hematologic profile, 1014–1015, 1015*t*
  hematopoiesis, 1010*t*
    lineages, 1012–1014
    normal parameters, 1014, 1015*t*
  inherited immunodeficiency disorders
    general considerations, 1020, 1020*f*
    platelet and megakaryocytic disorders, 1020–1021
    specific disorders, 1020, 1020*t*
  morphologic expectations, post-transplant, 1034
  myeloproliferative disorders, 1021
  neoplastic disorders
    acute leukemia, 1021–1022
    acute lymphoblastic leukemia, 1022–1025
    acute myelogenous leukemia, 1025–1031
    congenital leukemia, 1022
    myelodysplastic and chronic myeloproliferative disorders, 1032
    transient myeloproliferative disorders, 1021, 1022*f*
  neoplastic histiocytic disorders
    metastatic disorders, 1033–1034
    neoplastic histiocytoses, 1032–1033
  stem cells and progenitor cells, 1011, 1012*f*
  structure, 1011, 1011*f*
  transplantation, 1034
Boomerang dysplasia, 1205
Botulism, 231
Bowel, biopsy of, 47, 48*f*
Bowman membrane dystrophy, 416
Brachmann-de Lange syndrome, 111, 111*f*
Brain
  development, 360, 365–366
  edema
    trauma, 357
    types, 355
  hemorrhage, epidural, subarachoid, and subdural, 356–357
  herniation, 359
  hydrocephalus, 355–356, 356*f*
  increased intracranial pressure, 355–356
  trauma
    birth, 356, 356*f*
    infancy and childhood, 356–357
    inflicted injury, 357
  white matter of, metabolic disorder affecting, 369–370, 371*t*
Branched-chain ketoaciduria. *See* Maple syrup urine disease
Branchio-oto-renal syndrome, 108
Breast
  anomalies
    accessory breast tissue, 898
    breast asymmetry, 898
    congenital absence, 897
    supernumerary nipple, 898
  carcinoma, 25, 905–906, 905*f*
  epithelial-stromal lesions
    fibroadenoma and tubular adenoma, 902–903, 902*f,* 903*f*
    juvenile fibroadenoma, 903–904
    phyllodes tumor (cystosarcoma phyllodes), 904–905, 904*f,* 905*f*
  fat necrosis, 900
  fibroproliferative (fibrocystic) disease
    diabetic mastopathy, 899
    fibrocystic changes, 898–899
    juvenile papillomatosis, 899, 899*f,* 900*f*
    papillary duct hyperplasia, 899
  gynecomastia, 898*t,* 900–901, 900*t,* 901*t*
  hamartoma, 905
  infection, 899–900

Breast (*Continued*)
juvenile hypertrophy and macromastia, 901, 902*f*
mesenchymal lesions
fibromatosis, 906
granular cell tumor, 906–907, 907*f*
hematopoietic lesions, 907
lipoma, 906
sarcoma, 907
vascular tumors, 906, 906*f*
nipple duct adenoma, 905
Bronchial adenoma, 492
Bronchial-associated lymphoid tissue (BALT), 317
Bronchiectasis, 453
Bronchioloalveolar carcinoma, 494, 494*f*
Bronchitis, 455
Bronchobiliary fistulae, 453
Bronchoesophageal fistulae, 453
Bronchogenic carcinoma, 493–495, 494*f*–495*f*
Bronchogenic cyst, 454–455, 454*f*–455*f*
Bronchomalacia, 452
Bronchopulmonary dysplasia (BPD), 473–476
autopsy, 475
chronic lung disease of the premature, 475, 476*f*
features, 475
long-standing healed, 474, 474*f*
pathology, 473–474, 473*f*
surfactant replacement therapy, 474–475, 474*f*–475*f*
Bronchus(i), 450–455
abnormal branching and origin, 452–453, 452*f*–453*f*
atresia, 450–451
bronchiectasis, 453
bronchobiliary and bronchoesophageal fistulae, 453
bronchogenic cyst, 454–455, 454*f*–455*f*
bronchomalacia, 452
isomerism syndrome, 452
plastic bronchitis, 455
stenosis, 451–452
Brown fat, neglected child, 262
Brucellosis, 232
Bruck syndrome, 1200
Budd-Chiari syndrome, 692, 692*f*
Bullous diseases, 848
Bullous impetigo, 1120
Burkitt lymphoma
chromosome abnormalities in, 24*f*, 30
epidemiology, 988
Burns
abusive contact, 272
scalding, 271

C

Calcifying fibrous pseudotumor, 497
Call-Exner bodies, 840
Campylobacter jejuni, 605
CAN. *See* Chronic allograft nephropathy
Cancer predispostion (neurocutaneous) syndromes, 392, 392*t*
Candidiasis, 581
Cao gio (coin rubbing), child abuse *vs.,* 281
Capillary hemangioma, 406–407, 407*f*
Carbamoyl phosphate synthase I deficiency, 168–169
Carbohydrate metabolism disorders, 152–157
galactosemia, 152–153
glycogen storage diseases. *See* Glycogen storage disorders
hepatic involvement in, 658–662
fructosemia, 659
galactosemia, 658–659, 658*f*, 659*t*
glycogen storage disease, 659–662, 660*f*–662*f*
hereditary fructose intolerance, 153, 153*f*
Carbohydrate-deficient glycoprotein syndromes. *See* Congenital disorders of glycosylation
Carcinoid
lung, 492–493, 493*f*
testis, 888–889
Carcinoma, 905–906, 905*f*, 1134
Cardiac malformations
monosomy X, 67
trisomy 18, 66
trisomy 21, 66
VCF/DiGeorge syndrome, 88
Cardiomyopathy (CMP)
arrhythmogenic right ventricular dysplasia, 541–542, 541*f*
classification, 539*t*
dilated, 543–544, 543*f*, 543*t*
endocardial fibroelastosis, 544
fatty acid oxidation, 549*t*
histiocytoid, 568, 568*f*
hypertrophic, 539–541, 539*f*, 540*t*–541*t*
inflammatory, 544–547
maternal diabetes, 553
noncompaction, 542, 542*f*, 542*t*
restrictive, 544
skeletal myopathy associated with, 1174
Cardiopulmonary resuscitation (CPR), 277–280, 282–283
Cardiovascular disease
congenital malformation
aortic arch system, 533–536
classification, 517–518, 517*t*
conus and truncus, 521–526
coronary arteries, 536
etiology, 516
incidence, 516, 516*t*
pathophysiology, 516–517, 517*t*
position and situs, 537–538
septal malformation, 518–521
venous system, 536–537
ventricular inflow tract, 526–529
ventricular outflow tract, 529–533
hereditary and nonhereditary functional
arrhythmogenic right ventricular dysplasia, 541–542
conduction system abnormalities, 555–557
dilated cardiomyopathy, 543–544
endocardial diseases, 562–564
endocardial fibroelastosis, 544
endomyocardial biopsy and heart transplant, 554–555
Fabry disease, 549
fatty acid oxidation, 549
Friedreich ataxia, 550
gangliosidoses, 548–549
glycogen storage diseases, 547
histiocytoid cardiomyopathy, 568
infant of diabetic mother cardiomyopathy, 553
inflammatory/autoimmune disorders, 550–553
iron overload, 550
ischemic myocardial necrosis, 553–554
mitochondrial electron transport chain disorders, 549
mucolipidosis, 548
mucopolysaccaridoses, 547–548
myocardial disease, 538–541
myocarditis, 544–547
neuromuscular disorders, 550
N-glycosylation disorders, 549
noncompaction, ventricular myocardium, 542
pericardial diseases, 564–566
pulmonary hypertension, 557–558
restrictive cardiomyopathy, 544
systemic artery disease, 558–562
tumors, 566–569
Carnitine deficiency
hepatic involvement in, 679–680, 679*f*–680*f*
substrate transport defects, 159–160
Carnitine palmitoyltransferase (CPT), 159
Castleman disease/angiofollicular hyperplasia, 980, 980*f*
Cataracts
congenital, 419–421
Rubella, 420, 420*f*
toxic, 421, 421*f*
traumatic, 421
myotonic dystrophy, 419
polar, 419
posterior subcapsular, 419, 421*f*
pyramidal, 419
Catecholaminergic polymorphic ventricular tachycardia (CPVT), 556–557
Cat-scratch disease, 983, 983*f*
Cavernous hemangioma, 708
Cavernous transformation, portal vein, 692
Celiac disease, 608–612, 611*f*
Cell migration and specification disorders, 362–363
Cell surface antigens, flow cytometry of, 26
Central core disease, 550
Central hypotonia, 1154–1155, 1155*f*
Central nervous system (CNS)
autopsy, 14–17, 14*f*–16*f*
development, 358
infections, 392–399
inflicted injury trauma, 357
metabolic disorders, 367–373
neurodegenerative disorders, 373–377
neuropathology
axonal spheroids, 352, 353*f*
eosinophilic granular bodies, 353–354, 354*f*
microglia, 354, 355*f*
necrotic/dead neurons, 352, 353*f*
oligodendroglia, 354
pathologic reaction, 354
reactive gliosis, 352–353, 353*f*
Rosenthal fibers, 353–354, 354*f*
structural malformations

agenesis of the corpus callosum, 362, 362*f*
antenatal disruptive lesions, 366
axial mesodermal defects, 358–360, 360*f*
cell migration and specification disorders, 362–363
cerebral heterotopia, 364–365
Chiari and Dandy-Walker malformations, 366–367, 367*f*
cysts, 367, 368*t*
focal cortical dysplasia, 365–366, 365*f,* 365*t*
hindbrain malformations, 366
holoprosencephaly, 360–362, 361*f*
lissencephaly, 363–364, 363*f*
microcephaly and micrencephaly, 366
neural tube defects, 358–359
polymicrogyria, 364, 364*f*
tail bud defects, 358, 360
sudden infant death syndrome, 357–358
tumor, 381–392
clinical considerations, 377, 379
histology, 377, 377*t*
IHC stains, 380*t*
pathologic consideration, 379–381
signs and symptoms, 379*t*
WHO classification, 377, 378*t*–379*t*
vascular disorders, 399–402
Central odontogenic fibroma (COF), 1239
Cerebral edema
trauma, 357
types, 355
Cerebrohepatorenal syndrome. *See* Zellweger syndrome
Cerebro-oculo-facio-skeletal syndrome, 113–114
Cervical-thyroidal teratoma (CTT), 940–941
Chalazion, 407–408, 408*f*
Chediak-Higashi syndrome, 997
Chest wall hamartoma, 1228, 1230*f,* 1231*f*
Chiari malformations, 366–367, 367*f*
Child abuse
abdominal and thoracic blunt trauma, 278–280
characteristics of victims and perpetrators, 266–267
cutaneous evidence of, 256, 267–272
disorders mistaken for (mimicry), 280
documentation of, in forensic pathology, 253–255
head injuries, 272–277
homicidal suffocation, 266, 266*f*
Munchausen syndrome by proxy, 259
neglect as, 261–263
retinal hemorrhage, 277
skeletal evidence, 277–278
Chlamydia trachomatis, 846–847
Chlamydial infection, 237–238
C. pneumoniae, 237
C. trachomatis, 238
cell culture techniques, 238
childhood, 237, 238*t*
conjunctivitis, 238
Choanal atresia, 444–445
Cholangitis, primary sclerosing
diagnosis, 689
histopathology, 688–689, 689*f*
pathogenesis, 688
Cholecystitis, 736, 736*f*
Cholestasis
Alagille syndrome, 649–650, 651*f*
alpha-1-antitrypsin deficiency, 669, 672
extrahepatic biliary atresia, 645–649, 646*f*–649*f*
familial syndrome, 650*t*
neonatal, 644–646, 644*t,* 645*f,* 646*t*
nonsyndromic paucity of intrahepatic ducts, 653
persistent intrahepatic, 649–653, 650*t,* 651*f*–653*f*
progressive familial intrahepatic (Byler disease), 650–653, 652*f*–653*f*
recurrent intrahepatic
benign, 653
hereditary, with lymphedema, 654
total parenteral nutrition, 694–695, 694*f*
Cholesterol ester storage disease (CESD), 147, 148*f*
Chondroblastoma (CHB), 1226, 1228*f,* 1229*f*
Chondroma
bone, 1226, 1226*f*
lung, 489, 490*f*
Chondromatous hamartoma, 489, 490*f*
Chondromyxoid fibroma (CMF), 1226–1227, 1229*f,* 1230*f*
Chondrosarcoma (CS), 1228–1229
Chordoma, 1251
Choriocarcinoma, 883
Chorion
cytogenetic analysis, 58
in placental development, 324
Chorion sac, 102
Chorionic villi, 58
accelerated maturation of, 333
development of, 328, 329*f,* 332
edema, 327
hemorrhagic endovasculitis, 337
massive perivillous fibrin deposits, 338–339
maturation, 331
stromal hemorrhage, 345, 345*f*
Chorionic villitis
pathologic findings, 328
of unknown etiology, 330, 335–336
Choroid plexus tumors (CPTs), 391, 391*f*
Chromosomal abnormalities
acute lymphoblastic leukemia, 1024–1025
acute myelogenous leukemia, 1028, 1030–1032
CNS structural abnormalities, 360
cytogenetic analysis, 72–74
band resolution, 74*t*
banding techniques, 72, 73
cell types, 73, 74*t*
fetal autolysis, 73–74
incubation times, 73–74, 74*t*
nomenclature, 74*t*
routine cytogenetic studies, 72
tissue sources, 73, 74*t*
definition, 72
epigenetic modification and associated disorders, 89–90, 90*t*
karyotypic disorders, 74–88
aneuploidy. *See* Aneuploidy
autosomal monosomy, 79
autosomal trisomy. *See* Autosomal trisomy
chromosomal instability disorders, 86–88, 87*t,* 88*f*
confined placental mosaicism, 76–77, 76*f*
incidence, 74, 75*t*
mosaicism, 75–76
partial chromosomal aneuploidies, 85–86, 86*f,* 86*t*
polyploidy, 84–85, 85*t*
sex chromosome aneuploidy. *See* Sex chromosome aneuploidy
spontaneous abortion, 74, 75*t*
submicroscopic disorders, 88–89
submicroscopic chromosomal anomalies, 89*t*
subtelomeric deletions, 89
velocardiofacial/DiGeorge syndrome, 88–89
terminology, 73
translocations as, in solid tumors, 25*f,* 27*f,* 33
Chromosomal instability disorders, 86–88
cytogenetics and molecular genetics, 86–87, 87*t*
Fanconi anemia
complementation groups, 87–88, 88*f*
incidence, 87, 88*f*
Chronic allograft nephropathy (CAN), 305–306, 310
Chronic granulomatous disease, 984
Chronic lung disease of infancy, 487
Chronic lung disease of prematurity. *See* Bronchopulmonary dysplasia
Chronic lymphocytic thyroiditis (CLT), 932–933
Chronic progressive external ophthalmoplegia (CPEO), 163
Chronic synovitis, 1255
Cilia, nasal, electron microscopic examination of, 54, 54*f*
Cilia syndrome, immotile, 453
Cirrhosis, 695–696, 695*t,* 696*f. See also* Liver
Citrobacter infection, 224
Citrullinemia, 169
Clark dysplastic nevus, 1137
Clear cell sarcoma, 823–824, 824*f,* 1041*t,* 1091–1092
Cleft lip/palate, 60*f,* 66
incidence, 445
syndromes associated with, 445*t*
Clostridial infection, 231
Clostridial myonecrosis. *See* Gas gangrene
Clostridium difficile, 605–606
Cockayne syndrome, 112–113
Coenzyme Q_{10} deficiency (CoQ_{10}), 168
Coin rubbing *(cao gio),* child abuse *vs.,* 281
Colitis, 620–628, 620*t*
acute self-limited (infectious), 624–625
allergic, 627, 628*f*
associated with antibiotics, 625
causes, 620*t*
collagenous, 624
Crohn disease, 623–624, 623*f*
diversion, 625–626
indeterminate, 624
inflammatory bowel disease, 620–621
lymphocytic, 624
neonatal necrotizing enterocolitis, 626–627, 626*f*

Colitis (*Continued*)
pseudomembranous, 625, 625*f*
spontaneous perforation of the gastrointestinal tract, 627
typhlitis (neutropenic enterocolitis), 626
ulcerative, 621–623, 621*f*–622*f*
Collagen vascular diseases
lupus erythematosus, 25–26, 1129–1130, 1130*f*
scleroderma/progressive systemic sclerosus, 1130, 1130*f*
Collagenous colitis, 624
Common inlet ventricle, 529
Comparative genomic hybridization (CGH)
confined placental mosaicism, 76
early spontaneous abortion, 56
first trimester spontaneous abortion, 58
partial aneuploidy, 86
submicroscopic disorders, 88–89
Complete hydatidiform mole (CHM), 57, 62–63, 63*f*
Composite adrenal medullary neoplasms, 970
Conduction system abnormalities, 555–557
anatomy, 555
AV conduction disorder, 556
classification, 556*t*
histologic examination, 555
long QT syndrome, 556*t*
supraventricular tachycardia, 555–556
ventricular tachycardia, 556–557
Condylomata acuminata
anal, 66
female genitalia, 845
Confined placental mosaicism (CPM), 76–77
cytogenetic studies, 77
PCS-MVA, 77
placenta test, 76–77
trisomy, 16, 76
types, 76, 76*f*
uniparental disomy, 76
Congenital adrenal hyperplasia (CAH), 948–951
Congenital adrenal hypoplasia (CAHP), 948
Congenital alveolar capillary dysplasia, 469–470, 470*f*–471*f*, 470*t*
Congenital anomalies and malformation syndrome
abnormalities of unknown origin
nonimmune hydrops fetalis, 118–120, 118*f*, 119*t*
short-cord syndrome, 118
acrocephalosyndactyly syndrome, 109–111
Apert syndrome, 109
Brachmann–de Lange syndrome, 111
Crouzon craniofacial dysostosis, 110
features, 110*t*
Noonan syndrome, 111
Pfeiffer syndrome, 110
Robinow syndrome, 110
Stickler syndrome, 110–111
autosomal dominant conditions
branchiootorenal syndrome, 108
Holt-Oram syndrome, 109
mandibulofacial dysostosis, 109
nail-patella syndrome, 108
Opitz-Frias syndrome, 109
oral-facial-digital syndrome type I, 108
Townes-Brocks syndrome, 109
autosomal recessive conditions
Cockayne syndrome, 112–113
Dubowitz syndrome, 113
familial agnathia-holoprosencephaly, 114
hydrolethalus syndrome, 115
leprechaunism, 112
Meckel syndrome, 111–112, 112*f*
oral-facial-digital syndrome type II, 113
Pena-Shokeir phenotype type I, 113
Pena-Shokeir phenotype type II, 113–114
Robert syndrome, 114, 114*f*
Seckel syndrome, 113
Smith-Lemli-Opitz syndrome, 112
thrombocytopenia absent radius syndrome, 114–115
deformation, 96, 96*f*
disruption, 96–104
amnion rupture disruption sequence, 101–102, 102*f*, 103*t*
chorion and yolk sac rupture sequence, 102
diabetes mellitus, 100–101, 101*f*, 101*t*
dysplastic disruptions, 103
hyperthermia, 104
infectious disruptions, 101
ionizing radiation, 96–97
ischemic and vascular disruptions, 103
metabolic disruptions, 100–101
phenylketonuria, 100
teratogenic disruptions, 97–100, 97*t*, 98*t*
twin reversed arterial perfusion, 103, 104*f*
twin-twin transfusion syndrome, 103
etiology, 94
heterogenous autosomal dominant and recessive dysplasias
chondrodysplasia, 115
osteochondrodysplasia, 115, 116
metabolic dysplasia syndrome
Williams syndrome, 105
Zellweger syndrome, 105–106, 106*t*
morphogenesis, 94–96, 96*f*
MURCS association, 108
nonmetabolic dysplasia syndrome
Beckwith-Wiedemann syndrome, 104–105, 104*f*
Perlman syndrome, 105
pathogenesis, 54
Schisis association, 108
sequence
prune belly sequence, 107, 107*f*
Robin sequence, 106–107
sporadic abnormalities
Hallermann-Streiff syndrome, 117
hypomelanosis of Ito, 117–118
Klippel-Trenaunay-Weber vascular malformation, 117
Rubinstein-Taybi syndrome, 118
Sturge-Weber dysplasia, 117
terminology of, 94–96
VATER association, 107–108, 107*f*
X-linked mutations
Lesch-Nyhan syndrome, 117
Lowe syndrome, 116
Menkes syndrome, 116–117
Opitz-Kaveggia syndrome, 117
Pallister syndrome, 117
Congenital disorders of glycosylation (CDG), 176–177, 178*t*–179*t*, 373
Congenital hemidysplasia, ichthyosis, and limb defects (CHILD) syndrome, 177
Congenital hereditary corneal dystrophy (CHED), 416
Congenital infantile fibrosarcoma (CIFS), 1041*t*, 1061–1062, 1063*f*
Congenital infantile myofibromatosis, 1138, 1139*f*
Congenital intraspinal lipoma, 1070
Congenital lactic acidosis, 1173
Congenital malformations, kidney
bilateral renal agenesis, 780*t*, 781*t*, 783
hydronephrosis, 785, 785*f*
renal agenesis/hypoplasia, 782
renal duplication (duplex kidney), 784, 784*f*
renal ectopia, 781, 781*t*
renal fusion, 780*t*, 781–782, 782*f*
renal hypoplasia, 783–784
renal tubular dysgenesis, 784
renomegaly, 784
supernumerary kidney, 784–785
unilateral renal agenesis, 783
Congenital muscular dystrophy 1C (CMD1C), 1179
Congenital nevus, 1135
Congenital pseudarthrosis (CP), 1239
Congenital pulmonary airway malformation (CPAM), 464–469
acinar dysplasia/agenesis, 464–465, 465*f*
anomalies associated with, 468–469
classification, 464*f*
incidence, 464
large/predominant cyst type, 465–466, 465*f*–466*f*
medium cyst type, 466–467, 467*f*
peripheral acinar cyst type, 468, 469*f*
small cystic/solid type, 467, 468*f*
ultrasonography, 468
variants, 469
Congenital pulmonary lymphangiectasis (CPL), 463–464, 463*f*–464*f*
Congenital surfactant deficiency, 447*f*, 475–476
Conjunctiva
developmental abnormalities, 411, 411*f*–412*f*
inflammatory abnormalities, 410
melanocytic abnormalities, 411–413, 412*f*–413*f*
structure, 409–410, 410*f*
surgical procedures, 410
Conjunctival nevus, 412–413, 413*f*
Conradi-Hunermann syndrome, 177
Constitutional hematopoietic disorders, 1016, 1017*t*, 1018
B-cells and T-cells, 1021*t*
granulocytes, 1019*t*
Contact dermatitis, 1116
Contusions
cerebral, 273
dating, 256, 270–271
documentation, 254, 259
estimating age, 270
pattern injuries, 268, 268*f*
Conus and truncus malformation, 521–526
Cori-Forbe disease, 154, 156
Cornea
degeneration, 417, 418*f*
developmental abnormalities, 415

dystrophic abnormalities, 416–417, 416*f*–417*f*
hydrops, 417, 417*f*
inflammatory abnormalities, 415–416, 415*f*
plana, 415
structure, 413–414, 414*f*
surgical procedures, 414–415
Cornelia de Lange syndrome. *See* Brachmann-de Lange syndrome
Cortical cysts, 791–792, 791*f*
Cow's milk proteins induced enteropathy, 612–613, 613*f*
Coxsackie viruses infection, 216, 216*f*, 754
CPR. *See* Cardiopulmonary resuscitation
Craniopharyngioma (CPGs), 386–387
adamantinomatous, 386–387, 388*f*
papillary, 387
Craniopharyngiomas (CRPs), 921
Crescentic glomerulonephritis, 795*f*, 809
Crigler-Najjar syndrome (CNS), 643
Crohn disease, 608, 609*t*, 847
appendiceal, 63–65, 64–65
characteristics, 623–624, 623*f*
gastric, 584–585
malabsorption, 608, 609*t*
ulcerative colitis, 620–621
Crouzon craniofacial dysostosis, 110
Crown-heel length measurement, 2, 3*f*
Crypt apoptosis, 293–294, 294*f*
Cryptosporidium, 606–607, 607*f*
Cyst(s)
adrenal cysts, adrenal glands, 953
aneurysmal bone cyst, 1235, 1235*f*
bartholin, 848
central nervous system, 367, 368*t*
cortical, 791–792, 791*f*
cysts associated with syndromes, 792
dermoid
epidermoid, 881
Gartner duct, 848
medullary, 790
mucous, 848
Müllerian, 848
multiple follicular, 850
nonneoplastic cysts, pituitary gland, 919
parathyroid glands, 923
peritoneal lined cyst, 848
pineal gland, 914
simple cyst, 792
unicameral bone cyst, 1235, 1237*f*
Cystic dysplasia, 886
Cystic fibrosis, 502–503, 502*f*
appendiceal, 64, 64*f*
bronchiectasis, 453
gastrointestinal involvement, 593, 593*t*
hepatic involvement in, 671–672, 671*f*–672*f*
Cystic lymphangioma, 1048, 1048*f*
Cystinosis, 149, 150*f*
Cystitis
classification, 829
cystica and glandularis, 829–830
eosinophilic cystitis, 830
granulomatous, 829
hemorrhagic cystitis, 830
interstitial cystitis, 830
Cytogenetic studies, 32–34
applications of, 24*f*, 27*f*, 34
basis of methodology of, 32–34
compared with other molecular methods, 22*t*
limitations of, 34
Cytokeratin, 26
Cytomegalovirus (CMV), 65, 65*f*
causes, 193
central nervous system, 395–396, 396*f*
clinical features, 193, 197*f*, 198
diarrhea, 602, 602*f*
esophagitis, 581
hepatitis, 686, 687*f*
laboratory diagnosis, 198
Ménétrier disease, 583–584
pathology, 198
prognosis and outcome, 198
transmission, 198

D

Dandy-Walker malformations, 366–367, 367*f*
Danon disease, 138, 547
Darier disease, 1109, 1109*f*
D-bifunctional protein deficiency, 173
Death. *See also* Forensic pathology
accidental causes, 263–265
categories, forensic pathology, 264
scene of, investigation of, 252
utero, 260, 261, 281
Decomposition, of body, 248, 261
Deep lamellar keratoplasty (DLK), 414
Deep mycosis, 1124
Dehydration, neglected child, 262–263
del 1p36 deletion syndrome, 89
Dendritic cell (DC) neoplasms, 1068, 1069*f*
Denervation, fibers, 1156, 1157*f*
Denys-Drash syndrome, 875
Dermatitis
eczematous
atopic, 1116
contact, 1116
dyshidrotic, 1116
nummular, 1116
spongiotic, 1116–1117, 1117*f*
herpetiformis, 1114, 1114*f*
seborrheic, 1117
Dermatofibrosarcoma protuberans (DFSP), 104*t*, 1064, 1065*f*
Dermatopathia, 985, 986*f*
Dermoid cyst, 423–424, 424*f*
Dermoid cysts, 1132
Dermoid, limbal, 411, 411*f*
Desmin, 26
Desmoid-type fibromatosis, 1056–1057
Desmoplastic fibroma (DEF), 1238–1239
Desmoplastic infantile ganglioglioma (DIG), 390
Desmoplastic small round cell tumor, 1090–1091, 1091*f*
Developmental disorders
adrenal glands
adrenal cytomegaly, 947–948, 949*f*
adrenal fusion, 943
adrenocortical hyperplasia, 951
adrenocortical insufficiency, 952–953
adrenoleukodystrophy (ALD), 947, 947*f*
congenital adrenal hyperplasia (CAH), 948–951
congenital adrenal hypoplasia (CAHP), 948
ectopic adrenal tissue, 944–945
primary pigmented (micronodular) adrenocortical disease (PPAD), 951
Wolman disease, 945–947, 946*f*, 947*f*
parathyroid glands
agenesis-hypoplasia, 923
cyst(s), 923
ectopic parathyroid, 923
supernumerary parathyroid glands, 923
pineal gland
pineal agenesis, 913
pineal cysts, 914
pituitary gland
anencephaly, 917
anomalies, 916
duplication, 917
ectopia, 913*f*, 917
empty sella syndrome, 917–918
hypopituitarism, 916
thyroid gland
branchial apparatus–associated anomalies, 931–932
congenital hypothyroidism, 929–930
dysgenesis, 929
dysmorphism, 928–929
ectopia, 930–931, 930*f*
hemiagenesis, 930
thyroglossal duct cyst (TDC), 931, 931*f*
Dextrocardia, 537–538
Diabetes mellitus, 100–101, 101*f*, 101*t*
maternal, 553
maturity-onset diabetes of the young, 765
neonatal diabetes mellitus, 765
type 1, 763–764, 764*f*
type 2, 764–765, 764*f*
Diabetic mastopathy, breast, 899
Diabetic nephropathy, 799, 799*f*
Diaphanous dysplasia, 66
Diaphragm, 504–505
abnormalities, 504
accessory, 504
complete absence, 505
development, 504–505
eventration, 504*f*, 505
hernia, 503*f*, 505, 505*t*, 1149
anomalies associated with, 505*t*
Diffuse alveolar damage (DAD), 316–317
Diffuse large B-cell lymphoma (DLBCL), 988
Diffusely infiltrating astrocytoma, 382, 382*f*
DiGeorge anomaly, 1001
DiGeorge syndrome. *See* Velocardiofacial/DiGeorge syndrome
Dilated cardiomyopathy, 543–544, 543*f*, 543*t*
Diphenylhydantoin embryopathy, 99–100
Diphtheria, 224
Direct immunofluorescence (DIF)
applications, 29, 30*f*
methodology, 29, 29*f*
Dissection, forensic pathology autopsy, 256
Disseminated lipogranulomatosis. *See* Farber disease
Double inlet ventricle, 529
Double outlet ventricle
double outlet left ventricle, 524, 525*f*
double outlet right ventricle, 523–524, 524*f*, 524*t*
Down syndrome. *See* Trisomy 21
Drowning, accidental, 264

Dubin-Johnson syndrome, 643–644
Dubowitz syndrome, 113
Duplication, in pituitary gland, 917
Dysembryoplastic neuroepithelial tumor (DNT), 389–390, 390*f*
Dysgenesis, thyroid gland, 929
Dysgerminoma, 853–854
Dyshidrotic dermatitis, 1116
Dysmorphism, thyroid gland, 928–929
Dysostoses, 115
Dysplasia syndrome
  metabolic, 105–106, 106*t*
  nonmetabolic, 104–105, 104*f*
Dysplastic disruptions, 103
Dysplastic gangliocytoma of the cerebellum, 390

E

Early pregnancy
  anembryonic pregnancy, 328
  congenital infection, 330–331
  gestational trophoblastic disease, 326–328
  miscarriage, 328–330
  multiple, 324–326
Ecchymosis, periorbisal, in child abase, 254, 254*f*
Eccrine neoplasms, 1133–1134, 1134*f*
Echovirus infection, 215
Ectodermal dysplasias, 1110
Ectopia
  hepatic, 642, 642*f*
  in pituitary gland, 913*f*, 917
  renal, 781, 781*t*
  thyroid gland, 930–931, 930*f*
Ectopia cordis, 538, 538*f*
Ectopia lentis, 419–420, 420*f*
Ectopic pancreas, 746–747, 747*f*
Ectopic parathyroid, 923
Eczematous dermatitis
  atopic dermatitis, 1116
  contact dermatitis, 1116
  dyshidrotic dermatitis, 1116
  nummular dermatitis, 1116
  spongiotic dermatitis, 1116–1117, 1117*f*
Edema, cerebral. *See* Cerebral edema
Edwards syndrome. *See* Trisomy 18
Ehlers-Danlos syndrome, 559–560
Ehrlichiosis, 235–235
Electron microscopy, 47–54
  in diagnosis
    of leukemia, 51–52, 53*f*
    of peroxisomal disorders, 52*f*
  economics of, 48
  in examination
    of autopsy specimens, 49, 51*f*
    of cilia morphology, 54, 54*f*
    of fine-needle aspiration specimens, 51, 52*f*
    of frozen tissue, 49, 51*f*
  laboratory requirements for performing, 47–48
  specimen preparation for, 48
  suboptimal specimen processing and, 49–50, 50*f*
  surgical pathology specimens examined by, 47–48, 48*f*
  technique of, 48–54
  virus identification by, 54, 54*f*
  work load distribution and, 47, 48*f*
Embryo
  cleft lip and coloboma, 60*f*
  encephaloceles, 60*f*
  growth-disorganized. *See* Growth-disorganized embryo
  neural tube defects, 60–61
  normal development, 58–59, 59*f*
  triploid, 61, 61*f*, 63
  trisomy 13, 61, 61*f*
Embryonal carcinoma, 882
Embryonal rhabdomyosarcoma. *See* Rhabdomyosarcoma, embryonal
Embryonal sarcoma, undifferentiated, 728–731
Embryonal tumors, 384–386, 387*t*
Emery-Dreifuss muscular dystrophy, 550
Empty sella syndrome (ESS), 917–918
Encephalocele, 360*f*
Endocardial fibroelastosis, 544, 544*f*
Endocarditis
  bacterial and fungal, 562
  diagnosis, 564*t*
  features, 563*t*
  infective, 563–564, 563*t*–564*t*, 564*f*
  Libman-Sachs, 551
  nonbacterial thrombotic, 562
  noninfective, 562–563
  rheumatic, 552
  vegetations, 562
Endocrine pancreas
  abnormalities, 761–771, 761f, 763*f*, 764*f*, 765*t*, 767*t*, 771*f*
  aplasia and hypoplasia, 762
  diabetes mellitus, 763–765
  disorders, 773–774
  histogenesis, maturation, and morphology, 758–761, 760*f*, 761*f*
  hydrops fetalis, 762*f*, 763
  hyperinsulinism, 765–771, 765*t*, 768*f*, 769*f*
  infant of diabetic mother, 762–763, 762*f*
  islet hypertrophy, 761–762, 761*f*
  malformation syndromes, 771–773, 772*f*, 773*f*
  pancreatic islets in shock, 771
  tumors, 774
  viral infections, 771
Endodermal sinus tumor
  germ cell tumors, 854–855, 854*f*–855*f*
  lower female genital tract, 850, 850*f*
  yolk sac tumor, 878
Endometriosis/endometrioma, 851
Endoplasmic reticulum disorders, 175–177
  alpha-1-antitypsin (A1AT) deficiency, 175–176, 176*f*
  congenital disorders of glycosylation (CDG), 176–177
End-organ defects, testis, 870–872
Endothelial cushion formation, 336
Entamoeba histolytica, 244, 244*f*, 607
Enteric adenoviruses, 602
Enterobacteriaceae, 222–223, 222*f*
Enterococci infection, 221
Enteropathy
  AIDS, 618
  autoimmune, 615–616, 616*f*
  cow's milk proteins induced, 612–613, 613*f*
  postenteritis, 612
  tufting, 616, 617*f*
Enzyme deficiencies, of exocrine pancreas, 751
Eosinophilia
  esophagitis, 579–580, 579*f*
  gastroenteritis, 584, 584*f*
Eosinophilic cellulitis, 1125
Eosinophilic cystitis, 830
Eosinophilic granular bodies, 353–354, 354*f*
Ependymoma, 382–383, 383*f*
Epidermal inclusion cysts, 1132
Epidermal nevi, 1131–1132
Epidermoid cyst, 881
Epidermolysis bullosa, 1112–1113
Epidermolysis bullosa acquisita, 1115
Epididymal sarcoidosis, 880
Epididymoorchitis, 876
Epidural hemorrhage, head injuries, 276
Epigenetic chromosomal modifications, 89–90, 90*t*
Epilepsy, 374–375
Episcleral osseous choristoma, 411
Epithelial neoplasms, 859–861, 860*f*
Epithelial-stromal lesions
  fibroadenoma and tubular adenoma, 902–903, 902*f*, 903*f*
  juvenile fibroadenoma, 903–904
  phyllodes tumor (cystosarcoma phyllodes), 904–905, 904*f*, 905*f*
Epithelioid nevus, eyelid, 409
Epithelioid sarcoma, 1097
Epstein-Barr virus (EBV) infection, 211–214
  clinical features, 211
  infectious mononucleosis, 212–213, 213*f*
  lymph node, 980–981, 981*f*
  neoplasms, 213–214
  transmission, 211–212
Eruptive vellus hair cysts, 1132
Erysipelas, 1121–1122
Erythema multiforme, 1115–1116, 1115*f*
Erythema nodosum, 1127, 1127*f*
Erythema toxicum neonatorum, 1116
Erythroid disorders, benign, 1018–1019, 1019*f*
Erythropoiesis, 1012–1013, 1013*f*
Escherichia coli, 876
  diarrhea due to, 604–605
  enterohemorrhagic, 604
  enteropathogenic, 604
  histopathology, 604–605, 604*f*
  pancreatitis due to, 755
  screening, 605
Esophagitis
  candida, 581
  causes, 4*t*
  cytomegalovirus, 581
  eosinophilic, 579–580, 579*f*
  herpes simplex, 580–581, 580*f*
  infectious, 580
  reflux, 576–577, 577*f*
Esophagus
  acquired diseases, 576–581
  atresia, 449–450, 450*f*–451*f*, 451*t*
    tracheoesophageal fistula, 576, 576*f*
  Barrett, 578–579, 578*f*
  bronchoesophageal fistulae, 453
  congenital abnormalities, 575–576
  duplication, 575
  heterotopic gastric mucosa, 575
  mediastinal enteric cyst, 576
  persistent embryonic epithelium, 575

stenosis, 576
tracheoesophageal fistula, 449–450, 450*f*–451*f*, 451*t*
Eventration, diaphragm, 504*f*, 505
Ewing sarcoma-primitive neuroectodermal tumor, 1087–1090, 1089*t*, 1090*f*, 1240–1245, 1243*f*–1246*f*
Ewing sarcoma-primitive neuroectodermal tumor (EWS-PNET)
electron microscopic examination of, 51, 52*f*
Exocrine pancreas
abnormalities
with fibrosis, 752–754, 753*f*, 754*f*
without fibrosis, 751–752
atrophy without fibrosis, 751
cystic fibrosis, 752–753, 753*f*
drug-induced pancreatitis, 756, 756*t*
functional development, 750
hereditary pancreatitis, 756
idiopathic chronic pancreatitis, 756
infectious pancreatitis, 754–755, 755*f*
inflammatory pancreatitis, 755, 755*f*
inspissation and other changes, 753
isolated enzyme deficiencies, 751
Johanson-Blizzard syndrome, 751–752
neonatal hemochromatosis, 752, 752*f*
obstructive pancreatitis, 755
Pearson syndrome, 752
Shwachman-Diamond syndrome, 751
traumatic pancreatitis, 754, 754*f*
tumors, 756–758
Extracorporeal membrane oxygenation (ECMO), 481, 482*f*
Extraskeletal myxoid chondrosarcoma, 1041*t*, 1092–1093
Extravaginal torsion, 876
Eye(s)
abnormalities, 428–434
Fuchs adenoma, 434
medulloepithelioma, 433–434
retinoblastoma, 428–433
autopsy, 436, 436*f*–437*f*
glaucoma, 434
structure, 425–428, 426*f*–427*f*
surgical procedures, 428
trauma, 434–436
Eyelid
inflammatory abnormalities, 407–408, 407*f*–408*f*
neoplastic lesions, 408–409
structure, 406, 407*f*
surgical procedures, 406
vascular abnormalities, 406–407, 407*f*

F

Fabry disease, 131, 133*f*
cardiac involvement in, 549
hepatic involvement in, 666, 666*f*
lens, 419
Facial abnormalities, 66
Familial agnathia-holoprosencephaly, 114
Familial exudative vitreoretinopathy, 422
Fanconi anemia, 87–88
complementation groups, 87–88, 88*f*
incidence, 87, 88*f*
Fanconi syndrome, 88, 88*f*
Fanconi-Bickel syndrome, 157
Farber disease
characteristics, 147–149
hepatic involvement in, 665–666
Fat necrosis, breast, 900
Fatty acid oxidation disorders, 157–160
acyl-CoA dehydrogenase deficiency, 157–159, 159*f*
cardiac involvement in, 549, 549*t*
hepatic effects of, 679–680, 679*f*–680*f*
liver, 679–680, 679*f*–680*f*
substrate transport defects, 159–160
Female reproductive disease
acquired abnormalities
infections, 845–847, 846*f*
miscellaneous infectious diseases, 846
noninfectious inflammatory diseases, 847–848
anatomy and embryology
ductal system, 840–841, 840*f*
early gonadal development, 837–838, 838*f*
female external genitalia, 841
ovarian differentiation, 838–840, 838*f*, 839*f*
primordial germ cells, 837
intersex disorders
abnormal sex chromosomes, 843–845, 844*f*
female pseudohermaphroditism, 843
gonadal dysgenesis, 845, 845*f*
lower female genital tract maligancies
endodermal sinus tumor, 850, 850*f*
rhabdomyosarcoma, 849–850, 849*f*
non-neoplastic ovarian tumors, 851
ovarian neoplasms
epithelial neoplasms, 859–861, 860*f*
germ cell tumors, 851–857, 851*t*, 852*f*–854*f*, 856*f*
sex cord–stromal tumors, 857–859, 858*f*
premature ovarian failure, 841
structural abnormalities
ductal system, 842
external genitalia, 842
tumors of
benign cystic lesions, 848
benign solid tumors, 848–849
ovary, 850–851
Fetal akinesia deformation sequence, 113
Fetal akinesia-hypokinesia deformation (FAD) sequence, 1195–1196
Fetal alcohol syndrome (FAS), 99, 100*t*
Fetal face syndrome. *See* Robinow syndrome
Fetal hemorrhage, 347
Fetal rhabdomyoma, 1081, 1081*f*
Fetal vascular thrombo-occlusive disease, 336–338
background, 336
clinical correlation, 337–338
pathology, 338
Fetomaternal hemorrhage, 343–344
clinical correlation, 343
pathology, 343
Fetus
circulatory disorder of, 325
Hemorrhagic endovasculitis and villous stromal hemorrhage, 337
intrauterine death, 341
stem vessel thrombic and thrombotic vasculopathy, 337
Fibroadenoma, breast, 902–903, 902*f*
Fibroblastic-myofibroblastic tumors, 1052
Fibroepithelial polyp (mesodermal stromal polyp), 849
Fibrohistiocytic tumors
angiomatoid fibrous histiocytoma, 1041*t*, 1066–1067, 1067*t*
benign fibrous histiocytoma, 1065–1066
dendritic cell (DC) neoplasms, 1068, 1068*f*
giant cell tumor, 1066
pigmented villonodular synovitis, 1066
plexiform fibrohistiocytic tumor, 1067–1068, 1068*f*
Fibroma, cardiac, 567, 567*f*
Fibromatosis, breast, 906
Fibromatosis colli, 1059
Fibroproliferative (fibrocystic) disease
diabetic mastopathy, 899
fibrocystic changes, 898–899
juvenile papillomatosis, 899, 899*f*, 900*f*
papillary duct hyperplasia, 899
Fibrosarcoma (FS), 1060–1061, 1239
Fibrosis
atrophy of exocrine pancreas without, 751
exocrine pancreas abnormalities, 751–752
Fibrous dysplasia, 1221–1224
Fine-needle aspiration (FNA), 18–20
accuracy and sensitivity of, 20
advantages, 18, 18*t*
complications, 18
control of patient for, 19–20
papoose wrap, 19
electron microscopic examination of, 51, 52*f*
equipment for, 18, 19*t*
indications, 18, 19*t*
pitfalls in the diagnosis of lesions, 20
technique of, 18, 19*f*
First trimester spontaneous abortion, 57–63
examination
amnion and chorion, 58
chorionic villi, 58
complete hydatidiform mole, 62–63, 63*f*
early pregnancy loss, 58
embryo, normal development, 58–59, 59*f*
growth-disorganized embryo, 59–60, 59*f*–60*f*
GTN, 62–63
histological findings, 61–63
intervillositis, 62, 62*f*
isolated/focal abnormalities, 60–61, 60*f*
listeriosis, 62, 62*f*
partial hydatidiform mole, 62–63
perivillus fibrin, 62
p57kip2 and p57 staining, 63
placental tissues and decidua, 61–62
products of conception, 58
triploid embryo, 61, 61*f*, 63
trisomy 13, 61, 61*f*
trisomy 16, 62
trisomy 22, 62, 62*f*
viral and bacterial infections, 61, 62
indication, cytogenetic analysis
chromosome abnormality, 57–58
IVF and ICSI, 58
karyotype, 58
morphological abnormalities, 58
Fistulae
anal, 66
bronchobiliary, 453

Fistulae (*Continued*)
bronchobiliary and bronchoesophageal, 453
bronchoesophageal, 453
Flexner-Wintersteiner rosette, 431, 431*f*
Flow cytometry, 21–23
applications of, 23
basis of methodology in, 21–22
method, 22–23
Fluorescence *in situ* hybridization (FISH), 30–32, 31*f*, 32*f*
advantages, 30
applications of, 30–32
basis of methodology of, 30, 30*f*
confined placental mosaicism, 76
subtelomeric deletions, 89
VCF/DiGeorge syndrome, 88–89
FNA. *See* Fine-needle aspiration (FNA)
Focal cortical dysplasia (FCD), 365–366, 365*f*, 365*t*
Focal dermal hypoplasia, 1112
Focal fibrocartilaginous dysplasia (FFCD), 1224
Focal myositis, 1081
Focal nodular hyperplasia, 697–700
anomalies associated with, 699*t*
clinical features, 697–699
gross appearance, 699
histopathology, 699–700
molecular pathology, 700
pathogenesis, 697
prevalence, 697, 698*f*
treatment, 699
Focal segmental glomerulosclerosis (FSGS), 305, 310
Follicular hyperplasia
lymph nodes
Castleman disease/angiofollicular hyperplasia, 980, 980*f*
HIV-related adenopathy, 978–979, 979*f*
nonspecific germinal center hyperplasia, 978
progressively transformed germinal centers, 979, 979*f*
toxoplasmosis, 979, 979*f*
white pulp diseases, 999
Folliculitis, skin, 1129
Forensic pathology, 252–284
abrasion, 254, 254*f*
abusive head trauma, 273, 273*f*
accidental causes of death, 263–265
acute subdural hemorrhages, 273*f*
asphyxia, 265–266
autopsy, 253–257
blunt abdominal trauma and thorax, 280–281
crushing head injury, 276, 276*f*
cutaneous evidence
dating of concussions, 256, 270–271
scald burns and contact burns, 271–272
definition of, 252–253
epidural heat hematoma, 265, 265*f*
evidence and clothing, 253
external evidence of injury, 253–255
gunshot wounds, 283–284
head injuries, 272–277
contact injuries, 276
falls, 272
retinal hemorrhage, 277
homicidal suffocation, 266, 266*f*
investigation of death scene, 262–253
laceration, 254, 254*f*, 256*f*, 270, 279, 280, 282, 283
mimicry
cardiopulmonary resuscitation injuries, 282–284
findings, 281–282
Munchausen syndrome by proxy (MSBP), 259
neglect, 261–263
neonaticide
autopsy, 259–261
case history, 260
investigation, 260
periorbital ecchymosis, 254, 254*f*
physical child abuse, 266–267
polymerase chain reaction in, 44
satellite splash burns, 271, 271*f*
skeletal abuse, 256
skeletal injuries, 267, 277
smoke inhalation, 258, 265, 265*f*
sudden infant death syndrome, 257–258
techniques and procedures, 256–257
thermal injury, 265, 270*f*
vertical gluteal cleft, 269, 269*f*
Fractures
child abuse, 279
heat-related, 265
Frasier syndrome, 875
Friedreich ataxia (FA), 375, 375*f*, 550
Frozen tissue, electron microscopic examination of, 49, 51*f*
Fructosemia, 659
Fuchs adenoma, 434
Fuchs endothelial dystrophy, 416–417
Fucosidosis, 142, 142*f*
Fukuyama congenital muscular dystrophy (FCMD), 1179
Fulminant hepatic failure
liver biopsy, 686, 687*f*–688*f*
viral agents, 686, 686*f*–687*f*
Fungal infection
Aspergillosis, 240–241
Blastomycosis, 240
Candidiasis, 239–240, 240*f*
central nervous system, 397, 398*t*
Coccidioides immitis, 240, 241*f*
Cryptococcus neoforman, 240–242
diagnosis, 242
Histoplasmosis, 240, 240*f*
intestinal, 607
in-utero, 189–190
Malassezia furfur, 239
Mucormycosis, 241–242

G

Galactosemia
hepatic involvement in, 658–659, 658*f*, 659*t*
lens, 419
Galactosylceramide lipidosis, globoid cell leukodystrophy. *See* Krabbe disease
Galen aneurysms, 402
Gallbladder
abnormalities, 672
acquired disease, 736–737, 736*f*–737*f*
congenital anomalies, 736
development, 640–641
Ganglioglioma (GG), 389, 389*f*
Gangliosidoses, 143–146, 144*f*–146*f*
cardiac involvement in, 548–549
hepatic involvement in, 666, 666*f*
Gardner-nuchal fibroma, 1057
Gartner duct cyst, 848
Gas gangrene, 232
Gastritis, 581–583. *See also* Stomach
acute hemorrhagic, 582
erosive, 582
granulomatous, 585
Helicobacter heilmannii, 583, 583*f*
Helicobacter pylori, 582–583, 582*f*
Gastroenteritis, malabsorption, 612
Gastrointestinal stromal tumor, 1079
Gastrointestinal tract
anorectal disorders, 65–66
appendiceal disorder, 634–638
duplication, 590
embryology, 574–575, 574*f*–575*f*
esophageal disorders
acquired, 576–581
congenital, 575–576
gastric disorders
acquired, 581–586
congenital, 581
intestinal disorders
acquired, 598–634
congenital, 586–598
spontaneous perforation, 627
Gastroschisis, 587, 587*f*
Gaucher disease
hepatic involvement in, 667, 668*f*
types, 130–131, 131*t*, 132*f*
Gene expression arrays, 44
Genital differentiation disorder, 868–870
Genodermatoses
acrodermatitis enteropathica, 1113
aplasia cutis congenita, 1108
Darier disease, 1109, 1109*f*
ectodermal dysplasia, 1110
epidermolysis bullosa, 1112–1113
focal dermal hypoplasia, 1112
Hailey-Hailey disease, 1109–1110, 1110*f*
ichthyosis, 1108–1109, 1108*f*, 1109*f*
incontinentia pigmenti, 1113, 1113*f*
porokeratosis, 1110, 1110*f*
restrictive dermopathy, 1110, 1111*f*, 1112*f*
Germ cell tumors, 387–388, 388*f*
mixed, 883–884
ovaries
dysgerminoma, 853–854
endodermal sinus tumor, 854–855, 854*f*–855*f*
gliomatosis peritonei, 853, 853*f*
gonadoblastoma, 856, 856*f*
hematologic malignancies, 856–857
immature teratoma, 852–853, 852*f*, 853*f*
nongerminomatous tumors, 855–856, 855*f*
serologic markers, 856
teratomas, definition, 851–852, 852*f*
testis
embryonal carcinoma, 882
epidermoid cyst, 881, 881*t*
intratubular germ cell neoplasia, unclassified type, 882
mixed germ cell tumor, 883–884
seminoma, 882–883

teratoma, 879–881, 880*f*
yolk sac tumor, 878–879, 879*f*
Germinal matrix hemorrhage (GMH), 401, 401*f*
Gestational trophoblastic disease, 326–328
clinical correlation, 328
pathology, 326–328
Gestational trophoblastic neoplasia (GTN), 57, 62–63
Giant cell fibroblastoma, 1064, 1065, 1065*f*, 1139–1140, 1139*f*
Giant cell reparative granuloma (GCRG), 1232*t*, 1234
Giant cell tumor (GCT)
skeletal system, 1230, 1232*t*, 1233–1234, 1233*f*
soft tissue, 1066
Giardia lamblia, 606
Glaucoma, 434
Glial fibrillary acidic protein (GFAP), 26
Glioma
central nervous system, 381–382, 381*f*
low-grade, 383–384
optic nerve, 422
Gliomatosis cerebri, 384
Gliomatosis peritonei, 853, 853*f*
Glioneuronal heterotopia, 1077
Glioneuronal tumors, 389–391
Glomerular diseases
Alport syndrome, 803–804, 804*f*
collagen type III glomerulopathy, 801
crescentic glomerulonephritis, 795*f*, 809
diabetic nephropathy, 799, 799*f*
diffuse mesangial hypercellularity, 18–19, 796–797
focal segmental glomerulosclerosis, 18–19, 796–797
glomerulopathies, 801
Henoch-Schönlein purpura nephritis, 802–803
IgA nephropathy (Berger disease), 795*f*, 796*f*, 801–802
Loin Pain–Hematuria syndrome, 805
lupus nephritis, 808–809, 808*f*
membranoproliferative glomerulonephritis, 806–808, 807*f*
membranous glomerulonephritis, 796*f*, 797–799, 798*f*
minimal change disease, 795*f*, 796–797
Nail-Patella syndrome, 801
nephrotic syndrome, 799–801, 800*f*
Pierson syndrome, 801
postinfectious glomerulonephritis, 795*f*, 796*f*, 806–807, 806*f*
proteinuria/nephrotic syndrome, 794–796
thin glomerular basement membrane disease, 804–805, 804*f*
Glomerulopathies. *See* Glomerular diseases
Glomus tumor, 1049, 1049*f*
Glutaric acidemia
type I, 170
type II, 159, 159*f*
Glutaric aciduria, type II, 679
Gluteal cleft injury, child abuse, 269
Glycogen storage disorders
cardiac involvement in, 547
classification, 153, 154*t*
hepatic involvement in, 659–662, 659*t*
incidence and indication, 153
myopathy, 1166–1168, 1167*t*, 1168*f*
type I (von Gierke disease), 153–154, 155*f*–156*f*
hepatic involvement in, 659–660, 660*f*
type II, 135–136, 135*t*, 136*f*–137*f*, 154
type II (Pompe disease)
hepatic involvement in, 660, 660*f*–661*f*
type III (Cori or Forbes disease)
hepatic involvement in, 661
type III (Cori-Forbe disease), 154, 156
type IV (Andersen disease), 156, 157*f*
hepatic involvement in, 661, 662*f*
type IX, 157
type IX, X, and XI
hepatic involvement in, 661
type V (McArdle disease), 156
type VI (Hers disease), 156, 157*f*
hepatic involvement in, 661
type VII (Tarui disease), 157
type VIII, 157
hepatic involvement in, 661
type XI (Fanconi-Bickel syndrome), 157
Glycoprotein degradation disorders, 141–143, 142*f*–143*f*, 142*t*
Gonadal dysgenesis, mixed, 843
Gonadoblastoma
ovarian neoplasms, 856, 856*f*
testis, 887–888
Gorham-Stout disease, 1237
Gorlin and Gorlin-Goltz syndromes, 1134
Gorlin-Goltz syndrome, 409
Graft-*versus*-host disease, 619–620
Granular cell tumor, 1077, 1077*t*, 1078*f*
breast, 906–907, 907*f*
lung, 492, 492*f*
Granular corneal dystrophy, 416
Granulocytes, hematopoietic syndromes, 1019, 1019*t*
Granuloma
hepatic, 691, 692*t*
pyogenic, 407, 407*f*
Granuloma annulare, 1126, 1126*f*
Granulomatous cystitis, 829
Granulomatous gastritis, 585
Granulomatous hypophysitis, in pituitary gland, 918
Granulomatous synovitis, 1255
Granulopoiesis, 1012, 1012*f*
Graves disease, 934
Growth-disorganized embryo, 59–60
categories, 59
cylindrical embryo, 59, 59*f*
delayed organ development, 59, 60*f*
incidence, 59
intact empty sac, 59, 59*f*
nodular embryo, 59, 59*f*
ultrasound examination, 59–60
Gynecomastia, 898*t*, 900–901, 900*t*, 901*t*

H

Hailey-Hailey disease, 1109–1110, 1110*f*
Hallermann-Streiff syndrome, 117
Halo nevus, 1135–1136
Hamartoma
breast, 905
chest wall, 1228, 1230*f*, 1231*f*
chondromatous, 489, 490*f*
mesenchymal, 705–708, 706*f*
polyp, 630–631
Hand-Schüller-Christian syndrome, 1140
Head injuries
contact, 272, 276
crush type, 276, 276*f*
falls, 272
inflicted, 273*f*–276*f*
retinal hemorrhage, 277
Heart
biopsy, 554–555, 554*t*–555*t*
transplantation, 554–555
tumors, 566–569, 568*t*–569*t*
Heart disease, congenital
aortic arch system, 533–536
classification, 517–518, 517*t*
conus and truncus, 521–526
coronary arteries, 536
etiology, 516
incidence, 516, 516*t*
pathophysiology, 516–517, 517*t*
position and situs, 537–538
septal malformation, 518–521
venous system, 536–537
ventricular inflow tract, 526–529
ventricular outflow tract, 529–533
Hemangioma, 892, 1138
capillary, 406–407, 407*f*
cavernous, 708
lobular capillary, 1043, 1045*f*
sclerosing, 490, 492
tufted, 1138
Hemangiopericytoma (HPC), 1064
Hematologic disorders
constitutional, 1016, 1017*t*, 1018, 1019*t*, 1021*t*
neonate and infants, 1014–1015, 1015*t*
Hematologic malignancies, 856–857
Hematoma(s)
epidural heat, 265, 265*f*
placental
intervillous, 333*f*
marginal, 338
subamnionic, 347
Hematopoiesis
age-related physiologic variations, 1014, 1015*t*
breast, 907
constitutional disorders, 1016, 1017*t*, 1018
erythropoiesis, 1012–1013, 1013*f*
general features, 1010, 1010*t*
granulopoiesis, 1012, 1012*f*
inherited and congenital, granulocytes, 1019, 1019*t*
lymphopoiesis, 1014
malignancies
flow cytometry in diagnosis of, 21–22
polymerase chain reaction in diagnosis, 36
megakaryocytopoiesis, 1013
monopoiesis and dendritic cell development, 1013–1014
natural killer cells development, 1014
stem cells, 1011, 1012*f*
Hemiagenesis, 930
Hemochromatosis
cardiac, 550
neonatal, 752, 752*f*
Hemolytic uremic syndrome (HUS), 311, 812–813, 813*f*

Hemophagocytic lymphohistiocytosis, 985–986
Hemophilic arthropathy, 1255
Hemophilus influenza, 223–224, 223*f*
Hemorrhage
  adrenal, 953, 954*f*
  fetal, 347
  fetomaternal, 343–344
  germinal matrix, 401, 401*f*
  hepatic, 694
  pulmonary, 481–482
  retroplacental, 345
  subdural
    head injury, 273, 273*f*–274*f*, 276
  villous stromal, 324*f*, 337, 345, 345*f*, 346
Hemorrhagic cystitis, 830
Hemosiderosis, pulmonary, 482–483
  idiopathic, 483, 484*f*
  infant and childhood, 483*t*
Henoch-Schönlein purpura, 620, 620*f*
Henoch-Schönlein purpura nephritis, 802–803
Hepatic artery thrombosis (HAT), 296–297, 297*f*, 298–299, 301
Hepatic steatosis and steatohepatitis, 677–678, 678*f*
Hepatitis
  acute viral, 682, 684
  autoimmune, 688–690, 690*f*
  chronic, 685–686
    grading, 685*t*
    staging, 686*t*
  granulomatous, 691, 692*t*
  idiopathic neonatal, 644–645, 644*t*, 645*f*, 646*t*
  pathology, 682, 684–686
  systemic viral infection, 686
  viruses and liver disease, 681*t*
Hepatitis A, 680
Hepatitis B, 683*f*–684*f*
  acute and chronic, 681
  prevalence, 681
  transmission, 680–681
  treatment, 681
Hepatitis C, 681–682, 684*f*
Hepatitis D, 682
Hepatitis E, 682
Hepatitis G, 682
Hepatoblastoma, 713–723
  classification, 717*t*
  clinical features, laboratory studies, and imaging, 714–715
  clinical syndromes, congenital malformations and other conditions associated with, 714*t*
  cytogenetic findings, 723*t*
  gross appearance, 717
  histopathology, 717–721, 718*f*–720*f*
  immunohistochemistry, 721–722, 721*t*
  incidence, 713–714, 713*f*
  molecular pathology, 722
  pathogenesis, 714
  staging, 715–716, 716*t*
  treatment and outcomes, 716–717
Hepatocellular adenoma, 703–705
  clinical, laboratory, and imaging features, 703
  gross pathology, 704
  histopathology, 704
  molecular pathology, 704–705
  pathogenesis, 703
  prevalence, 703, 703*f*
  treatment and outcomes, 703–704
  typical, 704–705
  variants, 705
Hepatocellular carcinoma, 723–728
  children, 725*t*
  clinical features, laboratory studies, and imaging, 723–725
  gross appearance, 726
  histopathology, 726–727, 727*f*
  incidence, 723, 724*f*
  molecular pathology, 727–728
  pathogenesis, 723
  staging, 725
  treatment and outcome, 725–726
Hepatolenticular degeneration. *See* Wilson disease
Hepatorenal tyrosinemia, congenital tyrosinosis, 150–151
Hereditary arthroophthalmopathy. *See* Stickler syndrome
Hernia, diaphragmatic, 503*f*, 505, 505*t*, 1149
Herniation, brain, 359
Herniauteri inguinale. *See* Persistent müllerian duct syndrome
Herpes, 846
Herpes gestationis, 1114–1115
Herpes simplex virus (HSV), 199, 200*f*
  central nervous system, 395, 395*f*
  chorionic villitis, 328, 329*f*, 332
  cornea, 415
  diarrhea, 602
  esophagitis, 580–581, 580*f*
  herpes simplex, 1123
  human immunodeficiency virus, 1123
  varicella and herpes zoster, 1123, 1123*f*
Hers disease, 156, 157*f*
Heterotaxia. *See* Situs ambiguous
Heterotopia
  cerebral, 364–365
  pancreatic, 746–747, 747*f*
Heterotopic gastric mucosa, esophagus, 575
Hidradenoma papilliferum, 848
Hippocampal sclerosis. *See* Mesial temporal sclerosis
Hirschsprung disease
  biopsy, 593–596, 594*f*–596*f*
  enterocolitis, 625
Histiocytic disorders, bone marrow, 1032–1033, 1033*f*
Histiocytic synovitis, 1255
Histiocytoid cardiomyopathy, 568, 568*f*
Histiocytoses
  hematopoietic
    langerhans cell histiocytosis/histiocytosis X, 1140–1141, 1141*f*
    non-langerhans cell histiocytoses, 1141, 1141*f*
    sinus histiocytosis, 1142
  langerhans cell histiocytosis/histiocytosis X, 1140–1141, 1141*f*
  non-langerhans cell histiocytoses, 1141, 1141*f*
  sinus histiocytosis, 1142
Histone modifications, 90
Hodgkin lymphoma
  lymphocyte-depleted, 991, 992*t*
  lymphocyte-predominant, 992, 992*f*
  lymphocyte-rich classic, 992
  malignant lymphomas, 1003–1004
  mixed cellularity, 991, 992*t*
  nodular sclerosing, 990*f*, 991, 991*f*
Holoprosencephaly, 360–362, 361*f*
Holt-Oram syndrome, 109
Homicide
  definition of, 252
  incidences of, 256–257
  neonaticide as, 259–261
Homocystinuria, 151, 420
Homozygous achondroplasia, 1199
Hordeolum. *See* Sty
Horseradish peroxidase (HRP), 25
Horseshoe kidney
  monosomy X, 67, 82, 84*f*
  trisomy 18, 66
Human granulocytic anaplasmosis (HGA), 231
Human immunodeficiency virus (HIV), 203–210
  AIDS defining illness, 206*t*
  central nervous system, 397
  clinical features, 205–206, 207*f*
  clinical presentation, 204–205
  laboratory diagnosis, 209–210
  pathology
    central nervous system, 209
    frequency and distribution, 207
    kidney, 209
    liver disease, 209
    lungs, 209
    lymphoid organs, 209
    systemic, 208*t*
  surveillance case definitions, 204*t*–205*t*
  transmission, 205
  WHO and CDC staging, 210*t*
Human papillomavirus, 845–846, 846*f*, 1122, 1122*f*
Human parvovirus infection
  causes, 200
  clinical features, 200–201
  pathology, 201
  transmission, 200
Human T-lymphocytotropic virus-1 (HTLV), 191–192
Hyaline membrane disease (HMD), 470–473
  bacteria, 472–473
  characterization, 470
  examination, 471–472, 472*f*
  incidence, 471
  surfactant replacement therapy, 473
Hydrocephalus, 355–356, 356*f*
  Chiari malformation, 366–367
  ex vacuo, 355, 366, 373
  pathogenesis, 355–356
Hydrolethalus syndrome, 115
Hydronephrosis, 785, 785*f*
Hydrops, corneal, 417, 417*f*
Hydrops fetalis, 68, 68*f*, 762*f*, 763
  monosomy X, 82, 84*f*
  trisomy 21, 65–66, 66*f*
Hygroma, cystic
  conditions associated with, 100*t*
  fetal alcohol syndrome, 99
Hyperacute allograft rejection, 291
Hyperammonemia
  clinical presentation, 168
  hepatic involvement in, 676

metabolic disorders, 168–169
urea cycle disorder, 676–677
Hyperbilirubinemia
hereditary, 643–644
in physiologic jaundice, 643, 644*t*
Hypercalcemia, parathyroid gland, 924
Hyperinsulinism, 765–771, 765*t*, 768*f*, 769*f*
adenomas, 770
B-cell ATP-Sensitive potassium channel abnormalities (KATP-HI), 766–770, 768*f*, 769*f*
causes and defects, 770
nesidioblastosis, 770–771
Hyperlactatemia, lactic acidemia, 170–171, 171*f*
Hyperornithinemia, hyperammonemia, homocitrullinuria (HHH) disease, 169
Hyperoxaluria type I, 173
Hyperparathyroidism (HPT)
primary, 925
secondary, 925
Hyperphenylalaninemia. *See* Phenylketonuria
Hyperplasia
in pituitary gland, 919
thyroid gland, 933–934
Hypertension, pregnancy-induced, 334, 336, 344, 345
Hyperthermia, disruptive anomalies due to, 104
Hypertrophic cardiomyopathy, 539–541, 539*f*, 540*t*–541*t*
Hypertrophic pyloric stenosis, 581
Hypocalcemia, parathyroid glands, 926
Hypochondroplasia, 1198
Hypomelanosis of Ito, 117–118
Hypoparathyroidism, parathyroid glands, 926
Hypopituitarism, 916–917
Hypoplasia, 459, 461*f*, 461*t*, 1148–1149, 1149*f*, 1193
Hypothyroidism, congenital, 929–930
Hypotonia, central, 1154–1155, 1155*f*
Hypoxic-ischemic encephalopathy (HIE), 399–400

I

I-cell disease and pseudo-Hurler polydystrophy, 140–141, 141*f*
Ichthyoses, 1108–1109, 1108*f*
Ichthyosis, 1108–1109, 1108*f*, 1109*f*
Idiopathic inflammatory disease, 425
Idiopathic inflammatory myopathy, 1180–1181, 1181*f*–1183*f*, 1183
Idiopathic palmoplantar hidradenitis, 1125
IgA nephropathy (Berger disease), 795*f*, 796*f*, 801–802
Immature teratoma, 852–853, 852*f*, 853*f*
Immunodeficiency disorders
gastrointestinal
in AIDS, 618–619
graft-*versus*-host disease, 619–620
Henoch-Schönlein purpura and other systemic vasculitides, 620, 620*f*
primary immunodeficiency, 616–618, 618*f*
inherited, bone marrow
B-cells and T-cells, 1020, 1021*t*
general considerations, 1020
platelet and megakaryocytic disorders, 1020–1021
malabsorption, 613
Immunofluorescence, 29–30, 30*f*
Immunohistochemistry, 23–26. *See also* Antigens
applications, 25–26
automated stainers, 23
basics of methodology, 24–25
clinical interpretation, 25
primary antibody, 24
secondary antibody, 25
Imperforate anus, 65
In situ hybridization (ISH), 22*t*, 30–32
In vitro fertilization (IVF), 58
Inborn errors of metabolism (IEM), 126–181
aminoacidopathy, 150–152, 151*f*
carbohydrate metabolism abnormalities, 152–157, 153*f*, 154*t*, 155*f*–157*f*
clinical presentation, 126
databases, 126
diagnosis, 126–129
biochemical studies, 126–127
conjunctival and skin biopsy, 128*t*
liver biopsy, 127, 127*t*
muscle biopsy, 127
newborn screening, 127, 129*t*
placental lysosomal storage, 128*t*
transmission electron microscopy, 127, 127*t*
endoplasmic reticulum disorders, 175–177, 176*f*
fatty acid oxidation defects, 157–160, 158*t*, 159*f*
hyperammonemia/urea cycle disorders, 168–169
hyperlactatemia, lactic acidemia, 170–171, 171*f*
lipid metabolism disorders, 177, 178*t*–181*t*, 179–181, 179*f*–180*f*
lysosomal storage diseases, 129–150, 130*t*, 131*t*, 132*f*–150*f*, 133*t*, 135*t*, 140*t*, 142*t*
metal metabolism abnormalities, 173–175, 173*f*–175*f*
mitochondrial disorders, 160, 161*t*–163*t*, 163, 164*f*–166*f*, 166–168
organic acidemia, 169–170, 170*t*
peroxisomal disorders, 171–173, 172*t*
symptoms, 126*t*
Inclusion body fibromatosis, 1055–1056
Incontinentia pigmenti, 1113, 1113*f*
Indeterminate colitis, 624
Infantile cortical hyperostosis (ICH), 1254–1255
Infantile digital fibromatosis, 1138–1139
Infantile fibromatosis, 1053, 1055, 1055*f*
Infantile hemangioendothelioma, 708–712
clinical features, laboratory studies, and imaging, 708, 709*f*, 710–711
gross appearance, 711–712
histopathology, 712
molecular pathology, 712
pathogenesis, 708
treatment and outcomes, 711
Infantile (congenital) lobar emphysema (ILE), 459, 462–463
causes of, 459, 462*t*
classic patterns, 462–463, 463*f*
hyperinflated lung, 462, 462*f*
hyperplastic lungs, 463, 463*f*
symptoms, 462
Infantile myofibromatosis, 492, 1052–1053
Infantile neuroaxonal dystrophy, 374
Infantile Refsum disease, 172
Infantile spinomuscular atrophy (ISMA), 1157–1158
Infection
appendiceal, 63–64, 64*f*
bacterial infection. *See* Bacterial infection
causes, 186
central nervous system, 392–399
congenital
clinical correlation, 331
pathology, 330
conjunctiva, 410
esophagitis, 580
fetal infection evaluation, 192
fungal infection. *See* Fungal infection
incidence and severity, 188*t*–189*t*
lung
adenovirus, 485
Chlamydia trachomatis, 486
human metapneumovirus, 484–485
Legionella pneumonia, 485
respiratory syncytial virus, 483–484, 485*f*
mycobacteria, 983–984
pancreatitis due to, 754
parasitic diseases, 242
pathogenesis
environmental factors, 187, 189–192, 190*f*–192*f*
host genetic factors, 186–187, 187*t*–189*t*
placental
ascending, 330, 339, 340
hematogenous, 330, 340
protozoal infection. *See* Protozoal infection
systemic infectious agents, bioterrorism
anthrax, 246
differential diagnosis, 245–246, 245*t*
plague, 246–247
smallpox, 245–246, 245*f*
transmission
breast milk transmission, 191–192
fetal and neonatal infection, 192*t*
vertical transmission, 190–191
viral infection. *See* Viral infection
Infection-associated hemophagocytic syndrome, 215
Infectious disruptions, 101
Infectious mononucleosis, 212–213, 213*f*
clinical symptoms, 212
diagnosis, 212
histology, 212–213, 213*f*
Infectious myositis, 1180
Inflammatory and infiltrative disorders, 918
Inflammatory bowel disease, 620–621
Inflammatory cardiomyopathy, 544–547. *See also* Myocarditis
Inflammatory myofibroblastic tumor, 1059–1060–1060*t*, 1060*t*, 1061*f*. *See also* Inflammatory pseudotumor
Inflammatory pseudotumor, 488–489, 488*t*, 489*f*
Innervation, disorders of
denervated fibers, 1156, 1157*f*
motor neuron disease, 1157–1158
nutritional disorders, 1159–1160
peripheral neuropathy, 1158–1159, 1158*f*–1160*f*
spinal cord diseases, 1156–1157

Interfollicular granulomatous processes
cat-scratch disease, 983, 983*f*
chronic granulomatous disease, 984
dermatopathia, 985, 985*f*
foreign body sinusoidal histiocytic reactions, 985
hemophagocytic lymphohistiocytosis, 985–986
histiocytic proliferation, 984
langerhans cell histiocytosis, 986
mycobacterial infections, 983–984
sinus histiocytosis with massive lymphadenopathy, 984–985, 984*f*, 985*f*
Intermediate filaments, 26
Intermediate neoplasms, 860
Intermediate uveitis, 422
Interstitial cell tumor. *See* Leydig cell tumor
Interstitial cystitis, 830
Interstitial lung diseases, 486–487
Interstitial nephritis, 810
Interstitial pulmonary emphysema (IPE), 476–479
acute, 477, 479*f*
dissection, 476, 478*f*
incidence, 476–477
mechanical ventilation, 476, 478*f*
persistent, 478–479, 480*f*
Interval appendectomy, 63
Intervillositis, 62, 62*f*
Intestinal disorders
acquired diseases, 598–634
anorectal, 65–66
appendiceal, 634–638
atresia, 588–590, 589*f*
colitis, 620–628
congenital abnormalities, 586–598
cystic fibrosis, 593, 593*t*
duplication, 590, 590*f*
gastroschisis, 587, 587*f*
Hirschsprung disease, 593–596, 594*f*–596*f*
immunodeficiency syndromes, 616–620
infection, 600*t*–601*t*
bacterial, 602–606
fungal, 607
protozoal, 606–607, 607*f*–608*f*
viral, 599, 601–602, 602*f*
intestinal neuronal dysplasia, 597–598, 598*f*
intussusception, 598–599, 599*f*
malabsorption, 607–616
malrotation, 587–588, 588*f*
Meckel diverticulum, 19*f*, 591
meconium and meconium abnormalities, 591–592, 592*f*
neoplasms, 628–634
omphalocele, 586–587, 587*f*
pseudo-obstruction, 596–597, 597*t*
stenosis, 588–590, 589*f*
transplant pathology
acute rejection, 293–294, 294*f*
chronic rejection, 294–295
complications, 295, 295*f*, 296
graft-*versus*-host disease, 296
immunosuppression, 293
injury and hyperacute rejection, 293
vitelline duct anomalies, 591, 591*f*
Intestinal lymphangiectasia, 613
Intracytoplasmic sperm injection (ICSI), 58
Intratubular germ cell neoplasia, unclassified type (IGCNU), 882
Intravaginal torsion, 876
Intussusception, 598–599, 599*f*
Iron overload. *See* Hemochromatosis
Iron storage disease, 672–674
inherited and acquired, 672–673, 673*f*
neonatal, 673–674, 674*f*
Ischemic myocardial necrosis, 553–554
Islet hypertrophy, 761–762, 761*f*
Isotretinoin embryopathy, 99
Isovaleric acidemia, 170
Iysosomal storage diseases, 1208, 1210*f*

J

Jaundice, physiologic, 643, 644*t*
Johanson-Blizzard syndrome, 751–752
Juvenile fibroadenoma, breast, 903–904
Juvenile granulosa cell tumor, testis, 886–887, 887*f*
Juvenile granulosa cell tumors, 857–858
Juvenile hyaline fibromatosis (JHF), 1057–1058, 1058*f*, 1059*f*
Juvenile hypertrophy, breast, 901, 902*f*
Juvenile laryngotracheal papillomatosis, 490, 491*f*
Juvenile nasopharyngeal angiofibroma, 1059
Juvenile papillomatosis, 899, 899*f*, 900*f*
Juvenile rheumatoid arthritis, 982
Juvenile xanthogranuloma (JXG), 408, 882, 1251

K

Kaposi sarcoma (KS), 1047–1048
Kartagener syndrome, bronchiectasis, 453
Karyotype, in cytogenetics, 33
Kawasaki disease, 983
diagnosis, 561, 561*t*
epidemiology, 561*t*
pathology, 562, 562*f*
Kearns-Sayre syndrome (KSS)
CNS, 372–373
inborn errors of metabolism, 163, 166
pancreas, 752
Keratoconus, 417, 417*f*
Keratosis follicularis, 1109
Kidney(s)
angiomyolipomas, 826
clear-cell sarcoma, 823–824, 824*f*
congenital malformations
bilateral renal agenesis, 780*t*, 781*t*, 783
hydronephrosis, 785, 785*f*
renal agenesis/hypoplasia, 782
renal duplication (duplex kidney), 784, 784*f*
renal ectopia, 781, 781*t*
renal fusion, 780*t*, 781–782, 782*f*
renal hypoplasia, 783–784
renal tubular dysgenesis, 784
renomegaly, 784
supernumerary kidney, 784–785
unilateral renal agenesis, 783
congenital mesoblastic nephroma, 44–45, 44*f*, 45*f*
cystitis
classification, 829
cystica and glandularis, 829–830
eosinophilic cystitis, 830
granulomatous, 829
hemorrhagic cystitis, 830
interstitial cystitis, 830
embryology, 779–780, 780*f*
glomerular diseases
Alport syndrome, 803–804, 804*f*
Collagen Type III Glomerulopathy, 801
crescentic glomerulonephritis, 17*f*, 31, 795*f*, 809
diabetic nephropathy, 799, 799*f*
diffuse mesangial hypercellularity, 796–797
focal segmental glomerulosclerosis, 796–797
glomerulopathies, 801
Henoch-Schönlein purpura nephritis, 802–803
IgA nephropathy (Berger disease), 795*f*, 796*f*, 801–802
Loin Pain–Hematuria syndrome, 805
lupus nephritis, 808–809, 808*f*
membranoproliferative glomerulonephritis, 806–808, 807*f*
membranous glomerulonephritis, 18*f*, 19–21, 20*f*, 796*f*, 797–799, 798*f*
minimal change disease, 795*f*, 796–797
Nail-Patella syndrome, 801
nephrotic syndrome, 799–801, 800*f*
Pierson syndrome, 801
postinfectious glomerulonephritis, 795*f*, 796*f*, 806–807, 806*f*
proteinuria/nephrotic syndrome, 794–796
thin glomerular basement membrane disease, 804–805, 804*f*
metanephric tumors, 826
oncocytomas, 826
primitive neuroectodermal tumor, 826, 826*f*
renal cell carcinoma, 825, 825*f*
renal dysplasia/cystic diseases
autosomal dominant polycystic kidney disease, 790, 790*f*
autosomal recessive polycystic kidney disease, 788–790, 789*f*, 790*f*
cortical cysts, 791–792, 791*f*
cysts associated with syndromes, 792
juvenile nephronophthisis-medullary cystic kidney disease complex, 791
Meckel-Gruber Syndrome, 793
medullary cysts, 790
medullary sponge kidney, 790–791
polycystic kidney disease, 787–788
renal dysplasia, 785–787, 786*f*, 787*f*
simple cysts, 792
tuberous sclerosis, 792, 792*f*
Von Hippel-Lindau Disease, 792
renal neoplasms
cystic variants, 820, 820*f*, 821*f*
gross features, 817–818, 817*f*
microscopic features, 818–820, 819*f*, 820*f*, 820*t*
molecular and cellular biology, 816–817
nephroblastoma (Wilms tumor), 815
nephrogenic rests and nephroblastomatosis, 820–822, 823*f*
renovascular diseases
Bartter syndrome, 815
hemolytic uremic syndrome, 812–813, 813*f*
papillary necrosis, 814

radiation nephritis, 815
renal artery stenosis, 814
renal cortical necrosis, 814
systemic vasculitides, 813–814
rhabdoid tumor, 824–825, 824*f*, 825*f*
tubulointerstitial diseases
acute tubular necrosis, 810, 810*f*
hereditary diseases, 812
immune-mediated tubulointerstitial nephritis, 810–811
interstitial nephritis, 810
ureters, bladder, and urethra disease, 826–829, 827*f*, 828*f*
Kikuchi-Fujimoto disease, 982
Klinefelter syndrome (KS), 84, 874
Klippel-Trenaunay-Weber vascular malformation, 117
Krabbe disease, 149, 149*f*

L

Laceration, brain, 356, 356*f*
Lactic acidosis, 1173
Langerhans cell histiocytosis (LCH)
lymph node, 986
pituitary gland, 921–922
skeletal system, 1248–1251, 1250*f*
Large cell calcifying SCT (LCCSCT), 886, 887*f*
Laryngeal stenosis and atresia, 446–447, 446*f*
Laryngocele, 445
Laryngomalacia, 445–446
Laryngotracheoesophageal cleft, 447, 447*f*
Laser *in situ* keratomileusis (LASIK), 415
Late pregnancy
acute disease processes, 344–347
anatomy, 331–332
chronic disease processes, 332–339
subacute disease processes, 339–344
Lattice corneal dystrophy, 416
Leber hereditary optic neuropathy (LHON), 166
Leigh syndrome, 160, 163*t*, 166–167, 372
Leiomyoma, 490
Leiomyosarcoma, 496, 496*f*, 736
Leishmania, 244, 245*f*
Lens
cataract, congenital, 420–421, 420*f*–421*f*
congenital, 419
crystalline
developmental abnormalities, 418–419
dislocation, 420*f*
structure, 417–418
surgical procedures, 418
dislocation, 419–420, 420*f*
opacities, 419
zonules, 419–420
Lens notch, 419
Leprechaunism, 112, 773
Leptospirosis, 229
Lesch-Nyhan syndrome, 117
Lesions, breast
fibroproliferative (fibrocystic) disease
diabetic mastopathy, 899
fibrocystic changes, 898–899
juvenile papillomatosis, 899, 899*f*, 900*f*
papillary duct hyperplasia, 899
mesenchymal
fibromatosis, 906
granular cell tumor, 906–907, 907*f*
hematopoietic lesions, 907
lipoma, 906
sarcoma, 907
vascular tumors, 906, 906*f*
Letterer-Siwe disease, 1140
Leukemia, 1142
acute lymphoblastic
biologic basis, 1023–1025, 1024*f*
classification, 1022–1023, 1022*t*
clinical and laboratory features, 1025*t*
incidence, 1022, 1025*t*
morphologic basis, 1023, 1023*f*
phenotypic basis, 1023, 1024*t*
acute myelogenous
biologic basis, 1028, 1030–1032
classification, 1025, 1026*t*
FAB classification, 1026*t*
genotypic abnormalities, 1026, 1028*t*
incidence, 1025
inv (16), 1031, 1031*f*
monosomy 7, 1031
morphologic diagnosis, 1026, 1026*t*–1027*t*, 1027*f*
11q23 abnormalities, 1031, 1031*f*
t(8;21), 1028, 1030
t(15;17), 1030, 1030*f*–1031*f*
WHO classification, 1028*t*–1030*t*
chronic granulocytic, Philadelphia chromosome associated with, 34
chronic myelodysplastic and myeloproliferative, 1032, 1032*f*, 1032*t*
congenital acute, 1022
diagnosis of, electron microscopy in, 51–52, 54*f*
flow cytometty in diagnosis of, 22, 23
hematopoietic, 1142
immunohistochemistry, 25
Leukocoria, 429
Leukodystrophy
CNS, 369–370, 370*f*, 371*t*
metachromatic, 665, 665*f*
Leydig cell deficiency, 870
Leydig cell tumor (LCT), 884–885, 884*f*
Lhermitte Duclos disease. *See* Dysplastic gangliocytoma of the cerebellum
Lichen planus, 1117–1118
Lichen sclerosus, 847, 1119, 1120*f*
Ligneous conjunctivitis, 410
Limb reduction deficiency, 1191–1196
amelia, 1193
arthrogryposis/congenital contracture, 1195, 1195*f*
axial skeleton anomalies, 1194
caudal dysgenesis, 1193–1194
caudal regression syndrome, 1193–1194, 1194*f*
FAD sequence, 1195–1196
lower limb deficiencies, 1193
patellar aplasia and hypoplasia, 1193
polydactyly, 1194–1195, 1194*t*
sirenomelia, 1193–1194
split hand-foot limb defect, 1193
syndactyly, 1195
transverse limb defects, 1192–1193, 1192*t*
Limbal dermoid, 411, 411*f*
Limb–body wall complex (LBWC), 69, 69*f*
Linear IgA bullous dermatosis, 1113–1114, 1114*f*
Lipid metabolism disorders, 177–181
autopsy, 180–181, 180*t*–181*t*
CHILD syndrome, 177
Conradi-Hunermann syndrome, 177
Smith-Lemli-Opitz syndrome, 177, 179*f*
sudden unexpected death in infancy, 179–180
Lipoblastoma, 1070–1071
Lipoma, 906, 1070
Lipomatous atrophy, of exocrine pancreas, 751
Lipomatous atrophy/pseudohypertrophy, 751
Liposarcoma (LPS), 1041*t*, 1071–1072
Lissencephaly, 363–364, 363*f*
Listeriosis, 225, 225*f*
first trimester abortion, 62, 62*f*
second trimester abortion, 64, 64*f*–65*f*
Liver
abscess, 690–691
agenesis, 641
angiosarcoma, 734–736, 735*f*
bone marrow transplantation, 667, 693
cavernous hemangioma, 708
ciliated foregut cyst, 654
cirrhosis, 695–696, 695*t*, 696*f*
A1AT deficiency, 669, 671
causes, 695
cholestasis, 652, 652*f*
classification, 695–696
cystic fibrosis, 671–672
infant and child, 695*t*
macronodular, 672*f*, 675, 690*f*, 695–696, 726
micronodular, 648*f*–649*f*, 671, 695, 696, 726
congenital anomalies, 641–642, 641*f*–642*f*
congenital fibrosis, 656–657, 656*f*–657*f*
congenital hepatic fibrosis, 656–657, 657*f*
cystic abnormalities, 656, 656*t*
development, 640–641, 640*f*
ectopia/heteropia, 642, 642*f*
embryonal rhabdomyosarcoma, 733–734, 733*f*–734*f*
focal nodular hyperplasia, 697–700, 698*f*, 699*t*
fulminant hepatic failure, 686, 686*f*–688*f*
hemorrhage, 694
hepatic tumors, 697, 697*t*
hepatoblastoma, 713–723, 713*f*, 714*t*, 716*t*–717*t*, 718*f*–720*f*, 721*t*, 723*t*
hepatocellular adenoma, 703–705, 703*f*
hepatocellular carcinoma, 723–728, 724*f*, 725*t*, 727*f*
histology, 641, 641*f*
infantile hemangioendothelioma, 708, 709*f*–710*f*, 710–712
leiomyosarcoma, 736
mesenchymal hamartoma, 705–708, 706*f*
metabolic disorders, 657–680
alpha-1-antitrypsin deficiency, 669, 670*f*, 671
amino acid metabolism disorders, 662–663, 663*f*
bile acid metabolism disorders, 667–669
carbohydrate metabolism disorders, 658–662, 658*f*, 659*t*, 660*f*–662*f*
cystic fibrosis, 671–672, 671*f*–672*f*
fatty acid oxidation defects, 679–680, 679*f*–680*f*

Liver (*Continued*)
hepatic steatosis and steatohepatitis, 677–678, 678*f*
histologic features, 658*t*
iron storage disease, 672–674, 673*f*–674*f*
lysosomal storage diseases, 663–667, 664*f*–668*f*, 664*t*
porphyrias, 676
Reye syndrome, 678–679
urea cycle disorders, 676–677, 677*f*
Wilson disease, 674–676, 675*f*–676*f*
nested stromal epithelial tumor, 731–733, 732*f*
nodular regenerative hyperplasia, 700–702, 701*f*, 701*t*
parasitic diseases, 691
teratoma, 712–713, 713*f*
tissue triaging, 642–643, 643*f*
total parenteral nutrition, 694–695, 694*f*
transplant pathology
acute rejection, 299, 299*f*
biliary complications, 298
bone marrow, 303–304
chronic rejection, 300, 300*f*, 301
de novo and recurrent autoimmune hepatitis, 301
hepatic artery thrombosis, 298
hyperacute (humoral) rejection, 298–299, 299*f*
idiopathic posttransplantation chronic hepatitis, 302
posttransplant opportunistic infections, 302–303, 303*f*
preservation injury, 297, 297*t*, 298, 298*t*
recurrent diseases, 301
undifferentiated embryonal sarcoma, 728–731, 728*f*–729*f*
vascular disorder, 692–694, 692*f*–693*f*
viral infections of. *See* Hepatitis
Lobular capillary hemanioma, 1138
Local myositis, 1180
Loeys-Dietz syndrome, 559
Loin Pain–Hematuria syndrome, 805
Long QT syndrome, 556*t*
Lowe syndrome, 116, 418
Low-grade fibromyxoid sarcoma (LGFS), 1062–1064, 1063*f*
Lung(s)
abnormal lobation, location, and shape, 455–456
agenesis, 455
alveolar microlithiasis, 482
aspiration, 479–481, 481*f*–482*f*, 481*t*
asthma, 503–504, 503*f*
bronchopulmonary dysplasia, 473–475, 473*f*–476*f*
chronic lung disease of infancy, 487
congenital alveolar capillary dysplasia, 469–470, 470*f*–471*f*, 470*t*
congenital pulmonary airway malformation, 464–469, 464*f*–469*f*
congenital pulmonary lymphangiectasis, 463–464, 463*f*–464*f*
congenital surfactant deficiency, 475–476, 477*f*
cystic fibrosis, 502–503, 502*f*
development
acinar period, 441, 443*f*
alveolar period, 443, 444*f*
embryonic period, 441, 442*f*
phases, 441, 441*t*
pseudoglandular period, 441, 443*f*
saccular period, 442, 444*f*
vascular supply, 444
diaphragm
developmental anomalies, 504–505
eventration, 504*f*, 505
hernia, 503*f*, 505, 505*t*
eosinophilic pneumonia, 486–487
extracorporeal membrane oxygenation, 481, 482*f*
hemorrhage, 481–482
hemosiderosis, pulmonary, 482–483
idiopathic, 483, 484*f*
infant and childhood, 483*t*
hyaline membrane disease, 470–473, 472*f*
hypoplasia, 459, 461*f*, 461*t*
infantile (congenital) lobar emphysema, 459, 462–463, 462*f*–463*f*, 462*t*
infectious diseases. *See* Infection
interstitial glycogenosis, 487, 487*f*
interstitial lung diseases, 486–487
interstitial pulmonary emphysema, 476–479, 478*f*–480*f*
neuroendocrine cell hyperplasia of infancy, 487
peripheral cysts, 470, 471*f*
sarcoidosis, 497, 499, 501–502, 501*f*
sequestration
extralobar, 456, 457*f*
intralobar, 458–459, 458*f*, 460*f*
total, pulmonary hyperplasia, 456, 458, 458*f*
transplantation, 504
tumors
benign, 488–492, 488*t*, 489*f*–492*f*
malignant, 492–497, 493*f*–500*f*
veno-occlusive disease, 482
Lupus etythemarosus, systemic. *See* Systemic lupus erythematosis
Lyme disease
clinical features, 230
laboratory diagnosis, 230
piggyback infection, 231
prognosis and outcome, 230–231
transmission, 229–230
Lymph nodes
cytogenetic studies, 977, 977*t*
diagnostic approaches, 976, 976*t*
follicular hyperplasias
Castleman disease/angiofollicular hyperplasia, 980, 980*f*
HIV-related adenopathy, 978–979, 979*f*
nonspecific germinal center hyperplasia, 978
progressively transformed germinal centers, 979, 979*f*
toxoplasmosis, 979, 979*f*
immunophenotypic studies, 976–977, 977*t*
interfollicular granulomatous processes
cat-scratch disease, 983, 983*f*
chronic granulomatous disease, 984
dermatopathia, 985, 986*f*
foreign body sinusoidal histiocytic reactions, 985
hemophagocytic lymphohistiocytosis, 985–986
histiocytic proliferation, 984
langerhans cell histiocytosis, 986
mycobacterial infections, 983–984
sinus histiocytosis with massive lymphadenopathy, 984–985, 984*f*, 985*f*
interfollicular/paracortical reactions–immunoblastic
autoimmune lymphoproliferative syndrome, 982–983
Epstein Barr virus infection, 980–981, 981*f*
hypersensitivity-related lymphadenopathy, 981–982
juvenile rheumatoid arthritis, 982
Kawasaki disease, 983
Kikuchi-Fujimoto disease, 982
non-EBV viral adenopathy, 981
systemic lupus erythematosus, 982
lymphadenopathy in children, 976
malignant lymphadenopathy
anaplastic large cell lymphoma, 989–990, 990*f*, 991*f*
B-cell lymphomas, 988–989
burkitt lymphoma, 988
diffuse large B-cell lymphoma, 988
Hodgkin lymphoma, 990–992
peripheral T-cell lymphoma, 989, 989*t*
precursor B lymphoblastic lymphoma, 987–988, 987*f*, 988*f*
T-cell lymphoblastic lymphia, 989
tumors of monocyte/macrophage lineage, 992–993
reactive lymphadenopathy, 977, 978*t*
structure and function, 975–976, 975*f*, 976*f*
Lymphadenopathy
clinical significance, in children, 976
diagnostic approach, 976
reactive, 977, 978*t*
sinus histiocytosis, 984–985, 985*f*
Lymphangioleiomyomatosis, 490
Lymphangioma, 424–425
Lymphangiomatosis, 490
Lymphatic tumors
cystic lymphangioma, 1048, 1048*f*
glomus tumor, 1049, 1049*f*
Lymphocytic colitis, 624
Lymphocytic hypophysitis, 918
Lymphoma
anaplastic large cell, 989–990, 990*f*
B-cell lymphoblastic lymphoma
B-cell lymphomas, 988–989
Burkitt lymphoma, 988
diffuse large B-cell lymphoma (DLBCL), 988
flow cytometty in diagnosis of, 22, 23
hematopoietic, 1142
Hodgkin lymphoma
lymphocyte-depleted, 991, 991*t*
lymphocyte-predominant, 992, 992*f*
lymphocyte-rich classic, 992
mixed cellularity, 991, 992*t*
nodular sclerosing, 990*f*, 991, 991*f*
immunohistochemistry, 25
peripheral T-cell, 989, 989*t*
T-cell lymphoblastic lymphoma, 989
Lymphopoiesis, 1014

Lysinuric protein intolerance (LPI), 169
Lysosomal storage disorders
  central nervous system, 367–369, 368*f*, 369*t*
  cholesterol ester storage disease, 147, 148*f*
  classification, 129, 130*t*
  cystinosis, 149, 150*f*
  Danon disease, 138
  diagnosis, 128*t*, 129–130
  Fabry disease, 131, 133*f*
  Farber disease, 147–149
  gangliosidoses, 143–146, 144*f*–146*f*
  Gaucher disease, 130–131, 131*t*, 132*f*
  glycoprotein degradation disorders, 141–143, 142*f*–143*f*, 142*t*
  hepatic involvement in, 663–667, 664*f*–668*f*, 664*t*
  Krabbe disease, 149, 149*f*
  lens, 419
  metachromatic leukodystrophy, 146–147, 147*f*
  mucolipidoses, 140–141, 141*f*
  mucopolysaccharidoses, 138, 138*f*–140*f*, 140, 140*t*
  myopathy, 1165–1166, 1166*f*–1167*f*
  neuronal ceroid lipofuscinoses, 131, 133–135, 133*t*, 134*f*–135*f*
  Pompe disease, 135–136, 135*t*, 136*f*–137*f*
  symptoms, 129
  Wolman disease, 147, 148*f*

M

Maceration
  characteristics of, 253
  first trimester abortion, 58
  second trimester abortion, 64, 66
Macrodactyly, 1070
Macrodystrophia lipomatosa, 1070
Macromastia, breast, 901, 902*f*
Macular corneal dystrophy, 416
Maggots, forensic pathology, 253
Malabsorption
  abetalipoproteinemia, 614, 615*f*
  autoimmune enteropathy, 615–616, 616*f*
  causes, 607–608, 609*t*
  celiac disease, 608–612, 611*f*
  cow's milk proteins induced enteropathy, 612–613, 613*f*
  Crohn disease, 608, 609*t*
  gastroenteritis and postenteritis enteropathy, 612
  immunodeficiency disorders, 613
  intestinal biopsy, 608, 609*f*
  intestinal lymphangiectasia, 613
  malnutrition, 614
  microvillus inclusion disease, 614–615, 615*f*
  short-bowel syndrome and bacterial overgrowth, 614, 614*f*
  tufting enteropathy, 616, 617*f*
Male reproductive system
  epididymis, spermatic cord, and paratesticular tissues
    acquired abnormalities and lesions, 890–891
    congenital and developmental anomalies, 889–890
    tumor of paratesticular structures, 891–892
  penis, 892–893
  prostate
    acquired abnormalities and lesions, 893–894, 894*f*
    congenital and developmental anomalies, 893
  testis
    acquired abnormalities and lesions, 875–877, 876*f*
    congenital and developmental anomalies, 866–868, 867*f*
    end-organ defects, 870–872, 871*f*
    genital differentiation disorder, 868–870
    germ cell tumors, 878–884
    gonadoblastoma, 887–888
    miscellaneous tumor, 888–889
    neoplasms, 877, 877*t*
    sex cord-stromal tumors, 884–887
    sex development disorder (intersex disorders), 868, 869*t*
    sexual determination disorders, 872–875, 873*f*
    testicular development and disorders, 865–866
    Wilms tumor (WT1), 875
    XX male and XY female syndrome, 875
Malignant fibrous histiocytoma
  lung, 495
Malignant lymphadenopathy
  anaplastic large cell lymphoma, 989–990, 990*f*, 991*f*
  B-cell lymphomas, 988–989
  burkitt lymphoma, 988
  diffuse large B-cell lymphoma, 988
  Hodgkin lymphoma, 990–992
  peripheral T-cell lymphoma, 989, 989*t*
  precursor B lymphoblastic lymphoma, 987–988, 987*f*, 988*f*
  T-cell lymphoblastic lymphia, 989
  tumors of monocyte/macrophage lineage, 992–993
Malignant lymphoma
  Hodgkin lymphoma, 1003–1004
  large cell lymphoma, 1005
  lymphoblastic lymphoma, 1004–1005, 1004*f*
Malignant melanoma, 1135
Malignant mesothelioma, 497, 891–892
Malignant peripheral nerve sheath tumor
  lung, 495
Malignant peripheral nerve sheath tumor (MPNST), 1076–1077, 1076*f*
Malignant rhabdoid tumor, 1096–1097, 1096*t*
Malnutrition, 614
Malrotation, 587–588, 588*f*
Mandibulofacial dysostosis, 109
Mannosidosis, 141–142
Map-dot-fingerprint dystrophy, 416, 416*f*
Maple syrup urine disease (MSUD), 152
Marfan syndrome, 420, 559, 560*t*
Massive perivillous fibrin deposition
  clinical correlation, 339
  pathology, 338
Massive perivillous fibrin deposition/maternal floor infarction, 338–339
Mast cell diseases, 1140, 1140*f*
Maternal diabetes, 100–101, 101*f*, 101*t*
Maternal vascular under perfusion, 332–334
Maturity-onset diabetes of the young (MODY), 765
McArdle disease, 156
Measles, 210–211
  clinical features, 210
  pathology, 210–211, 211*f*
  transmission, 210
Mechanical ventilation
  bronchomalacia, 452
  bronchopulmonary dysplasia, 473–475
  hyaline membrane disease, 471
  infantile lobar emphysema, 462
  interstitial pulmonary emphysema, 476, 478*f*
  meconium aspiration syndrome, 480
Meckel diverticulum, 19*f*, 591
Meckel syndrome, 111–112, 112*f*
Meckel-Gruber syndrome, 748, 793
Meconium
  ileus, 591–592
  periorchitis, 891
  peritonitis, 592
  plug, 592
Meconium aspiration syndrome (MAS), 480, 481*f*
Mediastinal enteric cyst, 576
Medullary cysts, 790
Medulloblastoma, 384–386, 385*f*
  anaplastic, 385*f*
  D-N, 385
  grading, 385
  histology, 384–385, 385*f*
  IHC staining, 385
  LC-A, 385
  pathogenesis, 385–386
  survival rate, 386
Medulloepithelioma, 433–434
  benign and malignant acquired, 434
  congenital, 433
  teratoid, 433–434
Meesmann corneal dystrophy, 416
Megakaryocytic disorders, 1013, 1020–1021
Megalocornea, 415
Melanocytic neoplasms
  malignant melanoma, 1137, 1138*f*
  melanocytic nevi
    acquired melanocytic nevi, 1135
    blue nevus, 1136, 1136*f*
    clark dysplastic nevus, 1137
    congenital, 1134, 1134*f*, 1135*f*
    congenital nevus and malignant melanoma, 1135
    halo nevus, 1135–1136
    spitz nevus, 1135, 1136*f*
Melanocytic nevi, 408
  acquired melanocytic nevi, 1135
  blue nevus, 1136, 1136*f*
  clark dysplastic nevus, 1137
  congenital, 1134, 1134*f*, 1135*f*
  congenital nevus and malignant melanoma, 1135
  halo nevus, 1135–1136
  spitz nevus, 1135, 1136*f*
Melanoma, conjunctiva, 413
Melanosis
  acquired, 412
  conjunctiva, 411
  episclera and scleral tissue, 411, 412*f*
Melanotic neuroectodermal tumor, 892
Melanotic neuroectodermal tumor of infancy (MNTI), 1245–1246, 1247*f*

MELAR syndrome, 753
Melorheostosis, 1209
Ménétrier disease, 583–584
Meningioangiomatosis (MA), 402, 402*f*
Meningioma, 422
Menkes steely hair syndrome, 560
Menkes syndrome, 116–117
Mercury embryopathy, 99
Merosin, 1177–1178, 1178*f*
Mesenchymal chondrosarcoma, 1093
Mesenchymal cystic hamartoma, 490
Mesenchymal hamartoma, 705–708
  clinical features, laboratory studies, and imaging, 705–707, 706*f*
  gross appearance, 707
  histopathology, 707–708
  molecular pathology, 708
  pathogenesis, 705
  treatment and outcomes, 707
  undifferentiated embryonal sarcoma, 708
Mesenchymal hamartoma of the chest wall, 497
Mesenchymal lesions
  fibromatosis, 906
  granular cell tumor, 906–907, 907*f*
  hematopoietic lesions, 907
  lipoma, 906
  sarcoma, 907
  vascular tumors, 906
Mesenchymal neoplasms
  myogenic tumors
    congenital infantile myofibromatosis, 1138, 1139*f*
    giant cell fibroblastoma, 1139–1140, 1139*f*
    infantile digital fibromatosis, 1138–1139
  neurothekeoma, 1137, 1138*f*
  vascular tumors
    hemangioma, 1138
    pyogenic granuloma, 1138
    tufted hemangioma, 1138
Mesial temporal sclerosis (MTS), 374–375, 375*f*
Metabolic disorders. *See also* Inborn errors of metabolism
  calcinosis cutis, 1131
  cardiac involvement in, 547–550
  central nervous system, 367–373
  hepatic, 657–680
  mucopolysaccharidoses, 1131, 1132*f*
  vitamin deficiency, 373
Metabolic disruptions, 100–101
Metabolic dysplasia syndrome, 105–106, 106*t*
Metachromatic leukodystrophy (MLD), 146–147, 147*f*. *See also* Leukodystrophy, metachromatic
Metal metabolism abnormalities, 173–175
  Menkes disease, 174–175
  neonatal hemochromatosis, 173, 173*f*
  Wilson disease, 173–174, 174*f*–175*f*
Metanephric tumors, 826
Metaphyseal dysplasias, 1209–1211
Metastasis, bone marrow, 1033–1034, 1034*f*
2-Methylacyl-CoA racemase deficiency, 173
Methylmalonic acidemia, 169
Microarrays (gene chips), 44
Microcephaly and micrencephaly, 366
Microcornea, 415
Microdysgenesis, 365
Microglia, 354, 355*f*
Microlithiasis, pulmonary alveolar, 482
Microphakia, 418
Microvillus inclusion disease, 614–615, 615*f*
Miscarriage, 328–330
Mitochondrial disorders, 160–168
  central nervous system, 371–373, 372*f*
  characteristics of, 160, 164*f*–166*f*
  clinical presentation, 160, 161*t*–163*t*
  inner mitochondrial membrane defects, 168
  Leigh syndrome, 160, 163*t*
  mitochondrial DNA (mtDNA)
    abnormalities, 163
    maintenance disorder, 167
    rearrangements, 163, 166
  nuclear DNA mutation, 167–168
  point mutation
    mitochondrial structural proteins, 166–167
    transfer RNA, 167
Mitochondrial DNA (mtDNA)
  abnormalities, 163
  maintenance disorder, 167
  rearrangements, 163, 166
Mitochondrial DNA depletion syndrome, 167
Mitochondrial electron transport chain disorders, 549
Mitochondrial encephalopathy with lactic acidosis and strokes (MELAS), 167, 372
Mitochondrial myopathy, 1170–1173, 1171*f*–1173*f*
Mitochondrial neurogastrointestinal encephalopathy (MNGIE), 167
Mitral valve
  atresia, 528
  floppy mitral valve, 528–529
  malformation, 528*t*
  stenosis, 527–528
Mixed germ cell tumor (MGCT), 883–884
Mixed gonadal dysgenesis (MGD), 872–873
Mohr syndrome, 113
Molecular diagnostic techniques
  antigens, 26–29
  cytogenetics as, 31–32
  flow cytometry as, 21–23
  future directions, 45
  gene expression arrays as, 44–45
  immunofluorescence, 29–30
  immunohistochemistry, 23–26
  next-generation sequencing, 44–45
  nucleic acid hybridization as, 30–32, 31*f*
  polymerase chain reaction as, 34–44
  tissue handling, 21, 22*f*, 22*t*
Molluscum contagiosum, 408, 408*f*, 846, 847*f*, 1122, 1123*f*
Mongolian spot, child abuse *vs.*, 281, 281*f*
Monopoiesis, 1013–1014
Monosomy 7, acute myelogenous leukemia, 1031
Monosomy X, 80, 82–83
  aortic coarctation, 82, 84*f*
  gonadoblastoma, 83
  horseshoe kidney, 82, 84*f*
  hydrops and cystic hygroma, 82, 84*f*
  hypoplastic left heart, 82, 84*f*
  malformations and postnatal abnormalities, 82*t*
  mosaicism, 80
  second trimester spontaneous abortion, 67, 67*f*
  streak ovaries, 82, 84*f*
Mosaicism. *See also* Aneuploidy
  aneuploid:diploid mosaicism, 74, 75
  confined placental, 76–77, 76*f*
  definition, 73
  diagnosis, 75
  interorgan differences, 75
  monosomy X, 80
  phenotype, 75–76
Motor neuron disease, 1157–1158
MSBP. *See* Munchausen syndrome by proxy
Mucinous neoplasms, 860
Mucocutaneous lymph node syndrome. *See* Kawasaki disease
Mucoepidermoid carcinoma, 493, 493*f*
Mucolipidoses, 140–141, 141*f*
  cardiac involvement in, 548
  hepatic involvement in, 663–664
Mucopolysaccharidoses, 138, 138*f*–140*f*, 140, 140*t*, 1208–1209
  cardiac involvement in, 547–548, 548*f*, 548*t*
  hepatic involvement in, 666
Mucosal melanosis, 64
Mucous cyst, 848
Müllerian cyst, 848
Müllerian duct, renal, and cervicothoracic somite malformations (MURCS), 108
Müllerian/mesonephric papilloma, 848–849
Multiple follicular cysts, 850
Multiple myeloma-plasma cell dyscrasia, 1246–1247
Multiple pregnancy
  clinical correlation, 325–326
  complications of, 323
  pathology, 325
  placentation, 325*f*
  twinning, 325
Mumps, 754
Munchausen syndrome by proxy (MSBP), 259
Muscle(s)
  aplasia and hypoplasia, 1148–1149, 1149*f*
  atrophy, 1153, 1153*f*
  biopsy, 1151–1152
  biopsy of
    electron microscopic examination of, 47, 48*f*
  development, 1147–1148, 1147*f*–1148*f*
  fiber
    histopathology, 1153, 1153*t*
    maturation, steps in, 1147, 1147*f*
    small type I, congenital myopathy, 1164–1165, 1165*f*
    subtype, 1148, 1148*f*, 1152, 1152*f*
  maturation disturbances
    central hypotonia, 1154–1155, 1155*f*
    features, 1153–1154
    prototype, 1154, 1154*f*
Muscle-eye-brain (MEB) disease, 1179
Muscular dystrophy
  cardiac, 550
  congenital, 1177–1180, 1178*t*
    characteristics, 1177
    congenital polymyositis, 1180, 1180*f*
    α-dystroglycan glycosylation, 1179
    α_2-laminin deficiency, 1177–1178, 1178*f*–1179*f*
    pathological features, 1177

rigid-spine syndrome, 1179
Ullrich congenital muscular dystrophy, 1178–1179
Duchenne and Becker, 1175–1176, 1176f–1177f
fascioscapulohumeral, 1177
humeroperoneal, 1177
limb-girdle, 1176
Mycobacterial infections, 983–984
Mycoplasma infection, 236–237, 237f
Myelodysplastic disorder, 1032, 1032f, 1032t
Myelomeningocele, cervical, 359f
Myeloproliferative disorders
chronic, 1032
transient, Down syndrome, 1021, 1022f
Myoadenylate deaminase deficiency, 1173
Myocarditis, 544–547
agents and conditions associated with, 546t
bacterial, 545
criteria for diagnosis, 544–545, 545f
Dallas criteria, 545, 545t
idiopathic GC, 547
macroscopic appearance, 544–545
protozoal, 545–546
viral, 546–547
Myoclonic epilepsy with ragged-red fibers (MERRF), 167, 372
Myoepithelial tumor, 1093
Myofibrillar myopathy, 550
Myofibroma, 1238–1239
Myofibrosarcoma, 1239
Myogenic tumors
congenital infantile myofibromatosis, 1138, 1139f
giant cell fibroblastoma, 1139–1140, 1139f
infantile digital fibromatosis, 1138–1139
Myopathy
congenital, 550, 1161–1165
acquired, 1165, 1166f
central core disease, 1164, 1164f
central nuclear and myotubular myopathy, 1162, 1163f
charactersitics, 1162
cytoplasmic bodies, 1165, 1166f
fingerprint bodies, 1165
identification and classification, 1161–1162
minicore-multicore disease, 1164, 1165f
nemaline myopathy, 1163–1164, 1163f–1164f
small type I fibers, 1164–1165, 1165f
drug-induced, 1174–1175, 1175f
episodic myoglobinuria, 1173
inflammatory
idiopathic, 1180–1181, 1181f–1183f, 1183
infectious myositis, 1180
local myositis, 1180
malignant hyperthermia, 1173–1174
metabolic
congenital lactic acidosis, 1173
glycogen storage diseases, 1166–1168, 1167t, 1168f
lysosomal storage diseases, 1165–1166, 1166f–1167f
mitochondrial, 1170–1173, 1171f–1173f
myoadenylate deaminase deficiency, 1173
triglyceride storage diseases, 1169–1170, 1169f, 1169t
mitochondrial, 371, 372f
skeletal, associated with cardiomyopathy, 1174
Myositis ossificians (MO), 1050–1051
Myotonic dystrophy, 550
Myxoma, 567–568

N

Nail-Patella syndrome, 108, 801
Nasopharynx, 444–447
Natural killer cells, development of, 1014
Necrobiosis lipoidica, 1126
Necrotic/dead neurons, 352, 353f
Needles, gauge of, in fine-needle aspiration, 19t
Neisseria infection, 221, 221f, 222f
Neonatal adrenoleukodystrophy, 172
Neonatal diabetes mellitus, 765
Neonatal hemochromatosis, 173, 173f
Neonatal iron storage disease. *See* Neonatal hemochromatosis
Neonatal necrotizing enterocolitis, 626–627, 626f
Neonatal sepsis, 216–218
Neonaticide
autopsy, 260–261
case history, 260
scene investigation, 260–261f
Neoplasms. *See also* Tumors
pineal gland, 914–915
testis, 877, 877t
thyroid gland
cervical-thyroidal teratoma (CIT), 940–941
follicular, 938
medullary thyroid carcinoma (MTC), 939
papillary thyroid carcinoma (PTC), 936–938, 937f
Nephroblastoma, 888
Nephroblastoma (Wilms tumor), 815
Nephrotic syndrome, 799–801, 800f
Nerve sheath myxoma, 1077
Nerve sheath tumors, CNS, 391
Nervous system. *See* Central nervous system
Nesidioblastosis, 770–771
Nested stromal epithelial tumor, 731–733
clinical features, 731
gross appearance, 732
histopathology, 732–733, 732f
molecular pathology, 733
pathogenesis, 731
treatment and outcomes, 731–732
Neural tube defects (NTDs), 358–359
Neurilemoma, 492
Neuroaxonal dystrophy (NAD), 373–374
Neuroblastoma (NB), peripheral
biochemical markers, 960
clinical features, 958–959
epidemiology, 957–958
immunohistochemistry, 964–965
international NB pathology classification, 965–966
mass screening, 967–968
molecular diagnostics, 965
molecular/genetic alterations, 966
morphologic features, 960–964
MYCN amplification and status, 966
risk grouping, 967
ultrastructural features, 964
Neurocysticercosis, 398–399, 399f
Neurodegeneration with brain iron accumulation (NBIA), 374, 374f
Neurodegenerative disorders, 373–377, 374f–376f
Neuroendocrine cell hyperplasia of infancy, 487
Neurofibroma (NF), 492, 1072
Neurofibromatosis, 409
Neurofilament, 26
Neuromuscular diseases
aplasia and hypoplasia, 1148–1149, 1149f
arthrogryposis, 1149–1151, 1150f, 1151t
central hypotonia, 1154–1155, 1155f
congenital myopathy, 1161–1165
diagnostic evaluation
histochemistry, 1152–1153, 1152f
histopathology, 1153, 1153t
muscle atrophy, 1153
muscle biopsy, 1151–1152
disturbances of muscle maturation, 1153–155, 1154f–155f
episodic myoglobinuria, 1173
inflammatory myopathy, 1180–1183
innervation, 1156–1160
malignant hyperthermia, 1173–1174
metabolic myopathy, 1165–1173
muscular dystrophies. *See* Muscular dystrophy
primary types of, 1156, 1156t
skeletal myopathy associated with cardiomyopathy, 1174
transmission, 1160–1161
Neuronal ceroid lipofuscinoses (NCL), 131, 133–135, 133t, 134f–135f, 411, 412f
Neuronal dysplasia, intestinal, 597–598, 598f
Neuropathy, ataxia, and retinitis pigmentosa (NARP), 166–167
Neurothekeoma, 1077, 1137, 1138f
Neutropenic enterocolitis. *See* Typhlitis colitis
Neutrophilic dermatosis, acute febrile, 1125
Neutrophilic eccrine hidradenitis, 1125
Nevus flammeus, 407
Nevus of Ota, 412
Next-generation sequencing (NGS), 44–45
N-glycosylation disorders, 549
Niemann-Pick disease (NPD), 144–146, 145f–146f, 419, 666–667, 667f
Nipple duct adenoma, 905
Nodular fasciitis (NF), 1049–1050
Nodular mesothelial hyperplasia, 891
Nodular regenerative hyperplasia, 700–702
clinical features, 701
diagnosis, 701–702
management, 701
pathogenesis, 700
pathology, 702
prevalence, 700, 701f
Nonalcoholic fatty liver disease (NAFLD), 677–678, 678f
Nonbacterial osteitis (NBO), 1253–1254
Noncompaction cardiomyopathy, 542, 542f, 542t
Nongerminomatous tumors, 855–856, 855f
Nonketotic hyperglycinemia, 152
Nonneoplastic cysts, in pituitary gland, 919
Nonossifying fibroma, 1237–1238, 1239f, 1240f
Nonvenereal treponematoses, 231

Noonan syndrome, 111
North American Pediatric Renal Trials and Collaborative Studies (NAPRTCS), 305–306, 310
Norwalk virus, 601
Nummular dermatitis, 1116
Nutritional disorders, 1159–1160

O

Oculocutaneous tyrosinemia, 151, 151*f*
Oculodermal melanocytosis, 409
Oligodendroglia, 354
Oligodendroglioma, 384
Oligohydramnios, in twin-twin transfusion syndrome, 325
Oligosaccharidoses, hepatic involvement in, 664
Omphalocele, 66, 81*f*, 586–587, 587*f*
Opacity, lens, 419
Ophthalmic pathology. *See* Eye(s)
Opitz-Frias syndrome, 109
Opitz-Kaveggia syndrome, 117
Optic nerve
  structure, 422
  surgical procedures, 422
Oral-facial-digital syndrome type I, 108
Oral-facial-digital syndrome type II, 113
Orbit
  structure, 423
  surgical procedures, 423–425
Organic acidemia, 169–170, 170*t*
Ornithine transcarbamylase (OTC) deficiency, 168
Ossifying fibroma, 1221–1224
Osteoarthopathy (OAP), 1256
Osteoblastic proliferations, 1220
Osteochondroma (OCD), 1224–1226, 1225*f*
Osteofibrous dysplasia (OFD), 1221–1224
Osteogenesis imperfecta, 116
Osteoid osteoma and osteoblastoma, 1217–1220, 1218*f*–1220*f*
Osteoma, 1220–1221
Osteopathia striata, 1209
Osteopetrosis, 116
Osteopoikilosis, 1209
Osteosarcoma (OS), 1213–1217, 1214*f*, 1215*f*
Ovarian epithelial neoplasms, 859–860, 860*f*
Ovarian neoplasms
  epithelial neoplasms, 859–861, 860*f*
  germ cell tumors, 851–857, 851*t*, 852*f*–854*f*, 856*f*
  sex cord–stromal tumors, 857–859, 858*f*
Ovarian tumor
  benign cystic lesions, 850–851
  germ cell tumors
    dysgerminoma, 853–854
    endodermal sinus tumor, 854–855, 854*f*–855*f*
    gliomatosis peritonei, 853, 853*f*
    gonadoblastoma, 856, 856*f*
    hematologic malignancies, 856–857
    immature teratoma, 852–853, 852*f*, 853*f*
    mature teratoma, 851–852, 852*f*
    nongerminomatous tumors, 855–856, 855*f*
    serologic markers, 856
    teratomas, definition, 851–852, 852*f*
Oxalosis 1, 173

P

Palatal insufficiency/clefts, 88
Pallister syndrome, 117
Palmar-plantar fibroma, 1057
Pancreas
  congenital malformations
    agenesis and hypoplasia, 743, 745
    annular pancreas, 746, 746*f*
    cysts and cystic pancreatic dysplasia, 747–748, 747*f*, 748*f*
    ectopic pancreas, 746–747, 747*f*
    pancreatic enlargement, 745–746, 745*f*
    pancreatic pathology in trisomies, 748*f*, 749–750
    position abnormalities, 746
    variations in pancreatic ducts, 748–749
  endocrine
    abnormalities, 761–771, 761f, 763*f*, 764*f*, 765*t*, 767*t*, 771*f*
    aplasia and hypoplasia, 762
    diabetes mellitus, 763–765
    disorders, 773–774
    histogenesis, maturation, and morphology, 758–761, 760*f*, 761*f*
    hydrops fetalis, 762*f*, 763
    hyperinsulinism, 765–771, 765*t*, 768*f*, 769*f*
    infant of diabetic mother, 762–763, 762*f*
    islet hypertrophy, 761–762, 761*f*
    malformation syndromes, 771–773, 772*f*, 773*f*
    pancreatic islets in shock, 771
    tumors, 774
    viral infections, 771
  exocrine
    abnormalities
      with fibrosis, 752–754, 753*f*, 754*f*
      without fibrosis, 751–752
    atrophy without fibrosis, 751
    cystic fibrosis, 752–753, 753*f*
    drug-induced pancreatitis, 756, 756*t*
    functional development, 750
    hereditary pancreatitis, 756
    idiopathic chronic pancreatitis, 756
    infectious pancreatitis, 754–755, 755*f*
    inflammatory pancreatitis, 755, 755*f*
    inspissation and other changes, 753
    isolated enzyme deficiencies, 751
    Johanson-Blizzard syndrome, 751–752
    neonatal hemochromatosis, 752, 752*f*
    obstructive pancreatitis, 755
    Pearson syndrome, 752
    Shwachman-Diamond syndrome, 751
    traumatic pancreatitis, 754, 754*f*
    tumors, 756–758
  heterotopia, 581
  organogenesis and exocrine histogenesis, 743, 743*f*, 744*f*
Pancreas divisum, 748
Pancreas transplant pathology, 305
Pancreatic ducts
  inspissation, 753
  oncocytic changes, 753
Pancreatic secretory trypsin inhibitor, 756
Pancreaticoblastoma, 757
Pancreatitis
  drug-induced, 756, 756*t*
  hereditary, 756
  idiopathic chronic pancreatitis, 756
  infectious, 754–755, 754*f*, 755*f*
  inflammatory, 755, 755*f*
  obstructive, 755
  traumatic, 754, 754*f*
Pancreatoblastoma, 757–758, 757*f*
Panniculitis
  erythema nodosum, 1127, 1127*f*
  sclerema neonatorum, 1127
  subcutaneous fat necrosis of newborn, 1127, 1128*f*
Pantothenate kinase–associated neurodegeneration (PANK). *See* Neurodegeneration with brain iron accumulation
Papillary cystadenoma, 892
Papillary duct hyperplasia, 899
Papillary necrosis, 814
Papillary thyroid carcinoma (PTC), 936–938, 937*f*
Papular acrodermatitis of childhood, 1119
Parasitic infections
  central nervous system, 397–399
  hepatic, 691
Parathyroid adenomas, 925–926
Parathyroid glands
  acquired disorders
    hypercalcemia, 924
    hypocalcemia, 926
    hypoparathyroidism, 926
    parathyroid adenomas, 925–926
    primary hyperparathyroidism, 925
    secondary hyperparathyroidism, 925
  anatomy/physiology, 922–923
  developmental disorders, 923
    agenesis-hypoplasia, 923
    cyst(s), 923
    ectopic parathyroid, 923
    supernumerary parathyroid glands, 923
  imaging, 923, 924*f*
Parenteral nutrition, total
  cholestasis, 648, 694
  hepatic abnormalities associated with, 694–695, 694*f*
Pars planitis. *See* Intermediate uveitis
Partial androgen insensitivity syndrome, 872
Partial chromosomal aneuploidy, 85–86
  chromosomal rearrangements, 85, 86*f*
  genetic recombination sites, 85–86
  recognizable syndromes, 85, 86*t*
  Robertsonian translocation, 85
Partial hydatidiform mole (PHM), 62–63
Parvovirus infections, 328, 329*f*, 332
Patau syndrome. *See* Trisomy 13
Patellar aplasia, 1193
Paternal imprinting, 73, 90, 90*t*
Pearson marrow-pancreas syndrome, 166
Pediatric
  heart transplantation
    biopsy findings, 315
    complications, 312
    infections, 315
    outcome, 316
    rejection, 312–313, 313*f*
    surgical complications, 312
    volumes and indications, 312
  lung transplantation
    acute rejection, 316

airway anastomotic complications, 316
chronic rejection, 317–318
hyperacute rejection, 316–317, 317*f*
infections, 318–319
primary graft dysfunction, 316
rejection, 316
vascular complications, 316
volumes and indications, 316
Pediatric imprinting disorders, 89–90, 90*f*
Peliosis hepatis, 693, 693*f*
Pena-Shokeir phenotype
type I, 113
type II, 113–114
Penis, 28–29. *See also* Male reproductive system
Peptic ulcer(s), 583
Pericardial disorders
aplasia, 565
cysts, 565–566
pericardial effusion, 551
Pericarditis
causes, 565*t*
chronic or healed, 565
etiology, 565
purulent, 565
tuberculous, 565
Perifolliculitis, skin, 1129
Perineurioma, 1077
Peripheral cysts, 470, 471*f*
Peripheral nerve sheath tumors
glioneuronal heterotopia, 1077
granular cell tumor, 1077, 1077*t*, 1078*f*
malignant peripheral nerve sheath tumor, 1076–1077, 1076*f*
nerve sheath myxoma, 1077
neurofibroma, 1072–1073, 1074*f*, 1074*t*
neurothekeoma, 1077
perineurioma, 1077
schwannoma, 1073, 1074*t*, 1075, 1075*f*
schwannomatosis, 1075
Peripheral neuropathy, 1158–1159, 1158*f*–1160*f*
Peripheral T-cell lymphomas, 989, 989*t*
Peritoneal lined cyst, 848
Perivascular epithelioid cell neoplasm (PECOMA), 1079, 1079*f*
Periventricular leukomalacia (PVL), 400–401, 400*f*
Perivillus fibrin deposition, 62
Perlman syndrome, 105, 772, 773, 773*f*
Peroxisomal disorders, 171–173, 172*t*
central nervous system, 370–371
diagnosis of, by electron microscopy, 52
peroxisomal biogenesis disorders, 171–172
single peroxisomal enzyme deficiency, 172–173
Persistent embryonic epithelium, esophagus, 575
Persistent interstitial emphysema (PIPE), 478–479, 480*f*
Persistent Müllerian duct syndrome (PMDS), 870
Persistent truncus arteriosus, 524–525, 525*f*
Peters anomaly, 415
Pfeiffer syndrome, 110
Phakomatous choristoma, 419
Phenylketonuria (PKU), 100, 150
Pheochromocytoma, 968–970
Philadelphia chromosome, 33
Phosphatase, tensin homologue, and deleted on chromosome TEN (PTEN), 1069–1070
Photorefractive keratectomy (PRK), 415
Phthisis, 435, 435*f*
Phyllodes tumor (cystosarcoma phyllodes), 904–905, 904*f*, 905*f*
Physical child abuse
blunt trauma, 267–270*f*
dating of contusions, 270–271
scald burns and contact burns, 271–272
Pierson syndrome, 801
Pigmented villonodular synovitis, 1066
Pilocytic astrocytoma, 381–382, 381*f*
Pineal agenesis, 913
Pineal cysts, 914
Pineal germ cell neoplasms, 912
Pineal gland
acquired disorders, 913*f*, 914–915
anatomy and physiology, 911–912
developmental disorders, 913–914
pineal agenesis, 913
pineal cysts, 914
imaging, 912, 913*f*
Pineal parenchymal tumors (PPT), 914
pineoblastomas, 388
pineocytoma, 388–389, 389*f*
Pineoblastoma, 913*f*, 914
Pituitary adenoma (PA), 391, 919–921
Pituitary gland
acquired disorders
granulomatous hypophysitis, 918
inflammatory and infiltrative disorders, 918
lymphocytic hypophysitis, 918
nonneoplastic cysts, 919
pituitary hyperplasia, 919
salivary gland rests/heterotopia, 922
vascular lesions, 918–919, 919*f*
xanthogranulomatous inflammation, 918
anatomy and physiology, 915–916
developmental disorders
anencephaly, 917
anomalies, 916
duplication, 917
ectopia, 913*f*, 917
empty sella syndrome, 917–918
hypopituitarism, 916–917
imaging, 916–918
Pityriasis lichenoides, 1118–1119, 1119*f*
Pityriasis rosea, 1118, 1118*f*
Pityriasis rubra pilaris, 1118, 1118*f*
Placenta
abruption, 334–335
circumvallate, 335
diamnionic, dichorionic (DiDi), 325
diamnionic, monochorionic (DiMo), 325
early pregnancy
anembryonic pregnancy, 328, 329*f*
congenital infection, 330–331
development, 324*f*
gestational trophoblastic disease, 326–328
miscarriage, 328–330
multiple pregnancy, 324–326
infarcation, 339
infection and inflammation
ascending infection and chorioamniontis, 339
hematogenous infection, 340
villitis of unknown etiology, 330, 33
late pregnancy
acute disease processes, 344–346
anatomy, 331–332
chronic disease processes, 332–339
subacute disease processes, 339–344
maternal disease affecting, 329*f*
multiple pregnancy
complications, 323
placentation, 325*f*
zygosity, 325
pathologic correlates of common clinical syndrome, 331
thrombi and hematomas
fetal circulation, 340
maternal circulation, 343
vasa previa, 344
Placenta previa, 344
Placental aromatase deficiency, 868–869
Plague, 246–247
Plasmodium infection, 243–244
Plastic bronchitis, 455
Platelet, 1020–1021
Platelet peroxidases (PPO) identification of, by electron microscopy, 52, 53*f*
Pleomorphic xanthoastrocytoma (PXA), 384
Pleuropulmonary blastoma, 497, 498*f*–500*f*
Pleuropulmonary desmoid tumor, 497
Plexiform fibrohistiocytic tumor (PFHT), 1067–1068, 1068*f*
Polycystic disease
kidney, 787–788
pancreatic involvement, 748
Polycystic ovary syndrome (PCOS), 850
Polydactyly, 1194–1195, 1194*t*
Polymerase chain reaction (PCR), 34–44
applications, 36–44
forensic identification, 44
fusion gene transcripts detection, 17*t*–43*t*
genetic testing for mutations, 36, 44
molecular microbiology, 36
basis of methodology of, 34–36, 35*f*
compared with other molecular methods, 22*t*
limitations, 44
nested, 36
vs. NGS, 44
real-time, 28*f*, 36
reverse transcriptase
applications, 36
basis of, 34, 35*f*
Polymicrogyria, 364, 364*f*
Polymyositis, congenital, 1180, 1180*f*
Polyomavirus type BK (BKV) infection, 311–312, 312*f*
Polyp(s), 628–633
adenomatous, 632–633, 632*f*
gastric, 585
hamartoma, 630–631
juvenile, 628–630, 629*f*–630*f*
Peutz-Jeghers, 631–632, 631*f*–632*f*
Polyploidy
definition, 73*t*
triploidy. *See* Triploidy
Polysplenia syndrome, bronchial isomerism syndrome, 452
Pompe disease, 135–136, 135*t*, 136*f*–137*f*, 547
Porokeratosis, 110*f*, 1110

Porphyria, 676
Position and situs malformation, 537–538
Posterior polymorphous dystrophy, 417
Postprocedure pregnancy loss, 69
Pregnancy loss. *See* Spontaneous abortion
Premature chromatid separation with mosaic variegated aneuploidy (PCS-MVA), 77
Prenatal diagnosis, cytogenetics in, 22*t*, 34
Prepubertal teratoma, 880
Preseptal cellulitis, 408
Primary aphakia, 418
Primary intrathoracic rhabdomyosarcoma, 496
Primary lymphoma, 1246, 1248*f*
Primary pigmented (micronodular) adrenocortical disease (PPAD), 951
Primary pulmonary fibrosarcoma, 496, 496*f*
Primary pulmonary synovial sarcoma, 495
Primary vascular neoplasms, 1236–1237, 1237*f*
  fibrous and spindle cell tumors, 1237
  Gorham-Stout disease, 1237
Primitive neuroectodermal tumor, supratentorial, 386
Progestin, synthetic, fetal effects of, 99
Prolonged/repetitive antenatal hypoxia, 344
Propionic acidemia, 169
Prostate
  acquired abnormalities and lesions, 893
  congenital and developmental anomalies, 893–894, 894*f*
Proteinuria/nephrotic syndrome, 794–796
Protozoal infection
  category, 242*t*
  Entamoeba histolytica, 244, 244*f*
  intestinal
    cryptosporidium, 606–607, 607*f*
    Entamoeba histolytica, 607
    Giardia lamblia, 606
  leishmania, 244, 245*f*
  Plasmodium, 243–244
  Toxoplasmosis, 242–243, 244*f*
  Trypanosoma cruzi, 244
Prune belly sequence, 107
Pseudohermaphroditism
  female, 868
  male, 868
Pseudomembranous colitis, 231, 625, 625*f*
Pseudomonas aeruginosa, 224, 224*f,* 1121
Pseudo-obstruction of intestine, chronic, 596–597, 597*t*
Pseudorheumatoid nodule, 1126
Psoriasis vulgaris, 1117, 1117*f*
Pulmonary blastoma, 494–495
Pulmonary hypertension
  artery, 557, 558*t*
  familial and idiopathic, 558
  grading, 558*t*
  left right shunt, congenital heart disease, 558
  lung, 557
  obstructive left-heart disease, 558
  persistent, newborn, 557–558
  WHO classification, 557*t*
Pulmonary interstitial glycogenosis, 487, 487*f*
Pulmonary venous anomalies
  atresia/stenosis, 537
  cor triatriatum, 537
  partial anomalous connection, 536–537
  total anomalous connection, 537, 537*f,* 537*t*
Pure gonadal dysgenesis (PGD), 873
Pyknodysostosis, 1209
Pyoderma gangrenosum, 1125–1126
Pyogenic granuloma, 407, 407*f*
Pyramidal cataract, 419
Pyruvate carboxylase deficiency, 171
Pyruvate dehydrogenase (PDH) deficiency, 171, 171*f*

Q

22q11 deletion syndrome. *See* Velocardiofacial/DiGeorge syndrome

R

Radiation disruption, 96–97
Radiography
  full body, neglect, 261–263
  of skeleton, forensic pathology, 262, 278
Ragged red fibers (RRF), 371
Reactive gliosis, 352–353, 353*f*
Red pulp diseases
  congestion, 995
  hereditary hemolytic anemias, 995–996
  histiocytic proliferations, 996–997
  infection, 996
  langerhans cell histiocytosis, 997
  leukemia and myeloproliferative disorders, 997–998
  nonhematopoietic tumors, 998–999
  thrombocytopenia, 995
  vascular tumors, 998
  virus-associated hemophagocytic syndrome, 997
Refsum disease, 173
Renal agenesis/hypoplasia, 782
Renal artery stenosis, 814
Renal cortical necrosis, 814
Renal dysplasia/cystic diseases
  autosomal dominant polycystic kidney disease, 790, 790*f*
  autosomal recessive polycystic kidney disease, 788–790, 789*f,* 790*f*
  cortical cysts, 791–792, 791*f*
  cysts associated with syndromes, 792
  juvenile nephronophthisis-medullary cystic kidney disease complex, 791
  Meckel-Gruber Syndrome, 793
  medullary cysts, 790
  medullary sponge kidney, 790–791
  polycystic kidney disease, 787–788
  renal dysplasia, 785–787, 786*f,* 787*f*
  simple cysts, 792
  tuberous sclerosis, 792, 792*f*
  Von Hippel-Lindau Disease, 792
Renal ectopia, 781, 781*t*
Renal fusion, 780*t,* 781–782, 782*f*
Renal hypoplasia, 783–784
Renal neoplasms
  cystic variants, 820, 820*f,* 821*f*
  gross features, 817–818, 817*f*
  metanephric tumors, 826
  microscopic features, 818–820, 819*f,* 820*f,* 820*t*
  molecular and cellular biology, 816–817
  nephroblastoma (Wilms tumor), 815
  nephrogenic rests and nephroblastomatosis, 820–822, 823*f*
Renal transplant pathology
  acute rejection, 306, 307–308*t,* 309*f,* 310
  chronic allograft nephropathy (CAN), 310
  hyperacute, accelerated acute rejection and delayed graft function, 306
  immunosuppressive drug toxicity, 311
  polyomavirus type BK (BKV) infection, 311–312, 312*f*
  recurrent disease, 310
  vascular thrombosis, 310
Renovascular diseases
  bartter syndrome, 815
  hemolytic uremic syndrome, 812–813, 813*f*
  papillary necrosis, 814
  radiation nephritis, 815
  renal artery stenosis, 814
  renal cortical necrosis, 814
  systemic vasculitides, 813–814
Respiratory tract, 441–505
  bronchus, 450–455
  diaphragm, 504–505
  lung. *See* Lung(s)
  nasopharynx, 444–447
  trachea, 447–450
Restrictive cardiomyopathy, 544
Restrictive dermopathy, 1110, 1111*f,* 1112*f*
Retinal anlage tumor. *See* Melanotic neuroectodermal tumor
Retinoblastoma, 428–433
  clinical findings, 429–430, 429*f*–430*f*
  Flexner-Wintersteiner rosette, 431, 431*f*
  fluorescein angiography, 430
  genetic defect, 428
  growth patterns, 430–431
  heritable and nonheritable form, 429
  incidence, 428–429
  leukocoria, 429
  prognosis, 433
  radiography, 430
  spread, 431–432, 432*f*
  tumor cells, 432–433
Reverse transcriptase polymerase chain reaction (RT-PCR)
  applications, 36
  basis of, 34
Reye syndrome, hepatic involvement in, 678–679
Rhabdoid tumor, 824–825, 824*f,* 825*f*
Rhabdomyoma, 566–567, 566*f,* 1079, 1080*f*
Rhabdomyosarcoma, 849–850, 849*f,* 1055*f*–1057*f,* 1082–1087, 1082*f,* 1083*f*
  embryonal, 733–734, 733*f*–734*f*
  orbit, 425
Rheumatic fever
  diagnosis, 552*t*
  etiology, 551–552
  pathology, 552
Rheumatic heart disease
  diagnosis, 552*t*
  endocarditis, 552
  myocarditis, 553
  pericarditis, 553
Rheumatoid arthritis, 1126
Rhizomelic chondrodysplasia punctata, 172
Richner-Hanhart syndrome, 151

Rickettsial infection, 235–236
Ehrlichiosis, 235–236
epidemiologic features, 235*t*
human granulocytic anaplasmosis, 231
rocky mountain spotted fever, 235, 236*f*
Rigid-spine syndrome, 1179
Rigor morris, definition, 253
Ring chromosome, 73*t*
Robert syndrome, 114, 114*f*
Robertsonian translocation
balanced, 85
spontaneous abortion, trisomy 21, 66
Robin sequence, 106–107
Robinow syndrome, 110
Rocker bottom feet, 66, 81*f*
Rocky mountain spotted fever (RMSF), 235, 236*f*
Rokitansky technique, 9
Rosai-Dorfman disease (RDD), 1251, 1251*f*
Rosenthal fibers, 353–354, 354*f*
Rotaviruses, intestinal, 599, 601
Rotor syndrome, 644
Rubella
clinical features, 201
pathology, 202
prognosis amd outcomes, 202
transmission, 201
Rubella cataract, 420, 420*f*
Rubella infectious, pancreatitis, 754
Rubeola. *See* Measles
Rubinstein-Taybi syndrome, 118

S

Salivary gland rests/heterotopia, 922
Salmonella infection, 223, 603, 876
histology, 223
laboratory diagnosis, 223
symptoms and signs, 223
transmission, 223
Sandhoff disease, 144
Sanger method, 44
Sarcoidosis, 1127
Sarcoma. *See also* Rhabdomyosarcoma; Undifferentiated embryonal sarcoma, liver
breast, 907
lung, 495–496, 496*f*
Scald burns, 271–272
Schisis, 108
Schwannoma, 1073, 1074*t*, 1075, 1075*f*
Schwannomatosis, 1075
Sclerocornea, 415
Sclerosing epithelioid fibrosarcoma, 1064
Sclerosing hemangioma, 490, 492
Sclerosing stromal tumors, 858–859, 858*f*–859*f*
SCTAT. *See* Sex cord tumors with annular tubules
Seborrheic dermatitis, 1117
Seckel syndrome, 113
Second trimester spontaneous abortion, 63–65
ascending infection, 64
CMV infection, 65, 65*f*
cytogenetic studies, 64
hydrops fetalis, 68, 68*f*
internal and external examination, 64
limb–body wall complex, 69, 69*f*
listeriosis, 64, 64*f*–65*f*
maceration, 64
monosomy X, 67, 67*f*
nonchromosomal factors, 63
postprocedure pregnancy loss, 69
syphilis, 65
triploidy, 67–68, 67*f*–68*f*
trisomy 13, 66, 67*f*
trisomy 18, 66, 66*f*
trisomy 21, 65–66, 66*f*
twinning, 68–69, 68*f*–69*f*
umbilical cord compromise, 69, 69*f*
uterine anomalies, 64
Seitelberger disease. *See* Infantile neuroaxonal dystrophy
Seminoma, 882–883
Sepsis
classification, 217
congenital immunodeficiencies, 188*t*, 218
definition, 217, 217*t*
diagnosis, 217–218
early-onset, 217
incidence, 216
late-onset, 218
mortality, 216–217
pathology, 218
Septal malformation
aortopulmonary window, 525
atrial septum, 518
atrioventricular septum, 520–521
ventricular septum, 518–520
Serous neoplasms, 859
Serratia marcescens, 224
Sertoli cell tumor, 859, 885–886, 886*f*, 887*f*
Sertoli-Leydig cell tumors, 859
Severe acute respiratory syndrome (SARS), 216
Sex chromosome aneuploidy
monosomy X (Turner syndrome). *See* Monosomy X
sex chromosome polysomy, 83–84, 84*t*
Sex cord tumors with annular tubules (SCTAT), 858
Sex cord–stromal tumors, 857–859, 858*f*, 884
juvenile granulosa cell tumor, 886–887, 887*f*
leydig cell tumor, 884–885, 884*f*
sertoli cell tumor, 885–886, 885*f*, 887*f*
Sex development disorder (intersex disorders), 868, 869*t*
Sexual determination disorders, 872–875, 873*f*
Shigella infection, 603
Short-bowel syndrome, 614, 614*f*
Shwachman-Diamond syndrome, 751
Sialidosis, 142–143, 143*f*
Siderublastic anemia, with exocrine pancreatic insufficiency, 752
SIDS. *See* Sudden infant death syndrome
Sinus histiocytosis with massive lymphadenopathy (SHML), 984–985, 984*f*, 985*f*
Sirenomelia, 1193–1194
Situs ambiguous, 538
Skeletal and smooth muscle neoplasms
fetal rhabdomyoma, 1081, 1081*f*
rhabdomyomas, 1079, 1080*f*
rhabdomyosarcoma, 1055*f*–1057*f*, 1082–1087, 1082*f*, 1083*f*
smooth muscle tumors, 1081–1082
Skeletal dysplasia, 1196–1211
achondroplasia, 1198
bent bone dysplasias, 1207
bone density, 1207
bone density group, 1199
bruck syndrome, 1200
CDP group, 1205–1207, 1206*f*
defective mineralization group, 1200
FGFR3 group, 1198
filamin group, 1205
homozygous achondroplasia, 1199
hypochondroplasia, 1198
lysosomal storage diseases, 1208, 1210*f*
melorheostosis, osteopoikilosis, pyknodysostosis, and osteopathia striata, 1209
metaphyseal dysplasias, 1209–1211
mucopolysaccharidoses, 1208–1209
OI pathologic features, 1199–1200, 1200*f*
OP group, 1207–1208, 1209*f*
severe spondylodysplasias, 1202–1203
skeletal component group, 1211
spondylo-epi (-meta)physeal dysplasias, 1203–1204
SRD, polydactyly, 1201–1202, 1202*f*
sulphation disorder, 1204, 1204*f*, 1205*f*
TD occurance, 198–1199
type 2 collagen group, 1198*t*, 1200–1201
Skeletal metastasis, 1247–1248
Skeletal myopathy associated with cardiomyopathy, 1174
Skeletal system
acquired disorders
adamantinoma, 1239–1240
aneurysmal bone cyst, 1235, 1235*f*
central odontogenic fibroma, 1239
chest wall hamartoma, 1228, 1230*f*, 1231*f*
chondroblastoma, 1226, 1228*f*, 1229*f*
chondroma, 1226, 1226*f*
chondromyxoid fibroma, 1226–1227, 1229*f*, 1230*f*
chondrosarcoma, 1228–1229
chordoma, 1251
congenital pseudarthrosis, 1239
desmoplastic fibroma, 1238–1239
Ewing Sarcoma-primitive neuroectodermal tumor, 1240–1245, 1243*f*–1246*f*
fibrosarcoma, 1239
fibrous dysplasia, 1221–1224
focal fibrocartilaginous dysplasia, 1224
giant cell reparative granuloma, 1232*t*, 1234
giant cell tumor, 1230, 1232*t*, 1233–1234, 1233*f*
infection and inflammatory reaction, 1252–1256
juvenile xanthogranuloma, 1251
langerhans cell histiocytosis, 1248–1251, 1250*f*
melanotic neuroectodermal tumor of infancy, 1245–1246, 1247*f*
metabolic and nutritional conditions, 1211–1212
multiple myeloma-plasma cell dyscrasia, 1246–1247
myofibroma, 1238–1239
myofibrosarcoma, 1239
nonossifying fibroma, 1237–1238, 1239*f*, 1240*f*
ossifying fibroma, 1221–1224
osteoblastic proliferations, 1220
osteochondroma, 1224–1226, 1225*f*
osteofibrous dysplasia, 1221–1224

Skeletal system (*Continued*)
- osteoid osteoma and osteoblastoma, 1217–1220, 1218*f*–1220*f*
- osteoma, 1220–1221
- osteosarcoma, 1213–1217, 1214*f*, 1215*f*
- primary lymphoma, 1246, 1248*f*
- primary vascular neoplasms, 1236–1237, 1237*f*
- Rosai-Dorfman disease, 1251, 1251*f*
- round cell neoplasms, 1240–1251
- skeletal metastasis, 1247–1248
- tumor and tumor-like conditions, 1212–1229
- unicameral bone cyst, 1235, 1237*f*
- xanthoma, 1251

congenital and developmental disorders and malformations
- limb reduction deficiency, 1191–1196
- skeletal dysplasia, 1196–1211

Skin
- adnexal tumors, 1133–1134, 1133*f*
- algorithmic approach, 1106*t*, 1108
- bacterial infections
  - ecthyma, 1121
  - erysipelas, 1121–1122
  - impetigo, 1120, 1120*f*
  - staphylococcal scalded skin syndrome, 1120–1121, 1121*f*
  - toxic shock syndrome, 1121
- biopsy
  - electron microscopic examination of, 47, 48*f*
  - techniques, 1107
- carcinomas, 1134
- congenital diseases (genodermatoses)
  - acrodermatitis enteropathica, 1113
  - aplasia cutis congenita, 1108
  - Darier disease, 1109, 1109*f*
  - ectodermal dysplasia, 1110
  - epidermolysis bullosa, 1112–1113
  - focal dermal hypoplasia, 1112
  - Hailey-Hailey disease, 1109–1110, 1110*f*
  - ichthyosis, 1108–1109, 1108*f*, 1109*f*
  - incontinentia pigmenti, 1113, 1113*f*
  - porokeratosis, 1110, 1110*f*
  - restrictive dermopathy, 1110, 1111*f*, 1112*f*
- dermoid cysts, 1132
- eczematous dermatitis
  - atopic dermatitis, 1116
  - contact dermatitis, 1116
  - dyshidrotic dermatitis, 1116
  - nummular dermatitis, 1116
  - spongiotic dermatitis, 1116–1117, 1117*f*
- embryology, 1105–1107, 1107*f*
- epidermal inclusion cysts, 1132
- epidermal nevi, 1131–1132
- eruptive vellus hair cysts, 1132
- evidence of child abuse, 252–255
- folliculitis and perifolliculitis, 1129
- fungal infections, 1124, 1124*f*
- graft-*versus*-host disease, 1130–1131, 1131*f*
- hematopoietic
  - histiocytoses, 1140–1142
  - leukemia and lymphoma, 1142
  - mast cell diseases, 1140, 1140*f*
- infestations, 1124–1125
- injury manifestations
  - disorders that mimic child abuse, 280–283
  - documentation, 253–255
- leukocytoclastic vasculitis, 1128
- melanocytic neoplasms
  - malignant melanoma, 1137, 1137*f*
  - melanocytic nevi, 1134–1137
- mesenchymal neoplasms
  - myogenic tumors, 1138–1140, 1139*f*
  - neurothekeoma, 1137, 1138*f*
  - vascular tumors, 1137–1138
- metabolic disorders
  - calcinosis cutis, 1131, 1131*f*
  - mucopolysaccharidoses, 1131, 1132*f*
- noninfectious granulomatous dermatoses
  - granuloma annulare, 1126, 1126*f*
  - necrobiosis lipoidica, 1126
  - rheumatoid nodule, 1126–1127
  - sarcoidosis, 1127
- noninfectious inflammatory dermatoses
  - acute febrile neutrophilic dermatosis, 1125
  - eosinophilic cellulitis, 1125
  - idiopathic palmoplantar hidradenitis, 1125
  - neutrophilic eccrine hidradenitis, 1125
  - pyoderma gangrenosum, 1125–1126
- noninfectious papulosquamous dermatoses
  - lichen planus, 1117–1118
  - lichen sclerosus, 1119, 1120*f*
  - papular acrodermatitis of childhood, 1119
  - pityriasis lichenoides, 1118–1119, 1119*f*
  - pityriasis rosea, 1118, 1118*f*
  - pityriasis rubra pilaris, 1118, 1118*f*
  - psoriasis vulgaris, 1117, 1117*f*
  - seborrheic dermatitis, 1117
- noninffectious acquired vesiculobullous diseases
  - dermatitis herpetiformis, 1114, 1114*f*
  - epidermolysis bullosa acquisita, 1115
  - erythema multiforme, 1115–1116, 1115*f*
  - herpes gestationis, 1114–1115
  - linear IgA bullous dermatosis, 1113–1114, 1114*f*
  - Stevens-Johnson syndrome, 1115–1116, 1115*f*
  - toxic epidermal necrolysis, 1115–1116, 1115*f*
- normal histology, 1107
- panniculitis
  - erythema nodosum, 1127, 1127*f*
  - sclerema neonatorum, 1127
  - subcutaneous fat necrosis, newborn, 1127, 1128*f*
- routine processing, 1107–1108
- special processing, 1108
- steatocystoma multiplex, 1132–1133, 1132*f*
- systemic diseases, 1129–1130, 1130*f*
- transient neonatal pustular melanosis
  - infancy acropustulosis, 1116
- viral infections
  - herpes virus infection, 1122–1123, 1123*f*
  - human papillomavirus, 1122, 1122*f*
  - molluscum contagiosum, 1122, 1123*f*

Smallpox, 245–246, 246*f*

Smith-Lemli-Opitz syndrome, 112, 177, 179*f*

Smooth muscle tumors, 1081–1082

Smothering, sudden infant death syndrome, 258

Soft tissue
- adipocytic (lipomatous) tumors
  - congenital intraspinal lipoma, 1070
  - lipoblastoma, 1070–1071
  - lipomas, 1070
  - liposarcoma, 1071–1072
  - macrodystrophia lipomatosa and macrodactyly, 1070
  - phosphatase, tensin homologue, and deleted on chromosome TEN (PTEN), 1069–1070
- calcifying aponeurotic fibromatosis, 1058–1059
- congenital infantile fibrosarcoma, 1041*t*, 1061–1062, 1063*f*
- dermatofibrosarcoma protuberans, 1041*t*, 1064, 1065*f*
- desmoid-type fibromatosis, 1056–1057
- fibroblastic-myofibroblastic tumors, 1052
- fibrohistiocytic tumors
  - angiomatoid fibrous histiocytoma, 1041*t*, 1066–1067, 1067*t*
  - benign fibrous histiocytoma, 1065–1066
  - dendritic cell (DC) neoplasms, 1068, 1068*f*
  - giant cell tumor, 1066
  - pigmented villonodular synovitis, 1066
  - plexiform fibrohistiocytic tumor, 1067–1068, 1068*f*
- fibromatosis colli, 1059
- fibrosarcoma, 1060–1061
- fibrous hamartoma of infancy, 1055, 1055*f*
- Gardner-nuchal fibroma, 1057
- gastrointestinal stromal tumor, 1079
- giant cell fibroblastoma, 1064, 1065*f*
- hemangiopericytoma, 1064
- inclusion body fibromatosis, 1055–1056
- infantile fibromatosis, 1053, 1055, 1055*f*
- infantile myofibromatosis, 1052–1053
- inflammatory myfibroblastic tumor, 1059–1060, 1060*t*, 1061*f*
- juvenile hyaline fibromatosis, 1057–1058, 1058*f*, 1059*f*
- juvenile nasopharyngeal angiofibroma, 1059
- low-grade fibromyxoid sarcoma, 1062–1064, 1063*f*
- myositis ossificians, 1050–1051
- nodular fasciitis, 1049–1050
- palmar-plantar fibroma, 1057
- peripheral nerve sheath tumors
  - glioneuronal heterotopia, 1077
  - granular cell tumor, 1077, 1077*t*, 1078*f*
  - malignant peripheral nerve sheath tumor, 1076–1077, 1076*f*
  - nerve sheath myxoma, 1077
  - neurofibroma, 1072–1073, 1074*f*, 1074*t*
  - neurothekeoma, 1077
  - perineurioma, 1077
  - schwannoma, 1073, 1074*t*, 1075, 1075*f*
  - schwannomatosis, 1075
- perivascular epithelioid cell neoplasm (PECOMA), 1079, 1079*f*
- pseudosarcomatous proliferations, 1052
- sarcomas of uncertain histogenesis
  - alveolar soft part sarcoma, 1097–1099
  - clear cell sarcoma, 1041*t*, 1091–1092
  - desmoplastic small round cell tumor, 1090–1091, 1091*f*
  - epithelioid sarcoma, 1097
  - Ewing sarcoma-primitive neuroectodermal tumor, 1087–1090, 1089*t*, 1090*f*

extraskeletal myxoid chondrosarcoma, 1041*t*, 1092–1093
malignant rhabdoid tumor, 1096–1097, 1096*t*
mesenchymal chondrosarcoma, 1093
myoepithelial tumor, 1093
synovial sarcoma, 1093–1095, 1094*f*, 1095*f*
undifferentiated sarcoma, 1087, 1089*f*
scars, keloids, and fasciitis, 1049, 1049*f*
sclerosing epithelioid fibrosarcoma, 1064
skeletal and smooth muscle neoplasms
fetal rhabdomyoma, 1081, 1081*f*
rhabdomyomas, 1079, 1080*f*
rhabdomyosarcoma, 1055*f*–1057*f*, 1082–1087, 1082*f*, 1083*f*
smooth muscle tumors, 1081–1082
solitary fibrous tumor, 1064
vascular tumors
angiosarcoma, 1047
benign tumor, 1043
epithelioid hemangioendothelioma, 1047
hemangiomas, 1043–1046, 1045*f*
intermediate, 1044*t*, 1046
Kaposi sarcoma, 1047
kaposiform hemangioendothelioma, 1046–1047, 1047*f*
lobular capillary hemangioma, 1043, 1045*f*
lymphatic tumors, 1048–1049
Solid-pseudopapillary neoplasm, 758
Solitary fibrous tumor (SFT), 1064
Southern blotting, 36
Sphingolipidoses, 666–667, 667*f*–668*f*
Spinal cord diseases, 1156–1157
Spinal muscular atrophy (SMA), 376–377, 376*f*
Spindle cell tumors, 409, 1237
Spinocerebellar atrophy (SCA), 376
Spitz nevus, 409, 1135, 1136*f*
Spleen
congenital anomalies
accessory of, 994
asplenia, 994–995
cysts, 995
fusion, 995
hamartoma, 995
polysplenia, 994
embrology, 993
examination, 994, 994*t*
red pulp diseases
congestion, 995
hereditary hemolytic anemias, 995–996
histiocytic proliferations, 996–997
infection, 996
Langerhans cell histiocytosis, 997
leukemia and myeloproliferative disorders, 997–998
nonhematopoietic tumors, 998–999
thrombocytopenia, 995
vascular tumors, 998
virus-associated hemophagocytic syndrome, 997
structure and function, 993–994, 993*f*
white pulp diseases
follicular hyperplasia, 999
Hodgkin Lymphoma, 999
localized lymphoid hyperplasia, 999
non-Hodgkin lymphoma, 999
primary immunodeficiencies, 999
Split hand-foot limb defect, 1193
Spondylodysplasias, 1202–1203
Spongiotic dermatitis, 1116–1117, 1117*f*
Spontaneous abortion, 329*f*, 339
Spontaneous abortion (SA)
aneuploidy, 75
autosomal trisomy, 77
causes, 56–57
chromosomal abnormalities, 74
chromosomal anomalies, 75*t*
definition, 56
early, 1–2
aneuploidy, 56
autosomal monosomy, 57
CGH, 56
chromosome abnormality, 56–57
intrauterine death, 57
karyotype, 57
maternal age, 57
recurrent miscarriages, 57
structural rearrangement, 57
triploidy and monosomy X, 57
trisomy, 57
first trimester
examination, 58–63
indication, 57–58
in vitro fertilization, 74
incidence, 56
monosomy X, 80
pathologic examination, 56
second trimester, 63–65
hydrops fetalis, 68, 68*f*
limb–body wall complex, 69, 69*f*
monosomy X, 67, 67*f*
postprocedure pregnancy loss, 69
triploidy, 67–68, 67*f*–68*f*
trisomy 13, 66, 67*f*
trisomy 18, 66, 66*f*
trisomy 21, 65–66, 66*f*
twinning, 68–69, 68*f*–69*f*
umbilical cord compromise, 69, 69*f*
triploidy, 84
Sporadic congenital abnormalities, 117–118
Squamous cell carcinoma
conjunctiva, 413
lung, 494, 495*f*
Staphylococcal infection, 218–219, 219 *f*
Staphylococcal scalded skin syndrome, 1120–1121, 1121*f*
Staphylococcus aureus, 1120
Steatocystoma multiplex, 1132–1133, 1132*f*
Steatosis, hepatic, 677–678, 678*f*
Stem cells, 1011, 1012*f*
Stenosis
bronchial, 451–452
laryngeal, 446–447, 446*f*
trachea, 447, 449, 449*f*
Sterol carrier protein X deficiency, 173
Stevens-Johnson (S-J) syndrome, 1115–1116, 1115*f*
Stickler syndrome, 110–111
Stomach
acquired diseases, 581–586
antral web, 581
congenital anomalies, 581
Crohn disease, 584–585
duplication, 581
eosinophilic gastroenteritis, 584, 584*f*
gastritis, 581–583
granulomatous, 585
gastrointestinal stromal tumors, 585–586, 586*f*
hypertrophic pyloric stenosis, 581
Ménétrier disease, 583–584
pancreatic heterotopia, 581
peptic ulcer disease, 583
polyps and tumors, 585
spontaneous gastric perforation, 581
Storage disorders
glycogen storage diseases. *See* Glycogen storage disorders
lysosomal. *See* Lysosomal storage disorders
Strangulation, accidental, 266*f*
Streptococcal infection, 219–221
causes, 220
disease causing mechanism, 219
prevalence, 219
viridans group streptococci, 219–220
Sturge-Weber dysplasia, 117
Sty, 408
Subacute necrotizing encephalomyelopathy, 160, 163*t*
Subependymal giant cell astrocytoma (SEGA), 384
Submicroscopic disorders
submicroscopic chromosomal anomalies, 89*t*
subtelomeric deletions, 89
velocardiofacial/DiGeorge syndrome, 88–89
Substrate transport defects, 159–160
Subtelomeric deletion syndrome, 89
Sudanophilic gangliosides, 143
Sudden infant death syndrome (SIDS), 257–258, 357–358, 774
Sudden unexpected death in infancy (SUDI), 179–180
Sugar tumor, 490
Suicide, 252, 254, 283
Sulfatide lipidosis. *See* Metachromatic leukodystrophy
Sulphation disorder, 1204, 1204*f*, 1205*f*
Supernumerary kidney, 784–785
Supernumerary nipple, breast, 898
Supernumerary parathyroid glands, 923
Supratentorial primitive neuroectodermal tumor (sPNET), 386
Surfactant
congenital deficiency, 475–476, 477*f*
replacement therapy
bronchopulmonary dysplasia, 474–475, 474*f*–475*f*
hyaline membrane disease, 473
Swine influenza, 216
Sympathetic ophthalmia, 435, 435*f*
Syndactyly
acrocephalosyndactyly syndrome, 109–111, 110*t*
skeletal system, 1195
Synovial sarcoma, 1093–1095, 1094*f*, 1095*f*
Synovium
acute synovitis, 1255
chronic synovitis, 1255
granulomatous, 1255
hemophilic arthropathy, 1255
histiocytic synovitis, 1255
tumefactive lesions, 1255–1256

Syphilis, 65, 225–229, 846
clinical features, 226–228, 226*f*–227*f*
laboratory diagnosis, 229
pathology, 228–229
prognosis and outcome, 229
transmission, 226
Syringoma, 1133
Systemic artery disease
aneurysms, 559–560, 559*t*–560*t*
arteriopathy, 558–559
atherosclerosis, 560–561, 560*t*
Kawasaki disease, 561–562, 561*t*, 562*f*
Takayasu arteritis, 562
vasculitis, 561
Systemic lupus erythematosis (SLE), 982
immunologic aspects of, 550–551
myocarditis, 551
neonatal, 551
occurence, 550–551
pericarditis, 551, 565*t*
valves and endocardium, 551

T

Tail bud defects, 358, 360
Takayasu arteritis, 562
Tarui disease, 157
Tay-Sachs disease, 144
T-cell lymphoblastic lymphoma, 989
Teratogenic disruptions, 97–100
alcohol embryopathy, 99, 100*t*
diphenylhydantoin embryopathy, 99–100
fetal iodine deficiency, 98
folic acid deficiency, 98
isotretinoin embryopathy, 99
mercury embryopathy, 99
synthetic progestin embryopathy, 99
thalidomide embryopathy, 97
trimethadione syndrome, 98
valproic acid embryopathy, 98
warfarin embryopathy, 98–99
Teratogens
time of action, 98*t*
types, 97*t*
Teratoma
cardiac, 567
definition, 851–852, 852*f*
hepatic, 712–713, 713*f*
immature, 852–853, 852*f*, 853*f*
testis, 879–881, 880*f*
Testicular development and disorders, 865–866
Testicular microliths, 876
Testicular regression syndrome (TRS), 869–870
Testis
acquired abnormalities and lesions, 875–877, 876*f*
congenital and developmental anomalies, 866–868, 867*f*
end-organ defects, 870–872, 871*f*
genital differentiation disorder, 868–870
germ cell tumors, 878–884
embryonal carcinoma, 882
epidermoid cyst, 881, 881*t*
intratubular germ cell neoplasia, unclassified type, 882
mixed germ cell tumor, 883–884
seminoma, 882–883
teratoma, 879–881, 880*f*
yolk sac tumor, 878–879, 879*f*
gonadoblastoma, 887–888
miscellaneous tumor, 888–889
neoplasms, 877, 877*t*
sex cord–stromal tumors
juvenile granulosa cell tumor, 886–887, 887*f*
leydig cell tumor, 884–885, 884*f*
sertoli cell tumor, 885–886, 885*f*, 887*f*
sex development disorder (intersex disorders), 868, 869*t*
sexual determination disorders, 872–875, 873*f*
testicular development and disorders, 865–866
Wilms tumor (WT1), 875
XX male and XY female syndrome, 875
Testosterone synthesis, 870
Tetanus, 231
Thalidomide, 97
Thrombocytopenia absent radius (TAR) syndrome, 114–115
Thymic hypoplasia, 1001
Thymic tumors
Hodgkin lymphoma, 1003–1004
large cell lymphoma, 1005
lymphoblastic lymphoma, 1004–1005
malignant lymphomas, 1003
neoplastic proliferation, 1002–1003
Thymus
in AIDS, 1002
anatomy and histology, 1000
embryology, 1000
malignant lymphomas
Hodgkin lymphoma, 1003–1004
large cell lymphoma, 1005
lymphoblastic lymphoma, 1004–1005, 1004*f*
neoplastic proliferation, 1002–1003
thymic atrophy, 1000–1002, 1000*t*, 1001*t*
thymic tumors, 1002
Thyroglossal duct cyst (TDC), 931, 931*f*
Thyroid gland
acquired disorders
chronic lymphocytic thyroiditis, 932–933
Graves disease, 934
graves disease, 934
hyperplasia, 933–934
developmental disorders
branchial apparatus–associated anomalies, 931–932
congenital hypothyroidism, 929–930
dysgenesis, 929
dysmorphism, 928–929
ectopia, 930–931, 930*f*
hemiagenesis, 930
thyroglossal duct cyst (TDC), 931, 931*f*
imaging studies, 927–928, 928*f*, 929*f*
neoplasms, 934–941
cervical-thyroidal teratoma (CIT), 940–941
follicular, 938
medullary thyroid carcinoma (MTC), 939
papillary thyroid carcinoma (PTC), 936–938, 937*f*
Toddlers fractures, 267, 271*f*
Torsion, testis, 876
Townes-Brocks syndrome, 109
Toxic epidermal necrolysis, 1115–1116, 1115*f*
Toxic injury, 876–877
Toxic shock syndrome, 1121
Toxoplasmosis
acute, lymphadenopathy related to, 979, 979*f*
CNS, 397–398, 398*f*
fungal infection, 242–243, 244*f*
Trachea, 447–450
agenesis, 447, 448*f*
stenosis, 447, 449, 449*f*
Tracheobronchiomegaly, 449
Tracheoesophageal fistula, 449–451
anomalies associated with, 451*t*
esophageal atresia, 449–450, 451*f*, 576, 576*f*
postsurgical survival, 450
types of, 450*f*
Tracheomalacia, 449
Transient myeloproliferative disorder (TMD), 1021, 1022*f*
Translocation, 73*t*, 85
Transplant pathology
immunology
acute allograft rejection, 291–292
allograft tolerance, 292–293
chronic allograft rejection, 292
hyperacute allograft rejection, 291
intestine
acute rejection, 293–294, 294*f*
chronic rejection, 294–295, 295*f*
complications, 295–296
graft-*versus*-host disease, 296, 296*f*
preservation injury and hyperacute rejection, 293–294
liver
acute rejection, 293
biliary complications, 298
bone marrow transplantation, 303–304
chronic rejection, 10–11
de novo and recurrent autoimmune hepatitis, 301
hepatic artery thrombosis, 298
hyperacute (humoral) rejection, 298–299
idiopathic posttransplantation chronic hepatitis, 302
posttransplant opportunistic infections, 302
preservation injury, 297–298, 298*f*
recurrent diseases, 301
lung injury, 319
pancreas, 305
pediatric heart
biopsy findings, 315
complications, 312
infection, 315
outcome, 316
rejection, 312–313, 313*f*
surgical complications, 312
volumes and indications, 312
pediatric lung
acute rejection, 316
airway anastomotic complications, 316
chronic rejection, 317–318
infections, 318–319
primary graft dysfunction, 316
rejection and hyperacute rejection, 316
vascular complications, 316
volumes and indications, 316
renal
acute rejection, 306, 307–308*t*, 309*f*, 310

chronic allograft nephropathy (CAN), 310
hyperacute and accelerated acute rejection and delayed graft function, 306
immunosuppressive drug toxicity, 311
polyomavirus type BK (BKV) Infection, 311–312, 312*f*
recurrent disease, 310
vascular thrombosis, 310
Transplantation
bone marrow, 1034
lung, 504
Transposition of the great vessels
clinical groups, 523*t*
complete transposition, 522–523, 523*t*
corrected transposition, 523
normal blood flow, 522*f*
Transverse limb defects, 1192–1193, 1192*t*
Trauma, 280–284
blunt evaluation, 267–269, 267*f*, 268*f*, 270*f*
ocular, 434–436, 435*f*
pancreatitis, 754
Trichoepithelioma, 1133
Tricuspid valve
atresia, 526–527, 527*t*
Ebstein malformation, 527, 527*f*
Triglyceride storage diseases, myopathy, 1169–1170, 1169*f*, 1169*t*
Trilateral retinoblastoma syndrome, 914
Triploidy
common malformations, 85
complete syndactyly, 67
diandric triploid phenotype, 68, 68*f*
diandric *vs.* digynic, 84–85, 85*t*
digynic triploid phenotype, 67–68, 67*f*
imprinting, 67
second trimester abortion, 67–68, 67*f*–68*f*
spontaneous abortion, 84
Trisomy 13
appendiceal diverticula, 82*f*
cebocephaly, 82*f*
critical region, 77
malformations and postnatal disorders, 80*t*
placental mosaics, 77
second trimester abortion, 66, 67*f*
Trisomy 18
critical region, 77
malformations and postnatal disorders, 79*t*, 81*f*
second trimester abortion, 66, 66*f*
sensitivity and specificity, 77
Trisomy 21
detection rate, 77
life expectancy, 77, 79
malformations and postnatal disorders, 78*t*, 81*f*
spontaneous abortion
atrioventricular cardiac defect, 66
hydrops fetalis, 65–66, 66*f*
recurrence, 66
Trisomy, pancreatic pathology, 749–750
Trophoblast(s)
growth, 324
intermediate, 324*f*, 326, 327, 327*f*, 331, 338, 338*f*
True hermaphroditism (TH), 873–874
Truncus arteriosus, 524–525, 525*f*–526*f*
Trypanosoma cruzi, 244
Trypsinogen deficiency, 751
Tuberculosis, 232–235
clinical features, 233, 234*f*
incidence and prevalence, 232
laboratory diagnosis, 235
pathology, 233
transmission, 232–233
Tuberous sclerosis, 792, 792*f*
Tubular adenoma, 902–903
Tubulointerstitial diseases
acute tubular necrosis, 810, 810*f*
hereditary diseases, 812
immune-mediated tubulointerstitial nephritis, 810–811
interstitial nephritis, 810
Tufting enteropathy, 616, 617*f*
Tumors
appendiceal, 65
cardiac
benign, 566–569, 568*t*
malignant, 569, 569*t*
central nervous system, 377–392
chromosome abnormalities associated with, 33
cytogenetics associated with, 33–34
electron microscopy in diagnosis of, 47, 48*f*
eye, 428–434
gastric, 585
gastrointestinal, 585–586, 586*f*
lymphoma, 633–634, 634*f*
nonepithelial gastrointestinal, 633
polyps, 628–60, 629*f*–60*f*
hepatic, 697, 697*t*
immunohistochemistry, 23–26
lacrimal gland, 425
lung, 488–502
adenocarcinoma, 494
adenoid cystic carcinoma, 493
Askin tumor, 497
benign to malignant ratio, 487
bronchial adenoma, 492
bronchioloalveolar carcinoma, 494, 494*f*
bronchogenic carcinoma, 493–495, 494*f*–495*f*
calcifying fibrous pseudotumor, 497
carcinoid, 492–493, 493*f*
chondroma and chondromatous hamartoma, 489, 490*f*
granular cell tumor, 492, 492*f*
infantile myofibromatosis, 492
inflammatory pseudotumor, 488–489, 488*t*, 489*f*
juvenile laryngotracheal papillomatosis, 490, 491*f*
leiomyoma, 490
leiomyosarcoma, 496, 496*f*
lymphangioleiomyomatosis, 490
lymphangiomatosis, 490
malignant fibrous histiocytoma, 495
malignant mesothelioma, 497
malignant peripheral nerve sheath tumor, 495
mesenchymal cystic hamartoma, 490
mesenchymal hamartoma of the chest wall, 497
mucoepidermoid carcinoma, 493, 493*f*
neurofibroma and neurilemoma, 492
pleuropulmonary blastoma, 497, 498*f*–500*f*
pleuropulmonary desmoid tumor, 497
primary intrathoracic rhabdomyosarcoma, 496
primary pulmonary fibrosarcoma, 496, 496*f*
primary pulmonary synovial sarcoma, 495
primary pulmonary tumors, children, 488*t*
pulmonary blastoma, 494–495
sarcoma, 495–496, 496*f*
sclerosing hemangioma, 490, 492
squamous cell carcinoma, 55*f*, 494
sugar tumor, 490
medulloepithelioma, 433–434
retinoblastoma, 428–433
Turner syndrome, 844, 874. *See also* Monosomy X
Twin reversed arterial perfusion (TRAP), 69, 69*f*, 103, 104*f*
Twinning disruption, 103, 104*f*
Twin-twin transfusion syndrome, 68, 68*f*, 103
Typhlitis colitis, 626
Typhoid. *See* Salmonella infection
Tyrosinemia
hepatic involvement in, 662–663, 663*f*
inborn errors of metabolism, 150–151

U

Ulcer, peptic, 583
Ulcerative colitis
appendiceal, 64–65
gastrointestinal tract, 621–623, 621*f*–622*f*
Ullrich congenital muscular dystrophy (UCMD), 1178–1179
Umbilical cord compromise, spontaneous abortion, 69, 69*f*
Umbilical cord occlusion, 342, 345–346
Undifferentiated embryonal sarcoma, liver, 728–731
clinical features, laboratory studies, and imaging, 728–730, 728*f*–729*f*
gross appearance, 730
histopathology, 730–731
molecular pathology, 731
pathogenesis, 728
treatment and outcomes, 730
Unicameral bone cyst (UBC), 1235, 1237*f*
Uniparental disomy (UPD), 73*t*, 76
Univentricular atrioventricular connection, 529, 529*t*
Urea cycle disorders, 168–169
hepatic involvement in, 676–677, 677*f*
Ureteral ectopia, 826
Ureteral obstruction, 827, 827*f*
Ureterocele, 826

V

Valproic acid embryopathy, 98
Varicella zoster virus (VZV), 202–203
clinical features, 202–203, 203*f*
pathology, 203
prognosis and outcome, 203
transmission, 202
Vascular disorders
central nervous system, 399–402
hepatic, 692–694, 692*f*–693*f*
Vascular lesions, in pituitary gland, 918–919, 919*f*

Vascular tumors
breast, 906, 906*f*
mesenchymal neoplasms
hemangioma, 1138
pyogenic granuloma, 1138
tufted hemangioma, 1138
red pulp diseases, 998
soft tissue
benign tumor, 1043
epithelioid hemangioendothelioma, 1047
hemangiomas, 1043–1046, 1045*f*
intermediate, 1044*t*, 1046
Kaposi sarcoma, 1047
Kaposiform hemangioendothelioma, 1046–1047, 1047*f*
lobular capillary hemangioma, 1043, 1045*f*
lymphatic tumors, 1048–1049
Vasculitis, 561
leukocytoclastic vasculitis, 1128
lymphocytic vasculitis, 1128–1129
Vasculopathy, decidual, 335, 336*f*, 337
VATER association, 107–108, 107*f*
VATER/VACTERL association, 107*f*
Velocardiofacial/DiGeorge syndrome, 88–89
Veno-occlusive disease
hepatic, 692–693, 693*f*
pulmonary (PVOD), 482
Veno-occlusive disease (VOD), 303–304, 304*f*, 319
Venous system malformation
pulmonary, 536–537, 536*t*–537*t*
systemic, 536
Ventricular inflow tract malformation
mitral valve malformation, 527–529
tricuspid valve malformation, 526–527
univentricular atrioventricular connection, 529, 529*t*
Ventricular septal defects, 519*f*–520*f*
classification, 519*t*
clinical groups, 520*t*
clinical manifestations, 520
closure, 520
inlet, 519–520
muscular trabecular, 520
perimembranous, 519
Ventricular tachycardia, 556–557
Vibrio cholerae, 603–604
Villitis, unknown etiology, 335–336
Vimentin, 26
Viral hemorrhagic fevers, 214
Viral infection
adenovirus, 214
adverse fetal outcomes, 191*t*
central nervous system
arboviruses, 396
CMV, 395–396, 396*f*
encephalitis, 394
enteroviruses, 396
herpes simplex virus, 395, 395*f*
HIV, 397
measles, 396–397
meningitis, 394
VZV, 396
coxsackie viruses, 216, 216*f*
cytomegalovirus, 193, 197*f*, 198
echovirus, 215
Epstein-Barr virus, 211–214
fetus and neonate, 193, 194*t*–195*t*
herpes simplex virus, 199, 200*f*
HTLV, 215–216
human immunodeficiency virus, 203–210
human parvovirus infection, 200–201
infants and children, 193, 196*t*
infection-associated hemophagocytic syndrome, 215
intestinal
cytomegalovirus, 602
enteric adenoviruses, 602
herpes simplex virus, 602
rotaviruses, 599, 601
measles, 210–211
mumps, 215*f*, 216
rubella, 201–202
SARS, 216
skin
herpes simplex, 1123
human immunodeficiency virus, 1123
human papillomavirus, 1122, 1122*f*
molluscum contagiosum, 1122, 1123*f*
varicella and herpes zoster, 1123, 1123*f*
spontaneous abortion, 61, 62
swine influenza, 216
varicella zoster virus, 202–203, 203*f*
viral hemorrhagic fevers, 214
WNV infection, 216
Virus-associated hemophagocytic syndrome, 997
Viruses, identification of, by electron microscopy, 54, 54*f*
Vitelline duct anomalies, 591, 591*f*
Vitreous
aspiration of, forensic pathology, 263, 277
structure, 421
surgical procedures, 421–422
Vitreous fluid, determination of dehydration, 256
von Gierke disease, 153–154, 155*f*–156*f*
Von Hippel-Lindau Disease, 792

W

Walker-Warburg syndrome (WWS), 1179
Warfarin, 98–99
Weill-Marchesani syndrome, 420
West Nile virus (WNV) infection, 216
Whiplash shaken infant syndrome, 272, 276, 277
White pulp diseases
follicular hyperplasia, 999
Hodgkin Lymphoma, 999
localized lymphoid hyperplasia, 999
non-Hodgkin lymphoma, 999
primary immunodeficiencies, 999
Wilcott-Rallison syndrome, 772–773
Williams syndrome, 105
Williams-Campbell syndrome, bronchiectasis, 453
Wilms tumor (WT1), 888
Wilson disease
hepatic involvement in, 674–676, 675*f*–676*f*
inborn errors of metabolism, 173–174, 174*f*–175*f*
Wolman disease
adrenal glands, 945–947, 946*f*, 947*f*
hepatic involvement in, 663, 664*f*
inborn errors of metabolism, 147, 148*f*
Wounds and injuries
abdominal and thoracic trauma, 278, 279*f*, 280
burns, 271*f*
dating of contusions, 256, 270–271
documentation of, forensic pathology, 253*f*–255*f*
evaluation, 263, 284
gunshot wounds, 283–284
head injuries, 272*f*–276*f*
pattern injuries, 268*f*, 269*f*, 276, 284
skeletal evidence, 277–278
stab wounds, 255, 255*f*
wear and tear injuries, normal toddlers, 267, 267*f*

X

Xanthogranulomatous inflammation, 918
Xanthoma, 1251
Xeroderma pigmentosa, 409
X-linked adrenoleukodystrophy, 172
X-linked mutations, 116–117
X-linked vacuolar cardiomyopathy and myopathy, 138
XX male and XY female syndrome, 875

Y

Yersinia enterocolitica, 605
Yolk sac rupture sequence, 102
Yolk sac tumor. *See* Endodermal sinus tumor

Z

Zellweger syndrome
congenital anomalies and malformation syndrome, 105–106, 106*t*
hepatic involvement in, 668
inborn errors of metabolism, 172
Zoonoses, 232

CCS1110

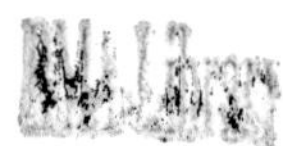